FITZPATRICK'S

DERMATOLOGY IN GENERAL MEDICINE

FIFTH EDITION

IRWIN M. FREEDBERG, MD

George Miller MacKee Professor and Chairman
The Ronald O. Perelman Department of Dermatology
New York University Medical Center
New York, New York

ARTHUR Z. EISEN, MD

Winfred A. and Emma R. Showman Professor of Medicine
Chairman, Division of Dermatology
Washington University School of Medicine
Dermatologist-in-Chief
Barnes Hospital
St. Louis, Missouri

KLAUS WOLFF, MD, DSc(Hon)

Professor and Chairman, Department of Dermatology
University of Vienna Medical School
Head, Division of General Dermatology
Vienna General Hospital
Vienna, Austria

K. FRANK AUSTEN, MD

Theodore Bevier Bayles Professor of Medicine
Harvard Medical School
Brigham and Women's Hospital
Boston, Massachusetts

LOWELL A. GOLDSMITH, MD

Dean
University of Rochester School of Medicine and Dentistry
Rochester, New York

STEPHEN I. KATZ, MD, PhD

Chief, Dermatology Branch, National Cancer Institute
Director, National Institute of Arthritis and Musculoskeletal and Skin Diseases
National Institutes of Health
Bethesda, Maryland

THOMAS B. FITZPATRICK, MD, PhD, DSc(Hon)

Edward C. Wigglesworth Professor of Dermatology, Emeritus
Chairman Emeritus, Department of Dermatology
Harvard Medical School
Chief Emeritus, Dermatology Service
Massachusetts General Hospital
Boston, Massachusetts

FITZPATRICK'S

DERMATOLOGY IN GENERAL MEDICINE

FIFTH EDITION

EDITORS

IRWIN M. FREEDBERG, MD

ARTHUR Z. EISEN, MD

KLAUS WOLFF, MD, DSc(Hon)

K. FRANK AUSTEN, MD

LOWELL A. GOLDSMITH, MD

STEPHEN I. KATZ, MD, PhD

THOMAS B. FITZPATRICK, MD, PhD, DSc(Hon)

VOLUME 2

McGRAW-HILL
Health Professions Division

New York   St. Louis   San Francisco   Auckland   Bogotá   Caracas   Lisbon
London   Madrid   Mexico   Milan   Montreal   New Delhi   Paris
San Juan   Singapore   Sydney   Tokyo   Toronto

McGraw-Hill
*A Division of The **McGraw·Hill** Companies*

FITZPATRICK'S DERMATOLOGY IN GENERAL MEDICINE

Fifth Edition

Copyright © 1999, 1993, 1987, 1979, 1971 by *The McGraw-Hill Companies, Inc.* All rights reserved. Printed in the United States of America. Except as permitted under the United States Copyright Act of 1976, no part of this publication may be reproduced or distributed in any form or by any means, or stored in a database or retrieval system, without prior written permission of the publisher.

1234567890   QPKQPK   998

Set Volume: ISBN 0-07-912938-2
  Volume I: ISBN 0-07-021942-7
  Volume II: ISBN 0-07-021943-5

This book was set in Times Roman by York Graphic Services, Inc. The editors were Martin Wonsiewicz, Mariapaz Ramos Englis, and Lucinda Bauer; the production supervisor was Richard Ruzycka. The index was prepared by Irving Condé Tullar. Text and cover were designed by Marsha Cohen/Parallelogram. Quebecor Printing/Kingsport was printer and binder.

Library of Congress Cataloging-in-Publication Data
Fitzpatrick's Dermatology in general medicine.—5th ed. / editors.
  Irwin M. Freedberg . . . [et al.]
      p.   cm.
    Rev. ed. of: Dermatology in general medicine. 4th ed. c1993.
    Includes bibliographical references and index.
    ISBN 0-07-912938-2 (set).—ISBN 0-07-021943-5 (v. 2).—ISBN
0-07-021942-7 (v. 1)
    1. Dermatology. 2. Skin—Diseases. 3. Cutaneous manifestations
of general diseases.   I. Freedberg, Irwin M.   II. Fitzpatrick,
Thomas B. (Thomas Bernard), date.
    [DNLM: 1. Skin Diseases. 2. Skin Manifestations.   WR 100F559
1999]
RL71.D46   1999
616.5—dc21
DNLM/DLC   98-37070
for Library of Congress   CIP

CONTENTS

v

PART THREE

Disorders Presenting in the Skin and Mucous Membranes

PART FOUR

Dermatology and Medicine

PART FIVE

Diseases due to Microbial Agents, Infestations, Bites, and Stings

PART SIX

Therapeutics

CONTRIBUTORS

A. Bernard Ackerman, MD

Professor of Dermatology and Dermatopathology, Director, Institute for Dermatopathology, Jefferson Medical College, Philadelphia, Pennsylvania [113]

Robert M. Adams, MD

Clinical Professor of Dermatology, Emeritus, Stanford University, Palo Alto, California [139]

David S. Aghassi

Clinical Fellow in Dermatology, Harvard Medical School, Boston, Massachusetts [248]

Steffen Albrecht, MD

Department of Pathology, Sir Mortimer B. Davis Jewish General Hospital, Montreal, Quebec, Canada [106]

Rex A. Amonette, MD

Clinical Professor of Dermatology, University of Tennessee, Memphis, Memphis, Tennessee [276]

Karl H. Anders, MD

Associate Clinical Professor of Pathology and Laboratory Medicine, University of California, Los Angeles School of Medicine, Los Angeles, California; Chief of Pathology and Director of Laboratories, SCPMG, Woodland Hills, California [113]

R. Rox Anderson, MD

Associate Professor of Dermatology, Harvard Medical School, Boston, Massachusetts [265]

Elliot J. Androphy, MD

Department of Dermatology, New England Medical Center, Boston, Massachusetts [224]

Grant J. Anhalt, MD

Professor of Dermatology and Pathology; Acting Chairman of Dermatology, The Johns Hopkins University, Baltimore, Maryland [261]

John C. Ansel, MD

Department of Dermatology, Emory University School of Medicine, Atlanta, Georgia [26]

Cheryl A. Armstrong, MD

Assistant Professor, Department of Dermatology, Emory University School of Medicine, Atlanta, Georgia [26]

Kenneth A. Arndt, MD

Chief of Dermatology, Beth Israel Deaconess Medical Center; Professor of Dermatology, Harvard Medical School, Boston, Massachusetts [269]

Eva Åsbrink, MD, PhD

Associate Professor of Dermatology, Department of Dermatology and Venereology, Karolinska Institute, Stockholm, Sweden [204]

Dalal Assaad, MD, FRCP(C)

Associate Professor, Department of Medicine, University of Toronto; Consultant Dermatologist and Dermatopathologist, Sunnybrook Health Science Centre, Toronto, Ontario, Canada [101]

K. Frank Austen, MD

Theodore Bevier Bayles Professor of Medicine, Harvard Medical School; Brigham and Women's Hospital, Boston, Massachusetts [1, 34]

Howard P. Baden, MD

Professor of Dermatology, Harvard Medical School; Dermatologist, Massachusetts General Hospital, Boston, Massachusetts [46, 54, 249]

Lynn A. Baden, MD, MPH

Instructor in Dermatology, Harvard Medical School; Brigham and Women's Hospital, Boston, Massachusetts [249]

Robert L. Baran, MD

Nail Disease Center, Cannes, France [72]

Raymond L. Barnhill, Jr.

Professor, Department of Dermatology and Pathology, The Johns Hopkins Medical Institutions, Baltimore, Maryland [92]

Eugene A. Bauer, MD

Carl and Elizabeth Naumann Professor, Vice-President for Medical Affairs, Dean of the School of Medicine, Stanford University Medical Center, Stanford, California [65]

Leslie S. Baumann, MD

Assistant Professor of Clinical Dermatology, Director of Cosmetic Dermatology, Department of Dermatology and Cutaneous Surgery, University of Miami, Miami, Florida [243]

Donald V. Belsito, MD

Professor of Medicine, Department of Dermatology, University of Kansas Medical Center, Kansas City, Kansas [122, 123]

Paul M. Benson, MD

Colonel, Medical Corp, USA; Acting Chief, Dermatological Serice, Walter Reed Army Medical Center; Director, Residency Program, National Capital Area Consortium, Dermatology Program, Washington, DC [246]

Timothy Berger, MD

Vice-Chair of Dermatology, School of Medicine, University of California, San Francisco, San Francisco, California [199]

Arthur P. Bertolino, MD, PhD

Associate Clinical Professor of Dermatology, Ronald O. Perelman Department of Dermatology, New York University Medical Center, New York, New York [17]

Jeffrey D. Bernhard, MD

Professor of Medicine, Director, Division of Dermatology, University of Massachusetts Medical Center, Worcester, Massachusetts [4]

David R. Bickers, MD

Chairman, Department of Dermatology, Columbia University, College of Physicians and Surgeons; Director of Service, Department of Dermatology, Presbyterian Hospital, New York, New York [151]

Clifton O. Bingham III, MD

Instructor in Medicine, Harvard Medical School; Associate in Rheumatology, Immunology, and Allergy, Brigham and Women's Hospital; Associate in Allergy, Massachusetts General Hospital, Boston, Massachusetts [34]

Alf Björnberg, MD

Associate Professor of Dermatology, Department of Dermatology, University of Lund, Lund, Sweden [47]

Andrew Blauvelt, MD

Investigator, Dermatology Branch, National Cancer Institute, National Institutes of Health, Bethesda, Maryland [121]

Mark Boguniewicz, MD

Staff Physician, National Jewish Medical and Research Center; Associate Professor of Pediatrics, University of Colorado Health Sciences Center, Denver, Colorado [124]

Numbers in brackets refer to chapters written or co-written by the contributor.

Edward E. Bondi, MD

Department of Dermatology and Dermatologic Surgery, Hospital of the University of Pennsylvania, Philadelphia, Pennsylvania [111]

Mark W. Bonner, MD

Major, Medical Corp, USA; Experimental Therapeutics Branch, Walter Reed Army Institute of Research, Washington, DC [246]

Kathryn E. Bowers, MD

Department of Dermatology, Beth Israel Hospital, Boston, Massachusetts [217]

Irwin M. Braverman, MD

Professor of Dermatology, Department of Dermatology, Yale Medical School, New Haven, Connecticut [24]

Stephen M. Breathnach, MD

Department of Dermatology, St. Thomas's Hospital, London, England [150]

Robert A. Briggaman, MD

Professor and Chairman, Department of Dermatology, University of North Carolina School of Medicine, Chapel Hill, North Carolina [66]

Harold J. Brody, MD

Clinical Associate Professor, Department of Dermatology, Emory University School of Medicine, Atlanta, Georgia [267]

June M. Brown, BS

Emerging Bacterial and Mycotic Diseases Branch, Division of Bacterial and Mycotic Diseases, National Center for Infectious Diseases, Centers for Disease Control and Prevention, Atlanta, Georgia [202]

Nigel W. Bunnett, PhD

Professor of Surgery and Physiology, University of California, San Francisco, San Francisco, California [26]

Denise M. Buntin, MD

Hermitage, Tennessee [228]

Walter H.C. Burgdorf, MD

Clinical Lecturer, Department of Dermatology, Ludwig Maximilian University, Munich, Germany [96, 98, 104, 105]

Robert E. Burgeson, PhD

Cutaneous Biology Research Center, Harvard Medical School, Boston, Massachusetts [21]

Ruggero Caputo, MD

Professor and Chair, Institute of Dermatological Science, University of Milan, Milan, Italy [160, 161]

Mary Wu Chang, MD

Assistant Professor of Dermatology and Pediatrics, New York University Medical Center, New York, New York [144]

Michelle Choucair, MD

Dermatology Fellow, Henry Ford Hospital, Detroit, Michigan [270]

Enno Christophers, MD

Professor and Chairman, Department of Dermatology, Venereology, and Allergology; Director, Clinic for Dermatology, University of Kiel, Kiel, Germany [43, 70]

Mon-Li Chu, PhD

Professor of Dermatology and Cutaneous Biology, Professor of Biochemistry and Molecular Pharmacology, Thomas Jefferson University, Philadelphia, Pennsylvania [19]

Chris Ciesielski-Carlucci, MD

Resident, Department of Internal Medicine, Stanford University Medical Center, Stanford, California [244]

Richard A.F. Clark, MD

Professor and Chair, Department of Dermatology, State University of New York at Stony Brook, Stony Brook, New York [27]

Beth D. Clayton, MD

Dermatology Associates, Greenville, South Carolina [165]

Jay D. Coffman, MD

Professor of Medicine, Section Head, Vascular Medical Section, Boston University Medical Center, Boston, Massachusetts [167]

Jeffrey I. Cohen, MD

Medical Virology Section, Laboratory of Clinical Investigation, National Institutes of Health, Bethesda, Maryland [218]

Philip R. Cohen, MD

Associate Professor, Departments of Dermatology and Pathology, University of Texas, Houston Medical School; Associate Professor, Department of Medical Specialties, Section of Dermatology, University of Texas, MD Anderson Cancer Center, Houston, Texas [93]

Suzanne M. Connolly, MD

Department of Dermatology, Mayo Clinic Scottsdale, Scottsdale, Arizona [86]

Louis Z. Cooper, MD

Director of Pediatrics, St. Luke's Roosevelt Hospital Center, New York, New York [211]

Lynn A. Cornelius, MD

Assistant Professor of Dermatology, Washington University School of Medicine, St. Louis, Missouri [177]

Thomas G. Cropley, MD

Associate Professor of Medicine, Division of Dermatology, University of Massachusetts Medical School, Worcester, Massachusetts [4]

Clyde S. Crumpacker, MD

Department of Medicine, Infectious Disease Division, Beth Israel Deaconess Medical Center, Boston, Massachusetts [215]

Ponciano D. Cruz, Jr., MD

Professor and Vice-Chair, Department of Dermatology, University of Texas Southwestern Medical Center; Chief of Dermatology, Dallas VA Medical Center, Dallas, Texas [186]

Mark V. Dahl, MD

Professor and Chair, Department of Dermatology, University of Minnesota Medical School, Minneapolis, Minnesota [99]

Jennifer Susan Daly, MD

Division of Infectious Diseases and Immunology, Department of Medicine, University of Massachusetts Medical Center, Worcester, Massachusetts [238]

Mazen S. Daoud, MD

Fellow, Dermatopathology and Immunodermatology, Department of Dermatology, Mayo Clinic, Rochester, Minnesota [49–51, 77]

Robert J. Desnick, PhD, MD

Professor and Chairman, Department of Human Genetics, Mount Sinai School of Medicine, New York, New York [153]

Charles H. Dicken, MD

Department of Dermatology, Mayo Clinic, Rochester, Minnesota [77]

John J. DiGiovanna, MD

Director, Dermatopharmacology Division, Department of Dermatology, Brown University School of Medicine, Providence, Rhode Island [52, 256]

Andrzej A. Dlugosz, MD

Associate Professor, Department of Dermatology and Comprehensive Cancer Center, University of Michigan, Ann Arbor, Michigan [38]

Raphael Dolin, MD

Dean for Clinical Programs, Harvard Medical School, Boston, Massachusetts [259]

Jeffrey S. Dover, MD

Associate Chairman, Department of Dermatology, Beth Israel Deaconess Medical Center; Associate Professor of Clinical Dermatology, Harvard Medical School, Boston, Massachusetts [269]

Donald T. Downing, PhD

Professor of Dermatology, Department of Dermatology, University of Iowa College of Medicine, Iowa City, Iowa [10]

Louis Dubertret, MD

Professor and Chair, Department of Dermatology, Hospital St. Louis, Paris, France [100]

Madeleine Duvic, MD

Professor of Dermatology, Department of Dermatology, University of Texas Health Science Center, Houston, Texas [29]

Richard L. Edelson, MD

Professor and Chair, Department of Dermatology, Yale University School of Medicine, New Haven, Connecticut [108]

Libby Edwards, MD

Carolinas Medical Center; Clinical Associate Professor of Dermatology, Wake Forest University School of Medicine, Winston-Salem, North Carolina [116]

Alfred R. Eichmann, MD

Associate Professor, Dermatologisches Ambulatorium des Stadtspitals Triemli, Zurich, Switzerland [231, 235]

Arthur Z. Eisen, MD

Winfred A. and Emma R. Showman Professor of Medicine, Chairman, Division of Dermatology, Washington University School of Medicine; Dermatologist-in-Chief, Barnes Hospital, St. Louis, Missouri [1, 23, 174]

Peter M. Elias, MD

Professor and Vice-Chair, Department of Dermatology, University of California, San Francisco, California [12, 196]

Dirk M. Elston, MD

Dermatology Service, Brooks Army Medical Center, Fort Sam Houston, Houston, Texas [132]

Christine M. Eng, MD

Assistant Professor of Human Genetics, Department of Human Genetics, Mt. Sinai School of Medicine, New York, New York [153]

Patricia G. Engasser, MD

Atherton, California [251]

Ervin H. Epstein, Jr., MD

Professor of Dermatology, Department of Dermatology, UCSF, San Francisco General Hospital, San Francisco, California [6, 112, 158]

Janet A. Fairley, MD

Associate Professor, Department of Dermatology, Medical College of Wisconsin, Milwaukee, Wisconsin [155]

David S. Feingold, MD

Professor and Chair, Department of Dermatology, Tufts University School of Medicine, New England Medical Center, Boston, Massachusetts [234]

Kenneth R. Feingold, MD

Professor of Dermatology and Medicine, University of California, San Francisco; Staff Physician, Veterans Affairs Medical Center, San Francisco, California [12]

David A. Fitzgerald, MB, ChB, MRCP(UK)

Salford Royal Hospitals, Worthington House, Hope Hospital, Salford, England [81]

James E. Fitzpatrick, MD

Associate Professor, Department of Dermatology, University of Colorado Health Sciences Center, Denver, Colorado [141, 247]

Thomas B. Fitzpatrick, MD, PhD, DSc(Hon)

Edward C. Wigglesworth Professor of Dermatology, Emeritus, Chairman Emeritus, Department of Dermatology, Harvard Medical School; Chief Emeritus, Dermatology Service, Massachusetts General Hospital, Boston, Massachusetts [1, 4, 15, 88, 89, 92, 138, 146, 248, 264]

Raul Fleischmajer, MD

Professor of Dermatology, Department of Dermatology, The Mount Sinai Medical Center, New York, New York [187, 188]

Genoveffa Franchini, MD

Chief, Section of Animal Models and Retroviral Vaccines, Basic Research Laboratory, Division of Basic Sciences, National Cancer Institute, Bethesda, Maryland [225]

Shoshana Frankenburg, MD

Research Associate, Department of Dermatology, The Hebrew University of Jerusalem, Jerusalem, Israel [236]

Andrew G. Franks, Jr., MD, FACP

Clinical Associate Professor of Dermatology, New York University School of Medicine, New York, New York [166]

Irwin M. Freedberg, MD

George Miller MacKee Professor and Chairman, The Ronald O. Perelman Department of Dermatology, New York University Medical Center, New York, New York [1, 9, 17, 45]

Ruth K. Freinkel, MD

Professor of Dermatology, Department of Dermatology, Northwestern University Medical School, Chicago, Illinois [169, 170]

Peter O. Fritsch, MD

Professor and Chair, Department of Dermatology and Venereology, University of Innsbruck, Innsbruck, Austria [58, 59, 78]

Lynn From, MD

Pathologist-in-Chief, Women's College Hospital; Associate Professor, University of Toronto, Toronto, Ontario, Canada [101]

Vincent A. Fulginiti, MD

Dean, College of Medicine, Tulane University, New Orleans, Louisiana [220]

George T. Gallagher, DMD, DMSc

Associate Professor, Department of Oral Pathology, Harvard School of Dental Medicine, Boston, Massachusetts [114]

Richard L. Gallo, MD

Assistant Professor of Dermatology, Harvard Medical School, Boston Children's Hospital, Boston, Massachusetts [22]

W. Ray Gammon, MD

Eastern Dermatology, Greenville, North Carolina [66]

Stephen E. Gellis, MD

Children's Hospital, Boston, Massachusetts [210]

Feroze N. Ghadially, MD

Canadian Reference Center for Cancer Pathology, Ottawa Civic Hospital, Ottawa, Ontario, Canada [82]

Ruby Ghadially, MB, ChB

VA Medical Center, San Francisco, California [82]

Irma Gigli, MD

Institute of Molecular Medicine for the Prevention of Human Diseases, University of Texas, Houston Health Science Center, Houston, Texas [35, 119]

Barbara A. Gilchrest, MD

Professor and Chair, Department of Dermatology, Boston University School of Medicine; Chief of Dermatology, Boston Medical Center, Boston, Massachusetts [145]

Mauricio Goihman-Yahr, MD, PhD

Professor, Immunology Section I, Institute of Biomedicine, Central University of Venezuela, Caracas, Venezuela [202]

Lowell A. Goldsmith, MD

Dean, University of Rochester School of Medicine and Dentistry, Rochester, New York [1, 6, 8, 11, 46, 54, 149, 192]

Robert W. Goltz, MD

Clinical Professor of Medicine and Dermatology, Division of Dermatology, University of California at San Diego Medical Center, San Diego, California [104]

Gloria F. Graham, MD

Atlantic Beach, North Carolina [275]

Robin A.C. Graham-Brown, BSc, MB, FRCP

Consultant Dermatologist, The Leicester Royal Infirmary; Honorary Senior Lecturer in Dermatology, University of Leicester, Leicester, England [68, 163, 164]

Richard D. Granstein, MD

Professor and Chair, Department of Dermatology, Cornell University Medical College, New York, New York [135]

Malcolm W. Greaves, MD, FRCP

St. Thomas's Hospital, St. John's Institute of Dermatology, London, England [42]

Joop M. Grevelink, MD, PhD

Director, MGH Dermatology Laser Center; Assistant Professor of Clinical Dermatology, Harvard Medical School; Associate Dermatologist, Massachusetts General Hospital, Boston, Massachusetts [265]

Scott M. Grundy, MD

Professor in Internal Medicine and Biochemistry, University of Texas Southwestern Medical Center, Dallas, Texas [152]

Anne R. Haake, PhD

Associate Professor, Department of Dermatology, University of Rochester School of Medicine and Dentistry, Rochester, New York [7]

Jennifer C. Haley, MD

Dermatopathology Fellow, Department of Pathology and Laboratory Medicine, Indiana University School of Medicine, Indianapolis, Indiana [212]

Russell P. Hall III, MD

Professor and Chief, Division of Dermatology, Duke University Medical Center, Durham, North Carolina [63]

Rudolf Happle, MD

Department of Dermatology, Philip University of Marburg, Marburg, Germany [189]

Christopher B. Harmon, MD

Clinical Instructor, Department of Dermatology, University of Alabama at Birmingham, Birmingham, Alabama; Major and Staff Dermatologist, Keesler AFB, Mississippi [268]

Ken Hashimoto, MD

Professor and Chair, Department of Dermatology, Wayne State University School of Medicine, Detroit, Michigan [84]

Conrad Hauser, MD

Hospital Cantanol, Department of Dermatology, Geneva, Switzerland [28]

Nancy Lyon Havlick

Dermatologist, Arnett Clinic, Lafayette, Indiana [146]

John L.M. Hawk, MD

Consultant Dermatologist, Photobiology Unit, St. Thomas's Hospital, London, England [134, 136]

R.J. Hay, MD

Professor of Cutaneous Medicine St. John's Institute of Dermatology, Guy's and St. Thomas's Hospital, London, England [208]

Harley A. Haynes, MD

Professor of Dermatology, Harvard Medical School; Department of Dermatology, Brigham and Women's Hospital, Boston, Massachusetts [185]

Peter W. Heald, MD

Professor of Dermatology, Yale School of Medicine, New Haven, Connecticut [108]

Peter J. Heenan, MD

The Queen Elizabeth II Medical Centre, Nedlands, Western Australia, Australia [55]

Robert Herd, MD

Royal Infirmary of Edinburgh, Edinburgh, Scotland [269]

G. Scott Herron, MD, PhD

Assistant Professor, Department of Dermatology, Stanford University School of Medicine, Palo Alto, California [65]

Jan V. Hirschmann, MD

Department of Veterans Affairs, Medical Center, Seattle, Washington [258]

Vincent C.Y. Ho, MD

Division of Dermatology, University of British Columbia, Vancouver, British Columbia, Canada [83]

Gary S. Hoffman, MD

Chair, Department of Rheumatic and Immunologic Diseases, The Cleveland Clinic Foundation, Cleveland, Ohio [175]

R. Hofmann-Wellenhof, MD

Assistant Professor of Dermatology, Department of Dermatology, University of Graz, Graz, Austria [85]

Karen A. Holbrook, PhD

Senior Vice-President for Academic Affairs and Provost, Professor of Cell Biology, University of Georgia, Athens, Georgia [7]

Steven M. Holland, MD

Investigator, Laboratory of Host Defenses, National Institute of Allergy and Infectious Diseases, National Institutes of Health, Bethesda, Maryland [33]

Karl Holubar, MD

Professor of Dermatology and of the History of Medicine; Chairman, Institute for the History of Medicine, University of Vienna, Vienna, Austria [2, 183]

Herbert Hönigsmann, MD

Professor of Dermatology, Department of Dermatology, Division of Special and Environmental Dermatology, University of Vienna Medical School, Vienna, Austria [69, 93, 264]

Antoinette F. Hood, MD

Professor of Pathology and Dermatology, Department of Dermatology, Indiana University Medical Center, Indianapolis, Indiana [141, 212]

Yoshiaki Hori, MD

Professor and Chairman, Department of Dermatology, Yamanashi Medical College, Yamanashi, Japan [88, 89]

Thomas D. Horn, MD

Professor and Chair, Department of Dermatology, University of Arkansas for Medical Sciences, Little Rock, Arkansas [120]

Karen R. Houpt, MD

Assistant Professor, Department of Dermatology, University of Texas Southwestern Medical Center at Dallas; Director, Dermatology Services, Parkland Memorial Hospital, Dallas, Texas [186]

Anders Hovmark, MD, PhD

Associate Professor of Dermatology, Department of Dermatology and Venereology, Karolinska Institute, Stockholm, Sweden [204]

George J. Hruza, MD

Associate Professor of Medicine, Surgery and Otolaryngology, Division of Dermatology, Washington University, St. Louis, Missouri [266]

Chung-Hong Hu, MD

Professor of Dermatology and Dean, Taipei Medical College, Taipei, Japan [48]

Robert J. Jacob, PhD

Associate Professor, Microbiology and Immunology, University of Kentucky Medical College, Lexington, Kentucky [221]

Sigbert Jahn, MD

Department of Dermatology, Medical Faculty, Humboldt University (Charité), Berlin, Germany [109]

William D. James, MD

Professor of Dermatology, Department of Dermatology, University of Pennsylvania Health System, Philadelphia, Pennsylvania [246]

Thomas Jansen, MD

Munich, Germany [74, 126]

Kowichi Jimbow, MD

Professor and Chair, Dermatology and Plastic Surgery Division, Department of Dermatology, Sapporo Medical University, Sapporo, Japan [15]

Richard Allen Johnson, MDCM

Instructor in Dermatology, Harvard Medical School; Clinical Associate in Dermatology, Massachusetts General Hospital; Dermatologist, Beth Israel Deaconess Medical Center, Boston, Massachusetts [115, 195, 197, 219, 226]

Joseph L. Jorizzo, MD

Professor and Chair, Department of Dermatology, The Bowman Gray School of Medicine, Wake Forest University, Winston-Salem, North Carolina [165, 179, 193]

Sewon Kang, MD

Associate Professor of Dermatology, Director of Dermatopharmacology Unit, Department of Dermatology, University of Michigan Medical Center, Ann Arbor, Michigan [245]

Stephen I. Katz, MD, PhD

Chief, Dermatology Branch, National Cancer Institute; Director, National Institute of Arthritis and Musculoskeletal and Skin Diseases, National Institutes of Health, Bethesda, Maryland [1, 64, 67, 94, 178, 253]

Paul Kechijian, MD

Clinical Associate Professor of Dermatology, Department of Dermatology; Chief, Nail Section, New York University Medical Center, New York, New York [277]

Francisco Kerdel, BSc, MBBS

Professor of Clinical Dermatology, Director of Inpatient Services, Department of Dermatology and Cutaneous Surgery, University of Miami, Miami, Florida [243]

Helmut Kerl, MD

Professor and Chair, Department of Dermatology, University of Graz, Graz, Austria [85]

Rebecca E.I. Kerr, MD, ChB

The University of Glasgow, The Royal Infirmary, Glasgow, Scotland [75]

Paul A. Khavari, MD, PhD

Associate Professor of Dermatology, Stanford University School of Medicine; Chief, Dermatology Service, VA Palo Alto Health Care System, Stanford, California [65]

Abdul-Ghani Kibbi, MD, FACP

Professor of Dermatology and Dermatopathology; Chairman, Department of Dermatology, Faculty of Medicine; President, Lebanese Dermatological Society, Lebanese Order of Physicians; Program Director, Residency Training Program, Active Medical Staff, American University of Beirut-Medical Center, Beirut, Lebanon [5]

Lloyd E. King, Jr., MD

Professor and Chair, Department of Dermatology, The Vanderbilt Clinic, Nashville, Tennessee [240]

Richard A. King, MD, PhD

Division of Genetics and Metabolism, Departments of Medicine and Pediatrics, Medical School, University of Minnesota, Minneapolis, Minnesota [87]

Jennifer E. Silverman-Kitchin, MD

Fellow, Department of Dermatology, New York School of Medicine, New York, New York [255]

Sidney N. Klaus, MD

The Aaron and Marie Blackman Department of Dermatology, Hadassah University Hospital, Kiryat Hadassah, Jerusalem, Israel [236]

Arnold William Klein, MD

Associate Clinical Professor of Medicine/Dermatology, University of California, Los Angeles; Center for Health Sciences, Beverly Hills, California [272, 273]

Jeffrey A. Klein, MD

Associate Clinical Professor of Dermatology, Department of Dermatology, University of California, Irvine, Irvine, California [272]

Albert M. Kligman, MD

Professor of Dermatology, University of Pennsylvania, Philadelphia, Pennsylvania [146]

Lorraine H. Kligman, PhD

Department of Dermatology, University of Pennsylvania, Philadelphia, Pennsylvania [146]

John H. Klippel, MD

Clinical Director, NIAMS, National Institutes of Health, Bethesda, Maryland [181]

Robert Knobler, MD

Department of Dermatology, University of Vienna, Austria [264]

Caroline S. Koblenzer, MD

Professor of Dermatology, Thomas Jefferson University; Faculty, Institute of Philadelphia Association for Psychoanalysis, Philadelphia, Pennsylvania [41]

George S. Kobayashi, PhD

Division of Dermatology, Washington University School of Medicine, St. Louis, Missouri [206, 207]

Irene E. Kochevar, PhD

Department of Dermatology, Massachusetts General Hospital, Boston, Massachusetts [16]

Alexandria S. Kongsiri, MD, MPH-TM, MSc

Resident, Department of Dermatology, St. Luke's Hospital, New York, New York [244]

Nellie Konnikov, MD

Senior Dermatologist, Department of Medical and Surgical Dermatology, New England Medical Center, Boston, Massachusetts [260]

Kenneth H. Kraemer, MD

Research Scientist, Laboratory of Molecular Carcinogenesis, National Cancer Institute, National Institutes of Health, Bethesda, Maryland [37, 157]

Margaret L. Kripke, MD

Vice-President for Academic Programs, Department of Immunology, The University of Texas, MD Anderson Cancer Center, Houston, Texas [40]

Jean Krutmann, MD

Department of Dermatology, University of Dusseldorf, Dusseldorf, Germany [263]

Thomas S. Kupper, MD

Chief, Division of Dermatology, Brigham and Women's Hospital; Thomas B. Fitzpatrick Professor of Dermatology; Director, Harvard Skin Disease Research Center, Harvard Medical School, Boston, Massachusetts [31]

Irene W. Lai, MD

Fellow, Dermatopharmacology, New York University Medical Center, New York, New York [250]

Alfred T. Lane, MD

Professor of Dermatology and Pediatrics, Department of Dermatology, Stanford University School of Medicine, Stanford, California [143]

Richard Langley, MD

Chief of Dermatology, Clinical Investigations Unit, Massachusetts General Hospital; Instructor in Dermatology, Department of Dermatology, Harvard Medical School, Boston, Massachusetts [92]

Charles M. Lapière, MD

Emeritus Professor of Dermatology, CHU Sart Tilman, Liège, Belgium [154]

Jo-Ann M. Latkowski, MD

Teaching Assistant, The Ronald O. Perelman Department of Dermatology, New York University Medical Center, New York, New York [9]

Robert M. Lavker, MD

Professor of Dermatology, Department of Dermatology, University of Pennsylvania School of Medicine, Philadelphia, Pennsylvania [17]

Thomas J. Lawley, MD

Dean, Emory University School of Medicine, Atlanta, Georgia [30, 168, 177]

Gerald S. Lazarus, MD

Professor of Dermatology, School of Medicine, University of California, Davis, Davis, California [111, 252]

Ullin W. Leavell, Jr., MD

Dermatology Associates of Kentucky, Lexington, Kentucky [221]

David J. Leffell, MD

Associate Professor of Dermatology, Plastic Surgery, and Otolaryngology, Dermatologic Surgery Unit, Yale University School of Medicine, New Haven, Connecticut [81]

Kristin M. Leiferman, MD

Professor of Dermatology, Dermatology Research Unit, Mayo Clinic, Rochester, Minnesota [95]

Irene M. Leigh, MD, FRCP

Professor of Dermatology, Centre for Cutaneous Research, St. Bartholomew's Royal London School of Medicine and Dentistry, London, England [53]

Donald Y.M. Leung, MD, PhD

Professor and Head, Pediatric Allergy-Immunology, Department of Pediatrics, National Jewish Health Center, Denver, Colorado [124, 205]

Walter F. Lever, MD†

[84]

Paul C. Levins, MD

Assistant Professor, Division of Dermatology, UCLA School of Medicine, Los Angeles, California [265]

S. William Levy, MD

Clinical Professor of Dermatology, University of California, San Francisco; Dermatologist, Children's Hospital and Mt. Zion-UCSF Hospital, San Francisco, California [131]

Henry W. Lim, MD

Chair, Department of Dermatology, Clarence S. Livingood Chair in Dermatology, Henry Ford Hospital and Medical Centers, Detroit, Michigan [137, 151]

Douglas R. Lowy, MD

Deputy Director, Division of Basic Sciences, National Cancer Institute, National Institutes of Health, Bethesda, Maryland [39, 209, 222–224]

Dolores J. Lucas, MD

Department of Dermatology, Vanderbilt University Medical Center, Nashville, Tennessee [228]

Leslie C. Lucchina, MD

Associate Physician, Department of Medicine, Brigham and Women's Hospital; Instructor in Dermatology, Harvard Medical School, Boston, Massachusetts [237]

Anne W. Lucky, MD

Adjunct Associate Professor of Dermatology and Pediatrics, University of Cincinnati College of Medicine; Director, Pediatric Dermatology Clinic, Children's Hospital Medical Center, Cincinnati, Ohio [205]

Thomas A. Luger, MD

Professor and Chairman, Department of Dermatology, University of Münster, Münster, Germany [26]

Howard I. Maibach, MD

Professor and Vice-Chairman, Department of Dermatology, University of California, San Francisco, San Francisco, California [239, 251]

Frederick D. Malkinson, MD

Department of Dermatology, Rush-Presbyterian-St. Luke's Medical Center, Chicago, Illinois [130]

---

†Deceased.

Brian F. Mandell, MD, PhD

Associate Professor of Medicine, Ohio State University School of Medicine; Cleveland Clinic Foundation, ASO-Rheumatic and Immunologic Diseases, Cleveland, Ohio [175]

David J. Margolis, MD, FACP

Director, Cutaneous Ulcer Center; Department of Dermatology, University of Pennsylvania, Philadelphia, Pennsylvania [111]

M. Peter Marinkovich, MD

Assistant Professor of Dermatology, Director, Blistering Disease Clinic, Stanford University School of Medicine; Attending Physician, Dermatology Service, VA Palo Alto Health Center System, Stanford, California [65]

J.M. Marks, MD

University of Newcastle, Newcastle-upon-Tyne, England [163]

Ann G. Martin, MD

Assistant Professor of Medicine, Department of Dermatology, Washington University School of Medicine, St. Louis, Missouri [206, 207]

Dieter Maurer, MD

Associate Professor of Immunology and Immunodermatology, Department of Dermatology, University of Vienna Medical School, Vienna, Austria [28]

Barbara McAlpine, MD

Associate Professor of Dermatology, Emory University, Atlanta, Georgia [30]

Jane M. McGregor, MD

Honorary Consultant and Senior Lecturer, St. John's Institute of Dermatology, St. Thomas's Hospital, London, England [134]

Donald S. McLaren, MD, PhD, FRCP

Associate Professor and Head, Nutritional Blindness Prevention Programme, International Centre for Eye Health, Institute of Ophthalmology, University of London, London, England [147]

David I. McLean, MD, FRCP

Professor and Head, Dermatology, University of British Columbia, Vancouver, British Columbia, Canada [185]

Michael M. McNeil, MD, MPH

Childhood and Respiratory Diseases Branch, Division of Bacterial and Mycotic Diseases, National Center for Infectious Diseases, Centers for Disease Control and Prevention, Atlanta, Georgia [202]

Dean D. Metcalfe, MD

Chief, Laboratory of Allergic Diseases, NIAID, National Institutes of Health, Bethesda, Maryland [162]

Martin C. Mihm, Jr., MD, FACP

Clinical Professor of Pathology, Harvard Medical School; Pathologist and Associate Dermatologist, Massachusetts General Hospital, Boston, Massachusetts [5, 92]

Robert L. Modlin, MD

Professor of Medicine/Dermatology, Division of Dermatology, UCLA School of Medicine, Los Angeles, California [32, 203]

David B. Mosher, MD

Clinical Instructor in Dermatology, Department of Dermatology, Harvard Medical School; Clinical Associate, Massachusetts General Hospital, Boston, Massachusetts [88, 89]

Janet A. Moy, MD

Assistant Professor, Department of Dermatology, New York University Medical Center, New York, New York [142]

Ulrich Mrowietz, MD

Assistant Professor of Dermatology, Department of Dermatology, University of Kiel, Kiel, Germany [43, 70]

John Butler Mulliken, MD

Associate Professor of Surgery, Harvard Medical School; Director, Craniofacial Centre, Division of Plastic Surgery, Children's Hospital, Boston, Massachusetts [102]

George J. Murakawa, MD, PhD

Chief of Dermatology, Residency Director, Assistant Professor, Department of Pathology, Albany Medical College, Albany, New York [199]

Rhoda S. Narins, MD

Clinical Associate Professor in Dermatology, New York University Medical Center, New York, New York [272]

Kenneth H. Neldner, MD

Professor of Dermatology, HSC Department of Dermatology, Texas Tech University, Lubbock, Texas [148]

Paul Nghiem, MD

Instructor in Dermatology, Department of Dermatology, Harvard Medical School, Boston, Massachusetts [138, 248]

W.C. Noble, PhD

Professor of Microbiology, Department of Microbial Diseases, University of London, St. Thomas's Hospital, London, England [14]

Paul G. Norris, MD

Photobiology Unit, St. Thomas's Hospital, London, England [136]

Hossein C. Nousari, MD

Department of Dermatology, Division of Dermatoimmunology, The Johns Hopkins University School of Medicine, Baltimore, Maryland [261]

William S. Oetting, MD

Department of Medicine, Genetics Division, University of Minnesota, Minneapolis, Minnesota [87]

John E. Olerud, MD

George F. Odland Professor of Medicine, Department of Medicine, Head, Division of Dermatology, University of Washington, Seattle, Washington [26]

Elise A. Olsen, MD

Associate Professor of Medicine, Duke University Medical Center, Division of Dermatology, Durham, North Carolina [71]

Milton Orkin, MD

Clinical Professor, Department of Dermatology, University of Minnesota, Minneapolis, Minnesota [239]

Seth J. Orlow, MD, PhD

Associate Professor of Dermatology and Cell Biology, New York University School of Medicine; Director of Pediatric Dermatology, New York University Medical Center, New York, New York [144]

Jean-Paul Ortonne, MD

Professor of Dermatology, Nice University School of Medicine; Chief, Department of Dermatology, Hospital Pasteur, Nice, France [88, 89]

Michael N. Oxman, MD

Professor of Medicine and Pathology, University of California at San Diego; Chief, Infectious Diseases and Clinical Virology Sections, VA Medical Center, San Diego, California [216]

Grace H. Pak, MD

Attending Physician, St. Vincent's Medical Center, New York Medical College, New York, NY [242]

Amy S. Paller, MD

Professor of Dermatology, Children's Memorial Hospital, Chicago, Illinois [117, 192]

John A. Parrish, MD

Professor and Chair, Department of Dermatology, Massachusetts General Hospital, Boston, Massachusetts [16]

Robert H. Parrott, MD

Department of Pediatrics, George Washington University School of Medicine, Washington, DC [213]

Madhu A. Pathak, MD, PhD

Senior Associate in Dermatology, Research Professor, Emeritus, Harvard Medical School; Department of Dermatology, Massachusetts General Hospital, Boston, Massachusetts [16, 138, 151, 248, 264]

Monica Peacocke

Associate Professor of Dermatology and Medicine, College of Physicians and Surgeons, Columbia University, New York, New York [234]

Gary L. Peck, MD

Washington Cancer Institute, Washington Hospital Center, Washington, DC [256]

Alice P. Pentland, MD

Professor and Chair of Dermatology, Department of Dermatology, University of Rochester School of Medicine and Dentistry, Rochester, New York [36]

Marco Petrazzouli, MD

Resident, Department of Dermatology, University of Rochester School of Medicine and Dentistry, Rochester, New York [8]

Peter Petzelbauer, MD

Associate Professor of Dermatology, Department of Dermatology, University of Vienna Medical School, Vienna, Austria [25]

Tania J. Phillips, MD

Associate Professor of Dermatology, Boston University School of Medicine, Boston, Massachusetts [270]

Warren W. Piette, MD

Department of Dermatology, University of Iowa Hospitals and Clinics, Iowa City, Iowa [159]

Bianca Maria Piraccini, MD, PhD

Department of Dermatology, University of Bologna, Bologna, Italy [18]

Mark R. Pittelkow, MD

Consultant, Department of Dermatology, Mayo Clinic; Professor of Dermatology and Biochemistry and Molecular Biology, Mayo Medical School, Rochester, Minnesota [49–51]

Enikö K. Pivnick, MD

Associate Professor, Department of Pediatrics, Division of Clinical Genetics, University of Tennessee School of Medical Science, Memphis, Tennessee [191]

Gerd Plewig, MD

Director, Dermatology Clinic, Ludwig-Maximilians University, Munich, Germany [74, 126]

Jordan S. Pober, MD, PhD

Professor of Pathology, Immunobiology, and Dermatology, Yale University School of Medicine; Director, Molecular Cardiobiology Program, Boyer Center for Molecular Medicine, New Haven, Connecticut [25]

Giuseppe Prota, MD

Professor, Department of Organic and Biological Chemistry, University of Naples, Naples, Italy [15]

Thomas T. Provost, MD

Professor of Dermatology, The Johns Hopkins University School of Medicine, Baltimore, Maryland [180]

Leena Pulkkinen, PhD

Department of Dermatology and Cutaneous Biology, Thomas Jefferson University, Philadelphia, Pennsylvania [19]

Walter C. Quevedo, Jr., MD

Professor, Dvision of Biology and Medicine, Brown University, Providence, Rhode Island [15]

Christopher J. Quirk, MD

Freemantle, Australia [55]

Klemens Rappersberger, MD

Professor of Dermatology, Department of Dermatology, University of Vienna, Vienna General Hospital, Vienna, Austria [103]

Curtis Raskin, MD

Resident in Dermatology, Department of Dermatology, Washington University School of Medicine, St. Louis, Missouri [213]

B.J. Rathbone, MD

Consultant Gastroenterologist, Leicester Royal Infirmary, Leicester, England [163]

Thomas H. Rea, MD
Section of Dermatology, LAC/USC Medical Center, Los Angeles, California [203]

Thomas E. Redelmeier, MD
President, Northern Lipids, Inc., Vancouver, British Columbia, Canada [241]

Marvin S. Reitz, Jr., PhD
Professor and Associate Director, Division of Basic Science, Institute of Human Virology, Baltimore, Maryland [225]

Steven D. Resnick, MD
Attending Dermatologist, Bassett Health Care Center, Cooperstown, New York [196]

Arthur R. Rhodes, MD
Professor of Dermatology and Medicine, University of Pittsburgh School of Medicine, University of Pittsburgh Medical Center, Pittsburgh, Pennsylvania [90, 91]

Vincent M. Riccardi, MD
The Neurofibromatosis Institute, La Crescenta, California [191]

Benjamin E. Rich, PhD
Instructor in Dermatology, Brigham and Women's Hospital, Harvard Medical School, Boston, Massachusetts [31]

Fred S. Rosen, MD
James L. Gamble Professor of Pediatrics, Center for Blood Research, Harvard Medical School, Boston, MA [119]

Joel Rosenbloom, MD, PhD
Professor of Biochemistry, School of Dental Medicine, University of Pennsylvania, Philadelphia, Pennsylvania [20]

E. Victor Ross, MD
Commander, Staff Physician, Naval Hospital; Assistant Clinical Professor, University of California at San Diego Medical School, San Diego, California [265]

Richard B. Rothenberg, MD
Assistant Director of Science, National Center for Chronic Disease Prevention and Health Promotion, Atlanta, Georgia [232, 233]

Ramon Ruiz-Maldonado, MD
Department of Pediatric Dermatology, National Institute of Pediatrics, Mexico City, Mexico [58, 59]

Bruce A. Russell, MD
Assistant Professor, Dermatology, Otolaryngology, Head and Neck Surgery, Oregon Health Sciences University, Portland, Oregon [276]

Terence J. Ryan, MD
Department of Dermatology, The Slade Hospital, Oxford, England [128]

Miguel R. Sanchez, MD
Associate Professor, Department of Dermatology, New York University Medical Center, New York, New York [229, 230]

Imrich Sarkany, MD, FRCP
Emeritus Consultant Dermatologist, The Royal Free Hospital, London, England [164]

Hans Schaefer, PhD
L'Oreal, Centre de Recherche Charles Zviac, Clichy, France [241]

William Schaffner, MD
Professor and Chair, Vanderbilt University School of Medicine, Department of Preventive Medicine, Nashville, Tennessee [227]

Mark Jordan Scharf, MD
Associate Professor of Medicine, University of Massachusetts Medical School, University of Massachusetts Memorial Health Care, Worcester, Massachusetts [238]

Jeffrey S. Schechner, MD
Assistant Professor of Dermatology, Department of Dermatology, Yale University School of Medicine, New Haven, Connecticut [25]

Thomas Scholzen, PhD
Department of Dermatology, Emory University, Atlanta, Georgia [26]

Robert A. Schwartz, MD, MPH, FACP
Professor and Head, Dermatology; Professor of Medicine, Pediatrics, Pathology, and Preventive Medicine and Community Health, UMDNJ, Newark, New Jersey [79, 80]

Karin Sege-Peterson, MD, PhD
Fellow in Pediatric Rheumatology, Department of Rheumatology, Hospital for Special Surgery, New York, New York [44]

Jo Louise Seltzer, PhD
Associate Professor of Medicine (Dermatology), Washington University School of Medicine, St. Louis, Missouri [23]

Om P. Sharma, MD
Professor, Department of Medicine, Pulmonary and Critical Care Medicine, USC Ambulatory Health Center, Los Angeles, California [184]

Elizabeth F. Sherertz, MD
Department of Dermatology, Bowman Gray-Wake Forest University Medical Center, Winston-Salem, North Carolina [147, 165]

Robert Sheridan, MD
Associate Professor of Clinical Surgery, Harvard Medical School; Assistant Chief of Staff, Shriner's Burn Hospital, Boston, Massachusetts [129]

Jerome L. Shupack, MD
Professor of Clinical Dermatology, Department of Dermatology, New York University Medical Center, New York, New York [242, 250, 255]

Mihael Skerlev, MD
Department of Dermatology and Venereology, Medical School of Zagreb University and KBC Salata, Zagreb, Yugoslavia [219]

Arthur J. Sober, MD
Department of Dermatology, Massachusetts General Hospital, Boston, Massachusetts [92]

Bhavik P. Soni, MD
Assistant Professor, Division of Dermatology, University of South Alabama, Mobile, Alabama [147]

Richard D. Sontheimer, MD
Professor and Chair, Department of Dermatology, The University of Iowa, Iowa City, Iowa [172, 173]

Nicholas A. Soter, MD
Professor of Dermatology, The Ronald O. Perelman Department of Dermatology, New York University School of Medicine, New York, New York [118, 125, 176, 257]

John R. Stanley, MD
Milton B. Hartzell Professor and Chair, Department of Dermatology, University of Pennsylvania, Philadelphia, Pennsylvania [60, 61]

Robert S. Stern, MD
Professor of Dermatology, Beth Israel Deaconess Medical Center, Harvard Medical School, Boston, Massachusetts [3, 140]

Wolfram Sterry, MD
Professor and Chair, Department of Dermatology, University of Berlin (Charité), Humboldt University, Berlin, Germany [109]

Howard P. Stevens, MA, MBBS, MRCP, PhD
Consultant Dermatologist, Barnet General Hospital, London, England [53]

Mary Ellen Stewart, PhD
Associate Research Scientist, Department of Dermatology, University of Iowa College of Medicine, Iowa City, Iowa [10]

Matthew J. Stiller, MD
Director, Clinical Pharmacology Unit, Columbia Presbyterian Medical Center; Associate Professor of Clinical Dermatology, Columbia University College of Physicians and Surgeons, New York, New York [244]

Georg Stingl, MD

Head, Division of Immunodermatology and Infectious Disease; Professor of Dermatology, Department of Dermatology, University of Vienna, Vienna, Austria [28, 97, 103]

Howard L. Stoll, Jr., MD

Department of Dermatology and Moh's Chemosurgery, Roswell Park Cancer Institute, Buffalo, New York [79, 80]

Stephen E. Straus, MD

Chief, Laboratory of Clinical Investigation, National Institutes of Health, Bethesda, Maryland [216]

John S. Strauss, MD

Professor, Department of Dermatology, University of Iowa Hospitals and Clinics, Iowa City, Iowa [10, 73]

Tung-Tien Sun, PhD

Rudolf A. Baer Professor of Dermatology, Professor of Pharmacology and Urology, New York University Medical School, New York, New York [17]

P.G. Sutej, MD

Assistant Professor of Medicine, Section on Rheumatology, Department of Internal Medicine, The Bowman Gray School of Medicine, Winston-Salem, North Carolina [179]

Gunnar Swanbeck, MD

Professor and Chair, Department of Dermatology and Venereology, Sahlgrenska University Hospital, Goteborg, Sweden [254]

Neil A. Swanson, MD

Professor and Chair, Department of Dermatology; Director, Cutaneous Surgery, Oregon Health Sciences University, Portland, Oregon [276]

Morton N. Swartz, MD, FACP

Professor of Medicine, Harvard Medical School; Chief, Infectious Disease Unit, Massachusetts General Hospital, Boston, Massachusetts [194, 197, 198, 200]

Rolf-Markus Szeimies, MD

Assistant Professor, Department of Dermatology, University of Regensburg, Regensburg, Germany [264]

Gerhard Tappeiner, MD

Associate Professor of Dermatology, Department of Dermatology, University of Vienna General Hospital, Vienna, Austria [201, 262]

Eva Tegner, MD

Associate Professor of Dermatology, Department of Dermatology, University of Lund, Lund, Sweden [47]

Michael Tharp, MD

The Clark W. Finnerod Professor and Chair, Department of Dermatology, Rush Presbyterian St. Luke's Medical Center, Chicago, Illinois [124]

Diane M. Thiboutot, MD

Associate Professor, Department of Medicine, Division of Dermatology, Pennsylvania State University Geisinger Health System, Hershey, Pennsylvania [73]

John Thomson, MD, FRCP

Consultant in Dermatology, The University of Glasgow, The Royal Infirmary, Glasgow, Scotland [75]

Ronald G. Tompkins, MD

Department of Surgery, Shriner's Burn Institute, Massachusetts General Hospital, Boston, Massachusetts [129]

Antonella Tosti, MD

Department of Dermatology, University of Bologna, Bologna, Italy [18, 72]

Franz Trautinger, MD

Associate Professor of Dermatology, Division of Special and Environmental Dermatology, Department of Dermatology, University of Vienna, Vienna, Austria [69]

Hensin Tsao, MD, PhD

Instructor in Dermatology, Harvard Medical School; Assistant in Dermatology, Massachusetts General Hospital, Boston, Massachusetts [197]

Erwin Tschachler, MD

Division of Immunology, Allergy and Infectious Diseases, Department of Dermatology, University of Vienna Medical School, Vienna, Austria [225]

John H. Tu, MD

Wellman Laboratories, Department of Dermatology, Massachusetts General Hospital, Boston, Massachusetts [174]

Jouni Uitto, MD, PhD

Chair, Department of Dermatology, Thomas Jefferson Medical School, Philadelphia, Pennsylvania [19, 20]

Walter P. Unger, MD, FRCP[C], FACP

Associate Professor of Medicine, Department of Dermatology, University of Toronto, Toronto, Ontario, Canada [274]

Sandy S. Urioste, MD

Laser and Cosmetic Surgery Fellow, Harvard Medical School, Boston, Massachusetts [219]

Suzanne Virnelli-Grevelink, MD

Division of Dermatology, Children's Hospital, Harvard Medical School, Boston, Massachusetts [102]

John J. Voorhees, MD

Professor and Chair of Dermatology, Department of Dermatology, University of Michigan, Ann Arbor, Michigan [245]

Patrick D. Wall, FRS, DM, FRCP

Professor of Physiology, St. Thomas's Hospital, London, England [42]

Daniel Wallach, MD

Maître de Conférences, Department of Dermatology, Hôpital Tarnier, Paris, France [2]

John S. Walsh, MD

Assistant Professor of Dermatology, Mayo Medical School, Jacksonville, Florida [155]

Ken Washenik, MD, PhD

Director of Dermatopharmacology, Assistant Professor of Clinical Dermatology, Department of Dermatology, New York University Medical Center, New York, New York [242, 250]

Guy F. Webster, MD

Jefferson Medical College, Philadelphia, Pennsylvania [255]

Arnold N. Weinberg, MD

Medical Director, Massachusetts Institute of Technology, Cambridge; Professor of Medicine, Harvard Medical School, Boston, Massachusetts [194, 198, 200]

Margaret A. Weiss, MD

Assistant Professor of Dermatology, The Johns Hopkins University School of Medicine, Baltimore, Maryland [271]

Robert A. Weiss, MD

Assistant Professor, Department of Dermatology, The Johns Hopkins University School of Medicine, Hunt Valley, Maryland [271]

C. Bruce Wenger, MD, PhD

Research Pharmacologist, Miltary Performance Division, U.S. Army Institute of Environmental Medicine, Natick, Massachusetts [13]

Richard J. Wenstrup, MD

Associate Professor of Pediatrics, Children's Hospital, Cincinnati, Ohio [156]

Victoria P. Werth, MD

Department of Dermatology, University of Pennsylvania, Philadelphia, Pennsylvania [252]

William L. Weston, MD

Professor of Pediatrics, University of Colorado Health Sciences Center, Denver, Colorado [143]

Jonathan K. Wilkin, MD

Director, Division of Dermatologic and Dental Drug Products, FDA, Rockville, Maryland [171]

John D. Wilkinson, MBBS, MRCS, FRCP

Consultant Dermatologist, Department of Dermatology, Amersham General Hospital, South Buckinghamshire, England [127]

Ifor R. Williams, MD, PhD

Assistant Professor, Department of Pathology and Dermatology, Emory University School of Medicine, Atlanta, Georgia [31]

David C. Wilson, MD

Central Virginia Dermatology, Inc., Lynchburg, Virginia [240]

Mary E. Wilson, MD

Chief of Infectious Diseases and Director, Travel Resource Center, Mount Auburn Hospital, Cambridge; Assistant Clinical Professor of Medicine, Harvard Medical School, Boston, Massachusetts [237]

Robert J. Winchester, MD

Director, Division of Autoimmune and Molecular Diseases, Department of Pediatrics, Columbia University College of Physicians and Surgeons, New York, New York [44, 182]

Bruce U. Wintroub, MD

Professor of Dermatology, School of Medicine, University of California, San Francisco, California [140]

Karen Wiss, MD

Dermatology Division, University of Massachusetts Medical Center, Worcester, Massachusetts [214]

Klaus Wolff, MD, DSc(Hon), FRCP

Professor and Chairman, Department of Dermatology, University of Vienna Medical School; Head, Division of General Dermatology, Vienna General Hospital, Vienna, Austria [1, 5, 28, 69, 93, 97, 103, 201, 262, 264]

Elisabeth Ch. Wolff-Schreiner, MD

Department of Dermatology, University of Vienna Medical School, Vienna General Hospital, Vienna, Austria [56, 57, 107]

Gary S. Wood, MD

Professor of Dermatology, Pathology, and Oncology, Case Western Reserve University; Chief of Dermatology, VA Medical Center, Cleveland, Ohio [48, 110]

David T. Woodley, MD

Walter J. Hamlin Professor and Chair, Department of Dermatology, University of Chicago, Chicago, Illinois [66]

Annette B. Wysocki, PhD

Director, Division of Intramural Research, National Institute of Nursing Research, Bethesda, Maryland [133]

Minna Yaar, MD

Professor of Dermatology, Boston Medical Center, Boston, Massachusetts [145]

Kim B. Yancey, MD

Senior Investigator, Dermatology Branch, National Cancer Institute, National Institutes of Health, Bethesda, Maryland [62, 168]

John M. Yarborough, Jr., MD

New Orleans, Louisiana [268]

Benjamin E. Yokel, MD

Department of Dermatology, The Johns Hopkins University School of Medicine, Baltimore, Maryland [141]

Stuart H. Yuspa, MD

Chief, Laboratory of Cellular Carcinogenesis and Tumor Promotion, National Cancer Institute, National Institutes of Health, Bethesda, Maryland [38]

PREFACE

Almost 35 years ago, before the age of computers and the revolution in science that has led to biomolecular medicine, much before the appearance of AIDS and even before the inauguration of Medicare during the years of the Great Society, five physicians, including three dermatologists, an immunologist, and a dermatopathologist, nurtured the first edition of *Dermatology in General Medicine (DIGM)*. Their concept was to present to the general medical community the thoughts and knowledge of a new generation of dermatologists who had grown up since World War II and whose training was focused on America rather than Europe; a generation whose strengths in morphologic dermatology continued although they were enhanced by knowledge and concern about the pathophysiology of dermatologic disease; and a generation whose focus was almost completely on medical dermatology.

In the preface to the first edition, the editors stated their conviction that dermatology was relevant and important to general medicine (hence, the title of their new volume) for three distinct reasons: the skin is an important window revealing clues to underlying diseases; the skin, when it is diseased, can cause significant morbidity and, in some cases, mortality, although the vast majority of skin diseases, in the hands of appropriately trained physicians, can be effectively treated; and, finally, because of its accessibility, the skin represents a unique source of research possibilities into fundamental aspects of disease.

Since that time in the mid-1960s, *Dermatology in General Medicine* has flourished as a textbook through three subsequent editions, each one bringing new editors, new authors, new areas of knowledge, and new techniques of presentation to the project. The book has been highly respected for the breadth and depth of its coverage, focusing on the entire spectrum of dermatologic disease, with contributing authors who are considered among the best in the world. Throughout this evolution of *DIGM* there have been two important constants—McGraw-Hill's commitment to make the work the best that there is and Thomas B. Fitzpatrick's dedication to the project as *DIGM's* senior editor.

As the editors began to consider the production of the 5th edition 4 years ago, several important decisions were made. The "veterans" felt it was important to expand the editorial board to continue the excellence not only of the 5th edition but also of the 6th, 7th, 8th, and all editions that will follow. To accomplish this goal, we asked two world-renowned dermatologists to join our team—Lowell A. Goldsmith, MD, of Rochester, New York, and Stephen I. Katz, MD, PhD, of Bethesda, Maryland. Their impact upon the quality of *DIGM, 5e,* has been extremely important in guaranteeing the excellence of this edition.

In addition, the entire editorial team concluded that the 5th edition must reflect all the progress that has been made in recent years in dermatology—in basic as well as clinical science. They decided that this edition must reflect the enormous breadth of dermatology. The specialty, which was based upon medical dermatology, has extended to pediatric dermatology, to dermatopathology, and, more recently, to dermatologic surgery. They also realized that aesthetic concerns regarding the skin and its diseases must be included if we are to appropriately serve our students, our colleagues, and, most importantly, our patients.

The other major change occurred when we recognized that *DIGM* had become a classic, assuming its position among the other greats in medicine—Osler's, Harrison's, Goodman & Gilman, and the rest. As Tom Fitzpatrick relinquished his role as the senior editor, we felt it appropriate to name the work *Fitzpatrick's Dermatology in General Medicine*—the name it has been known by throughout the world since 1965.

The editors also want to recognize those who preceded us on the editorial board. Kenneth A. Arndt, John Vaughn, and the late Wallace Clark gave generously of their time and produced the precursors of the work we now present. We thank them for their superb professional effort as we also thank, in absentia, Patricia K. Novak, a unique woman who made enormous contributions to the success of the first four editions. Pat died during the preparation of this edition, although her standards of excellence in production survive her.

Our gratitude is expressed to our families who had to have been stressed by the time and effort we put into the development of this edition. It is truly a new presentation. In addition to the change in the editorial board, the text has been reorganized to reflect current pathophysiologic knowledge, and we have completely altered and markedly expanded the sections on therapy and dermatologic surgery. We have produced over 50 new chapters and almost 60 more have been completely rewritten by new authors. We introduced color in the clinical photographs in the fourth edition and have now brought color into the dermatopathology and many of the diagrams.

We would also like to acknowledge the dedicated help of the following: Arlene Stolper Simon, in this as in previous editions; Reina Guzman; Renate Kosma; Ginger Roberts; Joanne Miccile; Cathi Gray; and Linda Nolan—of the editorial offices; Anna Ferrera, Marketing Manager; Cindy Bauer, Development Editor; and Richard Ruzycka, Production Supervisor—of the Health Professions Division, McGraw-Hill.

The staff at McGraw-Hill kept us on track and close to the production schedule throughout this endeavor. Our editor, Martin Wonsiewicz, has been very supportive, always ready to modify his conclusions if we were able to convince him that the book would be improved by such an alteration. Finally, it has been Mariapaz Ramos Englis, alternating between a comforting Den Mother and a stern task master, who has guaranteed the success of our venture.

Irwin M. Freedberg, MD
Senior Editor

PART FOUR

Dermatology and Medicine

CHAPTER 143

William L. Weston
Alfred T. Lane

Neonatal Dermatology

The newborn period is defined as the first 30 days of life. During the newborn period, skin conditions appear abruptly and frequently frighten parents and health care givers. Neonatal skin diseases evolve much more rapidly than adult skin diseases, and some conditions that initially appear to be serious turn out to be trivial, whereas in others the opposite is true.[1] A thorough knowledge of the fetal skin biology and of the cutaneous lesions of newborns is expected of those providing neonatal care.

This chapter is divided into five sections: newborn skin care, transient skin disease in the newborn, birthmarks, common congenital malformations, and hereditary skin conditions with dramatic newborn presentations. Many of the disorders of the newborn are considered by their clinical features, etiology and pathogenesis, clinical manifestations, pathology, diagnosis, course, and prognosis only, since no treatment is required of many self-limited problems. Many of the conditions are described in detail in other portions of this textbook, and only the aspects in newborns will be considered in this chapter.

NEWBORN SKIN CARE

The skin of a full-term newborn infant feels very soft and smooth. The smooth texture and softness are related to the hydration of the epidermis and the condition of the collagen and dermal matrix substances.[2] Although sweating may be inefficient, at birth the full-term infant's skin is otherwise functionally mature. The barrier portion of the epidermis, the stratum corneum, is intact and effectively protects the full-term infant.[2–4]

Even though the epidermal barrier function of the full-term baby may be normal at birth, the infant is at increased risk for systemic toxicity of topically applied compounds.[5] This is related to five factors, the most important being that the infant's surface area is great when compared to body mass. In addition, the infant's metabolism, excretion, distribution, and protein binding may be different from those of an adult.[5]

The premature infant is at much greater risk for skin complications than the mature newborn. The premature infant has markedly decreased epidermal barrier function and an even greater surface area to volume ratio.[6,7] In addition, the immature organs of the

premature infant may affect the metabolism, excretion, distribution, and protein binding of chemical agents.[5] Local or systemic toxicity can occur in the premature infant from soaps, lotions, or other cleansing solutions.[5,6]

The skin of the mature infant often appears dry and cracked shortly after birth.[6] The stratum corneum that has accumulated in utero has not yet shed. Following the first bath, fissures and bleeding may occur on the ankles and wrists, permitting infection to develop. During this time, topical care should include moisturizing lotions or creams. The goal of skin therapy in the newborn is to retain the soft flexible texture of the infant's skin and prevent bacterial superinfection by hydrating and lubricating the epidermis. For infants in a dry environment, moisturizers may need to be used indefinitely; infants in a more humid environment may need their use only intermittently.

The skin care of the premature infant is much more difficult and complex.[6,7] Not only is the barrier portion of the epidermis absent or defective, but the skin has markedly increased fragility. Because of epidermal and dermal injury, the infant may have significant cutaneous pain, which is accentuated by routine handling and nursing care. The premature infant is at risk for developing sepsis from skin-associated organisms entering through breaks in the thin and fragile skin. Sweating in the premature infant is functionally reduced and contributes to poor thermal regulation.[8] Heat regulation is dysfunctional also because of lack of a subcutaneous fat layer for insulation and poor autonomic control of cutaneous vessels.[9] Maintaining a humid environment will decrease the infant's transepidermal water loss and assist in skin hydration. This can be done by using a humidity-controlled isolet or by placing thin plastic tents over infants under infrared warmers.

Dry, flaking, fissured skin of premature infants should be treated with moisturizing creams or ointments. Petrolatum- or lanolin-based ointments with little or no preservatives appear to offer the greatest benefit and lowest risk.[6,7,10] Ointments placed on an infant's skin under an infrared warmer will usually not cause cutaneous burns, although infants who suffer asphyxia may be more susceptible to burns.[10] Semipermeable wound dressings may offer additional cutaneous pain relief and protection, but additional studies must be done to analyze the potential for bacterial growth under the dressings.[7] Removing wound dressings may tear fragile premature infant skin, thus selecting nonstick dressings is critical. The care of premature infants' skin is detailed in Table 143-1.

TABLE 143-1

Care of the Premature Infant's Skin

Gentle handling
  Use adhesive tape sparingly, over the smallest possible area
  Change cardiac monitor infrequently
  Use antibacterial cleansing solutions sparingly
  Avoid frictional trauma to the skin
Intervention
  Humidify infant environment
  Lubricate skin with awareness of possible absorption of preservatives and emulsifiers within the product used
  Use localized nontraumatic semipermeable wound dressings

TRANSIENT SKIN DISEASE

Skin diseases encountered in newborns that begin to resolve or are completely resolved by 30 days of age are considered to be transient. They are very common and almost expected in newborns.

Milia

Milia are multiple pinpoint papules seen over the forehead, cheeks, and nose of infants. They may be present in the oral cavity as well, where they are called *Epstein's pearls*.[11] They are expected findings in the newborn. Up to 40 percent of newborns have milia on the skin, and 64 percent on the palate.[1]

Etiology and pathogenesis Milia represent cystic retention of keratin within the superficial dermis. Trauma to the skin surface experienced during delivery or from intrauterine life may contribute.

Clinical manifestations Milia are 1- to 2-mm whitish, spherical papules within the outer layer of skin. They are seen prominently on the face and nose and on the cheeks as well. Usually, dozens are present. They are also found as 1- to 2-mm white papules on the gingiva and palate.

Pathology On histologic examination, milia appear as superficial epithelial, keratin-filled cysts in the upper dermis, just beneath the epidermis.

Diagnosis and differential diagnosis Molluscum contagiosum, an acquired viral infection, may mimic milia but does not appear in the immediate neonatal period. Sebaceous gland hyperplasia also occurs over the nose and cheeks of infants but is yellow, rather than whitish.

Course and prognosis The cystic spheres rupture onto the skin surface and exfoliate their contents within a few weeks of birth.[1]

Sebaceous Gland Hyperplasia

Sebaceous gland hyperplasia represents overgrowth of sebaceous glands in areas of sebaceous gland abundance. At least 50 percent of normal newborns have sebaceous gland hyperplasia. Premature infants often do not.

Etiology and pathogenesis Maternal androgens stimulate the overgrowth of sebaceous glands, and sebaceous hyperplasia is considered a feature of the "miniature puberty of the newborn." The stimulation occurs during the last month of pregnancy, and both the number of sebaceous cells and the individual cell volume increases.[2]

Clinical manifestations Tiny (1-mm) yellow macules or yellow papules are seen at the opening of each pilosebaceous follicle over the nose and cheeks of newborns.[1]

Pathology Sebaceous glands of large size with prominent secretory cells are observed surrounding the pilosebaceous follicle.

Diagnosis and differential diagnosis Milia may mimic sebaceous hyperplasia but are white and cystic in appearance, rather than yellow.

Course and prognosis They recede completely by 4 to 6 months of age.

Erythema Toxicum

Erythema toxicum is a transient, blotchy erythema seen in newborns. It occurs in about 50 percent of term infants and less commonly in premature infants.[12]

Etiology and pathogenesis The cause of erythema toxicum is unknown.

Clinical manifestations Blotchy erythematous macules 2 to 3 cm in diameter, with a tiny 1- to 4-mm central vesicle or pustule, are seen in erythema toxicum (Fig. 143-1). They usually begin at 24 to 48 h of age.[12] Lesions are seen on the chest, back, face, genitalia, and proximal extremities, sparing the palms and soles.

Pathology An intraepidermal vesicle is seen, which is filled with eosinophils.

Diagnosis and differential diagnosis A smear of the central vesicle or pustule contents will reveal numerous eosinophils on Wright-stained preparations. A peripheral blood eosinophilia up to 20 percent may accompany the tissue eosinophil accumulation, par-

FIGURE 143-1

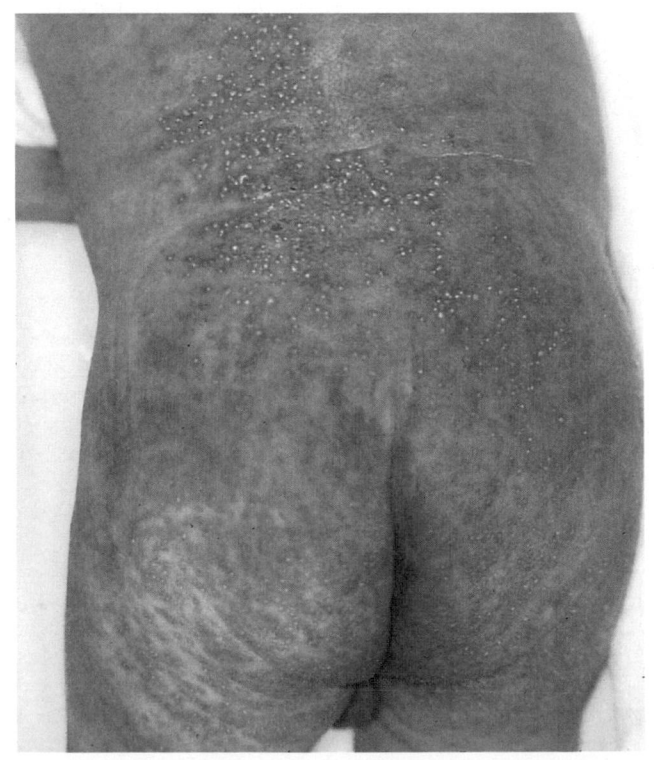

Erythema toxicum. Blotchy erythematous macules with tiny central vesicles and pustules in a newborn.

ticularly in infants with numerous lesions. Transient neonatal pustular melanosis (TNPM) mimics erythema toxicum, except that neutrophils rather than eosinophils are found within the pinpoint vesicles and individual lesions heal with residual pigmentation, not seen in erythema toxicum. Bacterial infections, *Pityrosporum* folliculitis, and congenital candidiasis may also mimic erythema toxicum. Bacterial and fungal culture of lesions and Gram staining will help differentiate.

Course and prognosis The individual lesions clear in 4 to 5 days, and new lesions may occur from birth to the tenth day of life. By 2 weeks of age, all lesions are resolved.

Transient Neonatal Pustular Melanosis

TNPM is a blotchy erythema of the newborn that heals with residual brown pigmentation. It is less common than erythema toxicum and is more prevalent among black newborns.

Etiology and pathogenesis The cause of the condition is unknown.

Clinical manifestations These lesions present at birth as vesicles, pustules, or ruptured vesicles or pustules with a collarette of surrounding scale (Fig. 143-2). Pigmented macules are also often present at birth or develop at the sites of resolving pustules or vesicles.[13] Most lesions occur on the trunk and proximal extremities, but the palms and soles may be involved.[13]

Pathology An intraepidermal vesicle filled with neutrophils is found.

Diagnosis and differential diagnosis Smear of the vesicle or pustule contents will reveal numerous neutrophils and an occasional eosinophil on Wright-stained preparations.

Miliaria rubra is frequently confused with erythema toxicum and TNPM. The erythema around miliaria rubra is small in area (1 to 2 mm versus 20 to 30 mm in erythema toxicum). The central vesicle or pustule of TNPM may mimic herpes simplex, congenital candidiasis, *Pityrosporum* folliculitis, or bacterial folliculitis lesions.[13,14] A Gram-stained slide of the pustules of erythema toxicum or TNPM will be negative. The Wright-stained slide from a pustule of erythema toxicum will show a predominance of eosinophils, while the slide of a pustule of TNPM will usually show a predominance of neutrophils.

Course and prognosis The vesicles and pustules usually disappear by 5 days of age, while the residual pigmented macules resolve over 3 weeks to 3 months.

Mottling

Mottling is a blotchy duskiness of skin that is temperature responsive. Virtually all babies demonstrate mottling at some time during the newborn period.

Etiology and pathogenesis Immaturity of the autonomic control of the skin vascular plexus is felt to be responsible for mottling, with constriction of the deeper plexus and opening of the superficial plexus.[9]

Clinical manifestations A lacelike pattern of dusky erythema appears over the extremities and trunk of neonates when exposed to a decrease in temperature.[1,9] This phenomenon may be sensitive to small increments of temperature change.

Diagnosis and differential diagnosis The mottling disappears on rewarming.[9] Mottling that persists beyond 6 months of life may

FIGURE 143-2

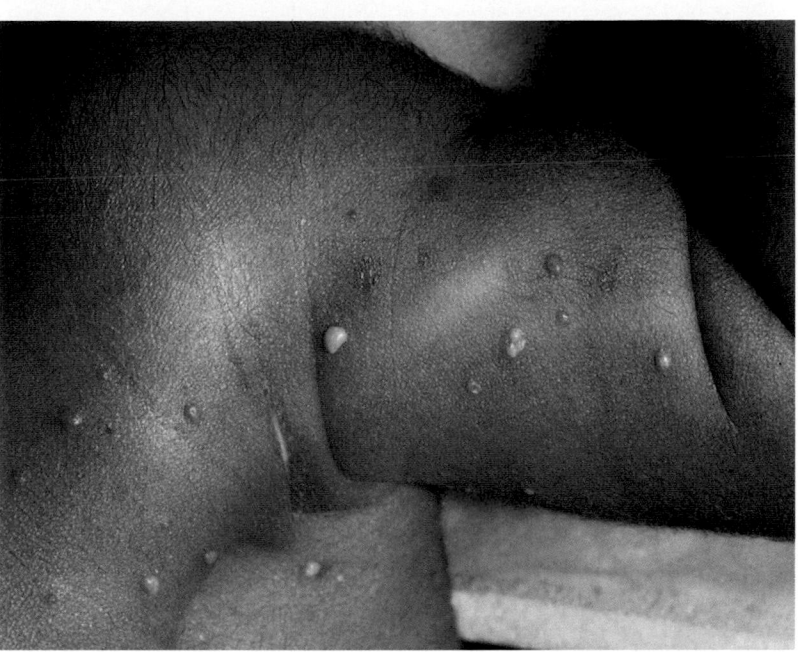

Transient neonatal pustular melanosis. Discrete pustules on trunk and back of black newborn.

be a sign of hypothyroidism or cutis marmorata telangiectatica congenita; these can be associated with musculoskeletal or vascular abnormalities and do not disappear with rewarming. Similarly, the livedo reticularis seen with collagen vascular disease such as neonatal lupus erythematosus will persist when the skin is warmed.

Course and prognosis The tendency to mottling upon cold exposure gradually diminishes and is no longer present after 6 months of age.

Harlequin Color Change

This distinct color change of one half of the body results from positioning. Harlequin color change is unusual in newborns and is usually seen in infants of low birth weight.

Etiology and pathogenesis The exact mechanism of this unusual phenomenon is not known, but immaturity of autonomic vasomotor control is felt to be responsible.

Clinical manifestations When a low-birth-weight infant is placed on one side, an erythematous flush with a sharp demarcation at the midline develops on the dependent side.[1] The upper half of the body becomes pale. The color change usually subsides within a few seconds of placing the baby in the supine position but may persist for as long as 20 min.

Diagnosis and differential diagnosis To observe the color change, the baby must be placed on one side. The harlequin color change is seldom confused with other vascular problems.

Course and prognosis The color change is seldom seen after 10 days of age.

Sucking Blisters

Sucking blisters are blisters apparent at birth as the result of intrauterine sucking; they are uncommon.

Etiology and pathogenesis   Vigorous sucking in utero has been postulated as the cause of these blisters.

Clinical manifestations   Sucking blisters are usually solitary, intact oval blisters or erosions on noninflamed skin in the newborn.[15] They occur on the dorsal aspect of forearms, wrists, or fingers or on the upper lip and resolve within a few days.

Diagnosis and differential diagnosis   Herpesvirus infection or bullous impetigo are often considered when sucking blisters are encountered, but lesions of the former appear on an erythematous base. Incontinentia pigmenti presents with multiple linear blisters, in contrast to the solitary sucking blister. Although epidermolysis bullosa may present with a solitary blister, multiple new blisters will develop after birth.

Course and prognosis   Sucking blisters are usually completely resolved by 14 days of age.

Subcutaneous Fat Necrosis

Subcutaneous fat necrosis is uncommon; it is caused by the rupture of lipocytes, resulting in a subcutaneous nodule.

Etiology and pathogenesis   Cold injury is felt to be responsible for subcutaneous fat necrosis. Compared to adults, the fat of the neonate contains more saturated fatty acids, which have a higher melting point. Once the temperature of the skin drops below the melting point of the fat, crystallization occurs within the dermal fat cells, followed by a granulomatous reaction.

Clinical manifestations   In subcutaneous fat necrosis of the newborn, firm, sharply circumscribed, reddish or purple nodules appear over the cheeks, buttocks, arms, and thighs.[16] The lesions usually begin within the first 2 weeks of life and resolve spontaneously over several weeks. Occasionally, the lesions heal with atrophy after several weeks, leaving a skin depression. Infrequently, hypercalcemia occurs with or without associated irritability, vomiting, weight loss, and failure to thrive.[16,17] Serum calcium evaluations should be repeated biweekly until the lesions have totally resolved for a month or more in infants who have either large plaques of involved skin or renal disease.[16,17]

Pathology   Granulomatous inflammation surrounding ruptured fat cells with necrotic amorphous debris is seen. Sometimes fat crystals are found within lipocytes.

Diagnosis and differential diagnosis   Bacterial cellulitis or septicemic lesions may be confused with subcutaneous fat necrosis at the onset. The infant with fat necrosis appears healthy and nurses vigorously, in contrast to those with bacterial infections. Several separate lesion sites are often seen with subcutaneous fat necrosis. This is extremely unusual with cellulitis.

Course and prognosis   Lesions evolve slowly over several months. The surface discoloration changes from red to bruiselike, then fades. A hard subcutaneous mass is felt. As more subcutaneous fat is deposited in the adjacent normal skin, the lesion appears more atrophic with time. Lesions resolve by 1 year, and the atrophy can often no longer be detected.

Sclerema

Sclerema is diffuse hardening of the skin in a sick premature newborn and is becoming rare as neonatal care improves worldwide.

Etiology and pathogenesis   Newborn exposure to low temperatures in the nursery or delivery room is felt to be responsible.

Clinical manifestations   Premature newborns who suffer hypothermia are susceptible to the development of sclerema, a diffuse hardening of the skin.[15,18] The trunk is always involved. The onset is characteristically after 24 h of age. The skin feels hard and immobile and looks yellow and shiny. Sclerema appears in severely ill premature newborns who have suffered sepsis, hypoglycemia, metabolic acidosis, or other severe metabolic abnormalities.

Pathology   Edema of fibrous septa surrounding fat lobules is found. There is no necrosis of fat.

Diagnosis and differential diagnosis   The thickening and hardening of the skin are so characteristic of sclerema that it is not confused with other disorders. The stiff-skin syndrome and other conditions characterized by contractions of extremities are present at delivery, whereas sclerema is acquired over several days.

Treatment   Careful monitoring of the skin surface temperature of ill newborns may prevent the development of sclerema. Supportive care includes temperature control, nutritional replacement, correction of metabolic acidosis, and possibly repeated exchange transfusions and will arrest the process.[18]

Course and prognosis   Sclerema is a sign of a severely ill newborn, and infant mortality is high. With successful supportive care of the premature infant, the thickening will reverse in several weeks.

Pustules in the Newborn

Pustules are discrete, yellow, 1- to 9-mm raised lesions that frequently display a red base. They are common in the newborn period. The incidence of bacterial sepsis is higher in the preterm infant than in the full-term infant, and overall sepsis is an uncommon cause of pustules in the newborn. However, the high mortality rate of unrecognized neonatal bacterial sepsis makes it imperative for the clinician to consider this possibility.

Etiology and pathogenesis   Although there are many causes of pustules in the newborn, their appearance should immediately bring to mind the possibility of bacterial sepsis (Table 143-2), especially when prolonged rupture of maternal membranes has occurred.[19]

Clinical manifestations   Pustules are discrete 1- to 9-mm yellow raised lesions with a red base. They may be observed anywhere on the skin. Pustules that appear during the first 7 days of life are of particular concern. Careful attention should be given to signs of illness in a newborn, such as low temperature, poor feeding, weak sucking, vomiting, irritability, or lethargy. If those signs are present, bacterial sepsis should be suspected.

Pathology   In bacterial infections, pustules arise as the result of accumulation of neutrophils within the skin, following dissemina-

TABLE 143-2

Symptoms and Signs of Bacterial Infection in the Newborn

SYMPTOM	SIGN
Lethargy	Pustules
Poor feeding	Jaundice
Irritability	Petechiae
Diarrhea	Pallor
	Cyanosis
	Omphalitis
	Conjunctivitis
	Enlarged liver or spleen
	Hypothermia

tion of bacteria from the blood to the skin or direct bacterial invasion of the skin.

Diagnosis and differential diagnosis Bacterial culture of pustules or of other body fluids such as blood, urine, and cerebrospinal fluid should be performed. There is no rapid, completely reliable method of determining whether or not a baby has bacterial sepsis, and one should always maintain a high index of suspicion. Other causes of pustules in the newborn may be considered after bacterial sepsis is eliminated as a possibility (Table 143-3). Erythema toxicum may occasionally be pustular, particularly if skin involvement is extensive.[12] TNPM mimics erythema toxicum and is characterized by pustules present at birth.[13] Skin infections from herpes simplex virus (HSV) may be pustular but are usually vesicular.[20–24] Acne neonatorum is usually not present in the first 14 days of life, and evolution to the pustular stage may require several more weeks.[1,25] Candidiasis, particularly of the diaper area or of other intertriginous areas, may be pustular, and satellite pustules are characteristically found at a distance from the margins of confluent areas of candidiasis. Congenital candidiasis, acquired in utero, may also be pustular, with discrete pustules at birth and subsequent development of diffusely eczematous skin.[26,27] Infantile acropustulosis may begin at birth or within the newborn period; it presents with discrete pustules limited to the distal extremities, with prominent involvement of the palms and soles.[28] Nevus comedonicus is a birthmark consisting of patulous follicular openings in which pustule formation, or even deeper abscesses, may occur.[29] Psoriasis rarely occurs in the newborn period, but it also may be extensive and pustular.[30]

Course and prognosis Bacterial sepsis in the newborn evolves within hours, and mortality is high if it is unrecognized.

Acne Neonatorum

Acne that develops within the first 30 days of life is termed *neonatal acne*. It is estimated that 50 percent of newborns may experience neonatal acne.

Etiology and pathogenesis Neonatal acne may be a part of the so-called miniature puberty of the newborn. Neonatal sebaceous glands are hyperplastic, and hydroxysteroid dehydrogenase activity in these structures is high in the 2 months just before birth and at birth.[2,3] There is evidence that newborns with acne experience transient increases in circulating androgens.[25]

Clinical manifestations Neonatal acne is rarely present at birth but may appear as multiple, discrete papules at 2 to 4 weeks of age.[25] The face, chest, back, and groin are the usual areas for cutaneous lesions (Fig. 143-3). Papules evolve into pustules after a few weeks. Neonatal acne may persist up to 8 months of age.[1] There is some suggestion that infants with extensive neonatal acne may experience severe acne as adolescents.

Pathology Findings are increased sebaceous gland volume and plugging of the pilosebaceous orifice with keratin. Rupture of dilated pilosebaceous structures will occur, with neutrophils or granulomatous inflammation.

Diagnosis and differential diagnosis The presence of microcomedones and inflammatory papules on the facial skin is seldom con-

TABLE 143-3

Differential Diagnosis of Pustules in the Newborn

Bacterial sepsis
Erythema toxicum
Transient neonatal pustular melanosis
Pityrosporum folliculitis
Herpes simplex infection
Acne neonatorum
Congenital candidiasis
Infantile acropustulosis
Nevus comedonicus
Pustular psoriasis

fused with other conditions. The differential diagnosis of acne neonatorum is the same as for pustules in the newborn.

Course and prognosis Neonatal acne usually resolves spontaneously without treatment. If the involvement is severe, topical therapy with 2.5% benzoyl peroxide gel can be used.[1]

Herpes Simplex Virus Infection

Neonatal herpes is a systemic infection with HSV acquired from a maternal genital herpes infection. The exact prevalence of neonatal HSV infection is unknown, but some estimates place it at 1 per 2000 live births.[20–24]

Etiology and pathogenesis Infection of the newborn with HSV is usually related to maternal infection in the birth canal.[20,21] Infected infants are likely to have been premature. Infants born to mothers with a primary herpes genital infection at the time of delivery are more likely to develop neonatal HSV infection than infants born to mothers with recurrent genital lesions.[23] Eighty percent of neonatal infections are HSV-2; the remainder are HSV-1.[20]

FIGURE 143-3

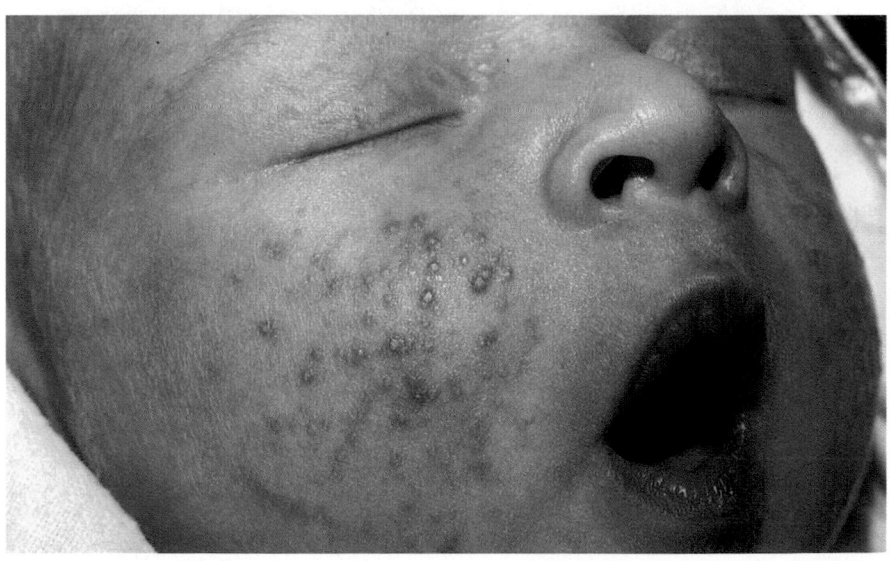

Neonatal acne. Microcomedones and red papules on cheek of 3-week-old.

Clinical manifestations Grouped vesicles on an erythematous base should bring to mind neonatal HSV infection (Fig. 143-4). Any area of skin may be involved, but vesicles on the scalp or buttock are particularly common.[20–24] Monitoring electrodes may produce sufficient skin trauma on involved skin sites to allow invasion by the virus and to induce HSV skin lesions. Vesicles may be present immediately at birth, but the onset after birth is more likely, with 6 days as the mean age of onset.[20–24] Some infants with neonatal HSV infection will not have skin lesions, but 70 percent of all infants infected with HSV display lesions.[20] Mucous membrane involvement is common.

Pathology HSV infection in skin reflects viral replication within keratinocytes. Ballooning degeneration of keratinocytes is seen in which the virus has destroyed the cells, and adjacent destruction results in an intraepidermal blister cavity. Some cells demonstrate nuclear fusion of adjacent keratinocytes, and large keratinocytes, which are mostly nuclear chromatin, form characteristic multinucleated giant cells. Inflammatory cells of all types are observed.

Diagnosis and differential diagnosis Other blistering diseases of the newborn such as congenital varicella, bullous impetigo, and incontinentia pigmenti may be considered in a differential diagnosis. A Wright-stained smear of cells scraped from a vesicle base will demonstrate multinucleated giant cells and balloon cells in HSV infection. Fluorescein-tagged anti-HSV-specific antibody may be used to examine vesicle smears or snap-frozen biopsy sections of skin to make a rapid diagnosis. Viral culture of HSV requires 12 to 120 h to grow, and in all infected or suspected neonates, cultures of skin lesions, urine, nasopharynx, eyes, and cerebrospinal fluid are indicated.[22] Serum antibodies for HSV are of little assistance in making the diagnosis. Rapid diagnosis of HSV infection is essential, and a high index of suspicion should be maintained.

FIGURE 143-4

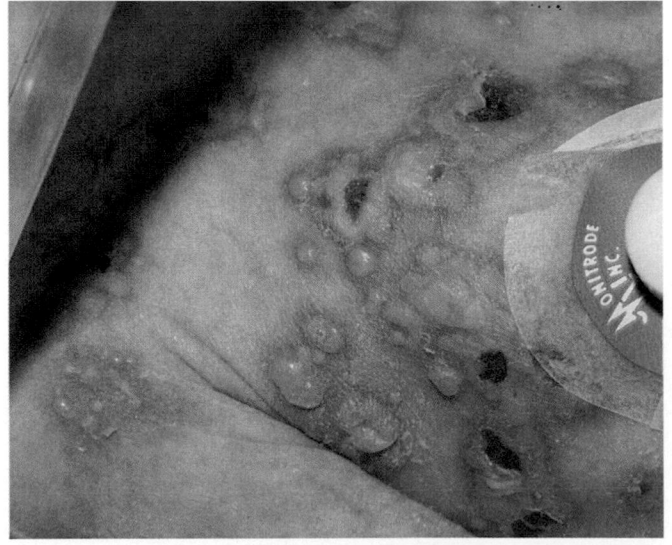

Herpes simplex infection. Grouped vesicles on an erythematous base. Pustules and erosions are also present. *(Courtesy of Alvin H. Jacobs, MD)*

Treatment Adenosine arabinoside or acyclovir administered intravenously have been demonstrated to be efficacious.[22] Prompt recognition and early therapeutic intervention appears to lead to an improved outcome in the infected infant.[22]

Course and prognosis Infected infants may have signs that mimic bacterial sepsis and may develop psychomotor retardation, even if obvious signs of dissemination of HSV are not evident in the newborn.

Varicella

Neonatal varicella is a systemic infection with varicella-zoster virus acquired during intrauterine life. Congenital varicella is quite rare.

Etiology and pathogenesis This infection is associated with maternal chickenpox 2 to 3 weeks before delivery.[20,31,32] Maternal infection with varicella-zoster virus, which may be unrecognized, results in dissemination of the virus to the newborn.[31,32] Varicella can also develop in neonates infected postnatally.

Clinical manifestations Lesions appear as crops of macules and papules that evolve into vesicles and then crust. Age of onset is within the first 10 days after birth, and a mortality rate of up to 20 percent has been reported in infants who develop skin lesions between 5 and 10 days of age.[20,31,32]

Pathology Pathologic changes in skin are identical to those observed for HSV infection.

Diagnosis and differential diagnosis Neonatal varicella may mimic HSV infection in the newborn.[20,31,32] A Wright-stained smear of cells from a blister base or a skin biopsy demonstrate the same changes as are seen in HSV infection. Maternal history of varicella and cutaneous lesions in the infant compatible with varicella are most useful in making the diagnosis. HSV infection and bullous impetigo are the two most important considerations in the differential diagnosis of congenital varicella. Fluorescein-tagged antiherpes-zoster-virus-specific antibody may be used to examine vesicle smears or snap-frozen biopsy sections of skin to make a rapid diagnosis. Culture identification of the virus from the vesicles may require 7 to 14 days.

Treatment Immediate administration of zoster immune globulin to the infant is recommended if maternal infection is present from 5 days before to 2 days after delivery.[32,33] Infected infants may require therapy with intravenous acyclovir. Passive immunization with varicella-zoster immunoglobulin should be considered for postnatal exposure of premature and term infants exposed to varicella.[32,33]

Course and prognosis Varicella may result in a severe infection, especially in premature infants. Mortality is low compared to HSV infection. A few infants will develop psychomotor retardation.

Impetigo

Impetigo is a superficial bacterial skin infection. Although uncommon, bacterial impetigo may be observed in the newborn period.

Etiology and pathogenesis *Staphylococcus aureus* is the predominant organism producing impetigo in the newborn, including those strains capable of producing the staphylococcal scalded skin syndrome. Occasionally group A streptococci or gram-negative bacteria can cause impetigo in the newborn period.

Clinical manifestations Flaccid, well-demarcated bullae may be seen that evolve into erosions.[1] Any area of skin may be involved, but the scalp, face, and diaper areas are the most common sites of infection. A collarette of scale around the erosion is characteristic of impetigo due to *S. aureus*.[34] Honey-colored crusts are less common in newborns than in older children.

Pathology Impetigo is characterized by a subcorneal neutrophilic abscess that contains bacteria.

Diagnosis and differential diagnosis Bacterial culture of skin lesions and culture of the nasopharynx will yield the organism within 24 h. Smear of vesicle contents and a Gram's stain will demonstrate the bacteria.

Treatment The appropriate systemic antibiotic should be administered promptly in order to prevent sepsis and diminish spread of bacteria to other patients and hospital personnel.

Course and prognosis Prompt treatment results in full recovery. Undetected impetigo may result in bacterial sepsis in the newborn or premature infant with an immature immune system.

Staphylococcal Scalded Skin Syndrome (Ritter's Disease) (See also Chap. 196)

This is an acute bacterial infection that results in red tender skin with subsequent desquamation. Ritter's disease is quite uncommon, although nursery epidemics have been well documented.

Etiology and pathogenesis Skin injury is the result of an intraepidermal cleavage through the granular layer of epidermis due to circulating exotoxin produced by *S. aureus*. Small amounts of staphylococci ($<10^8$ organisms) may produce enough toxin to exfoliate a neonate. Usually, hospital personnel carry the organism into the nursery.

Clinical manifestations Infants 2 to 30 days old may develop an abrupt onset of generalized erythema followed within 24 h by bullae. There is subsequent exfoliation of large sheets of skin within 48 h.[35] The lesions are commonly around the head, neck, buttocks, groin, axilla, and periumbilical area of the abdomen.

Pathology A subcorneal blister cavity is seen, but there is no necrosis of the overlying stratum corneum or inflammation.

Diagnosis and differential diagnosis Toxic shock syndrome and toxic epidermal necrolysis should be considered in the differential diagnosis of the staphylococcal scalded skin syndrome. However, they are rarely observed in the newborn period. The flushing and blistering of diffuse cutaneous mastocytosis may be confused with scalded skin syndrome. A skin biopsy that demonstrates excessive mast cells and the recurrence of episodes will distinguish between them. Cultures of the nasopharynx, rectum, and blisters are likely to yield the organism.

Treatment Isolation of the affected newborn to prevent nursery epidemics is essential.[35] Antistaphylococcal antibiotics should be administered systemically, and aggressive fluid and electrolyte replacement instituted, much like that provided for burn therapy.

Course and prognosis This is a life-threatening condition. Prompt recognition and aggressive therapy are essential.

Breast Abscess

Breast abscess is an acute bacterial infection of the breast tissue of a newborn, but is rare in the newborn period.

Etiology and pathogenesis *S. aureus* and gram-negative organisms are the most likely pathogens. It is believed that the bacteria enter through ductal tissue.

Clinical manifestations Swelling, erythema, and fluctuance in one breast of a newborn infant signifies the possibility of breast abscess. Onset usually begins 5 to 20 days after birth.[36] The infant may have fever but is usually asymptomatic otherwise.

Diagnosis and differential diagnosis A needle aspiration of the infection may be necessary to obtain a positive bacterial culture. Breast hyperplasia due to miniature puberty of the newborn may produce asymmetric enlargement of one breast.[36] On palpation, the breast is not red or fluctuant in breast hyperplasia, whereas it is when there is an abscess.

Treatment Systemic antibiotic therapy with the appropriate antistaphylococcal agent is usually necessary.

Course and prognosis With prompt antibiotic therapy, recovery is rapid. Unrecognized infection may eventuate in bacterial sepsis.

Omphalitis

Omphalitis represents bacterial infection of the tissues around the umbilical cord, and is uncommon in the newborn period.

Etiology and pathogenesis Bacterial infection through the cut surface of the umbilical cord is the usual cause. It is predominantly due to *S. aureus*.

Clinical manifestations Redness and induration of the umbilical region are characteristic of omphalitis. Often, the redness is not well localized and spreads diffusely beyond the umbilicus.[1]

Diagnosis and differential diagnosis An irritant dermatitis produced by the treatment of the umbilicus with various bacteriostatic agents may sometimes mimic omphalitis.

Treatment Prophylactic bacteriostatic agents applied to the cord in the newborn period have reduced the likelihood of this infection in many nurseries. Administration of systemic antistaphylococcal antibiotic is the treatment of choice.

Course and prognosis Omphalitis usually remains localized but, if untreated, may progress to bacterial sepsis.

Caput Succedaneum and Cephalohematoma

Caput succedaneum is subcutaneous edema over the presenting part of the head[1]; cephalohematoma is a subperiosteal collection of blood.[1] Caput succedaneum is common, whereas cephalohematoma is rare among newborns.

Etiology and pathogenesis Both lesions are due to shearing forces on the scalp skin and skull during labor.

Clinical manifestations Edema or hemorrhage of the scalp appears as deep swelling, with or without purpura. The swelling occurs primarily in vertex deliveries, particularly those with prolonged labor, and resolves spontaneously in 7 to 10 days. If the purpura is extensive, it can serve as a source of hyperbilirubinemia. Secondary bacterial infection of cephalohematoma may rarely occur, resulting in cellulitis.

Diagnosis and differential diagnosis The caput succedaneum tends to feel soft and lacks a well-defined outline. The cephalohematoma is bounded by the suture lines of the skull and often feels fluctuant. Both lesions can mimic cellulitis or bacterial abscess. Appropriate cultures may assist in the differential diagnosis.

Petechiae and Purpura

Petechiae are nonblanching macules, and purpura are bruiselike areas of skin; both are commonly encountered in the newborn period.

Etiology and pathogenesis Petechiae and purpura represent leakage of red blood cells from superficial cutaneous blood vessels into extravascular tissue. Often the result of birth trauma, they nonetheless, should alert the clinician because petechiae and purpura may be presenting features of congenital infection, particularly when the newborn is small for gestational age and has hepatosplenomegaly. Petechiae and purpura are the most common cutaneous symptoms for congenital infections and may be important clues to the diagnosis.[20] Toxoplasmosis, syphilis, rubella, cytomegalovirus, and congenital HSV infections are the usual congenital infections responsible for the production of petechiae and purpura, but many different congenital infections may also result in this finding.[19–21,37,38]

Clinical manifestations   Petechiae appear as pinpoint (<1 mm), nonblanching red macules, whereas purpura appear as larger areas of purple macules. Newborns with congenital infection may also demonstrate other features such as microophthalmia, congenital heart defects, cataracts, and psychomotor retardation.

Diagnosis and differential diagnosis   Congenital infection should be considered first as a possible cause. Serologic tests and viral cultures for the likely infections should be performed. Other causes of petechiae and purpura in the newborn include trauma, with face and scalp petechiae common in difficult vertex deliveries or in section-assisted deliveries. Neonatal thrombocytopenia due to maternal autoantibodies, as in idiopathic thrombocytopenic purpura, or systemic lupus erythematosus may also produce neonatal petechiae a few hours after birth. Hypoprothrombinemia may result in purpura in the newborn older than 2 or 3 days as a result of vitamin K deficiency. Protein C deficiency can also cause severe purpura in the neonate. Neonatal petechiae and purpura are unusual in the hemophilias, but bleeding from circumcision sites may be the first manifestation of hemophilia in the newborn period. Neonatal purpura secondary to platelet dysfunction may be observed in von Willebrand's disease or Wiskott-Aldrich syndrome.

Treatment   Treatment is guided by detection of the etiology of the petechiae or purpura.

BIRTHMARKS

Birthmarks represent an excess of one or more of the normal components of skin per unit area: blood vessels, lymph vessels, pigment cells, hair follicles, sebaceous glands, epidermis, collagen, or elastin. Birthmarks are collections of highly differentiated cells in tissue.

Congenital malformations are most frequently observed in skin. The vascular birthmarks are the most common.[39–41] The two most commonly seen birthmarks are flat capillary malformations of a faint red color, the so-called salmon patch, and Mongolian spots.[39,40,42] They are observed at least 100 times more frequently than any other skin birthmark. Salmon patches are observed with high frequency in infants, both in white infants (703 per 1000 live births) and black infants (592 per 1000 live births).[39,41] Mongolian spots are more frequently observed in Asians (910 per 1000 live births) and black infants (880 per 1000 live births), but are less common in white infants (48 per 1000 live births).[41,42]

Flat Capillary Malformations (See also Chap. 102)

Flat capillary malformations can be divided into those that are light red or pink in color [salmon patch (nevus flammeus)] and those that are deep red or purple-red (port-wine stain). A salmon patch is present over the back of the neck in over 40 percent of infants, and over the glabella or eyelids in 20 percent. Portwine stains are seen in 0.5 percent of newborns.

Clinical manifestations   The salmon patch appears as a light red macule over the nape of the neck, the upper eyelids, and the glabella.[42–44] Over the nape of the neck they may become inflamed and develop overlying dermatitis.[45] Port-wine stains appear as deep red or purple-red macules over the face or extremities; they are usually unilateral.[43,45–47] Occasionally, they are extensive and cover large areas of skin. Port-wine stains over the face or an extremity may be associated with soft tissue and bony hypertrophy.[43,44,47–50] A port-wine stain over the face may be a clue to the Sturge-Weber syndrome.[47–49] Overall, 8 percent of infants with facial port-wine stains will develop Sturge-Weber syndrome, but the incidence is higher if the lesion covers the upper and lower eyelid or is bilateral.[49] The Sturge-Weber syndrome is characterized by seizures, mental retardation, glaucoma, and hemiplegia.[47,49] Calcification of the capillary malformation in the brain in Sturge-Weber syndrome may be detected in childhood by skull x-ray.[48] Identification of cerebral vascular abnormalities and early calcification can be detected in infancy by computed tomography or magnetic resonance imaging. When port-wine stains are found over an extremity and are associated with soft tissue or bony hypertrophy of that extremity, the condition is called the Klippel-Trenaunay-Weber syndrome.[43,44,50] Elongation of an extremity can cause orthopedic deformity. Arteriovenous fistulas are present in 25 percent of such patients.[43,44] Absence of the deep venous channels in the affected limb may be detected by venography.[44]

Pathology   Numerous dilated capillaries without endothelial change are seen on a skin biopsy of lesions in an adolescent or adult.[44] The capillaries are mature and represent a developmental malformation. In infants and children, the skin biopsy may be indistinguishable from normal skin.

Diagnosis and differential diagnosis   In an older infant, capillary vascular malformations are so characteristic that they are seldom confused with other skin conditions, but in the first weeks of life the raised hemangioma may be flat and look like a port-wine stain. After several weeks of life, the raised hemangioma will begin to elevate the skin and be distinguished from a port-wine stain. Port-wine stain lesions usually cover a larger surface area and are unilateral.

Treatment   Recent data support use of a pulsed dye laser, which selectively causes thermal damage to cutaneous vasculature while sparing surrounding epidermal and dermal structures.[51–53] This therapy is best initiated during early infancy, and clearing is dependent on the size of the capillary malformation and the age when therapy is begun.[51] Therapy for the cutaneous lesion may reverse underlying soft tissue overgrowth, but bony hypertrophy or the neurologic progressions in Sturge-Weber syndrome are not affected. In addition, flat hemangiomas may be covered with make-up. If features of Sturge-Weber syndrome are present, ophthalmologic evaluation and follow-up should be obtained immediately.[48] Measurements of the length and girth of the extremities should be carefully recorded every 3 to 6 months if a port-wine stain is found over an extremity.[50] Since leg length differences can induce scoliosis, orthopedic evaluations and assistance may be required if one leg is longer than the other.

Course and prognosis   Flat vascular malformations tend to persist. Salmon patches may fade somewhat with time, but remnants persist well into adult life.[44] Generally, the eyelid lesions fade by 6 to 12 months of age. Lesions on the nape of the neck are likely to persist into adulthood.

Raised Hemangiomas (Superficial and Deep Hamangiomas) (See also Chap. 102)

Raised hemangiomas are vascular masses that appear red or purple-red; they are common and are seen in 2 percent of newborns.

Etiology and pathogenesis Most raised hemangiomas demonstrate both a superficial and deep component. They are mixtures of superficial dilated, proliferating capillaries and deep dilated venous channels.[54,55] The biologic behavior of the cavernous and mixed types is similar in children, however. Blood flow through such lesions is sluggish, and platelet aggregation can occur, followed by consumption of clotting factors in the Kasabach-Merritt syndrome.[56]

Clinical manifestations Raised hemangiomas may not be observed at birth, but a circumscribed area of blanched skin with a few fine telangiectases may be present, representing a developing raised hemangioma. By 2 to 4 weeks of age, the skin becomes raised, with red papules. This is followed a few weeks later by a dusky-blue, deep nodular component.[54,55] The lesions grow out of proportion to the baby for the first 8 to 12 months of life. Raised hemangiomas begin to show signs of involution around 15 months of age, when pale gray areas appear within the red nodule.[54,55] Soon the first sign of flattening appears. The raised lesion regresses to skin level by 5 years of age in 50 percent of the patients, and by puberty in almost all patients. Most often, only redundant loose skin that was stretched during the rapid growth phase remains. In large, raised hemangiomas, ulceration of the epithelial surface often occurs when secondary bacterial superinfection results (Fig. 143-5).

There are several major complications of raised hemangiomas: (1) platelet trapping, (2) airway obstruction, (3) visual obstruction, and (4) cardiac decompensation. Platelet trapping (Kasabach-Merritt syndrome) occurs within the sluggish circulation of the raised hemangioma.[56] It usually occurs in patients with a single large hemangioma, primarily within the first 6 months of life. Platelet trapping produces easy bruising and petechiae on areas of the body not involved with hemangioma and may progress to frank hemorrhage. Often the involved hemangioma will suddenly enlarge and become very firm at the onset of the platelet trapping.[56]

Obstruction of the airway results in respiratory stridor and is usually due to subglottic hemangiomas. Infants with such hemangiomas usually have multiple hemangiomas of the skin of the head and neck.[54] Visual acuity disturbances may occur either by growth of the hemangioma within the orbit, causing compression of the eyeball, or by swelling around the eyelid forcing the lid to close and obstructing vision. Large raised hemangiomas may pool sufficient blood to produce high-output cardiac failure. Internal hemangiomas may occur with or without cutaneous lesions.

Diagnosis and differential diagnosis Raised hemangiomas may be confused with pyogenic granulomas, malignant vascular tumors, and giant melanocytic birthmarks; the latter may be vascular at birth, with little pigment production. Usually, little confusion occurs, but occasionally, a biopsy is needed to help distinguish such lesions.

Treatment The indications for treatment are obstruction of a vital orifice (airway, excretory channel), visual obstruction, platelet trapping syndrome, and cardiac decompensation. The treatment of choice is prednisone, 2 to 6 mg/kg per day.[57] Alternate-day therapy may be sufficient. Treatment for 4 to 8 weeks is often necessary. Treatment initiated during the growing phase of the hemangioma (1 to 8 months of age) produces the best results. The mechanism of action of prednisone is unknown, but reduction of the capillary cell division by steroids has been postulated. Interferon-α2a may be considered in those babies who fail prednisone therapy, especially those with Kasabach-Merritt syndrome.[58] Response to interferon is slow. X-ray therapy produces poor cosmetic results, and squamous cell and basal cell carcinomas subsequently develop within the areas of radiodermatitis.[57] Surgical therapy results in significant blood loss and scarring. Newer methods of hemangioma control, such as the pulsed dye laser and the use of growth factors, are currently being tested. There is often great pressure to treat for cosmetic reasons, but strict adherence to the indications for therapy are advised except in small capillary hemangiomas or ulcerated hemangiomas, which may respond well to pulsed dye laser treatment.[51–53] Topical antibiotic or antiseptic agents will reduce secondary infection in ulcerated hemangiomas, but oral anti-staphylococcal therapy may often be necessary. The rapid growth of the tumor often convinces parents that such lesions will not disappear. Careful explanation of the natural history of these lesions is necessary.[54] Photographs and measurements are useful to follow the progress of a raised hemangioma. In infants treated with prednisone, patients should be seen every 2 weeks during therapy to monitor progress, then monthly thereafter until age 1. In other infants, a single follow-up visit in 2 weeks will allow reinforcement of the concept that treatment is not required. Monthly or bi-monthly follow-up visits are advised thereafter.

Cutis Marmorata Telangiectatica Congenita

Cutis marmorata is a rare, persistent mottling pattern due to a vascular birthmark.

Etiology and pathogenesis The disorder is considered to be a vascular ectasia of veins and, possibly, of capillaries.[59] Tortuous, dilated veins are found in the dermis and subcutaneous tissue on biopsy.

Clinical manifestations In cutis marmorata telangiectatica congenita, a mottled pattern of blue or dusky-red erythema is seen from birth.[59] It is unresponsive to skin warming. Often a single extremity is involved, but the lesions may occur bilaterally on the extremities or on the trunk.[59] The skin surface overlying such areas may be depressed. A gradual increase in the size of lesions is expected over

FIGURE 143-5

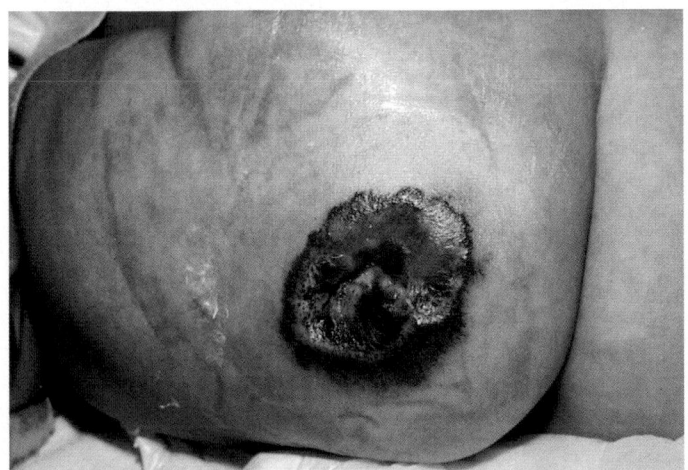

Ulcerated hemangioma. A four-week-old with large hemangioma of the buttock with central ulceration and crust.

the first few years of life, but most fade by adult life. Rigorous natural history studies of cutis marmorata telangiectatica congenita are not available. Associations with musculoskeletal or vascular abnormalities occur.[59]

Diagnosis and differential diagnosis   In contrast to cutis marmorata telangiectatica congenita, mottling of newborn skin is a transient vasodilation and is relieved by rewarming the skin. The livedo reticularis pattern of collagen vascular disease is flat, not depressed over the discolored areas, always bilateral, and associated with systemic signs and symptoms.

Treatment   There is no reliable treatment, but some lesions will respond to pulsed dye laser therapy.[52] Routine evaluations should include close inspection of the extremities for possible orthopedic deformity. It should be explained to parents that cutis marmorata telangiectatica congenita is a birthmark, and that some increase is expected in the area of skin involved. It should be emphasized that it is an unusual disorder and that few data are available for predicting the course. Associated deformities should be treated as necessary.

Diffuse Neonatal Hemangiomatosis and Blue Rubber Bleb Syndrome

These are vascular syndromes consisting of multiple raised hemangiomas. Both diffuse neonatal hemangiomatosis and blue rubber bleb syndrome are rare.

FIGURE 143-6

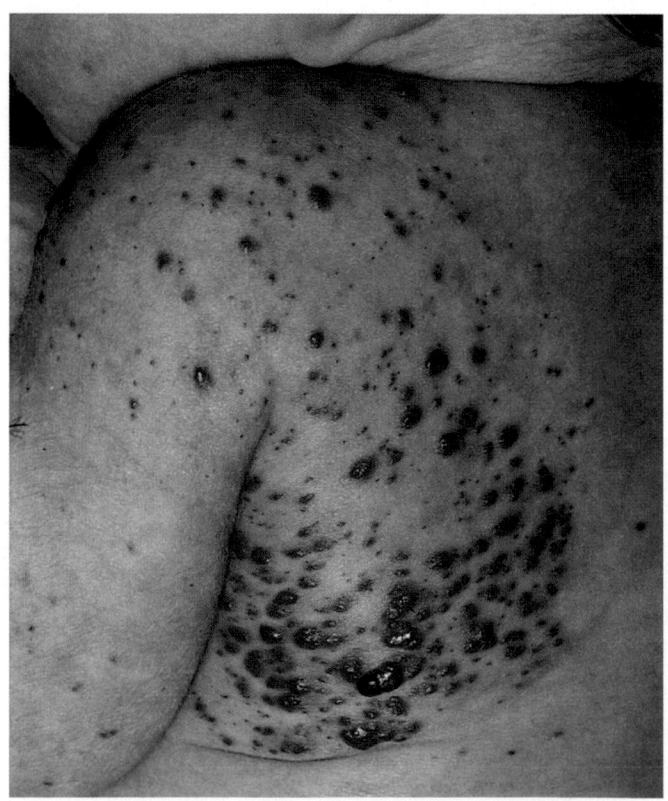

Diffuse neonatal hemangiomatosis. Dozens of hemangiomas grouped about the shoulder.

Etiology and pathogenesis   In diffuse neonatal hemangiomatosis, proliferating endothelial cells and numerous capillary lumens are observed within the middermis. This syndrome has been reported in twins, but insufficient data are available to determine whether it is hereditary. The blue rubber bleb nevus syndrome lesions are more similar to cavernous hemangiomas, with numerous dilated vascular channels.

Clinical manifestations   Diffuse neonatal hemangiomatosis consists of multiple, small, raised cutaneous hemangiomas, which may or may not be associated with hemangiomas in the liver, lungs, gastrointestinal tract, and central nervous system (CNS).[60,61] The raised hemangiomas may be present at birth, and more develop with time. The hemangiomas vary from 2 to 15 mm in diameter (Fig. 143-6). Spontaneous involution of the lesions has been reported.[60] Bleeding may occur into the gastrointestinal tract. The blue rubber bleb nevus syndrome is a rare disorder consisting of multiple cavernous hemangiomas of the skin and bowel.[62] The lesions are blue and 3 to 4 cm in diameter.

Diagnosis and differential diagnosis   The presence of skin hemangiomas is so characteristic that little difficulty in differential diagnosis is experienced. The lesions of blue rubber bleb nevus syndrome are compressible and may be painful or associated with excessive sweating. Monitoring stool samples for occult blood is helpful in identifying presence of intestinal lesions.

Treatment   Infants with diffuse neonatal hemangiomatosis who develop complications may respond to prednisone at a dose of 2 to 6 mg/kg per day, with appropriate attention to side effects.[60] The duration of treatment may exceed 8 to 12 weeks. The blue rubber bleb lesions are not responsive to systemic therapy and may require surgical resection.[62] Frequent stool examinations for blood will identify intestinal bleeding.

Lymph Vessel Birthmarks: Lymphangiomas

Lymphangiomas may be circumscribed, superficial skin papules or deep, cavernous nodules,[63] uncommon in the newborn period.

Etiology and pathogenesis   Dilated, tortuous lymph vessels appear within the dermis and subcutaneous fat. Most often, many channels are found spreading from the original lesion, so that the skin surface change reflects only the tip of a tetrahedral lesion. Cavernous lymphangiomas may involve the muscle as well.

Clinical manifestations   Circumscribed lymphangiomas appear as a solitary group of 2- to 4-mm, gelatinous skin-colored papules limited to a skin area less than 10 cm^2. They are often connected to underlying venous channels, and hemorrhage into one or more papules may occur, producing sudden darkening.[63] They may be present at birth but are often not noticed until late infancy or childhood.

Cavernous lymphangiomas are rubbery, skin-colored nodules that may result in grotesque enlargement of soft tissues. They are usually solitary and involve the face, trunk, and extremities.[63] They are particularly common over the parotid area, where they are called *cystic hygromas*. They may have a rapid growth phase similar to that of raised hemangiomas.

Diagnosis and differential diagnosis   Circumscribed lymphangioma may be mistaken for a disorder with grouped vesicles, such as herpes simplex, herpes zoster, or dermatitis herpetiformis. However, there is no erythematous base in circumscribed lymphangioma, and the lesions appear gelatinous, not fluid-filled. As noted, hemorrhage into such lesions results in darkening, which may be confused with malignant melanoma. Cavernous lymphangiomas may be confused with lipomas, neurofibromas, and other soft subcutaneous masses.

Treatment   There is no satisfactory treatment.[63] Surgical excision can result in defects two or three times larger than the observed skin lesion, and the recurrence rate is high. Often, the lymph channels are found to surround vital subcutaneous structures, such as major arteries or nerves. The lesions are not responsive to radiotherapy or systemic steroids. Monthly or bimonthly visits in which photographs of the lesions are taken and careful measurements made are indicated initially. Eventually, semiannual or annual visits are sufficient to evaluate the lesions and commence therapy for complications.

Mongolian Spots (See also Chap. 89)

Mongolian spots are blue-black macules found on the skin of dark-skinned newborns. Infants' skin is always light at birth, and becomes progressively darker with increasing age. Hyperpigmentation of the scrotum and of the linea alba is common in dark-skinned infants at birth. The most commonly observed pigmentary abnormality of infants is the Mongolian spot. Mongolian spots are found over the lumbosacral area in up to 90 percent of Asian, black, and American Indian babies.[40–42,64]

Etiology and pathogenesis   Mongolian spots consist of spindle-shaped pigment cells located deep within the dermis. The precise mechanism of this condition is not known.

Clinical manifestations   Mongolian spots are blue-black macules usually found in lumbosacral skin. They are occasionally noted over the shoulders and back and may extend over the buttocks and extremities.[64]

Course and prognosis   Mongolian spots fade somewhat with time, and the difference in pigmentation from normal skin pigment becomes less obvious as the newborn's pigment darkens. Some traces of Mongolian spots may persist into adult life.

Café au Lait Spots (See also Chap. 89)

Light-brown oval macules that may appear more dark brown on black skin are found anywhere on the body and are designated café au lait spots.[40–42] Black infants are far more likely (120 per 1000 live births) than white infants (3 per 1000 live births) to have a solitary café au lait spot. Café au lait spots persist through childhood and may increase in number with age.

Clinical manifestations   Café au lait spots are tan macules with distinct borders. They are usually 3- to 5-mm in diameter, although huge lesions may be seen in newborns. The presence of six or more café au lait spots, >5 mm at their greatest diameter, is considered by most authorities as a major clue to neurofibromatosis type 1 in prepubertal children.[65] However, newborns with neurofibromatosis type 1 may have only one or two café au lait spots and will not acquire numerous spots until 2 to 5 years of age.

Linear and Whorled Pigmentary Changes (See also Chap. 89)

Linear and whorled patterns of hyper- or hypopigmentation represent genetic mosaicism in which clones of melanocytes are producing more (or less) melanin than the normal skin. These patterns are uncommon, but their precise incidence is not known.[66]

Etiology and pathogenesis   Linear and whorled patterns of hyper- or hypopigmentation represent genetic mosaicism with two or more lines of genetically distinct melanocytes present in the skin.[66]

Clinical manifestations   Linear and whorled patterns follow the lines of Blaschko, with abrupt midline demarcation.[66] At birth, differences from normal skin color may be quite subtle and difficult to detect. Only after 1 to 6 months may the skin patterns become evident. Often the linear swirls are unilateral or segmental. The aberrant pigmentation may be brown, in which case the term *linear and whorled nevoid hypermelanosis* is used, or white, in which case the terms *hypomelanosis of Ito* or *nevus depigmentosis* are used. In approximately 30 percent of infants, extracutaneous, often CNS, manifestations are found.[66]

Junctional Nevocellular Nevi (See also Chap. 90)

Junctional nevocellular nevi are clones of pigment cells located at the junction of the epidermis and dermis. They are found in 5 per 1000 live births.

Etiology and pathogenesis   Clones of melanocytes are present in excess at the dermal-epidermal junction. The condition is considered to be a developmental defect.

Clinical manifestations   Dark-brown or black macules with distinct borders represent clones of melanocytes found at the junction of the epidermis and dermis.[67] As an infant ages, these nevi may become slightly raised and papular and develop intradermal melanocytes, creating a compound nevus. Often, the surface of the lesion at birth is slightly irregular.

Raised Nevocellular Nevi (See also Chap. 90)

Collections of pigment cells within the dermis produce raised nevocellular nevi. They are seen in 10 per 1000 live births.[67,68]

Etiology and pathogenesis   The cause of raised pigmented nevi is not known. There is no correlation with twinning, infant sex, parental consanguinity, parental age, birth order, radiation exposure, or drug intake.[68] They are more common in black infants.

Clinical manifestations   Intradermal nevi are skin-colored to tan or brown solitary papules with smooth surfaces.[67,68] Most nevi are small, measuring <1.5 cm at their greatest diameter.[67] When these localized, raised pigment cell lesions are >10 or 20 cm at their greatest diameter, there is a concern about their cancer potential (Fig. 143-7). Malignant melanoma may occur in such large

FIGURE 143-7

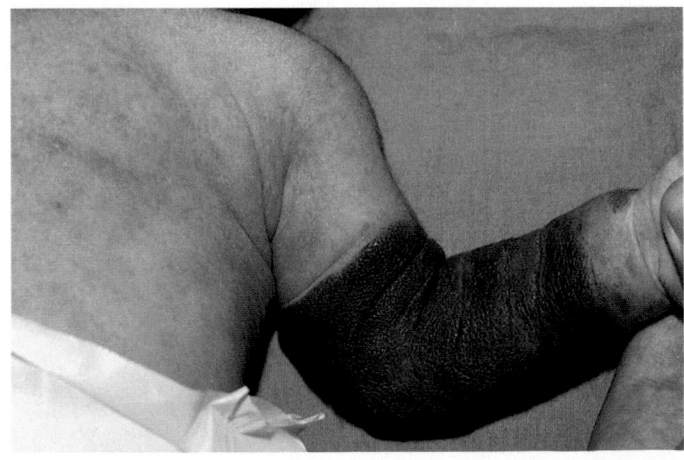

Giant congenital pigmented nevus. Raised pigmented lesion encircling the arm of a newborn.

nevi.[67] The precise estimate of cancer potential is unknown, but most authorities accept 1 percent or less.

Treatment Prophylactic removal of large congenital nevi within the first year of life has been recommended by many authorities, although the best age for removal is unknown.[67] Equal weight should be placed on the potential for cosmetic improvement and the cosmetic deformity produced by such surgical removal. Optimal surgical results may be best when the child is older. Whether smaller lesions have any malignant potential and require removal is not known.

Hypopigmentation

Hypopigmentation is seen as decrease in pigment from the normal skin. Localized areas of hypopigmented skin are uncommon in infants. A single hypopigmented area of skin is found in approximately 8 per 1000 live births, and a hypopigmented tuft of hair is found in 3 per 1000 live births.[40,42,43,66,69,70]

Albinism (See also Chap. 87)

Albinism is the congenital inability to produce pigment; it is rare and occurs 4 per 100,000 live births.

Etiology and pathogenesis All forms of albinism represent hereditary defects in the ability to produce or transfer melanin. The enzyme tyrosinase, which is pivotal in melanin production, is not functional in the most common types of albinism, and mutations in the tyrosinase gene have been identified.

Clinical manifestations Ten types of oculocutaneous albinism occur. Typically the newborns with albinism have fine, white hair and pink skin at birth.[71] They may also have nevi present at birth that are raised but not pigmented. Severe nystagmus and photophobia may also be present at birth.

Diagnosis and differential diagnosis Fair-skinned infants and infants with phenylketonuria as well as Chédiak-Higashi syndrome may be mistakenly diagnosed as having albinism. The presence of nystagmus is a clinical feature that often helps distinguish albinism.

Phenylketonuria (See also Chap. 149)

Phenylketonuria is a hereditary defect in phenylalanine metabolism. It is rare, occurring in 1 per 100,000 live births.

Etiology and pathogenesis Patients with phenylketonuria lack the enzymes needed to utilize phenylalanine. They develop hyperphenylalaninemia. Their hypopigmentation is thought to be related to the tight binding of phenylalanine to the receptor sites of tyrosinase so that the enzyme cannot oxidize tyrosine to melanin.

Clinical manifestations Newborns with phenylketonuria have blond hair, blue eyes, and light-colored skin. Routine screening tests for the presence of excessive amounts of phenylalanine in the blood will help detect this syndrome.

Diagnosis and differential diagnosis Phenylketonuria should be distinguished from albinism and Chédiak-Higashi syndrome. Analysis of blood for phenylalanine is the most useful differentiating test.

Epidermal Birthmarks

Increases in mature epidermal cells, hair follicles, or sebaceous glands may appear as birthmarks.[72] The majority of lesions are present at birth but new lesions can develop into adolescence.

EPIDERMAL NEVI (See also Chap. 83) Epidermal nevi are increases in mature epidermal cells in an area of skin, and are uncommon.

Etiology and pathogenesis Epidermal nevi are thought to be developmental.

Clinical features These lesions have a warty surface and appear anywhere on the body.[72] They are often linear or oval, with the long axis of the lesion parallel to the long axis of the dermatome. The majority of lesions are present at birth and up to 95 percent of the lesions are present by 7 years of age. Initially, the lesion is barely palpable and may be a confluence of smooth-topped papules. In time, the lesion becomes more wartlike and scaly. Most are 2 to 5 cm in length, but occasionally they may appear as long unilateral streaks involving an entire extremity or one side of the trunk (*nevus unius lateris*).[72] The lesions may be so extensive as to involve most of the body. The terms *ichthyosis hystrix* or *benign congenital acanthosis nigricans* have been applied to such extensive epidermal nevi. Epidermal nevi may become erythematous and itchy during the newborn period, with episodes of redness and inflammation, and may be designated *inflammatory linear verrucous epidermal nevi* (ILVEN).[72]

Patients with epidermal nevi may have associated abnormalities.[72] They have an increased number of cutaneous lesions, including café au lait spots, congenital hypopigmented macules, and congenital nevocellular nevi. They may have associated skeletal defects, seizure disorders, mental retardation, and ocular abnormalities. Patients with more extensive skin involvement have a higher association of other abnormalities than those with limited skin involvement. A birth defect clinic may be a good referral source for a multidisciplinary approach to such infants.

Pathology Epidermal nevi show thickening of the epidermis and hyperkeratosis.[72] In some lesions, a peculiar vacuolization of the granular layer appears, with separation of the cells in that layer, resulting in a microscopic blister cavity. This process is called *epidermolytic hyperkeratosis*. In inflammatory lesions, dermal accumulation of inflammatory cells and alternating bands of parakeratosis are described. Overgrowth of sebaceous glands and apocrine glands may be found underlying the epidermal proliferation.

Diagnosis and differential diagnosis Warts are commonly confused with epidermal nevi. The presence from birth and the linear arrangement will help distinguish epidermal nevi from warts. Extensive lesions may be confused with ichthyosis, and certain features of congenital bullous ichthyosiform erythroderma may exactly mimic epidermal nevi. Some investigators feel that congenital bullous ichthyosiform erythroderma is a variant of epidermal nevi. Inflammatory linear epidermal nevi may be confused with the warty stage of incontinentia pigmenti, with lichen striatus, or with a dermatitis.

Treatment For small lesions, surgical excision is the best treatment. Extensive lesions may be improved with the use of mild keratolytics, such as retinoic acid cream 0.05% once daily, 12% ammonium lactate lotion several times a day, or with bland lubricant therapy. The lesions revert to their hyperkeratotic state when treatments are discontinued.

SEBACEOUS NEVI (See also Chap. 83) Nevus sebaceous represent an excess of sebaceous glands in an area of skin. These are the most common of all epidermal birth marks and occur in 3 per 1000 live births.

Etiology and pathogenesis Like other epidermal nevi, nevus sebaceous is considered to be developmental.

Clinical manifestations Jadassohn's sebaceous nevus appears at birth as a slightly raised, oval or linear area with a yellow or orange color.[72,73] These nevi are common on the scalp and are devoid of hair, producing a congenital circumscribed hair loss. They may be seen on the face as well. Sebaceous nevus may be contiguous with an epidermal nevus and constitute part of the epidermal nevus syndrome.

Pathology Sebaceous nevus is a birthmark with an increased number of mature sebaceous glands without hair follicles. In addition, such lesions often have an increased number of apocrine glands.

Diagnosis and differential diagnosis Juvenile xanthogranulomas and xanthomas are yellow or orange lesions that may mimic sebaceous nevus. Skin biopsy will distinguish these lesions.

Treatment Surgical excision just prior to puberty is the treatment of choice because of the risk of basal cell carcinoma after puberty and for improved cosmetic appearance. Lesions excised before puberty may be incompletely excised and demonstrate warty growth along the surgical scar.

Course and prognosis At puberty, or with androgenic stimulation, the lesions enlarge and become warty on the surface and raised. Basal cell carcinomas have been reported to develop within the lesions after puberty on approximately 15 percent of children with sebaceous nevi.[73]

NEVUS COMEDONICUS (See also Chap. 83)
Nevus comedonicus is a birthmark consisting of pilosebaceous follicles with patulous openings.[29] It is the least common of epidermal birthmarks, but its prevalence is not precisely known.

Etiology and pathogenesis Nevus comedonicus is considered to be developmental.

Clinical manifestations In nevus comedonicus, linear or oval groups of widely dilated follicular openings plugged with keratin are present at birth on the face and scalp.[29] They may become inflamed and pustular as the child ages and mimic acne. The development of pustules within the lesions can occur as early as 2 to 4 weeks after birth. Bilateral and widespread lesions occur rarely.

Diagnosis and differential diagnosis In contrast to nevus comedonicus, neonatal acne begins at 1 month of age and involves discrete, single lesions rather than grouped arrangements of lesions.

Treatment In small lesions, simple surgical excision is the treatment of choice. Large or extensive lesions may be controlled with the application of topical retinoic acid cream once or twice daily.

APLASIA CUTIS CONGENITA
Aplasia cutis congenita is the failure to form certain layers of skin. This condition occurs in 1 per 3000 live births. It may be seen as an autosomal dominant trait in some families or associated with a variety of other malformations.[74,75]

Etiology and pathogenesis Aplasia cutis congenita is a developmental failure of skin fusion. Dermis, epidermis, and fat may all be missing, or single layers may be absent.[74]

Clinical manifestations In aplasia cutis congenita, oval, sharply marginated, 1- to 2-cm depressed areas are seen primarily in the midline of the posterior scalp.[74] They are hairless, may appear as an ulcer, or are covered by a smooth, finely wrinkled epithelial membrane (Fig. 143-8). Ulcerated defects heal with scar formation. Aplasia cutis congenita may be found as an isolated lesion or associated with other developmental defects, such as cleft palate or lip, syndactyly, absence of digits, eye anomalies, and congenital heart disease.[74,75] Although the majority of lesions appear on the scalp, lesions may be found on the trunk, face, or proximal extremities.

Diagnosis and differential diagnosis Scalp ulcers at birth may be mistaken for obstetric trauma, although a careful history will

FIGURE 143-8

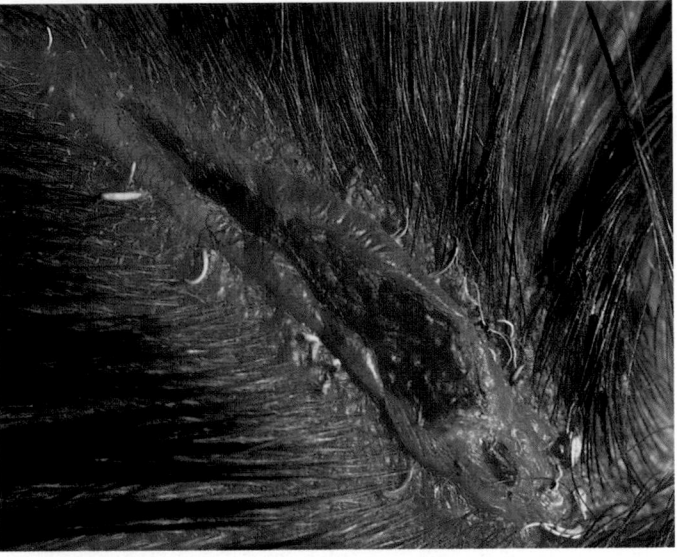

Aplasia cutis congenita. Newborn with a hairless crusted scalp defect.

distinguish between the two. Other forms of congenital circumscribed hair loss should be considered.

Treatment If the lesion is small, surgical excision, with mobilization of the scalp and simple closure, will correct the hairless defect.[74,75] Hair transplantation has been successful into large defects. Convincing the parents that this is not the result of obstetric trauma is critical.

CONNECTIVE TISSUE BIRTHMARKS (See also Chap. 101)
Connective tissue nevi are skin lesions consisting predominantly of the elements of extracellular collagen tissue and products of fibroblasts, such as collagen, elastin, and proteoglycans.[76] All connective tissue nevi are quite rare, although the precise incidence is not known.

Etiology and pathogenesis The etiology is unknown.

Clinical manifestations Connective tissue nevi are localized areas of thickened skin appearing as multiple skin-colored papules and plaques.[76] Stretching the overlying skin will give a yellowish discoloration to the areas. They may occasionally have increased vascularity and appear red. Collagenomas are localized areas of thickened skin with multiple skin-colored papules or plaques. They may be solitary or appear in a zosteriform segmental pattern. Elastomas are solitary plaques that are present at birth and contain increases in both elastic tissue and proteoglycans.[76] Elastomas may be solitary or they may be multiple in the Buschke-Ollendorff syndrome. This autosomal dominant syndrome appears as symmetrically distributed skin-colored papules or nodules with a predilection for the lower trunk or for the extremities.[76] Lesions may assume a thickened appearance of skin and develop a lacy pattern over the trunk. X-rays may show sclerotic densities of the ends of long bones, pelvis, and hands, although such lesions are often asymptomatic. The shagreen patch of tuberous sclerosis is a connective tissue nevus. The nevi are subtle at birth and may go unnoticed. They tend to persist throughout life.

Pathology Connective tissue nevi show thickened abundant collagen bundles, with or without associated increases in elastic tissue.[76] Such histologic changes are difficult to appreciate unless the skin biopsy includes adjacent normal skin for comparison.

Diagnosis and differential diagnosis The lesions are so characteristic that they are seldom misdiagnosed. Examinations for possible associated systemic disease may be necessary.

COMMON CONGENITAL MALFORMATIONS OF SKIN

Congenital malformations of skin are developmental defects in skin formation, and are frequently observed in newborns. They are observed in 7 per 100 live births.[77] Ear anomalies are found in 3 per 1000 live births, and simian crease as well as lip pits are seen in 2 per 1000 live births.

Ear Anomalies

Minor abnormalities in the formation of the ear constitute the most common congenital malformations. Loss of the fold of the skin in the superior part of the helix is the most common.[77] Low-set ears that angle away from the eye, periauricular skin tags, auricular or preauricular pits, or auricular sinuses and/or small ears are less common. Deafness may accompany congenital malformations of the external ear, or they may be associated with hemifacial microsomia (Goldenhar's syndrome).

Digital Abnormalities

A single crease on one or both upper palms is called a *simian crease*.[1,77] It is one feature of Down's syndrome but may also be observed in a variety of other syndromes, including trisomy 13, the Cornelia de Lange syndrome, Seckel's syndrome, and the cri du chat syndrome.[77] Clinodactyly with inward curvature of a digit is often observed in the fifth finger, and overlapping of the second and third toes is also a frequently observed malformation. Partial or complete fusion (syndactyly) of the second or third toes and clubfoot also occur with relative frequency.

Genital Abnormalities

Hydrocoele of one testis and hypospadias are the most common genital anomalies and malformations observed.[77] Malformations of the external genitalia may be clues to urinary tract anomalies, and investigation of the urinary tract may be indicated. They may also be clues to chromosomal abnormalities and may be associated with undescended testes.

Epicanthal Folds

Epicanthal folds of skin on the inner aspect of each eye are frequently observed. They are present in chromosomal abnormalities such as Down's, Turner's, and Klinefelter's syndromes.[77]

Neural Tube Defects

Primary defects in neural tube closures, such as meningomyelocele, encephalocoele, and anencephaly are relatively frequent congenital malformations.[77] In some instances, a tuft of hair that is longer and more pigmented than the adjacent scalp hair overlies the affected area of skull and is a cutaneous clue to an underlying neural tube defect.

Abnormalities of the Lip and Mouth

Pits in the lips are also quite common. Cleft lip and cleft palate or cleft lip alone are less common. The finding of lip pits or cleft lips and/or cleft palate may be a clue to the so-called first arch syndrome, which includes a small jaw and ocular hypertelorism.[77] A number of syndromes are associated with the first arch syndrome including the Pierre Robin syndrome, the orodigitofacial syndromes, and the Treacher-Collins syndrome.

Skin Dimpling

Infants may develop small dimple-like depressed scars secondary to injury during amniocentesis procedures.[78] The skin over the lesion appears to be pulled in by absent dermis. The lesion may not be noticed until the infant is several months old and has developed additional subcutaneous fat.

Major Chromosomal Abnormalities

Chromosomal abnormalities are phenotypic expressions of abnormal number or arrangement of chromosomes. They occur in 1 of 200 of all live births, in a higher percentage of births resulting in perinatal death, and in up to 50 percent of spontaneous abortions. Trisomy 21 is seen in 1 per 800 live births, trisomy 18 is observed in 1 per 3000 live births, and trisomy 13-15 occurs in 1 per 5000 live births.

TRISOMY 21 (DOWN'S SYNDROME) Mothers over 40 years of age have an increased chance of giving birth to a child with Down's syndrome. Cutaneous features are most useful in the recognition of this syndrome. These include prominent epicanthal folds, eyes slanting upward, small ears, simian palmar crease, excessive skin over the back of the neck, and clinodactyly of the fifth fingers.[77] The presence of these cutaneous features, plus muscular hypotonia and evidence of congenital heart disease, are the major clinical characteristic. Chromosomal analysis will confirm the diagnosis. Mental retardation may be severe, and growth failure associated with congenital heart disease makes the prognosis poor.[77]

TRISOMY 18 AND TRISOMY 13-15 In both of these chromosomal abnormalities, increased parental age has been an associated feature. Babies with trisomy 18 or trisomy 13-15 are small for gestational age, have low-set ears, simian creases, congenital heart disease, and severe mental retardation.[77] The presence of a cleft lip and palate associated with these features makes trisomy 13-15 more likely, while rocker-bottom feet and flexion contractures of the fingers makes trisomy 18 more likely to be diagnosed.[77] Chromosomal analysis is required for precise diagnosis.

TURNER'S SYNDROME The most common sex chromosome anomaly is Turner's syndrome, in which only one X chromosome is present (XO). Newborns with Turner's syndrome exhibit webbing of the neck and marked edema of the hands and feet.[77] The neck is often quite short. Coarctation of the aorta may be associated. Chromosomal analysis is necessary to confirm the diagnosis.

KLINEFELTER'S SYNDROME Extra sex chromosomes are characteristic of Klinefelter's syndrome (XXY, XXXY, or XXXXY). A low birth weight, undescended testes, and a small penis lead to suspicion of this syndrome.[77] Hypotonia and a variety of other anomalies may also be observed. Mental deficiency is usually severe in this syndrome, and chromosomal analysis is required to confirm the diagnosis.

Ichthyosis (See also Chap. 52)

Ichthyosis is a term used to describe excessive scaling of the skin which may be "fish-scale-like." It is thought to occur in 1 per 200 live births.[79]

Etiology and pathogenesis All forms of ichthyosis observed in the newborn period are hereditary.[79,80] Although normal infants born after 40 to 42 weeks of gestation display some scaling, as does the dysmature infant, the scaling in the forms of ichthyosis is usually generalized and characterized by thick scales. Four major types of ichthyosis have been described.[79] Lamellar ichthyosis and bullous ichthyosis usually present at birth with severe scaling.[79] Ichthyosis vulgaris and X-linked ichthyosis may be present in the neonate or may be expressed later in childhood.

Clinical manifestations ICHTHYOSIS VULGARIS Ichthyosis vulgaris is inherited as an autosomal dominant defect in the gene that encodes profilaggrin, which may be as frequent as 1 in 250 individuals.[79] The skin in ichthyosis vulgaris usually remains normal throughout the newborn period.

X-LINKED ICHTHYOSIS X-linked ichthyosis may appear at birth but usually appears later in infancy with scales over the posterior neck, upper trunk, and extensor surfaces of the extremities. As the child ages, the scales often become thicker and a dirty-yellow or brown color.[79] Scaling is usually mild during the first 30 days of life, and the skin is a normal color. Corneal opacities may be seen on slit-lamp examination of the eye of adults, both in patients and the carrier mothers. Palms and soles are spared, in contrast to the other forms of ichthyosis. Mutations in the gene encoding steroid sulfatase have been described in patients with X-linked ichthyoses.[80]

LAMELLAR ICHTHYOSIS AND CONGENITAL NONBULLOUS ICHTHYOSIFORM ERYTHRODERMA These two names are often used for the same condition and may cause confusion. Although both conditions appear to be an autosomal recessive trait, two separate disease entities may exist.[79,81] The nonbullous congenital ichthyosiform erythroderma patients have generalized fine scales on erythematous skin.[79] The lamellar ichthyosis patients have larger, darker, platelike scales with or without erythematous skin. Infants with either condition can be born with a collodion membrane (Fig. 143-9). The erythroderma may fade during childhood in some of these patients. Ectropion and eclabium may be present and appear shortly after birth in patients with lamellar ichthyosis.[79] The palms and soles in these patients may be greatly thickened. Skin biopsy after the collodion membrane is shed will demonstrate hyperkeratosis but is otherwise not diagnostic. Mutations in transglutaminase I genes have been demonstrated in lamellar ichthyosis.[81]

BULLOUS ICHTHYOSIS (CONGENITAL BULLOUS ICHTHYOSIFORM ERYTHRODERMA, EPIDERMOLYTIC HYPERKERATOSIS) Epidermolytic hyperkeratosis, an autosomal dominant disorder, is characterized by extensive scaling at birth, erythroderma, and recurrent episodes of bullae formation.

Increased epidermal turnover has been demonstrated in bullous ichthyosis, so that excessive numbers of stratum corneum cells are produced.[79,80] Vacuolization of suprabasilar epidermal cells with subsequent collapse and separation is seen. Mutations in the genes encoding one or the other of the paired keratins 1 and 10 has been reported.[80]

FIGURE 143-9

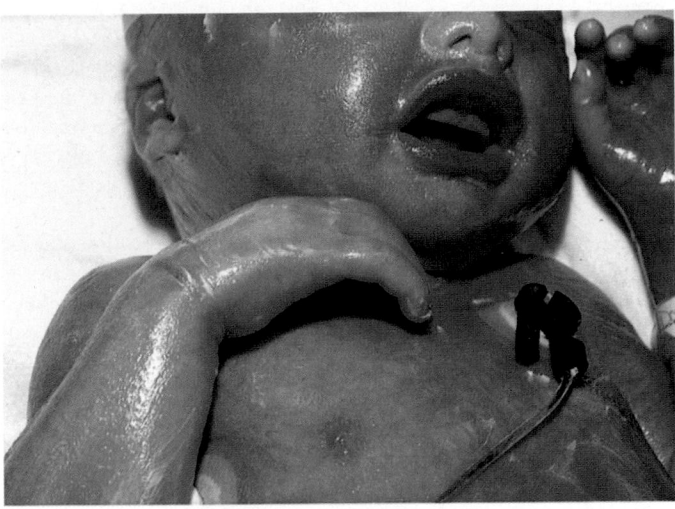

Collodion baby. Newborn encased in a tight membrane that restricts movement.

The blisters represent lysis of the epidermal granular layer, and secondary infection with *S. aureus* becomes a major difficulty in the neonatal period and during infancy.[79] As the child ages, the involvement becomes more limited in extent. By school age, thick, warty, dirty-yellow scales with malodorous excessive bacterial colonization of the skin will have developed on the palms, soles, elbows, and knees.[79] Skin biopsy will reveal enlargement of the granular cell layer with bizarre vacuolization of the epidermal granular cells.

Pathology Skin biopsy in the ichthyosis syndromes will often be of diagnostic value. In ichthyosis vulgaris there is a thin or absent granular cell layer in addition to the hyperkeratosis. X-linked ichthyosis demonstrates hyperkeratosis with an otherwise normal-appearing epidermis.[79] Vacuolization and separation of the granular cell layer with blister cavity formation are associated with the hyperkeratosis in bullous ichthyosis. Lamellar ichthyosis may demonstrate hyperkeratosis, acanthosis, and a mild chronic inflammatory infiltrate.

Diagnosis and differential diagnosis At birth, lamellar ichthyosis and bullous ichthyosis may be difficult to distinguish from one another.[79] The hereditary pattern and skin biopsy may help. As the infants age, the corneal opacities and sparing of the palms and soles will distinguish X-linked ichthyosis; the ectropion and eclabium will distinguish lamellar ichthyosis; and the recurrent bullous episodes will distinguish epidermolytic hyperkeratosis. Measurement of steroid sulfatase activity in red blood cells may be useful in the diagnosis of X-linked ichthyosis.[79] Scaling disorders similar to lamellar ichthyosis are present in many ichthyosis syndromes associated with neurologic disease.[79,80] In the Sjögren-Larsson syndrome, a defect in fatty alcohol dehydrogenase has been found.

Treatment There is no satisfactory treatment for the ichthyosis. In ichthyosis vulgaris and X-linked ichthyosis, hydration of the skin twice daily and the generous use of lubricants will control the dryness and scaling. The use of alpha-hydroxy acids such as lactic acid 5% ointment, citric acid 5% ointment, or 12% ammonium lactate lotion (Lac-Hydrin) applied once or more daily may be helpful in the more severe ichthyoses, although many such patients do as well with bland lubricants alone. In bullous ichthyoses, calcipotriol ointment may control the condition.[82] Systemic antistaphylococcal antibiotics are required to treat the bullous impetigo in the ichthyosis episodes.

Great caution must be used in applying any therapy to the skin of an infant or child. Because of their larger surface area relative to body weight, systemic toxicity and side effects can be seen in infants and children and acidosis can occur secondary to topical therapy.[82]

It should be recognized that both the active medication and the vehicle for the medication could cause significant toxicity in the infant with significant dermatitis or even normal skin. The synthetic retinoids given orally have shown promise in management of ichthyosis.[82]

HEREDITARY SKIN DISEASES WITH DRAMATIC NEONATAL PRESENTATIONS

The Red, Scaly Newborn

PHYSIOLOGIC SCALING AND REDNESS A scaling and often red newborn may be an enigma to the inexperienced observer. A postmature baby may exhibit desquamation that is marked over the hands, feet, and lower trunk. If observed during the first day of life when the newborn skin is quite red, this condition may result in an erroneous diagnosis of one of the ichthyoses.[1] Similarly, preterm infants born at 32 weeks of gestational age or earlier will have red or glistening skin that similarly may be confused with ichthyosis. Such changes are transient and are often resolved within the newborn period.

COLLODION BABY Newborns with an encasement of shiny, tight, inelastic scale are designated as having a collodion membrane (Fig. 143-9). Collodion babies are quite rare. The membrane is composed of greatly thickened stratum corneum that has been saturated with water.[79] As the water content evaporates in extrauterine life, large fissures appear in the membrane and the membrane is shed, revealing red skin underneath.

Collodion babies appear to be tightly encased in a membrane at birth. Their appearance is frightening to health care personnel. The presence of a collodion membrane does not allow one to predict that the affected baby will necessarily develop ichthyosis, and spontaneous healing may occur. Skin biopsy of the collodion membrane is usually not diagnostic. Most collodion babies do have a form of ichthyosis, and the majority of them develop features of lamellar ichthyosis. Bullous ichthyosis, X-linked ichthyosis and Gaucher's disease have also been reported to develop in collodion babies.[79,80]

HARLEQUIN FETUS A harlequin fetus is an infant born with massive plates of scales. Although this has been considered a more severe form of lamellar ichthyosis, most authorities now believe that it represents a distinct, rare autosomal recessive disease. It has been associated with defects in both lipid and protein metabolism.

Harlequin fetus is usually incompatible with extrauterine life. These infants have massive, dense, platelike scales, which produce severe deformities of skeletal and soft tissues that restrict respiration.[79] Recently, infants treated with systemic retinoids have survived, with residual severe ichthyosis.

Atopic Dermatitis and Seborrheic Dermatitis

Atopic dermatitis is said to have its onset after the newborn period, with the most frequently observed age of onset being 2 to 3 months.[83] If a dermatitis begins within the newborn period, many authorities designate it seborrheic dermatitis. It has now become clear, however, that infants who later develop typical atopic dermatitis may have the onset of their skin eruption within the newborn period.[1,83] There is significant overlap in infants who have seborrheic and atopic dermatitis, both in distributions of the lesions, which involve the scalp, diaper area, and extensor area, and in the history of pruritus, feeding patterns, food intolerance, and family members with atopic disease. In newborns, the dermatitis is usually acute, with crusting and oozing, and extensive. Physiologic overproduction of sebum occurs in the newborn period, giving any dermatitis a greasy feel to the skin surface. It is advisable to designate dermatitis seen in newborns as simply dermatitis.

Diaper Dermatitis

Diaper dermatitis occurring in the newborn period is primarily perianal in location and is related to the irritant substances found in stool.[83] It presents with a bright red perianal acute dermatitis. Superinfection with *Candida albicans* is frequent in neonatal perianal diaper dermatitis present for greater than 72 h. The role of diapers in the newborn period in preventing the perianal diaper dermatitis is unclear.[84]

Scabies

Newborns with scabies may present with a severe generalized dermatitis. They may have only a few or as many as thousands of lesions. Babies usually have involvement of the head and neck.[85] Individual burrows may be obscured and difficult to detect because of the confluence of dermatitis. The scabies mite can be recovered from papules or burrows, with the hands and feet the best sites of recovery.[85]

Histiocytosis X (See also Chap. 160)

A generalized dermatitis, particularly with purpuric papules or petechiae within the dermatitis and involvement of the head and neck, is characteristic of histiocytosis X (Fig. 143-10). The skin eruption may be present at birth or start during the first 30 days of life. The presence of chronic draining ears and enlargement of the liver and spleen are useful additional clues in the diagnosis.[86] Skin biopsy will demonstrate the characteristic infiltration with histiocytic cells containing Langerhans-like granules.

Congenital Candidiasis

Congenital candidiasis may present at birth with generalized eczematous, scaly skin.[27,28] Maternal infection of the birth canal with *Candida* is always present. Direct microscopic examination of scales scraped from the skin's surface will demonstrate yeast forms.

Epidermolysis Bullosa (See also Chap. 65)

Several types of epidermolysis bullosa are evident within the first 24 h of life. Hemorrhagic blisters and bleeding erosions may be extensive. Nursery personnel may induce numerous lesions while handling the baby before the diagnosis is recognized. Other forms of epidermolysis bullosa may begin slowly, with a few lesions be-

FIGURE 143-10

CHAPTER 143
Neonatal Dermatology   1679

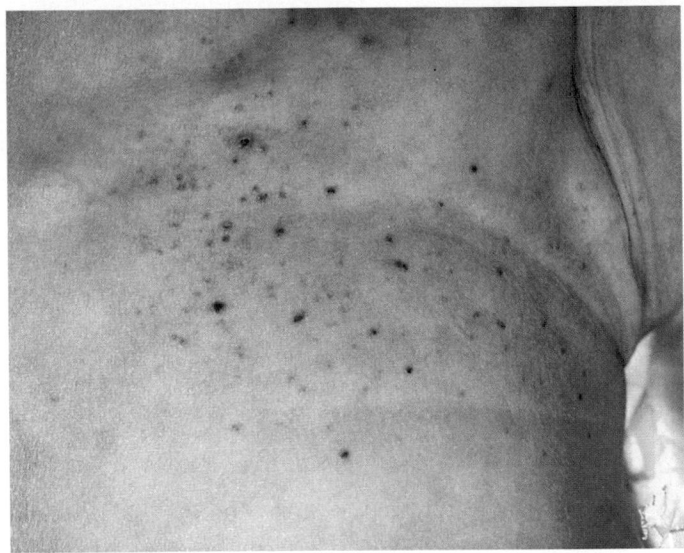

Histiocytosis X. A 4-week-old with enlarged inguinal lymph nodes and purpuric papules on the lower abdomen.

ginning 3 to 30 days after birth. Diagnosis of epidermolysis bullosa in the immediate newborn period may be quite difficult.[87,88] Many different types of epidermolysis bullosa exist that result in mild to lethal disease.[87,88] The final diagnosis of the patient depends upon characterization of the site of blister formation within the epidermis, basement membrane, or dermis and on molecular genetic analysis. Presence of few or many blisters in the neonate does not define the severity of the disease. Diagnosis should be made with a combination of biopsies for both light and electron microscopy and possibly with immunofluorescent mapping of antigenic sites within the basement membrane zone.[88] Extreme care must be taken in obtaining and interpreting skin biopsies from newborns to distinguish among these mechanobullous diseases. A shave or ellipse biopsy at the edge of a blister that is less than 12 h old is preferred. All forms of epidermolysis bullosa are related to adherence defects within the skin. Genetic mutations of type VII collagen are found in dystrophic forms of epidermolysis bullosa, laminin 5 in junctional epidermolysis bullosa, and keratins 5 or 14 in simplex forms of epidermolysis bullosa.[87,89] Mutations of the gene encoding plectin, a cornified envelope and skeletal muscle protein that binds keratins is the basis for epidermolysis bullosa simplex with muscular dystrophy.[90]

Acrodermatitis Enteropathica (See also Chap. 148)

Acrodermatitis enteropathica is an inherited disorder of zinc metabolism.

Etiology and pathogenesis   Depletion of body zinc stores due to faulty absorption of zinc is responsible for the symptoms and signs of acrodermatitis enteropathica. It is not known whether this is due to the lack of a zinc carrier protein or to some defect of zinc absorption in the intestine. Zinc is stored in the same tissues as iron and serves as an important cofactor for a variety of enzymes such as alkaline phosphatase and carbonic anhydrase.[91] It is thought that zinc deficiency results in impairment of metalloenzyme activity, which produces the clinical features.

Clinical manifestations   Acrodermatitis enteropathica is an autosomal recessive disorder of zinc metabolism.[91] It is not apparent

at birth but begins at 15 to 30 days of age, with acral skin erosions, diarrhea, and failure to thrive.[91] The erosions appear as red, moist areas over the distal extremities, including the hands and feet (Fig. 143-11), and in the perioral and perineal areas.

Often, the cutaneous features precede the diarrhea by several weeks to several months. As the disorder continues, weight loss occurs, as well as photophobia, apathy, alopecia, thrush, and paronychia due to *C. albicans*. If the child survives the infectious complications of malnutrition, the skin lesions become erythematous plaques with silvery scales that mimic psoriasis.

Diagnosis and differential diagnosis   The diagnosis is made by measuring serum or plasma zinc levels.[91] There are many sources of zinc contamination in rubber stoppers and glass tubes and other blood-collecting devices that produce falsely high zinc levels. Thus, the diagnosis may be obscured, and blood samples should be collected in acid-washed sterile plastic tubes, using acid-washed plastic syringes.

Zinc deficiency can also be seen in premature and term infants who are fed a diet deficient in zinc. Their clinical picture mimics acrodermatitis enteropathica. Occasionally, human breast milk can be low in zinc, allowing zinc deficiency in the totally breast-fed infant. The lesions are often mistaken for mucocutaneous candidiasis associated with immune deficiency. Plasma or serum zinc levels will distinguish between the two. Often, protein-calorie malnutrition states are considered, but lesions usually develop in such patients after 6 months of age, and the nutritional history may distinguish between the two. Histiocytosis X will present with intertriginous erosions in infancy. Acquired zinc deficiency states, such as seen with prolonged parenteral hyperalimentation, will mimic acrodermatitis enteropathica.[91]

Treatment   Oral zinc sulfate, 5 mg/kg per day given in two doses, produces rapid clinical improvement.[91] Apathy disappears within 24 h, and the skin lesions and diarrhea resolve within 7 to 14 days. Photophobia, alopecia, and growth failure are reversed over the ensuing months. It is not known whether or not lifetime maintenance with supplemental zinc is required.

FIGURE 143-11

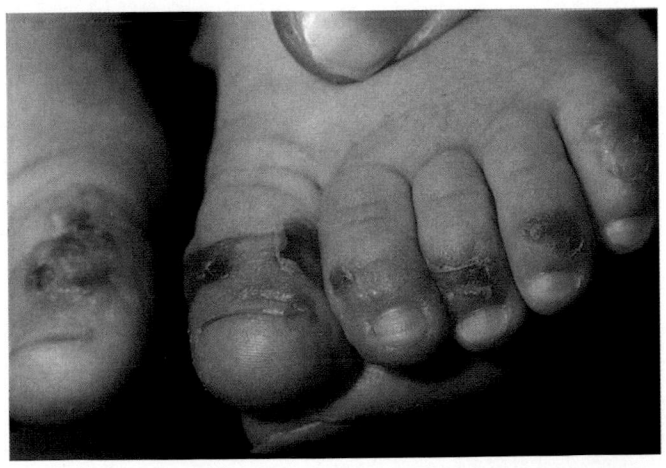

Acrodermatitis enteropathica. A zinc-deficient newborn with erosions and crusting around the toes.

Incontinentia Pigmenti

Incontinentia pigmenti is a hereditary condition characterized by linear rows of blisters on skin associated with ocular, CNS, and dental defects.

Etiology and pathogenesis Incontinentia pigmenti is an X-linked trait, usually lethal to the male, which explains the female predominance in this disorder.[92,93] The exact gene defect is unknown, but an unstable mutation may be responsible.[94]

Clinical manifestations Linear rows of blisters on the extremities are seen at birth in incontinentia pigmenti (Fig. 143-12). Occasionally the trunk is also involved. These blistering episodes recur over the first 3 months of life and are replaced by warty linear areas that may last until 1 year of age.[92] Rows of brown pigmentation are then left. In addition, whorls of brown pigmentation are found on the trunk and in areas where the blisters and warty lesions did not occur. The pigmentation fades as the child ages and is usually not seen after adolescence.[92] Mental retardation, seizures, microcephaly, and other CNS disorders occur in 30 percent of the patients. Ocular and skeletal anomalies may also be noted.[92,93]

Pathology Skin biopsy demonstrates an inflammatory dermatitis, with subcorneal vesicles filled with numerous eosinophils.[92] The warty stage merely demonstrates hyperkeratosis and chronic inflammation in the dermis. In the pigmentary stage, melanin is found free in the dermis or engulfed by dermal macrophages, which accounts for the name of the condition.

Diagnosis and differential diagnosis In the blistering stage, herpes simplex or bullous impetigo may be confused with incontinentia pigmenti, but the linear arrangement of its blisters and appropriate cultures will distinguish it from these two disorders. The warty phase may mimic linear epidermal birthmarks or warts. The hyperpigmentation is uniquely arranged in whorls and is unlikely to be confused with other causes of hyperpigmentation.

Treatment There is no satisfactory treatment.

FIGURE 143-12

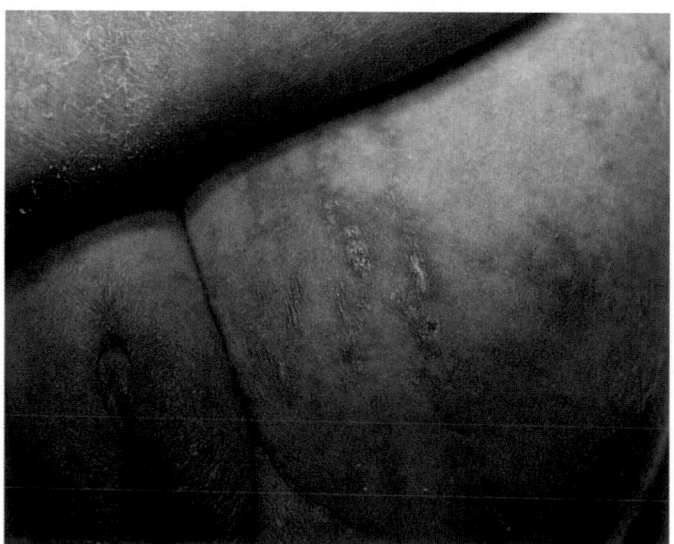

Incontinentia pigmenti. A newborn with linear rows of blisters.

REFERENCES

1. Weston WL et al: *Color Textbook of Pediatric Dermatology, 2d ed.* St. Louis, Mosby-Yearbook, 1996 p 326
2. Holbrook KA, Smith LT: Ultrastructural aspects of human skin during the embryonic, fetal, premature, neonatal and adult periods of life. *Birth Defects* **XVII**:9, 1981
3. Lane AT: Human fetal skin development. *Pediatr Dermatol* **3**:487, 1986
4. Fairley JA, Rasmussen JE: Comparison of stratum corneum thickness in children and adults. *J Am Acad Dermatol* **8**:652, 1983
5. Rutter N: The immature skin. *Eur J Pediatr* **155**: S18, 1996
6. Lane AT: Development and care of the premature infant's skin. *Pediatr Dermatol* **4**:1, 1987
7. Vernon HJ et al: The effect of a semi-permeable dressing on transepidermal water loss in premature infants. *Pediatrics* **86**:357,1990
8. Simonsen K et al: Iatrogenic heat burns in severely asphyxic newborns. *Acta Paediatr* **84**:1438, 1995
9. Smales ORC, Kime R: Thermoregulation in babies immediately after birth. *Arch Dis Child* **53**:58, 1978
10. Nopper AJ et al: Topical ointment therapy benefits premature infants. *J Pediatr* **128**:660, 1996
11. Jorgenson RJ et al: Intraoral findings and anomalies in neonates. *Pediatrics* **69**:577, 1982
12. Maffei A et al: An unusual presentation of erythema toxicum scrotal pustules present at birth. *Arch Pediatr Adolesc Med* **150**:649, 1996
13. Rapelanoro R et al: Neonatal *Malassezia furfur* pustulosis. *Arch Dermatol* **132**:2, 1996
14. Frieden IJ: Blisters and pustules in the newborn. *Curr Probl Pediatr* **11**:555, 1989
15. Murphy WF, Langley AL: Common bullous lesions—presumably self-inflicted—occurring in utero in the newborn infant. *Pediatrics* **32**:1099, 1963
16. Hicks J et al: Subcutaneous fat necrosis of the newborn and hypercalcemia: Case report and review of the literature. *Pediatr Dermatol* **10**:271, 1993
17. Cook JS et al: Hypercalcemia in association with subcutaneous fat necrosis of the newborn; Studies of calcium regulating hormones. *Pediatrics* **90**:93, 1992
18. Heilbron B, Saxe N: Scleredema in an infant. *Arch Dermatol* **122**:1417, 1986
19. Philip AGS, Hewit JR: Early diagnosis of neonatal sepsis. *Pediatrics* **65**:1036, 1980
20. Brown ZA et al: Neonatal herpes simplex virus infection in relation to asymptomatic maternal infection at the time of labor. *N Engl J Med* **324**: 1247, 1991
21. Kibrick S: Herpes simplex infection at term: What to do with mother, newborn, and nursery personnel. *JAMA* **243**:157, 1980
22. Whitley R et al: A controlled trial comparing vidarabine with acyclovir in neonatal herpes simplex virus infection. *N Engl J Med* **324**:444, 1991
23. Kulhanjian JA et al: Identification of women at unsuspected risk of primary infection with herpes simplex virus type 2 during pregnancy. *N Engl J Med* **326**:918, 1992
24. Randolph AG et al: Cesarean delivery for women presenting with genital herpes lesions. *JAMA* **270**:77,1993
25. Duke EMC: Infantile acne associated with transient increases in plasma concentrations of leutenizing hormone, follicle-stimulating hormone and testosterone. *Br Med J* **282**:1275, 1981
26. Stuart SM, Lane AT: *Candida* and *Malassezia* as nursery pathogens. *Semin Dermatol* **11**:19, 1992
27. Lane AT: Cutaneous candidiasis. *Pediatr Dermatol* **12**:369, 1995 Kam LA, Giacola GP: Congenital cutaneous candidiasis. *Am J Dis Child* **129**:1215, 1975
28. Jarratt M, Ramsdell W: Infantile acropustulosis. *Arch Dermatol* **115**:834, 1979
29. Cantu JM et al: Familial comedones. *Arch Dermatol* **114**:1807, 1978
30. Kalla G, Goyal AM: Juvenile generalized pustular psoriasis. *Pediatr Dermatol* **13**:45, 1996
31. Rubin L et al: Disseminated varicella in a neonate: implications for immunoprophylaxis of neonates postnatally exposed to varicella. *Pediatr Infect Dis J* **5**:100, 1986
32. Peter G (ed): Varicella-zoster infections, in *1997 Red Book: Report of the Committee on Infectious Diseases,* 24th ed. Elk Grove Village, IL, American Academy of Pediatrics, 1997, pp 573–585
33. Lipton SV, Brunell PA: Management of varicella exposure in a neonatal intensive care unit. *JAMA* **261**:1782, 1989

34. Darmstadt GL, Lane AT: Impetigo: An overview. *Pediatr Dermatol* **11**:293, 1994

35. Dancer SJ et al: Outbreak of staphylococcal scalded skin syndrome among neonates. *J Infection* **16**:87, 1988

36. Rudoy RC, Nelson JD: Breast abscess during the neonatal period. A review. *Am J Dis Child* **129**:1031, 1975

37. Fiumara NJ: Syphilis in newborn children. *Clin Obstet Gynecol* **18**:183, 1975

38. Dudgeon JA: Congenital rubella. *J Pediatr* **87**:1078, 1975

39. Jacobs AH, Walton RG: The incidence of birthmarks in the neonate. *Pediatrics* **58**:218, 1976

40. Nanda A et al: Survey of cutaneous lesions in Indian newborns. *Pediatr Dermatol* **6**:39, 1989

41. Alper JC, Holmes LB: The incidence and significance of birthmarks in a cohort of 4,641 newborns. *Pediatr Dermatol* **1**:58, 1983

42. Hidano A et al: Statistical survey of skin changes in Japanese neonates. *Pediatr Dermatol* **3**:140, 1986

43. Morelli JG: Hemangiomas and vascular malformations. *Pediatr Ann* **25**:91, 1996

44. Enjoras O, Mulliken JB: Vascular cutaneous anomalies in children: Malformations and hemangiomas. *Pediatr Surg Int* **11**:290, 1996

45. Tay Y-K et al: Inflammatory nuchal-occipital port wine stains. *J Am Acad Dermatol* **35**:811, 1996

46. Shamir R et al: Nevus flammeus. *Am J Dis Child* **145**:85, 1991

47. Enjolras O et al: Facial port-wine stains and Sturge-Weber syndrome. *Pediatrics* **76**:48, 1985

48. Paller AS: The Sturge-Weber syndrome. *Pediatr Dermatol* **4**:300, 1987

49. Talman B et al: Location of portwine stain and the likelihood of ophthalmologic or CNS complications. *Pediatrics* **87**:323, 1991

50. Lindenauer SM: The Klippel-Trenaunay syndrome. *Ann Surg* **162**:303, 1965

51. Morelli JG et al: Initial lesion size is a critical factor in determining the response of port wine stains in children treated with the pulsed [450 microseconds] dye [585 nanometers] laser. *Arch Pediatr Adolesc Med* **149**:142, 1995

52. Morelli JG et al: Treatment of congenital telangiectatic vascular malformations with the vascular specific pulsed dye laser. *Pediatrics* **93**:603, 1993

53. Lacour M et al: Role of the pulsed dye laser in the management of ulcerated capillary haemangiomas. *Br J Dermatol* **134**:161, 1996

54. Simpson JR: Natural history of cavernous hemangiomata. *Lancet* **2**:1057, 1959

55. Amir J et al: Strawberry hemangioma in preterm infants. *Pediatr Dermatol* **3**:331, 1986

56. Esterly NB: Kasabach-Merritt syndrome in infants. *J Am Acad Dermatol* **8**:504 1983

57. Sadan N, Wolach B: Treatment of hemangiomas in infants with high doses of prednisone. *J Pediatr* **128**:141, 1996

58. Eskowitz RAB et al: Interferon α-2a for life threatening hemangiomas in infancy. *N Engl J Med* **326**: 1456, 1992

59. Lewis-Jones MS et al: Cutis marmorata telangiectatica congenita—a report of two cases occurring in male children. *Clin Exp Dermatol* **13**:97, 1988

60. Esterly NB et al: Special symposia: The management of disseminated eruptive hemangiomata in infants. *Pediatr Dermatol* **1**:312, 1984

61. Stratte EG et al: Multimodal management of diffuse neonatal hemangiomatosis. *J Am Acad Dermatol* **34**:337, 1996

62. Oranje AP: Blue rubber bleb nevus syndrome. *Pediatr Dermatol* **3**:304, 1986

63. Flanagan BP, Helwig EB: Cutaneous lymphangioma. *Arch Dermatol* **113**:24, 1977

64. Goss BD et al: The prevalence and characteristics of congenital pigmented lesions in newborn babies in Oxford. *Paediatr Perinat Epidemiol* **61**:448, 1990

65. Gutmann DH: New insights into the neurofibromatoses. *Curr Opin Neurol* **7**:166, 1994

66. Nehal KS et al: Analysis of 54 cases of hypopigmentation and hyperpigmentation along the lines of Blaschko. *Arch Dermatol* **132**:1167, 1996

67. Maghoob AA et al: Large congenital melanocytic nevi and the risk for developing malignant melanoma: A prospective study. *Arch Dermatol* **132**:170, 1996

68. Dawson HA et al: A prospective study of congenital melanocytic naevi: Progress report and evaluation after 6 years. *Br J Dermatol* **134**:617, 1996

69. Fitzpatrick TB: History and significance of white macules, earliest visible sign of tuberous sclerosis. *Ann NY Acad Sci* **615**:26, 1991

70. Roach ES et al: Diagnostic criteria: Tuberous sclerosis complex. *J Child Neurol* **2**:221, 1992

71. Oetting WS, King RA: Molecular basis of oculocutaneous albinism. *J Invest Dermatol* **103**: 131s, 1994

72. Rogers M et al: Epidermal nevi and the epidermal nevus syndrome. *J Am Acad Dermatol* **20**:476, 1989

73. Domingo J, Helwig EB: Malignant neoplasms associated with nevus sebaceous of Jadassohn. *J Amer Acad Dermatol* **1**:545, 1979

74. Drolet B et al: "Membranous aplasia cutis" with hair collars—congenital absence of skin or neuroectodermal defect? *Arch Dermatol* **131**:1427, 1995

75. Gershonibaruch R, Leibo R: Aplasia cutis congenita, high myopia and cone-rod dysfunction in two sibs: A new autosomal recessive disorder. *Am J Hum Genet* **61**:42, 1996

76. Uitto J et al: Connective tissue nevi of the skin. *J Am Acad Dermatol* **3**:441, 1980

77. Holmes LB: Congenital malformations. *N Engl J Med* **295**:204, 1976

78. Bruce S et al: Skin dimpling associated with midtrimester amniocentesis. *Pediatr Dermatol* **2**:140, 1984

79. Schwader T, Ott F: All about ichthyosis. *Pediatr Clin North Am* **38**: 835, 1994

80. Bale SJ, Doyle SZ: The genetics of ichthyosis: A primer for epidemiologists. *J Invest Dermatol* **102**:49s, 1994

81. Huber M et al: Mutations of keratinocyte transglutaminase in lamellar ichthyosis. *Science* **267**:525, 1995

82. Kragballe K et al: Efficacy, tolerability and safety of calcipotriol ointment in disorders of keratinization: Results of a randomized, double-blind vehicle controlled right-left study. *Arch Dermatol* **131**:556, 1995

83. Yates VM et al: Early diagnosis of infantile seborrheic dermatitis and atopic dermatitis. Clinical features. *Br J Dermatol* **108**:633, 1983

84. Lane AT et al: Evaluations of diapers containing absorbent gelling material with conventional disposable diapers in newborn infants. *Am J Dis Child* **144**:315, 1990

85. Paller AS: Scabies in infants and small children. *Semin Dermatol* **12**:3, 1993

86. Leahy MA et al: Langerhans cell histiocytosis. *Curr Probl Dermatol* **6**:1, 1994

87. Uitto J et al: Molecular basis of the dystrophic and junctional forms of epidermolysis bullosa: Mutations of type VII collagen and kalinin (laminin 5) gene. *J Invest Dermatol* **103**:39s, 1994

88. Fine JD et al: Revised clinical and laboratory criteria for subtypes of inherited epidermolysis bullosa. *J Am Acad Dermatol* **24**:119,1991

89. Fuchs E et al: Genetic basis of epidermolysis bullosa simplex and epidermolytic hyperkeratosis. *J Invest Dermatol* **103**:25s, 1994

90. Smith FJD et al: Plectin deficiency results in muscular dystrophy with epidermolysis bullosa. *Nature Genet* **13**:450, 1996

91. Sandstrom B et al: Acrodermatitis enteropathica, zinc metabolism, copper status and immune function. *Arch Pediatr Adolesc Med* **148**:980, 1994

92. Landy SJ, Donnai D: Incontinentia pigmenti (Bloch-Sulzberger syndrome). *J Med Genet* **30**:53, 1993

93. Gorski JL, Burright EN: The molecular genetics of incontinentia pigmenti. *Semin Dermatol* **12**: 255, 1993

94. Hatchwell E: Unstable mutation in incontinentia pigmenti? *J Med Genet* **33**:349, 1996

Mary Wu Chang
Seth J. Orlow

Pediatric and Adolescent Dermatology

The subspecialty of pediatric dermatology is growing rapidly. Many, if not all, dermatologic diseases have different manifestations in children, and it is not possible to discuss the pediatric manifestations of all cutaneous diseases in one chapter. Instead, in this chapter we will focus on the methods and medical issues unique to the practice of pediatric dermatology. Within the chapter, three arbitrary age divisions are used. Infancy refers to patients less than 2 years of age, childhood includes patients aged 2 to 12 years, and adolescence, 12 to 18 years of age. Dermatology of the neonate (infants less than 30 days of age) has been discussed in Chap. 143. Within each age group, examination techniques will be discussed first, followed by psychosocial and developmental issues. Lastly, topics of special importance to pediatric dermatology, such as therapeutic issues (including a selected formulary), dysmorphology, issues surrounding correction of congenital disfigurement, and child abuse are discussed at the end of the chapter.

INFANCY

Examination Techniques

A complete evaluation of an infant includes obtaining gestational and perinatal information as well as family history. Information about exposures during pregnancy including medications and illicit drugs and infectious diseases such as varicella or sexually transmitted diseases are mandatory. Obstetrical data including placental cultures can be invaluable and are simple to obtain. Normal skin findings can vary greatly depending on the newborn's gestational age. For example, a baby born after 42 weeks' gestation may exhibit desquamation of skin and hyperlinearity of the palms and soles that may be confused with congenital ichthyosis. In Chap. 143 neonatal dermatology is discussed in more detail.

The most important element in the examination of an infant is to be thorough. Whether examined in the lap of the parent or on the examination table, all surfaces including the creases and valleys of body folds and the genitalia deserve close examination. A vascular stain or an erosion on a newborn can be the presenting sign of a hemangioma.[1] A benign finding such as an occult, stray hair may later strangulate an appendage and should be removed. Infants with digital tourniquet (pseudoainhum) and clitoral tourniquet have been described.[2,3] Congenital lesions of all classifications (e.g., pigmented, vascular, aplasias) warrant closer inspection to rule out associated findings. Midline lesions on the spine, scalp or face may have central nervous system (CNS) connections and should not be biopsied without prior evaluation (Table 144-1). The diaper area has its own unique set of problems and deserves examination at every visit.[8,9] Irritant contact dermatitis, candida diaper dermatitis,

impetigo, and seborrheic dermatitis are examples of common problems of this region and are addressed separately in this textbook. Nonhealing erosions or petechial lesions in the diaper area are presenting signs of Langerhans cell histiocytosis (Fig. 144-1) and should be biopsied (Langerhans cell histiocytosis is discussed in Chap. 160). Examination of the oral cavity is the most invasive part of the examination and is therefore best left to last.

Any infant with a history of suspected seizures or developmental delay should be examined for ash-leaf macules of tuberous sclerosis and other neurocutaneous syndromes. A Wood's lamp is helpful for examining infants with lightly pigmented skin. (Disorders of pigmentation and neurocutaneous disorders are discussed in Chap. 87 to 89 and 189, respectively.)

Jaundice, a common problem in healthy infants, can also be the presenting sign of certain metabolic or infectious disorders. In contrast, carotenemia is caused by a diet high in squash, carrots, or yams, leading to a reversible yellowish discoloration of the skin, accentuated in the palms and soles. The sclera are spared in carotenemia, but icteric in true jaundice. Carotenemia can be associated with diabetes mellitus and is seen in hypothyroid states; it is not uncommonly seen in children with hypothyroidism as a manifestation of Down's syndrome.

Medical and surgical decision making for the infant is based primarily on function rather than cosmesis. For example, while most hemangiomas require no intervention, those located on the lip or near the eye may compromise feeding or vision, and intervention is indicated (hemangiomas are addressed in Chap. 102). Similarly, extraction of a natal tooth is indicated if breast-feeding is impaired, whether or not the tooth is a sign of genetic syndrome. There are times when the parents' desire for treatment may not be in the best interest of the patient.[10] For example, treatment for neonatal acne may be more detrimental than the "disease."

Normal Skin Care

The infant's skin has a thinner stratum corneum[11] and contains lower levels of natural moisturizing factors[12] and sebum than that of adults.[13] For these reasons, frequent bathing of the infant leads to asteatosis and irritation of the skin. Bathing one or twice a week in plain water is sufficient for most infants; if bathing is more frequent, moisturization with unscented, simple moisturizers is recommended. The face, hands, and diaper area may be cleansed daily using a small amount of a mild, unscented soap. Baby powder on the diaper area offers no antimicrobial benefit to the infant; it adds a risk of aspiration and should not be used.[14] Well-meaning parents may use a multitude of products on their babies' skin. It has been estimated that the average newborn is exposed to approximately 10 skin care products in the first month of life, leading to exposure to

TABLE 144-1

Biopsy Pitfalls in Pediatric Dermatology

AGE GROUP	LESION AND SITE	DIAGNOSIS	DANGER	PROPER MANAGEMENT
Newborn	Erosion or vesicle on the scalp	Aplasia cutis congenita Differential diagnosis: herpes, fetal scalp electrode trauma	Possible intracranial connection, risk of meningitis with biopsy or scraping	Protect site, do not scrape lesion or biopsy. Consider ultrasound or MRI of head.
Infant	"Hair collar" sign surrounding lesion on scalp or midline lesion	Spina bifida occulta, meningomyelocoele	Possible intracranial connection, risk of meningitis	Preoperative imaging, consider neurosurgical consultation.
Infant	Tuft of hair over midline spine	Spina bifida occulta, meningomyelocoele	Possible intracranial connection, risk of meningitis	Preoperative imaging, consider neurosurgical consultation.
Infant	Preauricular "tag"	Accessary tragus	Risk of chondritis if removed by shave or snip excision. Risk of infection if ligated with suture.[4]	Appropriate closure if excised, if cartilaginous component present.[4]
Infant or child	Mass along midline scalp, glabella, side of forehead, or other embryonic fusion plane	Dermoid cyst	Intracranial connection in up to 25% for midline dermoids, risk is higher if sinus present.[5] Dermoids near the lateral eyebrows rarely have intracranial connections.[6]	Consider MRI and neurosurgical consultation.
Infant, young child	Nasal midline mass	Nasal glioma, encephalocele, or DDx: "hypertelorism" hemangioma	Intracranial connection 100% for encephaloceles. Gliomas may extend into oropharynx, or have intranasal connection.[5]	Consider MRI and neurosurgical consultation.
Infant, young child	Vascular mass with greatly increased warmth, often with pulsation or bruit	AV malformation DDx: hemangioma	Uncontrolled bleeding, problematic bony and/or soft tissue overgrowth	Consider Doppler studies, MRI, and surgical consultation.[7]

NOTE: MRI, magnetic resonance imaging; DDx, differential diagnosis; AV, arteriovenous

over 50 different chemicals, ranging from mildly toxic to toxic.[15] Parents should be taught that "less is best."[14]

Psychosocial and Developmental Issues

The social and cultural impact of a disfiguring birthmark should not be underestimated.[16] The age-old theory of maternal imprinting is widely believed in many countries, including the United States, and the mother may be actively blamed for congenital conditions in the newborn. With the selective photothermolysis offered by some lasers, and techniques in plastic surgery including tissue expansion, therapeutic options are increasing for vascular and pigmented birthmarks (see Chap. 102 and 265). Social, ethical, and health policy issues surrounding laser treatment for port-wine stains are discussed at the end of this chapter.

CHILDHOOD

Evaluation Techniques

When entering the room, prolonged or intense eye contact with the young child should be avoided, as this can be perceived as threatening. Observing the play of a child allows for a quick assessment of the neurologic development of the patient. Prefacing statements ("I'm going to look at your fingernails now,") are preferable to asking for permission ("May I look at your fingernails?"), because if the child refuses to be examined, trust is destroyed if the physician subsequently proceeds. If a language barrier exists between the parent and physician, it is best not to have the bilingual patient serve as an interpreter for her parents, as this responsibility creates additional anxiety in the child.

Examination of the perineum and genitalia is best accomplished with the child in the knee-chest position on the examination table (Fig. 144-2) or the parent's lap. Alternatively, the child may sit on the parent's lap with legs held apart by the parent. These positions minimize the anxiety of the child and enable better visualization. Figure 144-3 illustrates anatomic terminology of the young female genitalia for accurate documentation. Lichen sclerosus (discussed in Chap. 116), vitiligo, psoriasis, pinworms, and genital warts are but a few of the disorders of the anogenital region in childhood. An understanding of the developmental changes of the anogenital region from birth to adolescence is required for interpreting the physical examination, particularly of the female patient. Until very recently, basic normal female anatomy in children was unstudied. The advent of pediatric colposcopy has allowed objective study and definition of normal anogenital findings.[17–20] Ideally, colposcopic photographs will replace questionable parameters in current use (such as vaginal diameter[20,21]) and clarify nonstandard terminology. Still, caution must be used in interpreting the genital examination in the

FIGURE 144-1

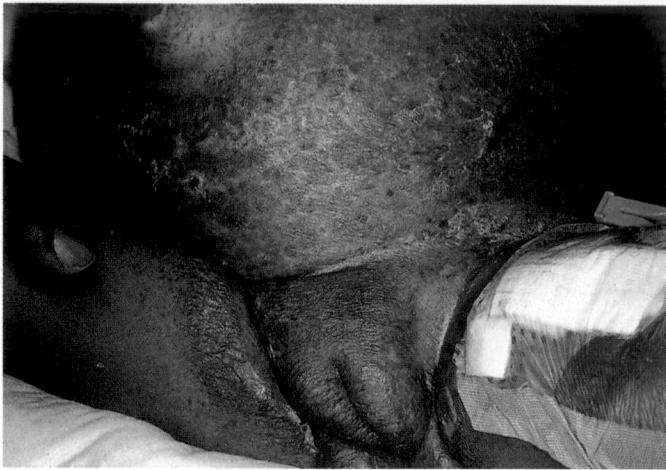

A.

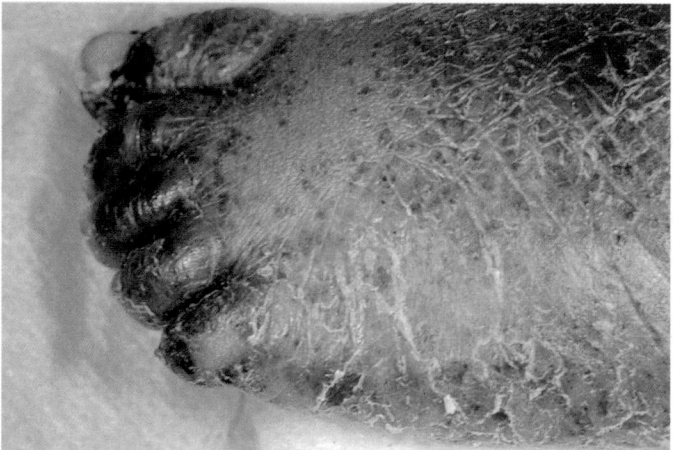

B.

A., B. Langerhans cell histiocytosis. Note erosions and petechiae.

FIGURE 144-2

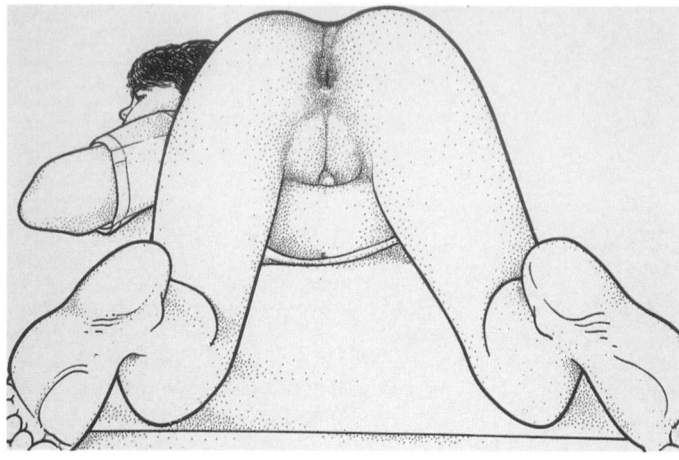

The knee-chest position allows visualization of the perineum and genitalia. (*From Finkel MA, DeJong AR: Medical findings in child abuse, in Child Abuse—Medical Diagnosis and Management, edited by RM Reece. Philadelphia, Lea & Febiger, 1994, Chap. 9, pp 185–247. Printed with permission.*)

young female so as not to underdiagnose or overdiagnose disease or abuse. For example, the presence of labia minora adhesions is not diagnostic of trauma or abuse, as they occur in as many as one-third of girls who are not abused.[17] The diastasis ani is a normal structure that can be mistaken for perianal scarring.[20] The infantile perianal pyramidal protrusion may be mistaken for condyloma acuminata, but is a harmless normal finding.[17,22] Child abuse is discussed in more detail later in this chapter.

Psychosocial Issues

Atopic dermatitis is the most common dermatologic disorder in the school-aged child, with prevalence estimated to be 5 percent (see Chap. 124). Moderate or severe childhood atopic dermatitis can profoundly affect the quality of life of the patient as well as the family. The psychosocial and financial impact of moderate or severe eczema on the patient's family can exceed that of children with insulin-dependent diabetes mellitus.[23] In one study, a 60 percent rate of psychological disturbance was found in children with moderate and severe eczema, which was significantly higher than in controls, even when scores for sleep disturbance were eliminated.[24]

Performing Procedures on the Young Child

Historically, there has been a widespread reluctance to biopsy skin lesions in children. This reluctance has led to a delay in diagnosis and proper management in many conditions such as blistering disorders in children.[25] With proper preparation of the parent and child, skin biopsies and other outpatient procedures are easily performed and should not be avoided if medically indicated. There are certain situations in pediatric dermatology in which a biopsy can be detrimental; examples of these "Pitfalls" are outlined in Table 144-1.

Children are fearful of needles and procedures because of experience with immunizations and an age-appropriate fear of bodily mutilation. A eutectic mixture of lidocaine and prilocaine (EMLA cream) is useful in minimizing pain of intralesional injections or local anesthetic injections for biopsies. The application of ice or cryospray are other options to numb the skin prior to injections. Alkalinizing local anesthetics to a pH of 7.0 (0.1 mEq/mL sodium bicarbonate or a 1:10 bicarbonate-to-anesthetic ratio by volume) minimizes the pain associated with cutaneous infiltration without limiting the anesthetic effect.[26–28] Alkalinization decreases the solution's shelf-life to approximately one week,[29] due to more rapid oxidation of epinephrine. Warming lidocaine has also been shown to lessen the pain of injection.[30,31]

Whether the parent(s) should be allowed to be present during a biopsy or procedure is a matter of physician preference, the age of the child, and the wishes of the parent. Observing a painful or invasive procedure on a baby is quite difficult for most parents, and it is often best that the parent is not present for the procedure. By contrast, a procedure on a young child often proceeds more efficiently if the parent is present and instructed on how to help calm the child. Separation anxiety can be great in young children, and the presence of a calm, reassuring parent can greatly increase cooperation in the child. However, if the parent is very anxious, the

FIGURE 144-3

CHAPTER 144
Pediatric and Adolescent Dermatology
1685

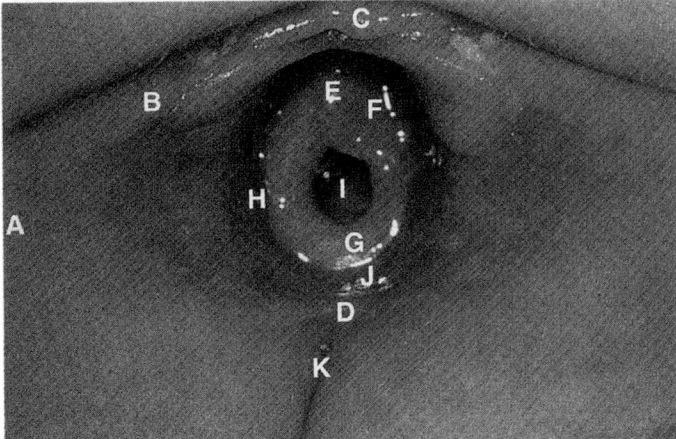

A.

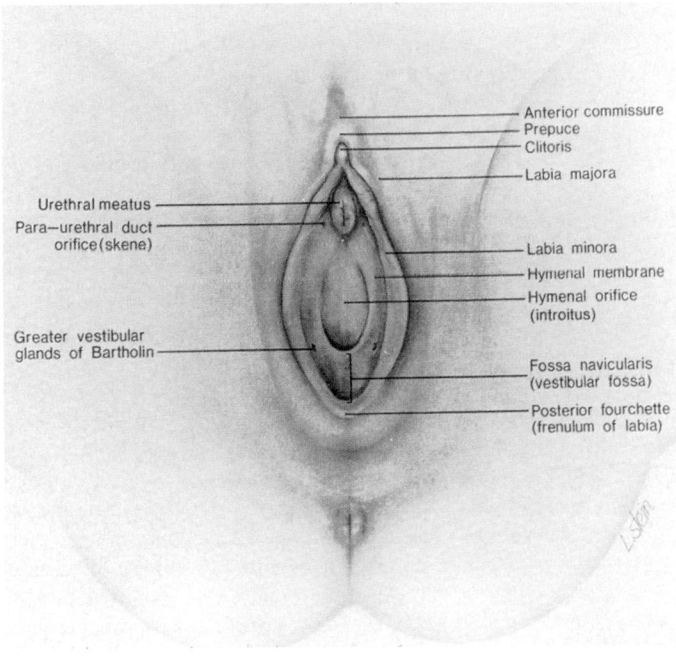

B.

A. Magnified view of a normal female child's genital anatomy. The following structures are labeled: A, labia majora; B, labia minora; C, clitoris; D, posterior fourchette; E, urethra; F, periurethral tissue; G, hymen; H, perihymenal sulcus; I, vagina; J, posterior navicular fossa (fossa navicularis); K, perineum. (*From Siegfried EC, Frasier LD,*[20] *with permission.*) B. Genital anatomy of an older female child. (*From Finkel MA, DeJong AR: Medical findings in child sexual abuse, in Child Abuse—Medical Diagnosis and Management, edited by RM Reece. Philadelphia, Lea & Febiger, 1994, Chap. 9, pp 185–247. Printed with permission.*)

child may have less fear if the parent is not present. The presence of a favorite stuffed animal or pillow is also helpful in allaying anxiety. Instruments and blood-stained gauze should be kept out of view of the patient and parent. Most importantly, all materials should be prepared before the child enters the room, to ensure rapid performance of the procedure.

Collection of specimens for fungal culture for tinea capitis is safely accomplished by the use of a toothbrush, ring curette, or moistened cotton swab, which are effective and less expensive than using a scalpel.[32,33] Alternatively, a media plate with non-slanted agar may be applied directly to the infected areas of the scalp to collect material.[33]

A parent's demand for surgical treatment of a young child's warts or molluscum poses an ethical dilemma, given that these benign viral diseases are generally self-resolving in a healthy child. Treatments are not curative, nor have they been proven to decrease transmission or to change the natural history of infection. Furthermore, many destructive treatments can be painful and may cause scarring. To complicate matters, if a dermatologist defers treatment of a single molluscum lesion, a parent may "blame" the physician for the spread of molluscum should this often unpreventable event occur. The risk-benefit ratio must be considered for each individual situation.[10,34] An initial trial of a destructive agent to a few lesions can be helpful in demonstrating to the parent what sequelae may occur (pigmentary changes being most common, with mild scarring a more remote possibility).

ADOLESCENCE

Though the dermatologic diagnoses of the adolescent overlap with general adult dermatology, caring effectively for the adolescent patient requires a different set of interviewing skills and different strategies in patient education. A discussion of interviewing techniques, treatment of acne, and eating disorders are included in this section. Sports dermatology is discussed in Chap. 132; cutaneous manifestations of drug abuse are discussed in Chap. 142; and sexually transmitted diseases are addressed in the chapters of Section 32.

Evaluation Techniques

Simple gestures such as greeting the adolescent first and the parents second and interviewing the adolescent patient alone at the beginning of the visit help to earn the patient's trust.[35–37] Confidentiality issues should be explicitly addressed during the interviews with both the teenager and the parents. Many states protect the adolescent's rights to confidential medical care for problems such as drug abuse, sexually transmitted diseases, contraception, pregnancy, and abortion. The laws of each state should be considered and the patient's right to privacy respected.[37]

The open-ended questioning style used for adults frequently fails with adolescents. Phrasings using the third person, and giving choices in the sentence are more effective techniques to obtain information. For example, "Many women on oral contraceptives forget to take their pill once in a while. How often do you forget to take your birth control pills: Often, sometimes, or almost never?" will yield a more accurate response than, "Do you take your birth control pills every day?"

Adolescents lack a well-developed sense of future time. Goals should be concrete, short-term, and relevant to the present, as long-term consequences are less often considered.[37] Rather than using goals related to more distant benefits, such as the reduction of potentially serious disease complications (e.g., smoking causes increased risk of lung cancer), emphasis should be on immediate and concrete effects (e.g., smoking causes your clothes, hair, and breath to smell bad, and your teeth to turn yellow.) Body image is a more powerful motivator (tanning salons cause premature wrinkles and ugly skin) than future health concerns (tanning salons increase your risk of skin cancer). Any treatment that is disfiguring or has visible side effects will meet with resistance.[37]

Physical development and psychosocial development may not be congruent. A sophisticated-appearing 15-year-old is not an adult and should not be expected, for example, to shoulder adult medical decisions or medical responsibilities for herself or her younger siblings. In an effort to establish rapport, the physician should be careful not to "overidentify" with the patient. The physician's role is not to befriend, nor is it to parent the adolescent patient, but is rather to be a trusted, valuable authority.

Acne and the Adolescent

Acne vulgaris is an extremely common and variable disorder. In the adolescent, it is a disorder than can have far-reaching detrimental effects on self-image and self-esteem. For example, sociologic investigation has demonstrated increased unemployment among patients with a history of severe acne.[38] Successful treatment of acne in the adolescent depends on addressing the patient's motivation and expectations. A single- or two-drug regimen can usually be selected to optimize compliance and cost-effectiveness.[39] A patient whose condition resists treatment must be reevaluated closely not only for incorrect or noncompliant use of medications, but also for an androgen-secreting tumor of the ovary, an incorrect diagnosis (e.g., pseudofolliculitis barbae or adenoma sebaceum), or a confounding agent (lithium or diphenylhydantoin-induced acne[39]). Monthly pregnancy tests, and emphasis on birth control, is mandatory for the adolescent female on isotretinoin therapy. Lastly, the adolescent should be instructed to resist sharing their medications with their friends. A discussion of acne is found in Chap. 73.

Anorexia Nervosa and Bulimia

The incidence of anorexia nervosa and bulimia is estimated to be 0.1 percent in young females in Western countries.[40,41] It has been estimated that 1 to 2 percent of young adult women in the United Kingdom have anorexia or bulimia.[42] It is also a serious problem in Japan.[43] Although more common in females, eating disorders do occur in males. Individuals involved in wrestling, weight-lifting, ballet, and other sports may incorporate vomiting or laxative use to reduce their weight and improve athletic performance.[44] Crude mortality rates for anorexia nervosa are approximately 5.9 to 6.6 percent.[45,46] Patients with eating disorders generally do not seek medical help; however, the astute physician can recognize warning signs during an unrelated office visit. Dermatologic manifestations of anorexia nervosa and bulimia nervosa are summarized in Table 144-2.

THERAPEUTICS

In this section, problems particular to the pediatric population, such as off-label prescription of medications, systemic absorption of topical medications, issues pertaining to systemic medications, and pediatric drug dosing are discussed. In addition, because many handbooks and textbooks do not contain adequate pediatric drug information, a selected formulary of frequently prescribed drugs in outpatient pediatric dermatology is presented at the end of the chapter (Table 144-3). Because no textbook can be all-inclusive, the primary literature should be consulted whenever possible.

Off-Label Prescriptions in Children

FDA guidelines for drug use in the pediatric age group are often inadequate. The thalidomide tragedy led to more stringent regulation of drugs in the early 1960s, and manufacturers began omitting drug studies in infants and children.[50] In the 1970s, pediatric dosage information in package inserts tended to exclude children from therapeutic benefit. Performing research in healthy children is problematic because of ethical and logistical questions (e.g., large blood volumes needed for assays), medicolegal risk, and cost. It has been estimated that three to four times the number of studies required for adults are necessary in children to cover the developmental continuum from neonates and infants through childhood and adolescence.[50] Often, because of these factors, the pediatric dosage is derived from simple body weight adjustment of the adult dosage, instead of pharmacokinetic studies. This may lead to toxicity or reduced efficacy in the pediatric population due to age-dependent differences in drug absorption, distribution, or elimination.[51]

What does this mean to the practicing dermatologist? "The lack of FDA approval for pediatric use does not imply the drug is contraindicated or disapproved; it simply means that insuf-

TABLE 144-2

Cutaneous Manifestations of Anorexia Nervosa (AN) and Bulimia

CUTANEOUS MANIFESTATIONS RELATED TO STARVATION AND/OR IDIOSYNCRATIC DIET (INCIDENCE IN PARENTHESES)	CUTANEOUS MANIFESTATIONS RELATED TO BINGING/PURGING
Lanugo-like body hair (29–50% of AN[47,48] patients)	Callus (single or multiple) on the dorsum of the dominant hand (Russel's sign)
Pedal or pretibial pitting without hypoproteinemia (26% of AN patients)	Dental enamel erosion and gingivitis
Dry skin with fine asteatotic scales (24–50%[47,48] of AN patients)	Parotidomegaly, usually bilateral and painless, mimicking Sjögren's syndrome or sarcoidosis
Hypercarotenemia (50–72% of AN[47–49] patients)	Transient facial purpura from increased intrathoracic pressure associated with vomiting
Pellagra, scurvy, and other hypovitaminoses	Fixed drug eruption (e.g., phenophthalein-containing laxatives)
Vitamin K deficiency with coagulopathy and bruising (due to decreased absorption of fat-soluble vitamins)	Photosensitivity with thiazide diuretics
Acne at times of weight gain, acne excoriée	Dermatomyositis-like syndrome (myopathy), secondary to ipecac usage
Factitial dermatoses	Finger clubbing associated with laxative abuse
Dermatoses related to obsessive-compulsive traits (e.g., hand dermatitis from repetitive hand washing)	Trichotillomania
Excessive loss of subcutaneous fat	

SOURCE: Modified from Gupta et al.[47]

TABLE 144-3

Pediatric Dermatology Formulary of Selected Systemic Drugs

Generic name (Trade name)	Dosage forms	Dose	Comment
Antiviral			
Acyclovir (Zovirax)	Caps: 200 mg Tabs: 800 mg Susp: 200 mg/5ml	Immunocompetent mucocutaneous HSV: Initial infection: 1200 mg/24 h ÷ q8h PO × 7–10 days. Recurrence: 1200 mg/24 h ÷ q8h PO × 5 days. Chronic suppressive therapy: 800–1000 mg/24 h ÷ 2–5 times/day PO for up to 1 yr. Zoster: 4000 mg/24 h ÷ 5 times/day PO × 5–7 days for patients > 12 yr Varicella: 80 mg/kg/24 h ÷ qid × 5 days (begin treatment at earliest signs/symptoms). Immunocompromised HSV, varicella or zoster: see *Red Book*.[119] Max. dose of oral acyclovir in children: 80 mg/kg/24 h.	Oral absorption unpredictable. See references for immunocompromised dosing, and parenteral dosing. Adequate hydration needed to prevent crystallization in renal tubules. Dose alteration necessary in patients with impaired renal function. Infrequent reports of headache, vertigo, insomnia, GI irritation, urticaria, fever. See *Red Book*[119] for further details.
Antibiotics			
Amoxicillin (Amoxil, Trimox, and others)	Drops: 50 mg/ml Susp: 125, 250 mg/5 ml Caps: 250, 500 mg Chewable tabs: 125, 250 mg	Children: 20–50 mg/kg/24 h ÷ q8h PO Adults: 250–500 mg/dose q8h PO. Max dose: 2–3 g/24 h	Rash and diarrhea may occur. Renal elimination. Serum levels about twice those achieved with equal dose of ampicillin.
Cephadroxil (Duricef, Ultracef, and others)	Susp: 125, 250, 500 mg/5 cc Tabs & caps: 500 mg, 1 g	Children: 30 mg/kg/day PO ÷ q12h Adult dose: 1 g/day PO ÷ qd bid.	1st-generation cephalosporin. See cephalexin.
Cephalexin (Keflex, Keftab, Cefanex and others)	Susp: 125 mg/5 mL, 250 mg/5 mL Drops: 100 ml/mL Tabs & caps: 250, 500 mg, 1 g	Children: 25–100 mg/kg/24 h PO ÷ q6–12. Adults: 1–4 g/h PO ÷ q6–12 h. Max dose 4 g/24 h.	Use with caution in renal insufficiency. Some cross-reactivity with penicillin.
Cephradine (Velocef, Anspor, and others)	Susp: 125, 250 mg/5 mL Cap: 250, 500 mg Tab: 1 g	Children: 25–50 mg/kg/day PO ÷ q6–12 h. Adults: 1–4 g/day PO ÷ q6h. Max dose 4 g/24 h.	1st-generation cephalosporin. See cephalexin.
Dicloxacillin (Dynapen, Dycill)	Cap: 125, 250, 500 mg Oral susp: 62.5/5ml	Children (<40 kg): Mild/moderate infections: 12.5–25 mg/kg/24 h ÷ q6h PO. Severe infections: 50–100 mg/kg/24 h ÷ q6h. Adults (≥40 kg): 125–500 mg/dose PO ÷ q6h h. Max dose 4 g/24 h.	Same side effects as other penicillins. Give on empty stomach.
Doxycycline (Vibramycin and others	Caps & tabs: 50, 100 mg Syrup: 50 mg/5 mL Susp: 25 mg/5 mL	Initial: ≤45 kg: 5 mg/kg/24 h ÷ bid PO × 1 day to max dose of 200 mg/24 h. >45 kg: 200 mg/24 h ÷ bid PO × 1 day. Maintenance: ≤45 kg: 2.5–5 mg/kg/24 h ÷ qd–bid PO. >45 kg: 100–200 mg/24 h ÷ qd–bid PO. Max adult dose: 300 mg/24 h.	For treatment of acne see Chap. 73. Use under age 9 years may cause discoloration of teeth. Use with caution in hepatic or renal disease. May cause increased intracranial pressure. GI symptoms and photosensitivity may occur. See also, tetracycline.

Erythromycin preparations (Erythrocin, Pediamycin, E-Mycin, Ery-Ped, and others)	Erythromycin base:
	  Tabs: 250, 333, 500 mg
	  Delayed release tabs: 333 mg
	  Delayed release caps: 250 mg
	
	Erythromycin ethyl succinate (EES):
	  Suspension: 200, 400 mg/5 mL
	  Drops: 100 mg/2.5 mL
	  Chewable tabs: 200 mg
	  Tabs: 400 mg
		Children: 30–50 mg/kg/24 h ÷ q6–8 h; max dose: 2 g/24 h.
		Adults: 1–4 g/24 h ÷ q6h; max dose: 4 g/24 h.
			GI side effects common. Give doses after meals. Use with caution in liver disease. May produce elevated digoxin, theophylline, carbamazepine, cyclosporine, methylprednisolone levels. Because of different absorption characteristics, higher oral doses of EES are needed to achieve therapeutic effects.

(continued)

TABLE 144-3 (*Continued*)

Pediatric Dermatology Formulary of Selected Systemic Drugs

GENERIC NAME (TRADE NAME)	DOSAGE FORMS	DOSE	COMMENT

	Erythromycin estolate:
	    Susp: 125 mg, 250 mg/5 mL
	    Tabs: 500 mg
	    Caps: 250 mg
	
	Erythromycin stearate:
	    Tabs: 250, 500 mg		

Minocycline (Minocin and others)	Tabs & caps: 50, 100 mg Oral susp: 50 mg/5mL	Children: (9–12 yr) 4 mg/kg/dose × 1 PO, then 2 mg/kg/dose q12h PO. Adolescents and adults: 200 mg/dose × 1 PO, then 100 mg q12h PO.	See Chap. 73 for treatment of acne. Nausea, vomiting, allergy, photophobia, injury to developing teeth, and hyperpigmentation may occur. High incidence of vestibular dysfunction. Do not take with milk or dairy products.
Penicillin V Potassium (Pen Vee K, V-Cillin K, and others)	Tabs: 125, 250, 500 mg Oral sol: 125 mg/5 mL, 250 mg/5 mL	Children: 25–50 mg/kg/24 h ÷ q6–8 h PO. Max dose: 3 g/24 h. Adults: 250–500 mg/dose PO q6–8 h.	Give 1 h before or 2 h after meals.
Tetracycline HCl (Achromycin, Terramycin, and others)	Susp: 125 mg/5 cc Tabs and caps: 100, 250, 500 mg	Children (9 yr and older): 25–50 mg/kg/24 h PO ÷ q6h. Max dose: 2 g/h. Adults: 1–2 g/24 h ÷ q6h PO. Max dose: 2 g/24 h.	For treatment of acne see Chap. 73. Discoloration of teeth in children less than age 9. May cause photosensitivity, GI upset, hepatotoxicity. Do not give with dairy products or with divalent cations (Fe^{2+}, Ca^{2+}, Mg^{2+}). Give 1 h before or 2 h after meals.
ANTIFUNGAL AGENTS			
Fluconazole (Diflucan)	Tabs: 50, 100, 150, 200 Susp: 10, 40 mg/ml	Children (3–13 yr): Loading dose: 10 mg/kg PO then Maintenance: (begin 24 h after loading dose) 3–6 mg/kg/24 h PO qd[132] Experimental dosage for tinea capitis: 6 mg/kg/day × 20 days[120] Adults: Oropharyngeal and esophageal candidiasis: Loading dose of 200 mg PO followed by 100 mg qd 24 h after, doses up to max dose of 400 mg/24 h may be used for esophageal candidasis. Vaginal candidiasis: 150 mg PO × 1.	Not FDA-approved for tinea capitis in children. May cause nausea, headache, rash, vomiting, abdominal pain, and diarrhea. Reduce maintenance dose in renal dysfunction. May increase effects or levels of cyclosporine, phenytoin, theophylline, warfarin, oral hypoglycemics, and AZT. Rifampin increases fluconazole metabolism. Cardiac arrythmia may occur when used with cisapride, terfenadine, astemizole. Concomitant administration of fluconazole with any of these drugs is contraindicated.

Griseofulvin (Grifulvin V, Grisactin, Fulvicin)	Microsize:
	    Susp: 125 mg/5 mL
	    Tabs: 250, 500 mg
	    Caps: 125, 250 mg
	
	Ultramicrosize:
	    Tabs: 125, 165, 250, 330 mg
		Microsize:
		    Children (>2 yr): 20 mg/kg/24 h PO ÷ qd–bid.
		    Adults: 500–1000 mg/24 h qd PO
		
		Ultramicrosize:
		    Children (> 2 yr): 7 mg/kg/24 h PO qd.
		    Adults: 330–750 mg/24 h PO ÷ qd–bid
			Give with milk or fatty food. Contraindicated in porphyria, hepatic disease. Penicillin allergy is not a contraindication. Not recommended in pregnancy because of possible teratogenicity. Reversible elevation of liver enzymes, photosensitivity may occur. May reduce effectiveness or decrease level of oral contraceptives, warfarin and cyclosporin. Phenobarbital may enhance clearance of griseofulvin. Not effective against Candida or other yeasts. See Chap. 206 and 208 for treatment of fungal infections.

(continued)

TABLE 144-3 (*Continued*)

Itraconazole (Sporonox)	Caps: 100 mg Solution: 10 mg/mL	All dosages given in capsules. Experimental dosages for tinea capitis in children[33,127–131]: 3–5 mg/kg/24 h × 4–6 wk. Or 10–20 kg: 100 mg qod; 20–30 kg: 100 mg/day; 30–50 kg: Alternate 100 mg/day, with 200 mg/day >50 kg: 200 mg/day	Not FDA-approved for use in pediatric patients. Solution is approved for treatment of oral and esophageal candidiasis in adults. Solution should not be used interchangeably with capsules, as the solution has greater bioavailability. Reversible elevation of liver enzymes, GI symptoms, headache, dizziness may occur. Do not use with terfenadine or other nonsedating antihistamines. See Chap. 206 and 208 for treatment of fungal infections.
Ketoconazole (Nizoral)	Tabs: 200 mg	Children (>2 yr): 5–10 mg/kg/24 h ÷ qd–bid PO. Adults: 200–400 mg/24 h PO. Max dose 800 mg/24 h.	Give with cranberry or orange juice or other acidic drink. Drugs that decrease gastric acidity will decrease absorption. Monitor liver function during long-term use. May cause nausea, vomiting, rash, headache, pruritis, and fever. Cardiac arrhythmia may occur when used with cisapride, terfenadine, astemizole. Concomitant administration of ketoconazole with any of these drugs is contraindicated. Not FDA-approved for the treatment of tinea capitis in children. See Chap. 206 and 208 for treatment of fungal infections.
Nystatin (Mycostatin, Nilstat and others)	Susp: 100,000 U/mL Tabs: 500,000 U Troches/Pastilles: 200,000 U	Infants: 1 mL (100,000 U) to each side of mouth qid. Children/adults: Susp: 4–6 ml (400,000–600,000 U) swish and swallow qid. Troche: 200,000–400,000 U 4–5 times/24 h.	May produce diarrhea and GI side effects. Treat until 48–72 h after resolution of symptoms. Drug poorly absorbed through the GI tract. Do not swallow troches whole.

CORTICOSTEROIDS AND NSAIDS

Acetaminophen (Tylenol, Tempra, Panadol, others)	Tabs: 325, 500, 650 mg Chewable tabs: 80, 160 mg Infant drops/solution/susp: 80 mg/0.8 mL Child solution/susp: 160 mg/5 mL Elixir: 80, 120, 130, 160, 325 mg/5 mL Caplet: 160, 325, 500 mg Suppository: 80, 120, 125, 325, 650 mg	10–15 mg/kg/dose PO/PR Or dosing by age: 0–3 mo: 40 mg/dose; 4–11 mo: 80 mg/dose; 1–2 yr: 120 mg/dose; 2–3 yr: 160 mg/dose; 4–5 yr: 240 mg/dose; 6–8 yr: 320 mg/dose; 9–10 yr: 400 mg/dose; 11–12 yr: 480 mg/dose Adults: 325–650 mg/dose; max dose: 4 g/24 h, 5 doses/24 h	Metabolized in the liver. Some preparations contain alcohol (7–10%) and/or phenylalanine. Contraindicated in patients with known G6PD deficiency. Shake suspensions before use.
Ibuprofen (Motrin, Advil, Nuprin and others)	Susp (OTC, Rx): 100 mg/5 mL Oral drops (Rx): 40 mg/mL Chew tabs (Rx): 50, 100 mg Caplets (Rx): 100 mg Tabs: 200 (OTC), 300, 400, 600, 800 mg	Children: Analgesic/Antipyretic: 5–10 mg/kg/dose q6–8 h PO. Max dose: 40 mg/kg/24 h PO. Adolescents/Adults: Pain/fever/dysmenorrhea: 200–400 mg/dose q4–6h PO. Max dose 3.2 g/24 h.	GI distress (lessened with milk), ocular problems, granulocytopenia, anemia may occur. Inhibits platelet aggregation. Use caution with aspirin hypersensitivity, hepatic or renal insufficiency, or dehydration.
Prednisone (many brand names)	Tabs: 1, 2.5, 5, 10, 20, 50 mg Syrup/sol: 1 mg/mL (5% alcohol) Conc sol: 5 mg/mL (30% alcohol)	Antiinflammatory/immunosuppressive: 0.5–2 mg/kg/24 h PO ÷ qd–qid.	Alternate daily dosing or single morning dosing lessens side effects. See Chap. 232 for relative steroid potencies, side effects and monitoring.

(continued)

TABLE 144-3 (*Continued*)

Pediatric Dermatology Formulary of Selected Systemic Drugs

Generic name (Trade name)	Dosage forms	Dose	Comment
Prednisolone (Prelone, Delta-Cortef, Pediapred)	Tabs: 5 mg Syrup: 5 mg/mL (Pediapred) or 15 mg per 5 mL (Prelone)	See Prednisone, above.	Syrup more palatable than prednisone syrup. See Prednisone, above.
Antihistamines/Sedatives			
Cetirizine HCl (Zyrtec)	Tabs: 10 mg Syrup: 5 mg/5 mL	6–11 yr: 5–10 mg PO qd >12 yr/Adults: 10 mg PO qd	Mild, dose-related sedation may occur. Dry mouth and other side effects common to antihistamines may occur. Decrease dose in patients with renal failure or hepatic insufficiency.
Chloral hydrate (Noctec, Somnos, Aquachloral)	Caps: 250, 500 mg Syrup: 250, 500 mg/5 mL Supp: 324, 500, 648 mg	Children: Sedative: 25–50 mg/kg/24 h PO/PR ÷ q6–8 h. Sedation for procedures: 25–100 mg/kg/dose PO/PR; max dose: 2 g/dose Adults: Sedative: 250 mg/dose tid PO/PR. Hypnotic: 500–1000 mg/dose PO/PR. Max dose: 2 g/24 h.	Not analgesic. May cause GI irritation, paradoxical excitement, hypotension, and myocardial/respiratory depression. Requires appropriate monitoring. Contraindicated in patients with hepatic or renal disease. Sudden withdrawal after chronic use may cause delirium tremens.
Chlorpheniramine maleate (Chlor-Trimeton and others)	Tabs: 4, 8, 12 mg Caps: 12 mg Sustained release caps and tabs: 8, 12 mg Chewable tab: 2 mg Syrup: 2 mg/5mL	Children: 0.35 mg/kg/24 h ÷ q4–6 h **or** 2–6 yr: 1 mg/dose PO q4–6 h, max dose 4 mg/24 h. 6–12 yr: 2 mg/dose PO q4–6 h, max dose 12 mg/24 h. Sustained release (6–12 yr): 8 mg/dose PO BID. >12 years/adults: 4 mg/dose q4–6 h PO, max dose 24 mg/24 h. Sustained release 8–12 mg PO bid.	May cause sedation, dry mouth, urinary retention, polyuria, disturbed coordination. Young children may be paradoxically excited. Sustained release forms not recommended in children less than 6 years old.
Cyproheptadine (Periactin)	Tabs: 4 mg Syrup: 2 mg/5 mL (5% alcohol)	Children: 0.25–0.5 mg/kg/24 h ÷ q8–12 h PO Adults: 12–32 mg/24 h ÷ tid PO Max dose: 2–6 yr: 12 mg/24 h; 7–14 yr: 16 mg/24 h; Adults: 32 mg/24 h	Contraindicated in neonates, patients on MAO inhibitors, patients with glaucoma, or GI/GU obstruction. May produce anticholinergic side effects, including appetite stimulation.
Diphenhydramine (Benadryl and others)	Elixir (14% alcohol): 12.5 mg/5 mL Syrup: 12.5 mg/5 mL (some contain 5% alcohol) Caps/tabs: 25, 50 mg	Children: 5 mg/kg/24 hr ÷ q6h PO, max dose 300 mg/24 h. Adults: 10–50 mg/dose q6–8 h PO, max dose: 400 mg/24 h.	Side effects common to antihistamines. CNS side effects more common than GI disturbances. May cause paradoxical excitement. Contraindicated in neonates, or with concurrent MAO inhibitor use.
Hydroxyzine (Atarax, Vistaril)	Tabs: 10, 25, 50, 100 mg Caps: 25, 50, 100 mg Syrup: 10 mg/5 mL Susp: 25 mg/5 mL	Children: 2 mg/kg/24 h ÷ q6h. Adults: 25–100 mg/dose ÷ tid-qid. Max adult dose: 600 mg/24 h.	May potentiate barbiturates, meperidine, and other depressants. Dry mouth, drowsiness, tremor, convulsions, blurred vision, hypotension, paradoxical excitement may occur.
Loratadine (Claritin)	Tabs: 10 mg Rapidly disintegrating tabs: 10 mg Syrup: 1 mg/mL	Children (>6 yr): 10 mg PO qd Adults: 10 mg PO qd	Reduce dose in hepatic failure or renal insufficiency. Low incidence of drowsiness. May cause dry mouth, dizziness, and other side effects common to antihistamines.

(*continued*)

TABLE 144-3 (*Continued*)

MISCELLANEOUS

Isotretinoin (Accutane)	Caps: 10, 20, 40 mg	Cystic acne: 0.5–2 mg/kg/24 h ÷ bid PO for 20 wk.	Known teratogen, contraindicated in pregnancy. Conjunctivitis, xerosis, pruritis, epistaxis, anemia, hyperlipidemia, pseudotumor cerebri, bone pain, muscle aches, skeletal changes, and other toxicities. Vitamin A or tetracyclines should not be given concomitantly. Monitor CBC, LFTS, triglycerides, and monthly pregnancy test. See Chap. 73 for treatment of acne.

NOTE: The drug information and doses listed above are given as guidelines only and are not intended to be comprehensive. Drug selection and dosage should be chosen according to the individual situation. Drug information may have changed since publication of this textbook. Parenteral dosages and neonatal dosages are not listed.

NOTE: Griseofulvin is the only FDA-approved drug for the treatment of tinea capitis in children at this time. The use of fluconazole,[120] terbinafine[121–126] and itraconazole[33,127–131] for tinea capitis in children, while promising, are still experimental and the reader should consult the primary literature before use.

NOTE: GI = gastrointestinal; GU = genitourinary; CBC = complete blood count; LFTS = liver function tests; G6PD = glucose-6-phosphate dehydrogenase.

ficient data are available to grant approval status. The clinician consequently has the option of either depriving the child of potential therapeutic benefits or using a drug despite disclaimers and pediatric inexperience."[50]

For example, hydrocortisone cream, an over-the-counter medication, does not have official FDA approval for use in children under 2 years of age.[52,53] Sunscreens, including titanium dioxide, are not approved for use in infants under 6 months of age.[52] There are no guidelines for the treatment of herpes zoster with acyclovir in children less than 12 years of age. Off-label use of medications is thus extremely common and, to some degree, unavoidable. The practicing physician must decide what clinical and medicolegal risks he or she is willing to accept.[51] Some physicians simply do not prescribe off-label medications for their pediatric patients, limiting their therapeutic options. However, many physicians choose the drugs and dosages that have been traditionally used in children, as the accumulation of individual experience provides some degree of safety and demonstrates conformity with perceived community standards. Reliance on tradition, however, is not always in the best interest of the child.

Topical Medications

Infants and small children have a greater risk of systemic toxicity from topical medications because of a greater surface to volume ratio coupled with decreased metabolic clearance of drugs. For this reason, special care must be used in choosing appropriate therapies and instructing parents on proper usage. Complications due to systemic absorption of topical agents are listed in Table 144-4.

TOPICAL CORTICOSTEROIDS The fact that topical application of corticosteroids can cause suppression of the hypothalamic-pituitary-adrenocortical (HPA) axis is well documented.[65,66] However, the clinical significance of this phenomenon and dosage limitations are not known. A study of 35 adults with severe childhood atopic dermatitis showed that full adult predicted height was attained despite long-term steroid use in childhood.[67]

The least potent topical steroid that is effective should be used, and the strength tapered as the condition improves. Topical steroid use in the diaper area should be limited to 7 to 10 days using a Class VII steroid, because percutaneous absorption is greatly enhanced due to moisture and warmth from occlusion in this region.[68] Traditionally it has been believed that dermatitis in children is more steroid responsive than in adults. Similarly, adverse effects such as hypopigmentation probably occur more readily in children than in adults. However, there are situations in which judicious short-term use of a Class I steroid is needed. Long-term topical steroid use in the ocular area is limited by the theoretical risk of developing glaucoma, but the actual risk is unknown. It is the responsibility of all dermatologists, and especially pediatric dermatologists, to educate primary care physicians on guidelines for topical steroid use.

TABLE 144-4

Topical Medications Reported to Cause Systemic Toxicity in Children

TOPICAL MEDICATION	COMPLICATION	REFERENCE
Benzocaine 3% (Lanacaine)	Methemoglobinemia in a 2 y.o. child	54
Iodoquinol, clioquinol (Vioform)	Neurotoxicity when used as treatment for diaper dermatitis	9, 55
Lindane	Neurologic toxicity in children with disrupted epidermal barrier, and/or excessive topical application, or ingestion	56, 57
N,N-diethyl-m-toluamide (DEET)	Slurred speech, tremors, seizures, and death in children after repeated and extensive application of high concentrations of DEET	58, 59
Povidone-iodine (Betadine)	Hypothyroidism in infants with spina bifida	60
Povidone-iodine (Betadine)	Decreased free thyroxine and elevated iodine levels in infants treated with diluted povidone-iodine during *Staphylococcus aureus* epidemic	61
Salicylic acid	7-year-old boy treated for ichthyosis vulgaris. Life-threatening salicylism, with neurologic sequelae lasting 6 months	62
Saline, sodium chloride	Fatalities in infants and children following ancient Turkish custom of "salting"	63
Viscous lidocaine, 2%	Lidocaine overdose following frequent application to oral lesions	64

Lindane (Kwell) was once the most common treatment for head lice and scabies. Its use is declining after reports of central nervous system toxicity including seizures and death. Adverse neurologic toxicity occurred in patients who ingested (392 g) of lindane or after excessive topical application.[56] Most, if not all of these patients had preexisting neurologic or intellectual compromise or extensive disruption of the epidermal barrier (one patient had non-bullous congenital icthyosiform erythroderma).[57] Because of these concerns, permethrin (Elimite) has become the drug of choice in the United States for infants and young children and for patients with preexisting neurologic disorders or compromised skin integrity.[69,70] However, lindane, which is safe when used properly in patients lacking the above risk factors,[70] is still a valuable scabicide in large-scale community control projects or in countries where public health funding is severely limited.

A eutectic mixture of lidocaine and prilocaine (EMLA cream) has revolutionized topical anesthesia and represents a welcome addition to the pediatric dermatologists' armamentarium. On using EMLA for the first time, many physicians are disappointed by the degree of anesthesia or the inconsistent efficacy. Common errors in the use of EMLA include applying the product too thinly, failing to occlude the medication, and not allowing sufficient contact time before the procedure (1 to 2 hours is usually sufficient, 3 to 4 hours is safe and more effective). Regional variation in percutaneous absorption may account in part for varying results.[71] An "EMLA patch" will soon be available in the United States, making occlusion unnecessary and home application much simpler. Systemic absorption is prevented by limiting the surface area of application, rather than limiting duration of application. EMLA is not approved for infants less than 1 month of age and for patients less than 1 year of age who are receiving methemoglobin-inducing agents, as the risk of methemoglobinemia is increased with EMLA use. The most commonly used methemoglobin-inducing agent in infants is acetaminophen. Other agents include sulfonamides, dapsone, benzocaine, chloroquine, phenobarbital, and phenytoin.

Tetracaine-adrenaline-cocaine (TAC) or adrenaline-cocaine (AC) in solution or gel forms are topical local anesthetics used by emergency room pediatricians for laceration repair[72] and in sinonasal surgery in the field of otolaryngology.[73] There is probably a role for TAC or AC in dermatologic surgery but it is largely unexplored. Increased absorption occurs at mucous membranes.[74] As with all anesthetics, drug interactions and dosage limits must be strictly monitored. Improper usage can lead to seizures and death, in large part due to the absorption of cocaine.[74,75] One study in a pediatric emergency room demonstrated that combination topical anesthetics with no cocaine were safe and effective.[76]

Systemic Medications

DRUG DOSAGES It is best to uphold the pediatric mg/kg dosing tradition for systemic medications to account for variation in size between young patients of the same age, and to account for increasing weight due to growth.[77] Equally important, the prescription must indicate concentration of syrups or suspensions (e.g., mg per teaspoon). Otherwise, overdosage is potentially a great problem. However, for the obese child, dosage calculated for body weight may lead to inappropriately high doses. Dosing in this situation must be solved on an individual basis, with consideration given to the goal of treatment, the age of the child, the toxicity, and the therapeutic window of the drug. Calculating a dose based on ideal weight for the obese patient's height is one alternative that may be acceptable.

SYSTEMIC GLUCOCORTICOIDS HPA axis suppression, osteonecrosis, and other adverse effects of systemic glucocorticoid therapy are reviewed in Chapter 252 of this textbook. The potential risk of growth suppression is unique to childhood. Exogenous glucocorticoids disrupt the secretion of growth hormone (GH), causing abnormal spontaneous GH secretion, with reduced pulse amplitude of GH release and reduced response to provocative stimuli.[78,79] There is also decreased local production of insulin-like growth factor-1. These and other effects of glucocorticoids act to cause delayed growth at the bony epiphyses, with the most noticeable reduction in growth velocity occurring during early childhood and adolescent growth spurts. There appears to be a linear relation between the daily dose and growth suppression. Alternate-day dosing, with the dose given in the morning, decreases the risk of glucocorticoid growth suppression. Most children will have adequate "catch-up" growth eventually with reduction of doses, alternate-day therapy, or cessation of therapy when possible.[66,80,81] For the pediatric patient on long-term systemic steroid therapy, plotting height and weight periodically on a standardized growth curve is the best method to screen for decreasing growth velocity.

Children on oral glucocorticoids should not be vaccinated with live virus vaccines (e.g., measles, oral polio, varicella). The American Academy of Pediatrics advises: "Children receiving 2 mg/kg/day or more of prednisone or its equivalent, or 20 mg or more daily if they weigh more than 10 kg, should not receive live-virus vaccines until steroid therapy has been discontinued for at least one month."[82] Systemic steroids should not be given to a healthy child if he or she has had recent varicella exposure and is not varicella-immune, since varicella infection can be fatal in this situation. Also, children with ocular herpes simplex and untreated tuberculosis should not be given systemic steroids, and patients with underlying diabetes, hypertension, peptic ulcer disease, renal insufficiency, or psychosis should be treated with great caution or with an alternative agent. Inactivated polio vaccine can substitute for the live attentuated vaccine if the patient or a household member is immunocompromised.[83]

ANTIMICROBIALS Tetracyclines cause brown discoloration of the teeth and decreased bone growth and should not be used in children younger than 8 to 10 years of age. Ciprofloxacin and quinolone use in children has been restricted because of studies demonstrating arthropathy, irreversible erosion and degeneration of joint cartilage, and noninflammatory joint effusion in laboratory dogs, rabbits, cats, and pigs after days to weeks of treatment.[84–86] Although there has been no clear causal relation between quinolones and arthropathy in children, it is recommended that their use be restricted to relatively serious pseudomonas infections for which intravenous antibiotics would be impractical.[87,88] Although studies with the itraconazole, fluconazole, and terbinafine are progressing, griseofulvin is the only FDA-approved drug for children with tinea capitis. Griseofulvin doses of 20 mg/kg/day of the liquid or 15 mg/kg/day of the ultramicrosized tablets for 2 to 4 months are recommended.[89] The dose may be given once daily or divided twice a day, and absorption is optimized when given with a fatty food. It is contraindicated in children with porphyria or decreased liver function. Griseofulvin is an inducer of the cytochrome P-450 enzyme system and can decrease blood levels of warfarin, oral contraceptives, and other drugs metabolized by the P-450 system.[90,91]

Cephalosporin suspensions are palatable, and compliance is superior to that seen with dicloxacillin suspension, which is extremely bitter. Prednisolone (Prelone) syrup tastes better and will be more successful than prednisone syrup. Note that while prednisolone has identical glucocorticoid and mineralocorticoid potencies as prednisone (i.e., equivalent milligram dosage), the concentrations of the two syrups may be different (i.e., prednisone syrup is 5 mg/mL, prednisolone is 5 or 15 mg/mL). If a bitter suspension is unavoidable, the taste can be masked by mixing in chocolate syrup or frosting.

Genodermatoses and Dysmorphology

The recognition of genodermatoses and dysmorphology are important elements of pediatric dermatology. Single minor anomalies occur in approximately 15 percent of all newborns. These include the supernumerary nipple and the accessory tragus, and are by definition of no functional significance. The occurrence of two is less common, however, and the presence of three or more is unusual, occurring in just 1 percent of all newborns. Such newborns should be carefully evaluated for possible hidden major malformations such as cardiac, renal, or vertebral defects, since 90 percent of them have an associated major malformation.[92,93] Forty-two percent of patients with idiopathic mental retardation have three or more malformations, 80 percent of which are minor.[94] Before ascribing significance to any minor anomaly, the patient's family members should be examined. Because minor anomalies are common in the general population, in some instances groupings of facial minor anomalies may represent variant additive patterns instead of true malformation syndromes.[92,95] The dysmorphic face is evaluated using subjective clinical impressions, soft-tissue measurements, and other simple methods. Techniques such as radiographic cephalometrics are time-consuming and expensive, and are more useful for planning and follow-up of craniofacial surgery.[92]

Medical photography is invaluable in documentation of dysmorphologic features. Furthermore, phenotypic features may change with time, and serial photographs may be crucial. In some conditions, such as the Cornelia de Lange syndrome or Down's syndrome, the facial features remain constant at all ages; however, the facial phenotype of Noonan syndrome may change significantly with age, making the diagnosis more challenging.[92,96] The phenotypic features of the cri-du-chat syndrome tend to become less distinct with time.[92,97] A complete review of dysmorphology and genodermatoses is beyond the scope of this chapter. The interested reader is referred to textbooks of dysmorphology and genodermatoses.[98–101]

CORRECTION OF DISFIGUREMENT IN CHILDREN

The port-wine stain (PWS) is a congenital malformation of capillaries and venules that commonly occurs on the face in a segmental distribution. Some lesions tend to darken with time to a reddish-purple color, and papular and nodular components may develop in adults (See Chap. 102). The most significant morbidity of PWS results from the negative psychosocial and developmental effects of growing up and living with facial disfigurement.[102] The advent of pulsed-dye laser treatment represents a significant milestone in the treatment of facial port-wine stains in children and is currently the treatment of choice. Dermatologic laser therapy in children has raised important social, ethical, and health policy issues. The parental decision to treat young children involves weighing the per-

ception of the future social risks of PWS against the pain of laser therapy and its costs.[102] Furthermore, the persistent concern and attention surrounding laser treatment may send a profound message to children that they are not acceptable the way they were born or that they are defective. Deferring treatment until children are old enough to decide for themselves if treatment is worthwhile is countered by the widely held, though unproven, belief that early treatment is more effective and that an optimal therapeutic window exists in late infancy and early childhood. In the future, now that PWS is a treatable condition, the pressure on parents and physicians to treat PWS will increase. Untreated PWS may become more "deviant" when most cases of PWS are being treated.[103]

On a societal level, does the possession of technology necessarily imply responsibility to correct all congenital deformity? The surgical normalization of faces of children with Down's syndrome stirred great controversy.[103,104] Access, cost, and equity represent additional issues. In the United States, insurance carriers or governmental agencies determine who receives expensive interventions such as laser therapy. It is clear that persons with visible birth defects or physical disfigurement have different social experiences,[105–107] but many citizens are unwilling to use taxpayers' money to fund expensive "cosmetic" treatments. Ultimately, will those children without insurance or personal wealth remain the most "deviant" in appearance? Humanists have argued that the values of society should change, not the faces of the affected children.[104]

CHILD ABUSE

Approximately 10 American children die each day from child abuse and 90 percent of all abused children are said to have suggestive or confirmative dermatologic findings.[108,109] The laws of all 50 states require that clinicians report any suspicions to child protective services. While each case must be considered individually, Table 144-5 lists factors that may raise the possibility of child abuse. Children with a history of prematurity or chronic illnesses or conditions are at higher risk for abuse (Fig. 144-4). Munchausen's syndrome by proxy is a specific form of child abuse in which the caretaker, most commonly the mother, secretly inflicts physical injury to the child in order to obtain psychological secondary gain from the medical establishment.[110,111] A high index of suspicion is needed in many situations to arrive at the correct diagnosis.

When abuse or neglect is suspected, the child's immediate safety should be the foremost priority. Hospitalization of the child may be appropriate. Examinations and interviews should be age-appropriate, and carefully documented. The history of sexual abuse as disclosed by a child is the single most important piece of evidence in a court of law.[112] More criminal convictions of sexual abuse have occurred in cases without physical evidence when the child's history was well documented than in cases that included physical evidence of abuse.[113,114] Fewer than 20 percent of girls and 10 percent of boys referred with a history of sexual abuse have abnormal examinations, particularly if examination occurs later than 72 h after the assault.[114,115] Thus, abuse cannot be excluded based on a normal physical examination alone. The subject of child abuse is large and complex and expert consultation for both interviews and examinations should always be considered.

FIGURE 144-4

TABLE 144-5

Criteria for Suspecting Child Abuse

Physical findings: Are there:
  Fresh bruises? Bruising of different ages? Unusual locations or shapes?
  Old scars? Unusual locations or shapes?
  Past or current burns? Unusual locations or shapes?
  Signs of rectal, genital, or oral injury or infection?
Medical experience: Is abuse or neglect suggested by:
  Prior emergency visits including accidents, ingestions or trauma?
  Prior hospitalizations or surgical interventions?
  Current or past sexually transmitted diseases (especially prepubertal)?
  Poor compliance with prior medical care or treatment?
  Incomplete immunizations for age?
  Poor mental or physical growth and development for age?
  Loss of previously attained developmental milestones?
Behavioral abnormalities: Is there evidence of:
  Withdrawal or hyperactivity?
  Overcompliance with physical examination or compliant posturing?
  Inappropriate affection or familiarity toward examiner?
  Phobias?
  Sleep problems?
  Recent onset of enuresis or encopresis?
  Sexualized play?
  Inappropriate sexual language?
  Excessive interest in genitalia?
Psychosocial conditions: Is there evidence of:
  Disturbed parent–child interaction?
  Violent interaction between parents? Between siblings?
  Violent interaction with friends and relatives?
  Parents being physically or sexually abused as children?
Extra stresses on the parent or family?
  Marital discord?
  Unemployment or financial hardship?
  Alcoholism or substance abuse?
  Recent death or illness in the family?
  History of prematurity in the child?
  Chronic disability in the child?
Inappropriate custodial care of the child?
  Daytime?
  After school?
  Evening?
  Nights?
  Weekends?
Inappropriate responsibilities for a child?
  Heavy chores, cooking, or housekeeping?
  Care of siblings?
Isolation of parent or family?
  Lack of telephone?
  Lack of supportive relatives, friends, or neighbors to whom they can turn in a crisis situation?
  Language barrier?
  Religious or cultural barriers?
Previous referrals for abuse or neglect?

SOURCE: Modified from Duarte et al.[108]

Anogenital Warts and Child Abuse

The incidence of anogenital warts among children is rising, yet the relationship to child abuse remains controversial.[116–118] While many cases of anogenital warts in children probably represent autoinoculation, vertical transmission, or nonsexual transmission, an-

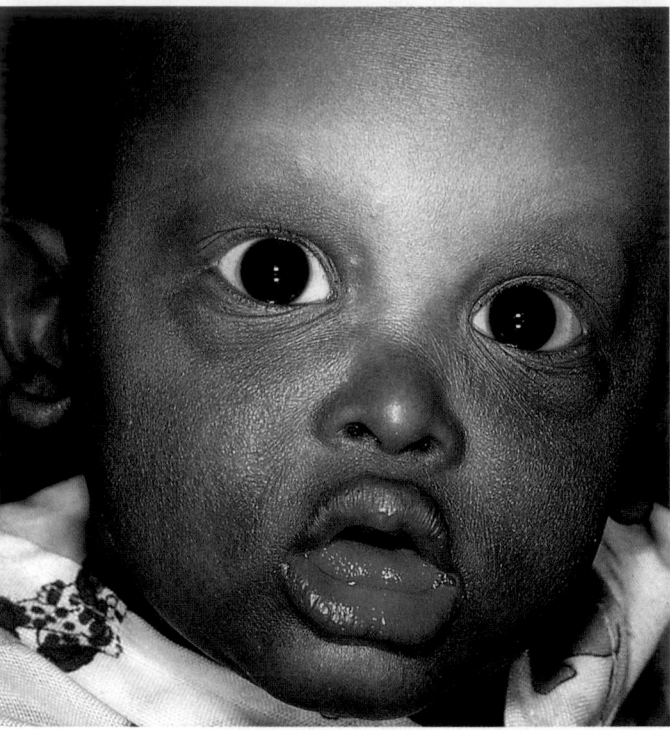

A.

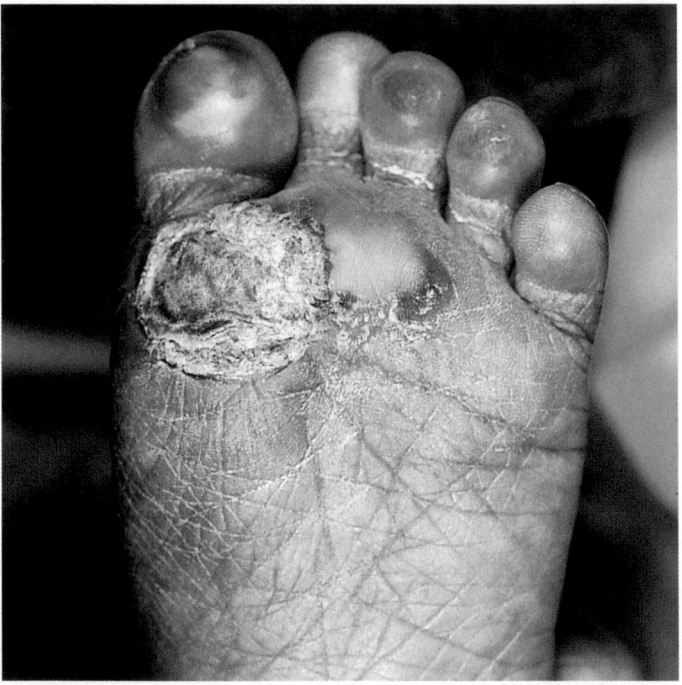

B.

A. A boy with hypohidrotic ectodermal dysplasia who was admitted for child abuse. B. Sole of foot with thermal burn.

ogenital warts can be the only manifestation of child sexual abuse. Although it is true that anogenital warts may not be equated with sexual abuse, the possibility must be considered in every case.[116] Unfortunately, there is no reliable test to distinguish benign from abusive situations. HPV typing does not provide definitive evidence for or against sexual abuse.[118] The potentially long incubation period of the HPV virus also confounds the picture. Vertical transmission may be common in newborns to 3-year-olds.[116,117] Some investigators believe that the appearance of warts before the age of 2 years is suggestive of perinatal transmission, and appearance either at birth or within the first week of life, is diagnostic of perinatal transmission.[117] Long-term follow-up is recommended in view of the oncogenic nature of some HPV types. Human papillomavirus infections are detailed in Chap. 224.

REFERENCES

1. Liang MG, Frieden IJ: Perineal and lip ulcerations as the presenting manifestation of hemangioma of infancy. *Pediatrics* **99**:256, 1997
2. Poole SR: The infant with acute, unexplained, excessive crying. *Pediatrics* **88**:450, 1991
3. Press S et al: Clitoris tourniquet syndrome. *Pediatrics* **66**:781, 1980
4. Frieden IJ et al: Suture ligation of supernumerary digits and accessory tragi: An outmoded practice? *Arch Pediatr Adolesc Med* **49**:1284, 1995
5. Paller AS et al: Nasal midline masses in infants and children: Dermoids, encephaloceles, and gliomas. *Arch Dermatol* **127**:362, 1991
6. Wagner A: Lumps and bumps in childhood. *Curr Probl Dermatol* **8**:137, 1996
7. Enjolras O: Classification and management of the various superficial vascular anomalies: Hemangiomas and vascular malformations. *J Dermatol* **24**:701, 1997
8. Berg RW: Etiology and pathophysiology of diaper dermatitis. *Advances in Dermatology* **3**:75, 1988
9. Singalavanija S, Frieden IJ: Diaper Dermatitis. *Pediatrics in Review* **16**:142, 1995
10. Orlow SJ: *Consultative Pediatric Dermatology.* New Haven, CT, Yale University/Glaxo Dermatology Lectureship Series in Dermatology, June 1996
11. Fairley J, Rasmussen J: Comparison of stratum corneum thickness in children and adults. *J Am Acad Dermatol* **8**:652, 1983
12. Yamamoto K: Soaps and detergents in children. *Clin Dermatol* **14**:81, 1996
13. Kawajiri Y et al: Physiological properties of infants' skin. *J Pediatr Dermatol* **12**:77, 1993
14. Malloy-McDonald MB, Lambert GH: Neonatal skin care. *Compr Ther* **19**:286, 1993
15. Cetta F et al: Newborn chemical exposure from over-the-counter skin care products. *Clin Pediatr* **30**:286, 1991
16. Shaw W: Folklore surrounding facial deformity and the origins of facial prejudice. *Br J Plast Surg* **34**:237, 1981
17. McCann J et al: Genital findings in prepubertal girls selected for nonabuse: A descriptive study. *Pediatrics* **86**:428, 1990
18. Kerns DL et al: Concave hymenal variations in suspected child sexual abuse victims. *Pediatrics* **90**:265, 1992
19. Berensen AB: A longitudinal study of hymenal morphology in the first three years of life. *Pediatrics* **95**:490, 1995
20. Siegfried EC, Frasier LD: The spectrum of anogenital diseases in children. *Curr Probl Dermatol* **9**:33, 1997
21. Paradise JE: Predictive accuracy and the diagnosis of sexual abuse: A big issue about a little tissue. *Child Abuse Negl* **13**:169, 1989
22. Kayashima K et al: Infantile perianal pyramidal protrusion. *Arch Dermatol* **132**:1481, 1996
23. Su JC et al: Atopic eczema: Its impact on the family and financial cost. *Arch Dis Child* **76**:159, 1997
24. Absolon CM et al: Psychological disturbance in atopic eczema: The extent of the problem in school-aged children. *Br J Dermatol* **137**:241, 1997
25. Weston WL et al: Misdiagnosis, treatments, and outcomes in the immunobullous diseases in children. *Pediatr Dermatol* **14**:264, 1997
26. Bartfield JM et al: Buffered versus plain lidocaine as a local anesthetic for simple laceration repair. *Ann Emerg Med* **19**:1387, 1990
27. Bartfield JM et al: Buffered versus plain lidocaine for digital nerve blocks. *Ann Emerg Med* **22**:216, 1993
28. Matsumoto AH et al: Reducing the discomfort of lidocaine administration through pH buffering. *J Vasc Intervent Radiol* **5**:171, 1994
29. Proudfoot J: Analgesia, anesthesia, and conscious sedation. *Emerg Med Clin North Am* **13**:357, 1995
30. Brogan GX Jr et al: Comparison of plain, warmed, and buffered lidocaine for anesthesia of traumatic wounds. *Ann Emerg Med* **26**:121, 1995
31. Mader TJ et al: Reducing the pain of local anesthetic infiltration: Warming and buffering have a synergistic effect. *Ann Emerg Med* **23**:550, 1994
32. Eichenfield LF et al: Cotton swab technique for obtaining cultures in patients with suspected tinea capitis (abstract). *Annal Dermatol Vénéréo* **125**(suppl 1):53, 1998
33. Elewski B: Tinea capitis. *Dermatol Clin* **14**:23, 1996
34. Ordoukhanian E, Lane AT: Warts and molluscum contagiosum: Beware of treatments worse than the disease. *Postgrad Med* **101**:223, 1997
35. Bowes G, Veit F: Clinical consultations with young people—some key considerations. *Aust Paediatr Rev* **5**:7, 1995
36. Sanci L, Young D: Engaging the adolescent patient. *Aust Fam Physician* **24**:2027, 1995
37. Blair S, Bowes G: Compliance issues in adolescence: Practical strategies. *Aust Fam Physician* **24**:2037, 1995
38. Cunliffe WJ: Acne and unemployment. *Br J Dermatol* **115**:386, 1986
39. Webster GE: Acne. *Curr Probl Dermatol* **8**:237, 1996
40. Fombonne E: Anorexia nervosa: No evidence of an increase. *Br J Psychiatry* **166**:462, 1995
41. Rooney B et al: The incidence and prevalence of anorexia nervosa in three suburban health districts in south west London, UK. *Int J Eat Disord* **18**:299, 1995
42. Siddiqui A et al: The cutaneous signs of eating disorders. *Acta Derm Venereol* **74**:68, 1994
43. Kuboki T et al: Epidemiological data on anorexia nervosa in Japan. *Psychol Res* **62**:11, 1996
44. Johnson MD: Disordered eating in active and athletic women. *Clin Sports Med* **13**:355, 1994
45. Sullivan PF: Mortality in anorexia nervosa. *Am J Psychol* **152**:1073, 1995
46. Eckert ED et al: Ten-year follow-up of anorexia nervosa: Clinical course and outcome. *Psychol Med* **25**:143, 1995
47. Gupta MA et al: Dermatologic signs in anorexia nervosa and bulimia nervosa. *Arch Dermatol* **123**:1386, 1987
48. Marshman GM et al: Cutaneous abnormalities in anorexia nervosa. *Australas J Dermatol* **31**:9, 1989
49. Robbay MS et al: The hypercarotenaemia in anorexia nervosa: A comparison of vitamin A and carotene levels in various forms of menstrual dysfunction and cachexia. *Am J Clin Nutr* **27**:362, 1974
50. Gilman JT, Gal P: Pharmocokinetic and pharmacodynamic data collection in children and neonates: A quiet frontier. *Clin Pharmacokinet* **23**:1, 1992
51. Wilson JT et al: Pediatric labelling requirements: Implications for pharmacokinetic studies. *Clin Pharmacokinet* **26**:308, 1994
52. *PDR for Nonprescription Drugs.* 18th ed. Montvale, NJ, Medical Economics, 1997.
53. *Physicians' Desk Reference.* 51st ed. Montvale, NJ, Medical Economics, 1997.
54. Eldadah M, Fitzgerald M: Methemoglobinemia due to skin application of benzocaine. *Clin Pediatr* **32**:687, 1993
55. AAP, Committee on Drugs, 1989–90: Clioquinol (Iodohydroxyquin, Vioform) and Iodoquinol (Diiodohydroxyquin): Blindness and neuropathy. *Pediatrics* **86**:797, 1990
56. Davies JE et al: Lindane poisonings. *Arch Dermatol* **19**:142, 1983
57. Friedman SJ: Lindane neurotoxic reaction in nonbullous congenital ichthyosiform erythroderma. *Arch Dermatol* **123**:1056, 1987
58. Osimitz TG, Grothaus RH: The present safety assessment of DEET. *J Am Mosq Control Assoc* **11**:274, 1995
59. Brown M, Hebert AA: Insect repellents: An overview. *J Am Acad Dermatol* **36**:243, 1997
60. Barakat M et al: Hypothyroidism secondary to topical iodine treatment in infants with spina bifida. *Acta Paediatr* **83**:741, 1994
61. Aihara M et al: Prevention and control of nosocomial infection caused by methicillin-resistant Staphylococcus aureus in a premature infant ward—preventive effect of a povidone-iodine wipe of neonatal skin. *Postgrad Med J* **69**(suppl 3):S117, 1993

62. Germann R et al: Lebensbedrohliche salicylatintoxikation durch per-kutane resorption bei einer schweren ichthyosis vulgaris. *Hautartzt* **47**:624, 1996

63. Yercen N et al: Fatal hypernatremia in an infant due to salting of the skin. *Am J Dis Child* **147**:716, 1993

64. Gonzalez del Rey J et al: Lidocaine overdose: Another preventable case? *Pediatr Emerg Care* **10**:344, 1994

65. Wolverton SE: Major adverse effects from systemic drugs: Defining the risks. *Curr Probl Dermatol* **7**:1, 1995

66. Wolverton SE: Glucocorticoids, in *Systemic Drugs for Skin Diseases*, edited by SE Wolverton, JK Wilkin. Philadelphia, Saunders, 1991, p 86

67. Patel L et al: Adult height in patients with childhood onset atopic dermatitis. *Arch Dis Child* **76**:505–508, 1997

68. Stoughton RB: Percutaneous absorption of drugs. *Annu Rev Pharmacol Toxicol* **29**:55, 1989

69. Paller AS: Scabies in infants and small children. *Semin Dermatol* **12**:3, 1993

70. Meinking TL: Safety of permethrin vs. lindane for the treatment of scabies. *Arch Dermatol* **132**:959, 1996

71. Larsson BA et al: Regional variations in skin perfusion and skin thickness may contribute to varying efficacy of topical, local anesthetics in neonates. *Paediatr Anaesth* **6**:107, 1996

72. Kendall JM et al: Topical anesthesia for children's lacerations: An acceptable approach? *J Accident Emerg Med* **13**:119, 1996

73. British Association of Otolaryngologists—Head and neck surgeons, Royal College of Surgeons of England. Questionnaire on the use of cocaine. *BAOL Newsletter*, p 11, 1991

74. Williamson P, Slack R: Dangers of cocaine and adrenaline paste: Accurate measurements of dose and patience are important. *BMJ* **311**:1089, 1995

75. Nicholson KEA, Rogers JEG: Cocaine and adrenaline paste: A fatal combination. *BMJ* **311**:250, 1995

76. Smith GA et al: New non-cocaine-containing topical anesthetics compared with tetracaine-adrenaline-cocaine during repair of lacerations. *Pediatrics* **100**:825, 1997

77. Lilley LL, Guanci R: Med errors: Caution with concentrations. *Am J Nurs* **96**:14, 1996

78. Brook CG et al: Growth and growth hormone secretion. *J Endocrinol* **119**:179, 1988

79. Fine RN: Corticosteroids and growth. *Kidney Int* **43**:S59, 1993

80. Lucky AW: Principles of the use of glucocorticoids in the growing child. *Pediatr Dermatol* **1**:226, 1984

81. Hughes IA: Steroids and growth. *Br Med J Clin Res* **295**:683, 1987

82. American Academy of Pediatrics. Active and passive immunization, in *1997 Red Book: Report of the Committee on Infectious Diseases,* 24th ed., edited by G Peter. Elk Grove Village, IL: American Academy of Pediatrics, 1997, p 50.

83. American Academy of Pediatrics. Poliovirus infections, in *1997 Red Book: Report of the Committee on Infectious Diseases,* 24th ed., edited by G Peter. Elk Grove Village, IL: American Academy of Pediatrics, 1997, p 426.

84. Burkhardt JE et al: Histologic and histochemical changes in articular cartilages of immature beagle dogs dosed with difloxacin and flu-oquinolone. *Vet Pathol* **27**:162, 1990

85. Periti P et al: Pharmacokinetic drug interactions of macrolides. *Clin Pharmacokinet* **23**:106, 1992

86. Wolfson JS, Hooper DC: Overview of fluoroquinolone safety. *Am J Med* **91**(suppl 6A):1535, 1991

87. Schaad UB et al: Use of fluoroquinolones in pediatrics: Consensus report of an International Society of Chemotherapy commission. *Pediatr Infect Dis J* **14**:1, 1995

88. Chapel KL, Rasmussen JE: Pediatric dermatology: Advances in therapy. *J Am Acad Dermatol* **36**:513, 1997

89. Presterl E, Graninger W: Efficacy and safety of fluconazole in the treatment of systemic fungal infections in pediatric patients: Multicentre study group. *Eur J Clin Microbiol Infect Dis* **13**:347, 1994

90. Cullin SI, Catalano PM: Griseofulvin-warfarin antagonism. *JAMA* **199**:482, 1967

91. Van Dijke CP, Weber JC: Interaction between oral contraceptives and griseofulvin. *BMJ* **288**:1125, 1984

92. Cohen MM Jr: Syndromology: An updated conceptual overview. IX. Facial dysmorphology. *Int J Oral Maxillofac Surg* **19**:81, 1990

93. Marden PM et al: Congenital anomalies in the newborn infant, including minor variations. *J Pediatr* **64**:358, 1984

94. Smith DW, Bostian KE: Congenital anomalies associated with idiopathic mental retardation. *J Pediatr* **65**:189, 1964

95. Cohen MM Jr, Cole DEC: Origins of recognizable syndromes: Etiologic and pathogenetic mechanisms and the process of syndrome delineation. *J Pediatr* **115**:161, 1989

96. Allanson JE et al: Noonan syndrome: The changing phenotype. *Am J Med Genet* **21**:507, 1985

97. Breg WR et al: The cri du chat syndrome in adolescents and adults: Clinical findings in 13 older patients with partial deletion of the short arm of chromosome number 5. *J Pediatr* **77**:782, 1970

98. Hall JG et al: *Handbook of Normal Physical Measurements.* New York, Oxford Medical Publications, 1989

99. Jones KL: *Smith's Recognizable Patterns of Human Malformation.* 5th ed. Philadelphia, W.B. Saunders, 1997

100. Spitz JL: *Genodermatoses: A Full-Color Clinical Guide to Genetic Skin Disorders.* Baltimore, Williams & Wilkins, 1996

101. Aase JM: *Diagnostic Dysmorphology.* New York, Plenum, 1990

102. Strauss RP, Resnick SD: Pulsed dye laser therapy for port-wine stains in children: Psychosocial and ethical issues. *J Pediatr* **122**:505, 1993

103. Höhler H: Changes in facial expression as a result of plastic surgery in mongoloid children. *Aesthetic Plast Surg* **1**:245, 1977

104. Mearig J: Facial surgery and an active modification approach for children with Down syndrome: Some psychological and ethical issues. *Rehabil Lit* **46**:72, 1985

105. MacGregor F: *Transformation and Identity—The Face and Plastic Surgery.* New York, Quadrangle/New York Times, 1974, p 119

106. Bersheid E: Overview of the psychological effects of physical attractiveness, in *Psychological Aspects of Facial Form,* edited by G Lucker, K Ribbens, J McNamara. Ann Arbor, Center for Human Growth and Development, 1980, p 1. (Craniofacial Growth Series Monograph No. 11.)

107. Cunningham M: Measuring the physical in physical attractiveness. *J Pers Soc Psychol* **58**:618, 1986

108. Duarte AM et al: Life-threatening dermatoses in pediatric dermatology. *Adv Dermatol* **10**:329, 1995

109. Raimer BG et al: Cutaneous signs of child abuse. *J Am Acad Dermatol* **5**:203, 1981

110. Byrk M, Siegel PT: My mother caused my illness: The story of a survivor of Munchausen by proxy syndrome. *Pediatrics* **100**:1, 1997

111. Weston WL, Morelli JG: Painful and disabling granuloma annulare: A case of Munchausen by Proxy. *Pediatr Dermatol* **14**:363, 1997

112. Myers J: The role of the physician in preserving verbal evidence of child abuse. *J Pediatr* **109**:409, 1986

113. DeJong AR, Rose M: Frequency and significance of physical evidence in legally proven cases of child sexual abuse. *Pediatrics* **84**:1022, 1989

114. Siegfried EC: The spectrum of anogenital diseases in children. *Curr Probl Dermatol* **9**:33, 1997

115. Rapps WR: Scientific evidence in rape prosecution. *Univ Missouri/Kansas City Law Review* **48**:216, 1980

116. Bingham EA: Significance of anogenital warts in children. *Br J Hosp Med* **52**:469, 1994

117. Handley J et al: Common association of HPV 2 with anogenital warts in prepubertal children. *Pediatr Dermatol* **14**:339, 1997

118. Gutman LT et al: Transmission of human genital papillomavirus disease: Comparison of data from adults and children. *Pediatrics* **91**:31, 1993

119. Peter G ed: 1997 Red Book: Report of the Committee on Infectious Diseases. 24th ed. Elk Grove, IL: American Academy of Pediatrics, 1997

120. Solomon BA et al: Fluconazole for the treatment of tinea capitis in children. *J Am Acad Dermatol* **37**:274, 1997

121. Kullavanijaya P et al: Randomized single-blind study of efficacy and tolerability of terbinafine in the treatment of tinea capitis. *J Am Acad Dermatol* **37**:272, 1997

122. Desgarennes MD et al: Therapeutic efficacy of terbinafine in the treatment of three children with tinea tonsurans. *J Am Acad Dermatol* **35**:114, 1996

123. Gruseck E et al: Oral terbinafine in tinea capitis in children. *Mycoses* **39**:237, 1996

124. Nejjam F et al: *Br J Dermatol* **132**:98, 1995

125. Jones TC: Overview of the use of terbinafine (Lamisil) in children. *Br J Dermatol* **132**:683, 1995

126. Haroon TS et al: A randomized double-blind comparative study of terbinafine for 1, 2 and 4 weeks in tinea capitis. *Br J Dermatol* **135**:86, 1996

127. Lopez-Gomez S et al: Itraconazole versus griseofulvin in the treatment of tinea capitis: A double-blind randomized study in children. *Int J Dermatol* **33**:743, 1994
128. Degreef H: Itraconazole in the treatment of tinea capitis. *Cutis* **58**:90, 1996
129. Greer DL: Treatment of tinea capitis with itraconazole. *J Am Acad Dermatol* **35**:637, 1996
130. Gupta AK et al: Itraconazole pulse therapy is effective in the treatment of tinea capitis in children: An open multicentre study. *Br J Dermatol* **137**:251, 1997
131. Ginter G: Microsporum canis infections in children: results of a new oral antifungal therapy. *Mycoses* **39**:265, 1996
132. Drug Doses, in *Harriet Lane Handbook.* 14th ed., edited by MA Barone. St. Louis, Mosby-Yearbook, 1996

CHAPTER 145

Mina Yaar
Barbara A. Gilchrest

Aging of Skin

In both developed and developing nations, the number and proportion of older people are increasing.[1] Twenty percent of the U.S. population and 27 percent of the Japanese population are expected to be 65 years or older by the year 2025. In the United States, depending on the population assumptions used, the number of elderly persons will double or triple during the first quarter of the twenty-first century. This demographic shift compels health care providers and government officials to confront the pathophysiology of aging and associated health issues.

THEORIES OF AGING

There are two basic theories of aging.[2] The programmatic theory states that aging, like development, is a preordained process due to an inherent genetic program, played out at a rate characteristic of each species. The stochastic theory states that random cumulative environmental damage to genes and proteins ultimately produces aging and homeostatic failure. Available data suggest that aging is in fact the interactive result of both a genetic program and cumulative wear and tear during the life span.

The Programmatic Theory

AGING GENES   Master aging genes, or "gerontogenes," responsible for the aging process have long been postulated, and supporting evidence is increasingly available, at least in lower organisms such as yeast. In humans, the only genes implicated in the rate of aging are those in which mutations are responsible for premature aging syndromes. For example, Cockayne syndrome patients display mutations in the DNA helicases encoded by the ERCC-6 or -3 genes,[3,4] and ataxia telangiectasia is caused by a mutation in the ATM gene, encoding a kinase that senses DNA damage.[5] The human ATM gene is homologous to a yeast gene involved in telomere

metabolism (see below).[6] Werner syndrome, caused by mutation in an apparent DNA helicase,[7] features elevated rates of DNA non-homologous recombination, rapid telomere shortening, and decreased repair of telomeres. A role for these genes in normal aging is suggested but certainly not established, since patients with so-called premature aging syndromes display some manifestations of aging at an accelerated rate but lack other features of normal aging and have characteristic findings that differ greatly from those of normal aging. Nevertheless, the striking effect of single gene mutations on aspects of the human aging process certainly argues for genetic determinants.

CELLULAR SENESCENCE   Cells have a limited capacity to undergo cell division, a phenomenon termed the *Hayflick limit*, or *cellular senescence*.[8] Senescence appears to involve a genetic program that ultimately inhibits DNA synthesis, in part by upregulating antiproliferative proteins.[9–12] Fusion studies in which young (early-passage) cells are fused with senescent cells indicate that senescence is dominant,[13] the effect of genes residing on human chromosomes 1, 4, and 7.[14]

The majority of genes overexpressed during in vitro cellular senescence contribute to blocking the cells in the G_1 phase of the cell cycle. Some encode DNA binding proteins that act as gene regulators.[15] Others, including statin[16] and the cyclin-dependent kinase inhibitors p21 (SDI-1)[17] and p16,[18] encode inhibitors of cell cycle regulatory nuclear proteins. Other overexpressed senescence-associated genes encode epitopes of extracellular matrix proteins such as fibronectin,[19] proteases involved in modulation of extracellular proteins such as collagenase and stromelysin,[20] or protease inhibitors such as plasminogen activator inhibitors 1 and 2,[21,22] suggesting that signals from extracellular matrix proteins regulate cellular proliferation and perhaps aging processes themselves.

TELOMERE SHORTENING   Telomeres, the terminal portions of eukaryotic chromosomes,[23] consist of up to many hundreds of tandem short sequence repeats (TTAGGG). During mitosis of somatic cells, DNA polymerase cannot replicate the final base pairs of each chromosome, resulting in progressive shortening with each round of cell division. A special reverse transcriptase, telomerase, can replicate these chromosomal ends, but, with few exceptions, the enzyme is normally expressed only in germ-line cells.[24] Telomere length shortens more than 30 percent during adulthood even in relatively quiescent skin fibroblasts.[25] Critically short telomeres appear to signal cell cycle arrest or apoptosis and to compromise DNA stability and transcription of subtelomeric genes,[26,27] perhaps contributing to the aged phenotype.

FAILURE OF APOPTOSIS At least in vitro, aging appears to be associated with refractoriness to apoptosis, the active cell death program that requires induction of several genes also required for entry into the cell cycle,[28] and late-passage fibroblasts express high levels of the antiapoptotic protein bcl-2.[29] Inability to eliminate damaged cells via apoptosis is speculated to decrease organ function, the phenomenon that defines aging.[29]

LONGEVITY GENES All characterized longevity genes encode proteins that assist in control of environmental stress. The *ras*-2 gene in yeast, whose overexpression delays senescence,[30] acts as an environmental sensor for response to a variety of stresses including starvation, UV irradiation, oxidative damage, and heat shock.

There are approximately 10 longevity genes identified to date in the nematode *Caenorhabditis elegans*, and all confer greater resistance to environmental stresses such as elevated temperature and UV irradiation.[31] Mutations in one or more of these genes doubles or triples maximal life span.

Expression of higher levels of antioxidative enzymes[32] or overexpression of genes associated with resistance to starvation, desication, or heat were identified in long-lived *Drosophilae*.[33]

Mice with extended life span show high expression of a small number of gene loci that control immune response,[34] a critical mammalian defense against environmental insults.

The Stochastic Theory

OXIDATIVE STRESS AND THE RATE OF LIVING THEORY It has long been speculated that oxygen utilization is somehow related to the process of aging.[35] Oxygen, required for survival of aerobic organisms, readily accepts single electron transfers, generating $\cdot O^{-2}$, H_2O_2, and $\cdot OH$, which further generate an array of reactive oxygen species (ROS) that damage biologic molecules.[36] Such damage includes peroxidation of membrane fatty acids, DNA base alterations, single-strand DNA breaks, sister chromatin exchange, DNA-protein cross-links, carbonyl modifications, and loss of sulfhydryl groups in proteins leading to inactivation of enzymes and increased proteolysis.[37] The antioxidative defense systems of the organism are not fully efficient, and hence throughout life cells accumulate molecular oxidative damage, sometimes leading to apoptotic cell death.[37,38] Several studies show that there is an age-associated increase in both ROS generation[39] and the level of oxidatively damaged proteins[37] and DNA.[38,40] Caloric restriction, which decreases the metabolic rate of the organism, reduces oxidative stress and extends life span in several species, including fish, spiders, rats, mice, and primates.[41] In addition to life span extension, lifelong caloric restriction is associated with improvement in learning ability, immune responses, gene expression, enzyme activities, hormonal action, glucose utilization, DNA repair capacity, and rate of protein synthesis in old rats. Moreover, mutation of one of

the longevity genes of *Caenorhabditis elegans* is associated with a hypometabolic state,[42] consistent with the free radical theory of aging that attributes the process primarily to oxidative stress.

AMINO ACID RACEMIZATION Racemization, a process that substitutes D-amino acids for L-amino acids within proteins, occurs during aging and may affect protein function. Furthermore, racemization affects the deamidation of the amino acids asparagine and glutamine, a process that decreases the rate of protein degradation. Thus, racemization may lead to accumulation of dysfunctional proteins in aged tissues.[43]

NONENZYMATIC GLYCOSYLATION Nonenzymatic glycosylation of proteins occurs when reducing sugar aldehydes condense with protein amino groups, resulting in brown discoloration, loss of function, and altered degradation.[43] Glycosylation of extracellular matrix proteins such as dermal collagen leads to cross-linking, with trapping and sequestration of other, unaffected proteins (see below).

AGING AND THE IMMUNE SYSTEM

The immune system has two major roles—defense against external insults and internal immunologic surveillance. Age-associated decrements in the function of B and T lymphocytes and a variety of accessory cells are postulated to contribute to the increased incidence of infections and malignancies in the elderly.[44]

SKIN AGING

Cutaneous aging includes two distinct phenomena: *True aging*, also termed *intrinsic aging*, is a universal, presumably inevitable change attributable to the passage of time alone; *photoaging* is the superposition on intrinsic aging of changes attributable to chronic sun exposure, which are neither universal nor inevitable. The former is manifested primarily by physiologic alterations with subtle but undoubtedly important consequences for both healthy and diseased skin. The latter has major morphologic as well as physiologic manifestations and corresponds more closely to the popular notion of "old skin."

Clinical and Histologic Skin Changes

The skin changes that occur with aging (Table 145-1) lead to a gradual physiologic decline (Table 145-2). Major age-related changes in the skin's appearance include "dryness" (roughness), wrinkling, laxity, and a variety of benign neoplasms. Early studies cited in the prior edition of this book and other comprehensive sources[45,46] will not be individually referenced.

THE EPIDERMIS The most striking and consistent histologic change is flattening of the dermal-epidermal junction with effacement of both the dermal papillae and epidermal rete pegs. This is accompanied by a more than 50 percent reduction in the number of these interdigitations per unit skin surface length between the third and ninth decades. This results in a considerably smaller surface between the epidermis and dermis and presumably less communication and nutrient transfer. Dermal-epidermal separation has been demonstrated to occur more readily in old skin, undoubtedly explaining the propensity of the elderly to torn skin and superficial abrasions following minor trauma such as bandage removal and to bulla formation in edematous sites. In females, a sharp decline in the number of interdigitations occurs between 40 and 60 years, while in males the rate of decline is more constant throughout adulthood.[47]

Average interrete epidermal thickness probably remains constant with advancing age, but variability in epidermal thickness and in individual keratinocyte size increases. At the electron microscopic level, sun-protected old skin is characterized by some widening of interkeratinocyte spaces, by reduplication of the lamina densa and anchoring fibril complex in the basement membrane zone, and by loss of the numerous microvillous projections of basal cell cytoplasm into the dermis.

Average thickness and degree of compaction of the stratum corneum appear constant with increasing age, although individual corneocytes are larger. The skin surface pattern, a patchwork of fine lines possibly determined by papillary dermal architecture, reveals slight age-associated loss of regularity. Age effects on percutaneous absorption depend in part on drug structure, with hydrophilic substances such as hydrocortisone and benzoic acid being less well absorbed through the skin of old versus young individuals but with hydrophobic substances such as testosterone and estradiol being equally well absorbed.[48] Of perhaps greater clinical importance, aging markedly delays the recovery of barrier function in damaged stratum corneum, apparently because of slow replacement of neutral lipids leading to decreased amount of lipids in the newly formed lamellar bodies.[49] Subtle changes in overall stratum corneum lipid prolile with aging may also affect barrier function.[47,50]

In the elderly, the skin often appears dry and flaky, especially over the lower extremities, an area in which a remarkable age-associated decrease in the content of epidermal filaggrin has been reported.[51] Filaggrin, required for binding of keratin filaments into macrofibrils, is also decreased in the skin of patients with ichthyosis vulgaris, and its lack has been postulated to cause the increased scaliness in both conditions.[51] Barrier function may also be affected by this structural change.

Epidermal turnover rate and thymidine-labeling index decrease approximately 30 to 50 percent between the third and eighth decades, with a corresponding prolongation in stratum corneum replacement rate. Linear growth rates also decrease for hair and nails. Epidermal repair rate after wounding likewise declines with age.

With increasing donor age, cultured keratinocytes and fibroblasts also show progressive decline in the response to growth factors,[52,53] associated with decrements in growth factor signal transduction.[54,55]

A decrease in the number of enzymatically active melanocytes per unit surface area of the skin, approximately 10 to 20 percent of the remaining cell population each decade, has been repeatedly documented, presumably reducing the body's protective barrier against UV radiation. The number of melanocytic nevi also progressively decreases with age, from a peak of 15 to 40 in the third and fourth decades to an average of four per person after age 50; such nevi are rarely observed in persons beyond age 80.

Between early and late adulthood there is a 20 to 50 percent reduction in the number of morphologically identifiable epidermal Langerhans cells, the skin's immune effector cells responsible for antigen presentation. The remaining cells display morphologic abnormalities including shorter dendrites. These changes, com-

TABLE 145-1

Histologic Features of Aging Human Skin

EPIDERMIS	DERMIS	APPENDAGES
Flattened dermal-epidermal junction	Atrophy (loss of dermal volume)	Depigmented hair
Variable thickness	Fewer fibroblasts	Loss of hair
Variable cell size and shape	Fewer mast cells	Conversion of terminal to vellus hair
Occasional nuclear atypia	Fewer blood vessels	Abnormal nailplates
Fewer melanocytes	Shortened capillary loops	Fewer glands
Fewer Langerhans cells	Abnormal nerve endings	

pounded by decreases in production of interleukin and perhaps other cytokines by keratinocytes, presumably contribute to the observed age-associated decrease in cutaneous immune responsiveness.

An endocrine function of human epidermis that declines with age is vitamin D production.[56] Some elderly individuals also have reduced serum levels of vitamin D and/or osteomalacia,[57,58] the decreased mineralization of bone classically associated with vitamin D deficiency. Although avoidance of dairy products (the principal dietary source of vitamin D), insufficient sun exposure, and sunscreen use undoubtedly contribute to vitamin D deficiency in the elderly, the level of epidermal 7-dehydrocholesterol per unit skin surface area also appears to decrease linearly by approximately 75 percent between early and late adulthood,[56] suggesting that lack of its immediate biosynthetic precursor may also limit vitamin D production. Indeed, in one study, old adult volunteers subjected to total-body UV irradiation produced far less vitamin D_3 than did complexion-matched young adult volunteers exposed to the same UV dose.[59]

With regard to susceptibility to oxidative damage, there is no consensus regarding age-associated changes in the activities of antioxidative enzymes including catalase, superoxide dismutase, glutathione peroxidase, or glutathione reductase.[60,61]

THE DERMIS Loss of dermal thickness approaches 20 percent in elderly individuals, although in sun-protected sites significant thinning occurs only after the eighth decade.[62] Old skin is relatively acellular and avascular. Precise histologic concomitants of wrinkling, if any, are unknown,[63] although the age-related loss of normal elastic fibers may be contributory, and increases in papillary dermal collagen are observed in photoaged skin after medical or surgical treatment that improves wrinkling.[64,65] Deep expression lines seem to result from contractions of connective tissue septae within the subcutaneous fat.[66]

TABLE 145-2

Functions of Human Skin that Decline with Age

Cell replacement	Immune responsiveness
Barrier function	Thermoregulation
Chemical clearance	Sweat production
Sensory perception	Sebum production
Mechanical protection	Vitamin D production
Wound healing	DNA repair

In one study, an approximately 50 percent reduction in mast cells and a 30 percent reduction in venular cross-sections were noted in the papillary dermis of buttock skin from elderly adults compared to that from young adult controls, associated with a corresponding reduction in histamine release and other manifestations of the inflammatory response following UV radiation exposure. The dermal microvasculature in middle-aged or elderly subjects may also show mild vascular wall thickening; vascular wall thinning to less than half the normal young adult measurement, associated with absent or reduced perivascular veil cells, has been reported in skin of very elderly subjects and probably contributes to vascular fragility. Electron microscopic studies also show sporadic degeneration of the elastic component of dermal arterioles. The striking age-associated loss of vascular bed, especially of the vertical capillary loops that occupy the dermal papillae in young skin, is felt to underlie many of the physiologic alterations in old skin, including palor, decreased skin temperature, and the approximately 60 percent reductions in basal and peak induced cutaneous blood flow.[67,68] Furthermore, reduction in the vascular network surrounding hair bulbs and eccrine, apocrine, and sebaceous glands may contribute to their gradual atrophy and fibrosis with age.

Age-associated decreases in wheal resorption and dermal clearance of transepidermally absorbed materials have been reported,[69] probably due to alterations in both the vascular bed and extracellular matrix. Conversely, the time required for development of a tense blister after topical ammonium hydroxide application is nearly twice as long in older individuals, suggesting a decreased transudation rate with age in injured skin. Impaired transfer of cells as well as solutes between the extravascular and intravascular dermal compartments is suggested by several studies; multiple factors undoubtedly contribute.

Decreased vascular responsiveness in the skin of older individuals has been documented by clinically assessing vasodilation and transudation after UV exposure, application of standardized irritants, histamine, and the mast cell degranulating agent 48/80. However, factors such as age-associated changes in percutaneous absorption or cytokine release may also contribute to the response.[69] Compromised thermoregulation, which predisposes the elderly to sometimes fatal heat stroke or hypothermia, may be due in part to reduced vasoactivity of dermal arterioles and, in the latter instance, to loss of subcutaneous fat as well.

Compared to young adult controls, healthy older subjects are less able to manifest skin sensitivity to dinitrochlorobenzene or standard recall antigens, undoubtedly reflecting the well-documented decrease in total number of circulating thymus-derived lymphocytes and in their responsiveness to standard mitogens,[44] as well as the above-mentioned local cutaneous changes.

Biochemical changes in collagen, elastin, and dermal ground substance during fetal and early postnatal development are far greater than those described with advancing age, but collagen content per unit area of skin surface decreases approximately 1 percent per year throughout adult life,[70] and the remaining collagen fibrils appear disorganized, more compact, and granular.[71] In rats, a gradual decline of collagen synthesis rate with advancing age was determined, and the rate at 24 months was only 10 percent that at 1 month of age.[70] In addition, approximately 50 percent of the newly synthesized collagen in old rats was degraded, versus only 6 percent in immature animals. Similarly, dermal fibroblasts derived from human donors of different ages have an age-associated increase in basal and induced levels of interstitial collagenase mRNA, due to increased transcriptional activity of the collagenase promoter,

as well as age-associated decreases in concentrations of procollagen type I and type III, a measure of collagen synthesis rate, in suction blister fluid.[72] In women, both bone mass (due primarily to collagen I) and skin collagen decline rapidly in the immediate postmenopausal years,[73–76] suggesting an estrogen influence on collagen synthesis and degradation. Such changes almost certainly contribute to impaired wound healing in the elderly.[77] Finally, a variety of biochemical analyses indicate increased cross-linkage of the collagen molecule with advancing age.[77,78]

Beginning in early adulthood, elastic fibers decrease in number and diameter; by old age, they often appear fragmented with small cysts and lacunae, especially in the dermal-epidermal junction.[79] Similar changes can be produced experimentally by incubation of dermal slices with elastase or chymotrypsin in vitro, suggesting that enzymatic degradation of elastin may be a mechanism for normal dermal aging. Elastic fibers also show progressive cross-linkage and calcification with age in adult skin.

The few reports concerning the possible postmaturational changes in mucopolysaccharides (glycosaminoglycans and proteoglycans) or other molecules of the ground substance in which collagen and elastic fibers are embedded suggest decreases relative to dry weight or collagen content of the skin, especially for hyaluronic acid,[80] or in hyaluronic acid extractability.[81] Electron-dense hyaluronic acid granules also decrease with age and are absent in those over age 60.[80] These changes may adversely influence skin turgor, as proteoglycans bind to 1000 times their own weight in water.

Changes with age during adulthood in mechanical properties of the skin include progressive loss of elastic recovery, consistent with gradual destruction of the dermal elastic network, and marked prolongation of the time required for excised skin to return to its original thickness after compression. In vivo studies of ventral forearm skin of 133 volunteers in each decade of life revealed linear declines during adulthood of approximately 25 percent in both men and women for elasticity and extensibility.[82] Loss of elasticity began in childhood and continued through the ninth decade, while extensibility was constant through the sixth decade and then declined more rapidly thereafter.[82]

Overall, a picture emerges of aging dermis as an increasingly rigid, inelastic, and unresponsive tissue, less capable of undergoing modification in response to stress.

NERVES AND APPENDAGES By the end of the fifth decade, approximately half the population has at least 50 percent gray (white) body hair with an even higher proportion of depigmented scalp hair, and virtually everyone has some degree of graying, due to progressive and eventually total loss of melanocytes from the hair bulb. Loss of melanocytes is believed to occur more rapidly in hair than in skin because the cells proliferate and manufacture melanin at maximal rates during the anagen phase of the hair cycle, while epidermal melanocytes are comparatively inactive throughout their life span. Scalp hair may gray more rapidly than other body hair because its anagen-to-telogen ratio is considerably greater than that of other body hair. Advancing age is also accompanied by a modest decrease in number of hair follicles, due in part to atrophy and fibrosis. Also, with aging there is an increase in the proportion of telogen hair follicles. Remaining hairs may be smaller in diameter and grow more slowly.

The process termed *balding* results primarily from the androgen-dependent conversion of the relatively dark, thick "terminal" scalp hairs to lightly pigmented short fine vellous hairs similar to those on the ventral forearm. Bitemporal hair line recession begins during late adolescence in most women and virtually all men. Assessment of baldness is hampered by lack of a precise definition, but by certain criteria, advanced bitemporal and occipital hair loss in men increases in prevalence from 20 percent and 3 percent at the end of the third decade to more than 60 percent and 25 percent by the seventh decade, respectively.

Eccrine glands decrease by approximately 15 percent in average number during adulthood in most body sites. Spontaneous sweating in response to dry heat is further reduced—more than 70 percent in healthy old subjects as compared to young controls—attributable primarily to a decreased output per gland. Maximal sweat production has not been quantified in the elderly but is almost certainly reduced and probably predisposes to heat stroke in this age group. Apocrine gland size and function also decrease with aging. Lipofuscin ("age pigment") gradually accumulates with age in the secretory cells of both eccrine and apocrine glands.

Sebaceous gland size and number appear not to change with age. The exponential decrease in sebum production of approximately 23 percent per decade beginning in the second decade in both men and women (approximately 60 percent over the adult life span) is attributed to the concomitant decrease in production of gonadal or adrenal androgens to which sebaceous glands are exquisitely sensitive.[83] The clinical effects of decreased sebum production, if any, are unknown. There is no direct relationship to xerosis or seborrheic dermatitis.

Pacinian and Meissner's corpuscles, the cutaneous end organs responsible for pressure perception and light touch, progressively decrease to approximately one-third their initial average density between the second and ninth decades of life, as determined histochemically in two body sites, and display greater size variation and structural irregularities. There are very few histologically demonstrable aging changes in Merkel's disks or in free nerve endings.

Decreased sensory perception in old skin encompasses optimal stimulus for light touch, vibratory sensation, and corneal sensation; ability to discriminate two points; and spatial acuity.[84,85] Cutaneous pain threshold increases up to 20 percent with advancing adult age. The available data do not permit differentiation among an age-associated increase in the prevalence of peripheral neuropathy, a true aging change in healthy subjects, increased rate of heat dispersion in old skin due to age-associated dermal alterations, an increased peripheral nerve threshold to painful stimuli, and an increased central threshold to pain perception. The many psychological and social factors influencing an individual's reaction to pain may also be presumed to vary with age. In any case, either decreased awareness of or reaction to noxious stimuli facilitates wounding and irritation of old skin.

Photoaging

Initially due to ignorance of its true pathophysiology and subsequently due to lack of an appropriate word, chronic sun damage has been widely mislabeled in both the lay and medical literature as "aging," "premature aging," or "accelerated aging." Clinical features of actinically damaged skin are listed in Table 145-3 and histologically contrasted with those of intrinsic aging in Fig. 145-1.

The relative severity of these changes varies considerably among individuals, undoubtedly reflecting inherent differences in vulnerability and repair capacity for the solar insult. All occur predominantly in fair-skinned whites with a history of ample past sun exposure and usually involve the face, neck, or extensor surface of the upper extremities most severely. These changes are exacerbated by cigarette smoking[86,87] and possibly other environmental factors. The apparent influence of sex on the prevalence of certain of these conditions undoubtedly reflects different hair styles, patterns of dress, and nature of sun exposure (occupational vs. recreational) between men and women over the past several generations; other sex differences such as epidermal thickness and sebaceous gland activity may also influence their development. The characteristic distribution of different lesions is a complex function of relative sun exposure for different body sites, anatomic distribution of the par-

TABLE 145-3

Features of Actinically Damaged Skin*

CLINICAL ABNORMALITY	HISTOLOGIC ABNORMALITY
Dryness (roughness)	Increased compaction of stratum corneum, increased thickness of granular cell layer, reduced epidermal thickness, reduced epidermal mucin content
Actinic keratoses	Nuclear atypia, loss of orderly, progressive keratinocyte maturation; irregular epidermal hyperplasia and/or hypoplasia; occasional dermal inflammation
Irregular pigmentation	
Freckling	Reduced or increased number of hypertrophic, strongly dopa-positive melanocytes
Lentigines	Elongation of epidermal rete ridges; increases in number and melanization of melanocytes
Guttate hypomelanosis	Reduced number of atypical melanocytes
Persistent hyperpigmentation	Increased number of dopa-positive melanocytes and increased melanin content per unit area and increased number of dermal melanophages
Wrinkling	
Fine surface lines	None detected
Deep furrows	Contraction of septae in the subcutaneous fat
Stellate pseudoscars	Absence of epidermal pigmentation, altered fragmented dermal collagen
Elastosis (fine nodularity and/or coarseness)	Nodular aggregations of fibrous to amorphous material in the papillary dermis
Inelasticity	Elastotic dermis
Telangiectasia	Ectatic vessels often with atrophic walls
Venous lakes	Ectatic vessels often with atrophic walls
Purpura (easy bruising)	Extravasated erythrocytes and increased perivascular inflammation
Comedones (maladie de Favre et Racouchot)	Ectatic superficial portion of the pilosebaceous follicle
Sebaceous hyperplasia	Concentric hyperplasia of sebaceous glands

*Basal cell carcinoma and squamous cell carcinoma also occur in actinically damaged skin but, unlike the table entries, affect only a small minority of individuals with photoaging.

FIGURE 145-1

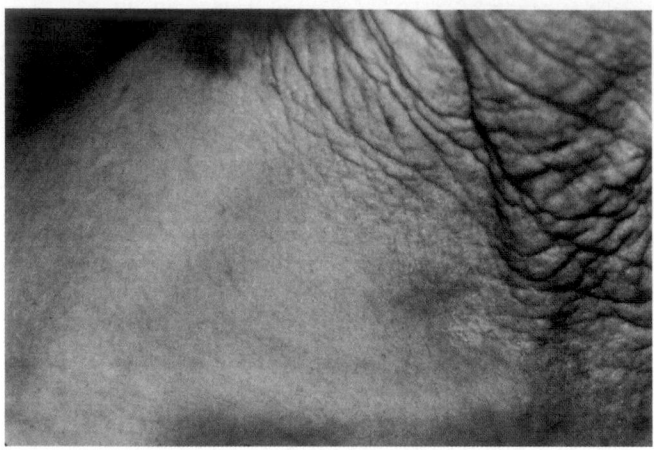

Photoaged vs. intrinsically aged skin of an elderly man. Habitually sun-exposed skin above the collar line is prominently wrinkled and lax, in contrast to the equally chronologically aged sun-protected skin of the shoulder. Despite the striking difference in appearance, both areas manifest age-associated functional decrements.

ticipating cutaneous structures (e.g., melanocytes and sebaceous glands), and other poorly understood factors.

The action spectrum for human photoaging has never been determined, and hence the relative contribution of the various spectral bands within sunlight is unknown. There is no truly appropriate animal model. In rodent skin, an elastosis-like condition can be produced by prolonged intense irradiation with a predominantly UVB source, but attempts to determine the action spectrum for murine elastosis have yielded conflicting results.[88-90] UVB photons are on average 1000 times more energetic than UVA photons and are overwhelmingly responsible for sunburn, suntanning, and photocarcinogenesis following sun exposure.[91] Nevertheless, in addition to UVB, UVA is suspected of playing a substantial role in photoaging because of its minimally 10-fold greater abundance in terrestrial sunlight, far greater year-round and day-long average irradiance, and greater average depth of penetration into the dermis compared to UVB. Moreover, human skin exposed daily for only 1 month to suberythemic doses of UVA alone demonstrates epidermal hyperplasia, stratum corneum thickening, Langerhans cell depletion, and dermal inflammatory infiltrates with deposition of lysozymes on the elastic fibers.[92,93] These latter changes in particular suggest that frequent casual exposure to sunlight containing principally UVA (e.g., while wearing a UVB-absorbing sunscreen) may eventually result in damage to dermal collagen and elastin in ways expected to produce photoaging.

Although the clinical manifestations of aging and chronic sun damage differ, in many instances these differences are subtle. Initially, histologic changes in elderly sun-exposed skin have been described by experienced investigators as differing only in degree from those in elderly sun-protected skin, at both the light microscopic and electron microscopic levels. Many of the age-associated physiologic decrements, such as slowed wound healing and loss of immunoresponsiveness, also appear to be accelerated in sun-exposed skin. Furthermore, cells cultured from chronically sun-exposed skin sites differ from cells cultured from sun-protected sites

of the same donors in having shortened culture life spans, slower growth rates, lower saturation densities, and altered responsiveness to retinoic acid,[94] all changes also observed as a function of advanced chronologic donor age. Only recently have qualitative differences in the dermal fibrous proteins and microvasculature of paired sun-exposed and sun-protected sites been documented. On a theoretical level, several of the mechanisms known to be involved in UV-mediated cellular damage are also postulated to underlie chronologic aging.[60,95,96] These include DNA injury and/or decreased DNA repair, oxidative damage, lysosomal disruption, and altered collagen structure.

Molecular mechanisms for some of the degenerative changes observed in photoaged skin, particularly the enzymatic breakdown of collagen and elastin, have been tentatively identified.[97] The overall clinical appearance of photodamaged skin suggests increased matrix degradation without compensatory increased matrix protein synthesis.[98,99] Indeed, very low dose UVB radiation induces dermal proteases such as collagenase, stromelysin, and gelatinase.[97]

UVA may also contribute to the process of photodamage. UVA induces the formation of reactive oxygen species that readily react with membrane lipids and amino acids.[91] Membrane damage results in the release of arachidonic acid and leads to activation of secondary cytosolic and nuclear messengers that activate "UV response" genes.

The histologic hallmark of dermal photoaging is elastosis, a quantitative and qualitative change in elastic fibers.[99] The precise composition of this material is unknown. It is speculated that fibroblasts, in response to chronic UV damage, produce abnormal elastin that is more susceptible to enzymatic degradation.

Smoking and Skin Aging

Cigarette smoking exacerbates photoaging,[86,87,100,101] particularly in women, with a direct correlation between the number of pack-years smoked and the severity of wrinkling and grayish discoloration. Histologic analysis of "smoker's skin" reveals elastic fiber thickening and fragmentation, similar to that found in sun-damaged skin.[102] However, solar elastosis is restricted in the papillary dermis, while elastic fiber changes of "smoker's skin" are also present in the reticular dermis. This dermal elastosis has been suggested to result from increased elastase activity in neutrophils,[103] chronic dermal ischemia, and prooxidant effects of cigarette smoke compounded by decreased levels of vitamin A, which reduce the capacity to quench free oxygen radicals.[87,100] Smoking has also been associated with decreased stratum corneum water content[87,100] and accelerated hydroxylation of estradiol, leading to decreased estrogens in the skin that may in turn contribute to dryness and atrophy.[87] Smokers have an increased incidence of skin cancers as well as increased severity of photoaging-like changes, compared to nonsmokers with otherwise similar risk factors,[86] and these facts suggest that mutagens present in cigarette smoke may also directly affect cells in the dermis and epidermis.

Relevance to Skin Disease

Disorders of the skin are known to be common and bothersome in the elderly,[104] and some occur predominantly in this age group. For example, age-specific incidence of skin cancer, including melanoma, increases exponentially with age,[105,106] presumably due to cumulative exposure to carcinogens over a lifetime as well as age-associated decreases in DNA repair capacity,[107] immunosurveillance,[108] and proliferative homeostasis. In addition, benign proliferative growths are especially characteristic of aging skin. Acrochordons, cherry angiomas, seborrheic keratoses, and lentigenes are numerous in nearly every adult beyond age 65 years. Also, pruritus is a common complaint of elderly patients.[104]

Bullous pemphigoid, characterized by subepidermal blister formation with fixation of complement and immunoglobulins along the basement membrane, is far more common in the elderly than in younger persons, a predilection that may be partially explained by the age-associated increases in circulating autoantibodies and ease of dermal-epidermal separation,[109] although many other autoimmune and blistering dermatoses are not more common in old age. Possibly age-associated changes in the basement membrane itself render it specifically vulnerable to the disease process.

The incidence rates for herpes zoster increase with age and peak at 1424 cases per 100,000 at ≥75 years.[110] Postherpetic neuralgia, uncommon in patients less than 40 years old, occurs frequently in older patients—in more than half of those beyond age 60 years in one large series.[111] No mechanism for this altered response to varicella virus has been established. Recurrent herpes simplex infection also involves reactivation of latent virus in regional ganglia and T cell–mediated host defenses but is more common in young adults and indeed rare among immunocompetent elders. The general phenomenon of impaired wound healing in the elderly may account for slower resolution of the acute eruption, but its relevance, if any, to postherpetic neuralgia is unclear. Age-associated muting of the inflammatory response might indeed be expected to reduce the risk of neuralgia, since prophylactic use of anti-inflammatory glucocorticoids is often successful.

Xerosis, the "dry" rough quality of old skin, may be attributed to a subtle disorder of epidermal maturation, such as inadequate filaggrin production[51] or altered lipid profile,[49,30] although histologic studies reveal little alteration of either the viable epidermis or the stratum corneum with age. Available data fail to support water loss, an overall decrease in stratum corneum lipids,[49] or altered amino acid composition as etiologic factors.[112] The surface irregularity may be attributed simply to slower transit of corneocytes through the stratum corneum, allowing accumulation of damage in situ. Similarly, there is no explanation for the pruritus that often accompanies xerosis.[105] Speculations include frequent penetration of irritants through an abnormal stratum corneum and an altered sensory threshold due to subtle neuropathy.

Many dermatoses more commonly observed in the elderly reflect the higher prevalence of systemic diseases such as diabetes, vascular insufficiency, and various neurologic syndromes in this population. Such disorders often appear to be compounded by age-associated intrinsic losses of cellular function, producing skin disease. The allegedly increased incidence of other disorders such as tinea pedis or seborrheic dermatitis may reflect reduced local skin care, with subsequent exacerbation of previously inapparent problems, rather than an age-associated change in the skin itself. Alternatively, subtle age-associated changes in immune status may be responsible, in analogy to the increased prevalence and severity of these disorders in patients with acquired immunodeficiency syndrome.

Reduced tolerance to systemically administered drugs is well documented in the elderly,[113] due to decrements in lean body mass and metabolism and renal excretion of the active ingredients. Comparable data for topically applied medications do not exist, but it is tempting to postulate that retarded dermal clearance of absorbed material, reduced dermal mass and cellularity, and possibly altered metabolic capacity may render old skin more susceptible to both beneficial and adverse effects of topical medications, or at least alter the optimal dosage frequency. In the case of glucocorticoid preparations, relative vascular unresponsiveness may render blanching of erythema an unreliable indicator of other effects in old skin.

TREATMENT

Treatment of age-associated skin diseases is covered in other chapters. The following discussion pertains only to prevention and treatment of the signs of skin aging and photoaging, until recently considered irreversible.

Photoprotection

Work in the rhino mouse model of photoaging first demonstrated deposition of new papillary dermal matrix, with downward compression of UV-induced elastosis after discontinuation of the daily irradiations required to produce the histologic changes; similar repair occurred despite continued irradiation if a highly protective sunscreen was applied to the mice.[114] Subsequently, patients in the control groups of large multicenter studies investigating topical tretinoin as a treatment for photoaging (see below) were found to have statistically significant improvement in fine wrinkling, roughness, dyspigmentation, and overall appearance after 6 months of daily sunscreen and moisturizer use, compared to their own baseline status,[64] changes presumably due principally to cessation of their ongoing photodamage. These data suggest an intrinsic repair capacity for photoaging and a central role for photoprotection in any treatment regimen.

All-*Trans*-Retinoic Acid

The ability of topical retinoic acid or tretinoin to improve photoaging changes in skin was suggested by studies in the rhino mouse model[115] and later definitively demonstrated in patients.[116] Clinically modest but highly statistically significant improvements in global appearance, surface roughness, fine and coarse wrinkling, mottled pigmentation, and sallowness were subsequently shown in several double-blind vehicle-controlled trials involving more than 700 subjects.[64] The beneficial effects are dose-dependent and increase with duration of therapy for at least 10 to 12 months. Accompanying epidermal acanthosis and hypergranulosis, as well as stratum corneum compaction, prominent in the first months of therapy,[64,116,117] regress within 12 months of continuous therapy, despite continued clinical improvement.[118] In contrast, reduction and redistribution of epidermal melanin parallels improvement in mottled hyperpigmentation and lentigenes.[64,118,119] Improvements in wrinkling are best attributed to increased papillary dermal collagen deposition in tretinoin-treated skin,[120] although increased anchoring fibrils[121] and improved ultrastructural characteristics of the epidermis and superficial dermis[64,122] probably also contribute. Increased vascularity of the papillary dermis, well documented in tretinoin-treated mouse skin and anecdotally reported in human skin, presumably reduces sallowness and renders the skin more responsive to environmental stimuli.[123] At a more fundamental level, tretinoin effects on photoaged skin, like all tretinoin effects, are presumed to be mediated through binding to the nuclear retinoic acid receptors (RARs) with subsequent binding of retinoic acid/RAR complexes to specific genes.[124] Tretinoin also appears capable of reversing histologic changes associated with intrinsic aging both in vivo[125] and in vitro.[126] Whether the retinoid effect on photoaged skin constitutes a true reversal of aging or age-associated environmental damage cannot be determined without a better understanding of these processes at the cellular and molecular levels.

Alpha-Hydroxy Acids

Alpha-hydroxy acids (AHA) are compounds derived from dairy products (lactic acid), fruit (malic acid, citric acid), or sugar cane (glycolic acid). Topical treatment of photodamaged skin with AHA has been reported to result in subtle clinical improvements in wrinkling, roughness, and depigmentation within months of daily application.[127,128] Histologically, after 6 months of daily applications of lotions containing 25 percent glycolic, lactic, or citric acids, an increase in total skin thickness of approximately 25 percent was reported, accompanied by increased thickness of viable epidermis and dermis, increased content of acid mucopolysaccharides, increased collagen density, and improved quality of the elastic fibers.[128]

Antioxidants

Antioxidants include vitamins A (retinol), C (ascorbic acid), and E (tocopherols); beta-carotene; and bioflavinoids. Although their role as endogenous protectors against oxidative stress is well documented, the ability of topically applied antioxidants to modify acute or chronic damage mediated by free radicals in skin is controversial.[129,130] In animals, topical application of α-tocopherol appears to decrease UVB-induced erythema and edema by approximately 50 percent, apparently by reducing the formation of free oxygen radicals. In some but not all human studies, topical application of α-tocopherol decreases sunburn cells after UV irradiation. Similarly, animal studies suggest that topical application of ascorbic acid decreases sunburn cell formation and erythema.[131] Some topical carotenoid preparations and synthetic phenolic antioxidants are similarly reported to reduce UV-induced erythema and retard development of squamous cell carcinomas in the hairless mouse model. Controlled human studies of possible beneficial effects of antioxidants on photoaging are lacking.

Hormone Therapy

Systemic treatment of postmenopausal women with conjugated estrogens or a combination of estrogen/glucocorticoids (paramethasone) significantly increases total skin and dermal thickness, dermal collagen content, and mitotic activity of keratinocytes.[132–136] These changes are said to be accompanied by decreased slackness of the skin, and a large epidemiologic study also strongly suggests that estrogen use by postmenopausal women mitigates against skin dryness and wrinkling.[137] Increased sebaceous gland activity, decreased roughness, and increased hydration of skin are also reported.[134] The cutaneous effects of topically applied estrogens, if any, are poorly documented.

Caloric Restriction

Caloric restriction, advocated to slow aging in general, significantly decreases dermal collagen glycation in rats severely restricted throughout their lifespan.[138] Skin appearance and function were not assessed.

REFERENCES

1. Winker MA, Glass RM: The aging global population. A call for papers. *JAMA* **276**:1758, 1996
2. Masoro EJ: Aging: Current concepts, in *Aging,* edited by EJ Masoro. Oxford, Oxford University Press, 1995, p 3
3. Weeda G et al: A presumed DNA helicase encoded by ERCC-3 is involved in the human repair disorders xeroderma pigmentosum and Cockayne's syndrome. *Cell* **62**:777, 1990
4. Troelstra C et al: ERCC6, a member of a subfamily of putative helicases, is involved in Cockayne's syndrome and preferential repair of active genes. *Cell* **71**:939, 1992
5. Savitsky K et al: A single ataxia telangiectasia gene with a product similar to PI-3 kinase. *Science* **268**:1749, 1995
6. Keith CT Schreiber SL: PIK-related kinases: DNA repair, recombination, and cell cycle checkpoints. *Science* **270**:50, 1995
7. Yu CE et al: Positional cloning of the Werner's syndrome gene. *Science* **272**:258, 1996
8. Hayflick L, Moorhead PS: The serial cultivation of human diploid cell strains. *Exp Cell Res* **25**:585, 1961
9. Porter MB, Smith JR: Role of endogenous proteins as negative growth modulators during in vitro cellular aging of human diploid fibroblasts. *Annu Rev Gerontol Geriatr* **10**:53, 1990
10. Smith JR: DNA synthesis inhibitors in cellular senescence. *J Gerontol* **45**:B32, 1990
11. Burmer GC et al: Evidence for endogenous polypeptide-mediated inhibition of cell-cycle transit in human diploid cells. *Cell Biol* **94**:187, 1982
12. Drescher-Lincoln CK, Smith JR: Inhibition of DNA synthesis in senescent-proliferating human cybrids is mediated by endogenous proteins. *Exp Cell Res* **153**:208, 1984
13. Smith JR, Pereira-Smith OM: Altered gene expression during cellular aging. *Genome* **31**:386, 1989
14. Golletz TJ et al: Molecular genetic approaches to the study of cellular senescence. *Cold Spring Harb Symp Quant Biol* **59**:59, 1994
15. Wistrom C, Villeponteau B: Cloning and expression of SAG: A novel marker of cellular senescence. *Exp Cell Res* **199**:355, 1992
16. Stein GH, Dulic V: Origins of G_1 arrest in senescent human fibroblasts. *Bioessays* **17**:537, 1995
17. Noda A et al: Cloning of senescent cell-derived inhibitors of DNA synthesis using an expression screen. *Exp Cell Res* **211**:90, 1994
18. Alcorta DA et al: Involvement of the cyclin-dependent kinase inhibitor p16 (INK4a) in replicative senescence of normal human fibroblasts. *Proc Natl Acad Sci USA* **93**:13742, 1996
19. Porter MB et al: Common senescent cell-specific antibody epitopes on fibronectin in species and cells of varied origin. *J Cell Physiol* **150**:545, 1992
20. Zeng G, Millis AJ: Differential regulation of collagenase and stromelysin mRNA in late passage cultures of human fibroblasts. *Exp Cell Res* **222**:150, 1996
21. West MD et al: Altered expression of plasminogen activator and plasminogen activator inhibitor during cellular senescence. *Exp Gerontol* **31**:175, 1996
22. Mu XC, Higgins PJ: Differential growth state–dependent regulation of plasminogen activator inhibitor type-1 expression in senescent IMR-90 human diploid fibroblasts. *J Cell Physiol* **165**:647, 1995
23. Blackburn EH: Structure and function of telomeres. *Nature* **350**:569, 1991
24. Sharma HW et al: Differentiation of immortal cells inhibits telomerase activity. *Proc Natl Acad Sci USA* **92**:12343, 1995
25. Allsopp RC: Telomere length predicts replicative capacity of human fibroblasts. *Proc Natl Acad Sci USA* **89**:10114, 1992
26. Vaziri H, Benchimol S: From telomere loss to p53 induction and activation of a DNA-damage pathway at senescence: The telomere loss/DNA damage model of cell aging. *Exp Gerontol* **31**:295, 1996
27. Sandell LL, Zakian VA: Loss of a yeast telomere: Arrest, recovery, and chromosome loss. *Cell* **75**:729, 1993
28. White E: Life, death, and the pursuit of apoptosis. *Genes Dev* **10**:1, 1996
29. Wang E: Senescent human fibroblasts resist programmed cell death, and failure to suppress bcl2 is involved. *Cancer Res* **55**:2284, 1995
30. Sun J et al: Divergent roles of RAS1 and RAS2 in yeast longevity. *J Biol Chem* **269**:18638, 1994
31. Johnson TE: Aging can be genetically dissected into component processes using long-lived lines of *Caenorhabditis elegans. Proc Natl Acad Sci USA* **84**:3777, 1987
32. Dudas SP, Arking R: A coordinate upregulation of antioxidant gene activities is associated with the delayed onset of senescence in a long-lived strain of *Drosophila. J Gerontol* **50**:B117, 1995
33. Jazwinski SM: Longevity, genes and aging. *Science* **273**:54, 1996
34. Covelli V et al: Inheritance of immune responsiveness, life span, and

disease incidence in interline crosses of mice selected for high or low multispecific antibody production. *J Immunol* **142**:1224, 1989

35. Cutler RG: Antioxidants, aging, and longevity, in *Free Radicals in Biology,* vol 6, edited by WA Pryor. New York, Academic Press, 1984, p 371

36. Davies KJ: Oxidative stress: The paradox of aerobic life. *Biochem Soc Symp* **61**:1, 1995

37. Stadtman ER: Protein oxidation and aging. *Science* **257**:1220, 1992

38. Ames BN et al: Oxidants, antioxidants, and the degenerative diseases of aging. *Proc Natl Acad Sci USA* **90**:7915, 1993

39. Sohal RS, Brunk UT: Mitochondrial production of pro-oxidants and cellular senescence. *Mutat Res* **275**:295, 1992

40. Agarwal S, Sohal RS: DNA oxidative damage and life expectancy in houseflies. *Proc Natl Acad Sci USA* **91**:12332, 1994

41. Sohal RS, Weindruch R: Oxidative stress, caloric restriction, and aging. *Science* **273**:59, 1996

42. Lakowski B, Hekimi S: Determination of life-span in *Caenorhabditis elegans* by four clock genes. *Science* **272**:1010, 1996

43. Balin AK, Allen RG: Molecular bases of biologic aging, in *Clinics in Geriatric Medicine,* vol 5/1, *Geriatric Dermatology,* edited by BA Gilchrest. Philadelphia, Saunders, 1989, p 1

44. Report of the Task Force on Immunology and Aging. US Department of Health and Human Services. National Institutes of Health: March, 1996

45. Gilchrest BA: *The Skin and Aging Processes.* Boca Raton, CRC Press, 1984

46. Balin AK, Kligman AM: *Aging and the Skin.* New York, Raven, 1989

47. Moragas A et al: Mathematical morphologic analysis of aging-related epidermal changes. *Anal Quant Cytol Histol* **15**:75, 1993

48. Roskos KV et al: The effect of aging on percutaneous absorption in man. *J Pharmacokinet Biopharm* **6**:617, 1989

49. Ghadially R et al: The aged epidermal permeability barrier. Structural, functional, and lipid biochemical abnormalities in humans and a senescent murine model. *J Clin Invest* **95**:2281, 1995

50. Denda M et al: Age- and sex-dependent change in stratum corneum sphingolipids. *Arch Dermatol Res* **285**:415, 1993

51. Tezuka T et al: Terminal differentiation of facial epidermis of the aged: Immunohistochemical studies. *Dermatology* **188**:21, 1994

52. Stanulis-Praeger BM, Gilchrest BA: Effect of donor age and prior sun exposure on growth inhibition of cultured human dermal fibroblasts by all *trans*-retinoic acid. *J Cell Physiol* **139**:116, 1989

53. Stanulis-Praeger BM, Gilchrest BA: Growth factor responsiveness declines during adulthood for human skin-derived cells. *Mech Ageing Dev* **35**:185, 1986

54. Reenstra WR et al: Aging affects epidermal growth factor receptor phosphorylation and traffic kinetics. *Exp Cell Res* **227**:252, 1996

55. Reenstra WR et al: Effect of donor age on epidermal growth factor processing in man. *Exp Cell Res* **209**:118, 1993

56. MacLaughlin J, Holick MF: Aging decreases the capacity of human skin to produce vitamin D$_3$. *J Clin Invest* **76**:1536, 1985

57. Matsuoko LY et al: Lower body stores of vitamin D among sunscreen users: A preliminary study. *Arch Dermatol* **124**:1802, 1988

58. Gloth FM III et al: Vitamin D deficiency in homebound elderly persons. *JAMA* **274**:1683, 1995

59. Holick MF et al: Age, vitamin D, and solar ultraviolet. *Lancet* **2**:1104, 1989

60. Lopez-Torres M et al: Effect of age on antioxidants and molecular markers of oxidative damage in murine epidermis and dermis. *J Invest Dermatol* **102**:476, 1994

61. Shindo Y et al: Changes in enzyme activities in skin fibroblasts derived from persons of various ages. *Exp Gerontol* **26**:29, 1991

62. de Rigal J et al: Assessment of aging of the human skin by in vivo ultrasonic imaging. *J Invest Dermatol* **93**:621, 1989

63. Kligman AM et al: The anatomy and pathogenesis of wrinkles. *Br J Dermatol* **113**:37, 1985

64. Gilchrest BA: A review of skin ageing and its medical therapy. *Br J Dermatol* **135**:867, 1996

65. Nelson BR et al: A comparison of wire brush and diamond fraise superficial dermabrasion for photoaged skin. A clinical, immunohistologic, and biochemical study. *J Am Acad Dermatol* **34**:235, 1996

66. Pierard GE, Lapiere CM: The microanatomical basis of facial frown lines. *Arch Dermatol* **125**:1090, 1989

67. Rooke GA et al: Maximal skin blood flow is decreased in elderly men. *J Appl Physiol* **77**:11, 1994

68. Tsuchida Y: The effect of aging and arteriosclerosis on human skin blood flow. *J Dermatol Sci* **5**:175, 1993

69. Roskos KV et al: Pharmacodynamic measurements of methyl nicotinate percutaneous absorption: The effect of aging on microcirculation. *Br J Dermatol* **122**:165, 1990

70. Shuster S et al: The influence of age and sex on skin thickness, skin collagen and density. *Br J Dermatol* **93**:639, 1975

71. Bernstein EF et al: Long-term sun exposure alters the collagen of the papillary dermis. Comparison of sun-protected and photoaged skin by northern analysis, immunohistochemical staining, and confocal laser scanning microscopy. *J Am Acad Dermatol* **34**:209, 1996

72. Burke EM et al: Altered transcriptional regulation of human interstitial collagenase in cultured skin fibroblasts from older donors. *Exp Gerontol* **29**:37, 1994

73. Castelo-Branco C et al: Relationship between skin collagen and bone changes during aging. *Maturitas* **18**:199, 1994

74. Sone T et al: Urinary excretion of type I collagen cross-linked *N*-telopeptides in healthy Japanese adults: Age- and sex-related changes and reference limits. *Bone* **17**:335, 1995

75. Garnero P: Genetic influence on bone turnover in postmenopausal twins. *J Clin Endocrinol Metab* **81**:140, 1996

76. Bolognia JL et al: Skin changes in menopause. *Maturitas* **11**:295, 1989

77. Gerstein AD et al: Wound healing and aging. *Dermatol Clin* **11**:749, 1993

78. Sell DR et al: Longevity and the genetic determination of collagen glycoxidation kinetics in mammalian senescence. *Proc Natl Acad Sci USA* **93**:485, 1996

79. Rongioletti F, Rebora A: Fibroelastolytic patterns of intrinsic skin aging: Pseudoxanthoma-elasticum-like papillary dermal elastolysis and white fibrous papulosis of the neck. *Dermatology* **191**:19, 1995

80. Ghersetich I et al: Hyaluronic acid in cutaneous intrinsic aging. *Int J Dermatol* **33**:119, 1994

81. Meyer LJ, Stern R: Age-dependent changes of hyaluronan in human skin. *J Invest Dermatol* **102**:385, 1994

82. Escoffier C et al: Age-related mechanical properties of human skin: An in vivo study. *J Invest Dermatol* **93**:353, 1989

83. Jacobsen E et al: Age-related changes in sebaceous wax ester secretion rates in men and women. *J Invest Dermatol* **85**:483, 1985

84. Shimokata H, Kuzuya F: Two-point discrimination test of the skin as an index of sensory aging. *Gerontology* **41**:267, 1995

85. Stevens JC, Patterson MQ: Dimensions of spatial acuity in the touch sense: Changes over the life span. *Somatosens Mot Res* **12**:29, 1995

86. Davis BE, Koh HK: Faces going up in smoke. A dermatologic opportunity for cancer prevention. *Arch Dermatol* **128**:1106, 1992

87. Smith JB, Fenske NA: Cutaneous manifestations and consequences of smoking. *J Am Acad Dermatol* **34**:717, 1996

88. Kligman LH, Sayre RM: An action spectrum for ultraviolet induced elastosis in hairless mice: Quantification of elastosis by image analysis. *Photochem Photobiol* **53**:237, 1991

89. Kligman LH: Photoaging. Manifestations, prevention, and treatment. *Clin Geriatr Med* **5**:235, 1989

90. Wulf HC et al: Narrow-band UV radiation and induction of dermal elastosis and skin cancer. *Photodermatology* **6**:44, 1989

91. Kochevar IE: Molecular and cellular effects of UV radiation relevant to chronic photodamage, in *Photodamage,* edited by BA Gilchrest. Cambridge, MA, Blackwell Science, 1995, p 51

92. Lavker RM et al: Quantitative assessment of cumulative damage from repetitive exposures to suberythemogenic doses of UVA in human skin. *Photochem Photobiol* **62**:348, 1995

93. Lavker RM et al: Cumulative effects from repeated exposures to suberythemal doses of UVB and UVA in human skin. *J Am Acad Dermatol* **32**:53, 1995

94. Gilchrest BA: In vitro studies of aging human epidermis: 1975–1990, in *Review of Biological Research in Aging,* edited by M Rothstein. New York, Alan R Liss, vol 41, 1990, p 281

95. Gilchrest BA, Bohr VA: Aging processes, DNA damage, and repair. *FASEB J* **11**:322, 1997

96. Schleicher ED et al: Increased accumulation of the glycoxidation product *N*(epsilon)-(carboxymethyl)lysine in human tissues in diabetes and aging. *J Clin Invest* **99**:457, 1997

97. Fisher GJ et al: Molecular basis of sun-induced premature skin aging and retinoid antagonism. *Nature* **379**:335, 1996

98. Brinckmann J et al: Collagen synthesis in (sun-) aged human skin

and in fibroblasts derived from sun-exposed and sun-protected body sites. *J Photochem Photobiol* 27:33, 1995

99. Bhawan J et al: Photoaging versus intrinsic aging: A morphologic assessment of facial skin. *J Cutan Pathol* 22:154, 1995

100. Joffe I: Cigarette smoking and facial wrinkling. *Ann Intern Med* 115:659, 1991

101. Ernster VL et al: Facial wrinkling in men and women, by smoking status. *Am J Public Health* 85:78, 1995

102. Frances C et al: Changes in the elastic tissue of the non-sun-exposed skin of cigarette smokers. *Br J Dermatol* 125:43, 1991

103. Weitz JI et al: Increased neutrophil elastase activity in cigarette smokers. *Ann Intern Med* 107:680, 1987

104. Fleisher AB Jr: Pruritus in the elderly. *Adv Dermatol* 10:41, 1995

105. Lin AN et al: Non melanoma skin cancers in the elderly, in *Clinics in Geriatric Medicine,* edited by BA Gilchrest. Philadelphia, Saunders, 1989, vol 5, p 161

106. Gallagher RP et al: Trends in basal cell carcinoma, squamous cell carcinoma, and melanoma of the skin from 1973 through 1987. *J Am Acad Dermatol* 23:413, 1990

107. Wei Q et al: DNA repair and aging in basal cell carcinoma: A molecular epidemiology study. *Proc Natl Acad Sci USA* 90:1614, 1993

108. Kessler II: Epidemiological considerations in the role of dendritic/Langerhans cells in human cancer. *In Vivo* 7:305, 1993

109. Yaar M, Gilchrest BA: Bullous pemphigoid: Disease of the aging immune system, in *Clinics in Dermatology,* edited by AR Ahmed. Philadelphia, Lippincott, 1987, vol 5, p 135

110. Donahue JG et al: The incidence of herpes zoster. *Arch Intern Med* 155:1605, 1995

111. de Moragas JM, Kierland RR: The outcome of patients with herpes zoster. *Arch Dermatol* 75:193, 1957

112. Jacobson TM et al: Effects of aging and xerosis on the amino acid composition of human skin. *J Invest Dermatol* 95:296, 1990

113. Vestal RE, Cusack BJ: Pharmacology and aging, in *Handbook of the Biology of Aging,* 3d ed, edited by EL Schneider, JW Rowe. San Diego, Academic, 1990, p 349

114. Kligman LH et al: Prevention of ultraviolet damage to the dermis of hairless mice by sunscreens. *J Invest Dermatol* 78:181, 1982

115. Kligman LH et al: Topical retinoic acid enhances the repair of ultraviolet damaged dermal connective tissue. *Connect Tissue Res* 12:139, 1984

116. Weiss JS et al: Topical tretinoin improves photoaged skin. A double-blind vehicle-controlled study. *JAMA* 259:527, 1988

117. Bhawan J et al: Effects of tretinoin on photodamaged skin. A histologic study. *Arch Dermatol* 127:666, 1991

118. Bhawan J et al: Histologic evaluation of the long-term effects of tretinoin on photodamaged skin. *J Dermatol Sci* 11:177, 1996

119. Rafal ES: Topical tretinoin (retinoic acid) treatment for liver spots associated with photodamage. *N Engl J Med* 326:368, 1992

120. Griffiths CE et al: Restoration of collagen formation in photodamaged human skin by tretinoin (retinoic acid). *N Engl J Med* 329:2038, 1993

121. Woodley DT et al: Treatment of photoaged skin with topical tretinoin increases epidermal-dermal anchoring fibrils. A preliminary report. *JAMA* 263:3057, 1990

122. Yamamoto O et al: Ultrastructural effects of topical tretinoin on dermo-epidermal junction and papillary dermis in photodamaged skin. A controlled study. *Exp Dermatol* 5:146, 1995

123. Griffiths CE et al: Two concentrations of topical tretinoin (retinoic acid) cause similar improvement of photoaging but different degrees of irritation. A double-blind, vehicle-controlled comparison of 0.1% and 0.025% tretinoin creams. *Arch Dermatol* 131:1037, 1995

124. Chambon P: A decade of molecular biology of retinoic acid receptors. *FASEB J* 10:940, 1996

125. Kligman AM et al: Effects of topical tretinoin on non-sun-exposed protected skin of the elderly. *J Am Acad Dermatol* 29:25, 1993

126. Varani J et al: All-*trans* retinoic acid (RA) stimulates events in organ-cultured human skin that underlie repair. Adult skin from sun-protected and sun-exposed sites responds in an identical manner to RA while neonatal foreskin responds differently. *J Clin Invest* 94:1747, 1994

127. Stiller MJ et al: Topical 8% glycolic acid and 8% L-lactic acid creams for the treatment of photodamaged skin. A double-blind vehicle-controlled clinical trial. *Arch Dermatol* 132:631, 1996

128. Ditre CM et al: Effects of alpha-hydroxy acids on photoaged skin: A pilot clinical, histologic, and ultrastructural study. *J Am Acad Dermatol* 34:187, 1996

129. Werninghaus KI: Role of antioxidants on reducing photodamage, in *Photodamage,* edited by BA Gilchrest. Cambridge, MA, Blackwell Science, 1995, p 249

130. Harman D: Role of free radical reactions in aging and disease. *J Geriatr Dermatol* 5:114, 1997

131. Darr D et al: Topical vitamin C protects porcine skin from ultraviolet radiation-induced damage. *Br J Dermatol* 127:247, 1992

132. Maheux R et al: A randomized, double-blind, placebo-controlled study on the effect of conjugated estrogens on skin thickness. *Am J Obstet Gynecol* 170:642, 1994

133. Pierard GE et al: Effect of hormone replacement therapy for menopause on the mechanical properties of skin. *J Am Geriatr Soc* 43:662, 1995

134. Vaillant L, Callens A: Hormone replacement treatment and skin aging. *Therapie* 51:67, 1996

135. Cortes-Gallegos V et al: Inverted skin changes induced by estrogen and estrogen/glucocorticoid on aging dermis. *Gynecol Endocrinol* 10:125, 1996

136. Brincat M et al: Skin collagen changes in postmenopausal women receiving different regimens of estrogen therapy. *Obstet Gynecol* 70:123, 1987

137. Dunn LB et al: Does estrogen prevent skin aging? *Arch Dermatol* 133:339, 1997

138. Cefalu WT et al: Caloric restriction decreases age-dependent accumulation of the glycoxidation products, *N*-epsilon-(carboxymethyl)lysine and pentosidine, in rat skin collagen. *J Gerontol* 50:B337, 1995

CHAPTER 146

Nancy Lyon Havlik
Thomas B. Fitzpatrick
Albert M. Kligman
Lorraine H. Kligman

Geriatric Dermatology

Skin Conditions and Diseases in Geriatric Patients

Nancy Lyon Havlik
Thomas B. Fitzpatrick

Have you not a moist eye, a dry hand, a yellow cheek, a white beard, a decreasing leg, an increasing belly?
William Shakespeare, King Henry IV
Part II, I, ii, 206

A person is generally judged to be aged based on the appearance of his or her skin. Most of the cutaneous changes attributed to aging are, in fact, due directly to ultraviolet (UV) light–induced effects on the skin. It has been estimated that 80 percent of these effects could be prevented by improving the protection against UV light during childhood and adolescence.[1–3] The more exaggerated the outwardly apparent aging appears to be, the less healthy a person is physiologically.[4] Additionally, lower self-esteem and less effective social relations seem to correlate directly with an exaggerated aged appearance.[5,6]

The aging process, unlike the specific diseases described throughout medical textbooks, inevitably affects all persons. Government and institutions arbitrarily define the geriatric population as those persons over 65 years of age. However, aging is a continuous process with a variable spectrum of manifestations. While chronologic age is a precise measurement, the physiologic age of an individual does not correlate strictly with chronologic age.[7] Pathologic aging refers to abnormal deterioration resulting from disease.

Outward appearance loosely correlates with chronologic age and, surprisingly, correlates more strongly with physiologic age.[8,9] Wrinkled and sagging skin are among the hallmarks of aging. These features are caused by an excessive laxity and loss of resiliency of the skin. In a study of 10,086 men (Longitudinal Study of the Gerontology Research Center in Baltimore, MD), Borkan and Norris[7] investigated the relationship between apparent age, chronologic age, and specific physiologic parameters (such as blood pressure, serum albumin and globulin, pulmonary function measurements). Individuals who appeared to be older than their chronologic age were biologically older, as determined by 19 out of 24 different measurements.[4] Grove et al. noted a relationship between the apparent age of a person as judged by outward appearance and the rate of chemical blistering provoked by a topical solution of 50% ammonium hydroxide.[10] They also noted that individuals who looked older took the longest time to heal.

A confounding variable in interpreting the intrinsic changes that occur with aging in the skin is the environmental effect of prolonged sun exposure. Increasingly it has been appreciated that the damage resulting from chronic UV radiation exposure is distinctly separate and may compound the changes seen in intrinsic aging (see Table 145-3). Excessive UV light exposure can overwhelm the antioxidant capability of the skin and lead to oxidative damage, resulting in immunosuppression, skin cancer, and cutaneous aging.[11] Several features of intrinsic aging have now been determined to contrast directly with sun-induced changes. The fine wrinkles of sun-protected aged skin contrast with the coarse furrows characteristic of cutaneous photodamage.[12] These morphologic differences can undoubtedly be explained, at least in part, by the connective tissue of the dermis. However, dermal changes with intrinsic aging have not yet been clearly delineated (see Chap. 145). It is known that the dermis becomes thinned and less dense.[13] Collagen fibers are coarser and less highly organized in three-dimensional array, in contrast to young dermis. The photoaged dermis appears to have a deficiency of superficial dermal collagen induced by UV light.[14] UV light induces expression of several matrix metalloproteinases capable of degrading collagen.[15] Glycosaminoglycans are greatly increased in photodamaged skin in contrast to skin protected from UV light.[12] Elastic tissue fibers in young sun-protected skin are delicate and organized vertically to the dermal-epidermal junction. However, these are lost in aged, sun-protected skin and are tremendously increased and clumped into amorphous masses in sun-exposed skin.[16] Truly aged skin uninfluenced by photochemistry and other extrinsic, environmentally imposed factors is most likely to be found in doubly protected areas such as the buttocks (see Table 145-1).

The various diseases and disorders in geriatric dermatology are listed in Table 146-1. Additionally, special reference should be made to Chap. 145.

Pruritus in Aging

Senile pruritus may be the most common disorder in elderly skin, particularly in persons over 80 years of age.[18] It is usually associated with dry, rough, scaly skin. The pruritus is frequently worse at night and after hot baths or after the change in temperature as-

TABLE 146-1

Geriatric Dermatology

	Chapter Cross Reference		Chapter Cross Reference
Pruritus in aging	145	Cellulitis, including post coronary artery bypass	197
Connective tissue changes in aging		Pyoderma	195
Wrinkling and sagging skin and fragility (not from sun exposure)	145	Herpes simplex: chronic herpetic ulcers, disseminated	215
Wound healing	9,145,266	Herpes zoster: postzoster neuralgia, disseminated	216
Disorders of altered epidermal kinetics	9		
Psoriasis vulgaris	43	Diphtheria: cutaneous, pharyngeal, and ocular	195
Xerosis	52,145		
Vesicular and bullous diseases	61	Lyme borreliosis and acrodermatitis chronica obliterans	204
Bullous pemphigoid	61,145	Infestations	
Acneform disorders	73	Scabies, including Norwegian	239
Rosacea	74	Pediculosis pubis	239
Benign neoplasia	83, 145	Pediculosis capita	239
Cherry angioma	83	Pediculosis corporis	239
Skin tags (acrochordons)	83	Disorders of the feet	
Colloid millium		Clavi, corns, calluses	
Cutaneous horns	79	Bursitis	
Fibroepithelioma		Bunions	
Keratoacanthoma	82	Intractable plantar keratoses	
Seborrheic keratoses	83	Neoplasia	
Sebaceous adenoma (hyperplasia)	83	Subungual exostosis	72
Clear cell acanthoma	83	Onychocryptosis	72
Disorders of nails	72	Onychauxis	72
Nail growth		Onycholysis	72
General aging-related nail changes	72	Onychogryphosis	72
Nail dystrophies	72	Onychophosis	
Disorders of mucous membranes	114	Cutaneous melanoma and its precursors	90, 92
Problems of edentulous mouth	114	Lentigo maligna	92
Cheilitis	114	Lentigo maligna melanoma	92
Perlèche	114	Superficial spreading melanoma	92
Leukoplakia	114	Desmoplastic melanoma	92
Oral cancer	114	Nodular melanoma	92
Eczematous dermatitis		Precancerous and malignant nonmelanoma cutaneous neoplasia	79–81
Nummular eczema	125		
Gravitational eczema	167	Angiosarcoma	102
Asteatotic eczema	125	Solar keratoses	79
Lichen simplex chronicus	125	Bowen's disease	79
Atopic eczema	124	Paget's disease of the breast	86
Autosensitization eczema	123	Extramammary Paget's disease	86
Prurigo nodularis		Basal cell carcinoma, including morpheic basal cell carcinoma	81
Disorders due to sun exposure	134–138		
Photoaging	146	Squamous cell carcinoma, including the lip	80
Cutis rhomboidalis nuchae	138	Cutaneous neuroendocrine carcinoma (Merkel cell carcinoma)	85
Solar lentigo	138		
Favre-Racouchot disease	138	Cutaneous metastasis to the skin	185
Solar purpura (Bateman's senile purpura)	138	Cutaneous manifestations of systemic malignancy paraneoplastic syndromes	185
Venous lakes	102		
Stellate scars of the hands and forearms	138	Cowden's disease	185
Radiodermatitis, acute and chronic	130	Paraneoplastic syndromes:	185
Photosensitivity disorders	136	dermatomyositis,	173
Actinic reticuloid	110, 136	paraneoplastic pemphigus,	60
Drug eruptions, phototoxic	137	acanthosis nigricans,	186
Drug eruptions, photoallergic	137	Basex syndrome	185
Adverse cutaneous drug reactions	140	Glucagonoma and migratory necrolytic erythema	185
Exanthematous	140		
Fixed eruptions	140	Disorders of hair	71
Warfarin necrosis	140	Age-related changes	71
Infections		Androgenetic alopecia	71
Dermatophyte infections	206	Graying	89
Candidiasis: cutaneous, mucosal, and invasive	207	Hair loss	71

(continued)

TABLE 146-1 (*Continued*)

Geriatric Dermatology

	Chapter Cross Reference		Chapter Cross Reference
Cutaneous lymphomas/leukemias	108	Disorders of heat and cold	
Parapsoriasis en plaque	48, 108	Erythema ab igne	13
Cutaneous T cell lymphoma (CTCL)	108	Chilblains	128
Sézary's syndrome	108	Metabolic, endocrine	
Cutaneous B cell lymphoma (CBCL)	109	Diabetes mellitus: diabetic dermopathy	170
Leukemia cutis	109	Hypothyroidism: myxedema	170
Multiple myeloma		Hyperthyroidism	170
Macroglobulinemia		Addison's disease	170
Disorders of the anogenitalia		Cushing's disease	170
Pruritus ani and vulvae	115,116	Gout	179
Atrophic vulvitis	116	Alkaptonuria	149
Leukoplakic vulvitis	116	Xanthomatoses	152
Balanitis xerotica obliterans	115	Disorders of nutrition	
Intraepithelial neoplasia	115,116	Calorie deficiency	147
Erythroplasia of Queyrat	115, 116	Zinc deficiency	148
Squamous cell carcinoma of the penis	115	Scurvy	147
Squamous cell carcinoma of the vulva	116	Pellagra	147
Complications of the immunocompromised host: organ transplantation, bone marrow transplantation, chemotherapy-induced		Circulatory disorders	
		Osler's disease	102
		Livedo reticularis	167
Graft-versus-host disease	120	Purpura, cortisone-induced	252
Chronic herpetic ulcers	121, 215	Ischemia and gangrene	167
Candidemia	121, 207	Chronic venous insufficiency	167
Neoplasia in the chronically immunosuppressed host	121	Varicose ulcers	167
		Dependent rubor	167
Immune, rheumatic disorders		Acrocyanosis	167
Amyloidosis	150	Sexually transmitted diseases	
Lupus erythematosus syndromes	172	Syphilis	229
Progressive systemic sclerosis	174	Gonorrhea	234
Morphea	174	Herpes simplex	215
Cryoglobulinemia	177	Condylomata acuminata	224
Sarcoidosis, lupus pernio	184	Intraepithelial neoplasia	224
Dermatomyositis	173	Cutaneous ulcers	
Rheumatoid arthritis	179	Leg ulcerations	167
Rheumatoid nodules	179	Pressure sores	133
Psoriatic arthritis	44	Miscellaneous	
Pemphigus vulgaris	60	Lichen sclerosus et atrophicus	115, 116
Livedo reticularis	167	Skin atrophy	204, 243
Giant cell arteritis temporal arteritis, Takayusu's arteritis	175	Seborrheic dermatitis	126
		Intertrigo	116
Hypersensitivity vasculitis, drug-induced	176		
Wegener's granulomatosis	175		
Erythroderma			
Psoriatic, pityriasis rubra pilaris, Sézary's syndrome, drug	45		

sociated with disrobing. Itch can be severe despite the lack of physical signs. It begins with xerosis, as described below, and is frequently aggravated during winter months when the humidity is low and indoor temperatures high. Frequent bathing without the use of emollients can dry the skin further. Initially, there may be only microfissures, but the sensation of itch can be intense. Excoriations can lead to eczematous changes and eventually to infection, which can be subtle and can increase the itch sensation. Contact dermatitis from topical medicaments may mimic xerosis, and the history is an important clue in differentiating these.

Connective Tissue Changes in Aging

WRINKLING AND SAGGING SKIN AND FRAGILITY (See Chap. 145) In distinct contrast to photoaged skin (see "Dermatoheliosis" below), sun-protected aged skin is uniformly pale and the wrinkles are quite fine.[19] Lines of facial expression are exaggerated, and there is laxity.[20] The skin of an aged person is less resilient and is easily disrupted, with less friction and shear required to disturb its integrity. The skin may tear or even develop bullae. Blood vessels, too, are easily disrupted, leading to purpura.[21]

Histologically, the stratum corneum of aged skin is unaltered, but there is flattening of the dermal-epidermal junction.[22] There is a slight increase in the quantity and thickness of elastic fibers in the dermis, and there is a loss of the delicate vertical elastic fibers at the dermal-epidermal junction.[23,24] Collagen fibers become larger and more randomly organized, and there is a relative decrease in the proportion of soluble collagen.[25] Glycosaminoglycans, so abundant in fetal skin, decrease rapidly early so that adult levels are low and relatively stable.[26] There appears to be a change in the localization of hyaluronic acid within tissue compartments in aged skin.[27] The vasculature is somewhat altered, with a relative loss of microvessels of the subepidermal capillary loops.[28,29] The conductance of the cutaneous vasculature and the vasoreactivity seems to be reduced in elderly men.[30,31]

WOUND HEALING   Wound healing occurs more slowly in old age. Epidermal kinetic studies demonstrate an age-related decrease in epidermal proliferation. Orentreich studied healing and epithelialization in a series of 12,000 full-face dermabrasion patients and found that healing was more efficient in younger patients, occurring in 10, 15, and 21 days, respectively, in 25-, 50-, and 75-year-old patients.[32] It must be remembered, however, that the face is chronically sun exposed and therefore photoaging may be involved as well.

Wound dehiscence increases with age following full-thickness surgical wounds.[33,34] It is not known whether the defect lies in reepithelialization, revascularization, connective tissue synthesis, or decreased wound contraction.[35] In vitro studies of response to cytokines have not shown differences in either collagen synthesis or collagen contraction between young and old tissue models when stimulated with transforming growth factor β.[36]

Disorders of Altered Epidermal Kinetics

PSORIASIS VULGARIS   A bimodal onset of psoriasis exists with reported cases beginning from birth to 108 years (see Chap. 43). Most patients present in the third decade, with another peak (11.8 percent of 2400 patients) occurring in those over 55. With increasing age of onset there is a decrease in familial associations. Although plaque type psoriasis seems to decrease with age, flexural psoriasis tends to be more frequent in persons older than 60 years. Based on a decrease in creatinine clearance, higher blood levels of methotrexate with lower doses are seen in older patients. Psoriatic arthritis peaks at 45 years, whereas psoriatic erythroderma peaks between 30 and 55 years. In the aged, psoriasis may lack its typical morphology, often appearing as a nonspecific eruption in unusual distributions. This blurred clinical appearance is consistent with the generalization that inflammatory reactions, regardless of cause, are muted in the aged.

XEROSIS   Rough, dry, scaling skin affects at least 75 percent of persons over the age of 64. Xerosis is esthetically unappealing, uncomfortable, pruritic, and can set the stage for eczematous eruptions and infection. The dryness has not been explained satisfactorily on a biochemical basis. The lipid alteration appears to be qualitative as opposed to quantitative.[37] Although the stratum corneum compartment, by some measurements, has less water, aged skin as a whole appears to have more, not less, water than younger skin.[38] The thickness of the stratum corneum, which is the major diffusion barrier of the skin, tends to be unchanged in the aged, although the mean corneocyte area increases. The functional ability of the stratum corneum to prevent water loss increases with age unless there is gross fissuring.

Although elderly persons sweat less, this is probably of little consequence in regard to dry skin. Water is not an effective therapy for xerosis, and prolonged bathing may worsen it. Sweat glands are greatly reduced in quantity and function.[21,39] The eccrine secretory coil becomes architecturally distorted, appearing shrunken, dilated, and surrounded by more fibrotic tissue.[40]

Too much emphasis has been placed on the effect of decreased sebum production as an etiologic factor. Except for the head, sebum production is quite low over the body surface owing to the sparcity of follicles. Besides, sebum is a poor "moisturizer." The skin of prepubertal children is smooth and soft despite very low levels of surface sebum. The real function of sebum is to lubricate and protect the pilage, no longer necessary for the "naked ape."

Vesicular and Bullous Disorders

BULLOUS PEMPHIGOID   This acute, severe, self-limited blistering disease, characterized by large, tense bullae, has also been called *pemphigus of the aged* and *senile pemphigoid* as most cases occur in the seventh and eighth decades[41] (see Chap. 61). Sixty-six percent of patients are older than 60 years at the onset. The disease is autoantibody-mediated with immune complexes, complement, and leukocytes activated at the basement membrane zone leading to cleft formation and bullae at the dermal-epidermal junction. The age-related changes probably involve both the skin and the immune system. There may be altered self-antigens or a loss of tolerance. B lymphocytes from bullous pemphigoid patients can be stimulated using mitogens to produce anti–basement membrane zone antibody, whereas lymphocytes from normal patients cannot be stimulated to produce these antibodies. Because aging is associated with a decline in T cell function, it has been suggested that perhaps there is a loss of B cell regulation, which normally keeps autoreactive B cell clones in check.

Benign Neoplasia

The epidermis exhibits an age-related decrease in proliferative activity. Thymidine-labeling studies exhibit a 50 percent reduction in thymidine-labeling index. There is a corresponding decrease in repair rate during wound healing. However, factors governing tissue homeostasis become less well regulated. The epidermis shows a loss in architectural hierarchy and increased cell-to-cell heterogeneity. Atrophy, hyperplasia, atypia, and neoplasia can all occur. Differentiation is disordered, focal proliferations of cells and tissues are commonplace in aged individuals, and increasing age strongly correlates with increased numbers of various benign neoplasms. Clinically, these appear as seborrheic keratoses, cherry angiomas, acrochordons, cutaneous horns, inverted follicular keratoses, clear cell acanthoma (Degos' acanthoma), lentigines, and sebaceous hyperplasia. Some are more prevalent on sun-damaged skin, increasing the probability of malignant transformations.

Disorders of Nails (See also "Disorders of the Feet," below)

NAIL GROWTH   Nail growth rate declines with increasing age. Bean's famous measurements of his own nail growth showed that it decreased to 0.52 mm per week in the eighth decade, as compared with 0.83 mm per week in the third decade.[42] Orentreich[32] correlated life expectancy with rate of decline in nail growth during aging and compared humans with beagles. The decrease in linear nail growth rate per year in humans is 0.5 percent per year from age 15 to 90 years, whereas with beagles, the decrease is 2.5 percent per year from age 1 to 14 years—a fivefold rate of decline in beagles, whose life expectancy is one-fifth that of humans.

GENERAL AGING-RELATED NAIL CHANGES Longitudinal ridges have been reported to occur in 67 percent of persons past 70 years of age.[43] Lamellar dystrophy, that is, brittle nails with split ends or layering is common in middle-aged women and most common in both sexes over 60 years of age.[44,45] Pigmentary changes occur with age but are confounded by disease states that may contribute to apparent nail color.[46] The lunulae become diffuse and poorly defined. There is a higher incidence of Terry's type of nails (whitish, opaque proximal nails).[47] One study of black persons' nails showed longitudinal pigment banding in 96 percent of persons over 50 years, as compared with 2.5 percent of 0- to 3-year-olds. Onychodystrophy may be misdiagnosed as a fungal infection. Dystrophic nails due to aging are most frequent in the toenails. Contributing factors include underlying orthopedic abnormalities and trauma from ill-fitting footwear. Aged nails are frequently more convex, the nail plate is thicker, and there may be subungual hyperkeratosis. These factors may combine to produce onychogryphosis. Grotesque malformations of the nails are common in the elderly, especially in women. Footwear is largely responsible for thickened, split, separated, rough, ridged, curved nails.

Disorders of Mucous Membranes

PERLÈCHE *Perlèche*, derived from the French, "to lick," simply refers to inflammation and fissures of the corners of the mouth. As laxity increases with the passage of time, the redundant skin creates a fold that becomes an intertriginous zone; it is then predisposed to retention of saliva and maceration. The lateral crevices deepen and become accentuated by a combination of factors. Among these are edentulousness with partial absorption of the alveolar ridge, sagging of the skin of the cheeks, loss of elasticity from photodamage, and excessive salivation. Misdiagnosis can occur. Candidiasis is often superimposed and can be readily diagnosed by culture, responding promptly to antifungal treatment. Vitamin deficiency is often blamed but rarely proved.

Eczematous Dermatitis

Eczematous dermatitis represented 38 percent of the chief presenting complaints in a study involving 330 geriatric patients (average age 69.95 years). A number of disease categories are involved (for cross-references, see Table 146-1).

NUMMULAR ECZEMA Coin-shaped eczema evolves as intensely pruritic discoid-shaped plaques. In men, the incidence rises in middle age, whereas nummular eczema may be more common in younger women. Extremities, most frequently the legs, are affected as well as the arms and hands. There may be several, coinlike patches 1 to 3 cm in diameter. Relapses can be expected. Nummular eczema may sometimes be a delayed manifestation of atopic dermatitis, but most patients do not have an atopic background. Xerosis is the background for the development of nummular eczema in the elderly. Bowen's disease and superficial basal cell cancer need to be considered in persistent lesions in this age group. Colonization by *Staphylococcus aureus* is a complicating factor that is often overlooked in the choice of therapy.

GRAVITATIONAL ECZEMA *Gravitational eczema* has replaced stasis dermatitis as a more appropriate term for the eczema that can accompany chronic venous hypertension. Actually there is an increase in blood flow within the venous circulation. The disorder is rarely seen prior to middle age. There is scaling, erythema, pigmentation, and fibrosis often associated with pruritus. Venous drain-

age has been compromised by a number of factors, some of which can be obesity, trauma, venous thrombosis, or multiple pregnancies. Heredity certainly plays a role by the presence of incompetent valves allowing back-flow of blood. The condition is common in the wheelchair-bound patient and in all situations where the muscle pump is not able to function in assisting blood return. Long-standing disease predisposes to ulceration with a predilection for the medial malleolus. When gravitational eczema and edema are acute in onset, an associated deep venous thrombosis must be excluded. Ischemia due to arterial impairment of blood flow is more common than is realized.

ASTEATOTIC ECZEMA Asteatotic eczema, or eczema craquelatum, is a transient dermatitis related to low ambient humidity, frequent bathing, and diminished use of emollients. It is essentially a complication of xerosis, which always precedes this type of eczema. The lesions have the appearance of a cracked river bed with poorly defined borders. Pruritic and frequently tender, the dermatitis is located predominantly on extensor limbs and trunk. Asteatotic eczema usually responds readily to emollient therapy with water-in-oil emulsions.

LICHEN SIMPLEX CHRONICUS Lichen simplex chronicus is a circumscribed, intensely pruritic plaque of eczema that results from habitual scraping and rubbing of the skin. Lichenification is a hallmark. The disorder is rarely seen in children and is most frequent in adults over 60 years of age. Usually there is but one lesion. Favored sites include occipital and nuchal areas in women, the perineum and scrotum in men. Wrist and leg involvement is frequent. Atopy is a predisposing factor; another is xerotic skin and its associated pruritus, which then inaugurates the itch-scratch cycle.

ATOPIC DERMATITIS In contrast to other types of eczema, atopic dermatitis is rare in the elderly, at least in its full form. Exacerbations decrease with the passage of time, fading away to less frequent exacerbations of eczema and less extensive lesions that become more limited to the extremities. The final clinical picture may be dry, scaly skin in which pruritus is disproportionately intense. When respiratory allergy and eczema coexist, the passage of time results in clearing of the dermatitis but without a corresponding relief of asthma. This may be partially related to an attenuated inflammatory response. Aged persons exhibit a measurable decrease in irritant reactions, cutaneous blister formation, and inflammatory conditions of all kinds.

Disorders Due to Sun Exposure (See also below)

PHOTOAGING Photoaging, or dermatoheliosis, is almost universal among the fair-skinned (Table 146-2). It is so common-place that it was previously misconceived as part of the aging process itself. Photoaging is covered in detail in the second part of this chapter.

CUTIS RHOMBOIDALIS NUCHAE Cutis rhomboidalis nuchae is an example of the profound textural and pigmentary changes that can occur on the neck of chronically sun-exposed persons. Coarse furrows lie in criss-cross fashion, dividing thickened, leathery, ruddy-colored skin.

SOLAR LENTIGO "Liver spots" (*les médaillons de cimetière*, sometimes called "coffin spots") are actinically induced and there-

TABLE 146-2

Dermatoheliosis ("Photoaging")

Anatomic Site	Process	Clinical Lesion
Keratinocyte	Variably increased	Roughness
		Solar keratosis
	Reduced	Translucence
Langerhans cell	Reduced	Altered and attenuated inflammatory and immune responses
Melanocyte	Variably increased	Irregular pigmentation
		Solar lentigo
	Reduced	Guttate hypomelanosis
		Actinic leukoderma
Extracellular matrix	Architectural alterations	
	Decreased collagen	Roughening, coarse furrowing
	Increased glycosamino-glycans	
	Increased elastin	Solar elastosis, yellowing
Blood vessel	Proliferation, permanent dilatation	Telangiectasia
		Bateman's purpura
	Fragility of blood vessel and supporting tissue	

fore should not be called senile lentigo. The appropriate term is *solar lentigo*; the term *liver spots* is misleading and should be discarded. The lesions may be present on UV-exposed skin in more than 90 percent of Caucasians over 70 years of age. Lesions are flat, have a uniform brown color, and are especially prominent on the dorsal hand of photodamaged older persons. The macules are usually larger than 1 cm, are multiple, and have circumscribed, well-defined round borders. Histologically, epidermal rete ridges are elongated with increased numbers of benign melanocytes.

FAVRE-RACOUCHOT DISEASE Favre-Racouchot disease, also known as nodular elastosis with cysts and comedones, occurs on facial sun-exposed skin and is characterized by huge open comedones (blackheads), predominantly on the temples of some older persons. The follicular orifices are greatly dilated and contain dense impacted horn. Sebaceous glands are atrophic. Dermatoheliosis is the necessary background for the development of solar comedones. The comedones respond to topical retinoic acid.

SOLAR PURPURA (BATEMAN'S SENILE PURPURA) Purpura frequently occurs following trauma to severely sun-damaged skin of the dorsal forearm of elderly persons. Torsional stresses rapidly lead to hemorrhages that may require months for the blood pigments to be resorbed.

VENOUS LAKE A venous lake is a venous ectasia that appears as a blue-black soft papule, typically on the lower lip and other sun-exposed areas such as the helix of the ear, the face, and the neck. Deteriorations in the three-dimensional network of connective tissue in the vascular adventitia as well as in the dermis contribute to their development. Venous lakes may be mistaken for melanomas or pigmented basal cell carcinomas. Diascopy is useful in making the diagnosis. Direct pressure created by a glass microscope slide

causes a vascular lesion to blanch, thereby differentiating it from a neoplasia.

STELLATE SCARS OF THE HANDS AND FOREARMS These have been mistakenly attributed to a preexisting purpura. The latter heals without scarring. Stellate scars have been incorrectly called pseudoscars (of Coulomb), but they are true scars resulting from tearing of fragile photodamaged skin.

Photosensitivity Disorders

ACTINIC RETICULOID (See Chaps. 110 and 136) This photosensitivity disorder occurs almost exclusively in elderly men and is associated with an exaggerated sensitivity to ultraviolet (UVA and UVB) and sometimes to visible light. Lichenified erythematous plaques occur on the forehead and the posterior nuchal area. With time the eruption becomes more deeply furrowed and intensely red, and there may be irregular areas of hyperpigmentation. There may be a gradual progression to an erythroderma. Leonine facies can develop. Itching can be intense, and there may be an associated lymphadenopathy. due to the dense dermal lymphohistiocytic infiltrate and the hyperchromatic cells similar in appearance to Sézary cells, actinic reticuloid is classified as a pseudolymphoma. It is important to recognize that malignant lymphoma may ultimately occur. T lymphocytes are chiefly suppressor T cells (OKT8 positive, in contrast to those in cutaneous T cell lymphoma, which are T helper cells). Some patients have demonstrated allergic contact hypersensitivity to oleoresin extracts from *Compositae* plants or common fragrances.

Adverse Cutaneous Drug Reactions

It is not known whether drug reactions are intrinsically more common in the elderly, because older patients are more likely to be receiving multiple drugs. Adverse cutaneous drug effects in the elderly have variable and ambiguous expression and may be more serious than in the young. In the elderly, drugs are more likely to incite autoimmune disorders such as pemphigus, bullous pemphigoid, and lupus erythematosus–like rashes. These are reversible upon discontinuation of the drug. Photosensitivity reactions also appear to be more prevalent in older age groups. A pseudoporphyria-like presentation can occur on light-exposed areas of patients taking naproxen or furosemide. Thiazide diuretics and sulfonamide-based hypoglycemic agents can cause photosensitivity. The elderly must always be closely questioned regarding drug intake, in view of age-associated forgetfulness. Resolution of the eruption upon withdrawal of the drug is often prolonged.

Infections

DERMATOPHYTE INFECTIONS (See Chap. 206) Superficial fungal infections, especially of the feet, are common. The usual dermatophytes prevail, often accompanied by onychomycosis. Superficial fungi are rarely acquired in old age. *Tinea pedis* is a lifelong disease, especially in men; it often worsens with age and is often misdiagnosed as dry skin. Decreased frequency of skin care, decreased epidermal turnover, and diminished immunologic function all play a role. As many as 80 percent of men over 64 years of age may have tinea pedis. The infection frequently exceeds the usual boundaries, with extension to beyond the fourth web space, creeping up onto the dorsum, invariably involving the nails. Sandal-type plantar involvement is common. There is often "one hand, two feet" involvement, which remains an unexplained presentation.

Maceration and white hyperkeratosis arise from cohabitation of dermatophyte and bacteria, frequently involving gram-negative organisms. *Tinea incognita* is a dermatophyte infection that eventuates from inappropriate, persistent use of topical glucocorticoids, which allow the fungus to grow unchecked by suppressing inflammation. Diagnosis is usually delayed or missed altogether as the typical signs are missing. *Tinea cruris* may be mistakenly diagnosed in elderly men when seborrheic dermatitis is the true culprit. *Tinea capitis* is very uncommon in the elderly.

CANDIDIASIS (See Chap. 207) *Candida albicans* can flourish in recesses created by redundant skin folds. Intertriginous zones are more common beneath the flabby, redundant tissues of elderly persons. For example, the inframammary creases beneath pendulous breasts, groins exposed to *Candida* from intestinal sources and kept moist with urine, and buttocks, which may rest atop plastic sheets to trap moisture, are all fertile ground for cutaneous candidiasis, which can extend onto the scrotum in men. *Candida* pustules can occur on the moist occluded back of bedridden patients, particularly those who have febrile sweats. Oral thrush may accompany severe illness. Exacerbating factors may include diabetes mellitus, systemic medications, nutritional factors, and diminished salivary function. The oral commissures may become intertriginous zones in the elderly, predisposed to *Candida* because of redundant labial skin folds and kept warm and moist with oral secretions. Colonization by *Candida* results in a mycotic perlèche. Vulvovaginal thrush and *Candida* balanitis can be promoted by combinations of the above factors.

CELLULITIS (See Chap. 197) Cellulitis in the aged may lack the classic signs and often goes undiagnosed. An indolent swelling in the older patient may be the only manifestation of a soft tissue infection that would have been warm, red, and associated with fever and leukocytosis in a younger person. Predisposing factors include chronic edema, poor arterial and venous circulation, diabetes mellitus, unrecognized trauma, and portals of entry created by tinea pedis or even xerosis with erythema cracquelatum.

Cellulitis may be related to significant underlying pathology, such as cholecystitis. The process may be retroperitoneal, as in a psoas muscle abscess, which may present with cellulitis of the groin or flank. Likewise, there may be an underlying incarcerated inguinal or umbilical hernia.

Patients undergoing coronary artery bypass can develop cellulitis at the saphenous vein donor site. Cellulitis can extend along the incision and rapidly evolve into a severe febrile illness. The site of origin of the causative group A streptococci is frequently an interdigital web space fissure secondary to tinea pedis. The perisaphenous tissues are fertile soil for infection, having been deprived of their normal lymphatic drainage. The lymphotropism of streptococcal infections and the consequent lymphatic scarring create more edema and set the stage for recurrent infections. Accordingly, there needs to be meticulous search for conditions, often seemingly minor, that provide a breach of skin through which streptoccci make their entrance.

Erysipelas is a special variant of cellulitis caused by beta-hemolytic streptococci and should be considered a life-threatening emergency that can evolve rapidly and dramatically. Face and scalp are favored locations, but lesions can occur anywhere, with organisms gaining entry in a web space fissure, a stasis ulcer, or from a small innocent-appearing scratch. Recurrences can occur in the same location and may warrant prophylactic antibiotic use. The sequelae of persistent livid edema on the face can produce disfiguring macrocheilia or persistent edematous periorbital tissue.

PYODERMA Pyoderma in the aged may be subtle and disguised. There may be only slight redness, tenderness, and warmth with no febrile response, even in severe infections such as carbuncles. A furuncle may simulate a cold abscess. The absence of overt clinical harbingers of infection leads to delay in recognition and treatment.

HERPES ZOSTER (See Chap. 216) In otherwise healthy persons, herpes zoster occurs more often in the elderly and is far more serious. This is principally because of postherpetic neuralgia, which is more frequent and severe in elderly persons, The risk of postherpetic neuralgia is as high as 20 percent in patients over 60 years of age; the actual figure may approach 50 percent. In one large follow-up study, postherpetic neuralgia was present 1 month after the onset of the rash in 60 percent, by 3 months there was some pain in 24 percent, and by 6 months 13 percent still had pain. The highest prevalence is in ophthalmic zoster. A recent preliminary study of older patients (age 60) demonstrated a reduced frequency of persistent pain when intravenous acyclovir, 10 mg/kg every 8 h for 5 days, was given within 4 days of the onset of the pain or within 48 h after the onset of the rash. It is important, however, to evaluate renal function prior to high-dose acyclovir therapy in elderly patients. While this is promising, prevention of neuralgia is not always achieved. An alternative is the addition of systemic glucocorticoids, starting with the onset of the eruption if no contraindications exist. The dosage is 60 mg of prednisone per day, tapered to zero over a course of 4 weeks; this allegedly prevents postherpetic neuralgia in the majority of patients. The mechanisms responsible for recrudescence of the varicella-zoster virus in healthy, aged persons are not known. The increased neuralgia likewise remains a mystery. In general, elderly persons have an increased tolerance to pain.

Infestations

SCABIES (See Chap. 239) The clinical presentation of scabies infestations in the elderly patient can be so varied that, although easily treated, diagnosis can be elusive. Casual skin contact can then innocently spread mites among family members or nursing home inhabitants. Three important clinical variations should be kept in mind. Cryptic cases can present with pruritus but only minimal lesions, as the hypersensitivity reaction responsible for cutaneous manifestations in younger patients may be muted in older persons. Scabies incognita can result from steroid treatment and lead to delay in diagnosis by masking signs and symptoms, which can be dramatically altered in extent and distribution. Subsequent superinfection can further confound the presentation. Nodules containing mites can persist after antiscabetic treatment. The associated histologic appearance can mimic lymphoid neoplasms. Norwegian scabies may occur in immunodepressed patients and in those who either cannot scratch effectively or who have depressed cutaneous sensation. These patients can present with extensive crusted accretions containing huge numbers of mites, creating a highly contagious situation. There may be an associated lymphadenopathy and eosinophilia. Epidemics are common in nursing homes.

Disorders of the Feet

The feet are frequently neglected by physicians and especially by patients who have impaired ability to care for their feet. In the elderly, the normal mechanical stresses affecting pedal anatomy, friction, compression, tension, shear, and torsion can be exaggerated and distorted by ill-fitting footwear, abnormalities in gait, and impaired sensory input.[48] Foot health is critically important in the elderly population to maintain mobility. Decreased physical activity may be the beginning of a vicious cycle of immobility and a decreased ability for self-care. A simple foot lesion could incapacitate the elderly person and foster further musculoskeletal atrophy and decline. Podiatrist geriatricians emphasize the necessity to "keep 'em walking." Toenails present a special geriatric problem, in large part associated with the impaired ability to maintain normal care; many elderly patients cannot cut their toenails.

CLAVI Fifty percent of podiatric visits are because of corns. A corn is a hyperkeratotic plaque, usually ring-shaped, caused by pressure and frictional forces from body weight, footwear, or digits pressing on each other. The differential diagnosis includes warts; however, a corn pared with a blade reveals only a central translucent core, devoid of the thrombosed capillaries characteristically seen in warts. Corns are of four types. They can be hard, soft, vascular, or neurovascular. Hard corns usually occur over dorsal interphalangeal joints. On the plantar surface, they are found underlying the metatarsal heads and on the great toe, beneath the interphalangeal joint or any area of increased pressure. Corns can occur subungually, between the toes, and in the nail bed sulcus. Onychoclavus is a subungual corn or heloma and usually occurs in the distal nail bed of the great toe, secondary to localized pressure on the hyponychium. The overlying nail may be distorted or split. Soft corns arise exclusively interdigitally, typically in the fourth web space. Most interdigital soft corns arise secondary to bony exostoses (usually condyles of the joints). Pressure is increased by shoes with pointed tips leading to crowding and compression of the toes. Podiatrists can supply a very effective molded plastic device that keeps the toes apart.

BURSITIS Bursae are anatomic cushions reducing stresses on tissues. The aged person may have extreme stresses on selected sites due to impaired mobility. Bursitis can develop beneath sites of shearing stress such as corns, hallux valgus, and near the Achilles tendon. Bursitis can be traumatic or infective. As the condition may be prolonged in the aged person, fluid can form fistulous tracks towards a joint space or a sinus tract to the skin, and the simultaneous occurrence of both processes can result in joint fluid leakage and the risk of serious infection.

BUNIONS A bunion is a deformity of the metatarsal phalangeal joint of the great toe. The pathophysiology is genetic and environmental. In the early stages, there is lateral deviation of the proximal phalanx over the first metatarsal head, pushing medially off the underlying sesamoids. Patients usually have a history of wearing inappropriate shoes with heels too high and/or toe boxes too narrow for the feet to operate naturally. As the proximal phalanx subluxates laterally, laxity increases medially, and ligament contracture causes the deformity to become progressive. The large, often painful medial prominence of a bunion is the first metatarsal head, which is exposed to increased pressure in shoes. This prominence enlarges as the bone reacts to the increased pressure. Often a bursa can form over the head medially, and this can become irritated and infected. The laterally subluxed proximal phalanx often causes an overriding second toe, which can be difficult to fit into shoes and can develop consequent painful keratoses.

INTRACTABLE PLANTAR KERATOSES Callus, or tyloma, commonly develops on the plantar surface below the middle three metatarsophalangeal joints. The thickened epidermis can greatly limit mobility. The callus can vary in size, depending on its underlying cause. There are usually bony deformities that lead to increased stresses on the soft tissue of the sole of the foot, creating hyperkeratotic plaques. The keratoses can be reduced by paring; however, the underlying biomechanics must be corrected in order to solve the problem. Treatment may require altering shoes, adding orthotics, and, sometimes, surgery.

NEOPLASIA The most common neoplasms are basal cell cancers and melanomas, which can be subungual and may be masked secondarily by traumatic hyperkeratosis. Epithelioma cuniculatum is squamous cell carcinoma of the foot that looks like a wart. Because warts are uncommon in the geriatric population, verrucous lesions mandate investigation. Epithelioma cuniculatum should not be treated with radiation, which can induce a more aggressive behavior pattern.

SUBUNGUAL EXOSTOSIS This is a small bony outgrowth typically on the great toe, three times as common on the hallux relative to the fifth toe. It occurs in women more frequently than in men. The diagnosis requires x-ray. The bony growth occurs secondary to trauma.

ONYCHOCRYPTOSIS Ingrown toenail occurs when a lateral portion of the nail edge, most frequently on the hallux, penetrates the neighboring soft tissue. It can be caused by improperly performed nail trimming. Other predisposing factors include ill-fitting footwear, distorted weight-bearing due to abnormalities in gait, and hyperhidrosis from occlusive footwear or overuse of foot baths. It can be complicated by insidious but serious infection that may go unnoticed in this population.

ONYCHAUXIS Onychauxis is a condition of hypertrophied nails secondary to trauma and chronic pressure. Neglect in nail trimming leads to increased forces from footwear as the nail grows. The nail plate is typically dull and opaque and may be discolored. The condition can be misdiagnosed as a fungal infection. Complicating sequelae can include pain, subungual hemorrhage, subungual ulceration, and predisposition to tinea unguium. Treatment includes partial or total debridement of the nail plate on a regular basis, nail plate evulsion, or matricectomy.

ONYCHOLYSIS In the elderly population, onycholysis may reflect systemically impaired peripheral circulation. dehiscence of the nail plate from the nail bed begins at the free nail margin and extends proximally. Onycholysis predisposes the nail bed to infection.

ONYCHOGRYPHOSIS Synonyms for onychogryphosis include ram's horn, Osler's toe, and Hippocratic nail. The nail is club-shaped with an exaggerated, laterally extended longitudinal curvature. The greatly distorted shape results from uneven nail growth. The nail may be a dark color. Trauma, poorly fitting footwear, and failure to trim nails aggravate the problem, may result in penetration of the distal nail tip into adjacent soft tissue, and lead to infection.

ONYCHOPHOSIS Onychophosis refers to hyperkeratotic tissue occurring either on or under nail folds or subungually. The hyperkeratosis can be focal or diffuse and occurs mainly on the first and fifth toes. It is seen frequently in elderly persons and results from local mild trauma to the nail plate. The setting usually includes several predisposing factors such as xerosis and nail fold and/or nail plate deformities. Treatment includes elimination of trauma-inducing factors and debridement of the hyperkeratotic tissue. Keratolytics can be useful.

Cutaneous Melanoma and Its Precursors

LENTIGO MALIGNA MELANOMA Lentigo maligna melanoma is a large, flat, irregular, pigmented lesion that typically develops in the sixth or seventh decade of life, usually on the face. Lentigo maligna melanoma is discussed in Chap. 92.

Precancerous and Malignant Nonmelanoma Cutaneous Neoplasia

Nonmelanoma skin cancers are common in older persons; however, the lesions occur principally on actinically damaged skin. Skin not exposed to sun may also have an increased tendency to develop malignancies, perhaps due to a diminished cellular immune function. Genetic factors also play a role. Certainly there are elderly persons with extensive dermatoheliosis and no cutaneous malignancies.

ANGIOSARCOMA Angiosarcoma is also known as malignant angioendothelioma. It is a rare tumor that, when cutaneous in origin, presents most typically on the scalp or face of elderly patients. Very rarely, angiosarcoma can arise in the setting of a chronic lymphedematous extremity. Postmastectomy lymphangiosarcoma, Stewart-Treves syndrome, occurs in the edematous upper extremity after radical mastectomy. Angiosarcoma can be mistakenly diagnosed as cellulitis or erysipelas.

EXTRAMAMMARY PAGET'S DISEASE (See Chap. 86) Extramammary Paget's disease is a well-circumscribed erythematous plaque that can be eczematous in appearance and may have erosions or ulcerations. The location is in areas having apocrine glands, and anogenital sites predominate. Extraperineal sites include axillae and periumbilical areas. Lesions can be pruritic and painful. Underlying carcinomas are usually apocrine in origin; however, 20 percent of anogenital lesions are associated with urogenital or rectal adenocarcinomas. The treatment is surgical. Lesions can be mistakenly diagnosed as psoriasis or eczema, and the diagnosis requires a biopsy.

CUTANEOUS NEUROENDOCRINE CARCINOMA (See Chap. 85) Cutaneous neuroendocrine carcinoma, known also as Merkel cell carcinoma, is a clinically subtle, underrecognized, highly aggressive tumor with a high rate of local recurrence following surgery. Average age at initial presentation is 68 years, with 91 percent of patients over age 50 years.[49] The precise histogenesis is not certain. Eighty-five percent of tumors arise in areas of actinic exposure, and other UV radiation–associated neoplasias seem to be associated. The actual incidence of Merkel cell carcinoma is underrepresented in the literature because of the difficulty in making the diagnosis. The tumor has frequently been confused with other neoplasms. Prognostic variables are not known, but the majority of patients are not alive 5 years after the diagnosis is made.

Disorders of the Anogenitalia (See Chaps. 115 and 116)

PRURITUS ANI AND VULVAE Cutaneous perineal inflammation is common in older persons. The diagnosis must exclude underlying skin disorders, such as tinea and candidiasis. Multiple factors can work in concert in these sensitive areas. They include poor hygiene,

moisture, and irritating excretions. Hemorrhoids commonly incite pruritus near the anus. Contact hypersensitivity to local preparations, residual cleansing agents, or cosmetics can play a role. There have been elderly women who responded to vulvar itching by applying a variety of household products including cleaning fluids and toothpaste. Patients are often embarrassed to talk about these problems, even though they certainly affect the quality of life.

Mild fecal incontinence can be an important cause of pruritus in persons who are scrupulous about removing feces following a bowel movement.[50] The prevalence of fecal incontinence has been estimated at slightly over 1 percent of persons over 65 years of age. The prevalence is much higher among nursing home residents (10 to 17 percent) and hospitalized elderly persons (10 to 47 percent). Fecal incontinence related to dysfunction of the anal sphincter can cause pruritus ani without clinically apparent skin manifestations. Pruritus results from the action of pruritogenic bacterial endopeptidases contained in feces. The diagnosis of a weak anal sphincter can be made with the aid of manometry, cinedefecography, and electromyography. Treatment includes limited short-pulse therapy with a potent class I glucocorticoid in severe cases having lichenification of the perianal skin. Harsh toilet paper should be replaced by cotton flannel pledgets soaked in witch hazel. Hygiene must be impeccable, and a bidet can be helpful. Topical menthol-camphor antipruritic lotions help relieve pruritis, and liberal application of talcum powder can help absorb the results of mild fecal incontinence. Dietary manipulation with high-fiber and stool-bulking supplements encourages formation of soft but solid stools as opposed to liquid stools, which are more easily leaked from a weak anal sphincter. Medical antidiarrheal agents, biofeedback training, and surgery may be indicated, depending on the etiology of the incontinence.

Circulatory Disorders

LIVEDO RETICULARIS In the geriatric population, livedo reticularis in a distal extremity represents atheroembolus until proved otherwise.

DEPENDENT RUBOR Intense dependent erythema occurs due to compensatory capillary dilatation and disappears with elevation. It is often mistaken for cellulitis. There may be associated dependent edema. If ulceration exists, revascularization procedures are required. Biopsy is contraindicated.

ACROCYANOSIS Acrocyanosis may indicate poor cardiac output and/or insufficient environmental temperature. Incontinent, semimobile patients have additional factors associated with heat loss.

Cutaneous Ulcers

PRESSURE SORES (See Chap. 133) Decubitus ulcer correctly refers to ulcers resulting from a prolonged supine, prone, or lateral position (Latin *decumbere*, "to lie down"). Seventy percent of patients with pressure sores are over 70 years of age. Mortality rate is estimated at 8 percent. Risk factors other than age include neurologic deficit, malnutrition, immobilization, and debilitating medical disease. Cutaneous changes reflect only the "tip of the iceberg." The skin overlying the evolving pressure sore belies the extent of tissue injury, which is cone-shaped with the apex directed toward the skin and the larger base adjacent to the bony pressure point.

When combined with friction, the force required to produce ulceration can be as small as 45 mmHg. Bony prominences may receive increased force due to loss of adipose cushioning. Sedentary habits, decreased ambulatory ability, and muscle atrophy prolong the time spent in any one position. Additionally, assistance and attempts at mobilization increase the chance that shearing forces act synergistically with pressure to create tissue ischemia. With the development of the first pressure sore, the risk is compounded for the development of additional sites, in an attempt to avoid pressure on the initial site.

Decubitus ulcers are serious lesions that require prompt attention at the earliest stage of erythema. With proper turning and relief of pressure, they are completely preventable. Decubitus ulcers are more than skin deep.

Miscellaneous

GENERAL SKIN CARE IN THE GERIATRIC POPULATION
The signs of cutaneous disorders in the elderly are not as pronounced as in younger persons. The degree of erythema is reduced, and the disease presentation of even cutaneous infections can be subtle. Prevention of common disorders should be stressed. Xerosis should be rigorously avoided in order to preclude asteatotic eczema. The use of emollients and proper methods of bathing should be emphasized. Foot care and treatment of tinea pedis can help to prevent the development of a life-threatening cellulitis. Intertrigo needs to be prevented as it can be a portal of entry for irritants and infectious agents. Prevention of venous ulcers and of allergic contact dermatitis needs to be meticulous in patients with gravitational eczema who are dangerously prone to both of these complications. Elderly skin is more prone to traumatic lacerations. Aged skin which is edematous is particularly susceptible to trauma and bulla formation.

SKIN ATROPHY
Skin atrophy can be compounded due to a poor understanding of the correct use of medications, leading to misuse of topical steroids in the elderly patient, who may have associated edema with vascular insufficiency. The geriatric dermal-epidermal interface is already compromised. The fragile skin of the poorly groomed foot is a setup for fissures, bullae, infection, and further loss of the ability to be mobile.

SEBORRHEIC DERMATITIS
(See Chap. 126) Although seborrheic dermatitis can affect all ages and both males and females, it becomes much more common with increasing age. The association with increasing age correlates best in men, whereas women have a peak in morbidity after puberty, after which it gradually declines. There appears to be a cephalocaudad progression of the location with increasing age. Although the face and head are the predominant sites in younger age groups and certainly can be severely affected in the elderly, genitocrural and lower extremity lesions increase with age. The pubis, crural folds, gluteal cleft, and penis (seborrheic balanitis) may be involved. Lesions may be misdiagnosed as tinea infections. Striking flares of seborrheic dermatitis have been associated with confining illnesses such as coronary infarction. Exacerbations may eventuate in a diffuse erythroderma, which is often misdiagnosed. Pathogenesis may be related to changes in the cutaneous microflora. A neurophysiologic role is suggested by the association of seborrheic dermatitis with mental retardation and with Parkinson's disease. Seborrheic dermatitis may appear abruptly in the elderly, heralding the onset of Parkinson's disease. The scalp is usually involved, often giving rise to a mistaken diagnosis of dandruff. Simple dandruff declines late in adult life.

INTERTRIGO
Intertrigo is more frequent in the elderly due to redundant skin folds and environmental factors, including temperature, moisture, friction, and inadequate hygiene. Polymicrobial secondary colonization and subsequent infection can occur. No one organism can be singled out as the main agent.

TREATMENT OF THE CUTANEOUS SIGNS OF AGING
Multiple medical and surgical therapeutic modalities are evolving for the treatment of the outward signs of intrinsic aging and photoaging. See Table 146-3.

Some publications still use the obsolete term *premature skin aging* to describe alterations in unprotected skin, notably the face and sun-exposed areas, implying that this is merely exaggerated manifestations of normal aging. However, the evidence is convincing that photoaging is not simply an acceleration of the inevitable age-dependent alterations. Photoaging denotes the gross and microscopic cutaneous changes that are a consequence of chronic solar radiation. Recent studies demonstrate that this spectrum of changes is often diametrically opposed to that which occurs in intrinsically aged skin.[4,64,65] Sun worshippers do look prematurely aged, and this is the basis for the common misconception. Those who scrupulously avoid the sun can reach the ninth decade with smooth, unblemished

TABLE 146-3

Treatment of the Cutaneous Signs of Aging*

Medical
  Chemical peels
    Alpha-hydroxy acids, beta-hydroxy acids, trichloroacetic acid, Jessner's, phenol
  Environment
    Eliminate actinic exposure
    Eliminate cigarette smoking and exposure
  Hormone replacement therapy
    Estrogen
    Growth hormone
  Injectable agents (includes soft tissue augmentation)
    Autologous fat transplantation
    Botulinum toxin
    Collagen
    Fibrel
  Topical agents
    Alpha-hyroxy acids
    Beta-hydroxy acids
    Dipyrimidine dithymidylic acid (experimental)
    Estrogen
    Melatonin
    Retinoids
    Sunscreens (broad spectrum)
    Vitamins C, E
Surgical
  Blepharoplasty
  Brow-lift
  Cervicofacial rhytidectomy (face-lift)
  Carbon dioxide laser resurfacing
  Dermabrasion
  Laser treatment of telangiectasias (585–595 nm)

*For complete details, see references 51–63.

skin that shows only mild thinning, loss of elasticity, and a deepening of normal expression lines. By contrast, at age 50, serious sun worshippers, especially those of skin phototype I (blue-eyed, fair-skinned, Celtic ancestry who burn easily and tan poorly), have a plethora of wrinkles, with yellowed, lax, dry, leathery, knobby, blotchy skin and a variety of benign, premalignant, and malignant neoplasms.

Late nineteenth century dermatologists, notably Unna and Dubreuilh, clearly recognized the baleful influence of sunlight by comparing the integument of farmers and sailors to that of indoor workers. This was at a time when the leisured class stayed out of the sun. Today, a tan is prized by Caucasians and is ironically equated with health and beauty. Because decades of extensive sun bathing can occur before the photoaging changes become apparent to the naked eye,[12] there is a lack of urgency concerning prevention. This latent period also reinforces the impressions that actinically damaged skin differs only quantitatively from intrinsic aging. However, photoaging has distinctive and unique features that are quite different from normal aging.

Photoaging

Albert M. Kligman
Lorraine H. Kligman

Elastosis, an overgrowth of abnormal elastic fibers, is a prototypical feature of actinically damaged skin[12]; it never occurs in the protected skin of even very old healthy persons. During adult life, the quantity of elastic fibers in unexposed skin increases slightly (Fig. 146-1A), and there is mild morphologic deterioration seen by electron microscopy.[19,23] However, the changes never reach the stage of coarse, tangled accretions of degraded elastic fibers that finally, in severe photoaging, degenerate into an amorphous mass (Fig. 146-1B). In actinically damaged skin, the glycosaminoglycans (GAGs) and proteoglycans comprising the ground substance are greatly increased, almost matching fetal skin in this regard. In protected aged skin, GAGs actually decrease.[24]

In the normal aging of unexposed skin, the cells of the dermis are depleted[66]; hypocellularity is the rule. Fibroblasts are scanty and shrunken and mast cells are much more scarce (see Chap. 145). This contrasts strikingly with photoaging, in which fibroblasts are numerous and hyperplastic.[67] Mast cells are abundant and partially degranulated. Histiocytes and other mononuclear cells are also increased. One might say that photoaged skin is chronically inflamed (Fig. 146-2), a process called *heliodermatitis*[67] or *dermatoheliosis*.

As elastin increases in photoaged skin, collagen proportionately decreases.[24,68] Histologically, a large portion of the dermis becomes

FIGURE 146-1

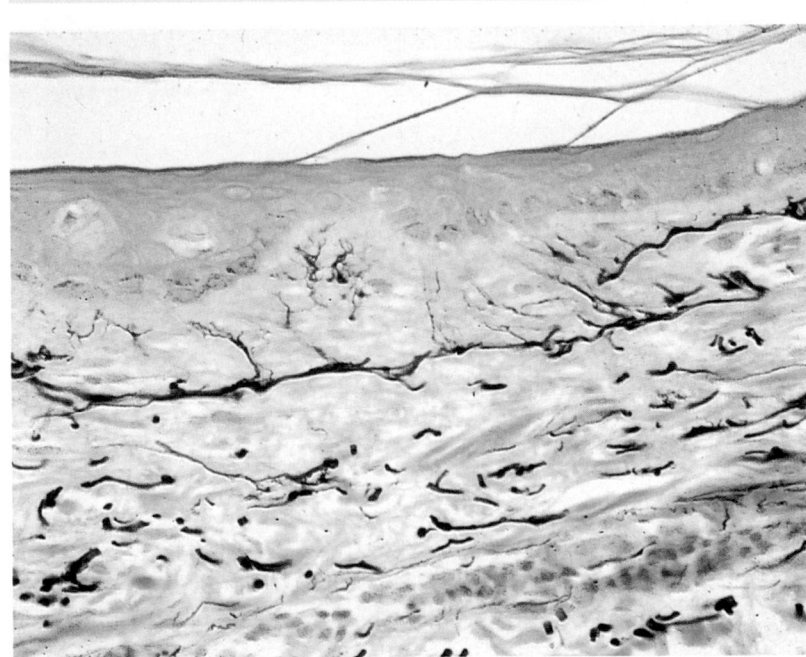

A.

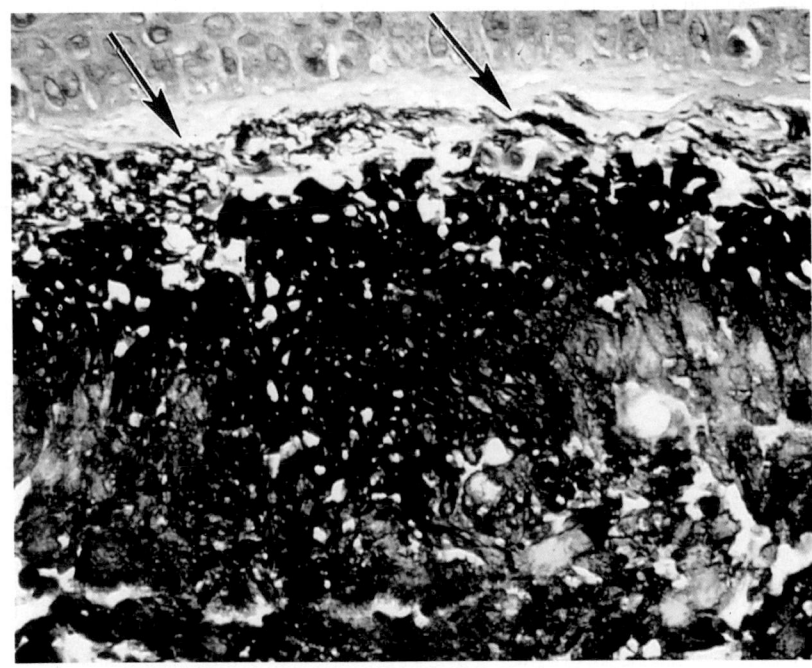

B.

A. Intrinsically aged skin. Protected abdominal skin from an 80-year-old woman shows a moderate increase and thickening of elastic fibers with resorption of most fine subepidermal fibers. The dermal-epidermal junction is flattened and dermal cells are sparse. *B.* Photodamaged facial skin. Large masses of deranged elastic fibers characterize solar elastosis. A thin subepidermal Grenz zone (*arrows*) is present, and the epidermis is acanthotic.

FIGURE 146-2

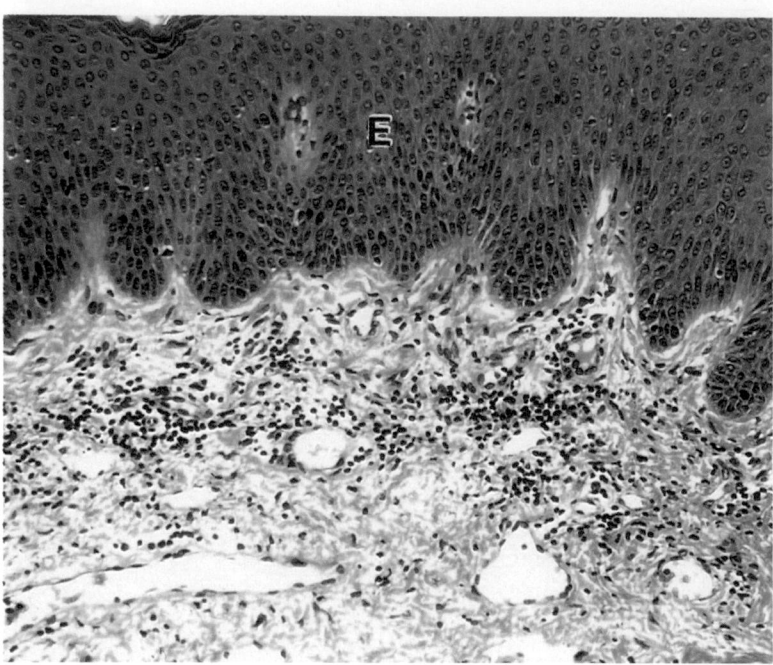

Marked dermal inflammatory infiltrate associated with the heliodermatitis (dermatoheliosis) that is characteristic of ongoing and chronic actinic exposure. E, epidermis.

occupied with material that was mistakenly believed to be a "basophilic degeneration" of collagen. It is now clearly recognized that this material consists of degraded elastin and microfibrillar proteins to which is bound fibronectin, a glycoprotein of the dermal matrix.[69] The massive loss of collagen and other degenerative matrix changes probably result from the metalloproteases and cytokines released by keratinocytes, fibroblasts, and inflammatory infiltrates as the result of sun exposure.[70,71] In normal aging, collagen, far from disappearing, becomes more stable and resistant to proteolysis.[72] The bundles become larger, forming ropelike structures.[73]

Epidermal thinning, with flattening of the dermal-epidermal junction, is characteristic of intrinsic aging. Again, the opposite holds in photoaging where the epidermis becomes thickened, a response to chronic stimulation.[74] It is only in end-stage photoaging that epidermal atrophy occurs. Acanthosis in photoaging is accompanied by cellular atypia, loss of polarity, and marked irregularities in cell size and staining properties. Melanocytes increase in size and number, whereas Langerhans cells decrease and become less functional.[75,76] In vitro, it has been shown that keratinocytes from photodamaged skin have a shorter lifespan than those from protected skin.[77] It is in this deranged milieu that various neoplasms arise, such as solar lentigines, seborrheic keratoses, keratoacanthomas, and actinic keratoses. Aside from malignant melanoma, tumors such as basal cell epitheliomas, squamous cell carcinomas, and lentigo maligna melanomas arise almost exclusively on actinically damaged skin of the face and dorsal hands and forearms. With the exception of senile (cherry) angiomas, which occur on the trunk area in nearly all aged persons, sometimes by the dozens, practically all of the important tumors that come to the attention of dermatologists originate in photoaged skin.

Finally, actinic radiation is exceedingly damaging to the microcirculation.[8] Many vessels are completely obliterated. The few that survive are variably dilated and scraggly; the normal horizontal plexuses are extinguished (Fig. 146-3). Ultrastructurally, it has been demonstrated that vascular basement membranes are greatly duplicated.[28,67] This does not occur in healthy, intrinsically aged protected skin. In protected skin, however, as in photodamaged skin, there is a considerable deletion of small vessels, especially subepidermally where the capillary loops regress. In contrast to photodamaged skin, the vessels are not dilated or tortuous, and the overall horizontal pattern of vascular plexuses is not greatly disturbed.[78]

Pigmented skin is only partially resistant to the ravages of the sun. Even the most darkly pigmented people have only about a 10-year period of grace with regard to elastosis.[79] Gross appearance is deceiving. Still, neoplasms are rare in the skin of blacks and even Asians.

THE ACTION SPECTRUM OF PHOTOAGING

Past accounts have focused on UVB (290 to 320 nm) as the portion of terrestrial solar radiation responsible for sunburning, dermal changes, and carcinogenesis. Recent experiments show that concern must be extended to UVA (320 to 400 nm). UVA can, like UVB, produce erythema, although a 500 to 1000 times greater dosage is required.[80,81] UVA also contributes, either additively or synergistically, to the sunburning effects of UVB in humans[81,82] and UVB tumorigenesis in animals.[83,84] Large single doses of UVA in humans can damage blood vessels, producing endothelial cell enlargement, vasodilatation, and extravascular infiltrates of neutrophils.[85] Chronic exposure of hairless mice to long-wavelength UVA (>340 nm) also results in vascular damage that includes excessive duplication of basement membranes, endothelial cell cytoplasmic vacuolization, thinning, gap formation, and mitochondrial damage.[86] Exploration of the multiple effects of chronic UV exposure has been greatly aided by the hairless mouse model for photoaging.[87] It has been shown that in addition to the induction of elastosis by UVB both the shorter (320 to 340 nm: UVA II) and longer (340 to 400 nm: UVA I) wavelength portions of UVA can produce elastosis, given a high enough dose.[88,89] The action spectrum for elastosis has been shown to be similar to that for a number of acute UV-induced damages, including erythema. As expected, UVB is the most damaging waveband because it is more energetic.[90] However, unlike clinical erythema, which requires up to a thousandfold more UVA than UVB, a 50 percent increase in elastic fibers requires only 20 times more full-spectrum UVA than UVB. However, UVB is capable of producing more severe ultrastructural damage to elastic fibers than is UVA.[86,91]

As knowledge develops from experimental animal studies, it becomes increasingly evident that the UV solar spectrum does not fully account for photoaging. Sunlight is, of course, polychromatic, extending into the visible (400 to 700 nm), infrared (IR) (700 to 1,000,000 nm), and, ultimately, radiowaves. The latter can probably be ignored with regard to skin. Visible light, seemingly innocuous, has been known to cause deleterious effects ranging from phototoxic reactions[92] and solar urticaria in susceptible persons[93] to DNA cross-links in vitro[94] and UVB tumor enhancement in animals.[95]

IR radiation is inseparably linked to sunlight. Historically, heat-induced skin cancers have long been known in China, India, and Japan. In northern regions of these countries, various devices ranging from hot bricks to pots of burning coal have been used in contact with skin to maintain body warmth.[96] The peat (turf) fires of rural Ireland are also implicated in heat-induced cancers.[97] In most of these cases, hydrocarbons are a likely co-carcinogen. Long recognized as an etiologic factor in erythema ab igne, IR radiation produces a typical reticulated pattern of pigmentation of the skin's surface that is a reflection of the underlying dilated, leaking blood vessels. In addition, heat produces many changes highly reminiscent of actinic damage, including elastosis (Fig. 146-4), telangiectasia, marked epidermal atypia, and keratoses, some of which advance to squamous cell carcinomas. IR radiation has also been shown to enhance UVB elastosis experimentally in guinea pigs.[98] Erythema ab igne differs from photoaged skin in having deposits of hemosiderin and in not showing the final amorphous stage of elastosis.

THE BIOCHEMISTRY AND IMMUNOCHEMISTRY OF PHOTOAGING

Early biochemical studies on photoaged human skin demonstrated increases in GAGs with a corresponding loss of insoluble collagen and an increase in soluble collagen.[24] The availability of sufficient quantities of human skin has limited research in this area. However, in recent studies, both acid-soluble (newly synthesized, non-cross-linked) and pepsin-soluble (partially cross-linked) collagen have been reported to be decreased in photodamaged skin.[68] Pepsin-insoluble collagen was not examined. Schwartz et al.[99] have reported a 20 percent loss of total collagen in severe photoaging (cutis rhomboidalis nuchae) and a 40 percent decrease in the content of the intact aminopropeptide moiety of type III procollagen, an indication of collagen degradation. In moderately damaged forearm skin, there is a 4 to 8 percent loss.[100] Thus, reports of increased type III collagen in photodamaged skin[101] have not been confirmed by more recent studies. A similar discrepancy is seen for fibronectin in immunofluorescence studies. Chen et al.[69] have reported large amounts of fibronectin associated with elastosis, but Oikarinen and Kallioinen[68] reported no increase. Because methodologies vary and especially because the degree of chronic sun exposure is difficult to estimate in humans, much more work will be needed before these discrepancies can be resolved.

Several studies using UV-exposed hairless mice have appeared recently.[87] Unfortunately, divergent results have been reported, again largely due to different methodologies and different cumulative UV doses. However, in these cases the doses administered are known. It has become possible to begin to separate out some of the differing effects of UVA and UVB. By examining biochemical changes in collagen over time, Kligman et al.[102] found that with chronic UVB exposure total collagen increased until week 20, after

FIGURE 146-3

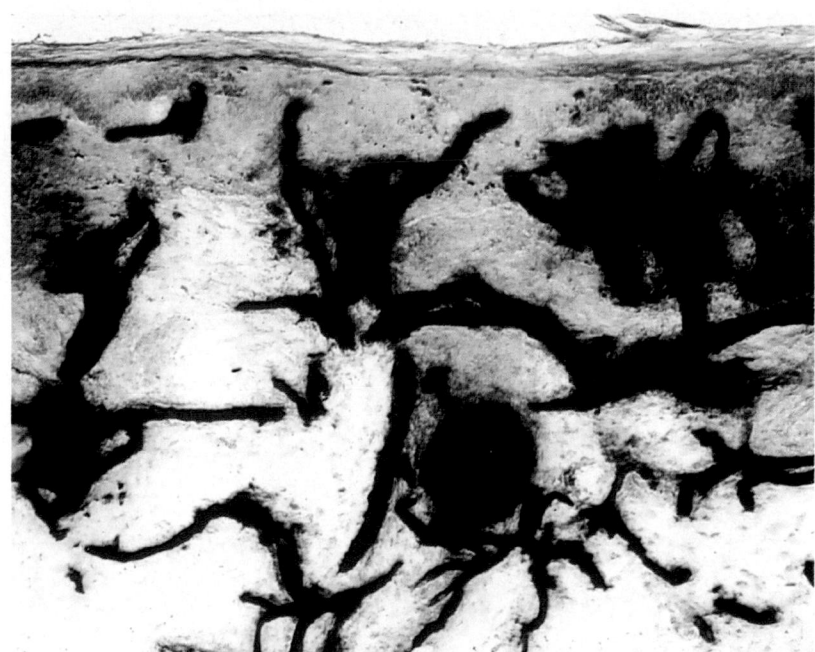

A.

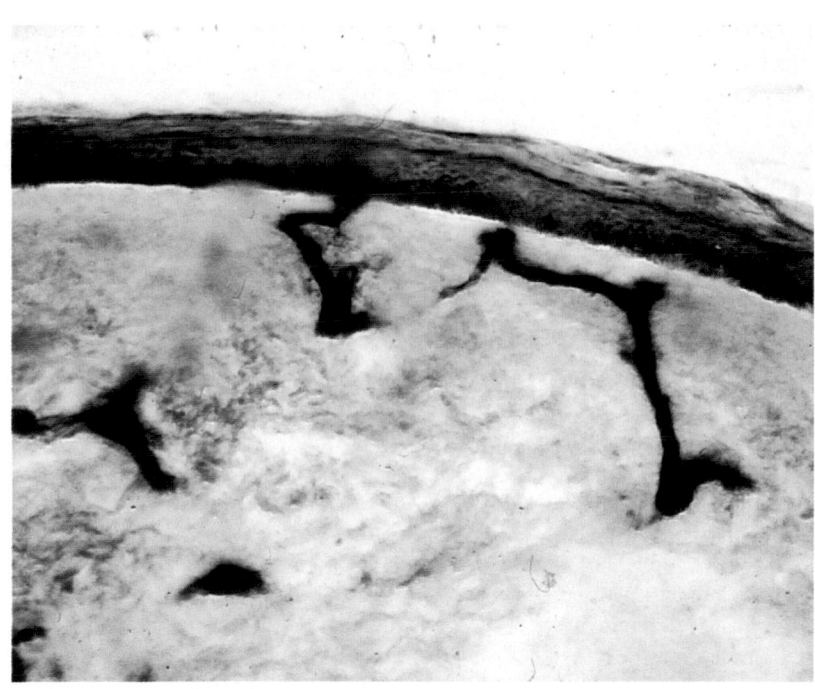

B.

A. Seen grossly as telangiectases, the vessels in photodamaged skin are dilated and tortuous, histologically. *B.* In end-stage, severe photoaging there is massive deletion of vessels.

REPAIR OF PHOTOAGED SKIN

FIGURE 146-4

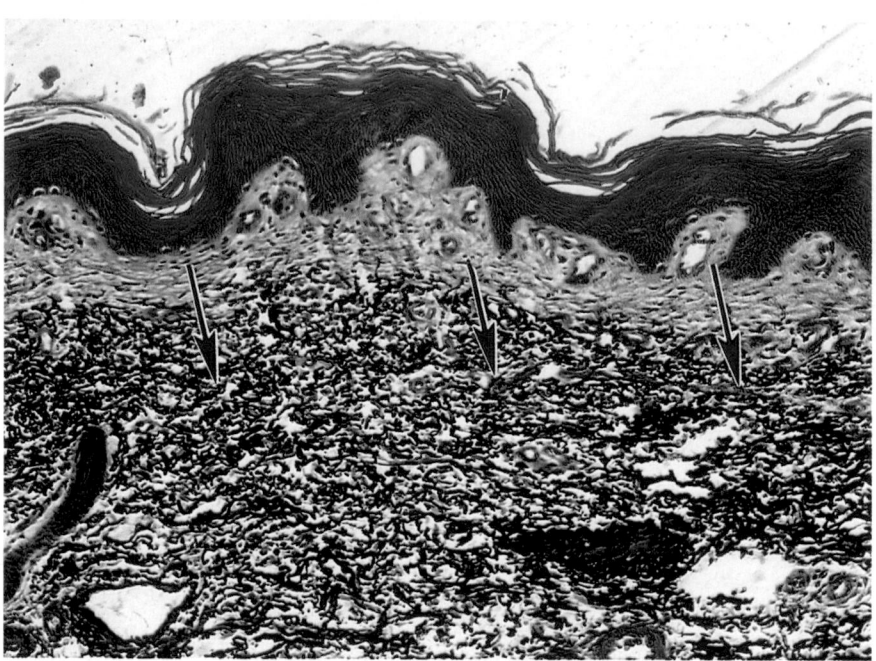

The deep elastosis (*arrows*) of infrared radiation-induced erythema ab igne.

Protection of skin against photoaging, as discussed in Chap. 248, is important because chronically sun-exposed skin was formerly thought to be irreversibly damaged. Recent studies require a revision of this pessimistic concept. It can be stated categorically that even in the most cruelly sun-damaged skin, dermal repair goes on continuously. The famous subepidermal Grenz zone, a zone of sparing from elastotic changes, affords the best evidence of ongoing repair. Long thought of as a "microscar" because of the parallel deposition of collagen,[111] the Grenz zone is actually an area where new procollagen I is constantly being synthesized.[112] In both humans and animals, discontinuation of radiation or proper protection by sunscreens is followed by widening of the Grenz zone.[113,114] As the deposition of new collagen continues, the expanding area of repair, or reconstruction zone, pushes the old elastotic dermis downward, so that a clear line of demarcation separates the newly created collagen from the degraded dermis (Fig. 146-5). The collagen bundles in the reconstruction zone are arranged parallel to the surface but should not be regarded as a scar on this account. This zone contains many fibroblasts that are actively synthesizing collagen, as revealed by an expanded cytoplasm filled with widely dilated rough endoplasmic reticulum.[113] The authors' findings indicate that destruction and repair go on simultaneously under continued assault by actinic radiation. The balance is shifted toward repair when the radiation stress is relieved. Both the epidermis and dermis are capable of moderate self-restoration when exogenous injury ceases.

Thus, it is never too late to advise older persons with actinically damaged skin to protect themselves from the sun. This not only favors repair of damaged dermis but also enables some regression of epithelial tumors. Clinicians in sunny areas have long realized that avoidance of sunlight may promote the disappearance of the flatter actinic keratoses.

The normal repair processes in photodamaged skin can be enhanced pharmacologically. Tretinoin (all-*trans*-retinoic acid) was the first to be assessed for this property.[115] Photodamaged hairless mice were treated topically for 10 weeks with tretinoin. In contrast to controls, the reconstruction zone of new collagen was significantly deeper in tretinoin-treated mice, with the enhanced repair being dose- and time-related.[115] The new collagen was histochemically, ultrastructurally, and biochemically normal.[115,116] As determined by radioimmunoassay, collagen content was increased twofold, and mRNAs for types I and III collagen were increased two- to threefold in the tretinoin-treated skin.[116] Immunofluorescence techniques located the new collagen synthesis in the histologically defined reconstruction zone and also showed the presence of new elastin and increased fibronectin in the region.[117] Isotretinoin (13-*cis*-retinoic acid) has also been demonstrated to enhance dermal repair in mice.[118] This repair activity remains retinoid-specific.

Studies on the effects of tretinoin on human photoaging have now progressed long enough to show dermal repair in addition to the earlier reported improvement in wrinkles, roughness, epidermal-

which loss occurred. This result mirrored the early histologic thickening of the upper dermis and the later loss of affinity for collagen-specific stains. Also in a time-course experiment, Plastow et al.[103] found an increase in type III collagen relative to type I. This change in ratio was not confirmed by Kligman et al.[102] or by Schwartz et al.[104] Immunochemical determination and radioimmunoassay have demonstrated that UVB radiation actually caused a loss of the aminopropeptide moiety of type III procollagen.[104] Photoaging alterations in other components of the dermal connective tissue were examined by Schwartz.[105] Immunofluorescence, biochemical, and enzyme-linked immunosorbent (ELISA) assays showed increases in elastin, microfibrillar proteins, GAGs, and fibronectin after chronic UVB exposure of hairless mice.

The most recent biochemical studies have centered on the effects of UVA radiation on hairless mouse collagen. After only a few low-dose exposures, Johnston et al.[106] reported a reduction in prolyl hydroxylase activity. UVB had no effect on this enzyme, which is involved in posttranslational modification of nascent collagen chains. Chronic UVA radiation appears to increase the resistance of collagen to digestion by pepsin significantly.[107,108] Compared to UVB-irradiated hairless mouse skin, in which 85 to 100 percent of the collagen can be digested, both full-spectrum (320 to 400 nm) and long-wavelength UVA (>340 nm) render up to 85 percent of the collagen indigestible. This phenomenon is UVA dose–dependent and may be the result of increased cross-linking of the collagen.[107] Similar effects on collagen solubility have been found in intrinsically aged human skin.[109] Total collagen content of mouse skin also decreased in a UVA dose-related fashion, perhaps related to the reduced prolyl hydroxylase activity reported by Johnston et al.[106] Fourtanier et al.[110] also found a decrease in total collagen after chronic exposure to full-spectrum UVA but not after long-wavelength UVA.

atypia, and pigmented lentigines.[119,120] Angiogenesis is stimulated,[119] anchoring fibrils at the dermal-epidermal junction are increased[121] and, after 2 to 5 years of treatment, a reconstruction zone of new collagen can be demonstrated.[122] Studies at the molecular level have shown that UVB radiation upregulates the collagen-degrading enzymes collagenase and gelatinase and that tretinoin reduces the mRNAs, protein, and activities of these enzymes by 50 to 80 percent.[123]

REFERENCES

1. Bergfeld WF: The aging skin. *Int J Fertil Womens Med* **42**:57, 1997
2. Guercio-Hauer C et al: Photodamage, photoaging and photoprotection of the skin. *Am Fam Physician* **50**:327, 1994
3. Naylor MF, Farmer KC: The case for sunscreens, a review of their use in preventing actinic damage and neoplasia. *Arch Dermatol* **133**:1146, 1997
4. Balin AK, Kligman AM: *Aging and the Skin.* New York, Raven, 1989
5. Kligman AM, Koblenzer C: Demographics and psychological implications for the aging population. *Dermatol Clin* **15**:549, 1997
6. Koblenzer CS: Psychologic aspects of aging and the skin. *Clin Dermatol* **14**:171, 1996
7. Borkan GA, Norris AH: Assessment of biological age using a profile of physical parameters. *J Gerontol* **35**:177, 1980
8. Kligman AM: Perspectives and problems in cutaneous gerontology. *J Invest Dermatol* **73**:39, 1979
9. Glogau RG: Aesthetic and anatomic analysis of the aging skin. *Semin Cutan Med Surg* **15**:134, 1996
10. Grove GL et al: Effect of aging on the blistering of human skin with ammonium hydroxide. *Br J Dermatol* **107**:393, 1982
11. Steenvoorden DP, van Henegouwen GM: The use of endogenous antioxidants to improve photoprotection. *J Photochem Photobiol* **41**:1, 1997
12. Kligman AM: Early destructive effect of sunlight in human skin. *JAMA* **210**:2377, 1969
13. Autio P et al: Collagen synthesis in human skin in vivo: Modulation by aging, ultraviolet B irradiation and localization. *Photodermatol Photoimmunol Photomed* **10**:212, 1994
14. Kang S et al: Photoaging and topical tretinoin: Therapy, pathogenesis, and prevention. *Arch Dermatol* **133**:1280, 1997
15. Fisher GJ et al: Pathophysiology of premature skin aging induced by ultraviolet light. *N Engl J Med* **337**:1419, 1997
16. Bernstein EF et al: Enhanced elastin and fibrillin gene expression in chronically photodamaged skin. *J Invest Dermatol* **103**:182, 1994
17. Marks R: *Skin Disease in Old Age.* London, Martin Dunitz, 1987
18. Beauregard SA, Gilchrest BA: Survey of skin problems and skin care regimens in the elderly. *Arch Dermatol* **123**:1638, 1987
19. Lavker RM: Structural alterations in exposed and unexposed aged skin. *J Invest Dermatol* **73**:59, 1979
20. Tsuji T: Ultrastructure of deep wrinkles in the elderly. *J Cutan Pathol* **14**:158, 1987
21. Montagna W, Carlisle K: Structural changes in aging human skin. *J Invest Dermatol* **73**:47, 1979
22. Katzberg A: The area of the dermal-epidermal junction in human skin. *Anat Rec* **131**:717, 1958
23. Braverman IM, Fonferko E: Studies in cutaneous aging. I. The elastic fiber network. *J Invest Dermatol* **78**:434, 1982
24. Smith JG, Davidson EA: Alterations in human dermal connective tissue with age and chronic sun damage. *J Invest Dermatol* **39**:347, 1962

FIGURE 146-5

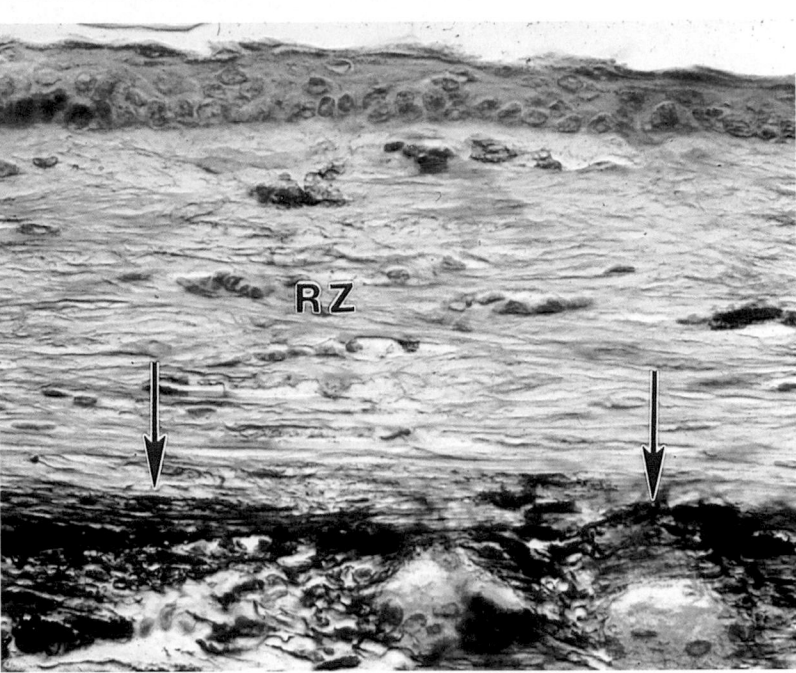

A.

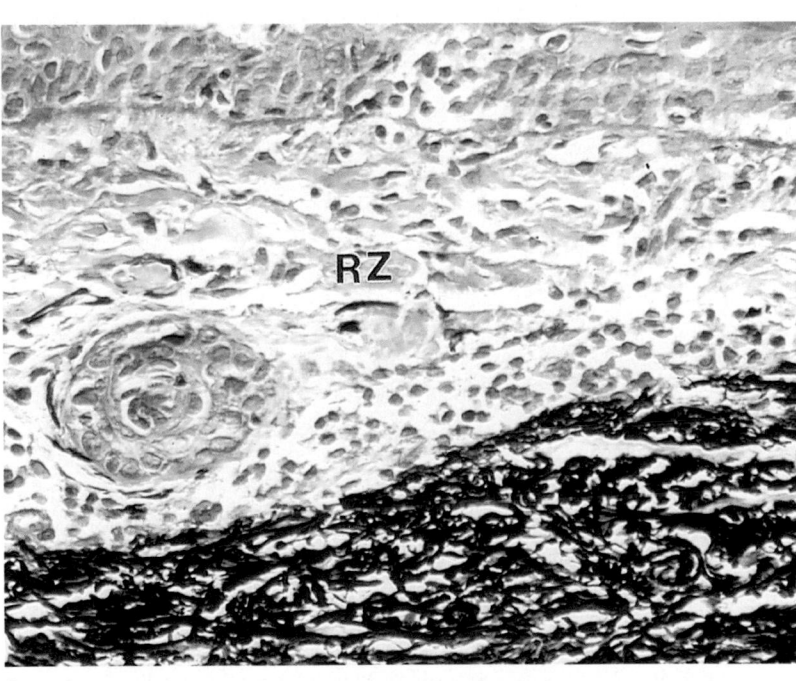

B.

A. Repair in hairless mouse skin. Fifteen weeks postirradiation, a reconstruction zone (RZ) of new parallel collagen compresses the elastotic fibers into a discrete band (*arrows*). *B.* Repair in human skin. Biopsy from the bald scalp of retired outdoor worker after 10 years of indoor residence in a home for the aged. As in the hairless mouse, a zone (RZ) of new connective tissue has been laid down subepidermally.

25. Shuster S, Black MM: The influence of age and sex on skin thickening, skin collagen and density. *Br J Dermatol* **93**:639, 1975

26. Fleischmajer R, Perlish JS: Human dermal glycosaminoglycans and aging. *Biochim Biophys Acta* **279**:265, 1972

27. Meyer LJ, Stern R: Age-dependent changes of hyaluronan in human skin. *J Invest Dermatol* **102**:385, 1994

28. Braverman IM, Fonferko E: Studies in cutaneous aging. II. The microvasculature. *J Invest Dermatol* **78**:444, 1982

29. Van den Brande P et al: Laser Doppler flux characteristics at the skin of the dorsum of the foot in young and in elderly healthy human subjects. *Microvasc Res* **53**:156, 1997

30. Rooke GA et al: Maximal skin blood flow is decreased in elderly men. *J Appl Physiol* **77**:11, 1994

31. Evans I et al: Thermally-induced cutaneous vasodilatation in aging. *J Gerontol* **48**:M53, 1993

32. Orentreich N, Selmanowitz VJ: Levels of biological functions with aging. *Trans NY Acad Sci* **31**:992, 1969

33. Halasz NA: Dehiscence of laparotomy wounds. *Am J Surg* **116**:210, 1968

34. Katlic MR(ed): *Geriatric Surgery: Comprehensive Care of the Surgical Patient.* Baltimore, Urban and Schwartzenberg, 1990

35. Holt DR, Kirk SJ: Effect of age on wound healing in healthy human beings. *Surgery* **112**:293, 1992

36. Reed MJ et al: TGF-beta 1 induces the expression of type I collagen and SPARC, and enhances contraction of collagen gels, by fibroblasts from young and aged donors. *J Cell Physiol* **158**:169, 1994

37. Saint-Leger D, Francois AM: Stratum corneum lipids in skin xerosis. *Dermatologica* **178**:151, 1989

38. Richard S et al: Characterization of the skin in vivo by high resolution magnetic resonance imaging: Water behavior and age-related effects. *J Invest Dermatol* **100**:705, 1993

39. Juniper J, Dykman RA: Skin resistance, sweat gland count and salivary flow. Age, race and sex differences. *Psychophysiology* **4**:216, 1967

40. Mackinnon PCB: Variations with age in the number of palmar digital sweat glands. *J Neurol Neurosurg Psychiatry* **17**:124, 1954

41. Lane CG, Rockwood EM: Geriatric dermatoses. *N Engl J Med* **241**:722, 1949

42. Bean W: Nail Growth: 30 years of observation. *Arch Intern Med* **184**:497, 1974

43. Lewin K: The finger nail in general disease. A macroscopic and microscopic study of 87 consecutive autopsies. *Br J Dermatol* **77**:431, 1965

44. Lewis BL, Montgomery H: The senile nail. *J Invest Dermatol* **24**:11, 1955

45. Lubach D et al: Incidence of brittle nails. *Dermatologica* **172**:144, 1986

46. Leyden JJ et al: Diffuse and banded melanin pigmentation in nails. *Arch Dermatol* **105**:548, 1972

47. Neale D, Adams IM: *Common Foot Disorders.* New York, Churchill Livingstone, 1985

48. Holzberg M, Walker HK: Terry's nails: Reviewed definition and new correlations. *Lancet* **1**:896, 1984

49. Pitale M et al: An analysis of prognostic factors in cutaneous neuroendocrine carcinoma. *Laryngoscope* **102**:244, 1992

50. Madoff RD et al: Fecal incontinence. *N Engl J Med* **326**:1002, 1992

51. Bangha E et al: Suppression of UV-induced erythema by topical treatment with melatonin. A dose response study. *Arch Dermatol Res* **288**:522, 1996

52. Blitzer A et al: The management of hyperfunctional facial lines with botulinum toxin. *Arch Otolaryngol Head Neck Surg* **123**:389, 1997

53. Callens A et al: Does hormonal skin aging exist? A study of the influence of different hormone therapy regimens on the skin of postmenopausal women using non-invasive measurement techniques. *Dermatology* **193**:289, 1996

54. Ditre CM et al: Effects of alpha-hydroxy acids on photoaged skin: A pilot clinical, histologic, and ultrastructural study. *J Am Acad Dermatol* **34**:187, 1996

55. Dunn LB et al: Does estrogen prevent skin aging? Results from the First National Health and Nutrition Examination Survey (NHANES 1). *Arch Dermatol* **133**:339, 1997

56. Gilchrest BA: Turning back the clock: Retinoic acid modifies intrinsic aging changes. *J Clin Invest* **94**:1711, 1994

57. Lewis AB, Gendler EC: Resurfacing with topical agents. *Semin Cutan Med Surg* **15**:139, 1996

58. Matarasso SL, Brody HJ: Deep chemical peeling. *Semin Cutan Med Surg* **15**:155, 1996

59. Orfanos CE et al: Current use and future potential role of retinoids in dermatology. *Drugs* **53**:358, 1997

60. Phillips CL et al: Effects of ascorbic acid on proliferation and collagen synthesis in relation to the donor age of human dermal fibroblasts. *J Invest Dermatol* **103**:228, 1994

61. Roenigk HH: The place of laser resurfacing within the range of medical and surgical skin resurfacing techniques. *Semin Cutan Med Surg* **15**:208, 1996

62. Sherris DA et al: Comprehensive treatment of the aging face—cutaneous and structural rejuvenation. *Mayo Clin Proc* **73**:139, 1998

63. Schmidt JB et al: Treatment of skin aging with topical estrogens. *Int J Dermatol* **35**:669, 1996

64. Lavker RM: Cutaneous aging: Chronologic versus photoaging, in *Photodamage,* edited by BA Gilchrest. Cambridge, MA, Blackwell Scientific, 1995, p 123

65. Gilchrest BA: *Skin and Aging Processes.* Boca Raton, FL, CRC Press, 1984, p 97

66. Andrews W et al: Changes with advancing age in the cell population of the human dermis. *Gerontologica* **10**:1, 1964

67. Lavker RM, Kligman AM: Chronic heliodermatitis: A morphologic evaluation of chronic dermal damage with emphasis on the role of mast cells. *J Invest Dermatol* **90**:325, 1988

68. Oikarinen A, Kallioinen M: A biochemical and immunohistochemical study of collagen in sunexposed and protected skin. *Photodermatology* **6**:24, 1989

69. Chen VL et al: Immunochemistry of elastotic material in sun-damaged skin. *J Invest Dermatol* **87**:334, 1986

70. Wlaschek M et al: UVA-induced autocrine stimulation of fibroblast-derived collagenase/MMP-1 by interrelated loops of interleukin-1 and interleukin-6. *Photochem Photobiol* **59**:550, 1994

71. Fisher GJ et al: Molecular basis of sun-induced premature skin aging and retinoid antagonism. *Nature* **379**:335, 1996

72. Bentley JP: Aging of collagen. *J Invest Dermatol* **73**:80, 1979

73. Lavker RM et al: Aged skin: A study by light, transmission electron and scanning electron microscopy. *J Invest Dermatol* **88**:44s, 1987

74. Kligman LH: Photoaging: Manifestations, prevention and treatment, in *Dermatology Clinics,* vol 4, *The Aging Skin,* edited by BA Gilchrest. Philadelphia, Saunders, 1986, p 517

75. Gilchrest BA et al: Effect of chronologic aging and ultraviolet radiation on Langerhans cells in human epidermis. *J Invest Dermatol* **79**:85, 1982

76. Räsänen L et al: Immediate decrease in antigen-presenting function and delayed enhancement of interleukin-1 production in human epidermal cells after in vivo UVB irradiation. *Br J Dermatol* **120**:589, 1989

77. Gilchrest BA: Relationship between actinic damage and chronologic aging in keratinocyte cultures in human skin. *J Invest Dermatol* **72**:219, 1979

78. Gilchrest BA et al: Chronologic aging alters the response to ultraviolet-induced inflammation in human skin. *J Invest Dermatol* **79**:11, 1982

79. Kligman AM: Solar elastosis in relation to pigmentation, in *Sunlight and Man: Normal and Abnormal Photobiological Responses,* edited by MA Pathak et al; consulting editor, TB Fitzpatrick. Tokyo, Univ of Tokyo Press, 1974, p 157

80. Kaidbey KH, Kligman AM: Acute effect of long wave ultraviolet irradiation on human skin. *J Invest Dermatol* **72**:253, 1979

81. Ying CY et al: Additive erythemogenic effects of middle (280–320 nm) and log-wave (320–400 nm) ultraviolet light. *J Invest Dermatol* **62**:273, 1974

82. Willis I et al: Effects of long ultraviolet rays on human skin: Photoprotective or photoaugmentative? *J Invest Dermatol* **59**:416, 1973

83. Willis I et al: The rapid induction of cancers in the hairless mouse utilizing the principle of photoaugmentation. *J Invest Dermatol* **76**:604, 1981

84. Kligman LH: UVA enhances low dose UVB tumorigenesis. *Photochem Photobiol* **47**:8s, 1988

85. Gilchrest BA et al: Histologic changes associated with ultraviolet-A-induced erythema in normal human skin. *J Am Acad Dermatol* **9**:213, 1983

86. Zheng P, Kligman LH: UVA radiation-induced ultrastructural changes in hairless mouse skin: A contrast to UVB-induced damage. *J Invest Dermatol* **96**:584, 1991

87. Kligman LH: The hairless mouse model for photoaging, in *Clinics in Dermatology,* edited by A Ledo. New York, Elsevier, 1996, p 183

88. Kligman LH et al: The contributions of UVA and UVB to connective tissue damage in hairless mice. *J Invest Dermatol* **84**:272, 1985

89. Kligman LH et al: Long wavelength (>340 nm) ultraviolet A induced skin damage in hairless mice is dose dependent, in *Human Exposure to Ultraviolet Radiation: Risks and Regulations,* edited by WF Passchier, BFM Bosnjakovic. Amsterdam, Elsevier, 1987, p 77

90. Kligman LH, Sayre RM: An action spectrum for ultraviolet induced elastosis in hairless mice: Quantification of elastosis by image analysis. *Photochem Photobiol* **53**:237, 1991

91. Hirose R, Kligman LH: An ultrastructural study of ultraviolet-induced elastic fiber damage in hairless mouse skin. *J Invest Dermatol* **90**:697, 1988

92. Kaidbey KH, Kligman AM: Identification of topical photosensitizing agents in humans. *J Invest Dermatol* **70**:149, 1978

93. Harber LC, Bickers DR: Solar urticaria, in *Photosensitivity Diseases: Principles of Diagnosis and Treatment,* edited by LC Harber, DR Bickers. Philadelphia, Saunders, 1981, p 160

94. Gantt R et al: Visible light induces DNA cross-links in cultured mouse and human cells. *Biochim Biophys Acta* **565**:231, 1970

95. Griffin AC et al: The effects of visible light on carcinogenicity of ultraviolet light. *Cancer Res* **10**:523, 1955

96. Kligman LH, Kligman AM: Reflections on heat. *Br J Dermatol* **110**:369, 1984

97. Cross F: On a turf (peat) fire cancer: Malignant change superimposed on erythema ab igne. *Proc R Soc Med* **60**:1307, 1967

98. Kligman LH: Intensification of ultraviolet induced dermal damage by infrared radiation. *Arch Dermatol Res* **272**:229, 1982

99. Schwartz E et al: Collagen alterations in chronically sun-damaged human skin. *Photochem Photobiol* **58**:841, 1993.

100. Kligman LH et al: Collagen loss in photoaging is overestimated by histochemistry (abstr). *J Invest Dermatol* **108**:627, 1997

101. Lovell CR et al: Collagen and elastin in actinic elastosis (abstr). *J Invest Dermatol* **82**:566, 1984

102. Kligman LH et al: Collagen metabolism in ultraviolet irradiated hairless mouse skin and its correlation to histologic observations. *J Invest Dermatol* **93**:210, 1989

103. Plastow SR et al: Early changes in dermal collagen of mice exposed to chronic UVB irradiation and the effects of a UVB sunscreen. *J Invest Dermatol* **91**:590, 1988

104. Schwartz E et al: Alterations in dermal collagen in ultraviolet irradiated hairless mice. *J Invest Dermatol* **93**:142, 1989

105. Schwartz E: Connective tissue alterations in the skin of ultraviolet irradiated hairless mice. *J Invest Dermatol* **91**:158, 1988

106. Johnston KJ et al: Ultraviolet radiation induced connective tissue changes in the skin of hairless mice. *J Invest Dermatol* **82**:587, 1984

107. Trautinger F et al: UVA- and UVB-induced changes in hairless mouse skin. *Arch Dermatol Res* **286**:490, 1994

108. Kligman LH, Gebre M: Biochemical changes in hairless mouse skin collagen after chronic exposure to UVA radiation. *Photochem Photobiol* **54**:233, 1991

109. Schnider SL, Kohn RR: Effects of age and diabetes mellitus on the solubility of collagen from human skin, tracheal cartilage and dura mater. *Exp Gerontol* **17**:185, 1982

110. Fourtanier A et al: In vivo evaluation of photoprotection against chronic ultraviolet-A irradiation by a new sunscreen Mexoryl SX. *Photochem Photobiol* **55**:549, 1992

111. Serri F et al: Studies on the pathomechanics of chronic actinic dermatosis, in *Research in Photobiology,* edited by A Castellani. New York, Plenum, 1977, p 547

112. Fleischmajer R et al: Immunofluorescence analysis of collagen, fibronectin and basement membrane protein in scleroderma skin. *J Invest Dermatol* **75**:270, 1980

113. Kligman LH et al: Prevention of ultraviolet damage to the dermis of hairless mice by sunscreens. *J Invest Dermatol* **78**:181, 1982

114. Kligman LH et al: Sunscreens promote repair of ultraviolet radiation-induced dermal damage. *J Invest Dermatol* **81**:98, 1983

115. Kligman LH et al: Topical retinoic acid enhances the repair of ultraviolet damaged dermal connective tissue. *Connect Tissue Res* **12**:139, 1984

116. Schwartz E et al: Topical all-*trans* retinoic acid stimulates collagen synthesis in vivo. *J Invest Dermatol* **96**:975, 1991

117. Schwartz E, Kligman LH: Topical tretinoin increases tropoelastin and fibronectin content of photoaged hairless mouse skin. *J Invest Dermatol* **104**:518, 1995

118. Kim et al: Effect of topical retinoic acids on the levels of collagen mRNA during the repair of UVB-induced dermal damage in the hairless mouse and the possible role of TGF-β as a mediator. *J Invest Dermatol* **98**:359, 1992

119. Kligman AM et al: Topical tretinoin for photoaged skin. *J Am Acad Dermatol* **15**:836, 1986

120. Weiss JS et al: Topical tretinoin improves photoaged skin: A double-blind, vehicle-controlled study. *JAMA* **259**:527, 1988

121. Woodley DT et al: Treatment of photoaged skin with topical tretinoin increases epidermal-dermal anchoring fibrils: A preliminary report. *JAMA* **263**:3057, 1990

122. Kligman AM, Graham GF: Histological changes in facial skin after daily application of tretinoin for 5 to 6 years. *J Dermatol Treat* **4**:113, 1993

123. Fisher GJ et al: Molecular basis of skin-induced premature skin aging and retinoid antagonism. *Nature* **379**:335, 1996

CHAPTER 147

Bhavik P. Soni
Donald S. McLaren
Elizabeth F. Sherertz

Cutaneous Changes in Nutritional Disease

Nutrition is defined as the process by which a living organism assimilates food or other substances (i.e., nutrients) and uses them for life, growth, and for the maintenance of health. Recently, the role of adequate nutrition, not only in the maintenance of well-being but also in the prevention and treatment of disease, has become the focus of increased attention. Clinical disease can be caused by nutrient deficiency or, less commonly, by nutrient excess. Nutrient deficiency can be due to inadequate intake, abnormal absorption, or improper utilization. Persons at greatest risk for inadequate nutrient intake include infants and the elderly, the impoverished and neglected, those in and from third world countries, those with chronic alcoholism, vegetarians, persons on parenteral nutrition, and those with eating disorders or unusual dietary habits. Inadequate intake can also be the result of hypercatabolic states, such as metastatic cancer, or other severe chronic illness (such as HIV disease). Abnormal absorption can be seen in patients with gastrointestinal diseases such as sprue or in those who have had gastrointestinal surgery. Prolonged antibiotic therapy can also produce a malabsorptive state. Improper utilization can be due to hepatic disease or drug-nutrient interactions. Genetic metabolic defects or enzyme deficiencies can also lead to nutrient deficiency, usually presenting early in life. Multiple factors may work together to produce nutrient deficiency in any given person. Nutrient excess is usually due to excess dietary or therapeutic intake.

Although the focus of this chapter is the cutaneous manifestations of nutritional disease, it is important to remember that nutritional disorders affect biochemical pathways in multiple organs, producing systemic consequences. Cutaneous findings in nutritional diseases can be very specific such as the changes seen in scurvy or pellagra. However, the skin findings are often nondiagnostic. Although certain physical findings are associated with inadequate amounts of specific nutrients, it is important to remember that inadequate dietary intake often leads to multiple deficiencies with overlapping clinical signs. The skin and its appendages can be very useful in the diagnosis of nutritional disease as cutaneous changes are often the chief complaint of the patient and the integumentary system is readily accessible to examination. The clinician must be careful to suspect and screen for nutritional disease, given the appropriate constellation of skin, hair, nail, mucous membrane, and systemic findings. Laboratory analysis of blood and urine nutrient levels can be helpful but should be interpreted cautiously as there is often poor correlation with tissue concentrations. Clinical improvement following replacement therapy may be the only way to confirm the clinical diagnosis. Several excellent reviews have recently discussed nutrition and the skin.[1-5]

ENERGY AND PROTEIN

Experimental Starvation in Adults

The most thorough study of the effects of inanition on the skin of human volunteers was made as part of the monumental Minnesota experiment.[6] The skin of the subjects, after 23 weeks on a diet providing only 1570 kcal, was thinner than normal, dry, inelastic, pallid, and grayish in color. It was described as being cold and "dead" to the touch, with a tendency to cyanosis in cold weather. All these signs were very suggestive of those commonly seen in old age. Less regular in occurrence was the rough gooseflesh appearance similar to the follicular hyperkeratosis associated by some workers with vitamin A deficiency (see "Vitamin A Deficiency," below). A patchy, dirty brownish pigmentation situated anywhere on the body, but most commonly on the face, was found to some degree but never sufficiently marked to resemble the skin changes of pellagra (see below). The hair was dry, dull, and "staring," with a tendency to cease growing and to fall out very easily, very much as described in protein-energy malnutrition in children (see "Kwashiorkor," below).

Privation Starvation in Adults

In times of famine and war many abnormal appearances of the skin have been described, in addition to the obvious loss of subcutaneous fat, which most noticeably affects normally prominent depots of fat (e.g., buttocks) and muscle masses (thighs, back) that waste, causing bones to protrude. Some of these changes may be attributed to starvation in terms of calories, but others are undoubtedly more closely related to the breakdown of sanitary and medical facilities at such times. Pallor of the skin is often more than can be explained by anemia, and the skin is abnormally cold as a result of vasoconstriction. In victims of famine and prisoners of war, the skin has frequently been described as dry, rough, scaly, thin, and inelastic— resembling the skin of old age. A similar appearance is found in any prolonged wasting disease, whatever the cause. In undernourished, dark-skinned people fine, mosaic-like fissuring of the skin is extremely common, particularly of the palms and soles, as are burnished, hyperpigmented lesions over the shins and dorsa of the feet. These appearances are probably related to repeated minor trauma in individuals with chronic marginal undernutrition resulting from habitually consuming a diet low in most essential nutrients.[7]

Follicular hyperkeratosis and folliculosis have been reputed to be associated with undernutrition. The former is recognized clinically as small, hard, elevated nodules around the hair follicles, giving the skin a "nutmeg grater" texture. The follicles may be filled with keratotic plugs. Exactly what is meant by *folliculosis* in nutrition survey reports is far from clear. It usually seems to mean a relative prominence of the hair follicle due to thinning of the epidermal, dermal, and subcutaneous layers of the skin; it is also called *follicular pouting* and *permanent gooseflesh*. The clinical significance of these appearances is unclear (see "Vitamin A Deficiency," below).

Pigmentary changes in the skin are characteristic in semistarvation. Their color is usually brownish, darker than ordinary suntan, and they usually manifest around the mouth and eyes and on the malar prominence. Less commonly, the hands, arms, and trunk are involved. The changes are not like those seen in pellagra.

Changes in the hair have also been reported to occur frequently in semistarvation. It is thin, brittle, grows slowly, falls out prematurely, and rapidly becomes gray. A pronounced development of downy lanugo hair all over the body, but especially on the face and nape of the neck, can be seen. The nails also grow slowly and are brittle. The nails can be fissured or layered, and intranail hemorrhages have been reported.

Cutaneous signs of starvation can also be seen in patients with underlying eating disorders such as anorexia nervosa and bulimia nervosa. Eating disorders should be on the "differential diagnosis" of starvation-related findings, particularly in industrialized nations. Additional findings include features of self-induced vomiting such as abrasions and scars on the hands (Russell's sign), dental enamel erosions, and gingivitis. Other psychiatric signs are also often present, and management by an appropriate psychiatric professional is critical.[8]

Starvation in Children (Marasmus)

Total inanition in the child, with intake of all nutrients greatly reduced but especially protein and energy, soon leads to suppression of growth, negative nitrogen balance due to catabolism of tissue protein for energy, and the state of *marasmus* (Greek, "wasting"). This is one form of what is now termed *protein-energy malnutrition* of early childhood (see also "Kwashiorkor," below). It is widely prevalent throughout the developing regions of the world and is to a large extent responsible for the high mortality in infancy and early childhood. The disturbed nutrition is usually secondary to weaning problems resulting from ignorance, poor hygiene, and economic and cultural factors.[9]

Both marasmus and kwashiorkor can occur in association with underlying HIV disease. The presence of HIV infection exacerbates the severity of the protein-energy malnutrition and leads to an extremely poor prognosis.[10]

In contrast to kwashiorkor, there is classically no clinical edema or dermatosis in marasmus. As in the undernourished, the skin is dry, wrinkled, and loose, due to marked loss of subcutaneous fat. The "monkey facies" with loss of the buccal fat pads is characteristic (Fig. 147-1). Emaciation may be extreme (Fig. 147-2). There is some evidence to suggest that pitting edema is seen only if the subcutaneous fat is largely preserved, as in kwashiorkor.

Kwashiorkor

This form of protein-energy malnutrition results from a diet quantitatively and qualitatively poor in protein and essential amino acids but with an adequate and often excessive intake of energy from carbohydrate sources such as starch or sugar. However, recent evidence suggests that the etiology of kwashiorkor is not wholly nutritional but is likely multifactorial in origin. Possible contributing factors include the presence of aflatoxins, underlying genetic enzyme deficiencies, and oxidant imbalance. The presence of aflatoxins is often associated with the consumption of significant quantities of maize contaminated with *Aspergillus flavus*.[11]

Characteristically, the weaning child is affected; in addition to the dermatosis and hair changes to be described below, there are typically retarded growth, hypoalbuminemia, edema, moon face, fatty liver, diarrhea, and psychomotor changes. Parkinsonian-like tremors known as *kwashi shakes* can be seen in the recovery phase

FIGURE 147-1

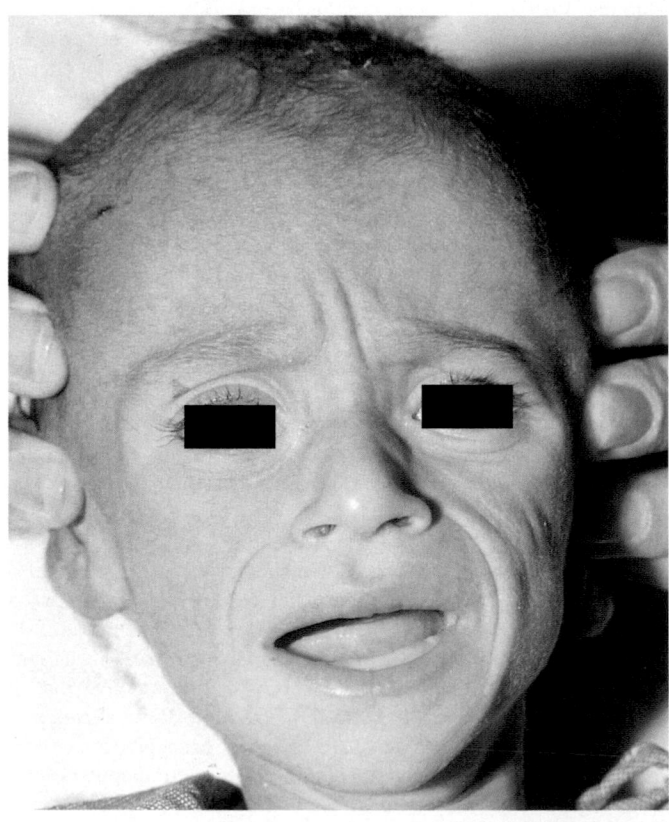

Marasmus. "Monkey facies" in an Arab infant with wrinkled skin and loss of subcutaneous fat.

FIGURE 147-2

FIGURE 147-3

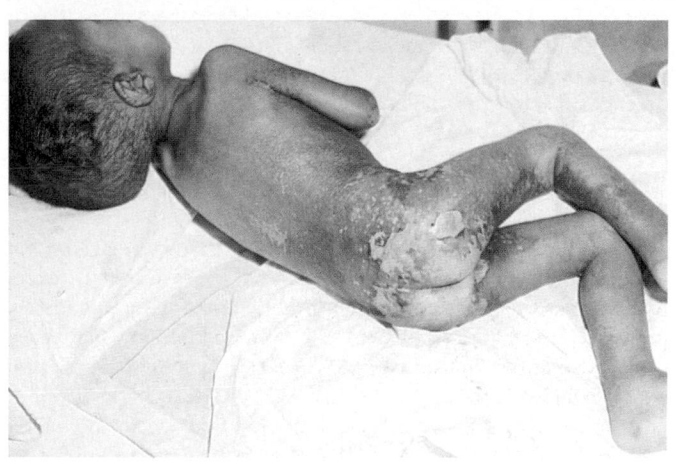

Kwashiorkor. "Flaky paint" dermatosis.

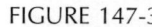

Marasmus. General appearance with advanced disease.

of kwashiorkor.[12] Much less commonly, a similar clinical picture has been reported in school-age children and young adults, and several cases are on record following extensive intestinal surgical treatment resulting in a secondary type of protein malnutrition. Although protein malnutrition is much more common in the third world, it is also the most common form of nutritional deficiency among hospitalized patients in the United States.

The skin lesions are not invariably present in kwashiorkor, but when present they are characteristic. They are more frequent and severe in dark-skinned races; the basic change is depigmentation. The first sign is circumoral pallor; pallor is also marked on the legs. The skin is stretched with edema, and the pallor may be due as much to thinning and distention of the skin as to actual loss of pigment. Localized losses of pigment may follow abrasions, wounds, ulceration, or other injuries (Fig. 147-3).

The characteristic dermatosis in white-skinned infants starts with erythema. At first the skin blanches on pressure, but this is rapidly followed by small, dusky, purple patches that do not blanch. On dark skins, purple areas darken within a few hours of appearing. They have a burnished surface and feel almost waxy to the touch. They have an absolutely sharp edge and appear raised above the surrounding skin, as if small particles of enamel paint had been applied. They are most common in areas subject to pressure, especially if combined with moisture resulting from sweat or any other secretions or discharge. The diaper area is affected early, as also are the trochanters, knees, ankles, elbows, and areas of pressure on the trunk. The dermatosis seldom appears on areas exposed to sunlight, and, in contrast to pellagra, it spares the feet and dorsa of the hands.

In mild cases patients show only a superficial desquamation, but in severe cases there are large areas of erosion in which much skin is lost. This characteristic dermatosis was given the descriptive names of "enamel paint," "flaky paint," and "crazy paving" dermatosis. Advanced cases may also show linear fissuring in the flex-

ures around the pinna, on the back of the knee, in front of the elbow, in the axilla, between the toes, at the edge of foreskin, and in the center of the lips. All these lesions appear to be precipitated by intermittent tension, and those occurring at the corners of the mouth should be distinguished from the angular stomatitis of riboflavin deficiency, in which there is usually a heaped-up, sodden appearance (Fig. 147-4, see also Fig. 147-13). Glossitis can be present. It has been observed that the skin changes of kwashiorkor bear a remarkable resemblance to those of acrodermatitis enteropathica (see Chap. 148). A well-controlled clinical trial to determine the relationship between kwashiorkor and zinc deficiency has not been carried out. Patients show multiple nutritional deficiencies, including that of zinc, and response of the skin and other abnormalities to a complete diet is often dramatic.

FIGURE 147-4

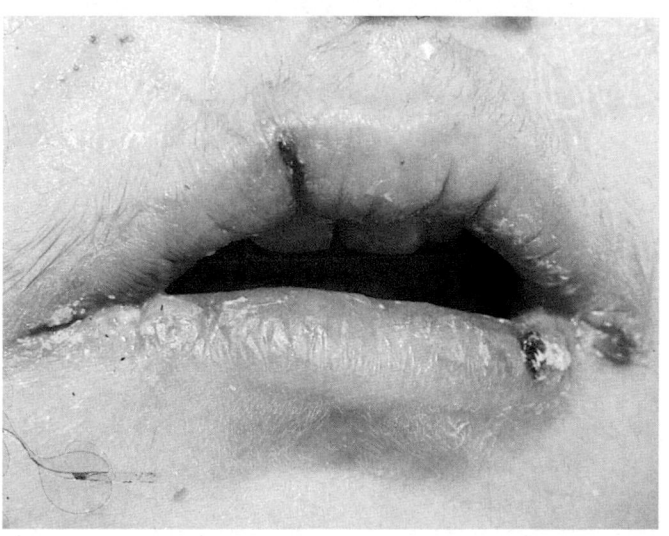

Kwashiorkor. Fissuring of lips in a child (compare with riboflavin in Fig. 147-13).

One of the milder skin changes in kwashiorkor, and the most commonly observed sign involving the skin in fair-skinned children, is a dry, fine desquamation with cracking along the natural lines to give "mosaic skin" or "cracked skin." The shins, outer sides of the thighs, and back of the trunk are among the other areas commonly affected. In fair Arab children, the changes are especially prone to affect the forehead with some hyperpigmentation (Fig. 147-5).

Occasionally on the dorsum of the foot, on the buttocks, or on sites not obviously related to pressure, a large bulla may form and break, leaving a shallow depression.

In advanced kwashiorkor the skin is very easily damaged. Bony points on the pelvis and over the elbows and knees are easily rubbed raw. Special care has to be taken in nursing these cases, most especially if metabolic experiments are being carried out that necessitate keeping the child on a special bed for continuous collection of stools and urine.

True pellagrous skin changes (see below) can occur in children with evidence of kwashiorkor. This is especially apt to arise when children are weaned onto a diet containing much maize flour, as in south and central Africa.

The nails are often thin and soft in kwashiorkor, and this may be particularly obvious when healthy new nails start to grow, forming a mass at the nail base that is completely separated from the old nail.

The hair in kwashiorkor shows depigmentation, is sparse and thin in texture, and comes out easily. None of these changes is specific to kwashiorkor; in malnourished Arab children they are seen about as frequently accompanying marasmus. Kwashiorkor

FIGURE 147-5

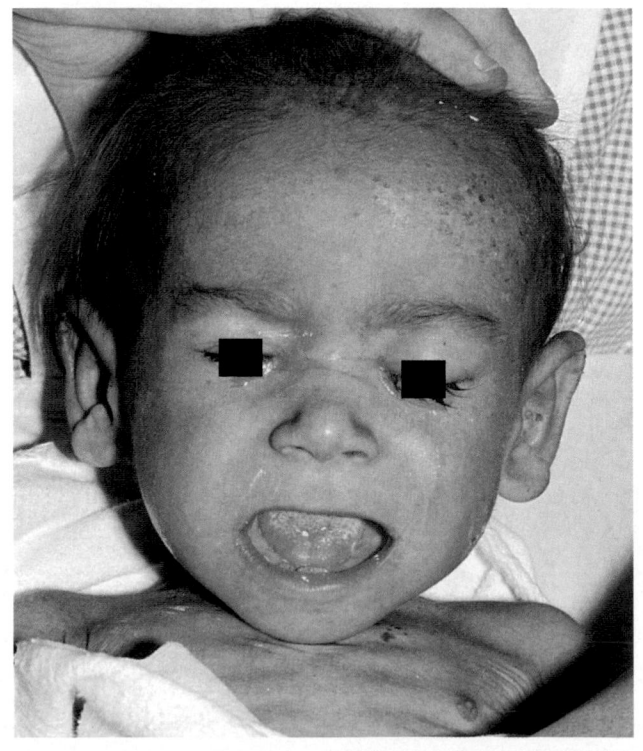

Kwashiorkor. Scaly hyperpigmented dermatosis of the forehead in an Arab child.

may be diagnosed without the presence of hair changes, although this is rather unusual. Hair that is normally black becomes brown or reddish, and brown hair turns blond. Somehow the idea has spread that kwashiorkor means "red boy," red referring to the hair change. The word *kwashiorkor*, however (taken from the Ga language of Ghana), means "the sickness of the weanling," an apt description of the pathogenesis of the condition. There are many causes of bleaching of the hair other than malnutrition—such as sunlight and oxidizing agents—and care must be taken in interpretation. Especially striking is the flag sign (*signe de la bandera*) affecting long and normally dark hair. The hair grown during periods of inadequate nutrition is pale, so that alternating bands of dark and pale hair can be seen along a single strand, recording alternating periods of adequate and inadequate nutrition (Fig. 147-6).

The other changes undergone by the hair are more constant and more reliable than the alterations in color described above. The growth of the hair is sparse and it comes out easily. There may be recession from the temporal region and loss from the back of the head, probably due to pressure when the child lies down. Loss of hair may be extreme in advanced cases. The texture of the hair becomes softer and finer than normal for a child of that age and culture. It tends to be unruly and to resemble the "staring" coat of some animals described in nutritional deficiency. The eyelashes may undergo the same change, having a so-called broomstick appearance.[13]

In health, most of the scalp hairs are in the anagen, or active, growth phase and a few in the telogen, or resting, phase. In early protein-energy malnutrition this is reversed, and analysis of the hair cycle has been advocated as a diagnostic procedure.

Treatment of kwashiorkor involves standard food with adequate protein and caloric intake, mineral and vitamin supplements, and antibiotics. Restoring electrolyte balance is also very important, particularly potassium balance.[14] Mortality in kwashiorkor tends to decrease with increased age of onset. However, severity of growth failure, amount of hypoproteinemia and hypoalbuminemia, and amount of electrolyte imbalance are predictors of poorer prognosis. Coexistent HIV disease, as mentioned, is associated with a very poor prognosis.

Cancrum Oris (Noma, Necrotizing Ulcerative Gingivitis)

Cancrum oris (Fig. 147-7) is a gangrenous disease of the tissues of the mouth, face, and surrounding areas. The disease primarily affects malnourished children from developing countries. Most reports have come from Africa, Southeast Asia, and tropical America. Recently, there have been reports of cases, often in adults, associated with AIDS in North America and Europe.[15] This would indicate that multiple local and systemic factors are implicated in the pathogenesis of noma, with the common denominator being a depressed immune system. Noma also used to be seen occasionally following measles, typhus, and typhoid fever.

The exact etiology of cancrum oris remains unclear. Vincent's organisms are usually present. Cancrum oris is likely due to an opportunistic mixed bacterial infection; however, one case has been reported to be caused by *Pseudomonas aeruginosa*.

Most cases probably start as an area of ulcerative gingivitis with a tender, firm swelling of the upper gum and underlying bone and some swelling of the overlying part of the face. Very soon, the teeth loosen and inflammation spreads into the underlying bone, with osteitis and a sequestrum. The cheek usually ulcerates, producing a cavity leading directly into the mouth. A strong putrid odor is usu-

FIGURE 147-6

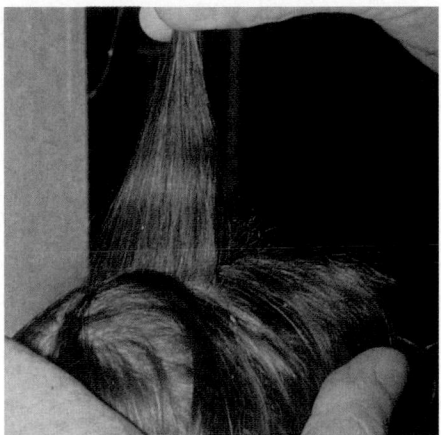

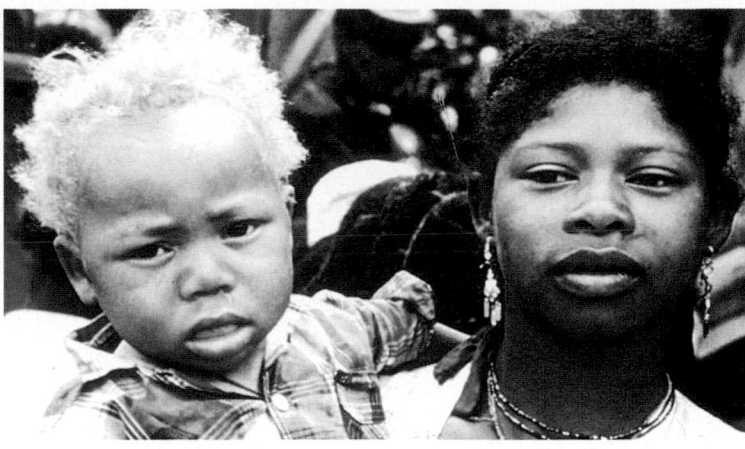

A.   B.

Kwashiorkor. A. Flag sign in a Salvadoran child. B. Hypomelanization of the hair and skin.

ally present. Occasionally the process originates in the nose, vulva, or elsewhere.

Without treatment there is rapid progress of the disease, frequently leading to death. Broad-spectrum antibiotics can halt the progression of the disease, although massive residual defects continue to present extremely difficult cosmetic surgery problems, particularly in relation to the relatively primitive medical facilities available where the disease occurs. A full diet is of great value, especially one rich in protein, high in energy value, and providing all vitamins and essential elements. Feeding difficulties can be overcome if total parenteral nutrition is available.[16,17]

FIGURE 147-7

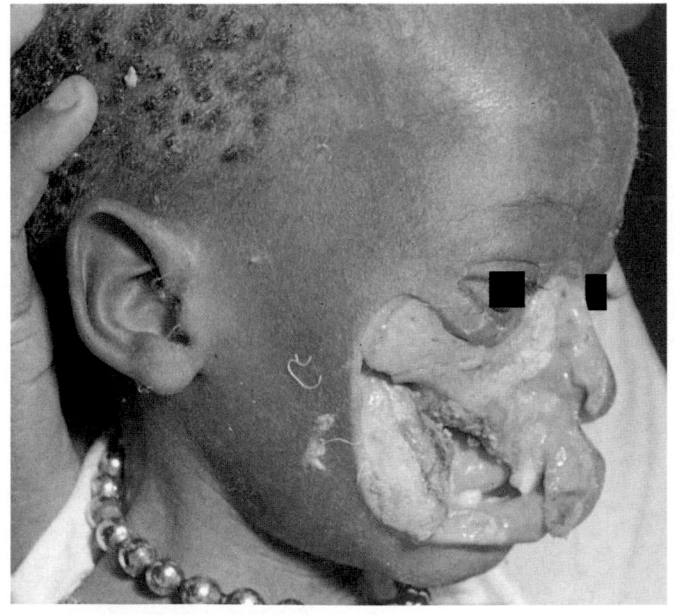

Cancrum oris (noma). Massive destruction of the face in a Tanzanian child.

Tropical Ulcer (Tropical Sloughing Phagedena)

This chronic condition, chiefly affecting the lower limbs above the malleoli, shares with cancrum oris the frequent background of general malnutrition of the patient and the occurrence of Vincent's organisms in the lesions. A survey[18] of 170 patients in Zambia, Gambia, South India, and Papua New Guinea found that children and teenagers were most commonly affected. There was no correlation between the development of an ulcer and nutritional status found in this survey. Nevertheless, a good diet, rest, and antibiotics give good results, and healing is usually complete within 6 months. Surgical debridement of dead tissue may be very helpful.[19]

The disease starts with the formation of a larger or smaller blister with serosanguineous contents. When the bulla ruptures, an ashgray moist slough is exposed. The sloughing process extends rapidly, until the skin and subcutaneous fascia over quite a large area may be converted into a yellowish, moist, foul-smelling ulcer. In extensive cases, muscles, tendons, nerves, vessels, and even the periosteum may have shared in the gangrenous process. Even after healing, deformity may ensue from ankylosis, and a contracting cicatrix may strangulate a vital part, necessitating amputation. Smaller healed tropical ulcers leave behind tissue-paper-like scars with pigmented edges. These are prone to break down.

Obesity

Skin disorders tend to be common in the obese. Excessive fat folds lead to intertrigo from friction between skin surfaces and to maceration of the skin from accumulated moisture in the folds. Infection frequently supervenes, particularly with staphylococci, dermatophytes, and yeast. The obese become overheated easily and sweat more profusely because of the thick layers of subcutaneous fat; areas of inflammation and skin rashes are thus exaggerated. Striae are more frequently seen in the obese. Common sites include the thighs, arms, abdomen, back, and buttocks. Obesity-associated acanthosis nigricans manifests as symmetric, velvety, papillomatous, hyperpigmented plaques in the axilla, groin, and sides of the neck. However, other sites can be involved. Skin tags are often seen in obesity, with or without associated acanthosis nigricans. Hirsutism is more common in the obese. Many obese patients have either a diabetic tendency or frank diabetes, with all the accompanying dermatoses. It is important in all these circumstances that due attention be paid during treatment to measures aimed at correction of the underlying obesity; otherwise, local treatment of the skin lesions will remain purely palliative.[20]

VITAMINS

Vitamin A (Retinol)

This fat-soluble vitamin is found only in the animal kingdom. Many plants contain one or more of the several provitamin carotenoids, of which beta-carotene is the most active. Vitamin A, as the aldehyde (retinal), has a well-defined role in night vision, and the earliest clinical manifestation of vitamin A deficiency is impairment of dark adaptation. In animals, deficiency of vitamin A has been shown to have profound effects, including cessation of growth, death, congenital malformations, and severe damage, especially to epithelial tissues. In both humans and animals, severe deficiency produces destructive eye lesions affecting the conjunctiva (xerosis conjunctivae, Bitot's spots) and cornea (xerosis corneae and keratomalacia). Recent work suggests that even subclinical deficiency of vitamin A is associated with increased morbidity from infections and mortality in young children.

VITAMIN A DEFICIENCY   There is general agreement that severely malnourished patients with the pathognomonic ocular lesions of vitamin A deficiency may also show changes in the skin attributable to the same cause. The skin over large areas of the body is dry, wrinkled, and covered with fine scales. These changes were described in China more than 60 years ago, together with deep, excavated lesions, which were termed *dermomalacia*. Marked changes of this type are extremely uncommon, even in children with bilateral keratomalacia (Figs. 147-8 and 147-9).

Histologically, those skin lesions that can confidently be attributed to vitamin A deficiency represent primary hyperkeratinization and hyperplasia of the epidermis, including the lining of the hair follicles and sebaceous glands. Most characteristically in the conjunctiva and cornea, vitamin A deficiency causes metaplasia, but in the skin there is an accentuation of a process of progressive keratinization normally inherent here.

In infants and very young children, before the pilosebaceous follicle has fully matured, simple xerosis, or xeroderma, is usually the characteristic feature.[21] The stratum corneum is usually several times its normal thickness, and there is blockage of sweat ducts and hyperkeratinization of the follicle lining.

Adults, especially those who have exhibited the advanced ocular manifestations, have shown grosser changes. The stratum corneum forms a broad network of horny plates, with abundant desquamation of fine scales. The stratum lucidum and stratum granulosum remain unchanged. The basal layers are unaltered except for increased melanin deposition. Sebaceous glands are reduced in number and sweat gland ducts are occluded by keratinous material; although the glands are normal in appearance, they are probably hypofunctional. Except for perifollicular infiltration, the dermis is normal.

It is significant that the follicular reaction is minimal in those cases with marked hyperkeratosis and pathognomonic eye lesions; this is in contrast to the pronounced reaction in the very common

FIGURE 147-8

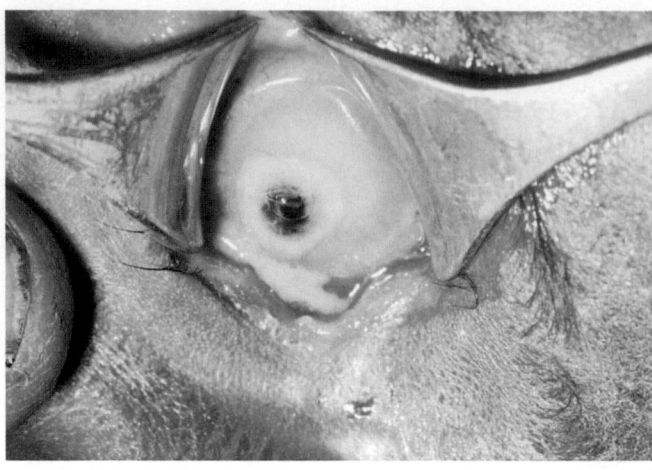

Vitamin A deficiency, advanced keratomalacia. 5-month-old Arab child. Note hyperkeratosis of facial skin. Serum vitamin A level was 2 μg/dL (normal, 20 to 50 μg).

follicular hyperkeratosis usually accompanied by generalized hyperkeratosis or eye changes.

It is a follicular eruption (Figs. 147-10 and 147-11), termed *follicular hyperkeratosis* by Frazier and Hu, that has proved to be so controversial. It is interesting to note that Pillat, the ophthalmologist, made no reference to such a finding, although he was working in the same hospital and the 14 cases that Frazier and Hu reported were drawn from a group of 209 soldiers with ocular lesions seen by Pillat. The follicular changes were described as occurring on a background of generally dry and rough skin. Spinous papules ap-

FIGURE 147-9

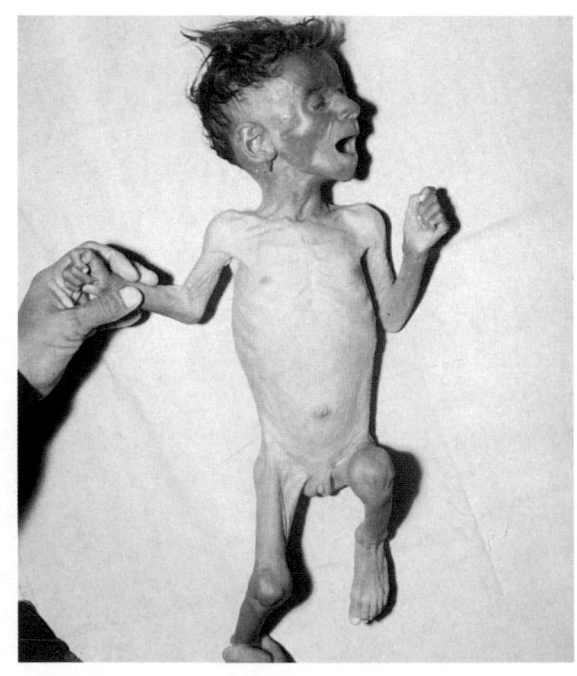

Vitamin A deficiency. General appearance in the same patient as Fig. 147-8.

FIGURE 147-10

CHAPTER 147
Cutaneous Changes in Nutritional Disease

1731

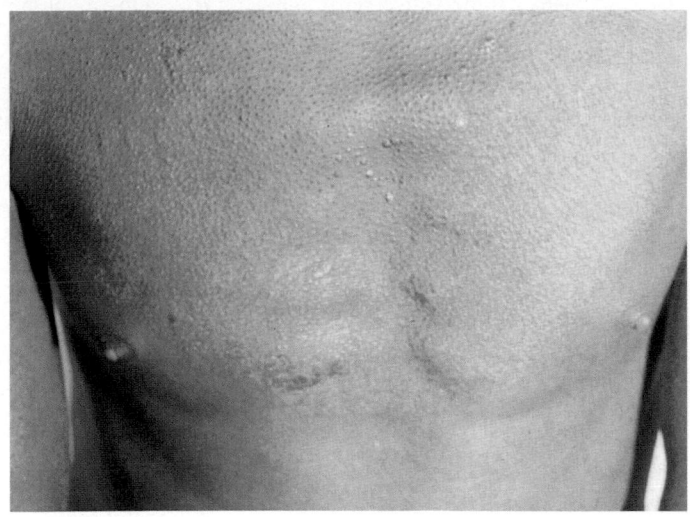

Vitamin A deficiency. Typical perifollicular hyperkeratosis of the chest in a Tanzanian adult male.

peared at the tips of the hair follicles. First affected were the anterolateral aspects of the thighs and the posterolateral parts of the upper forearms. The eruptions slowly spread to the extensor surface of upper and lower limbs; the shoulders; the lower part of the abdomen; and, to a lesser extent, the chest, back, and buttocks. Each papule had a keratotic plug at its apex, projecting as a hard spinous process. The eruption was usually abundant and symmetric. With a generally good diet and cod liver oil (up to 30 mL daily), the skin lesions improved slowly, but even after 2 months the skin had not regained its normal appearance.

Subsequently, under the name of *phrynoderma*, or "toad skin," such follicular changes, frequently of a much milder nature and more limited distribution, have been attributed to nutritional deficiency. Not only deficiency of vitamin A, but deficiency of linoleic acid or vitamins of the B complex have all been implicated.

The evidence from deprivation experiments in humans does not support the contention that follicular hyperkeratosis can be associated specifically with vitamin A deficiency. In the Sheffield experiment, 20 men and 3 women received a diet deficient in vitamin A and carotene for periods ranging from 6 1/2 to 25 months. With regard to the minimal skin changes observed, it was concluded that the enlargement and hyperkeratosis of the hair follicles that occurred among both the supplemented and the deprived group fluctuated in both extent and size of the eruption independently of the state of vitamin A nutrition. Vitamin A deficiency is confirmed by a low plasma retinol level. Administration of vitamin A leads to slow improvement.

In view of the lack of proof of nutritional deficiency as the cause of hyperfollicular keratosis, it is especially important to explore the possibility of other diagnoses. The distribution of the lesions and infrequency of pustulation should rule out acne vulgaris; the rarity of the eruption in postpubertal females and in adolescent children seems incompatible with keratosis pilaris, and the relatively rare Darier's disease may be excluded by the absence of familial tendency and the lack of dyskeratotic changes in the skin specimen.

Massive oral vitamin A therapy has been advocated for many skin conditions of unknown cause, including some mentioned above, that pose problems of differential diagnosis. Other conditions that have been treated with vitamin A include pityriasis rubra pilaris, keratosis palmaris et plantaris, ichthyosis, and pachyonychia. In none of these conditions has a deficiency of vitamin A been demonstrated.

Various synthetic vitamin A derivatives, known as *retinoids*, are effective in a variety of dermatologic diseases in which keratinization is disturbed. Prolonged use and high dosage of these compounds has led to toxic reactions, including severe fetal abnormalities in offspring of women who have become pregnant while receiving the drugs.

VITAMIN A TOXICITY (HYPERVITAMINOSIS A) The skin is frequently involved in both acute and chronic forms of vitamin A toxicity. Desquamation over large areas of the body, accompanied by severe headache and vomiting, has occurred in arctic explorers after a single meal of the liver of polar bear, bearded seal, or sledge dogs previously fed on the livers of these animals. Chronic poisoning results from injudicious therapeutic use of the vitamin or its derivatives. The bizarre symptomatology includes coarsening of the skin, with pruritus, exfoliative dermatitis, and loss of hair. Frequently the true diagnosis is made only when it occurs to someone to have the serum level of vitamin A checked by the laboratory. The unfortunate patients have been labeled as having brain tumors, psychoneurosis, generalized infectious arthritis, Addison's disease, hepatitis, or dermatomyositis before the true nature of the process has been determined.

Both acute and chronic manifestations of hypervitaminosis A must be watched for in young children; increasing numbers of such cases are being reported in the literature. Central nervous system and bone changes are especially common, but pruritus and desquamation are not infrequent.

Withdrawal of vitamin A brings about improvement over several weeks, and, in spite of the alarming manifestations of vitamin A poisoning, no fatalities have been reported to date.

CAROTENODERMA Carotenoid (beta-carotene) absorption is enhanced in the presence of dietary fat. Carotenoids have a long time constant for serum accumulation: 9 to 10 days. The time taken to produce clinically appreciable pigmentation depends to some extent on dietary consumption of carotenoids. Measurements of skin color

FIGURE 147-11

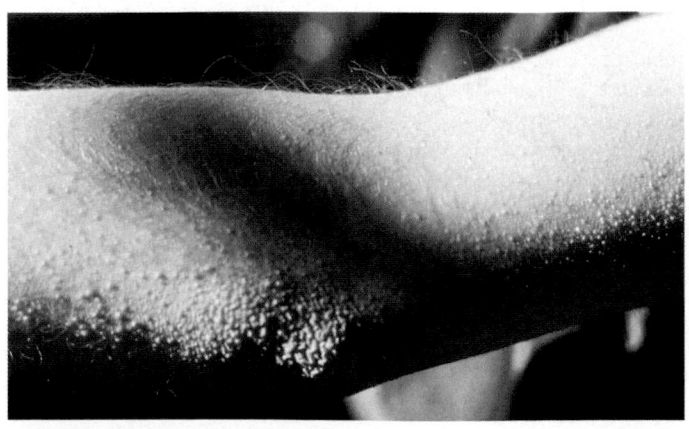

Vitamin A deficiency. Marked perifollicular hyperkeratosis on the arm in an undernourished Iranian child.

have shown that the accumulation of beta-carotene in skin is delayed by up to 2 weeks compared with serum accumulation.[22] Hypercarotenemia does not usually produce carotenoderma until the serum carotene level is usually three or four times normal. In one instance, 1.8 kg of carrots was consumed weekly for 7 months. Children develop carotenoderma more readily than adults. An infant showed the characteristic yellowish skin pigmentation after only 2 months on the breast milk of its carotenemic mother, while another, born pigmented to such a mother, remained yellow until weaned. Appropriate laboratory tests, including determination of total serum carotenoid (usual range for healthy adults: 40 to 150 μg/dL), will differentiate hypercarotenosis from such conditions as hemolytic anemia, pernicious anemia, or obstructive jaundice. Patients with high carotene levels in the blood will also often have slightly increased vitamin A levels. There is only a slight increase due to the slow conversion of carotene to vitamin A.[23] Carotenoderma is especially likely to occur during wartime, with rationing of meat, butter, and cheese and with increased consumption of fresh green leafy vegetables—rich sources of beta-carotene. It is endemic in parts of the world such as central and west Africa where red palm oil is used for cooking.[24]

Excess carotene is, in part, excreted in sweat and reabsorbed by the horny layer of the skin. Carotenoderma is said to develop more readily in those who sweat profusely. Deposition occurs first and predominantly in the nasolabial folds and over the forehead, where sebaceous glands abound, and on the palms and soles where the horny layer of the skin is thickest. It has to be borne in mind that some carotene is present in all normal skin. Carotene is found to a lesser degree on the upper eyelids, inner canthi, ears, and anterior folds of the axillae and over areas subject to pressure, e.g., the elbows, knees, and malleoli. This uneven distribution helps to distinguish carotenoderma from jaundice.

The color of the skin is canary yellow, ochre, or golden. It never has the bronze, orange, saffron, or green tint of jaundice. Mucous membranes, including the sclerae, are not stained by carotene. Subconjunctival or submucosal fat, if present, may be stained and lead to confusion. Other points of differentiation from jaundice are that hypercarotenosis does not cause itching and does not significantly change the color of urine or stools, although plasma is bright yellow. As far as is known, hypercarotenosis in all its forms appears to be harmless. If of dietary origin, it slowly disappears when the intake is reduced to normal levels. Resolution is slow due to the lipophilic character of carotenoids.

In diabetes mellitus there is frequently a raised serum carotene level, but carotenoderma develops in only about 10 percent of cases. In this disease it is probably due to a high dietary consumption, but there may possibly be impaired conversion of carotene to vitamin A. Some patients with hypothyroidism also have carotenoderma, and this may be related to the known function of thyroid hormone in facilitating carotene conversion. Hypercarotenemia has been consistently reported in anorexia nervosa. It occasionally results in carotenoderma and is of obscure origin.

Lycopenemia is a similar condition associated with orange-yellow skin pigmentation as a result of excess lycopene ingestion (e.g., excess tomatoes).

Vitamins of the B Complex

NIACIN (PELLAGRA)   The amide of niacin is an important constituent of coenzyme I (oxidized form of nicotinamide-adenine dinucleotide, NAD) and coenzyme II (reduced form of nicotinamide-adenine dinucleotide, NADP), which either donate or accept hydrogen ions in vital oxidation-reduction reactions. The essential amino acid tryptophan can be converted in the body to niacin, about 60 mg of tryptophan being the dietary equivalent of 1 mg of niacin. The cause of pellagra is still not entirely clear. It may arise from a diet deficient in niacin or tryptophan, or more commonly both, and amino acid imbalance may also play a part. A predominantly maize diet is usually implicated, but only if the maize is steamed or cooked. In parts of Latin America, maize flour is lime-treated and made into tortillas; this process releases niacin from an insoluble form called niacytin and usually prevents the occurrence of pellagra. Alterations in tryptophan metabolism secondary to carcinoid, Hartnup's disease, or ingestion of certain drugs (isoniazid, 5-fluorouracil, 6-mercaptopurine, or sulfapyridine) can also lead to niacin deficiency and pellagra.[25] Besides the dermatosis, there are important gastrointestinal and nervous system changes. Pellagra is characterized by the "three Ds": dermatitis, diarrhea, and dementia.[26]

The dermatosis is usually preceded by prodromal symptoms, especially of the digestive system. The skin changes are characteristic and pathognomonic, and their distribution is determined especially by exposure to the sun and by localized pressure. The diagnosis of pellagra is difficult in the absence of the dermatosis, which begins as erythema on the dorsa of the hands, with pruritus and burning. It is characteristically symmetric with slight edema of the skin. In some patients, several days after the onset of the erythema, blisters appear; these run together to form bullae and then break. In others, dry brown scales form. On the face, the scales are thicker, larger, and frequently become pustular.

In the second stage, the dermatosis becomes hard, rough, cracked, blackish, and brittle. The epidermis of the fingers thickens, and the articular folds disappear. Painful fissures develop in the palms and on the digits. The skin may look like that of a goose; hence the term *goose skin*. When the deficiency state is far advanced, the skin becomes progressively harder, drier, more cracked, and covered with scales and blackish crusts that are due to hemorrhages.

The usual sites are the face and neck and dorsal surfaces of the hands, arms, and feet. The changes are rarely seen elsewhere. The dorsa of the hands are the most frequent site; here the lesions may extend up the arms to form the "glove" or "gauntlet" of pellagra (Fig. 147-12*A*). The symmetry and clear line of demarcation from normal skin are especially striking. On the feet the lesions usually do not rise proximally to the malleoli, which are included; the heels remain free. Distally, the eruption ends at the toes or on the backs of the great toes. The front and back of the leg may be involved to form a "boot."

On the face the symmetry of the lesions is striking. They tend to spread from the sides to the rest of the nose, the forehead, cheeks, chin, lips, and, more rarely, eyelids and ears. The "butterfly" appearance, common to lupus erythematosus, is frequent. On the forehead there is always a narrow border of normal skin between the erythema and the hair. The face is often only slightly affected. The facial lesions never appear independently of lesions on the hands and elsewhere.

Casal's "necklace" extends as a fairly broad band, or collar, entirely around the neck (Fig. 147-12*B*). If the band is incomplete, the lesions are striking in their symmetry. The upper border reaches from somewhat below the hairline to the larynx anteriorly. The lower border begins under the vertebral prominences and extends to the edge of the manubrium. In many instances the necklace has an anterior continuation, or broad "cravat," extending from the manubrium over the sternum to the level of the nipples, ending in a point or square. Men, women, and children have the necklace, and it is always accompanied by the characteristic dermatosis elsewhere.

FIGURE 147-12

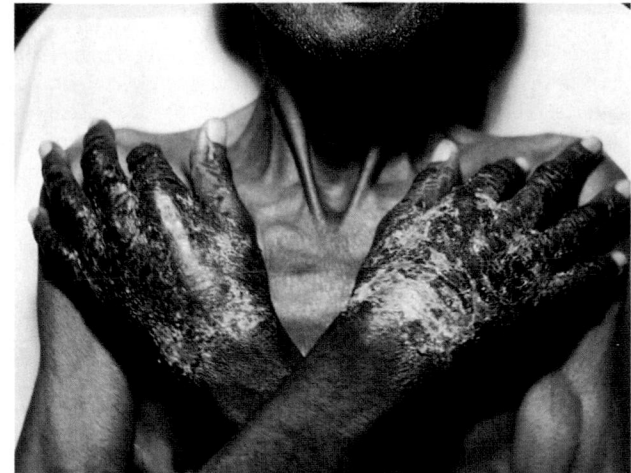

A.

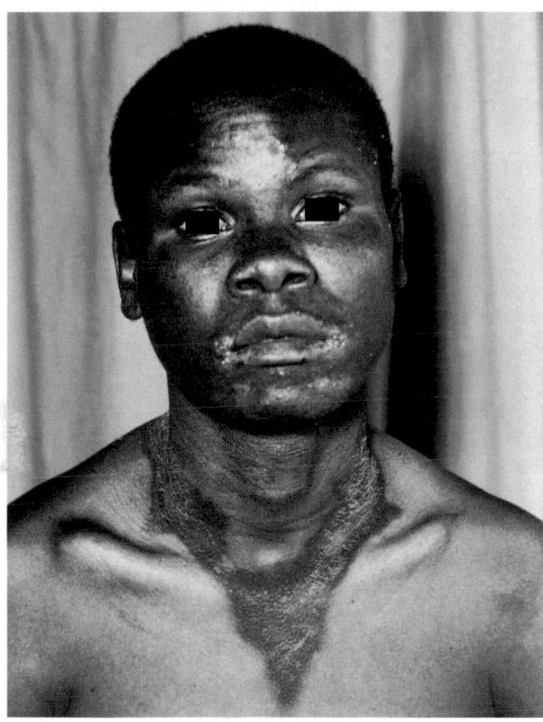

B.

Pellagra. Acute dermatosis: *A.* "Glove" or "gauntlet" exudative and crusted lesions on the hands. *B.* Casal's "necklace" on the neck with facial involvement.

Other sites occasionally affected are the shoulders, elbows, forearms, and knees. The so-called pellagrous vulvitis, vaginitis, and lesions of the perianal region and scrotum are dealt with as part of the "oro-oculo-genital" syndrome [see "Riboflavin (Oro-Oculo-Genital Syndrome)," below]. Features of the oro-oculo-genital syndrome can occur with niacin deficiency.

Healing usually takes place centrifugally, with the line of demarcation remaining actively inflamed after the center of the lesion has desquamated. The diagnosis can be confirmed by finding decreased levels of the urinary metabolites. Specific therapy consists of the oral administration of 100 to 300 mg of niacinamide daily in

divided doses. The amide is preferable since it does not precipitate the vasomotor disturbances resulting from administration of niacin in large doses. A similar dose is given subcutaneously when diarrhea or a noncooperative patient makes oral administration ineffective or difficult. Multivitamins (especially other vitamins of the B complex) and a high-quality protein diet should be given.

RIBOFLAVIN (ORO-OCULO-GENITAL SYNDROME)   This vitamin has coenzyme function in the chain of reversible oxidation-reduction reactions on which tissue respiration depends. A variety of lesions have been produced by animal experimental deficiency, but in humans the changes appear mainly in the skin and mucous membranes.

For many years a syndrome resembling pellagra but without the typical dermatosis had been known, going by the rather confusing name of *pellagra sine pellagra.* Sebrell and Butler studied a group of patients on a diet low in riboflavin and nicotinic acid and showed that the manifestations of pellagra sine pellagra were due to riboflavin deficiency. The changes commenced with pallor of the mucosa in the angles of the mouth. This was soon followed by an angular stomatitis with maceration and superficial linear fissures (Fig. 147-13). These fissures remained moist and became crusted. The skin of the nasolabial folds, on the alae nasi, in the vestibule of the nose, and sometimes on the ears and at the inner and outer canthi of the eyelids became rather greasy and scaly, producing a seborrheic dermatitis–like picture (Fig. 147-14).

In addition to these changes, other alterations of the skin and mucous membranes have been associated with riboflavin deficiency,[27] but it needs to be emphasized that none is pathognomonic. These changes include (1) soggy, white, angular lesions of the mouth, usually termed *perlèche* (French, perlècher, "to lick thoroughly with the tongue"), often associated with moniliasis; (2) involvement of the vermilion border of the lips including vertical fissuring, usually termed *cheilosis* (Greek, cheilos, "lip"); (3) a

FIGURE 147-13

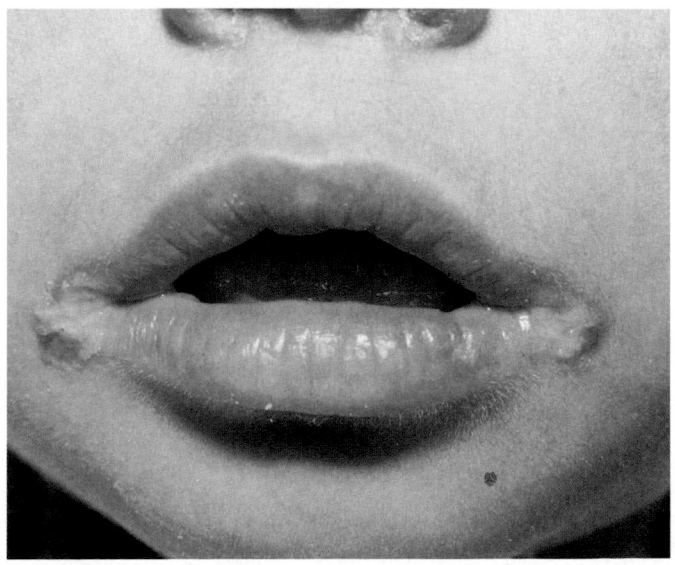

Riboflavin deficiency. Angular stomatitis with maceration in an Arab child. Riboflavin excretion in the urine was diminished.

FIGURE 147-14

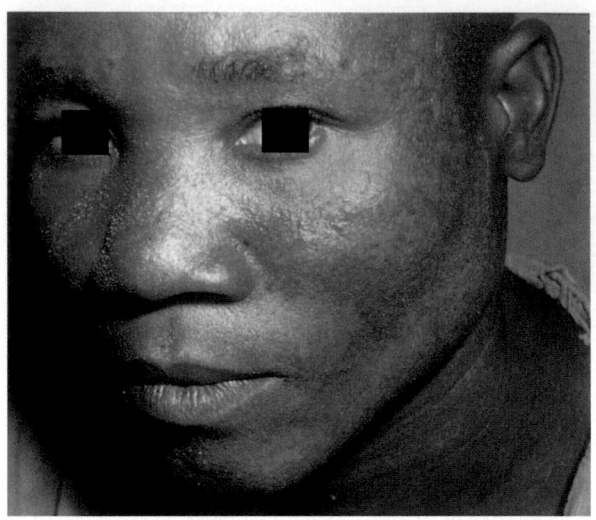

Riboflavin deficiency. Early nasolabial seborrhea in an African boy.

glossitis in which the tongue is smooth and has a magenta color; (4) rarely corneal vascularization and interstitial keratitis; and (5) lesions of the scrotum and vulva.

The dermatosis affecting the genital area has frequently been reported to be the earliest manifestation of riboflavin deficiency and also one of the most common. It may begin either as a patchy redness associated with scaling of the superficial epithelium or as a fine, powdery desquamation without any color change. In chronic cases lichenification is a characteristic feature, and far-advanced lesions are raw and extend up the shaft of the penis or onto the inner aspects of the thighs. When solitary, riboflavin deficiency usually promptly and dramatically responds to riboflavin supplementation (5 to 10 mg of riboflavin daily). However, riboflavin deficiency is usually a component of a mixed B-vitamin deficiency.

Sideropenic anemia with epithelial lesions (Plummer-Vinson syndrome), which has a little-understood relationship to postcricoid carcinoma, may be accompanied by evidence of riboflavin deficiency as well as deficiency of iron and other vitamins of the B complex.

PYRIDOXINE (VITAMIN B$_6$) Pyridoxine acts mainly as a coenzyme in the decarboxylation and transamination of a number of amino acids. It also plays a role in the conversion of linoleic to arachidonic acid and in adrenocortical function. It is now well established that occasional cases of both microcytic hypochromic and megaloblastic types of anemia may respond to pyridoxine therapy. In pyridoxine dependency, in which there is no deficiency of the coenzyme form of the vitamin but a defect in the apoenzyme itself, reversal of the clinical and biochemical changes is obtained only with massive doses of pyridoxine. One form of dependency is familial xanthurenic aciduria with urticaria as the main feature.

Adults may live on a pyridoxine-deficient diet for up to 2 months and remain symptom-free. However, symptoms of pyridoxine deficiency can occur after prolonged administration of an antimetabolite, desoxypyridoxine. In one study, the symptoms included seborrhea-like changes around the eyes, nose, and mouth; cheilosis; and glossitis. No response occurred with administration of thiamine,

riboflavin, or niacinamide, but the process cleared completely with pyridoxine. During the test period, there was increased excretion of xanthurenic acid.

Alcoholism and the intake of certain drugs can produce a pyridoxine deficiency state. Drugs that may impair pyridoxine metabolism include isoniazid, hydralazine, D-penicillamine, and oral contraceptives. The diagnosis may be confirmed by decreased serum levels of pyridoxine-t-phosphate. Replacement of pyridoxine leads to rapid improvement of oral lesions over days and cutaneous lesions over weeks.

VITAMIN B$_{12}$ (COBALAMIN) This vitamin, together with folic acid, is involved in the synthesis of DNA. Vegetarians can have insufficient vitamin B$_{12}$ intake. However, deficiency is usually due to malabsorption. A decrease in gastric intrinsic factor due to pernicious anemia or gastrectomy can produce vitamin B$_{12}$ deficiency. Vitiligo, alopecia areata, or premature graying of the hair can be seen with pernicious anemia. There are several reports of patients with vitamin B$_{12}$ deficiency having symmetric hyperpigmentation of the extremities and over the palms and dorsal aspects of the hands and around the wrists and forearms; it can also involve the lower limbs with a similar distribution.[28] In one case, epidermal cells in areas of pigmentation had abnormally large nuclei. Pigmented nail streaks can occur. A burning tongue is a characteristic finding. A macrocytic anemia can be seen, but the diagnosis is confirmed by decreased vitamin B$_{12}$ levels. There is a good response to treatment with parenteral vitamin B$_{12}$. Untreated pernicious anemia can lead to serious degenerative neurologic changes in the posterior columns and corticospinal tracts of the spinal cord.

VITAMIN B$_1$ (THIAMINE) Thiamine pyrophosphate is an enzyme involved in carbohydrate metabolism by decarboxylating alpha-keto acids. Thiamine is also a coenzyme in the pentose monophosphate pathway for glucose. Thiamine deficiency is known as *beriberi*. Thiamine deficiency can be due to inadequate intake, seen in persons subsisting on polished-rice diets. However, deficiency in the United States is most often seen in association with alcoholism. In alcoholism, there is a combination of decreased intake and impaired absorption and utilization, along with increased requirements.

Symptoms are predominantly neurologic and include a peripheral neuropathy with lower extremity paresthesia and burning of the feet. Korsakoff's syndrome (mental confusion and confabulation) and Wernicke's encephalopathy are seen. Mucocutaneous findings include edema and glossitis. Thiamine replacement is critical. However, thiamine deficiency is often seen associated with other B-complex vitamin deficiencies as well as folate deficiency. Broad nutritional support is usually required.

FOLIC ACID Folic acid acts as a coenzyme in purine and pyrimidine nucleotide biosynthesis. Folic acid deficiency produces a megaloblastic anemia. Dermatologic findings include glossitis and stomatitis. Vitiligo has been an associated finding in some patients. Serum levels of folic acid are low. Prior to treatment with folate, it is important to rule out a coexistent vitamin B$_{12}$ deficiency. Otherwise, the folate supplementation will alleviate the megaloblastic anemia, but the neurologic damage (from vitamin B$_{12}$ deficiency) will continue to progress.

BIOTIN Biotin deficiency occurs rarely. It can occur in neonatal or infantile forms as a result of genetic enzyme deficiencies (holocarboxylase synthetase or biotinidase enzymes).[29] Deficiency can also be seen with impaired absorption or from excessive raw egg-white intake. Raw egg-whites contain avidin, a biotin antagonist.

Patients who are receiving total parenteral nutrition without added biotin have also developed deficiency.

Biotin deficiency presents with scaling eczematoid and xerotic lesions on the arms, legs, and feet. Perioral and genital erosions and scaling are seen. There is also cheilosis, a waxy pallor of the face, and alopecia. Lethargy and hypotonia are among the neuropsychiatric changes seen. Symptoms will usually respond to biotin supplementation.[30]

PANTOTHENIC ACID   This is a component of coenzyme A and is involved in the process of acetylation. No deficiency symptoms have resulted during controlled human experiments in which volunteers were fed deficient diets. These results fail to substantiate frequent claims that have been made for the efficacy of pantothenic acid in the treatment of the "burning feet" syndrome.

Vitamin C (Ascorbic Acid)

Vitamin C plays an important role in the formation of collagen. Vitamin C is a necessary cofactor for prolyl hydroxylase, which catalyzes the hydroxylation of proline and lysine residues in procollagen. Nonhydroxylated collagen is weaker and more unstable

and does not adopt the usual triple helical structure. Vitamin C deficiency (*scurvy*) is usually seen in individuals with inadequate intake of fresh fruits or vegetables, such as the elderly or those who abuse alcohol. Clinical manifestations of vitamin C deficiency can be seen in the skin (Fig. 147-15), mucous membranes, bones, and blood. Poor wound healing is also seen in deficiency states. Scurvy often remains latent for several months following onset of severe vitamin C deficiency. Myalgias, malaise, and weakness often precede the cutaneous manifestations.[31]

Cutaneous manifestations of scurvy begin with follicular hyperkeratosis; the associated hair is often coiled or looped ("curly corkscrew hairs"). The main sites affected are the upper arms, back, buttocks, thighs, calves, and shins. Over time, blood vessels around the follicles proliferate and then bleed, producing perifollicular purpura. Perifollicular purpura are most often seen on the legs. Generalized ecchymoses can occur. Old scars can break down, and new wounds heal poorly. Bones can develop subperiosteal hemorrhage. Vitamin C deficiency also produces gum changes. The earliest signs are redness, swelling, and bleeding at the tips of the interdental papillae. Continued deficiency can lead to frank necrosis.

FIGURE 147-15

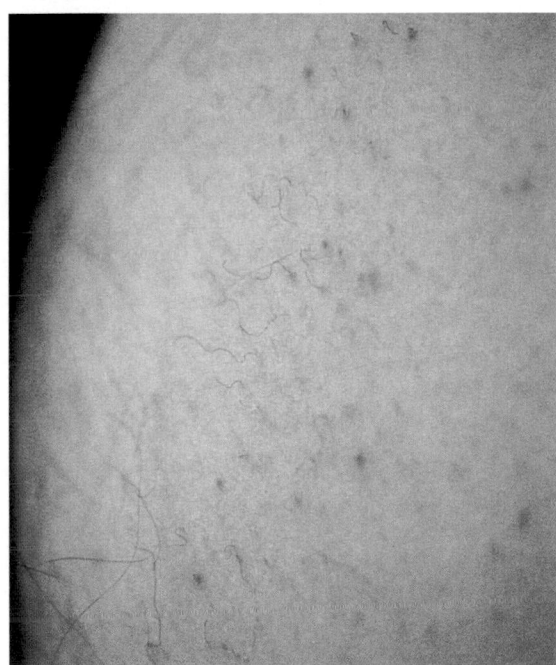

A.

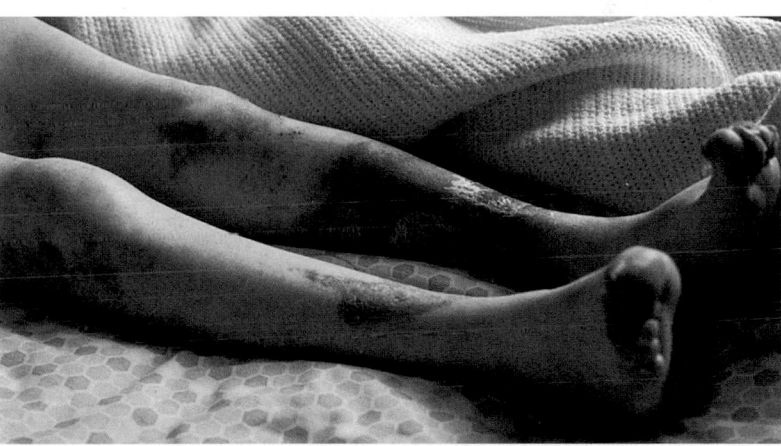

B.

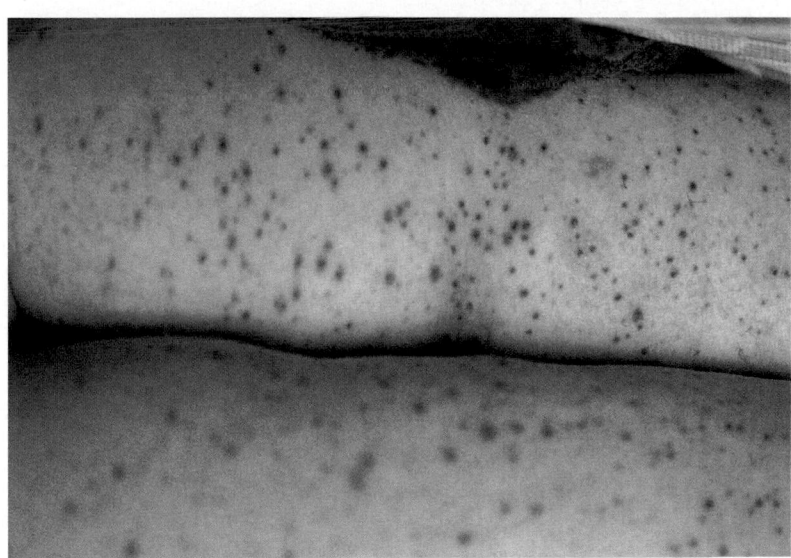

C.

Vitamin C deficiency (scurvy). 61-year-old male in Edinburgh, Scotland. *A.* "Swan neck" deformity of the hairs. *B.* Ecchymoses over the legs, especially around a varicose ulcer on the left. *C.* Numerous perifollicular petechial hemorrhages over the backs of the thighs.

Although perifollicular purpura and corkscrew hairs are virtually diagnostic of scurvy, the diagnosis is often missed due to a low index of suspicion. Scurvy can be mistaken for cutaneous vasculitis. Diagnosis is usually based on history, characteristic findings on physical examination, and determination of L-ascorbic acid levels. Biopsy is usually not necessary but can help to exclude cutaneous vasculitis. A positive capillary fragility test is also usually present.

Patients respond quickly to the administration of oral vitamin C. Adults may need up to 800 mg daily initially and then half this amount daily until recovery. Infants should receive 150 mg daily for up to a month. Thereafter, for both adults and infants, a daily intake of vitamin C in the form of fresh fruits or supplements should be ensured.[32]

Vitamin C excess can result from excessive intake. Manifestations are usually systemic. However, cutaneous manifestations of scurvy have been seen when excessive vitamin C intake has been abruptly discontinued.

Vitamin K

Vitamin K is a fat-soluble vitamin that is required for the synthesis of clotting factors II, VII, IX, and X. Vitamin K deficiency leads to hypoprothrombinemia and deficiency of other clotting factors, resulting in a coagulation-cascade impairment. Bleeding may occur anywhere in the body, including the skin. The presence of purpura is the major cutaneous finding. Massive hemorrhage can occur with vitamin K deficiency. In hemorrhagic disease of the newborn, areas of predilection include the umbilicus, skin, nose and mouth, intestines, and brain. The diagnosis can be confirmed by a prothrombin time measurement. Differentiation from scurvy, hemophilia, and thrombocytopenia can be made on the basis of differing clinical and laboratory features.

Intramuscular phytonadione (vitamin K_1) is the treatment. Dosage is 5 to 10 mg in adults, 2 mg in young children, and 1 mg in newborns, who usually receive it routinely. Skin reactions occurring after vitamin K_1 injection are rare but do occur. An acute eczematous reaction can be seen (a type IV allergic reaction) and more rarely a late-onset localized sclerosis and atrophy, which resembles morphea.[33]

Vitamin D

Vitamin D is a fat-soluble vitamin whose synthesis begins in the skin. Skeletal changes and muscle weakness are seen in vitamin D deficiency, but there are no cutaneous alterations. Recent advances in the understanding of the vitamin D receptor in the skin have led to an increased use of vitamin D analogues in the management of skin disease.[34]

ESSENTIAL FATTY ACIDS

Essential fatty acids are unsaturated fatty acids that the body cannot synthesize, and therefore they must be obtained from the diet. Linoleic acid and linolenic acid are essential fatty acids. Arachidonic acid is synthesized in the body from linoleic acid. Essential fatty acid deficiency can be seen in association with protein-energy malnutrition and low-fat diets. Although the total fat intake in many developing countries is low, fat of vegetable origin is very rich in linoleic acid. Essential fatty acid deficiency has also been associated with long-term parenteral nutrition.[35] However, the current use of a 10% fat emulsion prevents this complication.

Linoleic acid deficiency is associated with growth failure and a dry, scaly skin eruption, frequently on the legs. Alopecia can occur. Essential fatty acid deficiency has been associated with impaired inflammatory reactions, particularly delayed skin hypersensitivity.[36] Linolenic acid deficiency may also produce neurologic damage.

Deficiency is characterized by low plasma levels of linoleic and arachidonic acid. There are also increased levels of eicosatrienoic acid (upper limit of normal for ratio of eicosatrienoic acid to eicosatetraenoic acid is 0.4). Treatment is with essential fatty acid replacement.

ESSENTIAL ELEMENTS

Iron

Chronic iron deficiency is associated with glossitis, cheilosis, and koilonychia (spoon-shaped deformity of fingernails and toenails). In advanced cases, dysphagia associated with a postcricoid esophageal web is seen (Plummer-Vinson syndrome). Iron deficiency is the commonest cause of anemia. Iron replacement can be provided by ferrous sulfate or ferrous gluconate. However, a search for the cause of the iron deficiency is perhaps the most important aspect of management.

Chronic iron overload (*hemosiderosis*), when associated with tissue injury, is known as *hemochromatosis*. Typical findings include cirrhosis of the liver, a bronze pigmentation of the skin, diabetes mellitus, and cardiomyopathy. Iron overload is also a factor in the development of porphyria cutanea tarda. Phlebotomy is the treatment of choice. Early diagnosis and management can often prevent the end-organ damage.[37]

Zinc (See Chap. 148)

Acrodermatitis enteropathica is an autosomal recessive condition due to impaired absorption of zinc. Clinical features include a triad of dermatitis, diarrhea, and alopecia. The dermatitis usually includes an eczematous and erosive eruption around the mouth, acral, and genital areas. Pustular paronychia, angular stomatitis, glossitis, and a generalized alopecia are present. Other signs include diarrhea, growth retardation, poor appetite, mental lethargy, poor wound healing, decreased cell-mediated immunity, and neurosensory disorders including night blindness and impaired taste (hypogeusia). Lack of gonadal development can occur in males. The condition is fatal without zinc supplementation.[38]

Zinc deficiency can be seen in other settings. It has been reported in breast-fed preterm infants,[39] patients with cystic fibrosis, the elderly, and inhabitants of underdeveloped countries with diets high in cereal proteins.[40,41] It can also occur in patients with other chronic diseases. Cutaneous features are similar to acrodermatitis enteropathica.

Copper

Menkes' kinky (steely) hair disease is an X-linked recessive disorder caused by defective copper absorption (see Chap. 71). Affected infants have low levels of copper and ceruloplasmin. Many copper-dependent enzymes are affected, including lysyl oxidase, producing defective elastin.[42] Symptoms include growth retardation, cerebral degeneration, sparse and brittle hair, arterial lesions, and bone changes. The hair is hypopigmented and twisted like pili torti. Parenteral copper does not alter the course of the disease, and the outcome is fatal. Infants on an exclusively milk diet or prolonged parenteral nutrition can develop a similar syndrome, which is copper-responsive.[43]

Selenium

Several patients on prolonged parenteral nutrition in the United States developed a syndrome that included a white appearance of the fingernail beds and dyschromotrichia; these changes were reversed by administration of selenium.[44] Acute poisoning with selenium is often fatal, and skin changes include alopecia; paronychia; possible nail loss; and red pigmentation of nails, hair, and teeth.[45]

Manganese

A report exists of a single case of manganese deficiency, occurring in a volunteer who inadvertently received a deficient diet, developed transient dermatitis, changes in hair color, and slow growth of hair.[46]

REFERENCES

1. Ryan AS, Goldsmith LA: Nutrition and the skin. *Clin Dermatol* **14**:389, 1996
2. Brooke P: Diseases of nutrition and metabolism. *Adv Dermatol* **8**:155, 1993
3. Goskowicz M, Eichenfield LF: Cutaneous findings of nutritional deficiencies in children. *Curr Opin Pediatr* **5**:441, 1993
4. Prendiville JS, Manfredi LN: Skin signs of nutritional disorders. *Semin Dermatol* **11**:88, 1992
5. Miller SJ: Nutritional deficiency and the skin. *J Am Acad Dermatol* **21**:1, 1989
6. Keys A et al: *The Biology of Human Starvation,* 2 vols. Minneapolis, Univ of Minnesota Press, 1950
7. Lee BY, Thurmon TF: Nutritional disorders in a concentration camp. *J Am Coll Nutr* **16**:366, 1997
8. Gupta MA et al: Dermatologic signs in anorexia nervosa and bulimina nervosa. *Arch Dermatol* **123**:1386, 1987
9. McLaren DS: Skin in protein calorie malnutrition. *Arch Dermatol* **123**:1674, 1987
10. Prazuck T et al: HIV infection and severe malnutrition: A clinical and epidemiological study in Burkina Faso. *AIDS* **7**:103, 1993
11. Ramjee G et al: Aflatoxins and kwashiorkor in Durban, South Africa. *Ann Trop Paediatr* **12**:241, 1992
12. Thame M et al: Parkinsonian-like tremors in the recovery phase of kwashiorkor. *W Ind Med J* **43**:102, 1994
13. Albers SE et al: A case of kwashiorkor. *Cutis* **51**:445, 1993
14. Manary MJ, Brewster DR: Potassium supplementation in kwashiorkor. *J Pediatr Gastroenterol Nutr* **24**:194, 1997
15. Takkal AM et al: Noma (cancrum oris) associated with kwashiorkor: A case report and review of the literature. *Acta Chir Belg* **96**:179, 1996
16. Adolph HP et al: Noma: A review. *Ann Plast Surg* **37**:657, 1996
17. Costini B et al: Noma or cancrum oris: Etiopathogenic and nosologic aspects. *Med Trop* **55**:263, 1995
18. Robinson DC et al: The clinical and epidemiologic features of tropical ulcer (tropical phagedenic ulcer). *Int J Dermatol* **27**:49, 1988
19. Jackson R, Bell M: Phagedena: Gangrenous and necrotic ulcerations of skin and subcutaneous tissue. *Can Med Assoc J* **126**:363, 1982
20. Bray GA: Health hazards of obesity. *Endocrinol Metabol Clin North Am* **25**:907, 1996
21. Christiansen EN et al: Serum lipids in children with xeroderma from an inland district of Sri Lanka. *Ann Nutr Metab* **39**:9, 1995
22. Prince MR, Frisoli JK: Beta-carotene accumulation in serum and skin. *Am J Clin Nutr* **57**:175, 1993
23. Lascari AD: Carotenemia. A review. *Clin Pediatr* **20**:25, 1981
24. Stack KM et al: Xanthoderma: Case report and differential diagnosis. *Cutis* **41**:100, 1988
25. Oakley A, Wallace J: Hartnup disease presenting in an adult. *Clin Exp Dermatol* **19**:407, 1994
26. Dumitrescu C, Lichiardopol R: Particular features of clinical pellagra. *Rom J Intern Med* **32**:165, 1994
27. Roe DA: Riboflavin deficiency: Mucocutaneous signs of acute and chronic deficiency. *Semin Dermatol* **10**:293, 1992
28. Lin SH et al: Imerslund-Grasbeck syndrome in a Chinese family with distinct skin lesions refractory to vitamin B12. *J Clin Pathol* **47**:956, 1994
29. Livne M et al: Holocarboxylase synthetase deficiency: A treatable metabolic disorder masquerading as cerebral palsy. *J Child Neurol* **9**:170, 1994
30. Higuchi R et al: Biotin deficiency in an infant fed with amino acid formula and hypoallergenic rice. *Acta Paediatr* **85**:872, 1996
31. Adelman HM et al: Scurvy resembling cutaneous vasculitis. *Cutis* **54**:111, 1994
32. Ghorbani AJ, Eichler C: Scurvy. *J Am Acad Dermatol* **30**:881, 1994
33. Moreau-Cabarrot A et al: Cutaneous hypersensitivity at the site of injection of vitamin K1. *Ann Dermatol Venereol* **123**:177, 1996
34. Kragballe K: The future of vitamin D in dermatology. *J Am Acad Dermatol* **37**:572, 1997
35. Abushufa R et al: Essential fatty acid status in patients on long term home parenteral nutrition. *J Parenter Enteral Nutr* **19**:286, 1995
36. Cederholm TE et al: Low levels of essential fatty acids are related to impaired delayed skin hypersensitivity in malnourished chronically ill elderly people. *Eur J Clin Invest* **24**:615, 1994
37. Phatak PD, Cappucio JD: Management of hereditary hemochromatosis. *Blood Rev* **8**:193, 1994
38. Prasad AS: Zinc: An overview. *Nutrition* **11**:93, 1995
39. Heinen F et al: Zinc deficiency in an exclusively breast-fed preterm infant. *Eur J Pediatr* **154**:71, 1995
40. Prasad AS: Zinc deficiency in women, infants, and children. *J Am Coll Nutr* **15**:113, 1996
41. Prasad AS et al: Zinc deficiency in elderly patients. *Nutrition* **9**:218, 1993
42. Martins C et al: Menkes' kinky hair syndrome: Ultrastructural cutaneous alterations of the elastic fibers. *Pediatr Dermatol* **14**:347, 1997
43. Bennani-Smires C et al: Infantile nutritional copper deficiency. *Am J Dis Child* **134**:1155, 1980
44. Brown MR et al: Proximal muscle weakness and selenium deficiency associated with long term parenteral nutrition. *Am J Clin Nutr* **43**.549, 1986
45. Ruta DA, Haider S: Attempted murder by selenium poisoning. *Br Med J* **299**:316, 1989
46. Doisy EA: Human manganese deficiency, in *Trace Substances in Environmental Health,* VI, edited by DD Hemphill. Minneapolis, Univ of Minnesota Press, 1972, p 193

Kenneth H. Neldner

Acrodermatitis Enteropathica and Other Zinc-Deficiency Disorders

ACRODERMATITIS ENTEROPATHICA

Acrodermatitis enteropathica (AE) is a rare, inherited disorder, transmitted as an autosomal recessive trait. Prior to the discovery that the disorder was caused by an inability to absorb sufficient zinc from the diet, the disease was usually fatal in infancy or early childhood. It is now rapidly and dramatically cured by simple dietary supplementation with zinc salts.

The clinical syndrome is characterized by a phenotypic triad of acral dermatitis, alopecia, and diarrhea. The distribution of the rash (face, hands, feet, anogenital area) has become recognized as a virtually pathognomonic cutaneous marker for zinc deficiency, whether secondary to hereditary AE or to any of the numerous nonhereditary causes for zinc deficiency, which produces an identical clinical picture to that of classic hereditary AE.

Historic Aspects

Acrodermatitis enteropathica was originally described as a hereditary disorder by Danbolt and Closs[1] in 1943. In 1953, Dillaha et al.[2] reported modest therapeutic success with oral diiodohydroxyquin. While studying a patient with AE and associated lactose intolerance in 1973, Moynahan and Barnes[3] observed that alterations in zinc concentrations affected the well-being of the patient, leading to the discovery that AE was a disease of zinc deficiency.

Epidemiology

Hereditary acrodermatitis enteropathica has worldwide distribution with no apparent predilection for race or gender. Because of the early interest in the disease throughout Europe, particularly northern Europe, there are seemingly larger numbers of cases reported from these geographic areas. A recent Dutch study was able to find 226 patients with hereditary AE and 374 with nonhereditary zinc deficiency.[4]

Pathogenesis

After AE was discovered to be a disorder of zinc deficiency, the one missing link in the understanding of its pathogenesis was knowledge of the mechanism by which zinc is absorbed from the diet, a process that is not totally lacking in hereditary AE because the patients can absorb a small amount of zinc from an average diet. A simple increase in dietary zinc will rapidly raise plasma levels to normal and cure the disease. The fact that zinc in human milk is much more available biologically to infants with AE than zinc from bovine milk, with essentially equal zinc concentration, has led to much interest and speculation. The two milks have been compared in an effort to find a basic transport mechanism for zinc such as a possible species-specific zinc-binding ligand (ZBL) for humans that might be abnormal or deficient in AE. Thus far, the search has shown the process to be complex and controversial.

Eckert et al.[5] found the zinc in human milk to be associated primarily with a low molecular weight ligand ($\sim$10,000) and the zinc of bovine milk was contained in higher molecular weight fractions. Hurley et al.[6] and Casey et al.[7] have found a similarly sized low molecular weight zinc ligand in human duodenal-pancreatic secretions, adding to the impression that the size of the ZBL was critical. Casey and coworkers[8] also found that the low molecular weight ligand of duodenal-pancreatic secretions of patients with AE contained much less zinc than similar secretions from normal controls, suggesting that the ZBL in the duodenum of patients with AE was in some way less efficient in transporting zinc.

Cousins and Smith[9] found only 10 percent of the zinc in fat-free human milk to be associated with a low molecular weight ZBL (<2000). When additional zinc was added in vitro, almost all of it became associated with this fraction, suggesting that the overall concentration of zinc in milk determined how much of it appeared in which fraction. They postulated that the difference in total protein of human milk (5.3 mg/mL) compared to bovine milk (29.0 mg/mL) also influenced the bioavailability of zinc in some unknown way.

Lönnerdal et al.[10] and Menard and Cousins[11] found intestinal zinc to be complexed with citrate (molecular weight 600 to 650), which they believe to be a major intestinal ZBL. However, Oestreicher and Cousins[12] have since reported that the addition of citrate to milk does not enhance absorption of zinc in the rat.

To further complicate the picture, other ZBLs have been reported to exist. Song[13] proposed that prostaglandin E_2 has a role in zinc absorption from the gut. Evans and Johnson[14] found that picolinic acid, present in milk and duodenal contents, has a high affinity for zinc. On the other hand, Rebello et al.[15] found the intestinal concentration of picolinic acid to be normally so low that a significant role in zinc absorption was questioned.

Grider and co-workers have recently shown that human fibroblasts from AE patients have an impaired uptake of zinc in vitro, suggesting that the genetic defect in AE may not be limited to malabsorption from the gut.[16,17]

Other factors, such as the overall state of total-body zinc nurture of the host, will influence zinc absorption, i.e., the zinc-depleted individual will absorb zinc much more avidly than one in a zinc-adequate or -excess state. Poorly understood interactions with other trace elements, particularly copper, lead, iron, cadmium, and chelating drugs, are known to alter absorption.[18] Once zinc is absorbed by the intestinal villous brush border, another complex series of homeostatic events involving metallothioneines regulates the transport of zinc into the circulation and then on to the liver and kidneys, where a final, poorly understood homeostatic surveillance system operates to regulate how much zinc will be preserved and how much excreted. These mechanisms appear to function normally in AE. The defect, therefore, is believed to be somewhere in the early stages of zinc absorption, where the bioavailability of the chemical form and the structure in which dietary zinc is presented to the intestinal mucosal brush border in some way cause malabsorption.

Clinical Manifestations

HEREDITARY ZINC DEFICIENCY   Classic hereditary AE usually begins within days to a few weeks after birth in infants bottle-fed with bovine milk or soon after weaning from the breast in older infants. Acral dermatitis begins slowly with dry, scaly, eczematous plaques on the face, scalp, and anogenital areas (Figs. 148-1 and 148-2). Perlèche is a common early sign and has also been called a sign heralding relapse.[19] All lesions become progressively worse as vesicobullous, pustular, and erosive lesions develop. Superficial oral aphthous-like lesions may appear. The hands and feet are soon involved, commonly with paronychia and a brightly erythematous dermatitis of the palmar and finger creases plus annular lesions with collarette scaling. As the dermatitis worsens, secondary infections with bacteria and *Candida albicans* are common aggravating factors. Alopecia gradually worsens with time. Diarrhea is the most variable manifestation and may be only intermittent or totally absent. If diarrhea is severe and persistent, the clinical course will be further complicated by the loss of fluids, electrolytes, and other nutrients.

Within a few weeks, growth failure becomes measurable and becomes more apparent as the child approaches adolescence, when hypogonadism in males also becomes obvious. Emotional and mental disturbances are common manifestations of zinc deficiency, although difficult to evaluate. They are often best appreciated at the time when zinc supplementation is instituted, resulting in rapid im-

provement in mood, disposition, and overall mental status within 24 to 48 h.

Photophobia develops gradually and is believed to be due to malfunction of retinal binding protein, known to be zinc-dependent. Other manifestations include anorexia, hypogeusia, hyposmia, and anemia. A "zebra striped" light and dark banding of hair may be seen with polarized light microscopy.[20]

Prior to the use of zinc in AE, fertility was low in those who reached reproductive age, and congenital malformations were common, particularly neural tube defects. The disease was often fatal during infancy. In those with milder cases who survived and those who received larger amounts of dietary zinc for unrelated reasons, the manifestations were less severe but usually resulted in growth retardation and dwarfism, delayed puberty, hypogonadism in male adolescents, continuing skin problems (dry skin and/or acral dermatitis of varying degrees), frequent infections, delayed wound healing, and mental disturbances.[21] There are rare reports of spontaneous remission occurring in adolescence.[22]

FIGURE 148-2

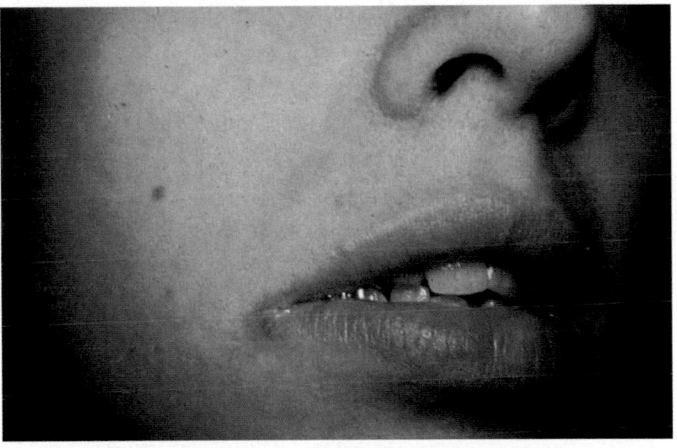

A.

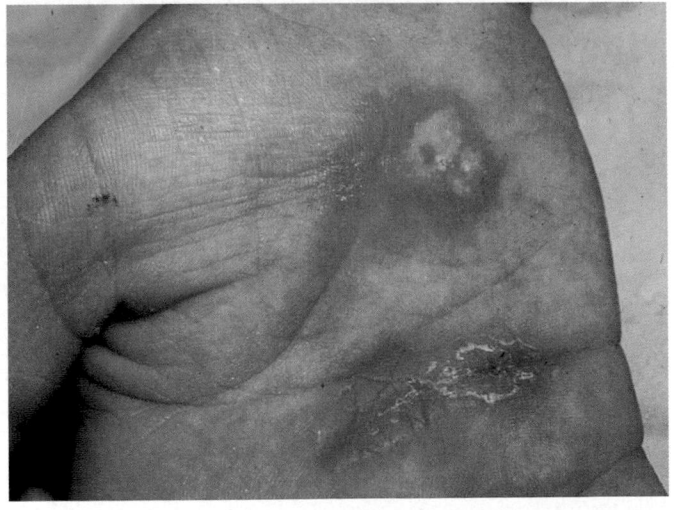

B.

Acrodermatitis enteropathica in older individuals showing typical lesions. *A.* Facial, and (*B*) palmar.

FIGURE 148-1

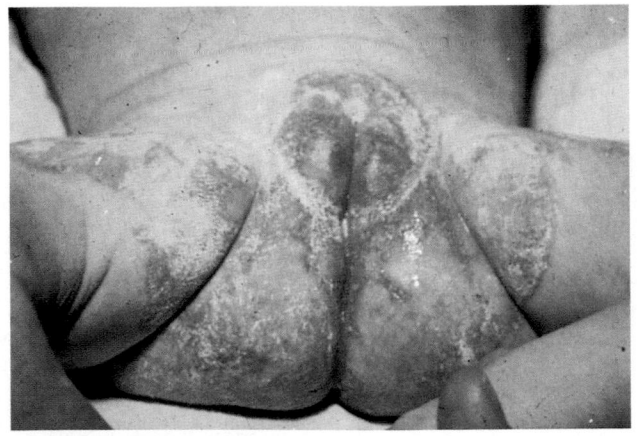

Acrodermatitis enteropathica. Erosive, eczematous, and secondarily infected lesions: genital area.

NONHEREDITARY ACQUIRED ZINC DEFICIENCY   As more is learned of the biochemical role of zinc in a vast array of physiologic functions, the subject of AE and zinc deficiency can no longer be viewed as a simple genetically determined event. Based on the knowledge gained from hereditary AE, it is now possible to recognize a similar pattern of signs and symptoms in patients with zinc deficiency from many other causes. In fact, the term *acrodermatitis enteropathica* is now being used in a general sense to include all patients with acral dermatitis due to zinc deficiency of hereditary or nonhereditary etiology. This anatomic distribution is now recognized as the sine qua non and hallmark of zinc deficiency, whether on a hereditary or nonhereditary basis (Fig. 148-3).

In recent years a number of infants with presumed hereditary AE have been reported who had all the typical findings of AE as outlined above, but who were found subsequently to have hypozincemia as a result of a very low concentration of zinc in their mother's milk.[23] Several new reports have been published documenting typical AE in infants who responded rapidly to supplemental zinc, and their condition was subsequently found to be due to low maternal milk zinc.[24–26] Unlike those with hereditary AE, as soon as the infants were weaned, they no longer required supplemental zinc, confirming that they suffered from simple acute dietary zinc deficiency and did not possess the hereditary defect in zinc absorption. No specific genetic reasons were found for the low maternal milk zinc levels. The mothers most likely became marginally zinc deficient due to the increased demands for zinc during pregnancy and lactation.

Such reports suggest that any breast-fed infant (especially premature infants) who develops an acral dermatitis of even mild degree should be checked for zinc status, and the maternal milk should also be checked.

A possible role for biotin in AE has been proposed, particularly in premature infants with zinc deficiency who responded better to a combination of zinc and biotin than to zinc alone.[27] There has been no evidence found for a biotinidase deficiency in these infants. Such a deficiency has been described recently in rare premature infants with a dermatitis that resembled AE to some extent but was found solely related to a defect in biotin metabolism.[28]

A list of disorders and postsurgical states that are now recognized to be causes for zinc deficiency is presented in Table 148-1. The most common are those involving the gastrointestinal tract, such as chronic inflammatory bowel disease with diarrhea and/or malabsorption, steatorrhea, pancreatic insufficiency, and cirrhosis or surgically induced conditions such as total or partial gastrectomies and bowel resections, with or without blind-loop syndromes. Any catabolic chronic disease is also likely to induce zinc deficiency. Alcoholics are particularly prone to zinc deficiency.[29,30] The clinical expression will depend on the severity and duration of the deficiency and the age of the patient. As expected, there is almost total overlap with hereditary AE. The potential manifestations are summarized in Table 148-2.

FIGURE 148-3

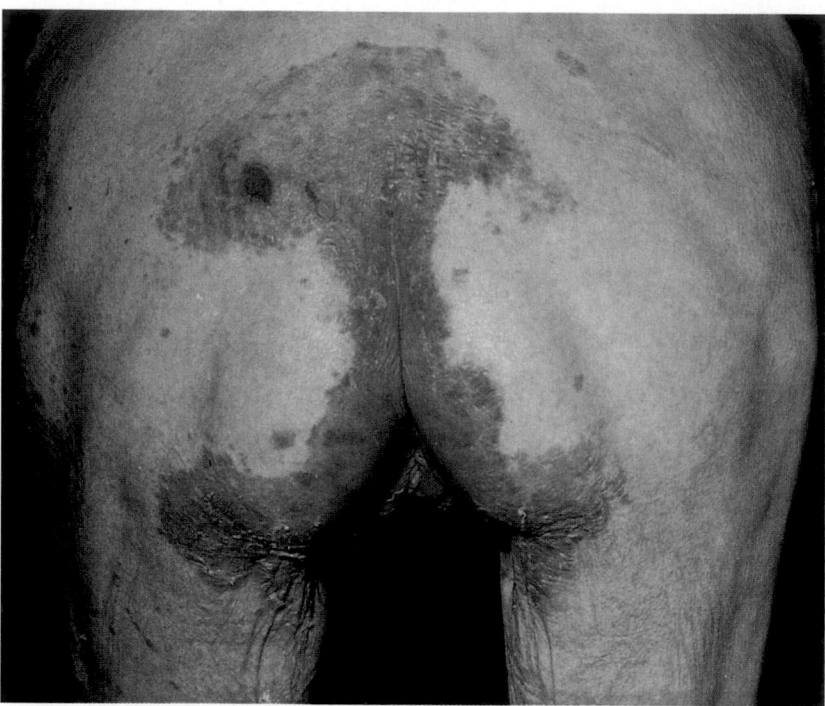

A.

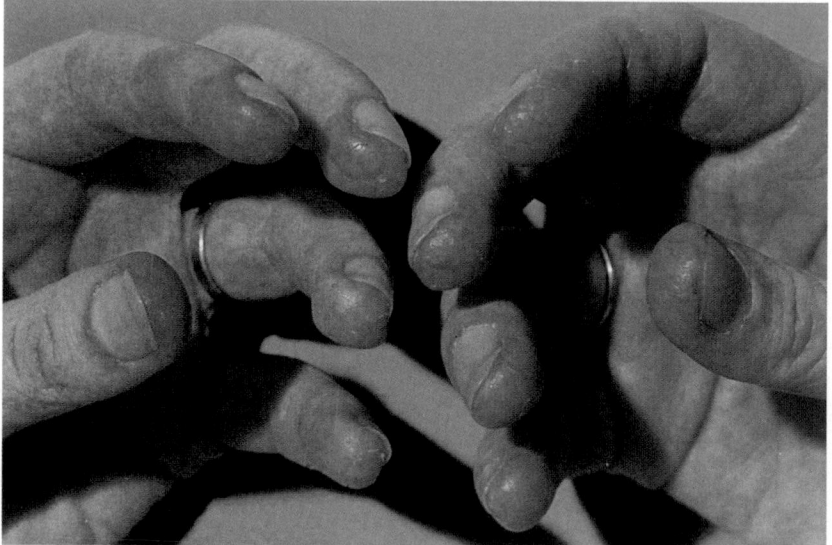

B.

Zinc deficiency. *A.* There are plaques of dry, scaly, eczematous skin around the buttocks. The lesions often become secondarily infected with *Candida albicans. B.* Hands. The fingers are enlarged, and there are paronychia and bright erythema on the terminal phalanges.

MARGINAL ZINC DEFICIENCY

A relatively new area of interest lies not at the obvious symptomatic end of the spectrum, but rather at the other end, i.e., individuals whose dietary zinc intake is marginal but still adequate to prevent overt

TABLE 148-1

CHAPTER 148
Acrodermatitis Enteropathica 1741

Conditions and Disorders that May Cause Zinc Deficiency

Disorder	Etiology
Gastrointestinal	
Mucosal diseases	Diarrhea
Malabsorption syndromes	Diarrhea
Pancreatic disorders	Reduced zinc ligands
Cirrhosis	Increased urinary loss
Postgastrectomy syndrome	Diarrhea
Blind-loop syndromes	Diarrhea
Dietary factors	
High dietary phytate	Chelation, ethnic diets
Alcoholism	Increased urinary loss
Total parenteral nutrition	Lack of zinc supplementation
Faddish weight reduction	Inadequate dietary zinc
Bulimia	Inadequate dietary zinc
Anorexia nervosa	Inadequate dietary zinc
Trauma	
Burns	Exudation, catabolism
Postsurgical procedure	Catabolism, anorexia
Malignancy	
All types	Catabolism, anorexia
Renal disorders	
Renal tubular disease	Failure to absorb zinc
Nephrotic syndrome	Proteinuria
Dialysis	Loss of zinc in dialyzate
Infection	
Parasitic	Chronic blood loss
Bacterial, viral	Redistribution, urinary loss
Miscellaneous	
Antimetabolite drug therapy	Catabolism
Chelation drug therapy	Chelation-urinary loss
Diabetes mellitus	Urinary loss
Hemolytic anemias	Urinary loss of erythrocyte zinc
Collagen-vascular diseases	Catabolism
Pregnancy/lactation	Increased fetal requirements

clinical manifestations. There is a growing body of evidence to suggest that such individuals are at significant long-term risk for a number of as yet ill-defined systemic and cutaneous disorders. In order to demonstrate more clearly the effects of this level of defi-

TABLE 148-2

Clinical Manifestations of Moderate to Severe Zinc Deficiency Observed in Nonhereditary Acquired Conditions

Rough dry skin
Progressively severe, patterned acral dermatitis (the diagnostic hallmark)
Perlèche (angular stomatitis)
Seborrheic dermatitis–like eruption
Alopecia
Diarrhea (variable)
Hypogeusia
Anorexia
Mental disturbances
Delayed wound healing
Growth retardation (children and adolescents)
Delayed puberty
Hypogonadism in developing males
Defective embryogenesis (neural tube defects)

ciency, animal studies are essential because it is almost impossible to maintain humans on a constant level of any nutrient for long periods and continue to monitor a broad range of possible physiologic consequences. On a global basis, the two most common causes for marginal (or symptomatic) zinc deficiency are probably chronic alcoholism and diets high in phytates where such diets are common for ethnic or geographic reasons.[31] Phytates are present in most cereal grains and are potent chelators of zinc. Several pieces of evidence to support the contention that marginal zinc deficiency may be a silent and unrecognized partner in the pathogenesis of diverse and seemingly unrelated skin and systemic diseases are summarized in Table 148-3.

Numerous human and animal studies have demonstrated T cell and immune dysfunction at all levels of zinc deprivation, including marginal levels, if extended over long periods of time.[32–35] The possibility for cause or aggravation of diseases of diverse nature seems very likely although difficult to prove. As immune function declines, an increased susceptibility to infection soon follows.[36] This is well demonstrated in the more severe forms of animal and human zinc deficiency. Marginal zinc deficiency in infants and children has been shown to cause failure to thrive across a broad range of anthropometric parameters.[37]

In both AE and an animal model of AE (Danish black pied Friesian breed of cattle), thymic atrophy is one consequence.[38] As a result, thymocytes and cellular immune functions, particularly a wide range of T cell functions, are depressed. This aspect of zinc deficiency has been reviewed by Good et al.[39] Neutrophils, peripheral blood monocytes, tissue macrophages, and mast cells are known to require optimal concentrations of zinc for normal function.[40] Zinc also plays an important, although not completely understood, role in essential fatty acid metabolism.[41,42] Reviews of the biochemistry and physiology of zinc metabolism have been written by Prasad[43,44] and Forbes.[45]

Wound healing requires many nutrients, one of which is zinc. Patients with low plasma zinc levels and poor wound healing decrease their healing time following zinc supplementation. However, there is believed to be no additional clinical benefit from high doses of oral zinc if zinc status is otherwise normal; indeed, prolonged high doses can be toxic (see "Zinc Toxicity"). A determination of the plasma zinc level is therefore indicated in patients with leg ulcers or other slow-healing wounds or infections.

A proven role for zinc in the treatment of other dermatologic disorders has been somewhat controversial. Claims for efficacy in acne have been made and disputed.[46,47] A recent study found epidermal zinc to be low in dermatitis herpetiformis, acne, psoriasis, and Darier's disease, but plasma levels were low only in dermatitis herpetiformis.[48] Brüske and Salfeld[49] found low serum levels in patients with vitiligo. Others found low serum and epidermal zinc in atopic eczema, but dietary zinc supplementation had no readily

TABLE 148-3

Potential Long-Term Effects of Low-Grade, Marginal Zinc Deficiency

Abnormal lymphocyte function
Increased susceptibility to infection
Delayed wound healing
Aggravation of other dermatologic disorders
Impaired free radical scavenging

apparent efficacy, indicating that if zinc does play a role, it is probably not primary, but one that could conceivably facilitate healing once the primary damage has been done.[50] It should be recalled that the topical use of zinc (calamine, zinc oxide) is one of the oldest dermatologic medications known, being recorded in a 2000 B.C. Ebers papyrus.

Superoxide dismutase is an important free radical scavenger and a zinc-copper-manganese metalloenzyme. Low concentrations of superoxide dismutase have been reported in the skin in severe zinc deficiency but have not been studied in marginally deficient humans or animals. Free radical scavengers as a group (vitamins A, C, and E, the carotenoids; catalases; zinc; selenium; and copper) protect against oxidative damage to all cell membranes, DNA macromolecules, and other vital cellular components. Free radicals are also potent carcinogens. The important role of zinc and other trace elements and vitamins in disease prevention has been thoroughly reviewed recently.[51]

BIOCHEMISTRY OF ZINC METABOLISM

Even though zinc has been known to be required for normal growth and development in the rat since 1934, it was not established as an essential human nutrient by the National Research Council until 1974, when a recommended dietary allowance (RDA) was set at 15 mg/day.

The adult body contains 2 to 3 g of zinc, which is about half the iron content and some 10 to 20 times more than other trace elements such as copper, magnesium, and nickel. The zinc cation exists almost totally in the Zn^{2+} oxidation state and does not readily undergo further oxidation or reduction, providing a stability that is believed to be significant in zinc biochemistry, such as hydrolysis and transfer or addition to double bonds.

The average diet in the United States provides approximately 12 to 15 mg of elemental zinc per day. Body stores and homeostatic mechanisms combine to ensure adequate supplies during times of reduced intake; however, during periods of dietary deprivation, the body will soon fall into a negative metabolic balance. In the rat, a negative balance develops within a few days after being fed a zinc-deficient diet, causing a rapid reduction in DNA synthesis.[52] Normally, about 30 percent of the daily intake is absorbed, although this figure is variable. Specific mechanisms of absorption have been discussed under "Etiology." The intravascular transport of zinc is primarily as a loosely bound complex with albumin (60 to 70 percent), and lesser amounts are more tightly bound to α_2-macroglobulin (10 to 20 percent), transferrin (1 to 5 percent), amino acid chelates (5 to 10 percent), and IgG (<1 percent).

All body tissues contain zinc. Muscle, bone, and the prostate gland have the richest stores. In the skin, zinc is concentrated in the epidermis, which contains up to five or six times greater concentration than the dermis.[53,54] Zinc also concentrates in hair, but changes in host zinc nutriture will be reflected in hair zinc concentration only after prolonged periods of deprivation (or excess), so its quantitation is unreliable for assessment of short-term or recent events.

The principal biochemical function of zinc is through its incorporation into a wide range of enzymes. Since zinc was discovered in 1940 to be present in carbonic anhydrase, the list of zinc metalloenzymes has grown to over 200, if those from nonhuman species

are included.[55] There are two basic types of zinc-activated enzymes; one is a metal-enzyme complex that readily dissociates but requires the presence of zinc for continued activity, and the other is one in which zinc is firmly bound to the active site so that it will not dissociate during isolation of the enzyme.

LABORATORY DIAGNOSIS OF ZINC DEFICIENCY

The laboratory verification of zinc deficiency is the same for hereditary deficiency (AE) or any of the acquired forms. Plasma or serum zinc levels are currently the easiest, best, and most commonly used method for assessing zinc status. However, it is well recognized that blood levels fluctuate rapidly following infection, injury, burns, or any sudden stressful stimuli, resulting in redistribution of zinc from the blood to other body compartments. Blood levels during such events may, therefore, not correctly reflect total zinc nutriture. Normal plasma levels are 70 to 110 μg/dL. Serum levels are 80 to 120 μg/dL. (For conversions to μmol/L, multiply by 0.153; 70 to 110 μg/L = 10.7 to 16.8 μmol/L.) Urinary zinc excretion is highly variable under normal circumstances but gradually decreases as zinc deficiency progresses. The normal urinary excretion ranges from 200 to 500 μg per 24 h. Hair zinc concentration is commonly measured but, again, reflects only the long-term zinc status. Its use and interpretation will therefore depend upon the clinical situation and type of information desired. Serum alkaline phosphatase activity is a moderately sensitive indicator of zinc status, although not a particularly early marker of deficiency. Its activity remains near normal until profound and prolonged deficiency exists. Leukocyte zinc levels have been shown to be quite sensitive to early minor changes in total-body zinc nutriture, but their measurement has the disadvantage of being a difficult and expensive assay.[56]

It should also be emphasized that specimen collections and laboratory technique are important. Contamination with environmental zinc in collecting tubes or containers plus laboratory contamination in the handling and transfer of specimens and in the preparation of laboratory chemicals and solutions are a constant threat. Spurious laboratory results will, therefore, almost always be on the side of higher than actual values, which may lead to a missed diagnosis of impending or borderline zinc deficiency. The time between collection of blood and separation of serum and plasma also affects zinc concentration, with increases in the plasma concentration of up to 6 percent during the first 2 h if not separated.[57] It is, therefore, recommended to use zinc-free vacuum tubes and stainless steel needles, avoid contact with rubber stoppers (they contain zinc), avoid hemolysis, separate plasma or serum from cells within 45 min, and use anticoagulants that are low in zinc or zinc-free. There is also a diurnal rhythm in plasma zinc concentration; morning fasting specimens are recommended for the most accurate results.

TREATMENT OF ZINC DEFICIENCY

The treatment of zinc deficiency is essentially that of dietary or intravenous supplementation with zinc salts, no matter what the etiology. In most instances, dietary supplementation with two to three times the RDA in doses of 30 to 55 mg of elemental Zn^{2+} daily will be adequate to restore a normal zinc status within days to a few weeks, depending on the degree of depletion. In all circumstances, a rapid clinical response will occur with dramatic reversal of many manifestations within hours to days.[18] Severe infected and erosive skin lesions will heal within 1 to 2 weeks without additional topical therapy. Diarrhea, if present, often stops within 24 h. Rapid improvement in mental disturbances is usually detectable within 24 to 48 h. In children, a surge of total-body and hair growth can be detected within 3 to 4 weeks after commencing zinc therapy.

Any of the zinc compounds available appear to work well (zinc sulfate, zinc acetate, zinc gluconate, zinc chloride, amino acid chelates). However, $ZnSO_4$ has been recommended more for oral supplementation, and $ZnCl_2$ for intravenous use. Dosage prescribed must be based on the amount of elemental zinc present in the preparation, which varies from one compound to another. For example, a standard capsule of 220 mg of $ZnSO_4 \cdot 7H_2O$ contains approximately 55 mg Zn^{2+}, which is an adequate daily dose for most deficient individuals.

High pharmacologic doses of oral zinc have been recommended by some investigators for the therapy of sickle cell anemia, acne, delayed wound healing, and leg ulcers. All of these conditions will improve with zinc therapy if a preceding zinc deficiency existed. However, in general, proof is lacking for a pharmacologic effect over and above that of restoration of a normal zinc nutritional status. Furthermore, the threat of zinc toxicity must be guarded against if prolonged high doses are ingested.[58]

ZINC TOXICITY

Most heavy metals, including zinc, become toxic if taken to excess. Moderate overdose is eliminated through homeostatic mechanisms involving decreased absorption and/or increased urinary and biliary excretions. However, plasma levels of 150 to 300 $\mu g/dL$ (22.9 to 45.9 $\mu mol/L$) are easily achieved by persons ingesting zinc supplements of 50 to 100 mg Zn^{2+} daily. Such doses usually produce no immediately apparent adverse effects, although the long-term safety of such a dose is unknown.

$ZnSO_4$ is listed in the *U.S. Pharmacopeia* as an emetic. Not surprisingly, its most common adverse effect is gastric irritation with nausea, vomiting, and mild gastric hemorrhage.

Acute and fatal zinc toxicity has been reported following large accidental oral and intravenous overdose.[59] Chronic toxicity among zinc smelter workers is known as "metal fume fever" and causes fevers, chills, gastroenteritis, and pulmonary symptoms.[60] Rats and mice fed moderate overdose for long periods have shown reduced growth rates, anemia, declining rates of reproduction, and hypertrophy of the adrenal cortex and pancreatic islets.[61] The finding that moderate to high (160 mg Zn^{2+} daily) overdose was atherogenic in humans was reported by Hooper et al,[62] but it has been found more recently that lower doses of zinc have no effect on high-density lipoprotein cholesterol.[63]

A reciprocal interaction with copper is well recognized.[64] Patients receiving prolonged oral zinc supplementation are prone to develop hypocupremia as a consequence of long-standing hyperzincemia. One adverse effect of hypocupremia is a refractory microcytic anemia that will not respond to iron therapy until the serum copper level is normalized.[65] Neutropenia, immune dysfunction, and hypoceruloplasminemia also occur with hypocupremia.[66]

It is recommended that patients on long-term zinc therapy should be monitored periodically with the following tests: plasma zinc concentrations taken as a fasting A.M. specimen to regulate dosage, complete hemogram with erythrocyte indices, leukocyte differential count, serum copper level, and a stool examination for occult blood.

RECENT ADVANCES

Considerable progress has been made recently regarding cellular zinc transport at a molecular genetic level.[67] Biologically active zinc is a highly charged species that cannot cross cell membranes by passive diffusion. Recent studies have therefore focused on a search for mechanisms for zinc to both enter and exit a cell. Some elemental zinc can probably cross cell membranes, but the process is greatly enhanced when zinc is complexed with zinc-binding ligands. Furthermore, zinc efflux from cells is believed to be a different process than that involved in zinc influx.

In brief, there is now a family of four mammalian zinc transporter genes identified and cloned that are designated zinc transporter 1 (ZnT-1) through ZnT-4. ZnT-1 is located in the plasma membrane of all cells and functions primarily as an exporter mechanism for zinc efflux.[68] ZnT-2 appears to function in cytoplasmic vesicular zinc uptake and efflux. ZnT-3 is associated with vesicular zinc uptake in neurons and in the testes. ZnT-4 is thus far found to be concentrated in the plasma membrane of cells in the mammary gland and the brain.[69]

A fifth metal transporter, called divalent cation transporter (DCT-1), is associated with the transport of several cations (Fe^{2+}, Cu^{2+}, Cd^{2+}, Mn^{2+}) in addition to zinc.[70] It is concentrated in the intestinal crypts and lower villi. The DCT-1 gene has a high homology to a family of mammalian genes called the macrophage Nramp group involved in host defense mechanisms.

Acrodermatitis enteropathica has thus far not been studied for a possible mutation in any of the zinc transporter genes.

REFERENCES

1. Danbolt N, Closs K: Acrodermatitis enteropathica. *Acta Derm Venereol (Stockh)* **23**:172, 1943
2. Dillaha CJ et al: Acrodermatitis enteropathica: Review of the literature and a report of a case successfully treated with Diodiquin. *JAMA* **152**:509, 1953
3. Moynahan EJ, Barnes PM: Zinc deficiency and a synthetic diet for lactose intolerance. *Lancet* **1**:676, 1973
4. Van Wouwe JP: Clinical and laboratory assessment of zinc deficiency in Dutch children. A review. *Biol Trace Elem Res* **49**:211, 1995
5. Eckert CD et al: Zinc binding: A difference between human and bovine milk. *Science* **195**:789, 1977
6. Hurley LS et al: Zinc binding ligands in milk and intestine: A role in neonatal nutrition. *Proc Natl Acad Sci USA* **74**:3547, 1977
7. Casey CE et al: Zinc binding in human duodenal secretions. *Lancet* **2**:423, 1978
8. Casey CE et al: Zinc binding in human duodenal secretions. *J Pediatr* **95**:1008, 1979
9. Cousins RJ, Smith KT: Zinc-binding properties of bovine and human milk in vitro: Influence of changes in zinc content. *Am J Clin Nutr* **33**:1083, 1980
10. Lönnerdal B et al: Isolation of a low molecular weight zinc binding ligand from human milk. *J Inorg Biochem* **12**:71, 1980
11. Menard MD, Cousins RJ: Effect of citrate, glutathione and picolinate on zinc transport by brush border membrane vesicles from rat intestine. *J Nutr* **113**:1653, 1983
12. Oestreicher P, Cousins RJ: Influence of intraluminal constituents on zinc absorption by isolated, vascularly profused rat intestine. *J Nutr* **112**:1978, 1982
13. Song MK: Evidence for an important role of prostaglandin E_2 and F_2 in the regulation of zinc transport in the rat. *J Nutr* **109**:2152, 1979
14. Evans GW, Johnson PE: Characterization and quantitation of a zinc binding ligand from human milk. *Pediatr Res* **14**:870, 1980
15. Rebello T et al: Picolinic acid in milk, pancreatic juice and intestine: Inadequate for role in zinc absorption. *Am J Clin Nutr* **35**:1, 1982

16. Grider A, Young EM: Acrodermatitis enteropathica mutation transiently affects zinc metabolism in human fibroblasts. *J Nutr* **126**:224, 1996

17. Vazquez F, Grider A: The effect of acrodermatitis enteropathica mutation on zinc uptake in human fibroblasts. *Biol Trace Elem Res* **50**:109, 1995

18. Solomons NW: Competitive mineral-mineral interaction in the intestine: Implications for zinc absorption in humans, in *Nutritional Bioavailability of Zinc,* edited by GE Inglett. Washington, DC, ACS Symposium Series, 1983, p 247

19. Mostafa WZ, Al-Zayer AA: Acrodermatitis enteropathica in Saudi Arabia. *Int J Dermatol* **29**:134, 1990

20. Traupe H et al: Polarizing microscopy of hair in acrodermatitis enteropathica. *Pediatr Dermatol* **3**:300, 1986

21. Neldner KH, Hambridge KM: Zinc therapy of acrodermatitis enteropathica. *N Engl J Med* **292**:879, 1975

22. Van Wouwe JP: Clinical and laboratory diagnoses of acrodermatitis enteropathica. *Eur J Pediatr* **149**:2, 1989

23. Lee MG et al: Transient symptomatic zinc deficiency in a full-term breast-fed infant. *J Am Acad Dermatol* **23**:375, 1990

24. Buehning LJ, Goltz RW: Acquired zinc deficiency in a premature breast fed infant. *J Am Acad Dermatol* **22**:499, 1993

25. Abitan R et al: Acquired zinc deficiency in a breast-fed premature infant (French). *Ann Dermatol Venereol* **121**:635, 1994

26. Heinen F et al: Zinc deficiency in an exclusively breast-fed preterm infant. *Eur J Pediatr* **154**:71, 1995

27. Lagier P et al: Zinc and biotin deficiency during prolonged parenteral nutrition in the infant. *Press Med* **31**:1795, 1987

28. Nyhan WL: Inborn errors of biotin metabolism. *Arch Dermatol* **123**:1696, 1987

29. Gaveau D et al: Cutaneous manifestations of zinc deficiency in ethylic cirrhosis. *Ann Dermatol Venereol* **114**:39, 1987

30. Taniguchi S et al: Acquired zinc deficiency associated with alcoholic liver cirrhosis. *Int J Dermatol* **34**:651, 1995

31. Ferguson EL et al: The zinc nutriture of preschool children living in two African countries. *J Nutr* **123**:1487, 1993

32. Fraber PJ et al: Zinc deficiency and immune function. *Arch Dermatol* **123**:1699, 1987

33. Anttila PH et al: Abnormal immune response during hypozincemia in acrodermatitis enteropathica. *Acta Paediatr Scand* **75**:988, 1986

34. Fraber PJ et al: Interrelationships between zinc and immune function *Fed Proc* **45**:1475, 1986

35. Couvreur Y et al: Zinc deficiency and lymphocyte subpopulations, a study by flow cytometry. *J Parenter Enterol Nutr* **10**:239, 1986

36. David TJ et al: Low serum zinc in children with atopic eczema. *Br J Dermatol* **111**:597, 1984

37. Walravens PA et al: Zinc supplementation in infants with a nutritional pattern of failure to thrive: A double-blind controlled study. *Pediatrics* **83**:532, 1989

38. Machen M et al: Bovine hereditary zinc deficiency: Lethal trait A46. *J Vet Diagn Invest* **8**:219, 1996

39. Good RA et al: Zinc and immunity, in *Clinical, Biochemical, and Nutritional Aspects of Trace Elements,* edited by AS Prasad. New York, Alan R Liss, 1982, p 189

40. Beisel WR: The role of zinc in neutrophil function, in *Clinical, Biochemical, and Nutritional Aspects of Trace Elements,* edited by AS Prasad. New York, Alan R Liss, 1982, p 203

41. Neldner KH et al: Acrodermatitis enteropathica. *Arch Dermatol* **110**:711, 1974

42. Walldius G et al: The effects of diet and zinc treatment of the fatty acid compositions of serum lipids and adipose tissue and/or serum lipoproteins in two adolescent patients with acrodermatitis enteropathica. *Am J Clin Nutr* **38**:512, 1983

43. Prasad AS: Chemical biochemistry and nutritional spectrum of zinc deficiency in human subjects: An update. *Nutr Rev* **41**:197, 1983

44. Prasad AS: Clinical endocrinologic and biochemical effects of zinc deficiency. *Spec Top Endocrinol Metab* **7**:45, 1985

45. Forbes RM: Use of laboratory animals to define physiological functions and bioavailability of zinc. *Fed Proc* **43**:2835, 1984

46. Michaëlsson G et al: A double-blind study of the effect of zinc and oxytetracycline in acne vulgaris. *Br J Dermatol* **97**:561, 1977

47. Orris L et al: Oral zinc therapy of acne. *Arch Dermatol* **114**:1018, 1977

48. Michaëlsson G, Ljunghall K: Patients with acne, psoriasis, dermatitis herpetiformis, and Darier's disease have low epidermal zinc concentrations. *Acta Derm Venereol (Stockh)* **70**:304, 1990

49. Brüske K, Salfeld K: Zinc and its status in some dermatologic diseases—a statistical assessment. *Z Hautkr* **62**(suppl):125, 1987

50. David TJ et al: Low serum zinc in children with atopic eczema. *Br J Dermatol* **111**:597, 1984

51. Slater TF, Block G (eds): Antioxidant vitamins and beta-carotene in disease prevention. *Am J Clin Nutr* **53**(suppl):1895, 1991

52. Prasad AS, Oberleas D: Thymidine kinase activity and incorporation of thymidine in DNA in zinc deficient tissues. *J Lab Clin Med* **83**:634, 1974

53. Michaëlsson G et al: Zinc in epidermis and dermis of normal subjects. *Acta Derm Venereol (Stockh)* **60**:295, 1980

54. Molokhia M, Portnoy B: Neutron activation and analysis of trace elements in skin: III. Zinc in normal skin. *Br J Dermatol* **81**:759, 1969

55. Vallee BL, Galdes A: The metallobiochemistry of zinc enzymes. *Adv Enzymol* **56**:284, 1984

56. Prasad AS et al: Experimental zinc deficiency in humans. *Ann Intern Med* **89**:483, 1978

57. English JL, Hambidge KM: Plasma and serum zinc concentration: Effect of time between collection and separation. *Clin Chim Acta* **175**:211, 1988

58. Prasad AS et al: Hypocupremia induced by zinc therapy in adults *JAMA* **240**:2166, 1978

59. Brocks A et al: Acute intravenous zinc poisoning. *Br Med J* **28**:1390, 1977

60. Papp JP: Metal fume fever. *Postgrad Med* **43**:160, 1968

61. Aughey E et al: The effect of oral zinc supplementation in the mouse. *J Comp Pathol* **87**:1, 1977

62. Hooper PL et al: Zinc lowers high-density lipoprotein-cholesterol levels. *JAMA* **244**:1960, 1980

63. Crounse SF et al: Zinc ingestion and lipoprotein values in sedentary and endurance-trained men. *JAMA* **252**:785, 1984

64. Kirchgessner M et al: Interactions of essential metals in human psychology, in *Clinical, Biochemical, and Nutritional Aspects of Trace Elements,* edited by AS Prasad. New York, Alan R Liss, 1982, p 477

65. Solomons NW et al: Studies on the bioavailability of zinc in humans: Mechanism of the intestinal interaction of non-heme iron and zinc. *J Nutr* **113**:337, 1983

66. Sandstrom B et al: Acrodermatitis enteropathica, zinc status, copper status and immune function. *Arch Pediatr Adolesc Med* **148**:980, 1997

67. McMahon RJ, Cousins RJ: Mammalian zinc transporters. *J Nutr* **128**:667, 1998

68. McMahon RJ, Cousins RJ: Regulation of the zinc transporter ZnT-1 by dietary zinc. *Proc Natl Acad Sci* **95**:4841, 1998

69. Huang L, Gitscher J: A novel gene involved in zinc transport is deficient in the lethal milk mouse. *Nat Genet* **17**:292, 1997

70. Gunshin H et al: Cloning and characterization of a mammalian proton-coupled metal-ion transporter. *Nature* (London) **388**:482, 1997

Cutaneous Changes in Errors of Amino Acid Metabolism: Tyrosinemia II, Phenylketonuria, Argininosuccinic Aciduria, and Alkaptonuria

An abnormality of amino acid metabolism may cause specific cutaneous syndromes, which are summarized in Table 149-1. The general aspects of amino acid metabolism are reviewed elsewhere.[1-3]

TYROSINEMIA TYPE II

Tyrosinemia type II (Richner-Hanhart syndrome) is a distinctive clinical syndrome involving the eyes, skin, and central nervous system. Tyrosine levels are elevated because of a deficiency of hepatic tyrosine aminotransferase.

General Features

Fewer than 100 patients with this clinical syndrome have been reported. All had tyrosinemia, phenolicaciduria, and inflammatory skin and eye lesions.[4] The sexes are affected equally; the disease is worldwide in distribution. Half the patients are of Italian descent. There is often consanguinity, which is strongly suggestive of autosomal recessive inheritance.[4] Recent case reports, in the past 6 years, have added no new features to the clinical descriptions.

DERMATOLOGIC FEATURES Patients have hyperkeratotic skin lesions limited to the palms and soles.[4-7] Lesions usually begin during the first year of life; in one patient, the first lesions appeared at age 6.[7] The skin lesions are painful, nonpruritic, and are frequently associated with hyperhidrosis (Fig. 149-1). The pain can be intense enough to cause patients to crawl rather than apply pressure to the lesions. Bullous lesions may occur and rapidly progress to erosions; these then become crusted and hyperkeratotic. Lesions are often linear. The fingertips and hypothenar eminences are commonly involved. One patient had hyperkeratotic subungual lesions; one patient may have been hyperpigmented.

OPHTHALMOLOGIC FEATURES Eye lesions occur weeks to months before the skin lesions. Eye symptoms start as early as 2 weeks of age and as late as 8 years. Tearing, redness, pain, and photophobia are early signs; late signs include corneal clouding and central or paracentral opacities, which are initially intraepithelial and can progress to superficial or deep dendritic ulcers (Fig. 149-2). Neovascularization is prominent. The eye disease may lead to scarring, nystagmus, and exodeviation. One patient had a persistent conjunctival plaque.[7] Topical therapy is ineffective, and herpes simplex and bacterial cultures are consistently negative.

NEUROLOGIC FEATURES Mental retardation of varying degrees is reported, as is normal mental development. Untreated tyrosinemia II during pregnancy may be associated with mental retardation or seizures in the children resulting from that pregnancy.[8]

OTHER ORGAN SYSTEM INVOLVEMENT Renal and liver function tests have been uniformly normal. One of the patients had multiple congenital anomalies, including microcephaly, cleft lip and palate, inguinal hernias, talipes equinovarus, and the absence of one kidney, associated with a chromosomal deletion.

Laboratory Findings

AMINO ACID ABNORMALITIES The blood and urine tyrosine levels of the affected patients are markedly elevated. Other amino acids have not been increased. Urinary tyrosine metabolites are elevated; these include p-hydroxyphenylpyruvic acid, p-hydroxyphenyllactic acid, p-hydroxyphenylacetic acid, tyrosine, and N-acetyltyrosine (Fig. 149-3). All of the metabolic effects are consequences of the deficiency of hepatic tyrosine aminotransferase.

Tyrosine aminotransferase (TAT) is a pyridoxal phosphate-dependent cytoplasmic enzyme that transaminates tyrosine, forming p-hydroxyphenylpyruvate (PHPPA). The human TAT gene contains 12 exons and transcribes a 3.0-kb mRNA, which codes for a 454–amino acid protein.[8] The liver is the richest source of TAT; this specific TAT is not present in skin. In tyrosinemia II, the liver biopsy shows little or no soluble TAT, although there is normal or slightly increased mitochondrial tyrosine (aspartate) transaminase activity.[9-11] In mitochondria, aspartate aminotransferase uses tyrosine as a substrate and is responsible for the production of increased amounts of PHPPA from the increased amounts of tyrosine available in tyrosinemia II. Since mitochondria do not have PHPPA oxidase activity, PHPPA and its metabolic products increase and ap-

TABLE 149-1

Inherited Disorders of Amino Acid and Organic Acid Metabolism with Skin Manifestations

DISEASE	SKIN MANIFESTATION	ENZYME DEFICIENCY/PATHOPHYSIOLOGY (MODE OF INHERITANCE)*
Alkaptonuria	Ochronosis	Homogentisic acid oxidase (AR)
	Black cerumen, eccrine and apocrine secretions	
Argininosuccinic aciduria	Trichorrhexis nodosa	Argininosuccinase (AR)
	Rough skin	
Aspartylglycosaminuria	Thick skin	Aspartylglycosamindase (AR)
	Coarsening of facies	
	Sagging skin folds	
	Increased acne	
	Photosensitivity	
Biotinidase deficiency	Erythematous rash	Biotinidase (AR)
	Alopecia	
	Oral candidiasis	
	Seborrheic dermatitis	
	Glossitis	
Citrullinemia	Light, short hair with interrupted cuticle	Argininosuccinate synthetase (AR)
Hartnup disease	Pellagra-like lesions	Defect of neutral amino acid transport in renal and intestinal brush border (AR); increased excretion of tryptophan metabolites
	Photosensitivity	
Histidinemia	Light-colored hair and eyes	Histidinase (AR)
		Decreased epidermal urocanic acid
Holocarboxylase synthetase deficiency	Seborrheic dermatitis	Holocarboxylase synthetase (AR)
	Alopecia	
Homocystinuria	Fine, sparse friable hair	Cystathionine β-synthetase (AR)
	Thin skin	
	Livedo reticularis	
	Malar flush	
	Vascular occlusions	
	Marfanoid habitus	
Hydroxykynureninuria	Chronic stomatitis	Kynureninase (AR)
	Ulcerated gums, gingivitis	
	Photosensitivity	
Hyperprolinuria I	Ichthyosis	? Proline dehydrogenase deficiency (AR)
Iminodipeptiduria (prolidase deficiency)	Chronic skin ulcers	Prolidase (AR)
	Recurrent infections	
Isovaleric acidemia	Odor of sweaty feet, alopecia	Isovaleryl-CoA dehydrogenase (?)
Methionine malabsorption syndrome	White hair	Defective methionine transport (?)
	Dried celery or oast house odor	
	Edema	
Phenylketonuria	Hypopigmentation	Phenylalanine hydroxylase (AR)
	Atopic dermatitis	Dihydropteridine reductase
	Scleroderma	Defective dihydrobiopterin synthesis
Tyrosinemia II	Painful, acral erosions	Tyrosine aminotransferase (AR)
	Hyperkeratosis	
	Corneal/conjunctival plaques and erosions	
Tryptophanuria with dwarfism	Photosensitivity	One patient (?)
Xanthurenic aciduria	Urticaria	Kynureninase (AD)
	Dermatitis	

*AR, autosomal recessive; AD, autosomal dominant; ?, unknown or unclear inheritance.

pear in the urine.[11] This creates the unusual situation in which metabolites are increased both proximally and distally to the defective enzyme (Fig. 149-4).

HISTOPATHOLOGY Routine histopathology is not diagnostic; it shows hyperkeratosis, parakeratosis, and acanthosis. In one patient, the biopsy was interpreted as showing epidermolytic hyperkeratosis[5]; however, review of the published biopsy does not support that specific diagnosis.

In one patient, the palmar papules showed parakeratosis with homogeneous, refractile, eosinophilic inclusions 2 to 3 μm in diameter in the stratum corneum and stratum spinosum.[7] Electron microscopy in one case suggested that the 2- to 3-μm inclusions were lipid-like granules. Discrete 10-nm filaments and myelin-like figures were intermixed with lipid-like droplets.[7] These electron microscopy results were interpreted as showing possibly lysosomal activation. Electron microscopy studies have shown increases in tonofibrils and keratohyalin, very tightly packed microtubular and

FIGURE 149-1

CHAPTER 149
Amino Acid Metabolism   1747

FIGURE 149-2

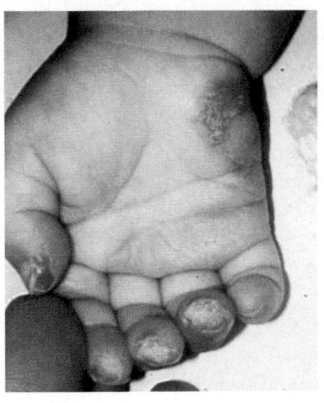 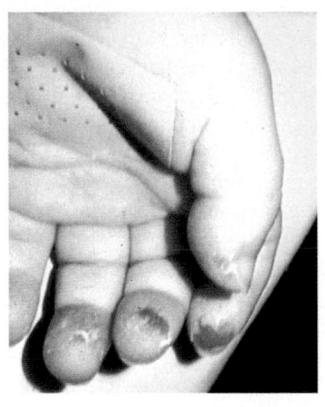

A.   *B.*

Hyperkeratotic and erosive lesions in a patient with tyrosinemia II.

microfibrillar masses, and minute tyrosine crystals in keratinocytes and Merkel cells.[12,13]

The conjunctival plaques of one patient showed eosinophilic inclusions in the superficial epithelial cells and a plasma cell infiltrate. Electron microscopy revealed aggregated clumps of chromatin and increased numbers of fibrils, forming bundles.[13] The superficial epithelial cells contained membrane-bound, alcian blue–positive inclusion bodies, 0.5 to 1.0 μm in diameter. Endothelial cells of the vessels contained similar inclusions and whorled membranous substances. In fibroblasts, dark bodies consisting of fine, needle-like crystals were found. A second conjunctival biopsy, 2 years after the initial biopsy, revealed no infiltration, but persistence of the inclusions in the epithelium and fibrocytes was seen.

GENETICS TAT maps to chromosome 16, the 16q22-q24 region. Detailed studies of one patient show her to be a double heterozygote with a contiguous deletion syndrome.[14] On her maternal 16q she has a deletion of least 11 of 12 TAT exons and a small de novo deletion in q22.1::q22.3. Her other somatic defects, which have not been part of the tyrosinemia syndrome, may be related to the deletions. Several point mutations scattered throughout the TAT gene have been associated with tyrosinemia type II.[15]

PATHOPHYSIOLOGY OF THE SKIN AND EYE LESIONS IN TYROSINEMIA II Rats fed a 12 percent protein diet with 0.5 to 2.0 percent tyrosine developed a syndrome resembling tyrosinemia II, with weight loss, a shortened life span, keratitis, conjunctivitis, alopecia, cheilitis, and inflammatory toe changes.[16] The high-tyrosine syndrome in rats was ameliorated by increasing the protein content of the diet or by adding threonine or thiouracil.[17] Inducers of TAT, such as glucagon, phenobarbital, glucocorticoids, and cataxic steroids devoid of glucocorticoid activity (e.g., pregnenolone-16-α-carbonitrile, or progesterone), prevented the syndrome.[18]

The affected animals had photophobia, corneal erosions, exudate, and panblepharitis. Microscopically, the initial lesion was epithelial edema associated with disorganization of the basal cells and polymorphonuclear leukocyte (PMNL) infiltration.[19] The PMNLs invaded the epithelium stroma and the anterior chamber. After 1 week, the cornea was opaque, thickened, and vascularized. By 2 to 3 weeks, the cornea was ulcerated.

The eyes contained birefringent crystals limited to the areas of corneal damage. The crystals were long (10 to 25 μm), slender (0.5 to 1.1 μm), and appeared to be membrane-bound; the crystals

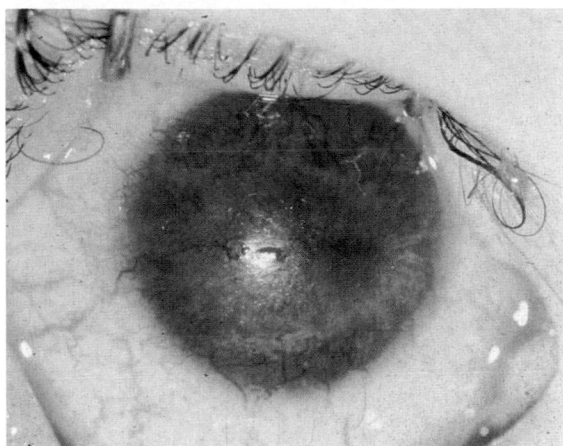

A.

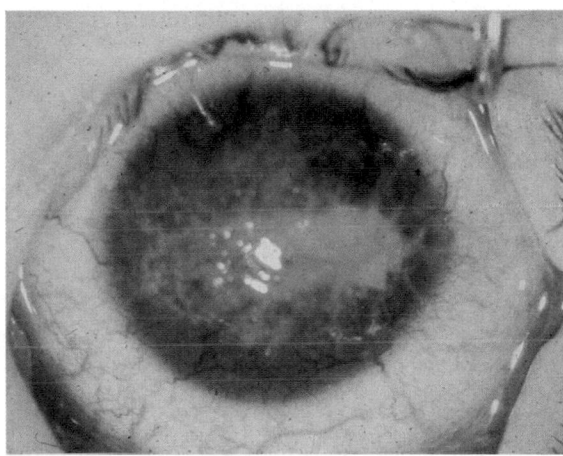

B.

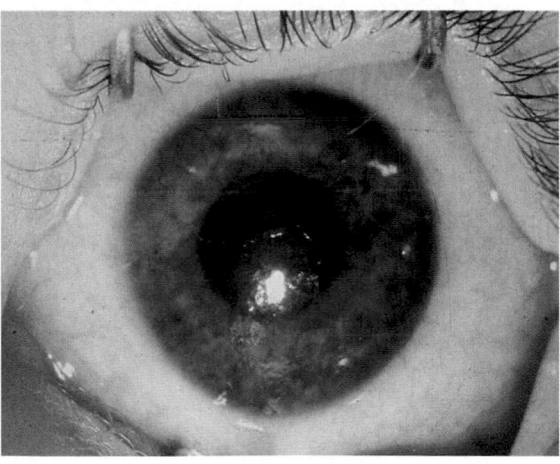

C.

Corneal changes in tyrosinemia II. Cornea before treatment, left eye (*A*) corneal opacity and neovascularization are prominent. The right eye (*B*) has even more extensive involvement. After 6 weeks of therapy, there is marked clearing of the lesions (*C*).

FIGURE 149-3

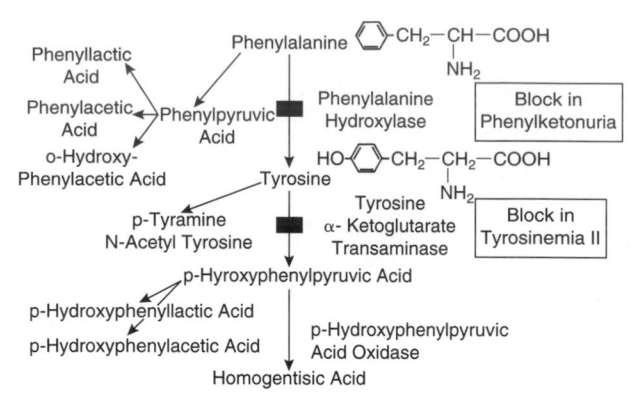

Metabolic scheme of phenylalanine, tyrosine, and their derivatives.

passed from cell to cell and penetrated nuclei. Multinucleate cells, vacuoles, autophagic vacuoles, and multivesicular bodies were present, which suggested lysosomal activation by the tyrosine crystals.

In unpublished studies, skin lesions in the rats were limited to the bottoms of the feet and the nail beds. The histologic changes were limited to the volar surfaces of the feet and the nail beds. Initially, there was dyskeratosis followed by local areas of intense PMNL infiltration, erosions, crusting, and hyperkeratosis. Subcorneal collections of PMNLs were seen first focally and then diffusely. By days 5 to 7, there were extravasated erythrocytes, basal cell vesiculation, subepidermal vesiculation, and necrotic epidermis. Biopsies of epidermis from the tail and back, even after epidermal cell division was stimulated, showed no evidence of inflammation.

FIGURE 149-4

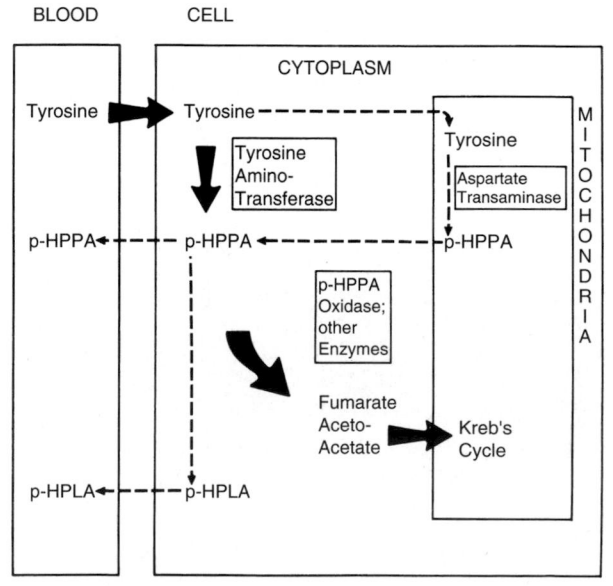

Tyrosine metabolism in normal subjects and in tyrosinemia II. The hepatic metabolism is depicted with the normal metabolic pathways in bold arrows. The pathway in disease is in broken arrows.

There are ranch mink and dogs with the clinical metabolic features of tyrosinemia.[20,21] The reason for the localization of the lesions to the eyes and volar skin in human, mink, and canine tyrosinemia II and in experimental tyrosinemia is unknown. Studies of the rat cornea showed that inflammation was limited to the location of crystal deposition, suggesting the importance of tyrosine crystals as a factor in the initiation of inflammation.[22] Electron microscopic studies of both human and rat tissues showed evidence of lysosomal activation and cytoskeletal disorganization.

In vitro studies showed that tyrosine crystals can cause release of lysosomal enzymes and as yet uncharacterized heat-labile chemotactic factors.[23,24] Crystal-induced inflammation has been studied in model systems using calcium pyrophosphate dihydrate and monosodium urate monhydrate. Phosphatidylinositol 3-kinase activation and tyrosine phosphorylation of several proteins occurred early in the activation process.[24] These studies have to be extended to tyrosine crystals.

Treatment

With a low-tyrosine, low-phenylalanine diet (Mead Johnson), there is a rapid decrease in tyrosine to normal levels (Fig. 149-5). Skin and eye lesions resolved within days in all individuals treated with the diet.[6] Normal growth and development took place in a patient when kept on the diet for 30 months starting at the age of 14 months. In this patient, 6 weeks after diet therapy was begun, the corneas were much clearer and less injected (see Fig. 149-2C), and the patient had sufficient vision to follow colored objects during play. At age 6 years, examination showed only remnants of vessels, and vision was normal except for myopia. Other patients have had slower resolution of symptoms. A 55-year-old man with tyrosinemia II had diffuse plantar hyperkeratosis (Fig. 149-6), which responded to a low-tyrosine, low-phenylalanine diet.[10]

Two adults have responded objectively to an aromatic retinoid (Ro 10-9359) (1.0 mg/kg per day). There was resolution without decrease in plasma tyrosine.[25] In none of the patients studied has there been response to cortisone acetate, ascorbic acid, pyridoxine, or folic acid, which are cofactors or known inducers of TAT and PHPPA oxidase.

Since the consequences of tyrosinemia II are serious, and a safe treatment is available, a patient presenting with any atypical bullous or hyperkeratotic disease on the palms and soles in the first months of life should be screened for tyrosine and its metabolites; simple screening tests (nitrosonaphthol in the presence of nitric acid and sodium nitrite) are available in most hospital laboratories. Amino acid analysis by ion-exchange chromatography is necessary to confirm the diagnosis and follow the response to diet therapy.

Differential Diagnosis

CLINICAL DISORDERS OF TYROSINE METABOLISM The disorders of tyrosine metabolism have a bewildering set of names. Tyrosinemia II (Richner-Hanhart syndrome) is distinct from the others; none of the others have any skin manifestations. These diseases are more completely reviewed elsewhere.[3,4]

Neonatal tyrosinemia is a common transient condition with decreased amounts of PHPPA oxidase apoenzyme and a relative deficiency of ascorbic acid contributing to the tyrosinemia, tyrosinuria, and increased excretion of tyrosine metabolites. Treatment is with ascorbic acid supplementation and a low-protein diet.

Hereditary tyrosinemia (tyrosinosis, tyrosinemia type I) is an autosomal recessive, severe liver and renal disease.[8] In the first 6 months of life, there are fever, edema, vomiting, a boiled-cabbage odor, hematuria, diarrhea, jaundice, hepatosplenomegaly, and the Fanconi syndrome. Long-term effects include hepatocellular carcinoma. Treatment includes liver transplantation. The basic biochemical defect is fumarylacetoacetate hydrolase deficiency with resulting increases in succinylacetone. Tyrosinemia, tyrosinuria, increased plasma PHPPA, hypermethioninemia, increased δ-aminolevulinic acid, increased catecholamines, and the renal findings of the Fanconi syndrome are present. Succinylacetone inhibits δ-aminolevulinic acid dehydratase and probably other enzymes, leading to the multiplicity of metabolic defects. Acute porphyria-related peripheral neuropathy (without skin lesions) may occur.

CLASSIC RICHNER-HANHART SYNDROME

The Richner-Hanhart syndrome classically (before amino acid analysis) consists of keratosis palmoplantaris, persistent dendritic lesions of the cornea with unaffected corneal sensitivity, photophobia, tearing, profound mental retardation, and autosomal recessive inheritance. In a review of the classic syndrome, 14 cases from 10 families are discussed.[26] All had corneal disease, 12 had keratosis palmoplantaris, and 8 were retarded. Consanguinity was common. Although none of the 14 patients had the extensive eye lesions of the patient in Fig. 149-2, it is suspected most of these patients had tyrosinemia II.

An autosomal dominant syndrome of volar keratosis and keratitis, which is clinically similar to tyrosinemia, was described in one family by Zmegac and Sarajlic.[27] The lesions were more extensive than those in the classic Richner-Hanhart syndrome but were similar to those seen in patients with tyrosinemia II. The keratitis of the Spanglang-Tappeiner syndrome, which is associated with palmar and plantar keratosis, appears to be related to lipid infiltration of the cornea.[28]

FIGURE 149-5

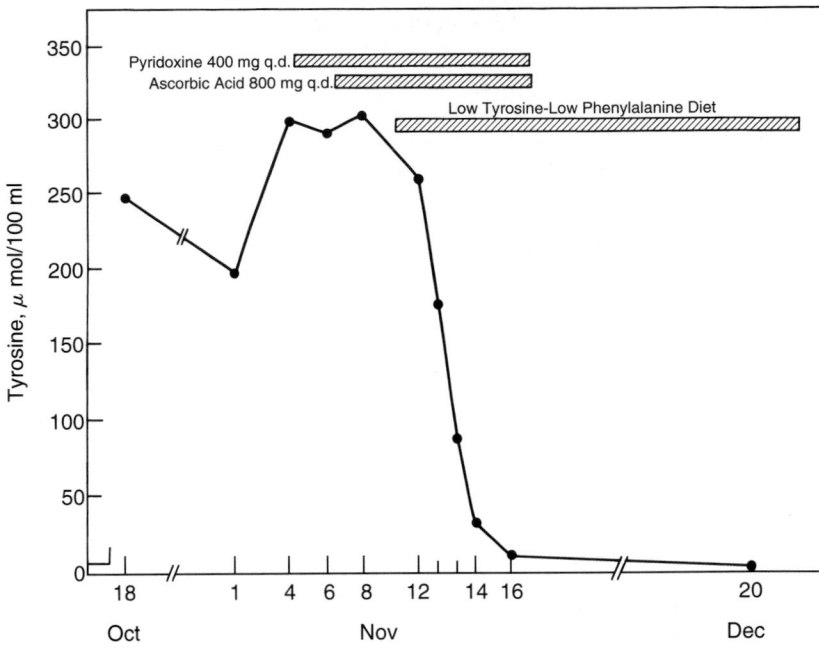

The response of elevated plasma tyrosine to a low-tyrosine, low-phenylalanine diet and failure of response to various cofactors in a patient with tyrosinemia II.

PHENYLKETONURIA

Phenylketonuria (PKU) is an autosomal recessive disease caused by a deficiency of hepatic phenylalanine hydroxylase or cofactors for phenylalanine hydroxylase. The increased levels of phenylalanine are associated with mental retardation; seizures; decreased pigmentation of the skin, hair, and eyes; and eczematous dermatitis.

FIGURE 149-6

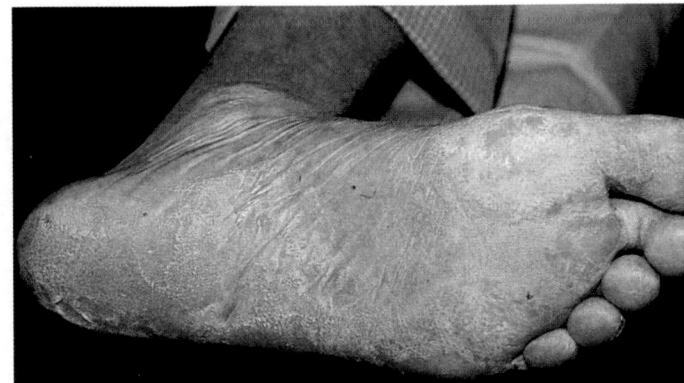

A.

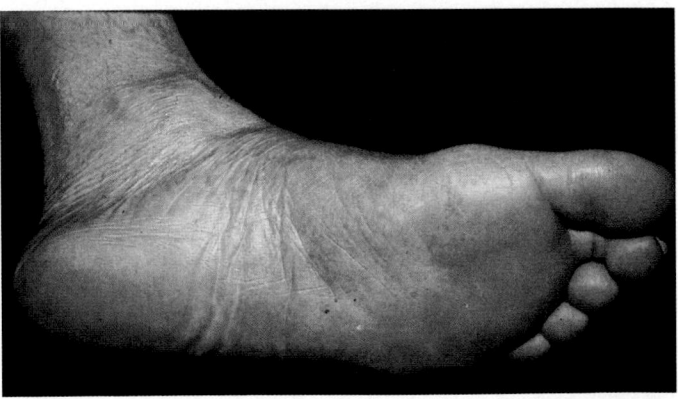

B.

Diffuse plantar hyperkeratosis in an adult with tyrosinemia (*A*). The hyperkeratosis cleared on a low-tyrosine, low-phenylalanine diet without topical treatment (*B*).

Clinical Features

This common metabolic defect occurs in 1 of 10,000 births and can be detected by screening procedures in neonatal life. One percent of institutionalized retarded patients have PKU. Mental retardation, athetosis, restlessness, increased tendon reflexes and muscle tone, hyperkinesis, tremors, and seizures accompany the untreated disease. The general features of the disease, its detailed genetics, biochemistry, heterozygote detection, prenatal diagnosis, and treatment are reviewed elsewhere.[29,30] Although there is a detailed understanding of the genetic abnormalities at the PKU focus and other related loci, there has been little research into the skin manifestations associated with PKU.

Patients with phenylketonuria have an increased incidence of eczematous dermatitis, pigment dilution of hair and skin color, and occasionally sclerodermatous skin changes. Other changes reported included a decreased number of pigmented nevi and an increased incidence of keratosis pilaris.[31] Skin phenylalanine levels are higher in PKU skin than in normal skin.[32]

Braun-Falco and Geissler and Fleisher and Zeligman found an increased incidence of atopic dermatitis in PKU.[31,33] In the former study, atopic dermatitis was present in 3 of 23 patients; in the latter, it was present in 15 of 25 patients. A potential mechanism suggested for the increased incidence of atopic disease is an increased tendency to vasoconstriction in PKU.[34] Dramatic clearing of eczema with a low-phenylalanine diet has been reported in some patients. It is possible that an inborn tendency to eczematous dermatitis has been nonspecifically triggered in these patients, although normal patients with eczema have no abnormality of phenylalanine metabolism detectable after a phenylalanine load.[35] Patients with PKU often have a lighter hair and eye color than their siblings.[36] The color changes may be especially striking in the rare black or Japanese patient with PKU whose eye or hair color may be very different from that of other members of the ethnic group. With a low-phenylalanine diet, or with aging alone, hair color darkens. When tyrosine is added to the diet of patients with PKU, hair darkens; if tyrosine is removed, the hair will lighten and banded hair is produced. The increased levels of phenylalanine and its oxidation products (phenylpyruvic acid, o-hydroxyphenylacetic acid, phenylacetic acid) inhibit the enzyme, tyrosinase, and therefore reduce melanization.[37]

The sclerodermatous changes in PKU are very striking and have been reviewed by Jablonska and Stachow.[38] Nine patients with PKU have had the onset of indurated areas of skin during the first year of life, most prominently on the thighs and associated with contractures. Acral areas of the body were least affected, in contradistinction to systemic sclerosis. Biopsy showed increased fibroblasts and histiocytes and atrophy of skin appendages. The elastic fibers were scanty and fragmented and were thus different from those found in true scleroderma. With dietary control, the sclerodermatous lesions cleared. The lesions may be due to alterations in tryptophan metabolism, which occur in patients with PKU; tryptophan absorption is decreased in the presence of high blood levels of phenylalanine.[39] Tryptophan and scleroderma-like skin lesions are associated in the eosinophilia-myalgia syndrome.[40] In two sibs with phenylketonuria, one had atrophoderma of Pasini and Pierini and the other localized scleroderma.[41] Pronounced skin lesions with skin dimpling are well documented in a recent report that reviews the literature.[42] In experimental PKU, there is an abnormal tubulin due to a decreased posttranslational addition of tyrosine to tubulin's α-chain.[43] This may explain some of the tissue effects in PKU.

Diagnosis

Phenylalanine can be quantitated by ion exchange chromatography. Increased levels of its metabolites in the urine are detected by a screening test in which $FeCl_3$ forms a bluish-green (olive-green) color in the presence of phenylpyruvic acid. The chemical determination distinguishes PKU from the various forms of oculocutaneous albinism and Chédiak-Higashi disease, which are also associated with pigment dilution.

Treatment

A low-phenylalanine diet results in increased pigmentation and, often, clearing of the eczema. Overrigorous control of diet can lead to protein deficiency and an eczematous dermatitis.

ARGININOSUCCINIC ACIDURIA

Definition and Clinical Features

Argininosuccinic aciduria (ASA) is characterized by hepatomegaly, mental retardation, seizures, episodic lethargy and ataxia, autosomal recessive inheritance, and friable, brittle hair with the morphology of trichorrhexis nodosa. The deficiency of an essential cytosolic enzyme in the urea cycle, argininosuccinase (argininosuccinate lyase), causes citrullinemia and an increase in blood ammonia. Argininosuccinate is increased in the blood and spinal fluid and is excreted in large amounts (2 to 9 g/day) in the urine.

The detailed clinical and biochemical features of the disease and the principles of therapy have been reviewed.[44] The disease presents in the neonatal period as failure to thrive and ammonia intoxication or, in the second year of age, with psychomotor retardation, seizures, and ataxia. The hair abnormality is more characteristic of the late-onset disease. Weaning and a change to a diet with higher protein content can be precipitating factors in clinical disease. Essential to current therapeutic regimens are diets providing adequate energy, protein, and arginine.[45]

The molecular pathology of the nucleic acids in this disease has been clarified, but the detailed pathophysiology of the hair defect remains to be studied.[45] Argininosuccinase cDNA has been cloned, sequenced, and mapped to chromosome 7 and is about 60 percent homologous to the δ-crystallins of the lens. Although there are at least 12 different mutant alleles, they all belong to one complementation group. Defining the molecular pathology allows prenatal diagnosis so that therapy can be instituted expeditiously.

Hair Defects

CLINICAL AND MORPHOLOGIC   About half of the reported patients have had abnormally friable hair with visible trichorrhexis nodosa; the other half have grossly normal hair.[44,46] Brushing and combing accentuate breaking (i.e., "brittle" hair).[46] No definite correlation can be made between liver ASase level, argininosuccinic acid levels, arginine levels, and the degree of hair abnormalities; some patients with severe ASA have had seemingly normal hair. Some patients' hair has improved with diet or without specific therapy.[47,48] One patient of Hartlage et al. had trichorrhexis nodosa at birth and improvement in her hair with the addition of increased amounts of arginine to the diet.[49] Eyelashes, eyebrows, and general body hair, as well as the nails, may be involved.[46,50]

There is variation in diameter within the same hair and torsion, grooving, and irregular contours of the intrafollicular portions of growing hairs.[46] With polarizing microscopy, there is no uniform cortical or medullary structure and no correlation of the lesion to polarized or nonpolarized regions.[46] Stains of the hair with acridine orange and subsequent fluorescent microscopy show red fluorescence instead of the green fluorescence seen in ordinary, mechanically induced trichorrhexis nodosa.[50]

MOLECULAR NATURE OF HAIR DEFECT During stress-strain testing in air, ASA hair broke prematurely at the end of the Hookean portion of the stress-strain curve, and Young's modulus of elasticity was less than 50 percent of normal.[51] In two patients, there was no argininosuccinic acid in the hair, and the only abnormality in amino acid content was a decreased serine level.[52] In another patient, the amino acid content was normal except for a cystine value one-half that of normal.[51]

The basic nature of the hair defect is not known. Are the brittle hair and the trichorrhexis nodosa a consequence of the deficiency of a product from the urea cycle, e.g., arginine, or is the hair defect related to an excess of one of the products that are increased due to argininosuccinate lyase deficiency? The administration of argininosuccinic acid to adult rats did not cause any specific effects, although there are no data on whether the argininosuccinic acid was absorbed from the gut.[48]

Increasing arginine in the diet aids hair growth and structure in this disease, suggesting that the decrease in arginine may be related to the defective hair. Since the urea cycle is depressed in ASA, the arginine required for protein synthesis would come predominantly from dietary sources. Hair protein is rich in arginine (up to 10 percent of the amino acid residues are arginine), and, furthermore, the citrulline present in certain specialized proteins in the medulla and internal root sheath is derived from arginine.[53] Increased ammonia levels also might inhibit ε-(γ-glutamyl) lysine bond formation, which is important for stabilization of the internal root sheath and medulla. The fumarate derived from ASA is important for the Krebs tricarboxylic acid cycle, and this cycle might be altered in ASA with consequent abnormalities of hair metabolism and growth.

Other Disorders of the Urea Cycle[44,45]

In citrullinemia, a rare recessive disease due to the absence of argininosuccinic acid synthetase, there are somatic and mental retardation and increased levels of blood, urine, and cerebral spinal fluid citrulline; low to normal values of plasma arginine; and increased blood ammonia.[44] Hair from a patient with citrullinemia was lightly pigmented, grew only to a length of 6 cm, and showed irregular areas of dystrophy and interruption of the cuticle.[54] The hair of an adult with the syndrome was said to be normal. More clinical details on the hair of these and similar patients and further studies of their hair would be of interest.

Deficiency of the cytosolic enzyme argininosuccinic acid synthetase is associated with trichorrhexis nodosa.[45] Its overall clinical presentation is almost identical to that of argininosuccinic aciduria, although the plasma citrulline levels are usually higher (>1 mM) in the former disease. Enzymatic and genetic analysis confirm the diagnosis.[45]

In lysinuric protein intolerance, which is due to defective transport, the skin may be hyperelastic, joints hypermobile, and the hair sparse and brittle.[43] One-half of the patients have been from Finland. Mice with deficiency in the X-linked urea cycle enzyme, ornithine carbamyl transferase, have sparse hair, but hair defects are not described in humans with the mutation.

Diagnosis

Retardation, ammonia intolerance, and abnormal hair will suggest these syndromes. The diagnosis is confirmed by high-voltage electrophoresis or ion-exchange chromatography of the urine, blood, or spinal fluid. Only a tiny percentage of the cases of trichorrhexis nodosa and brittle hair are due to ASA.

Microargininosuccinic Aciduria

In true ASA, urinary ASA ranges between 2 and 9 g/day. In contradistinction, there have been instances of normal individuals excreting a few milligrams of argininosuccinic acid a day, and some of these patients have had monilethrix, trichorrhexis nodosa, or pili torti.[55–57] In some of these cases ASA was not correctly identified, or there may have been dietary sources.[57] In any case, it is difficult to make a cause-and-effect relationship between these trivial levels of ASA and the associated hair defects.

ALKAPTONURIA

Alkaptonuria is a rare autosomal recessive disorder caused by deficiency of homogentisic acid oxidase (HGO), the sole catabolic enzyme for homogentisic acid (HGA). Excessive HGA is excreted in the urine, which often turns dark, and HGA accumulates in connective tissues, including the dermis.

Historic Aspects[58,59]

In 1859, Boedeker originally used the term *alcapton* to denote a urinary substance with great avidity for oxygen at an alkaline pH; later, he spelled the word *alkapton*. In 1866, Virchow saw the diffuse bluish-black pigmentation of connective tissue, in a presumably alkaptonuric individual, and called the condition *ochronosis* because of the ochre (yellow) hue seen microscopically. The prediction of Garrod, set forth in 1908, that alkaptonuria was caused by a specific enzyme deficiency was fully confirmed 50 years later when La Du and associates demonstrated the absence of hepatic HGA oxidase in an alkaptonuric patient.

Epidemiology

Alkaptonuria is inherited as an autosomal recessive trait. Pedigrees suggestive of a dominant mode of transmission contain a high degree of consanguinity and, when subjected to careful scrutiny, are actually "pseudodominants." In populations, alkaptonuria is rare (1:250,000), but clusters of high incidence are found in certain groups with inbreeding, e.g., in Slovakia and Santo Domingo. In Slovakian newborns the incidence is 1:25,000. Disease distribution is worldwide, and there is an approximately equal incidence in the sexes.

Etiology and Pathogenesis[59,60]

The HGO gene maps to 3q1-q23.[60] In two families, mutations in the exons have altered amino acids and led to loss of function mutations. The mutations change residues, which are conserved between *Aspergillus* HGO and human HGO, suggesting they are fundamental to HGO activity. Both compound heterozygotes and homozygotes have been detected.[60]

The biochemical pathway by which phenylalanine and tyrosine normally undergo oxidative degradation to acetoacetic acid is shown in Fig. 149-7. HGA (2,5-dihydroxyphenylacetic acid), the last molecule in the sequence to contain an intact aromatic ring, is cleaved to maleylacetoacetic acid. The enzyme catalyzing ring cleavage, HGA oxidase, is normally present in the soluble fraction of liver and kidney cells, but not in other cells. It is highly specific for HGA. HGO mRNA is found in liver, kidney, and prostate.[60] Atmospheric oxygen, ferrous ion, and sulfhydryl groups are required for enzymatic function. Quinones inhibit the enzyme. HGA oxidase activity is totally absent in both liver and kidney tissue from alkaptonuric subjects. In patients with alkaptonuria, HGA undergoes

FIGURE 149-7

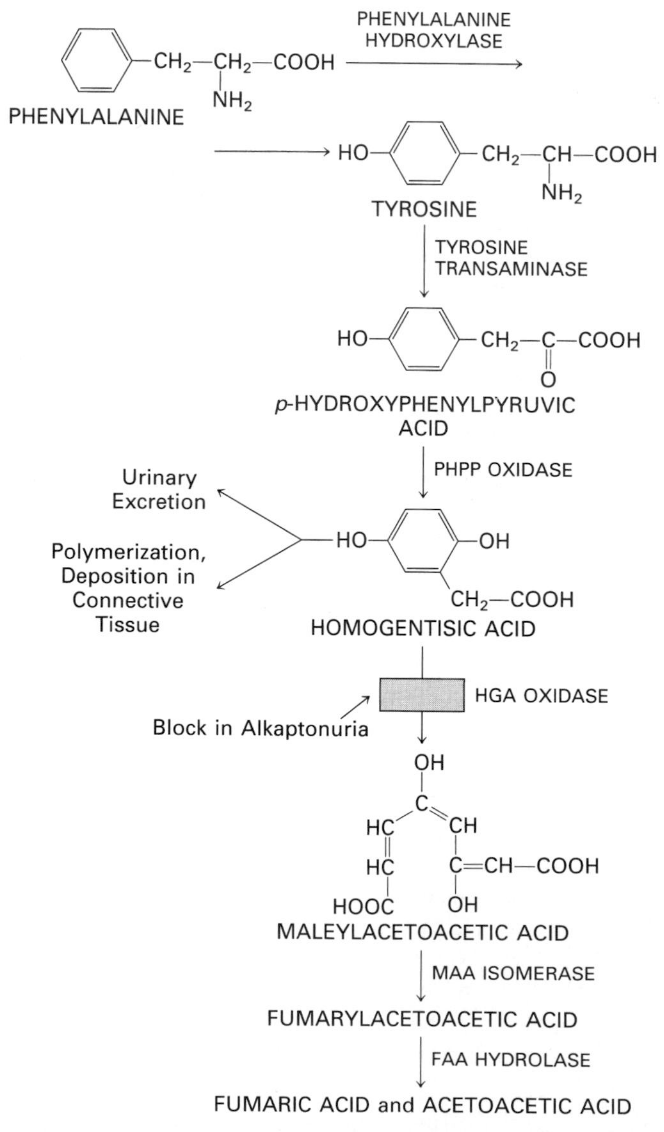

Metabolic pathway of phenylalanine and tyrosine degradation with homogentisic acid metabolites.

renal excretion or is transformed to ochronotic pigment within connective tissue. HGA may not be present in the first days of life due to the absence of enzymatic activity of other enzymes in the pathway of tyrosine catabolism.

The renal clearance of HGA is extremely high (up to 400 to 500 mL/min) in both normal and alkaptonuric subjects, indicating active tubular secretion of HGA.[59] This explains how with relatively low fasting plasma concentrations of HGA (in the range of 3 mg/dL), excretion may be up to 4 to 8 g/day in alkaptonuria. Compounds inhibiting this secretion may be an important factor in ochronosis. Once excreted, HGA (which is itself colorless in solution) gradually oxidizes to dark products. Oxidation occurs by degrees when the urine is exposed to air, but it can be markedly hastened by alkalinization. Urinary pH is the major variable causing the darkening of the urine, and some patients with acidic urine may *never* have spontaneously black urine. A diet high in protein or tyrosine increases the amount of HGA excreted in disease.

The precise manner by which HGA accumulation in tissues leads to ochronosis is only partially understood. A presumed HGA polymer has never been characterized. When HGA is injected into guinea pigs, it has a high predilection to localize in skin and cartilage; benzoquinoneacetic acid (BQA), the highly reactive quinone of HGA, binds irreversibly to connective tissue. Homogentisic acid polyphenol oxidase, a copper-containing enzyme in human, guinea pig, and rabbit skin and cartilage, catalyzes the oxidation of HGA into ochronotic pigment. In the presence of increased HGA, this enzyme may form BQA, which can then be polymerized by the same polyphenol oxidase.[61]

Alkaptonuric mice do not have black urine or deposition of pigment possibly related to the mouse's ability to synthesize ascorbic acid.[60] (Humans and guinea pigs are the only common mammals that are auxotrophs for ascorbic acid.)

Experimental ochronosis induced by prolonged feeding of high tyrosine diets to rats may delineate the precise interaction between HGA and its products and connective tissue.[62] Joint capsules, sternum, and trachea were affected, and there was increased nonsulfated acid mucopolysaccharides and decreased sulfated mucopolysaccharides. HGA and BQA were in the subcutaneous tissue. Alkaptonuria has also been produced in experimental animals by L-phenylalanine feeding and diets deficient in sulfur amino acids or tryptophan and the iron chelator, α,α'-dipyridyl.

HGA inhibits an enzyme crucial for collagen cross-linking, lysyl hydroxylase, in chick embryo calvaria, suggesting that a reduction of the structural integrity of collagen consequent to deficient hydroxylysine-derived cross-linkages may be responsible for cartilaginous degeneration in alkaptonuria.[63] The plasma level of HGA, approximately 0.1 m*M,* would cause 30 percent inhibition of lysyl hydroxylase. Milch has shown that autooxidized polymers of HGA combine with collagen chains to form significant cross-linking in vitro.[64]

Clinical Manifestations[58,59]

Dark urine is not always the initial manifestation of alkaptonuria. The urine is most apt to discolor rapidly at a pH above 7.0 and when reducing substances such as ascorbic acid, which normally protect HGA from oxidation, are not present in sufficient quantity. An early diagnosis of alkaptonuria is frequently made when: (1) it is specifically sought because of family history, (2) discoloration of diapers occurs after cleansing in (alkaline) soap, (3) the urinary pH favors the polymerization of HGA, or (4) testing for urinary glucose with Benedict's solution yields an orange precipitate (indicating a reducing substance) accompanied by a dark supernatant. A positive

Benedict's reaction and a negative glucose analysis with a glucose oxidase test reagent strongly suggest the diagnosis.

Although the diagnosis of alkaptonuria may be made during childhood, rare individuals are not detected until they develop pathologically significant changes in connective tissue in their third or fourth decade. If coincidental renal disease prevents effective HGA excretion, the development of ochronosis may be accelerated and diffuse hyperpigmentation result.[65,66]

Dark brown or black cerumen may be present in the first decade, even in those less than 5 years of age. Axillary skin pigmentation (greenish blue, blue, greenish yellow, or brown), in the pattern of glandular orifices, may be present late in the first decade; it may be accompanied by staining of underwear.

A grayish-blue tinge overlying ear cartilage occurs relatively early in the course of ochronosis. Later in the disease, structural changes result in loss of transillumination, stiffening, irregular contours, and eventually, in the third decade, calcification of the pinnae. The tympanic membrane may be blue. Tinnitus and variable degrees of deafness have been ascribed to ochronotic degeneration of the tympanic membrane and underlying ossicles. Laryngeal and tracheal cartilage become heavily pigmented but are asymptomatic.

The visible changes that occur with the passage of time are due primarily to the formation of ochronotic pigment granules in the dermis and sweat follicles and, most importantly, to the transmission of ochronotic discoloration through thin areas of skin overlying pigmented cartilage and tendon. The latter pigmentation, which is fairly uniform in ochronosis, is most apparent at the nose tip, ear (Fig. 149-8), costochondral junctions, and extensor tendons of the hands. Intrinsic pigmentation of the skin is typically less prominent but may occur in a butterfly pattern on the nose and cheeks. Rarely, bluish-gray fingernails and intensely dark nevi have been reported.[58]

Ochronotic pigment sometimes accumulates in the outer ocular tissues: sclerae (Fig. 149-9), corneas, conjunctivae, and tarsal plates. Scleral discoloration is generally restricted to that portion of the globe exposed by the palpebral fissure. The scleral pigmentation is usually triangular in shape, with the base of the triangle facing the cornea at the site of recti muscle insertion.[59] Tiny "oil droplets" of

ochronotic pigment appear at the inner and outer poles of the corneas in advanced ochronosis.

Insidious progression of ochronotic arthropathy, which generally begins in the third and fourth decades in males and about 10 years later in females, is the most disabling manifestation of alkaptonuria. The disease is more severe in males. Bouts of acute inflammation may occur. Hip, knee, and shoulder limitation are early signs. Lumbar pain, lordosis, kyphosis, and sciatica are common. X-rays show a characteristic appearance of early calcification of the intervertebral disc and later narrowing of the intervertebral spaces, with eventual disc collapse and progressive loss of height (Fig. 149-10). In addition to the spine, ochronotic arthropathy typically involves larger joints, such as the shoulders, knees, and hips. The hands and feet are generally spared. Pseudogout may coexist with ochronosis.[67]

There is some suggestion of an increased incidence of cardiovascular disease in ochronosis, but accelerated arteriosclerosis has not been clearly documented. At postmortem examination, pigmentation is commonly observed in the heart valves, annuli, and in arteriosclerotic plaques. A case of aortic valve stenosis has been attributed to the deposition of ochronotic pigment.[68]

Prostatic symptoms in older males are frequently due to the formation of soft pigmented calculi in the alkaline secretions of the ducts and sinuses of that gland. Porous black renal stones containing calcium, phosphate, and oxalate have also been reported. Prostate has high levels of HGO mRNA, which may explain the black prostate calculi that may be present in the disease.[60]

Laboratory Findings

Aside from the excretion of HGA, alkaptonuric patients show no abnormalities discernible on routine clinical laboratory tests. Normal individuals do not excrete HGA; therefore, darkening of the urine upon addition of sodium hydroxide is presumptive evidence of alkaptonuria.

Other tests based on the reducing properties of HGA include the black reaction after treatment with $FeCl_3$ and blackening of pho-

FIGURE 149-8

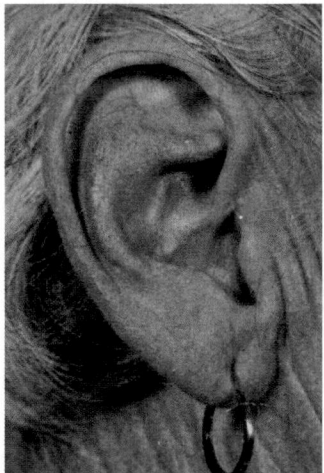

Ochronotic discoloration seen through the thin area of skin overlying the pigmented cartilage of the ear.

FIGURE 149-9

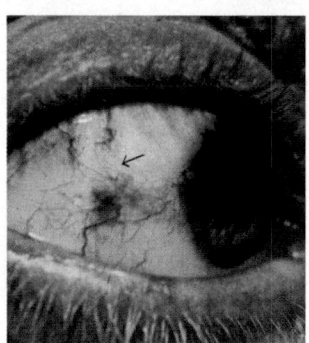

Ochronosis (alkaptonuria) has pathognomonic ocular signs. The first to appear is grayish-black scleral pigmentation (*arrow*) anterior to the tendon insertions of the horizontal recti muscles. At times pigmentation of the elastic tissue in pinguecula may be stained a dark brown or black and it usually has the configuration of small, dark rings. In advanced cases of ochronosis, Bowman's membrane, adjacent to the limbus, may have areas of black pigmentation.

FIGURE 149-10

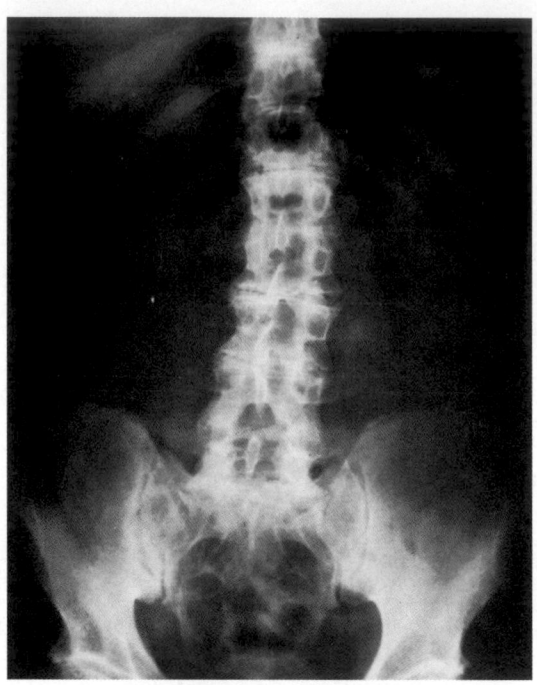

A.

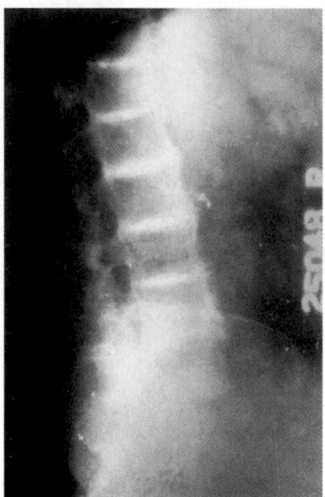

B.

Roentgenographic findings in ochronosis. Marked intervertebral disc calcification is present.

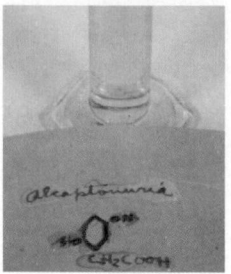

Urine from the patient with alkaptonuria. The urine itself was used to write on the photographic paper, then alkali was added. The homogentisic acid in the urine acted as a photographic developer.

Pathology

Yellow to light brown (ochre) color pigment granules, which gave the original designation of ochronosis, are present as free bodies and in dermal macrophages.[69] Irregular masses may be over 100 μm in diameter. The pigment is not bleached by 10% H_2O_2 after 72 h.[69] Routine special stains for melanin react with the ochronotic pigment.

Electron microscopic studies show smaller-sized homogeneous bodies fusing to form larger non-membrane-bound structures.[69] Although the original pigment is brown, Tyndall scattering of light makes involved skin appear blue.

The tendency of connective tissue, cartilage in particular, to darken gradually over the years constitutes the cardinal pathologic finding in alkaptonuria. Intervertebral discs are pigmented ("jet black") and darken when examined. Articular cartilage, when heavily pigmented, displays the degenerative changes of fibrillation, fissuring, fragmentation, and erosion to bare bone.[70] Phagocytosis of collagen fibrils is found in synovial macrophages.[71]

Diagnosis and Differential Diagnosis

The diagnosis of alkaptonuria may be made on the basis of typical urinary discoloration or may await the onset of ochronosis in adulthood. Inasmuch as the disease behaves in a quite stereotypical manner with few confusing variants in its mode of presentation, it has been concluded that the diagnosis need only be thought of to be made. Other causes of dark urine—melaninuria, porphyria, myoglobinuria, bilirubinuria, hematuria, etc.—ought not to be confused with alkaptonuria. An ochronotic-like pigmentation of skin and cartilage has been iatrogenically produced by quinacrine administration over a period of months and at the site of quinine injections.[72] Pigmentation due to antimalarial treatment is usually much more pronounced on mucosal surfaces and will fluoresce with a Wood's lamp.

Ochronotic pigmentation has also resulted from chronic application of carbolic acid to cutaneous ulcers, a form of therapy rarely used today. In a patient described by Osler and Garrod, the blue color was present on the sclera, the conchar concavity of the antihelix, and the extensor tendons of the hands.[73] The pigmentation on the eyes and ears regressed during hospitalization and upon discontinuation of carbolic acid. The light-related distribution of pigmentation was noted by the authors.

It is possible that the *reversible* ochronotic pigmentation caused by prolonged carbolic acid treatment is due to HGA polyphenol oxidase polymerizing the carbolic acid to an HGA-polymer-like

tographic emulsion paper upon application of a drop of alkaptonuric urine followed by a drop of sodium hydroxide (Fig. 149-11). Specific identification and quantitation of urinary (as well as blood) HGA can be achieved by the use of a direct spectrophotometric method employing HGA oxidase or with molecular techniques.[60]

With the development of ochronotic arthropathy, x-rays of the spine show characteristic disc calcification, which rarely occurs in other forms of spondylitis. Periostitis, ligament calcification, and sacroiliac sclerosis are not features of ochronotic spondylitis.

substance that differs from the polymer found in the genetic disease by its reversibility.

Exogenous ochronosis has been reported in a number of South Africans who used 2% or stronger hydroquinone bleaching creams for a prolonged period.[74,75] Forty-two percent of women and 15 percent of men who used hydroquinones had exogenous ochronosis.[75] A similar condition has been seen in American blacks.[76] The dermal material was autofluorescent, electron dense, and was phagocytosed, although another study emphasized the elastotic nature of the dermal fibers in the abnormal skin.[77] The precise etiology of the pigmentation remains to be determined. An occupationally induced blue-black dermal pigmentation resembling ochronosis has been described in a tiler who handled glues, varnishes, dyes, diluents, and stain removers.[78] Ochronotic arthropathy does not occur in these exogenous forms of hyperpigmentation.

Treatment

It is disappointing that despite advances in our biochemical understanding of alkaptonuria and the disposition of accumulated HGA to form ochronotic pigment in connective tissue, this information has yet to be translated into a successful therapeutic program for managing the disease. The treatment of ochronotic arthropathy centers about the proper balance of rest, physiotherapy, and analgesia. Prosthetic joint replacement is apt to be of considerable benefit for patients with advanced degenerative joint changes. Exogenous cutaneous ochronosis induced by hydroquinone has been treated with the carbon dioxide laser.[79]

Course and Prognosis

The ultimate course in adults with alkaptonuria is that of increasing pigmentation and skeletal incapacity. Little can be done to interrupt this progression; however, the disease is not incompatible with a normal life span, and the oldest patient on record lived to 99 years of age.

REFERENCES

1. Scriver CR et al: *Amino Acid Metabolism and Its Disorders.* Philadelphia, Saunders, 1973
2. Nyhan WL: *Heritable Disorders of Amino Acid Metabolism: Patterns of Clinical Expression and Genetic Variation.* New York, Wiley, 1974
3. Scriver CR et al (eds): *The Metabolic and Molecular Bases of Inherited Disease,* 7th ed. New York, McGraw Hill, 1995
4. Goldsmith LA, LaBerge C: Tyrosinemia and related disorders, in *The Metabolic Basis of Inherited Disease,* 6th ed, edited by CR Scriver et al. New York, McGraw-Hill, 1989, p 547
5. Zaleski WA et al: Skin lesions in tyrosinosis: Response to dietary treatment. *Br J Dermatol* **88**:335, 1973
6. Goldsmith LA, Reed J: Tyrosine-induced eye and skin lesions. A treatable genetic disease. *JAMA* **236**:382, 1976
7. Goldsmith LA et al: Tyrosinemia with plantar and palmar keratosis and keratitis. *J Pediatr* **83**:798, 1973
8. Mitchell GA et al: Hypertyrosinemia, in *The Metabolic and Molecular Bases of Inherited Disease*, 7th ed, edited by CR Scriver et al. New York, McGraw-Hill, 1995, p 1077
9. Burns RP: Soluble tyrosine aminotransferase deficiency: An unusual cause of corneal ulcers. *Am J Ophthalmol* **73**:400, 1972
10. Goldsmith LA et al: Hepatic enzymes of tyrosine metabolism in tyrosinemia II. *J Invest Dermatol* **73**:530, 1979
11. Fellman JH et al: Soluble and mitochondrial forms of tyrosine aminotransferase. Relationship to human tyrosinemia. *Biochemistry* **8**:615, 1969
12. Bohnert A, Anton-Lamprecht I: Richner-Hanhart's syndrome: Ultrastructural abnormalities of epidermal keratinization indicating a causal relationship to high intracellular tyrosine levels. *J Invest Dermatol* **79**:68, 1982
13. el-Shoura SM, Tallab TM: Richner-Hanhart's syndrome: New ultrastructural observations on skin lesions of two cases. *Ultrastruct Pathol* **21**:51, 1997
14. Natt E et al: Inherited and de novo deletion of the tyrosine aminotransferase gene locus at 16q22.1-q22.3 in a patient with tyrosinemia type II. *Hum Genet* **77**:352, 1987
15. Natt E et al: Point mutations in the tyrosine aminotransferase gene in tyrosinemia type II. *Genetics* **89**:9297, 1992
16. Schweizer W: Studies on the effect of L-tyrosine on the white rat. *J Physiol (Lond)* **106**:167, 1947
17. Alam SQ et al: Effect of threonine on the toxicity of excess tyrosine and cataract formation in the rat. *J Nutr* **89**:91, 1966
18. Selye H: Steroids influencing the toxicity of L-tyrosine. *J Nutr* **101**:515, 1971
19. Beard ME et al: Histopathology of keratopathy in the tyrosine-fed rat. *Invest Ophthalmol* **13**:1037, 1974
20. Goldsmith LA et al: Tyrosine aminotransferase deficiency in mink (*Mustela vison*): A model for human tyrosinemia II. *Biochem Genet* **19**:687, 1981
21. Jezyk PF et al: Screening for inborn errors of metabolism in dogs and cats, in *Animal Models of Inherited Metabolic Diseases,* edited by RJ Desnick. New York, Alan R. Liss, 1983, p 93
22. Gipson IK et al: Crystals in corneal epithelial lesions of tyrosine fed rats. *Invest Ophthalmol* **14**:937, 1975
23. Goldsmith LA: Hemolysis and lysosomal activation by solid-state tyrosine. *Biochem Biophys Res Commun* **64**:558, 1975
24. Jackson JK et al: The involvement of phosphatidylinositol 3-kinase in crystal induced human neutrophil activation. *J Rheumatol* **24**:341, 1997
25. Hunziker N et al: Richner-Hanhart syndrome (RHS)-tyrosinemia type II and oral aromatic retinoid (Ro 10-9359). Report of two cases, in *Retinoids. Advances in Basic Research and Therapy,* edited by CE Orfanos et al. New York, Springer, 1981, p 453
26. Franceschetti AT et al: Die cornea beim Richner-Hanhart Syndrom. *Ber Dtsch Ophthalmol Ges* **71**:109, 1971
27. Zmegac ZJ, Sarajlic MV: A rare form of an inheritable palmar and plantar keratosis. *Dermatologica* **130**:40, 1964
28. Geeraets WJ: *Ocular Syndromes,* 3d ed. Philadelphia, Lea & Febiger, 1976
29. Tourian A, Sidbury JB: Phenylketonuria and hyperphenylalaninemia, in *The Metabolic Basis of Inherited Disease,* 5th ed, edited by JB Stanbury et al. New York, McGraw-Hill, 1982, p 270
30. Scriver CR et al: The Hyperphenylalaninemias, in *The Metabolic and Molecular Bases of Inherited Disease,* 7th ed, edited by CR Scriver et al. New York, McGraw-Hill, 1995, p 1015
31. Braun-Falco O, Geissler H: Hauterscheinungen bei Phenylketonuric. *Med Welt* **37**:1941, 1964
32. Fisch RO et al: Studies of phenylketonuria with dermatitis. *J Am Acad Dermatol* **4**:284, 1981
33. Fleisher TL, Zeligman I: Cutaneous findings in phenylketonuria. *Arch Dermatol* **81**:898, 1960
34. Solomon LM, Desai K: Phenylketonuria. *Cutis* **4**:1233, 1968
35. Vickers CFH: Eczema and phenylketonuria. *Trans St Johns Hosp Dermatol Soc* **50**:56, 1964
36. Berg JM, Stern J: Iris color in phenylketonuria. *Ann Hum Genet* **22**:370, 1958
37. Miyamoto M, Fitzpatrick TB: Competitive inhibition of mammalian tyrosinase by phenylalanine and in relationship to hair pigmentation in phenylketonuria. *Nature* **179**:199, 1957
38. Jablonska S, Stachow A: Scleroderma-like lesions in phenylketonuria (PKU), in *Scleroderma and Pseudoscleroderma,* 2d ed, edited by S Jablonska. Warsaw, Polish Medical Publishers, 1975, p 489
39. Yarbro MT, Anderson JA: Tryptophan metabolism in phenylketonuria. *J Pediatr* **68**:895, 1966
40. Belongia AE et al: An investigation of the cause of the eosinophilia-myalgia syndrome associated with tryptophan use. *N Engl J Med* **323**:357, 1990
41. Lasser AE et al: Phenylketonuria and scleroderma. *Arch Dermatol* **114**:1215, 1978
42. Nova MP et al: Scleroderma-like skin indurations in a child with phenylketonuria: A clinicopathologic correlation and review of the literature. *J Am Acad Derm* **26**:329, 1992

43. Rodriguez JA, Borisy GG: Experimental phenylketonuria: Replacement of carboxyl terminal tyrosine by phenylalanine in infant rat brain tubulin. *Science* **206**:463, 1979

44. Walser M: Urea cycle disorders and other hereditary hyperammonemic syndromes, in *The Metabolic Basis of Inherited Disease,* 5th ed, edited by JB Stanbury et al. New York, McGraw-Hill, 1983, p 402

45. Brusilow SW, Horwich AL: Urea cycle enzymes, in *The Metabolic Basis of Inherited Disease,* 6th ed, edited by CR Scriver et al. New York, McGraw-Hill, 1989, p 629

46. Rauschkolb EW et al: Hair fragility—an important clue to aminoacidopathy in mental retardation. *Cutis* **4**:1315, 1968

47. Coryell ME et al: A familial study of a human enzyme defect, argininosuccinic aciduria. *Biochem Biophys Res Commun* **14**:307, 1964

48. Westall RG: Treatment of argininosuccinic aciduria. *Am J Dis Child* **113**:160, 1967

49. Hartlage RL et al: Argininosuccinic aciduria: Perinatal diagnosis and early dietary management. *J Pediatr* **85**:86, 1974

50. Levin B et al: Argininosuccinic aciduria. An inborn error of amino acid metabolism. *Arch Dis Child* **36**:622, 1961

51. Potter JL et al: Argininosuccinic-aciduria—the hair abnormality. *Am J Dis Child* **127**:724, 1974

52. Van Sande M: Hair amino acids: Normal values and results in metabolic errors. *Arch Dis Child* **45**:678, 1970

53. Rogers GE, Harding HWJ: Molecular mechanisms in the formation of hair, in *Biology and Disease of the Hair,* edited by T Kobofi, W Montagna. Baltimore, University Park Press, 1976, p 411

54. Porter PS: The genetics of human hair growth. *Birth Defects* **7**:69, 1971

55. Grosfeld JCM et al: Argininosuccinic aciduria in monilethrix. *Lancet* **2**:789, 1964

56. Winther A, Bundgaard L: Argininosuccinic aciduria in hereditary hair diseases. *Acta Derm Venereol (Stockh)* **48**:567, 1968

57. Efron ML, Hoefnagel D: Argininosuccinic acid in monilethrix. *Lancet* **1**:321, 1966

58. O'Brien WM et al: Biochemical, pathologic and clinical aspects of alkaptonuria, ochronosis and ochronotic arthropathy. *Am J Med* **34**:813, 1963

59. La Du BN: Alkaptonuria, in *The Metabolic and Molecular Bases of Inherited Disease,* 7th ed, edited by CS Scriver et al. New York, McGraw-Hill, 1995, p 1371

60. Fernandez-Canon JM et al: The molecular basis of alkaptonuria. *Nat Genet* **14**:19, 1996

61. Zannoni VG et al: Oxidation of homogentisic acid to ochronotic pigment in connective tissue. *Biochem Biophys Acta* **177**:94, 1969

62. Blivaiss BB et al: Experimental ochronosis: Induction in rats by long-term feeding with L-tyrosine. *Arch Pathol* **82**:45, 1966

63. Murray JC et al: *In vitro* inhibition of chick embryo lysyl hydroxylase by homogentisic acid. A proposed connective tissue defect in alkaptonuria. *J Clin Invest* **59**:1071, 1977

64. Milch RA: Studies of alkaptonuria: Mechanisms of swelling of homogentisic acid–collagen preparations. *Arthritis Rheum* **4**:253, 1961

65. Wyre CHW: Alkaptonuria with extensive ochronsis. *Arch Dermatol* **115**:461, 1979

66. Abreo K et al: Clinicopathologic conference: A fifty-year-old man with skin pigmentation, arthritis, chronic renal failure and methemoglobinemia. *Am J Med Genet* **14**:97, 1983

67. Rynes RI et al: Pseudogout in ochronosis. *Arthritis Rheum* **18**:21, 1975

68. Gould L et al: Cardiac manifestations of ochronosis. *J Thorac Cardiovasc Surg* **72**:788, 1976

69. Attwood HD et al: A histologic, histochemical and ultrastructural study of dermal ochronosis. *Pathology* **3**:115, 1971

70. O'Brien WM et al: Studies on the pathogenesis of ochronotic arthropathy. *Arthritis Rheum* **4**:137, 1961

71. Gaines JJ et al: An ultrastructural and light microscopy study of the synovium in ochronotic arthropathy. *Hum Pathol* **18**:1160, 1987

72. Bruce S et al: Exogenous ochronosis resulting from quinine injections. *J Am Acad Dermatol* **15**:357, 1986

73. Reid E et al: On ochronosis: Report of a case, the clinical features, the urine. *Q J Med* **1**:199, 1908

74. Findlay GH et al: Exogenous ochronosis and pigmented colloid milium from hydroquinone bleaching creams. *Br J Dermatol* **93**:613, 1975

75. Hardwick N et al: Exogenous ochronosis: An epidemiological study. *Br J Dermatol* **120**:229, 1989

76. Hoshaw RA et al: Ochronosis-like pigmentation from hydroquinone bleaching creams in American Blacks. *Arch Dermatol* **121**:105, 1985

77. Tidman MJ et al: Hydroquinone-induced ochronosis—light and electron-microscopic features. *Clin Exp Dermatol* **11**:224, 1986

78. Dupre A et al: Idiopathic pigmentation of the hands: Professional exogenous ochronosis? New entity? *Arch Dermatol Res* **266**:1, 1979

79. Diven DG et al: Hydroquinone-induced localized exogenous ochronosis treated with dermabrasion and CO_2 laser. *J Dermatol Surg Oncol* **16**:1018, 1990

CHAPTER 150

Stephen M. Breathnach

Amyloidosis of the Skin

DEFINITION AND CLASSIFICATION OF AMYLOIDOSIS

The generic term *amyloidosis* signifies the abnormal extracellular tissue deposition of one of a family of biochemically unrelated proteins that share certain characteristic staining properties, including apple-green birefringence of Congo red–stained preparations viewed under polarized light, and a fibrillar ultrastructure.[1–6] Paired, 7.5- to 10-nm, rigid, linear, nonbranching, aggregated, hollow fibrils of indefinite length constitute the bulk of amyloid deposits, regardless of clinicopathologic type or the tissue involved, and are arranged in a loose meshwork. Amyloid fibrils have been shown by x-ray diffraction crystallography and infrared spectroscopy to have, at least in part, a β-pleated sheet configuration, which probably accounts for their ability to bind Congo red.

TABLE 150-1

Classification of Amyloid and Biochemical Nature of Fibril Proteins

CLINICAL SYNDROME	FIBRIL PROTEINS AND PRECURSORS
Systemic Amyloidosis	
I. Associated with immunocyte dyscrasia	
A. Primary systemic (occult dyscrasia)	AL fibrils from monoclonal immunoglobulin light chains
B. Myeloma associated	
II. Associated with chronic active diseases (secondary or reactive systemic amyloidosis)	AA fibrils from serum amyloid A protein (SAA)
III. Hereditary syndromes	
A. Predominantly neuropathic forms (autosomal dominant)	Transthyretin variant *or*
1. Familial amyloid polyneuropathy	Apolipoprotein A1 *or*
	Gelsolin
B. Nonneuropathic forms (autosomal dominant)	Apolipoprotein A1 *or*
1. Ostertag type	Lysozyme or
	Fibrinogen α-chain
C. Predominantly nephropathic forms	
1. Familial Mediterranean fever (autosomal recessive)	AA fibrils from SAA
2. Muckle-Wells type	AA fibrils from SAA
D. Predominantly cardiomyopathic forms	Transthyretin variant
1. Cardiomyopathy with persistent atrial standstill	Unknown
IV. Senile systemic amyloidosis	Transthyretin from plasma
Localized (Organ-Limited) Amyloidosis	
I. Hereditary syndromes	
A. Hereditary cerebral hemorrhage with amyloidosis	
1. Icelandic type	Cystatin C fibrils
2. Dutch type	β-protein fibrils
II. Periarticular, bony, and renal amyloid in chronic hemodialysis patients	β_2-microglobulin from plasma
III. Cerebral amyloid angiopathy and cortical plaques in Alzheimer's disease, senile dementia, Down's syndrome	β-protein fibrils
IV. Sporadic Creutzfeldt-Jakob disease, kuru	Prion protein
V. Focal senile amyloidosis	
A. Heart atria	Atrial natriuretic peptide
B. Joints	Unknown
C. Seminal vesicles	Seminal vesicle exocrine protein
D. Prostate	β_2-microglobulin
VI. Ocular deposits (corneal, conjunctival)	Unknown
VII. Endocrine amyloidosis (APUD organs, APUDomas)	
A. Elderly non-insulin-dependent diabetics, benign insulinomas of the pancreas, normal aged pancreas	Islet amyloid polypeptide fibrils (homology with calcitonin gene–related peptides)
B. Medullary carcinoma of the thyroid	Precalcitonin-related fibrils
VIII. Nodular (skin, lung, genitourinary tract)	AL fibrils derived from monoclonal immunoglobulin light chains
IX. Primary localized cutaneous (macular amyloidosis and lichen amyloidosis)	?Keratin-derived
X. Secondary localized cutaneous (microscopic deposits secondary to a variety of cutaneous lesions)	?Keratin-derived

SOURCE: Derived from Hawkins.[1]

Amyloid deposition may occur throughout many organs of the body (systemic amyloidosis) or be restricted to a single tissue site (organ-limited or localized amyloidosis) (Table 150-1); it is usually associated with considerable tissue dysfunction. Interest in amyloidosis has increased tremendously with the realization that it is involved in the pathology of aging and of neurodegenerative diseases, including Alzheimer's disease and strokes.[4–6] Systemic types of amyloidosis include those associated with plasma cell dyscrasia, either overt as in multiple myeloma or occult as in "primary" systemic amyloidosis,[7] and amyloidosis secondary to a variety of chronic diseases.[8] The latter include acute recurrent and chronic infections, rheumatoid arthritis, juvenile chronic arthritis, ankylosing spondylitis, Reiter's syndrome, Behçet's syndrome, Sjögren's syndrome, systemic lupus erythematosus (very rarely), inflammatory bowel disease, Hodgkin's disease, some solid nonlymphoid tumors, and Castleman's disease.[9,10] Secondary systemic amyloidosis may also arise as a complication of a number of dermatoses.[11] These include recurrent venous ulceration[12]; generalized psoriasis and psoriatic arthritis[13,14]; lepromatous leprosy; hidradenitis suppurativa; chronically infected burns; chronic skin infection in drug addicts[15]; nodular nonsuppurative panniculitis[16]; giant, ulcerated, or metastatic basal cell carcinoma[17]; acne conglobata[18]; epidermolysis bullosa of dystrophic[19] and acquisita types; and X-linked anhidrotic ectodermal dysplasia.

Clinically evident involvement of the skin is frequent in primary systemic and myeloma-associated systemic amyloidosis but occurs only rarely, if at all, in secondary systemic amyloidosis. Although there is a degree of overlap, primary and myeloma-associated systemic amyloidosis typically involve the tongue, heart, gastrointestinal tract, skeletal and smooth muscle, carpal ligaments, nerves, and skin, whereas secondary systemic amyloidosis affects the liver, spleen, kidneys, and adrenals.[20] Skin manifestations are associated with a number of systemic heredofamilial syndromes of amyloid deposition including familial Mediterranean fever,[21] the Muckle-Wells syndrome,[22] and heredofamilial amyloid polyneuropathy.[23] Localized cutaneous amyloidosis may be of primary (nodular, and macular amyloid and lichen amyloidosis) or secondary type (Table 150-1).[24–26]

ETIOLOGY AND PATHOGENESIS

Amyloid material may accumulate as a result of a variety of different pathogenic mechanisms, and the biochemical composition of amyloid fibrils varies according to the clinicopathologic type of amyloidosis.[1–6] The various known amyloid fibril proteins are listed in Table 150-1. Only those relevant to cutaneous disease will be discussed further.

Systemic Amyloidosis

Amyloid deposition in primary and myeloma-associated systemic amyloidosis occurs as a result of plasma cell dyscrasia, and the fibrils are composed of immunoglobulin light chain material (*protein AL*)[1–3]: either intact light chains, light chain fragments (particularly the variable amino-terminal region), or both.[27–30] Abnormal light chain material is almost always present in the serum or urine, even in so-called primary systemic amyloidosis, and can be demonstrated on tissue culture of bone marrow cells from affected patients. Proteolytic digestion of only a proportion of Bence Jones proteins results in amyloid fibril formation,[31] which may account for the fact that amyloidosis develops in only about 15 percent of patients with myelomatosis. Amyloidogenic immunoglobulin AL monoclonal proteins appear to be preferentially of lambda type, of lower molecular weight, and of lower isoelectric point[32]; specific amino acid residue changes arising from point mutation may destabilize domains and render them susceptible to the formation of ordered, fibril-like aggregates in vitro.[28]

In secondary systemic amyloidosis and familial Mediterranean fever, the fibrils are composed of a nonimmunoglobulin protein designated *protein AA*.[1–3,8,33] A precursor of protein AA, known as *serum amyloid A protein* (protein SAA), is present in the serum of normal individuals as an apolipoprotein of high-density lipoprotein and behaves as an acute-phase reactant. A number of types of familial amyloidosis, which may manifest initially with progressive neuropathy, cardiomyopathy, or renal involvement, are related to a variant of transthyretin (prealbumin) inherited as a dominant trait, produced by a point mutation leading to an amino acid substitution in the transthyretin gene. This may destabilize the transthyretin tetramer in favor of a monomeric amyloidogenic intermediate under lysosomal (acidic) conditions.[1–3,34,35] However, in senile systemic amyloidosis, the amino acid primary structure of the transthyretin of which the fibrils are composed is normal, so that factors other than the primary structure must be involved in the amyloid depo-

sition.[4] In patients undergoing long-term hemodialysis, the amyloid fibrils are composed of beta$_2$-microglobulin.[36]

Localized Cutaneous Amyloidosis

SECONDARY LOCALIZED CUTANEOUS AMYLOIDOSIS Deposition of insignificant microscopic amounts of amyloid in relation to a variety of cutaneous lesions is the most common type of localized cutaneous amyloidosis. Reported predisposing conditions include intradermal nevi, sweat gland tumors, pilomatrixoma, dermatofibroma, seborrheic keratosis, solar elastosis, photosensitive annular elastolytic giant cell granuloma, actinic keratosis, porokeratosis of Mibelli, Bowen's disease, and basal cell carcinoma.[25,37–41] It can also occur following PUVA therapy.[42]

PRIMARY LOCALIZED CUTANEOUS AMYLOIDOSIS (PLCA) PLCA comprises macular, papular (lichen amyloidosis), and the rare nodular (tumefactive) forms.[24–26] Nodular PLCA may be regarded as akin to extramedullary plasmacytoma, since the fibrils are of immunoglobulin AL type and are thought to arise as a result of local aberrant light chain material production by clonally expanded plasma cells.[43,44] Fibrils in lichen and macular amyloidosis do not bind antibodies to protein AA or prealbumin,[45] and although immunoglobulins, kappa and lambda light chains, and complement are frequently observed in deposits of macular and papular PLCA,[46,47] they are not thought to be integral constituents of the fibrils since they are readily eluted. Instead, the concept has arisen of focal epidermal damage and filamentous degeneration of keratinocytes, followed by apoptosis and conversion of filamentous masses (colloid bodies) into amyloid material in the papillary dermis, perhaps with a contribution from the dermal-epidermal junction.[48–51] In support of this theory is the fact that dermal amyloid deposits in these forms of PLCA cross-react immunohistochemically with keratin.[49,50] However, the tertiary structure of epidermal keratin is of α-type, rather than the β-pleated sheet configuration typical of amyloid. Furthermore, the pathogenesis cannot be this simple, since colloid (keratin) bodies produced in other dermatoses such as lichen planus are not transformed into amyloid. One theory proposes that in lichen amyloidosis specific immunologic tolerance to the presence of colloid bodies in the papillary dermis favors their transformation into amyloid by macrophages or fibroblasts,[38] whereas in lichen planus a brisk inflammatory response ensures their removal.

Nonfibrillar Amyloid Proteins

In addition to the fibrillar component, amyloid deposits invariably contain up to 14 percent by dry weight of a protein termed *amyloid P (plasma) component* (AP),[1,52] which is derived from and identical to *serum amyloid P component* (SAP), a protein present in the blood of all normal individuals. AP is also constantly associated with the microfibrillar sheath of elastic fibers throughout the body in normal adults.[53] SAP prevents proteolysis of the amyloid fibrils of Alzheimer's disease, AA amyloidosis, and AL amyloidosis and may thereby contribute to their persistence in vivo.[52] In this regard, it is of interest that AP is absent from nonamyloidotic monoclonal immunoglobulin deposits. AP shows calcium-dependent binding to isolated amyloid fibrils in vitro, which may account for the frequent observation of amyloid deposition in the vicinity of elastic fibers.[54] Amyloid deposits also contain extracellular matrix components including glycosaminoglycans and proteoglycans, which may be involved in the pathogenesis.[55]

CLINICAL MANIFESTATIONS

Primary and Myeloma-Associated Systemic Amyloidosis

The field has been extensively reviewed.[1,3,7,20,24,56,57] These conditions are very rare in patients below the age of 40 years, the mean age of onset being about 65 years; there is a slight male preponderance. Diagnosis is often delayed because of nonspecific presenting symptoms; these include fatigue, weight loss, paresthesia, hoarseness, edema, dyspnea, and syncope secondary to orthostatic hypotension. The classic presentation with symptoms of carpal tunnel syndrome, macroglossia (which occurs in about 10 percent of patients and may result in painful dysphagia), specific mucocutaneous lesions, hepatomegaly, and edema should always alert the clinician to the presence of an underlying plasma cell dyscrasia.

SYSTEMIC REVIEW Hepatomegaly occurs in about 50 percent of patients at presentation, but splenomegaly in fewer than 10 percent. Pitting edema is common and may be the result of the nephrotic syndrome or of congestive cardiac failure, both of which occur in about 30 percent of patients; rarely, it may be a complication of protein-losing enteropathy from amyloid involvement of the small bowel. Ascites may develop. Angina, infarction, arrhythmias, or orthostatic hypotension may develop as a consequence of cardiac infiltration.[58] Congestive cardiac failure or arrhythmias account for death in about 40 percent of patients with AL type systemic amyloidosis. Pulmonary involvement is common but usually asymptomatic. Amyloid infiltration of blood vessels may lead to claudication of the legs or jaw, and gastrointestinal tract involvement may simulate inflammatory bowel disease with hemorrhage; malabsorption is found in 5 percent of cases. The carpal tunnel syndrome has been reported in up to 25 percent of patients with primary systemic amyloidosis. Peripheral neuropathy,[59] initially of the lower extremities, tends to pursue a chronic course and may be accompanied by superimposed autonomic neuropathy leading to orthostatic hypotension, diarrhea, loss of bladder control, or impotence. Muscle weakness may be caused by neuropathy or by direct infiltration of muscle or its vascular supply, and infiltration between muscle fibers leading to pseudohypertrophy is recognized.

Lymphadenopathy, which occurs in about 10 percent of patients, Sjögren's syndrome, or sicca syndrome[60] may occasionally be presenting features. Amyloid deposition in joints may mimic rheumatoid arthritis, and deposition around the shoulders may cause extensive soft tissue enlargement (the shoulder-pad sign).[61] Giant cell arteritis and polymyalgia rheumatica have been recorded.[62] Amongst the hematologic complications of systemic amyloidosis are isolated factor X deficiency,[63] disseminated intravascular coagulation, and fibrinolysis with severe bleeding.

MUCOCUTANEOUS FINDINGS Clinically evident mucocutaneous involvement occurs in up to 40 percent of patients (Table 150-2).[7,20,56,57] The surface of the tongue may be smooth and dry, or studded with waxy papules, nodules, plaques, or bullae; there may be fissuring, ulceration, and hemorrhage and tooth indentations on the lateral border.

The most common skin signs consist of petechiae, purpura, and ecchymoses, occurring spontaneously or after minor trauma, and are the result of amyloid infiltration of blood vessel walls. Purpuric lesions are found especially in flexural regions, such as the eyelids (Fig. 150-1), nasolabial folds, neck, axillae, umbilicus, and anogenital area, as well as in the mouth. Eyelid purpura following pinching

TABLE 150-2

Cutaneous Lesions in Primary and Myeloma-Associated Systemic Amyloidosis

COMMON	LESS COMMON
Petechiae, purpura, ecchymoses	Pigmentary changes
Waxy, translucent, or purpuric papules	Scleroderma-like infiltration
	Bullous lesions
Nodules	Alopecia
Plaques	Cordlike blood vessel thickening
Tumefactive lesions	Nail dystrophy
	Amyloid elastosis
	Cutis laxa

(pinch purpura) and periorbital purpura following coughing, vomiting, the Valsalva maneuver, forced expiration during spirometric testing, or proctoscopy (postproctoscopic palpebral purpura) are very characteristic. Target-like lesions may develop as transient purpuric haloes around Campbell de Morgan spots.[64] Pigmentary changes include jaundice due to hepatic disease, cardiac failure, or severe hemorrhage; pallor due to anemia; and hyperpigmentation due to hemorrhage.

Waxy, smooth, shiny papules (Fig. 150-2), nodules, and plaques, which may be skin- or amber-colored with a hemorrhagic appearance, are the most characteristic skin lesions. Translucent lesions may resemble vesicles. Flexural areas are sites of predilection, including the eyelids, retroauricular region, neck, axillae, umbilicus, and inguinal and anogenital regions. Lesions may also be found on the central face, lips, tongue, and buccal mucosa. Nodules, which occur at any site, may resemble condylomata lata on perianal and vulval skin and, when widespread, may appear like xanthomata.[65]

FIGURE 150-1

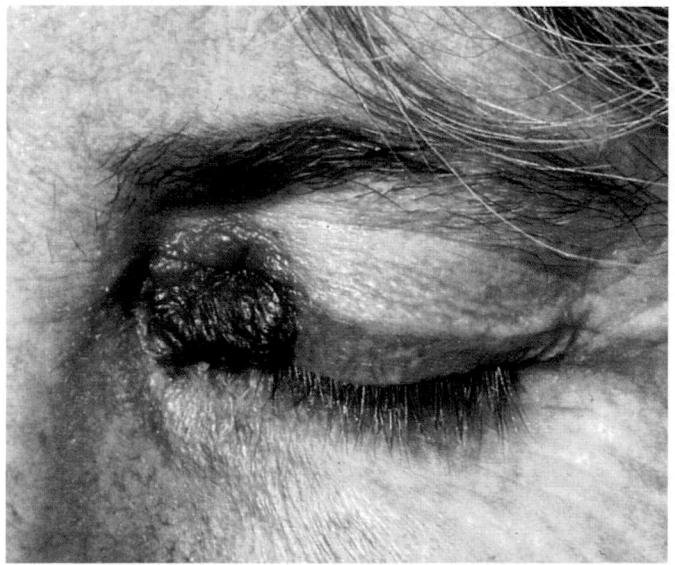

Amyloidosis of the eyelid with purpura.

FIGURE 150-2

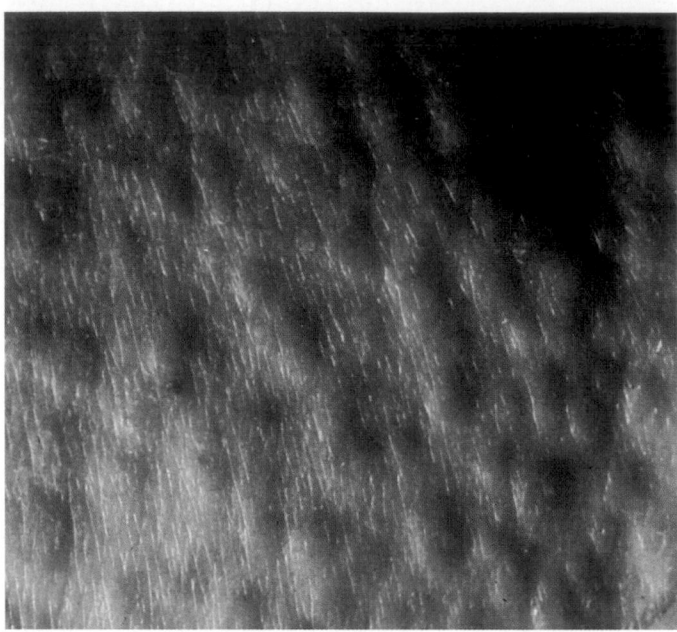

Papular lesions of cutaneous amyloidosis.

Plaques may be isolated or coalesce to produce large tumefactive lesions. Diffuse amyloid infiltration may produce a sclerodermatous appearance of the face, hands, and feet. Alternatively, a myxedema-like appearance may develop; scalp lesions may resemble cutis verticis gyrata or lead to patchy or universal alopecia.[66]

Signs that occur rarely include bullae of the skin or mucous membranes as a result of shearing within dermal amyloid deposits.[67] Extensive amyloid infiltration may lead to cordlike thickening of superficial blood vessels.[68] Dystrophic nail changes, including brittleness, crumbling, subungual striations, and partial or complete anonychia, may be a presenting sign.[69,70] Amyloid elastosis is an unusual syndrome in which papulonodular cutaneous lesions are associated with widespread amyloid infiltration of visceral and cutaneous blood vessels, particularly in relation to elastic fibers.[54,71] Acquired cutis laxa has also been described.[72]

Heredofamilial Amyloidosis

Familial Mediterranean fever, inherited as an autosomal recessive trait, may involve erysipelas-like lesions on the lower legs, urticaria, Henoch-Schönlein purpura, and vasculitic nodules.[21] Associated features are intermittent fevers and a tendency to peritonitis, pleurisy, synovitis, and renal amyloidosis. The Muckle-Wells syndrome, inherited as an autosomal dominant trait, is characterized by periodic attacks of urticaria, fever, and limb pains, associated with progressive perceptive nerve deafness and renal amyloidosis.[22] Trophic skin changes may develop in heredofamilial amyloid polyneuropathy.[23] The Finnish type of heredofamilial neuropathic amyloidosis, a gelsolin-related systemic amyloidosis characterized by cranial neuropathy and corneal lattice dystrophy, may be associated with cutis laxa, blepharochalasis, and lichen amyloidosis.[73,74]

Dialysis-Associated Amyloidosis

Dialysis-related amyloidosis with extensive tissue deposition of beta$_2$-microglobulin may rarely present as masses in the buttocks[75] or as lichenoid lesions.[36]

Localized Cutaneous Amyloidosis

NODULAR LOCALIZED CUTANEOUS AMYLOIDOSIS[43,44,76–78]

This presents clinically with single, or more commonly multiple, lesions on the limbs (Fig. 150-3), face, trunk, or genitalia. These appear indistinguishable from those associated with plasma cell dyscrasia–related systemic amyloidosis and vary in size from a few millimeters to several centimeters. The condition may follow a prolonged benign course over many years; however, some patients later develop paraproteinemia and overt systemic amyloidosis.[25,26]

MACULAR AND LICHEN AMYLOIDOSIS (PLCA)[25,26,56]

Macular amyloidosis, which tends to persist unchanged for many years, is a pruritic eruption of small brownish macules distributed typically in a rippled, symmetric fashion on the upper back (Fig. 150-4), limbs, and occasionally chest and buttocks; itching is not always present. Lichen amyloidosis is a persistent, pruritic eruption of multiple discrete hyperkeratotic papules, which may coalesce to form plaques, distributed principally on the shins. There may be spread to the calves, ankles, dorsa of the feet, and thighs, and the extensor aspects of the arms and abdominal or chest wall may also be involved.[79] Because macular and lichen amyloidosis may coexist in an affected individual (biphasic amyloidosis), they are regarded as variants of a single pathologic process.[80]

Lichen amyloidosis is more common among the Chinese,[79] and macular amyloidosis is more common among Central and South Americans,[81] Middle Easterners,[82] and Asians. This apparent racial incidence may, in the case of the Japanese, be partially contributed to by a habit of rubbing the skin vigorously with a nylon towel or brush ("friction amyloidosis").[83,84] There is a postulated association of PLCA with notalgia paresthetica.[85] The importance of genetic factors in the development of PLCA is emphasized by the occur-

FIGURE 150-3

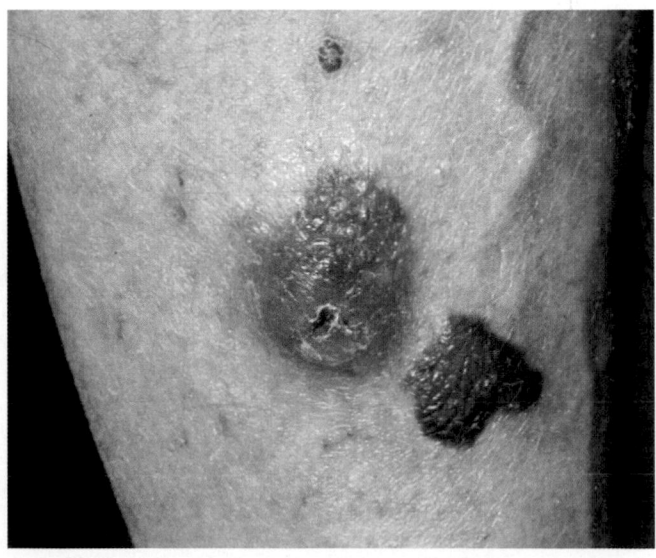

Nodular amyloidosis of the leg.

FIGURE 150-4

CHAPTER 150
Amyloidosis of the Skin

1761

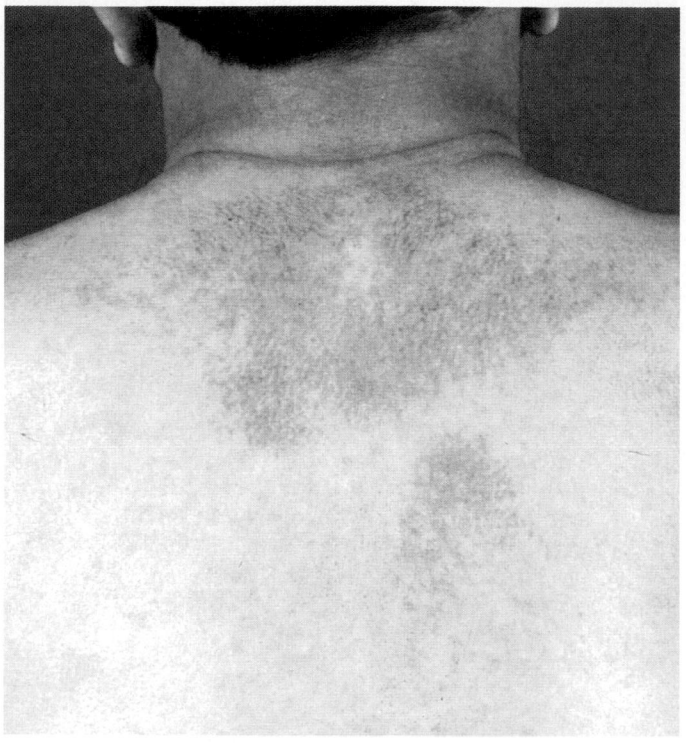

Macular amyloidosis of the upper back.

rence of familial cases.[86–88] PLCA has occasionally been reported to be associated with connective tissue diseases (including systemic sclerosis, primary biliary cirrhosis, and systemic lupus erythematosus)[26,89] and, in a few kindreds, with pachyonychia congenita[90] or multiple endocrine neoplasia type 2A.[91]

Unusual variants of PLCA include macular forms with diffuse hyperpigmentation,[92] simulating nevoid hyperpigmentation[93] or causing periocular hyperpigmentation,[94] and a poikiloderma-like form.[95] Amyloidosis cutis dyschromica is assumed to be a congenital disorder with hypersensitivity to UVB radiation, with possible DNA repair defects; hyperpigmented and hypopigmented xerotic lesions with deposits of amyloid in the papillary dermis occur in sun-exposed skin.[96] Primary cutaneous amyloidosis of the auricular concha, in which small papules are grouped on the concha of the ear, is also believed to be a variant of PLCA and may coexist with lichen amyloidosis.[97]

ANOSACRAL CUTANEOUS AMYLOIDOSIS This is a rare syndrome described in elderly Japanese males, in which pigmented macules and glossy hyperkeratotic lesions radiate out from the anus.[98]

LABORATORY AND SPECIAL EXAMINATION

Primary and Myeloma-Associated Systemic Amyloidosis[1,7,20,56,57,99]

Anemia is not a prominent feature, the leukocyte and differential counts are usually within normal limits, and the erythrocyte sedimentation rate is usually less than 50 mm/h (Westergren). Thrombocytosis of greater than $500,000/mm^2$ occurs in up to 10 percent of patients. Hepatic function abnormalities are usually minor apart from hypoalbuminemia, but the serum creatinine level is raised in 50 percent and proteinuria is present in about 80 percent of patients; hypercalcemia occurs in a third of myeloma patients but is rare in primary cases.

Immunoglobulin estimation reveals reduced IgG levels in half the primary and two-thirds of the myeloma-associated cases. Serum protein electrophoresis shows a spike pattern in slightly less than half the primary and two-thirds of the myeloma patients. However, the spike is usually of modest size and may be missed; monoclonal light chains rarely produce a recognizable band. Immunoelectrophoresis of serum reveals a monoclonal protein in two-thirds of patients with AL amyloidosis; only 45 percent have a monoclonal heavy chain, while 20 percent have free monoclonal light chains (Bence Jones proteinemia).

The heat test for Bence Jones protein is usually negative. Immunoelectrophoresis of concentrated urine reveals a monoclonal light chain in about two-thirds of cases (lambda to kappa ratio of 2:1). When screening of both serum and urine is performed, the frequency of patients with an identifiable monoclonal protein rises to about 86 percent. A combination of immunofixation on agarose gel electrophoresis and bone marrow plasma-cell–light-chain kappa/lambda ratio analysis improves diagnostic sensitivity.[99] Nevertheless, in some patients with the clinical features of AL amyloidosis, it is not possible to demonstrate a paraprotein, even after prolonged follow-up for as long as 24 years.[100]

HISTOPATHOLOGY

Systemic Amyloidosis

In primary and myeloma-associated systemic amyloidosis,[24,56,101,102] papular lesions contain amorphous, often fissured, faintly eosinophilic masses in the papillary dermis, and there is associated thinning or obliteration of the rete ridges. There may be diffuse amyloid deposition in the reticular dermis and subcutis in nodular lesions and plaques. There is usually little in the way of any associated inflammatory infiltrate. Amyloid infiltration of blood vessel walls, pilosebaceous units, arrector pili muscles, the lamina propria of sweat glands and ducts, and around individual fat cells in the subcutis as "amyloid rings" is characteristic. Amyloid deposits in the nail fold and bed of dystrophic nails has been reported.[69]

In secondary systemic amyloidosis, amyloid deposits may be found deep in the dermis in small blood vessels and around adnexal structures as well as surrounding individual cells in the subcuticular fat.[103] In the Swedish type of heredofamilial amyloid polyneuropathy, amyloid deposits are found in the dermis and subcutis associated with arrector pili muscles, sweat glands, and nerves in clinically normal skin.[104]

Localized Cutaneous Amyloidosis[25,26]

NODULAR PLCA The histopathology resembles that of primary systemic amyloidosis with the single exception that in nodular PLCA there is usually a marked infiltrate of plasma cells.[77,102,105]

MACULAR AND LICHEN AMYLOIDOSIS (PLCA) Amyloid deposits are usually confined to the papillary dermis and do not involve blood vessels or adnexal structures. Early lesions contain small multifaceted amorphous globules within the papillae, which are easily missed without the use of special stains. Later lesions show globules, which coalesce, expand the papillae, and displace the rete ridges laterally. In lichen amyloidosis, the deposits are slightly larger and are accompanied by irregular acanthosis and hyperkeratosis of the overlying epidermis.

Use of Special Stains[24,56,106]

The special stains for amyloid include the triphenyl-methane dyes methyl and cresyl violet for the demonstration of metachromasia, the PAS method, the substantive cotton dyes Congo red and Sirius red with or without fluorescence or polarized-light microscopy, and fluorescence with thiazole dyes such as thioflavine T. Alternative cotton dyes including Pagoda red, RIT scarlet no. 5, and RIT cardinal red no. 9 may be used; fluorescence methods using an optical brightener for cellulose (Phorwhite BBU) and immunohistochemical staining with anti-SAP have also been advocated. Unfortunately, methyl violet and Congo red staining may be equivocal and inadequate for detecting small deposits of amyloid; false-positive results occur in colloid milium and lipoid proteinosis. False-positive staining with Thioflavine T is seen with stromal hyaline deposits, collagen fibers, and colloid bodies in lichen planus; anti-SAP also stains colloid bodies and elastotic elastic fibers. Thus none of the existing stains is absolutely reliable, and ultrastructural examination may sometimes be necessary.

AL-type amyloid, unlike AA-type amyloid, retains its affinity for Congo red and its typical polarization characteristics after exposure to potassium permanganate.[107] Immunohistochemical staining with specific antisera is used to differentiate between the various types of fibril protein in amyloid deposits.[108,109]

DIAGNOSIS

The diagnosis of cutaneous amyloidosis evidently depends on the histochemical, immunohistochemical, or ultrastructural demonstration of amyloid material in a skin biopsy specimen. Biopsy of even clinically normal forearm skin has been reported positive in up to 50 percent of cases of primary and myeloma-associated disease.

Other Diagnostic Procedures in Systemic Amyloidosis[1,56,110]

Fine-needle biopsy of subcutaneous fat of clinically normal abdominal skin has become established as a simple, minimally invasive diagnostic test with a high positive yield in AL-type and AA-type systemic amyloidosis as well as in heredofamilial amyloidosis.[111] In AL- and AA-type amyloidosis, rectal biopsy is positive in up to 80 percent of cases, but the specimen must contain submucosal tissue; jejunal biopsy is positive in about two-thirds of patients; but gingival biopsy in only 19 percent. Gastric biopsy may produce a higher yield than rectal biopsy in AL-type amyloidosis. Ninety-six percent of hepatic and 90 percent of renal and of splenic percutaneous needle biopsies are positive. Bone marrow aspiration may be positive in up to 45 percent of cases. Electrocardiography, echocardiography,[58,112] angiocardiography, technetium scanning, and endomyocardial biopsy are useful in the diagnosis of amyloid heart disease. Computed tomography, ultrasound examination, and Doppler analysis of blood flow may be useful in renal amyloidosis.[10] Sural nerve biopsy in patients with peripheral neuropathy, synovial fluid analysis in patients with arthropathy, and examination of tissue removed at carpal tunnel decompression, may be helpful. Scanning with ^{123}I-labeled serum amyloid P component enables specific localization and imaging of amyloid deposits in vivo.[1,113]

Distinction between Primary and Myeloma-Associated Amyloidosis

Differentiation between the two ends of the spectrum of AL-type amyloidosis is of prognostic significance but is by no means clearcut. Most myeloma patients, and no primary systemic amyloidosis patients, have more than 15 percent plasma cells in the marrow. Similarly, 50 percent of myeloma patients show radiologic evidence of bone involvement, compared with only 6 percent of primary cases. In general, myeloma is not present if a patient has no lytic bone lesions, hypercalcemia, or anemia; has only a small serum or urine monoclonal component; and has fewer than 25 percent bone marrow plasma cells.

TREATMENT

Systemic Amyloidosis[1,56,114-117]

Assessment of response to therapy is hindered by (1) the lack of reliable methods for the quantification of the extent of amyloid in individual patients, and (2) the fact that apparent spontaneous clinical remissions of amyloid nephropathy may occur, despite histologic evidence of progressive amyloid infiltration. Liver transplantation in patients with familial amyloid polyneuropathy caused by transthyretin gene mutations leads to the disappearance of variant transthyretin from the plasma and halts progression of neurologic disease.

REACTIVE AA-TYPE (SECONDARY) AMYLOIDOSIS Resolution or remission has followed therapy of underlying disease, including nephrectomy for hypernephroma, antibiotic treatment of chronic infection, and etretinate and PUVA therapy for psoriasis.[1,56] Colchicine prevents the development of amyloidosis and deterioration of renal function in patients with familial Mediterranean fever.[118] Cytotoxic therapy has prolonged survival in patients with underlying rheumatic diseases; chlorambucil is particularly useful in juvenile rheumatoid arthritis with amyloidosis.[119] Dimethyl sulfoxide (DMSO) may improve renal function and is relatively nontoxic, but its use is limited because of the associated offensive breath odor.

AL-TYPE AMYLOIDOSIS Despite the relatively high risk of development of leukemia or a dysmyelopoietic syndrome,[120] it is reasonable for patients to receive a trial of chemotherapy, with or without autologous bone marrow transplantation, given the anecdotal reports of partial response.[56,121-123] Melphalan, prednisone, and/or colchicine are most commonly administered.[124,125] The new anthracycline 4'-iodo-4'-deoxydoxorubicin binds strongly to natural amyloid fibrils, inhibits in vitro fibrillogenesis, and can induce amyloid resorption in patients with immunoglobulin light chain amyloidosis.[126,127]

Diuretics are the mainstay of therapy for congestive cardiac failure, as digoxin may result in arrhythmias and calcium channel blockers are contraindicated. Cardiac transplantation has been used for intractable cases.[128] Renal failure may be treated with regular dialysis; hemodialysis membranes are nearly impermeable to the immunoglobulin light chain precursors of protein AL, so that peritoneal dialysis may be preferable.[129] Renal amyloidosis is not an absolute contraindication to transplantation, although amyloid may reaccumulate in the transplanted kidney; patients with AA-type amyloidosis seem to survive longer than those with AL-type.[129]

Localized Cutaneous Amyloidosis

Deposits of nodular PLCA may be excised surgically or treated with curettage and cautery,[78] cryotherapy, or the carbon dioxide laser[130]; they tend to recur. Macular and papular (lichen amyloidosis) forms of PLCA unfortunately respond poorly to topical steroids combined with systemic antihistamines to alleviate pruritus. Dermabrasion has been advocated for lichen amyloidosis.[131] There have been anecdotal reports of response to topical DMSO therapy in some cases,[132,133] but not in others.[134,135] Etretinate therapy may also be beneficial in some[136,137] but not all patients.[138]

PROGNOSIS

The prognosis of systemic amyloidosis, especially of the primary and myeloma-associated variants, remains poor as there is no very effective therapy; cardiac and renal failure are the major causes of death.[56] The median survival of patients with primary systemic amyloidosis without myeloma has been reported as from 12 to 20 months, and of patients with myeloma-associated amyloidosis is only 5 months.[139–141] The overall 5-year survival for primary systemic amyloidosis is about 20 percent. The median survival of 859 patients with primary systemic amyloidosis seen at the Mayo Clinic from 1982 to 1992 was 2.1 years.[115] The overall survival of 100 patients with primary amyloidosis in another study was 8.4 months[124]; survival was least for patients in the cardiac subgroup and longest in the renal group. Prognosis depends on response to therapy and the extent of disease; the median survival of patients with primary amyloidosis with response to chemotherapy was 28 months, compared to 7.5 months in nonresponders.[139,141] Patients presenting with amyloid neuropathy without associated cardiac, renal, or hepatic involvement have a significantly better prognosis (median survival 40 to 50 months; 5-year survival 31.6 percent).[59] Survival for more than 10 years has been recorded in a patient with primary systemic amyloidosis with sensorimotor polyneuropathy only.[142] Congestive heart failure indicates a very poor prognosis, with a median survival of approximately 6 months once symptoms develop.[128]

gene structure in senile systemic amyloidosis. *Lab Invest* **73**:703, 1995

5. Cornwell GG III et al: The age related amyloids: A growing family of unique biochemical substances. *J Clin Pathol* **48**:984, 1995

6. Selkoe DJ: Amyloid beta-protein and the genetics of Alzheimer's disease. *J Biol Chem* **271**:18295, 1996

7. Kyle RA et al: Primary systemic amyloidosis: Clinical and laboratory features in 474 cases. *Semin Hematol* **32**:45, 1995

8. Gertz MA: Secondary amyloidosis (AA). *J Intern Med* **232**:517, 1992

9. Brownstein MH, Helwig EB: Secondary systemic amyloidosis: Analysis of underlying disorders. *South Med J* **64**:491, 1971

10. Moon WK et al: Castleman disease with renal amyloidosis: Imaging findings and clinical significance. *Abdom Imaging* **20**:376, 1995

11. Brownstein MH, Helwig EB: Systemic amyloidosis complicating dermatoses. *Arch Dermatol* **102**:1, 1970

12. Landau M et al: Systemic amyloidosis secondary to chronic leg ulcers. *Cutis* **50**:47, 1992

13. Wittenberg GP et al: Secondary amyloidosis complicating psoriasis. *J Am Acad Dermatol* **32**:465, 1995

14. Tsuda S et al: Secondary amyloidosis complicating arthropathic psoriasis. *Clin Exp Dermatol* **21**:141, 1996

15. Neugarten J et al: Amyloidosis in subcutaneous heroin abusers ("skin popper's amyloidosis"). *Am J Med* **81**:635, 1986

16. Pallares R et al: Amyloidosis (AA type) associated with nodular nonsuppurative panniculitis. *Ann Intern Med* **99**:488, 1983

17. Yamamoto S et al: Giant basal cell carcinoma associated with systemic amyloidosis. *J Dermatol* **23**:329, 1996

18. Pérez-Villa F et al: Renal amyloidosis secondary to acne conglobata. *Int J Dermatol* **28**:132, 1989

19. Bourke JF et al: Fatal systemic amyloidosis (AA type) in two sisters with dystrophic epidermolysis bullosa. *J Am Acad Dermatol* **33**:370, 1995

20. Isobe T et al: Patterns of amyloidosis and their association with plasma cell dyscrasia, monoclonal immunoglobulins and Bence Jones proteins. *N Engl J Med* **290**:473, 1974

21. Sohar E et al: Familial Mediterranean fever: A survey of 470 cases and a review of the literature. *Am J Med* **43**:227, 1967

22. Nazzari G et al: Recurrent urticarial skin eruption since infancy. Muckle-Wells syndrome (MWS). *Arch Dermatol* **131**:81, 84, 1995

23. Rubinow A et al: Skin involvement in familial amyloidotic polyneuropathy. *Neurology* **31**:1341, 1981

24. Wong C-K, Breathnach SM (eds): Cutaneous amyloidosis. *Clin Dermatol* **8(2)**:1990

25. Brownstein MH et al: The cutaneous amyloidoses: I. Localized forms. *Arch Dermatol* **102**:8, 1970

26. Black MM: Primary localised amyloidosis of the skin: Clinical variants, histochemistry and ultrastructure, in *Amyloidosis,* edited by O Wegelius et al. London, Academic, 1976, p 479

27. Glenner GG et al: Amyloid fibril proteins: Proof of homology with immunoglobulin light chains by sequence analyses. *Science* **172**:1150, 1971

28. Helms LR et al: Specificity of abnormal assembly in immunoglobulin light chain deposition disease and amyloidosis. *J Mol Biol* **257**:77, 1996

29. Buxbaum JN et al: Monoclonal immunoglobulin deposition disease; light chain and light and heavy chain deposition diseases and their relation to light chain amyloidosis. Clinical features, immunopathology, and molecular analysis. *Ann Intern Med* **112**:455, 1990

30. Perfetti V et al: AL amyloidosis. Characterization of amyloidogenic cells by anti-idiotypic monoclonal antibodies. *Lab Invest* **71**:853, 1994

31. Glenner GG et al: Creation of "amyloid" fibrils from Bence-Jones proteins in vitro. *Science* **174**:712, 1971

32. Bellotti V et al: Relevance of class, molecular weight and isoelectric point in predicting human light chain amyloidogenicity. *Br J Haematol* **74**:65, 1990

33. Husby G et al: Serum amyloid A (SAA)—the precursor of protein AA in secondary amyloidosis. *Adv Exp Med Biol* **243**:185, 1988

34. McCutchen SL et al: Comparison of lethal and nonlethal transthyretin variants and their relationship to amyloid disease. *Biochemistry* **34**:13527, 1995

35. Reilly MM et al: Transthyretin gene analysis in European patients with suspected familial amyloid polyneuropathy. *Brain* **118**:849, 1995

REFERENCES

1. Hawkins PN: The diagnosis, natural history and treatment of amyloidosis. *J R Coll Physicians Lond* **31**:552, 1997

2. Cohen AS: Proteins of the systemic amyloidoses. *Curr Opin Rheumatol* **6**:55, 1994

3. Cohen AS: Clinical aspects of amyloidosis, including related proteins and central nervous system amyloid. *Curr Opin Rheumatol* **6**:68, 1994

4. Gustavsson A et al: Amyloid fibril composition and transthyretin

36. Sato KC et al: Lichenoid skin lesions as a sign of beta 2-microglobulin-induced amyloidosis in a long-term haemodialysis patient. *Br J Dermatol* **128**:686, 1993

37. Malak JA et al: Secondary localised cutaneous amyloidosis. *Arch Dermatol* **86**:465, 1962

38. Runne U et al: Amyloid production by dermal fibroblasts. Electron microscopic studies on the origin of amyloid in various dermatoses and skin tumours. *Br J Dermatol* **97**:155, 1977

39. Nojiri K et al: BCC-associated amyloidosis with a peculiar pattern of deposition. *J Dermatol* **19**:618, 1992

40. MacDonald DM et al: Secondary localised cutaneous amyloidosis in melanocytic naevi. *Br J Dermatol* **103**:553, 1980

41. Lee Y-S et al: Photosensitive annular elastolytic giant cell granuloma with cutaneous amyloidosis. *Am J Dermatopathol* **11**:443, 1989

42. Hashimoto K et al: Colloid-amyloid bodies in PUVA-treated human psoriatic patients. *J Invest Dermatol* **72**:70, 1979

43. Kitajima Y et al: Partial amino acid sequence of an amyloid fibril protein from nodular primary cutaneous amyloidosis showing homology to λ immunoglobulin light chain of variable subgroup III (A λ III). *J Invest Dermatol* **95**:301, 1990

44. Grünewald K et al: Gene rearrangement studies in the diagnosis of "primary" systemic amyloidosis and nodular localized cutaneous amyloidosis. *J Invest Dermatol* **97**:693, 1991

45. Breathnach SM et al: Primary localised cutaneous amyloidosis: Dermal amyloid deposits do not bind antibodies to amyloid A protein, prealbumin or fibronectin. *Br J Dermatol* **107**:453, 1982

46. MacDonald DM et al: Localised cutaneous amyloidosis: A clinical review of 100 cases including immunofluorescent studies, in *Amyloid and Amyloidosis,* edited by GG Glenner et al. Amsterdam, Excerpta Medica, 1980, p 239

47. Habermann MC et al: Primary cutaneous amyloidosis: Clinical, laboratorial and histopathological study of 25 cases: Identification of gammaglobulins and C3 in the lesions by immunofluorescence. *Dermatologica* **160**:240, 1980

48. Kumakiri M et al: Histogenesis of primary localized cutaneous amyloidosis: Sequential change of epidermal keratinocytes to amyloid via filamentous degeneration. *J Invest Dermatol* **73**:150, 1979

49. Kobayashi H, Hashimoto K: Amyloidogenesis in organ-limited cutaneous amyloidosis: An antigenic identity between epidermal keratin and skin amyloid. *J Invest Dermatol* **80**:66, 1983

50. Yoneda K et al: Immunohistochemical staining properties of amyloids with anti-keratin antibodies using formalin-fixed, paraffin-embedded sections. *J Cutan Pathol* **16**:133, 1989

51. Horiguchi Y et al: Lamina densa malformation involved in histogenesis of primary localized cutaneous amyloidosis. *J Invest Dermatol* **99**:12, 1992

52. Tennent GA et al: Serum amyloid P component prevents proteolysis of the amyloid fibrils of Alzheimer disease and systemic amyloidosis. *Proc Natl Acad Sci USA* **92**:4299, 1995

53. Breathnach SM et al: Amyloid P component is located on elastic fibre microfibrils in normal human tissue. *Nature* **293**:652, 1981

54. Sepp N et al: Amyloid elastosis: Analysis of the role of amyloid P component. *J Am Acad Dermatol* **22**:27, 1990

55. Husby G et al: Interaction between circulating amyloid fibril protein precursors and extracellular tissue matrix components in the pathogenesis of systemic amyloidosis. *Clin Immunol Immunopathol* **70**:2, 1994

56. Breathnach SM: Amyloid and amyloidosis. *J Am Acad Dermatol* **18**:1, 1988

57. Wong CK et al: Systemic amyloidosis: A report of 19 cases. *Dermatology* **189**:47, 1994

58. Lewis WR: Amyloid disease of the heart. *Clin Cardiol* **18**:241, 1995

59. Duston MA et al: Peripheral neuropathy as an early marker of AL amyloidosis. *Arch Intern Med* **149**:358, 1989

60. Schima W et al: Case report: Sicca syndrome due to primary amyloidosis. *Br J Radiol* **67**:1023, 1994

61. Edelson JG: Amyloid shoulder pads. Two cases of multiple myeloma. *Acta Orthopaed Scand* **66**:292, 1995

62. Salvarani C et al: Primary systemic amyloidosis presenting as giant cell arteritis and polymyalgia rheumatica. *Arthritis Rheum* **37**:1621, 1994

63. Marcatti M et al: Unusual bleeding manifestations in a case of primary amyloidosis with factor X deficiency but elevations of in vivo markers of thrombin formation and activity. *Thromb Res* **80**:333, 1995

64. Brear SG et al: Target-like skin lesions in primary amyloidosis. *Br J Dermatol* **112**:209, 1985

65. Chapman RS et al: Xanthoma-like skin lesions as a presenting feature in primary systemic amyloidosis. *Br J Clin Pract* **27**:271, 1973

66. Wheeler GE et al: Alopecia universalis: A manifestation of occult amyloidosis and multiple myeloma. *Arch Dermatol* **117**:815, 1981

67. Robert C et al: Bullous amyloidosis: Report of 3 cases and review of the literature. *Medicine* **72**:38, 1993

68. Breathnach SM et al: Amyloid vascular disease: Cord-like thickening of mucocutaneous arteries, intermittent claudication and angina in a case with underlying myelomatosis. *Br J Dermatol* **102**:591, 1980

69. Breathnach SM et al: Systemic amyloidosis with an underlying lymphoproliferative disorder. Report of a case in which nail involvement was a presenting feature. *Clin Exp Dermatol* **4**:495, 1979

70. Ostlere LS et al: Nail dystrophy. Systemic amyloidosis presenting with nail dystrophy. *Arch Dermatol* **131**:953, 1995

71. Winkelmann RK et al: Amyloid elastosis: A new cutaneous and systemic pattern of amyloidosis. *Arch Dermatol* **121**:498, 1985

72. Yoneda K et al: Elastolytic cutaneous lesions in myeloma-associated amyloidosis. *Arch Dermatol* **126**:657, 1990

73. Boysen G et al: Familial amyloidosis with cranial neuropathy and corneal lattice dystrophy. *J Neurol Neurosurg Psychiatry* **42**:1020, 1979

74. Ishiguchi H et al: Familial amyloidosis, Finnish type with marked anhidrosis [in Japanese]. *Rinsho Shinkeigaku* **36**:436, 1996

75. Lipner HI et al: Dialysis-related amyloidosis manifested as masses in the buttocks. *South Med J* **88**:876, 1995

76. Northcutt AD et al: Nodular cutaneous amyloidosis involving the vulva. Case report and literature review. *Arch Dermatol* **121**:518, 1985

77. Horiguchi Y et al: A case of nodular cutaneous amyloidosis. Amyloid production by infiltrating plasma cells. *Am J Dermatopathol* **15**:59, 1993

78. Vestey JP et al: Primary nodular cutaneous amyloidosis—long-term follow-up and treatment. *Clin Exp Dermatol* **19**:159, 1994

79. Wong C-K: Lichen amyloidosus: A relatively common skin disorder in Taiwan. *Arch Dermatol* **110**:438, 1974

80. Bourke JF et al: Diffuse primary cutaneous amyloidosis. *Br J Dermatol* **127**:641, 1992

81. Wolf M et al: Macular amyloidosis. *Arch Dermatol* **99**:73, 1969

82. Kurban AK et al: Primary localised macular cutaneous amyloidosis: Histochemistry and electron microscopy. *Br J Dermatol* **85**:52, 1971

83. Hashimoto K et al: Nylon brush macular amyloidosis. *Arch Dermatol* **123**:633, 1987

84. Onuma L et al: Friction amyloidosis. *Int J Dermatol* **33**:74, 1994

85. Pena-Penabad MC et al: Notalgia paraesthetica and macular amyloidosis: Cause-effect relationship? *Clin Exp Dermatol* **20**:279, 1995

86. De Pietro WP: Primary familial cutaneous amyloidosis: A study of HLA antigens in a Puerto Rican family. *Arch Dermatol* **117**:639, 1981

87. Rajagopalan K et al: Familial lichen amyloidosis. Report of 19 cases in 4 generations of a Chinese family in Malaysia. *Br J Dermatol* **87**:123, 1972

88. Newton JA et al: Familial primary cutaneous amyloidosis. *Br J Dermatol* **112**:201, 1985

89. Ogiyama Y et al: Cutaneous amyloidosis in patients with progressive systemic sclerosis. *Cutis* **57**:28, 1996

90. Tidman MJ et al: Pachyonychia congenita with cutaneous amyloidosis and hyperpigmentation—a distinct variant. *J Am Acad Dermatol* **16**:935, 1987

91. Kousseff BG: Multiple endocrine neoplasia 2 (MEN 2)/MEN 2A (Sipple syndrome). *Dermatol Clin* **13**:91, 1995

92. Wong CK et al: Macular amyloidosis with widespread diffuse pigmentation. *Br J Dermatol* **135**:135, 1996

93. Black MM, Maibach HI: Macular amyloidosis simulating naevoid hyperpigmentation. *Br J Dermatol* **90**:61, 1974

94. Van den Bergh WHHW et al: Macular amyloidosis, presenting as periocular hyperpigmentation. *Clin Exp Dermatol* **8**:195, 1983

95. Serna-Perez MJ et al: Extensive macular amyloidosis associated with poikiloderma. *Int J Dermatol* **31**:277, 1992

96. Moriwaki S et al: Amyloidosis cutis dyschromica. DNA repair reduction in the cellular response to UV light. *Arch Dermatol* **128**:966, 1992

97. Bakos L et al: Primary amyloidosis of the concha. *J Am Acad Dermatol* **20**:525, 1989

98. Ive FA et al: Diseases of the umbilical, perianal and genital regions: Anosacral cutaneous amyloidosis, in *Textbook of Dermatology,* 4th ed, edited by A Rook et al. Oxford, Blackwell Scientific, 1986, p 2173

99. Perfetti V et al: Diagnostic approach to and follow-up of difficult cases of AL amyloidosis. *Haematologica* **80**:409, 1995

100. Crow KD: Primary amyloidosis. *Br J Dermatol* **97**(suppl 15):58, 1977

101. Elder D et al (eds): *Lever's Histopathology of the Skin,* 8th ed. Philadelphia, Lippincott, 1997

102. Westermark P: Amyloidosis of the skin: A comparison between localized and systemic amyloidosis. *Acta Derm Venereol (Stockh)* **59**:341, 1979

103. Westermark P: Occurrence of amyloid deposits in the skin in secondary systemic amyloidosis. *Acta Pathol Microbiol Scand [A]* **80**:718, 1972

104. Shirahama T et al: Ultrastructure of skin biopsies from patients with heredo-familial amyloid polyneuropathy, in *Amyloid and Amyloidosis,* edited by GG Glenner et al. Amsterdam, Excerpta Medica, 1980, p 132

105. Masuda C et al: Histopathological and immunohistochemical study of amyloidosis cutis nodularis atrophicans—comparison with systemic amyloidosis. *Br J Dermatol* **199**:33, 1988

106. Elghetany MT et al: Methods for staining amyloid in tissues: A review. *Stain Technol* **63**:201, 1988

107. Wright JR et al: Potassium permanganate reaction in amyloidosis: A histologic method to assist in differentiating forms of this disease. *Lab Invest* **36**:274, 1977

108. Fujihara S et al: Identification and classification of amyloid in formalin-fixed, paraffin-embedded tissue sections by the unlabelled immunoperoxidase method. *Lab Invest* **43**:358, 1980

109. Linke RP et al: High-sensitivity diagnosis of AA amyloidosis using Congo red and immunohistochemistry detects missed amyloid deposits. *J Histochem Cytochem* **43**:863, 1995

110. Westermark P: Diagnosing amyloidosis. *Scand J Rheumatol* **24**:327, 1995

111. Blumenfeld W et al: Fine needle aspiration of abdominal fat for the diagnosis of amyloidosis. *Acta Cytol* **37**:170, 1993

112. Dubrey SW et al: Electrocardiography and Doppler echocardiography in secondary (AA) amyloidosis. *Am J Cardiol* **77**:313, 1996

113. Hachulla E et al: Prospective and serial study of primary amyloidosis with serum amyloid P component scintigraphy: From diagnosis to prognosis. *Am J Med* **101**:77, 1996

114. Pascali E: Diagnosis and treatment of primary amyloidosis. *Crit Rev Oncol Hematol* **19**:149, 1995

115. Gertz MA et al: Amyloidosis: Prognosis and treatment. *Semin Arthritis Rheum* **24**:124, 1994

116. Merlini G: Treatment of primary amyloidosis. *Semin Hematol* **32**:60, 1995

117. Kisilevsky R: Anti-amyloid drugs: Potential in the treatment of diseases associated with aging. *Drugs Aging* **8**:75, 1996

118. Livneh A et al: Colchicine treatment of AA amyloidosis of familial Mediterranean fever. An analysis of factors affecting outcome. *Arthritis Rheum* **37**:1804, 1994

119. Berglund K et al: Results, principles and pitfalls in the management of renal AA-amyloidosis: A 10–21 year follow-up of 16 patients with rheumatic disease treated with alkylating cytostatics. *J Rheumatol* **20**:2051, 1993

120. Gertz MA et al: Acute leukemia and cytogenetic abnormalities complicating melphalan treatment of primary systemic amyloidosis. *Arch Intern Med* **150**:629, 1990

121. van Buren M et al: Clinical remission after syngeneic bone marrow transplantation in a patient with AL amyloidosis. *Ann Intern Med* **122**:508, 1995

122. Moreau P et al: High-dose melphalan and autologous bone marrow transplantation for systemic AL amyloidosis with cardiac involvement. *Blood* **87**:3063, 1996

123. Dubrey S et al: Resolution of heart failure in patients with AL amyloidosis. *Ann Intern Med* **125**:481, 1996

124. Skinner M et al: Treatment of 100 patients with primary amyloidosis: A randomized trial of melphalan, prednisone, and colchicine versus colchicine only. *Am J Med* **100**:290, 1996

125. Livneh A et al: Colchicine in the treatment of AA and AL amyloidosis. *Semin Arthritis Rheum* **23**:206, 1993

126. Merlini G et al: Interaction of the anthracycline 4′-iodo-4′-deoxydoxorubicin with amyloid fibrils: Inhibition of amyloidogenesis. *Proc Natl Acad Sci USA* **92**:2959, 1995

127. Gianni L et al: New drug therapy of amyloidoses: Resorption of AL-type deposits with 4′-iodo-4′-deoxydoxorubicin. *Blood* **86**:855, 1995

128. Dubrey S et al: Recurrence of primary (AL) amyloidosis in a transplanted heart with four-year survival. *Am J Cardiol* **76**:739, 1995

129. Pasternack A et al: Renal transplantation in 45 patients with amyloidosis. *Transplantation* **42**:598, 1986

130. Truhan AP et al: Nodular primary localized cutaneous amyloidosis: Immunohistochemical evaluation and treatment with the carbon dioxide laser. *J Am Acad Dermatol* **14**:1058, 1986

131. Wong CK et al: Dermabrasion for lichen amyloidosus. Report of a long-term study. *Arch Dermatol* **118**:302, 1982

132. Monfrecola G et al: Lichen amyloidosus: A new therapeutic approach. *Acta Derm Venereol (Stockh)* **65**:453, 1985

133. Pravata G et al: Unusual localization of lichen amyloidosus. Topical treatment with dimethylsulfoxide. *Acta Derm Venereol (Stockh)* **69**:259, 1989

134. Bonnetblanc JM et al: Dimethyl sulphoxide and macular amyloidosus. *Acta Derm Venereol (Stockh)* **60**:91, 1980

135. Lim KB et al: Lack of effect of dimethyl sulphoxide (DMSO) on amyloid deposits in lichen amyloidosis. *Br J Dermatol* **119**:409, 1989

136. Helander I et al: Treatment of lichen amyloidosus by etretinate. *Clin Exp Dermatol* **11**:574, 1986

137. Marschalkó M et al: Etretinate for the treatment of lichen amyloidosis. *Arch Dermatol* **124**:657, 1988

138. Aram H: Failure of etretinate (RO 10-9359) in lichen amyloidosus. *Int J Dermatol* **25**:206, 1986

139. Kyle RA, Greipp PR: Amyloidosis (AL): Clinical and laboratory features in 229 cases. *Mayo Clin Proc* **58**:665, 1983

140. Cohen AS et al: Survival of patients with primary (AL) amyloidosis: Colchicine-treated cases from 1976 to 1983 compared with cases seen in previous years (1961 to 1973). *Am J Med* **82**:1182, 1987

141. Kyle RA et al: Primary systemic amyloidosis: Multivariate analysis for prognostic factors in 168 cases. *Blood* **68**:220, 1986

142. Rinaldi R et al: Primary systemic amyloidosis presenting with polyneuropathy characterized by very long survival. *Acta Neurol Scand* **91**:511, 1995

The Porphyrias

The porphyrias are among the most intriguing diseases of humans. Widely variable, even bizarre in their clinical manifestations, these disorders of porphyrin or porphyrin-precursor metabolism result from aberrations in the control of the porphyrin-heme biosynthetic pathway. Heme, the end product of the pathway, is a tetrapyrrole in which protoporphyrin (PROTO) is chelated with ferrous iron. Because of its special ability to bind and release oxygen, heme functions in numerous metabolic pathways of living organisms. Heme is the prosthetic group for a number of important cellular proteins, including hemoglobin; myoglobin; catalases; peroxidases; and cytochromes P_{450}, P_{448}, a_3, etc.; without this iron-chelated tetrapyrrole, most essential biochemical pathways in the body could not function. Heme is essential for oxygen binding and transport (as hemoglobin and myoglobin), for electron transport (as cytochromes), and for mixed-function oxidases such as cytochrome P_{450}, etc. Chlorophyll, a magnesium-chelated porphyrin, is another important tetrapyrrole and is critical for photosynthesis, the specialized energy-storing system found in plants in which the conversion of light energy into stabilized chemical energy is achieved with a sequence of oxidation-reduction reactions. The corrin ring, a cobalt-chelated tetrapyrrole, is a major constituent of vitamin B_{12}, the lack of which results in pernicious anemia. Porphyrins, therefore, are ubiquitous and essential biochemical constituents of living beings. The biologic importance of the porphyrins and their iron complexes in metabolism lies in their capacity to act as mediators of oxidation reactions, either as oxidative components in the metabolism of steroids, drugs, and environmental chemicals or as a means of exchanging gases, such as oxygen and carbon dioxide, between the environment and the tissues of the body.

Daily synthesis of porphyrins and heme in humans occurs in amounts sufficient to provide for the body's metabolic requirements. The control of heme synthesis is so precise that, under normal circumstances, microgram quantities or less of pathway intermediates are present in plasma, red blood cells (RBCs), urine, and stool (see Table 151-1).

Porphyria results from either inherited or acquired enzymatic abnormalities in heme synthesis. There are eight enzymes contributing to excessive accumulation of heme pathway intermediates in the body. Most of the human porphyrias appear to be characterized by deficient activity of specific enzymes, as shown in Table 151-2; each of these enzymes will be discussed separately. The different porphyrias arising from such derangements of normal heme synthesis manifest patterns of accumulation and excretion of specific porphyrins and/or their precursors.[1] In general, the major porphyrin excreted in a given porphyria is the oxidized substrate for the specific deficient or defective enzyme. The different porphyrias arising from such derangements of normal heme synthesis are also characterized by accumulation and excretion of specific intermediate porphyrins and/or their precursors (Table 151-3). These intermediates, when present in excess amounts, exert toxic effects that are likely responsible for the neurologic and cutaneous features of clinical porphyria.

The porphyrias are of particular dermatologic interest because several of them have distinct cutaneous manifestations that may permit diagnosis from clinical signs alone. Furthermore, simple laboratory procedures, easily performed in a physician's office, can confirm a clinically suspected diagnosis in many instances and can also help to initiate appropriate therapeutic measures for the amelioration of the biochemical derangements and the clinical symptoms of these diseases.

TABLE 151-1

Normal Values of Porphyrins and Porphyrin Precursors in Humans

Porphyrins or Precursors	Urine (μg/24 h)	RBC (μg/100 mL Packed Cells)	Plasma (μg/100 mL)	Feces (μg/g dry wt)
δ-Aminolevulinic acid (ALA)	<4000	—	15–23	—
Porphobilinogen (PBG)	<1500	—	—	—
Uroporphyrin (URO)	<40	0–2.0	0–2	10–50
Coproporphyrin (COPRO)	<280	0–2.0	0–1	10–50
Protoporphyrin (PROTO)	Absent	<90	0–2	0–20
X-porphyrin	Absent	Absent	Absent	Trace
Isocoproporphyrin (ISOCOPRO)	Absent	Absent	Absent	—
	(nmol/day)	(nmol/dL)	(nmol/dL)	(nmol/g dry weight)
δ-Aminolevulinic acid (ALA)	8.8×10^3	—	$1.1–1.8 \times 10^2$	—
Porphobilinogen (PGB)	4.6×10^4	—	—	—
Uroporphyrin (URO)	<40	—	24	
Coproporphyrin (COPRO)	<280	—	46	
Protoporphyrin (PROTO)	0	285	0.5	134

HISTORIC ASPECTS

One of the first known cases of cutaneous porphyria was that reported by Schultz,[2] who described a 33-year-old man with marked cutaneous photosensitivity and splenomegaly that he called pemphigus leprosus, a bullous disease. The excreted urine was red. Spectroscopic studies by Schultz and subsequently by Baumstark[3] identified abnormal urinary pigments, which were named urorubrohematin and urofuscohematin. This abnormal pigment was most likely uroporphyrin (URO), and this patient probably had porphyria, but of what type is disputed.[4] Anderson[5] reported two brothers with a scarring photosensitivity that he called hydroa aestivale. Beginning in childhood, this disease was said to be associated with "hematoporphyrin" in the urine. Anderson implied that the abnormal urinary pigment was related to the skin disease.

Detailed studies by Günther in 1911 led to the first classification of the porphyrias.[6] Günther felt that the dark pigment in the urine of patients with porphyria was the synthetic porphyrin, hematoporphyrin, but subsequent studies by Fischer proved that this pigment was a natural porphyrin, which he named URO as it was isolated from the urine of a patient with congenital porphyria.[7] The detailed study of Mathias Petry, the celebrated but unfortunate patient with congenital erythropoietic porphyria (EP), added greatly to modern knowledge of porphyria and of the cutaneous photosensitivity associated with it.[8] This is an excellent example of the interaction of basic science and clinical medicine leading to important new knowledge about the metabolic basis of a human disease.

Other types of porphyrias known as acute intermittent porphyria (AIP) and porphyria cutanea tarda (PCT) were first defined in Sweden by Waldenström in 1937.[9] The former, with abdominal and neurologic symptoms, was found to be very common in the northernmost provinces of Sweden, around Lapland, and to be comparatively rare in South Africa. Subsequently, Brunsting,[10] Waldenström,[11] and Schmid[12] further characterized PCT in various human populations and showed that environmental factors such as drugs and chemicals (xenobiotics) could influence the clinical expression of this disease. Barnes and Dean, separately and together, described a type of porphyria occurring predominantly in South Africans and characterized by cutaneous manifestations identical to those of PCT and acute attacks identical to those of AIP.[13–15] Defined as variegate porphyria (VP), this disease is now known to occur throughout the world.[16,17]

Another porphyria of bone marrow origin, erythropoietic protoporphyria (EPP), was described in 1961 by Magnus et al. in England,[18] and an extremely rare disorder, erythropoietic coproporphyria, was identified in Germany by Heilmeyer and Clotten in 1964.[19] In 1955, Berger and Goldberg in Scotland first described hereditary coproporphyria (HCP).[20] In 1969, hepatoerythropoietic porphyria (HEP) was described by Pinōl-Aguadé,[21] as was a type of porphyria associated with sideroblastic anemia.[22] Doss et al.[23] described hereditary aminolevulinic acid (ALA) dehydratase deficiency porphyria in 1979. This is also known as *plumboporphyria*.[24] In 1990, Poh-Fitzpatrick et al.[25] described a porphyria associated with Alagille syndrome, a familial form of cholestatic liver disease.

TABLE 151-2

Enzyme Activities in Various Porphyrias

ENZYME	TISSUE	DISEASE DISPLAYING ENZYMATIC DEFECT
δ-Aminolevulinic acid (ALA) synthase	Liver, kidney, fibroblasts, and lymphocytes	Increased activity in AIP, HCP, VP
δ-Aminolevulinic acid (ALA) dehydratase	Erythrocytes, liver, and kidney	Decreased in lead intoxication; decreased ALA-dehydratase deficiency porphyria
Porphobilinogen (PBG) deaminase	Erythrocytes, liver, fibroblasts, lymphocytes, and amnion cells	Decreased in AIP
Uroporphyrinogen III (UROGEN III) cosynthase	Erythrocytes and fibroblasts	Decreased in congenital EP
Uroporphyrinogen (UROGEN) decarboxylase	Erythrocytes and liver	Decreased in PCT (sporadic and familial) and HEP
Coproporphyrinogen (COPROGEN) oxidase	Fibroblasts, lymphocytes, and liver	Decreased in HCP
Protoporphyrinogen (PROTOGEN) oxidase	Liver and fibroblasts	Decreased in VP
Ferrochelatase	Bone marrow and fibroblasts	Decreased in EPP, lead poisoning, and ? in VP

NOTE: AIP, acute intermittent porphyria; EP, erythropoietic porphyria; EPP, erythropoietic protoporphyria; HCP, hereditary coproporphyria; HEP, hepatoerythropoietic porphyria; PCT, porphyria cutanea tarda; VP, variegate porphyria.

PORPHYRIN-HEME BIOSYNTHESIS

Most mammalian cells, including those in the epidermis and dermis, can synthesize the heme required for formation of essential hemeproteins; however, the major sites of heme synthesis in the body are the bone marrow and the liver. Heme is the prosthetic group for a number of hemoproteins, including hemoglobin, myoglobin, mitochondrial cytochromes, microsomal cytochromes (including cytochrome P_{450}), catalase, peroxidase, tryptophan pyrrolase, prostaglandin endoperoxide synthase, and the soluble form of guanylate cyclase. The two body organs that produce the vast majority of heme in humans are the liver and the bone marrow. Approximately 85 percent of heme synthesis occurs in bone marrow where it is utilized for the production of hemoglobin. Most remaining heme synthesis occurs in the liver for making cytochrome P_{450}, catalase, and various mitochondrial cytochromes. Heme is a critical cellular constituent essential for a variety of metabolic processes, primarily because of its unique ability to take up and release oxygen and to facilitate electron transport. Heme synthesis is regulated by the interplay of a number of factors and is directly dependent upon its concentration within cells and upon the requirements of the cell for production of the various hemoproteins described above. Many of these have rapid turnover times (minutes to hours), thereby necessitating continuously high rates of hepatic heme synthesis (e.g., cytochrome P_{450}, an important membrane-bound enzyme in the liver

TABLE 151-3

Biochemical Features of the Porphyrias

Type of Porphyria	Blood				Stool			Urine				
	RBC URO	RBC COPRO	RBC PROTO	Plasma	URO	COPRO	PROTO	Color	ALA	PBG	URO	COPRO
Erythropoietic												
Erythropoietic porphyria (EP)	++++	+++	+++	↑URO & COPRO	+	+++	+	Pink to red	N	N	++++*	++*
Erythropoietic protoporphyria (EPP)	N	N to +	++++	↑PROTO	N	++	++ to ++++	N	N	N	N	N
Hepatic												
Acute intermittent porphyria (AIP)												
Latent	N	N	N	N	N to +	N to +	N to +	Red to purple	+ to +++	+ to +++	N	N to +
Acute	N	N	N	N	N to +	N to +	N to +	Red to purple	++ to ++++	++ to ++++	+++	++
Porphyria variegata (VP)												
Latent	N	N	N	?N	N	+++	++++	N	N	N	N	N
Acute	N	N	N	?N	++	++	+++	Pink to red	++ to +++	++ to +++	+++	+++
Porphyria cutanea tarda (PCT)	N	N	N	↑URO	++	+++	+ ISOCOPRO	Pink to red	N	N	++++	++
Hereditary coproporphyria (HCP)												
Latent	N	N	N	?N	++	++++	N to +	N	N to +	N to +	N	N
Acute	N	N	N	?N	+	+++	N to +	Red	++ to N	++ to N	++	++++
Hepatoerythropoietic porphyria (HEP)	N	+/−	++++	↑URO	N	ISOCOPRO	N	Pink to red			+++	ISOCOPRO
ALA dehydratase deficiency porphyria	N	N	++	↑ALA ↑COPRO ↑PROTO	N	+	+	?	+++	N	+	++

NOTE: N, normal; +, above normal; ++, moderately increased; +++ and ++++, greatly increased; URO, uroporphyrin; COPRO, coproporphyrin; PROTO, protoporphyrin; ISOCOPRO, isocoproporphyrin. Findings of major diagnostic importance are boxed.
*Type I isomers.

involved in the detoxification and metabolism of drugs, has a half-life of 90 to 180 min). This regulation (and indeed the ability to synthesize heme at all) is dependent upon a series of eight intracellular enzymes, whose sequential catalytic activity accounts for heme synthesis. The first (ALA synthase) and the last three enzymes involved in heme synthesis (COPROGEN oxidase, PROTOGEN oxidase, and ferrochelatase) are localized in mitochondria, and the remaining intermediate enzymes [ALA dehydratase, porphobilinogen (PBG) deaminase, UROGEN III synthase, and UROGEN decarboxylase] are localized in the cytosol. Heme breakdown is catalyzed by the microsomal enzymes NADPH–cytochrome C reductase, heme oxygenase, and biliverdin reductase, which convert the cyclic tetrapyrrole to linear bile pigments. cDNAs for the eight enzymes in the heme synthesis pathway and the enzymes in the heme catabolic pathway have been cloned and defined in mammalian cells.[1] Abnormal control of heme synthesis may result from partial defects in enzymes of the pathway, and this may occur as the result of inherited and/or environmental factors. One result of such abnormal control is the accumulation in the body of one or more heme pathway intermediates, such as the porphyrins or their precursors, which are associated with the clinical disorders that are collectively referred to as the *porphyrias*. Although a diagnosis of porphyria can often be made from a careful history and physical examination, the definitive diagnosis rests upon measurements of porphyrin and/or porphyrin excretion or the activity of one or another of the enzymes in the heme pathway (see Table 151-3). Each porphyria demonstrates a unique pattern of porphyrin or porphyrin-precursor accumulation in blood or excretion in urine and/or feces. Molecular biology is emerging as a useful tool in further clarifying the nature of the porphyrias.[26] The steps involved in the biosynthesis of porphyrins and heme synthesis and its regulation are outlined in Figs. 151-1, 151-2, 151-3, and 151-4 and have recently been summarized with extensive references to the details of the individual steps.[1,26]

Delta-Aminolevulinic Acid Synthase (See Fig. 151-2)

Heme synthesis begins in the mitochondrion of the cell where succinate and glycine (single molecules of glycine and succinyl CoA) are conjugated to form a five-carbon aminoketone delta-ALA. The

FIGURE 151-1

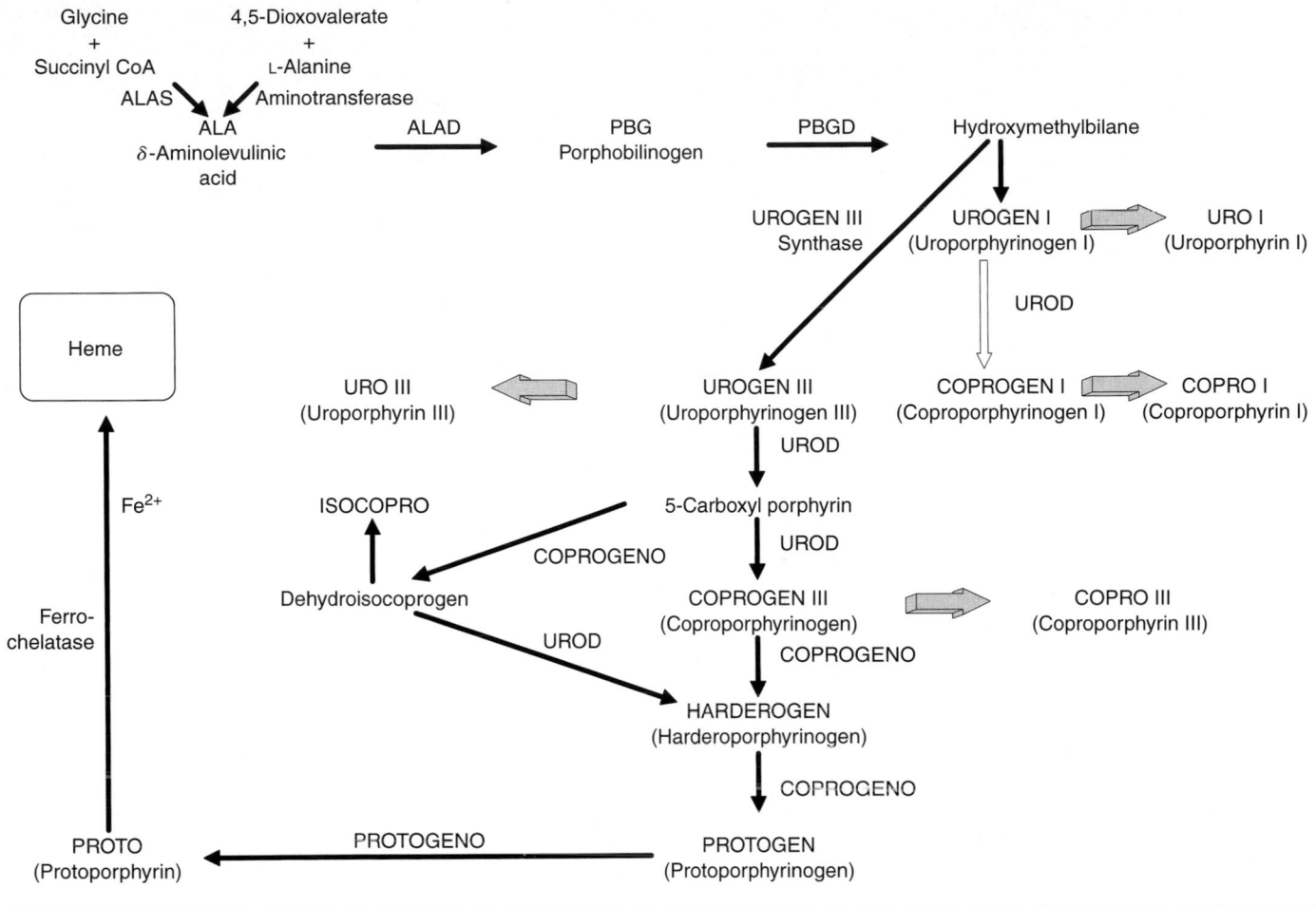

The porphyrin-heme biosynthetic pathway (see also legend for Fig. 151-2).

reaction requires pyridoxal 5′-phosphate as a cofactor. ALA synthase is the mitochondrial enzyme that catalyzes the formation of ALA and is a homodimer of two identical catalytically active subunits of molecular mass 55 kDa, linked to catalytically inactive substrates of higher molecular mass.[27]

The major significance of this enzyme is its regulatory role in controlling the rate of heme synthesis in the liver. Heme acts at multiple sites to regulate ALA synthase levels in the liver. It is thought that two pools, one cytosolic and one nuclear, regulate the isozymes. Heme represses transcription of the ALA synthase-1 gene and inhibits movement of its precursor into the mitochondria where it is proteolytically processed to produce the mature form. Heme can also reduce the stability of ALA synthase-1 mRNA. ALA synthase activity is increased in the liver of patients with those hepatic porphyrias in which acute attacks characterized by a neurologic–visceral symptom complex occur. This increase in ALA synthase is a major marker for AIP, VP, and HCP. It is also an inducible enzyme in the liver, and factors that lead to further increases in activity of ALA synthase are accompanied by exacerbation of the clinical manifestations of these types of porphyria. Conversely, factors that reduce ALA synthase activity are often useful therapeutically in those porphyrias characterized by elevated activity of the enzyme. The importance of ALA synthase for the regulation of heme synthesis will be discussed later in the chapter. ALA synthase in the erythroid compartment behaves in a rather different manner in that it is not inducible by xenobiotics that augment the synthesis of the hepatic enzyme. Immunochemical differences exist between the hepatic and erythroid enzyme in various animal species.[28]

Using chicken ALA synthase cDNA clones isolated from both liver and erythroid cells, Riddle et al.[27] have shown that at least two separate genes encode ALA synthase mRNAs found in these tissues and that the erythroid gene product is expressed exclusively in erythroid cells, whereas the hepatic form is expressed ubiquitously.

The two ALA isozymes show extensive amino acid identity in the C-terminal region encompassing about 75 percent of the mature proteins.[1] The region located at the N terminus is shorter in the erythroid protein. The exon-intron boundaries of the genes of ALA synthase are very similar and correlate with the putative domains of the protein. The human housekeeping gene is located on chromosome 3, and the erythroid gene on the X chromosome.

It should be pointed out that there is some evidence to suggest that a second mitochondrial enzyme in mammalian liver, known as L-alanine-4,5-dioxovalerate (DOVA) aminotransferase, can catalyze a transamination between L-alanine and DOVA, yielding ALA (Fig. 151-2) and pyruvate.[29] The importance of this reaction for production of tetrapyrroles in certain plants is well known, but its role in human heme synthesis remains to be defined.

FIGURE 151-2

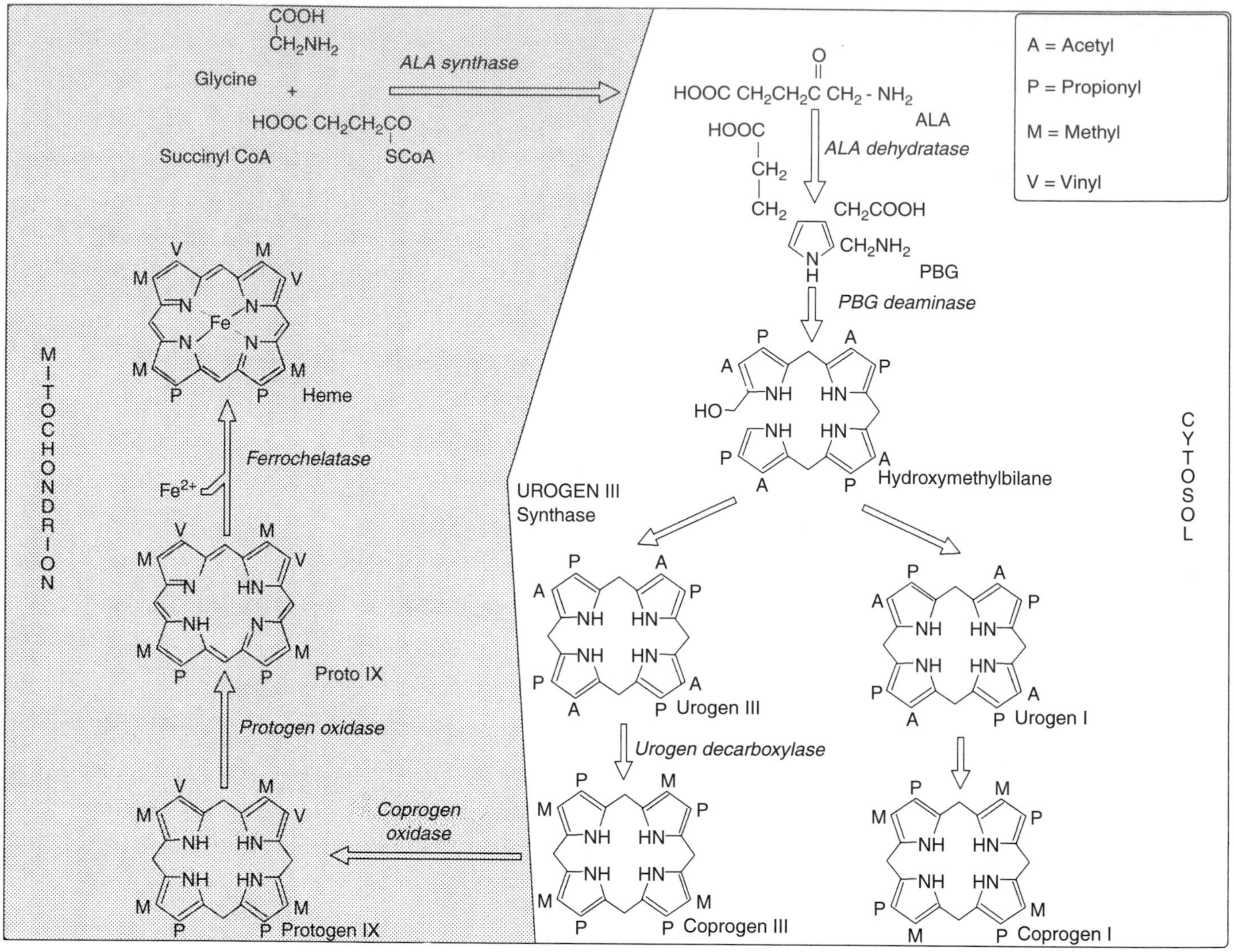

Major steps in the porphyrin-heme biosynthetic pathway: (*1*) Delta-aminolevulinic acid (ALA) synthase can be formed from glycine and succinyl CoA, which is the primary source in mammalian systems and is catalyzed by the mitochondrial enzyme δ-aminolevulinic acid synthase (ALAS). Two molecules of aminolevulinic acid form the monopyrrole porphobilinogen (PBG). (*2*) Four molecules of PBG are converted by PBG deaminase to a linear tetrapyrrole, hydroxymethylbilane, which can cyclize spontaneously to form uroporphyrinogen (UROGEN) I. (*3*) The four acetyl groups of UROGEN I are sequentially decarboxylated by UROGEN decarboxylase to form coproporphyrinogen (COPROGEN) I. (*4*) Hydroxymethylbilane can also be converted to URO-GEN III by the enzyme UROGEN III synthase. In this reaction one of the monopyrrole rings is "flipped over," thereby altering the sequence of the side chains. (*5*) The acetyl groups of UROGEN III are sequentially decarboxylated by UROGEN decarboxylase to form coproporphyrinogen III. (*6*) Coproporphyrinogen III is converted to protoporphyrinogen (PROTOGEN) IX by the enzyme COPROGEN oxidase, which oxidatively decarboxylates each of the propionyl groups. (*7*) PROTOGEN IX is converted to protoporphyrin (PROTO) IX by PROTOGEN oxidase. PROTO IX is converted to heme by ferrochelatase, which catalyzes the insertion of ferrous iron into the molecule.

Delta-Aminolevulinic Acid Dehydratase

In the next reaction, two molecules of ALA are combined in the presence of an enzyme known as ALA dehydratase to form the monopyrrole PBG (see Fig. 151-2). ALA dehydratase is present in the cytoplasm of the cell. Its activity is 50- to 100-fold higher than that of ALA synthase, so that virtually all of the ALA synthesized is converted to PBG.[30] While two distinct genes encode ALA synthase isozymes, all other heme pathway enzymes have a single structural gene.

Liver cDNA–expression libraries have been employed to isolate cDNA clones that encode for the rat and human enzyme.[1] ALA dehydratase from human liver was shown to be encoded by an open reading frame of 990 bp that possessed a high degree of homology with the enzyme in rats.[31] Genetic variation in the level of ALA dehydratase may be due to differences in copy number of the gene. The gene has separate housekeeping and erythroid-specific promoters.[32] mRNA isoforms for each arise by employing the specific promoters and alternative splicing. The isozymes are structurally identical.

Porphobilinogen Deaminase

This, the third enzyme in the pathway, combines four molecules of the monopyrrole PBG to form the linear tetrapyrrole, hydroxymethylbilane (see Fig. 151-2), which cyclizes spontaneously to form the initial porphyrinogen, or tetrapyrrole, known as uroporphyrinogen I (UROGEN I) (Fig. 151-2). Depending on the manner in which the PBG molecules are arranged, several different isomers of the tetrapyrroles are possible. The sole difference between type I and type III porphyrinogens is that one of the four pyrrole rings is "flipped over." Only two of them (labeled I and III) are known to occur in the mammalian heme synthetic pathway. PBG deaminase has been purified from human RBCs and shown to have a molecular mass of approximately 37 kDa and a pH optimum of 8.2.[33]

The PBG deaminase gene has been cloned and characterized.[34] Two isoforms, one ubiquitous and one erythroid-specific, are encoded by a single gene localized to chromosome 11.[35] It comprises 15 exons spread over 10 kb of DNA. The two isoforms of the enzyme are encoded by two distinct mRNAs that arise from two overlapping transcription units, the first of which (upstream) is active in all tissues, and its promoter has some features of a housekeeping promoter; the second, however, located 3 kb downstream, is active only in erythroid cells and displays structural homology with beta globin gene promoters.

PBG deaminase is present in the lowest concentration of any enzyme in the heme pathway except for ALA synthase. This suggests that factors (genetic or acquired) that influence PBG deaminase activity may have important regulatory influences on the rate of heme synthesis. Consequently, if excessive PBG is formed because of increased ALA synthase activity, as is often seen in the acute hepatic porphyrias, there may be only partial conversion of this monopyrrole to UROGEN I. These factors account for the elevated urinary PBG characteristic of attacks of the acute hepatic porphyrias. PBG deaminase activity is known to be reduced by about 50 percent in the tissues of patients with AIP and is currently thought to be the primary enzymatic abnormality in this autosomal dominant disorder. To

FIGURE 151-3

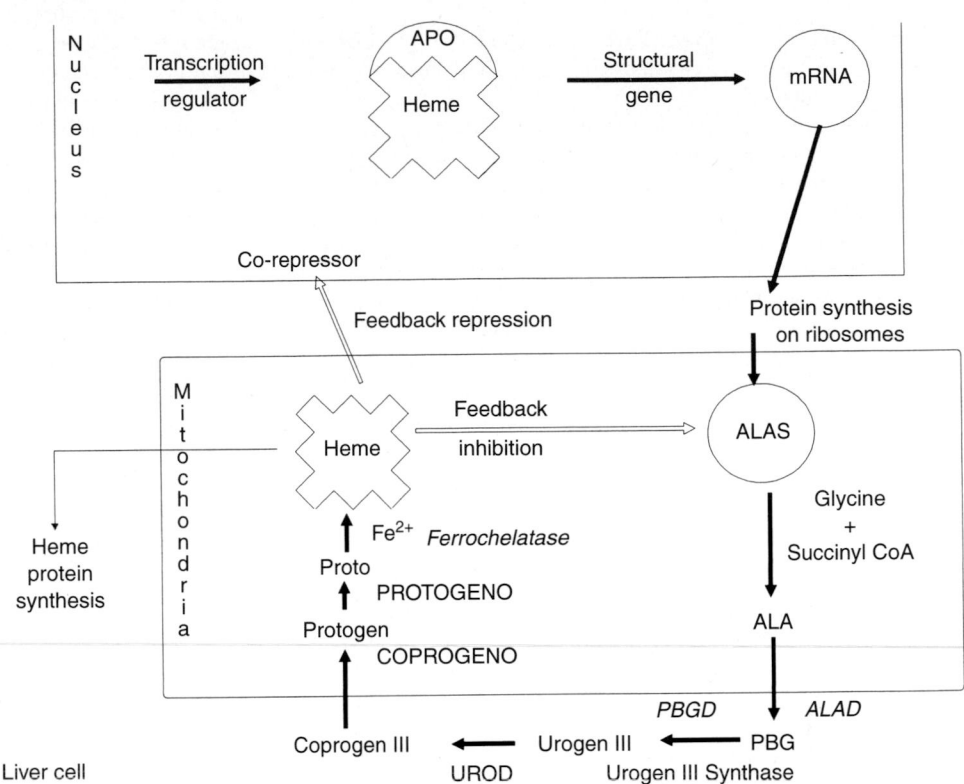

Heme is capable of regulating its synthesis by either directly inhibiting or repressing the synthesis of its rate-limiting enzyme, ALA synthase. The repression may result from the binding of heme, as a corepressor, to an aporepressor protein (APO) which, when combined with heme, becomes a functional unit that blocks transcription of ALA synthase mRNA. Heme may also block transport of the holoenzyme into the mitochondrion.

FIGURE 151-4

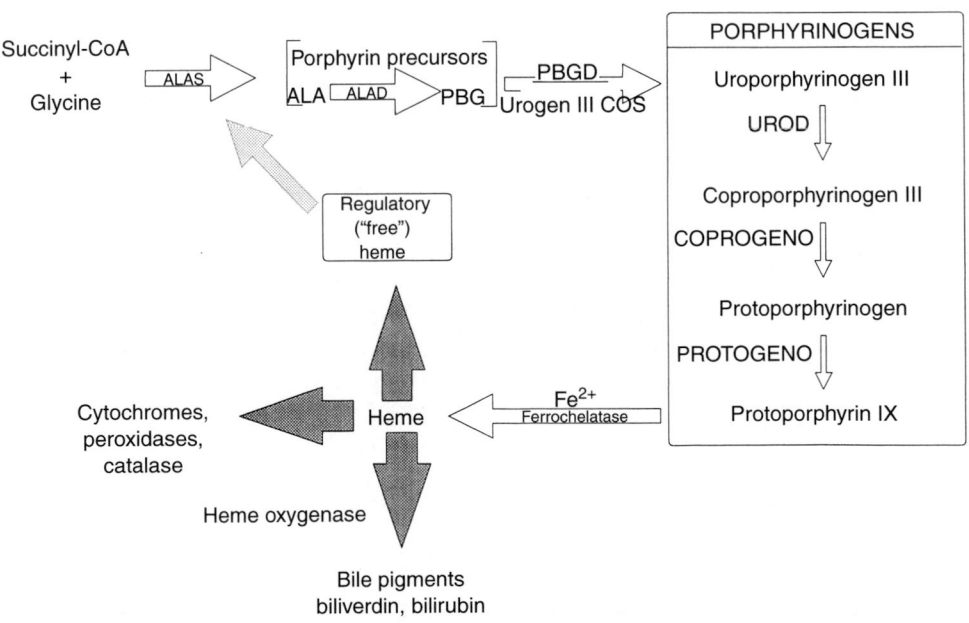

A regulatory pool of "free" heme unbound to apoproteins may be the critical determinant for regulation of synthesis of ALA synthase activity.

date, more than 60 mutations have been reported at the PBG deaminase locus, including deletions, insertions, missense, nonsense, and splicing mutations.[36]

ALA and PBG, the two aliphatic nonporphyrin precursors of heme, are excreted primarily in the urine; normally this amounts to less than 4000 and 1500 μg of each, respectively, per 24 h (see Table 151-1). However, in some types of porphyria (AIP and VP), there may be a 10- to 100-fold increase in urinary excretion of ALA and PBG, which can be detected using relatively simple diagnostic tests. For example, PBG reacts with Ehrlich's reagent, which contains p-dimethylaminobenzaldehyde in hydrochloric acid, to give a positive red-color reaction (Watson-Schwartz test) during attacks of AIP and VP.[37] The cherry-red chromogen is not extracted into chloroform or butanol and remains in the aqueous phase when PBG is elevated. The Hoesch test is a simpler modification of the Watson-Schwartz test that has found increasing application.[38]

Uroporphyrinogen III Synthase

The fourth enzyme in the heme pathway is UROGEN III synthase, which catalyzes the formation of uroporphyrinogen III from hydroxymethylbilane or from PBG if PBG deaminase is also present. By simple inversion of one PBG molecule during synthesis of UROGEN I, the III isomer is formed (see Fig. 151-2). This apparently minor structural alteration is of considerable biologic importance as only the III isomer can proceed to the formation of heme. Heme is a type III porphyrin, and no type I heme has been identified in nature, thus making production of the I isomer an essentially nonphysiologic pathway. The formation of UROGEN III is catalyzed by the cytoplasmic enzyme UROGEN III synthase, which is closely linked to PBG deaminase. This enzyme has been purified from human erythrocytes and has a molecular mass of approximately 30 kDa; it is thermolabile, exhibits maximum catalytic activity at pH 7.4,[39] and is inhibited by heavy metals such as zinc, cadmium, and copper.[40]

The human gene for UROGEN III synthase has also been cloned and sequenced and encodes a protein of 265 amino acids with a predicted mass of about 28.6 kDa.[41] In most tissues, UROGEN III synthase is present in considerable excess as compared to PBG deaminase, thus assuring efficient conversion of the I to the III isomer. The only difference between the I and III isomers of each of the porphyrinogens is the reversal of the side chains on the "D" ring of the tetrapyrrole molecule. The hepatic and erythroid forms of the enzyme are identical.

Uroporphyrinogen Decarboxylase

UROGEN I and III each contain eight carboxyl groups as side chains, four of which are acetate (—CH_2COOH) and four of which are propionate (—CH_2—CH_2—COOH) moieties (see Fig. 151-2). The soluble cytosolic enzyme UROGEN decarboxylase catalyzes the sequential decarboxylation of the four carboxyl groups of the acetic acid side chains to methyl groups to form coproporphyrinogen (acetate groups to methyl groups) (Fig. 151-2). Decarboxylation first occurs on ring D, then the enzyme turns around to decarboxylate rings A, B, and C in a clockwise fashion. This converts the original 8-carboxyl porphyrinogen (UROGEN I or III) first to 7-carboxyl, then to 6-carboxyl, and 5-carboxyl porphyrinogen. The 5-carboxyl porphyrinogen can then undergo decarboxylation of its last acetyl group to form the 4-carboxyl porphyrinogen that is known

as coproporphyrinogen (COPROGEN I or III) (Fig. 151-2). These intermediates are also referred to as hepta-, hexa-, penta-, and tetracarboxylate porphyrinogens. As discussed above, COPROGEN I cannot be further metabolized to heme. The purified human enzyme from erythrocytes has a molecular mass of about 42 kDa, and its activity is inhibited by metals such as copper, mercury, and lead. The human cDNA for UROGEN decarboxylase has been isolated, and the deduced sequence was found to be equivalent to 367 amino acids, consistent with the molecular mass and the amino acid composition of the purified protein.[1] Human UROGEN decarboxylase is encoded by a single gene on the short arm of chromosome 1, which contains 10 exons spread over 3 kb.[42]

UROGEN decarboxylase activity is reduced in the liver of patients with PCT and HEP.[43] Approximately 20 percent of patients with PCT have a 50 percent decrease in UROGEN decarboxylase concentration in all tissues; this form of PCT is inherited as an autosomal dominant trait with low penetrance (type II PCT). The molecular genetics of type II PCT have not been fully characterized, but at least three distinct mutations have been identified that either decrease the stability of the enzyme or produce defective pre-mRNA splicing.[42] In type I PCT, also known as the sporadic form, the enzyme deficiency is limited to the liver. A form of type II PCT in which the activity and concentration of erythrocyte enzyme is normal suggests that an autosomal gene, not necessarily at the UROGEN decarboxylase locus, could influence the expression of type II PCT.[44] Normal amounts of mRNA for the enzyme are present in type II PCT, and a splice-site mutation has been found in one pedigree with type II (familial) PCT that causes a deletion of exon 6 from the mRNA.[45] The resulting protein is shorter than the normal protein, missing the amino acids encoded by exon 6, and this aberrant protein lacks catalytic activity and is rapidly degraded.

In HEP, UROGEN decarboxylase activity is usually 5 to 10 percent of normal, and patients are either homozygotes or compound heterozygotes for mutations of the UROGEN decarboxylase gene. One mutation occurring in HEP homozygotes is also associated with overt PCT in heterozygotes.[46] The mutation that has been identified in some, but not all, families with HEP is a 281 (Gly→Glu) shift.[47,48]

Coproporphyrinogen Oxidase

This is a mitochondrial enzyme located in the intermembrane space. COPROGEN III has four carboxyl groups, each of which is part of a propionate side chain. COPROGEN oxidase, a mitochondrial enzyme of molecular mass 72 kDa, catalyzes the sequential oxidative removal of the carboxyl group from two of the propionate groups, forming first 3-carboxyl porphyrinogen, or harderoporphyrinogen (HARDEROGEN), and then 2-carboxyl porphyrinogen, or protoporphyrinogen IX (PROTOGEN) (see Fig. 151-2). Southern blot analysis of human restriction fragments suggests the presence of a single gene in the human genome.[49] The COPROGEN oxidase gene spans 14 kb and consists of seven exons and six introns. At least four mutations have been found in patients with HCP. These include point mutations resulting in base substitutions or exon skipping.[49]

A unique modification of normal heme synthesis can occur in PCT. No additional enzymes or enzymatic reactions are involved, but there is a reversal in the sequence of action of the enzymes UROGEN decarboxylase and COPROGEN oxidase. As shown in Fig. 151-1, UROGEN decarboxylase normally acts on 5-carboxyl porphyrinogen to decarboxylate the final remaining acetate group, forming a tetracarboxyl porphyrinogen known as COPROGEN III. This is subsequently converted to PROTOGEN by COPROGEN oxidase (see Figs. 151-1 and 151-2). However, in PCT where UROGEN decarboxylase is deficient, COPROGEN oxidase may first oxidatively decarboxylate a propionate group on 5-carboxyl porphyrinogen to form dehydroisocoproporphyrinogen (Fig. 151-1). The acetyl group on dehydroisocoproporphyrinogen can be decarboxylated by UROGEN decarboxylase to form HARDEROGEN, resulting in diversion back into the normal heme synthesis pathway (Fig. 151-1). Alternatively, dehydroisocoproporphyrinogen can undergo hydration to isocoproporphyrinogen (Fig. 151-1). These steps rarely, if ever, occur during the normal process of heme synthesis but become important in certain of the porphyrias such as PCT, where they provide one explanation for the increased isocoproporphyrin (ISOCOPRO) characteristically found in the feces of patients with this disease.

Protoporphyrinogen Oxidase

The oxidation of PROTOGEN IX to PROTO is catalyzed by the enzyme PROTOGEN oxidase, an integral protein of the inner mitochondrial membrane (Fig. 151-2). This reaction can also occur nonenzymatically, but the enzyme appears to be necessary for heme synthesis to proceed at a normal rate. PROTOGEN oxidase activity is reduced in patients with VP.[50,51] PROTOGEN oxidase isolated from rat liver mitochondria has been shown to have a molecular mass of 35 kDa and requires molecular oxygen to catalyze the oxidation of PROTOGEN to PROTO. The gene has been isolated and consists of 13 exons and about 8 kb and maps to chromosome 1.[52]

Ferrochelatase

The final step in the formation of heme, the incorporation of ferrous iron (Fe^{2+}) into PROTO, is catalyzed by the enzyme ferrochelatase at the matrix face of the inner mitochondrial membrane (Fig. 151-2). This enzyme is also referred to as heme synthase, or protoheme-ferro-lyase. Unlike other enzymes in the heme biosynthesis pathway, which require reduced forms of the porphyrins (porphyrinogens) as substrates, ferrochelatase can utilize oxidized PROTO. This lysine-rich enzyme has a molecular mass of 63 kDa and a pH optimum of 7.8. Ferrochelatase activity is decreased in various tissues of patients with EPP.

Murine ferrochelatase has been cloned, and two mRNA transcripts have been identified in multiple tissues.[53] The enzyme appears to be identical in both erythroid and hepatic cells. The protein has 367 amino acid residues and a molecular mass of about 41.7 kDa. The cDNA for human ferrochelatase has also been cloned, sequenced, and shown to have 88 percent identity to the mouse enzyme. Human ferrochelatase mRNA is encoded by a single nuclear gene that spans about 45 kb of chromosomal DNA.[54] The gene is located on chromosome 18 and consists of 11 exons and 10 introns. Molecular genetic studies have been conducted in patients with EPP and reveal at least 20 mutations of various types including exon skipping, missense, nonsense, and nucleotide deletions, resulting in encoding of truncated proteins that would be expected to have little or no catalytic activity.

The end product of the pathway, ferrous-PROTO (FePROTO) or heme, diffuses out of the mitochondrion into the cytoplasm, where it is available to function as a prosthetic group by combining with appropriate apoproteins.

It is important to emphasize that porphyrinogens (reduced porphyrins) are the true intermediates in heme synthesis. The irreversibly oxidized porphyrins, with the exception of PROTO, do not function as substrates for the enzymes of the pathway. Free porphyrins are not known to contribute any useful biologic function. These porphyrins exhibit an absorption spectrum with a major peak in the 400-nm region, the so-called Soret band, and smaller absorp-

tion peaks between 500 and 640 nm. These oxidized porphyrins induce photodynamic effects in skin tissue and subcellular elements when exposed to ultraviolet and short visible light (360 to 420 nm) or red wavelengths (640 to 700 nm). Thus, porphyrins are actually heme pathway by-products, which are of special interest to dermatologists because of their unique photosensitizing properties.

PATHOPHYSIOLOGY OF CUTANEOUS LESIONS IN PORPHYRIAS

One of the most common cutaneous manifestations of the porphyrias is photosensitivity; it is observed in patients with several of these disorders (EP, EPP, PCT, VP, HCP, and HEP) in whom plasma and tissue porphyrins are increased. Patients with AIP, in whom only nonphotosensitizing porphyrin precursors (ALA, PBG) are formed in substantially increased amounts, do not have photosensitivity. In addition, none of the four patients reported with ALA dehydratase–deficiency porphyria have exhibited photosensitivity.

Patients with the erythropoietic types of porphyria frequently complain of a burning sensation and pruritus following exposure to sunlight. A "primary" effect of sun exposure on cutaneous photosensitivity in EPP has been described in which threshold exposure on one day that evokes barely any symptoms, or none, will augment the reaction caused by additional sunlight on the following day.[55] The cause of this is unknown, but the phenomenon suggests that the repair of porphyrin photosensitization skin damage may be prolonged. These subjective symptoms are notably absent in patients with the chronic hepatic porphyrias such as PCT and VP. Although there is some information about the pathophysiology of photosensitivity and sclerodermoid skin changes in the chronic hepatic porphyrias, the causes of the pigmentary alterations and hypertrichosis seen in these patients remain to be elucidated.

Porphyrins have certain unique photobiologic and spectroscopic properties. The metal-chelated porphyrins (e.g., heme or FePROTO) show no fluorescence. Porphyrins that are chelated to other paramagnetic metals, such as Mn^{2+}, CO^{2+}, or Zn^{2+} (e.g., chlorophyll, ZnPROTO), also do not fluoresce. This is the reason that patients with lead intoxication, in which ZnPROTO is elevated, do not have photosensitivity.[56] However, metal-free porphyrins (e.g., URO, COPRO, PROTO) in acidic solutions show a major absorption peak in the 400- to 410-nm region (Soret band); they also exhibit four additional absorption bands with decreasing intensity between 500 and 700 nm. Exposure of porphyrins to the Soret band spectra results in two major fluorescence emission peaks at the 600- to 610-nm and 640- to 660-nm regions.[56]

The first experimental evidence for the photosensitizing property of porphyrins in human skin was provided by the heroic self-experiment of Meyer-Betz, reported in 1913.[57] After injecting himself intravenously with 200 mg of hematoporphyrin and exposing his skin to sunlight, he observed marked erythema and edema in light-exposed body areas, especially on his face and hands. With the increasing use of porphyrin derivatives for photodynamic therapy of human malignancy, porphyrin-induced photosensitivity is a frequent complication.[58]

Although there is no single clearly defined pathway that can currently explain the photosensitization evoked by porphyrins and light, there are a number of potential cellular and soluble factors that could be responsible. Among them, reactive oxygen species,

TABLE 151-4

Factors Contributing to the Development of Cutaneous Lesions in Porphyrias

Sunlight, especially blue and red light (380–760 nm)
Reactive oxygen species ($^1O_2$, $O_2^{\cdot-}$, H_2O_2, $\cdot OH$)
Cells
    Erythrocytes
    Mast cells
    Polymorphonuclear leukocytes
    Fibroblasts
Soluble mediators
    The complement system
    Factor XII-dependent pathways
    The eicosanoids
    Matrix metalloproteinases

certain cells (erythrocytes, mast cells, polymorphonuclear cells, and fibroblasts), and soluble mediators (the complement system, factor XII–dependent pathways, and the eicosanoids) will be discussed (Table 151-4). It is likely that interactions among these factors will prove to be responsible for the pathogenesis of the cutaneous lesions in the porphyrias.

Reactive Oxygen Species

Porphyrins such as URO, COPRO, and PROTO absorb light intensely in their Soret bands. Absorption of this radiant energy results in the generation of "excited"-state molecules (Fig. 151-5). The initial excited-state molecule generated is one that has an extremely short half-life, <0.01 μs. Singlet excited-state porphyrins may convert spontaneously to a triplet-state molecule, another excited-state molecule that has a lower energy level but a longer half-

FIGURE 151-5

	$PP_0 + h\nu$	⟶	^1PP	(Singlet state)
1	^1PP	⟶	a) $PP_0 + h\nu$	(Fluorescence)
2		⟶	b) PP_0	(Nonradiative decay)
3		⟶	c) ^3PP	(Triple-state transition)
4	^3PP	⟶	$PP_0 + h\nu$	(Phosphorescence)
5	$^3PP + {}^3O_2$	⟶	$PP_0 + {}^1O_2$	(Singlet-state oxygen)
6	$^1O_2 + A$	⟶	A (ox)	(Substrate oxidation, lipid peroxidation, and cell membrane damage)

Photoexcited porphyrins release energy in a variety of ways when returning to their ground state, and these may contribute to damaging reactions in biologic systems.

life (in the order of microseconds to milliseconds). Because of their long half-life, porphyrin molecules in their triplet state are more likely to react with biologic molecules and are likely candidates to mediate most porphyrin-associated photobiologic reactions. Excited-state porphyrin molecules subsequently return to their normal ground states by releasing their absorbed energy in the form of light (fluorescence is emitted by singlet-state molecules and phosphorescence by triplet states), heat, or by transferring energy to cell constituents (cell membranes, organelles, proteins, DNA) (Fig. 151-6).

Excited porphyrins in their singlet and triplet states can also transfer their absorbed energy to oxygen molecules, thereby creating reactive "excited" oxygen states.[59] Cellular and tissue damage induced by photoactivated porphyrins are believed to occur primarily as a result of the formation of reactive singlet oxygen ($^1O_2$), as illustrated in Figs. 151-5 and 151-7.[60,61] Various forms of reactive oxygen species capable of causing tissue damage are known to exist, including singlet oxygen ($^1O_2$) and superoxide anion ($O_2^{\cdot-}$). In some cases the sensitized porphyrin may react with oxygen to yield hydrogen peroxide (H_2O_2) or with water to form hydroxyl radicals ($\cdot OH$). Those processes in which activated oxygen species play a role in photosensitization are referred to as *photodynamic reactions*.[62] Most of the porphyrin-mediated cutaneous photosensitization reactions are essentially photodynamic and can be minimized or prevented if reactive oxygen is eliminated from the reaction system through inactivation processes known as *quenching* or *scavenging*.

Although these concepts regarding excited porphyrins and reactive oxygen species are valid in simple systems, their applicability to complex tissues such as the skin remains to be established. Several hypotheses have been advanced regarding the mechanism of porphyrin-induced photosensitivity. One hypothesis involves the transfer of energy from excited species of oxygen to water or to lipids, creating hydrogen and/or lipid peroxides. These peroxides, in turn, can evoke damage in lipid-rich cellular membranes (Fig. 151-7). Evidence for this type of reaction has come from the demonstration of porphyrin-UV–induced cross-linkage of proteins within RBC membranes[63] and destruction of fibroblast membrane sulfhydryl groups.[64] If such damage occurs in plasma membranes in cells in or adjacent to the skin, it could result in tissue destruction and possibly explain the photosensitivity seen in the cutaneous porphyrias. Goldstein and Harber showed that photoexcitation of PROTO-enriched RBCs resulted in the formation of hydrogen peroxide and lipid peroxides, each of which would be highly destructive to lipid-rich membranous structures.[65] There is evidence in RBCs of peroxidation of cholesterol groups in the cell membrane resulting in hemolysis following exposure to UV radiation and PROTO.[66]

Several other studies have also supported the participation of reactive oxygen species in porphyrin-induced phototoxicity. The release of inflammatory mediators from mast cells induced by photoexcited PROTO can be suppressed by catalase, which inactivates hydrogen peroxide by converting it to water and oxygen.[67] Singlet oxygen has been shown to mediate porphyrin-induced photodamage to hepatic and epidermal microsomal cytochrome P_{450}.[68] Porphyrin- and radiation-induced damage of lysosomal and mitochondrial membranes have also been reported.[69,70] DNA exposed to visible light and hematoporphyrin manifests selective degradation of the guanine moiety.[71] In vivo, beta-carotene, a scavenger of singlet oxygen, has been shown to be effective in diminishing the severity of cutaneous photosensitivity in patients with EPP.[72] In a murine model, it was demonstrated that xanthine oxidase–generated superoxide anions also play a significant role in the development of the phototoxicity induced by HPD.[73]

Erythrocytes

Erythrocytes have been used extensively in the study of porphyrin-membrane interactions. Photoexcited PROTO elicits peroxidation of cholesterol groups in cell membranes, whereas URO or COPRO has shown no such effect. This differential effect, also observed in studies using mast cells, polymorphonuclear leukocytes (PMLs), and fibroblasts, most likely relates to variations in lipid-water partitioning of the different porphyrins, which may relate to their polarity. The lipophilic PROTO, a 2-carboxyl porphyrin, is more damaging to membranes as compared to the more water-soluble COPRO and URO.[74,75]

Mast Cells

Mast cell degranulation occurs in the exposed skin of patients with EPP.[76] Irradiation of PROTO-treated mast cells in vitro induces release of mast cell–derived mediators, although exposure to lower doses of PROTO and radiation results in inhibition of secretagogue-induced histamine release from these cells.[67,77] In contrast, no mediator release is detectable when cells are radiated in the presence of URO.[67] These findings may help to explain the differences in the clinical presentation of patients with EPP and PCT. The elevated PROTO in patients with EPP may induce the release of mast cell mediators in vivo following sun exposure, resulting in painful, pruritic erythema and edema. The absence of these changes in patients with PCT may be explained by the apparent inability of photoexcited URO to damage cutaneous mast cells.

Studies conducted in animal models have further confirmed the participation of mast cells in porphyrin-induced phototoxicity. It has been shown that phototoxicity is associated with elevated serum histamine levels and dermal mast cell degranulation[78] and that the phototoxic response can be suppressed by pretreatment with antihistamines (H_1 blockers) and by intradermal injection of a mast cell secretagogue (compound 48/80).[79]

Polymorphonuclear Cells

Exposure of human PMLs to PROTO and radiation in vitro results in membrane damage, whereas photoexcited URO induces no such alterations.[80] These results are strikingly similar to those obtained in studies with mast cells (see above). In an animal model, the porphyrin-induced phototoxic response was associated with a dermal PML infiltrate,[78,81] and the phototoxicity was markedly suppressed in leu-

FIGURE 151-6

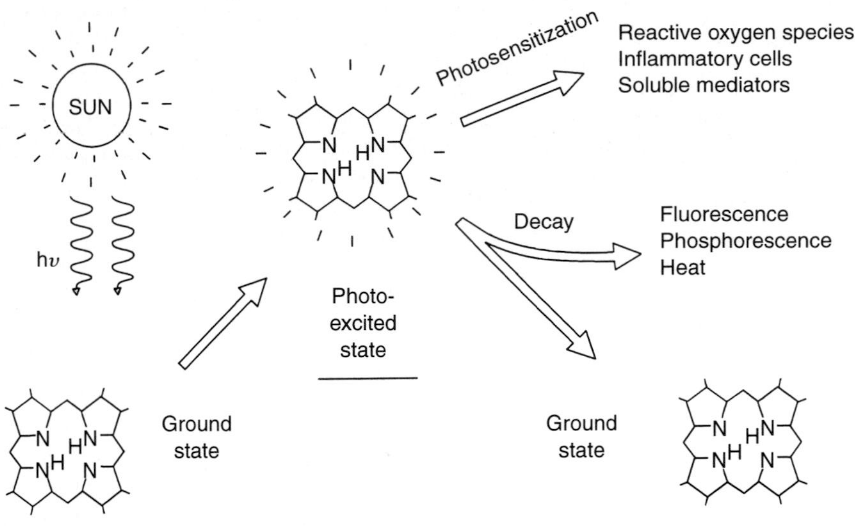

Porphyrins in ground state upon absorption of radiant energy (hv) undergo transition to photoexcited states. The photoexcited porphyrins generate reactive oxygen species, damaging cells by release of proinflammatory mediators; these in turn may contribute to damaging reactions in biologic systems such as skin.

FIGURE 151-7

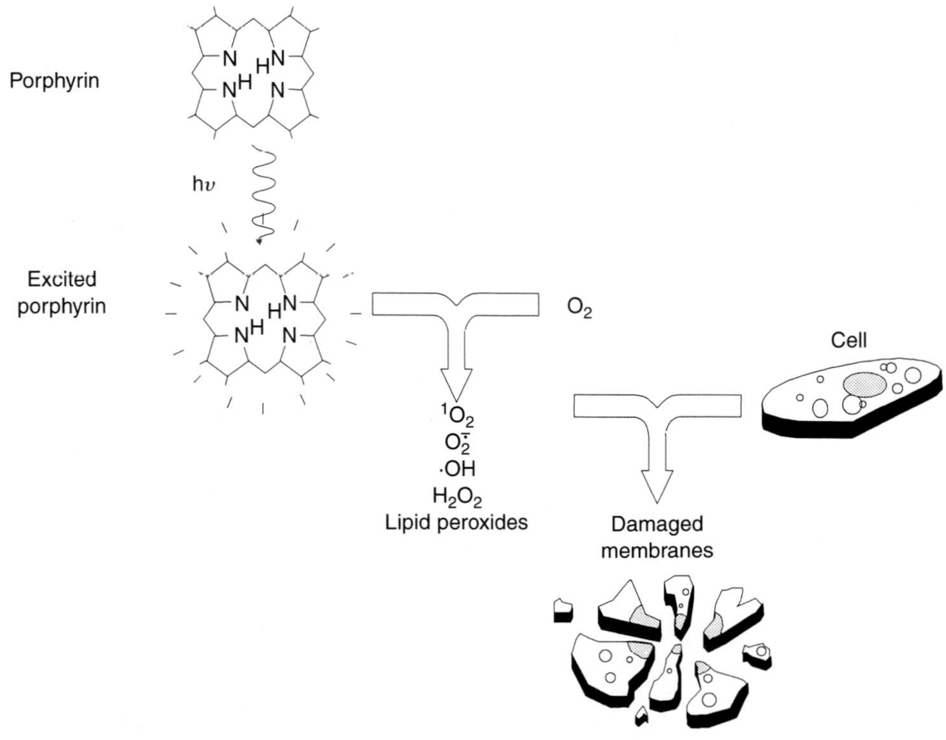

Photoexcited porphyrins in their triplet state transfer the absorbed energy to oxygen (O_2) molecules, thereby producing reactive oxygen species ($^1O_2$, $\cdot O_2^-$, $\cdot OH$, and lipid peroxides). These reactive oxygen species interact with cell membranes to cause tissue damage.

kopenic animals.[79] These results appear to suggest that PMLs may be necessary but not sufficient for the complete manifestation of phototoxicity induced by porphyrins.

Fibroblasts

Differential phototoxic effects of various porphyrins have also been verified in studies using dermal fibroblasts. An increase in collagen biosynthesis is observed following incubation of fibroblasts with URO.[82] This effect is independent of irradiation and may partly explain the sclerodermoid changes observed in patients with PCT, which can occur in sun-exposed and sun-protected areas. In contrast, PROTO induces photolysis of fibroblasts in vitro.[83,84]

The Complement System

The participation of the complement system in porphyrin-induced phototoxicity was initially suggested by immunofluorescent studies identifying selected complement components localized within vessel walls at the dermal-epidermal junction in patients with cutaneous porphyria.[85,86] In addition to endothelial cell damage, histologic changes consistent with those mediated by complement activation products, i.e., mast cell degranulation and infiltration of PMLs, are observed during the acute phase of photosensitivity in the skin of patients with EPP.[76] In vitro irradiation of sera obtained from patients with EPP and PCT results in complement activation.[87] In animal models, porphyrin-induced phototoxicity is associated with complement activation and is suppressed in complement-depleted animals as well as in animals congenitally deficient in the fifth component of complement.[88,89] Generation of complement-derived chemotactic activity is also seen following exposure of the skin of patients with EPP and PCT to Soret band radiation.[90]

Factor XII–Dependent Pathways of Coagulation

Activation of Hageman factor–dependent pathways in the presence of PROTO has been demonstrated in vitro.[91] In contrast, neither URO nor COPRO induces such activation. Whether this activation, which is independent of irradiation, contributes to the pathogenesis of porphyrin-induced phototoxicity remains to be determined.

The Eicosanoids

Porphyrins and radiation have been reported to affect eicosanoid metabolism. Incubation of mouse peritoneal macrophages or radiation-induced fibrosarcoma tumor cells in vitro with hematoporphyrin derivative PHOTOFRIN II, followed by 630-nm radiation, results in dose-dependent generation of prostaglandin E_2.[92]

Matrix Metalloproteinases

Photoexcited uroporphyrin has been shown to coordinately induce the matrix metalloproteinases (MMPs) interstitial collagenase (MMP-1), 72-kDa type IV collagenase (MMP-2), and stromelysin-1 (MMP-3) in human dermal fibroblasts in vitro.[93] The induction of the MMPs by porphyrin photosensitization suggests that their activation could contribute to the photocutaneous changes that occur in the photosensitizing porphyrias, particularly those associated with blistering.

Summary

Cutaneous phototoxicity in porphyrias is directly related to the interaction of porphyrins with light of the Soret and other bands, resulting in the generation of reactive oxygen species; this in turn can induce lipid peroxidation and cell membrane alterations. Release of mediators and enzymes from cells such as mast cells and PMLs contributes to the inflammatory response; the latter is modulated by the effects of porphyrins on the complement system, factor XII–dependent pathways, and the eicosanoids. Variations in solubility influenced by the lipid-water partitioning of porphyrins may account for the unique phototoxic manifestations observed in various types of porphyria.

CLASSIFICATION OF THE PORPHYRIAS

At present, most classifications of the porphyrias are based on the primary site of expression of the specific enzymatic defect and the abnormal porphyrin profile of patients with these disorders.

The porphyrias have been classified by Günther,[6] Waldenström,[9,11] and Watson et al.[75] The classification used here (Table 151-5) is an extension of that originally proposed by Watson et al.[75]

ERYTHROPOIETIC PORPHYRIA (Table 151-6)

Synomyms for EP include Günther's disease, congenital hematoporphyria, and erythropoietic uroporphyria.

Historic Aspects

This disease was originally named hematoporphyria congenita by Günther in 1911, and the first published case of porphyria was probably of this type.[2]

Between 1911 and 1936, Günther and Fischer performed a most detailed study of a patient with porphyria named Mathias Petry. In this study, an excessive excretion of a new type of porphyrin was identified, and because the porphyrin was in highest concentration in the urine, Fischer named it URO.[7] This was the first definite evidence that the type of porphyrin ob-

TABLE 151-5

Classification of Human Porphyria

Tissue Origin	Type	Inheritance
Erythropoietic	Erythropoietic porphyria (EP)	Autosomal recessive
	Erythropoietic protoporphyria (EPP)	Autosomal dominant
	Erythropoietic coproporphyria (ECP)	Autosomal dominant
Hepatic	Acute intermittent porphyria (AIP)	Autosomal dominant
	Variegate porphyria (VP)	Autosomal dominant
	Hereditary coproporphyria (HCP)	Autosomal dominant
	Porphyria cutanea tarda (PCT)	Variable, autosomal dominant
	ALA dehydratase porphyria	Autosomal recessive
Hepatoerythropoietic	Hepatoerythropoietic porphyria (HEP)	Autosomal recessive

served in excess in human porphyria was not hematoporphyrin. An excellent review of EP has recently been published by Fritsch et al.[94]

Etiology

EP is an autosomal recessive inborn error of metabolism that results from variably deficient activity of URO-GEN III synthase, the fourth enzyme in the heme synthetic pathway.

Genetics

The UROGEN III synthase gene has been cloned and its nucleotide sequence determined.[41] Multiple mutations have been identified.[95] The disease has also occurred in a child of non-consanguineous parents as a result of being a compound heterozygote and inheriting a separate and distinct mutation from each parent.[96] Studies comparing genotype and phenotype in EP have shown a correlation between certain mutations and the severity of the enzyme deficiency.[97]

TABLE 151-6

Erythropoietic Porphyria

Synonyms	Günther's disease, congenital hematoporphyria, erythropoietic uroporphyria
Inheritance	Autosomal recessive
Age of onset	Usually infancy or first decade
Incidence	Very rare (<250 reported cases)
Photosensitivity	Marked, early in childhood
Skin reactions	Early: Vesicles, bullae, erosions, hypertrichosis of lanugo hair and thickened brows and eyelashes, hypermelanosis, skin photosensitivity
	Late: Scarring with atrophy; mutilating deformities of hands, ears, face, and nose; cicatrizing alopecia; sclerodermoid changes
Clinical findings	Hemolytic anemia, erythrodontia, splenomegaly, skin photosensitivity, pink-red urine, fluorescent red blood cells and normoblasts, scleral ulceration of the eyes
Biochemical defects	Excretory: Mainly elevated URO I and COPRO I in urine and COPRO I in feces; URO > COPRO
	RBC and plasma: Increased URO I and PROTO
	Enzymatic: UROGEN III cosynthase deficiency primarily in bone marrow
	? Increased PBG deaminase activity
	? Decreased UROGEN decarboxylase in some cases
Management	Hemolysis may improve after splenectomy; avoidance of sunlight and treatment of secondary skin infections

Epidemiology

EP has been observed to occur in countries around the world. Fewer than 250 cases had been reported by 1998. Nearly all begin in childhood and only a few in adult life.[98] EP also occurs in a number of mammals, including swine, cattle, and cats,[99] and these animal models have greatly aided research in this disease.

Clinical Manifestations

The disease usually presents itself in the first few months of life with moderate to severe cutaneous photosensitivity associated with pinkish-red urine.[94,100] EP causes the most mutilating skin lesions of any of the porphyrias. The photosensitivity is due to the excessive URO I and COPRO I in RBCs, plasma, and skin, which may result in photolysis of porphyrin-rich cells.

The skin manifestations include skin fragility and vesicles and bullae, which may contain pink fluorescent fluid. Secondary infection, delayed healing, and scar formation may occur. This may lead to loss of acral tissue, such as the tips of the ears, the nose, and fingers (Fig. 151-8A, B), and facial mutilation. Hirsutism, with long, dark, lanugo-like hair, may occur and is particularly evident in light-exposed areas such as the face, neck, and extremities. The scalp may develop a cicatrizing alopecia. Other chronic findings include eye changes (photophobia, keratoconjunctivitis, ectropion, symblepharon, and even loss of vision) and irregular hyper- and hypopigmentation of the skin. Erythrodontia (red-stained teeth) is a common finding in both deciduous and permanent teeth and is virtually pathognomonic of EP. The urine also fluoresces reddish-pink.

In addition, splenomegaly, porphyrin-rich gallstones, and fluorescent bone marrow normoblasts are often observed. Hemolytic anemia associated with shortened erythrocyte life span and hypersplenism (36 vs. 120 days) is seen. Whether the hemolytic anemia is due to "photohemolysis" of circulating porphyrin-laden erythrocytes or to an associated intracorpuscular red cell defect is unresolved.[101]

Laboratory Findings

The primary defect in EP involves a decreased activity of UROGEN III synthase that results in accumulation of predominantly type I porphyrins in the tissues and increased excretion from the body. The pink to burgundy red color of the urine from excess URO I is often visible on inspection (Fig. 151-8C). Marrow normoblasts exhibit relatively stable fluorescence and contain markedly elevated URO I, COPRO I, and PROTO. Urinary excretion of ALA and PBG is normal. COPRO I may be present in large amounts in the feces. Typical biochemical findings of EP are summarized in Tables 151-3 and 151-6.

Histopathology

The bullous lesion of EP is subepidermal with minimal degrees of inflammation. Thickening of collagen bundles may be seen in areas of scarring. Perivascular deposits of porphyrin can be found when the unstained sections of skin or liver are viewed with a fluorescence microscope.

Differential Diagnosis

The diagnosis of EP can usually be made from the early onset of severe cutaneous photosensitivity associated with red-fluorescing urine and erythrodontia. Distinguishing EP from other congenital types of photodermatoses is important. Cutaneous findings in patients with xeroderma pigmentosum, epidermolysis bullosa, hydroa vacciniforme, and bullous pemphigoid may mimic those in patients with EP, but the porphyrin profiles of the former conditions are completely normal. Patients with chronic hepatic porphyrias such as PCT and VP can be differentiated from patients with EP by the

FIGURE 151-8

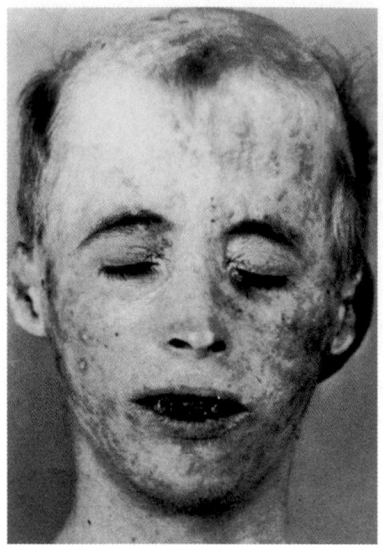

A.

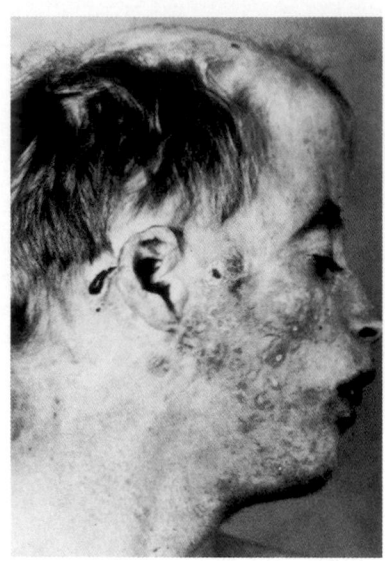

B.

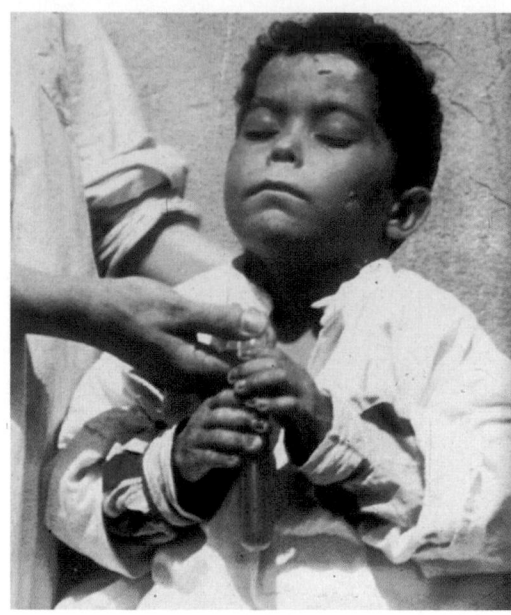

C.

Two cases of congenital erythropoietic porphyria (Günther's disease). A, B. Severe scarring, damage of the ear and nose cartilage, hair loss, and discolored teeth. (*Courtesy of A Wiskemann, MD, and J Kimmig, MD.*) C. Burgundy red urine of a patient with congenital porphyria.

normal PROTO content of their erythrocytes. The cutaneous manifestations of HEP may be strikingly similar to those of EP, and measurement of the enzymes UROGEN III synthase (decreased in EP) and UROGEN decarboxylase (decreased in HEP) will distinguish the two. The dual occurrence of HCP and EP in a single patient who inherited the HCP trait from her mother and the EP trait from both of her parents has been reported.[102]

Treatment

The treatment of EP is essentially preventive and symptomatic and includes avoidance of sun exposure, surveillance of the anemia, and treatment of recurrent skin infections. Protection from sunlight is absolutely essential, and this alone may be of substantial benefit. Patients should be instructed to wear broad-brimmed hats and other photoprotective clothing. Topical sunscreens are relatively little used as the only ones effective at wavelengths greater than 400 nm are light opaque (SPF > 30) and contain zinc oxide or titanium dioxide. Newer formulations with improved cosmetic properties may be helpful. The efficacy of oral administration of beta-carotene (120 to 180 mg daily) in EP is not proved, although there are reports that it may improve light tolerance (DJ Cripps, personal communication). Splenectomy because of intractable hemolytic anemia has occasionally resulted in marked improvement both in the anemia and in cutaneous photosensitivity. Suppression of erythropoiesis by transfusion of packed erythrocytes causes a marked decrease in porphyrin production and excretion[103]; however, iron overload is a drawback. Oral treatment of a single patient with activated charcoal (60 g three times a day) for 9 months was found to lower the porphyrin levels in plasma and skin, and there was complete remission of photosensitivity during the treatment period.[104] Charcoal is thought to interfere with the enterohepatic recirculation of the porphyrin and thereby enhance porphyrin clearance from the body.

However, this beneficial effect has been disputed.[105] Bone marrow transplantation has been performed and had beneficial effects on the abnormal porphyrin metabolism in at least one patient.[106]

ERYTHROPOIETIC PROTOPORPHYRIA

(Table 151-7)

Synonyms for EPP include erythrohepatic porphyria and protoporphyria.

Historic Aspects

EPP was first clearly defined and named by Magnus et al.[18] who, in 1961, showed a relationship between the protoporphyrinemia and the cutaneous photosensitivity in the Soret band manifested in the form of solar urticaria. This disease had escaped detection for many years for at least two reasons: (1) objective clinical signs of skin photosensitivity associated with EPP are much milder than those of EP, and (2) excessive porphyrins are almost never found in the urine of patients with EPP due to the virtual insolubility of PROTO in water.

Etiology

The specific enzyme defect in EPP is ferrochelatase, which has been shown to be decreased in RBCs, mitogen-stimulated lymphocytes, and cultured skin fibroblasts of patients and unaffected carriers of EPP.[54,107–109] Because the activity of ferrochelatase in cultured skin fibroblasts of EPP patients is only 10 to 25 percent of normal, questions have been raised about the dominant inheritance of the disease. In one study, several families with EPP were examined with respect to the mode of inheritance, and on the basis of erythrocyte ferrochelatase activity this was said to be either autosomal dominant or recessive.[108]

Genetics

Murine and human cDNAs for ferrochelatase have been cloned.[53,54] Norris et al.[110] studied 9 families including 14 patients with EPP. Two distinct inheritance patterns were identified: the first was autosomal dominant and the second was autosomal recessive. In some families studied, both parents had normal enzyme activity and the inheritance could not be determined. Goerz et al. showed similar findings in different families with EPP.[108] Deybach et al.[111] have reported a single patient with EPP with homozygous deficiency of the enzyme whose parents both manifest evidence of partially decreased ferrochelatase activity. This genetic heterogeneity requires further research to clarify the inheritance of EPP. More than 20 distinct ferrochelatase mutations have now been identified.

Epidemiology

Although the exact incidence of EPP is unknown, it has been reported with increasing frequency since 1961, indicating that it is likely the most common cutaneous porphyria except for PCT. Studies from one laboratory performing diagnostic tests for RBC porphyrins in patients with suspected cutaneous photosensitivity indicated that 8 percent of such samples demonstrate elevated RBC PROTO levels diagnostic of EPP. The disease has been reported from many countries around the world, and it is likely that no ethnic group is spared.[112]

Clinical Manifestations

The disease begins early in life and is characterized by cutaneous photosensitivity and by elevated PROTO in RBCs, feces, and plasma; there is no excess porphyrin excretion in the urine except when hepatic failure occurs as a terminal event. The acute episodes of cutaneous photosensitivity include burning, stinging (smarting), and pruritus in light-exposed skin, particularly of the nose, cheeks, and dorsal aspects of the hands. These are followed by erythema, edema (Fig. 151-9), urticarial lesions, and rarely purpura. Photosensitivity may occur within minutes of sun exposure; it often starts early in the spring, continues through the summer, and diminishes in the winter. The skin lesions may resolve slowly, leaving small, atrophic, waxy or pitted scars (Fig. 151-10A, B). There may be some pursing of perioral skin (pseudorhagades). The skin of the knuckles and fingers, particularly over the metacarpophalangeal and interphalangeal joints, often appears thickened, wrinkled, and waxy, suggesting a premature aging (so-called old knuckles) in a child. This subtle change is pathognomonic, particularly in children. Superficial scarring on the bridge of the nose and small circular shallow scars

TABLE 151-7

Erythropoietic Protoporphyria

Synonyms	Erythrohepatic protoporphyria, protoporphyria
Inheritance	Autosomal dominant, variable penetrance
Age of onset	Early childhood (1–4 years)
Photosensitivity	Mild to severe, onset immediate (in minutes)
Skin reactions	Early: Edematous plaques, erythema, urticaria (occasional), purpura, rare bullae on the nose and hands
	Late: Shallow waxy scars over nose and dorsa of hands; aged knuckles; skin thickening of exposed areas; erosions, crusts, and diffuse infiltration and wrinkling of the face
Differential diagnosis	Congenital EP, lipoid proteinosis, exaggerated sunburn
Clinical findings	Pruritus, burning, and stinging of skin during sun exposure; erythema and edema 12–24 h after exposure; waxy thickening of the knuckles and nose with fine linear scarring; nails may show onycholysis; gallstones may be present; cholelithiasis, terminal hepatic failure in a small percentage of patients; anemia uncommon
Biochemical defects	Excretory: Urine—normal porphyrins; feces—elevated PROTO
	RBC and plasma: Increased PROTO; RBC show orange-red fluorescence
	Enzymatic: Ferrochelatase deficiency in skin fibroblasts, liver, and bone marrow
Management	Beta-carotene (60–180 mg/day) to ameliorate photosensitivity; oral PUVA phototherapy when combined with beta-carotene may also improve sun tolerance

may be seen on the face. Vesicular or bullous lesions rarely occur in EPP in temperate climates, although they have occurred in patients exposed to tropical sunlight. The porphyrin abnormality persists throughout life, although some patients seem to be less symptomatic as they get older.

Controversy has existed concerning the tissue origin of the excessive PROTO. Some have shown that RBC PROTO levels alone are sufficient to explain the increased levels of PROTO,[113,114] whereas others have suggested that hepatic PROTO production contributes to the excessively high levels of circulating PROTO.[115]

Associated findings are few in most patients with EPP. There is no erythrodontia, hypertrichosis, milia, sclerodermoid change, or

FIGURE 151-9

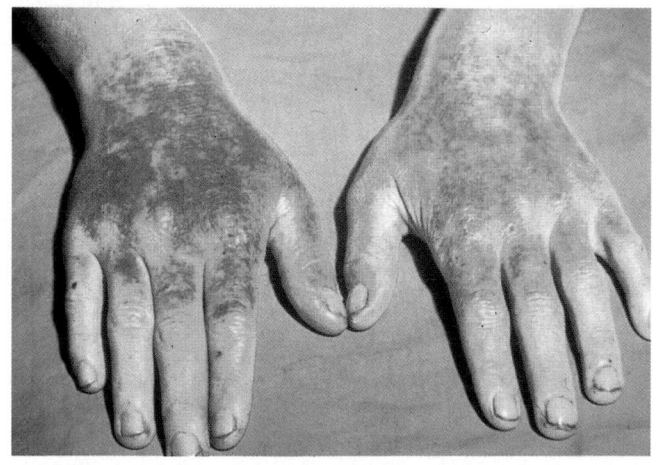

A case of erythropoietic protoporphyria showing swelling and purpura on dorsa of hands resulting from exposure to solar radiation.

FIGURE 151-10

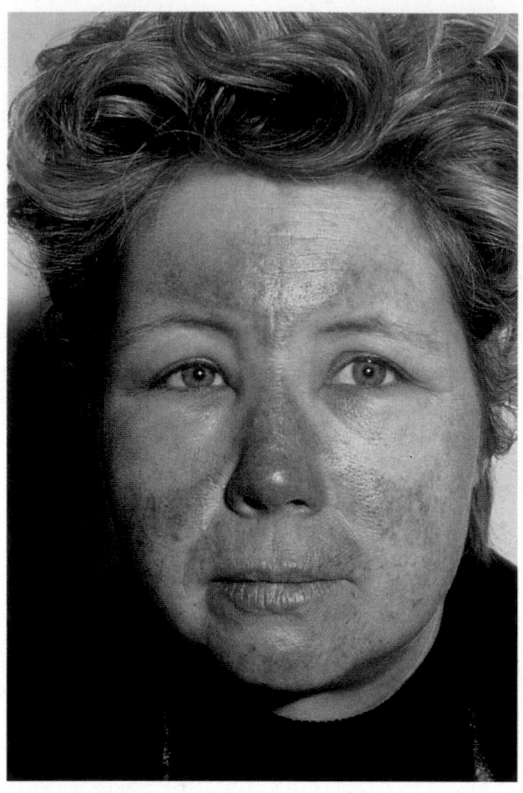

A.

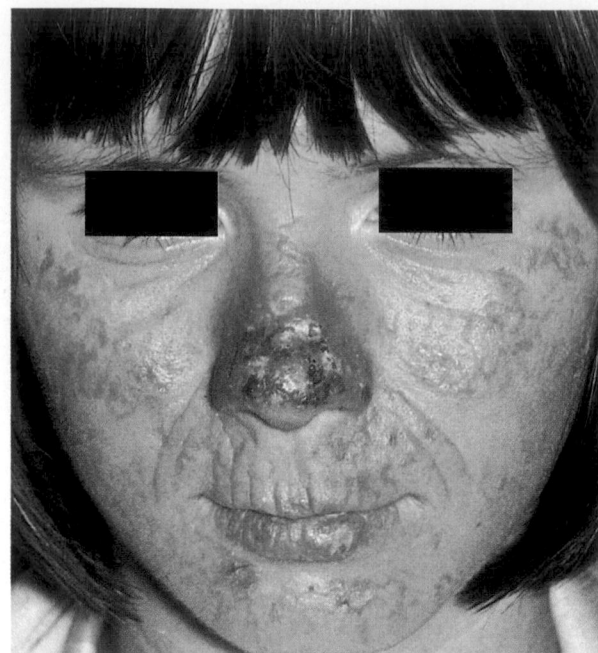

B.

A. One hour after exposure to sunlight, the face of this 35-year old female is edematous, erythematous, and there is purpura on the forehead, cheeks, and nose. The patient experiences severe burning sensations. *B.* A 15-year-old patient with erythropoietic protoporphyria with severe sensitivity to sunlight. The nose, lower lip, and chin show erythematous, in part erosive, and crusted lesions. Nose and cheeks show erythematous lesions, a few small slightly depressed scars, and peculiar waxy thickening of skin. Linear scars are seen between the nose and mouth.

hyperpigmentation. Hemolytic anemia is decidedly uncommon, although about 11 percent of patients with EPP have a mild anemia of unknown cause.[112]

Gallstones have been reported in some patients with EPP at a relatively early age; in one series, 12 percent of patients had cholelithiasis, of whom three underwent cholecystectomy.[116] Careful study of all gallstones obtained at surgery from two EPP patients showed that they contained large amounts of PROTO (Pathak and Bickers, unpublished observations).

Light microscopy of liver biopsies has revealed slight portal and periportal fibrosis and deposition of brown pigment, which may occlude bile canaliculi and ducts; it is also present in hepatocytes, in Kupffer cells, and in periportal macrophages. The pigment is birefringent on polarization microscopy.[117] Hepatocytes may also contain cytoplasmic or mitochondrial inclusions, which at the ultrastructural level appear as needle-like crystals, probably due to precipitated PROTO[118] (Fig. 151-11).

Terminal hepatic failure has been reported in about 5 percent of patients with EPP.[119] All these individuals were jaundiced, had hepatic cirrhosis, and died in hepatic coma or as a consequence of portal hypertension. Risk factors for this type of hepatic failure remain unknown, but it is likely that the deposits of crystalline PROTO lead to hepatocyte injury. Experimental studies have shown that perfusion of rat liver with PROTO induces a dose-dependent cholestasis that could contribute to the hepatotoxic effect of PROTO.[120] Liver failure has also occurred in two siblings who inherited EPP in an autosomal recessive pattern as compound heterozygotes, suggesting that this genotype may augment the risk of this complication.[121] However, this has been disputed since there are cases in which compound heterozygotes have had normal liver function and cases in which heterozygotes developed liver failure.[122]

Laboratory Findings

The diagnosis of EPP is made by detecting elevated levels of free PROTO in the RBCs and/or feces (see Tables 151-3 and 151-7). In addition, there may be increased plasma PROTO, increased fecal COPRO, and occasionally slightly increased RBC COPRO. In incomplete expression of EPP, only the fecal PROTO may be elevated. Examination of a blood smear under a fluorescent microscope reveals red-fluorescing RBCs (5 to 30 percent). This fluorescence is often transient and quite light sensitive, and the procedure should be carried out in subdued light or preferably in the dark. Poh-Fitzpatrick et al.[123] have devised a rapid quantitative microfluorometric assay for free erythrocyte and plasma PROTO that is useful as a screening test for suspected EPP. Finger-prick samples of blood collected on filter paper are used for this test. In one series of 32 patients with EPP, the RBC PROTO levels ranged from 131 to 1617 μg/dL of RBCs (normal < 90 μg/dL of RBCs).[112,124]

FIGURE 151-11

CHAPTER 151
The Porphyrias

1781

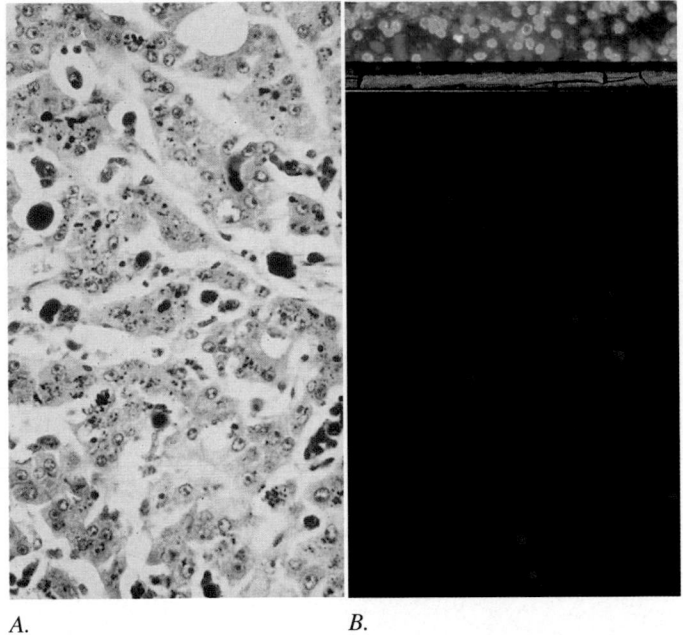

A. *B.*

A. Brown pigment deposits in the liver tissue found in bile canaliculy, hepatocytes, and Kupffer cells. *B.* Bright red fluorescence in red blood cells of a fresh smear of an EPP patient. Where all red blood cells contained in this smear are revealed by green fluorescence only (*top*), a few RBC contain increased amounts of protoporphyrins and thus fluorescence in red (*bottom*).

The photosensitizing activity of porphyrins is most probably related to the light absorption and emission characteristics of these tetrapyrroles (see Table 151-8). There is good evidence to suggest that unchelated (metal-free) PROTO is responsible for the skin photosensitivity reactions in EPP. Evidence for this has come from studies designed to explain the perplexing observation that in lead poisoning and in iron-deficiency anemia, conditions in which RBC PROTO levels are similar to those found in EPP, cutaneous photosensitivity does not occur. Studies by Piomelli et al.[113] and Lamola et al.[125] suggest that in these nonphotosensitizing disorders the excessive PROTO is probably chelated with zinc and bound to globin chains in the RBCs, which renders it incapable of diffusing into the plasma and then into cutaneous tissue. This explains why plasma PROTO is not elevated in these nonphotosensitizing disorders. In EPP, however, the majority of the excessive PROTO is probably unchelated or free. Free PROTO can diffuse out of the RBCs and is detectable in the plasma of patients with EPP who manifest cutaneous photosensitivity.[123] In one study, a patient with sideroblastic anemia had marked increases in free PROTO, both in the RBCs and in the plasma, but had no cutaneous photosensitivity.[126] Because ferrochelatase activity was normal in this patient, it is possible that the excessive free PROTO was either chelated with zinc or readily converted to heme in the skin, thereby precluding cutaneous accumulation of PROTO

and associated photosensitivity. It has also been suggested that the absence of hemolytic anemia in EPP is due to the unique capacity of PROTO to move out of the RBCs and to bind to albumin in the plasma.[127] The porphyrin does not remain within the lipid-rich cell membrane sufficiently long for light exposure to cause damage, and serum albumin has a potent inhibitory effect on photohemolysis in EPP.

Histopathology

Immediately following irradiation, endothelial cell damage, mast cell degranulation, and polymorphonuclear cells are seen in the dermis.[76] In sun-exposed areas, there is often marked eosinophilic homogenization and thickening of vessels in the papillary dermis due to the accumulation of an amorphous, homogeneous, slightly basophilic (hyaline-like) substance in and around the vessel walls.[112] The perivascular deposits of concentric eosinophilic layers of hyaline-like material stain strongly positive with PAS and are diastase-positive (see Fig. 151-12). Histochemical studies suggest that this material may be a neutral glycoprotein with smaller amounts of acid mucopolysaccharide and lipids.[128] The histologic findings are similar to those of lipoid proteinosis (hyalinosis cutis et mucosae).[129] Electron microscopic studies in EPP show that the amorphous material consists of a multilayered, partially fragmented basement membrane and finely fibrillar material of moderate density that permeates and surrounds the vessel walls.[130] Other studies have shown that type IV collagen and laminin as well as amyloid P and fibronectin are deposited in the walls of dermal blood vessels.[131]

Differential Diagnosis

EPP must be differentiated from other causes of photosensitivity, primarily hydroa aestivale, polymorphous light eruption (PMLE), idiopathic solar urticaria, and other types of porphyria. Contact dermatitis and angioedema should also be considered. In PMLE, the lesions are characteristically papules, plaques, and papulovesicles. A family history of photosensitivity is less common. Burning and smarting of the skin during or soon after sun exposure is unusual in PMLE, whereas it is a common occurrence in EPP. Porphyrin profile and skin biopsy with PAS staining may also be helpful in differentiating between PMLE and EPP. Idiopathic solar urticaria can be easily differentiated from EPP; it is not associated with elevated levels of RBCs or fecal PROTO. Contact dermatitis may

TABLE 151-8

Fluorescence Characteristics of Porphyrin-Containing Plasma Diluted with 1:10 Phosphate Buffered Solution

TYPE	EXCITATION, NM	EMISSION, NM	FLUORESCENT PORPHYRINS
Erythropoietic porphyria (EP)	398	619	URO I, COPRO I
Erythropoietic protoporphyria (EPP)	409	634	PROTO
Porphyria cutanea tarda (PCT)	398	619	URO I, III, COPRO III
Variegate porphyria (VP)	405	626	COPRO III, PROTO
Acute intermittent porphyria (AIP)	398	619	URO III
Hereditary coproporphyria (HCP)	398	619	COPRO III
Hepatoerythropoietic porphyria (HEP)	398	619	URO I

SOURCE: Modified from Poh-Fitzpatrick.[247]

FIGURE 151-12

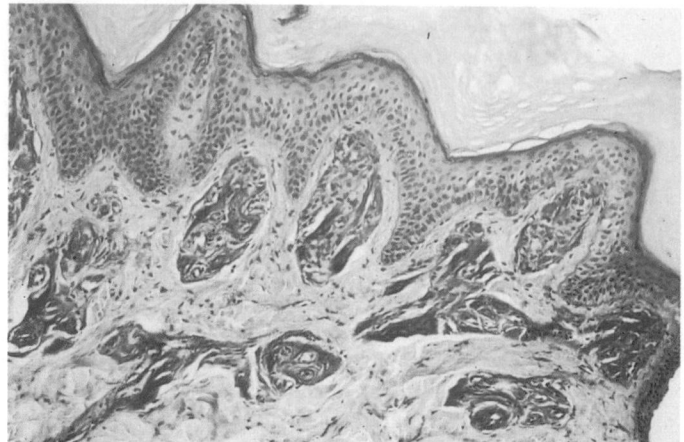

A.

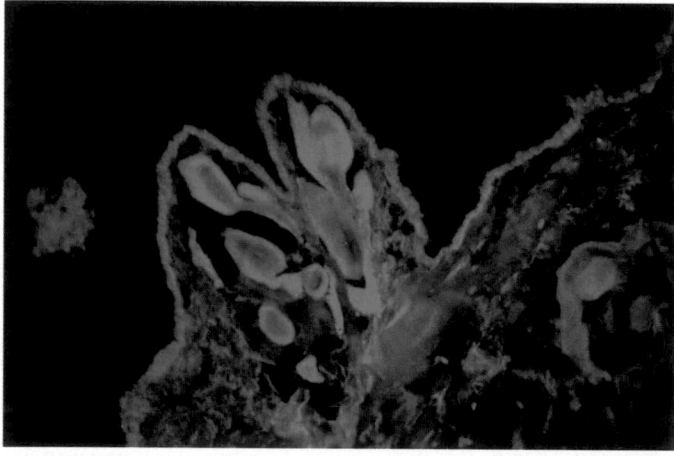

B.

C.

A. A biopsy of light-exposed skin from a patient with erythropoietic protoporphyria. There is marked thickening of the blood vessel walls of the upper dermis, which are surrounded by a hyaline-like material that stains brightly red with the PAS stain. B. Direct immunofluorescence reveals that the PAS-positive stain around papillary vessels contain immunoglobulins of classes. Immunoglobulins are also deposited along the dermo-epidermal junction. C. Electron micrograph of biopsy of chronically exposed skin from a patient with erythropoietic protoporphyria. Multiple concentric basal laminae surrounding dermal blood vessels and finely fibrillar material admixed with amorphous masses within perivascular tissue are shown.

involve non-light-exposed areas such as the skin folds and the submental areas. Patch testing with a suspected allergen and negative porphyrin values help to differentiate this condition. The lesions of angioedema may occur anywhere on the body, including the mucous membranes. Because discomfort is often disproportionate to visible lesions, EPP has been confused with psychoneurosis or even malingering. This problem in differential diagnosis is readily solved by porphyrin determinations. Erythropoietic coproporphyria (ECP), an extremely rare condition, should also be considered in the differential diagnosis.[19] Clinically, it resembles EPP and can only be diagnosed by chromatographic study of RBC porphyrins.

Treatment

The treatment of photosensitivity in EPP has been aided by the use of orally administered beta-carotene. Topical sunscreens, antimalarial drugs, cholestyramine, and vitamins E and C have all been suggested but have not been shown to be effective. As reported by Mathews-Roth et al.,[132] beta-carotene (60 to 180 mg per day by mouth) has been found helpful in preventing or minimizing the symptoms of skin photosensitivity reactions of EPP. Eighty-four percent of 133 patients claimed to triple their tolerance to sunlight after an adequate course of beta-carotene exceeding 2 months. The therapeutic effectiveness of the drug has been confirmed by several groups of investigators. These results are, however, based on limited controlled laboratory testing and uncontrolled clinical impressions; the one controlled trial failed to confirm the therapeutic effectiveness of beta-carotene.[133] To achieve optimal photoprotection, serum carotene levels should be maintained at a minimum of 600 μg/dL. In adult patients, this can usually be achieved by oral administration of 2 to 6 capsules of 30 mg each per day, which will produce serum carotene levels of 600 to 800 μg/dL after 4 to 6 weeks of therapy. Children under 12 years of age may receive 30 to 90 mg daily. Maximum effectiveness may not occur until 1 to 2 months after initiating therapy; hence patients should receive therapy in early spring through the fall season (February to October in the northern hemisphere). The drug is remarkably well tolerated at these doses, and there are no known toxic systemic effects of beta-carotene. Occasionally diarrhea occurs in a small number of patients. Orange or rusty discoloration of stools is common and is not an indication for discontinuing treatment. The only other side effect of note is the visible yellowing of the skin that occurs as a result of carotenoderma, and this is more noticeable on the palms and soles. Topical application of beta-carotene in cream form (1 to 5%) to light-exposed skin areas of EPP patients is totally ineffective; the photolability of carotenoid pigments results in rapid destruction of the applied beta-carotene (Pathak, unpublished observations).

The mechanism of the photoprotective effect of beta-carotene is not precisely known. Beta-carotene does not function as a sunscreen; it does, however, appear to be capable of quenching excited singlet oxygen and of trapping free radicals formed by the interaction of light with PROTO and molecular oxygen.

Uncontrolled studies have shown some clinical and biochemical improvement using the anionic-binding resin cholestyramine and the antioxidant vitamin E. Hematin infusions have been used to decrease the production of heme temporarily and are associated with a decrease in fecal and plasma PROTO in some patients.[114] The use of RBC exchange with autologous washed cells has also been explored for its ability to induce clinical and biochemical remission of EPP. Bechtel et al. showed that transfusion therapy in one patient with EPP resulted in a marked decrease in photosensitivity associated with a decline in free erythrocyte PROTO levels.[134] Management of the hepatic failure is particularly difficult. Orally administered bile salts have been used in an effort to diminish the enterohepatic circulation of the excessive PROTO[135] and to enhance the capacity of the liver to clear excess PROTO. Another approach was reported using large amounts of orally administered iron in a patient with EPP who manifested incipient hepatic failure as well as elevated erythrocyte and plasma PROTO levels and concomitant iron-deficiency anemia.[136] Oral iron therapy exacerbated the disease in another patient.[137] Liver transplantation has also been used successfully in some patients.[138] Future therapy could include replacement of defective ferrochelatase. Mathews-Roth et al. and Magness and Brenner have shown that it is possible to increase detectable levels of the enzyme in fibroblasts from EPP patients by adding the cDNA for normal ferrochelatase employing a retroviral vector.[139,140]

ERYTHROPOIETIC COPROPORPHYRIA

There are only three known cases of ECP that have been published. Heilmeyer and Clotten have described the disorder in some detail.[19] Elevated PROTO and COPRO were found in the RBCs of one patient. Topi et al.[141] described two brothers with cutaneous photosensitivity similar to that of EPP

but with elevated RBC PROTO and COPRO III in both. Very little is known about this disease.

PORPHYRIA CUTANEA TARDA (Table 151-9)

Synonyms for PCT include type I, symptomatic porphyria, acquired hepatic porphyria, and chemical porphyria.

Historic Aspects

PCT was originally classified by Günther as hematoporphyria chronica. He described it as a syndrome of skin lesions and darkly colored urine occurring later in life than either congenital or acute porphyria and without acute attacks of abdominal pain or neurologic dysfunction.[6] Waldenström[9,11] first named the disease PCT and observed that Swedish patients with acute attacks of porphyria (AIP) never developed cutaneous porphyria. He suggested that these two disorders were completely distinct, PCT being primarily acquired and AIP familial.

Following Waldenström's description of PCT in 1937, scattered case reports appeared in the literature. Early experience with this disorder in the United States was carefully described by Brunsting and his co-workers at the Mayo Clinic.[10,142] Later, patients with a comparable clinical picture were described in South Africa.[143] Finally, and even more confusing, it became clear that there were a small number of patients in the United States and a larger number in South Africa who manifested both the cutaneous changes of PCT as well as intermittent attacks of AIP. In South Africa, this was

TABLE 151-9

Porphyria Cutanea Tarda

Synonyms	Symptomatic porphyria, acquired hepatic porphyria, chemical porphyria
Inheritance	Mixed or variable autosomal dominant in approximately 20% of patients
Types	Acquired or type I; inherited (familial types II and III)
Age of onset	Usually in third or fourth decade; rare before puberty; prevalence: most common porphyria
Photosensitivity	Moderate to severe; bullae on dorsa of hands and feet
Skin reactions	Vesicular, bullous and ulcerative lesions, primarily on light-exposed skin; increased skin fragility to mechanical trauma; hyperpigmentation and sclerodermoid plaques; scarring alopecia, milia on fingers and hands, hypertrichosis, and periorbital violaceous suffusion; dystrophic calcification and photoonycholysis
Clinical findings	Diabetes mellitus in about 25% of patients; rare hepatic tumor; increased liver iron stores; increased serum iron; pink fluorescence in urine with Wood's lamp; unlike VP, acute attacks are absent in PCT
Biochemical defects	Excretory: Increased urinary URO (I > III) and 7-carboxyl porphyrins (III > I); increased COPRO in urine; increased ISOCOPRO in feces RBC: Normal porphyrins Plasma: Increased 8- and 7-carboxyl porphyrins Enzymatic: Deficiency of UROGEN decarboxylase in liver (type I) and RBCs (type II) and their families
Differential diagnosis	Pseudo PCT, VP, epidermolysis bullosa acquisita
Treatment or management	Stop ethanol or estrogens and other precipitating chemicals or drugs; phlebotomy (500 mL weekly or biweekly) until Hb is 10–11 g/dL and serum Fe is reduced to 50–60 µg/dL Alternative therapy: chloroquine 125 mg twice weekly

called VP, whereas initially in the United States it was known as mixed porphyria.[144] There is now agreement on the use of the term *VP* to describe this disorder throughout the world.[16,17]

Etiology

PCT is due to either an inherited or acquired UROGEN decarboxylase deficiency of the fifth enzyme in the heme pathway.[42] It is encoded by a single gene on the short arm of chromosome 1 and contains 10 exons spread over 3 kb.

Most classifications of PCT separate the disorder into at least two broad categories, both associated with decreased UROGEN decarboxylase activity: (1) PCT-symptomatic, or sporadic (also referred to as acquired or type I), and (2) PCT-hereditary, or type II. In symptomatic (sporadic) PCT, the enzyme is deficient only in the liver, which could be explained either by a different gene defect restricted to the liver or by exposure to chemicals that selectively inhibit the hepatic but not the RBC enzyme[145] (Table 151-10). Some of these substances (e.g., alcohol and estrogen) may provoke porphyria only in selected individuals, and others [e.g., hexachlorobenzene (HCB)] in practically all exposed individuals.

In hereditary (type II) PCT, UROGEN decarboxylase is decreased approximately 50 percent in all tissues, including RBCs and cultured skin fibroblasts.[43,44,146] The defect is inherited in an autosomal dominant fashion. Decreased enzyme concentration appears to follow a bimodal distribution, suggesting two overlapping groups of patients: a large group (>80 percent) with normal UROGEN decarboxylase concentration, and a small group (<20 percent) in whom the amount of detectable enzyme is about half normal. Some patients with type II PCT were found to have UROGEN decarboxylase activity at the lower end of the normal range. Penetrance of type II PCT is relatively low, so that the majority of individuals with the inherited enzyme defect do not manifest the disease.

On the other hand, it is important to emphasize that not every patient with a positive family history of PCT will have type II disease. Roberts et al.[147] showed that several patients with one or more relatives with clear-cut PCT had normal UROGEN decarboxylase concentrations and yet were clinically and biochemically indistinguishable from individuals with type I PCT. These patients could have inherited some form of UROGEN decarboxylase that is immunochemically indistinguishable from the normal enzyme but that is uniquely susceptible to inhibition in the liver, or they may have a second inherited enzyme deficiency unrelated to UROGEN decarboxylase. These possibilities require further investigation. This latter category of PCT has been designated as type III by some investigators.[148]

It is also unclear from some of the early studies whether patients who were reported as having hereditary PCT actually had VP, an autosomal dominant disorder. Studies by Watson et al. in the United States,[149] Day et al. in South Africa,[150] and Sieg et al.[151] in Europe have shown that PCT and VP may occur in different members of the same family, so-called dual porphyria. Another form of dual porphyria in which PCT and AIP coexist has been described.[152]

The most frequently incriminated agents that contribute to the development of PCT (type I, acquired, or sporadic) are alcohol, estrogens, iron, polychlorinated hydrocarbons, HCB, and hemodialysis in patients with renal failure. Some of these precipitating factors are discussed briefly below.

ALCOHOL   Heavy alcohol intake has long been recognized to exacerbate PCT. Ethanol has been shown to induce hepatic ALA synthase in patients with PCT.[153] Erythrocyte UROGEN decarboxylase activity is diminished in healthy subjects following acute ethanol ingestion and in chronic alcoholics.[154] Ethanol can also inhibit the activity of other enzymes in the heme pathway, including ferrochelatase and ALA dehydratase. Chronic alcoholism leads to suppression of erythropoiesis[155] and increased absorption of dietary iron, although whether the increased iron absorption of alcoholism contributes to the pathogenesis of the disease and to the characteristic hepatic siderosis of PCT is unknown. The fact that ALA synthase is increased in cirrhotic liver of individuals without porphyria raises questions concerning the relevance of alcohol effects on ALA synthase in the clinical expression of PCT.[156]

ESTROGENS   The widespread use of estrogens as contraceptive agents or as hormone supplements for postmenopausal replacement therapy in females and as adjunctive hormonal therapy in males with prostatic carcinoma has been associated with PCT.[157] The mechanism of the estrogen effect on the expression of PCT is not established. Diethylstilbesterol, an estrogen, induces hepatic ALA synthase,[158] but this would not explain the distinctive porphyrin excretion pattern found in PCT. The vast majority of patients receiving estrogens do not manifest the biochemical abnormalities associated with PCT.

HEXACHLOROBENZENE   This fungicide caused an "epidemic" of a PCT-like syndrome in southeastern Turkey in the 1950s.[159] It was added as a preservative to wheat intended for planting but, because of a famine, several thousand individuals of diverse ethnic origin, mostly children, ingested the seed wheat and subsequently developed typical PCT. Over 4000 cases of this syndrome were reported from 1956 to 1961. The porphyrin excretion pattern and the cutaneous findings in these patients were similar to those seen in PCT evoked by ethanol or estrogens. The outbreak of PCT in Turkey caused by ingestion of HCB indicated that the disease can be acquired in nongenetically predisposed individuals.

Twenty-five years after onset, the most common clinical findings in these HCB-poisoned individuals were those of chronic porphyria, including sclerodermoid scarring (84 percent), hyperpigmentation (78 percent), hirsutism (49 percent), thyromegaly, and increased skin fragility (38 percent).[160] A painless arthritis was seen in two out of three affected individuals, and a variety of neurologic signs and symptoms were seen in the majority. Stool and urine porphyrins remained elevated in many patients.

Studies have shown that the chronic administration of HCB to experimental animals produces excessive porphyrin accumulation in the liver in a pattern quite similar to that seen in PCT in humans.[161] These data are consistent with the hypothesis that chlorinated hydrocarbons, such as HCB, or their metabolites inhibit hepatic UROGEN decarboxylase, leading to excessive hepatic storage of URO and other acetate-substituted porphyrins.[162,163] Experimental studies have also shown that HCB can inactivate UROGEN decarboxylase by abolishing catalytic activity without changing the amount of im-

TABLE 151-10

Drugs and Chemicals Associated with the Clinical Expression of Porphyria Cutanea Tarda

Ethyl alcohol	Tetrachlorodibenzo-[*p*]-dioxin
Estrogenic hormones	Polychlorinated biphenyls (PCB)
Hexachlorobenzene	Herbicides 2,4-dichloro- and
Chlorinated phenols	trichlorophenoxyacetic acid
Iron	

munoreactive enzyme protein.[164] Additional studies on the porphyrinogenic effects of HCB, dioxin, and polychlorinated biphenyls suggest that metabolic activation of the compounds mediated by cytochrome P_{450} is associated with a decrease in UROGEN decarboxylase activity.[162,163] Chemical porphyria, similar to PCT, is caused by other chlorinated hydrocarbons such as the polychlorinated biphenyls and 2,3,7,8-tetrachlorodibenzo-*p*-dioxin (TCDD), a by-product in the synthesis of the herbicide 2,4,5-trichlorophenoxyacetic acid.[165]

TETRACHLORODIBENZO-*p*-DIOXIN   TCDD is a toxic environmental pollutant chemical. Among its numerous effects are chloracne, liver damage, and hepatic porphyria in experimental animals and perhaps also in humans.[166] It has been shown that the hepatic porphyrinogenic effect of TCDD can be abolished in mice by first depleting them of iron.[167] Furthermore, it is known that highly inbred mouse strains vary in their susceptibility to induction of hepatic porphyria by TCDD, indicating that the porphyrinogenic effect of this hydrocarbon is modulated by as yet undefined genetic factors.[168]

IRON   Serum iron and ferritin concentrations are elevated or in the upper range of normal in PCT, suggesting a possible role of iron in the pathogenesis of the disease.[169] Hepatic iron overload accompanies clinical PCT in practically all cases, and elevation of plasma iron is found in one-third to one-half of patients.[157] In PCT, the quantity of iron that can be mobilized by phlebotomy indicates that total iron stores are approximately twice normal. Ferrokinetic studies in patients with PCT are said to be normal. The long remissions that follow repeated phlebotomy and the apparent ineffectiveness of this treatment if supplemental iron is administered concomitantly suggest that iron plays a role in the excessive hepatic porphyrin production of PCT. PCT is particularly common where alcoholism and iron overload occur together.

The role of iron in the pathogenesis of PCT is undoubtedly a complex one, and several hypotheses have been proposed to explain it. Some believe that iron is capable of directly inhibiting UROGEN decarboxylase.[169] However, studies with purified UROGEN decarboxylase prepared from human erythrocytes have shown that the purified enzyme is not inhibited by Fe^{2+} or Fe^{3+}.[170] Chronic iron overload can produce peroxidative damage to lipid-rich mitochondrial and microsomal membranes in the liver of experimental animals, but the relationship of this toxic effect to changes in hepatic heme synthesis has not been clearly defined.[171] An increased frequency of the hemachromatosis CYS 282 → TYR mutation has been found in British patients with sporadic PCT.[172,173]

Iron may have a permissive effect on the inhibition by chlorinated phenols of UROGEN decarboxylase,[167,168] and it can also enhance the induction response of hepatic ALA synthase to drugs.[174] Although such an iron-augmented increase in ALA synthase activity could lead to enhanced porphyrinogenesis, this alone would not explain the porphyrin excretion pattern seen in PCT. Kushner et al. have shown that addition of ferrous iron to liver in vitro causes a marked increase in porphyrin synthesis and inhibits UROGEN III synthase activity.[175] This latter effect would explain the URO isomer I excess characteristic of PCT. From these known effects of alcohol, estrogens, chlorinated hydrocarbons, and iron on the heme pathway, it is clear that each of these could contribute to the excessive hepatic porphyrinogenesis characteristic of PCT. How the putative effects of alcohol, estrogens, and iron contribute to the hepatic UROGEN decarboxylase activity and associated porphyrin metabolism remains unclear. The clinical expression of PCT is therefore dependent upon the interaction of a number of factors, both genetic and environmental. However, it is important to note

that the ingestion of drugs usually associated with inducing attacks of the acute hepatic porphyrias (see Table 151-11) has not been reported to exacerbate PCT.

Genetics

UROGEN decarboxylase is the fifth enzyme in the heme pathway, and the cDNA and gene for the human enzyme have been isolated and sequenced. The human enzyme is a single polypeptide of 367 amino acids with a molecular mass of about 40.8 kDa. In one family with PCT, a specific mutation resulting in UROGEN decarboxylase deficiency was shown to be a glycine → valine substitution at amino acid 281.[176] This resulted in a marked decrease in the half-life of the enzyme from more than 100 h to around 4 h. The same mutation could not be identified in several other families, suggesting that there is genetic heterogeneity in PCT. In another study it was shown that PCT can occur in heterozygotes for the G281E mutation.[46]

Epidemiology

PCT occurs throughout the world,[177] and it is the most common of all the porphyrias. The disease most often begins in middle-aged individuals but can develop earlier. Prior to the widespread use of

TABLE 151-11

Examples of Drugs Potentially Hazardous in Patients with the Acute Hepatic Porphyrias

Amidopyrine	Hydralazine
Aminoglutethimide	Isopropylmeprobamate
Aminopyrine	Mephenytoin
Amphetamines	Meprobamate
Antipyrine	Methyldopa
Barbiturates	Methylprylon
Bemegride	*N*-butylscopolammonium bromide
Carbamazepine	Nalidixic acid
Carbromal	Nikethamide
Chloromethazone	Nitrazepam
Chloropropamide	Nortriptyline
Chloroquine	Novobiocin
Danazol	Pargyline
Dapsone	Pentazocine
Diclophenac	Pentylenetetrazole
Diethylpropione	Phenoxybenzamine
Diphenylhydantoin	Phenylbutazone
Dramamine	Primadone
Enflurane	Pyrazinamide
Ergot preparation	Rifampin
Erythromycin	Sedormid
Ethclorvynol	Succinimides
Ethinamate	Sulfonamides
Ethosuximide	Sulfonethylmethane
Ethyl alcohol	Sulfonylureas
Fentanyl	Synthetic estrogens, progestins
Furosemide	Theophylline
Furoxene	Tolazamide
Glutethimide	Tolbutamide
Griseofulvin	Trimethadione
Halothane	Valproic acid
Heavy metals	

FIGURE 151-13

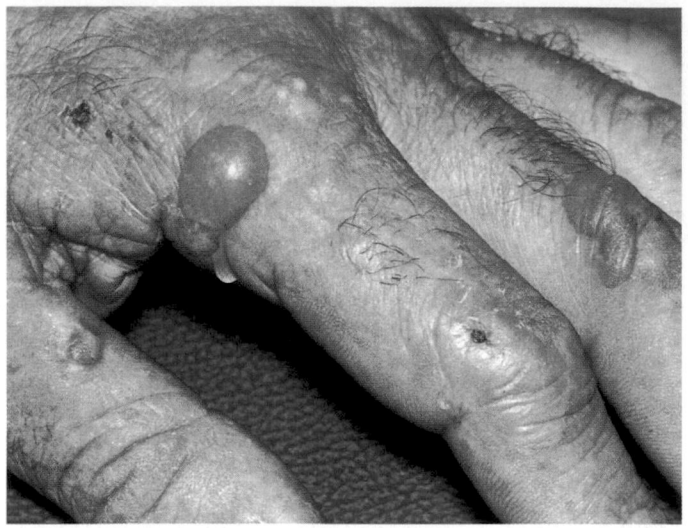

A case of porphyria cutanea tarda showing bullae filled with clear fluid. Elsewhere are remnants of blisters, and on the second metacarpophalangeal joint are small milia.

oral contraceptives, PCT developed predominantly in males. Brunsting's experience at the Mayo Clinic clearly illustrates this point because of 34 patients, 26 were male and more than 90 percent consumed moderate to heavy amounts of alcohol.[10]

In contrast, the experience of Grossman et al. indicates that the sex incidence is approximately equal[157]; in this series, 21 patients were male and 19 were female. The rising incidence of PCT in females is probably due to the widespread ingestion of estrogens in oral contraceptives or in hormone supplements.[178] It should be noted that males treated with estrogens, for example, as adjunctive therapy for carcinoma of the prostate, have also developed PCT.

FIGURE 151-14

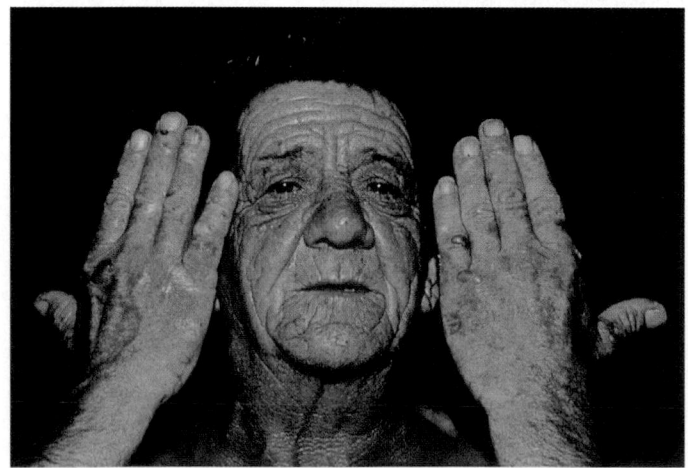

Periorbital and malar violaceous coloration, hyperpigmentation, and hypertrichosis. Bulla, crusts, and scars are seen on the dorsa of the hands.

Clinical Manifestations

Vesicles and bullae occur predominantly in areas subject to repeated trauma (Figs. 151-13, 151-14, and 151-15). There is increased skin fragility, usually on the dorsa of the hands but occasionally on the feet as well. The traumatized skin becomes crusted and, as the lesions resolve, areas of scarring may ensue. Numerous small milia can develop, particularly on the fingers and hands. These are pearly white to yellow, spherical subepidermal inclusions 1 to 5 mm in diameter, and characteristically they are present in each of the hepatic porphyrias with cutaneous photosensitivity (PCT and VP) (Figs. 151-14, 151-15). Although the cutaneous lesions are primarily seen on the light-exposed areas, patients are often unaware that sunlight plays a role in producing their lesions because the acute photosensitivity, so characteristic of the erythropoietic porphyrias, is rare in PCT (Fig. 151-16). However, most patients do recognize that their skin condition worsens in the spring and summer and seems to improve in the fall and winter. Porphyrin excretion in PCT appears to increase in summer months and decrease in winter months.[179] It remains unknown whether increased duration of sun exposure and photocatalyzed oxidation of porphyrin precursors account for this seasonal variation in porphyrin excretion and clinical expression of the disease.

Other skin changes seen in PCT include hyperpigmentation and hypopigmentation that may be mottled, resembling chloasma (Fig. 151-17). There may be an associated purplish-red ("heliotrope") suffusion of the central part of the face, particularly involving the periorbital areas, which may bear a striking resemblance to the plethora seen in polycythemia rubra vera (see Fig. 151-17). This is not seen in the porphyrias of bone marrow origin.

Hypertrichosis (nonvirilizing) is a useful diagnostic sign that often brings the female patient to the dermatologist (Fig. 151-18). Facial hypertrichosis develops gradually and is more apparent in females. The hair may vary in texture between fine and coarse and in color between light and dark. These hairs are particularly prominent along the temples and the cheeks but may occasionally involve

FIGURE 151-15

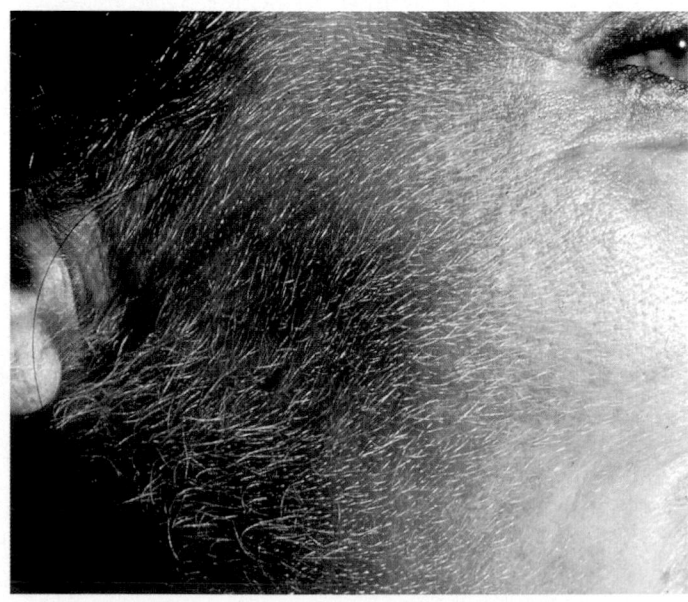

Hypertrichosis in a female with PCT; mostly pronounced on the zygomatic and malar skin.

FIGURE 151-16

CHAPTER 151
The Porphyrias

1787

FIGURE 151-17

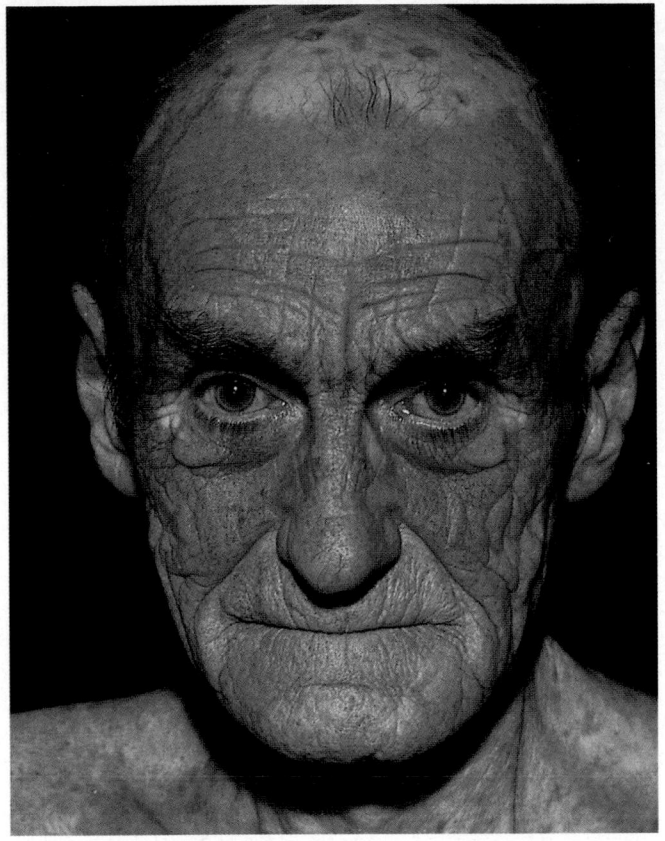

Porphyria cutanea tarda. Purple-red suffusion ("heliotrope") of central facial skin is most pronounced in the periorbital and frontal areas.

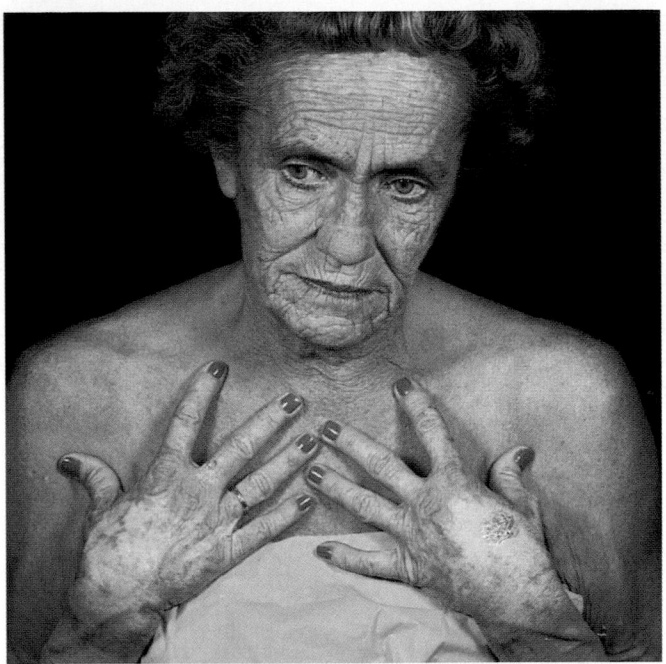

A.

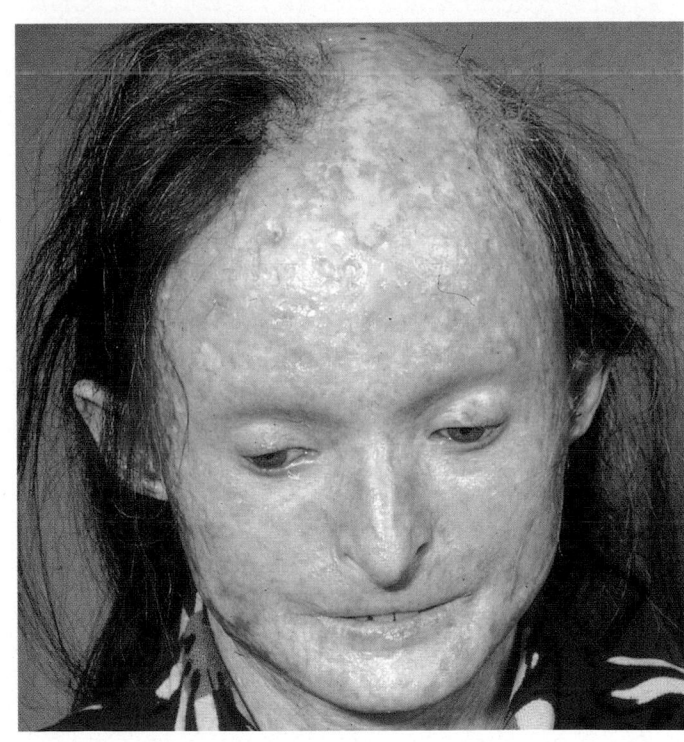

B.

A. Porphyria cutanea tarda. The patient exhibits marked photoaging changes on the face and depigmented scars on the dorsa of the hands. *B.* Sclerodermoid thickening, shrinkage of facial and scalp skin with ulcerations and scars in a patient with hepatoerythropoietic porphyria where these sclerodermoid changes are particularly pronounced.

the trunk and extremities in severe cases. Such hair may continue to grow, darken, and thicken, particularly on the cheeks, the forehead between the eyes, and at the hairline of the scalp. Males may complain that shaving is more difficult and that the growth pattern of their beard has changed. Hypertrichosis may be the presenting symptom in women, and a particularly severe form of hypertrichosis may occur in younger children with PCT. In the reports of HCB poisoning in Turkey, some of the children were described as "monkey-like" because of marked hypertrichosis.[180] The mechanism of this phenomenon is unknown; androgen levels are reported to be normal. It is possible that surface receptors or growth factors for hair bulb keratinocytes are activated by the dual action of light and porphyrins. The hypertrichosis of PCT usually improves slowly following appropriate treatment with phlebotomies.

Sclerodermoid plaques (Fig. 151-18) may develop on both light-exposed and light-protected body areas. These are usually scattered, waxy yellow to white, indurated plaques that closely resemble, both clinically and histopathologically, morphea or scleroderma. There is some evidence to indicate that PCT may occur concomitantly with true scleroderma, but this seems to be quite rare. As discussed earlier, URO I stimulates collagen synthesis in human skin fibroblasts.[82] In some patients, calcification has developed in these sclerodermoid plaques, necessitating excision and grafting.

PCT-like syndromes are occasionally seen in association with other conditions, including hepatic tumors,[181] hepatitis,[182] and lupus erythematosus.[183] Subepidermal bullous dermatoses mimicking PCT clinically and histologically have been described (see "Pseu-

FIGURE 151-18

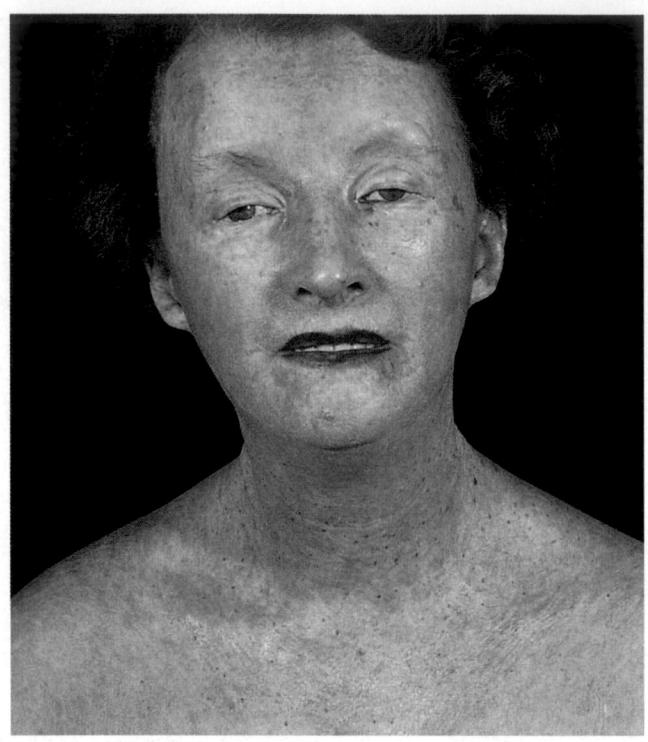

Porphyria cutanea tarda. Shiny, sclerodermoid plaques on the chest.

doporphyria," below). A number of cases have occurred in patients with renal failure undergoing hemodialysis.[184]

PCT and Human Immunodeficiency Virus/AIDS

In 1987, the first reported association between PCT and HIV was described in which three men with cutaneous symptoms and biochemical signs of PCT developed AIDS.[185] Since then, additional HIV-infected patients have been reported with PCT.[186] In many patients the signs and symptoms of PCT preceded the diagnosis of HIV infection, whereas in others they followed the diagnosis. The risk factors for HIV infection include homosexuality, transfusion, and intravenous drug abuse. Although the pathophysiology of this association is not understood, it has been suggested that the virus may lead to impairment of hepatic function, in combination with ongoing infection with the hepatitis C virus. In one study of patients with concomitant HIV infection and PCT, the vast majority were also seropositive for the hepatitis C virus, suggesting some joint role in the development of PCT.[187]

PCT and Hepatitis C

Several reports based predominantly on retrospective studies have shown a high prevalence (71 to 91 percent) of hepatitis C infection in PCT patients from Southern Europe, whereas a low prevalence was found in Germany and Ireland.[188] Although a strong link between the two diseases has been established, the mechanism of interaction between the virus and PCT is unknown.

Pseudoporphyria (Bullous Photosensitivity)

This term is used to describe patients who clinically exhibit cutaneous manifestations of PCT without the characteristic abnormal porphyrin profile. This disorder may develop in association with ingestion of certain drugs such as furosemide,[189] nalidixic acid,[190] tetracycline,[191] naproxen,[192] pyridoxine,[193] and isotretinoin.[194] In the drug-induced type of pseudoporphyria, the blistering process is subepidermal, with little or no dermal inflammation. Staining with PAS reveals little or no deposition around upper dermal blood vessels and capillary walls. Indirect immunofluorescence studies conducted on split skin reveal no dermal deposition of fluorescent material in pseudoporphyria.[192] Direct immunofluorescence studies have shown patchy granular deposition of IgG and C3 at the basement membrane zone in pseudoporphyria, PCT, and in epidermolysis bullosa acquisita.

In unpublished observations involving a severe cases of pseudoporphyria, homogeneous diffuse staining to all classes of immunoglobulins and albumin was also observed in the membrane propria of eccrine ducts, the perineurium, and around deeper vessels. Whether this is characteristic for pseudoporphyria or can be observed in PCT remains to be established.

A bullous dermatosis that is morphologically and histologically indistinguishable from PCT has also been observed in patients with chronic renal failure receiving maintenance hemodialysis.[195] Initially, porphyrin levels in urine, stool, and plasma were found to be in the normal range. Although it was believed that no porphyrin abnormalities occurred in these patients, subsequent studies revealed that true PCT with excess porphyrins can develop in some dialyzed patients.[184] Confirmation of the diagnosis rests on detection of elevated ISOCOPRO in the feces. An additional subset of patients undergoing long-term hemodialysis may exhibit increased plasma porphyrin levels, even though there is no clinical evidence of porphyria. This appears to be related to binding of porphyrins to nondialyzable plasma proteins.

Laboratory Findings

Virtually all patients with PCT have excessive total-body iron stores manifested as increased serum iron, ferritin, and/or hepatocellular iron. Occasionally, there is mild erythrocytosis. An abnormal glucose tolerance test occurs in 25 percent of patients.

Patients with PCT excrete increased amounts of porphyrins in the urine, which rarely may exhibit characteristic pink-red fluorescence when examined with a Wood's lamp. The porphyrin excretion pattern of PCT (see Table 151-9) has three main features: (1) increased urinary excretion of URO and of other acetate-substituted porphyrins, (2) a distinctive pattern of excretion of isomer series I and III porphyrins, and (3) increased excretion of fecal ISOCOPRO.[196,197] PCT patients excrete greatly increased amounts of urinary 8-carboxyl URO and also porphyrins with 7-, 6-, and 5-carboxyl groups; 4-carboxyl porphyrin (COPRO) is also increased, but to a lesser extent than URO, and rarely surpasses 600 μg per 24 h (see Table 151-3). In PCT, the hepatic UROGEN decarboxylase deficiency results in the accumulation of 5-carboxyl porphyrinogen III (see Figs. 151-1 and 151-2). This can be utilized as a substrate by the enzyme COPROGEN oxidase and it forms dehydroisocoproporphyrinogen, which in turn is oxidized to ISOCOPRO, resulting in the characteristic elevation of this compound in the feces of these patients.

The 8-carboxyl URO and 7-carboxyl porphyrins are the predominant urinary porphyrins in PCT (>90 percent of total porphyrins). The urinary porphyrin excretion pattern is a mixture of type I and type III isomers. URO is about 60 percent type I isomer and 40 percent type III; the 7- and 6-carboxyl porphyrins are >90 percent type III and <10 percent type I isomer; the 5- and 4-carboxyl porphyrins are about 50 percent each isomer. This distinctive isomer pattern is found consistently in patients with PCT.[197]

In general, only trace amounts of URO are present in the stools of normal individuals. The porphyrin content of stool is increased in PCT and consists primarily of ISOCOPRO (type III), 7-carboxyl porphyrin, and lesser amounts of URO and COPRO. The total daily 24-h fecal porphyrin excretion may exceed total urinary porphyrin excretion.

The ratio of URO to COPRO in the urine is often helpful in differentiating PCT and VP. Thus, in PCT, the URO:COPRO ratio is usually >3:1, whereas in VP the ratio is usually <1:1. Occasionally, 24-h urine porphyrins will be normal or only slightly increased in a patient with the cutaneous findings of PCT. This should alert the physician to evaluate stool porphyrins, as these are elevated in patients with VP (see "Variegate Porphyria," below).

The constellation of clinical and laboratory findings, including examination of the urine with a readily available Wood's lamp, often suffices to make the tentative diagnosis of PCT. Suspected PCT can frequently be confirmed by acidifying a random urine sample with a few drops of 10% hydrochloric acid or acetic acid and looking for orange-red fluorescence. The sensitivity of the screening test can be enhanced by addition of a small amount of talcum powder to a 5-mL sample of urine, shaking, centrifuging, and examining the talc pellet for fluorescence. If in doubt, this test can be modified as follows[198]: To 5 mL of urine (freshly voided or 24-h specimen), add 5 to 10 drops (0.5 mL) glacial acetic acid and 2.5 mL ethyl acetate. Shake and allow to settle. Examine the upper aqueous layer with a Wood's lamp for characteristic red-pink porphyrin fluorescence.

It should be emphasized that patients who appear clinically to have PCT may have a negative urine fluorescent screening test for porphyrins. In such patients, it is absolutely essential to perform quantitative 24-h urine URO and COPRO determinations and stool PROTO and COPRO determinations, which often permit differentiation of PCT from VP. However, some patients with VP will have normal fecal porphyrin excretion, and recent studies indicate that bile porphyrin measurements may be helpful in evaluating such patients.[199] Plasma porphyrin fluorescence testing is also useful.

Biochemical tests for liver function may be performed to identify liver disease. Elevated serum transaminases and γ-glutamyltranspeptidase levels may occur. Serum iron and ferritin concentrations may be elevated. The measurement of erythrocyte UROGEN decarboxylase is useful for detection of mutant-gene carriers in pedigrees having a proband with familial PCT.[200]

Histopathology

The characteristic histopathologic finding in PCT is a subepidermal bulla (Figs. 151-19 and 151-20). Bullae characteristically show a corrugated, undulating base that has been termed *festooned*.[201] There is little or no inflammatory infiltrate. PAS stain reveals a mild degree of thickening of the papillary vessel wall, not nearly so marked as that seen in patients with EPP. Reticulin staining demonstrates slight proliferation of fibers along the basement membrane. Direct immunofluorescence studies reveal deposition of C3 and IgG in a granular pattern at the dermal-epidermal junction and in and around vessel walls in affected individuals.[86] These changes are most apparent in sun-exposed areas of patients with active disease and high urinary porphyrin excretion, and they decrease sub-

FIGURE 151-19

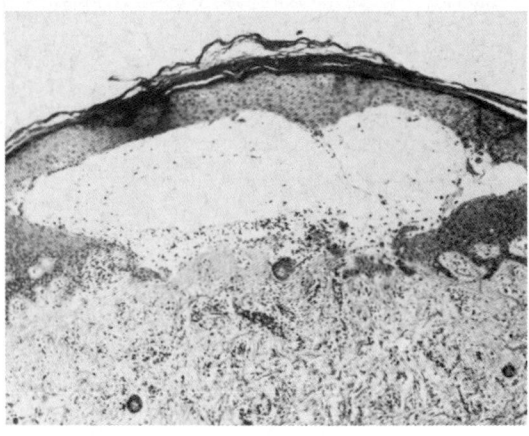

Porphyria cutanea tarda: subepidermal vesiculation in lesion. The subepidermal vesiculation of porphyria usually occurs with only a sparse, inflammatory cell infiltrate. (*Courtesy WH Clark, Jr, MD, University of Pennsylvania.*)

stantially in patients after appropriate treatment. It is also possible that the deposition of immunoglobulins and complement is a non-specific result of injury to the cutaneous tissue. The locus of damage to the upper dermal vessels and the dermal-epidermal junction suggests that damage to these areas evoked by porphyrin photosensitivity may be responsible for the unique skin fragility seen in PCT. Several studies have shown increased porphyrin concentrations in the skin of patients with PCT.[202,203] With rare exception, blisters have not been induced by phototesting; however, Rimington et al.,[204] using a monochromator, have been able to produce both erythema and delayed edema in the skin of patients with PCT.

FIGURE 151-20

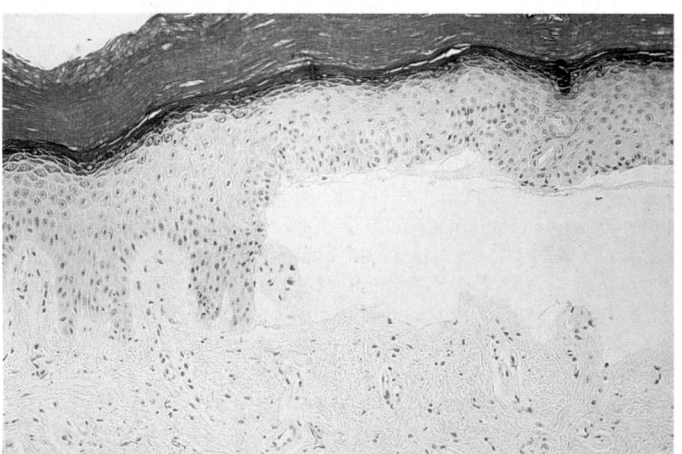

Porphyria cutanea tarda: subepidermal blistering in a late lesion. There is virtually no inflammatory response, but the form of the dermal papillae is partially preserved.

Differential Diagnosis

Other dermatoses that can be confused with PCT include VP, HEP, HCP, pseudoporphyria, scleroderma, and the acquired type of epidermolysis bullosa. Each of these can be differentiated on histopathologic grounds, by immunofluorescence tests, or by appropriate porphyrin studies. Careful evaluation of urine, stool, plasma, or bile porphyrins will almost always permit confirmation of the diagnosis of PCT. It should be emphasized that patients with PCT are not prone to the acute life-threatening attacks characteristic of the acute hepatic porphyrias. A very limited number of drugs and chemicals, particularly alcohol, estrogens, and selected halogenated hydrocarbons, seem capable of eliciting the disease in susceptible individuals (see Table 151-11). Drugs such as barbiturates, which are contraindicated in AIP, have been administered to PCT patients without untoward effect. Nonsteroidal anti-inflammatory drugs such as naproxen, antibiotics such as the tetracyclines and nalidixic acid, and a variety of other agents may rarely produce clinical signs of a bullous photosensitivity closely resembling PCT (see "Pseudoporphyria," above). VP has skin lesions identical to PCT. However, in VP, stool PROTO and COPRO excretion is usually increased (PROTO > COPRO), and urinary porphyrin levels are only moderately increased (COPRO > URO).[199,200] In PCT, stool ISOCOPRO is elevated, and total urinary porphyrin (URO > COPRO) is much higher than that observed in VP.

Treatment

Initially, a careful history should be taken in an effort to identify an environmental toxin, e.g., alcohol, estrogen, or chlorinated hydrocarbon, that may have triggered the disease. These should be strictly avoided if possible; often this alone can lead to gradual improvement. However, in most patients with PCT, more aggressive treatment is usually appropriate to accelerate the rate of clinical and biochemical improvement, and this currently consists of either repeated phlebotomy[205,206] or orally administered antimalarials, either chloroquine or hydroxychloroquine,[207,208] or a combination of both.[209] Other forms of treatment that have been described include administration of iron chelators,[210,211] oral administration of cholestyramine,[212] and the combination of genetically engineered erythropoietin combined with phlebotomy in patients with concomitant anemia secondary to chronic renal failure.[213]

PHLEBOTOMY   Phlebotomy is the treatment of choice for PCT. Numerous reports have emphasized the safety and efficacy of this form of therapy,[205,214] which was introduced by Ippen in 1961. Phlebotomy is effective because it depletes the excessive hepatic iron stores characteristic of PCT. Biochemical remission of PCT has occurred in patients treated with phlebotomy who had iron overload as well as in patients with quantitatively normal iron stores. Replenishment of iron following phlebotomy-induced remission of PCT may result in biochemical and clinical exacerbation of the disease.[169] Abstinence from the porphyrinogenic agent alone, especially alcohol, may induce a clinical and biochemical remission, although this may take months to years.

There are several interesting hypotheses concerning the mechanism whereby phlebotomy-induced depletion of excess iron leads to improvement in PCT, and these include the following:

1. *Iron effect on ALA synthase.* Iron can enhance the induction response of ALA synthase to drugs and the hepatic porphyrin-

ogenic response to HCB in experimental animals, and its depletion could render ALA synthase less inducible and thereby diminish hepatic porphyrinogenesis.

2. *Iron depletion effects on other heme pathway enzymes.* The studies of Kushner et al.,[169,175] showing that ferrous iron inhibits UROGEN decarboxylase and increases the rate of hepatic porphyrin synthesis from ALA or PBG, suggest that removal of iron can allow UROGEN decarboxylase activity to return to normal and/or reduce excessive porphyrinogenesis.

3. *Iron effects on hepatic lipid peroxidation.* Iron depletion could reverse this response of the liver to iron overload.[171]

4. *Iron effects on oxidation of URO.* Removal of iron could result in a diminished capacity of the ferrous metal to irreversibly oxidize the UROGEN substrate to nonmetabolizable porphyrins.[215]

Phlebotomy is a simple ambulatory procedure. The total amount of blood removed has varied widely, usually ranging from 1500 to 12,000 mL. It is most convenient to use plastic blood-drawing bags available in any blood bank. Approximately 500 mL of blood is removed at weekly or biweekly intervals until the hemoglobin decreases to approximately 10 g/dL or until the serum iron drops to 50 to 60 μg/dL. Patients are strongly encouraged to discontinue or decrease exposure to porphyrinogenic agents as this usually hastens clinical and biochemical remission.

It is particularly important to reassure the patient that clinical improvement may not become apparent for variable intervals after beginning the phlebotomies. Porphyrin excretion continues to fall long after phlebotomies are discontinued. Ramsay et al.[214] have shown that in more than 90 percent of patients treated with regular phlebotomy, urinary URO excretion reached normal levels (<100 μg per 24 h) after 5 to 12 months. Blistering is the first sign to disappear, followed by improvement in skin fragility and in hypertrichosis over a period of 3 to 18 months. Even sclerodermoid changes can resolve slowly, although this may take several years. There is little or no published information on long-term follow-up of treatment, but most relapsed patients have again responded to repeated courses of phlebotomies.[206] The length of remission induced by phlebotomy varies widely and ranges from 6 months to more than 10 years. At least 10 to 20 percent of patients will relapse within 1 year.

Phlebotomy is a safe, effective, and relatively simple form of therapy with minimum associated morbidity. A few patients may complain of mild to moderate fatigue and weakness during the treatment period, but this usually resolves as the hemoglobin returns to normal. Phlebotomy remains the treatment of choice for uncomplicated PCT.

ANTIMALARIALS   In some patients, phlebotomy is not recommended or is contraindicated owing to the presence of anemia or cardiopulmonary disorders or HIV infection. In such cases, low-dose antimalarial therapy may be useful. The antimalarial aminoquinolines, chloroquine (Aralen) and hydroxychloroquine (Plaquenil), have been recommended for treating PCT.[207,208] In 1957, London[216] first suggested that chloroquine was useful in treating PCT. The cutaneous signs of the disease cleared within 1 year in one patient who received 500 mg daily for several months. However, such doses will trigger severe hepatotoxicity in many PCT patients, and this is no longer an acceptable approach. Experience with low doses has proven that such a toxic response is not necessary for therapeutic benefit.[208,209] The clinical and biochemical remission of PCT obtained with chloroquine appears to be identical in all respects to that evoked by phlebotomy. However, it has been reported that rapid relapse occurred in several patients treated with hydroxychloroquine.[217] There is a marked increase in urinary URO excretion in patients receiving higher doses of the antimalarial. The effect of chloroquine seems to be due to rapid removal of a drug-porphyrin complex from the liver.[218] Taljaard et al.,[219] however, feel that chloroquine chelates iron in the hepatocyte and that the bound iron is then excreted.

Low-dose (125 mg twice weekly) chloroquine therapy has been shown to be effective in PCT. The concept of using low-dose chloroquine therapy to reduce the severity of the hepatotoxic effect in PCT was first suggested by Saltzer et al.[220] Remission of the disease was obtained in a single patient who received 50 mg of chloroquine twice weekly for 7 months. Taljaard et al.[219] extended these studies and reported good results in seven of eight PCT patients treated with chloroquine sulfate (330 mg base) twice weekly for several months. Kordac et al.[208] have reported the successful use of low-dose chloroquine (125 mg twice weekly for 8 to 18 months) in more than 100 patients with PCT. Complete clinical and biochemical remission occurred in all patients. Furthermore, the majority of these patients remained in remission for at least 4 years.

The authors suggest the following regimen for chloroquine administration in PCT. After obtaining baseline urinary porphyrin values and liver function tests, a single "test dose" of chloroquine base of 125 mg is administered. Liver function tests are repeated in 1 week, and if there are no abnormalities, the drug is then administered in doses of 125 mg twice weekly. Liver function tests and urinary prophyrins are monitored quarterly, and the medication continued until urinary URO is <100 μg per 24 h. This usually requires 6 to 12 months of treatment. Studies comparing the therapeutic efficacy of phlebotomy with that of low-dose chloroquine have verified the efficacy of each.[221,222]

Swanbeck and Wennersten[209] suggest that the combination of phlebotomy and chloroquine treatment may reduce the severity of the hepatotoxic response to chloroquine and also induce remission of the disease. Patients are treated with a series of one to four phlebotomies prior to starting chloroquine (250 mg daily for 7 days). The procedure is repeated when signs of biochemical or clinical relapse develop, which may occur in 1 to 2 years.

It should be emphasized that despite the tendency of the antimalarials to evoke hepatotoxic responses in patients with PCT, there is no evidence to suggest that the changes in hepatocellular pathology characteristic of PCT worsen as a result of treatment with these drugs.[223] The antimalarials may cause retinopathy, and the low-dose regimen helps to minimize the risk of this complication. Pretreatment and semiannual ophthalmologic examinations should be obtained on patients treated with these drugs.

ACUTE INTERMITTENT PORPHYRIA

(Table 151-12)

Synonyms include Swedish porphyria and pyrroloporphyria.

Historic Aspects

The disease has been known since the late nineteenth century. The first detailed clinical description of AIP was that of Waldenström,[9] who described a total of 179 cases in Sweden. Of these, 103 were said to have acute porphyria characterized by periodic attacks of abdominal pain with constipation, nervous and mental symptoms, and paralysis. This was accompanied by increased urinary excretion of PBG. Several excellent reviews have summarized the clinical and biochemical features of AIP.[26,35,224,225] The disease may affect the peripheral, autonomic, or central nervous systems with neuropathic symptoms and dysfunction.

Several groups showed that increased hepatic ALA synthase activity occurred in AIP.[36,225] It is now clear that the enzyme PBG deaminase, which converts PBG to UROGEN I, is deficient in various tissues of affected individuals and latent carriers of the disease. This helps to explain the excessive ALA and PBG excretion of AIP. PBG deaminase activity in AIP is approximately 50 percent of that in unaffected normal individuals, consistent with an autosomal dominant mode of inheritance. The decreased PBG deaminase may lead to a partial block in heme synthesis, which in turn decreases the regulatory heme pool and leads to derepression of the synthesis of mRNA for ALA synthase.

A most important concept is that, although AIP appears to be inherited as an autosomal dominant trait, fewer than 10 percent of latent carriers of the PBG deaminase defect overexpress the clinical phenotype.[200] The gene defect alone seems to be inconsequential unless the individual is exposed to precipitating factors, among which are drugs (see Table 151-11).[226,227]

Genetics

AIP has been thoroughly studied from the perspective of genetics using the techniques of molecular biology. The disease manifests considerable genetic pleomorphism that relates to more than 90 mu-

TABLE 151-12

Acute Intermittent Porphyria

Synonym	Swedish porphyria
Inheritance	Autosomal dominant
Age of onset	10 to 40; extremely rare prior to puberty
Incidence	1.5:100,000; more common in Scandinavia and Lapland
Photosensitivity	Absent
Skin reactions	None
Clinical findings	Acute attacks with a neurovisceral symptom complex; this includes abdominal pain, constipation, nausea, vomiting, abdominal distension, muscle weakness occasionally leading to paralysis and death; motor neuropathy; bizarre, neurotic or psychotic behavior; acute attacks often precipitated by drugs, hormones (progesterone, estrogen), and nutritional factors, including starvation
Biochemical defects	Excretory: Elevated ALA and PBG in the urine during and between attacks; stool porphyrins are normal
	Erythrocytes: Normal porphyrins
	Enzymatic: 50% PBG deaminase deficiency in liver, RBCs, lymphocytes, and skin fibroblasts; increased hepatic ALA synthase; hormones, drugs, and nutritional factors may increase ALA synthase; decreased hepatic sex steroid 5-α-reductase
Management	High carbohydrate diet, intravenous glucose, or hematin, and avoidance of drugs known to exacerbate porphyria

tations of the PBG deaminase gene that have been identified.[26,36,225] Grandchamp et al.[228] have shown tissue-specific expression of PBG deaminase in AIP. An additional peptide of 17 amino acid residues at the NH_2 terminus of the nonerythropoietic isoform accounts for its increased molecular mass. Identified mutations in AIP are distributed throughout the gene in exons common to both isozymes.[225]

Epidemiology

AIP is an autosomal dominant disease that rarely, if ever, manifests before puberty. Most published series emphasize the female predominance of affected patients, ranging from ratios of 1.5:1 to 2.0:1.[26] The incidence in the human population is approximately 1.5:100,000 in most areas of the world. However, in Scandinavia, particularly Lapland, Waldenström[9] showed that the incidence is much higher (1:1000).

Clinical Manifestations (See Table 151-12)

The clinical signs and symptoms of AIP may be related to the effects of porphyrin precursors on the autonomic nervous system.[2] The acute attack is characterized by abdominal pain and neurologic and psychiatric symptoms that can mimic various disorders.[229] Attacks are often precipitated by ingestion of drugs such as those listed in Table 151-11. Acute attacks of AIP are accompanied by seizures, especially in patients with hyponatremia resulting from vomiting and inappropriate fluid therapy.

There are no cutaneous lesions related to photosensitivity in AIP. This is logical as the abnormal excretion pattern of the disease consists mostly of the porphyrin precursors ALA and PBG, which are not photosensitizers.

These patients usually have abdominal pain (80 to 90 percent) during an acute attack (between attacks patients are often completely symptom free). The pain may be diffuse or localized and is often intermittent and spastic. Vomiting and constipation are frequently associated. Mild fever and leukocytosis may occur, making differential diagnosis extremely difficult. This is one reason many patients with AIP undergo repeated exploratory laparotomies before the diagnosis is finally established.

Peripheral neuropathy is a major part of the clinical syndrome in many patients.[230] This may vary from sensory (localized pain) to motor (weakness progressing to generalized flaccid paralysis). Patients may succumb to the disease, usually due to respiratory failure, or may improve slowly, although residual muscle weakness frequently persists for extended periods.

Laboratory Findings

The primary gene defect in AIP results in PBG deaminase deficiency, which causes excessive urinary excretion of ALA and PBG. Urinary porphyrins may also be elevated (see Table 151-3). Urinary excretion of ALA and PBG as high as 100 mg/24 h may occur during an acute attack. During clinical remission of the disease, urinary excretion of ALA and PBG decreases but usually remains above normal values. This is in contrast to patients with VP who often exhibit normal urinary excretion of ALA and PBG between acute attacks.

Two rapid screening tests are available to test freshly voided urine for increased PBG. The first is simply to expose the urine to bright sunlight for several hours. Darkening to a deep red color suggests that PBG is present but does not prove it. (Porphobilin, another dark pigment, can also be photocatalytically formed in urine.) The second rapid screening test, known as the Hoesch test, is also a simple procedure for detecting excessive urinary PBG.[231] To 2 mL of Ehrlich's reagent (3 g of p-dimethylaminobenzaldehyde dissolved in 125 mL of acetic acid and 24 mL of perchloric acid) 2 drops of fresh urine are added. A uniform cherry-red color of the sample indicates a positive reaction. This test is based upon the formation of a chromogen by PBG and Ehrlich's aldehyde reagent that produces a red pigment with strong absorbance at 552 nm. The well-known Watson-Schwartz test is based on this same principle, although a number of refinements have helped to enhance its accuracy.[232] In patients with suspected AIP, quantitative 24-h measurement of urinary ALA and PBG is essential.

Histopathology

Histopathologic findings of skin are unremarkable.

Differential Diagnosis

The clinical manifestations of AIP are so variable and resemble so many different diseases that Waldenström has used the term *little imitator* to describe it.[9,11,229] Several excellent reviews have summarized the differential clinical features of AIP.[26,225]

Treatment

Although there is still no specific treatment for AIP, several therapeutic modalities have been used, including glucose loading, hematin infusion, and administration of a gonadotropin-releasing hormone analogue.[233–235] Avoidance of precipitating factors such as drugs (Table 151-11), sex steroid hormones, starvation, etc., are important preventive measures. AIP patients should be provided with medical warning bracelets and with lists of drugs to avoid. A list of drugs thought to be safe for AIP patients is provided in Table 151-13.

VARIEGATE PORPHYRIA (Table 151-14)

Synonyms include South African porphyria, PCT hereditaria, mixed porphyria, and protocoproporphyria.

Historic Aspects

This disease has been a source of confusion among the human porphyrias. In 1957, Waldenström revised his original 1937 classification of the porphyrias and described two different types of PCT: PCT symptomatica and PCT hereditaria (protocoproporphyria).[11] PCT symptomatica was said to be the typical PCT with onset of cutaneous lesions in middle age or later, occurring predominantly in males who ingested moderate to heavy quantities of ethanol. PCT hereditaria was said to occur in individuals at a much younger age (15 to 30 years). Large amounts of PROTO and COPRO were excreted in the stool, and these patients had acute attacks indistinguishable from those of AIP. Waldenström suggested that this disease be named protocoproporphyria to separate it from PCT in which fecal porphyrins were usually elevated to a lesser extent.

TABLE 151-13

CHAPTER 151
The Porphyrias
1793

Drugs Considered to be Safe (or Probably Safe) in Patients with the Acute Hepatic Porphyrias

Acetaminophen	Insulin
Adrenaline	Labetalol
Amitryptyline	Lithium
Aspirin	Mandelate
Atropine	Methenamide
Bromide	Naproxen
Cephalosporins	Narcotic analgesics
Chloralhydrates	Neostigmine
Chloramphenicol	Nitrofurantoin
Chlordiazepoxide	Nitrous oxide
Colchicine	Oxazepam
Digoxin	Penicillin and derivatives
Diphenhydramine	Phenothiazines
EDTA	Propranolol
Ether	Prostigmine
Glucocorticoids	Rauwolfia alkaloids
Guanethidine	Streptomycin
Heparin	Succinylcholine
Hyocine	Tetracycline
Hypocine	Thiouracil
Ibuprofin	Thyroxine
Indomethacin	

Barnes[236] had described a similar disorder in South Africa. However, not being a physician, he found it difficult to pursue detailed clinical studies. Soon thereafter, Geoffrey Dean migrated to South Africa and in collaboration with Barnes began a careful evaluation of families affected with this type of porphyria.[14,15,237] Because it presents in a variety of forms, Dean and Barnes proposed the name porphyria variegata to describe the porphyria commonly seen in the South African white population. Dean has summarized this entire adventure in a fascinating book.[238] These patients manifest intermittent attacks typical of AIP, usually following ingestion of barbiturates or sulfonamides. These attacks, predominantly affecting females, are identical to those described in Waldenström's patients with AIP, and most, if not all, such acute attacks could be avoided by eliminating exposure to inducing drugs. Furthermore, Dean was able to obtain detailed histories and family trees from the patients and subsequently saw numerous family members, predominantly males, with a clinical picture practically identical to that of PCT, hence the name VP. The disease has now been recognized worldwide.[16,17]

Etiology

ALA synthase is elevated in the liver of patients with VP just as in those with AIP. This is a nonspecific finding as it occurs in each of the acute hepatic porphyrias.[225] A 50 percent decrease in PROTOGEN oxidase activity is now recognized as the primary enzyme defect in VP.[51] The enzyme acts specifically on PROTOGEN IX, the penultimate step in heme synthesis, and cannot catalyze the oxidation of CO-PROGEN I or III or UROGEN I.

Genetics

VP is due to mutations in the PROTOGEN oxidase gene. The cDNA sequence of the human gene contains 13 exons, is approximately 4.5 kb in length, and encodes a protein of 477 amino acids.[239] A C to T transition (codon 59, in exon 3, causing an arginine to tryptophan substitution) has been identified in 43 of 45 individuals with VP from 26 of 27 South African families but not in 9 unrelated British families with VP.[240] It was suggested that since at least one of the South African families studied was descended from the founder of the disease, this defect may represent the founder gene defect in VP. Additional mutations in the PROTOGEN oxidase gene have been identified.[241,242] Homozygous cases of VP, although rare, have been reported.[243]

Epidemiology

This form of porphyria is quite common among the white and so-called Cape-colored South Africans because of the "founder" effect described above. A high proportion of the present white population is descended from a pair of early Dutch settlers who emigrated to South Africa from Holland in 1680.[14,15] The disease is inherited as an autosomal dominant trait, and the incidence in South Africa is the highest in the world, approximately 1:300 individuals in the white population.

The cutaneous manifestations of PCT and VP are for the most part indistinguishable. Among the native black population of South Africa, typical PCT without associated acute attacks also occurs.[143] There is apparently no family history, and porphyrin excretion patterns are as for PCT, not VP. Excessive intake of home-brewed spirits (Kaffir beer) and dietary overload of iron from cooking vessels are considered important factors in the development of this disease. Thus, VP occurring in the descendants of the Dutch immigrants of South Africa is quite distinct from the PCT seen in the native black population. Finally, Dean has pointed out that the so-called Cape-colored, who are descendants of white European and Indian immigrants who intermarried with black natives, may have VP and PCT in the same family.[238] Factors that precipitate or lead

TABLE 151-14

Variegate Porphyria

Synonyms	Mixed porphyria; South African genetic porphyria; protocoproporphyria hereditaria; PCT hereditaria
Inheritance	Autosomal dominant
Age of onset	Usually between ages 15 to 30
Incidence	Common in South Africa (3/1000); relatively rare elsewhere
Photosensitivity	Similar to PCT (see Table 151-9)
Skin lesions	Similar to PCT (see Table 151-9)
Clinical findings:	Neurovisceral symptomatology similar to AIP; acute attacks similar to AIP precipitated by barbiturates, dapsone, and drugs (estrogens); history of acute episodes of abdominal pain, nausea, vomiting, behavioral disturbances, paralysis, and seizures
Biochemical defects	Excretory: Increased PROTO, COPRO (III > I), and X-porphyrins (ether-acetic–acid insoluble) in feces; PROTO > COPRO III; increased ALA and PBG in urine during acute attacks; normal between attacks
	Enzymatic: Decreased PROTOGEN oxidase in fibroblasts, some evidence for decreased ferrochelatase; increased hepatic ALA synthase
Management	Avoidance of precipitating factors (drugs); treatment for neurovisceral symptoms similar to AIP, photoprotection for photosensitivity

to activation of AIP also appear to induce VP (various drugs, starvation, etc.). All patients with suspected PCT should be screened for VP because VP has a life-threatening potential, and death can follow the ingestion of these drugs.

Clinical Manifestations

The clinical manifestations of VP include those of AIP and PCT, either or both of which may occur in the same individual. In general, females have more frequent acute attacks typical of AIP and males are more likely to have the cutaneous lesions of PCT. Two major differences between VP and PCT are: (1) the skin reactions, which usually develop at an earlier age (second and third decades) as compared to PCT (fourth and fifth decades); and (2) the neurovisceral symptomatology. The clinical features of VP are: (1) positive personal or family history of chronic skin involvement with or without attacks of abdominal pain, constipation, vomiting, muscle weakness, and neuropsychiatric manifestations of stupor and coma; and (2) photocutaneous lesions associated with minor mechanical trauma. The skin lesions of VP are indistinguishable from those of PCT. These include bullae, erosions, or ulcers following minor trauma of light-exposed skin (Fig. 151-21). Hyperpigmentation, milia, hypertrichosis, and increased skin fragility are also seen. They appear to be more common in the hot climate of South Africa and are less frequently seen in cold climates. Blisters are often blood-tinged, heal slowly, and form milia with some scarring. Occasionally the patient gives a history of acute sun sensitivity occurring during or soon after a period of exposure; this may include burning, erythema, and edema. In its chronic state, the skin changes include crusting, depigmented scarring, and hypertrichosis (Fig. 151-22). The skin manifestations do not correlate with the acute attacks in most patients. These clinical and biochemical features are usually seen after puberty, except in the homozygous patients who may develop signs and symptoms at or shortly after birth.[243,244]

Laboratory Findings

Urinary ALA and PBG are elevated during acute attacks of VP (when the Watson-Schwartz test may be positive) but characteristically fall to normal levels between attacks (see Table 151-3), whereas in AIP patients, the urinary ALA and PBG are elevated, both during and between attacks. Another distinguishing feature of the two disorders is the stool porphyrin excretion. Asymptomatic patients with VP usually, but not always, have marked elevations of stool PROTO and COPRO between attacks.[200] These may fluctuate somewhat during acute attacks. PROTO typically exceeds COPRO. In AIP, fecal porphyrins are not elevated between attacks and usually increase only slightly during attacks. Rimington et al.[244] have suggested that a markedly hydrophilic, ether-acetic acid–insoluble porphyrin-peptide conjugate is present in the stool of patients with VP. The name X-porphyrin was given to this peculiar porphyrin, as it could only be extracted from stool with a mixture of urea and the detergent, Triton-X. Elder et al.[245] have questioned the usefulness of measuring the X-porphyrin as it was also detected in the stools of patients with active PCT, and the levels overlapped considerably with those found in patients with VP.

Eales et al.[246] have suggested that certain patterns of fecal and urinary porphyrin excretion may help in distinguishing VP from PCT, e.g., urinary URO is only moderately elevated in VP and is usually less than COPRO. This is in marked contrast to active PCT where the reverse is seen, i.e., urinary URO is much higher than COPRO. Again in VP, fecal porphyrins exceed 500 μg/g dry weight in 92 percent of patients, whereas in PCT this amount of stool porphyrin is excreted by only 1 percent of patients. Furthermore, the ratio of stool PROTO to COPRO in VP usually exceeds 1.5:1, whereas in PCT the ratio is almost always <1:1 due to the increased ISOCOPRO content characteristic of this disease. Stool porphyrin excretion patterns consistent with both VP and PCT have been found in different members of single families.[150,151] These types of findings have led to the suggestion that measurement of bile porphyrins may be decisive in confirming a diagnosis of VP when excretory porphyrin patterns are ambiguous.[199]

Poh-Fitzpatrick has shown that saline-diluted plasma specimens from patients with VP have characteristic fluorescence emission spectra (626-nm emission peak) that can be used to differentiate this disease from other forms of acute porphyria, PCT, EPP, and lead poisoning (see Table 151-8).[247]

Histopathology

The skin lesions of VP are subepidermal bullae indistinguishable from those of PCT.

Differential Diagnosis

The differential diagnosis of VP should be considered from two perspectives. Acute attacks of abdominal pain and neurologic signs and symptoms are identical to those described for AIP. Fecal and biliary PROTO and COPRO determinations and plasma fluorescence spectra are decisive in making the diagnosis. The skin lesions of VP are identical to those of PCT, and, as such, the differential diagnosis includes the bullous diseases as well as other photosensitivity disorders. In HCP there may be identical acute attacks, but markedly elevated fecal COPRO III is diagnostic for this disease. HEP must also be considered, but this usually begins in childhood and is characterized by markedly deficient erythrocyte UROGEN decarboxylase and elevated erythrocyte PROTO as well as increased stool ISOCOPRO. The presence of skin lesions rules out AIP. The determination of urinary ALA and PBG concentrations may help to rule out PCT and HEP. Screening of family members by measuring fecal porphyrins may also be helpful in differentiating VP and PCT.

Treatment

Preventive treatment of VP is identical to that described in AIP, i.e., avoidance of inducing drugs (see Table 151-11). Glucose loading and hematin infusion have also been used with ill-defined success. Phlebotomy and the antimalarials are not effective.[248,249]

HEREDITARY COPROPORPHYRIA (Table 151-15)

Idiopathic coproporphyria is a synonym for HCP.

Historic Aspects

This rare disorder was first described by Watson et al.[250] in two completely asymptomatic individuals who excreted large amounts of COPRO III in the feces and to a lesser extent in the urine. The condition was named HCP by Berger and Goldberg,[20] who described similar findings in a 10-year-old Swiss boy and three relatives. These individuals were also completely asymptomatic.

FIGURE 151-21

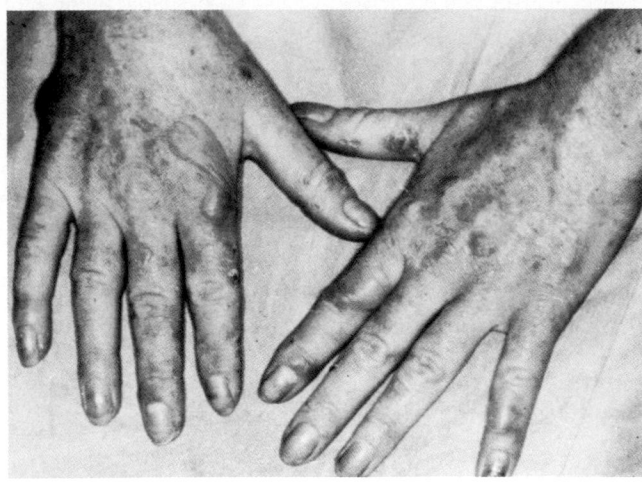

A.

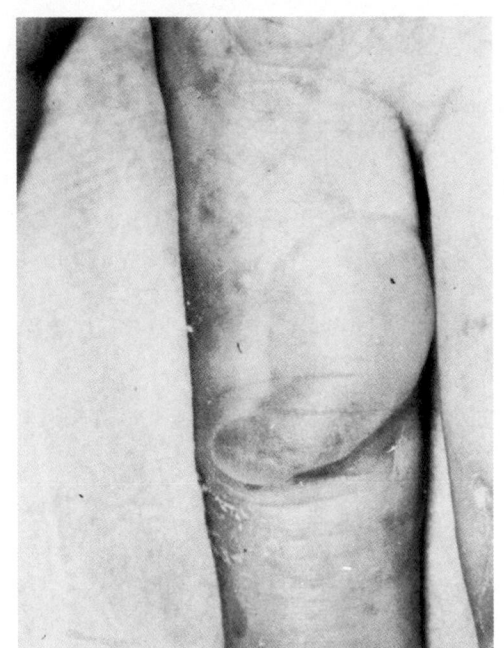

B.

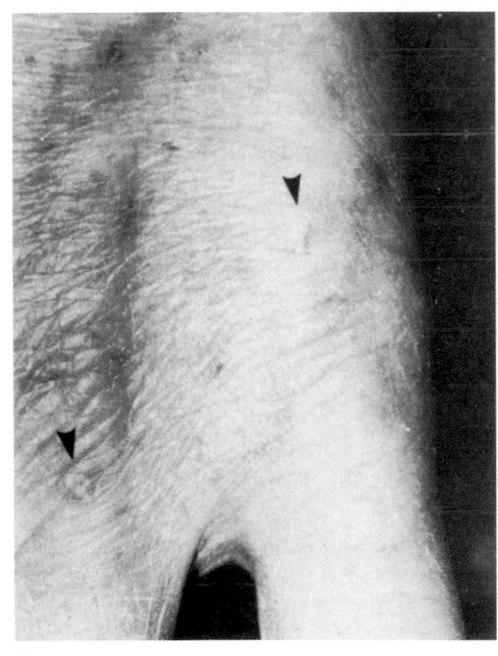

C.

D.

A case of variegate porphyria. *A.* Blisters, crusted erosions, and pigmentary changes over the dorsa of the hands and fingers. *B.* Close-up view of index finger shows an intact blister with milia and pigmentary changes. *C.* Healing phase shows milia (arrows) and pigmentary changes. *D.* Large bullae of dorsum of foot and toes. *Note:* Patients with porphyria cutanea tarda have indistinguishable cutaneous findings.

In 1967, Goldberg et al.[251] reported 10 cases of HCP and reviewed 20 more in the literature. They found that HCP was associated with acute attacks similar in many ways to those seen in AIP and VP, although severe neurologic sequelae seemed to occur less often. In addition, most acute attacks of HCP seemed to be precipitated by ingestion of drugs responsible for the exacerbation of AIP.

During acute attacks, urinary ALA and PBG are elevated just as in AIP and VP; however, a marked elevation of fecal COPRO is diagnostic of HCP.

Cutaneous photosensitivity has been reported in some patients; many of them have associated hepatocellular dysfunction and jaundice. Brodie et al.[252] reviewed the known cases of HCP and found

FIGURE 151-22

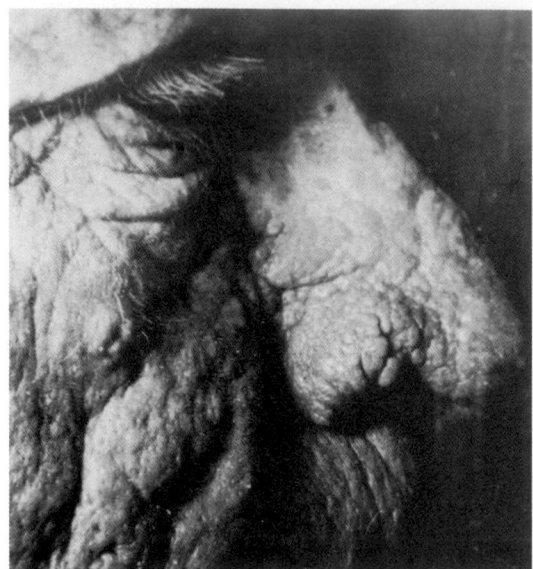

A.

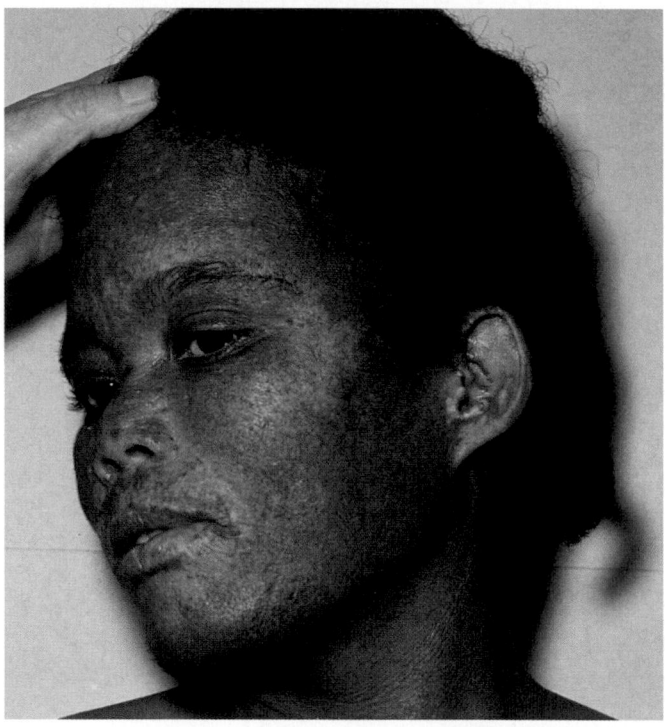

B.

Variegate porphyria. *A.* A peculiar leathery thickening of skin of the face of a patient chronically exposed to strong sunlight. A similar appearance has been noted in South African patients with erythropoietic protoporphyria. *(Courtesy of GH Findlay, MD, FP Scott, MD, and DJ Cripps, MD: Br J Dermatol 78:69, 1966.) B.* A South African pigmented patient showing less severe photodamage; the melanin appears to be photoprotective.

that 20 percent had suffered cutaneous photosensitivity reactions of an unspecified type and 35 percent acute attacks similar to those of AIP or VP.

Etiology

HCP is an autosomal dominant disorder due to mutations in the gene encoding COPROGEN oxidase.[49,253,254] There is deficiency of COPROGEN oxidase activity in cultured skin fibroblasts, in RBCs, and in leukocytes of affected individuals. Enzyme activity is approximately 50 percent of that of normal individuals or patients with other forms of porphyria. Hepatic ALA synthase is reported to be elevated in this disease.[225,256]

Epidemiology

The disease appears to occur worldwide and, like AIP, to have a female preponderance and probably also an autosomal dominant transmittance. Fewer than 200 cases have been reported. A patient with HCP who developed AIDS was reported.[257] An extremely rare form of porphyria known as *harderoporphyria* appears to be a variant of HCP in which COPROGEN oxidase activity is very low (10 percent of control values).[258] This disease has been identified in three siblings, and it is said that these patients may be homozygous for a gene that causes HCP in some families.

Clinical Manifestations

The acute attacks are similar to those of AIP, and neurovisceral symptomatology predominates in HCP. This includes abdominal pain, vomiting, constipation, neuropathies, and psychiatric symptoms. The oral hypoglycemic agent glipizide has been reported to exacerbate a coproporphyria-like syndrome that was reversible following discontinuation of the drug.[259] Cutaneous photosensitivity occurs in 20 percent of cases.[260] In general, it appears that this disorder is not associated with acute attacks as severe as those of AIP or VP.

Laboratory Findings

HCP is characterized by increased excretion of COPRO III in urine and feces. Markedly elevated fecal COPRO, more than 90 percent of which is the III isomer, is present at all times in these patients. In addition, the feces also contain increased amounts of hepta-, hexa-, and pentacarboxylic porphyrins. Urinary COPRO III is also raised, as are ALA and PBG, during attacks. The latter usually fall to near-normal levels in remission.

Histopathology

No histology has yet been reported.

Differential Diagnosis

Acute attacks are similar to those of AIP. The differential diagnosis rests on stool porphyrin determinations and measurement of COPROGEN oxidase in fibroblasts or leukocytes. The skin lesions are said to resemble PCT, although no definitive evidence for this has been reported. Fecal predominance of COPRO III is more suggestive of HCP than VP, in which PROTO and COPRO are usually increased.

Treatment

Avoidance of inducing drugs, glucose loading, and hematin infusions may be helpful.

HEPATOERYTHRO-POIETIC PORPHYRIA

(Table 151-16)

HEP is also known as hepatoerythrocytic porphyria.

Historic Aspects

In 1969, Pinõl Aguadé et al. first reported the occurrence of a new and at first biochemically unclassifiable type of porphyria in Spain.[21] Since that time, approximately 50 cases of a similar nature have been reported.[261–263] The skin manifestations resemble both PCT and EP and are characterized by severe photosensitivity, bullae, erosions, and mutilating scarring deformities that often begin in early childhood.

Etiology

HEP is due to a profound deficiency of UROGEN decarboxylase; in some cases this is due to inheritance of a mutant allele from each parent (compound heterozygote), and in other cases it is the result of inheriting a homozygous form of type II PCT. The primary enzyme defect is a profound deficiency of UROGEN decarboxylase activity.[42] Measurement of the enzyme in hemolyzed whole blood or skin fibroblasts from three unrelated patients with the disease showed that it was 7 to 8 percent of normal levels. The father of one HEP patient was heterozygous for the same enzyme defect, suggesting that patients with HEP are homozygous for the gene that causes PCT. There is no evidence, as yet, to show that clinical expression of HEP is related to exposure to environmental drugs or chemicals, as is true for PCT. Toback et al.[263] reported clinical, biochemical, and enzymatic studies in a three-generation family lineage in which a second-generation 31-year-old male was shown to have HEP. Both of the proband's parents and each of his three children had a moderate deficiency of UROGEN decarboxylase.

Epidemiology

Patients with HEP have been reported in Europe and America.

Genetics

deVerneuil et al.[47,48] cloned and sequenced a cDNA for UROGEN decarboxylase from a patient with HEP and identified a mutation consisting of a single base substitution, (Gly281Glu) that was present in some but not all families with the disease. In a further study, UROGEN decarboxylase cDNA was cloned from another patient, and comparison of the mutant and wild type sequences showed a single base difference within the coding sequence leading to replacement of glutamic acid by a lysine at codon 167 of the mutant protein.[264] This was not detected in six unrelated patients with type II PCT, indicating heterogeneity in the mutations responsible for PCT and HEP phenotypes.

Clinical Manifestations

This disease is usually manifest in early childhood with dark urine being the most frequently observed sign. Severe cutaneous photosensitivity includes blistering and pruritus. The photosensitivity seems to diminish with age and is followed by hypertrichosis, hyperpigmentation, and scleroderma-like scarring similar to that seen in Günther's disease. Ocular manifestations include ectropion as-

TABLE 151-15

Hereditary Coproporphyria

Synonym	Idiopathic coproporphyria
Inheritance	Autosomal dominant
Age of onset	Any age
Incidence	Rare (< 50 cases reported)
Photosensitivity	Occurs infrequently
Skin reactions	Usually blistering
Clinical findings	Neurovisceral symptomatology similar to but milder than that of AIP; acute attacks precipitated by barbiturates and other drugs
Biochemical defects	Excretory: Marked elevation of fecal and urinary COPRO III during and between attacks; fecal PROTO may be modestly elevated; ALA and PBG elevated during acute attacks
	Enzymatic: COPROGEN oxidase deficiency in lymphocytes and fibroblasts; increased hepatic ALA synthase
Management	Similar to AIP or VP (avoidance of precipitating factors)

TABLE 151-16

Hepatoerythropoietic Porphyria

Synonym	Hepatoerythrocytic porphyria
Inheritance	Autosomal recessive
Age of onset	Early infancy, before age 2
Incidence	Extremely rare (<50 cases)
Photosensitivity	Marked
Skin reactions	Early: Subepidermal vesicles, bullae, erosions, scarring, mutilation, hypertrichosis
	Late: Scleroderma-like scarring, hyperpigmentation, mutilating scarring deformities of acral areas such as hands, ears, face, and nose; cicatrizing alopecia
Clinical findings	Moderate normochromic anemia; ? hemolytic anemia; erythrodontia; pink urine; serum Fe normal
Biochemical defects	Excretory: Elevated URO (I–III) and 7-carboxyl porphyrin (III) in urine; elevated URO, COPRO, and ISOCOPRO in feces
	RBC: Elevated PROTO, usually Zn PROTO
	Enzymatic: Markedly decreased RBC UROGEN decarboxylase
Management	Avoidance of sun; phlebotomy not indicated, oral charcoal therapy may be attempted

sociated with cutaneous sclerosis and scleromalacia perforans. Splenomegaly has occurred in a small percentage of affected individuals, particularly after the age of 10, and hemolytic anemia has been documented as well. In some patients, liver function tests have been abnormal, but serum iron and iron binding are normal. In summary, the clinical manifestations of HEP resemble a combination of EP and PCT.

Laboratory Findings

Elevated urinary URO (I and III) and 7-carboxyl porphyrins (>90 percent III), elevated fecal COPRO and ISOCOPRO, and elevated RBC PROTO (zinc-chelated) have been observed in all patients. These findings suggest that there is abnormal porphyrin synthesis in both the liver and the bone marrow. In contrast to PCT patients, serum iron concentrations are usually normal in HEP.

Histopathology

Skin biopsies have shown subepidermal bullae similar to PCT. PAS-positive material in and around dermal capillaries has been observed.

Differential Diagnosis

The differential diagnosis is that of childhood porphyria and includes EP, PCT, and EPP. EP manifests erythrodontia and mutilating scarring, whereas EPP often presents with acute photosensitivity. Unlike EP, in which increased RBC URO is a characteristic finding, in HEP there is elevated RBC PROTO of the zinc-chelated type. The urinary porphyrin pattern is similar to that found in PCT with high URO (URO:COPRO ratio > 5:1). The elevated PROTO in RBC helps to distinguish HEP from PCT. Urinary porphyrin analysis can differentiate HEP and EPP because urinary porphyrins are normal in EPP.

Treatment

There is no known treatment aside from careful photoprotection.

ALA DEHYDRATASE DEFICIENCY PORPHYRIA
(Table 151-17)

This condition is also known as plumboporphyria.

This is a rare type of acute hepatic porphyria, and only a few patients have been reported.[23,265] Clinically, these patients have symptoms similar to AIP, and no skin lesions have been noted. Stress and ethanol ingestion have been reported to precipitate attacks. The patients have erythrocyte ALA dehydratase activity <5 percent of normal. Although it has been suggested that ALA dehydratase deficiency porphyria may represent a homozygous ALA dehydratase defect, recent cloning of a mutant ALA dehydratase cDNA in a patient showed that the patient was doubly heterozygous for two independent mutant alleles of ALA dehydratase.[266]

In the few patients studied, the urinary porphyrin profile revealed elevated levels of ALA, COPRO, and, to a lesser extent, URO. Fecal porphyrins revealed mildly elevated COPRO and PROTO in

TABLE 151-17

ALA Dehydratase Deficiency Porphyria

Inheritance	Autosomal recessive
Age of onset	Any age
Incidence	Extremely rare; <10 cases
Photosensitivity	None
Clinical findings	Symptoms similar to AIP
Biochemical findings	Excretory: Elevated ALA, COPRO, and URO in urine, COPRO and PROTO in feces
	RBC: Elevated PROTO
	Enzymatic: Markedly decreased ALA dehydratase activity
Management	Symptomatic; avoidance of known stimulating factors for acute hepatic porphyria

one patient, elevated COPRO in another, and a normal profile in two others. Erythrocyte PROTO was elevated in all patients. Increases of plasma ALA, COPRO, and PROTO have been reported.[265] The reason for the elevated porphyrins in these patients is not understood.

ABNORMAL PORPHYRIN PROFILE AND SIDEROBLASTIC ANEMIA

Some cases of sideroblastic anemia may be associated with an abnormal porphyrin profile.[22,267,268] Clinically, these patients may have photosensitivity most consistent with the features of EPP and subsequently develop sideroblastic anemia; in some, the two conditions may develop within a few months of each other. All patients have elevated PROTO in RBCs and/or plasma; many also have elevated stool PROTO levels. Urinary COPRO and URO are also elevated. The activities of ferrochelatase and, less frequently, of ALA synthase may be decreased. Chromosomal abnormalities, which include deletions in chromosomes 18 and 20, have been described.

PERSPECTIVE

The diagnosis of the human porphyrias has historically depended upon careful clinical observation and the performance of biochemical and enzyme assays, which, though quite helpful in many cases, have serious limitations. Overlapping values between normal and affected individuals can and do occur. It is rare for asymptomatic gene carriers to be identified by detection of porphyrin precursors in urine and/or stool specimens because excretion levels vary widely among individuals.[269] Similarly, enzyme activity can vary substantially, making these assays somewhat imprecise.

The more recent ability to identify the underlying genetic abnormalities in the human porphyrias portends the increasing usefulness of these modalities to confirm a suspected diagnosis in an affected individual and to detect asymptomatic carriers in the patient's family.

Similarly, the use of molecular technology will undoubtedly lead to the development of genetically engineered animals such as knock-out mice that will permit more intensive studies of the metabolic consequences of heme pathway enzyme derangements. Gene transfer experiments in vitro already indicate the feasibility of gene therapy for these disorders. As these methods are perfected, it is likely that gene therapy will become a new treatment option for human porphyria.[270]

REFERENCES

1. May BK et al: Molecular regulation of heme biosynthesis in higher vertebrates. *Prog Nucl Acid Res Mol Biol* **51**:1, 1995
2. Schultz JH: *Ein Fall von Pemphigus leprosus complicirt durch Lepra visceralis.* Greifswald, Kunike, 1874
3. Baumstark F: Zwei pathologische Harnfarbstoffe. *Arch Dtsch Ges Physiol* **9**:568, 1874
4. Taddeini L, Watson CJ: The clinical porphyrias. *Semin Hematol* **5**:335, 1968
5. Anderson TM: Hydroa aestivale in two brothers, complicated with the presence of haematoporphyrin in the urine. *Br J Dermatol* **10**:1, 1898
6. Günther J: Die Hamatoporphyrie. *Dtsch Arch Klin Med* **105**:89, 1911
7. Fischer H: Über das Urinporphyrin. *Z Physiol Chem* **95**:34, 1915
8. Fischer H et al: Zur Kenntnis der naturlichen. Porphyrine: Chemische Befund bei einem Fall von Porphyrinurie (Petry). *Z Physiol Chem* **150**:44, 1925
9. Waldenström J: Studien über Porphyrie. *Acta Med Scand* (suppl) **82**:1, 1937
10. Brunsting LA: Observations on porphyria cutanea tarda. *Arch Dermatol Syphilol* **70**:551, 1954
11. Waldenström J: The porphyrias as inborn errors of metabolism. *Am J Med* **22**:758, 1957
12. Schmid R: Cutaneous porphyria in Turkey. *N Engl J Med* **263**:397, 1960
13. Barnes HD: A note on porphyrinuria with a resumé of eleven South African cases. *Clin Proc* **4**:269, 1945
14. Dean G: Porphyria. *Br Med J* **2**:1291, 1953
15. Dean G, Barnes HD: Porphyria in Sweden and South Africa. *S Afr Med J* **33**:246, 1959
16. Fromke VL et al: Porphyria variegata. Study of a large kindred in the United States. *Am J Med* **65**:80, 1978
17. Mustajoki P: Variegate porphyria. *Ann Intern Med* **89**:238, 1978
18. Magnus IA et al: Erythropoietic protoporphyria: A new porphyria syndrome with solar urticaria due to protoporphyrinaemia. *Lancet* **2**:448, 1961
19. Heilmeyer L, Clotten R: Congenital erythropoietic coproporphyria. *German Med Monthly* **9**:353, 1964
20. Berger H, Goldberg A: Hereditary coproporphyria. *Br Med J* **2**:85, 1955
21. Piñol-Aguadé J et al: A case of biochemically unclassifiable hepatic porphyria. *Br J Dermatol* **81**:270, 1969
22. Rothstein G et al: Sideroblastic anemia with dermal photosensitivity and greatly increased protoporphyrin. *New Engl J Med* **280**:587, 1969
23. Doss M et al: New type of hepatic porphyria with porphobilinogen synthase defect and intermittent acute manifestation. *Klin Wochenschr* **57**:1123, 1979
24. Dyer J et al: Plumboporphyria (ALAD deficiency) in a lead worker: A scenario for potential diagnostic confusion. *Br J Ind Med* **50**:1119, 1993
25. Poh-Fitzpatrick MD et al: Cutaneous photosensitivity and coproporphyrin abnormalities in Alagille syndrome. *Gastroenterology* **99**:831, 1990
26. Ratnaike S, Blake D: The diagnosis and follow-up of porphyria. *Pathology* **27**:142, 1995
27. Riddle RD et al: Expression of δ-aminolevulinate synthase in avian cells: Separate genes encode erythroid specific and nonspecific isozymes. *Proc Natl Acad Sci USA* **86**:792, 1989
28. Yamamoto M et al: An immunochemical study of δ-aminolevulinate synthase and δ-aminolevulinate dehydratase in liver and erythroid cells of rat. *Arch Biochem Biophys* **245**:76, 1986
29. Morton KA et al: Biosynthesis of delta-aminolevulinic acid and heme from 4,5-dioxovalerate in the rat. *J Clin Invest* **71**:1744, 1983
30. Ben Ezzer J et al: Genetic polymorphism of delta-aminolevulinate dehydrase in several population groups in Israel. *Hum Genet* **37**:229, 1987
31. Wetmur JG et al: Molecular cloning of a cDNA for human δ-aminolevulinate dehydratase. *Gene* **43**:123, 1986
32. Kaya AH et al: Human delta-aminolevulinate dehydratase (ALAD) gene: Structure and alternate splicing of the erythroid and housekeeping mRNAs. *Genomics* **19**:242, 1994
33. Anderson PM, Desnick RJ: Purification and properties of uroporphyrinogen I synthase from human erythrocytes. Identification of stable enzyme-substrate intermediates. *J Biol Chem* **255**:1993, 1980
34. Chretien S et al: Alternative transcription and splicing of the human porphobilinogen deaminase gene result either in tissue-specific or in housekeeping expression. *Proc Natl Acad Sci USA* **85**:6, 1988
35. Deybach J-C, Puy H: Porphobilinogen deaminase gene structure and molecular defects. *J Bioenerg Biomembr* **27**:197, 1995
36. Lundin G et al: Four mutations in the porphobilinogen deaminase gene in patients with acute intermittent porphyria. *J Med Genet* **32**:979, 1995
37. Watson CJ, Schwartz S: A simple test for urinary porphobilinogen. *Proc Soc Exp Biol Med* **47**:393, 1941
38. Lamon J et al: The Hoesch test: Bedside screening for urinary uroporphyrinogen in patients with suspected porphyria. *Clin Chem* **20**:1438, 1974
39. Tsai SF et al: Purification and properties of uroporphyrinogen III synthase from human erythrocytes. *J Biol Chem* **262**:1268, 1987
40. Clement RP et al: Rat hepatic uroporphyrinogen III cosynthase: Purification, properties and inhibition of metal ions. *Arch Biochem Biophys* **214**:657, 1982
41. Tsai S-F et al: Human uroporphyrinogen III synthase: Molecular cloning, nucleotide sequence and expression of a full-length cDNA. *Proc Natl Acad Sci USA* **85**:7049, 1988
42. Elder GH, Roberts AG: Uroporphyrinogen decarboxylase. *J Bioenerg Biomembr* **27**:207, 1995
43. Kushner JP et al: An inherited enzymatic defect in porphyria cutanea tarda: Decreased uroporphyrinogen decarboxylase activity. *J Clin Invest* **58**:1089, 1976
44. Held JL et al: Erythrocyte uroporphyrinogen decarboxylase activity in porphyria cutanea tarda: A study of 40 consecutive patients. *J Invest Dermatol* **93**: 332, 1990
45. Garey JR et al: Uroporphyrinogen decarboxylase: A splice site mutation causes the deletion of exon 6 in multiple families with porphyria cutanea tarda. *J Clin Invest* **86**:1416, 1990
46. Roberts AG et al: A mutation (G281E) of the human uroporphyrinogen decarboxylase gene causes both hepatoerythropoietic porphyria and overt familial porphyria cutanea tarda. Biochemical and genetic studies on Spanish patients. *J Invest Dermatol* **104**:500, 1995
47. deVerneuil H et al: Uroporphyrinogen decarboxylase structural mutant(Gly^{281}→Glu) in a case of porphyria. *Science* **234**:732, 1986
48. deVerneuil H et al: Prevalence of the 281 (Gly→Glu) mutation in hepatoerythropoietic porphyria and porphyria cutanea tarda. *Hum Genet* **78**:101, 1988
49. Grandchamp B et al: Molecular abnormalities of coproporphyrinogen oxidase in patients with hereditary coproporphyria *J Bioenerg Biomembr* **27**:215, 1995
50. Deybach J-C et al: Mutations in the protoporphyrinogen oxidase gene in patients with variegate porphyria. *Hum Mol Genet* **5**:407, 1995
51. Lam H-M et al: Molecular basis of variegate porphyria: A de novo insertion mutation in the protoporphyrinogen oxidase gene. *Hum Genet* **99**:126, 1997
52. Teketani S et al: The human protoporphyrinogen oxidase gene (PPOX): Organization and location to chromosome 1. *Genomics* **29**:698, 1995
53. Taketani S et al: Molecular cloning, sequencing and expression of mouse ferrochelatase. *J Biol Chem* **265**:19377, 1990
54. Taketani S, Fujita H: The ferrochelatase gene structure and molecular defects associated with erythropoietic protoporphyria. *J Bioenerg Biomembr* **27**:231, 1995
55. Poh-Fitzpatrick MB: The "primary phenomenon" for acute phototoxicity in erythropoietic protoporphyria? *J Am Acad Dermatol* **21**:311, 1989
56. Lamola AA et al: Erythropoietic protoporphyria and lead intoxication: The molecular basis for difference in cutaneous photosensitivity. *J Clin Invest* **56**:1528, 1975
57. Meyer-Betz F: Untersuchungen über die biologische (photodynamische) Wirkung des Hamatoporphyrins und andere derivate des Blut und Gallenfarbstoffes. *Dtsch Arch Klin Med* **112**:476, 1913

58. Harty JI et al: Complications of whole bladder dihematoporphyrin ether photodynamic therapy. *J Urol* **141**:1341, 1989

59. Bodaness RS, Chan PC: Singlet oxygen as a mediator in the hematoporphyrin-catalyzed photooxidation of NADPH to NADP$^+$ in deuterium oxide. *J Biol Chem* **252**:8554, 1977

60. Kessel D, Rossi E: Determinants of porphyrin-induced photo-oxidation characterized by fluorescence and absorption spectra. *Photochem Photobiol* **35**:37, 1982

61. Bickers DR et al: Hematoporphyrin photosensitization of epidermal microsomes results in destruction of cytochrome P-450 and in decreased monooxygenase activities and heme content. *Biochem Biophys Res Commun* **108**:1032, 1982

62. Blum HF: *Photodynamic Action and Diseases Caused by Light.* Princeton, Reinhold, 1941

63. Girotti AW: Protoporphyrin-sensitized photodamage in isolated membranes of human erythrocytes. *Biochemistry* **18**:4403, 1979

64. Schothorst AA et al: Photochemical damage to skin fibroblasts caused by protoporphyrin and violet light. *Arch Dermatol Res* **268**:31, 1980

65. Goldstein BD, Harber LC: Erythropoietic protoporphyria: Lipid peroxidation and red cell membrane damage associated with photohemolysis. *J Clin Invest* **51**:892, 1972

66. Lamola AA et al: Cholesterol hydroperoxide formation in red cell membranes and photohemolysis in erythropoietic protoporphyria. *Science* **179**:1131, 1973

67. Lim HW et al: Differential effects of protoporphyrin and uroporphyrin on murine mast cells. *J Invest Dermatol* **88**:281, 1987

68. Dixit R et al: Destruction of cytochrome P-450 by reactive oxygen species generated during photosensitization of hematoporphyrin derivative. *Photochem Photobiol* **37**:173, 1983

69. Sandberg S, Romslo I: Phototoxicity of protoporphyrin as related to its subcellular localization in mice livers after short-term feeding with griseofulvin. *Biochem J* **198**:67, 1981

70. Coppola A et al: Ultrastructural changes in lymphoma cells treated with hematoporphyrin and light. *Am J Pathol* **99**:175, 1980

71. Canti G et al: Hematoporphyrin-treated murine lymphocytes: In vitro inhibition of DNA synthesis and light-mediated inactivation of cells responsible for GVHR. *Photochem Photobiol* **34**:589, 1981

72. Mathews-Roth MM et al: Beta-carotene as an oral photoprotective agent in erythropoietic protoporphyria. *JAMA* **228**:1004, 1974

73. Athar M et al: A novel mechanism for the generation of superoxide anions in hematoporphyrin derivative–mediated cutaneous photosensitization. Activation of the xanthine oxidase pathway. *J Clin Invest* **83**:1137, 1989

74. Emiliani C, Delmelle M: The lipid solubility of porphyrins modulates their phototoxicity in membrane models. *Photochem Photobiol* **37**:487, 1983

75. Watson CJ et al: The manifestations of the different forms of porphyria in relation to chemical findings. *Trans Assoc Am Physicians* **64**:345, 1951

76. Schnait FG et al: Erythropoietic protoporphyria—submicroscopic events during the acute photosensitivity flare. *Br J Dermatol* **92**:545, 1975

77. Yen A et al: Dual effects of protoporphyrin and long wave ultraviolet light on histamine release from rat peritoneal and cutaneous mast cells. *J Immunol* **144**:4327, 1990

78. He D et al: The late phase of hematoporphyrin derivative–induced phototoxicity in mice: Release of histamine and histologic changes. *Photochem Photobiol* **50**:91, 1989

79. Lim HW et al: Delayed phase of hematoporphyrin-induced phototoxicity: Modulation by complement, leukocytes and antihistamines. *J Invest Dermatol* **84**:114, 1985

80. Sandberg S et al: Porphyrin-induced photodamage to isolated human neutrophils. *Photochem Photobiol* **34**:471, 1981

81. Baart De La Faille H et al: Experimental protoporphyria in hairless mice, in *Photodermatitis,* in *Inflammation: Mechanisms and Treatment,* edited by DA Willoughby, JP Girouds. Baltimore, University Park Press, 1980, p 603

82. Varigos G et al: Uroporphyrin I stimulation of collagen biosynthesis in human skin fibroblasts. A unique dark effect of porphyrin. *J Clin Invest* **69**:129, 1982

83. Latham PS, Bloomer JR: Protoporphyrin-induced photodamage: Studies using cultured skin fibroblasts. *Photochem Photobiol* **37**:553, 1983

84. Wakulchik SD et al: Photolysis of protoporphyrin-treated human fibroblasts *in vitro.* Studies on the mechanism. *J Lab Clin Med* **96**:158, 1980

85. Cormane RH et al: Histopathology of the skin in acquired and hereditary porphyria cutanea tarda. *Br J Dermatol* **85**:531, 1971

86. Epstein JH et al: Cutaneous changes in the porphyrias. *Arch Dermatol* **107**:689, 1973

87. Lim HW et al: Generation of chemotactic activity in serum from patients with erythropoietic protoporphyria and porphyria cutanea tarda. *N Engl J Med* **304**:212, 1981

88. Lim HW, Gigli I: Role of complement in porphyrin-induced photosensitivity. *J Invest Dermatol* **76**:4, 1981

89. Torinuki W et al: Activation of the alternative complement pathway by 405-nm light in serum from porphyric rat. *Acta Derm Venereol (Stockh)* **64**:367, 1984

90. Lim HW et al: Activation of the complement system in patients with porphyrias after irradiation *in vivo. J Clin Invest* **74**:1976, 1984

91. Becker CG et al: Activation of factor XII–dependent pathways in human plasma by hematin and protoporphyrin. *J Clin Invest* **76**:413, 1985

92. Henderson BW, Donovan JM: Release of prostaglandin E$_2$ from cells by photodynamic treatment in vitro. *Cancer Res* **49**:6896, 1989

93. Herrmann G et al: Photosensitization of uroporphyrin augments the ultraviolet A–induced synthesis of matrix metalloproteinases in human dermal fibroblasts. *J Invest Dermatol* **107**:398, 1996

94. Fritsch et al: Congenital erythropoietic porphyria. *J Am Acad Dermatol* **36**: 594, 1997

95. Xu W et al: Molecular basis of congenital erythropoietic porphyria: Mutations in the human uroporphyrinogen III synthase gene. *Human Mutat* **7**:187, 1996

96. Nordmann Y et al: Molecular genetics of porphyrias. *Ann Med* **22**:387, 1990

97. Xu W et al: Congenital erythropoietic porphyria: Identification and expression of 10 mutations in the uroporphyrinogen III synthase gene. *J Clin Invest* **95**:905, 1995

98. Horiguchi Y et al: Late onset erythropoietic porphyria. *Br J Dermatol* **121**:255, 1989

99. Watson CJ et al: Some studies of the comparative biology of human and bovine erythropoietic porphyria. *Arch Intern Med* **103**:436, 1959

100. Nordmann Y, Deybach JC: Congenital erythropoietic porphyria. *Semin Liver Dis* **2**:154, 1982

101. Poh-Fitzpatrick MB: Erythropoietic porphyrias: Current mechanistic, diagnostic and therapeutic considerations. *Semin Haematol* **14**:211, 1977

102. Nordmann Y et al: Coexistent hereditary coproporphyria and congenital erythropoietic porphyria (Günther disease). *J Inherit Metab Dis* **13**:687, 1990

103. Piomelli S et al: Complete suppression of the symptoms of congenital erythropoietic porphyria by long term treatment with high level transfusions. *N Engl J Med* **314**:1019, 1986

104. Pimstone NR et al: Therapeutic efficacy of oral charcoal in congenital erythropoietic porphyria. *N Engl J Med* **316**:390, 1987

105. Minder EI et al: Lack of effect of oral charcoal in congenital erythropoietic porphyria. *N Engl J Med* **330**:1092, 1994

106. Thomas C et al: Correction of congenital erythropoietic porphyria by bone marrow transplantation. *J Pediatr* **129**:453, 1996

107. Bloomer JR: Characterization of deficient heme synthase activity in protoporphyria with cultured skin fibroblasts. *J Clin Invest* **65**:321, 1980

108. Goerz G et al: Ferrochelatase activities in patients with erythropoietic protoporphyria and their families. *Br J Dermatol* **134**:880, 1996

109. Sassa S et al: Studies in porphyria. Functional evidence for a partial deficiency of ferrochelatase activity in mitogen-stimulated lymphocytes from patients with erythropoietic protoporphyria. *J Clin Invest* **69**:809, 1982

110. Norris PG et al: Genetic heterogeneity in erythropoietic protoporphyria: A study of the enzymatic defect in nine affected families. *J Invest Dermatol* **95**:260, 1990

111. Deybach JC et al: Ferrochelatase in erythropoietic protoporphyria: The first case of a homozygous form of the enzyme deficiency, in *Porphyrins and Porphyrias,* edited by Y Nordmann. Paris, Colloque, INSERM, John Libbey EURO text, vol. 134, 1986, p 163

112. Schmidt H et al: Erythropoietic protoporphyria: A clinical study based on 29 cases in 14 families. *Arch Dermatol* **110**:58, 1974

113. Piomelli S et al: Erythropoietic protoporphyria and lead intoxication: The molecular basis for difference in cutaneous photosensitivity: I.

Different rates of disappearance of protoporphyrin from the erythrocytes, both in vivo and in vitro. *J Clin Invest* **56**:1519, 1975

114. Lamon JM et al: Hepatic protoporphyrin production in human protoporphyria. Effects of intravenous hematin and analysis of erythrocyte protoporphyrin distribution. *Gastroenterology* **79**:115, 1980

115. Scholnick P et al: Erythropoietic protoporphyria: Evidence for multiple sites of excess protoporphyrin formation. *J Clin Invest* **50**:203, 1971

116. Cripps DJ, Scheuer PJ: Hepatobiliary changes in erythropoietic protoporphyria. *Arch Pathol* **80**:500, 1965

117. Klatskin G, Bloomer JR: Birefringence of hepatic pigment deposits in erythropoietic protoporphyria: Specificity and sensitivity of polarization microscopy in the identification of hepatic protoporphyrin deposits. *Gastroenterology* **67**:295, 1974

118. Wolff K et al: Liver inclusions in erythropoietic protoporphyria. *Eur J Clin Invest* **5**:21, 1975

119. Romslo I et al: Erythropoietic protoporphyria terminating in liver failure. *Arch Dermatol* **118**:668, 1982

120. Avner DL et al: Protoporphyrin-induced cholestasis in the isolated in situ perfused rat liver. *J Clin Invest* **67**:385, 1981

121. Sarkany RPE, Cox TM: Autosomal recessive erythropoietic protoporphyria: A syndrome of severe photosensitivity and liver failure. *Q J Med* **88**:541, 1995

122. Schneider-Yin X et al: Recessive inheritance of erythropoietic protoporphyria with liver failure. *Lancet* **344**:337, 1994

123. Poh-Fitzpatrick MB et al: Rapid quantitative assay for erythrocyte porphyrins. *Arch Dermatol* **110**:225, 1974

124. Poh-Fitzpatrick MB, Lamola AA: Direct spectrofluorometry of diluted erythrocytes and plasma: A rapid diagnostic method in primary and secondary porphyrinemias. *J Lab Clin Med* **87**:362, 1976

125. Lamola AA et al: Erythropoietic protoporphyria and Pb intoxication: The molecular basis for difference in cutaneous photosensitivity. II. Differential binding of erythrocyte protoporphyrin to hemoglobin. *J Clin Invest* **56**:1528, 1975

126. Romslo I et al: Sideroblastic anemia with markedly increased free erythrocyte protoporphyrin without dermal photosensitivity. *Blood* **59**:628, 1982

127. Sandberg S, Brun A: Light-induced protoporphyrin release from erythrocytes in erythropoietic protoporphyria. *J Clin Invest* **70**:693, 1982

128. Peterka EA et al: Erythropoietic protoporphyria. II. Histological and histochemical studies of cutaneous lesions. *Arch Dermatol* **92**:357, 1965

129. Cripps DJ et al: Four cases of erythropoietic protoporphyria presenting as light-sensitive lipoid proteinosis. *Proc R Soc Med* **57**:1095, 1964

130. Ryan EA, Madill GT: Electron microscopy of the skin in erythropoietic protoporphyria. *Br J Dermatol* **80**:561, 1968

131. Breathnach SM et al: Immunohistochemical studies of amyloid P component and fibronectin in erythropoietic protoporphyria. *Br J Dermatol* **108**:267, 1983

132. Mathews-Roth MM et al: Beta-carotene therapy for erythropoietic protoporphyria and other diseases. *Arch Dermatol* **113**:1229, 1977

133. Corbett NF et al: The long term treatment with beta-carotene in erythropoietic protoporphyria: A controlled trial. *Br J Dermatol* **97**:653, 1977

134. Bechtel MA et al: Transfusion therapy in a patient with erythropoietic protoporphyria. *Arch Dermatol* **47**:99, 1981

135. McCullough AJ et al: Fecal protoporphyrin excretion in erythropoietic protoporphyria: Effect of cholestyramine and bile acid feeding. *Gastroenterology* **94**:177, 1988

136. Gordeuk VR et al: Iron therapy for hepatic dysfunction in erythropoietic protoporphyria. *Ann Intern Med* **105**:27, 1986

137. Milligan A et al: Erythropoietic protoporphyria exacerbated by iron therapy. *Br J Dermatol* **119**:63, 1988

138. Polson RJ et al: The effect of liver transplantation in a 13-year-old boy with erythropoietic protoporphyria. *Transplantation* **46**:386, 1988

139. Mathews-Roth MM et al: Amelioration of the metabolic defect in erythropoietic protoporphyria by expression of human ferrochelatase in cultured cells. *J Invest Dermatol* **104**:497, 1995

140. Magness ST, Brenner DA: Ferrochelatase cDNA delivered by adenoviral vector corrects biochemical defect in protoporphyric cells. *Human Gene Ther* **6**:1285, 1995

141. Topi G et al: Coproporphirie erithropoetique congenitales observée chez un frère et une soeur. *Ann Dermatol Venereol* **104**:68, 1977

142. Brunsting LA, Mason HL: Porphyria with cutaneous manifestations. *Arch Dermatol Syphilol* **60**:66, 1948

143. Eales L: Cutaneous porphyria: Observations on 111 cases in three racial groups. *S Afr J Lab Clin Med* **6**:63, 1960

144. Watson CJ: The problem of porphyria: Some facts and questions. *N Engl J Med* **263**:1205, 1960

145. Elder GH et al: Decreased activity of hepatic uroporphyrinogen decarboxylase in sporadic porphyria cutanea tarda. *N Engl J Med* **299**:274, 1978

146. Benedetto AV et al: Porphyria cutanea tarda in three generations of a single family. *N Engl J Med* **298**:358, 1978

147. Roberts AG et al: Heterogeneity of familial porphyria cutanea tarda. *J Med Genet* **25**:669, 1988

148. Held JL et al: Erythrocyte uroporphyrinogen decarboxylase activity in porphyria cutanea tarda: A study of 40 consecutive patients. *J Invest Dermatol* **93**:332, 1989

149. Watson CJ et al: Porphyria variegata and porphyria cutanea tarda in siblings: Chemical and genetic aspects. *Proc Natl Acad Sci USA* **72**:5126, 1975

150. Day RS et al: Coexistent variegate porphyria and porphyria cutanea tarda. *N Engl J Med* **307**:36, 1982

151. Sieg et al: Dual porphyria of coexisting variegata and cutanea tarda. *Eur J Clin Chem* **33**:405, 1995

152. Doss MO: New form of dual porphyria: Coexistent acute intermittent porphyria and porphyria cutanea tarda. *Eur J Clin Invest* **19**:20, 1989

153. Shanley BC et al: Effect of ethanol on liver and aminolevulinate synthetase activity and urinary porphyrin excretion in symptomatic porphyria. *Br J Haematol* **17**:389, 1969

154. McColl KEL et al: Abnormal haem biosynthesis in chronic alcoholics. *Eur J Clin Invest* **11**:461, 1981

155. Hourihane DO, Weir DG: Suppression of erythropoiesis by alcohol. *Br Med J* **1**:86, 1970

156. Kodama T et al: Changes in aminolevulinate synthase and aminolevulinate dehydratase activity and cirrhotic liver. *Gastroenterology* **84**:236, 1983

157. Grossman ME et al: Porphyria cutanea tarda. Clinical features and laboratory findings in 40 patients. *Am J Med* **67**:277, 1979

158. Levere RD: Stilbesterol-induced porphyria: Increase in hepatic delta-aminolevulinic acid synthetase. *Blood* **28**:569, 1966

159. Ochner RK, Schmid R: Acquired porphyria in man and rat due to hexachlorobenzene intoxication. *Nature* **189**:499, 1961

160. Cripps DJ et al: Porphyria turcica. Twenty years after hexachlorobenzene intoxication. *Arch Dermatol* **116**:46, 1980

161. Courtney KD: Hexachlorobenzene (HCB): A review. *Environ Res* **20**:225, 1979

162. Elder GH et al: The effect of the porphyrinogenic compound, hexachlorobenzene, on the activity of hepatic uroporphyrinogen decarboxylase in the rat. *Clin Sci Mol Med* **51**:71, 1976

163. Sinclair PR et al: Chlorinated biphenyls induce cytochrome P450IA2 and uroporphyrin accumulation in cultures of mouse hepatocytes. *Arch Biochem Biophys* **281**:225, 1990

164. Elder GH, Sheppard DM: Immunoreactive uroporphyrinogen decarboxylase is unchanged in porphyria caused by TCDD and hexachlorobenzene. *Biochem Biophys Res Commun* **109**:113, 1982

165. Poland AP, Glover E: 2,3,7,8-Tetrachlorodibenzo-*p*-dioxin: A potent inducer of delta-aminolevulinic acid synthetase. *Science* **179**:476, 1973

166. Schwartz BA et al: Toxicology of chlorinated dibenzo(*p*)dioxins. *Environ Health Perspect* **5**:87, 1973

167. Sweeney GD et al: Iron deficiency prevents liver toxicity of 2,3,7,8-tetrachlorodibenzo-*p*-dioxin. *Science* **204**:332, 1979

168. Jones KG, Sweeney GD: Dependence of the porphyrinogenic effect of 2,3,7,8-tetrachlorodibenzo(*p*)dioxin upon inheritance of aryl hydrocarbon hydroxylase responsiveness. *Toxicol Appl Pharmacol* **53**:42, 1980

169. Kushner JP et al: The role of iron in the pathogenesis of porphyria cutanea tarda. II. Inhibition of uroporphyrinogen decarboxylase. *J Clin Invest* **56**:661, 1975

170. deVerneuil H et al: Purification and properties of uroporphyrinogen decarboxylase from human erythrocytes. A single enzyme catalyzing the four sequential decarboxylations of uroporphyrinogens I and III. *J Biol Chem* **258**:2454, 1983

171. Feldman ES, Bacon BR: Hepatic mitochondrial oxidative metabolism and lipid peroxidation in experimental hexachlorobenzene-induced porphyria with dietary carbonyl iron overload. *Hepatology* 9:686, 1989

172. Roberts AG et al: Increased frequency of the haemochromatosis CYS 282TYR mutation in porphyria cutanea tarda. *Lancet* 349:321,1997

173. Santos M et al: Mutations of the hereditary hemochromatosis candidate gene HLA-H in porphyria cutanea tarda. *New Engl J Med* 336:1327, 1994

174. Bonkovsky HL: Mechanism of iron potentiation of hepatic uroporphyria: Studies in cultured chick embryo liver cells. *Hepatology* 10:354, 1989

175. Kushner JP et al: The role of iron in the pathogenesis of porphyria cutanea tarda: An in vitro model. *J Clin Invest* 51:3044, 1972

176. Garey JR et al: A point mutation in the coding region of uroporphyrinogen decarboxylase associated with familial porphyria cutanea tarda. *Blood* 73:892, 1989

177. Elder GH: The cutaneous porphyrias. *Semin Dermatol* 9:63, 1990

178. Enriquez de Salamanca R et al: Patterns of porphyrin excretion in female estrogen-induced porphyria cutanea tarda. *Arch Dermatol Res* 274:179, 1982

179. Burnett JW, Pathak MA: Effect of light upon porphyrin metabolism of rats. *Arch Dermatol* 89:257, 1964

180. Cam C, Nigogosyan G: Acquired toxic porphyria cutanea tarda due to hexachlorobenzene. *JAMA* 183:88, 1963

181. Solis JA et al: Association of porphyria cutanea tarda and primary liver cancer. *J Dermatol* 9:131, 1982

182. Burnett JW et al: Haemophilia, hepatitis and porphyria. *Br J Dermatol* 97:353, 1977

183. Clemmensen O, Thomsen K: Porphyria cutanea tarda and systemic lupus erythematosus. *Arch Dermatol* 118:160, 1982

184. Poh-Fitzpatrick MB et al: Porphyria cutanea tarda in two patients treated with hemodialysis for chronic renal failure. *N Engl J Med* 299:292, 1978

185. Wissel PS et al: Porphyria cutanea tarda associated with the acquired immune deficiency syndrome. *Am J Hematol* 25:107, 1987

186. Cohen PR et al: Porphyria cutanea tarda in human immunodeficiency virus–infected patients. *JAMA* 264:1315, 1990

187. O'Connor WJ et al: Porphyrin abnormalities in acquired immunodeficiency syndrome. *Arch Dermatol* 132:1443, 1996

188. Daoud MS et al: Chronic hepatitis C and skin diseases: A review. *Mayo Clin Proc* 70:559, 1995

189. Burry JN, Lawrence JR: Phototoxic blisters from high furosemide dosage. *Br J Dermatol* 94:495, 1976

190. Ramsay CA, Obreshkova E: Photosensitivity from nalidixic acid. *Br J Dermatol* 91:523, 1974

191. Epstein JH et al: Porphyria-like cutaneous changes induced by tetracycline hydrochloride photosensitization. *Arch Dermatol* 112:661, 1976

192. Girschich HJ et al: Naproxen-induced pseudoporphyria: Appearance of new skin lesions after discontinuation of treatment. *Scand J Rheumatol* 24:108, 1995

193. Baer RL, Stillman MA: Cutaneous skin changes probably due to pyridoxine abuse. *J Am Acad Dermatol* 10:527, 1984

194. Riordan CA et al: Isotretinoin-associated pseudoporphyria. *Clin Exp Dermatol* 18:69, 1993

195. Goldman CI, Taylor J: Porphyria cutanea tarda and bullous dermatoses associated with chronic renal failure. A review. *Cleve Clin Q* 50:151, 1983

196. Elder GH: Porphyrin metabolism in porphyria cutanea tarda. *Semin Hematol* 14:227, 1977

197. Elder GH et al: Laboratory investigation of the porphyrias. *Ann Clin Biochem* 27:395, 1990

198. Cripps DJ, Peters HA: Fluorescing erythrocytes and porphyrin screening tests on urine, blood and stool. *Arch Dermatol* 96:712, 1967

199. Logan GM et al: Bile porphyrin analysis in the evaluation of variegate porphyria. *N Engl J Med* 324:1408, 1991

200. Kushner JP: Laboratory diagnosis of the porphyrias. *N Engl J Med* 324:1432, 1991

201. Wolff K et al: Microscopic and fine structural aspects of porphyrias. *Acta Derm Venereol (Stockh)* 100(suppl):17, 1982

202. Pathak MA, Burnett JW: The porphyrin content of skin. *J Invest Dermatol* 43:119, 1964

203. Molina L et al: Skin porphyrin assay in porphyria. *Clin Chim Acta* 83:55, 1978

204. Rimington C et al: Porphyria and photosensitivity. *Q J Med* 36:29, 1967

205. Ippen H: Allgemeinsymptome der spaten Hautporphyrie (Porphyria cutanea tarda) als Hisweise fur deren Behandlung. *Dtsch Med Wochenschr* 86:127, 1961

206. Lundvall O: Phlebotomy treatment of porphyria cutanea tarda. *Acta Derm Venereol (Stockh)* 100(suppl):107, 1982

207. Vogler WR et al: Biochemical effects of chloroquine therapy in porphyria cutanea tarda. *Am J Med* 49:316, 1970

208. Kordac V et al: Chloroquine in the treatment of porphyria cutanea tarda. *N Engl J Med* 296:949, 1977

209. Swanbeck G, Wennersten G: Treatment of porphyria cutanea tarda with chloroquine and phlebotomy. *Br J Dermatol* 97:77, 1977

210. Rocchi E et al: Iron removal therapy in porphyria cutanea tarda—phlebotomy versus slow subcutaneous desferroxamine infusion. *Br J Dermatol* 114:621, 1986

211. Praga M et al: Treatment of hemodialysis-related porphyria cutanea tarda with desferroxamine. *N Engl J Med* 316:547, 1987

212. Stathers GM: Porphyrin-binding effect of chloestyramine. *Lancet* 2:780, 1966

213. Anderson KE et al: Erythropoietin for the treatment of porphyria cutanea tarda in a patient on long-term hemodialysis. *N Engl J Med* 322:315, 1990

214. Ramsay CA et al: The treatment of porphyria cutanea tarda by venesection. *Q J Med* 43:1, 1974

215. Mukerji SK, Pimstone NR: Free radical mechanism of oxidation of uroporphyrinogen in the presence of ferrous iron. *Arch Biochem Biophys* 281:177, 1990

216. London ID: Porphyria cutanea tarda: Report of a case successfully treated with chloroquine. *Arch Dermatol* 75:801, 1957

217. Malkinson FD, Levitt L: Hydroxychloroquine treatment of porphyria cutanea tarda. *Arch Dermatol* 116:1147, 1980

218. Scholnick PL et al: The molecular basis of the action of chloroquine in porphyria cutanea tarda. *J Invest Dermatol* 61:226, 1973

219. Taljaard JJF et al: Studies on low-dose chloroquine therapy and the action of chloroquine in symptomatic porphyria. *Br J Dermatol* 87:261, 1972

220. Saltzer EI et al: Porphyria cutanea tarda: Remission following chloroquine administration without adverse effects. *Arch Dermatol* 98:496, 1968

221. Malina L, Chlumsky J: A comparative study of the results of phlebotomy therapy and low-dose chloroquine treatment in porphyria cutanea tarda. *Acta Derm Venereol (Stockh)* 61:346, 1981

222. Cainelli T et al: Hydroxychloroquine versus phlebotomy in the treatment of porphyria cutanea tarda. *Br J Dermatol* 108:593, 1983

223. Chlumska A et al: Liver changes in porphyria cutanea tarda patients treated with chloroquine. *Br J Dermatol* 102:261, 1980

224. Mustajoki P: Acute intermittent porphyria. *Semin Dermatol* 5:155, 1986

225. Elder GH et al: The acute porphyrias. *Lancet* 349:1613, 1997

226. DeMatteis F: Disturbances of liver porphyrin metabolism caused by drugs. *Pharmacol Rev* 17:523, 1967

227. McColl KEL, Moore MR: The acute porphyrias—an example of pharmacogenetic disease. *Scott Med J* 26:32, 1981

228. Grandchamp B et al: Tissue-specific expression of porphobilinogen deaminase. Two isozymes from a single gene. *Eur J Biochem* 1621:105, 1987

229. Crimlisk HL: The little imitator—porphyria: A neuropsychiatric disorder. *J Neurol Neurosurg Psych* 62:319, 1997

230. McDougall AJ, McLeod JG: Autonomic neuropathy. II: Specific peripheral neuropathies. *J Neurol Sci* 138:1, 1996

231. Hoesch K: Über die Auswertung der Urobilinogenurie und die "umgekehrte" Urobilinogenurie. *Dtsch Med Wochenschr* 72:704, 1947

232. Tiepermann RV, Doss M: Simple diagnostic test for urinary porphobilinogen and porphyrins, in *Porphyrins in Human Diseases,* First International Porphyrin Meeting, Freiburg, edited by M Doss, P Nawrocki. Basel, Karger, 1976, p 249

233. Mustajoki P et al: Heme in the treatment of porphyrias and hematological disorders. *Semin Hematol* 26:1, 1989

234. Mustajoki P, Nordmann Y: Early administration of heme argmate for acute porphyric attacks. *Arch Intern Med* 153: 2004, 1993

235. Anderson KE et al: Gonadotropin releasing hormone analogue prevents cyclical attacks of porphyria. *Arch Intern Med* 150:1469, 1990

236. Barnes HD: Further South African cases of porphyrinuria. *S Afr J Clin Sci* 2:117, 1951

237. Dean G, Barnes HD: The inheritance of porphyria. *Br Med J* **2**:89, 1955
238. Dean G: *The Porphyrias*. Philadelphia, Lippincott, 1963
239. Dailey HA, Dailey TA: Characteristics of human protoporphyrinogen oxidase in controls and variegate porphyrias. *Cell Mol Biol* **43**:67, 1997
240. Meissner PN et al: A R59W mutation in human protoporphyrinogen oxidase results in decreased enzyme activity and is prevalent in South Africans with variegate porphyria. *Nat Genet* **13**:95, 1996
241. Warnich L et al: Identification of three mutations and associated haplotypes in the protoporphyrinogen oxidase gene in South African families with variegate porphyria. *Hum Mol Genet* **5**:981, 1996
242. Lam H-M et al: Molecular basis of variegate porphyria: A de novo insertion mutation in the protoporphyrinogen oxidase gene. *Hum Genet* **99**:126, 1997
243. Hift RJ et al: Homozygous variegate porphyria: An evolving clinical syndrome. *Postgrad Med J* **69**:781, 1993
244. Rimington C et al: The excretion of porphyrin-peptide conjugates in porphyria variegata. *Clin Sci* **35**:211, 1968
245. Elder GH et al: Faecal "X" porphyrin in the hepatic porphyrias. *Enzyme* **17**:29, 1974
246. Eales L et al: The place of screening tests and quantitative investigations in the diagnosis of the porphyrias, with particular reference to variegate and symptomatic porphyria. *S Afr Med J* **40**:63, 1966
247. Poh-Fitzpatrick MB: A plasma porphyrin fluorescence marker for variegate porphyria. *Arch Dermatol* **116**:543, 1980
248. Cramers M, Jepsen LV: Porphyria variegata: Failure of chloroquine treatment. *Acta Derm Venereol* **60**:89, 1980
249. Perrot H et al: La porphyrie variegata (à propos de 4 cas). *Lyon Med* **235**:905, 1976
250. Watson CJ et al: Studies of coproporphyrin III. Idiopathic coproporphyrinuria, a hitherto unrecognized form characterized by lack of symptoms in spite of the excretion of large amounts of coproporphyrin. *J Clin Invest* **28**:465, 1949
251. Goldberg A et al: Hereditary coproporphyria. *Lancet* **1**:632, 1967
252. Brodie NJ et al: Hereditary coproporphyria. *Q J Med* **46**:229, 1977
253. Fujita H et al: Characterization and expression of cDNA encoding coproporphyrinogen oxidase from a patient with hereditary coproporphyria. *Hum Mol Genet* **3**:1807, 1994
254. Sassa S et al: Molecular defects of the coproporphyrinogen oxidase gene in hereditary coproporphyria. *Cell Mol Biol* **43**:59, 1997
255. Elder GH et al: The primary enzyme defect in hereditary coproporphyria. *Lancet* **2**:1217, 1976
256. McIntyre N et al: Hepatic delta-aminolevulinic acid synthetase in an attack of hereditary coproporphyria and during remission. *Lancet* **1**:560, 1971
257. Herrero C et al: Acquired immunodeficiency syndrome in a patient affected by hereditary coproporphyria: Safety of zidovudine treatment. *Arch Dermatol* **126**:122, 1990
258. Lamoril J et al: A molecular defect in coproporphyrinogen oxidase gene causing harderoporphyria, a variant form of hereditary coproporphyria. *Hum Mol Genet* **4**:275, 1995
259. Moder KG: A coproporphyria-like syndrome induced by glipizide. *Mayo Clin Proc* **66**:312, 1991
260. Hunter JAA et al: Hereditary coproporphyria: Photosensitivity, jaundice and neuropsychiatric manifestations associated with pregnancy. *Br J Dermatol* **84**:301, 1971
261. Pinõl-Aguadé J et al: Hepato-erythrocytic porphyria: A new type of porphyria. *Ann Dermatol Syphiligr (Paris)* **102**:129, 1975
262. Lim HW, Poh-Fitzpatrick MB: Hepatoerythropoietic porphyria: A variant of childhood-onset porphyria cutanea tarda. *J Am Acad Dermatol* **11**:1103, 1984
263. Toback AG et al: Hepatoerythropoietic porphyria: Clinical, biochemical, and enzymatic studies in a three generation family lineage. *N Engl J Med* **316**:646, 1987
264. Romana M et al: Identification of a new mutation responsible for hepatoerythropoietic porphyria. *Eur J Clin Invest* **21**:225, 1991
265. Thunell S et al: Aminolevulinate dehydratase porphyria: A clinical and biochemical study. *J Clin Chem Clin Biochem* **25**:5, 1987
266. Ishida N et al: Message amplification phenotyping of an inherited δ-aminolevulinate dehydratase deficiency in a family with acute hepatic porphyria. *Biochem Biophys Res Commun* **172**:237, 1990
267. Sato Y et al: A case of sideroblastic anemia with dermal photosensitivity and increased erythrocyte protoporphyrin. *Jpn J Clin Hematol* **22**:1971, 1981
268. Lim HW et al: Photosensitivity, abnormal porphyrin profile, and sideroblastic anemia—a case report and review of the literature. *J Am Acad Dermatol* **27**:287, 1992
269. Frank J, Christiano AM: Genetic research strategies: A review of the acute porphyrias. *Retinoids* **13**:92, 1997
270. deVerneuil H et al: Porphyrias: Animal models and prospects for cellular and gene therapy. *J Bioenerg Biomembr* **27**:239, 1995

Xanthomatoses and Lipoprotein Disorders

XANTHOMAS, HYPERLIPIDEMIA, AND DYSLIPOPROTEINEMIAS

Lipoproteins consist of small particles that transport lipids in the circulation. The major lipids carried in lipoproteins include cholesterol, triglycerides, and phospholipids. An elevation of serum lipid levels is called *hyperlipidemia*, or *hyperlipoproteinemia*. The term *dyslipoproteinemia* signifies abnormalities in serum lipoproteins, whether or not serum lipid levels are categorically elevated. Several disorders of lipoprotein metabolism promote the development of coronary atherosclerosis, the precursor of coronary heart disease (CHD). The infiltration and deposition of lipoproteins into tissues, however, are not limited to the arterial tree. Lipoproteins can also enter into skin, subcutaneous tissues, and tendons, where lipids can accumulate to produce xanthomas. Of clinical interest, different species of lipoproteins typically produce different types of xanthomas. Thus, the pattern of xanthomas observed in a particular patient provides important clues as to the type of hyperlipoproteinemia (or dyslipoproteinemia) present. Before a discussion of specific dyslipoproteinemias, however, an overview of normal metabolism of lipoproteins is needed to set the stage for consideration of abnormalities in their metabolism.

LIPOPROTEINS AND THEIR METABOLISM

Chylomicrons

Most of the lipid consumed in the diet consists of triacylglycerol (triglyceride). In the intestine, triglycerides are hydrolyzed by pancreatic lipase into fatty acids and monoglycerides. These are solubilized by the bile and are taken up by the intestinal mucosa. In the enterocyte, fatty acids and monoglycerides are resynthesized into triglycerides and are incorporated into lipoproteins called *chylomicrons*. An enterocyte protein called *microsomal lipid transfer protein* is responsible for transferring triglycerides into chylomicron particles. Chylomicrons are particles composed of an inner core containing triglycerides plus small amounts of cholesterol ester and a surface coat composed of unesterified cholesterol, phospholipids, and proteins (apolipoproteins). The major apolipoprotein of chylomicron is called apo B-48; other apolipoproteins are named apo C-II, apo C-III, apo E, apo A-I, and apo A-IV. All of these apolipoproteins play special roles in the metabolism of chylomicrons.

Chylomicrons are secreted into the intestinal lymph and enter the systemic circulation through the thoracic duct (Fig. 152-1). They pass into the capillary bed of the peripheral circulation where they

FIGURE 152-1

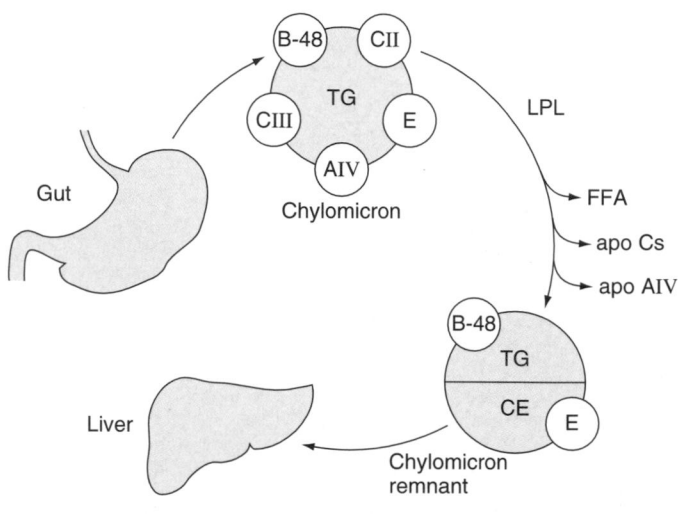

Metabolism of chylomicrons (see text for details).

come into contact with an enzyme, lipoprotein lipase (LPL). This enzyme, which is located on the endothelial surface of capillaries, hydrolyzes the triglycerides of chylomicrons into fatty acids. Several other surface components of chylomicrons are lost to the circulation during triglyceride lipolysis. When most triglycerides of chylomicrons have been hydrolyzed by LPL, a residual particle, called a *chylomicron remnant*, returns to the circulation. The core lipid of chylomicron remnants contains large amounts of cholesterol ester. Chylomicron remnants disappear quickly from the circulation because of uptake by the liver. Removal of chylomicron remnants is facilitated by the presence of apo Es.

Very Low Density Lipoproteins

Another class of triglyceride-rich lipoprotein derives from the liver. This class includes the very low density lipoproteins (VLDLs). VLDL particles contain less triglyceride than chylomicrons but relatively more cholesterol. Their synthesis in hepatocytes resembles chylomicron synthesis in enterocytes. In contrast to chylomicrons, however, VLDL particles contain apo B-100 as their major apolipoprotein; they also have apo Cs and apo Es. The total amount of triglyceride secreted daily associated with VLDL is only about one-fourth that entering with chylomicrons when dietary fat intake is that of the typical American diet. Newly secreted VLDL particles are named *nascent VLDLs*.

FIGURE 152-2

CHAPTER 152
Xanthomatoses and Lipoprotein Disorders

1805

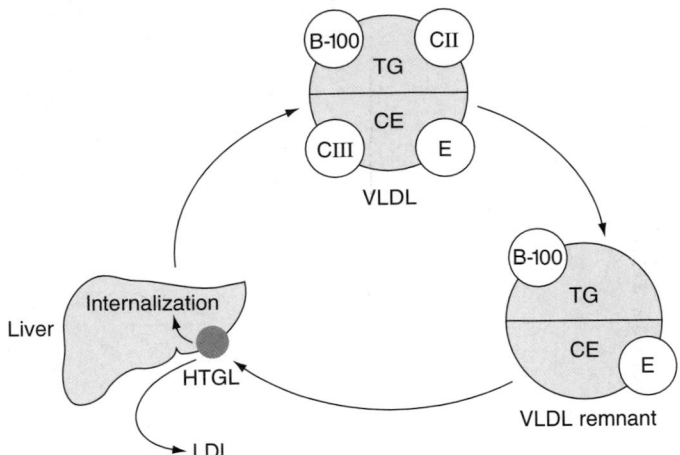

Metabolism of very low density lipoproteins (VLDL) (see text for details).

Like chylomicrons, circulating VLDLs pass into the peripheral circulation where they interact with LPL. This interaction hydrolyzes most of the VLDL triglycerides (Fig. 152-2). After much triglyceride is removed, a residual particle, called a *VLDL remnant,* returns to the circulation. Once VLDL remnants are formed, they can have two fates. About half of VLDL remnants are removed directly by hepatic uptake facilitated by apo E. A portion of VLDL remnant uptake occurs via receptors for low-density lipoproteins (LDL). The receptors are located on the surface of liver cells; they bind both to apo E and apo B-100 but not to apo B-48. When VLDL remnants attach to liver cells, many are internalized and degraded; however, a portion of these particles interacts with hepatic triglyceride lipase, which removes residual triglycerides and converts them into LDL (Fig. 152-3). Newly formed LDL particles are released from hepatocytes and returned to the circulation.

FIGURE 152-3

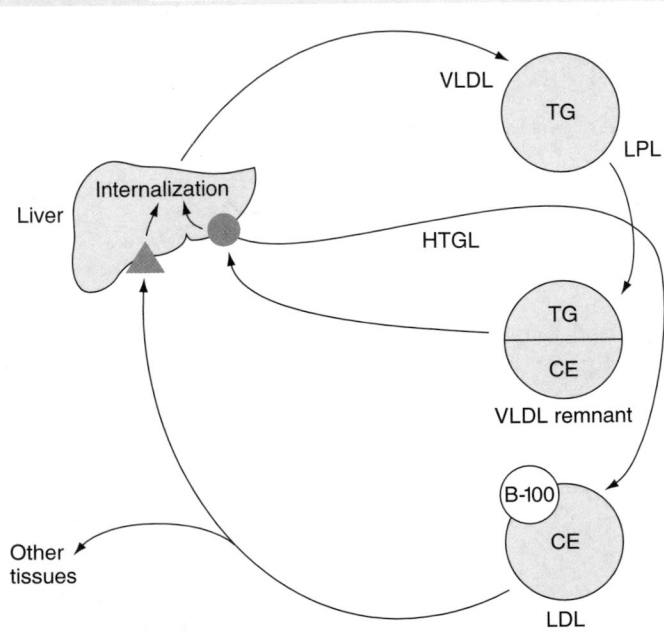

Metabolism of low-density lipoproteins (LDL) (see text for details).

Low-Density Lipoproteins

LDL particles carry most of the cholesterol present in the fasting serum (Fig. 152-3). LDLs are smaller than VLDLs and contain mostly cholesterol esters in their lipid cores. The only apolipoprotein of LDL is apo B-100. Removal rates of LDL from the circulation are slower than for VLDL; hence there is a tendency for LDL particles to accumulate in serum. This slow rate of removal for LDL explains why serum LDL concentrations typically exceed those of VLDL. About three-fourths of circulating LDL is removed through LDL receptors on liver cells. Lesser amounts of LDL are cleared via nonreceptor pathways or by extrahepatic tissues. When LDL particles bind to LDL receptors, they are internalized and pass into lysosomes, where they are degraded.

High-Density Lipoproteins

This category of lipoproteins has unique properties. High-density lipoproteins (HDLs) seem to have a "clean-up" function. During lipid transport through triglyceride-rich lipoproteins (chylomicrons and VLDL), many component molecules are released to the circulation (Fig. 152-4). They are taken up by HDL particles and are either removed from circulation or recycled to triglyceride-rich lipoproteins. Components of triglyceride-rich lipoproteins that are transferred to HDL during their catabolism include unesterified (free) cholesterol, phospholipids, apo Cs, apo Es, apo As, and small amounts of triglyceride. Some apo A-I and apo A-II molecules on HDL are also derived by direct secretion from the liver. Excess unesterified (free) cholesterol in the membranes of peripheral tissue cells may be taken up by HDL. This latter uptake is the first step of a process called *reverse cholesterol transport;* the process is so named because cholesterol synthesized in peripheral tissues is eventually returned to the liver for its disposal from the body. All of these components may be removed from the circulation through direct tissue uptake of HDL; alternatively, apo Cs, apo Es, and cholesterol esters can be shuttled back to nascent triglyceride-rich lipoprotein for reutilization in their catabolism.

FIGURE 152-4

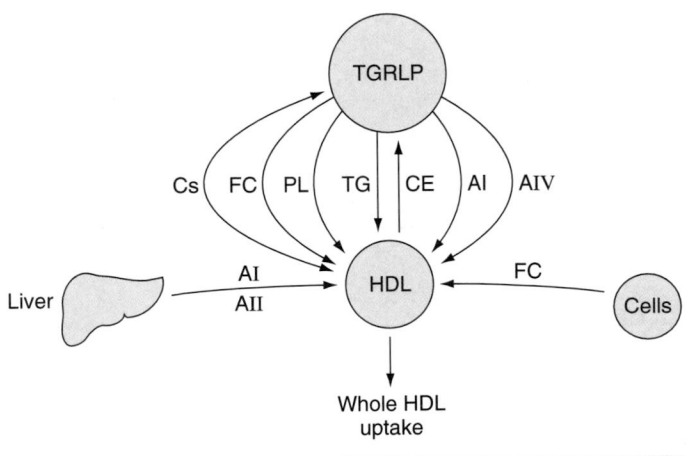

Metabolism of high-density lipoproteins (HDL) (see text for details).

HYPERCHOLESTEROLEMIA

The term *hypercholesterolemia* is usually taken to mean an increase in serum LDL-cholesterol concentrations. LDL has been identified as the major atherogenic lipoprotein by the National Cholesterol Education Program (NCEP).[1,2] Evidence of many types—epidemiologic, animal models, clinical forms of hypercholesterolemia, tissue culture studies, and clinical trials—supports the concept that elevated serum LDL concentrations are atherogenic and a major cause of CHD. The NCEP has classified both total cholesterol and LDL-cholesterol levels in terms of risk for CHD.[1,2] Approximate comparable values for total cholesterol and LDL cholesterol are shown in Table 152-1. In the discussion to follow, severe forms of hypercholesterolemia will be considered first. These forms illustrate clearly the mechanisms of hypercholesterolemia, and they are commonly accompanied by xanthomas.

Familial Hypercholesterolemia

The primary defect in familial hypercholesterolemia (FH) is a genetic deficiency of LDL receptors.[3] Normally, two functional alleles encoding for LDL receptors are inherited—one from each parent. Both inherited LDL receptors function in removal of LDL from the circulation. The synthesis and expression of cell surface receptors is a multistep process. Defects occurring at several of these multiple steps can produce the clinical picture of FH.[4] In some cases, the functional activity of the receptor produced by a defective allele is zero; in other cases, mutations in the receptor gene or associated genes produce defective receptor function.

In rare individuals, approximately 1 per 1 million persons in the general population, defective alleles for the LDL receptors are inherited from each parent. These doubly affected persons thus have *homozygous FH*.[4] They have either no LDL-receptor activity or only a very little activity. Their serum LDL-cholesterol levels are markedly elevated, often in the range of 800 to 1000 mg/dL. They commonly develop CHD or other forms of atherosclerotic disease before their teenage years. Patients with homozygous FH usually have severe xanthomatosis. Multiple types of xanthomas are found (Fig. 152-5). These include tuberous xanthomas (especially over the elbows), subperiosteal xanthomas (below the knees and over the olecranon process), tendon xanthomas (especially in the Achilles tendon and in the extensor tendon of the hand), and elevated xanthomatous plaques (over the extremities, buttocks, and hands).

Several forms of therapy have been proposed for homozygous FH. Since LDL-receptor function is largely absent, drugs that act by enhancing LDL-receptor activity produce little benefit. Such agents include bile acid sequestrants and lower doses of HMG-CoA reductase inhibitors (statins). High doses of statins, however, may cause moderate reductions in LDL-cholesterol levels in homozygous FH patients, probably by partial inhibition of VLDL secretion. A more radical approach to treatment of homozygous FH is liver transplantation.[5] This procedure supplies normal LDL receptors from the donor liver and markedly lowers LDL levels. A more practical approach is to remove LDL periodically from the circulation by plasmapheresis or LDL-apheresis.[6] The latter approach employs a variety of LDL-binding agents and is currently the preferred therapy.

A more common form of FH is *heterozygous FH*. This condition occurs from inheritance of a single abnormal allele for the LDL receptor. Serum LDL-cholesterol levels are approximately twice normal. The prevalence of heterozygous FH is about one in 500 people. Men with heterozygous FH commonly develop CHD in their thirties and forties; affected women typically manifest CHD in their fifties and sixties. In contrast to patients with homozygous FH, heterozygotes only rarely show tuberous xanthomas; tendon xanthomas, however, are common (Fig. 152-6). In fact, the majority of patients with tendon xanthomas will be found to have heterozygous FH. Less common causes of tendon xanthomas will be discussed later.

The statins have proven to be effective drugs for treatment of heterozygous FH.[7] These agents inhibit HMG-CoA reductase, the rate-limiting enzyme in cholesterol synthesis.[8] A reduction in cellular cholesterol content sends a signal to the nucleus of the cell to stimulate the synthesis of LDL receptors. In patients with heterozygous FH, the one functional allele for the LDL receptor is "upregulated" by statin therapy; this supplies more LDL receptors and reduces serum LDL levels. There are currently five statins available for treatment of hypercholesterolemia; these are listed, along with their approximate equivalent doses, in Table 152-2. All have a similar mechanism of action, although the dose required to produce a given LDL-cholesterol lowering varies among the drugs. Each of the doses shown in Table 152-2 produces an approximate 30 percent lowering of serum LDL-cholesterol levels. Each doubling of the dose above those shown leads to another 6 percent reduction of LDL-cholesterol levels. The frequency of side effects appears to correlate with LDL-lowering efficacy, i.e., higher doses cause more side effects. The major side effects of statins are myopathy and hepatotoxicity. These side effects are relatively rare but increase in frequency with increasing doses. The risk for myopathy is increased substantially when the statin is given with either a fibric acid (e.g., gemfibrozil) or cyclosporine. In patients with heterozygous FH, the lowering of LDL-cholesterol levels can be substantially enhanced by combining a statin with a bile acid sequestrant (e.g., cholestyramine or colestipol).

Familial Defective Apolipoprotein B-100

Familial defective apolipoprotein B-100 (FDB) is another cause of moderately severe hypercholesterolemia.[9,10] In this condition, the primary structure of apo B-100 is defective, and apo B thus binds poorly to LDL receptors. As a result, serum LDL levels are raised. Patients with FDB frequently resemble those with heterozygous FH except that they typically have somewhat lower LDL-cholesterol levels. Most patients with FDB are heterozygotes, and only half their LDL particles are defective in binding to LDL receptors. Rare patients are ho-

TABLE 152-1

Classification of Total Cholesterol and Low-Density Lipoprotein (LDL) Cholesterol

	TOTAL CHOLESTEROL		LDL CHOLESTEROL	
CATEGORY	CONCENTRATION, MG/DL	CATEGORY		CONCENTRATION, MG/DL
Desirable	<200	Desirable		<130
Borderline-high	200–239	Borderline–high risk		130–159
High	≥240	High risk		≥160

FIGURE 152-5

CHAPTER 152
Xanthomatoses and Lipoprotein Disorders   1807

FIGURE 152-6

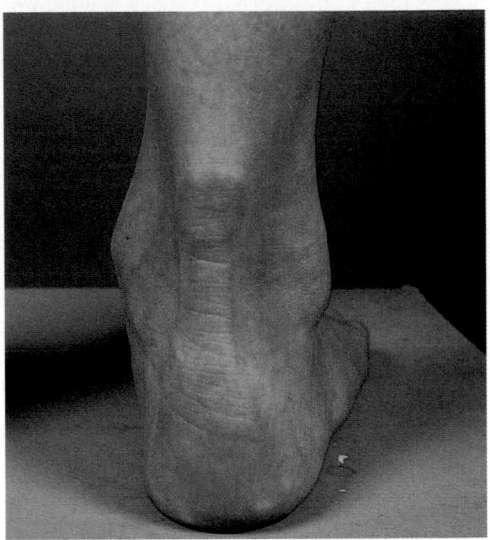

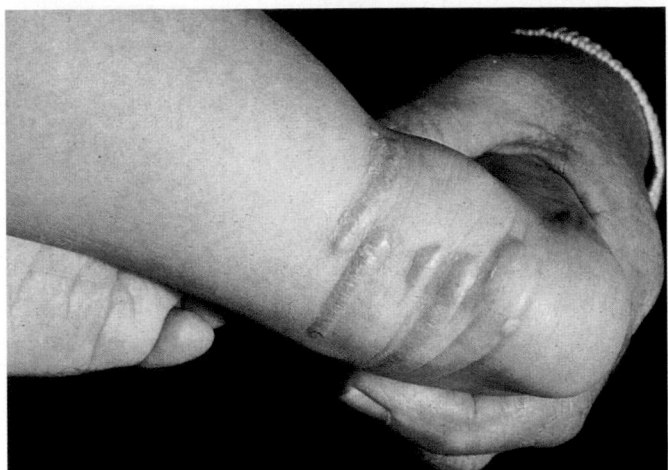

A.

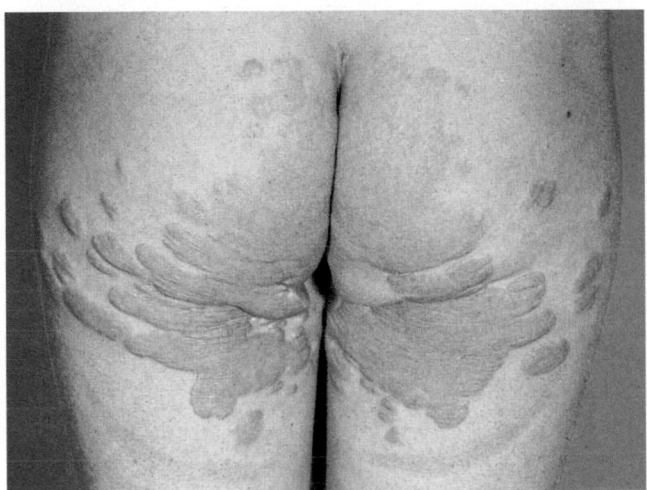

B.

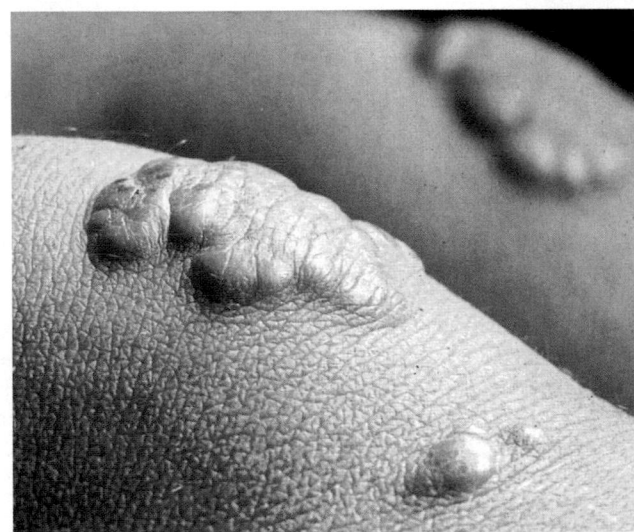

C.

Xanthomas typical of homozygous familial hypercholesterolemia.

Tendon xanthomas typical of heterozygous familial hypercholesterolemia. Similar xanthomas occur in patients with familial defective apolipoprotein B-100, cerebrontindinous xanthomatosis, and sitosterolemia.

mozygous and have more severe hypercholesterolemia, although usually not to the degree seen in patients with homozygous FH. Some patients with heterozygous FDB develop tendon xanthomas that are identical in appearance to those associated with heterozygous FH. Patients with FDB are prone to premature CHD,[11] and their hypercholesterolemia usually responds well to statin therapy.

Moderate Hypercholesterolemia

Most patients with primary hypercholesterolemia have only moderate elevations of serum LDL-cholesterol levels (e.g., 160 to 219 mg/dL). Multiple mechanisms appear to underlie primary moderate hypercholesterolemia; these include reductions in LDL-receptor activity, overproduction of lipoproteins containing apo B-100, and enrichment of LDL particles with cholesterol ester.[12,13] Approximately 20 percent of American adults have moderate hypercholesterolemia.[1,2] These persons are at increased risk for premature CHD, although less so than are those with severe forms of genetic hypercholesterolemia (i.e., FH and FDB). Patients with moderate hypercholesterolemia rarely have xanthomas, although one such patient

TABLE 152-2

HMG-CoA Reductase Inhibitors

Drug	Trade Name	Equivalent Dose, mg
Lovastatin	Mevacor	40
Pravastatin	Pravachol	40
Simvastatin	Zocor	20
Fluvastatin	Lescol	80
Atorvastatin	Lipitor	10

with severe xanthomas in the Achilles tendons has been studied.[14] Presumably, tissue susceptibility in patients of this type combines with moderately high LDL levels to produce xanthomas.

CHYLOMICRONEMIA

Another severe form of hyperlipidemia is one in which triglyceride levels are markedly elevated. When triglyceride levels are below 500 mg/dL, most of the triglycerides are carried in VLDLs. At higher concentrations, chylomicrons begin to accumulate in the serum. Some patients manifest severe chylomicronemia with triglyceride levels ranging from 1000 to 10,000 mg/dL. These marked elevations result from either severe genetic defects in triglyceride metabolism or moderate genetic defects combined with aggravating acquired factors.

Lipoprotein Lipase Deficiency

Rare patients are homozygous for genetic defects in LPL function.[15] A large series of mutations in the LPL gene that prevent the normal function of LPL has been identified. Patients who are homozygous for LPL defects typically manifest severe chylomicronemia. Triglyceride levels can be severely elevated from birth. When serum triglyceride concentrations exceed 2000 mg/dL, patients are at high risk for developing acute pancreatitis. Triglyceride levels in this range are often associated with eruptive skin xanthomas (Fig. 152-7). These lesions are white to yellow papules on a slightly erythematous base. Sometimes, they coalesce to form larger cutaneous plaques. Typical locations are over the buttocks, shoulders, and extensor surfaces of the extremities. Their rapid appearance usually signifies a striking rise of triglyceride concentrations. Patients with LPL deficiency generally are *not* at increased risk for CHD; the prevailing view has been that chylomicrons are too large to filter into the arterial wall to initiate atherogenesis. Although a few patients with LPL deficiency have manifested some atherosclerosis, premature CHD is rare. Patients who are heterozygous for LPL deficiency either have normal serum triglycerides or have mild hypertriglyceridemia.

There are no available drugs that can treat the severe chylomicronemia of LPL deficiency effectively. The most effective management is through dietary modification. The formation of chylomicrons can be curtailed by reducing the fat content of the diet. The intake of dietary fat should be reduced to less than 10 percent of total calories. Medium-chain triglycerides (MCTs) can be used as a substitute for dietary fat. The fatty acids of MCT are not incorporated into chylomicrons; thus, 10 to 15 percent of total calories can be safely consumed as MCTs. The goal of therapy is to keep total triglyceride levels below 1500 mg/dL, which will greatly reduce the risk for pancreatitis.

Apo C-II Deficiency

Apo C-II is carried on triglyceride-rich lipoproteins and is required for activation of LPL. Rare patients have a congenital absence of apo C-II. These patients develop severe chylomicronemia resembling that with LPL deficiency.[16] They also manifest skin xanthomas identical to those of patients deficient in LPL. Treatment of

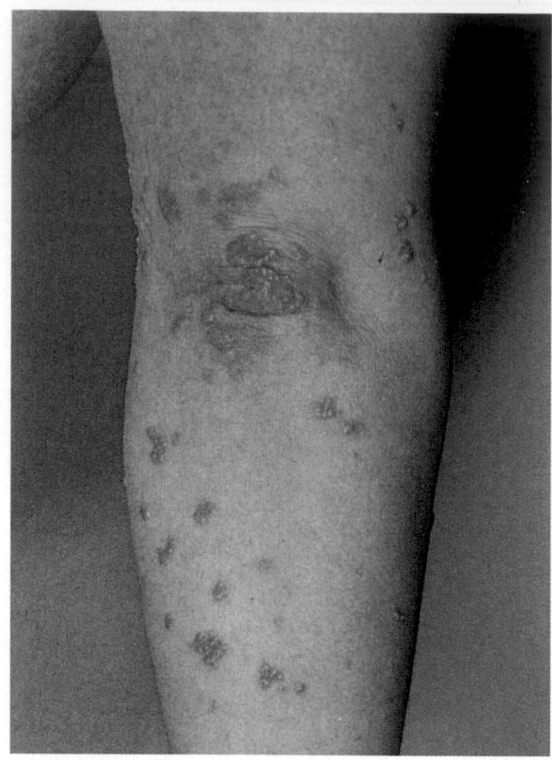

Eruptive skin xanthomas characteristic of severe chylomicronemia.

chylomicronemia associated with apo C-II deficiency is the same as in patients with LPL deficiency.

Chylomicronemia Combined with Endogenous Hypertriglyceridemia (Type 5 Hyperlipoproteinemia)

This disorder is defined by combined elevations in levels of chylomicrons and VLDL. Most cases appear to result from a dual defect in triglyceride metabolism, namely, overproduction of VLDL and defective lipolysis of triglyceride-rich lipoproteins.[17] Both abnormalities can have multiple causes. Overproduction of VLDL is commonly due to obesity and may be accentuated by non-insulin-dependent diabetes mellitus. There is growing evidence that hepatic overproduction of VLDL is frequently the result of insulin resistance; the latter in turn can be due to either a primary metabolic abnormality or obesity. Defective lipolysis of triglyceride-rich lipoproteins can occur in the heterozygous state for LPL mutations or from functional reduction of LPL activity.[15] Recent evidence also suggests that high serum levels of apo C-III, an inhibitor of LPL activity, can also cause defective lipolysis.[18] Elevated serum apo C-III levels may be secondary to insulin resistance.[19] Thus insulin resistance appears to cause *both* overproduction of VLDL and defective lipolysis of triglycerides in VLDL and chylomicrons; both defects are characteristic of type 5 hyperlipoproteinemia.[17] Patients with type 5 hyperlipoproteinemia appear to be at increased risk for CHD, and they commonly manifest peripheral arterial disease. The risk for acute pancreatitis rises sharply when triglyceride levels exceed 2000 mg/dL. At this triglyceride level, eruptive skin xanthomas also commonly appear. Treatment of type 5 hyperlipoproteinemia consists of a very low fat diet (<10 percent of total calories as fat) and fibric acids (e.g., gemfibrozil). In addition, weight reduction in obese patients will reduce triglyceride levels, as will improved glucose control in diabetic patients.

FIGURE 152-8

DEFECTIVE METABOLISM OF LIPOPROTEIN REMNANTS (DYSBETALIPOPROTEINEMIA)

Dysbetalipoproteinemia (type 3 hyperlipoprotienemia) denotes a category of lipid disorders defined by accumulation in serum of remnant lipoproteins, i.e., chylomicron remnants and VLDL remnants.[20] The usual abnormality is the presence of an abnormal isoform of apo E, named *apo E$_2$*. Normal isoforms are apo E$_3$ and apo E$_4$; these isoforms promote remnant uptake by the liver. When apo E$_2$ is present, especially in the homozygous form of the disease, remnant uptake is impaired; as a result, remnant lipoproteins are removed slowly and accumulate in the serum. Isolated homozygous apo E$_2$ typically produces mild remnant accumulation but not categorical hyperlipidemia. However, hyperlipidemia of the dysbetalipoproteinemic type can develop when lipoprotein metabolism is otherwise disturbed, i.e., in patients with obesity, diabetes mellitus, or endogenous hypertriglyceridedmia. Typically, in hyperlipidemic patients with dysbetalipoproteinemia, serum concentrations of cholesterol and triglycerides are about equally raised. The cholesterol-to-triglyceride ratio in the VLDL fraction usually exceeds 0.30. A definite diagnosis of dysbetalipoproteinemia is made by identifying the apo E$_2$ isoform.

Hyperlipidemic patients with dysbetalipoproteinemia are at increased risk for CHD and often have peripheral arterial disease. About two thirds of these patients have tuberoeruptive and tuberous xanthomas (Fig. 152-8). Also, they have a characteristic lipid deposition in the creases of the palms of the hands (xanthoma striata palmaris) (Figs. 152-8B, 152-9). Occasionally, patients manifest tendon xanthomas and xanthelasma. Some patients with dysbetalipoproteinemia exhibit tuberous xanthoma in the absence of raised serum levels of total cholesterol and triglyceride; in these patients, tissue susceptibility combined with increased remnant lipoproteins appear to be responsible for tuberous xanthomas. Tuberous xanthomas of the hands have been observed in two normolipidemic patients who were homozygous for apo E$_2$. In one patient, xanthomas apparently developed in the fingers because of heavy manual labor[21]; the other tuberous xanthomas resulted from the presence of apo E$_2$ combined with a form of histiocytosis. The hyperlipidemia in most patients with dysbetalipoproteinemia is responsive to fibric acids or nicotinic acid; however, if total cholesterol levels are markedly raised, statin therapy is more effective. Reducing serum lipids with drug therapy often causes xanthomas to regress.

DEFECTS IN HDL METABOLISM

Tangier Disease

This rare condition is characterized by profound deficiency of serum HDL.[22] The catabolism of HDL appears to be markedly increased in Tangier disease, which noticeably lowers serum HDL concentrations; the reasons for this excessive catabolism of HDL are unknown. Tangier homozygotes manifest accumulation of cholesterol esters in tonsils, spleen, lymph nodes, bone narrow, skin, thymus, and intestinal mucosa. These accumulations most commonly produce tonsillar hyperplasia, mild lymphadenopathy, and splenomeg-

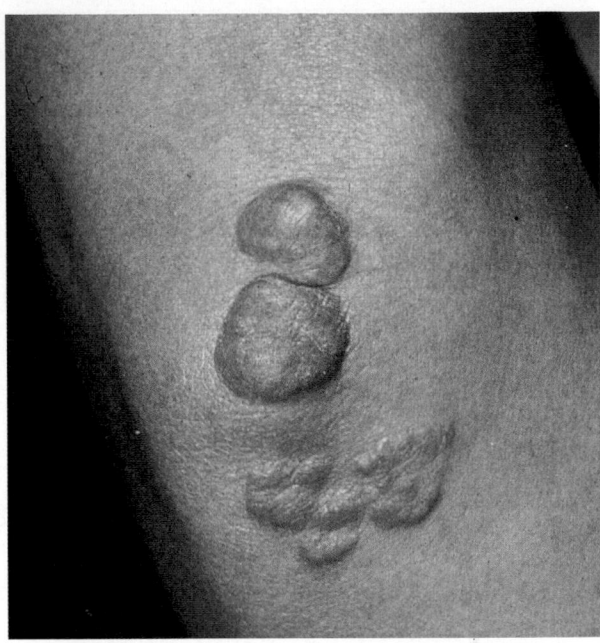

A.

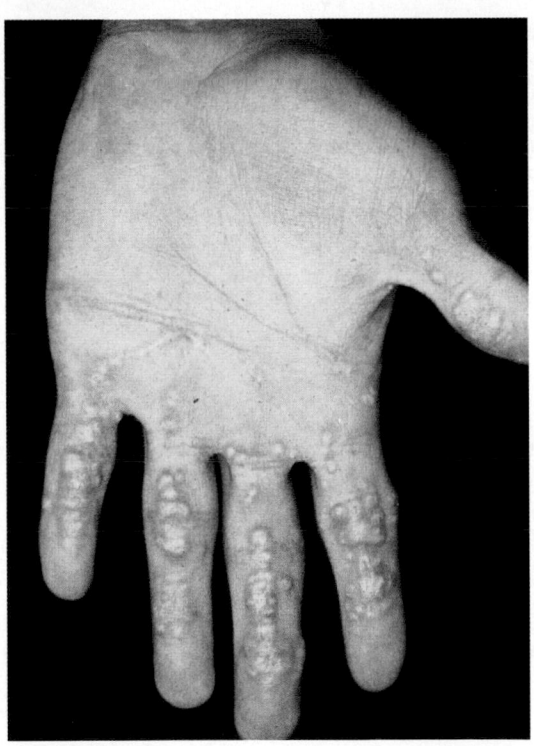

B.

Tuberoeruptive and tuberous xanthomas typical of familial dysbetalipoproteinemia.

aly. Older patients with Tangier disease often develop CHD. Despite widespread tissue accumulation of cholesterol esters, skin xanthomas are not prominent.

FIGURE 152-9

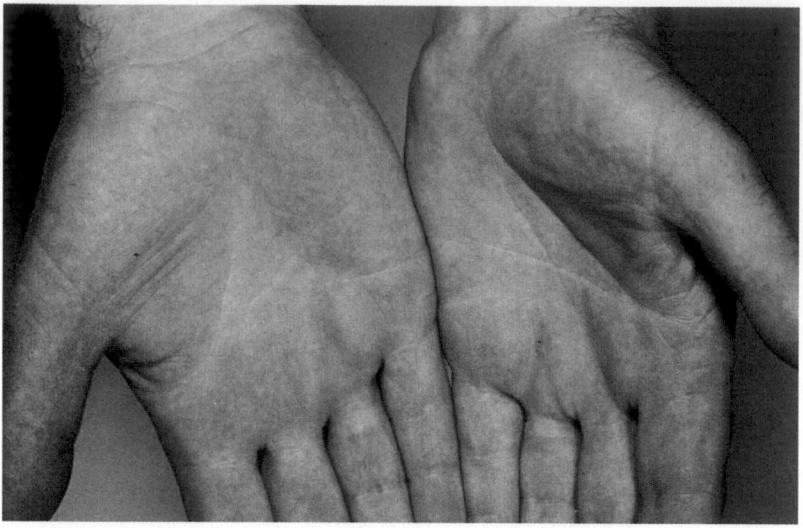

Xanthoma striata palmaris characteristic of familial dysbetalipoproteinemia.

HDL Deficiency with Plane Xanthomas

Mutations in apo A-I can reduce its synthesis and produce HDL deficiency.[23] In some cases, there is a concomitant defect in synthesis of apo C-III and apo A-IV. When the latter defects are present, complex abnormalities are present in lipoprotein metabolism, and affected patients are prone to premature CHD. Patients with defects limited to synthesis of apo A-I may manifest plane xanthomas.[24] It is uncertain whether these patients are prone to premature CHD; however, they do not appear to develop fulminant atherosclerosis, as do patients with homozygous FH.

LCAT Deficiency Syndrome

Lecithin-cholesterol acyl transferase (LCAT) is an enzyme responsible for esterification of cholesterol in plasma. Congenital defects in LCAT synthesis produce abnormalities in the metabolism of HDL and other lipoproteins.[25] Several such congenital defects have been discovered that produce related syndromes of varying degrees of clinical severity. The major clinical features include corneal infiltrates and opacity, anemia, and proteinemia. Xanthomatous deposits of the skin or tendons have not been reported with LCAT deficiency syndromes.

DISORDERS OF STEROL METABOLISM

Cerebrotendinous Xanthomatosis

Cerebrotendinous xanthomatosis (CTX) is a rare recessive disorder in which xanthomas occur in the tendons and brain.[26] The genetic abnormality is a defect in the conversion of cholesterol into bile acids in the liver. A by-product of this defect is an increased synthesis of a sterol named *cholestanol*. Accumulation of this abnormal sterol in the serum apparently is responsible for xanthomas in the brain and tendons. Cerebroxanthomatosis causes several neurologic manifestations. Patients with CTX also appear to be at increased risk for CHD. Treatment consists of replacement of the bile acid pool with oral chenodeoxycholic acid. This therapy reduces cholestanol synthesis and has been reported to alleviate neurologic symptoms.

Sitosterolemia

This rare disorder results from accumulation of plant sterols in the serum.[26] The major plant sterol in the serum is β-sitosterol; other plant sterols are increased as well, but to a lesser extent. The molecular defect in sitosterolemia is unknown; however, the metabolic abnormality appears to be a defective transfer of sterols into bile for excretion.[27] This defect causes retention of both cholesterol and plant sterols in the liver; in turn, serum cholesterol and plant sterol levels are raised. Early in life, serum cholesterol levels are extremely elevated, similarly to those of homozygous FH. Hence, sitosterolemia has been called *pseudohomozygous FH*. Later in life, cholesterol levels decline, but serum sitosterol levels remain elevated. Tendon xanthomas are common in sitosterolemia; they resemble those of patients with heterozygous FH. Seemingly, elevated serum sitosterol concentrations of a few milligrams per deciliter promote xanthoma formation, even without significant hypercholesterolemia. Treatment of sitosterolemia consists of a reduced intake of cholesterol and plant sterols. In addition, bile acid sequestrants promote conversion of cholesterol into bile acids and reduce serum levels of cholesterol.

DYSPROTEINEMIAS

A variety of forms of dysglobulinemia or paraproteinemias are accompanied by diffuse plane xanthomas that typically are macular, yellow-orange discolorations over the trunk.[28] Diffuse plane xanthomas have been reported in multiple myeloma, monoclonal gammopathy, cryoglobulinemia, leukemia, lymphoma, eosinophilic granulomatosis, and rheumatoid arthritis. The mechanism of production of xanthomas is typically the formation of a complex between an abnormal antibody globulin and a particular lipoprotein species. Cellular uptake of these complexes by macrophages in the skin produces plane xanthomas.

BILIARY OBSTRUCTION

Prolonged obstruction of the biliary tree leads to accumulation of cholesterol in the serum. Causes include primary biliary cirrhosis and secondary biliary obstruction. Serum cholesterol is high in unesterified cholesterol, which leads to the formation of an abnormal lipoprotein called *lipoprotein X*. Besides having hypercholesterolemia, patients with prolonged biliary obstruction usually manifest jaundice, pruritus, and hyperpigmentation of the skin. Prolonged hypercholesterolemia leads to plane xanthomas (beige-orange plaque on hands, feet, and trunk), xanthelasma, and occasionally tuberous xanthomas.

REFERENCES

1. Expert Panel on Detection, Evaluation, and Treatment of High Blood Cholesterol in Adults: Summary of the second report of the National Cholesterol Education Program (NCEP) Expert Panel on Detection, Evaluation, and Treatment of High Blood Cholesterol in Adults (Adult Treatment Panel II). *JAMA* **269**:3015, 1993

2. Expert Panel on Detection, Evaluation, and Treatment of High Blood Cholesterol in Adults, National Cholesterol Education Program: Second report of the Expert Panel on Detection, Evaluation, and Treatment of High Blood Cholesterol (Adult Treatment Panel II). *Circulation* **89**:1329, 1994

3. Brown MS, Goldstein JL: A receptor-mediated pathway for cholesterol homeostasis. *Science* **232**:34, 1986

4. Goldstein JL et al: Familial hypercholesterolemia, in *The Metabolic and Molecular Bases of Inherited Diseases,* 7th ed, edited by CR Scriver, AL Beaudet, WS Sly, D Valle. New York, McGraw-Hill, 1995, p 1981

5. Bilheimer DW et al: Liver transplantation to provide low-density-lipoprotein receptors and lower plasma cholesterol in a child with homozygous familial hypercholesterolemia. *N Engl J Med* **311**:1658, 1984

6. Uauy R et al: Treatment of children with homozygous familial hypercholesterolemia. Safety and efficacy of low density lipoprotein apheresis. *J Pediatr* **120**:892, 1992

7. Grundy SM: HMG-CoA reductase inhibitors for treatment of hypercholesterolemia. *N Engl J Med* **319**:24, 1988

8. Endo A: The discovery and development of HMG-CoA reductase inhibitors. *J Lipid Res* **33**:1569, 1992

9. Vega GL, Grundy SM: In vivo evidence for reduced binding of low density lipoproteins to receptors as a cause of primary moderate hypercholesterolemia. *J Clin Invest* **78**:1410, 1986

10. Innerarity TL et al: Familial defective apolipoprotein B-100: A mutation of apolipoprotein B that causes hypercholesterolemia. *J Lipid Res* **31**:1337, 1990

11. Tybjaerg-Hansen A, Humphries SE: Familial defective apolipoprotein B-100: A single mutation that causes hypercholesterolemia and premature coronary artery disease. *Atherosclerosis* **96**:91, 1992

12. Vega GL et al: Metabolic basis of primary hypercholesterolemia. *Circulation* **84**:118, 1991

13. Grundy SM: Multifactorial etiology of hypercholesterolemia: Implications for prevention of coronary heart disease. *Arterioscler Thromb* **11**:1619, 1991

14. Vega GL et al: Normocholesterolemic tendon xanthomatosis with overproduction of apolipoprotein B. *Metabolism* **32**:118, 1983

15. Brunzell JD: Familial lipoprotein lipase deficiency and other causes of the chylomicronemia syndrome, in *The Metabolic Basis of Inherited Diseases,* 6th ed, edited by CR Scriver, AL Beaudet, WS Sly, D Valle. New York, McGraw-Hill, 1989, p 1165

16. Breckenridge WC et al: Hypertriglyceridemia associated with deficiency of apolipoprotein C-II. *N Engl J Med* **298**:1265, 1978

17. Kesaniemi YA, Grundy SM: Dual defect in metabolism of very-low-density lipoprotein triglycerides. Patients with type 5 hyperlipoproteinemia. *JAMA* **251**:2542, 1984

18. Aalto-Setala K et al: Mechanism of hypertriglyceridemia in human apolipoprotein (apo) CIII transgenic mice. Diminished very low density lipoprotein fractional catabolic rate associated with increased apo CIII and reduced apo E on the particles. *J Clin Invest* **90**:1889, 1992

19. Dammerman M et al: An apolipoprotein CIII haplotype protective against hypertriglyceridemia is specified by promoter and 3' untranslated region polymorphisms. *Proc Natl Acad Sci USA* **90**:4562, 1993

20. Mahley RW, Rall SC Jr: Type III hyperlipoprotein (dysbetalipoproteinemia): The role of apolipoprotein E in normal and abnormal lipoprotein metabolism, in *The Metabolic and Molecular Bases of Inherited Diseases,* 7th ed, edited by CR Scriver, AL Beaudet, WS Sly, D Valle. New York, McGraw-Hill, 1995, p 1953

21. Abrams JJ et al: Normocholesterolemic dysbetalipoproteinemia with xanthomatosis. *Metabolism* **28**:113, 1979

22. Assmann G et al: Familial high density lipoprotein deficiency: Tangier disease, in *The Metabolic and Molecular Bases of Inherited Diseases,* 7th ed, edited by CR Scriver, AL Beaudet, WS Sly, D Valle. New York, McGraw-Hill, 1995, p 2053

23. Breslow JL: Familial disorders of high-density lipoprotein metabolism, in *The Metabolic Basis of Inherited Diseases,* 6th ed, edited by CR Scriver, AL Beaudet, WS Sly, D Valle. New York, McGraw-Hill, 1989, p 2031

24. Lackner KJ et al: High density lipoprotein deficiency with xanthomas. A defect in reverse cholesterol transport caused by a point mutation in the apolipoprotein A-I gene. *J Clin Invest* **92**:2262, 1993

25. Glomset JA et al: Lecithin: Cholesterol acyltransferase deficiency and fish eye disease, in *The Metabolic and Molecular Bases of Inherited Diseases,* 7th ed, edited by CR Scriver, AL Beaudet, WS Sly. New York, McGraw-Hill, 1995, p 1933

26. Björkhem I, Boberg KM: Inborn errors in bile acid biosynthesis and storage of sterols other than cholesterol, in *The Metabolic and Molecular Bases of Inherited Diseases,* 7th ed, edited by CR Scriver, AL Beaudet, WS Sly. New York, McGraw-Hill, 1995, p 2073

27. Bhattacharyya AK et al: Sluggish sitosterol turnover and hepatic failure to excrete sitosterol into bile cause expansion of body pools of sitosterol in patients with sitosterolemia and xanthomatosis. *Atheroscler Thromb* **11**:1287, 1991

28. Cruz PD Jr et al: Dermal, subcutaneous, and tendon xanthomas: Diagnostic markers for specific lipoprotein disorders. *J Am Acad Dermatol* **19**:95, 1988

CHAPTER 153

Robert J. Desnick
Christine M. Eng

Fabry Disease: α-Galactosidase A Deficiency (Angiokeratoma Corporis Diffusum Universale)

Fabry disease, an inborn error of glycosphingolipid metabolism, results from the defective activity of the lysosomal enzyme, α-galactosidase A. The enzymatic defect, transmitted by an X-linked recessive gene, leads to the progressive deposition of neutral glycosphingolipids (predominantly globotriaosylceramide) with terminal α-galactosyl moieties in most visceral tissues and fluids of the body (Fig. 153-1). The birefringent glycosphingolipids are primarily in the lysosomes of the vascular endothelium, in perithelial and smooth muscle cells of the cardiovascular-renal system, and, to a lesser extent, in reticuloendothelial, myocardial, and connective-tissue cells of the cornea, kidney, and other tissues, and in ganglion and perineural cells of the autonomic nervous system.

Clinically, hemizygous males have a characteristic skin lesion of *angiokeratoma corporis diffusum universale*. They also have acroparesthesias, episodic crises of excruciating pain, corneal and lenticular opacities, hypohidrosis, and cardiac and renal dysfunction. Death usually occurs in adult life from renal, cardiac, and/or cerebral complications of their vascular disease. Heterozygous females are usually asymptomatic and are most likely to show the corneal opacities.

HISTORIC ASPECTS

In 1898, two dermatologists, Anderson[1] in England and Fabry[2] in Germany, independently described the first patients with angiokeratoma corporis diffusum. Fabry originally made the diagnosis of purpura nodularis in a 13-year-old male whom he followed over the next 30 years (Fig. 153-2). He documented the presence of

FIGURE 153-2

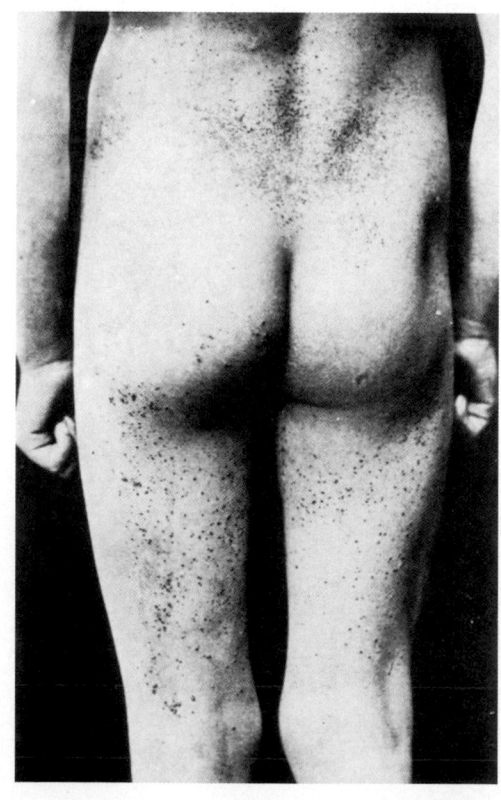

Distribution of angiokeratoma in a 30-year-old patient originally described by Fabry.[2]

FIGURE 153-1

Trihexosyl Ceramide

Galactose —α— Galactose —β— Glucose —β— Ceramide

α - Galactosodase A
(Ceramide Trihexosidase)

Lactosyl Ceramide

Galactose + Galactose —β— Glucose —β— Ceramide

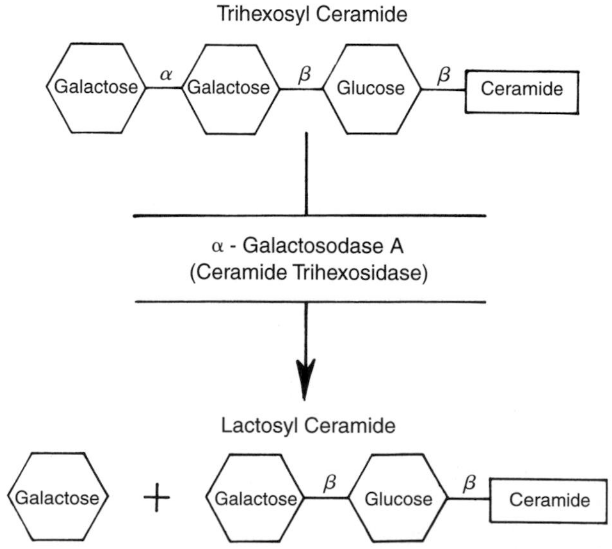

The metabolic defect in Fabry disease. Defective α-galactosidase A activity results in the accumulation of its major glycosphingolipid substrate, trihexosyl ceramide, which is also termed globotriaosylceramide.

albuminemia, further described the cutaneous lesions, noting the presence of small vessel aneurysms,[3] and subsequently classified his case to be one of *angiokeratoma corporis diffusum*, a designation that has persisted. Scriba definitively established the lipid nature of the storage material[4] and Hornbostel and Scriba were the first to confirm the diagnosis histologically by demonstrating the refractile lipid deposits in vessels of a skin biopsy specimen.[5] Opitz et al.[6] documented the X-linked recessive inheritance of the disorder by pedigree analysis.

In 1963, Sweeley and Klionsky[7] isolated and characterized the two major accumulated neutral glycosphingolipids—globotriaosylceramide (Gal-Gal-Glc-Cer) and galabiosylceramide (Gal-Gal-Cer)—from the kidney of a Fabry hemizygote obtained at autopsy, establishing Fabry disease as a sphingolipidosis. Subsequent chemical analyses of various Fabry tissues and fluids[5–7,9] have demonstrated the marked accumulation of Gal-Gal-Glc-Cer and, to a lesser extent, Gal-Gal-Cer. In addition, the accumulation of blood group B substances, glycosphingolipids with terminal α-galactosyl moieties, have been reported in affected individuals with B or AB blood types.[10]

In 1967, Brady et al.[11] demonstrated that the enzymatic defect was the defective activity of ceramide trihexosidase, a lysosomal galactosyl hydrolase required for the catabolism of Gal-Gal-Glc-Cer and Gal-Gal-Cer (see Fig. 153-1). Kint[12] characterized the defective enzymatic activity as an α-galactosyl hydrolase (designated α-galactosidase A). The accumulated glycosphingolipid substances, including blood group B substances, all had α-linked terminal galactosyl residues. The elucidation of the specific enzymatic defect permitted the enzymatic diagnosis of affected males, identification of heterozygous carrier females,[13,14] and the prenatal diagnosis of affected male fetuses.[15,16] Pilot trials of α-galactosidase A replacement for the experimental treatment of patients with this lysosomal storage disease have been reported.[17–19] The molecular cloning of the full-length cDNA and entire gene encoding human α-galactosidase A[20,21] has resulted in the characterization of the various mutations causing the disease, improved the accuracy of carrier diagnosis, and facilitated efforts to treat the disease using the recombinant enzyme.

In keeping with the terminology applied to other lipidoses and for the benefit of information retrieval, it would seem advisable to retain the commonly used eponym and to append the specific enzymatic defect. Thus, an appropriate designation is *Fabry disease: α-galactosidase A deficiency*. Comprehensive reviews on the clinical, pathologic, biochemical, and genetic aspects of the disease are available.[22]

CLINICAL MANIFESTATIONS

The Classically Affected Male

The clinical manifestations of Fabry disease predominantly result from the progressive deposition of Gal-Gal-Glc-Cer in the vascular endothelium (Table 153-1). Onset of the disease usually occurs during childhood or adolescence with periodic crises of severe pain in the extremities (acroparesthesias), the appearance of vascular cutaneous lesions (angiokeratoma), hypohidrosis, and the characteristic corneal and lenticular opacities. With advancing age, the progressive accumulation leads to early demise due to renal, cardiac, or cerebrovascular involvement.

PAIN The single most debilitating symptom of Fabry disease is the pain, of which two types have been described: episodic "crises"

TABLE 153-1

Major Clinical Manifestations in Hemizygotes with Fabry Disease*

VASCULAR GLYCOLIPID DEPOSITION	MANIFESTATION
Skin	Angiokeratoma
Peripheral nerves	Excruciating pain; acroparesthesias
Heart	Ischemia and infarctions
Brain	TIAs[†] and strokes
Kidney	Renal failure

*Average age at death, 41 years.
[†]TIA = transient ischemic attack.

consisting of agonizing, burning pain initially in the palms and soles. Attacks of abdominal or flank pain may simulate appendicitis or renal colic. The painful crises are usually triggered by exercise, fatigue, emotional stress, or rapid climatic changes in temperature and humidity. With increasing age, the periodic crises usually decrease in frequency and severity; however, in some patients, they may occur more frequently and the pain can be so excruciating that the patient may contemplate suicide. Because the pain is usually associated with a low-grade fever and an elevated erythrocyte sedimentation rate, these symptoms have frequently led to the misdiagnosis of rheumatic fever, neurosis, or erythromelalgia.[23] In addition to these intermittent crises, most patients complain of a nagging, constant discomfort in their hands and feet, characterized by burning, tingling paresthesias. These acroparesthesias may occur daily, usually during late afternoon, and may represent an attenuated form of the excruciating episodic crises. However, 10 to 20 percent of older patients deny any history of Fabry crises or acroparesthesias.

SKIN LESION There is a progressive increase in the number and size of these cutaneous vascular lesions with age. Classically, the angiokeratomas develop slowly as clusters of individual, punctate, dark red to blue-black angiectases in the superficial layers of the skin (Figs. 153-3, 153-4). The lesions may be flat or slightly raised and do not blanch with pressure; larger lesions may be hyperkeratotic. The clusters of lesions are most dense between the umbilicus and the knees and have a tendency toward bilateral symmetry. The hips, back, thighs, buttocks, penis, and scrotum are most commonly involved, but there is a wide variation in the pattern of distribution and density of the lesions. Involvement of the oral mucosa and conjunctiva is common, and other mucosal areas may also be involved. Variants without the characteristic skin lesions have been reported.[24–27] Although the angiectases may not be detected readily in some patients, careful examination of the skin, especially the scrotum and umbilicus, may reveal the presence of isolated lesions. In addition to these vascular lesions, anhidrosis or, more commonly, hypohidrosis is an early and almost constant finding.

CARDIAC, CEREBRAL, AND RENAL VASCULAR MANIFESTATIONS With increasing age, there is progressive infiltration of glycosphingolipid in the vascular system. Cardiac disease occurs in most hemizygotes, including anginal chest pain, myocardial infiltration, ischemia and infarction, mitral-valve prolapse, congestive heart failure, hypertension, mitral insufficiency, and cardiac enlargement.[28,29] These findings may be accentuated by systemic hy-

FIGURE 153-3

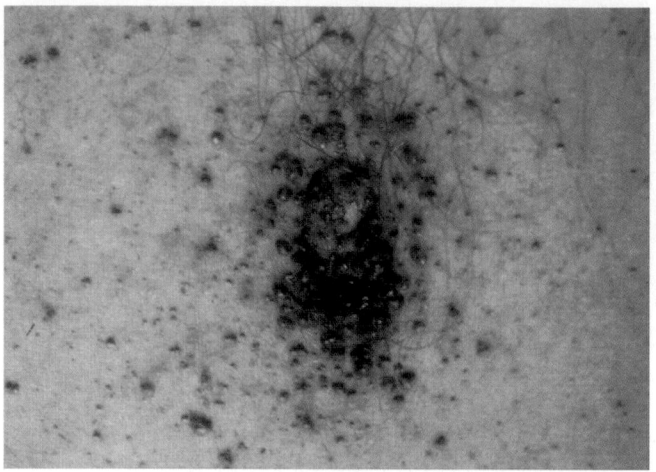

Clusters of dark red angiokeratomas in a hemizygote with Fabry disease.

pertension related to vascular involvement of renal parenchymal vessels. Hypertrophic obstructive cardiomyopathy,[30] as well as myocardial infarction secondary to occlusion of the coronary arteries due to glycolipid deposition[31] has been reported.

Cerebrovascular manifestations result primarily from multifocal small-vessel involvement and may include thromboses, basilar artery ischemia and aneurysm, seizures, hemiplegia, hemianesthesia, aphasia, labyrinthine disorders, or frank cerebral hemorrhage. Personality changes and psychotic behavior may become manifest with increasing age. Severe neurologic signs may be present without evidence of major thrombosis and are presumably due to multifocal small-vessel occlusive disease.

FIGURE 153-4

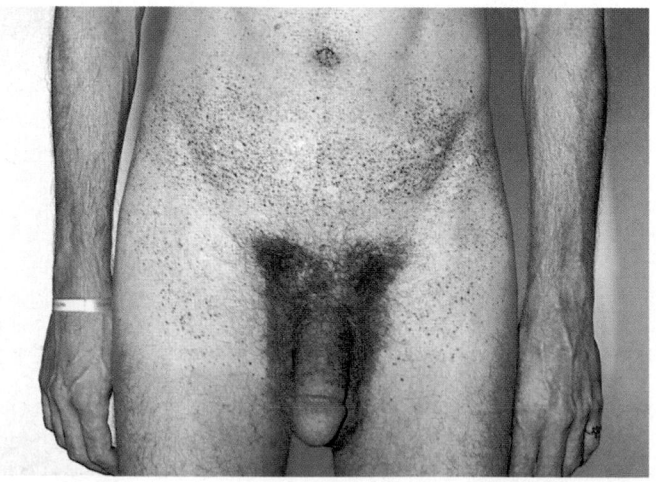

Angiokeratomas in a 28-year-old hemizygote with Fabry disease are seen in the "swimsuit" distribution.

Progressive glycosphingolipid deposition in the kidney results in proteinuria, with gradual deterioration of renal function and development of azotemia in middle age. During childhood and adolescence, protein, casts, red cells, and desquamated kidney and urinary tract cells may appear in the urine. Birefringent lipid globules with characteristic "Maltese crosses" can be observed free in the urine and within desquamated urinary sediment cells by polarization microscopy (Fig. 153-5). With age, progressive renal impairment is evidenced by significant proteinuria, isosthenuria (specific gravities of 1.008 to 1.012), and alterations of other renal tubular functions. Gradual deterioration of renal function and the development of azotemia usually occur in the third to fourth decades of life, although renal failure has been reported in the second decade. Death most often results from uremia unless chronic hemodialysis or renal transplantation is undertaken. The mean age at death of 104 hemizygous males who were not treated for uremia was 41 years,[32] but occasionally an affected individual has survived into his early 60s.

OCULAR FEATURES   Ocular involvement is most prominent in the cornea, lens, conjunctiva, and retina.[33–35] A characteristic corneal opacity, observed only on slit-lamp microscopy, is found in males with the disease and in most heterozygous females (Fig. 153-6). The earliest lesion is a diffuse haziness in the subepithelial layer. In more advanced cases, the opacities appear as whorled streaks extending from a central vortex to the periphery of the cornea. Typically, the whorllike opacities are inferior and cream-colored; however, they range from white to golden brown and may be very faint. An indistinguishable, drug-induced phenocopy of the Fabry corneal dystrophy occurs in patients on long-term chloroquine or amiodarone therapy (see "Genetics").

Two specific types of lenticular changes have been described. A granular anterior capsular or subcapsular deposit has been observed in about one-third of hemizygous males, but rarely in heterozygous females. Typically, these lenticular opacities are bilateral and inferior in position. They frequently appear in a "propeller-like" distribution, that is, wedge-shaped with their bases near the lenticular equator and aligned radially with the apices toward the center of the anterior capsule. A second, and possibly unique, lenticular opacity has been observed in both hemizygous and heterozygous individuals.[33,34] It may be the first ocular manifestation to appear. The opacity is posterior, linear, and appears as a whitish, almost translucent, spokelike deposit of fine granular material on or near the posterior cortex. This unusual opacity has been termed the *Fabry cataract*[33] and is best seen by retroillumination.

Conjunctival and retinal vascular lesions are common and represent part of the diffuse systemic vascular involvement. These vascular lesions occur early in life in normotensive individuals and are characterized by mild to marked tortuosity of the conjunctival and retinal vessels. There is an aneurysmal dilation of thin-walled venules as well as angulation and segmental, sausage-like dilatation of veins typically seen on the inferior bulbar conjunctiva. As the disease progresses, retinal changes associated with the development of hypertension and uremia may be superimposed. Vision is not impaired by the vascular lesions in the conjunctiva and retina or by the corneal dystrophy. However, acute visual loss has occurred in hemizygotes as a result of unilateral total central retinal artery occlusion.[33]

OTHER CLINICAL FEATURES   Because of the widespread visceral distribution of the glycosphingolipid deposits, signs and symptoms of this disorder arise in many other organs and systems. Several patients have had chronic bronchitis, wheezing respiration, or dyspnea with alveolar capillary block. Pulmonary function studies in older hemizygotes may show significant airflow obstruction, reduced diffusing capacity, and a reduction in the V_{max25} values.[36] In affected males, airway obstruction was found to occur commonly regardless of smoking history and to increase with age, most likely resulting from fixed narrowing of the airways by accumulated glycosphingolipid.[37]

Lymphedema of the legs may be present in adulthood without hypoproteinemia, varices, or any clinically manifest vascular disease and presumably reflects the progressive glycosphingolipid deposition in the lymphatic vessels and lymph nodes. Many patients have varicose leg veins and hemorrhoids. Priapism has also been reported.

Episodic diarrhea and, to a lesser extent, nausea, vomiting, and flank pain, are the most common gastrointestinal complaints[38]; these symptoms may be related to deposition of glycosphingolipid in intestinal small vessels and in the autonomic ganglia of the bowel. The symptomatology and pathophysiology of the gastrointestinal involvement have been reviewed.[38–40]

Anemia is probably due to decreased red-blood-cell survival. A decreased serum iron concentration, normal red-blood-cell fragility, and an elevated reticulocyte count have been reported.[22] Lipid-laden, foamy-appearing macrophages are present in the bone marrow. Many hemizygous males appear to have retarded growth or delayed puberty and sparse, fine facial and body hair. In some kindreds, an acromegalic-like appearance has been reported. Affected individuals may complain of fatigue and weakness and may be incapacitated for prolonged periods.

FIGURE 153-5

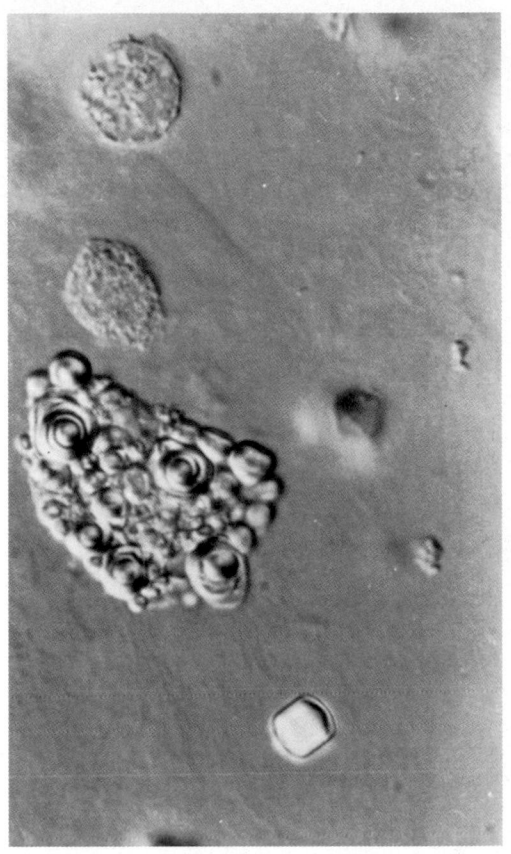 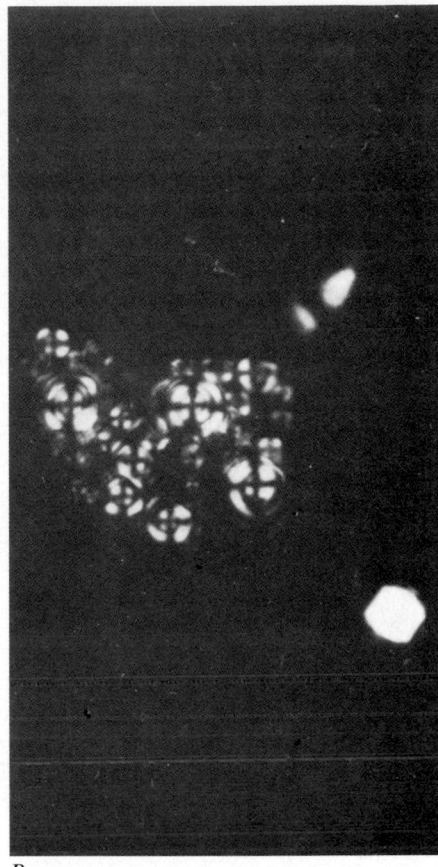

A.   B.

Photomicrographs of the urinary sediment from a heterozygote showing lipid accumulation by interference microscopy (A) and polarization light microscopy (B). Note that Maltese crosses are observed under polarization.

The Cardiac Variant

Affected males with a variant phenotype have been described who were essentially asymptomatic at ages when classical hemizygotes would be severely affected or would have died from the disease[22] (see Table 153-1). In contrast to patients with the classic phenotype who have no detectable α-galactosidase A activity, these variants have residual activity compatible with their milder phenotypes. Reports have described several patients with late-onset cardiac or cardiopulmonary disease.[41,42] These "cardiac variants" had cardiomegaly, typically involving the left ventricular wall and interventricular septum, and electrocardiographic abnormalities consistent with a cardiomyopathy. Others had hypertrophic cardiomyopathy and/or myocardial infarctions. They were essentially asymptomatic during most of their lives and did not experience the early classic manifestations, including acroparesthesia, angiokeratoma, corneal and lenticular opacities, and hypohidrosis. Most were diagnosed after the onset of cardiac manifestations and most had mild proteinuria.

The Heterozygote

The clinical course and prognosis of affected males and heterozygous females differ significantly.[22] Heterozygotes experience little difficulty in adult life at ages when hemizygous males already have severe renal and/or cardiac involvement, although with increasing age some manifest minor symptoms of the disease. Approximately 30 percent of heterozygotes have a few isolated skin lesions, fewer than 10 percent have acroparesthesias, and about 70 percent have the whorllike corneal dystrophy.[35] Renal findings in heterozygotes include hyposthenuria; the occurrence of erythrocytes, leukocytes, and granular and hyaline casts in the urinary sediment; proteinuria; and other signs of renal impairment. In some heterozygotes, cardiac involvement will develop with advanced age.[43] However, a few heterozygotes have been described with disease as severe as that observed in classically affected males.[44] In contrast, obligate heterozygotes (daughters of affected hemizygous males) without any clinical manifestations and with normal levels of leukocyte α-galactosidase A and urinary sediment glycosphingolipids have been reported.[45] Indeed, asymptomatic and symptomatic monozygotic female twins have been described.[46] Such markedly variable expres-

FIGURE 153-6

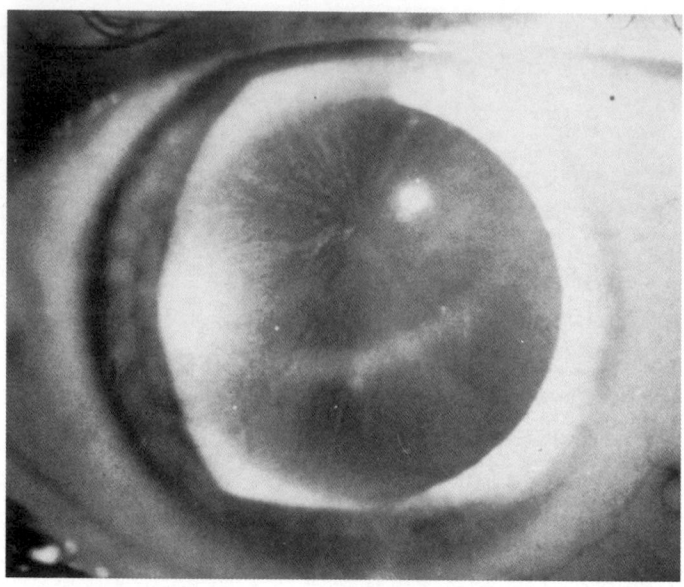

Corneal opacity in a heterozygote observed on slit-lamp microscopy. The corneal involvement results from subepithelial glycosphingolipid deposition.

sion is expected in females heterozygous for X-linked diseases due to random X-inactivation (see "Genetics").

PATHOLOGY

Morphologically, Fabry disease is characterized by widespread tissue deposits of crystalline glycosphingolipid that show birefringence with typical Maltese crosses under polarization microscopy (Fig. 153-5). The glycosphingolipid is deposited in all areas of the body, occurring predominantly in the lysosomes of endothelial, perithelial, and smooth muscle cells of blood vessels and, to a lesser degree, in histiocytic and reticular cells of connective tissue. Lipid deposits are also prominent in epithelial cells of the cornea and glomeruli and tubules of the kidney, in muscle fibers of the heart, and in ganglion cells of the autonomic system.

Pathology of the Skin

The skin lesions are telangiectases or small superficial angiomas (Fig. 153-7). After a silent period, cumulative vascular damage leads eventually to clinically apparent and progressive angiectases.[47,48] The pathologic involvement was observed in the vascular endothelium and perithelium of clinically normal skin from a 1-year-old affected male.[49]

Capillaries, venules, and arterioles contain pathologic lipid storage in the endothelium, perithelium, and smooth muscle. There is marked dilatation of the capillaries of the dermal papillae. Deeper vessels show less dilatation and aneurysm formation. Lipid stores have been noted in arrectores pilorum muscles, gingival tissues, sweat gland epithelium, and perineural cells.[49,50]

FIGURE 153-7

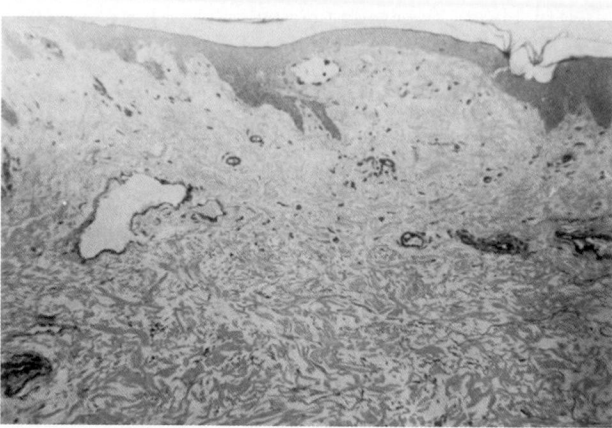

Telangiectatic vessels in the dermis that are typical of the changes seen in the skin.

The fully developed classic lesions are usually located in the upper dermis, where they may produce elevation, flattening, or hypertrophy of the epithelium. The larger lesions may have a slight to moderate keratosis, hence the term *angiokeratoma*.

Pathology of Other Systems

KIDNEY   The earliest lesions are due to the accumulation of glycosphingolipid in endothelial and epithelial cells of the glomerulus and of Bowman's space and in the epithelium of the loops of Henle and of distal tubules. Lipid-laden distal tubular epithelial cells desquamate and may be detected in the urinary sediment (see Fig. 153-5).

Concurrently, renal blood vessels are involved progressively and often extensively. An early finding is the presence of arterial fibrinoid deposits, which may result from the necrosis of severely involved muscular cells. Other histologic changes in the kidney are the sequelae of nonspecific, end-stage renal disease. The renal involvement has been the subject of comprehensive reviews.[51,52]

NERVOUS SYSTEM   Vascular involvement is also prominent in the nervous system[53–56] and presumably accounts for the observation of minor electroencephalographic and electromyographic abnormalities in these patients. In addition, vascular ischemia and lipid deposition in the perineurium may cause the peripheral nerve conduction abnormalities of slowed conduction velocities and distal latency, respectively. In both heterozygotes and affected males, glycosphingolipid deposition in nervous tissue appears to be limited to perineural sheath cells of peripheral nerves, neurons of the peripheral and central autonomic nervous system, and certain primary neurons of somatic afferent pathways.[54,55,57] Qualitative[55] and quantitative[58] studies of peripheral sensory neurons in sural nerves and spinal ganglia have shown preferential loss of small myelinated and unmyelinated fibers as well as small cell bodies of spinal ganglia.[58]

Multiple brainstem centers may be involved.[55,58] Hemisphere involvement has been noted in the amygdaloid, hypothalamic, and hippocampal nuclei. Lipid storage in neuronal cells of the anterior and posterior lobes of the pituitary has been described. Detailed reviews of the neurologic findings are available.[59]

EYE   Histologically, abnormal glycosphingolipid deposits are found in endothelial, perivascular, and smooth muscle cells of all ocular and orbital vessels, in smooth muscle of the iris and ciliary body, in perineural cells, and in connective tissue of the lens and cornea.[60,61] Inclusions have been localized in the epithelium of the conjunctiva, cornea, and lens, and, by electron microscopy, in the basal layer of conjunctival epithelial cells as well as in the surface epithelium. There may be hyperplasia and edema of corneal epithelial cells. Bowman's membrane appears normal and no deposits are observed in the stroma or endothelium. It has been suggested that the whorllike corneal dystrophic pattern may result from the formation of a series of subepithelial ridges or from the reduplication of the basement membrane.[60]

HEART The progressive deposition of glycosphingolipid in myocardial cells and valvular fibroblasts appears to be a primary cause of cardiac disease in affected males and some heterozygotes.[62,63] Most commonly, the left atrium and ventricle are enlarged, and the ventricular walls and septum are markedly thickened; right atrial and ventricular dilatation and enlargement are variable findings. Within the myocardial cells, there is extensive glycosphingolipid deposition around the nucleus and between myofibrils.

Histochemistry and Ultrastructure

The accumulated glycosphingolipids can be stained in frozen sections with lipid-soluble dyes and may be removed from tissues by the process of dehydration and embedding in paraffin. If lipid-solubilizing procedures are used, empty vacuoles are observed on light microscopy. Most of the lipid crystals are retained through alcohol dehydration but are lost on exposure to xylene or pyridine. Improved fixation of the lipid deposits can be achieved with 1% calcium formol. A comparison of various fixation and embedding techniques to preserve the storage material has been reported.[64] A modified periodic acid-Schiff (PAS) stain specific for neutral glycosphingolipids[65] and a positive test for sphingosine[66] have served to confirm the chemical identification of the accumulated glycosphingolipids. Peroxidase- or fluorescence-labeled *Banderiaea simplicifolia* lectin, which is specific for α-D-galactosyl residues, and antiglobotriaosylceramide antibodies also have been used to stain the glycosphingolipid substrates selectively.[64,67–68]

The ultrastructural characteristics of the lesions and of the lipid inclusions in various tissues from affected males have been described extensively.[69,70] At high resolution, a typical pattern of concentric or lamellar inclusions with alternating light- and dark-staining bands is observed (Fig. 153-8). The periodicity of these bands has been reported variably as 40 to 50 Å, 50 to 60 Å, 60 to 65 Å, or as great as 98 Å. The electron-dense component is 20 to 30 Å in thickness. These inclusions have coarser periods of 150 to 200 Å.

BIOCHEMICAL GENETICS OF FABRY DISEASE

The deficient activity of the lysosomal enzyme α-galactosidase A results in the accumulation of glycosphingolipids with terminal α-galactosyl moieties in most visceral tissues and body fluids. The predominant glycosphingolipid accumulated is globotriaosylceramide or galactosyl-($\alpha 1 \rightarrow 4$)-galactosyl-($\beta 1 \rightarrow 4$)-glycosyl-($\beta 1 \rightarrow 1'$)-ceramide. A second neutral glycosphingolipid, galabiosylceramide [Gal($\alpha 1 \rightarrow 4$)Gal($\beta 1 \rightarrow 1'$)Cer], also accumulates in Fabry hemizygotes to abnormally high concentrations. The deposition of galabiosylceramide, however, appears to be tissue-specific, since this substrate has been detected only in the kidney, pancreas, right heart, lung, and urinary sediment. In addition, the blood group B–

FIGURE 153-8

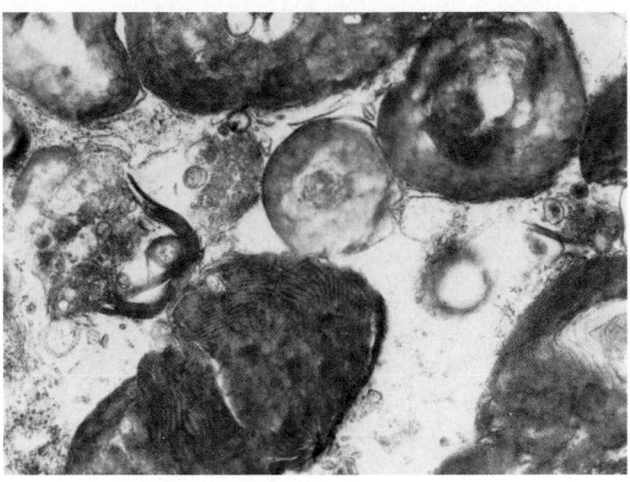

Electron photomicrograph of a section of the mitral valve from a hemizygote with Fabry disease, showing the concentric lamellar inclusions in lysosomes of fibrocytes. (*Courtesy of HL Sharp, MD.*)

specific substances, which have terminal α-galactosyl moieties, [Gal($\alpha 1 \rightarrow 3$)Gal($2 \leftarrow 1\alpha$Fuc)($\beta 1 \rightarrow 3$)GlcNac($\beta 1 \rightarrow 3$)Gal($\beta 1 \rightarrow 4$)Glc($\beta 1 \rightarrow 1'$)Cer] and the blood group B1 glycosphingolipid [Gal($\alpha 1 \rightarrow 3$)Gal($2 \leftarrow 1\alpha$Fuc)($\beta 1 \rightarrow 4$)GlcNac($\beta 1 \rightarrow 3$)Gal($\beta 1 \rightarrow 4$)Glc($\beta 1 \rightarrow 1'$)Cer] accumulate in patients who have the blood group B antigens. Thus, Fabry hemizygotes and heterozygotes who have blood group B and AB accumulate four major glycosphingolipid substrates (and generally have a more rapid disease course), whereas patients with A or O blood groups accumulate primarily globotriaosylceramide and galabiosylceramide.

Human α-galactosidase A is a homodimeric glycoprotein with native and subunit molecular masses of ~ 101 and ~ 46 kDa. The enzyme has a pH optimum of 4.6 and hydrolyzes the α-linked galactosyl moieties from glycolipids and glycopeptides. Isoelectric focusing studies of the enzyme from various sources reveals multiple forms with pI values ranging from 4.2 to 5.1, owing to glycoforms with varying sialylation and phosphorylation.[71] The α-galactosidase A subunit in cultured fibroblasts is normally synthesized as a precursor glycopeptide of ~ 50 kDa. After cleavage of the signal peptide and carbohydrate modifications in the Golgi apparatus and lysosomes, the mature enzyme subunits of ~ 46 kDa form the active, homodimeric enzyme, which contains complex, hybrid, and high-mannose type oligosaccharide moieties. A comprehensive review of glycosphingolipid metabolism, the biochemistry of α-galactosidase A, and the metabolic defect in Fabry disease is available.[22]

Classically affected hemizygotes with Fabry disease have no detectable α-galactosidase A activity. The physical and kinetic properties of the residual α-galactosidase activities (1 to 10 percent of normal) in atypical variants who are asymptomatic or have mild manifestations have been described.[22,32,52] Studies of α-galactosidase biosynthesis demonstrated several types of enzyme defects, suggesting the occurrence of allelic heterogeneity, including gene rearrangements and point mutations that affect α-galactosidase A synthesis, maturation, and stability.[22] In contrast to classically affected males, the atypical or cardiac variants have residual α-galactosidase A activity, consistent with the attenuation or absence of the characteristic clinical manifestations.[22,52]

α-GALACTOSIDASES A AND B Based on studies with synthetic substrates, the two activities initially thought to represent α-galactosidase isozymes were detected and designated α-galactosidases A and B.[72] The two "isozymes" were separable by electrophoresis, isoelectric focusing, and ion-exchange chromatography. Subsequently, the demonstration that polyclonal antibodies against α-galactosidase A or B did not cross react with the other enzyme,[73] that only α-galactosidase A activity was deficient in hemizygotes with Fabry disease, and that the genes for α-galactosidases A and B mapped to different chromosomes[22] clearly established that these enzymes were genetically distinct. Thus, it was not surprising when α-galactosidase B was shown in 1977 to be an α-N-acetylgalactosaminidase, a homodimeric glycoprotein that hydrolyzed artificial and natural substrates with terminal α-N-acetylgalactosaminyl moieties.[73] The gene has been subsequently identified and characterized.[74]

PATHOPHYSIOLOGY

The pattern of glycosphingolipid deposition in Fabry disease, particularly its predilection for vascular endothelial and smooth muscle cells, is uniquely different from that seen in other glycosphingolipidoses.[75] However, the origin of the accumulated glycosphingolipid substrates has not been fully clarified. Certainly there is a significant contribution from the endogenous synthesis and subsequent lysosomal accumulation of terminal α-galactosyl-containing glycosphingolipids following autophagy of cellular membranous material with these lipid substrates. Endogenous metabolism is presumably the major source of substrate accumulation in avascular sites, such as cornea, and in neural cells, which are presumably protected from the increased circulating levels of Gal-Gal-Glc-Cer by the blood–brain barrier. In addition, the turnover of Gal-Gal-Glc-Cer and particularly its precursor, globotriaosylceramide (globoside), which are present in higher concentrations in normal renal tissue than in any other tissue, is presumably responsible for the endogenous renal deposition of the Fabry substrate.

The unique cellular and tissue distribution of accumulated Gal-Gal-Glc-Cer, particularly in the vascular endothelium and smooth muscle, suggests that a significant intracellular contribution may be derived by the endocytosis or diffusion of Gal-Gal-Glc-Cer from the circulation, where the concentration is three- to tenfold higher than that of normal individuals. In Fabry hemizygotes and normal individuals, the circulating Gal-Gal-Glc-Cer is primarily transported in the low-density lipoprotein (LDL) and high-density lipoprotein (HDL) fractions.[22,76–78] In plasma from hemizygotes, the accumulated Gal-Gal-Glc-Cer is distributed in the LDL and HDL fractions in proportions similar to those in normal plasma, approximately 60 and 30 percent, respectively. The finding that little, if any, substrate deposition occurs in Fabry hepatocytes (in contrast to the accumulation in Kupffer cells,[64–79] supports the contention that Gal-Gal-Glc-Cer synthesized by the hepatocyte is associated with lipoprotein and secreted as a complex.[80] In support of this concept is the fact that patients with hypercholesterolemia have proportional plasma elevations of both LDL and neutral glycosphingolipids, including Gal-Gal-Glc-Cer.[76] The circulating Gal-Gal-Glc-Cer then presumably gains access to vascular endothelial and smooth muscle cells throughout the body by the high-affinity lipoprotein receptor-mediated uptake pathway.[81–83] Deposits in other tissues may also be derived to a lesser extent from receptor-independent diffusion or by nonabsorptive endocytosis of globoside- or Gal-Gal-Glc-Cer lipoprotein complexes from the plasma. Since lysosomes in all cells are deficient in the α-galactosidase A activity needed to degrade the accumulated glycosphingolipids, they accumulate within extended multivesicular bodies, or, in more advanced stages, as free intracytoplasmic masses, which may lead to cellular dysfunction or degeneration.

In addition to hepatocyte biosynthesis, glycosphingolipids are synthesized in the bone marrow, where they become incorporated into the membranes of the formed blood elements.[84,85] It has been postulated that erythrocyte globoside (GalNAc-Gal-Gal-Glc-Cer), the predominant glycosphingolipid of erythrocytes and the catabolic precursor of Gal-Gal-Glc-Cer, may be another major metabolic source of the circulating pathogenic lipid. Globoside is presumably released into the circulation from senescent erythrocytes,[84] and is subsequently catabolized (presumably in the spleen) to Gal-Gal-Glc-Cer. In Fabry disease, the Gal-Gal-Glc-Cer cannot be metabolized and may be partly released into the circulation, where it can be incorporated into both HDL and LDL fractions[80] and/or rapidly cleared by the liver, as has been shown for intravenously administered neutral glycosphingolipids.[86] Thus, the turnover of erythrocyte and other membrane glycosphingolipids may contribute significantly to the substrate load in Fabry disease. In addition, a minor amount of Gal-Gal-Glc-Cer may be "excreted" into the circulation from the secondary lysosomes of various cell types throughout the body. Because the glycosphingolipid cannot be catabolized in the circulation, it would slowly accumulate at a rate reflecting the turnover of various cells, the contribution from exocytosis, lipoprotein uptake, and/or diffusion.

The metabolism of at least two related compounds also is abnormal, as demonstrated by the accumulation of galabiosylceramide, Gal-Gal-Cer, and the blood group B antigenic substances. Affected males and heterozygous females who are blood group type B or AB appear to be more severely affected, presumably due to the additional accumulation of B-specific glycosphingolipids.[22] Thus, the total amount of glycosphingolipid stored in a given tissue depends on time, the rate of accumulation from intracellular and circulatory sources, the possibilities for excretion, the individual's ABO blood type, and the presence or absence of residual α-galactosidase A activity. The pattern of glycosphingolipid accumulation, predominantly in the cardiovascular-renal system, best correlates pathophysiologically with the major clinical manifestations of the disease as selectively described below.

Pathophysiology of the Vasculature

Narrowing, dilatation, motor unresponsiveness, and instability of blood vessels are major features of the altered physiology in Fabry disease. The swollen vascular endothelial cells, often accompanied by endothelial proliferation, encroach on the lumen, causing a focal increase of intraluminal pressure, dilatation, and angiectases as well as peripheral ischemia or frank infarction.[87] Such changes are frequently the precursors of thromboses and infarcts of the brain and other tissues. Muscle and peripheral nerve ischemia may contribute to the pain or fatigue.[88]

There may be progressive aneurysmal dilatation of the weakened vascular wall. This process is apparent in the progressive dilatation and microaneurysm formation of the retinal and conjunctival vessels and in the transition from normality to telangiectasia and frank angiokeratoma in the skin.

Observed alterations of vasomotor control may reflect either the vascular lesions themselves or the extensive glycosphingolipid deposits in autonomic ganglia and perineural sheath cells.[89,90] Both hemizygotes and heterozygotes with Fabry disease demonstrate an impaired ability to vasoconstrict, and the more severely involved hemizygotes show, in addition, inability to vasodilatate. Such a combined vascular and neural lesion may also explain the clinically observed temperature intolerance.[91]

Pathophysiology of Other Systems

NERVOUS SYSTEM The involvement of peripheral and central autonomic nerve cells may be responsible for the paresthesias, pain, hypohidrosis, such gastrointestinal symptoms as nausea and diarrhea, and a variety of vague neurologic signs and symptoms. Fukuhara et al.[88] found marked degeneration of the secretory cells and myoepithelial cells of sweat glands by electron microscopy and proposed that the hypohidrosis was due to local lipid deposition rather than autonomic nervous system involvement. The episodic fevers may be related to lesions of the hypothalamus.[57] The observations of a selective decrease in the number of unmyelinated and small myelinated fibers in peripheral nerves[54,55,59,92,93] have led to the suggestion that the selective damage to these fibers may account for the pain production and hypohidrosis in this disorder. Studies of autonomic function revealed sympathetic and parasympathetic dysfunction, particularly in distal cutaneous responses.[89] Alternatively, it has been suggested that the lipid deposition in the vasa nervorum may lead to the acroparesthesias, rather than involvement of the autonomic nervous system.[88,92]

KIDNEY The observed abnormalities in renal function have their basis in lesions of the nephron and of the renal vasculature, and possibly in disorders of the posterior pituitary and hypothalamus. Early glycosphingolipid deposits antedate clinical signs and symptoms. The observed mild proteinuria may be explained by alteration of the glomerular epithelial cells and their foot processes[51] or by increased desquamation of lipid-laden tubular epithelial cells.[67] Loss of renal concentrating ability with polyuria and polydipsia may occur well in advance of a significant decrease in glomerular filtration or evidence of renal failure.[94] The defect in concentrating ability may be due to decreased water permeability of the distal tubules and collecting ducts secondary to lipid deposition. The later and more severe renal changes are the result of vascular lesions and of hypertension.

HEART The progressive deposition of glycosphingolipids in the myocardial cells, the valvular fibroblasts, and the coronary vessels is the primary cause of cardiac disease in hemizygotes and some heterozygotes.[31,63] The left ventricular myocardium and the mitral valve are the sites of the most marked lipid deposition in the heart. The marked deposition of Gal-Gal-Glc-Cer in the coronary arteries leads to myocardial ischemia and frank infarction.[31,63]

OTHER INVOLVEMENT Pulmonary symptoms have been attributed to involvement of lung vasculature or bronchial and mucous gland epithelium.[36,37] The airflow obstruction may be due to the loss of elastic recoil secondary to lipid deposition in lung parenchyma. The lymphedema presumably results from lymphatic obstruction or venous insufficiency secondary to lipid-laden endothelial cells.

Abnormal Distribution in Tissues

Increased concentrations of globotriaosylceramide were found in all tissues analyzed except erythrocytes,[8,95] which indicates that most tissues are involved in the catabolism of these glycosphingolipids.

In one affected male, the magnitude of glycosphingolipid accumulation was 30- to 300-fold higher than normal levels.[95] The greatest levels of accumulation were observed in kidney, lymph nodes, vessels, prostate, and autonomic ganglia. Globotriaosylceramide accumulation in various tissues was compared in hemizygotes and heterozygotes.[96] Hemizygotes had markedly increased levels in the kidney, whereas a heterozygote had the highest accumulation in the heart. Accumulation of galabiosylceramide has been reported to occur only in the kidney, pancreas, heart, lungs, and urinary sediment.[7,9,62,95]

MOLECULAR GENETICS OF α-GALACTOSIDASE A AND FABRY DISEASE

α-Galactosidase A Gene and Transcript

Human α-galactosidase A is encoded by a single housekeeping gene, which has been localized to the chromosomal region Xq22.[22] The 12-kb α-galactosidase A gene has been completely sequenced.[20,21] It contains 7 exons ranging from 92 to 291 bp and 6 introns ranging from 0.2 to 3.8 kb. The gene is remarkably rich in *Alu* repetitive sequences with nine intronic repeats and three repeats in the immediate 3' flanking region; these sequences represent ~30% of the 12 kb gene, or ~1 *Alu*/kb. The full-length 1437-bp α-galactosidase A cDNA encodes a precursor peptide of 429 amino acids, including a 31-residue signal peptide. The mature 398 amino acid subunit contains four *N*-glycosylation consensus sequences.[20]

The Molecular Pathology of Fabry Disease

The availability of the full-length cDNA and genomic sequences for α-galactosidase A has facilitated investigation of the lesions causing Fabry disease. Southern hybridization analyses have identified gene rearrangements, Northern hybridization analyses and ribonuclease A studies have detected abnormalities in RNA processing and/or stability, and amplification and sequencing techniques have identified specific point mutations in the α-galactosidase A gene.[22,97] Over 125 molecular lesions of the α-galactosidase A gene in unrelated Fabry families have been identified emphasizing the molecular genetic heterogeneity of this disease. Most mutations have been private and occurred only in single pedigrees (see below). Characterization of these lesions provides information on the nature and frequency of the mutations causing this disease as well as insights into the structure–function relationships of this lysosomal hydrolase. More accurate carrier diagnosis has become possible by identification of the specific lesions in families or by analysis of closely linked polymorphisms (see "Diagnosis"). Eukaryotic expression of the full-length cDNA has resulted in the production of large amounts of active enzyme for characterization, crystallization, and future trials of enzyme replacement (see "Treatment"). Illustrations of the various classes of mutations are discussed below.

GENE REARRANGEMENTS The frequency of gene rearrangements in the α-galactosidase A gene causing Fabry disease has been assessed in 165 unrelated patients by Southern hybridization analysis using the full-length α-galactosidase A cDNA as a probe[98] or by multiplex polymerase chain reaction (PCR) amplification of the entire α-galactosidase A coding region.[99] One partial gene dupli-cation and five partial gene deletions were identified,[100] a frequency of 5 percent, which is similar to that reported for other X-linked diseases. Of note, no total gene deletions were identified. The partial duplication resulted from a recombination event between regions in introns 1 and 6 leading to the duplication of part of intron 1, exons 2 through 6, and part of intron 6. The five partial gene deletions ranged in size from 0.4 to 4.6 kb. Four of the five partial deletions had a breakpoint in intron 2 that contains three *Alu* repetitive ele-ments. The fifth deletion was unusual and involved two deletions (1.7 kb and 14 bp) that were separated by a 151-bp inverted se-quence.[100]

α-GALACTOSIDASE A SMALL INSERTIONS AND DELETIONS
Several examples of small insertions or deletions have been de-scribed.[101,102] Some of these rearrangements resulted in frameshift mutations that led to premature chain termination and were detected in classically affected hemizygotes, while some were in-frame de-letions or insertions that resulted in a qualitative change in the pro-tein. The postulated mechanism for several of the small rearrange-ments was slipped mispairing resulting from the presence of short direct repeats at the breakpoint junctions. Of interest, a mutation designated $1016\Delta11$ deletion[102] may have resulted from the pres-ence of polymerase α arrest sites upstream and immediately down-stream from the deleted sequence. Polymerase α has been shown to be the only polymerase that catalyzes DNA synthesis at repli-cation forks.[103]

RNA PROCESSING DEFECTS
Several mutations altering pro-cessing of the α-galactosidase A transcript have been described in classically affected hemizygotes.[102,104] These include a gt $\rightarrow$ gg single base substitution in the 5' donor consensus splice site of intron 2 (designated IVS2^{+2}),[102] a gt $\rightarrow$ tt substitution in the 5' donor consensus splice site of intron 6 (IVS6^{+1}),[104] and a 2-bp deletion, tcagΔt $\rightarrow$ g, that disrupted the 3' acceptor consensus splice site of intron 5 (IVS5$\Delta^{-2,3}$).[102] The IVS6^{+1} mutation, which has been the most fully characterized,[104] resulted from a gt $\rightarrow$ tt sub-stitution of the invariant 5' donor splice consensus site of intron 6, causing abnormal splicing of the α-galactosidase A pre-mRNA.

CODING REGION MUTATIONS
Approximately 75 percent of the mutations causing Fabry disease are missense or nonsense mu-tations. The majority of these coding region mutations occur in exons 5 through 7, although point mutations have been described in all seven exons. Although most of the missense and nonsense mutations were detected in classically affected hemizygotes, several missense mutations,[24,42,102] were identified in asymptomatic or mild variants of Fabry disease. Of the 14 CpG dinucleotides in the α-galactosidase A coding sequence, point mutations occurred at 5. The high frequency of mutations at CpG dinucleotides is consistent with their recognition as mutational hot spots due to the deamination of methylcytosine to thymine.

COMMON MOLECULAR LESIONS IN FABRY DISEASE
Most of the reported mutations have been private (i.e., confined to a sin-gle Fabry pedigree). In fact, the discovery that two presumably un-related families had identical mutations occasionally led to linking of two distant arms of the same pedigree. However, several muta-tions have been found in unrelated families of different ethnic or geographic backgrounds. These include N215S, R227Q, R227X and R342Q mutations. The N215S was a common mutation among

atypical hemizygotes who were asymptomatic or had mild disease manifestations.[102–105] R227Q and R227X, which occurred at a CpG nucleotide, were the most common mutations causing the classic phenotype.

GENOTYPE/PHENOTYPE CORRELATIONS
Of the reported mo-lecular lesions, affected hemizygotes with the classic disease man-ifestations and no detectable α-galactosidase A activity had a va-riety of α-galactosidase A lesions including large and small gene rearrangements, splicing defects, and missense or nonsense muta-tions. In contrast, all of the asymptomatic or mildly affected atypical hemizygotes had missense mutations, which expressed residual α-galactosidase A. However, efforts to establish genotype/phenotype correlations have been limited since most patients with Fabry dis-ease had private mutations, and attempts to predict the phenotype requires more extensive clinical information from unrelated patients with the same genotype.

GENETICS

Mode of Inheritance

Fabry disease is transmitted by an X-linked recessive gene, located at Xq2l.33-q22 (see "Molecular Genetics of α-Galactosidase A and Fabry Disease"), which normally encodes the gene product, α-ga-lactosidase A. The frequency of Fabry disease has not been deter-mined; the disease is rare, and it is estimated that the incidence is about 1:40,000. Of the over 400 described cases of affected hemi-zygous males, most are white; however, cases have been reported in blacks, Latin Americans, Native Americans, Egyptians, and Asians. The Fabry gene is highly penetrant in the hemizygote. Clin-ical onset is variable, occurring usually during childhood, but may be delayed until the second or third decade. Both intrafamilial and interfamilial variations in the clinical expression have been reported, the intrafamilial being less than the interfamilial variation.

Expressivity in the heterozygote is variable (see "The Hetero-zygote"). Proven heterozygotes may be completely asymptomatic throughout a normal life span. In contrast, complete clinical and biochemical expression of the disease, as severe as in affected males, has been documented in several heterozygotes.[22] The mark-edly variable expression of the Fabry gene in heterozygous females is anticipated for X-linked enzymatic deficiencies by the random X-inactivation hypothesis,[106] which predicts that heterozygotes for X-linked enzymatic defects will leave two populations of cells, one with mutant and the other with normal enzymatic activity. Two such populations have been isolated from individual cultured skin fibro-blasts from obligate heterozygotes, one with normal and the other with defective α-galactosidase A activities.[107]

Phenocopies

A phenocopy is a phenotypic mimic or simulation of a specific genetic trait that is usually the result of environmental factors and, thus, is not inherited. There are two such phenocopies for Fabry disease, one that mimics the characteristic corneal opacity and an-other that causes renal functional and ultrastructural changes resem-bling those in affected hemizygotes. Since the diagnosis of Fabry disease is often suspected from an eye examination or renal eval-uation for proteinuria, these phenocopies have significant diagnostic import.

The whorllike keratopathy of Fabry disease is readily distin-guishable from the corneal opacities of other lysosomal storage diseases, but is clinically and ultrastructurally identical to the corneal dystrophy associated with long-term chloroquine therapy.[108,109] Chloroquine has been shown to concentrate rapidly in lysosomes, increase the intralysosomal pH, decrease the activity of specific lysosomal hydrolases, alter the rate of proteolysis, and cause the formation of lysosomal inclusions. Based on these findings, it has been proposed that the chloroquine-induced keratopathy results from the pH inactivation of lysosomal α-galactosidase A and the subsequent accumulation of Gal-Gal-Glc-Cer.[86] In support of this concept is the finding that corneal α-galactosidase A is more sensitive to increasing pH in vitro than other lysosomal hydrolases.[110] More recently, amidarone has also been shown to cause a phenocopy of the Fabry keratopathy; although presumed to act like chloroquine, the mechanism underlying the amiodarone-induced pathology has not been elucidated.[111]

Another tissue-specific phenocopy of Fabry disease occurs in individuals who are environmentally exposed to silica dust. The pulmonary complications of silicolipoproteinosis have been described, but the renal manifestations of proteinuria and lipiduria have received little attention. Ultrastructural examination of renal tissue from these individuals has revealed the typical electron-dense lamellar inclusions in the lysosomes of glomerular epithelial and endothelial cells and proximal and distal tubular cells observed in Fabry disease.[112] The levels of α-galactosidase A and urinary sediment glycosphingolipids were normal in one such patient.[112] Although the mechanism responsible for the silica-induced phenocopy is unknown, the finding of such lesions in biopsied renal tissue should include silicosis as well as Fabry disease in the differential diagnosis.

Genetic Counseling

Genetic counseling should be made available to all families in which the diagnosis of Fabry disease is made. Inheritance of the Fabry gene from affected males and heterozygotes should be considered, since both genotypes transmit the gene. All sons of affected males will be unaffected, but all daughters will be obligate carriers of the gene. Heterozygous females have a 50 percent chance of transmitting the gene to sons who will have the disease and a 50 percent chance of transmitting the gene to daughters who will be carriers. On the average, half the sons of heterozygous females will have the disease and half the daughters will be carriers. All possible carriers among close female relatives should be examined clinically and biochemically for heterozygote identification. Fabry disease has been detected antenatally from cultured fetal cells and amniotic fluid obtained by amniocentesis as well as from chorionic villus samples (see "Prenatal Diagnosis").

DIAGNOSIS

Clinical Evaluation

The clinical diagnosis in affected males is most readily made from the history and by observation of the characteristic skin lesions and corneal dystrophy. The most common childhood symptom before the appearance of the cutaneous lesions is recurrent fever in association with pain in the hands and feet. The disorder has often been misdiagnosed as rheumatic fever, neurosis, erythromelalgia, or collagen vascular disease. Differential diagnosis of the cutaneous lesions must exclude the angiokeratoma of Fordyce,[113,114] angiokeratoma of Mibelli[115] and angiokeratoma circumscriptum,[116,117] none

of which have the typical histologic or ultrastructural pathology of the Fabry lesion (Figs. 153-3, 153-4). The angiokeratoma of Fordyce are similar in appearance to those of Fabry disease, but are limited to the scrotum and usually appear after age 30. The angiokeratoma of Mibelli are warty lesions on the exterior surfaces of extremities in young adults that are associated with chilblains. Angiokeratoma circumscriptum or naeviformis can occur anywhere on the body, are clinically and histologically similar to those of Fordyce, and are not associated with chilblains.

Angiokeratoma reportedly similar to or indistinguishable from the clinical appearance and distribution of the cutaneous lesions in Fabry disease have been described in patients with other lysosomal storage diseases, including fucosidosis, sialidosis (α-neuraminidase deficiency with or without α-galactosidase deficiency), adult-type β-galactosidase deficiency, aspartylglucosaminuria, a lysosomal disorder that presents with mental retardation and some features of the mucopolysaccharidoses, and an adult-onset variant of α-N-acetylgalactosaminidase deficiency. Ultrastructural examination of these lesions reveals lysosomal substrate deposition that differs in the fine structural appearance of the respective storage material. In addition, patients with classically appearing angiokeratoma, but no other clinical symptoms or morphologic evidence of lysosomal storage have been described; these patients have normal levels of α-galactosidase A and other lysosomal hydrolase activities. Clinical and pathologic details of the differential diagnosis of the skin lesion are available in reviews.[118–123]

Presumptive diagnosis of hemizygotes can be made by a careful ophthalmologic examination, demonstration of the birefringent inclusions in the urinary sediment, or by skin or bone marrow biopsy. The observation of the characteristic corneal dystrophy on slit-lamp examination should aid in the diagnosis. Biopsied skin will reveal the refractile lipid inclusions (Maltese crosses) in blood vessels.[49] Lipid-containing macrophages may also be observed in bone marrow aspirates. Women suspected of being heterozygous carriers of the Fabry gene should be carefully examined for evidence of the characteristic corneal opacity on slit-lamp microscopy and for isolated skin lesions, particularly on the breasts, back, trunk, and posterolateral thighs. Detection may also be accomplished by the histologic finding of lipid-laden cells in biopsied skin, tissues, or in the urinary sediment.

Biochemical Confirmation

All suspect hemizygotes should be confirmed biochemically by the demonstration of deficient α-galactosidase A activities in plasma or serum, leukocytes, tears, biopsied tissues, or cultured cells.[13,14,124] Alternatively, multiprocedural glycosphingolipid analyses can be accomplished to demonstrate the increased levels of Gal-Gal-Glc-Cer in urinary sediment, plasma, or cultured skin fibroblasts (Table 153-2).[9]

Suspected heterozygotes should be identified biochemically by their intermediate levels of α-galactosidase A activity in the above sources. Although many obligate heterozygous females can be detected by low or intermediate levels of α-galactosidase A activity in various sources, the biochemical identification of female carriers of the Fabry gene is problematic due to random X-chromosomal inactivation. Thus, heterozygotes can express levels of enzymatic activity ranging from essentially zero to normal, consistent with reports of obligate heterozygotes with normal α-galactosidase A activity and no keratopathy.[125,126] If borderline levels of enzymatic activity are obtained, then heterozygotes can be accurately diag-

TABLE 153-2

Mean Concentration of Globotriaosylceramide and Galabiosylceramide in Various Sources from Normal Individuals and Hemizygotes and Heterozygotes with Fabry Disease[8,9,121]

GLYCOSPHINGOLIPID SOURCE	NORMAL	HETEROZYGOTES	HEMIZYGOTES
Globotriaosylceramide			
Plasma	2.1*	4.5	7.6
Urinary sediment	26.1*	405	1570
Cultured fibroblasts	660*	2260	2430
Galabiosylceramide			
Plasma	nd†	nd	nd
Urinary sediment	trace	183	247
Cultured fibroblasts	nd	nd	nd

*Concentrations expressed as nmol/mL, nmol/24-h urine, nmol/g dry weight cultured fibroblasts.
†nd, not detectable.
SOURCE: Desnick et al.[22]

nosed by the identification of the specific molecular mutation present in affected males in the pedigree or by linkage analysis (see below).

Molecular Diagnosis of Heterozygotes

For families in which a specific α-galactosidase A gene lesion has been identified, heterozygote detection is specific. However, in the many Fabry families in which a gene lesion has not been identified, the use of RFLPs in or near the α-galactosidase A locus, or closely linked to it, is useful. Prenatal diagnosis requires sufficient quantities of chorionic villi or cultured fetal cells (i.e., enzyme protein) for accurate enzymatic assay. However, inadequate or slow cell growth can limit the rapidity and reliability of prenatal diagnosis by enzymatic assay. Even when fetal cells are available, DNA-based assays provide an important, and often diagnostic adjunct to the enzyme assay. Therefore, precise carrier detection and prenatal diagnosis require the identification of the specific α-galactosidase A mutation causing Fabry disease in each family. However, there are no common α-galactosidase A mutations causing this disease and almost every unrelated family has a different mutation,[97–102] necessitating a mutation study of the entire coding region in each Fabry family. Since mutation detection in this seven-exon gene spanning 12 kb is labor-intensive and time-consuming, accurate carrier detection and prenatal diagnosis may be problematic, especially in families whose α-galactosidase A mutations have not been identified prior to a pregnancy. Therefore, the availability of intragenic and closely linked polymorphisms for carrier detection and prenatal diagnosis by linkage analysis can be used to facilitate rapid molecular diagnoses. By the evaluation of highly informative short tandem repeats (DXS458, DXS454, DXS178, DXS101, DXS94, DXS17, and DXS7424), and two RFLPs that are closely linked to the α-galactosidase A gene, rapid, accurate molecular carrier and/or prenatal diagnoses have been achieved.[127] Three of these markers, DXS7424, DXS178, and DXS101, flank α-galactosidase A and lie within 1 cM of the gene; their proximity to the α-galactosidase A gene significantly limits the risk of misdiagnosis due to recombinational events. The other markers, DXS454 and DXS458 are estimated to lie between 3 and 5 cM proximal to the α-galactosidase

A gene, respectively, and DXS94 and DXS17 and are estimated to lie between 2.8 and 3.7 cM distal to the α-galactosidase A gene, respectively, and thus, would be predicted to have a 3 to 5 percent chance of recombination. These loci are all highly polymorphic, thereby increasing the likelihood that individuals will be informative and their genotypes can be assigned.

Prenatal Diagnosis

Prenatal diagnosis of Fabry disease can be accomplished by the assay of α-galactosidase A activity in chorionic villi obtained at 9 to 10 weeks of pregnancy[128] or in cultured amniotic cells obtained by amniocentesis at approximately 15 weeks of pregnancy.[16,129] The prenatal diagnosis of an affected hemizygous male fetus minimally requires the demonstration of deficient α-galactosidase A activity and an XY karyotype. For further confirmation of the prenatal diagnosis, molecular studies by direct mutation testing or indirectly by linkage analysis can be performed.

Biochemical and ultrastructural studies of tissues from fetuses with Fabry disease have been reported.[16,129] Consistent with the prenatal diagnosis, the α-galactosidase A activity was defective in all tissues studied; increased concentrations of globotriaosylceramide were found in all tissues analyzed with the exception of neural tissues.[130] Histologic and light microscopic examination of various tissues were unremarkable, but ultrastructural examination revealed electron-dense concentric lamellar inclusions in the lysosomes of vascular endothelium, myocardial cells, renal tubules, and epithelial and endothelial cells of renal glomeruli.[129,130]

TREATMENT

Medical Management

In Fabry disease, the chronicity of the clinical events causes severe debilitation and incapacity that extends over years. The single most debilitating and morbid aspect of Fabry disease is the excruciating pain. The pathophysiologic events that cause the incapacitating episodes of pain or the chronic burning acroparesthesias have not been clarified. The α-adrenergic blocking agent, phenoxybenzamine, which increases peripheral vascular flow, has been administered for pain relief; although this drug provided relief in a hemizygote on several occasions, priapism and epistasis were early complications in two other hemizygotes.[131] With the exception of centrally acting narcotic analgesics, which have been only partially effective, conventional analgesic agents have not been successful. However, prophylactic administration of low maintenance dosages of diphenylhydantoin have been found to provide relief from the periodic crises of excruciating pain and constant discomfort in hemizygotes and heterozygotes.[132] Carbamazepine also provides pain relief.[133] The combination of diphenylhydantoin and carbamazepine significantly reduced the pain in an affected hemizygote, and subsequent reports have further documented the effectiveness of diphenylhydantoin and/or carbamazepine in the prevention and amelioration of these debilitating pains.

Care of patients with regard to cardiac, pulmonary, and central nervous system manifestations remains nonspecific and symptomatic. Obstructive lung disease has been documented in older hemizygotes and heterozygotes, with more severe impairment in smokers; therefore, patients should be discouraged from smoking.

Because renal insufficiency is the most frequent late complication in patients with this disease, long-term hemodialysis or renal transplantation have become life-saving procedures. Successful transplantation will correct renal function. The α-galactosidase A in the allograft will catabolize the turnover of endogenous renal glycosphingolipid substrates. Renal transplantation also provides an in situ source of the normal enzyme.[134] Renal transplantation, however, should be undertaken only in patients with clinically significant renal failure.

Replacement therapy using partially purified human enzyme has proved biochemically effective in pilot trials[135,136]; however, sufficient enzyme has not been available to evaluate the clinical effectiveness in long-term replacement therapy. The high level expression of active human α-galactosidase A in mammalian cells has been achieved,[137] and the production of large amounts of the recombinant enzyme will permit trials of replacement therapy.

REFERENCES

1. Anderson W: A case of angiokeratoma. *Br J Dermatol* **10**:113, 1898
2. Fabry J: Ein Beitrag zur Kenntnis der Purpura haemorrhagica nodularis (Purpura papulosa hemorrhagica Hebrae). *Arch Dermatol Syphilol* **43**:187, 1898
3. Fabry J: Weiterer Beitrag zur Klinik des Angiokeratoma naeviforme (Naevus angiokeratosus). *Dermatol Wochenschr* **90**:339, 1930
4. Scriba K: Zur Pathogenese des Angiokeratoma corporis diffusum Fabry mit kardiovasorenalem Symptomenkomplex. *Verh Dtsch Ges Pathol* **34**:221, 1950
5. Hornbostel H, Scriba K: Zur Diagnostik des Angiokeratoma Fabry mit kardiovasorenalem Symptomenkomplex als Phosphatidspeicherungskrankheit dutch Probeexcision der Haut. *Klin Wochenschr* **31**:68, 1953
6. Opitz JM et al: The genetics of angiokeratoma corporis diffusum (Fabry's disease) and its linkage with Xg(a) locus. *Am J Hum Genet* **17**:325, 1965
7. Sweeley CC, Klionsky B: Fabry's disease: Classification as a sphingolipidosis and partial characterization of a novel glycolipid. *J Biol Chem* **238**:3148, 1963
8. Vance DE et al: Concentrations of glycosyl ceramides in plasma and red cells in Fabry's disease: A glycolipid lipidosis. *J Lipid Res* **10**:188, 1969
9. Desnick RJ et al: Diagnosis of glycosphingolipidoses by urinary sediment analysis. *N Engl J Med* **284**:739, 1971
10. Wherret JR, Hakomori S: Characterization of a blood group B glycolipid, accumulating in the pancreas of a patient with Fabry's disease. *J Biol Chem* **218**:3046, 1973
11. Brady RO et al: Enzymatic defect in Fabry's disease: Ceramide trihexosidase deficiency. *N Engl J Med* **276**:1163, 1967
12. Kint JA: Fabry's disease, α-galactosidase deficiency. *Science* **167**:1268, 1970
13. Desnick RJ et al: Fabry's disease. Enzymatic diagnosis of hemizygotes and heterozygotes. *J Lab Clin Med* **81**:157, 1973
14. Johnson DL et al: Fabry disease: Diagnosis of hemizygotes and heterozygotes by α-galactosidase A activity in tears. *Clin Chim Acta* **63**:81, 1975
15. Brady RO et al: Fabry's disease: Antenatal diagnosis. *Science* **172**:172, 1971
16. Desnick RJ, Sweeley CC: Prenatal detection of Fabry's disease, in *Antenatal Diagnosis,* edited by A Dorfman, Chicago, University of Chicago Press, 1971, p 185
17. Mapes CA et al: Enzyme replacement in Fabry's disease, an inborn error of metabolism. *Science* **169**:987, 1970
18. Brady RO et al: Replacement therapy for inherited enzyme deficiency: Use of purified ceramidetrihexosidase in Fabry's disease. *N Engl J Med* **289**:9, 1973
19. Desnick RJ et al: Enzyme therapy XII: Enzyme therapy in Fabry's disease: Differential enzyme and substrate clearance kinetics of plasma and splenic α-galactosidase isozymes. *Proc Natl Acad Sci USA* **76**:5326, 1979
20. Bishop EF et al: Human α-galactosidase A: Nucleotide sequence of a cDNA clone encoding the mature enzyme. *Proc Natl Acad Sci USA* **83**:4859, 1986
21. Kornreich R et al: Nucleotide sequence of the human α-galactosidase A gene. *Nucleic Acids Res* **17**:3301, 1989
22. Desnick RJ et al: α-Galactosidase A deficiency: Fabry disease, in *Metabolic and Molecular Bases of Inherited Disease,* 7th ed. edited

by CR Scriver, AL Beaudet, WS Sly, D Valle. New York, McGraw-Hill, 1995, pp 2741–2784
23. Lockman LA et al: Relief of pain of Fabry's disease by diphenylhydantoin. *Neurology* **23**:871, 1973
24. Urbain G et al: Fabry's disease without skin lesions. *Lancet* **1**:1, 1967
25. Clarke JTR et al: Ceramide trihexosidosis (Fabry's disease) without skin lesions. *N Engl J Med* **284**:233, 1971
26. Ainsworth SK, Smith RM: A case study of Fabry's disease occurring in a Black kindred without peripheral neuropathy or skin lesions. *Lab Invest* **38**:373, 1978
27. Wallace RD, Cooper WJ: Angiokeratoma corporis diffusum universale (Fabry). *Am J Med* **39**:656, 1965
28. Ferrans VJ et al: The heart of Fabry's disease: A histochemical and electron microscopic study. *Am J Cardiol* **24**:95, 1969
29. Becker AE et al: Cardiac manifestations of Fabry's disease: Report of a case with mitral insufficiency and electrocardiographic evidence of myocardial infarction. *Am J Cardiol* **36**:829, 1975
30. Colucci WS et al: Hypertrophic obstructive cardiomyopathy due to Fabry's disease. *N Engl J Med* **2**:926, 1982
31. Fisher E et al: Fabry disease: An unusual cause of severe coronary artery disease in a young man. *Ann Intern Med* **117**:221, 1992
32. Colombi A et al: Angiokeratoma corporis diffusum-Fabry's disease. *Helv Med Acta* **34**:67, 1967
33. Sher NA et al: The ocular manifestations in Fabry's disease. *Arch Ophthalmol* **97**:671, 1979
34. Spaeth GL, Frost P: Fabry's disease: Its ocular manifestations. *Arch Ophthalmol* **74**:760, 1965
35. Franceschetti ATh: La cornea verticillata (Gruber) et ses relations avec la maladie de Fabry (Angiokeratoma corporis diffusum). *Ophthalmologica* **156**:232, 1968
36. Bartinimon EE et al: Pulmonary involvement in Fabry's disease: A reappraisal: Follow up of a San Diego kindred and review of the literature. *Am J Med* **53**:755, 1972
37. Brown LK et al: Pulmonary involvement in Fabry disease. *Am J Respir Crit Care Med* **155**:1004, 1997
38. Rowe JW et al: Intestinal manifestations of Fabry's disease. *Ann Intern Med* **81**:628, 1974
39. Sheth KJ et al: Gastrointestinal structure and function in Fabry's disease. *Am J Gastroenterol* **76**:246, 1981
40. O'Brien BD et al: Pathophysiologic and ultrastructural basis for intestinal symptoms in Fabry's disease. *Gastroenterology* **82**:957, 1982
41. Nagao Y et al: Hypertrophic cardiomyopathy in late-onset variant of Fabry disease with high residual activity of α-galactosidase A. *Clin Genet* **39**:233, 1991
42. von Scheidt W et al: An atypical variant of Fabry's disease with manifestations confined to the myocardium. *N Engl J Med* **324**:395, 1991
43. Broadbent JC et al: Fabry cardiomyopathy in the female confirmed by endomyocardial biopsy. *Mayo Clin Proc* **56**:623, 1981
44. Desnick RJ et al: Correction of enzymatic deficiencies by renal transplantation: Fabry's disease. *Surgery* **72**:203, 1972
45. Avila JL et al: Fabry's disease: Normal α-galactosidase activity and urinary-sediment glycosphingolipid levels in two obligate heterozygotes. *Br J Dermatol* **89**:149, 1973
46. Levade T et al: Different phenotypic expression of Fabry disease in female monozygotic twins. *J Inherit Metab Disease* **14**:105, 1991
47. Sagebiel RW, Parker F: Cutaneous lesions of Fabry's disease: Glycolipid lipidosis-light and electron microscopic findings. *J Invest Dermatol* **50**:208, 1968
48. Tamowski WM, Hashimoto K: New light microscopic skin findings in Fabry's disease. *Acta Dermatol Venereol* **49**:386, 1969
49. Breathnach SM et al: Anderson-Fabry disease: Characteristic ultrastructural features in cutaneous blood vessels in a 1 year old boy. *Br J Dermatol* **103**:81, 1980
50. Hashimoto K et al: Angiokeratoma corpofis diffusum (Fabry): Histochemical and electron microscopic studies of the skin. *J Invest Dermatol* **44**:119, 1969
51. McNary W, Lowenstein LM: A morphological study of the renal lesion in angiokeratoma corporis diffusum universals (Fabry's disease). *J Urol* **93**:641, 1965
52. Burkholder PM et al: Clinicopathologic, enzymatic and genetic features in a case of Fabry's disease. *Arch Pathol Lab Med* **104**:17, 1980
53. Grunnet ML, Spilsbury PR: The central nervous system in Fabry's disease. *Arch Neurol* **28**:231, 1973

54. Kocen RS, Thomas PK: Peripheral nerve involvement in Fabry's disease. *Arch Neurol* **22**:81, 1970

55. Sung JH et al: Neuropathology of Fabry's disease: Proceedings of the VIIth International Congress of Neuropathology (ICS no. 362). Excerpta Medica Congress Series, vol 1, 1975, p 267

56. Sung JH: Autonomic neurons affected by lipid storage in the spinal cord of Fabry's disease: Distribution of autonomic neurons in the sacral cord. *J Neuropathol Exp Neurol* **38**:87, 1979

57. Rahman AN, Lindenberg R: The neuropathology of hereditary dystopic lipidosis. *Arch Neurol* **9**:373, 1963

58. Ohnishi A, Dyck PJ: Loss of small peripheral sensory neurons in Fabry disease: Histologic and morphometric evaluation of cutaneous nerves, spinal ganglia, and posterior columns. *Arch Neurol* **31**:120, 1974

59. de Veber GA et al: Fabry disease: Immunochemical characterization of neuronal involvement. *Ann Neurol* **31**:409, 1992

60. Witschel H, Mathyl J: Morphological elements of the specific ocular changes in Morbus Fabry. *Klin Monatsbl Augenheilkd* **154**:599, 1969

61. Font RF, Fine BS: Ocular pathology in Fabry's disease: Histochemical and electron microscopic observations. *Am J Ophthalmol* **73**:419, 1972

62. Desnick RJ et al: Cardiac valvular anomalies in Fabry's disease: Clinical, morphologic and biochemical studies. *Circulation* **54**:818, 1976

63. Goldman M et al: Echocardiographic abnormality and disease severity in Fabry disease. *Am J Coll Cardiol* **7**:1157, 1986

64. Faffagina T et al: Light and electron microscopic histochemistry of Fabry disease. *Am J Pathol* **103**:247, 1981

65. Lehner T, Adams CWM: Lipid histochemistry of Fabry's disease. *J Pathol Bacteriol* **95**:411, 1968

66. Van Mullem PJ, Ruiter M: Histochemical studies on lipid metabolism in so-called Fabry's disease (angiokeratoma corporis diffusum). *Arch Klin Exp Derm* **232**:148, 1968

67. Chatterjee S et al: Immunohistochemical localization of glycosphingolipid in urinary renal tubular cells in Fabry's disease. *Am J Clin Pathol* **82**:24, 1984

68. Robinson D, Khalfan HA: Fabry's disease: Identification of carrier status by fluorescenuelectron binding. *Biochem Soc Trans* **12**:1063, 1984

69. Van Mullem PJ, Ruiter M: Fine structure of the skin in angiokeratoma corporis diffusum (Fabry's disease). *J Pathol* **101**:221, 1970

70. Hashimoto K et al: Angiokeratoma corporis diffusum (Fabry disease). *Arch Dermatol* **112**:1416, 1976

71. Bishop EF, Desnick RJ: Affinity purification of α-galactosidase A from human spleen, placenta and plasma with elimination of pyrogen contamination. *J Biol Chem* **256**:1307, 1981

72. Beutler E, Kuhl W: Purification and properties of human α-galactosidases. *J Biol Chem* **247**:7195, 1972

73. Schram AW et al: The identity of α-galactosidase B from human liver. *Biochim Biophys Acta* **482**:138, 1977

74. Wang AE, Desnick RJ: Structural organization and complete sequence of the human α-N-acetylgalactosaminidase gene: Homology with the α-galactosidase A gene provides evidence for evolution from a common ancestral gene. *Genomics* **10**:133,1991

75. Johnson DL, Desnick RJ: Molecular pathology of Fabry's disease: Physical and kinetic properties of α-galactosidase A in cultured human endothelial cells. *Biochim Biophys Acta* **538**:195, 1978

76. Dawson G et al: Distribution of glycosphingolipids in the serum lipoproteins of normal human subjects and patients with hypo- and hyperlipidemias. *J Lipid Res* **17**:125, 1976

77. Clarke JTR et al: Neutral glycosphingolipids of serum lipoproteins in Fabry's disease. *Biochim Biophys Acta* **431**:317, 1976

78. Van den Bergh FAJTM, Tager JM: Localization of neutral glycosphingolipids in human plasma. *Biochim Biophys Acta* **441**:391, 1976

79. Meuweissen SGM et al: Ultrastructural and biochemical liver analyses in Fabry's disease. *Hepatology* **2**:263, 1982

80. Clarke JTR, Stoltz JM: Uptake of radiolabeled galactosyl-(α1-4)-galactosyl-(B1-4)-glucosylceramide by human lipoproteins in vitro. *Biochim Biophys Acta* **441**:165, 1976

81. Stein O, Stein Y: High density lipoproteins reduce the uptake of low density lipoproteins by human endothelial cells in culture. *Biochim Biophys Acta* **431**:363, 1976

82. Goldstein JL, Brown MS: The low density lipoprotein pathway and its relation to atherosclerosis. *Annu Rev Biochem* **46**:897, 1977

83. Voldavsky I et al: Role of contact inhibition in the regulation of receptor-mediated uptake of low density lipoprotein in cultured vascular endothelial cells. *Proc Natl Acad Sci USA* **75**:356, 1979

84. Dawson G, Sweeley CC: *In vivo* studies on glycosphingolipid metabolism in porcine blood. *J Biol Chem* **245**:410, 1970

85. Tao RVP: Biochemistry and metabolism of mammalian blood glycosphingolipids (Ph.D. thesis). Michigan State University, 1973

86. Barkai A, DeCesare JL: Influence of sialic acid groups on retention of glycosphingolipids in blood plasma. *Biochim Biophys Acta* **398**:287, 1975

87. Nakamura T et al: Angiokeratoma corporis diffusum (Fabry disease): Ultrastructural studies of the skin. *Acta Derm Venereol* **61**:37, 1981

88. Fukuhara N et al: Fabry's disease on the mechanism of the peripheral nerve involvement. *Acta Neuropathol* **33**:9, 1975

89. Dvorak AM et al: Diagnostic electron microscopy. Fabry's disease: Use of biopsies from uninvolved skin. Acute and chronic changes involving the microvasculature and small unmyelinated nerves. *Pathol Annu* **16**:139, 1981

90. Seino Y et al: Peripheral hemodynamics in patients with Fabry's disease. *Am Heart J* **105**:783, 1983

91. Morgan SH et al: The neurological complications of Anderson Fabry disease (α-galactosidase A deficiency)—investigation of symptomatic and presymptomatic patients. *Q J Med* **277**:491, 1990

92. Sheth KJ, Swick HM: Peripheral nerve conduction in Fabry disease. *Ann Neurol* **7**:319, 1980

93. Pelissier JF et al: Morphological and biochemical changes in muscle and peripheral nerve in Fabry's disease. *Muscle Nerve* **4**:381, 1981

94. Pabico RC et al: Renal pathologic lesions and functional alterations in a man with Fabry's disease. *Am J Med* **55**:415, 1973

95. Schibanoff JM et al: Tissue distribution of glycosphingolipids in a case of Fabry's disease. *J Lipid Res* **10**:515, 1969

96. Hozumi I et al: Biochemical and clinical analysis of accumulated glycolipids in symptomatic heterozygotes of angiokeratoma corporis diffusum (Fabry's disease) in comparison with hemizygotes. *J Lipid Res* **31**:335, 1990

97. Eng CM, Desnick RJ: Molecular basis of Fabry disease: Mutations and polymorphisms in the α-galactosidase A gene. *Hum Mutat* **3**:103, 1994

98. Bernstein HS et al: Fabry disease: Gene rearrangements and a coding region point mutation in the α-galactosidase A gene. *J Clin Invest* **83**:1390, 1989

99. Kornreich R, Desnick RJ: Fabry disease: Detection of gene rearrangements in the human α-galactosidase A gene by multiplex PCR amplification. *Hum Mutat* **2**:108, 1993

100. Kornreich R et al: α-Galactosidase A gene rearrangements causing Fabry disease: Identification of short direct repeats at breakpoints in an Alu rich gene. *J Biol Chem* **265**:9319, 1990

101. Madsen KM et al: Identification of mutations in Danish families with Fabry's disease. Proceedings of The Second International Duodecim Symposium: "Molecular Biology of Lysosomal Diseases," Majvik, Finland, May 23–26, 1993

102. Eng CM et al: Nature and frequency of mutations in the α-galactosidase A gene causing Fabry disease. *Am J Hum Genet* **53**:1186, 1993

103. DePamphilis ML, Wassarman PM: Replication of eukaryotic chromosomes: A close-up of the replication fork. *Annu Rev Biochem* **49**:627, 1980

104. Sakuraba H et al: Invariant exon skipping in the human α-galactosidase A pre-mRNA: A g to t substitution in a 5′ splice site causing Fabry disease. *Genomics* **12**:643, 1992

105. Davies JP et al: Mutation analysis in patients with the typical form of Anderson-Fabry disease. *Eur J Hum Genet,* **4**:219, 1996

106. Lyon M: Gene action in the X-chromosome of the mouse *(Mus musculus L).* Nature **190**:372, 1961

107. Romeo G, Migeon BR: Genetic inactivation of the α-galactosidase locus in carriers of Fabry's disease. *Science* **170**:180, 1970

108. Francois J, de Becker L: Les manifestations oculaires de l'intoxication chloroquine. *Ann Oculist* **198**:513, 1965

109. Desnick RJ et al: Fabry keratopathy: Molecular pathology of the chloroquine-induced phenocopy. *Am J Hum Genet* **26**:26a, 1974

110. Whitley CB: Studies of heritable and induced lysosomopathies (Ph.D. thesis). University of Minnesota, 1977

111. Whitley CB et al: Amiodarone phenocopy of Fabry's keratopathy. *JAMA* **249**:2177, 1983

112. Banks DE et al: Silicon nephropathy mimicking Fabry's disease. *Am J Nephr* **3**:279, 1983

113. Imperial R, Heliwig EB: Angiokeratoma of the scrotum (Fordyce type). *J Urol* **98**:379, 1967

114. Fordyce JA: Angiokeratoma of the scrotum. *J Cutan Genitourin Dis* **14**:81,1896

115. Traub EF, Tolmach JA: Angiokeratoma: Comprehensive study of the literature and report of a case. *Arch Derm Syph* **24**:39, 1931

116. Dammert K: Angiokeratosis naeviformis—a form of naevus telangiectatieus lateralis (naevus flammeus). *Dermatologica* **130**:17, 1965

117. Goldman L et al: Thrombotic angiokeratoma circumscriptum simulating melanoma. *Arch Dermatol* **117**:138, 1981

118. Holmes RC et al: Angiokeratoma corporis diffusum in a patient with normal enzyme activities. *J Am Acad Dermatol* **10**:384, 1984

119. Crovato F, Rebora A: Angiokeratoma corporis diffusum and normal enzyme activities. *J Am Acad Dermatol* **12**:885, 1985

120. Frost P et al: Fabry's disease: Glycolipidosis: Skin manifestations. *Arch Intern Med* **117**:440, 1966

121. Imperial R, Heliwig EB: Angiokeratoma: A clinicopathological study. *Arch Dermatol* **95**:166, 1967

122. Van Mullem PJ, Ruiter M: Electron microscopic study of the skin in angiokeratoma corporis diffusum. *Arch Klin Exp Derm* **226**:453, 1966

123. Elleder M et al: An atypical ultrastructural pattern in Fabry's disease: A study on its nature and incidence in seven cases. *Ultrastruct Pathol* **14**:467, 1990

124. Beutler E, Kuhl W: Biochemical and electrophoretic studies of ce-galactosidase in normal man, in patients with Fabry's disease, and *in Equidae*. *Am J Hum Genet* **24**:237, 1972

125. Avila JL et al: Fabry's disease: Normal α-galactosidase activity and urinary ediment glycolipid levels in two obligate heterozygotes. Br J Dermatol **89**:149, 1973

126. Francois J: Heterozygotes for sex-linked traits and mary Lyon's in-activation theory. XIV. Fabry's dysotpic lipidosis, in *Proceedings of the III International Congress of Human Genetics*. Baltimore, Johns Hopkins University Press, 1967, p 243

127. Caggana M et al: Fabry disease: Molecular carrier detection and prenatal diagnosis by analysis of closely-linked polymorphisms at Xq22.1. *Am J Med Genet* **71**:329, 1997

128. Desnick RJ et al: Prenatal diagnosis of glycosphingolipidoses: Sandhoff's (SD) and Fabry's diseases (FD). *J Pediatr* **83**:149, 1973

129. Kleijer W et al: Prenatal diagnosis of Fabry's disease by direct analysis of chorionic villi. *Prenat Diagn* **7**:283, 1987

130. Malouf M et al: Ultrastructural changes in antenatal Fabry's disease. *Am J Pathol* **82**:132, 1976

131. Funderbunk SJ et al: Pripaism after phenoxybenzamine in a patient with Fabry's disease. *N Engl J Med* **290**:630, 1974

132. Dupperrat B et al: Maladie de Fabry: Angiokeratomes presents a la naissance: Action del la diphenylhydantoine sur les crises douloureuses. *Ann Dermatol Syphilol* **102**:392, 1975

133. Filling-Katz M et al: Carbamazepine in Fabry's disease: Effective analgesia with dose-dependent exacerbation of autonomic dysfunction. *Neurology* **39**:598, 1989

134. Desnick RJ et al: Correction of enzymatic deficiencies by renal transplantation: Fabry's disease. *Surgery* **72**:203, 1972

135. Brady RO et al: Replacement therapy for inherited enzyme deficiency: Use of purified ceramidetrihexosidase in Fabry's disease. *N Engl J Med* **289**:9, 1973

136. Desnick RJ et al: Enzyme therapy XII: Enzyme therapy in Fabry's disease: Differential enzyme and substrate clearance kinetics of plasma and splenic α-galactosidase isozymes. *Proc Natl Acad Sci USA* **76**:5326, 1979

137. Ioannou YA et al: Overexpression of human α-galactosidase A results in its intracellular aggregation, crystallization in lysosomes, and selective secretion. *J Cell Biol* **119**:1137, 1992

CHAPTER 154

Ch. M. Lapière

Lipoid Proteinosis

Lipoid proteinosis, also called *hyalinosis cutis et mucosae* and *Urbach-Wiethe disease*, is an uncommon, recessively inherited disorder characterized by noninflammatory persistent papules on the skin and mucous membranes. The papules are produced by the accumulation of a basement membrane–like material in various connective tissues. The pathogenesis of the disease is not yet clear. Therapy is mainly symptomatic. For a complete review, see refs. 1 and 2.

HISTORY

In 1929, two Viennese, E. Urbach and C. Wiethe, a dermatologist and an otorhinolaryngologist, described an entity that they called *lipoidosis cutis et mucosae*[3] on the basis of histologic investigations demonstrating the deposition, in skin and mucous membranes, of a lipoid material associated with protein. The initial name was later modified to *lipoid proteinosis* to avoid confusion with other lipoidoses. At the present time, the most common names given to this syndrome are *lipoid proteinosis* or *hyalinosis cutis et mucosae*. It may be referred to as Urbach-Wiethe disease eponymously.

GENETICS

Parental consanguinity, affected siblings, and equal numbers of male and female patients suggest autosomal recessive transmission. Most of the reported patients have a European background, and more than half of them belong to or are related to the Germanic linguistic group. Interesting studies performed in the Afrikaaner population of South Africa suggest that most of the reported cases in that country derive from descendants of a brother and a sister who emigrated to South Africa from Germany in the middle of the seventeenth century.

CLINICAL PRESENTATION

The first clinical sign is often hoarseness, caused by infiltration of the laryngeal mucosa, that has developed by birth or in early childhood. Skin lesions usually appear shortly afterward or simultaneously. Clinical signs may be precipitated by an intercurrent disease as benign as, for example, vaccination.

Location of Lesions

Papular, nodular, or diffuse yellow waxy infiltrates are located on the face, the axillae, and the scrotum. Skin lesions resembling pitted acne scars may be located not only on the face but also in non-acneogenic regions. Other lesions of the face resemble solar elastosis because of the deposition of yellow material inducing a marked thickening of the skin with deep wrinkles (Fig. 154-1). The classic and most easily recognizable sign, although not always present, is the beaded arrangement of waxy papules along the eyelids (Fig. 154-1). Lesions on the scalp may occur and cause alopecia. Lesions on non-sun-exposed skin can be present, as well as alterations of the mucous membranes. The tongue is often firm, and its mobility may be limited (Fig. 154-2). The tonsils and other areas in the oral cavity may be infiltrated. A yellow discoloration of the lips is characteristic (Fig. 154-2). The skin lesions may be traumatized and present in the form of an oozing infiltrate leading to hyperkeratosis. Hyperkeratosis is also observed on the palm and dorsum of the hands (Fig. 154-3A and 154-3B), elbows, knees (Fig. 154-4), and buttocks, possibly related to frequent trauma in these locations.

FIGURE 154-1

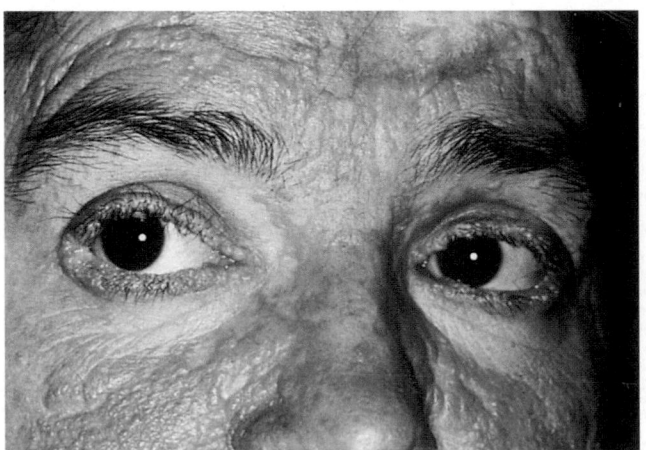

Lipoid proteinosis. Note the beaded arrangement of waxy papules along the margin of both eyelids and the pseudo solar elastosis of the cheeks and forehead. (*Courtesy of O. Braun-Falco, Munich.*)

FIGURE 154-2

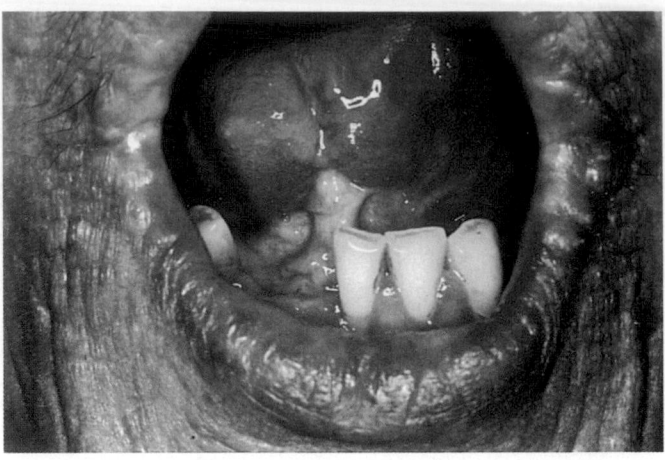

Discoloration of the lips in lipoid proteinosis. Limitation of mobility of the tongue is related to infiltration of the frenulum. (*Courtesy of O. Braun-Falco, Munich.*)

Involvement of Other Organs

Recurrent parotitis is related to occlusion of the salivary canal. The teeth are abnormal in almost 30 percent of patients: patients will lack permanent upper lateral incisors. Except for lesions in the oropharyngeal cavity, alterations of the digestive tract are uncommon[4] and reported only as autopsy findings in a few patients. The respiratory tract may be involved by infiltration of the vocal cords and obstruction.

A bilateral intracranial bean-shaped suprasellar calcification has been observed in 50 percent of the patients, but not all of them present with epilepsy or any other signs of cerebral dysfunction. This represents calcification in blood vessels of the hippocampal portions of the temporal lobes. Abnormalities of the peripheral nervous system are uncommon; four South African patients had peripheral nervous system lesions that may have been due to congenital analgesia.

Infiltration of the eyelids induces malfunction of the eyelashes, causing corneal ulceration. Alopecia of the eyelashes and eyebrows is observed. Focal degeneration of the macula has been found in a third of the examined patients.

Cardiac, endocrine, and urogenital disorders have been seen but are not clearly a part of the spectrum of this disease.

Deposition of hyaline material around the blood vessels is seen by microscopy to be present in internal organs. It indicates that the defect is a generalized disease. These changes appear to be asymptomatic.

CLINICAL COURSE AND PROGNOSIS

Except for the risk of respiratory obstruction in infancy, the disease is compatible with a normal life span. Lesions of the upper respiratory tract may cause problems in patients with tracheotomy or disease of the trachea. Quality of life is seriously impaired by the disfiguring lesions and the permanent hoarseness.

FIGURE 154-3

CHAPTER 154
Lipoid Proteinosis   1827

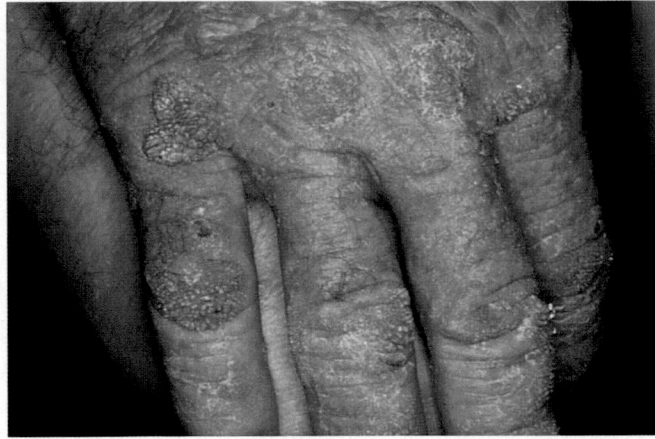

A.

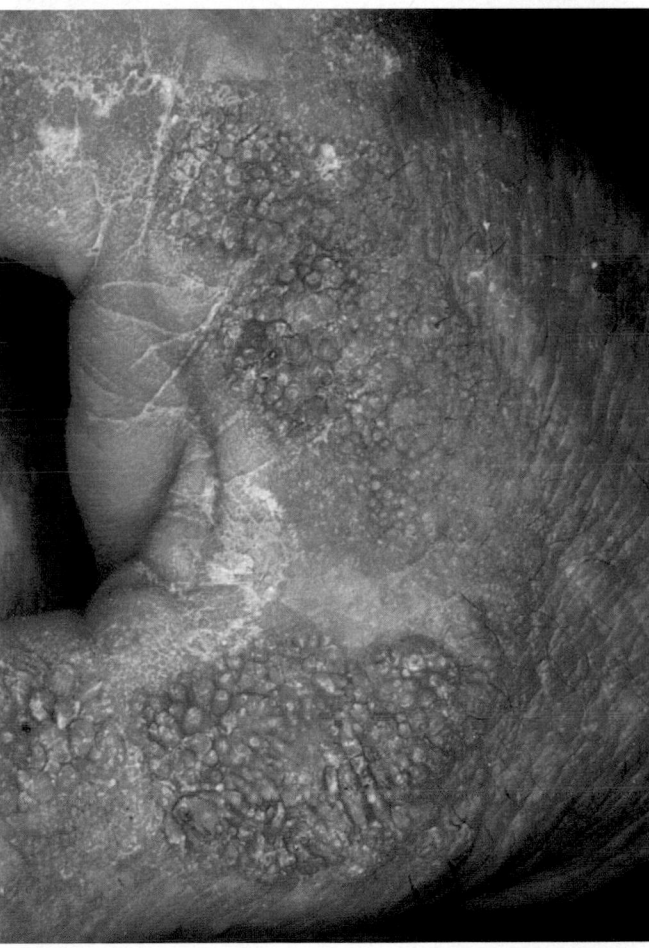

B.

Hyperkeratotic papular lesions on dorsum of hands (*A*), interdigital web, and the sides of the fingers (*B*) in lipoid proteinosis.

LABORATORY FINDINGS

No laboratory finding is typical of lipoid proteinosis. In some patients, abnormal glucose metabolism has been reported. Porphyrins, liver function, protein electrophoresis, lipids, and lipoproteins ar-

FIGURE 154-4

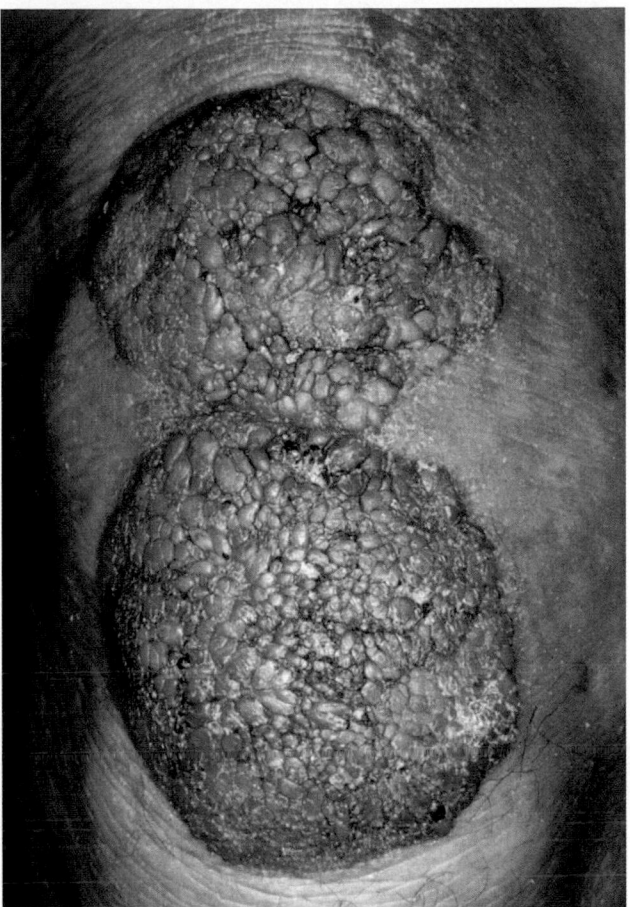

Verrucous nodular lesions on the knee in lipoid proteinosis.

enormal in the classic form of the disease. There may be signs of chronic or acute inflammation (increased alpha$_2$ or gamma globulins). Elevated serum calcium has been reported rarely.

DIFFERENTIAL DIAGNOSIS

Lipoid proteinosis has to be differentiated from other diseases related to the deposition of amorphous material in the dermis. The differential diagnosis applies at both clinical and histopathologic levels.

Porphyria, mainly erythropoietic protoporphyria, shows deposition of a PAS-positive material around the blood vessels, mainly in sun-exposed areas. Light sensitivity is not a feature of lipoid proteinosis, and the observation of lesions in nonexposed sites aids the diagnosis. The site of the biopsy should be provided to the pathologist for differential diagnosis.

Lipid deposition in the various forms of xanthomatosis is rarely a problem of differential diagnosis. Furthermore, xanthoma cells never occur in lipoid proteinosis.

Amyloidosis may resemble lipoid proteinosis. Its development is often more progressive and accompanied by involvement of the

FIGURE 154-5

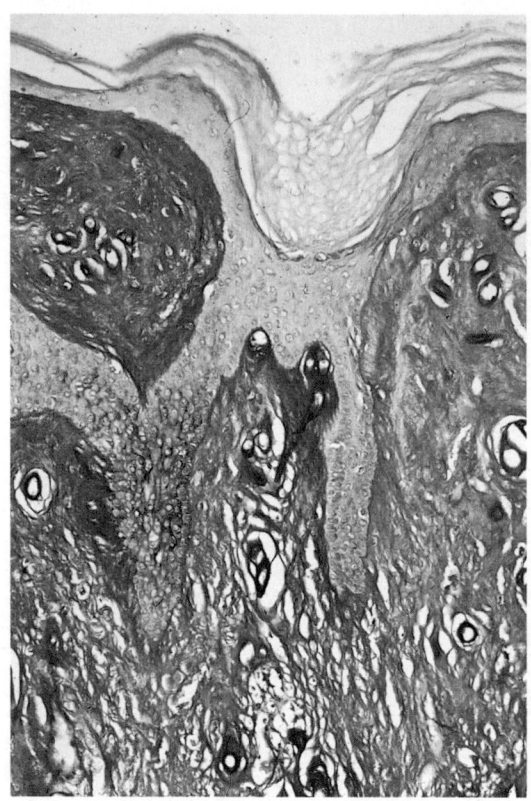

Extensive deposition of a PAS-positive material in the papillary dermis of a pitted acne scar lesion in lipoid proteinosis.

kidneys, heart, and other tissues. Amyloid deposition may occur in the skin of lipoid proteinosis patients. The clinical presentation of diabetic microangiopathy is often different from that of lipoid proteinosis, but the pathologic picture may be confusing.

A report of acquired hyalinosis cutis et mucosae in a patient with monoclonal immunoglobulinopathy requires attention.[5] This form of the syndrome can be differentiated by immunoelectrophoresis of the plasma proteins.

MORPHOLOGIC FINDINGS

The main manifestations of the disease are related to the deposition of an amorphous or laminated material in the connective tissues. The location and the immunohistochemical nature of the deposit support its relation to components of the basement membrane zone. It displays a PAS-positive reaction that resists digestion by enzymes and contains collagen type IV and laminin. The deposition of this material is progressive and often located next to cells that are known to synthesize a basement membrane.[6]

Little is known about the initial stage of the disease. Most often biopsy specimens are collected from obvious lesions and show deposition of the amorphous eosinophilic material initially around walls of the small and medium-sized blood vessels in the papillary dermis, which shows a pronounced "onion-skin" proliferation of the adventitia. The hyaline material is also found around the smooth muscle cells of the arrectores pilorum and ultimately involves the surrounding dermis of the sweat glands. The myoepithelial cells may also be involved in the development of these lesions. The amount of amorphous material increases with time to progressively encase the adnexae, filling up the dermis and pushing aside most of the normal collagen bundles (Fig. 154-5).

By electron microscopy, the deposit appears to be composed of small granules and short filaments of low electron density, 3 to 5 nm in diameter. Electron-dense bodies (mineralized) are located around the sweat glands.

The deposit in lipoid proteinosis is mainly composed of noncollagen protein, although the concentric layers of basement membrane–like material contain collagen types III and IV and laminin, as shown by immunodetection. A portion of this material, solubilized by reduction and injected to produce antibodies in rabbits, induced antibodies that recognize antigens also detectable in normal skin.[7] This indicates that the disease might be related to the overproduction and/or the lack of degradation of a normal component of the human skin.

The lipid nature of the deposit remains controversial. Solubilization in various solvents gave nonreproducible results. The deposit stains with lipophilic agents, suggesting that unsaturated hydrophobic lipids might be present.

The pathogenesis of the disease is still uncertain. Observations by Bauer et al.[8] of accumulations of cytoplasmic inclusions and vacuoles in culture of cells derived from lipoid proteinosis–afflicted skin suggest that the defect might be a storage disease. This intracellular material is rich in hexuronic acids and is sulphated. It has a lower than normal degradation rate, suggesting defective hydrolytic activity, as found in some mucolipidoses. In vitro, the fibroblasts collected from the affected skin also display an increased biosynthetic activity for collagen type IV (basement membrane collagen) and laminin.[9]

THERAPY

There is presently no effective therapy. Topical glucocorticoids have been extensively used with beneficial effect.

Plastic surgery and dermabrasion to remove lesions has been used in some patients. The use of these therapies is questionable because trauma has seemed to increase deposition of the pathologic material. Some beneficial effect has, however, been reported.

Treatment by oral dimethyl sulfoxide has been claimed to be successful.[10]

REFERENCES

1. Hofer PA: Urbach-Wiethe disease (lipoglucoproteinosis: lipoid proteinosis; hyalinosis cutis et mucosae). A review. *Acta Dermatol Venereol (Stockh)* **53**:71, 1973
2. Konstantinov K et al: Lipoid proteinosis. Review. *J Am Acad Dermatol* **27**:293, 1992
3. Urbach E, Wiethe C: Lipoidosis cutis et mucosae. *Virchows Arch Path Anat* **273**:285, 1929
4. Caccamo D et al: Lipoid proteinosis of the small bowel. *Arch Pathol Lab Med* **118**:572, 1994
5. Von der Helm D et al: Acquired hyalinosis cutis et mucosae in plasmacytoma with monoclonal IgG-lambda gammopathy. *Hautarzt* **40**(3):153, 1989
6. Pierard GE et al: A clinicopathologic study of six cases of lipoid proteinosis. *Am J Dermatopathol* **10**(4):300, 1989
7. Fleischmajer R et al: Ultrastructure and composition of connective tissue in hyalinosis cutis et mucosae skin. *J Invest Dermatol* **82**:252, 1984

8. Bauer EA et al: Lipoid proteinosis: In vivo and in vitro evidence for a lysosomal storage disease. *J Invest Dermatol* **76**:119, 1981
9. Olsen DR et al: Expression of basement membrane zone genes coding for type IV procollagen and laminin by human skin fibroblasts in vitro: Elevated alpha I (IV) collagen mRNA levels in lipoid proteinosis. *J Invest Dermatol* **90**:734, 1988

10. Wong CK, Lin CS: Remarkable response of lipoid proteinosis to oral dimethyl sulfoxide. *Br J Dermatol* **119**:541, 1988

CHAPTER 155

John S. Walsh
Janet A. Fairley

Cutaneous Mineralization and Ossification

CALCIUM

Calcium is involved in many physiologic processes. It is key to skeletal muscle and myocardial contraction, neurotransmission, and blood coagulation. In addition, it is the primary mineral in the bony skeleton. On the cellular level, its diverse functions include transmission of information into and between cells, regulation of plasma membrane potential, and exocytosis. Only over the past 15 years has the effect of calcium on skin been fully appreciated. Calcium was first discovered to influence epidermal cell growth and differentiation in 1980 when it was shown that the growth and differentiation of mouse epidermal cells in culture depended on extracellular calcium.[1] In cell culture, keratinocytes proliferate rapidly in low calcium conditions but do not differentiate.[2] With higher concentrations of extracellular calcium, keratinocytes begin to differentiate and express markers of terminal differentiation, such as transglutaminase activity and involucrin.[3,4] Calcium also plays an integral role in modulating cell-cell adhesion via the cadherin family of cell adhesion molecules.

REGULATORY HORMONES

Parathyroid Hormone

Parathyroid hormone (PTH) is an 84-amino acid, single chain polypeptide that is synthesized in the parathyroid glands. Under normal conditions, a decrease in the serum concentration of ionized calcium results in an increase in PTH production, whereas an increase in the serum concentration of ionized calcium results in a decrease in PTH production. An increased PTH plasma concentration causes an increased plasma concentration of calcium by its direct effects on the kidney and bone and its indirect effects on the intestine. In the kidney, PTH increases renal tubular reabsorption of calcium and increases renal clearance of phosphate. PTH also acts directly on the bone to increase the concentration of plasma calcium acutely by mobilizing calcium from bone into the extracellular fluid. Osteocytes and osteoblasts are the presumed target cells for this effect. PTH also stimulates osteoclastic bone resorption, possibly by stimulating osteoblasts to release factors that activate osteoclasts. PTH together with a decreased plasma phosphate concentration stimulates 1-α hydroxylase activity in the kidney, causing an increase in the plasma concentration of $1,25(OH)_2D_3$. $1,25(OH)_2D_3$ increases intestinal absorption of calcium.

The PTH-like peptide that is responsible for the humoral hypercalcemia of malignancy is produced by many malignant cells, particularly those derived from squamous epithelia. Cultured nonmalignant human keratinocytes also produce a similar protein called *parathyroid hormone–related peptide* (PTHrP).[5] The existence on dermal fibroblasts of receptors that recognize PTH and PTH-like peptides suggests that PTH and keratinocyte-produced PTHrP may contribute to normal skin physiology.

The levels of PTH are elevated in some patients with disorders of keratinization,[6] such as ichthyosis vulgaris, lamellar ichthyosis/nonbullous congenital ichthyosiform erythroderma, pityriasis rubra pilaris, ichthyosis linearis circumflexa, and Darier's disease. The cause and significance of this elevation are unknown.

Calcitonin

Calcitonin is a 32-amino acid polypeptide that is produced by parafollicular or C cells of the thyroid gland. Calcium is the primary stimulant for calcitonin secretion. Calcitonin lowers serum calcium concentration, primarily through osteoclast inhibition, but whether it plays a major role in serum calcium metabolism in vivo is unclear.

Vitamin D

Vitamin D_3, or cholecalciferol, is a secosteroid formed by the opening of the beta ring of 7-dehydrocholesterol. In humans, this formation occurs in the basal layer of the epidermis.[7] First there is a UVB-mediated conversion of 7-dehydrocholesterol to previtamin D_3, which then undergoes thermal isomerization to form vitamin D_3.

Vitamin D_3 is inert. To become biologically active, it must first be hydroxylated at carbon position 25 in the liver and then at carbon position 1-α by the enzyme 1-α hydroxylase in the kidney. 1-α Hydroxylase is tightly regulated. PTH and calcitonin increase its activity, whereas calcium, phosphate, and $1,25(OH)_2D_3$ inhibit it.[8]

$1,25(OH)_2D_3$, like PTH, increases plasma calcium. Its primary action is to stimulate the active transport of calcium across the intestine. $1,25(OH)_2D_3$ also increases plasma calcium by mobilizing calcium from bone.[9] The simultaneous presence of PTH appears to be necessary for this effect.

During the past decade it has been discovered that $1,25(OH)_2D_3$ not only is important in calcium regulation but also plays a major role in the growth and differentiation of tissues, including skin. Receptors for $1,25(OH)_2D_3$ have been found on epidermal keratinocytes, pilosebaceous structures, and in the dermis.[10–13] In human keratinocyte cultures, $1,25(OH)_2D_3$ causes a dose-dependent decrease in proliferation, an increase in morphologic differentiation, and an increase in the terminal differentiation markers transglutaminase activity and involucrin.[14] Cultured human keratinocytes can convert $25(OH)D_3$ to $1,25(OH)_2D_3$, suggesting that the epidermis may regulate its own growth and differentiation by endogenously produced $1,25(OH)_2D_3$.[14] The mechanism by which $1,25(OH)_2D_3$ may induce differentiation of epidermal cells may be through calcium, because calcium is required for terminal differentiation of keratinocytes. $1,25(OH)_2D_3$ may facilitate calcium entry into cells and, through induction of calcium-binding proteins, facilitate the ability of calcium to regulate a variety of cellular processes.[14] In addition $1,25(OH)_2D_3$ may effect terminal differentiation through its hormonal effects.

ABERRANT CALCIFICATION AND OSSIFICATION

Despite the careful regulation of serum calcium, calcification (mineralization)* and ossification of cutaneous and subcutaneous tissues may occur. Calcification is the deposition of insoluble calcium salts; when it occurs in cutaneous tissues it is known as *calcinosis cutis*. Ossification is the formation of true bony tissue by the deposition of calcium and phosphorus in a proteinaceous matrix as hydroxyapatite crystals. Cutaneous calcification may be divided into four major categories: dystrophic, metastatic, idiopathic, and iatrogenic (Table 155-1). Dystrophic calcification is the most common type of calcinosis cutis and occurs as a result of local tissue injury or abnormalities. Although calcium and phosphate metabolism and serum levels are normal, local tissue abnormalities, such as alterations in collagen, elastin, or subcutaneous fat, may precipitate calcification. The internal organs usually remain unaffected. Metastatic calcification is the precipitation of calcium salts in normal tissue secondary to an underlying defect in calcium and/or phosphate metabolism. The calcification is usually widespread and affects predominantly blood vessels, kidneys, lungs, and gastric mucosa. Cutaneous and subcutaneous tissues may also be involved. All patients presenting with signs of metastatic calcification should receive a

---

Mineralization is a universal term, whereas the more commonly applied term is *calcification*. As both a cation, usually calcium, and an anion, typically phosphate or carbonate, are deposited, the terms are used interchangeably.

TABLE 155-1

Causes of Cutaneous Calcification

Dystrophic
  Connective tissue disease
  Panniculitis
  Porphyria cutanea tarda
  Ehlers-Danlos syndrome
  Werner's syndrome
  Pseudoxanthoma elasticum
  Rothmund-Thomson syndrome
  Cutaneous neoplasms
  Infections
  Trauma
Metastatic
  Chronic renal failure
    Benign nodular calcification
    Calciphylaxis
  Hypervitaminosis D
  Milk-alkali syndrome
  Neoplasms
  Sarcoidosis
  Pseudoxanthoma elasticum
Idiopathic
  Idiopathic calcification of the scrotum
  Tumoral calcinosis
  Subepidermal calcified nodule
  Milia-like idiopathic calcinosis cutis in Down syndrome
Iatrogenic
  Intravenous calcium infusion
  Calcium chloride electrode paste

calcium and phosphate metabolic evaluation. Idiopathic calcification occurs without identifiable underlying tissue abnormalities or abnormal calcium and/or phosphate metabolism. Cutaneous calcification may also be iatrogenic. Cutaneous ossification most commonly occurs secondary to local tissue alteration or preexisting calcification. Any calcifying disorder of the skin may ossify secondarily. On rare occasions, primary cutaneous ossification may occur without underlying tissue abnormalities or preexisting calcification.

DYSTROPHIC CALCIFICATION

Connective Tissue Diseases

Dystrophic calcification frequently occurs in connective tissue diseases. Scleroderma and CREST syndrome (*c*alcinosis cutis, *R*aynaud's phenomenon, *e*sophageal dysfunction, *s*clerodactyly, *t*elangiectases) are notable examples that frequently show calcinosis cutis. In these disorders, nodules and plaques of calcium deposits may occur in the skin, subcutaneous tissue, muscle, or tendons, usually at least 10 years after disease onset.[15] The calcium deposits most commonly occur on the upper extremities, especially on the fingers and wrists, but may occur in any area subject to trauma or motion. As the calcifications enlarge, they may ulcerate and exude a chalky material. The successful use of long-term diltiazem therapy in patients with calcinosis cutis associated with scleroderma or CREST syndrome has been described.[16]

Dystrophic calcification also occurs in dermatomyositis. It is more commonly associated with juvenile rather than adult-onset dermatomyositis, occurring in 44 to 70 percent of children as opposed to 20 percent of adults.[17] The calcification tends to occur 2 to 3 years after disease onset.[18] The subcutaneous calcified nodules are most frequently seen on the elbows, knees, shoulders, and buttocks. The calcium deposits may be painful and can ulcerate. They may also exude a chalky material, form sinuses, and become chronically infected. Particularly in children, calcium salt deposition may become quite extensive, progressing along fascial planes of skin and muscle, forming an "exoskeleton," and leading to significant morbidity and mortality. Calcinosis cutis in dermatomyositis is difficult to treat; however, if the patient survives long enough, the calcified nodules usually improve spontaneously. A diet low in calcium and phosphate along with aluminum hydroxide may arrest or facilitate regression of the calcified nodules.[19] Disodium etidronate has also been used with some success, and intralesional glucocorticoids may have limited use.[20,21] Occasionally, surgical removal of calcium deposits is necessary to clear sinus tracts, ulcers, or chronic infections. Because high levels of vitamin K–dependent gamma-carboxyglutamic acid have been found in involved tissue of patients with calcinosis cutis, some investigators have treated patients with low-dose warfarin and found that it decreased the amount of extraskeletal ossification as measured by bone scan.[22] However, because none of the patients showed clinical improvement, the usefulness of this treatment remains uncertain. In advanced cases, glucocorticoid or immunosuppressant therapy may be indicated. Long-term use of diltiazem has been reported to improve calcinosis cutis.[23,24]

Although uncommon, calcinosis cutis has also been described in systemic lupus erythematosus[25,26] and discoid lupus erythematosus.[27]

Panniculitis

Pancreatic enzyme panniculitis is a type of lobular panniculitis that may undergo dystrophic calcification. Pancreatic enzyme panniculitis occurs in patients with pancreatitis or pancreatic adenocarcinoma and is presumably caused by the action of liberated pancreatic enzymes on subcutaneous fat. The fatty acids formed by lipolysis may combine with calcium and form calcium soaps.[28]

In subcutaneous fat necrosis of the newborn, erythematous, well-defined nodules and plaques characteristically occur during the first few weeks of life over the cheeks, back, buttocks, and extremities. The affected infants are generally otherwise healthy, and the nodules and plaques usually clear spontaneously. Occasionally, the lesions calcify, and in a small subset of patients symptomatic hypercalcemia may develop.[29,30]

Panniculitis may occur with connective tissue diseases and, like their cutaneous counterparts, may show dystrophic calcification. Lupus profundus and panniculitis associated with dermatomyositis may show calcification.[31]

Porphyria Cutanea Tarda

Dystrophic calcification has been observed in porphyria cutanea tarda (PCT). Sclerodermoid plaques with dystrophic calcification have occurred on the preauricular area, scalp, neck, and dorsa of the hands in patients with PCT.[32] In one case, a 78-year-old male with PCT developed extensive sclerodermoid changes with ulcerations on his torso, upper arms, and back.[33] The ulcerations showed transepidermally eliminated sheets of calcification.

Inherited Disorders

Ehlers-Danlos syndrome is a group of inherited disorders of collagen metabolism. The skin characteristically shows hyperelasticity and fragility with formation of pseudotumors and large gaping scars. In addition, particularly in Ehlers-Danlos syndrome type I, subcutaneous calcified spherules may appear.[34] Subcutaneous spherules are thought to represent calcified ischemic fat lobules.[35] Calcification of healing surgical incisions has also been reported in patients with Ehlers-Danlos syndrome.[36]

Werner's syndrome is an inherited disorder that leads to premature aging. The skin and subcutaneous tissue are often scleroderma-like in appearance and may show calcification. In one study, 12 of 24 patients with Werner's syndrome had soft tissue calcification.[37]

Dystrophic calcification is also observed in patients with pseudoxanthoma elasticum (PXE), a hereditary disorder characterized by abnormal elastin fibers affecting the skin, Bruch's membrane of the retina, and arteries. The specific genetic biochemical defect that allows for the calcification of elastin fibers is unknown. Less commonly, metastatic calcification may also occur with PXE.[38] Some patients with PXE have abnormal calcium, phosphate, and/or vitamin D metabolism and develop metastatic calcification in the form of calcific tumors, calcification of the falx cerebri, and arterial calcifications. This finding suggests that there may be a subset of patients with PXE who have an inborn error in both elastin fiber and calcium, phosphate, and vitamin D metabolism. The relation between the two remains unknown.

Calcinosis cutis presenting as numerous, small, yellow papules on the extremities has also been reported to occur in association with Rothmund-Thomson syndrome.[39]

Cutaneous Neoplasms

Dystrophic calcification occurs in association with a variety of benign and malignant cutaneous neoplasms. Often the neoplasms also show ossification in the surrounding stroma.

Pilomatricomas are the most common cutaneous neoplasms that manifest calcification and ossification. Approximately 75 percent show calcification, and 15 to 20 percent show ossification.[40,41] Some pilomatricomas perforate and exude a chalky material containing calcium.[42] Ossification usually occurs within the connective tissue adjacent to the shadow cells, probably through the metaplasia of fibroblasts into osteoblasts.[43]

Other neoplasms have been reported to be associated with calcification and ossification. Twenty-five percent of pilar cysts show foci of calcification.[44] Intradermal nevi may infrequently show ossification, probably as a result of inflammation or folliculitis.[45–47] Chondroid syringomas may also show calcification and ossification. However, unlike other neoplasms, the ossification occurs within the tumor via ossification of the chondroid cells, much like endochondral bone formation occurring in the epiphyses of bones.[45] Although rare, ossification has also been described in desmoplastic malignant melanomas and atypical fibroxanthomas.[48,49] Other neoplasms rarely associated with ossification include basal cell carcinomas, pyogenic granulomas, hemangiomas, neurilemmomas, trichoepitheliomas, and seborrheic keratoses.[45]

Infections

Infectious agents may produce enough cutaneous damage to cause dystrophic calcification. Notable parasitic infections that may result in calcinosis cutis include onchocerciasis,[50,51] caused by the filaria *Onchocerca volvulus*, and cysticercosis, caused by the tapeworm *Taenia solium*.[52] Calcinosis cutis has been reported as a complication of intrauterine herpes simplex infection.[53]

Trauma

Dystrophic calcification has been reported in a variety of situations where local tissue injury occurs, such as in scars caused by burns, trauma, neonatal heel sticks, and surgery.[54–57] One case report described calcification within abdominal keloids.[58]

METASTATIC CALCIFICATION

Chronic Renal Failure

Metastatic calcification most commonly occurs in chronic renal failure and takes the form of either benign nodular calcification or calciphylaxis. In chronic renal failure, the decreased clearance of phosphate results in hyperphosphatemia. In addition, the impaired production of $1,25(OH)_2D_3$ results in a decrease in calcium absorption from the intestine and decreased serum calcium levels. The hypocalcemia results in increased PTH production and secondary hyperparathyroidism. Elevated levels of PTH cause bone resorption and the mobilization of calcium and phosphate into the serum, leading to normalization of the serum calcium concentration but marked hyperphosphatemia. If the solubility product of calcium and phosphate is exceeded, metastatic calcification may occur. The calcifications typically occur at periarticular sites, and their size and number tend to correlate with the degree of hyperphosphatemia. The lesions disappear with normalization of calcium and phosphate levels.

Calciphylaxis is characterized by progressive vascular calcification, soft tissue necrosis, and ischemic necrosis of the skin. Clinically, calciphylaxis presents as firm, extremely painful, well-demarcated, violaceous plaques associated with soft tissue necrosis and ulceration. It is seen primarily in patients with chronic renal failure and prolonged secondary hyperparathyroidism. Most of the patients reported in the literature are female, and there may be a proportionately high number of patients with diabetes.[59,60] Calciphylaxis is considered a type of metastatic calcification, although the calcium and phosphate solubility product is not necessarily increased. The cause of calciphylaxis is unknown. One theory is based on the experimental studies of Selye[61] in which calciphylaxis was induced in rats by exposing them to a sensitizing agent, such as PTH, dihydrotachysterol, or vitamin D, and then exposing them to a challenging agent, such as metallic salts, egg albumin, or glucocorticoids. It is theorized that in human beings calciphylaxis may occur if tissues are previously sensitized and then challenged with a specific agent. Sensitizing agents may include increased levels of PTH or calcium and phosphate product (70 or higher). Suspected challenging agents include albumin and other blood infusions, glucocorticoids, and immunosuppressants.[62] Other investigators believe that patients with calciphylaxis have underlying small vessel disease, perhaps related to the etiology of their renal failure, and that this in conjunction with high serum levels of PTH predisposes them to small and medium artery medial calcification and soft tissue necrosis.[60]

Some patients with calciphylaxis have decreased function of protein C,[63] a potent anticoagulant synthesized in the liver that inhibits clotting factors V and VIII. Quantitative or functional protein C deficiency leads to hypercoagulable states. Whether this plays a direct role in the pathogenesis of calciphylaxis or is a marker for a coagulation defect that predisposes a subset of these patients to calciphylaxis is unknown.

Treating calciphylaxis is generally unrewarding. Removing the sensitizing and challenging agents, if possible, is recommended. Although not carefully studied, parathyroidectomy has helped some patients.[59] A total parathyroidectomy can be undertaken with autotransplantation of one gland in the forearm. The transplanted gland can be removed later if the patient's hyperparathyroidism persists.

Hypervitaminosis D

The chronic ingestion of vitamin D in supraphysiologic doses (50,000 to 100,000 units per day) may produce hypervitaminosis D. The initial signs and symptoms of hypervitaminosis D are attributable to hypercalcemia and hypercalciuria and include weakness, lethargy, headache, nausea, and polyuria. Metastatic calcification may also occur.[64]

Milk-Alkali Syndrome

Milk-alkali syndrome is characterized by the excessive ingestion of calcium-containing foods or antacids, leading to hypercalcemia. Complications other than the acute manifestations of hypercalcemia include irreversible renal failure, nephrocalcinosis, and subcutaneous calcification, occurring predominantly in periarticular tissues.[65]

Other Disorders

Other systemic disorders associated with hypercalcemia and/or hyperphosphatemia have been reported to cause metastatic calcification. These include the neoplasms associated with bony destruction, such as lymphoma, leukemia, multiple myeloma, and metastatic carcinoma,[66–68] as well as sarcoidosis.[69]

IDIOPATHIC CALCIFICATION

Idiopathic calcification of the scrotum is characterized by calcified nodules limited to the scrotum.[70] The lesions usually appear in otherwise healthy boys or young men and tend to increase in size and number with time. Eventually, they may break down and exude a chalky material. Controversy exists over its etiology. Many believe idiopathic calcification of the scrotum is truly idiopathic[71]; others maintain that calcified scrotal nodules are inflamed or ruptured epidermoid cysts that undergo dystrophic calcification.[72,73] Excision of the lesions is the treatment of choice, although patients may continue to develop nodules at other sites. Idiopathic calcification of the penis, vulva, and breast has also been reported.[74–76]

Tumoral calcinosis is a disorder characterized by the deposition of calcific masses around major joints, such as hips, shoulders, elbows, and knees. It generally occurs in otherwise healthy adolescents. The masses are intramuscular or subcutaneous and may enlarge to sizes causing significant impairment of joint function. Usually, the overlying skin is normal, but associated ulceration and calcinosis cutis may occur.[77] Familial occurrences among siblings and associated hyperphosphatemia in a subset of patients are well documented.[78] This has led some investigators to postulate that tumoral calcinosis is a form of metastatic calcification caused by an inborn error in phosphate metabolism. Others disagree, because hyperphosphatemia is not a universal finding and the calcification occurs only in periarticular regions. Surgical excision is the treatment of choice, but phosphate deprivation has met with some success.[79]

Subepidermal calcified nodules appear on the exposed area of the head and the extremities. They may be congenital or acquired and typically appear as a hard, 3- to 11-mm, solitary lesion, although multiple lesions may occur.[80] Some investigators believe the lesions represent calcified sweat gland hamartomas.[81]

Recent reports have described the appearance of milia-like idiopathic calcinosis cutis on the dorsa of hands and forearms of patients with Down syndrome.[82–84] Some of the calcifications were associated with lesional or palpebral syringomas.

IATROGENIC CALCIFICATION

Cutaneous calcification may be iatrogenic. Calcinosis cutis is a recognized complication of intravenous calcium chloride and calcium gluconate therapy. With extravasation of the calcium solution, calcified nodules may appear, probably as a result of an elevated tissue concentration of calcium and tissue damage at the site of the extravasation.[85] Minor trauma and prolonged contact with calcium salts can lead to calcinosis cutis in a variety of settings.[86,87] It has occurred in patients undergoing electroencephalography who had prolonged contact with saturated calcium chloride electrode paste.[88]

PRIMARY OSSIFICATION

Primary ossification of cutaneous and subcutaneous tissues rarely may occur without any underlying tissue abnormality or preexisting calcification. In addition to miliary osteoma of the face, there are four well-described ossifying syndromes: Albright's hereditary osteodystrophy, fibrodysplasia ossificans progressiva, progressive osseous heteroplasia, and platelike osteoma cutis. Other primary ossification disorders reported in the literature, such as isolated or widespread osteoma, are probably variants of the above or represent a group of poorly described primary ossification disorders.

Miliary osteoma cutis of the face most commonly occurs as multiple small, firm nodules on the faces of young women with a history of acne vulgaris. There are, however, reports of multiple miliary osteoma cutis occurring in older patients without acne vulgaris or other underlying skin disease.[89,90]

Albright's hereditary osteodystrophy is an X-linked or autosomal dominantly inherited syndrome characterized by the ossification of cutaneous and subcutaneous tissues in childhood.[90,91] The ossification can occur anywhere on the body. Albright's hereditary osteodystrophy generally follows a limited course, so that significant deformity or physical impairment is rare. In addition, patients typically have brachydactyly, dimpling over the metacarpophalangeal joints (Albright's sign), obesity, round or moon facies, and mental retardation. Most patients have a deficient end-organ response to PTH or "pseudohypoparathyroidism" with hypocalcemia, hyperphosphatemia, and elevated levels of PTH. Other patients with Albright's hereditary osteodystrophy have "pseudopseudohypoparathyroidism" with normal serum levels of calcium and phosphorus.[92]

Fibrodysplasia ossificans progressiva is an autosomal dominant syndrome characterized by the progressive ossification of deep connective tissues leading to significant morbidity and mortality.[93,94] Ossification of the skin occurs as a result of direct extension from underlying tissues. All patients have dysmorphic great toes. Other features include abnormal phalanges of the hands, deafness, baldness, and mental retardation. Although the genetic defect remains unknown, elevated levels of bone morphogenetic protein 4 have been identified in the preosseous lesional cells of patients.[95]

Progressive osseous heteroplasia is a recently described entity characterized by progressive ossification of skin and deep tissues occurring during infancy or childhood.[96,97] Most reported patients are female. Ossification usually begins within the dermis and progresses to involve deeper tissues, such as muscle, as well as overlying skin. Skin involvement has been described as a papular eruption resembling "rice grains" and having a "gritty" consistency. Unlike Albright's hereditary osteodystrophy or fibrodysplasia ossificans progressiva, there are no associated dysmorphic features.

Worret and Burgdorf[98] first described platelike osteoma cutis in a 4-month-old infant who had a slowly spreading bony plate within the dermis on the lateral thigh and knee. In addition, they described 12 other patients who had similar findings. Based on these cases, they coined the term *platelike osteoma cutis* and proposed the following as diagnostic criteria: lesion present at birth or within the first year of life; no evidence of abnormal calcium or phosphorus metabolism; no history of infection, trauma, or other predisposing events; and the presence of at least one bony plate with or without other cutaneous osteomas. Subsequent to their report, many patients with various findings were described under this heading of platelike osteoma cutis. It is likely, however, that many of these patients actually had progressive osseous heteroplasia or some other undefined ossification disorder.

REFERENCES

1. Hennings H et al: Calcium regulation on growth and differentiation of mouse epidermal cells in culture. *Cell* **19**:245, 1980
2. Yuspa SH: Chapter IV, in *Methods of Skin Research,* edited by D Skerrow, C Skerrow. Sussex, John Wiley, 1985, pp 213–249
3. Yuspa SH et al: Expression of murine epidermal differentiation markers is tightly regulated by restricted extracellular calcium concentrations in vitro. *J Cell Biol* **109**:1207, 1989
4. Milstone LM: Calcium modulates the growth of human keratinocytes in confluent culture. *Epithelia* **1**:129, 1987
5. Merendino J Jr et al: Parathyroid hormone–like protein from cultured human keratinocytes. *Science* **231**:388, 1986
6. Milstone LM et al: Serum parathyroid hormone level is elevated in some patients with disorders of keratinization. *Arch Dermatol* **128**:926, 1992
7. Holick MF et al: Photosynthesis of previtamin D_3 in human skin and the physiological consequences. *Science* **210**:203, 1980
8. Marx SJ: Vitamin D and other calciferols, in *Metabolic Basis of Inherited Disease,* 6th ed, edited by CR Scriver, AL Beaudet, WS Sly, D Valle. New York, McGraw-Hill, 1989, pp 2029–2045
9. Deluca HF, Schnoes HK: Vitamin D. Recent advances. *Annu Rev Biochem* **52**:411, 1983
10. Clemens TL et al: Interaction of 1,25 dihydroxyvitamin D with keratinocytes and fibroblasts from skin of normal subjects and a subject with vitamin D dependent rickets, type II: A model for the study of the mode of action of $1,25(OH)_2D_3$. *J Clin Endocrinol Metab* **56**:824, 1983
11. Eil C, Marx SJ: Nuclear uptake of 1,25 dihydroxy [^{3}H] cholecalciferol in dispersed fibroblasts cultured from normal human skin. *Proc Natl Acad Sci USA* **79**:2562, 1981
12. Feldman D et al: Vitamin D resistant rickets with alopecia: Cultured skin fibroblasts elicit defective cytoplasmic receptors and unresponsiveness to 1,25 dihydroxyvitamin D in rat skin. *Endocrinol Metab* **55**:1020, 1982
13. Simpson RU, DeLuca HF: Characterization of a receptor-like protein for 1,25 dihydroxyvitamin D in rat skin. *Proc Natl Acad Sci USA* **77**:5822, 1980

14. Pillai S et al: Vitamin D and epidermal differentiation. Evidence for a role of endogenously produced vitamin D metabolites in keratinocyte differentiation. *Skin Pharmacol* 1:149, 1988

15. Raimer SS: Calcinosis cutis. *Curr Concepts Skin Disorders* 6:9, 1985

16. Palmieri GM et al: Treatment of calcinosis with diltiazem. *Arthritis Rheum* 38:1646, 1995

17. Cook DC et al: Dermatomyositis and focal scleroderma. *Pediatr Clin North Am* 10:979, 1963

18. Bowyer SL et al: Childhood dermatomyositis. Factors predicting functional outcome and development of dystrophic calcification. *J Pediatr* 103:882, 1983

19. Wang WJ et al: Calcinosis cutis in juvenile dermatomyositis. Remarkable response to aluminum hydroxide therapy. *Arch Dermatol* 124:1721, 1988

20. Rabens SF, Bethune JE: Disodium etidronate therapy for dystrophic cutaneous calcification. *Arch Dermatol* 11:357, 1975

21. Lee SS et al: Calcinosis cutis circumscripta: Treatment with an intralesional corticosteroid. *Arch Dermatol* 114:1080, 1978

22. Berger RG et al: Treatment of calcinosis universalis with low-dose warfarin. *Am J Med* 83:72, 1987

23. Dolan AL et al: Diltiazem induces remission of calcinosis in scleroderma. *Br J Rheumatol* 34:576, 1995

24. Palmieri GMA et al: Treatment of calcinosis with diltiazem. *Arthritis Rheum* 38:1646, 1995

25. Rothe MJ et al: Extensive calcinosis cutis with systemic lupus erythematosus. *Arch Dermatol* 126:1060, 1990

26. Carette S, Urowitz MB: Systemic lupus erythematosus and diffuse soft tissue calcification. *J Dermatol* 22:416, 1983

27. Ueki H et al: Cutaneous calcinosis in localized discoid lupus erythematosus. *Arch Dermatol* 116:196, 1980

28. Levine N, Lazarus GS: Subcutaneous fat necrosis after paracentesis. Report of a case in a patient with acute pancreatitis. *Arch Dermatol* 112:993, 1976

29. Martin MM, Steven EM: Subcutaneous fat necrosis of the newborn associated with subcutaneous fat necrosis and calcification. *Am J Dis Child* 104:235, 1962

30. Shackelford GD et al: Calcified subcutaneous fat necrosis in infancy. *J Can Assoc Radiol* 26:203, 1975

31. Winkelmann RK: Panniculitis in connective tissue disease. *Arch Dermatol* 119:336, 1983

32. Grossman ME et al: Porphyria cutanea tarda. Clinical features and laboratory findings in 40 patients. *Am J Med* 67:277, 1979

33. Wilson PR: Porphyria cutanea tarda with cutaneous "scleroderma" and calcification. *J Dermatol* 30:39, 1985

34. Novice FM et al: Dysplasias and malformations, in *Handbook of Genetic Skin Disorders,* edited by FM Novice, DW Collison, WHC Burgdorf, NB Esterly. Philadelphia, Saunders, 1994, p 298

35. Linnemann MP, Johnson VW: Ehlers-Danlos syndrome presenting with torsion of stomach. *Proc R Soc Med* 68:330, 1975

36. Rees TD et al: The Ehlers-Danlos syndrome. *Plast Reconstr Surg* 32:39, 1963

37. Murata K, Nakashima H: Werner's syndrome. Twenty-four cases and review of the Japanese medical literature. *J Am Geriatr Soc* 30:303, 1982

38. Mallette LE, Mechanick JI: Heritable syndrome of pseudoxanthoma elasticum with abnormal phosphorus and vitamin D metabolism. *Am J Med* 83:1157, 1987

39. Aydemir EH et al: Rothmund-Thomson syndrome with calcinosis universalis. *J Dermatol* 27:591, 1988

40. Peterson WC, Hult AM: Calcifying epithelioma of Malherbe. *Arch Dermatol* 90:404, 1964

41. Forbis R, Helwig EB: Pilomatrixoma (calcifying epithelioma). *Arch Dermatol* 83:606, 1961

42. Arnold M, McGuire LJ: Perforating pilomatricoma. Difficulty in diagnosis. *J Am Acad Dermatol* 18:754, 1988

43. Geisr JD: L'epithelioma calcife de Malherbe. *Ann Dermatol Syphiligr* 86:383, 1959

44. Leppard BJ, Sanderson KB: The natural history of trichilemmal cysts. *Br J Dermatol* 116:113, 1980

45. Roth SI et al: Cutaneous ossification. Report of 120 cases and review of the literature. *Arch Pathol* 76:44, 1963

46. Duperant B: Osteomes cutanes. *Ann Dermatol Syphiligr* 88:11, 1961

47. Delacretaz J, Frank E: Zur Pathogenese des Osteo-naevus nanta. *Hautarzt* 15:487, 1964

48. Moreno A et al: Osteoid and bone formation in desmoplastic malignant melanoma. *J Cutan Pathol* 13:128, 1986

49. Chen KTK: Atypical fibroxanthoma of the skin with osteoid production. *Arch Dermatol* 116:113, 1980

50. Harman R et al: Helminthic diseases II, in *Clinical Tropical Dermatology,* edited by O Canizares, R Harman. Boston, Blackwell Scientific, 1992, p 348

51. Browne SG: Calcinosis circumscripta of the scrotal wall. The etiological role of *Onchocerca volvulus. Br J Dermatol* 74:136, 1962

52. Pastel A, Grupper C: Subcutaneous calcification, generalized calcinosis in nodular chains. Cysticercosis. *Bull Soc Fr Dermatol Syphligr* 76:28, 1969

53. Beers BB et al: Dystrophic calcinosis cutis secondary to intrauterine herpes simplex. *Pediatr Dermatol* 3:208, 1986

54. Coskey RJ, Mehregan AH: Calcinosis cutis in a burn scar. *J Am Acad Dermatol* 11:666, 1984

55. Ellis IO et al: Plumber's knee. Calcinosis cutis after repeated trauma in a plumber. *Br Med J* 288:1723, 1984

56. Leung A: Calcification following heel sticks. *J Pediatr* 106:168, 1985

57. Katz I, LeVine M: Bone formation in laparotomy scars. Roentgen findings. *Am J Radiol* 84:248, 1960

58. Redmond WJ, Baker SR: Keloidal calcification. *Arch Dermatol* 119:270, 1983

59. Hafner J et al: Uremic small-artery disease with medial calcification and intimal hyperplasia (so-called calciphylaxis): A complication of chronic renal failure and benefit from parathyroidectomy. *J Am Acad Dermatol* 33:954, 1995

60. Walsh JS, Fairley JA: Calciphylaxis. *J Am Acad Dermatol* 35:786, 1996

61. Selye H: *Calciphylaxis.* Chicago, University of Chicago Press, 1962, pp 1–16

62. Khafif RA et al: Calciphylaxis and system calcinosis. Collective review. *Arch Intern Med* 150:956, 1990

63. Mehta RL et al: Skin necrosis with acquired protein C deficiency in patients with renal failure and calciphylaxis. *Am J Med* 88:252, 1990

64. Wilson CW et al: Vitamin D poisoning with metastatic calcification. *Am J Med* 14:116, 1953

65. Werner P et al: Reversible metastatic calcification associated with excessive milk and alkali intake. *Am J Med* 14:108, 1953

66. Panicek DM et al: Calcification in untreated mediastinal lymphoma. *Radiology* 166:735, 1988

67. Raper RF, Ibels LS: Osteosclerotic myeloma complicated by diffuse arteritis, vascular calcification and extensive cutaneous necrosis. *Nephron* 39:389, 1985

68. Abe M et al: Hypercalcemia and metastatic calcification in adult T-cell leukemia—pathogenesis of hypercalcemia. *Fukushima J Med Sci* 31:85, 1985

69. Kroll JJ et al: Subcutaneous sarcoidosis with calcification. *Arch Dermatol* 106:894, 1972

70. Shapiro L et al: Idiopathic calcinosis of the scrotum. *Arch Dermatol* 102:199, 1970

71. Wright S et al: Idiopathic scrotal calcinosis is idiopathic. *J Am Acad Dermatol* 24:727, 1991

72. Sweinhart JW, Golitz LE: Scrotal calcinosis—dystrophic calcification of epidermoid cysts. *Arch Dermatol* 118:985, 1982

73. Bhawan J et al: The so-called idiopathic calcinosis. *Arch Dermatol* 119:709, 1983

74. Hutchinson IF et al: Idiopathic calcinosis cutis of the penis. *Br J Dermatol* 102:341, 1980

75. Balfour PJ, Vincenti AC: Idiopathic vulvar calcinosis. *Histopathology* 18:183, 1991

76. Kopans DB et al: Dermal deposits mistaken for breast calcification. *Radiology* 163:282, 1983

77. Pursley TV et al: Cutaneous manifestations of tumoral calcinosis. *Arch Dermatol* 115:1100, 1979

78. Baldursson H et al: Tumoral calcinosis with hyperphosphatemia. *J Bone Joint Surg* 51-A:913, 1969

79. Mozzafarian G et al: Treatment of tumoral calcinosis with phosphorus deprivation. *Ann Intern Med* 77:741, 1972

80. Woods B, Kellaway TD: Cutaneous calculi. Subepidermal calcified nodules. *Br J Dermatol* 75:1, 1963

81. Shmunes E, Wood MG: Subepidermal calcified nodules. *Arch Dermatol* 105:593, 1972

82. Smith ML et al: Milia-like idiopathic calcinosis cutis in Down's syndrome. *Arch Dermatol* 125:1586, 1989

83. Schepis C et al: Perforating milia-like idiopathic calcinosis cutis and periorbital syringomas in a girl with Down syndrome *Pediatr Dermatol* 11:258, 1994

84. Maroon M et al: Calcinosis cutis associated with syringomas. A transepidermal elimination disorder in a patient with Down syndrome. *J Am Acad Dermatol* **23**:372, 1990
85. Goldminz D et al: Calcinosis cutis following extravasation of calcium chloride. *Arch Dermatol* **124**:922, 1988
86. Wheeland RG, Roundtree JM: Calcinosis cutis resulting from percutaneous penetration and deposition of calcium *J Am Acad Dermatol* **12**:172, 1985
87. Clendenning WE, Auerbach R: Traumatic calcium deposition in the skin. *Arch Dermatol* **89**:360, 1964
88. Schoenfeld RJ et al: Calcium deposition in the skin. A report of four cases following electroencephalography. *Neurology* **15**:477, 1965
89. Goldminz D, Greenberg RD: Multiple miliary osteoma cutis. *J Am Acad Dermatol* **24**:878, 1991
90. Levell NJ, Lawrence CM: Multiple papules on the face. *Arch Dermatol* **130**(3):373, 1994
91. Brook CG, Valman HB: Osteoma cutis and Albright's hereditary osteodystrophy. *Br J Dermatol* **85**:471, 1971
92. Prendiville JS et al: Osteoma cutis as a presenting sign of pseudohypoparathyroidism. *Pediatr Dermatol* **9**(1):11, 1992
93. Cohen RB et al: The natural history of heterotopic ossification in patients who have fibrodysplasia ossificans progressiva. *J Bone Joint Surg Am* **75A**:215, 1993
94. Connor JM, Evans DAP: Fibrodysplasia ossificans progressiva: The clinical features and natural history of 34 patients. *J Bone Joint Surg Br* **64B**:76, 1982
95. Shafritz AB et al: Overexpression of an osteogenic morphogen in fibrodysplasia ossificans progressiva. *N Engl J Med* **335**:555, 1996
96. Kaplan FS et al: Progressive osseous heteroplasia: A distinct developmental disorder of heterotopic ossification. *J Bone Joint Surg Am* **76A**:425, 1994
97. Miller ES et al: Progressive osseous heteroplasia: Report of two cases. *Arch Dermatol* **132**:787, 1996
98. Worret WI, Burgdorf W: Angeborenes plattenartiges Oseoma cutis bei einem Saugling. *Hautarzt* **29**:590, 1978

CHAPTER 156

Richard J. Wenstrup

Heritable Disorders of Connective Tissue with Skin Changes

Heritable disorders of connective tissue are generalized defects due to mutations in the genes for components of connective tissues or in enzymes modifying them. They involve many tissues, reflecting organ distribution of those components. Virtually all are inherited in a simple Mendelian pattern.

MARFAN'S SYNDROME

Patients with Marfan's syndrome have major abnormalities primarily in three organ systems: the eye, most characteristically dislocation of the lenses; the skeletal system, excessive length of extremities, loose-jointedness, kyphoscoliosis, and anterior chest deformity; and the cardiovascular system, most characteristically aortic aneurysm and mitral valve redundancy.[1] Skin manifestations consist of striae distensae, a common finding, and elastosis perforans serpiginosa, a rare finding.

Clinical Manifestations

SKELETAL (Figs. 156-1 and 156-2) The skeletal features, particularly the long, narrow extremities, figured prominently in Marfan's initial description in 1896 of the syndrome that bears his name.

Some have suggested that Marfan's original patient, in fact, had congenital contractual arachnodactyly rather than the disorder now defined as Marfan's syndrome. Patients with Marfan's syndrome are usually taller than unaffected same-sex siblings. There is skeletal disproportion, with the most consistent and reliable measure being an abnormally low ratio of the upper segment (US) to the lower segment (LS). The segments are measured below and above the top of the pubic symphysis. In practice, two measurements are made with the patient standing: height and lower segment (top of the pubic symphysis to the floor). In adult Caucasians the mean ratio is about 0.92, and in adult American blacks it is about 0.87. The excessive length of the extremities is responsible for the abnormally low US:LS ratio in Marfan's syndrome. Shortening of the trunk by kyphoscoliosis exaggerates the low US:LS ratio. When kyphoscoliosis is more than minimal, the US:LS ratio should not be used. Another abnormal measurement includes the comparison of the arm span (fingertip to fingertip) with height; the arm span is usually longer by several centimeters.

The ribs appear to undergo the same excessive longitudinal growth as do the bones of the extremities. Depression (pectus excavatum) or projection (pectus carinatum) of the sternum or an asymmetric deformity of the anterior chest results.

Joint hyperextensibility is present in some but not all patients with Marfan's syndrome. Flat-footedness, hyperextensibility at the knees (genu recurvatum) and elbows, and occasional dislocation of

FIGURE 156-1

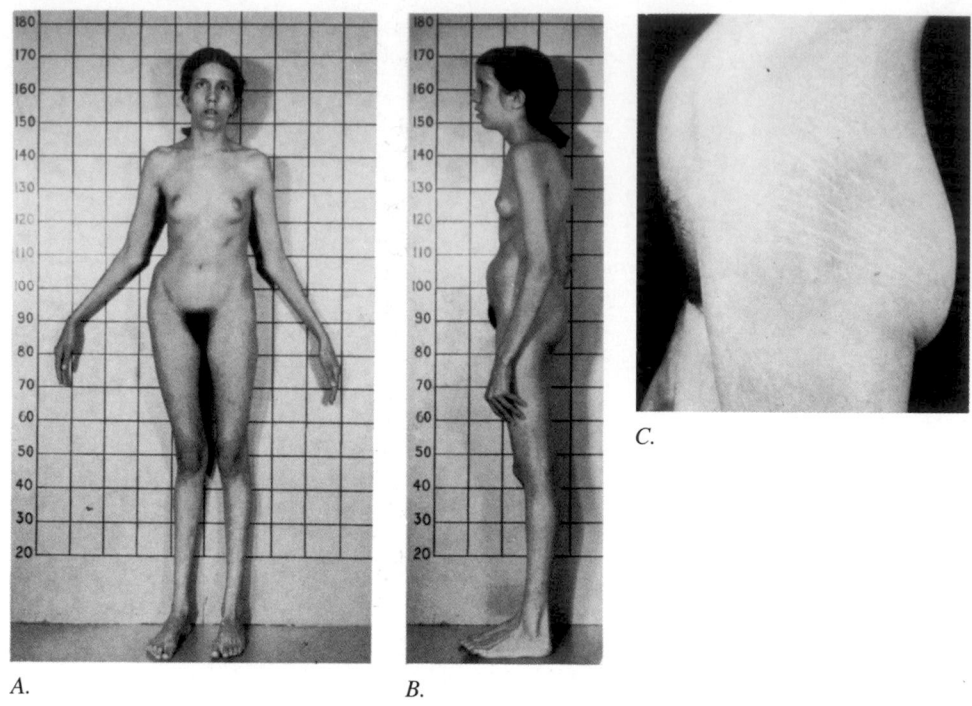

A. B. C.

joints are manifestations of the loose-jointedness. The patient is often able to touch his or her umbilicus with the right hand passed around the back and approaching the umbilicus from the left because of joint hyperextensibility and long, narrow extremities. A relatively narrow palm of the hand with a long thumb and hyperextensibility is the basis of Steinberg's sign: the thumb propped across the palm extends well beyond the ulnar margin of the hand.

OCULAR Virtually all patients with Marfan's syndrome have myopia since the orbit is abnormally long. In addition, about 70 percent of patients have ectopia lentis with the lens usually displaced upward. With significant dilation, the margin of the lens may be visible in the lower part of the pupil. Dislocation of the lens into the anterior chamber or trapping of the lens in the pupil sometimes occurs, and acute glaucoma may result. Detection of mild ectopia lentis requires full dilation of the pupils and slit-lamp examination for redundancy of the suspensory ligament of the lens. Therefore, clinical exclusion of ectopia lentis in an individual suspected of having Marfan's syndrome must include a slit-lamp ex-

Marfan syndrome. Frontal (A) and lateral views (B) of a 15-year-old girl with Marfan's syndrome. Note the tall stature, arachnodactyly, kyphoscoliosis, round shoulders, and strabismus. C. Striae distensae over the hips in the same patient.

FIGURE 156-2

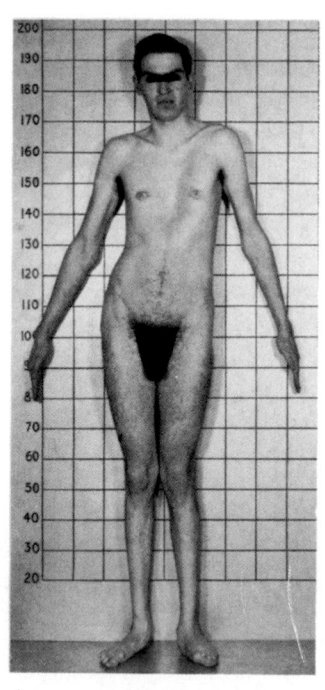

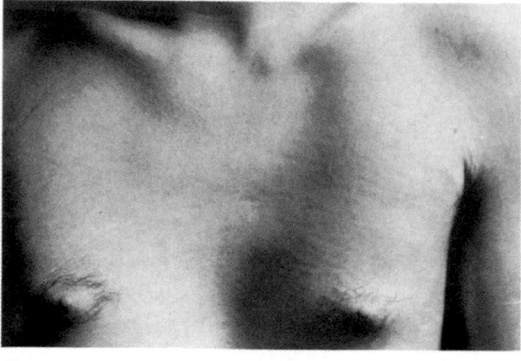

A. B. C.

Marfan's syndrome. Frontal (A) and lateral views (B) of a 20-year-old boy with Marfan's syndrome. Note the tall stature, depressed sternum, scoliosis, and arachnodactyly. The father and a younger brother were also affected. This patient falls among the approximately 30 percent who do not have ectopia lentis. His brother, however, did have ectopia lentis. C. Striae distensae over the pectoral and deltoid areas.

CARDIOVASCULAR   The most common serious cardiovascular
feature of Marfan's syndrome is a weakness of the aortic media.
This leads to diffuse aneurysm, which may develop in the first year
of life or not until the fifth or sixth decade. The ascending aorta is
the most severely affected region since it is exposed to more pulsatile fatigue, although the defect is clearly generalized. Abdominal
aneurysm without notable thoracic involvement has occurred in a
few patients.

Echocardiography of the proximal aorta is a very sensitive noninvasive diagnostic procedure for aortic root involvement. It must
be performed on any patient in whom the diagnosis of Marfan's
syndrome is considered, and patients with documented aortic dilation should be monitored yearly for progression. Echocardiography
can also determine the presence of prolapse of the mitral valve and
mitral regurgitation from redundancy of the valve and whether the
latter is hemodynamically significant.

OTHER FEATURES   A high-arched palate, crowding of the anterior teeth, and inguinal hernias are also common manifestations of
the syndrome. Pulmonary manifestations include cystic changes,
emphysema, and spontaneous pneumothorax. The skeletal musculature is often underdeveloped and hypotonic.

SKIN CHANGES   Although not often a conspicuous feature of
Marfan's syndrome, two types of skin change have been observed.
Most patients show striae distensae, particularly in the pectoral and
deltoid areas and over the buttocks and thighs. Elastosis perforans
serpiginosa has been described in some Marfan variants.[2]

Genetic Defect

Approximately 80 percent of patients with Marfan's syndrome have
a positive family history; in the remainder, the syndrome results
from de novo mutations in the sperm or ova of the parents. Thereafter, the syndrome is inherited as an autosomal dominant condition.
Marfan's syndrome is due to heterozygous mutations in the gene
for fibrillin (FBN1), a major constitutive element of extracellular
matrix microfibrils. Discovered in 1986,[3] it is abundant in tissues
prominently affected by Marfan's syndrome—the ascending aorta,
suspensory ligament of the lens, periosteum, and skin. Prefibrillin
is a 2871 residue protein with five distinct structural domains. The
largest of these, comprising 75 percent of the protein, is a series of
46 EGF domains, most of which are calcium-binding.[4] These EGF
repeats are interrupted by eight cysteine motifs that resemble those
found in latent transforming growth factor β binding protein type
1 (LTBP-1). Initial studies showed that there was dramatically decreased binding of fluorescent antibodies to fibrillin in skin and
dermal fibroblast matrix in patients with Marfan's syndrome,[5] and
the decreased antifibrillin staining cosegregated with the Marfan
clinical phenotype in several families with Marfan's syndrome.
Linkage studies by several investigators mapped Marfan's syndrome to 15q21.1, the chromosomal locus of the FBN1 gene.[6]

Over 80 mutations over the entire coding region of FBN1 have
been reported, nearly all of which occur within a single family.[7,8]
Some, though not all, mutations result in the classic features of
Marfan's syndrome, and a few genotype-phenotype correlations are
possible. Most missense mutations in the EGF domains generally
result in the classic form of the disease. Patients with dramatic structural rearrangements such as exon skipping (approximately 10 percent of the total) have comparatively severe forms of the disease.

Patients with mutations that lead to premature stop codons and reduced mRNA transcripts from the mutant allele have a surprisingly
wide range of clinical severity, which is unlike the clear differences
seen between patients with osteogenesis imperfecta (OI) who have
dominant-negative mutations and those with loss-of-function mutations (null alleles).

It has also become apparent that genetic alterations in FBN1
produce a spectrum of clinical abnormalities well beyond the classic
Marfan phenotype, the so-called fibrillopathies.[8–12] The spectrum
ranges from the severe neonatal Marfan phenotype at one end to
isolated aortic root dilatation to marfanoid skeletal features lacking
cardiovascular involvement or ectopia lentis at the other.

HOMOCYSTINURIA

Homocystinuria is by definition a biochemical abnormality, not a
specific disease entity. By far the most common cause of this condition is deficiency in the enzyme cystathionine β-synthase (CBS)
due to recessive mutations in the gene. Much less common causes
are defects in 5,10-methylenetetrahydrofolate reductase activity,
heritable vitamin B_{12} deficiency due to absorption abnormalities
(Immerslund syndrome), and transcobalamin II deficiency, leading
to defective cellular uptake of vitamin B_{12} (for review, see Mudd
et al.[13]).

The major clinical manifestations of CBS deficiency include dol-
ichostenomelia, ectopia lentis, and chest and spinal deformity; the
latter two findings make it superficially similar to Marfan's syndrome, but generalized osteoporosis, arteriovenous thrombosis, and
mental retardation are prominent features that allow differentiation
from Marfan's syndrome. The cutaneous manifestations include malar flush, thin hair and skin, and cutis reticulata.

Clinical Manifestations of CBS Deficiency

VASCULAR   The most serious complication of CBS deficiency is
arterial and venous thrombosis. Acute occlusion of the coronary
arteries can cause myocardial infarction, renal occlusion can cause
severe hypertension, occlusion of carotid or cerebral arteries can
cause stroke, and blindness can be caused by ophthalmic artery
occlusion. Venous thromboses may cause renal vein thrombosis or
portal vein thrombosis and pulmonary embolism. These manifestations are usually seen in patients homozygous for CBS deficiency.
However, heterozygotes for a mutation at the CBS locus may be at
increased risk for myocardial infarction. The vascular complications
of homocystinuria are the cause of increased mortality in these patients; at least 20 percent die prematurely from thrombotic complications.

OCULAR   Most patients with homocystinuria have ectopia lentis
in the first decade of life. It is progressive in CBS deficiency but
is stable in Marfan's syndrome. Rupture of the sclera and retinal
detachment have also been reported. Nearly all patients have significant myopia.

SKELETAL   Patients with homocystinuria have the same asthenic
habitus as those with Marfan's syndrome and have a high incidence
of scoliosis, thoracic asymmetry, and pectus excavatum. However,
joint hyperextensibility is not a feature of this disorder; more char-

acteristic is mild joint limitation. There is an increased incidence of pathologic fractures because of generalized osteopenia.

CUTANEOUS FEATURES   A prominent malar flush has been reported in many patients, most easily seen after vigorous exercise or after cold exposure. Hair is thinned. The dermis is usually thin, and dermis reticularis is commonly seen on the extremities. In patients with deep venous thromboses, collateral venous channels are rarely visible through the skin.

OTHER FEATURES   Mental retardation is a common but variable feature of CBS deficiency. Slightly over half of the patients have personality and psychiatric disorders including depression, chronic behavioral disorders, and obsessive-compulsive disorder.[14]

Metabolic Defect

CBS catalyzes the condensation of homocysteine and serine; in its absence, homocysteine is converted to homocystine, which is greatly increased in blood and appears in urine. Some homocysteine is converted back to methionine, which is also elevated in blood and urine. Cystine, which normally is supplied to the body by metabolism of methionine, becomes an essential amino acid in patients with CBS deficiency.

There has been considerable controversy over the mechanisms by which CBS deficiency and elevated homocysteine cause the clotting abnormality and the connective tissue findings characteristic of homocystinuria. With regard to the clotting abnormality, experimental work suggests that elevated homocysteine alters the aggregation of platelets, is toxic to endothelial surfaces, or alters the activity of soluble factors that regulate thrombosis, such as antithrombin III, but no widely accepted general explanation has taken hold.

With regard to the connective tissue findings of ectopia lentis, osteoporosis, and the vertebral and thoracic abnormalities, there is good evidence that elevated homocysteine inhibits cross-linking of collagen. Harris and Sjoerdsma[15] demonstrated a decrease of cross-linking of collagen in skin from two patients with homocystinuria. Specifically, they found an excess of monomeric collagen relative to the amount of dimerized collagen chains in reducing gels. The mechanism for decreased cross-linking in vivo is unknown, as is the biologic basis for mental retardation and psychiatric disturbance.

Genetics

The majority of patients with homocystinuria have primary deficiency of CBS. A minority have acquired (dietary) deficiency of cobalamin or heritable disorders that prevent conversion of dietary cobalamin to its biologically active forms; rarely, some have defects that cause decreased availability of 5-methyltetrahydrofolate, which is also required in the metabolism of methionine.

The clinical syndrome of homocystinuria due to CBS deficiency is inherited as an autosomal recessive trait. The gene for CBS has been located on the long arm of chromosome 21 (21q22.3),[16] and molecular analysis of the locus has identified several mutant alleles in patients with homocystinuria. Substitution of serine for glycine at amino acid position 370 (G370S) is the most common mutation in northern European populations, but most patients are compound heterozygotes for rare mutant alleles.[17]

Approximately one-half of patients with CBS deficiency respond clinically to very high doses of pyridoxine (250 to 500 mg/day) with

decreases of methionine in plasma and virtual elimination of homocysteine from urine.[13] Increases in responsiveness are likely due to increased production of pyridoxal-5' phosphate, which is the active form of vitamin B$_6$, a cofactor for CBS. Sensitivity to pyridoxine is constant in affected sibs and only occurs in the presence of residual CBS activity, indicating that the effect likely depends on the specific structural alteration of CBS.

OSTEOGENESIS IMPERFECTA

OI is a generalized connective tissue disorder in which the primary clinical manifestation is osseous fragility.[18,19] OI has an important place in the understanding of skeletal dysplasias because it was the first to have its molecular basis understood. Studies of type I collagen in OI fibroblasts have provided a conceptual framework that has been widely adaptable to other heritable disorders as well. Some of these guiding concepts include an illustration of dominant negative effects in human disease, the notion of a single heterozygous glycine substitution within the triple helix as a sufficiently ascertainable mutation within fibrillar collagens, and the molecular demonstration of somatic mutation/mosaicism as a common initiating event in the pathogenesis of autosomal dominant disorders.

There is an extremely wide range of clinical severity in OI, from mild osseous fragility in childhood with no bony deformities to a severe deforming disorder that is lethal in the perinatal period. The wide range of severity in OI is reflected in Table 156-1.[19] Nearly all cases of OI are due to heterozygosity for different kinds of mutations in the proα1(I) and proα2(I) genes of type I collagen (reviewed by Byers[7] and Prockop et al.[20]).

Clinical Description

SKELETAL   An increased incidence of fractures defines the clinical syndrome. Fractures are always present in utero in OI types II and III and may also occur in the milder forms. Skeletal deformity is a hallmark of all but the mildest forms; OI type II is so severe that it is readily detected by the beginning of the second trimester of pregnancy. Deformity of long bones at birth does not necessarily result from in utero fractures but may be the result of molding under the strain of normal muscle tone in the fetus. "Codfish vertebrae" (hollowing out of vertebral bodies by pressure from expansile intervertebral disks) or flat vertebrae are observed in some patients, particularly older patients in whom senile or postmenopausal changes exaggerate the change or younger patients who are immobilized after fractures or osteotomies.

Fracture frequency usually decreases after puberty, but there is a second fracture peak in late adulthood. Patients with OI types III and IV also have dentinogenesis imperfecta, which presents as graying, opalescent teeth prone to erosion.

HEARING   Deafness develops in many patients by the third decade of life. There appears to be a mixture of otosclerosis and sensorineural deafness involved in OI hearing loss.

SKIN   Patients with OI, particularly type I, have thin skin with wider scars than normal after incisions. This same subset of patients also has increased bruisability after mild trauma, probably because of abnormal collagen fibril structure in the walls of small blood vessels or in the supporting connective tissues.

OTHER CONNECTIVE TISSUE   Because type I collagen is found in nearly all tissues, it is not surprising that clinical problems stem-

TABLE 156-1

Clinical Subtypes and Associated Defects in Osteogenesis Imperfecta (OI)

OI TYPE	CLINICAL FEATURES	INHERITANCE	BIOCHEMICAL DEFECTS
I	Normal stature; little or no deformity; blue sclerae; hearing loss in about 50% of individuals; dentinogenesis imperfecta rare and may distinguish a subset	AD	Decreased production of type I procollagen; Substitution for residue other than glycine in triple helix of $\alpha1(I)$
II	Lethal in the perinatal period; minimal calvarial mineralization; beaded ribs, compressed femurs, marked long bone deformity, platyspondylisis	AD (new mutation) AR (rare)	Rearrangements in the COL1A1 and COL1A2 genes; substitutions for glycyl residues in the triple-helical domain of the $\alpha1(I)$ or $\alpha2(I)$ chain Small deletion in $\alpha2(I)$ on the background of a null allele
III	Progressively deforming bones, usually with moderate deformity at birth; sclerae variable in hue, often lighten with age; dentinogenesis common; hearing loss common; stature very short	AR (rare) AD	Frameshift mutation that prevents incorporation of pro$\alpha2(I)$ into molecules (noncollagenous defects) Point mutations in the $\alpha1(I)$ or $\alpha2(I)$ chain
IV	Normal sclerae; mild to moderate bone deformity and variable short stature; dentinogenesis common; hearing loss occurs in some	AD	Point mutations in the $\alpha2(I)$ chain; rarely, point mutations in the $\alpha1(I)$ chain; small deletions in the $\alpha2(I)$ chain

NOTE: AD, autosomal dominant; AR, autosomal recessive.
SOURCE: Sillence et al.[19]

ming from dysfunction of other connective tissues are increased in patients with OI. Joint laxity and occasional joint dislocation are relatively common in milder forms of OI. Tendon rupture and, rarely, rupture of blood vessels are probably increased in patients with OI compared with the general population.

Biochemical and Molecular Genetics

Linkage studies and biochemical and molecular characterizations of OI cell strains indicate that almost all patients with OI are heterozygous for mutations in the genes for the pro$\alpha1(I)$ and pro$\alpha2(I)$ chains of type I collagen on chromosomes 17 and 7, respectively. Although earlier clinical genetic studies of OI suggested that the most severe forms (types II and III) were autosomal recessive because of recurrences in the offspring of clinically unaffected parents, there is direct evidence that these recurrences are in most cases caused by germline mosaicism for a type I collagen mutation. A relatively minor subset of OI types II and III may be caused by an autosomal recessive mutation at a different locus.[21]

There are two general classes of type I collagen mutations distinguished by their biochemical effects on cultured dermal fibroblasts.[7,22–25] One class, almost always associated with mild OI (type I, Table 156-1), results in loss of expression of one pro$\alpha1(I)$ allele and half-normal production of type I collagen from cultured dermal fibroblasts (Fig. 156-3). The second class of mutations, usually associated with more severe OI (types II, III, and IV), results in type I collagen molecules with an altered triple-helical structure. Some of these structural mutations are deletions or insertions of peptidyl material, but the great majority are single amino acid substitutions for glycine residues in $\alpha1(I)$ or $\alpha2(I)$ chains that disrupt the Gly-X-Y repeat structure of the triple-helical domain.

Biochemical studies of abnormal type I collagen molecules synthesized by OI fibroblasts have consistently shown that molecules have increased posttranslational modifications—primarily lysyl hydroxylation and glycosylation—that are limited to the portion of the molecule that is amino-terminal to the site of a glycine substitution (reviewed by Byers[7]). Molecules assemble and wind from the carboxyl- to the amino-terminal end, but winding is slowed through the region of the substitution. Unwound chains are either further modified before molecular assembly, or else the final conformation of the helix amino-terminal to the mutation is altered sufficiently to allow posttranslational modifications after the helix is formed. These biochemical features form the basis of current methods of biochemical screening for this form of OI. In addition, abnormal molecules are secreted more slowly from cultured fibroblasts and have decreased thermal stability.

EHLERS-DANLOS SYNDROMES

The Ehlers-Danlos syndromes (EDS) are a genetically, biochemically, and clinically diverse group of heritable connective tissue disorders having joint laxity and dermal features in common.[26–28] Prior classifications of EDS have included up to eleven disorders. Recently, a simplified classification has been proposed that takes into account recent advances in our understanding of the molecular pathogenesis of these disorders. Table 156-2 provides the currently accepted classification; footnotes to the Table indicate the proposed changes. Many patients with features of EDS do not fit readily into one of the well-defined subtypes.

Clinical Description

EDS TYPE I EDS type I, also known as the *gravis* form, is characterized by joint laxity, hyperextensibility of skin, poor wound healing, and autosomal dominant inheritance (Figs. 156-4, 156-5, 156-6). The skin is soft and velvety and can be stretched easily. The dermis is fragile and is easily bruised. Scars after trauma or

FIGURE 156-3

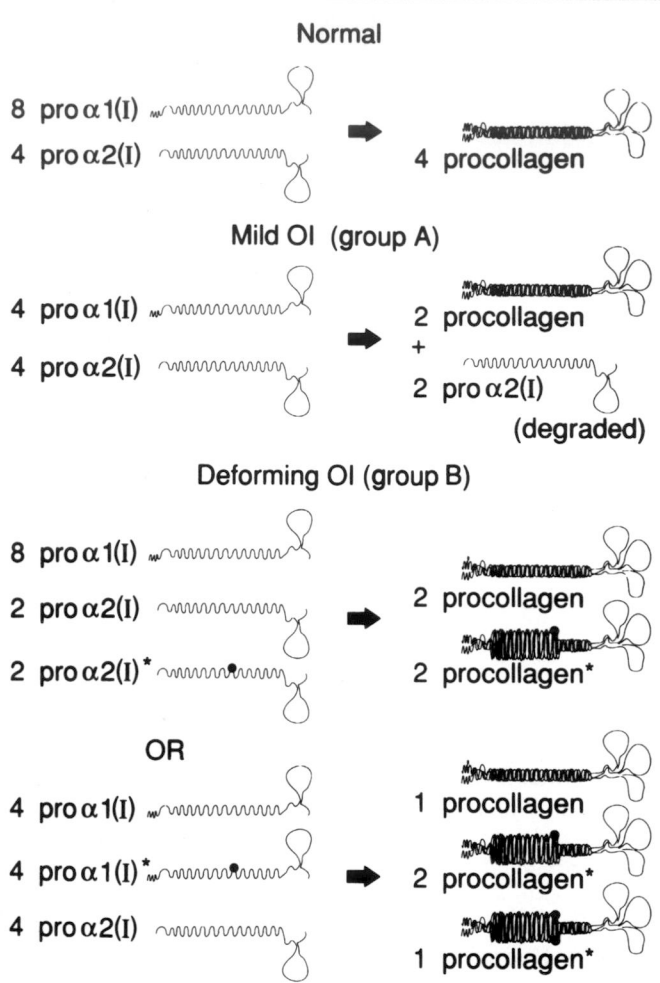

Stoichiometric relationship of normal and abnormal α chains of type I collagen resulting from dominant mutations that produce the observed biochemical phenotypes of OI. Mild OI is caused by 50 percent reduction of proα1(I) chains. More severe OI is caused by production of molecules that contain mutant chains (the site of mutation is indicated by the black dot in the triple-helical domain). Proα chains in these molecules undergo increased posttranslational modification aminoterminal to the site of the mutation, may be inefficiently secreted with increased degradation within cells, and result in defective collagen fibrillogenesis. The broadened area of the triple helix depicts overmodification.

surgical procedures are thinned and atrophic and may stretch considerably after healing, having a characteristic "cigarette paper" appearance. Molluscoid pseudotumors are present at the extensor surfaces of joints, in the foot, and on the shins. About half of affected individuals are delivered prematurely as infants because of premature rupture of fetal membranes, presumably due to abnormalities in structure of fetal tissues. A significant number of individuals with EDS type I have cardiac defects, most commonly mitral valve prolapse. A few patients have dilation and occasionally rupture of the ascending aorta or proximal pulmonary artery. Musculoskeletal features include joint hyperextensibility in all patients and a fairly high frequency of scoliosis and pes planus (flat feet). The joint hyper-

mobility can be associated with the onset of osteoarthritis in the third or fourth decade.

EDS TYPE II   EDS type II is clinically similar to EDS type I, except that the skin is less fragile and scar formation more closely approximates normal. Ultrastructural findings show thickened collagen fibril in skin, similar to findings in the dermis in patients with EDS type I. Since the molecular basis of this disorder is similar to EDS type I, it has been proposed that EDS types I and II be merged as a single entity.

EDS TYPE III   EDS type III is characterized primarily by hyperextensibility of large and small joints, soft velvety skin, and autosomal dominant inheritance. Individuals with EDS type III have normal scarring and do not have stretchy skin. Molluscoid pseudotumors are absent.

EDS TYPE IV   EDS type IV is a condition characterized by thin, translucent skin with easy bruisability but normal scar formation.[29,30] In fair-skinned individuals, subcutaneous vasculature is easily visible beneath the skin. Affected individuals are at high risk for life-threatening rupture of the large intestine, uterus, or medium-sized arteries. The most common sites of arterial rupture are the mesenchymal arteries in the abdomen, the splenic artery, renal arteries, and the descending aorta. There may also be an increased incidence of stroke in patients with EDS type IV. Another life-threatening complication is uterine rupture in the peripartum period. EDS type IV is clinically distinct from other EDS subtypes in that skin hyperextensibility is not as prominent a finding as in other forms of EDS.

EDS type IV was initially thought to be autosomal recessive in inheritance, but most EDS type IV individuals have family histories compatible with autosomal dominant inheritance, and linkage analysis has documented dominant inheritance in several EDS type IV families.

EDS TYPE V   EDS type V is a rare X-linked disorder characterized by mild skin hyperelasticity, mildly abnormal scarring, and joint hyperextensibility. Female carriers are asymptomatic. There is only a single large, well-documented family with EDS type V in the literature. This disorder clinically resembles EDS type II except that the latter disorder has autosomal dominant inheritance. Thus, in clinical situations in which diagnosis of EDS types V and II are both possible, the much more common EDS type II should be considered unless family history clearly suggests X-linked inheritance.

EDS TYPE VI   The cardinal features of lysyl hydroxylase deficiency are neonatal onset of joint laxity, kyphoscoliosis, and hypotonia.[31] These features are found in virtually all patients. Ocular fragility, which was observed in the original reports of lysyl hydroxylase deficiency, was found in only a minority of patients. Skin fragility, easy bruisability, and dermal hyperextensibility occur to some extent in most patients, although it is much less prominent a feature than in patients with EDS type I. Individuals with EDS type VI, like those with EDS IV, are at risk of having a potentially catastrophic arterial rupture.

EDS TYPE VII   EDS type VII (*arthrochalasia multiplex*) is characterized by extreme joint laxity, multiple joint dislocations, and congenital hip dislocations that are difficult to repair surgically. Dermal features in these patients include tissue fragility and widened scars; in EDS types VIIA and VIIB, these dermal findings are less prominent than in EDS types I/II. On the other hand, patients with EDS type VIIC, or *human dermatosparaxis*, have striking dermal fragility. Their skin is lax, but not stretchy, and joint dislocation is usually not a feature of this subtype.

CHAPTER 156
Heritable Disorders of Connective Tissue

1841

EDS TYPE VIII Ehlers-Danlos type VIII is a rare autosomal dominant condition characterized by soft, hyperextensible skin, abnormal scarring, easy bruising, hyperextensible joints, and generalized periodontitis. It resembles the gravis form of EDS (type I), but in the few available clinical reports it is distinguished from the latter disorder by periodontitis with early loss of teeth and by the characteristic purplish discoloration of scars on the shins. The molecular basis of EDS type VIII is unknown. It is unclear as to whether this is an entity that is truly distinct from EDS types I/II.

EDS TYPE X Arneson and coworkers[32] reported a single family in which two siblings of unaffected parents had joint hyperextensibility, mitral valve prolapse, easy bruisability, and poor wound healing. Clotting studies performed to evaluate excessive bleeding at incision sites were normal except for a striking defect in the platelet adhesion that is normally observed in response to exposure of platelets to collagen. Addition of purified fibronectin to the patients' plasma improved platelet adhesiveness. The authors suggested that this disorder may be due to a defect in fibronectin.

Basic Defect

Virtually all forms of EDS for which the molecular basis is well established are the result of mutations that code for fibrillar collagen genes or for enzymes that catalyze their intracellular or extracellular posttranslational modifications.[7] EDS type VI is due to deficiency of lysyl hydroxylase as a result of two abnormal alleles.[33] EDS type VII is due either to recessive mutations in the gene for type I collagen N-proteinase or to dominant mutations that affect the N-peptidase cleavage site in proα1(I) or proα2(I) chains, or the N-peptidase enzyme itself. EDS type IV is due to dominant mutations in the gene for the proα1(III) chain of type III collagen (COL3A1).[34]

EDS TYPES I/II For both these types, genetic abnormalities that result in abnormal type I collagen fibril structure have been suspected because electron micrographs have detected abnormally thick type I collagen fibrils[35] in the skin of some patients with EDS I and II and fiber bundles are abnormally small. There have been rare reports of individuals with type I collagen abnormalities and a phenotype similar to EDS type I or type II, but linkage studies have excluded type I collagen genes themselves as the genetic defect in some families with EDS types I and II.[36,37]

TABLE 156-2

Current Classification of Ehlers-Danlos Syndromes

TYPE	CLINICAL FEATURES	INHERITANCE	BIOCHEMICAL DEFECTS
I Gravis*	Soft, hyperextensible skin; easy bruising; thin, atrophic scars; hypermobile joints; varicose veins; prematurity of affected newborns	AD	Mutations in proα1(V) or proα2(V) chains of type V collagen (COL5A1, COL5A2) in some families
II Mitis*	Similar to EDS type I but less severe	AD	Same as EDS I
III Familial hypermobility	Soft skin; large and small joint hypermobility	AD	Not known
IV Arterial	Thin, translucent skin with visible veins; easy bruising; absence of skin and joint extensibility; arterial, bowel, and uterine rupture	AD	Mutations in COL3A1: abnormal type III collagen synthesis, secretion, or structure
V X-linked†	Similar to EDS type II	XLR	Not known
VI	Soft skin muscle hypotonia; scoliosis: joint laxity; hyperextensible skin	AR	Lysyl hydroxylase deficiency; mutations in PLOD gene
VII Arthrochalasia multiplex			
Type VIIA, B	Congenital hip dislocation, severe joint hypermobility; soft skin with normal scarring	AD (type VIIA,B)	Deletion of exons from type I collagen genes that encode the amino-terminal propeptide cleavage site of COL1A1 (type VIIA) or COL1A2 (type VIIB)
Type VIIC	Severe skin fragility; sagging, redundant skin	AR (type VIIC)	Recessive mutations in type I collagen N-peptidase (type VIIC)
VIII Periodontal‡	Generalized periodontitis; soft hyperextensible skin; chronic purple-hued scarring over shins	AD	Not known
X†	Similar to EDS type II, with abnormal clotting studies	AR	Proposed defect in fibronectin

*In proposed new classification, merged as a single entity.
†Found only in a single family.
‡May be a variant of EDS type I/II rather than a distinct entity.
NOTE: AD, autosomal dominant; AR, autosomal recessive; XLR, X-linked recessive.

Interest in type V collagen as a candidate molecule in EDS came about because type V collagen and type I collagen molecules form heterotypic collagen fibrils.[38] There is both in vitro[39] and in vivo[40] evidence that type V collagen may regulate fibril diameter. Transgenic mice that synthesized type V molecules containing mutant proα2(V) chains that lack the N-proteinase cleavage site exhibited some features of EDS, including dermal fragility and skin distensibility, and had electron microscopic evidence of collagen fibril disruption.[40] A single patient with Ehlers-Danlos syndrome and hypomelanosis of Ito had a balanced translocation with breakpoints at Xq21.1 and 9q34, and the latter breakpoint was shown by Toriello et al.[41] to interrupt COL5A1 and result in haploinsufficiency of proα1(V) chains. There are now several published reports of linkage to COL5A1 and/or mutations in the coding regions of proα1(V) chains in EDS families.[42–44] Also, there is evidence of locus heterogeneity, because mutations in the triple-helical domain of proα2(V) chains of type V collagen can also cause the classic EDS

FIGURE 156-4

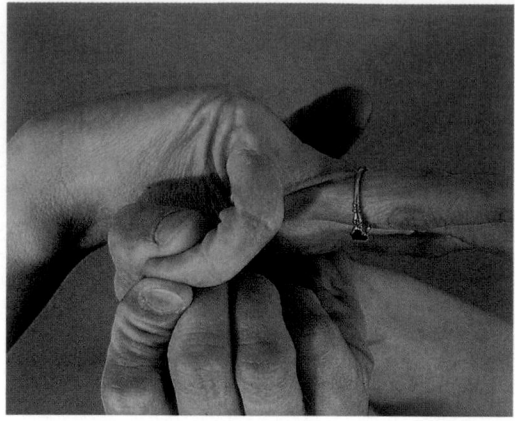

A.

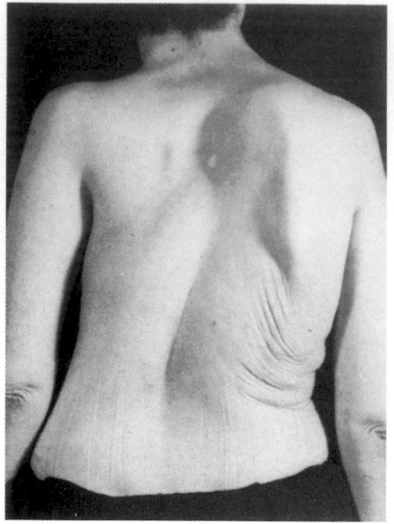

B.

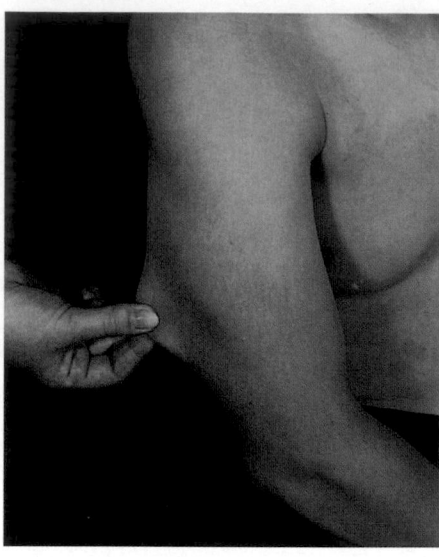

C.

The Ehlers-Danlos syndrome in a 37-year-old woman. *A.* Loose-jointedness is demonstrated. *B.* Note the severe scoliosis as well as the loose, puckered skin over the elbows. *C.* Loose skin is demonstrated over the elbow. The patient is blind from retinal detachment, as is a brother with the Ehlers-Danlos syndrome.

type I/II phenotype.[45] A minority of EDS type I/II families have had COL5A1 and COL5A2 loci excluded, indicating that mutations at other loci are responsible for the EDS type I/II clinical phenotype as well.

EDS TYPE IV Type IV is defined by abnormal synthesis, structure, or secretion of type III collagen.[27–30] Collagen fibers are small and irregular in skin and blood vessels, and several mutations have been described in the triple-helical region of the molecule. These include multiexon deletions, single point mutations, and splicing defects. In contrast to mutations of type I collagen that result in OI, mutations that result in EDS type IV are equally likely to be single exon splicing defects as substitutions for glycine residues in the triple-helical domain. Surprisingly, splicing defects and multiexon deletions do not result in more severe disease phenotypes than glycine substitutions, as they often do in OI. All mutations associated with EDS type IV appear to affect type III collagen structure deleteriously. In part due to the difficulties in standardizing conditions for

FIGURE 156-5

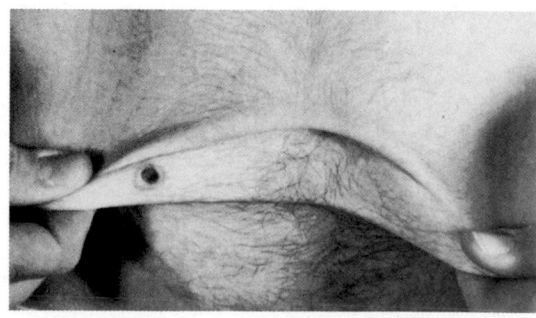

Abnormally stretchable skin of a patient with Ehlers-Danlos syndrome.

FIGURE 156-6

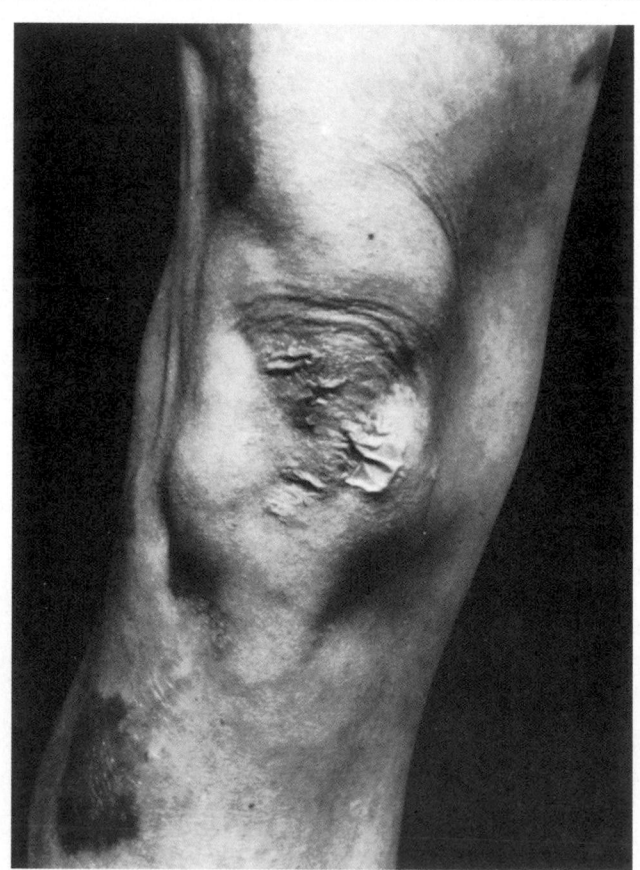

Atrophic scarring and a pseudotumor in a patient with the Ehlers-Danlos syndrome.

measurement of type III collagen synthesis in fibroblasts, there are no convincing data indicating that null mutations resulting in loss of expression of one COL3A1 allele result in EDS. Rather, they may be responsible for isolated aortic aneurysms or stroke later in life.

EDS TYPE VI Collagen is hydroxylysine-deficient because of a deficiency of lysyl hydroxylase (PLOD: procollagen lysyl 2-oxo-glutarate 5-dioxygenase).[46] Many of the cross-links that normally occur between adjacent collagen monomers within a fibril begin as chemical modifications of hydroxylysyl residues. Therefore, although hydroxylysine-deficient collagen is secreted from cells efficiently, it is not capable of normal cross-linking.

All patients with EDS type VI have decreased hydroxylysine content in dermal tissues. Hydroxylysine content in dermal collagen is typically less than 10 percent of normal, or <0.5 per 1000 residues in all patients with EDS type VI. The deficiency is highly tissue- and collagen type–specific, apparently affecting only types I and III collagens.[47,48] Most patients have a reduction of lysyl hydroxylase activity in cultured dermal fibroblasts in assays that use ^{14}C [lysine]-labeled underhydroxylated collagen; prolyl 4-hydroxylase activity is used as a positive control. Unfortunately, values for enzyme activity differ considerably from assay to assay and from laboratory to laboratory, so maximum activity values consistent with the disease phenotype cannot be uniformly stated. More recently, measurement of the ratio of urinary excretion of pyridinium cross-links have become widely used as a screen for EDS type VI. Patients diagnosed with EDS type VI by either analysis of skin hydroxylysine or lysyl hydroxylase activity demonstrate a narrow range of deoxypyridinoline : pyridinoline ratios that is at least one order of magnitude greater than those seen in age-matched controls.[49,50] This method shows great promise in providing a rapid, inexpensive diagnostic test for EDS.

The isolation and DNA sequence analysis of human lysyl hydroxylase[51,52] has allowed for molecular analysis of patients to determine the cause of its deficiency. Several patients have been reported who have defined molecular defects at both PLOD alleles. Hyland et al.[33] reported homozygosity for a single base pair substitution that resulted in an Arg319Ter change in two sisters who were products of a consanguineous mating. One patient who was reported to be ascorbate-responsive was a compound heterozygote for a single nucleotide substitution (Gly678Arg) in one allele and a 3-bp deletion (Glu532Del) in the other allele.[53,54] Hautala et al.[55] reported homozygosity for an intragenic duplication of exons 9 to 15 in two patients. The duplication, which is probably caused by Alu-Alu recombination in introns 9 and 16, appears to be the only common mutant allele, with an allele frequency of 19.1 percent in 35 EDS type VI families for the duplication.[56]

It has also been suggested that EDS type VI be divided into two subtypes: types VIA and VIB. EDS type VIA is due to mutations in the gene for lysyl hydroxylase that lead to deficiency of the enzyme. EDS type VIB is a clinically indistinguishable phenocopy that has normal lysyl hydroxylase activity and normal hydroxylysyl content in skin.[28,57]

EDS TYPE VII The biochemical defect that results in EDS type VII is the retention of amino-terminal propeptide of type I collagen in all tissues. Electron micrographs of collagen fibrils from skin of a patient with this disorder show abnormal collagen fibrils that are irregular in outline and vary widely in diameter. Because the disease is often sporadic, it was assumed that the disorder was usually due to reduction in collagen N-peptidase activity.[58] However, it is now evident that most patients with EDS type VII have dominant mutations that remove the exon containing the N-peptidase recognition sequence in proα1(I) (EDS type VIIA) or proα2(I) (EDS type VIIB) chains. This recognition sequence is contained in exon 6 of both COL1A1 and COL1A2, which are highly homologous and have well-conserved intron-exon boundaries. The molecular mechanisms for EDS types VIIA and VIIB are almost always mutations that disrupt the splice acceptor or splice donor sequences 5' or 3' to exon 6, causing removal of that exon during processing of mRNA.[7,26,28,59]

In skin from patients with the recessively inherited EDS type VIIC, procollagen metabolites that contain the N-propeptides are present and cultured dermal fibroblasts secrete procollagens in which the N-propeptide but not the C-propeptide is retained. Procollagen molecules from mutant cell strains are normally cleaved when placed into control cultures, indicating that the defective processing is not due to abnormalities in the procollagen substrate as in EDS types VIIA and VIIB.

PSEUDOXANTHOMA ELASTICUM

Pseudoxanthoma elasticum is a genetic disorder of connective tissue characterized by progressive mineralization of elastic fibers.[60] The disorder consists of characteristic skin lesions involving flexural sites, ocular involvement (angioid streaks and retinal hemorrhage), and cardiovascular manifestations (gastrointestinal hemorrhage, hypertension, and occlusive vascular disease). The disease may be inherited as an autosomal dominant or autosomal recessive trait and has a prevalence estimated at 1 in 100,000. The cause of the disorder is unknown. Progressive calcification and fragmentation of elastic fibers in skin, in Bruch's membrane in the eye, and in blood vessels appear to be responsible for the clinical manifestations of the disorder.

Clinical Manifestations

SKIN Yellowish papules giving a "plucked chicken" appearance in flexural skin occur at an average age of 13.5 years.[61] Commonly affected areas include antecubital, popliteal, inguinal, neck, axillae, and periumbilical areas, as well as oral, vaginal, and rectal mucosa (Fig. 156-7). Involvement may be progressive and involve the entire skin. In time, the skin may become lax and hang in folds, particularly in the neck, axillae, and groin. Plastic surgery can ordinarily be undertaken without complication, although calcium-containing material may be extruded. Diagnosis can be made by biopsy of affected skin. The characteristic histology consists of fragmentation and calcification of elastic fibers in the middle and lower third of the dermis (Fig. 156-8). Although normal elastic fibers do not stain with hematoxylin/eosin, altered elastic fibers from patients with pseudoxanthoma elasticum stain blue because of their calcium content. Elastosis perforans serpiginosa may coexist in patients with pseudoxanthoma elasticum.[61]

OCULAR Angioid streaks, the characteristic ocular lesion of pseudoxanthoma elasticum, are red to brown curvilinear bands radiating from the optic disk. Although they are irregular and generally wider, they are often mistaken for blood vessels. They occur commonly in patients with pseudoxanthoma elasticum (85 percent) but may be

Basic Defect

Although the basic defect in pseudoxanthoma elasticum is unknown, there is a progressive calcification of elastin with fragmentation of elastic fibers in the area of calcification.[64] In dermal blood vessels, abnormal elastin in the internal elastic lamina may be detected in the absence of mineralization. Abnormal amounts of proteoglycans have been detected in skin and urine of patients with pseudoxanthoma elasticum.[65] Abnormal proteolytic and elastolytic[66] activity have been reported in dermal fibroblasts from patients with the disorder. Skin changes consistent with pseudoxanthoma elasticum have been reported in patients with cystinuria who are taking D-penicillamine,[67] possibly due to inhibition of intermolecular cross-linking of collagen and elastin. The severity of pseudoxanthoma elasticum may be influenced by calcium ingestion.

Genetics

Two autosomal dominant and three autosomal recessive forms of pseudoxanthoma elasticum have been reported (Table 156-3).[68,69] Most patients appear to inherit their disorder as an autosomal recessive trait, although new dominant mutations cannot be excluded. The least common form of the disorder involves skin only and presents with generalized skin sagging clinically similar to cutis laxa.[70]

FIGURE 156-7

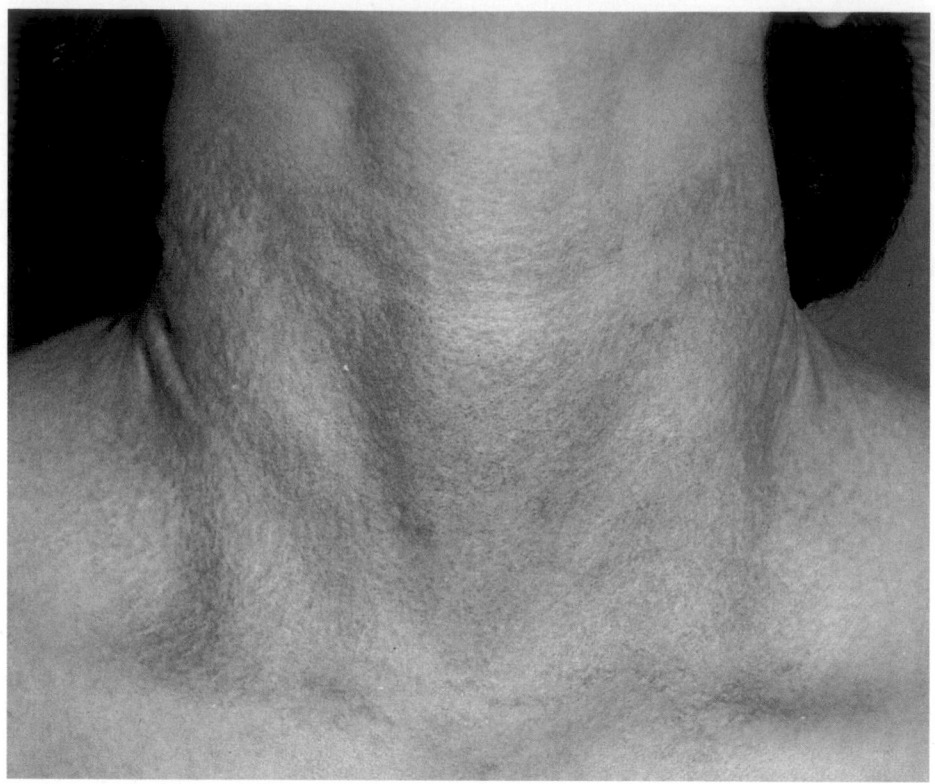

Pseudoxanthoma elasticum. Papules on the neck. There is a distinct yellowish hue. Loose, thickened skin with a pebbled appearance on the neck.

found in those with other conditions, including Paget's disease of bone and sickle cell disease. Angioid streaks apparently result from breaks in Bruch's membrane associated with faulty elastic fibers in its outer portion, the lamina elasticum. Fibrovascular ingrowth may result in retinal hemorrhage, detachment, and severe visual loss. Because laser repair may be sight-sparing, early diagnosis and regular examination are critically important. Other ocular lesions include a characteristic yellowish mottling of the posterior pole, called "leopard spotting," and a reticular pigmentary pattern in the retina.[62]

VASCULAR DISEASE Calcification of the elastic media of blood vessels with subsequent intimal proliferation leads to serious complications in this disorder. Claudication is the most common problem; pulses in adults are often obliterated. Angina pectoris or abdominal angina may become incapacitating. Hypertension is prevalent in adults[60] and appears to be associated with renal artery involvement. It may occur early in the disease. Gastrointestinal hemorrhage, apparently due to fragile submucosal vessels, may occur early and often is the presenting sign. Bleeding may also occur in the urinary tract. For unknown reasons, cerebrovascular disease appears to be less common than expected.

OTHER Despite an abundance of elastic tissue, lungs are not prominently affected in pseudoxanthoma elasticum. Pregnancy is surprisingly uncomplicated, but the rate of first trimester miscarriage may be increased.[63]

CUTIS LAXA (DERMATOCHALASIS, GENERALIZED ELASTOLYSIS)

Cutis laxa is the name given to a group of rare disorders that have in common loose, redundant skin and widespread manifestations in other organs. Autosomal dominant, autosomal recessive, and X-linked recessive forms are recognized. The dominant form is primarily a cosmetic problem, and the prognosis is good. Onset may be delayed, and the disease may appear to be an acquired defect. One autosomal recessive form of cutis laxa is associated with severe cardiorespiratory complications and early death.[71] Another, less severe form is characterized by growth retardation, developmental delay, and ligamentous laxity.[72] X-linked cutis laxa is characterized by mild joint laxity, bladder diverticula, hernias, and cranial occipital exostoses or horns.[7,73,74] Acquired forms have been reported, often following an ill-defined febrile illness.[75,76] Other inherited disorders with cutis laxa as an associated feature include DeBarsy's syndrome, Patterson's syndrome, "wrinkly skin" syndrome, geroderma osteodysplastica, and pseudoxanthoma elasticum. Cutis laxa may also be associated with amyloidosis and plasma cell dyscrasias.

The best characterized form of cutis laxa, and the only form for which the molecular pathogenesis is well understood, is the X-linked recessive form, formerly known as Ehlers-Danlos syn-

FIGURE 156-8

CHAPTER 156
Heritable Disorders of Connective Tissue 1845

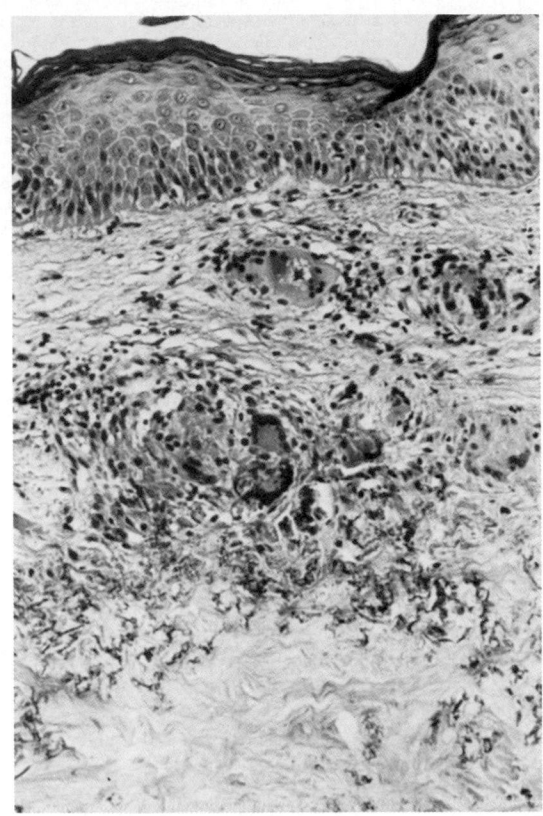

Pseudoxanthoma elasticum. The pathology affects the connective tissue of most of the reticular dermis. Even in routine hematoxylin and eosin preparations one may see the tightly, but irregularly coiled, basophilic elastic fibers. The collagen associated with the fibrils is also abnormal; the broad collagen bundles so characteristic of the reticular dermis are replaced by irregular and rather confluent collagen fibrils. (*Micrograph by Wallace H. Clark, Jr., MD.*)

drome type IX and now known as *X-linked cutis laxa* or the *occipital horn syndrome.*

Clinical Manifestations

SKIN In all forms of cutis laxa, the skin gives the appearance of being too large for the rest of the body.[77] It tends to sag in areas where the skin is normally loose, e.g., around the face and eyes (Fig. 156-9). Sagging jowls may result in a "bloodhound" look. The skin may be excessively wrinkled and appear prematurely aged. At birth, the skin may be noticeably soft, loose, and hyperextensible; in contrast to the skin of patients with EDS, it returns very slowly to its normal position after being stretched. Skin fragility, easy bruisability, joint hypermobility, and poor wound healing are not usually associated with cutis laxa. Cosmetic surgery can ordinarily be undertaken without complication.

OTHER FEATURES In the X-linked form, characteristic facial features include a hooked nose, inverted nostrils, and a long upper lip.[78] The cry of an affected infant may be hoarse, and a low-pitched voice is often associated with redundancy of the vocal chords. Diagnostic skeletal features of this condition can be identified on plain x-rays and include short flat clavicles, fused carpal bones, and occipital horns, which may not be present until a few years of age. Other manifestations of systemic connective tissue defects, including hernias (inguinal, umbilical, and obturator) as well as diverticula of the gastrointestinal and genitourinary tracts, are common. Chronic diarrhea is a widely reported complication. Diverticula of the genitourinary tract may lead to ureteral obstruction and secondary kidney damage. Angiographic studies in patients have revealed tortuous blood vessels with a peculiar corkscrew appearance. Aortic dilation, occasionally leading to rupture, and peripheral pulmonary artery stenosis have been described. The most severe manifestation of cutis laxa is progressive emphysema, which may lead to early death from cor pulmonale. Many patients have mild mental retardation.

Basic Defect—X-Linked Cutis Laxa

A systemic defect in copper metabolism has long been suspected in X-linked cutis laxa.[74] Low levels of ceruloplasmin and serum copper are a characteristic feature. In a study of cultured dermal fibroblasts, there was reduced activity of lysyl oxidase, which catalyzes a key initiation step in type I collagen cross-linking. Decreased lysyl oxidase activity is probably the reason that conversion of newly synthesized procollagen molecules to insoluble collagen was reduced in cultured cells. Since lysyl oxidase requires copper as a cofactor, it has been hypothesized that diminished activity of that enzyme mediates the generalized connective tissue manifestations.

Some investigators thought that X-linked cutis laxa was an allelic variant of Menkes' syndrome, another disorder of copper metabolism with connective tissue features. The subsequent identification of mutations in the copper-transporting ATPase (MNK) in both disorders has confirmed that hypothesis.[79] Connective tissue abnormalities similar to X-linked cutis laxa were found in the mottled "blotchy" mouse *(Mo-blo)*, which has been shown to carry similar mutations in the mouse homologue of the copper-transporting ATPase.[79–82]

TABLE 156-3

Pseudoxanthoma Elasticum

CLINICAL CHARACTERISTICS		AD1 (*n*=12)	AD2 (*n*=52)	AR1 (*n*=54)	AR2 (*n*=3)	AR3 (*n*=39)
Skin	Classic flexural	100%	4%	77%	—	100%
	Generalized	—	—	100%	—	—
Cardiovascular system	Hypertension	75%	7.8%	19.7%	—	41%
	Angina/claudication	56%	—	—	—	20.5%
Ophthalmic manifestations	Angioid streaks	34%	47%	47%	—	76.9%
	Retinal deterioration	75%	7.8%	35%	—	51.3%
Marfanoid features	High arched palate, loose jointedness, blue sclerae	—	50%	10%	—	—

NOTE: AD, autosomal dominant; AR autosomal recessive.
SOURCE: Adapted from Viljoen et al.[63]

FIGURE 156-9

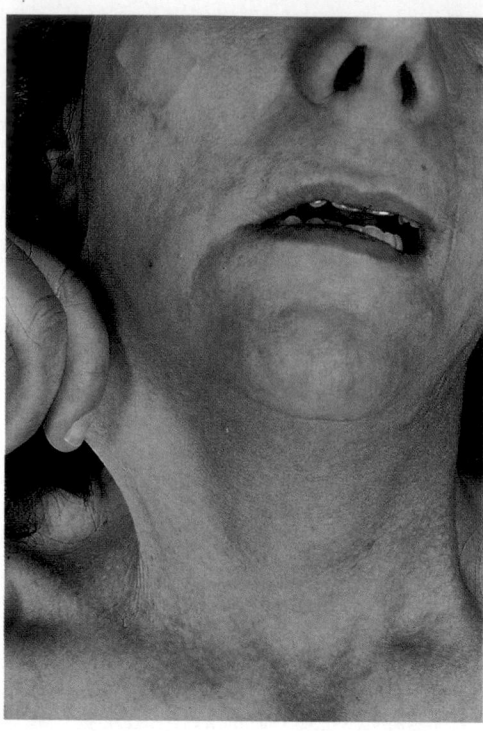

Cutis laxa. The skin hangs in loose folds, giving the appearance of premature aging.

REFERENCES

1. Godfrey M: The Marfan syndrome, in *McKusick's Heritable Disorders of Connective Tissue,* 5th ed, edited by P Beighton. St. Louis, Mosby, 1992, p 51
2. Haber J: Miescher's elastoma (elastoma intrapapillare perforans verruciforme). *Br J Dermatol* **71**:85, 1959
3. Sakai LY et al: Fibrillin, a new 350-kD glycoprotein, is a component of extracellular microfibrils. *J Cell Biol* **103**:2499, 1986
4. Corson GM et al: Fibrillin binds calcium and is coded by cDNAs that reveal a multidomain structure and alternatively spliced exons at the 5-prime end. *Genomics* **17**:476, 1993
5. Hollister DW et al: Immunohistologic abnormalities of the microfibrillar-fiber system in the Marfan syndrome. *N Engl J Med* **323**:152, 1990
6. Magenis RE et al: Localization of the fibrillin (FBN) gene to chromosome 15, band q21.1. *Genomics* **11**:346, 1991
7. Byers PH: Disorders of collagen biosynthesis and structure, in *The Metabolic and Molecular Bases of Inherited Diseases,* 7th ed, edited by CR Scriver et al. New York, McGraw-Hill, 1995, chap 134, p 4029
8. Deitz HC, Pyeritz PE: Mutations in the human gene for fibrillin-1 (FBN1) in the Marfan syndrome and related disorders. *Hum Mol Genet* **4**:1799, 1995
9. Aoyama T et al: Fibrillin abnormalities and prognosis in Marfan syndrome and related disorders. *Am J Med Genet* **58**:169, 1995
10. Francke U et al: A Gly1127Ser mutation in an EGF-like domain of the fibrillin-1 gene is a risk factor for ascending aortic aneurysm and dissection. *Am J Hum Genet* **56**:1287, 1995
11. Dietz HC et al: Clustering of fibrillin (FBN1) missense mutations in Marfan syndrome patients at cysteine residues in EGF-like domains. *Hum Mutat* **1**:366, 1992
12. Dietz HC et al: The phenotypic continuum associated with FBN1 mutations includes the Shprintzen-Goldberg syndrome. *Am J Hum Genet* **57**:A211, 1995
13. Mudd SH et al: Disorders of transsulfuration, in *The Metabolic and Molecular Bases of Inherited Disease,* 7th ed, edited by CR Scriver et al. New York, McGraw-Hill, 1995, p 1279
14. Abbott MH et al: Psychiatric manifestations of homocystinuria due to cystathionine beta-synthase deficiency: Prevalence, natural history, and relationship to neurologic impairment and vitamin B6-responsiveness. *Am J Med Genet* **26**:959, 1987
15. Harris ED Jr, Sjoerdsma A: Effect of penicillamine on human collagen and its possible application to treatment of scleroderma. *Lancet* **2**:996, 1966
16. Munke M et al: The gene for cystathionine beta-synthase (CBS) maps to the subtelomeric region on human chromosome 21q and to proximal mouse chromosome 17. *Am J Hum Genet* **42**:550, 1988
17. Kraus JP: Molecular basis of phenotype expression in homocystinuria. *J Inherit Metab Dis* **17**:383, 1994
18. Smith R: *The Brittle Bone Syndrome: Osteogenesis Imperfecta.* London, Butterworths, 1983
19. Sillence DO et al: Genetic heterogeneity in osteogenesis imperfecta. *J Med Genet* **16**:101, 1979
20. Prockop DJ et al: Mutations in type 1 procollagen that cause osteogenesis imperfecta: Effects of the mutations on the assembly of collagen into fibrils, the basis of phenotypic variations, and potential antisense therapies (review). *J Bone Miner Res* **8**(suppl 2):S489, 1993
21. Sillence DO et al: Osteogenesis imperfecta type III. Delineation of the phenotype with reference to genetic heterogeneity. *Am J Med Genet* **23**:821, 1986
22. Wenstrup RJ et al: Distinct biochemical phenotypes predict clinical severity in nonlethal variants of osteogenesis imperfecta. *Am J Hum Genet* **46**:975, 1990
23. Rowe DW et al: Diminished type I collagen synthesis and reduced alpha 1(I) collagen messenger RNA in cultured fibroblasts from patients with dominantly inherited (type I) osteogenesis imperfecta. *J Clin Invest* **76**:604, 1985
24. Barsh GS, Byers PH: Reduced secretion of structurally abnormal type I procollagen in a form of osteogenesis imperfecta. *Proc Nat Acad Sci USA* **78**:5142, 1981
25. Bonadio J, Byers PH: Subtle structural alterations in the chains of type I procollagen produce osteogenesis imperfecta type II. *Nature* **316**:363, 1985
26. Beighton P: The Ehlers-Danlos Syndromes, in *McKusick's Heritable Disorders of Connective Tissue,* 5th ed, edited by P Beighton. St. Louis, Mosby, 1992, p 189
27. Beighton P et al: International Nosology of Heritable Disorders of Connective Tissue, Berlin, 1986. *Am J Med Genet* **29**:581, 1988
28. Steinmann B et al: The Ehlers-Danlos Syndrome, in *Connective Tissue and Its Heritable Disorders,* edited by PM Royce, B Steinmann. New York, Wiley-Liss, 1993, p 351
29. De Paepe A: Ehlers-Danlos syndrome type IV. Clinical and molecular aspects and guidelines for diagnosis and management. *Dermatology* **189**(suppl 2):21, 1994
30. Byers PH et al: X-linked cutis laxa: Defective collagen crosslink formation due to decreased lysyl oxidase activity. *N Engl J Med* **303**:61, 1980
31. Wenstrup RJ et al: Ehlers-Danlos syndrome type VI: Clinical manifestations of collagen lysyl hydroxylase deficiency. *J Pediatr* **115**:405, 1989
32. Arneson MA et al: A new form of Ehlers-Danlos syndrome. Fibronectin corrects defective platelet function. *JAMA* **244**:144, 1980
33. Hyland J et al: A homozygous stop codon in the lysyl hydroxylase gene in two siblings with Ehlers-Danlos syndrome type VI. *Nat Genet* **2**:228, 1992
34. Kuivaniemi H et al: Identical G+1 to A mutations in three different introns of the type III procollagen gene (COL3A1) produce different patterns of RNA splicing in three variants of Ehlers-Danlos syndrome IV. An explanation for exon skipping some mutations and not others. *J Biol Chem* **265**:12067, 1990
35. Hausser I, Anton-Lamprecht I: Differential ultrastructural aberrations of collagen fibrils in Ehlers-Danlos syndrome types I–IV as a means of diagnostics and classification. *Hum Genet* **93**:394, 1994
36. Wordsworth BP et al: Segregation analysis of the structural genes of the major fibrillar collagens provides further evidence of molecular heterogeneity in type II Ehlers-Danlos syndrome. *Br J Rheumatol* **30**:173, 1991
37. Sokolov BP et al: Exclusion of COL1A1, COL1A2, and COL3A1 genes as candidate genes for Ehlers-Danlos syndrome type I in one large family. *Hum Genet* **88**:125, 1991
38. Birk DE et al: Collagen type I and type V are present in the same fibril in the avian corneal stroma. *J Cell Biol* **106**:999, 1988

39. Birk DE et al: Collagen fibrillogenesis in vitro: Interaction of types I and V collagen regulates fibril diameter. *J Cell Sci* **95**:649, 1990

40. Andrikopoulos K et al: Targeted mutation in the col5a2 gene reveals a regulatory role for type V collagen during matrix assembly. *Nat Genet* **9**:31, 1995

41. Toriello HV et al: A translocation interrupts the COL5A1 gene in a patient with Ehlers-Danlos syndrome and hypomelanosis of Ito. *Nat Genet* **13**:361, 1996

42. De Paepe A et al: Mutations in the COL5A1 gene are causal in the Ehlers-Danlos syndromes I and II. *Am J Hum Genet* **60**:547, 1997

43. Wenstrup RJ et al: A splice-junction mutation in the region of proα1(V) chains results in the gravis form of the Ehlers-Danlos syndrome (type I). *Hum Mol Genet* **5**:1733, 1996

44. Nicholls AC et al: An exon skipping mutation of a type V collagen gene (COL5A1) in Ehlers-Danlos syndrome. *J Med Genet* **33**:940, 1996

45. Michalickova K et al: Mutations of the α2(v) chain of type V collagen impair matrix assembly and produce Ehlers-Danlos syndrome type I. *Hum Mol Genet* **7**:249, 1998

46. Heikkinen J et al: Structure and expression of the human lysyl hydroxylase gene (PLOD): Introns 9 and 16 contain Alu sequences at the sites of recombination in Ehlers-Danlos syndrome type VI patients. *Genomics* **24**:464, 1994

47. Eyre DR, Glimcher MJ: Reducible crosslinks in hydroxylysine-deficient collagens of a heritable disorder of connective tissue. *Proc Nat Acad Sci USA* **69**:2594, 1972

48. Ihme A et al: Ehlers-Danlos syndrome type VI: Collagen type specificity of defective lysyl hydroxylation in various tissues. *J Invest Dermatol* **83**:161, 1984

49. Pasquali M et al: Urinary pyridinium cross-links: A noninvasive diagnostic test for Ehlers-Danlos syndrome type VI (letter). *N Engl J Med* **331**:132, 1994

50. Steinmann B et al: Urinary pyridinoline cross-links in Ehlers-Danlos syndrome type VI (letter). *Am J Hum Genet* **57**:1505, 1995

51. Hautala T et al: Cloning of human lysyl hydroxylase: Complete cDNA-derived amino acid sequence and assignment of the gene (PLOD) to chromosome 1p36.3—p36.2. *Genomics* **13**:62, 1992

52. Yeowell HN et al: Characterization of a partial cDNA for lysyl hydroxylase from human skin fibroblasts: Lysyl hydroxylase mRNAs are regulated differently by minoxidil derivatives and hydralazine. *J Invest Dermatol* **99**:864, 1992

53. Elsas L et al: Inherited human collagen lysyl hydroxylase deficiency: Ascorbic acid response. *J Pediatr* **92**:378, 1978

54. Ha VT et al: A patient with Ehlers-Danlos syndrome type VI is a compound heterozygote for mutations in the lysyl hydroxylase gene. *J Clin Invest* **93**:1716, 1994

55. Hautala T et al: A large duplication in the gene for lysyl hydroxylase accounts for the type VI variant of Ehlers-Danlos syndrome in two siblings. *Genomics* **15**:399, 1993

56. Heikkinen J et al: Duplication of seven exons in the lysyl hydroxylase gene is associated with longer forms of a repetitive sequence within the gene and is a common cause for the type VI variant of Ehlers-Danlos syndrome. *Am J Hum Genet* **60**:48, 1997

57. Ogur G et al: Clinical, ultrastructural and biochemical studies in two sibs with Ehlers-Danlos syndrome type VI-B-like features. *Clin Genet* **46**:417, 1994

58. Lichtenstein JR et al: Defect in conversion of procollagen to collagen in a form of Ehlers-Danlos syndrome. *Science* **182**:298, 1973

59. Barabas AP: Heterogenity of the Ehlers-Danlos syndrome: Description of three clinical types and a hypothesis to explain the basic defect. *Br Med J* **2**:612, 1967

60. Neldner KH: Pseudoxanthoma elasticum. *Int J Dermatol* **27**:98, 1988

61. Neldner KH: Pseudoxanthoma elasticum. *Clin Dermatol* **6**:1, 1988

62. McDonald HR et al: Reticular-like pigmentary patterns in pseudoxanthoma elasticum. *Ophthalmology* **95**:306, 1988

63. Viljoen DL et al: The obstetric and gynaecological implications of pseudoxanthoma elasticum. *Br J Obstet Gynaecol* **94**:884, 1987

64. Tsuji T: Three-dimensional architecture of altered dermal elastic fibers in pseudoxanthoma elasticum: Scanning electron microscopic studies. *J Invest Dermatol* **82**:518, 1984

65. Longas MO et al: Glycosaminoglycans of skin and urine in pseudoxanthoma elasticum: Evidence for chondroitin 6-sulfate alteration. *Clin Chim Acta* **155**:227, 1986

66. Schwartz E et al: Elastase-like protease and elastolytic activities expressed in cultured dermal fibroblasts derived from lesional skin of patients with pseudoxanthoma elasticum, actinic elastosis, and cutis laxa. *Clin Chim Acta* **176**:219, 1988

67. Meyrick Thomas RH, Kirby JD: Elastosis perforans serpiginosa and pseudoxanthoma elasticum-like skin change due to D-penicillamine. *Clin Exp Dermatol* **10**:386, 1985

68. Pope F: Autosomal dominant pseudoxanthoma elasticum. *J Med Genet* **11**:152, 1974

69. Pope F: Two types of autosomal recessive pseudoxanthoma elasticum. *Arch Dermatol* **110**:209, 1974

70. Rongioletti F et al: Generalized pseudoxanthoma elasticum with deficiency of vitamin K-dependent clotting factors. *J Am Acad Dermatol* **21**:1150, 1989

71. Beighton P: The dominant and recessive forms of cutis laxa. *J Med Genet* **9**:216, 1972

72. Ogur G et al: Syndrome of congenital cutis laxa with ligamentous laxity and delayed development: Report of a brother and sister from Turkey. *Am J Med Genet* **37**:6, 1990

73. Ross UH et al: Osteogenesis imperfecta: Clinical symptoms and update findings in computed tomography and tympano-cochlear scintigraphy. *Acta Otolaryngol* **113**:620, 1993

74. Kuivaniemi H et al: Abnormal copper metabolism and deficient lysyl oxidase activity in a heritable connective tissue disorder. *J Clin Invest* **69**:730, 1982

75. Reed WB et al: Acquired cutis laxa. Primary generalized elastolysis. *Arch Dermatol* **103**:661, 1971

76. Koch SE, Williams ML: Acquired cutis laxa: Case report and review of disorders of elastolysis. *Pediatr Dermatol* **2**:282, 1985

77. Pope FM: Cutis laxa, in *McKusick's Heritable Disorders of Connective Tissue,* 5th ed, edited by P Beighton. St. Louis, Mosby, 1992, p 253

78. Beighton P: Other heritable and generalized disorders of connective tissue, in *McKusick's Heritable Disorders of Connective Tissue,* 5th ed, edited by P Beighton. St. Louis, Mosby, 1992, p 519

79. Petrukhin K, Gilliam TC: Genetic disorders of copper metabolism. *Curr Opin Pediatr* **6**:698, 1994

80. Levinson B et al: A repeated element in the regulatory region of the MNK gene and its deletion in a patient with occipital horn syndrome. *Hum Mol Genet* **5**:1737, 1996

81. Reed V, Boyd Y: Mutation analysis provides additional proof that mottled is the mouse homologue of Menkes' disease. *Hum Mol Genet* **6**:417, 1997

82. Kaler SG et al: Occipital horn syndrome and a mild Menkes' phenotype associated with splice site mutations at the MNK locus. *Nat Genet* **8**:195, 1994

CHAPTER 157

Kenneth H. Kraemer

Heritable Diseases with Increased Sensitivity to Cellular Injury

A group of heritable diseases with differing clinical features share the common characteristics of in vitro or in vivo cellular hypersensitivity to damage by certain physical or chemical agents (Table 157-1). Diseases with autosomal recessive, X-linked, and autosomal dominant inheritance fall in this group. These diseases include xeroderma pigmentosum, Cockayne syndrome, trichothiodystrophy, Bloom syndrome, Fanconi anemia, dyskeratosis congenita, basal cell nevus syndrome, ataxia-telangiectasia, and familial melanoma with dysplastic nevi. Clinical abnormalities involve the cutaneous, ocular, nervous, immune, hemopoietic, skeletal, or gastrointestinal systems. Some are associated with increased incidence of neoplasia. Several have a major feature of progressive degeneration of previously normal bodily function.

The cellular hypersensitivity is often of diagnostic utility. Further, it may suggest pathogenic mechanisms and measures for therapeutic or prophylactic intervention. The molecular basis of the cellular hypersensitivity is currently being clarified in some of these disorders.

In this chapter, the clinical features and laboratory abnormalities of the first six of the heritable diseases with cellular hypersensitivity listed above are presented. Basal cell nevus syndrome, ataxia-telangiectasia, and familial melanoma with dysplastic nevi are reviewed in Chaps. 81, 90, 91, 92, 157, and 192. The diseases are discussed in terms of the systems affected, the cellular hypersensitivity, and the relevance of the cellular abnormality to the clinical symptoms. The major tests used to measure cellular hypersensitivity and to assess DNA repair are described in Chap. 37 ("Cellular Hypersensitivity and DNA Repair").

XERODERMA PIGMENTOSUM

Xeroderma pigmentosum (XP) serves as the prototype heritable disease with increased sensitivity to cellular injury.[1-4] XP is an autosomal recessive disease with sun sensitivity, photophobia, early onset of freckling, and subsequent neoplastic changes on sun-exposed surfaces. There is cellular hypersensitivity to UV radiation and to certain chemicals in association with abnormal DNA repair. Some of the patients have progressive neurologic degeneration.[2,5]

Frequency

Xeroderma pigmentosum occurs with an estimated frequency of 1: 1,000,000 in the United States. It is more common in Japan.[1,3] Patients have been reported worldwide in all races including whites, Asians, blacks, and Native Americans.[2] Consanguinity is common.

Clinical Features

SKIN Approximately half of the patients with XP have a history of acute sunburn reaction on minimal UV exposure. The other patients apparently tan normally without excessive burning. In all patients, numerous freckle-like hyperpigmented macules appear (Fig. 157-1). The median age of onset of the cutaneous symptoms is between 1 and 2 years (Fig. 157-2).[2] These abnormalities are strikingly limited to sun-exposed areas (Fig. 157-1E). Continued sun exposure causes the patient's skin to become dry and parchment-like, with increased pigmentation, hence the name *xeroderma pigmentosum* ("pigmented dry skin") (Fig. 157-1A). Premalignant actinic keratoses develop at an early age (Fig. 157-1B). XP is an example of accelerated photoaging, and the appearance of sun-exposed skin in children with XP is similar to that occurring in farmers and sailors after many years of extreme sun exposure.

CANCER Patients with XP under 20 years of age have a greater than 1000-fold increased risk of cutaneous basal cell or squamous cell carcinoma or melanoma.[2,6] The median age of onset of non-melanoma skin cancer reported in patients with XP was 8 years, in comparison to 60 years in the general population (Fig. 157-2).[2,6] Multiple primary cutaneous neoplasms, including melanomas, commonly occur.

Review of the world literature has revealed a substantial number of cases of oral cavity neoplasms, particularly squamous cell carcinoma of the tip of the tongue—a presumed sun-exposed location.[2,6] Brain (sarcoma and medulloblastoma), central nervous system (astrocytoma of the spinal cord), lung, uterine, breast, pancreatic, gastric, renal, and testicular tumors and leukemias have been reported in a few patients with XP.[2,6,7] Overall, these reports suggest an approximate ten to twenty-fold increase in internal neoplasms in XP.

EYES Ocular abnormalities are almost as common as the cutaneous abnormalities and are an important feature of XP[2,6] (Fig. 157-1C). The posterior portion of the eye (retina) is shielded from UV radiation by the anterior portion (lids, cornea, and conjunctiva). Clinical findings are strikingly limited to these anterior, UV-exposed structures. Photophobia is often present and may be associated with prominent conjunctival injection. Continued UV exposure of the eye may result in severe keratitis leading to corneal opacification and vascularization. The lids develop increased pigmentation and loss of lashes. Atrophy of the skin of the lids results in ectropion, entropion, or, in severe cases, complete loss of the lids. Benign conjunctival inflammatory masses or papillomas of the

TABLE 157-1

Heritable Diseases with Cellular Hypersensitivity

DISEASE AUTOSOMAL RECESSIVE	CLINICAL ABNORMALITIES					CELLULAR ABNORMALITIES	
	CUTANEOUS	OCULAR	NEUROLOGIC	HEMATOPOIETIC	NEOPLASIA	TYPE	MECHANISM
Xeroderma pigmentosum	Sun sensitivity, atrophy, freckling	Photophobia, UV conjunctivitis, UV keratitis	Deafness progressive mental deterioration	Normal	BCC, SCC, melanoma	UV-induced cell killing, mutagenesis, chromosome breakage, SCE	Abnormal DNA repair
Ataxia-telangiectasia	Telangiectasia, x-ray sensitivity	Conjunctival telangiectasia, oculomotor dyspraxia	Progressive ataxia	Humoral and cellular immune defects	Lymphoreticular, GI	Spontaneous chromosome breakage; x-ray-induced cell killing and chromosome breakage	Abnormal ATM gene (cell cycle regulation)
Cockayne syndrome	Sun sensitivity	Retinal pigmentation	Progressive mental deterioration, deafness	Normal	None	UV-induced cell killing, SCE	Abnormal DNA repair
Trichothiodystrophy	Sun sensitivity	Normal	Mental retardation	Normal	None	UV-induced cell killing	Abnormal DNA repair
Bloom syndrome	Telangiectasia, sun sensitivity	Normal	Normal	Defective immunity	Leukemia, GI	Spontaneous chromosome breakage	Abnormal DNA helicase
Fanconi anemia	Hyperpigmentation	Normal	Normal	Anemia, pancytopenia	Leukemia, liver	Spontaneous chromosome breakage; diepoxybutane-induced chromosome breakage	Abnormal DNA cross-link repair
X-LINKED							
Dyskeratosis congenita	Poikiloderma, nail dystrophy	Stenosis of lacrimal duct	Normal	Anemia	GI	Psoralen-induced SCE	?
AUTOSOMAL DOMINANT							
Basal cell nevus syndrome	Palmar pits, x-ray sensitivity	Cataract, coloboma	Mental retardation (some patients)	Normal	BCC, medulloblastoma, ovarian tumors	?	Defective *PTCH* gene (cell differentiation)
Familial melanoma with dysplastic nevi	Dysplastic nevi	Normal	Normal	Normal	Cutaneous melanoma	UVB-induced mutagenesis	Defective p16 gene (cell cycle regulation)

NOTE: BCC, basal cell carcinoma; SCC, squamous cell carcinoma; SCE, sister chromatid exchange; GI, gastrointestinal.

lids may be present. Epithelioma, squamous cell carcinoma, and melanoma of UV-exposed portions of the eye are common.[2,6,8]

NEUROLOGIC SYSTEM Neurologic abnormalities have been reported in approximately 30 percent of the patients[1,2,5,6]; their onset may be early in infancy or, in some patients, delayed until the second decade. The neurologic abnormalities may be mild (e.g., isolated hyporeflexia) or severe, with progressive mental retardation, sensorineural deafness (beginning with high-frequency hearing loss), spasticity, or seizures[1,2,5,6] (Fig. 157-1D). The most severe

form, known as the *DeSanctis-Cacchione syndrome*, involves the cutaneous and ocular manifestations of classic XP plus additional neurologic and somatic abnormalities including microcephaly, progressive mental deterioration, low intelligence, hyporeflexia or areflexia, choreoathetosis, ataxia, spasticity, Achilles tendon shortening leading to eventual quadraparesis, dwarfism, and immature sexual development.[1,2,5,6] The complete DeSanctis-Cacchione syndrome has been recognized in very few patients; however, many patients with XP have one or more of its neurologic features. In clinical practice, deep tendon reflex testing and routine audiometry can usually serve as a screen for the presence of XP-associated

FIGURE 157-1

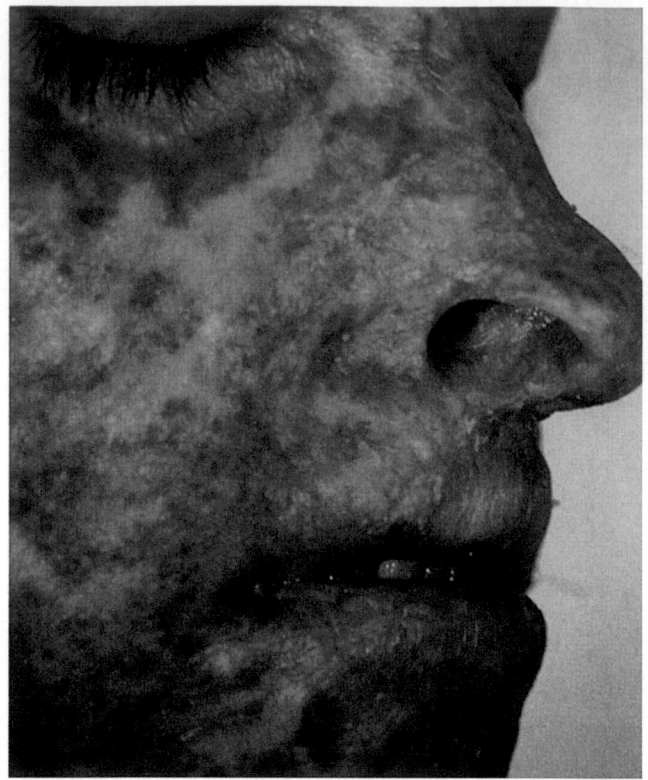

A.

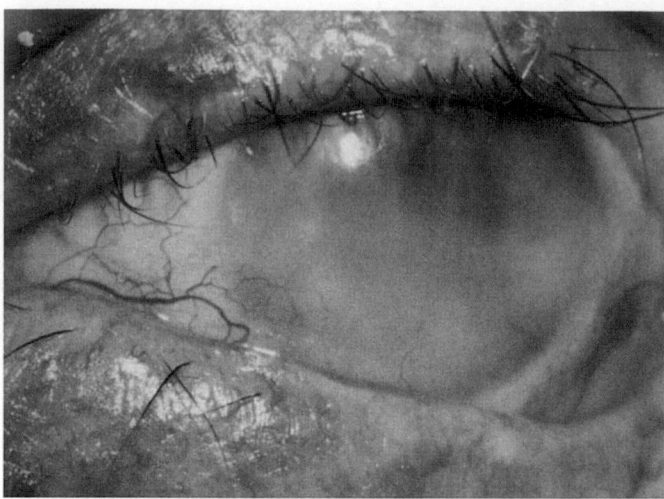

C.

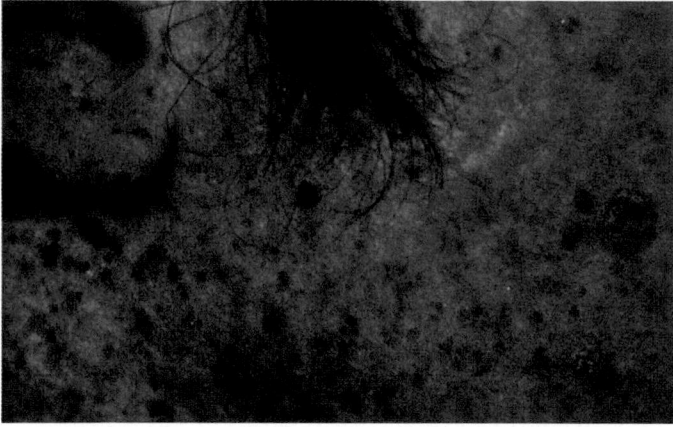

B.

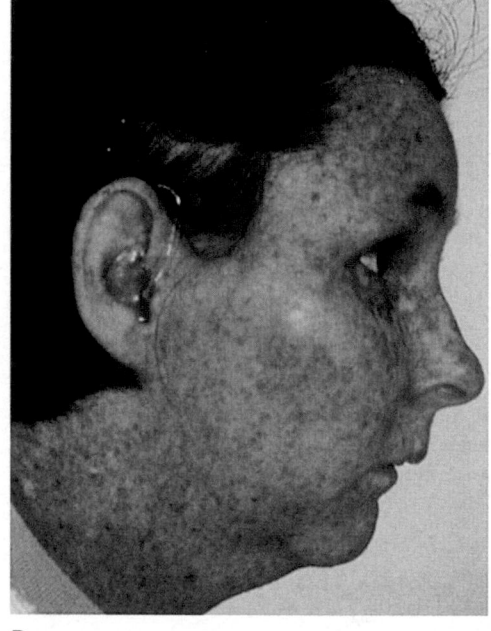

D.

Xeroderma pigmentosum. *A.* Pigmentary changes, atrophy, dryness, and cheilitis in a 16-year-old patient. *B.* Cheek of a 14-year-old patient with pigmented macules of varying size and intensity, actinic keratosis, basal cell carcinoma, and a surgical scar. *C.* Corneal clouding, prominent conjunctival blood vasculature, and loss of lashes. *D.* A 26-year-old patient with deafness and mental retardation. *E.* Myriads of pigmented macules of varying size and intensity and scattered achromic areas on the back, with marked sparing of sun protected buttocks of a 14-year-old patient.

neurologic abnormalities. Clinically asymptomatic neurodegeneration in an adult has been described.[9]

The predominant neuropathologic abnormality found at autopsy in patients with neurologic symptoms was loss (or absence) of neurons, particularly in the cerebrum and cerebellum. There is evidence for a primary axonal degeneration in these patients.[1,5,10–12]

Laboratory Abnormalities

There have been no consistent routine clinical laboratory abnormalities in patients with XP. Tests of cellular hypersensitivity to UV damage, however, have shown uniformly abnormal results.[1,4,13,14] One patient was reported with hypoglycinemia.[15]

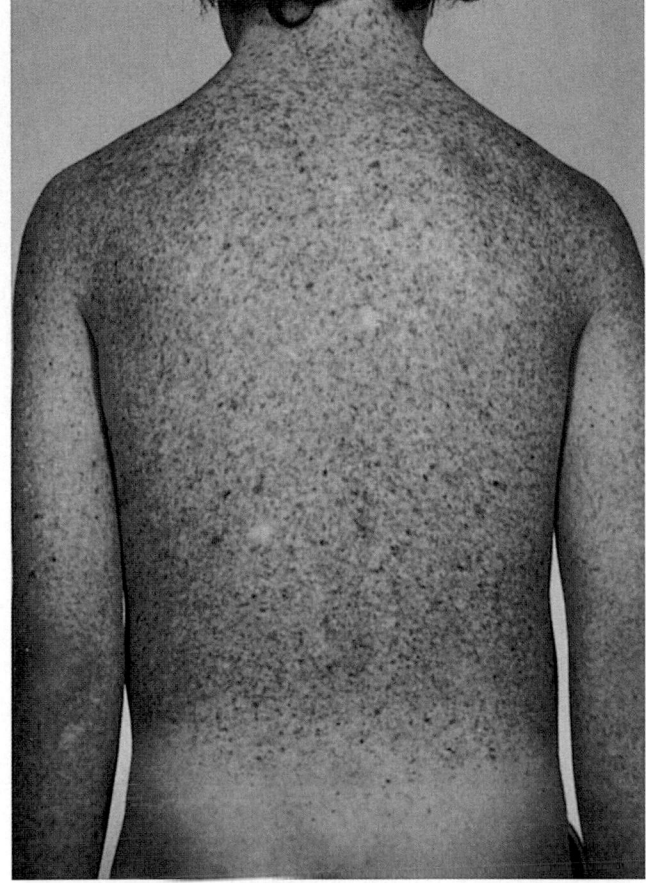

E.

large increases in chromosome breakage and in sister chromatid exchanges have been observed.[4,14,17] The extent of this induced abnormality varies in different patients.

DNA REPAIR In 1968, hypersensitivity of cultured XP cells to UV damage was reported by Cleaver[18] to be the result of defective DNA repair. He found defective UV-induced repair replication, indicating a defect in the nucleotide excision repair system. Most XP cells have a normal response to treatment with x-rays, indicating the specificity of the DNA repair defect. The defective genes for the seven excision repair–defective forms of XP have been cloned,[4,14] and their functions are being investigated.

COMPLEMENTATION GROUPS Genetic heterogeneity among the XP DNA repair defects was found by fusing cultured fibroblasts from two different patients then measuring UV-induced unscheduled DNA synthesis. The unfused cells had the typical low level of UV-induced unscheduled DNA synthesis seen in most XP fibroblasts. Fusion of cells from certain pairs of patients resulted in the presence of fused cells with nearly normal levels of unscheduled DNA synthesis. In these "heterokaryons," each cell provides components that the other was lacking, resulting in enhanced DNA repair. These "complementing cells" thus have different DNA repair defects. Fibroblasts from patients with the same DNA repair defect do not correct each other when fused and are said to be in the same complementation group. Up to 1998, seven such DNA excision repair–deficient complementation groups have been identified (named XP-A to XP-G) and the corresponding genes have been identified (Table 157-2).[4,14]

There has been a report of a patient, whose condition has been called "XP variant," with clinically severe xeroderma pigmentosum who had normal unscheduled DNA synthesis in his fibroblasts, lymphocytes, and even his tumor cells.[1] Studies of cellular hypersensitivity revealed a slightly increased sensitivity to UV-induced in-

CELLULAR HYPERSENSITIVITY Cultured cells from patients with XP generally grow normally when not exposed to damaging agents. The population growth rate or single-cell colony-forming ability is reduced to a greater extent than normal, however, following exposure to UV radiation. A range of post-UV colony-forming abilities has been found with fibroblasts from patients, some having extremely low post-UV colony-forming ability and others having nearly normal survival.[1,2,4]

XP fibroblasts are deficient in their ability to repair some UV-damaged viruses or plasmids to a functionally active state.[4,14,16] These "host cell reactivation" assays have detected an abnormality in every form of XP tested.

UV-irradiated XP fibroblasts produce more mutations per survivor than normal fibroblasts. XP cells also introduce more mutations into UV-damaged plasmids than do normal cells.[4,14,16]

CHROMOSOME ABNORMALITIES XP cells generally are found to have a normal karyotype without excessive chromosome breakage or increased sister chromatid exchanges. Following exposure to UV radiation, however, abnormally

FIGURE 157-2

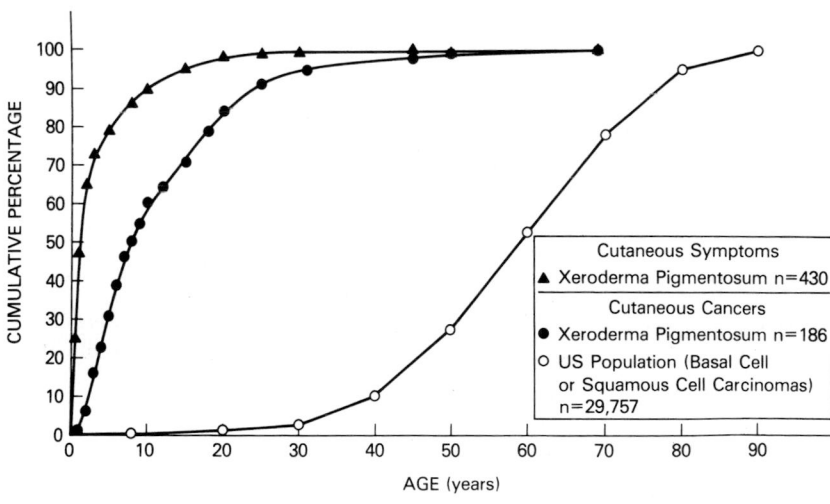

Xeroderma pigmentosum. Age at onset of clinical symptoms and skin cancers. Age at onset of cutaneous symptoms (generally sun sensitivity or pigmentation) was reported for 430 patients. Age at first skin cancer was reported for 186 patients and is compared with the age distribution for 29,757 patients with basal cell carcinoma or squamous cell carcinoma in the U.S. general population. (From Kraemer et al.[2])

TABLE 157-2

Xeroderma Pigmentosum: Characteristics of DNA Repair Complementation Groups

COMPLEMENTATION GROUP	SKIN CANCER	NEUROLOGIC ABNORMALITIES	NUMBER OF PATIENTS, LOCATION	DNA REPAIR, % OF NORMAL
A	Yes	Severe or mild	63, Japan	<2
B	Yes	XP/CS	3, US, Europe	3–7
	No	TTD	1, Italy	
C	Yes	No	62, US, Europe, Egypt	10–25
D	Yes	Moderate	28, US, Europe	25–50
	No	TTD	6, US, Europe	
	Yes	XP/CS	2, Europe	
E	Yes	No	10, Europe, Japan	40–50
F	Yes	No	16, Japan, Europe	10–20
G	Yes	Yes	5, Europe, Japan	<5
	No	XP/CS	4, US, Europe	
Variant	Yes	No	54, US, Europe, Japan	100

NOTE: XP/CS, patient with xeroderma pigmentosum–Cockayne syndrome complex; TTD, patients with trichothiodystrophy (without xeroderma pigmentosum).
SOURCE: References 1,2,3,4, and 31–42 and personal communications.

hibition of cell growth and colony-forming ability, to adenovirus host-cell reactivation, and to UV-induced mutations in vitro. DNA repair studies revealed the presence of a defect in a second DNA repair system, that of postreplication repair.[4,14,19] Cells from this patient had a delayed rate of increase of the molecular weight of newly replicating DNA following UV-irradiation. Further, these cells were especially sensitive to inhibition of this process by caffeine. XP variant patients have also been identified in Japan[3] and Europe.

PRENATAL DIAGNOSIS This has been reported by measuring UV-induced unscheduled DNA synthesis in cultured amniotic fluid cells[20] and, more recently, by use of DNA diagnosis of trophoblast cells obtained early in pregnancy.[21]

DRUG AND CHEMICAL HYPERSENSITIVITY A number of DNA-damaging agents other than UV radiation have been found to yield hypersensitive responses with XP cells (Table 157-3).[4,14,22] These agents include drugs (psoralens, chlorpromazine), cancer chemotherapeutic agents (cisplatin, carmustine), and chemical carcinogens (benzo[a]pyrene derivatives). Presumably, these agents induce DNA damage whose repair involves portions of the DNA repair pathways that are defective in XP.

Treatment

Management of patients with XP is based on early diagnosis, lifelong protection from UV radiation exposure, and early detection and treatment of neoplasms. Diagnosis rests on recognition of the characteristic clinical features and is confirmed by laboratory tests of cellular hypersensitivity.

SUN PROTECTION Patients should be educated to protect all body surfaces from UV radiation by wearing protective clothing and UV-absorbing glasses and long hair styles. They should adopt a life-style to minimize UV exposure and use sunscreens with high sun protective factor (SPF) ratings (minimum SPF 15) daily. Cells from patients with XP are hypersensitive to killing by UVC, UVB,

and UVA.[13] Patients should be examined frequently by a family member who has been instructed in recognition of cutaneous neoplasms. A set of color photographs of the entire skin surface with close-ups of lesions (including a ruler) is often extremely useful to both the patient and the physician in detecting new lesions. A physician should examine patients at frequent intervals (about every 3 to 6 months depending on severity of skin disease). Premalignant lesions such as actinic keratoses may be treated by freezing with liquid nitrogen or with topical 5-fluorouracil. Larger areas have been treated with therapeutic dermatome shaving or dermabrasion to remove the more damaged superficial epidermal layers.[23–25] This procedure permits repopulation by relatively UV-shielded cells from the follicles and glands.

Since cells from patients with XP are also hypersensitive to environmental mutagens, such as benzo[a]pyrene found in cigarette smoke (Table 157-3), prudence dictates that patients should be protected against these agents. A patient who smoked cigarettes for more than 10 years died of bronchogenic carcinoma of the lungs at age 35.[2]

CANCERS Cutaneous neoplasms are treated in the same manner as in patients who do not have XP. This involves electrodesiccation and curettage, surgical excision, or chemosurgery. Since multiple surgical procedures are often necessary, removal of undamaged skin should be minimized. Extremely severe cases have been treated by excision of large portions of facial surface and grafting with uninvolved skin.[23,24] Most patients with XP are not abnormally sensitive to therapeutic x-rays.[26] However, cultured cells from a few XP-G patients were found to be hypersensitive to x-rays,[27] so that when x-ray therapy is indicated, an initial small dose is advisable to test for clinical hypersensitivity.

High-dose oral isotretinoin has been shown to be effective in preventing new neoplasms in patients with multiple skin cancers.[28] Because of its toxicity (hepatic, hyperlipidemic, teratogenic, calcification of ligaments and tendons, premature closure of the epiphyses) oral isotretinoin should be reserved for patients with XP who have had multiple skin cancers.

A bacterial DNA repair enzyme, denV T4 endonuclease in a topical liposome-containing preparation, is currently under investi-

TABLE 157-3

Xeroderma Pigmentosum: DNA-Damaging Agents Inducing Cellular Hypersensitivity

Drugs	Carcinogens
Psoralens plus long-wavelength UV radiation (PUVA)	Aflatoxin
Chlorpromazine	Benzo[a]pyrene
Nitrofurantoin	Nitroquinoline oxide derivatives (4NQO)
Mitomycin C	Acetoaminofluorene derivatives (AAF)
Anthramycin	Phenanthrene derivatives
Cisplatin	
Carmustine	

gation in a phase III trial for prevention of actinic keratoses in XP patients.[29]

EYES The eyes should be protected by wearing UV-absorbing glasses with side shields. Methyl cellulose eye drops or soft contact lenses have been used to keep the cornea moist and to protect against mechanical trauma in patients with deformed eyelids. Corneal transplantation has restored vision in patients with severe keratitis with corneal opacity. Neoplasms of the lids, conjunctiva, and cornea are usually treated surgically.[8]

Clinical-Laboratory Correlations

Patients with XP are hypersensitive to UV radiation, as are their cultured cells. Cutaneous and ocular abnormalities are strikingly limited to UV-exposed areas and usually spare such UV-shielded locations as the axillae, buttocks, and retina.

COMPLEMENTATION GROUPS
At least eight different molecular defects are associated with the clinical abnormalities recognized as XP, as indicated by the existence of seven DNA excision repair–deficient complementation groups [A to G] and the variant form (Table 157-2). A discussion of the seven cloned XP genes and their function can be found in Chap. 37.

Complementation group A contains patients with the most severe neurologic and somatic abnormalities (the DeSanctis-Cacchione syndrome) as well as patients with minimal or no neurologic abnormalities.[1,3,4] This form is seen in the United States, Europe, and the Middle East. It is the most common form of XP in Japan. Approximately 90 percent of the Japanese XP-A patients have the same single base substitution mutation in this gene.[30] This finding has served as the basis for development of a rapid diagnostic assay for Japanese XP-A patients using polymerase chain reaction analysis of a small sample of DNA.[21]

Complementation group B is composed of three patients in two kindreds who had the cutaneous abnormalities characteristic of XP (including neoplasms) in conjunction with neurologic and ocular abnormalities typical of Cockayne's syndrome (CS).[1,31] Surprisingly, a patient with trichothiodystrophy (TTD) was also found to have a defect in the XP-B gene.[32]

Patients in complementation group C, with rare exceptions, have XP with skin and ocular involvement but without neurologic abnormalities.[1,4,33] This is the most common group in the United States, Europe, and Egypt but has rarely been found in Japan.

Patients in complementation group D have been described with four different clinical phenotypes. They may have cutaneous XP with late onset of neurologic abnormalities in their second decade of life or XP with no neurologic abnormalities.[1,4,33,34] Two XP-D patients have been reported with clinical symptoms of both XP and CS.[35,36] Finally, cells from patients with a photosensitive form of TTD (without XP) were also assigned to XP complementation group D.[37]

Complementation group E was found in one kindred in Europe and several in Japan.[4,33,34] These patients had relatively mild cutaneous abnormalities without neurologic involvement.

Complementation group F patients have been found mainly in Japan.[34,38] These patients have mild clinical symptoms without neurologic abnormalities or skin cancer. The residual rate of DNA repair, however, is very low (only 10 to 20 percent of normal).

Five patients in complementation group G have been identified in Europe and Japan. Several had neurologic abnormalities without skin cancer. Fibroblasts from one of the patients were found to be hypersensitive to killing by x-rays as well as by UV radiation.[27]

Four other patients in XP complementation group G had clinical features of both XP and severe CS.[39–42]

XP variant cells have normal DNA nucleotide excision repair and thus do not fall into any of the complementation groups of cells with defective DNA excision repair.[1,4,33] There is, however, defective postreplication repair. XP variant patients have been identified in the United States, Europe, and Japan.[3,7] Very few have neurologic abnormalities. The cutaneous and ocular abnormalities have been severe in some patients and mild in others. A family with four affected individuals was described in Germany. The affected individuals had extensive sun exposure and late onset of cutaneous cancers. They had originally been thought to represent a separate disorder (pigmented xerodermoid). Subsequent laboratory studies showed the findings typical of XP variants.[43]

ENVIRONMENTAL-GENETIC INTERACTION
The cutaneous and ocular changes in patients with XP are consistent with the notion that repeated insults by environmental agents, particularly UV radiation, produce repeated bouts of DNA damage. Because of defective DNA repair, this damage results in cell death, diminished cell growth, or somatic cell mutations. Through mechanisms that are not completely understood, these cellular alterations lead to atrophy, hyper- and hypopigmentation, and telangiectasia as well as to a 1000-fold increase in malignant neoplasms. Thus XP provides strong support for the somatic mutation theory of carcinogenesis. In addition, rigorous protection from UV radiation from early infancy in a few patients has been shown to prevent most of the serious cutaneous and ocular abnormalities.

Some patients with XP demonstrate progressive neurologic degeneration.[1,4,5] Severely affected patients lose their ability to walk and talk. Histologically, the picture is of a primary neuronal degeneration with loss (or absence) of neurons, without evidence of vascular abnormality, deposition of abnormal material, or inflammatory reaction. It has been hypothesized, in analogy to the cutaneous degenerative changes, that the neurologic degeneration is a manifestation of unrepaired DNA damage. Since mature neurons do not divide, unrepaired DNA damage would lead to cell death without replacement by other neurons. This process would lead to progressive loss of neurologic function. The specific cause of such damage, whether by exogenous or endogenous agents, and the explanation of why some neurons are more severely affected than others are not known. The severity of the neurologic symptoms in patients with XP with associated neurologic disease has been shown to correlate with the UV sensitivity of their skin fibroblasts.[1,4,5]

HETEROZYGOTES
XP heterozygotes (parents and some other relatives) are carriers of the gene for XP but are clinically normal. There is limited epidemiologic evidence to indicate that such persons have an increased risk of developing skin cancer.[44] Most tests of cell function or DNA repair yield normal responses with cells from XP heterozygotes. A nonspecific test of hypersensitivity to x-ray-induced chromosome breakage has been reported to be abnormal with cells from obligate heterozygotes for XP.[45] Cloning of the defective genes in different XP complementation groups should provide a direct assay for detection of XP heterozygotes.[46]

REGISTRY AND PATIENT SUPPORT GROUP
In order to gather information on clinical abnormalities in XP and to provide information to physicians a registry has been established. Patients with

XP should be reported to and additional clinical information is available from

Xeroderma Pigmentosum Registry
c/o Department of Pathology
Medical Science Building, Room C520
CMDNJ- New Jersey Medical School
185 South Orange Avenue
Newark, NJ 07103

The Xeroderma Pigmentosum Society is an educational, advocacy, and support organization for helping patients with XP and their families. Their address is 57 Sleight-Plass Rd, Poughkeepsie, NY 12603; e-mail: xps@mhv.net; web site: http://www.xps.org.

COCKAYNE SYNDROME

CS is a very rare autosomal recessive degenerative disease with cutaneous, ocular, neurologic, and somatic abnormalities[39,47,48] (see Table 157-1). A review published in 1992 described 140 cases reported in the literature.[49]

Clinical Features

In l936, Cockayne described a syndrome characterized by cachectic dwarfism, deafness, and pigmentary retinal degeneration with a characteristic "salt and pepper" appearance of the retina. The skin had photosensitivity[50] without the excessive pigmentary abnormalities seen in XP. There was marked loss of subcutaneous fat, resulting in a "wizened," appearance with typical "bird-headed" facies and prominent "Mickey Mouse" ears. Other ocular findings included cataracts and optic atrophy.[51] Neurologic abnormalities, in addition to deafness, include peripheral neuropathy, normal pressure hydrocephalus, and microcephaly. Birth weight and early development are usually normal. The disease onset is usually in the second year of life with slowly progressive neurologic degeneration. Intellectual deterioration may be nonuniform, with some functions preserved better than others. A severe infantile form has been described[39,52] as well as a milder form with late onset.[53,54] Cerebro-oculo-facio-skeletal (COFS) syndrome[55] with microcephaly and severe mental retardation and CAMFAK syndrome of congenital cataracts, microcephaly, failure to thrive, and kyphoscoliosis[56] have some similar features.

CS is not associated with an increased incidence of neoplasia.

Laboratory Abnormalities

Clinical laboratory testing often shows sensorineural deafness, neuropathic electromyogram, and slow motor nerve conduction velocity.[39,47–49,57–59] The electroencephalogram may be abnormal, and x-ray examination may show thickened skull and microcephaly. CT may be diagnostically useful in the detection of normal pressure hydrocephalus[57] and showing calcification of the basal ganglia and other structures[60] (Fig. 157-3). Magnetic resonance imaging (MRI) of the brain shows atrophy and dysmyelination of the cerebrum and cerebellum.[60,61] Bone age is usually normal. Height and weight are usually well below the third percentile for the age.

CELLULAR HYPERSENSITIVITY As with XP, cultured cells (fibroblasts or lymphocytes) from patients with CS are hypersensitive to UV-induced inhibition of growth and colony-forming ability.[4,62]

Host cell reactivation of UV-damaged adenovirus or plasmids is reduced, although generally to a lesser extent than in XP.[63] The mutant frequency was elevated in circulating lymphocytes from two donors with CS.[50]

CHROMOSOME ABNORMALITIES Chromosome karyotype and sister chromatid exchange frequency is usually normal in untreated cells, but one patient was described with deletion of a part of chromosome 10[54] and another with 47XXX.[64] UV treatment of CS cells results in a greater than normal increase in sister chromatid exchanges[62,65] and a delayed recovery of chromosome damage after near UV light exposure.[66]

CS cells do not have the same DNA repair defects as XP cells. The usual tests of DNA excision repair are normal. In 1990, Venema et al.[67] reported that normal cells repair the DNA of UV-damaged active genes at

FIGURE 157-3

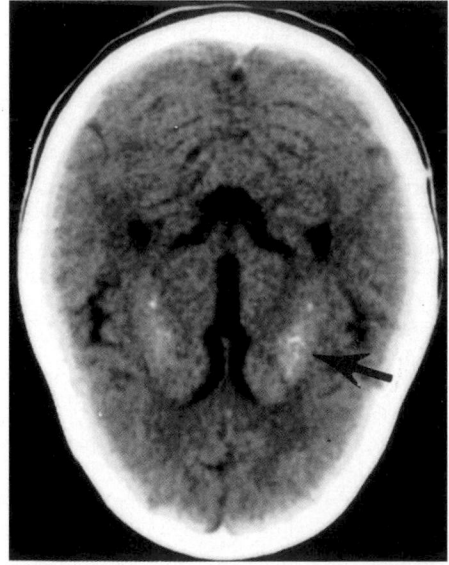

A.

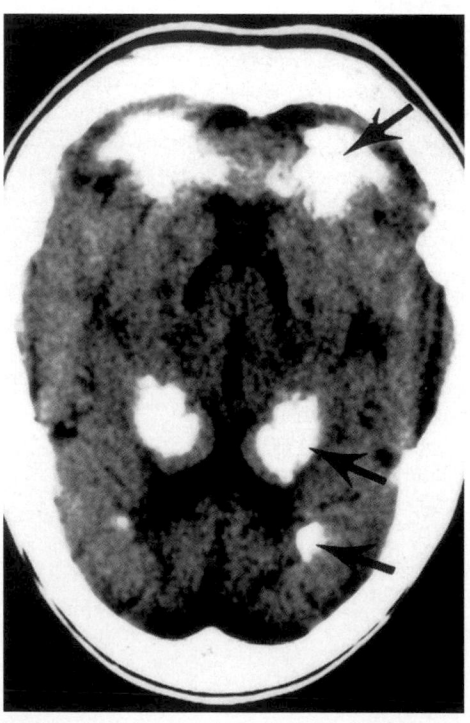

B.

Cockayne syndrome. Calcification of brain visualized on CT scan. A. 2-year-old patient with bilateral calcification of basal ganglia (arrow). B. 15-year-old patient with extensive calcification involving basal ganglia, cerebellum, and cerebral hemispheres (arrows).

a faster rate than inactive genes, and this preferential repair is absent in CS cells. There is also evidence that CS cells are unable to repair photoproducts of the cyclobutane dimer type but are able to repair nondimer photoproducts.[63]

CS cells have a prolonged decrease in the rate of RNA synthesis following UV irradiation.[68] There are two complementation groups (A, B) in CS and their genes have been cloned.[69,70]

PRENATAL DIAGNOSIS Prenatal diagnosis of CS has been performed[71] based on the delay in recovery of post-UV RNA synthesis and the increased cell killing by UV radiation.

Clinical-Laboratory Correlation

CS, like XP, is a disease of progressive neurologic degeneration. Pathologically, CS shows abnormal (dys)myelinization of neurons, whereas XP shows primary axonal degeneration. These findings are consistent with the theory that the myelin-producing cells in CS or neurons in XP are damaged repeatedly but do not recover fully and die.[1,5] Since mature neurons cannot divide, the dead neurons are not replaced, resulting in progressive loss of neurologic functioning. As in XP, the cause of this damage in CS and the reason for the precise anatomic location of the damage is not known.

Despite similar UV-hypersensitivity to cell killing in CS as in XP, patients with CS do not have an increased frequency of cutaneous (or internal) neoplasia. The few patients with CS in the literature with multiple skin cancers also had XP (the XP-CS complex—see below). Thus cellular UV hypersensitivity does not

necessarily result in increased neoplasia. The neoplastic process may be more closely related to the DNA excision repair defects present in XP but absent in CS.

Patient Support Group

There is an educational, advocacy, and support organization for helping patients with CS and their families:

The Share and Care Cockayne Syndrome Network
Box 552
Stanleytown, VA 24168
Tel: 540-629-2369; FAX: 540-647-3728;
    e-mail: cockayne@kimbanet.com

Xeroderma Pigmentosum–Cockayne Syndrome Complex

Nine patients with CS have been found to have, in addition, clinical features of XP. These features include freckling on sun-exposed skin and cutaneous neoplasms (Fig. 157-4). Cells from these XP/CS patients have reduced DNA excision repair characteristic of XP. Clinically, these patients may be distinguished from XP patients with neurologic abnormalities by the presence of the CS features of pigmentary retinal degeneration, calcification of the basal ganglia,

FIGURE 157-4

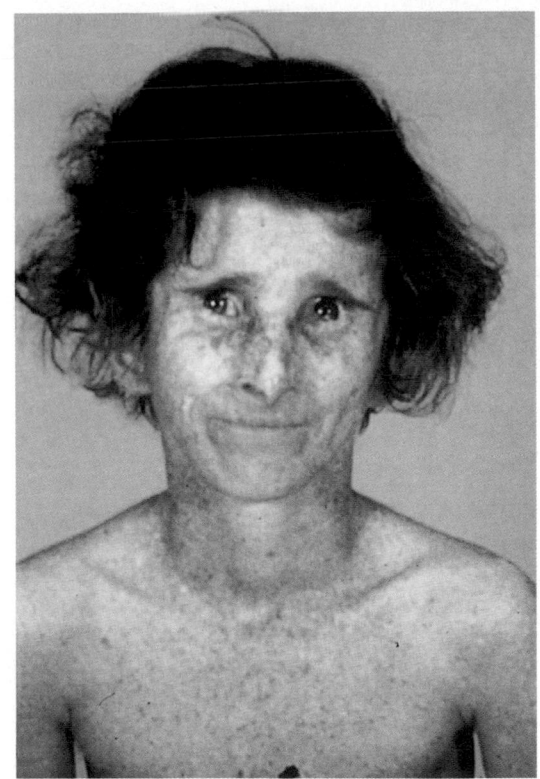
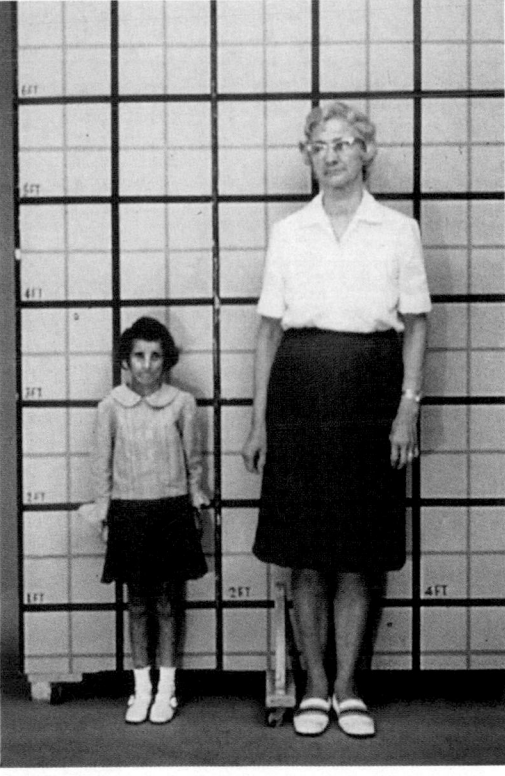

Xeroderma pigmentosum–Cockayne syndrome complex. *Left.* A 28-year-old patient (XP11BE) in XP complementation group B with cutaneous changes of xeroderma pigmentosum, including pigmentary changes and atrophy. She has the beaklike nose and loss of subcutaneous tissue typical of Cockayne syndrome. *Right.* The patient is of short stature (less than 4 ft tall). Her mother, an obligate heterozygote, is clinically normal.

normal-pressure hydrocephalus, and hyperreflexia. Cells from patients with this complex have been found to be in three different XP complementation groups: XP-B,[1,31] -D,[35,36] and -G,[39–42] implying that several different genes are implicated in this disorder (see Table 157-2).

TRICHOTHIODYSTROPHY

Patients with TTD,[72–75] also called Tay syndrome or IBIDS syndrome, have ichthyosis, sulfur-deficient brittle hair,[76] intellectual impairment, decreased fertility, and short stature. Some patients are also sun-sensitive (see Table 157-1 and Chap. 71). TTD is not associated with cancer. It is autosomal recessive, and a small number of affected families have been described in Italy[77] and elsewhere. TTD may be part of a group of similar rare disorders[75] known variously as Amish brittle hair syndrome, Sabinas brittle hair syndrome, or Pollitt syndrome; they all have low cystine content of hair and in addition may have brittle nails, cataracts, hypogonadism, microcephaly, or ataxia. Patients may have abnormal brain myelin on MRI, a finding similar to that in CS.[78,79]

Laboratory Abnormalities

Diagnosis is based on microscopic observation of broken hair shafts with characteristic light and dark bands visible in polarized light ("tiger tail"), although this may not be present at birth.[80] The sulfur content of the hairs is reduced due to low cystine content. It is not known whether other proteins also have low sulfur content. Fibroblasts from some TTD patients with sun sensitivity have been found to have similar abnormalities to fibroblasts from patients with XP in complementation groups D[37,77,81] or B,[32] whereas others form a unique TTD complementation group.[82] The cells are hypersensitive to killing by UV radiation and have reduced unscheduled DNA synthesis. Fibroblasts from TTD patients without sun sensitivity have normal UV survival and normal unscheduled DNA synthesis.[83]

BLOOM SYNDROME

Bloom syndrome (BS) is an autosomal recessive disease characterized by sun sensitivity, facial telangiectasia, short stature, and immunodeficiency[84–91] (see Table 157-1). Patients have an increased frequency of various internal neoplasms including acute leukemia and carcinomas of skin, breast, and gastrointestinal tract.[91] About 150 patients have been reported.[90] BS is most frequent among Ashkenazi Jews where the carrier rate has been estimated as 1:120.[90] Fourteen patients have been reported from Japan[87] and 10 from Germany.[92]

Clinical Features

Facial erythema and telangiectasia superficially resembling lupus erythematosus are often present within the first few weeks after birth in the malar area, nose, and around the ears.[85–87,90,91] Sun exposure accentuates these abnormalities and may induce bullae, bleeding, and crusting of the lips and eyelids. The telangiectatic lesions often involve the ears and dorsa of the hands but characteristically spare the trunk, buttocks, and lower extremities. The intensity of the facial lesions may vary from minimal telangiectasia around the lips to severe erythema of the malar area, cheeks, and nose (Fig. 157-5). Café au lait spots are common, at times accompanied by adjacent depigmented areas.

Affected children are generally born at full term but are of low birth weight, averaging approximately 2000 g. Patients are well proportioned but small. Adult height is usually under 150 cm. Patients have a long, narrow head, with a characteristic facies consisting of a narrow prominent nose, relatively hypoplastic malar areas, and a receding chin. Major skeletal abnormalities are unusual, neurologic abnormalities are uncommon, and intelligence is generally normal.

Patients with BS are predisposed to multiple severe infections of the respiratory or gastrointestinal tracts. There is a tendency for the frequency of infections to decrease with advancing age. There is immune dysfunction.[86,88] Diabetes mellitus is common. Sexual development generally appears to be normal, but male infertility due to defective sperm is the rule.[84]

Approximately 20 percent of patients with BS develop neoplasms.[91] Half occur before age 20 years. Patients with Bloom syndrome have been estimated to have a 150- to 300-fold increased frequency of development of lymphatic and nonlymphatic leukemia, lymphosarcoma, lymphoma, and carcinoma of the oral cavity and digestive system.

FIGURE 157-5

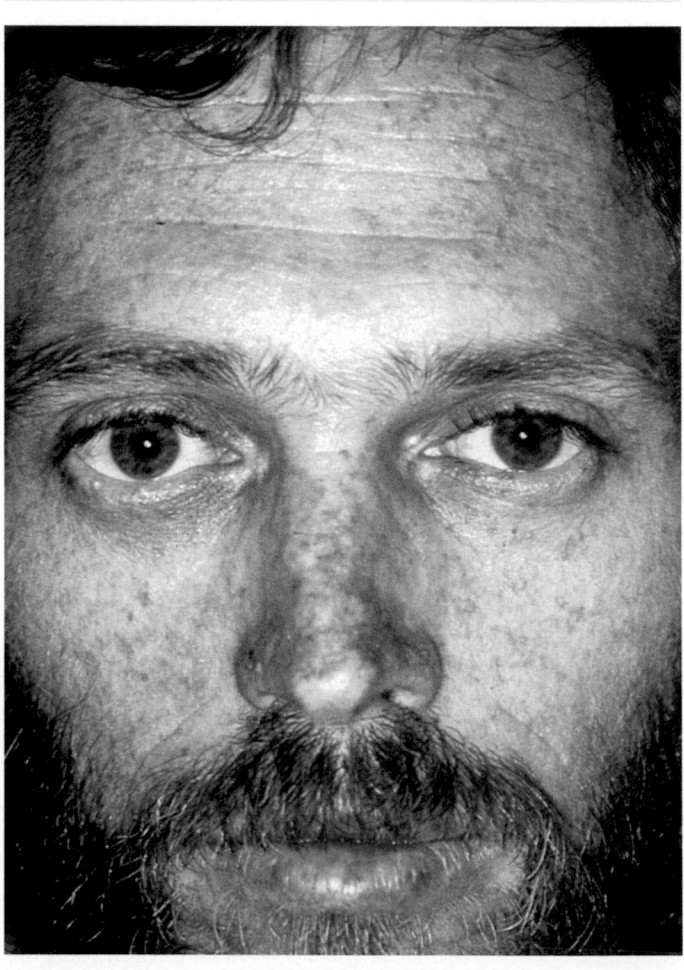

Bloom syndrome. Prominent telangiectasia in malar distribution.

Laboratory Studies

Laboratory studies of immunity have shown diminished immunoglobulin levels, reduced cellular proliferative response to mitogens, and decreased proliferation in the mixed leukocyte reaction.[86,88]

Studies of gonadal function in males revealed azoospermia and a high follicle-stimulating hormone (FSH) response to luteinizing hormone–releasing hormone (LHRH).[84] The studies indicated primary hypogonadism mainly affecting the tubular element of the testis. There was relative sparing of the androgen-secreting Leydig cells, resulting in puberty within normal limits.

CHROMOSOME ABNORMALITIES BS cells have a characteristic elevated frequency of chromosome abnormalities, accompanied by a markedly elevated rate of spontaneous sister chromatid exchanges (Chap. 37) and spontaneous hypermutability of circulating blood cells.[17,93,94] The chromosome abnormalities include a high frequency of chromosomal breakage and rearrangements. The most characteristic of these aberrations, the quadriradial configuration, was found in 0.5 percent to 14.0 percent of all dividing phytohemagglutinin-stimulated lymphocytes from patients with BS.[93] Quadriradials are believed to be the result of a rearrangement before the onset of mitosis resulting from the exchange of chromatid segments of two homologous chromosomes. The quadriradial is almost never found in cells from normal individuals. Increased sister chromatid exchanges and the presence of quadriradials are considered essential for the diagnosis of BS. BS cells show an abnormally large increase in chromosome aberrations when treated with x-rays in the G2 phase of the cell cycle.[95]

CELL KILLING AND MUTAGENESIS There are a few reports of cellular hypersensitivity to agents such as UVB, but this has not been a consistent finding.[13] BS cells were reported to have an eight- to tenfold increase in the spontaneous mutation rate and a 50- to 100-fold increase in frequency of in vivo mutations at the glycophorin A (MN blood group) locus,[96] hypermutability at a tandem-repeat locus,[97] and a 100-fold increase in hypoxanthine-guanine phosphoribosyltransferase (HGPRT) mutations.[98]

BLOOM SYNDROME GENE The defective gene in BS (BLM)[99,100] was identified on chromosome 15q26.1 as a helicase that serves to unwind DNA. An identical deletion/insertion mutation in the BLM gene was identified in several Ashkenazi Jews.[99,100] This mutation may be used for DNA diagnosis of BS patients and carriers among Ashkenazi Jews.

Clinical-Laboratory Correlation

The clinical diagnosis of BS is confirmed by the findings of increased sister chromatid exchange and increased chromosome breakage, including the presence of quadriradials.

The high frequency of neoplasia in BS may be related to the chromosome breakage or the immune deficiency, as in ataxia-telangiectasia. The observation of an increased spontaneous mutation rate in cultured cells suggests that somatic mutations may play a role in the neoplasia. Homologous chromosome exchange (as in quadriradials) or genetic recombination may be a mechanism whereby heterozygous (recessive) traits become homozygous within somatic cells and thereby result in mutation or neoplasia.[100]

FANCONI ANEMIA

Fanconi anemia (FA) is an autosomal recessive disease with progressive loss of all the formed elements of the blood (pancytopenia) (see Table 157-1). Patients may also have malformations of the heart, kidney, or limbs,[101,102] although about one-third may not have congenital malformations.[103] Internal neoplasms such as leukemia occur with increased frequency.[104] Blood cells show increased spontaneous chromosome breakage. More than 700 patients have been reported to the Fanconi Anemia Registry.[103,105]

Clinical Features

Cutaneous abnormalities are present in almost 80 percent of patients.[106,107] Hyperpigmentation is present from birth or early childhood and is diffuse and accentuated over the neck, joints, and trunk. Café au lait spots and achromic lesions are present. Following repeated blood transfusions, hyperpigmentation due to iron overloading may be present.

Hemopoietic manifestations usually have their onset before age 10 years. These consist of a hypocellular bone marrow, with progressive decrease in the number of circulating platelets, granulocytes, and erythrocytes. A late-onset form has been described.[108,109] Of 129 patients with FA, 66 percent had skeletal malformations.[101] These included aplasia or hypoplasia of the thumb, metacarpals, or radius; less frequently, hip dislocation or scoliosis were reported. About 60 percent of the patients had short stature; most had low birth weight. Malformations of other organ systems were also observed: 28 percent of the patients had renal deformities including renal aplasia and horseshoe kidney, 21 percent had ocular abnormalities including strabismus and microphthalmia and 20 percent had hypogonadism. Central nervous system abnormalities (hyperreflexia and mild mental retardation) were observed in fewer than 20 percent of the patients, and deafness due to deformities of the ear anatomy was present in fewer than 10 percent. Heart defects (patient ductus arteriosus, aortic stenosis, auricular septum defect) were observed in eight patients.

Patients with FA have a high incidence of neoplasia, particularly nonlymphatic leukemia.[102,104] In recent years, hepatomas have been noted with increasing frequency.[104]

The course is often progressively downhill, with death from infection, hemorrhage, or neoplasia. Bone marrow transplantation has been attempted in more than 200 patients.[110,111]

Laboratory Abnormalities

Clinical laboratory abnormalities reflect the bone marrow failure. There is a hypocellular marrow with thrombocytoplasia, leukopenia, and anemia.

CHROMOSOME ABNORMALITIES FA is associated with a high frequency of spontaneous chromosomal abnormalities,[94,112] including gaps, breaks, and translocations.[113] With FA cells, the chromosomal abnormalities are increased to a greater extent than with normal cells following treatment with diepoxybutane,[112,114] mitomycin C, psoralen plus UVA, or isonicotinic acid hydrazide (INH), and chromosome abnormalities persist longer than normal after damage by x-irradiation in the G2 phase of the cell cycle.[112,115]

The baseline frequency of sister chromatid exchanges is normal. However, following treatment with psoralen plus UVA, the increase in sister chromatid exchanges in FA lymphocytes is less than in normal fibroblasts.

CELL KILLING   The colony-forming ability of cultured fibroblasts is hypersensitive to inhibition by treatment with agents that form cross-links in DNA.[106] These include mitomycin C, busulfan, nitrogen mustard, psoralen plus UVA, and cisplatin.[106,116] Colony-forming ability has a normal response to killing by UV radiation.

The mechanism of the cellular hypersensitivity to DNA cross-linking agents is thought to involve defective DNA repair[106,117,118] or increased DNA damage.[119] A detailed understanding of this defect has not yet been attained[113] The FA group C protein may play a role in cross-link-induced apoptosis[120] or cell cycle arrest.[121]

FANCONI ANEMIA GENE   Eight FA complementation groups have been described.[122] The genes for FA group A[123,124] and group C[125] have been cloned. Replacement therapy with retroviral vectors is being considered.[126,127] Of nearly 400 FA patients, 15 percent had a mutation in the FA group C gene.[105] Patients with FA group C mutations in IVS4 or exon 14 appeared to have earlier onset of hematologic abnormalities and poorer survival than patients with exon 1 mutations or those in other complementation groups.[105]

HETEROZYGOTES   Cells from heterozygous carriers of FA have an abnormal chromosomal response to damage with diepoxybutane or with nitrogen mustard intermediate between the homozygotes and normal individuals. The carrier frequency of a particular base substitution mutation in the FA group C gene is greater than 1 percent among Ashkenazi Jews and thus may be used for carrier detection.[114]

PRENATAL DIAGNOSIS   The chromosomal aberrations induced by diepoxybutane have been used successfully as a test for prenatal diagnosis of FA.[128] Many more chromosome aberrations are induced by diepoxybutane in cultured amniotic fluid cells from fetuses with FA than from normal fetuses.

Clinical-Laboratory Correlation

FA is a progressive, degenerative disease with major involvement of the hematologic system. There is a high frequency of spontaneous chromosomal breakage in association with a high rate of neoplasia, particularly nonlymphatic leukemia. Immunodeficiency is not prominent. Cells are hypersensitive to killing and to induction of chromosome aberrations by DNA cross-linking agents. Two of the defective genes have recently been cloned.[123–125]

At present, incorporating these diverse observations into a unitary theory involves considerable speculation: The progressive nature of the disease is similar to XP and ataxia-telangiectasia and suggests the presence of accumulated cellular damage. "Spontaneous" chromosomal breakage may be a manifestation of this damage. FA shows more chromosome aberrations than BS, but in the latter most aberrations are between homologous chromosomes, while in FA they are between nonhomologous chromosomes. The neoplasia may be related to the chromosome breakage. There appears to be a common molecular signal for deletions in spontaneous HGPRT mutations in FA cells.[113] However, when considering two diseases with spontaneous chromosome breakage (FA and ataxia-telangiectasia)

lymphoid leukemia is absent in FA and predominant in ataxia-telangiectasia. In contrast, nonlymphoid leukemia predominates in FA and is absent in ataxia-telangiectasia. Thus other modifying factors, perhaps the immune defects in ataxia-telangiectasia, may be at work.

Registry

In order to gather information on clinical abnormalities in FA and to provide information to physicians a registry has been established. Patients with FA may be reported to

Fanconi Anemia Registry
c/o Dr. Arleen D. Auerbach
Laboratory of Human Genetics and Hematology
Rockefeller University Box 77
1230 York Ave
New York, NY 10021

DYSKERATOSIS CONGENITA

Dyskeratosis congenita, the Zinsser-Engman-Cole syndrome, is an X-linked multisystem disease with cutaneous, mucosal, ocular, gastrointestinal, and hematologic abnormalities and an increased incidence of cancer (see Table 157-1). More than 100 cases are recorded in the literature, including some female cases.[129–132] Patients have been reported from the United States, Europe, Japan,[129,133,134] China,[135] and India.

Clinical Features

The most common features are reticulated hyperpigmentation, dystrophic nails, and leukoplakia.[129,131,136–138] During the first decade of life, patients develop reticulated poikiloderma of sun-exposed areas, with hyperpigmentation and, occasionally, bullae. Nail dystrophy is present in virtually all patients beginning at approximately age 2 to 5 years. The nails initially split easily, then develop longitudinal ridging with irregular free edges. Eventually the nails become smaller, resulting in rudiments remaining. The fingernails are usually involved before the toenails. Other skin abnormalities include atrophic, wrinkled skin over the dorsum of hands and feet and hyperhidrosis and hyperkeratosis of palms and soles with disappearance of dermal ridges (absence of fingerprints).

Leukoplakia may be present in any mucosal site. The oral mucosa is the most frequent, but leukoplakia is also found in the urethra, glans penis, vagina, and rectum. Lingual hyperkeratosis may be present.[139] Mucosal surfaces such as the esophagus, urethra, and lacrimal duct may become constricted and stenotic, resulting in dysphagia, dysuria, and epiphora. Multiple dental caries and early loss of teeth are common. Approximately half of the patients have subnormal intelligence. Patients may have multiple infections, especially in the lungs.[133]

There is an increased incidence of neoplasia, particularly squamous cell carcinoma of the mouth, rectum, cervix, vagina, esophagus, and skin. A large British kindred had Hodgkin's disease and adenocarcinoma of the pancreas.[130] Several patients had multiple primary neoplasms[133]; most neoplasms occurred in the third or fourth decade. However, a gastric carcinoma was reported in an adolescent.[140] None of the patients had leukemia.

Half of the patients develop anemia secondary to bone marrow failure in the second or third decade. Leukopenia and thrombocytopenia may also be present, resulting in a hematologic picture similar to FA. Patients have been treated with bone marrow transplantation[141] or with granulocyte colony-stimulating factor and erythropoietin.[134,142]

Laboratory Studies

Immune function has been studied in only a small number of patients. Defects in immunoglobulin levels and in cell-mediated immunity were found in some patients.[133]

There have been several reports of intracranial calcifications, especially of the basal ganglia.[143]

Chromosomes are usually normal in untreated cells; however, chromosomal abnormalities have been found in fibroblasts and bone marrow cells from a few patients.[144] The leukoplakia cells may show chromosomal changes presaging malignancy.[145] Peripheral blood lymphocytes show abnormally large numbers of chromosome breaks following treatment with bleomycin[144,146] or x-rays.[147]

Clinical Laboratory Correlation

A gene for dyskeratosis has been assigned to the q28 region of the X chromosome by linkage analysis.[148,149] The gene has been cloned and motif analysis suggests nucleolar function and a role in the cell cycle.[148] There is also evidence for an autosomal form.[132,149]

Dyskeratosis congenita, like FA, is associated with anemia and increased incidence of neoplasia. However, patients with dyskeratosis congenita do not have the developmental malformations or spontaneous chromosomal breakage seen in FA. In both disorders there is a suggestion of an abnormal chromosomal response to the DNA cross-linking induced by psoralens.

As in ataxia-telangiectasia, dyskeratosis congenita has increased neoplasia and immune deficiency. However, the types of neoplasia most commonly seen in ataxia-telangiectasia, lymphoma and leukemia, have not been reported in dyskeratosis congenita. The mechanism and the extent of cellular abnormalities in dyskeratosis congenita are presently not understood.

CONCLUSION

Increased sensitivity to some physical and chemical agents has been recognized in a number of heritable diseases in recent years (see Table 157-1). Clinical hypersensitivity to sunlight or to radiotherapy has been shown to be manifested by a corresponding cellular hypersensitivity in XP, CS, TTD, and ataxia-telangiectasia. In patients with XP and CS and in some patients with TTD, the cellular hypersensitivity has been shown to be related to defective DNA repair.

Spontaneous chromosomal breakage is a feature of BS, FA, and ataxia-telangiectasia. As with most of these disorders, the molecular mechanisms involved in these chromosomal abnormalities is just beginning to be understood.

There has been remarkable progress in identifying and cloning the genes responsible for XP, CS, TTD, BS, and FA. These genes may be useful for DNA diagnosis. Understanding their functioning should provide insights into the mechanism of disease and may provide opportunities for new therapeutic approaches.

Although these heritable diseases are rare, it can be calculated that carriers of the affected genes comprise several percent of the general population. These individuals are usually free of clinical symptoms. However, epidemiologic studies have suggested that they may have an increased risk of neoplasia. In particular, heterozygous carriers of ataxia-telangiectasia may have a six-fold in-

creased risk of developing breast cancer.[150] Since they may comprise 1 percent of the general population they may thus represent 6 percent of the women with breast cancer. There is a similar suggestion that persons heterozygous for XP have an increased risk of developing skin cancer.[44] Many of these individuals may be at an increased risk from exposure to environmental agents. There are thus implications for cancer control, preventive medicine, and occupational medicine. At present, however, there is no laboratory test that can reliably detect the asymptomatic carriers of most of these disorders. However, as the defective genes are identified, molecular biologic techniques should permit carrier identification.

REFERENCES

1. Robbins JH et al: Xeroderma pigmentosum: An inherited disease with sun sensitivity, multiple cutaneous neoplasms, and abnormal DNA repair. *Ann Intern Med* **80**:221, 1974
2. Kraemer KH et al: Xeroderma pigmentosum: Cutaneous, ocular, and neurologic abnormalities in 830 published cases. *Arch Dermatol* **23**:241, 1987
3. Takebe H et al: Genetics and skin cancer of xeroderma pigmentosum in Japan. *Jpn J Cancer Res* **78**:1135, 1987
4. Cleaver JE, Kraemer KH: Xeroderma pigmentosum and Cockayne syndrome, in *The Metabolic and Molecular Bases of Inherited Disease,* 7th ed, edited by CR Scriver et al. New York, McGraw-Hill, 1995, p 4393
5. Robbins JH et al: Neurological disease in xeroderma pigmentosum. Documentation of a late onset type of the juvenile onset form. *Brain* **114**:1335, 1991
6. Kraemer KH et al: The role of sunlight and DNA repair in melanoma and nonmelanoma skin cancer: The xeroderma pigmentosum paradigm. *Arch Dermatol* **130**:1018, 1994
7. Mamada A et al: Xeroderma pigmentosum variant associated with multiple skin cancers and a lung cancer. *Dermatology* **184**:177, 1992
8. Calonge M et al: Management of corneal complications in xeroderma pigmentosum. *Cornea* **11**:173, 1992
9. Robbins JH et al: Clinically asymptomatic xeroderma pigmentosum neurological disease in an adult: Evidence for a neurodegeneration in later life caused by defective DNA repair. *Eur Neurol* **33**:188, 1993
10. Mimaki T et al: Neurological manifestations in xeroderma pigmentosum. *Ann Neurol* **20**:70, 1986
11. Mimaki T et al: EEG and CT abnormalities in xeroderma pigmentosum. *Acta Neurol Scand* **80**:136, 1989
12. Kanda T et al: Peripheral neuropathy in xeroderma pigmentosum. *Brain* **113**:1025, 1990
13. Smith PJ, Paterson MC: Lethality and the induction and repair of DNA damage in far, mid or near UV-irradiated human fibroblasts: Comparison of effects in normal, xeroderma pigmentosum and Bloom's syndrome cells. *Photochem Photobiol* **36**:333, 1982
14. Friedberg EC et al: *DNA Repair and Mutagenesis.* Washington, DC, ASM Press, 1995, p 698
15. Khan SG et al: Xeroderma pigmentosum with hypoglycinemia and intron expansion—a new syndrome? *J Invest Dermatol* **108**:596, 1997
16. Gözükara EM et al: The human DNA repair gene, *ERCC2* (XPD), corrects ultraviolet hypersensitivity and ultraviolet hypermutability of a shuttle vector replicated in xeroderma pigmentosum group D cells. *Cancer Res* **54**:3837, 1994
17. Mamada A et al: Different sensitivities to ultraviolet light–induced cytotoxicity and sister chromatid exchanges in xeroderma pigmentosum and Bloom's syndrome fibroblasts. *Photodermatology* **6**:124, 1989
18. Cleaver JE: Defective repair replication of DNA in xeroderma pigmentosum. *Nature* **218**:652, 1968
19. Boyer JC et al: Defective postreplication repair in xeroderma pigmentosum variant fibroblasts. *Cancer Res* **50**:2593, 1990
20. Ramsay CA et al: Prenatal diagnosis of xeroderma pigmentosum. Report of the first successful case. *Lancet* **2**:1109, 1974
21. Kore-eda S et al: A case of xeroderma pigmentosum group A diagnosed with a polymerase chain reaction (PCR) technique. Usefulness

of PCR in the detection of point mutation in a patient with a hereditary disease. *Arch Dermatol* **128**:971, 1992

22. Mello JA et al: DNA adducts of *cis*-diaminedichloroplatinum(II) and its trans isomer inhibit RNA polymerase II differentially *in vivo*. *Biochemistry* **34**:14783, 1995

23. Atabay K et al: Facial resurfacing in xeroderma pigmentosum with monoblock full-thickness skin graft. *Plast Reconstr Surg* **87**:1121, 1991

24. Leal-Khouri S et al: Management of a young patient with xeroderma pigmentosum. *Pediatr Dermatol* **11**:72, 1994

25. Nelson BR et al: The role of dermabrasion and chemical peels in the treatment of patients with xeroderma pigmentosum. *J Am Acad Dermatol* **32**:623, 1995

26. DiGiovanna JJ et al: Spinal cord astrocytoma in a patient with xeroderma pigmentosum: 9-year survival with radiation and isotretinoin therapy. *J Cutan Med Surg* **2**:153, 1998

27. Arlett CF et al: Studies of a new case of xeroderma pigmentosum (XP3BR) from complementation group G with cellular sensitivity to ionizing radiation. *Carcinogenesis* **1**:745, 1980

28. Kraemer KH et al: Prevention of skin cancer in xeroderma pigmentosum with the use of oral isotretinoin. *N Engl J Med* **318**:1633, 1988

29. Yarosh DB, Klein J: DNA repair enzymes in prevention of photocarcinogenesis. *Photochem Photobiol* **63**:445, 1996

30. Nishigori C et al: Gene alterations and clinical characteristics of xeroderma pigmentosum group A patients in Japan. *Arch Dermatol* **130**:191, 1994

31. Scott RJ et al: Xeroderma pigmentosum–Cockayne syndrome complex in two patients: Absence of skin tumors despite severe deficiency of DNA excision repair. *J Am Acad Dermatol* **29**(suppl):883, 1993

32. Weeda G et al: A mutation in the *XPB/ERCC3* DNA repair transcription gene, associated with trichothiodystrophy. *Am J Hum Genet* **60**:320, 1997

33. Thielmann HW et al: Clinical symptoms and DNA repair characteristics of xeroderma pigmentosum patients from Germany. *Cancer Res* **51**:3456, 1991

34. Kondo S et al: Late onset of skin cancers in 2 xeroderma pigmentosum group F siblings and a review of 30 Japanese xeroderma pigmentosum patients in groups D, E and F. *Photodermatology* **6**:89, 1989

35. Vermeulen W et al: Xeroderma pigmentosum complementation group H falls into complementation group D. *Mutat Res* **255**:201, 1991

36. Broughton BC et al: Molecular and cellular analysis of the DNA repair defect in a patient in xeroderma pigmentosum complementation group D who has the clinical features of xeroderma pigmentosum and Cockayne syndrome. *Am J Hum Genet* **56**:167, 1995

37. Taylor EM et al: Xeroderma pigmentosum and trichothiodystrophy are associated with different mutations in the XPD (ERCC2) repair/transcription gene. *Proc Natl Acad Sci USA* **94**:8658, 1997

38. Yamamura K et al: Clinical and photobiological characteristics of xeroderma pigmentosum complementation group F: A review of cases from Japan. *Br J Dermatol* **121**:471, 1989

39. Jaeken J et al: Clinical and biochemical studies in three patients with severe early infantile Cockayne syndrome. *Hum Genet* **83**:339, 1989

40. Vermeulen W et al: Xeroderma pigmentosum complementation group G associated with Cockayne syndrome. *Am J Hum Genet* **53**:185, 1993

41. Hamel BCK et al: Xeroderma pigmentosum–Cockayne syndrome complex: A further case. *J Med Genet* **33**:607, 1996

42. Moriwaki SI et al: DNA repair and ultraviolet mutagenesis in cells from a new patient with xeroderma pigmentosum group G and Cockayne syndrome resemble xeroderma pigmentosum cells. *J Invest Dermatol* **107**:647, 1996

43. Somos S et al: Xeroderma pigmentosum variant or pigmented xerodermoid. *Anticancer Res* **17**:753, 1997

44. Heim RA et al: Heterozygous manifestations in four autosomal recessive human cancer-prone syndromes: Ataxia telangiectasia, xeroderma pigmentosum, Fanconi anemia, and Bloom syndrome. *Mutat Res* **284**:25, 1992

45. Parshad R et al: Carrier detection in xeroderma pigmentosum. *J Clin Invest* **85**:135, 1990

46. Moriwaki S et al: Absence of DNA repair deficiency in the confirmed heterozygotes of xeroderma pigmentosum group A. *J Invest Dermatol* **101**:69, 1993

47. Cantani A et al: Rare syndromes. I. Cockayne syndrome: A review of the 129 cases so far reported in the literature. *Riv Eur Sci Med Farmacol* **9**:9, 1987

48. Özdirim E et al: Cockayne syndrome: Review of 25 cases. *Pediatr Neurol* **15**:312, 1996

49. Nance MA, Berry SA: Cockayne syndrome: Review of 140 cases. *Am J Med Genet* **42**:68, 1992

50. Norris PG et al: Abnormal erythemal response and elevated T lymphocyte HRPT mutant frequency in Cockayne's syndrome. *Br J Dermatol* **124**:453, 1991

51. Traboulsi EI et al: Ocular findings in Cockayne syndrome. *Am J Ophthalmol* **114**:579, 1992

52. Patton MA et al: Early onset Cockayne's syndrome: Case reports with neuropathological and fibroblast studies. *J Med Genet* **26**:154, 1989

53. Kennedy RM et al: Cockayne syndrome: An atypical case. *Neurology* **30**:1268, 1980

54. Fryns JP et al: Apparent late-onset Cockayne syndrome and interstitial deletion of the long arm of chromosome 10 (del(10)(q11.23q21.2)). *Am J Med Genet* **40**:343, 1991

55. Del Bigio MR et al: Neuropathological findings in eight children with cerebro-oculo-facio-skeletal (COFS) syndrome. *J Neuropathol Exp Neurol* **56**:1147, 1997

56. Talwar D, Smith SA: CAMFAK syndrome: A demyelinating inherited disease similar to Cockayne syndrome. *Am J Med Genet* **34**:194, 1989

57. Brumback RA et al: Normal pressure hydrocephalus. Recognition and relationship to neurological abnormalities in Cockayne's syndrome. *Arch Neurol* **35**:337, 1978

58. Vos A et al: The neuropathy of Cockayne syndrome. *Acta Neuropathol (Berl)* **61**:153, 1983

59. Schenone A et al: Peripheral neuropathy in Cockayne syndrome. *Ital J Neurol Sci* **7**:447, 1986

60. Demaerel P et al: Cranial CT and MRI in diseases with DNA repair defects. *Neuroradiology* **34**:117, 1992

61. Boltshauser E et al: MRI in Cockayne syndrome type I. *Neuroradiology* **31**:276, 1989

62. Marshall RR et al: Increased sensitivity of cell strains from Cockayne's syndrome to sister-chromatid-exchange induction and cell killing by UV light. *Mutat Res* **69**:107, 1980

63. Parris CN, Kraemer KH: Ultraviolet-induced mutations in Cockayne syndrome cells are primarily caused by cyclobutane dimer photoproducts while repair of other photoproducts is normal. *Proc Natl Acad Sci USA* **90**:7260, 1993

64. Hayashi M et al: A neuropathological study of early onset Cockayne syndrome with chromosomal anomaly 47XXX. *Brain Dev* **14**:63, 1992

65. Seguin LR et al: Ultraviolet light-induced chromosomal aberrations in cultured cells from Cockayne syndrome and complementation group C xeroderma pigmentosum patients: Lack of correlation with cancer susceptibility. *Am J Hum Genet* **42**:468, 1988

66. Price FM et al: Radiation-induced chromatid aberrations in Cockayne syndrome and xeroderma pigmentosum group C fibroblasts in relation to cancer predisposition. *Cancer Genet Cytogenet* **57**:1, 1991

67. Venema J et al: The genetic defect in Cockayne syndrome is associated with a defect in repair of UV-induced DNA damage in transcriptionally active DNA. *Proc Natl Acad Sci USA* **87**:4707, 1990

68. Mayne LV, Lehmann AR: Failure of RNA synthesis to recover after UV irradiation: An early defect in cells from individuals with Cockayne's syndrome and xeroderma pigmentosum. *Cancer Res* **42**:1473, 1982

69. Henning KA et al: The Cockayne syndrome group A gene encodes a WD repeat protein that interacts with CSB protein and a subunit of RNA polymerase II TFIIH. *Cell* **82**:555, 1995

70. Gool AJ et al: The Cockayne syndrome B protein, involved in transcription-coupled DNA repair, resides in an RNA polymerase II–containing complex. *EMBO J* **16**:5955, 1997

71. Lehmann AR et al: Prenatal diagnosis of Cockayne's syndrome. *Lancet* **1**:486, 1985

72. Price VH et al: Trichothiodystrophy: Sulfur-deficient brittle hair as a marker for a neuroectodermal symptom complex. *Arch Dermatol* **116**:1375, 1980

73. Itin PH, Pittelkow MR: Trichothiodystrophy: Review of sulfur-deficient brittle hair syndromes and association with the ectodermal dysplasias. *J Am Acad Dermatol* **22**:705, 1990

74. McCuaig C et al: Trichothiodystrophy associated with photosensitivity, gonadal failure, and striking osteosclerosis. *J Am Acad Dermatol* **28**:820, 1993

75. Tolmie JL et al: Syndromes associated with trichothiodystrophy. *Clin Dysmorphol* **3**:1, 1994

76. Kleijer WJ et al: Intermittent hair loss in a child with PIBI(D)S syndrome and trichothiodystrophy with defective DNA repair–xeroderma pigmentosum group D. *Am J Med Genet* **52**:227, 1994

77. Mondello C et al: Molecular analysis of the *XP-D* gene in Italian families with patients affected by trichothiodystrophy and xeroderma pigmentosum group D. *Mutat Res DNA Repair* **314**:159, 1994

78. Chen E et al: Trichothiodystrophy: Clinical spectrum, central nervous system imaging, and biochemical characterization of two siblings. *J Invest Dermatol* **103**(suppl):154S, 1994

79. Ostergaard JR, Christensen T: The central nervous system in Tay syndrome. *Neuropediatrics* **27**:326, 1996

80. Brusasco A et al: The typical "tiger tail" pattern of the hair shaft in trichothiodystrophy may not be evident at birth. *Arch Dermatol* **133**:249, 1997

81. Takayama K et al: Defects in the DNA repair and transcription gene ERCC2(XPD) in trichothiodystrophy. *Am J Hum Genet* **58**:263, 1996

82. Stefanini M et al: A new nucleotide-excision-repair gene associated with the disorder trichothiodystrophy. *Am J Hum Genet* **53**:817, 1993

83. Broughton BC et al: Relationship between pyrimidine dimers, 6-4 photoproducts, repair synthesis and cell survival: Studies using cells from patients with trichothiodystrophy. *Mutat Res* **235**:33, 1990

84. Kauli R et al: Gonadal function in Bloom's syndrome. *Clin Endocrinol (Oxf)* **6**:285, 1977

85. Gretzula JC et al: Bloom's syndrome. *J Am Acad Dermatol* **17**:479, 1987

86. Van Kerckhove CW et al: Bloom's syndrome. Clinical features and immunologic abnormalities of four patients. *Am J Dis Child* **142**:1089, 1988

87. German J, Takebe H: Bloom's syndrome. XIV. The disorder in Japan. *Clin Genet* **35**:93, 1989

88. Weemaes CM et al: Immunological studies in Bloom's syndrome. A follow-up report. *Ann Genet* **34**:201, 1991

89. Kondo N et al: Long-term study of the immunodeficiency of Bloom's syndrome. *Acta Paediatr* **81**:86, 1992

90. German J: Bloom syndrome: A mendelian prototype of somatic mutational disease. *Medicine (Baltimore)* **72**:393, 1993

91. German J. Bloom's syndrome.20. The first 100 cancers. *Cancer Genet Cytogenet* **93**:100, 1997

92. Passarge E: Bloom's syndrome: The German experience. *Ann Genet* **34**:179, 1991

93. Chaganti RS et al: A manyfold increase in sister chromatid exchanges in Bloom's syndrome lymphocytes. *Proc Natl Acad Sci USA* **71**:4508, 1974

94. Sakamoto Hojo ET et al: Spontaneous chromosomal aberrations in Fanconi anaemia, ataxia-telangiectasia fibroblast and Bloom's syndrome lymphoblastoid cell lines as detected by conventional cytogenetic analysis and fluorescence in situ hybridisation (FISH) technique. *Mutat Res Environ Mutagen Rel Subj* **334**:59, 1995

95. Sanford KK et al: Factors affecting and significance of G2 chromatin radiosensitivity in predisposition to cancer. *Int J Radiat Biol* **55**:963, 1989

96. Langlois RG et al: Evidence for increased in vivo mutation and somatic recombination in Bloom's syndrome. *Proc Natl Acad Sci USA* **86**:670, 1989

97. Groden J, German J: Bloom's syndrome. XVIII. Hypermutability at a tandem-repeat locus. *Hum Genet* **90**:360, 1992

98. Tachibana A et al: Large deletions at the *HPRT* locus associated with the mutator phenotype in a Bloom's syndrome lymphoblastoid cell line. *Mol Carcinog* **17**:41, 1996

99. Ellis NA et al: The Bloom's syndrome gene product is homologous to RecQ helicases. *Cell* **83**:655, 1995

100. Ellis NA, German J: Molecular genetics of Bloom's syndrome. *Hum Mol Genet* **5**:1457, 1996

101. Gmyrek D, Syllm-Rapoport I: Fanconi's anemia: Analysis of 129 described cases. *Z Kinderheilkd* **91**:294, 1964

102. Auerbach AD, Allen RG: Leukemia and preleukemia in Fanconi anemia patients. A review of the literature and report of the International Fanconi Anemia Registry. *Cancer Genet Cytogenet* **51**:1, 1991

103. Giampietro PF et al: Diagnosis of Fanconi anemia in patients without congenital malformations: An International Fanconi Anemia Registry study. *Am J Med Genet* **68**:58, 1997

104. Alter BP: Fanconi's anemia and malignancies. *Am J Hematol* **53**:99, 1996

105. Gillio AP et al: Phenotypic consequences of mutations in the Fanconi anemia *FAC* gene: An International Fanconi Anemia Registry Study. *Blood* **90**:105, 1997

106. Fujiwara Y et al: Heritable disorders of DNA repair: Xeroderma pigmentosum and Fanconi's anemia. *Curr Probl Dermatol* **17**:182, 1987

107. Auerbach AD: Fanconi anemia. *Dermatol Clin* **13**:41, 1995

108. Zatterale A et al: Identification and treatment of late onset Fanconi's anemia. *Haematologica* **80**:535, 1995

109. Kwee ML et al: An atypical case of Fanconi anemia in elderly sibs. *Am J Med Genet* **68**:362, 1997

110. Gluckman E et al: Bone marrow transplantation for Fanconi anemia. *Blood* **86**:2856, 1995

111. Zanis-Neto J et al: Bone marrow transplantation for patients with Fanconi anemia: A study of 24 cases from a single institution. *Bone Marrow Transplant* **15**:293, 1995

112. Auerbach AD et al: International Fanconi Anemia Registry: Relation of clinical symptoms to diepoxybutane sensitivity. *Blood* **73**:391, 1989

113. Laquerbe A et al: The molecular mechanism underlying formation of deletions in Fanconi anemia cells may involve a site-specific recombination. *Proc Natl Acad Sci USA* **92**:831, 1995

114. Seyschab H et al: Comparative evaluation of diepoxybutane sensitivity and cell cycle blockage in the diagnosis of Fanconi anemia. *Blood* **85**:2233, 1995

115. Parshad R et al: Chromatid damage after G2 phase x-irradiation of cells from cancer-prone individuals implicates deficiency in DNA repair. *Proc Natl Acad Sci USA* **80**:5612, 1983

116. Dijt FJ et al: Formation and repair of cisplatin-induced adducts to DNA in cultured normal and repair-deficient human fibroblasts. *Cancer Res* **48**:6058, 1988

117. Sun Y, Moses RE: Reactivation of psoralen-reacted plasmid DNA in Fanconi anemia, xeroderma pigmentosum, and normal human fibroblast cells. *Somat Cell Mol Genet* **17**:229, 1991

118. Zhen W et al: Deficient gene specific repair of cisplatin-induced lesions in xeroderma pigmentosum and Fanconi's anemia cell lines. *Carcinogenesis* **14**:919, 1993

119. Youssoufian H: Cytoplasmic localization of FAC is essential for the correction of a prerepair defect in Fanconi anemia group C cells. *J Clin Invest* **97**:2003, 1996

120. Marathi UK et al: The Fanconi anemia complementation group C protein corrects DNA interstrand cross-link-specific apoptosis in HSC536N cells. *Blood* **88**:2298, 1996

121. Kruyt FAE et al: Involvement of the Fanconi's anemia protein FAC in a pathway that signals to the cyclin B/cdc2 kinase. *Cancer Res* **57**:2244, 1997

122. Joenje H et al: Evidence for at least eight Fanconi anemia genes. *Am J Hum Genet* **61**:940, 1997

123. Ten Foe JRL et al: Expression cloning of a cDNA for the major Fanconi anaemia gene, *FAA*. *Nat Genet* **14**:320, 1996

124. Ianzano L et al: The genomic organization of the Fanconi anemia group A (FAA) gene. *Genomics* **41**:309, 1997

125. Strathdee CA et al: Cloning of cDNAs for Fanconi's anaemia by functional complementation [published erratum appears in *Nature*, 1992, Jul 30; **358**(6385):434]. *Nature* **356**:763, 1992

126. Fu KL et al: Functional correction of Fanconi anemia group A hematopoietic cells by retroviral gene transfer. *Blood* **90**:3296, 1997

127. Liu JM et al: Retroviral mediated gene transfer of the Fanconi anemia complementation group C gene to hematopoietic progenitors of group C patients. *Hum Gene Ther* **8**:1715, 1997

128. Auerbach AD et al: Fanconi anemia: Prenatal diagnosis in 30 fetuses at risk. *Pediatrics* **76**:794, 1985

129. Sirinavin C, Trowbridge AA: Dyskeratosis congenita: Clinical features and genetic aspects. Report of a family and review of the literature. *J Med Genet* **12**:339, 1975

130. Connor JM, Teague RH: Dyskeratosis congenita. Report of a large kindred. *Br J Dermatol* **105**:321, 1981

131. Davidson HR, Connor JM: Dyskeratosis congenita. *J Med Genet* **25**:843, 1988

132. Pai GS et al: Etiologic heterogeneity in dyskeratosis congenita (see comments). *Am J Med Genet* **32**:63, 1989

133. Kawaguchi K et al: Dyskeratosis congenita (Zinsser-Cole-Engman syndrome). An autopsy case presenting with rectal carcinoma, noncirrhotic portal hypertension, and *Pneumocystis carinii* pneumonia. *Virchows Arch A Pathol Anat Histopathol* **417**:247, 1990

134. Yel L et al: Dyskeratosis congenita: Unusual onset with isolated neutropenia at an early age. *Acta Paediatr Jpn* **38**:288, 1996

135. Ho CL, Chong LY: Dyskeratosis congenita in an ethnic Chinese girl. *Int J Dermatol* **35**:659, 1996
136. Drachtman RA, Alter BP: Dyskeratosis congenita: Clinical and genetic heterogeneity. Report of a new case and review of the literature. *Am J Pediatr Hematol Oncol* **14**:297, 1992
137. Drachtman RA, Alter BP: Dyskeratosis congenita. *Dermatol Clin* **13**:33, 1995
138. Limmer RL et al: Abnormal nails in a patient with severe anemia. Dyskeratosis congenita. *Arch Dermatol* **133**:97, 1997
139. McKay GS et al: Lingual hyperkeratosis in dyskeratosis congenita: Ultrastructural findings. *J Oral Pathol Med* **20**:196, 1991
140. Chatura KR et al: Case report: Gastric carcinoma as a complication of dyskeratosis congenita in an adolescent boy. *Dig Dis Sci* **41**:2340, 1996
141. Langston AA et al: Allogeneic marrow transplantation for aplastic anaemia associated with dyskeratosis congenita. *Br J Haematol* **92**:758, 1996
142. Alter BP et al: Treatment of dyskeratosis congenita with granulocyte colony-stimulating factor and erythropoietin. *Br J Haematol* **97**:309, 1997

143. Derex L et al: [Striato-pallido-dentate calcifications and acquired facial atrophy]. *Rev Neurol (Paris)* **151**:559, 1995
144. Dokal I et al: Dyskeratosis congenita fibroblasts are abnormal and have unbalanced chromosomal rearrangements. *Blood* **80**:3090, 1992
145. Kehrer H, Krone W: Chromosome abnormalities in cell cultures derived from the leukoplakia of a female patient with dyskeratosis congenita. *Am J Med Genet* **42**:217, 1992
146. Ning Y et al: Heterozygote detection through bleomycin-induced G2 chromatid breakage in dyskeratosis congenita families. *Cancer Genet Cytogenet* **60**:31, 1992
147. DeBauche DM et al: Enhanced G2 chromatid radiosensitivity in dyskeratosis congenita fibroblasts. *Am J Hum Genet* **46**:350, 1990
148. Heiss NS et al: X-linked dyskeratosis congenita is caused by mutations in a highly conserved gene with putative nucleolar functions. *Nat Genet* **19**:32, 1998
149. Devriendt K et al: Skewed X-chromosome inactivation in female carriers of dyskeratosis congenita. *Am J Hum Genet* **60**:581, 1997
150. Athma P et al: Molecular genotyping shows that ataxia-telangiectasia heterozygotes are predisposed to breast cancer. *Cancer Genet Cytogenet* **92**:130, 1996

CHAPTER 158

Ervin H. Epstein, Jr.

Basal Cell Nevus Syndrome

The basal cell nevus syndrome (BCNS) (nevoid basal cell carcinoma syndrome, Gorlin syndrome, McKusick Mendelian Inheritance in Man 109400) is a rare autosomal dominant abnormality with a panoply of phenotypic abnormalities that can be divided into developmental anomalies and postnatal tumors, especially basal cell carcinomas (BCCs). Although individual aspects had been reported previously, their syndromic association was appreciated widely only in the late 1950s.[1,2] As in many dominant conditions, new mutations are common, and so patients frequently have no affected ancestors or siblings.

ETIOLOGY AND PATHOGENESIS

Genetic Abnormality

The BCNS is caused by mutations in the *PATCHED (PTCH)* gene.[3,4] This gene is the human homologue of the *Drosophila* patched (ptc) gene, which is essential for the establishment of normal body and limb patterning in the developing fly embryo. Efforts to identify this gene began in the mid-1980s when the following

became apparent: (1) the appearance of BCCs in small numbers at an older age in sporadic cases and in larger numbers at a younger age in patients with BCNS is reminiscent of the sporadic and hereditary development of retinoblastoma, (2) BCCs therefore follows the Knudson "two-hit" model for familial cancers,[5] and (3) a tumor suppressor gene important in the common sporadic BCCs might be identified by study of the rare BCNS. Numerous laboratories participated in efforts to identify the BCNS gene, and its cloning allowed verification of the prediction that the same gene is mutated in BCCs—by two somatic "hits" in the same cell in sporadic cases or by one somatic hit plus the inheritance of one defective allele in BCNS patients. Mutations in *PTCH* have been identified in other sporadic tumors as well, including those known to be present in greater than expected numbers in BCNS patients (e.g., medulloblastomas and meningiomas) and those not found in increased incidence in BCNS patients (e.g., breast cancers). Screening has identified *PTCH* somatic mutations in a minority of BCCs and constitutional mutations in a minority of BCNS patients, but it is not yet clear whether this relatively low "yield" is due simply to the relative insensitivity of the methods used thus far. The *PTCH* gene resides on chromosome 9q, and no family with BCNS has been reported in which the causative gene does not map to this site.

PTCH Function

The PTCH protein's single known function is as a participant in the "hedgehog" signaling pathway. Genetic evidence suggests that PTCH protein functions to inhibit this signaling pathway and that the extracellular ligand hedgehog functions to alleviate this inhibition. That alleviation allows signaling by the 7-transmembrane protein SMOOTHENED (SMO), and members of the intracellular pathway, at least in *Drosophila,* include costal 2, fused, protein kinase A, and the transcription factor cubitis interruptus (vertebrate homologues of which are the *GLI* genes, so named because of *GLI*'s initial identification as a gene upregulated in some cases of glioblastoma multiforme). Activation of the hedgehog signaling pathway leads to upregulation of expression of several genes, including members of the transforming growth factor β and the *wingless/wnt* families of signaling molecules, as well as of *PTCH* itself. Thus for *PTCH,* the hedgehog signaling pathway appears to form a negative feedback loop: "insufficient" PTCH protein function activates the pathway and thus stimulates the production of more PTCH mRNA and protein, which in turn blocks the pathway.

In addition to the finding of homozygous *PTCH* mutations in tumors, heterozygous apparently activating mutations in the genes encoding sonic hedgehog (the most widely distributed of the three vertebrate hedgehog molecules) and SMO have also been identified in BCCs. Thus in BCCs, mutations may occur in any of the three peripheral components of the hedgehog signaling pathway; hence it appears that it is activation of the pathway rather than mutation of a specific gene that is important for BCC development.

Since activation of the pathway causes increased *PTCH* gene expression, the observation of consistently increased *PTCH* mRNA in BCCs argues that this activation uniformly accompanies transformation of keratinocytes into BCCs and hence is of fundamental importance in their initiation and/or maintenance. Further support for this view comes from the production of BCC-like proliferations in experimental models in which the keratinocyte hedgehog signaling pathway is activated experimentally.

PTCH is normally expressed not only postnatally but also, in vertebrates as well as in insects, during development. Experimental models with abnormalities of the hedgehog signaling pathway cause significant developmental anomalies in mice and flies. The resemblance of some of these anomalies to those characteristic of the BCNS gives evidence that activation of the hedgehog signaling pathway is a sufficient explanation for the developmental anomalies of the BCNS, even if the precise pathogenic mechanism has yet to be elucidated.

CLINICAL FEATURES

Patients with BCNS sustain multiple abnormalities, none of which are unique to this syndrome. The three abnormalities traditionally considered to be most characteristic of the syndrome are BCCs, pits of the palms and soles, and cysts of the jaw.

BCCs in patients with the BCNS cannot be distinguished individually from those in sporadic cases, which is not surprising in view of the similar pathogenesis in familial and sporadic cases. What is distinguishing is their appearance in large numbers starting at an early age. They may be banal-appearing and confused grossly with nevocytic nevi—hence the name *basal cell nevus.* They may also have the more characteristic translucent, papulonodular appearance and may invade locally and even, rarely, metastasize and cause the patient's death. Although the ratio of sun-protected to sun-

exposed BCCs may be higher in BCNS than in sporadic cases, sunlight clearly accelerates BCC formation in BCNS patients, and darkly pigmented BCNS patients may have few to no BCCs (see Fig. 81-6A).

Palmoplantar pits are small defects in the stratum corneum and may be pink or, if dirt has accumulated, dark in color (see Fig. 81-6B). Jaw cysts are often the first detectable abnormality, and they may be asymptomatic and therefore diagnosed only radiologically. However, they also may erode enough bone to cause pain, swelling, and loss of teeth (see Chap. 114 and Fig. 114-34).

Tissue overgrowth, which also is a feature of hedgehog signaling pathway activation in *Drosophila,* is often manifested by an overall body size larger than that of other family members; limbs may be particularly long, giving a Marfanoid appearance, and a large head circumference (at least in probands) and frontal bossing are often described.

Table 158-1 lists the phenotypic abnormalities that have been reported often enough that they are probably true aspects of the syndrome. Variation in clinical severity is typical even within a single kindred, and this heterogeneity likely is due both to environmental differences (e.g., exposure to ultraviolet and ionizing radiation) and to genetic background differences.

Pathology

Histologic examination cannot differentiate abnormalities that arise sporadically from those that arise in the context of BCNS.

Diagnosis

Since the individual abnormalities are not unique to BCNS patients, it is possible to diagnose the BCNS only when multiple, typical defects are present. The severity of abnormalities may differ markedly among members of a single kindred, and diagnostic certainty may be difficult for individuals even if they are known to belong to a BCNS kindred.

Generally, the diagnosis is suggested to the dermatologist in a patient with multiple BCCs arising at an unexpectedly early age and in unexpectedly large numbers. Further evaluation should include the following: (1) questions about whether other family members have had abnormalities consistent with the BCNS (although perhaps 25 to 30 percent of patients with BCNS have no affected ancestors) and whether the patient is taller and heavier than his or her relatives; (2) examination for palmoplantar pits and skin cysts, and assessment of body and head size; and (3) radiologic evaluation for jaw cysts, calcification of the falx (which occurs in nearly all adults with BCNS), and abnormalities of the ribs, spine, and phalanges (flame-shaped lucencies), each of which are present in one-third to one-half of BCNS patients[6–8] (Fig. 158-1). Identification of *PTCH* gene mutations should become the "gold standard" for diagnosis, but for now it is only a research, not a clinical, tool.

DIFFERENTIAL DIAGNOSIS

Several very rare syndromes that include the development of multiple BCCs have been described—the Bazex-Dupré-Christol syndrome; the Rombo syndrome; and a family with BCCs, milia, and coarse, sparse hair.[9–11] Hair abnormalities are present in all three

three syndromes are uncertain, but patients with the BCNS have normal hair, and all three syndromes seem quite different from the BCNS.

Patients with chronic arsenic ingestion may have multiple BCCs; their dyschromia and lack of other phenotypic abnormalities differentiate them from BCNS patients. Patients with xeroderma pigmentosa develop multiple BCCs but are readily differentiated from BCNS patient by their severe photosensitivity and other phenotypic abnormalities. Finally, patients with a marked propensity to develop multiple BCCs, sometimes sporadically and rarely following therapeutic irradiation (e.g., for Hodgkins disease), occasionally produce diagnostic confusion, and it is not known whether their defect is related to the hedgehog pathway, to DNA repair, to an unknown toxin, or to undescribed mechanisms.

TABLE 158-1

Diagnostic Findings in Adults with Basal Cell Nevus Syndrome

DEVELOPMENTAL	HYPER/NEOPLASTIC
FREQUENCY ≥ 50 PERCENT	
Enlarged occipitofrontal circumference (macrocephaly, frontoparietal bossing, in index cases only?)	Multiple basal cell carcinomas
High-arched palate	Odontogenic keratocysts of jaws
Palmar or plantar pits	Epidermal cysts of skin
Rib anomalies (e.g., splayed, fused, partially missing, bifid)	
Spina bifida occulta of cervical or thoracic vertebrae	
Calcified falx cerebri	
Calcified diaphragma sellae (bridged sella, fused clinoids)	
Hyperpneumatization of paranasal sinuses	
FREQUENCY 15 TO 49 PERCENT	
Calcification of tentorium cerebelli and petroclinoid ligament	Calcified ovarian fibromas
Short fourth metacarpals	Pseudocystic lytic lesion of bones (hamartomas)
Kyphoscoliosis or other vertebral anomalies	
Lumbarization of sacrum	
Narrow sloping shoulders	
Prognathism	
Pectus excavatum or carinatum	
Strabismus (exotropia)	
FREQUENCY < 14 PERCENT BUT NOT RANDOM	
Inguinal hernia (?)	Medulloblastoma
True ocular hypertelorism	Meningioma
Ovarian fibrosarcoma	Lymphomesenteric cyst
Marfanoid build	Cardiac fibroma
Anosmia	Fetal rhabdomyoma
Agenesis of corpus callosum	
Cyst of septum pellucidum	
Cleft lip and/or palate	
Low-pitched female voice	
Polydactyly, postaxial in hands or feet	
Sprengel deformity of scapula	
Syndactyly	
Congenital cataract, glaucoma, coloboma of iris, retina, optic nerve, medullated retinal nerve fibers	
Subcutaneous calcifications of skin (possibly underestimated frequency)	
Minor kidney malformations	
Hypogonadism in male subjects	
Mental retardation	

SOURCE: Adapted from Gorlin,[2] with permission.

TREATMENT

Therapy must be directed at the individual lesions as they arise, and the most important aspect of management is frequent examination and early treatment of small tumors. Clinicians caring for BCNS patients generally become confident enough of their clinical acumen that they treat tiny BCCs, e.g., with cryotherapy, without histopathologic confirmation, since obtaining tissue for the latter produces more scarring. Since the key is to convince the patient to accept frequent treatments, minimization of discomfort and of scarring is a major concern.

X-irradiation of BCCs should be avoided if possible, since enhanced radiation-induced carcinogenesis (e.g., in the skin of the portals of irradiation of childhood medulloblastomas) is characteristic of BCNS (Fig. 158-2).

Genetic counseling is appropriate—50 percent of children of affected individuals are expected to develop the BCNS, and prenatal diagnosis is potentially achievable for many families, if they desire this option.

syndromes; a finding of interest in view of the often repeated suggestion that BCCs arise from hair follicles rather than from interfollicular epidermis. The exact nosologic relationships among these

FIGURE 158-1

CHAPTER 158
Basal Cell Nevus Syndrome

1865

FIGURE 158-2

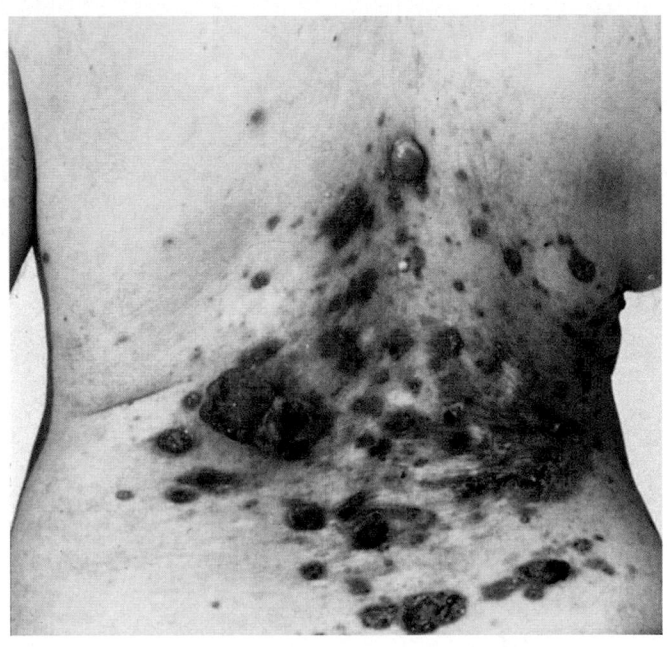

Basal cell nevus syndrome. Multiple, large, fungating basal cell carcinomas arising in a portion of the lower back treated years earlier with superficial x-ray for therapy of basal cell carcinomas.

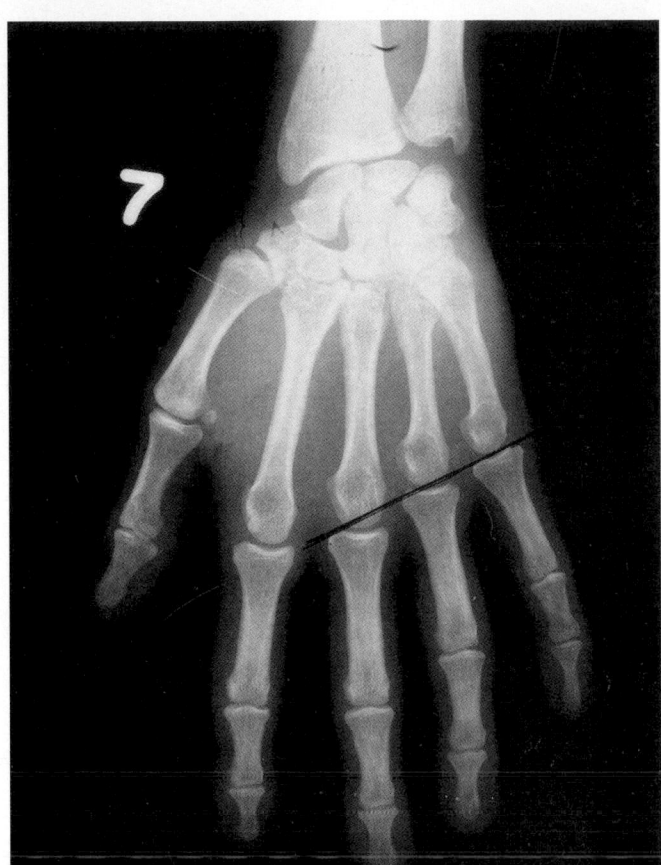

A.

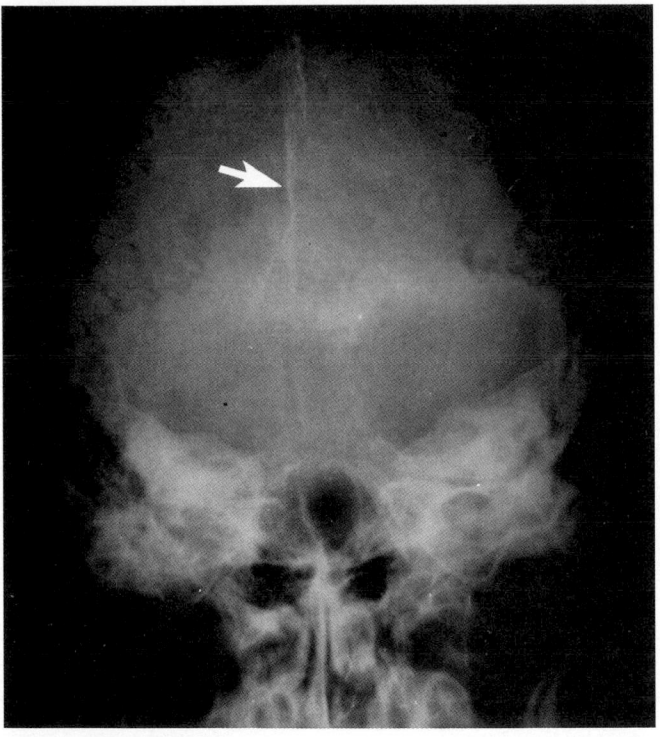

B.

Basal cell nevus syndrome. *A.* Short fourth, metacarpal (Albright's sign). A line drawn through the distal ends of the fifth and fourth metacarpals, intersects the third metacarpal proximal to its end. *B.* Lamellar calcification of the falx (*arrow*).

REFERENCES

1. Howell JB, Caro MR: Basal cell nevus: Its relationship to multiple cutaneous cancers and associated anomalies of development. *Arch Dermatol* **79**:67, 1959
2. Gorlin RJ: Nevoid basal-cell carcinoma syndrome. *Medicine* **66**:98, 1987
3. Hahn H et al: Mutations of the human homologue of *Drosophilia patched* in the nevoid basal cell carcinoma syndrome. *Cell* **85**:841, 1996
4. Johnson RL et al: Human homolog of *patched,* a candidate gene for the basal cell nevus syndrome. *Science* **272**:1668, 1996
5. Howell JB: Nevoid basal cell carcinoma syndrome: Profile of genetic and environmental factors in oncogenesis. *J Am Acad Dermatol* **11**:98, 1984
6. Dunnick NR et al: Nevoid basal cell carcinoma syndrome: Radiographic manifestations including cystlike lesions of the phalanges. *Radiology* **127**:331, 1978
7. Ratcliffe JF et al: The diagnostic implication of falcine calcification on plain skull radiographs of patients with basal cell naevus syndrome and the incidence of falcine calcification in their relatives and two control groups. *Br J Radiol* **68**:361, 1995
8. Ratcliffe JF et al: The prevalence of cervical and thoracic congenital skeletal abnormalities in basal cell naevus syndrome: A review of cervical and chest radiographs in 80 patients with BCNS. *Br J Radiol* **68**:596, 1995
9. Goeteyn M et al: The Bazex-Dupré-Christol syndrome. *Arch Dermatol* **130**:337, 1994
10. Ashinoff R et al: Rombo syndrome: A second case report and review. *J Am Acad Dermatol* **28**:1011, 1993
11. Oley CA et al: Basal cell carcinomas, coarse sparse hair, and milia. *Am J Med Genet* **43**:799, 1992

CHAPTER 159

Warren W. Piette

Hematologic Diseases

Hematology includes the study of blood and blood-forming tissues. Given the large number and variety of hematologic disorders, it is not surprising that mucocutaneous manifestations of hematologic disorders are common. Many hematologic malignancies and malignancy-mimicking diseases can involve the skin through tumor infiltration (specific lesions), and some of these may present preferentially in the skin. These conditions, such as T and B cell cutaneous lymphomas, other leukemias and lymphomas, plasma cell dyscrasias, and Langerhans and non-Langerhans histiocytoses, are discussed in other chapters. Likewise, patients with serious or chronic hematologic diseases are often at risk for complications of therapy, especially chemotherapy, certain cytokine therapies, radiation therapy, or marrow transplantation. Any of these interventions may affect skin and mucous membranes; these associations are also discussed elsewhere.

The first major section of this chapter is directed to nonspecific (non-tumor-containing) cutaneous findings that may be associated with hematologic disorders. Although the ready availability of laboratory testing has made early recognition of such conditions as anemia and polycythemia common and much less dependent on physical findings, cutaneous associations still may aid in the diagnosis of a hematologic condition or complicate its management. A comprehensive listing of these associations is presented in Table 159-1. Selected associations are covered in more detail in the text.

The second section of the chapter focuses on the differential diagnosis of purpura with an emphasis on those subsets of purpura with important underlying hematologic abnormalities.

CUTANEOUS SIGNS AND SYMPTOMS ASSOCIATED WITH HEMATOLOGIC DISEASES

Pallor

Cutaneous pallor results from a drop in the hemoglobin content of the cutaneous microvasculature. This decrease can occur either with a drop in the overall cutaneous blood flow due to emotion, epi-nephrine, cold exposure, or shock, or with physiologic adjustments to severe anemia.

Patients with acute severe anemia usually present with constitutional signs and symptoms such as dyspnea on exertion and occasionally at rest, faintness, dizziness, or hypotension and shock secondary to hypovolemia. Such acute severe anemia most commonly follows major bleeding or brisk hemolysis. Patients whose severe anemia develops more slowly often have surprisingly few complaints, presumably due to gradual physiologic adaptation. Nonetheless, dyspnea, especially on exertion, and palpitations are common in individuals with severe anemia. Malaise and fatigue are also common, although with nutritional anemias these symptoms may be much more evident in retrospect after replacement therapy.

A measurable increase in the resting cardiac output does not occur until the hemoglobin concentration is also below 7 g/dL, and clinical signs of cardiac hyperactivity are not usually present until the hemoglobin concentration reaches even lower levels.[1] In human chronic anemia, oxygenation of oxygen-sensitive areas such as brain, heart, and muscle is maintained by a selective increase in blood flow, at the expense of perfusion to less oxygen-sensitive tissues.[1] The skin and kidneys appear to be the first sites of reduced perfusion. Although vasoconstriction and oxygen deprivation in the subcutaneous tissue seem well tolerated, they are partly responsible for the anemic pallor. In the fully opened hand, the palmar creases appear pink until the hemoglobin level is less than 7 g/dL.[2]

Severe anemia due to marrow failure, fibrosis, or infiltration is typically accompanied by infections or bleeding secondary to associated neutropenia or thrombocytopenia. Development of a chronic anemia with the hemoglobin concentration below 7 g/dL and no other cytopenias is usually slow and due to nutritional deficiencies or to severe hypothyroidism, each of which may produce distinctive clinical syndromes. In any anemic patient, examination of the peripheral blood smear can reveal important clues to the pathogenesis of the anemia.[3] Further testing (including Coombs' tests for antibody-mediated hemolysis; specific assays for vitamin B_{12}, folate, or iron; or a bone marrow aspirate or biopsy) will generally lead to a correct diagnosis.

IRON DEFICIENCY Fatigue, irritability, and headaches are common complaints in iron-deficiency anemia. The severity of symp-

TABLE 159-1

Cutaneous Findings with Hematologic Associations[51–54]

I. Pigmentary changes
  A. Generalized hyperpigmentation
    1. POEMS syndrome (polyneuropathy, organomegaly, endocrinopathy, M-protein, skin lesions)[55,56]
      a. Hyperpigmentation, 93–98%; apparent skin thickening, 77–85%; hypertrichosis, 78–81%; peripheral edema, ~90%; digital clubbing, 56%; white fingernails; verrucous angiomata; telangiectasia
    2. Hemochromatosis may have bronze or grayish pigmentation of the skin
    3. Megaloblastic anemia of vitamin B_{12} or folate deficiency (see text)
    4. Fanconi's anemia[57,58]
      a. Begins age 4–10 years with skin or heme presentation
      b. Generalized hyperpigmentation, especially lower trunk, flexures, neck, 85%
      c. Scattered darker and lighter macules within hyperpigmented areas
      d. Progressive hypoplastic anemia with pancytopenia
      e. Death from leukemia, other neoplasms, or infections 2–5 years after onset
    5. Dyskeratosis congenita[59]
      a. Nail dystrophy, beginning 5–13 years of age
      b. Fine reticulate gray-brown hyperpigmentation, especially neck, thighs, and trunk
      c. Atrophic skin with telangiectasias
      d. Oral leukoplakia
      e. Mucocutaneous carcinomas, occasional pancreatic carcinoma, Hodgkin's disease
      f. Frequent blood dyscrasias, aplasias, refractory anemias, pancytopenias
  B. Localized hyperpigmentation
    1. Hypermelanosis and hemosiderosis may develop on the lower legs in hemolytic anemias
    2. Porphyria cutanea tarda, variegate porphyria, erythropoietic porphyria, occasionally hereditary coproporphyria cause hyperpigmentation, primarily in sun-exposed areas (see Chap. 151)
  C. Generalized hypopigmentation
    1. Chédiak-Higashi (see Section II)
    2. Hermansky-Pudlak[60]
      a. White, red, or brown hair; cream-gray to light normal skin
      b. Blue-gray to brown iris
      c. Platelet bleeding diathesis
      d. Ceroid-like deposits in reticuloendothelial system, gastrointestinal tract, lung, and kidney that lead to pulmonary interstitial fibrosis, nephritis, granulomatous colitis
  D. Localized hypopigmentation
    1. POEMS syndrome (see Section I, A)
    2. Pernicious anemia with vitiligo (see text)
    3. Vitamin B_{12} deficiency associated with poikilodermatous hypopigmentation[10]
    4. Anemia of autoimmune hypothyroidism may be associated with vitiligo
    5. Adult Gaucher's disease[61]
      a. Brown chloasma-like macules on face, neck, and hands
      b. Symmetric hyperpigmentation of lower legs
    6. Niemann-Pick disease[62,63]
      a. Indurated discolored patches, especially on cheeks; café au lait spots
      b. Mongolian spots on skin and oral mucosa
    7. Porphyria cutanea tarda, variegate porphyria, erythropoietic porphyria, mostly in areas of scarring
II. Recurrent cutaneous infections
  A. Neutropenia
    1. Severe neutropenia (counts of 500/μL usually associated with fever, erythema without pus, painful ulcers). Causes include congenital and cyclic neutropenia; leukemia, lymphoma; marrow toxicity, failure, infiltration; and immune and autoimmune neutropenias.
  B. Functional leukocyte defects (counts may be low, normal, or elevated; defects identified in adherence, chemotactic response, phagocytosis, and killing)[64,65]
    1. Chédiak-Higashi syndrome[60,66]
      a. Autosomal recessive
      b. Defect in cytoplasmic granule function
      c. Fair skin, light blond or silvery hair, and pale retina; translucent irides due to abnormal melanosomes
      d. Large neutrophil inclusion on Wright-stained blood smear
      e. Usually die in childhood
    2. Griscelli's syndrome[67] (Chap. 117)
      a. Pigmentary dilution with silvery-gray hair
      b. Autosomal recessive
      c. Hypogammaglobulinemia, defective cell-mediated immunity
      d. Neutropenia, thrombocytopenia, lymphohistiocytosis, hepatosplenomegaly
      e. Neurologic deterioration

(continued)

TABLE 159-1 (*Continued*)

3. Chronic granulomatous disease of childhood (Chap. 143)
    a. Leukocytes ingest bacteria normally but fail to kill them because of defects in H_2O_2 and oxygen radical production
    b. Multiple types, most X-linked; overall sex ratio, male:female 6:1
    c. Skin lesions eczematous and purulent initially, transition to chronic cutaneous granulomas
    d. Catalase-positive microbes (e.g., *Staphylococcus aureus, Salmonella, Aspergillus*) can multiply intracellularly, while catalase-negative microbes (e.g., pneumococci or streptococci) that generate their own H_2O_2 are killed
    e. Nitroblue tetrazolium (NBT) dye helpful in diagnosis
    f. X-linked carriers may develop lupus-like skin lesions, aphthous stomatitis, or granulomatous cheilitis
4. Myeloperoxidase deficiency
    a. Autosomal recessive affecting neutrophils but not eosinophils
    b. Functional impairment not severe
    c. Occasional difficulty with pyogenic infections, persistent fungal infection more common
C. Membrane and cytoskeletal defects (see Chap. 117)
    1. Leukocyte adherence disorders due to congenital lack or defect of some component of CD11/CD18 surface glycoproteins
        a. Neutrophils unable to adhere firmly to surfaces or complement-opsonized microorganisms
        b. Possible persistent leukocytosis
        c. Failure to develop much neutrophil response at inflammatory or infectious sites
    2. Cytoskeletal defect in polymerizable actin[68]
        a. Similar presentation to leukocyte adherence defects, but with normal CD11/CD18 but impaired motility
    3. Complement abnormalities
        a. C3 deficiency, C3b inactivator deficiency
    4. Hyperimmunoglobulin E syndrome
        a. Job's and Buckley's syndromes are subsets
        b. Elevated IgE, defective neutrophil chemotaxis
        c. No clear relationship between IgE levels and neutrophil motility defect
        d. Cold abscesses
    5. Leiner's disease
        a. Severe seborrheic dermatitis
        b. Diarrhea, failure to thrive
        c. Gram-negative bacterial and candidal infections during infancy
    6. Wiskott-Aldrich syndrome[69,70]
        a. X-linked
        b. Thrombocytopenia, small and dysfunctional platelets, hemorrhage
        c. Eczema
        d. Recurrent infections: initially bacteria such as pneumococcus, *Haemophilus influenzae, Neisseria meningitidis*; over time, T cell function deteriorates and patient becomes susceptible to opportunistic viral, bacterial, and fungal infections
        e. Immunologic abnormalities and lymphoreticular malignancies
        f. CD43, a ligand of ICAM-1, is defective; however, probably not primary defect because CD43 gene is on chromosome16, not X
    7. Persistent or extensive herpes simplex or recurrent or disseminated herpes zoster suggest underlying immune defect or hematologic malignancy
III. Neutrophilic cutaneous reactions
    A. Acute febrile neutrophilic dermatosis (Sweet's syndrome): Under 10% of reported patients have heme association, usually acute myelogenous leukemia, myeloproliferative disorder, myelodysplastic syndrome, multiple myeloma, or monoclonal gammopathy
    B. Pyoderma gangrenosum: Often atypical or bullous—hematologic associations similar to those in Sweet's syndrome
    C. Antineutrophil cytoplasmic autoantibody (ANCA)-positive neutrophilic dermatosis
        1. Polymorphic disease with monoclonal IgA ANCA[71]
    D. Erythema elevatum diutinum (see Section VI)
    E. Leukocytoclastic vasculitis (see Section VI)
IV. Vesiculobullous disease
    A. Pemphigus vulgaris: lymphoproliferative diseases[19,72]
    B. Paraneoplastic pemphigus: lymphoproliferative diseases, thymoma[73]
    C. Acquired immunobullous disease with skin fragility: Waldenström's macroglobulinemia[74]
    D. Linear IgA dermatosis: associations include Hodgkin's lymphoma, non-Hodgkin's lymphoma, polycythemia vera, chronic lymphocytic leukemia, plasmacytoma[75]
    E. IgA pemphigus: occasional monoclonal gammopathy or myeloma, most often IgA
    F. Subcorneal pustular dermatosis: IgG or IgA monoclonal gammopathy or myeloma[55,56]
    G. Dermatitis herpetiformis: frequent polyclonal IgA gammopathy, occasional myeloma, lymphomas, angioimmunoblastic lymphadenopathy
    H. Porphyria cutanea tarda, variegate porphyria, hereditary coproporphyria, and erythropoietic porphyria (see Sections XII and I,A)
    I. Bullous mastocytoma, bullous urticaria pigmentosa of infancy[18]
    J. Hypereosinophilic syndrome can induce vesiculobullous lesions[20]
V. Skin cancers
    A. Basal cell and squamous cell carcinoma increased in non-Hodgkin's lymphoma and chronic lymphocytic leukemia (CLL)[76]
    B. Kaposi's sarcoma increased in lymphoma, CLL, some immune deficiencies

(*continued*)

TABLE 159-1 (*Continued*)

Cutaneous Findings with Hematologic Associations[51-54]

VI. Vascular disorders and coagulopathies
    A. Vasculitis
        1. Usually cutaneous leukocytoclastic vasculitis (including urticarial vasculitis) and polyarteritis nodosa; about 5% of patients with vasculitis have an underlying malignancy[77]; lymphoproliferative disease most common, especially hairy cell leukemia; other hematologic associations include cryoglobulinemia, Hodgkin's disease, non-Hodgkin's lymphoma, myelodysplastic syndrome, chronic myelogenous leukemia, and multiple myeloma[19,78]
        2. Erythema elevatum diutinum: gammopathy or myeloma, frequently IgA[55,56]
        3. Urticaria and angioedema
            a. Lymphoproliferative disease, sometimes with decreased C1-esterase inhibitor function[55]
            b. Cryoglobulinemia; can also cause cold-induced urticaria[55]
            c. Lymphocytic vasculitis: angioblastic lymphadenopathy, non-Hodgkin's lymphoma, CLL[79]
            d. Vasculitis panniculitis: children, non-Hodgkin's lymphoma[80]
            e. Hypereosinophilic syndrome[20]
    B. Vasculopathies and altered vascular reactivity
        1. Flushing, erythroderma: see text
        2. Plethora, ruddy cyanosis: see text
        3. Erythema annulare centrifugum: lymphoma, "malignant histiocytosis," hypereosinophilic syndrome[20]
        4. Erythralgia/erythromelalgia[81-83]
            a. Polycythemia vera, essential thrombocythemia; less commonly myelofibrosis, chronic myelogenous leukemia, cryoglobulinemia
        5. Raynaud's phenomenon
            a. Waldenstrom's macroglobulinemia[55]
            b. Cryoglobulinemia[55]
        6. Livedo reticularis[84,85]
            a. Plasma cell dyscrasias with hyperviscosity, cryoglobulinemia, or cold agglutinin disease, macroglobulinemia[86]
            b. Hyperleukocytosis
            c. Polycythemia vera, thrombocythemia[87]
(For the following, see also Tables 159-2 to 159-7)
            d. Antiphospholipid antibody, lupus anticoagulant[48,88]
            e. Hereditary protein C deficiency[89]
            f. Antithrombin III deficiency[89,90]
            g. Heparin-associated thrombocytopenia[91]
        7. Acral cyanosis
            a. Coumadin or other anticoagulant enhanced tendency for cholesterol embolization: blue toe syndrome
            b. Polycythemia vera, thrombocythemia, rarely with myeloblast leukostasis syndrome of chronic myelogenous leukemia[92]
            c. Cryoglobulinemia[55,93]
            d. Cold agglutinins[55,86]
            e. Crystalglobulin vasculopathy: multiple myeloma[94,95]
    C. Vascular changes
        1. POEMS syndrome: telangiectasias or angiomas
        2. Langerhans cell histiocytosis: telangiectasias, petechial hemorrhage
        3. Telangiectasia macularis eruptiva perstans (TMEP) variant of urticaria pigmentosa[18]
    D. Bleeding or coagulopathy secondary to dysproteinemia
        1. Mucocutaneous hemorrhage
            a. Hyperviscosity syndrome, usually Waldenström's macroglobulinemia, occasionally myeloma, cryoglobulinemia[55]
            b. Abnormal platelet function from dysproteinemias[55]
            c. Factor deficiencies or inhibitors: Factor V or VIII with IgM or IgA[55]; Factor VII with IgG[55]; Factor X adsorptive depletion in amyloidosis[96]
            d. Low-grade disseminated intravascular coagulation (DIC) with protein C dysfunction secondary to IgG gammopathy[55]
VII. Cutaneous deposition/induration[55,56]
    A. AL (light-chain related) systemic amyloidosis: papules, plaques, nodules, bullae, sclerotic plaques, urticaria-pigmentosa-like lesions, alopecia, macroglossia; occurs with idiopathic or disease-associated monoclonal gammopathies
    B. Nodular cutaneous amyloidosis: local monoclonal plasma cell infiltrate; atrophic outpouchings of abdominal skin[97]
    C. Storage papule disease (translucent, often crusted or purpuric centers, buttocks and lower extremities): Waldenström's macroglobulinemia[98]
    D. Cutaneous swelling associated with crystalline protein deposition: myeloma[99]
    E. Follicular spicules of the nose: multiple myeloma, cryoglobulinemia[100]
    F. Scleromyxedema variant of lichen myxedematosus: usually IgGλ gammopathy[101]
    G. Scleredema: usually IgG monoclonal gammopathy, occasionally myeloma
    H. Niemann-Pick: waxy induration with transient xanthomas overlying enlarged lymph nodes[63,102]
    I. Thickened, doughy skin of diffuse cutaneous mastocytosis[103]
    J. Anetoderma: cutaneous plasmacytoma, benign lymphoid hyperplasia[104]
VIII. Xanthomas[55,56]
    A. Necrobiotic xanthogranuloma with paraproteinemia
        1. Usually periorbital xanthoma, typically ulcerative

(*continued*)

TABLE 159-1 (*Continued*)

      2. Leukopenia
      3. Monoclonal gammopathy or multiple myeloma
   B. Xanthoma disseminatum—occasional association with monoclonal gammopathy, multiple myeloma, Waldenström's macroglobulinemia
   C. Generalized plane xanthomatosis
      1. Multiple myeloma, monoclonal gammopathies, leukemias
      2. Xanthomas and café au lait spots: juvenile chronic granulocytic leukemia
      3. Eruptive or tuberous xanthomas rarely reported with dysproteinemias
IX. Cutaneous sarcoidal or histiocytic tissue reactions
   A. Cutaneous sarcoidal reactions: lymphoma[105]
   B. Multicentric reticulohistiocytosis: lymphoproliferative disorders[106]
X. Epidermal changes
   A. Acquired ichthyosis: lymphoproliferative malignancies, primarily Hodgkin's disease[107]
   B. Sign of Leser-Trelat: lymphomas comprise one-fifth of cases[108]
XI. Hypertrichosis
   A. Porphyria cutanea tarda, erythropoietic porphyria
XII. Pruritus, prurigo, burning
   A. Severe itching occurs in 1–11% of patients with Hodgkin's disease even in the absence of any visible skin lesions; occasional complication of non-Hodgkin's lymphoma and leukemia[19]
   B. Mycosis fungoides, Sézary syndrome, or other lymphomas with skin involvement may also present as itching
   C. Eosinophilic folliculitis following marrow transplant or chemotherapy for heme malignancies[109]
   D. Aquagenic pruritus: polycythemia vera, hypereosinophilic syndrome, myelodysplastic syndrome, juvenile xanthogranuloma[26]
   E. Hypereosinophilic syndrome: pruritic, erythematous papules or nodules, and angioedematous or urticarial plaques common[20]
   F. Mastocytosis: pruritic and usually pigmented papules or diffuse pruritus[18]
   G. Erythropoietic protoporphyria: pruritus and burning within minutes of sun exposure; may develop urticaria, edema, erythema, purpura
   H. Angioimmunoblastic lymphadenopathy: macular and papular eruptions, petechial, purpuric, nodular, ulcerative and erythrodermic eruptions described[21,110]
XIII. Ulcerations[111]
   A. Nonmalignant red blood cell disorders and leg ulcers
      1. α and β thalassemias
      2. Hb SS, Hb S-β thal, Hb SC
      3. Hereditary spherocytosis and elliptocytosis
      4. Paroxysmal nocturnal hemoglobinuria
   B. Cutaneous lesions of leukemia, lymphoma, and some histiocytoses may ulcerate
   C. Lymphomatoid papulosis
   D. Polycythemia vera and essential thrombocythemia
   E. Kaposi's sarcoma
   F. Reactive hemophagocytic syndrome
   G. Angioimmunoblastic lymphadenopathy[21]
   H. Necrobiotic xanthogranuloma with paraproteinemia, xanthoma disseminatum
   I. Sweet's syndrome
   J. Cryoglobulinemia[55]
   K. Hypereosinophilic syndrome, especially mucosal ulcerations and erosions[20,112]
   L. Protein C deficiency, inherited and acquired (including coumadin necrosis, some DIC)
   M. Heparin necrosis
   N. Antiphospholipid antibody syndrome
   O. Neutropenic and immune deficiency–related infections
   P. Pyoderma gangrenosum or pyoderma gangrenosum-like ulcers,[55,111] Chédiak-Higashi
   Q. Leukocyte adhesion deficiency
   R. Chronic granulomatous disease
   S. Hyperimmunoglobulinemia E
   T. Felty's syndrome
   U. Acute myelogenous leukemia

toms correlates poorly with the blood hemoglobin concentration.[4,5] The depletion of storage iron and often of tissue iron precedes the appearance of anemia. Some of the symptoms of iron deficiency may be due to impaired function of iron-containing enzymes or proteins other than hemoglobin. For example, headache, paresthesia, and a burning sensation of the tongue are symptoms of iron deficiency that are likely due to tissue cell iron depletion. Pica, the craving to eat substances such as dirt, clay, ice, laundry starch, salt, or cardboard, is a classic manifestation of iron deficiency and is usually cured promptly by iron therapy.[4,6]

The physical findings of iron-deficiency anemia, in their approximate order of frequency, include pallor, glossitis (smooth, red tongue), stomatitis, and angular cheilitis.[4] Skin dryness and coarsening; brittle nails; and dry, fine, and brittle hair may also be seen. Koilonychia (spooning of nails) is now rare. Retinal hemorrhages and exudates occur in severely anemic patients (hemoglobin ≤5g/dL), and proliferative retinopathy may accelerate in iron-deficient diabetic patients.

The differential diagnosis of microcytic anemias includes the thalassemias and some other hemoglobinopathies, chronic inflammatory disorders, benign or malignant neoplasms, chemical blockade of heme synthesis (lead, pyrazinamide, isoniazid), and sideroblastic anemias.[4] Although serum levels of iron, iron binding capacity (transferrin), and ferritin are useful in the diagnosis of iron deficiency, none of these is uniformly reliable when compared to stainable iron in marrow biopsies. For example, serum iron levels characteristically drop in patients after an acute myocardial infarction, with acute or chronic inflammatory disorders, or with malignancies, despite marrow evidence of sufficient iron.[4,7] Likewise, even in iron-deficient individuals, disorders such as hepatitis, chronic inflammatory diseases (e.g., rheumatoid arthritis, chronic infections), chronic renal disease, and malignancies can elevate serum ferritin into the normal range. Therefore, as with all laboratory values, the proper interpretation of serum indices of iron stores requires correlation with the clinical setting.

MEGALOBLASTIC ANEMIAS Megaloblastic anemias result from impaired DNA synthesis.[8] The most common causes of megaloblastic anemia are folate or cobalamin (vitamin B_{12}) deficiency. Acute megaloblastic anemia can result from nitrous oxide exposure or severe illness combined with extensive transfusion, dialysis, total parenteral nutrition, or weak folate antagonist exposure (e.g., trimethoprim). Other causes of more chronic megaloblastosis include certain medications (especially antimetabolites, inhibitors of dihydrofolate reductase or deoxynucleotide synthesis, some anticonvulsants, oral contraceptives) and a variety of inborn metabolic errors.

Megaloblastic anemias share certain clinical features. The slowly developing anemia produces few symptoms until the hematocrit is severely depressed. Symptoms of weakness, palpitation, fatigue, light-headedness, and shortness of breath are due to anemia. Hyperbilirubinemia secondary to ineffective erythropoiesis with hemolysis can lead to a mild jaundice. Severe anemic pallor and slight jaundice combine to produce a lemon-yellow skin. Hyperpigmentation is commonly noted, particularly in dark-skinned individuals, in both folate- and vitamin B_{12}–deficient patients.[9–11] In the latter, the hyperpigmentation frequently localizes to the face, hands, and feet but occasionally only to the fingers.[12] Poikilodermatous pigmentary change has also been described in vitamin B_{12} deficiency[10]; replacement typically reverses the hyperpigmentation. When pernicious anemia is the etiology, there is an increased incidence of vitiligo and of premature graying.[13] Cheilosis and atrophy of filiform papillae of the tongue may develop with folate or cobalamin deficiency. Leukopenia and thrombocytopenia may occur but are seldom severe enough to be symptomatic. Characteristic findings on peripheral blood smear are red cell oval macrocytosis and neutrophil hypersegmentation.

Folate deficiency typically results from poor nutrition (common in elderly, poor, or alcoholic individuals), from decreased absorption (such as with sprue), or from increased metabolic requirements due to pregnancy or increased cell turnover (chronic hemolytic anemia, exfoliative dermatoses).[8,14] Cobalamin deficiency results from impaired absorption or decreased intake of vitamin B_{12}. Dietary deficiency is uncommon but is most likely to develop in vegetarians who avoid dairy products, eggs, and B_{12} supplements (vegans). Impaired absorption is usually the cause of cobalamin deficiency and may be due to gastric causes (pernicious anemia, gastrectomy, Zollinger-Ellison syndrome), intestinal causes (ileal resection or disease, blind loop syndrome, fish tapeworm), or pancreatic insufficiency.

The most common disorder of impaired vitamin B_{12} absorption is pernicious anemia, an autoimmune disease of insidious onset producing gastric atrophy and impaired intrinsic factor production. Absorption of cobalamin is severely impaired by the absence of intrinsic factor. In addition to anti–(gastric) parietal cell antibodies,

many patients with pernicious anemia also develop antibodies to intrinsic factor or the intrinsic factor–cobalamin complex. Anti–parietal cell antibodies occur in 90 percent of patients with pernicious anemia but also in 60 percent of patients with other forms of atrophic gastritis and in 5 percent of a random 30- to 60-year-old population. Although anti-intrinsic factor antibodies are found in only about 70 percent of patients with pernicious anemia, they are highly specific for this condition. Other autoimmune diseases occurring more often than expected in patients with pernicious anemia include thyroid disease, type I diabetes, hypoparathryroidism, Addison's disease, postpartum hypophysitis, ulcerative colitis, vitiligo, acquired agammaglobulinemia, and certain forms of infertility.[8,13]

The hematologic manifestations of vitamin B_{12} or folate deficiency are indistinguishable, but it is critical to determine the deficient nutrient because of the often serious neurologic complications of severe vitamin B_{12} deficiency. With folate deficiency, physiologic replacement of folate (200 μg daily) should result in a full hematologic response, while a pharmacologic dose of folate (5 mg daily) will correct the hematologic abnormalities of cobalamin deficiency.[8] However, this replacement should not be used as a diagnostic test to distinguish the two, because any folate replacement may accelerate the neurologic damage of cobalamin deficiency.[8] Neurologic complications include paresthesia in the feet and fingers; changes in vibratory sense and proprioception; and progression to spastic ataxia, somnolence, altered taste, smell, and vision, dementia, psychotic depression, or paranoid schizophrenia.[8,15] In some patients, the neurologic findings may appear in the absence of megaloblastic changes. Since numbness or dysesthesia are perceived by some patients as skin problems, it is possible that a patient might present with these findings to a dermatologist.

ANEMIA OF ENDOCRINE DISORDERS Pituitary deficiency, adrenal dysfunction, gonadal dysfunction, and thyroid dysfunction are the endocrine disorders in which hormonal deficiency is most likely to lead to anemia. The absence of androgen in men is followed by a drop in hemoglobin levels to those of women. The lowest hemoglobin levels are associated with myxedema, which may present with dry, coarse, and scaly skin and anemia. Hemoglobin levels in hypothyroidism are seldom below 8 to 9 g/dL.[16] Uncomplicated thyroid hormone deficiency produces a normochromic, normocytic anemia. However, for reasons only partly understood, iron deficiency frequently accompanies severe hypothyroidism, producing a hypochromic and microcytic anemia. To further complicate matters, pernicious anemia, with vitamin B_{12} deficiency and a megaloblastic anemia, is also associated with autoimmune thyroid disease at a rate higher than chance alone.

Flushing and Erythroderma (Generalized Erythema)

Just as emotional factors or cold may trigger cutaneous vasoconstriction and pallor, so may emotion or heat stimulate vasodilatation and flushing. Rosacea or actinic damage can cause facial redness. Rarely, the POEMS syndrome with idiopathic flushing may mimic carcinoid syndrome.[17] Patients with cutaneous mastocytosis may also develop flushing episodes lasting ≥ 30 min, unlike the typical carcinoid flush of ≤ 10 min.[18] Widespread erythroderma occurs in cutaneous T cell lymphoma, in some cases of chronic lymphocytic leukemia, lymphocytic lymphoma, and rarely in angioimmunoblastic lymphadenopathy or hypereosinophilic syndrome.[19–21] The skin is often involved, sometimes severely enough to produce erythroderma, in both acute and chronic graft-versus-host disease.

A sustained increase in red cell production will lead to an increase in both hematocrit and blood volume, directly raising blood viscosity and vascular volume. These in turn are responsible for many of the signs and symptoms of polycythemia.[1,22] A ruddy cyanosis or acrocyanosis is seen in conditions associated with abnormally high levels of hemoglobin and sluggish flow of deoxygenated blood through dilated cutaneous vessels. An increased red cell mass may be compensatory, as in chronic hypoxic states, or it may be primary, as in polycythemia vera.

POLYCYTHEMIA VERA Ruddy cyanosis or plethora is probably the best known cutaneous finding in polycythemia vera (PV), but this myeloproliferative disease may present to the dermatologist with a variety of cutaneous findings. This disorder involves all hematopoietic stem cell lines, even though erythroid proliferation is usually dominant. It occurs most commonly after age 50.[23] Bleeding and thrombosis are frequent and often serious complications of this disease, including stroke and Budd-Chiari syndrome (hepatic vein occlusion). A cerebral event may precede the diagnosis of PV in up to 35 percent of patients. Signs and symptoms involving the peripheral vasculature are frequent (34 to 62 percent), including peripheral vascular disease (6 to 22 percent), erythromelalgia (18 percent), peripheral gangrene (16 percent), deep venous thrombosis (7 to 13 percent), digital artery occlusion (7.5 percent), Raynaud's phenomenon (1 to 3 percent), and leg ulcers (2 percent). Erythromelalgia, a syndrome of burning erythema in the feet or hands triggered by warmth, may precede the diagnosis of PV by several years. PV-associated erythromelalgia is probably due to the platelet abnormalities that occur in PV, may result in cutaneous necrosis, and should respond well to treatment with aspirin.

Other possible cutaneous findings include paresthesia (29 percent) and pruritus (14 to 50 percent).[23,24] Aquagenic pruritus is distinct from various forms of water-related urticaria, is characterized by intense itching after water exposure without visible skin changes, and is usually of unknown origin. Recognized associations include PV and rarely myelodysplastic syndromes or juvenile xanthogranuloma.[25–27] The pruritus is often sudden in onset after a warm bath or shower and must be distinguished from transient pruritus after bathing or aquagenic pruritus of the elderly. True aquagenic pruritus is characterized by intense, constant, disabling, and often progressive symptoms.[26] There is no clear relationship between the degree of pruritus and the severity of the disease, with roughly 20 percent of patients continuing to itch despite adequate control of their PV.[24] Although the pathogenesis of pruritus has been tied to elevated blood and urine histamine levels, H_1-antagonists are generally of little value. Occasional patients may respond to aspirin, cholestryramine, H_2-receptor antagonists, oral iron, or PUVA.[24,28] Recombinant interferon-α may be an effective therapy in PV and in one study provided greater than 50 percent improvement in pruritus control in 77 percent of patients.[24] Suberythemal UVB and PUVA may also induce at least temporary remissions.[26]

The diagnosis of PV depends on an increased red cell mass ($\geq$36 mL/kg in males or $\geq$32 mL/kg in females) and arterial O_2 saturation ($\geq$92%). In addition, patients must have either splenomegaly or any two numerically defined minor criteria, which include thrombocytosis, leukocytosis, an elevated leukocyte alkaline phosphatase score, and a greatly elevated serum vitamin B_{12}–binding capacity.[23] Phlebotomy is the treatment of choice for relief of symptoms of hypervolemia and hyperviscosity, but it does not relieve pruritus or thrombocytosis. Beyond phlebotomy, there is no single best treatment for PV. Myelosuppressive therapy or radioactive phosphorus (^{32}P) is indicated to reduce the incidence of thrombosis but may be complicated by the development of acute leukemia or other secondary malignancies.

Cyanosis

In patients with normal hemoglobin levels, peripheral cyanosis indicates at least 5 g/dL of reduced hemoglobin in capillary blood. Peripheral cyanosis has multiple etiologies, including vasoconstriction with resulting slow acral flow. Only central cyanosis (tongue and sublingual region) reliably indicates significant arterial deoxygenation or altered hemoglobin. Cyanosis is best observed in fluorescent lighting.[29] Thin skin areas are the best places to look for cyanosis: in adults these include the lips, earlobes, nailbeds, and oral mucous membranes; and in newborns the highly vascular palms and heels.[30] However, multiracial studies suggest that the tongue is the most sensitive site for detection of central cyanosis.

Lingual cyanosis as the earliest manifestation of central cyanosis is reliably detectable at a level of 3.4 g/dL of reduced arterial hemoglobin, resulting in a level of 5 g/dL of reduced capillary hemoglobin.[30] The total concentration of hemoglobin determines the level of arterial deoxygenation that this lower limit of detectable cyanosis represents. For example, in a patient with a hemoglobin of 15 g/dL, 3.4 g/dL corresponds to an Sa_{O_2} of 77% and a Pa_{O_2} of 43 mmHg. This same level of reduced hemoglobin in a patient with 12 g/dL hemoglobin corresponds to a Pa_{O_2} of 39 mmHg. A severely anemic patient with a hemoglobin of $\leq$7 g/dL may never manifest cyanosis despite fatal hypoxia. In contrast, a polycythemic patient with 18 g/dL hemoglobin with 3.4 g/dL of reduced hemoglobin will develop central cyanosis with an Sa_{O_2} of 84% and a Pa_{O_2} of 49 mmHg. Because cyanosis depends on the absolute amount of reduced hemoglobin, patients with PV can rather easily manifest peripheral cyanosis despite normal arterial saturation, explaining their ruddy cyanosis.

Central cyanosis in an individual with normal hemoglobin levels and an acceptable Pa_{O_2} implies an abnormal hemoglobin or related problem. These include inherited methemoglobinemia (hemoglobins M), toxic methemoglobinemia, inherited NADH-diaphorase (cytochrome b_5 reductase) deficiency, cytochrome b_5 deficiency, acquired sulfhemoglobinemia, and low oxygen affinity hemoglobins.[31] At least 34 hemoglobins M or low oxygen affinity hemoglobins are recognized.

Methemoglobinemia occurs naturally as 1 percent of total hemoglobin. At a 1.5-g/dL concentration (roughly 10 percent in men), cyanosis is easily detectable. At 20 percent, a chocolate cyanosis is seen, turning the tongue and sublingual area brown. Levels >60 percent methemoglobinemia are a medical emergency and should be treated with IV methylene blue or exchange transfusion. Many medications may cause methemoglobinemia, including dapsone, phenazopyridine (pyridium), sulfamethoxazole, nitroglycerin, nitrites, and the local anesthetics benzocaine and prilocaine.[31] Nitrates in drinking water and aniline dyes in diapers are important and easily overlooked causes of this condition in infants.[31,32] NADH-diaphorase deficiency and the very rare cytochrome b_5 deficiency impair the ability of the red cells to reduce iron to the divalent form and thereby increase the formation of methemoglobinemia.

Sulfhemoglobinemia produces cyanosis at levels of only 0.5 g/dL capillary blood and cannot be reversed. Medications (especially sulfonamides, phenacetin, acetanilid, and phenazopyridine) are the usual cause of sulfhemoglobinemia, but this condition has occurred independent of drug use in association with chronic constipation and with purging.

Hemoglobins with altered oxygen affinity produce cyanosis through different mechanisms, but the predominant abnormalities are either lowered oxygen affinity with higher levels of reduced hemoglobin, or increased formation of methemoglobin. Cyanosis of the ears or fingertips is observed after exposure to cold in some individuals with cryoglobulins or cold agglutinins. Raynaud's phenomenon and acrocyanosis are nonhematologic causes of peripheral cyanosis with characteristic clinical presentations.

Jaundice

Jaundice is due to staining of the skin by bile pigment. Bilirubin glucuronide (direct-reacting or conjugated bilirubin) stains the skin more readily than does the unconjugated form.[2] Jaundice of the skin may not be visible if the bilirubin level is below 2 to 3 mg/dL. Unconjugated hyperbilirubinemia suggests hemolytic anemia or inefficient hematopoiesis, as in megaloblastosis. Usually, total bilirubin is only modestly increased (<5 mg/dL), with unconjugated bilirubin comprising at least 85 percent of the total amount.[33] Urinary urobilinogen is increased regularly, but bile is not detected in the urine unless serum conjugated bilirubin is increased. Usually, serum haptoglobin levels are low, and lactate dehydrogenase (LDH) levels are elevated. Hemoglobinuria is encountered in rare patients with hyperacute hemolysis who develop significant hemoglobinemia.

Infiltrative Lesions/Extramedullary Hematopoiesis

Specific (tumor-containing) lesions occur in many leukemias, lymphomas, and related disorders and are detailed elsewhere. Some of these same conditions induce non-tumor-containing extramedullary hematopoiesis, with the skin being an occasional and sometimes presenting site. Lesions of extramedullary hematopoiesis may present as red, pink, or violaceous papules or plaques, hemangioma-like nodules, bullae, or leg ulcerations; they may occasionally be surrounded by a hemorrhagic border.[34–36] Such extramedullary hematopoiesis usually occurs in idiopathic myelofibrosis but has been seen rarely in other myeloproliferative disease. Neonatal cases are associated with congenital infections, erythroblastosis fetalis, and, even more rarely, conditions such as twin transfusion syndrome.[36]

HEMOSTASIS AND THE DIFFERENTIAL DIAGNOSIS OF PURPURA

Hemostasis

Hemostasis is divided into two components, primary and secondary. Primary hemostasis depends both on vasoconstriction of the injured vessel and on the development of a platelet plug at the site of injury. This is a critical homeostatic mechanism for repair of small defects and is a sufficient mechanism for most focal injury in the microcirculation. Because the skin is richly endowed with microcirculatory vessels, presumably in part to support its heat exchange function, the skin is a sensitive early warning site for problems in primary hemostasis, especially with problems in platelet function or numbers. Defects larger than can be sealed by a platelet plug alone and defects in larger vessels require secondary hemostasis. This involves the cascade pathway of coagulation factors and results in fibrin clot reinforcement for the platelet plug. Whereas platelet problems are an important cause of purpuric skin lesions, defects

or deficiency of a single procoagulant clotting factor are an uncommon cause of cutaneous hemorrhage, usually leading instead to soft tissue hemorrhage, particularly into joints.

Differential Diagnosis of Purpura

The differential diagnosis of purpura can be confusing, and etiologies encompass hematologic, rheumatologic, dermatologic, infectious, and traumatic. Although it is the pathogenesis or etiology of the purpura that we usually most want to know, many approaches to the differential diagnosis of purpura begin with classifications by etiology. That is, many differential trees begin by requiring that which we ultimately wish to know. To circumvent this requirement, we must understand what the morphology of purpura can reveal about its likely pathogenesis. At the most basic level, purpura in the skin can be due to simple hemorrhage, inflammatory hemorrhage, or microvascular occlusion with ischemic hemorrhage. Careful inspection of purpuric lesions is essential for the bedside sorting of lesions into one of these fundamental categories as well as for providing an initial focus for history taking, further clinical examination, and laboratory assessment.

Morphologic differentiation can be extremely helpful in sorting through the differential diagnosis, but this approach requires a definition of terms not always used in a standard fashion and the addition of terms to categorize important morphologic subsets not previously distinguished. In this text, the term *purpura* refers to visible hemorrhage in skin or mucous membranes. Morphologic subsets of purpura include petechia (pl. petechiae), ecchymosis (pl. ecchymoses), contusions (bruises), classic palpable purpura, target lesions, inflammatory retiform purpura, and noninflammatory retiform purpura.[37]

The morphologic diagnosis of purpura begins with three P's: Is the lesion *p*urpuric, is it *p*rimary, and is it *p*alpable? For a lesion to qualify as purpuric, it must have a color that is compatible with hemorrhage—usually some shade of red, blue, or purple, but sometimes yellow-brown, green, or black—and at least some of this color must persist on compression of the skin. If the vessels are compressible, and if the color is caused by red cells free to move, then the color should completely blanch on compression. False-positive results occur if the lesion contains tortuous vessels that kink or constrict each other on compression, or if the lesion is difficult to compress sufficiently because of lesional firmness or because it is located in an area of dermis overlying a particularly soft subcutis, such as on the abdomen.

Red cells that have extravasated or are trapped within thrombi or vascular plugs will not be free to move, and therefore some of the color will persist. In addition to defining purpura, compression of a lesion can be used to determine the ratio of erythema to hemorrhage. A lesion due solely to the erythema of inflammation or flushing should blanch completely. A lesion consisting of some inflammation and some hemorrhage, such as vasculitis, should blanch partially. A lesion of simple hemorrhage or extravasation of red cells or one related to ischemic or thrombotic hemorrhage usually has no blanchable component. Lesions due to microvascular occlusion alone appear to induce visible purpura through ischemic extravasation of red cells around the vessel, inasmuch as thrombosis within the dermal microvasculature itself is too small to be seen directly.

Next, one must decide if purpura is primary, that is, caused by the same process that induces the lesion. With simple extravasation, the entire visible lesion is due solely to red cells in the dermis, and macular, nonerythematous purpura is the lesion. In contrast, a mosquito bite is not a clinically evident hemorrhagic event for most people, but sufficient scratching can induce purpura in such a lesion.

This purpura would be secondary and not primary. Vasculitis as vessel-directed injury can induce both a papule and hemorrhage as part of the same vessel injury, producing a primary purpura lesion.

Finally, palpability must be determined. Red cells alone do not determine palpability, since simple hemorrhage in the dermis is usually not palpable. Extravasation of blood into or beneath the panniculus can produce a palpable hematoma, which may or may not be purpuric (the overlying dermis may or may not show visible hemorrhage). Edema confers palpability to purpuric lesions, usually secondary to inflammation but sometimes to occlusion with preceding microvascular ischemia.

The color of lesions provides additional clues. Red implies saturated hemoglobin, while blue implies desaturated hemoglobin. Usually, color due to blood flow is red, whereas color due to hemorrhage is blue. However, hemorrhage may remain bright red even without an inflammatory component, most often when small and superficial—for example, petechial hemorrhage. Presumably, it is possible for the hemoglobin in the extravasated cells to remain saturated through simple diffusion of oxygen from the dermis or through the epidermis. Likewise, slow flow in the skin commonly produces the bluish-purple discoloration of livedo reticularis. The term *livedo reticularis* should be limited to a completely blanchable, netlike discoloration of the skin; defined in this way livedo reticularis is a sign of slowed or restricted cutaneous blood flow. Another nonpurpuric cause of bluish discoloration discussed previously is cyanosis.

Finally, a very important morphologic feature is the presence of retiform features. Retiform purpura without inflammation suggests microvascular occlusion as the etiology of the lesion, whereas prominent erythema in early retiform lesions suggests vasculitis due either to IgA or to mixed–vessel size inflammatory syndromes.[37,38] It is presumed that the reticulate or livedoid patterning of such lesions is due to the same microvascular anatomy of the skin responsible for the localization of the livedo reticularis pattern in slow-flow states. This bedside approach is summarized in Fig. 159-1.

NONPALPABLE PURPURA Petechial, nonpalpable hemorrhage in the skin and mucous membranes raises concerns about two general categories of hematologic syndromes, hemostatically relevant thrombocytopenia, usually less than 50,000 platelets per microliter, and abnormal platelet function (Table 159-2). There are also nonhematologic causes of nonpalpable petechial hemorrhage. The most common include spiking elevations of intravascular pressure (e.g., straining during childbirth, repetitive vomiting, and paroxysmal coughing), which usually result in petechial hemorrhage above the clavicles, and the syndromes of chronic pigmented purpura. The clinical features of the chronic pigmented purpuras typically include clustered petechiae within patches of orange-brown discoloration. This color results from a mix of mild erythema with hyperpigmen-

FIGURE 159-1

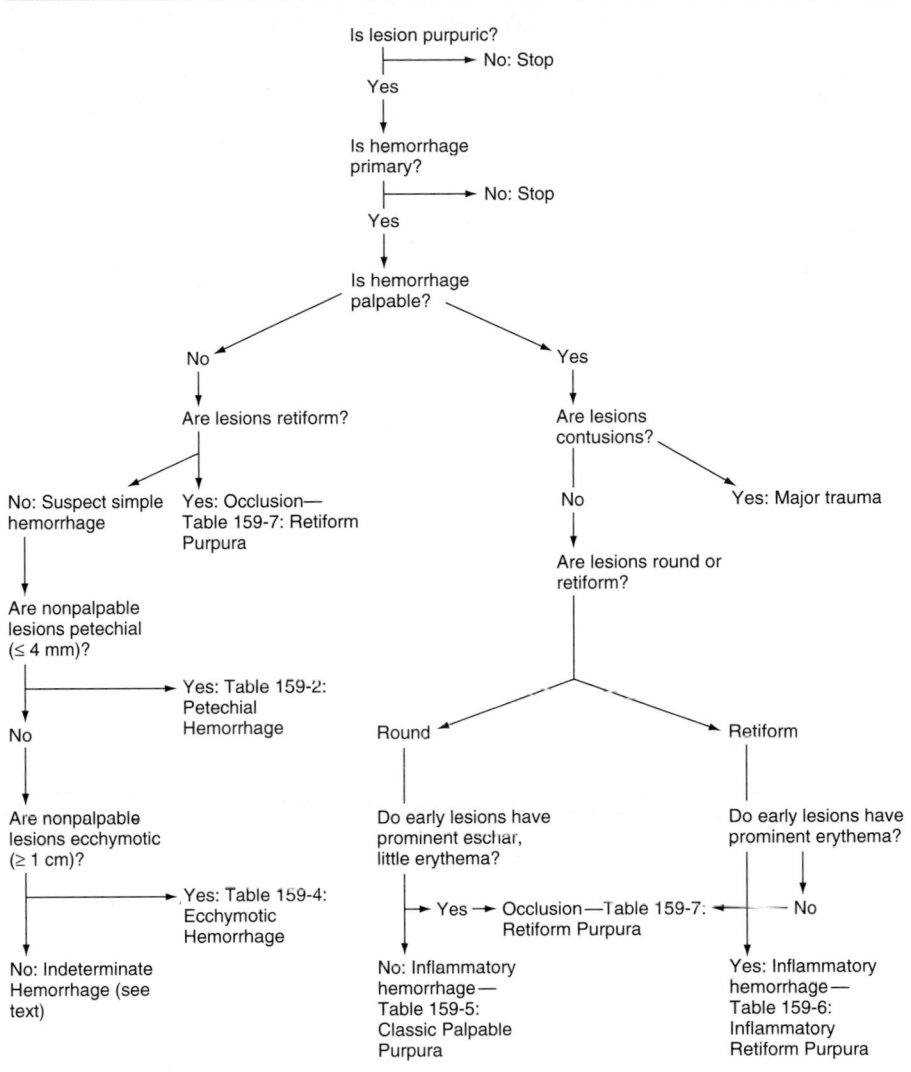

Algorithm for assessing purpura.

tation from hemosiderin and melanin in dermis. In many patients with the Schamberg's disease variant, the petechiae are not palpable. Clinical features that distinguish the subsets of pigmented purpura are summarized in Table 159-3. Occasionally, viral syndromes may present with widespread petechiae, which in some patients are not palpable. Enteroviral syndromes seem most likely to produce this outcome. Very rarely, benign hypergammaglobulinemic purpura can present as nonpalpable petechiae.

Macular hemorrhage >4 mm and <1 cm in diameter (intermediate or indeterminate hemorrhage) can be due to most of the causes of either petechial or ecchymotic hemorrhage. Laboratory studies are therefore less directed, and physicians must screen for both platelet and procoagulant problems. Patients who are immunocompromised may have little or no inflammatory response to organisms, and therefore septic lesions may lack palpability in these patients. Another disorder that often presents with similar-sized macular lesions is benign hypergammaglobulinemic purpura of Waldenström.[39,40] This syndrome is seen most characteristically as an idiopathic syndrome in young women, with recurring crops of

TABLE 159-2

Differential Diagnosis of Nonpalpable Petechiae[37,113]

I. Hemostatically relevant thrombocytopenia*
  A. Diminished platelet production
    1. Congenital and childhood defects (e.g., Wiskott-Aldrich syndrome, May-Hegglin anomaly)[114]
    2. Acquired defects
      a. Acute viral infections: rubella, cytomegalovirus, Epstein-Barr virus
      b. Nutritional deficiencies: vitamin B_{12}, folate, iron
      c. Marrow infiltration, fibrosis, or failure
      d. Drug- or toxin-related marrow toxicity or idiosyncratic reaction
  B. Altered distribution
    1. Hypersplenism/congestive splenomegaly (platelet count rarely <50,000/μL)
  C. Increased destruction
    1. Immune thrombocytopenias
      a. (Auto) immune thrombocytopenia (ITP)
    2. Secondary immune thrombocytopenia
      a. Lupus, lymphoma, CLL
      b. Drug: quinine, quinidine, heparin, many others[113]
      c. Infection-induced: posttransfusion; neonatal isoimmune; alloimmune
    3. Disseminated intravascular coagulation
    4. Thrombotic thrombocytopenia purpura
    5. Thrombocytopenia of extracorporeal circulation (cardiopulmonary bypass)
II. Abnormal platelet function
  A. Congenital or hereditary platelet function defects
  B. Acquired platelet function defects
    1. Aspirin
    2. Renal or hepatic insufficiency
    3. Monoclonal gammopathy
  C. Thrombocytosis in myeloproliferative disease (often >1,000,000/mL)
III. Nonplatelet etiologies
  A. Spiking elevations of intravascular venous pressure (Valsalva-like maneuvers such as repeated vomiting, childbirth, paroxysmal coughing)
  B. Chronic pigmented purpuras
  C. Benign hypergammaglobulinemic purpura

*While the differential diagnosis of thrombocytopenia is extensive, the differential diagnosis of the most common settings in which the thrombocytopenia is low enough to explain hemorrhage is much more limited.

macular hemorrhage, most often on the legs, frequently after exercise or prolonged standing. In women middle-aged and older, it may be associated with Sjögren's or sicca syndrome, lupus, rheumatoid arthritis, or rarely a lymphoproliferative syndrome or monoclonal gammopathy.[40] A polyclonal gammopathy is the typical finding, but the most distinctive finding is an IgG rheumatoid factor that marks as a 12- to 15-s immune complex on analytic ultracentrifugation.

Ecchymoses have multiple etiologies and are probably the most common form of hemorrhage (Table 159-4). They are almost always localized by minor trauma and therefore typically develop in areas prone to trauma (dorsum of hand, pretibial area, extensor forearm, lateral or anterior thighs) and in a geometric pattern, usually linear or rectangular (Figs. 159-2 and 159-3). Petechial hemorrhage arranged linearly, often with skip areas, may have the same significance as ecchymoses, especially when the petechiae are themselves asymmetric or linear rather than symmetric and round. Easy bruising is a common complaint, most often due to the dermal effects of chronic sun injury, glucocorticoids, or (in some geographic areas) scurvy. In some individuals, usually women, no abnormalities may be found after detailed study, leaving the etiology uncertain. Less commonly, ecchymoses may result from a mild hereditary bleeding disorder.

Contusions and hematomas are usually due to trauma significant enough to be remembered. Such lesions are often swollen and therefore palpable and tender; they may also show erythema or abrasions, depending on the degree of trauma.

Determining the age of ecchymoses and contusions can be a critical aspect of forensic medicine and in suspected abuse, but recent studies have suggested that dating hemorrhage is far less precise than reported earlier.[41–43] A bruise may become more prominent with the passage of hours or days due to continued bleeding from the ruptured vessels or to a delay in reaching the surface because of deflection by fascial planes and other anatomic structures. Additionally, bruises may move under gravity, such as those related to a laceration on the upper forehead. The subcutaneous hemorrhage can slide downwards over the eyebrow ridge and appear in the orbit, to give a "black eye." Similarly, a bruise of the upper arm or thigh may surface lower down around the elbow or knee.[41] Another factor in the delayed prominence of hemorrhage is hemolysis of the extravasated cells, inasmuch as free hemoglobin stains tissues more diffusely than intact red blood cells.

Chemical degradation of hemoglobin into hemosiderin, biliverdin, and bilirubin causes a sequence of color changes from purple or bluish brown, to greenish brown or green, and finally to yellow before completely fading. Variables affecting color changes in bruising include the size of the extravasation (a larger bruise may contain more color changes due to delay in resolution from the margin inward), the age and constitution of the individual (severely sun-damaged skin resolves purpura much more slowly), and individual idiosyncrasies such as persistent coagulation defects.

Hemosiderin does not usually appear within the first 2 or 3 days. Hematoidin, another breakdown product of blood pigment, can appear in old bruises and in hematomas after the first week.

The capillaries of the subcutaneous tissues make the greatest contribution to bruising. Data are sparse regarding the reliability of wound dating by appearance. There was a consensus that red, blue, and purple are early colors; greens show after 4 to 7 days; and yellow color is delayed until after the seventh day. In experiments with cattle, the sequence of color development was red from 15 min to 2 days (due to red cells and free hemoglobin), green on days 3 and 4, and yellow and orange from days 4 to 6 (due to bilirubin). Recent studies have challenged this consensus with the demonstration that red, blue, purple, or black coloration can develop from within 1 h of bruising up to 21 days.[42,43] A bruise with yellow color is at least 18 h old in any individual, although the development of a yellow color occurs significantly faster in persons younger than 65 years of age.[42]

PALPABLE OR RETIFORM PURPURA The differential diagnosis of inflammatory hemorrhage, including vasculitis, is extensive. Summarized in Tables 159-5 and 159-6, such syndromes have been reviewed and are covered elsewhere in this text. Examples of classic palpable purpura, target lesions, and inflammatory retiform purpura are provided in Figs. 159-4, 159-5, and 159-6.

It is critical to distinguish vascular injury in which inflammation predominates from processes in which microvascular thrombosis or occlusion is the primary mechanism. Table 159-7 summarizes the major differential possibilities for microvascular occlusion, characterized clinically by noninflammatory retiform purpura (Fig. 159-7) and histologically by bland (noninflammatory) occlusion of

TABLE 159-3

Chronic Pigmented Purpura*

	Schamberg's Disease	Itching Purpura	Pigmented Purpuric Lichenoid Dermatosis of Gougerot and Blum	Lichen Aureus	Purpura Annularis Telangiectodes (Majocchi's Disease)
Male/Female	Usually male	Usually male	Male	—	Either sex
Age	Childhood upward	Adult	40–60 years old	—	Adolescent, young adult
Usual site	Lower legs	Ankles, spreading to lower body, more prominent in areas of friction with clothing	Legs	Anywhere, often solitary lesions	Anywhere
Lesional appearance	Irregular patches, orange-brown, cayenne pepper spots	Erythematous, orange, purpuric macules, may become confluent	Similar to Schamberg's, but also has lichenoid papules	Rust- to purple-colored (seldom golden); zosteriform lesions reported	1–3 cm plaques, usually annular initially; telangiectasias, purple, yellow, or brown with cayenne pepper spots
Lesional course	Lesions may clear while new ones develop	Lesions may clear	Same as Schamberg's	Lesion often persists for years	Lesions persist for years, may slowly extend or develop central atrophy
Disease course	Chronic	Remission after a few months	Chronic	Chronic	Chronic
Symptoms	Occasionally pruritic	Pruritus prominent	Asymptomatic	Asymptomatic	Usually asymptomatic

*Common histologic picture: extravasation of red cells, hemosiderin in macrophages, superficial small vessels may show lumenal narrowing, endothelial swelling, perivascular lymphocytic infiltrate.

dermal vessels. Space precludes discussion of the syndromes important in microvascular occlusion. References are appended to listings in Table 159-7. Medicine has seen important advances in understanding hypercoaguable states in recent years, especially in the areas of the protein C–thrombomodulin pathway, factor V Leiden,

antiphospholipid antibody syndrome, and homocystinuria.[44–50] It is important to recognize that the causes of microvascular thrombosis or occlusion overlap, but are not identical to, the causes of thrombotic disorders of larger vessels. For example, antithrombin III deficiency is an important risk factor for large vein thrombosis but

TABLE 159-4

Differential Diagnosis of Nonpalpable Ecchymotic Hemorrhage

I. Procoagulant defect[115,116]
   A. Hemophilia
   B. Anticoagulant use
   C. Disseminated intravascular coagulation
   D. Vitamin K deficiency
   E. Hepatic insufficiency with poor procoagulant synthesis
II. Poor dermal support of vessels[117–119]
   A. Actinic (senile) purpura
   B. Glucocorticoid therapy, topical or systemic
   C. Vitamin C deficiency (scurvy)
   D. Systemic amyloidosis (light chain–related, some familial types)
   E. Ehlers-Danlos syndrome (some types)
   F. Pseudoxanthoma elasticum
III. Other
   A. Benign hypergammaglobulinemic purpura
   B. Psychogenic purpura

SOURCE: Modified from Piette,[37] with permission.

FIGURE 159-2

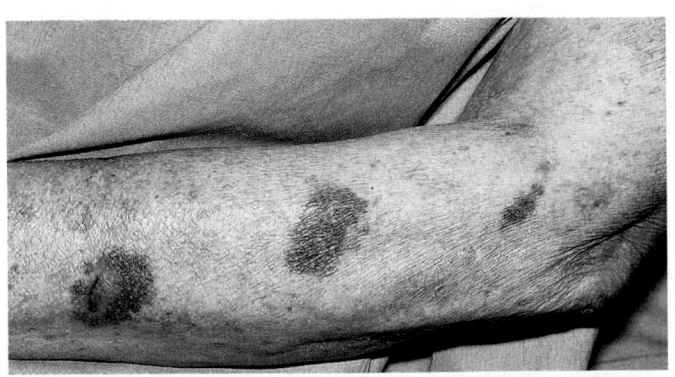

Nonpalpable ecchymoses in a patient on chronic oral glucocorticoid therapy. Note the rectangular and linear lesions that suggest the minor trauma component. (*From Piette,[37] used with permission.*)

FIGURE 159-3

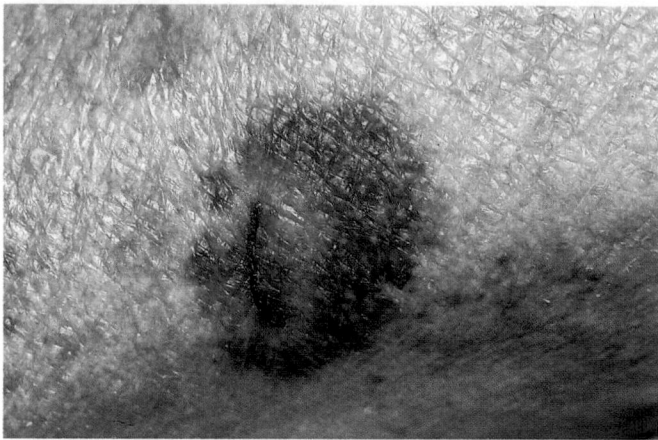

Close-up of one of the ecchymotic areas in Fig. 159-2, showing a linear traumatic injury, with surrounding ecchymosis. (*From Piette,*[37] *used with permission.*)

rarely, if ever, is responsible for occlusion of the dermal microvasculature. Likewise, monoclonal cryoglobulins are a distinctive and important cause of dermal vessel occlusion in acral areas but do not occlude major veins. Therefore, expertise in this area of cutaneous disease can be critical not only in interpreting the cutaneous changes but also in suggesting likely individual syndromes responsible for occlusion. The proper interpretation of morphologic findings of purpura can be an important aid in the timely and accurate evaluation of causes of cutaneous hemorrhage.

TABLE 159-5

Partial Differential Diagnosis for Discrete, Round Palpable Purpura with Early Prominent Erythema

Classic palpable purpura: Inflammatory hemorrhage[37,120]
A. Small vessel leukocytoclastic vasculitis[120,121]
    1. Idiopathic, drug- or infection-related
        a. IgG or IgM small vessel vasculitis ("hypersensitivity" vasculitis)
        b. IgA dermal vessel vasculitis (Henoch-Schönlein purpura)[38,122]
        c. Erythema elevatum diutinum
        d. Septic vasculitis
B. Small vessel component of leukocytoclastic or granulomatous vasculitides that may affect both small and medium-size cutaneous vessels
    1. ANCA-positive vasculitides
        a. Wegener's granulomatosis
        b. Microscopic polyarteritis nodosa
        c. Churg-Strauss syndrome
    2. Mixed cryoglobulinemia
    3. Lupus or rheumatoid vasculitis
C. Small vessel injury, not leukocytoclastic
    1. Erythema multiforme
    2. Pityriasis lichenoides et varioliformis acute (PLEVA)
    3. Chronic pigmented purpuras (occasionally)
    4. Benign hypergammaglobulinemic purpura
Target lesions: Classic three-zone target lesions are almost always due to erythema multiforme

SOURCE: Modified from Piette,[37] with permission.

TABLE 159-6

Differential Diagnosis of Inflammatory Retiform Purpura

   I. Dermal vessel leukocytoclastic vasculitis
      A. IgA vasculitis[38,123]
  II. Dermal vessel inflammation and occlusion or constriction
      A. Livedoid vasculitis
      B. Septic vasculitis
      C. Chilblains (pernio)
 III. Dermal and subcutaneous vessels usually involved
      A. Wegener's granulomatosis
      B. Allergic granulomatosis of Churg-Strauss syndrome
      C. Microscopic polyarteritis nodosa
      D. Benign cutaneous polyarteritis nodosa
      E. Pyoderma gangrenosum

NOTE: Many of these syndromes or diseases present with classic palpable purpura morphologies.
SOURCE: Modified from Piette,[37] with permission.

FIGURE 159-4

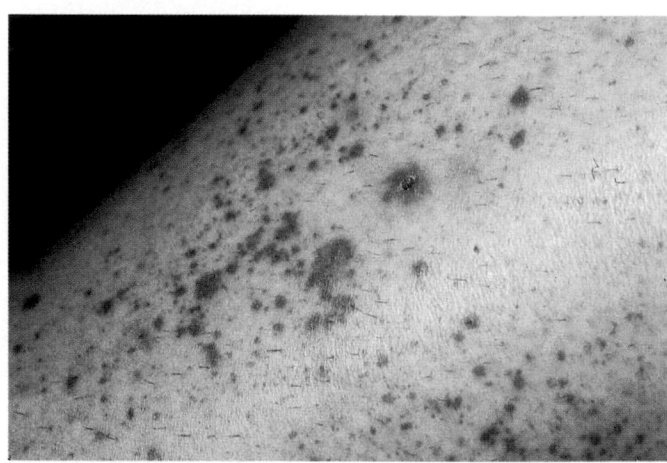

Classic palpable purpura on the leg of a patient with IgA vasculitis. Partial blanching of an early lesion on compression supports the clinical impression of inflammatory hemorrhage.

FIGURE 159-5

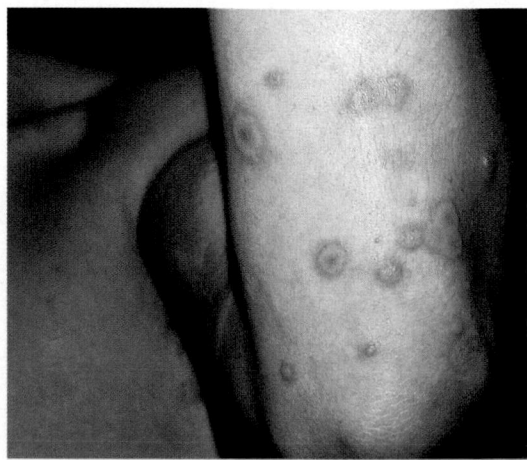

Target lesions with central hemorrhage in a patient with erythema multiforme (EM). Unfortunately, many patients with EM do not develop target lesions, and some may develop lesions clinically identical to those in Fig. 159-4.

FIGURE 159-6

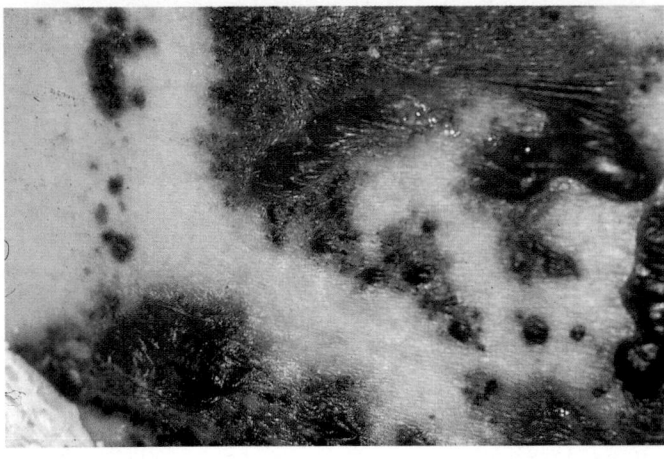

Inflammatory retiform palpable purpura in a patient with IgA vasculitis. The initial erythematous phase is still present but fading in these lesions.

FIGURE 159-7

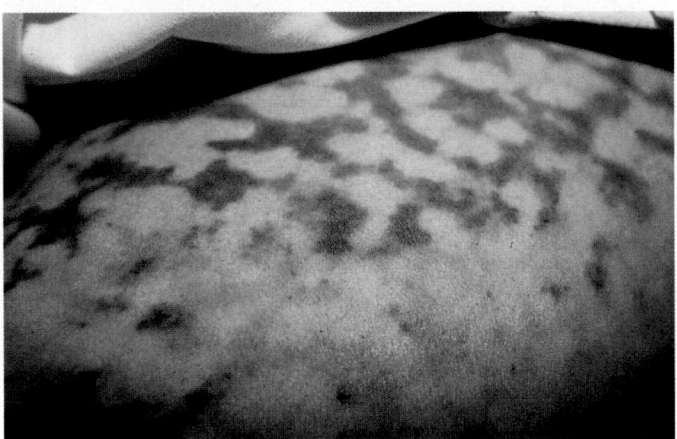

Noninflammatory retiform palpable purpura on the thigh in a patient with disseminated intravascular coagulation secondary to sepsis. None of the lesional color faded on compression. The biopsy showed multiple dermal vessels occluded by clot without inflammation.

TABLE 159-7

Differential Diagnosis of Noninflammatory Retiform Purpura

I. Occlusion due to microvascular platelet plugs
  A. Heparin necrosis[91,124]
  B. Thrombotic thrombocytopenic purpura (idiopathic, drug, post–bone marrow transplantation[125]; platelet plugs form primarily in visceral vessels; cutaneous hemorrhage, while occasionally related to dermal vessel plugging, is due more often to thrombocytopenia and simple hemorrhage
  C. Myeloproliferative disease, usually with thrombocytosis[126]
II. Cold-related gelling or agglutination
  A. Cryoglobulinemia, monoclonal or mixed[93,127]; many lesions of mixed cryoglobulinemia are inflammatory palpable purpura secondary to immune complex complement activation
  B. Cryofibrinogenemia[128,129]; most cryofibrinogens are incidental findings in hospitalized patients
  C. Cold agglutinins[130]; rarely cause occlusion; usually cause hemolysis or are asymptomatic
III. Occlusion due to organisms living in vessels
  A. Vessel-invasive fungi; *Mucormycosis, Aspergillus, Cephalosporum,* and others, usually in immunocompromised patients
  B. Ecthyma gangrenosum[131]; usually due to *Pseudomonas* species proliferating in adventitia of subcutaneous supply arteriole
  C. Disseminated strongyloidiasis[132]
IV. Local or systemic alterations in control of coagulation
  A. Disseminated intravascular coagulation[133]
  B. Homozygous protein C or protein S deficiency[134,135]
  C. Acquired protein C or protein S deficiency[136,137]
  D. Coumadin necrosis[138,139]
  E. Antiphospholipid antibody (lupus anticoagulant) syndrome[48,49]
  F. Paroxysmal nocturnal hemoglobinuria[140,141]
  G. Atrophie blanche or livedoid vasculitis[142,143]
V. Embolization or crystal embolization
  A. Cholesterol emboli[144]
  B. Oxalate crystal deposition[145]
  C. Thrombus from atrial myxoma, marantic or septic endocarditis
  D. Crystalglobulin vasculopathy: multiple myeloma[94,95]
VI. Other
  A. Cutaneous calciphylaxis[146–148]
  B. Sickling, complicated by reticulocyte adhesion
  C. Hypereosinophilic syndrome: cutaneous microthrombi[20]

SOURCE: Modified from Piette,[37] with permission.

REFERENCES

1. Erslev A: Clinical manifestations and classification of erythrocyte disorders, in *Williams Hematology,* 5th ed, edited by E Beutler, M Lichtman, B Coller, T Kipps. New York, McGraw-Hill, 1995, pp 441–447
2. Williams W: Approach to the patient, in *Williams Hematology,* 5th ed, edited by E Beutler, M Lichtman, B Coller, T Kipps. New York, McGraw-Hill, 1995, pp 3–8
3. Bull B, Breton-Gorius J: Morphology of the erythron, in *Williams Hematology,* 5th ed, edited by E Beutler, M Lichtman, B Coller, T Kipps. New York, McGraw-Hill, 1995, pp 349–363
4. Fairbanks V, Beutler E: Iron deficiency, in *Williams Hematology,* 5th ed, edited by E Beutler, M Lichtman, B Coller, T Kipps. New York, McGraw-Hill, 1995, pp 490–511
5. Wood M, Elwood P: Symptoms of iron deficiency anemia: A community survey. *Br J Prev Soc Med* **20**:117, 1966
6. Callinan V, O'Hare J: Cardboard chewing: Cause and effect of iron deficiency anemia. *Am J Med* **85**:449, 1988
7. Sears D: Anemia of chronic disease. *Med Clin North Am* **76**:567, 1992
8. Babior B: The megaloblastic anemias, in *Williams Hematology,* 5th ed, edited by E Beutler, M Lichtman, B Coller, T Kipps. New York, McGraw-Hill, 1995, pp 471–489
9. Baker S et al: Hyperpigmentation of skin. *Br Med J* **1**:1713, 1963
10. Gilliam J, Cox A: Epidermal changes in vitamin B$_{12}$ deficiency. *Arch Dermatol* **107**:231, 1973
11. Downham T et al: Hyperpigmentation and folate deficiency. *Arch Dermatol* **112**:562, 1976
12. Ridley C: Pigmentation of fingertips and nails in vitamin B$_{12}$ deficiency. *Br J Dermatol* **97**:105, 1977
13. Howitz J, Schwartz M: Vitiligo, achlorhydria, and pernicious anemia. *Lancet* **1**:1331, 1971
14. Hild D: Folate losses from the skin in exfoliative dermatitis. *Arch Intern Med* **123**:51, 1969
15. Beck W: Neuropsychiatric consequences of cobalamin deficiency. *Adv Intern Med* **36**:33, 1991
16. Erslev A: Anemia of endocrine disorders, in *Williams Hematology,* 5th ed, edited by E Beutler, M Lichtman, B Coller, T Kipps. New York, McGraw-Hill, 1995, pp 462–466
17. Myers B et al: POEMS syndrome with idiopathic flushing mimicking carcinoid syndrome. *Am J Med* **90**:646, 1991
18. Longley J et al: The mast cell and mast cell disease. *J Am Acad Dermatol* **32**(4):545, 1995
19. Kurzrock R, Cohen P: Mucocutaneous paraneoplastic manifestations of hematologic malignancies. *Am J Med* **99**(2):207, 1995
20. Weller PF: The idiopathic hypereosinophilic syndrome. *Blood* **83**(10):2759, 1994

21. Schmuth M et al: Cutaneous involvement in prelymphomatous angioimmunoblastic lymphadenopathy. *J Am Acad Dermatol* **36**:290, 1997

22. Dintenflass I: A preliminary outline of the blood high viscosity syndromes. *Arch Intern Med* **118**:427, 1966

23. Bilgrami S, Greenberg B: Polycythemia rubra vera. *Semin Oncol* **22**(4):307, 1995

24. Taylor P et al: Efficacy of recombinant interferon-alpha (rIFN-α) in polycythaemia vera: A study of 17 patients and an analysis of published data. *Br J Haematol* **92**:55, 1996

25. Kligman A et al: Water-induced itching without cutaneous signs. Aquagenic pruritus. *Arch Dermatol* **122**:183, 1986

26. de Peloux Menagé H, Greaves M: Aquagenic pruritus. *Semin Dermatol* **14**:313, 1995

27. Handfield-Jones S et al: Aquagenic pruritus associated with juvenile xanthogranuloma. *Clin Exp Dermatol* **18**:253, 1993

28. Swerlick R: Photochemotherapy treatment of pruritis associated with polycythemia vera. *J Am Acad Dermatol* **13**:675, 1988

29. Barnette H et al: When does central cyanosis become detectable? *Clin Invest Med* **1**:39, 1990

30. Carpenter K: A comprehensive review of cyanosis. *Crit Care Nurse* **13**:66, 1993

31. Beutler E: Methemoglobinemia and other causes of cyanosis, in *Williams Hematology,* 5th ed, edited by E Beutler, M Lichtman, B Coller, T Kipps. New York, McGraw-Hill, 1995, pp 654–663

32. Johnson C, Kross B: Continuing importance of nitrate contamination of groundwater and wells in rural areas. *Am J Ind Med* **18**:449, 1990

33. Packman C, Leddy J: Acquired hemolytic anemia due to warm-reacting autoantibodies, in *Williams Hematology,* 5th ed, edited by E Beutler, M Lichtman, B Coller, T Kipps. New York, McGraw-Hill, 1995, pp 677–685

34. Levine L et al: Extramedullary hematopoiesis. *Arch Dermatol* **120**:1282, 1984

35. Pedro-Botet J et al: Cutaneous myeloid metaplasia with dysplastic features in idiopathic myelofibrosis. *Int J Dermatol* **27**:179, 1988

36. Patel B et al: Cutaneous extramedullary hematopoiesis. *J Am Acad Dermatol* **32**:805, 1995

37. Piette WW: The differential diagnosis of purpura from a morphologic perspective. *Adv Dermatol* **9**:3, 1994

38. Piette WW, Stone MS: A cutaneous sign of IgA-associated small dermal vessel leukocytoclastic vasculitis in adults (Henoch-Schönlein purpura). *Arch Dermatol* **125**:53, 1989

39. Finder KA et al: Hypergammaglobulinemic purpura of Waldenström. *J Am Acad Dermatol* **23**:669, 1990

40. Habib G et al: Hypergammaglobulinemic purpura of Waldenström associated with systemic lupus erythematosus: Report of a case and review of the literature. *Lupus* **4**:19, 1995

41. Knight B: The pathology of wounds, in *Forensic Pathology,* 2d ed. London, Arnold, 1996, pp 133–169

42. Langlois N, Gresham G: The ageing of bruises: A review and study of the colour changes with time. *Forensic Sci Int* **50**:227, 1991

43. Stephenson T, Bialas Y: Estimation of the age of bruising. *Arch Dis Child* **74**:53, 1996

44. Thomas D, Roberts H: Hypercoagulability in venous and arterial thrombosis. *Ann Intern Med* **126**:638, 1997

45. Cadroy Y et al: The thrombodulin/protein C/protein S anticoagulant pathway modulates the thrombogenic properties of the normal resting and stimulated endothelium. *Arterioscler Thromb Vasc Biol* **17**(3):520, 1997

46. Ridker P et al: Age-specific incidence rates of venous thromboembolism among heterozygous carriers of factor V Leiden mutation. *Ann Intern Med* **126**:528, 1997

47. Hille E et al: Mortality and causes of death in families with the factor V Leiden mutation (resistance to activated protein C). *Blood* **89**:1963, 1997

48. Asherson R, Cervera R: Antiphospholipid syndrome. *J Invest Dermatol* **100**:21s, 1993

49. Nahass GT: Antiphospholipid antibodies and the antiphospholipid syndrome. *J Am Acad Dermatol* **36**:149, 1997

50. Mandel H et al: Coexistence of hereditary homocystinuria and factor V Leiden—effect on thrombosis. *N Engl J Med* **334**:763, 1996

51. Kurzrock R et al: Clinical manifestations of vasculitis in patients with solid tumors: A case report and review of the literature. *Arch Intern Med* **154**:334, 1994

52. Piette W: An approach to cutaneous changes caused by hematologic malignancies. *Dermatol Clin* **7**:467, 1989

53. Piette W: Leukemia and lymphoma, in *Dermatological Signs of Internal Disease,* 2d ed, edited by J Callen, J Jorizzo, K Greer, N Penneys, W Piette, J Zone, Philadelphia, Saunders, 1995, pp 129–136

54. Cohen P: Paraneoplastic dermatopathology: Cutaneous paraneoplastic syndromes. *Adv Dermatol* **11**:215, 1996

55. Dominey A, Tschen J: Cutaneous manifestations of dysproteinemias. *Dermatol Clin* **7**:449, 1989

56. Piette W: Myeloma, paraproteinemias, and the skin. *Med Clin North Am* **70**:155, 1986

57. Farell G: Fanconi's familial hypoplastic anaemia with some unusual features. *Med J Aust* **1**:116, 1976

58. Fanconi G: Familial constitutional panmyelocytopathy, Fanconi's anemia (FA) 1. Clinical aspects. *Semin Hematol* **4**:233, 1967

59. Tchou P, Kohn T: Dyskeratosis congenita: An autosomal dominant disorder. *J Am Acad Dermatol* **6**:1034, 1982

60. Bolognia J, Pawelek J: Biology of hypopigmentation. *J Am Acad Dermatol* **19**:217, 1988

61. Goldblatt J, Beighton P: Cutaneous manifestations of Gaucher disease. *Br J Dermatol* **111**:331, 1984

62. Mardini M et al: Niemann-Pick disease: Report of a case with skin involvement. *Am J Dis Child* **136**:650, 1982

63. Joliffe D, Sarkany I: Niemann-Pick type III and Crohn's disease. *J R Soc Med* **76**:307, 1983

64. Etzioni A: Adhesion molecules—their role in health and disease. *Pediatr Res* **39**:191, 1996

65. Wahl S et al: Regulation of leukocyte adhesion and signaling in inflammation and disease. *J Leuk Biol* **59**:789, 1996

66. Blume R, Wolff S: The Chédiak-Higashi syndrome: Studies in four patients and a review of the literature. *Medicine* **51**:247, 1977

67. Griscelli C et al: A syndrome associating partial albinism and immunodeficiency. *Am J Med* **65**:691, 1978

68. Howard T et al: The 47-kD protein increased in neutrophil actin dysfunction with 47- and 89-kD protein abnormalities is lymphocyte-specific protein. *Blood* **83**:231, 1994

69. Ormerod A: The Wiscott-Aldrich syndrome. *Int J Dermatol* **24**:77, 1985

70. Rosenstein Y et al: CD43, a molecule defective in Wiskott-Aldrich syndrome, binds ICAM-1. *Nature* **354**:233, 1991

71. Bayle P et al: Neutrophilic dermatosis: A case of overlapping syndrome with monoclonal antineutrophil cytoplasmic autoantibody activity. *Dermatology* **189**:69, 1994

72. Younus J, Ahmed A: The relationship of pemphigus to neoplasia. *J Am Acad Dermatol* **23**:498, 1990

73. Anhalt G: Paraneoplastic pemphigus. *Adv Dermatol* **12**:77, 1997

74. Whitworth S et al: Acquired immunobullous disease: A cutaneous manifestation of IgM macroglobulinaemia. *Br J Dermatol* **135**:283, 1996

75. McEvoy M, Connolly S: Linear IgA dermatosis: Association with malignancy. *J Am Acad Dermatol* **22**:59, 1990

76. Levi F et al: Non-Hodgkin's lymphomas, chronic lymphocytic leukemias and skin cancers. *Br J Cancer* **74**:1847, 1996

77. Sanchez-Guerrero J et al: Vasculitis as a paraneoplastic syndrome. Report of 11 cases and review of the literature. *J Rheumatol* **17**:1458, 1990

78. Milone G et al: Cutaneous vasculitis in non Hodgkin's lymphoma. *Haematologica* **80**:529, 1995

79. Pavlidis N et al: Cutaneous lymphocytic vasculopathy in lymphoproliferative disorders—a paraneoplastic lymphocytic vasculitis of the skin. *Leuk Lymphoma* **16**:477, 1995

80. Ruiz-Maldonado R et al: Edematous, scarring vasculitic panniculitis: A new multisystem disease with malignant potential. *J Am Acad Dermatol* **32**:37, 1995

81. Freeman R, Dover J: Autonomic neurodermatology (part I): Erythromelalgia, reflex sympathetic dystrophy, and livedo reticularis (review). *Semin Neurol* **12**:385, 1992

82. Drenth J, Michiels J: Erythromelalgia and erythermalgia: Diagnostic differentiation. *Int J Dermatol* **33**:393, 1994

83. Michiels J, Drenth J: Erythromelalgia and erythermalgia: Lumpers and splitters. *Int J Dermatol* **33**:412, 1994

84. Fleischer Jr AB, Resnick SD: Livedo reticularis. *Dermatol Clin* **8**:347, 1990

85. Picascia DD, Pellegrini JR: Livedo reticularis. *Cutis* **39**:429, 1987

86. Pereira A et al: Anti-Sa cold agglutinin of IgA class requiring plasma-exchange therapy as early manifestation of multiple myeloma. *Ann Hematol* **66**:315, 1993

87. Maroon M: Polycythemia rubra vera presenting as livedo reticularis. *J Am Acad Dermatol* **26**:264, 1992

88. Eng A: Cutaneous expressions of antiphospholipid syndromes. *Semin Thromb Hemost* **20**:71, 1994

89. Weir N et al: Livedo reticularis associated with hereditary protein C deficiency and recurrent thromboembolism. *Br J Dermatol* **132**:283, 1995

90. Donnet A et al: Cerebral infarction, livedo reticularis, and familial deficiency in antithrombin-III (letter). *Stroke* **23**:611, 1992

91. Gross A et al: Heparin-associated thrombocytopenia and thrombosis (HATT) presenting with livedo reticularis. *Int J Dermatol* **32**:276, 1993

92. Frankel D et al: Acral lividosis—a sign of myeloproliferative diseases. Hyperleukocytosis syndrome in chronic myelogenous leukemia. *Arch Dermatol* **123**:921, 1987

93. Speight E, Lawrence C: Reticulate purpura, cryoglobuliaemia and livedo reticularis. *Br J Dermatol* **129**:319, 1993

94. Hasegawa H et al: Multiple myeloma–associated systemic vasculopathy due to crystalglobulin or polyarteritis nodosa. *Arthritis Rheum* **39**:330, 1996

95. Ball N et al: Crystalglobulinemia syndrome. A manifestation of multiple myeloma. *Cancer* **71**:1231, 1993

96. Furie R et al: Syndrome of acquired factor X deficiency and systemic amyloidosis. *N Engl J Med* **297**:81, 1977

97. Carroll C et al: Atrophic outpouchings of abdominal skin. *Arch Dermatol* **132**:223, 1996

98. Lipsker D et al: Examination of cutaneous macroglobulinosis by immunoelectron microscopy. *Br J Dermatol* **135**:287, 1996

99. Jenkins R et al: Cutaneous crystalline deposits in myeloma. *Arch Dermatol* **130**:484, 1994

100. Requena L et al: Follicular spicules of the nose: A peculiar cutaneous manifestation of multiple myeloma with cryoglobulinemia. *J Am Acad Dermatol* **32**:834, 1995

101. Dineen A, Dicken C: Scleromyxedema. *J Am Acad Dermatol* **33**:37, 1995

102. Crocker A, Farber S: Niemann-Pick disease: A review of 18 patients. *Medicine* **37**:1, 1958

103. Griffiths W, Daneshbod K: Pseudoxanthomatous mastocytosis. *Br J Dermatol* **93**:91, 1975

104. Jubert C et al: Anetoderma may reveal cutaneous plasmacytoma and benign cutaneous lymphoid hyperplasia. *Arch Dermatol* **131**:365, 1995

105. Kahn L et al: Florid sarcoid reaction associated with lymphoma of the skin. *Cancer* **33**:1117, 1974

106. Rapini R: Multicentric reticulohistiocytosis. *Clin Dermatol* **11**:107, 1993

107. Van Dijk E: Ichthyosiform atrophy of the skin with internal malignant diseases. *Dermatologica* **127**:413, 1963

108. Ellis D, Yates R: Sign of Leser-Trélat. *Clin Dermatol* **11**:141, 1993

109. Bull R et al: Eosinophilic folliculitis: A self-limiting illness in patients being treated for haematological malignancy. *Br J Dermatol* **129**:178, 1993

110. Gross A et al: Fever, maculopapular eruption, and lymphadenopathy. Angioimmunoblastic lymphadenopathy (AILD). *Arch Dermatol* **130**(12):1551, 1994

111. Piette W: Hematologic associations of leg ulcers. *Clin Dermatol* **3/4**:66, 1990

112. Aractingi S et al: Specific mucosal erosions in hypereosinophilic syndrome. Evidence for eosinophil protein deposition. *Arch Dermatol* **132**:535, 1996

113. Rutherford CJ, Frenkel EP: Thrombocytopenia: Issues in diagnosis and therapy. *Med Clin North Am* **78**:555, 1994

114. Najean Y, Lecompte T: Hereditary thrombocytopenias in childhood. *Semin Thromb Hemost* **21**:294, 1995

115. Kottke-Marchant K: Laboratory diagnosis of hemorrhagic and thrombotic disorders. *Hematol Oncol Clin North Am* **8**:809, 1994

116. Sham R, Francis C: Evaluation of mild bleeding disorders and easy bruising. *Blood Rev* **8**(2):98, 1994

117. Champion RH, Rook A: Idiopathic thrombocythemia—cutaneous manifestations. *Arch Dermatol* **87**:302, 1963

118. Piette WW: Purpura, in *Dermatological Signs of Internal Disease,* 2d ed, edited by JP Callen, JL Jorizzo, KE Greer, NS Penneys, WW Piette, JJ Zone. Philadelphia, Saunders, 1995, pp 87–95

119. Sams W Jr: Macular purpuras, in *Principles and Practice of Dermatology,* 2d ed, edited by W Sams Jr, P Lynch. New York, Churchill Livingstone, 1996, pp 559–564

120. Piette WW: Primary systemic vasculitis, in *Cutaneous Manifestations of Rheumatic Diseases,* edited by RD Sontheimer, TT Provost. Baltimore, Williams & Wilkins, 1996, pp 177–232

121. Jennette CJ et al: Vasculitis affecting the skin: A review. *Arch Dermatol* **130**:899, 1994

122. Tancrede-Bohin E et al: Schönlein-Henoch in adult patients: Predictive factors for IgA glomerulonephritis in a retrospective study of 57 cases. *Arch Dermatol* **133**(4):438, 1997

123. Piette WW: What is Schönlein-Henoch purpura, and why should we care? *Arch Dermatol* **133**:515, 1997

124. Warkentin T: Heparin-induced skin lesions. *Br J Haematol* **92**:494, 1996

125. Moake J, Byrnes J: Thrombotic microangiopathies associated with drugs and bone marrow transplantation. *Hematol Oncol Clin North Am* **10**:485, 1996

126. Sams W Jr: Diseases presenting with a livedo or stellate pattern, in *Principles and Practice of Dermatology,* 2d ed, edited by W Sams Jr, P Lynch. New York, Churchill Livingstone, 1996, pp 565–573

127. Cohen SJ et al: Cutaneous manifestations of cryoglobulinemia: Clinical and histopathologic study of seventy-two patients. *J Am Acad Dermatol* **25**:21, 1991

128. Smith S, Arkin C: Cryofibrinogenemia: Incidence, clinical correlations, and a review of the literature. *Am J Clin Pathol* **58**:524, 1972

129. McKee P, Kalbfleisch J: Incidence and significance of cryofibrinogenemia. *J Lab Clin Med* **61**:203, 1963

130. Stone MS et al: Cutaneous necrosis at sites of transfusion: Cold agglutinin disease (letter). *J Am Acad Dermatol* **19**:356, 1988

131. Greene S et al: Ecthyma gangrenosum: Report of clinical, histopathologic, and bacteriologic aspects of eight cases. *J Am Acad Dermatol* **11**:781, 1984

132. Ronan S et al: Disseminated strongylodiasis presenting as purpura. *J Am Acad Dermatol* **21**:1123, 1989

133. Robboy S et al: The skin in disseminated intravascular coagulation: Prospective analysis of thirty-six cases. *Br J Dermatol* **88**:221, 1973

134. Marlar RA, Neumann A: Neonatal purpura fulminans due to homozygous protein C or protein S deficiencies. *Semin Thromb Hemost* **16**:333, 1990

135. Dreyfus M et al: Treatment of homozygous protein C deficiency and neonatal purpura fulminans with a purified protein C concentrate. *N Engl J Med* **325**:1565, 1991

136. Frances RB Jr: Acquired purpura fulminans. *Semin Thromb Hemost* **16**:310, 1990

137. Manco-Johnson MJ et al: Lupus anticoagulant and protein S deficiency in children with postvaricella purpura fulminans or thrombosis. *J Pediatr* **128**:319, 1996

138. Schramm W et al: Treatment of coumarin-induced skin necrosis with a monoclonal antibody purified protein C concentrate. *Arch Dermatol* **129**:753, 1993

139. Gladson C et al: Coumarin necrosis, neonatal purpura fulminans, and protein C deficiency. *Arch Dermatol* **123**:1701a, 1987

140. Rietschel R et al: Skin lesions in nocturnal paroxysmal hemoglobinuria. *Arch Dermatol* **114**:560, 1978

141. Draelos Z, Hansen R: Hemorrhagic bullae in an anemic woman. *Arch Dermatol* **122**:1325, 1986

142. Bard J, Winkelman R: Livedo vasculitis: Segmental hyalinizing vasculitis of the dermis. *Arch Dermatol* **96**:489, 1967

143. Shornick J et al: Idiopathic atrophie blanche. *J Am Acad Dermatol* **8**:792, 1983

144. Falanga V et al: The cutaneous manifestations of cholesterol crystal embolization. *Arch Dermatol* **122**:1194, 1986

145. Greer KE et al: Primary oxalosis with livedo reticularis. *Arch Dermatol* **116**:213, 1980

146. Ivker R et al: Calciphylaxis in three patients with end stage renal disease. *Arch Dermatol* **131**:63, 1995

147. Hafner J et al: Uremic small-artery disease with medial calcification and intimal hyperplasia (so-called calciphylaxis): A complication of chronic renal failure and benefit from parathyroidectomy. *J Am Acad Dermatol* **33**:954, 1995

148. Rostaing L et al: Calciphylaxis in a chronic hemodialysis patient with protein S deficiency. *Am J Nephrol* **15**:524, 1995

Ruggero Caputo

Langerhans Cell Histiocytosis

Langerhans cell histiocytosis (LCH), previously called histiocytosis X, is a disease of unknown cause characterized by the proliferation of a distinct cell type that is S-100 and CD1a positive and contains cytoplasmic Langerhans granules.[1] LCH includes four main clinical forms: Letterer-Siwe disease (LSD), Hand-Schüller-Christian disease (HSCD), eosinophilic granuloma, and Hashimoto-Pritzker disease (HPD).[1,2]

In 1953, Lichtenstein[3] integrated the three previously described clinical conditions LSD, HSCD, and eosinophilic granuloma into one single nosologic entity called *histiocytosis X*; self-healing reticulohistiocytosis, a condition characterized by nodular, self-healing lesions restricted to the skin, was described by Hashimoto and Pritzker[4] in 1978. In 1969, Basset and Nezelof[5,6] demonstrated that the proliferating cells present in the lesions of these conditions share the ultrastructural characteristics of Langerhans cells. Thus, these conditions are now designated as *Langerhans cell histiocytosis*.[7]

CLINICAL FINDINGS

Letterer-Siwe Disease

LSD is the acute, disseminated multisystemic form of LCH. LSD begins within the first 6 months of life in one-third of cases and before 2 years of age in most of the others.[1,8] More than 20 congenital cases[9,10] and approximately 30 adult cases have been documented.[11–14]

Cutaneous manifestations are very common in LSD. The cutaneous lesions are characteristic and may represent the earliest sign of the disease. The typical lesion is a small translucent papule (1 to 2 mm in diameter), slightly raised, rose-yellow in color (Fig. 160-1A, -1B), and usually located on the trunk (Fig. 160-1A, -C, -D) and scalp (Fig. 160-1B).[1,8] The lesions frequently show scaling (Fig. 160-1A) and may become crusted and ulcerate (Fig. 160-1C, -D). Vesicles and pustules may occur,[1,15] simulating eczema, miliaria, scabies,[16] and varicella.[17] Purpura represents a poor prognostic sign.[1]

Cutaneous lesions appear in successive crops. The lesions tend to merge on the scalp, displaying a seborrheic dermatitis-like appearance, and on the folds (retroauricular, axillary, and genital) mimicking intertrigo.[1,8,15] In LSD, mucous membrane involvement, consisting of erosions and ulcerations, is rare. Nail changes including paronychia, nail fold destruction, onycholysis, subungual hyperkeratosis, and purpuric striae of the nail bed (Fig. 160-2)[18] are considered an unfavorable prognostic sign. Cutaneous manifestations in elderly patients (Fig. 160-3) are similar to those seen in LSD of early childhood.[11–14]

Systemic manifestions of LSD are extremely variable.

Pulmonary involvement can be detected in more than half of affected children.[1,2,8,9,13] Functional symptoms consist of dyspnea, cyanosis, and pneumothorax. The lungs may show a classic "honeycomb" appearance (Fig. 160-4). Pulmonary lesions can be asymptomatic, but can also cause death.[9]

Hepatosplenomegaly is never the initial sign of the disease. Marked hepatomegaly is a frequent complication and is a prognostically unfavorable sign, particularly when accompanied by jaundice.[1,2,8,19] Splenomegaly is less frequent. *Lymphadenopathy* is rarely prominent but has been noted in 25 to 75 percent of fatal cases.[19] In the later stages of the disease, *bone lesions* occur in about 60 percent,[1,2,8] and more frequently flat bones, vertebral bones, and cranial bones are involved. Osteolytic lesions, either asymptomatic or accompanied by pain and functional impairment, are generally multiple and appear gradually. Their presence is more frequent in cases with a favorable course. Teeth may be lost prematurely. Chronic otitis media is frequent.[8] *Hemopoietic involvement* is rare.[1,2] When spontaneous thrombocytopenia and severe anemia occur, death is almost certain.[2] Bone marrow involvement is characterized by the presence of numerous histiocytic cells.[2,8] *Fever* is frequently present.

Hand-Schüller-Christian Disease

HSCD is the chronic, progressive, multifocal form of LCH. HSCD begins between the second and sixth year of life in 70 percent of cases and before the age of 30 in 91 percent.[1] The disorder is characterized by the following four findings: bone lesions, diabetes insipidus, exophthalmos, and mucocutaneous lesions.[1,2,8,19–21] It is uncommon for all four manifestations to be seen together in the same patient.[1]

Bone lesions are the most frequent manifestations of HSCD (80 percent of cases). They preferentially involve the calvarium, especially in the temporoparietal region, where the infiltrate causes well-limited osteolytic areas that merge to give a typical "map" appearance (Fig. 160-5). Osteolysis of the lower maxillary bones is also frequent, and therefore on x-ray the teeth appear to be floating in the mouth.[22] Bone lesions of the mastoidal region may cause otitis media. These lesions are usually painful but not tender.[2]

Diabetes insipidus is present in over 50 percent of cases and is easily controlled by vasopressin. It occurs more often in children and in patients with involvement of the skull and the orbits.[23] Diabetes insipidus is considered a prognostically favorable symptom.

Exophthalmus[1,8] usually appears later on; it is present in 10 to 30 percent of cases and may be unilateral or bilateral. Since it is infrequent, it has little diagnostic significance.

Mucocutaneous lesions occur in about one-third of the cases. In the early stage, cutaneous lesions are papular with the same mor-

FIGURE 160-1

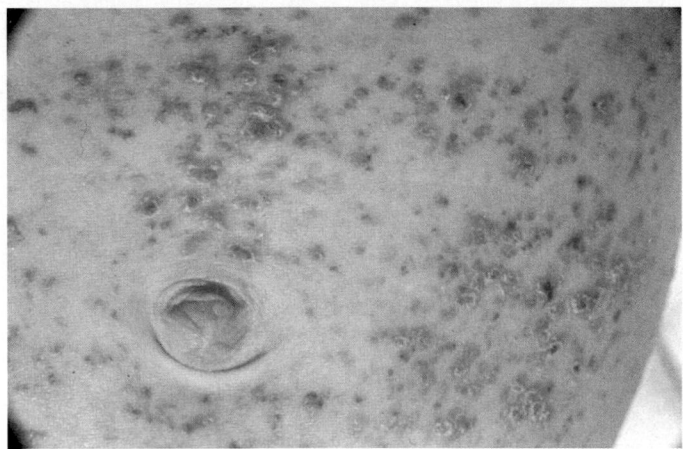

A.

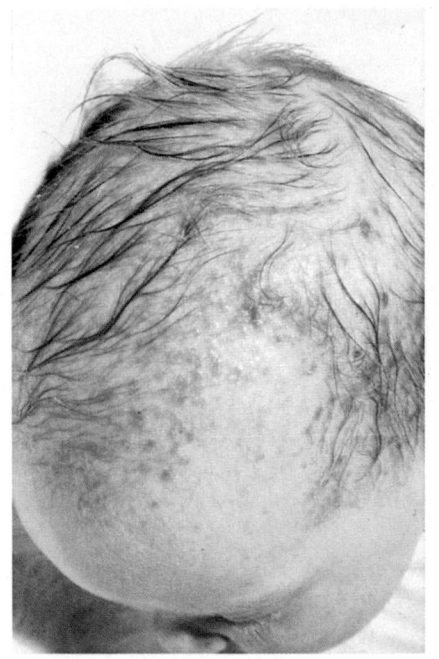

B.

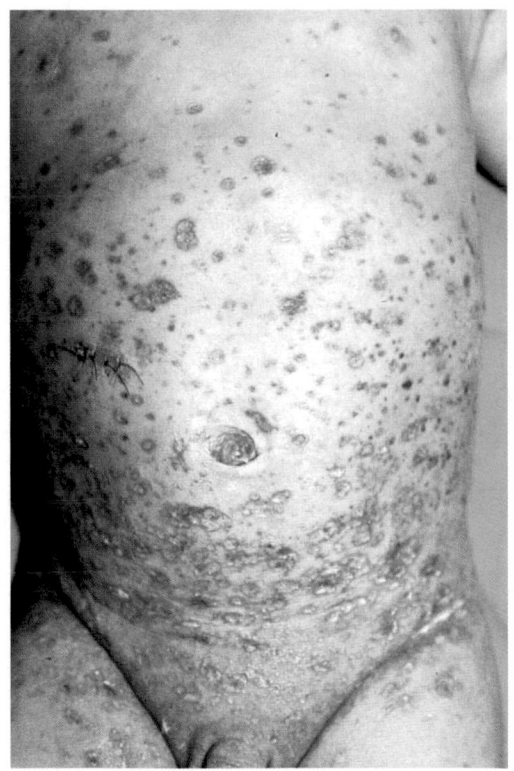

C.

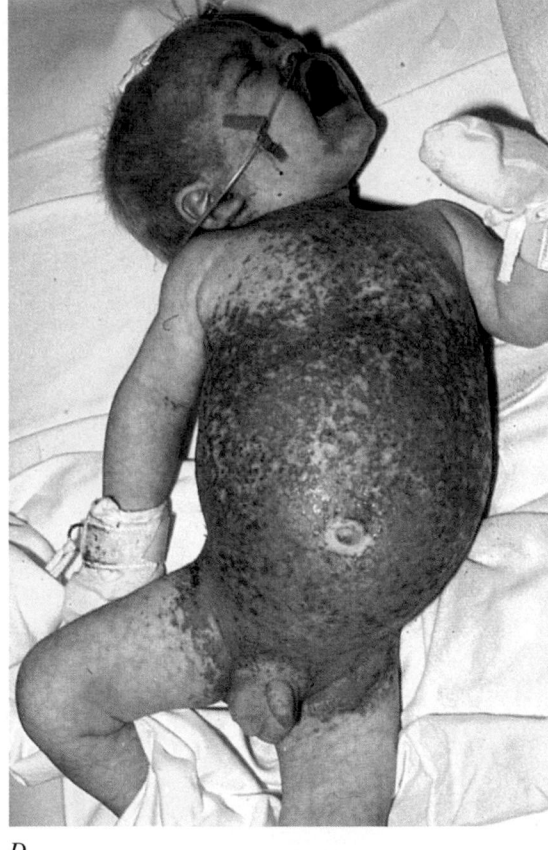

D.

Langerhans cell histiocytosis, Letterer-Siwe diseases. *A.* Abdominal area of infant with multiple yellowish erythematous papules covered by scale or crust. *B.* Seborrheic papules on the scalp mimicking seborrheic dermatitis. *C.* Infant with multiple ulcerated skin lesions on the trunk. *D.* Severe Letterer-Siwe disease with confluent erosive and crusted lesions forming ulcers; distension of abdomen reflects hepatospleno-megaly.

FIGURE 160-2

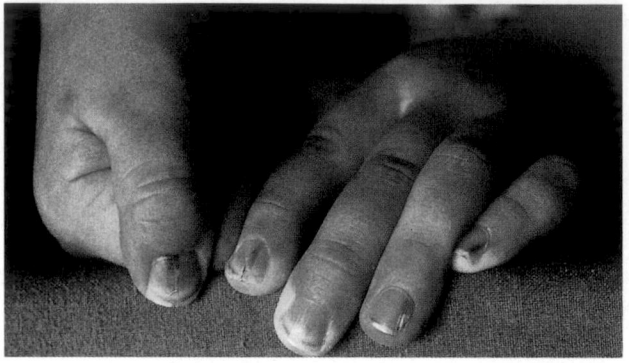

Letterer-Siwe disease. All nails, save one, show purpuric striae of the nail bed. Nail changes are considered an unfavorable prognostic sign.

phologic characteristics as those observed in LSD. In the later phases, skin lesions are frequently grouped on the medial aspect of the chest (Fig. 160-6), back, and temporoparietal regions,[1,8,19] and they may become xanthomatous.[14] Occasionally the lesions tend to merge into plaques (Fig. 160-7). The involvement of the large body

FIGURE 160-3

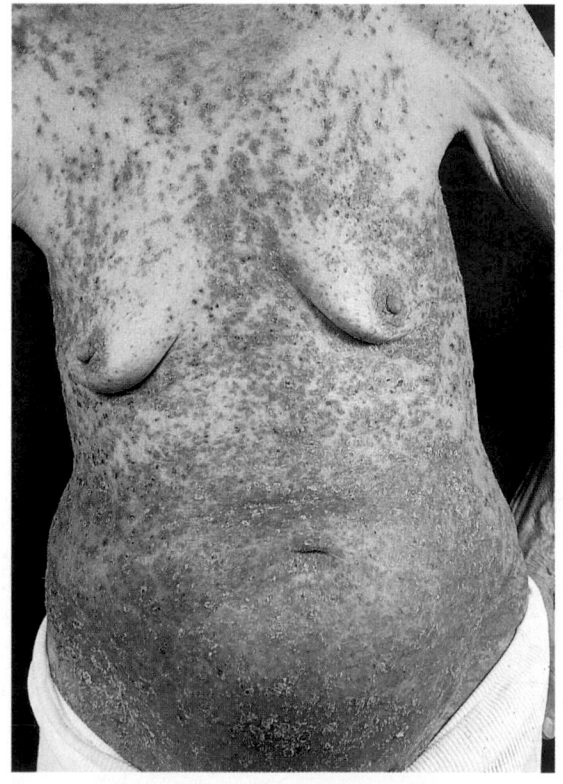

Letterer-Siwe disease in an 81-year-old woman. The diffuse papuloscaling and papulocrusted lesions on the trunk are similar to those seen in early childhood. Systemic involvement consists of hepatosplenomegaly and pulmonary lesions. (*From Caputo et al,*[14] *with permission.*)

folds may mimic intertrigo (Fig. 160-7), while on the scalp the lesions may look like seborrheic dermatitis (Fig. 160-6) or folliculitis. Mucous membrane lesions are commonly noduloulcerative[19–21] and mainly involve the gingiva (Fig. 160-8) and the vulva.

Pulmonary infiltrates can be found in fewer than 20 percent of HSCD cases, and *hepatomegaly* and *lymphadenopathy* are rare.[1,2]

The initial manifestations of the disease most frequently are diabetes insipidus, chronic otitis media, or skin lesions.[19]

Eosinophilic Granuloma

Eosinophilic granuloma is the localized, benign form of LCH. It occurs between the ages of 5 and 30 and is more common in males.[1,8] The granulomatous lesions affect the *bones* in the following decreasing order of frequency[24,25]: cranial vault, ribs, vertebral column, pelvis, scapulae, and long bones (Fig. 160-9). The onset is insidious. The osseous lesion is frequently single and may go undetected until spontaneous fracture and/or otitis media occur. When the lesions do become symptomatic, there will be localized pain, tenderness, and soft tissue swelling.

Mucocutaneous lesions[1,13,26,27] are rare and noduloulcerative and preferentially involve the mucous membranes and the perigenital, perioral, or perianal regions (Fig. 160-10).

Hashimoto-Pritzker Disease

HPD, or congenital self-healing reticulohistiocytosis,[28] is the benign self-healing variant of LCH. HPD is usually present at birth or may appear during the first few days of life.[28–35] Typically, the disease is characterized by the eruption of multiple disseminated, elevated, firm, red-brown nodules (Fig. 160-11).[29] These lesions can grow in size and number in the first few weeks of life, and some may become quite large; they then form brown crusts, which are shed and occasionally leave whitish atrophic scars. In a few cases, solitary lesions have been reported (Fig. 160-12).[32,36–38] The absence of mucous membrane lesions is a key feature of HPD. Systemic signs are usually absent except for occasional hepatomegaly.[30] No significant hematologic abnormalities have been observed. Physical and mental development is normal. The salient features of HPD are multiple or solitary papulonodular lesions, sparing of mucous membranes, absence of systemic involvement, and rapid spontaneous regression.

INCIDENCE

The annual incidence of LCH has been estimated at 0.5 per 100,000 children in the United States[2,8] and at 1 per 2 million children worldwide.[8] The male to female ratio is 1.8:1.[1]

COURSE AND PROGNOSIS

LCH presents a very wide clinical spectrum and runs a variable course; manifestations range from isolated self-healing lesions to generalized and fatal destructive disease of tissue. Classically, the course of LSD is rapid and fatal; for HSCD, it is protracted but progressive (and fatal in about 50 percent of untreated patients); for

is self-healing.[1] The most frequent causes of death are pulmonary and bone marrow involvement and intercurrent infections.[1,9,11,19]

Single-system disease is usually associated with a good prognosis, whereas multisystem disease may be fatal.[15,39–41] However, some patients with LSD have been reported to recover spontaneously.[2]

The appearance of *xanthomatous lesions* in the course of LCH in children[15] and adults[11] is considered by some authors to be an expression of a shift from a disseminated subacute form (LSD) into a progressive chronic form (HSCD)[11]; others believe that these lesions may represent a distinct clinical entity independent of the primary disease.[1]

Intercurrent infections (mainly candidiasis) are frequently observed in LSD.[1,15] Multiple staging systems have been proposed on the basis of prognostic factors derived from retrospective case studies. Nezelof et al.[42] relate prognosis to the number of organs involved, Oberman[39] to bone and soft tissue involvement, Lahey[40] to age of appearance and number of involved tissues, and Komp et al.[41] to the age at diagnosis and the presence or absence of vital organ dysfunction. Thus, the age of patients at diagnosis, the number of organs involved, and organ dysfunction are the three main parameters on which evaluation of prognosis is based.[2]

It is impossible to attribute prognostic significance to any single symptom, but jaundice, thrombocytopenia, spontaneous anemia, biologic signs of hepatic failure, and nail involvement are considered unfavorable prognostic signs.[1,42] A favorable prognosis can be ascribed to a small number of lesions, nodular lesions (as in HPD), their prompt resolution, and the involvement of only one organ system (skin or bones).[1,38,42] Multisystem LCH in adults carries a better prognosis than in children.[43]

FIGURE 160-4

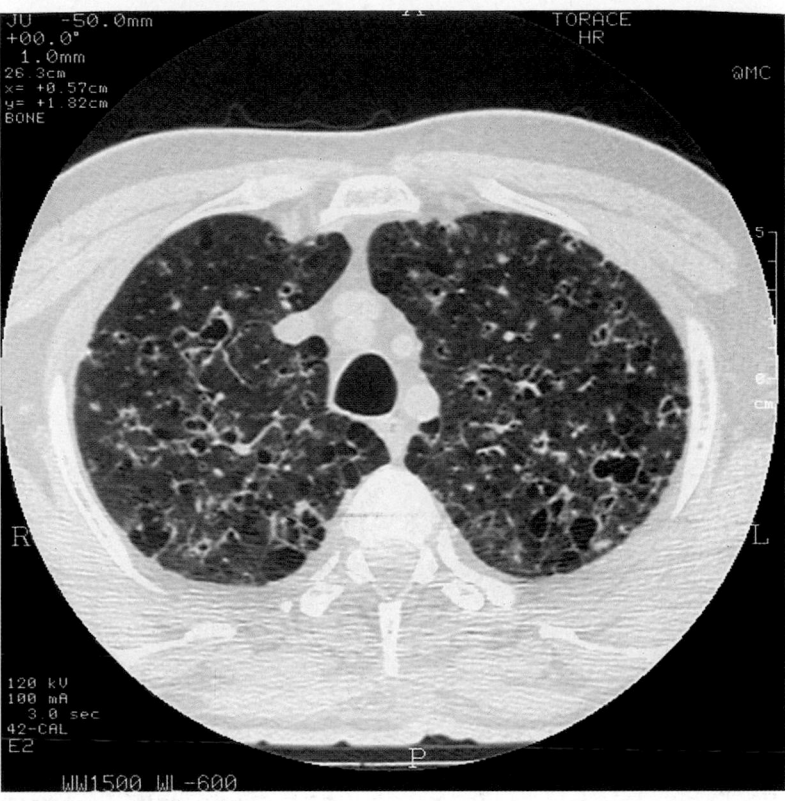

Letterer-Siwe disease. Bilateral involvement of lungs characterized by multiple cystic cavities (honeycomb appearance). (*Courtesy of E.De Juli, MD*)

LABORATORY FINDINGS

The laboratory evaluation of a patient with LCH should include complete blood count, platelet count, prothrombin time and partial thromboplastin time, liver function tests, urinalysis, serum protein electrophoresis, T and B cell counts and T cell subset analysis for immunologic evaluation, chest x-ray, complete skeletal radiographic survey, and biopsy of the most accessible area of involvement.[2] In specific cases the following examinations are required: abdominal sonography, computed tomography of the head, pulmonary function tests, and bone marrow aspirate.

Lahey's concept of organ dysfunction[40,41,44] may be evaluated as follows. Liver dysfunction is considered present if there is hypoproteinemia (<5.5 mg/dL total protein and/or <2.5 g/dL of albumin) or edema or ascites and/or hyperbilirubinemia (total serum bilirubin >1.5 mg/dL). Lung dysfunction is considered present if there is tachypnea and/or dyspnea, cyanosis, pneumothorax, or pleural effusion attributable to the disease rather than to infection. The presence of radiographic densities alone is not interpreted as evidence of dysfunction. Hemopoietic dysfunction is considered present if there is anemia (<10 g/dL hemoglobin not due to iron deficiency or superimposed infection), leukopenia (white blood count <4000/μL), or thrombocytopenia (<100,000 platelets/μL). The presence of excessive numbers of histiocytes in the marrow aspirate is not considered per se as evidence of dysfunction.

HISTOPATHOLOGIC, IMMUNOHISTOCHEMICAL, AND ULTRASTRUCTURAL FINDINGS

The unifying aspect of the entire spectrum of LCH lies in its pathologic features. The linking histologic element of the different lesions is the typical "LCH cell," a cell easily identified and differentiated from the nonspecific elements of the infiltrate by its size and configuration. This cell is about four to five times larger than small lymphocytes; has an irregular and vesiculated nucleus; is often reniform (kidney shaped); and has abundant, slightly eosinophilic cytoplasm.[1,2]

The histologic patterns observed in LCH are of three types[1,8,45,46]: proliferative (Figs. 160-13 and 160-14), granulomatous (Fig. 160-15), and xanthomatous (Fig. 160-16). A proliferative reaction is seen in early papules. It consists of an extensive LCH cell infiltration in the upper dermis close to the epidermis, which soon becomes compressed, thinned, invaded, and even destroyed

FIGURE 160-5

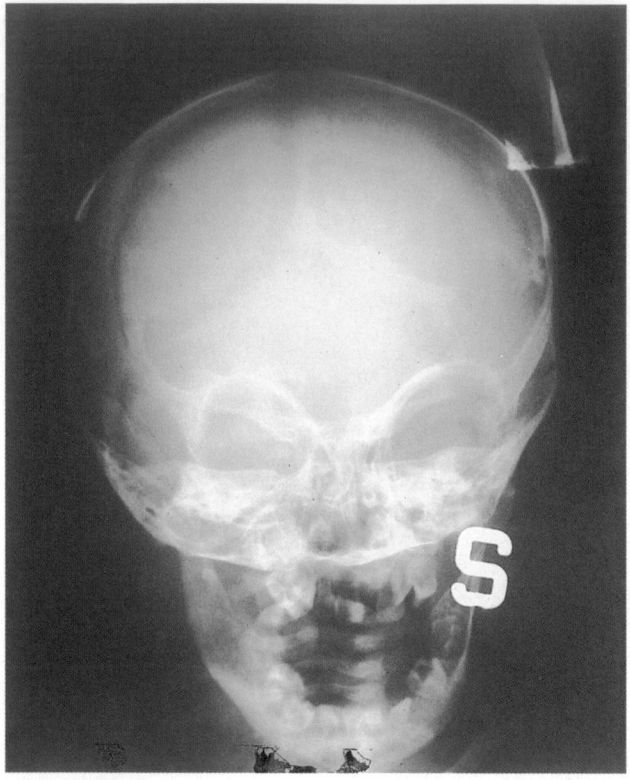

Hand-Schüller-Christian disease. X-ray of the skull shows well-circumscribed osteolytic areas resulting in a typical "map" appearance.

FIGURE 160-6

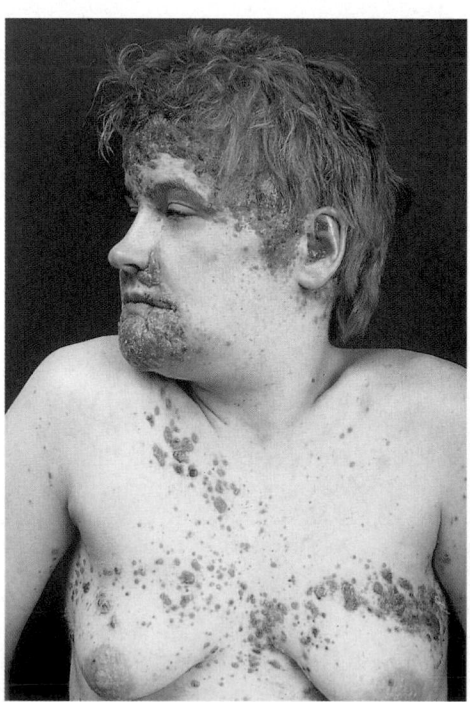

Hand-Schüller-Christian disease. The papuloscaling and papulocrusted lesions show a typical distribution on the trunk and the scalp. The involvement of the face in the patient is unusual.

FIGURE 160-7

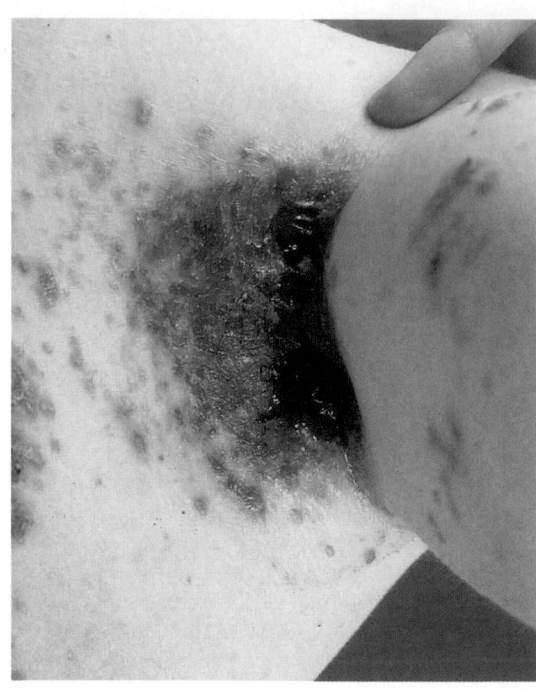

Hand-Schüller-Christian disease. In the axillae of the same patient as in Fig. 160-6, the lesions merge into a red, ulcerated malodorous plaque.

(Fig. 160-14). In the upper dermis, LCH cells are typically separated by edema, whereas in the lower dermis their cell membranes coalesce. In the deep dermis, the infiltrate is often localized around vessels and may invade the hypodermis. A few mitotic figures may occasionally be found.[46] Cytologic examination of LCH cells is easily performed by scraping early papules.[1] The granulomatous reaction (Fig. 160-15) consists of an aggregation of LCH cells with some multinucleated histiocytes and a varying number of eosinophils, generally in clusters. Neutrophils, lymphocytes, and plasma cells may also be present in the infiltrate. This type of reaction is

FIGURE 160-8

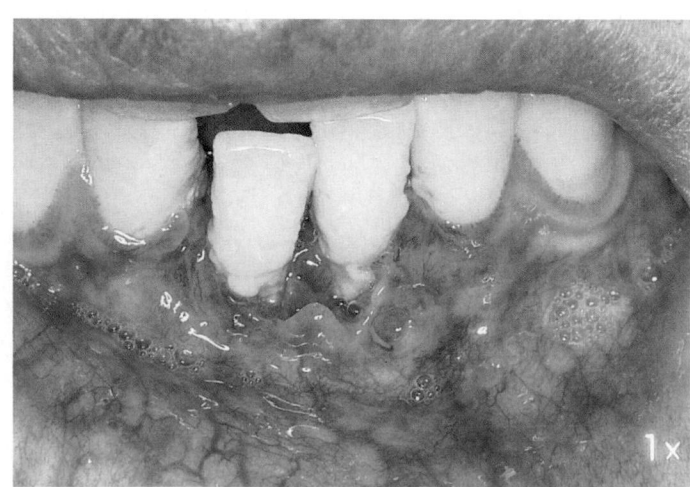

Hand-Schüller-Christian disease. Infiltrating lesions of the gingival tissue, frequently leading to loss of teeth.

FIGURE 160-9

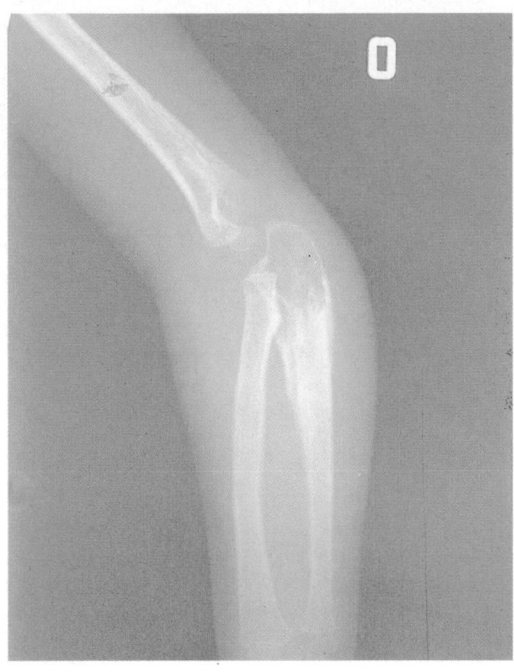

Eosinophilic granuloma. The bones of the elbow reveal well defined osteolytic lesions. These lesions manifest by swelling of soft tissue and localized pain.

FIGURE 160-10

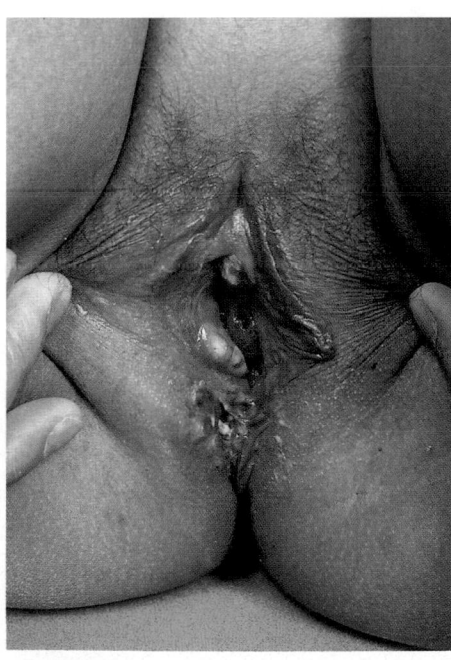

Eosinophilic granuloma. Noduloulcerative lesions in the vulva and on the perianal area. These lesions, although rare, are as unique as the bone lesions.

FIGURE 160-11

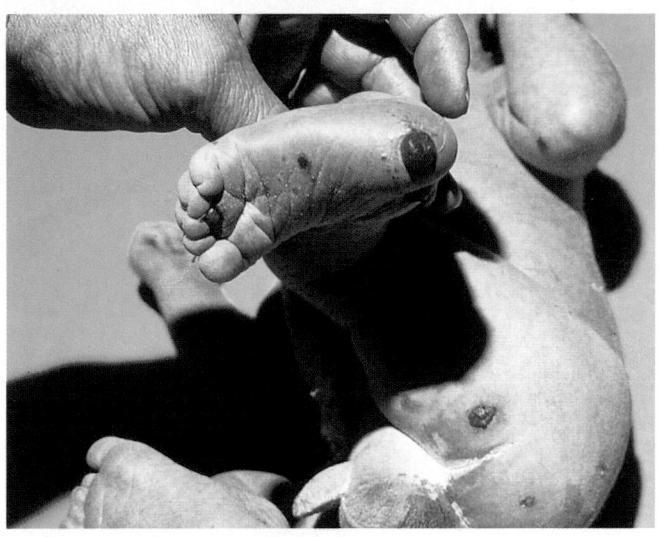

Hashimoto-Pritzker disease. Multiple, disseminated, elevated, firm red-brown or dark red nodules (multiple form) present at birth. (*From Bonifazi et al,*[29] *with permission.*)

seen in the chronic stages of the disease. The xanthomatous reaction is encountered mainly in HSCD and consists of numerous foam cells intermingled with LCH cells and eosinophils (Fig. 160-16). Multinucleated giant cells are frequently seen. They are mainly of the foreign body type but occasionally may have the appearance of Touton giant cells (Fig. 160-16). Lipid accumulation is considered to be a late secondary phenomenon.[1]

These different types of histologic reactions may be found simultaneously in the same patient,[1] and the visceral lesions present in LCH show the same three types of reactions observed in the skin.[2,8]

FIGURE 160-12

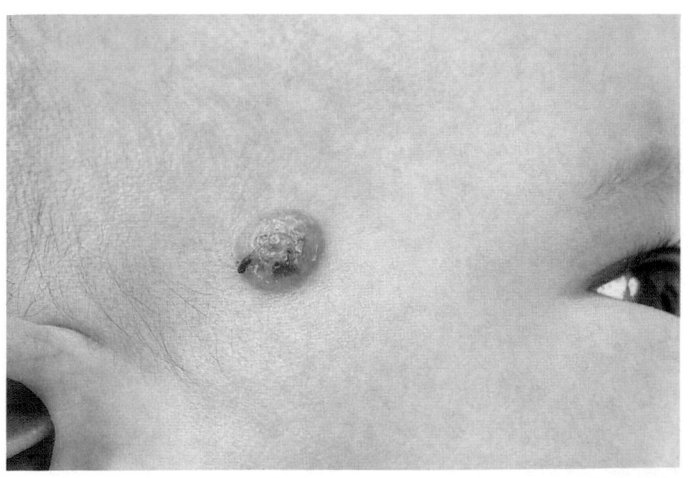

Hashimoto-Pritzker disease. Solitary nodule on the temple. The central crust is an expression of rapid spontaneous regression (solitary form).

FIGURE 160-13

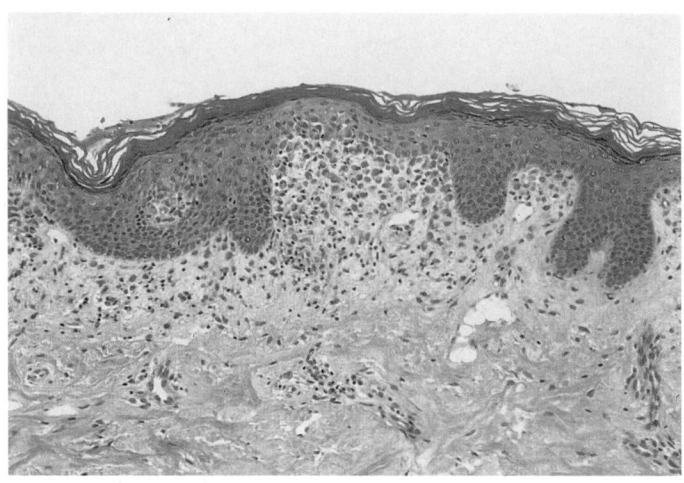

Langerhans cell histiocytosis. Conventional microscopy. An early papule composed mainly of LCH cells located in the upper dermis (pure proliferative reaction).

In HPD,[28–35] the infiltrate appears to consist mostly of large multinucleated giant cells intermingled with typical LCH cells. The cytoplasm of the giant cells is either acidophilic or has a "ground glass" appearance. It is usually localized in the mid and deep dermis; occasionally the epidermis may be infiltrated and ulcerated.

The LCH cells show the immunophenotype of normal Langerhans cells. These cells constitutively express high levels of major histocompatibility complex (MHC) class II molecules, S-100 protein, CD1a complex (Fig. 160-17), and CD4 molecules; however, in contrast to Langerhans cells, LCH cells also express several macrophage-associated markers including CD11c, CDW32, and CD68.[2,47–50] Morever, heterogeneity with respect to the expression of various cell markers has been reported.[48,49] There are few reliable

FIGURE 160-14

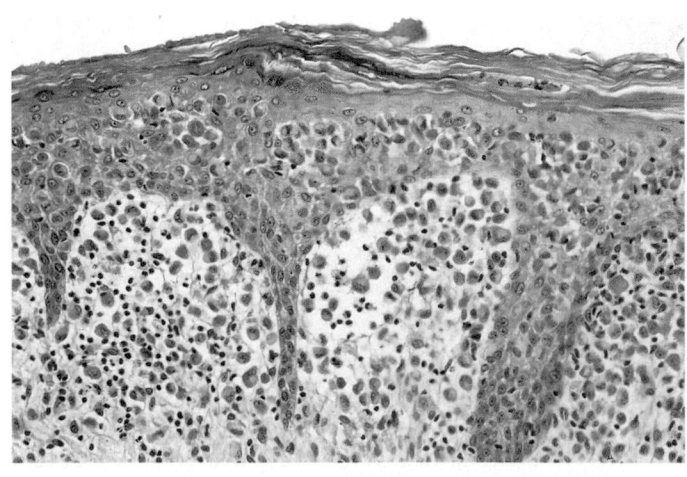

Langerhans cell histiocytosis. Conventional microscopy. A pure LCH cell infiltrate invades and destroys the epidermis.

FIGURE 160-15

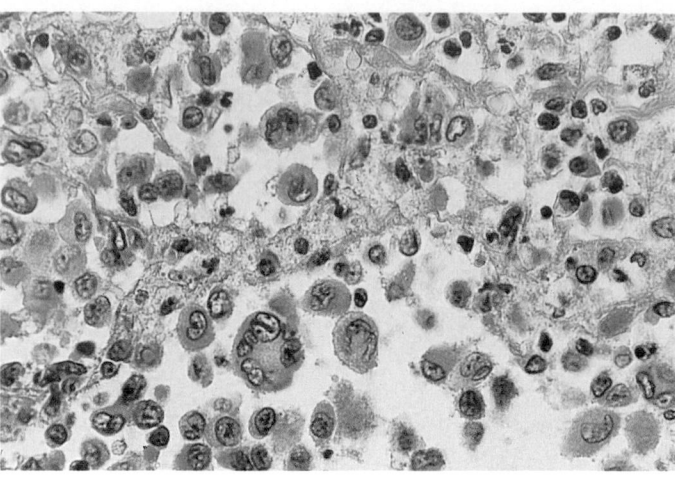

Langerhans cell histiocytosis. Conventional microscopy. The granulomatous reaction consists of an aggregation of LCH cells with some multinucleated histiocytes, as well as with varying numbers of eosinophils, neutrophils, lymphocytes, and plasma cells. This type of reaction is seen in the chronic stage of the disease.

markers capable of distinguishing LCH cells from Langerhans cells of normal skin. Three markers, placental alkaline phosphatase (PLAP), peanut agglutinin (PNA), and interferon-γ receptor (IFN-γ R), are especially valuable in differentiating normal Langerhans from LCH cells.[51]

Electron microscopic studies show that approximately 50 percent of the histiocytes of LCH contain Birbeck's granules (Fig. 160-17).[52–54]

In HPD, LCH cells are less numerous (10 to 25 percent of tumor cells) and may contain dense and regularly laminated bodies.[31]

FIGURE 160-16

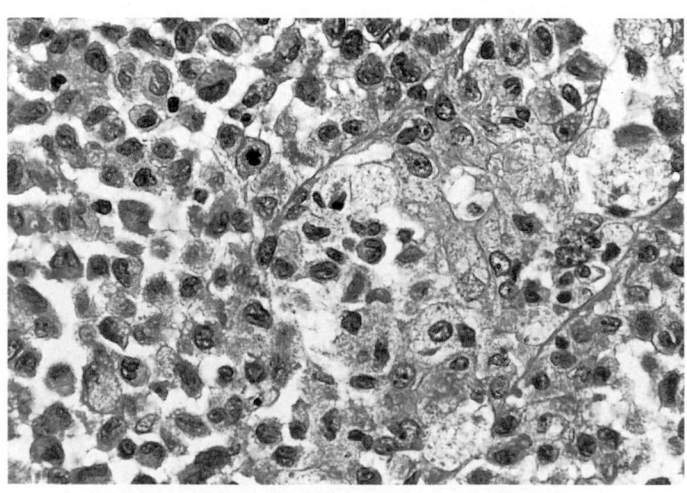

Langerhans cell histiocytosis. Conventional microscopy. The xanthomatous reaction consists of numerous foam cells intermingled with LCH cells and is encountered mainly in Hand-Schüller-Christian disease. Mitotic figures may occasionally be seen.

FIGURE 160-17

CHAPTER 160
Langerhans Cell Histiocytosis   1889

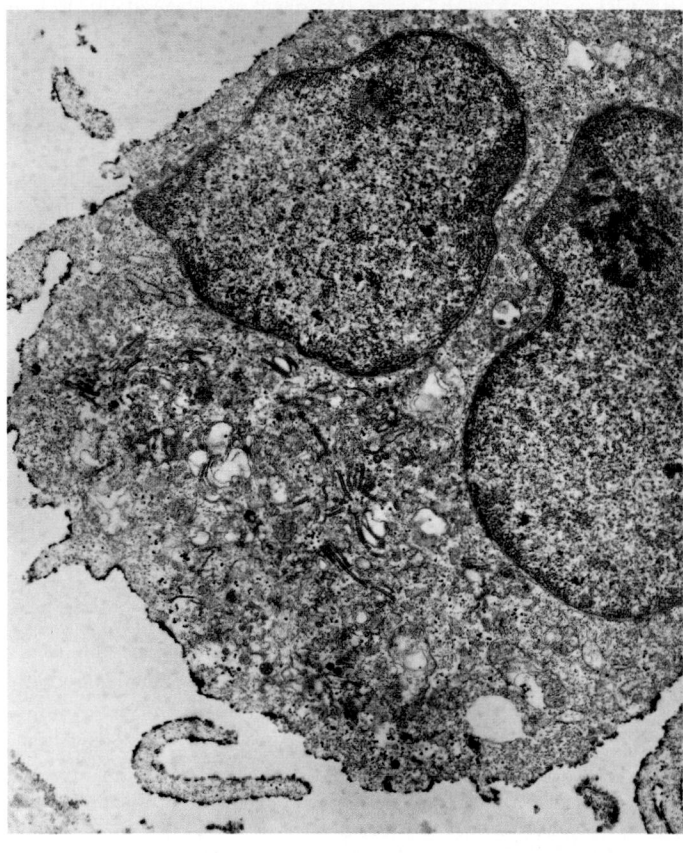

Langerhans cell histiocytosis. Immunoelectronmicroscopy. A CD1a-positive LCH cell with indented nucleus containing typical Birbeck's granules.

ETIOPATHOGENESIS

The etiopathogenesis of LCH remains a mystery despite numerous investigative efforts. Viral, immunologic, and neoplastic pathogenic mechanisms have been considered, but none has been proven.

Viruses have long been suspected as potential etiologic agents of LCH, and the abnormal proliferation of LCH cells has been interpreted as an altered response to viral infections.[2,55] Favara[55] suggests the following hypothesis: (1) Viruses induce activation of histiocytes; (2) viral-specific antigens appear on the surface of activated histiocytes; (3) antiviral antibodies react with these cell-surface antigens; (4) receptor-mediated endocytosis of these complexes induces the pathologic LCH phenotype; and (5) a subsequent cytokine-mediated, positive-feedback loop results in the clinicopathologic syndrome recognized as LCH.

The human herpesvirus (HHV) type 6 has been suspected of playing a role in the pathogenesis of LCH by Lahey et al.,[56] who detected HHV-6 DNA in lesions from 14 (47 percent) of 30 patients with LCH. In contrast to these findings McClain et al.[57] failed to find genomic evidence for adenovirus, cytomegalovirus, Epstein-Barr virus, herpes simplex virus, HHV-6, human T cell leukemia viruses types I and II, and parvovirus. The literature suggests that, at present, none of the viruses mentioned above are responsible for LCH.

Immunologic testing of patients with LCH performed during the past 20 years[58–60] has failed to show consistent defects in immune

function. Several cytokines, such as interleukin 1, tumor necrosis factor α, granulocyte-macrophage colony stimulating factor, interleukin 8, and leukemia inhibitory factor, have been detected in significant amounts in cultured cells of LCH lesions.[61] These molecules may play a crucial role in inducing/promoting the growth of LCH cells, but it is not known how these cytokines relate to different clinical features of the disorder.[62] Although LCH cells are probably of clonal origin, as suggested by an X-chromosome inactivation assay,[63,64] they do not show clonal T cell receptor gene rearrangements.[65] These findings together with flow cytometric DNA analysis of lesions[66] and the spontaneous regression in LCH suggest that LCH is a nonneoplastic disease.

DIFFERENTIAL DIAGNOSIS[67] (See also Chap. 161)

Skin lesions of disseminated LCH are similar to those of seborrheic dermatitis, moniliasis, and miliaria, but the presence of purpura indicates that the diagnosis is LCH. When a condition thought to be banal, such as seborrheic dermatitis, does not respond to proper therapy, LCH should be suspected. The diagnosis may be confirmed promptly by a cytologic examination performed by scraping an early papule.

In Darier's disease, the lesions appear between ages 8 and 15 years, and the papules are hyperkeratotic and may involve the extremities.

Lichen nitidus is differentiated from LCH by the presence of shiny, skin-colored, nonscaling papules and the Koebner phenomenon, which cannot be included in LCH.

Chronic and persistent xanthomatous lesions of LCH must be differentiated from urticaria pigmentosa and non-Langerhans cell histiocytosis. In urticaria pigmentosa, the lesions are macular, papular, or nodular and wheal immediately after they have been rubbed.

Benign cephalic histiocytosis is characterized by flat-topped, low-domed, nonscaling papules that involve preferentially the head. The scalp, trunk, mucous membranes, and viscera are spared by the process.

Histopathologic examination is necessary to differentiate some lesions of juvenile xanthogranuloma and xanthoma disseminatum from the xanthomatous lesions of LCH; in juvenile xanthogranuloma, bone lesions are not present, and in xanthoma disseminatum, cutaneous xanthomas are distributed symmetrically and tend to coalesce.

In sinus histiocytosis with massive lymphadenopathy, cervical lymphadenopathy is a prominent feature and is usually accompanied by fever, leukocytosis with neutrophilia, and polyclonal hypergammaglobulinemia.

Papules of generalized eruptive histiocytosis are differentiated from those of LCH by absence of scales and crusts, presence of red-brown or red-blue hue, and symmetric distribution.

The presence of violaceous plaques or nodules with patulous follicular ostia on the face distinguishes granuloma faciale from eosinophilic granuloma. HPD must mainly be differentiated from nodular forms of LCH such as eosinophilic granuloma, juvenile xanthogranuloma, generalized eruptive histiocytosis, and urticaria pigmentosa. The distinction of HPD from nodular lesions present in the disseminated form of LCH may be difficult because of the histologic, ultrastructural, and immunologic similarities. HPD is distinctive in that the skin alone is involved and the lesions are rapidly

TABLE 160-1

Treatment of Langerhans Cell Histiocytosis

SINGLE-SYSTEM DISEASE			MULTISYSTEM DISEASE
SKIN		**BONE**	
CHILDREN	**ADULTS**		
Observation or topical nitrogen mustard	Topical nitrogen mustard PUVA CO_2 laser Thalidomide Isotretinoin	Surgery Glucocorticoid injections Radiotherapy Monochemotherapy (in multiple bone lesions)	Monochemotherapy with vinblastine or etoposide, preceded or not by glucocorticoid administration Nonresponders may be treated with polychemotherapy

self-healing. Nodular lesions of juvenile xanthogranuloma may be present at birth. However, they rapidly become yellow, do not tend to ulcerate, and heal spontaneously within several years but never in a few months. Histologically, the lesions are composed of foamy cells and multinuclear giant cells; S-100 and CD1a positive cells are absent, and no cells containing Langerhans granules are detected by electron microscopy.

Generalized eruptive histiocytosis consists of numerous, discrete papules appearing in successive crops and involving mainly the trunk and proximal limbs. The disease is rare in children and has never been seen at birth. Histologically, the infiltrate is monomorphous and the histiocytes are S-100 and CD1a negative and do not contain Langerhans granules (see also Chap. 161). The absence of urtication and, as shown by histology, of mast cells rules out urticaria pigmentosa.

MANAGEMENT

Treatment strategies of LCH are chosen on the basis of the age of patients, extent of disease, and location of lesions[2,15] (Table 160-1).

In "single-system disease" involving skin or bone, management is nonaggressive. In children with skin involvement only, observation is the best option[15]; if the lesions are persistent, topical nitrogen mustard may be an effective treatment.[68,69] Therapy consists of application of nitrogen mustard diluted in water to a concentration of 20 mg/dL and applied daily for 5 days.

The use of systemic glucocorticoids or antimitotic drugs is suggested for resistant cases.[15] In adults with skin involvement only, topical treatment with nitrogen mustard may be an effective treatment strategy. Significant improvement has been obtained with conventional PUVA treatment in a considerable number of cases.[70,71] CO_2 laser therapy has been suggested in periorificial eosinophilic granuloma.[72] The use of thalidomide may induce a remission of skin lesions.[73–75] The suggested dose is 100 mg/day for 1 month and then 50 mg/day for 1 or 2 months (see Chap. 261). Usually the disease recurs after stopping treatment. The effect of this drug seems to be due to its immunomodulatory and anti-inflammatory properties. In one case, a complete remission of skin lesions was obtained after oral isotretinoin therapy.[76] The patient was treated with 1.5 mg/kg daily for a period of 8 months and remained free of recurrence and visceral involvement for 5 years.

In patients with bone involvement only, surgery (excision or curettage) is the treatment of choice if the lesions are accessible.[2,15,77] In children, glucocorticoid injections into selected sites may be successful to avoid surgical trauma to developing teeth or the growth plate of long bones.[15,78] In adults, radiotherapy is indicated for involvement of vertebrae, the sella turcica, and weight-bearing bones with risk of spontaneous fracture.[2,19,79] In children, radiotherapy must be reserved for cases that fail to respond to other measures in order to avoid the risk of long-term effects.[15] In the case of multiple bone lesions, monochemotherapy is suggested as with multiorgan involvement.

The management of patients with multisystem disease is, however, controversial.[79] At the current time, monochemotherapy with vinblastine or etoposide with or without glucocorticoids is probably the most suitable treatment.[80–82] Vinblastine is given intravenously at doses of 0.1 to 0.2 mg/kg once weekly (6.5 mg/m^2) for 1 to 3 months. Readministration of the alkaloid should be instituted only when new lesions appear.[1,80,82] Etoposide[81–85] is administered at a dose of 200 mg/m^2 orally or intravenously for 3 consecutive days every 3 to 4 weeks for at least three to four courses. Etoposide gave approximately a 90 percent response rate in one study.[81,82] Both vinblastine and etoposide are well tolerated and cause only a few toxic effects. In case of relapses, retreatment with the same type of monochemotherapy may result in complete clearing in 60 percent of cases.[2] Finally, methylprednisolone (30 mg/kg intravenously on 3 consecutive days) may be the initial therapeutic approach.

Only nonresponders to monochemotherapy should be given multiagent regimens including vincristine, cyclophosphamide, doxorubicin, and chlorambucil.[2,80,82,86] In refractory and advanced cases of LCH, cyclosporine[87,88] and interferon-α_2 have been used.[89] Allogeneic bone marrow transplantation was successful in one child with a very poor prognosis.[90]

REFERENCES

1. Gianotti F, Caputo R: Histiocytic syndromes: A review. *J Am Acad Dermatol* **13**:383, 1985
2. Lahey MA et al: Langerhans' cell histiocytosis. *Curr Probl Dermatol* **6**:1, 1994
3. Lichtenstein L: Histiocytosis X: Integration of eosinophilic granuloma of bone. Letterer-Siwe disease and Hand-Schüller-Christian disease as related manifestations of a single nosologic entity. *Arch Pathol* **56**:84, 1953
4. Hashimoto K, Pritzker MS: Electron microscopic study of reticulohistiocytoma. An unusual case of congenital self healing reticulohistiocytosis. *Arch Dermatol* **107**:263, 1978
5. Basset F, Nezelof C: Anatomie pathologique de l'histiocytose X. Ultrastructure et approche étiologique. *Polmon Coeur* **25**:651, 1969
6. Basset F, Nezelof C: Les histiocytoses. *Presse Med* **12**:2809, 1983
7. Chu T et al: Histiocytosis syndromes in children. *Lancet* **1**:208, 1978
8. Belaich S: Langerhans cells histiocytosis. *Dermatology* **189** (suppl):2, 1994
9. Bingham EA et al: Letterer-Siwe disease: A study of thirteen cases over a 21-year period. *Br J Dermatol* **106**:205, 1982
10. Katz AM et al: Langerhans cell histiocytosis in monozygotic twins. *J Am Acad Dermatol* **24**:32, 1991
11. Chevrant-Breton J: La maladie de Letterer-Siwe de l'adulte: Revue de la litterature. *Ann Dermatol Venereol* **105**:301, 1978

12. Caputo R et al: Letterer-Siwe disease in an octogenarian. *J Am Acad Dermatol* **10**:226, 1984

13. Winkelmann RK: Adult histiocytic skin diseases. *G Ital Dermatol Venereol* **115**:67, 1980

14. Caputo R et al: Mucocutaneous expressions of Langerhans cell histiocytosis in adults. *Eur J Dermatol* **4**:528, 1994

15. Esterly NB et al: Histiocytosis X: A seven-year experience at a children's hospital. *J Am Acad Dermatol* **13**:481, 1985

16. Talanin NY et al: Cutaneous histiocytosis with Langerhans cell features induced by scabies: A case report. *Pediatr Dermatol* **11**:327, 1994

17. Johno M et al: Langerhans cell histiocytosis presenting as a varicelliform eruption over the entire skin. *J Dermatol* **21**:197, 1994

18. De Berker D et al: Nail features in Langerhans cell histiocytosis. *Br J Dermatol* **130**:523, 1994

19. De Lacharriere O, Ougier E: Histiocytose Langerhansienne de l'adulte à expression cutanée. Revue genérale. *Ann Dermatol Venereol* **117**:303, 1990

20. Dolezal JF, Thomson ST: Hand-Schüller-Christian disease in a septuagenarian. *Arch Dermatol* **114**:85, 1978

21. Takata M et al: An adult case of histiocytosis X with vulvar ulcer and multiple bone lesions. *J Dermatol* **21**:259, 1994

22. Sigala JL et al: Dental involvement in histiocytosis X. *Oral Surg* **33**:42, 1972

23. Dunger DB et al: The frequency and natural biopsy of diabetes insipidus in children with Langerhans-cell histiocytosis. *N Engl J Med* **321**:1157, 1989

24. McGavian MH, Spady HA: Eosinophilic granuloma of bone: A study of 28 cases. *J Bone Joint Surg* **42**:979, 1960

25. Sparbaro JL, Francis KC: Eosinophilic granuloma of bone. *JAMA* **178**:706, 1961

26. Cavender PA, Bennett RG: Perianal eosinophilic granuloma resembling condyloma latum. *Pediatr Dermatol* **5**:50, 1988

27. Otis CN et al: Histiocytosis X of the vulva. A case report and a review of the literature. *Obstet Gynecol* **75**:555, 1990

28. Hashimoto K, Pritzker MS: Electron microscopic study of reticulohistiocytoma: An unusual case of congenital self-healing reticulohistiocytosis. *Arch Dermatol* **107**:263, 1978

29. Bonifazi L et al: Congenital self-healing histiocytosis. *Arch Dermatol* **118**:267, 1982

30. Hashimoto K et al: Self-healing reticulohistiocytosis. *Cancer* **49**:331, 1982

31. Hashimoto K et al: Congenital self-healing reticulohistiocytosis. Report of the seventh case with histochemical and ultrastructural studies. *Arch Dermatol* **11**:447, 1984

32. Berger TG et al: A solitary variant of congenital self-healing reticulohistiocytosis: Solitary Hashimoto-Pritzker disease. *Pediatr Dermatol* **3**:230, 1986

33. Cambazard F et al: Hashimoto-Pritzker congenital self-healing histiocytosis. *Pediatrics* **148**:29, 1988

34. Alexis JB et al: Congenital self-healing reticulohistiocytosis. Report of case with 7 year follow-up and a review of the literature. *Am J Dermatopathol* **13**:189, 1991

35. Enjolras O et al: Congenital cutaneous Langerhans histiocytosis. A propos of 7 cases. *Ann Dermatol Venereol* **119**:111, 1992

36. Taieb A et al: Solitary Langerhans cell histiocytoma. *Arch Dermatol* **122**:1033, 1986

37. Ofuji S et al: Congenital self-healing reticulohistiocytosis (Hashimoto-Pritzker): A case report with a solitary lesion. *J Dermatol* **14**:182, 1987

38. Bonifazi E et al: Langerhans cell histiocytosis. I. Cutaneous self-healing congenital variety. *Eur J Pediatr Dermatol* **1**:6, 1991

39. Oberman HA: Idiopathic histiocytosis: A clinicopathologic study of 40 cases and review of literature on eosinophilic granuloma of bone, Hand-Schüller-Christian disease and Letterer-Siwe disease. *Pediatrics* **58**:307-326, 1961

40. Lahey ME: Histiocytosis X: An analysis of prognostic factors. *J Pediatr* **87**:184, 1975

41. Komp DM et al: A staging system for histiocytosis X: A Southwest Oncology Group study. *Cancer* **47**:798, 1981

42. Nezelof C et al: Disseminated histiocytosis X: Analysis of prognostic factors based on retrospective study of 50 cases. *Cancer* **44**:1824, 1979

43. McLelland J, Chu AC: Multisystemic Langerhans cell histiocytosis in adults. *Clin Exp Dermatol* **15**:79, 1990

44. Lahey ME: Prognostic factors in histiocytosis X. *Am J Pediatr Hematol Oncol* **3**:57, 1981

45. Lever WF, Schaumburg-Lever G: *Histopathology of the Skin,* 6th ed. Philadelphia, Lippincott, 1983, p 392

46. Pierard GE et al: Proliferation of the characteristic histiocyte of histiocytosis X in the skin. *Am J Dermatopathol* **4**:215, 1982

47. Cambazard F et al: Identification immunohistologique des cellules de l'histiocytosis X. Intérnet diagnostique. *Ann Dermatol Venereol* **110**:33, 1983

48. Bos JD et al: Acute disseminated histiocytosis X: In situ immunophenotyping with monoclonal antibodies. *J Cutan Pathol* **11**:59, 1984

49. Groh V et al: The phenotypic spectrum of histiocytosis X cells. *J Invest Dermatol* **90**:441, 1988

50. Hage C et al: Langerhans' cell histiocytosis (histiocytosis X): Immunophenotype and growth fraction. *Hum Pathol* **24**:840, 1993

51. Chu T, Jaffe R: The normal Langerhans cell and the LCH cell. *Br J Cancer* **70**:4, 1994

52. Tarnowski W, Hashimoto H: Langerhans' cell granules in histiocytosis X. *Arch Dermatol* **96**:298, 1976

53. Eady RAJ: Letterer-Siwe disease in elderly patient: Histological and ultrastructural findings. *Clin Exp Dermatol* **4**:413, 1979

54. Caputo R, Gianotti F: Cytoplasmic markers and unusual ultrastructural features in histiocytic proliferations of the skin. *G Ital Dermatol Venereol* **115**:107, 1980

55. Favara BE: Langerhans cells histiocytosis pathobiology and pathogenesis. *Semin Oncol* **18**(1):3, 1991

56. Lahey MA et al: Human herpes virus 6 is present in lesions of Langerhans cell histiocytosis. *J Invest Dermatol* **101**:642, 1993

57. McClain K et al: Langerhans cell histiocytosis: Lack of a viral etiology. *Am J Hematol* **47**:16, 1994

58. Cederbaum SD et al: Combined immunodeficiency presenting as Letterer-Siwe syndrome. *J Pediatr* **85**:466, 1974

59. Nesbit ME Jr et al: The immune system and the histiocytosis syndromes. *Am J Pediatr Hematol Oncol* **3**:141, 1981

60. Newton WA et al: Role of the thymus in histiocytosis X. *Hematol Oncol Clin North Am* **1**:63, 1987

61. Kannourakis G, Abbas A: The role of cytokines in the pathogenesis of Langerhans cell histiocytosis. *Br J Cancer* **70**:37, 1994

62. Jenney MEM: Langerhans cell histiocytosis: Where do we go from here? *Lancet* **344**:1717, 1994

63. Yu RC et al: Clonal proliferation of Langerhans cell in Langerhans cell histiocytosis. *Lancet* **1**:767, 1994

64. William CI et al: Langerhans cell histiocytosis (histiocytosis X): A clonal proliferative disease. *N Engl J Med* **331**:154, 1994

65. Yu RC, Clin AC: Lack of T cell receptor gene rearrangements in cell involved in Langerhans cell histiocytosis. *Cancer* **75**:1162, 1995

66. Ornvold K et al: Flow cytometric DNA analysis of lesions from 18 children with Langerhans cell histiocytosis. *Am J Pathol* **136**:1301, 1990

67. Caputo R et al: Histiocytosis X, in *Pediatric Dermatology and Dermatopathology,* vol II edited by R Caputo, AB Ackerman, and ES Torre. Philadelphia, Lea & Febiger, 1993, p 471

68. Atherton DJ et al: Topical use of mustine hydrochloride in cutaneous histiocytosis X. *Med Pediatr Oncol* **14**:112, 1986

69. Sheehan MP et al: Topical nitrogen mustard: An effective treatment for cutaneous Langerhans' cell histiocytosis. *J Pediatr* **119**:317, 1991

70. Kaudewitz P et al: Cutaneous lesions in histiocytosis X: Successful treatment with PUVA. *J Invest Dermatol* **86**:324, 1986

71. Sakai H et al: Satisfactory remission achieved by PUVA therapy in Langerhans cell histiocytosis in an elderly patient. *J Dermatol* **23**:42, 1996

72. Truong Tt et al: Granulome éosinophile: Essai de traitement avec le laser au CO_2. *Nouv Dermatol* **9**:850, 1990

73. Bensaid P et al: Histiocytose Langerhansienne de l'adulte: Localisation parotidienne régressive après traitement par thalidomide. *Ann Dermatol Venereol* **119**:281 1992

74. Misery L et al: Remission of Langerhans cell histiocytosis with thalidomide treatment. *Clin Exp Dermatol* **18**:487, 1993

75. Thomas L et al: Successful treatment of adults Langerhans cell histiocytosis with thalidomide. *Arch Dermatol* **129**:1261, 1993

76. Tsambaos D et al: Langerhans' cell histiocytosis: Complete remission after oral isotretinoin therapy. *Acta Derm Venereol* **75**:62, 1995

77. McLelland J et al: Langerhans' cell histiocytosis: The case for conservative treatment. *Arch Dis Child* **65**:301, 1990

78. Cohen M et al: Direct injection of methylprednisolone sodium succinate in the treatment of solitary eosinophilic granuloma of bone: A report of 9 cases. *Radiology* **136**:289, 1980

79. Broadbent V, Pritchard J: Histiocytosis X—current controversies. *Arch Dis Child* **60**:605, 1985

80. Lahey ME: Histiocytosis X—comparison of three treatment regimens. *Pediatrics* **87**:179, 1975

81. Ceci A et al: Etoposide in recurrent childhood Langerhans' cell histiocytosis: An Italian cooperative study. *Cancer* **82**:2528, 1988

82. Ceci A et al: Langerhans' cell histiocytosis: Results from the Italian cooperative group AIEOP-CNR-HX 83 study. *Med Pediatr Oncol* **21**:259, 1993

83. Broadbent V et al: Etoposide (VP16) in the treatment of multisystem Langerhans' cell histiocytosis (histiocytosis X). *Med Pediatr Oncol* **17**:97, 1989

84. Viana MB et al: Etoposide in the treatment of six children with Langerhans' cell histiocytosis (histiocytosis X). *Med Pediatr Oncol* **19**:289, 1991

85. Shaehan MP, Chu AC: Oral, skin and bone multisystem Langerhans' cell histiocytosis and its response to etoposide—a case report. *Clin Exp Dermatol* **16**:463, 1991

86. Komp DM et al: Combination therapy in histiocytosis X. *Med Pediatr Oncol,* **3**:267, 1977

87. Mahmoud HH et al: Cyclosporine therapy for advanced Langerhans' cell histiocytosis. *Blood* **77**:721, 1991

88. Arico M: Cyclosporine therapy for refractory Langerhans' cell histiocytosis. *Blood* **78**:3107, 1991

89. Bellmunt J et al: Interferon and disseminated Langerhans' cell histiocytosis. *Med Pediatr Oncol* **20**:336, 1992

90. Stoll M et al: Allergic bone marrow transplantation for Langerhans' cell histiocytosis. *Cancer* **66**:284, 1990

CHAPTER 161

Ruggero Caputo

Cutaneous Nonhistiocytoses X

Nonhistiocytoses X,[1] or non-Langerhans cell histiocytoses, are characterized by the proliferation of histiocytes that always lack Langerhans granules (LG) and are usually S-100 and CD1a negative. Nonhistiocytoses X include a series of nonaggressive, frequently self-healing diseases, affecting both children and adults.[2–4]

JUVENILE XANTHOGRANULOMA

Definition and Historic Aspects

Juvenile xanthogranuloma (JXG) is a benign, self-healing disorder of infants, children, and occasionally adults, characterized by yellowish papulonodular lesions located in the skin and other organs and consisting of an infiltrate of histiocytes with a progressively greater degree of lipidation in the absence of metabolic disorders.

Nevoxanthoendothelioma[5] was the name first used in 1912 to describe this disease. Since there was no evidence for a relationship to nevi or endothelial cells, in 1954 Helwig and Macknay[6] proposed the term *juvenile xanthogranuloma.* Laurb and Lain[7] reported the first case of JXG with visceral involvement in 1937; in 1949, Blank et al[8] first described ocular involvement.

Incidence

JXG is the most common form of nonhistiocytosis X.[9] The author has observed 117 cases in the past 30 years. There is no sexual or racial predilection.

Age of Onset

JXG appears within the first year of life in about 80 percent of cases[10,11]; in 20 to 30 percent it is present at birth.[6,11] About 25 adult cases have been collected in the literature.[1,12]

Clinical Findings

Two main clinical forms can be distinguished: a papular form and a nodular form.[2,10] The *papular form* (Fig. 161-1) is characterized by numerous (up to 100), firm, hemispheric lesions, 2 to 5 mm in diameter, that are a red-brown color at first and quickly turn yellowish. These lesions are irregularly scattered throughout the skin but are located mainly on the upper part of the body. Mucous membranes are seldom involved. The *nodular form* (Fig. 161-2) is less frequent and occurs as one or a few lesions. Such nodules are generally round, 10 to 20 mm in diameter, translucent, red or yellowish, and may show telangiectases on their surface. The term *giant JXH* is used to indicate lesions larger than 2 cm.[13,14] Mucous membrane lesions are more commonly seen in the nodular form than in the papular form. Both types of lesions are generally asymptomatic. Unusual clinical variants have been recently reported.[15] The *mixed form* is characterized by the simultaneous presence of both small and large nodules. The term *JXG en plaque* is used to define a group of JXG lesions with a tendency to coalesce into a plaque as the only expression of the disease. The *subcutaneous form*[16,17] consists of a solitary deep-seated congenital or perinatal lesion, 1 to 2 cm in diameter, usually located on the head.

FIGURE 161-1

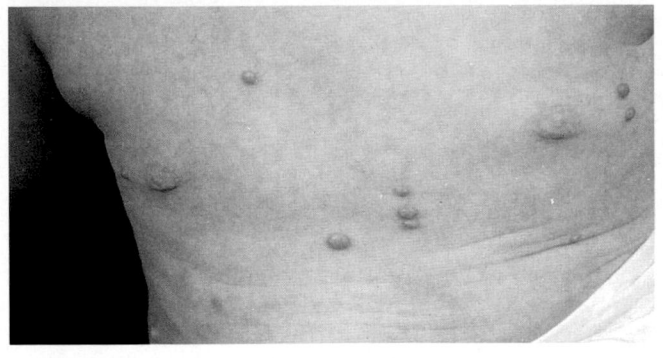

Juvenile xanthogranuloma. Papular form.

Associations

Café au lait macules of neurofibromatosis may be noted in about 20 percent of patients with the papular form of JXG.[11,18] In the papular form, ocular involvement[11,19] is the most typical extracutaneous manifestation; it may precede or follow the cutaneous lesions. Such lesions are usually unilateral and may lead to hemorrhage and glaucoma. An extremely rare extracutaneous manifestation of the papular variant is central nervous system involvement.[20]

The nodular form of JXG may occasionally be related to systemic lesions of lungs, bones, kidneys, pericardium, colon, ovaries, and testes.[10,11] Juvenile chronic myeloid leukemia has been observed in association with this variant of JXG.[21]

Histopathologic Findings

Early lesions are characterized by a monomorphous, non-lipid-containing histiocytic infiltrate[1,2,9,12] that occupies at least the upper half, and sometimes the entire thickness, of the dermis. Mature lesions (Fig. 161-3) contain foamy cells, foreign body giant cells, and Touton giant cells, mainly distributed in the superficial dermis and on the border of the infiltrate. Lymphocytes, eosinophils, and neutrophils are variably associated. Older lesions may show fibrosis. In mature lesions fat stains are positive. The histiocytes forming the

FIGURE 161-2

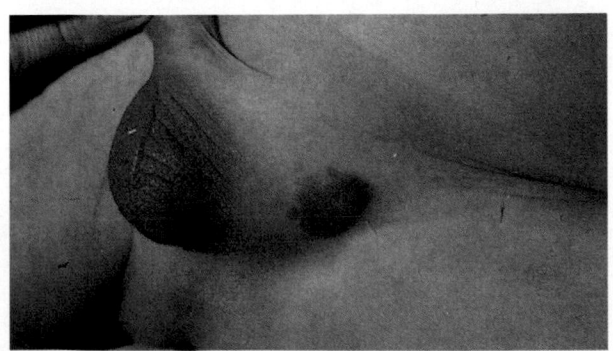

Juvenile xanthogranuloma. Nodular form.

FIGURE 161-3

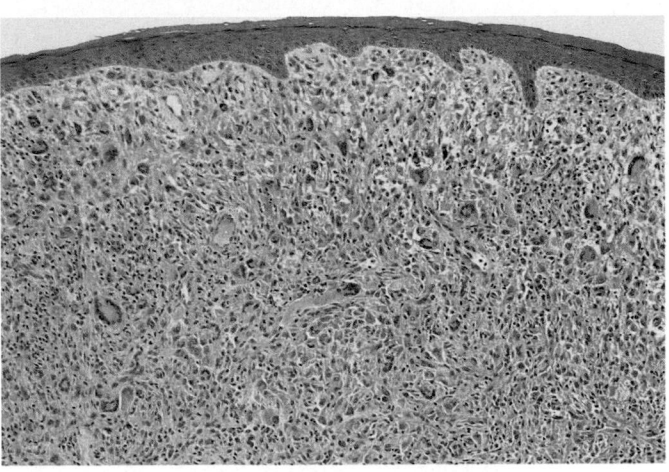

Juvenile xanthogranuloma. Histopathologic findings. A mature lesion containing foamy cells, foreign body giant cells, and Touton giant cells.

infiltrate are CD15, CD36, CD116, and CD4 positive and S-100 negative.

Under the electron microscope,[2,22,23] the histiocytes that characterize the early stage of the disease exhibit pleomorphic nuclei, are rich in pseudopods, and contain many elongated and irregular dense bodies.

Clusters of comma-shaped bodies, but no LG, can occasionally be observed. In older lesions there is a predominance of foamy cells, the cytoplasm of which is completely filled with lipid vacuoles, cholesterol clefts, and myeloid bodies. The cells corresponding to Touton giant cells are extremely large and sometimes contain more than 10 nuclei. At their periphery, such cells are rich in lipid material, whereas in their center, mitochondria and lysosomes predominate.

Differential Diagnosis

JXG can be differentiated from nodular urticaria pigmentosa, in which lesions become urticarial immediately after rubbing and histologically have many mast cells. Benign cephalic histiocytosis (BCH) differs from JXG by its papular lesions, which are located only on the head and neck. Its infiltrate lacks foamy cells and multinucleated giant cells. Generalized eruptive histiocytoma (GEH) is not granulomatous, and lipidation of the cells never occurs; histiocytes are monomorphous and are rich in dense and regularly laminated bodies on electron microscopic examination. In self-healing reticulohistiocytoma, the cutaneous lesions persist for only the first few months of life, and 10 to 25 percent of the cells are S-100 protein-positive and show LG. Tuberous xanthoma appears only in hyperlipidemic states. Papular xanthoma (PX) is distinguishable from JXG and xanthoma disseminatum (XD), from a histologic point of view, only because the primitive pure histiocytic phase is lacking. The nodular forms of histiocytosis X can be differentiated because of the different histologic, immunocytochemical, and ultrastructural characteristics (i.e., the presence of histiocytosis X cells, which are S-100 positive and contain LG). Single JXG may be clinically difficult to distinguish from Spitz nevus, which is characterized by the presence of spindle and epithelial nevus cells. Histologically, however, they are distinct.

Course and Prognosis

The cutaneous lesions tend to flatten with time. Each lesion evolves separately; thus, lesions at different stages of evolution may be seen on the same patient.[1,2,10,11] Both cutaneous and visceral lesions disappear spontaneously within 3 to 6 years. The patient's general health is not impaired, and physical and mental development is normal. Metabolic disturbances have not been identified. Prognosis is good, in the absence of associated conditions.

GENERALIZED ERUPTIVE HISTIOCYTOSIS

Definition and Historic Aspects

GEH[24,25] is a papular, nonlipidic, self-healing histiocytosis affecting mainly adults. The first adult case of this disease was described by Winkelmann and Müller[24] in 1963; Caputo et al.[26] in 1987 reported a series of pediatric cases.

FIGURE 161-4

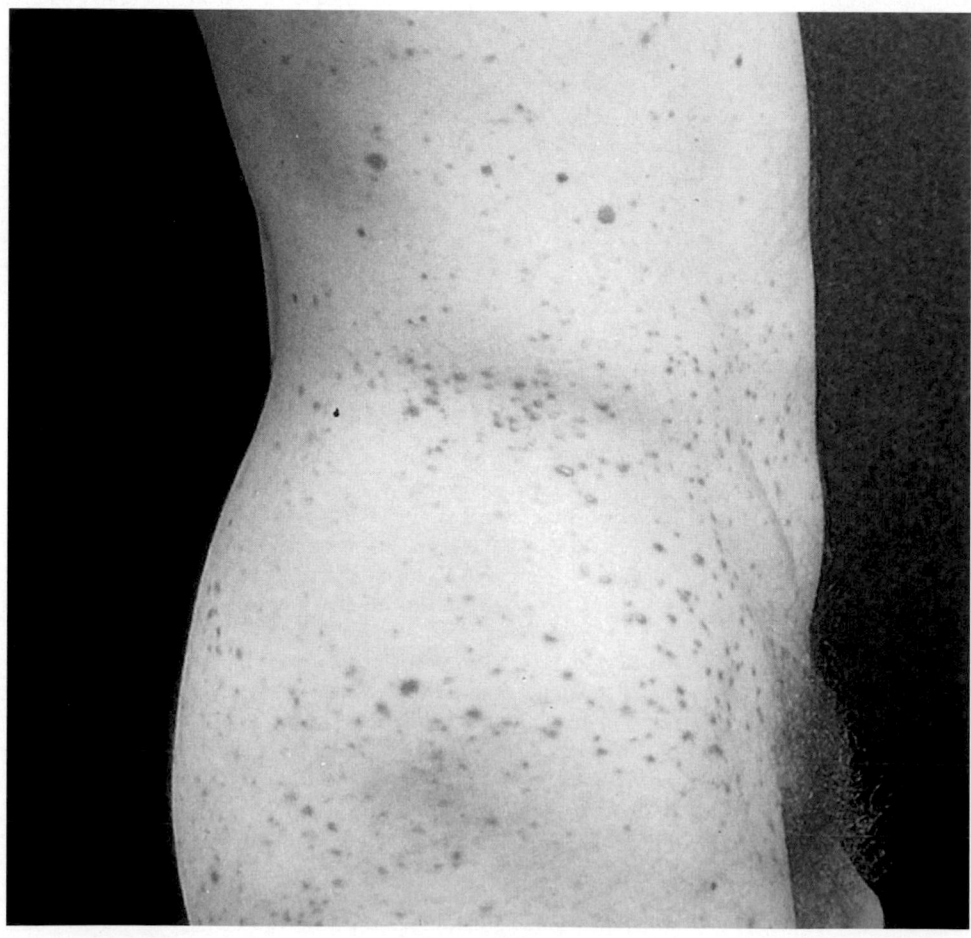

Generalized eruptive histiocytosis in an adult.

Incidence

GEH is an extremely rare disease. Approximately 30 cases[24–33] have been described, of which 7 were in children.[2,26,27,32,33]

Age of Onset

GEH may start at any age, from 3 months[27] to 58 years.[24]

Clinical Findings

The skin lesions consist of an asymptomatic eruption of round or oval papules that are firm, dark red or dark blue, and range in size from 3 to 10 mm (Fig. 161-4). These lesions appear in successive crops and are usually numerous (hundreds). In adults the lesions are symmetrically distributed and may involve mucous membranes, while in children the lesions are irregularly scattered over the entire body and mucous membranes are spared.[26] In both children and adults, no visceral lesions have been observed.

Histopathologic Findings

The lesions (Fig. 161-5) consist of a dense, monomorphous, histiocytic infiltrate in the papillary and midportion of the dermis, with a few lymphocytes.[24,26,28] The histiocytes contain a nucleus with scanty chromatin and an abundant, light, poorly limited cytoplasm. These cells are often arranged in nests around vessels. Older lesions in children may contain foamy cells.[26]

In all the cases studied with immunologic techniques,[26] the histiocytes of the infiltrate were negative for S-100 protein and CD1a and positive for CD11b and CD4, except for the case described by Sigal-Nahum et al.[32] in which many cells of the infiltrate were S-100 negative and CD1a positive. Electron microscopy shows the tumor cells to contain a large number of dense and regularly laminated bodies, often clustered together. Occasionally, wormlike bodies are found, whereas LG are always absent.[2,22,26,28]

Differential Diagnosis

JXG and PX can be excluded in view of the color of the lesions and the presence of both foamy cells and Touton giant cells. Multicentric reticulohistiocytosis can be ruled out because of the absence of arthritis and the lack of multinucleated giant cells. Benign cephalic histiocytosis (BCH) has lesions localized on the face and affects only children; nevertheless, this disease may represent a problem in differential diagnosis because it is histologically closely related to GEH.

Histiocytosis X is easily excluded not only on the basis of its clinical features but because of its typical histologic, immunocytochemical, and ultrastructural features.

FIGURE 161-5

CHAPTER 161
Cutaneous Nonhistiocytoses X   1895

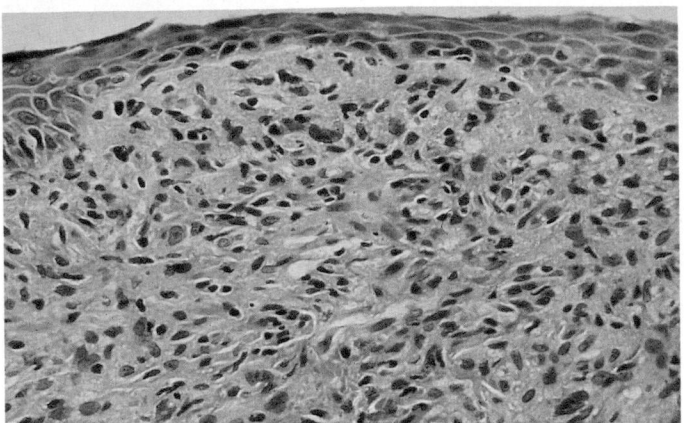

Generalized eruptive histiocytosis. Histopathologic findings. Dense monomorphous histiocytic infiltrate in the papillary and mid-dermis intermingled with a few lymphocytes.

Course and Prognosis

New crops of lesions may continue for years. Slowly the disease subsides spontaneously without a trace or leaving anetoderma-like macules. General health is always normal. Winkelmann[1] suggests that this syndrome could represent the primitive form of other, more developed, nonhistiocytoses X [JXG, papular xanthoma (PX), BCH, multicentric reticulohistiocytosis]. The appearance of xanthomatous lesions in children with the disease[26,33] may support this hypothesis.

BENIGN CEPHALIC HISTIOCYTOSIS

Definition and Historic Aspects

BCH is self-healing, cutaneous, nonhistiocystosis X, characteristically occurring on the head, especially the face.

First described in 1971 by Gianotti et al,[34] it was named "histiocytosis with intracytoplasmic wormlike bodies" because of the presence of such particles in the cytoplasm. Ultrastructural examination of specimens from many different histiocytopathies has shown comma-shaped bodies. Therefore the name *benign cephalic histiocytosis* was suggested,[2] focusing on its most typical clinical feature. The first two cases observed in the United States were reported by Barsky et al.[35] in 1984 and Eisemberg et al.[36] in 1985.

Incidence

The condition is very rare. Since 1971, about 30 cases have been described.[37–45] The incidence in boys and girls is about the same.

Age of Onset

The age of onset is 5 to 34 months (mean, 13.5 months).

Clinical Findings

The eruption consists of asymptomatic, slightly raised, round or oval, pinkish and brownish-yellow papules, 2 to 8 mm in diameter, localized first on the upper part of the face, mainly around the

FIGURE 161-6

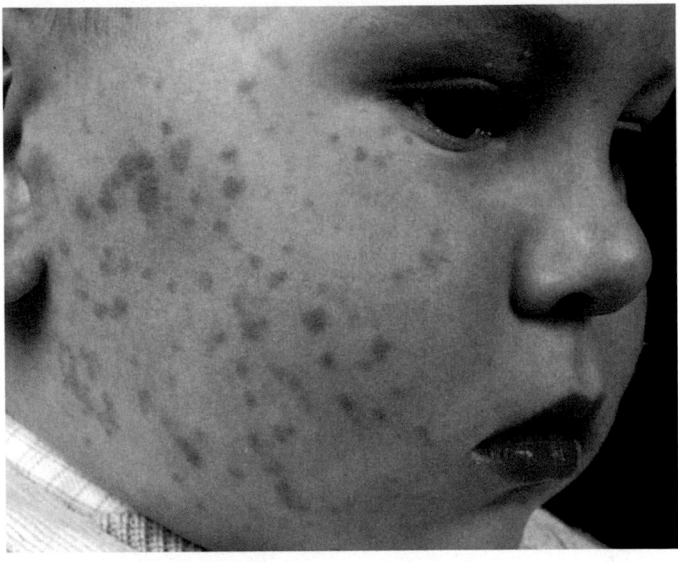

Benign cephalic histiocytosis.

eyelids, forehead, and cheeks (Fig. 161-6). Other lesions subsequently appear over the entire head, the auricles (particularly on the posterior side), the occipital region, and the neck; a few other lesions may appear on the shoulders and arms. Mucous membranes and viscera are always spared. The number of lesions at the beginning of the disease varies considerably, from 2 to more than 100. New lesions continue to appear for many months.

Histopathologic Findings

By conventional microscopy,[37,45] early lesions show a well-circumscribed infiltrate, closely attached to the lower surface of the epidermis, which is thin and flattened. Most of the cells in the infiltrate are histiocytes with pleomorphic nuclei, sparse chromatin, and barely recognizable, sometimes glassy, cytoplasm. Scattered or grouped lymphocytes and a few eosinophils are found among the histiocytes. Old lesions have few multinucleated giant cells with peripheral nuclei. The histiocytes are S-100 and CD1a negative and CD11b and CD4 positive. By electron microscopy,[22,34,35,37,38] many coated vesicles with a diameter ranging from 500 to 1500 mm are seen in all the histiocytes. Clusters of comma-shaped bodies (Fig. 161-7) are present in nearly one-fourth of the histiocytes. The comma-shaped bodies are formed by two electron-dense membranes of approximately 6 mm, separated by a light space of about 8 mm. Where the infiltrate is more dense, desmosome-like junctions may be observed among the histiocytes. These cells always lack LG.

Differential Diagnosis

BCH can be differentiated from JXG (particularly the small nodular type), in which the nodules are pleomorphic and not limited to the head and neck. Histologically, the latter nodules appear to be composed of many multinucleated giant cells and foamy cells. Electron microscopy demonstrates lipid droplets without limiting membranes in the cytoplasm of the macrophages. The nodular type of urticaria

pear without leaving scars. Both the mental and the physical development of the patients are normal.

FIGURE 161-7

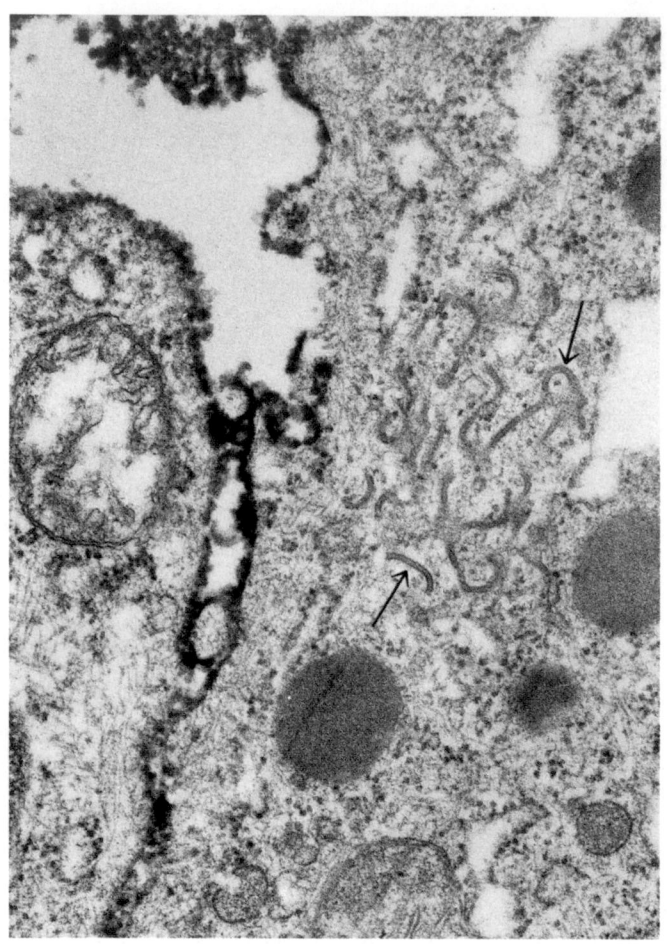

Benign cephalic histiocytosis. Ultrastructural findings. Comma-shaped bodies may be seen in the cytoplasm (*arrows*); they consist of two electron-dense membranes separated by a less dense space.

pigmentosa is distinguishable because of the wheal that follows immediately after the lesions are rubbed; mast cells are an obvious histopathologic marker. The lichenoid form of sarcoidosis can be diagnosed by its islands of epithelioid cells permeated and surrounded by reticulum fibers. GEH is distinguishable because of the age of onset (mainly adults) and the sites involved. Electron microscopy demonstrates many dense and regularly laminated bodies clustered together in the macrophages. PX can be differentiated because the lesions are widespread and show foamy cells and Touton giant cells, even in the early stage. Histiocytosis X, especially the chronic disseminated form (Hand-Shüller-Christian disease), is distinguishable because its papular lesions spread to the scalp and the trunk. Histopathology, S-100 protein staining, and electron microscopy confirm the diagnosis.

Course and Prognosis

Spontaneous regression of lesions occurs 8 months to 4 years after the onset of the eruption. Regression of lesions starts characteristically where papules first appeared. The papules begin to flatten and then, after a short period of hyperpigmentation, the lesions disap-

SINUS HISTIOCYTOSIS WITH MASSIVE LYMPHADENOPATHY

Definition and Historic Aspects

Sinus histiocytosis with massive lymphadenopathy (SHML)[46,47] is a benign, generally self-limited disease confined mainly to cervical lymph nodes. It is usually accompanied by fever, elevated erythrocyte sedimentation rate, leukocytosis with neutrophilia, and polyclonal hypergammaglobulinemia. Cutaneous manifestations are observed in about 10 percent of patients.[48–52]

SHML was first described in 1969 by Rosai and Dorfman[46] (Rosai-Dorfman syndrome). Thawerani et al.[49] emphasized its cutaneous manifestations in 1978.

Incidence

SHML is a relatively rare disease; about 365 cases have been studied and followed.[53] The disease has a worldwide distribution with a predilection for blacks from Africa and the West Indies. There is no sexual predilection.

Age of Onset

Any age group may be affected, but 80 percent of cases occur in the first or second decades of life.[52,53]

Clinical Findings

Cutaneous lesions are polymorphic[50–52] (Fig. 161-8). They may occur as yellowish macules and patches, reddish-brown papules, plaques, and nodules that may become eroded or ulcerated. In one patient,[49] firm purple nodules and tumors, as large as 10 cm in

FIGURE 161-8

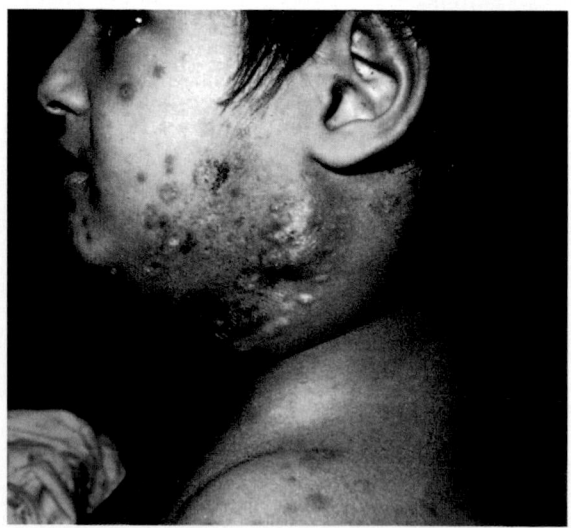

Sinus histiocytosis with massive lymphadenopathy.

diameter, were noted, but in most instances the lesions are much smaller. Most lesions are multiple, widespread, and asymptomatic. A special presentation of SHML on the skin can be misinterpreted when periocular involvement results in a lobulated induration of the eyelids.[54] Cutaneous manifestations may be the initial presentation of the disease and may constitute its sole presenting feature.[52] A massive bilateral cervical lymphadenopathy, usually painless, is the hallmark of the condition. Less commonly, axillary, mediastinal, inguinal, and preauricular lymph nodes may be affected.

Associations

Extranodal disease occurs in about 25 percent of patients[52] and may be the initial manifestation of the disorder. The extranodal non-cutaneous sites most commonly affected are the eye,[54] upper respiratory tract,[55] liver, spleen, testes, skeleton,[56] and nervous system.[57] Fever, an elevated erythrocyte sedimentation rate, leukocytosis with neutrophilia, and polyclonal hypergammaglobulinemia are common (90 percent of tested patients).[53] Less frequent findings include moderate anemia (60 percent), lymphopenia, elevated titers of Epstein-Barr virus,[53] and, in one case, elevated *Klebsiella* antibody titers.[52]

Histopathologic Findings

Histopathologically,[49,50,52] the skin lesions are characterized by a dermal infiltrate composed predominantly of histiocytes with large vesicular nuclei and abundant pale cytoplasm. Some histiocytes are foamy, multinucleated, or both. Lymphophagocytosis has been described. Histiocytes are sometimes aggregated in clusters resembling lymph node sinuses. Lymphocytes, plasma cells, and polymorphonuclear leukocytes may be intermixed in the infiltrate. Recent reports[53,58] have shown that most of the histiocytes of SHML lesions are S-100 positive and CD1a negative. Electron microscopy[50] shows that most histiocytes forming the infiltrate are rich in phagosomes and may contain clusters of comma-shaped bodies. LG are absent.

Etiology

The cause of SHML remains obscure. Two main hypotheses have been proposed: a disturbance of cell-mediated immunity or a primary infection (Epstein-Barr virus, *Klebsiella*).[52,53]

Differential Diagnosis

The absence of characteristic cutaneous clinical aspects and the variety of the lesions observed in patients with SHML require a differential diagnosis with many diseases, both proliferative and inflammatory, mainly based on histopathologic and immunologic findings. The histopathologic combination of histiocytes with abundant pale cytoplasm, a mixed-cell infiltrate, and karyophagocytosis is an important criterion of differentiation. The observation that histiocytes forming the infiltrate of SHML are mainly S-100 positive and CD1a negative, if confirmed, could be another distinctive feature of this disease.

Treatment

Because the vast majority of lesions of SHML heal spontaneously, no treatment is necessary as a rule. In rare instances, a space-occupying lesion may interfere with the function of an organ and then

treatment with systemic glucocorticoids or with various chemotherapeutic regimens may be useful.[52]

Course and Prognosis

In most patients, SHML has a benign course[52] with a spontaneous regression over a period of months to years. Usually the extranodal lesions regress first, whereas adenopathy may persist for years.[47] A worse prognosis results mainly from associated immunologic abnormalities.[59]

XANTHOMA DISSEMINATUM

Definition and Historic Aspects

XD, or Montgomery's syndrome, is a rare, benign, normolipemic form of histiocytoxanthomatosis affecting the skin and mucous membranes, frequently associated with diabetes insipidus.

Montgomery and Osterberg[60] in 1938 first recognized this distinct type of cutaneous xanthomatosis. Altman and Winkelmann[61] reviewed the literature and confirmed this syndrome.

Incidence

The condition is rare (about 100 cases)[62–64] and affects males more frequently than females.[60] The apparently random nature of this disorder does not permit an exact evaluation of either familial involvement or morbidity.

Age of Onset

In about 60 percent of the patients, onset is before age 25 years.[61]

Clinical Findings

The cutaneous manifestations consist of an eruption of hundreds of papules that are red-brown at first and then become yellowish (Fig. 161-9). They symmetrically involve the trunk, face, and proximal

FIGURE 161-9

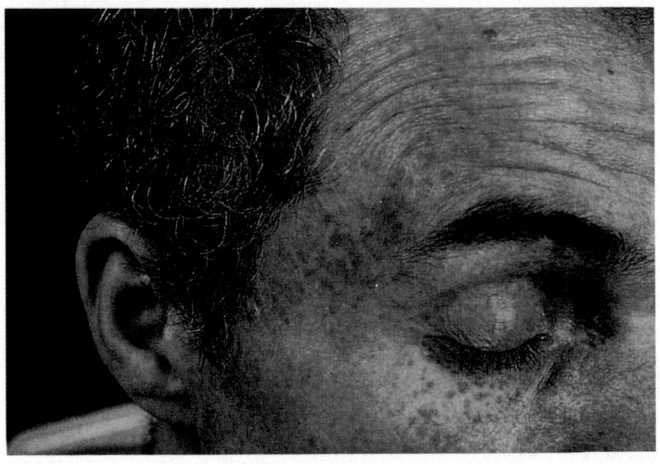

Xanthoma disseminatum.

extremities and, in flexures and folds, tend quickly to merge, forming verrucous plaques.[61,64] In about 50 percent of the cases,[61,63] xanthomatous lesions may also be observed on the mucous membranes of the mouth, pharynx, and larynx and on the conjunctiva and cornea. Symptoms of dyspnea and dysphagia are not uncommon. Vasopressin-sensitive transitory diabetes insipidus is present in less than 50 percent of cases.[61,63] The polyuria and polydipsia are generally mild. The specific gravity of the urine may be relatively high (more than 1003).[61] A normal lipid profile is present in this disease; nevertheless, slightly elevated values of serum cholesterol or triglycerides have been found in a few cases.[63]

Associations

Osteolytic lesions have been reported in only a few patients.[65] XD may be associated with multiple myeloma,[66] Waldenström's macroglobulinemia,[67] and monoclonal gammopathy.[68]

Histopathologic Findings

In the early stage, histopathologic study shows a mixture of histiocytes, foamy cells, and inflammatory cells; later, foamy cells predominate and Touton giant cells are frequently present.[63] Siderosis is often observed[61] (Fig. 161-10). The proliferating cells are S-100 and CD1a negative.[62] Ultrastructurally,[22] the cells are similar to those present in JXG and in PX, but the plasma membranes of foamy cells show many microvilli. LG are absent.

Differential Diagnosis

In hyperlipemic xanthomatoses, the metabolic disorder is primary and it affects the appearance of the lesions; moreover the distribution of xanthomas is completely different. XD differs from PX in the tendency of its lesions to merge into plaques, the typical mucous membrane involvement, and its associated diabetes insipidus. JXG

FIGURE 161-10

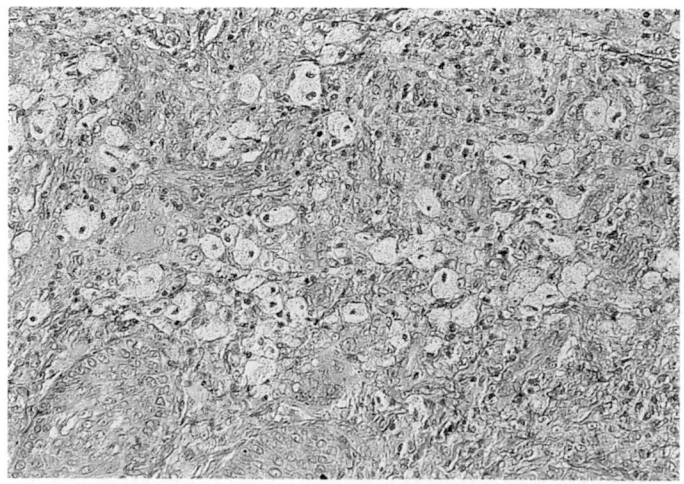

Xanthoma disseminatum. Histopathologic findings. The lesions are characterized by a mixture of histiocytes, inflammatory cells, and foamy cells. Touton giant cells are present.

mainly affects children, and the lesions do not merge into plaques; there may be visceral involvement, but diabetes insipidus is absent. Multicentric reticulohistiocytosis occurs mainly in adults, is associated with destructive joint lesions, and is not self-limited. The lesions of GEH never contain lipids, and there is a tendency of the lesions to coalesce. The chronic disseminated form of histiocytosis X (Hand-Schüller-Christian disease) is distinguishable because its papular lesions spread to the scalp and trunk, and bone lesions are the most frequent manifestation. Histiocytosis X cells are S-100 and CD1a positive and contain LG.

Treatment

Treatment is usually not helpful.[61,63] Systemic glucocorticoids and antimitotic agents have been used for the more disfiguring forms. Vasopressin injection is necessary to check associated diabetes insipidus.

Course and Prognosis

Based on the evolution and prognosis of reported cases, Caputo et al.[64] have distinguished three clinical variants of XD: a self-healing form, a persistent form, and a progressive form. The persistent form is the most frequent one; mucocutaneous lesions, even if discrete, may persist forever in patients in good general condition. XD could represent the evolution of other, less developed nonhistiocytoses X–like generalized eruptive histiocytoses.[61,69] Prognosis is usually good, but the involvement of the respiratory tract may induce dyspnea and dysphagia. Tracheotomy has been required in a few cases.[61]

PAPULAR XANTHOMA (See also Chap. 152)

Definition and Historic Aspects

PX is a normolipidemic papular xanthomatosis histologically different from other normolipidemic xanthomatoses such as JXG and XD.

This disease was first described by Winkelmann[1] in 1981 in adults. The first pediatric cases were reported by Caputo et al.[70] in 1990.

Incidence

PX is a rare disorder; fewer than 20 cases have been described.[1,70]

Age of Onset

The onset of PX in children is usually during the first year of life[70] (9 of 10 cases reported to date). The disease seems to be more frequent in males.

Clinical Findings

PX is characterized by the eruption of 2- to 12-mm, rounded, yellowish, asymptomatic, papulonodular lesions in a generalized distribution with no tendency to merge into plaques (Fig. 161-11). Occasionally mucous membranes may be involved. No visceral involvement can be found; the lipid profile is normal; diabetes insipidus is absent.

FIGURE 161-11

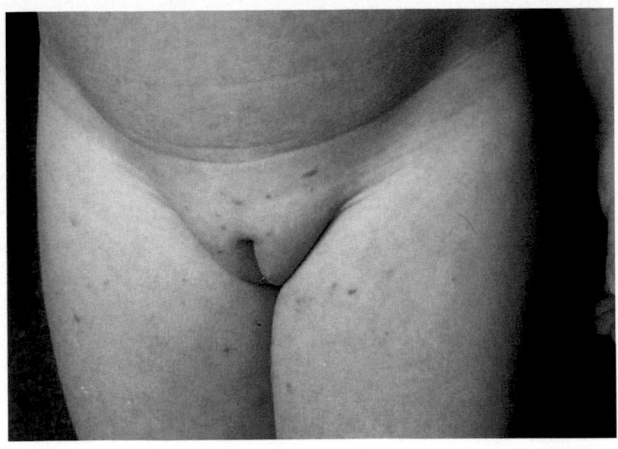

Papular xanthoma in a child.

Histopathologic Findings

The lesions are composed almost entirely of foamy cells and Touton giant cells. There is no evidence of a primitive histiocytic phase and inflammatory cells are absent[1,70] (Fig. 161-12). The foamy cells are S-100 and CD1a negative.[70–72] Ultrastructurally,[70,71] the cytoplasm is completely filled with lipid vacuoles that lack a limiting membrane, myeloid bodies, and lysosomal inclusions. Neither LG nor comma-shaped bodies are found in these histiocytes.

Differential Diagnosis

PX differs from XD in that the lesions do not tend to merge into plaques and do not turn red-brown, the skin folds are spared, and there is no diabetes insipidus. Histologically, inflammatory cells are absent. JXG can be recognized by its pure primitive histiocytic phase and, in mature lesions, by the presence of inflammatory cells. Benign cephalic histiocytosis differs in localization and never shows lipidation. GEH does not have lipid-containing cells. PX is clini-

FIGURE 161-12

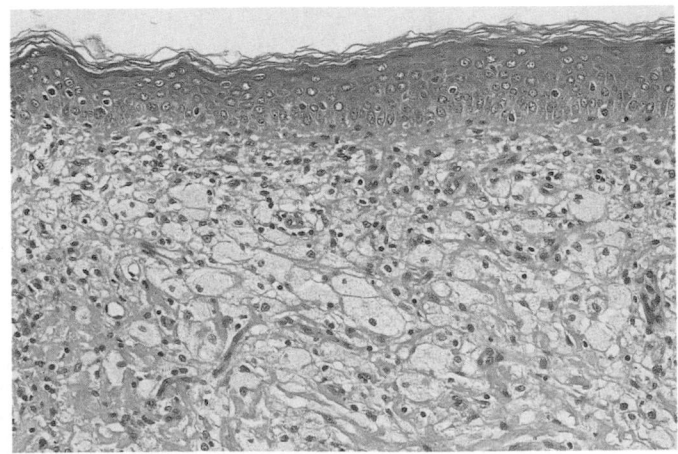

Papular xanthoma. Histopathologic findings. The lesion is composed almost entirely of foamy cells. Inflammatory cells are absent.

cally and histologically difficult to differentiate from the xanthomatous lesions that may appear in histiocytosis X, but history and the absence of lesions typical of histiocytosis X (S-100 positive cells and LG) are discriminating factors. It is clinically and histologically indistinguishable from disseminated papular xanthomas with hyperlipoproteinemia, but here serum lipids provide the correct diagnosis.

Course and Prognosis

In most of the cases involving children the lesions regressed within 1 to 5 years[70]; thus PX seems to be, at least in children, a self-healing xanthomatosis. A progressive course has also been described in several cases.[71,73,74]

NECROBIOTIC XANTHOGRANULOMA

Definition

Necrobiotic xanthogranuloma (NXG) was first recognized as a separate entity by Kossard and Winkelmann in 1980.[75] It is an inflammatory histiocytoxanthomatosis involving the dermis and subcutaneous tissue primarily of the face and less frequently of the trunk and extremities. Clinically, the disorder is characterized by indurated yellow-red nodules or plaques, often ulcerated; histologically, by xanthogranulomatous features with various amounts of necrobiosis or hyalin necrosis and the presence of lymphoid nodules. There is frequently paraproteinemia, and occasionally there are elevated erythrocyte sedimentation rate, cryoglobulinemia, anemia, and leukopenia.[75–90]

Incidence

Approximately 60 cases have been described in the literature.[89]

Age of Onset

The age of onset of NXG ranges from 17 to 85 years, and the disease has no sex predilection.[83,85]

Clinical Findings

Early cutaneous lesions consist of firm papulonodules varying in color from red-orange to violaceous.[75,81,85] These lesions slowly enlarge into plaques with well-demarcated edges, ranging in size from a few centimeters to 25 cm in diameter; the color may assume a yellow, xanthomatous hue. Often these plaques may show central atrophy with telangectasias or areas of ulceration (Fig. 161-13). Most cases are asymptomatic, but pain or a burning sensation may be noted.[85] The lesions are usually multiple and involve, in order of frequency, the face, trunk, and extremities. The periorbital area is the site of predilection (85 percent of cases).[85] The oral mucosa is occasionally involved.[88] Hepato- and splenomegaly have been observed in approximately 20 percent of patients.[85]

Associations

NXG may be associated with myeloma,[76,82,90] arthropathy,[85] hypertension,[85] neuropathy,[85] neoplastic syndrome,[82] primary biliary cirrhosis,[81] and Graves' disease.[85]

FIGURE 161-13

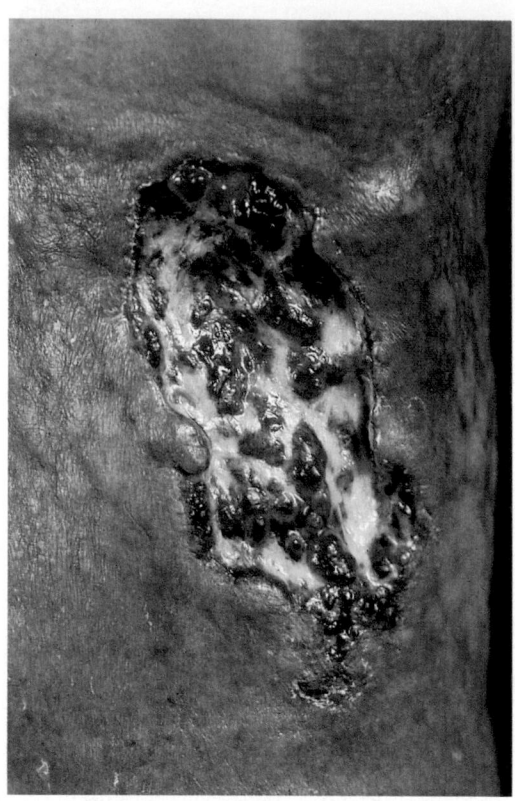

Necrobiotic xanthogranuloma on the calf. Note "granulomatous" periphery of the lesion, with central ulceration and necrotic material at the base.

Complications

The periorbital involvement may lead to important ocular complications such as lagophthalmos, conjunctivitis, keratitis, scleritis, uveitis, corneal ulceration and even loss of ocular function.[77,78,82,85]

Laboratory Findings

Ninety percent of patients have paraproteinemia (IgG κ or λ), while cryoglobulinemia has been found in about 40 percent of cases.[81,82,85,87,88] Other abnormal laboratory tests include an elevated sedimentation rate (57 percent), neutropenia (30 percent), leukopenia (35 percent), and decreased CH50 (47 percent).

Histopathologic Findings

The histopathologic picture of NXG is characteristic and consists of a granulomatous infiltrate involving the whole dermis and the subcutis and comprising a mixture of lymphocytes, epithelioid cells, foamy cells, and Touton giant cells.[76,81,82,85,90] Areas of severe, clearly defined necrobiosis are sharply marginated from the surrounding granuloma. Cholesterol crystals may be located within the necrobiotic areas. Numerous, atypical, very large, bizarrely angulated, multinucleated giant cells may be seen adjacent to the areas of necrobiosis. Dense, well-defined lymphoid nodules, occasionally containing a germinal center, may be present in the dermis or pan-

niculus. A Touton cell panniculitis may involve the entire fat lobules. Occasionally, a granulomatous infiltrate may surround some vessels.

Immunohistochemically, the cells constituting the infiltrate are CD15 and CD4 positive and CD1a and S-100 negative.[85,90] Ultrastructurally, cells are rich in lipid droplets, cholesterol clefts, and myeloid bodies[84,90] and are similar to those observed in JXG.

Etiopathogenesis

The pathogenesis of NXG is unclear and so is its link to paraproteinemia.

Differential Diagnosis

The differential diagnosis of NXG includes necrobiosis lipoidica diabeticorum, granuloma annulare, XD, and multicentric reticulohistiocytosis.

In necrobiosis lipoidica diabeticorum, facial and scalp lesions are exceptional and are not associated with any serum protein abnormalities but are with diabetes. Histologically, the necrobiotic changes and the granulomatous infiltrate are less prominent, lymphoid nodules are absent, and cholesterol clefts are rare.

The subcutaneous form of granuloma annulare occurs mainly in children and does not tend to ulcerate. Giant cells are rare, and lymphoid nodules and cholesterol clefts are absent.

In XD, the large body folds are the main sites of predilection and the periorbicular lesions are less firm and infiltrated and do not tend to ulcerate.

In multicentric reticulohistiocytosis, the lesions do not tend to ulcerate and do not merge into plaques; they are frequently associated with a severe arthropathy and histologically feature large histiocytes with a typical "ground glass" cytoplasm and no necrobiosis.

Treatment

Intermittent glucocorticoid treatment can induce partial response without complete disappearance of the lesions.[81,90] Low-dose alkylating agents, such as chlorambucil or melphalan, produced remission of the paraproteinemia and skin lesions in several cases.[81,82,85] These treatments did not prevent the evolution to multiple myeloma.[82] Temporary remissions of skin lesions have been obtained with radiation therapy[91] and with plasmapheresis.[92]

Course and Prognosis

NXG has a chronic, often progressive course characterized by the appearance of new lesions and ulcerations.[82,85] The prognosis of patients is difficult to predict and depends on extracutaneous involvement, multiple myeloma, or visceral tumors.

REFERENCES

1. Winkelmann RK: Cutaneous syndromes of non-X histiocytosis. A review of the macrophage-histiocyte diseases of the skin. *Arch Dermatol* **117**:667, 1981
2. Gianotti F, Caputo R: Histiocytic syndromes: A review. *J Am Acad Dermatol* **13**:383, 1985
3. Ringel E, Moschella S: Primary histiocytic dermatoses. *Arch Dermatol* **121**:1531, 1985
4. Roper SS, Spraker MD: Cutaneous histiocytosis syndromes. *Pediatr Dermatol* **3**:19, 1985
5. McDonough JFR: A contribution to our knowledge of naevo xanthoendothelioma. *Br J Dermatol Syphilol* **24**:85, 1912

6. Helwig EB, Macknay VC: Juvenile xanthogranuloma. *Am J Pathol* **30**:625, 1954

7. Laurb HM, Lain ES: Nevoxanthoendothelioma: Its relationship to juvenile xanthomas. *S Afr Med J* **30**:585, 1937

8. Blank M et al: Nevoxanthoendothelioma with ocular involvement. *Pediatrics* **4**:349, 1949

9. Cohen BA, Hood A: Xanthogranuloma: Report on clinical and histologic findings in 64 patients. *Pediatr Dermatol* **6**:262, 1989

10. Gianotti F, Zina G: Xanthogranulomatoses juvenile, in *XIIIé Congrès de l'Association des Dermatologistes et Syphiligraphes de Langue Française, Turin, 1969*. Paris, Masson, 1971, p 103

11. Guinnepin MT, Puissant A: Juvenile xanthogranulome. *G Ital Dermatol Venereol* **115**:101, 1980

12. Malbos G et al: Le xanthogranulome de l'adulte: Étude anatomo clinique d'un cas. *Dermatologica* **158**:334, 1979

13. Campbell L et al: Giant juvenile xanthogranuloma. *Arch Dermatol* **124**:1723, 1988

14. Cohen BA, Hood A: Xanthogranuloma: Report on clinical and histologic findings in 64 patients. *Pediatr Dermatol* **6**:262, 1989

15. Caputo R et al: Unusual aspects of juvenile xanthogranuloma. *J Am Acad Dermatol* **29**:868, 1993

16. Janney CG et al: Deep juvenile xanthogranuloma. Subcutaneous and intramuscular forms. *Am J Surg Pathol* **15**:150, 1992

17. Sanchez Yus E et al: Subcutaneous juvenile xanthogranuloma. *J Cutan Pathol* **22**:460, 1995

18. Newell GB et al: Juvenile xanthogranuloma and neurofibromatosis. *Arch Dermatol* **107**:262, 1973

19. Zimmerman E: Ocular lesions of juvenile xanthogranuloma. *Am J Ophthalmol* **60**:1011, 1965

20. Flach DB, Winkelmann RK: Juvenile xanthogranuloma with central nervous system lesions. *J Am Acad Dermatol* **14**:405, 1986

21. Cooper PM et al: Association of juvenile xanthogranuloma with juvenile myeloid leukemia. *Arch Dermatol* **120**:371, 1984

22. Caputo R, Gianotti F: Cytoplasmic markers and unusual ultrastructural features in histiocytic proliferations of the skin. *G Ital Dermatol Venereol* **115**:107, 1980

23. Török E, Daròczy J: Juvenile xanthogranuloma: An analysis of 45 cases by clinical follow-up, light- and electron microscopy. *Acta Derm Venereol (Stockh)* **65**:167, 1985

24. Winkelmann RK, Müller SA: Generalized eruptive histiocytoma: A benign papular histiocytic reticulosis. *Arch Dermatol* **88**:586, 1963

25. Müller SA et al: Generalized eruptive histiocytoma: Enzyme histochemistry and electron microscopy. *Arch Dermatol* **96**:11, 1967

26. Caputo R et al: Generalized eruptive histiocytoma in children. *J Am Acad Dermatol* **17**:449, 1987

27. Winkelmann RK et al: Eruptive histiocytoma of childhood. *Arch Dermatol* **166**:565, 1980

28. Caputo R et al: Generalized eruptive histiocytoma. A clinical, histological, ultrastructural study. *Arch Dermatol* **117**:216, 1981

29. Arnold ML et al: Generalisierte eruptive histiozytome. *Hautarzt* **33**:428, 1982

30. Bobin P et al: Histiocytome eruptive généralizé. *Ann Dermatol Venereol* **110**:817, 1983

31. Vignon-Pennamen MD et al: Histiocytome éruptif généralisé: Histiocytose cutanée non X marquée par l'OKT6. *Ann Dermatol Venereol* **113**:1027, 1986

32. Sigal-Nahum M et al: Histiocytose non X (histiocytome éruptive généralisé?) marquée par l'OKT6, à filaments de vimentine. *Ann Dermatol Venereol* **114**:211, 1987

33. Repiso T et al: Generalized eruptive histiocytoma evolving into xanthoma disseminatum in a 4-year-old boy. *Br J Dermatol* **132**:978, 1995

34. Gianotti F et al: Singulière histiocytose infantile à cellules avec perticules vermiformes intracytoplasmiques. *Bull Soc Fr Dermatol Syphilol* **72**:232, 1971

35. Barsky BL et al: Benign cephalic histiocytosis. *Arch Dermatol* **120**:650, 1984

36. Eisemberg EL et al: Benign cephalic histiocytosis. *J Am Acad Dermatol* **12**:328, 1985

37. Gianotti F, Caputo R: Unknown histiocytosis with intracytoplasmic worm-like particles in 2 children, in *Dermatology Proceedings of the XIV International Congress*. Amsterdam, Excerpta Medica, 1972, p 47

38. Gianotti F et al: Benign cephalic histiocytosis. *Arch Dermatol* **122**:1038, 1986

39. Ayala F et al: Benign cephalic histiocytosis. *Acta Dermatol Venereol (Stockh)* **68**:264, 1988

40. Larralde de Luna M et al: Benign cephalic histiocytosis: Report of four cases. *Pediatr Dermatol* **6**:198, 1989

41. Godfrey KM, James MP: Benign cephalic histiocytosis: A case report. *Br J Dermatol* **123**:245, 1990

42. Aoki N et al: A case of benign cephalic histiocytosis (abstr). *Nippon Hifuka Gakkai Zasshi* **101**:469, 1991

43. Goday JJ et al: Benign cephalic histiocytosis. Study of a case. *Clin Exp Dermatol* **18**:280, 1993

44. Lucky AW, Prendville JS: An 18-month-old boy with a persistent papular eruption. *Pediatr Dermatol* **10**:195, 1993

45. Pena-Penabad C et al: Benign cephalic histiocytosis: Case report and literature review. *Pediatr Dermatol* **11**:164, 1994

46. Rosai J, Dorfman RF: Sinus histiocytosis with massive lymphadenopathy: A newly recognized benign clinicopathological entity. *Arch Pathol* **87**:63, 1969

47. Rosai J, Dorfman RF: Sinus histiocytosis with massive lymphadenopathy: A pseudolymphomatous benign disorder. Analysis of 34 cases. *CA* **30**:1174, 1972

48. Pickering LK, Phelan E: Sinus histiocytosis. *J Pediatr* **86**:745, 1974

49. Thawerani H et al: The cutaneous manifestations of sinus histiocytosis with massive lymphadenopathy. *Arch Dermatol* **114**:191, 1978

50. Avril MF et al: Manifestations cutanées du syndrome de Rosai et Dorfman. *Ann Dermatol Venereol* **111**:661, 1984

51. Lorette G et al: Histiocytose sinusale avec manifestations cutanées. *Ann Dermatol Venereol* **114**:1430, 1987

52. Olsen EA et al: Sinus histiocytosis with massive lymphadenopathy. *J Am Acad Dermatol* **18**:1322, 1988

53. Foucar E et al: Sinus histiocytosis with massive lymphadenopathy. Current status and future directions. *Arch Dermatol* **124**:1211, 1988

54. Friendly DS et al: Orbital involvement in "sinus" histiocytosis. A report of four cases. *Arch Ophthalmol* **95**:2006, 1977

55. Foucar E et al: Sinus histiocytosis with massive lymphadenopathy. Ear, nose and throat manifestations. *Arch Otolaryngol* **104**:687, 1978

56. Walker PD et al: The osseous manifestations of sinus histiocytosis with massive lymphadenopathy. *Am J Clin Pathol* **75**:131, 1981

57. Foucar E et al: The neurologic manifestations of sinus histiocytosis with massive lymphadenopathy. *Neurology* **32**:365, 1982

58. Bonetti F et al: Immunohistological analysis of Rosai-Dorfman histiocytosis: A disease of S 100$^+$ CDl$^-$ histiocytes. *Virchows Arch [A]* **411**:129, 1987

59. Foucar E et al: Sinus histiocytosis with massive lymphadenopathy. An analysis of 14 deaths occurring in a patient registry. *CA* **54**:1834, 1984

60. Montgomery H, Osterberg AE: Xanthomatosis. Correlation of clinical, histopathologic and chemical studies of cutaneous xanthoma. *Arch Dermatol Syphilol* **208**:373, 1938

61. Altman J, Winkelmann RK: Xanthoma disseminatum. *Arch Dermatol* **85**:582, 1962

62. Chanudet MM et al: Xanthomatose cutaneo-muqueuse de Montgomery. *Ann Dermatol Venereol* **114**:1360, 1987

63. Beury J et al: Xantoma disseminatum (sindrome de Montgomery). *Ann Dermatol Venereol* **106**:353, 1979

64. Caputo R et al: The various clinical patterns of xanthoma disseminatum. *Dermatology* **190**:19, 1995

65. Mishkel MA et al: Xanthoma disseminatum. Clinical, metabolic, pathologic and radiologic aspects. *Arch Dermatol* **13**:1094, 1977

66. Maize JC et al: Xanthoma disseminatum and multiple myeloma. *Arch Dermatol* **110**:758, 1974

67. Goodemberger ME et al: Xanthoma disseminatum and Waldenstrom's macroglobulinemia. *J Am Acad Dermatol* **23**:1015, 1990

68. Vignon-Pennamen MD et al: Xanthomatose cutaneomuqueuse de Montgomery et gammopathie monoclonale. *Ann Dermatol Venereol* **18**:821, 1991

69. Coldiron BM et al: Benign non X histiocytosis: A unique case bridging several non X histiocytic syndromes. *J Am Acad Dermatol* **18**:1282, 1988

70. Caputo R et al: Papular xanthoma in children. *J Am Acad Dermatol* **22**:1052, 1990

71. Sanchez RL et al: Papular xanthoma. *Arch Dermatol* **121**:626, 1985

72. Bundino S et al: Papular xanthoma. Clinical, histological and ultrastructural study. *Dermatologica* **177**:382, 1988

73. Tauriton OD et al: Progressive nodular histiocytoma. *Arch Dermatol* **114**:1505, 1978

74. Burgdorf WH et al: Progressive nodular histiocytoma. *Arch Dermatol* **117**:644, 1981

75. Kossard S, Winkelmann RK: Necrobiotic xanthogranuloma. *Australas J Dermatol* **21**:85, 1980

76. Finan MC, Winkelmann RK: Necrobiotic xanthogranuloma with paraproteinemia: A review of 22 cases. *Medicine (Baltimore)* **65**:376, 1986

77. Kocsard E: Xantogranuloma necrobiotico con paraproteinemia. *G Ital Dermatol Venereol* **118**:219, 1983

78. Codère F et al: Necrobiotic xanthogranuloma of the eyelid. *Arch Ophthalmol* **101**:60, 1983

79. Hunter L, Burry AF: Necrobiotic xanthogranuloma—a systemic disease with paraproteinemia. *Pathology* **17**:533, 1985

80. MacFarlane AW, Verbov JL: Necrobiotic xanthogranuloma with paraproteinaemia. *Br J Dermatol* **113**:339, 1985

81. Holden CA et al: Necrobiotic xanthogranuloma: A report of four cases. *Br J Dermatol* **114**:241, 1986

82. Venencie PY et al: Necrobiotic xanthogranuloma with myeloma: A case report. *Cancer* **59**:588, 1987

83. Venencie PY et al: Le xanthogranulome nécrobiotique. *Ann Dermatol Venereol* **115**:1297, 1988

84. Bourlond A et al: Xanthogranulome nécrobiotique et myélome. *Dermatologica* **179**:139, 1989

85. Mehregan DA, Winkelmann RK: Necrobiotic xanthogranuloma. *Arch Dermatol* **123**:94, 1992

86. Venencie PY et al: Xanthogranulome nécrobiotique avec paraprotéinémie. *Ann Dermatol Venereol* **119**:825, 1992

87. Tomasini C et al: Xantogranuloma nacrobiotico. *G Ital Dermatol Venereol* **128**:61, 1993

88. Forstson JS, Schroeter AL: Necrobiotic xanthogranuloma with IgA paraproteinemia and extracutaneous involvement. *Am J Dermatopathol* **12**:579, 1990

89. Umbert I, Winkelmann RK: Necrobiotic xanthogranuloma with cardiac involvement. *Br J Dermatol* **133**:438, 1995

90. Plotnick H et al: Periorbital necrobiotic xanthogranuloma and stage I multiple myeloma. *J Am Acad Dermatol* **25**:373, 1991

91. Char DH et al: Radiation therapy for ocular necrobiotic xanthogranuloma. *Arch Ophthalmol* **105**:174, 1987

92. Finelli LG, Ratz JL: Plasmapheresis: A treatment modality for necrobiotic xanthogranuloma. *J Am Acad Dermatol* **17**:351, 1987

CHAPTER 162

Dean D. Metcalfe

The Mastocytosis Syndrome

Mastocytosis is a condition characterized by mast cell hyperplasia in the bone marrow, liver, spleen, lymph nodes, gastrointestinal tract, and skin. Clinically, the disease is often accompanied by evidence of mast cell activation, which includes pruritus, flushing, urtication, abdominal pain, nausea, vomiting, diarrhea, bone pain, vascular instability, headache, and neuropsychiatric difficulties. Mastocytosis can occur at any age and demonstrates a slight male-to-female predominance (1.5:1.0). The prevalence of the disease is unknown, and familial occurrence appears unusual.

Mastocytosis is divided into distinct clinicopathologic entities on the basis of clinical presentation, pathologic findings, and prognosis. A consensus-based classification for mastocytosis is shown in Table 162-1.[1] Patients in the indolent category have a good prognosis, while patients in the other three groups do poorly. Most children diagnosed with mastocytosis are in the group with good prognosis. Indolent mastocytosis is delineated on the basis of the presence of syncope, cutaneous disease, ulcer disease, malabsorption, bone marrow involvement, skeletal disease, hepatosplenomegaly, and lymphadenopathy. In most cases, patients with indolent disease are managed successfully with medications that provide symptomatic relief.

The second most common form of mastocytosis is that associated with a hematologic disorder and is not often observed in children. In this group, examination of the bone marrow and peripheral blood reveals the hematologic abnormality. The prognosis in these patients is determined by the course of the associated hematologic disorder.

Patients in the third category have an aggressive form of mastocytosis; these individuals, usually adults, have poor prognostic features but do not have a distinctive hematologic disorder or mast cell leukemia. There exists a subset of patients with aggressive mastocytosis who have a distinct syndrome termed *lymphadenopathic mastocytosis with eosinophilia* because of the pronounced eosino-

TABLE 162-1

Consensus Revised Classification

I. Indolent
   A. Syncope
   B. Cutaneous disease
   C. Ulcer disease
   D. Malabsorption
   E. Bone marrow mast cell aggregates
   F. Skeletal disease
   G. Hepatosplenomegaly
   H. Lymphadenopathy
II. Hematologic disorder
   A. Myeloproliferative
   B. Myelodysplastic
III. Aggressive
   A. Lymphadenopathic mastocytosis and eosinophilia
IV. Mastocytic leukemia

philia, hepatosplenomegaly, and lymphadenopathy. Patients with aggressive disease have rapidly increasing mast cell numbers and are difficult to manage medically. Their prognosis is less favorable than that of patients with indolent mastocytosis.

The fourth category of mast cell disease is mast cell leukemia; it is the rarest form and has the most fulminant behavior. The peripheral blood smear shows numerous immature mast cells. Mast cell leukemia is distinguished from the other categories by its unique pathologic and clinical picture.

ETIOLOGY AND PATHOGENESIS

Human mast cells originate from pluripotent (CD34+) bone marrow cells[2] and circulate through the bloodstream[3] to specific sites in the body where they mature into fully granulated cells. The targeting of mast cells to defined locations appears to be determined by the sequential expression of cell surface adhesion molecules, predominantly members of the integrin family.[4]

The regulation of mast cell number and mast cell differentiation is under the control of factors produced both in the bone marrow and by cells in the tissues in which mast cells finally reside. For example, human mast cell differentiation depends on c-kit ligand, also known as stem cell factor (SCF).[2,5] Final maturation and granule composition depend on factors produced in the tissue microenvironment,[6] including SCF produced by fibroblasts and stromal cells. Inhibition of local production of SCF leads to mast cell apoptosis.[7]

The receptor for SCF is c-kit. Mutations have now been identified in c-kit in peripheral blood cells and tissues from patients with mastocytosis. These mutations are associated with enhanced receptor function and may contribute to the increase in mast cell number that is characteristic of mastocytosis. The first and most common mutation identified in patients with mastocytosis consists of an A to T substitution at nucleotide 2468 of c-kit mRNA that causes an aspartic acid to valine substitution at amino acid 816.[8] This appears to be a somatic mutation,[9] which is observed in all patients with mastocytosis associated with a hematologic disorder and in patients with indolent mastocytosis. Other mutations have now been described in individual patients at amino acids 560 (Val to Gly) and 820 (Asp to Gly).[10] The relationship of these mutations to chromosomal abnormalities is unknown. However, fluorescent in situ hybridization has been used to identify trisomy 8 in five patients and trisomy 9 in one patient with unspecified patterns of mastocytosis.[11]

The pathogenesis of mastocytosis is largely the result of the increased production of mast cell mediators, which have effects both at the site of their production and remote from their origin, irrespective of the etiology of the increased burden of mast cells or the category of disease. Mast cell mediators are of three categories; all may circulate through the bloodstream and lymphatics to produce biologic effects observed in patients with mastocytosis (Table 162-2).

CLINICAL FEATURES

The four categories of mastocytosis share clinical features that are due to the excess production of mast cell–dependent mediators, although some aspects of disease may predominate in a specific cat-

TABLE 162-2

Mast Cell Mediators and Their Contribution to Pathogenesis

MEDIATORS	EFFECTS
GRANULE-ASSOCIATED	
Histamine	Pruritus, urticaria, increased vasopermeability, gastric hypersecretion, bronchoconstriction
Heparin	Local anticoagulation, osteoporosis
Tryptase, chymotryptic proteases	Bone lesions
LIPID-DERIVED	
Cysteinyl leukotrienes	Increased vasopermeability, bronchoconstriction, vasoconstriction (LTC_4); increased vasopermeability, bronchoconstriction, vasodilation (LTD_4 and LTE_4)
Prostaglandin D_2	Vasodilation, bronchoconstriction
Platelet-activating factor	Increased vasopermeability, vasodilation, bronchoconstriction
CYTOKINES	
Proinflammatory factor	Fibrosis (TGF-β); activation of vascular endothelial cells, cachexia (TNF-α)
Growth enhancing	Mast cell growth factors (IL-3, SCF); eosinophilia (IL-5)

egory. The skin, gastrointestinal tract, lymph nodes, liver, spleen, bone marrow, and skeletal system contribute the most significant management problems. The respiratory tract and endocrine systems are seldom if ever involved. Also, patients with mastocytosis do not suffer from recurrent bacterial, fungal, or viral infections even though mast cells release mediators such as histamine that can inhibit immune responses in vitro.

Urticaria pigmentosa is the most common skin manifestation of mastocytosis in both children (Fig. 162-1) and adults (Fig. 162-4). It is seen in over 90 percent of patients with indolent mastocytosis, and in fewer than 50 percent of patients with mastocytosis with an associated hematologic disorder or those with lymphadenopathic mastocytosis with eosinophilia. The lesions of urticaria pigmentosa appear as small, yellow-tan to reddish-brown macules or slightly raised papules scattered over the body. The palms, soles, face, and scalp may be free of lesions. Mild trauma, including scratching or rubbing of the lesions, usually causes urtication and erythema around the macules; this is known as *Darier's sign*. Urticaria pigmentosa is associated with a variable amount of pruritus, which may be exacerbated by changes in climatic temperature, skin friction, ingestion of hot beverages or spicy foods, ethanol, and certain drugs. The diagnosis is confirmed by characteristic skin histopathology.[12]

Diffuse cutaneous mastocytosis consists of a diffuse mast cell infiltration of the skin without discrete lesions. It usually occurs before the age of 3 years. The entire cutaneous integument is involved. The skin is normal to yellow-brown in color and is diffusely thickened.[13]

Solitary lesions called *mastocytomas* (Fig. 162-2) do occur but are quite rare. Their onset is generally before 6 months of age. In most cases such lesions involute spontaneously.

FIGURE 162-1

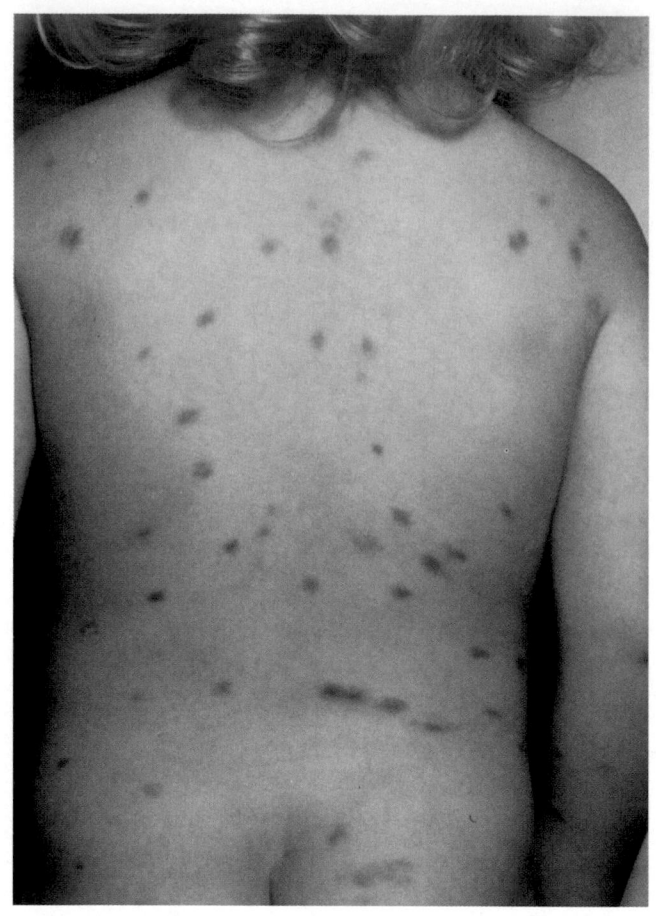

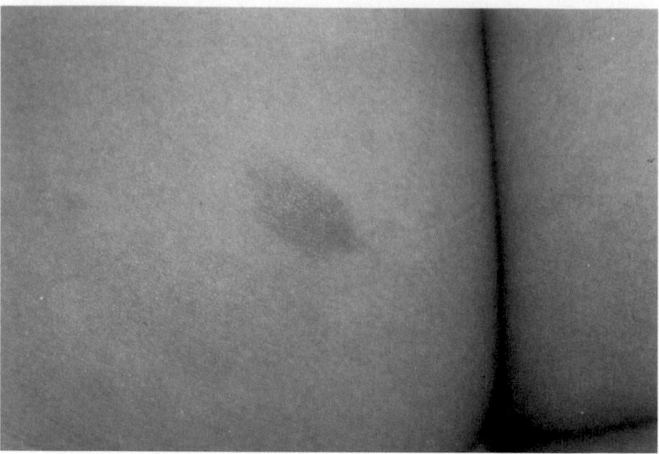

A.

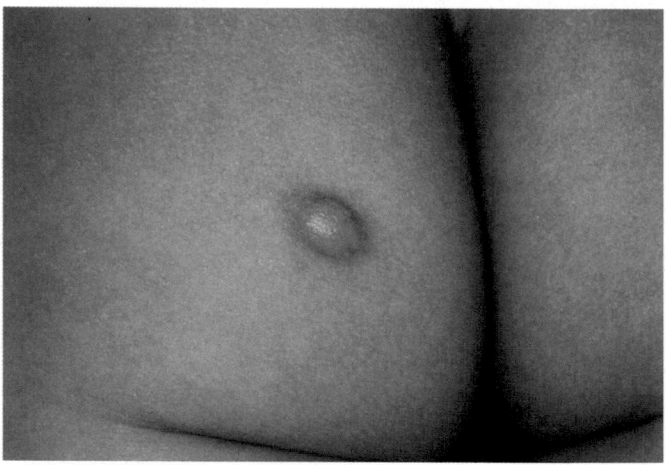

B.

Urticaria pigmentosa in a child with cutaneous disease only.

Solitary mastocytoma. *A.* A tan macule is seen on the buttocks of an 18-month-old child. *B.* After the child's diaper was changed, the lesion became an urticarial plaque.

Young children with urticaria pigmentosa or diffuse cutaneous mastocytosis may have bullous eruptions with hemorrhage (Fig. 162-3). Blisters may erupt spontaneously or in association with infection or immunization. Blisters may occur at birth and thus are in the differential diagnosis of neonatal disorders with blisters.

Telangiectasia macularis eruptiva perstans is observed in fewer than 1 percent of patients with mastocytosis (Fig. 162-4). It appears as tan to brown macules and patchy erythema. Telangiectasias are observed. This form of cutaneous disease in mastocytosis is observed exclusively in adults.[14]

Both children and adults with mastocytosis may develop gastrointestinal disease. Gastric hypersecretion due to elevated plasma histamine with resultant gastritis and peptic ulcer disease is the most common problem.[15] Diarrhea and abdominal pain are also common and are followed by the onset of malabsorption in approximately one in three patients. Roentgenographic abnormalities fall into three major categories: peptic ulcers; abnormal mucosal patterns such as mucosal edema, multiple nodular lesions, coarsened mucosal folds, or multiple polyps; and motility disturbances. Histologic sections of jejunal biopsies have shown moderate blunting of the villi; however, significant mast cell hyperplasia is uncommon.

Significant hepatic disease in indolent systemic mastocytosis in adults is relatively infrequent, although liver function tests are abnormal in about half of patients. The most common chemical ab-

FIGURE 162-3

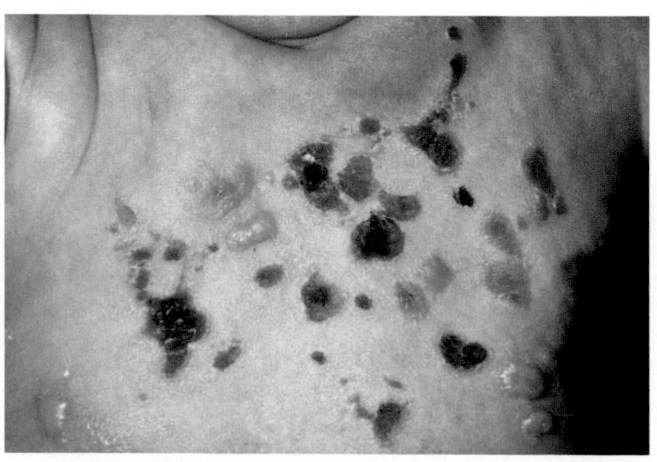

Bullous eruption on the back of a child with diffuse cutaneous mastocytosis and indolent mastocytosis.

FIGURE 162-4

CHAPTER 162
The Mastocytosis Syndrome   1905

FIGURE 162-5

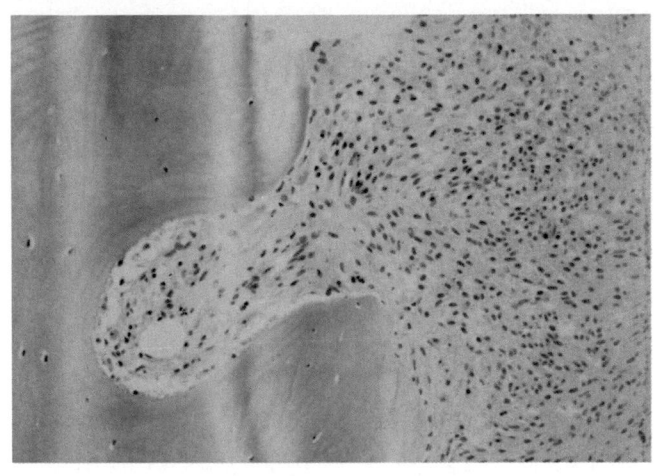

Bone marrow biopsy shows a characteristic lesion of systemic mastocytosis with paratrabecular infiltrates of mast cells and bony erosion.
Mast cells are spindle-shaped, resembling fibroblasts or histiocytes.

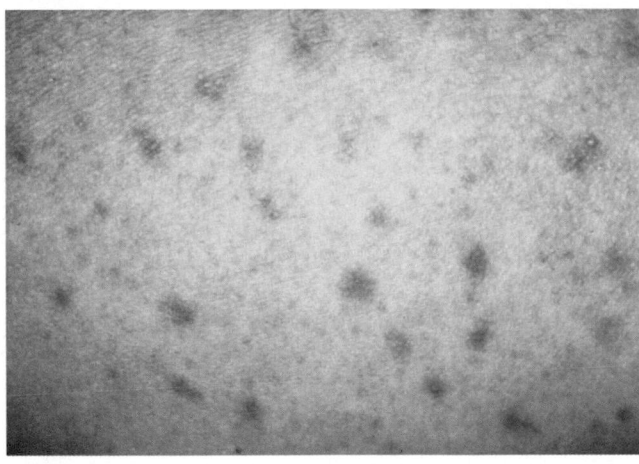

A.

B.

Urticaria pigmentosa in an adult with indolent systemic mastocytosis.
A. Hundreds of lentigo-like macules are seen on the back of this adult.
If vigorously rubbed, these lesions will show urtication and become
erythematous, raised, and pruritic. B. Close-up.

normality is an elevated level of alkaline phosphatase, which must
be distinguished from bone-derived alkaline phosphatase (which
may also be elevated). Serious manifestations of hepatic and splenic
involvement, including portal hypertension and ascites associated
with liver fibrosis,[16] are more common in patients who have mastocytosis with an associated hematologic disorder or in those with
aggressive mastocytosis.

Splenic involvement is also observed in about half of patients
with mastocytosis.[17] A paratrabecular distribution of mast cell infiltrates and fibrosis is most common. Eosinophilic infiltrates are
also noted, as are areas of extramedullary hematopoiesis. Markedly
increased splenic weights (greater than 700 g) generally occurred in
patients who fit into unfavorable categories of mastocytosis, i.e.,

aggressive mastocytosis or mastocytosis with an associated hematologic disorder.

Bone marrow lesions consist of focal and paratrabecular aggregates of spindle-shaped mast cells, often mixed with eosinophils,
lymphocytes, and occasional plasma cells, histiocytes, and fibroblasts (Fig. 162-5).[18–21] These lesions are rarely seen in children.[21]
Anemia, leukopenia, thrombocytopenia, and eosinophilia may occur
in association with systemic disease.[18,20] Bone marrow infiltration
with mast cells may induce bone changes that cause radiographically detectable lesions in the majority of patients. The proximal
long bones are most often affected, followed by the pelvis, ribs, and
skull. Skeletal scintigraphy (bone scan) is more sensitive than a
radiographic survey in detecting and locating active lesions.[22] Bone
pain affects 19 to 28 percent of patients. In patients with severe or
advanced disease, pathologic fractures may occur.

Patients in every category of mastocytosis sometimes experience
flushing or vascular collapse.[20] In occasional patients, such reactions may be provoked by alcohol, aspirin, narcotics, iodinated contrast media, insect stings, exercise, or infections.

Neuropsychiatric abnormalities have been reported.[23,24] Problems include decreased attention span, memory impairment, and
irritability. Depression as a consequence of chronic disease or possibly mediated by mast cell products is a possibility.

DIAGNOSIS

The diagnosis of mastocytosis is suspected on clinical grounds and
confirmed by histology. Supporting evidence is derived from biochemical and radiographic data (Table 162-3).[15,20,21] Mast cells may
be overlooked on histologic sections depending on the fixation and/
or stain employed. The most useful stains for mast cells include
metachromatic stains, such as toluidine blue and Giemsa; enzymatic
stains, such as chloroacetate esterase and aminocaproate esterase;

TABLE 162-3

Consensus Diagnostic Workup for Mastocytosis Suspected on Clinical Grounds

Routine studies
  Skin examination—gross and microscopic
  Bone marrow biopsy and aspiration
  24-h urine for mediators
Additional studies
  Bone scan/skeletal survey
  GI workup—upper GI series, small bowel x-ray,
    CT scan, endoscopy
  EEG, neuropsychiatric workup

and avidin, which binds to heparin.[12,25] These procedures highlight the granules in the cytoplasm of the mast cell, thereby facilitating identification. In trephine core bone marrow biopsies, decalcification interferes with subsequent attempts to visualize mast cell granules, making their identification more difficult.[21]

Fortunately, most patients with mastocytosis have either urticaria pigmentosa or diffuse cutaneous mastocytosis, which can be recognized on physical examination.[14] These diagnoses should be confirmed by skin biopsy. Blind skin biopsies must be interpreted with caution because other skin conditions including eczema and chronic urticaria are associated with a two- to fourfold increase in dermal mast cells.[12]

In patients with urticaria pigmentosa, mast cells are found in increased numbers in the dermal papillae, particularly near blood vessels.[12,25,26] Mast cells may distribute in a bandlike infiltrate of the papillary dermis (Fig. 162-6) or appear as nodular infiltrates from the papillary dermis to subcutaneous tissues. Analysis of the relationship between mast cells and blood vessels has suggested that mast cells in patients with mastocytosis first increase around blood vessels and later appear in tissues distant from vessels.[12] Mast cells may also be found in increased numbers in skin between lesions of

FIGURE 162-6

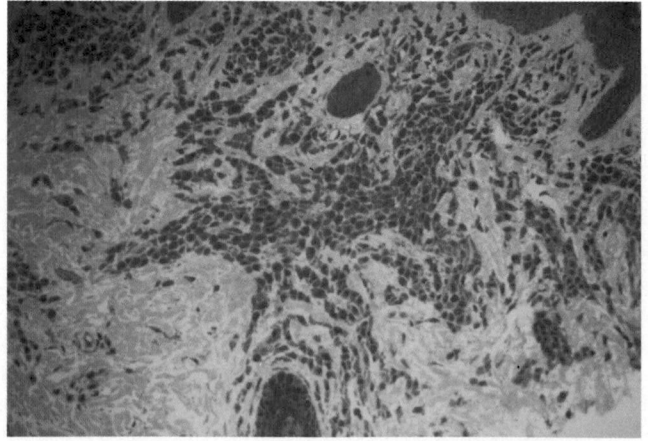

Mast cell hyperplasia in the dermis of a patient with systemic mastocytosis.

urticaria pigmentosa. The greatest increases in mast cell number do occur beneath urticaria pigmentosa macules and papules where, on average, there is a fifteen- to twentyfold increase in mast cells. However, in occasional patients, only a two- to fourfold increase in mast cells is found beneath these lesions. Two- to fourfold increases in mast cell number have also been documented in patients with recurrent episodes of flushing or anaphylaxis[12] or in other skin involved in scleroderma,[27] chronic urticaria,[28] and prolonged antigenic contact.[29] These observations document the need to correlate the gross skin examination with skin mast cell numbers and to avoid the diagnosis of urticaria pigmentosa based solely on small increases in dermal mast cells. Cutaneous responses to intradermal histamine are unchanged in patients with urticaria pigmentosa.[30]

In patients with diffuse cutaneous mastocytosis, prominent bandlike infiltrates are observed, which may be indistinguishable from some lesions of urticaria pigmentosa or from tissue obtained from mastocytomas. Cutaneous mast cell hyperplasia in patients with telangiectasia macularis eruptiva perstans is observed around the capillary venules of the superficial plexus.

Dermal mast cells in patients with mastocytosis have been examined by both light and electron microscopy. When mast cells were examined for tryptase and chymase with specific antibodies to these proteases, only tryptase-positive, chymase-positive mast cells (MC_{TC}) were identified.[31] Because MC_{TC} are by far the predominant mast cell type in normal skin, the observation that MC_{TC} also predominate in mastocytosis skin is consistent with the conclusion that this is a nonmalignant hyperplasia. On electron microscopy and morphometric analysis, lesional mast cells from adults with systemic mastocytosis had a larger mean cytoplasmic area, nuclear size, and granule diameter than mast cells from normal individuals.[26] Bilobed or highly identical nuclei were more numerous.

Mastocytosis should be suspected in patients without skin lesions if they have one or more of the following: unexplained ulcer disease or malabsorption, radiographic or ^{99m}Tc bone scan abnormalities, hepatomegaly, splenomegaly, lymphadenopathy, peripheral blood abnormalities, or unexplained flushing or anaphylaxis. Elevated levels of plasma[32,33] or urinary histamine or histamine metabolites,[34] prostaglandin D_2 metabolites in the urine,[35] or plasma mast cell tryptase[36] are not diagnostic but do raise the index of suspicion of mastocytosis. However, reliable tests for these substances are not generally available except in research laboratories.

In the absence of skin lesions, patients suspected of having mastocytosis should have a bone marrow biopsy and aspirate for diagnosis and categorization of the type of mastocytosis. Patients with urticaria pigmentosa or diffuse cutaneous mastocytosis should also have this procedure, particularly if they have peripheral blood abnormalities, hepatomegaly, splenomegaly, or lymphadenopathy, to determine if they have an associated hematologic disorder. Other tissue specimens, such as lymph nodes, spleen, liver, and gastrointestinal mucosa, define the extent of mast cell involvement but are usually obtained only as dictated by necessity. For example, gastrointestinal biopsies are obtained only if a gastrointestinal workup is indicated, and lymph nodes are biopsied only if lymphoma is considered.

Patients suspected of having mastocytosis should have 24-h urine 5-hydroxyindoleacetic acid (5-HIAA) and urinary metanephrines measured to help eliminate the possibility of a carcinoid tumor or pheochromocytoma. The fact that patients with mastocytosis do not excrete increased amounts of 5-HIAA suggests that serotonin, present in the mast cells of some species, is not synthesized by human mast cells. Idiopathic anaphylaxis and flushing must also be ruled out. Patients with these disorders do not have histologic evidence of significant mast cell proliferation and should have normal plasma histamine levels between episodes of anaphylaxis.[33]

TREATMENT

The primary objective of treatment in all categories of mastocytosis is to control mast cell mediator–induced signs and symptoms such as vascular collapse, gastric hypersecretion, gastrointestinal cramping, and pruritus. H_1 receptor antagonists such as hydroxyzine, loratadine, and doxepin are helpful in reducing pruritus, flushing, and tachycardia. If insufficient relief occurs, the addition of an H_2 antagonist such as ranitidine or cimetidine may be beneficial. However, many patients continue to complain of bone pain, headaches, and flushing, resulting in part from the inability to block the effects of high levels of histamine with histamine antagonists and the presence of other mast cell mediators.

Disodium cromoglycate (cromolyn sodium) inhibits the degranulation of mast cells and may have some efficacy in the treatment of mastocytosis, particularly in relieving gastrointestinal complaints.[37,38] Cromolyn sodium does not lower plasma or urinary histamine levels in patients with mastocytosis.[37] Both ketotifen and azelastine, antihistamines with mast cell–stabilizing properties, help by relieving the pruritus and whealing associated with mastocytosis. However, neither drug appears to offer an advantage over a standard antihistamine such as hydroxyzine.[39,40]

Epinephrine is used to treat episodes of vascular collapse.[41] All patients should be prepared to self-administer this drug. If subcutaneous epinephrine is insufficient, intensive therapy for vascular collapse should be instituted. Patients with recurrent episodes of vascular collapse may be placed on H_1 and H_2 antihistamines to lessen the severity of attacks. Episodes of vascular collapse may be spontaneous but have also been observed after stings from insects.

Methoxsalen with long-wave ultraviolet radiation (PUVA) has been shown to relieve pruritus and whealing after 1 to 2 months of treatment.[42,43] Improvement is associated with a temporary decrease in dermal mast cells. Pruritus recurs within 3 to 6 months after stopping treatment. Photochemotherapy should be used only in instances of extensive cutaneous disease unresponsive to other forms of therapy. Some patients report a diminution in the number or intensity of cutaneous lesions after exposure to natural sunlight.

Topical glucocorticoids, such as 0.05 percent betamethasone dipropionate ointment, under plastic-film occlusion for 8 h per day over 8 to 12 weeks can be used to treat extensive urticaria pigmentosa or diffuse cutaneous mastocytosis. Mast cell numbers decrease as the lesions clear. These lesions eventually recur after discontinuation of therapy,[44,45] although the treatment may lead to improvement in the cutaneous lesions for up to 1 year.

Treatment of gastrointestinal disease is directed to controlling peptic symptoms, diarrhea, and malabsorption.[15] Gastric acid hypersecretion leading to peptic symptoms and ulcerations is controlled with H_2 antagonists. Diarrhea is difficult to manage, and H_2 antagonists are generally not effective. Anticholinergics may give partial relief. In patients with severe malabsorption, systemic glucocorticoids have been effective. Ascites is also difficult to control. Portal hypertension in one patient was successfully managed with a portacaval shunt.[46] Another patient with an exudative ascites was treated successfully with systemic glucocorticoid therapy.[47]

Patients with mastocytosis and an associated hematologic disorder are managed as dictated by the specific hematologic abnormality. Interferon alpha-2b has been used to treat patients with aggressive forms of mastocytosis with apparent mixed results.[48–50] In some cases, there was response; in others, there was none. In patients with mast cell leukemia, chemotherapy has not yet been shown to produce remission or to prolong survival.[19] Chemotherapy has no place in the treatment of indolent mastocytosis. Splenectomy may improve survival in patients with forms of mastocytosis that have a poor prognosis.[51] Radiotherapy has been used to treat refractory bone pain in advanced disease.[52]

PROGNOSIS

Prognosis must be addressed separately for each category of mastocytosis. One study[20] found seven variables that were strongly associated with poor survival: constitutional symptoms, anemia, thrombocytopenia, abnormal liver function tests, a lobated mast cell nucleus, a low percentage of fat cells in the bone marrow biopsy, and an associated hematologic disorder. Other poor prognostic variables include absence of urticaria pigmentosa, male sex, absence of skin and bone symptoms, hepatomegaly, splenomegaly, and normal bone x-ray findings.

As a group, patients with indolent mastocytosis and skin involvement alone have the best prognosis. Among children with isolated urticaria pigmentosa, at least 50 percent of cases reportedly resolve by adulthood.[53,54] Adults with urticaria pigmentosa usually progress gradually to systemic disease and rarely may develop hematologic disease. Diffuse cutaneous mastocytosis is usually associated with indolent systemic disease. Patients with mastocytosis with an associated hematologic disorder have a variable course dependent on the prognosis of their hematologic disorder. With mast cell leukemia, mean survival is less than 6 months. Survival with lymphadenopathic mastocytosis with eosinophilia is 2 to 4 years without therapy. The prognosis appears to improve with aggressive symptomatic management.

REFERENCES

1. Metcalfe DD: Conclusions. *J Invest Dermatol* **96**:64S, 1991
2. Kirshenbaum AS et al: The effect of IL-3 and stem cell factor on the appearance of mast cells and basophils from CD34+ pluripotent progenitor cells. *J Immunol* **148**:772, 1992
3. Castells MC et al: The presence of membrane-bound stem cell factor in highly immature nonmetachromatic mast cells in the peripheral blood of a patient with aggressive systemic mastocytosis. *J Allergy Clin Immunol* **98**:831, 1996
4. Vliagoftis H, Metcalfe DD: Cell adhesion molecules in mast cell adhesion and migration, in *Adhesion Molecules in Allergic Disease,* edited by BS Bochner. New York, Marcel Dekker, 1997, p 151
5. Zsebo KM et al: Stem cell factor is encoded at the Sl locus of the mouse and is the ligand for the c-kit tyrosine kinase receptor. *Cell* **63**:213, 1990
6. Gurish MF et al: Tissue-regulated differentiation and maturation of a v-*abl*-immortalized mast cell–committed progenitor. *Immunity* **3**:175, 1995
7. Finotto S et al: Glucocorticoids decrease tissue mast cell number by reducing production of the c-*kit* ligand, stem cell factor, by resident cells: In vitro and in vivo evidence in murine systems. *J Clin Invest* **99**:1721, 1997
8. Nagata H et al: Identification of a point mutation in the catalytic domain of the proto-oncogene c-*kit* in the peripheral blood mononuclear cells of patients with mastocytosis. *Proc Natl Acad Sci USA* **92**:10560, 1995
9. Longley BJ et al: Somatic c-*kit* activating mutation in urticaria pigmentosa and aggressive mastocytosis: Establishment of clonality in a human mast cell neoplasm. *Nature Genetics* **12**:312, 1996
10. Pignon JM et al: A new c-*kit* mutation in a case of aggressive mast cell disease. *Br J Haematol* **96**:374, 1997
11. Lishner M et al: Trisomies 9 and 8 detected by fluorescence in situ hybridization in patients with systemic mastocytosis. *J Allergy Clin Immunol* **98**:199, 1996

12. Garriga MM et al: A survey of the number and distribution of mast cells in the skin of patients with mast cell disorders. *J Allergy Clin Immunol* **82**:425, 1988

13. Orkin M et al: Bullous mastocytosis. *Arch Dermatol* **101**:547, 1970

14. Soter N: The skin in mastocytosis. *J Invest Dermatol* **96**:32S, 1991

15. Cherner JA et al: Gastrointestinal dysfunction in systemic mastocytosis: A prospective study. *Gastroenterology* **95**:657, 1988

16. Mican JM et al: Hepatic involvement in mastocytosis: Cinicopathologic correlations in 41 cases. *Hepatology* **22**:1163, 1995

17. Travis WD, Li C-Y: Pathology of the lymph node and spleen in systemic mast cell disease. *Modern Pathol* **1**:4, 1988

18. Lawrence JB et al: Hematologic manifestations of systemic mast cell disease: A retrospective study of laboratory and morphologic features and their relation to prognosis. *Am J Med* **91**:612, 1991

19. Travis WD et al: Mast cell leukemia: Report of a case and review of the literature. *Mayo Clin Proc* **61**:957, 1986

20. Travis WD et al: Systemic mast cell disease: Analysis of 58 cases and literature review. *Medicine* **67**:345, 1988

21. Kettelhut BV et al: Hematopathology of the bone marrow in pediatric cutaneous mastocytosis: A study of seventeen patients. *Am J Clin Pathol* **91**:558, 1989

22. Chen CC et al: A retrospective analysis of bone scan abnormalities in mastocytosis: Correlation with disease category and prognosis. *J Nucl Med* **35**:1471, 1994

23. Rogers MO et al: Mixed organic brain syndrome as a manifestation of systemic mastocytosis. *Psychosomatic Med* **48**:437, 1986

24. McFarlin KE et al: A preliminary assessment of behavioral problems in children with mastocytosis. *J Psych Med* **21**:281, 1991

25. Kasper CS, Tharp MD: Quantification of cutaneous mast cells using morphometric counting and a conjugated avidin stain. *J Am Acad Dermatol* **16**:326, 1987

26. Tharp MD et al: Ultrastructural morphometric analysis of lesional skin: Mast cells from patients with systemic and nonsystemic mastocytosis. *J Am Acad Dermatol* **18**:298, 1988

27. Nishioka K et al: Mast cell numbers in scleroderma. *Arch Dermatol* **123**:205, 1987

28. Elias J et al: Studies of the cellular infiltrate of chronic idiopathic urticaria: Prominence of T-lymphocytes, monocytes, and mast cells. *J Allergy Clin Immunol* **78**:914, 1986

29. Mitchell EB et al: Increase in skin mast cells following chronic house dust mite exposure. *Br J Dermatol* **114**:65, 1986

30. Keffer JM et al: Analysis of the wheal and flare reactions that follow the intradermal injection of histamine and morphine in adults with recurrent unexplained anaphylaxis and systemic mastocytosis. *J Allergy Clin Immunol* **83**:595, 1989

31. Irani A-M et al: Mast cells in cutaneous mastocytosis: Accumulation of the MC_{TC} type. *Clin Exp Allergy* **20**:53, 1990

32. Kettelhut BV, Metcalfe DD: Plasma histamine in the evaluation of pediatric mastocytosis. *J Pediatr* **111**:419, 1987

33. Friedman BS et al: Analysis of plasma histamine levels in patients with mast cell disorders. *Am J Med* **87**:649, 1989

34. Van Gysel D et al: Value of urinary N-methylhistamine measurements in childhood mastocytosis. *J Am Acad Dermatol* **35**:556, 1996

35. Morrow JD et al: Improved diagnosis of mastocytosis by measurement of the major urinary metabolite of prostaglandin D_2. *J Invest Dermatol* **104**:937, 1995

36. Schwartz LB et al: The α form of human tryptase is the predominant type present in blood at baseline in normal subjects, and is elevated in those with systemic mastocytosis. *J Clin Invest* **96**:2702, 1995

37. Frieri M et al: Comparison of the therapeutic efficacy of cromolyn sodium with that of combined chlorpheniramine and cimetidine in systemic mastocytosis: Results of a double-blind clinical trial. *Am J Med* **78**:9, 1985

38. Horan RF et al: Cromolyn sodium in the management of systemic mastocytosis. *J Allergy Clin Immunol* **85**:852, 1990

39. Kettelhut BV et al: A double blind placebo controlled trial of ketotifen versus hydroxyzine in the treatment of pediatric mastocytosis. *J Allergy Clin Immunol* **83**:866, 1989

40. Friedman BS et al: Comparison of azelastine and chlorpheniramine in the treatment of mastocytosis. *J Allergy Clin Immunol* **92**:520, 1993

41. Turk J et al: Intervention with epinephrine in hypotension associated with mastocytosis. *J Allergy Clin Immunol* **71**:189, 1983

42. Vella-Briffa D et al: Photochemotherapy (PUVA) in the treatment of urticaria pigmentosa. *Br J Dermatol* **109**:67, 1983

43. Czarnetski PM et al: Phototherapy of urticaria pigmentosa: Clinical response and changes of cutaneous reactivity, histamine, and chemotactic leukotrienes. *Arch Dermatol Res* **277**:105, 1985

44. Laoker RM, Schechter NM: Cutaneous mast cell depletion results from topical corticosteroids usage. *J Immunol* **135**:2368, 1985

45. Barton J et al: Treatment of urticaria pigmentosa with corticosteroids. *Arch Dermatol* **121**:1516, 1985

46. Bonnet P et al: Intractable ascites in systemic mastocytosis treated by portal diversion. *Digestive Dis Sci* **32**:209, 1987

47. Reisberg IR, Oyakawa S: Mastocytosis and malabsorption, myelofibrosis and massive ascites. *Am J Gastroenterology* **82**:54, 1987

48. Kluin-Nelemans HC et al: Response to interferon alpha-2b in a patient with systemic mastocytosis. *N Engl J Med* **326**:619, 1992

49. Lehmann T et al: Severe osteoporosis due to systemic mast cell disease: Successful treatment with interferon alpha-2b. *Br J Rheumatol* **35**:898, 1996

50. Worobec AS et al: Treatment of three patients with systemic mastocytosis with interferon alpha-2b. *Leukemia Lymphoma* **18**:179, 1995

51. Friedman B et al: Splenectomy in the management of systemic mast cell disease. *Surgery* **107**:94 1990

52. Johnstone PA et al: Radiotherapy of refractory bone pain due to systemic mast cell disease. *Am J Clin Oncol* **17**:328, 1994

53. Sondergaard J, Asbo-Hansen E: Mastocytosis in childhood, in *Pediatric Dermatology,* edited by R Happle et al. Berlin, Springer-Verlag, 1987, pp 148–154

54. Kettelhut BV, Metcalfe DD: Pediatric mastocytosis *J Invest Dermatol* **96**:15S, 1991

SKIN MANIFESTATIONS OF GASTROINTESTINAL AND RENAL DISORDERS

CHAPTER 163

Robin A.C. Graham-Brown
B. Rathbone
J. Marks

The Skin and Disorders of the Alimentary Tract

Diseases of the skin and alimentary tract frequently occur together and, just as a full examination should be part of a full dermatologic assessment, it is important to examine the skin in someone presenting with a gastrointestinal problem.

This chapter deals with skin changes associated with diseases of the pharynx, esophagus, stomach, pancreas, and intestines and their main presenting signs and symptoms, including dysphagia, gastrointestinal bleeding, abdominal pain, diarrhea, and malabsorption. Investigation and treatment of the gastrointestinal aspects of combined disease will require a gastroenterologist, especially for specialized procedures such as endoscopy and laser surgery. However, the expertise of the dermatologist can be important in diagnosis and when, for example, skin and gastrointestinal disease respond to the same or similar treatment.

DYSPHAGIA

Dysphagia may occur when dermatologic diseases extend into the pharynx and esophagus, in oro-oculogenital syndromes, esophageal cancer, and collagen vascular disease (Table 163-1).

TABLE 163-1

Skin Abnormalities That Occur with Dysphagia

Rashes that may extend to the esophagus	Carcinoma of the esophagus
Infections	Iron deficiency
Blistering diseases, congenital and acquired	Dermatitis herpetiformis
Lichen planus	Tylosis
Darier's disease	Inorganic arsenic ingestion
Acanthosis nigricans	Collagen vascular diseases
Oro-oculo-genito-cutaneous syndromes	Systemic sclerosis
Stevens-Johnson syndrome	Dermatomyositis
Behçet's disease	

Rashes that Extend to the Pharynx and Esophagus

INFECTIONS Infections of the skin and mouth are discussed elsewhere (see Sections 29, 30, and 31). Symptoms resulting from infections of the esophagus occur in patients on oral and inhaled glucocorticoids or in those with immunodeficiency (e.g., AIDS) (see Chap. 226). *Candida albicans* is the most frequent pathogen, although opportunistic viruses can also be responsible.[1] Ulcerative hairy leukoplakia in the esophagus is a rare cause of dysphagia[2] (see Chap. 226).

BLISTERING DISEASES *Congenital epidermolysis bullosa* (See Chap. 65) Serious esophageal involvement with blisters, erosions, and strictures occurs, particularly in the recessive dystrophic and junctional forms. Treatment involving high-dosage glucocorticoids is not advocated as much as it once was,[3] but reconstructive surgery (including esophageal) can be successful. Prenatal diagnosis is now possible, and some pregnancies with an affected fetus are terminated.

Acquired "immunologic" blistering diseases Pemphigus, bullous pemphigoid, acquired epidermolysis bullosa, and dermatitis herpetiformis (DH) can affect mucosae (Fig. 163-1), but dysphagia is most troublesome in mucous membrane or cicatricial pemphigoid (see Chap. 62). Esophageal stenosis is relatively common: in one study of 81 patients with mucous membrane pemphigoid, 35 patients had lesions in the pharynx and 6 in the esophagus, with 2 needing dilation for strictures.[4]

OTHER CONDITIONS One endoscopic study of 19 patients with oral lichen planus showed that 5 had visible esophageal changes: papules in 4 and severe ulceration in 1. The histologic changes were consistent with lichen planus.[5] Esophageal involvement has been reported in Darier's disease and in acanthosis nigricans.

Oro-Oculo-Genito-Cutaneous Syndromes

The mucosae may be extensively involved in Stevens-Johnson syndrome and Behçet's disease, resulting in dysphagia. Intestinal involvement, usually due to vasculitis, sometimes coexists in Behçet's

FIGURE 163-1

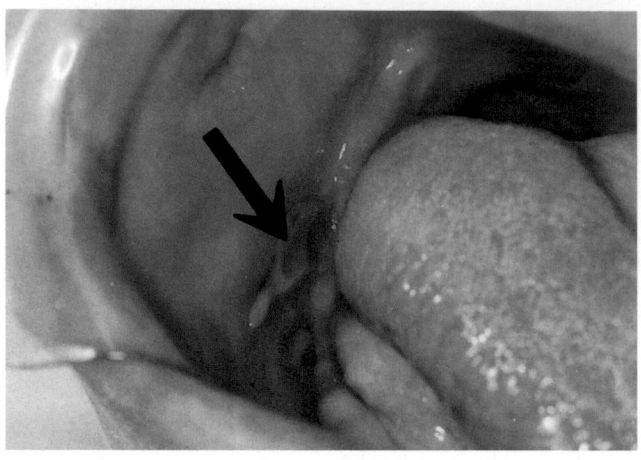

Ulceration of the mouth in a patient with mucous membrane pemphigoid.

disease and can be difficult to distinguish from Crohn's disease with mouth ulceration.

Carcinoma of the Esophagus

In the Plummer-Vinson (Paterson-Kelly) syndrome, a postcricoid web is associated with koilonychia, angular stomatitis, a sore tongue, and, usually, iron deficiency. Between 5 and 10 percent of patients with a postcricoid web develop carcinoma at the site. Patients with celiac disease may be at an increased risk of developing carcinoma of the esophagus,[6] but this does not appear to be the case with DH.[7,8] The syndrome of tylosis and carcinoma of the esophagus[9] is exceedingly rare, but 95 percent of those with tylosis eventually develop cancer. Two families have been described in whom both were inherited as dominant traits. Finally, inorganic arsenic can increase the risk of malignancy. Useful dermatologic markers are skin cancers and palmoplantar keratoses.

Collagen Vascular Diseases

Vasculitic ulcers in the mouth and pharynx occur, though relatively infrequently, in systemic lupus erythematosus. Dysphagia also occurs, particularly in systemic sclerosis and dermatomyositis.

SYSTEMIC SCLEROSIS (See Chap. 174) The esophagus is often involved in systemic sclerosis. Heartburn and dysphagia are common, and radiologic or manometric abnormalities are found in up to 70 percent of cases.[10] Decreased peristalsis, dilation, and stricture formation are thought mainly to be due to fibrosis similar to that in the skin. Abnormalities at the gastroesophageal junction lead to acid regurgitation with its complications and are another cause of dysphagia. H_2 blockers or proton pump inhibitors may relieve symptoms and limit mucosal damage. Esophageal dilation and other surgical procedures are sometimes necessary.

DERMATOMYOSITIS (See Chap. 173) In dermatomyositis and polymyositis, the muscles of swallowing can be affected in a fashion similar to the proximal skeletal muscles. Myopathy, especially when it involves muscles of swallowing, is an indication for urgent treatment with systemic glucocorticoids and immunosuppressive drugs such as azathioprine or cyclosporine.

GASTROINTESTINAL BLEEDING

Gastrointestinal bleeding may present as hematemesis, melena, or passing of fresh blood in the stools. The skin may give diagnostic clues in a number of causes (Table 163-2). Some of these may also present as abdominal pain or disturbances of bowel habit and will be dealt with later.

Vascular Abnormalities

HEREDITARY HEMORRHAGIC TELANGIECTASIA The characteristic vascular dilations occur on the skin and on oral, nasal, and gastrointestinal mucosa. Bleeding may occur from any of these sites. Treatment can be difficult, but local lesions can be controlled with cautery, laser ablation, or embolization. The results of systemic treatment with antifibrinolytic therapy and other procoagulant drugs, such as danazol and estrogens, are mixed.[11]

BLUE RUBBER BLEB NEVUS SYNDROME This condition is also an autosomal dominant trait. The cavernous hemangiomas look and feel as their name suggests and project into the gut lumen, particularly of the small intestine.

Inherited Defects of Connective Tissue

EHLERS-DANLOS SYNDROME (See Chap. 156) Many clinical and pathologic variants have now been described within this group of disorders.[12] Rupture of vessels in the gastrointestinal tract occurs mainly in Ehlers-Danlos syndrome type IV, in which type III collagen is defective.[13] Diverticula and hiatus and inguinal hernias may also occur.

PSEUDOXANTHOMA ELASTICUM Six types have now been recorded,[14] and gastrointestinal bleeding and arterial damage are seen in some (see Chap. 156).

Kaposi's Sarcoma

This tumor of the vascular endothelium and pericapillary cells presents clinically with vascular macules, papules, and nodules in skin and mucosae. The gut is a common site; involvement may be asymptomatic, but severe bleeding may occur[1] (see Chap. 103).

TABLE 163-2

Skin Abnormalities in Patients with Gastrointestinal Bleeding

Congenital malformations of blood vessels	Kaposi's sarcoma
Hereditary hemorrhagic telangiectasia	Vasculitis
	Polyposis
Blue rubber bleb nevi	Ulcerative colitis and Crohn's disease
Inherited defects of connective tissue	Gastrointestinal tumors
Ehlers-Danlos syndrome	Drugs used to treat skin disease
Pseudoxanthoma elasticum	

Vasculitis, Polyposis, Ulcerative Colitis and Crohn's Disease, and Gastrointestinal Tumors

See below.

Drugs Used in Dermatology

Gastrointestinal bleeding in a patient with a dermatologic disease may be due to therapy and is an important cause of morbidity and mortality. Systemic glucocorticoids and methotrexate are major culprits.

ABDOMINAL PAIN

Skin signs may occasionally help in the diagnosis of abdominal pain (Table 163-3). Vasculitis, polyposis, inflammatory bowel disease, and cancers have several possible gastrointestinal presentations.

Herpes Zoster

Involvement of the sensory roots of T_6-L_1 may produce abdominal pain, even before skin lesions appear. Occasionally herpes zoster in the distribution of S_2, S_3, and S_4 is associated with perineal pain and disturbances of urination and defecation[15] (see Chap. 216).

Angioedema

Acute attacks of urticaria and angioedema may present as abdominal pain due to gut edema. This is more common in familial hereditary angioedema, an important diagnosis because fatalities occur from laryngeal edema and unnecessary operations are undesirable. Clues include an autosomal dominant inheritance, subcutaneous and

TABLE 163-3

Skin Abnormalities in Patients with Abdominal Pain

Herpes zoster
Angioedema
Porphyria
Anderson-Fabry disease
Vasculitis
   Henoch-Schönlein disease
   Collagen vascular diseases
   Malignant atrophic papulosis
Polyposis
   Gardner's syndrome
   Peutz-Jeghers syndrome
   Canada-Cronkhite syndrome
   Neurofibromatosis
   Ulcerative colitis
Inflammatory bowel disease: ulcerative colitis and Crohn's disease
Pancreatitis
Gastrointestinal tumors
   Signs of wasting
   Metastases
   Dermatomyositis
   Acanthosis nigricans
   Hypertrichosis lanuginosa
   Carcinoma of esophagus, stomach, small bowel, large bowel, and pancreas

other mucosal edema *often without urticaria*, and low levels of C1 esterase inhibitor in the blood (see Chap. 119).

Porphyria Variegata

It is only in the rare porphyria variegata that skin involvement and attacks of abdominal pain coexist. The skin shows changes identical to those in porphyria cutanea tarda. Acute attacks may be precipitated by drugs such as estrogen and griseofulvin[16] (see Chap. 151). The diagnosis is made by estimation of porphyrins in urine and, particularly, in feces. Simple "screening" tests on urine will not rule out the diagnosis, especially between attacks (see Chap. 151).

Anderson-Fabry Disease (Angiokeratoma Corporis Diffusum)

This rare disease is a sex-linked recessive trait resulting in a deficiency of the lysosomal enzyme α-galactosidase. Similar changes may occur with other defects, such as fucosidosis.[17] Internal signs and symptoms are many and varied, and pains at various sites are one form of presentation. The diagnosis is easily missed if skin signs are missed. The angiokeratomas may not appear until adolescence and, even then, can be very unimpressive. The diagnostic enzyme assay is possible prenatally as well as in established cases, and female carriers can often be identified. Renal transplantation has been successful, but characterization of the α-galactosidase gene offers the possibility of enzyme replacement (see Chap. 153).

Vasculitis (See Chaps. 175 and 176)

ANAPHYLACTOID PURPURA (HENOCH-SCHÖNLEIN DISEASE) Palpable purpura, especially on the legs and buttocks, is accompanied by joint swelling, hematuria, and abdominal colic with blood in the stools. In children, intussusception may occur.

COLLAGEN VASCULAR DISEASES Acute involvement of vessels in the small and large intestines occurs in this group of diseases and may be fatal. Chronic obliteration of small intestinal vessels can result in malabsorption.[18]

MALIGNANT ATROPHIC PAPULOSIS (See Chap. 100) It is difficult to know whether this subacute vasculitis of skin, brain, and gut vessels[19] is a separate disease entity, but the histologic finding of endarteritis with thrombosis is said to be diagnostic. Patients usually die from vascular disease or perforation of the bowel, but skin lesions can be present for years with apparent fitness in other respects.[20]

Polyposis

True polyps are rare except in the colon and rectum. Polypoid lesions which are hamartomatous or inflammatory occur in all parts of the gut.[21] All may have dermatologic associations.

GARDNER'S SYNDROME Premalignant adenomatous polyps, particularly in the colon, occur in this autosomal dominant disorder,[22] along with epidermoid cysts, fibromas, lipomas, and facial osteomas. Skin lesions occur early in life and are an important marker. Regular colonoscopy is essential for patients at risk.

PEUTZ-JEGHERS SYNDROME (See Chap. 89) In this syndrome,[23] hamartomatous polyps occur mainly in the small intestine. Malignant change with metastasis has been overstressed but does occur. There is also an increased risk of malignancy in general.[24] Small dark freckles occur around the mouth, on the lips, and on the digits. Patchy pigmentation also occurs inside the mouth. The freckles tend to disappear over time, leaving pigmentary mouth changes indistinguishable from those due to racial factors or Addison's disease. The syndrome is an autosomal dominant trait, but in some families the skin signs and the intestinal changes may appear alone in some individuals.

CANADA-CRONKHITE SYNDROME In this rare acquired disease there is a patchy alopecia and characteristic, but not diagnostic, nail changes.[25] Inflammatory polyps are present in the stomach and bowel, and a protein-losing enteropathy may occur. However, the hair and nail changes precede the bowel trouble and cannot be due to lack of protein.

NEUROFIBROMATOSIS Gastrointestinal neurofibromatosis is a feature of von Recklinghausen neurofibromatosis (NF1) (see Chap. 191). Twenty-five percent of patients have gastrointestinal involvement, usually in the form of polypoid tumors.[26] Most are neurofibromas, but leiomyomas and other tumors (both benign and malignant) also occur.

ULCERATIVE COLITIS Inflammatory polyposis occurs in ulcerative colitis.

Inflammatory Bowel Disease: Ulcerative Colitis and Crohn's Disease

Both of these inflammatory bowel diseases can present with abdominal pain, gastrointestinal bleeding, or diarrhea. Ulcerative colitis predisposes to carcinoma of the colon. The skin complications of the two diseases are similar, although some occur with different frequencies; in particular, granulomas are much more common in Crohn's disease (Table 163-4).

PYODERMA GANGRENOSUM (See also Chap. 97) Pyoderma gangrenosum occurs in inflammatory bowel disease, rheumatoid disease, myeloma, and leukemias and in patients who are otherwise well. Figures about associated diseases vary, partly as a result of the source of patients studied and partly because of different diagnostic criteria.[27] One study found that half of the patients with pyoderma gangrenosum had ulcerative colitis, but fewer than 10 percent of patients with ulcerative colitis had pyoderma gangrenosum.

TABLE 163-4

Skin Lesions in Ulcerative Colitis and Crohn's Disease

Pyoderma gangrenosum
Granulomas
Erythema nodosum
Aphthous ulcers
Malnutrition
Erythemas, lichen planus, vascular thrombosis
Rashes at ileostomy and colostomy sites

Another found that a third of 86 patients with pyoderma gangrenosum had inflammatory bowel disease, ulcerative colitis, and Crohn's disease featuring almost equally.[28] Investigation of the bowel may be worthwhile in the absence of symptoms, because relevant disease has been found in some patients with pyoderma gangrenosum. Pyoderma gangrenosum can be triggered by trauma and may appear around scars or stoma sites.[29] The severity and extent of ulceration may be linked to the activity of the underlying disease, but this is not always the case. Pyoderma gangrenosum usually heals with effective treatment of the bowel disease but is occasionally very resistant.

GRANULOMAS Oral granulomatous nodules are quite common in Crohn's disease, where they may coalesce to give a "cobblestone" appearance. Crohn's disease is one cause of granulomatous cheilitis (see Chap. 114), and this may predate bowel disease by several years. Such patients should be given a guarded prognosis. Granulomas may also occur in the perineum; at colostomy and ileostomy sites; and in association with scars, sinuses, and fistulas. Very rarely, metastatic granulomas occur at sites remote from the bowel.

ERYTHEMA NODOSUM Flares of ulcerative colitis and Crohn's disease are an uncommon cause of erythema nodosum.

APHTHOUS ULCERS These lesions are reported to occur in 8 percent of patients with ulcerative colitis[30] and in 6 percent of patients with Crohn's disease[31]; they may be the presenting feature of either (or, indeed, of celiac disease). Appropriate investigation of the bowel should be considered in any patient with intractable mouth ulcers.

MALNUTRITION Signs of deficiencies can arise from inflammatory bowel disease or its treatment with elemental diets (see below).

MISCELLANEOUS SKIN CONDITIONS Annular erythemas, vascular thromboses, erythema multiforme, lichen planus, and rosacea have all been described with inflammatory bowel disease, but it is far from clear that they are true associations.

RASHES AT COLOSTOMY AND ILEOSTOMY SITES These rashes are most common in patients with inflammatory bowel disease but are seen regardless of the primary disease. They are worst with ileostomies in which gut enzymes digest the skin and in those who have ureters transplanted into the bowel. The following factors are important:

- *Siting and fashioning of the stoma:* Stomas must be sited and fashioned so that bowel contents are directed away from the skin into the bag. Resiting and refashioning may be necessary.
- *Fluidity of bowel contents:* It may be possible to improve fluidity by drugs and dietary manipulation.
- *Ill-fitting appliance:* Appliances should not leak and adhesives must be effective. Some skin protection may come from silicone barrier creams or aluminum paint, as long as they do not interfere with adhesion.
- *Infection:* C. albicans or bacteria from the gut are best cleared by systemic therapy. Topical applications may sensitize the skin.
- *Koebner's phenomenon:* Peristomal lesions may occur in psoriasis; peristomal pyoderma gangrenosum[29] is probably also due to this phenomenon.

- *Contact eczema:* Contact eczema may be irritant or allergic.[32] *There are many potential allergens:* rubber or plastic of bags, adhesives, deodorants, skin cleansers, applied medicaments.
- *Patient attitude and support:* The management of difficult cases depends on close cooperation between surgeon, physician, dermatologist, stoma nurse, and patient. A number of ileostomy and colostomy "clubs" exist for patient self-help.

Acute and Chronic Pancreatitis

Skin signs may help in establishing pancreatic disease as the cause of abdominal symptoms.

ACUTE PANCREATITIS Bruising of the skin around the umbilicus (Cullen's sign) or in the flanks (Grey Turner's sign) are well known, if rare, features of acute pancreatitis.

CHRONIC PANCREATITIS Chronic pancreatitis may cause tender, subcutaneous nodular areas of fat necrosis that may ulcerate (see Chap. 111).

Gastrointestinal Cancer and Other Malignancies

Many skin changes occur in association with gastrointestinal malignancies.

SIGNS OF WEIGHT LOSS OR CACHEXIA Dry skin (acquired ichthyosis) with cracking and eczematization (eczema craquelé), poor hair and nails, and hyperpigmentation are not specific to malignancy and may occur with malabsorption syndromes (see below).

METASTASES Any tumor may metastasize to the skin. The scalp is a common site. Metastases at the umbilicus (Sister Joseph nodules) occur particularly with carcinoma of the stomach, colon, and ovary (Fig. 163-2). Metastases do not always produce symptoms, but they may be massive and can cause bleeding, anemia, and ulceration.

DERMATOMYOSITIS (See Chap. 173) When seen in adults, dermatomyositis is said to be associated with underlying malignant

disease in 15 to 34 percent of cases.[33] Gastric and colonic cancers are less frequent than bronchogenic and breast cancers in Europe and North America. In China, nasopharyngeal carcinoma is a common tumor and is also most often associated with dermatomyositis. The rash and myopathy can regress after removal of the tumor, and, since dermatomyositis may be an early sign, its recognition is potentially life-saving. However, investigation of patients for malignancy gives a poor return in finding cancers not detectable clinically or by simple tests, and this should temper the vigor of investigation.[34]

ACANTHOSIS NIGRICANS (See Chap. 186) This clinical (Fig. 163-3) and histologic change may be due to a number of conditions, including obesity, several developmental or nevoid disorders accompanied by insulin resistance and/or hyperandrogenism, and some acquired conditions such as acromegaly. It may also be seen in malignancy. In two-thirds of patients with acanthosis nigricans and cancer, the tumor is gastric. The changes may regress if the

FIGURE 163-3

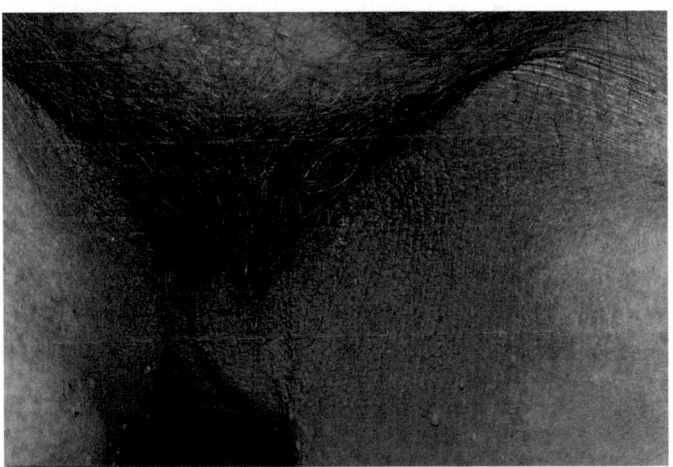

A.

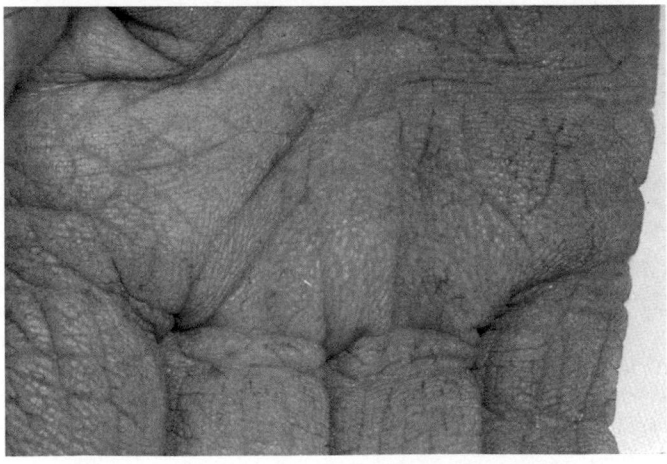

B.

Patient with acanthosis nigricans due to adenocarcinoma of jejunum. *A.* Velvety, hyperpigmented skin in groin. *B.* "Tripe hands."

FIGURE 163-2

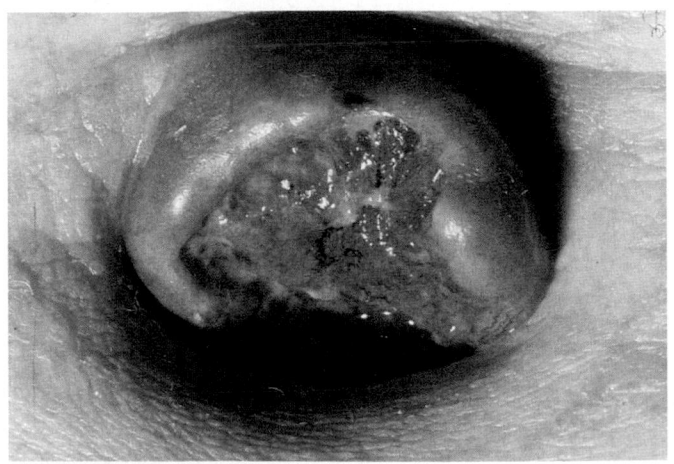

Umbilical metastasis (Sister Joseph nodule) from intraabdominal adenocarcinoma.

tumor, usually an adenocarcinoma of the stomach or bowel, is removed. However, recognition of the disorder is more important diagnostically than therapeutically, since the tumor is already well established in 80 to 90 percent of patients at the time of diagnosis.

HYPERTRICHOSIS LANUGINOSA Excessive growth of lanugo hair (Fig. 163-4) is a rare complication of malignant disease, including gastrointestinal cancer.

OTHER RASHES Urticarias, erythemas (including erythema gyratum repens), and vasculitis are among the rashes that occur occasionally, apparently as a result of malignant disease.

SIGNS OF SPECIAL GASTROINTESTINAL TUMORS *Carcinoma of the esophagus* See above.

Carcinoma of the stomach Atrophic gastritis may lead to gastric carcinoma and is associated with pernicious anemia. Patients with pernicious anemia may develop vitiligo and alopecia areata.

Small bowel tumors CARCINOID TUMORS (See Chap. 171) These tumors produce a number of vasoactive substances. It is likely that several may be required to produce the typical carcinoid flush (Fig. 163-5). The most common tumors (appendix and small bowel) do not produce flushing until the vasoactive substances reach the systemic circulation. Flushing therefore usually indicates metastasis to the liver or a primary tumor at a different site, e.g., lung or ovary.

MASTOCYTOSIS (See Chap. 162) Urticaria pigmentosa may involve organs other than the skin. The rarer diffuse cutaneous mast cell infiltration is usually accompanied by infiltration of internal organs. The small bowel and pancreas may be affected, resulting in malabsorption. Celiac disease has also been described in patients with mastocytosis.[35] Gastrointestinal effects of mastocytosis may also result from the liberation of large amounts of histamine and other pharmacologically active substances, leading to diarrhea and abdominal pain.

LYMPHOMA (See below) Lymphoma can be difficult to diagnose early because the clinical signs are often vague and nonspecific. Patients with lymphomas, including those of the bowel, are prone to complications of immunosuppression from the disease or its treatment. In the skin this results in infection with various organisms, including those that are not normally pathogenic.

Carcinoma of the large bowel Skin signs occur with the potentially malignant forms of polyposis and in ulcerative colitis (a premalignant condition). Paget's disease (see Chap. 186) in the perianal skin is often associated with an underlying carcinoma. This tumor is not always in adjacent tissue but is most commonly in rectal mucosa, apocrine glands, or cloacal remnants. A very rare presentation is chronic anal fistula.

Carcinoma of the pancreas CARCINOMA OF EXOCRINE CELLS Migratory superficial thrombophlebitis occurs in association with neoplasia, particularly carcinoma of the pancreas.

GLUCAGONOMA (See Chap. 185) This neoplasm is one of the APUD (*A*mine *P*recursur *U*ptake and *D*ecarboxylation) cell tumors. Those that produce glucagon usually arise in the islet cells of the pancreas, though not invariably so. Glucagonomas are usually malignant.

The distinctive necrolytic migratory erythema associated with glucagonoma[36] is occasionally seen with tumors that produce other peptides and rarely in patients who apparently have no tumor at all.[37,38] The rash is most common around orifices (Fig. 163-6*A*), in

FIGURE 163-4

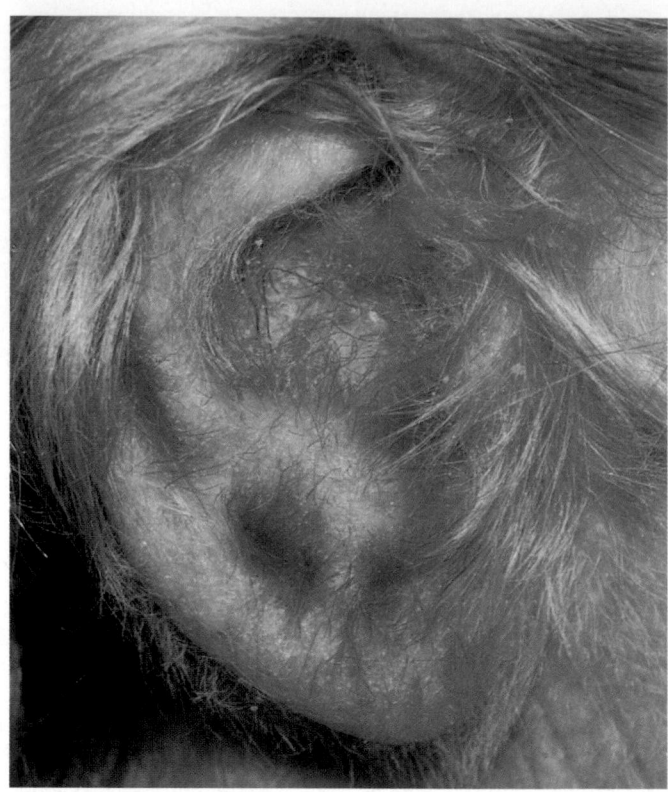

Hypertrichosis lanuginosa in a patient with metastatic adenocarcinoma.

FIGURE 163-5

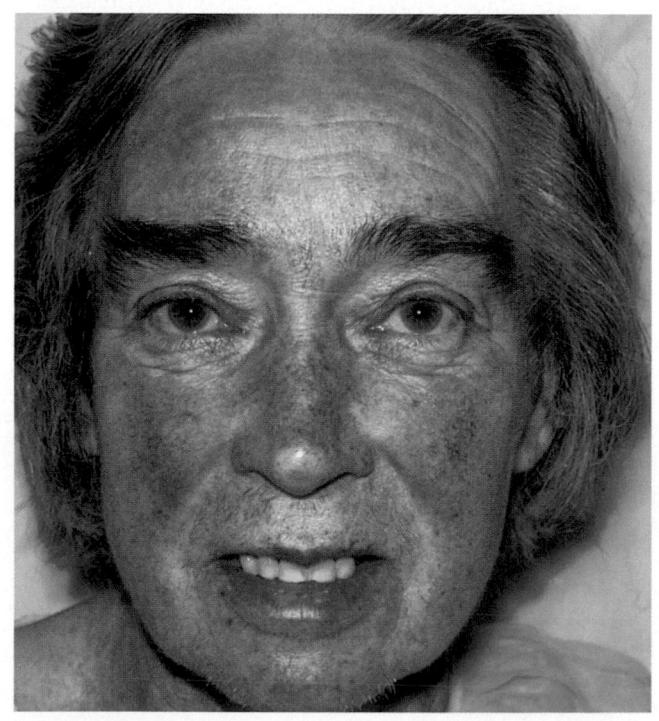

Facial rash in a patient with liver metastases from a carcinoid tumor of the small bowel.

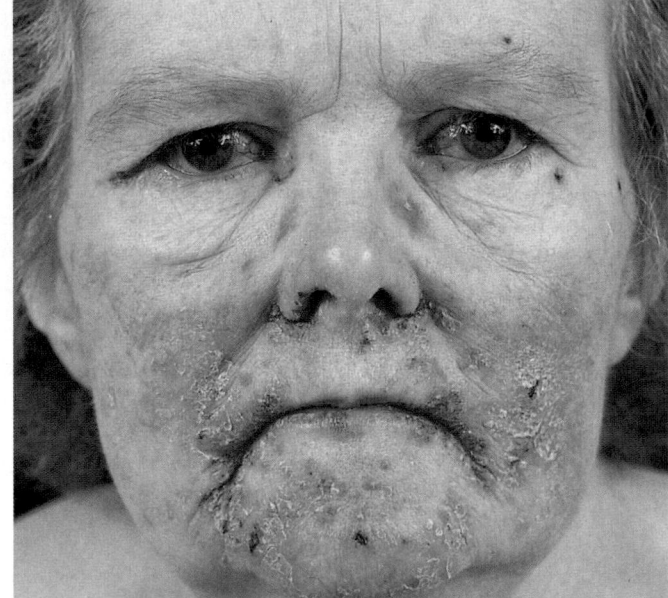

A.

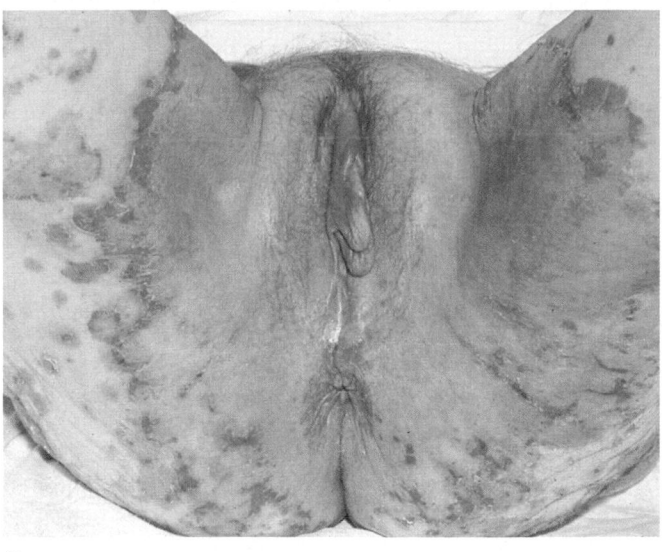

B.

The glucagonoma syndrome. Papulovesicular lesions (*A*) with erosions, crusting, and fissures around the orifices and (*B*) appearing as geographic, circinate "necrolytic migratory erythema" in the groin.

flexures (Fig. 163-6*B*), and on the fingers. Erythematous papules coalesce and spread outward; vesicles appear in the center and proceed through crusting to postinflammatory pigmentation. The eventual appearance is a geographic circinate pattern (Fig. 163-6*B*). Histologic examination shows superficial necrolysis with separation of the outer layers of the epidermis and infiltration with lymphocytes and histiocytes. Suprabasal acantholysis has been reported.[39]

Patients with glucagonoma are usually ill with any or all of the following: weight loss, diarrhea, malabsorption, sore mouth, diabetes, psychiatric disturbance, anemia, hypoaminoacidemia, and hypozincemia. In a few, however, the rash is an early sign and is an important diagnosis in benign or slow-growing tumors.

Diagnosis is by detection of excess glucagon in the blood. If specimens of tumor are available, immunochemical stains specific to the peptide will provide additional confirmation. The tumor may be localized by ultrasound, isotope scan, or CT scan.

If the tumor can be removed, the rash will disappear. If removal is not possible, the peptide antagonist streptozotocin has been given with good results. Somatostatin, a peptide that inhibits the release of a number of gastrointestinal peptides, has also been used. Symptomatic treatment of the rash with topical glucocorticoids and anti-yeast preparations may help, as may potassium permanganate baths.

The similarity of the rash to that of zinc deficiency, essential fatty acid (EFA) deficiency, and hypoaminoacidemia has led to speculation that these deficiencies are to blame, but correcting them does not usually help.

DIARRHEA AND MALABSORPTION

Some of the skin associations of gastrointestinal disease that produce diarrhea have already been mentioned. When the diarrhea is due to steatorrhea, additional possibilities must be considered. Many skin changes occur in association with malabsorption, some as a result of it, some due to a disease process that affects the bowel as well as the skin, and some because of a genetic susceptibility to two different diseases. In addition, skin disease can actually cause malabsorption.[40]

Skin Changes due to Malabsorption

Some skin changes due to malabsorption (Table 163-5) are quite specific (e.g., the rash of zinc deficiency), whereas others are nonspecific (e.g., those that occur as a result of wasting illnesses).

NONSPECIFIC CUTANEOUS EFFECTS   Nonspecific effects do not depend on the nature of the underlying disease. By the time the skin is involved it is usually apparent that the patient is systemically

TABLE 163-5

Malabsorption and Skin Disease

Skin changes due to malabsorption
  Nonspecific
    Acquired ichthyosis and pruritus
    Hair and nail changes
    Hyperpigmentation
    Skin texture and elasticity
    Eczematous and psoriatic rashes
    Jejunoileal and jejunocolic anastomoses
  Specific nutrients
    Zinc
    Essential fatty acids
    Vitamins
Malabsorption due to skin disease
  Dermatogenic enteropathy
Collagen vascular disease
Dermatitis herpetiformis and celiac disease

ill, but this is not invariable: patients with lymphoma may itch long before they have clinical evidence of underlying disease.

Acquired ichthyosis and pruritus The skin of sick people often feels "dry" (i.e., slightly roughened and scaly); this is one of the causes of the itch about which they may complain. The skin may resemble that seen in ichthyosis of mild degree. The skin may also become eczematized, and the resulting clinical picture is described as eczema craquelée, or "crazy-paving eczema." The presence of this sign in patients with malabsorption, cancer, chronic renal disease, or chronic hepatic disease has led to speculation the common factor might be flattening of the intestinal mucosa, such as has been described in malignant disease. Villous atrophy has been found with acquired ichthyosis due to lymphoma.[40] An alternative possibility is EFA deficiency or a comparable defect due to malabsorption or abnormal metabolism. Some patients itch without any visible abnormality of their skin. The mechanism for this is not understood. Despite the well-known causes, investigation for systemic disease in a patient who is apparently well and yet suffers from pruritus is an exercise of few returns. However, hypoferremia is a rare cause, and a group of male patients with pruritus and hypoferremia who subsequently developed lymphoma has been described.[41]

Hair and nails Marked reductions in both linear growth and diameter of hair shafts occur in kwashiorkor, and there is an increase in the percentage of hairs in telogen.[42] The nails are generally poor and brittle, and there may be episodic slowing of growth resulting in horizontal ridges (Beau's lines). When koilonychia occurs in malnourished patients, it usually indicates iron deficiency, even without anemia.

Skin color One curious skin change associated with malabsorption and malignant disease is hypermelanization. The abnormal pigmentation may be gross. It is not due to an increase in circulating melanocyte-stimulating hormone peptide.

Skin texture and elasticity In the course of wasting diseases, the skin becomes thinner from loss of collagen. The skin is also less elastic and does not spring back normally after stretching.

Eczematous and psoriasiform rashes due to malabsorption These rashes occur in association with malabsorption, regardless of its cause. Treatment of the malabsorption is always effective in curing the rash, but definitive links to particular nutrients are hard to establish. Although atypicality of the eczematous and psoriasiform rashes has been stressed in the past, there do not seem to be any special diagnostic features in the rashes occasionally associated with malabsorption. In the absence of other clear reasons, investigation of the bowel in atypical eczematous or psoriasiform eruptions is not necessary. No cases of celiac disease were found by small-intestinal mucosal biopsy of 100 unselected consecutive patients with eczema and psoriasis (personal observations).

Jejunoileal and jejunocolic anastomoses Patients with gross obesity are occasionally treated by various bypass operations. Dryness of the skin and hair loss, presumably due to malabsorption, and inflammatory and vasculitic skin lesions have been described, together with fever, leukocytosis, and arthralgia.[43]

CUTANEOUS EFFECTS OF MALABSORPTION OF SPECIFIC NUTRIENTS ***Zinc deficiency*** (See Chap. 148) Zinc deficiency can occur from malabsorption or when elemental feeds are deficient in zinc. Although there are theoretical reasons for believing that deranged zinc metabolism may have adverse effects on the skin, it has been difficult to confirm in common skin conditions. Low plasma zinc concentrations have been found in patients with pso-

riasis, leg ulcers, and many other unrelated diseases,[44] but this does not indicate a tissue deficiency or that zinc is helpful in therapy.

Acrodermatitis enteropathica (See Chap. 148) This usually presents at the time of weaning or in very early infancy. There is blistering on the hands and feet and around the mouth and anus; alopecia and "failure to thrive" are other features. Similar changes occur in zinc deficiency, whatever the cause.

Essential fatty acid deficiency The appearance of a scaly rash in experimental animals with EFA deficiency is well known, and dry skin with cracking of the horny layer has been reported in children fed diets low in linoleic acid. Adults receiving parental nutrition had similar skin problems until the cause was recognized and rectified. Other information comes from patients who have scaly skin as a result of malabsorption from small gut resection.[45] They have low levels of linoleic acid and an abnormal metabolite, 5,8,11-eicosatrienoic acid, in the plasma. Clinically their skin is improved by topical linoleic acid such as that found in sunflower seed oil. In other conditions, including celiac disease, levels of plasma linoleic acid are again low but the abnormal metabolite is not found. It is not certain how specific this finding is to EFA deficiency.

How EFA deficiency leads to scaliness is not clear. Barrier function is impaired, with an increase in transepidermal water loss. There is an increase in total lipid synthesis in the skin, with qualitative changes in the lipid classes. EFA deficiency also impairs prostaglandin synthesis. The role claimed for EFA deficiency in dermatoses such as eczema and psoriasis will not be discussed here, but the links are tenuous.

Malabsorption of vitamins and other nutrients The rashes due to deficiency of vitamins A, B, C, and K, usually in combination, may occur in severe small bowel abnormalities. In addition, malabsorption of vitamin K occurs in obstructive jaundice.

Folate, iron, and zinc deficiency may contribute to the poor hair growth of malnutrition.

Malabsorption due to Skin Disease

DERMATOGENIC ENTEROPATHY[46] A large proportion of patients with extensive skin disease develop mild malabsorption. In one study of 30 patients with erythroderma, steatorrhea was found in 22. In patients with eczema and psoriasis, steatorrhea is proportional to the extent of the skin disease and responds rapidly to topical treatment of the rash. Structural changes, if they occur at all, are minimal.[47] The mechanism of production of dermatogenic enteropathy is unknown, but it is one of the systemic effects of skin disease; similar malabsorption appears to occur in other chronic diseases.

Symptoms are rare, and their importance lies in the confusion that can occur if they are not recognized in a patient with a rash and malabsorption. If in doubt, a small intestinal biopsy should be performed: a flat biopsy will exclude a dermatogenic cause and point to celiac disease. No treatment is necessary for dermatogenic enteropathy, other than clearing the skin disease.

Malabsorption in Collagen Vascular Diseases

Malabsorption can occur as a result of poor intestinal peristalsis in systemic sclerosis or by chronic obliteration of mesenteric vessels in polyarteritis and other forms of vasculitis.[18] The small intestinal changes in systemic sclerosis are structurally similar to those that occur in the esophagus and the large bowel. This interferes with peristalsis and results in malabsorption by allowing bacterial colonization higher up the bowel than is usual and produces, in effect, a blind loop syndrome. There is also some evidence of a primary enterocyte defect that may contribute to the malabsorption.[48] Symptoms and signs may be severe but can be improved, at least for a time, by broad-spectrum antibiotics.

Dermatitis Herpetiformis (See Chap. 67)

When malabsorption occurs in DH, it is due to gut abnormalities of an identical character to those seen in celiac disease. Diagnosing DH thus has gastrointestinal implications. It is important to take account of the numerous characteristic (but not necessarily pathognomonic) features.[49] Immunofluorescence is probably the most valuable single diagnostic aid in reliable hands but should not be the sole criterion for diagnosis; it is inadvisable to label a rash as DH from the immunofluorescence findings alone.[50] A combination of clinical and histologic features and response to treatment is as good as immunofluorescence alone. In linear IgA disease (see Chap. 63), celiac disease occurs but is much less common. A number of clinical features and the different frequencies of the HLA types suggest that most linear IgA disease is different from classic DH.[51] There are, however, reports of patients with linear IgA disease who have developed complications typical of DH, including lymphoma.[52]

CELIAC DISEASE IN DERMATITIS HERPETIFORMIS
Severe celiac disease does occur in patients with DH but is rare. Most cases are mild, subclinical, or latent. The structural abnormalities are, as in celiac disease, sometimes patchy, worse in the proximal small bowel, and responsive to withdrawal of gluten.

DIAGNOSIS AND INCIDENCE OF CELIAC DISEASE IN COMBINATION WITH DERMATITIS HERPETIFORMIS
Only 10 to 20 percent of patients with overt celiac disease have rashes, and only a proportion of these are DH. By contrast, the proportion of patients with DH who have celiac disease is high. The precise number depends on the criteria used for diagnosing celiac disease. In one series, 33 percent of patients had clinical or biochemical evidence of celiac disease, but 58 percent had structural abnormalities.[49]

Attempts have been made to extend the diagnostic criteria of celiac disease, and, if a raised interepithelial lymphocyte count in the small bowel is taken as indicating celiac disease, the incidence in DH becomes 81 percent.[53] Whatever criteria are used, the percentage of patients with DH in whom celiac-type gut abnormalities can be demonstrated still falls short of 100 percent, at least with current techniques.

RELATIONSHIP OF DERMATITIS HERPETIFORMIS AND CELIAC DISEASE
It is clear that the presence of clinical celiac disease is not necessary for the development of DH, and that malabsorption cannot be the cause of the rash. Likewise the role of gluten, although probably important, is not fully understood. Although the gut almost always responds to gluten withdrawal, the response of the skin is less clear and its time course can be remarkably prolonged. Moreover, the responses of the skin and gut can occur independently of one another.[54] Patients with both DH and celiac disease have a significant increase in the incidence of HLA-B8, -DRw3, and -DQw2. The presence of anti-reticulin,[55] anti-gliadin,[56,57] and anti-endomyseal antibodies in both provides additional links but does not explain why some patients develop the rash and others do not.

TREATMENT OF DERMATITIS HERPETIFORMIS WITH A GLUTEN-FREE DIET
There are several reasons for treating DH with a gluten-free diet. First, it is obviously necessary for patients with clinical and biochemical evidence of celiac disease, but it can be more difficult to advise DH patients who have only structural changes in the bowel, or who have no detectable changes at all, to stick to what is, at times, a difficult diet.

There is also the question of prescribing a diet for the rash. Although patients can develop DH on a gluten-free diet for celiac disease, the general view is that gluten avoidance helps DH to be controlled without dapsone or with a much reduced dose. In one series, 85 percent of 251 patients had been able to reduce the dose of dapsone, and 47 percent were off the drug completely.[8] However, control by diet alone may take months or years, and some patients prefer taking tablets to lifelong dietary restriction. This is especially true in the elderly.

The third consideration, however, is in the prevention of gastrointestinal lymphoma, which can occur in patients with DH, with[58] or without[8] celiac disease. Gluten consumption can increase the risk of lymphoma in celiac disease,[59] and, since this is likely to be true of patients with DH, gluten withdrawal should probably be advised.

REFERENCES

1. Gazzard BG: HIV disease and the gastroenterologist. *Gut* **29**:1497, 1988
2. Kitchen V et al: Ulcerating pharyngo-esophageal leukoplakia, in *Advanced HIV Disease*. Montreal, 5th International Conference on AIDS, **244**:262, 1989
3. Moynahan E: The treatment and management of epidermolysis bullosa. *Clin Exp Dermatol* **7**:665, 1982
4. Hardy KM et al: Benign mucous membrane pemphigoid. *Arch Dermatol* **104**:467, 1971
5. Dickens C et al: The oesophagus in lichen planus: Endoscopic studies. *Br Med J* **300**:84, 1990
6. Holmes GKT et al: Malignancy in coeliac disease—effect of a gluten-free diet. *Gut* **30**:333, 1989
7. Swerdlow AJ et al: Mortality and cancer incidence in patients with dermatitis herpetiformis: A cohort study. *Br J Dermatol* **129**:140, 1993
8. Collin P et al: Malignancy and survival in dermatitis herpetiformis: A comparison with coeliac disease. *Gut* **38**:528,1996
9. Howel-Evans W et al: Carcinoma of the oesophagus with keratosis palmaris et plantaris (tylosis). *Q J Med* **27**:413, 1958
10. Weihrauch TR, Korling GW: Manometric assessment of oesophageal involvement in progressive systemic sclerosis, morphoea and Raynaud's disease. *Br J Dermatol* **107**:325, 1982
11. Phillips MD: Stopping bleeding in hereditary telangiectasia. *N Engl J Med* **330**:1822, 1994
12. Beighton P: The Ehlers-Danlos syndrome, in *McKusick's Heritable Disorders of Connective Tissue*, 5th ed, edited by P Breighton and VA McKusick. St Louis, Mosby-Year Book, 1993, p 189
13. Pope FM et al: Patients with Ehlers-Danlos syndrome type IV lack type III collagen. *Proc Natl Acad Sci USA* **72**:1314, 1975
14. Mallory SB: *An Illustrated Dictionary of Dermatologic Syndromes*. New York, Parthenon, 1994, p 186
15. Jellinek EH, Tulloch WS: Herpes zoster with dysfunction of bladder and anus. *Lancet* **2**:1219, 1976
16. Moore MR et al: Drugs and the acute porphyrias. *Trends Pharmacol Sci* **2**:330, 1981
17. George S, Graham-Brown RAC: Angiokeratoma corporis diffusum in fucosidosis. *J R Soc Med* **87**:707, 1994
18. Carron DB, Douglas AP: Steatorrhoea in vascular insuffciency of the small intestine. *Q J Med* **34**:331, 1963
19. Degos R et al: Dermatite papulosquameuse atrophiante. *Bull Soc Fr Dermatol Syphiligr* **52**:60, 1942
20. Hall-Smith P: Malignant atrophic papulosis (Degos' disease). *B J Dermatol* **81**:817, 1969
21. Bussey H, Morson B: Familial polyposis coli, in *Gastrointestinal Tract Cancer*, edited by M Lipkin, R Good. New York, Plenum, 1978, p 275

22. Gardner EJ: A genetic and clinical study of intestinal polyposis, a predisposing factor for carcinoma of the colon and rectum. *Am J Hum Genet* **3**:167, 1951

23. Jeghers H et al: Generalized intestinal polyposis and melanin spots of the oral mucosa, lips and digits. *N Engl J Med* **241**:993, 1961

24. Spieglman AD et al: Cancer and the Peutz-Jeghers syndrome. *Gut* **30**:1588, 1989

25. Cunliffe W, Anderson J: Case of Cronkhite-Canada syndrome with associated jejunal diverticulosis. *Br Med J* **4**:601, 1967

26. Davis GB, Berk RN: Intestinal neurofibromas in von Recklinghausen's disease. *Am J Gastroenterol* **60**:410, 1973

27. Hickman JG, Lazarus GS: Pyoderma gangrenosum: A reappraisal of associated systemic diseases. *Br J Dermatol* **102**:235, 1980

28. Powell FC et al: Pyoderma gangrenosum: A review of 86 patients. *Q J Med* **55**:173 1985

29. Cairns BA et al: Peristomal pyoderma gangrenosum and inflammatory bowel disease. *Arch Surg* **129**:769, 1994

30. Edwards FC, Truelove SC: The course and prognosis of ulcerative colitis. *Gut* **5**:1, 1964

31. Croft CB, Wilkinson AR: Ulceration of mouth, pharynx and larynx in Crohn's disease of the intestine. *Br J Surg* **59**:249, 1972

32. Cronin E: In *Contact Dermatitis.* Edinburgh, Churchill Livingstone, 1980, p 886

33. Rowell NR: The connective tissue diseases, in *Textbook of Dermatology,* 5th ed, edited by A Rook et al. Oxford, Blackwell, 1992, p 2163

34. Cox NH et al: Dermatomyositis and malignancy in an audit of the value of extensive investigation. *Br Med J* **121**:47, 1989

35. Scott BB et al: Involvement of the small intestine in systemic mast cell disease. *Gut* **16**:918, 1975

36. Malinson et al: A glucagonoma syndrome. *Lancet* **2**:l, 1974

37. Choksi VA et al: An unusual skin rash associated with a pancreatic polypeptide–producing tumour of the pancreas. *Ann Intern Med* **108**:64, 1988

38. Thivolet J: Necrolytic migratory erythema without glucagonoma. *Arch Dermatol* **117**:4, 1981

39. Long CC et al: Suprabasal acantholysis—an unusual feature of necrolytic migratory erythema. *Clin Exp Dermatol* **18**:464, 1993

40. Shuster S: The gut and the skin, in *Third Symposium of Advanced Medicine. Proceedings of a Conference held at Royal College of Physicians, London,* edited by AM Dawson. London, Pitman Medical, 1967, p 349

41. Vickers CFH: Nutrition and the Skin, in *Tenth Symposium on Advanced Medicine.* London, Pitman Medical, 1974

42. Sims RT: Hair as an indicator of incipient and developed malnutrition and response to therapy—principles and practice, in *An Introduction to the Biology of the Skin,* edited by RH Champion et al. Oxford, Blackwell, 1970, p 387

43. Kennedy C: The spectrum of inflammatory skin disease following jejuno-ileal bypass for morbid obesity. *Br J Dermatol* **105**:425, 1981

44. Greaves MW, Boyd TRC: Plasma-zinc concentrations in patients with psoriasis, other dermatoses and venous leg ulceration. *Lancet* **2**:1019, 1967

45. Prottey C et al: Correction of the cutaneous manifestations of essential fatty acid deficiency in man by application of sunflower seed oil to the skin. *J Invest Dermatol* **64**:918, 1975

46. Shuster S, Marks J: Dermatogenic enteropathy—a new cause for steatorrhoea. *Lancet* **1**:1367, 1965

47. Marks J, Shuster S: Small intestinal mucosal abnormalities in various skin diseases—fact or fancy. *Gut* **11**:281, 1970

48. Hendel L et al: Enterocyte function in progressive systemic sclerosis. *Gut* **28**:435, 1987

49. Marks J: Dogma and dermatitis herpetiformis. *Clin Exp Dermatol* **2**:189, 1977

50. Karlsson I et al: Absence of cutaneous IgA in coeliac disease without dermatitis herpetiformis. *Br J Dermatol* **99**:621, 1978

51. Sachs J et al: A comparative serological and molecular study of linear IgA disease and dermatitis herpetiformis. *Br J Dermatol* **118**:759, 1988

52. Kapur A et al: Linear IgA dermatosis, coeliac disease, and extraintestinal B cell lymphoma. *Gut* **37**:731, 1995

53. Fry L et al: Lymphocytic infiltration of epithelium in diagnosis of gluten-sensitive enteropathy. *Br Med J* **3**:371, 1972

54. Fry L et al: Long-term follow up of dermatitis herpetiformis with and without gluten withdrawal. *Br J Dermatol* **107**:631, 1982

55. Ljunghall K et al: Circulating reticulin auto-antibodies of IgA class in dermatitis herpetiformis. *Br J Dermatol* **100**:173, 1979

56. Kumar PJ et al: Food antibodies in patients with dermatitis herpetiformis and adult coeliac disease. *Scand J Gastroenterol* **11**:5, 1976

57. Menzel EJ et al: Demonstration of antibodies to wheat gliadin in dermatitis herpetiformis using 14C-radio-immunoassay. *Clin Immunol Immunopathol* **10**:193, 1978

58. Leonard JN et al: Increased incidence of malignancy in dermatitis herpetiformis. *Br Med J* **286**:16, 1983

59. Holmes GKT et al: Malignancy in coeliac disease—effect of a gluten free diet. *Gut* **35**:1215, 1994

CHAPTER 164

Robin A.C. Graham-Brown
Imrich Sarkany

The Hepatobiliary System and the Skin

An association between the skin and the liver has been recognized for centuries (Fig. 164-1) and is part of folklore. For example, in medieval times females with vascular skin blemishes were labeled as witches, a "bottlenose" is still seen as a sign of alcoholic liver trouble, and a variety of pigmented skin lesions are often known as "liver spots." The term *spider* is said to have originated in the New York underworld, where barmaids spotted "spiders" as evidence of advanced liver disease in their customers.

Several types of interaction between the skin and the hepatobiliary system are encountered in clinical practice:

FIGURE 164-1

CHAPTER 164
The Hepatobiliary System and the Skin   1919

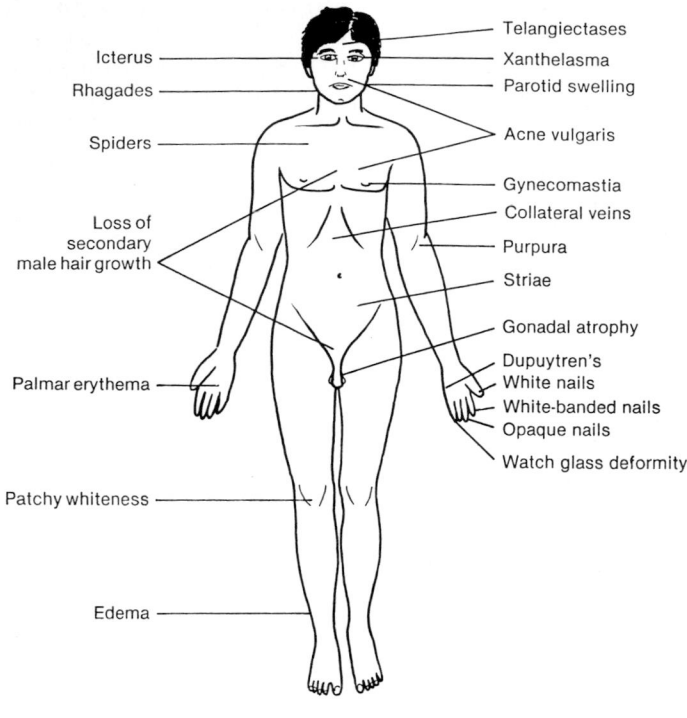

Icterus
Rhagades
Spiders
Loss of secondary male hair growth
Palmar erythema
Patchy whiteness
Edema

Telangiectases
Xanthelasma
Parotid swelling
Acne vulgaris
Gynecomastia
Collateral veins
Purpura
Striae
Gonadal atrophy
Dupuytren's
White nails
White-banded nails
Opaque nails
Watch glass deformity

The main skin changes in liver disease.

1. Liver disease may cause skin changes.
2. The skin and the liver may be involved by the same pathologic process or by exposure to exogenous chemicals.
3. Skin disease may cause liver abnormalities and/or disturbances of hepatic function.
4. The liver may be damaged by drugs used to treat skin disease.

SKIN LESIONS DUE TO HEPATOBILIARY DISEASE

When skin lesions occur in association with liver disease, they are generally not specific to a particular hepatic pathology, but the most florid cutaneous lesions are generally seen in patients with chronic active hepatitis and in alcoholics. However, the changes seen in the skin, nails, and hair of patients with hepatobiliary disease may also occur in its absence or in association with physiologic states. For example, spider nevi may be seen in normal children and in pregnant women, and male alcoholics may develop gynecomastia, vascular spiders, and changes in body hair and fat distribution even in the absence of cirrhosis.[1]

It is also possible for there to be no visible skin changes in patients with severe or advanced liver disease, and dramatic cutaneous manifestations may be seen in those with minimal hepatic dysfunction. Severe itching may antedate other features of biliary cirrhosis by months or years.

Jaundice

Jaundice, or icterus, is the generalized yellow or ocher coloration of the skin, mucous membranes, and other body tissues imparted by the bile pigment bilirubin. Both jaundice and pigmentation are most prominent in disease states that produce extrahepatic biliary obstruction and in primary biliary cirrhosis. Clinically detectable jaundice is always indicative of disease and must be distinguished from olive or sallow skin complexions, carotenemia, the yellowish skin pigmentation produced by quinacrine and busulfan, and lycopenemia due to ingestion of tomato juice.

PATHOGENESIS No system of classification is perfect, but a functional approach is given in Table 164-1.

Jaundiced skin, varying in hue from faint golden to dark greenish yellow, results from increased local cellular or connective tissue binding of the bilirubin (or its metabolites). The tissue pigment has

TABLE 164-1

Functional Classification of Jaundice

Unconjugated ("indirect") hyperbilirubinemia
  Newborn and infant
    "Physiologic"—functional hepatic immaturity
    Hemolysis—Rh, ABO, sepsis, drug factors
    Prematurity
    Transient familial hyperbilirubinemia—maternal steroid inhibitors
    Crigler-Najjar syndrome—glucuronyl transferase deficiency (hereditary)
  Adult
    Excess bilirubin production
      Hemolysis
        Congenital
        Acquired
      Dyserythropoietic—"shunt" hyperbilirubinemia
    Deficient conjugation
      Familial
        Constitutional hepatic dysfunction (Gilbert's syndrome)
        Crigler-Najjar syndrome type II
      Acquired
        Posthepatic
        Associated disease—cardiac, enteric, metabolic
        Drug-induced
  Diagnostic features
    Serum-conjugated bilirubin less than 15% of total
    Absence of bilirubinuria
    Low to normal urine urobilinogen
    Absence of other liver function disturbances
    Normal morphologic features of liver

Conjugated ("direct-reacting") hyperbilirubinemia
  Hepatic cell damage
    Acute—viral, toxic, anoxic, metabolic
    Chronic—cirrhosis, metabolic
  Impaired bile excretion
    Extrahepatic obstruction
    Intrahepatic cholestasis—atresias, viral, drugs, hormones, pregnancy, benign recurrent cholestasis
  Familial (defect confined to bilirubin excretion)
    Dubin-Johnson syndrome—excretory defect and cell pigment
    Rotor's syndrome—excretory defect and no pigment
  Diagnostic features
    Serum-conjugated bilirubin more than 15% of total
    Bilirubinuria common
    Urine uribilinogen often elevated
    Other liver functions often abnormal in hepatic cell damage and impaired bile excretion
    Characteristic morphologic abnormalities of liver

a special affinity for elastin but circulates almost exclusively as a tightly bound complex with albumin. Elevation of serum bilirubin level results from an imbalance between overall pigment production and excretion, 80 to 90 percent being derived from the degradation of heme.

Tissue-serum equilibration is slow and the intensity of clinical icterus often fails to reflect the concurrent serum bilirubin level. Hyperbilirubinemia may therefore antedate the onset of detectable jaundice by 1 day or more and, conversely, icterus may persist despite falling or normal serum bilirubin levels. Local changes in vascular permeability may "sequester" bile pigment or impair its equilibration—hence the occasional finding of jaundice of different intensity in areas of edema. The correlation between cutaneous staining and serum pigment levels is especially poor in newborns. A further discrepancy between tissue and serum pigment levels in infants may result from the administration of drugs that uncouple protein-bound bilirubin and favor its passage into body tissues.[2] Clinically detectable jaundice appears when sufficient bilirubin has become tissue-bound, generally when total serum levels have exceeded 2.5 to 3.0 mg/dL in adults or 6.0 to 8.0 mg/dL in infants.

CLINICAL FEATURES   Jaundice is a cardinal sign of disease and requires careful evaluation, but hyperbilirubinemia and cutaneous icterus themselves produce neither symptoms nor harmful effects in adults.

Slight jaundice is frequently unremarked by patients and family: poor lighting, dark skin coloration, and subtle progression often combine to delay the clinical diagnosis for days or weeks. Careful inspection of the sclerae in natural or bluish light is the best method for detecting jaundice; the high elastic tissue content of sclerae apparently accounts for this preferential staining. Prolonged and deep jaundice may assume a greenish-tan quality, probably due to melanosis and the oxidation of pigments.

The intensity of jaundice and levels of serum bilirubin in patients with biliary atresia, acquired bile duct obstruction, or defective bilirubin conjugation tend to stabilize despite continued pigment production. The fate or disposition of the excess pigment is still uncertain. Some degradation of bilirubin has been shown to occur with exposure to ultraviolet radiation. This phenomenon is the basis for phototherapy of babies to prevent kernicterus in severe neonatal jaundice: colorless breakdown products are probably excreted in the urine. The urine becomes dark yellow and then brown as conjugated serum bilirubin exceeds an inconstant "threshold" value of 0.4 to 0.6 mg/dL. Bilirubinemia is not a feature of unconjugated hyperbilirubinemic states. Since most of the brown color of normal feces is produced by urobilins derived from degradation of bilirubin in the intestine, the jaundice of impaired pigment excretion or bile obstruction is associated with "clay-colored" stools.

DIAGNOSIS   The diagnosis of jaundice requires a methodical consideration of the factors that may be responsible (Table 164-1). History and clinical examination should indicate the cause in 60 to 70 percent of cases; liver function tests should afford a diagnosis in another 10 to 15 percent; special procedures may be required in the remainder.

TREATMENT AND COURSE   Jaundice in patients with acute hepatitis resolves spontaneously. A small percentage, especially those with hepatitis types A and C, may enter a cholestatic phase with jaundice and severe itching. The jaundice of chronic liver disease may improve when the underlying liver involvement improves. Pa-

tients with chronic active hepatitis often lose their jaundice to a large extent after successful therapy with glucocorticoids, and patients with primary biliary cirrhosis may also show lessening of jaundice after treatment. The jaundice of biliary obstruction resolves when the obstruction is relieved. In addition to phototherapy in babies, help may be offered to patients with Gilbert's and the Crigler-Najjar syndromes, in which benign unconjugated hyperbilirubinemia is found in association with otherwise normal liver function. Microsomal enzyme inducers, such as phenobarbital, result in a lowering of bilirubinemia.

Melanosis and Other Pigmentary Changes

Apart from jaundice, both diffuse and circumscribed color changes may occur in chronic liver disease. A *diffuse* muddy gray color in patients with long-standing cirrhosis is largely due to basal cell melanin.

Melanosis is common in primary biliary cirrhosis and initially involves exposed areas, but it gradually becomes generalized. It may be an early presenting sign.[3] Pigmentation is generally mild in other forms of chronic liver disease and is not a feature of secondary biliary cirrhosis.

Blotchy, *circumscribed* areas of dirty brown pigmentation are also occasionally seen, and accentuation of normal freckling and areolar pigmentation may appear. Localized linear pigmentation may be found in the creases of the fingers and palms. Pigmentation resembling chloasma may localize to the perioral and periorbital areas (sometimes called *chloasma hepaticum* or *masque biliaire* by Francophones.[4] White, pea-sized flecks—guttate hypomelanosis, sometimes with a central spider—on the skin of the buttocks, back, thighs, and forearms may occur in cirrhosis.[5]

The skin pigmentation in hemochromatosis (an inherited condition in which excess iron is deposited in the liver, pancreas, heart, and joints) is so striking that its alternative name is *bronzed diabetes*. The metallic gray or bronze-brown color of hemochromatosis is usually generalized,[6] with accentuation over sun-exposed sites. Buccal mucosal and conjunctival pigmentation may affect 20 percent of patients.

ETIOLOGY AND PATHOGENESIS   The etiology and pathogenesis of hyperpigmentation in chronic liver disease are obscure. The slow progression of generalized brownish pigmentation in some conditions suggests a humoral mechanism, perhaps comparable to that seen with excessive adrenocorticotropic hormone (ACTH) or melanocyte-stimulating hormone (MSH),[7] but MSH levels are not raised.

A different mechanism for pigmentation in primary biliary cirrhosis was suggested by Burton and Kirby,[8] who suggested that the continued release of proteolytic enzymes in the skin could account for both the pigmentation and the pruritus of patients with chronic obstructive jaundice.

A histologic and ultrastructural study of cutaneous pigmentation in primary biliary cirrhosis showed that pigmentation was predominantly due to excess melanin, no stainable iron being demonstrable.[9] Similar changes were seen in a patient with alcoholic cirrhosis and skin pigmentation. It is not clear whether the excess melanin results from increased melanogenesis or defective melanin degradation.

In hemochromatosis, cutaneous pigmentation is caused not only by the presence of hemosiderin in the skin but also by excess melanin. Hemosiderin granules are seen in macrophages within the dermis and its appendages and probably do contribute to the striking color of hemochromatotic skin.[10] After phlebotomy, histologic siderosis and clinical skin pigmentation decrease, even though melanosis remains histologically. However, the important role of melanin is illustrated by a patient with both vitiligo and hemochromatosis.[11] Histochemically there was iron in the areas of vitiligo as well as in the remainder of the skin, but the vitiliginous areas remained completely white while the remainder of the skin showed the expected hyperpigmentation.

Other cutaneous pigmentary changes associated with liver disease may be due to derangement of porphyrin or cholesterol metabolism. In porphyria cutanea tarda, healed sites show residual pigmentation and there may be a variable degree of generalized hyperpigmentation on the face and hands. The yellow and orange lesions of xanthomatosis and xanthelasma are common in biliary cirrhosis, especially in the primary form.

DIAGNOSIS AND MANAGEMENT OF PIGMENTATION A number of conditions should be considered in the differential diagnosis of generalized pigmentation: primary adrenal insufficiency (Addison's disease) and some pituitary tumors produce pigmentary changes of the skin and mucous membranes; chronic diseases—such as lymphoma, tuberculosis, and malabsorption syndromes—may produce both pigmentation and hepatic dysfunction. Liver biopsy may be essential in making the definitive diagnosis.

Once the liver is chronically damaged, as in cirrhosis, it never regains its normal structure. However, liver cells retain such enormous regenerative capacity that functional compensation may be attained. Bed rest in acute cases, control of alcoholism, improved nutrition, appropriate medication, and surgical correction of mechanical biliary obstruction may arrest or reverse secondary cutaneous pigmentary changes.

Vascular Changes

Patients with chronic liver disease often have telangiectatic changes, mainly over the areas of the body exposed to light. They resemble the vascular changes seen in sailors and farmers. Numerous tiny telangiectases sometimes give the impression of a diffuse, almost exanthematic redness. They are known as "dollar paper markings," after the small threads in paper money held up against the light. They fade on pressure with a glass slide and rarely pulsate.

SPIDER NEVUS The vascular spider, arterial spider, or spider angioma is the most representative and classical vascular lesion of chronic liver disease, although it may also be seen in alcoholics without liver involvement. Its name reflects a resemblance to a spider, with a central arteriole represented by a red point from which numerous small, twisted vessels radiate (Fig. 164-2). Spiders range in size from a pinhead to 2 cm. When sufficiently large, it can be seen or felt to pulsate, especially when pressed with a glass slide. Pressure on the central arteriole with the head of a pin or a matchstick causes blanching of the whole lesion.

Spider nevi are most common on the face, necklace area, forearms, hands, and upper part of the chest (Fig. 164-2), i.e., mainly over the region drained by the superior vena cava. Only rarely are they found in the mucous membranes of the nose, mouth, and pharynx. The reasons for this selective distribution are not understood. They fade after death.[12]

Spider nevi may be seen in 10 percent of the normal general population and not infrequently in children. They may appear in large numbers during pregnancy, usually disappearing after parturition, although some persist. They may also be seen in patients with thyrotoxicosis, those with rheumatoid arthritis receiving estrogen therapy, and in women taking oral contraceptives. A familial incidence of spider nevi has also been reported. It has been suggested that the rare association of unilateral nevoid telangiectasia

FIGURE 164-2

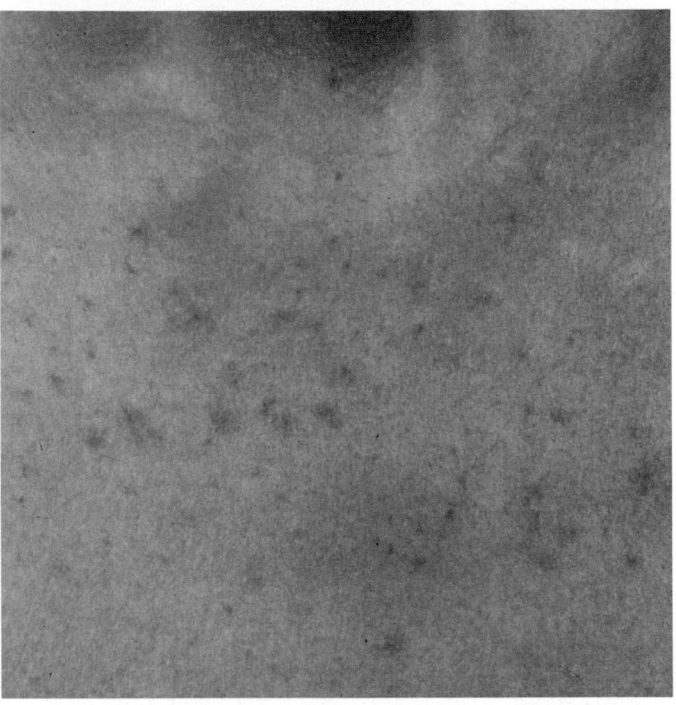

Spider nevi in a patient with cirrhosis.

and liver disease could be manifestations of a disease involving skin and liver vessels, as in hereditary hemorrhagic telangiectasia.[13]

Regression of spiders in patients with liver disease is possible with improvement of the underlying condition, although persistence is more likely.

The blood pressure in these small arteries has been measured at 50 to 70 mmHg, and the temperature is 2 to 3°C higher than that of the surrounding skin. Morphologic studies with the help of reconstruction methods[14] demonstrated that spiders represent an arterial end organ with five separate parts: (1) a cutaneous arterial net, (2) a central spider arteriole, (3) a subepidermal ampulla, (4) a star-shaped arrangement of efferent spider vessels, and (5) capillaries. The central spider vessel comes from the subcutis, winds up to the epidermis, and there branches out as an end artery.[15] However, the efferent branches show no evidence of a transition into veins. The spider is not, therefore, an arteriovenous anastomosis.

Traditionally, vascular spiders and palmar erythema have been attributed to estrogen excess, particularly since they are also found during pregnancy and because estrogens have an enlarging, dilating effect on the spiral arterioles of the endometrium. This would also explain cutaneous spiders in men receiving estrogen therapy for prostatic cancer, although this very rare. However, it may be more complex than this. The relationship of vascular spiders to sex hormone levels and to capillary circulation in the nail fold has been examined.[16] There were structural and functional differences between patients with cirrhosis and control subjects, but nothing separated patients with cirrhosis with spiders from those without. Serum estradiol and total testosterone were comparable in patients with cirrhosis and controls, but free serum testosterone was reduced in male patients with cirrhosis, particularly in those with spiders, and the estradiol/free testosterone ratio was highest in male patients with spiders.

PALMAR ERYTHEMA   Palmar erythema or "liver palm" occurs in two clinical forms:

- In one (Fig. 164-3) there is an exaggeration of normal mottling, the hands are warm and bright red, especially on the palm, on the dorsa of the hands, and on fingers and the bases of nails.
- In the second, there is well-demarcated redness of the hypothenar eminence, which gradually spreads to other parts of the hand.

The soles of the feet may show similar changes. The mottling blanches on pressure and, when a glass slide is pressed on the palm, it flushes synchronously with the pulse rate. Patients may complain of throbbing or tingling. "Liver palms" occur not only in liver disease but also in pregnancy, thyrotoxicosis, and a number of chronic diseases.

It has been suggested that palmar erythema in liver disease and pregnancy is also related to estrogen levels, but the high incidence of palmar erythema in patients with an alcoholic fatty liver has been blamed on direct effects of ethanol on the vasculature.[17] In a number of individuals, the characteristic mottling and blotchy redness are of no clinical significance and palmar flushing may be familial.

OTHER VASCULAR CHANGES   Corkscrew scleral vessels (tortuous small arteries that traverse the margins of the ocular sclerae) have been described in patients with chronic liver disease and are possibly due to increased local cutaneous arterial perfusion and vasodilatation. Cardiac output is frequently increased in cirrhosis, total peripheral resistance may be decreased, and arteriovenous shunting may occur within the lungs, liver, and extremities. Some patients (so-called *Child's A*) have warm hands and some (*Child's B*) have cold hands. The cause of this is unknown but it does not seem to be related to autonomic dysfunction.[18]

Portal-systemic collateral vessels may develop and may be an important clue to the existence of portal hypertension. Often the umbilical vein is dilated and visible in the epigastrium, an occurrence more common than the oft-quoted *caput Medusae*.

Purpuric lesions ranging from pinpoint size to large ecchymoses may occur with acquired clotting defects of liver disease. They occur mainly on the lower limbs, may be transient and recurrent, are sometimes accompanied by follicular hyperkeratosis, but are not usually associated with vitamin C deficiency. Bruising is common at the sites of venipuncture.

Hormone-Induced Changes of the Skin

Hormonal disturbances have been claimed to be responsible for many of the skin and hair changes in patients with cirrhosis. There may be a decrease in the rate of growth of facial hair in men, but loss of forearm, axillary, and pubic hair may occur in both sexes. Pectoral alopecia and female pubic hair distribution may be seen in men, as may loss of libido and potency, testicular atrophy, and oligospermia. Striae distensae occur in both men and women in association with chronic liver disease (Fig. 164-4), especially chronic active hepatitis, with or without ascites or systemic corticosteroid therapy. Gynecomastia (often with Dupuytren's contracture and swelling of the parotid gland) is also associated with cirrhosis. However, although it has been generally assumed that these and many other changes are due to hyperestrogenism due to failure

FIGURE 164-3

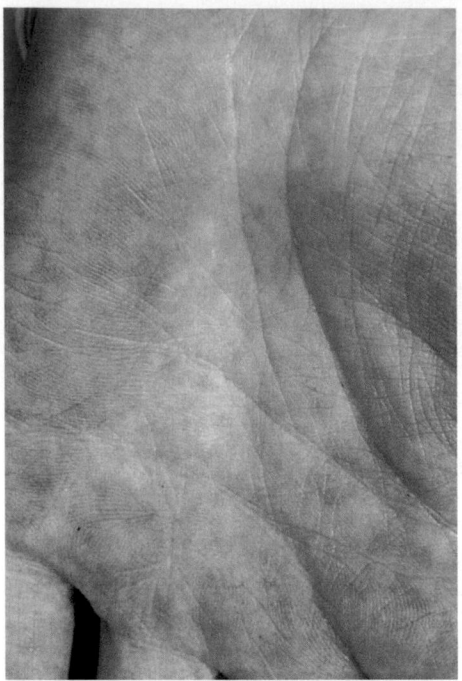

Palmar erythema or "liver palms" showing the characteristic blotchy redness.

of inactivation of estrogens, it has been pointed out that many of these so-called hormonal changes occur more commonly in alcoholic cirrhotics.[5] It may be that, as with vascular spiders, the ratio of estrogens to free testosterone is important. Chronic alcoholics also develop other "pseudoendocrine" effects even in the absence of liver disease,[19] including facial mooning, truncal obesity, and proximal muscle wasting, all features reminiscent of Cushing's syn-

FIGURE 164-4

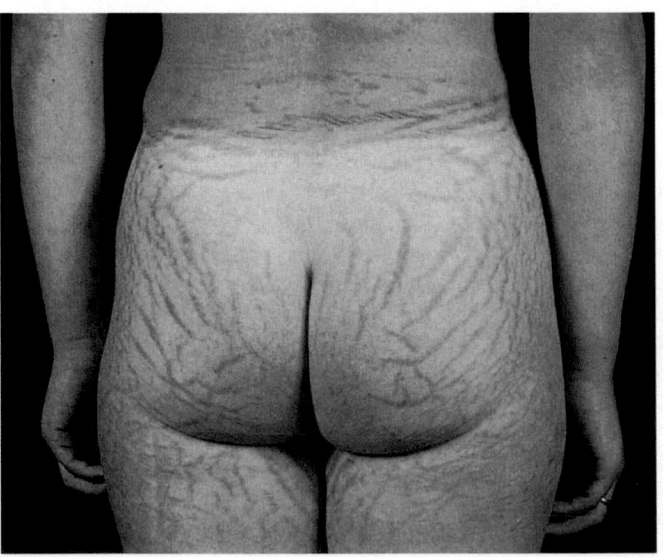

Widespread stretch marks in a 16-year-old boy with chronic active hepatitis.

drome. This "pseudo-Cushing's syndrome" reverts to normal when alcohol is discontinued.

An exuberant growth of condylomata acuminata of the vulva and vagina has been described in women with cirrhosis[20] and has been linked to the occasional appearance of large, moist warts in pregnancy.

Immunologic Manifestations of Liver Disease

Abnormal immunologic mechanisms have been implicated in some forms of hepatitis and cirrhosis, especially chronic active hepatitis and primary biliary cirrhosis. These diseases may show evidence of nonspecific cutaneous involvement encountered in other forms of hepatic dysfunction but may also be accompanied by skin changes that form part of a multisystem autoimmune process.

Around one-third of patients with hepatitis B develop urticaria in the 2 weeks before overt liver damage occurs, and various erythemas and purpura are also seen in some.[21]

We have seen a patient with localized scleroderma and chronic active hepatitis and several patients with scleroderma in association with primary biliary cirrhosis, as have others.[22–26] More recently the acronym PACK (*p*rimary biliary cirrhosis, *a*nticentromere antibody, CREST (*c*alcinosis cutis, *R*aynaud's phenomenon, *e*sophageal dysfunction, *s*clerodactyly, and *t*elangiectasia) syndrome, and keratoconjunctivitis sicca) has been suggested for a somewhat expanded version of this relationship.[27]

CHRONIC ACTIVE HEPATITIS AND THE SKIN As mentioned above, cutaneous striae were present in about one-quarter of 81 patients with chronic active hepatitis, even before glucocorticoid therapy (Fig. 164-4).[28] Acne, "erythematous" rashes, lupus erythematosus–type changes, localized scleroderma, purpura, and splinter hemorrhages of the nails were also found.[28] An allergic capillaritis of the skin was first described by Sarkany.[29] The lesions occur mainly on the trunk (Fig. 164-5) and may erupt over many years, fluctuating with the severity of the disease and with therapy. There are active inflammatory papules with a central pustular element, later forming a crust, leading to atrophy and formation of a characteristically depressed scar. Eventually the pink color fades, leaving a persistent, pale, depressed, circular or oval lesion resembling a postvaccination scar. Systemic glucocorticoids have a suppressive effect.

Histopathologically, the epithelium contains a crater in which there is a parakeratotic plug. There is a dermal infiltrate consisting of lymphocytes, histiocytes, and eosinophils. Many capillaries show edema and cuffing, with a periodic acid–Schiff (PAS)-positive fibrin-like material. There appears to be increased permeability of small vessels, associated with endothelial swelling, permeation of plasma fibrin formation, and hyalinosis.

Pyoderma gangrenosum[30] and a wide range of less uniform clinical and histologic skin reaction patterns have also been reported in patients with chronic active hepatitis. These patterns included urticarial, macular, and papular rashes and raised purpuric lesions,[31] which histologically showed various degrees of cutaneous vasculitis. Some were primarily a lymphocytic venulitis with focal necrosis, while the purpuric lesions were represented by neutrophilic necrotizing vasculitis involving small vessels. The presence of perivascular deposits of immunoglobulins, complement, and fibrin in these patients suggests an immune complex–mediated vascular injury.

CUTANEOUS MANIFESTATIONS AND PRIMARY BILIARY CIRRHOSIS The diagnosis of primary biliary cirrhosis is based on a typical clinical picture, liver function tests suggesting chole-

FIGURE 164-5

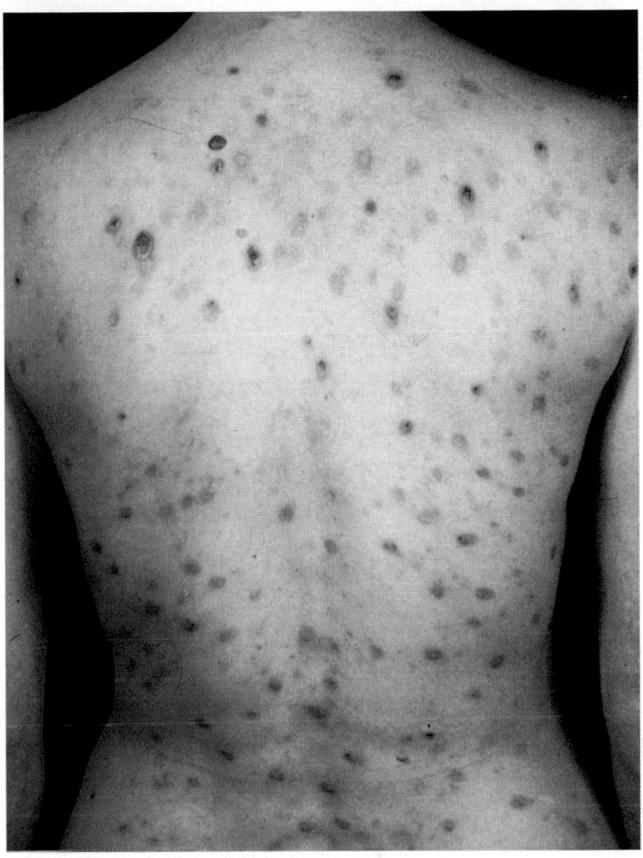

Eruption of red papules with central crusts and depressed scars caused by allergic capillaritis in a patient with chronic active hepatitis.

stasis, antimitochondrial antibodies, and characteristic histology. Various cutaneous changes may be seen, including the nonspecific skin changes usually associated with liver disease.

Scleroderma and systemic sclerosis have been mentioned earlier.

An IgM-associated membranous glomerulonephritis has been reported in association with primary biliary cirrhosis and cutaneous capillaritis.[32]

Another skin disease that has been reported in association with primary biliary cirrhosis is lichen planus. A group of five patients with lichen planus and primary biliary cirrhosis was reported by the authors.[33] We suggested that this coexistence might be due to the fact that both conditions involve altered immune function. A report from the Mayo Clinic at about the same time recorded a larger number of patients in whom lichen planus appeared to develop after the administration of penicillamine, although in some, the skin lesions developed in the absence of the drug.[34]

Immunopathologic mechanisms play an important role in both lichen planus and primary biliary cirrhosis, and it has also been pointed out that primary biliary cirrhosis shares features with chronic graft-versus-host disease: similar changes are seen in the liver, and damage to the lacrimal and salivary glands in both gives rise to the sicca syndrome.[35] Lichen planus–like lesions are often seen in cutaneous features of graft-versus-host reactions, and the appearance of lichen planus in patients with primary biliary cirrhosis strongly suggests common pathogenic mechanisms.[33] The relationship between lichen planus and liver disease is also discussed briefly below.

Another immunopathologic link between primary biliary cirrhosis and the skin is provided by cutaneous immunofluorescence.[36-38] IgM has been demonstrated at the basement membrane zone and around blood vessels, in a pattern similar to that seen in lupus erythematosus. C3, fibrin, IgA, and IgG have also been found, but less frequently. Such positivity is not related to high IgM levels and is not a washout effect.[39] This may represent an additional accessible immunologic marker and diagnostic aid in primary biliary cirrhosis. Some authors have reported that penicillamine altered or abolished the immunofluorescence,[36] but we did not find this.[36]

Miscellaneous Changes of the Skin

Porphyria cutanea tarda and erythropoietic protoporphyria are considered in Chap. 151. Liver disease is frequently associated with the former and the liver may rarely be seriously damaged by the latter. A wide range of xanthomatous lesions may be seen in patients with biliary cirrhosis and other hyperlipemic states. These lesions are described in detail in Chap. 152.

Nail Changes in Liver Disease

Although a variety of changes have been described, the nails of many patients with liver disease are normal and nail abnormalities are a less constant physical sign than spiders or liver palms. However, in cirrhotic patients a number of changes may occur: clubbing, white nails, watch-glass deformity, flat nails, white bands, striations, and brittleness.

Although it is a more constant sign of certain cardiopulmonary disorders, *clubbing* of the fingers is quite common in all forms of cirrhosis. This is especially true of primary biliary cirrhosis (18 of 106 cases in one series) and chronic active hepatitis (5 of 35 cases).[40] Martini[41] noted an association between the incidence of clubbing and palmar erythema. Cirrhosis and the cardiopulmonary disorders associated with clubbing disease share an increased blood flow,[42] but the pathogenesis of clubbing is still not understood.

Anatomically there is increased thickness of the nail bed. This may be due to edema, cellular infiltration, an increase in connective tissue, increased vascularity, or a combination of all or some of these. The importance of the vascular element is demonstrated by the findings of Mendlowitz,[43-45] who found that the blood flow of the distal portion of the fingers in patients with clubbing was greater than in normal digits and that the gradient of pressure, diminishing toward the periphery of the finger, was lost. There was also a marked increase in blood pressure in the digital arteries compared with controls. It has also been shown that when clubbing disappears, a reduction in blood flow follows.

White nails may occasionally be seen in normal individuals and in a variety of diseases, especially cryoglobulinemia, Raynaud's syndrome, and systemic sclerosis. However, intensely white nails are characteristic of cirrhosis (Figs. 164-6 and 164-7): Terry (after whom the sign is named) reported white nails in 82 of 100 patients with cirrhosis.[46] The whiteness does not alter with nail growth or with compression of digital vessels and is likely to be due to opacity of the nail plate itself. In severe cases, all fingernails may be affected, showing opacity of almost the entire nail bed (Fig. 164-7), although there may be a pink zone at the distal edge of the nail. The so-called *watch-glass deformity* may accompany white nails (Fig. 164-6). In one patient with alcoholic liver disease, the finger-

FIGURE 164-6

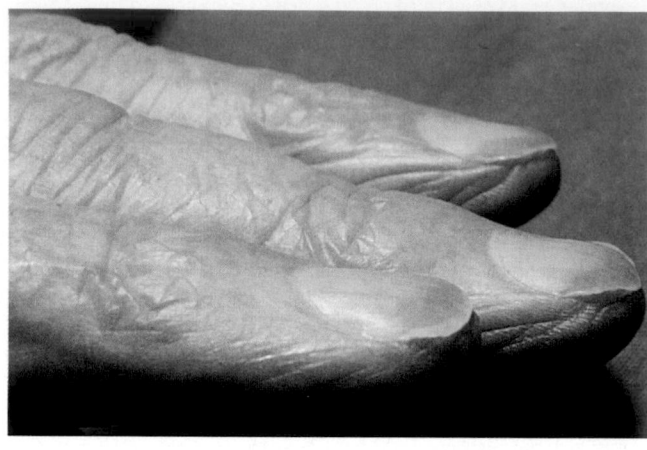

Flat white nails with slight convex watchglass deformity showing a distal pink band in a patient with liver disease.

nails showed multiple transverse white bands that evolved into typical white nails.[49] *Opaque nails* and thinned nail folds with a wide cuticle have also been reported in patients with alcoholic liver disease.[48,49]

Flat or *spoon nails*[50] are less common in patients with liver disease. The nails are either flat or concave, pale in color, and frequently show longitudinal ridging. In hemochromastosis, koilonychia is probably the most common of the nail abnormalities, but it is not related to anemia.[6] *Brittle nails* have also been blamed on liver disease, often without adequate documentation.

Azure lunulae, a bluish color of the lunular portion of nails, occur in hepatolenticular degeneration (Wilson's disease).[51] Azure lunulae and corneal changes resembling Kayser-Fleischer rings may also be seen in patients with argyria.[51,52]

The characteristic nail changes of lichen planus—including longitudinal ridging, pterygium formation, and permanent nail loss—have been reported in primary biliary cirrhosis.[54] (See Chap. 72 for further discussion of nail changes.)

FIGURE 164-7

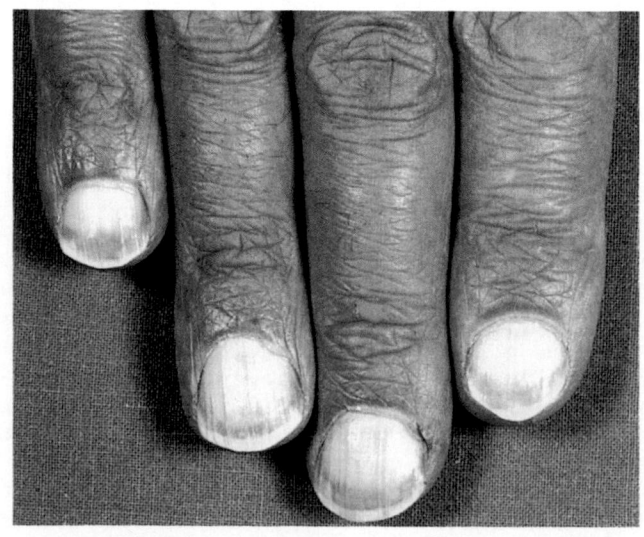

Terry's white nails in a patient with cirrhosis.

Itching

Pruritus is one of the commonest and most distressing symptoms of hepatobiliary disease. It may be mild and transient or so severe and prolonged that it dominates the clinical picture of the disease. It is predominantly associated with those conditions causing cholestasis.

In hepatitis, itching is frequently missed as an early sign of the disease, but it may occur in the later, icteric, phase. Some drugs may also induce cholestasis and hence pruritus: erythromycin, oral contraceptives, phenothiazines, chlorpropamide, paraaminosalicylic acid, and nitrofurantoin. Pruritus is the presenting symptom in over 50 percent of cases of primary biliary cirrhosis and may precede jaundice by months or even years. One important point is that, whatever the cause, if hepatocellular failure supervenes, even previously intolerable itching may subside.

PATHOGENESIS OF PRURITUS (See also Chap. 42)   The physiologic basis of pruritus is still not completely understood. Itch is carried by slow-conducting C fibers to the spinal cord and from there, in the anterolateral spinothalamic tracts, to the thalamus, and to the posterior central gyrus. Mechanical, electrical, and thermal stimuli can cause itching; histamine release may cause itching, but proteolytic enzymes and prostaglandins have also been shown to be involved in the chemical mediation of pruritus.

In jaundice, the association of itching with the absence of bile from the feces, whether as a result of cholestasis or hepatitis, suggests that something normally excreted in the bile is responsible. Bile acids have been identified in the skin of patients with pruritus, but no direct relationship has yet been found between itching and the concentration of any particular conjugated or free bile acid: a great overlap of bile acid levels has been shown in cholestatic patients with and without pruritus. Moreover, when pruritus stops in terminal liver failure, serum bile acids may still be elevated. Thus, retained bile acids may not have a *direct* role,[55] but the relief of itching by bile salt–chelating resins and the disappearance of pruritus when liver cells fail suggest that bile salts are implicated or at least that the responsible agent(s) is manufactured by the liver.

One reason for the poor correlation between serum bile salt concentration and pruritus may be variation in bile salt composition. The pruritic effect of purified bile salts has been tested by applying them to blister bases.[56] All salts tested caused itching, but dihydroxy salts (especially unconjugated chenodeoxycholate) were more potent than trihydroxy salts.

Chemical mediators of itching, whether bile salts or not, may act directly on cutaneous nerves or by releasing endogenous pruritogens. However, although bile salts liberate small amounts of histamine on perfusion of animal skin[57] and blood histamine levels increase in experimental obstructive jaundice,[58] there is a poor correlation between pruritus and plasma histamine in liver disease.[59] This, and the poor response to antihistamines, suggests that histamine is not the major mediator in liver disease. The inhibition of cholestatic itch by opiate antagonists suggests that endogenous opioids may be important.[60]

CLINICAL FEATURES   Itching in hepatobiliary disease may be transient or continuous and may or may not be accompanied by jaundice. Although usually most marked on the extremities, severe pruritus may affect the trunk, but the neck and face are rarely and the genitalia hardly ever involved. Pruritus may be debilitating in patients with primary biliary cirrhosis, mechanical biliary obstruction, or other causes of cholestasis and is usually generalized. There may be no visible skin change, but more often there are scratch marks and excoriations. Macular, papular, or urticarial lesions may

be present; in long-standing cases, lichenified plaques or the nodules of prurigo are found. Histologically, these changes are nonspecific. In the differential diagnosis, a whole range of systemic diseases and skin conditions must be considered. Itching of pregnancy has been found to be associated with cholestasis with or without jaundice and has tended to recur in subsequent pregnancies in half the cases.

MANAGEMENT   The itching of acute viral hepatitis and of mild drug-induced cholestasis requires sympathetic understanding, reassurance, mild sedation and local applications such as calamine lotion with 1% phenol or 0.25% menthol. The persistent and troublesome itching of primary biliary cirrhosis may require more effective topical antipruritics such as Eurax cream or lotion (crotamiton 10%), topical corticosteroids, or systemic phenothiazines. More effective are anion-exchange resins, which sequester bile acids within the intestine and lower levels in serum (and tissue).

These drugs need to be administered with care, however. Patients with cirrhosis often have vitamin deficiencies and exchange resins may bind vitamins and drugs.

Although infusions have no place in the management of chronic cholestatic pruritus, it has recently been suggested that newer, orally effective opiate antagonists may prove useful.[61] Itching due to mechanical obstruction of bile requires surgical correction. Plasmapheresis has also been tried in the treatment of cholestatic pruritus with variable results.[62–63] Rifampicin reduced pruritus in primary biliary cirrhosis in a double-blind, crossover trial,[64] although the mechanism of action remains unknown. A combination of phototherapy and cholestyramine seemed to work in a patient when the drug alone had failed.[65]

Hepatitis and the Skin

Hepatitis A is largely spread by fecal-oral contamination and is most common in young adults who have visited countries with poor standards of hygiene. In the early phase a discrete, transient, maculopapular, urticarial, or petechial rash may develop, together with joint symptoms.[66]

Hepatitis B infection is a worldwide problem, accounting for a large burden of morbidity, mortality, and economic consequences, whether due to its acute effects or to its chronic sequelae, including primary hepatoma.[67]

Hepatitis B has a marked tendency to induce a chronic infective state, with 10 percent of infected subjects becoming carriers. Furthermore, 90 percent of infants born of mothers infected with the virus will develop an ongoing infection.[68] This prevalence has implications for health professionals. The risk of infection to dermatologists has been discussed,[69–71] but there are also issues for the patients of hepatitis B–positive health care workers. It is generally accepted that health care workers, including dermatologists, should always wear gloves while carrying out invasive procedures and that screening and/or vaccination with evidence of serologic conversion should be carried out. Indeed, these are now legal requirements for practicing in many countries.

There are four well-documented cutaneous associations of hepatitis B:

- A serum sickness–like syndrome
- Essential mixed cryoglobulinemia
- Polyarteritis nodosa
- Papular acrodermatitis of childhood (Gianotti-Crosti syndrome)

A *serum sickness–like syndrome* occurs in about 20 to 30 percent of patients with hepatitis B infection. Urticaria may be the predominant or sole feature, but polyarthralgia, a true arthritis, proteinuria, and hematuria may also occur. The skin changes may become vasculitic. This phase usually lasts from 1 to 6 weeks before jaundice appears.[72] The skin lesions are associated with the perivascular deposition of immune complexes containing HBsAg, IgM or IgG, and C3[72–74] (see also Chap. 176).

In *essential mixed cryoglobulinemia*, patients develop purpura, acropathy, and weakness, and renal involvement is common.[75,76] Histopathologically there is a necrotizing vasculitis. Cryoglobulins are present with IgG and IgM in near equal amounts.[77] It is more common to find circulating antibodies than the antigen itself in these patients (in contrast to the situation in polyarteritis nodosa; see below) (see also Chap. 177).

Polyarteritis nodosa has been well documented in association with hepatitis B infection.[78,79] The disease may present soon after an attack of hepatitis B, but there may be a delay of years.[80] Electron microscopy has shown the virion of the hepatitis B virus in the serum of these patients, and circulating immune complexes containing hepatitis B surface antigen (HBsAg) and immunoglobulin have been demonstrated. A leukocytoclastic vasculitis may develop when immunofluorescence for HBsAg in dermal vessels is often positive[80,81] (see also Chaps. 175 and 176).

Papular acrodermatitis of childhood (Gianotti-Crosti syndrome) affects children aged 2 to 6 years and is characterized by the appearance of a papular eruption on the face and limbs. This eruption usually lasts 2 to 3 weeks and is accompanied by lymphadenopathy and acute hepatitis, which is anicteric and usually lasts for about 2 months.[82] However, antigenemia (usually of a subtype known as "ayw") may persist for months or years in a third of patients, accompanied by continuously elevated liver enzymes.[83] (See also Chap. 144.)

Hepatitis C accounts for many cases of posttransfusion hepatitis but also occurs sporadically and epidemically. Several cutaneous manifestations have been reported, including leukocytoclastic vasculitis, cryoglobulinemia,[84,85] pruritus,[86] porphyria cutanea tarda, erythema nodosum, urticaria, erythema multiforme, polyarteritis nodosa, and lichen planus.[84] There is some debate about the latter, however, as one group found no significant association in a careful case-controlled study.[87]

Disorders in which Both Skin and Liver May Be Involved

There are many systemic diseases that involve both the skin and the liver but in which the changes are not dependent on one another, do not always both occur, or may appear separated by an interval of months or years. A list of some of the more important ones is given in Table 164-2.

Argininosuccinic aciduria (See Chap. 149) is a rare autosomal recessive disorder characterized by ataxia, seizures, severe mental retardation, hepatomegaly and liver dysfunction, and brittle hair.

Cutaneous and ocular telangiectases are associated with cerebellar ataxia and immunologic defects in *ataxia telangiectasia* (see Chap. 192). There has also been report of a hepatoma in one patient.[88] It is of interest, therefore, that alpha fetoprotein levels are often raised in ataxia telangiectasia. *Dermatomyositis* is not asso-

TABLE 164-2

Disorders in which Both Skin and Liver May Be Involved

Argininosuccinic aciduria	Neurofibromatosis
Ataxia telangiectasia	Pityriasis rotunda with hepatoma
Dermatomyositis	
Drug reactions	Porphyrias
Eruptive neonatal angiomastosis	Porphyria cutanea tarda
Graft-versus-host disease	Variegate porphyria
Hereditary hemorrhagic telangiectasia (Osler-Weber-Rendu disease)	Erythropoietic (erythrohepatic) porphyria
	Hereditary coproporphyria
Histiocytoses	Sarcoidosis
Immunodeficiency states	Syphilis
Mastocytosis	Systemic lupus erythematosus
Mucocutaneous lymph node syndrome	Tuberous sclerosis
	Vinyl chloride disease (Kawasaki disease)

ciated with any specific hepatic changes but may be the presenting sign of an underlying cancer with hepatic secondaries. In *eruptive neonatal angiomatosis* multiple angiomata may occur anywhere on the skin surface and vascular lesions may also occur in internal organs, including the liver. Both liver and skin may be prominently involved in both acute and chronic phases of *graft-versus-host reactions*. Although these features are most commonly seen in patients receiving bone marrow transplants, similar states have been described in association with disseminated cancers.[89] Laparoscopic examination of patients with *hereditary hemorrhagic telangiectasia* has revealed small vascular lesions on the surface of the liver. Ateriovenous fistulas and cirrhosis have also been described. Both skin and liver may be involved in several of the *histiocytoses*, including Langerhans cell histiocytosis (Chap. 160), malignant histiocytosis, and cytophagic histiocytic panniculitis (Chaps. 109 and 111). Any *immunodeficiency* state may result in multiple infections of skin and liver, and some have significant cutaneous markers. Examples include congenital disorders such as ataxia telangiectasia (see above), Chédiak-Higashi syndrome and chronic granulomatous disease, and acquired immunodeficiency states, including AIDS.

Hepatomegaly is relatively common in *mastocytosis* (Chap. 162). Ten to fifteen percent of children with *mucocutaneous lymph node syndrome* (Kawasaki disease) (Chap. 205) develop upper abdominal pain associated with hepatobiliary changes, usually nonspecific elevation of liver enzymes, due to vasculitic changes or bile duct inflammation. Hydrops of the gallbladder may also develop. Extrahepatic biliary obstruction due to neural masses has been reported in patients with *neurofibromatosis*, and there are reports of hepatoma,[92] polycystic liver disease,[93] and unexplained pruritus and cholestasis.[94] The *porphyrias* are covered in detail elsewhere (Chap. 151).

Sarcoidosis may cause many different skin changes, and sarcoidal infiltration of the liver may accompany many of them (Chap. 184). Hepatic granulomata may also occur in tuberculosis, glandular fever, syphilis, and as a result of the administration of several drugs (phenylbutazone, sulfonamides, and allopurinol). True syphilitic hepatitis is rare but well documented[95] and presents with pruritus and cholestatic jaundice.

Of 238 patients with *systemic lupus erythematosus* (SLE), 43 were found to have liver disease, including cirrhosis, chronic active hepatitis, and fatty change[96] (Chap. 172). In one patient a granulomatous hepatitis was associated with an exacerbation of the SLE.[97] Autopsy in some patients with SLE has revealed multiple nodular hyperplasia without cirrhosis.[98] Hepatic lesions are well described in *tuberous sclerosis* (Chap. 190). These are usually hamartomatous malformations involving fat, smooth muscle, and blood vessels, but portal fibrosis may occur. There is one report of clumps of large, abnormal hepatocytes.[99] Liver function abnormalities are common in patients with *vinyl chloride disease,* and there may be hepatosplenomegaly and frank cirrhosis. Angiosarcomas of the liver may develop.[100]

The association of hepatocellular carcinoma in 10 South African blacks with *pityriasis rotunda* has been reported.[101]

THE EFFECTS OF SKIN DISEASE ON THE LIVER

A number of metabolic and other disturbances occur as a consequence of skin disease, and some of them reflect abnormalities of hepatic function.

Extensive Loss of Skin

Large areas of skin may be lost after thermal burns, in severe pemphigus, staphylococcal scalded skin syndrome, and toxic epidermal necrolysis. Autopsies reveal degenerative changes in the livers of severely burned patients, and liver enzyme abnormalities are common during acute shock immediately after a bad burn.[102] A more significant finding is cholestatic jaundice, which generally occurs in more severely affected patients with complications. This is preceded by a gradual rise in the alkaline phosphatase, and liver biopsies confirm cholestasis and nonspecific inflammatory changes. The mortality remains very high.[103]

Exfoliative Dermatitis

The systemic effects of exfoliative dermatitis are considerable. Patients with exfoliative dermatitis may develop hypoalbuminemia, gynecomastia, and hepatomegaly—features suggestive of hepatic dysfunction. However, these seem likely to be due to a combination of protein loss from shed scale and, more importantly, hemodilution.[104] The hepatomegaly seen in exfoliative dermatitis is probably largely due to congestion. Liver enzymes are generally normal, and, when liver biopsies have been performed, the liver architecture is unaffected in most instances (see also Chap. 45).

Psoriasis

Features suggesting hepatic dysfunction, similar to the changes described above in exfoliative dermatitis, may occur in severe, widespread psoriasis. Some patients with generalized pustular psoriasis develop jaundice, which has been attributed to a combination of oligemia, general toxicity, and drugs.[105] However, abnormalities in liver architecture have been described in several patients with uncomplicated plaque psoriasis.[106] The most common finding is fatty change, but focal necrosis, periportal inflammation, and fibrosis have also been found. There has been controversy over what these changes represent, as they seem unlikely to be due to psoriasis alone. Alcohol consumption may be one factor, because several studies have shown a relationship between psoriasis and alcohol intake.[107–109] It remains unclear whether alcohol has a direct pharmacologic role in determining the severity of a patient's psoriasis or whether severe psoriasis leads to excessive drinking, which would tend to reduce patient compliance with treatment and followup, establishing a vicious circle of poor disease control and increased alcohol abuse (see also Chap. 43).

Dermatitis Herpetiformis

Abnormalities of liver function tests were found in a significant proportion of patients with dermatitis herpetiformis.[110] Concomitant autoimmune liver disease was specifically excluded, but patients on a gluten-free diet generally had a lower incidence of abnormalities than those on a normal diet (see Chap. 67).

Lichen Planus

The occurrence of lichen planus in patients with primary biliary cirrhosis has already been mentioned. Similar claims have been made for chronic active hepatitis[111,112] and one large epidemiologic study has found a remarkably high incidence of liver abnormalities in patients with lichen planus.[113] This remains an area of controversy, however, because others have been unable to substantiate this[114–116] (see Chap. 50).

Cancers of the Skin

Some skin cancers are capable of producing hepatic metastases, especially melanoma and Kaposi's sarcoma.

TABLE 164-3

Potentially Hepatotoxic Drugs Used in the Treatment of Skin Disease

DRUG	THERAPEUTIC USE	HEPATIC COMPLICATIONS
Azathioprine	Immunosuppression	Liver enzyme elevation; severe injury rare
Cyproterone acetate	Acne	May worsen preexisting liver dysfunction
Danazol	Hereditary angioedema	May worsen preexisting liver dysfunction and porphyrias; cholestatic jaundice (rare)
Griseofulvin	Fungal infections	May worsen preexisting liver dysfunction
Ketoconazole	Fungal infections	Severe hepatitis (rare)[117]
Methotrexate	Psoriasis; sarcoidosis; miscellaneous skin disorders	Hepatic fibrosis[106]
Psoralens	Psoriasis; T-cell lymphoma; vitiligo	Hepatitis (rare)[118]
Retinoids	Disorders of keratinization; psoriasis; acne	Liver enzyme elevation,[119,120] hepatitis (rare)
Stanozolol	Venous disease; Behçet's syndrome	Liver enzyme elevation, exacerbation of porphyrias

HEPATOTOXIC EFFECTS OF DRUGS USED IN THE TREATMENT OF SKIN DISEASE

Several drugs used frequently in managing patients with skin disease, and some hardly used for anything else, are known to be hepatotoxic. Table 164-3 lists some of the most important. Of these, the one drug that has caused most concern over the years is methotrexate. Patients with diabetes, the obese, the elderly, and those with high alcohol consumption are at higher risk than others.[106] The main method of assessing possible liver damage with methotrexate has been regular liver biopsy, but other, less invasive techniques may be adequate.[121]

REFERENCES

1. Morgan MY: Sex and alcohol. *Br Med Bull* **38**:43, 1982
2. Diamond I, Schmid R: Experimental bilirubin encephalopathy: The mode of entry of bilirubin-^{14}C into the central nervous system. *J Clin Invest* **45**:678, 1966
3. Schaffner F: Primary biliary cirrhosis. *Clin Gastroenterol* **4**:351, 1975
4. Bohnstedt RM: Haut und Leber, in *Leber, Haut und Skelett,* edited by L. Wannagat. Stuttgart, George Thieme, 1964
5. Martini GA: Leber und Haut, in *Leber, Haut und Skelett,* edited by L Wannagat. Stuttgart, George Thieme, 1964.
6. Chevrant-Breton J et al: Cutaneous manifestations of idiopathic hemochromatosis. *Arch Dermatol* **113**:161, 1977
7. Lerner AB, McGuire JS: Melanocyte-stimulating hormone and adrenocorticotrophic hormone. *N Engl J Med* **270**:539, 1964
8. Burton JL, Kirby J: Pigmentation and biliary cirrhosis. *Lancet* **1**:458, 1975
9. Mills PR et al: Melanin pigmentation of the skin in primary biliary cirrhosis. *J Cutan Pathol* **8**:404, 1981
10. Finch SC, Finch CA: Idiopathic hemochromatosis, an iron storage disease: A. Iron metabolism in hemochromatosis. *Medicine (Baltimore)* **34**:381, 1955
11. Perdup A, Poulson H: Hemochromatosis and vitiligo. *Arch Dermatol* **90**:34, 1964
12. Bean WB: The arterial spider and similar lesions of the skin and mucous membrane. *Circulation* **8**:117, 1953
13. Capron JP et al: Unilateral nevoid telangiectasia and chronic liver disease. *Am J Gastroenterol* **76**:47, 1981
14. Schirren C: Hautveränderungen beie inneren Erkrankungen, in *Handbuch der Haut- und Geschleschtskrankheiten,* edited by HA Gottron. Berlin, Springer-Verlag, 1967, p 569
15. Martini GA, Staubesand J: Zur Morphologie der Gefässpinnen ("vascular spiders") in der Haut Leberkranker. *Virchows Arch Pathol Anat* **324**:147, 1953
16. Pirovino M et al: Cutaneous spider nevi in liver cirrhosis: Capillary, microscopical and hormonal investigations. *Klin Wochenschr* **66**:289, 1988
17. Tarao K et al: The incidence of palmar erythema in patients with alcoholic fatty liver. *Jpn J Gastroenterol* **83**:2365, 1986
18. Steele D et al: Hand skin temperature changes in patients with chronic liver disease. *J Hepatol* **21**: 927, 1994
19. Morgan MY: Alcohol and the endocrine system. *Br Med Bull* **38**:35, 1982
20. Blank H: Common viral diseases of the skin. *Med Clin North Am* **43**:1401, 1959
21. Veyre B, Brette R: L'hépatite B à la phase prémonitoire. *Nouv Presse Med* **4**:1349, 1975
22. Murray-Lyon IM et al: Scleroderma and primary biliary cirrhosis. *Br Med J* **3**:258, 1970
23. Rau R et al: Liver involvement in scleroderma. *Schweiz Med Wochenschr* **104**:1877, 1974
24. McCoy DG: Spontaneous rupture of the liver in a case of scleroderma. *J Irish Med Assoc* **60**:474, 1967
25. De Graaf P et al: Princire bilaire cirrose met sclerodermie en hypothyreidie. *Tijdschr Gastroenterol* **18**:151, 1975
26. Reynolds TB et al: Primary biliary cirrhosis with scleroderma, Raynaud's phenonemon and telangiectasis: New syndrome. *Am J Med* **50**:302, 1971
27. Powell FC et al: Primary biliary cirrhosis and the CREST syndrome—new terminology? *Q J Med* **62**:75, 1987
28. Read AE et al: Active "juvenile" cirrhosis considered as part of a systemic disease and the effect of corticosteroid therapy. *Gut* **4**:378, 1963
29. Sarkany I: Juvenile cirrhosis and allergic capillaritis of the skin: A hepato-cutaneous syndrome. *Lancet* **2**:666, 1966
30. Burns DA, Sarkany I: Active chronic hepatitis and pyoderma gangrenosum: Report of a case. *Clin Exp Dermatol* **4**:465, 1979
31. Popp JW et al: Cutaneous vasculitis associated with acute chronic hepatitis. *Arch Intern Med* **141**:623, 1981
32. Rai GS et al: Primary biliary cirrhosis, cutaneous capillaritis, and IgM-associated membranous glomerulonephritis. *Br Med J* **1**:817, 1977
33. Graham-Brown RAC et al: Lichen planus and primary biliary cirrhosis. *Br J Dermatol* **106**:600, 1982
34. Seehafer JR et al: Lichen planus-like lesions caused by penicillamine in primary biliary cirrhosis. *Arch Dermatol* **117**:140, 1981
35. Epstein O et al: Primary biliary cirrhosis is a dry gland syndrome with features of chronic graft-versus-host disease. *Lancet* **1**:1166, 1980
36. Randle HW et al: Cutaneous immunofluorescence in primary biliary cirrhosis. *JAMA* **246**:1679, 1981
37. Hendricks AA et al: Cutaneous immunoglobulin deposition in primary biliary cirrhosis. *Arch Dermatol* **118**:634, 1982
38. Graham-Brown RAC, Sarkany I: Positive cutaneous immunofluorescence in primary biliary cirrhosis. Personal observations, 1983
39. Lindgren S et al: IgM deposition in skin biopsies from patients with primary biliary cirrhosis. *Acta Med Scand* **210**:317, 1981
40. Cook GC: Active chronic hepatitis and its response to corticosteroid therapy. MD thesis. University of London, 1965
41. Martini GA: Über Gefässveränderungen der Haut bei Leberkranken. *Z Klin Med* **153**:470, 1955
42. Martini GA, Hagemann JE: Über Fingernagelveränderungen bei Lebercirrhose als Folge veränderter peripherer Durchblutung. *Klin Wochenschr* **34**:25, 1956
43. Mendlowitz M: Some observations on clubbed fingers. *Clin Sci* **3**:387, 1938
44. Mendlowitz M: Measurements of blood flow and blood pressure in clubbed fingers. *J Clin Invest* **20**:113, 1941
45. Mendlowitz M: *Digital Circulation.* New York, Grune & Stratton, 1954
46. Terry RB: White nails in hepatic cirrhosis. *Lancet* **1**:757, 1954
47. Jenssen O: White fingernails preceded by multiple transverse white bands. *Acta Derm Venereol (Stockh)* **61**:261, 1981
48. Lewin K: The finger nail in general disease: A macroscopic and microscopic study of 87 consecutive autopsies. *Br J Dermatol* **77**:431, 1965
49. Young AW: Cutaneous stigmata of alcoholism. *Alcohol Health Res World,* Summer 1974, p 24
50. Kleeberg J: Flat finger-nails in cirrhosis of the liver. *Lancet* **2**:248, 1951
51. Bearn AG, McKusick VA: Azure lunulae: An unusual change in the fingernails in two patients with hepatolenticular degeneration (Wilson's disease). *JAMA* **166**:904, 1958
52. Sarkany I: The skin lesions associated with liver disease. *Prog Dermatol* **4**:1, 1969
53. Whelton MJ, Pope FM: Azure lunules in argyria. *Arch Intern Med* **121**:267, 1968
54. Sowden JM et al: Isolated lichen planus of the nails associated with primary biliary cirrhosis. *Br J Dermatol* **121**:659, 1989
55. Freedman MR et al: Pruritus in cholestasis: No direct causative role for bile acid retention. *Am J Med* **70**:1011, 1981
56. Kirby J et al: Pruritic effect of bile salts. *Br Med J* **4**:693, 1974
57. Schachter M: The release of histamine by pethidine, atropine, quinine and other drugs. *Br J Pharmacol* **7**:646, 1952
58. Anrep GV, Barsoum GS: Blood histamine in experimental obstruction of the common bile duct. *J Physiol (Lond)* **120**:427, 1953
59. Mitchell RG et al: Histamine metabolism in diseases of the liver. *Clin Invest* **33**:1199, 1954
60. Bergasa NV et al: Effects of naloxone infusions in patients with pruritus of cholestasis: A double-blind, randomized controlled trial. *Ann Intern Med* **123**:161, 1995

61. Bergasa NV, Jones EA: The pruritus of cholestasis: Potential pathogenic and therapeutic implications of opioids. *Gastroenterology* **108**:1582, 1995

62. Garden JM et al: Pruritus in hepatic cholestasis. *Arch Dermatol* **121**:1415, 1985

63. Lauterburg BH et al: Treatment of pruritus of cholestasis by plasma perfusion through USP-charcoal-coated glass beads. *Lancet* **2**:53, 1980

64. Ghent CN, Carruthers SG: Treatment of pruritus in primary biliary cirrhosis with rifampicin. *Gastroenterology* **94**:488, 1988

65. Cerio R et al: A combination of phototherapy and cholestyramine for the relief of pruritus in primary biliary cirrhosis. *Br J Dermatol* **116**:265, 1987

66. Doutre MS, Beylot C: Les signes cutanes lies aux virus de l'hepatite. *Ann Dermatol Venereol* **110**:647, 1983

67. Rogers RB et al: Hepatitis and the skin. *J Am Acad Dermatol* **7**:552, 1981

68. Thomas HC, Scully LJ: Antiviral therapy in hepatitis B infection. *Br Med Bull* **41**:374, 1985

69. Pegum JS: Wound suturing without gloves. *Lancet* **2**:269, 1982.

70. Armati RP, McCullagh RB: Hepatitis in dermatologists. *Med J Aust* **142**:78, 1983

71. Leydon JJ et al: Serologic survey for markers of hepatitis B infection in dermatologists. *J Am Acad Dermatol* **12**:676, 1985

72. Dienstag LJ et al: Urticaria associated with acute viral hepatitis type B: Studies of pathogenesis. *Ann Intern Med* **89**:34, 1978

73. Popp JW et al: Cutaneous vasculitis associated with acute and chronic hepatitis. *Arch Intern Med* **141**:623, 1981

74. Neumann HAM et al: Hepatitis B surface antigen deposition in the blood vessel walls of urticarial lesions in acute hepatitis B. *Br J Dermatol* **104**:383, 1981.

75. Levo Y et al: Association between hepatitis B virus and essential mixed cryoglobulinemia. *N Engl J Med* **296**:1501, 1977

76. Heim LR: Cryoglobulins: Characterizations and classification. *Cutis* **23**:259, 1979

77. McElgunn PSJ: Dermatologic manifestations of hepatitis B virus infection. *J Am Acad Dermatol* **8**:539, 1983

78. Gocke DJ et al: Association between polyarteritis nodosa and Australia antigen. *Lancet* **2**:1149, 1970

79. Trepo CG et al: The role of circulating hepatitis B antigen/antibody immune complexes in the pathogenesis of vascular and hepatic manifestations in polyarteritis nodosa. *J Clin Pathol* **27**:863, 1974

80. Cohen RO et al: Clinical features, prognosis and response to treatment in polyarteritis. *Mayo Clin Proc* **55**:146, 1980

81. Sams WM Jr: Necrotizing vasculitis. *J Am Acad Dermatol* **3**:1, 1980

82. Gianotti F: Papular acrodermatitis of childhood: An Australia antigen disease. *Arch Dis Child* **48**:794, 1973

83. Colombo M et al: Immune response to hepatitis B virus in children with papular acro-dermatitis. *Gastroenterology* **73**:1103, 1977

84. Daoud MS et al: Chronic hepatitis C and skin diseases: A review. *Mayo Clin Proc* **70**:559, 1995

85. Daoud MS et al: Chronic hepatitis C, cryoglobulinemia, and cutaneous necrotizing vasculitis. *J Am Acad Dermatol* **34**:219, 1996

86. Fisher D, Wright T: Pruritus as a symptom of hepatitis C. *J Am Acad Dermatol* **30**:629, 1995

87. Cribier B et al: Lichen planus and hepatitis C virus infection: An epidemiologic study. *J Am Acad Dermatol* **31**:1070, 1994

88. Weinstein S et al: Ataxia telangiectasia with hepatocellular carcinoma in a 15-year old girl and studies of her kindred. *Arch Pathol Lab Med* **109**:1000, 1985

89. Graham-Brown RAC et al: A graft-versus-host-disease-like eruption with carcinomatosis. *Br J Dermatol* **116**:249, 1987

90. Solis-Herruzo JA et al: Laparascopic findings in hereditary haemorrhage telangiectasia (Osler-Weber-Rendu disease). *Endoscopy* **16**:137, 1984

91. Melish M et al: Kawasaki syndrome: An update. *Hosp Practice* **16**:137, 1982

92. Ettinger LJ, Freeman AI: Hepatoma in a child with neurofibromatosis. *Am J Dis Child* **133**:528, 1979

93. Varma SC et al: Association of von Recklinghausen's neurofibromatosis with adult polycystic disease of kidneys and liver. *Postgrad Med J* **58**:117, 1982

94. Monk BE et al: Neurofibromatosis, generalised pruritus and cholestatic liver function—report of two cases. *Clin Exp Dermatol* **10**:590, 1985

95. Sarkany I: Pruritus and cholestatic jaundice due to secondary syphilis. *Proc R Soc Med* **66**:237, 1973

96. Runyon BA et al: The spectrum of liver disease in systemic lupus erythematosus. *Am J Med* **69**:187, 1980

97. Feurle GE et al: Granulomatous hepatitis in systemic lupus erythematosus: Report of a case. *Endoscopy* **14**:153, 1982

98. Kuramochi S et al: Systemic lupus erythematosus associated with multiple nodular hyperplasia of the liver. *Acta Pathol Jpn* **32**:547, 1982

99. Grasso S et al: Unusual liver lesion in tuberous sclerosis. *Arch Pathol Lab Med* **106**:49, 1982

100. Walker A: Occupational acro-osteolysis (two cases). *Proc R Soc Med* **68**:343, 1975

101. Di Bisceglie AM et al: Pityriasis rotunda. *Arch Dermatol* **122**:802, 1986

102. Czaja AJ et al: Acute liver disease after cutaneous thermal injury. *J Trauma* **15**:887, 1975.

103. Pruitt BA: Other complications of burn injury, in *Burns: A Team Approach,* edited by CP Artz et al. Philadelphia, Saunders, 1979, p 523

104. Shuster S, Wilkinson P: Protein metabolism in exfoliative dermatitis and erythroderma. *Br J Dermatol* **75**:344, 1963

105. Ryan TJ, Baker H: Systemic corticosteroids and folic acid antagonists in the treatment of generalized pustular psoriasis. *Br J Dermatol* **81**:134, 1969

106. Zachariae H: Psoriasis and the liver, in *Psoriasis,* edited by HH Roegnigk, HI Maibach. New York, Marcel Dekker, 1985, p 45

107. Chaput JC et al: Psoriasis, alcohol and liver disease. *Br Med J* **291**:25, 1985

108. Morse RM et al: Alcoholism and psoriasis. *Alcohol Clin Exp Res* **9**:396, 1985

109. Monk BE, Neill SM: Alcohol consumption and psoriasis. *Dermatologica* **173**:57, 1986

110. Wojnarowska F, Fry L: Hepatic injury in patients with dermatitis herpetiformis. *Acta Dermatovenereol* **61**:165, 1981

111. Rebora A, Rongioletti F: Lichen planus and chronic active hepatitis. *J Am Acad Dermatol* **10**:840, 1984

112. Korkij W et al: Liver abnormalities in patients with lichen planus. *J Am Acad Dermatol* **11**:609, 1984

113. Gruppo Italiano Studi Epidemiologici in Dermatologia (GISED): Lichen planus and liver diseases: A multicentre case-control study. *Br Med J* **300**:227, 1990

114. Mobacken H et al: Lichen planus and the liver. *Acta Dermatovenereol* **64**:570, 1984

115. Shuttleworth D et al: The autoimmune background in lichen planus. *Br J Dermatol* **115**:199, 1986

116. McDonagh AJG et al: Lichen planus is not commonly a skin marker of primary biliary cirrhosis. *Dermatologica* **180**:111, 1990

117. Heiberg JK et al: Toxic hepatitis during ketoconazole treatment. *Br Med J* **183**:825, 1981

118. Pariser DM, Wyles RJ: Toxic hepatitis from oral methoxalen photochemotherapy (PUVA). *J Am Acad Dermatol* **3**:248, 1980

119. Orfanos CE: Laboratory investigations in psoriasis under oral retinoid treatment. *Dermatologica* **159**:62, 1979

120. Marsden JR et al: Effects of isotretinoin on serum lipids and lipoproteins, liver and thyroid function. *Clin Chim Acta* **143**:243, 1984

121. Zachariae H et al: Serum aminoterminal propeptide of type III procollagen: A non-invasive test for liver fibrogenesis in methotrexate treated psoriatics. *Acta Dermatovenereol* **69**:241, 1989

Cutaneous Changes in Renal Disorders

A number of diseases are characterized by distinctive cutaneous and renal manifestations. These diseases are covered extensively elsewhere in this volume and a partial list is outlined in Table 165-1. Occasionally a skin biopsy may be helpful in establishing a diagnosis of renal disease, such as IgA nephropathy.[1,2] The remainder of this discussion will be devoted to a review of cutaneous changes related to chronic renal failure, changes seen in patients on dialysis, and changes seen in patients who have undergone renal transplantation.

CUTANEOUS CHANGES RELATED TO CHRONIC RENAL FAILURE

The sequelae of chronic renal failure are complex and involve multiple systems. Careful examination of the skin, hair, nails, and mucous membranes reveals many abnormalities in these patients, which may be important components of the first impression made by these patients.

Changes in skin color may be striking. Pallor is usually present and results from anemia. A sallow, yellowish cast to the skin is caused by urochrome deposition in the skin.[3] Diffuse hyperpigmentation in sun-exposed areas has been attributed to an increase in β-melanocyte-stimulating hormone (β-MSH), which leads to increased deposition of melanin in the basal layer and superficial dermis.[4] Extensive ecchymoses are a sequela of platelet and other hemostatic abnormalities. Dry skin and poor skin turgor are related to the dehydration that accompanies chronic renal failure.

Calcinosis cutis seen in the setting of chronic renal failure occurs with secondary hyperparathyroidism.[5] Hard papules, nodules, or plaques, which typically occur around large joints, may produce a chalky discharge. Calcium deposits in blood vessels may result in cutaneous ulceration. Calciphylaxis is a rare, life-threatening complication of chronic renal failure manifest by rapidly progressive calcification of small and medium-sized blood vessels. Lesions are typically described as a violaceous pattern of livedo reticularis found primarily on the trunk and extremities, which results in extensive cutaneous necrosis. Benefits from parathyroidectomy in this condition are controversial.[6,7] Primary oxalosis, a rare disorder resulting in renal failure, has been associated with livedo reticularis in which oxalate crystals may be found on biopsy.[8]

"Half-and-half" nails have been described in patients with chronic renal failure; they consist of a proximal white half of the nail due to edema of the nail bed and a distinct normal distal portion (Fig. 165-1). Uremic frost is a classic manifestation of chronic renal failure consisting of white deposits on the skin of the face and neck in patients dying of uremia, but it is rarely found today.

TABLE 165-1

Some Examples of Diseases with Prominent Cutaneous and Renal Manifestations

Immunologic/rheumatologic diseases
  Poststreptococcal glomerulonephritis
  Systemic lupus erythematosus
  Scleroderma
  Necrotizing vasculitis
    Small-vessel necrotizing venulitis
    Larger vessels
      Polyarteritis nodosa
      Wegener's granulomatosis
Hematologic/oncologic diseases
  Thrombotic thrombocytopenic purpura
  Dysproteinemia
  Leukemia/lymphoma
  Solid tumors
Genetic/metabolic diseases
  Diabetes mellitus
  Gout
  Tuberous sclerosis
  Neurofibromatosis
  Nail-patella syndrome
  Angiokeratoma corporis diffusum universale (Fabry's disease)
Other diseases
  Familial Mediterranean fever
  Amyloidosis
  Sarcoidosis

FIGURE 165-1

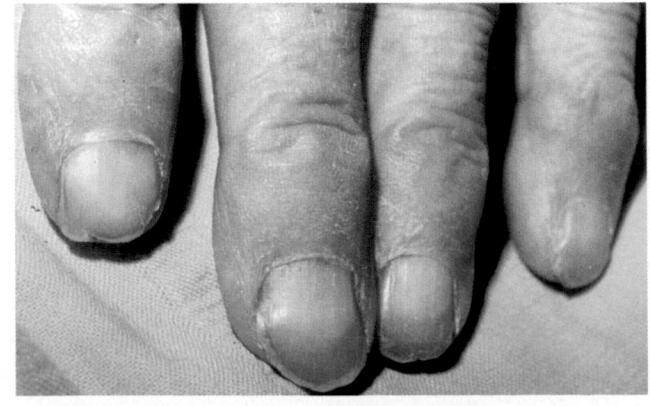

Half-and-half nails in a patient with chronic renal failure.

CUTANEOUS CHANGES PARTICULARLY PREVALENT IN PATIENTS ON DIALYSIS

Pruritus

Generalized pruritus without a primary cutaneous eruption can be a sign of underlying systemic disease in as many as 50 percent of patients who present with this cutaneous sign. Chronic renal failure is probably the most important known cause of generalized pruritus. The prevalence of itch in patients on long-term hemodialysis has been shown to be as high as 86 percent,[9] and pruritus is experienced by 60 to 80 percent of patients with end-stage renal disease.[10] Several etiologies for pruritus in patients with renal disease have been suggested, but the pathogenesis remains unclear. Pruritus is not a feature of acute renal failure.

Xerosis is a common finding in patients with chronic renal failure. Several studies have linked xerosis to atrophy of sebaceous and eccrine glands. A positive correlation between the degree of xerosis and the severity of pruritus has been reported, but other studies have shown no difference in the hydration of the stratum corneum or the transepidermal water loss between patients on chronic dialysis and controls.[11–13] However, simple emollient therapy has been shown to improve symptoms of pruritus in patients on chronic dialysis, perhaps through rehydration of the stratum corneum.[14]

Hyperparathyroidism is a commonly proposed etiology of pruritus, and some patients have had relief of symptoms following parathyroidectomy. Histamine release from mast cells is less likely to be the promotor of itching response in end-stage renal disease[15] but may activate other inflammatory mediators that lead to pruritus.[16] Studies are conflicting as to whether there are higher plasma levels of histamine in patients with end-stage renal disease as opposed to healthy controls.[17,18] Erythropoietin lowers plasma histamine concentrations during therapy and has been shown to be beneficial in some patients suffering from pruritus,[19] but antihistamines are usually not effective in treatment of pruritus in this patient population.

Hyperphosphatemia is associated with uremic pruritus, and a lowering of serum phosphorus levels is often associated with control of pruritus. The mechanism by which ultraviolet B ameliorates uremic pruritus may involve a decrease in skin phosphorus content, possibly via an effect of vitamin D.[20] It is also possible that ultraviolet B has direct effects on mast cells or other inflammatory cells. Levels of vitamin A may be increased in the epidermis of patients with uremia. The epidermal retinol content may be reduced after ultraviolet B therapy.[21] Previous studies have suggested that precipitation of calcium or magnesium phosphate salts may lead to pruritus.[22] Immunohistochemical studies have shown neuron-specific enolase immunoreactive nerve fibers sprouting through the epidermis in dialysis patients but not in control subjects, raising the question of whether abnormal patterns of cutaneous innervation may occur in dialysis patients and account for their pruritus.[23] However, other studies have shown no difference in the pattern of positive nerve fibers but found a reduction of skin nerve terminals in uremic patients as compared with control subjects.[24] In summary, despite ongoing investigation, the cause of uremic pruritus remains undefined. A multifactorial etiology is likely.

Treatment of uremic pruritus can be difficult. Ultraviolet B therapy has become a mainstay of therapy. Treatment of half of the body produces generalized improvement, implying a systemic effect.[25] Various other described systemic therapies including oral activated charcoal, cholestyramine, mexiletine, naloxone, and intravenous lidocaine may be ineffective or have undesirable side effects.[26] Adjunct therapies consisting of emollients and topical anesthetics such as pramoxine may be helpful. Topical capsaicin has recently been explored as a treatment modality.[27]

BULLOUS DISEASE

A bullous dermatosis resembling porphyria cutanea tarda has been well described in patients undergoing chronic hemodialysis and is sometimes termed *pseudoporphyria*. Clinical presentation of this eruption is similar to porphyria cutanea tarda, with skin fragility and bullae on sun-exposed skin that heal with scarring and milia formation (Fig. 165-2). Histologically the bullae are indistinguishable from lesions of porphyria cutanea tarda.[28] Drug-induced bullous dermatoses can occur in patients taking furosemide, tetracycline, or nalidixic acid, and these patients may also have renal failure.[29] The absence of urine output has complicated the evaluation of patients with chronic renal failure for true porphyria, which, not surprisingly, can also occur in this setting.[30] Elevated plasma porphyrin levels are sometimes found in patients with end-stage renal disease due to lack of urinary excretion of porphyrins, which can make the diagnosis of porphyria cutanea tarda difficult.[31,32] Normally utilized treatments of porphyria cutanea tarda, such as phlebotomy or chloroquine therapy, are not usually advisable or effective in patients with chronic renal failure. Erythropoietin has been shown to be an effective treatment for porphyria cutanea tarda in this patient population, either alone or in combination with phlebotomy.[33–35]

FIGURE 165-2

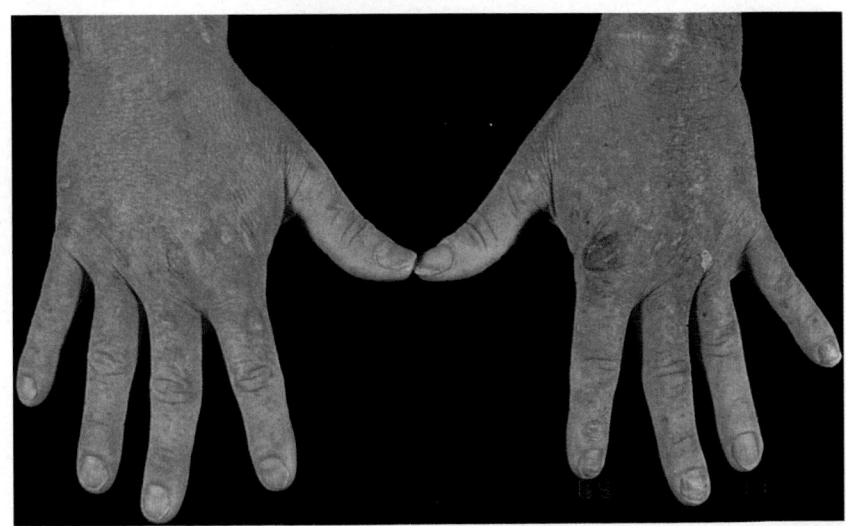

Bullous dermatosis in a patient undergoing chronic hemodialysis.

PERFORATING DISEASE

Anywhere from 4 to 10 percent of patients with chronic renal failure develop various perforating disorders such as Kyrle's disease, perforating folliculitis, or reactive perforating collagenosis[36] (see Chap. 57). Clinical and histopathologic similarities among these cases of perforating disease associated with uremia are striking, and an argument has been made to unify them as acquired perforating disease of chronic renal failure.[37] Diabetes mellitus is a frequent finding in these patients. The pathogenesis of these disorders has been theorized to be dermal microdeposition of substances such as uric acid or hydroxyapatite, followed by an inflammatory response which allows transepidermal elimination of degraded dermal deposits.[38] Local trauma such as scratching may also play a role.

Various therapies have been described for perforating disorders, including keratolytics, topical 5-fluorouracil, topical glucocorticoids, and topical retinoic acid. Aggressive control of uremic pruritus with ultraviolet B and control of the serum phosphorus level are also beneficial.

OTHER SKIN DISEASES

Contact dermatitis to dialysis tubing, nickel (needles), and topical medicaments may occur in patients on dialysis. Acroangiodermatitis, or pseudo-Kaposi's sarcoma, is a benign vascular proliferation that develops distal to an arteriovenous shunt (Fig. 165-3) and may resolve following thrombus or surgical ligation of the shunt.[39] Increased carriage of *Staphylococcus aureus* has been found in pa-

FIGURE 165-3

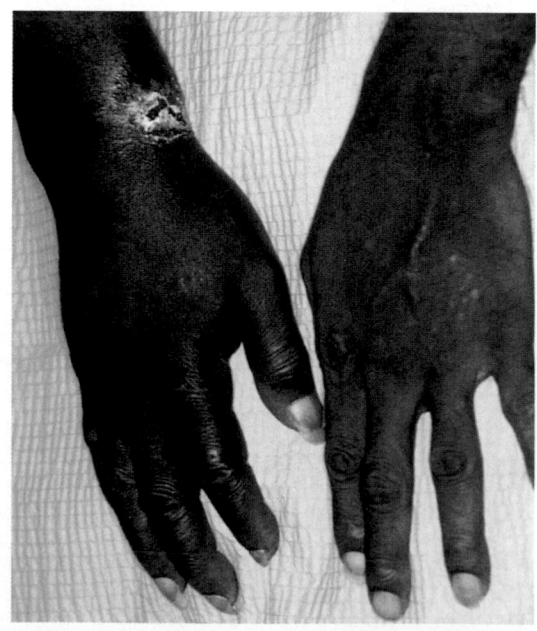

Acroangiodermatitis (pseudo-Kaposi's sarcoma) due to vascular proliferation distal to the site of an arteriovenous fistula.

tients undergoing peritoneal dialysis and hemodialysis and may predispose patients to folliculitis, furunculosis, or catheter-site infections.

CUTANEOUS CHANGES IN RENAL TRANSPLANT PATIENTS

Patients with renal and other transplants have many cutaneous problems, including reactions to medication, infections occurring in the setting of the iatrogenic immunosuppression required in these patients, and neoplasms occurring in the setting of immunosuppression. A review of the direct cutaneous sequelae of systemic glucocorticoids is beyond the scope of this chapter, as is a review of the sequelae of other types of therapy, but they are described elsewhere.[40]

Cutaneous infections are well described in renal transplant patients. Cutaneous mycoses including dermatophytes, tinea versicolor, and candidiasis are common and may be widespread.[41] Human papillomavirus infections are particularly problematic.[42] Molluscum contagiosum is not uncommon. Septic vasculitis or other cutaneous manifestations of disseminated infection with unusual bacteria, virus, acid-fast organisms, and fungi are unfortunately not rare in this patient population. Systemic infections with *Pneumocystis carinii*, *Candida*, *Aspergillus*, *Nocardia*, and cytomegalovirus may be associated with significant morbidity in these patients.

Squamous cell carcinomas, actinic keratoses, and keratoacanthomas may occur with increased frequency, which is a feature of chronic immunosuppression.[43] Human papillomavirus may play a role in the development of cutaneous malignancies in this population.[44] There is controversy over whether there is an increased incidence of basal cell carcinoma in this patient population. The incidence of Kaposi's sarcoma may be increased, and there appears to be an increased occurrence of non-Hodgkin's lymphoma in patients following renal transplant.[45] Acitretin, an oral retinoid given for periods ranging from 6 to 12 months, has been shown to prevent the development of squamous cell carcinomas and reduce the number of actinic keratoses when compared with placebo in a group of renal transplant patients.[46,47] The dermatologist should be involved in the pretransplantation evaluation of patients with kidney failure to treat warts and actinic keratoses, to educate patients about sun protection, and to establish cutaneous surveillance as part of the follow-up.

REFERENCES

1. Zawada GT, Ramirez G: The skin in IgA nephropathies. *Cutis* **36**:341, 1985
2. Hené RJ et al: The relevance of IgA deposits in vessel walls of clinically normal skin. *Arch Intern Med* **146**:745, 1986
3. Kopple JD, Massry SG: Uremic toxins: What are they? How are they identified? *Semin Nephrol* **3**:263, 1983
4. Pico MR et al: Cutaneous alterations in patients with chronic renal failure. *Int J Dermatol* **31**:860, 1992
5. Poesen N et al: Chronic renal failure and skin calcifications. *Dermatology* **190**:321, 1995
6. Hafner J et al: Uremic small-artery disease with medial calcification and intimal hyperplasia (so-called calciphylaxis): A complication of chronic renal failure and benefit from parathyroidectomy. *J Am Acad Dermatol* **33**:954, 1995
7. Ivker RA et al: Calciphylaxis in three patients with end stage renal disease. *Arch Dermatol* **131**:63, 1995
8. Winship IM et al: Primary oxalosis—an unusual case of livedo reticularis. *Clin Exp Dermatol* **16**:367, 1991

9. Young AW et al: Dermatologic evaluation of pruritus in patients on hemodialysis. *NY State J Med* **73**:2670, 1973

10. Ståhle-Bäckdahl M et al: Experimental and immunohistocompatibility studies in the role of parathyroid hormone in uraemic pruritus. *J Intern Med* **225**:411, 1989

11. Yosipovitch G et al: Skin surface pH, moisture, and pruritus in haemodialysis patients. *Nephrol Dial Transplant* **8**:1129, 1993

12. Osterle LS et al: Relationship between pruritus, transepidermal water loss, and biochemical markers of renal itch in haemodialysis patients. *Nephrol Dial Transplant* **9**:1302, 1994

13. Deleixhe-Mauhin F et al: Biometrological evaluation of the stratum corneum texture in patients under maintenance hemodialysis. *Nephron* **64**: 110, 1993

14. Morton CA et al: Pruritus and skin hydration during dialysis. *Nephrol Dial Transplant* **11**:2031, 1996

15. Mettang T et al: Uremic pruritus in patients on hemodialysis or continuous ambulatory peritoneal dialysis (CAPD): The role of plasma histamine and skin mast cells. *Clin Nephrol* **34**:136, 1990

16. Balaskas EV, Oreopoulos DG: Uremic pruritus. *Dial Transplant* **21**:192, 1992

17. Piazza V et al: Uraemic pruritus and plasma histamine concentrations. *Nephrol Dial Transplant* **8**:670, 1993

18. De Filippi C et al: Uraemic pruritus is not related to plasma histamine concentrations. *Clin Exp Dermatol* **20**:294, 1995

19. De Marchi S et al: Relief of pruritus and decreases in plasma histamine concentrations during erythropoietin therapy in patients with uremia. *N Engl J Med* **326**:969, 1992

20. Blackley JD et al: Uremic pruritus and skin ion content. *Am J Kidney Dis* **5**:236, 1985

21. Berne B et al: UV treatment of uraemic pruritus reduces the vitamin A content of the skin. *Eur J Clin Invest* **14**:203, 1984

22. Ponticelli C, Bencini PL: Uremic pruritus: A review. *Nephron* **60**:1, 1992

23. Ståhle-Bäckdahl M: Uremic pruritus: Clinical and experimental studies. *Acta Derm Venerol (Stockh)* **145**(suppl):1, 1989

24. Fantini F et al: Cutaneous innervation in chronic renal failure patients. *Acta Derma Venerol (Stockh)* **72**:102, 1992

25. Gilchrest BA et al: Ultraviolet phototherapy of uremic pruritus: Long-term results and possible mechanism of action. *Ann Intern Med* **91**:17, 1979

26. Balaskas EV, Oreopoulos DG: Uremic pruritus. *Dial Transpl* **21**:282, 1992

27. Breneman DL et al: Topical capsaicin for treatment of hemodialysis-related pruritus. *J Am Acad Dermatol* **26**:91, 1992

28. Gilchrest BA et al: Bullous dermatosis of hemodialysis. *Ann Intern Med* **83**:480, 1975

29. Harvey E et al: Pseudoporphyria cutanea tarda: Two case reports on children receiving peritoneal dialysis and erythropoietin therapy. *J Pediatr* **121**:749, 1992

30. Poh-Fitzpatrick MB et al: Porphyria cutanea tarda associated with chronic renal disease and hemodialysis. *Arch Dermatol* **116**:191, 1980

31. Gafter U et al: Bullous dermatosis of end stage renal disease: A possible association between abnormal porphyrin metabolism and aluminum. *Nephrol Dial Transplant* **11**:1787, 1996

32. Gebril M et al: Plasma porphyrins in chronic renal failure. *Nephron* **55**:159, 1990

33. Sarkell B, Patterson JW: Treatment of porphyria cutanea tarda of end-stage renal disease with erythropoietin. *J Am Acad Dermatol* **29**:499, 1993

34. Yaqoob M et al: Haemodialysis-related porphyria cutanea tarda and treatment by recombinant erythropoietin. *Nephron* **60**:428, 1992

35. Anderson KE et al: Erythropoietin for the treatment of porphyria cutanea tarda in a patient on long term hemodialysis. *N Engl J Med* **322**:315, 1990

36. Eral A, Gurer MA: Acquired reactive perforating disorder associated with chronic renal failure. *Int J Dermatol* **33**:42, 1994

37. Patterson JW: The perforating disorders. *J Am Acad Dermatol* **10**:561, 1984

38. Haftek M et al: Acquired perforating dermatosis of diabetes mellitus and renal failure: Further ultrastructural clues to its pathogenesis. *J Cutan Pathol* **20**:350, 1993

39. Rashkovsky I et al: Acro-angiodermatitis: Review of the literature and report of a case. *Acta Derm Venereal (Stockh)* **75**:475, 1995

40. Abel EA: Cutaneous manifestation of immunosuppression in organ transplant recipients. *J Am Acad Dermatol* **21**:167, 1989

41. Lugo-Janer G et al: Prevalence and clinical spectrum of skin diseases in kidney transplant recipients. *J Am Acad Dermatol* **24**:410, 1991

42. Dyall-Smith D et al: Benign human papillomavirus infection in renal transplant recipients. *Int J Dermatol* **30**:785, 1991

43. Blohmé I, Larkö O: Skin lesions in renal transplant patients after 10–23 years of immunosuppressive therapy. *Acta Derm Venereol (Stockh)* **70**:491, 1990

44. Euvrard S et al: Association of skin malignancies with various and multiple carcinogenic and noncarcinogenic HPV in renal transplant recipients. *Cancer* **72**:2198, 1993

45. Opelz G: Are post-transplant lymphomas inevitable? *Nephrol Dial Transplant* **11**:1952, 1996

46. Bavinck JN et al: Prevention of skin cancer and reduction of keratotic skin lesions during acitretin therapy in renal transplant recipients: A double-blind, placebo-controlled study. *J Clin Oncol* **13**:1933, 1995

47. Yuan Z et al: Use of acitretin for the skin complications in renal transplant recipients. *NZ Med J* **108**:255, 1995

CHAPTER 166

Andrew G. Franks, Jr.

Cutaneous Aspects of Cardiopulmonary Disease

Descriptions of abnormalities of the skin in association with diseases of the heart and lungs are among those first recorded in medical antiquity. While many are familiar and easily recognizable by the physician, others are unique and may remain a diagnostic challenge (Table 166-1). The primary objective of this chapter is to present the cutaneous manifestations of selected cardiopulmonary diseases; however, in addition, interesting associations between the skin, heart, and lung are also included.

A number of situations in which the skin and the cardiopulmonary system are both involved are described elsewhere in this volume. These conditions include pruritus associated with cardiac failure or pulmonary insufficiency, pigmentary changes associated with hemochromatosis or endocrine abnormalities (see Chaps. 164, 169, and 170), the hyperlipidemias (see Chap. 152), mucocutaneous lymph node syndrome (see Chap. 205), lipoid proteinosis (see Chap. 154), and amyloidosis (see Chap. 150).

TABLE 166-1

Diseases with Heart and Skin Involvement

Joint and connective tissue diseases	Nevoid or genetic disorders
Rheumatoid arthritis	Progressive lentigines
Systemic lupus erythematosus	(Moynahan syndrome)
Reiter's syndrome	Watson syndrome
Behçet's syndrome	Neurofibromatosis
Systemic scleroderma	Tuberous sclerosis
Dermatomyositis	LEOPARD syndrome
Rheumatic fever	LAMB syndrome
Ehlers-Danlos syndrome	NAME syndrome
Cutis laxa	Danoff syndrome
Marfan's syndrome	Infectious diseases
Periarteritis nodosa	Varicella
Multicentric	Gonococcemia
reticulohistiocytosis	Subacute and acute bacterial
Metabolic diseases	endocarditis
Hemochromatosis	Chagas' disease
Amyloidosis	Diphtheria
Fabry's disease	Miscellaneous (protozoal,
Carcinoid tumors	viral, rickettsial, and
Myxedema	bacterial infections)
Hyperlipidemias	Diseases of uncertain etiology
Hyperthyroidism	Sarcoidosis
	Whipple's disease
	Kawasaki disease
	Degos' disease

NOTE: See Table 166-4 for definitions of LEOPARD, LAMB, and NAME syndromes.
SOURCE: Modified and reprinted with permission from *Dermatologic Capsule & Comment,* edited by TB Fitzpatrick. September 1987, p 9.

ALTERATIONS IN SKIN QUALITY

The skin may be warm in patients with erythroderma or exfoliative dermatitis due to shunting or increased metabolism with or without high-output congestive failure. Hyperthyroidism with increased cardiac output and vasodilation may lead to increased skin temperature. Conversely, the temperature may be reduced in patients with hypothyroidism and low-output congestive failure secondary to atherosclerotic disease or myocardial infarction.

Systemic amyloidosis may cause waxy induration of the skin, and when stroked it may become hemorrhagic ("pinch purpura"). Cardiac conduction disturbances, myocardial disease, and orthostatic hypotension are common.

Hyperelastic velvety skin that rebounds to the original position after being stretched, "cigarette-paper" scars, and hyperextensible joints are characteristic of the Ehlers-Danlos syndrome (see Chap. 156). Mitral and tricuspid prolapse, dilatation of the aorta and pulmonary artery, arterial rupture, a variety of congenital heart diseases, and panacinar emphysema may accompany this syndrome.[1]

A progressive looseness of the skin with pendulous folds and droopy eyelids can be a clue to cutis laxa (see Chap. 156). This condition may be associated with generalized hyperelastosis that may cause aortic dilatation and rupture, congestive heart failure, or

FIGURE 166-1

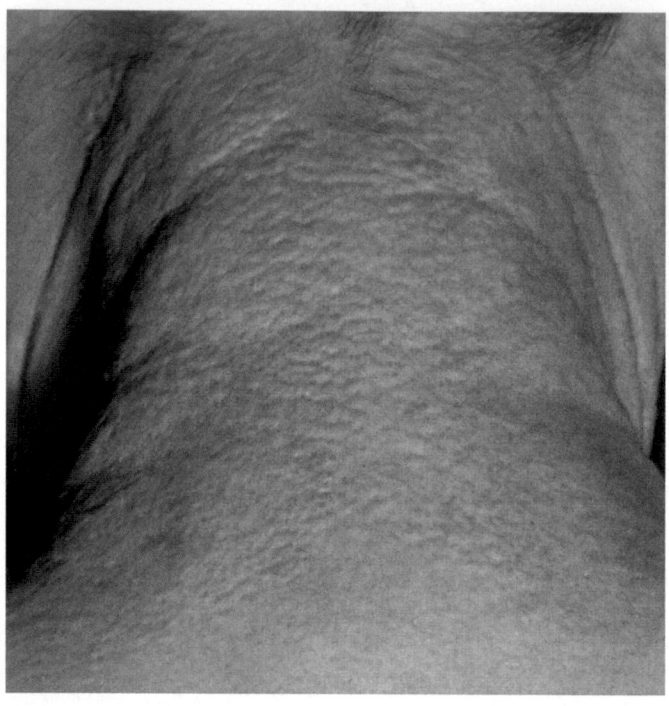

Pseudoxanthoma elasticum. Thickened, pebbly, yellowish lesions on the neck.

pulmonale with pulmonary artery stenosis and progressive emphysema.

The skin of patients with pseudoxanthoma elasticum (see Chap. 156) is thick, lax, and yellowish, especially over the axillae, antecubital area, and neck (Fig. 166-1). The skin around the mouth may sag. Yellow patches may occur on mucous membranes, especially the labia. The arteries may be calcified, and the aortic and mitral valves thickened. Angina pectoris and claudication are frequent symptoms.[2]

In Werner's syndrome (progeria), the skin appears atrophic and tight: there is marked loss of subcutis, with ulcerations of the legs and severe coronary atherosclerosis; death by myocardial infarction is frequent at an early age.

CHANGES IN SKIN COLOR

Changes in skin color are due to a number of variables including hemoglobin, melanin, carotene, vasoactivity, metals, and miscellaneous other phenomena.

Cyanosis

An increase in the absolute amount of desaturated (reduced) hemoglobin results in a purplish or bluish discoloration of the skin. By definition, cyanosis is divided into "central" and "peripheral" types, the latter being the more common. Conceptually, the terms refer to the level of arterial oxygen saturation and not to the ana-

tomic source of the cyanosis. Thus central cyanosis occurs in states that produce low arterial oxygen saturation, such as congenital heart disease with intracardiac or intrapulmonary right-to-left shunting, as well as most severe pulmonary diseases. Peripheral cyanosis occurs in states that have normal arterial oxygen saturation but reduced blood flow, such as low-output cardiac failure of any etiology, and local vasospastic phenomena. Pulmonary embolism may result in a combination of central cyanosis due to intrapulmonary shunting and peripheral cyanosis due to low cardiac output.

Central cyanosis is usually present on the warm areas of the skin such as the tongue, oral mucosae, and conjunctivae. Peripheral cyanosis is usually seen on the cool areas such as the nose, lips, earlobes, and fingertips. However, this distinction is not absolute since both central and peripheral cyanosis may affect any of the aforementioned areas of the body. Detection of cyanosis may be difficult, even to the experienced observer. Although the tongue is probably the area where it is most easily detected, a number of false-positive evaluations may occur. Therefore examination of the fingertips and conjunctivae, while less sensitive, may reflect the underlying condition more clearly. In the anemic patient, detection of cyanosis may be impossible since the absolute amount of reduced hemoglobin is not increased. To avoid confusion with staining of the skin, either topically or from systemic deposits of heavy metals or other chemicals, it is important to note that cyanosis fades when pressure is applied since the color is within the blood vessels.

Cyanosis that is more intense in the fingers than in the toes suggests complete transposition of the great vessels, with either a preductal coarctation or complete interruption of the aortic arch, pulmonary hypertension, and a reversed shunt through a patent ductus arteriosus. If the cyanosis is slightly more on the right hand, coarctation of the aorta is more likely. Equal cyanosis of both hands suggests complete aortic interruption.

Cyanosis and clubbing of the toes associated with cyanosis in the left hand and a normal right hand suggest pulmonary hypertension with a reversed shunt through a patent ductus arteriosus bringing saturated blood to the left arm and both legs.

Redness/Flushing

Redness of the skin may be due to an increase in the amount of saturated hemoglobin, an increase in the diameter or actual number of skin capillaries, or a combination of these factors.

Erythroderma or exfoliative dermatitis with intense redness may be associated with so much capillary dilatation that high-output cardiac failure occurs, especially in compromised patients (see Chap. 45).

Polycythemia may produce the characteristic "ruddy" complexion, but may also cause a peculiar coloration termed *erythremia*, which is a combination of redness and cyanosis. The tongue, lips, nose, earlobes, conjunctivae, and fingertips especially demonstrate this coloration. Erythremia results when increased amounts of saturated hemoglobin produce the redness and when increased amounts of desaturated hemoglobin produce cyanosis because of the inability of the body to oxygenate fully the increased absolute amounts of hemoglobin. The absence of nail clubbing may help differentiate patients with polycythemia vera from those patients with cardiopulmonary disease who develop secondary polycythemia. In addition, the hypervolemic state of polycythemia vera is associated with increased stroke volume and may lead to high-output cardiac failure, while pulmonary infarction may result from venous thrombosis and embolization caused by hyperviscosity.

Paroxysmal intense flushing of the face, neck, chest, and abdomen, often with telangiectases of the face and neck, may occur in patients with carcinoid tumors that have metastasized to the liver and thereby produce increased amounts of serotonin (see Chap. 171). Serotonin and histamine are responsible for the bronchospasm seen in this syndrome. Fibrosis of the right side of the heart may lead to a combination of stenosis and regurgitation at the tricuspid valve and pulmonary stenosis. If cyanosis occurs, the combination of flushing and cyanosis may produce the reddish, cyanotic erythremia seen in some patients with polycythemia. Occasionally patients in whom this syndrome develops have a patent ductus arteriosus or foramen ovale, and metastases occur in the lung. In this setting, left-sided cardiac lesions may also occur.

Systemic mastocytosis may produce flushing as a result of vasodilatation and may be associated with telangiectasia (see Chap. 162). Histamine release from degranulated mast cells is the pathogenetic mechanism. Cardiopulmonary alterations include hypotension and bronchospasm.

Pheochromocytomas may cause flushing of the face and forehead as well as redness and cyanosis of the hands (see Chap. 171). Generalized, extreme flushing, mimicking carcinoid, may occur in Sipple's syndrome, in which levels of prostaglandin, serotonin, and catecholamine are increased.

Edema of the face, arms, and hands associated with redness and/or cyanosis may indicate obstruction of the superior vena cava due to mediastinal disease.

ERYTHROMELALGIA (LABILE HYPERTHERMIA) Atherosclerosis, hypertension, and polycythemia may produce this peculiar pattern of erythema on the hands and feet, or it may be idiopathic. During the episodes, and especially when exposed to heat, patients complain of pain, warmth, and swelling of the areas, which sometimes extend to the elbows and knees. The pulse is either normal or slightly increased in intensity.[3]

PALMAR ERYTHEMA Palmar erythema may occur in many healthy women, but recent onset or increased intensity of this condition raise the possibility of liver involvement (see Chap. 164). Palmar erythema may be associated with high-output cardiac failure. The erythema primarily involves the hypothenar eminence but may also affect the thenar eminence and the fingertips. Other factors, including pregnancy and hyperthyroidism, may cause this condition.

Jaundice (See also Chap. 164)

Hyperbilirubinemia and jaundice may occur in patients in heart failure as a result of raised intrahepatic pressure due to passive congestion. Hemorrhagic pulmonary infarction with destruction of red cells and hemoglobin may also produce jaundice, especially in patients with passive congestion of the liver. Constrictive pericarditis and tricuspid valvular disease may produce jaundice secondary to cardiac cirrhosis. Under fluorescent light, jaundice may be difficult to assess.

ALTERATIONS IN SWEATING

Sweating may be prominent in a number of cardiopulmonary states such as acute myocardial infarction, cardiogenic shock, left ventricular failure, massive pulmonary emboli, and pulmonary edema. Pallor and clamminess or coldness of the extremities and exposed surfaces are also often found. When associated with hypertension, excessive sweating may suggest pheochromocytoma. There may also be additional features such as flushing, most prominent in those

patients with Sipple's syndrome in whom prostaglandin and serotonin production by the tumor may simulate carcinoid. Myocardial infarction may occur or cardiac failure may develop due to a metabolic cardiomyopathy. Neurofibromatosis and café au lait macules have been found in as many as 10 percent of patients, especially those with bilateral pheochromocytoma.

The sodium and chloride content of sweat is increased in patients with cystic fibrosis and may lead to an increase in skin wrinkling after immersion, as when bathing.[4]

ALTERATIONS OF NAILS, HANDS, AND ARMS

Nail Clubbing

Nail clubbing and osteoarthropathy are distinct entities that may be associated with significant cardiopulmonary abnormalities (Fig. 166-2).

Clinically, nail clubbing has various manifestations. Beaking or distal curvature of the nail may occur. There may be loss of the normal 15° angle between the nail and cuticle (unguophalangeal angle). Sponginess or "floating" of the nail when pressure is applied is also characteristic. Finally, the size of the terminal tuft may increase. This change may be quantified by measuring the depth of the finger at the base of the nail and dividing by the depth of the finger at the distal interphalangeal (DIP) joints. The ratio should normally be less than 1.0.

Clubbing most commonly occurs in patients with bronchogenic carcinoma, suppurative lung disease, endocarditis, and congenital heart disease, but it may be idiopathic or familial.

Quincke Pulse

Flushing of the nail beds synchronous with the heartbeat is one sign of aortic regurgitation called *Quincke pulsation*.

In addition, the fingernail beds may be used to evaluate the microcirculation. Capillary "fill" is estimated by pressing down on the

FIGURE 166-2

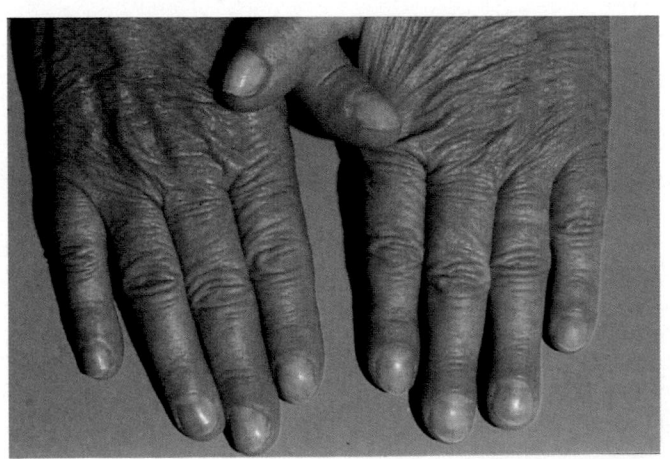

Clubbing of fingernails.

nail bed until blanching occurs. Following release, there should be immediate filling and a pink appearance. However, perfusion of the skin may not reflect perfusion of internal organs.

Hypertrophic Osteoarthropathy

Hypertrophic osteoarthropathy often has clubbing as a feature, but in addition there is an associated arthralgia and/or arthritis of the fingers, wrists, knees, and ankles, as well as painful periostitis revealed as subperiosteal new bone formation on x-ray. Suffusion of the digits may be prominent, with pitting edema. Shiny skin with increased sweating and paronychial thickening are sometimes noted.

Although hypertrophic osteoarthropathy is most often associated with malignant tumors of the chest, there are numerous other disorders that produce this syndrome. In addition, some cases are primary or idiopathic. Pachydermoperiostosis, a primary form, is frequently familial. Its onset is around puberty, and it has a number of cutaneous manifestations. Distinctive thickening and furrowing of the skin of the scalp, forehead, and cheeks may create a leonine facies. Other features include excessive sweating, especially of the hands and feet, severe seborrhea of the scalp and face, and dermatitis of the hands and feet. Familial clubbing alone may also be found and may represent a partial expression of this syndrome. Thyroid acropachy (Chap. 170) may mimic osteoarthropathy but is most often painless.

SHOULDER-HAND SYNDROME

The shoulder-hand syndrome is a painful periarthritis or adhesive capsulitis of the shoulder ("frozen shoulder"), usually on the left side, associated with erythema, sweating, shiny induration, edema, tenderness, pain, and immobility of the ipsilateral hand. Neurotrophic ulcerations of the fingers and thickening of the palmar aponeurosis with nodules and/or Dupuytren's contracture may be late sequelae. This syndrome was observed in up to 15 percent of patients with myocardial infarction in the past when bed rest was prolonged, but it is now uncommon. Other predisposing conditions include arterial embolization, cerebrovascular accidents, and protective disuse of the arms for any reason.[5]

THE HEART AND THE SKIN

Coronary Heart Disease

FAMILIAL HYPERLIPIDEMIA The risk of coronary artery disease (CAD) may increase with elevation of plasma cholesterol and triglyceride concentrations. Familial hyperlipidemias comprise a group of metabolic disorders with elevated plasma cholesterol and/or triglycerides, and some may be associated with a high incidence of CAD. Xanthomatosis may be present in patients with these disorders, and they have been associated for many years with a high incidence of CAD. As noted previously, the lipidoses are discussed in Chap. 152.

EARLOBE CREASE A number of reports relate CAD to the presence of a diagonally positioned skin crease along the earlobe. These creases may be unilateral or bilateral. It is not known whether such creases are congenital or acquired, nor is the mechanism of their formation understood.

Their association with other risk factors including hyperlipidemia has not been evaluated. However, their presence suggests an increased risk for CAD based on clinical, angiographic, and post-mortem studies.[6]

CHOLESTEROL EMBOLI (See Chap. 167) In patients with advanced atherosclerosis of the abdominal aorta, cholesterol crystals may microembolize to the lower extremities, particularly after invasive vascular procedures or surgery. The pulses may remain normal. In addition to complaints of pain in the legs, buttocks, and low back, as well as myalgia, restless legs, or abdominal symptoms, both renal insufficiency and various skin lesions frequently develop. Livedo reticularis may affect the lower abdomen and back, buttocks, and legs, and ulcerations on the legs and feet, surrounded by an erythematous or violaceous halo and a small scab, may be present. Cyanosis and digital gangrene may simulate necrotizing vasculitis.[7]

Indurated plaques and nodules and their association with livedo reticularis and ulceration may mimic polyarteritis nodosa. These plaques and nodules are firm, violaceous, painful, and necrotic in the center. Deep skin and muscle biopsy reveals occlusions of arterioles by multinucleated foreign-body giant cells and fibrosis surrounding biconvex, needle-shaped clefts corresponding to the cholesterol crystal microemboli.[8]

POST-BYPASS SKIN CHANGES Coronary artery bypass surgery is commonly performed using the superficial veins of the legs as donor-graft sites. A dermatitis has been reported to occur along the saphenous vein graft scars on the medial aspect of the legs.[9] Patients have no history of venous stasis, thrombophlebitis, ankle edema, or skin disease. Examination generally reveals a reddish-brown, slightly scaling, and fissured dermatitis along the distal part of a well-healed saphenous vein graft scar. Dermatitis develops 2 to 6 months after surgery and the patients' return to full activity. The cause is unclear but may be related to the high incidence of postoperative thrombophlebitis and resultant stasis dermatitis. The dermatitis responds to topical glucocorticoids. Recurrence is usual and most patients have required continued treatment.

Recurrent cellulitis may develop in the healed vein graft many months after surgery. These patients present with fever and chills; erythema may extend along the entire vein graft site, accompanied by pain and tenderness. Swelling may be significant, and often the patients are initially considered to have thrombophlebitis. Although cultures are not always positive, beta-hemolytic streptococcus was isolated in a number of cases.

The presence of an associated tinea pedis in patients with this complication has been reported and it has been recommended that all patients considered for vein graft surgery be examined carefully for evidence of tinea infections of the feet, which, if found, should be treated vigorously with antifungal medication prior to surgery.

Cardiomyopathy

Cutaneous abnormalities may aid in the diagnosis and subsequent treatment of some kinds of cardiomyopathy. These disorders of the myocardium affect ventricular function and may produce cardiac failure. A useful classification divides cardiomyopathies into dilated, nondilated, and hypertrophic types. It has recently been stressed that each type of cardiomyopathy has a distinct differential diagnosis and that little etiologic overlap occurs.[10,11]

Thus a specific cutaneous finding in conjunction with the appropriate studies to determine the type of cardiomyopathy may be very important in making the correct diagnosis. Either radionuclide ventriculography or two-dimensional echocardiography estimates ventricular volume and left ventricular ejection fraction. These measurements are utilized to distinguish among the three types of cardiomyopathy. Tables 166-2 and 166-3 list the causes of cardiomyopathy according to type.

Myxoma

Atrial myxomas, the most common primary tumors of the heart, are benign hamartomatous intracardiac tumors that may produce a wide variety of clinical symptoms and signs and may simulate a number of disease states.

The cardiopulmonary findings include in order of frequency: congestive heart failure, mitral murmur, chest pain, pulmonary edema, and embolic phenomena.

Additionally, valvular insufficiency, constrictive pericarditis, conduction blocks, arrhythmias, and intracardiac shunts may occur. Variable murmurs may be an important clue.

Pulmonary emboli and pulmonary hypertension may also occur in addition to other systemic findings, including fever, cachexia and malaise, arthralgias, arthritis, clubbing, hypergammaglobulinemia, anemia or polycythemia, thrombocytosis or thrombocytopenia, and leukocytosis.

The cutaneous manifestations of atrial myxomas may be dramatic. In addition to biphasic digital color changes on cold exposure, various cutaneous lesions have been described that simulate collagen vascular disease or vasculitis: tender, violaceous, nonblanching, annular, and serpiginous lesions of the digital pads, as well as splinter hemorrhages presenting as a systemic vasculitis or infective endocarditis. Characteristic pruritic, erythematous papules as well as cyanosis and ecchymosis of the extremities may also occur.

The diagnosis may be made by biopsy of the skin and subcutaneous tissue in an area of embolic infarct. Myxomatous emboli

TABLE 166-2

Causes of Cardiomyopathy by Type

Dilated	Neoplastic*
Coronary artery disease with multiple infarcts*	Melanoma*
Alcoholic*	Ventricular thrombosis
Peripartum	Polycythemia vera*
Valvular*	Mitral valve prosthesis
Infectious acute inflammatory myocarditis*	Idiopathic
Chagas' disease*	Hypertrophic
Sarcoid*	Genetic form (? autosomal dominant)
Doxorubicin toxicity	Acquired or secondary forms
Uremia*	Neurofibromatosis*
Hemochromatosis*	Lentiginosis*
Pheochromocytoma*	Hyperthyroidism*
Hypocalcemia	Hypothyroidism*
Diabetes mellitus*	Noonan's syndrome
Nutritional (? selenium)	Hypertension
Idiopathic	Valvular or subvalvular obstruction of
Nondilated	left ventricular outlet tract
Amyloid heart disease*	Pompe's disease
Endomyocardial diseases	Friedreich's ataxia
Löffler's disease*	In infants of diabetic mothers
Pseudoxanthoma elasticum*	
Endomyocardial fibrosis (Davies' disease)	

*May have significant cutaneous features.
SOURCE: Modified from Johnson and Palacios.[10]

TABLE 166-3

Infectious Causes of Acute Dilated Cardiomyopathy*

Coxsackie virus B	Cytomegalovirus
Coxsackie virus A	Mumps
Echo virus	Psittacosis
Poliovirus	*Cryptococcus neoformans*
Arbovirus (dengue, chikungunya fever)	*Candida albicans*
Toxoplasma gondii	*Trichinella spiralis*
Trypanosoma cruzi	*Schistosoma mansoni*
Mycoplasma pneumoniae	*Corynebacterium diphtheriae*
Varicella	*Neisseria meningitidis*
Variola	*Leptospira*
Influenza	Polymicrobial bacterial
Rabies	myocarditis

*Most have cutaneous features.
SOURCE: Modified from Johnson and Palacios.[10]

with large pale-staining cytoplasms and stellate nuclei may be found among occluded blood vessels.

Before the introduction of the echocardiogram in 1960, over 80 percent of patients were undiagnosed at postmortem. The diagnosis may now be made earlier and more frequently during routine echocardiography, allowing successful surgical intervention.[12]

Various associations of atrial myxoma with mucocutaneous pigmented lobules, including lentigines (Fig. 166-3), nevomelanocytic nevi and blue nevi, as well as dermal myxomatous nodules, have been described[13] (Table 166-4).

LEOPARD Syndrome

Multiple lentigines syndrome, an autosomal dominant disorder, has been associated with numerous abnormalities of variable clinical expression including disturbances of the heart. Each letter of the mnemonic represents a feature of the syndrome (see Table 166-4): *l*entigines, multiple; *e*lectrocardiogram conduction defects; *o*cular telorism; *p*ulmonary stenosis; *a*bnormalities of genitalia; *r*etardation of growth; *d*eafness, sensorineural (see Chap. 89).

The types of cardiac involvement include electrocardiogram conduction disturbances and anatomic malformation. Axis deviation, prolonged P-R intervals, left anterior hemiblock, bundle branch block, and complete heart block have been reported.

Hypertrophic cardiomyopathy appears to be the most common anatomic abnormality. Subaortic stenosis is the most common valvular lesion. Although earlier reports suggested that pulmonary stenosis was frequent, some of the clinical and physiologic features of hypertrophic cardiomyopathy mimic pulmonary stenosis and were clarified only after catheterization or echocardiography.

Because the clinical expression of the conduction disturbances and the anatomic malformation vary in onset and severity, frequent cardiac evaluation should be performed.

FIGURE 166-3

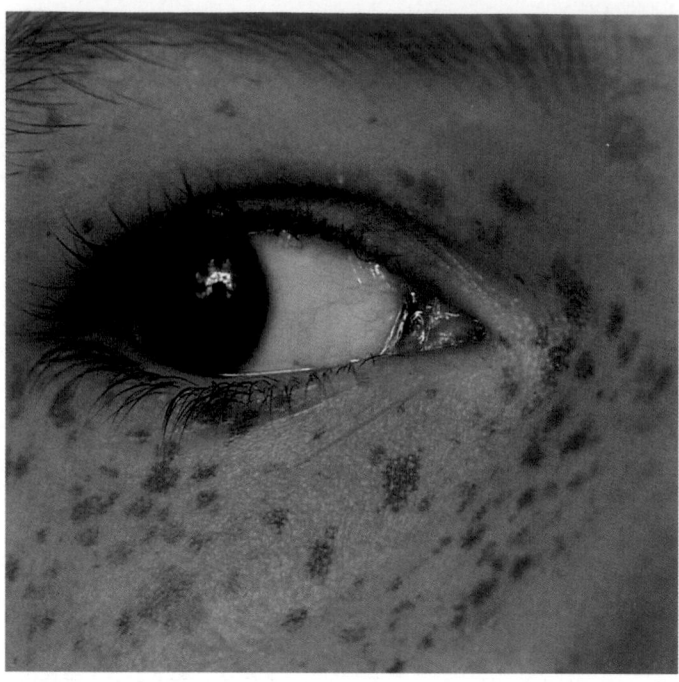

Lentiginous lesions in the atrial myxoma syndrome complex. This child has the LAMB syndrome (see Table 166-4).

Subacute Bacterial Endocarditis

The cutaneous manifestations of bacterial endocarditis are important clues to the diagnosis, although less frequently than in the preantibiotic era. They include Osler's nodes, Janeway lesions, subungual

TABLE 166-4

Clinical Findings Associated with Lentigines

LEOPARD syndrome*[†]	NAME syndrome[‡]
Lentiginosis	Nevi
Electrocardiographic	Atrial myxoma
abnormalities	Myxoid neurofibrotoma
Ocular hypertelorism	Ephelides
Pulmonic stenosis	Danoff syndrome[§]
Abnormal genitalia	Adrenocortical micronodular
Retardation	dysplasia
Deafness	Lentigines
LAMB syndrome[‡]	Atrial myxoma
Lentigines	Spindle cell tumors
Atrial myxoma	
Mucocutaneous myxomas	
Blue nevi	

*Skeletal deformities can occur frequently.
[†]Autosomal dominant inheritance.
[‡]Inheritance pattern not determined.
[§]Possible autosomal dominant inheritance.
SOURCE: Reprinted with permission from *Dermatologic Capsule & Comment,* Fitzpatrick TB (ed), September 1987, p 10.

splinter hemorrhages, cutaneous purpura and petechiae, and conjunctival petechiae (Roth's spots) (see also Chap. 195).

Petechiae are the most common mucocutaneous manifestation of bacterial endocarditis, their incidence varying from 20 to 40 percent of patients with both acute and subacute bacterial endocarditis. Small, red or violaceous macules that do not blanch subsequently become brownish and fade. Purpuric lesions, both flat and elevated, have also been associated with subacute endocarditis without evidence of platelet dysfunction and may represent a leukocytoclastic vasculitis. The petechiae may be observed on the skin, especially on the heels, shoulders, and legs, but the conjunctiva and oral mucosa must also be evaluated.

Osler's nodes and Janeway lesions may both present as erythematous or hemorrhagic macules, papules, or nodules (Fig. 166-4). However, while Osler's nodes are exquisitely painful, tender, and located distally on the digital tufts, Janeway lesions are nontender and located proximally on the palms and soles. Osler's original description in 1885 did not specify the tenderness of these lesions, but his later report did emphasize the findings noted above.

Histologically, Osler's nodes are a perivasculitis or necrotizing vasculitis without microabscess formation or other evidence of infection or emboli. Cultures have generally been negative, although more recent reports have reemphasized the possibility of septic microemboli with microabscess formation. Janeway lesions have also been described histologically as a vasculitis with microabscess formation. The cutaneous and conjunctival petechiae are histologically similar.[14]

Current theories regard the pathogenesis of both Osler's nodes and Janeway lesions as immunologic or allergic due to immune complex deposition. Some reports dispute this concept, suggesting that the initial event is a septic microembolism that subsequently causes the endothelial swelling and perivasculitis seen in older lesions. Thus organisms may be occasionally cultured initially, but later the lesions become sterile.[15]

That infected arterial catheters may precipitate clinical lesions comparable to Osler's nodes, Janeway lesions, and splinter hemorrhages supports the concept that these lesions are infectious in etiology. Osler's nodes and Janeway lesions have been found in patients with other conditions, particularly systemic lupus erythematosus (SLE), gonococcemia, hemolytic anemia, and typhoid fever.

FIGURE 166-4

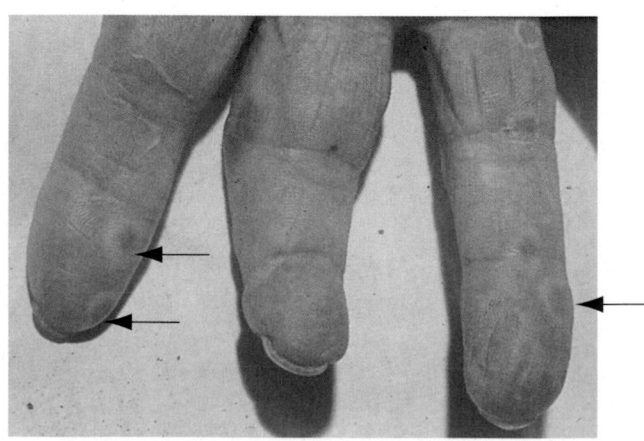

Osler nodes (*arrows*).

THE LUNGS AND THE SKIN

Yellow Nail Syndrome

Yellow nails with primary lymphedema were described in 1964. Separately, primary lymphedema and pleural effusion were reported. The triad of yellow nails, primary lymphedema, and pleural effusion was then recognized, followed by a number of reports with partial or complete features.

The characteristics of nails include thickening, transverse ridging, diminished growth, increased curvature with a "hump," and onycholysis. The lunulae and cuticles may be absent. The color may vary from pale yellow to green (Fig. 166-5). The nail changes are secondary to congenitally hypoplastic lymphatics.[16]

The lymphedema in this disorder is also due to congenitally hypoplastic lymphatics. It is characteristically slowly progressive and somewhat asymmetric, with induration and hyperkeratosis extending to the thighs. Periodic lymphangitis is frequent and may contribute to the swelling.

Respiratory findings include sinusitis, bronchiectasis, and pleural effusions. Symptoms vary from mild to severe, and some patients require repeated thoracentesis, treatment for pneumonia secondary to bronchiectasis, and drainage of the sinusitis. Patients may have a productive or nonproductive cough, dyspnea, frequent upper respiratory infections, and pneumonia. Chest x-rays may be normal but generally reveal evidence of fibrosis and/or effusion at the bases.[17]

Pulmonary features and lymphedema may not occur until late in the course; therefore follow-up of patients who present with this type of nail dystrophy is recommended. Finally, a number of patients have developed lymphomas or sarcomas with metastases.

Pulmonary Arteriovenous Fistulas

Pulmonary arteriovenous fistulas are congenital abnormalities of capillary development that may not become clinically apparent until late adolescence. Osler-Rendu-Weber disease (hereditary hemorrhagic telangiectasia), an autosomal dominant trait, may be present in one-third to one-half of such patients (see Chap. 102). It is characterized clinically by punctate, linear, or spider-like telangiectasias of the skin, especially the upper body, oral and nasal mucous membranes, and nail beds (Fig. 166-6). The radiating arms about an elevated punctum are the most characteristic feature, especially on the lips and tongue. They are distinguished from true spider telangiectasis in that they do not pulsate.

Recurrent epistaxis is the most frequent presenting symptom and may begin in early childhood or adolescence. Other organ systems besides the lungs may be involved, including the liver, gastrointestinal and genitourinary tracts, and central nervous system, and recurrent hemorrhage may result. Bleeding may be enhanced by an associated von Willebrand's disease.

The pulmonary findings in those patients with an arteriovenous fistula of the lungs include dyspnea, hemoptysis, cyanosis, clubbing, polycythemia, and pulmonary bruits accentuated by inspiration. Chest x-rays reveal nodular "coinlike" lesions, sometimes initially considered to be metastatic disease.

Chronic Pulmonary Diseases

Chronic obstructive pulmonary disease (COPD) is actually a group of disorders including chronic bronchitis, bronchiectasis, emphysema, and asthma. The incidence and mortality of COPD have in-

FIGURE 166-5

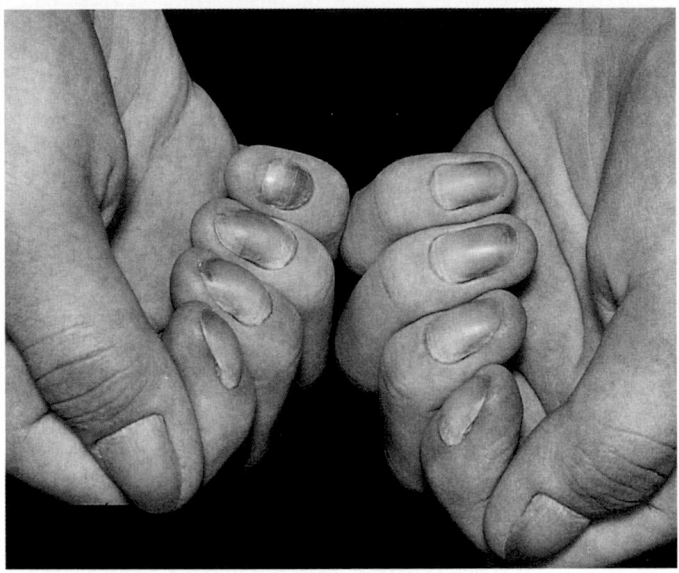

Yellow nail syndrome. There is thickening, increased curvature, and yellowish discoloration of all fingernails. This patient had lymphedema of the extremities and bronchiectasis with multiple recurrent respiratory infections.

FIGURE 166-6

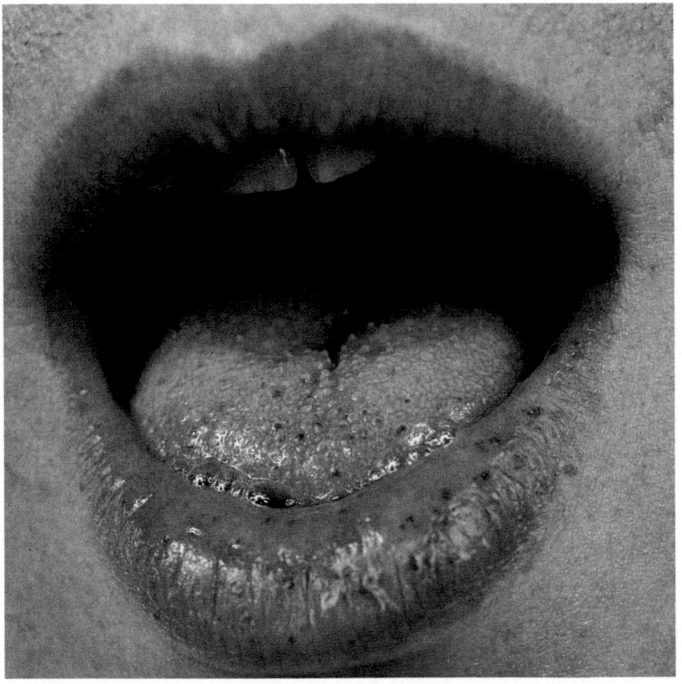

Osler-Rendu-Weber disease. Note the punctate and splinter-like telangiectasia on the lips.

creased recently and approach that of heart disease in the United States. Smoking habits as well as increased longevity of the population may be responsible, in part, for this increase. Genetic, infectious, occupational, and environmental factors also contribute.

Two basic types of COPD have been described: type A, or emphysematous, and type B, or bronchial. Clinically both may present with dyspnea, cough, wheezing, and recurrent respiratory infections. Type A patients have been termed "pink puffers" since they usually hyperventilate and maintain arterial oxygen tension. Type B patients have been termed "blue bloaters" since they frequently are hypoxic with cyanosis and associated right congestive heart failure. These patients, especially if young, should be evaluated for the possibility of cystic fibrosis.

Cystic Fibrosis

Cystic fibrosis is an autosomal recessive disorder of the exocrine glands that subsequently involves the tracheobronchial tree, pancreas, and gastrointestinal tract. The basic alteration of mucus is unknown, but viscid mucous plugs may cause fecal impaction, intussusception, and rectal prolapse in infancy. Pancreatic insufficiency may subsequently predominate, but it is the pulmonary disease that is the most significant feature. Progressive lung disease with chronic bronchitis, emphysema, and cor pulmonale from cystic fibrosis is a leading cause of death among patients with genetic disorders in the United States.

The cutaneous features of this disorder result from increased amounts of electrolyte in the sweat, which leads to excessive skin wrinkling when the palms and soles are immersed in water. Although this feature is not always present, it may be a valuable clue to the disease. Parents are often aware of, but not disturbed by, the wrinkling.[18]

Larva Migrans and Pulmonary Involvement (See also Chap. 237)

Cutaneous larva migrans, or creeping eruption, may occasionally cause minimal respiratory symptoms and be associated with transient pulmonary infiltrates and a peripheral eosinophilia (Löffler's syndrome).

Visceral larva migrans, or toxocariaris, may lead to granulomatous involvement of the liver, lungs, heart, muscle, brain, and eyes. Marked eosinophilia, hyperglobulinemia, pneumonitis with wheezing, recurrent bronchitis, fever, and tender hepatomegaly frequently occur. Skin lesions may present as patchy urticaria or erythematous papular eruptions.

Fat Embolism Syndrome

Petechiae, respiratory insufficiency, and cerebral dysfunction after long bone fracture are termed the *fat embolism syndrome*. Petechiae alone after fractures should suggest this syndrome. Histologically, fat globules are present within the dermal and pulmonary vessels. Additional factors such as hyperglycemia, diabetes, or elevated beta-lipoproteins may play a contributing role.

The petechiae are most commonly on the neck, axillae, shoulder, chest, and conjunctivae and often appear before other manifestations. They begin about the second or third day after injury, appear in crops, and are almost never found on the face or posterior aspects of the body. When widespread, they tend to herald more significant

cerebral and pulmonary dysfunction. In addition, cyanosis may be prominent.

The respiratory involvement may begin with dyspnea, tachypnea, or hemoptysis. Tachycardia, fever, and pulmonary edema may occur. X-rays may show patchy densities or linear streaks progressing to the bilateral opacities characteristic of the adult respiratory distress syndrome.

Cerebral dysfunction includes restlessness, irritability, delirium, and coma. Additional features include jaundice, renal involvement, anemia, thrombocytopenia, and elevated sedimentation rate.[19]

SELECTED DISEASES AFFECTING THE CARDIOPULMONARY SYSTEM

Lipoid Proteinosis (Hyalinosis Cutis et Mucosae)
(See also Chap. 154)

Oropharyngeal and laryngeal mucous membranes are usually affected early in the course of the disease, during infancy or childhood. The tongue enlarges and acquires a firm consistency and a smooth, glistening surface (Fig. 166-7A). Hoarseness due to laryngeal infiltration is often the initial finding and may be present at birth. Laryngeal and tracheal infiltration may progress to obstruction and cause respiratory insufficiency requiring tracheostomy. The trachea and main-stem bronchus may be thickened and studded with wartlike hyaline projections. An increased risk of aspiration pneumonia has been reported, as well as repeated upper respiratory infections. Cardiovascular involvement is rare, but conduction defects and arrhythmias have been reported. Skin changes include confluent, waxy papules, acne-like scarring and plaques, particularly on the face (Fig. 166-7B).

Multicentric Reticulohistiocytosis (See also Chap. 183)

Multicentric reticulohistiocytosis is an uncommon disorder presenting with characteristic mucocutaneous lesions and a deforming arthritis in association with systemic symptoms such as fever, malaise, weight loss, and myopathy. The cardiopulmonary complications include pulmonary infiltrates, pleural effusions, pericarditis, cardiomegaly, congestive heart failure, angina pectoris, myocardial infarction, and pulmonary infarction.[20]

An association of multicentric reticulohistiocytosis with malignancy has been recorded in a few reports, suggesting the need for complete evaluation of these patients.[21]

Sarcoidosis (See also Chap. 184)

Sarcoidosis is a multisystem granulomatous disease with unknown cause and widespread manifestations. Cardiac involvement consisting of myocardial or conduction system granulomata may be occult, but it may be clinically evident in about 20 percent of the patients. Ventricular arrhythmias and conduction disturbances are responsible for the palpitations, presyncope, and syncope reported. Congestive heart failure and chest pain occur less frequently and may be due to cardiomyopathy or cor pulmonale. Additionally, prolapsed mitral valves, papillary muscle dysfunction, and aneurysm formation may be found rarely. The prognosis for patients with cardiac involvement is unfavorable.[22]

Sarcoidosis affecting the pulmonary system may be suggested by lupus pernio, with involvement of the hilar nodes, bronchi, and/or alveoli resulting in obstructive and/or restrictive dysfunction.

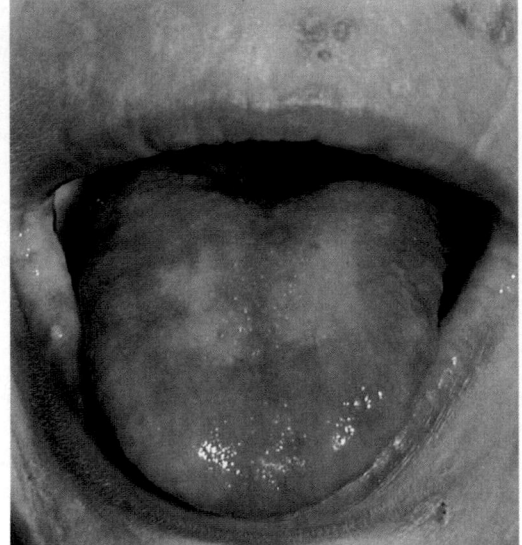

A.

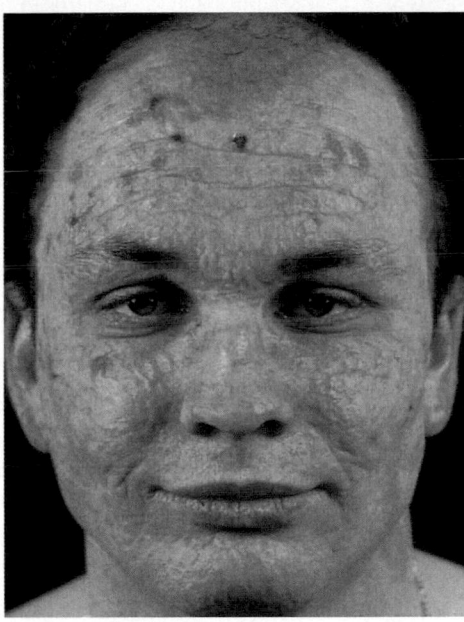

B.

Lipoid proteinosis. *A.* The tongue is hard and shows a smooth, waxy surface. Note also the pitted, acne-like scars on the lips. *B.* Multiple waxy papules and plaques and pitted, acne-like scarring in the face. Note also the alopecia in this 20-year-old man.

Respiratory failure is often the most difficult clinical problem, characterized by shortness of breath, dyspnea, and hypoxemia.[23]

The cutaneous features of sarcoidosis may not be clinically apparent at the time of cardiac involvement but occur in about 30 percent of patients. Lesions are found especially about the eyes, nose, nasolabial folds, and mouth (lupus pernio).[24]

While there are at least two forms of sarcoidosis, acute (transient) and chronic (persistent), no definite correlation between skin and internal involvement has been made. However, those patients who present abruptly with hilar adenopathy and nonspecific skin involvement, such as erythema nodosum (Löfgren's syndrome), ap-

pear to respond to glucocorticoid therapy and have fewer recurrences and a more favorable prognosis.

Amyloidosis (See also Chap. 150)

Involvement of the heart may be associated with all three systemic forms of amyloidosis but appears to be clinically predominant in the primary myeloma-associated types. Senile amyloidosis may also affect the heart but is often asymptomatic. Clinical findings include dizziness, palpitations, syncope, orthostatic hypotension, and congestive heart failure. Chest x-ray may reveal cardiomegaly. ECGs may show low-voltage, abnormal Q waves, conduction defects, and arrhythmias. Echocardiography may reveal a restrictive cardiomyopathy with enlargement of the left ventricular wall and obstruction of the outflow tract. Pathologically, infiltration of the endocardium, myocardium, pericardium, valves, and coronary vessels may occur.[25]

Upper and lower respiratory tract involvement also occurs in all systemic forms of amyloidosis but is clinically predominant in primary and myeloma-associated types. Macroglossia may impede respiration, especially when complicated by bleeding. The larynx and trachea may become infiltrated, causing hoarseness, cough, and respiratory stridor. Bronchial and lung parenchymal involvement may cause asthma-like symptoms, hemoptysis, and severe pulmonary disease. Chest x-rays may reveal interstitial type involvement and occasionally amyloid nodules may mimic a malignant tumor. Pulmonary function studies may reveal obstructive or restrictive dysfunction depending on the location of the amyloid deposition.[26]

Cutaneous involvement occurs most often in the primary and myeloma-associated types and therefore serves as a marker for cardiopulmonary involvement. A skin biopsy of clinically normal skin in a patient suspected of having amyloidosis may thus demonstrate deposition within the vessels in as many as 50 percent of patients.

Lymphomatoid Granulomatosis (See also Chap. 109)

This infiltrative systemic disease affects the skin, lungs, central nervous system, kidneys, and other organs in a characteristic histologic pattern. Pulmonary involvement may begin with transient alveolar or interstitial infiltrates and effusions on chest x-ray, which subsequently may progress to nodular, masslike densities. These lesions may cavitate and be responsible for profuse hemoptysis. Although many patients remain asymptomatic, cough, dyspnea, and chest pain may occur. Cardiac involvement is uncommon but, when present, may involve the coronary vessels with subsequent myocardial ischemia.[27]

Skin lesions are found in up to half of all patients and are varied in appearance, often not suggestive of vasculitis. Erythematous papules, nodules, and plaques are found and sometimes ulcerate. These lesions usually reveal the characteristic histologic pattern of lymphoreticular cells surrounding and infiltrating blood vessels.[28]

COLLAGEN VASCULAR DISEASES

The cardiopulmonary complications of the various collagen vascular diseases may sometimes be associated with a specific cutaneous sign or constellation of features.

Rheumatoid Arthritis (See also Chap. 179)

Extraarticular manifestations of rheumatoid arthritis, especially in the pulmonary system, appear to correlate with subcutaneous nodules and vasculitic skin lesions. The nodules may become necrobiotic and ulcerate, causing pain, secondary infection, and poor healing. The vasculitic lesions include palpable purpura, splinter hemorrhages, digital pitting, ulceration, or gangrene, sometimes in association with Raynaud's phenomenon, and pyoderma gangrenosum.[29]

In addition, laboratory evidence of high-titer rheumatoid factor, hypocomplementemia, cryoimmunoglobulinemia, and hypereosinophilia may be associated with the extraarticular manifestations including cardiopulmonary disease. These manifestations occur more commonly in men with long-standing disease but may not necessarily correlate with arthritis activity at the time. The pulmonary disease consists of pleural effusions, localized or diffuse parenchymal infiltrates, or, rarely, lung nodules. Complaints include dypsnea, cough, pleuritic chest pain, and hemoptysis. Cardiac involvement may not be clinically apparent, although autopsy studies have revealed a high incidence of cardiac lesions related to granuloma or vasculitis.[30]

Systemic Lupus Erythematosus (See also Chap. 172)

Cutaneous manifestations of SLE appear in over 75 percent of patients during the course of their disease. While the extent of the cutaneous features in SLE may not correlate with the severity of visceral disease, the trend toward serologic and clinical subsets has suggested certain associations.

PLEUROPULMONARY DISEASE IN SLE Pleuritis may be present during the course of the disease in about half of patients with SLE. Chest pain may become subacute or chronic because of adhesions and may be confused with costochondritis. Pleural effusions with or without a friction rub may also occur. Parenchymal lung involvement in SLE is usually due to secondary factors such as infections or pulmonary emboli. Primary lung involvement in SLE may be classified as follows: (1) diffuse interstitial pneumonitis, (2) acute pneumonitis, (3) intrapulmonary hemorrhage, (4) diaphragm dysfunction with decreased lung volume (shrinking lung syndrome), (5) pulmonary hypertension with cor pulmonale, and (6) fibrosing alveolitis.[31]

Respiratory difficulty may also be due to acute epiglottitis, necrotic and ulcerative laryngitis, and tracheobronchitis.

CARDIAC DISEASE IN SLE Cardiac involvement in patients with SLE is frequently subclinical. Pericarditis may be more common in patients with drug-induced syndromes or those with photosensitive discoid lesions. Chest pain may be present, especially when associated with effusion. A friction rub may be heard. The ECG changes primarily are T-wave abnormalities.

Myocarditis is often undiagnosed and may be associated with prolonged P-R intervals, heart block, and arrhythmias. Since the introduction of glucocorticoid therapy, an increased incidence of atherosclerotic-related myocardial infarction has been reported.

Valvular heart disease in patients with SLE is most often of the Libman-Sacks type, is frequently associated with antiphospholipid antibodies, and is manifested by systolic murmurs, which may occur in almost one-half of all patients. These murmurs are rarely clinically significant.[32] Although diastolic murmurs may occur due to noninfectious mitral stenosis or aortic insufficiency, the onset of a new diastolic murmur should provoke a search for subacute bacterial endocarditis. The cutaneous clues of this disease, such as splinter hemorrhages, Osler's nodes, Janeway lesions, and Roth's spots, should be sought, although they may occur in SLE without infection. It appears that SLE, as well as other cutaneous vascular diseases, may be associated with complete heart block in newborn infants. In SLE this may be due to placental transfer of maternal antibodies, especially anti-Ro antibody.[33] The newborn infants of patients with SLE or of clinically normal but Ro-antibody-positive mothers may also have distinctive evanescent cutaneous eruptions, including prominent telangiectasia and periorbital erythema (neonatal lupus erythematosus).[34]

Systemic Sclerosis (See also Chap. 174)

Microvascular abnormalities are among the earliest pathologic changes seen in patients with systemic sclerosis, a finding supporting the concept of a primary vascular defect in the disease. Typically, the vascular lesions are characterized by intimal proliferation with loose connective tissue at the internal elastic membrane, medial thinning, and adventitial fibrosis.

Many of the cutaneous features of this disorder are directly attributable to vascular abnormalities and occur early in the disease. They include vasospastic episodes (Raynaud's), telangiectases, and nail fold capillary changes appearing as dilated and distorted capillary loops alternating with avascular areas on wide-field capillary microscopy.

PULMONARY ABNORMALITIES Dypsnea on exertion, occurring in about half the patients, is usually the most common symptom. Chronic, nonproductive cough and pleuritic chest pain may also occur. Examination may reveal dry rales, especially at the bases, as well as diminished breath sounds and pleural rubs. Chest x-ray may show a diffuse reticulonodular interstitial pattern, cystic changes, calcification, pleural effusion, or scarring. Pulmonary function tests reveal diminished diffusing capacity, decreased volume, and decreased compliance characteristic of restrictive disease.[35]

Abnormalities of the respiratory system may not be due only to parenchymal lung disease. For example, pulmonary hypertension with cor pulmonale and congestive heart failure may develop independently of parenchymal disease. Biopsies of the lung show the typical changes described earlier around the small pulmonary arteries and arterioles. Esophageal dysmotility may cause aspiration pneumonia and acute respiratory insufficiency. Finally, abrupt changes in respiratory function suggest the possibility of a bronchoalveolar carcinoma in association with long-standing pulmonary fibrosis.

CARDIOVASCULAR DISEASE Acute or chronic pericarditis is an important feature of the disease and, when associated with congestive heart failure, may be a marker for incipient renal failure. Pericardial effusions may be occult, and constrictive pericarditis and tamponade may occur.

Transient vasospasm may involve the coronary vessels and cause myocardial ischemia with angina. Additionally, small-vessel involvement of the myocardium may lead to fibrosis (scleroderma heart).

Fibrosis of the conduction system may cause arrhythmias and sudden death. Right ventricular hypertrophy due to cor pulmonale with congestive heart failure and pulmonary hypertension is observed. The presence of the CREST variant (*c*alcinosis cutis, *R*aynaud's phenomenon, *e*sophageal dysfunction, *s*clerodactyly, and *tel*angiectasia) may be associated with biliary cirrhosis and may not imply diminished cardiopulmonary or renal involvement in all cases as originally described.[36]

In 1976 an attempt to correlate nail fold capillary abnormalities with visceral manifestations was reported. The increased tortuosity of capillaries and areas of avascularity suggest an increased probability of cardiopulmonary and renal disease.

Relapsing Polychondritis (See also Chap. 178)

Relapsing polychondritis is characterized by inflammation and destruction of cartilage and connective tissues, including those of the cardiopulmonary system. The pathogenesis is unknown, although it appears to be an autoimmune process frequently associated with other immunologic disorders such as SLE and rheumatoid arthritis.

Auricular chondritis with pain, swelling, and redness of the pinna but complete sparing of the lobes is characteristic.

Respiratory tract involvement may begin with hoarseness or tenderness of the anterior trachea. Degeneration of the laryngeal, tracheal, and/or bronchial rings may lead to progressive insufficiency or sudden collapse requiring emergency tracheostomy. Adequate ventilatory support may not be possible if advanced scarring and deformity are present.

Cardiac involvement includes degeneration of the aortic ring with valvular insufficiency and aneurysmal dilatation. "Floppy" mitral valve syndrome also occurs. Pericardial and myocardial abnormalities have been reported.[37]

REFERENCES

1. Dolan AL et al: Clinical and echocardiographic survey of the Ehler-Danlos syndrome. *Br J Rheumatol* **36**:459, 1997
2. Kevorkian JP et al: New report of severe coronary artery disease in an eighteen-year-old girl with pseudoxanthoma elasticum. Case report and review of the literature. *Angiology* **48**:735, 1997
3. Hart JJ: Painful, swollen, and erythematous hands and feet. *Arthritis Rheum* **39**:1761, 1996
4. Mascaro JM Jr et al: Congenital generalized follicular hamartoma associated with alopecia and cystic fibrosis in three siblings. *Arch Dermatol* **131**:454, 1995
5. Wilson PR: Post-traumatic upper extremity reflex sympathetic dystrophy. Clinical course, staging, and classification of clinical forms. *Hand Clin* **13**:367, 1997
6. Gutiu IA et al: Diagonal earlobe crease: A coronary risk factor, a genetic marker of coronary heart disease, or a mere wrinkle. Ancient Greco-Roman evidence. *Rom J Intern Med* **34**:271, 1996
7. Rosman HS et al: Cholesterol embolization: Clinical findings and implications. *J Am Coll Cardiol* **15**:1296, 1990
8. Sijpkens Y et al: Vasculitis due to cholesterol embolism. *Am J Med* **102**:302, 1997
9. Hruza LL, Hruza GJ: Saphenous vein graft donor site dermatitis. Case reports and literature review. *Arch Dermatol* **129**:609, 1993
10. Johnson RA, Palacios I: Dilated cardiomyopathies of the adult. *N Engl J Med* **307**:1051, 1119, 1982
11. Coughlin SS et al: Descriptive epidemiology of idiopathic dilated cardiomyopathy in Washington County, Maryland, 1975–1991. *J Clin Epidemiol* **46**:1003, 1993
12. Akbos H et al: Surgical treatment of left-atrial myxoma in Carney's complex. *Thorac Cardiovasc Surg* **45**:148, 1997
13. Rhodes AR et al: Mucocutaneous lentigines, cardiomucocutaneous myxomas, and multiple blue nevi: The "LAMB" syndrome. *J Am Acad Dermatol* **10**:72, 1984
14. Vinson RP et al: Septic microemboli in a Janeway lesion of bacterial endocarditis. *J Am Acad Dermatol* **35**:984, 1996
15. Parikh SK et al: The identification of methicillin-resistant *Staphylococcus aureus* in Osler's nodes and Janeway lesions of acute bacterial endocarditis. *J Am Acad Dermatol* **35**:767, 1996
16. Bull RH et al: Lymphatic function in the yellow nail syndrome. *Br J Dermatol* **134**:307, 1996
17. Morandi U et al: "Yellow nail syndrome" associated with chronic recurrent pericardial and pleural effusions. *Eur J Cardiothorac Surg* **9**:42, 1995
18. Johns MK: Skin wrinkling in cystic fibrosis. *Med Biol Illus* **25**:205, 1975
19. Bulger EM et al: Fat embolism syndrome. A 10-year review. *Arch Surg* **132**:435, 1997
20. Yee KC et al: Cardiac and systemic complications in multicentric reticulohistiocytosis. *Clin Exp Dermatol* **18**:555, 1993
21. Kocanaogullari H et al: Multicentric reticulohistiocytosis. *Clin Rheumatol* **15**:62, 1996
22. Sekiguchi M et al: Cardiac sarcoidosis: Diagnostic, prognostic, and therapeutic considerations. *Cardiovasc Drugs Ther* **10**:495, 1996
23. Mana J et al: Cutaneous involvement in sarcoidosis. Relationship to systemic disease. *Arch Dermatol* **133**:882, 1997
24. Jorizzo JL et al: Sarcoidosis of the upper respiratory tract in patients with nasal rim lesions. *J Am Acad Dermatol* **22**:439, 1990
25. Patel AR et al: Right ventricular dilation in primary amyloidosis: An independent predictor of survival. *Am J Cardiol* **80**:486, 1997
26. Takashi S et al: Diffuse pulmonary amyloidosis with monoclonal IgG-kappa gammopathy. *Intern Med* **36**:357, 1997
27. Wilson WH et al: Association of lymphomatoid granulomatosis with Epstein-Barr viral infection of B lymphocytes and response to interferon-alpha 2b. *Blood* **87**:4531, 1996
28. McNiff JM et al: Lymphomatoid granulomatosis of the skin and lung. An angiocentric T-cell-rich B-cell lymphoproliferative disorder. *Arch Dermatol* **132**:1464, 1996
29. Anaya JM et al: Pulmonary involvement in rheumatoid arthritis. *Semin Arthritis Rheum* **24**:242, 1995
30. McRorie ER et al: Rheumatoid constrictive pericarditis. *Br J Rheumatol* **36**:100, 1997
31. Zamora MR et al: Diffuse alveolar hemorrhage and systemic lupus erythematosus. Clinical presentation, histology, survival, and outcome. *Medicine(Baltimore)* **76**:192, 1997
32. Metz D et al: Prevalence of valvular involvement in systemic lupus erythematosus and association with antiphospholipid syndrome: A matched echocardiographic study. *Cardiology* **85**:129, 1994
33. Tseng CE, Buyon JP: Neonatal lupus syndromes. *Rheum Dis Clin North Am* **23**:31, 1997
34. Borrego L et al: Neonatal lupus erythematosus related to maternal leukocytoclastic vasculitis. *Pediatr Dermatol* **14**:221, 1997
35. Kane GC et al: Lung involvement in systemic sclerosis (scleroderma): Relation to classification based on extent of skin involvement or autoantibody status. *Respir Med* **90**:223, 1996
36. Deswal A, Follansbee WP: Cardiac involvement in scleroderma. *Rheum Dis Clin North Am* **22**:841, 1996
37. Del Rosso A et al: Cardiovascular involvement in relapsing polychondritis. *Semin Arthritis Rheum* **26**:840, 1997

Cutaneous Changes in Peripheral Vascular Disease

OBSTRUCTIVE ARTERIAL DISEASES

Arteriosclerosis Obliterans

Arteriosclerosis obliterans is characterized by muscle pain or fatigue with exercise or by rest pain, ulcers, or gangrene of the distal lower extremities due to stenosis or obstruction of large arteries by atheroma and thrombosis.

EPIDEMIOLOGY Intermittent claudication due to arteriosclerosis obliterans affects about 1 percent of the population over 35 years of age. It occurs predominantly in males. Most patients have superficial femoral artery disease and develop symptoms in the seventh decade, but symptoms from aortoiliac disease usually occur a decade earlier.[1]

ETIOLOGY AND PATHOGENESIS The arteriosclerosis is similar to vascular disease that occurs in other areas of the body. Arteriosclerosis obliterans develops at twice the frequency in patients who smoke compared with nonsmokers.[2] About 50 percent of patients have hyperlipoproteinemia. It is very common in patients with hypertension. Patients with diabetes mellitus develop the disease at an earlier age than nondiabetics and have more severe and progressive disease. The distribution of the disease is different in that diabetics have less aortoiliac disease and more disease of the vessels between the knees and the ankles than nondiabetics; superficial femoral artery disease is similar in both populations.[2]

The cause of atheromas is not known, but progressive buildup of cholesterol plaques narrows the vessel lumen, and finally occlusion may occur by thrombosis. Since the disease progresses slowly, collateral blood vessels develop to supply the extremity distal to the stenosis or obstruction. Therefore, the blood supply to the limb is usually adequate at rest, but the blood pressure distal to the lesions is decreased due to the high resistance of the collateral vessels.[2] When skin lesions develop, the blood supply to the limb is severely compromised.

CLINICAL MANIFESTATIONS *History* The patient complains of pain, fatigue, or a tiredness in the muscles distal to the diseased segment on walking (intermittent claudication). The distance covered before symptoms appear is quite constant for each patient, except that shorter distances can be covered when walking up inclines or carrying heavy bundles. The symptoms are usually relieved within 5 min by rest, even while standing. Patients with inadequate collateral circulation will complain of coldness, hyperesthesias, rest pain, discolored toes, or skin breakdown. Rest pain may be so severe that patients cannot sleep or sleep with the leg in a dependent position; they then may develop edema of the lower parts of the extremity.

Physical examination The limbs in patients with only intermittent claudication may appear normal, although there may be hair loss, coldness, and thickened or malformed toe nails. In aortoiliac disease, there may be global atrophy of the lower limbs. Pulses will be decreased or absent distal to the diseased arterial segment, and there may be bruits over the distal vessels. In patients with severe ischemia, the skin is apt to be atrophic, dry, and shiny. In patients with rest pain, the foot is usually bright red and cold in dependency. Rest pain occurs in the foot; the muscles rarely have rest symptoms. Ulcerations most often start at the tips of the toes and are extremely painful except when a diabetic neuropathy is present. Ulcers occasionally start on the lower calves (Fig. 167-1). The ulcers have a sloughing gray or black base. The heels may show cracks in the skin. When gangrene occurs, usually one or more toes become black, dry, and mummified.

LABORATORY AND SPECIAL EXAMINATIONS The collateral circulation to limbs affected by arteriosclerosis obliterans can be evaluated by simple tests.[2] With the patient supine, elevation of the limb at a 45° angle for 2 min should not produce pallor. The collateral circulation is not adequate if the toes and feet become pale. If the patient then assumes a sitting position with the legs dependent, the times for filling of the foot veins and flushing of the feet

FIGURE 167-1

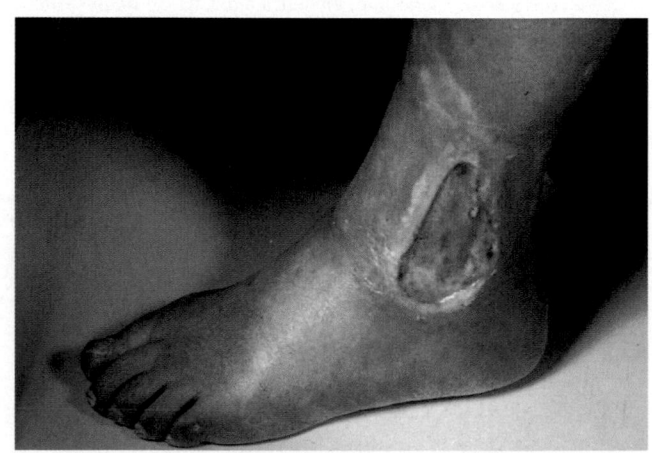

An ischemic ulcer in a patient with arteriosclerosis obliterans. The location on the lateral aspect of the ankle is typical. The base of the ulcer shows fibrous tissue with scant granulation tissue and the outline of tendons. The distal foot and toes are cyanotic from ischemia.

can be measured. The veins should fill within 20 s and the feet flush immediately in a warm environment. When these times exceed 30 s, the collateral circulation is inadequate and the patient must be observed frequently for the development of rest pain, ulcers, or gangrene. Venous filling times are not of value in the presence of varicose veins.

An objective test to document the disease is the measurement of ankle systolic blood pressure. The ankle systolic pressure in the supine position should be equal to or greater than the brachial artery systolic pressure. An ankle-to-arm systolic pressure index is usually calculated; values greater than 0.95 are considered normal, while those less than 0.4 are indicative of severe disease.

Arteriography can be used to demonstrate the location and extent of disease in the arteries but supplies no hemodynamic information. It is usually used only before vascular surgery and not as a diagnostic test.

PATHOLOGY There is a focal accumulation of lipids, mucopolysaccharides, blood and blood products, fibrous tissue, and calcium deposits in the intima of arteries. Localized areas of thickening of the intima by fibroblastic proliferation and phagocytes laden with lipid material are seen. The media is atrophic with thin strands of smooth muscle, disrupted elastic lamella, collagen tissue, and calcium deposits. Enlarging plaques encroach on the lumen despite dilation of the artery, and the plaques may ulcerate. Hemorrhages occur in the arterial wall. Thrombi may form and occlude the narrowed arterial lumen.

DIAGNOSIS AND DIFFERENTIAL DIAGNOSIS The diagnosis of arteriosclerosis obliterans can usually be made by the typical history of intermittent claudication and palpation of all pulses in the limbs. In questionable cases, ankle systolic blood pressures should be measured at rest and, if needed, after exercise.

In patients with diabetes mellitus, ulcers may develop on the heel, toes, or anterior calf in the presence of normal pulses. These painless ulcers are due to repetitive trauma not noticed by the patient because of peripheral neuropathy (Fig. 167-2; see also Fig. 169-3). Other causes of neuropathy also lead to neurotropic ulcers. Surrounding callus formation is typical of these ulcers.

Thromboangiitis obliterans also causes intermittent claudication, ulcers, and gangrene. It occurs in a younger age group and is often associated with superficial thrombophlebitis and vasospasm. It affects medium and smaller arteries and the upper extremities more commonly than does arteriosclerosis obliterans. Neurogenic clau-

FIGURE 167-2

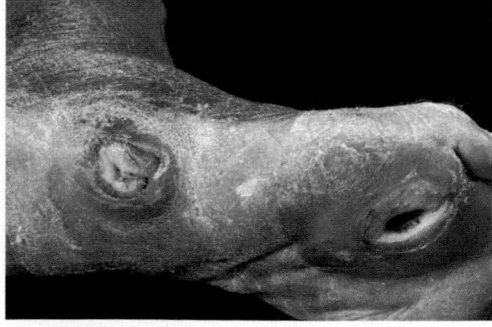

Two neurotropic ulcers over the metatarsal head and on the heel in a patient with diabetes mellitus and neuropathy. The ulcers are painless, and deep, surrounded by callus.

dication is often a difficult differential diagnosis and is due to compression or intermittent ischemia of the lower spinal cord or corda equina with exercise. Etiologic factors are prolapsed intervertebral discs, congenital stenosis, or hypertrophic bony ridging of the spinal canal. In contrast to arteriosclerosis obliterans, leg pain may occur in the erect position without exercise, neurologic signs may be present before or after exercise, and peripheral pulses are normal. Magnetic resonance imaging (MRI) or CT scan will confirm the diagnosis.

TREATMENT For patients with intermittent claudication and an adequate collateral circulation, an exercise regime is the treatment of choice.[3] Patients are instructed to exercise to tolerable pain, rest, and then exercise again for 30 to 60 min a day in excess of their normal activity. The exercise period must be performed in one session, and any type of exercise is beneficial as long as it is in the upright position. In several studies, about 80 percent of patients have increased their walking distance. Patients must also quit smoking, for smokers have a greater amputation[1] and vascular graft occlusion rate than nonsmokers. Patients should also be instructed to keep their feet warm, clean, and dry; extremes of temperature should be avoided, as ischemic tissue is more susceptible to burning at lower temperatures and to frostbite than normal tissue. Cuts or severe bruises of the limbs or feet should be reported to a physician immediately. Vasodilator drugs have not been shown to be of value in treatment.[2] Pentoxifylline, an agent that has hemorheologic effects, has improved treadmill walking distance in some studies.[4]

Surgical or angioplasty procedures are usually reserved for patients with intermittent claudication that interferes with employment, ischemic symptoms at rest, or ulcers and gangrene. Sympathectomy is not of value for intermittent claudication but may allow small ulcers or areas of gangrene to heal.

In patients with rest pain, ulcers, or gangrene who cannot undergo revascularization procedures, treatment is difficult. A period of rest with legs dependent may help some patients, but amputation is a frequent outcome. Parenterally administered prostacyclin or prostaglandin E_1 has had favorable reports but has not yet been adequately evaluated.

Arterial ulcers should be soaked twice a day with bandages soaked with warm 0.9% saline solution for 20 to 30 min. If debridement is necessary, the saline-soaked bandages should be allowed to dry overnight. Removal of the dry bandage will cleanse the ulcer of dead tissue. Enzymatic debriding agents often cause inflammatory reactions and should not be used. Patients should sleep with the limb dependent by elevating the head of the bed 18 cm. Ulcers should be cultured and appropriate systemic antibiotics used when indicated. Elastic bandages should never be applied to an ischemic limb. The lesion should be protected from trauma by loose wrapping bandage. Pain medication may be needed, but care must be exercised to prevent addiction to narcotics. When good granulation tissue covers the whole base of the ulcer, skin grafting can be considered.

Dry gangrene of the digits or lower limbs should be allowed to demarcate by itself. Soaking or ointments are unnecessary. The edges of the gangrenous areas should be kept open if possible and observed frequently for infection. Pain medication is usually necessary for 2 to 3 months with digital gangrene. Conservatism and patience will save many digits and extremities. Infected (wet) gangrenous areas must be debrided and appropriate antibiotics administered. Amputations may be necessary.

PREVENTION   Preventive measures that may help avoid arteriosclerosis obliterans are targeted at the risk factors.[3] It is very important not to smoke tobacco. Hypertension and diabetes mellitus should be controlled, and hyperlipoproteinemias should be treated. Evidence is accumulating that control of hypercholesterolemia will prevent progression of atherosclerotic complications. In patients with diabetic neuropathy, trauma to the limbs must be avoided and special shoes may be needed.

COURSE AND PROGNOSIS   In most studies, 60 to 90 percent of patients with intermittent claudication due to arteriosclerosis obliterans remained stable over a period of 5 to 9 years. Patients with diabetes mellitus, however, have progressive disease, and their amputation rate is fourfold greater than for patients without diabetes.

FIGURE 167-3

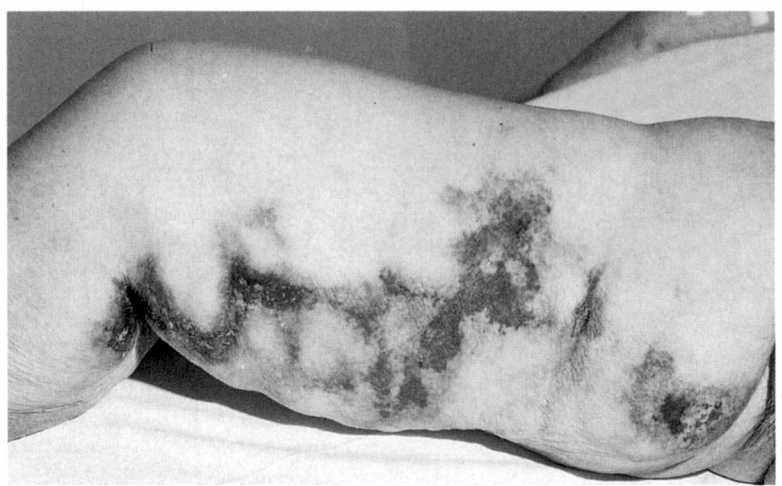

A.

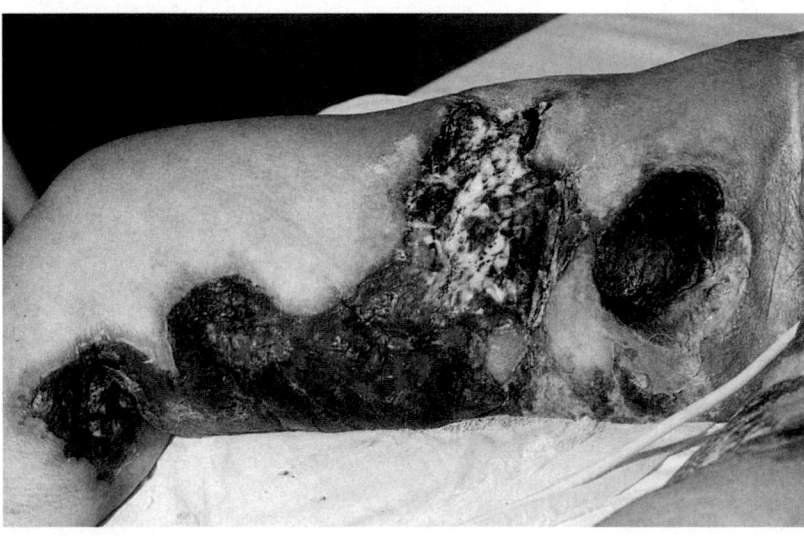

B.

Multiple atheromatous emboli to the lower body and limbs in a patient with extensive atheromatous disease of the aorta. *A.* Livedoid vascular pattern with early infarcts. *B.* Within several days the initial infarction and necrosis has become much more extensive.

Atheromatous Embolism

Atheromatous embolism is the embolization of small pieces of atheromatous debris from arteries to the extremities or body organs. This disease has also been called the *blue toe syndrome* or the *trash foot syndrome*.

EPIDEMIOLOGY   In 100 consecutive autopsies of patients predominantly greater than 50 years old, 4 percent revealed artherosclerotic emboli.[5] In another autopsy series, only 0.79 percent of 2126 patients over 60 years of age had such emboli, but many cases may have been missed. Usually patients are males over 50 years of age.

ETIOLOGY AND PATHOGENESIS   Instigating causes are often absent, but coughing or straining has been postulated as a factor in breaking loose the emboli. Catheterization of blood vessels has been associated with embolization.[5] Coumarin derivatives have also been blamed, but it is more likely that they aggravate the lesions and prevent healing. The emboli usually originate from the aorta or proximal blood vessels that are severely involved with atherosclerotic lesions. An aneurysm can also be the source. The vessel lining of the atherosclerotic vessels is usually irregularly ulcerated and shaggy. The clinical picture is caused by ischemia of the skin and muscle due to the emboli, although all organs of the body may be involved.

CLINICAL MANIFESTATIONS   *History*   Patients will present with unilateral or bilateral discolored or ulcerated painful toes.[5] They may complain of painful and tender calf muscles and a rash on the lower calf or foot. If the entire aorta is involved, transient ischemic attacks or strokes, renal failure, hemorrhagic pancreatitis, and gastrointestinal ulcerations and bleeding may occur. In these patients, almost all organs except the lung have been shown to contain cholesterol crystals.[5]

Physical examination   Physical examination reveals tender, blue toes, and there may be ecchymoses of the sole and lateral aspects of the feet. In some patients, the entire extremities and trunk may show ecchymotic lesions and petechiae. Livedo reticularis and petechiae may be present on the calf and feet. Ulcers or gangrene may be present (Fig. 167-3*A, B*). Surrounding the ischemic areas is normally perfused tissue. The calf muscles are often tender. The upper extremities are involved in patients with disease of the entire aorta (Fig. 167-4). Occasionally there are elevated plaques of skin. Pedal and proximal pulses are usually normal, but there may be systolic bruits over the aorta or common femoral arteries. Fever may be present.

LABORATORY AND SPECIFIC EXAMINATIONS   Eosinophilia is common and has been described in up to 80 percent of patients with renal atheromatous emboli.[6] Thrombocytopenia, hypocomplementemia, and anemia may occur. The sedimentation rate is often elevated. In patients with multisystem involvement, there may be elevated renal function tests, increased amylase levels, blood in the urine or stool, and anemia. Angiography demonstrates diffuse atherosclerotic involvement of the vessels proximal to the lesions.

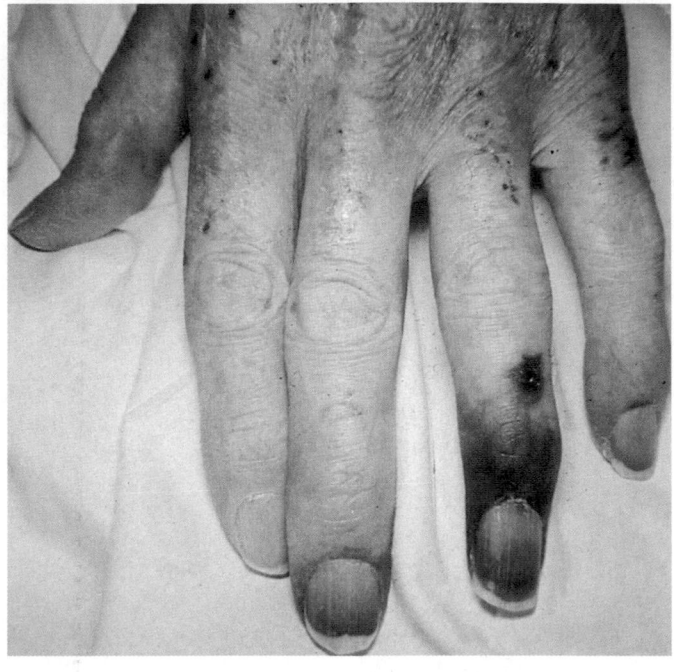

Atheromatous emboli to the fingers in an elderly patient with extensive atheromatous disease of the aorta. There is gangrene of the third and fourth distal fingers and ecchymotic discrete areas proximally. Radial and ulnar pulses were normal.

PATHOLOGY   Skin or muscle biopsies may reveal the characteristic elongated, needle-shaped clefts of cholesterol crystals in small arterial vessels. There may be inflammatory infiltrates, intimal thickening, and perivascular fibrosis. Giant cells may also be present.

DIAGNOSIS AND DIFFERENTIAL DIAGNOSIS   The diagnosis of atheromatous emboli is suggested by the blue or ulcerated painful digits, livedo reticularis, petechiae, tender calf muscles, and elevated skin plaques in the presence of normal pulses. A definite diagnosis can be made by skin, muscle, or renal biopsies. Occasionally, cholesterol emboli may be visualized in the retinal arterioles.

In the differential diagnosis of the blue toe syndrome, several other entities must be considered (Table 167-1). Biopsy of skin or muscle showing cholesterol crystals will usually rule out other causes.

TREATMENT   Atheromatous emboli can be stopped by surgical bypasses or endarterectomy to remove or exclude the source. However, many of these patients have contraindications to major sur-

TABLE 167-1

Differential Diagnosis of the Blue Toe Syndrome

Atheromatous emboli	Vasculitis
Emboli from the heart	Polyarteritis
Connective tissue diseases	Malignancy with or without
Primary Raynaud's disease	cryoglobulins or macroglobulins
Thrombocytosis	Antiphospholipid and anti-
Polycythemia	cardiolipin antibodies

gery. In these cases, therapeutic doses of subcutaneous heparin or aspirin and dipyridamole can be tried and, if successful, should be continued for at least 1 year.[5] Warfarin is usually avoided, especially if toe ulcers are present. Many patients will not respond to any therapy except surgery.

PREVENTION   One way of prevention is to avoid catheterization of severely atherosclerotic blood vessels.

COURSE AND PROGNOSIS   The syndrome usually subsides and lesions heal following successful surgical or medical treatment. Sometimes the emboli cease spontaneously. When surgery cannot be performed and emboli continue, amputations may result. In the malignant multisystem disease, patients usually die within a year if treatment is unsuccessful.

Thromboangiitis Obliterans

Thromboangiitis obliterans (also known as Buerger's disease) is an inflammatory occlusive disease affecting medium and small arteries and veins.

EPIDEMIOLOGY   The prevalence of the disease is greatest in eastern Europe, the Mediterranean area, and Asia. Males are afflicted in much greater number than females, although an increased incidence in females has occurred in recent years. Patients are usually between the age of 20 and 40 years.

ETIOLOGY AND PATHOGENESIS   The etiology of thromboangiitis obliterans remains unknown. Almost all patients who develop this disease are smokers, and the syndrome sometimes abates with the cessation of tobacco smoking. An increased frequency of HLA-A9 and HLA-B5 or HLA-B8 has been reported but not found by all investigators.[7] For some reason, there has been a marked decline in the prevalence of the disease in the United States. The pathogenesis involves the production of tissue ischemia and all its manifestations by an inflammatory reaction of medium and small arteries of the extremities and obstruction by thrombi. Veins may also be involved. Occasionally cardiac, intestinal, and cerebral vessels are involved.

CLINICAL MANIFESTATIONS   *History*   The most common initial complaints are claudication of the foot or lower calf, digital cyanosis or gangrene, or rest pain. Patients may present with ulcers of the toes or fingers, for although the lower extremities are affected most often, more than a third of patients have upper extremity involvement. Ulcerations or gangrenous areas are characteristically extremely painful. Vasospasm or migratory superficial thrombophlebitis may occur in 40 percent of patients.

Physical examination   Physical examination may reveal cyanotic, ulcerated, or gangrenous, very painful digits. The dorsalis pedis and posterior tibial pulses may be absent. In the upper extremity, the ulnar pulse is often absent. During episodes of thrombophlebitis, small indurated red, tender nodules will be found, which follow the course of superficial veins and are common on the thigh or calf. Typical changes of Raynaud's phenomenon, with well-demarcated pallor or cyanosis of the digits, may be seen on exposure to cold; one or more extremities may be involved.

LABORATORY AND SPECIAL EXAMINATIONS   There are no specific blood studies. Arteriography is sometimes typical, showing segmental occlusions of medium and small blood vessels with normal vessel walls between diseased areas, no arteriosclerosis of proximal vessels, and corkscrew configuration of collateral vessels originating from occluded vessels.[8]

PATHOLOGY   In the acute stage, there is a panvasculitis of arteries and veins; the diagnostic finding is arterial thrombi with foci of microabscesses and giant cells. In the chronic stage, only fibrotic obliteration of the arteries is seen, and the diagnosis can only be surmised since arteriosclerosis is absent.

DIAGNOSIS AND DIFFERENTIAL DIAGNOSIS   The diagnosis should be considered in young male smokers presenting with symptoms and signs of distal extremity ischemia, migratory thrombophlebitis, and Raynaud's phenomenon. Arteriography may suggest the diagnosis, but only a biopsy of an artery during the active phase of the disease that shows the characteristic pathologic picture is diagnostic.

Arteriosclerosis obliterans occurs in an older age group, larger vessels are involved, Raynaud's phenomenon is infrequent, and the upper extremities are rarely involved. In diabetes mellitus, the arteriosclerosis may affect medium-sized vessels, but the blood sugar is normal in thromboangiitis obliterans. Raynaud's phenomenon associated with scleroderma may present with a similar picture, but systemic symptoms, proximal skin changes, and antinuclear antibodies will help in the diagnosis.

TREATMENT   There is no specific treatment. Patients must give up smoking, and in some the disease will abate. Otherwise, the treatment of the disease is the same as for arteriosclerosis obliterans or Raynaud's phenomenon. Glucocorticoids have not been of benefit. Sympathectomy may be of value in patients with a prominent vasospastic component.

PREVENTION   The only preventive measure is never to smoke.

COURSE AND PROGNOSIS   The course of the disease is marked by exacerbations and remissions, but finally the disease usually quiesces after many years. Cessation of tobacco smoking sometimes hastens the disappearance of the disease. Amputations of digits or even extremities may be necessary, especially in patients who continue to smoke. Patients often have a normal life expectancy.

ERYTHROMELALGIA (ERYTHERMALGIA) (See Chap. 128)

VASOSPASTIC DISEASES AND DISEASE DUE TO COLD EXPOSURE (See also Chap. 128)

Raynaud's Disease and Phenomenon

Raynaud's phenomenon is the occurrence of episodic attacks of well-demarcated blanching or cyanosis of one or more digits on exposure to cold.

EPIDEMIOLOGY   Primary Raynaud's disease usually occurs in patients 15 to 40 years of age but may occur in young children and patients over 50 years of age.[9] There is a strong 4:1 female to male predominance. Raynaud's phenomenon occurs in 4.6 to 30 percent of randomized questioned populations.[10]

ETIOLOGY AND PATHOGENESIS   The pathogenesis of Raynaud's phenomenon or episodic vasospastic attacks is unknown. A local fault at the digital artery level in which the blood vessels are abnormally sensitive to cold and an overactivity of the sympathetic nervous system are the two proposed theories. The local fault theory has the most scientific backing. The local fault may be at the α_2-adrenoceptor level, because there are increased levels of α_2 adrenoceptors in platelets of patients with primary Raynaud's disease[11] and patients show an increased digital vasoconstrictor response to an intraarterial α_2-adrenoceptor and not an α_1-adrenoceptor agonist.[12] Vasospastic attacks are probably due to a combination of factors, including the following: (1) normal vasoconstriction due to reflex sympathetic activity and local cold, (2) low systemic and intravascular blood pressure, (3) external pressure on the digit, (4) increased sensitivity of certain receptors (α_2 adrenoceptors, S_2-serotonergic receptors), and (5) release of vasoactive agents from platelets.[9]

The connective tissue diseases are the most common cause of secondary Raynaud's phenomenon (Table 167-2). Between 80 and 90 percent of patients with scleroderma manifest Raynaud's phenomenon and/or persistent vasospasm. It is the presenting symptom in about one-third of patients and may be the only manifestation of the disease for years. Raynaud's phenomenon occurs in 10 to 35 percent of patients with systemic lupus erythematosus and in about 30 percent with dermatomyositis. It is also sometimes present in rheumatoid arthritis and the vasculitides. Arteriograms in patients

TABLE 167-2

Causes of Raynaud's Phenomenon

Connective tissue disease	Trauma
Scleroderma	Vibratory tools
Systemic lupus erythematosus	Hypothenar hammer
Dermatomyositis and polymyositis	syndrome
Mixed connective tissue disease	Pianists, typists
Rheumatoid arthritis	Meat cutters
Sjögren's syndrome	Hematologic causes
Obstructive arterial disease	Cryoproteins
Arteriosclerosis obliterans	Cold agglutinins
Thromboangiitis obliterans	Macroglobulins
Arterial embolism	Polycythemia
Neurogenic disorders	Miscellaneous
Thoracic outlet syndrome	Hypothyroidism
Carpa; tunnel syndrome	Vinyl chloride disease
Reflex sympathetic dystrophy	Neoplasms
Hemiplegia	Vasculitis and hepatitis B
Poliomyelitis	antigenemia
Multiple sclerosis	Intraarterial injections
Syringomyelia	
Drug	
β-Adrenergic blockers	
Ergot preparations	
Methysergide	
Bleomycin and vinblastine	
Clonidine	
Bromocriptine	
Cyclosporine	

with connective tissue diseases show digital and sometimes ulnar or radial artery obstructions.

Raynaud's phenomenon may be occupational in origin and is especially common in people who use vibratory tools to cut stones or wood. Arteriograms have shown digital, radial, ulnar, or palmar arch thromboses.

Any neurologic condition that produces permanent disuse of a limb can produce a sympathetic nervous system disturbance to that limb. This is usually manifested by persistent vasospasm with coldness, paleness or cyanosis, and even ulcerations, but Raynaud's phenomenon may occur. Nerve root pressure or nerve entrapment may produce Raynaud's phenomenon. It is often present in the carpal tunnel syndrome and may occur secondary to neurovascular compression at the thoracic outlet.

Several drugs have been implicated as causing Raynaud's phenomenon. Propranolol, one of the most widely used β-adrenoceptor blockers in cardiovascular diseases and migraine headaches, is probably the most frequent offender. The exact mechanism is not known, but cardioselective β-adrenoceptor blocking drugs have not been shown to be free of this side effect. Ergot preparations and methysergide used in the treatment of migraine headaches also cause the phenomenon. Ergotamine is a powerful α-adrenoceptor vasoconstrictor agonist and may produce gangrene of the fingers. Methysergide, a serotonin antagonist and agonist, produces peripheral vascular symptoms or signs in about 7 percent of patients. Industrial exposure to the vinyl chloride polymerization process may produce acroosteolysis of the distal phalanges of the fingers in a small percentage of workers, and Raynaud's phenomenon may also occur. Arteriograms in these patients show digital artery obstructions. The chemotherapeutic agents bleomycin and vinblastine may also cause the phenomenon.

Patients with cryoglobulins, macroglobulins, and polycythemia can exhibit Raynaud's phenomenon, probably secondary to rheologic disturbances or actual occlusion of small vessels. Cold agglutinins may occasionally cause the syndrome due to blockage of the vessels by agglutinated erythrocytes. The most common hormonal disturbance causing Raynaud's phenomenon is hypothyroidism, and the condition usually remits with thyroid replacement.

CLINICAL MANIFESTATIONS *History* Patients complain of episodic attacks of well-demarcated, white or blue digits on exposure to cold and sometimes induced by emotional stimuli (Fig. 167-5). During the attacks, one or more fingers or toes may be numb and may be described as "dead." The thumbs are often spared. On rewarming, the digits may become bright red and throbbing pain may occur. When pain is a prominent symptom in the ischemic phase, a secondary cause should be suspected. Attacks may last minutes to hours. Patients may experience one or more attacks per cold season or multiple attacks throughout the year. The fingers are most commonly involved, but vasospastic attacks may occur in the toes in 40 percent of patients.

Physical examination Examination is usually normal in patients with primary disease, and vasospastic attacks are difficult to induce in the office. If an attack is witnessed, there is well-demarcated blanching or cyanosis of the digits extending from the tips to varying levels of the digits. The digits distal to the line of ischemia are cold, while the proximal skin is pink and warmer. The hands and feet are not involved except in some secondary etiologies. On rewarming, blanched digits may become cyanotic due to the slow blood flow and then bright red due to reactive hyperemia. The digits appear normal between attacks but may be cool and moist with excess perspiration. The radial and ulnar pulses are normal. Patients may show the nail change known as *pterygium*, which refers to a cuticle widened to several millimeters with a proximal skin

FIGURE 167-5

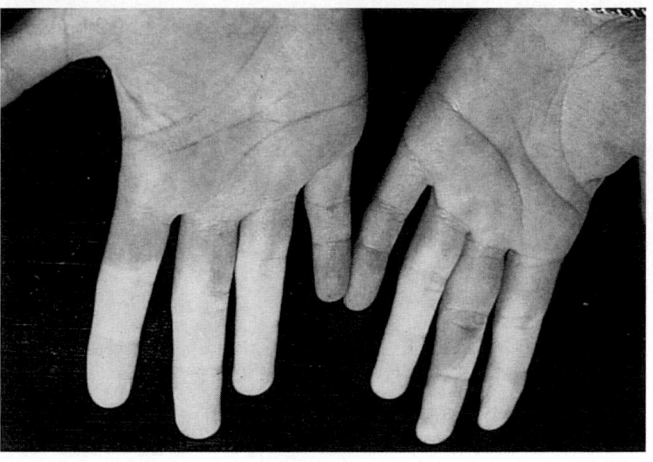

A vasospastic attack in a young woman with Raynaud's phenomenon. Well-demarcated blanching of the fingers on exposure to cold is present. Ulnar and radial pulses were normal. The hand is not involved. The attacks were episodic.

fold thin and merging with the cuticle. Trophic changes with tense and atrophic skin, deformity of nails, and shortening and contracture of digits (sclerodactyly) may also be present. Gangrene is rare and only affects the tips of fingers. Patients with secondary Raynaud's phenomenon may show other manifestations of their underlying disease; persistent ischemic discoloration of digits suggests a secondary cause.

LABORATORY AND SPECIAL EXAMINATIONS Blood and urine studies are normal in patients with primary Raynaud's disease. The effect of local cooling with an ischemic stimulus has been used as a diagnostic test for Raynaud's phenomenon but does not differentiate primary from secondary disease.[13] Compared to normal individuals, patients with Raynaud's phenomenon have a greater reduction in finger systolic pressure with cooling and many show a loss of pressure or digital artery closure.

Nailfold capillary microscopy may be valuable to diagnose secondary causes of Raynaud's phenomenon but is normal in the primary disease. In scleroderma, mixed connective tissue disease, and dermatomyositis, there may be enlarged, deformed capillary loops surrounded by avascular areas.[14] Abnormal capillary loops and a prominent subpapillary venous plexus occur in lupus erythematosus, while bushy capillary formations are most prominent in mixed connective tissue disease.

PATHOLOGY Histologic examination of digital arteries has been performed in a few patients with mild primary Raynaud's disease and has been normal. In patients with more severe disease, intimal hyperplasia, narrowing or total occlusion of arteries, or thrombi are present.

DIAGNOSIS AND DIFFERENTIAL DIAGNOSIS The diagnosis is usually made from the history of typical episodic attacks of well-demarcated white or blue discoloration of the digits on cold exposure.[9] Patients with sufficient symptoms to seek a physician's advice should have a complete workup to exclude secondary causes.

The history will elicit symptoms of connective tissue disease (arthralgias, arthritis, dysphagia, heartburn, facial rash from the sun, persistent tans), a drug etiology, symptoms of obstructive arterial diseases (intermittent claudication, migratory thrombophlebitis), and exposure to vibratory tools or continuous finger trauma. During the physical examination, the physician should pay attention to all pulses, blood pressure in both the arms, telangiectasis, subcutaneous nodules, swollen or deformed joints, skin texture, discoloration of the eyelids, bruits in the neck, thyroid size, relaxation time of reflexes, neurologic deficits, and organomegaly. The thoracic outlet maneuvers should be performed, and Tinel's sign (distal tingling or pain on percussion of the median nerve at the wrist) sought. Blood analyses for anemia, polycythemia, leukopenia, sedimentation rate, serum protein electrophoresis, antinuclear antibodies, rheumatoid factor, cryoglobulins, and cold agglutinins are necessary. Proteinuria and red blood cell casts should be specifically looked for in the urinalysis. A chest film will rule out the presence of cervical ribs. The history, physical examination, and laboratory tests should all be normal before a patient is reassured that the benign, idiopathic disease is probably the diagnosis.

The main differential diagnoses are patients complaining of cold digits and acrocyanosis. Many patients complain of cold, sometimes painful digits but color changes are absent. This may be one extreme of the spectrum of normal sympathetic nerve activity. In acrocyanosis (see Chap. 128), the hands and feet are involved compared to only the digits in Raynaud's phenomenon, the color change is persistent and not episodic, a pallor phase is absent, and there is no sex predilection.

TREATMENT Most patients with Raynaud's disease respond to reassurance that they have a benign disease, to instructions to wear loose fitting warm clothes covering as much of the body as possible to prevent reflex sympathetic vasoconstriction, and to avoid cold especially with pressure on the digits.[9] Tobacco smoking should be discouraged since nicotine induces cutaneous vasoconstriction; smokers are more numerous among patients with Raynaud's disease and with traumatic vasospastic disease. The underlying cause must be treated in patients with secondary Raynaud's phenomenon.

Drug therapy can be used in the more severe cases of the disease or phenomenon but is only successful in about two-thirds of patients.[9] The calcium channel blocking agent nifedipine has had the most success. Several studies have shown that nifedipine decreases the frequency, duration, and severity of attacks in about two-thirds of patients with primary or secondary Raynaud's phenomenon. The long-acting preparations have fewer side effects and are just as beneficial. Diltiazem, but not verapamil, may also be beneficial. Both reserpine and guanethidine have been shown to increase capillary blood flow during cold exposure in patients. Prazosin, an α_1-adrenoceptor agonist, has been shown to produce moderate benefit. Nitrates or their ointments have their proponents but are usually used in combination with other agents. Parenteral prostacyclin has been reported of benefit, but oral preparations are not available. Either biofeedback or pavlovian conditioning may provide some benefit to patients, but they require a time commitment by the patient. Upper extremity sympathectomy is not of value in the disease or the phenomenon; its benefit only lasts from 6 months to 2 years. Lumbar sympathectomy does produce lasting relief for lower extremity Raynaud's phenomenon.

PREVENTION Moving to a warmer climate alleviates symptoms in about 50 percent of patients. Some of the secondary causes can be prevented. Measures have been instituted to decrease the vibration of tools and to shorten hours for workers to prevent traumatic vasospastic disease. Vasoconstrictor drugs must be used with care to prevent overdoses. Mechanics and meat cutters should be warned not to use the hand as a hammer.

COURSE AND PROGNOSIS In patients with primary Raynaud's disease, approximately 38 percent have no change in symptoms over time, 36 percent improve, 16 percent develop more severe attacks, and in 10 percent the syndrome disappears.[15] Sclerodactyly develops in 3.3 percent. Fewer than 1 percent have digital amputations, although digital trophic changes occur in 13 percent. Although trophic changes of the fingers may develop in many patients, the prognosis is fairly good.[16] Unfortunately, scleroderma is difficult to diagnose, and some patients will develop manifestations of this disease many years after the onset of Raynaud's phenomenon.

Acrocyanosis (See Chap. 128)

Livedo Reticularis (See also Chap. 128)

Livedo reticularis is characterized by a reddish-blue mottling of the skin in a "fishnet" reticular pattern.

EPIDEMIOLOGY All types of livedo reticularis occur most commonly in young women less than 40 years of age.

ETIOLOGY AND PATHOGENESIS Livedo reticularis has been called by many names including idiopathic livedo reticularis, cutis marmorata, livedo annularis, livedo racemosa, sympathetic livedo reticularis, and asphyxia reticularis. Livedo reticularis with ulceration is also known as livedo or livedoid vasculitis and *atrophie blanche*. A variety of names usually reflects an unknown etiology.

Secondary livedo reticularis is most commonly seen accompanying vasospastic conditions such as primary and secondary Raynaud's phenomenon, acrocyanosis, and vasculitis. It is often a manifestation of an underlying disease and may be a clue to its diagnosis. It has been reported in association with connective diseases, especially lupus erythematosus, obstructive arterial disease, endocrine disorders, neurogenic diseases, drug reactions, hyperviscosity states, hypertension, and lymphomas. It has been shown to be induced by amantadine, a drug used for Parkinson's disease and influenza. It is an important diagnostic manifestation in atheromatous embolization. Livedo reticularis with cerebrovascular lesions has been described (*Sneddon's syndrome*)[17]; this may be part of a syndrome with arterial and venous thromboses, spontaneous abortions, and anticardiolipin or antiphospholipid antibodies[18] (Fig. 167-6).

Livedo reticularis with ulceration may be secondary to a localized vasculitis.[19] Immunofluorescence studies have shown IgM deposits. Complement factors, fibrin, and sometimes IgA have also been found in the vessel walls, which suggests an immune complex pathogenesis. Other investigators consider that this disease may be due to blood or tissue abnormalities that induce thromboses of arterioles. A defect in the fibrinolytic system may be present. Abnormalities of platelet aggregation or increased platelet adhesiveness have also been reported.

Amantadine causes livedo reticularis and is known to release norepinephrine from central and peripheral nerves in addition to enhancing the action of norepinephrine and dopamine on several peripheral tissues. These actions with amantadine's ability to inhibit uptake of dopamine and norepinephrine in neurons could lead to arteriolar constriction.

FIGURE 167-6

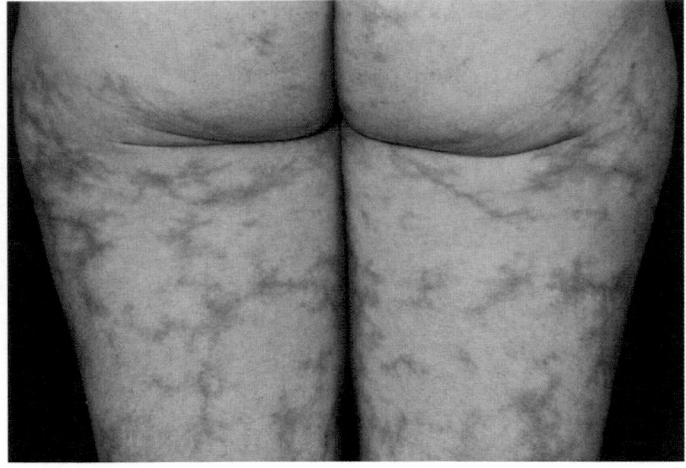

Livedo reticularis of the buttocks and thighs in a woman who had a cerebrovascular thrombosis. This is an example of Sneddon's syndrome.

Vasospasm or obstruction of the small perpendicular arterioles in the dermis is the probable cause of the fishnet appearance of the skin. The red to blue periphery of each web of the net would be due to deoxygenated blood in surrounding horizontally arranged venous plexuses.[20] Elevation of the extremity therefore decreases the intensity of the color changes by emptying the veins. The reversibility of the color pattern with warming, the frequent association with vasospastic diseases of the digits, and the beneficial response to sympathetic blocking agents suggest an increased sympathetic nerve activity as the cause of benign livedo reticularis.

CLINICAL MANIFESTATIONS *History* Patients with benign livedo reticularis have no complaints except for the cosmetic appearance of the cutaneous fishnet. Numbness and pain are rare, but a subjective feeling of coldness is common. Patients with secondary livedo reticularis may complain of symptoms of their underlying disease. Persistence of the fishnet pattern during warming and purpuric macular lesions or skin nodules that ulcerate are the complaints in patients with livedo reticularis with ulceration. Most patients have the painful ulcers only in the winter, while others have them in the summer also.

Physical examination In the benign form, a fishnet pattern affects mainly the extremities and the webs are rose, violet, red, or blue. Between the webs, the skin appears pale. The colors are aggravated by exposure to cold and may disappear on warming. The examination is normal except for the skin. In livedo reticularis with ulceration (livedoid vasculitis), purpuric lesions, cutaneous papules, or ulcers may be found (Fig. 167-7A). The ulcers are usually covered with eschars and surrounded by red inflammation; they are very tender. About 50 percent of patients have edema of the legs, which often occurs before the ulcerations. Healed ulcers have a smooth ivory-white plaque of atrophic skin surrounded by hyperpigmented borders and telangiectatic blood vessels (*atrophie blanche*) (Fig. 167-7B). Most ulcers are found on the lower part of the legs, ankles, and dorsa of the feet.

In patients with secondary livedo reticularis, other manifestations of their underlying disease may be present.

LABORATORY AND SPECIAL EXAMINATIONS In livedo reticularis with or without ulceration, no specific blood or urine tests are abnormal.[19]

FIGURE 167-7

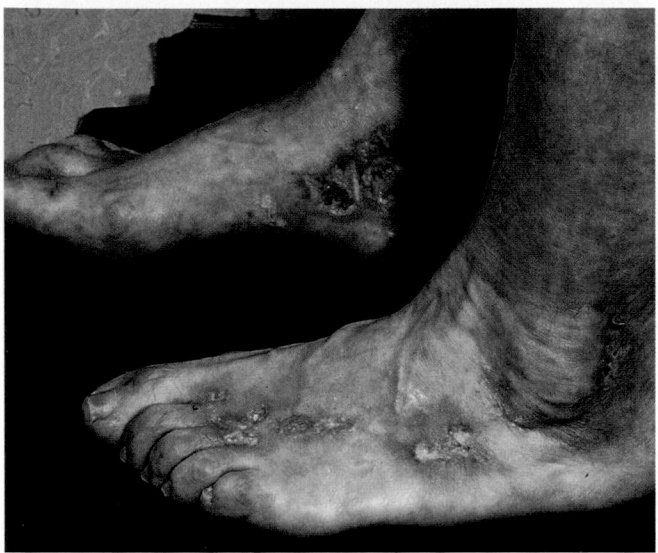

A.

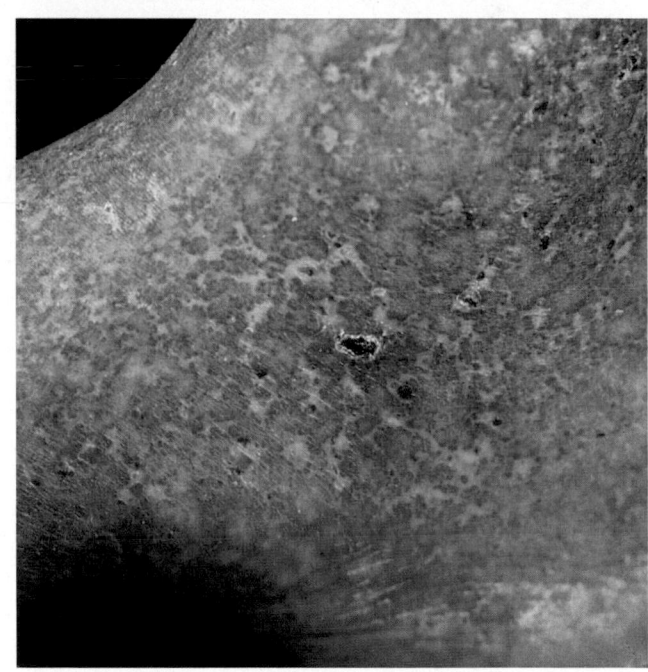

B.

A. Recurrent irregular, extremely painful ulcers of the feet and lower legs in a 32-year-old woman with livedo reticularis with ulceration. Pigmented areas of healed ulcers are present. Ulcerations had been recurrent since age 16 with no relation to seasons. Pedal pulses were normal. *B.* Close up of *atrophic blanche* with irregular porcelain-white atrophic scars, ulcerations, and crusting in a similar patient.

PATHOLOGY In benign livedo reticularis and that due to drug therapy, biopsies have shown nonspecific changes or increased numbers of dilated capillaries. A segmental hyalinizing vasculitis of the middle dermal vessels has been described in the ulcerative disease.[19] In Sneddon's syndrome, there are also a noninflammatory hyalinization and thickening of vessel walls and vascular occlusions, which are seen only in biopsies obtained from the center of the mesh of the fishnet pattern.

DIAGNOSIS AND DIFFERENTIAL DIAGNOSIS The diagnosis is made easily from the typical fishnet pattern on the skin in the benign form. In patients with ulcers, other causes of lower extremity ulcers must be ruled out. Secondary causes must be sought before the diagnosis is considered to be benign livedo reticularis or with ulceration. It is therefore a diagnosis by exclusion of underlying diseases.

TREATMENT The benign type of livedo reticularis needs no treatment. The skin discoloration can be covered with cosmetics or, as a last resort, sympatholytic agents can be tried for patients bothered by the social stigma.

In secondary causes, the underlying disease should be treated. Patients with anticardiolipin antibodies and thromboses should be treated with anticoagulants. In livedo reticularis with ulceration, treatment has been unsuccessful. Saline soaks and analgesic ointments are helpful. Antiplatelet agents and agents that induce fibrinolysis[21] are the most recently recommended therapies. Dextran infusions, nicotinic acid, pentoxifylline, nifedipine, heparin, glucocorticoids, cytoxan, methotrexate, radiotherapy, sympathetic blocking agents, and other therapies have all been reported to benefit some patients. Since the disease is rare, there are no large controlled studies of treatment modalities.

PREVENTION Only measures to keep the body and extremities warm may be of preventive benefit.

COURSE AND PROGNOSIS The benign condition has an excellent prognosis. In livedo reticularis with ulceration, the painful ulcers are often recurrent and may be disabling. The lower limbs and feet become scarred; amputations have been necessary for deep ulcers and severe pain.

Frostbite (See Chap. 128)

DISEASES OF THE VEINS

Thrombophlebitis

Thrombophlebitis or deep venous thrombosis is due to thrombotic obstruction of veins with or without an inflammatory response to the thrombus.

ETIOLOGY AND PATHOGENESIS Deep venous thrombosis occurs due to slow blood flow, hypercoagulability, or changes in the venous walls. The most common causes are shown in Table 167-3. Some malignancies, such as those of the lung, pancreas and stomach, are associated with thrombophlebitis, and it may be of the migratory variety. Oral contraceptives significantly reduce activated factor X inhibitory activity and induce venous thrombosis. In recent years, coagulation factor deficiencies predisposing to thrombophlebitis have been discovered. These are often hereditary and include the common resistance to activated protein C (Leiden factor 5 mutation) and the rarer antithrombin III, protein C or S, and fibrinolytic

TABLE 167-3

Predisposing Factors in Deep Venous Thrombosis

COMMON FACTORS

Major surgery	Oral contraceptives
Fractures	Malignancies
Congestive heart failure	Venous varicosities
Acute myocardial infarction	Previous history of venous thrombosis
Stroke	Leiden factor 5 mutation
Pregnancy and postpartum	Severe pulmonary insufficiency
Spinal cord injuries	Prolonged immobilization
Shock	

LESS COMMON FACTORS

Sickle cell anemia	Antithrombin III deficiency
Homocystinuria	Antiphospholipid antibodies
Protein C or S deficiency	Ulcerative colitis

factor deficiencies. Thrombophlebitis and arterial thrombus may occur in patients with antiphospholipid antibodies and is most common in lupus erythematosus.

Superficial thrombophlebitis is usually due to infections of or trauma to superficial veins from needles or catheters. A migratory variety is seen in thromboangiitis obliterans and malignancies. Mondor's disease is an inflamed subcutaneous vein from the breast to the axillary region, which has no special associations.[22]

The thrombus originates in an area of low or no venous flow, and the extrinsic pathway for blood coagulation is probably most important.[23] An occlusion of a vein by thrombus imposes a block to venous return, which leads to increased venous pressure and edema in the distal limb. An inflammatory response to the thrombus causes pain and tenderness. Prominent collateral veins appear early to bypass the obstruction and relieve the edema; recanalization may occur in several weeks. If the venous pressure is too high, arterial inflow may rarely be compromised and ischemia of the distal limb occurs. The thrombus within the vein often has a free-floating tail, which may break off to produce a pulmonary embolus. The free-floating tail is bound down to the vein wall in about 10 days. Organization of the thrombus in the vein destroys the venous valves, which leads to the postphlebitic syndrome.

CLINICAL MANIFESTATIONS *History* Patients may complain of pain or aching in the involved limb, have no symptoms, or notice limb swelling. Some patients present with the symptoms of pulmonary emboli without extremity symptoms.

Physical examination The clinical picture is very variable, varying from subtle signs of swelling to a tensely swollen, warm, tender limb with prominent, distended collateral veins. Swelling may first be detected by an increased turgor of the muscles or careful measurement of limb circumference compared to the opposite limb. Pitting edema may occur but is not always present. A tender cord may be felt where the vein is thrombosed. With iliofemoral thrombophlebitis, the limb is swollen from the foot to the inguinal region (Fig. 167-8), tenderness is not present in the limb because the thrombus is proximal, and collateral veins may form from the thigh to the abdominal wall. The limb may be very pale (*phlegmasia alba dolens*) or may be cyanotic with cold digits if the arterial inflow is compromised (*phlegmasia cerulea dolens*). In thrombosis of calf veins, the calf and foot are swollen and warm; there is deep tenderness with or without a palpable cord. Increased resistance to dorsiflexion of the foot may be present (Homans' sign). Thrombophlebitis of a superficial vein or varicosity is evidenced by pain-

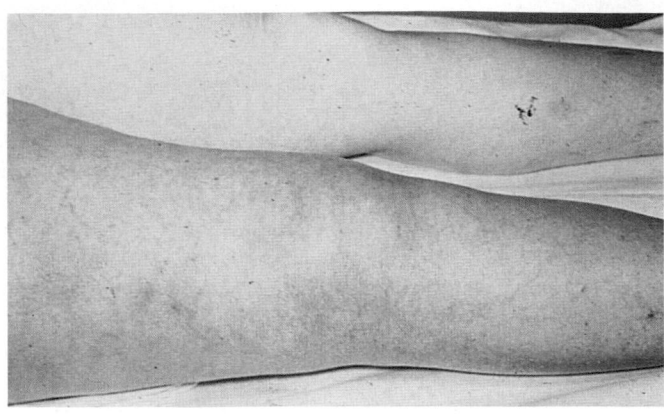

Acute iliofemoral deep venous thrombosis in a woman postpartum. The thigh and calf are very swollen compared to the opposite limb and have a blotchy cyanotic discoloration.

ful induration of the vein with redness and increased heat. Migratory cases have successive areas of superficial veins involved over a variable period of time. Mondor's disease is manifested by a tender cord from the breast to the axillary region; during healing, the venous cord shortens and puckers the skin.[22]

LABORATORY AND SPECIAL EXAMINATIONS Venous imaging by B-mode duplex ultrasound scanning combined with Doppler examination is an extremely valuable test that can diagnose proximal venous thrombi by indirect means (noncompressibility of the vein) or actual visualization of the thrombi.[24] With proximal venous occlusions, pulsed-wave Doppler ultrasound will reveal an absence of flow or the normal respiratory venous flow variation. These tests have a high sensitivity and specificity but only for proximal venous thrombosis and not for calf disease. For thrombophlebitis of the calf veins, the localization in the leg of intravenously administered ^{125}I fibrinogen is the only definitive test besides venography. White blood counts and sedimentation rates are usually normal but may be high in extensive or inflammatory thrombophlebitis.

PATHOLOGY The thrombus is composed of fibrin, red blood cells, and platelets. The thrombus propagates proximally and then consists predominantly of fibrin interspersed with red cells. The underlying vein wall may show minimal to marked inflammatory changes with infiltration of white blood cells and loss of endothelium. The thrombus may also undergo the same process and thereby become adherent to the vein wall. Some thrombi recanalize. The venous valves within the area of the thrombus are permanently damaged as the thrombus becomes adherent to the vein wall.

DIAGNOSIS AND DIFFERENTIAL DIAGNOSIS Thrombophlebitis is difficult to diagnose clinically. The symptoms and signs are nonspecific; studies have shown that the clinical diagnosis is incorrect in about 50 percent of patients.[25] Definitive tests by Doppler, impedance plethysmography, or preferably venous scanning and Doppler ultrasound are necessary to make the diagnosis. A venogram is only necessary when these tests give indeterminate results. Although a diagnosis is often not found for the cause of a painful or swollen extremity, these patients have a benign prognosis if noninvasive tests are negative for deep venous thrombosis. Superficial thrombophlebitis can be diagnosed by the characteristic clinical picture, although lymphargitis and cellulitis must be considered; the

former usually has red streaking up the limb and tender lymph nodes proximally, while the latter presents a more diffuse involvement of the extremity.

The most common differential diagnoses of thrombophlebitis include rupture of the plantar muscle, which produces an ecchymotic area in the dependent ankle area and sometimes a tender knot over the muscle. Ruptured synovial membrane of the knee joint can imitate thrombophlebitis; knee joint fluid, inflammation, or arthritis are clues to the diagnosis, but an arthrogram may be needed.

TREATMENT The treatment of deep venous thrombosis is anticoagulation.[23] Heparin is given by intravenous infusion at approximately 1000 U/h after a loading dose of 5000 U. The aim is to keep the partial thromboplastin time (PTT) at 1.5 or 2 times normal, but it is very important to reach this level within the first day.[26] Low molecular weight heparins have also been shown to be effective in the treatment of thrombophlebitis without the inconvenience of blood tests. Warfarin can be started orally at the same time at 10 mg daily to prolong the international normalized ratio (INR) to 2.0 to 3.0 times normal. Warfarin should overlap heparin for 5 days until the necessary blood factors for blood clotting are depressed by the warfarin. Patients are then usually treated with warfarin for 3 months, which is the time of high frequency of recurrence of thrombophlebitis or pulmonary emboli. Thrombolytic agents have been used in acute deep venous thrombosis but have not been very successful; this may be due to patients presenting late in the course of the disease. They should be given a trial in iliofemoral or subclavian venous thrombosis when possible. Ambulation is usually allowed when symptoms and signs subside, but elastic stockings with 30 mmHg pressure should be worn for 3 months. In patients who have a contraindication to anticoagulation, hemorrhage during anticoagulation, or pulmonary emboli while adequately anticoagulated, the therapy of choice is insertion of an inferior vena cava filter.

When gangrene of the toes is impending in iliofemoral venous thrombosis, removal of the thrombus surgically will often alleviate the condition, even though there is rethrombosis of the vein. Septic thrombophlebitis is treated by removal of catheters and appropriate antibiotic therapy. However, resistant cases may require removal of the affected area of the vein.

PREVENTION Minidose heparin (5000 U subcutaneously every 8 to 12 h) has been shown to be effective prophylaxis against deep venous thrombosis for surgical patients and for patients with myocardial infarctions, strokes, and congestive heart failure. Minidose heparin does not protect patients undergoing orthopedic procedures or with fractures, but low molecular weight heparin is effective. Elastic stockings and early ambulation after surgery are also excellent preventive measures in combination with the above methods.

COURSE AND PROGNOSIS Most cases of thrombophlebitis subside within 10 days, but many patients have persistent limb swelling especially with iliofemoral and subclavian venous thrombosis. The postphlebitic syndrome may develop in some patients within 2 years, whereas it may not occur for 20 years in others.

Varicose Veins

Varicose veins are dilated, distended, tortuous veins with incompetent valves.

EPIDEMIOLOGY Varicose veins are more common in women than men and usually appear in women during the child-bearing

FIGURE 167-9

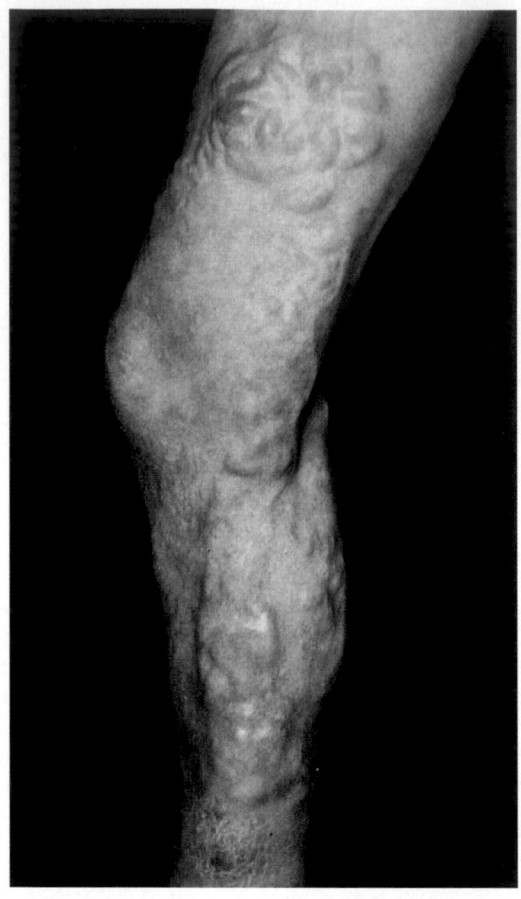

Extensive superficial varicose veins of the thigh and calf.

years. They are more common in countries where the population eats a low-fiber diet than in African countries where the diet is high in fiber.[27]

ETIOLOGY AND PROGNOSIS A hereditary influence in some patients with varicose veins is suggested by the presence of the disorder in several members of the same family and the appearance of varices during adolescence. Because varicosities, hemorrhoids, and diverticulae of the colon are infrequent in countries subsisting on a high-fiber diet, constipation, and hence increased intraabdominal pressure, has been incriminated for all three entities.[27] Pregnancy is one of the prime causes of varicose veins due to vein relaxation by the increased hormones, expansion of blood volume, and increased venous pressure, especially in the limb whose iliac vein is compressed by the enlarged uterus. Thrombophlebitis leads to the formation of varicosities by the destruction of venous valves. Arteriovenous communications also cause varices.

The first abnormality inducing varicosities is a weakening of the commissures of the valves with dilation.[28] The dilation leads to incompetence of the valves and increased venous pressure distally. The increased venous pressure creates a vicious cycle because it causes further dilation of the vein and valves. The increased venous pressure is transmitted to the capillaries, which results in leakage of fluid into the subcutaneous tissues and muscles.

CLINICAL MANIFESTATIONS *History* Most patients have no symptoms but seek medical advice because of the cosmetic appearance. Some patients do complain of fatigue or aching in the calves or swelling of the ankles at the end of the day. The swelling disappears with bed rest overnight. Rarely, patients with very large varicosities will complain of lightheadedness or blurry vision on standing due to venous pooling.

Physical examination Varicose veins can be seen as dilated, tortuous, sacculated superficial veins (Fig. 167-9). They are often thick walled. The greater saphenous vein is most commonly involved, but varicosities may be found anywhere on the legs and feet without involvement of the saphenous veins. There may be pitting edema at the ankle area or increased turgor of the calf muscles. In patients with very large varicosities, systemic blood pressure may fall on standing. Many patients have prominent, multiple, fine cutaneous veins on the thigh, which are not varicose veins; they usually appear after age 20 in females and increase in number.

LABORATORY AND SPECIAL EXAMINATIONS The incompetent valves of varicose veins can be demonstrated by applying a tourniquet on an elevated extremity so that the superficial veins are empty (Fig. 167-10). On the patient's assuming the erect posture, release of the tourniquet will allow rapid filling of a varicose vein if the valves are incompetent. Venography is seldom necessary but will show the dilated, tortuous veins and incompetent valves. Air plethysmography can document the degree of venous insufficiency (see "Postphlebitic Syndrome," below). Duplex scanning can visualize

FIGURE 167-10

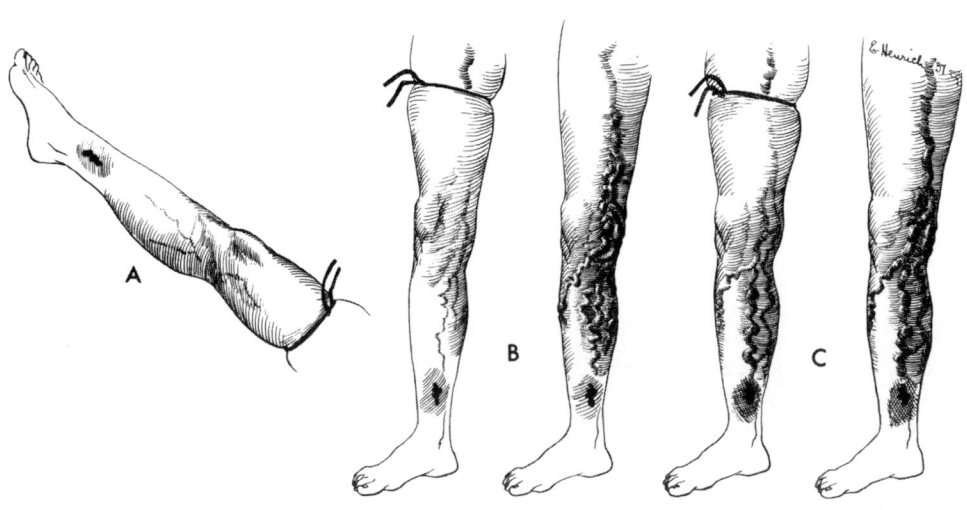

Varicose veins. Demonstration of venous reflux by the Trendelenburg test. *A.* Elevation of the leg empties the varices and a tourniquet is applied. *B.* While the patient is standing, varices remain empty until the tourniquet is removed, showing reflux from the saphenous vein. *C.* Reflux takes place via communicating veins before removal of the tourniquet, with additional reflux from the saphenous vein when the tourniquet is removed.

the valves, and color flow scanning can show reversal of venous flow during distal muscle compression.

PATHOLOGY The pathology is variable, with some varicose veins appearing normal but dilated so that the venous valves no longer are in opposition. Others show damaged, deformed valves and fibrotic vein walls.

DIAGNOSIS The diagnosis of varicose veins rests primarily on seeing and palpating the varices. The above tourniquet test will delineate the incompetent valves.

TREATMENT (See also Chap. 271) Symptoms from varicose veins respond to heavy-gauge elastic stockings (≥30 mmHg). Such stockings will prevent further enlargement of veins and edema but will not reverse the size of varicosities. Panty girdles or garters should never be worn. Ligation and stripping of vein are usually reserved for patients with very large and symptomatic varicosities. The operation has markedly decreased in popularity, since the veins may be needed in the future for arterial bypass. Small to medium-sized varicosities can be injected with a sclerosing solution [0.5 to 1 mL of sodium tetradecyl sulfate (Sotradecol) or concentrated saline solutions]. These solutions cause an inflammation and then fibrosis of the vein. Stab avulsion has been used successfully to remove clusters of varicose veins and to interrupt perforating veins in the leg; this method usually involves small incisions.

PREVENTION Many varicose veins would be prevented if women wore elastic support hose during pregnancy. Chronic constipation should always be avoided.

COURSE AND PROGNOSIS Without adequate external support, varicose veins continue to enlarge in most but not all patients. New varicose veins usually appear in a 10-year period after stripping or sclerosing injections. Some patients will develop a postphlebitic syndrome.

Postphlebitic Syndrome

The postphlebitic syndrome is characterized by edema, stasis pigmentation, and ulcers of the lower extremities due to venous stasis.

EPIDEMIOLOGY Studies are lacking on the epidemiology, but it is more common in females than males. Whites and blacks appear equally affected.

ETIOLOGY AND PATHOGENESIS The postphlebitic syndrome may occur soon after an episode of deep venous thrombosis or up to 20 years later.[29,30] It has been a common belief that most patients have had thrombophlebitis, although many do not give a history of the disease. It can occur in patients with superficial varicosities or incompetent deep veins; the perforating veins may also have defective valves.

Valve destruction occurs with thrombophlebitis and is the main factor in causing increased venous pressure in the leg. The edema is due to leakage of fluid from the capillaries. Stasis pigmentation is the result of red blood cell escape into the tissues, which results in an inflammatory reaction to the deposited hemoglobin. The exact mechanism of spontaneous ulcer formation is unknown. A reasonable explanation is that there is ischemia in the area in the erect state from the high venous pressure preventing capillary blood flow. Venous blood drawn from the ulcer area is often "black" from desaturation. Marked fibrosis in the subcutaneous tissue may develop,

and channels can be palpated where veins course in the fibrotic tissue.

CLINICAL MANIFESTATIONS *History* The patient complains of swelling of the limb, discoloration of the calf and ankle area, and breakdown of skin or ulcers. Since the ulcers are often painless, patients may not see a physician for several weeks to months after the beginning of an ulcer. A history of thrombophlebitis may or may not be obtained. Some patients will present with fever, chills, and redness of the involved extremity due to cellulitis.

Physical examination Pitting edema of the extremity is usually present, but varicose veins are not always apparent. There is brownish to dark pigmentation and often extensive scaling of the skin, especially on the medial side of the ankle and lower calf. Although cellulitis may occur, the leg may also be red, warm, and tender from an inflammatory reaction to the pigment in the dermis. Small erosions to very large but usually not deep ulcers may develop (Fig. 167-11). The ulcers usually have a red base of granulation tissue. They also occur on the medial ankle or lower calf in the majority of cases. Sometimes a fluctant area denoting an incompetent perforating vein can be palpated at the base or near an ulcer or a varicosity can be traced draining the ulcer area. The subcutaneous tissue may be indurated, and retraction of the subcutaneous tissue of the lower third of the leg may occur with pitting edema above it. One or both legs may be involved with signs of the postphlebitic syndrome.

LABORATORY AND SPECIAL EXAMINATIONS Incompetence of the superficial or deep venous system can be determined by tourniquet tests as described in the preceding section on varicose veins. Incompetent perforators can be detected by applying two tourniquets at various levels of an extremity with the veins empty (see

FIGURE 167-11

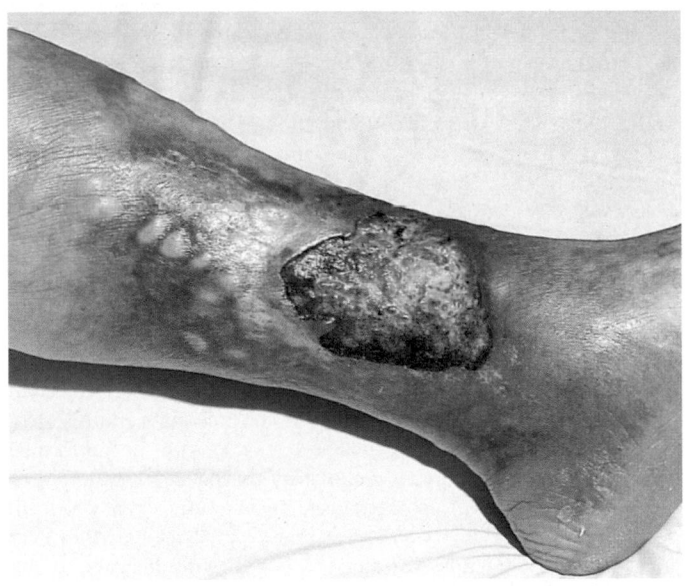

A large venous ulcer in a patient with the postphlebitic syndrome. This painless ulcer is shallow with good granulation tissue. Surrounding tissue shows typical stasis pigmentation, varicous veins, and subcutaneous tissue fibrosis and contraction.

Fig. 167-10). When the patient assumes the standing position, the segment of the superficial vein between the two tourniquets will fill when the underlying perforator has an incompetent valve. Before surgery, air plethysmography (APG) or high-resolution real-time ultrasonic imaging combined with Doppler pulsed-wave ultrasound should be performed. APG gives a measure of overall limb valvular incompetence and the effectiveness of the calf muscle pump. It measures calf venous volume changes in response to passive and active leg maneuvers in the supine and erect position. A venous filling index is calculated that indicates the volume of blood refluxing into the calf. Duplex scanning shows the diameter and location of the main venous trunks, evidence of obstruction or old venous disease, and actual visualization of the valves. Color flow scanning can image forward and reverse flow during muscle compression. Ascending venography with tourniquets as described above visualizes the incompetent perforator veins, and descending venography documents reflux; both are often used before surgery.

PATHOLOGY   In the area of postphlebitic changes there may be edema, inflammation, fibrosis, hemosiderin deposits, and tissue breakdown of the skin and subcutaneous tissues. In late cases, venous walls are thickened, and endothelial proliferation and fragmentation of the walls of venules and arterioles of the skin may be seen.

DIAGNOSIS AND DIFFERENTIAL DIAGNOSIS   The characteristic picture of edema, stasis pigmentation, and ulcers is diagnostic of the postphlebitic syndrome. The differential diagnosis includes lymphedema, which does not have stasis pigmentation or ulcers. Other causes of ulcers discussed below are usually painful, while venous ulcers are painless or only tender. Demonstration of superficial or deep venous valvular incompetence by plethysmography, Doppler, duplex scanning, or venography may be needed when varicosities are absent.

TREATMENT (See also Chap. 271)   The treatment of the postphlebitic syndrome is elastic compression to prevent venous stasis. Ace bandages or elastic stockings ($\geq$30 mmHg compression) must be worn throughout the day whenever the patient is sitting or standing. It also helps to sleep with the foot of the bed elevated 18 cm so that the patient starts the day with as little tissue fluid as possible. Itching or inflammation of stasis dermatitis usually yields to the application of glucocorticoids in cream or ointment. Unna boots are a very successful treatment method for venous ulcers and can be left in place for up to a week. The limb is encased in zinc oxide–impregnated bandages from the foot to above the ulcer and then wrapped with elastic compression bandage. Additional compression of the ulcer-bearing area or an obvious perforating vein is often necessary. Sponge rubber pieces can be cut to fit the area and applied under the elastic bandage. Systemic antibiotics may be needed for obviously infected ulcers or for a surrounding cellulitis. Debridement of fibrin covering material may have to be performed weekly. Patients can remain ambulatory during treatment. Hydrocolloid dressings have also been used successfully. It may help to perform sclerosing injections of varicose veins feeding the ulcer area. Small to moderate-size ulcers will heal with this regime, but large ulcers often need skin grafts. In the treatment of venous ulcers, surgery has been advocated but may be no better than conservative therapy.[31] With only superficial venous insufficiency, ligation and stripping of the greater or lesser saphenous system with or without subfascial ligation of incompetent perforating veins are effective in

healing venous ulcers. For deep venous insufficiency, valvuloplasty (with or without angioscopic visualization) of the proximal superficial femoral vein, vein transplantation or transfer, or replacement of the popliteal vein with an axillary vein with a competent valve has been advocated. A femorofemoral crossover graft has been used to bypass iliac vein obstruction.

PREVENTION   Elastic stockings with suitable venous compression will prevent progression of venous insufficiency to the postphlebitic syndrome. Similarly, elastic compression may prevent recurrence of venous ulcers late in the disease.

COURSE AND PROGNOSIS   Without treatment, stasis dermatitis will usually progress to venous ulceration. The course is then recurrent ulcers and episodes of cellulitis. With adequate elastic compression and sometimes surgical procedures to decrease venous pressure in the area, the course will stabilize. However, the prognosis depends on great effort and cooperation by the patient.

LYMPHEDEMA

Lymphedema is the occurrence of chronically swollen extremities due to an inadequate drainage of interstitial tissue fluid by the lymphatic vessels.

EPIDEMIOLOGY   The prevalence of primary lymphedema is less than 1 in 6000,[32] and it has a 1:3 male to females predominance. Secondary lymphedema is more common in countries with warm climates because of their higher prevalence of filariasis.

ETIOLOGY AND PATHOGENESIS   Primary lymphedema is most often seen in women and appears between ages 10 and 25 years.[33] It may be congenital, appear at puberty (praecox), or occur after age 35 (tardum) (Table 167-4). Milroy's disease is both familial and congenital. Other lymphatic defects causing yellow finger and

TABLE 167-4

Classification of Lymphedema

PRIMARY

Congenital
Familial (Milroy's disease)
Idiopathic
    Praecox
    Tardum
    Variant with yellow nails and pleural effusions

SECONDARY

Infection
    Bacterial
    Filariasis
Bartonella (cat-scratch fever)
Radical lymph node excision or surgical scarring
Malignant infiltration
Fibrosis
    Radiation therapy
    Stasis
    Localized myxedema
    Panniculitis
    Idiopathic or pharmacologic retroperitoneal fibrosis

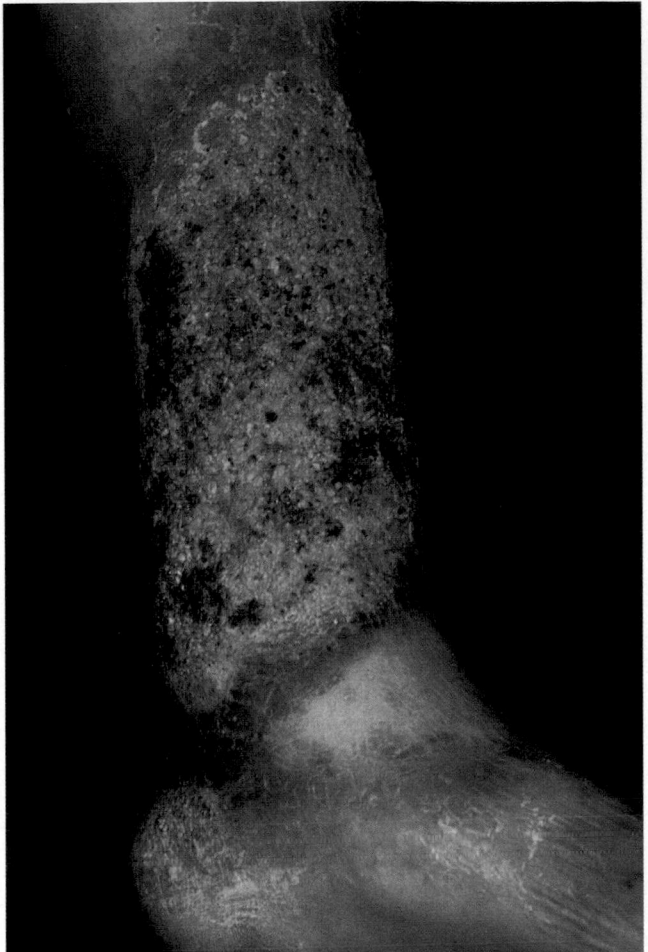

A.

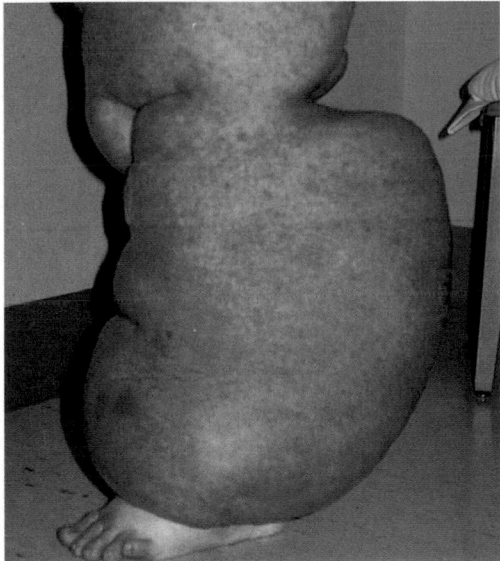

B.

A. Elephantiasis nostras verucosa. Edema has been replaced by fibrosis, pseudopapillomatosis, hyperkeratosis, and hyperpigmentation. *B.* Lymphedema of the left leg in a 47-year-old fireman. The extreme swelling began at birth and was painless. Note the lack of stasis pigmentation or ulceration. The patient functioned normally at work and wanted no treatment.

toe nails (yellow nail syndrome), chylous pleural effusions or ascites, malabsorption, or intrahepatic cholestasis may rarely accompany primary lymphedema. A genetic defect causing distichiasis and lymphedema affects males more than females.

Secondary lymphedema is due to obstruction of lymphatic flow by surgical removal or radiation fibrosis of lymph nodes, infiltration by malignancies of lymph vessels or nodes, or destruction of lymphatics by recurrent infections or filariasis.

The pathogenesis is the accumulation of tissue fluid due to a failure of lymphatic drainage.

CLINICAL MANIFESTATIONS *History* The patient often does not notice the swelling of the limb as the onset is very gradual and the edema is painless. The swelling may also disappear overnight, which leads to delay in seeking medical advice. The abdomen may swell with ascites. Intestinal lymphangiectasis may produce pale-colored stools and diarrhea. Secondary lymphedema will have symptoms of the underlying disease.

Physical examination There is soft, pitting edema of the distal extremity in the beginning. In the later stages, the swelling becomes indurated and nonpitting. The skin may thicken and resist wrinkling; hair follicles are prominent. A pebbled surface may develop and may lead to pseudopapillary growths and hyperkeratosis (Fig. 167-12A). Some patients proceed to develop disfigured extremities with thick folds of skin (Fig. 167-12B). Patients may present with cellulitis of the involved extremity because lymphedematous limbs are susceptible to infection.

In primary lymphedema, the lower extremities are involved most often and bilateral swelling occurs in about 50 percent of patients. In secondary lymphedema, usually only one extremity is involved. Discoloration of nails, distichiasis, jaundice, and signs of pleural effusion or ascites may occur rarely in patients with primary lymphedema.

LABORATORY AND SPECIAL EXAMINATIONS Invasive diagnostic tests are not usually necessary. Blood and urine studies are normal in primary and most cases of secondary lymphedema. Lymphoscintigraphy with radioisotope preparations is useful in differentiating lymphedema from other causes of extremity edema.[34] Lymphangiography is usually avoided since it is painful and involves an incision with the chance of infection.

PATHOLOGY The pathologic picture as determined by lymphangiography varies from aplasia or hypoplasia to varicosities of the lymphatic channels.[33] Primary lymphedema with distichiasis is associated with bilateral hyperplasia of the lymphatic vessels. In secondary cases, there may be neoplastic involvement of lymph nodes or fibrosis of lymph nodes and lymph vessels.

DIAGNOSIS AND DIFFERENTIAL DIAGNOSIS The diagnosis of lymphedema can usually be made by physical examination; the patient has a swollen, painless limb without varicosities, stasis pigmentation, or collateral veins (Table 167-5). Invasive tests are not necessary in most patients. Noninvasive studies of the venous system or venography may be indicated to rule out venous disease. Lymphoscintigraphy and rarely lymphangiography are used to distinguish the lipomatous nodular masses of lipodystrophy.

Secondary lymphedema should be considered in most patients before a diagnosis of primary lymphedema is made. A history of radiation or radium treatment, surgery of lymph nodes, or symptoms of malignancy should be ascertained. Patients from endemic areas

TABLE 167-5

Differential Diagnosis of Lymphedema

Postphlebitic syndrome	Idiopathic or cyclic edema
Edema of inactivity (old age)	Arthritis and synovitis
Hereditary "piano" legs	Panniculitis
Edema of constitutional disease	Localized myxedema
Lipodystrophy	

may need blood tests or biopsies for filariasis. Males should be carefully examined for prostate cancer, which often presents with a unilateral swollen limb due to lymph node invasion. An ultrasound examination of the abdomen is usually performed, especially in females, to rule out tumors or enlarged lymph nodes. Occasionally, women present complaining of swollen legs, but no edema or other pathology can be found in the large legs. This configuration of the legs is usually familial. Clues to the absence of pathology are symmetric measurements of the ankles, calves, and thighs; small ankles in comparison to the calves and thighs; and lack of edema.

TREATMENT It is important to minimize extremity edema to prevent subcutaneous fibrosis, skin thickening, and recurrent episodes

of cellulitis. Elastic garments with at least 30 mmHg pressure but sometimes as high as 60 mmHg must be worn from morning to bedtime. The elastic garments should have graded pressure from the distal to the proximal extremity. The patient should also sleep with the foot of the bed elevated 18 cm to promote drainage of tissue fluid overnight. A low-sodium diet and occasional but not continuous use of diuretics may be helpful. Administration of 5,6-benzo-[α]-pyrone (coumarin) has been shown to decrease the size of the arms and legs slowly and to improve symptoms in patients with primary and secondary lymphedema.[35] In patients with edema resistant to conservative measures, a sequential pneumatic compression device may be used. However, these machines must be used for at least 4 h on the extremity each night, are uncomfortable, and only move the fluid more proximally in some patients. Decongestive physical therapy may also help.

In very large incapacitating limbs or for the development of lymphangiosarcoma, various surgical procedures have been performed including removal of the subcutaneous tissue[33] and lymphovenous anastomoses.[36] Removal of the subcutaneous tissue leaves a very scarred but more usable limb. Lymphovenous anastomosis is less successful in primary than in secondary lymphedema. Lymphatic grafts are also being used with some benefit.[37]

PREVENTION In some patients, recurrent episodes of cellulitis and lymphangitis occur in the involved limb. Each attack destroys more lymphatic vessels and aggravates the lymphedema. These patients should be treated with antibiotic prophylaxis, usually

TABLE 167-6

Differential Diagnosis of Ulcers

TYPE	CAUSE	LOCATION	PAIN	CHARACTERISTICS
Venous	Postphlebitic syndrome Arteriovenous shunts	Medial lower leg–ankle	Absent to mild	Red base of granulation tissue; surrounding pigmentation, induration, edema; warm foot
Arterial				
Large vessel	Arteriosclerosis obliterans Thromboangiitis obliterans	Usually toes or foot	Severe	Black or gray base; shallow, irregular; no granulation tissue; cold foot with dependent rubor
Small vessel	Raynaud's phenomenon Vasculitis Atherosclerotic emboli	Toes, fingers, or lower legs	Severe	Irregular, inflamed edges, whitish base
Neurotrophic	Diabetes mellitus and other neuropathies; spinal cord lesions	Over metatarsal arch, heel, toes	None	Often deep and infected; surrounded by thick callus
Hypertensive	Hypertension	Lateral or posterior calf	Severe	Black to white base surrounded by purpura
Infectious	Bacterial, fungal, syphilis, tuberculosis	Arms or legs	Absent to moderate	Purulent, erythematous margins, raised edges, linear—may be multinodular in lymphatic distribution
Hematologic	Sickle cell anemia Thalassemia	Lower legs	Moderate	Often punched-out with sharp edges and deep; white base; can also resemble small vessel arterial ulcers
Neoplastic	Cancer, sarcoma	No predilection	Usually not painful	Raised edges above skin level; nonhealing
Pyoderma gangrenosum	Ulcerative colitis and unknown etiologies	Calves and thighs	Often severe	Black base with rolled edges of violaceous red color; often purulent

penicillin. The acute attacks produce a red, warm extremity with increased swelling; red streaks may be seen on the proximal extremity extending from the inflamed area, and regional lymph nodes may be enlarged and tender. Fever and leukocytosis may accompany the infection. The most common offending organisms are the coagulase-positive staphylococcus and the hemolytic streptococcus. Even when organisms cannot be cultured, therapy should be directed to these bacteria.

COURSE AND PROGNOSIS Primary lymphedema usually progresses to a chronically swollen limb. Some patients with primary, and many patients with secondary, lymphedema remain stable and do not progress. Malignant degeneration of the lymphatic vessels, called *lymphangiosarcoma,* develops in 1 percent of cases and is more common in secondary lymphedema due to mastectomies (Stewart-Treves syndrome). In lymphedema associated with Turner's syndrome, the edema has abated in some patients.

DIFFERENTIAL DIAGNOSIS OF ULCERS

Table 167-6 lists the common and some of the uncommon etiologies and characteristics of extremity ulcers. The most common ulcer is due to venous stasis. Arterial ulcers due to large vessel disease are next in frequency; then the neurotropic ulcers of diabetic neuropathy. Normal pulses are usually present in the limbs except in ulcers due to large vessel arterial disease. Pain is characteristically absent to mild in venous, neurotropic, and neoplastic ulcers. An ulcer with a red granulating base is usually venous. Excess callus formation around a painless ulcer on pressure points suggests a neuropathic ulcer (see Fig. 167-2). Very painful, often serpiginous ulcers occur on the feet and legs in vasculitis, connective tissue diseases, and livedo reticularis with ulceration (see Fig. 167-7). Most secondary

FIGURE 167-13

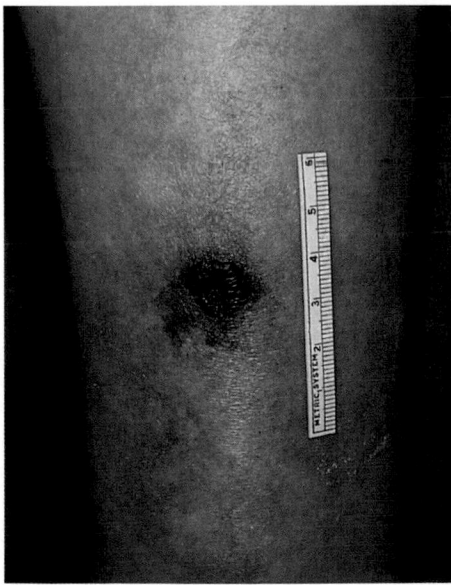

A hypertensive ulcer in a 56-year-old woman. The usual location is the lateral aspect of the calf. The base has a black eschar with surrounding ecchymotic tissue. Pain was extreme. All pulses in the extremity were normal.

causes of Raynaud's phenomenon may lead to digital ulcers. Ulcers may also occur in scleroderma over subcutaneous calcification and will not usually heal until the calcium is extruded. These ulcerations usually occur on the digits, wrists, elbows, knees, or ankles.

A painful ulceration may occur on the posterolateral aspect of the calf in hypertensive patients.[38] These lesions may start as purplish blebs and then ulcerate with a black eschar that is surrounded by purpura (Fig. 167-13). The etiology is unknown, but biopsy of surrounding tissue shows thrombosis and hyalinization of arterioles. A variety of infections may cause ulcerations, and diagnosis is usually difficult without a culture or biopsy. Ulceration of the nonischemic lesion of necrobiosis lipoidica in diabetes mellitus is uncommon. Malignancies of the skin must always be considered in indolent, nonhealing ulcers.

REFERENCES

1. Juergens JL et al: Arteriosclerosis obliterans: Review of 520 cases with special reference to pathogenic and prognostic factors. *Circulation* **21**:188, 1960
2. Coffman JD: Intermittent claudication and rest pain: Physiological concepts and therapeutic approaches. *Prog Cardiovasc Dis* **22**:53, 1979
3. Coffman JD: Principles of conservative treatment of occlusive arterial disease, in *Clinical Vascular Disease,* edited by JA Spittell Jr. Philadelphia, FA Davis, 1983, pp 1–13
4. Hood SC et al: Management of intermittent claudication with pentoxifylline. Meta-analysis of randomized controlled trials. *Can Med Assoc J* **155**:1053, 1996
5. Coffman JD: Atheromatous embolism. *J Vasc Med Biol* **1**:267, 1996
6. Kasinath BS et al: Eosinophilia in the diagnosis of atheroembolic renal disease. *Am J Nephrol* **7**:173, 1987
7. Mills JL et al: Buerger's disease in the modern era. *Am J Surg* **154**:123, 1987
8. Suzuki S et al: Buerger's disease (thromboangiitis obliterans): An analysis of the arteriograms of 119 cases. *Clin Radiol* **33**:235, 1982
9. Coffman JD: *Raynaud's Phenomenon.* New York, Oxford University Press, 1989
10. Maricq HR et al: Geographic variation in the prevalence of Raynaud's phenomenon—Charleston, S.C., U.S.A. vs Tarentaise, Savoie, France. *J Rheumatol* **20**:70, 1993
11. Edward JM et al: α_2-Adrenergic receptor levels in obstructive and spastic Raynaud's syndrome. *J Vasc Surg* **5**:38, 1987
12. Coffman JD, Cohen RA: α_2-Adrenergic and $5HT_2$-receptor hypersensitivity in Raynaud's phenomenon. *J Vasc Med Biol* **2**.100, 1990
13. Nielsen SL: Raynaud's phenomenon and finger systolic pressure during cooling. *Scand J Clin Lab Invest* **38**:765, 1978
14. Maricq HR et al: Diagnostic potential of in vivo capillary microscopy in scleroderma and related disorders. *Arthritis Rheum* **23**:183, 1980
15. Gifford RW, Hines EA: Raynaud's disease among women and girls. *Circulation* **16**:1012, 1957
16. Farmer RG et al: Raynaud's disease with sclerodactylia. *Circulation* **23**:13, 1961
17. Sneddon IB: Cerebrovascular lesions and livedo reticularis. *Br J Dermatol* **77**:180, 1965
18. Weinstein C et al: Livedo reticularis associated with increased titers of anticardiolipin antibodies in systemic lupus erythematosus. *Arch Dermatol* **123**:596, 1987
19. Winkelmann RK et al: Clinical studies of livedoid vasculitis (segmental hyalinizing vasculitis). *Mayo Clin Proc* **49**:746, 1974
20. William CM, Goodman H: Livedo reticularis. *JAMA* **85**:955, 1925
21. Milstone LM et al: Classification and therapy of atrophie blanche. *Arch Dermatol* **119**:963, 1983
22. Abramson DJ: Mondor's disease and string phlebitis. *JAMA* **196**:1087, 1966
23. Coffman JD: Deep venous thrombosis and pulmonary emboli: Etiology, medical treatment and prophylaxis. *J Thorac Imag* **4**:4, 1989
24. Lensing AWA et al: Detection of deep vein thrombosis by real-time B-mode ultransonography. *N Engl J Med* **320**:342, 1989

25. Barnes RW et al: The fallibility of the clinical diagnosis of venous thrombosis. *JAMA* **234**:605, 1975

26. Hull RD et al: Continuous intravenous heparin compared with intermittent subcutaneous heparin in the initial treatment of proximal vein thrombosis. *N Engl J Med* **315**:1109, 1986

27. Burkitt DP: Varicose veins: Facts and fantasy. *Arch Surg* **111**:1327, 1976

28. Edward EA, Edwards JE: The effects of thrombophlebitis on the venous valve. *Surg Gynecol Obstet* **65**:310, 1937

29. Jacobs P: Pathogenesis of the postphlebitic syndrome. *Annu Rev Med* **34**:91, 1983

30. McEnroe CS et al: Correlation of clinical findings with venous hemodynamics in 386 patients with chronic venous insufficiency. *Am J Surg* **156**:148, 1988

31. Rodriquez AA, O'Donnell TF Jr: Surgical management of chronic venous insufficiency, in *Current Therapy in Vascular Surgery,* edited by CB Ernst, JC Stanley. St. Louis, Mosby, 1995, pp 914–919

32. Dale RF: The inheritance of primary lymphoedema. *J Med Genet* **22**:274, 1985

33. Kinmonth JB: *The Lymphatics: Diseases, Lymphography, and Surgery.* Baltimore, Williams & Wilkins, 1972

34. Weisseleder R, Thrall JH: The lymphatic system: Diagnostic imaging studies. *Radiology* **172**:315, 1989

35. Casley-Smith JR et al: Treatment of lymphedema of the arms and legs with 5,6-benzo-[α]-pyrone. *N Engl J Med* **329**:1158, 1993

36. Glovickzki P et al: Microsurgical lymphovenous anastomosis for treatment of lymphedema: A critical review. *J Vasc Surg* **7**:647, 1988

37. Baumeister RG, Siuda S: Treatment of lymphedemas by microsurgical lymphatic grafting: What is proved? *Plastic Reconstr Surg* **85**:64, 1990

38. Schnier BR et al: Hypertensive ischemic ulcer: A review of 40 cases. *Am J Cardiol* **17**:560, 1966

CHAPTER 168

Thomas J. Lawley
Kim B. Yancey

Skin Changes and Diseases in Pregnancy

Cutaneous changes and eruptions during pregnancy are exceedingly common and in some cases a cause for substantial anxiety on the part of the prospective mother. These alterations may range from normal cutaneous changes that occur with almost all pregnancies, to common skin diseases that are not associated with pregnancy, to eruptions that appear to be specifically associated with pregnancy. Likewise, the concerns of the patient may range from cosmetic appearance, to the chance of recurrence of the particular problem during a subsequent pregnancy, to its potential effects on the fetus in terms of morbidity and mortality. In this chapter the cutaneous changes that are specifically associated with pregnancy are reviewed.

HORMONAL CHANGES

Pregnancy is a time of significant and complex physiologic changes. Some of these changes are due to the de novo production of a variety of protein and steroid hormones by the fetoplacental unit as well as by the increased activity of the maternal pituitary, thyroid, and adrenal glands. The currently recognized hormones produced by the placenta include the protein hormones human chorionic gonadotropin (HCG), human placental lactogen (HPL) or human somatomammotropin, human chorionic thyrotropin, and human chorionic corticotropin, as well as the steroid hormones progesterone and estrogen.[1,2] A description of the chemistry, function, and metabolism of these hormones is beyond the scope of this chapter, but it should be kept in mind that the production and the serum levels of these hormones are dynamic. For instance, HCG levels peak between the 10th and 12th weeks of gestation, although they remain elevated throughout pregnancy. The levels of progesterone and estrogen rise throughout the first and second trimesters of pregnancy and plateau during the third trimester. The levels of these hormones are of diagnostic significance in certain obstetric conditions and complications, but their exact impact on cutaneous physiology as well as their influence on the immunology of the skin and the inflammatory response are essentially unknown.

Cutaneous Changes Commonly Associated with Pregnancy

Although the influences that the individual hormones have on the skin are incompletely understood, it is thought that they are responsible, either primarily or secondarily, for many of the cutaneous changes that normally occur during pregnancy.

PIGMENTATION The nipples, areolae, and external genitalia become hyperpigmented during pregnancy. The linea alba becomes the pigmented linea nigra. Occasionally hyperpigmentation is noted in the axillae and the proximal medial portions of the thighs. The most noticeable pigmentary change during pregnancy is the development of a masklike hyperpigmentation of the face, known as chloasma or melasma, in over 50 percent of women[3] (Fig. 168-1). This tendency is exacerbated by sun exposure in susceptible individuals and may also be exacerbated by birth control pills in nonpregnant women. Additionally, preexisting nevi or ephelides frequently darken during pregnancy. The degree of hyperpigmentation tends to be related to the skin type of the individual, with lightly complected individuals developing less intense pigmentation. In all of these instances there is usually partial, and at times complete, regression of the hyperpigmentation occurring gradually after termination of pregnancy. The physiology of the hyperpigmentation appears to be related to the increased production of estrogens and perhaps to increased levels of progesterone or melanocyte stimulating hormone.

HAIR Mild to moderate hirsutism is frequently seen during pregnancy. The hirsutism tends to resolve shortly after delivery or in some instances in the third trimester. After delivery, the resulting telogen effluvium may be severe, resulting in significant hair loss from 1 to 5 months postpartum. In these instances regrowth, usually within 1 year, is the rule.

CONNECTIVE TISSUE The most common change in connective tissue is the development of striae distensae over the abdomen, hips, buttocks, and sometime the breasts (Fig. 168-2). Striae distensae occur in up to 90 percent of pregnant women.[4] The exact cause of

FIGURE 168-1

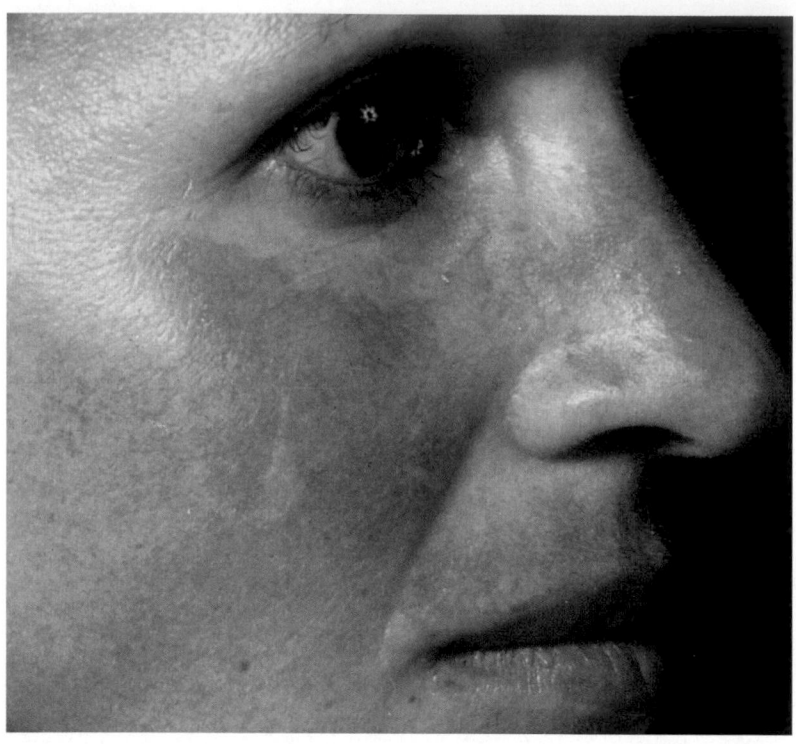

Melasma.

FIGURE 168-2

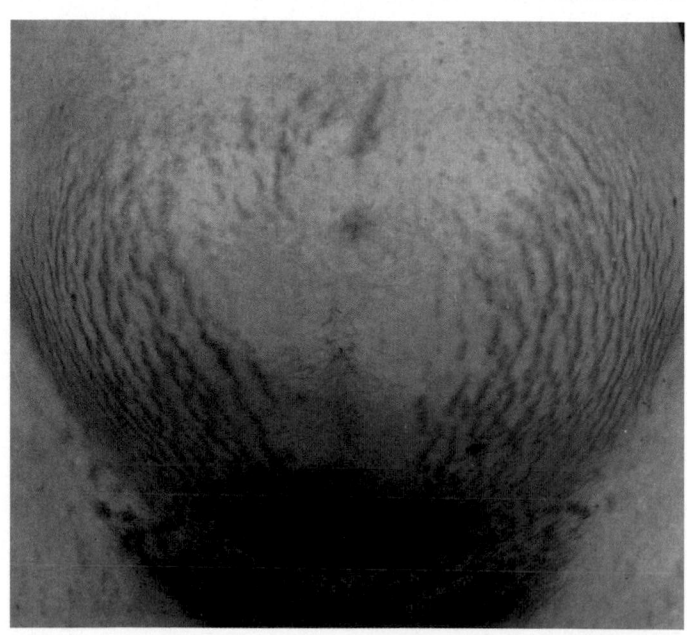

Striae distensae.

striae is unknown, although a combination of increased adrenal cortical activity associated with increased lateral stress on the connective tissue due to increased size of the various portions of the body is thought to be important. Striae distensae initially appear as pink to purple atrophic bands (Fig. 168-2) sometimes associated with mild pruritus. Following delivery, they become pale and less apparent. Skin tags, also known as molluscum fibrosum gravidarum, often appear on the lateral portions of the neck and axillae during pregnancy and may persist after delivery.

VASCULAR Hyperemia is physiologic during pregnancy. This, combined with a tendency toward vascular proliferation, results in a number of common cutaneous changes during pregnancy. Up to two-thirds of women develop palmar erythema and/or spider angiomas during pregnancy.[5] Vascular distention resulting in part from increased intraabdominal pressure is thought to be responsible for the edema and venous varicosities that commonly occur on the legs and feet. Hemorrhoids also occur for the same reasons. Vascular tumors such as glomus tumors or hemangiomas may appear or enlarge during pregnancy. The pregnancy tumor of the gingiva is a pyogenic granuloma that may appear in the second or third trimester and resolves shortly after delivery.

WELL-DEFINED DERMATOSES ASSOCIATED WITH PREGNANCY

A variety of cutaneous diseases have been reported to be associated with pregnancy (Table 168-1). Most of these "diseases" are poorly characterized both clinically and pathophysiologically. In a number of instances their very existence as disease entities is in doubt. Even with diseases that are reasonably well-defined clinically, there is some dispute with regard to nomenclature. The section that follows describes the best-known and most common of these dermatoses.

Pemphigoid (Herpes) Gestationis

Pemphigoid (herpes) gestationis is an extremely pruritic, recurrent, bullous dermatosis of pregnancy and the immediate postpartum period. Herpes gestationis is a misnomer, since it is not related to any active or prior viral infection. Pemphigoid gestationis has been suggested as an alternative name for this disease and will be used

TABLE 168-1

Dermatoses of Pregnancy

Well-defined eruptions
   Pemphigoid (herpes) gestationis
   Pruritic urticarial papules and plaques of pregnancy (PUPPP)
   Recurrent cholestasis of pregnancy
   Impetigo herpetiformis
Poorly defined eruptions
   Prurigo gestationis (Besnier)
   Papular dermatitis of pregnancy (Spangler)
   Follicular eruption of pregnancy
   Autoimmune progesterone dermatitis

throughout this chapter. Pemphigoid gestationis is immunologically mediated. This disease is discussed in Chap. 64.

Pruritic Urticarial Papules and Plaques of Pregnancy

Pruritic urticarial papules and plaques of pregnancy (PUPPP) is a common, intensely pruritic dermatosis that usually occurs late in the third trimester of pregnancy. It typically affects primigravidas.

HISTORY The eruption was first described in detail and named by Lawley et al. in 1979.[6] Previously Nurse[7] and Bourne[8] reported similar eruptions that probably represented PUPPP. Nurse termed these eruptions *prurigo of pregnancy–late type,* and Bourne used the term *toxemic rash of pregnancy.* Subsequently, Holmes et al.[9] used the name *polymorphous eruption of pregnancy* to describe a somewhat similar group of patients.

CLINICAL FEATURES PUPPP is characterized by the onset of tiny (1- to 2-mm) erythematous papules on the abdomen, most often in the latter part of the third trimester of pregnancy.[6,10–15] The papules frequently begin in the striae distensae (Fig. 168-3A) but soon coalesce to form large erythematous plaques centered on the umbilicus. The lesions are extraordinarily itchy, and patients frequently are unable to sleep at night. Curiously, despite the intense pruritus, excoriations are extremely unusual. The urticarial papules and plaques spread over the course of a few days to involve the buttocks and thighs (Fig. 168-3B). The morphology of the lesions as well as their anatomic progression is in general rather uniform from patient to patient. In some instances, lesions also occur on the arms, forearms, and legs. Lesions on or above the breasts are rare, and lack of involvement of the face is a characteristic feature. Close observation of the primary erythematous papules often reveals a surrounding narrow pale halo. Occasionally some papules are so edematous as to appear as papulovesicles.

Almost all reported cases have begun in the third trimester and most after the 35th week. The onset of PUPPP in the immediate postpartum period is rare. Although this eruption can occur in any pregnancy, it is most frequently seen in primigravidas. In the experience at the National Institutes of Health with 25 patients, 19 (76 percent) were primigravidas.[10] All of these patients had their onset of disease in the third trimester except one, who developed lesions in the immediate postpartum period. The average time of onset was the 36th week of gestation, and the most frequent week of onset was the 39th. In all 25 patients, lesions began on the abdomen, and nearly one half specifically indicated onset in their periumbilical striae distensae. One study found an increased maternal weight gain, increased neonatal birth weight, and an increased incidence of twinning in 30 patients with PUPPP. These findings suggested that abdominal distention or a reaction to it may play a role in the development of this disorder.[16] In contrast, these features were not documented in 22 patients studied by Roger and co-workers.[17]

HISTOPATHOLOGY AND IMMUNOFLUORESCENCE The histopathologic findings in PUPPP are not specific. Biopsy of skin reveals a superficial and often mid-dermal perivascular lymphohistiocytic infiltrate associated, in some cases, with a variable number of eosinophils and edema of the papillary dermis. Epidermal changes may include mild focal spongiosis and parakeratosis.

Direct immunofluorescence microscopy of lesional or perilesional skin shows no specific immunoreactants.

FIGURE 168-3

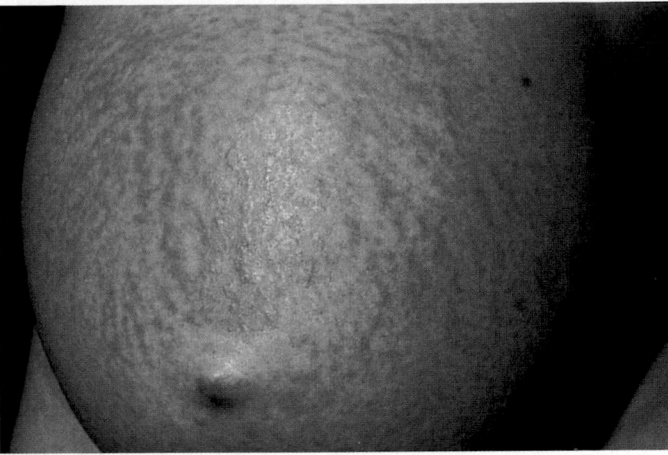

A.

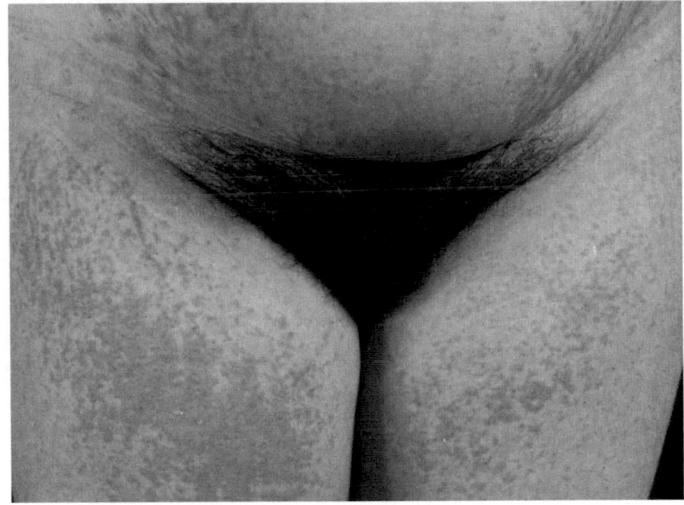

B.

Pruritic urticarial papules and plaques of pregnancy. *A.* The earliest lesions are tiny erythematous papules frequently localized to the striae distensae. *B.* They then coalesce to form erythematous plaques and spread to involve buttocks and thighs.

COURSE The natural history of PUPPP appears to be spontaneous resolution of most cases within a few days after delivery. Unlike pemphigoid gestationis, postpartum onset or exacerbation of PUPPP is exceptional. It tends not to recur in subsequent pregnancies, although a few cases have been reported. Moreover, there does not appear to be an increased incidence of fetal morbidity or mortality associated with it.[10] There is one report of an infant being born with lesions.[11] In our series of patients with PUPPP, follow-up revealed that eight patients had subsequent pregnancies and that none was complicated by PUPPP.[10]

DIFFERENTIAL DIAGNOSIS In most instances the diagnosis of PUPPP is not difficult. The classic presentation is a primigravida late in the third trimester with an extraordinarily pruritic eruption of papules and plaques that began in periumbilical striae distensae and then spread to involve the buttocks and thighs, yet spared the upper chest and face. Pemphigoid gestationis must be considered as a diagnostic possibility in some instances, although usually prominent vesicular and/or bullous lesions are found in these patients. Direct immunofluorescence microscopy of perilesional skin should be performed if pemphigoid gestationis is considered.

It must be kept in mind that all of the eruptions that occur in nonpregnant individuals may also occur in pregnancy and should not be confused with those dermatoses that are apparently pregnancy-specific. Thus erythema multiforme, drug eruptions, contact dermatitis, urticaria, and insect bites can at times be confused with PUPPP (or other pregnancy-related dermatoses).

TREATMENT   Intense (five or six times per day) therapy with potent topical glucocorticoids provides symptomatic relief in almost all cases. New lesions usually stop appearing within 2 to 3 days, and most patients can then begin to taper the frequency of applications. In many instances patients are able to stop all therapy before delivery. Brief tapering courses of systemic corticosteroids also provide relief. H_1 antihistamines are not as effective as potent topical glucocorticoids.

Recurrent Cholestasis of Pregnancy (Prurigo Gravidarum)

Recurrent cholestasis of pregnancy, also known as *prurigo gravidarum* or *benign recurrent intrahepatic cholestasis,* is a hepatic condition usually occurring late in pregnancy and first manifested by severe generalized pruritus followed by the appearance of clinical jaundice. It is thought to be hormonally induced in susceptible individuals. Its incidence has been estimated at 0.02 to 2.4 percent of pregnancies.[18]

HISTORY   Recurrent cholestasis of pregnancy was first separated from other causes of jaundice in pregnancy by Svanborg and Ohlsson.[19]

CLINICAL FEATURES   Recurrent cholestasis of pregnancy has no primary cutaneous lesions although secondary excoriations may occur. The first symptom of recurrent cholestasis of pregnancy is pruritus. The severity may vary from moderate to severe, and in the early stages the pruritus may manifest itself only at night. Although often localized at first, the pruritus tends to become generalized.[20] The pruritus may precede the onset of clinical jaundice by up to 4 weeks although, rarely, it can be much longer. Patients may complain of fatigue and anorexia and, in some instances, may develop nausea and vomiting. Most cases occur during the third trimester, although the onset has been reported as early as the first trimester. In fully developed cases numerous excoriations may be seen in conjunction with icterus. Patients may complain of right quadrant fullness or tenderness as well as dark urine and light colored stools. Although the diagnosis of this disorder is largely clinical, laboratory studies may reveal elevations in hepatic transaminases and total serum bile salts. Postprandial determinations of the latter are probably one of the most sensitive indicators of this disorder.[14,21]

COURSE   The pruritus associated with recurrent cholestasis of pregnancy usually remits within a few days after delivery. The disorder tends to recur in subsequent pregnancies, and there have been reports of several members of families being affected, suggesting a genetic predisposition in some instances.[22] There have also been documented instances where patients who had developed recurrent cholestasis of pregnancy developed cholestatic jaundice while taking synthetic estrogens and progestational agents for contraception.[22] It is not entirely clear whether estrogen or progesterone is the primary inciting agent; they may work synergistically. The precise pathophysiology of the cholestasis is unknown. There have been patients who have been diagnosed with recurrent cholestasis of pregnancy who did not develop clinical jaundice.

The incidence of prematurity and low birth weights is increased in the offspring of patients with recurrent cholestasis of pregnancy.[14] Postpartum hemorrhage is also more likely in these women. The incidence of untoward events seems to be highest in patients with both jaundice and pruritus.[23]

TREATMENT   Attempts should be made to control pruritus with bland emollients and topical antipruritic regimens. In many instances these provide adequate relief. Antihistamines are at times of some benefit. Cholestyramine may occasionally be effective.[24] Some have advocated the administration of vitamin K before delivery to diminish the risk of postpartum hemorrhage (and offset deficiency of this fat-soluble vitamin).

Impetigo Herpetiformis

Impetigo herpetiformis is a form of pustular psoriasis that occurs during pregnancy and may be life-threatening (see also Chap. 43). It is exceedingly rare and only approximately 100 cases have been reported.[25]

HISTORY   This disorder was first reported in 1872 by von Hebra in five pregnant women, four of whom died.[26]

CLINICAL MANIFESTATIONS   Impetigo herpetiformis tends to occur in the third trimester of pregnancy, although cases have been reported as early as the first trimester. Many of the affected women have had no personal or family history of psoriasis. Reoccurrences in subsequent pregnancies have been reported.

The earliest lesions are erythematous patches occurring in the groin, axillae, and anterior as well as posterior neck.[27] At their margins these erythematous patches are studded with tiny superficial pustules (Fig. 168-4). The lesions expand by peripheral extension, with new pustules occurring at the leading edges while the old pustules at the interior of the expanding lesions break down, resulting in crusting or in some cases impetiginization. Pruritus is unusual in impetigo herpetiformis. Large areas of the body may be affected eventually, and in flexural areas the lesions may become vegetative. In some cases mucous membranes may be affected and subungual pustules can cause onycholysis.

Most patients also have constitutional signs and symptoms, the most common being fever and chills accompanied at times by nausea, vomiting, and diarrhea. In the past, delirium, convulsions, and tetany secondary to hypocalcemia were often reported; but these complications as well as bacterial sepsis are infrequently seen in the modern era.

HISTOLOGY   The histopathology of impetigo herpetiformis is the same as that of pustular psoriasis. The characteristic finding in an early lesion is the presence of collections of polymorphonuclear neutrophils in spongiotic foci in the epidermis, known as *spongiform pustules of Kogoj.* In mature lesions, the spongiform pustules become quite large and may assume a subcorneal location. Parakeratosis and elongation of rete ridges are often found.

FIGURE 168-4

CHAPTER 168
Skin Changes and Diseases in Pregnancy 1967

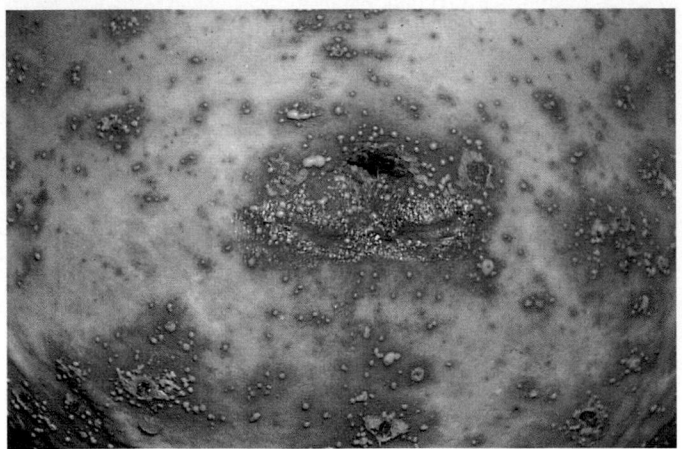

Impetigo herpetiformis. This is pustular psoriasis occurring in pregnancy. Erythematous patches are studded with tiny superficial pustules.

LABORATORY RESULTS Elevated white blood cell counts and sedimentation rates are quite common in impetigo herpetiformis. When these occur in the presence of fever, infection must be ruled out. The unopened pustules are sterile, but the skin may become secondarily infected. Decreased serum calcium and serum albumin levels are sometimes found.

COURSE The disease tends to remit promptly after delivery but may recur in subsequent pregnancies.[28] There may be an increased risk of fetal morbidity and mortality associated with placental insufficiency.

TREATMENT Systemic glucocorticoids are the treatment of choice in impetigo herpetiformis, with prednisone in doses of up to 60 mg per day being necessary at times to control the eruption.[28–31] Once under control, the prednisone can be tapered judiciously, but there is a risk of sudden exacerbation of disease if it is tapered too rapidly.

Patients should be monitored for systemic and cutaneous infections and treated with appropriate antibiotics when indicated. Serum calcium and albumin levels should also be followed, and replacement therapy undertaken if levels become too low.

POORLY DEFINED ERUPTIONS ASSOCIATED WITH PREGNANCY

Prurigo Gestationis (Besnier)

Prurigo gestationis is a pruritic dermatosis that may occur any time in the fourth to ninth months of gestation but has peak incidence between the 20th and 34th weeks of pregnancy. It is characterized by the occurrence of small papules, most of which are excoriated, on the proximal limbs and upper trunk. In some instances the limb lesions tend to be distributed on extensor surfaces. Although Costello estimated a 2 percent incidence of prurigo gestationis in otherwise normal pregnancies, this is clearly a large overestimation.[32] Nurse[7] suggested an incidence of 0.5 percent, but this also is probably much too high. Moreover, as much as 25 percent of Nurse's series of patients probably had PUPPP.

The eruption tends to resolve quickly after delivery, although postinflammatory hyperpigmentation may persist for some time. Therapy with topical glucocorticoids is helpful. It is uncommon for prurigo gestationis to recur in subsequent pregnancies, and there is no known increased incidence of fetal morbidity or mortality associated with it.

Papular Dermatitis of Pregnancy

Papular dermatitis of pregnancy is a rare, controversial eruption described by Spangler et al. in 1962.[33] The very existence of this disease is in doubt owing to the paucity of subsequent reports of well-described cases. Spangler estimated the incidence to be 1 case in 2400 pregnancies, but this is surely a vast overestimation.

CLINICAL MANIFESTATIONS As described by Spangler, papular dermatitis of pregnancy is a pruritic eruption that may begin at any time during pregnancy. It is characterized by the appearance of small erythematous papules, usually 3 to 5 mm in diameter, that are often surmounted by a 1- to 2-mm central papule or central crust. Spangler indicated that the lesions were excoriated so rapidly that it was extremely rare to find an intact papule. The distribution of the lesions was generalized with no predilection for any area.

HISTOLOGY Spangler did not report biopsies of any of his cases. A biopsy of an unexcoriated papule in a case reported by Michaud et al.[34] showed hyperkeratosis, spongiosis, exocytosis, elongation of the rete ridges, and a perivascular infiltrate of lymphocytes in the papillary dermis. Direct immunofluorescence testing of skin for deposits of IgG, IgA, IgM, and C3 was negative.

LABORATORY RESULTS Patients with papular dermatitis of pregnancy are said to have markedly elevated levels of urinary chorionic gonadotropin. Some patients have also been reported to have low levels of urinary estriol[35] and plasma hydrocortisone. The half-life of plasma hydrocortisone is said to be decreased for the group as a whole.

TREATMENT Therapy with systemic glucocorticoids reportedly controls the eruption.[4,18] Doses of up to 100 mg of prednisone per day have been reported to be necessary in some patients.

Diethylstilbestrol, once recommended by Spangler and Emerson,[35] should not be used due to the increased risk of vaginal carcinoma in offspring born to mothers treated with this agent. Spangler later withdrew his therapeutic recommendation.[36]

COURSE The disease has been reported to recur in subsequent pregnancies. Spangler reported a 27 percent incidence of fetal death in untreated cases, whereas there was no fetal loss in treated cases. A recent careful reevaluation of these data has demonstrated a 12 percent incidence of fetal loss in patients with papular dermatitis of pregnancy.[3] The previously reported higher incidence was caused by the inclusion of fetal wastage in pregnancies in which there was no cutaneous eruption. Several of these mothers would almost surely be classified as habitual aborters today. The exact basis and existence of the disorder has been in doubt for many years.

Miscellaneous Disorders

Six patients with an eruption termed *pruritic folliculitis of pregnancy* were described by Zoberman and Farmer.[37] The onset of their eruption ranged from the fourth to the ninth month of gestation and their lesions consisted of 3- to 5-mm excoriated, erythematous papules. The lesions were generalized in five patients and confined to the extremities and abdomen in one. The striking feature of the histopathology of five of these cases was the presence of folliculitis, with the hair follicles showing intraluminal pustule formation. The skin biopsy of one patient did not reveal folliculitis but only a mild perivascular infiltrate in the upper dermis and parakeratosis at the edges of the acrotrichium. Direct immunofluorescence microscopy was negative in all four patients tested. Two patients reported similar eruptions in previous pregnancies. All of the offspring born of these pregnancies were healthy. Of the five patients available for follow-up, the eruption resolved in two at delivery, in two one month after delivery, and in one spontaneously within a week of onset.

An eruption termed *autoimmune progesterone dermatitis of pregnancy* has been reported in one patient.[38] The eruption was characterized by the appearance of papules and pustules on the extensor surfaces of the thighs, arms, forearms, hands, and buttocks. The eruption began early in pregnancy and the patient experienced a spontaneous abortion in the third month. The patient reported a similar eruption associated with a previous pregnancy that also terminated in a spontaneous abortion in the second month. The eruption was exacerbated by an oral contraceptive. Intradermal skin tests with aqueous progesterone produced delayed hypersensitivity reactions whose histology was similar to that found in naturally occurring lesions. However, the patient did not develop an exacerbation of her skin lesions premenstrually, a time during which progesterone levels are elevated. The exact relation of progesterone to this eruption as well as the existence of autosensitivity to progesterone is unclear.[3]

In 1988, Alcalay and colleagues described a patient who developed an intensely pruritic eruption of firm erythematous papules on the forearms, legs, thighs, and abdomen in the third trimester of pregnancy.[39] The patient had no vesicles, bullae, urticarial plaques, or erosions; histologic finds were nonspecific. Immunoflorescence microscopy studies showed dense, continuous deposits of IgM in the epidermal basement membrane; there was no evidence of circulating IgM, IgG, or IgA anti-basement membrane autoantibodies in the patient's serum. The eruption cleared after delivery. Based on the findings in this patient, the authors proposed that this eruption be termed *linear IgM dermatosis of pregnancy*. The relationship of this patient to those described by Velthuis and co-workers remains to be determined.[40]

In 1992, Zurn and colleagues[41] described five third-trimester patients with a pruritic, erythematous papular and/or urticarial eruption of the trunk who had low levels of circulating IgM autoantibodies directed against the epidermal side of $1\,M$ NaCl split skin. Three of five patients examined had no evidence of immunoreactants in their epidermal basement membranes by direct immunofluorescence microscopy. IgM in these patients' sera did not immunoblot any proteins in epidermal extracts. The eruption in four of five patients resolved within 4 to 10 days. In subsequent studies Borradori and co-workers[42] found that the frequencies of circulating IgM anti–basement membrane antibodies in 52 patients with the polymorphic eruption of pregnancy, 69 healthy pregnant controls, and 42 nonpregnant women were the same (12, 10, and 14 percent of these groups, respectively). These investigators also found that 12 to 14 percent of pregnant patients (both those with polymorphic eruption of pregnancy and those with normal gestations) had IgM reactive with epidermal proteins by immunoblotting. Such reactivity was seen only in 2 percent of the sera from normal, nonpregnant women.

These workers concluded that there is no evidence for the existence of an *IgM anti-basement membrane autoantibody dermatosis of pregnancy,* and that pregnancy may be associated with low levels of IgM reactivity against epidermal (and perhaps other) proteins.

REFERENCES

1. Jaffe RB: Endocrine physiology of normal pregnancy, in *Obstetrics and Gynecology,* edited by DN Danforth. Philadelphia, Harper & Row, 1982, p 342
2. Osathanondoh R, Tulchinsky D: Placental polypeptide hormones, in *Maternal-Fetal Endocrinology,* edited by D Tulchinsky, KJ Ryan. Philadelphia, Saunders, 1980, p 17
3. Winton GB, Lewis CV: Dermatoses of pregnancy. *J Am Acad Dermatol* **6**:977, 1982
4. Scoggins RB: Skin changes and diseases in pregnancy, in *Dermatology in General Medicine,* 2d ed, edited by TB Fitzpatrick et al. New York, McGraw-Hill, 1979, p 1363
5. Demis DJ: Skin conditions during pregnancy, in *Clinical Dermatology,* edited by DJ Demis et al. Hagerstown, MD, Harper & Row, 1980, p 1
6. Lawley TJ et al: Pruritic uritcarial papules and plaques of pregnancy. *JAMA* **241**:1696, 1979
7. Nurse DS: Prurigo of pregnancy. *Australas J Dermatol* **9**:258, 1968
8. Bourne G: Toxemic rash of pregnancy. *Proc R Soc Med* **55**:462, 1962
9. Holmes RC et al: A comparative study of toxic erythema of pregnancy and herpes gestationis. *Br J Dermatol* **106**:499, 1982
10. Yancey KB et al: Pruritic urticarial papules and plaques of pregnancy (PUPPP): Clinical experience in 25 patients. *J Am Acad Dermatol* **10**:473, 1984
11. Ulhin SR: Pruritic urticarial papules and plaques of pregnancy. *Arch Dermatol* **117**:238, 1981
12. Ahmed AR, Kaplan R: Pruritic urticarial papules and plaques of pregnancy. *J Am Acad Dermatol* **4**:679, 1981
13. Callen JP, Hanno R: Pruritic urticarial papules and plaques of pregnancy (PUPPP): A clinicopathologic study. *J Am Acad Dermatol* **5**:401, 1981
14. Roger D et al: Specific pruritic diseases of pregnancy: A prospective study of 3192 pregnant women. *Arch Dermatol* **130**:734, 1994
15. Aronson IK et al: Immunopathology of pruritic urticarial papules and plaques of pregnancy. *J Invest Dermatol* **94**:504, 1990
16. Cohen LM et al: Pruritic urticarial papules and plaques of pregnancy and its relationship to maternal-fetal weight gain and twin pregnancy. *Arch Dermatol* **125**:1534, 1989
17. Roger D et al: Pruritic urticarial papules and plaques of pregnancy are not related to maternal or fetal weight gain (letter). *Arch Dermatol* **126**:1517, 1990
18. Sasseville D et al: Dermatoses of pregnancy. *Int J Dermatol* **20**:223, 1981
19. Svanborg A, Ohlsson S: Recurrent jaundice of pregnancy. *Am J Med* **27**:40, 1939
20. Holzbach RT: Jaundice in pregnancy. *Am J Med* **61**:367, 1976
21. Laatikainen TJ, Tulenheimo A: Maternal serum bile acid levels and fetal distress in cholestasis of pregnancy. *Int J Gynaecol Obstet* **22**:91, 1984
22. DePagter AGF et al: Familial benign recurrent intrahepatic cholestasis. *Gastroenterology* **71**:202, 1976
23. Johnston WG, Baskett TF: Obstetric cholestasis: A 14-year review. *Am J Obstet Gynecol* **133**:299, 1979
24. Laatikainen T: Effect of cholestyramine and phenobarbital on pruritus and serum bile levels in cholestasis of pregnancy. *Am J Obstet Gynecol* **132**:501, 1978
25. Braverman IM: Pregnancy and the menstrual cycle, in *Skin Signs of Systemic Disease.* Philadelphia, Saunders, 1981, p 761
26. von Hebra F: On some affections of the skin occurring in pregnant and puerperal women. *Wien Med Wochenschr* **48**:1197, 1872. Abstracted in *Lancet* **1**:399, 1872
27. Baker H, Ryan TJ: Generalized pustular psoriasis: A clinical and epidemiological study of 104 cases. *Br J Dermatol* **80**:771, 1968
28. Beveridge GW et al: Impetigo herpetiformis in two successive pregnancies. *Br J Dermatol* **78**:106, 1966
29. Sauer G: Impetigo herpetiformis. *Arch Dermatol* **83**:119, 1961
30. Oosterling RJ et al: Impetigo herpetiformis. *Arch Dermatol* **114**:1527, 1978
31. Oumeish OY et al: Some aspects of impetigo herpetiformis. *Arch Dermatol* **118**:103, 1982

32. Costello MJ: Eruptions of pregnancy. *NY State J Med* **41**:849, 1941
33. Spangler AS et al: Papular dermatitis of pregnancy. *JAMA* **181**:577, 1962
34. Michaud RM et al: Papular dermatitis of pregnancy. *Arch Dermatol* **118**:1003, 1982
35. Spangler AS, Emerson K: Estrogen levels and estrogen therapy in papular dermatitis of pregnancy. *Am J Obstet Gynecol* **110**:534, 1971
36. Spangler AS: Letter to the editor. *Am J Obstet Gynecol* **113**:570, 1972
37. Zoberman E, Farmer E: Pruritic folliculitis of pregnancy. *Arch Dermatol* **112**:1534, 1976
38. Bierman SM: Autoimmune progesterone dermatitis. *Arch Dermatol* **107**:896, 1973
39. Alcalay J et al: Linear IgM dermatosis of pregnancy. *J Am Acad Dermatol* **18**:412, 1988
40. Velthuis PJ et al: Is there a linear IgM dermatosis? Significance of linear IgM junctional staining in cutaneous immunopathology. *Acta Dermatol Venereol (Stockh)* **68**:8, 1988
41. Zurn A et al: A prospective immunofluorescence study of 111 cases of pruritic dermatoses of pregnancy: IgM anti-basement membrane zone antibodies as a novel finding. *Br J Dermatol* **126**:474, 1992
42. Borradori L et al: IgM autoantibodies to 180- and 230- to 240-kDa human epidermal proteins in pregnancy. *Arch Dermatol* **131**:43, 1995

CHAPTER 169

Ruth K. Freinkel

Diabetes Mellitus

Diabetes mellitus is a metabolic disorder characterized by disturbances in traffic of fuels, primarily as affected by insulin. The abnormalities arise from heterogeneous mechanisms that fall into two major groups: insulin-dependent diabetes mellitus (IDDM), also known as type 1, and non-insulin-dependent diabetes mellitus (NIDDM), also known as type 2. IDDM, which frequently but not always begins in younger life, is characterized by absolute deficiency in pancreatic and circulating insulin. Patients commonly (60 to 90 percent) have circulating antibodies to pancreatic islet cells and distinctive patterns of major histocompatibility antigens. NIDDM occurs in older populations, is often linked to obesity, and frequently has a hereditary pattern. Pancreatic and circulating insulin are not lacking but are insufficient to meet the needs of peripheral tissues.

Disposition of ingested nutrients and recall of endogenous fuels are faulty in all types of diabetes. The common denominator is insufficient action of insulin on peripheral tissues. Whereas this is due to lack of pancreatic insulin in IDDM, in NIDDM the problem is one of relative insufficiency despite the presence of insulin stores in the pancreas and even high levels of circulating insulin. Sluggish release of insulin from the pancreas in response to glucose challenge, peripheral resistance to insulin action at the level of tissue receptors,[1] and abnormal insulin[2] are among the pathogenic mechanisms operative in NIDDM.

The acute derangements resulting in hyperglycemia, hyperlipidemia, symptomatic diabetes, and ketoacidosis are usually correctable by appropriate therapy. However, all forms of diabetes are associated in the long term with multiple degenerative disorders affecting the cardiovascular system, nervous system, eyes, and skin. Effects on large and small blood vessels (macro- and microangiopathy) are the cardinal pathologic factors, although direct effects of the metabolic derangements on certain tissues may play a sig-

nificant role. It is generally accepted that the changes are all due to chronic metabolic derangements that are not entirely regulated by available hypoglycemic strategies. Although there is some evidence that prolonged "tight" control may lessen degenerative complications or even induce regression of vascular changes (e.g., thickened capillary basement membranes), practical long-term therapeutic regimens have not been developed to meet such ends.

The skin shares both in the effects of acute metabolic derangements and in the chronic degenerative complications of diabetes. This is not surprising, as the skin is an actively metabolizing tissue depending on insulin and circulating fuels for metabolic and biosynthetic activity.

Insulin affects the utilization of glucose in skin, even though it is not required to facilitate the entry of glucose into epidermal cells. The increase in apparent intracellular content of glucose in diabetic skin suggests that insulin regulates glucose disposition in cutaneous cells.

Insulin profoundly affects various cutaneous compartments. It is required for growth and differentiation of keratinocytes in culture systems. Healing of experimental wounds, which involves both dermis and epidermis, is delayed in diabetic animals until they are treated with insulin. However, the most pronounced effects of insulin may be on the dermal fibroblasts. In experimental diabetes there is less soluble dermal collagen and it is more cross-linked.[3] These changes parallel the findings in dermal collagen of diabetic individuals, which shows a decrease in acid-soluble collagen and more glycosylation than in age-matched controls.[4] Dermal fibroblasts from diabetic mice produce more fibronectin than do control cells.[5]

Consideration of the cutaneous manifestations of diabetes may be divided into those that accompany acute metabolic derangements and those that correlate with the presence of chronic degenerative complications. In addition, there are dermatologic disorders that occur more frequently in diabetic patients but that do not correlate with either acute metabolic derangements or degenerative changes.

CUTANEOUS MANIFESTATIONS CORRELATED WITH GROSS METABOLIC DERANGEMENTS

Certain cutaneous disorders occur in diabetic patients specifically in relation to hyperglycemia and hyperlipidemia and are reversible when these abnormalities are corrected.

Infections

Poorly controlled diabetes may be associated with bacterial and fungal infections of the skin. The infections most frequently encountered are staphylococcal pyodermas, candidiasis, erythrasma, and epidermophytosis. Although the prevalence of the latter two appears to be increased in diabetic patients, such a correlation has not been established for staphylococcal and candidal infections. Moreover, it is not clear whether the diabetic host is more susceptible to infection or less able to deal with it once the infection is established.

Abnormalities in leukocyte function, including diminished chemotaxis, phagocytosis, and killing of organisms, have been demonstrated in diabetic individuals who are hyperglycemic.[6] Such effects may also include the consequences of insulin lack on insulin-dependent action of cytokines such as interleukins.[7] The diminished leukocyte response may also be due to the inability of leukocytes to migrate through thickened capillary walls as well as to the diminished diffusion of nutrients to sustain extravascular inflammatory cells. Furthermore, repair of minor trauma may be affected both by delayed wound healing and compromised dermal vasculature, thereby providing access for pathogenic organisms.

Vulvovaginitis due to *Candida albicans* is a common complication of poorly controlled diabetes. Involvement of other intertriginous skin and nails is frequently seen together with the vaginal infection. The candidiasis responds readily to control of hyperglycemia and does not occur more frequently in aglycosuric diabetic patients than in the normal population. Although generalized pruritus is not a feature of diabetes,[8] vulvar itching with candidiasis should alert the clinician to the possible presence of diabetes unless other obvious precipitating causes can be invoked.

Pyodermas, especially furunculosis, were formerly a more serious complication of diabetes. The availability of antibiotics and better control of diabetes has lessened both the morbidity and incidence of septic skin infections in the diabetic population. Nonetheless, pyogenic infections do occur more frequently in patients whose diabetes is poorly controlled; conversely, control of well-regulated diabetes can be interrupted by intercurrent pyogenic infection.

Infections of the lower extremities constitute a particular hazard for the diabetic patient. The presence of atherosclerosis and peripheral neuropathy leads to ulceration and gangrene as well as poor wound healing. The damaged and devitalized skin provides a fertile breeding ground for secondary infections. Moreover, the increased incidence of epidermophytosis of the feet provides portals of entry for pathogenic organisms.

Prevention of such infections requires meticulous care of the feet. Such care should be incorporated into every diabetic regimen and includes the regular services of a podiatrist and twice-daily foot washing with tepid water followed by thorough drying and use of emollients. Prompt attention to foot wounds, blisters, minor infections, and epidermophytosis is indicated.

Xanthomatosis (See also Chap. 152)

Hyperlipidemia involving triglycerides and cholesterol more than phospholipids is common in diabetic individuals, even in those with rather mild elevations of blood glucose. Xanthomas, secondary to the chylomicronemia, are characteristically multiple and tend to occur rapidly in crops. Small reddish-yellow nodules up to 0.5 cm in diameter present in clusters primarily on extensor surfaces and buttocks. They may be pruritic initially and are much smaller and more inflammatory than the tendon and tuberous xanthomas associated with hypercholesterolemia. They are clinically indistinguishable from xanthomas secondary to other states associated with chylomicronemia.

The lesions are laden with neutral lipid–rich histiocytes. Ultrastructural studies have demonstrated that chylomicrons migrate through the dermal capillary walls and are phagocytosed by tissue macrophages and perithelial cells. In freshly erupted xanthomas, the lipid composition of the lesion reflects that of plasma chylomicrons, containing about 45 percent triglycerides. Resolving or evolving lesions gradually lose triglycerides and become relatively richer in cholesterol. Rapid regression occurs when diabetes is brought under control.

Xanthelasma occurs in most hyperlipidemic states, including diabetes, but it may occur without demonstrable abnormality of plasma lipids; it does not usually regress when therapy for diabetes is instituted. Hyperlipidemia is sometimes accompanied by yellowish discoloration of the palms, soles, and nasolabial folds due to deposition of carotene.

CUTANEOUS MANIFESTATIONS OF DIABETES CORRELATED WITH CHRONIC DEGENERATIVE COMPLICATIONS

It is now generally accepted that microangiopathy characteristic of diabetes occurs in the dermal vasculature as well as in other small blood vessels and may result in decreased cutaneous blood flow. Reduplication and thickening of basement membranes have been shown in diabetic skin.[9] Veil cells are seen more frequently surrounding cutaneous vessels. It has been postulated that these cells produce excessive amounts of basement membrane–like material, accounting for vascular thickening (see Chap. 24). In addition to changes in blood vessels, there are changes in dermal connective tissue and in cutaneous innervation. Thus, the cutaneous manifestations that appear to correlate with multisystem degenerative complications are probably attributable to biochemical and anatomic disturbances within the skin itself.

Diabetic Dermopathy

These lesions were first described as atrophic, circumscribed, brownish lesions of the lower extremities.[10] The presence of small blood vessel changes led to the term *diabetic dermopathy*,[11] although the pathogenic significance of vascular changes in relation to the lesions remains to be established. The lesions are asymptomatic, irregularly shaped patches occurring primarily over the anterior lower legs; their surfaces are depressed and they have a light brown color (Fig. 169-1). Lesions appear in crops and gradually resolve over 12 to 18 months; however, the constant appearance of new lesions gives the impression of a stationary course. Although the initial reports[10,11] did not note antecedent cutaneous changes, other authors[12,13] have noted the presence of red patches, sometimes with scaling and erosion, prior to the development of the pigmented atrophic patches. Despite their resemblance to scars, recall of antecedent trauma is seldom elicited.

Histologically, dermal arterioles and capillaries display intimal thickening and deposition of periodic acid–Schiff (PAS)-positive fibrillar material in vessel walls. Capillary basement membranes are thickened with focal deposition of PAS-positive material. Hemosiderin and extravasated red cells are often present, and accumulation of leukocytes around vessels has been described.

Although these lesions are not clinically distinguishable from posttraumatic scarring on the legs of older patients with compromised circulation, they appear more frequently and in greater numbers in diabetic individuals. They are more common in men than women (2:1) and are often accompanied by evidence of significant microangiopathy elsewhere.

Erythema and Necrosis

Reddening of the face (rubeosis faciei) and of the extremities has been described in long-standing diabetes. Erysipelas-like areas on the lower legs and feet, which may or may not eventuate in frank necrosis, and destructive lesions of underlying bone have also been described.[14] These painless areas are often edematous and do not differ clinically from the erythema that accompanies gangrene of the toes and feet due to arterial insufficiency. Cardiac failure, unilateral edema from venous occlusion, and arterial insufficiency have been cited as precipitating factors.

Bullous Lesions

Although the appearance of bullae in diabetic individuals was noted earlier, the first carefully studied series of 15 patients was presented in 1963.[15] In this and subsequent reports, the bullae appeared spontaneously, usually on the extremities, especially the feet (Fig. 169-2). Generally the bullae heal in several weeks without significant scarring, although they may recur. The bullae are subepidermal, and ultrastructural studies have demonstrated the plane of separation to be in the basement membrane zone above the basal lamina. In some cases distribution of the lesions in light-exposed areas suggests porphyria cutanea tarda, but abnormalities of porphyrin metabolism have not been found. Neither trauma nor immunologic mechanisms have been implicated.

The cause of this rare manifestation of diabetes is unknown. At least 75 percent of patients have significant diabetic retinopathy, and in one series of three patients dermopathy and cutaneous angiopathy were present.[11] The localization of the plane of separation suggests that weakness in the basement membrane zone is an underlying factor. That this may be the case is suggested by the presence of a reduced threshold to formation of suction blisters on the forearms of insulin-dependent diabetics.[16]

Thickened Skin, Stiff Joints, and Scleredema Adultorum

As many as one-third of diabetic patients (both IDDM and NIDDM) have tight, thickened, and waxy skin over the dorsa of the hands.[17] An associated change is the presence of multiple, minute, flesh-

FIGURE 169-1

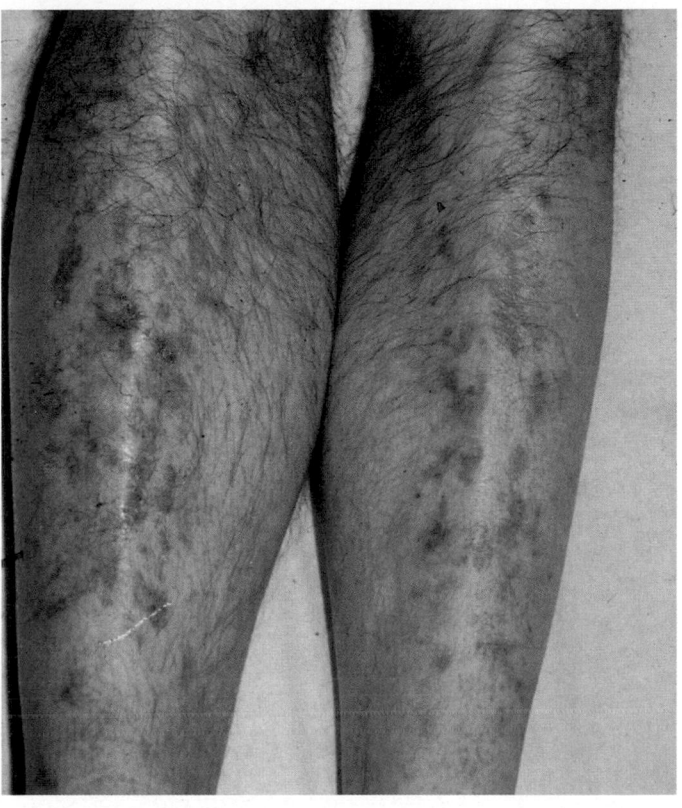

Diabetes mellitus with diabetic dermopathy. Hyperpigmented scars are seen on the anterior lower leg at sites of trauma. The absence of hair on the lower legs is associated with peripheral vascular disease.

FIGURE 169-2

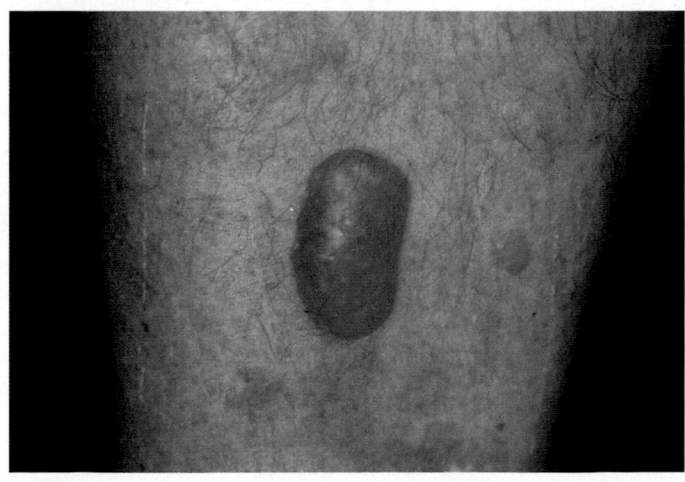

Diabetes mellitus with bullous dermatosis. Two intact bullae are seen on the anterior lower leg.

FIGURE 169-3

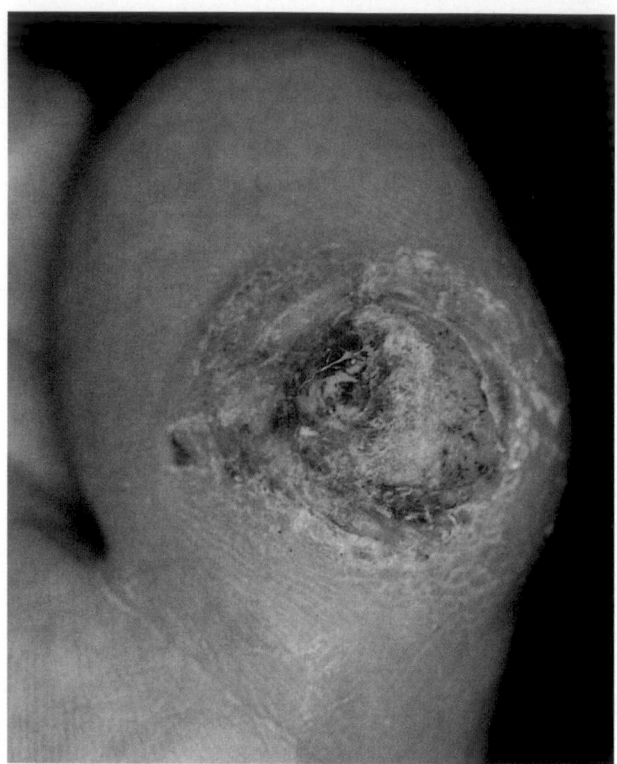

Diabetes mellitus with neuropathy and neuropathic ulcer. A large ulcer is present on the plantar aspect of the great toe, surrounded by a ring of callus and associated with diminished sensation. Osteomyelitis of the underlying bone is common.

colored papules (pebbles) on the dorsum of the fingers, knuckle pads, and periungual areas. A possibly related connective tissue change is limited mobility of joints, especially of the proximal interphalangeal joints of patients with IDDM. The contractures can be demonstrated by an inability to approximate the palmar surfaces of the fingers when the palms are pressed together. The changes are strongly correlated with an increased risk for microangiopathy.

Scleredema adultorum, a well-defined entity (see Chap. 187), has been recognized as a cutaneous manifestation of diabetes. It consists of induration of the skin beginning on the posterior and lateral neck. The painless swelling may gradually spread to the face, shoulders, anterior neck, and upper torso; it may eventually involve the abdomen, arms, and hands. The hard skin does not pit on pressure. Demarcation from normal skin may be sharp or poorly defined.

Histologically there are thickened collagen bundles and deposition of glycosaminoglycans, chiefly hyaluronic acid, in the dermis.

In contrast to the identical changes occurring after infection (especially streptococcal), scleredema associated with diabetes may not remit even after long periods of time. Diabetic scleredema occurs mainly in obese diabetic individuals with evidence of vascular complications.

Although the underlying mechanisms for these various connective tissue abnormalities remain to be elucidated, it may be postulated that they represent the clinical manifestations of altered metabolism of collagen and mucopolysaccharide due to insulin deprivation.

Cutaneous Neuropathy

Autonomic disturbances may accompany the sensory neuropathy that is a common degenerative complication (Fig. 169-3). This may manifest as anhydrosis, either confined to extremities or generalized. Involved areas of skin show abnormalities in autonomic fibers adjacent to eccrine sweat glands.[18]

CUTANEOUS DISORDERS THAT ARE MORE COMMON IN DIABETES WITHOUT REGARD TO METABOLIC DERANGEMENTS OR DEGENERATIVE CHANGES

Certain skin disorders are more frequently associated with diabetes. Although the literature abounds with reports of well-defined cutaneous diseases occurring more frequently in diabetics, only a few of these associations have withstood careful scrutiny.

Necrobiosis Lipoidica Diabeticorum

This very distinctive skin disease is perhaps the best example of such an association, occurring in about 0.3 percent of diabetic patients. These relatively asymptomatic lesions, which are three times more common in women than in men, are characteristically found on the anterior and lateral surfaces of the lower legs. They may also be present on the face, arms, and trunk. There may be one or several lesions, either unilaterally or bilaterally. The lesion begins as a small, dusky-red elevated nodule with a sharply circumscribed border. It slowly enlarges, becoming a plaque irregular in outline, flattened, and eventually depressed as the dermis becomes more atrophic (Fig. 169-4). The color becomes more brownish yellow except for the border, which may remain red. Coalescing or enlarging lesions may in time encompass the entire anterior tibial area. The epidermis is smooth or slightly scaly and atrophic. Delicate vessels can be seen through the surface (Fig. 169-4). The lesions may be anesthetic due to destruction of cutaneous nerves.[19] The lesions of necrobiosis lipoidica diabeticorum (NLD) are extremely chronic and indolent; shallow, often painful ulcers frequently appear in long-standing lesions. In the early stages, NLD may resemble granuloma annulare or sarcoid, but the well-developed plaque is characteristic and easily recognized.

The primary pathologic changes are in the lower dermis, where collagen is markedly altered with focal areas of loss of normal structure, swelling, basophilia, and distortion of the bundles (necrobiosis). Cross-striations and diameters of collagen fibers are irregular. Although the amount of collagen is actually decreased, the relative proportions of types I and III are preserved. Fibroblasts cultured from lesional skin have been reported to make less collagen.[20] There is also loss and fragmentation of elastic fibers. There is increased collagenase in the lesional skin.[21]

In these areas, there are aggregations of inflammatory cells including epithelioid cells, histiocytes, and multinucleated giant cells, sometimes containing asteroid bodies. The late appearance of foam cells accounts for the designation *lipoidica*. The vasculature is always involved, with endothelial proliferation and occlusion of the lumina of arterioles and venules. Capillary walls are thickened with

FIGURE 169-4

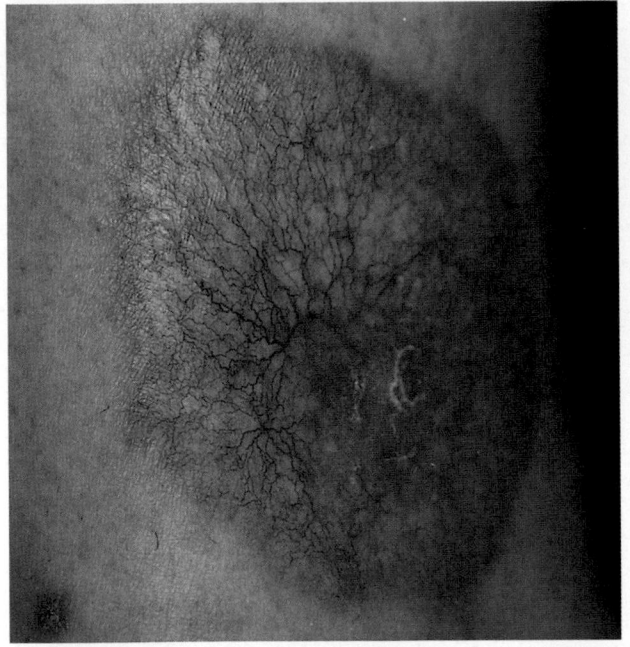

A.

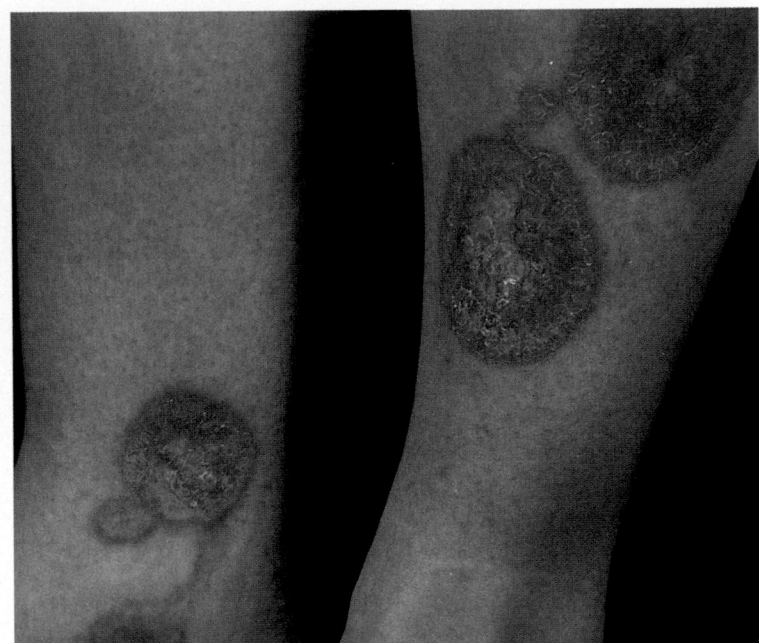

B.

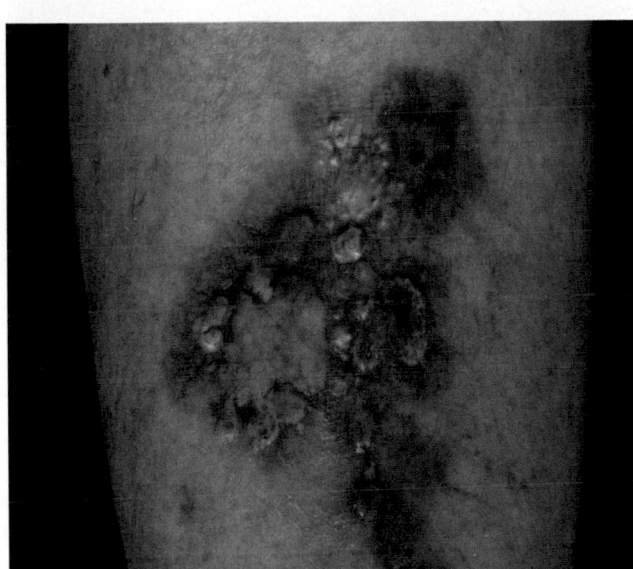

C.

Diabetes mellitus with necrobiosis lipoidica diabeticorum (NLD). *A.* A single orange plaque with atrophy of the overlying epidermis and arborizing telangiectasis is seen on the lower leg of a juvenile diabetic; the crust marks an area of early ulceration. *B.* Older lesions with striking central atrophy involving both the epidermis and dermis. *C.* NLD of longstanding duration with sharply demarcated atrophic areas, sites of healed ulcerations.

focal deposits of PAS-positive material that may also be present in the lumen.

The precise correlation between NLD and diabetes remains somewhat controversial. The disease was first described in patients with well-established diabetes but subsequently reported in patients without evident diabetes. In a study of 171 patients,[22] the majority had diabetes when NLD developed; in most of the rest, diabetes developed later, or there were other stigmata such as a close relative with the disease or abnormal cortisone-glucose tolerance tests. Only about 10 percent of patients with NLD do not fall into any of these categories. The induction of abnormal carbohydrate tolerance with glucocorticoids has been demonstrated in most patients with NLD and without evident diabetes.[23]

Thus, despite the lack of full concordance, NLD seems to be a valid marker for diabetes. However, the nature of the association and the pathogenesis remain unclear. Because NLD occurs in both IDDM and NIDDM, its pathogenesis cannot be related to genetic factors, underlying autoimmune disease, or other causes of diabetes. It can be reasonably assumed that the granulomatous response is secondary to alterations in dermal collagen. The controversy concerns the nature of the degenerative change in collagen. It is not clear whether this is secondary to an underlying vascular disease or develops independently. The latter would ascribe the changes in dermal collagen and vasculature to some primary disorder of connective tissue (as yet unknown). However, the invariable presence of arteriolar changes deep into and within the areas of collagen degeneration suggests an interrelation between the two components of NLD. It has been hypothesized that increased platelet aggregation may be a trigger factor in the vascular changes.

Immunoglobulins, complement (C3 and C4), and fibrinogen are present in blood vessels in lesional and, in some cases, nonlesional skin.[24] These findings are in concordance with the presence of inflammatory changes in adjacent clinically normal skin. Whether or not an immune process is a factor in the pathogenesis of NLD has not been resolved.

Treatment of NLD is not very satisfactory. Progression of lesions does not correlate with normalization of hyperglycemia. Local therapy with topical applications of glucocorticoids under occlusion or by intralesional injection may afford some improvement of active lesions. There have been some enthusiastic reports on the use of aspirin and dipyridamole, but these were not confirmed in a rigorous double-blind trial.[25] In rebuttal it has been pointed out that the dose of aspirin is a critical factor in achieving an optimal effect on platelet aggregation, and that favorable effects were obtained with very small doses of aspirin: 3.5 mg/kg every 48 to 72 h.[26] Among other agents that have been reported to be helpful are clofazimine, nicotinamide, and pentoxifyllin.

Granuloma Annulare (See Chap. 99)

Similarity between the pathologic changes of NLD and granuloma annulare and sporadic reports of diabetes in patients with granuloma annulare have led to a search for the presence of an abnormal carbohydrate metabolism in the latter disease. Although there is little evidence to support association of overt diabetes with granuloma annulare, abnormal carbohydrate metabolism after cortisone administration has been reported by some authors. Others have failed to confirm such findings in patients with typical disease.

Vitiligo (See Chap. 88)

Vitiligo occurs with greater than expected incidence (4.8 percent) in patients with NIDDM. It may precede the onset of clinically evident diabetes. Vitiligo has also been reported in association with IDDM; in one series, four out of five children also had autoantibodies to adrenal, thyroid, or gastric parietal cells. Such autoantibodies have not been reported in patients with NIDDM and vitiligo in the absence of other endocrine disease. The association of the pigment disorder and diabetes per se thus requires further clarification.

Acanthosis Nigricans (See also Chap. 186)

This disorder is characterized by velvety papillomatous hyperplasia of the epidermis with intense hyperpigmentation most prominently displayed in axillary, inguinal, and inframammary folds and in creases of the neck (Fig. 169-5). In more severe forms it may be more generalized and accompanied by verrucous patches on knuckles and other extensor surfaces, hyperkeratosis of the palms and soles, and other hyperplastic lesions. Acanthosis nigricans is associated with two types of disorders. The more severe form is usually

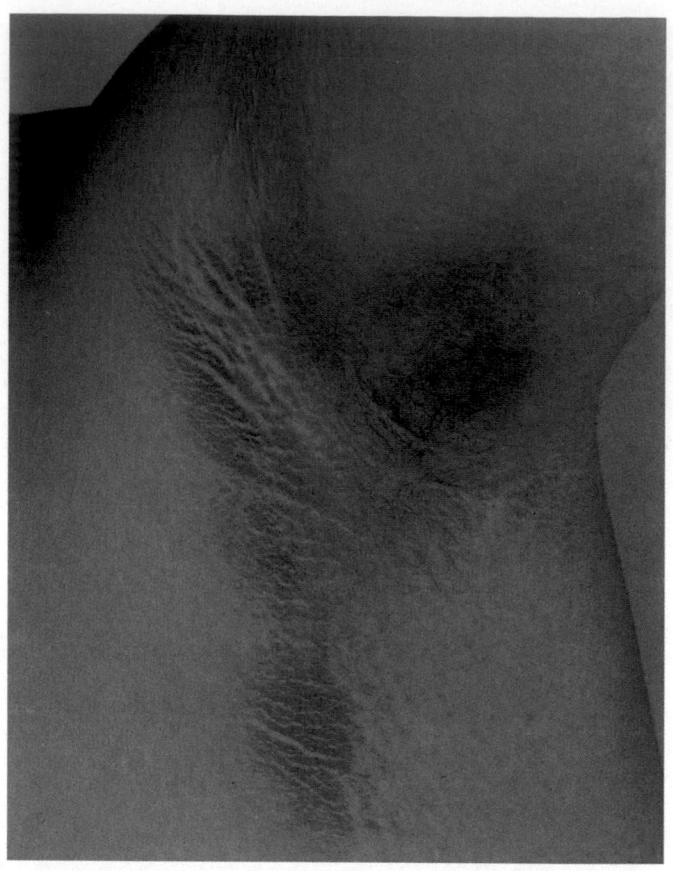

Diabetes mellitus with acanthosis nigricans. Velvety, papillomatous hyperplasia of the skin with hyperpigmentation is seen in the axilla of the patient with insulin-resistant diabetes mellitus.

found in patients with advanced malignant disease. The more limited form is more frequently found in association with a variety of endocrinopathies,[27] including acromegaly, Cushing's syndrome, polycystic ovary disease (Fig. 169-5), and diabetes. Mild forms also occur in obesity without evident endocrine disorder.

It appears likely that a common pathogenetic mechanism accounts for acanthosis nigricans linked to endocrinopathy. Studies of patients with a variety of endocrine diseases and acanthosis nigricans suggest that insulin resistance is a common denominator even in the absence of overt diabetes. It was first shown to be associated with insulin resistance in patients with the rare syndrome of lipoatrophic diabetes.[28] Subsequently, acanthosis nigricans has been associated with all three types of insulin resistance: type A, in which insulin resistance is due to receptor defects resulting in decreased binding of insulin; type B, in which insulin resistance is conferred by effects of circulating antireceptor antibodies; and type C, in which postreceptor defects—including abnormalities in signal transduction, such as autophosphorylation of the receptor and activation of tyrosine kinase—inhibit insulin action.[29,30]

The mechanism for pathogenesis in insulin-resistant states has been proposed to involve the action of insulin on the insulin-like growth factor (IGF) receptor. Hyperinsulinemia, induced by insulin resistance, provides excess insulin that may then compete for IGF receptors on keratinocytes and thus stimulate growth.[31] The fact that hypercortisolism induces insulin resistance may explain acanthosis nigricans in cushingoid states and is probably relevant in other endocrinopathies.

Kyrle's Disease/Reactive Perforating Collagenosis
(See Chap. 57)

This uncommon skin disease is characterized by hyperkeratotic follicular and perifollicular papules. The pathologic process involves transepidermal elimination of dermal material that may represent altered collagen. The perforating disease occurs in diabetics with renal failure but is also associated with renal failure without diabetes.[32,33]

GLUCAGONOMA SYNDROME (See also Chap. 185)

An unusual and striking cutaneous disease is found in patients with glucagon-secreting islet cell tumors. Although there is hyperglycemia as a consequence of excess glucagon secretion, the cutaneous findings are not a manifestation of diabetes.

The glucagonoma syndrome was first recognized as such by Mallinson et al.[34] Although the eruption may begin as a recalcitrant nonspecific eczematous dermatitis, the typical pattern consists of migrating marginated areas of erythema with blisters that heal with hyperpigmentation. The eruption waxes and wanes, involving different areas, especially the lower abdomen, buttock, perineum, and legs. A beefy red tongue, angular cheilitis, and nail dystrophy may be present. The somewhat diverse clinical features may also suggest various bullous dermatoses, pustular psoriasis, or acrodermatitis enteropathica. Histologically there is necrosis and cleft formation in the upper epidermis. This picture, known as *necrolytic migratory erythema*, is considered to be characteristic of an underlying glucagonoma.

However, the relationship of the cutaneous lesions and the tumor are still obscure. About 75 percent of the associated tumors are malignant, and widespread metastases are often present when the tumor is diagnosed. Regression of the cutaneous lesions follows removal of the tumor. Somatostatin, which depresses glucagon levels, may also suppress the skin lesions. Because skin lesions do not accompany many of the tumors despite elevated levels of circulating glucagon, it is not yet clear what role the hormone plays. Possibly some other factor secreted by the tumor is responsible. In this regard, clinically and histologically typical necrolytic migratory erythema has been reported in a number of patients with normal glucagon levels and without pancreatic tumors. Hepatocellular dysfunction has been the common denominator in many of these cases.[35]

REFERENCES

1. Flier JS et al: Antibodies that impair insulin receptor binding in an unusual diabetic syndrome with severe insulin resistance. *Science* **190**:63, 1975
2. Shoelson S et al: Three mutant insulins in man. *Nature* **302**:1, 1983
3. Chang KJ et al: Increased cross linkages in experimental diabetes. *Diabetes* **29**:778, 1980
4. Schnider SL, Kohn RR: Effects of age and diabetes mellitus on the solubility and nonenzymatic glycosylation of human skin collagen. *J Clin Invest* **67**:1630, 1981
5. Phan Than L et al: Increased biosynthesis and processing of fibronectin in fibroblasts from diabetic mice. *Proc Natl Acad Sci USA* **84**:1911, 1987
6. Sabin JA: Bacterial infections in diabetes mellitus. *Br J Dermatol* **91**:481, 1974
7. Lang CH et al: IL-1 induced increases in glucose utilization are insulin mediated. *Life Sci* **45**:2127, 1989
8. Neilly JB et al: Pruritus in diabetes mellitus: Investigation of prevalence and correlation with diabetes control. *Diabetes Care* **9**:273, 1986
9. Braverman I: Ultrastructural features of aging in the skin of normal adults and juvenile diabetes. *Clin Res* **28**:247A, 1980
10. Melin H: An atrophic circumscribed skin lesion in the lower extremities of diabetics. *Acta Med Scand* **423**(suppl):1, 1964
11. Binkley GW: Dermopathy in the diabetic syndrome. *Arch Dermatol* **92**:625, 1965
12. Kurwa A et al: Concurrence of bullous and atrophic skin lesions in diabetes mellitus. *Arch Dermatol* **103**:607, 1971
13. Bauer M, Levan NE: Diabetic dermangiopathy. *Br J Dermatol* **83**:528, 1970
14. Lithner F: Lesions of the legs in diabetics. *Acta Med Scand* **589**(suppl):1, 1976
15. Rocca FF, Pereyra E: Phlyctenar lesions in the feet of diabetic patients. *Diabetes* **12**:220, 1963
16. Bernstein JE et al: Reduced threshhold to suction-induced blister formation in insulin dependent diabetics. *J Am Acad Dermatol* **8**:790, 1983
17. Clark CV et al: Decreased skin wrinkling in diabetes mellitus. *Diabetes Care* **7**:224, 1984
18. Faerman I et al: Autonomic neuropathy in the skin: A histological study of the sympathetic nerve fibers in diabetic anhydrosis. *Diabetologica* **22**:96, 1982
19. Mann JR, Harman RRM: Cutaneous anesthesia in necrobiosis lipoidica diabeticorum. *Br J Dermatol* **110**:323, 1984
20. Oikarinen A et al: Necrobiosis lipoidica: Ultrastructural and biochemical demonstration of a collagen defect. *J Invest Dermatol* **88**:227, 1987
21. Ulpu KS et al: Expression of interstitial collagenase, 92-kDa gelatinase and tissue inhibitor of metalloproteinase in granuloma annulare and necrobiosis lipoidica diabeticorum. *J Invest Dermatol* **100**:335, 1993
22. Muller SA, Winkelmann RK: Necrobiosis lipoidica diabeticorum, a clinical and pathological investigation of 171 cases. *Arch Dermatol* **93**:272, 1966
23. Narva WM et al: Necrobiosis lipoidica diabeticorum with apparently normal diabetic tolerance. *Arch Intern Med* **115**:718, 1965
24. Quimby SR et al: Cutaneous immunopathology of necrobiosis lipoidica diabeticorum. *Arch Dermatol* **124**:1364, 1983
25. Statham B et al: A randomized double blind comparison of an aspirin-dipyridamole combination versus a placebo in the treatment of necrobiosis lipoidica. *Acta Derm Venereol* **61**:270, 1981
26. Karkavitsas K et al: Aspirin in the management of necrobiosis lipoidica. *Acta Derm Venereol* **62**:183, 1982
27. Matsuoka LY et al: Spectrum of endocrine abnormalities associated with acanthosis nigricans. *Am J Med* **83**:719, 1985
28. Kahn CR et al: Syndromes of insulin resistance and acanthosis nigricans. *N Engl J Med* **294**:739, 1976
29. Accili D et al: Mutations in the insulin receptor gene in patients with genetic syndromes of insulin resistance. *J Invest Dermatol* **98**:77S, 1992
30. Cruz PD, Hud JA: Excess insulin binding to insulin-like growth factor receptors: Proposed mechanism for acanthosis nigricans. *J Invest Dermatol* **98**:82S, 1992
31. Geffner ME, Golde DW: Selected insulin action on skin, ovary, heart in insulin resistant states. *Diabetes Care* **11**:500, 1988
32. Poliak SC et al: Reactive perforating collagenosis is associated with diabetes mellitus. *N Engl J Med* **306**:81, 1982
33. Zarate AR et al: Hyperkeratosis penetrans (HKP), a rare dermatological disease with high incidence in patients on hemodialysis. Proceedings of the Dialysis Transplant Forum 1978, p 99.
34. Mallinson CN et al: A glucagonoma syndrome. *Lancet* **2**:1, 1974
35. Marinkovich MP et al: Necrolytic migratory erythema in patients with liver disease. *J Am Acad Dermatol* **32**:604, 1995

CHAPTER 170

Ruth K. Freinkel

Other Endocrine Diseases

Hormones regulate physiologic processes by modification of existing activities rather than by initiation of reactions de novo. Thus, in the skin as elsewhere, excesses or deficiencies of hormones generally result in quantitative rather than qualitative changes in cutaneous function and morphology. However, the expression of altered hormonal balance is determined to some extent by intrinsic properties of skin in various areas. The capacity of cutaneous structures to respond, local hemodynamics, and extrinsic factors such as light and trauma influence the distribution as well as the quantity of hormonally induced changes in the skin.

The expression of endocrine disorders in the skin may reflect both alterations in total body economy and direct actions on cutaneous structures. For example, abnormalities in fluid and electrolyte balance resulting from endocrine abnormalities produce changes in skin turgor. As a major site for dissipation and conservation of heat, the skin may reflect derangements in thermogenesis in endocrine disease; skin temperature, vascular dilatation, and sweating reflect such changes.

Intermediary metabolism is controlled by balanced actions of hormones. Control is exerted by both direct effects on cells and indirect effects via circulating fuels and other regulatory substances. Expression of hormonal effects at the cellular level is a function of circulating levels of hormones and the ability of the tissue to respond. Excessive amounts of hormones accentuate activity of a cutaneous structure to the degree that it can respond. Hormone deficiency may result in diminished function of a responsive structure or be expressed by effects of unbalanced or excessive activity of other hormones [e.g., excess adrenocorticotropic hormone (ACTH) in adrenal insufficiency].

For certain hormones (e.g., sex hormones) the skin displays the responsiveness of a specific target tissue; other hormones (e.g., thyroid hormone) have global effects on tissues that are expressed also in skin; still other hormones (e.g., adrenal mineralocorticoids) have little or no discernible effects on the skin. Because cell turnover, synthesis of structural proteins, lipids, and mucopolysaccharides, and a vast network of blood vessels are affected by hormones, the skin affords a sensitive barometer of endocrine disease. In subsequent sections, the effects of various endocrinopathies on the skin will be considered in detail. In keeping with the concept that hormones regulate rather than initiate functions, the discussion will be formulated in terms of *too little* and *too much* of given hormones.

Finally, not all of the cutaneous manifestations of endocrine disorders can be attributed to direct effects of hormones on the skin itself. Thus, vitiligo in Addison's disease and pretibial myxedema in Graves' disease appear to reflect underlying pathologic processes that also initiate the endocrinopathy.

THYROID HORMONE

Effects of Thyroid Hormone on the Skin

Thyroid hormones act on fundamental mechanisms of energy metabolism, fuel metabolism, and biosynthetic and degradative processes at the cellular level. They appear to have diverse primary sites of action at the level of cell membranes, mitochondria, and gene transcription that enhance substrate availability and oxidative metabolism and regulate functional properties, including those of keratinocytes and fibroblasts.[1,2]

Thyroid hormone plays a pivotal role in embryonic development of mammalian skin as well as in maintenance of normal cutaneous function in adult skin. Ablation of the thyroid gland of sheep in utero retards formation of hair follicles and other adnexal structures as well as development of the dermis and epidermis.[3] Extrapolation from experiments in amphibian skin suggests that the effects of thyroid hormone on fetal development involve stimulation of mitotic activity as well as differentiation. Oxygen consumption, epidermal mitotic activity, and protein synthesis are increased by thyroid hormone. Thyroid hormone appears to be necessary for both the initiation and the maintenance of hair growth and for normal secretion of sebum.

Thyroid hormones affect production of collagen and mucopolysaccharides by dermal fibroblasts. Acid-soluble collagen is increased, insoluble collagen is decreased, and accumulation of glycosaminoglycans is retarded by thyroid hormone.

Lack of thyroid hormone is expressed by changes in all of the above functions in the skin. However, excess amounts of thyroid hormone do not correlate with abnormal acceleration of these functions.

Thyroid hormones also appear to affect pigmentation, and both hyper- and hypopigmentation are seen in hyperthyroidism.

Some of the effects of thyroid hormones on the skin are mediated indirectly by generalized effects on heat production and cardiovascular dynamics. Excessive sweating and increased cutaneous blood flow result from hyperthyroidism. To what extent these changes impinge on local cutaneous metabolism cannot be assessed.

Finally, it should be pointed out that some of the cutaneous changes in thyroid disease cannot be attributed directly to the effects of thyroid hormones. Altered activity in neurotransmitters may be responsible for actions that appear to result from altered levels of thyroid hormones. The autoimmune states that underlie Graves' disease and Hashimoto's thyroiditis appear to be responsible for some of the more striking cutaneous changes.

Cutaneous Manifestations of Too Much Thyroid Hormone

Thyrotoxicosis is the syndrome that results from excessive amounts of thyroid hormone. It may be due to Graves' disease, toxic nodular goiter, administration of excessive amounts of thyroid hormone, or as a transient phase in subacute thyroiditis.

The skin is warm, moist, and smooth. The warmth, which is due to peripheral vasodilatation and increased blood flow, is often accompanied by a persistent flush of the face, redness of the elbows, and palmar erythema. There is excessive sweating generally, but this is particularly pronounced on the palms and soles, where eccrine glands are under sympathetic control. Other evidence of vasomotor instability is seen in evanescent blushing over the head and neck.

The epidermis is thin but not atrophic, and the stratum corneum is well hydrated. Altered texture of the hair and diffuse alopecia are commonly observed. Nails exhibit a characteristic onycholysis in which the free edge of the nail curves upward (Plummer's nail).

Other cutaneous manifestations may include generalized pruritus, chronic urticaria, and alopecia areata.[4] Hyperpigmentation of a diffuse or patchy nature is not uncommon and generally occurs on the face. Vitiligo occurs in approximately 7 percent of patients with Graves' disease but is not abnormally more frequent in other forms of hyperthyroidism.[5] It may antedate the endocrine disorders and is not improved by treatment of the thyrotoxicosis.

GRAVES' DISEASE Graves' disease is an autoimmune disorder manifesting goiter and thyrotoxicosis, infiltrative ophthalmopathy, acropachy, and an infiltrative dermopathy (pretibial myxedema) (Fig. 170-1). Although these features can occur independently, pretibial myxedema almost always occurs in the presence of ophthalmopathy and usually develops late in the course of the disease.[6] Correction of the thyrotoxicosis has no effect on the skin lesions, which are found in about 5 percent of patients with Graves' disease. Indeed, half of the cases of pretibial myxedema occur after the patient has been rendered euthyroid. The clinical picture may not be pathognomonic, as similar lesions have been reported in patients with primary hypothyroidism and Hashimoto's thyroiditis.

The lesions occur most frequently on the anterior tibia and dorsa of the feet and are morphologically varied. They are usually bilateral but not symmetric. The lesions commonly consist of pink, flesh-colored, or purplish nodules (Fig. 170-2). A diffuse brawny edema may be present without nodules. Less common is an elephantiasis nostras variant, in which the extremity becomes enlarged and covered with verrucous nodules. Thickening of the skin of the extensor surface of the forearm (preradial myxedema) has been reported.[7] The dermal changes are like those of myxedema proper. Excessive amounts of hyaluronic acid and chondroitin are present in lesions as well as in clinically normal skin and have a characteristic distribution.[8]

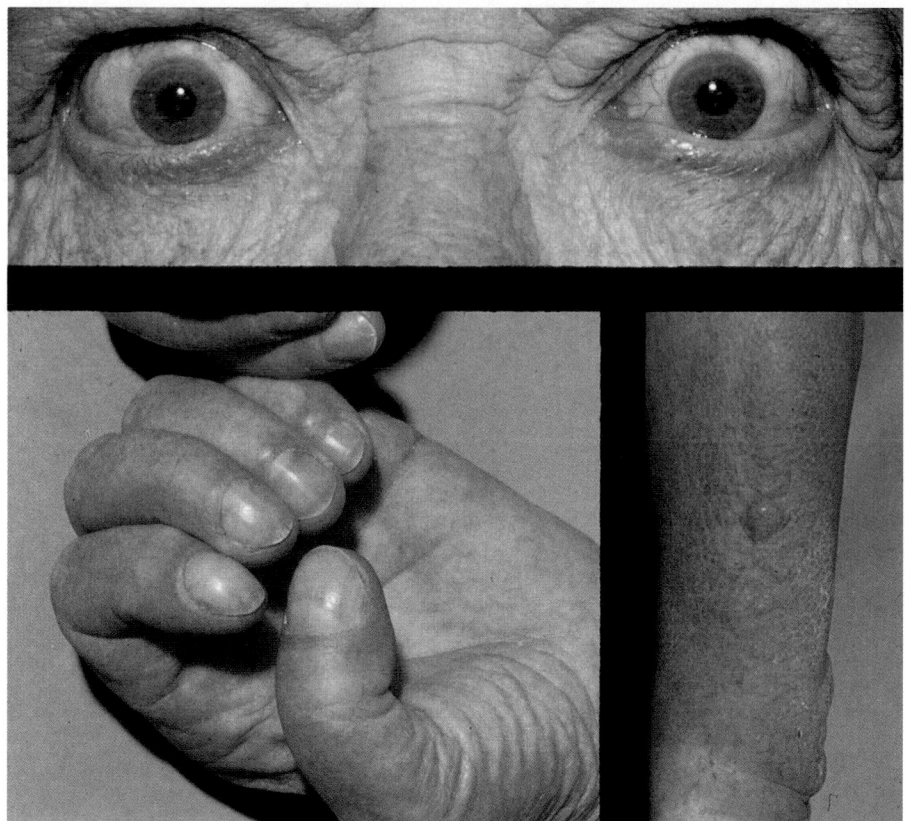

Fibroblasts in the eye and pretibial dermis are extrathyroidal targets for the autoimmune process that causes Graves' disease. The thyroid-stimulating hormone (TSH) receptor is the primary autoantigen, and activated T cells are the effectors that induce fibroblast proliferation and the elaboration of glycosaminoglycans. Ocular and dermal fibroblasts appear to share antigenic sites with the primary target in the thyroid.[9]

Treatment of pretibial myxedema is not very successful. Systemic or intralesional glucocorticoids or topical application of potent steroids under occlusion may afford some relief.

Cutaneous Manifestations of Too Little Thyroid Hormone

Thyroid deficiency occurs when there is decreased production of thyroid hormone due to loss of functioning thyroid tissue, inadequate stimulation of the thyroid gland due to failure of the pituitary or hypothalamus, or absolute or relative impairment in biosynthesis of thyroid hormone due to either extrinsic or intrinsic factors. The resultant endocrine disorder derives its name, *myxedema*, from its most prominent manifestation in the skin.

In hypothyroidism, the skin is cold, xerotic, and pale. The coldness is due to reduced core temperature and cutaneous vasoconstriction. The latter is also in part responsible for the pallor. Xerosis is

FIGURE 170-1

Hyperthyroidism. This composite illustrates the proptosis, acropathy, and pink or skin-colored papules, plaques, and nodules of pretibial myxedema.

FIGURE 170-2

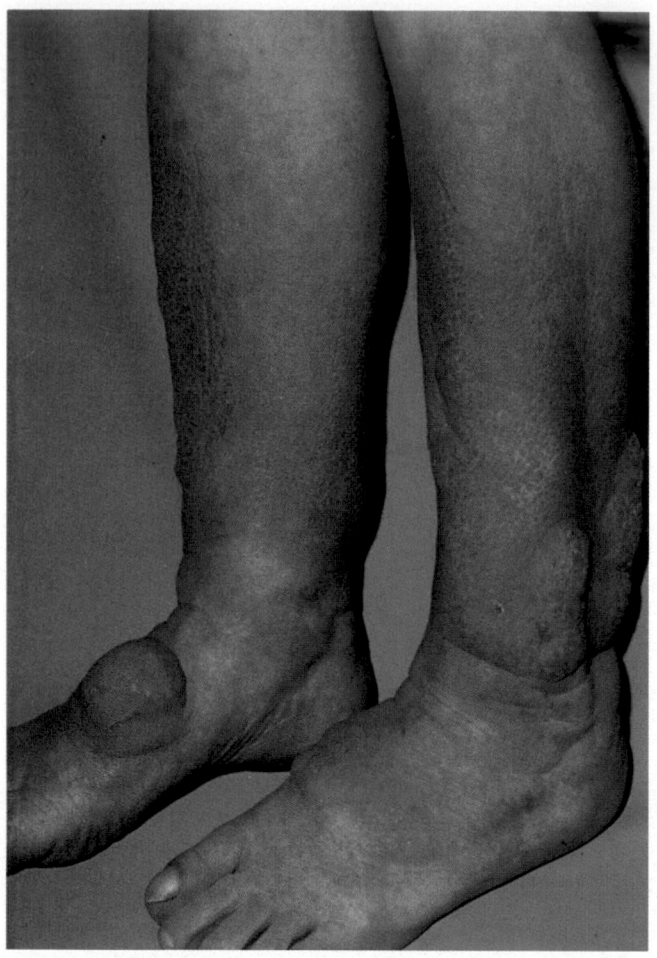

Hyperthyroidism with pretibial myxedema. Note infiltrated plaques that also extend to the calf and are partially hyperkeratotic. There is also an isolated nodule on the dorsum of the right foot.

due to a change in skin texture and poor hydration of the stratum corneum. The epidermis is thin and hyperkeratotic, and there is follicular plugging. Because the changes are generalized, they can be differentiated from similar alterations in the skin of atopic individuals and in keratosis pilaris, where the findings are more prominent on the extremities. Fine wrinkling imparts a parchment-like quality to the skin, especially in hypothyroidism secondary to pituitary failure.

A yellowish discoloration of the skin is sometimes present and is accentuated on the palms and soles and nasolabial folds. This is due to the accumulation of carotene in stratum corneum, secondary to carotenemia. Elevated blood levels of carotene have been attributed to a hepatic defect in the conversion of β carotene to vitamin A.

The hair is dry, coarse, and brittle, and it grows slowly. There is both patchy and diffuse loss of scalp hair, a very characteristic loss of the outer third of the eyebrow, and diminished body hair. Massive telogen effluvium may occur when there is abrupt onset of hypothyroidism, and the percentage of scalp hairs in telogen is generally increased in hypothyroid states. The chronology of the

reversal of these changes when thyroid hormone is administered suggests that hair loss is due to both premature anagen arrest and failure in initiation of anagen.[10] Hypothyroid patients, especially children, frequently develop long, lanugo-type hair on the back, shoulders, and extremities.

Diminished sebum secretion contributes to the coarse appearance of the hair. Nails grow slowly and tend to be brittle.

The most striking change in the skin is due to dermal accumulation of mucopolysaccharides (myxedema). Although these accumulations are more striking in acral parts, the distribution of myxedema is not affected by a dependent position. Generally myxedema is diffuse, but focal mucinous papules, responsive to L-thyroxine, have been described.

The facial changes are especially characteristic (Fig. 170-3). The nose is broadened and lips are thickened. The tongue is large, smooth, and clumsy. There may be sticky secretions on the eyelids, which show fine wrinkling and a flaccid and translucent puffiness. Drooping of the upper lid may occur in the absence of edema due to decreased sympathetic stimulation of the superior palpebral muscle. At rest, the face lacks expressiveness, and changing emotions are registered slowly because of the concomitant lethargy. These facies are almost pathognomonic, although they may be simulated in untreated pernicious anemia and the nephrotic syndrome.

The hypothyroid skin heals slowly, and this tendency is proportional to the degree of hormone deficiency.

The mucopolysaccharides that accumulate in the dermis are hyaluronic acid and chondroitin sulfate. They appear first in the pap-

FIGURE 170-3

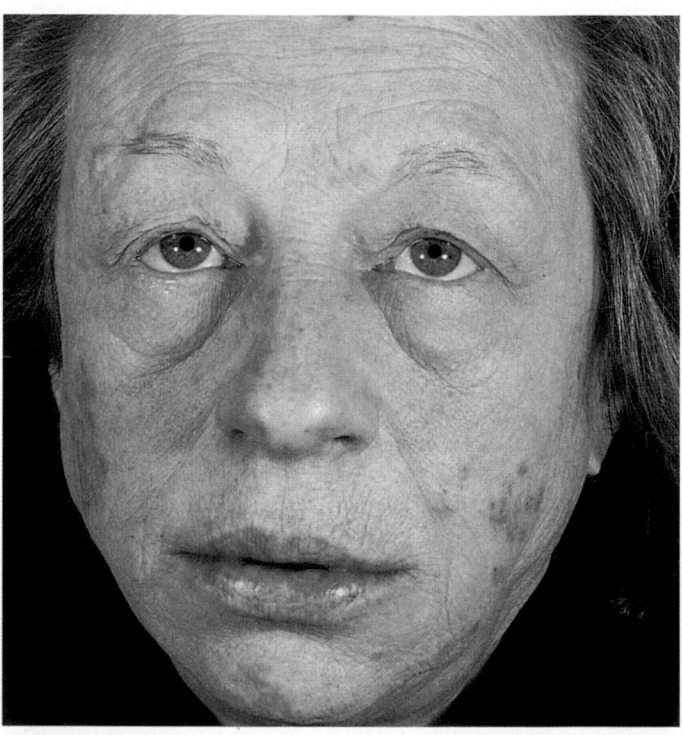

Hypothyroidism. This patient has many of the typical features of hypothyroidism: a cold, dry, pale skin; absence of hair in the lateral third of the eyebrows; and a puffiness of the face and lips due to the accumulation of water and mucopolysaccharides in the dermis. The hair is dry, coarse, and brittle. The nose is broadened; the tongue is large, smooth, red, and clumsy; and there is drooping of the eyelids. The face lacks expression and is the most pathognomonic of any of the features.

illary dermis and are most prominent around hair follicles and vessels. They separate the collagen bundles and there may be some secondary degeneration of collagen.

All of the changes are reversible by judicious use of thyroid hormone. Mobilization of myxedematous deposits is one of the earliest indications of the action of thyroid hormone replacement and is characterized by a rise in serum sodium and a fall in hematocrit due to the conjoint release of water and electrolytes bound to the hydrophilic mucopolysaccharides.

The mechanism that causes myxedema is not clear. There is evidence in animals and tissue culture supporting actions of thyroid hormone on both restraint of synthesis and catabolism of mucopolysaccharides. Thyrotropic hormone has been reported to cause dermal accumulation of mucopolysaccharides, suggesting a role for pituitary factors, which are elevated in primary thyroid failure. However, while myxedema is less prominent in hypothyroidism secondary to pituitary failure, it need not be absent. Thus, it is likely that lack of thyroid hormone is the primary factor in causing myxedema but that interactions with pituitary and/or other hormones may play a facilitating role.

PARATHYROID HORMONE

Effects of Parathyroid Hormone on the Skin

Parathyroid hormone regulates the flux of calcium between extra- and intracellular compartments in responsive tissues (i.e., kidney and bone) and the metabolism of vitamin D. A role for this hormone in the skin has not been established. However, receptors for parathyroid hormone have been identified in dermal fibroblasts, and the hormone affects collagen synthesis in dermal fibroblasts in vitro. The possible role of parathyroid hormone in the skin is clouded by the presence of a parathyroid hormone-like protein (parathyroid hormone–related protein) in keratinocytes that stimulates adenylcyclase and acts on dermal fibroblasts.[11] Recent studies suggest that parathyroid hormone–related protein plays a role in hair follicle development and may function in the regulation of cellular differentiation.[12]

Hypercalcemia may result in calcium deposits in the skin, irrespective of its cause. Moreover, clinical experience suggests[13] that abnormalities of calcium and phosphate per se produce profound changes in the skin, attesting to the importance of these ions in normal skin physiology.

Cutaneous Manifestations of Too Much Parathyroid Hormone

Primary hyperparathyroidism is not associated with any cutaneous manifestation except, rarely, pruritus and deposition of calcium. Because of this, intractable pruritus in renal disease has been attributed to the presence of secondary hyperparathyroidism. An increased amount of calcium has been reported in the skin of such patients, and some, but not all, have experienced relief of itching after parathyroidectomy. However, it should be noted that such patients are usually being treated with chronic dialysis and that itching is frequently intensified by the treatment. Furthermore, itching in uremic patients may be alleviated by irradiation of the skin with ultraviolet B (UVB). Thus, the mechanism of pruritus in chronic renal disease and in hyperparathyroidism has not been elucidated.

Cutaneous Manifestations of Too Little Parathyroid Hormone

Primary failure of the parathyroid glands may occur as an isolated phenomenon or as part of an autoimmune syndrome of multiple endocrine failure. In the latter case, it may be associated with Hashimoto's thyroiditis, Addison's disease, ovarian failure, or pernicious anemia; alopecia areata and vitiligo may be present in this syndrome. The least common cause of hypoparathyroidism is peripheral refractoriness to parathyroid hormone (pseudohypoparathyroidism). The most common cause is ablation of the parathyroids as a complication of thyroidectomy.

In all types of hypoparathyroidism the skin is dry, scaly, hyperkeratotic, and puffy. Nails become opaque and brittle and develop transverse ridges. Hair may be coarse and sparse. Eczematous dermatitis and hyperkeratotic and maculopapular eruptions have been reported. Since these changes are reversed when calcium levels are normalized, they appear to relate directly to the lack of calcium rather than to the level of parathyroid hormone.

Primary hypoparathyroidism may be associated with chronic mucocutaneous candidiasis. The infection commonly involves the nails and oral mucosa, but there may be vulvovaginitis and candidal intertrigo. Candidiasis may present on glabrous skin as an annular or scaling eruption resembling a dermatophytosis.

These infections are not altered by regulation of blood calcium and phosphorus levels and are attended by defects in cellular immune mechanisms. They may antedate the onset of hypoparathyroidism by years. The presence of autoantibodies to parathyroid tissue and other endocrine tissues has suggested that the fungal infections are related to the disturbance of immune function that underlies the endocrinopathy.[14]

GLUCOCORTICOIDS

Effects of Glucocorticoids on the Skin

The effects of glucocorticoids on the skin are best appreciated by observation of the changes produced by excess hormone. Although endogenous hypercortisolism is uncommon, the iatrogenic disease has become all too familiar due to the common use of synthetic glucocorticoids in nonendocrine disorders. These will be discussed in detail elsewhere but do not differ qualitatively from those produced by endogenous hormone (see Chaps. 243 and 252).

The actions of glucocorticoids on the skin have been extensively studied both in vivo and in vitro. Cortisol decreases the mass of dermal connective tissue due to direct effects on dermal fibroblasts. The hormone decreases synthesis as well as accumulation of glycosaminoglycans and alters their composition,[15] possibly via receptor-mediated mechanisms. Glucocorticoid increases collagen cross-linking and decreases the activity of collagenase,[16,17] but it does not affect the relative proportions of types I and III collagen. Although glucocorticoid inhibits the production of collagen,[18] dermal atrophy may also reflect diminished numbers of dermal fibroblasts.[19]

Glucocorticoid appears to regulate diurnal variations in mitotic activity of the epidermis. Mitotic peaks correlate inversely with serum cortisol levels,[20] and these effects may be mediated via adenylcyclase. Differentiation of epidermal cells is accelerated by the hormone in vitro.[21,22]

Glucocorticoid retards growth of hair in experimental animals, possibly owing to effects on initiation of anagen and mitotic activity. However, excess endogenous glucocorticoid produces hypertrichosis, whereas deficiency of the hormone causes loss of axillary hair, suggesting that the hormone plays a physiologic role in maintaining hair growth, at least in some sites. There is little clear evidence of an effect on sebaceous glands; however, follicular hyperkeratosis is frequently observed and plays a role in steroid-induced acne.

Glucocorticoids profoundly affect the immune system and inflammatory reactions. While the immunosuppressive actions are at least partially the basis of their use as anti-inflammatory agents, steroid-induced immunomodulation may play a role under physiologic conditions and in some of the manifestations of endogenous hypercortisolism. Among the effects are constraints on the production of interleukins and other cytokines, neutrophil chemotaxis, the numbers of Langerhans cells, the actions of growth factors such as epidermal growth factor and platelet-derived growth factor, and the synthesis of prostanoids due to inhibition of phospholipase A. Antiinflammatory effects are also abetted by stabilization of lysosomes, with resulting inhibition of release of proteases and other mediators.

The skin is a major site for degradation and interconversion of glucocorticoids and other steroid hormones, as established by numerous studies. In particular, interconversion of cortisone and cortisol is relevant to the effects of hormone excess. Cortisol has much greater effects on the skin and inflammatory reactions than cortisone. Exquisite regulation of interconversion of these two endogenous hormones, which has been shown in such physiologic events as wound healing, may provide control of proliferative events.[23]

Despite all of the above, it is not clear what role glucocorticoids play in maintenance of normal structure and function of the adult skin. In contrast to the effects of hormone excess, hormone lack seems to result in no clinically discernible changes in cutaneous integrity. However, the protean nature of glucocorticoid effects on the skin suggests that they play a regulatory role here as elsewhere. Indeed, high-affinity receptors for these hormones have been demonstrated in dermal fibroblasts as well as in keratinocytes. Perhaps the absence of gross structural and functional changes in the presence of too little glucocorticoid attests to the ability of the skin to function without fine tuning of such varied activities as mitotic division and collagen synthesis.

Effects of ACTH on the Skin

Effects of glucocorticoids on the skin cannot be discussed without mentioning the extraadrenal actions of pituitary corticotropin. Although glucocorticoids do not directly affect pigmentation, corticotropin and its structurally related pituitary peptides, melanocyte-stimulating hormones (MSH)-α and -β, stimulate melanogenesis. These hormones belong to a series of peptides arising from the prohormone pro-opiomelanocortin, which also includes the endorphins.

Cutaneous Manifestations of Too Much Glucocorticoid

Hypercortisolism can arise from functioning tumors of the adrenal cortex (Cushing's syndrome) or adrenal hyperplasia due to inappropriate secretion of ACTH by the pituitary (Cushing's disease) or by nonpituitary neoplasia (ectopic ACTH syndrome). In all types the effects of excess glucocorticoids may be mixed, but in varying degrees, with those of excess mineralocorticoids and androgenic steroids.

The skin becomes generally atrophic. The epidermis is thin and shiny and may show slight scaling. The dermis is also thin and loose, especially where subcutaneous fat is diminished. The skin becomes friable and easily damaged. Wound healing is markedly impaired; even slight injuries may fail to heal and become ulcerated and secondarily infected. Patients are prone to develop dermatophytosis as well as tinea versicolor.

There is increased vascular fragility, and patients often display petechiae and ecchymoses from slight trauma, especially in dependent parts. Decreased vascular tone is evident in purplish mottling of the lower extremities (cutis marmorata).

Among the characteristic lesions of glucocorticoid excess are the broad, purple striae that usually appear in areas of stretched skin on the trunk as well as elsewhere. They differ from the commonly found striae of adolescence, pregnancy, and obesity only with respect to their inordinate depth and breadth and intense color. The color fades when the disease is arrested, but the atrophy remains. The lesions represent another index of the loss of integrity of the dermal connective tissue and the failure of normal regenerative powers.

Hyperpigmentation is unusual in Cushing's syndrome but may occur in Cushing's disease in which production of ACTH (and related peptides) is increased; it has also been reported with ectopic ACTH production. Acanthosis nigricans occurs but is usually mild.

Plethora is common and accompanied by telangiectasia on the face (Fig. 170-4). This is usually attributed to associated polycy-

FIGURE 170-4

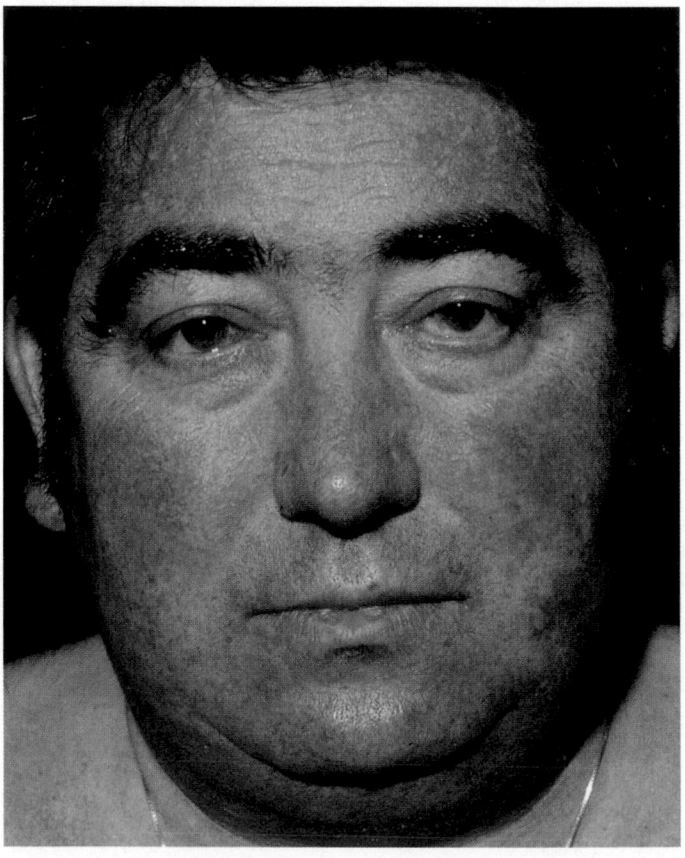

Hypercortisolism (Cushing's disease). Plethoric moon facies.

themia, although it occurs in the absence of increased red cell mass (personal observation).

Hypertrichosis and acne are common. The excess hair is usually found on the face—on the upper lip, chin, and lateral cheeks. Pure hypercortisolism (as seen in iatrogenic Cushing's syndrome) does not induce true beard growth; rather, the hair tends to be more lanugo-like. Intense hirsutism, involving body hair as well and accompanied by male-pattern alopecia, is sufficiently unusual in bilateral adrenal hyperplasia to justify suspicion of an adrenal tumor producing androgenic steroids.

One of the striking features of excess glucocorticoids is the change in appearance and body habitus. Excessive deposits of fat over the clavicles and back of the neck (buffalo hump) and abdomen are accompanied by loss of subcutaneous fat over the extremities. In addition, there is deposition of fat in the cheeks, giving the face a rounded appearance (moon facies). The central obesity may be associated with muscle wasting. Reduced height and kyphosis as a result of osteoporosis and compression fractures of the vertebrae may add to the altered appearance.

Cutaneous Manifestations of Too Little Glucocorticoid

Deficiency of glucocorticoids (i.e., Addison's disease) can occur when the adrenal cortex is (1) atrophic, either idiopathically or secondary to destructive disease (e.g., tuberculosis) or surgical ablation, or (2) inadequately stimulated by ACTH or when glucocorticoid synthesis is thwarted by abnormality in the biosynthetic sequence (e.g., adrenogenital syndrome). Although the clinical manifestations of these disorders vary to some extent with causative factors, glucocorticoid deficiency is common to all. Except in adrenogenital syndrome, there is also a lack of adrenal androgens. This produces clinical stigmata of androgen deficiency only when gonadal function is also diminished (e.g., after menopause).

Although large amounts of glucocorticoids have a marked effect on the skin, their absence causes surprisingly little change. Unless the patient is severely debilitated, texture of the skin appears normal. Loss of body hair, however, is common and is most striking in the axillae. Since replacement with cortisone may partly restore axillary hair, some of the effect may be ascribable to glucocorticoid per se. Except for fibrosis and calcification of the pinnae, mesenchymal changes are not apparent in the dermis.

The most striking cutaneous change of chronic adrenal insufficiency is hyperpigmentation, which occurs almost uniformly. In 20 to 40 percent of cases it is the first sign of the disease. Hyperpigmentation that results from excess ACTH is one of the chief differentiating features between adrenal insufficiency due to pituitary disease and that due to primary adrenal failure.

The hyperpigmentation is generalized and represents an accentuation of normal pigment distribution. It is often noted as the persistence of a tan acquired in the summer, and it is always darker in sun-exposed areas (Fig. 170-5A). Darkening also occurs in areas of trauma, recent scars, and points of pressure and friction (elbows, knees, skin folds, and palmar creases) (Fig. 170-5B). Skin in sexual areas (nipples, areolae, axillae, perineum, and genitalia) becomes darker. In parous females, the linea alba darkens. Hair may darken and longitudinal pigmented bands appear on the nails. Pigmentation appears on mucosal surfaces, especially the buccal mucosa, gums, and tongue. Such pigmentation is normally present in non-Caucasians and may darken. From the above description it is obvious that the hyperpigmentation is relative and can be evaluated only in terms of the patient's previous skin color (see also Chap. 89). Replacement therapy produces a gradual diminution of the color. In the

FIGURE 170-5

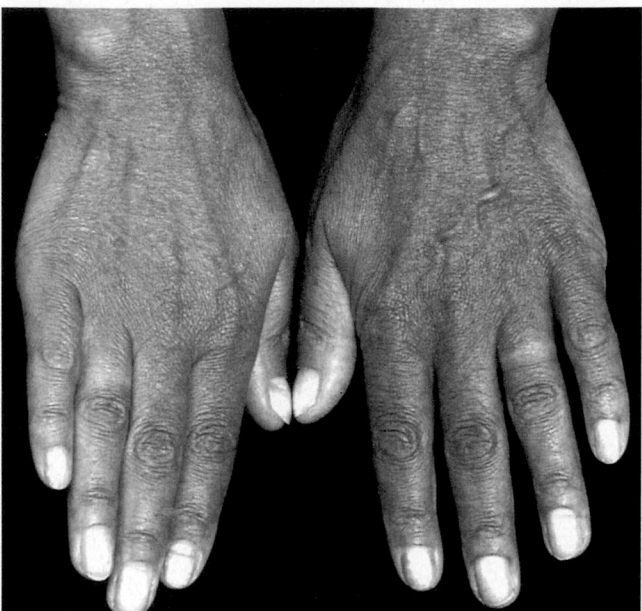

A.

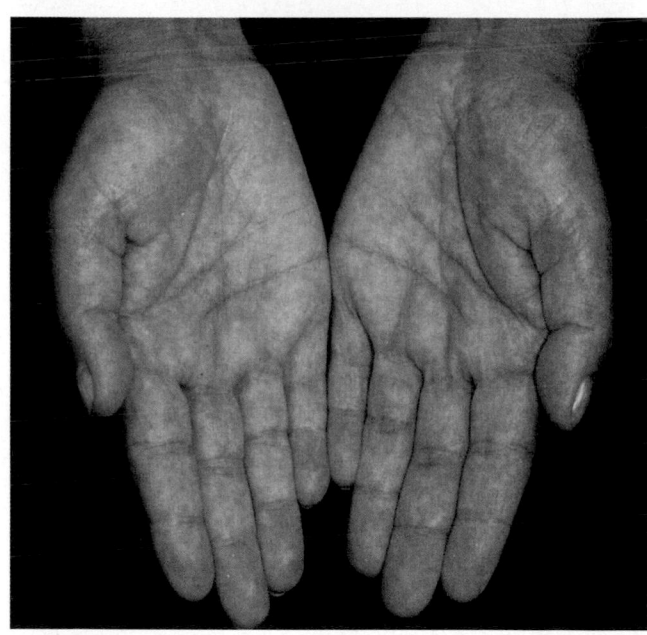

B.

Addison's disease. Hyperpigmentation of the hands: *A.* dorsa; *B.* palmar creases.

treated patient with Addison's disease, waxing and waning of the intensity of pigmentation may be one of the most sensitive indices of changing requirements for maintenance doses of glucocorticoids.

Other pigmentary changes are also observed. An early and sometimes prominent change is darkening of pigmented nevi and the appearance of lentigo-like lesions. Vitiligo is associated with primary adrenal failure in as many as 15 percent of cases and may precede clinical manifestations of adrenal cortical insufficiency.

FIGURE 170-6

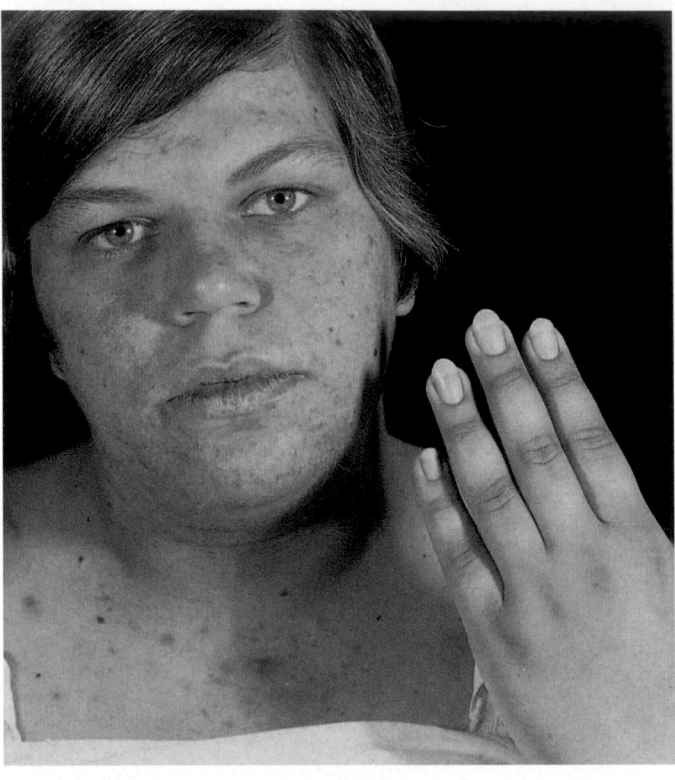

Pituitary adenoma with Nelson's syndrome. This patient is a skin phototype II who became markedly hyperpigmented as the result of a functioning tumor of the pituitary. The patient had a chromophobe adenoma that excreted large amounts of ACTH and associated peptides.

Some studies have suggested that vitiligo associated with Addison's disease is limited to patients with multiglandular deficiency syndromes,[24] as is the association with mucocutaneous candidiasis.

One of the more unusual variants of hyperpigmentation due to pituitary stimulation occurs after bilateral adrenalectomy for adrenal hyperplasia. This syndrome (Nelson's syndrome, Fig. 170-6) is characterized by intense hyperpigmentation as well as amenorrhea and signs of an expanding pituitary lesion (see also Chap. 89).[25] The pituitary adenomas in this condition produce extremely high levels of ACTH/MSH. Because the neoplasms are not usually observed before adrenalectomy, some theories ascribe their development to loss of feedback to the pituitary that follows the loss of glucocorticoids after adrenalectomy.

SEX HORMONES

Effect of Sex Hormones on the Skin

Androgenic hormones have trophic actions on the skin as a whole, but certain parts of the skin, such as sexual zones, are particularly sensitive. Moreover, hair follicles and sebaceous glands appear to be particularly responsive. Under the influence of androgenic hormones, mitotic activity, cell turnover time, and thickness of epidermis are increased. Growth of sebaceous glands is enhanced, and measurements of sebum production are sensitive indices of androgenicity. Hair growth is markedly affected by androgens (see Chaps. 17 and 71). Pigmentation is increased by androgens not only in sexual skin but generally. Androgens also cause thickening of the dermis with an increase in skin collagen content.

The nature of the effects appears to be identical for all androgenic hormones, irrespective of their source (adrenal or gonadal). Of circulating hormones, testosterone is the most potent. However, other androgens have trophic effects on cutaneous structures and may be quantitatively more important, either because they are more abundant in the circulation (as may be the case for adrenal androgens in women) or because of target tissue sensitivity.

A detailed review of the mechanism of action of androgens and other steroid hormones is beyond the scope of this chapter. Briefly, testosterone and other sex steroids circulate in association with transport proteins (sex hormone–binding globulin) and enter the cell in free form. Within cells, testosterone may be converted into dihydrotestosterone (DHT) by 5α-reductase. Conversions of other androgens by reductases, dehydrogenases, and isomerases produce intermediates that may be converted to DHT. For certain cutaneous structures, androgen responsiveness appears to depend more upon the availability of DHT rather than testosterone itself.

DHT and other active androgenic steroids are bound to specific high-affinity receptor proteins in the cytosol and translocated into the nucleus. The receptor-hormone complex bound to nuclear proteins initiates protein synthesis and sets the anabolic machinery into motion. Thus anabolic effects of androgenic hormones are determined by specificity and prevalence of receptors and nuclear binding sites and in certain sites by conversion to DHT. As the skin itself is an important site for the metabolism of sex steroids, adrenal and ovarian androgens (such as androstenedione and dehydroepiandrosterone) may be more important sources of androgenic stimulation in the female than the limited amounts of circulating testosterone.

A considerable body of evidence suggests that there are marked differences in the sensitivity of various portions of the skin to androgenic stimulation. These differences may reside in differences in the activity and distribution of androgen-metabolizing enzymes, such as hydroxy steroid dehydrogenases and isomerases as well as α-reductases,[26] and in intracellular androgen-binding proteins.[27] Thus, sebocytes from the face respond differently from those from the legs to testosterone and DHT.[28] While hair growth is stimulated in most follicles by androgens, only scalp, pubic, and axillary hair grows in men with 5α-reductase deficiency, suggesting that DHT is an active intracellular androgen in all other locations. The exception is posterior scalp hair, which grows independently of androgens. Androgen receptors have been identified in androgen-responsive follicles but not in posterior scalp.[29]

Studies in animals have suggested that anterior pituitary hormones may facilitate the effects of testosterone. Although the mechanisms remain controversial, such studies have shown that pituitary hormones facilitate the uptake and/or conversion of testosterone to DHT.

Estrogens likewise have significant effects on skin, mainly in the sexual zones. They may accelerate the rate of maturation of epidermal cells even as they induce cornification of vaginal mucosa. It has been demonstrated that there are increases in both mitotic division and thickness of the epidermis in estrogen-treated women after castration[30] and alterations in collagen formation in the skin.[31]

For the most part, however, the effect of estrogens on skin under physiologic conditions remains poorly defined. The suppression of sebaceous glands by pharmacologic amounts of estrogen is a well-known phenomenon that can be only partially explained by suppression of the pituitary-ovarian axis and reduced production of ovarian androgen. Some direct effect on the target tissue must be invoked to explain the increased response of sebaceous glands to dosages of estrogen in excess of those required for suppression of ovarian function. The presence of high-affinity estrogen receptors in the skin suggests a role for the direct effects of these hormones.

Cutaneous Manifestations of Too Much Sex Hormone

TOO MUCH ANDROGEN The clinical manifestations of androgen excess are recognized as virilization when they occur in the adult female and as precocious puberty when present in preadolescent children. Although the cutaneous changes are similar for various endocrine disorders in which virilization occurs, diagnostic differentiation can be made on the basis of additional features.

In virilizing syndromes, the skin becomes thickened and coarse. Pores on the face enlarge, and there is excessive oiliness. Typical acne vulgaris may develop. In children, the straight hairline is molded to conform to the adult configuration (calvities frontalis adolescentium); androgenetic alopecia may develop (see Chap. 71). Growth of body hair is accelerated, so that coarse hair appears on the extremities, on the anterior chest, and in the beard area. Pubic and axillary hair develops in children. The genitalia show masculinization; the clitoris enlarges in women, and in prepubertal males there is penile hypertrophy and increasing folding of the scrotal skin. If virilization occurs during fetal life in females, pseudohermaphroditism may result. Hyperpigmentation of the perineum, external genitalia, axillae, aureolae, and nipples is present.

The skin changes are accompanied by effects on musculature and distribution of body fat characteristic of the male. In children, excess androgens initially accelerate growth of the long bones but also cause premature closure of the epiphyses, resulting in short stature.

The adrenogenital syndrome is one of the more common of the hereditary disorders characterized by virilization. The biochemical lesion is a defect in the synthesis of glucocorticoids and mineralocorticoids, most commonly due to defective hydroxylation of carbon-21 or -11 of the steroid nucleus. Pituitary secretion of ACTH is then not restrained by negative feedback because of the relative absence of hydroxylated steroids. As a result the adrenal cortex is driven to secrete increased amounts of androgenic steroids. The resulting disorder is a combination of adrenal glucocorticoid and mineralocorticoid deficiency in the face of virilization. Moreover, the increased availability of ACTH may effect generalized hyperpigmentation (as in Addison's disease). Partial deficiencies of 3β-hydroxylase steroid dehydrogenase, as well as 11- or 21- hydroxylases, have also been recognized to underlie hirsutism and recalcitrant acne in postadolescent women.[32] A number of syndromes have been described in which hirsutism, androgenetic alopecia, and acne occur and for which the pathogenesis is not clearly established (see Chap. 73). Elevated levels of free testosterone, dehydroepiandrosterone, and urinary ketosteroids may be present even without polycystic ovaries in such patients. Such rather milder signs of hyperandrogenization should provoke an investigation of androgenic hormone levels.

TOO MUCH ESTROGEN Excess estrogen may result from estrogen-producing tumors of the ovary or testes or rarely from hypothalamic disorders. It results in precocious puberty in the female. In males, gynecomastia may be the only manifestation. However, testicular atrophy may follow, with diminished androgen-dependent functions.

The widespread use of oral contraceptive agents containing combinations of synthetic estrogens and progestins has introduced a spectrum of cutaneous changes due to prolonged exposure to sex hormones. Many of these are similar to the cutaneous changes encountered in pregnancy (see Chap. 168). Vaginal candidiasis is common, some patients develop melasma, and hair loss during or after withdrawal of these drugs may occur. Telangiectasia, spider angioma, and palmar erythema may appear. Some agents ameliorate acne whereas others make it worse, depending on the androgenicity of the progestin and the quantity of estrogen. Other cutaneous disorders are occasionally precipitated or worsened by oral contraceptive agents; these include erythema nodosum, porphyria cutanea tarda, herpes gestationis, and systemic lupus erythematosus.

Cutaneous Manifestations of Too Little Sex Hormone

Absolute or relative lack of sex hormone may result from (1) congenital disorders in which gonads fail to develop; (2) end-organ unresponsiveness in the target tissue due to defects in metabolism or receptors of sex hormones; (3) destruction of gonads by disease or castration; (4) suppression of gonadal function by hormone administration; or (5) pituitary disturbance resulting in lack of gonadotrophic hormones.

It should be noted, however, that while gonadal testosterone is the prime source of androgens in the male, adrenal androgens may provide some androgenicity for the skin in the male and a major source for androgens in females. Skin changes due to lack of gonadal hormones are therefore not as complete as they might be if there were only a single source for androgenization. Moreover, peripheral metabolism of steroid hormones may provide some minimal sources in the absence of gonadal function.

The skin changes that result from lack of androgens depend in large measure upon the age and sex of the individuals. If males are deprived of testosterone before puberty, the fully developed picture of eunuchoidism or infantilism results; the skin remains thin and fine, and sebaceous glands, apocrine glands, and sexual hair remain dormant. Facial pores are small, and there is neither oiliness nor acne. As time goes on, the skin around the eyes and lips develops the fine wrinkling characteristic of aging. The hairline remains straight over the forehead and low over the temples. Beard, axillary, and pubic hair do not develop and neither does androgenetic alopecia. Pallor of the skin is an outstanding feature. There is less pigment not only in sexual zones but generally. Reduced cutaneous blood flow may contribute to the pallor.

The penis remains small, and scrotal skin does not develop deep furrows. Delayed somatic maturation is evident in poor muscular development and in excessive subcutaneous fat in the pectoral and girdle regions. Delayed closure of the epiphyses results in prolonged growth of the long bones, so that normal height may be achieved by virtue of disproportionate length of the extremities.

The picture is modified if hypoandrogenicity develops after puberty. Although initiation of growth of body hair and beard requires androgens, maintenance of some growth usually persists. Thus, in the postpubertal male castrate, axillary and pubic hair usually remains although it may be sparse and slow-growing. Terminal hair on the body and beard shows even less change. Regular shaving of the beard may still be necessary, but at longer intervals.

Because sebaceous glands require constant androgenization, sebum secretion is markedly reduced. Although the texture of the skin is less coarse and may be finely wrinkled, it does not revert to a prepubertal state. Replacement therapy with androgens will reverse all these changes.

PITUITARY HORMONES

Effect of Pituitary Hormones on the Skin

The adenohypophysis and neurohypophysis are the sources of a number of hormones, some of which regulate activity of endocrine glands: ACTH, gonadotropins, and thyrotropin (TSH). They also include somatotropin (growth hormone, GH), prolactin, MSH, and lipotropin, which seem not to stimulate endocrine glands but to act on other tissues. Peptides that are indistinguishable from their pituitary counterparts may be produced ectopically by solid tumors. To what extent ectopic production of pituitary-like tropic hormones may occur under other physiologic or pathologic conditions is not known; however, it has been shown that keratinocytes produce ACTH and MSH.

The implications of disordered adenohypophyseal function for the skin must be formulated in terms of direct actions mediated via target-gland hormones stimulated by tropic pituitary hormones. The latter introduce multiple potentialities so that alterations of the skin in pituitary disorders usually present a composite of endocrine effects. For example, hyperandrogenicity is often seen in women with excess prolactin. The prolactin inhibits gonadotropin and may precipitate the development of polycystic ovary disease, with increased levels of adrenal androgens resulting in hirsutism and acne.

With the exception of MSH and ACTH, direct effects of pituitary hormones on the skin have not been convincingly demonstrated in humans. However, numerous studies in animals have indicated that GH, prolactin, and TSH as well as ACTH and MSH may facilitate response of sebaceous glands to androgenic stimulation, suggesting that pituitary peptides have subtle effects directly on the skin.

FIGURE 170-7

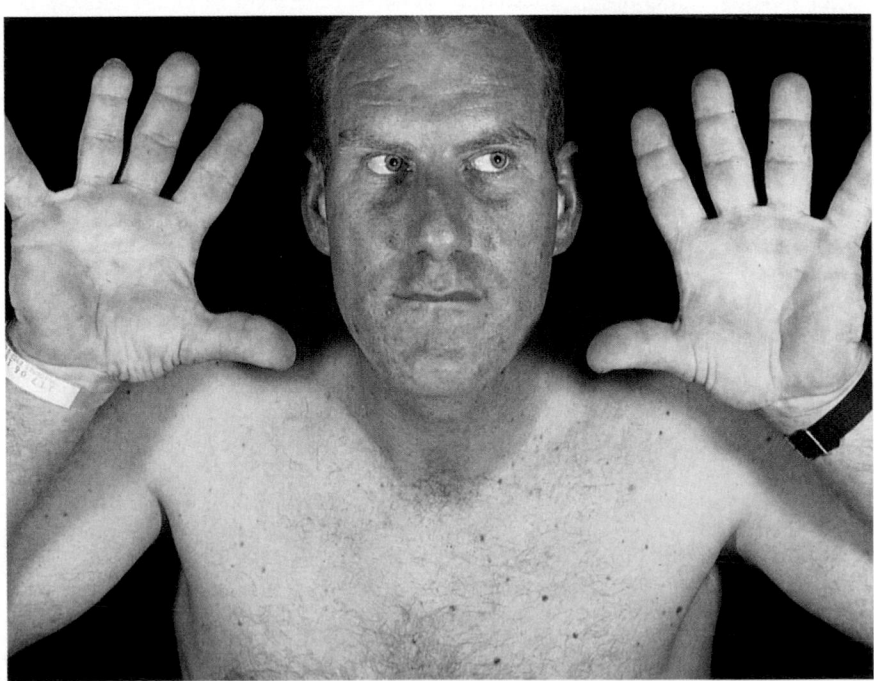

Acromegaly. Coarse facies with enlargement of the nose, chin, hands, and fingers.

The next two sections deal with two disorders of pituitary function that are well defined and illustrate the complexity of composite endocrine effects on the skin, that is, too much GH (acromegaly) and too little of all anterior pituitary hormones (panhypopituitarism).

Cutaneous Manifestations of Too Much Growth Hormone: Acromegaly

Excessive GH elaboration is commonly associated with eosinophilic adenomas of the pituitary. Although elaboration of other hormones such as gonadotropins may be compromised, the preponderant changes in the skin and the rest of the body are those due to excessive amounts of GH. The cutaneous changes are most pronounced in the dermis, with hyperplasia due to increased amounts of glycosaminoglycans[33] and an attendant retention of water. Whether collagen is also increased remains controversial.

These effects, like those on skeletal tissue, are mediated by growth factors, collectively known as *somatomedins,* which have been identified to be the circulating insulin-like growth factor(s) (IGF). Of the two major IGFs responsible for growth and insulin-like effects, IGF-1 is more responsive to stimulation by GH than IGF-2. IGF-1 and IGF-2 both promote sulfation of collagen and affect synthesis of RNA and DNA. Although circulating somatomedin is made primarily in the liver, many other tissues, such as fibroblasts, produce somatomedin-like peptides under control of GH (and other growth factors) that act via autocrine and paracrine mechanisms. It is possible that acanthosis nigricans, a frequent feature of acromegaly, may result from circulating or even locally produced IGF.

In acromegaly there is also hyperplasia of the epidermis and dermal appendages. Whether this is an effect on epidermal cells per se or secondary to alterations of the connective tissue is not yet clear. For example, in certain nonendocrine conditions characterized by similar mesenchymal hyperplasia, changes in the epidermis and its appendages are quite analogous to those in acromegaly—for example, pachydermaperiostosis.

GH may also exert effects on pilosebaceous structures by potentiating the effectiveness of androgens. Such actions have been demonstrated in animals; data in humans are not definitive. Thus, isolated deficiency of GH in sexual ateliotic dwarfs may not be associated with significant depression of sebaceous gland activity, but pilosebaceous functions are usually sustained in acromegaly even after hypogonadism develops.

Although the most striking clinical expression of acromegaly is due to effects on bone and cartilage, there are usually prominent changes in the skin (Fig. 170-7). Clinically, the effect on the integument can be described as "too much skin." The skin is thickened and has a doughy feel; this is most marked over the face and on the extremities, where skeletal changes are also most prominent. Furrowing and accentuation of folds contributes to the coarsening of the facial features. Deepening of creases on the forehead and nasolabial folds gives the patients a scowling, somber expression. In some cases, overgrowth of the dermis results in bizarre ridging of the skin of the scalp (cutis vertices gyrata). Eyelids become thick and edematous. The lower lip is enlarged and protruding and there is macroglossia. The nose becomes elongated, and the exuberant hypertrophy of soft tissue usually exceeds the cartilaginous overgrowth. Increased soft tissue in the alae nasi gives the nose an unmistakable triangular configuration. Similar changes occur on the hands and feet. Folds of skin over bony prominences on the hands are accentuated. The pads of the digits become fleshy, and fingers assume a blunted shape. The heel pads on the feet are predictably thickened. The overgrowth of fibrous tissue leads to production of small sessile or pedunculated fibromas that are found in 20 to 30 percent of patients.

There is thickening of the epidermis with accentuation of markings and enlarged pores. Nails become thick and hard. Excessive eccrine and apocrine sweating occurs in the majority of patients and may be implicated in the heightened incidence of abscesses in the axillae and intergluteal cleft. Although breast tissue often becomes atrophic in women, along with other stigmata of hypogonadism, galactorrhea may occur, probably because many of the somatotropic adenomas associated with acromegaly elaborate both GH and prolactin.[34]

Hypertrichosis occurs in about half of the patients. However, it differs from that in virilizing syndromes in that it does not affect the beard area. The skin is said to be oily, but acne is not a common feature.

Hyperpigmentation has been observed in about 40 percent of patients. The increase in color is generalized but not marked.

As activity of the disease diminishes, skin changes become stationary and may even regress. Occasionally, in the late stages of the disease, a predominating hypogonadism may contribute to regression of changes, especially in hair growth.

Acanthosis nigricans is found in a small percentage of patients.

Cutaneous Manifestations of Too Little of All Pituitary Hormones: Panhypopituitarism

A variety of conditions may compromise the anterior pituitary and thereby the elaboration of all pituitary hormones. Acute infarction may occur, as in postpartum hemorrhage (Sheehan's syndrome). Slower failure may be due to destruction of the gland by chronic infection (syphilis and tuberculosis), granulomatous inflammation (sarcoid), neoplastic invasion (histiocytosis X, metastatic cancer), or by tumors arising within the pituitary (chromophobe adenomas) or contiguous structures (craniopharyngioma).

The alterations of the skin in panhypopituitarism depend on how much pituitary tissue has been destroyed and the effects of integrated deprivation of those hormones that have been considered singly in earlier portions of the chapter. Individual hormonal deficits may not be as pronounced as in primary failure of the target glands, as some autonomous function of target glands may persist in the absence of tropic stimulation. Moreover, the effects of the lack of one hormone may be modified by the lack of others. For example, although the patient with panhypopituitarism may have severe hypothyroidism, myxedema is often mild. This may be due to the lack of other hormones that stimulate synthesis of mucopolysaccharides.

Pallor of the skin with a yellowish tinge is a prominent feature. Melanin content is apparently diminished, especially in the sexual areas. There may be increased sensitivity to sunlight and less pigmentation of traumatized and inflamed skin. Lack of the normal pink color of the cheeks, earlobes, and palms contributes to the pallor, but mucous membranes retain their normal hue unless the patient is anemic. The texture of the skin is dry but smoother and softer than in primary hypothyroidism. The face may be puffy. The facies tend to be less expressive because of a diminution in skin folds. Thinness of the skin and subcutaneous tissues results in fine wrinkling around the eyes and mouth, making the patient look older.

Loss of body hair occurs in all patients early in the course. Axillary hair is affected first, and a reduced need for axillary shaving may be an initial symptom. Pubic hair loss takes longer to develop and is less consistent. Beard growth slows but is not altogether lost in adult males. Scalp hair tends to be fine and dry and there may be generalized thinning. Sebaceous secretions and sweating also decrease.

REFERENCES

1. Holt PJ: In vitro responses of epidermis to triiodothyronine. *J Invest Dermatol* **71**:202, 1978
2. Smith TJ et al: The effect of thyroid hormone in glycosaminoglycans accumulation in human skin fibroblasts. *Endocrinology* **108**:2397, 1981
3. Chapman RE et al: The effects of fetal thyroidectomy and thyroxin: A demonstration on the development of skin and wool follicles of sheep fetuses. *J Anat* **117**:419, 1974
4. Barrow MV, Bird ED: Pruritus in hyperthyroidism. *Arch Dermatol* **93**:237, 1966
5. Ochi Y, deGroot LJ: Vitiligo in Graves' disease. *Ann Intern Med* **71**:935, 1969
6. Fatourechi V et al: Dermopathy of Graves' disease (pretibial myxedema): Review of 150 cases. *Medicine* **73**:1, 1994
7. Wortsman J et al: Preradial myxedema in thyroid states. *Arch Dermatol* **117**:635, 1981
8. Sumach SC et al: Pretibial mucin: Histological patterns and clinical correlation. *Arch Dermatol* **129**:1152, 1993
9. Heufelder AE et al: Antigen receptor variable region repertoires expressed by T cells infiltrating thyroid, retroorbital and pretibial tissue in Graves' disease. *J Clin Endocrinol Metab* **81**:3733, 1996
10. Freinkel RK, Freinkel N: Hair growth and alopecia in hypothyroidism. *Arch Dermatol* **106**:349, 1972
11. Wu TL et al: Skin-derived fibroblasts respond to human parathyroid hormone like adenylcyclase stimulating protein. *J Clin Endocrinol Metab* **651**:105, 1987
12. Wysolmerski JJ et al: Overexpression of parathyroid hormone related protein in the skin of transgenic mice interferes with hair follicle development. *Proc Natl Acad Sci USA* **91**:1133, 1994
13. Hirano K et al: Cutaneous manifestations in idiopathic hypoparathyroidism. *Arch Dermatol* **109**:242, 1975
14. Blizzard RM, Gibbs JH: Candidiasis: Studies pertaining to its association with endocrinopathies and pernicious anemia. *Pediatrics* **42**:231, 1968
15. Sarnstrand B et al: Effect of glucocorticoids on glycosaminoglycans metabolism in cultured skin fibroblasts. *J Invest Dermatol* **79**:412, 1982
16. Oxlund H et al: Changes in the mechanical properties, thermal stability, reducible cross-links and glycosyl-lysines in rat skin induced by corticosteroid treatment. *Acta Endocrinol* **101**:312, 1982
17. Koob TJ et al: Hormonal interactions in mammalian collagenase regulation. Comparative studies in human skin and rat uterus. *Biochim Biophys Acta* **629**:13, 1980
18. Oikarinen AP et al: Systemic glucocorticoids decrease the synthesis of type I and type III collagen in human skin in vivo whereas isotretinoin has little effect. *Br J Dermatol* **131**:660, 1994
19. Booth BA et al: Steroid induced dermal atrophy: Effects of glucocorticoids on collagen metabolism in human skin fibroblast cultures. *Int J Dermatol* **21**:333, 1982
20. Schell H et al: Evidence of diurnal variation of human epidermal cell proliferation. *Arch Dermatol Res* **271**:41, 1980
21. Laurence EB, Christophers E: Selective action of hydrocortisone on post mitotic epidermal cells in vivo. *J Invest Dermatol* **66**:222, 1976
22. Monzon RI et al: Regulation of involucrin gene expression by retinoic acid and glucocorticoids. *Cell Growth Differ* **7**:1751, 1996
23. Nabors CJ, Berliner DL: Corticosteroid metabolism during wound healing. *J Invest Dermatol* **52**:465, 1969
24. McGregor BC et al: Vitiligo and multiglandular insufficiencies. *JAMA* **219**:724, 1972
25. Nelson DH et al: ACTH-producing pituitary tumors following adrenalectomy for Cushing's syndrome. *Ann Intern Med* **52**:561, 1960

26. Hay JB, Hodgins MB: Distribution of androgen metabolizing enzymes in isolated tissues of human forehead and axillary skin. *J Endocrinol* **79**:29, 1978

27. Sawaya ME et al: Increased androgen binding capacity in scalp of male pattern baldness. *J Invest Dermatol* **92**:91, 1989

28. Zouboulis CC et al: Androgens affect the activity of human sebocytes in a manner dependent on the localization of the sebaceous glands and their effect is antagonized by spironolactone. *Skin Pharmacol* **7**:33, 1994

29. Itami S et al: Interaction between dermal papilla cells and follicular epithelial cells in vitro: Effect of androgen. *Br J Dermatol* **132**:527, 1995

30. Puonnen R: Effect of castration and peroral estrogen treatment on the skin. *Acta Obstet Gynecol Scand* **21**(suppl):3, 1972

31. Yang SL et al: The effect of estrogens on collagen synthesis at the site of a skin graft. *Am J Obstet Gynecol* **116**:694, 1973

32. Rose LI et al: Adrenocortical hydroxylase deficiencies in acne vulgaris. *J Invest Dermatol* **66**:324, 1976

33. Matsuoka LY et al: Histochemical characterization of cutaneous involvement of acromegaly. *Arch Intern Med* **142**:1820, 1982

34. Trouillas J et al: Relationships between pathological diagnosis and clinical parameters in acromegaly. *Metab Clin Exp* **45**(81 suppl 1):53, 1996

CHAPTER 171

Jonathan K. Wilkin

Skin Changes in the Flushing Disorders and the Carcinoid Syndrome

FLUSHING DISORDERS

Flushing is a transient reddening of the face and frequently other areas, including the neck, upper chest, and epigastric areas. The erythema is easily extinguished with direct pressure, and the redness subsides between flushing episodes. The latter feature excludes patients with a "red face," for example, due to drug photosensitivity, in whom the erythema is much longer-lived (fixed) and not subject to transient, pronounced changes in intensity.

Despite the limited distribution of the erythema, flushing is the visible sign of a generalized increase in cutaneous blood flow.[1] The greater visibility of the superficial cutaneous vasculature and the greater capacity of these vessels for erythrocytes provide for this limited distribution of observed erythema. This also explains the limited flush distribution seen after obviously systemic stimuli.

Pathophysiology: Two Basic Mechanisms

Because flushing is a phenomenon of transient vasodilation, the mechanisms of vasodilation provide a physiologic scheme for classifying flushing reactions.[2] There is a dual control of vascular smooth muscle by autonomic nerves and by circulating vasoactive agents. Autonomic nerves also control the eccrine sweat glands, so that whenever vasodilation is mediated by autonomic nerves, it is accompanied by eccrine sweating.

Accordingly, two mechanisms of flushing can be distinguished at the bedside or in the office: neural-mediated flushing, which includes eccrine sweating ("wet flush"), and flushing from agents that act directly on vascular smooth muscle ("dry flush"). An important caveat to the clinician is that the presence or absence of eccrine sweating is specifically associated contemporaneously with the actual flushing, that is, the transient reddening. It is not rare for a patient with carcinoid syndrome to have a flushing reaction of such intensity that it is *followed* by coexisting pallor and diaphoresis. The "wet pallor" does not invalidate the clinical significance of the preceding dry flush.

Consequences: The Cutaneous Stigmata

In susceptible persons, frequent, intense flushing leads to a cluster of physical signs, called *rosacea*. Rosacea is characterized by erythema or cyanosis in the flush distribution, telangiectasia, papules, pustules, and eventually connective tissue hypertrophy, including rhinophyma (see Chap. 74). Frequent, intense flushing may lead to loss of vascular tone, resulting in the permanent background erythema. That the venules in the superficial plexus are involved, and not the superficial collecting veins, is compatible with infrared studies of rosacea.[3] Thus, the shunting of a considerable volume of blood during a flushing reaction directly into the venules of the subpapillary plexus, leading to loss of tone, may represent a significant step in the pathogenesis of the erythematotelangiectatic component of rosacea.

Various observations support the view that flushing is an important factor in the pathogenesis of rosacea.[4] There is a correlation between the severity of ocular rosacea (which is largely vascular) and the tendency to strong flushing. Patients with severe flushing due to carcinoid develop all of the various rosacea stigmata, including ocular rosacea, facial telangiectasia, and severe connective tissue hypertrophy. Patients with severe flushing due to mastocytosis can similarly develop rosacea in less than a year after the onset of flushing episodes. Mild rosacea is more common in women and usually appears after age 35, when the frequency of hot flashes and flushing increases. Flushing is typically the earliest component of rosacea to be apparent. Rosacea is exacerbated during vasodilator therapy accompanied by flushing. Finally, extrafacial rosacea may occur in extrafacial areas of flushing.

The pathophysiologic mechanism by which flushing leads to rosacea probably involves edema formation.[4] This edema is usually subclinical or only barely perceptible, although the frequent occurrence of overt facial edema in the course of rosacea has been documented. It follows a severe flushing episode and may last only a day initially. Over time it can become more persistent. Rosacea stigmata are typically in those areas of the face overlying relatively inactive musculature, where the edema fluid tends to persist. Rosacea responds to massage therapy, thereby supporting the pathologic role for edema.

Evaluation of the Patient with a Flushing Disorder

It is important to consider the clinical characteristics of the patient with flushing before embarking on an expensive laboratory evaluation. Four key elements of information must be obtained: provocative and palliative factors, morphology, associated features, and temporal characteristics.

Provocative and palliative factors should be sought first. This information may permit a more focused differential diagnosis—for example, alcohol-related, drug-related, or eating-related flushing (Table 171-1).

Morphology of the flushing reaction may suggest not only the cause of the flushing but also, in the case of carcinoidosis, the anatomic origin of the disorder. Important points to consider include one basic feature that comes and goes versus discrete phases or stages; patchy versus confluent; bright pink to cyanotic; pallor, preceding or following; and dry skin versus perspiration.

Associated findings, when present, aid in the differential diagnosis. Bronchospasm, abdominal cramps, diarrhea, headaches, urticaria, and pruritus can provide important clues.

Temporal characteristics include the timing of the specific features during each flushing reaction and the frequency of the flushing reactions. Since this is often the weakest part of the patient's account, a 2-week diary will provide data of better quality. The patient should record qualitative and quantitative aspects of the flushing reaction and list all occupational exposures, physical exercise, and exogenous agents, especially food, beverages, and drugs. In a patient with caffeine-withdrawal flushing, it was the absence of an exogenous agent at the critical time in a 2-week diary that led to the diagnosis.[5] The 2-week diary should be considered whenever the cause of the flushing is not immediately obvious.

When the diagnosis remains obscure after evaluation of the 2-week diary, the patient is given an exclusion diet listing foods high in histamine, foods and drugs that affect urinary 5-hydroxyindoleacetic acid (5-HIAA) tests, and foods and beverages that cause flushing. If the flushing reactions completely disappear, restoring the excluded items individually can identify the causative agent. If the flushing reactions continue unchanged, then histamine and urinary 5-HIAA may be assayed.

Occasionally, the exclusion diet will eliminate nonspecific factors that lower the threshold for flushing, perhaps by additive effects. Careful attention must be directed to a variety of such nonspecific factors, which must be avoided as much as possible. Examples are legion: menopause exacerbates flushing in the dump-

ing syndrome; warming augments gustatory flushing; and alcohol can enhance a menopausal flush.

Hyperthermic Flushing

Hyperthermic stress can be exogenous, such as a hot day, or endogenous, for example, resulting from exercise. In many patients heat can cause flushing or overheating can lower the threshold to flushing from other causes, such as menopausal flushing. Although hyperthermia is usually considered in the context of the total body thermal economy, the actual physiologic thermostat resides in the anterior hypothalamus. Thus, the ingestion of hot beverages and the resultant increased heat in the oral cavity may cause flushing by a countercurrent heat-exchange mechanism.[6]

Menopausal (Climacteric) Flushing

Although the name suggests the cessation of menses, some women develop menopausal-like symptoms in their middle thirties while still having cyclic menses. They have flushing just before or during their periods each month, when the estrogen levels are lowest. Hot beverages, physical exertion, and emotional upsets can provoke menopausal flushing. Although natural climacteric flushing is extremely rare in men, surgical climacteric flushing in men is not uncommon after orchiectomy.[7] Pharmacologic menopause with flushing can be induced by a variety of drugs: 4-hydroxyandrostenedione, danazol, tamoxifen, clomiphene citrate, decapeptyl, and leuprolide.

Surgical menopause with flushing can occur any time after puberty when there is surgical loss of ovarian function. Bilateral tubal ligation can also compromise the vascular supply to the ovaries, possibly resulting in menopausal symptoms.

Several characteristics of climacteric flushing suggest the clinical diagnosis. First, drenching perspiration, which is often the most distressing component of the climacteric flush, implicates a neural-mediated mechanism. Second, waking episodes at night accompanied by flushing and sweating are typical. Third, the prodromal sensation of overheating before the onset of flushing and sweating suggests a dysfunction in the thermoregulatory mechanism. Several lines of recent evidence indicate that the site of dysfunction lies in the central catecholaminergic system.[4]

Most women choose hormonal replacement therapy for menopausal flushing. However, nonhormonal alternatives exist, such as clonidine hydrochloride. The smallest dosage form of clonidine hydrochloride marketed in the United States is the 0.1-mg tablet. The patient should be instructed to crush one tablet daily. Half the powder is taken in the morning and the other half in the evening before bed. This regimen of 0.05 mg twice daily is sufficient for many patients.[8] Some patients may require 0.1 mg twice daily.

Emotional Flushing

Some people with fair skin and a readily visible superficial cutaneous vasculature of the face are extremely troubled by blushing. It is critical to discern at the outset whether the blushing is simply intense and the emotional dynamics are normal or whether there is a significant emotional disturbance that is accompanied by frequent blushing.

Therapies for flushing attending normal emotional responses include biofeedback, hypnosis, paradoxical intention, and nadolol.

TABLE 171-1

Differential Diagnosis of Flushing Reactions

I. Flushing reactions related to alcohol
  Increased susceptibility in Asian and Native American populations
  Occupational "degreaser's" flush in workmen drinking beer after exposure to industrial solvents
    Trichloroethylene vapor
    N,N-dimethylformamide
    N-butyraldoxime
    Carbon disulfide
    Xylene
  Fermented alcoholic beverages (beer, sherry) may contain tyramine or histamine, which induce flushing.
  Drugs
    Disulfiram
    Chlorpropamide
    Calcium carbamide
    Phentolamine
    Griseofulvin
    Metronidazole
    Ketoconazole
    Chloramphenicol
    Quinacrine
    Beta-lactams with methyltetrazolethiol side chain (cephalosporin antibiotics)
      Cefamandole
      Cefoperazone
      Moxalactam
  Eating *Coprinus* mushrooms
  Carcinoid flushing
  Mastocytosis flushing
II. Flushing related to food additives
  Monosodium glutamate (MSG) putatively provokes flushing, but this is not verified.
  Sodium nitrite in cured meats (frankfurters, bacon, salami, ham) may cause headache and flushing.
  Sulfites (potassium metabisulfite) may cause wheezing and flushing.
III. Flushing associated with eating
  Hot beverages cause flushing through countercurrent heat exchange into blood vessels leading to the anterior hypothalamus.
  Auriculotemporal flushing, especially after cheese, chocolate, lemon, highly spiced foods.
  Gustatory flushing, especially after chewing a chili pepper.
  Dumping syndrome, especially after a meal or ingestion of hot liquids or hypertonic glucose.
  Spoiled scombroid (tuna, mackerel, skipjack, and bonito) and non-scombroid (mahi-mahi, bluefish, amberjack, herring, sardines, and anchovies) fishes and cheeses. Histamine is the probable toxin.

IV. Neurologic flushing
  Anxiety
  Simple blushing
  Brain tumors
  Spinal cord lesions (autonomic hyperreflexia)
  Migraine headaches
  Parkinson's disease
  Climacteric (menopausal) flushing: "hot flashes"
  Cholinergic erythema
V. Flushing due to drugs
  All vasodilators (e.g., nitroglycerin, prostaglandins, synthetic calcitonin-gene-related peptide)
  All calcium channel blockers
    Nifedipine
    Verapamil
    Diltiazem
  Nicotinic acid (not nicotinamide)
  Morphine and other opiates
  Amyl nitrite and butyl nitrite (recreational drugs)
  Cholinergic drugs, e.g., metrifonate, an anthelminthic
  Bromocriptine used in Parkinson's disease
  Thyrotropin-releasing hormone (TRH)
  Tamoxifen
  Cyproterone acetate
  Oral triamcinolone used with psoriatic arthritis
  Cyclosporine
  Rifampin
VI. Flushing due to systemic diseases
  Carcinoid syndrome
  Male hypogonadism (pseudocarcinoid syndrome)
  Mastocytosis
  Basophilic chronic granulocytic leukemia
  Pheochromocytoma
  Medullary carcinoma of thyroid
  Pancreatic tumors (e.g., VIPoma)
  Renal cell carcinoma
  Horseshoe kidneys (Rovsing's syndrome)

Nadolol is a nonselective beta blocker that can attenuate the vascular response to anxiety in most patients at a dose of 40 to 80 mg daily. The long plasma half-life (14 to 24 h) permits a once-daily dose. Nadolol is a convenient therapy for patients with rosacea who have flushing associated with anxiety or who otherwise describe emotional flushing.[9]

Rosacea Flushing

Although the term *rosacea flushing* has been used, there is no evidence to date that suggests that flushing in rosacea is qualitatively different from flushing in the general population. However, quantitative differences based on such factors as the reactivity of the vasculature, the visibility of the vasculature, and the enhanced release of endogenous mediators are quite likely.[4]

Monosodium Glutamate Flushing

Monosodium glutamate (MSG) is widely regarded as a cause of flushing in the "Chinese restaurant syndrome." However, a true MSG-induced flushing reaction must be extremely rare, if it occurs at all.[10] Patients should be encouraged to look beyond MSG at other dietary agents, such as red pepper (capsaicin), other spices, nitrites and sulfites (additives in many foods), thermally hot food and beverages, and alcohol.

Pheochromocytoma

Flushing is so rare in patients diagnosed as having pheochromocytoma that its presence casts doubt on the diagnosis.[11] If flushing occurs at all, it is seen after a paroxysm of hypertension, tachycardia, palpitations, chest pain, severe throbbing headaches, and excessive perspiration. Pallor is present during the attack, and mild flushing may occur after the attack as a rebound from the facial cutaneous vasoconstriction.

Mastocytosis See Chap. 162

CARCINOID SYNDROME

Pathology

Although malignant carcinoid neoplasms are not rare, the carcinoid syndrome is. Less than 4 percent of 3718 patients with abdominal carcinoid tumors had the carcinoid syndrome.[12] The lack of neuroendocrine product–related symptomatology in most patients may be related to the detoxifying effect of the liver or to low levels of bioactive hormone produced by the tumors. The presence of the carcinoid syndrome implies either hepatic metastases, extraabdominal carcinoid tumor, or large or multiple primary intraabdominal lesions with sufficient biomass to produce more hormone than the liver can degrade.

Carcinoid tumors, which are derived from enterochromaffin (Kulchitsky) cells, produce a variety of humoral agents, even within a single tumor. Carcinoid tumors develop different histologic patterns and biochemical characteristics according to primary growth sites and embryonic derivation.[13,14] The appendix is the most common site, and the ileum is the second most common site. Ileal tumors are the most common source of the classic carcinoid syndrome, and the ileum is the most frequent origin for metastasizing carcinoid. Other sites for carcinoid tumors include the rectum, duodenum, stomach, colon, biliary tract, and pancreas. Less than 10 percent of carcinoid tumors originate outside the gastrointestinal tract, in sites such as ovary, testis, skin, and bronchus.[15]

The carcinoid syndrome and tumors have important characteristics that correlate with the site of origin.[13,14] Most important is the comparison between those tumors that originate in the embryologic foregut (bronchus, stomach, pancreas) and the carcinoids of the midgut (small intestine to midcolon). Although tumors from both sites produce serotonin, foregut carcinoid tumors also produce histamine, which may explain the associations of peptic ulcer disease with foregut rather than midgut carcinoid tumors. Furthermore, the flushing reaction associated with foregut tumors as compared with midgut tumors is brighter (salmon pink to red), more persistent, and more intense; shows a geographic pattern; and has prominent associated findings, including lacrimation, sweating (with pallor), vomiting, and asthma. Bronchial carcinoids show a closer relationship to foregut tumors and have a similar associated type of flushing, which is also of considerable intensity. Midgut tumors are associated with a cyanotic flush, giving an appearance of mixed cyanosis, erythema, and pallor. This flush occurs more frequently and is regarded as the classic pattern for carcinoid syndrome. Hypotension and bronchoconstriction are more common with the flushing reactions associated with midgut tumors. Hindgut (descending colon and rectal) tumors do not lead to flushing or other manifestations of carcinoid syndrome.

Clinical Manifestations

Cutaneous findings are multiple, and many can be grouped according to probable pathogenesis. Thus, pellagra-like lesions result from the excessive utilization of tryptophan by the carcinoid tumor, leaving little for the daily niacin requirement. These lesions include hyperkeratosis; xerosis; scaling of the legs, forearms, and trunk; angular cheilitis; and glossitis.

Severe carcinoid flushing can explain the rosacea stigmata, including ocular rosacea, scleral reddening, facial telangiectasia and cyanosis, and severe frontophyma, rhinophyma, and zygophyma.[4,15] The flushing, found in nearly all patients with carcinoid syndrome, can be especially intense, with facial edema occurring during the attacks.

Additional skin manifestations associated with carcinoid syndrome include yellow-brown or brown-gray patches on the forehead, back, and wrists; pruritus; pruritus with pressure-induced "orange blotches"[16]; scleroderma-like changes[17,18]; acropachyderma and pachyperiostitis[19]; cutaneous metastatic nodules[19]; erythematous, telangiectatic, atrophic patches with central ulceration[20]; pyoderma gangrenosum[21]; erythema annulare centrifugum and white banding of the toenails[22]; blisters that heal leaving white scarlike lesions and white macular lesions surrounded by an erythematous halo[23]; and reddish cyanotic, hyperkeratotic papules.[24]

Gastrointestinal manifestations may precede or coexist with the carcinoid syndrome. Chronic watery diarrhea occurs in 85 percent of patients.[25] Abdominal pain, constipation, nausea, vomiting, malabsorption, anorexia, weight loss, small bowel obstruction, and rectal bleeding may also precede the full carcinoid syndrome.

Respiratory manifestations include wheezing, stridor, dyspnea, coughing, and bronchospasm.[25] Additional findings include arthritis, psychiatric symptoms, osteoblastic bone lesions associated with bronchial carcinoid metastases, acromegaly, neurofibromatosis, Cushing's disease, and a unique retinal lesion consisting of very small, punched-out areas of postischemic changes in the peripheral retina.[15]

Fibrotic reactions are curious manifestations occurring in collagenous and elastic tissues. Endocardial fibrosis with valve damage is classically on the ventricular surface of the tricuspid valve and the pulmonary arterial surface of the pulmonic valve, producing valvular stenosis followed by insufficiency.[25] Hypotensive episodes, edema of the lower limbs, murmurs, and congestive heart failure can occur. Less commonly, the fibrotic valvular damage is left-sided due to either bronchial carcinoids or the combination of hepatic metastases with an atrial septal defect.[26]

The fibrotic reactions to surgery, fibrosis of the bladder, and fibrosis of the peritoneum may be of the same nature as the valvular lesions, that is, young fibrous tissue hyperproliferation that is purely collagenous and not elastic. A distinctly different type of reaction is the elastic vascular sclerosis of mesenteric blood vessels. This unique process, which occurs only with ileal carcinoid tumors, can lead to ischemic ileal necrosis. Serotonin may have a direct role in the fibrotic processes.[15]

Diagnosis and Serotonin Metabolism

The essential diagnostic criterion of carcinoid syndrome is biochemical evidence of serotonin overproduction.[7] This is usually established by an elevated output of urinary 5-HIAA, which is normally 2 to 10 mg per day. In carcinoid syndrome it is often over 40 mg per day. Various foods and drugs can affect the urinary excretion of 5-HIAA (Table 171-2), and specimens for determination of uri-

TABLE 171-2

Foods and Drugs That Affect Urinary Excretion of 5-Hydroxyindoleacetic Acid

Foods

Avocados	Red plums
Bananas	Tomatoes
Eggplant	Walnuts
Pineapples	

Drugs

ACTH	Mephenesin
Acetaminophen	Methamphetamine
Acetanilid	Methenamine
Bromocriptine	Methocarbamol
Caffeine	Methyldopa
Chlorpromazine	Methysergide
Fluorouracil	Monoamine oxidase inhibitors
Guaifenesin	Phenacetin
Glyceryl guaiacolate	Phenmetrazine
Heparin	Phenothiazines
Imipramine	Promethazine
Isoniazid	Reserpine
Lugol's solution	Somatostatin analogues (e.g., octreotide)
Melphalan	

nary 5-HIAA excretion should be collected during the third day of an exclusion diet. It cannot be overemphasized that a qualitative (screening, or "spot") test for urinary 5-HIAA is of value only when positive. If carcinoid tumor is suspected clinically and the qualitative test is negative, a quantitative assay should be performed on a sample from a 24-h urine collection. Excretion fluctuates, so that repeated measurements may be necessary. Occasional patients are reported with carcinoid syndrome and normal 5-HIAA excretion.[27] These patients have hyperserotoninemia, and they lack the metabolic machinery to convert serotonin to 5-HIAA. In addition, men have been reported with increased urinary 5-HIAA levels, secondary hypogonadism, and flushing. Resolution of flushing and normalization of 5-HIAA levels may be achieved with testosterone treatment.[28]

Provocative tests, which should be performed in an appropriate clinical setting, can also be valuable. Epinephrine, 5 μg, or calcium gluconate, 10 to 15 mg/kg, administered intravenously over 4 h, may produce a flush mimicking a spontaneous attack.[29] Selective abdominal vein catheterization with blood sampling for serotonin determination in a platelet-poor plasma fraction can both determine whether carcinoid tumor is present and identify the site in cases in which urine 5-HIAA levels and liver scintiscan are negative and angiograms are inconclusive.[30] A radiolabeled octreotide scanning technique has been shown to be a rapid and safe procedure for the visualization of primary tumors or metastases in patients with carcinoid tumors.[31] A positive scan can also predict the ability of octreotide therapy to control symptoms of hormonal hypersecretion.

It is important to remember that the tissue diagnosis of carcinoid tumor in a patient with flushing does not unequivocally establish the diagnosis of carcinoid syndrome.[7]

Management and Prognosis

Even though carcinoid syndrome may appear relatively homogeneous clinically, biochemical and pharmacologic heterogeneity is present. Serotonin may affect the qualitative nature of the flush, that is, the cyanotic aspect, but it is not the mediator of the flushing reaction. In fact, the hypersecretion of serotonin and the flushing reaction can be pharmacologically dissociated.[4] Corticosteroids and bromocriptine have been effective in patients with bronchial carcinoid tumors.[32,33] Serotonin antagonists and depleters, such as methysergide and parachlorophenylalanine, respectively, may effectively control the diarrhea but have no effect on the flushing.[34–36] Another serotonin antagonist, ketanserin, has been successful perioperatively in a patient with the carcinoid syndrome undergoing hepatic artery embolization.[37] Cyproheptadine, which is a serotonin antagonist among other properties, has been helpful in controlling flushing.[34] Antihistamines may be especially useful in patients with foregut carcinoid tumors that produce histamine. Clonidine controls carcinoid flushing in some patients in whom the release of catecholamines, which act on the tumor cells, may be an important factor.[38,39] Thus, the pharmacologic basis for management of carcinoid flushing reactions is complex.

Importantly, somatostatin is a potent antagonist of the flushing reaction associated with both gastric and ileal carcinoid tumors.[40–42] Since somatostatin is effective in midgut carcinoid flushing, where histamine is without a major role, it is likely that somatostatin does more than simply inhibit the release of histamine. However, clinical use of somatostatin is limited because of its short half-life and intravenous delivery.

The somatostatin analogue octreotide has pharmacologic effects similar to those of somatostatin but a much longer half-life, making subcutaneous therapy possible. Octreotide not only controls the flushing and diarrhea of carcinoid syndrome but also may suppress cancerous cell growth.[43] Octreotide must be given by subcutaneous injection at least once a day and usually twice a day. Octreotide has also been used intravenously with success to treat carcinoid crisis during anesthesia.[44]

In addition to the specific pharmacologic agents used to control flushing, the dermatologist should determine that the patient is receiving an adequate niacin supplement (as nicotinamide, not nicotinic acid, since the latter causes flushing). Patients should avoid foods, agents, and activities that precipitate symptoms (Table 171-3).

TABLE 171-3

Factors That Precipitate Flushing in the Carcinoid Syndrome

Foods and beverages
    Hot (thermal) food/beverages
    Spicy food
    Chocolate
    Cheeses
    Tomatoes
    Avocados
    Red plums
    Walnuts
    Eggplant
    Ingestion of any food
    Alcohol
Emotional stress
Valsalva maneuver
    Straining during defecation
    Vigorous coughing
Sudden, direct pressure on a large carcinoid tumor
    Physical examination
    Intraoperative manipulation
Spontaneous

At present, antitumor drugs and subtotal tumor resection lead to variable results in the patient with carcinoid syndrome. Only total surgical removal can offer cure, and this is, unfortunately, seldom feasible.

REFERENCES

1. Wilkin JK: Why is flushing limited to a mostly facial cutaneous distribution? *J Am Acad Dermatol* **19**:309, 1988
2. Burnstock G, Iwayama T: Fine-structural identification of autonomic nerves and their relation to smooth muscle. *Prog Brain Res* **34**:389, 1971
3. Wilkin JK, Josephs JA: Infrared photographic studies of rosacea. *Arch Dermatol* **116**:678, 1980
4. Wilkin JK: Flushing reactions, in *Recent Advances in Dermatology,* No. 6, edited by AJ Rook, HI Maiback. New York, Churchill Livingstone, 1983, p 157
5. Wilkin JK: The caffeine withdrawal flush: Report of a case of "weekend flushing." *Mil Med* **151**:123, 1986
6. Wilkin JK: Oral thermal-induced flushing in erythematotelangiectatic rosacea. *J Invest Dermatol* **76**:15, 1981
7. Wilkin JK: Climacteric flushing in a patient with carcinoid tumour. *Br J Dermatol* **112**:357, 1985
8. Edington RF et al: Clonidine (Dixarit) for menopausal flushing. *Can Med Assoc J* **123**:23, 1980
9. Wilkin JK: Effect of nadolol on flushing reactions in rosacea. *J Am Acad Dermatol* **20**:202, 1989
10. Wilkin JK, Fortner G: Does monosodium glutamate cause flushing? *J Am Acad Dermatol* **15**:225, 1986
11. Bravo EL, Gifford RW: Pheochromocytoma: Diagnosis, localization and management. *N Engl J Med* **311**:1298, 1984
12. Wilson H: Carcinoid syndrome. *Curr Probl Surg* **11**:36, 1970
13. Williams ED, Sandler M: The classification of carcinoid tumors. *Lancet* **1**:238, 1963
14. Soga J, Tazawa K: Pathologic analysis of carcinoids. *Cancer* **28**:990, 1971
15. Wilkin JK, Demis DJ: Carcinoidosis (carcinoid syndrome), in *Clinical Dermatology,* edited by DJ Demis, RL Dobson, JS McGuire. Philadelphia, Harper & Row, 1985, pp 1, 4-12
16. Mengel C: Cutaneous manifestations of malignant carcinoid syndrome. *Ann Intern Med* **58**:989, 1963
17. Zarafonetis C, Lorber S: Association of functioning carcinoid syndrome and scleroderma. *Am J Med Sci* **236**:1, 1958
18. Fries JF et al: Scleroderma-like lesions and the carcinoid syndrome. *Arch Intern Med* **131**:550, 1973
19. Walker J: Metastasizing argentaffinomas from dermatologist's point of view. *S Afr Med J* **31**:1271, 1957
20. Bean SF, Fusaro RM: An unusual manifestation of the carcinoid syndrome. *Arch Dermatol* **98**:268, 1968
21. Lee SS et al: Pyoderma gangrenosum with carcinoid tumor. *Cutis* **18**:791, 1976
22. Everall JD et al: Unusual cutaneous associations of a malignant carcinoid tumour of the bronchus: Erythema annulare centrifugum and white banding of the toe nails. *Br J Dermatol* **93**:341, 1975
23. Smith AS, Greaves MW: Blood prostaglandin activity associated with noradrenaline-produced flush in the carcinoid syndrome. *Br J Dermatol* **90**:547, 1974
24. Lachapelle J-M et al: Syndrome carcinoide: Manifestations cutanées chroniques florides. *Ann Dermatol Venereol* **104**:66, 1977
25. Beaton H, Dineen P: Gastrointestinal carcinoids and the malignant carcinoid syndrome. *Surg Gynecol Obstet* **152**:268, 1981
26. Waldenstrom J, Ljungberg E: Studies on the functional circulatory influence from metastasizing carcinoid tumours and their possible relation to enteramine production. *Acta Med Scand* **152**:293, 1955
27. Davis RB, Rosenberg JC: Carcinoid syndrome associated with hyperserotoninemia and normal 5-hydroxyindoleacetic acid excretion. *Am J Med* **30**:167, 1961
28. Shakir KMM et al: Pseudocarcinoid syndrome associated with hypogonadism and response to testosterone therapy. *Mayo Clin Proc* **71**:1145, 1996
29. Kaplan EL et al: A new provocative test for the diagnosis of the carcinoid syndrome. *Am J Surg* **123**:173, 1972
30. Nobin A et al: Selective mesenteric vein catheterization and plasma serotonin determination in patients with carcinoid tumors. *World J Surg* **7**:223, 1983
31. Lamberts SWJ et al: Somatostatin-receptor imaging in the localization of endocrine tumors. *N Engl J Med* **323**:1246, 1990
32. Reith PR et al: Prolonged suppression of a corticotropin-producing bronchial carcinoid by oral bromocriptine. *Arch Intern Med* **147**:989, 1987
33. Sebastian A et al: The spectrum produced by malignant carcinoid tumor. *Calif Med* **106**:64, 1967
34. Brown H et al: Functioning carcinoid tumors, in *Cancer of the Gastrointestinal Tract.* Chicago, Year Book, 1967, p 155
35. Satterlee WG et al: The carcinoid syndrome: Chronic treatment with parachlorophenylalanine. *Ann Intern Med* **72**:919, 1970
36. Engelman K et al: Inhibition of serotonin synthesis by para-chlorophenylalanine in patients with the carcinoid syndrome. *N Engl J Med* **277**:1103, 1967
37. Houghton K, Carter JA: Peri-operative management of carcinoid syndrome using ketanserin. *Anaesthesia* **41**:596, 1986
38. Wilkin JK, Rountree CB: Blockade of carcinoid flush with cimetidine and clonidine. *Arch Dermatol* **118**:109, 1982
39. Metz SA et al: Suppression of plasma catecholamines and flushing by clonidine in man. *J Clin Endocrinol Metab* **46**:83, 1978
40. Roberts LJ et al: Carcinoid: Provocation by pentagastrin and inhibition by somatostatin. *Gastroenterology* **84**:272, 1983
41. Thulin L et al: Efficacy of somatostatin in a patient with carcinoid syndrome. *Lancet* **2**:43, 1978
42. Quatrini M et al: Effects of somatostatin infusion in four patients with malignant carcinoid syndrome. *Am J Gastroenterol* **78**:149, 1983
43. Maton PN: Use in patients with gut neuroendocrine tumors, p 41, in Gordon P, moderator: Somatostatin and somatostatin analogue (SMS 201-995) in treatment of hormone-secreting tumors of the pituitary and gastrointestinal tract and non-neoplastic diseases of the gut. *Ann Intern Med* **110**:35, 1989
44. Marsh HM et al: Carcinoid crisis during anesthesia: Successful treatment with a somatostatin analogue. *Anesthesiology* **66**:89, 1987

CHAPTER 172

Richard D. Sontheimer

Lupus Erythematosus

Lupus erythematosus (LE) is the root designation for a diverse array of illnesses that are linked together by distinctive clinical findings and characteristic patterns of polyclonal B cell autoimmunity. Some patients present with life-threatening manifestations of systemic LE (SLE); whereas others, who are affected with what likely represents the same basic underlying disease process, express little more than discoid LE (DLE) skin lesions throughout their illness. Many have found it convenient to conceptualize LE as a clinical spectrum ranging from mildly affected patients with only localized DLE skin lesions to those at risk of dying from the systemic manifestations of LE such as nephritis, central nervous system disease, or vasculitis. The pattern of skin involvement expressed by an individual patient with LE can provide insight about the position on the spectrum where the patient's illness might best be placed.

The nomenclature and classification system originally devised by James N. Gilliam divides the cutaneous manifestations of LE into those lesions that are histopathologically specific for LE (*LE-specific skin disease*) and those that are not histopathologically specific for LE (*LE-nonspecific skin disease*). The rationale behind this system of nosology and classification has recently been discussed in depth.[1] The term *cutaneous LE* is often used synonymously with LE-specific skin disease as an umbrella designation for the three major categories of LE-specific skin disease—acute cutaneous LE (ACLE), subacute cutaneous LE (SCLE), and chronic cutaneous LE (CCLE). This framework will be used to discuss the extraordinarily diverse set of cutaneous lesions that occur in patients with LE (Table 172-1).

The essence of LE is in its heterogeneity, and the challenge for those who treat it is to recognize clinically useful patterns within the mosaic of features that constitute this protean illness. The focus of this presentation will be on the cutaneous features of this disorder, especially the LE-specific skin lesions. (The LE-nonspecific skin lesions will be summarized at the end of the chapter.) The systemic manifestations of LE and their management are covered in current monographs.[2–4] An overview of the systemic manifestations of LE can be surmised from the American College of Rheumatology's classification criteria for SLE,[5] which are presented in Table 172-2, and from the outline of the systemic manifestations of SLE presented in Table 172-3. In addition, the cutaneous manifes-

tations of LE with comprehensive citations have been reviewed elsewhere.[6–16]

HISTORIC ASPECTS

Cazenave is credited for first using the term *lupus érythèmateaux* in 1851 to refer to Biett's earlier description of DLE skin lesions. The use of this term helped to distinguish cutaneous LE from cutaneous tuberculosis (lupus vulgaris) with which it had been earlier confused. Kaposi expanded Hebra's description of what is now recognized as SLE in 1875. Kaposi employed the "butterfly" simile, which had first been used by Hebra to describe the facial skin lesions associated with SLE. Jonathan Hutchinson in 1880 and William Osler at the turn of the century emphasized the multisystem nature of LE. Even until 1936 it was felt to be unusual for the systemic features of LE to be present in the absence of skin lesions. Comprehensive historic perspectives on the cutaneous manifestations of LE have been written.[6,17,18]

EPIDEMIOLOGY

The epidemiology and socioeconomic impact of LE in general[19,20] and cutaneous LE specifically[6,8,21] have been reviewed. Skin disease is the second most frequent clinical manifestation of LE after joint inflammation. As many as 45 percent of patients with cutaneous LE experience some degree of vocational handicap.

Demographics

Malar, or butterfly, rash (localized ACLE) has been reported in 20 to 60 percent of large cohorts of patients with LE. Limited data suggest that the maculopapular, or SLE, rash of generalized ACLE

TABLE 172-1

The Gilliam Classification of Skin Lesions Associated with LE

I. LE-specific skin disease (cutnaeous LE [CLE])*
  A. Acute cutaneous LE [ACLE]
    1. Localized ACLE (malar rash; butterfly rash)
    2. Generalized ACLE (lupus maculopapular lupus rash, SLE rash, rash, photosensitive lupus dermatitis)
  B. Subacute cutaneous LE [SCLE]
    1. Annular SCLE (lupus marginatus, symmetric erythema centrifugum, autoimmune annular erythema, lupus erythematosus gyratus repens)
    2. Papulosquamous SCLE (disseminated DLE, subacute disseminated LE, superficial disseminated LE, psoriasiform LE, pityriasiform LE, and maculopapular photosensitive LE)
  C. Chronic cutaneous LE (CCLE)
    1. Classic discoid LE [DLE]
      a. Localized DLE
      b. Generalized DLE
    2. Hypertrophic/verrucous DLE
    3. Lupus profundus/lupus panniculitis
    4. Mucosal DLE
      a. Oral DLE
      b. Conjunctival DLE
    5. Lupus tumidus (urticarial plaque of LE)
    6. Chilblains LE (chilblains lupus)
    7. Lichenoid DLE (LE/lichen planus overlap, lupus planus)
II. LE-nonspecific skin disease
  A. Cutaneous vascular disease
    1. Vasculitis
      a. Leukocytoclastic
        (1) Palpable purpura
        (2) Urticarial vasculitis
      b. Periarteritis nodosa–like cutaneous lesions
    2. Vasculopathy
      a. Degos' disease-like lesions
      b. Secondary atrophie blanche (livedoid vasculitis, livedo vasculitis)
    3. Periungual telangiectasia
    4. Livedo reticularis
    5. Thrombophlebitis
    6. Raynaud's phenomenon
    7. Erythromelalgia (erythermalgia)
  B. Nonscarring alopecia
    1. "Lupus hair"
    2. Telogen effluvium
    3. Alopecia areata
  C. Sclerodactly
  D. Rheumatoid nodules
  E. Calcinosis cutis
  F. LE-nonspecific bullous lesions
  G. Urticaria
  H. Papulonodular mucinosis
  I. Cutis laxa/anetoderma
  J. Acanthosis nigricans (type B insulin resistance)
  K. Erythema multiforme
  L. Leg ulcers
  M. Lichen planus

*Alternative or synonymous terms are listed in parentheses; abbreviations are indicated in brackets.
SOURCE: Reprinted from Sontheimer[1] with permission from Stockton Journals, Macmillian Press, Ltd.

is present in about 35 to 60 percent of patients with SLE. ACLE, like SLE in general, is much more common in women than men (8:1). All races are affected; however, the early clinical manifestations of ACLE can be overlooked in a dark-skinned individual.

Patients presenting with SCLE lesions have constituted 7 to 27 percent of LE patient populations. SCLE is primarily a disease of white females, with the mean age of onset in the fifth decade.

The most common form of CCLE, classic DLE skin lesions, is present in 15 to 30 percent of SLE populations selected in various ways. Approximately 5 percent of patients presenting with isolated localized DLE subsequently develop SLE. It has been suggested that SLE is sevenfold more common than DLE. Although DLE can occur in infants and the elderly, it is most common in individuals between 20 and 40 years of age. DLE has a female:male ratio of 3:2 to 3:1, which is much lower than that of SLE. All races are affected, but recent investigation has suggested that DLE might be more prevalent in blacks.

Genetic Associations

ACLE is usually encountered in patients having overt SLE, and SLE is known to be associated with HLA-DR2 and -DR3. A genetic component for SLE has been suggested by concordance in monozygotic twins and familial associations.

SCLE has been most strongly associated with the HLA-B8, DR3 haplotype. Patients with SCLE and overlapping features of Sjögren's syndrome are more likely to have the HLA-B8, DR3, DRw6, DQ2, and DRw52 extended haplotype. The HLA-DR antigen associations of SCLE may reflect the genetic contribution to anti-Ro/SS-A antibody production; patients with the extended haplotype HLA-B8, DR3, DRw6, DQ1/2, and DRw52 produce the highest levels of Ro/SS-A autoantibodies. Genetic deficiencies of various complement components, including C2, C3, C4, and C5 as well as the C1 esterase inhibitor, have been associated with both SCLE and DLE.

Significant increases of HLA-B7, B8, Cw7, DR2, DR3, and DQw1 and a significant decrease in HLA-A2 have been reported for patients with DLE. The combinations of HLA-Cw7, DR3, and DQw1 and HLA-B7, Cw7, and DR3 conferred the maximum relative risk (7.4) for DLE. DLE also occurs with increased frequency in female carriers of X-linked chronic granulomatous disease.

Environmental Factors

Exposure to natural (sunlight) or artificial sources of UV radiation (unshielded fluorescent lighting, some photocopiers) is a frequent precipitating factor for ACLE. The presence of anti-Ro/SS-A autoantibody is an additional risk factor for such photosensitivity. Numerous drugs have been implicated in inducing various features of SLE (e.g., procainamide, hydralazine, isoniazid, chlorpromazine, dilantin). However, it is curious that the skin is often spared in such classic drug-induced SLE states. L-Canavanine in alfalfa sprouts can induce an SLE-like illness. Infections of all types are capable of exacerbating SLE, and subtle viral infections (e.g., retroviruses) have long been implicated as an etiologic factor.

Patients with SCLE are highly sensitive to UV radiation. Increasing evidence suggests that UVA as well as UVB radiation can elicit SCLE lesions. SCLE lesions have been reported to be precipitated by exposure to certain drugs including hydrochlorothiazide, procainamide, D-penicillamine, sulfonylureas, oxyprenolol, griseofulvin, piroxicam, naproxen, diltiazem, cilazapril, and PUVA.

DLE skin lesions, in approximately half of patients, are precipitated or aggravated by UV radiation, especially UVB. Although drug-induced DLE lesions are extremely rare, we have observed patients whose previously refractory DLE lesions improved spontaneously in a dramatic fashion after the cessation of cigarette smoking, which has been implicated as an etiologic factor in cutaneous LE.[22]

ETIOLOGY AND PATHOGENESIS

The cause(s) of and pathogenetic mechanisms responsible for LE-specific skin disease are poorly understood. What is known about this subject and speculations about possible pathogenetic mechanisms have been presented elsewhere in more detail than is possible here.[6,23–26]

Increasing evidence suggests that many of the SLE-associated humoral autoimmune responses such as those directed at Ro/SS-A ribonucleoprotein particles are the result of conventional antigen-driven CD4 T cell immune responses triggered by environmental stimuli such as UV radiation, infection, and/or chemical exposure. These conventional immune responses are thought to become cross-reactive with homologous autoantigens because of genetically determined immune dysregulation. Through physiologic B cell mechanisms of somatic mutation, affinity maturation, and epitope spreading, these autoantibody responses then spread to other autoantigens that are physically linked to the initially targeted cross-reactive autoantigen.[27–31]

Etiologic factors implicated in LE-specific skin disease include UV radiation, viral infections, drug and chemical exposure, and cigarette smoking. Early studies demonstrated that cutaneous LE lesions could be provoked in the clinically normal skin of patients with both SLE and cutaneous LE by repeated delivery of high doses of UVB radiation to the same test site. More recent studies have argued that UVA radiation can also induce cutaneous LE lesions. Mononuclear cell accumulation in dermal perivascular areas has been the first recognizable pathologic change in UV-induced LE skin lesions. The deposition of immunoglobulin and complement components at the dermal-epidermal junction after the appearance of perivascular cellular inflammation in UV-challenged skin argues against a primary, initiating role for such immune deposits in the pathogenesis of LE-specific skin disease.

The pathogenetic effects of UV light in cutaneous LE are poorly understood. Proposed mechanisms include neoantigen formation/ autoantigen modulation, exaggerated release of immune mediators, and the perturbation of cutaneous immunoregulatory circuits. UV light has been suggested to induce the expression of "neoantigens" that could become the target of a dysregulated immune attack. It has been shown that UVB radiation can displace autoantigens such as Ro/SS-A and related autoantigens, La/SS-B and calreticulin, from their normal locations inside epidermal keratinocytes to the

TABLE 172-2

The 1982 Revised Criteria for Classification of Systemic Lupus Erythematosus*

CRITERION	DEFINITION
1. Malar rash	Fixed erythema, flat or raised, over the malar eminences, tending to spare the nasolabial folds
2. Discoid rash	Erythematous raised patches with adherent keratotic scaling and follicular plugging; atrophic scarring may occur in older lesions
3. Photosensitivity	Skin rash as a result of unusual reaction to sunlight, by patient history or physician observation
4. Oral ulcers	Oral or nasopharyngeal ulceration, usually painless, observed by a physician
5. Arthritis	Nonerosive arthritis involving two or more peripheral joints, characterized by tenderness, swelling, or effusion
6. Serositis	a. Pleuritis—convincing history of pleuritic pain or rub heard by a physician or evidence of pleural effusion *or* b. Pericarditis—documented by ECG or rub or evidence of pericardial effusion
7. Renal disorder	a. Persistent proteinuria—>0.5 g/day or greater than 3+ if quantitation not performed *or* b. Cellular casts—may be red cell, hemoglobin, granular, tubular, or mixed
8. Neurologic disorder	a. Seizures—in the absence of offending drugs or known metabolic derangements, e.g., uremia, ketoacidosis, or electrolyte imbalance *or* b. Psychosis—in the absence of offending drugs or known metabolic derangements, e.g., uremia, ketoacidosis, or electrolyte imbalance
9. Hematologic disorder	a. Hemolytic anemia—with reticulocytosis *or* b. Leukopenia—<4000/μL total on two or more occasions *or* c. Lymphopenia—<1500/μL on two or more occasions *or* d. Thrombocytopenia—<100,000/μL in the absence of offending drugs
10. Immunologic disorder	a. Anti-DNA antibody to native DNA in abnormal titer *or* b. Anti-Sm—presence of antibody to Sm nuclear antigen *or* c. Positive finding of antiphospholipid antibodies based on (1) an abnormal serum level of IgG or IgM anticardiolipin antibodies, (2) a positive test result for lupus anticoagulant using a standard method, or (3) a false-positive serologic test for syphilis known to be positive for at least 6 months and confirmed by *Treponema pallidum* immobilization or fluorescent treponemal antibody absorption test
11. Antinuclear antibody	An abnormal titer of antinuclear antibody by immunofluorescence of an equivalent assay at any point in time and in the absence of drugs known to be associated with "drug-induced lupus" syndrome

*The proposed classification is based on 11 criteria. For the purpose of identifying patients in clinical studies, a person shall be said to have SLE if any 4 or more of the 11 criteria are present, serially or simultaneously, during any interval of observation.
SOURCE: Reprinted from Tan et al,[5] *Arthritis Rheumatism,* copyright 1982. Used by permission of the American College of Rheumatology.

TABLE 172-3

Overview of the Extracutaneous Manifestations of SLE

General
  Fever, fatigue, malaise, weight loss
Musculoskeletal
  Symmetric small joint arthralgia, arthritis (nondeforming and
    deforming), morning stiffness
  Myalgia, myositis
  Tendinitis
  Avascular (aseptic) bone necrosis
Hematologic
  Anemia
    Normocytic, normochromic
    Hemolytic
  Leukopenia
    Lymphopenia
    Granulocytopenia
  Thrombocytopenia
Cardiopulmonary
  Pleurisy, pleural effusions, aseptic pneumonitis, pulmonary
    hemorrhage
  Pericarditis, tachycardia, cardiomegaly, congestive heart failure,
    arrhythmias, conduction defects, coronary arteritis,
    Libman-Sacks endocarditis
Renal
  Mesangial glomerulitis [World Health Organization (WHO) class II]
    Mild proteinuria
  Focal proliferative glomerulonephritis (WHO class III):
    Proteinuria, hematuria, occasionally nephrotic syndrome
  Diffuse proliferative glomerulonephritis (WHO class IV):
    Proteinuria, hematuria, red cell casts, renal insufficiency,
      nephrotic syndrome, hypertension
  Membranous glomerulonephritis (WHO class V):
    Severe proteinuria, nephrotic syndrome
Neuropsychiatric
  Peripheral neuropathy, transverse myelitis, Guillain-Barré syndrome
  Chorea, choreoathetosis
  Seizures
  Headaches (severe, migraine-like)
  Brain infarcts secondary to cerebral arteritis
  Organic brain syndrome
    Psychosis due to diffuse cerebritis
  Psychological
    Depression
Gastrointestinal
  Anorexia, nausea, vomiting, abdominal pain
  Bowel infarction/perforation secondary to mesenteric vasculitis
  Pancreatitis
  Peritonitis, ascites
  Hepatomegaly, chronic active hepatitis
Ocular
  Conjunctivitis, episcleritis
  Blindness secondary to central retinal artery occlusion
  Cytoid bodies
  Keratoconjunctivitis sicca
Lymphatic system
  Lymphadenopathy
  Splenomegaly

cell surface. Evidence suggests that UV-induced keratinocyte apoptosis is a major mechanism responsible for this aberrant pattern of cell surface autoantigen expression.[24] Cell surface expression would allow Ro/SS-A, La/SS-B, and calreticulin autoantibodies in the cir-

culation to bind to these autoantigens that are normally sequestered from the humoral immune response inside cells. Autoantibody binding to the exposed antigens could result in tissue injury through complement-mediated lysis or antibody-dependent cell-mediated cytotoxicity. Infection by alphaviruses such as sindbis and rubella appears able to induce cell surface expression of Ro/SS-A and related autoantigens in cells undergoing virus-induced apoptosis. Other viruses such as cytomegalovirus also trigger cell surface expression of Ro/SS-A and related autoantigens. It is possible that humoral factors other than anti-Ro/SS-A might be involved in the pathogenesis of LE photosensitivity.

UV light may cause an exaggerated release of immune mediators such as interleukin (IL) 1, tumor necrosis factor (TNF) α, prostaglandin E, proteases, oxygen free radicals, and histamine in genetically predisposed individuals with LE. IL-1 receptor antagonist and TNF-α gene polymorphism has been implicated as a genetic factor in cutaneous LE. The aberrant expression of adhesion molecules such as intercellular adhesion molecule (ICAM) 1 could play a role in the pathogenesis of LE photosensitivity. UV light may directly affect immunoregulatory cells such as cutaneous T cells, which normally help suppress "abnormal" patterns of cutaneous inflammation.[23,25,26,32,33]

Evidence suggests that autoantigen-specific T cells play a role in the pathogenesis of other organ-specific autoimmune disorders such as autoimmune thyroiditis and multiple sclerosis. Autoreactive T cells could play a role in the pathogenesis of forms of cutaneous LE, such as DLE, that are not associated with specific autoantibodies. The fact that T cells in cutaneous LE lesions are oligoclonal supports the idea that antigen-driven T cell proliferation is occurring within such lesions.[34] The recognition by T cells of autoantigens being presented by epidermal Langerhans cells might help explain the decreased numbers of Langerhans cells in areas of active cutaneous LE inflammation. Epidermal keratinocytes in cutaneous LE lesions often express class II histocompatibility antigens as well as adhesion molecules involved in T cell binding interactions such as ICAM-1. Epidermal basal cell CD40 ligation by infiltrating T cells could contribute to the altered epidermal kinetics in cutaneous LE lesions (hyperproliferation, normal early differentiation, premature terminal differentiation).

CLINICAL MANIFESTATIONS

The clinical aspects of LE-specific skin disease are extremely varied.[6–16,35] The key clinical, histopathologic, and laboratory features of patients presenting with ACLE, SCLE, and classic DLE skin lesions are compared in Table 172-4.

ACLE

Although ACLE localized to the face is the usual pattern of presentation, ACLE can assume a generalized distribution. Localized ACLE has commonly been referred to as the classic *butterfly rash* or *malar rash* of SLE (Fig. 172-1). In localized ACLE, confluent symmetric erythema and edema is centered over the malar eminences and bridges over the nose (unilateral involvement with ACLE has been described). The nasolabial folds are characteristically spared. The forehead, chin, and V area of the neck can be involved, and severe facial swelling may occur. Occasionally, ACLE begins as small macules and/or papules on the face that later may become confluent and hyperkeratotic. Generalized ACLE presents as a widespread morbilliform or exanthematous eruption often

TABLE 172-4

CHAPTER 172
Lupus Erythematosus   1997

Comparison of the Major Types of LE-Specific Skin Disease

DISEASE FEATURES	ACLE	SCLE	CLASSIC DLE
Clinical features of skin lesions			
Induration	0*	0	+++
Dermal atrophy	0	0	+++
Pigment changes	+	++	+++
Follicular plugging	0	0	+++
Hyperkeratosis	+	++	+++
Histopathology			
Thickened basement membrane	0	+	+++
Lichenoid infiltrate	+	++	+++
Periappendageal inflammation	0	+	+++
Lupus band			
Lesional	++	++	+++
Nonlesional	++	+	0
Antinuclear antibodies	+++	++	+
Ro/SS-A antibodies			
By immunodiffusion	+	+++	0
By ELISA	++	+++	+
Anti-double-stranded DNA antibodies	+++	+	0
Hypocomplementemia	+++	+	+
Risk for developing SLE	+++	++	+

*+++, Strong association; ++, moderate association; +, weak association; 0, negative, no association.
SOURCE: Reprinted from Sontheimer and Provost,[6] with permission from Williams & Wilkins Publishers.

FIGURE 172-1

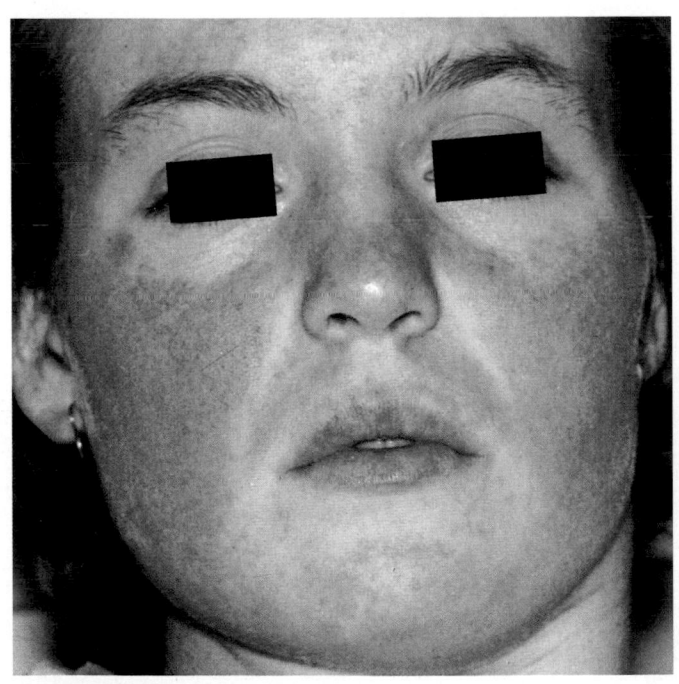

Localized acute cutaneous LE (ACLE). Erythematous, slightly edematous, sharply demarcated erythema is seen on the malar areas in a "butterfly" distribution.

focused over the extensor aspects of the arms and hands and characteristically sparing the knuckles (Fig. 172-2). Although perivascular nailfold erythema and telangiectasia can occur (Fig. 172-2), they are considerably more common and occur in more exaggerated forms in dermatomyositis (see Fig. 173-3). Generalized ACLE has been indiscriminately referred to as *the maculopapular rash of SLE*, *photosensitive lupus dermatitis*, and *SLE rash*. An extremely acute form of ACLE is rarely seen that can simulate toxic epidermal necrolysis. This form of bullous LE results from dissolution of the epidermal basal cell layer due to very intense lichenoid inflammation.

ACLE is typically precipitated or exacerbated by exposure to UV light. This form of cutaneous LE can be quite ephemeral, lasting only hours, days, or weeks; however, some patients experience more prolonged periods of activity. Postinflammatory pigmentary change is most prominent in patients with heavily pigmented skin. Scarring does not occur in ACLE unless the process is complicated by secondary bacterial infection. ACLE occasionally occurs in conjunction with SCLE; however, the simultaneous occurrence of ACLE and active DLE is unusual.[11] Both localized and generalized ACLE wax and wane in parallel with underlying SLE disease activity, including LE nephritis.

SCLE

A number of names have been used to describe SCLE skin lesions: symmetric erythema centrifugum, disseminated DLE, autoimmune annular erythema, subacute disseminated LE, superficial disseminated LE, psoriasiform LE, pityriasiform LE, maculopapular photosensitive LE, and lupus erythematosus gyratum repens. A disease presentation dominated by SCLE lesions marks the presence of a distinct subset of LE having characteristic clinical, serologic, and genetic features. Although a finding of circulating autoantibodies to the Ro/SS-A ribonucleoprotein particle strongly supports a diagnosis of SCLE, the presence of this autoantibody specificity is not required to make a diagnosis of SCLE.

SCLE initially presents as erythematous macules and/or papules that evolve into hyperkeratotic papulosquamous or annular/polycyclic plaques (Fig. 172-3). Whereas patients have either annular or papulosquamous SCLE, a few develop elements of both morphologic varieties. SCLE lesions are characteristically photosensitive and occur in predominantly sun-exposed areas (i.e., upper back, shoulders, extensor aspects of the arms, V area of the neck, and less commonly the face). SCLE lesions typically heal without scarring but can resolve with long-lasting if not permanent vitiligo-like leukoderma and telangiectasias.

Several variants of SCLE have been described. On occasion, SCLE lesions present initially with an appearance of erythema multiforme, and such cases can simulate the appearance of Rowell's syndrome (erythema multiforme–like lesions occurring in patients with SLE in the presence of La/SS-B autoantibodies). As a result of intense injury to epidermal basal cells, the active edge of an annular SCLE lesion occasionally undergoes a vesiculobullous change that can subsequently produce a strikingly crusted appearance. Such lesions mimic toxic epidermal necrolysis. Rarely, SCLE presents with exfoliative erythroderma or displays a curious acral distribution of annular lesions. Pityriasiform and exanthematous variants of SCLE have been reported. In one case, annular SCLE lesions were observed to evolve over time to plaques of morphea. The skin lesions of neonatal LE (transient, photosensitive, nonscarring LE-specific skin lesions in neonates who have received IgG

FIGURE 172-2

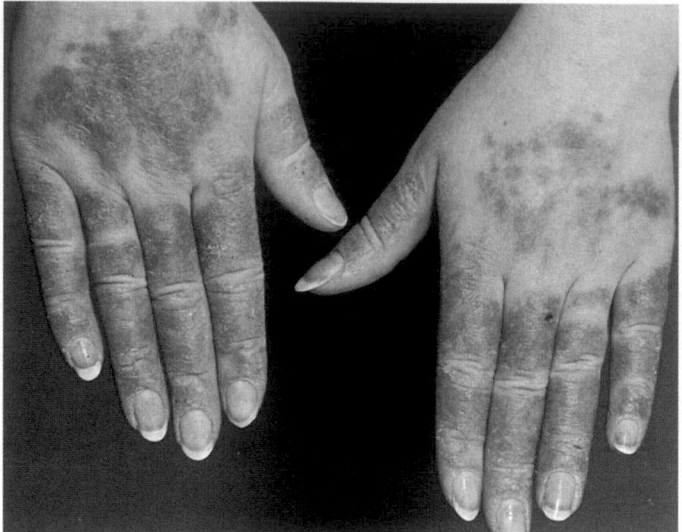

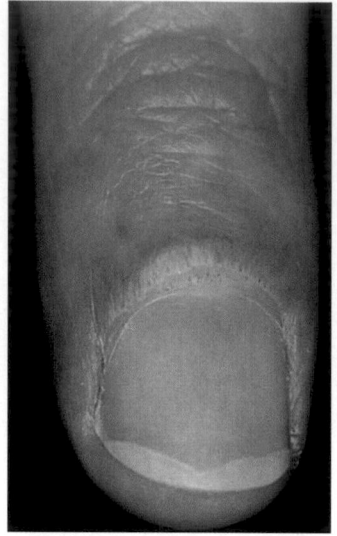

A.

B.

Generalized ACLE. *A.* Well-demarcated patches of erythema with fine overlying scale on the dorsal aspect of the hands, fingers, and periungual areas. Note the characteristic sparing of the knuckles. *B.* Closeup view of periungual erythema and grossly visible telangiectasia. Although these lesions can be seen in LE, they are more typical of dermatomyositis.

anti-Ro/SS-A and occasionally other autoantibody specificities transplacentally) share many features with SCLE.[35]

Between 15 and 20 percent of patients with SCLE lesions may also develop ACLE or classic DLE at some point. ACLE skin lesions tend to be more transient than SCLE lesions and heal with less pigmentary change. They are also more edematous and less hyperkeratotic than SCLE lesions. ACLE more commonly affects the malar areas of the face, whereas SCLE focuses more on the neck, shoulders, upper extremities, and trunk. DLE lesions occurring in the context of SCLE are generally associated with a greater degree of hyper- and hypopigmentation, atrophic dermal scarring, follicular plugging, and adherent scale. A consistent clinical differ-

ence is that DLE lesions are characteristically indurated, whereas SCLE lesions are not; this reflects the greater depth of inflammation seen histopathologically in DLE lesions.

Other skin lesions that are not histopathologically specific for LE can be found in patients with SCLE. These include nonscarring alopecia, painless mucous membrane lesions, livedo reticularis, periungual telangiectasias, leukocytoclastic vasculitis, and Raynaud's phenomenon. Cutaneous sclerosis and calcinosis may rarely be seen in patients with SCLE.

Approximately half of patients with SCLE meet the American College of Rheumatology's revised criteria for the classification of SLE. However, manifestations of severe SLE such as nephritis, cen-

FIGURE 172-3

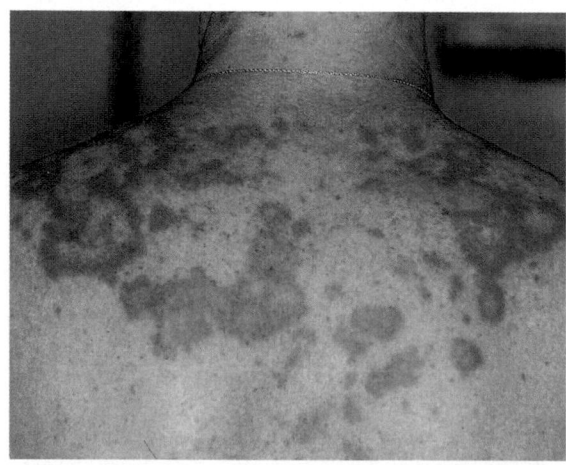

A.

B.

Subacute cutaneous LE (SCLE). *A.* Annular SCLE on the upper back of a 38-year-old woman. Note the central areas of hypopigmentation in which no dermal atrophy is present. *B.* Papulosquamous SCLE over the extensor aspect of the forearm of a 26-year-old woman.

tral nervous system disease, and systemic vasculitis develop in only 10 to 15 percent of patients with SCLE. It has been suggested that the papulosquamous type of SCLE, leukopenia, high titer of antinuclear antibody (ANA) (<1:640) and anti-double-stranded DNA antibodies are risk factors for the development of SLE in a patient presenting with SCLE lesions.

SCLE can overlap with other autoimmune diseases including Sjögren's syndrome, rheumatoid arthritis, and Hashimoto's thyroiditis. Other disorders that have been anecdotally related to SCLE are Sweet's syndrome, porphyria cutanea tarda, gluten-sensitive enteropathy, and Crohn's disease. There has also been the suggestion that SCLE can be associated with internal malignancy (carcinoma of the breast, lung, gastrointestinal tract, uterus; Hodgkin's disease).

CCLE

Classic DLE lesions, the most common form of CCLE, begin as red-purple macules, papules, or small plaques and rapidly develop a hyperkeratotic surface. Early classic DLE lesions typically evolve into sharply demarcated, coin-shaped (i.e., discoid) erythematous plaques covered by a prominent, adherent scale that extends into the orifices of dilated hair follicles (Fig. 172-4).

Early DLE lesions typically expand with erythema and hyperpigmentation at the periphery, leaving atrophic central scarring, telangiectasia, and hypopigmentation (Fig. 172-5). DLE lesions at this stage can merge to form large, confluent, disfiguring plaques. DLE in certain ethnic backgrounds such as Indians can present clinically as isolated areas of macular hyperpigmentation. Follicular involvement is a prominent feature. Keratotic plugs accumulate in dilated follicles that soon become devoid of hair. When the adherent scale is lifted from more advanced lesions, keratotic spikes similar in appearance to carpet tacks can be seen to project from the undersurface of the scale (i.e., the "carpet tack" sign).

DLE lesions are most frequently encountered on the face, scalp, ears, V area of the neck, and extensor aspects of the arms. Any area

FIGURE 172-5

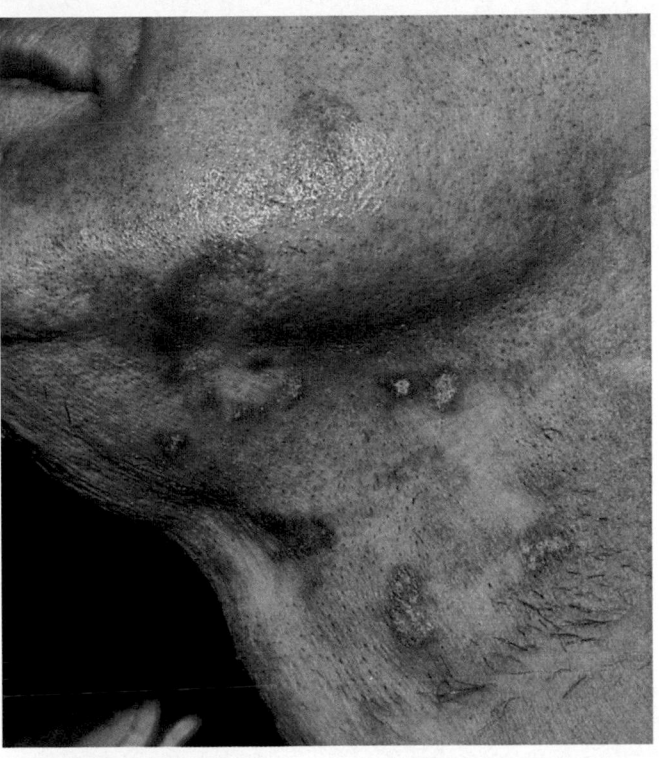

Classic DLE. Sharply demarcated, round-to-ovoid, slightly indurated, erythematous plaques on the neck and face. Most plaques show a mild degree of hyperkeratosis and some show dermal atrophy. Noninflamed areas of hypopigmentation and scarring mark the sites of prior lesions that have resolved.

of the face including the eyebrows, eyelids, nose, and lips can be affected. A symmetric, hyperkeratotic, butterfly-shaped DLE plaque is occasionally found over the malar areas of the face and bridge of the nose. Such lesions should not be confused with the more transient, edematous, minimally scaling ACLE erythema reactions that occur in the same areas. DLE, like ACLE and SCLE, usually spares the nasolabial folds. When DLE lesions occur periorally, they resolve with a striking acneiform pattern of pitted scarring. DLE characteristically affects the external ear including the outer portion of the external auditory canal (Fig. 172-6). Such lesions often present initially as dilated, hyperpigmented follicles. The scalp is involved in 60 percent of patients with DLE, and irreversible, scarring alopecia resulting from such involvement has been reported in one-third of patients (Fig. 172-6). The *irreversible, scarring alopecia* resulting from DLE differs from the *reversible, nonscarring alopecia* that patients with SLE often develop during periods of systemic disease activity.

Localized DLE lesions occur only on the head or neck, whereas generalized DLE lesions occur both above and below the neck. DLE lesions below the neck most commonly occur on the extensor aspects of the arms, forearms, and hands, although they can occur at virtually any site on the body. The palms and soles can be the sites of painful and at times disabling erosive DLE lesions. On occasion, small DLE lesions occurring only around follicular orifices can be seen at the elbow and elsewhere (*follicular DLE*). DLE activity can localize to the nail unit. The nail can be impacted by other forms

FIGURE 172-4

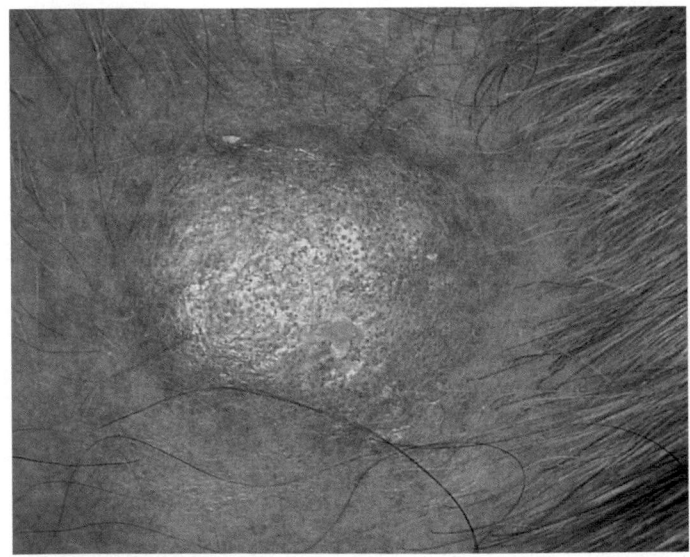

Classic discoid LE (DLE). Typical early erythematous plaque on the forehead demonstrating hyperkeratosis and accentuation of follicle orifices in a 60-year-old male with a 25-year history of cutaneous LE. The lesion had been present for 3 months; no dermal atrophy was present at this stage.

FIGURE 172-6

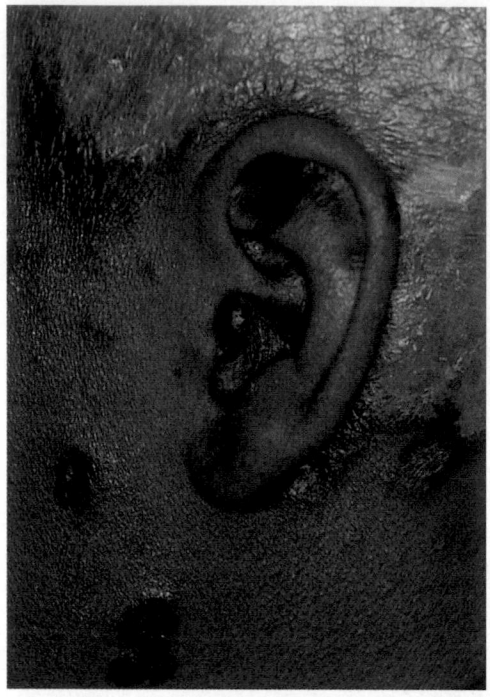

A.

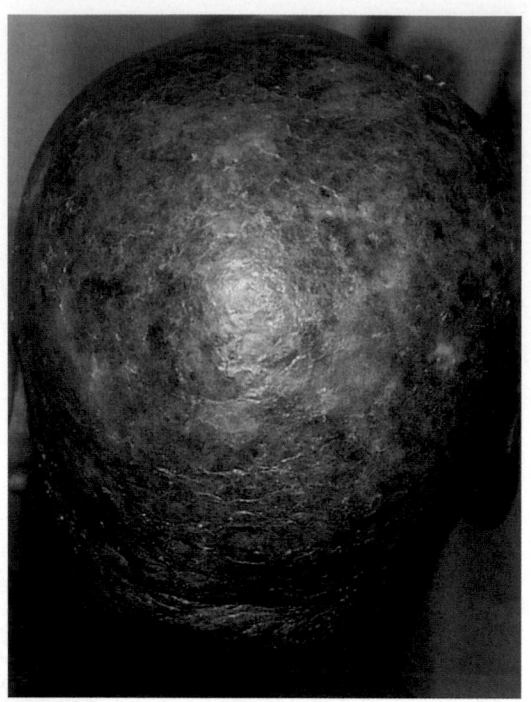

B.

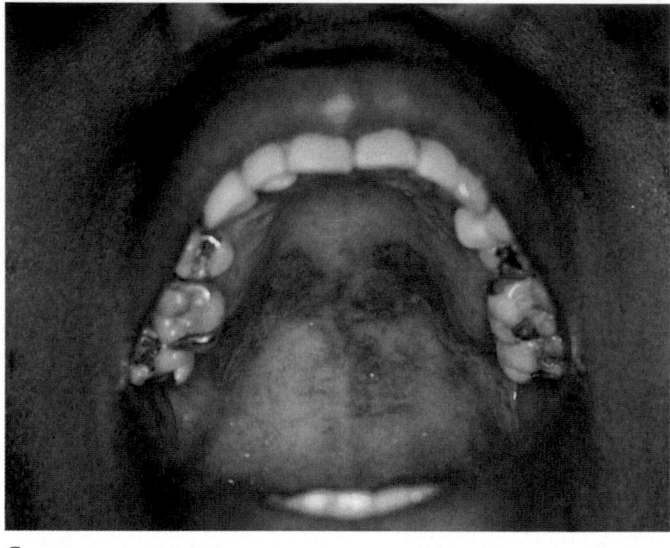

C.

Classic DLE and mucosal DLE in a 45-year-old African-American female with a 20-year history of untreated cutaneous LE. *A.* Characteristic involvement of the ear shows lesions with atrophy and postinflammatory hyperpigmentation as well as inflammatory red plaques on the scalp with postinflammatory hypopigmentation. *B.* Confluent lesions on the scalp have resulted in extensive scarring alopecia. *C.* Plaques of DLE on the palatal mucosa showing similar morphologic features to cutaneous lesions.

of cutaneous LE as well as SLE, producing nail fold erythema and telangiectasia, red lunulae, clubbing, paronychia, pitting, leukonychia striata, and onycholysis.

DLE lesions can be potentiated by sunlight exposure but to a lesser extent than ACLE and SCLE lesions. DLE as well as other forms of LE skin disease activity can be precipitated by any form of cutaneous trauma (i.e., the Koebner or isomorphic response).

The relationship between classic DLE and SLE has been the subject of much debate.[6,36] The following summary points can be made: (1) 5 percent of patients presenting with classic DLE lesions subsequently develop unequivocal evidence of SLE; and (2) patients with generalized DLE (i.e., lesions both above and below the neck) have somewhat higher rates of immunologic abnormalities, a higher risk for progressing to SLE, and a higher risk for developing more severe manifestations of SLE than patients with localized DLE.

The following have been suggested to be risk factors for the development of SLE in a patient with DLE: diffuse nonscarring alopecia; generalized lymphadenopathy; periungual nail fold telangiectasia; Raynaud's phenomenon; SCLE/ACLE skin lesions; LE-nonspecific skin lesions such as vasculitis; unexplained anemia; marked leukopenia; false-positive tests for syphilis; persistently positive high-titer ANA assay; anti-single-stranded DNA antibody; hypergammaglobulinemia; an elevated erythrocyte sedimentation rate (especially >50 mm/h); positive, sun-protected, non-lesional lupus band test; and elevated levels of soluble IL-2 receptor.

Roughly one-fourth of patients with SLE develop DLE lesions at some point in the course of their disease, and such patients tend to have less severe forms of SLE. The relative risks for systemic disease activity that are associated with the clinical varieties of LE-specific skin disease are illustrated in Fig. 172-7.

FIGURE 172-7

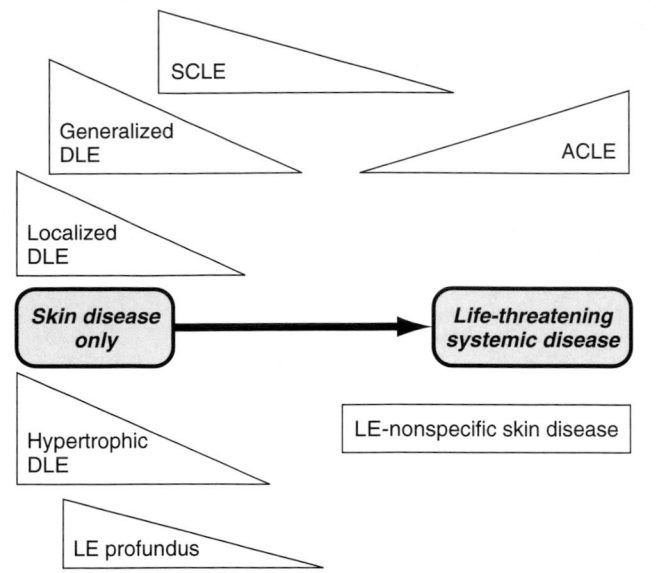

Relative risk for coexistence of or progression to SLE in patients presenting with various forms of LE-specific skin disease. The spectrum of LE is depicted as a disease continuum ranging from skin disease alone to life-threatening systemic disease.

Hypertrophic DLE, also referred to as hyperkeratotic or verrucous DLE, is a rare variant of CCLE in which the hyperkeratosis normally found in classic DLE lesions is greatly exaggerated. The extensor aspects of the arms, the upper back, and the face are the areas most frequently affected. Overlapping features of hypertrophic LE and lichen planus have been described under the rubric *lupus planus*. The entity *lupus erythematosus hypertrophicus et profundus* appears to represent a rare form of hypertrophic DLE affecting the face with the additional features of violaceous/dull red, indurated, rolled borders and striking central, crateriform atrophy. The name for this clinical entity is ambiguous because LE panniculitis is not characteristic of its histopathology. Patients with hypertrophic DLE probably do not have a greater risk for developing SLE than do patients with classic DLE lesions.

LE profundus/LE panniculitis (Kaposi-Irgang disease) is a rare form of CCLE typified by inflammatory lesions in the lower dermis and subcutaneous tissue. Approximately 70 percent of patients with this type of CCLE also have typical DLE lesions, often overlying the panniculitis lesions. The term *LE profundus* is used to designate those patients who have both LE panniculitis and DLE lesions, whereas *LE panniculitis* refers to those having only subcutaneous involvement. Typical subcutaneous lesions present as firm nodules, 1 to 3 cm in diameter. The overlying skin often becomes attached to the subcutaneous nodules and is drawn inward to produce deep, saucerized depressions (Fig. 172-8). The head, proximal upper arms, chest, back, breasts, buttocks, and thighs are the sites frequently affected. LE panniculitis in the absence of overlying DLE may produce breast nodules that can mimic carcinoma clinically and radiologically (*lupus mastitis*). Confluent facial involvement can simulate the appearance of lipoatrophy. Dystrophic calcification frequently occurs within older lesions of LE profundus/LE panniculitis, and pain associated with such calcification can at times be the dominant clinical problem. Roughly 50 percent of patients with LE profundus/panniculitis have evidence of SLE. The systemic features of patients with LE panniculitis/profundus tend to be less se-

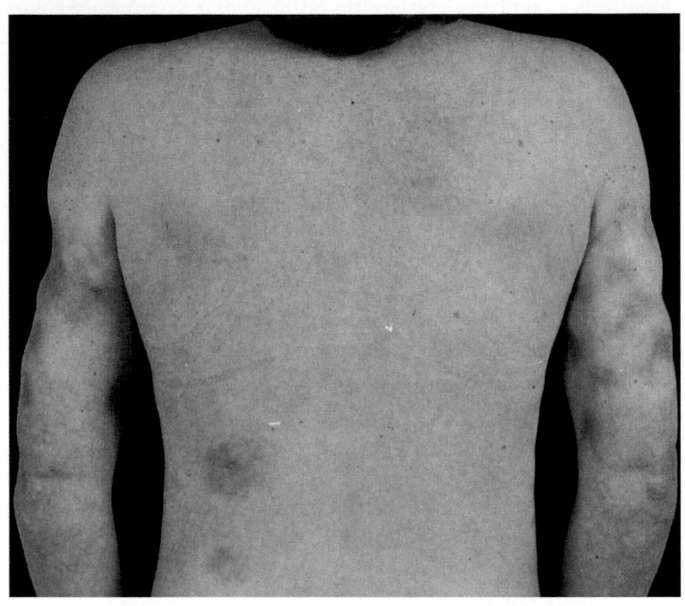

LE panniculitis. Lupus panniculitis has resulted in large, sunken areas of overlying skin; erythema and atrophy of the skin are present.

vere, similar to those of patients with SLE who have DLE skin lesions.

Mucosal DLE occurs in approximately 25 percent of patients with CCLE.[37] The oral mucosa is most frequently affected; however, nasal, conjunctival, and genital mucosal surfaces can be targeted. In the mouth, the buccal mucosal surfaces are most commonly involved, with the palate (see Fig. 172-6), alveolar processes, and tongue being sites of less frequent involvement. Lesions begin as painless, erythematous patches that evolve to chronic plaques that can be confused with lichen planus. Chronic buccal mucosal plaques are sharply marginated and have irregularly scalloped, white borders with radiating white striae and telangiectasia. The surfaces of these plaques overlying the palatal mucosa often have a honeycomb appearance. Central depression often occurs in older lesions, and painful ulceration can develop. Oral mucosal DLE lesions can degenerate into squamous cell carcinoma, similar to longstanding cutaneous DLE lesions. Any degree of nodular asymmetry within a mucosal DLE lesion should be evaluated for the possibility of malignant degeneration. Chronic DLE plaques also appear on the vermillion border of the lips. At times, DLE involvement of the lips can present as a diffuse cheilitis, especially on the more sun-exposed lower lip.

The nasal, conjunctival, and anogenital mucosa can be sites of DLE lesions. Nasal septum perforation is more often associated with SLE than DLE. Conjunctival DLE lesions affect the lower lid more often than the upper lid. Lesions begin as focal areas of nondescript inflammation most commonly affecting the palpebral conjunctivae or the lid margin. Scarring becomes evident as lesions mature, and the permanent loss of eyelashes and ectropion can develop, producing considerable disability.

The risk for systemic disease activity in patients with LE and mucosal involvement is a function of the type of mucosal lesion present. Chronic mucosal DLE plaques are seen most commonly in patients with LE who do not have life-threatening manifestations of SLE. However, transient superficial oral or nasal mucosal ulcerations with a relatively nonspecific histopathology occur in patients with active SLE. Mucosal lesions of this type represent 1 of the 11 revised classification criteria for SLE of the American College of Rheumatology.

Chilblains LE/perniotic LE lesions initially develop as livid patches and plaques on the toes, fingers, and face that are precipitated by cold, damp climates. As they evolve, these lesions usually assume the appearance of DLE lesions clinically and pathologically. Patients with chilblains LE often have typical DLE lesions on the face and head. Approximately 20 percent of patients presenting with chilblains LE later develop SLE.

Lupus tumidus (tumid LE) is a rare variant of CCLE in which excessive dermal mucin accumulates early in the disease process. The characteristic epidermal histologic changes of LE-specific skin disease are only minimally expressed, if at all. This results in succulent, edematous, urticaria-appearing plaques with little surface change. The paucity of epidermal change often produces confusion concerning the diagnosis of lupus tumidus as a form of cutaneous LE. A European center has reported a very high rate of photosensitivity in patients with LE tumidus.

Vesiculobullous Skin Change in LE

Vesiculobullous skin change in LE is a very confusing subject.[6,38] As with nonbullous LE skin disease, vesiculobullous skin lesions in patients with LE can be divided on the basis of histopathology into those that are LE-specific and those that are LE-nonspecific (Table 172-5). Bullae may develop in ACLE and SCLE as a manifestation of particularly aggressive liquefactive degeneration of the

TABLE 172-5

Proposed Classification Scheme for Vesiculobullous Skin Disorders Encountered in Patients with LE

LE-Specific Vesiculobullous LE

Acute cutaneous LE
  Toxic epidermal necrolysis–like ACLE
Subacute cutaneous LE
  Toxic epidermal necrolysis–like SCLE
  Vesiculobullous annular SCLE
Chronic cutaneous LE
  Bullous DLE

LE-Nonspecific Vesiculobullous LE

"Bullous SLE" [proposed alternative terms: dermatitis herpetiformis (DH)–like LE-nonspecific skin disease, epidermolysis bullosa acquisita (EBA)–like LE-nonspecific skin disease; LE-nonspecific vesiculobullous eruption of SLE]
Vesiculobullous skin disorders anecdotally reported to occur in LE patients but whose relationship to LE has not yet been firmly established
  Bullous pemphigoid
  Dermatitis herpetiformis
  Pemphigus erythematosus
  Porphyria cutanea tarda

SOURCE: Reprinted from Sontheimer,[1] with permission from Stockton Journals, Macmillian Press, Ltd.

epidermal basal layer, resulting in basal cell dissolution and simulating the clinical and histopathologic appearance of toxic epidermal necrolysis. Vesiculobullous changes can develop at the active edge of annular SCLE lesions, and subepidermal bullous changes occasionally develop in DLE lesions.

The cutaneous entity described as *bullous SLE* is an example of LE-nonspecific bullous skin change. Patients who typically have or subsequently develop active SLE including nephritis occasionally develop a severe vesiculobullous eruption. Histopathologically, marked neutrophilic infiltration with papillary microabscess formation is present similar to dermatitis herpetiformis (DH) and the inflammatory variant of epidermolysis bullosa acquisita (EBA). However, the direct immunofluorescence findings are more typical of those seen in LE. Type VII collagen autoantibodies are present in some patients. Although the vague term bullous SLE has most often been used to describe such lesions, more descriptive terms such as *DH-like cutaneous LE* or *EBA-like cutaneous LE* would seem more appropriate inasmuch as other forms of bullous skin lesions can occur in patients with SLE, as noted above.

Other bullous skin diseases that have been linked anecdotally to LE include bullous pemphigoid, pemphigus erythematosus (the Senear-Usher syndrome), DH, and porphyria cutanea tarda. It is not clear whether there is a primary association between these bullous skin disorders and LE or whether their coexistence is the result of chance alone.

LABORATORY FINDINGS

The major laboratory findings associated with the varieties of LE-specific skin disease are summarized in Table 172-4 and the autoantibody associations of SLE are presented in Table 172-6. Because of the strong association between ACLE and SLE, the laboratory features of ACLE are those associated with SLE (high-titer ANA, anti-double-stranded DNA, anti-Sm, hypocomplementemia).

The laboratory markers for SCLE are the presence of a-Ro/SS-A (70 to 90 percent) and, less commonly, a-La/SS-B (30 to 50 percent) autoantibodies. ANA are present in 60 to 80 percent of patients with SCLE, and rheumatoid factor is present in approximately one-third. Other autoantibodies seen in SCLE include false-positive reactions (7 to 33 percent), anticardiolipin antibodies (10 to 16 percent), antithyroid (18 to 44 percent), anti-Sm (10 percent), anti-double-stranded DNA (10 percent), and anti-U_1 ribonucleoprotein (RNP) antibodies (10 percent). Patients with SCLE, particularly those with systemic involvement, may have a number of laboratory abnormalities including anemia, leukopenia, thrombocytopenia, elevated erythrocyte sedimentation rate, hypergammaglobulinemia, proteinuria, hematuria, urine casts, elevated serum creatine and BUN, and depressed complement levels (resulting from genetic deficiency or increased complement consumption).

ANA is present in low titer in 30 to 40 percent of patients with DLE; however, fewer than 5 percent have the higher ANA levels that are characteristically seen in patients with overt SLE ($\geq 1:320$). Antibodies to single-stranded DNA are not uncommon in DLE, but antibodies to double-stranded DNA are distinctly uncommon. Precipitating antibodies to U_1RNP are sometimes found in patients whose disease course is dominated by DLE lesions; however, such patients usually have only mild manifestations of SLE or overlapping connective tissue disorders such as mixed connective tissue disease. Precipitating Ro/SS-A and La/SS-B autoantibodies are rare in patients with DLE; low levels of anti-Ro/SS-A antibody detected by enzyme-linked immunoassay are more common. A small percentage of patients with DLE have low-grade anemia, biologic false-positive serologic tests for syphilis (VDRL, rapid plasma reagin), positive rheumatoid factor tests, slight depressions in serum complement levels, modest elevations in gamma globulin, and modest leukopenia. It has been suggested that such findings are risk factors for the development of SLE. ANA are present in 70 to 75 percent of patients with LE profundus/panniculitis, but anti-double-stranded DNA antibodies are distinctly uncommon.

The laboratory findings associated with cutaneous LE in adults and newborns have been reviewed,[6,35] and the subject of SLE-associated autoantibodies has also been reviewed.[39,40]

HISTOPATHOLOGY

The LE-specific skin disease histopathology is a distinctive constellation of hyperkeratosis, epidermal atrophy, liquefactive/vacuolar basal cell degeneration, dermal-epidermal junction basement membrane thickening, dermal edema, and mononuclear cell infiltration of the epidermis, dermal-epidermal junction, and dermis focused in a perivascular and periappendageal distribution (Fig. 172-9). Variable degrees of these features are encountered in the different forms of LE-specific skin disease. Differences of opinion exist as to whether ACLE, SCLE, and DLE lesions can be distinguished reliably based on their histopathologic appearances alone. These and related issues have been reviewed.[6,41]

ACLE

The histopathologic changes in ACLE lesions are generally less impressive than those in SCLE and DLE lesions. The lymphohistiocytic cellular infiltrate is relatively sparse. A mild degree of focal liquefactive degeneration of the epidermal basal cell layer can be seen. Mucinous edema of the upper dermis may be prominent. In its most severe form, ACLE can display extensive epidermal necrosis similar to toxic epidermal necrolysis.

SCLE

Epidermal changes include focal epidermal basal cell injury, disorientation, liquefaction degeneration, and mild atrophy. Rarely, frank epidermal necrosis is seen. Dermal changes include edema and sparse mononuclear cell infiltration usually limited to the perivascular areas and adnexal structures in the upper third of the dermis. Vesiculation changes can occur in SCLE lesions, particularly at the active border of annular SCLE lesions. Lesser degrees of hyperkeratosis, follicular plugging, mononuclear cell infiltration of adnexal structures, and dermal melanophages are seen in SCLE lesions when compared to DLE lesions. It has not been possible to differentiate papulosquamous from annular SCLE by histopathologic criteria alone.

TABLE 172-6

Autoantibodies Associated with Unselected SLE

ANTIGEN	AUTOANTIBODY FREQUENCY, %		MOLECULAR SPECIFICITY	CLINICAL ASSOCIATION
	ID	SPA/RIA		
HIGH DISEASE SPECIFICITY FOR SLE				
dsDNA		60	Native DNA	LE nephritis
Sm	25		Ribonucleoprotein	—
rRNP	10		Ribosomal P protein	CNS LE
PCNA	3		Cyclin	—
LOW DISEASE SPECIFICITY FOR SLE				
ssDNA		60	Denatured DNA	Risk for SLE in patients with DLE
Histones		50	Histones	Drug-induced SLE
U$_1$RNP	25		Ribonucleoprotein	Overlap CTD (MCTD)
Ro/SS-A	25	50	Ribonucleoprotein	SCLE, SSj, neonatal LE
La/SS-B	10	20	Ribonucleoprotein	SSj, SCLE
Ku	10		Transcription factor	Overlap CTD

NOTE: ID, immunodiffusion; SPA, solid phase immunoassay (i.e., ELISA); RIA, radioimmunoassay; CTD, connective tissue disease; MCTD, mixed CTD; SSj, Sjögren's syndrome.
SOURCE: Reprinted from Sontheimer and Provost,[6] with permission from Williams and Wilkins Publishers.

CCLE

In classic DLE lesions, epidermal changes include hyperkeratosis, atrophy, and basal layer abnormalities similar to those described for SCLE. The epidermal basement membrane is markedly thickened. Dermal changes include a dense mononuclear cell infiltrate composed primarily of CD4 T lymphocytes and macrophages predominantly in the periappendageal and perivascular areas, melanophages, and dermal mucin deposition. Chronic scarring DLE lesions often have a dense inflammatory cell infiltrate that extends well

FIGURE 172-9

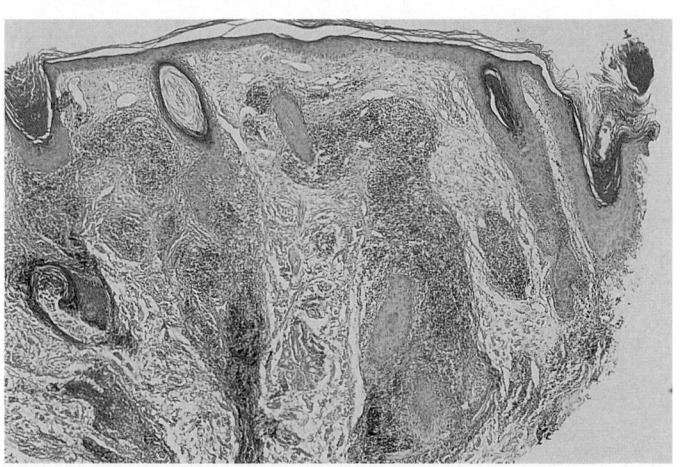

Histopathology of LE-specific skin disease. Histology of a DLE lesion demonstrating marked basal cell layer damage with vacuolization and irregularity of basal cell size. Mild hyperkeratosis is present.

into the deeper reticular dermis and/or subcutis. In contrast, ACLE and SCLE lesions contain a less dense inflammatory infiltrate that is confined to the upper dermis but still shows the distinctive pattern of injury along the dermal-epidermal junction. The periappendageal inflammation characteristic of DLE is less prominent in SCLE and ACLE.

The histopathology of hypertrophic DLE lesions is similar to that of classic DLE lesions except for a much greater degree of epidermal acanthosis and hyperkeratosis. In LE panniculitis, the absence of the characteristic epidermal and dermal changes of LE can make the histologic diagnosis difficult. In LE panniculitis, subcutaneous tissue displays a lobular lymphocytic panniculitis with perivascular infiltration with lymphocytes, plasma cells, and histiocytes in the deep dermis and subcutaneous fat (including lymphoid nodule formation); vessel wall thickening and invasion by mononuclear cells (*lymphocytic vasculitis*); absence of polymorphonuclear leukocytes; hyaline fat necrosis; prominent fibrinoid degeneration of collagen; and mucinous degeneration and calcification in old, established lesions. Except for the differences related to the absence of hair follicles and stratum corneum in mucous membranes, the microscopic changes of mucosal DLE are highly reminiscent of those seen in cutaneous DLE lesions.

IMMUNOHISTOLOGY

Immunoglobulins (IgG, IgA, IgM) and complement components (C3, C4, Clq, properdin, factor B, and the membrane attack complex, C5b-C9) deposited in a continuous granular or linear bandlike array at the dermal-epidermal junction have been observed in the lesional and nonlesional skin of patients with LE since the early 1960s (Fig. 172-10). However, debate about terminology in this

FIGURE 172-10

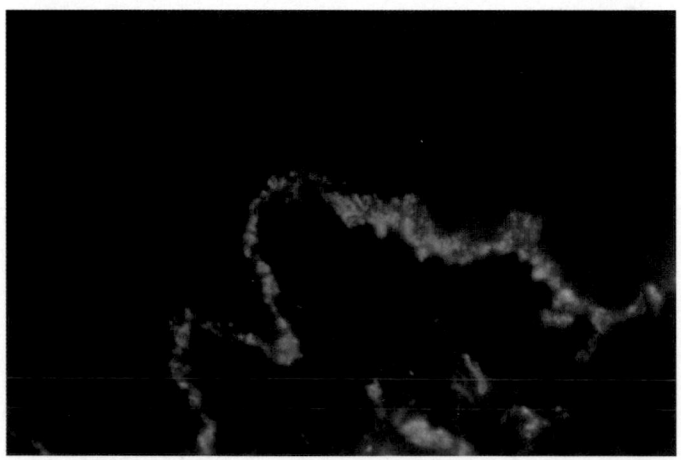

Immunopathology of LE-specific skin disease. Direct immunofluorescence examination of a DLE lesional skin biopsy showing a continuous band of granular fluorescence at the dermal-epidermal junction as a result of staining with fluorescein isothiocyanate-conjugated goat anti-IgG.

area continues to cloud the field.[6] Some restrict the use of the term *lupus band test* (LBT) to refer to the examination of *nonlesional* skin biopsies for the presence of this bandlike array of immunopathologic findings at the dermal-epidermal junction. Others qualify the LBT as being either "lesional" or "nonlesional." Less confusion might exist if the terms *lesional LBT* or *lesional lupus band* and *nonlesional LBT* or *nonlesional lupus band* were uniformly adopted.

ACLE

The sparse data that exist suggest that 60 to 100 percent of ACLE lesions display a lesional lupus band. However, the realization that sun-damaged skin from otherwise healthy individuals can display similar immunopathology has diluted the clinical value of this finding.

SCLE

Initial studies indicated that approximately 60 percent of patients with SCLE had lesional lupus bands. A "dustlike particle" pattern of IgG deposition focused around epidermal basal keratinocytes has been suggested to be more specific for SCLE by reflecting the presence of in vivo–bound a-Ro/SS-A autoantibody.

CCLE

Early reports suggested that over 90 percent of classic DLE lesions had lesional immunoreactants at the dermal-epidermal junction, often extending along the basement membrane of the hair follicle; but subsequent studies have reported somewhat lower rates. Lesions on the head, neck, and arms are positive more frequently (80 percent) than those on the trunk (20 percent). The lesional lupus band also appears to be a function of the age of the lesion being examined, with older lesions (i.e., >3 months) being positive more often than younger ones. Ultrastructural localization of immunoglobulin at the dermal-epidermal junction has confirmed that these proteins are deposited on the upper dermal collagen fibers and along the lamina densa of the epidermal basement membrane zone.

In LE profundus, immunoglobulin and complement deposits are usually found in blood vessel walls of the deep dermis and subcutis. Immunoglobulin deposits at the dermal-epidermal junction may or may not be present depending on the site biopsied, the presence or absence of accompanying SLE, and the presence or absence of overlying changes of DLE at the dermal-epidermal junction.

Nonlesional Lupus Band Test

Much debate over the past three decades has centered on the diagnostic and prognostic significance of an immunoglobulin/complement band at the dermal-epidermal junction of nonlesional skin taken from patients with LE.[6,41] When totally sun-protected nonlesional skin (e.g., buttocks) is sampled, the diagnostic specificity for SLE appears to be very high when three or more immunoreactants are present at the dermal-epidermal junction. Prospectively ascertained follow-up data also suggest that the presence of a nonlesional LBT correlates positively with risk for developing LE nephritis. However, the nonlesional LBT has fallen out of favor as a clinical tool largely because the information gained from this invasive procedure has not been proven to be of significantly greater value than the results of more readily available serologic assays such as antibody to double-stranded DNA.

DIAGNOSIS AND DIFFERENTIAL DIAGNOSIS

ACLE

A number of unrelated dermatoses that can produce a red face, such as acne rosacea, dermatomyositis, seborrheic dermatitis, polymorphous light eruption, and photoallergic contact dermatitis, can be confused with localized ACLE. Routine histopathologic examination of a lesional skin biopsy is the most definitive way to make this distinction, since each of these red face look-alikes except for dermatomyositis has a pathology quite different from that of LE-specific skin disease (dermatomyositis can be distinguished from cutaneous LE by its nonfacial clinical features). Generalized ACLE can be confused with other causes of widespread exanthematous reactions such as drug hypersensitivity and viral infections.

SCLE

Papulosquamous SCLE can be simulated by the photosensitive variant of psoriasis. Annular SCLE lesions can be confused with erythema multiforme and other figurate erythemas such as erythema annulare centrifugum, erythema gyratum repens, and granuloma annulare. The photodistribution of SCLE lesions and the LE-specific histopathology are often crucial in helping the clinician differentiate SCLE from these other conditions. Seborrheic dermatitis, polymorphous light eruption, dermatophyte infections, nummular eczema, contact dermatitis, dermatomyositis, pityriasis rubra pilaris, disseminated superficial actinic porokeratosis, and cutaneous T cell lymphoma/mycosis fungoides have also been confused with SCLE. The presence of circulating Ro/SS-A autoantibodies further supports a diagnosis of SCLE.

CCLE

Although fully evolved classic DLE lesions are unlikely to be confused with other dermatoses, DLE lesions lacking all of the classic clinical findings might be confused with other disorders that produce persistent red plaques on the face such as plaque-type polymorphous light eruption, granuloma faciale, sarcoidosis, Jessner's benign lymphocytic infiltration of the skin, pseudolymphoma of Spiegler-Fendt (synonymous with Spiegler-Fendt sarcoid), lymphocytoma cutis, lymphoma cutis, angiolymphoid hyperplasia with eosinophilia, lupus vulgaris, and tertiary syphilis. The histopathologies of these conditions are quite distinct from that of DLE and would be expected to be negative for immunoglobulin and complement components at the dermal-epidermal junction on direct immunofluorescence microscopic examination. Hypertrophic DLE can be mistaken for keratoacanthoma, squamous cell carcinoma, prurigo nodularis, or hypertrophic lichen planus. The differential diagnosis of patients with lupus panniculitis includes Weber-Christian panniculitis, factitial panniculitis, meperidine (Talwin)-induced panniculitis, pancreatic panniculitis, traumatic panniculitis, morphea profundus, eosinophilic fasciitis, sarcoidosis, subcutaneous granuloma annulare, and rheumatoid nodules. Deep excisional biopsy may be required to distinguish LE panniculitis from these other disorders, particularly when classic DLE lesions are not present. With respect to the differential diagnosis, oral lichen planus presents the closest clinical appearance to that of oral mucosal DLE.

TREATMENT

The initial management of patients with any form of cutaneous LE should include an evaluation to rule out underlying SLE disease activity at the time of diagnosis. All patients with cutaneous LE should receive instruction about protection from sunlight and artificial sources of UV radiation and should be advised to avoid the use of potentially photosensitizing drugs such as hydrochlorothiazide, griseofulvin, and piroxicam. With regard to specific medical therapy, local measures should be maximized and systemic agents employed if significant local disease activity persists or systemic activity is superimposed.

ACLE lesions usually respond to the systemic immunosuppressive measures required to treat the underlying SLE disease activity that so frequently accompanies this form of cutaneous LE (e.g., systemic glucocorticoids, azathioprine, cyclophosphamide). Increasing evidence suggests that aminioquinoline antimalarial agents such as hydroxychloroquine can have a steroid-sparing effect on SLE, and these drugs can be of value in ACLE. The local measures discussed below can also be of value in treating ACLE. Because the lesions of SCLE and CCLE are often found in patients who have little or no evidence of underlying systemic disease activity, unlike the lesions of ACLE, nonimmunosuppressive treatment modalities are required for SCLE and CCLE (Table 172-7). For the most part, SCLE and CCLE lesions respond equally to such agents.

Local Therapy

SUN PROTECTION Patients should be advised to avoid direct sun exposure, wear tightly woven clothing and broad-brimmed hats, and regularly use broad-spectrum, water-resistant sunscreens [SPF ≥ 15 with an efficient UVA blocking agent such as Parsol 1789

TABLE 172-7

Options for Systemic Therapy in Cutaneous LE

First line
  Hydroxychloroquine (Plaquenil, Quineprox)
  Hydroxychloroquine + quinacrine (Atabrine)
  Chloroquine (Aralen) + quinacrine
Second line
  Dapsone, retinoids [isotretinoin (Accutane), etretinate (Tegison), acitretin (Soriatane)], thalidomide
Third line
  Clofazimine, gold
Fourth line
  Systemic glucocorticoids
    Oral prednisone
    Pulse intravenous methylprednisolone
  Azathioprine (Imuran)
  Methotrexate
  Cyclophosphamide (Cytoxan)
Evolving/experimental
  Sulfasalazine, phenytoin (Dilantin), danazol, dehydroepiandrosterone, interferon-alpha, cytosine arabinoside (Cytarabine), cyclosporine, immunotherapy (high dose IV gamma globulin, CD4 T cell–depleting monoclonal antibody), phototherapy (UVA-I phototherapy, photopheresis)

(avobenzone) or micronized titanium dioxide]. UV-blocking films should be applied to home and automobile windows, and acrylic diffusion shields should be placed over fluorescent lighting. Corrective camouflage cosmetics such as Dermablend and Covermark offer the dual benefit of being highly effective physical sunscreens as well as aesthetically pleasing cosmetic masking agents.

LOCAL GLUCOCORTICOIDS Although some prefer intermediate strength preparations such as triamcinolone acetonide 0.1% for sensitive areas such as the face, superpotent topical class I agents such as clobetasol propionate 0.05% or betamethasone dipropionate 0.05% produce the greatest benefit in cutaneous LE. Twice-daily application of the superpotent preparations to lesional skin for 2 weeks followed by a 2-week rest period can minimize the risk of local complications such as steroid atrophy and telangiectasia. Ointments are more effective than creams for more hyperkeratotic lesions such as hypertrophic DLE. Occlusive therapy with glucocorticoid-impregnated tape (e.g., flurandrenolide) or glucocorticoids with plastic food wrap (Saran) can potentiate the beneficial effects of topical glucocorticoids but also carry a higher risk of local side effects. Class I or class II topical steroid solutions and gels are best for treating the scalp. Unfortunately, even the most aggressive regimen of topical glucocorticoids alone does not provide adequate improvement for most patients with SCLE and CCLE.

INTRALESIONAL GLUCOCORTICOIDS Intralesional glucocorticoids (e.g., triamcinolone acetonide suspension, 2.5 to 5 mg/mL for the face with higher concentrations allowable in less sensitive sites) are more useful in the management of DLE than SCLE. Intralesional glucocorticoids themselves can produce cutaneous and subcutaneous atrophy (deep injections into the subcutaneous tissue enhances this risk). A 30-gauge needle is preferred since it produces only mild discomfort upon penetration, especially when injected perpendicularly to the skin. The active borders of lesions should be thoroughly infiltrated. Intralesional therapy is indicated for particularly hyperkeratotic lesions or lesions that are unresponsive to topical glucocorticoids, but most patients with cutaneous LE have too many lesions to be managed exclusively by intralesional glucocorticoid injections.

Systemic Therapy

ANTIMALARIALS One or a combination of the aminoquinoline antimalarials can be effective for approximately 75 percent of patients with cutaneous LE who have failed to benefit adequately from the local measures described above.[42] The risks of retinal toxicity should be discussed with the patient, and a pretreatment ophthalmologic examination should be performed. However, the risk of antimalarial retinopathy is extremely rare if recommended daily dose maximum levels of these agents are not exceeded (hydroxychloroquine, 6.5 mg/kg per day; chloroquine, 4 mg/kg per day). Patients should have follow-up ophthalmologic evaluations every 6 to 12 months while on therapy.

Hydroxychloroquine sulfate (Plaquenil), 400 mg/day by mouth, should be given for the first 6 to 8 weeks of treatment to reach equilibrium blood levels. Once an adequate clinical response has been achieved, the daily dose should be decreased to a maintenance dose of 200 mg/day for at least a year to minimize chances of recurrence (some authorities recommend even longer periods of inductive treatment). If no response is seen after 8 to 12 weeks, quinacrine hydrochloride, 100 mg/day (currently available in the United

States only through compounding pharmacies), can be added to the hydroxychloroquine without enhancing the risk of retinopathy (quinacrine does not cause retinopathy). If after 4 to 6 weeks adequate clinical control has not been achieved, consideration should be given to replacing the hydroxychloroquine with chloroquine diphosphate (Aralen), 250 mg/day. In Europe, chloroquine is generally felt to be more efficacious than hydroxychloroquine in treating cutaneous LE, perhaps due to the earlier therapeutic responses that might occur as a result of the shorter time period required to reach equilibrium blood levels with chloroquine compared to hydroxychloroquine. Hydroxychloroquine and chloroquine should not be used simultaneously because of enhanced risk for retinal toxicity.

A number of side effects other than retinal toxicity are associated with the use of antimalarials. Quinacrine is associated with a higher incidence of side effects, such as headache, gastrointestinal intolerance, hematologic toxicity, pruritus, lichenoid drug eruptions, and mucosal or cutaneous pigmentary disturbance, than is either hydroxychloroquine or chloroquine. Quinacrine commonly produces a yellow discoloration of the entire skin in fair-skinned individuals, which is completely reversible upon discontinuation of the drug. Quinacrine can produce significant hemolysis in patients with glucose-6-phosphate dehydrogenase (G6PD) deficiency (this has also been reported to occur rarely with hydroxychloroquine and chloroquine). Each of the aminoquinoline antimalarials can produce bone marrow suppression including aplastic anemia, although this effect is exceedingly rare with the dosage regimens used currently. Toxic psychosis, grand mal seizures, neuromyopathy, and cardiac arrhythmias were observed with the use of high doses of these drugs in the past; these reactions are uncommon with the lower daily dose regimens used today.

Before beginning therapy with hydroxychloroquine and chloroquine, complete blood counts as well as liver and renal function tests should be performed; these tests should be repeated 4 to 6 weeks after therapy has been initiated, and every 4 to 6 months thereafter. A screen for hematologic toxicity when using quinacrine is recommended more often. To reduce the risk of acute hemolysis, some authorities advocate confirming that patients are not deficient in G6PD activity before beginning treatment with antimalarials, especially quinacrine. Patients with overt or subclinical porphyria cutanea tarda are at particularly high risk for developing acute hepatotoxicity, which often simulates an acute surgical abdomen, when treated with therapeutic doses of antimalarials for cutaneous LE. It is also recommended to check urine levels of beta-human chorionic gonadotropin initially in women having childbearing potential, although recent evidence indicates that the risk to pregnant women of currently recommended dose regimens of antimalarials is minimal.

NONIMMUNOSUPPRESSIVE OPTIONS FOR ANTIMALARIAL-REFRACTORY DISEASE Some patients with refractory cutaneous LE (SCLE more than DLE) respond to diaminodiphenylsulfone (Dapsone). An initial dose of 25 mg by mouth twice daily can be increased up to 200 to 300 mg/day if necessary. Significant dose-related hemolysis and/or methemoglobinemia can result from the use of diaminodiphenylsulfone, especially in individuals deficient in G6PD activity, and therefore complete blood counts and liver function tests should be performed regularly. Isotretinoin (Accutane), etretinate (Tegison), and acitretin (Soriatane) (0.5 to 2 mg/kg per day) have also been used in this setting, but their efficacy is limited by their prevalent side effects (teratogenicity, mucocutaneous dryness, hyperlipidemia). In addition, breakthrough of cutaneous LE activity has also been a problem with long-term use of retinoids. Thalidomide (100 to 300 mg/day) is effective for cutaneous LE that is refractory to antimalarials. However, because of its teratogenicity it is available in the United States only through a compassionate-use investigational new drug approval that is issued on a case-by-case basis by the U.S. Food and Drug Administration. Sensory neuropathy from thalidomide has also been reported in patients with cutaneous LE. Other drugs reported to be of value in the treatment of refractory cutaneous LE are gold (Auranofin, Myochrysine) and clofazimine (Lamprene); however, the benefit varies from case to case and both of these agents are associated with the risk of significant side effects. Inferferon α, vitamin E, phenytoin (Dilantin), sulfasalazine, danazol, dehydroepiandrosterone (DHEA), and phototherapy (UVA-I phototherapy, photopheresis) have also been reported in uncontrolled trials to be of value in cutaneous LE.

SYSTEMIC GLUCOCORTICOIDS Every effort should be made to avoid the use of systemic glucocorticoids in patients with LE limited to the skin. However, occasionally patients are encountered who have especially severe and symptomatic skin disease. In particularly difficult cases, intravenous pulse methylprednisolone has been used. In less acute cases, moderate daily doses or oral glucocorticoids (prednisone, 20 to 40 mg/day, given as a single morning dose) can be used as supplemental therapy during the loading phase of therapy with an antimalarial agent. The dose of glucocorticoids should be reduced at the earliest possible time because of the complications of long-term steroid therapy in patients with LE, especially avascular (aseptic) bone necrosis. When the disease activity is controlled, the daily dosage should be reduced by 5- to 10-mg decrements until activity flares again or until a daily dosage of 20 mg/day is achieved. The daily dose should then be lowered by 2.5-mg decrements (some prefer to use 1-mg dose decrements below 10 mg/day). Alternate-day glucocorticoid therapy has not been successful in suppressing disease activity in most patients with cutaneous LE or SLE. Prednisolone rather than prednisone should be used in patients who have significant underlying liver disease, since prednisone requires hydroxylation in the liver to become biologically active. Any amount of prednisone given as a single oral dose in the morning will have less adrenal-suppressing activity than the same amount given in divided doses throughout the day. However, any given amount of this drug, taken in divided doses, has a greater LE-suppressing activity than does the same amount of drug given as a single morning dose.

OTHER IMMUNOSUPPRESSIVES Azathioprine (Imuran) (1.5 to 2.0 mg/kg per day orally) can play a steroid-sparing role in the severely affected patient with cutaneous LE. Methotrexate (7.5 to 25 mg orally one day per week) is also gaining popularity in this regard. The physician should become thoroughly familiar with the proper use of these drugs, including side effects and drug interactions, before using them. T cell–depleting anti-CD4 monoclonal antibody therapy has been reported to be of value in refractory cutaneous LE. Other immunosuppressives that have been used anecdotally include cytosine arabinoside (Cytarabine) and cyclosporine. Immunotherapy with high dose IV gamma globulin has also been used.

Surgical and Cosmetic Therapy

DLE lesions can produce permanent scarring alopecia, cosmetically disturbing dermal atrophy, and pigmentary changes. Patients so affected often ask about the possibility of cosmetic correction of these changes. Surgical interventions such as hair transplantation and dermabrasion carry finite risks since cutaneous LE is characterized by a tendency for nonspecific mechanical trauma, including surgical incision or laser ablation, to exacerbate disease activity (i.e., Koebner phenomenon/isomorphic phenomenon). Some patients tolerate

scar revision techniques including dermabrasion if they are on maintenance systemic therapy (e.g., antimalarials) to blunt trauma-induced skin disease flares. Anecdotal reports of the successful management of cutaneous LE with argon laser therapy and split-thickness skin grafting have appeared. The injection of atrophic lesions with collagen or other similar materials should be avoided. Reviews of the management of cutaneous LE are available.[6,7,43–45]

PROGNOSIS

ACLE

Both localized and generalized forms of ACLE lesions flare and abate in parallel with underlying SLE disease activity. Therefore, the prognosis for any given patient with ACLE is dictated by the pattern of the underlying SLE. Both 5-year (80 to 95 percent) and 10-year (70 to 90 percent) survival rates for SLE have progressively improved over the past four decades due to both earlier diagnosis made possible by more sensitive laboratory testing and improved immunosupressive treatment regimens. Ominous prognostic signs in SLE are hypertension, nephritis, systemic vasculitis, and central nervous system disease.

SCLE

Because SCLE has been recognized as a separate disease entity for only two decades, the long-term outcome associated with SCLE lesions has yet to be determined. It is the author's experience that most patients with SCLE have intermittent recurrences of skin disease activity over long periods of time without significant progression of systemic involvement (the author is aware of only one death directly attributable to SLE in approximately 150 patients with SCLE that he has personally examined). Others patients enjoy long-term if not permanent remissions of their skin disease activity. A few patients have experienced unremittant cutaneous disease activity.

It has also been the author's experience that approximately 15 percent of the patients with SCLE developed active SLE including lupus nephritis. This subgroup of patients was marked by the presence of papulosquamous SCLE, localized ACLE, high-titer ANA, leukopenia, and (or) antibodies to double-stranded DNA. Long-term follow-up studies of SCLE are required to determine the true risk of severe systemic disease progression in patients presenting with SCLE skin lesions. CCLE lesions, typically classic DLE, have also been seen to arise in patients initially presenting with SCLE.

Evidence suggests that overlap occurs between SCLE and Sjögren's syndrome. Patients with SCLE who develop Sjögren's syndrome are at risk for developing the extraglandular systemic complications known to be associated with Sjögren's syndrome, including vasculitis, peripheral neuropathy, autoimmune thyroiditis, renal tubular acidosis, myositis, chronic hepatitis, primary biliary cirrhosis, psychosis, lymphadenopathy, splenomegaly, and B cell lymphoma.

CCLE

Most patients with untreated classic DLE lesions suffer indolent progression to large areas of cutaneous dystrophy and scarring alopecia that can be psychosocially devastating and occupationally disabling. However, with treatment, skin disease can be largely controlled. Spontaneous remission is occasionally observed, and the disease activity can recrudesce at the sites of older, inactive lesions. Squamous cell carcinoma occasionally develops in chronic smoldering DLE lesions.

Death from SLE disease activity is distinctly uncommon in patients who present initially with localized DLE. As previously discussed, patients presenting with localized DLE have only a 5 percent chance of subsequently developing clinically significant SLE disease activity. Generalized DLE and persistent, low-grade laboratory abnormalities appear to be risk factors for such disease progression.

LE-NONSPECIFIC SKIN LESIONS

LE-nonspecific skin lesions are lesions that can be seen in clinical settings other than LE. For the most part, LE-nonspecific skin lesions are seen in the setting of SLE. It is not possible to present here a comprehensive discussion of the numerous LE-nonspecific skin lesions that have been described, but such discussions can be found elsewhere.[6,8]

From 20 to 70 percent of patients with SLE develop vasculitic lesions that range from palpable purpura to urticaria-like lesions to large ulcers. Most frequently, such lesions are the result of cutaneous small vessel leukocytoclastic vasculitis. Urticarial vasculitis (and chronic urticaria) is occasionally the presenting manifestation of SLE. However, some vessel-based skin lesions in patients with LE result from thrombotic vasculopathies rather than vasculitis. Skin lesions resulting from thrombotic occlusion of cutaneous vessels (livedo reticularis with or without ulceration, acral cyanosis, cutaneous infarction, Degos'-like lesions, *atrophie blanche*- or "livedo vasculitis"-like lesions) often occur in the setting of antiphospholipid antibody production (i.e., anticardiolipin antibodies and/or lupus anticoagulant). The antiphospholipid syndrome (Hughes syndrome) has recently been reviewed.[46]

Other vessel-based skin lesions occur in patients with SLE. Approximately 10 to 15 percent of patients with SLE demonstrate nail fold erythema and/or telangiectasia; however, this finding is more frequent in patients with dermatomyositis. The incidence of Raynaud's phenomenon in patients with SLE ranges between 18 and 46 percent and often occurs in LE patients who have features of an overlapping connective tissue disease associated with anti-U$_1$RNP antibodies such as mixed connective tissue disease. Erythromelalgia (erythermalgia) has been found on rare occasion to be associated with SLE.

Several forms of nonscarring alopecia occur in patients with SLE. They may demonstrate a transient, diffuse, nonscarring hair loss associated with exacerbations of their systemic disease process that appears to be a form of telogen effluvium. Another form of nonscarring alopecia seen in patients with SLE, especially at the periphery of the scalp has been termed *lupus hair* or *wooly hair*. Alopecia areata has occasionally been detected.

Other LE-nonspecific skin lesions include sclerodactyly, rheumatoid nodules, erythema multiforme–like lesions seen in the context of Rowell's syndrome, cutaneous mucinosis, anetoderma, cutis laxa, lichen planus, acanthosis nigricans, and cytophagic histiocytic panniculitis.

Nail changes, including pitting, horizontal and longitudinal ridging, leukonychia, onycholysis, dyschromia, nail bed atrophy, and telangiectasia of the cuticle nail fold, have been observed in patients with SLE.

REFERENCES

1. Sontheimer RD: The lexicon of cutaneous lupus erythematosus—a review and personal perspective on the nomenclature and classification of the cutaneous manifestations of lupus erythematosus. *Lupus* **6**:84, 1997
2. Lahita RG (ed): *Systemic Lupus Erythematosus,* 2d ed., New York, Churchill Livingstone, 1992
3. Schur PH (ed): *The Clinical Management of Systemic Lupus Erythematosus,* 2d ed., Philadelphia, Lippincott-Raven, 1996.
4. Wallace DJ, Hahn BH (eds): *Dubois' Lupus Erythematosus,* 5th ed., Baltimore, Williams & Wilkins, 1997
5. Tan EM et al: The 1982 revised criteria for the classification of systemic lupus erythematosus. *Arthritis Rheum* **25**:1271, 1982
6. Sontheimer RD, Provost TT: Lupus erythematosus, in *Cutaneous Manifestations of Rheumatic Diseases,* edited by RD Sontheimer, TT Provost. Baltimore, Williams & Wilkins, 1996, p 1
7. McCauliffe DP, Sontheimer RD: Cutaneous lupus erythematosus, in *The Clinical Management of Systemic Lupus Erythematosus,* 2nd ed, edited by PH Schur. Philadelphia, Lippincott-Raven, 1996, p. 67
8. Sontheimer RD, Provost TT: Cutaneous manifestations of lupus erythematosus, in *Dubois' Lupus Erythematosus,* 5th ed, edited by DJ Wallace, BH Hahn. Baltimore, Williams & Wilkins, 1997, Chap 34, p 569
9. Sontheimer RD (guest ed): Skin disease in lupus erythematosus (special issue). *Lupus* **6**(2):1997
10. Yell JA et al: Cutaneous manifestations of systemic lupus erythematosus. *Br J Dermatol* **135**:355, 1996
11. Watanabe T, Tsuchida T: Classification of lupus erythematosus based upon cutaneous manifestations. Dermatological, systemic and laboratory findings in 191 patients. *Dermatology* **190**:277, 1995
12. Healy E et al: Cutaneous lupus erythematosus—a study of clinical and laboratory prognostic factors in 65 patients. *Ir J Med Sci* **164**:113, 1995
13. Laman SD, Provost TT: Cutaneous manifestations of lupus erythematosus. *Rheum Dis Clin North Am* **20**:195, 1994
14. David-Bajar KM: Subacute cutaneous lupus erythematosus. *J Invest Dermatol* **100**:2S, 1993
15. Wallace DJ: Cutaneous manifestations of SLE, in *Dubois' Lupus Erythematosus,* 4th ed, edited by DJ Wallace, BH Hahn. Philadelphia, Lea & Febiger, 1993, p 356
16. Donnelly AM et al: Discoid lupus erythematosus. *Australas J Dermatol* **36**:3, 1995
17. Rowell NR: Some historical aspects of skin disease in lupus erythematosus. *Lupus* **6**:76, 1997
18. Talbott JH: Historical background of discoid and systemic lupus erythematosus, in *Lupus Erythematosus,* 4th ed, edited by DJ Wallace, BH Hahn, Philadelphia, Lea and Febiger, 1993, p 3
19. Hopkinson N: Epidemiology of systemic lupus erythematosus. *Ann Rheum Dis* **51**:1292, 1992
20. Hochberg MBP-CR: The epidemiology of systemic lupus erythematosus, in *Dubois' Lupus Erythematosus,* 4th ed, edited by DJ Wallace, BH Hahn. Philadelphia, Lea & Febiger, 1993, p 49
21. Tebbe B, Orfanos CE: Epidemiology and socioeconomic impact of skin disease in lupus erythematosus. *Lupus* **6**:96, 1997
22. Brown K et al: Cutaneous manifestations of SLE: Associations with other manifestations of SLE and with smoking [abstract]. *Arthritis Rheum* **39**(suppl):S291, 1996
23. Bennion SD, Norris DA: Ultraviolet light modulation of autoantigens, epidermal cytokines and adhesion molecules as contributing factors of the pathogenesis of cutaneous LE. *Lupus* **6**:181, 1997
24. Casciola-Rosen L, Rosen A: Ultraviolet light–induced keratinocyte apoptosis: A potential mechanism for the induction of skin lesions and autoantibody production in LE. *Lupus* **6**:175, 1997
25. Sontheimer RD: Photoimmunology of lupus erythematosus and dermatomyositis: A speculative review. *Photochem Photobiol* **63**:583, 1996
26. Norris DA: Pathomechanisms of photosensitive lupus erythematosus. *J Invest Dermatol* **100**:58S, 1993

27. Harley JB, Scofield RH: Systemic lupus erythematosus: RNA–protein autoantigens, models of disease heterogeneity, and theories of etiology. *J Clin Immunol* **11**:297, 1991

28. Drake CG, Kotzin BL: Genetic and immunological mechanisms in the pathogenesis of systemic lupus erythematosus. *Curr Opin Immunol* **4**:733, 1992

29. Mohan C, Datta SK: Lupus: Key pathogenic mechanisms and contributing factors. *Clin Immunol Immunopathol* **77**:209, 1995

30. Harley JB, James JA: Autoepitopes in lupus. *J Lab Clin Med* **126**:509, 1995

31. Casiano CA, Tan EM: Recent developments in the understanding of antinuclear autoantibodies. *Int Arch Allergy Immunol* **111**:308, 1996

32. Kind P et al: Phototesting in lupus erythematosus. *J Invest Dermatol* **100**:53S, 1993

33. Walchner M et al: Phototesting and photoprotection in LE. *Lupus* **6**:167, 1997

34. Furukawa F et al: Selective expansions of T cells expressing Vbeta8 and Vbeta13 in skin lesions of patients with chronic cutaneous lupus erythematosus. *J Dermatol* **23**:670, 1996

35. Lee LA, Weston WL: Cutaneous lupus erythematosus during the neonatal and childhood periods. *Lupus* **6**:132, 1997

36. Wallace DJ: The relationship between discoid and systemic lupus erythematosus, in *Dubois' Lupus Erythematosus,* 4th ed, edited by DJ Wallace, BH Hahn. Philadelphia, Lea & Febiger, 1993, p 310

37. Burge SM et al: Mucosal involvement in systemic and chronic cutaneous lupus erythematosus. *Br J Dermatol* **121**:727, 1989

38. Yell JA, Wojnarowska F: Bullous skin disease in lupus erythematosus. *Lupus* **6**:112, 1997

39. von Muhlen CA, Tan EM: Autoantibodies in the diagnosis of systemic rheumatic diseases. *Semin Arthritis Rheum* **24**:323, 1995

40. Sontheimer RD et al: Antinuclear antibodies: Clinical correlations and biologic significance. *Adv Dermatol* **7**:3, 1992

41. David-Bajar KM, Davis BM: Pathology, immunopathology, and immunohistochemistry in cutaneous lupus erythematosus. *Lupus* **6**:145, 1997

42. Costner M, Sontheimer RD: Antimalarial therapy in photosensitive dermatoses. *Dermatol Ther* **4**:86, 1997

43. Callen JP: Management of antimalarial–refractory cutaneous lupus erythematosus. *Lupus,* **6**:203, 1997

44. Duna GF, Cash JM: Treatment of refractory cutaneous lupus erythematosus. *Rheum Dis Clin North Am* **21**:99, 1995

45. Rothe MJ, Kerdel FA: Treatment of cutaneous lupus erythematosus. *Lupus* **1**:351, 1992

46. Frances C, Piette JC: Cutaneous manifestations of Hughes syndrome occurring in the context of lupus erythematosus. *Lupus* **6**:139, 1997

CHAPTER 173

Richard D. Sontheimer

Dermatomyositis

Dermatomyositis is a disease in which characteristic patterns of autoimmune inflammatory injury occur in striated muscle and skin. A subgroup of dermatomyositis exists in which the classical cutaneous manifestations of dermatomyositis occur for extended periods of time without accompanying muscle disease (amyopathic dermatomyositis or dermatomyositis siné myositis). Dermatomyositis has traditionally been classified as one of the idiopathic inflammatory myopathies.[1] Polymyositis and inclusion-body myositis are also included in this disease grouping. Patients with polymyositis have the same clinical pattern of muscle disease as those suffering from dermatomyositis but lack skin changes. Patients with inclusion-body myositis have a fundamentally different type of muscle disorder from that of patients with dermatomyositis/polymyositis and suffer no accompanying skin lesions.[2]

The classic Bohan classification scheme of 1977[3] (Table 173-1) and its revision presented by Dalakas[1] in 1991 both failed to include amyopathic dermatomyositis, a form of this disease of special interest to the dermatologist. Later attempts at classifying this group of clinical disorders[4] have been criticized for not including amyopathic dermatomyositis.[5] The classification scheme that includes amyopathic dermatomyositis (Table 173-2) will be used for the discussion in this chapter.[2,6]

Both the cutaneous manifestations of dermatomyositis[2] and the extracutaneous manifestations of dermatomyositis/polymyositis have been reviewed in detail.[7,8] Drugs such as hydroxyurea, penicillamine, niflumic acid/diclofenac, tryptophan, and practolol are capable of inducing skin changes that can mimic both classical dermatomyositis (skin plus muscle involvement) and amyopathic dermatomyositis (skin disease alone).[2]

HISTORIC ASPECTS

Classic Dermatomyositis

Wagner in 1863[9] and Unverricht in 1887[10] first recognized dermatomyositis as a distinct entity (i.e., Wagner-Unverricht disease). Gottron was among the first to characterize the cutaneous manifestations of dermatomyositis.[11] Pearson laid the groundwork in the 1960s and 1970s for our current understanding of the spectrum of disorders that is now recognized as dermatomyositis/polymyositis.[3,12] His work facilitated subsequent efforts, including those of Bohan, that led to the modern classification systems.[1,13] The dif-

TABLE 173-1

The Bohan Classification of Polymyositis/Dermatomyositis

Clinical subgroups
1. Polymyositis
2. Dermatomyositis
3. Polymyositis or dermatomyositis associated with malignancy
4. Childhood dermatomyositis
5. Polymyositis or dermatomyositis with an associated connective tissue disorder

Diagnostic criteria
1. Typical skin rash
2. Symmetric proximal muscle weakness with or without dysphagia or respiratory muscle involvement
3. Abnormal muscle biopsy specimen
4. Elevation of skeletal muscle–derived enzymes
5. Abnormal electromyogram

Confidence limits for diagnosis of dermatomyositis
1. Definite dermatomyositis—rash and three of the four other diagnostic criteria
2. Probable dermatomyositis—rash and two of the four other diagnostic criteria
3. Possible dermatomyositis—rash and one of the four other diagnostic criteria

SOURCE: Bohan et al.,[3] with permission.

ferences between the juvenile and adult forms of dermatomyositis were first emphasized by Everett and Curtis in 1957[14] and Banker and Victor in 1966.[15] These workers emphasized that severe vasculopathy/vasculitis, calcification, and disability are more often suf-

TABLE 173-2

A Comprehensive Classification of Idiopathic Inflammatory Dermatomyopathies

Dermatomyositis
1. Adult-onset classic dermatomyositis*
2. Classic dermatomyositis with malignancy
3. Juvenile-onset classic dermatomyositis
4. Classic dermatomyositis as part of an overlap connective tissue disorder
5. Amyopathic dermatomyositis (adult and juvenile onset):
    Confirmed
        Biopsy-confirmed hallmark cutaneous manifestations without muscle weakness and with normal muscle enzymes for 2 years or longer
    Provisional
        Biopsy-confirmed hallmark cutaneous manifestations without muscle weakness and with normal muscle enzymes for more than 6 months but less than 2 years

Polymyositis
1. Isolated polymyositis
2. Polymyositis as part of an overlap connective tissue disorder

Inclusion-body myositis

*The term *classic dermatomyositis* is used here to denote the combination of both cutaneous and muscle manifestations of dermatomyositis as opposed to the term *amyopathic dermatomyositis,* which is used here to signify the presence of only the hallmark cutaneous manifestations of dermatomyositis for prolonged periods of time.
SOURCE: Adapted from the work of Bohan et al., 1977[3]; Dalakas, 1991[1]; and Euwer and Sontheimer, 1991.[24,25] Reprinted from Euwer and Sontheimer[2,6] with permission from the publishers, Current Sciences and Williams & Wilkins.

FIGURE 173-1

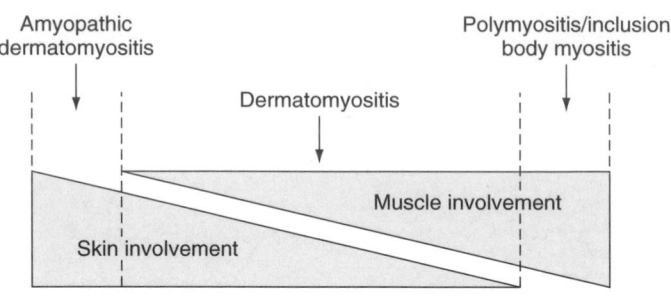

Graphic representation of the relationship between the cutaneous and muscular manifestations of the idiopathic inflammatory myopathies, including the nosologic entities found within this spectrum of illness.

fered by children with this disease than by adults. Shy in 1962 debated a purported relationship between dermatomyositis/polymyositis and occult malignancy.[16] More recent population-based studies have confirmed that patients with dermatomyositis are at increased risk for malignancy.[17,18]

Amyopathic Dermatomyositis

Although most patients with dermatomyositis develop weakness within 6 months after the onset of cutaneous inflammation, a small percentage of patients express the hallmark cutaneous manifestations of dermatomyositis for much longer periods of time without clinical evidence of muscle disease.[19–23] The term *dermatomyositis siné myositis* has been used to refer to this pattern of disease, and attention has recently been focused on this subgroup of patients under the designation *amyopathic dermatomyositis*.[5,24,25] Thus, the idiopathic inflammatory myopathies comprise a disease spectrum extending from isolated inflammatory myositis (polymyositis and inclusion-body myositis) to exclusively cutaneous dermatomyositis (amyopathic dermatomyositis)[24] (Fig. 173-1).

EPIDEMIOLOGY

Classic Dermatomyositis

Cutaneous involvement occurs in 30 to 40 percent of adults[3,26] and 95 percent of children with dermatomyositis/polymyositis.[27,28] Skin disease by definition is absent in patients with polymyositis and present in 100 percent of patients with classic dermatomyositis and amyopathic dermatomyositis. Skin disease commonly precedes muscle disease in classic dermatomyositis by as much as 6 months.[3,22]

The incidence of dermatomyositis/polymyositis between 1963 and 1982 was 5.5 cases per million.[29] The incidence probably is higher, inasmuch as this study was based on hospital-based diagnoses only and did not include cases of amyopathic dermatomyositis. Black women during their childbearing years were affected most frequently, and dermatomyositis might be underdiagnosed in blacks because of the more subtle coloration of inflammatory changes in their skin.[30] Females are affected twice as often as males. Polymyositis/dermatomyositis can occur from infancy to adult life, most frequently presenting in the fifth and sixth decades. Familial concordance occurs rarely, and concordant disease expression has been reported in identical twins.

Polymyositis is extremely rare in children. Cutaneous ulceration occurring as a result of infarctive vasculopathy and calcification is more common in the childhood form of the disease.[31]

Polymyositis and dermatomyositis have been associated with HLA-B8, DR3, and DRw52, especially in Caucasian patients.[32,33] This association is likely due to linkage disequilibrium with HLA-DQA1*0501.[34] The production of anti-synthetase antibodies such as Jo-1 is strongly linked to HLA-DR3[35] and even more so with its supertypic specificity, HLA-DRw52.[36]

Environmental factors have been implicated as disease triggers. Seasonality, suggesting the possibility of an infectious etiology, has been noted in both childhood-onset[37] and adult-onset polymyositis/dermatomyositis.[33] Dermatomyositis- and polymyositis-like syndromes have been reported in patients with X-linked immunodeficiency[37] as well as with the acquired immunodeficiency syndrome and human T-cell leukemia virus type I infection.[38] Other environmental factors that have been implicated include certain drugs,[1,39–42] silicone breast implants,[43] silicon,[44] and bovine collagen implants.[45] However, the links to silicone implants and bovine collagen implants have been seriously questioned.[43,46]

Amyopathic Dermatomyositis

Although there are no population-based prevalence/incidence data, small case series have suggested that amyopathic dermatomyositis occurs in approximately 10 to 20 percent of dermatomyositis patient series reported by dermatologists.[22,24] This form of the disease appears to have even a stronger female preponderance than the classical form. Amyopathic dermatomyositis was initially described in adults, but evidence indicates that it affects children as well.[47] Human leukocyte antigen (HLA) typing data have not yet been reported for amyopathic dermatomyositis. The author has observed a familial constellation of amyopathic dermatomyositis in a father and his two adult daughters (unpublished personal observation).

ETIOLOGY AND PATHOGENESIS

The etiology and pathogenesis of dermatomyositis/polymyositis are unknown. The inflammatory nature of the muscle and skin manifestations coupled with the characteristic humoral autoimmune abnormalities have led to the hypothesis that this disorder results from a genetically determined, aberrant autoimmune response to environmental agents such as myotropic infectious agents.[7] Candidates include RNA viruses such as coxsackievirus, echovirus, human retroviruses [human T-cell leukemia/lymphoma virus type I (HTLV-1) and HIV], and nonviral pathogens such as *Toxoplasma gondii*. However, attempts to confirm persistent myotropic virus infection have not

been successful.[48] Myxovirus-like structures observed by electron microscopy in lesional skin of patients with dermatomyositis[49] probably represent artifacts.[50] Cell-mediated immunity against muscle autoantigens is thought to be responsible for the muscle injury that occurs in polymyositis, whereas humoral autoimmune mechanisms have been implicated in the pathogenesis of muscle and skin injury in dermatomyositis. Several types of myositis-specific autoantibody responses are seen in dermatomyositis/polymyositis (Table 173-3). Whether these autoantibodies are pathogenetic or represent only a by-product of muscle injury is not known.

The histopathology of cutaneous dermatomyositis is similar to that of certain forms of cutaneous lupus erythematosus (LE). Some forms of photosensitive cutaneous LE, such as subacute cutaneous LE and neonatal LE, are associated with Ro/SS-A autoantibody, implicating a mechanism of antibody-dependent cell-mediated cytotoxicity.[51] Although photosensitive cutaneous dermatomyositis does not have a known autoantibody marker, humoral factors have been implicated in the pathogenesis of dermatomyositis.[52,53] Epidermal Langerhans cell alterations differ between cutaneous LE and dermatomyositis skin lesions.[54]

The immunopathology of cutaneous dermatomyositis includes a variable degree of immunoglobulin and complement deposition at the dermal-epidermal junction and within the dermal microvasculature. The deposition of the membrane attack complex (C5-9) in the walls of dermal microvessels occurs more frequently in cuta-

TABLE 173-3

Autoantibodies Encountered in Patients with Dermatomyositis/Polymyositis

NAME	FREQUENCY (%)	BINDING SPECIFICITY	CLINICAL ASSOCIATION
High specificity			
56 kDa	85	56-kDa nuclear protein	—
Jo-1	20	Histidyl tRNA synthetase	Antisynthetase syndrome
Mi-2	8	Nuclear protein	Shawl sign, cuticular overgrowth
SRP	4	Signal-recognition particle	Fulminant dermatomyositis/polymyositis, cardiac involvement
PL-7	3	Threonyl tRNA synthetase	Antisynthetase syndrome
PL-12	3	Alanyl tRNA synthetase	Antisynthetase syndrome
OJ	Rare	Isoleucyl tRNA synthetase	Antisynthetase syndrome
EJ	Rare	Glycyl tRNA synthetase	Antisynthetase syndrome, increased frequency of skin changes
Fer	Rare	Elongation factor 1-α	—
Mas	Rare	Small RNA	—
KJ	Rare	Translation factor	—
Low specificity			
U$_1$RNP	12	Ribonucleoprotein	Overlap connective tissue disease
Ro/SS-A	10	Ribonucleoprotein	Overlap with Sjögren's syndrome, subacute cutaneous lupus erythematosus, systemic lupus erythematosus
PM-Scl	8	Nucleolar proteins	Overlap with scleroderma
Ku	3	DNA binding protein	Overlap with scleroderma
U2RNP	1	Ribonucleoprotein	Overlap with scleroderma

SOURCE: Adapted from Euwer and Sontheimer[2] and Targoff.[7,94] Reprinted with permission of the publisher, Williams & Wilkins.

neous dermatomyositis than cutaneous LE.[55] The predominate infiltrating cell types in cutaneous dermatomyositis are activated macrophages and CD4 T cells, arguing for a cell-mediated pattern of immune injury.[56] Wakino and co-workers have reported that the peripheral blood lymphocyte subpopulations in a single patient with amyopathic dermatomyositis were different from those reported for patients with classic dermatomyositis/polymyositis.[57]

The dermal microvasculature is more prominently altered in cutaneous dermatomyositis than cutaneous LE.[53] It has been suggested that humoral factors could produce microvascular injury by triggering local activation of complement with deposition of C5-9,[52,53] perhaps through endothelial-specific autoantibodies.[58] Class II histocompatibility antigen expression by dermal endothelial cells is decreased[56] in dermatomyositis skin lesions, and this cell type appears to display an activation phenotype with respect to adhesion molecule expression [intercellular adhesion molecule 1 (ICAM-1), vascular cell adhesion molecule 1 (VCAM-1), E-selectin].[59]

Dermal mucin is a prominent finding in biopsies of dermatomyositis skin lesions. It has been suggested that this might be due to the increased production of glycosaminoglycans by dermal fibroblasts as a result of immunologic stimulation.[60] Evidence suggesting that mononuclear cells from patients with dermatomyositis can be cytotoxic for cultured dermal fibroblasts does exist.[61] Serum factors in patients with LE can stimulate the production of glycosaminoglycans by dermal fibroblasts.[62] The limited observations pertaining to the etiology and pathogenesis of dermatomyositis/polymyositis continue to be assessed.[2,7,8,63–65]

CLINICAL MANIFESTATIONS

Cutaneous Features

HALLMARK SKIN LESIONS The hallmark cutaneous manifestations of dermatomyositis and amyopathic dermatomyositis are presented in Table 173-4 (to date, no recognizable differences in the cutaneous manifestations of classic dermatomyositis and amyopathic dermatomyositis have been reported).[2] Some of these lesions, such as Gottron's sign (Fig. 173-2) and Gottron's papules (Figs. 173-2 and 173-3), are virtually pathognomic of this disease, whereas others are highly characteristic, such as periorbital confluent macular violaceous (heliotrope) erythema/edema and grossly visible periungual telangiectasia/dystrophic cuticles. The primary skin change of dermatomyositis is a highly characteristic, intensely pruritic, symmetrical, confluent, macular violaceous erythema overlying the extensor aspect of the fingers, hands, forearms, arms, deltoid areas, posterior shoulders, and neck (the shawl sign), the V area of the anterior neck and upper chest, the central aspect of the face, the forehead, and the scalp (Fig. 173-4, 173-5). Lesions such as poikiloderma atrophicans vasculare (poikilodermatomyositis) (Fig. 173-6) and calcinosis cutis are often seen in patients with dermatomyositis, but can also be seen in patients with cutaneous T-cell lymphoma (poikiloderma atrophicans vasculare) and scleroderma (calcinosis cutis).

Several other types of skin lesions have recently been suggested to also be characteristic of dermatomyositis/polymyositis; however, there is not yet enough published experience to determine their true disease specificity or prevalence. The mechanic's hand lesion consists of a nonpruritic, hyperkeratotic eruption accompanied by scaling, fissuring, and hyperpigmentation, giving the false appearance

TABLE 173-4

Classic Cutaneous Manifestations of Dermatomyositis

Pathognomonic
1. Gottron's papules
   Papules having a violaceous hue overlying the dorsal-lateral aspect of interphalangeal and/or metacarpophalangeal joints. When fully formed, these papules become slightly depressed at the center, which can assume a white, atrophic appearance. Associated telangiectasia can be present.
2. Gottron's sign
   Symmetric confluent macular violaceous erythema with or without edema overlying the dorsal aspect of the interphalangeal/metacarpophalangeal joints, olecranon processes, patellae, and medial malleoli.

Characteristic
1. Periorbital confluent macular violaceous (heliotrope) erythema with or without associated edema of the eyelids and periorbital tissue.
2. Grossly visible periungual telangiectasia with or without dystrophic cuticles and cuticular hemorrhage.
3. Symmetric confluent macular violaceous erythema overlying the dorsal aspect of the hands and fingers (where it can track along the extensor tendons), extensor aspects of the arms and forearms, deltoids, posterior shoulders and neck (shawl sign), V area of anterior neck and upper chest (V sign), central aspect of the face and forehead, and scalp.
4. Mechanic's hand lesion—bilaterally symmetric confluent hyperkeratosis having the appearance of that produced by manual labor distributed along the ulnar aspect of the thumb and radial aspect of the fingers; also prominent on the index and middle fingers with occasional extension to the palmar surfaces

Compatible with dermatomyositis
1. Poikiloderma atrophicans vasculare (poikilodermatomyositis)
   Circumscribed violaceous erythema with associated telangiectasia, hypopigmentation, hyperpigmentation, and superficial atrophy most commonly found over the posterior shoulders, back, buttocks, and V area of the anterior neck and chest. Often asymmetric.
2. Calcinosis cutis

SOURCE: Adapted from Euwer and Sontheimer.[2,6] Reprinted with permission from the publishers, Current Sciences and Williams & Wilkins.

of the callused hands of a laborer. These changes are bilaterally symmetrical and distributed along the ulnar aspect of the thumb and radial aspect of the fingers; they are prominent on the index and middle fingers with occasional extension to the palmar surfaces.[33,66,67] There appears to be a strong association between this skin lesion and the presence of antisynthetase antibodies such as Jo-1 and active myositis. Mucinous plaques centered over the flexural creases of the palms and fingers have also been seen in the context of dermatomyositis/polymyositis.

The characteristic anatomic distribution of the hallmark cutaneous manifestations of dermatomyositis are presented in Table 173-5. There is very little published information on the prevalence of involvement in these different anatomic locations. In some series reported by dermatologists, Gottron's papules have been more commonly seen than periorbital heliotrope erythema,[24,68] which, by many outside of dermatology, is felt to be the hallmark cutaneous manifestation of dermatomyositis.

The violaceous hue of the cutaneous inflammation is a striking clinical finding that usually is evident from the outset of disease activity. This violaceous hue helps to distinguish cutaneous dermatomyositis from cutaneous LE, in which it is a late finding when present. It has been suggested that edema associated with this dis-

FIGURE 173-2

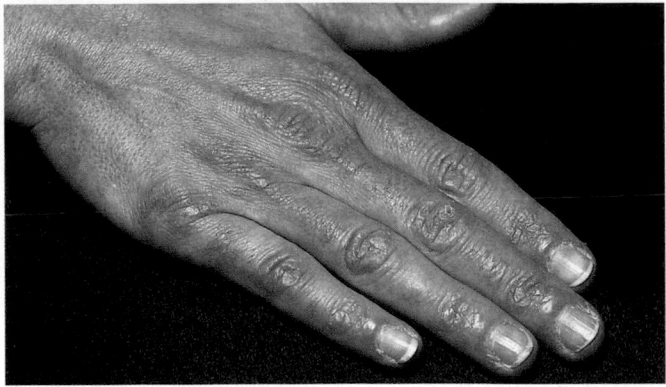

Hand of a 30-year-old female with a 15-year history of amyopathic dermatomyositis. Note the confluent macular violaceous erythema, most pronounced over the metacarpophalangeal/interphalangeal joints, extending in a linear array over the extensor tendons overlying the hand and fingers. These changes, referred to as *Gottron's sign,* are a hallmark cutaneous feature of dermatomyositis. Early Gottron's papules, an extension of Gottron's sign, can be seen over the distal interphalangeal joints along with periungual erythema and dystrophic cuticles. Contrast this appearance with that of LE involving the same anatomic site illustrated in Fig. 172-2A. In dermatomyositis the violaceous erythema is centered over the metacarpophalangeal/interphalangeal joints, whereas in LE these areas are relatively spared.

FIGURE 173-3

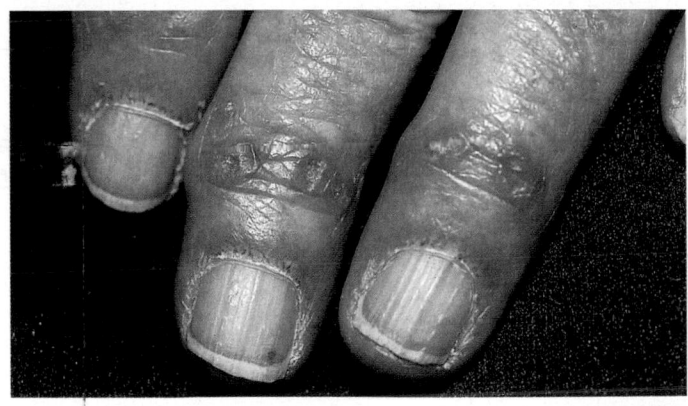

Fingers of an elderly female with classic dermatomyositis. Note the fully formed Gottron's papules over the distal interphalangeal joints, a hallmark cutaneous feature of dermatomyositis. Prominent, grossly visible nail fold telangiectasias are also present, along with dystrophic cuticles. The combination of Gottron's papules and nail fold changes such as these is pathognomic for dermatomyositis. Such changes are seen to an equal degree in classic dermatomyositis and amyopathic dermatomyositis. (*Photograph reprinted from Euwer and Sontheimer,*[2] *with permission of the publisher, Williams & Wilkins.*)

ease process indirectly produces the violaceous hue by displacing the hyperemic cutaneous vasculature more deeply into the dermis.[69] It could also result from the deoxygenation of blood flow through an abnormal dermal microvascular bed. A striking clinical feature that helps to distinguish cutaneous dermatomyositis from cutaneous LE is pruritus, which can be so severe in dermatomyositis as to be disabling even in the absence of systemic involvement.

FIGURE 173-4

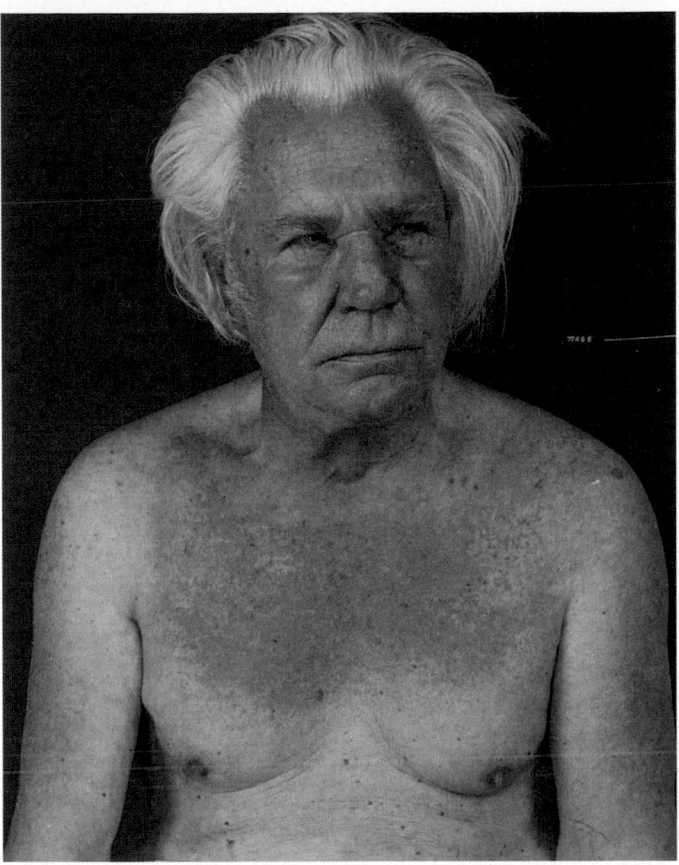

The confluent, macular, violaceous erythema of the V area of the upper chest and neck (V sign), when persistent over time, can evolve to poikilodermatous skin changes. Less evident in this photograph are periorbital edema and confluent, macular, violaceous (heliotrope) erythema of the upper eyelids. Note the absence of involvement of the malar areas, which are often involved in LE.

FIGURE 173-5

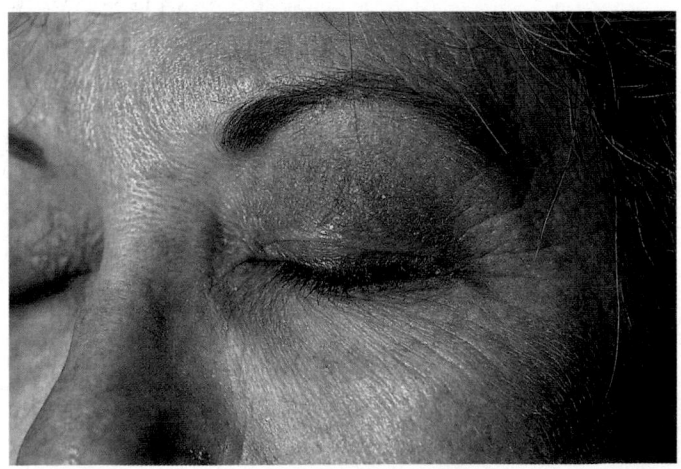

Periorbital confluent, macular, violaceous (heliotrope) erythema most prominent on the upper eyelids. Like Gottron's papules and Gottron's sign, this is a hallmark cutaneous feature of dermatomyositis.

FIGURE 173-6

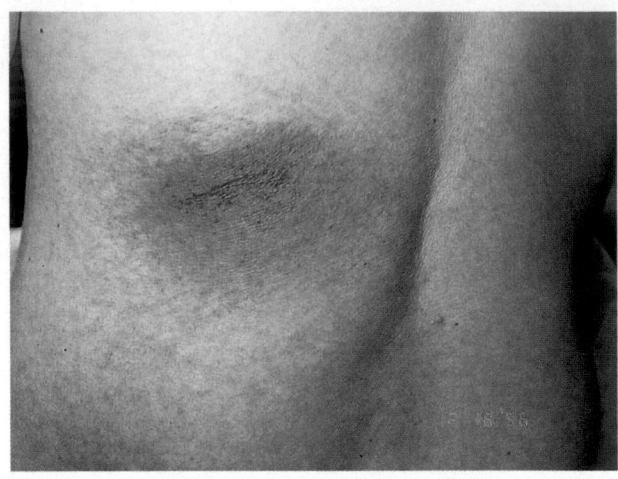

An asymmetrical plaque of poikiloderma atrophicans vasculare on the flank of a 55-year-old male with classic dermatomyositis.

A number of other skin changes can be encountered in patients with dermatomyositis. Hyperkeratosis can follow the onset of the confluent, macular, violaceous erythema; however, the scale in dermatomyositis skin lesions is usually less prominent than that in subacute cutaneous LE and discoid LE. Secondary skin changes in dermatomyositis skin lesions include excoriation with secondary infection and ulceration. Subepidermal vesicles and/or bullae occasionally occur in areas of particularly intense cutaneous inflammation. Post-inflammatory pigmentary changes, both hyperpigmentation and hypopigmentation, can be seen. Older lesions can display white lacy markings somewhat similar to those of lichen planus (Wickham's striae). Other similarities between cutaneous dermatomyositis and lichen planus, such as the characteristic violaceous hue, have been pointed out.[70] Mucinous infiltration, a common histologic finding in the dermis of dermatomyositis skin lesions, can be clinically prominent, producing an infiltrated, glistening appearance. Superficial erosions and ulcers can subsequently develop over the face and eyelids as well as in other areas affected by intense and protracted inflammation. Deep, irregular retiform ulcers can also develop in areas of poikiloderma in both adults and children.

The cutaneous manifestations of dermatomyositis are precipitated or exacerbated by natural and artificial sources of ultraviolet light.[65] Approximately 50 percent of patients with dermatomyositis experience photosensitivity.[14,68] The action spectrum appears to include both ultraviolet B (UVB) and ultraviolet A (UVA).[68] As with LE, clinical experience suggests that the activity of dermatomyositis/polymyositis can be precipitated or exacerbated by emotional and physical stress, although there is scant published evidence to support this idea. Strenuous physical exertion can be detrimental to patients suffering from active myositis.

Cutaneous calcification is less common in adults than in children with dermatomyositis.[71] In adults it often presents as firm dermal and/or subcutaneous papules or nodules that are often most prominent around the elbows and hands. Large subcutaneous tumoral deposits can also occur over the trunk; such lesions can be filled with a liquid suspension of calcium crystals (i.e., "milk of calcium"). Four types of calcification have been described in children

with dermatomyositis: a superficial pattern consisting of small, firm nodules and plaques in the skin, periarticular subcutaneous nodules (calcinosis circumscripta), deposition along fascial planes in muscles (calcinosis universalis) (Fig. 173-7), and a severe "exoskeleton" pattern of deposition in the subcutaneous tissue. Calcinosis cutis or calcium deposition in muscles and tendons is more common in the late phases of the disease in children.

Dermatomyositis can develop as a component of an overlap connective tissue disorder. Most common are overlaps with systemic lupus erythematosus (SLE) and systemic sclerosis. Raynaud's phenomenon, sclerodactyly, sclerosis of the skin, and the characteristic hyperpigmentation can all be present in the latter setting. The term *sclerodermatomyositis* has been used to describe patients who present with dermatomyositis and develop striking features of scleroderma 6 months to 3 years later.[72,73] In addition, myositis occurs in approximately 5 percent of anti-Ro/SS-A autoantibody–positive patients (most of whom have Sjögren's syndrome). The cutaneous

TABLE 173-5

Anatomic Distribution of Hallmark Cutaneous Manifestations of Dermatomyositis

Anatomic Location	Lesions
Scalp	Confluent, macular, violaceous, erythema (CMVE); nonscarring diffuse alopecia
Face	
Periorbital region	CMVE (usually most intense on the upper eyelids), edema
Malar eminences	CMVE sparing the nasolabial fold
Forehead, chin	CMVE
Neck and shoulders	
Anterior	CMVE evolving to poikiloderma
Posterior	CMVE (shawl sign)
Upper extremities	
Arms, forearms	CMVE on the extensor aspects
Elbows	CMVE usually most intense in this location (Gottron's sign)
Hands, fingers	
Dorsal aspect	CMVE usually most intense over the extensor tendons and metacarpophalangeal/interphalangeal joints (Gottron's sign), Gottron's papules overlying the dorsal-lateral aspect of the metacarpophalangeal/interphalangeal joints, relative sparing of the dorsal aspects of the phalanges, periungual nailfold telangiectasia (often grossly visible), cuticular microvascular hemorrhage, dystrophic/ragged cuticles
Palmar aspect	Mechanic's hand lesion, mucinous plaques centered over the flexural creases
Trunk	CMVE evolving to large areas of poikiloderma (poikiloderma atrophicans vasculare) commonly seen over the flanks and lower back
Lower extremities	
Thighs	CMVE
Knees	CMVE (Gottron's sign)
Lower legs, feet	CMVE often focal centered over the medial malleoli, Gottron's sign overlying the medial malleoli

FIGURE 173-7

CHAPTER 173
Dermatomyositis

2015

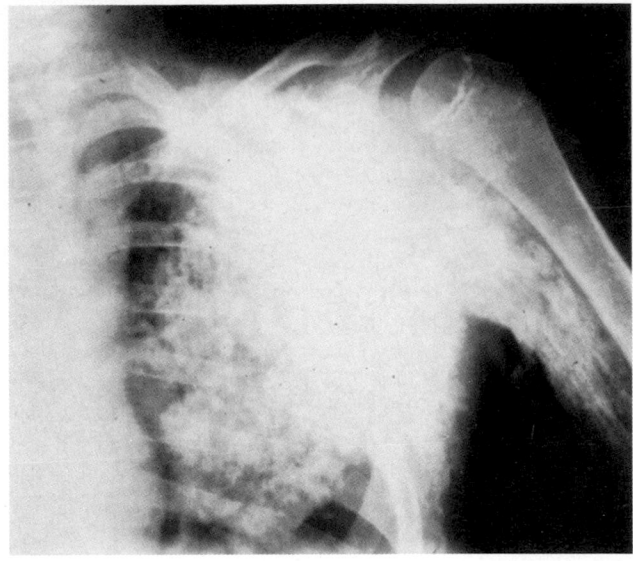

Calcinosis universalis. Calcification of subcutaneous tissue and pectoralis fascia in a child with dermatomyositis.

manifestations of dermatomyositis are usually not found in this setting.

UNCOMMON CUTANEOUS ASSOCIATIONS A number of rare cutaneous associations have been reported in patients with dermatomyositis, including acquired ichthyosis, erythroderma, facial swelling without erythema, follicular hyperkeratosis, hypertrichosis, lichen planus, linear IgA bullous dermatosis, malakoplakia, malignant erythema (suffusion), mucous membrane lesions, nasal septal perforation, panniculitis, cutaneous mucinosis, glucocorticoid-induced acanthosis nigricans, uticaria/urticarial vasculitis, cutaneous vasculitis, vulvar and scrotal involvement, zebra-like stripes, malignant atrophic papulosis, and partial lipodystrophy.

Systemic Features

The systemic manifestations and associations of classic dermatomyositis/polymyositis[7,8] are outlined in Table 173-6. Most of the extramuscular systemic features associated with classic dermatomyositis have not been reported in amyopathic dermatomyositis except for fatal interstitial pneumonitis in several patients with amyopathic dermatomyositis.[57,74,75]

MUSCLE DISEASE Muscle involvement typically presents as symmetrical weakness of the proximal muscles of the extremities. Lower extremity weakness manifesting as difficulty with routine activities of daily living, such as rising from a chair or bathtub and climbing stairs, is often the initial clinical finding. Weakness of the upper extremities soon follows, often manifest by difficulty in raising the arms above the head to perform routine activities such as combing the hair. Pain or tenderness in the affected muscle groups commonly occurs. Some patients experience a fulminant course, resulting in disabling weakness within a few weeks. Confirmation that proximal muscle weakness is due to the inflammatory myositis of dermatomyositis/polymyositis can be difficult because so many other clinical disorders produce proximal muscle weakness[7] (Table 173-7). The diagnosis can be supported by demonstrating the pres-

TABLE 173-6

Systemic Manifestations/Associations of Dermatomyositis/Polymyositis

Musculoskeletal
  Myositis with proximal weakness
  Muscle atrophy and contracture*
  Muscular calcification*
Cardiac
  Cardiomyopathy
  Conduction defects
Respiratory
  Dysphonia
  Diffuse interstitial pneumonitis/fibrosis
  Aspiration pneumonia
  Respiratory failure from muscle weakness
Gastrointestinal
  Proximal dysphagia
  Large bowel infarction/perforation secondary to vasculopathy*
Ophthalmologic
  Retinopathy*
Internal malignancy[†]

*Usually limited to juvenile dermatomyositis.
[†]Not significantly increased in juvenile dermatomyositis.

TABLE 173-7

Conditions That Can Simulate the Proximal Muscle Weakness of Dermatomyositis/Polymyositis

Infectious myopathies
  HIV-1, HTLV-I, coxsackievirus, echovirus, influenza, adenovirus, hepatitis B, Epstein-Barr virus
Other myopathies
  Inclusion-body myositis, rheumatic disease vasculitis, muscular dystrophies, metabolic myopathies
Neurologic disorders
  Myasthenia gravis, amyotrophic lateral sclerosis, Guillain-Barré syndrome
Endocrine disorders
  Hypothyroidism and hyperthyroidism, Cushing's syndrome, diabetic neuropathy, hypokalemia
Drug-induced myopathies
  Alcohol, antimalarials (vacuolar myopathy), colchicine, glucocorticoids, cyclosporine, street drugs (cocaine, heroin), lipid-lowering agents (lovastatin, simvastatin, gemfibrozil, clofibrate, niacin), D-penicillamine, zidovudine, isotretinoin/etretinate

SOURCE: Adapted from Euwer and Sontheimer[2] and Targoff.[7] Reprinted with permission of the publisher, Williams & Wilkins.

ence of characteristic serum muscle enzyme elevations as well as identifying diagnostic electromyographic (EMG) and muscle biopsy changes (see further discussion below).

Myositic inflammation can be highly focal. A number of noninvasive techniques are currently being examined for their ability to localize affected muscle groups. These include magnetic resonance imaging (MRI) of muscles,[76,77] phosphorus-31 spectroscopy,[78] muscle ultrasound,[79] and thallium scanning.[80] The possibility that MRI-guided needle biopsy could obviate the need for the more costly and invasive open muscle biopsy is also being explored.[81]

It is possible that some patients with amyopathic dermatomyositis suffer from low grade, subclinical muscle disease. However, the overall clinical significance of such mild muscle involvement can be questioned when no symptoms of muscular weakness develop in some patients who express the hallmark cutaneous manifestations of dermatomyositis for 10 to 20 years, as has been personally observed by the author.

Inclusion-body myositis is a pathologically distinctive type of steroid-resistant myositis that more commonly affects the distal muscle groups of men in an asymmetrical pattern. Cutaneous involvement is not seen with this disorder or with classical polymyositis.

INTERNAL MALIGNANCY The association between dermatomyositis/polymyositis and malignancy was suggested by Shy in 1962.[16] In 1980, Callen and colleagues found a relationship between dermatomyositis and malignancy in 25 percent of their patients.[82] However, the validity of such an association has been debated due to the retrospective nature of the earlier studies addressing this issue.[83,84] Several more recent population-based studies have documented that patients with dermatomyositis have a higher than expected risk for malignancy. One of these studies demonstrated a relative risk for malignancy of 2.4 in male patients with dermatomyositis and 3.4 in females with dermatomyositis.[17] The risk for malignancies was negligible in patients with polymyositis. The mortality rates from cancer were 3.8 in the patients with dermatomyositis and 0.9 for the patients with polymyositis. During the 5-year period after the diagnosis of dermatomyositis, the risk of a woman developing ovarian cancer in this study was 16.7-fold higher than the risk for women without dermatomyositis. In a more recent study, the standardized incidence ratio for malignancy in patients with dermatomyositis was 6.5.[18] In the first year following diagnosis, the relative risk for malignancy in patients with dermatomyositis was 26.0. Females with dermatomyositis in this study had a 32-fold higher risk of developing ovarian carcinoma. This study also found that polymyositis was not associated with an increased risk of cancer and that cytotoxic drug treatment of dermatomyositis did not increase the risk of malignancy. Because of the risk of ovarian cancer in females with dermatomyositis,[17,85,86] Whitmore and colleagues[86] have suggested that all women with dermatomyositis (classic dermatomyositis and amyopathic dermatomyositis) undergo an initial and repeat comprehensive gynecologic examination at 6- to 12-month intervals for the first 2 years after the diagnosis of dermatomyositis.[86] In addition to a bimanual pelvic examination, these authors have recommended that cancer antigen 125 (CA-125) serum level determination and transvaginal ultrasonography be carried out on all women having their ovaries.

Solid tumors other than ovarian carcinoma have been associated with dermatomyositis, including melanoma,[87] mycosis fungoides,[88] and Kaposi's sarcoma.[89] Carcinomas are more frequent than sarcomas, and lymphoproliferative malignancies are uncommon. Except for ovarian cancer in women, no preponderance of specific types of cancer is seen in dermatomyositis/polymyositis. The diagnosis of cancer is most often made by following leads discovered in a comprehensive history, review of systems, physical examination, and routine laboratory/radiologic testing. Debate exists about the routine use of surveillance imaging techniques such as chest or abdominal computed tomography and/or MRI in this setting. Age appears to be a factor concerning malignancy risk; there is not a significant risk of occult malignancy in juvenile-onset dermatomyositis, whereas individuals 50 years or older at the time of onset of dermatomyositis appear to have an increased risk of malignancy. The leading cause of death in patients with dermatomyositis/polymyositis who have malignancy is metastatic spread of the malignancy rather than complications directly related to the myositis. In patients with malignancy, the myositis and cutaneous manifestations are less responsive to systemic glucocorticoid therapy. In a few well-documented cases, definitive therapy for the malignancy has resulted in resolution of the dermatomyositis, and a recurrence of the cancer has been associated with the reappearance of the dermatomyositis.[84] Winklemann has suggested that a very bright vascular flush of the face, scalp, neck, and shoulders, which he designated as *malignant erythema*, occurs more commonly in patients with dermatomyositis who have an associated malignancy.[72]

Some workers have suggested that patients with amyopathic dermatomyositis have the same risk of malignancy as patients with classic dermatomyositis,[86,90,91] but others have not found an equal degree of risk.[92] There are not yet enough published data to determine the risk of internal malignancy in patients with amyopathic dermatomyositis.

Relationship between Cutaneous and Systemic Manifestations

There is little correlation between skin and muscle disease activity in dermatomyositis. It is not unusual for patients having skin and muscle disease at the outset of their illness to have their skin disease activity return unaccompanied by muscle involvement once immunosuppressive treatment has been withdrawn.

Attempts have been made to correlate the periungual microvascular changes that are seen in adult and juvenile dermatomyositis by nail fold capillaroscopy (i.e., dilatation, tortuosity, budding or arborization, and avascularity) with the systemic manifestations of this disease process, including myositis. In our experience the periungual nail fold capillary changes in patients with amyopathic dermatomyositis are qualitatively similar and as prominent as those in patients with classic dermatomyositis. Similar changes can be seen in patients with systemic sclerosis and to a lesser degree in those with systemic LE and mixed connective tissue disease.

LABORATORY FINDINGS

Classic Dermatomyositis

MUSCLE ENZYMES An elevation in the level of serum creatine kinase (CK) is the most sensitive and specific laboratory indicator of muscle disease activity in dermatomyositis/polymyositis. Ninety percent of patients with classic dermatomyositis/polymyositis have elevated levels of CK at some point. The elevated CK activity is due predominately to the CK-MM isoenzyme; however, elevations due to the CK-MB isoenzyme are also seen.[7] Elevated levels of CK can be associated with some of the disorders listed in Table 173-7 (e.g., other myopathies, hypothyroidism, and drug ingestions) as well as with strenuous physical exertion and needle trauma (intramuscular injection, EMG needle insertion). Enzymatic detection of CK activity can at times be inhibited by serum factors. Levels of CK may become elevated before the development of weakness and can normalize several weeks before the return of normal strength during treatment. Patients with dermatomyositis/polymyositis who present with normal CK levels may have a worse prognosis with

Serum aldolase is a somewhat less sensitive indicator than CK for active myositis in dermatomyositis/polymyositis; however, aldolase levels are occasionally elevated in the presence of a normal CK level.[7] Transaminases (AST, ALT) and lactic dehydrogenase can also be elevated in active myositis, but these values are less useful clinically because of their low degree of specificity. Elevations of transaminases during treatment with methotrexate could reflect the activity of myositis as well as drug-induced hepatotoxicity.

Urinary creatine excretion can also be used to monitor the status of myositis. However, the specificity is low in that urinary creatine excretion can also be elevated in steroid myopathy. Serum myoglobin levels can also be elevated in dermatomyositis/polymyositis.

AUTOANTIBODIES Elevated antinuclear antibody (ANA) levels with human tumor cell substrates are found in 60 to 80 percent of patients with classic dermatomyositis/polymyositis. A number of autoantibodies[2,7,8,64,94,95] having both diagnostic and prognostic value have been identified by Ouchterlony double immunodiffusion; these autoantibodies are directed against a disparate group of nuclear and cytoplasmic antigens (Table 173-3). The most frequently encountered autoantibodies in this group are those that target the various aminoacyl transfer RNA synthetases. Of these "antisynthetase" autoantibodies, autoantibodies to Jo-1 (histidyl transfer RNA synthetase) are the most common, being found in 20 percent of patients with classic dermatomyositis/polymyositis overall and 30 to 40 percent of adult patients with polymyositis. Fever, interstitial lung disease, polyarthritis, Raynaud's phenomenon, and incomplete response to therapy occur more often in patients who produce these antibodies (the "antisynthetase syndrome") as does the mechanic's hand skin lesion. Patients who produce Jo-1 antibodies less frequently display the classic cutaneous manifestations of dermatomyositis; but another antisynthetase autoantibody, anti-EJ, may be more strongly associated with these typical skin changes.[7]

Signal-recognition particle (SRP) antibodies occur in 5 percent of patients with polymyositis and are more common in those who exhibit acute-onset, severe, treatment-resistant forms of classic dermatomyositis/polymyositis with cardiac involvement. Such patients rarely have any type of skin involvement. Autoantibodies to Mi-2, a nuclear protein complex, are seen almost exclusively in patients with classic dermatomyositis. Mi-2 antibody has been found in 5 to 10 percent of patients with classic dermatomyositis/polymyositis overall and in 15 to 20 percent of patients with classic dermatomyositis. This autoantibody has been associated with more treatment-responsive forms of classic dermatomyositis as well as with the shawl sign and prominent cuticular changes. The clinical correlations of the myositis-specific autoantibodies found in adults also occur in juvenile patients with classic dermatomyositis/polymyositis. Dermatomyositis/polymyositis autoantibodies that currently have less clinical significance are also listed in Table 173-3.

OTHER LABORATORY ABNORMALITIES The erythrocyte sedimentation rate is elevated in about half of patients with classic dermatomyositis/polymyositis, but it does not correlate with disease activity to the degree that it does in patients with SLE.[7] Rheumatoid factor is elevated in 20 percent of cases, more often in patients with overlap disease. Other serum factors such as neopterin[96] and factor VIII–related antigen (von Willebrand factor)[97] have been reported to correlate with disease activity in juvenile patients with classic dermatomyositis.

ELECTROMYOGRAPHY The EMG changes of myositis include a myopathic pattern of the motor unit action potential, a myopathic recruitment pattern, increased insertional activity, and increased spontaneous activity.[7,98] The paraspinous muscles can be abnormal by EMG when the limb girdle musculature is normal. As many as 10 percent of patients with biopsy-documented myositis have a normal EMG.

Amyopathic Dermatomyositis

By definition, the levels of CK and other muscle enzymes are normal in amyopathic dermatomyositis. ANA are detected in most patients with amyopathic dermatomyositis when human tumor cell substrates are used.[24,86,92] Mi-2 antibody has been found in a single patient who had the skin changes of dermatomyositis but no muscle disease[7]; however, none of the six patients with amyopathic dermatomyositis reported by another group[24] had such antibodies. There has been no mention of myositis-specific autoantibodies in other series of patients with amyopathic dermatomyositis.[86,91,92]

HISTOPATHOLOGY

Skin

The histopathologic changes in three clinical categories of cutaneous dermatomyositis have been reviewed.[99] The earliest histologic appearance is similar to normal skin except for PAS-positive thickening of the basement membrane, a smudgy, homogeneous appearance of the papillary dermis, and increased dermal mucin and edema. No lymphocytic infiltrate is seen at this stage, and vacuolar alteration of basal keratinocytes, pigment incontinence, and colloid body formation are variably present. Biopsy specimens from more advanced lupus-like skin lesions (i.e., scaling violaceous erythema) have changes similar to or indistinguishable from those seen in LE. These changes include hyperkeratosis, epidermal atrophy, and effacement of the rete ridges. An interface dermatitis with vacuolar degeneration of the basal keratinocytes and a sparse, superficial, patchy, or bandlike perivascular lymphocytic infiltration can also be seen, along with thickening of the basement membrane and pigment incontinence. The dermis is often pale as a result of the accumulation of edema and mucin. In poikiloderma, these same features are encountered except that ectatic dermal vessels are present. Hyperkeratosis, acanthosis, undulating papillomatosis, vacuolar alteration of basal keratinocytes, thickened basement membrane, variable lymphocytic exocytosis, and increased mucin deposition in the epidermis are seen in Gottron's papules. The cutaneous histologic changes of amyopathic dermatomyositis have been reported to be indistinguishable from those of classic cutaneous dermatomyositis.[24] Lipomembranous (membranocystic) changes previously thought to be specific for panniculitis have been noted in the histopathology of punched-out ulcers of dermatomyositis. No differences in the histopathology or immunopathology of the cutaneous manifestations of classic and amyopathic dermatomyositis have been observed.

Muscle

Muscle fiber degeneration/regeneration, perifasicular atrophy, and capillary injury are frequently present in the muscle biopsies of patients with dermatomyositis/polymyositis. A perivascular infiltrate of T lymphocytes and histiocytes and occasionally B lymphocytes, plasma cells, and eosinophils is also seen.[99] Biopsies from patients with dermatomyositis often show CD4 T cells and B cells in the perivascular areas, whereas CD8 T cells preferentially associate with damaged muscle fibers in patients with polymyositis.[100] A decreased capillary density in muscle specimens from patients with dermatomyositis has been observed.[101] Inflammation may be absent in up to 25 percent of biopsy specimens from patients with otherwise typical muscle disease by clinical, electromyographic, or biochemical criteria.[3]

An occlusive vasculopathy is a striking aspect of the pathology of childhood dermatomyositis/polymyositis.[15] Phlebitis and arteritis leading to intimal hyperplasia, fibrinous occlusion of vessels, and infarction of the involved tissues can be seen. The muscles, gastrointestinal tract, and nerves are particularly affected. This vasculopathy in muscles is noninflammatory and occurs predominately in the capillaries. There is a spectrum of endothelial changes from swelling to obliteration to necrosis.

IMMUNOHISTOLOGY

Skin

Bandlike granular deposits of immunoglobulin and complement along the dermal-epidermal junction, subepidermal cytoid bodies, dermal connective tissue staining, and epidermal cytoplasmic staining have been described in dermatomyositis skin lesions.[102,103] Lesional dermal-epidermal junction immunoglobulin and complement bands have been reported to occur in 5 to 86 percent of patients, depending on the site of biopsy, with the nail fold being a high-prevalence area. However, similar findings can be observed in actinically exposed skin of otherwise normal individuals. The observation that components of the membrane attack complex (C5-9) are more often present in the dermal microvessels than at the dermal-epidermal junction in cutaneous dermatomyositis lesions whereas the opposite occurs in cutaneous LE lesions[55] was not confirmed.[103]

The dermal infiltrate of cutaneous dermatomyositis lesions contains predominately macrophages and CD4 T lymphocytes, some of which demonstrate an activation phenotype.[56] Focal HLA-DR antigen expression has been noted on lesional keratinocytes while being reduced on dermal endothelial cells.

Muscle

Immunoglobulin and complement deposition occurs in affected muscle tissue, albeit inconsistently and unrelated to disease activity. The presence of the complement membrane attack complex in muscle capillaries has suggested that local activation of complement with resulting endothelial cell toxicity could be related to the microvascular abnormalities of this disorder.[52,101]

DIAGNOSIS AND DIFFERENTIAL DIAGNOSIS

The diagnosis of classic dermatomyositis is based on the presence of hallmark skin lesions (Table 173-4) in the context of proximal muscle weakness that can be confirmed to result from active myositis. Amyopathic dermatomyositis is diagnosed when the biopsy-confirmed hallmark cutaneous lesions of dermatomyositis are present for longer than 6 months (provisional) or 2 years (confirmed) in the absence of muscle weakness, elevated muscle enzymes, immunosuppressive drug therapy (which could suppress the development of muscle disease activity), and drugs such as hydroxyurea that can produce dermatomyositis-like cutaneous hypersensitivity changes.

In the earlier stages, cutaneous dermatomyositis might be confused with contact dermatitis, seborrheic dermatitis, lichen planus, psoriasis, polymorphic light eruption, and atopic dermatitis. In the later stages, when the more typical cutaneous manifestations of dermatomyositis have had a chance to evolve, the greatest challenge can be to distinguish the skin involvement of dermatomyositis from that of LE (Table 173-8). Periorbital heliotrope erythema and edema can occasionally be seen in SLE, but Gottron's papules are never seen as a cutaneous manifestation of LE. The pattern of involvement over the hands also differs; in LE the skin over the dorsal interphalangeal and metacarpophalangeal joints is spared, and the skin between these joints is preferentially involved (Fig. 172-2A). The exact opposite is true for dermatomyositis; the skin overlying the dorsal interphalangeal and metacarpophalangeal joints is usually affected first (Fig. 173-2). However, when extensive, the linear streaking of violaceous erythema along the track of the extensor tendons of the hands and fingers can sometimes obscure this point of differential diagnosis.

As previously noted, certain drugs can produce an eruption with clinical similarities to cutaneous dermatomyositis. Such agents include hydroxyurea,[39,104] niflumic acid/diclofenac,[41] tryptophan,[1] penicillamine,[1,40] and practolol.[42]

Multicentric reticulohistiocytosis has been reported to masquerade as dermatomyositis. However, the "string of pearls" papules occurring in the periungual areas in multicentric reticulohistiocytosis can be clearly distinguished from the periungual inflammatory changes of dermatomyositis by close clinical and pathologic examination.

Conditions other than dermatomyositis/polymyositis can be associated with proximal muscle weakness. These disorders are outlined in Table 173-7.

TREATMENT

Local

Patients with either classic or amyopathic dermatomyositis should avoid excessive sun exposure and use substantive broad-spectrum sunscreens. Topical glucocorticoids (classes I and II) dampen cutaneous inflammation and pruritus, but these agents alone usually cannot fully suppress the disease. Daily use of a tar-containing shampoo followed by application of a topical glucocorticoid solution, gel, or spray to the affected areas can provide relief for the scalp pruritus. Xerosis is often present, especially in the elderly, and effective moisturization regimens can be of value in managing the difficult pruritus often experienced by patients with dermatomyositis. Topical antipruritic agents such as combinations of menthol/phenol/camphor, pramoxine, and doxepin can provide short-term relief.

CHAPTER 173
Dermatomyositis

2019

TABLE 173-8

Systemic

When possible, nonsteroidal systemic therapy should be maximized. Doxepin, a tricyclic antidepressant, is also an extremely potent H1- and H2-blocking antihistamine; when given at bedtime in doses of 10 to 30 mg, it can ameliorate pruritus and excoriation experienced during the evening. Conventional or nonsedating antihistamines can be used during the day. Hydroxychloroquine sulfate (400 mg/day) has been successfully used to treat dermatomyositis skin disease.[105] Some patients respond better to a combination of hydroxychloroquine, 400 mg/day, and quinacrine, 100 mg/day, or to chloroquine, 250 mg/day, and quinacrine, 100 mg/day. However, the author's experience has been that even with combination therapy, only a minority of patients respond really well, and there is a report of two patients with dermatomyositis whose cutaneous lesions worsened on hydroxychloroquine. Appropriate precautions should be taken to minimize the risk of retinal toxicity with hydroxychloroquine or chloroquine and hematologic toxicity with quinacrine. Dapsone has also recently been suggested to be of value for the cutaneous manifestations of dermatomyositis.[106]

Systemic glucocorticoids remain the traditional first line therapy for classic dermatomyositis. Early inter-

Comparative Features of Skin Involvement in Dermatomyositis and Lupus Erythematosus

	DERMATOMYOSITIS	LUPUS ERYTHEMATOSUS
Distribution		
Face		
Malar eminences	+	++
Eyelids, periorbital areas	++	+
Scalp	++	++
Oral mucosa	+	++
Extensor arms, forearms	++	++
Hands		
Dorsal aspect	++	++
Palmar aspect	+	+
Dorsal fingers	+	++
Knuckles	++	+
Periungual telangiectasia	++	+
Color of skin lesions		
Violaceous	++	+
Red, pink	+	++
Alopecia	+	++
Hyperkeratosis	+	++
Gottron's papules	++	0
Pruritus	++	+
Pathology		
Dermal mucinosis	++	++
Intense mononuclear cell infiltrate	+	++
Immunopathology		
D-E junction Ig, complement band	+	++
Dermal microvessel C5-9 deposits	++	+
Laboratory findings		
ANA	++	++
anti-Ro/SS-A	+	++
anti-native DNA	0	++
anti-Sm	0	++
Elevated ESR	+	++
Malignancy association	++	0

KEY: ++ Frequently seen; + occasionally seen; 0 absent.
SOURCE: Euwer and Sontheimer.[2] Reprinted with permission of the publisher, Williams & Wilkins.

vention with systemic glucocorticoids has been associated with a better overall prognosis. In adults prednisone (prednisolone for those with decreased liver function) is given orally in divided doses of 1 to 1.5 mg/kg per day,[7] while children are given 1 to 2 mg/kg per day.[107] Significant improvement of muscle strength, normalization of muscle enzyme levels, and improvement in cutaneous inflammation are the end points of therapy. Most patients require 1 to 3 months of full-dose prednisone treatment. With improvement, the dose can be consolidated from a divided dose to a single daily dose given in the morning to reduce the risk of adrenal suppression and other glucocorticoid side effects. The glucocorticoid dose can then be progressively decreased (e.g., 10 percent every 2 weeks). Treatment should be continued for a consecutive 12-month period to minimize the chance for recurrence of disease activity. Attention should be paid to managing the side effects of long-term systemic glucocorticoids.[108] In acutely ill patients, intravenous pulse therapy with methylprednisolone can be used; this approach has become increasingly popular in the management of juvenile dermatomyositis. Alternate-day glucocorticoids usually do not provide adequate relief. If no response to high-dose oral glucocorticoid therapy has occurred after 2 months or if maintenance doses of glucocorticoids are too high, other forms of immunosuppressive therapy should be

considered. Adjunctive therapy with drugs such as methotrexate or azathioprine can also be used at the outset of prednisone treatment to minimize the debilitating side effects of high-dose, long-term systemic glucocorticoid therapy. The cutaneous lesions of dermatomyositis can be refractory to high-dose, long-term glucocorticoids in some patients. In addition, other patients have recrudescent disease activity only in their skin after complete suppression of their muscle disease with systemic glucocorticoid therapy.

Systemic glucocorticoids have also been used for disabling skin disease activity in patients with amyopathic dermatomyositis.[24] It remains to be determined whether early aggressive immunosuppressive treatment of amyopathic dermatomyositis might prevent the development of clinically significant myositis later.

Approximately 25 percent of patients with classic dermatomyositis/polymyositis do not respond adequately to systemic glucocorticoids. Azathioprine (1 to 2 mg/kg per day),[3] cyclophosphamide (1 to 2 mg/kg per day),[3] methotrexate (10 to 25 mg/week),[109] chlorambucil (2 to 6 mg per day),[110] and cyclosporine (5 mg/kg per day)[111] have been used in this setting and for patients who cannot tolerate the numerous side effects of high-dose glucocorticoids. Extracorporeal photochemotherapy has been explored as an adjunctive therapy.

Methotrexate given orally at doses of 15 to 25 mg/week is most often used to treat adults with classic dermatomyositis. Higher doses can be given subcutaneously or intravenously; the intramuscular route may spuriously elevate muscle enzyme levels. Oral methotrexate (10 to 25 mg) given in pulse fashion once weekly has also been successful in some patients primarily affected by the cutaneous manifestations of dermatomyositis.[109] Oral azathioprine given at 2 mg/kg per day can also be of benefit. Chlorambucil has been used in some patients with dermatomyositis whose disease is refractory to glucocorticoids. Combination therapy with glucocorticoids, methotrexate, and chlorambucil has been advocated for such resistant cases.[112]

In children, oral cyclophosphamide (2 to 4 mg/kg per day) has traditionally been used in cases that could not be satisfactorily managed by systemic glucocorticoids. High-dose intravenous gamma globulin therapy has been used in both children and adults in this setting, with the advantage of low toxicity. A controlled clinical trial has indicated that plasmapheresis and leukopheresis have little additional value in the management of dermatomyositis/polymyositis.

Medical treatment of cutaneous calcium deposits that occur most commonly in the juvenile form of the disease has been virtually impossible.[113] Numerous approaches have been tried, including aluminum hydroxide suspension (15 to 20 mL four times per day), probenecid (250 mg/day), potassium para-amino benzoic acid (15 to 25 g/day), warfarin (1 mg/day), EDTA, colchicine (1.2 to 1.8 mg/day), and, most recently, diltiazem.[114] The surgical removal of symptomatic cutaneous or subcutaneous calcium deposits can be considered as a last resort.

Passive range-of-motion exercise should be provided early in the disease course to prevent disabling joint contractures, especially in children. After disease activity is suppressed medically, an active exercise program can facilitate the return of normal strength.

Surveillance for the detection of occult malignancy has been discussed above. In addition, changes in the clinical status of the respiratory, cardiovascular, or gastrointestinal system should be evaluated carefully for the possibility of systemic disease activity in these target organs.

Initial observations suggested that pregnancy outcome in patients with dermatomyositis/polymyositis could be quite risky (data reviewed in reference 210). However, subsequent reports have suggested that patients can do well under these circumstances. Various issues related to the management of dermatomyositis have been reviewed.

PROGNOSIS

Classic Dermatomyositis

Reports of mortality have varied from 25 to 80 percent, depending greatly on the case mix and medical era in which the cases were collected. In the past two decades, mortality has decreased because of the more aggressive use of glucocorticoids and other immunosuppressives and better supportive medical care. The 5- and 8-year survival rates for 76 patients with dermatomyositis/polymyositis studied in the 1980s were 80 and 73 percent, respectively.[26] The early and aggressive use of glucocorticoids has reduced the mortality rate in children to less than 10 percent. The most common causes of death in dermatomyositis/polymyositis are malignancy, infection, and cardiac and pulmonary disease.

Some adults with classic dermatomyositis respond quickly to treatment with systemic glucocorticoids and enjoy treatment-free intervals of various durations after these drugs have been tapered. The majority of such patients eventually experience a recurrence of disease activity. Others do not respond fully to systemic glucorticoids or to other immunosuppressive agents and have a long-term, unremitting course. Some patients have a fulminant course with early death. Factors suggested to be associated with a poor prognosis include older age at onset, fulminant disease onset, dysphagia, interstitial lung disease, cardiac involvement, associated malignancy, glucocorticoid resistance, and delay in treatment.

Certain types of skin lesions have also been said to correlate with a poor outcome. Ulcers arising over violaceous indurated plaques on the trunk with or without indurated papules were reported to be more frequent in adult patients with dermatomyositis who developed a malignancy. Necrotic/ulcerative skin disease has been noted to be a bad prognostic feature. The "mechanic's hand" lesion has been associated with risk for interstitial lung disease.

Prognosis in both adult and juvenile patients with classic dermatomyositis/polymyositis is associated with the types of autoantibodies produced. Antisynthetase autoantibodies (Jo-1, PL-7, PL-12) have been correlated with incomplete response to therapy and interstitial lung disease. Signal-recognition particle antibodies have been found in patients with more acute onset, severe, and treatment-resistant forms of disease with frequent cardiac involvement. Autoantibodies to Mi-2 have been associated with more treatment-responsive forms of dermatomyositis.

Amyopathic Dermatomyositis

There are insufficient long-term follow-up data available to assess prognosis in patients with amyopathic dermatomyositis. All six of the patients in one cohort who initially presented with only skin disease and were treated conservatively ultimately developed muscle disease.[19] In another cohort, none of the five adult patients with amyopathic dermatomyositis treated aggressively with high-dose systemic glucocorticoids developed clinical evidence of myositis.[24] While fatal malignancies have been reported to occur in patients with amyopathic dermatomyositis, the statistical significance of such an association has not yet been determined. Based on the reports to date, there appears to be a low frequency of systemic organ involvement in patients with amyopathic dermatomyositis.

REFERENCES

1. Dalakas MC: Polymyositis, dermatomyositis and inclusion–body myositis. *N Engl J Med* **325**:1487, 1991
2. Euwer RL, Sontheimer RD: Dermatomyositis, 2, in *Cutaneous Manifestations of Rheumatic Diseases,* edited by Sontheimer RD, Provost TT. Baltimore, Williams & Wilkins, 1996
3. Bohan A et al: Computer–assisted analysis of 153 patients with polymyositis and dermatomyositis. *Medicine* **56**:255, 1977
4. Tanimoto K et al: Classification criteria for polymyositis and dermatomyositis. *J Rheumatol* **22**:668, 1995
5. Zuber M: Tanimoto's classification and diagnostic criteria for polymyositis and dermatomyositis do not recognize the variant of amyopathic dermatomyositis. *J Rheumatol* **23**:191, 1996
6. Euwer RL, Sontheimer RD: Dermatologic aspects of myositis. *Curr Opin Rheumatol* **6**:583, 1994
7. Targoff IN: Dermatomyositis and polymyositis, in *Current Problems in Dermatology,* edited by WL Weston, RM MacKie, TT Provost. St. Louis, Mosby-Year Book, 1991, p 131
8. Plotz PH et al: Myositis: Immunologic contributions to understanding cause, pathogenesis, and therapy. *Ann Intern Med* **122**:715, 1995

9. Wagner E: Fall einer seltuen Muskelkranheit. *Arch Heilkd* **4**:282, 1863

10. Unverricht H: Polymyositis acuta progressiva. *Zeitschr Klin Med* **12**:533, 1887

11. Gottron H: Haut Veranderungen bei Dermatomyositis, in *VIII Congres International de Dermatologie; 1930; Copenhagen,* edited by S Lomholt. Copenhagen, Engelsen and Schroder, 1931

12. Pearson CM, Bohan A: The spectrum of polymyositis and dermatomyositis. *Med Clin North Am* **61**:439, 1977

13. Bohan A, Peter JB: Polymyositis and dermatomyositis. *N Engl J Med* **292**:344, 1975

14. Everett MA, Curtis AC: Dermatomyositis: A review of 19 cases in adolescents and children. *Arch Intern Med* **100**:70, 1957

15. Banker BQ, Victor M: Dermatomyositis (systemic angiopathy) of childhood. *Medicine* **45**:261, 1966

16. Shy GM: The late onset myopathy: A clinicopathologic study of 131 patients. *World Neurol* **3**:149, 1962

17. Sigurgeirsson B et al: Risk of cancer in patients with dermatomyositis or polymyositis: A population-based study. *N Engl J Med* **326**:363, 1992

18. Airio A et al: Elevated cancer incidence in patients with dermatomyositis: A population based study. *J Rheumatol* **22**:1300, 1995

19. Krain L: Dermatomyositis in six patients without initial muscle involvement. *Arch Dermatol* **111**:241, 1975

20. Pearson CM: Polymyositis and dermatomyositis, in *Arthritis (and Allied Conditions),* 9th ed, edited by DJ McCarty. Philadelphia, Lea & Febiger, 1979, p 742

21. Caro I: A dermatologist's view of polymyositis/dermatomyositis. *Clin Dermatol* **6**:9, 1988

22. Rockerbie NR et al: Cutaneous changes of dermatomyositis precede muscle weakness. *J Am Acad Dermatol* **20**:629, 1989

23. Braverman I: Connective tissue (rheumatic) diseases, 7, in *Cutaneous Signs of Systemic Disease,* 2d ed. Philadelphia, Saunders, 1981, p 299

24. Euwer RL, Sontheimer RD: Amyopathic dermatomyositis (dermatomyositis siné myositis): Presentation of six new cases and review of the literature. *J Am Acad Dermatol* **24**:959, 1991

25. Euwer RL, Sontheimer RD: Amyopathic dermatomyositis: A review. *J Invest Dermatol* **100**:124S, 1993

26. Hochberg MC et al: Adult onset polymyositis/dermatomyositis: An analysis of clinical and laboratory features and survival in 76 patients with a review of the literature. *Semin Arthritis Rheum* **15**:168, 1986

27. Crowe WE et al: Clinical and pathogenetic implications of histopathology in childhood polydermatomyositis. *Arthritis Rheum* **25**:126, 1982

28. Pachman LM, Marykowski MC: Juvenile dermatomyositis and polymyositis. *Clin Rheum Dis* **10**:95, 1984

29. Oddis CV et al: Incidence of polymyositis-dermatomyositis: A 20-year study of hospital diagnosed cases in Allegheny County, PA, 1963–1982. *J Rheumatol* **17**:1329, 1990

30. Bridges BF: The rashes of dermatomyositis in a black patient. *Am J Med* **91**:661, 1991

31. Lee LA, Weston WL: Special considerations concerning the cutaneous manifestations of rheumatic diseases in children, 12, in *Cutaneous Manifestations of Rheumatic Diseases,* edited by RD Sontheimer, TT Provost. Baltimore, Williams & Wilkins, 1996, p 323

32. Arnett FC et al: Major histocompatibility complex genes in systemic lupus erythematosus, Sjögren's syndrome, and polymyositis. *Am J Med* **85**:38, 1988

33. Love LA et al: A new approach to the classification of idiopathic inflammatory myopathy: Myositis-specific autoantibodies define useful homogeneous patient groups. *Medicine (Baltimore)* **70**:360, 1991

34. Reed AM et al: Molecular genetic studies of major histocompatibility complex genes in children with juvenile dermatomyositis: Increased risk associated with HLA-DQA1 *0501. *Hum Immunol* **32**:235, 1991

35. Arnett FC et al: The Jo-1 antibody system in myositis: Relationships to clinical features and HLA. *J Rheumatol* **8**:925, 1981

36. Goldstein R et al: HLA-D region genes associated with autoantibody responses to Jo-1 (histidyl-tRNA synthetase) and other translation-related factors in myositis. *Arthritis Rheum* **33**:1240, 1990

37. Webster ADB: Echovirus disease in hypogammaglobulinemic patients. *Clin Rheum Dis* **10**:189, 1984

38. Wiley CA et al: HTLV-1 polymyositis in a patient also infected with the human immunodeficiency virus. *N Engl J Med* **320**:992, 1989

39. Thomas L et al: Dermatomyositis-like eruption complicating hydroxyurea therapy of chronic myelogenous leukemia: Report of a case and literature review. *Eur J Dermatol* **2**:492, 1992

40. Simpson NB, Golding JR: Dermatomyositis induced by penicillamine. *Acta Derm Venereol* **59**:543, 1979

41. Grob JJ et al: Dermatomyositis-like syndrome induced by nonsteroidal anti-inflammatory agents. *Dermatologica* **178**:58, 1989

42. Cox NH et al: Dermatomyositis: Disease associations and an evaluation of screening investigations for malignancy. *Arch Dermatol* **126**:61, 1990

43. Houpt KR, Sontheimer RD: Autoimmune connective tissue disease and connective tissue disease-like illnesses after silicone gel augmentation mammoplasty. *J Am Acad Dermatol* **31**:626, 1994

44. Koeger AC et al: Occupational exposure to silicon and dermatopolymyositis: Three cases. Observations [French]. *Ann Med Interne* **142**:409, 1991

45. Cukier J et al: Association between bovine collagen dermal implants and a dermatomyositis or a polymyositis-like syndrome. *Ann Intern Med* **118**:920, 1993

46. Rosenberg MJ, Reichlin M: Is there an association between injectable collagen and polymyositis/dermatomyositis? *Arthritis Rheum* **37**:747, 1994

47. Eisenstein DM et al: Juvenile dermatomyositis presenting as rash alone: Late onset of myositis. *Arthritis Rheum* **39**:S192, 1996

48. Jongen PJ et al: Polymyositis and dermatomyositis: No persistence of enterovirus or encephalomyocarditis virus RNA in muscle. *Ann Rheum Dis* **52**:575, 1993

49. Hashimoto K et al: Dermatomyositis: Electron microscopic, immunologic, and tissue culture studies of paramyxovirus-like inclusions. *Arch Dermatol* **103**:120, 1971

50. Luu J et al: Tubuloreticular structures and cylindrical confronting cisternae: A review. *Hum Pathol* **20**:617, 1989

51. Norris DA: Pathomechanisms of photosensitive lupus erythematosus. *J Invest Dermatol* **100**:58S, 1993

52. Kissel JT et al: Microvascular deposition of complement membrane attack complex in dermatomyositis. *N Engl J Med* **314**:329, 1986

53. Basta M, Dalakas MC: High-dose intravenous immunoglobulin exerts its beneficial effect in patients with dermatomyositis by blocking endomysial deposition of activated complement fragments. *J Clin Invest* **94**:1729, 1994

54. Sontheimer RD, Bergstresser PR: Epidermal Langerhans cell involvement in cutaneous lupus erythematosus. *J Invest Dermatol* **79**:237, 1982

55. Crowson AN, Magro CM: The role of microvascular injury in the pathogenesis of cutaneous lesions of dermatomyositis. *Hum Pathol* **27**:15, 1996

56. Hausmann G et al: Immunopathologic study of skin lesions in dermatomyositis. *J Am Acad Dermatol* **25**:225, 1991

57. Wakino S et al: Serial lymphocyte subpopulation analysis in peripheral blood from a patient with amyopathic dermatomyositis [letter]. *Br J Rheumatol* **33**:498, 1994

58. Cervera R et al: Antibodies to endothelial cells in dermatomyositis: Association with interstitial lung disease. *BMJ* **302**:880, 1991

59. Hausmann G et al: Cell adhesion molecule expression in cutaneous lesions of dermatomyositis. *Acta Derm Venereol* **76**:222, 1996

60. Igarashi M et al: Dermatomyositis with prominent mucinous skin change: Histochemical and biochemical aspects of glycosaminoglycans. *Dermatologica* **170**:6, 1985

61. Saito E et al: Damaging effect of peripheral mononuclear cells of dermatomyositis on cultured human skin fibroblasts. *J Rheumatol* **14**:936, 1987

62. Pandya AG et al: Papulonodular mucinosis associated with systemic lupus erythematosus: Possible mechanisms of increased glycosaminoglycan accumulation. *J Am Acad Dermatol* **32**:199, 1995

63. Sontheimer RD, Ziff M: Questions pertaining to the etiology and pathophysiology of polymyositis/dermatomyositis. *Clin Dermatol* **6**:105, 1988

64. Targoff IN: Humoral immunity in polymyositis/dermatomyositis [review]. *J Invest Dermatol* **100**:116S, 1993

65. Sontheimer RD: Photoimmunology of lupus erythematosus and dermatomyositis: A speculative review. *Photochem Photobiol* **63**:583, 1996

66. Stahl NI et al: A cutaneous lesion associated with myositis. *Ann Intern Med* **91**:577, 1979

67. Mitra D et al: Clinical and histological features of "mechanic's hands" in a patient with antibodies to Jo-1—a case report. *Clin Exp Dermatol* **19**:146, 1994

68. Cheong W-K et al: Cutaneous photosensitivity in dermatomyositis. *Br J Dermatol* **131**:205, 1994
69. Stone OJ: Dermatomyositis/polymyositis associated with internal malignancy: A consequence of how neoplasms alter generalized extracellular matrix in the host [review]. *Med Hypotheses* **41**:48, 1993
70. Al-Najjar A et al: Dermatomyositis and lichen planus—An association or manifestation? *Clin Exp Dermatol* **10**:174, 1985
71. Cohen MG et al: Calcification is rare in adult-onset dermatopolymyositis. *Clin Reumatol* **5**:512, 1986
72. Winkelmann RK: The cutaneous diagnosis of dermatomyositis, lupus erythematosus, and scleroderma. *NY State J Med* **63**:3080, 1963
73. Corson JK: Sclerodermatomyositis. *Arch Dermatol* **96**:596, 1967
74. Fernandes L, Goodwill CJ: Dermatomyositis without apparent myositis, complicated by fibrosing alveolitis. *J R Soc Med* **72**:777, 1979
75. Tokiyama K et al: Two cases of amyopathic dermatomyositis with fatal rapidly progressive interstitial pneumonitis [Japanese]. *Ryumachi* **30**:204, 1990
76. Fraser DD et al: Magnetic resonance imaging in the idiopathic inflammatory myopathies. *J Rheumatol* **18**:1693, 1991
77. Reimers CD et al: Magnetic resonance imaging of skeletal muscles in idiopathic inflammatory myopathies of adults. *J Neurol* **241**:306, 1994
78. King LE Jr et al: Evaluation of muscles in a patient with suspected amyopathic dermatomyositis by magnetic resonance imaging and phosphorus-31-spectroscopy. *J Am Acad Dermatol* **30**:137, 1994
79. Stonecipher MR et al: Dermatomyositis with normal muscle enzyme concentrations: A single-blind study of the diagnostic value of magnetic resonance imaging and ultrasound. *Arch Dermatol* **130**:1294, 1994
80. Osmanagaoglu K et al: Thallium-201 accumulation in myositis ossificans and in juxta-articular ossification. *J Nucl Med* **36**:2239, 1995
81. Pitt AM et al: MRI-guided biopsy in inflammatory myopathy: Initial results. *Magn Reson Imaging* **11**:1093, 1993
82. Callen JP et al: The relationship of dermatomyositis and polymyositis to internal malignancy. *Arch Dermatol* **116**:295, 1980
83. Callen JP: Malignancy in polymyositis/dermatomyositis. *Clin Dermatol* **6**:55, 1988
84. Callen JP: Dermatomyositis and malignancy. *Clin Dermatol* **11**:61, 1993
85. Cherin P et al: Dermatomyositis and ovarian cancer: A report of 7 cases and literature review. *J Rheumatol* **20**:1897, 1993
86. Whitmore SE et al: Ovarian cancer in patients with dermatomyositis. *Medicine* **73**:153, 1994
87. Sunnenberg TD, Kitchens CS: Dermatomyositis associated with malignant melanoma: Parallel occurrence, remission, and relapse of the two processes in a patient. *Cancer* **51**:2157, 1983
88. Connor B: Mycosis fungoides with dermatomyositis. *Proc R Soc Med* **65**:251, 1972
89. Weiss VC, Serushan M: Kaposi's sarcoma in a patient with dermatomyositis receiving immunosuppressive therapy. *Arch Dermatol* **118**:183, 1982
90. Whitmore SE et al: Dermatomyositis *sine* myositis: Association with malignancy. *J Rheumatol* **23**:101, 1996

91. Gallais V et al: Prognosis factors and predictive signs of malignancy in dermatomyositis [French]. *Ann Dermatol Venereol* **123**:722, 1996
92. Cosnes A et al: Dermatomyositis without muscle weakness—long-term follow-up of 12 patients without systemic corticosteroids. *Arch Dermatol* **131**:1381, 1995
93. Fudman EJ, Schnitzer TJ: Dermatomyositis without creatine kinase elevation: A poor prognostic sign. *Am J Med* **80**:329, 1986
94. Targoff IN: Laboratory manifestations of polymyositis/dermatomyositis. *Clin Dermatol* **6**:76, 1988
95. Sontheimer RD et al: Antinuclear antibodies: Clinical correlations and biologic significance. *Adv Dermatol* **7**:3, 1992
96. Malleson PN: Controversies in juvenile dermatomyositis. *J Rheumatol Suppl* **23**:1, 1990
97. Bowyer SL et al: Factor VIII related antigen and childhood rheumatic diseases. *J Rheumatol* **16**:1093, 1989
98. Greenlee R Jr: The neurologist's approach to polymyositis [review]. *Clin Dermatol* **6**:23, 1988
99. Kasper CS et al: Pathology and immunopathology of polymyositis/dermatomyositis. *Clin Dermatol* **6**:64, 1988
100. Engel AG, Arahata K: Monoclonal antibody analysis of mononuclear cells in myopathies: II. Phenotypes of autoinvasive cells in polymyositis and inclusion body myositis. *Ann Neurol* **16**:209, 1984
101. Emslie-Smith AM, Engel AG: Microvascular changes in early and advanced dermatomyositis: A quantitative study. *Ann Neurol* **27**:343, 1990
102. Nesbitt LT Jr: Cutaneous immunofluorescence in dermatomyositis. *Int J Dermatol* **19**:270, 1980
103. Mascaro JM Jr et al: Membrane attack complex deposits in cutaneous lesions of dermatomyositis. *Arch Dermatol* **131**:1386, 1995
104. Bahadoran P et al: Pseudo-dermatomyositis induced by long-term hydroxyurea therapy: Report of two cases. *Br J Dermatol* **134**:1161, 1996
105. Woo TY et al: Cutaneous lesions of dermatomyositis are improved by hydroxychloroquine. *J Am Acad Dermatol* **10**:592, 1984
106. Konohana A, Kawashima J: Successful treatment of dermatomyositis with dapsone. *Clin Exp Dermatol* **19**:367, 1994
107. Roberts LJ, Fink CW: Childhood polymyositis/dermatomyositis. *Clin Dermatol* **6**:36, 1988
108. Werth VP: Systemic glucocorticoids and the skin: Dermatologists can prevent steroid-induced osteoporosis. *Med Surg Dermatol* **3**:343, 1996
109. Zieglschmid-Adams ME et al: Treatment of dermatomyositis with methotrexate: Presentation of ten cases and review of the literature. *J Am Acad Dermatol* **32**:754, 1995
110. Sinoway PA, Callen JP: Chlorambucil: An effective corticosteroid-sparing agent for patients with recalcitrant dermatomyositis [comments]. *Arthritis Rheum* **36**:319, 1993
111. Grau JM et al: Cyclosporin A as first choice therapy for dermatomyositis. *J Rheumatol* **21**:381, 1994
112. Cagnoli M et al: Combined steroid, methotrexate and chlorambucil therapy for steroid-resistant dermatomyositis. *Clin Exp Rheumatol* **9**:658, 1991
113. Ansell B: Is there a treatment for the calcinosis of juvenile dermatomyositis? *Br J Rheumatol* **29**:263, 1990
114. Oliveri MB et al: Regression of calcinosis during diltiazem treatment in juvenile dermatomyositis. *J Rheumatol* **23**:2152, 1996

John H. Tu
Arthur Z. Eisen

Scleroderma

Scleroderma is a chronic disease of unknown etiology that affects the microvasculature and loose connective tissue and is characterized by fibrosis and obliteration of vessels in the skin, lungs, gastrointestinal tract, kidneys, and heart.[1–4] It may occur in a localized form or as a systemic disease, systemic sclerosis (systemic scleroderma, SSc), that is often progressive and fatal. SSc is characterized clinically by induration and thickening of the skin. The fibrous deposition and vascular obliteration seen in the skin also occur in certain internal organs.

CLASSIFICATION

Several clinical forms of localized scleroderma are recognized, including morphea, generalized morphea, guttate morphea (which may be a variant of lichen sclerosus et atrophicus, LSA), nodular (keloidal) morphea, subcutaneous morphea (morphea profunda), and linear scleroderma. Localized scleroderma is not a life-threatening disease but can cause disfigurement. The most common type is morphea, in which the lesions are usually single or few in number. In the generalized form of morphea, symmetric and bilateral lesions occur. The absence of Raynaud's phenomenon, acrosclerosis, and organ involvement differentiates generalized morphea from SSc. In linear scleroderma the lesions are arranged in a band-like linear distribution and may involve the deeper layers of the skin and underlying structures. Deformities, such as hemiatrophy, may be associated with linear scleroderma.

It has been proposed[1–3] that SSc be divided into two distinct subsets: limited SSc (lSSc) and diffuse SSc (dSSc). Several other minor scleroderma subtypes are also recognized (Table 174-1). Sixty percent of patients with SSc are in the lSSc group, which includes individuals with the CREST syndrome, so-called for its features of *c*alcinosis cutis, *R*aynaud's phenomenon, *e*sophageal dysfunction, *s*clerodactyly, and *t*elangiectasia. Patients with lSSc typically are women who are older than patients with dSSc and have a long history (10 to 15 years) of Raynaud's phenomenon; skin involvement limited to the digits or hands, face, feet, and forearms; nail fold capillary dilatation; and early onset of facial and digital telangiectasias. In addition, they have a high incidence of anticentromere antibodies (ACA) (70 to 80 percent). Systemic involvement (notably pulmonary hypertension) may not appear for years (often decades), and many patients outlive their disease and die of other causes. Miners, users of vibrating machines, and those exposed to chemicals or plastics may develop a seronegative form of lSSc.

The typical patient with dSSc is well until the abrupt onset of swelling (nonpitting) of the hands and feet associated with Raynaud's phenomenon and hidebound changes in the skin, often sparing only the back and buttocks. Polyarticular symmetric synovitis, tenosynovitis, and tendon friction rubs are often present. Nail fold capillary dilatation and destruction are common, and there is an early onset of internal organ involvement. ACA are uncommon, but antitopoisomerase 1 antibodies (Scl-70) are present in approximately 30 percent of the patients. In some patients, skin involvement progresses rapidly initially and then subsides slowly over years.[1] Some patients with dSSc do not develop extensive or severe internal organ involvement. These patients form a subset whose disease is termed *chronic dSSc*. The subsets of SSc are classified in detail in Table 174-1.[4]

TABLE 174-1

Classification of Systemic Scleroderma Subsets

"Pre-scleroderma"
    Raynaud's phenomenon plus nail fold capillary changes
    Disease-specific circulating antinuclear autoantibodies [antitopoisomerase-I, anticentromere (ACA), or nucleolar]
    Digital ischemic changes
Diffuse cutaneous SSc (dSSc)
    Onset of skin changes (puffy or hidebound) within 1 year of onset of Raynaud's phenomenon
    Truncal and acral skin involvement
    Tendon friction rubs
    Early and significant interstitial lung disease, oliguric renal failure
    Diffuse gastrointestinal disease
    Myocardial involvement
    Nail fold capillary dilatation and drop out
    Antitopoisomerase-I (Scl-70) antibodies (30% of patients)
Limited cutaneous SSc (lSSc)
    Raynaud's phenomenon for years (occasionally decades)
    Skin involvement limited to hands, face, feet, and forearms (acral)
    A significant (10–15%) late incidence of pulmonary hypertension, with or without interstitial lung disease, skin calcification, telangiectasia, and gastrointestinal involvement
    High prevalence of ACA (70–80%)
    Dilated nail fold capillary loops, usually without capillary dropout
Scleroderma sine scleroderma
    Raynaud's phenomenon
    No skin involvement
    Presentation with pulmonary fibrosis, scleroderma, renal crisis, cardiac or gastrointestinal disease
    Antibodies may be present (Scl-70, ACA, nucleolar)

EPIDEMIOLOGY

Localized scleroderma is relatively uncommon. Women are affected about three times as often as men. The disease appears much more common in whites than in blacks, and in 75 percent of patients with morphea the onset is between ages 20 and 50. In linear scleroderma, the age of onset is earlier, with a significant number occurring in the first two decades of life.

SSc is four times more common in women than in men and is more frequent among black women than white women. The incidence rate in the adult population is approximately 17 per million, with a prevalence rate of 240 per million in adults.[4] Age-specific incidence rates are higher in black women than in white women. The greatest difference is in the young to mid-adult (<54 years) age group. Diffuse disease also occurs more commonly in the black population, and the age of onset is younger than the age of onset of limited disease. The disease incidence increases with age in white women but remains stable among black women throughout adulthood. It may occur at any age but is relatively uncommon in childhood. In most patients, onset is between ages 30 and 50.

In patients with SSc, the 7-year survival from the time of diagnosis is approximately 75 percent. There is a significantly decreased survival rate in older patients. Women have a significantly better survival rate than men, and the mortality from scleroderma for black women is significantly greater, due to their predilection for diffuse disease, than for white women. In a study of 177 patients,[1] the 10-year survival was 71 percent in patients with sclerodactyly alone, 58 percent in patients with skin stiffness proximal to the metacarpophalangeal joint but sparing the trunk, and only 21 percent in those with diffuse skin stiffness including the trunk. ACA positivity correlated strongly with patients having sclerodactyly alone and may be a marker for milder disease. The classification of SSc into the lSSc and dSSc subsets is important prognostically. It has been estimated that the survival rates for 1, 6, and 12 years for patients with dSSc are 80 percent, 30 percent, and 15 percent, respectively; whereas for those patients with lSSc, the corresponding survival rates are 98 percent, 80 percent, and 50 percent, respectively.[2]

Scleroderma-Like Disorders

SSc is more common in underground coal and gold miners. In male patients with silicosis who are over 40 years of age, the likelihood of developing SSc is approximately 190 times greater than in males not exposed to silica and is 50 times greater than in males without silicosis but exposed to silica dust.[5] Silica exposure itself seems to be a principal factor in the cause of the disease.

An unusual form of scleroderma characterized by Raynaud's phenomenon, morphea-like skin changes, capillary abnormalities of the nail fold (similar to those seen in SSc), osteolysis of the distal phalanges, and hepatic and pulmonary fibrosis may occur in workers exposed to polyvinyl chloride. The relationship of this disorder to SSc remains unclear. Bleomycin also produces pulmonary fibrosis, Raynaud's phenomenon, and cutaneous changes indistinguishable from those of SSc.[5] The development of these changes appears to be dose dependent and is reversible upon discontinuation of the drug. Other agents connected with sclerodermatous disease include epoxy resins, metaphenylenediamine, pentazocine, and denatured rapeseed oil. Whether SSc can occur after augmentation mammo-

plasty with silicone gel implants remains controversial, and no well-controlled study has convincingly demonstrated causation.[5] Removal of the silicone implant in an uncontrolled study was associated with an apparent remission, and this approach was suggested for patients developing hypertension.[6] Scleroderma-like skin changes may be associated with scleromyxedema, porphyria cutanea tarda, and graft-versus-host (GVH) disease. Similar skin changes, primarily in the legs, have been described in the carcinoid syndrome; but these entities, although related, are clearly separable from scleroderma per se. Familial cases of SSc have been reported,[4] but a clear-cut genetic predisposition for the disease has not been established. It is clear that inherited genetic factors play a role in the tendency and/or ability to produce autoantibodies. However, the major factor in developing SSc involves an acquired environmental exposure that remains unknown.[4]

CLINICAL MANIFESTATIONS

Localized morphea is characterized by circumscribed sclerotic plaques with ivory-colored centers and, if the disease is in an active state, violaceous borders (Fig. 174-1). The lesion often begins as a reddened or lilac-colored area that may show some nonpitting edema. The center gradually becomes white or yellowed. There may be a diminished sweat response and an absence of hair in the lesion. The plaques, whether slightly elevated or depressed, are indurated but not bound to the deeper structures. Most commonly, the lesions are single or few in number, but they may be multiple, ranging in size from 1 to 30 cm. Uncommonly, localized morphea may occur after radiation therapy at the site of treatment. Its development is not related to dosage or to the severity of the acute reaction. Whether it results from the well-recognized fibroblastic response to irradiation is unknown.

Generalized morphea is a severe form of the local disease. Involvement of the skin is widespread, with multiple indurated plaques and hyperpigmentation. The plaques may be larger than the lesions of localized morphea, but in early stages they are often indistinguishable. They involve the upper trunk, abdomen, buttocks, and legs. Generalized morphea is not associated with systemic disease.

FIGURE 174-1

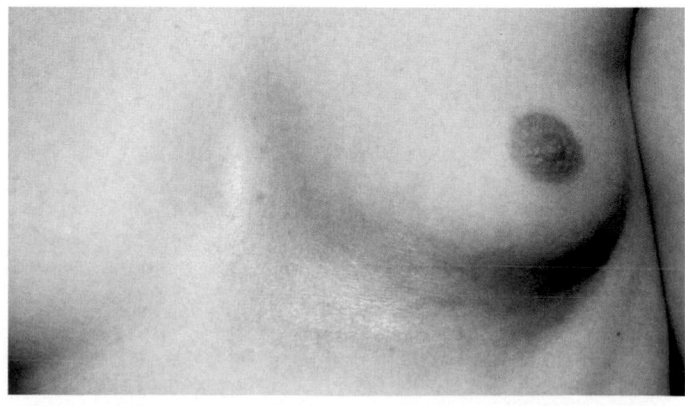

Morphea. There is an indurated, poorly defined plaque under the left breast. The lesion is multicolored with a central, yellow, "carnauba-wax" area surrounded by a lilac border.

Antinuclear antibodies (ANA), elevated immunoglobulin levels, and rheumatoid factor have been reported in all forms of localized scleroderma, but the overall incidence is uncertain. The prognosis is good; the disease often becomes inactive in 3 to 5 years. Slight atrophy, often with hyperpigmentation, may be the only persisting sequela of either form of morphea. However, disability from muscle atrophy may be a sequela of severe morphea.

Guttate morphea may be a variant of localized morphea or of LSA. Morphea and LSA can occur simultaneously in the same patient. The coexistence of these two disorders in 10 patients has been reported, with the same lesion frequently showing histologic evidence of both diseases.[7] Guttate morphea is characterized by multiple small chalk-white lesions that lack the firm character of morphea, involving primarily the neck and upper trunk.

Nodular (keloid) morphea is a rare variant of morphea. It is characterized by the presence of nodular lesions resembling keloids. The coexistence of typical lesions of localized morphea may aid in the diagnosis.

Subcutaneous morphea (morphea profunda) is characterized by deep, bound-down, sclerotic plaques. Since inflammation is in the subcutaneous fat and facia, the typical color changes that occur in the skin of localized morphea are absent.

Atrophoderma of Pierini and Pasini is an uncommon superficial form of localized morphea in which several oval, hyperpigmented, atrophic plaques develop on the trunk. The unusual feature is the absence of sclerosis. The well-defined lesions have a slightly depressed center; the defined border has been described as having a cliff-drop appearance. Whether this disorder is an end stage of morphea is unclear.

Linear scleroderma is a form of the disease that occurs as a linear band, usually with a single unilateral lesion. The lower extremities are most often involved, followed in frequency of occurrence by the upper extremities, frontal areas of the head, and anterior thorax. If the upper and lower extremities are involved, the lesions are homolateral. Calcinosis within a linear lesion occurs rarely. Frontal or frontoparietal linear scleroderma, called *coup de sabre,* is characterized by atrophy and a furrow in the skin (Fig. 174-2). The depression may be extensive, causing facial hemiatrophy, sometimes with atrophy of the tongue on the same side. Linear frontal lesions and active morphea plaques may coexist on the same side of the face. An important distinction between linear scleroderma and morphea is that linear scleroderma involves not only superficial but also deeper layers of the skin, with fixation to underlying structures. Because linear scleroderma occurs most often during the first two decades of life, it may cause severe deformities, such as hemiatrophy of an extremity or a side of the face, or contractures. Linear scleroderma may also be associated with anomalies of the vertebral column, the most common being spina bifida occulta.

Melorheostosis is an unusual linear, dense, cortical hyperostosis that occurs rarely. It usually affects an involved limb but occasionally is widespread.

The tick-borne spirochete *Borrelia burgdorferi,* the etiologic agent of Lyme disease, has been reported[8] to play a role in the pathogenesis of morphea and LSA in Europe and Japan but not in North America. The coexistence of morphea and acrodermatitis chronica atrophicans, a disorder in which *B. burgdorferi* is known to be the causative agent, does occur.[9] *B. burgdorferi* has been divided into three genospecies, whose distribution is different in Eurasia and America. A small study[8] of morphea and LSA using the polymerase chain reaction for the genotype-specific amplification of all known types of *B. burgdorferi* yielded positive signals in the cases from Germany and Japan. No American cases were positive for *Borrelia.* The results were consistent with the different geographic distributions of *Borrelia* genospecies. Because not all cases of morphea and LSA result from *Borrelia* infection, other factors must be involved in their etiology. In the experience of the authors, there is no evidence that the antibiotic therapy used successfully in treating Lyme disease is effective in treating morphea.

Eosinophilia may occur in localized scleroderma. In one such study,[10] eosinophilia (>400 cells/μL) was most common in generalized morphea and linear scleroderma and uncommon in morphea. Eosinophilia signified active disease. ANA are commonly present in localized scleroderma and are found in 50 percent of cases when HEp-2 cells are used as the substrate.[11] The incidence of ANA is greatest in linear scleroderma, being present in at least 67 percent of the patients examined in one study.[12] Antibodies to single-stranded DNA (ssDNA) have been reported in 59 percent of cases, with the highest levels in patients with generalized morphea, especially those with clinically active disease.[11]

The *Parry-Romberg syndrome* (facial hemiatrophy) may be a form of linear scleroderma, but this has not been established. The syndrome is characterized by hyperpigmentation followed by atrophy of the dermis, subcutaneous fat, muscle, and sometimes the underlying bone. The atrophy is usually deeper than that seen in *coup de sabre,* but the skin is less often bound down. It may be impossible to distinguish the two disorders. Whether scleroderma-like hemiatrophy of the face that spreads to the homolateral or contralateral side of the body forms a variant of the Parry-Romberg syndrome has not been established. There has been one report[13] of progressive facial hemiatrophy with the presence of ANA, rheumatoid factor, and elevated gamma globulin levels, findings that may be associated with linear scleroderma.

The clinical manifestations of SSc depend on the sites involved.[14] The initial complaints are usually related either to Raynaud's phenomenon or to chronic, usually nonpitting, edema of the hands and fingers. As many as one-third of patients first have pain and stiffness of the fingers and knees. In some patients, the first manifestation is active, often migratory, polyarthritis. In others, severe erosive digital osteoarthritis (related to the CREST syndrome, particularly in females) occurs first. Flexion contractures and sclerodactyly are present; on x-ray, digital tuft resorption, subcutaneous calcification, joint space narrowing, and focal erosions of the peri-

FIGURE 174-2

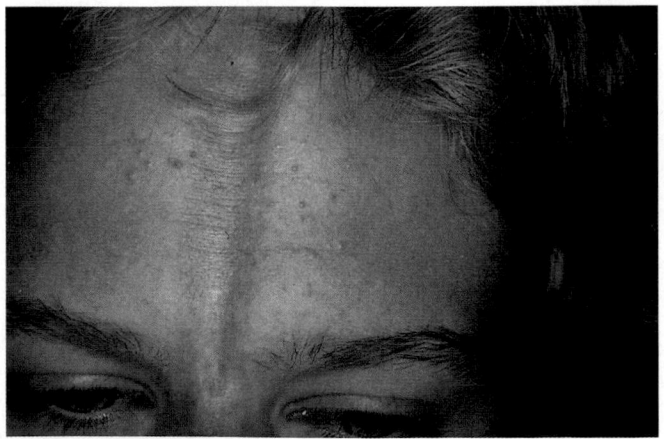

Coup de sabre. Linear, atrophic depression involving the forehead.

FIGURE 174-3

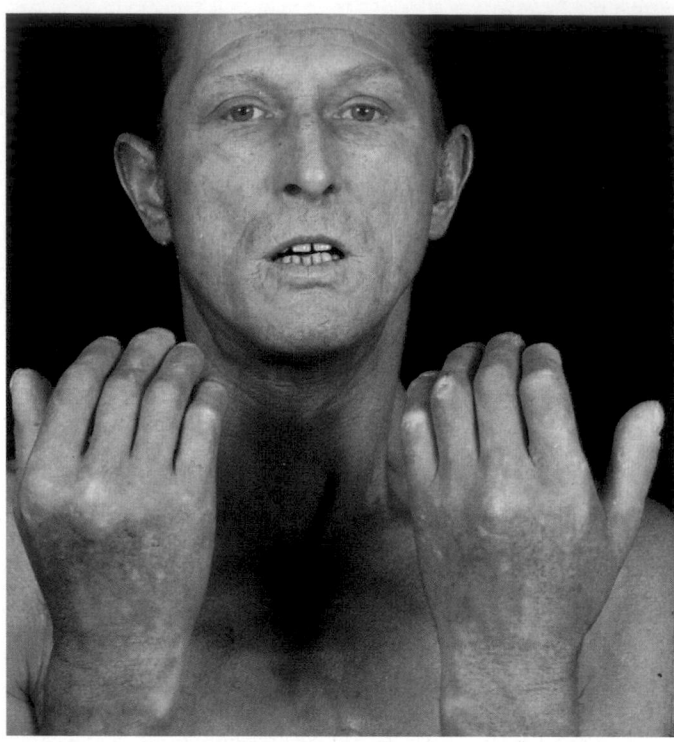

Scleroderma. The connective tissue changes in the face result in loss of the normal facial lines producing a masklike appearance, a thinning of the lips, and a perioral furrowing (rhagades). The hands exhibit a sclerodactylia with tapering of the fingers and a waxy, shiny, atrophic skin. There are flexion contractures and ulceration of the skin overlying the bony prominences on the right hand.

articular bone are seen. Usually, skin changes precede visceral involvement by several years, but occasionally this order is reversed.

The disease then extends to involve the upper extremities (Fig. 174-3), trunk, face, and finally the lower extremities, which may sometimes be spared. In the early stages, the painless slightly pitting edema often lasts several months before tightening of the skin occurs. Isolated periorbital edema may occur in the early edematous phase in patients with few other manifestations of SSc. Often the skin feels indurated and stiff; as it progresses to the atrophic state, it becomes tense, smooth, hardened, and eventually firmly bound to the underlying structures (Fig. 174-4). The skin of the face becomes masklike and expressionless, with loss of the normal facial lines and then thinning of the lips and constriction of the opening of the mouth (microstomia). Radial furrowing around the mouth is seen (Fig. 174-5). Uncommonly, the mucous membranes are involved, with painful induration of the gums and tongue. A prominent feature is tightening of the skin over the nose, giving it a small sharp appearance. The neck sign, ridging and tightening of the skin of the neck on extending the head, is common. Matlike telangiectases may develop (Fig. 174-5), especially about the face and upper trunk. There may be thinning or complete loss of hair and anhidrosis in the affected areas. Generalized hyperpigmentation, like that of Addison's disease but with no evidence of adrenal insufficiency or elevated plasma levels of melanocyte-stimulating hormone β, can occur and may antedate the sclerosis. Focal hyper- or hypopigmen-

FIGURE 174-4

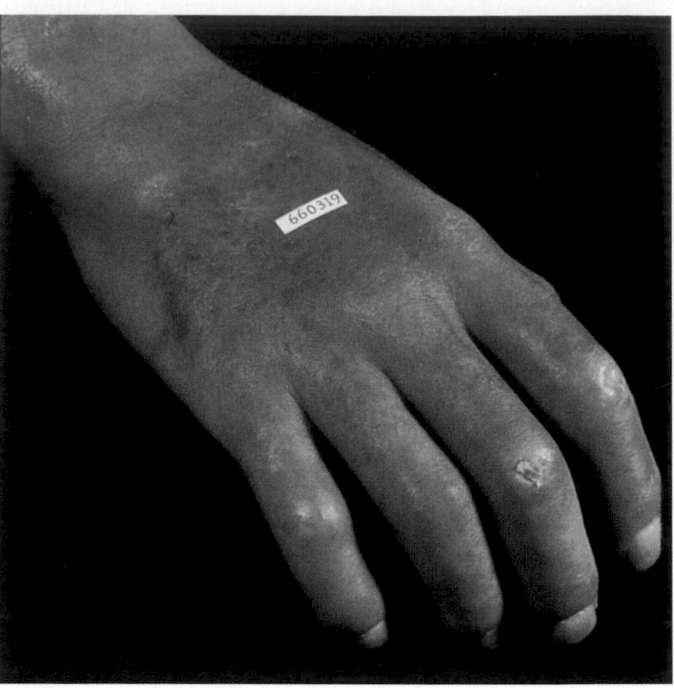

Scleroderma. Skin is atrophic, appears tense and smooth, and has become firmly bound to the underlying structures.

tation may represent a postinflammatory response in the areas of sclerosis.

Sclerodactyly causes the fingers to become tapered, with marked skin atrophy. As in systemic lupus erythematous and dermatomyositis, periungual telangiectasia occurs. In as many as 75 percent of patients with SSc, enlarged, dilated nail fold capillaries forming "giant" or sausage-shaped loops can be seen by capillary microscopy of nail folds (done with an ophthalmoscope),[15] and this examination can be useful in confirming the diagnosis.[16] The pattern in scleroderma can be distinguished from the changes in systemic

FIGURE 174-5

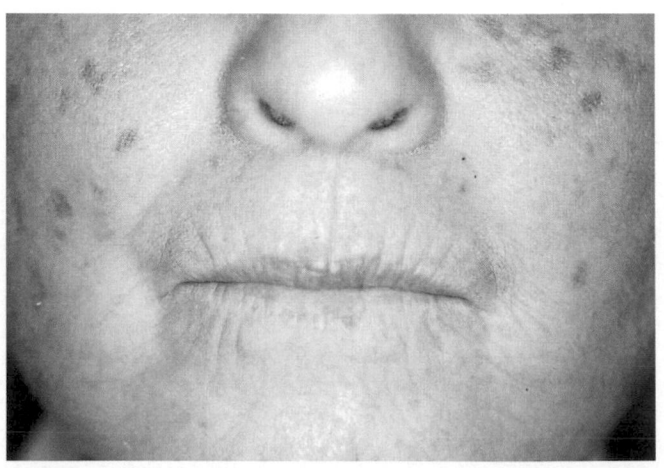

Radial furrowing around the mouth and matlike telangiectases are prominent on the cheeks in a patient with scleroderma.

lupus erythematosus but not from those in dermatomyositis. Capillary microscopy may be of prognostic value in Raynaud's disease, because if nail fold capillary changes are present, the patient is more likely to develop SSc later. Another common problem is recurrent painful ulceration of the fingertips (Fig. 174-6). Slow-healing ulcers over the knuckles may also occur. These ulcers may heal with stellate scarring, become chronic, or, rarely, become gangrenous. Flexion contractures of the stiff fingers trouble many patients. Resorption of bone may cause dissolution of terminal phalanges, and cutaneous calcification develops in some cases, especially around fingertips and bony prominences but also in any area involved with scleroderma. These calcifications may ulcerate, extrude calcified material, and reepithelialize very slowly.

Dental x-rays of patient with SSc often show widening of the periodontal membrane and loss of the lamina dura. Bone absorption at the angle of the mandible may occur, perhaps secondary to tightness of facial skin and atrophy of the underlying muscles.

Systemic involvement manifests itself in many ways. Esophageal dysfunction is the most common internal manifestation (over 90 percent). Dysphagia is due to diminished peristalsis, especially in the distal two-thirds of the esophagus, easily seen on radiologic or manometric study. Heartburn from reflux esophagitis due to a loss of tone in the lower esophageal sphincter occurs commonly, but hemorrhage is rare. Dysphagia may occur long before skin involvement, thereby giving rise to the idea of *systemic sclerosis sine scleroderma*. Abnormal esophageal motility has also been reported in Raynaud's phenomenon, dermatomyositis, and lupus erythematosus. In SSc, the small intestine may be involved, producing symptoms of constipation, diarrhea, bloating, and sometimes malabsorption. Common findings on x-ray include delayed transit with prolonged retention of barium and distention of the small bowel, all secondary to atonia.

Another important feature of SSc is pulmonary involvement with fibrosis. Patients complain of exertional dyspnea, and small airway disease is an early sensitive indicator of pulmonary involvement that often proceeds measurable impairment of gas diffusion. Alveolitis, which can be detected by bronchoalveolar lavage, occurs frequently in SSc and results in progressive reduction in pulmonary function over time. Early treatment with prednisone and cyclophosphamide may produce significant clinical improvement. Early pulmonary involvement, functionally characterized by a lowered diffusing capacity of the alveolocapillary membrane, correlates with morphologic changes of the nail fold capillaries.[17] Cardiac involvement in SSc may cause conduction defects, heart failure, or pericarditis; the latter is often associated with pericardial effusion and sometimes with tamponade. The overall prevalence of myocardial fibrosis in SSc is approximately 50 to 70 percent. Myocardial fibrosis is associated with microvascular coronary vasospasm, which has been linked to a myocardial Raynaud's phenomenon.

Renal involvement occurs in about 45 percent of patients with SSc. Some patients have slowly progressive uremia, but for most the renal failure is abrupt and associated with a malignant form of hypertension. Although there has been some suggestion that the acute renal failure and hypertension were induced by glucocorticoids, these findings have occurred in patients who had never received glucocorticoids.

CREST SYNDROME

A clinical variant of scleroderma is the CREST syndrome. The telangiectasias are most evident on the skin of the face (see Fig. 174-5), upper trunk, and hands but also occur on the lips and oral mucosa and throughout the entire gastrointestinal tract. Gastrointestinal bleeding from the lesions occurs uncommonly. The CREST syndrome is a more slowly progressive form of scleroderma; it develops later in life than dSSc and so has a more favorable prognosis. It is not entirely a benign syndrome, because the esophageal dysfunction is identical to that of the more severe forms of the disease, and occasionally pulmonary hypertension and biliary cirrhosis occur. ACA have been identified in 50 to 96 percent of patients with CREST syndrome but in only 12 to 25 percent of patients with dSSc.[18] Because ACA may appear before the development of the full CREST syndrome and are associated with less systemic involvement, they have prognostic value. Scl-70 are more frequently associated with dSSc (approximately 30 percent), and patients with these antibodies appear to have a less favorable prognosis than patients with ACA.[18]

Patients with combined features of scleroderma, lupus erythematosus, and myositis have been grouped under the heading of *mixed connective tissue disease*. The patients have high titers of antibody to a ribonucleoprotein, the extractable nuclear antigen. Patients with SSc have not been found to have this antibody.

EOSINOPHILIC FASCIITIS AND EOSINOPHILIA-MYALGIA SYNDROME

Other syndromes that cause scleroderma-like skin changes, such as eosinophilic fasciitis (Shulman's syndrome) and the eosinophilia-myalgia syndrome are discussed in Chap. 95.

TOXIC OIL SYNDROME

The toxic oil syndrome occurred in epidemic form in Spain in 1981 and affected approximately 25,000 people.[19–23] It resulted from the consumption of denatured rapeseed oil sold as olive oil for cooking.

FIGURE 174-6

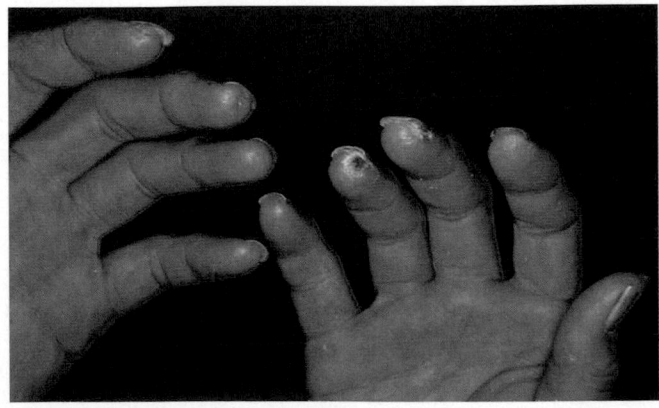

Ulceration of the fingertips in a patient with Raynaud's phenomenon and scleroderma.

To date, ingestion of the denatured rapeseed oil has caused approximately 600 deaths and has left 300 individuals disabled by a chronic multisystem disease. This syndrome has the features of a toxic allergic reaction, with an acute phase associated with a morbilliform-type eruption, pruritus, fever, interstitial pneumonitis, myalgia, and liver function abnormalities. Serum IgE levels were elevated in 37 to 50 percent of the cases. Approximately 5 percent of those affected presented with seizures and encephalopathy. Several months after onset, a chronic phase began that was characterized by severe neuromuscular abnormalities, generalized edema, scleroderma-like skin lesions, joint contractures, Sjögren-like syndrome, and pulmonary hypertension. The histopathology of the skin lesions is similar to that described in the eosinophilia-myalgia syndrome (see Chap. 95). In both processes, the primary injury is vascular, with evidence of perivascular inflammation, intimal proliferation, reduplication of the basal lamina, endothelial damage, and luminal obliteration.[23] Immunofluorescence with antiprocollagen and antifibronectin antibodies and electron microscopy confirmed the vascular damage.

The exact cause of the syndrome remains obscure, but it appears that the ingestion of aniline-degraded, reprocessed rapeseed oil leads to a chronic autoimmune disease. An oil of comparable chemical composition to case-related oils has been produced, and an in vitro toxicologic assay with mouse neuroblastoma and rat liver epithelial cells has been developed.[24] Extracts from aniline-treated rapeseed oil and several high-performance liquid chromatography fractions were toxic to these cells when compared to appropriate controls. It appears that at least some of the puzzling aspects of this syndrome may be solved.

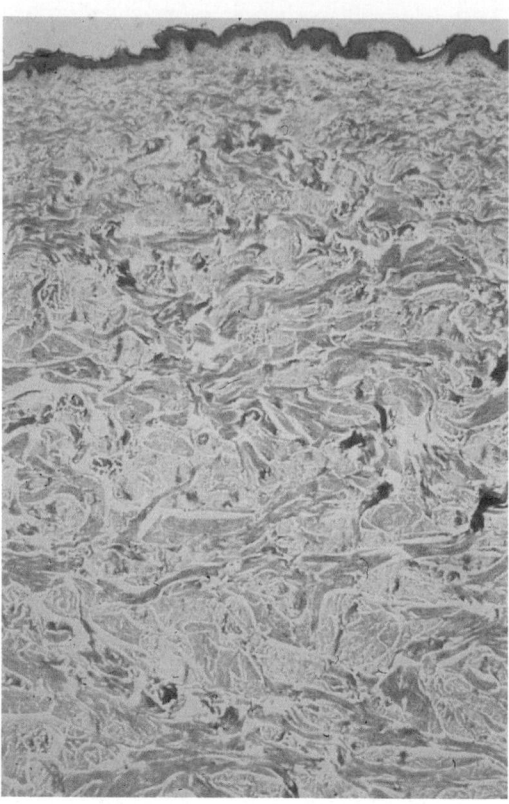

Scleroderma. The changes of generalized scleroderma and localized scleroderma (morphea) overlap; the former, however, is dominated by dense, acellular sclerosis, and the latter shows varying degrees of inflammation with some extension into the subcutis. Fig. 174-7 shows the pathologic changes of scleroderma and Fig. 174-8 shows the pathologic changes of morphea. In this photomicrograph one sees broad collagen bundles that tend to parallel each other, diminished interbundle spaces, and few cells of any kind.

CUTANEOUS HISTOPATHOLOGY

The features of morphea or SSc in histologic sections of a skin biopsy depend on the stage of the disease and the biopsy site (Figs. 174-7 and 174-8). In morphea, specimens from the peripheral violaceous border show many inflammatory cells among collagen bundles of the lower two-thirds of the reticular dermis, the fibrous trabeculae of the subcutaneous tissue. Usually lymphocytes and histocytes predominate, but there may be large numbers of plasma cells, and occasionally there are mast cells. Formation of typical lymphoid follicles with germinal centers may be seen. Mononuclear cell infiltrates are much less common in SSc than in localized scleroderma and are often less prominent.

Associated with the inflammatory infiltrate are collagen changes that first occur in the lower third of the dermis and in the fibrous trabeculae of the subcutaneous tissues. Later in the disease, the changes extend to the upper portion of the dermis and consist of a markedly increased eosinophilia of collagen, broadening of collagen bundles, and decreased space between collagen bundles. Biopsies from the central region of well-developed lesions of morphea may show only collagen changes and no inflammation. In these later stages of morphea the pathology is similar to that of SSc. The collagen bundle pattern is altered so that most bundles appear to parallel the dermal-epidermal junction. The inflammatory stage is followed by the replacement of the subcutaneous tissue by hyalinized connective tissue. On electron microscopy, the fibrous trabeculae of the subcutaneous tissue are increased in thickness by deposition of immature collagen fibrils smaller in diameter than normal, suggesting increased collagen synthesis.

In morphea profunda, the lesions are associated with a subcutaneous, dense, mononuclear cell infiltrate with abundant plasma cells. There is extensive sclerosis and hyalinization of the connective tissue and occasional involvement of the underlying fascia. Lymphoid aggregates with germinal center formation have been described in some of the solitary lesions.

The pathology of SSc is similar to that of morphea. The lower two-thirds of the dermis and the subcutaneous fibrous trabeculae are sclerosed. Panniculitis may also be a prominent feature in the early stages. Subcutaneous fat is replaced by hyalinized connective tissue, and this process is particularly evident around eccrine sweat glands. The collagen bundles appear pale, homogeneous, and swollen, but the collagen bundle swelling, increased numbers of eosinophils, and inflammation are not as prominent as in morphea. In the late stages of SSc, secondary changes, such as absence of pilosebaceous units, eccrine ducts, and glands, and effacement of the rete ridges of the epidermis may be evident. Electron microscopy has revealed randomly arranged "immature" collagen fibrils, from 10 to 40 nm in diameter, in contrast to mature collagen fibrils, from 70 to 80 nm in diameter. Whether the immature fibrils represent newly synthesized collagen remains speculative.

FIGURE 174-8

CHAPTER 174
Scleroderma

2029

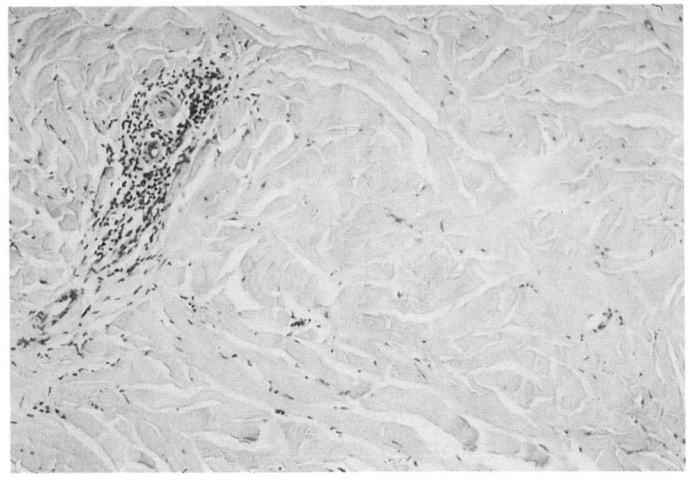

Morphea. The connective tissue changes in morphea seem to extend from the lower reticular dermis outward and are usually indistinguishable from the changes of generalized scleroderma. Biopsies taken from the margins of morphea lesions, however, frequently show extensive inflammation; such inflammation may be patchy, as one sees here, or it may involve the reticular dermis rather diffusely, presenting some difficulty in histologic diagnosis.

Vessels of all sizes may be involved in SSc, and vascular involvement is an important, although inconsistent, feature. In the early stages, there may be only dilatation of capillaries and lymphatics. Then intimal proliferation and complete occlusion of the vessel can occur. These changes also appear in muscle capillaries. Occlusive vascular changes are not found in morphea, but the precise implications of the difference are unclear; possibly they are related to the spontaneous involution of morphea. In morphea, skeletal muscle fibers underlying affected skin may be structurally damaged in the absence of histologic changes in muscle capillaries.

PATHOGENESIS

Three processes have been identified in pathogenesis: damage to vascular endothelium, immunologic and inflammatory activation, and dysregulated extracellular matrix metabolism. The temporal relationship between vascular damage and immunologic activation is unclear, and the primary etiologic agents or events preceding progression to end-stage sclerosis have not yet been ascertained. Furthermore, the association of scleroderma-like syndromes with toxins (e.g., toxic oil, silica, L-tryptophan) may provide valuable clues to the pathogenetic mechanisms leading to end-stage fibrosis and sclerosis.

The intriguing finding of autoimmune antibodies directed at cellular targets in both localized and diffuse forms of SSc point to a role for autoantibodies as clinically valuable prognostic indicators. ACA and Scl-70 found in SSc have a 50 to 80 percent prevalence with greater than 90 percent specificity for CREST and dSSc, respectively.[25] The major target of ACA activity is a complex of centromeric proteins (CENP) composed of at least six polypeptide subunits, CENP-A through CENP-F. More than 90 percent of ACA-positive sera react against CENP-A, -B, and -C.[26] The injection of antibodies specific for CENP-A, -B, or -C into nuclei disrupts mi-

tosis.[27] The minor 17-kDa CENP-A antigen bears structural similarity to histone H3, and the 140-kDa CENP-C antigen is a component of the inner kinetochore plate.[28,29] Affinity-purified antibodies to the major 80-kDa CENP-B antigen bind to both CENP-A and CENP-C.[30] True to their nomenclature, these antigens are localized to the centromere/kinetochore regions of chromosomes and may be involved in critical aspects of cell division and mitosis. Epitope mapping of recombinant CENP-B antigen has revealed DNA binding by CENP-B that can be abrogated by antibodies to CENP-B. Furthermore, ACA were directed against highly conserved regions of CENP-B.[25,31,32]

Scl-70 are directed against the 70-kDa degradation fragment of the 100-kDa DNA topoisomerase I (topo I) involved in relaxation of supercoiled DNA, a prerequisite to DNA synthesis and transcription. The murine homologue of Scl-70 is also found in tight skin (Tsk) mice, a putative model of human cutaneous scleroderma.[33] It has been suggested that the 5' flanking regions of dermal collagen genes are particularly susceptible to binding by Scl-70-associated antigen. The association of Scl-70 provides a tentative link between the major histocompatibility complex and collagen gene expression.[34] A survey of sequences corresponding to the topo I binding sequence in 4 fibrillar collagen genes and 16 noncollagen genes showed a marked presence of the canonical tetrameric sequences in the fibrillar collagen genes. Nonrandom clustering of three potential topo I–binding sites is seen within 350 base pairs of 5' flanking DNA in the dermal collagen $\alpha2(I)$ gene, and a fourth site is seen in the promoter region of the collagen $\alpha I(III)$ gene. The findings suggest that selective vulnerability to the action of Scl-70 may be built into the structure of dermal collagen genes.[35] Autoantibody reactivities in SSc are summarized in Table 174-2.

The consistent finding of autoantibody reactivities associated with SSc has always suggested a pathogenetic role for these autoantibodies. Autoantigens targeted in SSc, but not lupus, seem to be particularly susceptible to fragmentation in the presence of reactive oxygen species generated during tissue ischemia and when certain metals are present (e.g., iron, copper).[36] Vascular injury leading to autoantigen fragmentation uncovers cryptic epitopes on autoantigens that help to break immunologic tolerance and generate autoantibodies. Autoantibodies are proposed to propagate vascular injury by as yet unclear mechanisms. Vascular injury and breaking of immunologic tolerance are then part of a vicious circle. The association of scleroderma-like syndromes with environmental toxins that may further autoantigen fragmentation fits nicely into this hypothesis. Autoantibodies, even if not pathogenetic per se, are rather specific immunologic markers of preexisting cellular damage.[37]

Sclerodermatous GVH disease shares clinical and histologic features with SSc. Remission and progression of the sclerotic phenotype correlate with the amount of immunosuppressive chemotherapy, clearly demonstrating that the sclerotic phenotype is mediated by immune cells in the bone marrow transplant.[38] Development of chronic scleroderma-like GVH disease is associated not only with Scl-70 and polymyositis-scleroderma overlap syndrome antigen (PM-Scl), but also with La/SSB and antibodies to nucleolar antigen C23 (nucleolin), which are not usually associated with SSc.[39]

The almost invariable presence of Raynaud's phenomenon before the development of SSc strongly supports vascular pathology as an early event in pathogenesis. Plasma concentrations of von Willebrand factor (vWF) and endothelin-1 are significantly elevated in some but not all patients with SSc.[40,41] Elevated levels of vWF are found in a number of disease entities in which endothelial cells

TABLE 174-2

Autoantibodies in Scleroderma

ANTIBODY REACTIVITY	PREVALENCE, %	NATURE OF ANTIGEN	FUNCTION OF ANTIGEN
Scl-70	40–70 in dSSc	100-kDa topoisomerase I [70-kDa degradation fragment (Scl-70) = major antigen]	Relaxation of supercoiled DNA: DNA synthesis and repair
Centromere	55–96 in CREST	17- to 400-kDa proteins at centromeric regions of chromosomes	Cell division (mitosis)
RNA pol 1	0.04	11- to 210-kDa subunits of RNA polymerase 1	Transcription of rDNA
PM-Scl	0.03	20- to 110-kDa subunits of a particle of unknown function	?
Fibrillarin (U3-RNP)	0.08	34-kDa component of U3-RNP	Processing of RNA pol 1 transcripts
To/Th	Rare	40-kDa protein complexed with 7-2 and 8-2 RNA	?
NOR-90	Rare	89- and 94-kDa protein doublet associated with nucleolus organizer region (NOR)	Promoter of RNA pol 1 transcripts
Mitochondrial 70 kDa	0.08	70-kDa protein of ATPase complex	?

are damaged. Furthermore, tissue plasminogen activator release is deficient in patients with Raynaud's phenomenon and SSc. These procoagulant or prothrombotic endothelial cell changes can be reproduced in vitro by treatment of endothelial cells with cytokines such as interleukin (IL)1 and tumor necrosis factor (TNF) α.[42,43]

Various immunologic changes occur in SSc. CD4+ T cells are increased in number in mononuclear cell infiltrates; CD8+ T cells and natural killer cells are decreased in number in peripheral blood.[44] HLA-DR expression is increased, as are circulating levels of lymphocyte- and monocyte-derived cytokines such as IL-1, -2, -4, and -6, suggesting lymphocyte activation.[45,46] Levels of these lymphokines and of the soluble IL-2 receptor correlate with disease activity.[47,48]

Fibroblast activity is markedly altered by interaction with activated inflammatory cells and their elaborated cytokines. IL-1 and -4 stimulate fibroblast proliferation and collagen synthesis. IL-6 stimulates matrix metalloproteinase enzymes. Vascular injury and activation of the coagulation cascade lead to the release of platelet-derived growth factor (PDGF) and transforming growth factor (TGF) β, which also activate fibroblasts. These activated fibroblasts in turn release IL-1, prastaglandin E, TGF-β, and PDGF.[49] TGF-β increases type I collagen mRNA and protein synthesis in fibroblasts.[50] TGF-β can increase collagen $\alpha2(I)$ promoter activity in transfected fibroblasts and can stimulate the transcription of type I collagen genes in vitro via DNA-binding *trans*-acting nuclear factors.[51,52] However, these effects are modulated by the presence of other cytokines such as TNF-α, IL-1, and the interferons (IFNs). IFNs, especially IFN-γ, are potent suppressors of collagen synthesis.

Activation of lymphocytes is associated with modulation of the expression of adhesion ligands on lymphocytes, endothelial cells, fibroblasts, and connective tissue. Endothelial cells have increased expression of MadCAM11, CD34, selectins, and intercellular adhesion molecule (ICAM) 1. Upregulated lymphocyte and monocyte ligands L-selectin, sialated glycoproteins, leukocyte function associated antigen (LFA) 1 (CD11a, CD18), and Mac 1 (CD11B, CD18) mediate cellular adhesion to vascular endothelium. Egress into the perivascular tissue requires fibroblast activation and expression of ICAM-1 to mediate lymphocyte-fibroblast interaction.[53] Noncellular integrins associated with collagen and fibronectin via cell-surface very late activation antigen (VLA) 1 (CD49a, CD29) and VLA-4 (CD49d, CD29) further localize immune cells to the perivascular tissue.[54] Increased mast cell numbers and activity are seen in chronic murine GVH disease and in active scleroderma itself.[55]

Multiple toxins have been implicated in SSc-like disorders. These include solvents (vinyl chloride, benzene, toluene), drugs (bleomycin, carbidopa, pentazocine, cocaine, docetaxel), and miscellaneous agents (silica, rapeseed oil, L-tryptophan). Vibration-induced endothelial cell damage and associated cytotoxic activity cause the connective tissue disease seen in some patients. Although bleomycin is known to be a clastogenic (chromosome-breaking) agent, it is unknown if the SSc-like symptoms that appear after bleomycin exposure are related to this activity. Evidence of clastogenic activity can be found in the sera and cell extracts of patients with SSc.[56,57] The common thread among these disparate agents may be that they cause a primary assault on vascular tissue, which progresses to the SSc-like syndrome. Removal of the offending agent usually but not always results in cessation of the progression of the disease.

The loss of long stretches of telomeric repeat at the ends of linear chromosomes in patients with SSc reveals a possible susceptibility to chromosomal instability. There was an average loss of 3 kb in patients with SSc and family members that was not related to age or duration of disease.[58] HLA-DR and -DQ genes control the autoimmune response to DNA topoisomerase in SSc.[59] HLA haplotypes shared by affected siblings in the same family are also present in family members without disease. Major histocompatibility complex genes are required but not sufficient for the development of SSc.[60] HLA-DR3 is linked to CREST, and HLA-DR5 is linked to diffuse disease.[61] HLA-DR1 and -DR5 are linked to nondiffuse disease.[62] Family members of patients with scleroderma or related disease share the A2, B8, DR3 haplotype.[63] Polar amino acids at position 26 in the second hypervariable region of HLA-DQB1 may form a candidate epitope associated with the production of ACA.[64]

Work on the genetics of SSc has been hampered by the relative rarity of SSc among first-degree family members. SSc differs from many other autoimmune disorders in that there is no strong primary HLA association. However, the expression of ACA is associated with DR1 and DR4, whereas the expression of Scl-70 is associated with DQB1 and DPB1.[60,65] There is a strong association between the development of lung fibrosis and the B8-DR3-DR52-DQB2 haplotype. In particular, DR52a and Scl-70 permit the prediction of pulmonary disease (i.e., severe pulmonary hypertension or pulmonary fibrosis).[66] Concordance studies of first-degree relatives diagnosed with lSSc or dSSc demonstrate a shared cutaneous subset of disease severity and autoantibody profiles. The timing of onset of SSc in these studies suggested an environmental trigger in genetically predisposed individuals.

Animal models of SSc include the Tsk mouse and the UCD-200 and UCD-206 chickens. Tsk mice have connective tissue changes but no vascular changes characteristic of human SSc. The human counterpart for this mutant animal is believed to be congenital fascial dystrophy (stiff skin syndrome), which is differentiated from SSc in that the skin is rock-hard and firmly bound to underlying tissues, especially in areas with abundant fascia. The skin is immovable but normal in appearance and texture.[67] UCD-200 and -206 chickens develop a hereditary systemic connective tissue disease resembling human SSc and permit study of disease stages not accessible in humans. Studies in these animals have shown that endothelial cells are the first cells to undergo apoptosis in the skin, a process that seems to be induced by antiendothelial cell antibodies. In human fibrotic skin diseases, apoptotic endothelial cells could be detected only in early inflammatory disease stages of SSc and lSSc.[68]

COURSE

In patients with morphea or linear scleroderma, the disease may last from a few months to many years. In the 50 percent of patients in whom lesions disappear or soften, areas of hypo- or depigmentation are left. *Coup de sabre* lesions may remain unchanged or become more extensive.

Limited SSc rarely progresses to dSSc. In dSSc, visceral involvement is found to develop in most patients if they are followed for sufficient duration. The overall 5-year mortality rate in dSSc is 40 to 50 percent. The main causes of death are pulmonary fibrosis and renal hypertensive crisis in dSSc and isolated pulmonary hypertension in lSSc.[69] Clinical parameters associated with poor prognosis include proximal sclerosis, trunk skin involvement, presence of anti-Scl-70 autoantibody, pulmonary and/or heart involvement, and advanced age at time of diagnosis (45 or older).[70,71] ACA are predictive for lSSc including CREST (sensitivity 60 percent, specificity 98 percent). Scl-70 are predictive for dSSc (sensitivity 38 percent, specificity 100 percent).[25] Findings of ACA and Scl-70 are positively associated with the development of telangiectasias and tight skin, respectively.[72] Scl-70 and HLA-DR3/DR52a are associated with increased risk of pulmonary fibrosis, a major cause of morbidity and mortality in SSc.[34] Antibodies to RNA-polymerases seem to correlate with severe renal or lung disease.[73] Laboratory methods to track disease activity include measurement of soluble IL-2 receptor levels and vWF levels, which correlate with clinical disease activity and vascular damage, respectively.[47,48]

MANAGEMENT

The treatment of localized scleroderma remains unsatisfactory, but since the disease is generally self-limited, most cases require little or no treatment. When treatment is attempted, it usually involves application of high- to ultrahigh-potency topical glucocorticoids to the lesions. This may be augmented by intralesional injections of steroids. Antimalarials, phenytoin, colchicine, and systemic glucocorticoids have been used in generalized morphea but provide little proven benefit. In one study of 11 patients with severe localized scleroderma treated with D-penicillamine, 6 improved after 3 to 6 months of therapy, with skin softening, resumption of growth in affected limbs, and absence of new lesions. The mean length of treatment was 21 months (range 15 to 53) at a daily dose of 2.0 to 5.0 mg/kg. Careful monitoring for renal and hematologic toxicity is essential.[74] The use of high dose UVA 1 (340 to 450 nm) produced marked clinical improvement of treated lesions in patients with morphea.[75] Relapse did not occur once therapy was discontinued, but a longer period of observation will be required to determine whether the results of treatment are long lasting.

Many agents have been tried in the therapy of SSc, and most have been found wanting. Global immunosuppression with such agents as azathioprine, chlorambucil, methotrexate, and cyclophosphamide has had variable success. Cyclophosphamide may be useful in treatment of SSc lung fibrosis, but long-standing fibrosis does not appear to be affected significantly by global immunosuppression. Systemic glucocorticoids may be of some benefit early in the disease or for specific inflammatory lesions (e.g., myositis, alveolitis, myocarditis) but do not alter the overall disease course. Chlorambucil, 5-fluorouracil, and ketotifen (a mast cell stabilizer) are ineffective. Cyclosporine has been shown in some studies to result in a 40 percent decrease in mean skin thickness scores over 1 year. Pulmonary diffusing capacity remains unchanged. However, the use of cyclosporine is limited at higher doses by hypertension and renal insufficiency, which may be attributable to either the drug or SSc and may confound clinical assessment of efficacy.[76] Plasmapheresis removes circulating immune mediators. Small studies have demonstrated equivocal results. Three patients had reduction of skin scores after 2 months of therapy in combination with low-dose (4 mg/day orally) prednisone.[77]

In extracorporeal photopheresis, patients receive oral 8-methoxypsoralen that is absorbed by lymphocytes and photoactivated extracorporeally by UVA irradiation. Treated lymphocytes with covalently cross-linked DNA are then reinfused into the patient in the hopes of evoking an immune response to specific pathogenetic T cell clones.[78] In early studies, the mean skin severity score, mean percentage of skin involvement, and mean oral aperture measurements were significantly improved from baseline among those who received photochemotherapy compared with those receiving D-penicillamine.[79] Considerable controversy still surrounds the efficacy of this therapeutic modality. Long-term studies with untreated and sham photopheresis controls are in progress. Photopheresis has yet to be approved by the U.S. Food and Drug Administration.[80,81]

D-Penicillamine, which interferes with intermolecular cross-linking of collagen, has shown some promise in the treatment of early aggressive dSSc, decreasing body surface area involvement from 65 to 16 percent.[82] It is administered orally at 250 mg/day on an empty stomach, and the dosage is increased every 2 to 3 months to a maximum of 750 to 1500 mg/day. In patients with a disease duration of less than 3 years, significant reductions in skin thickness and joint contractures are seen after 18 to 30 months of therapy. Patients demonstrate improved survival, due in part to a lower incidence of renal disease. However, long-term use is limited by side effects that include hematologic abnormalities as well as autoimmune syndromes such as pemphigus, nephrotic syndrome, lupus/polymyositis-like syndrome, Goodpasture syndrome, and myasthenia gravis.

One early trial series of 18 patients with rapidly progressive SSc treated with an 18-week course of IFN-γ showed a decrease in the mean skin thickness score from a baseline of 25.9 to 19.1, and a decrease of the mean area scores from 33.1 to 19.6. Ten patients had more than a 25 percent decrease in the area score, five patients had more than a 70 percent decrease in the area score, and three had not experienced disease recurrence 6 to 17 months after cessation of IFN-γ.[83]

Tissue-specific aspects of SSc should be treated to ameliorate morbidity and potential mortality. Inflammatory lung disease, which has a "ground-glass" appearance on high-resolution CT scan, responds to cyclophosphamide and prednisolone.[84,85] Renal crises should be treated with an angiotensin-converting enzyme inhibitor; captropril markedly improves survival and, in some patients, may permit discontinuation of dialysis.[86]

The peripheral vasospasm in lSSc occasionally improves with oral vasodilators such as diltiazem. Intravenous prostacyclin infusion or radical microarteriolysis has been advocated for critically ischemic digits.[87] In patients with calcinosis in both CREST and dSSc, there is some suggestion that calcium channel blockers may alleviate the calcinosis.[88] Reflux esophagitis with spasm responds to omeprazole and cisapride. Bacterial overgrowth, identifiable by a positive hydrogen breath test, can be treated with courses of broad-spectrum antibiotics. Octreotide (30 to 100 μg/day subcutaneously) stimulates intestinal motility in patients with dSSc and reduces abdominal symptoms, small-bowel dysfunction, intestinal pseudoobstruction, and bacterial overgrowth.[89]

Physical therapy is paramount in minimizing the loss of function in sclerotic digits and limbs. The cessation of smoking provides a significant decrease in morbidity in those patients with documented Raynaud's phenomenon.

REFERENCES

1. Barnett AS et al: A survival study of patients with scleroderma diagnosed over 30 years (1953–1983): The value of a simple cutaneous classification in early stages of the disease. *J Rheumatol* **15**:276, 1988
2. Leroy EC et al: Scleroderma (systemic sclerosis): Classification, subsets and pathogenesis. *J Rheumatol* **15**:202, 1988
3. Denton CP, Black CM: Systemic sclerosis: Current pathogenetic concepts and future prospects for targeted therapy. *Lancet* **22**:1453, 1996
4. Mayes MD: Scleroderma epidemiology. *Rheum Dis Clin North Am* **22**:751, 1996
5. Silman AJ: Occupational and environmental influences on scleroderma. *Rheum Dis Clin North Am* **22**:739, 1996
6. Gutierrez FJ, Espinoza LR: Progressive systemic sclerosis complicated by severe hypertension: Reversal after silicone implant removal. *Am J Med* **89**:390, 1990
7. Uitto J et al: Morphea and lichen sclerosis et atrophicus. *J Am Acad Dermatol* **3**:271, 1980
8. Fujiwara H et al: Detection of *Borrelia burgdorferi* DNA (*Bgorinis* or *Bafzelii*) in morphea and lichen sclerosis et atrophicus tissues of German and Japanese but not US patients. *Arch Dermatol* **133**:41, 1997
9. Coulson IH et al: Acrodermatitis chronica atrophicans with coexisting morphea. *Br J Dermatol* **121**:263, 1989
10. Falanga V, Medsger TA: Frequency, levels, and significance of blood eosinophilia in systemic sclerosis, localized scleroderma, and eosinophilic fasciitis. *J Am Acad Dermatol* **17**:648, 1987
11. Falanga V, Medsger TA: Antinuclear and anti-single-stranded DNA antibodies in morphea and generalized morphea. *Arch Dermatol* **123**:350, 1987
12. Takehara K et al: Antinuclear antibodies in localized scleroderma. *Arthritis Rheum* **26**:612, 1983
13. Hickman JW, Shiels WS: Progressive facial hemiatrophy. *Arch Intern Med* **113**:716, 1964
14. Mitchell H: Scleroderma and related conditions. *Med Clin North Am* **81**:129, 1997
15. Minkin W, Rabban NB: Office nail fold capillary microscopy using ophthalmoscope. *J Am Acad Dermatol* **7**:190, 1982
16. Maricq HR et al: Predictive value of capillary microscopy in patients with Raynaud's phenomenon. *Arthritis Rheum* **23**:716, 1980
17. Groen H et al: Pulmonary diffusing capacity disturbances are related to nail fold capillary changes in patients with Raynaud's phenomenon with and without an underlying connective tissue disease. *Am J Med* **89**:34, 1990
18. Weiner ES et al: Clinical association of anticentromere antibodies and antibodies to topoisomerase 1: A study of 355 patients. *Arthritis Rheum* **31**:378, 1988
19. Tabuenca JM: Toxic-allergic syndrome caused by ingestion of rapeseed oil denatured with aniline. *Lancet* **2**:567, 1981
20. Rigau-Perez JG et al: Epidemiologic investigation of an oil-associated pneumonic paralytic eosinophilic syndrome in Spain. *Am J Epidemiol* **119**:250, 1984
21. Kilbourne EM et al: Clinical epidemiology of toxic-oil syndrome: Manifestations of a new illness. *N Engl J Med* **309**:1408, 1983
22. Castroviejo-Pascual I: A multisystem disease caused by adulterated rapeseed oil. *Brain Dev* **10**:84, 1988
23. Phelps RG et al: Clinical, pathologic, and immunopathologic manifestations of the toxic oil syndrome: Analysis of fourteen cases. *J Am Acad Dermatol* **18**:313, 1988
24. Slack PT et al: Toxic oil disaster. *Nature* **345**:583, 1990
25. Kallenberg CG: Antitopoisomerase and anticentromere antibodies in the sclerodermatosus complex. *Clin Rev Allergy* **12**:222, 1994
26. Earnshaw W et al: Three human chromosomal autoantigens are recognized by sera from patients with anti-centromere antibodies. *J Clin Invest* **77**:426, 1986
27. Bernat RL et al: Injection of anticentromere antibodies in interphase disrupts events required for chromosome movement at mitosis. *J Cell Biol* **11**:1519, 1990
28. Palmer DK et al: Purification of the centromere-specific protein CENP-A and demonstration that it is a distinctive histone. *Proc Natl Acad Sci USA* **88**:3734, 1991
29. Saitoh H et al: CENP-C, an autoantigen in scleroderma, is a component of the human inner kinetochore plate. *Cell* **70**:115, 1992
30. Earnshaw WC et al: Analysis of anticentromere autoantibodies using cloned autoantigen CENP-β. *Proc Natl Acad Sci USA* **84**:4979, 1987
31. Cooke CA et al: CENP-β: A major human centromere protein located beneath the kinetochore. *J Cell Biol* **100**:1475, 1990
32. Tan EM: Antibody markers in systemic autoimmunity, in *Diagnostic Studies in Rheumatology,* series edited by Brandt KD. Summit, NJ, CIBA-GEIGY, 1992
33. Bona C et al: Autoantibodies in scleroderma and tightskin mice. *Curr Probl Immunol* **6**:931, 1994
34. Briggs D et al: Genetic factors in scleroderma. *Rheum Dis Clin North Am* **16**:31, 1990
35. Douvas A: Does Scl-70 modulate collagen production in systemic sclerosis? *Lancet* **2**:475, 1988
36. Casciola-Rosen L et al: Scleroderma autoantigens are uniquely fragmented by metal-catalyzed oxidation reactions: Implications for pathogenesis. *J Exp Med* **185**:71, 1997
37. Peng SL et al: Scleroderma: A disease related to damaged proteins? *Nature Med* **3**:276, 1997
38. Chosidow O et al: Sclerodermatous chronic graft-versus-host disease. Analysis of seven cases. *J Am Acad Dermatol* **26**:49, 1992
39. Bell SA et al: Specificity of antinuclear antibodies in scleroderma-like chronic graft-versus-host disease: Clinical correlation and histocompatibility locus antigen association. *Br J Dermatol* **134**:848, 1996
40. Blann AD et al: Mechanisms of endothelial cell damage in systemic sclerosis and Raynaud's phenomenon. *J Rheumatol* **20**:1325, 1993
41. Vancheeswaran R et al: Circulating endothelin-1 levels in systemic sclerosis subsets—a marker of fibrosis or vascular dysfunction? *J Rheumatol* **21**:1838, 1994
42. Kahaleh MB: The vascular endothelium in scleroderma. *Int Rev Immunol* **12**:227, 1995
43. Pearson JD: The endothelium: Its role in scleroderma. *Ann Rheum Dis* **50**:866, 1991
44. Roumm AD et al: Lymphocytes in the skin of patients with progressive systemic sclerosis. Quantification, subtyping, and clinical correlations. *Arthritis Rheum* **27**:645, 1984
45. Needleman BW: Immunologic aspects of scleroderma. *Curr Opin Rheumatol* **4**:862, 1992
46. Ihn H et al: Demonstration of interleukin-2, interleukin-4, and interleukin-6 in sera from patients with localized scleroderma. *Arch Dermatol Res* **287**:193, 1995
47. Ihn H et al: Clinical significance of serum levels of soluble interleukin-2 receptor in patients with localized scleroderma. *Br J Dermatol* **134**:843, 1996
48. Patrick MR et al: Circulating interleukin 1β and soluble interleukin 2 receptor: Evaluation as markers of disease activity in scleroderma. *J Rheumatol* **22**:654, 1995

49. Postlethwaite AE: Connective tissue metabolism including cytokines in scleroderma. *Curr Opin Rheumatol* **7**:535, 1995

50. Slack JL et al: Regulation of expression of the type I collagen genes. *Am J Med Genet* **45**:140, 1993

51. Rossi P et al: A nuclear factor 1 binding site mediates the transcriptional activation of a type I collagen promoter by TGF-β. *Cell* **52**:405, 1988

52. Trevisan G et al: *Borrelia burgdorferi* and localized scleroderma. *Clin Dermatolol* **12**:475, 1994

53. Sollberg S et al: New aspects in scleroderma research. *In Arch Allergy Immunol* **11**:330, 1996

54. Anonymous: Systemic sclerosis: Current pathogenetic concepts and future prospects for targeted therapy (clinical conference). *Lancet* **347**:1453, 1996

55. Claman HN: Mast cells and fibrosis. The relevance to scleroderma. *Rheum Dis Clin North Am* **16**:141, 1990

56. Emerit I et al: Chromosomal breakage in diffuse scleroderma. A study of 27 patients. *Rev Eur Etudes Clin Biol* **16**:684, 1971

57. Wolff DJ et al: Spontaneous and clastogen-induced chromosomal breakage in scleroderma. *J Rheumatol* **18**:837, 1991

58. Artlett CM et al: Telomere reduction in scleroderma patients: A possible cause for chromosomal instability. *Br J Rheumatol* **35**:732, 1996

59. Kuwana M et al: The HLA-DR and -DQ genes control the autoimmune response to DNA topoisomerase I in systemic sclerosis (scleroderma). *J Clin Invest* **92**:1296, 1993

60. Manolios N et al: Immunogenetic analysis of 5 families with multicase occurrence of scleroderma and/or related variants. *J Rheumatol* **22**:85, 1995

61. Livingston JZ et al: Systemic sclerosis (scleroderma): Clinical, genetic, and serologic subsets. *J Rheumatol* **14**:512, 1987

62. Black CM et al: HLA antigens, autoantibodies and clinical subsets in scleroderma. *Br J Rheumatol* **23**:267, 1984

63. Hietarinta M et al: Familial scleroderma: HLA antigens and autoantibodies. *Br J Rheumatol* **32**:336, 1993

64. Reveille JD et al: Association of polar amino acids at position 26 of the HLA-DQB1 first domain with the anticentromere autoantibody response in systemic sclerosis (scleroderma). *J Clin Invest* **89**:1208, 1992

65. Briggs D et al: A molecular and serologic analysis of the major histocompatibility complex and complement component C4 in systemic sclerosis. *Arthritis Rheum* **36**:943, 1993

66. Black CM et al: Genetics of scleroderma. *Clin Dermatol* **12**:337, 1994

67. Jablonska S et al: Congenital fascial dystrophy: Stiff skin syndrome—a human counterpart of the tight-skin mouse. *J Am Acad Dermatol* **21**:943, 1989

68. Sgonc R et al: Endothelial cell apoptosis is a primary pathogenetic event underlying skin lesions in avian and human scleroderma. *J Clin Invest* **98**:785, 1996

69. Arroliga AC et al: Pulmonary manifestations of scleroderma. *J Thorac Imaging* **7**:30, 1992

70. Vayssairat M et al: Long-term follow-up study of 164 patients with definite systemic sclerosis: Classification considerations. *Clin Rheumatol* **11**:356, 1992

71. Silman AJ: Scleroderma and survival. *Ann Rheum Dis* **50**:267, 1991

72. Weiner ES et al: Prognostic significance of anticentromere antibodies and antitopoisomerase I antibodies in Raynaud's disease. A prospective study. *Arthritis Rheum* **34**:68, 1991

73. Hirakata M et al: Identification of autoantibodies to RNA polymerase II. Occurrence in systemic sclerosis and association with autoantibodies to RNA polymerases I and III. *J Clin Invest* **91**:2665, 1993

74. Falanga V et al: D-Penicillamine in the treatment of localized scleroderma. *Arch Dermatol* **126**:609, 1990

75. Stege H et al: High-dose UVA₁ radiation therapy for localized scleroderma. *J Am Acad Dermatol* **36**:938, 1997

76. Clements PJ et al: Cyclosporine in systemic sclerosis. Results of a forty-eight week open safety study in ten patients. *Arthritis Rheum* **36**:75, 1993

77. Wach F et al: Treatment of severe localized scleroderma by plasmapheresis—report of three cases. *Br J Dermatol* **133**:605, 1995

78. Edelson RL: Photopheresis: A clinically relevant immunobiologic response modifier. *Ann NY Acad Sci* **636**:154, 1991

79. Rook AH et al: Treatment of systemic sclerosis with extracorporeal photochemotherapy. Results of a multicenter trial. *Arch Dermatol* **128**:337, 1992

80. Fries JF et al: Photopheresis for scleroderma? *J Rheumatol* **19**:1011, 1992

81. Rook AH et al: Photopheresis for scleroderma? Let's abandon the innuendos and get to the data. *J Rheumatol* **20**:1081, 1993

82. Jimenez SA et al: A 15-year prospective study of treatment of rapidly progressive systemic sclerosis with D-penicillamine. *J Rheumatol* **18**:15496, 1991

83. Freundlich B et al: Treatment of systemic sclerosis with recombinant interferon-gamma. A phase I/II clinical trial. *Arthritis Rheum* **35**:1134, 1992

84. Wells AU et al: High resolution computed tomography as a predictor of lung history in systemic sclerosis (corrected and republished article originally printed in *Thorax* **47**:508, 1992). *Thorax* **47**:738, 1992

85. Silver RM et al: Cyclophosphamide and low-dose prednisone therapy in patients with systemic sclerosis (scleroderma) with interstitial lung disease. *J Rheumatol* **20**:838, 1993

86. Steen VD et al: Outcome of renal crisis in systemic sclerosis: Relation to availability of angiotensin-converting enzyme (ACE) inhibitors. *Ann Intern Med* **113**:352, 1990

87. O'Brien BM et al: Radical microarteriolysis in the treatment of vasospastic disorders of the hand, especially scleroderma. *J Hand Surg [Br]* **17**:447, 1992

88. Dolan AL et al: Diltiazem induces remission of calcinosis in scleroderma. *Br J Rheumatol* **34**:576, 1995

89. Sjögren RW: Gastrointestinal motility disorders in scleroderma. *Arthritis Rheum* **37**:1265, 1994.

Brian F. Mandell
Gary S. Hoffman

Systemic Necrotizing Arteritis

Blood vessels may be affected by a number of diverse processes including the hypercoagulability syndromes, Raynaud's vasospasm, coagulopathies, myointimal proliferation with occlusion (e.g., scleroderma), embolic occlusion, congenital or acquired dysplasias (e.g., Marfan's syndrome, fibromuscular dysplasia), and atherosclerosis. This chapter focuses on the primary inflammatory disorders that have been grouped together as the systemic vasculitides. Diseases characterized by primary isolated cutaneous vasculitis, the necrotizing capillaritis/venulitis syndromes, are discussed in greater detail in Chap. 176.

The inflammatory process per se is often associated with laboratory and clinical abnormalities; but these, however prominent, tend to be nonspecific (e.g., elevated erythrocyte sedimentation rate, anemia, fatigue, fevers) and do not substantially aid in distinguishing vasculitis from other inflammatory or proliferative diseases. Blood vessels have limited ways of responding to injury: increased permeability may lead to edema and purpura, attenuation of the vessel wall may lead to aneurysm formation or hemorrhage, and intimal proliferation or thrombosis may cause stenosis or occlusion with tissue ischemia or infarction. The definitive diagnosis of a primary "vasculitis" remains dependent upon histopathologic documentation of vasculitis in conjunction with the appropriate clinical picture and the exclusion of diseases that can cause secondary vascular inflammation such as infection (e.g., meningococcemia, rickettsial diseases, and endocarditis). The principal clinical clue to diagnosis of a specific vasculitic disorder is the pattern of organ involvement. Identification of qualitative pathologic changes in affected organs (pattern of necrosis, presence of granulomas, eosinophilic infiltration) further delineates the differential diagnosis. The primary determinants of prognosis and selection of therapy include whether critical organs are involved, the severity of involvement, and the rate of disease progression. The toxic nature of the therapies for severe systemic vasculitis emphasizes the need for an accurate diagnosis.

Cutaneous involvement in systemic vasculitis may lead to consultation with a dermatologist. However, it is the symptomatic or asymptomatic involvement of other organ systems that is generally more ominous. Consequently, the dermatologist must be familiar with the clinical spectrum of vasculitic disorders. Conversely, not all cases of cutaneous vasculitis are part of a systemic process.

GENERAL PRINCIPLES OF DIAGNOSIS

The evaluation of the patient with a potentially life-threatening systemic disease process warrants considerable thought before a diagnostic workup is begun. The physician should not be reluctant to pursue invasive testing before initiating potentially toxic therapy. Once the diagnosis of a systemic vasculitis is seriously considered, less specific tests should be eschewed as they may only muddle the diagnostic waters, postpone appropriate therapy, or be used to encourage inappropriate therapies. The differential diagnosis of the systemic vasculitides often includes distinct or coexistent coagulopathy, occult malignancy, or infection—particularly deep-seated abscess, viral hepatitis, or bacterial endocarditis. Thus, an approach directed towards *ruling in* a specific form of vasculitis should be pursued, in addition to *ruling out* specific alternatives.

Cutaneous involvement can occur in any of the primary systemic vasculitic syndromes. However, the cutaneous features are often not sufficient to provide a complete diagnosis. Histopathology and immunofluorescent evaluation of skin biopsies may be invaluable in supporting the diagnosis of systemic inflammatory diseases such as Henoch-Schönlein purpura (HSP), sarcoidosis, Sweet's syndrome, or systemic lupus erythematosus (SLE); in diagnosing proliferative disorders (T cell lymphomas, leukemia cutis, Kaposi's sarcoma) and emboli from atherosclerosis or atrial myxomas; and occasionally in diagnosing specific infections (syphilis, cytomegalovirus, fungemia). Angiographic and selected serologic studies may provide support for certain diagnoses, but are not by themselves pathognomonic for any specific form of vasculitis. In general, the diagnosis of a specific form of systemic arteritis will come from a careful documentation of the pattern of organ involvement and histopathology.

Several classification schemes have been proposed in attempts to organize the systemic vasculitic disorders into a consistent paradigm.[1–3] Such schemes are useful in providing a diagnostic framework to distinguish clinical disorders with distinct differences in prognosis and response to treatment. Although no scheme is perfect or universally accepted, classification systems such as that shown in Fig. 175-1 provide useful constructs for communication and the design of research protocols.

The most widely used diagnostic classification systems are based on the caliber of affected blood vessels, the pattern of organ involvement, and the presence or absence of granulomas and/or eosinophilic infiltration. Some authors have proposed a prime diagnostic role for the presence or absence of specific serum antineutrophil cytoplasmic antibodies (ANCAs), particularly antibodies to PR3 and myeloperoxidase. We believe that the role of these tests at the present time is to support a rationally developed clinical diagnosis, not to define one. In patients who do not fit neatly into a well-defined diagnostic category, these serologic tests should not supplant an attempt to obtain a tissue diagnosis, if the latter is feasible. In patients who present with symptoms and findings shared by several diseases, such as cutaneous venulitis, targeted physical examination and serologic testing for potential etiologies may be valuable. Examples include studies for Sjögren's syndrome, hepatitis B or C infection, HIV, and cryoglobulinemia. The value

FIGURE 175-1

CHAPTER 175
Systemic Necrotizing Arteritis

2035

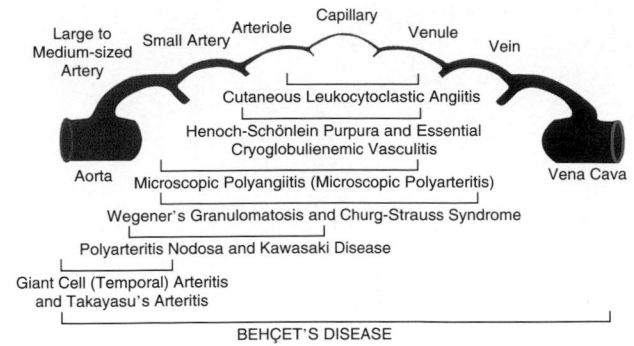

A classification scheme for the vasculitides. (*Adapted from Jennette et al.,[2] with permission.*)

Although multiple consultants commonly become involved in the initial evaluation of patients with multisystem disease, it is crucial that a single physician accept primary responsibility for the patient's management. This role should be made apparent to the patient and to the other members of the management team.

SPECIFIC VASCULITIC SYNDROMES

Small Vessel Vasculitis

The most common form of vasculitis exclusively affects capillaries and venules,[4,5] almost invariably involves the skin, and is extensively discussed in Chap. 176. It is frequently, although not always, associated with immune complex deposition. This form of vasculitis has also been termed *hypersensitivity vasculitis*. It can occur in the following circumstances: (1) as an isolated primary cutaneous disorder; (2) secondary to drug allergy, bacterial endocarditis, viral infections (such as hepatitis B or C,[6] parvovirus B19, cytomegalovirus, or Epstein-Barr virus), or disseminated neisserial and rickettsial infection; (3) as part of defined systemic autoimmune disorders (e.g., Sjögren's syndrome, SLE, dermatomyositis, rheumatoid arthritis); or (4) in association with hematologic,[7,8] lymphoid,[9,10] and solid organ[11] malignancies. Primary small vessel vasculitis may be limited to the skin[12] or may be associated with visceral involvement including pulmonary hemorrhage,[13] intestinal ischemia or hemorrhage,[14] and glomerulonephritis. Visceral involvement may or may

of indiscriminate testing for antinuclear antibodies, rheumatoid factor, and angiotensin-converting enzyme to look for the presence of possible "immune" disease is arguable, at best. These studies should be utilized primarily as aids in supporting a tenable clinical diagnosis.

The first step in the diagnosis of a vasculitic syndrome is to obtain a detailed patient history and perform a physical examination to seek or document specific organ involvement. Special attention should be paid to finding evidence of inflammation in the eyes, ears, nose, paranasal sinuses, mouth, trachea, joints, intestine, or peripheral nerves. The presence of adenopathy, periungual capillary abnormalities, cardiac abnormalities, asymmetric peripheral pulses, or abdominal and subclavian bruits provides other diagnostic clues. It is reasonable to include a few "basic" laboratory tests in the initial evaluation; more specialized studies should be obtained only after a focused differential diagnosis is generated. Initial studies should include a complete blood count with differential, measurement of serum creatinine and liver enzyme levels, and a dipstick and microscopic urinalysis. The urinalysis should ideally be performed immediately by a physician on a fresh morning sample; urine that has been allowed to sit for several hours before analysis will not permit identification of cellular casts that may rapidly degenerate ex vivo. Red blood cell casts are highly suggestive of the presence of glomerulonephritis. A clinical axiom is that the primary vasculitides are almost never associated with leukopenia or thrombocytopenia. The presence of these laboratory findings should suggest alternative diagnoses such as SLE, vasculitis associated with malignancy, disseminated intravascular coagulation, infection, or drug-induced cytopenias. Some disorders that may mimic or be associated with a vasculitis are shown in Table 175-1.

TABLE 175-1

Selected Conditions That May Mimic or Be Associated with* Systemic Arteritis

Infections
Endocarditis*
Histoplasmosis
Syphilis*
Borrelia burgdorfer (Lyme disease)
Viral
Hepatitis (A,B,C)*
HIV*
CMV*
Pneumonia *(Legionella, Streptococcus pneumoniae)*
Mycobacteria
Parasites
Trichinella
Toxoplasma
Plasmodium (malaria)
Strongyloides
Vasoocclusive processes
Sickle cell anemia
Disseminated intravascular coagulation
Antiphospholipid antibody syndrome
Thromboangiitis obliterans
Protein C or S deficiency
Warfarin-induced skin necrosis
Thrombotic thrombocytopenic purpura

Neoplastic diseases
Atrial myxoma
Carcinoma (disseminated, renal cell, colon, lung)*
Lymphoma*
Hairy cell leukemia*
Myelogenous leukemias/myelodysplasia*
Drug reactions, toxicities, and abuse
Phencyclidine
Cocaine
Amphetamines*
Warfarin
Ergotamine
Others
Amyloidosis
Cryoglobulinemia*
Sarcoidosis*
Anti–glomerular basement membrane disease
Multiple sclerosis
Familial Mediterranean fever
Heavy metal poisoning
Hepatic porphyrias
Systemic lupus erythematosus*
Hypereosinophilic syndrome
Hyperviscosity syndrome
Still's disease
Occult cirrhosis
Rheumatoid arthritis*
Fabry's disease

FIGURE 175-2

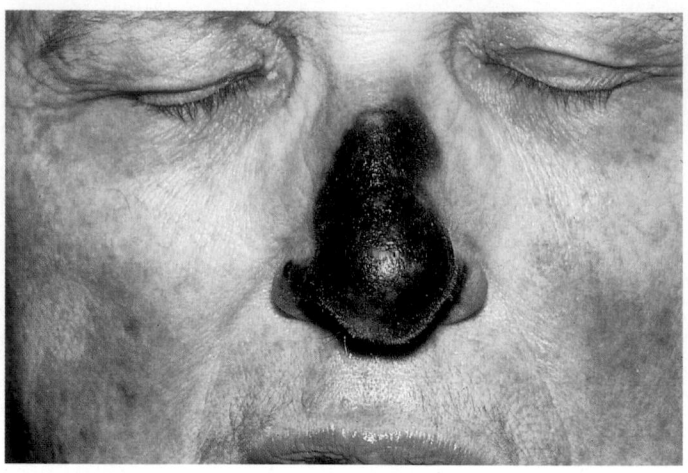

Nasal purpura in a patient with lymphoma-associated cryoglobulinemia.

not be part of the syndrome of HSP, which occurs in adults as well as children and is usually associated with vascular and renal deposition of IgA-containing immune complexes. Common manifestations include purpura and/or urticaria, abdominal pain, gastrointestinal bleeding or intussusception, arthralgias, arthritis or periarthritis, and glomerulonephritis. Visceral symptoms may precede the skin lesions, leading to diagnostic confusion. Delayed skin involvement may be misinterpreted to be a drug reaction. Purpura tends to occur in crops of lesions of similar age. Small vessel vasculitis/purpura is generally more pronounced in gravity-dependent areas. One exception is vasculitis due to cryoglobulinemia, especially in association with lymphoma. Figures 175-2 and 175-3 show nasal and digital purpura in a patient with B cell lymphoma–related (IgG) cryoglobulinemic purpura; similar extensive purpura also involved her ears and legs. Cutaneous vasculitis may be associated with such striking edema that nephrotic syndrome is suggested. Punch biopsy is useful in excluding infiltrative causes of nonvasculitic purpura. Immunofluorescent staining for IgA can support the diagnosis of HSP in the appropriate clinical setting.

The most important principles in the evaluation of patients with cutaneous vasculitis are the following:

1. It must be established that the vasculitis is not due to a process that may not benefit from, or may be aggravated by, immunosuppressive therapy. Examples include infections such as disseminated gonorrhea, bacterial endocarditis, and viral-related vasculitides.
2. The finding of small vessel vasculitis in the skin does not exclude concurrent medium or larger vessel arteritis. For example, purpura may occur in Wegener's granulomatosis (WG),[15] Churg-Strauss syndrome (CSS), polyarteritis, Behçet's disease, and Cogan's syndrome.

Therapy of isolated cutaneous vasculitis is directed at the underlying process, if one can be identified. Documented infections should be treated. Suspected offending antigens such as drugs should be withdrawn. If no precipitants are apparent, low-risk therapy can be attempted with nonsteroidal anti-inflammatory drugs, colchicine, pentoxifylline, dapsone, or short-term, low-dose glucocorticoids. However, if visceral involvement with organ dysfunction is present, a more aggressive approach is usually required. In the latter case, higher dose glucocorticoids are generally effective. In the setting of severe visceral involvement, methotrexate, azathioprine, cyclophosphamide, or other immunosuppressive agents may be required. When treating disease that is not organ- or life-threatening, close attention must be paid to the risk-versus-benefit ratio of selected therapies.

Urticarial vasculitis[16] represents a peculiar subset of small vessel vasculitis. The clinical presentation is that of typical wheals or serpentine papules, sometimes with surrounding or geographically separate angioedema. Individual lesions are slower to resolve than typical urticaria and often last for several days. There is frequently a burning, dysesthetic quality to the discomfort from the lesions. They often heal with skin discoloration—hyperpigmentation or an ecchymotic area. Most cases are idiopathic, although they may be associated with an underlying autoimmune disorder such as SLE or Sjögren's syndrome,[17] IgM paraproteinemia (Schnitzler's syndrome[18]), viral infections (hepatitis, acute Epstein-Barr), and HSP. Joint and, less commonly, abdominal pain may occur. There may be an association with ocular inflammatory disease and obstructive pulmonary disease. A form of urticarial vasculitis with neutrophil infiltration and destruction of the postcapillary venules has been

described[19] occurring in association with hypocomplementemia. The lesions are generally responsive to moderate doses of daily glucocorticoids. However, this approach is fraught with long-term toxicity. Anecdotal reports have noted improvement with colchicine, dapsone, nonsteroidal agents, and the antimalarials.[16]

Wegener's Granulomatosis

WG is a relatively uncommon, potentially lethal disease characterized by necrotizing granulomatous inflammation and vasculitis of small- and medium-sized vessels. Multiple organs are often involved, with a predilection for the upper and lower respiratory tracts, the eye, and the kidney.[20–22] Males and females of all ages can be affected. Upper airway disease tends to be particularly striking but is often initially attributed for months or even years to "rou-

FIGURE 175-3

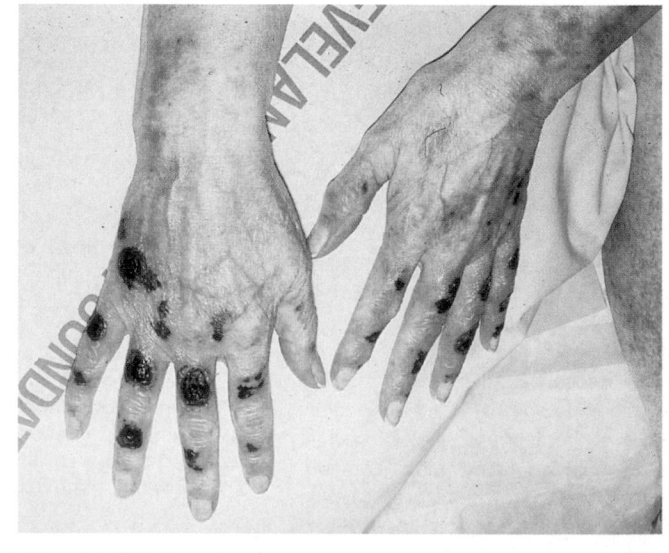

Digital purpura (leukocytoclastic angiitis) in the same patient shown in Fig. 175-2.

tine" sinus disease until other manifestations of WG are recognized. In addition to pansinusitis, WG can cause septal perforations and saddle nose deformities. Ear involvement is common, particularly otitis media. Auricular destruction similar to that in polychondritis has rarely been reported and may represent an overlap syndrome.[23] Occult involvement of the inner ear and nose must be sought. Sinus disease is often destructive and may be recalcitrant to therapy because of superinfection of the necrotic tissue by *Staphylococcus aureus*.[22] Laryngotracheal involvement may result in subglottic stenosis, especially in young patients.[20] Orbital pseudotumors and nasolacrimal duct stenosis occur frequently in WG. Orbital pseudotumors may cause proptosis with intractable pain and loss of vision; these inflammatory and fibrous masses may be refractory to anti-inflammatory, immunosuppressive, and even radiation therapy. Isolated uveitis and retinal disease are less common.

Lower respiratory tract involvement is part of the WG diagnostic triad (upper and lower respiratory tract and glomerulonephritis). However, it may not be clinically evident at the outset of disease or even at the time of diagnosis. Pulmonary involvement may be dramatic with diffuse alveolar hemorrhage. More commonly, patients present with mild or no symptoms, and chest radiographs or computed tomography scans are necessary to demonstrate the infiltrates or nodules. Nodules may undergo necrosis, leading to cavity formation. Pleural involvement occurs, but bronchospasm is not characteristic of WG. It is frequently necessary to rule out infectious causes of the pulmonary infiltrates, and bronchoscopy is useful in this regard. However, tissue obtained from transbronchial biopsy is usually quantitatively insufficient to make the pathologic diagnosis of WG. Open lung biopsy generally provides the optimal opportunity to demonstrate the typical pathologic findings of WG (Figs. 175-4 and 175-5) and to exclude malignancies and atypical infections. Biopsy of alternative tissues may not have the same likelihood of revealing the specific diagnosis. Nasal tissue, although readily available, has a far lower likelihood of yielding the correct diagnosis[24] than lung tissue obtained by thoracoscopy-guided or open biopsy. Renal biopsy may reveal focal and segmental glomerulonephritis with variable proliferative changes, in the absence of significant immune-complex deposition. Although supportive of the diagnosis of WG, these are not specific histopathologic findings. "Typical" open lung biopsies contain areas of necrosis (frequently in a "geographic pattern"), giant cell granulomas in the parenchymal tissue, and vasculitis. Not all histopathologic components may be present in the same section. Because these findings may also occur in chronic mycobacterial or fungal infections, special stains and cultures are essential.

Glomerulonephritis is a common cause of morbidity and mortality in WG. Its presence or absence defines the "generalized" or "limited" forms of the disease. When present, its expression may be relatively indolent or, more frequently, aggressive. It may be clinically and pathologically indistinguishable from idiopathic rapidly progressive crescentic glomerulonephritis. The evolution from subclinical to dialysis-dependent renal disease may take place over a period of several weeks.[20,25] Glomerulonephritis may be present at the outset or initial recognition of the disease or may develop only after the patient has been ill with an apparently limited form of the disease for long periods of time.[20–22,25] The importance of frequent microscopic urinalyses in the initial and follow-up evaluation of patients with WG cannot be overemphasized. Occasional 24-h urine collections, to establish a more accurate estimate of the glomerular filtration rate than the serum creatinine measurement alone can provide, may be valuable, especially in elderly or debilitated patients.

Musculoskeletal involvement probably occurs in over half of patients with WG. Most note only arthralgias or myalgias, but some

FIGURE 175-4

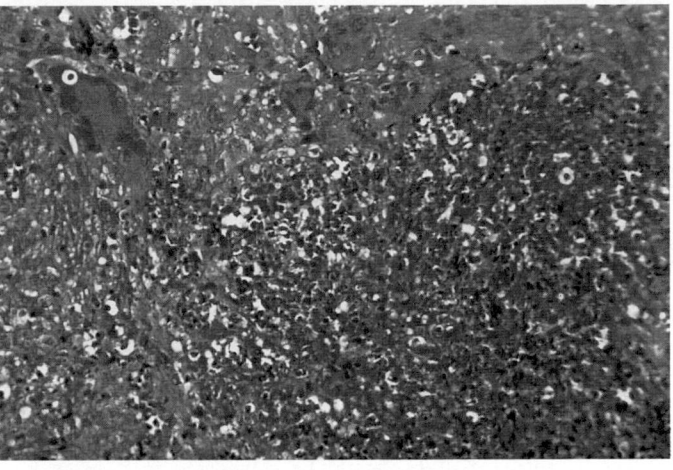

Lung histopathology from a patient with Wegener's granulomatosis demonstrating necrosis, giant cells, and mixed cellular inflammation.

may experience true polyarthritis or migratory or fixed inflammatory mono- or oligoarthritis.[20,26] Rheumatoid factor, which is frequently present in patients with WG, may cause some diagnostic confusion with rheumatoid arthritis when joint symptoms are significant. The joint disease of WG, however, only rarely produces bone erosions.[27] Neurologic signs and symptoms occur in fewer than 50 percent of patients, peripheral neuropathy in fewer than 20 percent, and involvement of the central nervous system in fewer than 10 percent.[20,28] Oculomotor involvement may occur due to the presence of retroorbital mass impingement. Gastrointestinal ulcerations and ischemic syndromes can occur,[29] as can cardiac ischemia, conduction disease, and pericarditis.[20,30]

Cutaneous involvement has been reported in up to 50 percent of patients with WG.[21] The authors have seen several patients who

FIGURE 175-5

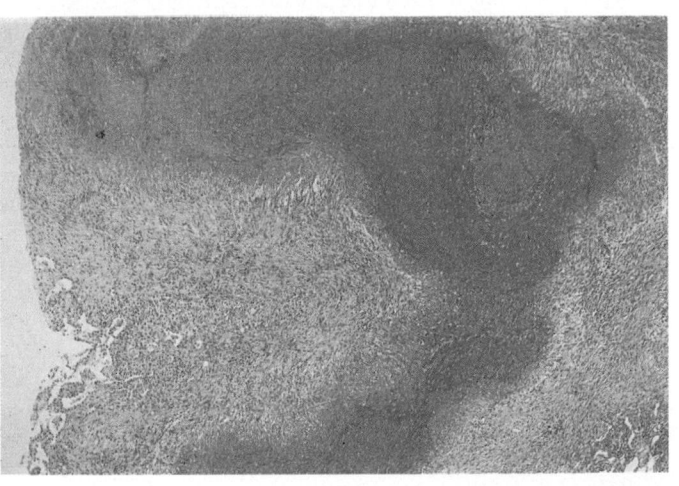

"Geographic necrosis" in a low-power view of an open lung biopsy specimen from a patient with Wegener's granulomatosis.

experienced acute or indolent deep inflammatory skin masses as the initial manifestation of their disease. Reported manifestations include palpable purpura,[15,31] pyoderma-like ulcerations,[31,32] gingival hyperplasia,[33] inflammatory papules, small ulcers, panniculitis, and subcutaneous nodules.[21,31,33,34] The activity of the skin disease generally parallels systemic disease activity. No skin histopathology is pathognomonic for WG. Leukocytoclastic angiitis is most apparent in the presence of purpura or inflammatory papules but is clearly not sufficient to make the diagnosis of WG. Granulomatous vasculitis[34] may be seen, occasionally in the presence of soft tissue necrosis or panniculitis, which may suggest the diagnosis of WG. Skin biopsies are not usually sufficient to confirm the diagnosis. Cutaneous granulomatous vasculitis, similar to that seen in patients with WG, has been described in patients with isolated skin involvement, Crohn's disease, sarcoidosis, or lymphoproliferative disorders.[5] Oral and nasal ulcerations are common. Several patients with orbital WG and a treatment-responsive yellow discoloration of the eyelids have been described.[35]

The diagnosis of WG should be considered in patients with otherwise unexplained inflammation of the upper or lower respiratory tract or eye or with glomerulonephritis. Suspicion of WG should be increased when multiple organ involvement is demonstrated, the upper airway disease is destructive, or pulmonary nodules (especially with cavities) are demonstrated by radiography. Any combination of organ involvement is conceivably possible, but most patients exhibit upper airway involvement at the time of diagnosis.[20] If the entire clinical picture is compatible with WG, and alternative diagnoses have been appropriately ruled out, the finding of C-ANCA with anti-PR3 specificity in the patient's serum is sufficient to make the diagnosis and initiate therapy. However, if there are any atypical features or special concerns regarding the initiation of immunosuppressive therapy or if the patient does not respond appropriately to therapy, tissue documentation of the diagnosis is mandatory. Since WG generally requires glucocorticoid plus cytotoxic drug therapy, it should be distinguished from other inflammatory disorders, including other vasculitic syndromes, which may be effectively treated with a less toxic approach.

Treatment of systemic WG virtually always requires dual-drug immunosuppressive therapy. Glucocorticoids may induce symptomatic improvement in the upper airway, lungs, skin, and musculoskeletal system but only rarely produce remission. Glucocorticoids alone essentially never control aggressive renal disease. Even if improvement follows single-drug treatment with glucocorticoids, tapering usually results in a flare in the disease. Consequently, serious disease, particularly renal disease, is treated initially with glucocorticoids and daily cyclophosphamide, with subsequent tapering of the steroids. There are some strong relative contraindications to the use of cyclophosphamide, including bladder outlet obstruction and leukopenia. In patients with milder or limited WG, weekly methotrexate (0.20 to 0.30 mg/kg, adjusted for renal function) with folic acid or leucovorin may be substituted for the cyclophosphamide.[21,36] Patients treated with either regimen must be continuously monitored for flares in disease or side effects of therapy. Side effects include cytopenias; hepatic or pulmonary toxicity from methotrexate; and pulmonary toxicity, cystitis, bladder cancer, or pancytopenia from cyclophosphamide. Some authors have suggested using trimethoprim-sulfamethoxazole as adjunctive therapy for treatment of the WG and/or for prevention of bacterial infections that may promote upper airway disease flares, but this approach remains controversial.[37] Three times weekly therapy with trimethoprim-sulfamethoxazole is of use, however, to protect patients against *Pneumocystis carinii* pneumonia while they are receiving high doses of glucocorticoids or a cytotoxic agent. The authors do not routinely utilize sequential C-ANCA measurements to dictate changes in immunosuppressive therapy. Local nasal and sinus care and otolaryngoscopic evaluations are a routine part of the therapy of patients with WG and upper airway disease.

Churg-Strauss Syndrome (Allergic Angiitis and Granulomatosis)

CSS, like WG, affects small- to medium-sized arteries and veins. Clinically, CSS and WG have similar patterns of organ involvement and pathology, especially in regard to upper and lower airway disease and glomerulonephritis. CSS differs most strikingly from WG by its usual occurrence in patients with a history of atopy, asthma, or allergic rhinitis, which is often ongoing. In the prevasculitic atopy phase, as well as during the systemic phase of the illness, eosinophilia is characteristic and often of striking degree ($\geq$1000 eosinophils/μL). When eosinophilia is present in WG, it is usually more modest ($\leq$500/μL). Systemic features of CSS include some combination of pulmonary infiltrates, cardiomyopathy, coronary arteritis, pericarditis, polyneuropathy (symmetric or mononeuritis multiplex), ischemic bowel disease, eosinophilic gastroenteritis, ocular inflammation, nasal perforations, glomerulonephritis, and cutaneous nodules and/or purpura.

The pulmonary infiltrates of CSS are usually transient and patchy,[38] and may be associated with alveolar hemorrhage. Pulmonary nodules are uncommon; when present, they rarely cavitate.[39] Pleural effusions are common and often contain abundant eosinophils. Clinical distinction of CSS from hypersensitivity pneumonitis, allergic aspergillosis, and pulmonary lymphoma is at times difficult. Cardiac disease can be severe and is a leading cause of mortality in these patients. It often does not manifest itself until late in the course of the illness. Valvular heart disease is not as striking or as common as in the hypereosinophilic syndrome. Neurologic involvement occurs in >60 percent of patients, may be severe, and is generally attributable to arteritis of the vasa nervorum. Purpura is the most common cutaneous feature. Urticaria and polymorphous erythematous eruptions also occur.[40] Cutaneous nodules occur in approximately one-third of patients, primarily on the extensor surfaces of the arms and scalp.[41–43] The nodules may be tender and occasionally infarct. Gastrointestinal involvement is due to ischemic vasculitis and/or eosinophilic gastroenteritis, which can cause pain, cramping, and diarrhea.

Histopathology of involved skin, nerve, lung, heart, and gastrointestinal tract typically exhibits a vascular or extravascular granulomatous inflammation, with a prominent eosinophilic infiltrate and vasculitis. Vasculitis in a given tissue section may be granulomatous or nongranulomatous. Granulomas can be found in tissue at areas separate from the demonstrable vasculitis. Eosinophilic infiltrates are more striking than those in WG. Eosinophils, granulomas, and giant cells are not found in abundance in classic polyarteritis nodosa (PAN). It has been suggested that the initial small vessel vasculitis in the skin evolves into a pattern of inflammation with granulomas that coalesce into the palpable nodules.[44] However, the pathology of these nodules is not by itself sufficient to make a diagnosis of CSS because similar pathology can be seen in lymphoma and sarcoidosis.[43,45] Glomerulonephritis is not as common as in WG but, when present, is usually focal and segmental, occasionally with crescents.[46] The glomerulonephritis of CSS is often milder than that of WG or microscopic polyangiitis.

CSS generally responds to treatment with glucocorticoids. Some patients are able to be tapered from steroids. However, the presence of bronchial asthma and sinus disease may require ongoing therapy, even if the vasculitic component of the disease has remitted. Patients with severe or refractory visceral organ involvement are treated with additional agents, such as cyclophosphamide,[47,48] methotrexate, or azathioprine.

Polyarteritis Nodosa and Microscopic Polyangiitis

Attempts to neatly separate these two forms of necrotizing small- and medium-sized vessel arteritis have not been universally accepted.[2,48,49] A recent international consensus conference proposed that the diagnosis of these disorders be based on the absence of granulomatous inflammation in both and the lack of involvement of arterioles, capillaries, venules, and glomerular capillaries in classic PAN. Microscopic polyangiitis (MPA) involves vessels ranging in size from capillaries and venules to medium-sized arteries (Fig. 175-1). Glomerulonephritis, especially rapidly progressive glomerulonephritis, and alveolar hemorrhage are particularly common in MPA and uncommon in PAN. Antibody to myeloperoxidase, a type of P-ANCA, is detected in sera from 60 percent of patients with MPA. It may well be that some cases of classic PAN do involve the smaller vessels, and until it can be demonstrated that the two syndromes have distinct pathophysiologies, attempts to clearly distinguish MPA from PAN will remain imperfect. Hepatitis B and C infections have been associated with a classic PAN-like syndrome[48] as well as with MPA-like disease.

Given the diagnostic nuances and disagreements, it is not surprising that a clear-cut distinction between the two syndromes cannot be provided in terms of prognosis or response to therapy. Most importantly, because the distinction between these two syndromes is still being defined, it is difficult to interpret the clinical descriptions in the older studies of PAN, which included patients with both classic PAN and MPA. This accounts for some of the wide variation in the reported frequency of pulmonary[50] or glomerular involvement in PAN.

Constitutional symptoms such as fever, asthenia, and myalgias are often present in both PAN and MPA. Elevated acute-phase reactants, thrombocytosis, leukocytosis, and the anemia of inflammatory disease are common, although not uniformly present. MPA is typically manifest by crescentic necrotizing, segmental glomerulonephritis and/or alveolar hemorrhage in conjunction with small and medium-sized vessel vasculitis in other organ systems.

Anti-glomerular basement membrane antibodies are generally absent. Alveolar hemorrhage may manifest as dyspnea, pulmonary infiltrates, and anemia, with or without hemoptysis. Peripheral neuropathy with symmetric mixed motor and sensory components, or mononeuritis multiplex pattern is common. Upper airway and ocular inflammation may occur[51] and may occasionally make the distinction from WG difficult. Purpura and/or splinter hemorrhages are commonly found[51,52] in MPA.

Classic PAN may present with hypertension and/or renal insufficiency with a bland urine sediment on microscopic analysis. Renal ischemia may result from inflammation, stenosis, or occlusion of preglomerular muscular arteries. Peripheral neuropathy, testicular pain/epididymitis, ischemic myalgias, and livedo reticularis occur fairly frequently. Both PAN and MPA may cause ischemia in the heart and gastrointestinal tract. PAN is associated with the development of microaneurysms, 1 to 5 mm in size, in the mesenteric, hepatic, or renal arteries in perhaps 40 percent of patients. Microaneurysms can also occur in patients with MPA, WG, CSS, Behçet's disease, SLE, and other disorders affecting medium-sized vessels (Fig. 175-1).

When PAN or MPA is recognized clinically, it is imperative to be certain that it is not secondary to or associated with infection

with hepatitis B and C. The presence of hepatitis B or C infection does not seem to alter the presentation of the PAN or MPA syndrome dramatically, although membranous glomerulonephritis, liver failure, and thrombocytopenia are more likely to occur with viral hepatitis infection. Infection with parvovirus B19 and HIV should also be excluded.

The diagnosis of these disorders should ideally be based on histopathology and clinical pattern of disease. In the patient with a urine sediment analysis suggestive of glomerulonephritis or with neuropathy, a renal biopsy or biopsy of a clinically involved nerve may provide the diagnosis of MPA. The presence of serum P-ANCA with antimyeloperoxidase specificity further supports the clinical diagnosis but is not specific for this disease. The renal biopsy tissue in MPA, as in WG, is negative for immune complexes by immunofluorescent staining and electron microscopy (so-called pauci-immune glomerulonephritis). Lung biopsy in the setting of pulmonary infiltrates or hemorrhage reveals "capillaritis" but yields less specific pathology than in WG. Biopsy is useful to rule out alternative pulmonary diagnoses. The diagnosis of classic PAN is more difficult in the setting of dominant, but nonspecific, constitutional symptoms and the absence of easily accessible disease-affected tissue such as nerve. Biopsy of clinically uninvolved tissue (e.g., asymptomatic muscle) is not usually fruitful. Several diagnostic algorithms have been proposed.[4,53,54] If biopsy is not indicated due to the absence of accessible involved tissue, complete abdominal angiography should be considered to evaluate the medium-sized vessels. The sensitivity and specificity of this procedure is not well defined, especially in the absence of abdominal complaints. Angiography is generally avoided, whenever possible, in the setting of progressive or significant renal insufficiency.

Treatment of both PAN and MPA is somewhat empirical, although recent work by Guillevin et al. has provided valuable information.[55] Glucocorticoids in high doses remain the initial mainstay of therapy for both PAN and MPA. Glucocorticoids alone may be sufficient therapy for patients who do not have critical organ involvement, defined as renal insufficiency, gastrointestinal ischemia, cardiomyopathy, dense peripheral neuropathy, and central nervous system involvement. Such patients have increased risk of morbidity or mortality and are usually treated with glucocorticoids and an additional immunosuppressive agent such as cyclophosphamide. Although this is the common practice, the usefulness of initial combination therapy in this setting has not been formally studied.

When active hepatitis B or C infection is present, a relatively short course of steroids should be considered, based on disease severity, in conjunction with antiviral therapy and perhaps apheresis.[55] Controlled studies have not been conducted to assess objectively the value of adding apheresis to the combination of antiviral and glucocorticoid therapy.

Kawasaki Disease

Kawasaki disease (KD) was first described in 1967 as *mucocutaneous lymph node syndrome*.[56,57] The presence of characteristic clinical features[58] has permitted the establishment of diagnostic criteria, which are listed in Table 175-2. KD typically affects infants and young children with dominant cutaneous manifestations. The vascular component of the disease may involve vessels ranging in size from venules to the aorta. The inflammation is noted primarily in the larger coronary arteries, which results in aneurysm formation in approximately 25 percent of untreated patients. It has been postulated, but not proved, that there is an infectious trigger for KD.

TABLE 175-2

Diagnostic Criteria for Kawasaki Disease

Persistent fever (>5 days)

Plus 4 of the following 5 conditions:

Bilateral conjunctivitis (nonpurulent)
Oral mucosal involvement (erythematous pharynx, red or fissured
  lips, strawberry tongue)
Soft tissue abnormalities of hands and feet (edema/erythema,
  desquamation)
Rash (polymorphous but nonvesicular)
Cervical adenopathy

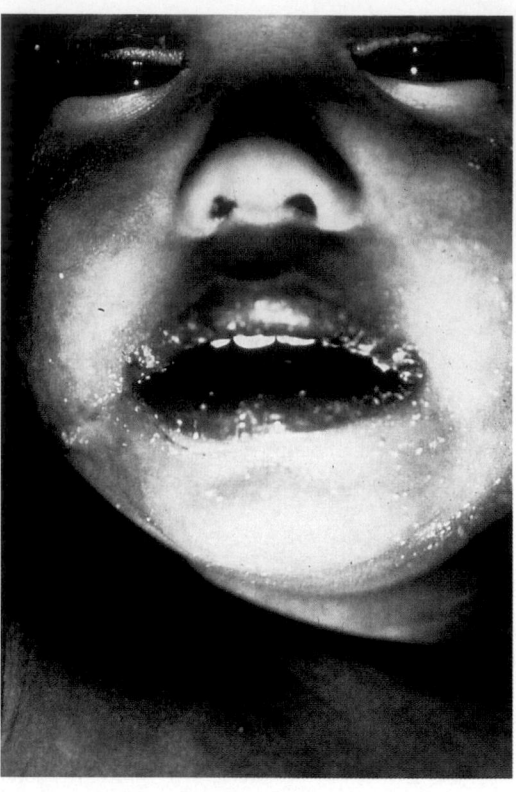

Kawasaki disease: lip and facial involvement. (*Courtesy of B. Singsen, MD.*)

No specific diagnostic tests exist. However, the immediate and delayed life-threatening cardiac complications of the disease, coupled with its unique therapy (intravenous gamma globulin, IVIg), mandate prompt clinical diagnosis.

Fever is usually high and spiking and may persist for 1 to 2 weeks if untreated, but rapid defervescence is usually observed with the initiation of appropriate therapy. Conjunctivitis, usually nonexudative, often appears concurrent with the fever. Uveitis occurs less frequently. Aseptic (lymphocytic) meningitis may contribute to the photophobia as well as headache and prominent irritability. Oral involvement includes erythema, dryness and fissuring of the lips, nonexudative pharyngitis, and tongue erythema with very prominent papillae (Figs. 175-6 and 175-7). Mucosal ulcerations do not characteristically occur.

Distal limb swelling often begins several days after the fever. The hands and feet may have associated erythema and tenderness that is not limited to the joints. Desquamation (Fig. 175-8), often in sheets, may begin days to a few weeks after the onset of the fever. When desquamation occurs early in KD, it may appear concurrently with a truncal rash and with eye and lip changes and may mimic a drug reaction or Stevens-Johnson syndrome. The rash is usually diffuse and polymorphous (Fig. 175-9), with urticarial, morbilliform, annular, or plaque components; but it is not vesicular. It is generally less evanescent and more readily apparent than the rash of Still's disease (systemic pattern juvenile rheumatoid arthritis). However, it may not be present at the time of initial presentation or concurrent with the febrile component of the illness. Distal vasculitis has been described, and digital necrosis may occur.[59]

Adenopathy, which is present in 75 percent of patients, is generally most apparent in the cervical region and ranges from mild to extensive.[60] Other less common (noncardiac) aspects of the disease include abdominal cramping and diarrhea, hydrops of the gall bladder, synovitis of large and small joints, hepatitis, pulmonary infiltrates, otitis media, thrombocytopenia with evidence of disseminated intravascular coagulation, and urethritis.

The morbidity and mortality (<3 percent) of KD are overwhelmingly associated with the development of inflammatory coronary artery aneurysms, most of which are asymptomatic at the time of formation. Many aneurysms can be detected by echocardiography. Cardiac involvement occurs in at least 20 percent of unsuccessfully treated patients. Thrombosis occurs in some of the aneurysms, resulting in direct or embolic coronary occlusion syndromes, including sudden death. Clinical coronary events often do not occur until weeks or years after the onset of febrile illness. The focus of initial prompt therapy is on the prevention of aneurysm formation and

coronary thrombosis. A baseline echocardiogram should be obtained at the time of the acute illness and repeated 2 and 6 weeks later. If abnormalities are identified, additional studies are warranted.[61] Early recognition of the disease and treatment with IVIg and aspirin have significantly decreased the frequency of aneurysm formation and thrombotic coronary events.

Histopathology of the conjunctiva or skin is not specific, revealing edema and vessel dilatation with a mixed mononuclear infiltrate of predominantly CD4+ cells and macrophages.[62,63] Lymph node pathology demonstrates variable necrosis and occasional areas of vasculitis.

Treatment should be initiated with IVIg (2 g/kg as a single dose) and aspirin (80 to 100 mg/kg per day, given every 6 h) as soon as the disease is suspected.[64] It has been suggested that the early administration of IVIg therapy is most effective at preventing aneurysm formation. Aspirin has been shown to be more effective than glucocorticoids in preventing aneurysms. Glucocorticoid therapy is usually unnecessary. Fever, conjunctivitis, and rash tend to respond within several days to aspirin and IVIg. Patients who do not respond to aspirin and IVIg therapy may benefit from high-dose glucocorticoid therapy.[65]

Large Vessel Arteritis (Takayasu's Arteritis and Temporal Arteritis)

Takayasu's arteritis (TA) and temporal (giant cell) arteritis (GCA) are the most common inflammatory diseases of the aorta and its major branches. Similar vascular targeting may occur in Behçet's disease, Cogan's syndrome, and sarcoidosis. These diseases are readily distinguished by their associated extravascular features.

FIGURE 175-7

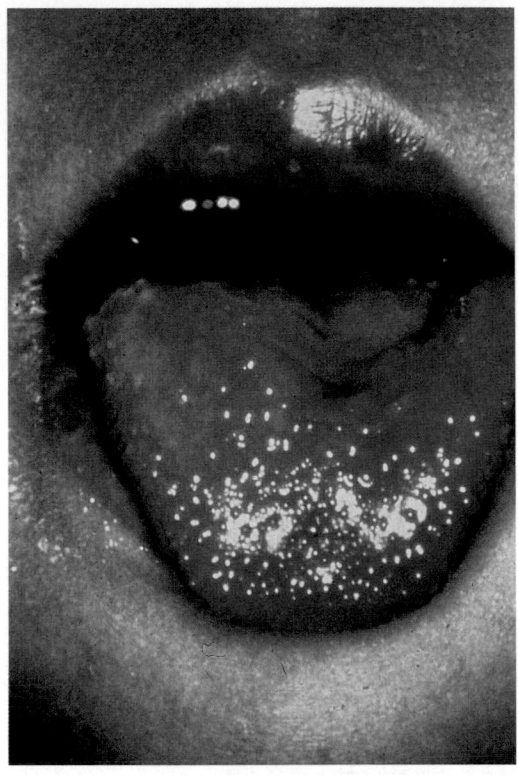

Kawasaki disease: strawberry tongue. (*Courtesy of B. Singsen, MD.*)

GCA generally affects individuals older than 50 years of age. It is associated in some patients with polymyalgia rheumatica, a syndrome characterized by proximal muscle pain that is more severe at night and in the early morning. There may be a subjective sense of weakness, without true weakness on examination or elevation of serum muscle enzyme levels. GCA is variably associated with fever, headache, masticatory muscle claudication, peripheral vascular disease, inflammatory aortic aneurysms, and retinal ischemic syndromes. Cutaneous manifestations include rare cases of scalp or tongue ischemia and necrosis and, in a minority of cases, cyanosis or pallor due to distal extremity ischemia arising from proximal

FIGURE 175-8

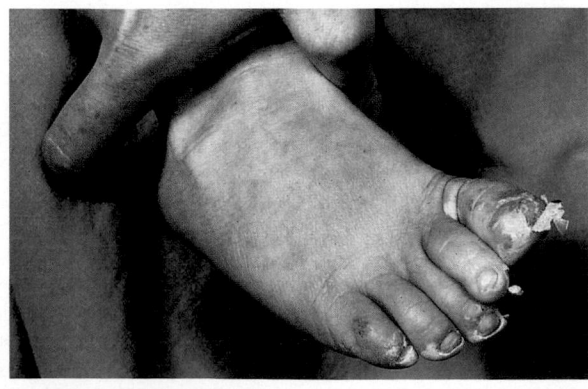

Kawasaki disease: distal extremity desquamation. (*Courtesy of B. Singsen, MD.*)

FIGURE 175-9

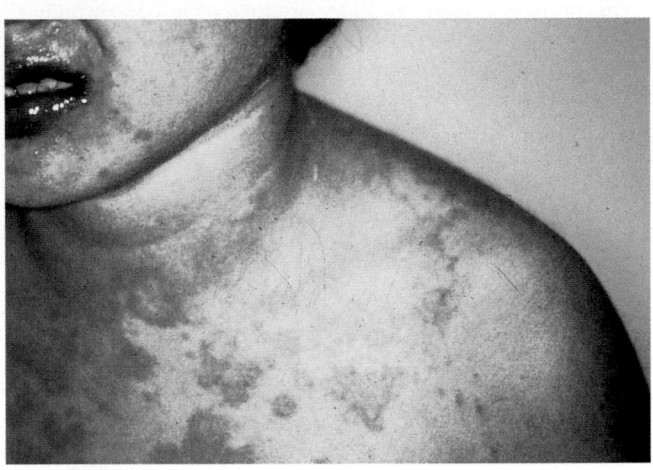

Kawasaki disease: rash on trunk. (*Courtesy of B. Singsen, MD.*)

large vessel occlusive disease. Symptoms and signs in the extremities may be clinically indistinguishable from those occurring in arteriosclerotic obliterative disease.

GCA is generally diagnosed by biopsy of the superficial temporal artery. The pathology of GCA usually includes chronic mononuclear cell infiltrates and giant cells. There are isolated reports of GCA overlap syndromes also involving medium-sized vessels of the viscera, but generally this disease is not associated with small (capillary, venule) blood vessel inflammation.[4,66]

Takayasu's arteritis (pulseless disease) is also a chronic inflammatory disease affecting the aorta and its major branches. Although it is usually recognized in younger, predominantly female patients of reproductive age, it can also occur in young children and older patients of either sex. TA is more commonly associated with aortic and aortic branch vessel stenoses and aneurysms than GCA. It is uncertain whether TA and GCA are distinct disorders or the same disorder, with modified expression in different age groups. TA has been associated with erythema nodosum or rarely pyoderma-like lesions more frequently than has GCA.[67–69] The presenting clinical syndrome may include prolonged flulike illness, with a polymyalgia rheumatica pattern of muscle pain. Other patients present only with evidence of limb, cerebral, or cardiac ischemia. Renal ischemia can elicit high renin hypertension. The characteristic features of the disease reflect the ischemia produced by the inflammatory stenoses of the aorta and its major branches. Predominant sites of involvement are the aortic arch vessels, particularly the subclavian artery. Arm claudication is common. Bruits are frequently detectable. Superficial artery pain and tenderness (e.g., carotidynia) may be found on examination but are not diagnostic of TA. Severe central hypertension due to renal artery stenosis may not be recognized because of coexistent arm artery stenosis; thus, four extremity blood pressures must be evaluated initially and monitored on a frequent basis. Stroke is not uncommon and is often related to hypertension. It is extremely difficult to assess the activity of TA; the presence or absence of constitutional features or of elevated acute-phase reactants are poor measures of disease activity. This impression is supported by histopathologic studies of vessel tissue obtained at the time of reconstructive surgery.[67,70,71] More than 40 percent of specimens from patients thought to be in remission revealed active inflammation.

Diagnosis is usually made by arteriographic demonstration of stenotic and obstructive lesions. Aneurysms are less commonly observed. The entire arch as well as abdominal aorta and renal vessels should be evaluated; central arterial pressure should be obtained at the time of angiography and compared with simultaneously obtained arm and leg arterial pressures. The role for vascular magnetic resonance imaging in the evaluation and follow-up of these patients is currently under investigation. Pathologic documentation is more difficult to obtain in TA, but the histopathology is similar to that described above in GCA.

Sarcoidosis may involve the large arteries and occasionally may mimic the vascular disease of TA.[4] As noted above, a full physical examination and chest radiograph are requisite components of the evaluation of any patient with suspected systemic vasculitic syndrome. Careful examination may reveal subtle findings such as lacrimal enlargement (Fig. 175-10) to suggest the diagnosis of sarcoidosis. Atherosclerotic disease often presents a more difficult diagnostic distinction in patients with obliterative arterial disease and certainly can coexist with a primary form of large vessel arteritis. Livedo reticularis (Fig. 175-11) may be seen in patients with peripheral vascular disease of various etiologies.

The initial therapy of both TA and GCA is with glucocorticoids. GCA is generally quite steroid responsive, although the most appropriate initial dose remains controversial. Different authors have advocated different initial daily doses, ranging from 20 mg to 1 mg/kg body weight, with tapering of the glucocorticoids over 8 to 12 months. The measurement of acute-phase reactants provides an imperfect index of disease activity and an imperfect guide to steroid tapering. If significant steroid-induced side effects occur, or if patients relapse during tapering, a second-line agent such as methotrexate is usually (empirically) added to the glucocorticoid regimen. TA appears to respond less consistently to initial glucocorticoid therapy than GCA, but this observation has not been carefully studied. Some authors have advocated the earlier use of methotrexate therapy in TA to reduce the toxicity risks of long-term glucocorticoid therapy.[72] Vascular reconstructive surgery or angioplasty is an adjunctive therapeutic option for some patients.[73]

FIGURE 175-10

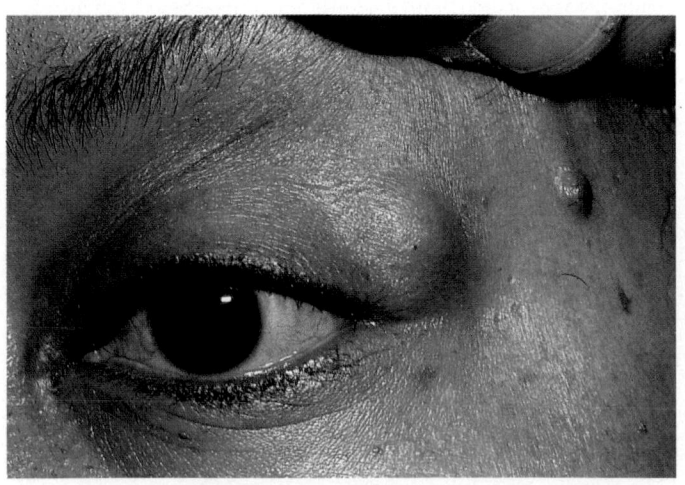

Sarcoidosis: lacrimal gland enlargement.

FIGURE 175-11

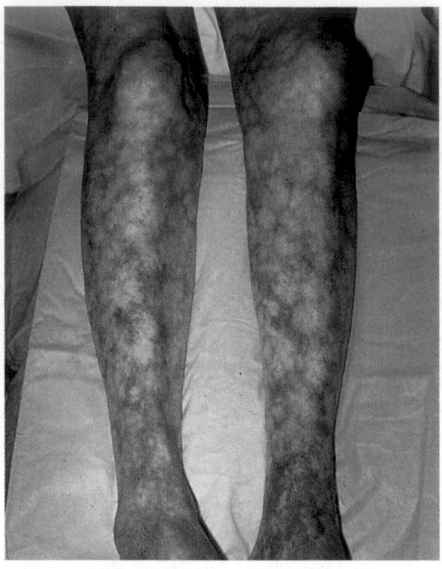

Livedo reticularis.

GENERAL COMMENTS ON THE TREATMENT OF PATIENTS WITH SYSTEMIC ARTERITIS

The systemic vasculitides are potentially life-threatening and often require potent anti-inflammatory and immunosuppressive therapy. Diagnoses should be made with as much certainty as possible. However, questions regarding alternative diagnoses or coexistent diseases may linger. Hence, even after therapy is initiated, physicians need to maintain a high degree of vigilance to detect unrelated medical problems and/or complications of therapy. After the initiation of potent immunosuppressive therapy, there is increased susceptibility to opportunistic infection. The greatest risks occur in patients with marked neutropenia or lymphopenia. Physicians must be particularly wary about attributing new problems to "flares" in the underlying disease without considering the possibility of a new or recrudescent infection. Varicella-zoster may present with fever and pain before the appearance of the tell-tale vesicles. Infections from *P. carinii* and cytomegalovirus, systemic fungal infections, and the reactivation of mycobacterial disease occur more frequently than in the normal host. Significant immunosuppression from glucocorticoids and the other medications is frequently associated with mucosal candidiasis, less commonly with molluscum contagiosum, and rarely with Kaposi's sarcoma. Methotrexate may cause a flulike illness after each dose. Methotrexate, azathioprine, and cyclophosphamide may cause leukopenia and, less often, other cytopenias. Glucocorticoids can cause a significant amount of facial and truncal acne, which, especially in younger patients, must be addressed to encourage compliance with therapy. Cutaneous complications, including allergic purpura, can also result from adjunctive medications for hypertension, epilepsy, or arthritis. Reactions to thrombolysis or angiographic studies may include urticaria as well as the cholesterol embolization syndrome in patients with atherosclerosis. Drug-induced pneumonitis has been reported with the use of immunosuppressive agents, especially methotrexate and cyclophosphamide.

1. Fauci AS et al: The spectrum of vasculitis: Clinical, pathologic, immunologic and therapeutic considerations. *Ann Intern Med* **89**:660, 1978

2. Jennette C et al: Nomenclature of systemic vasculitides. Proposal of an international consensus conference. *Arthritis Rheum* **37**:187, 1994

3. Zeek PM: Periarteritis nodosa: A critical review. *Am J Clin Pathol* **22**:777, 1952

4. Mandell BF, Hoffman GS: Differentiating the vasculitides. *Rheum Dis Clin North Am* **20**:409, 1994

5. Gibson EL, Su WPD: Cutaneous vasculitis. *Rheum Dis Clin North Am* **21**:1097, 1995

6. Karlsberg PL et al: Cutaneous vasculitis and rheumatoid factor positivity as presenting signs of hepatitis C virus–induced mixed cryoglobulinemia. *Arch Dermatol* **131**:1119, 1995

7. Castro M et al: Rheumatic manifestations in myelodysplastic syndromes. *J Rheumatol* **18**:721, 1991

8. Stahl RL, Silver R: Vasculitic leg ulcers in chronic myelogenous leukemia. *Am J Med* **78**:869, 1985

9. Kesseler ME, Slater DN: Cutaneous vasculitis: A presenting feature in Hodgkin's disease. *J R Soc Med* **79**:485, 1986

10. Means RT et al: Leukocytoclastic vasculitis and multiple myeloma. *Ann Intern Med* **106**:329, 1987

11. Lacour JP et al: Cutaneous leukocytoclastic vasculitis and renal cancer: Two cases. *Am J Med* **94**:104, 1993

12. Cupps TR et al: Chronic recurrent small vessel cutaneous vasculitis. *JAMA* **247**:1994, 1982

13. Carbone L et al: Goodpasture's syndrome complicating Henoch-Schönlein purpura. *J Clin Rheum* **1**:350, 1995

14. Szer IS: Henoch-Schönlein purpura: When and how to treat. *J Rheumatol* **23**:1661, 1996

15. Mangold MC et al: Cutaneous leukocytoclastic vasculitis associated with active Wegener's granulomatosis. *J Am Acad Dermatol* **26**:579, 1992

16. O'Donnell B et al: Urticarial vasculitis. *Int Angiol* **14**:166, 1995

17. Asherson RA et al: Urticarial vasculitis in a connective tissue disease clinic: Patterns, presentations, and treatment. *Semin Arthritis Rheum* **20**:285, 1991

18. Morita A et al: A case of urticarial vasculitis associated with macroglobulinemia (Schnitzler's syndrome). *J Dermatol* **22**:32, 1995

19. Zeiss CR et al: A hypocomplementemic vasculitis urticarial syndrome. *Am J Med* **68**:867, 1980

20. Hoffman GS et al: Wegener's granulomatosis: An analysis of 158 patients. *Ann Intern Med* **116**:488, 1992

21. Duna G et al: Wegener's granulomatosis. *Rheum Dis Clin North Am* **21**:949, 1995

22. Fauci AS et al: Wegener's granulomatosis: Prospective clinical and therapeutic experience with 85 patients for 21 years. *Ann Intern Med* **98**:80, 1983

23. Diaz-Jouanen E et al: Chondritis of the ear in Wegener's granulomatosis. *Arthritis Rheum* **20**:1288, 1977

24. Devaney KO et al: Interpretation of head and neck biopsies in Wegener's granulomatosis. A pathologic study of 126 biopsies in 70 patients. *Am J Surg Pathol* **14**:555, 1990

25. Pinching AJ et al: Wegener's granulomatosis: Observations on 18 patients with severe renal disease. *Q J Med* **208**:435, 1988

26. Noritake DT et al: Rheumatic manifestations of Wegener's granulomatosis. *J Rheumatol* **14**:949, 1987

27. Jacobs RP et al: Wegener's granulomatosis presenting with erosive arthritis. *Arthritis Rheum* **30**:943, 1987

28. Nishino H et al: Neurological involvement in Wegener's granulomatosis: An analysis of 324 consecutive patients at the Mayo Clinic. *Ann Neurol* **33**:4, 1993

29. Hoffman GS et al: Gastrointestinal emergencies: Vasculitis and the gut, in *Current Topics in Gastroenterology and Hepatology,* edited by GNJ Tytgat, M Van Blankenstein. New York, Thieme, 1990, p 36

30. Forstot JZ et al: Cardiac complications of Wegener's granulomatosis: A case report of a complete heart block and review of the literature. *Semin Arthritis Rheum* **10**:148, 1980

31. Frances C et al: Wegener's granulomatosis. Dermatological manifestations in 75 cases with clinicopathologic correlations. *Arch Dermatol* **130**:861, 1994

32. Handfield-Jones SE et al: Wegener's granulomatosis presenting as pyoderma gangrenosum. *Clin Exp Dermatol* **17**:197, 1992

33. Patten SF et al: Wegener's granulomatosis: Cutaneous and oral mucosal disease. *J Am Acad Dermatol* **28**:710, 1993

34. Barksdale SK et al: Cutaneous pathology in Wegener's granulomatosis. A clinicopathologic study of 75 biopsies in 46 patients. *Am J Surg Pathol* **19**:161, 1995

35. Tullo AB et al: Florid xanthelasmata in orbital Wegener's granulomatosis. *Br J Ophthalmol* **79**:453, 1995

36. Sneller MC et al: An analysis of 42 Wegener's granulomatosis patients treated with methotrexate and prednisone. *Arthritis Rheum* **38**:608, 1995

37. Leavitt RY et al: The role of trimethoprim/sulfamethoxazole in the treatment of Wegener's granulomatosis. *Arthritis Rheum* **31**:1073, 1988

38. Chumbley LC et al: Allergic granulomatosis and angiitis. *Mayo Clinic Proc* **52**:477, 1977

39. Desgys GE et al: Allergic granulomatosis. Churg-Strauss syndrome. *Am J Radiol* **135**:1821, 1980

40. Abe-Matsuura Y et al: Allergic granulomatosis (Churg-Strauss) associated with cutaneous manifestations: Report of two cases. *J Dermatol* **22**:46, 1995

41. Crotty CP et al: Cutaneous clinicopathologic correlation of allergic granulomatosis. *J Am Acad Dermatol* **5**:571, 1981

42. Finan MC et al: The cutaneous extravascular necrotizing granuloma and systemic disease. A review of 27 cases. *Medicine (Baltimore)* **62**:142, 1983

43. Gibson LE et al: The spectrum of cutaneous granulomatous vasculitis: Histopathologic report of eight cases with clinical correlation. *J Cutan Pathol* **21**:437, 1994

44. Lanham JG et al: Churg-Strauss syndrome, in *Systemic Vasculitides,* edited by A Churg, J Churg. New York, Igaku-Shoin, 1991, p 101

45. Calonje JE et al: Cutaneous extravascular necrotizing granuloma (Churg-Strauss) as a paraneoplastic manifestation of non-Hodgkin's B-cell lymphoma. *J R Soc Med* **86**:549, 1993

46. Gaskin G et al: Renal disease in the Churg-Strauss syndrome. *Contrib Nephrol* **94**:58, 1991

47. Guillevin L et al: Systemic necrotizing angiitis with asthma: Causes and precipitating factors in 43 cases. *Lung* **65**:165, 1987

48. Lhote F et al: Polyarteritis nodosa, microscopic polyangiitis and Churg-Strauss syndrome. *Rheum Dis Clin North Am* **21**:911, 1995

49. Lie J: Nomenclature and classification of vasculitis: Plus ça change, plus c'est la meme chose (editorial). *Arthritis Rheum* **37**:181, 1994

50. Matsumoto T et al: The lung in polyarteritis nodosa: A pathologic study of 10 cases. *Hum Pathol* **24**:717, 1993

51. Lhote F et al: Microscopic polyangiitis: Clinical aspects and treatment. *Ann Med Interne (Paris)* **147**:165, 1996

52. Penas PF et al: Microscopic polyangiitis. A systemic vasculitis with a positive P-ANCA. *Br J Dermatol* **134**:542, 1996

53. Dahlberg PJ et al: Diagnostic studies for systemic necrotizing vasculitis. Sensitivity, specificity, and predictive value in patients with multisystem disease. *Arch Intern Med* **149**:161, 1989

54. Albert DA et al: The diagnosis of polyarteritis nodosa. II. Empirical verification of a decision analysis model. *Arthritis Rheum* **31**:1128, 1988

55. Guillevin L et al: Polyarteritis nodosa related to hepatitis B virus. A prospective study with long-term observation of 41 patients. *Medicine (Baltimore)* **74**:238, 1995

56. Kawasaki T: Acute febrile mucocutaneous syndrome with lymph node involvement with specific desquamation of the fingers and toes in children. *Arerugi* **16**:178, 1967

57. Kawasaki T et al: A new infantile acute febrile mucocutaneous lymph node syndrome. *Pediatrics* **54**:271, 1974

58. Wortman DW et al: Kawasaki syndrome. *Rheum Dis Clin North Am* **16**:363, 1990

59. Ames EL et al: Bilateral hand necrosis in Kawasaki syndrome. *J Hand Surg* **10**:391, 1985

60. Kim-Stamos J et al: Lymphadenitis as the dominant presentation of Kawasaki disease. *Pediatrics* **93**:525, 1994

61. Committee on Rheumatic Fever, Endocarditis and Kawasaki Disease, American Heart Association: Guidelines for long-term management of patients with Kawasaki disease. *Circulation* **89**:916, 1994

62. Burns JC et al: Conjunctival biopsy in patients with Kawasaki disease. *Pediatr Pathol Lab Med* **15**:547, 1995

63. Sato N et al: Immunopathology and cytokine detection in the skin lesions of patients with Kawasaki disease. *J Pediatr* **122**:198, 1993

64. Shulman ST et al: Kawasaki disease. *Pediatr Clin North Am* **21**:1013, 1995

65. Wright DA et al: Treatment of immune globulin resistant Kawasaki disease with pulsed doses of corticosteroids. *J Pediatr* **128**:146, 1996
66. Nordberg E et al: Giant cell arteritis. *Rheum Dis Clin North Am* **21**:1013, 1995
67. Kerr G et al: Takayasu arteritis. *Ann Intern Med* **120**:919, 1994
68. Nikolic J et al: Takayasu arteritis preceded by cardiac and cutaneous lesions. A case report. *Vasa* **22**:347, 1993

69. Frances C et al: Cutaneous manifestations of Takayasu's arteritis: A retrospective study of 80 cases. *Dermatologica* **181**:266, 1990
70. Hoffman GS: Treatment resistant Takayasu's arteritis. *Rheum Dis Clin North Am* **21**:73, 1995
71. Lagneau G et al: Surgical treatment of Takayasu's disease. *Ann Surg* **205**:157, 1987
72. Hoffman GS et al: Treatment of glucocorticosteroid resistant or relapsing Takayasu's arteritis with methotrexate. *Arthritis Rheum* **37**:578, 1994
73. Giordano JM: Takayasu's disease—current status. *Eur J Vasc Endovasc Surg* **11**:1, 1996

CHAPTER 176

Nicholas A. Soter

Cutaneous Necrotizing Venulitis

Necrotizing angiitis or vasculitis comprises a diverse group of disorders that combine segmental inflammation with necrosis of the blood vessels. The vascular damage results from immunologic and/or inflammatory mechanisms. Clinical syndromes are based on criteria that include the gross appearance and the histologic alterations of the vascular lesions, the caliber of the affected blood vessels, the frequency of involvement of specific organs, and the presence or absence of laboratory abnormalities. Necrotizing vasculitis may be a primary disease, may develop as a feature of a systemic disorder, or may be idiopathic.

Although all sizes of blood vessels may be involved in the skin, necrotizing vasculitis predominantly involves venules and is known as *cutaneous necrotizing venulitis* (CNV) *or leukocytoclastic vasculitis.* CNV may occur in association with an underlying chronic disease, may be precipitated by infections or drugs, or may develop for unknown reasons (Table 176-1).

Systemic involvement of the small blood vessels in concert with cutaneous lesions has been classified as *hypersensitivity angiitis* or *hypersensitivity vasculitis.* Hypersensitivity vasculitis includes CNV and microscopic polyangiitis.[1] Systemic necrotizing vasculitis involving blood vessels of various sites, but not fitting any diagnostic category and accompanied by skin lesions, is termed *systemic polyangiitis.*[2] Although IgA-mediated small-vessel necrotizing vasculitis has been proposed as a nosologic entity, at the present time an immunopathobiologic classification of CNV is not possible. Other systemic forms of systemic necrotizing vasculitis are considered in Chap. 175.

TABLE 176-1

Cutaneous Necrotizing Venulitis

Associated chronic disorders
   Rheumatoid arthritis
   Sjögren's syndrome
   Systemic lupus erythematosus
   Hypergammaglobulinemic purpura
   Paraneoplastic vasculitis
   Cryoglobulinemia
   Ulcerative colitis
   Cystic fibrosis
   Antineutrophil cytoplasmic or antiphospholipid antibody syndromes
Precipitating events
   Bacterial, viral, and mycobacterial infections
   Therapeutic and diagnostic agents
Idiopathic disorders
   Henoch-Schönlein syndrome
   Acute hemorrhagic edema of childhood
   Urticarial vasculitis and variants
   Erythema elevatum diutinum
   Nodular vasculitis
   Livedoid vasculitis
   Genetic complement deficiencies
   Eosinophilic vasculitis
   Idiopathic

PATHOGENESIS

Experimental studies in animal models and observations in humans implicate immune complexes as a major pathobiologic mechanism in the production of CNV. The mechanism of the localization of circulating immune complexes to a specific vessel site in human disease remains speculative; however, data obtained in animals suggest that the localization in venules is related to vasoactive amines and subsequent vasopermeability alterations. Additional factors that are operative in the localization of immune complexes include endothelial cell surface receptors and the defective clearance of complexes by the reticuloendothelial system.

The most frequently postulated mechanisms in the production of CNV are the local deposition of circulating immune complexes formed during antigen excess or the formation of immune complexes in situ in the skin. Certain types of immune complexes activate the complement system and lead to the generation of C5a anaphylatoxin, which attracts neutrophils. The neutrophils, in turn, release lysosomal enzymes that damage tissue. The neutrophil superoxide-generating system may produce reactive oxygen products, which also cause tissue injury. The generation of the chemoattractant leukotriene B$_4$ (LTB$_4$) from infiltrating neutrophils further enhances the influx of neutrophils. An infiltrate composed predominantly of neutrophils in the lesional skin of patients with CNV is consistent with tissue damage induced by immune complexes that activate the complement system.

In patients with CNV, circulating immune complexes have been demonstrated in serum directly as mixed-type cryoglobulins and indirectly by assays that detect C1q precipitins, materials that bind to complement receptors on human lymphocytoid (Raji) cells, materials that bind to monoclonal rheumatoid factor, and substances that function in the antibody-dependent cellular cytotoxicity inhibition assay. The presence of immune complexes is inferred also from the occurrence of serum hypocomplementemia with activation of the classic activating pathway. Further evidence implicating complement activation is provided by the detection of increased plasma levels of C4a and C3a anaphylatoxins and of C3 nephritic factor, an IgG autoantibody that results in C3 consumption.[3]

Immune complexes have been detected in lesional tissues by ultrastructural observation as electron-dense subendothelial deposits; and the membrane-attack complex, C5b-9, of the complement system has been detected on the surface of endothelial cells and infiltrating neutrophils. Decay-accelerating factor, a regulatory complement protein that prevents the assembly of the membrane-attack complex, was not present on the surface of endothelial cells of the upper dermal microvasculature. Tissue immune complexes have also been detected by direct immunofluorescence techniques as deposited immunoglobulins and complement proteins. In time-course studies of the evolution of cutaneous vascular lesions, immune reactants have been detected almost exclusively in lesions less than 24 h old. The antigens have been identified in only a few instances as bacterial, viral,[4] mycobacterial, or rickettsial proteins detected by direct immunofluorescence techniques or the polymerase chain reaction (PCR).

A role for lymphocytes and mononuclear cells in the production of CNV is suggested by a perivenular infiltrate in skin lesions that is rich in lymphocytes with large and hyperchromatic nuclei and by a prominence of mononuclear cells in the vascular skin lesions of patients with CNV and Sjögren's syndrome. Lymphocytes may be activated by immune complexes, by cellular immune mechanisms, or directly in autoimmune disease to produce lymphokines. Endothelial cells may also present antigens to and activate T lymphocytes. Activated macrophages secrete chemokines and lysosomal enzymes. Gamma/delta T cells have been detected in CNV with a neutrophil-rich pattern and with a documented infectious etiology.[5,6] In these specimens, the simultaneous expression of a 72-kDa heat shock protein was expressed by endothelial cells and antigen-presenting cells.

The participation of mast cells in CNV is suggested by the presence of hypogranulated mast cells, often with shed extracellular granules, and the decreased number of mast cells in histologic sections prepared from biopsy specimens of skin lesions and stained with toluidine blue as well as by the development of vascular lesions after the intracutaneous injection of histamine in patients with active episodes of CNV. Through the release of histamine and the generation and release of vasopermeability eicosanoids, the mast cell could alter venular permeability; interendothelial cell gaps have been noted in venules in patients with CNV. Eosinophils and neutrophils could be attracted by mast cell–derived chemotactic factors. The neutral proteases and acid hydrolases of mast cells could further facilitate tissue damage. The mast cell may also release tumor necrosis factor (TNF) α that could increase expression of E-selectin on endothelial cells.[7]

Additional evidence for the role of the mast cell is provided by a time-course analysis of the sequential histopathologic changes in an individual with circulating immune complexes and hypocomplementemia, in whom cold and trauma elicited CNV.[8] After initial mast cell degranulation, the infiltration by neutrophils was followed by an influx of eosinophils and basophils, the deposition of fibrin, and venular alterations including necrosis. A postulated sequence of events would be the activation of the mast cell by physical stimuli, the release of vasoactive mediators, the deposition of circulating immune complexes with activation of the complement system, the influx of neutrophils, and the development of CNV.

The time-course of necrotizing vasculitis in human skin has been studied in an individual with exercise-induced vasculitis.[9] At 3 h, the number of identifiable mast cells decreased and the eosinophil was the first cell to appear around the venules with the deposition of eosinophil peroxidase. TNF-α levels were elevated, and E-selectin was expressed on endothelial cells. Subsequently, an influx of neutrophils appeared with the deposition of neutrophil elastase and the development of CNV.

Early in the course of necrotizing vasculitis, endothelial cells show increased expression of intercellular adhesion molecule (ICAM) 1 and E-selectin without the expression of vascular cell adhesion molecule (VCAM) 1. Endothelial cells may show increased expression of ICAM-1, VCAM-1, and E-selectin in response to TNF-α.[10] Because E-selectin is an adhesion molecule for neutrophils and for skin-homing, memory T lymphocytes that display lymphocyte function–associated antigen 3, CD58, and lymphocyte common antigen,[11] the increase in E-selectin is consistent with a neutrophilic infiltrate within the first 24 h.[12] CD11b on neutrophils (Mac-1) may bind to ICAM-1.[12] VCAM-1 acts as an adhesion molecule for lymphocytes, monocytes, and eosinophils.

In skin biopsy specimens from patients with idiopathic cutaneous vasculitis, hypersensitivity vasculitis, urticarial vasculitis, and Henoch-Schönlein purpura, E-selectin was detected on endothelial cells of lesions less than 48 h old and was associated with an infiltrate of neutrophils bearing CD11b. The endothelial cells expressed HLA-DR and very late activating antigen 1 (VLA-1) but not P-selectin. The perivascular cells demonstrated VCAM-1 and HLA-DR.[12] Further evidence of endothelial cell activation was demonstrated by increased plasma levels of tissue plasminogen activator antigen and von Willebrand factor antigen in some patients with livedoid vasculitis.[13] Diminished fibrinolysis occurs in patients with CNV, and the subsequent reduction in fibrinolytic activity leads to fibrin deposition.

Cutaneous nerve fibers can release neuropeptides, such as substance P, neurokinin A, and calcitonin gene–related peptide (CGRP), that cause vasodilation. Substance P activates mast cells and macrophages and increases fibrinolytic activity mediated by plasminogen activator. CGRP induces expression of endothelial E-selectin and is chemotactic for T lymphocytes.

Eosinophils are minor infiltrating cells in necrotizing vasculitis. Eosinophils produce leukotriene C$_4$ (LTC$_4$) and platelet-activating factor, which increase vascular permeability. Eosinophil granule proteins are toxic to endothelial cells and cause further release of chemical mediators from mast cells.

Associations have been recognized between small-vessel necrotizing vasculitis and autoantibodies termed *antineutrophil cytoplasmic autoantibodies* (ANCAs), which have specificity for proteins of the cytoplasmic granules of neutrophils and the lysosomes of monocytes. Two staining patterns on neutrophils are recognized: cytoplasmic (C-ANCA) and perinuclear (P-ANCA). In patients with necrotizing vasculitis, most C-ANCAs are specific for proteinase 3 and most P-ANCAs are specific for myeloperoxidase. Experimental models suggest that ANCAs induce necrotizing vasculitis by activating circulating neutrophils and monocytes, which then adhere to blood vessels, degranulate, and release toxic oxygen metabolites to cause vascular injury.[14] Antiendothelial cell antibodies cause experimental vasculitis in BALB/c mice,[15] and these antibodies have been detected in the sera of patients with systemic vasculitis, rheumatoid arthritis with vasculitis, microscopic polyangiitis,[16] and Sneddon's syndrome.[17]

An increased prevalence of the HLA haplotype HLA-A11, Bw35 in patients with CNV and associated connective tissue disorders suggests that genetic factors may be operative.

CLINICAL MANIFESTATIONS

The age of patients has a limited influence on CNV. The associated chronic disorder usually determines the age of the affected individual. In children, CNV is most commonly described as the Henoch-Schönlein syndrome or acute hemorrhagic edema of childhood. ANCA-associated vasculitides are most common in patients older than 50 years.

The skin lesions of CNV are polymorphous; however, erythematous papules that do not blanch when the skin is pressed, known as *palpable purpura*, are the signature lesions (Fig. 176-1A). Papules, urticaria/angioedema, pustules, vesicles, ulcers, necrosis, and livedo reticularis may be seen. Occasionally there is subcutaneous edema below the area of the dermal lesions.

The vascular eruption most often appears on the lower extremities or over dependent areas, such as the back and gluteal regions. The lesions may occur anywhere on the skin but are uncommon on the face, palms, soles, and mucous membranes. They are episodic and may recur over weeks to years. Palpable purpura persists from 1 to 4 weeks and resolves at times with transient hyperpigmentation and/or atrophic scars. Lesional symptoms include pruritus or burning and, less commonly, pain.

An episode of cutaneous vascular lesions may be attended by fever, malaise, arthralgias, or myalgias irrespective of a defined underlying or associated disease. Systemic involvement of the small blood vessels most commonly occurs in the synovia, gastrointestinal tract, voluntary muscles, peripheral nerves, and kidneys.

Associated Chronic Disorders

CNV has been associated with certain connective tissue diseases, notably rheumatoid arthritis, Sjögren's syndrome, systemic lupus erythematous (SLE), and hypergammaglobulinemic purpura. It rarely occurs in mixed connective tissue disease, relapsing polychondritis, and scleroderma. In patients with rheumatoid arthritis and CNV, the development of vascular lesions is related to the severity of the disease, which is generally but not always seropositive. Subcutaneous nodules as well as cutaneous ulcers may be present. Patients with rheumatoid arthritis often have involvement of larger vessels with associated peripheral neuropathy, nail fold infarcts, and digital gangrene.

In patients with SLE, the vasculitis is associated with exacerbations of the underlying disease. Vasculitis, however, is rare in patients with subacute cutaneous lupus erythematosus.[18] Approximately 5 percent of women with necrotizing vasculitis without connective tissue disease have anti-Ro antibodies, and their infants may be born with neonatal lupus erythematosus.[19–21]

In patients with Sjögren's syndrome, the vascular lesions are located predominantly on the lower extremities and appear after exercise. Both hyperpigmentation and cutaneous ulcers are common features. Hypergammaglobulinemic purpura occurs in older women and may be associated with Sjögren's syndrome, SLE, or a lymphoproliferative disorder. Dermatomyositis in children, but not in adults, may be associated with systemic vasculitis, especially of the gastrointestinal tract.

Paraneoplastic vasculitis is a term used to describe CNV with associated malignant conditions, including Hodgkin's disease, lymphosarcoma, adult T cell leukemia, mycosis fungoides, myelofibrosis, acute and chronic myelogenous forms of leukemia, IgA myeloma, diffuse large cell leukemia, hairy cell leukemia, squamous cell bronchiogenic carcinoma, prostatic carcinoma, renal carcinoma, and colon carcinoma.

Cryoglobulins, especially mixed types II and III, may be found in patients with CNV and associated connective tissue diseases; lymphoproliferative disorders; and hepatitis A, B, and C virus infections. Cryoglobulins also occur in patients with idiopathic CNV, and CNV has been noted in patients with cystic fibrosis, inflammatory bowel diseases of the colon, and Behçet's disease.[22]

Both ANCAs and antiphospholipid antibodies have been associated with various forms of necrotizing vasculitis.[23] ANCAs are present in patients with microscopic polyangiitis and cutaneous vasculitis associated with hepatitis C virus infection.[24] The most common cutaneous feature in patients with ANCAs is palpable purpura. Microscopic polyangiitis is associated with small-vessel systemic vasculitis that also involves the skin, in which venules and arterioles are involved.[25] It is associated with necrotizing and crescentic glomerulonephritis and P-ANCAs with antimyeloperoxidase specificity.[1,25,26] A single male patient has experienced microscopic polyangiitis restricted to the skin and ANCAs for 20 years without progression to systemic vascular disease.[27]

Antiphospholipid antibodies, either anticardiolipin antibodies and/or lupus anticoagulant, occur in patients with autoimmune and connective tissue diseases and as an idiopathic disorder. Livedo reticularis is the most frequently recognized cutaneous finding.[28,29] Antiphospholipid antibodies of the IgA class were detected in 6 of 10 patients with idiopathic cutaneous necrotizing vasculitis,[30] and antiphospholipid antibodies have been detected in some individuals with livedoid vasculitis.[31] A female patient with antiphospholipid antibodies and cutaneous nodules that demonstrated vasculitis and thrombosis has been reported.[32]

Precipitating Infections and Drugs

Infections[33] and drugs precipitate episodes of CNV. The most commonly recognized infectious agents are group A hemolytic streptococci, *Staphylococcus aureus*, *Mycobacterium leprae*, and hepatitis B virus. Transient episodes of urticaria may occur early in the course of hepatitis B virus infection and represent immune complex–induced vasculitis; episodes of palpable purpura may occur in

FIGURE 176-1

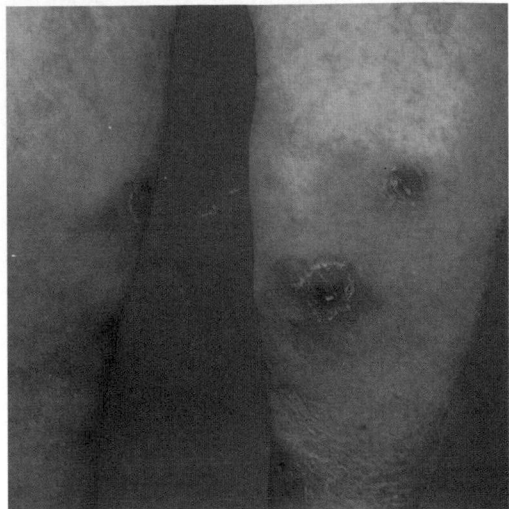

A.

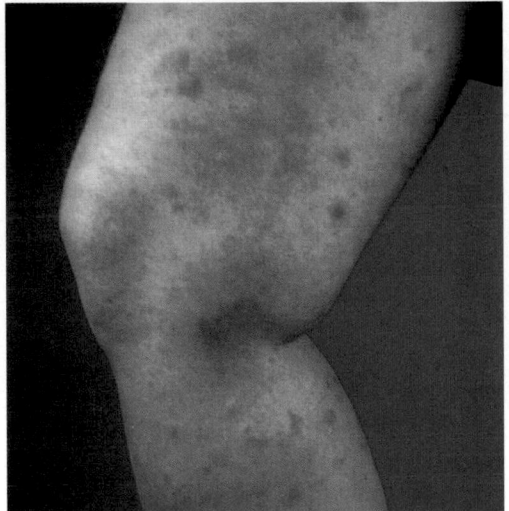

B.

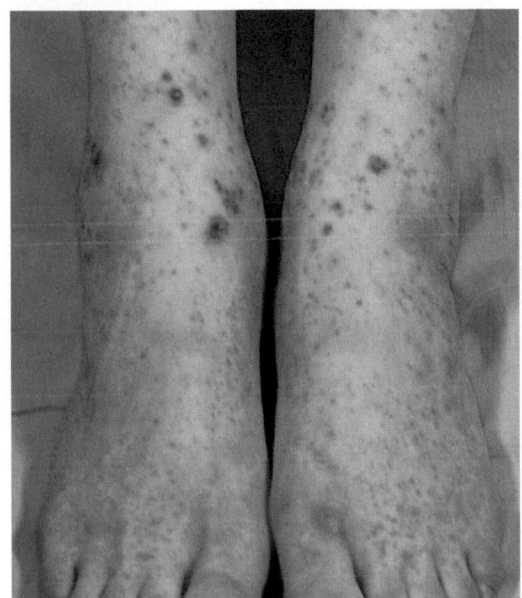

C.

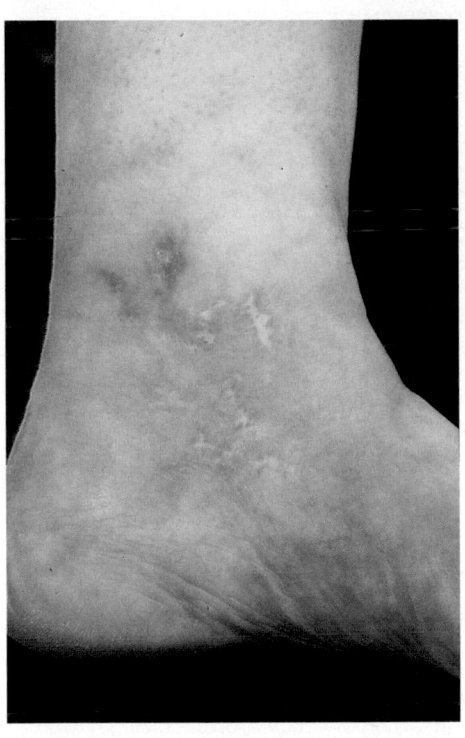

D.

A. Palpable purpura over the lower legs of a patient with Henoch-Schönlein syndrome. B. Idiopathic urticarial vasculitis over the leg. C. Nodular vasculitis over the feet and ankles. Note ulcers. D. Atrophie blanche over the medial malleolus with atrophic areas, telangiectases, punctate ulcers, and hyperpigmentation.

patients with chronic active hepatitis. Cutaneous vasculitis was identified in patients with hepatitis A and C infections[34–41] and cryoglobulins. HIV infection has been recognized in a limited number of individuals with cutaneous vasculitis,[42] including homosexual men, one girl who had received a transfusion, and one patient with a history of intravenous drug use. The skin lesions consisted of palpable purpura, at times with a follicular localization and cutaneous ulcers.

Erythema nodosum leprosum, which appears as cutaneous nodular lesions in lepromatous leprosy, is a form of necrotizing vasculitis involving capillaries, venules, arterioles, small- to medium-sized arteries, and veins. The vascular lesions, which occur spontaneously or are precipitated by the administration of chemotherapeutic agents, develop on the extremities, trunk, and face and may be accompanied by fever, malaise, arthralgias, lymphadenopathy, and polyneuritis.

Necrotizing vasculitis caused by the direct invasion of the blood vessel walls occurs with various microorganisms, such as in *Neisseria meningitidis* bacteremia, in Rocky Mountain spotted fever, and in infections localized at the site of a catheter.

Urticaria occurs in about 70 percent of patients with serum sickness after the administration of drugs; often a necrotizing vasculitis is present in skin biopsy specimens. Inasmuch as palpable purpura is one of the less common forms of drug reaction, the literature consists of case reports rather than of prospective or retrospective studies. The most frequently incriminated therapeutic agents are penicillin, sulfonamides, thiazides, allopurinol, phenytoins, and nonsteroidal anti-inflammatory agents. Propylthiouracil and hydralazine may cause vasculitis in association with ANCAs. Cutaneous vasculitis has occurred after the administration of streptokinase,[43] radiocontrast media, monoclonal antibodies, granulocyte colony-stimulating factor,[44,45] staphylococcal protein A column immuno-absorption therapy,[46] and drug additives,[47] and after exposure to fumes released from heat-activated photocopy paper.

Idiopathic Disorders

HENOCH-SCHÖNLEIN SYNDROME The most widely recognized subgroup of idiopathic CNV is the Henoch-Schönlein syndrome, formerly known as anaphylactoid purpura. It occurs predominantly in children, with a peak incidence at 5 years of age, but does occur in adults.[48] A history of a recent upper respiratory tract infection is obtained in up to 75 percent of individuals. One adult patient had associated *Helicobacter pylori* infection.[49] The syndrome includes involvement of the skin, synovia, gastrointestinal tract, and kidneys. The skin lesions of adults but not children may show blisters and necrosis. Endoscopic examination may demonstrate red, raised lesions, areas of intense redness, or ulcers, especially in the descending duodenum.[50,51] Long-term morbidity is from progressive renal disease and occurs in 5 percent of patients.[52] The spread of purpura to the upper parts of the trunk is a predictive factor for renal involvement.[48]

ACUTE HEMORRHAGIC EDEMA OF CHILDHOOD This uncommon disorder, which often goes unrecognized or has been confused with Henoch-Schönlein syndrome, affects infants and children less than 2 years of age, but it has been reported in one adult.[53] The lesions appear as painful, edematous petechiae and ecchymoses that affect the head and distal portions of the extremities.[54] Facial edema may be the initial sign. The skin lesions may be associated with a target-like appearance and may develop bullae[55] and necrosis. Infection, drugs, ingestion, or immunization may be triggering factors. Acute hemorrhagic edema of childhood is distinguished from Henoch-Schönlein syndrome by its occurrence in children aged 4 months to 2 years, lack of systemic features, and resolution within 1 to 3 weeks without sequelae.

URTICARIAL VASCULITIS Episodes of recurrent urticaria and angioedema may be a clinical manifestation of CNV.[56] Known as urticarial vasculitis, this edematous form of necrotizing venulitis occurs in patients with serum sickness, connective tissue disorders, an IgM_κ M component, infections, physical urticarias, and colon carcinoma; after the administration of potassium iodide, fluoxetine,[57] and nonsteroidal anti-inflammatory agents; and as an idiopathic disorder. Infections include hepatitis B and C[58] viruses and infectious mononucleosis. In the idiopathic group, the variety of skin lesions and systemic manifestations has led to a plethora of diagnostic appellations, such as atypical erythema multiforme, chronic urticaria as a manifestation of venulitis, unusual SLE-like syndrome, hypocomplementemic vasculitis, and hypocomplementemic-urticaria-vasculitis syndrome.

The skin lesions appear as erythematous, occasionally indurated, wheals (see Fig. 176-1*B*). Other skin manifestations include angioedema, macular erythema, foci of purpura in the wheals, livedo reticularis, nodules, and bullae. Although the individual urticarial lesions may last for less than 24 h, they often persist for up to 3 to 5 days. The lesions are pruritic or possess a burning or painful quality; they usually resolve without residua, although certain individuals develop hyperpigmentation. The episodes of urticaria are chronic, range in duration from months to years, and vary in frequency from daily to monthly. Approximately 70 percent of the afflicted individuals are women. The prevalence of this disorder remains unknown. General features include fever, malaise, and myalgia; the lymph nodes, liver, and spleen may be enlarged (Table 176-2).

Episodic arthralgias with associated stiffness are a major clinical manifestation and affect the elbows, wrists, fingers, knees, ankles, and toes. Arthritis with necrotizing venulitis apparent in biopsy specimens of the synovial tissue occasionally develops. It has been associated with Jaccoud's syndrome.[59] Renal involvement occurs as a diffuse glomerulitis or glomerulonephritis; however, progression to severe impairment of renal function is rare. Gastrointestinal tract manifestations include nausea, vomiting, diarrhea, and pain. The upper airway may be affected with laryngeal edema. Chronic obstructive pulmonary manifestations and interstitial lung disease may develop.[58] Conjunctivitis, episcleritis, and uveitis occur in some individuals. There is one report of an individual becoming blind. Central nervous system involvement occurs as headaches and pseudotumor cerebri (benign intracranial hypertension).

The natural history of urticarial vasculitis is unknown, although individuals have been described with historic episodes of cutaneous lesions for up to 25 years. In one series of patients followed for 1 year, 40 percent experienced complete resolution of skin lesions; in another series of individuals followed for as long as 14 years, resolution occurred in only one patient. Sjögren's syndrome and SLE have developed. Deaths have been reported from pulmonary disease, sepsis, and myocardial infarction.

Necrotizing vasculitis of cutaneous venules has been described in isolated instances of dermographism, cold urticaria,[60] delayed-pressure urticaria, solar urticaria, and exercise-induced urticaria.[9] However, the prevalence of necrotizing vasculitis in patients with physical urticaria is unknown, and the importance of this histologic finding for prognosis and therapy remains to be elucidated. Individuals with these physical urticarias have provided experimental

TABLE 176-2

Extracutaneous Manifestations of Urticarial Vasculitis

General features
  Fever
  Malaise
  Myalgia
Specific organ involvement
  Lymphadenopathy
  Hepatosplenomegaly
  Synovia (arthralgia, arthritis)
  Kidneys (glomerulitis, glomerulonephritis)
  Gastrointestinal tract (nausea, vomiting, pain, diarrhea)
  Respiratory tract (laryngeal edema, shortness of breath, chronic obstructive pulmonary disease)
  Eyes (conjunctivitis, episcleritis, uveitis)
  Central nervous system (headache, benign intracranial hypertension)

models for time-course studies of the evolution of necrotizing vasculitis in human skin.

Schnitzler's syndrome[61] consists of episodes of urticarial vasculitis that occur in association with a monoclonal IgM$_\kappa$ M component. Associated features include fever, lymphadenopathy, hepatosplenomegaly, bone pain, and a sensorimotor neuropathy.[62]

ERYTHEMA ELEVATUM DIUTINUM Erythema elevatum diutinum (see Chap. 94) presents as symmetric, persistent, red-purple or red-brown plaques that are predominantly disposed over the joints of extensor surfaces and over the gluteal area. Arthralgia of the associated joints may be a feature. Systemic manifestations are lacking. A history of recurrent streptococcal infections of the pharynx and sinuses is frequently obtained. This condition may be associated with IgA monoclonal gammopathy,[63] multiple myeloma, myelodysplasia,[64] celiac disease,[65] relapsing polychondritis,[66] and HIV infection.[67,68] Biopsy specimens of the acute lesions exhibit necrotizing venulitis; specimens of the chronic lesions exhibit fibrosis and an infiltrate containing macrophages.[69,70]

NODULAR VASCULITIS Nodular vasculitis (see Fig. 176-1C) occurs as recurrent, tender, red, subcutaneous nodules over the lower extremities, especially the calves, without systemic manifestations. At times lesions occur on the thighs, buttocks, trunk, and arms, and ulcerated nodules are present. It is more common in women and has a peak incidence in individuals between 30 and 40 years of age. Erythema induratum is a form of nodular vasculitis that has been associated with *M. tuberculosis*, as demonstrated by PCR amplification for *M. tuberculosis* DNA in skin biopsy specimens.[71,72] Various sizes of blood vessels including venules are affected in this disorder.[73]

LIVEDOID VASCULITIS This disorder (see Fig. 176-1D), also known as livedo reticularis with summer/winter ulceration, segmental hyalinizing vasculitis, and atrophie blanche, occurs in women as recurrent, painful ulcers of the lower extremities in association with a persistent livedo reticularis (*livedo racemosa*) that is often deep purple in color. Healing results in sclerotic pale areas surrounded by telangiectases that are designated *atrophie blanche*. Many patients have arteriosclerosis or stasis of the lower extremities. Livedoid vasculitis also may occur in patients with SLE who develop central nervous system features. Atrophie blanche, however, probably represents the end stage of a variety of forms of vascular damage in the skin. Blood fibrinopeptide A levels are elevated.[74] Pathogenesis has focused on the fibrin thrombi in the lumens of the superficial blood vessels. Some consider this condition a thrombogenic vasculopathy rather than a small-vessel vasculitis.[74] Antiphospholipid antibodies have been detected in a few individuals.[31]

Sneddon's syndrome[75,76] is a condition in which livedo reticularis and livedoid vasculitis are associated with ischemic cerebrovascular lesions, hypotension, and extracerebral arterial and venous thromboses. Antiendothelial cell antibodies were detected in the serum in 35 percent of individuals,[17] and antiphospholipid antibodies and anti-β_2-glycoprotein antibodies[77] were detected in some patients.

GENETIC COMPLEMENT DEFICIENCIES Genetic C2 deficiency has been recognized in association with CNV in three children and with C4 deficiency in one child. Deficiencies of C4a and C4b isotypes were found in some children and adults with Henoch-Schönlein syndrome. A partial C4b deficiency with allotyping C4a1,a3,b1 and a null allele B*QO was reported in a 51-year-old woman with CNV.[78]

EOSINOPHILIC VASCULITIS Eosinophilic vasculitis has been described as an idiopathic syndrome in three individuals with recurrent pruritic and purpuric papular skin lesions and angioedema.[79] Urticarial plaques and palpable purpura were also present. Skin biopsy specimens showed an infiltrate composed of eosinophils with VCAM-1 on endothelial cells of involved vessels. Eosinophilic vasculitis also has been described in some individuals with connective tissue disorders.[80]

IDIOPATHIC Some individuals with idiopathic CNV who do not meet the criteria for recognized idiopathic syndromes are listed as idiopathic.

LABORATORY FINDINGS

The laboratory evaluation of patients with CNV depends on information from the history and physical examination (Table 176-3). An elevated erythrocyte sedimentation rate is the most consistent abnormal laboratory finding. The platelet count is usually normal. Other abnormalities reflect either a coexistent underlying disorder or the involvement of additional organ systems. Occasionally, leukocytosis, anemia, thrombocytosis, an abnormal urine sediment, circulating immune complexes, rheumatoid factor, and antinuclear antibodies have been reported in idiopathic disease.

Serum complement levels are usually normal. Acquired hypocomplementemia may develop in patients with concomitant connective tissue diseases or cryoglobulinemia. Rheumatoid factor may be present in serum. In these instances, the complement abnormalities reflect the associated disease or the composition of the cryoglobulin. Hypocomplementemia also occurs in some individuals with idiopathic CNV and in 40 percent of individuals with urticarial vasculitis.

In rheumatoid arthritis with CNV, serum levels of the early complement components C1, C4, and C2 are reduced, and IgM with a sedimentation coefficient of 7S has been noted. In patients with SLE and CNV, there may be low serum levels of C1q, C4, C2, C3b, and C9. In Sjögren's syndrome with CNV, complement abnormalities reflect the presence and nature of the associated cryoglobulin.

TABLE 176-3

Laboratory Evaluation of Cutaneous Necrotizing Venulitis

Erythrocyte sedimentation rate
White cell count with differential analysis
Platelet count
Urinalysis
24-h urine protein and creatinine clearance
Blood chemistry profile
Serum protein electrophoresis
Hepatitis B antigens and hepatitis A and C antibodies
Cryoglobulins
CH50
Antinuclear antibody
Rheumatoid factor
Antineutrophil cytoplasmic antibodies
Antiphospholipid antibodies
Circulating immune complexes
Skin biopsy

In some patients with urticarial vasculitis and hypocomplementemia, a low molecular weight 7S C1q precipitin identified as an IgG autoantibody against the collagen-like region of C1q was detected.[81] In Henoch-Schönlein syndrome, serum IgA₁ levels are elevated.[82] Various types of putative circulating immune complexes have been described. IgG autoantibodies against IgE also have been identified in four of eight patients with urticarial vasculitis and normal serum IgE levels.

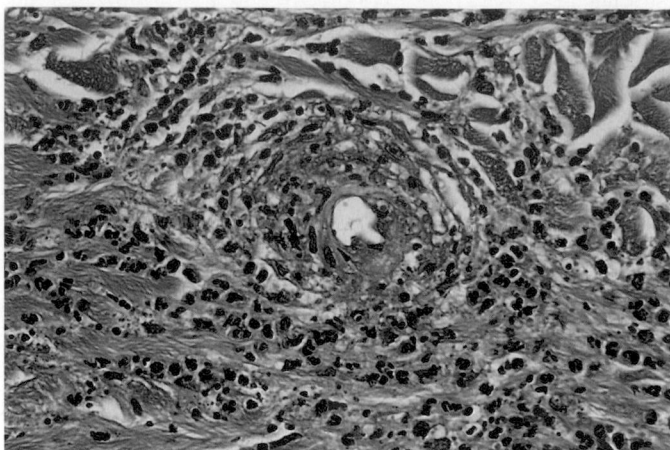

A.

PATHOLOGY

In routinely prepared skin biopsy specimens of palpable purpura and urticarial vasculitis stained with hematoxylin-eosin (Fig. 176-2A), the histologic criteria requisite for the diagnosis of CNV include necrosis of the blood vessels with the deposition of fibrinoid material and dermal cellular infiltrates that consist of various numbers of neutrophils with nuclear debris, mononuclear cells, and extravasated erythrocytes. The dermal inflammatory infiltrates vary in intensity and are usually perivenular in location but at times are dispersed widely. The fibrinoid material consists predominantly of fibrin but also contains necrotic endothelial cells and deposited immunoreactants.

Studies with 1-μm sections (Fig. 176-2B) of lesional skin show two distinct cellular patterns in CNV—one rich in neutrophils and the other in lymphocytes. Neither pattern appears to be the result of evolution of the tissue changes with the dynamic nature of the inflammatory infiltrate. In a time-course study over 6 days of the evolution of experimental human CNV in a patient with physical urticarias, the number of infiltrating neutrophils decreased without a concomitant increase in lymphocytes, although the number of monocyte-macrophages was increased at 48 and 72 h. Other features in both cell patterns include hypogranulated mast cells, macrophages containing debris, and the perivenular and interstitial deposition of fibrin. Venular alterations in both cell patterns consist of endothelial cell swelling, activation of nuclei, wrinkling of nuclear membranes, necrosis (Fig. 176-2B), and basement membrane reduplication and thickening. The arterioles are not affected. Some patients with connective tissue disorders and cutaneous vasculitis have an inflammatory infiltrate composed predominantly of eosinophils with deposited major basic protein and decreased numbers of mast cells.[80]

Ultrastructural studies of CNV have shown endothelial alterations consisting of interendothelial cell gaps and pinocytotic activity. Also observed were thickening of the basement membrane and coating of collagen fibers with fibrillar material interpreted to be fibrin. The membrane-attack complex, C5b-9, has been localized by ultrastructural study to the surface of the endothelial cells and infiltrating neutrophils.

By direct immunofluorescence techniques, fibrin deposition in venules has been identified routinely in biopsy specimens of skin lesions, whereas the deposition of immunoglobulins and complement proteins has varied widely. When present in lesions, immunoglobulins and C3 were occasionally detected in adjacent, clinically uninvolved skin. IgG is the most commonly deposited immunoglobulin, although IgM and IgA have also been detected. IgA is deposited about blood vessels in the skin, intestine, and kidney in the Henoch-Schönlein syndrome and has become an immunopathologic marker of this condition.[83] In the skin, IgA is depos-

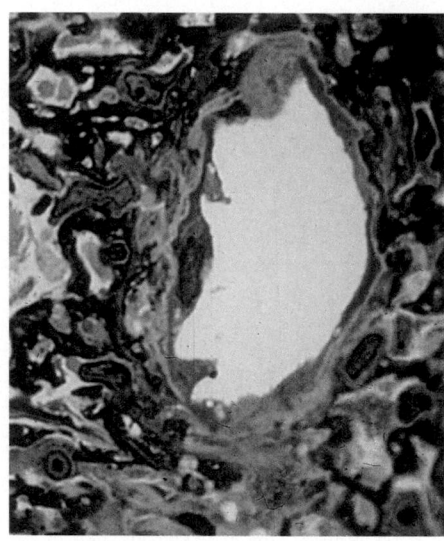

B.

A. Perivenular infiltrate of neutrophils with fibrin deposition. *B.* Endothelial cell necrosis of venule with perivenular fibrin and neutrophils. 1-μm section, Giemsa.

ited with equal frequency in clinically normal and lesional sites. C3 is the only complement protein that has been sought with any frequency. In some lesions, it has been possible to identify bacterial or viral antigens, including streptococcal, staphylococcal, mycobacterial, and hepatitis B virus, combined into complexes with immunoglobulins and complement.

DIAGNOSIS AND DIFFERENTIAL DIAGNOSIS

Thrombocytopenia may result in purpura; however, these lesions are flat. Other causes of nonpalpable cutaneous purpura include local trauma to the skin of aged individuals with vascular fragility, chronic sun exposure, and endogenous or iatrogenic hypercorticism. Erythema elevatum diutinum may resemble Kaposi's sarcoma. Scurvy may appear as hemorrhagic follicular papules over the lower extremities. Various infectious agents may be associated with hemorrhagic skin lesions that arise from disseminated intravascular coagulation or septic emboli. The cutaneous manifestations of disseminated intravascular coagulation appear as extensive areas of purpura with a slate-gray color and may or may not be palpable. These lesions, often called *purpura fulminans*, are seen especially in patients with acute meningococcemia; skin biopsy specimens show thrombosis but not necrotizing venulitis. Septic emboli occur as finite numbers of hemorrhagic pustules, papules, and vesicles that are distributed over acral areas in gonococcemia, for example. Rarely, certain echo- and coxsackievirus infections cause purpuric papules. Rocky Mountain spotted fever typically begins as purpuric papules over the ankles and wrists that spread to include the trunk. Cholesterol embolization includes purpura, livedo reticularis, ulcers, and nodules.

The progressive pigmentary purpuric dermatoses (*purpura simplex*) include a number of disorders that share similar clinical and histologic features. The common clinical findings are macular, petechial, pigmented, or lichenoid lesions. The lesions occur on the lower extremities but may also be present on the trunk and upper extremities. In Schamberg's disease, pigment predominates in the center of the lesion and red puncta are located at the periphery. Purpura annularis telangiectodes (Majocchi's disease) is characterized by annular lesions with telangiectases at the periphery. Lichenoid papules in addition to purpura are noted in pigmented purpuric lichenoid dermatitis of Gougerot and Blum. A rare form is lichen aureus, which is characterized by yellow lichenoid papules. The biopsy specimens show an infiltrate of lymphocytes with extravasated erythrocytes and hemosiderin deposition around the capillaries of the papillary dermis. The endothelial cells are enlarged, but necrosis and fibrin deposition are absent.

The differential diagnosis of cutaneous nodules includes erythema nodosum, panniculitis, superficial forms of thrombophlebitis, fat necrosis associated with pancreatic disease, and systemic vasculitides such as polyarteritis nodosa, Wegener's granulomatosis, and Churg-Strauss syndrome.

TREATMENT

Therapeutic approaches may be divided into removal of the antigen, treatment of an underlying disease, and treatment of the CNV. Treatment of necrotizing vasculitis consists of preventing the deposition of immune complexes, suppressing the inflammatory response, modulating underlying immunopathologic mechanisms, and empiric and miscellaneous therapy. When the eruption is associated with a precipitating event, withdrawal of the medication or treatment of the infection results in resolution of the cutaneous lesions. If a coexistent chronic disease is present, treatment of the underlying disease may be associated with improvement in the cutaneous vascular lesions.

The treatment of CNV can be divided into two phases (Table 176-4), each of which depends on an analysis of the cutaneous disability as well as the toxicity and side effects of the therapeutic agents. H_1 antihistamines are used in patients with palpable purpura to alleviate lesional symptoms and perhaps to prevent tissue deposition of circulating immune complexes. Nonsteroidal anti-inflammatory agents are combined with the H_1 antihistamine. Depending on the therapeutic response, colchicine or hydroxychloroquine sulfate can be added to or substituted for these agents. If there is no benefit, dapsone should be used. If there is still no therapeutic response, a major decision must be made, since the medications to

TABLE 176-4

Algorithm for Treatment of Cutaneous Necrotizing Venulitis

Phase one
  H_1 antihistamines
  Nonsteroidal anti-inflammatory agents
  Colchicine
  Hydroxychloroquine sulfate
  Dapsone
Phase two
  Systemic glucocorticoids
  Azathioprine
  Cyclophosphamide
  Intravenous gamma globulin
  Cyclosporine
  Plasmapheresis

be considered in the second phase, systemic glucocorticoids,[84] azathioprine, cyclophosphamide, plasmapheresis, and cyclosporine,[85] are associated with more serious side effects. Although all of these agents have been reported to benefit some patients, controlled clinical trials are not available except with colchicine, which had no significant therapeutic effect in a prospective, randomized controlled trial.[86] The administration of interferon-α has been associated with clearing of cutaneous vasculitis in patients with hepatitis C virus infection.[87] High-dose intravenous immunoglobulin therapy was associated with improvement in Henoch-Schönlein syndrome.[88]

The treatment of urticarial vasculitis is similar to that of palpable purpura. H_1 antihistamines may be administered to alleviate the pruritus. Both skin and joint manifestations may respond to indomethacin. The oral administration of systemic glucocorticoids may relieve the urticaria, uveitis, episcleritis, abdominal pain, arthritis, and renal disease. Isolated reports exist on the treatment of patients with colchicine, hydroxychloroquine, dapsone, methotrexate,[89] intramuscular gold therapy, and cyclophosphamide.

In patients with erythema elevatum diutinum, dapsone is the drug of choice. Plasma exchange plus chlorambucil was a successful treatment in one individual with erythema elevatum diutinum and a monoclonal IgA paraprotein.[90] The treatment of nodular vasculitis consists of empirical trials of a variety of therapeutic agents including a saturated solution of potassium iodide, nonsteroidal anti-inflammatory drugs, colchicine, and systemic glucocorticoids. Thalidomide is the treatment of choice for erythema nodosum leprosum.

In the treatment of livedoid vasculitis, empirical trials of aspirin and dipyridamole, colchicine, low-dose heparin, systemic glucocorticoids, nicotinic acid, low molecular weight dextran, phenphormin and ethylestranol, nifedipine,[91] and pentoxifylline are used.[91] Low-dose recombinant tissue plasminogen activator therapy was reported to be successful in one study[92] but not in another.[93] Infusions of prostacyclin[94] and of prostaglandin E_1[95] have been used successfully in one patient each.

Successful treatment of common variable immunodeficiency and concomitant cutaneous vasculitis with intravenous immunoglobulin was reported in a single patient.[96]

REFERENCES

1. Jeanette JC et al: Nomenclature of systemic vasculitides: Proposal of an international consensus conference. *Arthritis Rheum* **37**:187, 1994

2. Leavitt RY, Fauci AS: Polyangiitis overlap syndrome: Classification and prospective experience. *Am J Med* **81**:79, 1986

3. Carmichael AJ, Marsden JR: Urticarial vasculitis: A presentation of C3 nephritic factor. *Br J Dermatol* **128**:589, 1993

4. Durand JM et al: Cutaneous vasculitis in a patient infected with hepatitis C virus: Detection of hepatitis C virus RNA in the skin by polymerase chain reaction. *Br J Dermatol* **128**:359, 1993

5. Ghersetich I et al: γ/δ TCR lymphocytes in cutaneous necrotizing vasculitis (CNV): A clue to the infective etiology. *J Invest Dermatol* **100**:465, 1993

6. Ghersetich I et al: Immunohistochemical and ultrastructural aspects of leukocytoclastic cutaneous necrotizing vasculitis (CNV). *J Invest Dermatol* **100**:545, 1993

7. Wedi B et al: Modulation of intercellular adhesion molecule-1 (ICAM-1) expression on the human mast cell line (HMC-1) by inflammatory mediators. *Allergy* **51**:676, 1996

8. Soter NA et al: Cutaneous necrotizing vasculitis: A sequential analysis of the morphological alterations occurring after mast cell degranulation in a patient with a unique syndrome. *Clin Exp Immunol* **32**:46, 1978

9. Kano Y et al: Cellular and molecular dynamics in exercise-induced urticarial vasculitis lesions. *Arch Dermatol* **134**:62, 1998

10. Norris P et al: The expression of endothelial leukocyte adhesion molecule-1 (ELAM-1), intercellular adhesion molecule-1 (ICAM-1), and vascular cell adhesion molecule-1 (VCAM-1) in experimental cutaneous inflammation. *J Invest Dermatol* **96**:763, 1991

11. Rohde D et al: Infiltration of both T cells and neutrophils in the skin is accompanied by the expression of endothelial leukocyte adhesion molecule-1 (ELAM-1). *J Invest Dermatol* **98**:794, 1992

12. Sais G et al: Adhesion molecule expression and endothelial cell activation in cutaneous leukocytoclastic vasculitis: An immunohistologic and clinical study of 42 patients. *Arch Dermatol* **133**:443, 1997

13. Jurd KM et al: Endothelial cell activation in cutaneous vasculitis. *Clin Exp Dermatol* **21**:28, 1996

14. Jennette C et al: Do antineutrophil cytoplasmic autoantibodies cause Wegener's granulomatosis and other forms of necrotizing vasculitis? *Rheumatol Clin North Am* **19**:1, 1993

15. Damianovich M et al: Pathogenic role of anti-endothelial cell antibodies in vasculitis: An idiotypic experimental model. *J Immunol* **156**:4946, 1996

16. Chan TM et al: Clinical significance of anti-endothelial cell antibodies in systemic vasculitis: A longitudinal study comparing anti-endothelial cell antibodies and anti-neutrophil cytoplasm antibodies. *Am J Kidney Dis* **22**:387, 1993

17. Francès C et al: Prevalence of anti-endothelial cell antibodies in patients with Sneddon's syndrome. *J Am Acad Dermatol* **33**:64, 1995

18. Sanchez-Perez J et al: Leukocytoclastic vasculitis in subacute cutaneous lupus erythematosus. *Br J Dermatol* **128**:469, 1993

19. Waltuck J, Buyon JP: Autoantibody-associated congenital heart block: Outcome in mothers and children. *Ann Intern Med* **120**:544, 1994

20. DeArgila D et al: Cutaneous vasculitis with anti-Ro SSA antibodies not associated to connective-tissue disease. *Acta Dermatol Venereol (Stockh)* **86**:499, 1995

21. Borrego L et al: Neonatal lupus erythematosus related to maternal leukocytoclastic vasculitis. *Pediatr Dermatol* **14**:221, 1997

22. Chen K-R et al: Cutaneous vasculitis in Behçet's disease: A clinical and histopathologic study of 20 patients. *J Am Acad Dermatol* **36**:689, 1997

23. Burrows NP, Lockwood CM: Antineutrophil cytoplasmic antibodies and their relevance to the dermatologist. *Br J Dermatol* **132**:173, 1995

24. Romani J et al: Detection of antineutrophil cytoplasmic antibodies in patients with hepatitis C virus-induced cutaneous vasculitis with mixed cryoglobulinemia. *Arch Dermatol* **132**:974, 1996

25. Homas PB et al: Microscopic polyarteritis: Report of a case with cutaneous involvement and antimyeloperoxidase antibodies. *Arch Dermatol* **128**:1223, 1992

26. Peñas PF et al: Microscopic polyangiitis: A systemic vasculitis with a positive P-ANCA. *Br J Dermatol* **134**:542, 1996

27. Irvine AD et al: Microscopic polyangiitis: Delineation of a cutaneous-limited variant associated with antimyeloperoxidase autoantibody. *Arch Dermatol* **133**:474, 1997

28. Naldi L et al: Cutaneous manifestations associated with antiphospholipid antibodies in patients with suspected primary antiphospholipid syndrome: A case-controlled study. *Ann Rheum Dis* **52**:219, 1993

29. Nahass GT: Antiphospholipid antibodies and the antiphospholipid syndrome. *J Am Acad Dermatol* **36**:149, 1997

30. Burden AD et al: IgA class anticardiolipin antibodies in cutaneous leukocytoclastic vasculitis. *J Am Acad Dermatol* **35**:411, 1996

31. Stephansson EA, Scheynius A: Immunological studies of cutaneous vasculitis and primary antiphospholipid syndrome. *Eur J Dermatol* **3**:289, 1993

32. Renfro L et al: Painful nodules in a young female. *Arch Dermatol* **128**:847, 1992

33. Somer T, Finegold SM: Vasculitides associated with infections, immunization, and antimicrobial drugs. *Clin Infect Dis* **20**:1010, 1995

34. Marcellin P et al: Cryoglobulinemia with vasculitis associated with hepatitis C virus infection. *Gastroenterology* **104**:272, 1993

35. Pakula AS et al: Cryoglobulinemia and cutaneous leukocytoclastic vasculitis associated with hepatitis C virus infection. *J Am Acad Dermatol* **28**:850, 1993

36. Revenga Arranz F et al: Cryoglobulinemic vasculitis associated with hepatitis C infection. *Acta Derm Venereol (Stockh)* **75**:234, 1995

37. Karlsberg PA et al: Cutaneous vasculitis and rheumatoid factor positivity as presenting signs of hepatitis C virus-induced mixed cryoglobulinemia. *Arch Dermatol* **131**:1119, 1995

38. Dupin N et al: Essential mixed cryoglobulinemia: A comparative study of dermatologic manifestations in patients infected or noninfected with hepatitis C virus. *Arch Dermatol* **131**:1124, 1995

39. Pawlotsky J-M et al: Hepatitis C virus in dermatology: A review. *Arch Dermatol* **131**:1185, 1995

40. Daoud MS et al: Chronic hepatitis C, cryoglobulinemia, and cutaneous necrotizing vasculitis: Clinical, pathologic, and immunopathologic study of twelve patients. *J Am Acad Dermatol* **34**:219, 1996

41. Abe Y et al: Leukocytoclastic vasculitis associated with mixed cryoglobulinaemia and hepatitis C infection. *Br J Dermatol* **136**:272, 1997

42. Watkins KV, Ittman MM: Necrotizing vasculitis in a patient with acquired immunodeficiency syndrome. *J Oral Maxillofac Surg* **50**:1003, 1992

43. Lantin JP et al: Anaphylactoid purpura-like vasculitis following fibrinolytic therapy: Role of the immune response to streptokinase. *Clin Exp Rheumatol* **12**:429, 1994

44. Jain KK: Cutaneous vasculitis associated with granulocyte colony-stimulating factor. *J Am Acad Dermatol* **31**:213, 1994

45. Johnson ML, Grimwood RE: Leukocyte colony-stimulating factors: A review of associated neutrophilic dermatoses and vasculitides. *Arch Dermatol* **130**:77, 1994

46. Arbiser JL et al: Leukocytoclastic vasculitis following staphylococcal protein A column immunoabsorption therapy: Two cases and a review of the literature. *Arch Dermatol* **131**:707, 1995

47. Lowry MD et al: Leukocytoclastic vasculitis caused by drug additives. *J Am Acad Dermatol* **30**:854, 1994

48. Tancrede-Bohin E et al: Henoch-Schönlein purpura in adult patients: Predictive factors for IgA glomerulonephritis in a retrospective study of 57 cases. *Arch Dermatol* **133**:438, 1997

49. Reinauer S et al: Schönlein-Henoch purpura associated with gastric *Helicobacter pylori* infection. *J Am Acad Dermatol* **33**:876, 1995

50. Kato S et al: Gastrointestinal endoscopy in Henoch-Schönlein purpura. *Eur J Pediatr* **11**:482, 1992

51. Jeong YK et al: Gastrointestinal involvement in Henoch-Schönlein syndrome: CT findings. *Am J Roentgenol* **168**:965, 1997

52. Goldstein AR et al: Long-term follow-up of childhood Henoch-Schönlein nephritis. *Lancet* **339**:280, 1992

53. Cribier B et al: Cutaneous vasculitis with edema: Acute hemorrhagic edema of the skin in an adult? *Eur J Dermatol* **5**:286, 1995

54. Tomaç N et al: Acute haemorrhagic oedema of infancy: A case report. *Clin Exp Dermatol* **21**:217, 1996

55. Ince E et al: Infantile acute hemorrhagic edema: A variant of leukocytoclastic vasculitis. *Pediatr Dermatol* **12**:224, 1995

56. Mehregan DR et al: Urticarial vasculitis: A histopathologic and clinical review of 72 cases. *J Am Acad Dermatol* **26**:441, 1992

57. Roger D et al: Urticarial vasculitis induced by fluoxetine. *Dermatology* **191**:164. 1995

58. Lin RY et al: Hypocomplementaemic urticarial vasculitis, interstitial lung disease and hepatitis C. *Br J Dermatol* **132**:821, 1995

59. Ishikawa O et al: Hypocomplementaemic urticarial vasculitis associated with Jaccoud's syndrome. *Br J Dermatol* **137**:804, 1997

60. Demierre M-F, Winkelmann WJ: Idiopathic cold-induced urticarial vasculitis and monoclonal IgG gammopathy. *Int J Dermatol* **35**:151, 1996

61. Baty V et al: Schnitzler's syndrome: Two case reports and review of the literature. *Mayo Clin Proc* **70**:570, 1995

62. Lebbe C et al: Schnitzler's syndrome associated with sensorimotor neuropathy. *J Am Acad Dermatol* **30**:316, 1994
63. Yiannias JA et al: Erythema elevatum diutinum: A clinical and histopathologic study of 13 patients. *J Am Acad Dermatol* **26**:38, 1992
64. Oueipo de Llano MP et al: Myelodysplastic syndrome in association with erythema elevatum diutinum. *J Rheumatol* **19**:1005, 1992
65. Rodriguez-Serna M et al: Erythema elevatum diutinum associated with coeliac disease: Response to a gluten-free diet. *Pediatr Dermatol* **10**:125, 1993
66. Bernard P et al: Erythema elevatum diutinum in a patient with relapsing polychondritis. *J Am Acad Dermatol* **26**:312, 1992
67. LeBoit PE, Cockerell CJ: Nodular lesions of erythema elevatum diutinum in patients infected with human immunodeficiency virus. *J Am Acad Dermatol* **28**:919, 1993
68. Dronda F et al: Erythema elevatum diutinum in human immunodeficiency virus-infected patients: Report of a case and review of the literature. *Clin Exp Dermatol* **21**:222, 1996
69. Wilkinson SM et al: Erythema elevatum diutinum: A clinicopathological study. *Clin Exp Dermatol* **17**:87, 1992
70. Sangüeza OP et al: Erythema elevatum diutinum: A clinicopathological study of eight cases. *Am J Dermatopathol* **19**:214, 1997
71. Schneider JW et al: Erythema induratum of Bazin: A clinicopathological study of 20 cases and detection of *Mycobacterium tuberculosis* DNA in skin lesions by polymerase chain reaction. *Am J Dermatopathol* **17**:357, 1995
72. Baselga E et al: Detection of *Mycobacterium tuberculosis* DNA in lobular granulomatous panniculitis (erythema induratum-nodular vasculitis). *Arch Dermatol* **133**:457, 1997
73. Schneider JW et al: The histopathologic spectrum of erythema induratum of Bazin. *Am J Dermatopathol* **19**:323, 1997
74. McCalmont CS et al: Livedo vasculitis: Vasculitis or thrombotic vasculopathy? *Clin Exp Dermatol* **17**:4, 1992
75. Zelger B et al: Life history of cutaneous vascular lesions in Sneddon's syndrome. *Hum Pathol* **23**:668, 1992
76. Zelger B et al: Sneddon's syndrome: A long-term follow-up of 21 patients. *Arch Dermatol* **129**:437, 1993
77. Francès C et al: Anti-β2 glycoprotein in Sneddon's syndrome. *Dermatology* **186**:273, 1993
78. Lilic D, Carmichael AJ: Cutaneous vasculitis with partial C4 deficiency responsive to dapsone. *Br J Dermatol* **137**:467, 1997
79. Chen K-R et al: Recurrent cutaneous necrotizing eosinophilic vasculitis. *Arch Dermatol* **130**:1159, 1994
80. Chen K-R et al: Eosinophilic vasculitis in connective-tissue diseases. *J Am Acad Dermatol* **35**:173, 1996
81. Wisnieski JJ, Jones SM: IgG autoantibody to the collagen-like region of C1q in hypocomplementemic urticarial vasculitis syndrome, systemic lupus erythematosus, and 6 other musculoskeletal or rheumatic diseases. *J Rheumatol* **19**:884, 1992
82. Saulsbury FT: Heavy and light chain composition of serum IgA and IgA rheumatoid factor in Henoch-Schönlein purpura. *Arthritis Rheum* **35**:1377, 1992
83. Helander SD et al: Henoch-Schönlein purpura: Clinicopathologic correlation of cutaneous vascular IgA deposits and the relationship to leukocytoclastic vasculitis. *Acta Dermatol Venereol (Stockh)* **75**:125, 1995
84. Cupps TR et al: Chronic, recurrent small-vessel cutaneous vasculitis: Clinical experience in 13 patients. *JAMA* **247**:1994, 1992
85. Tosca AD et al: Cyclosporin A in the treatment of cutaneous vasculitis: Clinical and cellular effects. *J Eur Acad Dermatol Venereol* **6**:135, 1996
86. Sais G et al: Colchicine in the treatment of cutaneous leukocytoclastic vasculitis: Results of a prospective, randomized controlled trial. *Arch Dermatol* **131**:1399, 1995
87. Misiani R et al: Interferon alfa-2a therapy in cryoglobulinemia associated with hepatitis C virus. *N Engl J Med* **330**:751, 1994
88. Rostoker G et al: High-dose immunoglobulin therapy for severe IgA nephropathy and Henoch-Schönlein purpura. *Ann Intern Med* **120**:476, 1994
89. Stack PS: Methotrexate for urticarial vasculitis. *Ann Allergy* **72**:36, 1994
90. Chow RKP et al: Erythema elevatum diutinum associated with IgA paraproteinemia successfully controlled with intermittent plasma exchange. *Arch Dermatol* **132**:1360, 1996
91. Nikolova K et al: Leg ulcerations due to livedo vasculitis: Successful combined therapy with pentoxifylline and nifedipine. *J Eur Acad Dermatol Venereol* **5**:54, 1995
92. Klein KL, Pittelkow MR: Tissue plasminogen activator for treatment of livedoid vasculitis. *Mayo Clin Proc* **67**:923, 1992
93. Murrell DF et al: Failure of livedoid vasculitis to respond to tissue plasminogen activator. *Arch Dermatol* **131**:231, 1995
94. Hoogenberg K et al: Successful treatment of ulcerating livedo reticularis with infusions of prostacyclin. *Br J Dermatol* **127**:64, 1992
95. Uchida M et al: Successful treatment of ulcerating livedo vasculitis with infusions of prostaglandin E₁. *Eur J Dermatol* **5**:365, 1995
96. Sais G et al: Leukocytoclastic vasculitis and common variable immunodeficiency: Successful treatment with intravenous immunoglobulin. *J Allergy Clin Immunol* **98**:232, 1996

CHAPTER 177

Lynn A. Cornelius
Thomas J. Lawley

Cryoglobulinemia and Cryofibrinogenemia

CRYOGLOBULINEMIA

Cryoglobulins are circulating immunoglobulins complexed with other immunoglobulins or proteins that reversibly precipitate in the cold. The symptoms of type I cryoglobulinemia are caused by vascular occlusion resulting from protein precipitation; mixed cryoglobulinemia (type II or type III) is an immune complex disease (see below).

The existence of cryoproteinemia as a clinical entity was first noted by Wintrobe and Buell in 1933.[1] The immunoglobulin composition of these cryoproteins was recognized by Waldenström in

1943.[2] Four years later, Lerner and Watson[3] performed the first large-scale examination of pathologic sera for cryoglobulins and found them in 11 percent of the sera examined.

Classification

The classification of cryoglobulinemia consists of three distinct groups initially described by Brouet et al.[4] based on immunoglobulin type. Type I cryoglobulins consist of a single monoclonal immunoglobulin, usually an IgG or an IgM. Patients with type I cryoglobulinemia usually have an underlying B cell malignancy such as multiple myeloma or a B cell lymphoma. Type II and type III cryoglobulins consist of rheumatoid factors (usually IgM) complexed with IgG and thus constitute immune complexes. Type II cryoglobulins are single monoclonal immunoglobulins (usually IgG). Type III cryoglobulins are polyclonal immunoglobulins that form cryoprecipitates with polyclonal IgG or a nonimmunoglobulin serum component. Types I, II, and III cryoglobulins may be associated with various disease states (Table 177-1).

Isolation Techniques

The isolation and characterization of cryoglobulins are described in detail by Gorevic.[5] In brief, cryoproteins are isolated from blood that has clotted at 37°C. Most type I cryoprecipitates will be evident within 24 h, whereas mixed type III cryoglobulins may require several days of cold incubation for precipitation. Therefore, it is important to hold serum for approximately 1 week before final determination is made of the presence of a cryoprecipitate. The reversibility of the formation of the serum cryoprecipitate is confirmed through rewarming to 37°C. The cryoprecipitate is purified by repeated washing and low-speed cold centrifugation. Of note is that cryoglobulins may become associated with serum lipids and remain suspended during centrifugation, thereby obscuring the formation of a visible precipitate.[6]

The concentration of cryoglobulins may be expressed as a percentage of the volume of the total collected serum, milligrams per milliliter, or as a cryocrit. Type I cryoglobulins are typically present in concentrations greater than 5 mg/mL. In contrast, type III cryoglobulins are usually present in lesser amounts, i.e., cryocrits less than 1 percent.[7] Alternatively, quantitation may be accomplished by determining the protein concentration of the dissolved cryoprecipitate. A method for rapid cryoglobulin screening has been described[8]; this method uses centrifugation, incubation of paired se-

TABLE 177-1

Selected Diseases Associated with Cryoglobulins

CRYOGLOBULIN	DISEASE STATE
Type I	Multiple myeloma, chronic lymphocytic leukemia, Waldenström's macroglobulinemia
Type II	Multiple myeloma, Waldenström's macroglobulinemia, chronic lymphocytic leukemia, rheumatoid arthritis, Sjögren's syndrome, hepatitis C
Type III	Systemic lupus erythematosus, rheumatoid arthritis, Sjögren's syndrome, infectious mononucleosis, cytomegalovirus infections, biliary cirrhosis, hepatitis B, hepatitis C

rum samples at 37°C and 4°C for 1 h, and comparison of optical densities via spectrophotometry of the sera held at the two temperatures. Symptom severity may reflect cryoprotein concentration in the serum as well as the temperature at which cryoprecipitation takes place; some reports, however, have described dramatic clinical symptoms at relatively low cryoglobulin concentrations.[9] The components of the cryoprecipitate are identified by use of specific antibodies against suspected protein components such as immunoglobulin, complement, or viral antigen.

Cryoglobulin Characteristics

TYPE I MONOCLONAL CRYOGLOBULINS Type I cryoglobulins are monoclonal immunoglobulins, typically IgM or IgG, although IgA and Bence Jones proteins have been identified. In a review of 86 patients with cryoglobulinemia, Brouet et al.[4] reported that 25 percent of patients had only monoclonal cryoglobulins. Further characterization of these cryoglobulins revealed a predominance of IgM immunoglobulin. IgG and IgM light chain types did not differ significantly from normal serum immunoglobulin types with respect to specific immunoglobulin characteristics. Amino acid abnormalities as well as changes in the composition of carbohydrate side chains have been noted in monoclonal as well as in mixed cryoglobulins.[10] The carbohydrate abnormalities have been hypothesized to contribute to the decreased solubility of the immunoglobulins.[11] However, such abnormalities are not invariably found, and the precipitation of cryoglobulins most likely results from varied interactions of the constituent molecules at decreased temperatures.[12] The large molecular size of IgM monoclonal cryoglobulins may predispose these immunoglobulins to precipitation; in fact, it has been postulated that, in some instances, cryoprecipitation may be an extension of normal immunoglobulin solubility.[13] In certain monoclonal IgG cryoprecipitates, the cryoprecipitate determinant resides in the variable region of the immunoglobulin, since the activity may be retained in the F(ab')2 fragment.[5]

Some idiotypic relatedness may exist among monoclonal IgG cryoglobulins; the finding in one study of cross-reactivity among 5 of 15 IgG cryoglobulins suggested similar variable region structures and, possibly, antigenic specificities.[14] Complement components are not routinely found as components of type I cryoprecipitates.

MIXED CRYOGLOBULINS Type II cryoglobulins consist of two immunoglobulin components, one of which is monoclonal. The most common composition is that of a monoclonal IgM rheumatoid factor complexed with a polyclonal IgG. Although the serum concentration of type II cryoglobulin is often very high, a typical monoclonal spike is not always apparent on immunoelectrophoresis. IgG monoclonal rheumatoid factors are identified in about 10 percent of cases with type II cryoglobulinemia, and IgA monoclonal rheumatoid factors are rare. Some evidence suggests that there is an increased prevalence of kappa light chains in the monoclonal IgM, and that the monoclonal IgM has restricted specificity for IgG.

The most common type (approximately 50 percent) of cryoglobulins identified are type III mixed cryoglobulins. These cryoglobulins usually occur in low concentration and consist of polyclonal immunoglobulin complexes or polyclonal immunoglobulin–nonimmunoglobulin cryoprecipitates. These cryoglobulins are found in association with diseases that may involve the formation of immune complexes. Again, IgM-IgG cryoglobulins are most frequent.[4] The finding of complement system components in these cryoprecipitates, in particular C1q,[15] provides substantial evidence for the immune complex nature of this phenomenon. Indeed, these cryoglobulins activate complement in vitro, and patients with type III cryoglobulinemia often have decreased serum complement levels.

Various antigens, both autologous and exogenous, have been found associated with polyclonal immunoglobulins in this disease. Polyclonal IgG-antilipoprotein autoantibodies,[16] IgM antihepatitis A virus,[17] antihepatitis C,[18] and antifibronectin antibodies[19] have been described. DNA has been identified in the cryoglobulins of patients with systemic lupus erythematosus (SLE).[20] Additionally, DNA and anti-DNA antibodies have been found in the cryoglobulins of patients with glomerulonephritis who do not have SLE.[21]

"Essential" mixed cryoglobulinemia describes the presence of cryoglobulins and the concomitant manifestation of symptoms without an identifiable connective tissue, neoplastic, or infectious process. In early studies, Levo et al.[22] recognized the high frequency of liver involvement in these patients and identified hepatitis B surface antigen, hepatitis B surface antibody, or Dane particles associated with most of their sera or cryoprecipitates. At that time, these researchers postulated that most of these cases resulted from hepatitis B virus or other viral infections. In fact, recent evidence has demonstrated a striking and significant association of essential mixed cryoglobulinemia with hepatitis C virus (HCV) infection. In chronic HCV infection, both types II and III cryoglobulins have been found, with a predominance of type III.[23] In a review of the literature on the extrahepatic manifestations of hepatitis C,[24] the prevalence of HCV antibody and/or RNA in serum samples of patients with the diagnosis of essential mixed cryoglobulinemia was found to range between 42 and 91 percent of patients studied, as documented by recombinant immunoblot assay or polymerase chain reaction, respectively. Patients with type I cryoglobulinemia may be seropositive for HCV[25,26] at a much lower incidence[26]; by definition, however, the cryoprecipitate does not contain the virus/antibody. In light of these findings, it is imperative that patients with mixed cryoglobulinemia, without previously identified associated disease, be evaluated for HCV infection.

Pathophysiology

Type I cryoglobulins demonstrate a self-association of monoclonal immunoglobulins at temperatures ranging from 0 to 30°C or more. Monoclonal cryoglobulins are present in substantial amounts, often ranging from 1 to 30 mg/mL.[4] They may precipitate as a gel, a flocculent precipitate, or in some instances as crystals. The specific physical forces involved in causing precipitates of type I cryoglobulins seems to include temperature-induced conformational changes, deficient carbohydrate side chains, and nucleation reactions.[5] In some instances, type I cryoglobulins, even when present in large amounts, may not result in signs or symptoms of disease. Clinical manifestations of type I disease usually consist of occlusive peripheral vascular phenomena such as Raynaud's phenomenon, cutaneous ulcers, or gangrene. Renal disease and peripheral neuropathy are much less common (see "Clinical Features," below).

Types II and III cryoglobulins are typically present in relatively small amounts. These monoclonal (type II) or polyclonal (type III) rheumatoid factor–IgG complexes usually occur with a concomitant disease process such as connective tissue disease, infection, hepatic disease, or lymphoproliferative disease. As mentioned, the exception is the occurrence of mixed cryoglobulins in "essential" mixed cryoglobulinemia, where an underlying disease process cannot be identified. Mixed cryoglobulins function as immune complexes and in many instances are effective activators of complement. Therefore, analysis of types II and III cryoglobulins often reveals the presence of complement in addition to immunoglobulins. The characterization of the cryoglobulin composition in one patient with type II cryoglobulinemia associated with hepatitis C revealed that the cryoprotein was composed of monoclonal IgM rheumatoid factor, polyclonal IgG (almost 50 percent anti-HCV), HCV RNA, and C3.[27]

Additionally, patients with mixed cryoglobulinemia not only have immune complexes composed of cryoprecipitable material but may also have distinctive circulating immune complexes that are noncryoprecipitable (predominantly composed of IgG)[28]; these latter immune complexes may contribute to the disease presentation.

Earlier studies of the complement system in cryoglobulinemia revealed decreased levels of "whole complement" (CH50), C1, C4, and C2.[29] Normal levels of C3 and elevated levels of later components were sometimes found, leading to the hypothesis of hyposynthesis and/or hypercatabolism of the early complement components in this disease.[30,31] However, a number of clinical studies since have identified patients with mixed cryoglobulinemia who typically evidence depressed levels of C3 along with decreased levels of CH50, C2, and C4.[32]

Immunoglobulins and complement deposits in involved tissues have been evaluated for their contribution to disease presentation. The immunoglobulins in the serum cryoprecipitate of patients with mixed cryoglobulinemia have been identified, along with complement, in involved renal vessels; the histologically normal vasculature may evidence immunoglobulin deposition without complement.[33] Gorevic et al.[32] performed immunofluorescence studies on the skin of patients with cryoglobulinemia and found immune reactants and complement in the vessel walls of 50 percent of the patients studied but did not find immunoglobulin or complement in the uninvolved skin. Studies such as these have been cited as evidence for the pathogenic role of immune complex deposition in cryoglobulinemia. In fact, recent investigations evaluating the localization of HCV antigen in the skin of patients with HCV infection and mixed cryoglobulinemia found evidence of HCV antigens in 6 of 15 skin biopsy specimens studied by indirect immunohistochemistry, with immunoglobulin deposition showing features comparable to the HCV antigen deposition.[34] Such cutaneous histologic findings are not invariable, and immunohistochemical studies may be negative.[5]

Clinical Features

The classic presentation of a patient with cryoglobulinemia is the appearance of purpura. Cold sensitivity is not an invariable feature of cryoglobulinemia. Patients may also evidence serum cryoprecipitates in the absence of clinical symptoms. Some patients with type I cryoglobulins may present initially with cutaneous lesions and ultimately may develop significant vascular compromise with subsequent visceral injury.[4]

The usual organ systems affected in cryoglobulinemia are the skin, kidneys, liver, and musculoskeletal and nervous systems. In general, type I cryoglobulins are typically associated with acrocyanosis, retinal hemorrhage, Raynaud's phenomenon, and arterial thrombosis.[5] Types II and III cryoglobulins are associated with arthritis or arthralgias and vascular purpura.[5] Renal and neurologic symptoms may be found in patients with types II and III cryoglobulins.[4] In an early series of 40 patients with mixed cryoglobulins,[32] 100 percent had recurrent palpable purpura, 73 percent had polyarthralgias, and 55 percent had renal disease. A recent prospective study of 115 patients with mixed cryoglobulinemia found that 45 percent had underlying identifiable diseases or "nonessential" cryoglobulinemia.[18] Of the remaining patients ("essential" mixed cryoglobulinemia), approximately one-half had anti-HCV antibodies, associated with cutaneous and systemic signs and symptoms of greater severity than those patients who were HCV antibody negative. Cutaneous disease included Raynaud's phenomenon, purpura, livedo, distal ulcerations, and "gangrenous" changes (see below). This cohort also had higher serum alanine aminotransferase levels, higher cryoglobulin levels, and lower complement (CH50, C4) levels. These findings suggest that patients with hepatitis C–related mixed cryoglobulinemia have more severe cutaneous and systemic disease than their HCV seronegative cohort.

CUTANEOUS FEATURES　Purpura is considered to be a cutaneous hallmark of cryoglobulinemia. It is usually located distally, most typically on the lower extremities. Showers of these lesions may occur spontaneously, may be provoked by cold exposure, and may be induced by long periods of standing or sitting.[4] Noninflammatory purpura, with histologic evidence of an amorphous eosinophilic precipitate within the vasculature, is seen characteristically in type I cryoglobulinemia[35] and less commonly in types II and III.[36] Leukocytoclastic vasculitis, presenting clinically as palpable purpura, is the characteristic hallmark of the mixed cryoglobulinemias (Fig. 177-1). The lesions are intermittent in nature (typically lasting 3 to 10 days) and are usually nonpruritic.[32] In comparative studies, the incidence of palpable purpura has been found to be higher in patients with mixed cryoglobulinemia who are HCV antibody positive[37] but may present late after initial infection.[38]

Synovitis, serositis, digital ulcerations, and gangrene have been described. Urticaria, urticarial vasculitis, and cold urticaria may also occur in association with cryoglobulinemia.[39–41] As previously mentioned, Raynaud's phenomenon and ulcerations of the lower extremities have also been reported.[32]

RENAL DISEASE　Early reports indicated that 30 to 60 percent of patients with essential mixed cryoglobulinemia had, or would develop, renal involvement.[5] Pathologic evaluation reveals a predominantly membranoproliferative glomerulonephritis.[42] In a study that compared patients with "essential" mixed cryoglobulinemia associated with glomerulonephritis, 94 percent of patients were found to have HCV antibodies in their cryoprecipitates in contrast to 2 percent of patients with glomerulonephritis without cryoglobulin-

FIGURE 177-1

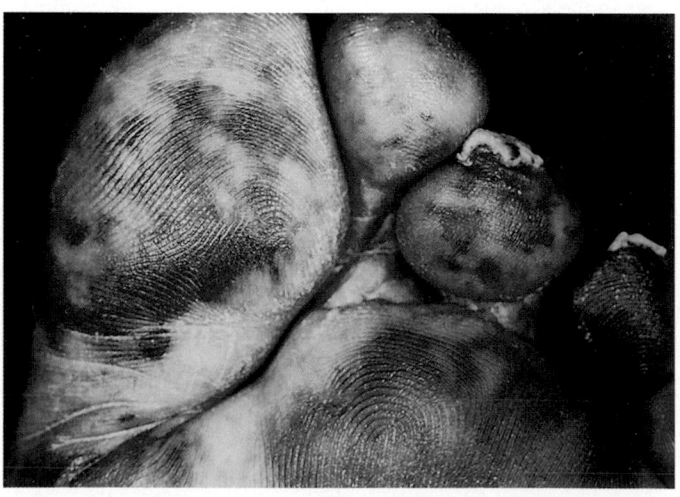

Leukocytoclastic vasculitis in a patient with mixed cryoglobulinemia manifested as palpable purpura; the patient also had tuberculosis, positive antinuclear antibodies, and hepatitis.

emia.[43] In fact, a specific membranoproliferative "cryoglobulinemic glomerulonephritis" has been recognized that has characteristic renal findings and occurs in association with HCV-induced type II cryoglobulinemia.[44] In general, the initial clinical presentation of membranoproliferative glomerulonephritis may include diastolic hypertension, edema, or frank renal failure. Laboratory findings may include proteinuria, hematuria, pyuria, and red cell casts.[32] In contrast to skin, immunofluorescence is characteristically positive and reflects the immunoglobulin and/or complement components identified in the isolated cryoglobulin.

OTHER　Neurologic symptoms may occur in a small percentage of patients and typically consist of a peripheral sensorimotor polyneuropathy, which may present as paresthesia or foot drop.[32] Articular manifestations, more common in types II and III cryoglobulinemias, rarely involve a distinct arthritis[5]; arthralgias are more commonly reported.[45] Hepatic signs consist of hepatomegaly and splenomegaly, while the most common liver function abnormality is elevation of alkaline phosphatase levels.[32] As previously described, serologic studies for hepatitis B and C may be positive. In patients with mixed cryoglobulinemia and HCV seropositivity, HCV infection of bone marrow and peripheral blood mononuclear cells has been found.[46] Other manifestations of vascular occlusive phenomena or immune complex disease may affect the eyes and the gastrointestinal system.

Associated Diseases

Lymphoproliferative disorders, autoimmune disorders, and infectious etiologies are the most frequently associated diseases. Lymphoproliferative diseases such as macroglobulinemia and lymphomas are associated with types I and II cryoglobulins, and autoimmune disorders and hepatitis C are associated with types II and III (see above). Autoimmune disorders most typically include rheumatoid arthritis, SLE, and Sjögren's syndrome. Other less common immunologic disorders such as epidermolysis bullosa acquisita have also been described in association with mixed cryoglobulins.[47]

Treatment

Treatment of cryoglobulinemia is based on the severity of disease presentation. Mild cutaneous symptoms may not require therapeutic intervention. Dermatologic and articular manifestations may be improved by nonsteroidal anti-inflammatory agents. More severe visceral involvement, particularly renal disease, may require glucocorticoid therapy in conjunction with cytotoxic agents. Melphalan, chlorambucil, or cyclophosphamide may benefit some patients.[5] Plasmapheresis has been used to treat patients with rapidly progressive disease refractory to conventional therapy, but a postpheresis rebound in disease activity may occur. Plasma exchange is usually instituted together with immunosuppressive or cytotoxic agents in an attempt at better disease control as well as avoidance of rebound. Cryofiltration is a recently described method of combining a refrigerated membrane unit with pheresis and has been used to treat patients refractory to more conventional therapy.[48]

Patients with hepatitis C–associated cryoglobulinemia have been successfully treated with interferon (IFN)α.[49,50] Following allograft transplantation, however, IFN-α therapy is relatively contraindicated.[51]

CRYOFIBRINOGENEMIA

Cryofibrinogens are cryoproteins in anticoagulated blood or plasma that reversibly precipitate in the cold and are composed of fibrinogen. In the evaluation of cryofibrinogens, it is imperative that blood collection be performed in citrate, oxalate, or ethylenediamine-tetraacetic acid. Heparin may produce false-positive precipitates (heparin-precipitable fraction) through the formation of heparin fibronectin cryoprecipitable complexes, the formation of which may be further enhanced by the presence of fibrinogen.[5]

Many earlier investigators found evidence of cryofibrinogens in a small percentage of normal individuals. Some reports describe cryofibrinogen complexes composed of fibrin, fibrinogen, and fibrin split products together with albumin, fibronectin, and von Willebrand factor.[52] These reports may reflect the formation of cryoprecipitates composed of these normal plasma proteins upon freeze-thawing of plasma.[5] Cutaneous manifestations of cryofibrinogenemia may include purpura, ecchymoses, gangrene, and ulcerations.[53] Associated disease states most commonly include malignancies and thromboembolic diseases. Diabetes and hyperglycemia have been described, as have pregnancy, oral contraceptive agents, and pseudotumor cerebri.[54] The treatment of cryofibrinogenemia is that of the underlying disease or associated condition.

REFERENCES

1. Wintrobe NM, Buell MV: Hyperproteinemia associated with multiple myeloma: With report of a case in which an extraordinary hyperproteinemia was associated with thrombosis of the retinal veins and symptoms suggesting Raynaud's disease. *Bull Johns Hopkins Hosp* **52**:156, 1933
2. Waldenström J: Klinska metoder for pavisande and hyperproteinam: Oc deras praktiska for diagnostiken. *Nord Med* **20**:2288, 1943
3. Lerner AB, Watson CJ: Studies of cryoglobulins. II. The spontaneous precipitation of protein from serum at 5°C in various disease states. *Am J Med Sci* **214**:416, 1947
4. Brouet JC et al: Biological and clinical significance of cryoglobulinemia: Report of 86 cases. *Am J Med* **57**:775, 1974
5. Gorevic PD: Cryopathies: Cryoglobulins and cryofibrinogenemia, in *Immunological Diseases*, edited by M Samter et al. Boston/Toronto, Little, Brown, 1978, p 1687
6. Winfield JB: Cryoglobulinemia. *Hum Pathol* **14**:350, 1983
7. Lospalluto J et al: Cryoglobulinemia based on interaction between a macroglobulin and 7S gammaglobulin. *Am J Med* **32**:142, 1962
8. Kalovidouris AE, Johnson L: Rapid cryoglobulin screening: An aid to the clinician. *Ann Rheum Dis* **37**:444, 1978
9. Letendre L, Kyle RA: Monoclonal cryoglobulinemia with high thermal insolubility. *Mayo Clin Proc* **57**:629, 1982
10. Zinneman HH, Caperton E: Cryoglobulinemia in a patient with Sjögren's syndrome, and factors of cryoprecipitation. *J Lab Clin Med* **89**:483, 1997
11. Levo Y: Nature of cryoglobulinaemia. *Lancet* **1**:285, 1980
12. Litman G et al: Molecular basis for the temperature-dependent insolubility of cryoglobulins. IX. Physiochemical characterization of an IgG1 K monoclonal cryoglobulin exhibiting marginal low temperature-dependent insolubility. *Mol Immunol* **17**:337, 1980
13. Middaugh CR et al: Physiochemical characterization of six monoclonal cryoimmunoglobulins: Possible basis for cold dependent insolubility. *Proc Natl Acad Sci USA* **75**:3440, 1978
14. Abraham GN et al: Idiopathic relatedness of human monoclonal IgG cryoglobulins. *Immunology* **48**:315, 1983
15. Stastny P, Ziff M: Cold-insoluble complexes and complement levels in systemic lupus erythematosus. *N Engl J Med* **280**:1376, 1969
16. Kodama H: Determination of cryoglobulins as lipoprotein-autoantibody immune complexes and antigenic determinants against antilipoprotein autoantibody. *Clin Exp Immunol* **28**:437, 1977
17. Ilan Y et al: Vasculitis and cryoglobulinemia associated with persisting cholestatic hepatitis A virus infection. *Am J Gastroenterol* **85**:586, 1990
18. Munoz-Fernandez S et al: Evidence of hepatitis C virus antibodies in the cryoprecipitate of patients with mixed cryoglobulinemia. *J Rheumatol* **21**:229,1994
19. Beaulieu AD et al: The influence of fibronectin on cryoprecipitate formation in rheumatoid arthritis and systemic lupus erythematosus. *Arthritis Rheum* **24**:1383, 1981
20. Winfield JB et al: Specific concentration of polynucleotide complexes in the serum cryoprecipitates of patients with SLE. *J Clin Invest* **56**:563, 1975
21. Roberts JL, Lewis EJ: Immunochemical demonstration of cryoprecipitable anti-native DNA antibody in the serum of patients with glomerulonephritis. *J Immunol* **124**:127, 1980
22. Levo YL et al: Association between hepatitis B virus and essential mixed cryoglobulinemia. *N Engl J Med* **296**:1501, 1977
23. Wong VS et al: Incidence, character, and clinical relevance of mixed cryoglobulinemia in patients with chronic hepatitis C virus infection. *Clin Exp Immunol* **104**(1):25,1996
24. Gumber SC, Chopra S: Hepatitis C: A multifaceted disease. *Ann Intern Med* **123**:615,1995
25. Agnello V et al: A role of hepatitis C infection in type II cryoglobulinemia. *N Engl J Med* **327**:1490, 1992
26. Willems M et al: Hepatitis C virus and its genotypes in patients suffering from chronic hepatitis C with or without a cryoglobulinemia-related syndrome. *J Med Virol* **44**:226, 1994
27. Sczmanski IO et al: Electron microscopic and immunochemical studies in a patient with hepatitis C virus infection and mixed cryoglobulinemia type II. *Am J Clin Pathol* **102**:278, 1994
28. Lawley TJ et al: Multiple types of immune complexes in patients with mixed cryoglobulinemia. *J Invest Dermatol* **75**:297, 1980
29. Linscott WD, Kane JP: The complement system in cryoglobulinaemia: Interaction with immunoglobulins and lipoproteins. *Clin Exp Immunol* **21**:510, 1975
30. Tarantino A et al: Serum complement pattern in essential cryoglobulinaemia. *Clin Exp Immunol* **32**:77, 1978
31. Haydey RP et al: A newly described control mechanism of complement activation in patients with mixed cryoglobulinemia (cryoglobulins and complement). *J Invest Dermatol* **74**: 328, 1980
32. Gorevic PD et al: Mixed cryoglobulinemia: Clinical aspects and long-term follow-up of 40 patients. *Am J Med* **69**:287, 1980
33. Feiner HD: Relationship of tissue deposits of cryoglobulin to clinical features of mixed cryoglobulinemia. *Hum Pathol* **14**:710, 1983
34. Sansonno D et al: Localization of hepatitis C virus antigens in liver and skin tissues of chronic hepatitis C virus–infected patients with mixed cryoglobulinemia. *Hepatology* **21**:305, 1995
35. Elder D et al: *Lever's Histopathology of the Skin*, 8th ed. Philadelphia, Lippincott, 1997, pp 196–197
36. Cattaneo R et al: The cryoglobulinemic vasculitis. *Ricera Clinica Laboratorio* **16**:327, 1986
37. Dupin N et al: Essential mixed cryoglobulinemia: A comparative study of dermatologic manifestations in patients infected or noninfected with hepatitis C virus. *Arch Dermatol* **131**:1124, 1995
38. Daoud MS et al: Chronic hepatitis C, cryoglobulinemia, and cutaneous necrotizing vasculitis. *J Am Acad Dermatol* **34**:219, 1996
39. Costanzi JJ et al: Activation of complement by a monoclonal cryoglobulin associated with cold urticaria. *J Lab Clin Med* **74**:902, 1969
40. Rawnsley HM, Shelley WB: Cold urticaria with cryoglobulinemia. *Arch Dermatol* **98**:12, 1968
41. Kuniyuki S, Katoh H: Urticarial vasculitis with papular lesions in a patient with type C hepatitis and cryoglobulinemia. *J Dermatol* **23**:279, 1996
42. Tarantino A et al: Renal disease in essential mixed cryoglobulinemia. *Q J Med* **197**:1, 1981
43. Miasiani R et al: Hepatitis virus infection in patients with essential mixed cryoglobulinemia. *Ann Intern Med* **117**:573, 1992
44. D'Amico G, Fornasieri A: Cryoglobulinemic glomerulonephritis: A membranoproliferative glomerulonephritis induced by hepatitis C virus. *Am J Kidney Dis* **25**:361, 1995
45. Weinberger A et al: Articular manifestations of essential cryoglobulinemia. *Semin Arthritis Rheum* **10**:224, 1981
46. Gabrielli A et al: Active hepatitis C virus infection in bone marrow and peripheral mononuclear cells from patients with mixed cryoglobulinemia. *Clin Exp Immunol* **97**:87, 1994
47. Krivo JM, Miller F: Immunopathology of epidermolysis bullosa acquisita. *Arch Dermatol* **114**:1218, 1978

48. Siami GA et al: Cryofiltration apheresis for treatment of cryoglobulinemia associated with hepatitis C. *ASAIO J* **41**:M315, 1995

49. Abe K et al: Anti-liver/kidney microsome-1 positive chronic hepatitis C with type I cryoglobulinemia responding to interferon. *Intern Med* **34**:1114, 1995

50. Wener MH et al: Hepatitis C virus and rheumatic disease. *J Rheumatol* **23**:953, 1996

51. Marcellin P et al: Interferon alpha therapy for chronic hepatitis C in special patient populations. *Dig Dis Sci* **41**:126S, 1995

52. Ireland TA et al: Cutaneous lesions in cryofibrinogenemia. *Clin Lab Obstet* **105**:67, 1984

53. Martin S: Cryofibrinogenemia, monoclonal gammopathy, and purpura. *Arch Dermatol* **115**:208, 1979

54. Smith SB, Arkin C: Cryofibrinogenemia: Incidence, clinical correlations and a review of the literature. *Am J Clin Pathol* **58**:524, 1972

CHAPTER 178

Stephen I. Katz

Relapsing Polychondritis

Relapsing polychondritis is a rare disease manifested by recurring episodes of inflammation in cartilagenous tissues throughout the body.

HISTORIC ASPECTS

The disease was first described by Jaksch-Wartenhorst in 1921[1] and given the name polychondropathia in 1923.[2] In 1960, Pearson et al.[3] suggested the name *relapsing polychondritis* to emphasize its episodic nature, which leads to degeneration and replacement of cartilagenous structures by fibrous tissue. In 1976, McAdam et al. reviewed 159 reported cases of relapsing polychondritis, including 23 patients whom they had seen over the 15-year period of 1960 to 1975.[4] They also empirically defined diagnostic criteria that included the most common clinical features.

ETIOLOGY AND PATHOGENESIS

Considerable evidence suggests that relapsing polychondritis is an autoimmune disease mediated by immunity to type II collagen. In humans, type II collagen is restricted to cartilage and constitutes more than 50 percent of the proteins of cartilage.

The concurrence of relapsing polychondritis with various rheumatic and autoimmune diseases initially led to the suggestion that an immunologic dysfunction might play a role in the pathogenesis of relapsing polychondritis.[4] Indeed, several investigators had reported abnormal cellular and humoral immunologic phenomena in relapsing polychondritis.[5–10] However, most of the reported findings lacked specificity for relapsing polychondritis, and the antigens used were not well characterized. Foidart et al.[11] detected antibodies to type II collagen in the sera of 6 of 23 patients with relapsing polychondritis. All patients in whom antibodies were detected had active disease. Subsequently, Terato et al.,[12] using an enzyme-linked immunosorbent assay (ELISA), found antibodies to type II collagen in the sera of 50 percent of patients with relapsing polychondritis but in only 15 percent of patients with rheumatoid arthritis and 4 percent of normal individuals.

The demonstration of antibodies to type II collagen in sera of patients with relapsing polychondritis raises the question of whether these antibodies are functionally active in vivo or whether they simply represent an epiphenomenon secondary to injury to cartilage and consequent exposure to the relevant antigens. That the antibodies are directed mainly against native rather than denatured collagen would favor the former possibility.[11] Also, the epitope specificity of the antibodies is different in patients with rheumatoid arthritis and those with relapsing polychondritis.[12] The clinical manifestations may then be influenced by this specificity. Experimentally induced autoimmunity to type II collagen in rats[13,14] results in acute arthritis, suggesting that immune responses to type II collagen may play a role in inciting an inflammatory reaction in cartilage. Moreover, some rats sensitized with type II collagen also develop inflammatory ear lesions characterized by an intense, destructive chondritis, which resembles relapsing polychondritis histologically.[15] Although relapsing polychondritis is not usually observed in neonates born of mothers with the disease,[16] the observation that relapsing polychondritis may be transferred from an afflicted mother to her newborn child and that the child may then recover completely from the disease[17] suggests an important role for antibodies in the pathogenesis of relapsing polychondritis. Finally, the finding in vivo of deposits of immunoglobulin and complement in inflamed cartilage in two patients with relapsing polychondritis[18] supports the likelihood that immunity to type II collagen plays a role in the pathogenesis of relapsing polychondritis. Further evidence that immunologic mechanisms play a role in the pathogenesis of relapsing polychondritis comes from immunogenetic studies demonstrating a significant association between relapsing polychondritis and HLA-DR4.[19]

CLINICAL MANIFESTATIONS

The most frequent presenting manifestations are auricular chondritis and arthritis.[4,20] The chondritis is characterized by the sudden onset of redness, warmth, swelling, and tenderness limited to the cartilagenous portion of the external ears. Often only one ear is involved initially, and the ear lobe is typically uninvolved. The acute inflammation usually subsides spontaneously in 1 to 2 weeks. It is characterized by recurrences that appear after highly variable periods—from weeks to months. Eventually 85 to 90 percent of patients with relapsing polychondritis develop auricular chondritis.[4,20] Nasal chondritis follows the same pattern as the auricular chondritis and eventually occurs in 54 to 70 percent of patients. The recurrent episodes of chondritis usually result in the destruction of normal cartilagenous structures and their fibrotic replacement. Clinically this process results in floppy or cauliflower ears and nasal deformities (Figs. 178-1 and 178-2).

Arthritis, which may involve only one or many small or large joints, is the second most frequent presenting sign and is eventually manifested in 52 to 80 percent of patients. At its onset, the arthritis is often migratory and is frequently associated with effusions, but it may be monoarticular and difficult to distinguish from gouty or infectious arthritis.

Other organ system involvement includes the eyes, where the inflammation may involve almost every part of the eye and adnexal structures,[4,21] manifesting as conjunctivitis, episcleritis, keratitis, and iritis (Fig. 178-3); the respiratory tract, where symptoms may include hoarseness, aphonia, and dyspnea; the inner ear, where symptoms may include nausea, vomiting, tinnitus, and deafness as a result of audiovestibular damage; and, less frequently, the cardiovascular system, where the most frequent abnormalities are aortic regurgitation and aortic aneurysm.[22] Aortic valve replacement may become necessary.[23] Approximately 30 to 35 percent of patients

FIGURE 178-2

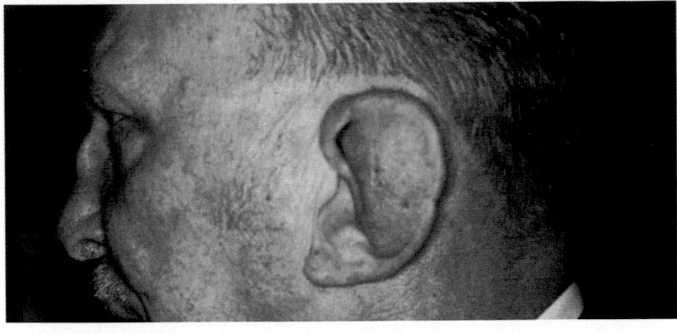

Relapsing polychondritis. "Cauliflower" ear and nasal deformity.

FIGURE 178-3

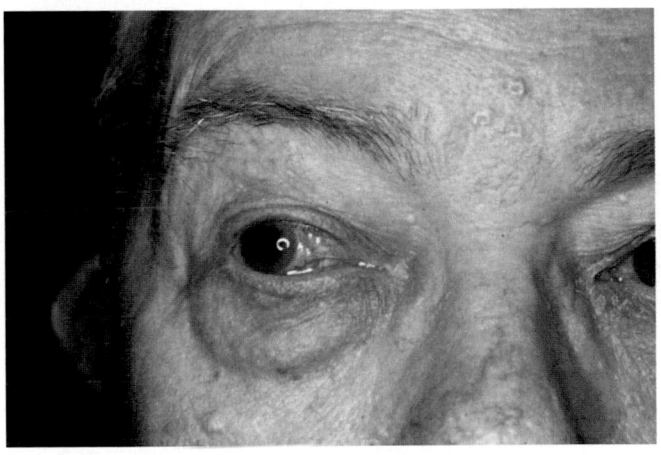

Relapsing polychondritis. Acute episcleritis.

have an associated rheumatic or autoimmune disease, and a significant percent of patients also have leukocytoclastic vasculitis.[4,20,24] Myelodysplastic syndromes are also associated with relapsing polychondritis.[25,26]

LABORATORY FINDINGS

The only laboratory finding that is consistently abnormal is an elevated erythrocyte sedimentation rate. The white blood count is elevated and/or the hemoglobin or hematocrit is decreased in more than half of patients.[4] Indirect immunofluorescence and ELISA studies have detected circulating antibodies to type II collagen in one-third to one-half of patients.[11]

PATHOLOGY

Relapsing polychondritis is characterized by a loss of the normal basophilia of cartilage with a perichondral inflammatory infiltrate (Fig. 178-4). The earliest of the inflammatory cells are thought by

FIGURE 178-1

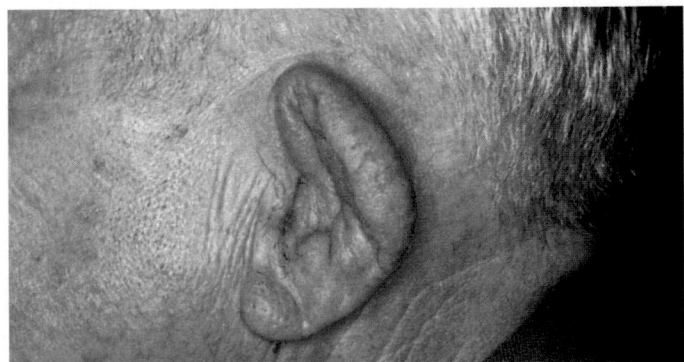

Relapsing polychondritis. Cartilagenous portion of ear is deformed and fibrotic.

FIGURE 178-4

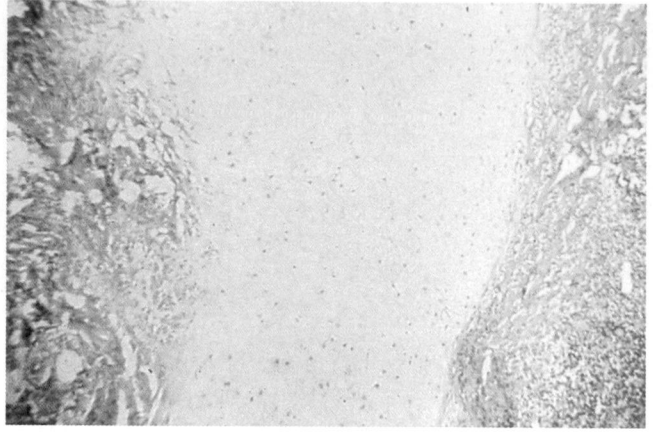

Relapsing polychondritis. Histopathology showing loss of basophilic staining of cartilage and perichondrial inflammatory infiltrate.

some to be neutrophils and by others to be mononuclear cells. The end stage of the disease is characterized by the fibrotic replacement of cartilage.

DIAGNOSIS

McAdam et al.[4] suggested that the diagnosis of relapsing polychondritis can be made when three of the following criteria are present along with histologic confirmation of the chondritis:

1. Bilateral auricular chondritis
2. Nonerosive seronegative inflammatory polyarthritis
3. Nasal chondritis
4. Ocular inflammation
5. Respiratory chondritis
6. Audiovestibular damage

Ordinarily, relapsing polychondritis presents little problem in diagnosis. However, there are patients who have only auricular and nasal chondritis and none of the other manifestations of relapsing polychondritis. If the histology shows perichondrial inflammation and the loss of the normal cartilagenous basophilia and if other conditions are excluded, a diagnosis of relapsing polychondritis should be made.

Concurrent rheumatologic diseases may, at times, obscure the diagnosis of relapsing polychondritis. Cellulitis of the ear or nose may be confused on rare occasion with relapsing polychondritis; however, sparing of the ear lobe favors the diagnosis of relapsing polychondritis.

TREATMENT

Because of the highly variable course of relapsing polychondritis, individualized therapy is the key to optimum management. Systemic glucocorticoids are helpful in controlling the acute inflam-

mation. Seventy-five percent of patients in McAdam's series required chronic glucocorticoid therapy; the average dose of prednisone was 25 mg/day.[4] Immunosuppressive therapy, including cyclosporine, may also be efficacious in severe progressive disease,[4,27,28] and methotrexate has been helpful as a steroid-sparing agent.[29] Dapsone has also been reported to be an effective treatment[30,31]; however, our experience and that of others[20] with dapsone in relapsing polychondritis have been disappointing. Although dapsone may be effective in some patients with diffuse anterior scleritis, it does not control the destructive scleral inflammation.[32] The frequent spontaneous remissions that occur during the acute episodes have made evaluation of most treatments difficult. The more chronic manifestations of relapsing polychondritis can be managed with indomethacin in some patients.

COURSE AND PROGNOSIS

The course of relapsing polychondritis is unpredictable. The acute chondritis in most patients lasts for 1 to 4 weeks, but in a few it may be more prolonged. Some patients have a relatively mild course with few episodes of chondritis. Other patients may have multiple episodes of chondritis. The degree of tissue destruction and fibrosis is difficult to predict early in the course of the disease. The presence of peripheral arthritis is said to be associated with widespread disease and a poorer prognosis.[33] About one-third of the patients die as a result of relapsing polychondritis. The most frequent causes of death are airway collapse or obstruction, cardiovascular complications including systemic vasculitis and ruptured aneurysms, and infections (probably secondary to glucocorticoid-induced immunosuppression).[4,20,22,34]

REFERENCES

1. Jaksch-Wartenhorst R: Arztliche vortragsabende. *Prag Med Klin* **17**:342, 1921
2. Jaksch-Wartenhorst R: Polychondropathia. *Wien Arch Inn Med* **6**:93, 1923
3. Pearson CM et al: Relapsing polychondritis. *N Engl J Med* **263**:51, 1960
4. McAdam LP et al: Relapsing polychondritis. Prospective study of 23 patients and a review of the literature. *Medicine* **55**:193, 1976
5. Herman JH, Dennis MV: Immunopathologic studies in relapsing polychondritis. *J Clin Invest* **52**:549, 1973
6. Rajapakse DA, Bywaters EGL: Cell-mediated immunity to cartilage proteoglycan in relapsing polychondritis. *Clin Exp Immunol* **16**:497, 1974
7. Dolan DL et al: Relapsing polychondritis. *Am J Med* **41**:285, 1966
8. Hundeiker M et al: Infiltrat und Knorpelzerstorung bei polychondritis (Histochemische und immunofluoreszenz-histologische Befunde). *Z Haut Geschl Kr* **45**:437, 1970
9. Hughes RAC et al: Relapsing polychondritis. *Q J Med* **41**:363, 1972
10. Rogers PH et al: Relapsing polychondritis with insulin resistance and antibodies to cartilage. *Am J Med* **55**:243, 1973
11. Foidart JM et al: Antibodies to type II collagen in relapsing polychondritis. *N Engl J Med* **299**:1203, 1978
12. Terato K et al: Specificity of antibodies to type II collagen in rheumatoid arthritis. *Arthritis Rheum* **33**:1493, 1990
13. Trentham DE et al: Autoimmunity to type II collagen: An experimental model of arthritis. *J Exp Med* **146**:857, 1977
14. Trentham DE et al: Humoral and cellular sensitivity to collagen in type II collagen-induced arthritis in rats. *J Exp Med* **154**:535, 1981
15. Cremer MA et al: Auricular chondritis in rats: An experimental model of relapsing polychondritis induced with type II collagen. *J Exp Med* **154**:535, 1981
16. Papo T et al: Pregnancy in relapsing polychondritis: Twenty-five pregnancies in eleven patients. *Arthritis Rheum* **40**:1245, 1997

17. Arundell FW, Haserick JR: Familial chronic atrophic polychondritis. *Arch Dermatol* **82**:439, 1960
18. Valenzuela R et al: Relapsing polychondritis: Value of immunomicroscopic examination of ear biopsy. *Hum Pathol* **11**:19, 1980
19. Zeuner M et al: Relapsing polychondritis: Clinical and immunogenetic analysis of 62 patients. *J Rheumatol* **24**:96, 1997
20. Michet CJ et al: Relapsing polychondritis—survival and predictive role of early disease manifestations. *Ann Intern Med* **104**:74, 1986
21. Isaak BL et al: Ocular and systemic findings in relapsing polychondritis. *Ophthalmology* **93**:681, 1986
22. Del Rosso A et al: Cardiovascular involvement in relapsing polychondritis. *Semin Arthritis Rheum* **26**:840, 1997
23. Lang-Lazdunski L et al: Cardiac valve replacement in relapsing polychondritis: A review. *J Heart Valve Dis* **4**:227, 1995
24. Michet CJ: Vasculitis and relapsing polychondritis. *Rheum Dis Clin North Am* **16**:441, 1990
25. Hebbar M et al: Association of myelodysplastic syndrome and relapsing polychondritis. Further evidence. *Leukemia* **9**:731, 1995
26. Diebold L et al: Bone marrow pathology in relapsing polychondritis: High frequency of myelodysplastic syndromes. *Br J Haematol* **89**:820, 1995
27. Anstey A et al: Relapsing polychondritis: Autoimmunity to type II collagen and treatment with cyclosporin A. *Br J Dermatol* **125**:588, 1991
28. Diercks K et al: Cyclosporin A therapy of chronic recurrent polychondritis. *Hautartz* **47**:376, 1996
29. Park J et al: Steroid-sparing effect of methotrexate in relapsing polychondritis. *J Rheumatol* **23**:937, 1996
30. Barranco VP et al: Treatment of relapsing polychondritis with dapsone. *Arch Dermatol* **112**:1286, 1976
31. Martin J et al: Relapsing polychondritis treated with dapsone. *Arch Dermatol* **112**:1272, 1976
32. Hoang-Xaun T et al: Scleritis in relapsing polychondritis. Response to therapy. *Ophthalmology* **97**:892, 1990
33. Balsa A et al: Joint symptoms in relapsing polychondritis. *Clin Exp Rheumatol* **13**:425, 1995
34. Eng J, Sabanathan S: Airway complications in relapsing polychondritis. *Ann Thorac Surg* **51**:686, 1991

CHAPTER 179

Paul Sutej
Joseph L. Jorizzo

Rheumatoid Arthritis, Rheumatic Fever, and Gout

In this chapter, we deal with common rheumatologic ailments that ordinarily have prominent musculoskeletal presentations. Common to all of these ailments is an often pronounced extraskeletal manifestation that may be cutaneous in nature.

RHEUMATOID ARTHRITIS

Rheumatoid arthritis (RA), perhaps better known as rheumatoid disease, is a systemic inflammatory disease characterized by a chronic, symmetric polyarthritis and significant extraarticular manifestations, which include rheumatoid nodules, vasculitic lesions, systemic features, and internal organ involvement. The disease process may be progressive and destructive of joint function, with a resultant decline in functional status and premature mortality. Permanent remission is extremely unusual. The initial joint manifestation may be quite asymmetric in terms of involvement of the proximal interphalangeal and metacarpophalangeal joints, but eventually a symmetrical process ensues with predominant and prominent involvement of the hands and feet. It has been estimated that between 1 and 2 percent of the adult population in most parts of the world is affected with definite or classic RA.

In the early stages of the disease process, a diagnosis may be difficult. In spite of an excellent history, thorough musculoskeletal and general medical examination, and serologic and radiologic workups, the diagnosis may be in doubt. Guidelines for the diagnosis of RA appear in Table 179-1. For a patient to be diagnosed with definite RA, four of the seven criteria need to be present. Criteria 1 through 4 need to have been present for at least 6 weeks.

There is considerable anxiety as both physician and patient strive for an early diagnosis, with a view to controlling the synovial inflammatory response and ultimately limiting long-term joint deformity and subsequent loss of function. Several studies have suggested that the bulk of significant joint damage occurs within the first 2 years of the disease process, placing a burden on the managing physician to start appropriate therapy early.[1–3] Rheumatoid factor and antinuclear antibody profiling should be viewed as being predominantly screening, particularly in the early phases of the disease process. Extra-articular manifestations may help delineate the disease process early and may signify a more serious disease process requiring the initiation of aggressive therapy.

Epidemiology

The prevalence of RA varies from 0.5 to 1 percent in developed countries. The disease frequency has not significantly changed during the last century, but there are indications that it may have been lower before the onset of the industrial revolution. Rheumatoid arthritis is two to three times more common in women. The incidence of the disease increases with age until about the seventh decade.

TABLE 179-1

1987 American College of Rheumatology Revised Criteria for the Classification of Rheumatoid Arthritis (Modified)

CRITERION	DEFINITION
Morning stiffness	Morning stiffness in and around the joints, lasting at least 1 h before maximal improvement
Arthritis of three or more joint areas	At least three joint areas simultaneously afflicted with soft tissue swelling or joint fluid observed by a physician. The 14 possible areas are (right or left): PIP, MCP, wrists, elbow, knee, ankle, and MTP joints
Arthritis of hand joints	At least one area swollen in a wrist, MCP, or PIP joint
Symmetric arthritis	Simultaneous involvement of the same joint areas on both sides of the body (bilateral involvement of PIP, MCP, or MTP acceptable without perfect symmetry)
Rheumatoid nodules	Subcutaneous nodules over bony prominences or extensor surfaces or in juxtaarticular regions (observed by a physician)
Serum rheumatoid factor	Abnormal amount of serum rheumatoid factor by any method for which the result has been positive in <5% of control subjects
Radiographic changes	Erosions or unequivocal bony decalcification localized in or most marked adjacent to the involved joints

KEY: PIP, proximal interphalangeal; MCP, metacarpophalangeal; MTP, metatarsophalangeal.

Etiology and Pathogenesis

Recent evidence suggests that the susceptibility and severity of RA are controlled differently. The initial onset of joint symptoms may be induced by a variety of factors with genetic constraints, while the immunogenetic background of the patient may then determine whether the inflammation regresses or progresses.

Joints have unique anatomic and physiologic qualities that render them targets for immune and inflammatory attack. Cartilage is responsible for the retention of antigens and proinflammatory cytokines, has a limited capacity for regeneration, and is subject to repeated mechanical injury. The capacity of chondrocytes to regenerate decreases with age, although the ability to produce proinflammatory cytokines, nitric oxide, prostaglandins, and matrix metalloproteinases is retained.[4] The inflammatory process in a joint is difficult to extinguish. The restimulation of T lymphocytes by sequestered self antigens—such as heat-shock proteins overexpressed in response to stress, deposition of immune complexes in the synovial microvasculature, and dysregulation of the tachykinins and cytokines—can override the control mechanisms that place limits on the physiologic inflammatory response. Once proteolytic enzymes cause erosions, narrowing of the joint space, and mechanical instability, rheumatoid inflammation may become self-sustaining.

The concordance of RA in monozygotic twins is no more than 15 percent, which would seem to suggest that RA might also be attributable to superimposed nongenetic factors. Patients with more severe RA are much more likely to have an affected twin than patients with mild RA. Patients expressing HLA DR4 subtypes 01 and 04 have the highest risk of developing severe disease.[5] It has been felt that the HLA class II molecules that predispose to RA potentially can influence the immunoresponses by selecting and deleting particular subsets of T lymphocytes during thymus development and by binding selectively self and non-self peptides. HLA molecules, rheumatoid factors, and cytokines interact and enable a host to maintain an early and vigorous immune reaction to non-self antigens with changes in joint structure and cellular function sufficient to produce self-sustaining synovitis.

Clinical Features

ARTICULAR MANIFESTATIONS The most common mode of onset is the insidious development of symptoms over a period of several weeks. However, an explosive, acute polyarticular onset also occurs. Articular manifestations of RA can be categorized into reversible signs and symptoms related to inflammatory synovitis and irreversible structural damage brought on by the chronic synovitis. Structural damage usually begins somewhere between the first and second years of the disease. It is not uncommon for RA to begin in a single joint, but the usual early manifestations are polyarticular. The developing pattern of joint involvement is very suggestive of the diagnosis, with sparing of the distal interphalangeal joints of the hands. Although the initial manifestations in the hand may be asymmetric, the clinical course subsequently takes on a very symmetric diffuse involvement of the proximal interphalangeal joint.

Involvement of the thoracic and lumbar spine in RA is exceptional. When low back pain exists, unrelated mechanical back pain should be considered, as well as the possibility of osteoporosis-related fractures. Involvement of the cervical spine is of particular concern. Instability of C1-C2 is not universally accompanied by neck pain. Frequently, the course of neck pain and neurologic symptoms are not synchronous. While the shoulder joint is often involved, it is soft tissue structures that include the rotator cuff tendons and muscles and the subacromial bursa that are usually involved in the patient's symptomatology. The patient may complain of pain in the shoulder muscles rather than close to the glenohumeral joint. Separating these specific disease entities may require an MRI or arthroscopy. RA is characterized by synovitis; and tendons, bursae, and joints are all lined by synovial tissue. Hence, the bursae and tendons are an integral part of the process, as can be evidenced by shoulder manifestations.

Hand and foot involvement forms the basis of the disease in most patients with RA. Sparing of the distal interphalangeal joints is usual. When these joints are involved, superimposed osteoarthritis, gout, or psoriasis should be considered as part of the differential diagnosis. Symptoms of carpal tunnel entrapment should alert the clinician to the possibility of an underlying inflammatory arthritis of the wrist. The foot is essentially divided into four compartments, to include the true ankle joint, the subtalar joint, the multiple midfoot joints, and the forefoot area. Rheumatoid arthritis may affect all of these simultaneously, with a resultant effect on function. These joints need to be closely examined and may demand specific and very different management plans.

DERMATOLOGIC MANIFESTATIONS The characteristic rheumatoid nodule occurs in 25 to 50 percent of patients with RA (Fig. 179-1). Rheumatoid factor is inevitably found with nodules. These nodules tend to occur during active phases of the disease process and form subcutaneously, in bursae, and along tendon sheaths. The usual location is over pressure points such as the olecranons, the extensor surface of the forearms, and Achilles' tendons. However,

FIGURE 179-1

FIGURE 179-2

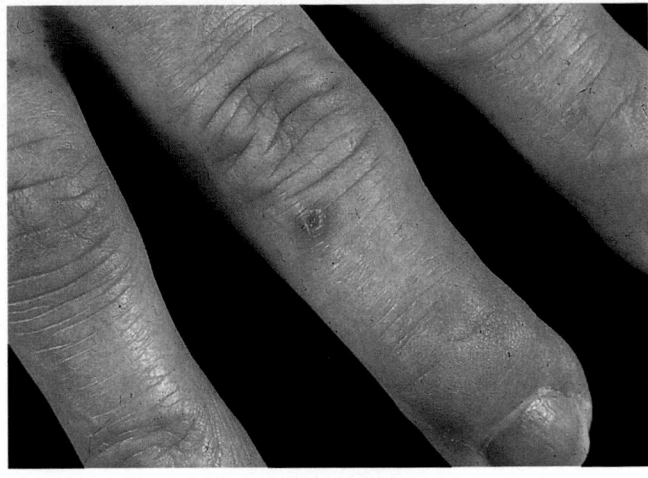

Bywater's lesions. Note the purpuric papules in the finger.

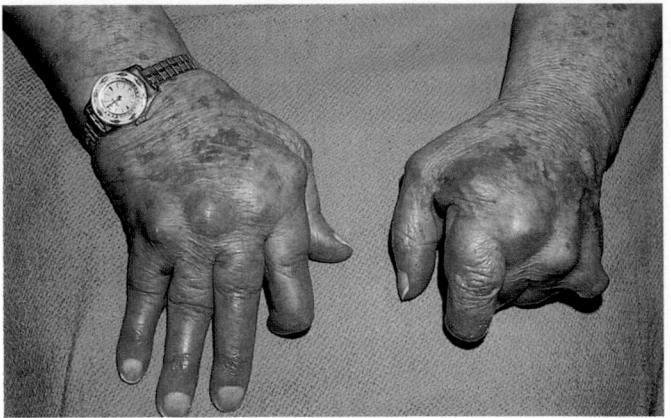

Patient with severe rheumatoid arthritis. Note the dramatic erosions in the nodules over several joints.

they have been described in almost every location, including viscera. Nodules are associated with a more aggressive outcome of the rheumatoid disease.

Rheumatoid vasculitis is typically of small to medium-sized vessels with associated peripheral neuropathy (quite often motor), digital gangrene, nail fold infarcts, and palpable purpura.[5] Histologic examination of skin biopsy specimens usually shows leukocytoclastic vasculitis with neutrophilic infiltration of the vessel wall, fibrinoid necrosis, and hemorrhage. Some patients may have nail fold telangiectasias, with minute digital ulcerations or petechiae and digital pulp papules (Bywater's lesions) (Fig. 179-2). These papules are considered a manifestation of mild rheumatoid vasculitis because they usually occur without systemic signs of vasculitis. These lesions usually show leukocytoclastic vasculitis and differ from rheumatoid nodules in that no palisading granulomatous response is found.[6] The spectrum of clinical lesions reported in rheumatoid vasculitis is wide and varies with the size and location of the vessels involved and with the extent of the disease. Leukocytoclastic vasculitis usually involves small venules of the skin, but the same fibrinoid process may occur in arterioles and in larger vessels of the viscera, heart, and central nervous system. There is an association with HLA Dr 4.

An increased frequency of pyoderma gangrenosum is suspected in the presence of liquefying ulcers and a characteristic purple, undermined border in patients with RA. The ulcers may occur at any site but are most common in the abdomen and lower extremities. Leg ulcers are also a feature of Felty's syndrome in patients who also have hypersplenism (Fig. 179-3).

Lesions that resemble necrobiosis lipoidica diabeticorum have been called *superficial ulcerating rheumatoid necrobiosis*. These are usually symmetric, on the lower extremities, and occur as multiple, yellow-red, well-circumscribed ulcers that do not become confluent. Telangiectasias as well as local atrophy may occur. The lesions are often confused with venostasis ulcers. Subclinical vasculitis is thought to initiate the palisading granuloma process when the RA is in an acute phase. A papular eruption with clinical and pathologic features of both granuloma annulare and leukocytoclastic vasculitis has been described. These lesions begin fairly superficially and occur in crops, quite often during a flare of arthritis and occasionally in association with pyoderma gangrenosum.

Rheumatoid neutrophilic dermatosis is a very rare cutaneous manifestation in patients with severe RA. First described by Ack-

erman in 1978,[7] these lesions are usually chronic, erthematous, and urticaria-like plaques and papules that are sharply marginated. It may be difficult to differentiate rheumatoid neutrophilic dermatosis from acute febrile neutrophilic dermatosis (Sweet's syndrome).

Other vasculitis syndromes such as erythema elevatum diutinum and livedo vasculitis (segmental hyalinizing vasculitis) have also been described in patients with RA.[8]

NONDERMATOLOGIC, EXTRAARTICULAR MANIFESTATIONS
Manifestations of RA in other systems are presented in Table 179-2.

Laboratory Findings

There is no specific histologic, radiographic, or laboratory test that conclusively permits the diagnosis of RA. Rheumatoid factor is found in the serum of 85 percent of patients with RA. High titers

FIGURE 179-3

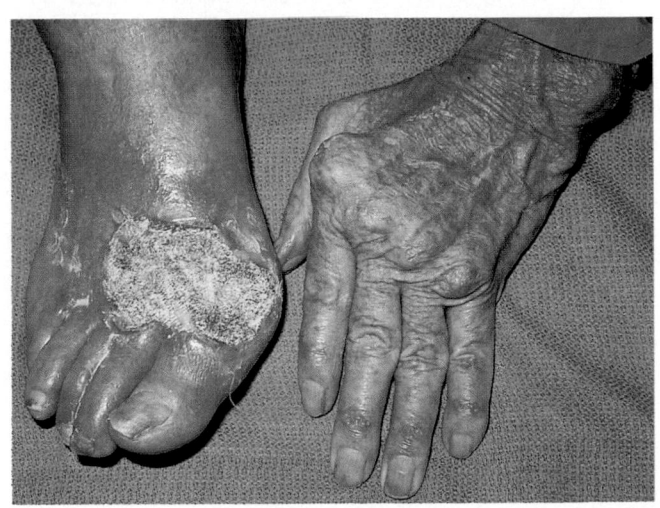

Felty's syndrome. Note the refractory ulcer on the foot in this patient with rheumatoid arthritis and hypersplenism.

TABLE 179-2

Nondermatologic, Extraarticular Manifestations of Rheumatoid Arthritis

TYPE	MANIFESTATIONS
Ocular	Keratoconjunctivitis sicca, scleritis, episcleritis, scleromalacia, retinal toxicity due to hydroxychloroquine sulfate (Plaquenil)
Renal	Amyloidosis and vasculitis
Hematologic	Anemia, thrombocytosis, lymphadenopathy, Felty's syndrome
Neurologic	Entrapment neuropathy, cervical myelopathy, mononeuritis multiplex (vasculitis), peripheral neuropathy
Lung	Pleural effusions, pulmonary fibrosis, bronchiolitis obliterans, rheumatoid nodules, vasculitis
Cardiac	Pericarditis, premature atherosclerosis, vasculitis, nodules, aortic root dilatation

are associated with severe disease. Serial titers are of no useful value. A false-positive rheumatoid factor can be caused by many factors, including chronic bacterial infections such as infective endocarditis, tuberculosis, and Lyme disease as well as by viral diseases such as rubella and infectious mononucleosis. Chronic inflammatory diseases (sarcoidosis), liver diseases, and pulmonary fibrotic disease processes are all associated with the presence of rheumatoid factor. Cryoglobulinemia is also associated with rheumatoid factor.

Treatment

Because the exact cause of RA is unknown, treatment has been directed against various components of the chronic inflammatory process rather than at a specific cause. There is no single therapy that is the treatment of choice. Many drugs, frequently in combination, are used to treat the disease. The major change in the therapy of RA over the past decade is the more rapid institution of drugs to attempt to modify the clinical course of disease activity. For many years, the initial approach was a traditional therapeutic pyramid. In this model, patients would initially be educated and receive salicylates or nonsteroidal anti-inflammatory drugs (NSAIDs). Then they would have their therapy upgraded gradually with antimalarials, gold salts, penicillamine, methotrexate, or azathioprine and eventually would be treated with experimental drugs and procedures and/or other cytotoxic agents. With the knowledge that joint erosions are closely linked to long-term disability and that they develop within the first few years of disease onset, it is now felt that a more aggressive approach is necessary. Wilske and Healey recommended the "step-down bridge approach," in which patients initially receive 10 to 20 mg of prednisone and then begin multiple drug combinations including methotrexate, azathioprine, intramuscular gold salts, and hydroxychloroquine.[9] As the disease process is suppressed, drugs are sequentially withdrawn. Most clinicians take an intermediate approach as they attempt to control the synovitis by whatever strategies are appropriate at the given time.

Nevertheless, first-line therapy remains the standard initial approach in the treatment of RA. Specifically, this includes salicylates or other NSAIDs, the purpose of which is to control some aspect of joint inflammation and pain, while disease-modifying drugs (second-line therapies) are presumably taking hold over time. Recent focus on NSAIDs has changed to their effect on cyclooxygenase

(COX), with particular emphasis on the isoenzymes COX-1 and COX-2. These isoenzymes have similar affinities for and capacities to convert arachidonic acid to endoperoxides, but they differ in their regulation and expression. COX-1 is constitutively expressed in most tissues, with vascular endothelial cells, platelets, kidney collecting tubules, and stomach and smooth muscles expressing high levels. COX-2 is nearly undetectable in most tissues but is increased during inflammation up to 100 times the normal level. Thus, COX-1 seems necessary for the regulation of normal cellular processes, such as the maintenance of gastric and renal function. It is quite logical that NSAIDs are being developed predominantly to affect COX-2 levels, with the ultimate goal of reducing nephrotoxicity and gastrointestinal side effects.

Second-line anti-RA drugs are currently being used much earlier in the course of the disease process. Whether they reduce disease progression detected by radiography remains controversial. Drugs may be used singly or in combination. Some of these medications are reviewed briefly below.

ANTIMALARIALS Clinical responses may not occur for 3 to 6 months after the initiation of therapy. Although hydroxychloroquine is generally well tolerated, the seemingly serious ocular toxicity requires ophthalmologic monitoring. This side effect represents an extremely unusual clinical event. Hydroxychloroquine is often used in combination with other agents.

SULFASALAZINE This medication takes 15 to 20 weeks to produce a response. The drug is usually used in patients with mild to moderate disease or in combination with other agents. Limiting side effects are usually mucocutaneous and gastrointestinal.

METHOTREXATE (MTX) This agent has become one of the most popular therapies for RA. A response is often seen by 12 weeks. Liver biopsies are recommended by the American College of Rheumatology only for patients who have persistent abnormalities of the liver function profile. MTX pneumonitis, the most feared of adverse effects, has been estimated to occur in one case per 276 patient-years[10] but generally can be reversed with treatment after the MTX is discontinued.

GOLD SALTS Parenteral gold is still used and is an effective drug for the therapy of RA. Patients do need to be monitored for bone marrow (especially platelets) and renal toxicity to permit early termination of this therapy if indicated. Cutaneous eruptions from gold salts may require that this therapy be discontinued due to the possibility of exfoliation.

AZATHIOPRINE This drug is usually reserved for patients who have failed conventional therapy including MTX. The onset of action is slow. Aggressive squamous cell carcinomas have been described in rare patients receiving long-term therapy.[11]

CYCLOSPORINE This drug has been studied for the use in RA over the past 10 years and has become an earlier alternative for patients with refractory disease. However, because of the associated renal toxicity, sometimes with hypertension, the drug is generally used in combination to focus on a minimum useful dose.

Biologic response modifiers such as monoclonal antibodies to tumor necrosis factor alpha (TNF-α) or interleukin 6 (IL-6), soluble receptors such as TNF-R, or natural receptor inhibitors such as that for the IL-1 receptor are of significant interest. Most of the clinical responses have been observed in open pilot studies, and results from long-term randomized, placebo-controlled studies are needed. It is likely that these agents will be used in combination with standard therapy in the future.

The decision about which drug to use and when to use it in the therapy of RA is somewhat individualized and determined by the clinical involvement, onset of loss of functional status, and concerns about the safety profile in a given patient.

GOUT

Gout is a disease in which crystals of monosodium urate from supersaturated extracellular fluids are deposited in tissue, leading to one or more clinical manifestations. These include (1) attacks of acute or chronic joint or periarticular inflammation (gouty arthritis); (2) accumulation of tophi; (3) renal impairment (gouty nephropathy); and (4) uric acid calculi in the urogenital tract. The classic presentation is that of an acute lower extremity peripheral joint monoarthritis. Although hyperuricemia is a common pathogenetic denominator, this abnormality is most often insufficient for the expression of gout. Therefore, asymptomatic hyperuricemia in the absence of gout is not a disease state.

Epidemiology

The prevalence of gout seems to have increased over the last few decades in the United States. The peak incidence is in the fifth decade. Gout rarely occurs in men before late adolescence or in women before menopause. Gout is primarily a disease of males (95 percent of cases).

Pathogenesis

Uric acid is the end product of the catabolism of purines. Humans lack the enzyme uricase. Uric acid renal clearance sufficient to balance production is usually achieved in plasma concentrations below the limit of solubility of monosodium urate in plasma (about 7 mg/dL). This remains a very narrow margin of safety.

Causes and Classification of Hyperuricemia

A classification of hyperuricemia is presented in Table 179-3.

Probably less than 10 percent of patients with hyperuricemia or gout excrete excessive quantities of uric acid in a 24-h urine collection (more than 1000 mg on a normal diet). It is usually in this group that one can find identifiable and inherited derangements in mechanisms regulating protein nucleotide synthesis, specifically a deficiency of hypoxanthine-guanine phosphoribosyltransferase (HGPRT), either partial or complete. In these instances, family history or early presentation may be a clue. The Lesch-Nyhan syndrome, well described but very infrequent, is an extremely severe form of HGPRT deficiency associated with mental retardation, gout, and self-mutilation.

Uric acid underexcretion occurs in 90 percent of patients with primary hyperuricemia. No specific mechanism has been identified at the glomerulus, in the proximal tubule, or in the collecting ducts. The kidney appears normal. Many pharmacologic agents affect tubular function and include diuretics, cyclosporine at a low dose, and salicylates (which are frequently used for antiplatelet effect).

TABLE 179-3

Classification of Hyperuricemia

Overproduction of uric acid
  Primary hyperuricemia
    Idiopathic
    Hypoxanthine-guanine phosphoribosyltransferase deficiency
    Phosphoribosylpyrophosphate synthetase superactivity
  Secondary hyperuricemia
    Excessive dietary purine intake
    Increased nucleotide turnover (e.g., myeloproliferative and lymphoproliferative disorders, hemolytic diseases, psoriasis)
Diminished excretion of uric acid
  Primary hyperuricemia
    Idiopathic
  Secondary hyperuricemia
    Diminished renal function
    Inhibition of tubular urate secretion by competitive anions (e.g., keto- and lactic acidosis)
  Enhanced tubular urate reabsorption
    Dyhydration, diuretics
  Miscellaneous
    Hypertension
    Hyperparathyroidism
    Certain drugs (e.g., cyclosporine, pyrazinamide, ethambutol, low dose salicylates)
    Lead nephropathy

Stages of Gouty Arthritis

1. *Asymptomatic hyperuricemia* does not necessitate any specific management unless there is a strong family history of gout, uric acid levels are exceedingly high, or there is a history of renal calculi.

2. *Acute gouty arthritis* usually occurs in the lower extremities. The metatarsophalangeal joint is affected in approximately 75 percent of patients at some time. The first episode of acute gout usually has a dramatic presentation with a warm, red, tender joint. Early attacks may subside spontaneously in 3 to 10 days. Occasionally there is desquamation of the skin overlying the affected joint.

3. *Intercritical gout* describes the interval that occurs between attacks of gout. Initially, these periods are asymptomatic.

4. *Chronic tophaceous gout* describes the presence of tophi in fairly advanced gout. They are usually noted some time after the onset, often up to 10 years after the initial episode of gout. These tophi usually occur in the olecranon bursa, infrapatella, and Achilles' tendons, subcutaneous tissues on the extensor surface of the forearms, overlying joints, and occasionally around the helix of the ear. These tophi may be found around Heberden's nodes in postmenopausal women. Less frequently, they have been described around the tricuspid and mitral valves, nasal cartilage, eyelids, and cornea. They may be confused with rheumatoid nodules and aspiration or biopsy may prove useful.

While an acute presentation of podagra (with involvement of the first tarsometatarsophalangeal joint) is very suggestive of the diagnosis of gout, most clinicians would feel more comfortable confirming the presence of crystals within the joint. The finding of negative birefringent crystals (within or outside of macrophages) is specific for gout. The synovial fluid usually contains from 20 to

100,000 white cells. There is limited value in the serum uric acid level at the time of the acute diagnosis. Normal serum uric acid does not exclude the diagnosis of gout. Roentgenograms are usually not helpful in an acute early presentation. However, in a patient who has had recurrent episodes, particularly in a given joint, erosions with an overhanging margin may be suggestive of the diagnosis of gout.

Treatment

ACUTE GOUT In acute gout, the drugs of choice probably still are short-acting NSAIDs. These are often used for about 1 week and are discontinued when the episode has resolved. Because of the age and other factors of patients with gout, contraindications to the use of these agents often exist, namely, history of peptic ulceration, renal insufficiency, or a condition requiring anticoagulation. In this setting, glucocorticoids and adrenocorticotropic hormone (ACTH) are increasingly being used. Colchicine remains an alternative to NSAIDs but has a high incidence of gastrointestinal toxicity.

PROPHYLAXIS Prescribing lifelong therapy for a patient should be done only when the diagnosis is absolutely established. The usual reasons for such therapy include the following: recurrent acute attacks (particularly if they occur within a short time interval); chronic tophaceous gout; renal calculi; extremely high values of serum uric acid (particularly in the young); high serum uric acid levels in the setting of a known familial history of gout (for example, where there is a known deficiency of one of the relevant enzymes previously described); and prophylaxis for patients receiving acute courses of chemotherapy.

Before placing patients on such therapy, it is important to attempt to discontinue or change the doses of drugs that potentially might increase uric acid levels, for example, low-dose aspirin or thiazide diuretics. Alcohol intake should be decreased, and the patient should be provided with information on diet. Such behavioral modification on its own is occasionally adequate without relying on drug therapy. Protracted use of small doses of colchicine, to a dose of 0.6 mg twice daily, is safe. This has been shown to be prophylactic against recurrent acute attacks without necessarily creating a need to address the issue of hyperuricemia.

The goal of urate-lowering drugs is to consistently maintain the serum urate at less than 6 mg/dL. As previously stated, 90 percent of patients with gout and hyperuricemia are underexcretors of uric acid, which can be confirmed by a 24-h urine test.

Uricosurics include probenecid, at a dose of 500 to 1000 mg/day. Sulfinpyrazone is another potent uricosuric agent. Contraindications to this class of drug include renal calculi and renal insufficiency. The xanthine oxidase inhibitor allopurinol is the drug of choice by convention because the uricosuric agents increase attacks of gouty arthritis. The dose of allopurinol is usually 300 mg/day but should be tapered down in the elderly and in those with renal insufficiency. Side effects of allopurinol include dyspepsia, headache, diarrhea, a pruritic papular rash, thrombocytopenia, and hepatic function abnormalities. The syndrome of allopurinol hypersensitivity is well described and has a significant mortality. It usually occurs in an elderly patient with some renal dysfunction, often with poorly defined gout. Characteristic clinical toxic features include fever, urticaria, leukocytosis, eosinophilia, interstitial nephritis, acute renal failure, granulomatous hepatitis, and toxic epidermal necrolysis.

Gout in Unusual Situations

Cyclosporine, used in the treatment of transplant patients, causes significant rises in serum uric acid and may precipitate an attack of gout. These patients are difficult to manage because they are often on diuretics, have some renal insufficiency, and may be receiving low doses of glucocorticoids. It is extremely unusual for gout to coexist with RA, even though both of these disease processes are common ailments. The coexistence of systemic lupus erythematosus and gout has been described.[12]

RHEUMATIC FEVER

The prevalence of rheumatic fever and rheumatic heart disease would seem to be a reflection of the inadequacy of preventative medical care in a given community. These diseases have become quite rare in developed countries and communities but are more common in developing countries. Inadequate prevention may lead to strikingly different trends within the same country. In South Africa, for example, the prevalence of rheumatic fever has decreased substantially among a white minority, whereas in the schoolchildren of Soweto, a large black community, the reported prevalence in 1996 was 6.9 per 1000 children.[13]

Clinical Features

The diagnostic criteria have not changed since they were initially described by Chettle in 1889. Duckett-Jones assembled the major signs of polyarthritis, carditis, chorea, subcutaneous nodules, and erythema marginatum into a set of specific diagnostic criteria. Minor signs of systemic inflammation, to include fever, a high erythrocyte sedimentation rate, and concentrations of C-reactive protein, were organized into specific criteria. There have been few modifications except for those to include supporting evidence of an antecedent infection with a group A streptococcus. Echocardiography has greater sensitivity and specificity than auscultation for the assessment of valvular regurgitation.[14,15] This procedure is not an integral part of the tools for the diagnosis of rheumatic fever at the primary care level or in settings where the disease is common and medical resources are limited. A right ventricular endomyocardial biopsy provides little useful additional clinical information but may be used to confirm the presence of underlying carditis in cases of unexplained congestive heart failure.

The diagnosis of chorea is based entirely on clinical signs, which include fleeting local muscular weakness, emotional lability, personality changes, and erratic, jerky, purposeless movements. Chorea does not occur in adult men. Subcutaneous nodules and erythema marginatum are characteristic but rare. The nodules are small, painless, and localized over bony prominences and in tendon sheaths and may be seen in the back of the scalp and over the vertebral spine. Erythema marginatum is usually apparent in fair-skinned individuals. The eruption has a serpiginous pink border and is not usually indurated; it blanches on pressure and changes its shape to the clinician's observation. It is unusual on the face and on the lower extremities and is often hidden by the clothing. Patients are often unaware of its presence.

Changes in Epidemiology

Not all group A streptococcal infections cause rheumatic fever. Extrapharyngeal infections with group A streptococci, specifically pyodermas and soft tissue infections, are not rheumatogenic precursors. Serotypes M24 and M28 do not seem to be associated with rheumatic fever, whereas a more clear association occurs with M5 and perhaps M3, M6, and M14. Antibiotics seem to have resulted in a decline of rheumatogenic strains in African communities. However, there was a resurgence of rheumatic fever in focal epidemics in the mid-1980s in separate military and civilian populations in the United States. These were associated with M3, M5, and M18 serotypes.[16]

Treatment

The anti-inflammatory treatment has not changed since the control studies with glucocorticoids in the 1950s. Lingering doubts remain about the possible long-term benefits of glucocorticoids over salicylates. Some 80 percent of patients who fulfill the criteria for this disorder exhibit spontaneous healing. For prevention in communities where there is a high prevalence, intramuscular injection of penicillin G and benzathine is usually the first treatment. For those who have recurrences, a monthly intramuscular injection of 1.2 million units of penicillin G benzathine is recognized as the most effective regimen. Recommended alternatives include oral penicillin G or V or sulfadiazine. Successful vaccination against rheumatic fever may not require inclusion of all M-protein serotypes but rather those already known to be harmful.[13]

REFERENCES

1. Eberhardt K et al: The occurrence and significance of hand deformities in early rheumatoid arthritis. *Br J Rheumatol* **30**:211, 1991
2. Brook A, Corbett M: Radiographic changes in early rheumatoid disease. *Ann Rheum Dis* **36**:71, 1977
3. van der Heijde DMFM et al: Three-year prospective follow-up of patients with early rheumatoid arthritis. *Arthritis Rheum* **35**:26, 1992
4. Guerne P-A et al: Growth factor responsiveness of human articular chondrocytes in aging and development. *Arthritis Rheum* **38**:960, 1995
5. Weyand CM et al: The influence of HLA-DRBI genes on disease severity in rheumatoid arthritis. *Ann Intern Med* **117**:801, 1992
6. Craig SD et al: Cutaneous signs of rheumatic disease: Acral purpuric papules in a patient with rheumatoid arthritis. *Arthritis Rheum* **36**:957, 1994
7. Ackerman AB: Histological diagnosis of inflammatory skin disease. Philadelphia, Lea & Febiger, 1978, p 449
8. Jorizzo JL, Daniels E: Dermatologic conditions report in patients with rheumatoid arthritis. *J Am Acad Dermatol* **8**:439, 1983
9. Wilske KR, Healey LA: Remodeling the pyramid-a concept of whose time has come. *J Rheumatol* **16**:565, 1989
10. Beyeler C et al: Pulmonary function in rheumatoid arthritis treated with low-dose methotrexate: A longitudinal study. *Br J Rheumatol* **35**:446, 1996
11. Bottomley WW et al: Aggressive squamous cell carcinomas developing in patients receiving long-term azathioprine. *Br J Dermatol* **133**:460, 1995
12. DeCastero P et al: Coexistent systemic lupus erythematosus and tophaceous gout. *J Am Acad Dermatol* **13**:650, 1985
13. McLaren MJ, Markowitz MM: Rheumatic heart disease in developing countries: The consequence of inadequate prevention. *Ann Intern Med* **120**:243, 1994
14. Vasan RS et al: Echocardiographic evaluation of patients with acute rheumatic fever and rheumatic carditis. *Circulation* **94**:73, 1996
15. Wilson NJ, Neutze JM: Echocardiographic diagnosis of subclinical carditis in acute rheumatic fever [editorial]. *Int J Cardiol* **50**:1, 1995
16. Centers for Disease Control: Acute rheumatic fever—Utah. *MMWR* **36**:108, 1987

CHAPTER 180

Thomas T. Provost

Sjögren's Syndrome

Sjögren's syndrome (SS) is a rheumatologic disease characterized by dryness of the mucous membranes of the eyes, mouth, and vagina. A patchy lymphocytic infiltrate composed predominantly of CD4+ T lymphocytes and an admixture of histiocytes and plasma cells invading the minor and major salivary glands and lacrimal glands is characteristic.[1,2] Destruction of these glands produces xerostomia and keratoconjunctivitis sicca. The etiology is unknown. SS may occur alone (primary SS) or in association with other connective tissue diseases such as rheumatoid arthritis, progressive systemic sclerosis, and systemic lupus erythematosus (SLE) (secondary SS).

Primary SS is a heterogeneous disease. Some patients have only mucous membrane dryness. Others, especially those with anti-Ro(SS-A) and anti-La(SS-B) antibodies, frequently have extraglandular manifestations including cutaneous vasculitis[3] (Tables 180-1 and 180-2). Patients with SS and cutaneous vasculitis are at increased risk for the development of peripheral and central nervous system manifestations.[4] The early recognition of SS patients with

TABLE 180-1

Extraglandular Manifestations of Primary Sjögren's Syndrome

Arthritis
Pulmonary disease
  Interstitial
  Necrotizing bronchoalveolitis
Chronic active hepatitis
Primary biliary cirrhosis
Renal disease
  Interstitial disease
  Glomerulonephritis
Myositis
Thyroiditis
Vasculitis (cutaneous)
Peripheral nervous system disease
Central nervous system disease
B cell lymphoma

TABLE 180-2

Association of Clinical and Laboratory Features in anti-Ro(SS-A) Antibody-Positive Sjögren's Syndrome

| | PATIENTS WITH ANTI-RO(SS-A) | | |
FEATURES	POSITIVE (n = 33)	NEGATIVE (n = 42)	P VALUE
Clinical			
Vasculitis	24	4	0.0005
Lymphadenopathy	19	4	0.0005
Hematologic			
Anemia	19	6	0.0005
Leukopenia	14	3	0.001
Thrombocytopenia	7	1	0.025
Serologic			
Hypergammaglobulinemia	21	8	0.0005
Rheumatoid factor	29	17	0.0005
Cryoglobulinemia	7/13	0/22	0.001
Hypocomplementemia	11	2	0.005

SOURCE: Adapted from Alexander et al. Ro(SS-A) and La(SS-B) antibodies in the clinical spectrum of Sjögren's syndrome. *J Rheumatol* **9**:239, 1982, with permission.

cutaneous vasculitis identifies individuals at risk for the development of a chronic relapsing disease process (decades) associated with a great deal of morbidity.

Diagnostic criteria for SS have been published.[5–9] In the author's experience, the European diagnostic criteria for SS have been most satisfactory[10] (Table 180-3).

HISTORY

Sjögren's syndrome was first described by Hadden in 1888. In 1892, Mikulicz described a patient with bilateral enlargement of the parotid glands. On biopsy, the glands demonstrated focal lymphocytic infiltrates. In 1933, Henrik Sjögren described the triad of keratoconjunctivitis sicca, xerostomia, and arthritis. In 1953, Castleman and Morgan reported the pathologic features of Mikulicz disease and Sjögren's syndrome were identical (reviewed in ref. 11).

In the early 1960s Anderson et al.[12] demonstrated the presence of two precipitin antibodies (detected by gel double diffusion) in the sera of patients with SS. These were termed SjD and SjT antibodies. Rowell et al. in 1963 described erythema multiforme-like lesions in anti-SjT antibody positive patients with SLE [this is the first description of subacute cutaneous lupus erythematosus (SCLE)-like lesions associated with anti-Ro(SS-A) and anti-La(SS-B) antibodies (see below)].[13]

In 1969 Clark et al.[14] described anti-Ro(SS-A) antibodies, and in 1974 Mattioli and Reichlin[15] described anti-La(SS-B) antibodies in patients with SLE. Alspaugh and Tan[16] in 1975 described two precipitin antibody systems (anti-SS-A and anti-SS-B) in patients with SS. Subsequently, an interlaboratory collaboration by Alspaugh and Maddison[17] established the identity of anti-Ro with anti-SS-A and of anti-La with anti-SS-B.

EPIDEMIOLOGY

SS occurs with approximately the same frequency as rheumatoid arthritis. It affects approximately 4 million Americans. In Greece and the United Kingdom, a frequency of SS in elderly patients ranging from 3 to 5 percent has been reported.[18,19] The disease most commonly occurs in women (9:1 female/male ratio). Male patients with SS generally have a more benign disease with fewer extraglandular manifestations and lower frequencies of anti-Ro(SS-A) and anti-La(SS-B) autoantibodies.[20] Although SS usually occurs in the fourth and fifth decades of life, it has been described in children (albeit uncommonly).[21,22] Elderly individuals have an increased frequency of both SS and anti-Ro(SS-A) antibodies. In one U.S. study, approximately 12 percent of 103 elderly patients (>70 years) had definite or probable SS; and of these patients with SS, 7 possessed anti-Ro(SS-A) antibodies.[23]

IMMUNOGENETIC STUDIES

In recent years, immunogenetic, autoantibody, and viral studies have provided important information possibly related to the pathogenesis of SS.

Immunogenetic studies have described a variety of autoimmune diseases in relatives of SS patients, as well as various autoantibodies. The autoimmune diseases found in 98 primary and secondary SS probands are presented in Table 180-4.[24] Furthermore, first degree relatives of patients with SS demonstrate an increased frequency of antinuclear, anti-ssDNA, biological false-positive test for syphilis (BFP-STS), and anti-Ro(SS-A) antibodies.

Two antibody response patterns have been noted: anti-Ro(SS-A) and anti-La(SS-B) and anti-Ro(SS-A) without anti-La(SS-B). The combination of anti-Ro and anti-La occurs more frequently in patients with primary SS than in those with SLE. This coupled antibody response is associated with the serologically defined HLA-B8, DR3, DQw2, DRw52 haplotype (Table 180-5). The second antibody response, anti-Ro(SS-A) without anti-La(SS-B) antibodies, is detected primarily in patients with SLE and is associated with the HLA-DR2, DQw1 haplotype. Heterozygosity (HLA-DQw1/DQw2) is associated with the highest anti-Ro(SS-A) antibody titers.[25,26] Subsequent studies with restriction fragment length polymorphism have determined that the highest anti-Ro(SS-A) and anti-La(SS-B) antibody titers are associated with heterozygosity for HLA-DQw2.1/DQw6 (subtypes of HLA-DQw2 and DQw1, respectively) (Table 180-5).[27]

Nucleotide sequence analysis of the DQA1 and DQB1 chain alleles reveals 100 percent of anti-Ro(SS-A) antibody-positive patients with SS or SLE possess a glutamine residue at position 34 of the outermost domain of the DQA1 chain and/or a leucine at position 26 of the outermost domain of the DQB1 chain. A dosage effect of these alleles is present. For example, patients with anti-Ro(SS-A) plus anti-La(SS-B) antibodies are more likely to have all four of their DQA1-DQB1 chains (one set on each haplotype) containing these amino acid residues than are anti-Ro(SS-A) antibody-negative patients with SLE, patients with SS, or controls. Theoretically, these data indicate that the glutamine and leucine residues, located in the floor of the antigen-binding cleft of the HLA-DQA1/DQB1 heterodimer, may be important in binding the antigenic peptide(s) responsible for the anti-Ro(SS-A) and anti-La(SS-B) antibody responses.[28]

These studies also indicate that the HLA associations in SS are not disease specific but are associated with the anti-Ro(SS-A) and anti-La(SS-B) antibody responses (see Table 180-5).

ANTIBODY STUDIES

By gel double diffusion, 40 to 45 percent of patients with primary SS evaluated on a rheumatology service possess anti-Ro(SS-A) antibodies and approximately 20 percent demonstrate anti-La(SS-B) antibodies.[3,29] However, ELISA techniques revealed that approximately 90 percent of this same population have anti-Ro(SS-A) antibodies and approximately 70 percent have anti-La(SS-B) antibodies [anti-La(SS-B) antibodies are almost never found in the absence of anti-Ro(SS-A) antibodies]. Thus, the frequency of anti-Ro(SS-A) and anti-La(SS-B) antibodies in patients with SS depends, at least in part, on the study techniques employed.

Primary SS is a very heterogeneous disease with respect to the expression

TABLE 180-3

European Community Criteria for Diagnosis of Sjögren's Syndrome

CRITERION	DEFINITION
1. Ocular symptoms Positive response to any of these questions	Daily dry eyes for more than 3 months Recurrent sensations of sand or gravel in the eyes Tear substitutes employed >3X/day
2. Oral symptoms Positive response to any of these questions	Daily dry mouth for >3 months Recurrent or persistently swollen salivary glands in an adult Frequent drinking of liquids to swallow food
3. Ocular signs Objective evidence of dryness in one of these tests	Schirmer's test (≤5 mm in 5 min) Rose Bengal score (≥4 according to van Bÿsteweld scoring system)
4. Histopathology	A focus score ≥1 in a minor salivary gland (a focus defined as an aggregate of at least 50 mononuclear cells around an intralobular duct; the focus score is defined by the number of foci in 4 mm^2 of glandular tissue)
5. Salivary gland involvement One of following test positive	Salivary scintigraphy Parotid sialography Unstimulated salivary flow (≤1.5 mL/15 min)
6. Autoantibodies One of three antibodies present	Antibodies to La(SS-B) and/or Ro(SS-A) Antinuclear antibodies Rheumatoid factor

Sjögren's syndrome present if 4/6 criteria positive (93 percent sensitivity; 93 percent specificity).

SOURCE: Adapted from Vitali C et al. Preliminary criteria for the diagnosis of Sjögren's syndrome. Results of a prospective concerted action supported by the European community. *Arth Rheum* **36:**340, 1993, with permission.

TABLE 180-4

Autoimmune Diseases in Family Members of Probands with Primary or Secondary Sjögren's Syndrome

	PROBAND DIAGNOSES			
	PRIMARY SJÖGREN'S (%)	SLE SJÖGREN'S (%)	RA SJÖGREN'S (%)	UCTD SJÖGREN'S (%)
Proband #	51	20	20	7
Positive family history of autoimmune disease	18(35)	6(30)	4(20)	3(43)
Autoimmune diagnoses of family members				
Sjögren's syndrome	6(12)	1(5)	0	0
SLE	2(5)	2(10)	0	0
Rheumatoid arthritis	7(14)	3(15)	2(10)	2(29)
Multiple sclerosis	1(2)	0	0	0
Systemic sclerosis	1 (2)	0	0	0
Myasthenia gravis	1(2)	0	0	0
Discoid LE	0	0	1(5)	0
Thyroid disease	7(14)	1(5)	1(5)	2(29)

ABBREVIATIONS: SLE, systemic lupus erythematosus; RA, rheumatoid arthritis; UCTD, undifferentiated connective tissue disease
SOURCE: Adapted from Reveille JD et al. Primary Sjögren's syndrome and other autoimmune diseases in families. *Ann Intern Med* **101:**748, 1984, with permission.

TABLE 180-5

HLA-DR and DQ Specificities in Anti-Ro(+) Caucasian and Anti-Ro(−) Patients with Primary Sjögren's Syndrome

	ANTI-RO(+) SS PATIENTS (n = 24)	ANTI-RO(−) SS PATIENTS (n = 13)	CONTROLS (N = 79)
HLA			
DR3 (17)*	67%[†][‡]	23%[†]	20%[‡]
DRw52a (DW24)*	75%[¶]	38%	39%[¶]
DQw2.1	67%[†][‡]	23%[†]	20%[‡]
DQw2.1/DQw6	29%[§]	0%	3%[§]

*Splits of broader HLA specificities
[†]$P = 0.03$; RR = 6.7
[‡]$P = 0.00005$; RR = 7.9
[¶]$P = 0.004$; RR = 4.6
[§]$P = 0.0002$; RR = 16
SOURCE: Adapted from Reveille JD, Arnett RD. The immunogenetics of Sjögren's syndrome. *Rheum Dis Clin North Am* **18:**539, 1992, with permission.

of these autoantibodies. In a study of 50 patients with SS documented by minor salivary gland lip biopsy who were referred from dermatologists, rheumatologists, general internists, allergists, and obstetricians/gynecologists, a 30 percent frequency of anti-Ro(SS-A) and a 15 percent frequency of anti-La(SS-B) antibodies were detected with both gel double diffusion and ELISA techniques.[30] These studies indicate that selection bias occurs in the evaluation of patients with SS and that those patients with primary SS with many extraglandular manifestations are most commonly evaluated by rheumatologists, whereas those with only mucous membrane involvement are generally seen by allergists, ophthalmologists, dentists, and obstetricians/gynecologists. Dermatologists may see a sicker primary SS patient population because of the frequent presence of cutaneous vasculitis in anti-Ro(SS-A) antibody-positive patients with SS who also have other extraglandular manifestations (see Table 180-2).

Immunoblotting studies have demonstrated that the anti-Ro(SS-A) antibody in patients with SS recognizes predominantly the 52-kDa protein (reviewed in ref. 31). In contradistinction, the anti-Ro(SS-A) antibody in patients with SLE predominantly recognizes the 60-kDa protein. Mothers of neonatal lupus infants possess anti-Ro(SS-A) antibodies that predominantly recognize the 52-kDa protein.[32,33] This observation plus the clinical observation of mothers with SS giving birth to infants with neonatal lupus erythematosus (NLE) has promoted the idea that NLE syndrome may be more closely related to SS than to lupus erythematosus. Moreover, evidence suggests that 52-kDa anti-Ro(SS-A) antibodies may be etiologically significant in the pathogenesis of the isolated congenital heart block of the NLE syndrome.[34]

The 52-kDa and 60-kDa nuclear and cytoplasmic proteins are associated with small RNAs known as hY1, hY3, hY4, and hY5 RNAs. Molecular cloning studies of the Ro(SS-A) autoantigens have determined that the 52 kDa and the 60 kDa are different proteins, with little, if any, sequence homology. The 60-kDa polypeptide has an RNA binding domain as well as a zinc finger motif. The RNA binding domain presumably binds with the hY RNAs, whereas the putative zinc finger motif of the 60-kDa protein may interact with the 52-kDa protein.[31]

The 52-kDa Ro protein contains a zinc finger as well as leucine zipper domains. Because zinc fingers and leucine zippers are motifs found in proteins involved in gene regulation, it has been proposed that the 52-kDa Ro(SS-A) may be involved in the regulation of gene expression.[31]

Anti-Ro(SS-A) antibody positive sera also react with a synthetic polypeptide construct of the calcium binding protein, calreticulin (CR). The exact relationship of CR to Ro(SS-A) is unknown, but recent immunization studies in mice have demonstrated spreading of immunity from Ro52 and Ro60 to CR. This finding suggests that CR or CR particles must associate under certain circumstances with Ro52 and Ro60 in vivo.[35]

Anti-La(SS-B) antibodies are directed against an RNA binding protein that transiently binds all RNA polymerase III transcripts, as well as precursors of tRNA and 5sRNA. Studies by Gottesfeld et al.[36] and by Gottlieb and Steitz[37,38] indicate that the in vivo transcription of RNA polymerase III genes is inhibited if the La(SS-B) ribonucleoprotein is depleted with anti-La(SS-B) antibodies from the transcription extract. Furthermore, the few RNA transcripts produced in the La(SS-B)-depleted extract are truncated (loss of several uridylate residues at the 3' end). Therefore, the La(SS-B) protein is a transcription, as well as a termination factor for all RNA polymerase III transcripts. Because the La(SS-B) and the hY5 Ro(SS-A) ribonuclear protein may be at least transiently complexed, it has been hypothesized, but not proved, that the Ro(SS-A) polypeptide may also be involved in RNA polymerase III transcription.[39]

Studies indicate that cells undergoing ultraviolet-induced apoptosis express a species of the Ro(SS-A) and La(SS-B) autoantigens on the cell surface membranes. Furthermore, keratinocytes cultured in the presence of 17β-estradiol express these antigens on the keratinocyte cell surface. These studies suggest possible immune-mediated cellular injury mechanisms involving anti-Ro(SS-A) and anti-La(SS-B) autoantibodies (reviewed in ref. 31).

Epitope mapping of the Ro and La peptides has thus far failed to establish a definite relationship of one or several epitopes with clinical disease expression (LE or SS). Tertiary protein structures rather than linear protein sequences may be responsible for epitopes that correlate with disease expression.[40]

VIRAL STUDIES

A possible viral pathogenesis of SS is an area of active study (reviewed in ref. 41). The salivary gland, the main site of mucous membrane involvement in SS, contains a number of viruses in their latent state. At present, all herpesviruses are possible candidates, but the strongest candidate is the Epstein-Barr virus. Biopsies of salivary glands from patients with SS contain increased Epstein-Barr viral DNA. This finding, however, is not specific for SS and has been detected in organ transplant patients receiving immune suppressive medication without evidence of SS.

The possible role of retroviruses in the pathogenesis of SS has received attention. Talal et al.[42] found that sera from some patients with SS contain an antibody reactive against the retroviral protein p24. Furthermore, studies of the human acquired immunodeficiency syndrome (AIDS) have detected diffuse infiltrative lymphocytosis syndrome (DILS), a syndrome associated with HIV-1 infection (most commonly, AIDS) that may present with sicca features (reviewed in ref. 43). Clinically, most patients with DILS demonstrate bilateral parotid gland enlargement and xerostomia. Xerophthalmia and keratoconjunctivitis sicca occur less frequently.

Although these clinical features are reminiscent of SS, there are many immunologic differences in DILS. For example, CD8 T cells predominate in the lymphocytic tissue infiltrate and blood lymphocytosis. In contradistinction, the inflammatory infiltrate in Sjögren's syndrome is predominantly CD4+. In addition, the frequency of autoantibody formation is much higher in SS, and the HLA associations in SS are markedly different from those found in DILS.

CLINICAL MANIFESTATIONS

Mucous membrane dryness (eyes, mouth, vagina) is universally present in patients with SS. However, dryness of only one or two mucous membranes may predominate, and the disease may be heralded for several years by dryness involving only one mucous membrane.

Xerostomia

Xerostomia is caused by a chronic progressive destruction of the major and minor salivary glands by the lymphocytic inflammatory infiltrate. Dryness of the mouth is insidious in onset and progressively gets worse. As a consequence, patients may have difficulty swallowing and may be unable to carry on a conversation without the frequent ingestion of fluids.

Physical examination during the early phase of SS may fail to uncover dryness in the oral cavity. However, with progression of the disease, an absence of the infralingual salivary pool becomes evident, and the patient may fail to produce any saliva or the saliva may be cloudy and stringy.

Several complications of xerostomia occur. Oral candidiasis is frequent, especially in those patients who wear dentures, and approximately one-third of patients with SS develop this complication. The oral candidiasis may manifest itself as perleche or as a burning mouth. Physical examinations may or may not reveal a beefy red appearance of the oral mucosa. A potassium hydroxide (KOH) examination or fungal culture from the corners of the mouth or mucosal surface of the denture will generally exhibit Candida albicans. Exotoxins released by Candida albicans produce a primary irritant reaction responsible for the burning sensation and the red appearance.

Patients with SS also have an increased frequency of dental caries. Caries along the gingival margin are common. These caries are difficult to repair, making tooth restoration problematic. Many patients with SS have partial plates or are completely edentulous.

The major salivary glands are enlarged in approximately 20 percent of patients. Enlargement is generally transient and unilateral but on occasions is bilateral and, uncommonly, permanent. Both the parotid and submandibular glands are affected. Blockage of the salivary gland ducts by inspissated mucous is responsible for the transient enlargement. Secondary infection is uncommon.

The diagnosis of the oral component of SS is problematic. Various drugs including sedatives, antipsychotics, antidepressants, antihistamines, anticholinergics, and diuretics may produce dryness. Also to be considered in the differential diagnosis are viral infections such as mumps and human immunodeficiency virus (HIV). Radiation therapy to the neck, graft-versus-host disease, sarcoidosis, and amyloidosis may induce dryness. Furthermore, neoplasms, cirrhosis, and gonadal hypofunction may be associated with salivary gland enlargement.

Although it is possible to investigate salivary gland function with sialometry and sialography, the most common technique is a lip biopsy to examine the minor salivary gland pathology. The lower lip is injected with a local anesthetic and a 1-in. vertical incision is made (Fig. 180-1). The vermilion border is identified at all times

FIGURE 180-1

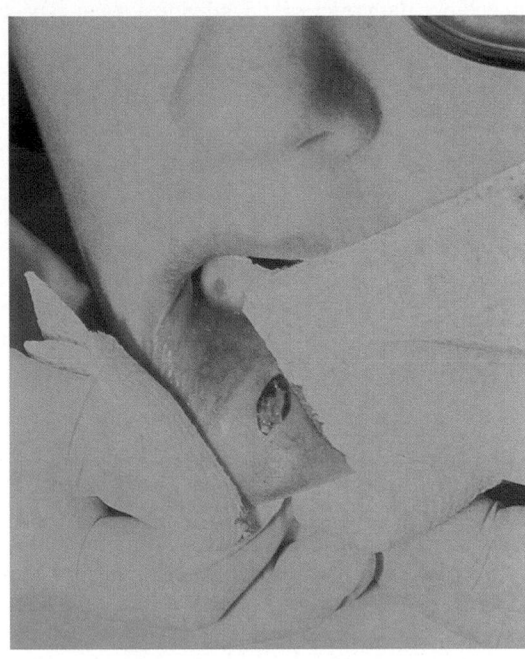

Lip biopsy technique exposing minor salivary glands (see text for description).

and avoided. After the incision, five minor salivary glands are identified and excised with straight scissors. The incision is then closed with two or three absorbable sutures.

The classic pathology associated with SS is a patchy inflammatory infiltrate composed of mononuclear cells involving both the ductal and acinar tissue (Fig. 180-2). Most classifications are based on the detection of aggregates of 50 or more mononuclear cells.[44,45] Although the lip biopsy is proported to be "the gold standard" for

FIGURE 180-2

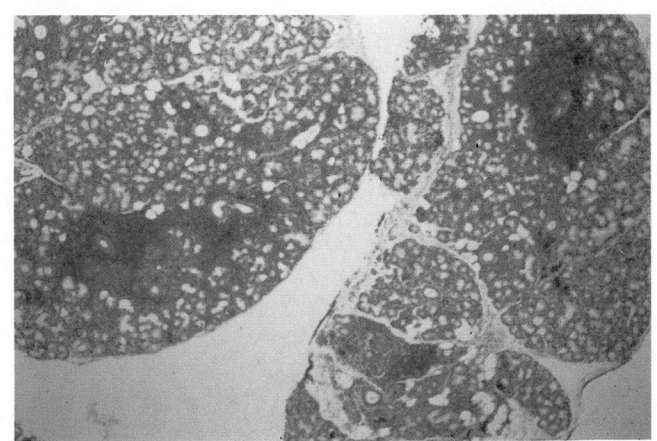

Pathology of Sjögren's syndrome in a minor salivary gland biopsy. Note patchy aggregates of lymphocytes involving glandular and ductal regions of the gland. Also note large areas of gland are free of disease.

the diagnosis of SS, several caveats are important. Initially, the inflammatory infiltrate is patchy and may involve only one of several glands. In addition, large areas of an individual gland may be totally uninvolved; thus, sampling error is problematic.

In addition, with longstanding SS, fatty metamorphosis and fibrosis of minor salivary glands occur, producing total destruction. No allowance for this end-stage SS is accommodated by the present minor salivary gland SS diagnostic criteria.

Xerophthalmia

The first symptoms of ocular dryness include a foreign body sensation secondary to repeated blinking and rubbing of the eyes, which produces minor corneal abrasions. The minor corneal abrasions may produce photophobia. With severe dryness, a deep aching sensation may occur.[46]

Ocular SS is commonly manifested by conjunctival injection. Filiform defects along the inferior portion of the cornea adjacent to the conjunctiva may occur and are detected by the Rose Bengal dye test. Patients with advanced SS may display a marked decrease in the aqueous component and an increased viscosity of their tears. Some can pull long strings of mucin from their eyes. Testing for ocular SS includes the Schirmer's test. The inferior eyelid is anesthetized and a Whatman paper wick is folded over the lower eyelid. The migration of fluid along the wick is measured during a 5-min time period. Values of 5 mm or less are highly suggestive of SS.

In addition to the Rose Bengal dye test and the Schirmer's test, lysosome, lactoferrin, and β_2-macroglobulin assays have been used to evaluate ocular SS. These tests are more investigational and have not achieved widespread clinical acceptance.

Vaginal Dryness

Vaginal dryness in patients with SS is much more common than realized. It is not a symptom freely volunteered by the patient and generally must be elicited by direct questioning. Dyspareunia may be the initial manifestation of SS, antedating the development of other mucous membrane involvement by years.[47] Yeast and bacterial vaginal infections are common.

Xeroderma

The cutaneous manifestations of SS are listed in Table 180-6. Xerosis is a common complaint. In their classic paper, Block et al.[48] reported an approximate 50 percent frequency. Pruritus frequently

TABLE 180-6

Cutaneous Manifestations of Sjögren's Syndrome

Xerosis
Palpable and nonpalpable purpura
Urticaria-like vasculitic lesions
Erythema multiforme-like, erythema perstans, erythema nodosum lesions
Cutaneous lymphoma
Nodular amyloidosis
Sweet's syndrome
Annular erythematosus lesion (donut lesion) described in Japanese patients

accompanies the xerosis, and hyperpigmentation may occur in areas subjected to repeated scratching.[48,49] Patients with SS also complain of dryness of the hair and loss of luster as well as of severe dryness of the external ear canal with impaction of dried cerumen.

The pathogenesis of the xerosis is unknown. A lymphohistiocytic infiltrate of eccrine sweat glands has been reported.[50] A decreased sweating response to pilocarpine has been observed in some patients with SS.[51] It should be emphasized, however, that the major lubrication of the skin is provided by sebaceous glands. Whether or not the lymphohistiocytic infiltrate detected in the salivary glands and in other organs in SS also involves the sebaceous glands is not known.

Inflammatory Dermatoses

In addition to xerosis, approximately 20 percent of patients with SS have Raynaud's phenomenon. Furthermore, SS patients uncommonly demonstrate erythematous nodules on the lower extremities, persistent plaque-like lesions (erythema multiforme-like lesions), as well as superficial, ill-defined, persistent erythematous patches (erythema perstans).[52] Sweet's syndrome has been detected in patients with SS.[53,54] Cutaneous lymphomas, as well as nodular amyloidosis, have also been reported in patients with SS.[55,56] The author has seen one anti-Ro(SS-A) antibody-positive patient with a cutaneous B-cell lymphoma and adjacent nodular amyloidosis.

Japanese investigators have reported an erythematous, elevated, plaque-like lesion with central clearing resembling a "donut" in patients with SS.[57,58] In the author's experience with several hundred Caucasian and African-American anti-Ro(SS-A) antibody-positive patients with SS and LE, no similar lesion has been seen.[59] The occurrence of this erythematous, edematous, plaque-like lesion in anti-La(SS-B) and/or anti-Ro(SS-A) antibody-positive Japanese patients with SS may indicate a racial difference in the cutaneous expression of SS. Large quantities of mucin, a hydroscopic substance, has been reported in these erythematous, indurated, plaque-like lesions. This mucin may be responsible for the thickened, plaque-like nature of the lesion.

Vasculitis

The most important cutaneous feature associated with SS is vasculitis. The most common vasculitic lesions are palpable and nonpalpable purpura of the lower extremities (Fig. 180-3; Table 180-6).[60] The purpuric lesions on the lower extremities in SS are indistinguishable from the lesions of Waldenström's benign hypergammaglobulinemic purpura.[61,62] Approximately 25 to 30 percent of patients with Waldenström's benign hypergammaglobulinemic purpura have been previously reported to have SS. Many of the patients with SS and vasculitis also have mixed cryoglobulinemia and rheumatoid factor positivity (Table 180-2). The patients reported with mixed cryoglobulinemia vasculitis by Meltzer and Franklin frequently had vasculitic lesions on the lower extremities,[63,64] and many of these patients probably had SS.

The second most common type of vasculitic lesion seen in patients with SS is urticaria-like vasculitic lesions (Fig. 180-4; Table 180-6). Urticaria-like vasculitic lesions have been seen in SLE and in the syndrome termed hypocomplementemic urticarial vasculitis; in the latter syndrome patients not only have urticaria-like vasculitic lesions but also may develop obstructive lung disease.[65-68] Urticaria-like lesions are now a well-recognized cutaneous manifestation of vasculitis.[69] These urticaria-like vasculitic lesions, unlike common hives, which usually come and go over a period of 3 to 6 h, may persist for days or weeks. In addition, these vasculitic lesions may demonstrate petechiae (an indication of compromise of the

FIGURE 180-3

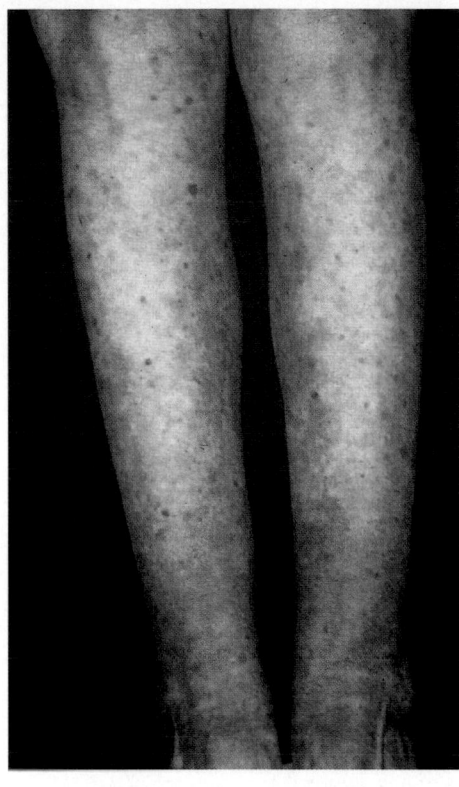

Palpable purpuric lesions of the lower extremities. Note, in addition to new lesions, the widespread deposition of hemosiderin (brownish patches), evidence of previous vasculitic lesions.

vascular integrity) as well as hyperpathia and a burning sensation elicited by the application of light touch.

Two types of histopathology have been detected in the SS vasculitic lesions. One is a neutrophilic inflammatory vascular insult indistinguishable from a leukocytoclastic angiitis; the other is a mononuclear inflammatory vascular disease characterized by lym-

FIGURE 180-4

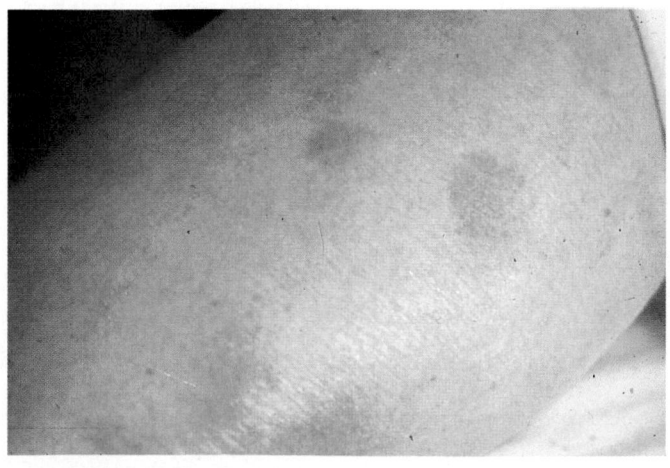

Urticaria-like vasculitic lesion in an anti-Ro(SS-A) antibody-positive patient with SS.

FIGURE 180-5

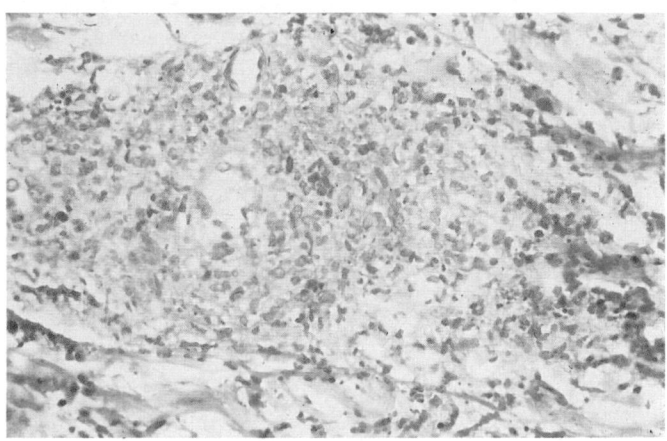

Leukocytoclastic vasculitis characterized by destruction of blood vessel in an anti-Ro(SS-A) antibody-positive patient with SS with palpable purpura on lower extremity.

phocyte invasion and destruction of blood vessel integrity (Figs. 180-5 and 180-6). The neutrophilic inflammatory infiltrate is composed predominantly of neutrophils, many of which are fragmented. In addition, the lesions frequently demonstrate fibrinoid necrosis, lumen occlusion, and extravasation of red blood cells. The mononuclear inflammatory vascular disease is characterized by an invasion and destruction of blood vessel walls. Fibrinoid necrosis is present, but less prominent than the neutrophilic inflammatory infiltrate.

Other investigators have previously recognized two histopathologic forms of necrotizing vasculitis.[70] The cutaneous expressions of urticaria-like vasculitis and palpable and nonpalpable purpura of the lower extremities, despite two different histopathologies, are indistinguishable. In other words, we were unable to detect morphologic differences between the cutaneous expression of the leukocytoclastic and mononuclear vasculopathies.

FIGURE 180-6

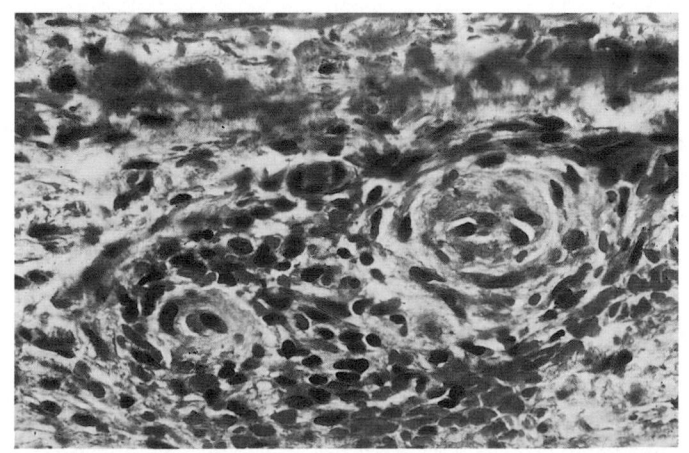

Histopathology of a palpable purpuric lesion of the lower extremity demonstrating a mononuclear vasculopathy.

Relationship of Vascular Disease to Serologic Abnormalities

Anti-La(SS-B) and/or anti-Ro(SS-A) antibodies, rheumatoid factor, antinuclear antibodies, cryoglobulins, hypocomplementemia, and hypergammaglobulinemia are found to be statistically significantly increased in patients with SS with the neutrophilic inflammatory vascular disease (Tables 180-2 and 180-7).[71] Lawley et al. have previously demonstrated the presence of circulating immune complexes in SS.[72] The mononuclear inflammatory vasculopathy occurring in patients with SS generally fails to demonstrate these serologic associations.[71]

Nervous System Involvement

The inflammatory vascular disease in patients with SS recurs over time. In general, small blood vessels (postcapillary venules and arterioles) are involved. Both histopathologic types of vascular insult may be associated with peripheral and central nervous system (CNS) disease, most likely resulting from a systemic small vessel vasculopathy (Table 180-8).[73] In addition, physical examination, spinal fluid studies, evoked sensory response testing, magnetic resonance imaging (MRI), and autopsy studies have all documented the presence of peripheral and central nervous system disease in SS.[74–78] The autopsy and MRI data suggest diffuse small cerebral vascular disease (vasculitis).

The peripheral and central nervous system manifestations that occur in patients with SS are listed in Table 180-9. The presence of central nervous system disease associated with SS has been until recently controversial.[79–81] Spanish investigators have now confirmed the presence of a multiple sclerosis-like central nervous system disease process in association with SS, and a recent study from a Finnish group has confirmed the presence of central nervous system disease in their SS population.[82,83] These latter investigators have described a higher frequency of CNS complications in patients with SS than previously reported from the United States.

TABLE 180-7

Serologic Correlation with Histopathologic Type of Vascular Disease in Sjögren's Syndrome

PATHOLOGY	ANA%	GLOB%	RF%	ANTI-RO%	ANTI-LA%
Leukocytoclastic angiitis (%), n = 27	21(78)	14(52)	18(67)	20(74)	12(44)
Mononuclear? vasculopathy (%), n = 18	7(39)	2(11)	3(17)	2(11)	2(11)
P-value	0.02	0.01	0.002	0.00006	0.036

ABBREVIATIONS: ANA, antinuclear antibody; Glob, hypergammaglobulinemia; RF, rheumatoid factor
SOURCE: Adapted from Molina R et al: Two histopathologic prototypes of inflammatory vascular disease in Sjögren's syndrome: Differential association with seroreactivity to rheumatoid factor and antibodies to Ro(SS-A) and with hypocomplementemia. *Arth Rheum* **28:**1251, 1985, with permission.

TABLE 180-8

Central and Peripheral Nervous System Disease in Patients with Sjögren's Syndrome with Peripheral Vascular Disease

	NUMBER (%) OF SS PATIENTS WITH NERVOUS SYSTEM DISEASE		
PATHOLOGY (n)	CENTRAL ALONE	PERIPHERAL ALONE	BOTH
Leukocytoclastic angiitis (17)	3 (18)	6 (35)	8 (47)
Mononuclear vasculopathy (16)	2 (12)	3 (18)	11 (70)
Total (33)	5 (15)	9 (28)	19 (58)

SOURCE: Adapted from Molina R et al: Peripheral inflammatory vascular disease in Sjögren's syndrome: Association with nervous system complications. *Arth Rheum* **28:**1341, 1985, with permission.

TABLE 180-9

Some of the Neurologic Features Associated with Sjögren's Syndrome

Brain
    Cognitive dysfunction[94]
    Alzheimer-like disease[94]
    Multiple sclerosis-like disease[95]
    Aseptic meningitis[96]
    Focal neurologic disease[97]
    Intranuclear ophthalmoplegia
Spinal cord
    Transverse myelopathy
    Neurogenic bladder
    Rectal incontinence
Peripheral nervous system
    Trigeminal neuropathy[97]
    Sensory neuronopathy[98]
    Sensorineural hearing defect[99]

B Cell Lymphomas

Patients with SS frequently have B cell proliferation characterized by hypergammaglobulinemia. Monoclonal light chains and heavy chains have been detected in SS patients with very sensitive immunofixation techniques. Patients with SS are also at increased risk for developing B cell lymphomas (relative risk 32–44).[84,56] The lymphomas in some cases have involved the parotid gland; in others, the skin. Anti-Ro(SS-A) antibody-positive patients with SS appear to be at greater risk to develop B cell proliferative responses (Table 180-2).

RELATIONSHIP OF ANTI-RO(SS-A) POSITIVE SS WITH SLE

A close association between the phenotypic expression of SS and lupus erythematosus occurring in HLA-DR3, anti-Ro(SS-A) positive female patients has been demonstrated. This interrelationship is depicted in Fig. 180-7. Approximately 0.5 percent of asymptomatic females of childbearing age possess anti-Ro(SS-A) antibodies.[85–87] In the author's experience, these patients, with heavy sun

FIGURE 180-7

CHAPTER 180
Sjögren's Syndrome

2075

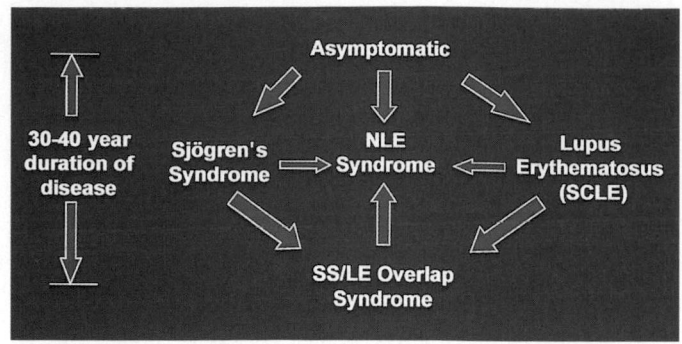

Schematic representation of the interrelationship between the various clinical presentations of HLA-DR3, anti-Ro(SS-A) antibody-positive female patients (see text for discussion).

exposure, may develop transiently a phototoxic reaction that on biopsy demonstrates an interface dermatitis suggestive of lupus erythematosus. The phototoxic dermatitis may completely disappear, but with time the patients may develop clinical features of lupus erythematosus. Most prominent in these anti-Ro(SS-A) female patients with SLE is an exquisite photosensitivity. Many of these patients relate burning through window glass (reviewed in refs. 88–90).

These asymptomatic anti-Ro(SS-A) antibody-positive patients may alternatively develop dryness of their mucous membranes and demonstrate a phenotypic expression of SS. With time, both the anti-Ro(SS-A) antibody-positive SS patients and the anti-Ro(SS-A) antibody-positive SLE patients may develop features of both SS and SLE. These SS/SLE patients have a high frequency of cutaneous disease including subacute cutaneous lupus lesions and cutaneous vasculitis.[91] Central nervous system manifestations and pulmonary interstitial disease are prominent features. Renal disease is also a significant manifestation.

The factors that determine the phenotypic expression of these anti-Ro(SS-A) antibody-positive HLA-DR3 positive female patients are unknown. Certainly, ultraviolet light precipitates and exacerbates the cutaneous lupus disease process in anti-Ro(SS-A) antibody-positive patients with LE. However, intriguing is the fact that clinical experience indicates that those HLA-DR3 positive, anti-Ro(SS-A) antibody-positive female patients with the SS phenotype are not photosensitive.

Despite these phenotypic differences, all of these HLA-DR3, anti-Ro(SS-A) antibody-positive females with asymptomatic SS, lupus erythematosus, or SS/lupus erythematosus patients during their childbearing years are at risk to give birth to children demonstrating the NLE syndrome. These HLA-DR3, anti-Ro(SS-A) antibody-positive women may have a dynamic disease process associated with a great deal of morbidity and cutaneous features of vasculitis or SCLE lesions extending over a 30- to 40-year period.

TREATMENT

Oral Manifestations

The treatment of xerostomia is problematic. Methylcellulose saliva substitutes are generally a poor substitute with low patient acceptance. The frequent ingestion of water or other sugarless fluids is generally the most acceptable form of therapy. Chewing sugarless gum helps massage the minor and major salivary glands, resulting in increased fluid production. Oral pilocarpine (Salagen) may also effectively stimulate saliva production.

Oral candidiasis is treated by removal of dentures and cleaning at night. Scouring the mucosal surface of the denture with Nystatin powder and a toothbrush is effective. The prophylactic use of Nystatin oral suspension (one teaspoon, two to three times a day; swish and swallow) or clotrimazole troches (four to five times daily) is also effective.

Prophylactic fluoride treatment and frequent routine dental examinations are indicated because of the increased frequency of dental caries.

Ocular Manifestations

Ocular SS is treated successfully with artificial tears. Many preservative-free artificial tear preparations are now commercially available. Lubricant ointments, applied at night, are also of value.

According to patients, the use of a humidifier in the bedroom to increase ambient humidity helps with both the ocular and the oral symptomatology. Patients also have indicated the use of underwater goggles containing water-soaked soft cotton at night is an effective means of combating ocular dryness. Occlusion of the nasal lacrimal duct is a common therapeutic approach to preserve moisture in the eye. A temporary punctal occlusion is first tried; if successful, a permanent ductal occlusion after local anesthesia can be achieved with either an argon laser or electrocautery.[46]

Vaginal Manifestations

Vaginal dryness is problematic. Vaginal moisturizers (e.g., Replens) are commercially available but in the author's experience are of limited value. The application of vaseline after bathing has some benefit. The frequent use of Nystatin vaginal suppositories at night is helpful in combating yeast infections.

Cutaneous Manifestations

Xeroderma can be combated with the use of moisturizing creams (e.g., Eucerin, Aquaphor). After bathing, the patient pats himself or herself dry, leaving a residue of moisture on the skin. A liberal amount of cream is applied to predetermined areas of xerosis, trapping moisture between the moisturizer and the skin.

As a general measure to combat mucous membrane dryness and xeroderma, the ambient humidity should be increased in the patient's living area by placing a humidifier on the heating system or, as noted above, using a humidifier in the bedroom. Large leafy plants, watered regularly, help to create a greenhouse-like atmosphere in the living area.

Systemic Manifestations

Patients with primary SS frequently complain of myalgias and arthralgias; in recent years, hydroxychloroquine has been employed with some success in the treatment of these symptoms.[92] In addition, some patients with SS have noted a decrease in ocular and oral dryness. A recent retrospective study with hydroxychloroquine for at least a 2-year period of time demonstrated an approximate 50 percent improvement in ocular symptoms of pain and dryness, as well as an improvement in the Rose Bengal dye staining. The Schirmer's test improved by 2 mm or more for 5 min in approximately 50 percent of patients. The salivary flow rate increased in at least 82 percent of patients, and the physician global assessment indicated an improvement in more than 62 percent of the patients.

The presence of cutaneous vasculitis should prompt a search for evidence of systemic involvement in which rheumatologists and/or neurologists participate. Cerebral involvement or peripheral nervous system involvement detected by MRI or proton emission tomography (PET) may warrant the need for long-term suppression of the vascular insult. The risk/benefit ratio of high dose steroids, pulse steroids, and immunosuppressive agents such as Imuran and pulse Cytoxan must be evaluated.[93]

REFERENCES

1. Adamson TC III et al: Immunohistologic analysis of lymphoid infiltrates in primary Sjögren's syndrome using monoclonal antibodies. *J Immunol* **120**:203, 1983
2. Andrade RE: Distribution of an immunophenotype of the inflammatory cell population in benign lymphoepithelial lesions (Mikulicz disease). *Hum Pathol* **19**:932, 1988
3. Alexander EL et al: Ro(SS-A) and La(SS-B) antibodies in the clinical spectrum of Sjögren's syndrome. *J Rheumatol* **9**:239, 1982
4. Alexander EL et al: Neurologic complications of primary Sjögren's syndrome. *Medicine* **61**:245, 1982
5. Fox RI et al: Sjögren's syndrome. Proposed criteria for classification. *Arthritis Rheum* **29**:577, 1986
6. Manthorpe R et al: The Copenhagen criteria for Sjögren's syndrome. *Scand J Rheumatol* **(suppl)61**:19, 1986
7. Skopouli F et al: Preliminary diagnostic criteria for Sjögren's syndrome. *Scand J Rheumatol* **(suppl)6**:22, 1986
8. Homma M et al: Criteria for Sjögren's syndrome in Japan. *Scand J Rheumatol* **(suppl)61**:26, 1986
9. Daniels TE, Talal N: Diagnosis and differential diagnosis of Sjögren's syndrome, in *Sjögren's Syndrome. Clinical and Immunological Aspects*, edited by N Talal, HM Moutsopoulos, SS Kassan. Berlin, Springer, 1987, p 193
10. Vitali C et al: Preliminary criteria for the diagnosis of Sjögren's syndrome. Results of a prospective concerted action supported by the European community. *Arthritis Rheum* **36**:340, 1993
11. Talal N: Sjögren's syndrome: Historical overview and clinical spectrum of disease. *Rheum Dis Clin North Am* **18**:507, 1992
12. Anderson JR et al: Precipitating autoantibodies in Sjögren's disease. *Lancet* **2**:456, 1961
13. Rowell MR et al: Lupus erythematosus and erythema multiforme-like lesions. *Arch Dermatol* **88**:176, 1963
14. Clark G et al: Characterization of a soluble cytoplasmic antigen reactive with sera from patients with systemic lupus erythematosus. *J Immunol* **102**:117, 1969
15. Mattioli M, Reichlin M: Heterogeneity of RNA protein antigens reactive with sera of patients with systemic lupus erythematosus. *Arthritis Rheum* **17**:421, 1974
16. Alspaugh MA, Tan EM: Antibodies to cellular antigens in Sjögren's syndrome. *J Clin Invest* **55**:1067, 1975
17. Alspaugh MA, Maddison P: Relation of the identity of certain antigen/antibody systems in systemic lupus erythematosus and Sjögren's syndrome: An interlaboratory collaboration. *Arthritis Rheum* **22**:796, 1979
18. Whaley K et al: Sjögren's syndrome and autoimmunity in a geriatric population. *Age Ageing* **1**:197, 1972
19. Drosos AA et al: The prevalence of primary Sjögren's syndrome in an elderly population. *Br J Rheumatol* **27**:123, 1988
20. Molina R et al: Primary Sjögren's syndrome in men: Clinical, serologic, and immunogenetic features. *Am J Med* **80**:23, 1986
21. Drosos AA et al: Subgroups of primary Sjögren's syndrome: Sjögren's syndrome in male and pediatric Greek patients. *Ann Rheum Dis* **56**:333, 1997
22. Tomiita M et al: The clinical features of Sjögren's syndrome in Japanese children. *Acta Paediatr Jpn* **39**:268, 1997
23. Strickland RW et al: The frequency of Sjögren's syndrome in an elderly female population. *J Rheumatol* **14**:766, 1985
24. Reveille JD et al: Primary Sjögren's syndrome and other autoimmune diseases in families. Prevalence and immunogenetic studies in six kindreds. *Ann Int Med* **101**:748, 1984
25. Harley JB et al: Gene interaction at HLA-DQ enhances autoantibody production in primary Sjögren's syndrome. *Science* **232**:1145, 1986
26. Hamilton RG et al: Two Ro(SS-A) autoantibody responses in systemic lupus erythematosus. Correlation of HLA-DR/DQ specificities with quantitative expression of Ro(SS-A) autoantibody. *Arthritis Rheum* **31**:496, 1988
27. Reveille JD et al: Specific amino acid residues in the second hypervariable region of HLA-DQA1 and DQB1 chain genes promote the Ro(SS-A)/La(SS-B) autoantibody responses. *J Autoimmun* **146**:3871, 1991
28. Reveille JD, Arnett FC: The immunogenetics of Sjögren's syndrome. *Rheum Dis Clin North Am* **18**:539, 1992
29. Harley JB et al: Anti-Ro/SSA and anti/La/SSB in patients with Sjögren's syndrome. *Arthritis Rheum* **29**:196, 1986
30. Provost TT et al: Detection of anti-Ro(SS-A) antibodies by gel double diffusion and a "sandwich" ELISA in systemic and subacute cutaneous lupus erythematosus and Sjögren's syndrome. *J Autoimmun* **4**:87, 1991
31. Chan EKL, Andrade LEC: Antinuclear antibodies in Sjögren's syndrome. *Rheum Dis Clin North Am* **18**:551, 1992
32. Buyon JP et al: Identification of mothers at risk for congenital heart block and other neonatal lupus syndromes in their children. *Arthritis Rheum* **36**:1263, 1993
33. Julkunen H et al: Isolated congenital heart block: Fetal and infant outcome and familial incidence of heart block. *Obstet Gynecol* **82**:11, 1993
34. Boutdjir M et al: Arrhythrogenicity of IgG and anti-52 kD SSA/Ro affinity purified antibodies from mothers of children with congenital heart block. *Circ Res* **80**:354, 1997
35. Kinoshita G et al: Spreading of the immune response from 52 kDa and 60 kDa Ro to calreticulin in experimental autoimmunity. *Lupus* **7**:7, 1998
36. Gottesfeld JM et al: Association of an RNA polymerase III transcription factor with a ribonuclear protein complex recognized by autoimmune sera. *Nucl Acid Res* **12**:3185, 1984
37. Gottlieb E, Steitz JA: The RNA binding protein La influences both the accuracy and the efficiency of RNA polymerase III transcription in vitro. *EMBO J* **8**:841, 1989
38. Gottlieb E, Steitz JA: Function of mammalian La protein: Evidence for its action in transcription termination by RNA polymerase III. *EMBO J* **8**:851, 1989
39. Boire G, Craft J: Human Ro ribonuclear protein particles: Characterization of native structure and stable association with La polypeptide. *J Clin Invest* **85**:1182, 1990
40. Boire G et al: Sera from patients with autoimmune disease recognized confirmational determinants on the 60 kD Ro/SS-A protein. *Arthritis Rheum* **34**:722, 1991
41. Venables PJW, Rigby SP: Viruses in the etiopathogenesis of Sjögren's syndrome. *J Rheumatol* **24**:3, 1997
42. Talal N et al: Detection of serum antibodies to retroviral proteins in patients with primary Sjögren's syndrome (autoimmune exocrinopathy). *Arthritis Rheum* **33**:774, 1990
43. Itescu S, Winchester R: Diffuse infiltrative lymphocytosis syndrome: A disorder occurring in human immune deficiency virus-1 infection that may present as a sicca syndrome. *Rheum Dis Clin North Am* **18**:683, 1992
44. Greenspan JS et al: The histopathology of Sjögren's syndrome and labial salivary gland biopsies. *Oral Surg* **37**:217, 1974
45. Daniels TE, Fox PC: Salivary and oral components of Sjögren's syndrome. *Rheum Dis Clin North Am* **18**:571, 1992
46. Friedlaender M: Ocular manifestations of Sjögren's syndrome: Keratoconjunctivitis sicca. *Rheum Dis Clin North Am* **18**:591, 1992
47. Mulherin M et al: Sjögren's syndrome in women presenting with chronic dyspareunia. *Br J Obstet Gynecol* **104**:1019, 1997
48. Bloch KJ et al: Sjögren's syndrome: A clinical, pathological, and serologic study of 62 cases. *Medicine* **44**:187, 1965
49. Markusse HM et al: Primary Sjögren's syndrome: Clinical spectrum and mode of presentation based on an analysis of 50 patients selected from a department of rheumatology. *Netherlands J Med* **40**:125, 1992
50. Whaley K et al: Sjögren's syndrome. I. Sicca components. *Q J Med* **166**:279, 1973
51. Ellman P et al: A contribution to the pathology of Sjögren's disease. *Q J Med* **77**:33, 1951

52. Alexander EL, Provost TT: Cutaneous manifestations of primary Sjögren's syndrome: A reflection of vasculitis in association with anti-Ro(SS-A) antibodies. *J Invest Dermatol* **80**:386, 1983

53. Prystowsky SD et al: Acute febrile neutrophilic dermatoses associated with Sjögren's syndrome. *Arch Dermatol* **114**:1234, 1978

54. Provost TT et al: The relationship between anti-Ro(SS-A) precipitin antibody positive Sjögren's syndrome and anti-Ro(SS-A) precipitin antibody positive lupus erythematosus. *Arch Dermatol* **124**:63, 1988

55. Talal N: The development of malignant lymphoma in the course of Sjögren's syndrome. *Am J Med* **36**:529, 1964

56. Kassan SS et al: Increased risk of lymphoma in Sjögren's syndrome. *Ann Int Med* **89**:888, 1978

57. Teramoto N et al: Annular erythema: Possible association with Sjögren's syndrome. *J Am Acad Dermatol* **20**:596, 1989

58. Katayama I et al: Annular erythema associated with primary Sjögren's syndrome: Analysis of T cell subsets in cutaneous infiltrates. *J Am Acad Dermatol* **21**:1218, 1989

59. Nishikawa T, Provost TT: Differences in clinical, serologic, and immunogenetic features of White versus Oriental anti-SSA/Ro positive patients (editorial). *J Am Acad Dermatol* **25**:6563, 1991

60. Tsokos M et al: Vasculitis in primary Sjögren's syndrome: Histologic classification and clinical presentation. *Am J Clin Pathol* **88**:26, 1987

61. Strauss WG: Purpura, hypergammaglobulinemia of Waldenstrom. *N Engl J Med* **260**:857, 1959

62. Kyle RA et al: Benign hypergammaglobulinemic purpura of Waldenstrom. *Medicine* **50**:113, 1971

63. Meltzer M et al: Cryoglobulinemia: A clinical and laboratory study. II. Cryoglobulins and rheumatoid factor. *Am J Med* **40**:837, 1966

64. Meltzer M, Franklin EC: Cryoglobulinemia. A study of 29 patients: IgG and IgM cryoglobulins and factors associated with cryoprecipitability. *Am J Med* **40**:828, 1966

65. O'Laughlin S et al: Chronic urticaria-like lesions in systemic lupus erythematosus. *Arch Dermatol* **114**:879, 1978

66. Provost TT et al: Unusual cutaneous manifestations of systemic lupus erythematosus. I. Urticaria-like lesions: Correlation with clinical and serologic abnormalities. *J Invest Dermatol* **75**:495, 1980

67. McDuffie FC et al: Hypocomplementemia with cutaneous vasculitis and arthritis: Possible immune complex syndrome. *Mayo Clin Proceed* **48**:340, 1973

68. Schwartz HR: Hypocomplementemic urticarial vasculitis: Association with chronic obstructive pulmonary disease. *Mayo Clin Proceed* **57**:231, 1982

69. Monroe EW et al: Vasculitis and chronic urticaria: An immunopathologic study. *J Invest Dermatol* **76**:103, 1981

70. Soter NA et al: Two distinct cellular patterns in cutaneous necrotizing angiitis. *J Invest Dermatol* **66**:344, 1976

71. Molina R et al: Two histopathologic prototypes of inflammatory vascular disease in Sjögren's syndrome: Differential association with seroreactivity to rheumatoid factor antibodies to Ro(SS-A) and with hypocomplementemia. *Arthritis Rheum* **28**:1251, 1985

72. Lawley TJ et al: Demonstration of circulating immune complexes in Sjögren's syndrome. *J Immunol* **123**:1282, 1979

73. Molina R et al: Peripheral inflammatory vascular disease in Sjögren's syndrome. Association with nervous system complications. *Arthritis Rheum* **28**:1341, 1985

74. Alexander EL et al: Magnetic resonance imaging of cerebral lesions in patients with Sjögren's syndrome. *Ann Int Med* **108**:815, 1988

75. Alexander EL et al: Serum complement activation in central nervous system disease in Sjögren's syndrome. *Am J Med* **85**:513, 1988

76. DeLaMonte SM et al: Polymorphous meningitis with atypical mononuclear cells in Sjögren's syndrome. *Ann Neurol* **14**:455, 1983

77. Alexander EL et al: Necrotizing arteritis and spinal subarachnoid hemorrhage in Sjögren's syndrome. *Ann Neurol* **11**:632, 1982

78. Ferreiro JE, Robalino BD: Primary Sjögren's syndrome with diffuse cerebral vasculitis and lymphocytic interstitial pneumonitis. *Am J Med* **82**:1227, 1987

79. Noseworthy JH et al: The prevalence of primary Sjögren's syndrome in a multiple sclerosis population. *Ann Neurol* **25**:95, 1989

80. Andronopoulos AP et al: The spectrum of neurologic involvement in Sjögren's syndrome. *Br J Rheumatol* **29**:21, 1990

81. Binder A et al: Sjögren's syndrome: A study of its neurologic complications. *Br J Rheumatol* **27**:275, 1988

82. Miro J et al: Prevalence of primary Sjögren's syndrome in patients with multiple sclerosis. *Ann Neurol* **22**:582, 1990

83. Heitaharju A et al: Nervous system manifestations in Sjögren's syndrome. *Acta Neurol Scan* **81**:144, 1990

84. Valesini G et al: Differential risk of non-Hodgkins lymphoma in Italian patients with primary Sjögren's syndrome. *J Rheumatol* **24**:2376, 1997

85. Maddison PJ: The clinical significance of autoantibodies to soluble cytoplasmic antigen in systemic lupus erythematosus and other connective tissue diseases. *J Rheumatol* **6**:189, 1979

86. Harmon CE et al: The frequency of autoantibodies to the SS-A/Ro antigen in pregnancy sera. *Arthritis Rheum* **28**:S20, 1984

87. Fritzler M et al: Antinuclear, anticytoplasmic, and anti-Sjögren's syndrome antigen A (SS-A/Ro) antibodies in female blood donors. *Clin Immunol Immunopathol* **36**:120, 1985

88. Provost TT et al: Significance of the anti-Ro(SS-A) antibody in the evaluation of patients with cutaneous manifestations of connective tissue diseases. *J Am Acad Dermatol* **35**:147, 1996

89. Provost TT, Watson RM: Anti-Ro(SS-A), HLA-DR3 positive females: The interrelationship between some ANA negative, SS, SCLE, NLE mothers and SS/LE overlap female patients. *J Invest Dermatol* **100(suppl)**:14S, 1993

90. Simmons-O'Brien E et al: 100 anti-Ro(SS-A) antibody positive patients: A 10 year follow-up. *Medicine* **74**:109, 1995

91. Provost TT: Anti-Ro(SS-A) antibody positive Sjögren's/lupus erythematosus overlap syndrome. *Lupus* **6**:105, 1997

92. Fox RI et al: Treatment of primary Sjögren's syndrome with hydroxychloroquine: A retrospective open label study. *Lupus* **5(suppl 1)**:S31, 1996

93. Alexander E: Central nervous system disease in Sjögren's syndrome: New insights in immunopathogenesis. *Rheum Dis Clin North Am* **18**:637, 1992

94. Malinow KL et al: Neuropsychiatric dysfunction in primary Sjögren's syndrome. *Ann Int Med* **103**:344, 1985

95. Alexander EL et al: Primary Sjögren's syndrome with central nervous system dysfunction mimicking multiple sclerosis. *Ann Int Med* **104**:323, 1986

96. Alexander EL, Alexander GE: Aseptic meningitis in primary Sjögren's syndrome. *Neurology* **33**:593, 1982

97. Kaltreider HB, Talal N: The neuropathy of Sjögren's syndrome: Trigeminal nerve involvement. *Ann Int Med* **70**:751, 1969

98. Griffin JW et al: Ataxic sensory neuronopathy and dorsal root ganglionitis associated with Sjögren's syndrome. *Ann Neurol* **27**:304, 1990

99. Tumiati B et al: Hearing loss in Sjögren's syndrome. *Ann Int Med* **126**:450, 1997

CHAPTER 181

John H. Klippel

Raynaud's Phenomenon

Raynaud's phenomenon is the occurrence of episodic attacks of digital ischemia provoked by exposure to cold or emotional stress. The condition was originally described by the French physician Maurice Raynaud in 1862,[1] and the term *Raynaud's phenomenon* was suggested by Hutchinson, who recognized that multiple disorders were associated with attacks of digital vasospasm.[2] The classic episode of Raynaud's phenomenon is characterized by a triphasic color change of pallor, cyanosis, and hyperemia of the fingers. Symptoms of numbness or tingling during the attack or actual pain with recovery are common, although patients may be totally asymptomatic throughout an attack. Raynaud's phenomenon is generally divided into primary (idiopathic) and secondary forms, based on whether an underlying cause or disease associated with peripheral vasospasm can be identified.

EPIDEMIOLOGY

Studies of the epidemiology of Raynaud's phenomenon are complicated owing to underreporting, since most patients with primary Raynaud's are otherwise asymptomatic and never seek medical evaluation, and biases of studies done by investigators interested in the secondary forms of the disorder. Surveys indicate that Raynaud's phenomenon affects up to 20 percent of the general population.[3–6] Primary Raynaud's is estimated to be approximately twice as common as secondary Raynaud's phenomenon.[7] Symptoms most often develop in the teenage years, although onset after the age of 40 is not infrequent.[8] Most series show a female predominance of the disorder (female:male = 4:1), and increases in the frequency and severity of attacks during the menses suggest that female sex hormones are involved in the pathogenesis.[9] Familial aggregation has been noted to suggest the contribution of genetic factors to the disorder.[10] Other reported associations identified in epidemiology studies include living in a cold climate, occupation, smoking history, cardiovascular disease, low body-mass index, and use of vibratory tools.[11,12]

PATHOPHYSIOLOGY

There are multiple causes of Raynaud's phenomenon, and the pathophysiology of the vasospasm is complex and only partially understood. Studies have shown significant reductions of peripheral blood flow throughout all phases of central body cooling and rewarming, suggesting impairments of central thermoregulatory control mechanisms.[13,14] The principal mechanisms thought to contribute to the development of Raynaud's phenomenon include (1) a local defect of a digital blood vessel causing abnormal vascular reactivity or reduced blood flow; (2) an enhanced localized production of vasoconstrictors or reduced production of vasodilators; (3) hyperreactivity of the sympathetic nervous system; and (4) abnormal properties of the blood that compromise distal perfusion.

Gross histologic examinations of digital arteries in patients with primary Raynaud's phenomenon are normal. Structural abnormalities of the digital microvasculature play a far more important role in patients with secondary forms of Raynaud's phenomenon, particularly in the connective tissue diseases. Studies have shown a range of pathology including intimal hyperplasia, narrowing or total occlusion of arteries, or thrombi. In most patients with systemic sclerosis, evidence of activation and damage of the endothelium, fibrinolysis, and platelet activation are present.[15] Microcirculatory flow studies with laser Doppler in scleroderma have shown marked reductions in flow and hand temperature during an attack, with prominent abnormalities during rewarming; these findings suggest a failure of the arteriovenous anastomoses to open.[16]

Peripheral vascular resistance is primarily controlled by the interaction between α_1- and α_2-adrenergic receptors. In vivo studies indicate that α_2-adrenoceptors are more important than α_1-adrenoceptors during reflex sympathetic vasoconstriction and that α_2-adrenoceptors predominantly affect arteriovenous anastomoses in the finger. Skin blood flow is especially sensitive to α_2-adrenergic receptor antagonism. Intraarterial infusions of clonidine are associated with greater vasoconstriction in patients with Raynaud's phenomenon than in unaffected control subjects.[17,18] Studies of brachial artery infusions of α_1- and α_2-adrenergic antagonists in patients with primary Raynaud's phenomenon have shown that activation of α_1-adrenergic receptors is necessary for the production of the vasospastic attacks.[19] The finding of increased levels of α_2-adrenergic receptors on platelets of patients with Raynaud's phenomenon[20] raises the possibility of an increased density or sensitivity of the receptor on vascular endothelium.

Studies have revealed the importance of neurotransmitters in the control of vessel tone. Increased levels of endothelin-1, a potent vasoconstrictor peptide present in the digital cutaneous microvasculature, and reductions of calcitonin gene–related peptide, a powerful vasodilator in digital cutaneous nerves, have been found in patients with Raynaud's phenomenon.[21] Infusion of magnesium sulfate further decreases circulating levels of calcitonin gene–related peptide.[22] The deficit of calcitonin gene–related peptide has been hypothesized to result in a functional deficit of vasodilation by nitric oxide synthetase.[23] Serotonin has also been incriminated as an important mediator in the induction of ischemic attacks of Raynaud's phenomenon. Patients have an increased sensitivity to intraarterial infusions of serotonin,[18] and an S2-serotonergic antagonist relieves vasospastic attacks but does not prevent their induction.[24]

The evidence of direct central sympathetic nervous system hyperactivity is strongest in vibration-induced injury, in which the use of a vibration tool in one hand has been shown to produce vasospasm in the contralateral hand.[25] Similarly, vasospasm can be inhibited by proximal nerve blockade in patients with vibration-induced injury. In general, most studies of the sympathetic nervous system in patients with primary or other secondary forms of Raynaud's phenomenon have failed to detect evidence of sympathetic hyperactivity. The results of microelectrode studies of skin sympathetic nervous activity during cold pressor tests are normal, and plasma levels of catecholamines are not increased in the venous drainage of the hands of patients with Raynaud's phenomenon.[26]

Consistent abnormalities in plasma fibrinogen, cold agglutinins, or cryoglobulins have not been demonstrated in primary Raynaud's phenomenon but are important in certain secondary cases, particularly scleroderma. Levels of von Willebrand factor and soluble thrombomodulin, thromboxane B2 and beta-thromboglobulin, and tissue plasminogen activator inhibitor-1 are increased in patients with scleroderma compared to levels in patients with primary Raynaud's phenomenon.[15]

CLASSIFICATION

The classification of Raynaud's phenomenon begins with separation into a primary (idiopathic) form and a secondary form in which an underlying cause or disease association can be identified.

Primary Raynaud's Phenomenon

Primary Raynaud's phenomenon is a disorder in which known causes of attacks of peripheral vasospasm are absent. Criteria for the diagnosis of primary Raynaud's phenomenon have been developed by Allen and Brown[27] and LeRoy and Medsger[28] (Table 181-1). Patients with primary Raynaud's phenomenon are typically otherwise totally asymptomatic with the exception of perhaps an increase in migraine headaches and variant angina pectoris.[29]

Several studies have examined the long-term outcome of patients with primary Raynaud's phenomenon.[7,30,31] Progression to a secondary form of Raynaud's phenomenon, most commonly a connective tissue disease such as scleroderma, occurs in approximately 15 percent of patients over the first decade following the onset. Variables predictive of a transition to a secondary form include nail fold capillary abnormalities, hand swelling, positive Allen's test, and antinuclear antibodies.

Secondary Raynaud's Phenomenon

CONNECTIVE TISSUE DISEASES The connective tissue diseases are the most common cause of secondary Raynaud's phenomenon (Table 181-2). Among patients with scleroderma, 80 to 90 percent manifest Raynaud's phenomenon and/or persistent vasospasm. It is the presenting symptom in about one-third of patients and may be the only manifestation of the disease for years. Raynaud's phenomenon occurs in about one-third of patients with systemic lupus erythematosus and the idiopathic inflammatory myopathies and is commonly seen in patients with systemic vasculitis. Although patients with rheumatoid arthritis often complain of cold hands with mottled red and white areas, true Raynaud's phenomenon appears to be no more common among these individuals than in the general population.[32] Arteriograms of patients with connective tissue dis-

TABLE 181-1

Criteria for Primary Raynaud's Phenomenon*

1. Vasospastic attacks precipitated by exposure to cold or emotional stimuli
2. Bilateral involvement of extremities
3. Normal vascular examination with symmetric peripheral pulses and normal nail fold capillary microscopy
4. Absence of gangrene or, if present, limited to the skin of the fingertips
5. No evidence of an underlying disease, drug, or occupational exposure that could be responsible for vasospastic attacks
6. Negative antinuclear antibody
7. Normal erythrocyte sedimentation rate
8. History of symptoms for at least 2 years

*Combined criteria of Allen and Brown[27] and Le Roy and Medsger.[28]

eases usually show digital and sometimes ulnar or radial artery obstructions.

OCCUPATIONAL Raynaud's phenomenon may be occupational in origin and is especially common in individuals who use vibratory tools (e.g., air hammers, chain saws, riveters) or whose occupation requires prolonged exposure of the extremities to cold temperatures (e.g., butchers, ice cream workers, fish packers). Prevalence rates correlate with the vibration level of the tool and duration of the exposure and can be as high as 90 percent in high-risk occupations such as logging or mining.[33] Other working conditions associated with the development of Raynaud's phenomenon include use of plastic gloves, continuous repetitive movements of an extremity, and work breaks in an unheated environment.[34] Arteriograms in patients with occupation-induced Raynaud's phenomenon often reveal digital, radial, ulnar, or palmar arch thromboses.

NEUROLOGIC DISORDERS Any neurologic condition that produces permanent disuse of a limb can be associated with sympathetic nervous system disturbances to that limb. Patients often develop persistent vasospasm with coldness, paleness or cyanosis, and even ulcerations of the limb, and Raynaud's phenomenon may occur. Thermoregulatory abnormalities may be a prominent feature of reflex sympathetic dystrophy syndrome.[35] Nerve root pressure or nerve entrapment may produce Raynaud's phenomenon. It is often present in patients with the carpal tunnel syndrome[36] and typically involves the first, index, and middle fingers, digits innervated by the median nerve. Tapping the median nerve at the wrist (Tinel's sign) or wrist flexion for 60 s (Phalen's sign) may produce shooting pain in the distribution of the median nerve. Demonstration of a prolonged conduction time in the median nerve is the definitive diagnostic test. Raynaud's phenomenon may occur secondary to neurovascular compression at the thoracic outlet.[37] Such compression may be due to cervical ribs; abnormalities of the scalenus anticus muscle; bony abnormalities of the cervical vertebrae, clavicle, or first rib; or shoulder compression syndromes (the costoclavicular or hyperabduction syndrome). To confirm the diagnosis, assumption of postures to exaggerate the abnormality—such as the Adson test, in which the patient holds a deep breath, extends his neck, and then turns toward the side being examined—must reproduce the symptoms or produce a pale hand from which the radial pulse disappears. Loss of the pulse is not diagnostic, neither are nerve conduction studies.

chronic infections, leukemia, and lymphoblastoma and as an idiopathic condition.

TABLE 181-2

Secondary Raynaud's Phenomenon

Connective tissue disease
  Scleroderma
  Systemic lupus erythematosus
  Dermatomyositis and polymyositis
  Undifferentiated connective tissue disease
  Systemic vasculitis
  Sjögren's syndrome
  Eosinophilic fasciitis
Obstructive arterial disease
  Atherosclerosis
  Thromboangiitis obliterans (Buerger's disease)
  Thromboembolism
  Thoracic outlet syndrome
Neurologic disorders
  Carpal tunnel syndrome
  Reflex sympathetic dystrophy
  Hemiplegia
  Poliomyelitis
  Multiple sclerosis
  Syringomyelia
Drugs and toxins
  Beta-adrenergic blockers
  Ergotamines
  Oral contraceptives
  Methysergide
  Bleomycin and vinblastine
  Clonidine
  Bromocriptine
  Cyclosporine
  Amphetamines
  Fluoxetine
  Alpha interferon

Occupation/environmental exposure
  Vibration injury (lumberjacks, pneumatic hammer operators)
  Posttraumatic injury (hypothenar hammer syndrome, crutch pressure)
  Vinyl chloride disease
  Cold injury
Hyperviscosity disorders
  Cryoproteins
  Cold agglutinins
  Macroglobulins
  Polycythemia
  Thrombocytosis
Miscellaneous
  Hypothyroidism
  Infections (bacterial endocarditis, Lyme disease, viral hepatitis)
  Neoplasms
  Primary pulmonary hypertension
  Arteriovenous fistula
  Intraarterial injections

MISCELLANEOUS The most common endocrine disturbance associated with Raynaud's phenomenon is hypothyroidism; symptoms usually remit with thyroid replacement. Raynaud's phenomenon may be a feature of various infectious disorders including subacute bacterial endocarditis, Lyme disease, and viral hepatitis, presumably a reflection of systemic vasculitis. Manifestations of peripheral vasospasm may also be seen in association with malignant tumors, including pheochromocytoma, carcinoid, and ovarian carcinoma.[44]

DIFFERENTIAL DIAGNOSIS

The main differential diagnoses are cold digits, chilblain (pernio), livedo reticularis, and acrocyanosis (see Chap. 128). Many patients complain of cold, sometimes painful digits without color changes. This condition likely represents one extreme of the spectrum of normal sympathetic nervous system activity. Chilblain is an inflammatory condition of the skin of the extremities induced by cold. Patients develop a bluish-red discoloration and edema, typically involving the lower limb and associated with warmth, erythema, and burning. In severe cases, hemorrhagic lesions, bullae, or ulcers may develop, and secondary infections may supervene. The lesions last from 7 to 10 days, often leaving a residual pigmentation of the skin. Livedo reticularis is a bluish discoloration of the skin of the extremities with a characteristic lacy, irregular appearance. The bluish discoloration becomes more intense on exposure to cold and may disappear in a warm environment. Most patients are entirely asymptomatic, although livedo reticularis may be a feature of the antiphospholipid syndrome, in which patients are at increased risk for venous and arterial thromboses, thrombocytopenia, and pregnancy losses. In acrocyanosis, the hands and less commonly the feet develop a persistent bluish discoloration. The blue color is intensified by exposure to cold and converted into a purplish or red color by warming; a pallor phase is absent. The skin is cold and the palms are often wet and clammy from sweat. Trophic changes or ulcerations are rarely observed.

DRUGS AND TOXINS Drugs and toxins have been implicated as causing Raynaud's phenomenon. Propranolol, one of the most widely used beta-adrenergic blockers for cardiovascular diseases and migraine headaches, is probably the most frequent offender. Ergot preparations and methysergide used to treat migraine headaches may also cause the phenomenon.[38,39] Intraarterial use of many medications has been associated with vasospasm and gangrene of the fingers. Drug-induced toxicity to endothelial cells may produce irreversible structural damage to the microvasculature of the extremities and be responsible for severe Raynaud's phenomenon. Industrial exposure to vinyl chloride polymerization processes may produce Raynaud's phenomenon, as well as acroosteolysis of the distal phalanges of the fingers; arteriograms show digital artery obstructions.[40] The chemotherapeutic agents bleomycin and vinblastine also may cause the phenomenon.[41-43]

HYPERVISCOSITY Patients with cold-perceptible plasma proteins, macroglobulins, cold agglutinins, and polycythemia can exhibit Raynaud's phenomenon as a result of flow disturbances or actual occlusion of small vessels. These episodes are usually associated with monoclonal gammopathies, particularly macroglobulinemia, or polyclonal gammopathies, as with rheumatoid arthritis. Cryoglobulins are most commonly present in patients with multiple myeloma, but they also occur in patients with rheumatic diseases,

HISTORY AND PHYSICAL EXAMINATION

The history is important in order to elicit a clear description of the attacks, which is necessary to establish the diagnosis of Raynaud's phenomenon and to screen for evidence of signs and symptoms suggestive of a secondary cause. Patients complain of episodic attacks of well-demarcated, white or blue digits induced by exposure to cold and sometimes by emotional stimuli (Fig. 181-1). Often only a portion of the digit is affected, and the thumbs are typically spared. A classic tricolor change (white to blue to red) described in most textbooks is rarely volunteered by patients; most describe only blanching of the digits accompanied by numbness. During the attacks, one or more fingers or toes may be numb and be described as "dead." On rewarming, the digits may become bright red, and throbbing pain may occur. When pain is a prominent symptom in the ischemic phase, a secondary cause should be suspected. Attacks last minutes to hours. Patients may experience one or more attacks per cold season or multiple attacks throughout the year. The fingers and toes are most commonly involved; however, the attacks may involve the nose, earlobes, or nipples. A systemic form of Raynaud's phenomenon with vasospasm of major organ systems such as the heart, lungs, kidneys, esophagus, gastrointestinal tract, and cerebral circulation has been documented in patients with connective tissue disorders and may be an important contributory factor to pathology. There is no evidence, however, to suggest that there is a systemic vasospastic component in patients with primary Raynaud's phenomenon.[45]

A careful review of systems is important to screen for symptoms of connective tissue disease (arthralgias, arthritis, dysphagia, heartburn, rash, photosensitivity, skin changes, muscle weakness, or sicca), a drug-related etiology, symptoms of obstructive arterial diseases (intermittent claudication), and exposure to vibratory tools or continuous finger trauma. In patients with primary Raynaud's phenomenon, a review of systems is entirely unrevealing with the exception of occasional complaints of migraine headaches or variant angina pectoris.

Attacks of Raynaud's phenomenon, presumably stress-induced, are commonly witnessed during the course of the history or physical examination. There is well-demarcated blanching or cyanosis of the digits extending from the tip to varying levels of the digit. The

digits distal to the line of ischemia are cold, while the proximal skin is pink and warmer. On rewarming, blanched digits may become cyanotic, because of the slow blood flow, and then bright red, because of reactive hyperemia. Persistent ischemic discoloration of digits suggests a secondary cause.

The digits should be carefully examined for trophic or ischemic changes, which are signs of prolonged or severe attacks of Raynaud's phenomenon. The skin may become atrophic, thin, and tight (sclerodactyly) with loss of hair over the dorsal surfaces. The nails may become brittle and deformed. Ulcerations may develop on the finger pads or around the nail bed, which can be extremely painful, particularly at night. These heal slowly, leave characteristic small, pitted scars (Fig. 181-2) and may become infected. Gangrene of the distal aspects of the digit is rare.

In general, the physical examination is unrevealing in patients with primary Raynaud's phenomenon. Patients with secondary Raynaud's phenomenon would be expected to have features of their underlying disease. The physical examination should pay attention to all pulses, and blood pressure should be obtained in both arms. Allen's test is useful to assess arterial and capillary function of the hands; abnormalities imply structural disease of the microcirculation and raise the suspicion of a secondary form of Raynaud's phenomenon. The radial and ulnar arteries are simultaneously compressed by the examiner's thumbs while the patient opens and closes the fist to induce blanching of the palm. Selective arterial filling is judged by the rate of color return as pressure is sequentially released from the radial and ulnar arteries. Vascular obstruction from the thoracic outlet syndrome should be assessed by the Adson maneuver, which tests for diminution in the radial pulse with exaggerated movements of the neck and shoulder. A careful neurologic examination should be performed to detect evidence of sympathetic hyperactivity, abnormal reflexes, muscular weakness or atrophy, or compression of the median nerve within the carpal tunnel. Skin changes such as telangiectases, changes in skin texture, rashes, or purpura provide valuable clues to the presence of a connective tissue or hyperviscosity disorder.

FIGURE 181-1

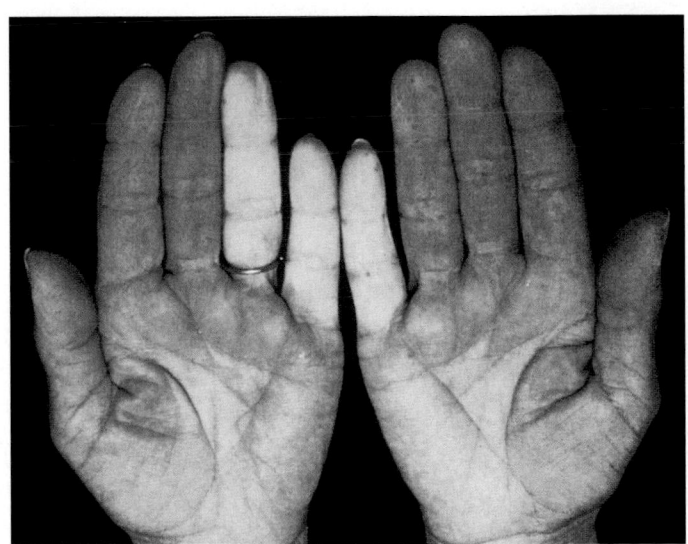

Ischemic phase of attack of Raynaud's phenomenon with marked pallor of the ring and little fingers of the left hand and little finger of the right hand.

FIGURE 181-2

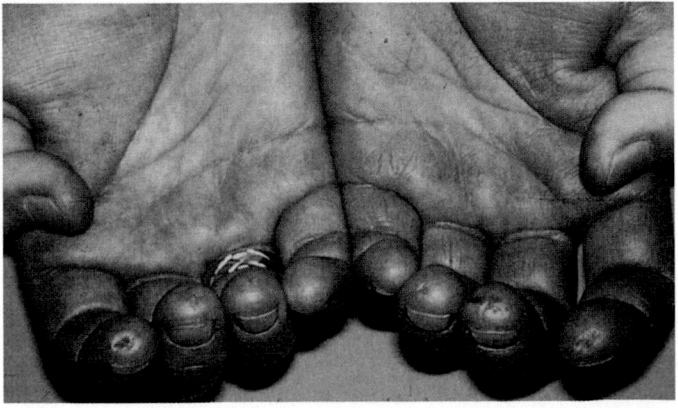

Loss of pulp of the pad of the digit with pitting scars and ulcerations from chronic, severe Raynaud's phenomenon.

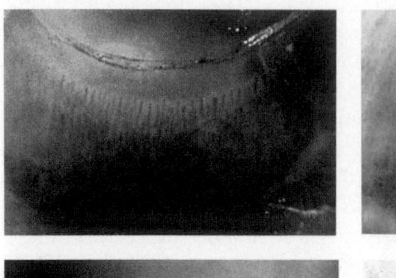
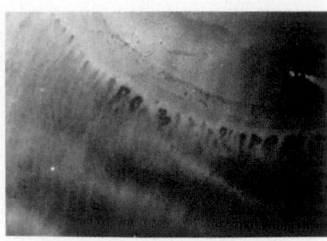
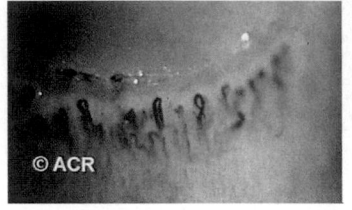
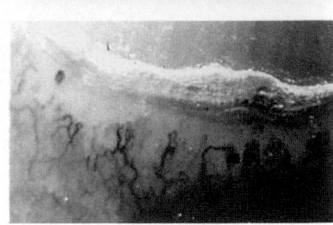

INVESTIGATIONS

Although differences in the vascular response to cooling have been reported between patients with primary and secondary Raynaud's phenomenon,[14] there is no need to attempt to induce an attack as by immersing the patient's hand in ice water. In all patients, a complete blood count, erythrocyte sedimentation rate, urinalysis, and antinuclear antibody test should be obtained. Additional laboratory studies should be directed by findings elicited by the history and physical examination. In patients with abnormal antinuclear antibodies, tests for antibodies to specific nuclear antigens such as topoisomerase or centromere antigens or the Smith (Sm) antigen are helpful to detect early scleroderma or systemic lupus erythematosus. A routine chest radiograph should be obtained to look for a cervical rib.

Nail fold capillary microscopy is a useful procedure to distinguish primary from secondary Raynaud's phenomenon and should be done as part of the routine evaluation of all patients. Capillary microscopy is easily performed with a hand-held ophthalmoscope at powers of less than 20 diopters with water-soluble gels such as K-Y jelly as the moisturizing agent to increase translucency of the epidermis.[46] Although mild capillary abnormalities may be observed in patients with primary Raynaud's phenomenon, patients with connective tissue diseases may have enlarged, deformed capillary loops surrounded by avascular areas (Fig. 181-3).[47] Serial studies reveal progressive decreases in the total number of nail fold capillary loops in secondary but not primary forms of Raynaud's phenomenon.[48] The patency of small arteries can be assessed by Doppler techniques with a 10-MHz pencil transducer. Digital subtraction arteriography should be reserved for selected patients with prolonged, severe ischemia for whom arterial reconstruction is a consideration.

TREATMENT

The management of Raynaud's phenomenon is guided by the frequency and severity of attacks and the complications from ischemia (Table 181-3). Secondary forms of Raynaud's phenomenon require treatment directed at the underlying medical disorder, discontinuation of drugs implicated in causing the vasospasm, or occupational modifications.

General Measures

Mild Raynaud's phenomenon is generally easy to control with lifestyle changes to minimize exposure to the cold; dressing warmly with loose-fitting, layered clothing; and keeping the thermostat a few degrees higher than normal. Limiting time spent outdoors in winter or wearing insulated gloves and using hand or foot warmers are usually helpful. Patients should be taught to recognize and terminate attacks promptly by returning to a warmer environment and applying local heat to the hands (e.g., placing their hands in warm water or using a hair dryer). Patients should be strongly encouraged to stop smoking and to avoid secondhand smoke, since nicotine induces cutaneous vasoconstriction.[49] Stress modification and social support are valuable aspects of treatment to minimize vasoconstriction induced by hyperactivity of the sympathetic nervous system.

Nail fold capillary microscopy in a patient with scleroderma, showing capillary drop out with enlarged, dilated, tortuous capillary loops.

Counseling, training in relaxation, or medications may be helpful. Some patients benefit from conditioning programs such as biofeedback training.[50]

Dietary therapy with fish-oil supplements containing the omega-3 fatty acids, eicosopentaenoic acid, and docosahexaenoic acid has been studied in Raynaud's phenomenon.[51] These fatty acids serve as alternate substrates for cyclooxygenase and 5-lipoxygenase pathways to produce vasodilation, inhibit platelet aggregation, and alter red cell deformability. The study showed improvements in digital systolic pressures and digital artery flow in patients with primary but not secondary Raynaud's phenomenon.

Drug Therapy

A wide variety of drugs have been used to treat Raynaud's phenomenon, including vasodilators, platelet inhibitors, serotonin antagonists, and fibrinolytics.[52] Drug therapy is usually reserved for

TABLE 181-3

Management of Raynaud's Phenomenon

Infrequent or mild attacks	Preventative measures
	Cessation of smoking
Frequent or severe attacks	Calcium channel blockers (nifedipine, diltiazem)
	Antiadrenergic drugs (prazosin, reserpine)
	Topical nitroglycerin
Acute, severe ischemia	Intravenous prostaglandin E_1 or prostacyclin
	Digital sympathectomy
	Microvascular surgery
Digital ulcers	Antiseptic soaks, antibiotic ointments, occlusive dressing
	Calcium channel blockers (maximal doses)
	Intravenous prostaglandin E_1 or prostacyclin
Gangrenous, infected ulcers	Analgesics
	Antibiotics
	Surgical debridement
	Amputation

patients with prolonged or frequent attacks that fail to respond to conservative measures. In general, improvements with drug therapy are more pronounced in patients with primary Raynaud's phenomenon, presumably as a consequence of fixed, structural damage in patients with secondary forms.

The calcium channel blockers are by far the most widely used and effective drugs for treating Raynaud's phenomenon. Vasodilating properties vary among different agents. Nifedipine (10 to 20 mg tid or qid) reduces the severity and frequency of attacks; the long-acting preparation of nifedipine is better tolerated but may be less effective. Diltiazem (60 mg tid or qid) may be substituted if nifedipine is ineffective or not well tolerated. Side effects of calcium channel blockers include fluid retention, light-headedness, and heartburn; these may limit therapy. Both reserpine (0.1 to 0.5 mg daily) and guanethidine (10 to 40 mg daily) increase capillary blood flow during cold exposure and have the advantage of once-a-day administration. Painful ulcerations or gangrene have been reported to respond to intraarterial reserpine (0.5 to 1.0 mg). Prazosin (1 to 5 mg tid), an α_1-adrenoceptor agonist, produces a moderate benefit. Other sympatholytic drugs—including methyldopa, phenoxybenzamine, and tolazoline—have been recommended. Ketanserin, a selective antagonist of the S2-serotonergic receptor, blocks serotonin-mediated vasoconstriction and platelet aggregation. In a large, international randomized trial, ketanserin was shown to reduce the frequency of vasospastic attacks; however, there were no differences in the severity or duration of attacks or increases in finger blood flow.[53] Stanozolol, which has fibrinolytic properties, has been reported to be beneficial in Raynaud's phenomenon.[54] Topical nitroglycerine paste (2%) as well as a sustained-release transdermal glyceryl patch may be helpful.[55] Topical minoxidil, a potent vasodilator, did not increase the blood flow in patients with primary Raynaud's phenomenon.[56]

Prostaglandin E_1 (PGE$_1$) and prostacyclin (PGI$_2$), administered intravenously, have beneficial effects in Raynaud's phenomenon[57]; however, the vasodilatory effects are not sustained.[58] Oral prostaglandins are currently available only as investigational agents, although preliminary results from studies of a prostaglandin I_2 analogue (beraprost) and misoprostol, an analogue of PGE$_1$, have been disappointing.[59–61] Agonists of endothelial receptors[62] and calcitonin gene-related peptide[63] appear to be promising future approaches to drug therapy.

Digital Ulcers

Digital ulcers from Raynaud's phenomenon can be extremely painful and typically take weeks or months to heal completely. Pain control is an important part of therapy, since pain can lead to additional vasospasm and more ischemia. On occasion, narcotic pain medications may be necessary to control symptoms. The finger should be soaked in a tepid antiseptic solution (e.g., half-strength hydrogen peroxide) twice daily to soften or loosen the crust or eschar. After drying, an antibiotic ointment is applied to the ulcer and the digit covered with an occlusive dressing. Maximum drug therapy with a calcium channel blocker should be used throughout treatment. Infection is a common complication of digital ulcers and is typically manifest by increasing pain, erythema, swelling, or purulent drainage. Cultures usually demonstrate *Staphylococcus* species, and treatment with dicloxacillin or cephalosporins is usually effective.

Sympathectomy

Sympathectomy may be a consideration for the management of patients with refractory disabling attacks or with an acutely ischemic digit that is unresponsive to other measures. A positive vasodilator response to a stellate ganglion block or epidural infusion should be documented before a permanent procedure is done. Lumbar sympathectomy has an important role in the management of severe Raynaud's phenomenon of the feet, and selective digital sympathectomy may be used to relieve pain and heal digital ulcers in patients with ischemic digits.[64,65] Sympathectomies for the management of Raynaud's phenomenon of the upper extremities have largely been abandoned because of poor long-term results, with up to two-thirds of patients reporting no benefit at the end of 1 year.[66] Newer procedures for thoracic sympathectomy, including percutaneous radiofrequency[67] and thoracoscopic procedures,[68,69] have been advocated as technically easier to perform, with fewer complications and more promising long-term results.

Severe Vasospasm

Severe vasospasm with prolonged ischemia (dead white finger) poses a threat of gangrene and amputation; it is considered a medical emergency. The patient should be hospitalized and the affected extremity put to rest. Nifedipine (10 to 20 mg tid) should be started immediately, as well as prostaglandin E_1 (6 to 10 ng/kg per min) or prostacyclin (0.5 to 2 ng/kg), given by continuous intravenous infusion for several hours over 3 consecutive days. Intraarterial phentolamine or tolazoline may reverse acute vasospasm, but monitoring of vital signs is essential and these drugs need to be used with great caution. A digital (or stellate ganglion) block with lidocaine hydrochloride or bupivicaine hydrochloride (without epinephrine) relieves pain and produces a chemical sympathectomy that may reverse vasoconstriction. Sympathectomy (thoracic, lumbar, or digital) should be considered in patients who have a positive response. Arterial reconstruction should be reserved for patients with angiographically documented occlusive vascular disease.

REFERENCES

1. Raynaud M: *On Local Aphyxia and Symmetrical Gangrene of the Extremities,* 1862, and *New Research on the Nature and Treatment of Local Asphyxia of the Extremities,* 1877, translated by T. Barlow. In selected monographs, vol 121. London, New Syndenham Society, 1888
2. Hutchinson J: Raynaud's phenomenon. *Med Press Circ* **23**:403, 1901
3. Silman A et al: Prevalence of symptoms of Raynaud's phenomenon in general practice. *Br Med J* **301**:590, 1990
4. Weinrich MC et al: Prevalence of Raynaud phenomenon in the adult population of South Carolina. *J Clin Epidemiol* **43**:1343, 1990
5. O'Keeffe ST et al: Color chart assisted diagnosis of Raynaud's phenomenon in an unselected hospital employee population. *J Rheumatol* **19**:1415, 1992
6. Maricq HR et al: Geographic variation in the prevalence of Raynaud's phenomenon: Charleston, SC, USA, vs. Tarentaise, Savoie, France. *J Rheumatol* **20**:70, 1993
7. Hirschl M, Kundi M: Initial prevalence and incidence of secondary Raynaud's phenomenon in patients with Raynaud's symptomatology. *J Rheumatol* **23**:302, 1996
8. Planchon B et al: Primary Raynaud's phenomenon: Age of onset and pathogenesis in a prospective study of 424 patients. *Angiology* **45**:677, 1994
9. Greenstein D et al: The menstrual cycle and Raynaud's phenomenon. *Angiology* **47**:427, 1996
10. Freedman RR, Mayes MD: Familial aggregation of primary Raynaud's disease. *Arthritis Rheum* **39**:1189, 1996
11. Maricq HR et al: Geographic variation in the prevalence of Raynaud's phenomenon: A 5 region comparison. *J Rheumatol* **24**:879, 1997
12. Valter I, Maricq HR: Prevalence of Raynaud phenomenon in Tartu and Tartumaa, southern Estonia. *Scand J Rheumatol* **26**:117, 1997

13. Greenstein D et al: Impaired thermoregulation in Raynaud's phenomenon. *Angiology* **46**:603, 1995

14. Maricq HR et al: Digital vascular responses to cooling in subjects with cold sensitivity, primary Raynaud's phenomenon, or scleroderma spectrum disorders. *J Rheumatol* **23**:2068, 1996

15. Herrick AL et al: Von Willebrand factor, thrombomodulin, thromboxane, beta-thromboglobulin and markers of fibrinolysis in primary Raynaud's phenomenon and systemic sclerosis. *Ann Rheum Dis* **55**:122, 1996

16. Toms SL, Cooke ED: A comparison of the functioning of arteriovenous anastomoses in secondary Raynaud's phenomenon and control subjects in response to local hand warming. *Int Angiol* **14**:74, 1995

17. Freedman RR et al: Increased α-adrenergic responsiveness in idiopathic Raynaud's disease. *Arthritis Rheum* **32**:61, 1989

18. Coffman JD, Cohen RA: α_2-adrenergic and 5-HT2 receptor hypersensitivity in Raynaud's phenomenon. *J Vasc Med Biol* **2**:100, 1990

19. Freedman RR et al: Blockade of vasospastic attacks by alpha 2-adrenergic but not alpha 1-adrenergic antagonists in idiopathic Raynaud's disease. *Circulation* **92**:1448, 1995

20. Bennett RM et al: Symptoms of Raynaud's syndrome in patients with fibromyalgia: A study utilizing the Nielsen test, digital photoplethysmography, and measurement of platelet α_2-adrenergic receptors. *Arthritis Rheum* **34**:264, 1991

21. Bunker CB et al: Calcitonin gene-related peptide, endothelin-1, the cutaneous microvasculature and Raynaud's phenomenon. *Br J Dermatol* **134**:399, 1996

22. Myrdal U et al: Magnesium sulphate infusion decreases circulating calcitonin gene-related peptide (CGPR) in women with primary Raynaud's phenomenon. *Clin Physiol* **14**:539, 1994

23. Dowd P et al: Raynaud's phenomenon. *Lancet* **346**:283, 1995

24. Siebold JR, Terregino CA: Selective antagonism of S2-serotonergic receptors relieves but does not prevent cold-induced vasoconstriction in primary Raynaud's phenomenon. *J Rheumatol* **13**:337, 1986

25. Chen GS et al: Responses of cutaneous microcirculation to cold exposure and neuropathy in vibration-induced white finger. *Microvasc Res* **47**:21, 1994

26. Fagius J, Blumberg H: Sympathetic outflow to the hand in patients with Raynaud's phenomenon. *Cardiovasc Res* **19**:249, 1985

27. Allen EV, Brown GE: Raynaud's disease: A critical review of minimal prerequisites for diagnosis. *Am J Med Sci* **183**:187, 1932

28. LeRoy EC, Medsger TA Jr: Raynaud's phenomenon: A proposal for classification. *Clin Exp Rheumatol* **10**:485, 1992

29. Koh KK et al: Does prevalence of migraine and Raynaud's phenomenon also increase in Korean patients with proven variant angina? *Int J Cardiol* **51**:37, 1995

30. Luggen M et al: The evolution of Raynaud's phenomenon: A long-term prospective study. *J Rheumatol* **22**:2226, 1995

31. Landry GJ et al: Long-term outcome of Raynaud's syndrome in a prospectively analyzed patient cohort. *J Vasc Surg* **23**:76, 1996

32. Grassi W et al: Raynaud's phenomenon in rheumatoid arthritis. *Br J Rheumatol* **33**:139, 1994

33. Mirod SM et al: Prevalence of Raynaud's phenomenon in different groups of workers operating hand-held vibrating tools. *Int Arch Occup Environ Health* **66**:13, 1994

34. Kaminski M et al: Risk factors for Raynaud's phenomenon among workers in poultry slaughterhouses and canning factories. *Int J Epidemiol* **26**:371, 1997

35. Herrick AL et al: Abnormal thermoregulatory responses in patients with reflex sympathetic dystrophy syndrome. *J Rheumatol* **21**:1319, 1994

36. Pal B et al: Raynaud's phenomenon in idiopathic carpal tunnel syndrome. *Scand J Rheumatol* **25**:143, 1996

37. Pistorius MA, Planchon B: Incidence of thoracic outlet syndrome on the epidemiology and clinical presentation of apparently primary Raynaud's phenomenon: A prospective study in 570 patients. *Int Angiol* **14**:60, 1995

38. Cranley JJ et al: Impending gangrene of four extremities secondary to ergotism. *N Engl J Med* **269**:727, 1963

39. Graham JR: Methysergide for prevention of headache. *N Engl J Med* **270**:67, 1964

40. Falappa P et al: Angiographic study of digital arteries in workers exposed to vinyl chloride. *Br J Ind Med* **39**:169, 1982

41. Berger CC et al: Secondary Raynaud's phenomenon and other late vascular complications following chemotherapy for testicular cancer. *Eur J Cancer* **31A**:2229, 1995

42. Fossa SD et al: Clinical and biochemical long-term toxicity after postoperative cisplatin-based chemotherapy in patients with low-stage testicular cancer. *Oncology* **52**:300, 1995

43. Doll DC, Yarbro JW: Vascular toxicity associated with chemotherapy and hormonotherapy. *Curr Opin Oncol* **6**:345, 1994

44. Kohli M, Bennett RM: Raynaud's phenomenon as a presenting sign of ovarian adenocarcinoma. *J Rheumatol* **22**:1393, 1995

45. Limburg AJ et al: Esophageal hypomotility in primary and secondary Raynaud's phenomenon: Comparison of esophageal scintigraphy with manometry. *J Nucl Med* **36**:451, 1995

46. McKierman FE: Water-soluble gels in narrowfield capillary microscopy. *Arthritis Rheum* **29**:304, 1986

47. Bukhari M et al: Increased nailfold capillary dimensions in primary Raynaud's phenomenon and systemic scleroderma. *Br J Rheumatol* **35**:1127, 1996

48. ter Borg EJ et al: Serial nailfold capillary microscopy in primary Raynaud's phenomenon and scleroderma. *Semin Arthritis Rheum* **24**:40, 1994

49. Goodfield MJD et al: The acute effects of cigarette smoking on cutaneous blood flow in smoking and non-smoking subjects with and without Raynaud's phenomenon. *Br J Rheumatol* **29**:89, 1990

50. Yocum DE et al: Use of biofeedback training in treatment of Raynaud's disease or phenomenon. *J Rheumatol* **12**:90, 1985

51. DiGiacomo RA et al: Fish-oil dietary supplementation in patients with Raynaud's phenomenon: A double-blind controlled prospective study. *Am J Med* **86**:158, 1989

52. Belch JJ, Ho M: Pharmacotherapy of Raynaud's phenomenon. *Drugs* **52**:682, 1996

53. Coffman JD et al: International study of ketanserin in Raynaud's phenomenon. *Am J Med* **87**:264, 1989

54. Helfman T, Falanga V: Stanozolol as a novel therapeutic agent in dermatology. *J Am Acad Dermatol* **33**:254, 1995

55. The LS et al: Sustained-release transdermal glyceryl trinitrate patches as a treatment for primary and secondary Raynaud's phenomenon. *Br J Rheumatol* **34**:636, 1995

56. Whitmore SE et al: Acute effect of topical minoxidil on digital blood flow in patients with Raynaud's phenomenon. *J Rheumatol* **22**:50, 1995

57. Wigley FM et al: Intravenous iloprost infusion in patients with Raynaud's phenomenon secondary to systemic sclerosis. A multicenter placebo-controlled double-blind study. *Ann Intern Med* **120**:199, 1994

58. Kingma K et al: Double-blind, placebo-controlled study of intravenous prostacyclin on hemodynamics in severe Raynaud's phenomenon: The acute vasodilatory effect is not sustained. *J Cardiovasc Pharmacol* **26**:388, 1996

59. Vayssairat M: Controlled multicenter double blind trial of an oral analog of prostacyclin in the treatment of primary Raynaud's phenomenon. *J Rheumatol* **23**:1917, 1996

60. Wise RA, Wigley F: Acute effects of misoprostol on digital circulation in patients with Raynaud's phenomenon. *J Rheumatol* **21**:80, 1994

61. Belch JJ et al: Oral iloprost as a treatment for Raynaud's syndrome: A double blind multicentre placebo controlled study. *Ann Rheum Dis* **54**:197, 1995

62. Ferro CJ, Webb DJ: The clinical potential of endothelin receptor antagonists in cardiovascular medicine. *Drugs* **51**:12, 1996

63. Bunker CB et al: Calcitonin gene-related peptide in treatment of severe peripheral vascular insufficiency in Raynaud's phenomenon. *Lancet* **342**:80, 1993

64. Koman LA et al: The microcirculatory effects of peripheral sympathectomy. *J Hand Surg* **20**:709, 1995

65. Gammal EL, Blair WF: Digital periarterial sympathectomy for ischemic digital pain and ulcers. *J Hand Surg* **16**:382, 1991

66. de Trafford JC et al: An epidemiologic survey of Raynaud's phenomenon. *Eur J Vasc Surg* **2**:167, 1988

67. Wilkinson HA: Percutaneous radiofrequency upper thoracic sympathectomy. *Neurosurgery* **40**:216, 1997

68. Bonjer HJ et al: Advantages of limited thorascopic sympathectomy. *Surg Endosc* **10**:721, 1996

69. Ahn SS et al: Thoracoscopic cervicovesal sympathectomy: Preliminary results. *J Vasc Surg* **20**:511, 1994

Reiter's Syndrome

Reiter's syndrome is a genetically determined and often protracted immune response focused on the skin and joints that usually develops several weeks after infection of the gut or urinary tract with certain microorganisms. The disorder is recognized by a set of clinical manifestations that are usually highly distinctive: mouth ulcers; conjunctivitis; balanitis; keratoderma blennorrhagicum; onychodystrophy; acute oligoarthritis, primarily involving the knee and ankle; enthesopathy (inflammation of the tendon and ligament insertions), especially of the Achilles tendon; dactylitis; and urethritis or cervicitis. Because there is no specific diagnostic test, diagnosis is sometimes complicated by a *forme fruste* expression of the features of the illness or by a protracted evolution of the full illness.

Reiter's syndrome is a member of a family of diseases termed the *seronegative spondyloarthropathies* that have in common varying degrees of arthrocutaneous and sometimes ocular manifestations (Table 182-1). They exhibit familial clustering, an inherited predisposition associated with the presence of certain major histocompatibility gene complex (MHC) class I alleles, such as HLA-B27, and are frequently precipitated by infection with certain microorganisms. The presence of enthesopathy is a diagnostic hallmark in each of these entities. Nail involvement is often prominent. The mechanism of disease in the spondyloarthropathies appears to involve an as yet imprecisely characterized cellular immune response centered on the CD8 T cell. It is clearly distinguished from the immune reaction of rheumatoid arthritis by the absence of immunoreactants, such as rheumatoid factor, and by its occurrence with undiminished, and often enhanced, intensity in the setting of the frank immunosuppression of advanced HIV infection. Reiter's syndrome and pustular psoriasis with arthritis are increasingly being considered as related entities, a finding emphasized by the arthrocutaneous syndromes of HIV infection. *Reactive arthritis* is a name sometimes used to describe incomplete forms of Reiter's syndrome affecting only the joints. There is disagreement whether Behçet's syndrome and Whipple's disease are included among the spondyloarthropathies.

HISTORIC ASPECTS

The earliest mentions of the characteristic triad of arthritis, conjunctivitis, and urethritis following enteric or venereal infections were in 1776 by Stoll and in 1818 by Brodie. The differentiation of this triad from the similar findings in gonococcal infection was difficult. Indeed, the term *keratoderma blennorrhagicum* was introduced at the end of the nineteenth century to refer to a supposed complication of gonococcal infection. Reiter's syndrome was independently described by Reiter and by Feissinger and Leroy in the setting of the appalling sanitary conditions of the Balkan and Western fronts in World War I that led to epidemics of dysentery. Again during World War II, the distinctive epidemiology of Reiter's syndrome was documented in a study of more than 150,000 Finns who developed shigellosis, of whom Reiter's syndrome was found in 344, and of 602 similarly infected sailors on the cruiser *Little Rock*, of whom Reiter's syndrome developed in 9. The understanding of the importance of ligament and tendon insertional inflammation, or enthesopathy, as a general manifestation of Reiter's syndrome was advanced by the work of Ball.

The fundamental observation in 1973 by Brewerton et al.[1] that susceptibility to Reiter's syndrome was strongly associated with the MHC class I specificity HLA-B27 ushered in the intense period of current interest in this disease and made Reiter's syndrome the first instance of a human immune response to a bacterial infection that was genetically regulated by allelic forms of MHC molecules. This observation pointed to the role of the human MHC as the site of immune response genes. The role of HLA-B27 in Reiter's syndrome was confirmed by returning to the survivors of the two epidemiologic studies and identifying this HLA specificity in approximately 80 percent of the 50 Finns and 5 sailors with Reiter's syndrome who were available for study; the expected low levels were found in the unaffected controls. The recognition that Reiter's syndrome can occur in persons with advanced AIDS emphasized that the CD4 T cell lineage was not involved in its pathogenesis. Attention was therefore directed to the role of the residual T cells of the CD8 lineage, introducing the notion of a CD8 T cell–driven disease process.[2,3]

TABLE 182-1

The Spondyloarthropathies

DISEASE	HLA MARKER OF SUSCEPTIBILITY	MUCOCUTANEOUS INVOLVEMENT
Reiter's syndrome	HLA-B27, HLA-B7	Marked
Reactive arthritis	HLA-B27, HLA-B7	No
Psoriatic arthritis	HLA-Cw6, -Bw13, etc., HLA-B27, HLA-B44(?)	Marked
Ankylosing spondylitis	HLA-B27	No
Enteric arthritis (ulcerative colitis, Crohn's disease)	HLA-B27 (axial disease)	Occasional
Behçet's syndrome?	HLA-B51	Marked
Whipple's disease?	HLA-B27(?)	No

EPIDEMIOLOGY AND GENETIC FACTORS

There are two epidemiologically distinct forms of Reiter's syndrome. One, the venereal or endemic form, follows a sexually transmitted route and is initiated by urethritis. The other is the epidemic or postdysenteric form that follows enteric infection. The analysis of Reiter's syndrome is made difficult by the fact that both urethritis and bowel inflammation can be components of the Reiter's syndrome reaction as well as antecedent inducing factors associated with a predisposing infection. The sex ratio is approximately equal in the postdysenteric form but is greatly male-biased in the clinically equivalent form that follows urethritis, perhaps because nonspecific urethritis is much more common among men. Reiter's syndrome develops in from 1 to 3 percent of individuals with nonspecific urethritis.[4] Since epidemic enteric infections are relatively uncommon in the United States, Reiter's syndrome is largely a disease of males, and male predominance ranges from 85 to 88 percent. The most frequent age of onset is in the early twenties, but Reiter's syndrome has been recognized from childhood into the sixth decade.[5,6]

Reiter's syndrome is more prevalent among Caucasians, perhaps because the frequency of HLA-B27 is relatively high among this ethnic group. In addition, other incompletely defined genetic factors appear to be involved. HLA-B27 is the major determinant of susceptibility to both Reiter's syndrome and ankylosing spondylitis. However, in some families with HLA-B27 there is a strong concentration of Reiter's syndrome without ankylosing spondylitis, whereas in others the opposite is the case.[7,8] In general, Reiter's syndrome is found in 1 of 10 relatives of the proband. A similar divergence between Reiter's syndrome and ankylosing spondylitis is evident among certain groups of American Indians and Inupiat Eskimos in whom HLA-B27 is prevalent. For example, the Haida and Pima have a high frequency of ankylosing spondylitis, and the Navaho and Inupiat have a high frequency of Reiter's syndrome.

As would be anticipated in a disorder with an infectious etiology, characteristic modes of transmission, a genetic susceptibility associated with an allele that has a complex distribution, and no specific diagnostic test to identify atypical clinical presentations, it is difficult to arrive at a reliable estimate of the prevalence or incidence of Reiter's syndrome. In the rural midwestern United States, the annual age-adjusted incidence[9] is reported to be 3.5 per 100,000. This figure varies greatly according to socioeconomic status, lifestyle, and various other factors. Reiter's syndrome is considered to be the most common cause of arthritis in young males. However, it is found in the pediatric age group, typically after enteric infections, where it has been encountered after cryptosporidial enteritis.[10]

ETIOLOGY AND PATHOGENESIS

Infectious Etiology

The postdysenteric form of Reiter's syndrome is initiated by infections with a specific set of gram-negative enteric organisms that are designated as arthritogenic. These include *Salmonella enteritidis*, *S. typhimurium*, and *S. heidelberg*; *Shigella flexneri*, types 1b and 2a, and *S. dysenteriae* but not *S. sonnie*; *Yersinia enterocolitica* and *Y. pseudotuberculosis*; and *Campylobacter fetus* and *Clostridium difficile*. Among the *Salmonella* and *Shigella* infections that result in Reiter's syndrome there is a very close connection between the ability to induce Reiter's syndrome and the presence of a distinctive plasmid. In contrast, the infectious etiology of the endemic or venereal form of Reiter's syndrome has been more difficult to define. *Chlamydia trachomatis* has been implicated as a possible agent. This agent can be cultured from over one-third of men with nonspecific urethritis regardless of whether or not they develop Reiter's syndrome, and elementary bodies of the organism have been observed in the synovial membrane.[11] Identification of the chlamydial ribosomal RNA operon by polymerase chain reaction (PCR) analyses is proving to be a more efficient means of identification of relevant infection by this organism. This identification is enhanced if synovial tissue obtained on needle biopsy is used, as opposed to only synovial fluid.[12]

In contrast to the clear epidemiologic implication of microorganisms, in individual cases it is often difficult to establish a role of a specific microorganism because the clinical response of Reiter's syndrome follows the apparent inciting infection by 1 to 4 weeks, and cultures are usually negative. For this reason, primary emphasis has been placed on analyzing the serologic and cellular responses to microorganisms present in the blood and joint fluids of the patient with Reiter's syndrome. In infection with *Yersinia*, elevated titers of IgA antibodies correlate with the development of Reiter's syndrome, and these antibodies are primarily directed to lipopolysaccharide components of the organism.[13] Similar antibodies are found in instances of Reiter's syndrome incited by other microorganisms.[14] Paradoxically, the T cell proliferative response to microbial antigens in the blood of those who develop Reiter's syndrome is lower than in others who are similarly infected but who do not develop Reiter's syndrome; however, there is a much greater response in the lymphocytes of the joint fluid compared to those in the blood of those who develop the disease.[15,16] These findings again raise the question of whether microbial antigens persist, possibly because the cellular component of the immune response in susceptible individuals is incapable of effectively eliminating them. Such strain-related persistence is associated with the development of *Yersinia*-induced reactive arthritis in a rat model,[17] and there is increasing evidence, by PCR, for the demonstration of *Yersinia, Chlamydia,* and *Salmonella* antigens or portions of their genome in the tissue or, less efficiently, the joint fluids of affected persons.[11,12,18-20]

Genetic Factors

In the Caucasian population at large, cross-sectional studies demonstrate a close association between HLA-B27 and Reiter's syndrome. In one study this HLA specificity was found in 80 percent of 906 patients and 9 percent of 13,477 ethnically matched controls.[21] The relative risk is 37, showing that the presence of HLA-B27 marks the potential for an untoward immune response. Other studies observe a somewhat lower frequency, in the range of 50 to 80 percent. In general, the intensity of the association between Reiter's syndrome and HLA-B27 is appreciably less than that observed between the same specificity and ankylosing spondylitis. Furthermore, among the 20 percent or more of HLA-B27-negative patients with Reiter's syndrome, many have one of a group of HLA class I specificities termed *HLA-B27 cross-reacting antigens* (CREGs).[5,22] The CREGs include HLA-B7, HLA-Bw22, HLA-Bw40, and HLA-Bw42, and they share structural and antigenic similarities with

HLA-B27. Among non-Caucasians the association with HLA-B27 is weaker. From 14 to 37 percent of non-Caucasian patients with Reiter's syndrome have HLA-B27, whereas the frequency of the HLA specificity in healthy controls is only 2 percent or less. When Reiter's syndrome occurs in individuals infected with HIV, the same genetic predisposition is found that is primarily defined by the presence of HLA-B27.[23] In a study of HIV-infected individuals developing Reiter's syndrome in Zimbabwe, HLA-B27 was not found, but half of the individuals had a recognized CREG.[24] While the relationship to HLA-B27 and the CREG alleles strongly suggests that the class I HLA molecule is the driving element in determining susceptibility, the chromosomal region around the HLA-B and HLA-C loci contains several additional polymorphic genes including MICA, HLA-17, and BAT1, which could also be relevant.[25,26] These polymorphisms have not been studied in Reiter's disease, although a related polymorphism in the nearby MICA gene was shown to have a weaker association than HLA-B27 in ankylosing spondylitis,[27] in which the relative risk is over 90 and susceptibility is not associated with CREG specificities. Therefore, ankylosing spondylitis may be related more directly to a particular structure in the HLA-B27 molecule itself, while Reiter's syndrome is most probably developed in response to a shared determinant encoded by the HLA-B27 alleles[28] and several evolutionarily related alleles of the CREG group (Fig. 182-1). The risk of developing Reiter's syndrome in an HLA-B27-positive person in an epidemic setting has been calculated to be as high as 20 percent,[29] but in other epidemics, such as that among the Finns, the risk is as much as an order of magnitude lower.[6]

Immunologic Mechanisms

Several features discussed previously suggest the following overall model of the immunopathogenesis of Reiter's syndrome, although some of the details still remain conjectural. The immune response underlying the syndrome is initiated by particular antigens encoded by certain microorganisms that mimic self peptides.[30] This immune response involves the CD8 T cell lineage and recognition of antigen presented by the class I MHC molecules. While the response is initially directed to the antigen of the microorganism, the immune reactivity spreads to target autoantigens. It is this CD8 T cell response that initiates the inflammation and alteration of the pattern of gene expression in target tissues through the release of cytokines and other inflammatory mediators by the responding lymphocytes.

Three experimental models are particularly relevant to the pathogenesis of Reiter's syndrome. Adjuvant arthritis in rats resulting from the administration of inactivated *Mycobacterium tuberculosis* is a strain-specific response characterized by tendinitis, keratoderma blennorrhagicum, urethritis, and ophthalmitis, which resembles Reiter's syndrome.[31] Similarly, the 57-kDa heat-shock protein of *Chlamydia* induces experimental eye inflammation that mimics the reactive, inflammation induced by the whole organism and, in turn, that in Reiter's syndrome.[32] The expression of the HLA-B27 molecule in mice at levels from five to ten times those of the mouse MHC molecules resulted in phenotypically normal animals which, however, had enhanced susceptibility to *Yersinia* infection.[33] Taken together with the previous information, this finding reinforces the paradigm that Reiter's syndrome is a specific immunologic reaction to a microorganism antigen presented by MHC molecules to T cells.

The central immune recognition event in Reiter's syndrome appears to involve the recognition of a peptide presented by a class I molecule to a CD8 lineage T cell. This observation is based on three main lines of evidence: (1) Reiter's syndrome occurs with

FIGURE 182-1

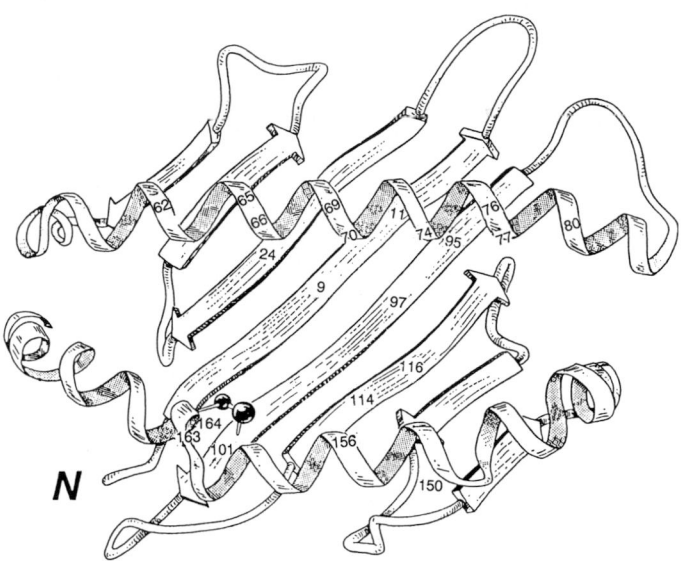

A.

B.

A. The conformation of the MHC class I molecule as described by Bjorkman et al.[51] from the perspective of a T cell receptor looking down at the antigen-binding portion of the molecule. The polypeptide backbone of the class I molecule consists of two α helices that form the walls of the antigen-presenting cleft and the eight strands of antiparallel β-pleated sheet that form the base. *B.* The dark areas indicate the location of the amino acid substitutions that define the HLA-B27 specificities.

undiminished intensity in those with advanced AIDS and loss of CD4 T cell function, (2) the response does not involve classic autoantibodies that reflect the action of CD4 T cell help occurring in diseases such as systemic lupus erythematosus and rheumatoid arthritis, and (3) susceptibility is determined by the presence of certain class I alleles that act as immune response genes. The nature of the antigen and the specificity of the T cell receptor remain unknown.

The nature and method of regulation of the CD8 T cell immune response also remain unknown. It could develop through one of at least three quite dissimilar mechanisms. One possibility is that the HLA-B27 molecule and its CREG species induce a highly specific immunologic tolerance to the arthritogenic organisms through a process of deleting specific T cell clones during the formation of the T cell repertoire, thereby creating a hole in the T cell repertoire. These clones would be necessary for the elimination of the organism, which does not occur in the HLA-B27-positive person. In this model of microbial persistence, the resulting sustained immune response to the organism would be incapable of eliminating the organism, similar to the situation in leprosy, but would be of sufficient intensity to give rise to the clinical disease. The pathogenic immune response would be both induced and sustained by the persisting foreign microorganism. Two alternative possibilities exist to account for the clinical phenomena: dissemination of microbial antigen to target tissues or development of an autoimmune response by breach of a tolerance mechanism.

A second, less likely, possibility involves nonantigen-specific stimulation of T lymphocytes by bacterial superantigens.[34] Superantigens are molecules encoded either by a microorganism such as certain heat shock proteins or by endogenous genes such as the integrated murine mouse mammary tumor retrovirus. They bind to particular $V\beta$ gene segment products that comprise a portion of the T cell receptor β chain and interact with MHC molecules. The interactions are nonclonal, are nonantigen specific, and are not restricted by specific MHC types. The chronicity of this mechanism involves the sustained drive of particular T cell clones that then become stimulated by a self antigen through loss of tolerance.

A third "autoimmune" model postulates that upon stimulation by arthritogenic microorganisms, the immune system loses tolerance for self molecules through mimicry of specific self antigens by molecules of the microorganism. This model differs from the first model in that the principle immune perturbation occurs in the regulation of peripheral tolerance by the class I allele involved in determining the susceptibility state. This loss of tolerance most likely would arise through an induced response to minor antigenic determinants on self molecules for which tolerance does not exist (*clonal ignorance*) and which are usually not seen as antigenic. The resulting pathogenic immune response, occurring at the CD8 T cell level, is autoimmune in character, with its persistent driving element a component of self. It differs from the other two mechanisms in that microbial antigens only induce the abnormality but play no part in its sustained presence.

While clear differences exist between Reiter's syndrome and psoriasis/psoriatic arthritis at multiple levels, certain elements in the pathogenesis of these two entities appear to be quite similar, if not identical. T cells of the CD8 lineage and immune recognition events involving class I MHC molecules appear centrally involved in both illnesses. The presence of HLA-B27 alters the host response in psoriasis/psoriatic arthritis to resemble more the pattern of skin and joint involvement in Reiter's syndrome, with axial disease and pustular lesions indistinguishable from keratoderma blennorrhagicum.

Similarly, the clinical findings in Reiter's syndrome associated with HIV infection form a continuum with those of psoriasis/psoriatic arthritis. A diagram of the role of the CD8 T cell applicable to the pathogenesis of Reiter's syndrome is found in Chap. 44, "Psoriatic Arthritis."

PATHOLOGY

Skin

Histologically, the appearance of established keratoderma blennorrhagicum is indistinguishable from that of pustular psoriasis, with hyperkeratosis and parakeratosis, elongation and hypertrophy of the rete pegs, general epidermal hyperplasia, and extensive neutrophilic infiltration with formation of microabscesses and spongiform pustules. The initial lesion is a vesicular, pustular, or erythematous macule. Balanitis in circumcised individuals has a similar histologic appearance, whereas the moist lesion of uncircumcised males and the mouth ulcers are otherwise similar but are not keratinized. Differentiation from psoriasis may by helped by the presence of a greatly thickened horny layer in Reiter's syndrome.

Musculoskeletal System

The characteristic lesions of the entheses have not been studied in great detail but contain small numbers of lymphocytes and proliferating fibroblasts. The appearance of the synovium is typical of any nonspecific chronic synovitis but with rather more marked vascular involvement and fibroblast proliferation. Edema, vascular congestion, increased surface fibrin, lining cell proliferation, infiltration with neutrophils and lymphocytes, and considerable fibroblast proliferation are found. Occlusion by platelet and fibrin thrombi, simulating that caused by endotoxins, is common.[11] The inciting antigen may be demonstrable.

Systemic

Sixty-seven percent of patients with Reiter's syndrome are reported to have either acute ileocolitis or evidence of Crohn's disease upon biopsy, with most having no gastrointestinal symptoms.[35] Five percent of patients have granulomatous lesions found at the aortic root and annulus that may cause abnormalities in conduction, including complete heart block and frank atonic regurgitation. Secondary amyloidosis with AA protein deposition is a rare complication usually found after a long course of illness.

CLINICAL MANIFESTATIONS

Natural History

The chronologic evolution of Reiter's syndrome is a distinctive feature that often provides the clue to diagnosis. The enteric or genitourinary infection that initiates Reiter's syndrome is followed by a characteristic latent period of 1 week to 1 month, during which the initial symptoms attributable to the infection subside. Urethritis and conjunctivitis are usually the first manifestations of Reiter's syndrome; they are followed within several days by the often abrupt and diagnostically characteristic onset of arthritis. The mucocutaneous involvement occurs independently, sometimes coinciding with or preceding the phase of urethritis and conjunctivitis and sometimes developing after the onset of arthritis. During the acute phase of Reiter's syndrome, constitutional symptoms and signs are prominent, including fever, fatigue, malaise, and weight loss that can be profound.

Skin Disease

Circinate balanitis is the most common cutaneous finding, being reported in about 36 percent of patients with Reiter's syndrome.[36] The lesion is initially vesicular with little or no surrounding erythema. Irregular moist superficial ulcers form in the uncircumcised male and may coalesce to give a circinate distribution (Fig. 182-2). These ulcers may occasionally become secondarily infected. In the circumcised male, the lesions evolve to form hard crusts and plaques. Painless mucosal ulcers of varying size on the tongue, palate, buccal mucosa, and lips are found in 17 percent of cases and are usually transient and cause little or no morbidity.

The initial lesions of keratoderma blennorrhagicum are small vesicles or erythematous macules that may coalesce and are usually surrounded by an erythematous base. The vesicle wall becomes progressively thickened, forming a small papule, nodule, or even a horny excrescence (Fig. 182-3). The appearance of the lesions varies from a scaling plaquelike process that resembles pustular psoriasis to combinations of crusting, exudation, and erosion associated with erythema. Lesions of keratoderma blennorrhagicum are found in an average of 15 percent of patients. Keratoderma blennorrhagicum is most commonly found on the soles, toes, and palms where the lesions are often densely scattered. More isolated lesions occur

FIGURE 182-3

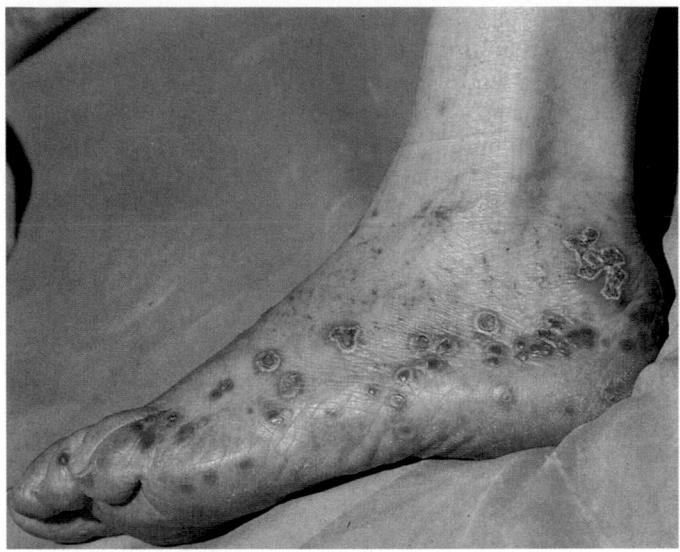

Reiter's syndrome, keratoderma blennorrhagicum. Red-to-brown papules, vesicles, and pustules, with central erosion and confluence of lesions on the foot.

on the glans penis, scrotum, trunk, limbs, and scalp. In severe cases, notably those associated with HIV infection, the keratoderma blennorrhagicum may be distributed over the entire body, with an intensification on the digits in a pattern that resembles the lesions of pustular psoriasis and in the groin in the pattern of inverse psoriasis or sebopsoriasis. The soles may exhibit unusually marked keratotic changes (Fig. 182-4). The keratoderma blennorrhagicum lesions may last for weeks to months, disappear, and then recur.[37] In patients with HIV infection, the initial Reiter's syndrome–like illness may gradually assume the chronic features of pustular psoriatic arthritis.

FIGURE 182-2

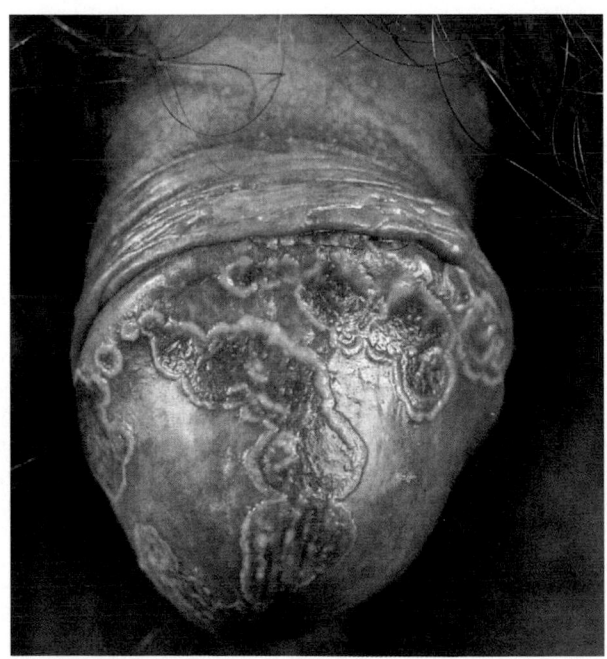

Reiter's syndrome, balanitis circinata. Illustrated in this patient is circinate balanitis with moist, well-demarcated erosions with a slightly raised border.

FIGURE 182-4

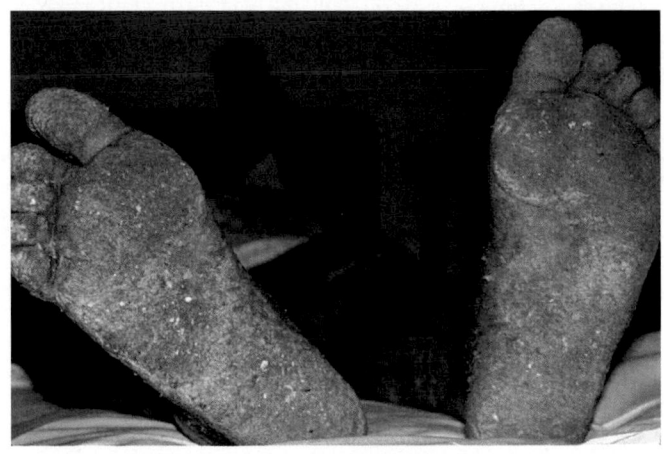

Severe keratodermia blennorrhagicum with marked dyskeratotic change in an HIV-positive person. The margins of the dyskeratotic process are intensely inflamed.

Joint Disease

The foot, ankle, and knee are the principal sites of musculoskeletal involvement. Joint disease includes both enthesopathy, mainly of the plantar fascia and Achilles tendon, and arthritis of the subtalar, ankle, and knee joints. The arthritis is generally abrupt in onset and may be florid, particularly in the knee joint where massive effusion may lead to rupture of the popliteal Baker's cyst and the syndrome of pseudothrombophlebitis. The joint inflammation occasionally subsides and does not recur; more commonly, it remains as a chronic problem, manifesting itself as either sustained or recrudescent arthritis. The small or large joints of the upper limbs may be involved, but only in association with predominant arthritis of the large joints of the legs. In the instances of Reiter's syndrome associated with HIV infection, the course of the joint disease is sometimes slowly cumulative and ultimately results in an extensive polyarthritis involving the small and large joints of the arms and legs in a pattern more similar to that of psoriatic arthritis. This cumulative pattern is usually accompanied by sustained joint disease that leads to erosions and marked periarticular osteoporosis (Fig. 182-5).

Inflammation at the sites of insertion of ligaments and tendons is a striking feature of Reiter's syndrome. In addition to the plantar fasciitis and Achilles and posterior tibial tendinitis, the enthesopathy results in chest wall and lower back pain, tenderness over ischial tuberosities and iliac crests, and dactylitis, or "sausage digits." In addition to the back pain directly attributable to enthesopathy that is usually manifest as transient pain or stiffness, approximately one-quarter of patients with chronic Reiter's syndrome develop chronic sacroiliitis or a characteristic asymmetric spondylosis that limits back mobility.[38] The characteristic symptoms include stiffness and pain after periods of rest, such as in the early morning, with improvement upon exercise. Enthesopathy may be more florid in instances of juvenile onset.[39]

Nail Disease

Involvement of the nail may begin as erythema of the nail fold or more insidiously as subungual hyperkeratosis, a diagnostic finding in psoriasis and Reiter's syndrome that distinguishes these entities from rheumatoid arthritis. The nail becomes thickened, yellowed, and brittle. Frank onycholysis with shedding of the nail often occurs. The acral portion of the digit may be hyperkeratotic with erythema and scaling and may exhibit the appearance of pseudoparonychia. The tendency to extensive acral disease is pronounced in HIV-associated cases. In some cases of HIV-associated Reiter's syndrome, yellowing of the nails has been the first manifestation of the syndrome. Pitting of the nails, characteristic of psoriasis, is not seen in Reiter's syndrome.

Other Manifestations

Urethritis and prostatitis are frequently associated findings. They may present only as sterile pyuria in the first voided specimen or range up to moderately severe dysuria with frank mucopurulent discharge. The dominant ocular lesion in Reiter's syndrome is conjunctivitis of varying intensity that usually resolves quickly. A smaller proportion of patients also exhibits uveitis, initially manifest as acute anterior iritis, which may progress to chronic iridocyclitis and visual impairment. The uveitis resembles that of ankylosing spondylitis in that it is acute in onset, frequently unilateral, and

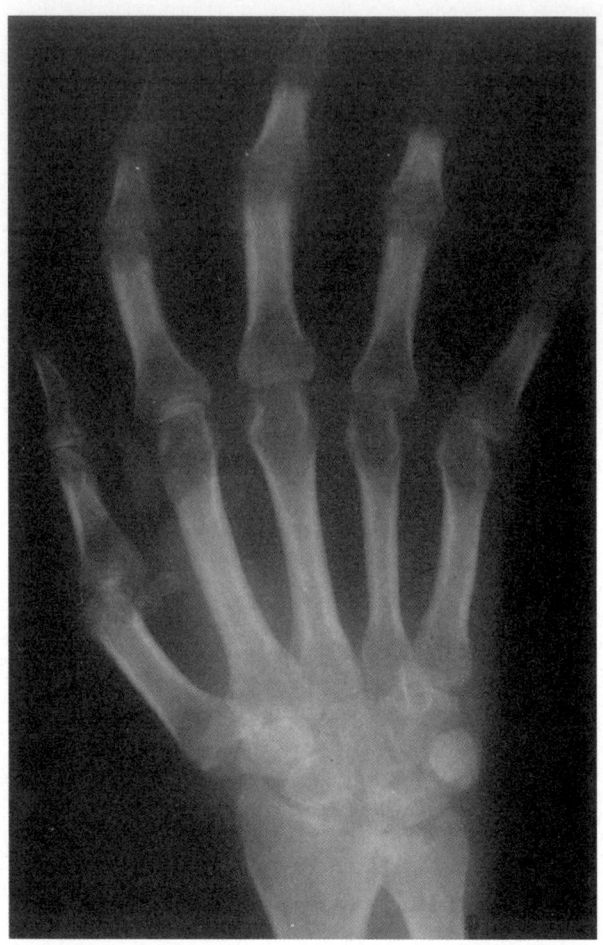

Juxtaarticular osteoporosis in an HIV-positive person who presented with typical Reiter's syndrome, but who exhibited a cumulative pattern of joint involvement indistinguishable from that of psoriatic arthritis. The involvement of the small joints in the hands is also more typical of psoriatic arthritis.

spares the choroid and retina.[40] Uveitis is a potentially serious problem that must be carefully evaluated and treated.

The cardiac symptoms in Reiter's syndrome include palpitations, pericardial type chest pain, and, relatively rarely, symptoms of aortic valve incompetence. Findings present in 5 percent of the patients include first-, second-, and third-degree heart block; ST-segment and T- and Q-wave changes on electrocardiography; pericardial rubs; and varying degrees of aortic and occasionally mitral valve incompetence from granulomatous involvement at the aortic root.[41,42] Atrioventricular conduction disturbances may appear early in the course. Relatively rare manifestations include peripheral neuropathy and other neurologic findings, pleuritic and pulmonary parenchymal inflammation, erythema nodosum, and amyloidosis.

LABORATORY FINDINGS

High levels of cytokines associated with the inflammation of Reiter's syndrome are reflected by the elevation in acute-phase reactants, a variably elevated erythrocyte sedimentation rate, hypochromic or normochromic anemia, and mild hypoalbuminemia. There are no diagnostically specific antimicrobial antibodies, although elevated antibody titers to specific enteric pathogenic agents or *Chlamydia* often help with differential diagnosis. Rheumatoid factor and classic autoantibodies are absent. Urine and stool cultures are usually nonrevealing, although the persistence of *Salmonella* carriage would be important to determine. The demonstration of persistent microorganismal components in tissue biopsies is still an experimental technique, but identification of the chlamydial ribosomal RNA operon by PCR analyses is an efficient means of identification of relevant infection by this organism.[12] Testing for HIV should be considered in view of the fact that HIV infection is also a sexually acquired disease.

Much has been written about whether or not to perform HLA typing for diagnostic reasons.[43] The sensitivity and specificity of determinations of the presence of HLA-B27 are approximately those of tests for antinuclear antibodies in lupus erythematosus. In a classic but mild case, where Reiter's syndrome is an obvious clinical diagnosis, the test seems unnecessary. However, since HLA-B27 positivity is associated with more severe and protracted disease (including the occurrence of uveitis, carditis, and sacroiliitis) and the presence of CREG specificities alone is associated with milder disease,[44,45] testing may be useful in difficult cases for diagnostic or prognostic reasons.

The joint fluid cell count varies from occasional to over 50,000 neutrophils per μL, a level that in conjunction with the intense inflammation might otherwise suggest a septic joint and is designated *pseudosepsis*. Occasionally "Reiter's cells" are observed, which are macrophages that have ingested a neutrophilic leukocyte. Total joint fluid protein levels are elevated in proportion to the degree of inflammation, and because there is little or no intraarticular consumption of complement, the joint fluid complement component levels are about two-thirds of their levels in serum when normalized on a per gram of serum protein basis. Glucose levels are normal, and bacteriologic cultures are uniformly negative.

RADIOGRAPHIC FEATURES

Frank arthritis may initially only show signs of an effusion. Periarticular osteoporosis develops after several weeks of inflammation, and in some instances where the arthritis becomes chronic, erosions and loss of the cartilaginous joint space are seen. Enthesopathy is characterized by a combination of erosions about tendon and ligament insertions, bone lucency, and new bone formation, often in the form of spurs extending into the tendon or fascia. Widespread periosteal new bone formation can be found, especially on the bones of the pelvis and feet. Calcaneal enthesopathy is also found in psoriatic arthritis and certain metabolic arthropathies. Sacroiliitis is typical in appearance but may be only asymmetric, distinguishing it from the uniformly bilateral form in ankylosing spondylitis. Similarly, the frank spondyloarthropathy, when present, is often asymmetric without the uniformity in extension from the lower lumbar vertebrae that occurs in psoriatic arthritis.[38] Indeed, neck involvement is rather more common in Reiter's syndrome.

DIAGNOSIS

The diagnosis of Reiter's syndrome can be simple or exceedingly challenging. The classic presentation is a young male with an antecedent nonspecific urethritis or one of many individuals with an epidemic enteric infection. After a few days to weeks, fever, conjunctivitis, characteristic mucocutaneous disease, urethritis, florid arthritis of the knees, ankles, and feet, and extensive enthesopathy develop. However, in the majority of patients a variable number of these features are absent. In the absence of the distinctive mucocutaneous findings, a careful differential diagnosis must be made among entities such as other spondyloarthropathies (including especially ankylosing spondylitis and psoriatic arthritis), infectious arthritis (notably that due to the gonococcus or Lyme disease), the crystal-induced arthropathies (primarily gout), and other rheumatic diseases such as rheumatoid arthritis, Behçet's syndrome, and rheumatic fever. Difficulties may arise in those with skin disease because elements of the early history are ignored or suppressed. The history of a sexual contact or risk factors leading to the acquisition of HIV infections may be concealed, or an episode of dysentery may be disregarded unless the patient is specifically questioned. Similarly, many of the features of the illness may be mild so that mouth ulcers, if noticed at all, are passed off as "cold sores," and transient dysuria is dismissed. The remaining signs and symptoms may add up to a relatively perplexing entity.

Although gonococcal arthritis and Reiter's syndrome may superficially resemble one another in that urethritis, skin rash, oligoarthritis, and tenosynovitis occur in both, the character and natural history of the two illnesses are usually readily distinguishable. Gonococcal arthritis is more common in females, and upper limb joint involvement predominates. The arthritis is not florid and is usually preceded by insidiously developing migratory arthralgia. Enthesopathy, keratoderma blennorrhagicum, balanitis, and back pain are absent. Culture may be helpful but can be negative. That both entities can coexist should be emphasized.

The differential diagnosis between psoriatic arthritis and Reiter's syndrome is discussed in detail in the chapter on psoriatic arthritis (Chap. 44). The presence of mouth ulcers, urethritis, predominant foot or lower extremity disease, and antecedent infection favor Reiter's syndrome; an insidious onset, extensive skin disease, primary upper limb arthritis, and especially distal interphalangeal joint involvement are characteristic of psoriatic arthritis. Examination of the nails, especially those of the fingers, can be of great importance in the diagnosis of either entity. Nail involvement is prevalent but distinctive in both diseases. HLA type can often be useful. In HIV infection, the differential diagnosis between pustular psoriatic arthritis and Reiter's syndrome may in principle be impossible because the entities appear to be interrelated if not identical, as discussed in detail in Chap. 44.

In any florid arthritis, the fluid should be studied for the presence of microorganisms by culture and staining and examined for urate crystals by polarized light microscopy. Rheumatic fever remains a rare but strong simulator of Reiter's syndrome. The antecedent pharyngitis and characteristic rash of streptococcal infection are points of differentiation, but similar cardiac and joint findings can prove problematic. Behçet's syndrome is another rare entity in North America, but the combination of mucocutaneous disease and arthritic disease in this syndrome can cause diagnostic difficulties. Neurologic findings and the pustulonecrotic pathergic lesions at injury sites, as well as extensive, painful genital and oral ulcers, suggest the diagnosis of Behçet's syndrome.

The complications of the effusive inflammatory arthritis include ruptured popliteal cysts and thrombophlebitis. The rupture of popliteal cysts with the syndrome of pseudothrombophlebitis should be differentiated from true thrombophlebitis, which can also be found in this setting due to pressure on the popliteal vein by the joint effusion and the contiguous inflammation.

The special problems of the radiologic diagnosis of juvenile-onset Reiter's syndrome and its distinction from the other spondyloarthropathies and from forms of juvenile chronic arthritis have been reviewed.[39]

TREATMENT

Therapy of Reiter's syndrome is difficult when the illness is sustained or severe because there are no agents capable of eliminating the inflammatory host response definitively and safely. The cutaneous manifestations and the systemic concomitant of intense inflammation (fever, mild anemia) are often the most obvious features of the illness; but despite their significant psychological impact, they are usually in themselves not the cause of significant morbidity. In contrast, arthritis, uveitis, and the more uncommon visceral manifestations, especially those of the heart, while often less overt to the patients, may require intensive drug therapy to prevent serious complications or disability. Certainly, physical therapy is very important to maintain range of motion and prevent joint fibrosis.

The pharmacologic agents potentially available for the treatment of Reiter's syndrome may be placed in three theoretical groups: (1) Antibiotics to eliminate persistent infection by the inciting organism; (2) anti-inflammatory agents that blunt the chemokine-mediated entry or consequences of leukocytes into sites of immunologic response or that downmodulate other late pathways of inflammation; and (3) immunomodulatory or immunosuppressive agents that attenuate the CD8 T cell arm of specific immune recognition underlying the lymphocyte component of the inflammation.

Antibiotic therapy is still a controversial topic. The traditional view has been not to treat, although newer data about microbial persistence in the synovial tissues, described above, support a role for antibiotics. Reiter's syndrome following chlamydial urethritis and chronic Reiter's syndrome in a setting of colonization by an arthritogenic organism are situations where short-term antibiotics appear quite appropriate. It is still a matter of discussion whether well-tolerated docytetracycline or tetracycline preparations are appropriate in severe, recent-onset Reiter's syndrome in HLA-B27-positive persons. In the absence of carefully controlled studies on this subject with PCR follow-up to monitor persistence of infection, the physician's judgment of all factors remains the deciding factor. Clearly, any suggestion that an individual had an impaired immune system with the question of enhanced microbial persistence would suggest that antibiotics be used if a specific inciting organism were documented by culture or by molecular biologic diagnostics. Because advanced HIV infection is associated with microbial persistence, it is felt that therapy of documented inciting infectious agents in an HIV-positive individual with Reiter's syndrome is clearly appropriate. This is especially so because the inflammatory response of Reiter's syndrome may transactivate the virus, leading to an increase in viral load and consequent increased viral cytopathogenic effect. For this reason, HIV-positive individuals with Reiter's syndrome should have a program of monitoring viral load and initiation of effective antiviral agents.

The choice of the use of anti-inflammatory and immunomodulatory therapy is discussed below in the context of each therapeutic situation. In general, the anti-inflammatory agents have a high benefit-to-risk ratio, and the decision to use them is usually not complex. In contrast, the use of immunomodulatory/immunosuppressive agents is associated with considerably greater risks. Since the evidence that the CD8 T cell plays a central role in the pathogenesis of Reiter's syndrome is mounting, it might be of interest to have an agent that selectively acts on T cells of this lineage and avoids the concomitant suppression of the CD4 T cell compartment. Currently, there is little to suggest that any available agents exhibit a sparing of the CD4 T cell.

All patients with Reiter's syndrome must be informed about the sometimes difficult nature of the illness and its variable outcome. It is important to engender both an optimistic mentality on the ultimate outcome and a sense of realism about the potential problems. Psychological support is particularly important for this type of arthrocutaneous syndrome because of anxiety associated with sexually transmitted routes of infection and the fact that these younger patients often have not had a prior major and potentially chronic illness. Moreover, public health aspects involve other individuals in the identification of enteric or sexually transmitted routes. Available evidence suggests that reinfection may induce a recrudescence that is sometimes more severe than the original episode. Therefore, counseling must be offered on prevention by avoidance of reexposure to microorganisms, including the avoidance of travel in areas of the world with unreliable hygiene, and attention to measures that reduce the likelihood of acquiring a sexually transmitted disease.

Skin Disease

The management of the acute mucocutaneous lesions of uncomplicated Reiter's syndrome is usually limited to the general measures discussed above because the lesions are rarely severe enough to mandate specific therapeutic attention. The severe, extensive, and chronic cutaneous reactions that are more common in the form of Reiter's syndrome associated with HIV infection present a much more difficult challenge. Moderate success has been obtained by treating these lesions in the same manner as pustular psoriasis. UVB irradiation, coal tar, and etrinate administration, combined with very judicious use of topical steroids, are the mainstay of therapy. When HIV infection is excluded, extremely severe skin lesions can be treated with immunosuppressive agents including methotrexate, PUVA therapy, or cyclosporine.

Eye Disease

Conjunctivitis is a common short-lived occurrence and can be adequately managed by nonspecific local therapy. Topical antibiotics have no established efficacy. In marked contrast, the development, actual or suspected, of uveitis is a threatening complication. Eye pain, ciliary flush, and other symptoms of early iritis should prompt immediate referral to an ophthalmologist for definitive evaluation and therapy. Treatment includes the use of agents that diminish intraocular tension and intraocular or occasionally systemic steroid therapy.

Visceral Disease

The development of cardiac involvement is a potentially life-threatening complication that can either appear as a part of the initial presentation or develop in otherwise clinically stable individuals.

Conduction disturbances and aortic or mitral valvular involvement mandate immediate medical evaluation. Systemic glucocorticoid therapy is useful in this specialized situation.

Musculoskeletal Disease

Arthritis and enthesopathy are the symptoms that necessitate treatment in most patients. Exercise and physical therapy are important. Nonsteroidal anti-inflammatory drug (NSAID) therapy is the first line of treatment. Five NSAIDs, indomethacin, sulindac, diclofenac, naproxen, and phenylbutazone, are generally considered to be the most efficacious of this large class of agents for the therapy of Reiter's syndrome. Because of idiosyncratic reactions (including cytopenias) phenylbutazone, the most effective of the agents, has fallen out of use, with the major exception of treating HIV-associated cases of Reiter's syndrome. Therapy with indomethacin or naproxen is begun at the lowest dose and increased. Naproxen, 200 to 375 mg, is administered two to three times a day and is increased to the maximum recommended dose of 1500 mg over a 1- to 2-week period. Indomethacin, 25 mg, is administered two to three times a day and increased to a total of 225 mg daily. Three weeks or more should be allowed before an agent is deemed ineffective. Change to another drug should include at least a 1-week taper of the initial drug to prevent "rebound" activation, while the alternative drug is begun concomitantly.

The untoward effects of NSAIDs include erosive and irritative gastrointestinal effects, bronchial asthma exacerbations, headache, depression, nephropathy, antihemostatic action on platelets, salt retention with attendant congestive heart failure and hypertension, and idiosyncratic allergic responses such as cytopenias and rash.

Sulfasalazine is reported to be effective in the therapy of Reiter's syndrome unresponsive to NSAIDs when given at 2 g daily in divided doses, but in one study one in five patients had to discontinue the agent because of side effects.[46] The drug is initially given at 250 to 500 mg one to two times a day to minimize the prominent untoward gastrointestinal effects of nausea and vomiting. The maintenance dose of 2 g is approached slowly over 1 to 2 months by weekly increments in dosage. Because it is slow-acting, its therapeutic effect may not be seen until after 5 months of maintenance therapy, although most patients respond by 2 months. Most untoward effects resemble those of aspirin and sulfonamides, including gastrointestinal irritation, hematologic cytopenias, central nervous system disturbances, nephrotoxicity, oligospermia, and hypersensitivity responses. A large double-blind study of 134 individuals who failed to respond to NSAIDs further documented the efficacy of sulfasalazine at a dosage of 2 g daily.[47]

Agents such as methotrexate or azathioprine remain choices of last resort for intractable, severe disease not associated with HIV infection. Oral or parenteral methotrexate is given in weekly doses beginning at 2.5 mg and increasing in weekly or biweekly steps of 2.5 mg to a maximum of 20 mg, if necessary. The weekly dosage is divided into two or three units and given every 12 h. Methotrexate appears to be devoid of the mutagenic effects that characterize alkylating agents, for example; but both immunosuppression, which can be fatal even on low-dose therapy, and a set of idiosyncratic parenchymal disorders, including liver injury and fibrosis and lung disease, are recognized untoward effects (discussed in Chaps. 43 and 44). Cyclosporine has been reported as being effective in severe recurrent Reiter's syndrome.[48] This agent, used at a daily dose of 3 to 5 mg/kg, has been shown to improve both the psoriatic skin and joint disease in about 50 percent of patients with psoriasis. Improvement in the skin disease was usually noted after 2 to 6 weeks of treatment, whereas the joint involvement took up to 24 weeks to improve.[49] Within 4 weeks of discontinuing the drug, exacerbations of both skin and joint disease were seen. Untoward effects of cyclosporine include renal toxicity and the potential for the development of B cell lymphomas.

Methotrexate or other immunosuppressive agents should be used with particularly great caution, if at all, in those individuals with concurrent HIV infection.[2,50] The potential efficacy of these agents must be balanced against the possibility of inducing further immune suppression and either enhancing viral replication through reduction of the CD8 antiviral immune response or increasing the likelihood of opportunistic infections. Anecdotal reports of their safe use must be balanced against reports where the agents appeared to accelerate immune deficiency. In theory, the same T cell lineage involved in the pathogenesis of Reiter's syndrome is involved in mediating host immunity to HIV, a fact that should temper the use of these agents unless there is no alternative.

COURSE AND PROGNOSIS

Increasingly, Reiter's syndrome is being recognized as an illness that may result in a relatively unfavorable outcome. Sixty-three percent of patients with Reiter's syndrome in a rural midwest setting had a prolonged or relapsing course.[9] Often, the mucocutaneous aspect of the illness remits while the arthritic manifestations persist. However, in a smaller proportion of patients, persistent dermal lesions such as balanitis can be extremely troublesome. Patients with chronic or recrudescent illness require progressive escalation of therapy to agents that have more harmful side effects.

A few patients with chronic disease progress into other forms of spondyloarthropathy. The HIV-associated forms of Reiter's syndrome usually illustrate the worst features of this illness. The tendency of these patients to develop chronic arthritis and skin disease indistinguishable from pustular psoriasis is a most troublesome feature. Similarly, the evolution of individuals who present with a psoriasiform picture to an illness with features of Reiter's syndrome has been emphasized.[50]

REFERENCES

1. Brewerton DA et al: Ankylosing spondylitis and HL-A 27. *Lancet* 1:904, 1973
2. Winchester R et al: The co-occurrence of Reiter's syndrome and acquired immunodeficiency. *Ann Intern Med* 106:19, 1987
3. Winchester R: Psoriatic arthritis (review). *Dermatol Clin* 13:779, 1995
4. Keat AC et al: Role of *Chlamydia trachomatis* and HLA-B27 in sexually acquired reactive arthritis. *Br Med J* 1:605, 1978
5. Arnett FC: Incomplete Reiter's syndrome: Clinical comparisons with classical triad. *Ann Rheum Dis* 38(suppl 1):73, 1979
6. Paronen I: Reiter's disease: A study of 344 cases observed in Finland. *Acta Med Scand* 131(suppl 212):1, 1948
7. Hochberg MD et al: Family studies in HLA-B27 associated arthritis. *Medicine (Baltimore)* 57:463, 1978
8. Calin A et al: The nature and prevalence of spondylarthritis among relatives of probands with ankylosing spondylitis and Reiter's syndrome. *Arthritis Rheum* 24:S78, 1981
9. Michet CJ et al: Epidemiology of Reiter's syndrome in Rochester, Minnesota: 1950–1980. *Arthritis Rheum* 31:428, 1988
10. Cron RQ, Sherry DD: Reiter's syndrome associated with cryptosporidial gastroenteritis. *J Rheumatol* 22:1962, 1995
11. Schumacher HR Jr et al: Light and electron microscopic studies on the synovial membrane in Reiter's syndrome. Immunocytochemical iden-

tification of chlamydial antigens in patients with early disease. *Arthritis Rheum* **31**:937, 1988

12. Branigan PJ et al: Comparison of synovial tissue and synovial fluid as the source of nucleic acids for detection of *Chlamydia trachomatis* by polymerase chain reaction [published errata appear in *Arthritis Rheum* **40**:387, 1997 and **40**:782, 1997. *Arthritis Rheum* **39**:1740, 1996

13. Granfors K et al: Analysis of IgA anti-lipolysaccharide antibodies in *Yersinia*-triggered reactive arthritis. *J Infect Dis* **159**:1142, 1989

14. van Bohemen CG et al: HLA-B27M1M2 and high immune responsiveness to *Shigella flexneri* in post-dysenteric arthritis. *Immunol Lett* **13**:71, 1986

15. Gaston JS et al: In vitro responses to a 65-kilodalton mycobacterial protein by synovial T cells from inflammatory arthritis patients. *J Immunol* **143**:2494, 1989

16. Inman RD et al: HLA class I-related impairment in IL-2 production and lymphocyte response to microbial antigens in reactive arthritis. *J Immunol* **142**:4256, 1989

17. Wright V: Rheumatism and psoriasis. *Am J Med* **27**:454, 1959

18. Keat A et al: *Chlamydia trachomatis* and reactive arthritis: The missing link. *Lancet* **1**:72, 1987

19. Granfors K et al: *Yersinia* antigens in synovial fluid cells from patients with reactive arthritis. *N Engl J Med* **320**:216, 1989

20. Li F et al: Molecular detection of bacterial DNA in venereal-associated arthritis (see comments). *Arthritis Rheum* **39**:950, 1996

21. Tiwari JL, Terasaki PI: *HLA and Disease Associations*. New York, Springer, 1985

22. Inman RD: Postdysenteric reactive arthritis. A clinical and immunogenetic study following an outbreak of salmonellosis. *Arthritis Rheum* **31**:1377, 1988

23. Winchester R et al: Implications from the occurrence of Reiter's syndrome and related disorders in association with advanced HIV infection. *Scand J Rheumatol* **74**:89, 1988

24. Stein CM, Davis P: Arthritis associated with HIV infection in Zimbabwe. *J Rheumatol* **23**:506, 1996

25. Mizuki N et al: Nucleotide sequence analysis of the HLA class I region spanning the 237-kb segment around the HLA-B and -C genes. *Genomics* **42**:55, 1997

26. Mizuki N et al: Triplet repeat polymorphism in the transmembrane region of the MICA gene: A strong association of six GCT repetitions with Behçet disease. *Proc Nat Acad Sci USA* **94**:1298, 1997

27. Goto K et al: MICA gene and ankylosing spondylitis: Linkage analysis via a transmembrane-encoded triplet repeat polymorphism. *Tissue Antigens* **49**:503, 1997

28. Lopez de Castro JA: HLA-B27 and HLA-A2 subtypes: Structure, evolution and function. *Immunol Today* **10**:239, 1989

29. Calin A, Fries JF: An "experimental" epidemic of Reiter's syndrome revisited: Follow-up evidence on genetic and environmental factors. *Ann Intern Med* **84**:564, 1976

30. Porcelli S: Molecular mimicry and the generation of autoimmune diseases. *Rheumatol Rev* **2**:41, 1993

31. Battisto JR et al: Susceptibility to adjuvant arthritis in DA and F344 rats: A dominant trait controlled by an autosomal gene locus linked to the MHC. *Arthritis Rheum* **25**:1194, 1982

32. Morrison RP et al: Chlamydial disease pathogenesis. The 57-kD chlamydial hypersensitivity antigen is a stress response protein. *J Exp Med* **170**(4):1271, 1989

33. Nickerson CL et al: Role of enterobacteria and HLA-B27 in spondyloarthropathies: Studies with transgenic mice. *Ann Rheum Dis* **49**:426, 1990

34. Kappler J et al: Vβ-specific stimulation of human T cells by staphylococcal toxins. *Science* **244**:813, 1989

35. Cuvelier C et al: Histopathology of intestinal inflammation related to reactive arthritis. *Gut* **28**:394, 1987

36. Aho K et al: HLA B27 in reactive arthritis following infection. *Ann Rheum Dis* **34**(suppl 1):29, 1975

37. Hancock JAH: Surface manifestations of Reiter's disease in the male. *Br J Venereal Dis* **36**:36, 1960

38. McEwen C et al: Ankylosing spondylitis and spondylitis accompanying ulcerative colitis, regional enteritis, psoriasis, and Reiter's disease. *Arthritis Rheum* **14**:291, 1971

39. Azouz EM, Duffy CM: Juvenile spondyloarthropathies: Clinical manifestations and medical imaging (review). *Skeletal Radiol* **24**:399, 1995

40. Belz J et al: Characterization of uveitis associated with spondyloarthritis. *J Am Acad Dermatol* **20**:898, 1989

41. Csonka GW, Oates JK: Pericarditis and electrocardiographic changes in Reiter's syndrome. *Br Med J* **1**:866, 1957

42. Tucker CR et al: Aortitis in ankylosing spondylitis: Early detection of aortic root abnormalities with two-dimensional echocardiography. *Am J Cardiol* **9**:680, 1982

43. Calin A: HLA-B27 in 1982. Reappraisal of a clinical test. *Ann Intern Med* **96**:114, 1982

44. Brewerton DA et al: HL-A 27 and arthropathies associated with ulcerative colitis and psoriasis. *Lancet* **1**:956, 1974

45. Leirisalo-Repo M et al: Follow-up study of Reiter's disease and reactive arthritis. Factors influencing the natural course and the prognosis. *Clin Rheumatol* **6**(suppl 2):73, 1987

46. Stroehmann I et al: Therapy of seronegative oligoarthritis with salazopyrine. *Z Rheumatol* **46**:79, 1987

47. Clegg DO et al: Comparison of sulfasalazine and placebo in the treatment of reactive arthritis (Reiter's syndrome). A Department of Veterans Affairs Cooperative Study. *Arthritis Rheum* **39**:2021, 1996

48. Kiyohara A et al: Successful treatment of severe recurrent Reiter's syndrome with cyclosporine. *J Am Acad Dermatol* **36**:482, 1997

49. Mahrle G et al: Anti-inflammatory efficacy of low-dose cyclosporin A in psoriatic arthritis. A prospective multicentre study. *Br J Dermatol* **135**:752, 1996

50. Romani J et al: Reiter's syndrome–like pattern in AIDS-associated psoriasiform dermatitis. *Int J Dermatol* **35**:484, 1996

51. Bjorkman PJ et al: Structure of the human class I histocompatibility antigen, HLA-A2. *Nature* **329**:506, 1987

Multicentric Reticulohistiocytosis

Multicentric reticulohistiocytosis (MR) is a rare systemic granulomatous disease of unknown cause characterized by a distinct histopathology. Skin, mucosa, synovia, bone, and internal organs may be involved. Cutaneous nodules and destructive arthritis are the most prominent clinical features. MR is a paraneoplastic process in a portion of the patients afflicted.

HISTORIC ASPECTS

In 1952, Caro and Senear[1] first studied histopathologic skin sections of a patient with these features and called the syndrome *reticulohistiocytic granuloma.* Goltz and Laymon in 1954[2] created the term *multicentric reticulohistiocytosis,* which most authors now use, because of the multifocal origin and the systemic nature of the process. At least a dozen synonyms appear in the literature, including lipoid dermatoarthritis, giant cell (reticulo)histiocytosis, (giant cell) reticulohistiocytoma, and nondiabetic cutaneous xanthomatosis. By the early 1950s, the entity of MR was established.[3]

EPIDEMIOLOGY

Two comprehensive reviews are available.[3,4] More than 100 cases have been reported, but many others may have gone undiagnosed. There appears to be no geographic area of prevalence. White patients predominate, but this finding may merely reflect the higher number of reports from North America, Australia, and Europe. Patients of African, South American, Japanese, and American-Indian ancestry have also been identified. In one study, a greater number of women were found to be affected[3]; in another, an equal distribution was found between the sexes.[4] The mean age of onset was found to be 43 years. After an average of 8 years, the disease burns out and becomes inactive. Children and adolescents with the disease have been identified,[5–8] and a case of MR diagnosed during pregnancy has been reported.[9]

During the past four decades, most investigators considered MR to be of histiocytic rather than lymphocytic origin. In 1996, however, Zelger et al.[10] proposed a new concept of *non-Langerhans cell histiocytoses* and included MR as an oncocytic type among more than a dozen types of these histiocytoses. They claim that each of the mononuclear and multinucleate histiocytic types reveals characteristic, but as yet not diagnostic, immunophenotypic features. They consider the KiM1p marker (CD68 family) to be the most reliable marker of the non-Langerhans cell histiocytoses. Although this scheme is tempting to follow, it has yet to stand the test of time. Therefore, this discussion will adhere to the findings and interpretations of the original authors.

ETIOLOGY AND PATHOGENESIS

The etiology of MR remains obscure, and its pathogenesis can only be speculated on.[3,4] The hallmark of the disease is a granulomatous, proliferative process of histiocytes, some of which are multinucleated and laden with lipids. The stimulus is not known, and no specific metabolic defect has been found. There is no evidence of an infectious agent, and there are no convincing data on a compromise of the immune status of the host. Little if any evidence exists to permit the categorization of MR with disorders of deranged lipid metabolism.

CLINICAL MANIFESTATIONS

Skin and joint symptoms dominate the clinical picture. Almost two-thirds of patients note arthritis first; one-fifth note skin nodules first; and in another fifth, skin and joint changes appear simultaneously. About half of the patients develop mucous membrane manifestations.[3]

Skin Changes

The face (particularly the nose and paranasal areas), hands (particularly the nail folds; Fig. 183-1), ears, forearms, scalp (especially behind the ears), neck, eyelids,[11] the limbus and the cornea,[12] and the trunk are involved in decreasing order of frequency. The hemispherical, nontender nodular lesions have a reddish-brown hue; they vary in size from a few millimeters to conglomerate nodules measuring several centimeters. Ulceration is uncommon. Erythema may precede the formation of nodules. Pruritus may be a prominent symptom.

Articular Changes

There is symmetric involvement of the interphalangeal joints, knees, shoulders, wrists, hips, ankles, feet, elbows, vertebral and temporomandibular joints, in decreasing order of frequency. The arthritis is destructive (arthritis mutilans); bone and cartilage are destroyed, and severe deformation ensues. The disease progresses rapidly in

FIGURE 183-1

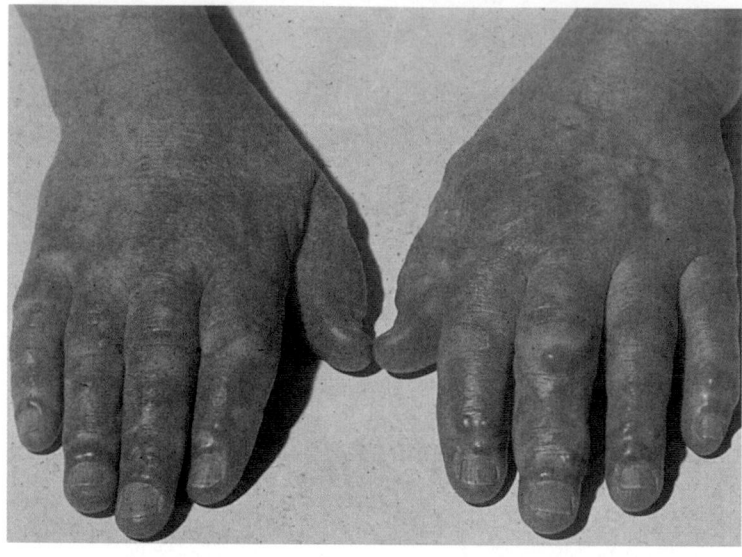

Hands of a patient with active skin lesions of multicentric reticulohistiocytosis. Note periungual array of some of the nodules. (*From Barrow and Holubar,[3] with permission of Hautarzt.*)

the beginning, tapers, and finally burns out. There is a marked discrepancy between the severity of the radiographic findings and the underlying bone destruction, and the relatively mild clinical symptoms. In far-advanced cases the fingers are considerably shortened but can be pulled out to their full length, leading to such designations as *la main en lorgnette*, opera-glass hand, telescope fingers, and concertina-hand. There is no periostal reaction or osteoporosis.

Mucosal Changes

Roughly half the patients have mucosal lesions; the lips, buccal mucosa, tongue, gingiva, nasal septum, larynx, and trachea are involved. Physically, the nodules mimic those in the skin (Fig. 183-2).

Other Clinical Manifestations

Patients may also exhibit xanthelasma, lesions along tendon sheaths, lesions in the myocardium and the lungs, adenopathy, pathologic fractures, hypertension, and hyperextensible joints. In some cases a definitive diagnosis of MR could not be substantiated, and the association of unusual findings may have been fortuitous, as in patients with carpal tunnel syndrome, Dupuytren's contracture, and pleural effusion; cardiopulmonary complications; splenomegaly and pancytopenia; gamma heavy-chain paraprotein; and involvement of the salivary glands and pericardial effusion. Chevrant-Breton in her review[4] quoted reports of neurologic and (terminal) hematologic changes.

LABORATORY FINDINGS

One report cites an association of MR with type IV hyperlipidemia[13]; another considers MR a "lipid disorder with normolipidemic xanthomatosis."[14] These are chance findings. Otherwise, only non-specific laboratory findings have become known in individual cases: anemia, elevated sedimentation rate, leukocytosis, eosinophilia, hypo- and hypercholesterolemia, hypergammaglobulinemia, and the presence of cold agglutinins and cryoglobulins.

PATHOLOGY

Skin and Mucous Membranes

The histopathology of skin lesions is fairly uniform.[3,4] The nodules are nonencapsulated, moderately well circumscribed, and occupy the entire dermis or parts of it. Frequently a narrow zone of noninfiltrated connective tissue is present between the infiltrates and the slightly atrophic epidermis. Lesions consist of histiocytic cells that are irregular in size and shape (Fig. 183-3A). Many have transformed into multinucleated giant cells, generally up to 250 μm in diameter but occasionally larger (Fig. 183-3B). They contain up to 20 or more aggregated nuclei with a distinct nuclear membrane and prominent nucleoli. The cytoplasm is slightly eosinophilic, has a granular appearance ("ground-glass cytoplasm"), and may be foamy or show tiny vacuoles. There are no Touton giant cells. MR nodules contain lymphocytes, which are more numerous in early lesions, and plasma cells, eosinophils, mast cells, and, occasionally, extravasated erythrocytes. With increasing age of the lesions, lymphocytes and giant cells decrease in number, fibroblasts appear, and fibrosis ensues. Lesions are well vascularized, and capillaries show endothelial hypertrophy. In places, histiocytes and giant cells have a perivascular arrangement. Elastic fibers are fragmented, clumped, and thickened, particularly in early lesions.

FIGURE 183-2

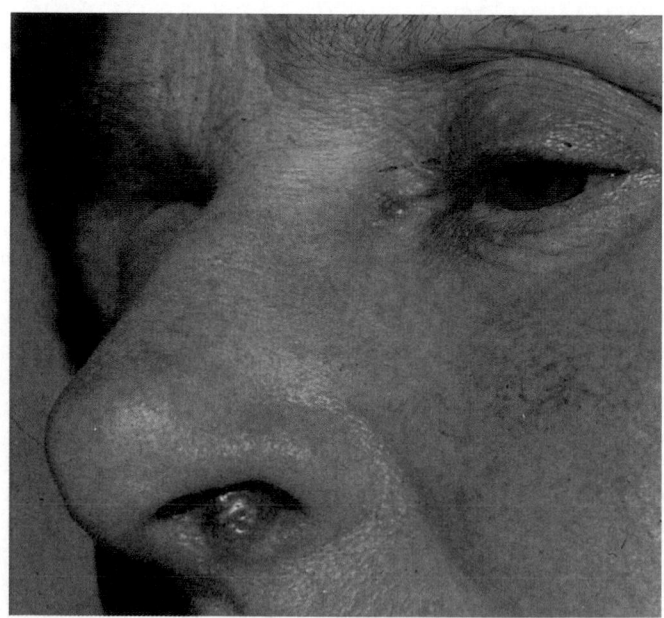

Multicentric reticulohistiocytosis. Mucocutaneous nodular infiltrate on nasal mucosa and adjoining skin.

FIGURE 183-3

CHAPTER 183
Multicentric Reticulohistiocytosis

2097

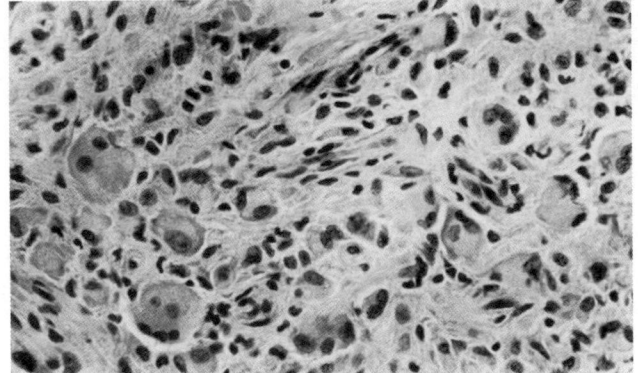

A.

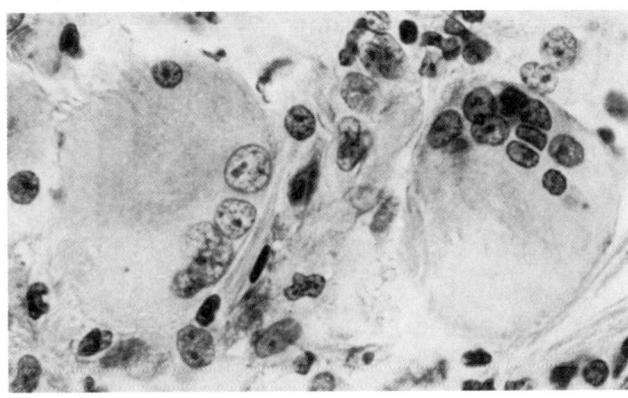

B.

Microphotograph of a lesion from the patient shown in Fig. 183-1. Note histiocytic infiltrate (A) and multinucleated giant cells with aggregated nuclei and "ground glass" cytoplasm (B). (*From Holubar K, Mach K: Histiocytosis giganto-cellularis. Hautarzt 17:440, 1966, with permission of Hautarzt.*)

Histochemical Investigations

The cytoplasm of histiocytes and giant cells is PAS-positive and hyaluronidase- and diastase-resistant, suggesting the presence of glycoproteins. It contains phospholipids, neutral fats, and iron. Biochemical studies have not revealed an isolated enzyme defect responsible for lipid accumulation.

Electron Microscopy

There are no Langerhans cell granules in the histiocytic cells. Both histiocytes and giant cells have lobulated nuclei with indented contours and margination of nuclear chromatin, an enlarged Golgi apparatus, and hyperplastic endoplasmic reticulum with dilated cysternae. Lipid-laden vacuoles are present, and numerous small, electron-dense, ovoid or rod-shaped cytoplasmic granules, up to 250 nm in size, have been described. These granules are positive for acid phosphatase, as are autophagic vacuoles. A characteristic feature is the complex interdigitation of membranes of adjacent histiocytic cells. In addition, collagen phagocytosis has been observed, and intra- and extracellular fragments of collagen VI in histiocytes have been documented.[15] The histiocytes of MR have been characterized by their iron uptake, positivity of acid phosphatase, un-

specific esterase, and lysozyme. The histopathology of synovial lesions is identical to that of skin lesions.

Lesions in Other Tissues

The morphology and localization of cutaneous nodules, the typical articular symptoms, and the radiographic findings (symmetric involvement of distal interphalangeal joints) are highly suggestive of MR, but histopathologic examination of a nodule permits the diagnosis. Various disorders have to be differentiated from MR: rheumatoid arthritis, the various types of xanthomas, Farber's disseminated lipogranulomatosis, lepromatous leprosy, lipoid proteinosis, sarcoidosis, histiocytosis X, juvenile and adult xanthogranuloma, solitary reticulohistiocytoma, generalized eruptive histiocytoma of Hashimoto and Pritzker, and Zayid and Farraj's familial histiocytic dermatoarthritis. MR is not familial or congenital. The newly proposed grouping[10] into Langerhans and non-Langerhans types of histiocytic and lymphocytic proliferations may make many of these previously detailed diagnoses obsolete.

ASSOCIATED CONDITIONS

Concomitant diseases have been mentioned: thyroid disorders; tuberculosis; diabetes; hemoblastoses; cancer of the colon, breast, bronchus, cervix, ovary, and stomach; mesothelioma; and melanoma.[16] An association with sarcoma and lymphomas has also been reported. The tumors may progress and MR may remit; in contrast, MR may progress despite removal of the tumor. Many investigators therefore remain skeptical about the alleged paraneoplastic nature of MR. Others claim that such a paraneoplastic character exists in up to 28 percent of cases.[17] A careful tumor search is always warranted in MR.

TREATMENT

Gianotti and Caputo state that "treatment is usually not helpful."[18] Glucocorticoids (administered also as pulse therapy), ACTH, antimalarials, salicylates, indomethacin, pyrazolone, clofibrate, penicillamine, and, increasingly, various antimitotic compounds such as azathioprin, methotrexate, cyclophosphamide, and systemic and topical nitrogen mustard have been used; but no controlled studies have been performed. Antimitotic agents appear to be a rational choice for therapy. However, because MR may be a paraneoplastic condition, antimetabolites might be harmful when malignancies are associated. Surgical measures have also been used.

COURSE AND PROGNOSIS

Skin nodules and arthritis do not necessarily run in parallel. Articular changes may wax and wane and finally evolve into mutilating arthritis, whereas skin nodules may not appear at all or may erupt in successive crops with new infiltrates being superimposed on older, regressing ones. The course of MR is capricious, and prediction is difficult; about half the patients will eventually suffer from prominent destructive arthritis. Most commonly, the disease burns out after 5 to 8 years, leaving the patient with severe articular deformations and disfigurement of the hands, face, and scalp.

REFERENCES

1. Caro MR, Senear FE: Reticulohistiocytoma of the skin. *Arch Dermatol* **65**:701, 1952
2. Goltz RW, Laymon CW: Multicentric reticulohistiocytosis. *Arch Dermatol* **69**:717, 1954
3. Barrow MV, Holubar K: Multicentric reticulohistiocytosis. *Medicine (Baltimore)* **48**:287, 1969
4. Chevrant-Breton J: La réticulo-histiocytose multicentrique. Revue de la litterature récente (dupuis 1969). *Ann Dermatol Venereol* **104**:745, 1977
5. Omdal M et al: Multicentric reticulohistiocytosis in a 9-year-old boy. *Arthritis Rheum* **31**:1588, 1988
6. Kuramoto Y et al: Multicentric reticulohistiocytosis in a child. *J Am Acad Dermatol* **20**:329, 1989
7. Raphael SA et al: Multicentric reticulohistiocytosis in a child. *J Pediatr* **114**:266, 1989
8. Kuramoto Y et al: Development of a Ki-1 lymphoma in a child suffering from multicentric reticulohistiocytosis. *Acta Derm Venereol* **71**:448, 1991
9. Conaghan P et al: A unique presentation of multicentric reticulohistiocytosis in pregnancy. *Arthritis Rheum* **36**:269, 1993
10. Zelger BWH et al: Non-Langerhans cell histiocytoses. A new unifying concept. *Am J Dermatopathol* **18**:490, 1996
11. Eagle RC Jr et al: Eyelid involvement in multicentric reticulohistiocytosis. *Ophthalmology* **102**:426, 1995
12. Allaire GS et al: Reticulohistiocytoma of the limbus and cornea. A clinicopathologic study of two cases. *Ophthalmology* **97**:1018, 1990
13. Gharpuray MB et al: Multicentric reticulohistiocytosis. *Int J Dermatol Venerol Leprol* **55**:253, 1989
14. Kesäniemi YA et al: Multicentric reticulohistiocytosis, another lipid disorder with normolipidemic xanthomatosis? *Atherosclerosis* **68**:179, 1987
15. Fortier-Beaulieu M et al: New electron microscopic findings in a case of multicentric reticulohistiocytosis. Long spacing collagen inclusions. *Am J Dermatopathol* **15**:587, 1993
16. Gibson G et al: Multicentric reticulohistiocytosis associated with recurrence of malignant melanoma. *J Am Acad Dermatol* **32**:134, 1995
17. Campbell DA, Edwards NL: Multicentric reticulohistiocytosis: Systemic macrophage disorder. *Clin Rheumatol* **5**:301, 1991
18. Gianotti F, Caputo R: Histiocytic syndromes. A review. *J Am Acad Dermatol* **13**:383, 1985

CUTANEOUS MANIFESTATIONS OF DISEASES IN OTHER ORGAN SYSTEMS

CHAPTER 184

Om P. Sharma

Sarcoidosis of the Skin

More than a century ago, Jonathan Hutchinson, a surgeon-dermatologist, described the first case of sarcoidosis at King's College Hospital in London. Jonathan Hutchinson's intellectual discourses, discussions, and lectures greatly impressed his contemporaries, including Sir Arthur Conan Doyle. Thus, it is not surprising that a skin disease, very much like cutaneous sarcoidosis, became a basic ingredient of the plot of *Adventures of the Blanched Soldier,* one of the Sherlock Holmes mysteries.

During most of the twentieth century, sarcoidosis remained confined to the domain of the chest physician, but its multisystem nature is now universally recognized. The clinical and radiologic features of the disease are relatively clear-cut, but the diagnosis is often delayed or completely missed because of the resemblance of sarcoidosis to tuberculosis, leprosy, blastomycosis, coccidioidomycosis, berylliosis, brucellosis, and other granulomas. In this chapter, the clinical features, pathogenesis, biochemical changes, and immunologic alterations are described, and the diagnostic criteria and management of patients suffering from cutaneous as well as multisystem sarcoidosis are discussed.

SARCOID GRANULOMA

The lesion of sarcoidosis is a well-defined round or oval granuloma made up of compact, radially arranged epithelioid cells with pale nuclei. The typical giant cell of the sarcoid granuloma is of the Langhans' type in which the nuclei are arranged in an arc or a circular pattern around a central granular zone. Lymphocytes are usually seen at the periphery. Caseation is absent; fibrinoid necrosis may occasionally be seen in areas where several granulomas have coalesced (Fig. 184-1).

Monoclonal antibody techniques and indirect immunofluorescence methods have uncovered the dynamic relationship between the various components of the granuloma. The center of the granuloma is composed of macrophage-derived cells and CD4+ helper lymphocytes, whereas the periphery of the granuloma has a large number of interdigitating macrophages and CD8+ suppressor lymphocytes. The lymphokines from the inflammatory cells recruit blood-borne monocytes, prevent macrophage migration, and keep the chronic inflammatory reaction alive and efficient. It is probable that this arrangement of interdigitating CD8+ cells on the periphery and the epithelioid cell–CD4+ pattern in the center provides an efficient perimeter defense to a persistent, poorly degradable "antigen" of low potency. This architectural arrangement is also found in cases of tuberculoid leprosy, in which an efficient immune system keeps the bacillary load to a minimum; in lepromatous leprosy, in contrast, the arrangement of the immune cells is disorganized and haphazard, and bacteria abound (see Chap. 203).

The mechanisms regulating the formation and course of granulomas are not well understood. It appears that a T cell–mediated response to an antigen that has been processed and presented by macrophages to antigen-specific T lymphocytes is a fundamental step. Activated T cells orchestrate the accumulation and differentiation of mononuclear phagocytes by releasing a number of cytokines. The important cytokines released by lung T cells include interleukin (IL) 2, interferon (IFN) γ, monocyte chemotactic factor, and migration inhibitory factor. Activated T cells also express surface markers, including IL-2 and HLA-DR class II major histocompatibility complex molecules.[1] The macrophage not only processes the antigen but also influences the granuloma formation and fibrosis by releasing a number of mediators, including IL-1, macrophage-derived fibroblast growth factor (which activates fibroblasts), fibronectin, and biologically active factor VII. Neutrophils recruited from blood by a macrophage-derived factor may participate in the development of fibrosis either by producing superoxide anion or by influencing the local concentration of immune complexes.[2]

CUTANEOUS SARCOIDOSIS

Skin lesions occur in about a quarter of patients with sarcoidosis. However, the incidence varies considerably. The lesions may be specific or nonspecific. The important specific lesions are lupus pernio, plaques, and maculopapular eruptions. The important non-specific lesion is erythema nodosum. Other skin changes include alopecia, erythroderma, subcutaneous nodules, erythema multiforme, itching ichthyotic dryness, dystrophic calcifications, and verrucous outgrowths. Nail involvement is rare in sarcoidosis.

Lupus pernio, the most characteristic of all sarcoid skin lesions, is a chronic, violaceous, indurated skin lesion with a predilection for the nose, ears, lips, and face (Fig. 184-2). It occurs commonly in women with persistent sarcoidosis characterized by extensive pulmonary infiltration and fibrosis, chronic uveitis, and bone lesions. Occasionally, only a few tiny button-like papules or nodules may be seen involving the nasal rim. The nose lesion is often associated with granulomatous infiltration of the nasal mucosa and the upper respiratory tract.[3] Occasionally, the bony nasal septum may be destroyed. A bulbous or sausage-shaped finger in a patient with lupus pernio indicates the presence of an underlying bone lesion. Rarely, the nails may become dystrophic and brittle.

Skin plaques, like lupus pernio, are purplish, elevated, indurated patches commonly located on the limbs, face, back, and buttocks (Fig. 184-3). The distribution is usually symmetric. The center of the plaque is pale and atrophic; the periphery indurated, elevated, and dark. In the presence of large telangiectatic vessels, the lesions are called *angiolupoid*. Occasionally, the plaques, particularly in black patients, have a hypopigmented appearance—"hypomelanotic umbrella." The plaques are often associated with chronic features of sarcoidosis including pulmonary fibrosis, bone cysts, peripheral lymphadenopathy, and uveitis. Rarely, sarcoidosis plaques may present a crusty, scaly appearance indistinguishable from psoriasis. These benignly deceptive lesions may be diagnosed in time if a biopsy specimen is obtained.

The *papular eruptions* are the most common skin manifestation of sarcoidosis in black patients. The waxy translucent lesions with a distinct flat top vary from 2 to 6 mm in diameter. They characteristically occur on the face, lids, around the orbits (Fig. 184-4), in the nasolabial folds, and on the nape and upper back.

Subcutaneous nodules, also called *Darier-Roussy sarcoidosis*, are oval, firm, painless structures that arise deep in the dermis and

FIGURE 184-1

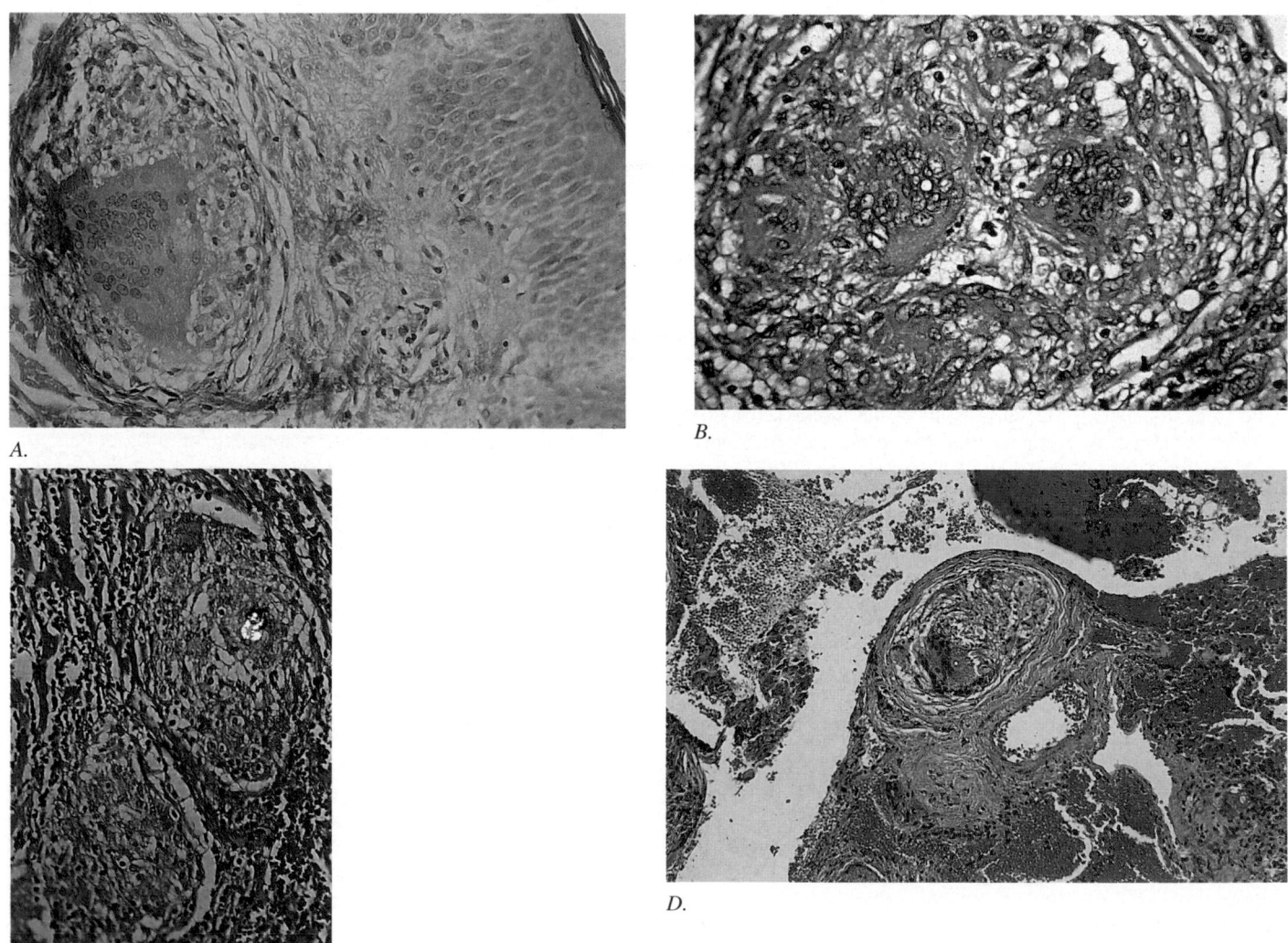

A.

B.

C.

D.

A. An oval, cutaneous sarcoidosis granuloma composed of epithelioid cells, a multinucleated giant cell, and a few lymphocytes. H & E. *B.* A conglomerate of epithelioid granulomas with multiple, multinucleated giant cells in a lymph node biopsy in sarcoidosis. H & E. *C.* Crystalline inclusions in a sarcoid granuloma. H & E. *D.* Late stage sarcoidosis granuloma showing hyalinization. H & E.

FIGURE 184-2

CHAPTER 184
Sarcoidosis of the Skin

2101

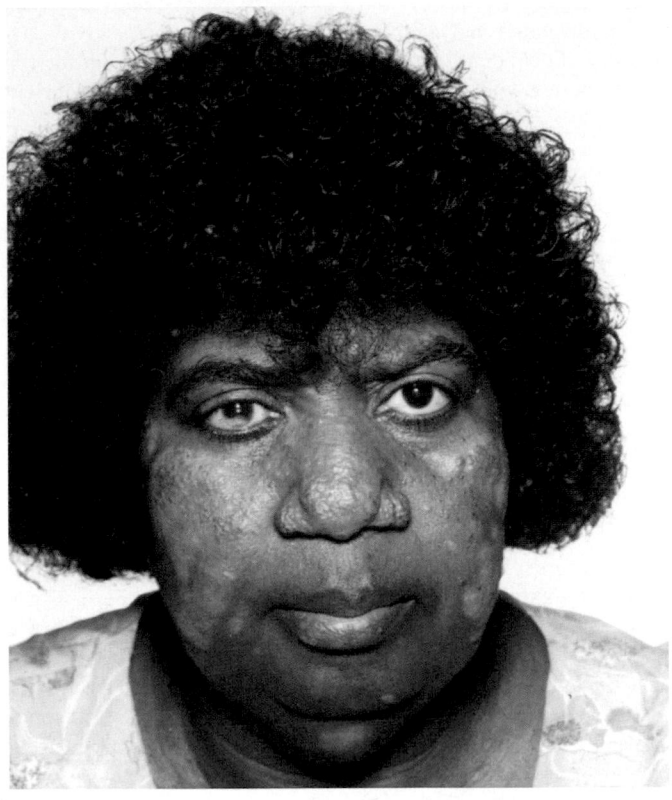

Lupus pernio in a black patient with chronic sarcoidosis of more than 25 years.

FIGURE 184-3

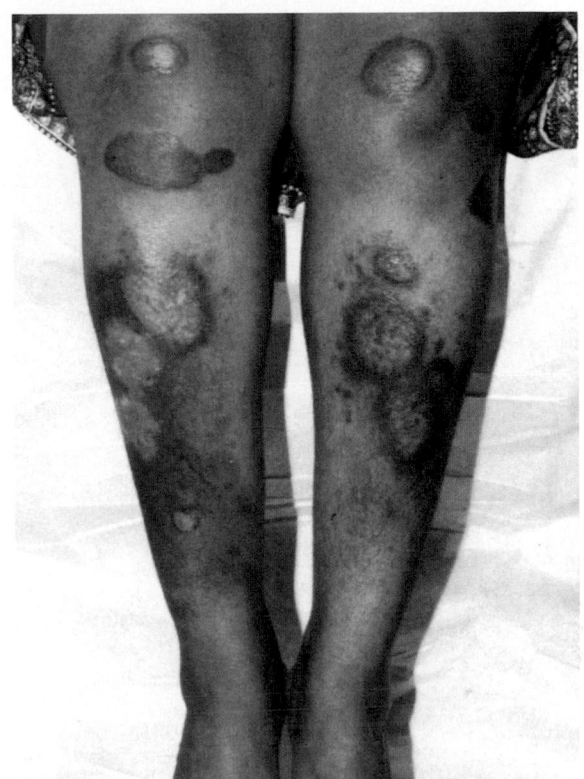

A.

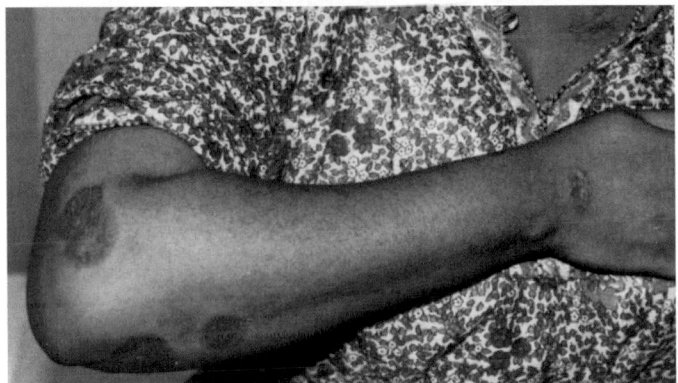

B.

Chronic sarcoidosis skin plaques on the legs (A) and the arm (B). Occasionally, these lesions may ulcerate.

subcutaneous tissue of the trunk and extremities. On biopsy they show noncaseating granulomas. Rarely, these lesions may ulcerate.

Scars from atrophy, trauma, surgery, or venipuncture may become purple, swollen, and tender either at the time the patient presents or during reactivation of the disease. Biopsies of these areas show noncaseating granulomas. Ulcerative sarcoidosis is rare. Occurring most frequently in black women, the lesions usually involve the legs (Fig. 184-5). The biopsy may show typical noncaseating granulomas as well as necrotic changes.

Erythema nodosum is a hypersensitivity reaction that results from exposure to many bacterial, fungal, and chemical antigens. It is the most common nonspecific cutaneous manifestation of sarcoidosis and is the hallmark of acute sarcoidosis, predominantly in women of childbearing age (see Chap. 111). Systemic manifestations such as fever, malaise, and polyarthralgia occur in about 50 percent of patients with erythema nodosum. Because of the high rate of spontaneous resolution, patients with erythema nodosum seldom require glucocorticoid therapy.

Cutaneous Sarcoidosis in Children

Sarcoidosis is infrequent among children. James and Kendig[4] have constructed a picture of childhood sarcoidosis based on data collected from Yugoslavia, France, Great Britain, Scandinavia, Hungary, Japan, and many areas in the United States. Intrathoracic involvement appears to be consistently present. Bilateral hilar adenopathy with and without paratracheal adenopathy is a common finding. Peripheral lymphadenopathy occurs in about two-thirds and eye involvement in about one-third to one-fourth of children in the

United States. Cutaneous lesions are frequently found, but erythema nodosum is unusual. The clinical picture in children below 4 years of age is different from the presentation in older children. Skin rash, uveitis, and arthritis are more common in children under 4 years of age. The rash, usually macular and papular, starts peripherally and may precede the other manifestations by several months. Intrathoracic involvement is absent in this group. The disease should be distinguished from the more common polyarticular juvenile rheumatoid arthritis (JRA), which has a later age of onset of 5 to 15 years. Thus, the diagnosis of sarcoidosis should be entertained in a

FIGURE 184-4

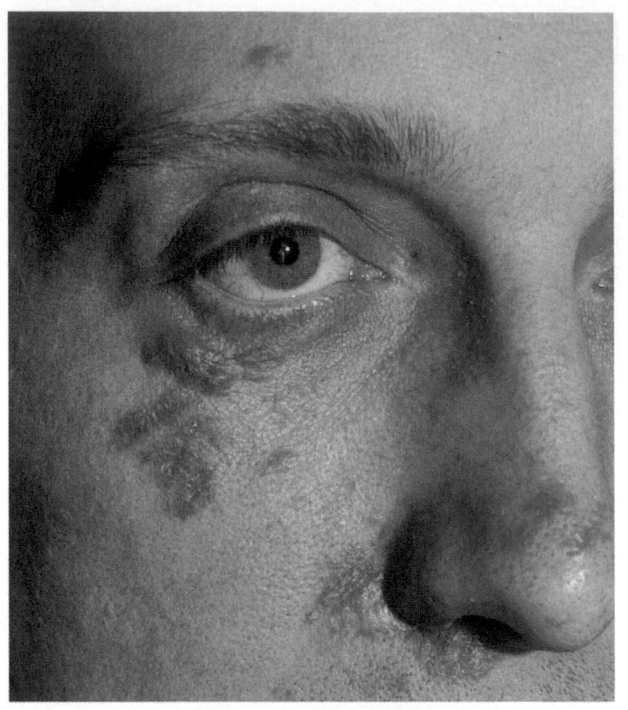

Sarcoidosis. Yellowish-brown plaques and papules on the face. On diascopy these lesions exhibit a pale brownish-red color.

FIGURE 184-5

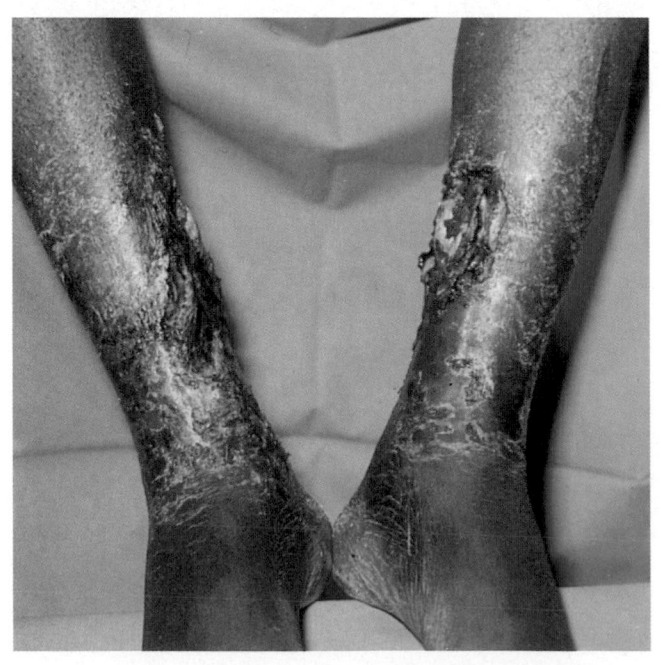

Chronic skin ulcers in a young black woman with sarcoidosis.

child with skin rash, uveitis, lymphadenopathy, and pulmonary involvement. A rise in serum angiotensin-converting enzyme (ACE) level, although not specific for sarcoidosis, may be helpful in making the diagnosis and monitoring the granulomatous activity. The prognosis in children is more favorable than in adults, but for very young children with symptomatic multisystem involvement, the outlook is less favorable.

THE MULTISYSTEM NATURE OF SARCOIDOSIS

Because of its diverse manifestations, patients with sarcoidosis present to clinicians of many different specialties. Clinical manifestations depend on age, race, duration of the illness, site and extent of tissue involvement, and activity of the granulomatous process.

Nonspecific Constitutional Manifestations

About a third of patients with sarcoidosis complain of such nonspecific symptoms as fever, fatigue, and weight loss. Fever is generally mild, but temperatures are occasionally elevated to 39.5 or 40°C (103 to 104°F). Weight loss is generally limited to 2 to 7 kg (5 to 15 lb) during the 10 to 12 weeks before presentation. Night sweats sometimes occur. Constitutional symptoms are present more frequently in blacks and Asians from the Indian subcontinent than in whites.

Lungs

RESPIRATORY SYMPTOMS More than one-third of patients with sarcoidosis complain of dyspnea, cough, chest pain, and tightness of the chest. The cough is usually dry. Chest pain, generally confined to the retrosternal area, may be severe and indistinguishable from cardiac pain. Occasionally, the pain may become intensified after drinking alcohol.

CHEST RADIOGRAPHIC ABNORMALITIES The following radiographic staging system is useful in sarcoidosis: stage 0, normal chest roentgenogram; stage I, bilateral hilar lymphadenopathy without pulmonary infiltrates; stage II, bilateral hilar lymphadenopathy with pulmonary infiltrates; stage III, pulmonary infiltrates without hilar adenopathy; and stage IV, end-stage fibrosis, bullae, and honeycombing.

LUNG FUNCTION ABNORMALITIES Extensive physiologic studies emphasize functional changes characteristic of "restrictive impairment" in patients with sarcoidosis. Vital capacity, residual volume, and total lung capacity are reduced. The loss of diffusing capacity remains perhaps the most common abnormality in sarcoidosis. The diffusing capacity is reduced even in patients with hilar adenopathy without any associated parenchymal infiltrates on chest x-ray film (stage I). Severe abnormalities of gas exchange are also more frequent than is generally realized. The obstruction of airways, large and small, is quite common, particularly in black patients.

Eyes

Any structure of the eye may be involved in sarcoidosis, but granulomatous uveitis is the most common eye lesion. Uveitis may be acute, subacute, or chronic.

Acute uveitis presents suddenly with redness of the eyes, watering, cloudy vision, and photophobia. Circumcorneal ciliary congestion is present, pupils are irregular, and "mutton fat" keratotic precipitates may be prominent in the anterior chamber. The patient may have other manifestations of early sarcoidosis, including erythema nodosum and bilateral hilar lymphadenopathy and arthralgias.

Chronic uveitis, in contrast, develops slowly and may lead to adhesions between the iris and the lens, glaucoma, cataracts, and blindness. Ciliary congestion is absent, but keratotic precipitates are present. The patient complains of pain and blurred vision. Other manifestations of chronic sarcoidosis include lupus pernio, plaques, bone and joint lesions, and interstitial pulmonary fibrosis.

Other ocular lesions include conjunctival follicles, retinal periphlebitis, retinal hemorrhages, retinitis proliferans, cataracts, band keratopathy, proptosis, and exophthalmos.

Peripheral Lymph Nodes

The most frequently involved nodes are cervical, axillary, epitrochlear, and inguinal. In the neck, the nodes in the posterior triangle are more commonly affected than those in the anterior triangle. Enlarged nodes are discrete, shotty, mobile, painless, and free from the surrounding structures.

Spleen

Although the spleen is infiltrated by sarcoid granulomas in more than 50 percent of patients, the incidence of a clinically palpable spleen is only about 15 percent. Splenic enlargement is usually silent, but, as the disease progresses, pressure symptoms, anemia, leukopenia, and thrombocytopenia are likely to occur.

Gastrointestinal Tract

Asymptomatic granulomas occur in the gastric mucosa in 10 percent of patients, and hematemesis may occur. There are only a few documented cases of intestinal and esophageal involvement. It should be emphasized, however, that the distinction between sarcoidosis confined to the intestinal tract and Crohn's or Whipple's disease may be difficult. Joints may be involved in all three conditions. Unexplained abdominal pain in a patient with sarcoidosis may be due to pancreatic involvement.[5] The liver is palpable in about 20 percent of patients, and granulomas are found in 63 to 87 percent, depending on the stage and activity of the disease. Alkaline phosphatase and serum bilirubin levels may be mildly elevated in as many as 80 percent of patients. Portal hypertension is rare.

Heart

Heart involvement is clinically recognizable in about 5 percent of the patients with sarcoidosis; however, at autopsy granulomas are found in as many as 27 percent. Myocardial involvement may present in many ways, including conduction disturbances, disturbances of rhythm, sudden death, congestive heart failure, valvular involvement, pericardial disease, and myocardial infarction. Endomyocardial biopsy is of limited value because of the patchy distribution of the disease.

Musculoskeletal System

The incidence of joint involvement ranges from 25 to 39 percent in various series, and it may precede other manifestations by many years.[6] The onset of articular symptoms has occurred as early as 4 months and as late as 59 years of age.

The joints most commonly affected by sarcoidosis are the knees, ankles, elbows, wrists, and small joints of the hands. The affected joints are usually swollen, warm, tender, and painful; effusions are common, particularly in patients with chronic disease. Sarcoid arthritis may be indistinguishable from that observed in rheumatic fever, rheumatoid disease, and JRA. Cystic lesions may occur in the small bones of the hands and feet leading to bottle-like deformation of one of more digits (Fig. 184-6).

Kidneys

Renal involvement in sarcoidosis may result from one or more of the following mechanisms: hypercalcemia/hypercalciuria, granulomatous infiltration of the renal parenchyma, glomerular disease, or renal arteritis secondary to granulomas. The incidence of renal granulomas varies from 4 to 40 percent.

Salivary Glands

Although the parotid gland is palpable in only about 6 percent of patients, subclinical involvement is more common and may be detected by technetium-99m scan and by measuring salivary volume and amylase. Granulomas in minor salivary glands occur in as many as 50 percent of patients with mediastinal sarcoidosis but seldom occur without hilar adenopathy or other evidence of multisystem involvement.

Upper Respiratory Tract

Nasal involvement is an indicator of chronic disease, and the presence of nasal granulomas even in the early stage of the disease constitutes an indication for glucocorticoid therapy. Intralesional

FIGURE 184-6

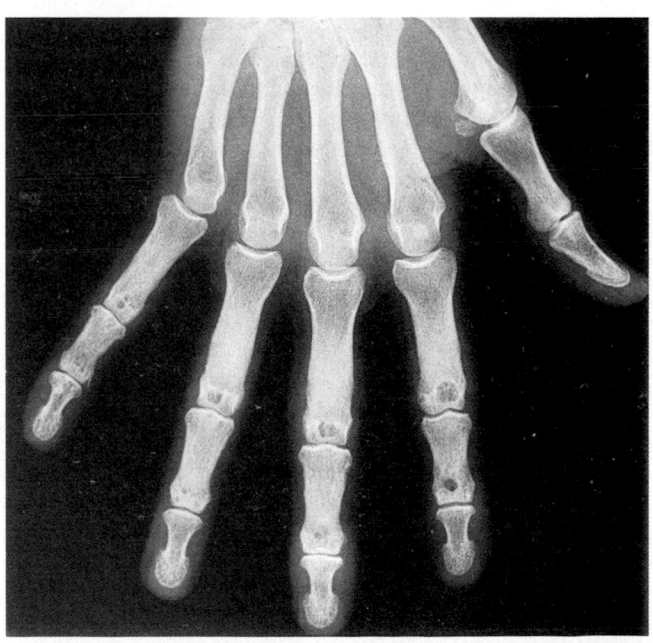

"Bone cysts" involving the small bones of a hand. These cysts, which typically involve the small bones of the feet as well as the hands, almost always are associated with chronic skin lesions.

glucocorticoid injections may be beneficial for polypoidal growths. Laryngeal involvement occurs in about 5 percent of patients. The granulomatous lesions most commonly affect the epiglottis, aryepiglottic folds, arytenoids, and false cords. Ulceration is rare. A large exophytic lesion may produce severe airway obstruction.

Endocrine Glands

The pituitary and hypothalamus are the most commonly affected endocrine glands in sarcoidosis. An elevated prolactin level may be a sensitive marker of hypothalamic sarcoidosis. The thyroid, parathyroid, and adrenal glands are rarely involved.

Nervous System

Sarcoidosis may involve the nervous system in 1 to 29 percent of patients, with an average of about 5 percent. The clinical diagnosis of neurosarcoidosis depends on the finding of neurologic involvement in a patient with histologically proven multisystem disease. The cranial nerves, meninges, hypothalamus, and pituitary gland are the most frequently involved sites in the central nervous system. Peripheral neuropathy, spinal cord involvement, and psychiatric manifestations are infrequent.

LABORATORY INVESTIGATIONS

The incidence of anemia (hemoglobin <11 g) in sarcoidosis is about 5 percent. Hemolytic anemia is rare. Although glucocorticoid therapy is useful in some cases, spontaneous correction of hemolytic anemia may occur. Leukopenia is a frequent finding. It may occur in the absence of splenomegaly and reflect bone marrow involvement. Leukemoid reactions and polycythemia are rare. The mean incidence of eosinophilia is about 24 percent. In many patients, thrombocytopenia is associated with an enlarged spleen, but there is some evidence that it may be an expression of a generalized immune reaction. The erythrocyte sedimentation rate is high in about two-thirds of patients, but this finding does not carry any diagnostic or prognostic complications.

Hypercalcemia

Hypercalcemia may occur in any stage of sarcoidosis. The available evidence indicates that it is due to increased intestinal calcium absorption. In normal individuals, vitamin D is converted by the liver to 25-hydroxyvitamin D, which in turn undergoes 1-hydroxylation in the kidney to form 1-25-dihydroxyvitamin D [$1,25(OH)_2$ D], the most potent metabolite of vitamin D. In sarcoidosis, endogenous overproduction of $(3H)1,25(OH)_2$ D_3 by activated pulmonary macrophages seems to be the cause of increased intestinal absorption of calcium. Glucocorticoids lower the raised calcium level by inhibiting the peripheral action of $1,25(OH)_2$ D_3 and stimulating its metabolism to an inactive metabolite.[7]

Serum Angiotensin-Converting Enzyme

In sarcoidosis, the serum ACE level is raised in about 60 percent of patients. ACE activity is higher in patients with hilar adenopathy and pulmonary infiltration (stage II) than in those with either hilar adenopathy alone (stage I) or pulmonary infiltrate/fibrosis (stages III/IV). The test is positive in patients with extrathoracic sarcoidosis. Because ACE is derived from the epithelioid cells of the granulomas, it reflects the granuloma load in the body.

The diagnostic value of the serum ACE level is limited because the test has a false-negative incidence of 40 percent and a false-positive incidence of 10 percent. The test is most useful in monitoring the clinical course of the disease.[8]

IMMUNOLOGY

Cutaneous Anergy

The depression of cutaneous delayed-type hypersensitivity reactions is a cardinal immunologic feature of sarcoidosis. Approximately two-thirds of patients do not respond to the tuberculin test in any of the conventional strengths. However, this cutaneous anergy does not correlate with the activity of the disease, and the immunologic defect persists in most patients despite clinical and radiographic recovery.

Lymphopenia and Helper/Suppressor T Lymphocyte Ratio

Cutaneous anergy in sarcoidosis appears to be due to the unavailability of immune effector lymphocytes. Lymphopenia is a prominent feature of the disease. In normal individuals, the helper/suppressor cell ratio in the peripheral blood is 1.8:1. In patients with low-activity sarcoidosis, the ratio is somewhat lower (1.4:1), and in patients with high-intensity alveolitis, it is significantly lower (0.8:1). The relatively high number of suppressor cells in the peripheral blood may explain in part the cutaneous and in vitro anergy in sarcoidosis.

The helper/suppressor cell ratio is significantly higher (10.5:1) at the site of tissue granulomas. The cells bearing the suppressor-cytotoxic antigen are located in a mantle surrounding the granuloma, whereas the helper-inducer cells are distributed throughout the granuloma among the aggregated epithelioid cells.

Humoral Responses and Immune Complexes

Circulating antibody production is exaggerated in sarcoidosis. Hypergammaglobulinemia occurs in perhaps half the patients and is more frequent among blacks. The prevalence of immune complexes also varies. Circulating immune complexes are present in about half the patients with acute sarcoidosis, particularly in those with erythema nodosum. In chronic disease, immune complexes are less frequent. Direct immunofluorescence techniques have demonstrated the complexes in cutaneous granulomas. It has been suggested that they alter the distribution and function of the helper and suppressor cells and macrophages.

Kveim Test

Although the Kveim test (intradermal injection of homogenized tissue from a patient with sarcoidosis) is considered specific for sarcoidosis, the potent validated antigen is not widely available. It requires 4 to 6 weeks for the Kveim nodule to mature.

Bronchoalveolar Lavage

In normal nonsmokers, the effector population of the alveolar cells consists of 93 ± 3 percent alveolar macrophages, 3 to 7 percent lymphocytes, and fewer than 1 percent polymorphonuclear leukocytes. In smokers, the proportion of polymorphonuclear leukocytes increases to 2 to 8 percent.

In patients with active sarcoidosis there is a significant increase in the number of T lymphocytes. The T cell/B cell ratio in the lung approaches 18:1, whereas the T cell/B cell ratio in the blood is only about 3:1. T lymphocytes in bronchoalveolar lavage fluid are also increased in other conditions, including hypersensitivity pneumonitis, pulmonary lymphoma, and miliary tuberculosis. The expansion of the T lymphocyte population in sarcoidosis is due to an increase in CD4 (helper) T cells, whereas in hypersensitivity pneumonitis the expansion is due to the preferential increase of CD8 (suppressor) subsets. Other cell types, including $\gamma\delta+$ T cells, are also found in larger proportion in bronchoalveolar lavage fluids, suggesting the presence of a persistent yet unknown antigenic stimulus. B cell activation in sarcoidosis is reflected by the increased concentration of immunoglobulins in blood and bronchoalveolar lavage fluid.[9]

DIAGNOSIS

The criteria for establishing the diagnosis of sarcoidosis include (1) a compatible clinical or radiologic picture, or both; (2) histologic evidence of noncaseating granulomas; and (3) negative special stains and cultures for other entities (e.g., acid-fast bacilli or fungi in sputum or tissue biopsy specimens).

Recently developed tests, including serum ACE levels, lysozyme, the gallium 67 lung scan, and the bronchoalveolar lavage fluid lymphocyte count, have provided us with a better understanding of biochemical and immunologic changes of sarcoidosis but are of little help in establishing the specific diagnosis. The definitive diagnosis of sarcoidosis still requires the demonstration of noncaseating granulomas in the involved tissue.

TREATMENT

Glucocorticoids

At present, glucocorticoids are the most effective agents for influencing the course of cutaneous sarcoidosis. The skin lesions in sarcoidosis are not dangerous to life, and the patients should be treated on the basis of the severity and progression of the involvement. Oral prednisone, 20 to 40 mg daily in divided doses, is the treatment of choice. The total daily dose is then gradually reduced to maintenance levels, usually to about 10 mg daily. In many cases, after the initial 4 to 6 weeks of daily treatment, the dose may be reduced to 10 to 20 mg every other day. The alternate-day use of prednisone for maintenance therapy seems to be at least as effective as daily administration. The use of systemic glucocorticoids is detailed in Chap. 252.

Disfiguring skin lesions can also be treated by intralesional injection of triamcinolone acetonide. Intralesional injection of triamcinolone acetonide diluted with 1% procaine to a final concentration of 2 to 5 mg/mL may be repeated at weekly intervals. On occasion, glucocorticoid cream or lotion applied three to four times daily and

massaged in well, are helpful. Topical glucocorticoid therapy is detailed in Chap. 243.

Antimalarials: Chloroquine and Hydroxychloroquine

These agents are particularly useful in the management of chronic skin lesions.[10,11] Chloroquine is administered in dosages of 250 mg twice a day for 6 months. Hydroxychloroquine is given in dosages of 200 mg twice a day for periods longer than 6 months. Antimalarials may also be used together with glucocorticoids to reduce the dosage of the latter. The drugs are described in Chap. 254.

Immunosuppressive Drugs

Of all the immunosuppressive drugs, methotrexate seems, so far, to have the best track record in the treatment of cutaneous as well as disseminated sarcoidosis. Symptomatic and objective improvement occurred in 13 of 14 patients with refractory sarcoidosis treated with low-dose methotrexate. Four patients experienced a greater than 50 percent reduction in skin lesions.[12] Azathioprine and chlorambucil have also been tried but with limited success. For details of use of these agents, see Chap. 255.

Other Drugs

Oxyphenbutazone, colchicine, allopurinol, levamisole, and radiation have also been tried in the management of sarcoidosis.[13]

Cosmetic Surgery

Surgical treatment may involve excision of small lesions or skin grafting of extensive sarcoid ulcers. In either case, caution should be exercised because of the risk of keloid formation, particularly in black patients

Miscellaneous

The creative use of available cosmetic preparations and laser surgery in patients with disfiguring skin plaques and refractory lupus pernio can improve the quality of life both socially and psychologically.[14]

Clinical Caution

Antimalarial drugs, especially chloroquine but rarely hydroxychloroquine as well, can lead to retinopathy and blindness. Therefore, regular ophthalmologic examinations are mandatory. Methotrexate may cause liver damage, and liver biopsies may be needed if the therapy is long term.

Antituberculosis therapy is not indicated routinely in patients with sarcoidosis. However, those patients who show a positive tuberculin test, if given glucocorticoids, immunosuppressive drugs, or radiation, should receive prophylactic isoniazid.

REFERENCES

1. du Bois RM et al: Granulomatous processes, in *The Lung: Scientific Foundations,* edited by RG Crystal et al. New York, Raven, 1991, p 1925

2. Semenzato G: The immunology of sarcoidosis. *Semin Respir Med* **8**:17, 1986
3. Jorizzo JL et al: Sarcoidosis of upper respiratory tract in patients with nasal rim lesions: A pilot study. *J Am Acad Dermatol* **22**:439, 1990
4. James DG, Kendig EL Jr: Childhood sarcoidosis. *Sarcoidosis* **5**:57, 1988
5. Garcia C et al: Pancreatic sarcoidosis. *Sarcoid Vasc Diff Lung Dis* **13**:28, 1996
6. Rizzato G, Montemurro L: The locomotor system, in *Sarcoidosis and Other Granulomatous Disorders. Lung Biology in Health and Disease,* vol 73, edited by DG James. New York, Marcel Dekker, 1994, p 349
7. Sharma O: Vitamin D, calcium and sarcoidosis. *Chest* **109**:535, 1996
8. Allen RKA: Angiotensin-converting enzyme, in *Sarcoidosis and other Granulomatous Disorders. Lung Biology in Health and Disease,* vol 73, edited by DG James. New York, Marcel Dekker, 1994, p 529
9. Kunkel SL et al: Th1 and Th2 responses regulate experimental lung granuloma development. *Sarcoid Vasc Diff Lung Dis* **13**:120, 1996
10. Siltzbach LE, Teirstein AS: Chloroquine therapy in 43 patients with intrathoracic and cutaneous sarcoidosis. *Acta Med Scand* **176** (suppl 425):302, 1954
11. Adams J et al: Effective reduction in the serum 1-25-dihydroxyvitamin D and calcium concentration in sarcoidosis-associated hypercalcemia with short chloroquine therapy. *Ann Intern Med* **111**:437, 1989
12. Lower EE, Baughman RP: The use of low-dose methotrexate in refractory sarcoidosis. *Am J Med Sci* **299**:153, 1990
13. Brechtel B et al: Allopurinol—a therapeutic alternative for disseminated cutaneous sarcoidosis. *Br J Dermatol* **135**:307, 1996
14. Stack BC Jr et al: CO_2 laser excision of lupus pernio of the face. *Am J Otolaryngol* **17**:260, 1996

CHAPTER 185

David I. McLean
Harley A. Haynes

Cutaneous Manifestations of Internal Malignant Disease

Changes in the skin can be a marker for an internal malignant neoplasm. The specific relationship of the cancer with the marker can be variable. For instance, hypertrichosis lanuginosa acquisita can be a marker for many different malignant neoplasms, whereas necrolytic migratory erythema is quite specific for a glucagon-producing tumor of the pancreas.

An attempt has been made to group these manifestations in a useful manner (Table 185-1). Where possible, these groupings have been made by the major clinical manifestation. Unfortunately, our lack of knowledge does not allow us to classify these diseases by a pathophysiologic approach in all cases. Indeed, there is a very large group where the biochemical relationship to the neoplasia is not understood.

There must be a proven association of the cutaneous eruption with a tumor. This is not difficult when the supposed manifestation is very rare and the tumor is also very uncommon. It becomes a major problem, however, when the manifestation is very common, such as the seborrheic keratoses in the sign of Leser-Trélat, and the presumed association is with a wide spectrum of commonly occurring neoplasms. In this situation the literature becomes replete with anecdotal reports, which may or may not be an indication of whether there is a true association with the malignant neoplasm.

There is an evolving consensus of what constitutes a true paraneoplastic syndrome.[1] There are two essential criteria: (1) the dermatosis must develop only after the development of the malignant tumor, and (2) both the dermatosis and the malignant tumor should follow a parallel course. The second criterion means that removal of the cancer results in clearing of the dermatosis, and recurrence of the cancer can cause relapse of the dermatosis (certainly relapse of the dermatosis cannot occur in the absence of the cancer). These criteria have been amplified more fully.[1]

COLOR CHANGES SECONDARY TO THE DEPOSITION OF SUBSTANCES IN THE SKIN

Icterus (See also Chap. 164)

Icterus as a manifestation of internal malignancy is generally a late sign. It is usually secondary to obstruction of the bile duct or gross intrahepatic obstruction. Extrahepatic obstruction can be secondary to malignant disease of the gall bladder, pancreas, bile duct, or adjacent bowel.

Melanosis (See also Chap. 89)

Melanosis is a condition caused by the abnormal deposition of melanin pigments in tissue. It is externally manifested by a diffuse gray-brown pigmentation of the skin (Fig. 185-1), but the pigment can be deposited in most of the organs of the body. A mild darkening of the skin may be seen with adrenal insufficiency, with ACTH-producing tumors such as primary tumors of the pituitary gland, or with other malignant tumors metastatic to the pituitary gland.[2]

Diffuse melanosis can also be secondary to malignant melanoma (see also Chap. 92). Usually occurring late in the disease course, melanosis can, however, be the presenting sign. The pigment of the skin has been attributed to the presence of melanin granules in both the circulation and tissue macrophages[3] or to the presence of single-cell metastases from the primary melanoma.[4] Diffuse micrometastases can also appear in the nail matrix, leading to pigment streaks in the nail plate. Circulating tumor cells have also been found in patients with melanosis.[4] Melanuria is frequently associated with melanosis of the skin. Urine from patients who have melanuria is usually not black when voided, but gradually darkens to a deep brown and later a black color when exposed to the air for several hours. It would appear that intermediary metabolites of tyrosine are oxidized spontaneously to melanin. Highly increased amounts of 5-S-cysteinyldopa have been reported in the urine of such patients.[5]

Andreev and Petkov noted a melasma (chloasma) type of hyperpigmentation on the face of five patients with "brain tumors."[6] In three patients the hyperpigmentation resolved after the surgical removal of the tumor.

A diffuse gray-brown pigmentation of the skin can also be produced by hemochromatosis.

Hemochromatosis

Hemochromatosis is an iron-storage disorder resulting predominantly from increased iron absorption from the gut. There is deposition of iron in the form of hemosiderin in many tissues. A third of untreated patients with hemochromatosis will develop hepatocellular carcinoma.[7]

TABLE 185-1

Cutaneous Manifestations of Internal Malignant Disease

I. Lesions secondary to the deposition of substances in the skin
  A. Icterus
  B. Melanosis
  C. Hemochromatosis
  D. Xanthomas
  E. Systemic amyloidosis
II. Vascular and blood abnormalities
  A. Flushing
  B. Palmar erythema
  C. Telangiectasia
  D. Purpura
  E. Vasculitis
  F. Cutaneous ischemia
  G. Thrombophlebitis
III. Bullous disorders
  A. Bullous pemphigoid
  B. Pemphigus vulgaris
  C. Paraneoplastic pemphigus
  D. Dermatitis herpetiformis
  E. Herpes gestationis
  F. Erythema multiforme
  G. Epidermyolysis bullosa acquisita
  H. Linear IgA dermatosis
IV. Infections and infestations
  A. Herpes zoster
  B. Herpes simplex
  C. Bacterial infections
  D. Fungi and yeast infections
  E. Scabies
V. Disorders of keratinization
  A. Acanthosis nigricans
  B. Acquired ichthyosis
  C. Palmar hyperkeratosis
  D. Tripe palm
  E. Erythroderma
  F. Paraneoplastic acrokeratosis of Bazex

VI. Collagen-vascular disease
  A. Dermatomyositis
  B. Lupus erythematosus
  C. Progressive systemic sclerosis
VII. Skin tumors and internal malignant disease
  A. Muir-Torre syndrome
  B. Gardner's syndrome
  C. Cowden disease
  D. Mucosal neuroma syndrome
  E. Neurofibromatosis
VIII. Hormone-related conditions
IX. Disorders associated with primary skin cancer
  A. Nevoid basal cell carcinoma syndrome
  B. Arsenical manifestations
X. Other disorders associated with internal malignant disease
  A. Pruritus
  B. Erythema gyratum repens
  C. Subcutaneous fat necrosis
  D. Sweet's syndrome
  E. Hypertrichosis lanuginosa acquisita
  F. Necrolytic migratory erythema
  G. Clubbing
  H. Leukoderma
  I. Peutz-Jeghers syndrome
  J. Tuberous sclerosis
  K. Multiple eruptive seborrheic keratoses
  L. Porphyria cutanea tarda
XI. Direct tumor involvement in the skin

Xanthomas (See also Chap. 152)

The predominant type of xanthoma associated with internal malignant disease is the plane xanthoma. The most common association of diffuse plane xanthoma is with multiple myeloma. Xanthomas, as well as atypical eruptive histiocytosis with lipid deposition, have also been associated with myelocytic leukemia, myelomonocytic leukemia, leukemic lymphocytic reticuloendotheliosis, diffuse histiocytic lymphoma, and in the cutaneous T cell lymphoma.[8,9] Juvenile xanthogranuloma can be associated with juvenile chronic myeloid leukemia.[10]

Patients with xanthomas associated with cancer may be normolipidemic[11] or they may, more commonly, have a hyperlipoproteinemia. Type 2A hyperlipoproteinemia has been described in association with IgG L type myeloma, as has type 4 or type 5 hyperlipoproteinemia. Type 3 (broad beta) and pre-beta hyperlipoproteinemia have been described in association with IgA myeloma.

Purpura may be a feature of diffuse plane xanthomas associated with malignant disease. Pinch purpura has been noted in a normolipidemic patient with myeloma. Hemorrhagic bullae have been associated with xanthoma disseminatum and IgG K type multiple myeloma.[12]

Systemic Amyloidosis (See also Chap. 150)

Systemic amyloidosis of both the primary type and that associated with multiple myeloma commonly have skin lesions. It is important to differentiate skin lesions of systemic amyloidosis from the far more commonly seen purely cutaneous variants of amyloidosis. All patients with skin lesions of systemic amyloidosis should be thoroughly investigated for multiple myeloma. Acute nonlymphocytic leukemia has also been reported in association with systemic amyloidosis treated with melphalan.[13]

Intradermal bullae have been associated with myeloma-related amyloidosis. These bullae are the result of extensive dermal infiltration with amyloid, resulting in cleavage of the uppermost dermis from the lower dermis.

Familial cutaneous lichen amyloidosus has been reported in a large kindred in association with multiple endocrine neoplasia (MEN) type 2A.[13]

FIGURE 185-1

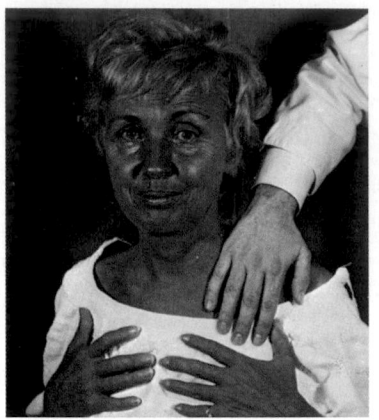

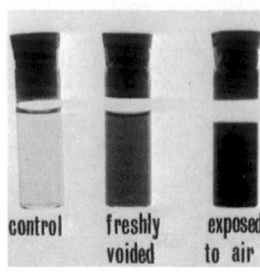

B.

A.

Slate gray dermal pigmentation with metastatic melanoma and melanogenuria. *A.* Diffuse blue argyria-like hypermelanosis. This patient died 1 month after this photograph was taken, illustrating that this bizarre argyria-like blue pigmentation is a terminal complication. *B.* Dark urine from a patient with melanogenuria, compared with normal urine.

VASCULAR AND BLOOD ABNORMALITIES

Flushing (See Chap. 171)

Acquired pronounced flushing, usually of the central face and upper trunk, may be a manifestation of carcinoid syndrome, caused by carcinoid tumors.[14]

One study compared the symptomatology of patients with idiopathic flushing with that of patients with carcinoid syndrome.[15] That study showed that palpitations, syncope, and hypotension occurred only in patients with idiopathic flushing, whereas wheezing and abdominal pain occured only in patients with carcinoid. Diarrhea occurred in both.

Vasoactive substances can also be released in patients with extensive localized or systemic mastocytosis (see Chap. 162) and in patients with pheochromocytoma. Unilateral flushing and sweating (harlequin syndrome) have been associated with a contralateral lung cancer invading the spine, in a patient with Pancoast's syndrome, and with Horner's syndrome.[16]

Palmar Erythema (See Chap. 164)

Palmar erythema can be associated with advanced liver failure. Such liver failure may be secondary to either a primary or a metastatic tumor in the liver.

Telangiectasia

Localized, grouped telangiectatic vessels on the anterior chest wall may be a marker for breast cancer. There is often a clinically palpable, indurated, warm, subcutaneous plaque immediately beneath the telangiectatic area. Telangiectatic vessels may also be the first evidence of dermal or subcutaneous metastases of breast cancer as well as of other malignant tumors.

Generalized telangiectasia can be a presenting factor of malignant angioendotheliomatosis (see Chap. 109). Biopsy of the telangiectatic vessels will confirm the diagnosis.

Progressive telangiectases have been associated with carcinoid tumors (see "Flushing") and with adenocarcinoma of the hepatic bile duct.[17]

Telangiectasia may also be a manifestation of a genodermatosis, which in turn can be associated with systemic malignant disease such as lymphoma. These genodermatoses include ataxia-telangiectasia (see Chap. 192), Bloom's disease, and xeroderma pigmentosum and its variant de Sanctis-Cacchione syndrome (see Chap. 157). In addition to the well-known association of lymphocytic leukemia and non-Hodgkin's lymphoma in patients with ataxia-telangiectasia, there appears to be an increased incidence of solid tumors of the oral cavity, breast, stomach, pancreas, ovary, and bladder, as well as others.[18] Female heterozygotes of ataxia-telangiectasia have a significantly increased risk of breast cancer.[19]

Telangiectasia can also be a marker for the collagen-vascular group of diseases including progressive systemic sclerosis, which can be associated with an increased cancer risk (see Chaps. 172, 173, and 174).

Purpura

Lymphoma is the most common cause of idiopathic thrombocytopenic purpura (ITP) associated with malignant disease. Hodgkin's disease is the most common associated lymphoma, and the diagnosis of ITP may precede other evidence of lymphoma.

Purpura related to cancer can occur from a wide variety of mechanisms: thrombocytopenia, consumption coagulopathy, hyper- or dysglobulinemia, vascular fragility, and vasculitis.

Disseminated intravascular coagulation (DIC) as a cause of purpura in malignant disease is most commonly associated with acute lymphocytic or myelomonocytic leukemia, in particular T cell acute lymphocytic leukemia.[20] Many patients may not have full-blown DIC, having only biochemical or mild clinical manifestations of the process.

Thrombotic thrombocytopenic purpura, when associated with cancer, is usually a late sign.

Purpura can also be associated with the hyperglobulinemia seen in multiple myeloma or lymphoma. When purpura is secondary to the presence of cryoglobulins, lesions are often found in acral areas and may be associated with Raynaud's phenomenon. Benign hyperglobulinemic purpura can be associated with Sjögren's syndrome, which in turn can be associated with malignant disease.

Purpura, usually palpable, is a clinical sign of cutaneous vasculitis (see Chap. 176), which in turn can be associated with cancer. It is important not to forget that a bacterial septicemia can present as a palpable purpuric eruption in patients with cancer.

Vasculitis (See also Chap. 176)

Leukocytoclastic vasculitis, such as can be seen in Henoch-Schönlein purpura, can be very rarely associated with malignant neoplasms. The vasculitis seen in patients with malignant neoplasms does not differ clinically from that which occurs much more commonly secondary to nonneoplastic causes. It can be a presenting sign in squamous cell carcinoma, particularly of the bronchus,[21] and in renal carcinoma.[22] Leukocytoclastic vasculitis can also be associated with leukemia and leukemic lymphoma.[23]

A periarteritis nodosa–like syndrome has also been reported in association with hairy cell leukemia, acute lymphocytic leukemia, and multiple myeloma.[24,25]

Cutaneous Ischemia

Evidence of compromised peripheral circulation can be a marker for many malignant neoplasms. It is frequently manifested by evidence of digital ischemia, either as Raynaud's phenomenon or frank gangrene.

Peripheral ischemia has been associated with many malignant neoplasms, including carcinoma of the pancreas, stomach, small bowel, ovary, and kidney, as well as lymphoma and leukemia.[26]

There may be associated splinter hemorrhages of the nail bed, suggestive of an underlying vasculitic process. The etiology, though, is rarely apparent.

The peripheral cutaneous ischemia of polycythemia rubra vera appears to be secondary to the increased viscosity of the peripheral circulation associated with this disease.[27] This increased viscosity may lead to frank venous thrombosis. Similarly, some patients with leukemia can develop leukostasis secondary to very high white blood cell concentrations.

The ischemia seen in cryoglobulinemia appears also to be secondary to increased blood viscosity. Cryoglobulinemia may be associated with multiple myeloma or with lymphoma.

Thrombophlebitis (See also Chap. 167)

Isolated vein thrombophlebitis is uncommonly associated with internal malignant disease. Multiple-lesion "migratory" superficial thrombophlebitis is much more often seen in association with cancer, and when this syndrome is present the patient should be examined carefully for occult malignant disease. The association of peripheral thrombophlebitis (phlebothrombosis) with gastric carcinoma was noted by Trousseau in the nineteenth century. Migratory superficial thrombophlebitis as a marker for cancer has been confirmed, and the association has been extended to include tumors of the pancreas, prostate, lung, liver, bowel, gallbladder, and ovary, as well as to lymphoma and leukemia. The migratory nature of the thrombophlebitis probably relates to a generalized hypercoagulable state.

Mondor's disease is thrombophlebitis of the anterior chest wall presenting as a tender or nontender cord. Usually benign, it may be associated with primary[28] or recurrent breast cancer.

Patients with deep venous thrombosis who are younger than 50 years of age appear to have a very significant risk of occult cancer (relative risk 19.0)[29] and thus should have an appropriately thorough examination and laboratory investigation. Those at greatest risk for cancer had a low hemoglobin and an eosinophilia.

BULLOUS DISORDERS

Bullous Pemphigoid (See also Chap. 61)

There is probably no significantly increased risk of a malignant tumor in patients with bullous pemphigoid, other than that associated with the age of the patient,[30] although a Japanese cohort of patients with bullous pemphigoid had a 5.8 percent prevalence of neoplasia, versus 0.61 percent of controls.[31] Also, there have been anecdotal reports showing that some patients with bullous pemphigoid clear when the concomitant tumor is treated, indicating a possible causal relationship in some patients.

Pemphigus (See also Chap. 60)

Pemphigus vulgaris can be associated with Hodgkin's disease, in which case the two diseases can run a parallel course.[32] The relationship of solid tumors to pemphigus vulgaris is less well defined, although in one series 5 percent of pemphigus vulgaris patients had cancer, a higher rate than in controls.[31] Pemphigus vulgaris has been reported in association with many solid tumors, but, other than for lung cancer,[31] these associations have been in small series or isolated case reports.

There is a well-defined association of pemphigus with thymoma, with or without clinical myasthenia gravis.[33-36] Paraneoplastic pemphigus[37] is clinically, histopathologically, and immunopathologically a distinct form of pemphigus with features of erythema multiforme (see Chap. 58). It has been described in association with lymphoma, chronic lymphocytic leukemia, thymoma, sarcoma, and Waldenström's macroglobulinemia; it has a very poor prognosis.

Dermatitis Herpetiformis (See also Chap. 67)

Dermatitis herpetiformis is occasionally associated with intestinal lymphoma. The relative risk of non-Hodgkin's lymphoma associated with dermatitis herpetiformis is 5.4 (2.2 to 11.1) in males, less in females.[38] Patients with dermatitis herpetiformis have gluten sensitivity, and the presumed etiology of the lymphoma is the resulting chronic antigenic stimulation. The lymphoma, when it occurs, is usually a diffuse histiocytic lymphoma.[39] There is no indication that there are a greater than expected number of patients with dermatitis herpetiformis developing tumors other than intestinal lymphoma.[40]

Herpes Gestationis (See also Chap. 64)

Herpes gestationis has been described in association with a hydatidiform mole[41] and germ cell tumor.[42]

Erythema Multiforme (See also Chap. 58)

Erythema multiforme does not appear to be a specific marker for any internal neoplasm. It appears to occur more frequently in patients with acute leukemia, but whether this relates to the leukemia or to its treatment has not been well defined.

Erythema multiforme can occur in cancer patients secondary to drug or radiation therapy, and it has been suggested to be particularly common in patients on phenytoin and receiving radiation therapy for intracranial tumors.[43]

Erythema multiforme–like lesions can sometimes be evident in paraneoplastic pemphigus (see Chap. 60).

Epidermolysis Bullosa Acquisita (See Chap. 66)

Epidermolysis bullosa acquisita is a very rare disorder that has been described rarely in association with carcinoma of the bronchus and with amyloidosis and multiple myeloma.[44] Most cases of epidermolysis bullosa acquisita are not associated with cancer.

Linear IgA Dermatosis (See also Chap. 63)

Linear IgA dermatosis has been reported in association with lymphoma, chronic lymphocytic leukemia, myeloma, carcinoma of the bladder and esophagus, and with hydatidiform mole.[45,46]

INFECTIONS AND INFESTATIONS

Herpes Zoster (See also Chap. 216)

Only a small percentage of patients with localized herpes zoster have a concurrent malignant disease, and investigation for malignant disease in otherwise healthy patients is not indicated. Patients with leukemia or lymphoma do have an increased risk of herpes zoster, but the herpes zoster usually occurs late in the course of their disease. The incidence of herpes zoster in patients with lymphoma is approximately 10 percent, possibly even higher in patients with Hodgkin's disease.[47]

Localized herpes zoster can also occur in association with solid tumors such as breast cancer. In the case of breast cancer, the dermatomal distribution of the herpes zoster may indicate involvement of the nerve root area with metastatic tumor. The site of the primary tumor correlates with the site of herpes zoster in patients with breast cancer, cancer of the respiratory tract, and gynecologic cancer. Segmental herpes zoster can also occur after radiation therapy, presumably secondary to nerve damage with subsequent viral activation.

Disseminated herpes zoster is commonly associated with underlying malignant disease. Any patient with disseminated herpes zoster that is otherwise unexplained should be carefully examined for evidence of cancer. The most commonly associated malignant diseases are lymphoma and leukemia.[48] The development of herpes zoster in a previously treated lymphoma patient can be evidence of the recurrence of a lymphoma. This sign is of particular value in patients who develop the herpes zoster more than 6 months after clinical remission.[47]

Herpes Simplex (See Chap. 215)

Typical localized herpes simplex is rarely a marker for cancer. Extensive, often chronic, local herpes simplex with massive ulceration and destruction of tissue (Fig. 185-2), generalized cutaneous herpes simplex, and disseminated systemic herpes simplex are indeed associated with malignant disease, which is often far advanced. Lymphoma and leukemia are most often the associated cancers, but any advanced malignant tumor can produce the compromised host immune response associated with these conditions.[49]

Bacterial Infections

Bacterial infection of the skin as a marker for the presence of internal malignancy is very uncommon, and when it is associated with malignancy, it is usually associated with very advanced disease.

Fungi and Yeast

Dermatophyte infections of the skin are not associated with internal malignant disease. Deep fungal infections, with their associated skin lesions, can be associated with malignant disease. Similarly, mucosal candidiasis usually indicates a severely compromised host immune response, which can be secondary to advanced malignant disease or to chemotherapy.

Scabies

Norwegian scabies, a severe generalized form of scabies, is associated with the leukemia-lymphoma group of neoplasms, but it can be seen in any severely immunocompromised host. The scabies is frequently manifested by a minimal inflammatory response and should always be considered in patients who have advanced malignant disease associated with pruritus.

DISORDERS OF KERATINIZATION

Acanthosis Nigricans (See Chap. 186)

Acanthosis nigricans can be classified into two major groups: benign and malignant. Malignant acanthosis nigricans is usually of sudden onset and is rapidly progressive, but it is otherwise clinically indistinguishable from benign acanthosis nigricans (Fig. 185-3). Diffuse keratoderma involving the palms, soles, and flexor surfaces of the fingers and toes may be more common in malignant acanthosis nigricans than in the benign form. Such changes can be early.

Malignant acanthosis nigricans is usually secondary to an adenocarcinoma. The adenocarcinoma is usually intraabdominal (70 to 90 percent) and gastric (55 to 61 percent).[50,51] There is evidence that malignant acanthosis nigricans is linked to an enhanced secretion by the cancer of transforming growth factor α.[52]

Acquired Ichthyosis

The sudden onset of ichthyosis in an adult may indicate an occult malignant tumor, most often lymphoma. The ichthyosis is a true hyperkeratosis and can be differentiated clinically and histologically from simple dry skin (xerosis). Although the ichthyosis usually occurs as a late manifestation of a lymphoma, it may precede the diagnosis by several years.

Palmar Hyperkeratosis

There are two groups of patients with palmar hyperkeratosis and associated malignant tumors: those patients with diffuse palmar hyperkeratosis and those with punctate palmar hyperkeratosis.

In 1958, diffuse hyperkeratosis, or tylosis, was reported by Howel-Evans et al.[53] to be associated in two families with an almost

FIGURE 185-2

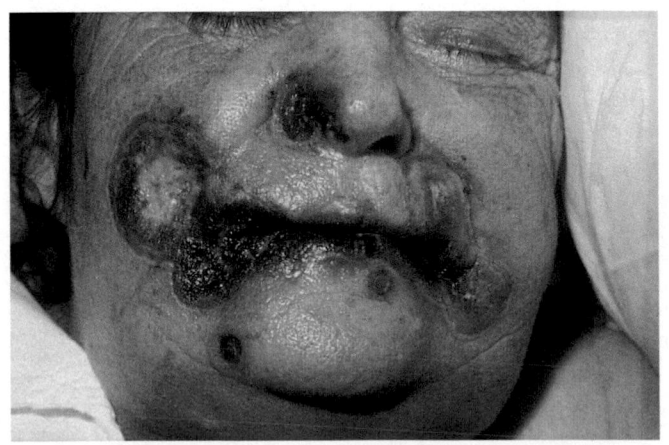

Female with advanced non-Hodgkin's lymphoma and chronic, ulcerative herpes simplex involving lips, cheek, and nose.

FIGURE 185-3

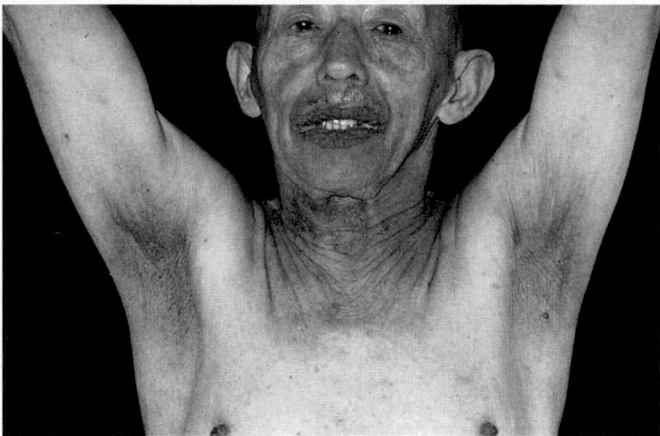

A.

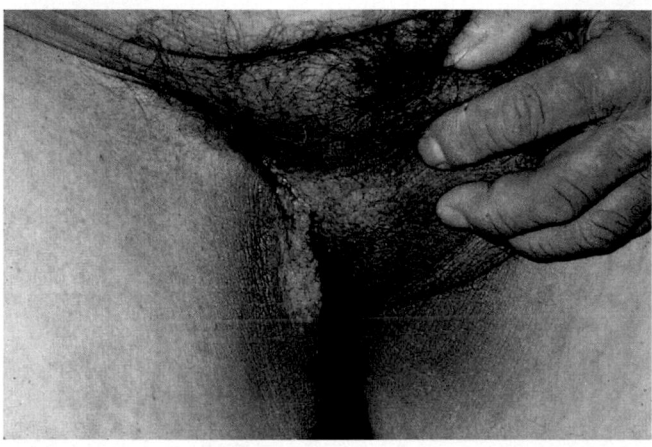

B.

A. Malignant acanthosis nigricans with pigmented, velvety, papillo-matous lesions in both axillae and the neck, and papillomatous, ver-rucous lesions on the vermilion border of the lips. *B.* Acanthosis nigri-cans in the groin and scrotal area. (*Courtesy of Fritz Gschnait, MD.*)

certain development of esophageal carcinoma by age 65. The tylosis in these patients can be separated clinically from the benign form of tylosis, which occurs at an earlier age (early childhood), has sharply delimited edges, and is of uniform thickness. In addition to the Howel-Evans families, there would appear to be a greater than expected incidence of esophageal carcinoma in other families with a pedigree of tylosis.[54]

A large kindred has been described with palmoplantar kerato-derma in association with breast or ovarian carcinoma, or both.[55] The clinical lesions cover the entire surface of the palms and soles and show a yellowish uniform hyperkeratosis surrounded by a red border. Histologically, the lesions show features of epidermolytic hyperkeratosis. (see Chap. 53)

The second type of palmar hyperkeratosis that may be associated with neoplasia consists of discreet hyperkeratotic papules on the palms. These patients have been reported to have a greater than expected risk of cancer of the breast and uterus, among other tu-mors.[56,57] While some kindreds have been described, arsenic, known to be associated with punctate palmar hyperkeratosis and an increased risk of cancer, may be responsible for other cases,[58] al-though studies have failed to show increased arsenic exposure on

history. Other authors question the existence of the relationship of punctate palmar hyperkeratosis and internal cancer. It appears that the association, if present, is not very strong.

Palmar hyperkeratosis is also seen in paraneoplastic acrokera-tosis of Bazex (see below).

Tripe Palm

Tripe palm is a rugose thickening of the palms that is strongly associated with internal cancer.[59] The honeycombed and corrugated thickening of the palms may be associated with periungual tender-ness.[60] Normal dermatoglyphic ridges are accentuated. The most common cancers associated with tripe palms are carcinomas of the stomach and lung, with fewer occurrences being noted with other solid tumors.[61] There may be an associated acanthosis higricans (see Chap. 186).

Erythroderma

Erythroderma, a diffuse erythema of the skin surface usually asso-ciated with induration and scaling, is not uncommonly associated with malignancy, most commonly hematologic, in particular leu-kemia and lymphoma where there is direct infiltration of the skin by the malignant cells. The cells are most frequently lymphocytes of T cell type. These malignancies include Sézary syndrome and mycosis fungoides (see Chap. 108).

Among solid tumors, erythroderma has been associated with car-cinoma of the lung, liver, prostate, thyroid, colon, pancreas, and stomach. The erythroderma associated with solid tumors usually occurs at a relatively late stage of the disease and may resolve after resection of the tumor. The etiology of the erythroderma associated with solid tumors is not known, (see Chap. 45).

Paraneoplastic Acrokeratosis of Bazex

Paraneoplastic acrokeratosis of Bazex is a symmetric dermatosis that most commonly affects the hands, feet, ears, and nose with an erythematous psoriasiform eruption. The eruption is of a bluer hue than in psoriasis.[62] Later changes involve the cheeks, elbows, and knees, with still later changes often involving the central trunk, where bullae may be seen. Acanthosis nigricans may be an asso-ciated finding. In acrokeratosis of Bazex, the nails are involved early and severely. There is subungual hyperkeratosis as well as a flaky white surface to the nail. The nails may be shed. The distal digits show an erythematous scaling eruption, often fissured and often with suppuration.[63,64] Biopsy of the skin lesions of one patient showed diffuse deposition of IgA, IgM, and IgG along the basement membrane.[65] Nails appeared to have an abnormal amino acid com-position.[66]

Bazex syndrome is almost always associated with cancer, and is overwhelmingly seen in males.[67] It is usually associated with neo-plasia of the upper respiratory system, which includes the pharynx, esophagus, tongue, and lungs, although rarely other solid tumors have been reported in association. Lung tumors have included car-cinoid. The eruption predates evidence of the cancer in 67 percent of patients,[67] with the cancer often not being diagnosed until the later stages of the syndrome.[62,68] Bazex syndrome has been reported to respond to etretinate, even though the primary lesion was left untreated.

This syndrome should not be confused with follicular atrophoderma associated with basal cell carcinoma, hypotrichosis, and localized or generalized hypohidrosis, also described by Bazex.[69]

COLLAGEN-VASCULAR DISEASE

Dermatomyositis (See also Chap. 173)

Dermatomyositis can be a marker for internal neoplasia, and the development of the dermatomyositis can predate the diagnosis of the cancer. Studies combining polymyositis patients with those with dermatomyositis show a lower prevalence of cancer[70,71] than those that examine patients with dermatomyositis alone. There is probably no significant relationship of polymyositis to cancer. The slightly higher than expected rate in some studies of polymyositis cohorts might be due to cancer detection bias, as the increase is noted only after polymyositis diagnosis.[72] The cancers are usually identifiable by history and physical examination.[73] It would appear that adults with dermatomyositis, but not polymyositis, should be examined thoroughly for evidence of an associated malignant tumor. In children, dermatomyositis is not statistically linked to malignancy.

The clinical manifestations of dermatomyositis appear to be the same with and without a malignant tumor, although Basset-Sequin et al.[74] noted that cutaneous necrosis and an elevated erythrocyte sedimentation rate appeared to be markers for those with cancer and, also, a reduced survival.

Lupus Erythematosus

Systemic lupus erythematosus (SLE) is only rarely associated with malignant neoplasia, most often with lymphoma or thymoma. Pemphigus erythematosus has been noted in association with malignant thymoma and myasthenia gravis, as has a pemphigus vulgaris–like eruption and positive LE cell test (see Chap. 60).

Scleroderma (See also Chap. 174)

Systemic scleroderma is not commonly associated with internal malignancy. In 727 cases of systemic scleroderma, only 2.6 percent had an internal malignant lesion.[75] The only tumor that has been found to be consistently associated with scleroderma is carcinoma of the lung.[76] Almost all patients with associated lung tumors have very advanced systemic scleroderma. The association is most likely one of a lung tumor developing secondary to the chronic pulmonary fibrosis.

SKIN TUMORS AND INTERNAL MALIGNANT DISEASE

Muir-Torre Syndrome

First described by Muir et al. in 1967 and by Torre in 1968, the essential features of the Muir-Torre syndrome are sebaceous tumors of the skin (Fig. 185-4), with or without keratoacanthomas, in association with visceral neoplasms, which are often multiple.[77,78] The sebaceous tumors are usually on the face or trunk and are usually multiple; and whereas most are sebaceous adenomas, they can include sebaceous hyperplasia, sebaceous epithelioma, and sebaceous carcinoma. Often the same patient will have the complete histologic spectrum of sebaceous tumors. Some skin lesions have histologic features of both keratoacanthoma and sebaceous proliferation.[79] Keratoacanthomas, if present, can be very large.

The visceral neoplasms are often multiple and include a wide variety of tissues. Colon cancers are particularly common and may be associated with colonic polyposis.[77-81] Other neoplasms include other tumors of the gastrointestinal tract and tumors of the larynx and endometrium. There has been one report of an associated lymphoma. Patients with Muir-Torre syndrome appear to have a reasonably good survival, despite the profusion of neoplasms.[82] It has been suggested that a solitary benign sebaceous gland tumor of the eyelid is a good marker for the Muir-Torre syndrome and that its presence warrants review for systemic cancer.

The Muir-Torre syndrome is inherited as autosomal dominant. There is an association of the Muir-Torre syndrome with cancer family syndrome,[83] and markers have been identified in chromosome 2P, a site linked to Lynch II cancer family syndrome.[84]

Long-term treatment with isotretinoin appears to be useful in some patients,[85] and immunosuppression apparently exacerbates the cutaneous manifestations.[86]

FIGURE 185-4

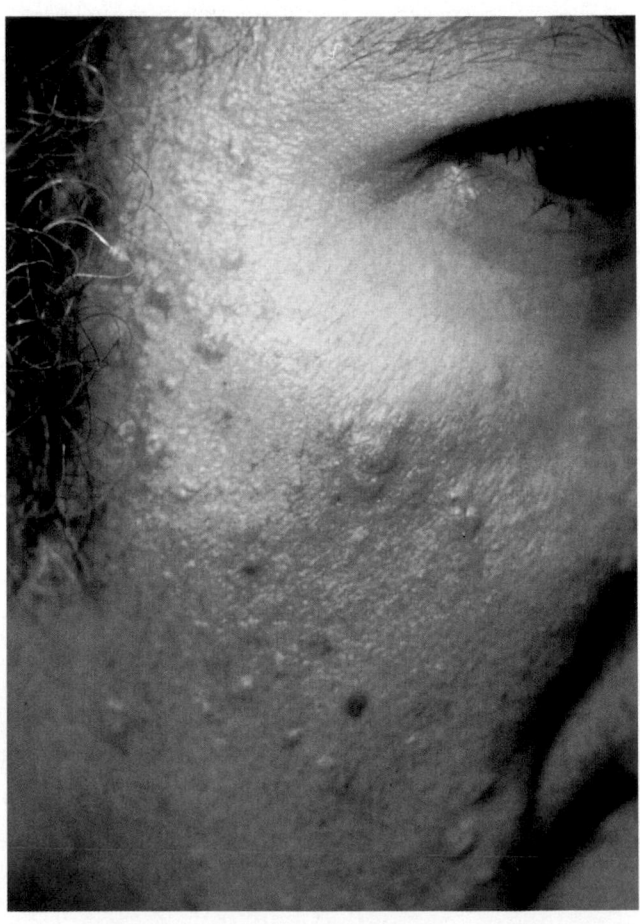

Muir-Torre syndrome showing typical sebaceous adenomas, in association with colonic polyposis and carcinoma in situ. (*Courtesy of T. Christensen, MD, and R. Wilkinson, MD.*)

Gardner's Syndrome

The essential features of Gardner's syndrome are intestinal polyposis (usually colonic), with a high rate of malignant transformation; epidermoid cysts, particularly of the face, scalp, and trunk; osteomatosis of the maxilla, mandible, and cranial bones; and fibromas, desmoids, and other fibrous tumors of the skin and subcutaneous tissue.[87] Histologically, the epidermoid cysts may show areas of pilomatrixoma or a hybrid cyst with epidermal keratinization and inner root sheath keratinization. The desmoids often occur in wounds and can be deeply invasive, requiring chemotherapy or radical surgery. At times, erroneously called sebaceous cysts, the epithelioid cysts of Gardner's syndrome often precede the development of bowel cancer.

There is a virtual certainty of malignant transformation of the gastrointestinal tract polyps. Some of the polyps are almost always visible by proctoscope examination, but they can be found up to the stomach.[88] There is an association of hepatoblastoma, a rare neoplasm of infants and children with Gardner's syndrome, and there may be some overlap of the features of Gardner's syndrome and nevoid basal cell carcinoma syndrome.[89] Gardner's syndrome is inherited as an autosomal dominant condition.

Cowden Disease (See Chap. 114)

Cowden disease, or multiple hamartoma syndrome, was first described in 1963 by Lloyd and Dennis and was named after the propositus.[90] Inherited as an autosomal dominant trait, the distinctive cutaneous lesions are multiple tricholemmomas (Fig. 185-5A). These lesions are grouped around the mouth, nose, and ears and clinically resemble warts. Some patients also show closely set papules with a cobblestone pattern that have a fibromatous histology and also occur on the oral mucosa (Fig. 185-5B). Small keratotic lesions resembling plane warts occur on the acral skin. Patients may have an adenoid facies and high arched palate. Other cutaneous lesions can include lipomas, hemangiomas, neuromas, vitiligo, café au lait lesions, and acromelanosis.[91] Angioid streaks may be present in the retina.

Patients with Cowden disease have a greatly increased risk of breast and thyroid carcinoma. The breast changes seen in women range from fibrocystic disease to adenocarcinoma and can occur at a young age. Prophylactic mastectomy may be indicated.[99] Thyroid adenoma is the most common thyroid tumor, but thyroid carcinoma can develop. Gastrointestinal tract polyposis is common.[93] There may also be an increased risk of gastrointestinal malignancy. One patient has been reported with a T lymphocyte defect who eventually developed acute myelogenous leukemia. Female reproductive tract hamartomas and benign tumors are common. Squamous carcinoma of the tongue and basal cell carcinoma of the perianal skin have been reported.

The facial tricholemmomas respond well to carbon dioxide laser vaporization.

Mucosal Neuroma Syndrome

Mucosal neuroma syndrome is probably a variant of multiple endocrine neoplasia, type 2 (MEN 2 or 2A, Sipple's syndrome). Also designated MEN 3 or MEN 2B, the typical features include oral, nasal, upper gastrointestinal tract, and conjunctival neuromas, associated with medullary thyroid carcinoma (MTC) and pheochromocytoma. The lesions are typically soft to firm intradermal nodules. Corneal nerves may be highly visible.[94] The appearance of the neuromas usually precedes the development of cancer, but the MTC can appear in early childhood. The major cause of death in patients

FIGURE 185-5

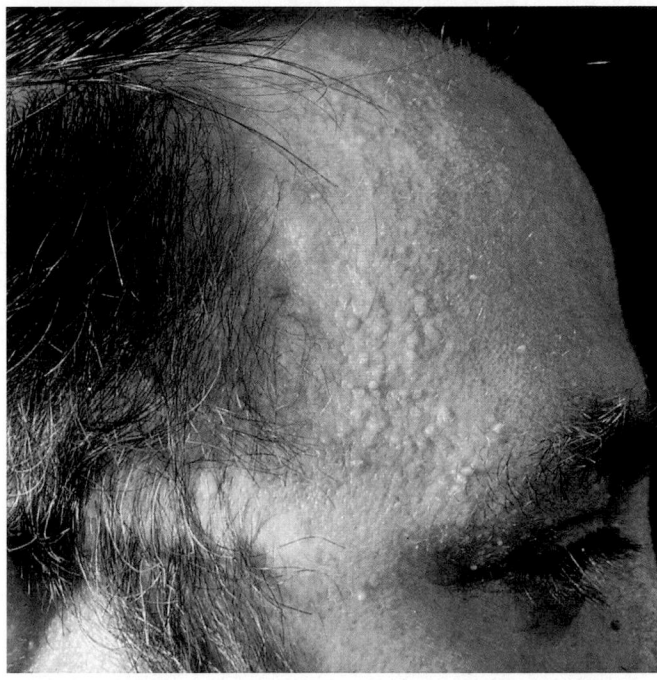

A.

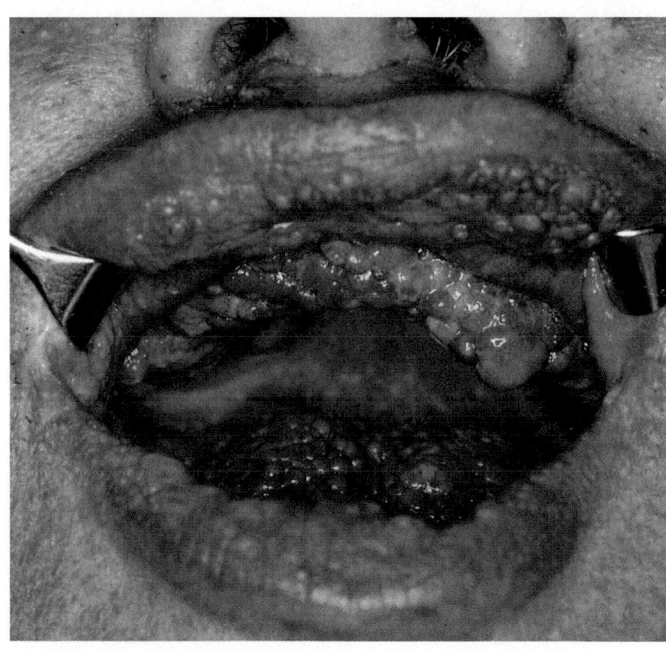

B.

A. Cowden disease with papular lesions on the forehead that histologically proved to be tricholemmomas. *B.* Oral mucosa of same patient with multiple fibropapillomas. (*Courtesy of Peter Fritsch, MD.*)

with MEN 3 is MTC, as metastases are common. The pheochromocytomas are often bilateral. Unlike MEN 2, parathyroid hyperplasia is rare.

In addition to the mucosal neuromas, other abnormalities can include "blubbery" lips, a marfanoid habitus, lax joints, kyphoscoliosis, lentigines, café au lait lesions, medullated corneal nerve fibers, diverticulosis, and megacolon.[95] Localized intense itching may be a feature in some patients.

Neurofibromatosis (See Chap. 191)

Von Recklinghausen's neurofibromatosis has many associated malignant tumors.[96] Malignant schwannoma is the most common, occurring in one series in 29 percent of patients.[97] These patients were usually over the age of 30. Other tumors include fibrosarcoma, rhabdomyosarcoma, nephroblastoma (Wilms' tumor), and acute and chronic myelogenous leukemia. There is an increased incidence of ocular melanoma, with anecdotal reports of cutaneous melanoma. Benign neural tumors, peripheral and intracranial, are common.

HORMONE-RELATED CONDITIONS (See Chap. 170)

Malignant tumors may release hormones into the circulation, and such hormones can produce skin manifestations. The manifestation of such hormone excess is not specific to the tumor and can occur secondarily from an excess of that hormone from any cause.

Hirsutism may be a manifestation of an increase in circulating androgens. Such androgen excess is most typically seen with testicular or ovarian tumors. Non-androgen-regulated hair increase, hypertrichosis, may result from porphyria cutanea tarda, which may be associated with internal malignancy, or may appear as hypertrichosis lanuginosa acquisita (see Chap. 163), also secondary to internal malignant disease.

Gynecomastia in the male can be produced by an excess of estrogens. Such estrogens may be produced by a tumor of the testis. Lung tumors can also produce gynecomastia.

Cushing's syndrome is generally secondary to excessive ACTH production. Tumors from widely diverse sites can produce excessive ACTH. Many of these are derived from APUD tissue. The most common site is the lung, with the pancreas being the next most common.

Acne can be caused by the same tumors that produce hirsutism. Acne may also be a marker for internal malignancy in another way. Female patients with severe acne show an apparent increase in the incidence of breast cancer. Patients with breast cancer have increased sebum production.[98] It may well be that the stimulus for breast cancer and for increased sebum production may result from a similar mechanism.

OTHER DISORDERS ASSOCIATED WITH PRIMARY SKIN CANCERS

Nevoid Basal Cell Carcinoma Syndrome (See also Chap. 158)

Nevoid basal cell carcinoma syndrome, or Gorlin-Goltz syndrome, is a syndrome consisting of multiple basal cell carcinomas, jaw cysts, skin pitting, skeletal abnormalities, and a tendency to malignant disease.[99] The most common malignant tumor is medulloblas-

toma.[100] These tumors can occur in patients without any cutaneous basal cell carcinomas but with a family history of nevoid basal cell carcinoma syndrome. Other tumors include astrocytomas, meningiomas, and craniopharyngiomas. Nevoid basal cell carcinoma syndrome is the result of a defective patched gene.[101]

Arsenical Manifestations

Chronic arsenic toxicity can be manifested by arsenical melanosis, plantar and palmar keratoses (Fig. 185-6), and Bowen's disease. There would also appear to be an increased risk of internal neoplasia. The increased cancer risk was originally estimated to be to nine times the expected incidence, with approximately one-third of patients with Bowen's disease developing an internal malignancy 6 to 10 years after their initial diagnosis.[102] Malignancies have included tumors of the urogenital region, mouth, esophagus, and lung. There is now evidence that not all patients with Bowen's disease, including both on sun-exposed and non-sun-exposed sites, have an increased risk of internal malignancy. When a large series of general Bowen's disease was compared to controls, no significant difference in systemic malignancy was found.[103] Arsenical keratoses on the palms (Fig. 185-6) and soles, a more specific finding, did correlate with an apparent increase in internal malignancy.[104]

Oral retinoids may be useful as chemopreventive drugs.

OTHER DISORDERS ASSOCIATED WITH INTERNAL MALIGNANT DISEASE

Pruritus

Pruritus, often accompanied by excoriations, can be a nonspecific marker of internal malignant disease. Although often associated with xerosis, the pruritus of malignant disease can occur in apparently normal skin. It can be continuous or paroxysmal. It is usually generalized.

When occurring with malignant diseases, pruritus is most commonly associated with leukemia and lymphoma, including drug-induced lymphoma.[105] The pruritus of Hodgkin's disease will often

FIGURE 185-6

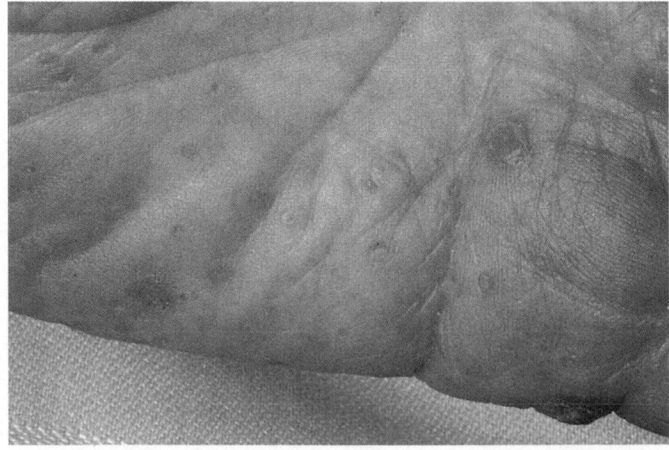

Punctate palmar keratoderma in a patient with previous arsenic exposure.

start on the legs, is usually continuous, and may be associated with a burning feeling. Pruritus is one of the most common cutaneous manifestations of leukemia, probably exceeded only by purpura. It is usually less severe than that associated with lymphoma and is more often generalized. Although the pruritus of both leukemia and lymphoma can precede the diagnosis, it is usually a sign of late disease. Its severity tends to parallel the course of the disease, with severe pruritus heralding a poor prognosis.[106]

Pruritus associated with bathing is a marker for polycythemia rubra vera and is present in half of patients.[107] This itch can be severe and paroxysmal. Patients with polycythemia rubra vera can also have chronic continuous pruritus unrelated to bathing.

Severe pruritus can be a feature of Fanconi's anemia and myeloma.

Pruritus associated with visceral neoplasia is most commonly associated with pancreatic and stomach tumors[108] but may also be associated with most other solid tumors. The appearance of severe pruritus after treatment of the primary tumor may herald a tumor recurrence. Renal and liver involvement with primary or metastatic cancer can also produce pruritus secondary to the accumulation in the skin of pruritogenic metabolites.

Erythema Gyratum Repens

Erythema gyratum repens is a cutaneous eruption consisting of concentric raised erythematous bands moving in waves over the body surface in a "wood-grain" pattern.[109] The erythematous bands may be flat or raised. They are frequently surmounted by a fine marginal desquamation and may move at a speed of approximately 1 cm/day. Removal of the malignant tumor usually results in complete resolution of erythema gyratum repens within 6 weeks.

Almost all cases of erythema gyratum repens, which is extremely rare, are associated with internal malignancy. Although first described with carcinoma of the breast,[109] erythema gyratum repens has also been found in association with tumors of the lung,[110] bladder, prostate, cervix, stomach, and esophagus and with multiple myeloma.

Subcutaneous Fat Necrosis (See also Chap. 111)

Subcutaneous fat necrosis is a cutaneous marker for acinar cell carcinoma of the pancreas. Identical lesions can also occur with pancreatitis[111] and pancreatic pseudocyst. Subcutaneous fat necrosis associated with pancreatic disease frequently has an associated polyarthralgia, which can affect most of the joints of the body. Ankle involvement is common. Intraosseus fat necrosis can also occur,[112] with the production of osteolytic lesions visible on x-ray examination. The polyarthralgia is presumably the result of fat necrosis of the periarticular tissue. There is frequently a concomitant associated fever and eosinophilia.

Sweet's Syndrome (See also Chap. 93)

In 1964, Sweet described a syndrome, which he termed *acute febrile neutrophilic dermatosis*.[113] Malignancy-associated Sweet's syndrome is most commonly seen with acute myelocytic leukemia but may also be observed in acute myelomonocytic leukemia, myelodysplastic syndrome, chronic myelogenous leukemia, acute lymphoblastic leukemia, chronic lymphocytic leukemia, hairy cell leukemia, multiple myeloma, and lymphoma. Much less commonly, it is seen with solid tumors such as embryonal carcinoma of the testes, ovarian carcinoma, gastric carcinoma, and adenocarcinoma of the breast, prostate, and rectum.

Hypertrichosis Lanuginosa Acquisita

Hypertrichosis lanuginosa acquisita (HLA) is an acquired excessive growth of lanugo (vellus) hairs. Soft downy hairs initially cover the face and ears, but eventually all hair-bearing skin may be involved (Fig. 185-7). Associated abnormalities include a glossitis that is often painful. The tongue is studded with red papules.[114] Fully expressed HLA is usually secondary to malignant tumors, but excessive lanugo hair growth can also be caused by drugs such as exogenous steroids, phenytoin, diazoxide, streptomycin, penicillamine, cyclosporine, and minoxidil or by conditions such as anorexia nervosa.

HLA secondary to malignancy is usually abrupt in its onset and is rapidly progressive. Associated tumors reported include tumors of the colon (including carcinoid tumors), rectum, bladder, lung, pancreas, gallbladder, uterus, and breast and lymphoma.[115–117] The excessive lanugo hair growth is presumably secondary to a circulating factor produced by the tumor, but has also occurred after cytotoxic chemotherapy for cancer.[118] Most of the tumors capable of producing HLA would appear to be of the APUD group.

FIGURE 185-7

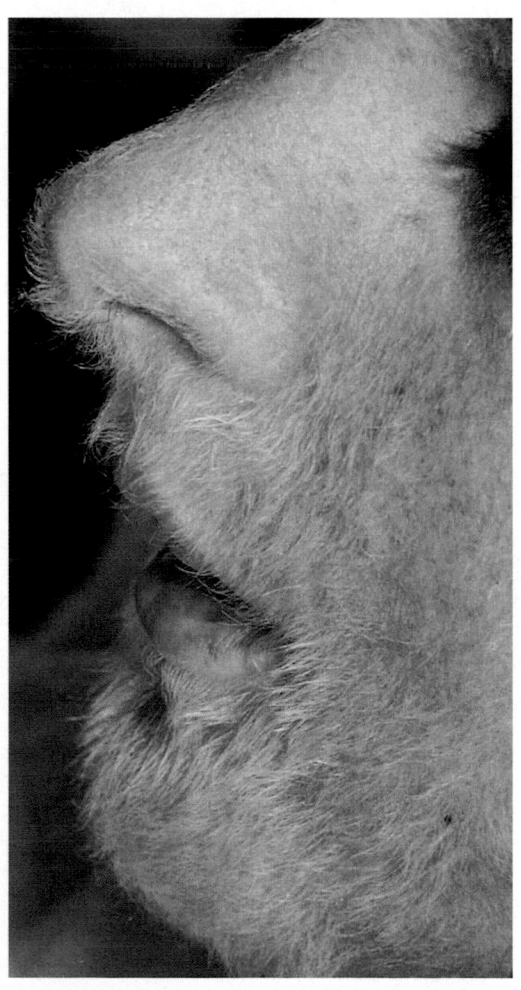

Hypertrichosis lanuginosa acquisita in a 19-year-old woman with pancreatic carcinoma.

Necrolytic Migratory Erythema

Necrolytic migratory erythema is a marker for an alpha-2-glucagon-producing islet cell tumor of the pancreas.[119–121] It is manifested by erythema, vesicles, pustules, bullae, and erosions, which typically involve the face, the intertriginous areas, in particular the groin, and the perigenital region (Fig. 185-8). It also involves the shins, ankles, and feet as well as the fingertips. The vesicles are often very superficial and tend to become confluent. Patients can also have brownish-red papules scattered over much of the skin surface. Associated abnormalities include a glossitis, stomatitis, dystrophic nails, alopecia, weight loss, anemia, and diabetes.

Most patients with necrolytic migratory erythema have a pancreatic tumor of the glucagon-producing type. Resection of the tumor clears the eruption, sometimes within 48 h. These patients have high blood glucagon levels. Infusion of amino acids has been reported to clear the dermatitis, as has an infusion of somatostatin or dacarbazine.[122]

The dermatitis has also occurred in patients without cancer but who have hepatitic cirrhosis and hyperglucagonemia, pancreatitis, celiac sprue, or zinc deficiency.[122,123]

FIGURE 185-8

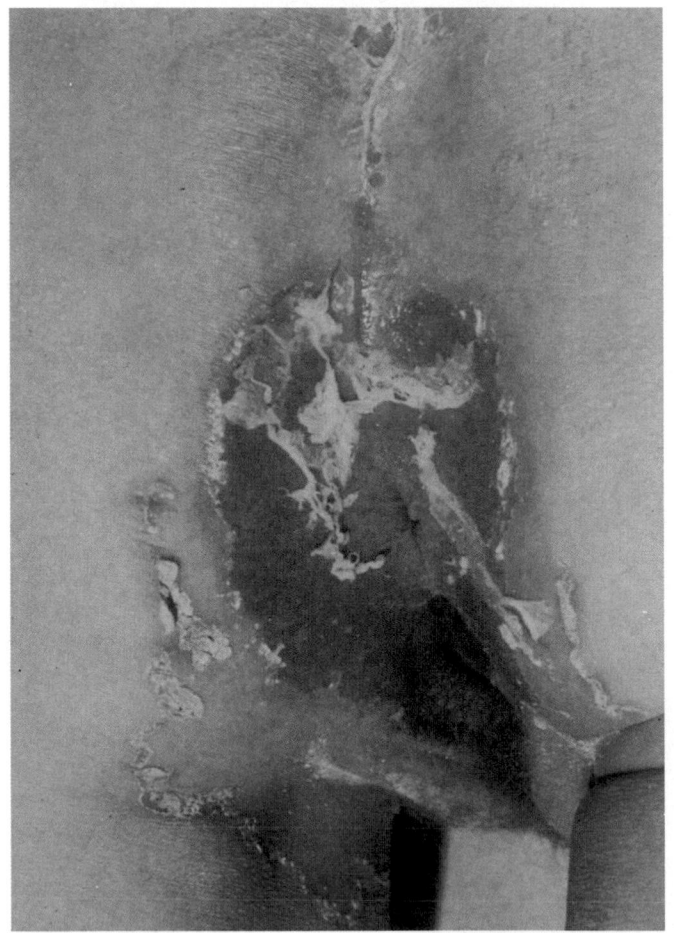

Necrolytic migratory erythema (glucagonoma syndrome). Flaccid vesicles and erosions in the perigenital and perianal region.

Clubbing

Clubbing is the soft tissue enlargement of the tips of the fingers and toes. More typically associated with chronic lung disease, it can also be associated with neoplasms of the chest, usually bronchogenic carcinoma.

Clubbing can also be associated with intestinal polyposis of the Cronkhite-Canada types and with schistosomal colonic polyposis. Clubbing is manifested by an enlargement of the distal digits. Clubbing accompanied by subperiosteal new bone formation is called *hypertrophic osteoarthropathy*. A more florid expression of this, accompanied by acromegalic features, is called *pachydermoperiostosis*. Patients with these latter two conditions can have diffusely painful bones. Pachydermoperiostosis is usually idiopathic but can be secondary to lung cancer.[124] The clubbing and associated bone changes can be either insidious or abrupt.

The most common tumor associated with clubbing is bronchogenic carcinoma. Five to ten percent of patients with bronchogenic carcinoma develop clubbing.[125] Mesothelioma can also produce similar changes. Clubbing can also be produced by other solid tumors metastatic to the thorax and has been reported in Hodgkin's disease of the lung. Clubbing can also be seen with diffuse intestinal lymphoma.

Some patients with clubbing secondary to pulmonary disease can develop an associated thickening and yellowing of the nails—the yellow nail syndrome.

Leukoderma (See Chap. 89)

Leukoderma is the acquired complete loss of normal skin pigment. The most common cause of leukoderma is vitiligo. Vitiligo is usually unassociated with malignant disease but has been reported rarely in association with thyroid carcinoma. Far more significant is the association of leukoderma and malignant melanoma. The appearance of leukoderma in patients after resection of their primary tumor may herald occult metastatic disease. Despite this, there is growing evidence that melanoma patients with metastatic disease and leukoderma may have a relatively prolonged survival.[126]

Peutz-Jeghers Syndrome (See also Chaps. 89 and 163)

First described by Hutchinson in 1900, the association of cutaneous and mucosal hyperpigmentation with gastrointestinal tract polyposis is now well known.[127] These gastrointestinal tract polyps can be associated with malignant tumors. The pigmentary changes involve both the skin and mucous membrane. The skin hyperpigmented macules are usually present at birth or early infancy and frequently fade at puberty. They can be typically grouped around the mouth, eyes, and nostrils, with pigmented macules also located on the fingers, palms, toes, periumbilical skin, or diffuse over the skin surface. Mucosal pigmented lesions are similar but persist for life. Buccal mucosal pigmented papillomas have also been described.

The most common malignancy associated with the Peutz-Jeghers syndrome is duodenal carcinoma. These malignant tumors are frequently associated with hamartomatous polyps. The lifetime risk of a patient with Peutz-Jeghers syndrome developing an upper gastrointestinal tract malignancy carries an overall cancer relative risk of up to 18.[127] Granulosa theca cell tumors may be present in as many as 20 percent of females with the Peutz-Jeghers syndrome and may be associated with precocious puberty. Peutz-Jeghers syndrome is inherited as an autosomal dominant condition.

Tuberous Sclerosis (See Chap. 190)

Tuberous sclerosis can be associated with tumors within many organ systems. Most of these are hamartomatous, and some of these can become malignant. However, malignant transformation in tuberous sclerosis is uncommon, occurring in probably no more than 5 percent of patients.

Multiple Eruptive Seborrheic Keratoses

Multiple eruptive seborrheic keratoses, also known as the sign of Leser-Trélat, have been mentioned in association with multiple internal malignancies.[128] These malignancies have included tumors of the stomach, breast, prostate, lung, and colon and malignant melanoma, as well as many references to their occurrence in lymphoma, primary lymphoma of the brain, and mycosis fungoides, including Sézary syndrome. They have also been mentioned in association with hyperkeratosis of the palms and soles associated with malignant disease and with acanthosis nigricans.

Evidence to support the presumed relationship of seborrheic keratoses to malignant disease is meager.[129] Most of the cancers described in association are common; seborrheic keratoses are common. Proving an uncommon causal relationship between a common cancer and a common skin sign is difficult. Reports of solitary cases abound.

A hallmark of many patients with so-called eruptive seborrheic keratoses is a cutaneous eruption that is also inflammatory. It may well be that the inflammatory dermatosis is centering around skin papillomas and seborrheic keratoses, making them suddenly "appear." Indeed, it is a common clinical experience to see an increase in the prominence of seborrheic keratoses in patients with generalized dermatitis from any cause. The sign of Leser-Trélat may or may not be a paraneoplastic syndrome.

If there is a relationship with cancer, it could be explained via growth factor or hormone effects on keratinocytes; perhaps a similar mechanism to that involved in the production of acanthosis nigricans, or by the removal of the immune suppression of precursor lesions possibly of papilloma virus origin.

Porphyria Cutanea Tarda (See Chap. 151)

Porphyria cutanea tarda has been associated with the development of malignant tumors, predominantly of the liver. The relative risk of hepatocellular carcinoma in patients with porphyria cutanea tarda has been estimated at 61,[130] a truly significant association. The porphyria cutanea tarda can predate or antedate the apparent development of the primary liver tumor.

DIRECT TUMOR INVOLVEMENT IN THE SKIN

Solid Tumors

Direct involvement of the skin by metastatic spread from a distant primary tumor is perhaps the most unquestioned marker for the internal malignancy. In a large review by Lookingbill et al.[131] skin involvement was the first sign of cancer in 0.8 percent of systemic cancer patients. Of this group, approximately equal numbers had direct extension to the skin, local metastases, or distant skin metastases. Direct extension was most common in patients with breast and oral cancer. Local metastases were most common in patients with breast cancer or pelvic cancer. Distant metastases were from many tumor types and sites.

Generally such a metastatic lesion is obvious, being an erythematous cutaneous or subcutaneous mass, and is frequently rapidly growing. At times, though, it can be difficult to diagnose metastatic lesions. This is especially true with metastases from breast cancer.

Most commonly breast cancer lesions metastasize to the anterior chest wall. They can typically show up as small nodules ranging from tiny 1- to 2-mm lesions to large masses of tumor (Fig. 185-9C). The tiny nodules can be erythematous or can be frankly hemorrhagic. The hemorrhage can be present within the nodules or in the field surrounding the nodules. Metastatic breast cancer can also present as an erysipelas-like eruption (carcinoma erysipelatodes, Fig. 185-9A, B). A diffuse, warm, indurated plaque appears on the skin surface. Frequently, it is asymptomatic but can be painful. Even more uncommon is the leatherlike skin change of sclerosing metastatic breast cancer known as carcinoma en cuirasse, which may later develop nodules and ulcerate (Fig. 185-10). Carcinoma en cuirasse can be progressive for many years, even decades, in the absence of any apparent systemic involvement.

Metastases from malignant melanoma are usually pigmented. Often there is a bluish tint to the lesion, even if it is deep in the skin. Even if the primary tumor was pigmented, the metastases can be amelanotic. The reverse is also true.

Other tumors that commonly metastasize to skin include tumors of the lung, stomach, kidney, and ovary. The scalp is quite commonly involved by metastases from lung, kidney, and breast tumors. Alopecia may result. The face and neck may be involved by metastases from oropharyngeal carcinomas.

Metastases to the skin can appear many years after extirpation of the primary tumor. Progression, as in the case of carcinoma en cuirasse, can be very slow and may indeed not appreciably shorten life expectancy. Generally, though, cutaneous metastases herald a poor prognosis, as evidence of systemic spread to other sites is usually quickly apparent.

Metastases from renal and thyroid carcinoma may be pulsatile and may have a bruit.

Lymphoma-Leukemia (See Chaps. 108 and 109)

Involvement of the skin with lymphoma cells is quite common, particularly in the case of a T cell lymphoma. T cell leukemias frequently have skin involvement, and this involvement may manifest itself as a diffuse erythroderma as is seen in Sézary syndrome.

B cell lymphomas can also involve the skin, with Hodgkin's disease being the most common. B cell lymphoma involvement of the skin is usually manifested by the development of one or more papules or nodules that may be ulcerated and form arcuate lesions (see Chap. 109). Alopecia can also be caused by lymphoma. Alopecia mucinosa is involvement of the hair follicles by lymphoma, with associated mucin deposition.

Aside from the erythroderma seen in T cell leukemia, other lymphocytic, myeloid, and myelomonocytic leukemias can have cutaneous manifestations. The most common of these are the infiltrations of the skin produced by monocytic or myelomonocytic leukemia, which can produce a leonine facies in addition to other infiltrative plaques. Involvement of the skin can be a presenting feature in myelomonocytic leukemia, although it generally occurs late in the course of the disease (see Chap. 109).

Multiple myeloma can appear as small red nodules on the skin surface with a diagnostic myeloma histology.

When assessing a solitary nodule that is histologically lymphoma but in the absence of any definable systemic disease, it is important

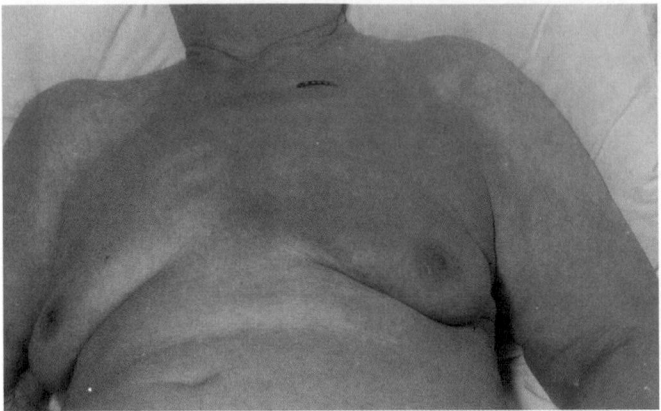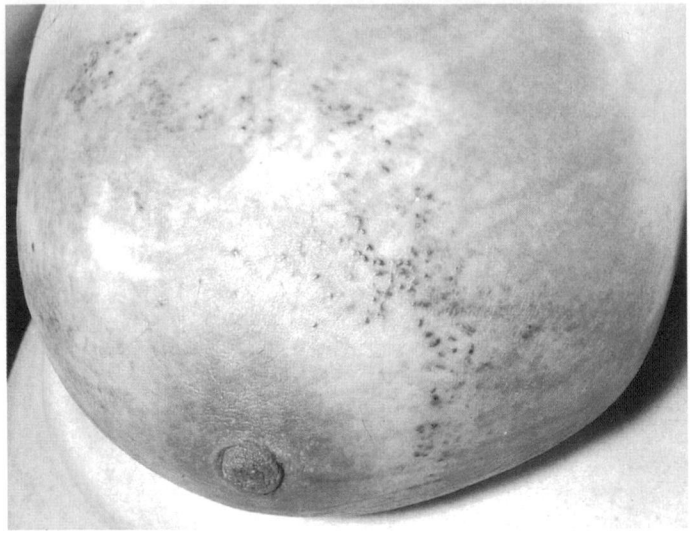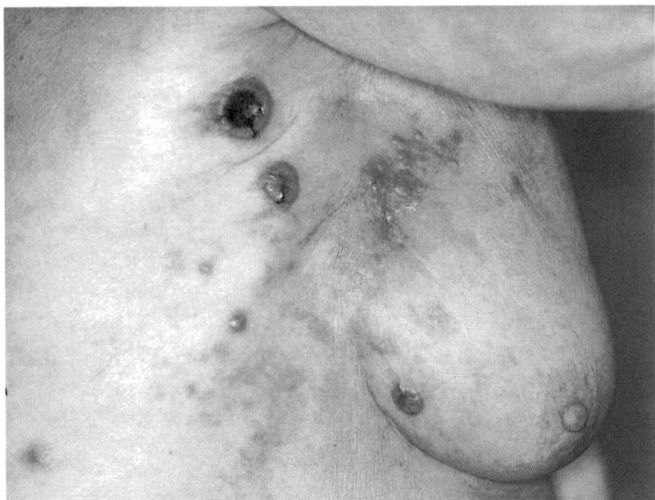

FIGURE 185-9

A.

B.

C.

Involvement of skin by metastatic breast cancer. *A.* Carcinoma erysipelatodes. Intralymphatic spread of mammary carcinoma that manifests as erysipelas-like erythema. *B.* In this close-up of another patient, the erysipelas-like quality of the erythema is even more evident. In addition, there are small, bright red lenticular metastases. *C.* Metastatic breast cancer can also present as nodules. These may ulcerate and can be very painful.

to consider the benign cutaneous lymphoid infiltrates in the differential diagnosis.

FIGURE 185-10

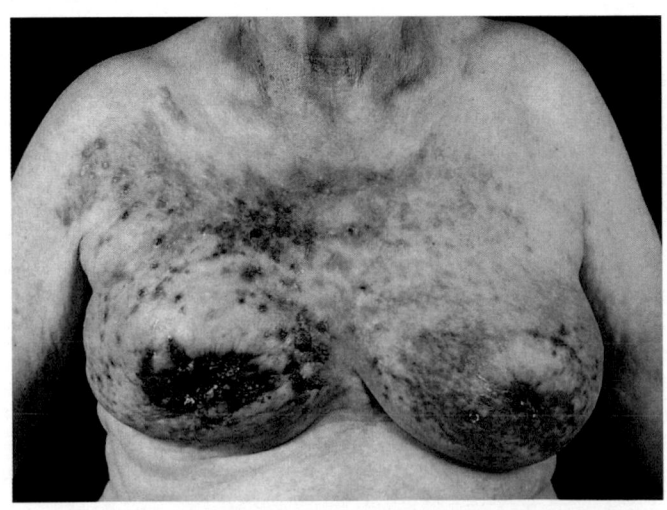

Cancer en cuirasse involving both breasts and thoracic wall.

Paget's Disease (See Chap. 86)

Paget's disease of the nipple is an erythematous scaling eruption that indicates ductal carcinoma of the underlying breast. Extramammary Paget's disease, which can occur in the anogenital skin, similarly may be associated with an underlying adenocarcinoma. The underlying carcinoma may be of apocrine or eccrine sweat gland origin, or can be from the rectum or urethra.

REFERENCES

1. McLean D: Cutaneous paraneoplastic syndromes. *Arch Dermatol* **122**:765, 1986
2. Nelson DH et al: ACTH-producing pituitary tumors following adrenalectomy for Cushing's syndrome. *Ann Intern Med* **52**:560, 1960
3. Silberberg I et al: Diffuse melanosis in malignant melanoma. *Arch Dermatol* **97**:671, 1968
4. Konrad K, Wolff K: Pathogenesis of diffuse melanosis secondary to malignant melanoma. *Br J Dermatol* **91**:635, 1974
5. Rorsman H et al: Trichochromuria in melanosis of melanoma. *Acta Derm Venereol (Stockh)* **66**:468, 1986
6. Andreev VC, Petkov I: Skin manifestations associated with tumours of the brain. *Br J Dermatol* **92**:675, 1975

7. Powell LW, Isselbacher KJ: Hemochromatosis, in *Harrison's Principles of Internal Medicine,* 14th ed, edited by AS Fauci et al. New York, McGraw-Hill, 1998, p 2149

8. Lynch PJ, Winkelmann RK: Generalized plane xanthoma and systemic disease. *Arch Dermatol* **93**:639, 1966

9. McCadden ME et al: Mycosis fungoides associated with dystrophic xanthomatosis. *Arch Dermatol* **123**:91, 1987

10. Cooper PH et al: Association of juvenile xanthogranuloma with juvenile myeloid leukemia. *Arch Dermatol* **120**:371, 1984

11. Feingold KR et al: Cutaneous xanthoma in association with paraproteinemia in the absence of hyperlipidemia. *J Clin Invest* **83**:796, 1989

12. Maize JC et al: Xanthoma disseminatum and multiple myeloma. *Arch Dermatol* **110**:758, 1974

13. Gertz MA, Kyle RA: Acute leukemia and cytogenetic abnormalities complicating melphalan treatment of primary systemic amyloidosis. *Arch Intern Med* **150**:629, 1990

13. Gagel RF et al: Multiple endocrine neoplasia type 2A associated with cutaneous lichen amyloidosis. *Ann Intern Med* **111**:802, 1989

14. Kaplan LM: Endocrine tumors of the gastrointestinal tract and pancreas, in *Harrison's Principles of Internal Medicine,* 14th ed, edited by AS Fauci et al. New York, McGraw-Hill, 1998, p 584

15. Aldrich LB et al: Distinguishing features of idiopathic flushing and carcinoid syndrome. *Arch Intern Med* **148**:2614, 1988

16. Umeki S et al: Harlequin syndrome (unilateral flushing and sweating attack) due to spinal invasion of the left apical lung cancer (in Japanese). *Rinsho* Shinkeigaku **30**:94, 1990

17. Rosenbaum FF et al: Essential telangiectasia, pulmonic and tricuspid stenosis, and neoplastic liver disease: A possible new clinical syndrome. *J Lab Clin Med* **42**:941, 1953

18. Morrell D et al: Mortality and cancer incidence in 263 patients with ataxia-telangiectasia. *J Natl Cancer Inst* **77**:89, 1986

19. Swift M et al: Breast and other cancers in families with ataxia-telangiectasia. *N Engl J Med* **316**:1289, 1987

20. French AJ, Lilleyman JS: Bleeding tendency of T-cell lymphoblastic leukemia. *Lancet* **2**:469, 1979

21. Cairns SA et al: Squamous cell carcinoma of bronchus presenting with Henoch-Schönlein purpura. *Br Med J* **2**:474, 1978

22. Lacour JP et al: Cutaneous vasculitis and renal cancer: Two cases. *Am J Med* **94**:104, 1993

23. Greer JM et al: Vasculitis associated with malignancy. *Medicine (Baltimore)* **67**:220, 1988

24. Hughes GRV et al: Polyarteritis nodosa and hairy-cell leukemia. *Lancet* **1**:678, 1979

25. Gerber MA et al: Periarteritis nodosa, Australia antigen and lymphatic leukemia. *N Engl J Med* **286**:14, 1972

26. Palmer HM: Digital vascular disease and malignant disease. *Br J Dermatol* **91**:476, 1974

27. Fagrell B, Mellstedt H: Polycythemia vera as a cause of ischemic digital necrosis. *Acta Chir Scand* **144**:129, 1978

28. Vieta JO, Heymann AD: Mondor's disease. *N Y State J Med* **77**:120, 1977

29. Goldberg RJ et al: Occult malignant neoplasm in patients with deep venous thrombosis. *Arch Intern Med* **147**:251, 1987

30. Lindelöf B et al: Pemphigoid and cancer. *Arch Dermatol* **126**:66, 1990

31. Ogawa H et al: The incidence of internal malignancies in pemphigus and bullous pemphigoid in Japan. *J Dermatol Sci* **9**:136, 1995

32. Sood VD, Pasricha JS: Pemphigus and Hodgkin's disease. *Br J Dermatol* **90**:575, 1974

33. Stillman MA, Baer RL: Pemphigus and thymoma. *Acta Derm Venereol (Stockh)* **52**:393, 1972

34. Vetters JM et al: Pemphigus vulgaris and myasthenia gravis. *Br J Dermatol* **88**:437, 1973

35. Safai B et al: Pemphigus vulgaris associated with a syndrome of immunodeficiency and thymoma: A case report. *Clin Exp Dermatol* **3**:129, 1978

36. Imamura S et al: Pemphigus foliaceus, myasthenia gravis, thymoma and red cell aplasia. *Clin Exp Dermatol* **3**:285, 1978

37. Anhalt GJ et al: Paraneoplastic pemphigus: An autoimmune mucocutaneous disease associated with neoplasia. *N Engl J Med* **323**:1729, 1990

38. Sigurgeirsson B et al: Risk of lymphoma in patients with dermatitis herpetiformis. *BMJ* **308**:13, 1994

39. Reunala T et al: Lymphoma in dermatitis herpetiformis: Report on four cases. *Acta Derm Venereol (Stockh)* **62**:343, 1982

40. Swerdlow AJ et al: Mortality and cancer incidence in patients with dermatitis herpetiformis: A cohort study. *Br J Dermatol* **129**:140, 1993

41. Dupont C: Herpes gestationis with hydatidiform mole. *Trans St John's Hosp Dermatol Soc* **60**:103, 1974

42. Halkier-Sorensen L et al: Herpes gestationis in association with neoplasma malignum generalisatum. *Acta Derm Venereol (Stockh)* **120**(suppl):96, 1985

43. Delattre JY et al: Erythema multiforme and Stevens-Johnson syndrome in patients receiving cranial irradiation and phenytoin. *Neurology* **38**:194, 1988

44. Trump DL et al: Epidermolysis bullosa acquisita. *JAMA* **243**:1461, 1980

45. Green ST, Natarajan S: Linear IgA disease and oesophageal carcinoma. *J R Soc Med* **80**:48, 1987

46. McEvoy MT, Connolly SM: Linear IgA dermatosis: Association with malignancy. *J Am Acad Dermatol* **22**:59, 1990

47. Wilson JF et al: Herpes zoster in Hodgkin's disease. *Cancer* **29**:461, 1972

48. Rusthoven JJ et al: Varicella-zoster infection in adult cancer patients. A population study. *Arch Intern Med* **148**:1561, 1988

49. Shneidman DW et al: Chronic cutaneous herpes simplex. *JAMA* **241**:592, 1979

50. Rigel DS, Jacobs MI: Malignant acanthosis nigricans: A review. *J Dermatol Surg Oncol* **6**:923, 1980

51. Ollendorff-Curth H: Significance of acanthosis nigricans. *Arch Dermatol* **66**:80, 1952

52. Wilgenbus K et al: Further evidence that acanthosis nigricans maligna is linked to enhanced secretion by tumor of transforming growth factor alpha. *Arch Dermatol Res* **284**:266, 1992

53. Howel-Evans W et al: Carcinoma of the oesophagus with keratosis palmaris et plantaris (tylosis). *Q J Med* **27**:413, 1958

54. Harper PS et al: Carcinoma of the oesophagus with tylosis. *Q J Med* **30**:317, 1970

55. Blanchet-Bardon C et al: Hereditary epidermolytic palmoplantar keratoderma associated with breast and ovarian cancer in a large kindred. *Br J Dermatol* **117**:363, 1987

56. Dobson RL et al: Palmar keratoses and cancer. *Arch Dermatol* **92**:553, 1965

57. Mortimer P et al: Palmar keratoses and internal malignancy. *Br J Dermatol* **109**:21, 1983

58. Andreev VC: Skin manifestations in visceral cancer, in *Current Problems in Dermatology,* series editor, H Mali. Basel, Karger, 1978

59. Breathnach SM, Wells GC: Acanthosis palmaris: Tripe palms. A distinctive pattern of palmar keratoderma frequently associated with internal malignancy. *Clin Exp Derematol* **5**:181, 1980

60. Lawrence N et al: A palmar dermatosis linked to occult carcinoma of the upper thorax, head and neck: Bazex's syndrome and tripe palm. *Laryngoscope* **100**:1323, 1990

61. Lo WL, Wong CK: Tripe palms: A significant cutaneous sign of internal malignancy. *Dermatology* **185**:151, 1992

62. Jacobsen F et al: Acrokeratosis paraneoplastica (Bazex syndrome). *Arch Dermatol* **120**:502, 1984

63. Bazex A, Griffiths A: Acrokeratosis paraneoplastica—a new cutaneous marker of malignancy. *Br J Dermatol* **102**:301, 1980

64. Baran R: Paraneoplastic acrokeratosis of Bazex. *Arch Dermatol* **113**:1613, 1977

65. Pecora A et al: Acrokeratosis paraneoplastica (Bazex syndrome). *Arch Dermatol* **119**:820, 1983

66. Juhlin L, Baran R: Abnormal amino acid composition of nails in Bazex's paraneoplastic acrokeratosis. *Acta Derm Venereol (Stockh)* **64**:31, 1984

67. Bolognia JL: Basex syndrome: Acrokeratosis paraneoplastica. *Semin Dermatol* **14**:84, 1995

68. Richard M, Giroux JM: Acrokeratotis paraneoplastica (Bazex syndrome). *J Am Acad Dermatol* **16**:178, 1987

69. Bazex A et al: Génodermatose complexe de type indéterminé associant une hypotrichose, un état atrophodermique généralisé et des dégénérescence cutanées multiples (épithéliomas basocellulaires). *Bull Soc Fr Dermatol Syphiligr* **71**:206, 1964

70. Manchul LA et al: The frequency of malignant neoplasms in patients with polymyositis-dermatomyositis. A controlled study. *Arch Intern Med* **145**:1835, 1985

71. Lakhanpal S et al: Polymyositis, dermatomyositis and malignant lesions: Does an association exist? *Mayo Clin Proc* **61**:645, 1986

72. Zantos D et al: The overall and temporal association of cancer with polymyositis and dermatomyositis. *J Rheumatol* **21**:1855, 1994

73. Richardson JB, Callen JP: Dermatomyositis and malignancy. *Med Clin North Am* **73**:1211, 1989

74. Basset-Sequin N et al: Prognostic factors and predictive signs of malignancy in adult dermatomyositis. *Arch Dermatol* **126**:633, 1990

75. Tuffanelli DL, Winkelmann RK: Systemic scleroderma. *Arch Dermatol* **84**:359, 1961

76. Haggani MT, Holti G: Systemic sclerosis with pulmonary fibrosis and oat cell carcinoma. *Acta Derm Venereol (Stockh)* **53**:369, 1973

77. Muir EG et al: Multiple primary carcinomata of the colon, duodenum and larynx associated with kerato-acanthomata of the face. *Br J Surg* **54**:191, 1967

78. Torre D: Multiple sebaceous tumours. *Arch Dermatol* **98**:549, 1968

79. Burgdorf WH et al: Muir-Torre syndrome. Histologic spectrum of sebaceous proliferations. *Am J Dermatopathol* **8**:202, 1986

80. Housholder MS, Zeligman I: Sebaceous neoplasms associated with visceral carcinomas. *Arch Dermatol* **116**:61, 1980

81. Schwartz RA et al: The Torre syndrome with gastrointestinal polyposis. *Arch Dermatol* **116**:312, 1980

82. Bitran J, Pellettiere EV: Multiple sebaceous gland tumors and internal carcinoma: Torre's syndrome. *Cancer* **33**:835, 1974

83. Fusaro RM et al: Torre's syndrome as phenotypic expression of cancer family syndrome. *Arch Dermatol* **116**:986, 1980

84. Hall NR et al: Genetic linkage in Muir-Torre syndrome to the same chromosomal regions as cancer family syndrome. *Eur J Cancer* **30A**:180, 1994

85. Spielvogel RL et al: Oral isotretinoin therapy for familial Muir-Torre syndrome. *J Am Acad Dermatol* **12**:475, 1985

86. Stone MD et al: Torre's syndrome: Exacerbation of cutaneous manifestations with immunosuppression. *J Am Acad Dermatol* **15**:1101, 1986

87. Gardner EJ: A genetic and clinical study of intestinal polyposis, a predisposing factor for carcinoma of the colon and rectum. *Am J Hum Genet* **3**:167, 1951

88. Golitz LE: Heritable cutaneous disorders which affect the gastrointestinal tract. *Med Clin North Am* **64**:829, 1980

89. Lynch PJ: Nevoid basal cell carcinoma syndrome with features of Gardner's syndrome. *Cutis* **16**:905, 1975

90. Lloyd KM, Dennis M: Cowden's disease. *Ann Intern Med* **58**:136, 1963

91. Gentry WC et al: Multiple hamartoma syndrome (Cowden's disease). *Arch Dermatol* **109**:521, 1974

92. Brownstein MH et al: Cowden's disease. *Cancer* **41**:2393, 1978

93. Taylor AJ et al: Alimentary tract lesions in Cowden's disease. *Br J Radiol* **62**:890, 1989

94. Aine E et al: Visible corneal nerve fibers and neuromas of the conjunctiva—a syndrome of type-3 multiple endocrine adenomatosis in two generations. *Graefes Arch Clin Exp Ophthalmol* **225**:213, 1987

95. Gorlin RJ et al: Multiple mucosal neuroma, pheochromocytoma and medullary carcinoma of the thyroid—a syndrome. *Cancer* **22**:293, 1968

96. Bader JL: Neurofibromatosis and cancer. *Ann N Y Acad Sci* **486**:57, 1986

97. Das Gupta TK, Brasfield RD: von Recklinghausen's disease. *Cancer* **21**:174, 1971

98. Burton JL et al: Increased sebum excretion in patients with breast cancer. *Br Med J* **1**:665, 1970

99. Gorlin RJ: Nevoid basal cell carcinoma syndrome. *Medicine (Baltimore)* **66**:98, 1987

100. Gorlin RJ et al: The multiple basal cell nevi syndrome. *Cancer* **18**:89, 1965

101. Johnson RL et al: Human homolog of patched, a candidate gene for the basal cell nevus syndrome. *Science* **272**:1668, 1996

102. Graham JH, Helwig EB: Bowen's disease and its relationship to systemic cancer. *Arch Dermatol* **80**:133, 1959

103. Andersen SLC et al: Relationship between Bowen's disease and internal malignant tumors. *Arch Dermatol* **108**:367, 1973

104. Reymann F et al: Relationship between arsenic intake and internal malignant neoplasms. *Arch Dermatol* **114**:378, 1978

105. Rubinstein N et al: Generalized pruritus as a presenting symptom of phenytoin-induced Hodgkin's disease. *Int J Dermatol* **24**:54, 1985

106. Feiner AS et al: Prognostic importance of pruritus in Hodgkin's disease. *JAMA* **240**:2738, 1978

107. Wasserman LR: The treatment of polycythemia vera. *Semin Hematol* **13**:57, 1976

108. Newbold PCH: Skin markers of malignancy. *Arch Dermatol* **102**:680, 1970

109. Gammel JA: Erythema gyratum repens. *Arch Dermatol Syphilol* **66**:494, 1952

110. Appell ML et al: Erythema gyratum repens. *Cancer* **62**:548, 1988

111. Hughes PSH et al: Subcutaneous fat necrosis associated with pancreatic disease. *Arch Dermatol* **111**:506, 1975

112. Radin DR et al: Pancreatic acinar cell carcinoma with subcutaneous and intraosseous fat necrosis. *Radiology* **158**:67, 1986

113. Sweet RD: An acute febrile neutrophilic dermatosis. *Br J Dermatol* **76**:349, 1964

114. Hegedus SI, Schorr WF: Acquired hypertrichosis lanuginosa and malignancy. *Arch Dermatol* **106**:84, 1972

115. Hensley GT, Glynn KP: Hypertrichosis lanuginosa as a sign of internal malignancy. *Cancer* **24**:1051, 1969

116. McLean DI, Macaulay JC: Hypertrichosis lanuginosa acquisita associated with pancreatic carcinoma. *Br J Dermatol* **96**:313, 1977

117. Jemec GBE: Hypertrichosis lanuginosa acquisita. *Arch Dermatol* **122**:805, 1986

118. Gaffney CC, Roberts JT: Hypertrichosis lanuginosa acquisita following cytotoxic chemotherapy. *Clin Oncol (R Coll Radiol)* **4**:267, 1992

119. McGavran MH et al: A glucagon-secreting alpha-cell carcinoma of the pancreas. *New Engl J Med* **274**:1408, 1966

120. Wilkinson DS: Necrolytic migratory erythema with carcinoma of the pancreas. *Trans St John's Dermatol Soc* **59**:244, 1973

121. Mallinson CN et al: A glucagonoma syndrome. *Lancet* **2**:1, 1974

122. Rappersberger K et al: Das Glukagonom—Syndrom. *Hautarzt* **38**:589, 1987

123. Sinclair SA, Reynolds NJ: Necrolytic migratory erythema and zinc deficiency. *Br J Dermatol* **136**:783, 1997

124. Braverman IM: *Skin Signs of Systemic Disease,* 2d ed. Philadelphia, Saunders, 1981

125. Minna JD: Neoplasms of the lung, in *Harrison's Principles of Internal Medicine,* 14th ed, edited by AS Fauci et al. New York, McGraw-Hill, 1998, p 552

126. Nordlund JJ et al: Vitiligo in patients with metastatic melanoma: A good prognostic sign. *J Am Acad Dermatol* **9**:689, 1983

127. Giardiello FM et al: Increased risk of cancer in the Peutz-Jeghers syndrome. *N Engl J Med* **316**:1511, 1987

128. Venencie PY, Perry HO: Sign of Leser-Trélat: Report of two cases and review of the literature. *J Am Acad Dermatol* **10**:83, 1984

129. Rampen HJ, Schwengle LE: The sign of Leser-Trélat, does it exist? *J Am Acad Dermatol* **21**:50, 1989

130. Kauppinen R, Mustajoki P: Acute hepatic porphyria and hepatocellular carcinoma. *Br J Cancer* **57**:117, 1988

131. Lookingbill DP et al: Skin involvement as the presenting sign of internal carcinoma—a retrospective study of 7616 cancer patients. *J Am Acad Dermatol* **22**:19, 1990

CHAPTER 186

Karen R. Houpt
Ponciano D. Cruz, Jr.

Acanthosis Nigricans

Acanthosis nigricans is a cutaneous marker, most commonly of insulin resistance and less frequently of a malignancy. It is recognized clinically by hyperpigmented, hyperkeratotic, verrucous plaques that bestow a velvety texture on involved skin. Typically symmetric in distribution, it usually involves intertriginous areas, including the neck, axillae, groin, antecubital and popliteal fossae, and umbilicus[1,2]; occasionally, it involves the oral, esophageal, pharyngeal, laryngeal, conjunctival, and anogenital mucosae.[3–9]

HISTORIC ASPECTS

The term *acanthosis nigricans* was originally proposed by Unna, although the first cases were described independently in 1891 by Pollitzer and by Janovsky. Other patients have since been reported, many of whom have been classified into malignant, benign, or syndromic acanthosis nigricans or pseudoacanthosis nigricans, as suggested by Curth.[10–13] A key advance toward understanding the pathogenesis was made in 1976 by Kahn et al.,[14] who described two syndromes of insulin resistance: the *type A syndrome*, seen in younger women with acanthosis nigricans, masculinization, and hyperandrogenism, is characterized by defective insulin receptors; whereas the *type B syndrome*, seen in older women with acanthosis nigricans and autoimmune diseases, is associated with circulating anti-insulin receptor autoantibodies. Although the concept of acanthosis nigricans as a marker of malignancy remains valid, most cases are related to insulin resistance.[15–25]

EPIDEMIOLOGY

The incidence and prevalence of acanthosis nigricans in the general population is not known, although its frequency in selected subpopulations has been studied. Stuart et al.[18] identified the skin disorder in 7 percent of public school children in the sixth and eighth grades. This prevalence rose to 28 percent among children judged to be obese based on ideal body weight, with boys and girls affected equally. A relatively high frequency was noted in blacks (13 percent) compared to Hispanics (6 percent) and whites (0.5 percent)[18]; in a separate study, an even higher prevalence was documented in Native-American children (32 percent).[26] Hud et al.[19] observed acanthosis nigricans in 74 percent of adult patients treated for obesity; black patients in this study also had a higher frequency of the skin disorder than did other ethnic groups.

Malignancy-associated acanthosis nigricans is quite rare. In one study it was present in only 1 of 35 patients with intrathoracic or intraabdominal malignancies,[27] and in another, in only 2 out of 12,000 cancer patients examined.[28] It has been reported in patients of all age groups but more commonly in middle-aged and older individuals of either gender.[8,9,27]

PATHOGENESIS

Although the precise basis for the development of acanthosis nigricans remains unclear, there is ample evidence to implicate an etiologic role for insulin.[29–31] At normal concentrations, insulin binds preferentially to classic receptors through which it transduces effects on glucose metabolism. By contrast, at higher concentrations, it binds with greater affinity to insulin-like growth factor (IGF) receptors through which it promotes effects on cellular proliferation.[17,32] Insulin can reach the skin, where it may affect fibroblasts and keratinocytes, both of which have been shown to express classic insulin and IGF receptors.[33] Tissue resistance to insulin leads to hyperinsulinemia, which should favor increased binding of insulin to IGF receptors, which in turn may stimulate the proliferation of keratinocytes and dermal fibroblasts in a manner that produces acanthosis nigricans.[32,33]

Hyperinsulinemia may also trigger the ovarian hyperandrogenism that commonly coexists with acanthosis nigricans in women with severe insulin resistance (e.g., type A syndrome of insulin resistance and polycystic ovarian syndrome).[32] The prevalence of the skin eruption in hyperandrogenic women has been reported to be between 5 and 29 percent.[29,30] An etiologic role for androgens has been suggested by the improvement of acanthosis nigricans in two hyperandrogenic women who were treated with antiandrogen medications.[34] Other studies have provided contrary evidence, showing that antiandrogen treatments reversed hirsutism but had no effect on the acanthosis nigricans.[35]

The pathogenesis of malignancy-associated acanthosis nigricans is even less clear. A humoral factor produced by the tumor is likely, given that the skin disorder can improve or even resolve following treatment of the malignancy.[11] Elevated levels of transforming growth factor α in urine and of its receptor (epidermal growth factor receptor) in lesional skin were noted in a patient with acanthosis nigricans, acrochordons, the sign of Leser-Trélat, and melanoma. The enhanced expression of this cytokine and its receptor normalized after surgical treatment of the melanoma, and the acanthosis nigricans, acrochordons, and seborrheic keratoses improved postoperatively.[36] In a separate case, a gastric cancer was also shown to express transforming growth factor α and epidermal growth factor receptors.[37]

CLINICAL MANIFESTATIONS

The clinical hallmark of acanthosis nigricans is the development of grayish-brown, velvety plaques that may start merely as a dirty appearance. The hyperpigmentation is later accompanied by hypertrophy, increased skin markings, and papillomatosis. The most commonly involved locations in order of decreasing frequency are the axillae (Fig. 186-1), neck (Fig. 186-2), external genitalia, groin, face, inner thighs, antecubital and popliteal fossae, umbilicus (Fig.

FIGURE 186-1

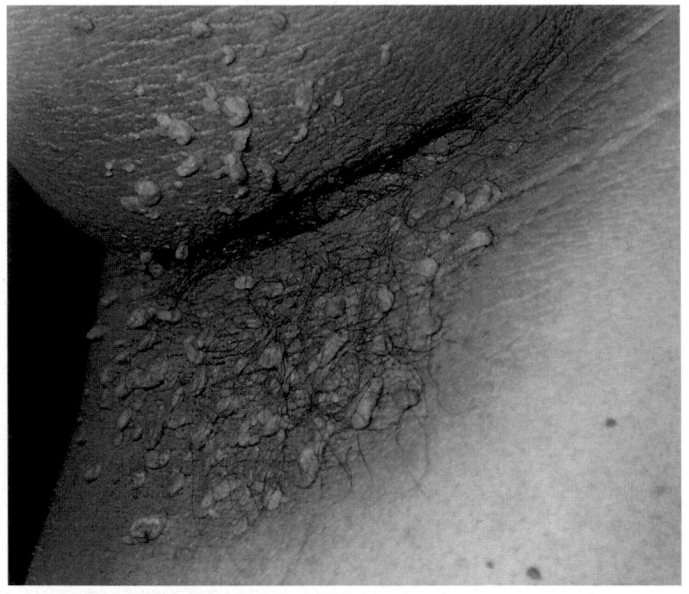

Acanthosis nigricans involving the axilla, with numerous acrochordons.

FIGURE 186-2

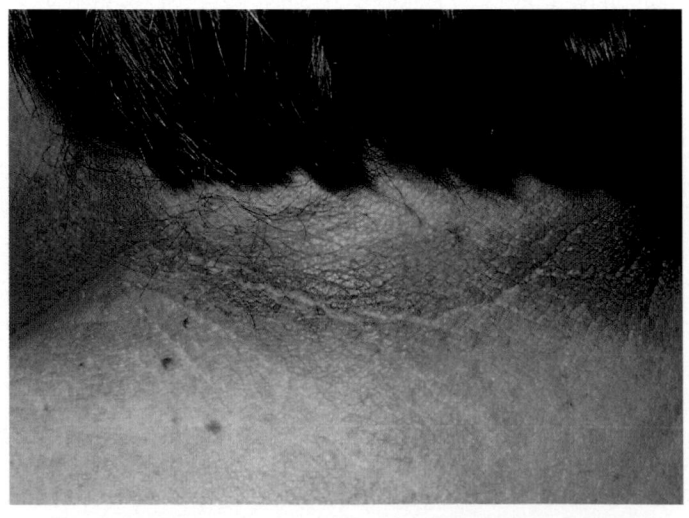

Acanthosis nigricans involving the neck.

FIGURE 186-3

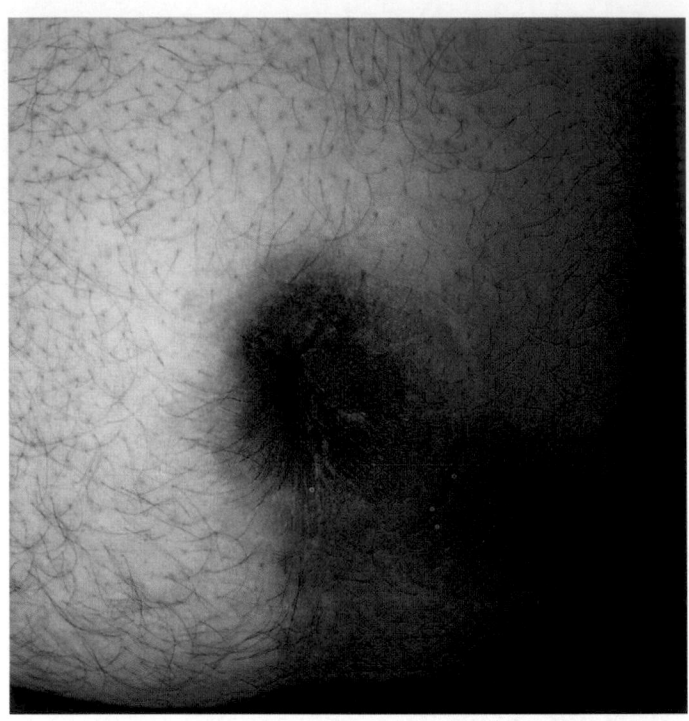

Acanthosis nigricans involving the umbilicus.

186-3), and perianal area.[2] Acrochordons may develop, either superimposed on the acanthosis nigricans (Fig. 186-1) or in other locations. Tylosis (palmoplantar hyperkeratosis) and acanthosis palmaris or pachydermatoglyphy (exaggeration of fingerprints) may also occur. The latter condition is also called "tripe palms" because of its similarity to the rugose appearance of bovine foregut (Fig. 186-4).[9] Mucocutaneous surfaces may also be affected, and the eruption can be generalized, particularly in cases associated with malignancy.[9,38,39] Mucosal involvement may consist of thickening and papillomatosis with minimal hyperpigmentation (Fig. 186-5).[3–7,15,40,41]

ASSOCIATED CONDITIONS

From a management standpoint, acanthosis nigricans is best classified based on the underlying problem or cause (Table 186-1).

INSULIN RESISTANCE Acanthosis nigricans is a common feature of several insulin-resistant states. *Insulin resistance* is defined as hyperinsulinemia inappropriate for the concurrent plasma glucose level.[8,9,42,43] Obesity, previously categorized by Curth as pseudoacanthosis nigricans, is the most commonly associated condition.[13] Moreover, a positive correlation has been shown between the development of acanthosis nigricans and the severity of obesity.[18,19] The skin changes often parallel the development of obesity; conversely, these changes can regress following appropriate weight reduction. Insulin resistance in obese individuals is most likely due to reduced affinity of the classic receptors for insulin and/or to postreceptor defects.[33]

Mutations of the insulin receptor gene or postreceptor defects have been implicated in other insulin-resistant states, such as lepre-

FIGURE 186-4

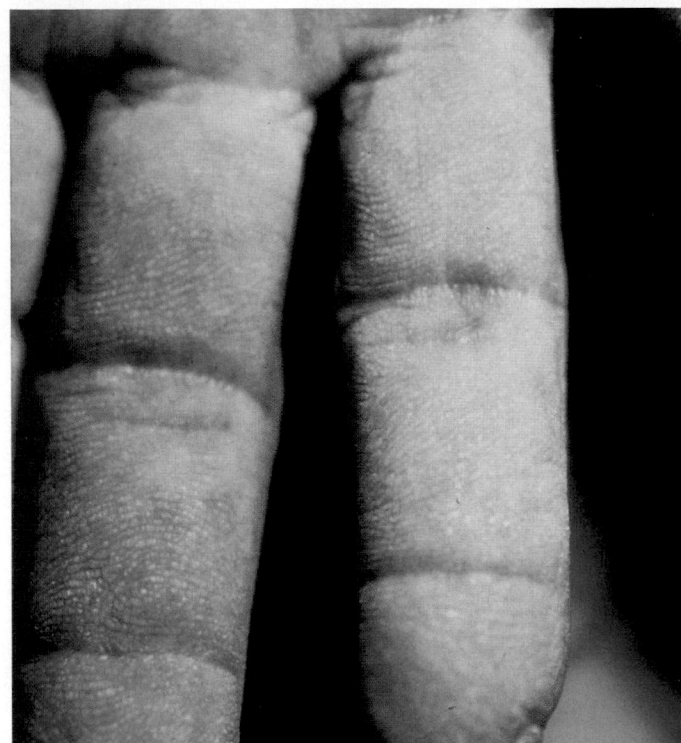

Acanthosis palmaris, pachydermatoglyphy, or tripe palm.

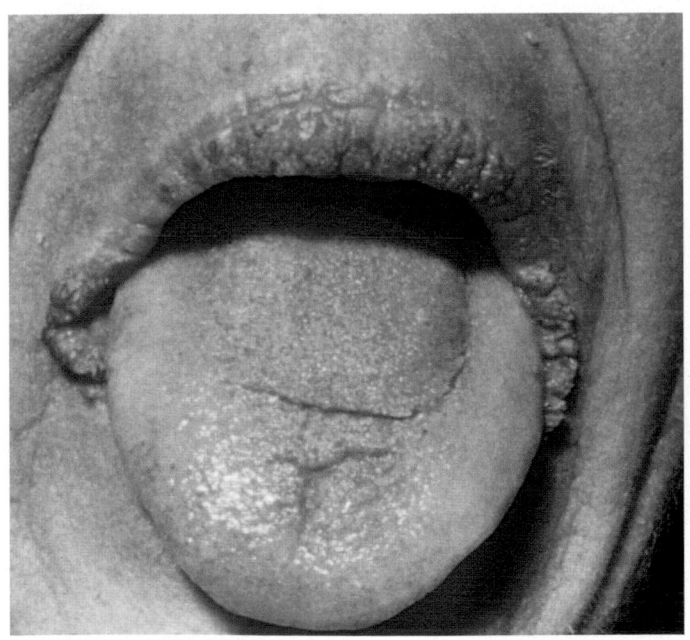

Acanthosis nigricans involving the lips, with minimal hyperpigmentation. *(All rights reserved. Reprinted with permission from the American Academy of Dermatology.)*

FIGURE 186-5

TABLE 186-1

Classification of Acanthosis Nigricans Based on the Most Common Associations

Insulin resistance–related
  Leprechaunism (Donohue syndrome)
  Lipodystrophies
  Obesity
  Polycystic ovarian disease (Stein-Leventhal syndrome)
  Pseudoacromegaly
  Rabson-Mendenhall syndrome
  Rud syndrome
  Type A syndrome
  Type B syndrome
Malignancy-related (see Table 186-2)
Drug-induced
Idiopathic
  Familial
  Nonfamilial
Other
  Syndromic (see Table 186-3)
  Acral acanthotic anomaly
  Nevoid form

chaunism, Lawrence-Seip syndrome (congenital lipodystrophy), pseudoacromegaly, Rabson-Mendenhall syndrome, and the type A syndrome.[16,17,20,23–25,44–50]

The lipodystrophies are acquired or congenital syndromes that differ in the extent of fat atrophy. The congenital form is also known as Lawrence-Seip syndrome. The generalized form has been equated with lipoatrophic diabetes mellitus and is characterized by an almost complete absence of body fat. The more common partial form exhibits atrophy of fat localized to the head, upper trunk, and upper extremities. Patients may develop hepatosplenomegaly, cardiomegaly, lymphadenopathy, muscle hypertrophy, and acanthosis nigricans. Mental retardation is common, hirsutism and hypertrophied external genitalia may be present, and renal disease may develop. In addition to hyperinsulinemia, hyperglycemia and hypertriglyceridemia may be present.[33]

Leprechaunism is characterized by an elfin appearance of the face, thickened skin, absence of subcutaneous fat, and hirsutism. The Rabson-Mendenhall syndrome consists of dental dysplasia, dystrophic nails, premature puberty, and acanthosis nigricans.[33]

Patients with the type A syndrome usually have generalized and severe acanthosis nigricans. Reported cases have been overwhelmingly in black women, with the onset of signs and symptoms in infancy or early childhood. Associated features include hirsutism, clitoromegaly, and masculine habitus.[33,51]

Patients with the type B syndrome have also been mostly black women. Unlike type A patients, however, these patients tend to manifest acanthosis nigricans after their teens, and the skin changes are less extensive and less severe. Furthermore, in contrast to the progressive nature of acanthosis nigricans in the type A syndrome, patients with type B symptoms may exhibit waxing and waning of the skin changes in parallel with worsening and improvement of their underlying immunologic diseases, the most common of which has been systemic lupus erythematosus. Insulin resistance in these patients is due to circulating anti-insulin receptor autoantibodies that compete with insulin for binding to classic receptors.[33,51]

TABLE 186-2

Malignancies Reported in Association with Acanthosis Nigricans

Adenocarcinomas	Lung carcinomas
Gastric	Bronchoalveolar
Other	Squamous cell
Endocrinologic malignancies	Small cell
Carcinoid	Lymphoreticular
Pheochromocytoma	Lymphomas
Pinealoma	Cutaneous T cell lymphoma
Testicular	Other carcinomas
Thyroid	Cervical
Melanoma	Urinary bladder
Sarcomas	

MALIGNANCY Acanthosis nigricans may precede, occur simultaneously with, or develop following the clinical onset of the malignancy.[9,11] Malignancy-associated acanthosis nigricans tends to be more extensive and to involve mucosal surfaces.[9] The vast majority of associated malignancies documented by Curth were adenocarcinomas, most commonly gastric in origin.[11] Other associated malignancies are listed in Table 186-2.[8,9,52–54]

DRUGS Acanthosis nigricans has been reported in association with systemic administration of testosterone, nicotinic acid, diethylstilbestrol, oral contraceptives, triazinate, glucocorticoids, and with topical application of fusidic acid.[8,9,55] Acanthosis nigricans developing at sites of subcutaneous insulin injections has also been described.[56]

TABLE 186-3

Syndromes Associated with Acanthosis Nigricans

Acromegaly	Laurence-Moon-Bardet-Biedel syndrome
Addison disease	Lawrence-Seip syndrome (congenital
Alstrom syndrome	lipodystrophy)*
Ataxia-telangiectasia	Lipoatrophic diabetes*
Barter syndrome	Lupoid hepatitis
Beare-Stevenson syndrome	Lupus erythematosus
Benign encephalopathy	MORFAN syndrome (mental retardation, over-
Bloom syndrome	growth, remarkable facies, acanthosis nigricans)
Capozucca syndrome	Phenylketonuria
Chondrodystrophy with dwarfism	Pituitary hypogonadism
Costello syndrome	Pituitary tumors
Crouzon syndrome	Prader-Willi syndrome
Cushing's syndrome	Pseudoacromegaly*
Dermatomyositis	Pyramidal tract degeneration
Diabetes insipidus	Rud syndrome*
Donohue syndrome (leprechaunism)*	Scleroderma
Edwards syndrome*	Stein-Leventhal syndrome (polycystic ovarian
Gigantism	disease)*
HAIR-AN syndrome (hyperandrogenemia,	Streak gonads
insulin resistance, acanthosis nigricans)*	Type A syndrome of insulin resistance*
Hashimoto thyroiditis	Type B syndrome of insulin resistance*
Hepatic cirrhosis	Werner syndrome
Hirschowitz syndrome	Wilson disease (hepatolenticular degeneration)
Hypothyroidism	

* Shown to be associated with insulin resistance.

IDIOPATHIC True idiopathic acanthosis nigricans requires the exclusion of an underlying cause (insulin resistance, obesity, endocrinopathy, malignancy, or drug).[9,11,13] Familial cases of idiopathic acanthosis nigricans have been reported, with onset at birth, during childhood, or more commonly at puberty.[9,57] These cases appear to be inherited as an autosomal dominant trait with variable penetrance.[9,57] Because obesity is commonly familial, it may be difficult to differentiate obesity-related familial acanthosis nigricans from the idiopathic familial form. Two distinguishing features of the latter are worsening of the acanthosis nigricans during puberty and irreversibility of the skin changes despite weight reduction.[13]

OTHER Numerous other syndromes have been reported in association with acanthosis nigricans (Table 186-3).[8,9,42,58,59] Insulin resistance appears to be the pathogenic link in many syndromes, but it has not been documented in others.

An atypical case, termed *acral acanthotic anomaly*, was noted in a nonobese 60-year-old black man with velvety skin on the backs of his hands and feet that worsened after renal dialysis. The possibility of drug-induced acanthosis nigricans in this case was raised by a remote history of oral testosterone treatment for impotence.[8,60] A transient form of acanthosis nigricans was reported following bone marrow transplantation in a patient with lymphoblastic lymphoma, who developed graft-versus-host disease that was treated with prednisolone.[61] Finally, an idiopathic, unilateral (nevoid) form of acanthosis nigricans has been described.[8,62,63]

DIFFERENTIAL DIAGNOSIS

The distinctive clinical appearance and distribution of acanthosis nigricans renders the diagnosis readily apparent. Occasionally, however, acanthosis nigricans may simulate a hyperpigmented nevus (Becker's, epidermal, or melanocytic), reticulate pigmented flexural anomaly (Dowling-Degos disease), or confluent and reticulated papillomatosis (Gougerot-Carteaud syndrome).[8,64] Mycosis fungoides has been reported to mimic acanthosis nigricans.[65] Oral acanthosis nigricans may be confused with Cowden's disease, dyskeratosis congenita, hereditary benign intraepithelial dyskeratosis, lipoid proteinosis, pachyonychia congenita, pyostomatitis vegetans, and Wegener's granulomatosis.[6]

HISTOPATHOLOGY

The histology of acanthosis nigricans is consistent regardless of its clinical associations. Characteristic features include hyperkeratosis and slight acanthosis undulating with dermal papillomatosis (Fig. 186-6). The clinical brown color is likely a result of hyperkeratosis (rather than of hypermelanosis, which is usually minimal to nil). Thus, the name acanthosis nigricans has little histologic justifica-

FIGURE 186-6

CHAPTER 186
Acanthosis Nigricans

2125

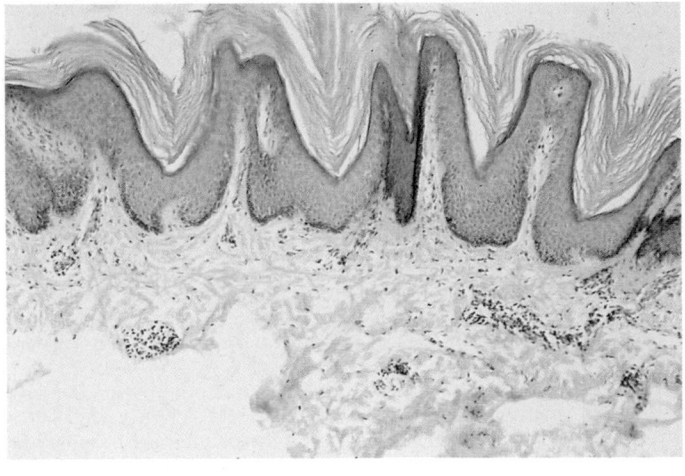

Histology of acanthosis nigricans demonstrating hyperkeratosis and slight acanthosis alternating with dermal papillomatosis.

tion.[6,9,64] Mucous membrane involvement may display focal parakeratosis, greater acanthosis, and epithelial papillary hyperplasia.[6]

LABORATORY TESTS

The underlying cause may be suggested by historic information and physical examination findings. It is important to exclude a malignancy, especially in nonobese patients with no readily discernible cause of acanthosis nigricans. In these cases, screening tests appropriate for the patient's age, risk factors, and other leading features should be performed. Because insulin resistance is the most common etiologic factor, the authors recommend concurrent fasting plasma determinations of insulin and glucose. Inappropriate hyperinsulinemia for the corresponding plasma glucose level supports a diagnosis of insulin resistance. Hyperandrogenic women should be tested for plasma testosterone and dehydroepiandrosterone sulfate. Patients with rheumatic diseases should be tested for antinuclear and anti-insulin receptor autoantibodies.

TREATMENT

Whenever possible, the underlying cause should be identified and treated. Obese patients can reverse the skin changes with weight loss. Systemic and topical retinoids have been used with varying success.[66–69] Patients with the type A syndrome have been treated with ovarian wedge resection, with or without cyclical norethindrone and mestranol,[34,70,71] oral contraceptives,[34,72] ketoconazole,[73,74] or cyproterone acetate.[75] In some patients, infusion of IGF improved the acanthosis nigricans and hyperinsulinemia but aggravated the hyperandrogenism.[76,77] The management of cases with type B syndrome should be directed primarily toward the underlying autoimmune disease. In one case of lipodystrophic diabetes, the acanthosis nigricans improved following dietary fish oil supplementation.[78] Malignancy-associated acanthosis nigricans may regress following effective treatment of the underlying cancer.[11] In

one case, cyproheptadine improved the skin condition, despite progression of the metastatic disease.[79]

REFERENCES

1. Chuang SD et al: Familial acanthosis nigricans with madarosis. *Br J Dermatol* **133**:104, 1995
2. Pollitzer S: Acanthosis nigricans. *JAMA* **53**:1369, 1909
3. Tabandeh H et al: Conjunctival involvement in malignancy-associated acanthosis nigricans. *Eye* **7**:648, 1993
4. Lamba PA, Lal S: Ocular changes in benign acanthosis nigricans. *Dermatologica* **140**:356, 1970
5. Pindborg JJ, Gorlin RJ: Oral changes in acanthosis nigricans (juvenile type): Survey of the literature and report of a case. *Acta Derm Venereol* **42**:63, 1962
6. Hall JM et al: Oral acanthosis nigricans: Report of a case and comparison of oral and cutaneous pathology. *Am J Dermatopathol* **10**:68, 1988
7. Kozlowski LM, Nigra TP: Esophageal acanthosis nigricans in association with adenocarcinoma from an unknown primary site. *J Am Acad Dermatol* **26**:348, 1992
8. Schwartz RA: Acanthosis nigricans. *J Am Acad Dermatol* **31**:1, 1994
9. Brown J, Winkelmann RK: Acanthosis nigricans: A study of 90 cases. *Medicine* **47**:33, 1968
10. Curth HO et al: The site and histology of the cancer associated with malignant acanthosis nigricans. *Cancer* **15**:364, 1962
11. Curth HO: Cancer associated with acanthosis nigricans: Review of literature and report of a case of acanthosis nigricans with cancer of the breast. *Arch Surg* **47**:517, 1943
12. Curth HO: Benign type of acanthosis nigricans: Etiology. *Arch Dermatol* **34**:353, 1936
13. Curth HO, Aschner BM: Genetic studies on acanthosis nigricans. *Arch Dermatol* **79**:55, 1959
14. Kahn CR et al: The syndromes of insulin resistance and acanthosis nigricans: Insulin-receptor disorders in man. *N Engl J Med* **294**:739, 1976
15. Grasinger CC et al: Vulvar acanthosis nigricans: A marker for insulin resistance in hirsute women. *Fertil Steril* **59**:583, 1993
16. Moller DE, Flier JS: Insulin resistance—mechanisms, syndromes, and implications. *N Engl J Med* **325**:938, 1991
17. Flier JS: Lilly Lecture: Syndromes of insulin resistance: From patient to gene and back again. *Diabetes* **41**:1207, 1992
18. Stuart CA et al: Prevalence of acanthosis nigricans in an unselected population. *Am J Med* **87**:269, 1989
19. Hud JA et al: Prevalence and significance of acanthosis nigricans in an adult obese population. *Arch Dermatol* **128**:941, 1992
20. Garcier F, Claudy AL: Acanthosis nigricans in monozygotic twins with post receptor defects causing insulin resistance. *Clin Exp Dermatol* **10**:358, 1985
21. Minaker KL et al: Phenytoin-induced improvement in muscle cramping and insulin action in three patients with the syndrome of insulin resistance, acanthosis nigricans, and acral hypertrophy. *Arch Neurol* **46**:981, 1989
22. Flier JS et al: Familial insulin resistance with acanthosis nigricans, acral hypertrophy, and muscle cramps. *N Engl J Med* **303**:970, 1980
23. Reddy SS-K et al: Molecular defects in the insulin receptor in patients with leprechaunism and in their parents. *J Lab Clin Med* **114**:165, 1989
24. Goodman PA et al: Growth factor receptor regulation in the Minn-1 leprechaun: Defects in both insulin receptor and epidermal growth factor receptor gene expression. *Metabolism* **41**:504, 1992
25. Maddux BA et al: Inhibitors of insulin receptor tyrosine kinase in fibroblasts from diverse patients with impaired insulin action: Evidence for a novel mechanism of postreceptor insulin resistance. *J Clin Endocrinol Metab* **77**:73, 1993
26. Stuart CA et al: Acanthosis nigricans among native americans: An indicator of high diabetes risk. *Am J Public Health* **84**:1839, 1994
27. Kierland RH: Acanthosis nigricans: An analysis of data in twenty-two cases and a study of its frequency in necropsy material. *J Invest Dermatol* **9**:299, 1947
28. Andreev VC: Malignant acanthosis nigricans. *Semin Dermatol* **3**:265, 1984

29. Flier JS et al: Acanthosis nigricans in obese women with hyperandrogenism: Characterization of an insulin-resistant state distinct from the type A and B syndromes. *Diabetes* **34**:101, 1985

30. Dunaif A et al: Characterization of groups of hyperandrogenic women with acanthosis nigricans, impaired glucose tolerance and/or hyperinsulinemia. *J Clin Endocrinol Metab* **65**:499, 1987

31. Peters EJ et al: Acanthosis nigricans and obesity: Acquired and intrinsic effects in insulin action. *Metabolism* **35**:807, 1986

32. Flier JS: Metabolic importance of acanthosis nigricans. *Arch Dermatol* **121**:193, 1985

33. Cruz PDJ, Hud JAJ: Excess insulin binding to insulin-like growth factor receptors: Proposed mechanism for acanthosis nigricans. *J Invest Dermatol* **98**:82s, 1992

34. Givens JR et al: Remission of acanthosis nigricans associated with polycystic ovarian disease and a stromal luteoma. *J Clin Endocrinol Metab* **38**:347, 1974

35. Corenblum B, Baglis BM: Medical therapy for the syndromes of familial virilization, insulin resistance and acanthosis nigricans. *Fertil Steril* **53**:421, 1990

36. Ellis DL et al: Melanoma, growth factors, acanthosis nigricans, the sign of Leser-Trélat, and multiple acrochordons: A possible role for alpha-transforming growth factor in cutaneous paraneoplastic syndromes. *N Engl J Med* **317**:1582, 1987

37. Wilgenbus K et al: Further evidence that acanthosis nigricans maligna is linked to enhanced secretion by the tumour of transforming growth factor alpha. *Arch Dermatol Res* **284**:266, 1992

38. Azizi E et al: Generalized malignant acanthosis nigricans (letter). *Arch Dermatol* **116**:381, 1980

39. Mikhail GR et al: Generalized malignant acanthosis nigricans. *Arch Dermatol* **115**:201, 1979

40. Pinto GL, Meyer DR: Ophthalmic manifestations of acanthosis nigricans. *Ophthal Plast Reconstr Surg* **10**:49, 1994

41. Groos EB et al: Eyelid involvement in acanthosis nigricans. *Am J Ophthalmol* **115**:42, 1993

42. Ober KP: Acanthosis nigricans and insulin resistance associated with hypothyroidism. *Arch Dermatol* **121**:229, 1985

43. Panidis D et al: Association of acanthosis nigricans with insulin resistance in patients with polycystic ovary syndrome. *Br J Dermatol* **132**:936, 1995

44. Accili D et al: Mutations in the insulin receptor gene in patients with genetic syndromes of insulin resistance and acanthosis nigricans. *J Invest Dermatol* **98**:77s, 1992

45. Taylor SI: Lilly Lecture: Molecular mechanisms of insulin resistance. Lessons from patients with mutations in the insulin-receptor gene. *Diabetes* **41**:1473, 1992

46. Bar RS et al: Insulin resistance, acanthosis nigricans and normal insulin receptors in a young woman: Evidence for a post-receptor defect. *J Clin Endocrinol Metab* **47**:620, 1978

47. Seemanova E et al: Autosomal dominant insulin resistance syndrome due to postbinding defect. *Am J Med Genet* **44**:705, 1992

48. Moller DE et al: Prevalence of mutations in the insulin receptor gene in subjects with features of the type A syndrome of insulin resistance. *Diabetes* **43**:247, 1994

49. Podskalny JM, Kahn CR: Cell culture studies on patients with extreme insulin resistance. I. Receptor defects on cultured fibroblasts. *J Clin Endocrinol Metab* **54**:261, 1982

50. Moller DE, Flier JS: Detection of an alteration in the insulin-receptor gene in a patient with insulin resistance, acanthosis nigricans, and the polycystic ovary syndrome (type A insulin resistance). *N Engl J Med* **319**:1526, 1988

51. Rendon MI et al: Acanthosis nigricans: A cutaneous marker of tissue resistance to insulin. *J Am Acad Dermatol* **21**:461, 1989

52. Gross G et al: Acanthosis nigricans maligna: Clinical and virological investigations. *Dermatologica* **168**:265, 1984

53. Cottoni F et al: Follicular mucinosis plus mycosis fungoides and acanthosis nigricans plus alveolar bronchiolar carcinoma. *Int J Dermatol* **34**:867, 1995

54. Gohji K et al: Acanthosis nigricans associated with transitional cell carcinoma of the urinary bladder. *Int J Dermatol* **33**:433, 1994

55. Teknetzis A et al: Acanthosis nigricans-like lesions after local application of fusidic acid. *J Am Acad Dermatol* **28**:501, 1993

56. Fleming MG, Simon SI: Cutaneous insulin reaction resembling acanthosis nigricans. *Arch Dermatol* **122**:1054, 1986

57. Tasjian D, Jarratt M: Familial acanthosis nigricans. *Arch Dermatol* **120**:1351, 1984

58. Seemanova E et al: Morfan: A new syndrome characterized by mental retardation, pre- and postnatal overgrowth, remarkable face and acanthosis nigricans in 5-year-old boy. *Am J Med Genet* **45**:525, 1993

59. Edwards JA et al: A new familial syndrome characterized by pigmentary retinopathy, hypogonadism, mental retardation, nerve deafness and glucose intolerance. *Am J Med* **60**:23, 1976

60. Schwartz RA: Acral acanthotic anomaly (AAA). *J Am Acad Dermatol* **5**:345, 1981

61. Ifrah N et al: Transient acanthosis nigricans following bone marrow transplantation for lymphoid malignancy. *Bone Marrow Transplant* **5**:281, 1990

62. Curth HO: Unilateral epidermal naevus resembling acanthosis nigricans. *Br J Dermatol* **95**:433, 1976

63. Krishnaram AS: Unilateral nevoid acanthosis nigricans. *Int J Dermatol* **30**:452, 1991

64. Lever WF, Schaumburg-Lever G: Metabolic diseases, in *Histopathology of the Skin,* 7th ed, edited by WF Lever, G Schaumburg-Lever et al. Philadelphia, Lippincott, 1990, p 477

65. Willemze R et al: Mycosis fungoides simulating acanthosis nigricans. *Am J Dermatopathol* **7**:365, 1985

66. Berger BJ, Gross PR: Another use for tretinoin—pseudoacanthosis nigricans. *Arch Dermatol* **108**:133, 1973

67. Darmstadt GL et al: Treatment of acanthosis nigricans with tretinoin. *Arch Dermatol* **127**:1139, 1991

68. Katz RA: Treatment of acanthosis nigricans with oral isotretinoin. *Arch Dermatol* **116**:110, 1980

69. Akovbyan VA et al: Successful treatment of acanthosis nigricans with etretinate. *J Am Acad Dermatol* **31**:118, 1994

70. Barth JH et al: Acanthosis nigricans, insulin resistance and cutaneous virilism. *Br J Dermatol* **118**:613, 1988

71. Imperato-McGinley J et al: Primary amenorrhea associated with hirsutism, acanthosis nigricans, dermoid cysts of the ovaries, and a new type of insulin resistance. *Am J Med* **65**:389, 1978

72. Friedman CI et al: Familial acanthosis nigricans: A longitudinal study. *J Reprod Med* **32**:531, 1987

73. Tercedor J et al: Effect of ketoconazole in the hyperandrogenism, insulin resistance and acanthosis nigricans (HAIR-AN) syndrome. *J Am Acad Dermatol* **27**:786, 1992

74. Pepper GM et al: Ketoconazole reverses hyperandrogenism in a patient with insulin resistance and acanthosis nigricans. *J Clin Endocrinol Metab* **65**:1047, 1987

75. Tatnall FM et al: The syndrome of acanthosis nigricans, hyperandrogenism and insulin resistance. *Clin Exp Dermatol* **9**:526, 1984

76. Kuzuya H et al: Trial of insulinlike growth factor I therapy for patients with extreme insulin resistance syndromes. *Diabetes* **42**:696, 1993

77. Ishihama H et al: Long-term follow up in type A insulin resistant syndrome treated by insulin-like growth factor I. *Arch Dis Child* **71**:144, 1994

78. Scheretz EF: Improved acanthosis nigricans with lipodystrophic diabetes during dietary fish oil supplementation. *Arch Dermatol* **124**:1094, 1988

79. Greenwood R, Tring FC: Treatment of malignant acanthosis nigricans with cyproheptadine. *Br J Dermatol* **106**:697, 1982

CHAPTER 187

Raul Fleischmajer

Scleredema

Scleredema is a connective tissue disease that was recognized as a distinct entity by Buschke in 1902. The disease affects all races and appears to be more prevalent among females. In a review of 209 cases by Greenberg et al.[1] 29 percent were children under 10 years, 22 percent were between 10 and 20 years old, and 49 percent were adults.

PATHOGENESIS

The cause of scleredema is unknown. Streptococcal hypersensitivity, injury of lymph channels, alterations of pituitary function, and peripheral nerve abnormalities have been proposed as hypotheses, but none has been substantiated. The dermis is markedly increased in thickness, although it appears that this finding is due in part to the replacement of subcutaneous tissue by connective tissue (Fig. 187-1). Chemical analysis of the dermis reveals an increase in hydroxyproline and hexosamines proportional to the increase in skin thickness.[2] Cultured fibroblasts reveal increased synthesis of total proteins and collagen and the elevation of mRNA levels of procollagens I and III.[3] Fractionation of acid mucopolysaccharides shows a normal distribution of hyaluronic acid and dermatan sulfate. The water content of the skin is normal.[2] Teller and Vester,[4] using electron microscopy, noted clumping of collagen fibrils, increase in

FIGURE 187-1

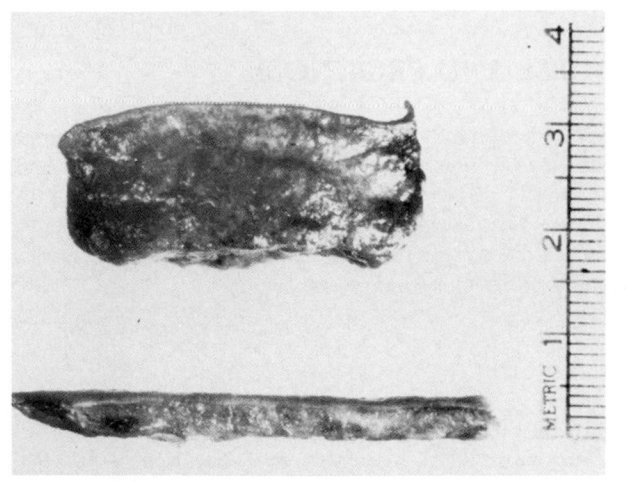

Scleredema skin from the back (*top*) and normal control. Note marked increase in thickness. (*From Fleischmajer et al.* [2])

ground substance, and collagen fibrils with reduced diameter. The urinary excretion of hydroxyproline and hydroxylysine appears normal.[5] Scleredema has been found in association with a monoclonal gammopathy. Serum immunoglobulins are usually of the IgG type, although IgA and IgM have also been reported. The chains are either of the kappa or lambda type.[6,7] The association of multiple myeloma and scleredema has been documented.[8–10] There is some evidence that the serum of scleredema patients may contain a factor that stimulates collagen synthesis.[7]

CLINICAL MANIFESTATIONS

Skin involvement may be preceded by a prodrome of low-grade fever, malaise, myalgia, and arthralgia. A few days to 6 weeks before the onset, 65 percent of patients develop an infection, usually of streptococcal origin.[1] Influenza, scarlet fever, measles, mumps, tonsillitis, pharyngitis, otitis, furuncles, erysipelas, and impetigo have been observed.

The onset is frequently sudden and consists of marked, nonpitting, symmetric induration of the skin, usually affecting the posterior and lateral aspects of the neck and spreading to the face, shoulders, back, arms, and thorax (Fig. 187-2). The buttocks, legs, and abdomen are less frequently involved, and the hands and feet are affected in about 10 percent of the cases. The disease usually reaches maximal involvement in about 1 to 2 weeks, although it may continue to spread for 2 to 3 additional months.

The induration is of wooden-like consistency, waxy white or shiny in appearance, and rather diffuse so that there is no sharp line

FIGURE 187-2

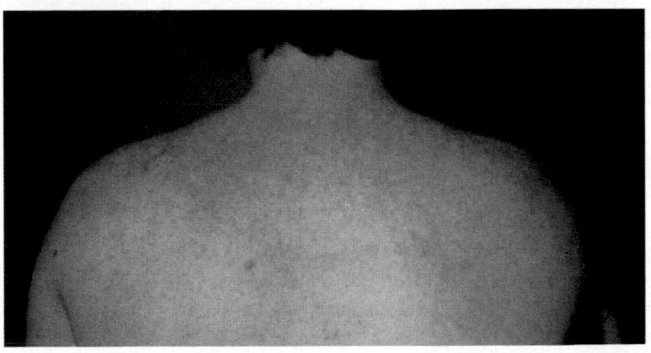

Scleredema of 41-year duration affecting the neck and back.

of demarcation between involved and noninvolved areas. Folding of the skin is almost impossible, and the normal markings are lost. When the face is involved, there is lack of expression and often difficulty in opening the mouth. Curtis and Shulak[11] described a transient, erythematous, macular or papular eruption during the early stage of the disease. Pain is absent, although paresthesia may occur. Heart abnormalities occur; in children the most common are diastolic gallop without evidence of cardiac failure, a nonspecific S-T depression, and T-wave inversion, usually reverting to normal in 3 to 9 months. Carditis secondary to rheumatic fever has been noted.[5]

In 1970, a syndrome was recognized that consists of scleredema of long duration, obesity, maturity onset, latent or overt diabetes, and a high incidence of cardiovascular disease.[2,12] Diabetic retinopathy is not uncommon.[2,12] Most patients are quite resistant to antidiabetic therapy, including insulin, chlorpropamide, and phenformin. Antidiabetic therapy has no effect on the evolution of the scleredema.

LABORATORY FINDINGS

Most laboratory tests are usually normal except for an increase in anti-streptolysin O titer in some patients. A glucose tolerance test should be performed to rule out diabetes mellitus. Hyperinsulinism may be present.[2]

PATHOLOGY

The epidermis and its appendages are normal. The dermis reveals collagen bundles separated by large interfascicular spaces (Fig. 187-3). The papillary layer is prominent and slightly edematous. In the upper dermis, there may be mild perivascular or scattered infiltrates consisting mostly of lymphocytes and histiocytic type cells. An increase in the numbers of mast cells has also been noted.[7,13] The secretory coils of the eccrine sweat glands are found in the upper third or mid-dermis. The subcutaneous tissue is reduced, probably due to its replacement by connective tissue.[2] The ground substance reveals an increase in metachromatic material when stained with toluidine blue.[14] This material also stains positive with alcian blue at pH 2.5 but not with alcian blue at pH 5.0, which stains sulfated acid mucopolysaccharides. Hyaluronidase digestion completely removes the alcian blue–positive material, suggesting an increase in hyaluronic acid. However, this increase is only temporary and does not appear in all patients.[14]

DIFFERENTIAL DIAGNOSIS

Scleredema has to be differentiated from the early edematous stage of systemic scleroderma. In systemic scleroderma Raynaud's phenomenon, a predilection for hands, abnormal pigmentation, telangiectasia, ischemia, and atrophic skin changes are usually present (see Chap. 174); these findings are not seen in scleredema. Scleredema should also be differentiated from trichinosis, dermatomyo-

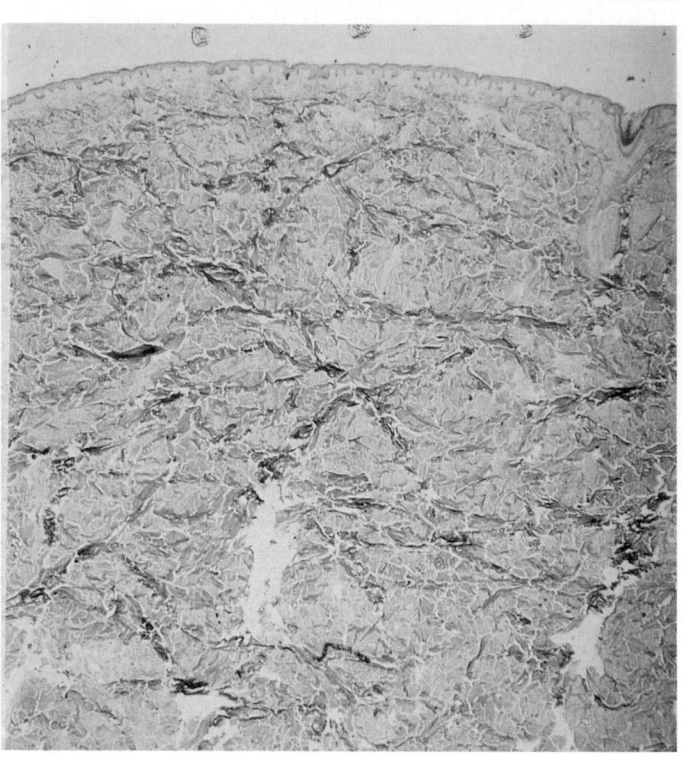

Scleredema. Edematous papillary layer, thick dermis, and large collagen bundles separated by interfascicular spaces. Trichrome, ×5.

sitis, scleromyxedema, myxedema, progeria, sclerema neonatorum, edema neonatorum, primary systemic amyloidosis, and edema from cardiac or renal origin.

TREATMENT

There is no effective treatment, although significant improvement was reported recently with the use of electron-beam therapy.[15]

COURSE AND PROGNOSIS

Prognosis is usually good, and the disease undergoes spontaneous resolution in 6 months to 2 years. However, Curtis and Shulak[11] noted that 25 percent of the patients showed no tendency toward resolution. The disease persists indefinitely in those patients with associated diabetes mellitus. In the Fleischmajer et al.[2] series, duration ranged from 2 to 41 years.

REFERENCES

1. Greenberg LM et al: Scleredema adultorum in children. *Pediatrics* **32**:1044, 1963
2. Fleischmajer R et al: Scleredema and diabetes mellitus. *Arch Dermatol* **101**:21, 1970
3. Varga J et al: Scleredema adultorum: Case report and demonstration of abnormal expression of extracellular matrix genes in skin fibroblasts "in vivo" and "in vitro." *Br J Dermatol* **132**:992, 1995

4. Teller H, Vester G: Elektronenmikroskopische Untersuchungsergebnisse an der Interzellularsubstanz des Coriums beim Skleroedema adultorum Buschke. *Z Haut Geschlechskr* **23**:142, 1957

5. Yogman M, Echeverria P: Scleredema and carditis: Report of a case and review of the literature. *Pediatrics* **54**:108, 1974

6. Kovary PM et al: Monoclonal gammopathy in scleroderma: Observations of three cases. *Arch Dermatol* **117**:536, 1981

7. Ohta A et al: Paraproteinemia in patients with scleredema: Clinical findings and serum effects on skin fibroblasts in vitro. *J Am Acad Dermatol* **16**:96, 1987

8. Schmidt KT et al: Scleredema and smoldering myeloma. *J Am Acad Dermatol* **26**:319, 1992

9. Sansom JE et al: A fatal case of scleredema of Buschke. *Br J Dermatol* **130**:669, 1994

10. Pujol JA: Improvement of scleredema associated with IgA multiple myeloma after chemotherapy. *Clin Exp Dermatol* **20**:149, 1995

11. Curtis AC, Shulak BM: Scleredema adultorum. *Arch Dermatol* **92**:526, 1965

12. Cohn BA et al: Scleredema adultorum of Buschke and diabetes mellitus. *Arch Dermatol* **101**:27, 1970

13. Breinin GM: Scleredema adultorum: Ocular manifestations. *Arch Ophthalmol* **50**:155, 1953

14. Fleischmajer R, Lara JV: Scleredema: A histochemical and biochemical study. *Arch Dermatol* **92**:643, 1965

15. Besson CA et al: Electron-beam therapy in scleredema adultorum with associated monoclonal hypergammaglobulinemia. *Br J Dermatol* **130**:394, 1994

CHAPTER 188

Raul Fleischmajer

Papular Mucinosis

Papular mucinosis, or lichen myxedematosus, is a rare disease characterized by a papular-lichenoid eruption, mucin deposition, and paraproteinemia. A clinical variant of papular mucinosis is scleromyxedema, in which the disease is more generalized and is accompanied by erythema and sclerosis.[1]

PATHOGENESIS

The pathogenesis of papular mucinosis remains unknown. This disease is frequently associated with paraproteinemia that consists of a myeloma-like, homogeneous serum globulin of the IgG type with predominantly lambda light chains, although kappa light chains have also been noted.[2,3] Less commonly, paraproteins of the IgM and IgA types have been identified. The paraprotein in papular mucinosis is a 7S, papain-sensitive globulin, which is strongly basic due to its high content of lysine.[3] Its molecular mass of about 110 kDa (normal IgG has a molecular mass of 160 kDa) suggests that this IgG globulin is incomplete, missing a significant antigenic portion of the Fc fragment.[4,5] The initial suggestion that papular mucinosis represents a plasma cell dyscrasia has never been substantiated. Its association with multiple myeloma is rare, if it occurs at all. Furthermore, the paraprotein in multiple myeloma is usually a monoclonal IgG with kappa light chains. Serum from patients with papular mucinosis can stimulate DNA synthesis and the proliferation of normal human fibroblasts in vitro.[6] However, the removal of the paraprotein from the culture medium does not decrease fibroblast mitosis, suggesting that another serum factor may be responsible for the proliferative effect.

CLINICAL MANIFESTATIONS

The disease affects adults from 30 to 70 years of age, has no sex predilection, and usually runs a chronic course. The primary lesion is a dome-shaped papule, skin color or erythematous, 2 to 4 mm in diameter; the lesions may be densely grouped in a lichenoid fashion or may show a linear arrangement. The areas most frequently affected are the dorsa of the hands and fingers, the axillary folds, and the external surfaces of the arms and legs. The coalescence of papules on the face, particularly in the glabella area, results in longitudinal folding, giving the appearance of leonine facies (Fig. 188-1). The lesions are usually asymptomatic, although mild pruritus may be present. In scleromyxedema, large parts of the body may be involved; the skin shows erythematous, scleroderma-like induration accompanied by reduced mobility of the lips, hands, arms, and legs (Fig. 188-2). Other skin lesions include urticaria, nodules, and cysts.[7] Although the disease primarily affects the skin, systematic manifestations have been described such as severe proximal myopathy,[8–10] inflammatory polyarthritis, central nervous system symptoms resembling acute organic brain syndrome,[11] esophageal aperistalsis, and hoarseness.[12,13] Ophthalmic findings consist of corneal opacities, lagophthalmos, ectropion, choroidal folds, and papilledema.[14]

FIGURE 188-1

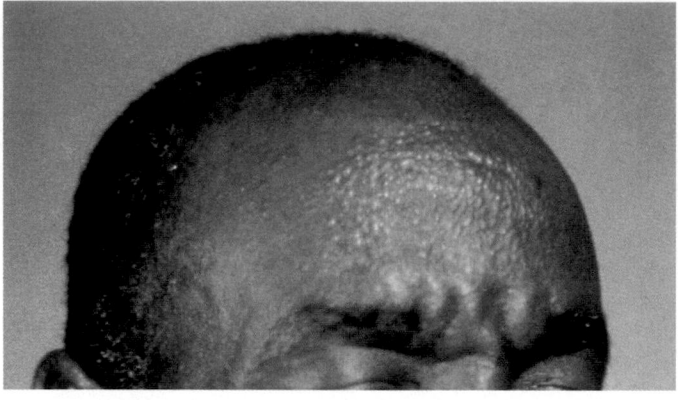

Papular mucinosis. Note discrete papules on the forehead and longitudinal folding of the glabella. (*Courtesy of L. Shapiro, MD.*)

FIGURE 188-2

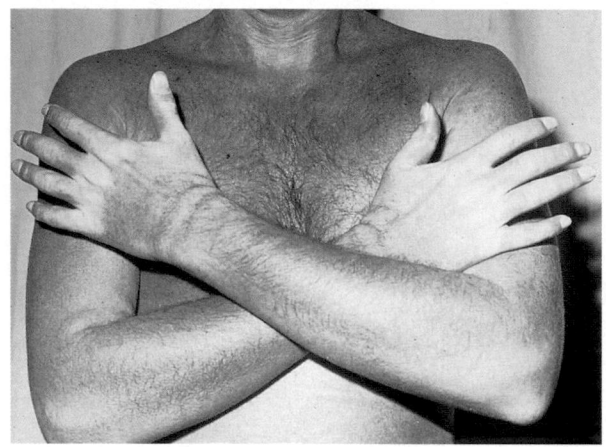

Scleromyxedema. Diffuse skin induration and erythema involving chest, arms, and dorsum of hands.

LABORATORY FINDINGS

Paraproteinemia, usually an IgG with lambda light chains, is present in most patients, particularly in those with the clinical form of scleromyxedema. Immunofluorescence microscopy of the skin lesions occasionally shows deposits of IgG with or without IgM in the papillary and upper reticular dermis.[4] However, others have failed to reproduce these findings.[15] Other inconsistent findings include elevated sedimentation rate, leukocytosis with eosinophilia, albuminuria, and plasma cell aggregates in the bone marrow.

PATHOLOGY

The most striking changes are in the upper dermis, which shows a horizontal band of mucinous material between collagen bundles. This material is a glycosaminoglycan that stains with alcian blue at

pH 2.5 and is susceptible to hyaluronidase digestion (Fig. 188-3). The epidermis may appear thinner due to pressure from the mucinous deposits. There is an increase in the number of fibroblasts, which appear plump and stellate, and dermal fibrosis. Cellular infiltrates may be present around the small blood vessels and appendages and consist mostly of lymphocytes with some histiocytic types and polymorphonuclear cells.[15] An increase in the number of plasma cells has also been noted. Electron microscopy reveals fibroblasts with long cytoplasmic processes and dilated rough endoplasmic reticulum. In addition, there are numerous thin collagen fibrils, suggestive of young collagen.[16] Muscle biopsies reveal an atypical necrotizing myopathy with fiber necrosis, severe type II fiber atrophy, and vacuolization.[10] Mucin deposits have also been reported in the adventitia of blood vessels in kidney, heart, adrenal glands, pancreas, and kidney papillae. Papular mucinosis has to be differentiated histologically from follicular mucinosis, amyloidosis, hyalinosis cutis et mucosae, scleredema, scleroderma, cutaneous focal mucinosis, pretibial myxedema, and colloid degeneration.

DIAGNOSIS AND DIFFERENTIAL DIAGNOSIS

Diagnosis is based on the presence of papular lesions, the demonstration of mucin in the dermis, and the presence of paraproteinemia. Clinically, papular mucinosis should be differentiated from scleredema, scleroderma, amyloidosis, disseminated granuloma annulare, malignant lymphomas, and dermatomyositis. The more localized forms should be differentiated from colloid degeneration,

FIGURE 188-3

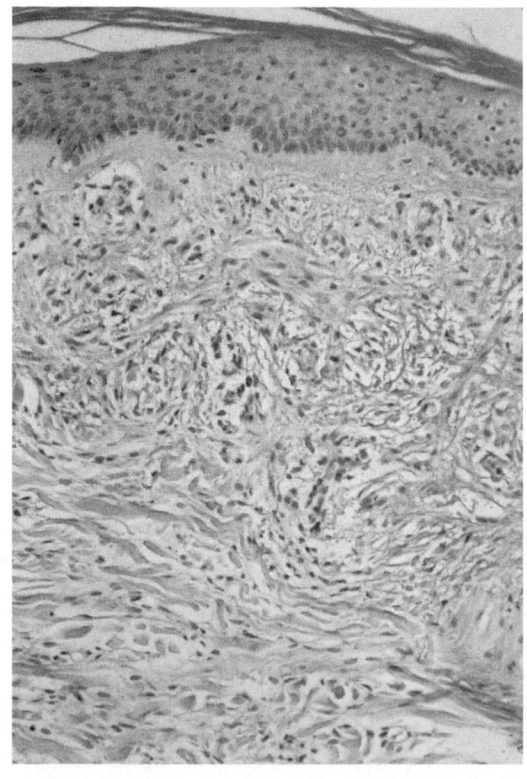

Scleromyxedema. Mucin and numerous plump fibroblasts in the upper dermis. Alcian blue, pH 2.5. (*Courtesy of L. Shapiro, MD.*)

lichen planus, morbus moniliformis, and epithelioma adenoides cysticum.

TREATMENT

The treatment of papular mucinosis remains unsatisfactory. Topical therapy is of no help. Complete clearance of lesions has been reported with melphalan (1 to 10 mg per day) and cyclophosphamide (200 mg per day) alone or in combination with prednisone.[17–20] However, since side effects can be severe, these drugs should be restricted to patients with widespread disease. Recently, electron-beam therapy was found to improve skin lesions.[21]

COURSE AND PROGNOSIS

The disease runs a chronic course and usually has no tendency toward spontaneous resolution. The prognosis is poor.[22] Reported causes of death appear to be unrelated to the disease and include tuberculosis, pneumonia, and vascular thrombosis.

REFERENCES

1. Gottron HA: Skleromyxodem (Eine eigenartige Erscheinungsform von Myxothesaurodermie). *Arch Dermatol Syphilol* **199**:71, 1954
2. Osserman EF, Takatsuki K: Role of an abnormal myeloma-type, serum gamma globulin in the pathogenesis of the skin lesions of papular mucinosis (lichen myxedematosus). *J Clin Invest* **42**:962, 1963
3. McCarthy JT et al: An abnormal serum globulin in lichen myxedematosus. *Arch Dermatol* **89**:446, 1964
4. Lawrence DA et al: Immunochemical analysis of the basic immunoglobulin in papular mucinosis. *Immunochemistry* **9**:41, 1972
5. Kitamura W et al: Immunochemical analysis of the monoclonal paraprotein in scleromyxedema. *J Invest Dermatol* **70**:305, 1978
6. Harper RA, Rispler J: Lichen myxedematosus serum stimulates human skin fibroblast proliferation. *Science* **188**:545, 1978
7. Wright RC et al: Scleromyxedema. *Arch Dermatol* **112**:63, 1976
8. Taylor AL et al: Scleromyxoedema associated with synovitis and myopathy. *Br J Rheumatol* **33**:872, 1994
9. McAdam LP et al: Papular mucinosis with myopathy, arthritis, and eosinophilia: A histopathologic study. *Arthritis Rheum* **20**:989, 1977
10. Verity MA et al: Scleromyxedema myopathy: Histochemical and electron microscopic observations. *Am J Clin Pathol* **69**:446, 1978
11. Webster GF et al: The association of potentially lethal neurologic syndromes with scleromyxedema. *J Am Acad Dermatol* **28**:105, 1993
12. Braverman IM: *Skin Signs of Systemic Disease,* 3d ed. Philadelphia, Saunders, 1998, p 172
13. Alligood TR et al: Scleromyxedema associated with esophageal aperistalsis and dermal eosinophilia. *Cutis* **28**:60, 1981
14. Davis ML et al: Ophthalmic findings in scleromyxedema. *Ophthalmology* **101**:252, 1994
15. Farmer ER et al: Papular mucinosis: A clinicopathologic study of four patients. *Arch Dermatol* **118**:9, 1982
16. Perry HO et al: Further observations on lichen myxedematosus. *Ann Intern Med* **53**:955, 1960
17. Feldman P et al: Scleromyxedema: A dramatic response to melphalan. *Arch Dermatol* **99**:51, 1969
18. Harris RB et al: Treatment of scleromyxedema with melphalan. *Arch Dermatol* **115**:295, 1979
19. Jessen RT et al: Lichen myxedematosus: Treatment with cyclophosphamide. *Int J Dermatol* **17**:833, 1978
20. Howsden SM et al: Lichen myxedematosus: A dermal infiltrative disorder responsive to cyclophosphamide therapy. *Arch Dermatol* **111**:1325, 1975
21. Koeppel MC et al: Electron-beam therapy in Arndt-Gottron's scleromyxedema. *Br J Dermatol* **129**:733, 1993
22. Dinneen AM, Dicken CH: Scleromyxedema. *J Am Acad Dermatol* **33**:37, 1995

CHAPTER 189

Rudolf Happle

Neurocutaneous Diseases

GENERAL CONSIDERATIONS

Neurocutaneous disease can be defined in various ways: a rather broad definition would include all diseases that may show both cutaneous and neurologic lesions. For the purpose of this chapter, however, a more strict definition will be applied. *Neurocutaneous diseases* are genetically determined disorders showing both cutaneous and neurologic involvement. This definition includes both hereditary and nonhereditary phenotypes but excludes acquired disorders.

In the past, neurocutaneous disorders have been classified according to their clinical morphology, and some of them have been called *phacomatoses*, although it was never quite clear which neurocutaneous disease should belong to this particular group. Progress in molecular genetics supports the view that neurocutaneous diseases can be reasonably classified according to formal genetics. Either they follow the established Mendelian modes of inheritance, or they represent lethal mutations surviving by mosaicism, or they belong to the group of chromosomal disorders. Clinically similar disorders may follow different modes of Mendelian inheritance, but this does not constitute a major problem.

Classification according to formal genetics will confirm the well-established differences between autosomal dominant, autosomal recessive, and X-linked gene expression.[1,2] The list of autosomal recessive phenotypes is particularly long, and, in general, these diseases are more severe than the diseases inherited as autosomal dominant traits. The group showing X-linked dominant inheritance with lethality for male embryos is of particular interest because the lethal effect on hemizygous male embryos may be largely due to a diffuse involvement of the central nervous system (CNS). In those phenotypes that are generally categorized as X-linked recessive traits, such as Fabry's disease, the Lyon effect of X-inactivation tends to blur the difference between the terms *dominant* and *recessive* because female gene carriers may show a more or less widespread clinical involvement, reflecting functional X-chromosome mosaicism.[3] The group of neurocutaneous phenotypes that can be explained by a lethal mutation surviving in a mosaic state contains some disorders that have been classified in the past as autosomal dominant traits showing low penetrance or variable expressivity. Today, their sporadic occurrence can be explained reasonably.[4] Some of these disorders, however, may exceptionally affect several members of a family, and for this phenomenon the concept of *paradominant inheritance* has been proposed (see below).[4] Chromosomal disorders showing both neurologic and cutaneous involvement are Turner's syndrome and trisomy 21.

Some clinicians still use "phacomatosis" to categorize particular neurocutaneous diseases characterized by patchy lesions involving the skin and the nervous system. Unfortunately, this term has diminished rather than increased our understanding of these disorders because the group of phacomatoses has never been well defined. Today, this term should no longer be used for the classification of neurocutaneous diseases but may be applied, together with a specifying adjective, to some genetically determined diseases characterized by the presence of multiple nevi, such as phacomatosis pigmentovascularis.

AUTOSOMAL DOMINANT PHENOTYPES

A list of autosomal dominant neurocutaneous traits is presented in Table 189-1. Some of these phenotypes are presented in detail in separate chapters of this book, e.g., neurofibromatosis 1 and 2 in Chap. 191. There are at least two different phenotypes of tuberous sclerosis (Chap. 190) that can be distinguished at the molecular level but not clinically.[7–9]

NEVOID BASAL CELL CARCINOMA SYNDROME   This disorder is described in Chap. 158. The major CNS anomalies observed in this syndrome are presented in Table 189-1. In the author's experience, a remarkable neurologic feature observed in many patients with nevoid basal cell carcinoma syndrome is their good-natured easy friendliness, or bonhomie. This good-naturedness should not be taken as a sign of mental deficiency. On the other hand, mental deficiency has been reported in about 3 percent of the cases; it probably occurs more frequently in a mild form.

LEOPARD SYNDROME   This syndrome has also been called multiple lentigines syndrome or cardiomyopathic lentiginosis,[11] but the term *LEOPARD syndrome* has been firmly entrenched in the clinicians' language. The acronym was coined by Gorlin et al.[1] and stands for *l*entiginosis, *e*lectrocardiographic conduction abnormalities, *o*cular hypertelorism, *p*ulmonic stenosis, *a*bnormal genitalia, *r*etardation of growth, and sensorineural *d*eafness. Patients usually have a characteristic facial appearance with a triangular shape due to frontal bossing, hypertelorism, and low-set ears. The underlying autosomal dominant gene has a high penetrance, but the expression may vary to a large degree, often resulting in rather mild involvement or incomplete phenotypes. The typical lentigines usually develop in childhood, and their number increases with age (Fig. 189-1). In contrast to ordinary freckles, the number of melanocytes is definitely increased. They contain giant pigment granules similar to those seen in the café au lait spots of neurofibromatosis.[12] Electrocardiographic conduction abnormalities are almost always found. They appear to result from right or left ventricular hypertrophy. Typical findings are interventricular conduction delays with a substantial left axis deviation. The electrocardiographic findings may be present without any structural cardiac defect, but severe involvement with a complete heart block may likewise occur. In male patients, the penis may be small, and hypospadias is present in about 50 percent of cases. Moreover, unilateral or bilateral cryptorchidism may be present. Female patients may show absence or hypoplasia of an ovary. Most patients tend to remain below average for height and weight. Various skeletal defects have been noted, such as pectus excavatum or carinatum, scoliosis, absence of ribs, or defects of the elbow joints.[1] Encephalographic examination may show a disturbed wave activity. In some patients, mild mental retardation is present, but intellectual capacity may be completely normal in this syndrome.

PIEBALD TRAIT WITH NEUROLOGIC DEFECTS   A piebald trait, consisting of unpigmented areas of skin showing smaller spots of hyperpigmentation in combination with a white forelock, has been described by Telfer et al.[13] in two families showing an autosomal dominant mode of transmission. Affected family members showed, in addition, defective motor coordination, cerebellar ataxia, as well as mental retardation of varying degree. Moreover, several affected family members suffered from hearing loss. Apparently, this association of anomalies is extremely rare, and this raises the question whether these families were affected with a contiguous gene syndrome. In this way, the unusual co-occurrence of anomalies could be explained as a defect involving two neighboring genes.

WAARDENBURG SYNDROME   This phenotype has been mapped to 2q37.3. The mutation involves the PAX3 gene, a homeobox gene that has been highly conserved during phylogenesis.[14] Various allelic mutations have been described.

NOONAN'S SYNDROME (CARDIOFACIOCUTANEOUS SYNDROME)   In the past, Noonan's syndrome and cardiofaciocutaneous syndrome have been considered to represent different entities, but when the signs and symptoms of the two phenotypes are compared, it appears difficult to find any rhyme or reason to distinguish the disorders.[15–17] Therefore, the two designations are considered synonyms. Noonan's syndrome includes retarded growth and congenital cardiac defects and a peculiar facial appearance showing ptosis, hypertelorism, down-slanting palpebral fissures, thick lips, and low-set ears (Fig. 189-2). The nose shows a bullous tip. Characteristically, the scalp hair becomes more curly or woolly during childhood and adolescence. The skin may show many small melanocytic nevi, and keratosis pilaris is likewise frequently noted.

TABLE 189-1

Neurocutaneous Syndromes: Autosomal Dominant Phenotypes

DISORDER	MIM No.*	CUTANEOUS ANOMALIES	NEUROLOGIC ANOMALIES	OTHER ANOMALIES	COMMENTS
Neurofibromatosis 1	162200	Café au lait macules, neurofibroma, axillary freckling	Mental retardation of varying degree	Lisch nodules	17q11.2[5] (see Chap. 191)
Neurofibromatosis 2	101100	Café au lait spots (less than 6), schwannomas of flat or spherical appearance	Bilateral acoustic neuromas, menigioma, schwannoma	No Lisch nodules; cataracts, macular hamartomas	22q12.2[6] (see Chap. 191)
Tuberous sclerosis 1 Tuberous sclerosis 2	191100 191092	Hypopigmented macules, facial angiofibromas, poliosis, shagreen patches, parungual fibromas	Cerebral hamartomas (cortical tubers), seizures, mental deficit	Gingival fibromatosis, pit-shaped enamel defects, renal angiomyolipomas	9q34[8] 16p13.3[9](see Chap. 190)
Nevoid basal cell carcinoma syndrome	109400	Multiple basal cell carcinoma, palmar and palmar pits, milia, epidermoid cysts	Intracerebral calcifications, hydrocephalus internus, agenesis of corpus callosum, medulloblastoma, mild mental deficiency, "bonhomie"	Jaw cysts, hypertelorism, bone anomalies (spine, ribs, fingers), ovarian fibromas	9q22 Homology between humans and *Drosophila*[10] (see Chap. 158)
LEOPARD syndrome	151100	Generalized lentigines	Disturbed EEG wave activity, diffuse encephalopathy, deafness, mild mental retardation	Genital hypoplasia, cardiac defects, ECG abnormalities, ocular hypertelorism, pulmonic stenosis, retardation of growth	
Piebald trait with neurologic defects	172850	Patchy leukoderma containing smaller spots of hyperpigmentation, white forelock	Defective motor coordination, cerebellar ataxia, mental retardation, hearing loss		
Waardenburg's syndrome	193500	Patchy leukoderma containing smaller spots of hyperpigmentation, white forelock, synophrys	Neurosensory hearing loss	Dystopia canthorum, broad nasal root, heterochromia of the irides	2q37.3 PAX3 gene, a homeobox gene[14]
Noonan's syndrome (cardio-facio-cutaneous syndrome)	115150; 163950	Curly or woolly hair, multiple melanocytic nevi, keratosis pilaris, lymphedema	Mild mental retardation	Retarded growth, cardiac defects, hypertelorism, down-slanting palpebral fissures, thick lips, bullous tip of nose	
Osler-Weber-Rendu disease	187300	Multiple vascular dilations	Vascular lesions of the brain or the spinal cord, cerebral abscesses	Angiodysplastic lesions of oral mucosa, esophagus, lungs, liver, etc.	See Chap. 102
Variegate porphyria	176200	Light sensitivity, blisters, erosions, crusts, hypertrichosis	Neuropathic features such as abdominal pain, muscle weakness, sensory disturbances; psychosis during attacks		1q21 (see Chap. 151)
KID syndrome	148210	Sharply demarcated erythemato-squamous plaques, often with a rippled aspect; leather-like hyperkeratosis of the palms	Neurosensory deafness	Bilateral keratitis	See Chap. 52
HID syndrome	no entry	Hystrix-like ichthyosis	Neurosensory deafness		
Verbov-Sharland syndrome	148350	Palmoplantar keratoderma of diffuse type	Neurosensory hearing loss		
Preaxial anonychia with neurologic defects	no entry	Anonychia of the thumbs, the great toes and the 2nd toes	Choreoathetosis, seizures, developmental delay		Autosomal dominant inheritance not proven but very likely[27]

*MIM, Mendelian inheritance in man.

FIGURE 189-1

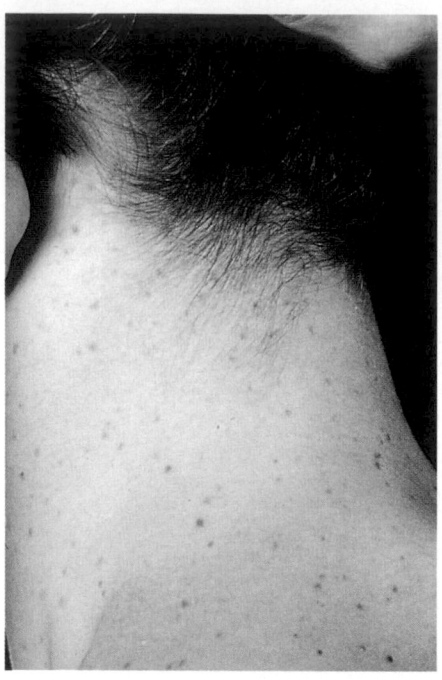

Multiple lentigines as a feature of LEOPARD syndrome.

Another cutaneous abnormality associated with this syndrome is lymphedema resulting from hypoplasia or aplasia of lymphatic vessels. The most common heart defects are pulmonic stenosis and atrial septal defect. Mild mental retardation is often noted, but the syndrome may also be associated with normal intelligence.

OSLER-WEBER-RENDU DISEASE (HEREDITARY HEMOR-RHAGIC TELANGIECTASIA) This disorder is described in Chap. 102.

VARIEGATE PORPHYRIA For a detailed description of this disorder, the reader is referred to Chap. 151. Due to a founder effect, variegate porphyria is particularly frequent in South Africa. It has been estimated that currently about 800 South African citizens are suffering from this disease. Apparently, all of them are descendants of Gerrit Jansz, a Dutch settler in the Cape, and of Ariaantje Jacobs, who was sent from an orphanage in Rotterdam to become his wife.[18] The high prevalence of variegate porphyria in Finland can be explained by a similar founder effect. In addition to the well-known cutaneous signs of porphyria, affected individuals may suffer from neuropathic features such as abdominal pain, muscle weakness, or sensory disturbances. During attacks they may be disoriented or even frankly psychotic. These attacks are often triggered by medication. Remarkably, several patients homozygous for the underlying gene defect have been described.[19,20] In the affected families, both parents were shown, by biochemical testing, to be heterozygous. The patients described by Korda et al.[19] developed severe neurologic symptoms with seizures and mental deficiency.

KID SYNDROME This phenotype is described in Chap. 52.

HID SYNDROME (HYSTRIX-LIKE ICHTHYOSIS WITH DEAFNESS) In 1989, Traupe[21] proposed the term *HID syndrome* for a phenotype characterized by hystrix-like ichthyosis associated with bilateral neurosensory deafness (Fig. 189-3). Similar cases were published earlier under the designation "ichthyosis hystrix gravior, type Rheydt."[22] Previously the genetic basis was not clear because all cases were sporadic, but recently father-to-son transmission of this trait has been observed.[23]

FIGURE 189-2

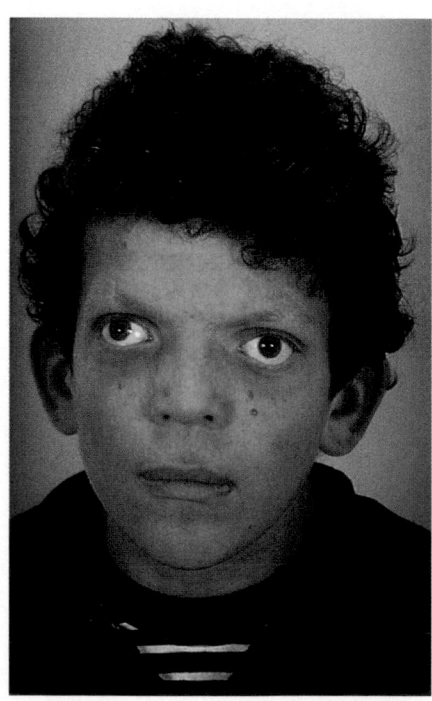

Noonan's syndrome: peculiar facies showing hypertelorism, low-set ears, thick lips, and curly hair.

FIGURE 189-3

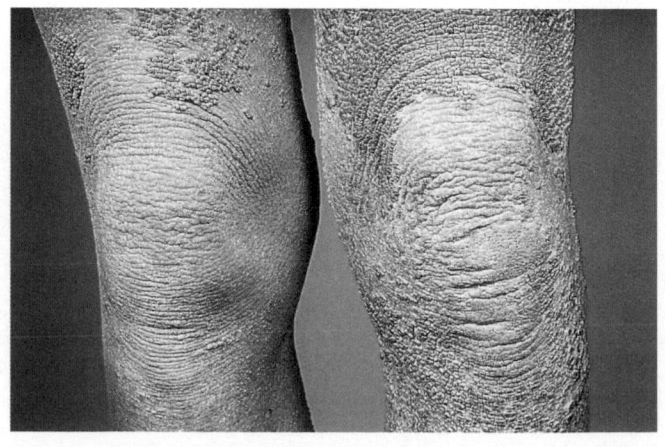

HID syndrome (hystrix-like ichthyosis with deafness).

VERBOV-SHARLAND SYNDROME (PALMOPLANTAR KERATODERMA WITH NEUROSENSORY DEAFNESS)

Verbov[24] and Sharland et al.[25] described families with diffuse palmoplantar keratoderma and bilateral, progressive, high-frequency sensorineural hearing loss occurring in several consecutive generations. Molecular studies have so far not been performed in these families.[26]

PREAXIAL ANONYCHIA WITH NEUROLOGIC DEFECTS

Lynch et al.[27] described a syndrome of anonychia, involving the thumbs as well as the first and the second toes, combined with neurologic defects in a family showing vertical transmission of the trait.

AUTOSOMAL RECESSIVE PHENOTYPES

A list of autosomal recessive neurocutaneous traits is given in Table 189-2. For a more detailed description of the various ichthyoses associated with neurologic anomalies, such as neutral lipid storage disease, Refsum's disease, Sjögren-Larsson syndrome (Fig. 189-4), as well as Tay's syndrome and Amish brittle hair syndrome (BIDS syndrome) (Fig. 189-5), the reader is referred to Chap. 52.

MULTIPLE SULFATASE DEFICIENCY Multiple sulfatase deficiency is a neurodegenerative disorder that usually leads to death in early childhood. The disorder is caused by a mutation that results in enhanced degradation of various sulfatases.[28] In spite of some clinical similarities, the disease can be separated from metachromatic leukodystrophy on the basis of different metabolic features. Psychomotor retardation usually becomes manifest during the second year of life. A child that has already learned to walk begins to show an unsteady gait and needs help to stand upright; simultaneously, speech begins to deteriorate. In the final stage, the children are blind and unable to eat or drink. Microscopic examination of biopsies obtained from peripheral nerves shows metachromatic degeneration of myelin. Affected children usually die before their tenth year. The disease is associated with mild ichthyosis resulting from steroid sulfatase deficiency. It is usually less severe than observed in classic X-linked recessive ichthyosis. This difference may be explained by a residual activity of steroid sulfatases.[29]

STEIJLEN'S SYNDROME A syndrome consisting of congenital atrichia (Fig. 189-6), transgradient palmar and plantar keratoderma (Fig. 189-7), early loss of teeth, and severe mental retardation was observed by Steijlen et al.[30] The disease occurred in four siblings. The mother had had five miscarriages. Autosomal recessive inheritance is most likely.

BJØRNSTAD'S SYNDROME Bjørnstad's syndrome is an autosomal recessive disorder characterized by pili torti and nerve deafness.[31]

SHAPIRA'S SYNDROME Shapira et al.[32] described a syndrome consisting of sparse, brittle, and light-colored scalp hair; developmental delay; short stature; and mild to moderate neurologic abnormalities. Further clinical observations may show whether this combination of features represents a new entity.

ELEJALDE'S SYNDROME Elejalde's syndrome is a phenotype belonging to the group of silvery hair syndromes (Fig. 189-8). The disease should be distinguished from Chediak-Higashi syndrome and Griscelli's syndrome.[33] Elejalde's syndrome, which has also

been called "neuroectodermal melanolysosomal disease,"[34] is characterized by frequent occurrence of fatal neurologic alterations. Psychomotor impairment is a constant feature and may be observed in the newborn or during infancy. In contrast to other silvery hair syndromes, microscopical examination of hair shafts shows an irregular distribution of abnormally small or large clumps of melanin (Fig. 189-9). Neuromuscular alterations consist of hypotonia, hemiplegia, quadriplegia, ataxia, and mental retardation that is usually of a severe degree.

CROSS' SYNDROME This phenotype belongs likewise to the silvery hair syndromes.[35] It is characterized by generalized hypopigmentation, ocular anomalies, and neurologic defects such as mental and physical retardation, ataxia, and spasticity.[36]

XERODERMA PIGMENTOSUM Several types of xeroderma pigmentosum are associated with neurologic abnormalities (see Chap. 157). In the past, the term *De Sanctis-Cacchione syndrome* has been used to designate this association, but this term should no longer be used because neurologic defects are not characteristic of a particular complementation group.[37] However, groups A and D appear to be especially prone to neurologic involvement including mental retardation, electroencephalographic changes, microcephaly, cortical atrophy, ventricular dilation, or peripheral neuropathy.[38]

COCKAYNE'S SYNDROME Cockayne's syndrome is a progeroid phenotype characterized by short stature and markedly increased photosensitivity resulting in dermatitis with blistering, scarring, and pigmentary disturbances.[39,40] The subcutaneous fatty tissue is diminished. Associated neurologic features include microcephaly and progressive impairment of neurologic and mental functions such as sitting, walking, and speaking. Pathologic examination has shown severe demyelinization of the subcortical structures.

ACRODERMATITIS ACIDEMICA Some enzyme defects such as methylmalonic acidemia[41] or propionic acidemia[42] are characterized by lethargy, failure to thrive, vomiting, dehydration, dyspnea, and hypotonia. The affected infants often die in coma. These metabolic defects are usually associated with cutaneous features reminiscent of acrodermatitis enteropathica. Sharply demarcated erythemas with desquamation are usually observed in a periorificial localization.[43] The scalp hair is sparse, brittle, and hypopigmented.

HARTNUP DISEASE Hartnup disease is a metabolic disorder characterized by a transportation defect involving certain amino acids (see Chap. 149).[44] Affected children show photosensitivity resulting in skin changes reminiscent of pellagra and progressive cerebellar ataxia.

TANGIER DISEASE The disease is caused by a deficieny of high-density lipoproteins resulting in xanthomatosis of various tissues and recurrent neuropathy.[45] The disorder is named after Tangier Island in the Chesapeake Bay, where affected individuals are descendants from a small founder population. The skin may show xanthomatous papules resulting from abnormal deposition of cholesterol esters.

CHIME SYNDROME The term *CHIME* is an abbreviation for *co*lobomas of the eye, *h*eart defects, *i*chthyosiform dermatosis, *m*ental retardation, and *e*ar defects.[46] The condition is characterized by a

TABLE 189-2

Neurocutaneous Syndromes: Autosomal Recessive Phenotypes

Disorder	MIM No.*	Cutaneous Anomalies	Neurologic Anomalies	Other Anomalies	Comments
Neutral lipid storage disease	275630	Congenital ichthyotic erythroderma; mild ichthyosis with fine scaling in older children and adults	Muscular weakness, abnormal EMG, ataxia, neurosensory hearing loss, nystagmus	Fatty degeneration of the liver	See Chap. 52
Refsum disease	266500	Very mild ichthyosis; accentuated palmar creases; yellowish hue of melanocytic nevi	Anosmia, neurosensory hearing loss, peripheral neuropathy, diminished tendon reflexes, cerebellar ataxia, intention tremor	Retinopathia pigmentosa, night blindness, cardiac involvement (AV block, bundle-branch block)	See Chap. 52
Sjögren-Larsson syndrome	270200	Ichthyosis with areas of lichenification (Fig. 189-4)	Pathologic reflexes, muscular hypertonus, spastic paraplegia or tetraplegia, mental retardation	Glistening dots in the macular region of retina	Deficiency of fatty alcohol: NAD+ oxido-reductase (see Chap. 52)
Multiple sulfatase deficiency	272200	Mild ichthyosis, similar to X-linked recessive ichthyosis (see text)	Severe psychomotor retardation; metachromatic leukodystrophy	The disorder usually leads to death in early childhood	The mutation causes rapid degradation of various sulfatases[28]
Tay's syndrome (IBIDS syndrome)†	601675	Congenital ichthyosis developing into mild scaling; sulfur-deficient brittle hair (trichothiodystrophy), dysplastic nails, hypoplasia of subcutaneous tissue	Mental retardation, microcephaly, intracerebral calcifications, EEG anomalies, mild hearing loss, coordination deficit, spasticity, ataxia, hemiparesis, intention tremor	Low birth weight, short stature, progeroid facial appearance, hypogenitalism, cataracts, hoarse or high-pitched voice	See Chap. 52
Amish brittle hair syndrome (BIDS syndrome)†	234050	Sulfur-deficient brittle (hair trichothiodystrophy) (Fig. 189-5)	Mental retardation, EEG anomalies, ataxia, intention tremor	Low birth weight, short stature, hypogenitalism, decreased fertility	
Steijlen's syndrome	No entry	Congenital atrichia, palmoplantar keratoderma extending to the dorsal aspect of hands or feet	Mental retardation of moderate or severe degree	Early loss of teeth	
Bjørnstad's syndrome	262000	Pili torti	Neurosensory deafness		
Shapira's syndrome	261900	Sparse, brittle, light-colored hair	Developmental delay, short stature, ataxia, unsteady gait		
Elejalde's syndrome	256710	Silvery hair showing irregular distribution of melanin clumps, peculiar bronzed skin color	Hypotonia, hemiplegia, tretraplegia, ataxia, severe mental retardation, nystagmus, blindness, EEG anomalies	Pigmentary disturbance of retina	The disorder should be distinguished from Chediak-Higashi syndrome and Griscelli's syndrome
Cross' syndrome	257800	Silvery hair, generalized hypopigmentation	Microcephaly, mental retardation, spasticity, ataxia, cerebellar hypoplasia, posterior fossa cyst, EEG anomalies	Growth retardation, hypopigmented fundus, ERG anomalies	
Xeroderma pigmentosum	278730 278780 278799 278800	Photosensitivity, diffuse freckled hyper- and hypopigmentation, multiple skin cancers	Mental retardation, microcephaly, EEG anomalies, cortical atrophy, ventricular dilation, peripheral neuropathy		"De Sanctis-Cacchione syndrome" is no longer considered a particular entity (see text). See Chap. 157

(continued)

TABLE 189-2 (*Continued*)

DISORDER	MIM NO.*	CUTANEOUS ANOMALIES	NEUROLOGIC ANOMALIES	OTHER ANOMALIES	COMMENTS
Cockayne's syndrome	257800	Increased photosensitivity with dermatitis, blistering, scarring and pigmentary disturbances; diminished subcutaneous tissue	Microcephaly, progressive deterioration of mental and neurologic functions, demyelinization of subcortical structures		
Acrodermatitis acidemica	251000 251110 251120 232050	Sharply demarcated periorificial and acral erythema and desquamation; sparse, brittle, hypopigmented scalp hair	Lethargy, vomiting, hypotonia	Dehydration, dyspnea	Acrodermatitis acidemica is a cutaneous feature of various enzymatic defects involving the branched chain amino acid metabolism (see text)
Hartnup disease	234500	Increased photosensitivity, pellagroid skin changes	Progressive cerebellar ataxia		See Chap. 149
Lipoid proteinosis	247100	Numerous yellowish nodules on the face and elsewhere on the body; pearly papules at the eyelid margins	Intracranial calcification; seizures	Hoarse voice, involvement of oral mucosa resulting in "cobblestone" appearance	See Chap. 154
Tangier disease	205400	Xanthomatous papules	Recurrent neuropathy	Large, orange-yellow tonsils; splenomegaly	
Ataxia-telangiectasia	208900	Telangiectasia in sun-exposed areas; hyper- and hypopigmentation	Progressive cerebellar ataxia, muscular weakness, peripheral neuropathy	Telangiectasia of conjunctiva, immune deficiency, increased chromosome breakage, leukemia	See Chap. 192
Oculocutaneous albinism	203100	Absence of pigment in skin and hair	Nystagmus, photophobia, strabismus, reduced visual acuity		See Chap. 87
CHIME syndrome	280000	Ichthyosiform skin changes	Mental retardation	Coloboma, cardiac defects, ear defects	
De Barsy syndrome	219150	Diminished subcutaneous tissue resulting in wrinkling, pronounced nasolabial folds, and progeroid facial appearance	Mental retardation, microcephaly	Growth retardation, large dysplastic ears, corneal opacities, cataracts, hypermobility of joints	
Dubowitz's syndrome	223370	Eczematous lesions during infancy, sparse scalp hair, diminished subcutaneous tissue	Mental retardation, usually of mild degree	Typical facial appearance, epicanthal folds, ptosis, broad nasal tip, micrognathia	The phenotype is so far rather ill-defined[48]

*MIM, Mendelian inheritance in man.
†IBIDS, ichthyosis, brittle hair, intellectual impairment, decreased fertility, short stature.

congenital migratory ichthyosiform dermatosis, hyperkeratotic palms and soles, and sparse, fine hair.

DE BARSY SYNDROME This phenotype is characterized by growth retardation, progeroid facial appearance with pronounced nasolabial folds, and diminished subcutaneous tissue resulting in wrinkling, large dysplastic ears, corneal opacities, cataracts, hypermobility of joints, and mental retardation.[47] Microcephaly is often present.

X-LINKED MALE-LETHAL PHENOTYPES

Some X-linked neurocutaneous disorders occur almost exclusively in girls because the underlying genes exert a lethal effect on male embryos (Table 189-3).[49] In female embryos, the Lyon effect of X-inactivation[3] accounts for survival. Exceptionally, however, male patients may be observed, and this can be explained either by a gonosome constitution XXY, by an early postzygotic mutation, or by a gametic half-chromatid mutation.[4]

FOCAL DERMAL HYPOPLASIA (GOLTZ'S SYNDROME) The main features include widespread lesions of dermal hypoplasia with herniation of adipose tissue, streaks of pigmentary disturbance following the lines of Blaschko, and severe absence deformities of bones.[50,51] Some patients may show mental retardation, which is usually mild, and others may suffer from hearing loss. The spectrum of ocular anomalies includes defects of the optic nerve.

INCONTINENTIA PIGMENTI Incontinentia pigmenti is a syndrome characterized by skin lesions that are arranged in a linear pattern.[52] During the first months of life, an episode of inflamma-

FIGURE 189-4

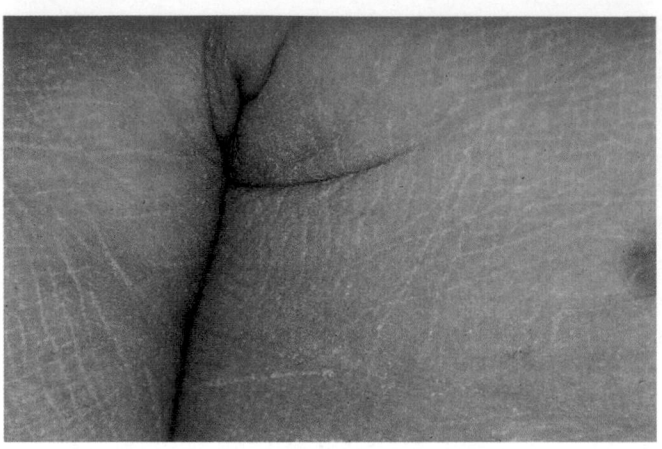

Sjögren-Larsson syndrome: characteristic rippled appearance of hyper-keratotic skin. (*Courtesy of Peter M. Steijlen, MD, Nijmegen, The Netherlands.*)

FIGURE 189-5

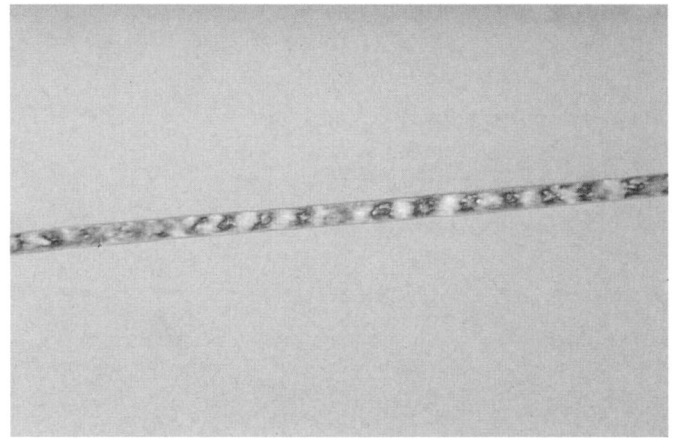

Trichothiodystrophy as found in Tay's syndrome and Amish brittle hair syndrome. Hair shaft shows a characteristic tiger-tail pattern when examined between polarizing filters.

tion and blistering occurs and apparently reflects a selection against the functionally defective cell clone.[53] The blisters are filled with eosinophils. Later on, these lesions are replaced by hyperkeratotic verrucous areas, whereas in the older child a linear or patchy pattern of hyperpigmentation is found (Fig. 189-10). In women, a fourth stage in the form of linear hypopigmentation involves the lower legs predominantly. The disorder is associated with ocular defects such as coloboma, retinal detachment, strabismus, cataracts, optic atrophy, or corneal opacities. Dental abnormalities include absence of deciduous or permanent teeth and crown deformities. Involvement of the CNS occurs rather frequently, but it appears impossible to present the incidence in terms of percentages because all case reports and reviews contain a considerable bias of ascertainment. Neurologic abnormalities comprise psychomotor retardation, micro-

FIGURE 189-6

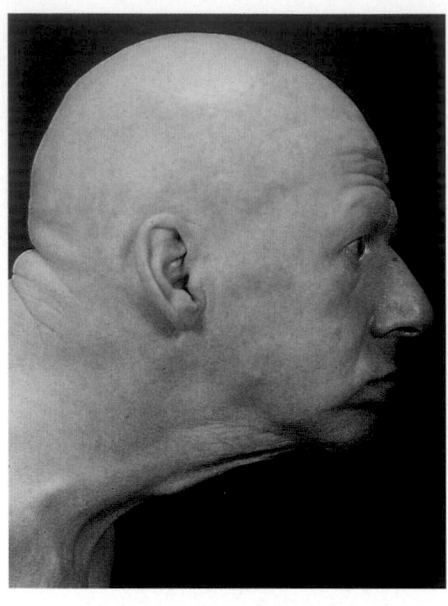

Microcephaly as a feature of Steijlen's syndrome (atrichia, palmoplantar keratoderma, and mental retardation).

FIGURE 189-7

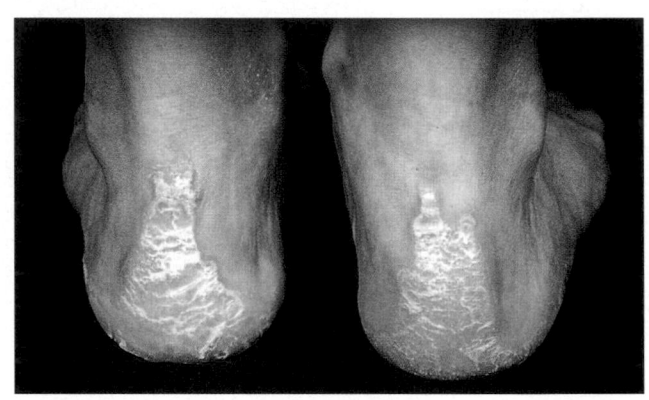

Steijlen's syndrome: plantar keratoderma extending to the heels.

cephaly, seizures, spasticity, and cerebellar ataxia. The great variability of these phenotypic associations can be explained by the Lyon effect of random X-inactivation.[3] Morphologic evidence of functional X-chromosome mosaicism involving the brain has been provided.[54]

CHILD SYNDROME   The term *CHILD* is an acronym for *c*ongenital *h*emidysplasia with *i*chthyosiform nevus and *l*imb *d*efects[55] (see Chap. 52). (The term *ichthyosiform erythroderma* is misleading and should no longer be used.) The phenotype is characterized by a unique inflammatory nevus that has been called *CHILD nevus*.[56] Usually this nevus shows a striking lateralization with a sharp midline demarcation (Fig. 189-11). However, a streaky arrangement following the lines of Blaschko may also be present.[55] Ipsilateral limb defects may vary from mild hypoplasia of one finger or toe to complete absence of an arm or leg. The nails are often replaced by keratotic, clawlike material. Ipsilateral CNS abnormalities in-

FIGURE 189-8

CHAPTER 189
Neurocutaneous Diseases

2139

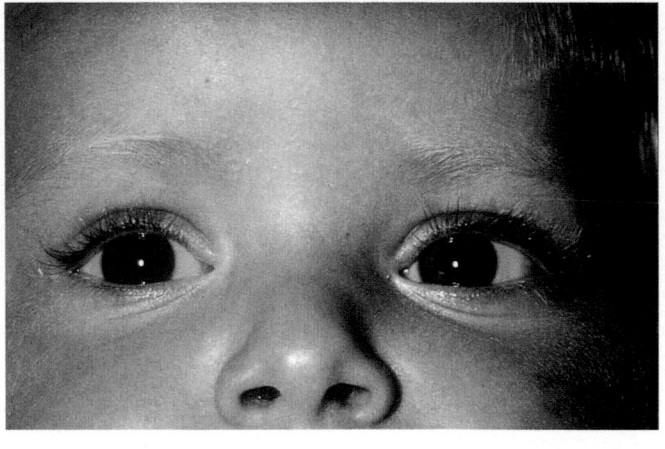

Elejalde's syndrome: bronzed skin and silvery hair.

FIGURE 189-9

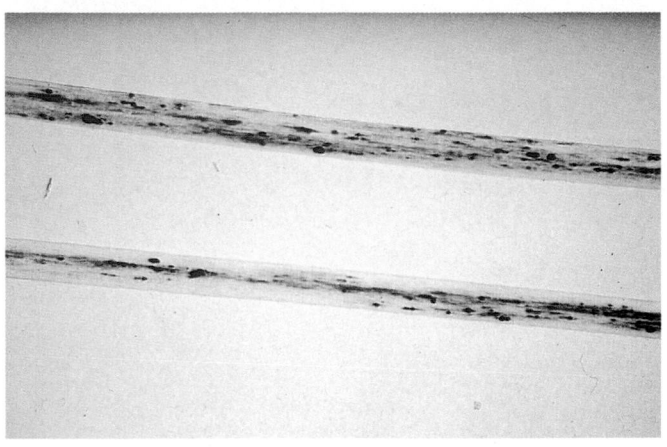

Elejalde's syndrome: hair shafts show irregular distribution of melanin clumps.

TABLE 189-3

Neurocutaneous Syndromes: X-linked Male-Lethal Phenotypes

DISORDER	MIM No.*	CUTANEOUS ANOMALIES	NEUROLOGIC ANOMALIES	OTHER ANOMALIES	COMMENTS
Focal dermal hypoplasia	305600	Linear and patchy lesions of dermal hypoplasia, herniation of fatty tissue, poikiloderma; periorificial papillomas	Mild mental retardation, meningomyelocele, hydrocephalus, defects of optic nerve	Striation of long bones, absence deformities of bones, diaphragmatic hernia, hypodontia, cleft lip/palate	
Incontinentia pigmenti	308310	Linear lesions of inflammation resulting in pigmentary disturbance (see text)	Psychomotor retardation, microcephaly, seizures, spasticity, cerebellar ataxia	Coloboma, retinal detachment, cataracts, corneal opacities; absence of teeth	Xq28 "Incontinenti pigmenti type 1" ("sporadic type," MIM no. 308 300)[2] does not exist. All cases belong to MIM no. 308 310.
CHILD syndrome	308050	CHILD nevus (see text)	Hypoplasia of ipsilateral hemisphere, hypoplasia of cranial nerves, defects of spinal cord, reduced sensation to touch and heat	Ipsilateral absence deformities of limbs (see text), ipsilateral absence of lung or kidney, cardiac defects	Many cases have so far been erroneously taken as inflammatory linear verrucous epidermal nevus (ILVEN). See Chap. 52
MIDAS syndrome	309801	Linear lesions of dermal aplasia involving mainly the face and neck	Microcephaly, focal dysplasia of brain, absence of septum pellucidum, agenesis of corpus callosum	Microphthalmia, sclerocornea, anterior chamber eye abnormalities, cardiac defects	All cases are caused by a deletion at Xp22.3[62]
OFD I syndrome	311200	Linear or patchy areas of hairlessness; multiple facial milia	Porencephaly, partial agenesis of corpus callosum, hydrocephalus, mental retardation	Broad nasal root, midfacial clefting defects, lobulated tongue, fibrous bands traversing the mucobuccal fold, syndactyly, brachydactyly, clinodactyly	Xp22.3–p22.2[64]

*MIM, Mendelian inheritance in man.

FIGURE 189-10

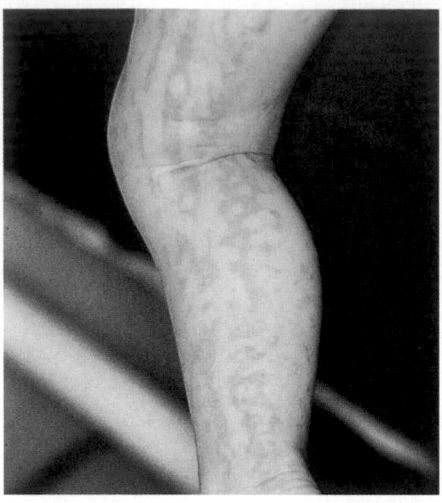

Incontinentia pigmenti: linear arrangement of hyperpigmented skin lesions.

FIGURE 189-11

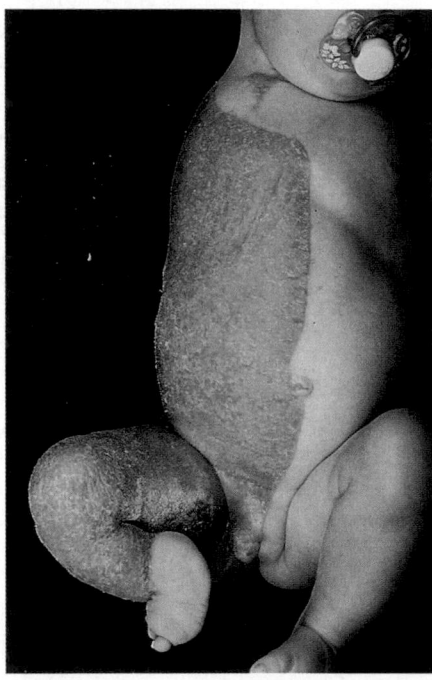

CHILD syndrome: CHILD nevus showing striking lateralization and ipsilateral limb defects.

clude hypoplasia of a hemisphere or hypoplasia of cranial nerves or the spinal cord; there may be reduced sensation to touch and heat on the affected side.[57] However, in most of these girls the mental development is completely normal. Apparently, the unaffected hemisphere can take over all of the necessary functions. In one case, mild intellectual impairment was reported.[58]

FIGURE 189-12

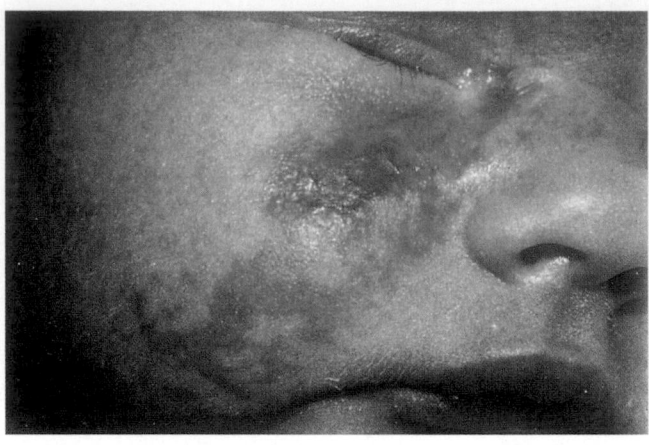

MIDAS syndrome: microphthalmia and dermal aplasia showing linear arrangement.

MIDAS SYNDROME The term *MIDAS* is an acronymic designation that stands for *mi*crophthalmia, *d*ermal *a*plasia, and *s*clerocornea.[59] All of the associated defects reflect functional X-chromosome mosaicism. Microphthalmia is usually bilateral, but unilateral involvement has also been reported. Dermal aplasia typically involves the face (Fig. 189-12), the scalp, and the neck, but other body areas may also be affected. In contrast to focal dermal hypoplasia, these lesions never show herniation of the underlying fatty tissue.[60] In some of the affected girls, neurologic defects such as focal dysplasia of the brain with absence of the septum pellucidum, microcephaly, or agenesis of the corpus callosum have been reported.[59] However, the latter may also result from a deletion that involves a neighboring gene, producing a contiguous gene syndrome that includes Aicardi's syndrome in addition to the MIDAS syndrome.[61,62]

OFD I SYNDROME (ORAL-FACIAL-DIGITAL SYNDROME) This syndrome includes midfacial clefting defects, lobulation of the tongue, hypoplasia of the nose, syndactyly, brachydactyly, clinodactyly, and circumscribed hairlessness that visualizes the lines of Blaschko on the scalp.[63,64] The upper lip is short, and the nasal root is broad. During infancy, many milia may be present on the cheeks or the ears. Typical oral manifestations are large hyperplastic fibrous bands traversing the mucobuccal fold. Many of the affected girls show mild mental retardation. Neurologic examination of the brain may reveal porencephaly, partial agenesis of the corpus callosum, or hydrocephalus.

X-LINKED NONLETHAL PHENOTYPES

In this group of disorders, women are usually more mildly affected because of the Lyon effect of X-inactivation (Table 189-4). Remarkably, however, several X-linked genes located at different regions of the X chromosome escape inactivation, and one example may be the gene for bullous dystrophy of Mendes da Costa.[65]

PARTINGTON'S SYNDROME This syndrome is characterized by generalized reticulate hyperpigmentation, failure to thrive, recurrent pneumonia, seizures, and hemiplegia.[66,67] Female gene carriers are

TABLE 189-4

Neurocutaneous Syndromes: X-Linked Nonlethal Phenotypes

DISORDER	MIM NO.*	CUTANEOUS ANOMALIES	NEUROLOGIC ANOMALIES	OTHER ANOMALIES	COMMENTS
Partington's syndrome	301220	Generalized reticular hyperpigmentation in men; female carriers are mildly affected and show linear skin lesions	Seizures, hemiplegia	Failure to thrive, recurrent pneumonia	Xp22-p21[67]
Menkes disease	309400	Brittle hair showing characteristic kinking, light skin complexion	Mental retardation, seizures, hypothermia	Bone defects; affected boys usually die during infancy	Xq13 Female carriers show a mixture of normal and defective hair shafts. Prenatal diagnosis of affected boys is possible
Bullous dystrophy of the Mendes da Costa type	302000	Generalized macular hyper- and hypopigmentation, total hair loss	Microcephaly, mental retardation		Xq27.3-qter[75] Female carriers are phenotypically normal (see text)
Albinism-deafness syndrome	300700	Pigmentary disorder of the piebald type	Neurosensory deafness		Xq26.3-q27.1[78] Female carriers may show mild hearing loss (see Chap. 87)
Lesch-Nyhan syndrome	308000	Severe lesions of self-mutilation, mainly on the lips and the fingers	Delayed motor development, choreoathetosis		Neuropsychiatric manifestations may result from dopaminergic deficits[84]
Adrenoleukodystrophy	300100	Bronzed discoloration of skin, diminished hair growth	Spastic paresis, sensory disturbances, urinary incontinence	Endocrinopathy	The putative gene encodes a transmembrane transporter protein regulated by ATP[85]
Fabry's disease	301500	Multiple pinpoint-sized vascular lesions, increasing in number with age	Attacks of burning pain in fingers and toes	Gastrointestinal involvement with nausea and vomiting; conjunctival and retinal vascular lesions, cloudy cornea, lenticular opacities	See Chap. 153

*MIM, Mendelian inheritance in man.

only mildly affected and show a patchy or linear pattern of hyperpigmentation.

MENKES DISEASE (See Chap. 71)   The disorder includes sparse, brittle hair showing characteristic kinking, mental retardation, seizures, hypothermia, and bone defects. The disease is caused by a defect of copper transport.[68] Affected boys usually die during infancy. Early copper-histidine treatment has been advocated but is still a matter of controversy.[69] Due to the Lyon effect of X-inactivation, female gene carriers show a mixture of normal and defective hair shafts and may be otherwise affected.[70,71] There is a murine homologue of Menkes disease.[72,73]

BULLOUS DYSTROPHY OF THE MENDES DA COSTA TYPE
Affected boys show macular hyperpigmentation and depigmentation, total hair loss, microcephaly, and mental retardation.[74,75] Women heterozygous for this X-linked mutation are phenotypically normal. For this reason, it has been assumed that the underlying gene escapes X-inactivation.[65]

ALBINISM-DEAFNESS SYNDROME   This X-linked form of albinism represents a pigmentary disorder of the piebald type in combination with a profound deafness that results in deaf-mutism.[76] A less severe hearing impairment has been found in female carriers.[77]

KALLMANN'S SYNDROME   Kallmann's syndrome is characterized by anosmia, due to agenesis of the olfactory lobes, and hypogonadotropic hypogonadism.[79] The underlying gene defect does not involve the skin. However, several patients affected with Kallmann's syndrome display a contiguous gene syndrome that involves several neighboring gene loci, including that of steroid sulfatase.[80,81] Consequently, these patients are also affected with X-linked recessive ichthyosis.

LESCH-NYHAN SYNDROME   This phenotype is caused by a deficiency of hypoxanthine-guanine phosphoribosyl-transferase.[82,83] During the first months of life, neurologic anomalies such as delayed motor development and choreoathetosis become manifest. Affected boys usually show severe self-mutilation. The lips and fingers are most frequently involved.

and endocrinopathy.[87] The cutaneous features consist of a bronzed discoloration of the skin and diminished hair growth.

ADRENOLEUKODYSTROPHY   Adrenoleukodystrophy is a peroxisomal disorder characterized by progressive demyelination and adrenocortical insufficiency.[85] Affected male individuals show increased levels of long-chain fatty acids.[86] Clinical symptoms include spastic paresis, sensory disturbances, urinary incontinence,

LETHAL AUTOSOMAL MUTATIONS SURVIVING BY MOSAICISM

Some autosomal mutations, when present in a zygote, cause early death of the embryo (Table 189-5). Cells carrying the mutation can

TABLE 189-5

Neurocutaneous Syndromes: Lethal Autosomal Mutations Surviving by Mosaicism

DISORDER	MIM NO.*	CUTANEOUS ANOMALIES	NEUROLOGIC ANOMALIES	OTHER ANOMALIES	COMMENTS
Sturge-Weber–Klippel-Trenaunay syndrome	149000 185300	Telangiectatic nevi showing lateralization	Leptomeningeal angiomatosis, spinal angiomatosis, seizures, hemiplegia	Glaucoma, buphthalmos, hypertrophy of related limbs	See also Chap. 166 Familial aggregation may be explained by paradominant inheritance (see text)
Van Lohuizen's syndrome	219250	Reticular livedo-like lesions, telangiectatic nevi with and without lateralization	Developmental delay, seizures	Macrocephaly, syndactyly and other growth abnormalities of limbs	
Encephalocraniocutaneous lipomatosis	No entry	Hairless fatty tissue nevus of the scalp	Multiple intracranial lipomas, porencephaly, vascular dysplasia, mental retardation, seizures	Lipodermoid of conjunctiva, protuberances of cranial bones	
Schimmelpenning's syndrome	163000 165000	Sebaceous nevus	Mental retardation	Lipodermoid of conjunctiva, coloboma, bone defects	
Delleman's syndrome	164180	Periorbital skin tags, focal aplastic skin lesions (see text)	Porencephaly	Eyelid coloboma, focal skull defects	
Phacomatosis pigmentokeratotica	No entry	Speckled lentiginous nevus of papular type, sebaceous nevus	Segmental dysesthesia, segmental hyperhidrosis, mild mental retardation, seizures, deafness, ptosis, strabismus, muscular weakness		Cooccurrence of the two nevi may reflect twin spotting (see text)
Nevus comedonicus syndrome	No entry	Nevus comedonicus	EEG abnormalities	Ipsilateral cataract, absence deformities of bones	
Proteus syndrome	176920	Epidermal nevus of nonepidermolytic, non-organoid type; cerebriform hyperplasia of plantar tissue, subcutaneous hamartomas, telangiectatic nevi	Mental retardation, seizures	Partial gigantism of hands or feet, macrocephaly, hemihypertrophy	Recent reports suggest that patchy areas of dermal or subcutaneous hypoplasia may also be present
Neurocutaneous melanosis	249400	Giant melanocytic nevus	Leptomeningeal melanocytosis		Increased risk of malignant melanoma
Pigmentary mosaicism of the Ito type	146150 (see text)	Mosaic lesions of hypopigmentation	See comments and text	See comments and text	It should be noted that "hypomelanosis of Ito" no longer exists as an entity (see text)
Pallister-Killian syndrome	601803	Circumscribed areas of hypopigmentation on the cranium or elsewhere on the body, sparse eyebrows and lashes; scalp hair is sparse and fine during infancy	Severe mental retardation, hearing loss, seizures, ptosis	High forehead, puffy eyelids, hypertelorism, small nose with anteverted nostrils, down-turned mouth with thin upper lip	The disorder is caused by mosaic tetrasomy 12p (see text)

*MIM, Mendelian inheritance in man.

survive only in a mosaic state, in close proximity with normal cells.[88] Such mosaics usually result from an early postzygotic mutation. The following neurocutaneous phenotypes can be best explained by this concept.

STURGE-WEBER–KLIPPEL-TRENAUNAY SYNDROME According to conventional rules of classification, the Sturge-Weber syndrome and the Klippel-Trenaunay syndrome are separate entities, but from a genetic point of view it is obvious that they are caused by the same gene defect.[88] For a detailed description of the Sturge-Weber phenotype, which is characterized by lateral telangiectatic nevi of the face (Fig. 189-13), see Chap. 102. Bilateral involvement occurs rather frequently.[89] Klippel-Trenaunay syndrome differs with regard to the location of the lesions and is characterized by lateral telangiectatic nevi associated with hypertrophy of related bones and soft tissues of one or several limbs. Again, bilateral involvement is frequently observed, and a combination of Sturge-Weber and Klippel-Trenaunay syndrome has sometimes been described.[90,91]

Remarkably, this syndrome may exceptionally show a familial aggregation.[92,93] To explain this phenomenon, paradominant inheritance has been proposed.[94] Heterozygous individuals would be phenotypically normal, and the trait would only be expressed when loss of heterozygosity occurs at an early stage of embryogenesis, giving rise to a mosaic population of cells that have become either homozygous or hemizygous for the underlying mutation.[94]

VAN LOHUIZEN'S SYNDROME (CUTIS MARMORATA TELANGIECTATIA CONGENITA) The disease is characterized by reticular vascular lesions resulting in a bluish-red, livedo-like network that may involve large parts of the body. Extracutaneous symptoms comprise macrocephaly, seizures, and developmental delay, as well as growth anomalies of the limbs.[95,96] Vascular nevi similar to those observed in Sturge-Weber–Klippel-Trenaunay syndrome may like-

FIGURE 189-13

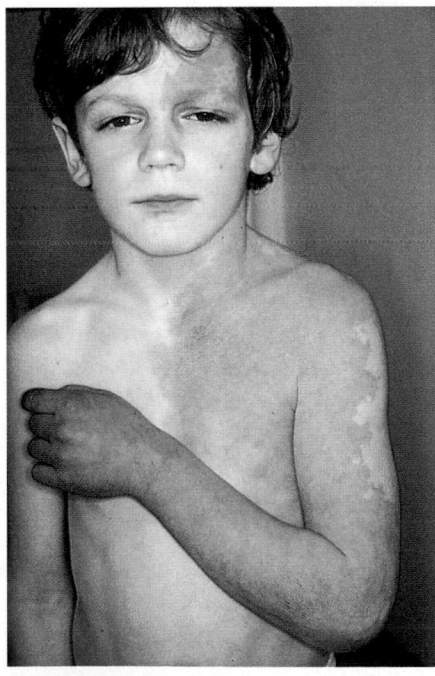

Sturge-Weber–Klippel-Trenaunay syndrome. (*Courtesy of Jean Maleville, MD, Bordeaux, France.*)

wise be present, but, remarkably, do not always show lateralization. Virtually all cases so far observed were sporadic, and for this reason they may originate from a lethal mutation surviving by mosaicism.

ENCEPHALOCRANIOCUTANEOUS LIPOMATOSIS This syndrome includes an extensive fatty tissue nevus of the scalp, protuberances of the cranial bones, lipodermoid of the conjunctiva, multiple intracranial lipomas, and porencephaly.[97] It has been proposed that the associated fatty tissue nevus of the scalp should be distinguished from other connective tissue nevi such as the Hoffmann-Zurhelle nevus.[98] Involvement of the CNS may include vascular dysplasia, mental retardation, and epileptic seizures. All cases so far reported have been sporadic.[97]

DELLEMAN'S SYNDROME This phenotype includes orbital cysts, porencephaly, skull defects, eyelid coloboma, and multiple skin tags, which are usually arranged in the periorbital region; in addition, there are widespread aplastic skin lesions that never show herniation of the fatty tissue, as observed in focal dermal hypoplasia.[99] All of these lesions suggest a mosaic arrangement, and all observations are sporadic.[88]

SCHIMMELPENNING'S SYNDROME This syndrome is characterized by the presence of a systematized sebaceous nevus associated with various cerebral defects causing mental retardation and seizures, ocular anomalies including conjunctival lipodermoids or colobomas, as well as bone defects.[88,100] The combination of these mosaic anomalies may vary to a large degree. There are two reports suggesting familial occurrence of this syndrome. If the clinical diagnosis was correct in these cases, they can be explained either by a coincidence or by paradominant inheritance.[94]

PHACOMATOSIS PIGMENTOKERATOTICA This disorder is defined by the co-occurrence of a speckled lentiginous nevus of a papular type and an epidermal nevus of a nonepidermolytic, organoid type, usually in the form of sebaceous nevus (Fig. 189-14). The coexistence of the two cutaneous lesions has been explained as a twin-spot phenomenon.[101] Associated neurologic defects include segmental dysesthesia, segmental hyperhidrosis, mild mental retardation, seizures, deafness, ptosis, strabismus, and muscular weakness of varying degrees.[102]

NEVUS COMEDONICUS SYNDROME This syndrome is characterized by a nevus comedonicus in combination with ipsilateral cataract and skeletal defects.[100] Electroencephalographic abnormalities have likewise been reported.[88]

PROTEUS SYNDROME This phenotype includes partial gigantism of hands or feet and other forms of hemihypertrophy including macrocephaly; multiple subcutaneous hamartomas such as lymphangioma, hemangioma, lipoma, or fibroma; cerebriform hyperplasia of plantar connective tissue; and a linear epidermal nevus of the nonepidermolytic, nonorganoid type (Fig. 189-15).[103] Because of the marked variability of all these defects, the disorder was named after the Greek god Proteus, who was said to be able to change his outward appearance in many ways. Paradoxically, patchy areas of dermal hypoplasia or lipohypoplasia have been observed in many cases.[104] Intelligence may be normal, but there is an increased incidence of mental retardation and seizures.[1]

NEUROCUTANEOUS MELANOSIS Neurocutaneous melanosis is characterized by giant melanocytic nevus in combination with

FIGURE 189-14

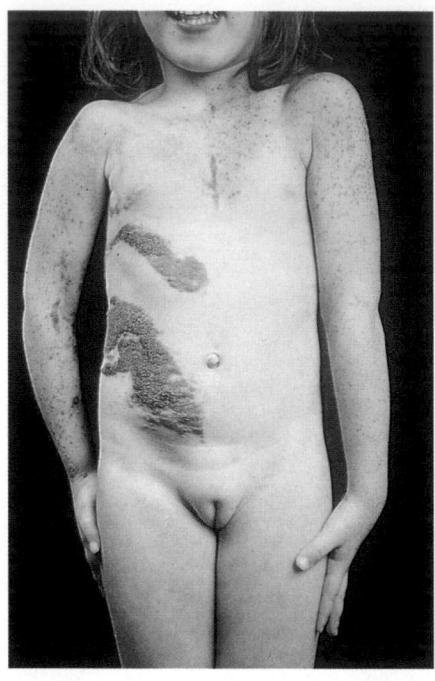

Phacomatosis pigmentokeratotica: speckled lentiginous nevus and contralateral sebaceous nevus.

leptomeningeal melanocytosis. The giant cutaneous lesion may be associated with widespread small congenital melanocytic nevi. The risk of malignant melanoma developing from either cutaneous or

FIGURE 189-15

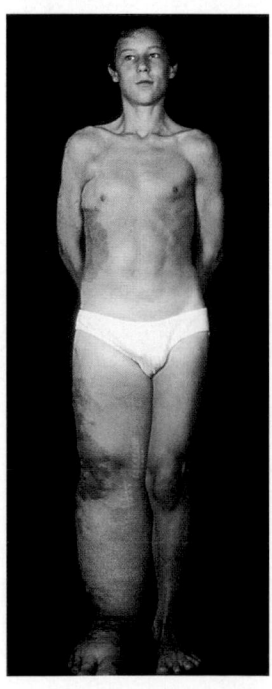

Proteus syndrome.

cerebral lesions is markedly increased.[105] Because all cases are sporadic, mosaicism of a lethal gene has been suggested.[88]

PIGMENTARY MOSAICISM OF THE ITO TYPE   Previously, such phenotypes were often described under the designation *hypomelanosis of Ito*, but it is important to realize that this is an outdated term that does not refer to any specific neurocutaneous syndrome.[106,107] On the contrary, it simply describes a cutaneous symptom as observed in many different states of genetic mosaicism that may or may not involve, in addition, extracutaneous organs such as the brain or eyes.[107] The associated neurologic anomalies vary to a large degree. Because virtually all cases are sporadic, they most likely represent mosaicism of a lethal mutation that may be a numerical chromosome aberration, a deletion, or a point mutation. Cytogenetic or molecular analysis to find one of the underlying defects is advisable.

PALLISTER-KILLIAN SYNDROME   The disorder is caused by mosaic tetrasomy for the short arm of chromosome 12 (isochromosome12p syndrome).[108,109] From a heuristic point of view, the disease can be taken as a specific entity within the spectrum of so-called hypomelanosis of Ito. Clinical features are postnatal growth deficiency and severe mental retardation and a characteristic facial appearance with a high forehead, sparse eyebrows and lashes, puffy eyelids, ptosis, hypertelorism, hypoplastic nose with anteverted nostrils, and a down-turned mouth with a thin upper lip.[1] During infancy the hair is markedly sparse and fine, but later on, hair growth becomes normal. Circumscribed hypopigmented areas are often present on the cranium and sometimes elsewhere on the body. Apparently, these hypopigmented lesions do not follow the lines of Blaschko.

CHROMOSOMAL DISORDERS

Some phenotypes characterized by numerical chromosome aberrations are associated with characteristic cutaneous features (Table 189-6).

ULLRICH-TURNER SYNDROME   This syndrome was described in 1930 by Ullrich[110] and in 1938 by Turner.[111] The chromosome constitution 45,X results in a female phenotype with short stature, sexual infantilism, webbed neck, and various other anomalies.[1] Remarkably, the intelligence deficit present in this syndrome does not refer to all brain functions. In general, affected women have a handicap in visual-spatial orientation and perceptual organization, whereas language skills are normal. Newborn girls may show marked lymphedema of the feet with hypoplastic toenails. Affected women show large numbers of melanocytic nevi.[1]

KLINEFELTER'S SYNDROME   The clinical features of Klinefelter's syndrome result from the chromosome constitution 47,XXY. Affected men are relatively tall and, characteristically, the arm span exceeds the height.[1] The testes are small, and gynecomastia is often present in adult individuals. Mental development is only mildly retarded. Typical cutaneous features are varicose veins and hypostatic leg ulcers.[112]

TRISOMY 21   Trisomy 21 is a well-known syndrome[1] that will not be described in detail in this chapter. Rather, the cutaneous signs and symptoms observed in this phenotype will be mentioned. A more or less widespread ichthyosiform hyperkeratosis is often ob-

TABLE 189-6

Neurocutaneous Syndromes: Disorders Caused by Numerical Chromosome Aberrations

DISORDER	NUMERICAL CHROMOSOME ABERRATION	CUTANEOUS ANOMALIES	NEUROLOGIC ANOMALIES	OTHER ANOMALIES	COMMENTS
Ullrich-Turner syndrome	45,XO	Lymphedema in new-born girls, multiple melanocytic nevi in women	Intelligence deficit regarding specific functions (see text)	Short stature, webbed neck, sexual infantilism, cardiovascular defects	In about 45% of cases, mosaicism such as 46,XX/45,XO is found
Klinefelter's syndrome	47,XXY	Varicose veins, leg ulcers	Mild mental retardation	Gynecomastia, small testes	In about 20% of cases, mosaicism such as 46,XY/47,XXY is found
Trisomy 21	47,XY,+21 47,XX,+21	Single palmar crease, ichthyosiform hyperkeratosis, elastosis perforans serpiginosa, multiple syringomas, alopecia areata	Microcephaly, mental retardation of varying degree	Characteristic facial appearance, macroglossia, immune deficiency	?Causative role of superoxide mutase (21q22)[2]

served in adults.[113] Other typical features are elastosis perforans serpiginosa[114] and milia-like calcinosis cutis.[115] Syringomas occur far more frequently than in the general population.[116] Moreover, trisomy 21 individuals show a markedly increased proneness to alopecia areata.[117]

PHENOTYPES STILL UNCLASSIFIABLE ACCORDING TO FORMAL GENETICS

Some neurocutaneous disorders are obviously genetically determined but can so far not be categorized according to formal genetics (Table 189-7).

BRACHMANN–DE LANGE SYNDROME This phenotype is characterized by low birth weight, delayed growth, and mental re-

tardation. Affected children have a typical facial appearance with microcephaly, low frontal hair line, synophrys, hypoplastic nose with anteverted nostrils, and protruding philtrum.[118] Absence deformities of hands or feet may be noted. As a characteristic cutaneous feature, pronounced hypertrichosis may be found in many areas of the body.[119] Additional cutaneous anomalies include cutis marmorata, hypoplastic nipples, hypoplastic umbilicus, and simian crease of the palm. The genetic basis of this syndrome has so far not been elucidated.[120,121] Discordant monozygotic twins have been described.[122]

SATOYOSHI'S SYNDROME Satoyoshi's syndrome is of interest for the dermatologist because this genetically determined disorder is associated with early onset of alopecia areata (see Table 189-7).[123]

NICOLAIDES-BARAITSER SYNDROME This syndrome includes mental retardation, sparse hair, prominent lower lip, and brachy-

TABLE 189-7

Neurocutaneous Syndromes: Disorders Still Unclassifiable According to Formal Genetics

DISORDER	MIM NO.*	CUTANEOUS ANOMALIES	NEUROLOGIC ANOMALIES	OTHER ANOMALIES	COMMENTS
Brachmann–de Lange syndrome	122470	Low frontal hairline, synophrys, hypertrichosis of various areas of the body	Microcephaly, mental retardation	Small nose with anteverted nostrils, protruding philtrum, absence of deformities of hands or feet	A mild form may be inherited as an autosomal dominant trait[121,122]
Satoyoshi's syndrome	No entry	Alopecia areata of early onset	Painful intermittent muscle spasms	Short stature, skeletal defects, malabsorption	Pathogenesis involves an autoimmune mechanism[123]
Nicolaides-Baraitser syndrome	No entry	Sparse hair	Mental retardation	Prominent lower lip, brachydactyly, short metacarpals	
Johnston's syndrome	No entry	Diffuse ichthyotic hyperkeratosis, contractures with skin fissuring	Hypoplasia of dorsal roots and posterior columns, absent sensory response	Death in early infancy	Pedigree is compatible with either autosomal or X-linked recessive inheritance[125]

*MIM, Mendelian inheritance in man.

dactyly.[124] Further clinical research should show whether the concept of a new syndrome holds true.

JOHNSTON'S SYNDROME   Hyperkeratotic skin changes reminiscent of collodion baby were observed by Johnston et al.[125] in two brothers suffering from severe arthrogryposis. The two boys died shortly after birth. Autopsy performed in one of them showed severe hypoplasia of the posterior columns. The syndrome is most likely inherited as either a monogenic autosomal or an X-linked recessive trait.

REFERENCES

1. Gorlin RJ et al: *Syndromes of the Head and Neck,* 3d ed. New York, Oxford Univ Press, 1990
2. McKusick VA: *Mendelian Inheritance in Man: A Catalog of Human Genes and Genetic Disorders,* 11th ed. Baltimore, Johns Hopkins Univ Press, 1994
3. Lyon MF: Gene action in the X-chromosome of the mouse (*Mus musculus* L). *Nature* **190**:372, 1961
4. Happle R: Mosaicism in human skin: Understanding the patterns and mechanisms. *Arch Dermatol* **129**:1460, 1993
5. Friedman JM, Birch PH: Type 1 neurofibromatosis: A descriptive analysis of the disorder in 1,728 patients. *Am J Med Genet* **70**:138, 1997
6. Mautner VF et al: Skin abnormalities in neurofibromatosis 2. *Arch Dermatol* **133**:1539, 1997
7. Carbonara C et al: Apparent preferential loss of heterozygosity at TSC2 over TSC1 chromosomal region in tuberous sclerosis hamartomas. *Genes Chromosom Cancer* **15**:18, 1996
8. European Chromosome 16 Tuberous Sclerosis Consortium: Identification and characterization of the tuberous sclerosis gene on chromosome 16. *Cell* **75**:1305, 1993
9. Povey S et al: Two loci for tuberous sclerosis: One on 9q35 and one on 16p13. *Ann Hum Genet* **58**:107, 1994
10. Bale AE: Variable expressivity of patched mutations in flies and humans. *Am J Hum Genet* **60**:10, 1977
11. Ruiz-Maldonado R et al: Progressive cardiomyopathic lentiginosis: Report of six cases and one autopsy. *Pediatr Dermatol* **1**:146, 1983
12. Selmanowitz VJ: Lentiginosis profusa syndrome. IV. Giant pigment granules (light microscopy). *Acta Derm Venereol (Stockh)* **55**:481, 1975
13. Telfer MA et al: Dominant piebald trait (white forelock and leukoderma) with neurological impairment. *Am J Hum Genet* **23**:383, 1971
14. Asher JH Jr et al: Effects of Pax3 modifier genes on craniofacial morphology, pigmentation, and variability: A murine model of Waardenburg syndrome variation. *Genomics* **34**:285, 1996
15. Krajewska-Walasek M et al: The cardio-facio-cutaneous (CFC) syndrome—two possible new cases and review of the literature. *Clin Dysmorphol* **5**:65, 1996
16. Leichtman LG: Are cardio-facio-cutaneous syndrome and Noonan syndrome distinct? A case of CFC offspring of a mother with Noonan syndrome. *Clin Dysmorphol* **5**:61, 1996
17. Wieczorek D et al: Cardio-facio-cutaneous (CFC) syndrome—a distinct entity? Report of three patients demonstrating the diagnostic difficulties in delineation of CFC syndrome. *Clin Genet* **52**:37, 1997
18. Jenkins T: The South African malady. *Nat Genet* **13**:7, 1996
19. Korda V et al: Increased erythrocyte protoporphyrin in homozygous variegate porphyria. *Photodermatology* **2**:257, 1984
20. Murphy GM et al: Homozygous variegate porphyria: Two similar cases in unrelated families. *J R Soc Med* **79**:361, 1986
21. Traupe H: *The Ichthyoses: A Guide to Clinical Diagnosis, Genetic Counseling, and Therapy.* Berlin, Springer, 1989
22. Schnyder UW: Ichthyosis hystrix Typus Rheydt (Ichthyosis hystrix gravior mit praktischer Taubheit). *Z Hautkr* **52**:763, 1977
23. König A et al: Autosomal dominant inheritance of HID syndrome (hystrix-like ichthyosis with deafness). *Eur J Dermatol* **7**:554, 1997
24. Verbov J: Palmoplantar keratoderma, deafness and atopy. *Br J Dermatol* **116**:881, 1987
25. Sharland M et al: Autosomal dominant palmoplantar hyperkeratosis and sensorineural deafness in three generations. *J Med Genet* **29**:50, 1992
26. Fitzgerald DA, Verbov J: Hereditary palmoplantar keratoderma with deafness. *Br J Dermatol* **134**:939, 1996
27. Lynch SA et al: Absent nails, kinesogenic choreoathetosis, epilepsy and developmental delay—a new autosomal dominant disorder? *Clin Dysmorphol* **6**:133, 1997
28. Schmidt B et al: A novel amino acid modification in sulfatases that is defective in multiple sulfatase deficiency. *Cell* **82**:271, 1995
29. Castaño Suárez E et al: Ichthyosis: The skin manifestation of multiple sulfatase deficiency. *Pediatr Dermatol* **14**:369, 1997
30. Steijlen PM et al: Congenital atrichia, palmoplantar hyperkeratosis, mental retardation, and early loss of teeth in four siblings: A new syndrome? *J Am Acad Dermatol* **30**:893, 1994
31. Cremers CW, Geerts SJ: Sensorineural hearing loss and pili torti. *Ann Otol Rhinol Laryngol* **88**:100, 1979
32. Shapira SK et al: Unknown syndrome in sibs: Pili torti, growth delay, developmental delay, and mild neurological abnormalities. *J Med Genet* **29**:509, 1992
33. Elejalde BR et al: Mutations affecting pigmentation in man: I. Neuroectodermal melanolysosomal disease. *Am J Med Genet* **3**:65, 1979
34. Duran C et al: Neuroectodermal melanolysosomal disease: Silvery hair as a marker of neurologic pathology. *Arch Dermatol* 1998 (in press)
35. Lerone M et al: Oculocerebral syndrome with hypopigmentation (Cross syndrome): Report of a new case. *Clin Genet* **41**:87, 1992
36. Tezcan I et al: A new case of oculocerebral hypopigmentation syndrome (Cross syndrome) with additional findings. *Clin Genet* **51**:118, 1997
37. Greenhaw GA et al: Xeroderma pigmentosum and Cockayne syndrome: Overlapping clinical and biochemical phenotypes. *Am J Hum Genet* **50**:677, 1992
38. Kanda T et al: Peripheral neuropathy in xeroderma pigmentosum. *Brain* **113**:1025, 1990
39. Nance MA et al: Cockayne syndrome: Review of 140 cases. *Am J Med Genet* **42**:68, 1992
40. Stefanini M et al: Genetic analysis of twenty-two patients with Cockayne syndrome. *Hum Genet* **97**:418, 1996
41. Ledley FD, Rosenblatt DS: Mutations in mut methylmalonic acidemia: Clinical and enzymatic correlations. *Hum Mutat* **9**:1, 1997
42. Gravel RA et al: Mutations participating in interallelic complementation in propionic acidemia. *Am J Hum Genet* **55**:51, 1994
43. Koopman RJJ, Happle R: Cutaneous manifestations of methylmalonic acidemia. *Arch Dermatol Res* **282**:272, 1990
44. Symula DJ et al: A candidate mouse model for Hartnup disorder deficient in neutral amino acid transport. *Mamm Genome* **8**:102, 1997
45. Schmitz G et al: Tangier disease: A disorder of intracellular membrane traffic. *Proc Nat Acad Sci USA* **82**:6305, 1985
46. Shashi V et al: Neuroectodermal (CHIME) syndrome: An additional case with long term follow up of all reported cases. *J Med Genet* **32**:465, 1995
47. Karnes PS et al: De Barsy syndrome: Report of a case, literature review, and elastin gene expression studies of the skin. *Am J Med Genet* **42**:29, 1992
48. Winter RM: Dubowitz syndrome. *J Med Genet* **23**:11, 1986
49. Happle R: Lyonization and the lines of Blaschko. *Hum Genet* **70**:200, 1985
50. Kore-Eda S et al: Focal dermal hypoplasia (Goltz syndrome) associated with multiple giant papillomas. *Br J Dermatol* **133**:997, 1995
51. Bellosta M et al: Focal dermal hypoplasia: Report of a family with 7 affected women in 3 generations. *Eur J Dermatol* **6**:499, 1996
52. Jouet R et al: Incontinentia pigmenti. *Eur J Hum Genet* **4**:168, 1997
53. Parrish JE et al: Selection against mutant alleles in blood leukocytes is a consistent feature in incontinentia pigmenti type 2. *Hum Mol Genet* **5**:1777, 1996
54. Rott HD, Koniszewski G: L'analogie des lignes de Blaschko à l'oeil. *J Génét Hum* **35**:19, 1987
55. Happle R: Psychotropism as a cutaneous feature of the CHILD syndrome. *J Am Acad Dermatol* **23**:763, 1990
56. Happle R et al: The CHILD nevus: A distinct skin disorder. *Dermatology* **191**:210, 1995
57. Pereiro Miguens M et al: Lesiones psoriasiformes de distribución linear acompañadas de malformaciones congénitas. *Actas Dermo-Sifiliogr (Madrid)* **51**:213, 1960

58. Baden HP, Rex IH: Linear ichthyosis associated with skeletal abnormalities: ?New entity. *Arch Dermatol* **102**:126, 1970

59. Happle R et al: MIDAS syndrome (microphthalmia, dermal aplasia and sclerocornea): An X-linked phenotype distinct from Goltz syndrome. *Am J Med Genet* **47**:710, 1993

60. Mücke J et al: MIDAS syndrome (microphthalmia, dermal aplasia and sclerocornea): An autonomous entity with linear skin defects within the spectrum of focal hypoplasias. *Eur J Dermatol* **5**:197, 1995

61. Naritomi K et al: Combined Goltz and Aicardi syndromes in a terminal Xp deletion: Are they a contiguous gene syndrome? *Am J Med Genet* **43**:839, 1992

62. Wapenaar MC et al: The genes for X-linked ocular albinism (OA1) and microphthalmia with linear skin defects (MLS): Cloning and characterization of the critical regions. *Hum Mol Genet* **2**:947, 1993

63. Happle R et al: Wie verlaufen die Blaschko-Linien am behaarten Kopf? *Hautarzt* **35**:366, 1984

64. Feather SA et al: The oral-facial-digital syndrome type 1 (OFD1), a cause of polycystic kidney disease and associated malformations, maps to Xp22.2-Xp22.3. *Hum Mol Genet* **6**:1163, 1997

65. Happle R: Cutaneous manifestation of X-linked genes escaping inactivation. *Clin Exp Dermatol* **17**:69, 1992

66. Partington MW et al: Familial cutaneous amyloidosis with systemic manifestations in males. *Am J Med Genet* **10**:65, 1981

67. Gedeon AK et al: Localization of the gene for X-linked reticulate pigmentary disorder with systemic manifestations (PDR), previously known as X-linked cutaneous amyloidosis. *Am J Med Genet* **52**:75, 1994

68. Kelly EJ, Palmiter RD: A murine model of Menkes disease reveals a physiological function of metallothionein. *Nat Genet* **13**:219, 1996

69. Tumer Z et al: Early copper-histidine treatment for Menkes disease. *Nat Genet* **12**:11, 1996

70. Collie WR et al: Hair in Menkes disease: A comprehensive review, in *Hair, Trace Elements, and Human Illness*, edited by AC Brown, RG Crounse. New York, Praeger, 1980, pp 197–209

71. Gerdes AM et al: Clinical expression of Menkes syndrome in females. *Clin Genet* **38**:452, 1990

72. George AM et al: Analysis of Mnk, the murine homologue of the locus for Menkes disease, in normal and mottled (Mo) mice. *Genomics* **22**:27, 1994

73. Grimes A et al: Molecular basis of the brindled mouse mutant (Mo(br)): A murine model of Menkes disease. *Hum Mol Genet* **6**:1037, 1997

74. Lungarotti MS et al: X-linked mental retardation, microcephaly, and growth delay associated with hereditary bullous dystrophy, macular type: Report of a second family. *Am J Med Genet* **51**:598, 1994

75. Wijker M et al: The gene for hereditary bullous dystrophy, X-linked macular type, maps to the Xq27.3-qter region. *Am J Hum Genet* **56**:1096, 1995

76. Zlogotora J: X-linked albinism-deafness syndrome and Waardenburg syndrome type IIa: A hypothesis. *Am J Med Genet* **59**:386, 1995

77. Fried K et al: Hearing impairment in female carriers of the sex-linked syndrome of deafness with albinism. *J Med Genet* **6**:132, 1969

78. Shiloh Y et al: Genetic mapping of X-linked albinism-deafness syndrome (ADFN) to Xq26.3-qH27.1. *Am J Hum Genet* **47**:20, 1990

79. Quinton R et al: The neuroradiology of Kallmann's syndrome: A genotypic and phenotypic analysis. *J Clin Endocrinol Metab* **81**:3010, 1996

80. Bick D et al: Male infant with ichthyosis, Kallmann syndrome, chondrodysplasia punctata, and an Xp chromosome deletion. *Am J Med Genet* **33**:100, 1989

81. Meindl A et al: Analysis of a terminal Xp22.3 deletion in a patient with six monogenic disorders: Implications for the mapping of X-linked ocular albinism. *J Med Genet* **30**:838, 1993

82. Davidson BL et al: Identification of 17 independent mutations responsible for human hypoxanthine-guanine phosphoribosyltransferase (HPRT) deficiency. *Am J Hum Genet* **48**:951, 1991

83. Nyhan WL: The recognition of Lesch-Nyhan syndrome as an inborn error of purine metabolism. *J Inherit Metab Dis* **20**:171, 1997

84. Ernst M et al: Presynaptic dopaminergic deficits in Lesch-Nyhan disease. *N Engl J Med* **334**:1568, 1996

85. Dodd S et al: Mutations in the adrenoleukodystrophy gene. *Hum Mutat* **9**:500, 1997

86. Krasemann EW et al: Identification of mutations in the ALD-gene of 20 families with adrenoleukodystrophy/adrenomyeloneuropathy. *Hum Genet* **97**:194, 1996

87. Laureti S et al: X-linked adrenoleukodystrophy is a frequent cause of idiopathic Addison's disease in young adult male patients. *J Clin Endocrinol Metab* **81**:470, 1996

88. Happle R: Lethal genes surviving by mosaicism: A possible explanation for sporadic birth defects involving the skin. *J Am Acad Dermatol* **16**:899, 1987

89. Sujansky E et al: Outcome of Sturge-Weber syndrome in 52 adults. *Am J Med Genet* **57**:35, 1995

90. Teller H, Lindner B: Über Mischformen der phakomatösen Syndrome von Sturge-Weber und Klippel-Trenaunay. *Z Hautkr* **13**:113, 1952

91. Harper PS: Sturge-Weber syndrome with Klippel-Trenaunay-Weber syndrome. *Birth Defects* **7**(8):314, 1971

92. Aelvot GE et al: Genetic aspects of Klippel-Trenaunay syndrome. *Br J Dermatol* **126**:603, 1992

93. Ceballos-Quintal JM et al: A new case of Klippel-Trenaunay-Weber (KTW) syndrome: Evidence of autosomal dominant inheritance. *Am J Med Genet* **63**:426, 1996

94. Happle R: Klippel-Trenaunay syndrome: Is it a paradominant trait? *Br J Dermatol* **128**:465, 1993

95. Stephan MJ et al: Macrocephaly in association with unusual cutaneous angiomatosis. *J Pediatr* **87**:353, 1975

96. Clayton-Smith J et al: Macrocephaly with cutis marmorata, haemangioma and syndactyly—a distinctive overgrowth syndrome. *Clin Dysmorphol* **6**:291, 1997

97. Happle R, Steijlen PM: Enzephalokraniokutane Lipomatose: Ein nichterblicher Mosaikphänotyp. *Hautarzt* **44**:19, 1993

98. Happle R, Küster W: Nevus psiloliparus: A distinct fatty tissue nevus. *Dermatology* **197**, 1998 (in press)

99. Moog U et al: Oculocerebrocutaneous syndrome: A case report, a follow-up, and differential diagnostic considerations. *Genet Counsel* **7**:257, 1996

100. Happle R: Epidermal nevus syndromes. *Semin Dermatol* **14**:111, 1995

101. Happle R: Phacomatosis pigmentokeratotica: A melanocytic-epidermal twin nevus syndrome. *Am J Med Genet* **65**:363, 1996

102. Tadini G et al: Phacomatosis pigmentokeratotica: Report of 3 cases and further delineation of the syndrome. *Arch Dermatol* **134**:333, 1998

103. Clark RD et al: Proteus syndrome: An expanded phenotype. *Am J Med Genet* **27**:99, 1987

104. Happle R et al: Patchy dermal hypoplasia as a characteristic feature of Proteus syndrome. *Arch Dermatol* **133**:77, 1997

105. Demirci A et al: MR of parenchymal neurocutaneous melanosis. *AJNR* **16**:606, 1995

106. Donnai D et al: Hypomelanosis of Ito: A manifestation of mosaicism or chimerism. *J Med Genet* **12**:809, 1988

107. Küster W et al: "Hypomelanosis of Ito": No entity, but a cutaneous sign of mosaicism, in *The Pigmentary System and its Disorders*, edited by JJ Nordlund et al. New York, Oxford Univ Press, 1998, pp 594–601

108. Cormier-Daire V et al: Prezygotic origin of the isochromosome 12p in Pallister-Killian syndrome. *Am J Med Genet* **69**:166, 1997

109. Schubert R et al: Report of two new cases of Pallister-Killian syndrome confirmed by FISH: Tissue-specific mosaicism and loss of i(12p) by in vitro selection. *Am J Med Genet* **72**:106, 1997

110. Ullrich O: Über typische Kombinationsbilder multipler Abartungen. *Z Kinderheilk* **49**:271, 1930

111. Turner HH: A syndrome of infantilism, congenital webbed neck and cubitus valgus. *Endocrinology* **23**:566, 1938

112. Spier C et al: Recurrent leg ulcerations as the initial clinical manifestation of Klinefelter's syndrome. *Arch Dermatol* **131**:230, 1995

113. Wentscher U, Happle R: Ichthyosiform hyperkeratosis as a characteristic feature of trisomy 21. *Eur J Dermatol* **5**:417, 1995

114. Scherbenske JM et al: Cutaneous and ocular manifestations of Down syndrome. *J Am Acad Dermatol* **22**:933, 1990

115. Schepis C et al: Milia-like idiopathic calcinosis cutis: An unusual dermatosis associated with Down syndrome. *Br J Dermatol* **134**:143, 1996

116. Schepis C et al: Perforating milia-like idiopathic calcinosis cutis and periorbital syringomas in a girl with Down syndrome. *Pediatr Dermatol* **11**:258, 1994

117. Carter DM, Jegasothy BV: Alopecia areata and Down syndrome. *Arch Dermatol* **112**:1397, 1976

118. Jackson L et al: De Lange syndrome: A clinical review of 310 individuals. *Am J Med Genet* **47**:940, 1993

119. Schuster DS, Johnson SAM: Cutaneous manifestations of the Cornelia de Lange syndrome. *Arch Dermatol* **93**:702, 1966

120. Chodirker BN et al: Male-to-male transmission of mild Brachmann–de Lange syndrome. *Am J Med Genet* **52**:331, 1994

121. Feingold M, Lin AE: Familial Brachmann–de Lange syndrome: Further evidence for autosomal dominant inheritance and review of the literature. *Am J Med Genet* **47**:1064, 1993

122. Carakushansky G et al: Identical twin discordance for the Brachmann–de Lange syndrome revisited. *Am J Med Genet* **63**:458, 1996

123. Ehlayel MS, Lacassie Y: Satoyoshi syndrome: An unusual postnatal multisystemic disorder. *Am J Med Genet* **57**:620, 1995

124. Krajewska-Walasek M et al: Another patient with an unusual syndrome of mental retardation and sparse hair? *Clin Dysmorphol* **5**:183, 1996

125. Johnston K et al: Joint contractures, hyperkeratosis, and severe hypoplasia of the posterior columns: A new recessive syndrome. *Am J Med Genet* **47**:246, 1993

CHAPTER 190

Lowell A. Goldsmith

Tuberous Sclerosis Complex

Tuberous sclerosis complex (TSC) is an autosomal dominant disease attributable to mutations in one of two different genes. Lesions occur predominantly in the skin, nervous system, heart, and kidney. The most commonly recognized clinical manifestations are ash-leaf hypopigmented macules, adenoma sebaceum, seizures, and mental retardation.[1] The hypopigmented skin lesions and their differential diagnosis are discussed in Table 89-5; a precis definition of the disease is given in Table 89-4.

HISTORY

Although Virchow recognized scleromas of the cerebrum in the 1860s and von Recklinghausen found a similar case with multiple myomata of the heart in 1862, Bourneville's articles, appearing between 1880 and 1900, presented the first systematic account of the disease and related the cerebral and skin lesions. Vogt, in 1908, delineated the classic triad of adenoma sebaceum, epilepsy, and mental retardation.[2,3]

EPIDEMIOLOGY

The prevalence of the disease is estimated to be approximately 3 to 10 per 100,000.[4–6] There is no difference in frequency among whites, blacks, and Asians; both sexes are affected equally although some symptoms are more predominant in women. Heredity is evident in approximately one-third of cases; the remaining cases are attributed to a *de novo* mutation. Probably, prevalence data drawn from surveys of mental hospital populations magnified the overall incidence of mental retardation in this disorder.[2,7] There is no increase in paternal age in patients with new mutations. There is an instance of germinal mutation with three affected siblings with no somatic mutation in the parents. There are multiple instances of mutations limited to the germline in parents with multiple affected children and no clinical evidence of parental disease.[3]

ETIOLOGY AND PATHOGENESIS

Mutations in two genes, *TSC1* and *TSC2,* each account for about half the cases of tuberous sclerosis. No third gene has been linked to the disease. Tuberous sclerosis 1 (*TSC1*) maps to 9q34, is a 8.6-kb gene and codes a 130-kDa protein, hamartin, which is probably a tumor-suppressor gene with a nuclear localization signal and a cdc2 kinase site.[8,9]

The *TSC2* gene maps to 16p13.3 and codes for a 1784 amino acid protein, tuberin, which has homologies to a GTPase-acclerating protein (GAP) and has intrinsic GTPase activity. It localizes with Rap1 (a GTPase member of the ras superfamily of GTP-binding proteins) in the Golgi apparatus.[10] Inhibition of *TSC2* up-regulates cyclin, thus placing tuberin in the G_1 GDK-dependent control steps, regulating entrance into the S phase of the cell cycle from G_1 or G_0. *TSC2* mutations include deletions, insertions, missense duplications and tandem repeats. There were no mutational hot spots in the GTPase-activating protein–related domain.[11]

In the subependymal giant-cell astrocytomas and angiomyolipomas associated with TSC there was loss of heterozygosity in the

Portions of this chapter are based on sections of Chapter 184 by Raymond Adams, MD, and Priscilla Short, MD, in the fourth edition of this book.

16p13 region supporting a two-hit cancer-suppressor model for the pathogenesis of those tumors and supporting the role of *TSC2* as a tumor-suppressor gene.[12]

FIGURE 190-1

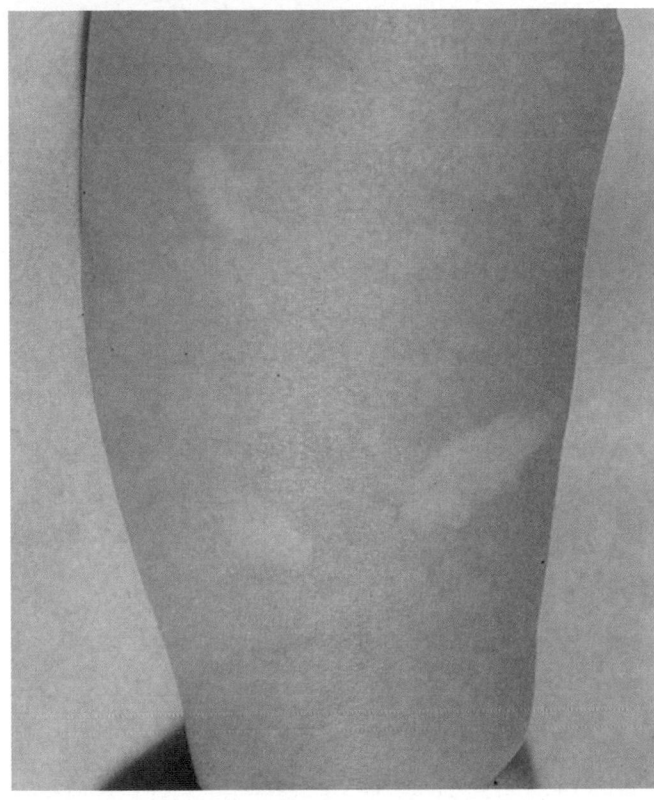

Hypomelanotic "ash-leaf" macules on the lower leg in a child with the tuberous sclerosis complex.

CLINICAL MANIFESTATIONS

The disease may be present at birth, but not recognized. Careful examination often will reveal hypopigmented macules. Focal or generalized seizures with or without developmental delay is often the first symptom of the disease. Adenoma sebaceum appears later in childhood, usually between the 4th and 10th years.

Seizures, a reliable index of cerebral lesions, in the first year to two take the form of infantile spasms with characteristic EEG pattern of hypsarrhythmia. Different seizure types may develop with age.

There is often a lack of parallelism between the epilepsy, mental deficit, and skin abnormalities. Less than a third of the patients have the complete Vogt triad. Some patients with recurrent seizures retain relatively normal mental function; however, those with mental retardation nearly all have epilepsy. When only a few skin lesions or a retinal phakoma are present, the diagnosis may require additional studies such as renal ultrasound and/or cranial neuro-imaging (CT or MRI).

Gray or yellow plaques (single or multiple) may be found in the retina (often in or near the optic disk) in about 50 percent of cases. It is from this lesion, called phakoma, that van der Hoeve derived the term, phakomatoses, applied to all neurocutaneous diseases of this class. Benign rhabdomyomas of the heart are common and may be associated with Wolff-Parkinson-White syndrome. Eighty percent of all children presenting with rhabdomyomas have TSC.[13] Up to 60 percent of patients have kidney angiomyolipomas, although symptomatic lesions predominate in women. The lesions present early, are often multiple and bilateral, and in contrast to nontuberous sclerosis-associated angiomyolipoma that are seen in older women. Cystic renal disease is seen in association with tuberous sclerosis, more frequently in patients with mutations in TSC2. In some cases, this is related to a contiguous gene syndrome related to mutations involving the TSC2 gene and the adjacent polycystic kidney disease gene (PKD).[14] Benign tumors have been found in the liver, thyroid, testes, and gastrointestinal tract. Pulmonary lymphangiomyomatosis, a proliferation of smooth muscle cells, is a rare complication of TSC in women, can occur without other findings of TSC, and may represent a form of segmental TSC with lower reproductive risk for TSC.[15]

SKIN LESIONS

In approximately 87 percent of the patients with tuberous sclerosis, congenital hypomelanotic macules lesions are present (Fig. 190-1). These are discussed in detail in Chap. 89. 4.7 percent of the general population has at least one hypopigmented macule; none has more than three. These data and the relative incidence of tuberous sclerosis mean that one macule per se should not prompt an extensive evaluation to rule out tuberous sclerosis.[16]

Facial angiofibromas, diagnostic of tuberous sclerosis, are present in 50 percent of patients over 4 years of age.[2,3,17,18] The earliest manifestation of facial angiofibromatosis may be a mild erythema over cheeks and forehead, which is intensified by crying. Although called adenoma sebaceum, the sebaceous glands are only passively involved. Typically they are red to pink papules with a smooth, glistening surface, localized to the nasolabial folds, cheeks, chin, and sometimes the forehead and scalp (Fig. 190-2). Segmental forms of the disease occur.[19] The differential diagnosis for angiofibroma includes acne vulgaris, acne rosacea, multiple trichoepitheliomas, and syringomas. Trichoepitheliomas have a similar centrofacial distribution of papules and nodules that lack the pink vascular aspect of angiofibromas. The occurrence of large plaques of connective tissue on the forehead represents another diagnostic feature. These are similar to adenoma sebaceum except for the absence of vascular elements.

A characteristic truncal lesion is the shagreen patch, most often in the lumbosacral region (Fig. 190-3). It is a flat, slightly elevated, flesh-colored plaque with a "pigskin," "elephant hide," or "orange peel" appearance; they vary from less than 1 cm up to 10 cm in diameter.

Periungual fibromas (Koenen tumors), most often appearing after puberty, are common (50 percent) in tuberous sclerosis.[20] They may also be subungual (Fig. 190-4). Fibromas in the matrix or nail bed lead to thinning or even destruction of the nail plate. Excision is usually curative. Gingival fibromas also occur, as do fibromas on the palate or lips.

Other skin changes seen not infrequently, but not in themselves diagnostic, include fibroepithelial tags (soft fibromas), café au lait spots, and port-wine hemangiomas.

FIGURE 190-2

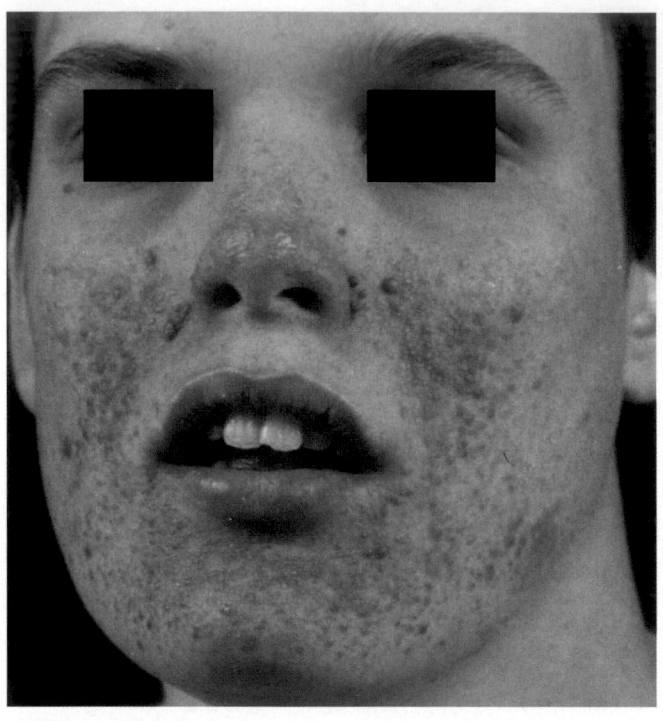

Adenoma sebaceum, the classic facial lesions in the tuberous sclerosis complex. These angiofibromas are typically localized on the cheeks and the nasolabial folds; they are pink or red and have a smooth surface.

FIGURE 190-3

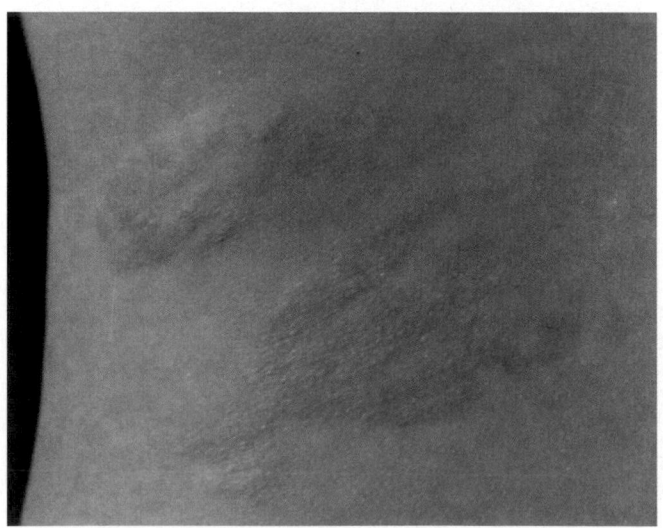

Shagreen patch in tuberous sclerosis. This is a flat, elevated lesion with an "orange peel" appearance. It corresponds to circumscribed subepidermal fibrosis.

FIGURE 190-4

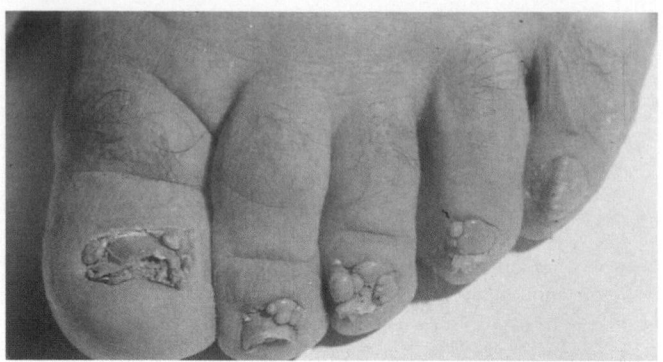

Koenen tumors in the tuberous sclerosis complex. These peri- and subungual fibromas are characteristic.

BRAIN PATHOLOGY

The brain exhibits a number of diagnostic features that include cortical tubers, areas of increased firmness on the cortical surface that on cut surface reveal loss of normal gray-white junction. These can vary in size from several millimeters to several centimeters. Microscopically, the cortical tubers show loss of the normal cortical cytoarchitecture and presence of abnormal neuronal and glial cells. The number and size of cortical tubers correlate with occurrence of seizures and mental retardation in TSC. Subependymal nodules along the ventricular surface, particularly at the level of the caudate nuclei and close to the foramen of Monro, are another typical neuropathologic finding in TSC. Historically, these lesions have accounted for the phrase "candle guttering" on gross examination. The nodules consist of large irregular cell of more glial histology although occasional bizarre neuronal type cells are seen. Some subependymal nodules may enlarge and obstruct the outflow of the lateral ventricles with the development of obstructive hydrocephalus. These are referred to as subependymal giant cell astrocytomas; however, they are distinctly different than the typical astrocytoma with rare malignant transformation. Both cortical tubers and subependymal nodules can calcify over time and account for earlier use of plain skull radiographs for diagnosis. Currently, magnetic resonance imaging and computed tomography are preferred neuroimaging for diagnosis and management.

The phakomas of the retina are generally asymptomatic and consists of neuronal and glial elements. Clinically the translucent forms in contrast to the calcified "mulberry" form need to be distinguised from retinoblastoma when first encountered.

SKIN PATHOLOGY (See Chap. 101)

The skin and nail lesions contain interlacing strands of fibroblasts and collagen with numerous blood vessels. The shagreen plaque is composed of a relatively avascular, dense, sclerotic mass of bundles of collagen fibers.

DIAGNOSIS AND DIFFERENTIAL DIAGNOSIS

When the mental, convulsive, and dermal abnormalities are conjoined, the diagnosis is clear. Epilepsy (i.e., spasms infantile and developmental delay are by no means diagnostic of tuberous sclerosis. It is in these cases, especially when the family history is unrevealing, that a thorough examination of the skin for hypomelanotic ash-leaf macules, adenoma sebaceum, collagenous patches, or subungual or gingival fibromas is so rewarding. The hypopigmented macules, as the earliest manifestation of the disease, are most helpful. The history of seizures and/or mental retardation is supportive in the presence of other diagnostic features of tuberous sclerosis. The radiographic demonstration of cortical tubers and subependymal nodules by either computed tomography or magnetic resonant imaging are more specifically diagnostic.

TREATMENT

Prenatal counseling can be recommended for a couple when one is affected, given the 50 percent risk for each pregnancy with the caveat that the clinical phenotype can be quite variable. If the affected individual has been informative on molecular testing for a mutation in either TSC1 or TSC2, a molecular prenatal test may be available. The test, although informative that a fetus is affected, is not prognostic for the severity of possible symptoms. The presence of cardiac rhabdomyomas may be detected by prenatal echocardiography and the pregnancy monitored for fetal cardiac compromise. Medical therapy is recommended when possible for complications of these lesions and over time the lesions disappear on sequential echocardiography. Seizure management is important in eventual intellectual outcome in children who present with early onset seizures. Neurosurgery for epilepsy control is a consideration in children who have intractable seizures to medical management and have a demonstrable dominant electroconvulsive focus. Obstructive hydrocephalus related to enlarged subependymal giant cell astrocytomas obstructing the outflow of the lateral ventricles is quite successful with limited morbidity in centers with experience. There are many patients, not mentally deficient, who can be helped by dermabrasion, electrodesiccation, or laser surgery (CO_2, copper vapor) of their facial lesions, with the knowledge that they will slowly regrow.[22,23]

COURSE AND PROGNOSIS

There is increased morbidity and mortality with patients with TSC with decreased survival curves compared to the general public that varies depending on different systemic involvement. The sources of mortality vary in different age groups with cardiovascular involvement predominant in the first decade of life, followed by brain tumors in the second decade. Mortality related to complications of renal involvement, angiomyolipomas that can be symptomatic on the basis of size with the development renovascular hypertension, decreased renal function, catastrophic hemorrhage, and, in a smaller percentage, malignant transformation represent an increasing source of morbidity through an affected individual's lifespan. Status epilepticus as a source of morbidity remains a significant source of mortality. Complications of pulmonary lymphangiomyomatosis contribute to mortality in the fourth decades and beyond.

REFERENCES

1. Gomez MR (ed.): *Tuberous Sclerosis,* 2d ed. New York, Raven, 1988, p 14
2. Reed WB et al: Internal manifestations of tuberous sclerosis. *Arch Dermatol* **87**:715, 1963
3. Yates JR et al: Female germline mosaicism in tuberous sclerosis confirmed by molecular genetic analysis. *Hum Mol Genet* **6**:2265, 1997
4. Hunt A, Lindenbaum RH: Tuberous sclerosis: A new estimate of prevalence within the Oxford region. *J Med Genet* **23**:272, 1984
5. Sampson JR et al: Genetic aspects of tuberous sclerosis in the west of Scotland. *J Med Genet* **26**:28, 1989
6. Wiederholt WC et al: Incidence and prevalence of tuberous sclerosis in Rochester, Minnesota, 1950 through 1982. *Neurology* **35**:600, 1985
7. Lagos JE, Gomez MR: Tuberous sclerosis: Reappraisal of a clinical entity. *Mayo Clinic Proc* **42**:26, 1967
8. Kwiatkowska J et al: Human XPMC2H: cDNA cloning, mapping to 9q34, genomic structure, and evaluation as TSC1. *Genomics* **44**:350, 1997
9. van Slegtenhorst M et al: Identification of the tuberous sclerosis gene TSC1 on chromosome 9q34. *Science* **277**:805, 1997
10. Soucek T et al: Role of the tuberous sclerosis gene-2 product in cell cycle control. *J Biol Chem* **272**:29301, 1997
11. Au K et al: Germ-line mutational analysis of the TSC2 gene in 90 tuberous sclerosis patients. *Am J Hum Genet* **62**:286, 1998
12. Henske EP et al: Loss of tuberin in both subependymal giant cell astrocytomas and angiomyolipomas supports a two-hit model for the pathogenesis of tuberous sclerosis tumors. *Am J Pathol* **151**:1639, 1997
13. Webb D et al: Cardiac rhabdomyomas and their association with tuberous sclerosis. *Arch Dis Chil* **68**:367, 1993
14. Sampsom JR et al: Renal cystic disease in tuberous sclerosis: Role of the polycystic kidney disease 1 gene. *Am J Hum Genet* **61**:843, 1997
15. Smolarek TS et al: Evidence that lymphangiomyomatosis is caused by TSC2 mutations: Chromosome 16p13 loss of heterozygosity in angiomyolipomas and lymph nodes from women with lymphangiomyomatosis. *Am J Hum Genet* **62**: 1998
16. Vanderhooft SL et al: Prevalence of hypopigmented macules in a healthy population. *J Pediatr* **129**:355, 1996
17. Butterworth T, Wilson M Jr: Dermatologic aspects of tuberous sclerosis. *Arch Dermatol Syphilol* **43**:1, 1941
18. Gomez MR: Neurologic and psychiatric features, in *Tuberous Sclerosis,* 2d ed, edited by MR Gomez. New York, Raven, 1988, p 9
19. McGrae JD et al: Unilateral facial angiofibromas—a segmental form of tuberous sclerosis. *Br J Dermatol* **134**:727, 1996
20. Nickel WR, Reed WB: Tuberous sclerosis: Special reference to the microscopic alterations in the cutaneous hamartomas. *Arch Dermatol* **85**:209, 1962
21. Roach E et al: Diagnostic criteria: Tuberous sclerosis complex. *J Child Neurol* **7**:221, 1992
22. Bellack GS, Shapshay SM: Management of facial angiofibromas in tuberous sclerosis: Use of the carbon dioxide laser. *Otolaryngol Head Neck Surg* **94**:37, 1986
23. Kaufman AJ et al: Treatment of adenoma sebaceum with the copper vapor laser. *J Am Acad Dermatol* **33**:770, 1995
24. Shepherd CW et al: Causes of death in patients with tuberous sclerosis. *Mayo Clin Proc* **66**:792, 1991

CHAPTER 191

Enikö K. Pivnick
Vincent M. Riccardi

The Neurofibromatoses

The neurofibromatoses are a heterogeneous set of genetic disorders having clinical manifestations that involve the skin, the nervous system, or both. Clinically, at least two distinct autosomal dominant disorders (with somewhat overlapping features) have been recognized. The most common type of neurofibromatosis (NF) is type 1 (NF1) (85 percent of patients), which should be distinguished from type 2 (NF2) (10 percent of patients). Molecular biologic studies have confirmed that these two conditions are genetically distinct: NF1 results from defects in the NF1 gene on chromosome 17, and NF2 results from defects in the NF2 gene on chromosome 22. The nomenclature, definition, and diagnosis of NF1 and NF2 are currently based on the clinical criteria of the National Institutes of Health Consensus Developmental Conference[1] (Table 191-1).

TABLE 191-1

Diagnostic Criteria for Neurofibromatosis Type 1 and Type 2

NEUROFIBROMATOSIS TYPE 1

(The diagnostic criteria are met if two or more of the features listed
are present)
Six or more café au lait macules over 5 mm in greatest diameter in
  prepubertal individuals and over 15 mm in greatest diameter in post-
  pubertal individuals
Two or more neurofibromas of any type or one plexiform neurofi-
  broma
Freckling in the axillary or inguinal regions
Optic glioma
Two or more Lisch nodules (iris hamartomas)
A distinctive osseus lesion such as sphenoid dysplasia or thinning of
  long bone cortex with or without pseudoarthrosis
A first-degree relative (parent, sibling, or offspring) with NF1 by the
  above criteria

NEUROFIBROMATOSIS TYPE 2

(The criteria are met by an individual who satisfies condition 1 or 2)
1. Bilateral masses of the eighth cranial nerve seen with appropriate
   imaging techniques (e.g., computed tomography or MRI)
   or
2. A first-degree relative with NF2 and either:
   a. Unilateral mass of the eighth cranial nerve, or
   b. Two of the following:
      Neurofibroma
      Meningioma
      Glioma
      Schwannoma
      Juvenile posterior subcapsular lenticular opacity

SOURCE: From Stumf et al.[1]

NEUROFIBROMATOSIS TYPE 1

NF1, or von Recklinghausen neurofibromatosis, is one of the most common autosomal dominant disorders in humans, primarily affecting cells of neural crest origin and resulting in developmental, pigmentary, and neoplastic abnormalities. NF1, also one of the most distinctive inherited diseases, has caused great fascination among physicians and scholars for many centuries. The earliest known representation of NF1 appears in a statue, which has been dated to Hellenistic times.[2] Aristic illustrations of individuals presumed to have NF1 have been portrayed in medieval woodcarving,[3] in Renaissance drawings,[4] and in the literature of the nineteenth century.[5] The disease was first recorded by Tilesius in 1793,[6] and von Recklinghausen gave the first organized description of the syndrome in 1882.[7] Unfortunately, due to misdiagnosis, NF1 has erroneously earned the reputation of being identical with the "Elephant Man's disease," thereby causing enormous stress among the individuals affected with NF1.[8] A posthumous diagnosis of John Merrick, the "Elephant Man," revealed that he suffered from a disorder known as Proteus syndrome.[9]

NF1 is a dynamic pathologic process, with physical manifestations often present at birth and becoming more apparent with age. Although the age at which NF1 is diagnosed is not predictive of the possible serious consequences of the disorder, an earlier age of onset of serious problems means a higher lifetime burden. Early diagnosis of NF1 is important in that it provides the opportunity for genetic counseling and education of the patient and family about neurofibromatosis, awareness of the serious consequences of this disorder, appropriate medical follow-up, and early intervention.

Clinical Features

The cardinal features of NF1 are multiple neurofibromas, café au lait spots (CLS), axillary and inguinal freckling, and pigmented iris hamartomas (Lisch nodules).[10] In addition, the disease can be confounded by a broad spectrum of complications, such as various kinds of osseous lesions, stenosis of the renal arteries, aqueduct stenosis, optic glioma, and learning disabilities. Malignant progression of tumors developing in NF1 patients is a major cause of morbidity and mortality.[11]

Skin involvement in NF1 is common. Patches of cutaneous pigmentation and multiple cutaneous tumors create the most conspicuous findings. There are two basic types of NF1 hyperpigmentation abnormalities: focal and diffuse. The latter involves virtually all the skin.[10]

CLS have long been known as part of the syndrome. In fact, the first sign of this condition may be the presence of CLS. In most patients, CLS are obvious at birth, though their number and definition tend to increase during the first year of life. Subsequent increases in pigmented macules are largely related to freckling.[10] In older patients with NF1, fading of the CLS may take place.[12] It is important to recognize that a few CLS do not establish the diagnosis of NF1, since about 10 percent of the normal population have from one to five CLS.[13] When there are multiple pigmented spots, a diagnosis of neurofibromatosis must be seriously considered.

The CLS of NF1 are randomly distributed on the body except for the eyebrows, scalp, palms, and soles. When CLS are limited to a single unilateral segment, other forms of NF should be considered, for example, segmental NF.[14]

The CLS vary in size, shape, and hue but are darker than the normal color of the surrounding skin (Fig. 191-1). The typical CLS are 10 to 30 mm in diameter, ovoid in shape, and of uniform color intensity (proportionate to background skin coloration), with sharp, well-defined borders that are usually smooth. In some instances in NF1, a CLS alters the appearance of the "Mongolian spot" on which it may be superimposed.[15]

There are a number of disorders other than NF1 in which multiple CLS may occur. These include NF2, Watson's syndrome, McCune-Albright syndrome, multiple lentigines syndrome, multiple neuroma syndrome (multiple endocrine neoplasia, type IIB), Bannayan-Riley-Ruvalcaba syndrome, tuberous sclerosis, Maffucci's syndrome, and familial multiple CLS. Most can be distinguished from NF1 by other clinical features, although this can be difficult in young children. The importance of examining parents must be emphasized.[16]

The other form of characteristic skin pigmentation in NF1 is axillary freckling. Freckling of the inguinal region and other areas limited to intertriginous zones or sites of skin-to-skin contact also appears to be a feature unique to NF1. Freckling is usually acquired later in childhood and adulthood.[10] This freckling is found in 81 percent of children with NF1 before 6 years of age.[17] In some patients with NF1, there may be innumerable freckles over the entire body.[18] The timely appearance and location of freckles suggest that freckling develops by a different mechanism than CLS.[19]

It has been reported that CLS of NF1 patients have more melanocytes than does the surrounding skin. There is also increased activity of the melanocytes, and giant pigment (melanin) granules can be found in the majority of cases. Patients with NF1 also have a higher melanocyte count in their normally pigmented skin, compared to normal individuals.[20] The higher melanin content of NF1

FIGURE 191-1

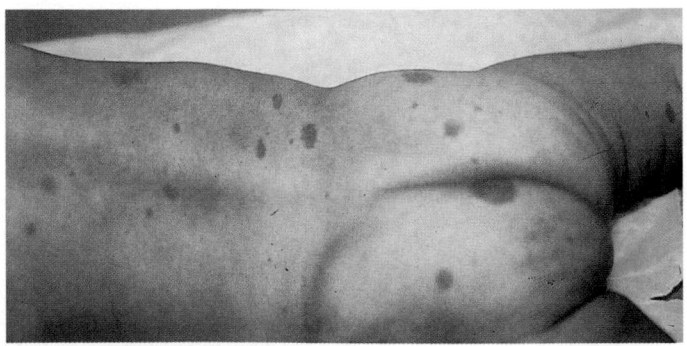

Multiple café au lait spots distributed over the trunk of an infant.

melanocytes is a result of aberrant regulation of melanogenesis.[21] It is unknown, however, how the altered function of neurofibromin (NF1 gene product) leads to increased melanogenesis in the skin melanocytes.[22] It should be noted that giant melanin granules are not unique to neurofibromatosis and can be found in conditions such as McCune-Albright syndrome and multiple lentigines syndrome.[18] Therefore, biopsy of the CLS has little or no utility in making the diagnosis of NF1.

In another type of *hyperpigmentation* in NF1, the edges of the hyperpigmented patch are concordant with or extend the borders of an underlying plexiform neurofibroma. These patches are darker than typical CLS. Congenital localized *hypertrichosis* of varying degrees may be present simultaneously.[23] The recognition of an *aberrant hair whorl* pattern overlying a paraspinal neurofibroma or vertebral dysplasias may assist the clinician in early diagnosis of these potentially severe complications of NF1. Scalp *hypotrichosis* or *alopecia* may be seen occasionally in association with tumors of the scalp.[10]

Although *hypopigmentation* is not specific for NF1, it may occur as small punctate macules and local areas of skin hypoplasia or as *pseudoatrophic macules*. Histopathologic examination of these macules suggests that these macules are variants of neurofibromas.[24]

Individuals with NF1 maintain a velvety quality of the skin even in adulthood.[25] Laxity of the skin often gives the face a prematurely aged appearance. Patients with NF1 often show secondary creases in their fingertip and palmar crease pattern.[26]

Juvenile xanthogranuloma (JXG) is a rare, benign cutaneous abnormality in childhood and occurs in 1 percent of young children with NF1. The presence of this lesion should raise the clinician's concern since there may be an excess of juvenile chronic myelogenous leukemia in children with JXG and NF1.[27,28]

Multiple *neurofibromas* are a distinctive feature in patients with NF1. The sometimes impressive number and size of these tumors resulted in the original term *neurofibromatosis*. Neurofibromas virtually always involve the skin. They may become evident as skin tags or nodules located in cutaneous or subcutaneous tissues or as masses involving deep tissues. Neurofibromas are benign tumors of nerve sheath origin. They consist of Schwann cells, nerve fibers, fibroblasts, vascular elements, mast cells, and mixoid matrix.[29] There is no histologic difference between the neurofibromas of neurofibromatosis and solitary neurofibromas in persons without the syndrome. Although the tumors are often seen in small number in childhood, they tend to appear more extensively around puberty in both sexes and during pregnancy.[17,30] Areolar neurofibromas occur in 80 percent or more of postpubertal women.[10]

There are four distinct types of neurofibromas. *Cutaneous neurofibromas* are literally in the skin and move with the skin. These are the most common tumors in NF1, appearing as early as 4 or 5 years of age, though their occurrence in the 8- to 12-year-old range is more typical.[31] They are soft, flesh-colored tumors that range in size from several millimeters to many centimeters in diameter and are not painful (Fig. 191-2). They can invaginate into the underlying dermal defect with light digital pressure ("button-holing").[13] This feature is a useful sign in distinguishing the lesions of this disease from other surface tumors, e.g., multiple lipomas. Their clinical consequences include cosmetically distressing appearance and, in about 10 percent of patients, varying degrees of pruritus.

Subcutaneous neurofibromas are firm, rubbery, often painful tumors that are deeply seated in the dermis. They may be small (a

FIGURE 191-4

few millimeters in diameter) or as large as 8 cm (Fig. 191-2). About 20 percent of patients with NF1 have at least one subcutaneous neurofibroma, and of these, about one-quarter will have serious problems as a result.

Nodular plexiform neurofibromas are a network clustering of large subcutaneous neurofibromas. They may be palpated as firm, usually tender, nodules along nerve plexuses or dorsal nerve roots (Fig. 191-3). As a consequence of neurofibromas extending through the vertebral foramina, disfigurement of the vertebra, scoliosis, vertebral collapse, and compression of the cord may occur and may result in severe neurologic deficits. Involvement of the dorsal nerve roots and major nerves may be associated with severe pain and neurologic compromise.[10]

About 5 percent of NF1 patients have *diffuse plexiform neurofibromas*; they are virtually always of congenital origin (though often not immediately visible) and are thought to be the hallmark of this condition (Fig. 191-4). Diffuse plexiform neurofibromas are highly vascular and may involve all the layers of the skin, the immediately adjacent fascia, and deeper elements—at times even re-

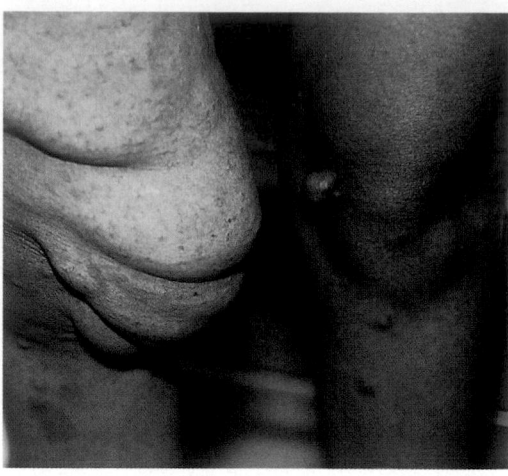

Right knee of a NF1 patient, showing large diffuse plexiform neurofibroma.

placing whole sections of muscles, eroding bony structures, and infiltrating visceral elements. A key consideration is that what appears to be only a small or modest-sized neurofibroma on the outside may actually be very large, involving extensive regions of the mediastinum or retroperitoneum.[31] A common feature of plexiform neurofibroma is localized or segmental hypertrophy of adjacent connective tissues, including enlargement of the underlying bone.[18] Diffuse plexiform neurofibroma is often associated with overlying hyperpigmentation and hypertrichosis. When these skin changes overlap the neuroaxis, evaluation of spinal involvement is mandatory. Visceral involvement with diffuse plexiform neurofibromas may lead to various complications such as constipation, bleeding, and obstruction.[10]

Plexiform neurofibromas tend to infiltrate the nerve diffusely and progress to neurofibrosarcoma, also termed *malignant peripheral nerve sheath tumor* (MPNST), in as many as 5 to 6 percent of affected individuals. These tumors are highly malignant and carry a poor prognosis.[11] Such malignant transformation in a known neurofibroma is often heralded by either physical or radiologic evidence of sudden growth or a rapid progression in clinical symptoms (pain and neurologic deficit).

Other tumors that commonly lead to confusion in the differential diagnosis of NF1 are schwannomas, lipomas, and angiolipomas. Multiple schwannomas require the consideration of NF2, regardless of the presence or absence of skin pigmentation abnormalities, although multiple schwannomatosis may be the diagnosis.[32,33] Multiple lipomas, often associated with other tumors including central nervous system tumors, are exemplified in Bannayan-Riley-Ruvalcaba syndrome. This syndrome may be similarly confused with NF1.[34]

There are no specific treatments for neurofibromas. Surgery is palliative, not curative, and multiple procedures are expected due to the progressive nature of these tumors. Surgical removal of these tumors solely for cosmetic reasons is inappropriate and unnecessary. However, there are many reasons for removing neurofibromas, including excessive size, pain, and/or prominent cosmetic disfigurement. This is true for superficial as well as deep tumors, but in the latter case, a diagnostic biopsy may be another consideration since the tumor cannot be visualized or palpated for characterization.[10]

Some of the symptoms associated with these tumors are more bothersome than the tumors themselves. Generalized itching or itch-

FIGURE 191-2

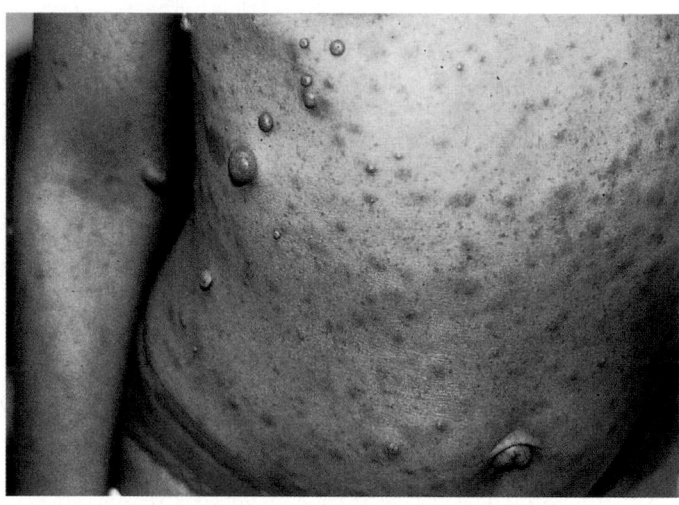

Large number of neurofibromas (cutaneous, subcutaneous) scattered over the entire torso of a patient.

FIGURE 191-3

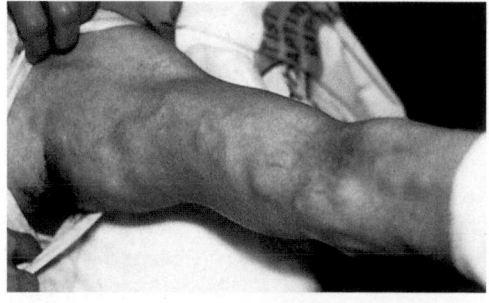

The left arm of a NF1 patient demonstrating extensive nodular plexiform neurofibroma.

ing localized to newly developing neurofibromas has been described.[10] There is a significant increase in mast cells in neurofibromas. Mast cells influence the growth of neurofibromas because some of their mediators also act as growth factors.[35] One study has shown that a mast cell stabilizer, ketotifen, decreased the rate of neurofibroma growth, pruritus, pain, and tenderness.[36] Another interesting observation is that trauma seems to be the initiating or aggravating event in the growth of neurofibromas.[10]

Certain ophthalmic manifestations (Lisch nodules, optic glioma, and sphenoid dysplasia) account for three of the six diagnostic criteria of NF1. *Lisch nodules* (multiple iris melanocytic hamartomas), presenting as small yellow-brown lesions on the surface of the iris, are the most common manifestation and have crucial diagnostic value. Lisch nodules are the only ocular findings that do not cause visual dysfunction, but they are useful for confirming or discounting the diagnosis of NF1. They are present in 94 percent of patients who are 6 years of age or older.[37]

Optic gliomas, a form of astrocytoma, are the most frequent central nervous system complications in NF1 during early childhood, with an incidence of 10 to 15 percent.[38] These tumors may arise anywhere along the optic pathway.[39] The natural history is not well understood. Two-thirds are asymptomatic, their mitotic activity is low, and they generally do not undergo malignant progression. A small subgroup of patients with optic gliomas, however, presents with progressive vision loss and/or proptosis associated with the expanding tumor. Mass lesions of the optic nerve and tract are neither biopsied nor treated unless clinical progression is documented. Optic gliomas are best demonstrated by magnetic resonance imaging (MRI).[40]

A characteristic congenital, and usually unilateral, bony defect in the posterior wall of the orbit is due to *sphenoid dysplasia* and often results in pulsating exophthalmos. One may mistake this condition for an orbital tumor.

The skeletal involvement in NF1 is exemplified by the relatively high frequency of macrocephaly and short stature. *Pseudoarthrosis* of long bones (usually the tibia or fibula) is an infrequent but distinctive congenital skeletal abnormality in NF1.[41] Appreciation of its significance should be helpful to the clinician who is faced with a patient who has subtle manifestations of this complex disease. The spectrum of this bony anomaly may range from mild bowing of the tibia to thinning of the cortex, which eventually predisposes to pathologic fractures and false joint formation (Fig. 191-5). Early detection of this complication allows early treatment and prevents severe compromise of the affected limb.

Complications of NF1, other than pigmentary- or tumor-related, include endocrine disturbances, hypertension, and vascular headaches.

Frank mental retardation is uncommon in NF1. By far the most common neurologic complications of NF1 in childhood are specific learning disabilities and neuropsychological deficits, estimated to occur in 30 to 50 percent of affected children.[42] The pathogenesis of the learning disabilities remains obscure. These special deficits may or may not be related to the severity of the clinical manifestations of NF1; therefore, mildly affected NF1 children should also be monitored for specific learning disabilities and behavioral problems.

A common neuroradiologic abnormality—high-signal abnormalities on T2-weighted MRI, called *u*nidentified *b*right *s*ignals (UBSs)—is found in the basal ganglia, cerebellum, and brainstem of over 60 percent of patients with NF1.[43] These lesions are not visible with computed tomography scans. The impact of UBSs on measures of cognitive and academic performance has been the subject of controversy.[44,45]

FIGURE 191-5

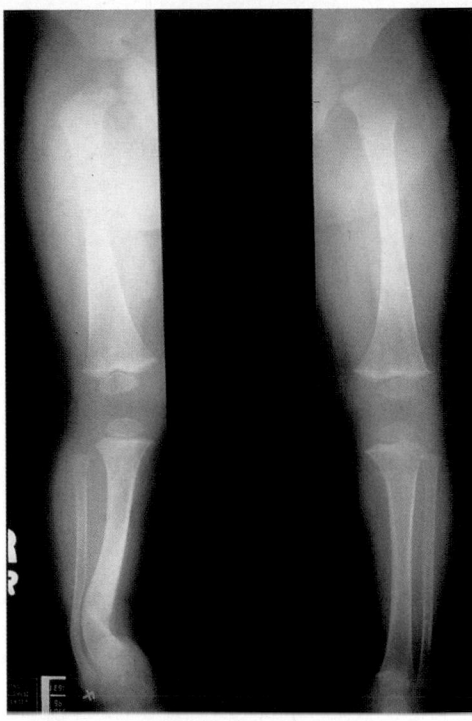

Plain radiographs of the lower extremities of a NF1 patient. Note moderately severe tibial bowing.

There is an increased incidence of specific cancers in approximately 2 to 5 percent of individuals affected with NF1. These include MPNST and Triton tumor (a variant of MPNST), malignant gliomas, and extraneural malignancies such as pheochromocytoma, carcinoid tumors, rhabdomyosarcoma, and juvenile chronic myeloid leukemia.[27,46,47] The absence of an increased incidence of malignant melanoma is worth noting since melanomas are of neural crest origin. Meningiomas, so characteristic of NF2, are not seen in NF1.[10]

Genetics of NF1

NF1 exemplifies many of the fundamental principles of classic genetics. It is inherited in an autosomal dominant manner; therefore, affected individuals have a 50 percent risk of transmitting the disorder to their offspring. NF1 appears to affect all races, ethnic groups, and both sexes, with an estimated incidence of 1 in 3000. NF1 has a rate of new mutations of approximately 1 in 10,000, one of the highest described for a human disorder. Approximately half of all index cases of NF1 have no family history of NF1 and thus are thought to arise due to mutation in the sperm or egg of the parents.[13] Gene penetrance is virtually 100 percent by the age of 5 years.[48] The pleiotropic and protean manifestations of NF1 affect many different organ systems. The variable expression is inter- and intrafamilial, which makes it difficult to predict clinical severity and complications of the disease in offsprings of an affected parent.[49]

The NF1 gene is located on chromosome 17 at band q11.2.[50] The gene has been cloned and characterized as a tumor-suppressor gene. Neurofibromin, the protein product of the nonmutated gene, has the activity of a GTPase-activating protein and is capable of downregulation of the cellular p21-*ras* proto-oncogene.[51] The loss of neurofibromin function may lead to uncontrolled cell growth or tumor formation.

Numerous types of mutation in different parts of the NF1 gene have been detected to date. There is no indication that the mutations are concentrated in any region of the gene (NF1 Genetic Analysis Consortium). The majority of the mutations give rise to a diminished function of neurofibromin in affected persons. No phenotype-genotype correlation has been established except for cases where deletion has removed the entire NF1 gene, resulting in facial dysmorphia, early onset of a large number of neurofibromas, and dull intelligence.[52]

Diagnosis and Management

A definite diagnosis of NF1 is commonly made on clinical grounds, based on the National Institutes of Health diagnostic criteria. Young children who present with six or more CLS but without other physical findings or family history of NF1 may pose clinical dilemmas. Such children must be followed to look for the appearance of other manifestations of NF1. Most of these children turn out to have NF1.

Routine clinical application of DNA analysis in the diagnosis of NF1 is not yet a reality. Linkage studies using DNA markers in the molecular diagnosis of certain families with NF1 are feasible, but such studies are not possible when there is only one affected individual in the family, as is often the case for NF1.[53] New molecular technology (protein truncation assay) has great potential for use as a direct diagnostic or presymptomatic test for NF1. At the present time, the assay's diagnostic utility lies in providing bases for prenatal, preimplantation diagnosis and for further evaluation in cases when the diagnosis is problematic. Genetic counseling should be provided for anyone who is tested, so that the limitations of the assay are clearly understood.[54]

The effect of the complications in NF1 on many organ systems often leads to involvement of a multitude of subspecialists in the care of these patients. It is in the best interest of patients with NF1 to improve the coordination of their care by using clinicians who have an expertise with the disease. Since there is no cure for NF1 at the present time, the main goal is the early detection of the various complications, intervention, and genetic counseling. Routine follow-up is necessary, with the interval of these visits dependent on pertinent medical problems.

Related Conditions

Segmental NF should be considered in individuals who have features of neurofibromatosis confined to a particular region of the body.[14] Segmental NF is postulated to arise from a somatic mutation in the NF1 gene early in embryonic development. Segmental NF is less common than NF1 and is also more easily overlooked. Patients with segmental NF may have a child with classic NF1 due to germinal mosaicism.[55]

Watson's syndrome is a variant of NF1 that features multiple CLS, only a small number of neurofibromas, short stature, pulmonary valvular stenosis, and dull intelligence. Molecular analysis in a few cases of Watson's syndrome has shown a large deletion in the NF1 gene.[52]

Certain features of *Noonan's syndrome* (characteristic face, pectus excavatum, short stature) have been observed in a subset of patients with NF1. While it is likely that some features of these two common syndromes may overlap, a recent linkage study of several families showed that NF1 and Noonan's syndrome are genetically distinct.[56]

NEUROFIBROMATOSIS TYPE 2

NF2, previously known as central neurofibromatosis or bilateral acoustic neuroma, is characterized by multiple slow-growing nervous system tumors, particularly schwannomas and meningiomas. The hallmark of NF2 is the development of bilateral vestibular schwannomas. NF2 is much less common than NF1 and has an estimated frequency of 1 in 50,000.[32] NF2 is an autosomal dominant disease with penetrance over 95 percent, so that for any offspring of an affected parent, the risk that these tumors will develop is about 50 percent.[57] In up to 50 to 75 percent of NF2 cases there is no family history of the disease, and these may represent spontaneous mutations.[58] NF2 was once thought to be a form of NF1.[59] The National Institutes of Health Consensus Developmental Conferences (1987), however, provided clear guidelines on nomenclature, recommending the use of the term *neurofibromatosis type 2*. It also suggested substitution of the term *vestibular schwannoma* in place of the term *acoustic neuroma*, so as to reflect the anatomic origin of these tumors.[1] Preliminary evidence suggests that there are two subtypes of NF2: a milder (Gardner) variant, and an intermediate or severe (Whishart) type.[60]

The skin manifestations in NF2 are less prominent than in NF1. CLS in NF2 tend to be fewer in number and show less distinct hyperpigmentation. Intertriginous freckling is not present. Other skin findings in NF2 include cutaneous and subcutaneous schwannomas. The most common of these is a superficial, discrete, slightly raised papule. The surface of the papule is rough and is often pigmented and covered by excess hair.[32] Subcutaneous schwannomas are often spherical tumors that occur on peripheral nerves. The thickened nerve can often be palpated at either end of the tumor.[58] The least common cutaneous manifestations in NF2 are neurofibromas. Peculiarly, the palm of the hand and the lateral alae nasi are frequent sites of these tumors. Plexiform neurofibromas are distinctly unusual in NF2.

Dorsal nerve root paraspinal schwannomas are a relatively constant feature of NF2. They are the major source of morbidity from direct compromise of the involved nerves and by centripetal growth and compromise of the spinal cord.[61]

Schwannomas may occur on any of the cranial nerves except for the olfactory nerve.[58] Patients with NF2 tend to develop vestibular schwannomas, which are acoustic tumors arising from neural covering. Symptoms related to vestibular schwannomas are usually due to pressure on the vestibulocochlear and facial nerve complex. In NF2, symptoms usually begin in the second or third decade. However, occasional patients may present as early as the first or as late as the seventh decade.[32] The first symptom is usually loss of hearing, which may be accompanied by intermittent tinnitus, unsteadiness, and facial weakness. Other tumors in NF2 include intracranial meningiomas, gliomas, and ependymomas. Spinal cord meningiomas and astrocytomas are common, in contrast to NF1. Meningiomas in NF2 tend to be bilateral and occur at a younger age than their sporadic counterparts. It is of interest that malignancies do not appear to be prevalent in NF2.[61] There is no evidence to suggest that mental function is impaired due to NF2.

The spectrum of ocular abnormalities of NF2 has only recently received attention. Presenile posterior cortical cataracts are highly specific for NF2. These lens opacities have little visual significance; however, their presence in an individual at risk may give a clue to the diagnosis of NF2. A host of other ocular manifestations including retinal hamartomas, optic disk glioma, optic nerve meningioma, and eyelid ptosis can impair the vision of patients with NF2.[62] Lisch nodules are extraordinarily rare in NF2.

The genetic defect that underlies NF2 has been localized to the long arm of chromosome 22.[63] The gene responsible for NF2 has been cloned and characterized. It codes for a protein designated as *merlin*, or *schwannomin*, which belongs to a superfamily of membrane-organizing proteins.[64] Analysis of tumoral DNA from both NF2-associated and sporadic meningiomas and schwannomas has demonstrated chromosome 22 deletions and inactivation of the merlin protein. This strengthens the argument that the NF2 gene acts as a tumor suppressor.[65] However, the role of merlin in tumor suppression is still obscure. There is some evidence that genotype-phenotype correlation exists for certain NF2 mutations.[66,67]

As the course of NF2 is variable, once a patient is diagnosed as having NF2, a number of tests and procedures may be helpful to define the nature and progression of the disease in that individual. These include regular monitoring for central nervous system tumors (particularly, vestibular schwannoma, meningiomas, and spinal cord tumors) and for related functional impairments (hearing loss, focal neurologic signs). MRI of the head and spine is the neurodiagnostic modality of choice in patients with known or suspected NF2. The natural history of NF2 is such that the onset of auditory and visual symptoms is often delayed, not infrequently until childbearing age.[68] Examination of high-risk patients may suggest the diagnosis before symptomatic central nervous system tumors arise, allowing genetic counseling and family planning.

Early detection of NF2 gene mutation carriers has become possible by using linkage analysis in familial NF2.[69] Direct gene test is becoming increasingly available.[70]

Treatment of vestibular schwannomas is aimed at preserving hearing. Currently, the only treatments that are available for the tumors of NF2 are surgery and specialized radiation therapy. The timing of surgery is difficult to determine. However, early diagnosis allows for earlier surgical intervention and resection of subclinical vestibular schwannomas.

Multiple schwannomatosis is a disorder characterized by the development of multiple schwannomas in a variety of anatomic locations involving the skin, the spinal cord, or both, in the absence of CLS, neurofibromas, or other stigmata of NF1, and without evidence of vestibular tumor diagnostic of NF2.[71] In addition, various types of multiple schwannomatosis exist, including *multiple cutaneous plexiform schwannomas*. These tumors have a growth pattern similar to that seen in plexiform neurofibroma but do not have an association with progression to MPNST.[72]

Recent molecular studies have shown that some, but not all, forms of multiple schwannomatosis are variant forms of NF2, but not all instances of multiple schwannomas are necessarily NF2.

Familial meningioma, without other features of NF2, represents yet another distinct entity, with its separate gene locus on the long arm of chromosome 22 (not too distant from the NF2 locus).[73]

REFERENCES

1. Stumf DA et al: NIH Consensus Development Conference: Neurofibromatosis conference statement. *Arch Neurol* 45:575, 1988
2. Ragge NK, Munier FL: Ancient neurofibromatosis. *Nature* 368:815, 1994
3. Madigan P, Masello MJ: Report of a neurofibromatosis-like case: Monstrorum Historica, 1642. *Neurofibromatosis* 2:53, 1988
4. Madigan P, Shaw RV: Neurofibromatosis in thirteenth century Austria. *Neurofibromatosis* 1:339, 1988
5. Solomon LM: Quasimodo's diagnosis. *JAMA* 204:190, 1968
6. Tilesius WG, cited by Worster-Drought C et al: Multiple meningeal and perineural tumours with analogous changes in the glia and ependyma (neurofibromatosis), with report of two cases. *Brain* 60:85, 1937
7. von Recklinghausen FD: *Ueber die Multiplen Fibrome der Haut und Ihre Beziehung zu den Multiplen Neuromen. Festschrift fur Rudolf Virchow.* Berlin, August Hirschwald, 1882
8. Ablon J: 'The Elephant Man' as 'self' and 'other': The psychosocial costs of a misdiagnosis. *Soc Sci Med* 40:1481, 1995
9. Cohen MM Jr: Understanding Proteus syndrome, unmasking the elephant man, and stemming elephant fever. *Neurofibromatosis* 1:260, 1988
10. Riccardi VM: *Neurofibromatosis: Phenotype, Natural History, and Pathogenesis,* 2d ed. Baltimore, The Johns Hopkins University Press, 1992
11. Kleihues P et al: *Histological Typing of Tumours of the Central Nervous System,* 2d ed. New York, Springer, 1993
12. Huson SM: Recent development in the diagnosis and management of neurofibromatosis. *Arch Dis Child* 64:745, 1989
13. Crowe FW et al: *A Clinical, Pathological and Genetic Study of Multiple Neurofibromatosis.* Springfield, II, Charles C Thomas, 1956
14. Calzavara PG et al: Segmental neurofibromatosis: Case report and review of the literature. *Neurofibromatosis* 1:318, 1988
15. Niimura M: Life cycle of Recklinghausen's disease. *J Pediatr Dermatol* 12:146, 1983
16. Korf BR: Diagnostic outcome in children with multiple cafe au lait spots. *Pediatrics* 90:924, 1992
17. Obringer AC et al: The diagnosis of neurofibromatosis in the child under the age of 6 years. *Am J Dis Child* 143:717, 1989
18. Riccardi VM: Von Recklinghausen neurofibromatosis. *N Engl J Med* 305:1617, 1981
19. Riccardi VM: Cutaneous manifestation of neurofibromatosis: Cellular interaction, pigmentation, and mast cells. *Birth Defects* 17:129, 1981
20. Johnson BL, Charneco DR: Cafe au lait spot in neurofibromatosis and in normal individuals. *Arch Dermatol* 102:442, 1970
21. Suzuki H et al: Activation of the tyrosinase gene promoter by neurofibromin. *Biochem Biophys Res Commun* 205:1984, 1994
22. Kaufmann D et al: Increased melanogenesis in cultured epidermal melanocytes from patients with neurofibromatosis 1 (NF1). *Hum Genet* 87:144, 1991
23. Riccardi VM: The pathophysiology of neurofibromatosis IV. Dermatologic insights into heterogeneity and pathogenesis. *J Am Acad Dermatol* 3:157, 1980
24. Pique E et al: Pseudoatrophic macules: A variant of neurofibroma. *Cutis* 57:100, 1996
25. Hall BD, Cadle RG: Extremely soft skin and hyperextensible joints in adult male with thousands of neurofibromas. Cause/effect relationship in possible connective tissue aberration. Annual NNFF Clinical Care Symposium 10, 1990
26. Vormittag W et al: Dermatoglyphics and creases in patients with neurofibromatosis of von Recklinghausen. *Am J Med Genet* 25:389, 1986
27. Bader JL, Miller RW: Neurofibromatosis and childhood leukemia. *J Pediatr* 92:925, 1978
28. Zvulunov A et al: Juvenile xanthogranuloma, neurofibromatosis, and juvenile chronic myelogenous leukemia: World statistical analysis. *Arch Dermatol* 131:904, 1995
29. Harkin JC: Pathology of nerve sheath tumors. *Ann NY Acad Sci* 486:147, 1986
30. Jarvis GJ, Crompton AC: Neurofibromatosis and pregnancy. *Br J Obstet Gynaecol* 85:844, 1978
31. Riccardi VM: Type 1 neurofibromatosis and the pediatric patient. *Curr Probl Pediatr* 22:66, 1992
32. Martuza FL, Eldridge R: Neurofibromatosis 2 (bilateral acoustic neurofibromatosis). *N Engl J Med* 318:684, 1988
33. Rongioletti F et al: Multiple cutaneous plexiform schwannomas with tumors of the central nervous system. *Arch Dermatol* 125:431, 1989
34. Cohen MM Jr: Bannayan-Riley-Ruvalcaba syndrome: Renaming three formerly recognized syndromes as one etiologic entity. *Am J Med Genet* 35:291, 1990

35. Nurnberger M, Moll I: Semiquantitative aspects of mast cells in normal skin and in neurofibromas of neurofibromatosis types 1 and 5. *Dermatology* **188**:296, 1994

36. Riccardi VM: A controlled multiphase trial of ketotifen to minimize neurofibroma-associated pain and itching. *Arch Dermatol* **129**:577, 1993

37. Lewis RA, Riccardi VM: Von Recklinghausen neurofibromatosis: Prevalence of iris hamartomas. *Ophthalmology* **88**:348, 1981

38. Lewis RA et al: Von Recklinghausen neurofibromatosis. II: Incidence of optic gliomata. *Ophthalmology* **91**:929, 1984

39. Packer RJ et al: Intracranial visual pathway gliomas in children with neurofibromatosis. *Neurofibromatosis* **1**:212, 1988

40. NIH Consensus Conference: Magnetic resonance imaging. *JAMA* **259**:2132, 1988

41. Andersen KS: Congenital pseudoarthrosis of the tibia and neurofibromatosis. *Acta Orthop Scand* **47**:108, 1976

42. Riccardi VM: Neurofibromatosis update. *Neurofibromatosis* **2**:284, 1989

43. Duffner PK et al: The significance of MRI abnormalities in children with neurofibromatosis. *Neurology* **39**:373, 1989

44. Ferner RE et al: MRI in neurofibromatosis: The nature and evolution of increased intensity T2-weighted lesions and their relationship to intellectual impairment. *J Neurol Neurosurg Psychiatry* **56**:492, 1993

45. North K et al: Specific learning disability in children with neurofibromatosis type 1: Significance of MRI abnormalities. *Neurology* **44**:878, 1994

46. von Deimling A et al: Neurofibromatosis type 1: Pathology, clinical feature and molecular genetics. *Brain Pathol* **5**:153, 1995

47. Shannon KM et al: Loss of the normal NF1 allele from the bone marrow of children with type 1 neurofibromatosis and malignant myeloid disorders. *N Engl J Med* **330**:597, 1994

48. Riccardi VM, Lewis RA: Penetrance of von Recklinghausen neurofibromatosis: Distinction between predecessors and descendants. *Am J Hum Genet* **42**:284, 1988

49. Easton DF et al: An analysis of variation in expression of neurofibromatosis type 1 (NF1): Evidence for modifying genes. *Am J Hum Genet* **53**:305, 1993

50. Barker D et al: Gene for von Recklinghausen neurofibromatosis is in the pericentric region of chromosome 17. *Science* **236**:1100, 1987

51. Xu G et al: The neurofibromatosis type 1 gene encodes a protein related to GAP. *Cell* **62**:599, 1990

52. Kayes LM et al: Deletions spanning the neurofibromatosis 1 gene: Identification and phenotype of five patients. *Am J Hum Genet* **54**:424, 1994

53. Ward K et al: Diagnosis of neurofibromatosis 1 by using tightly linked, flanking DNA markers. *Am J Hum Genet* **46**:943, 1989

54. Heim RA et al: Distribution of 13 truncating mutations in the neurofibromatosis 1 gene. *Hum Mol Genet* **4**:975, 1995

55. Rubinstein AE et al: Familial transmission of segmental neurofibromatosis. *Neurology* **33**(suppl 2):76, 1983

56. Colley A et al: Neurofibromatosis/Noonan phenotype: A variable feature of type 1 neurofibromatosis. *Clin Genet* **49**:59, 1996

57. Eldridge R: Central neurofibromatosis with bilateral acoustic neuroma. *Adv Neurol* **29**:57, 1981

58. Evans DGR et al: A genetic study of type 2 neurofibromatosis in the United Kingdom. I: Prevalence, mutation rate, fitness, and confirmation of maternal transmission effect on severity. *J Med Genet* **29**:841, 1992

59. Wishart JH: Case of tumours in the skull, dura mater, and brain. *Edinburgh Med Surg J* **18**:393, 1822

60. Huson SM, Thrush DC: Central neurofibromatosis. *Q J Med* **55**:213, 1985

61. Riccardi VM: The neurofibromatoses. *Hem/Onc Ann* **2**(2):119, 1994

62. Rettele GA et al: Blindness, deafness, quadriparesis, and a retinal malformation: The ravages of neurofibromatosis 2. *Surv Ophthalmol* **41**:135, 1996

63. Wolff R et al: Analysis of chromosomal deletions in neurofibromatosis type 2 related tumors. *Am J Hum Genet* **51**:478, 1992

64. Trofatter JA et al: A novel moezin-, ezrin-, radixin-like gene is a candidate for the neurofibromatosis 2 tumor suppressor. *Cell* **72**:791, 1993

65. Sanson M: Un nouveau gene supresseur de tumeur responsable de la neurofibromatose de type 2, est altere dans les neuromes et les meningiomes. *Rev Neurol (Paris)* **152**:1, 1996

66. Parry DM et al: Neurofibromatosis 2 (NF2): Clinical characteristics of 63 affected individuals and clinical evidence for heterogeneity. *Am J Med Genet* **52**:450, 1994

67. Parry DM et al: Germline mutations in the neurofibromatosis 2 gene: Correlation with disease severity and retinal abnormalities. *Am J Hum Genet* **59**:529, 1996

68. Mautner VF et al: Neurofibromatosis 2 in the pediatric age group. *Neurosurgery* **33**:92, 1993

69. Rouleau GA et al: Genetic linkage of bilateral acoustic neurofibromatosis to a DNA marker on chromosome 22. *Nature* **329**:246, 1987

70. MacCollin M et al: DNA diagnosis of neurofibromatosis 2. Altered coding sequence of the merlin tumor suppressor in an extended pedigree. *JAMA* **270**:2316, 1993

71. Shishiba T et al: Multiple cutaneous neurilemmomas as a skin manifestation of neurilemmomas. *J Am Acad Dermatol* **10**:744, 1984

72. Reith JD, Goldblum JR: Multiple cutaneous plexiform schwannomas. Report of a case and review of the literature with particular reference to the association with types 1 and 2 neurofibromatosis and schwannomatosis. *Arch Pathol Lab Med* **120**4:399, 1996

73. Pulst SM et al: Familial meningioma is not allelic to neurofibromatosis 2. *Neurology* **43**:2096, 1993

Ataxia Telangiectasia

Ataxia telangiectasia (AT) (OMIM 208900), first described by Mme. Louis Bar in 1941, is an autosomal recessive disorder (incidence 1:40,000) characterized by cerebellar ataxia, oculocutaneous telangiectases, recurrent sinopulmonary infections including bronchiectasis, immunodeficiency, and the development of lymphorecticular malignancies.[1]

ETIOLOGY AND PATHOGENESIS[2]

In normal mammalian cells, exposure to ionizing radiation results in a delay in both progression from G1 to S phase and G2 into mitosis as well as inhibition of DNA synthesis. AT cultured cells have abnormal radioresistant DNA synthesis and fail to activate either G1/S or G2/M checkpoints in response to ionizing irradiation. AT cells demonstrate chromosomal instability and hypersensitivity to DNA-damaging agents such as x-rays and radiomimetic agents such as bleomycin. Responses to ultraviolet irradiation are normal. Several immunological defects in both T- and B-cell function are associated with the clinical immune defects in ATM.

The identification of the ATM gene and the functions of the proteins that it codes allow a more complete understanding of the molecular and clinical pathophysiology of the disease. The gene for the ataxia-telangiectasia phenotype is located on chromosome 11q22.3, a site involved in the chromosome translocations in some nonlymphoid leukemias.[3] Five AT complementation groups, all mapping to 11q22.3, have been identified.

ATM protein is 350 kDa phosphoprotein of the nucleus and cytoplasmic microsomes with similarities to the phosphatidyl-inositol-3-kinases, which participate in checkpoint regulation. The gene has 66 exons and spans 150 kb of genomic DNA.[2] Over 100 different ATM mutations have been identified.

ATM mutations truncate or destabilize the ATM proteins. ATM interacts with c-Abl and p53 proteins, which control a cell's stress response.[4]

p53 has a major role in allowing passage through the G1/S checkpoint, which tests DNA integrity before initiation of new DNA synthesis and protects against strand breaks after immunoglobulin gene rearrangement. The lack of induction of p53 in AT cells may explain why intrachromosomal recombinant rates are 30 to 200 times higher than normal in such cells.[5] ATM is also associated with the synaptonemal complex of meiotic chromosomes, which may explain gonadal atrophy in AT.[6]

Portions of this chapter are derived from Chapter 184, "Neurocutaneous Diseases," by M. Priscilla Short, MD, and Raymond D. Adams, MD, in the fourth edition of this book.

Clinical Features

Characteristic oculocutaneous telangiectases begin near the ocular canthi and progress across the bulbar conjunctivae (Fig. 192-1) and usually appear at 3 to 6 years of age (after degenerative changes in the cerebellum and basal ganglia occur). The lower tarsal conjunctiva is involved. Cutaneous telangiectases subsequently may develop on the malar prominences, ears, eyelids, anterior chest, and popliteal and antecubital fossae and the dorsa at the hands and feet (Fig. 192-2). The telangiectases may be subtle and resemble fine petechiae, especially in the flexural areas. The development of telangiectases may be related to sun exposure, since ocular but not cutaneous telangiectases develop in affected black children.[1]

Progeric changes of the skin, including xerosis and gray hair, occur in 90 percent of patients.[1] During adolescence, the facial skin may become progressively more atrophic and sclerotic, causing a masklike appearance. Occasionally the ears, arms, and hands also become sclerodermatous. The hair may be diffusely gray by adolescence, and subcutaneous fat is generally lost in childhood. Recurrent severe impetigo often develops in patients with AT. Seborrheic dermatitis occurs in many patients, and the associated blepharitis may lead to a diagnosis of blepharoconjunctivitis rather than ocular telangiectasia. Mottled hyper- and hypopigmentation frequently occur and, together with the telangiectases and atrophy, can resemble the poikiloderma of radiodermatitis, actinic damage, or scleroderma.[7] Other pigmentary changes include café au lait spots that may be found in a dermatomal distribution,[7] multiple ephilides, and vitiligo. Hirsutism of the arms and legs, alopecia areata, multiple warts, atopic dermatitis, keratosis pilaris, nummular eczema, and acanthosis nigricans have been described in association with AT. Among the most common cutaneous manifestations of AT

FIGURE 192-1

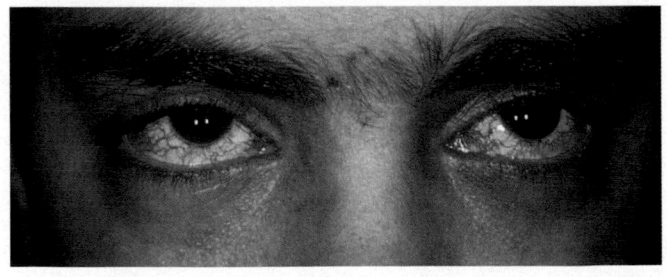

Bulbar conjunctival telangiectases in a patient with ataxia telangiectasia. (*From Paller AS: Hereditary immunodeficiency disorders, in Genetic Disorders of the Skin, edited by JC Alper. Chicago, Mosby Year Book, 1991, Chap 7, pp 105–123, with permission.*)

FIGURE 192-2

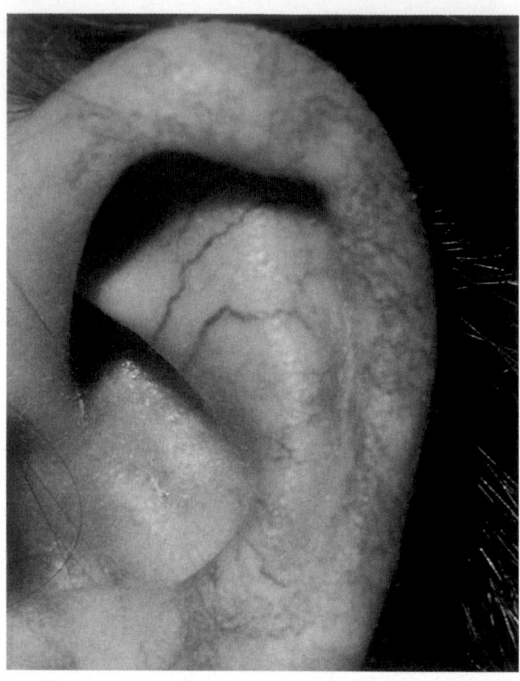

Ataxia telangiectasia. Telangiectases inside and on the helix.

are noninfectious cutaneous granulomas.[8,9] These persistent, atrophic, and often ulcerative lesions are often mistaken for other granulomateus processes, including sarcoidosis, necrobiosis lipoidica diabeticorum, granuloma annular, and granulomatous dermatitis. Intralesional injections of triamcinolone have helped to promote healing of the painful associated ulcerations, although the lesions do not clear completely with treatment.

Usually, the progressive cerebellar ataxia first becomes apparent during infancy (medium age, 1.2 years) with swaying of the head and trunk and apraxia of eye movements long before skin or conjunctival abnormalities. In childhood, dysarthric speech, drooling, choreoathetosis, and myoclonic jerks become prominent. The gradual development of a persistent cerebellar ataxia, appearing in the first few years of life, should alert the clinician to ataxia-telangiectasia. Close inspection of the limbs shows none of the usual features of cerebellar ataxia, i.e., dysmetria, lack of synergism of component muscle groups involved in skilled acts, hypotonia, or intention tremor. The diagnosis of AT is usually made at a median age of 7 years. Once fully developed, the syndrome includes slow, dysarthric speech, impassive face, nystagmus, choreoathetosis, occasionally myoclonic jerks of the limbs, difficulty in initiating ocular deviation from the central position, and poor voluntary control of eye movements (apraxia of gaze). Tendon reflexes are diminished or absent; intelligence may deteriorate as the disease advances. Patients usually require a wheelchair by their teenage years.

Recurrent bacterial and viral sinopulmonary infections occur in up to 80 percent of patients; these are the most common cause of death, which is usually from bronchiectasis and respiratory failure. Approximately three-quarters of patients with AT may have growth retardation and endocrine disorders, especially ovarian agenesis or testicular hypoplasia and insulin-resistant diabetes. Malignant lymphoreticular neoplasms develop in 10 to 15 percent of patients, usu-

ally by adolescence; the lymphomas tend to be of B-cell origin and the leukemias T-cell chronic lymphocytic leukemia.[10,11]

Heterozygotes for the AT gene (1 percent of the U.S. population) are at high risk for neoplasia, especially female breast cancer (up to five-fold relative risk).[10] Heterozygotes show increased risk of chromosomal breaks after exposure to irradiation in vitro, suggesting that mammograms in known carriers of AT are contraindicated.

Pathology

Autopsy findings indicate that about half the patients die from pulmonary disease and most of the remainder die from lymphoreticular or other malignant tumors; the thymus is absent or hypoplastic, and the spleen may be reduced in size. The significant pathologic abnormalities in the central nervous system are severe degeneration in the cerebellar cortex, loss of myelinated fibers in the posterior columns, and degenerative cell changes in the posterior root and sympathetic ganglia.[12]

Differential Diagnosis

Ataxia telangiectasia is one of a group of diseases characterized by defects in the repair process of DNA damage. The others are xeroderma pigmentosum, Bloom's syndrome, and Cockayne's syndrome. In fibroblast cultures from patients with ataxia-telangiectasia, several complementation groups have been found, suggesting clinical heterogeneity. The Nijmegen breakage syndrome, a condition similar to AT, is due to alteration in an as yet unknown protein that may be part of the ATM complex.

Laboratory Findings

Patients with AT tend to have both humoral and cellular immunologic abnormalities. Serum IgA and IgE are absent or deficient in the majority of patients. Circulating anti-IgA antibodies are common in patients with IgA deficiency. Defective cell-mediated immunity is found in 70 percent of patients. There is an increase in T cells bearing gamma/delta receptors. Virtually all patients have elevated levels of α-fetoprotein, and many have detectable carcinoembryonic antigen. Patients with AT often have elevated hepatic transaminases (40–50%), and glucose intolerance.

Spontaneous chromosomal abnormalities (fragments, breaks, gaps, and translocations) occur 2 to 18 times more frequently in patients with AT than in normal individuals and mainly involve chromosomes 2, 7, and 14. Rearrangements of chromosomes 7 and 14, and especially 14;14 translocations, seem to predict the development of lymphoreticular malignancy including leukemia.

Treatment

The therapy for AT is supportive and includes administration of antibiotics for infection, physiotherapy for pulmonary bronchiectasis, physical therapy to prevent contractures in patients with neurologic dysfunction, and sunscreens and sun avoidance to diminish actinic-like changes. Lymphoreticular malignancies, including lymphoid leukemia, are the second most common cause of death, leading to the deaths of 15 percent of patients with AT. Therapeutic radiation and radiomimetic chemotherapeutic agents, especially bleomycin, may lead to extensive tissue necrosis. The administration of small doses of other chemotherapeutic drugs and low-dose, fractionated radiation is the least harmful means of managing these malignancies. Death usually occurs by late childhood or early adolescence; however, the oldest surviving patient died at the age of 50 years.

Prenatal diagnosis has been achieved by measurement of amniotic α-fetoprotein levels, by increased spontaneous breakage of chromosomes of fetal ammocytes, and by the presence of a clastogenic factor in the amniotic fluid[13] as well in some instances of the mutated DNA itself.

REFERENCES

1. Boder E: Ataxia-telangiectasia: An overview, in *Ataxia-Telangiectasia: Genetics, Neuropathology, and Immunology of a Degenerative Disease of Childhood*, edited by RA Gatti, M Smith. New York, Alan R Liss, 1985, p 1
2. Lavin MF et al: The genetic defect in ataxia-telangiectasia. *Annu Rev Immunol* **15**:177, 1997
3. Lange E et al: Localization of an ataxia-telangiectasia gene to an 850 kb interval on chromosome 11q 23.1 by linkage analysis of 176 families in an international consortium. *Am J Hum Genet* **57**:112, 1995
4. Baskaran R et al: Ataxia telangiectasia mutant protein activates c-Abl tyrosine kinase in response to ionizing radiation. *Nature* **387**:516, 1997
5. Barlow C et al: ATM selectively regulates distinct p53-dependent cell-cycle checkpoint and apoptotic pathways. *Nat Genet* **17**:453, 1997
6. Plug AW et al: ATM and RPA in meiotic chromosome synapsis and recombination. *Nat Genet* **17**:457, 1997
7. Cohen LE et al: Common and uncommon cutaneous findings in patients with ataxia-telangiectasia. *J Am Acad Dermatol* **10**:431, 1984
8. Fleck RM et al: Ataxia-telangiectasia associated with sarcoidosis. *Pediatr Dermatol* **3**:339, 1986
9. Paller AS et al: Granulomatous lesions in patients with ataxia-telangiectasia. *J Pediatr* **119**:917, 1991
10. Swift M et al: Cancer predisposition of ataxia-telangiectasia heterozygotes. *Cancer Genet Cytogenet* **46**:21, 1990
11. Hecht F, Hecht BK: Cancer in ataxia-telangiectasia patients. *Cancer Genet Cytogenet* **46**:9, 1990
12. Aguilar MJ et al: Pathological observations in ataxia-telangiectasia: Report of 5 cases. *J Neuropathol Exp Neurol* **27**:659, 1968
13. Schwartz S et al: Tests appropriate for the prenatal diagnosis of ataxia-telangiectasia. *Prenat Diagn* **5**:9, 1985

CHAPTER 193

Joseph L. Jorizzo

Behçet's Disease

Behçet's disease is a complex multisystem disease characterized clinically by the presence of oral aphthae and at least two of the following: genital aphthae, synovitis, cutaneous pustular vasculitis, posterior uveitis, or meningoencephalitis. The absence of inflammatory bowel disease and collagen vascular diseases must be documented.

HISTORIC ASPECTS

About 2400 years ago Hippocrates used the designation *aphthai* to refer to common oral aphthae (canker sores), and he may have described the first patient with Behçet's disease.[1] Hulusi Behçet, a Turkish dermatologist, described his patients with recurrent orogenital ulcerations and uveitis in 1937, and in 1940 he added four patients with the "triple symptom complex."[2,3] The first international multidisciplinary conference on Behçet's disease was organized by two dermatologists, Drs. Monacelli and Nazarro, in Rome in 1964. The most recent conference was held in Tunis in 1996.

EPIDEMIOLOGY

The prevalence of Behçet's disease is highest in Japan, Southeast Asia, the Middle East, and southern Europe.[4,5] The disease is not common in northern Europe and the United States. Behçet's disease most often affects patients in their twenties and thirties, and men are more frequently affected than women, but pediatric cases are often reported.[6,7]

ETIOLOGY AND PATHOGENESIS

Genetics

Several large series in Britain, Japan, Korea, and the Middle East have shown a significant association between Behçet's disease and HLA-B51.[8] Familial clustering of Behçet's disease is not common but is reported.[9]

Infectious Precipitants

Early theories of the pathogenesis of Behçet's disease proposed a viral or other infectious etiology.[2,3] Extensive investigation has failed to substantiate a primary infectious etiology. The possibility that infectious agents might trigger an immunoregulatory defect in genetically predisposed individuals has been investigated by several research groups. Hybridization studies have demonstrated homology between the DNA of herpes simplex virus type 1 and the ribonucleic acid of peripheral blood lymphocytes from patients with Behçet's disease.[10] Recent investigations, especially in Japan, have focused on immunologic alterations related to exposure to streptococcal strains such as *Streptococcus oralis* and *S. pyogenes*.[11,12]

Immunologic Aspects

Important early studies demonstrated autoantibodies reactive to oral mucosal antigens in patients with Behçet's disease. Rogers and associates demonstrated lymphocytoxicity to oral epithelial cells.[13] Various studies have suggested that nonspecific abnormalities of cellular immunity are relevant in the pathogenesis of Behçet's disease.[14–16] Newer studies have focused on a possible role for $\gamma\delta$ T cells[17] and on late expression of Fas antigen on CD4 and CD8 T cells[18] in Behçet's disease.

Studies have also focused on a role for circulating immune complexes and neutrophils in the pathogenesis of mucocutaneous lesions in Behçet's disease. Nazzaro[19] demonstrated that the earliest histology from aphthae, pustular vasculitic lesions, and erythema nodosum–like lesions is what we would now call a neutrophilic vascular reaction or even fully developed leukocytoclastic vasculitis, and these findings have been confirmed.[20,21] Antigen nonspecific assays for circulating immune complexes are reported to be positive in about half of patients, and they seem to correlate with disease activity.[22] Light, immunofluorescence, and electron microscopic studies support a neutrophilic vascular reaction or even fully developed leukocytoclastic vasculitis as the earliest finding in mucocutaneous lesions.[19–21,23] Pathergy lesions (cutaneous pustular vasculitis lesions induced by intradermal trauma) have been studied with a modification of Braverman's histamine trap test.[20,21] Patients with active disease show a neutrophilic vascular reaction or leukocytoclastic vasculitis in a biopsy specimen obtained 24 h after histamine injection and on direct immunofluorescence usually show immunoreactants in biopsy specimens obtained 4 h after histamine injection.[20,21] Studies have repeatedly suggested increased migration of neutrophils to chemoattractants in Boyden chamber or subagarose assays.[24] Recent experiments in HLA-B51 transgenic mice show a similar phenomenon.[25] This may be due to a heat-stable serum factor.[20] Neutrophil adhesion to endothelial cells has been another important area of investigation.[26] The therapeutic benefit of colchicine, but not of thalidomide, may be due to a blockade of the ability of neutrophils to hyperrespond to serum from patients with Behçet's disease.[20,24]

Lehner's group in London has presented data to support the theory that various infectious agents could trigger a defect in immunoregulation in genetically predisposed individuals.[10] Disagreement exists as to whether subsequent tissue injury might be mediated by lymphoid cells or by circulating immune complex–mediated, neutrophil-induced vessel damage.

CLINICAL MANIFESTATIONS

Mucocutaneous Lesions

The oral aphthae that occur in patients with Behçet's disease are like those that occur in simple recurrent aphthosis, although they may be more extensive and may occur more frequently (Fig. 193-1A).[4,27] Genital aphthae are similar lesions that occur in the genital area (Fig. 193-1B). Herpes simplex should be excluded with appropriate Tzanck preparation, viral culture, or even skin biopsy.

In the author's opinion, cutaneous lesions that should be accepted as being diagnostically relevant in Behçet's disease should be confined to cutaneous pustular vasculitis lesions (including pathergy lesions), erythema nodosum–like lesions, Sweet's-like lesions, pyoderma gangrenosum–like lesions, and palpable purpuric lesions of necrotizing venulitis (Fig. 193-2). All of these are characterized by a neutrophilic vascular reaction in their early stages.[28] Acneiform lesions or follicle-based pustules should not be considered relevant.[29,30]

Systemic Lesions

Ocular involvement is the major cause of morbidity in patients with Behçet's disease. The most diagnostically relevant lesion is *posterior uveitis* (called *retinal vasculitis* in Great Britain). Other ocular lesions include anterior uveitis, hypopyon (now uncommon), and secondary cataracts, glaucoma, and neovascular lesions.[31]

The characteristic arthritis is a nonerosive, asymmetric oligoarthritis.[4,5,32] Patients with HLA-B27–positive, erosive sacroiliitis have been included in some series of patients with Behçet's disease, but their condition is more appropriately considered as a part of the Reiter's enteropathic arthritis spectrum of disease.[32]

Significant neurologic manifestations occur in fewer than one-fourth of patients and may be delayed in onset. Meningoencephalitis, benign intracranial hypertension, cranial nerve palsies, brainstem lesions, and pyramidal or extrapyramidal lesions have all been described.[33,34]

Vascular involvement can be significant and includes aneurysms, arterial occlusions, venous occlusions, and varices that can be fatal.[35] Hemoptysis can occur due to vessel-based pulmonary lesions and is also potentially fatal.[36] Cardiac involvement can include myocarditis, coronary arteritis, endocarditis, and valvular disease.[37] Renal disease may be mild or asymptomatic, but in a recent series a majority of patients with active Behçet's disease had evidence of glomerular immunoreactant deposition.[38] Aphthae may occur throughout the gastrointestinal tract. Some patients with inflammatory bowel disease have been included in series of patients with Behçet's disease, but these cases are best excluded.

LABORATORY EVALUATION

There are no pathognomonic laboratory abnormalities in patients with Behçet's disease. Laboratory abnormalities may occur in association with dysfunction of various organ systems, depending on clinical disease manifestations.

FIGURE 193-1

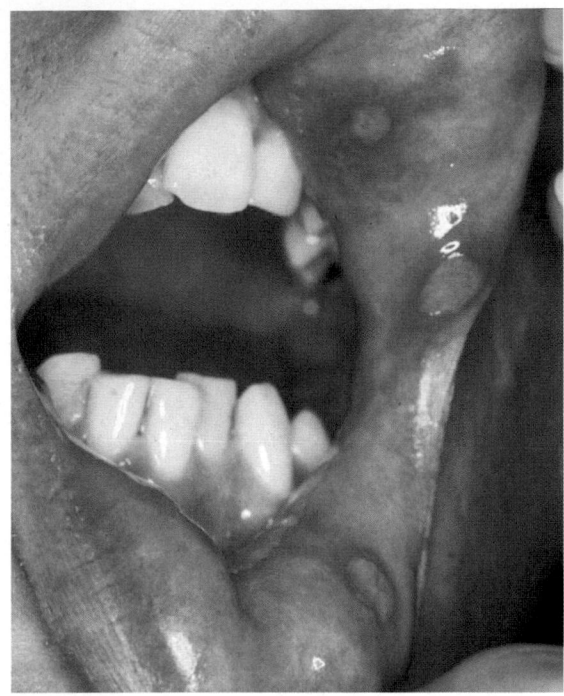

A.

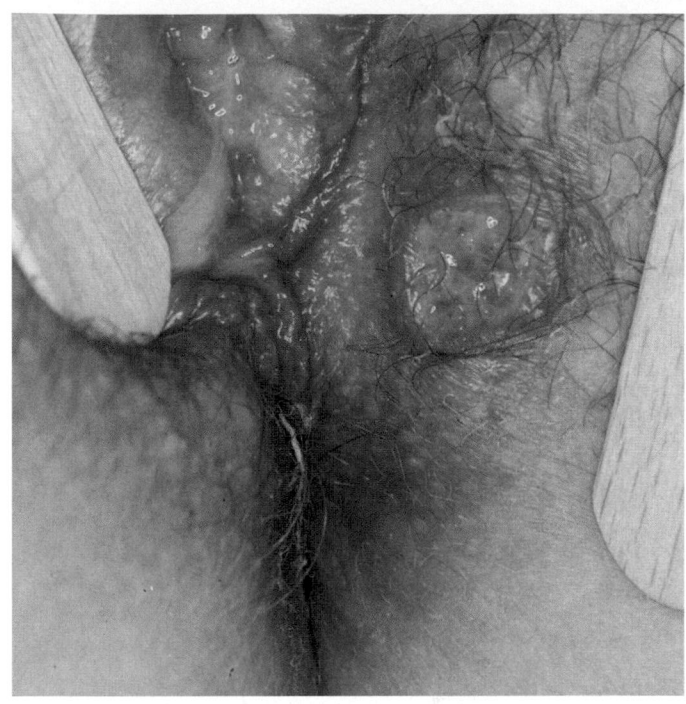

B.

Behçet's syndrome. *A.* On the labial mucosa there are painful aphthous-type ulcerations. *B.* Large, painful aphthous-type ulcer on the vulva.

FIGURE 193-2

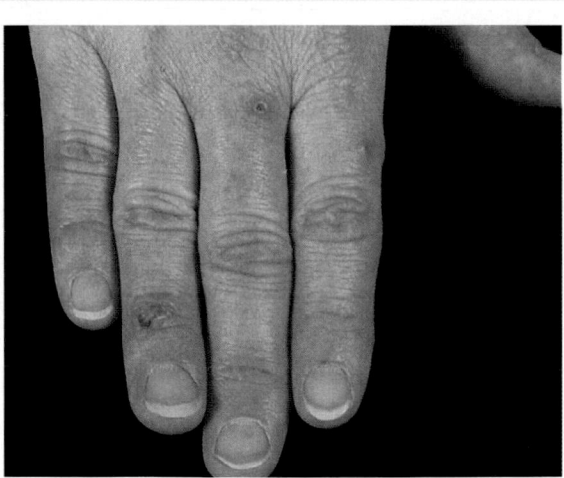

Pustular vasculitic lesions on the hand of a patient with Behçet's disease.

HISTOPATHOLOGY

Traditional histopathologic interpretations of various types of lesions sampled in patients with Behçet's disease describe primarily a lymphocytic perivasculitis. These reports usually have focused on late lesions and on autopsy data.[39] Biopsies from the earliest mucocutaneous lesions show a neutrophilic vascular reaction with endothelial swelling, extravasation of erythrocytes, and leukocyto-clasia or fully developed leukocytoclastic vasculitis with these features plus fibrinoid necrosis of blood vessel walls.[19,21,23,29,30] Others have reported more lymphocytes with fewer numbers of neutrophils from such lesions.[40]

DIAGNOSIS

Behçet's disease is a complex multisystem disease that must be diagnosed by clinical criteria in the absence of a pathognomonic laboratory test. Various sets of criteria have been published; the preferred North American criteria have been those of O'Duffy and associates.[41] Patients must have oral aphthae plus at least two of the following: genital aphthae, synovitis, posterior uveitis, cutaneous pustular vasculitis (a modification by the author and associates[20] from original pathergy) (see Fig. 193-2), or meningoencephalitis in the absence of inflammatory bowel disease or collagen vascular disease.

International criteria have been published,[42] and their usefulness validated.[43] These new criteria require the presence of oral aphthae plus two of the following: recurrent genital aphthae, eye lesions, skin lesions, or a positive pathergy test. An explanation of these criteria is given in Table 193-1. There are several problems with the new criteria. The omission of synovitis and of meningoencephalitis makes four of the five criteria variations of the same basic mucocutaneous lesion. We would require histologic confirmation that the cutaneous pustular lesions are indeed vessel-based and neutrophilic. Because 20 percent of normal young adults have oral aphthae and almost all adolescents have at least one acneiform lesion, they could practically meet the criteria if "acneiform skin le-

TABLE 193-1

International Criteria for Behçet's Disease*

CRITERIA	DESCRIPTION
Oral	Minor aphthae, major aphthae, or herpetiform ulcers observed by physicians or reported reliably by patient. Recurrent at least three times in one 12-month period.
Genital	Recurrent genital aphthae or scarring, especially scrotal in males, observed by physician or reliably reported by patient.
Eye	Anterior uveitis, posterior uveitis, cells in vitreous on slit-lamp examination, or retinal vasculitis, observed by qualified physician.
Skin	Erythema nodosum–like lesions observed by physicians or papulopustular lesions consistent with Behçet's disease, observed by a physician.
Pathergy	Positive pathergy test (neutrophilic vascular reaction or leukocytoclastic vasculitis) read by a physician at 24 or 48 h, performed with oblique insertion of a 20-gauge or smaller needle under sterile conditions.

*Findings are applicable if no other clinical explanation is present.

sions" are not excluded! Exclusion of inflammatory bowel disease as in the O'Duffy criteria should also be mandatory.

Reiter's disease is often confused with Behçet's disease by nondermatologists. Reiter's disease and the HLA-B27–positive spectrum of disease are characterized by an axial erosive arthritis and by psoriasiform mucocutaneous lesions and not by aphthae or pustular vasculitis. Patients with inflammatory bowel disease have an increased incidence of oral aphthae. These patients or those who have had bowel bypass or Bilroth II surgery can have a dermatosis-arthritis syndrome that mimics Behçet's disease, including an indistinguishable pustular vasculitis.[24] Eye disease is generally absent in these patients. Patients with complex aphthosis have recurrent oral and genital aphthae or almost ever present, multiple (>3) oral aphthae, but no other features of Behçet's disease.[44] Patients with pustular vasculitis alone may have gonococcal or even chronic meningococcal sepsis, or the pustular vasculitis may occur as an idiopathic syndrome.[45]

TREATMENT

Therapy for patients with Behçet's disease can generally be divided into treatment regimens for patients with primarily mucocutaneous disease and for patients with ocular or neurologic manifestations. Palliative therapy of aphthae has included a host of agents, such as counterirritant antipruritic agents, potent topical glucocorticoids, intralesional glucocorticoids, and local anesthetics. Colchicine, 0.6 mg orally two to three times daily as tolerated by the gastrointestinal tract, can reduce the frequency and severity of mucocutaneous lesions.[21,46] Patients should be monitored for the infrequent neutropenia that can complicate therapy. Thalidomide therapy is dramatically beneficial. Dapsone therapy has been used,[24,47] as has pentoxifylline.[48] Therapeutic options available for systemic disease, particularly for severe ocular manifestations, include prednisone,

prednisone plus azathioprine, cyclophosphamide (including a pulse regimen), azathioprine alone,[49] chlorambucil,[50] and cyclosporine.[51]

COURSE AND PROGNOSIS

The clinical course of Behçet's disease is variable. Mucocutaneous and arthritic manifestations usually occur first. Ophthalmic involvement is the leading course of morbidity. Skin lesions may be a predictive factor in vision loss as is posterior as opposed to anterior uveitis.[52] Blindness can often be prevented with early aggressive therapy of posterior uveitis. If neurologic involvement occurs at all, it is usually delayed. Death may occur from neurologic involvement, vascular disease, bowel perforation, cardiopulmonary disease, or as a complication of immunosuppressive therapy.

REFERENCES

1. Feigenbaum A: Description of Behçet's syndrome in the Hippocratic third book of endemic diseases. *Br J Ophthalmol* **40**:355, 1956
2. Behçet H: Uber rezidivierende Aphthöse, durch ein Virus verusachte Geschwüre am Mund, am Auge und an den Genitale. *Dermatol Wochenschr* **105**:1152, 1937
3. Behçet H: Some observations on the clinical picture of the so-called triple symptom complex. *Dermatologica* **81**:73, 1940
4. Shimuzu T et al: Behçet's disease (Behçet's syndrome). *Semin Arthritis Rheum* **8**:223, 1979
5. Chajek T, Fainaru M: Behçet's disease: Report of 41 cases and review of the literature. *Medicine (Baltimore)* **54**:179, 1975
6. Ammann AJ et al: Behçet syndrome. *J Pediatr* **107**:41, 1985
7. Pivetti-Pezzi P et al: Behçet's disease in children. *Jpn J Ophthalmol* **39**:309, 1995
8. Yazici H et al: HLA antigens in Behçet's disease: A reappraisal by a comparative study of Turkish and British patients. *Ann Rheum Dis* **39**:344, 1980
9. Dundar SV et al: Familial cases of Behçet's disease. *Br J Dermatol* **113**:319, 1985
10. Lehner T: The role of a disorder in immunoregulation associated with herpes simplex virus type I in Behçet's disease, in *Recent Advances in Behçet's Disease,* edited by T Lehner, CG Barnes, London, Royal Society of Medicine Services, 1986, p 31
11. Niwa Y, Mizushima Y: Neutrophil-potentiating factors released from stimulated lymphocytes: Special reference to the increase in neutrophil-potentiating factors from streptococcus-stimulated lymphocytes of patients with Behçet's disease. *Clin Exp Immunol* **79**:353, 1990
12. Narikawa S et al: *Streptococcus oralis* previously identified as uncommon *"Streptococcus sanguis"* in Behçet's disease. *Arch Oral Biol* **40**:685, 1995
13. Rogers RS III et al: Lymphocytotoxicity for oral epithelial cells in recurrent aphthous stomatitis and Behçet's syndrome. *Arch Dermatol* **109**:361, 1974
14. Victorino RMM et al: Cell mediated immune functions and immunoregulatory cells in Behçet's syndrome. *Clin Exp Immunol* **48**:121, 1982
15. Sakane T et al: Functional aberration of T-cell subsets in patients with Behçet's disease. *Arthritis Rheum* **25**:1343, 1982
16. Valesini G et al: Evaluation of T-cell subsets in Behçet's syndrome using anti-T-cell monoclonal antibodies. *Clin Exp Immunol* **60**:55, 1985
17. Hasan A et al: Role of gamma delta T cells in pathogenesis and diagnosis of Behçet's disease. *Lancet* **347**:789, 1996
18. Nakamura S et al: Insufficient expression of Fas antigen on helper T cells in Behçet's disease. *Br J Ophthalmol* **80**:174, 1996
19. Nazzaro P: Cutaneous manifestations of Behçet's disease, in *International Symposium on Behçet's Disease in Rome,* edited by M Monacelli, P Nazzaro. Basel, Karger, 1966, p 15
20. Jorizzo JL et al: Behçet's syndrome: Immune regulation, circulating immune complexes, neutrophil migration and colchicine therapy. *J Am Acad Dermatol* **10**:205, 1984
21. Jorizzo JL et al: Behçet's syndrome: Immunopathologic and histopathologic assessment of pathergy lesions is useful in diagnosis and follow up. *Arch Pathol Lab Med* **109**:747, 1985

22. Valesini G et al: Circulating immune complexes in Behçet's syndrome: Purification, characterization and cross reactivity studies. *Clin Exp Immunol* **44**:522, 1981

23. Muller W, Lehner T: Quantitative electron microscopic analysis of leukocyte infiltration in oral ulcers of Behçet's syndrome. *Br J Dermatol* **106**:535, 1982

24. Jorizzo JL et al: Thalidomide effects in Behçet's syndrome and pustular vasculitis. *Arch Intern Med* **146**:878, 1986

25. Takeno M et al: Excessive function of peripheral blood neutrophils from patients with Behçet's disease and from HLA-B51 transgenic mice. *Arthritis Rheum* **38**:426, 1995

26. Sahin S et al: Neutrophil adhesion to endothelial cells and factors affecting adhesion in patients with Behçet's disease. *Ann Rheum Dis* **55**:128, 1996

27. Rogers RS: Recurrent aphthous stomatitis: Clinical characteristics and evidence for an immunopathogenesis. *J Invest Dermatol* **69**:499, 1977

28. Jorizzo JL et al: Neutrophilic vascular reactions. *J Am Acad Dermatol* **19**:983, 1988

29. Jorizzo JL et al: Mucocutaneous criteria for the diagnosis of Behçet's disease: An analysis of clinicopathologic data from multiple international centers. *J Am Acad Dermatol* **32**:968, 1995

30. Mangelsdorf HC et al: Behçet's disease: Report of twenty-five patients from the United States with prominent mucocutaneous involvement. *J Am Acad Dermatol* **34**:745, 1996

31. Bhisitkuk RB, Foster CS: Diagnosis and ophthalmological features of Behçet's disease. *Int Ophthalmol Clin* **36**:127, 1996

32. Yurdakul S et al: The arthritis of Behçet's disease: A prospective study. *Ann Rheum Dis* **42**:505, 1983

33. O'Duffy JD, Goldstein NP: Neurologic involvement in seven patients with Behçet's disease. *Am J Med* **61**:170, 1976

34. Parisi L et al: Pre-symptomatic neurological involvement in Behçet's disease: The diagnostic role of magnetic transcranial stimulation. *Electroencephalogr Clin Neurophysiol* **101**:42, 1996

35. Sagdic K et al: Venous lesions in Behçet's disease. *Eur J Vasc Endovasc Surg* **11**:437, 1996

36. Efthimiou J et al: Pulmonary disease in Behçet's syndrome. *Q J Med* **58**:259, 1986

37. James DG, Thomson A: Recognition of the diverse cardiovascular manifestations of Behçet's disease. *Am Heart J* **30**:457, 1982

38. Herreman G et al: Behçet's syndrome and renal involvement: A histological and immunofluorescence study of eleven renal biopsies. *Am J Med Sci* **284**:10, 1982

39. Lakanpal S et al: Pathologic features of Behçet's syndrome: A review of Japanese autopsy registry data. *Hum Pathol* **16**:790, 1985

40. Gul A et al: Immunohistology of skin pathergy reaction in Behçet's disease. *Br J Dermatol* **132**:901, 1995

41. O'Duffy JD et al: Behçet's disease: Report of 10 cases, 3 with new manifestations. *Am J Intern Med* **75**:561, 1971

42. International study group for Behçet's disease: Criteria for diagnosis of Behçet's disease. *Lancet* **335**:1078, 1990

43. Ferraz MB et al: Sensitivity and specificity of different diagnostic criteria for Behçet's disease according to the latent class approach. *Br J Rheumatol* **34**:932, 1995

44. Jorizzo JL et al: Complex aphthosis: A forme fruste of Behçet's syndrome? *J Am Acad Dermatol* **13**:80, 1985

45. McNeely MC et al: Primary idiopathic cutaneous pustular vasculitis. *J Am Acad Dermatol* **14**:939, 1986

46. Miyachi Y et al: Colchicine in the treatment of cutaneous manifestations of Behçet's disease. *Br J Dermatol* **104**:67, 1981

47. Sharquie K: Suppression of Behçet's disease with dapsone. *Br J Dermatol* **110**:493, 1984

48. Yasui K et al: Successful treatment of Behçet disease with pentoxifylline. *Ann Intern Med* **124**:891, 1996

49. Yazici H et al: A controlled trial of azathioprine in Behçet's syndrome. *N Engl J Med* **322**:281, 1990

50. O'Duffy JD et al: Chlorambucil in the treatment of uveitis and meningoencephalitis of Behçet's disease. *Am J Med* **76**:75, 1984

51. Nussenblatt RB et al: Effectiveness of cyclosporine therapy for Behçet's disease. *Arthritis Rheum* **28**:671, 1985

52. Sakamoto M et al: Prognostic factors of vision in patients with Behçet disease. *Ophthalmol* **102**:317, 1995

Diseases due to Microbial Agents, Infestations, Bites, and Stings

CHAPTER 194

Morton N. Swartz
Arnold N. Weinberg

General Considerations of Bacterial Diseases

The patient with a fever and cutaneous lesions presents one of the most challenging and frequently rewarding problems in medicine. The question of a treatable etiology (bacterial, fungal, herpes virus) should always be raised initially. The physician must actively and thoughtfully consider these possibilities and seek confirmation by appropriate studies to ensure early optimal antimicrobial therapy.

Bacterial infection involving the skin may manifest itself in either of two major forms: (1) as a primarily cutaneous process, or (2) as a secondary manifestation in the skin of infection in some other organ. The cutaneous changes associated with infection are not always suppurative but may present as a vasculitis or a hypersensitivity response (e.g., lesions in subacute bacterial endocarditis or erythema nodosum).

The importance of the skin as a mirror of systemic infection cannot be overemphasized, especially when classic clinical findings are distorted as in immunocompromised patients. The timely recognition of the cutaneous clues of bacteremia may provide the early warning to consider life-threatening infections due to organisms such as *Pseudomonas aeruginosa*, *Vibrio vulnificus*, *Salmonella typhi*, *Staphylococcus aureus*, and *Neisseria meningitidis*.

NATURAL RESISTANCE OF THE SKIN

The normal skin of healthy individuals is highly resistant to invasion by the wide variety of bacteria to which it is constantly exposed. It is difficult to produce localized infections such as impetigo, furunculosis, or cellulitis in laboratory animals[1] or human volunteers[2] if the integument is intact. Pathogenic organisms such as *Streptococcus pyogenes* (group A streptococcus) and *S. aureus* produce characteristic lesions of cellulitis and furunculosis in the absence of any obvious impairment of host defenses via disruption of the intact integument, i.e., by alcohol sponging, insect bites, an abrasion, or the introduction of a foreign body. For example, Elek[3] demonstrated that the presence of a silk suture reduces by a factor of 10,000, in the case of *S. aureus,* the number of organisms needed to produce an abscess in the human skin. Treatment with immu-

nosuppressive agents can predispose patients to infections by the same organisms or by others of much lower intrinsic pathogenicity (e.g., *Corynebacterium jeikeium*). The basis for this enhanced susceptibility of the compromised host is not understood but undoubtedly involves specific and nonspecific factors such as immunocompetence, nutritional state, and integrity of the cutaneous barrier.[4]

Bacteria are unable to penetrate the keratinized layers of normal skin and, when applied to the surface, rapidly decrease in number.[2] The nature and the relative importance of the factors thought to be involved in this local resistance to bacterial multiplication and to infection are not clear.[5] The low pH (approximately 5.5) of the skin environment has been suggested as one of these properties, but it does not appear to have an important role. Many virulent bacteria are capable of growing at pHs below that of normal skin. The presence of natural antibacterial substances in the sebaceous secretions may be a factor in bacterial elimination from the skin. Streptococci appear to be particularly sensitive, in vitro, to the unsaturated long-chain fatty acids of the skin lipids, but in controlled studies in humans *S. pyogenes* (gpA streptococci) grow equally well in high- or low-lipid-containing regions.[2] Areas such as the palms and soles, lacking in sebaceous glands, remain relatively free of streptococci as well. On the other hand, reduction of skin surface lipids with topical solvent treatment has prolonged the survival time of *S. aureus* on the skin.[6] Several free fatty acids (linoleic and linolenic acids) among skin lipids are more inhibitory for *S. aureus* than for coagulase-negative staphylococci, a component of the normal skin flora.[7] The role of circulating immunoglobulins, cellular immunity, and delayed hypersensitivity in the defense of the skin against certain organisms is under intense investigation (See Chap. 28). IgM has not been found in normal sweat, and IgA, IgG, and IgD have been found only in minute amounts (0.01 percent of the level in serum). However, the greater frequency with which a specific cutaneous and mucous membrane mycotic infection, moniliasis, occurs in patients with severe combined immunodeficiency (e.g., Swiss type of congenital lymphopenic agammaglobulinemia) suggests a relationship. Experimental and clinical observations, summarized by Kligman et al.,[5] consistently support the importance of moisture content and the indigenous cutaneous microflora (see Chap. 14) in limiting colonization of the skin by potential pathogens. The relative dryness of normal skin contributes to the marked limitation of growth of bacteria, especially gram-negative bacilli with their higher moisture requirements (*Escherichia coli, Pseudomonas, Proteus*). Whereas application of 10^6 *P. aeruginosa* alone on normal skin produced no lesions, the presence of a similar inoculum under dressings increasing local skin hydration led to a superficial papular and pustular infection.[8] Bacterial interference (the suppressive effect of one bacterial strain or species on colonization by another) exerts a major influence on the overall complexion of the skin flora. Although this effect is somewhat difficult to define, its relevance, at least in the case of colonization of the nose and skin by *S. aureus,* appears clear.[9] Profound changes in these bacterial interactions may be effected by the use of antibiotics.

All of these factors allow certain bacterial species to colonize the skin surface successfully while others are rapidly excluded. The organisms that characteristically survive and multiply in various ecologic niches of the skin constitute the "normal cutaneous flora." An appreciation of the composition of this flora and the attributes of its major elements is important in understanding and treating many bacterial infections of the skin (see Chap. 14).

PATHOGENESIS OF BACTERIAL INFECTION OF THE SKIN

The host-bacteria relationship in infections of the skin, as in infectious disease in general, involves three major elements: (1) the pathogenic properties of the organism, (2) the portal of entry, and (3) the host defense and inflammatory response to microbial invasion of the anatomic region.

Pathogenicity of the Microorganism

The disease-producing capacity of bacteria is determined to a large measure by (1) the invasive potential (often based on antiphagocytic surface components), and (2) the toxigenic properties of the organism. A few species of bacteria (e.g., pneumococcus) appear to owe their pathogenicity solely to their ability to multiply extensively and invade tissues while resisting phagocytosis. No definable extracellular products or toxins that might contribute to their invasiveness have been discovered. Conversely, a few species have toxigenic properties that account for the local lesion (*C. diphtheriae, Bacillus anthracis*) or systemic manifestations (*Clostridium tetani*) of a local infection. In the case of *C. perfringens*, elaboration of a variety of extracellular toxins and enzymes (alpha toxin or lecithinase, proteases, collagenases) appears to play an important role in the rapidly spreading skin lesions and the systemic manifestations of clostridial myonecrosis. Though it is useful to distinguish between these two major pathogenic mechanisms whenever possible, most bacterial infections result from the combination of the invasive and toxigenic properties of the organism. Local invasiveness (dependent to a considerable extent on the antiphagocytic M protein of the bacterial cell envelope) is an important element in streptococcal pharyngitis, but the clinical features of scarlet fever result from the elaboration of the erythrogenic toxin. For most disease-producing bacteria, including *S. aureus* suppurative lesions, a clear understanding of the basis for pathogenicity has been lacking. Recently, evidence has accumulated indicating that the capsular polysaccharides of 2 (types 5 and 8) of the 11 known *S. aureus* capsular types are both virulence

factors and protective antigens.[10] This evidence is both epidemiologic (80 percent of *S. aureus* bloodstream isolates in hospitalized patients belong to types 5 and 8) and derived from in vitro testing (types 5 and 8 resist opsonophagocytosis). *S. aureus* toxins have roles in the pathogenesis of a variety of entities such as the staphylococcal toxic shock syndrome (*S. aureus* toxic shock syndrome toxin, or TSST-1) and staphylococcal scalded skin syndrome (exfoliatin A and B). The increasing prevalence of serious infections in compromised hosts, due to "traditionally" nonpathogenic bacteria that include the resident skin flora, supports the concept that pathogenicity is the result of microorganism and host interactions.

Gram-negative bacteria (*E. coli, S. typhi, N. meningitidis, N. gonorrhoeae, Brucella melitensis,* and others) contain endotoxin, complex phospholipid-polysaccharide macromolecules [lipopolysaccharides (LPS)], as an integral part of the bacterial cell envelope. Endotoxins, unlike exotoxins, are released only upon breakdown of the bacterial cell. Their toxicity appears to be linked principally to the lipid fraction, whereas their antigenic determinants reside with the polysaccharide component.[11] Although the biologic effects of LPS in experimental animals are numerous (shock, fever, gastrointestinal hemorrhages, leukopenia, abortion) and well studied, their role in invasiveness and the pathogenesis of localized bacterial diseases until recently remained ill defined.[12] In the past 15 years this has changed considerably. Much is now known of the mechanisms by which LPS exerts its biologic effects, in systemic infections due to gram-negative bacteria or in major localized infections that may also be capable of producing the sepsis syndrome.[13] The effects are both toxic (lethality, shock, fever, anorexia and cachexia, somnolence, complement activation, disseminated intravascular coagulation, and capillary thrombosis) and immunologic (adjuvant function, polyclonal B cell stimulation, macrophage activation, cytokine production). The two cytokines most relevant to the toxic and proinflammatory effects of LPS are produced by LPS-activated macrophages: tumor necrosis factor (TNF) and interleukin (IL) 1, the latter formerly known as leukocytic pyrogen.[14,15]

After it enters the circulation, TNF, among its many biologic effects, acts as an endogenous pyrogen on hypothalamic centers to induce fever.[16,17] It also acts on mononuclear phagocytes to stimulate production of IL-1 (another endogenous pyrogen), IL-6 (an inducer of production of serum amyloid A and other proteins of the "acute phase response"), and IL-8 (an inflammatory cytokine stimulating leukocyte chemotaxis and activation) (see Chap. 31). Thus, TNF initiates a proinflammatory cytokine cascade. TNF itself acts on the liver to increase synthesis of acute phase reactants, including fibrinogen. It also activates the coagulation system through its effects on vascular endothelium and decreases blood pressure and tissue perfusion by reducing myocardial contractility and relaxing smooth muscle.

High circulating levels of TNF are demonstrable in patients with meningococcemia and other forms of severe sepsis.[18,19] Its direct role as a mediator of circulatory collapse in gram-negative bacillary bacteremia is supported by the fact that pretreatment with antibody to TNF can prevent mortality in animals (associated with hypotension and cardiac and renal failure) from experimental *E. coli* bacteremia.[20] In addition, infusion of high concentrations of purified TNF alone can produce shock and death.

LPS can directly trigger release of IL-1 from activated macrophages as well as act indirectly through initial induction of TNF. Like TNF, IL-1 acts on endothelial cells as a procoagulant and as a stimulator of leukocyte adhesion. It can cause fever, stimulate production of acute phase proteins, and initiate (in combination with TNF) muscle wasting and cachexia. IL-1 also acts in an immunomodulatory role to enhance proliferation of CD4+ T cells and to stimulate B cell growth and differentiation.

The Shwartzman reaction is an intensified response in experimental animals to bacteria containing LPS or to purified LPS itself. LPS injected intravenously twice, 24 h apart, causes disseminated intravascular coagulation in rabbits (systemic Shwartzman reaction); LPS injected intradermally, followed by a second (intravenous) injection, produces hemorrhagic necrosis of the skin (localized Shwartzman reaction) at the site of intradermal introduction. The necrosis stems from poor tissue perfusion as a consequence of capillary blockage by neutrophils and platelets and by local fibrin formation. TNF is the major mediator of the Shwartzman reaction; unlike TNF, IL-1 cannot directly mediate this reaction. The ability of LPS, through TNF production, to induce leukocyte adherence to capillary endothelium and to induce fibrin deposition has been suggested as the basis for development of the hemorrhagic necrotic skin lesions (with or without direct bacterial invasion) that sometimes occur during the course of gram-negative bacillary bacteremias and meningococcemia.

CHANGING PATTERNS OF BACTERIAL INFECTIONS OF THE SKIN

In addition to the usual pathogens, a variety of "nonpathogenic" members of the cutaneous, intestinal, or respiratory tract flora are capable of producing acute disease in debilitated patients and in individuals with altered humoral or cellular defenses and with a variety of skin defects. A patient receiving immunosuppressive therapy, for example, may have an atypical streptococcal or staphylococcal lesion due to impairment of the normal inflammatory response, or an unusual organism may be causal. Pain can be the most prominent feature, and etiologic considerations should include, in addition to streptococci and staphylococci, members of the Enterobacteriaceae (*E. coli, Klebsiella-Enterobacter-Serratia, Proteus* spp.); a variety of nonfermentative gram-negative bacilli (*Pseudomonas, Aeromonas, Acinetobacter* spp., etc.); halophilic vibrios (e.g., *V. vulnificus*); and the indigenous anaerobic flora (peptostreptococci, *Bacteroides* spp., *C. perfringens*, etc.)[4,21-25]

Portal of Entry

In laboratory animal models the pathogenic potential of many microorganisms depends, to a considerable extent, on the route of administration. Similarly, the character of the cutaneous inflammatory response to certain bacteria will be influenced by how the organisms reached the involved area. Thus, the vascular wall is often the primary site of skin involvement during bacteremic infection; hemorrhage or thrombosis with infarction is the initial manifestation. This is followed somewhat later by the cellular reaction expected from direct inoculation of the bacteria into the skin. Local inflammation and suppuration commonly accompany direct bacterial invasion of the skin, and these may, in turn, give rise to systemic spread via the rich cutaneous vascular network. Certain bacteria can produce bacteremia or distant lesions without evoking an obvious inflammatory response at the portal of entry [e.g., *Yersinia pestis, Streptobacillus moniliformis* (rat-bite fever)], even in a nonimmunosuppressed host. Occasionally a devastating *S. pyogenes* septicemia has followed closely upon an innocuous pinprick or abrasion that has not induced a significant local lesion. Table 194-1 lists those bacterial species most frequently involved in pyogenic infections of the skin.

Specific Features of Host Inflammatory Response to Cutaneous Infection

MORPHOLOGIC ASPECTS In view of the relatively few cell types present in the skin, it is surprising that such a variety of rather

distinctive clinical responses to various bacterial infections have been catalogued. In most instances it is the anatomic site of the infection and the attendant inflammatory response pattern, rather than the specific pathogen, that provide the characteristic clinical picture. The following brief examples are expanded upon in Chaps. 195 and 197.

Impetigo The very superficial location of the infection, with vesicopustule formation just beneath the stratum corneum, is the specific clinical feature.

Folliculitis This represents a circumscribed infectious process that originates in the hair follicle and is defined by its anatomic features. It may be located superficially in the follicle or may extend more deeply to produce perifollicular inflammation.

Furuncle (boil) This infection either complicates an antecedent folliculitis or develops as a deep-seated nodule about a hair follicle. The distinctive pathologic change results from its relation to the hair follicle; thus it does not occur in glabrous areas such as the palms. The deep location and its containment by the relatively thick dermis prevent spontaneous early drainage to the surface and contribute to the hard, nodular, painful character of the lesion.

Carbuncle This is a larger, more deep-seated extension of a furuncle, with infection spreading under and between fibrous tissue septa, forming a whole series of interconnected abscesses. Drainage occurs through a number of projecting necrotic points in the skin.

Cellulitis This is an acute, inflammatory process in the skin, particularly in the deeper subcutaneous tissues. Because of the subcutaneous location, the borders of the lesion are usually indistinct, in contrast to the sharply defined margin of erysipelas (see below).

Interplay of Morphology and Specific Bacterial Properties

ERYSIPELAS This is a superficial inflammatory process of the skin and subjacent lymphatics, characterized by marked edema of the dermis and extensive invasion of connective tissue usually, but not exclusively, caused by *S. pyogenes* (gpA streptococci). The rapid progression of the process and the prominence of edema of the affected skin relate to the involvement of superficial lymphatics and the biologic properties of the microorganisms.

Influence of Hypersensitivity to Bacterial Antigens on Inflammatory Reaction in Skin

Although the introduction of certain bacteria in large numbers into the skin will elicit a local inflammatory reaction, the character and extent of this response may be modified by various host factors (e.g., leukopenia). In the case of skin infections due to *S. aureus*, the tendency to recur is often quite striking. Initial lesions are usually suppurative and localized, whereas subsequent infections, when due to the same antigenic strain, may have more prominent surrounding cellulitis. The immunologic response to *S. aureus* has been suggested as a factor in this altered inflammatory response.[26]

Vasculitis as a Cutaneous Response to Systemic Infection

Inflammatory changes in and about small blood vessels in the skin may occur in a variety of bacteremic infections in the absence of obvious localization of bacteria at these sites. The macular, papular,

TABLE 194-1

Bacteria Involved in Cutaneous Infection*

I. Primary cutaneous inflammation
  A. Gram-positive bacteria
    1. *Staphylococcus aureus*
    2. Streptococci
      a. Group A
      b. Groupable streptococci other than group A (groups B, C, D, G, particularly)
      c. *Streptococcus iniae*
      d. Anaerobic streptococci (peptostreptococci) alone or mixed infection
    3. *Bacillus anthracis*
    4. *Corynebacterium diphtheriae*
    5. Anaerobic diphtheroids (*Propionibacterium acnes*)
    6. Aerobic diphtheroids (*Corynebacterium minutissimum*; various coryneform bacteria)
    7. *Clostridium perfringens*
    8. *Erysipelothrix rhusiopathiae* (erysipeloid)
    9. *Borrelia burgdorferi* (Lyme disease)
    10. *Bartonella henselae* and *B. quintana* (cat scratch disease, bacillary angiomatosis)
  B. Gram-negative bacteria
    1. *Francisella tularensis* (tularemia)
    2. *Pasteurella multocida* (infected animal bites)
    3. Enterobacteriaceae (*Escherichia coli, Klebsiella-Enterobacter*)
    4. Nonfermentative gram-negative bacilli (*Pseudomonas, Acinetobacter, Aeromonas*)
    5. *Burkholderia* (formerly *Pseudomonas*) *mallei* (glanders)
    6. *Burkholderia* (formerly *Pseudomonas*) *pseudomallei*
    7. *Bacteroides* spp.
    8. *Haemophilus influenzae*
    9. Halophilic vibrios (*Vibrio vulnificus, V. alginolyticus, V. cholerae*)

II. Bacteremic spread to skin
  A. Gram-positive bacteria
    1. *S. aureus*
    2. Group A streptococci
    3. In bacterial endocarditis (acute)
      a. *S. aureus*
      b. Streptococci (group A, group B especially)
      c. *Enterococcus* spp.
    4. *Listeria monocytogenes*
    5. Histotoxic clostridia, primarily *Clostridium septicum*
  B. Gram-negative bacteria
    1. *Neisseria meningitidis*
    2. *Neisseria gonorrhoeae*
    3. *Pseudomonas aeruginosa*
    4. *Salmonella typhi*
    5. *Brucella* spp.
    6. *H. influenzae*
    7. *Streptobacillus moniliformis*
    8. *B.* (formerly *Pseudomonas*) *pseudomallei* (melioidosis)
    9. *Bartonella bacilliformis*

III. Bacteremia or systemic manifestation from innocuous skin portal
  A. Gram-positive bacteria
    1. Group A streptococci
    2. *S. aureus*
    3. *B. anthracis* (rarely)
    4. *Clostridium tetani*
    5. *Leptospira interrogans* serotypes
  B. Gram-negative bacteria
    1. *Yersinia pestis* (plague)
    2. *F. tularensis*
    3. *S. moniliformis* (rat-bite fever)
    4. *Brucella* spp.
    5. *B.* (formerly *Pseudomonas*) *pseudomallei*

*Exclusive of mycobacterial and treponemal infections.

nodular, and petechial lesions of chronic meningococcemia (see Chap. 198) show such histologic changes. The lesions of erythema nodosum (see Chap. 111) have a prominent element of vasculitis, even though the initiating infection (e.g., streptococcal pharyngitis) is distant and has a suppurative character. The Osler nodes and petechiae of subacute bacterial endocarditis, due to viridans streptococci, probably provide the best examples of this association of small-vessel vasculitis with bacteremia (see Chaps. 166 and 195). Histologically, these lesions are more suggestive of vasculitis than of emboli. The occasional development of such lesions in profusion, localized to the lower extremities, supports the concept of cutaneous vascular inflammation rather than embolization.

Shwartzman Phenomenon in Bacteremia due to Gram-Negative Bacteria

The experimental production of a characteristic hemorrhagic necrotic reaction in the skin and in certain other organs (e.g., kidney) of the rabbit has been a subject of considerable interest for many years.[27-29] This interest has been heightened because of the gross similarity of these lesions to those that occur during the course of meningococcemia. The Shwartzman reaction is divided into two types: local and generalized (see "Pathogenicity of the Microorganism," above). Following the preparatory injection, there is polymorphonuclear leukocyte "cuffing" about the small veins locally. The intravenous eliciting reaction produces peripheral vasoconstriction, particularly in the veins at the prepared skin site. Leukocyte-rich thrombi form, with ensuing occlusion of capillaries and small veins, producing necrosis of vessel walls and resulting hemorrhage. This form of response probably represents a type of hyperreactivity to LPS that can be neutralized by homologous antiserum.[30] Results of treatment of gram-negative bacteremia with human antiserum to LPS core have been encouraging in one limited clinical study.[31]

The typical histologic lesion of the generalized Shwartzman reaction consists of fibrin deposition within capillaries, which is the lesion of disseminated intravascular coagulation. This is particularly striking in the kidney, where characteristic bilateral renal cortical necrosis occurs. Alterations in levels of fibrinogen and other clotting factors have been found, and it appears that intravascular coagulation is the initiating event in this generalized phenomenon. Polymorphonuclear leukocytes appear to have a central role in the pathogenesis of this process, as prior induction of leukopenia with nitrogen mustard will prevent both the local and generalized reaction. Circulating fibrin monomers and inhibition of fibrinolysis appear to be essential, as their absence will obviate the reaction.[28]

It is tempting to attribute the hemorrhagic necrotic lesions that occur in meningococcemia (and gram-negative bacillary bacteremias) to this phenomenon.

CLASSIFICATION OF BACTERIAL INFECTIONS OF THE SKIN

The introduction of a variety of specific antibiotic and chemotherapeutic agents has effected rather striking changes in the management of bacterial infections. Indeed, with the availability of such drugs, the focus of attention has been on the determination of the specific bacterial cause so that the proper choice of antibacterial agent can be made. This has rendered unnecessary, and even obsolete, descriptions of some of the dermatologic entities whose status depended on imprecise morphologic criteria rather than on etiologic considerations. Consequently, from the pragmatic (therapeutic) viewpoint, the approach has been to consider and classify these infections by bacterial causation, e.g., infections due to gram-positive organisms and infections due to gram-negative organisms. Although the foregoing classification is helpful from the therapeutic point of view, there is still need for a system of categorizing bacterial infections of the skin so that the dermatologic picture will provide the basis for consideration of the most likely bacterial etiologies. To this end, the classification of skin infections as (1) primary infections (pyodermas), (2) secondary infections, and (3) cutaneous manifestations of systemic bacterial disease seems warranted. Primary bacterial infections are produced by the invasion of ostensibly normal skin by a *single* species of pathogenic bacteria. In such infections there is usually no doubt as to the primary etiologic role of the specific agent in the pathogenesis of the lesion. Treatment aimed at the bacterial pathogen almost universally results in cure of the lesion. Impetigo, erysipelas, and furunculosis are familiar examples of primary cutaneous infections. Contrastingly, secondary infections develop in areas of already damaged skin. Although the bacteria present did not produce the underlying skin disorder, their proliferation and subsequent invasion of surrounding areas may aggravate and prolong the disease. Such secondary infection may occur when the skin has been broken or bruised, primarily involved with mycotic or viral infections, or altered by sensitivity reactions or medications. In contrast to the primary infections, the secondary infections often show a *mixture* of organisms on culture, and not infrequently it is impossible to determine which plays the major role. Pathogenic organisms such as *S. aureus* and *S. pyogenes* (gpA), generally considered transients on the skin, can colonize such lesions and sometimes produce active secondary infection. The appearance of these lesions is not characteristic, in comparison to the primary pyodermas, but is largely dependent on the nature of the underlying skin condition. The result of antibacterial treatment is much less clear-cut, as it has no effect on the underlying process.

Table 194-2 presents an outline of infections involving the skin in a classification based upon the appearance of the lesions. In this outline, specific entities that will be discussed elsewhere in detail are described only by the appropriate chapter reference, and the more common bacterial etiologic agents are noted. This table refers exclusively to bacterial infections. Two of the categories identified in Table 194-2 present a broad differential diagnosis and warrant special consideration. These consist of infectious gangrene/gangrenous cellulitis (Table 194-3) and crepitant soft tissue wounds and cellulitis (Table 194-4). In addition, an uncommon group of infections present as chronic nodular, and sometimes ulcerative, granulomatous lymphangitis (with or without an evident initiating chancriform lesion) of a distinctive character. Because definition of the specific microbial etiology may be difficult without careful epidemiologic history, biopsy with culture, special stains of histologic

sections, and an awareness of the broad variety of microorganisms (fungi, bacteria, mycobacteria, protozoa) that may be involved, a listing of the possible causes is presented separately (Table 194-5).

DIAGNOSTIC STRATEGIES

Direct Examination of Aspirates and Biopsies

Identification of bacteria from skin lesions may provide important information as to the cause of cutaneous infections, whether primary or secondary to systemic processes. The presence of "normal skin flora" can confuse interpretation of these cultures. All too often, the finding of a potential pathogen such as *S. aureus* or *P. aeruginosa* is equated with the presence of disease. It is important to recall that damaged skin (operative incisions, exudative dermatoses, etc.) provides a medium for proliferation of certain bacteria. Only by correlating the clinical appearance of the lesion (local suppuration, cellulitis, etc.) with the bacteriologic data can one reach the proper decision concerning the presence of a bacterial disease. Examination of a Gram-stained smear of material from a suspected skin infection can guide decisions on early antibiotic therapy before a cultural diagnosis is made. For these reasons, bacteriologic investigation is an important part of the initial evaluation of patients with skin lesions and includes: (1) appropriate sampling, (2) interpretation of Gram-stained smears, and (3) use of selective growth media for culturing.

Gram staining provides a very rapid method for examining a sample for number and type of bacteria as well as for the character of the inflammatory exudate. Skin contaminants are usually recognized by being present in low concentration, often clumped in characteristic microcolonies (growth in skin crypts) and usually not associated with polymorphonuclear leukocytes. Obtaining an appropriate specimen for microscopic study and culture requires care to avoid contamination. Results of needle aspiration of superficial erysipelas lesions have been generally unrewarding. Slightly better, but still limited, results have been obtained on aspiration culture of lesions of cellulitis. Aspirates from the advancing edge of cellulitis yielded positive cultures in only 10 percent of patients, and culture of skin punch biopsy specimens taken from the leading edge were positive in only 20 percent of patients in the study by Hook et al.[32] Positive cultures (beta-hemolytic streptococci and coagulase-positive *S. aureus*) were more likely in patients with apparent primary sites of infection associated with the cellulitis. In another study of needle aspiration cultures of the leading edge of erythema in patients with cellulitis, the yield of pathogenic bacteria was low (15 percent) as well.[33] Others have suggested a greater yield on needle aspiration of the leading edge of cellulitis when performed in patients with underlying conditions such as diabetes mellitus and neoplastic disease.[34] A higher yield (about 50 percent) for positive cultures has been reported in aspirates obtained from the point of maximal inflammation than that (5 percent) obtained from the leading edge of cellulitis in children.[35] The authors' personal experience is in accord with published results for sampling *deeper* cellulitic lesions and bullae associated with acute infections. Findings on needle aspiration when positive can provide an immediate useful guide to therapy. If sterile saline is injected into a lesion that initially yields no aspirate, bacteriostatic agent–free solutions should be employed. In circumstances where no data are available from needle

TABLE 194-2

Bacterial Infections Involving the Skin*

I. Primary pyodermas
  A. Impetigo—group A streptococci and *Staphylococcus aureus* (see Chap. 195)
    1. Impetigo contagiosa—primarily due to group A streptococci in the past; now increasingly due to *S. aureus*
    2. Impetigo bullosa—primarily due to *S. aureus* of phage group II
  B. Folliculitis (see Chap. 195)
    1. Superficial
      a. Follicular impetigo (Bockhart's impetigo)—usually due to *S. aureus* but in conditions of lowered host resistance (glucocorticoid and antibiotic therapy, etc.) may be due to a variety of opportunistic organisms (gram-negative coliform bacilli, particularly). The lesions consist of small globular pustules, each located about a hair.
      b. *Pseudomas aeruginosa*—associated with water exposure (see Chap. 198)
    2. Deep
      a. Sycosis barbae (usually *S. aureus*)
      b. Pyoderma faciale (usually *S. aureus*)
      c. Folliculitis decalvans—rare condition, producing a scarring type of alopecia of the scalp, attributed to chronic infection with *S. aureus,* but this etiologic role is not clearly established
  C. Furuncles and carbuncles (*S. aureus*) (see Chap. 195)
  D. Paronychia—usually of bacterial origin due to *S. aureus* or group A streptococci; (see Chap. 195); rarely, a chronic form of the disease is due to *P. aeruginosa*
  E. Ecthyma—group A streptococci initially (see Chap. 195); may also be due to *Pseudomonas* (see Chap. 198), but should be distinguished from ecthyema gangrenosum
  F. Erysipelas—group A streptococci (see Chap. 197)
  G. Cellulitis—group A streptococci, *S. aureus,* and, less commonly, a variety of other organisms, especially in compromised hosts (see Chap. 197)
  H. Lymphangitis—usually group A streptococci, but occasionally *S. aureus* and other organisms (see Chap. 197)
  I. Erythrasma—*Corynebacterium minutissimum* (see Chap. 195)
  J. Bacillary angiomatosis—*Bartonella henselae* (rarely, *B. quintana*) in patients with AIDS (see Chap. 199)
II. Secondary bacterial infections
  A. Complicating preexisting skin lesions, such as:
    1. Burns (see information in Chap. 129)
    2. Eczematous dermatitis, including exfoliative erythrodermas—*S. aureus* or group A streptococci (see Chaps. 45, 122, 123, 124)
    3. Chronic ulcers [varicose, traumatic—these are particularly liable to invasion by gram-negative organisms (*Escherichia coli, Proteus, Pseudomonas*) as well as by anaerobic streptococci, *Bacteroides* or *Clostridium perfringens* (either alone or as a "synergistic" infection)] (see Chap. 167)
    4. Dermatophytoses—usually *S. aureus* or groups A, B, C, G streptococcal infection
    5. Traumatic lesions (abrasions, infestations, animal or insect bites, etc.)—*Pasteurella multocida, Corynebacterium diphtheriae, S. aureus,* gpA streptococcus
    6. Vesicular or bullous eruptions (varicella, pemphigus, etc.)—*S. aureus,* gpA streptococcus
  B. Distinctive dermatologic clinical entities
    1. Secondary folliculitis
      a. Acne conglobata—*Propionibacterium acnes, S. aureus, Proteus,* and other coliforms (particularly after antibiotic therapy)
      b. Hidradenitis suppurativa—*S. aureus, Proteus* and other coliforms, peptostreptotocci, *Bacteroides*
      c. Perifolliculitis capitis abscedens et suffodiens (dissecting cellulitis of the scalp)—essentially the same process as acne conglobata or hidradenitis suppurativa pathogenetically, but occurring on the scalp; secondary infection occurs with similar varieties of bacteria to the other two entities
    2. Infectious eczematous dermatitis (usually *S. aureus;* occasionally group A streptococci)
    3. Intertrigo (*S. aureus;* occasionally group A streptococci)
    4. Pilonidal and sebaceous cysts—in addition to coliform organisms, particularly in infected pilonidal cysts, there is a high incidence of anaerobic streptococci and *Bacteroides* spp.
    5. Infectious gangrene
      a. Clostridial gas gangrene (see Chap. 197)
      b. Streptococcal gangrene [also known as necrotizing fasciitis (type II) due to group A streptococci] (see Chap. 197)
      c. Necrotizing fasciitis (type I)—a synergistic necrotizing mixed infection due to anaerobic organisms such as *Fusobacteria, Bacteroides, Peptostreptococcus,* enteric bacteria, and *Vibrio* spp. and usually associated with malnutrition, diabetes, agranulocytosis, other debilitating diseases or local injury, or with "skin popping"

(continued)

aspiration, a surgical biopsy may yield information that is life-saving. Local lesions of the skin and subcutaneous tissues in immunocompromised patients should always be biopsied if aspiration fails to define a pathogen.[4] Encouraging results have been reported in a series of patients with suspected necrotizing fasciitis who had biopsies done to confirm the diagnosis early in the course of this devastating infection.[36]

Methods of Culture of Skin Material

All samples for culture should be planted routinely on blood agar and inoculated into a tube of thioglycollate (anaerobic) broth. Additional, more selective media should be used as indicated by clinical findings and evaluation of the Gram-stained smear and frozen sections if a biopsy is done. If cutaneous diphtheria is a consider-

TABLE 194-2 (*Continued*)

   5. Infectious gangrene (*continued*)
       d. †Synergistic necrotizing cellulitis—mixed anaerobic and facultative infection often involving skin and muscle in addition to fascia, seen in diabetic and debilitated elderly patients
       e. Gangrenous balanitis and perineal phlegmon (Fournier's gangrene)—an acute cellulitis with gangrene located in the area of the genitalia, usually due to group A streptococci, enteric bacteria (*E. coli, Klebsiella, Proteus*) or anaerobes, and most commonly seen in diabetic patients
   6. Necrotizing ulcers
       a. Pyoderma gangrenosum (see Chap. 97)—many organisms (*S. aureus,* microaerophilic streptococci, *Proteus, E. coli,* and *Pseudomonas*) may be found secondarily in such lesions, which complicate ulcerative colitis. Proof of a primary bacterial cause of the lesions of pyoderma gangrenosum is lacking. In fact, cultures of early lesions are usually sterile.
       b. Progressive bacterial synergistic gangrene (Meleney) (See Chap. 197)—peptostreptococci or microaerophilic streptococci plus a second organism (*S. aureus, Proteus*)
       c. Decubitus ulcer (*S. aureus,* coliforms, *Pseudomonas, Bacteroides, C. perfringens*)
       d. Tropical ulcer
       e. Phagedenic ulcers—small, circumscribed ulcers with black necrotic centers and erythematous areolas complicating preexisting lesions (e.g., varicella); lesions look like end stage of ecthyma; usually *S. aureus* or *Pseudomonas* cultured from lesions
III. Cutaneous involvement in systemic bacterial infections (exclusive of venereal diseases and mycobacterial infections)
   A. Bacteremia (see II in Table 194-1)
   B. Cutaneous lesions without direct microbial involvement of the skin
       1. Bacterial endocarditis (see Chap. 166, 195)
           a. Subacute (usually viridans streptococci or other non-group A streptococci): petechiae; Osler's nodes; Janeway lesions, uncommonly
           b. Acute (most commonly *S. aureus*): petechiae; purulent purpura; Janeway lesions
       2. Streptococcosis (group A)
           a. Scarlet fever (see Chap. 195)
           b. Streptococcal toxic shock syndrome (see Chap. 195)
           c. Purpura fulminans (see Chap. 195)
       3. Chronic meningococcemia—a variety of sterile macular, papular, nodular, and hemorrhagic lesions occurring intermittently (see Chap. 198)
       4. *S. aureus* including toxin-mediated syndromes—"scalded skin" (see Chap. 196) and "toxic shock" (see Chap. 195)
       5. Erythema nodosum (see Chap. 111) associated with a variety of drugs and infections; among the latter are those due to group A streptococci, *Mycobacterium tuberculosis,* M. *leprae, Yersinia enterocolitica, Legionella pneumophila,* also associated with fungal infections (e.g., coccidioidomycosis and histoplasmosis)
       6. Bacterids
       7. Purpura (other than purpura fulminans and disseminated intravascular coagulation) associated with bacteremias (*S. aureus;* gram-negative bacteria)
IV. Infections due to unusual organisms (see Chap. 200)
   A. Cutaneous diphtheria
   B. Listeriosis (*Listeria monocytogenes*)
   C. Animal-borne or associated diseases
       1. *Bacillus anthracis*—cutaneous anthrax (malignant pustule)
       2. Pasteurelloses and related organisms
           a. *Francisella tularensis* (tularemia)
           b. *P. multocida*—produces infection at site of animal (usually cat) bite
           c. *Yersinia pestis* (plague)
       3. Brucellosis (*Brucella abortus, B. suis,* or *B. melitensis*)—skin lesions are rare in this systemic disease
       4. Rat-bite fever
           a. *Streptobacillus moniliformis* (Haverhill fever)
           b. *Spirillum minus* (sodoku)—exanthem with primarily erythematous macules, some papules, and nodules
       5. Erysipeloid (*Erysipelothrix rhusiopathiae*)
       6. Leptospirosis, including Weil's disease—*Leptospira interrogans* serotypes
       7. *Streptococcus iniae* (produces cellulitis and bacteremia in handlers of fish raised by aquaculture)
       8. Infections due to *Capocytophaga canimorsus* (following dog bite)
       9. *Rhodococcus equis* infection
       10. Glanders (*Burkholderia mallei;* formerly *Pseudomonas mallei*)
   D. Diseases associated with particular geographic locations
       1. Bartonellosis (Carrion's disease)—due to *Bartonella bacilliformis*
       2. Melioidosis (*Burkholderia pseudomallei;* formerly *Pseudomonas pseudomallei*)
       3. Infections due to *Vibrio* spp. (*V. vulnificus, V. cholerae* non 01)
       4. Rhinoscleroma (*pneumoniae Klebsiella* subspec. *rhinoscleromatis*)

---

*The localization and morphologic changes seen often constitute the initial clue in arriving at a specific etiologic cause of the skin lesion(s). It is important to recognize that the morphology of specific infectious lesions as seen in immunocompetent individuals may have an altered appearance when the same infectious lesions occur in an immunosuppressed host (see Chap. 226).
†A term sometimes used in the past to describe necrotizing fasciitis (due to mixed infection with aerobes and anaerobes) with involvement of subjacent muscle as well. Currently, this process would be included under the designation of "necrotizing fasciitis."

TABLE 194-3

Differential Diagnosis of Infectious Gangrene and Gangrenous Cellulitis

	PROGRESSIVE BACTERIAL SYNERGISTIC GANGRENE	NECROTIZING FASCIITIS (TYPE I)	NECROTIZING FASCIITIS (TYPE II) (STREPTOCOCCAL GANGRENE)	CLOSTRIDIAL MYONECROSIS (GAS GANGRENE)	NECROTIZING CUTANEOUS MUCORMYCOSIS	BACTEREMIC PSEUDOMONAS GANGRENOUS CELLULITIS	PYODERMA GANGRENOSUM
Predisposing conditions	Surgery; draining sinus	Diabetes common	Occasionally diabetes or myxedema; after abdominal surgery	Local surgery or trauma; carcinoma of colon (*Clostridium septicum*)	Diabetes; glucocorticoid therapy	Burns, immunosuppression	Ulcerative colitis; rheumatoid arthritis
Pain	Prominent	Prominent	Prominent	Prominent	Minimal	Mild	Moderate
Systemic toxicity	Minimal	Marked	Marked	Very marked	Variable	Marked	Minimal
Course	Slow	Rapid	Very rapid	Extremely rapid	Rapid	Rapid	Slow
Fever	Minimal or absent	Moderate	High	Moderate or high	Low grade	High	Low grade
Anesthesia of lesion	−	−	±	−	+	±	−
Crepitus	−	Often present	−	+	−	−	−
Appearance of the involved area	Central shaggy, necrotic ulcer surrounded by dusky margin and erythematous periphery	Crepitant cellulitis; thick, copious, foul-smelling "dishwater" drainage from scattered areas of skin necrosis	Necrosis of subcutaneous tissue and fascia; black necrotic "burned" appearance of overlying skin	Marked swelling; yellow-bronzed discoloration of skin; gray-brown bullae; green-black patches of necrosis; serosanguinous discharge	Usually a central black necrotic area with purple raised margin; also may be present as just a black ulcer	A sharply demarcated necrotic area with black eschar and surrounding erythema, resembling a decubitus ulcer; may evolve from initial hemorrhagic bulla; cellulitis with fasciitis	Begin as bullae, pustules, or erythematous nodules that ulcerate deeply; often multiple, large and coalesce; usually on lower extremities or abdomen
Etiology	Microaerophilic streptococcus plus *S. aureus* (or *Proteus* sometimes)	Usually a mixture of organisms (e.g., *Bacteroides*, peptostreptococci, *E. coli*, etc.)	Primarily group A streptococci; when develops secondary to abdominal surgery, enteric bacteria also involved	*C. perfringens* (occasionally other histotoxic clostridia)	*Rhizopus*, *Mucor*, *Absidia*	*P. aeruginosa*	Not an infection; may be confused with such due to secondary colonization by Enterobacteriaceae, microaerophilic streptococci, *P. aeruginosa*, *S. aureus*

SOURCE: GL Mandell et al (eds): *Principles and Practice of Infectious Diseases*, 4th ed. New York, Churchill Livingstone, 1995, chap 72, with permission.

ation, Loeffler or tellurite agar should be inoculated. When gram-negative rod infection is suspected, an EMB or MacConkey plate is used; a chocolate agar or modified Thayer-Martin plate incubated in a CO_2 atmosphere is indicated for suspected meningococcal or gonococcal lesions; a blood agar plate incubated in an oxygen-free atmosphere should be used if anaerobic streptococci, clostridia, or *Bacteroides* are suspected. When the skin lesions are thought to be part of a generalized infection, blood cultures should also be obtained prior to institution of antibiotic therapy.

Other Diagnostic Procedures

FLUORESCENT ANTIBODY The practical use of this procedure in bacterial diseases of the skin is of limited availability at this time. Spirochetes can be demonstrated (by the direct or indirect techniques) in chancres, but dark-field examinations are easier to perform and more reliable (see Chap. 229). *N. gonorrhoeae, Actino-myces israelii, Legionella* spp., *Franciscella tularensis*, and *Y. pestio* have been identified by this rapid method. At the present time, these techniques are still in the stage of experimental development for identifying the etiologic agent in most infections of the skin.[37]

OTHER IMMUNOLOGIC METHODS A variety of serologic tests may be helpful in the diagnosis of bacterial infections of the skin, particularly in those where the cutaneous manifestations are secondary to systemic disease (e.g., "rose spots" of typhoid fever). In general, these tests have proved of value in confirming a diagnosis that has already been made by direct bacteriologic identification of the offending organism (e.g., *Salmonella* agglutination, *Brucella* agglutination, agglutination reaction for tularemia, leptospirosis complement fixation or agglutination tests). As in any serologic test, a fourfold or greater rise in titer during the course of the illness is considered significant.

TABLE 194-4

Differential Diagnosis of Crepitant Soft Tissue Wounds*

	CLOSTRIDIAL CELLULITIS	NONCLOSTRIDIAL ANAEROBIC CELLULITIS	CLOSTRIDIAL MYONECROSIS (GAS GANGRENE)	STREPTOCOCCAL MYOSITIS	NECROTIZING FASCIITIS TYPE I†	INFECTED VASCULAR GANGRENE	SYNERGISTIC NECROTIZING CELLULITIS‡	NONINFECTIOUS CAUSES OF GAS IN TISSUES
Predisposing conditions	Local trauma or surgery	Diabetes mellitus; preexisting localized infection	Local trauma or surgery	Local trauma	Diabetes mellitus; abdominal surgery; perineal infection; drug addiction	Peripheral arterial insufficiency	Diabetes mellitus; cardiorenal disease; obesity; perirectal infection	Mechanical effects of penetrating trauma; injuries involving use of compressed air; entrapment of air under loosely sutured wounds or under ulcers; irrigation of wounds with hydrogen peroxide; intravenous catheter placement
Incubation period	Usually over 3 days	Several days	1–2 days	3–4 days	1–4 days	>5 days	3–14 days	Less than an hour
Onset	Gradual	Gradual or rapid	Acute	Not as rapid as gas gangrene	Acute	Subacute	Acute	Usually present immediately after trauma or manipulation; may not be recognized until examined several hours later
Pain	Mild	Mild	Marked	Occurs late; marked	Moderate or severe	Variable	Moderate or severe	Mild
Swelling	Moderate	Moderate	Marked	Moderate	Marked	Moderate or marked	Moderate or marked	Slight or absent
Skin appearance	Minimal discoloration	Minimal discoloration	Yellow-bronze; dark bullae; green-black patches of necrosis	Erythema	Erythematous cellulitis; areas of skin necrosis	Discolored or black	Scattered areas of skin necrosis	Only those due to initiating trauma
Exudate	Thin, dark	Dark pus	Serosanguinous	Abundant, seropurulent	Seropurulent	0	"Dishwater" pus	0
Gas	++++	++++	++	±	++	+++	++	Variable but present; does not extend
Odor	Sometimes foul	Foul	Variable; slightly foul or peculiar sweet	Slight; "sour"	Foul	Foul	Foul	0
Systemic toxicity	Minimal	Moderate	Marked	Only late in course	Moderate or marked	Minimal	Marked	0
Muscle involvement	0	0	++++	+++	0	Dead	++	0

*In addition to the causes of crepitant infections in this table, *Aeromonas hydrophila* myositis may be associated with gas in soft tissues.
†The term *necrotizing fasciitis* is employed here to designate forms of this syndrome other than streptococcal (group A) gangrene.
‡Synergistic necrotizing cellulitis is essentially the same process as type I necrotizing fasciitis. Since the former occasionally extends to involve muscle, it is given a separate designation here; however, the two processes are clinically indistinguishable in most instances.
NOTE: ±, rarely present; ++, present to mild extent; +++, present to moderate extent; ++++, extensive.
SOURCE: GL Mandell et al (eds): *Principles and Practice of Infectious Diseases,* 4th ed. New York, Churchill Livingstone, 1995, chap 72, with permission.

ANTIBIOTIC THERAPY (See also Chap. 258)

The selection of the appropriate antibiotic should be made initially on the basis of the appearance of the skin lesion, the characteristics of any systemic illness, and a Gram-stained smear of material from a lesion if available to sample. Culture results and susceptibility testing of the isolated pathogen(s) are usually available within 48 h (Table 194-6).

Additional epidemiologic factors (current hospitalization or residence in a nursing home, recent antibiotic use, neutropenia, and immunocompromise) should be considered in the choice of initial antimicrobial therapy. Also, it is important to make the choice based on the latest data from the local area and from frequently updated

TABLE 194-5

Causes of Chronic Nodular (Granulomatous) Sporotrichoid Lymphangitis

PRINCIPAL CONSIDERATIONS	RELATIVE FREQUENCY AS ETIOLOGY
Fungi	
Sporothrix schenkii (causative agent of sporotrichosis) (see Chap. 208)	Occasional
Mycobacteria	
Mycobacterium marinum (causative agent of "swimming pool granuloma" (see Chap. 201)	Occasional
M. kansasii	Rare
Bacteria	
Nocardia brasiliensis	Rare
N. asteroides	Very rare
Francisella tularensis	Very rare
Staphylococcus aureus	Very rare
Botryomycosis (*S. aureus*)	Very rare
Protozoa	
Leishmania brasiliensis and *L. mexicana* (causative agents of new world cutaneous leishmaniasis (see Chap. 236)	Occasional

sources (e.g., *Medical Letter*) in view of the rapidly changing patterns of antimicrobial resistance of various bacterial species, requiring alterations in the previous drugs of choice and the use of newer drugs or drug combinations.

Dosage: Methods of Administration—Excretion

Primary cutaneous infections of mild to moderate severity can be treated with local measures, topical drugs, oral antibiotics, or by a combination of these methods. In recent years there has been a proliferation of oral cephalosporins with activity against group A streptococci and methicillin-susceptible. *S. aureus,* which cause infections of the skin and soft tissues such as impetigo, cellulitis, subcutaneous abscesses, and wound infections (Table 194-7). Extensive infections of the skin, with or without systemic manifestations, should be vigorously treated with parenteral antibiotics in adequate dosage.

A number of factors must be considered in administering antibiotics: oral treatment may be limited by absorption and gastrointestinal disturbances; hypotension, severe thrombopenia, and extensive skin disease can prohibit the intramuscular route; the proper drug selected may be suitable for administration only by a specific route. Caution must be exercised in administering intramuscular medications to avoid sterile or infected abscesses. When the intravenous route is used, a needle or "heparin-lock" is preferred. Percutaneous catheters should be changed frequently (every 2 to 3 days), and all line-skin sites kept clean with a topical antibiotic ointment and sterile dressing that is changed daily.

The excretory pattern of a given antibiotic should always be considered in order to avoid toxic accumulation in the face of specific organ malfunction (e.g., use of aminoglycosides or vancomycin in the presence of renal impairment).

Toxicity

The toxicity of antibiotics should be considered on an individual basis, but some problems are applicable to all antibiotics. Hypersensitivity reactions are relatively common and may include skin rashes, fever, or more severe manifestations such as acute anaphylaxis or exfoliative erythrodermas. The penicillins and sulfonamides are particularly likely to produce these problems. Questions regarding previous drug allergy should be asked whenever any antibiotic is to be administered. All antibiotics alter the relative kinds and absolute numbers of the indigenous flora, and superinfection may result from their use, especially with broad-spectrum agents like the cephalosporins. Gastrointestinal disturbances and oral mucous membrane lesions are the major nonspecific types of problems encountered with alteration of the flora, although changes also occur on burn surfaces and other lesions. There are numerous other untoward reactions (renal, hematologic, hepatic, nervous system) to antibiotics that may represent acceptable risks if the reasons for use of these drugs are compelling (see footnotes, Table 194-6). The responsibility is the physician's, however, to be aware of the usual and unusual manifestations of toxicity to any of the antibiotics used and to be alert to possible novel effects in individual patients.

Antibiotic Resistance due to "R" Factors

Transferable resistance to multiple antibiotics has emerged as a widespread problem. Extrachromosomal genetic elements (R plasmids) in bacteria are the basis for much of such resistance.[38,39] Prolonged antibiotic therapy, especially in a closed environment like a hospital, may select R-factor-carrying members of the indigenous flora (e.g., in the gastrointestinal tract), which may subsequently transfer this property to a recently acquired organism. In this way, antibiotic resistance to chloramphenicol, tetracycline, and kanamycin conferred by a plasmid in *E. coli* can be transferred during mating to a *Klebsiella* or *Salmonella* strain. As a consequence, organisms with greater intrinsic pathogenicity can become antibiotic-resistant as well. This phenomenon and its practical consequences have been verified in a number of studies.[40]

R plasmids (R factors) have been found in most pathogenic gram-negative bacteria, including *E. coli, Klebsiella, Proteus, Pseudomonas, Salmonella,* and *Shigella.* They are responsible also for high-level resistance to the penicillins (penicillinase plasmids) and cephalosporins.

R-factor-associated antibiotic resistance has been identified in *S. aureus* and *Enterococcus* spp. as well as in *Haemophilus influenzae* and *N. gonorrhoeae,* all important pathogens in skin as well as systemic infection.

Topical Antibacterial Agents

Topical antibacterial agents have frequently been used to prevent, as well as to suppress, bacterial growth in burns and other open lesions (see Chap. 246). Their greatest usefulness has been when employed along with strict aseptic techniques in preventing percutaneous line sepsis. These agents are capable of inhibiting the local flora, but, as is true of all antibiotics, they have a relatively limited spectrum of activity, which favors the emergence of bacterial resistance during treatment. In addition, topical drugs may precipitate contact dermatitis and can be absorbed to toxic levels. Furthermore, there has been very little evidence that they add a great deal therapeutically.[41] An exception to this is the result, in burn patients, of the use of sulfamylon (mafenide) acetate cream or of 0.5% silver nitrate solution. However, even with these broad-spectrum agents, resistant species, such as *C. perfringens, Klebsiella,* and *Entero-*

TABLE 194-6

Selection of Antibiotics

INFECTING AGENT	DRUG OF CHOICE[a,b]	
	FIRST	ALTERNATIVES
Gram-positive cocci:		
Staphylococcus aureus or coagulase-negative staphylococci		
Non-penicillinase-producing	Penicillin G[c] (or V)	Cephalosporins,[d] erythromycin and other macrolides (clarithromycin, azithromycin),[e] vancomycin,[f] clindamycin[g]
Penicillinase-producing	Penicillinase-resistant penicillin[i]; cephalosporin[d]	Same as above for non-penicillinase-producing strains; also a fluoroquinolone[h]
Methicillin-resistant[j]	Vancomycin(± rifampin or gentamicin)[k]	Teicoplanin, fluoroquinolone, trimethoprim-sulfamethoxazole[l] + rifampin
Streptococci		
Groupable (groups A, B, C, G)	Penicillin G or V	Erythromycin (clarithromycin or azithromycin), clindamycin, cephalosporin, vancomycin
Enterococcus spp[m] (systemic infection)	Penicillin G (or ampicillin) + gentamicin	Vancomycin + gentamicin
Nongroupable (viridans streptococci, etc.)	Penicillin G	Cephalosporin, erythromycin (clarithromycin or azithromycin), vancomycin
Streptococcus bovis	Penicillin G	Cephalosporin, erythromycin (clarithromycin or azithromycin), vancomycin
Anaerobic	Penicillin G	Clindamycin, erythromycin, chloramphenicol,[n] cephalosporin, vancomycin
Gram-positive bacilli:		
Bacillus anthracis (anthrax)	Penicillin G	Tetracycline[o] (or doxycycline), erythromycin, ciprofloxacin
Borrelia burgdorferi (Lyme disease spirochete)	Amoxicillin, doxycycline	Penicillin G, ceftriaxone, erythromycin
Clostridium perfringens (gas gangrene)	Penicillin G + clindamicin	Chloramphenicol, metronidazole,[p] imipenem
Corynebacterium, including *C. diphtheriae*	Erythromycin	Penicillin G, vancomycin
Erysipelothrix rhusiopathiae	Penicillin G (or ampicillin)	Cephalosporin (3d generation), fluoroquinolone, erythromycin
Leptospira spp.	Doxycycline	Penicillin G
Listeria monocytogenes	Ampicillin (or penicillin G) ± gentamicin	Trimethoprim-sulfamethoxazole
Gram-negative cocci:		
Neisseria gonorrhoeae	Ceftriaxone	Cefixime, fluoroquinolone, cefoxitin[q] spectinomycin
Neisseria meningitidis (meningococcus)	Penicillin G or ampicillin	Cefotaxime, ceftriaxone, chloramphenicol, a sulfonamide (only if sulfonamide susceptibility of organisms is proved by appropriate quantitative methods), cefuroxime
Gram-negative bacilli:		
Aeromonas hydrophilia	Trimethoprim-sulfamethoxazole	Fluoroquinolone, imipenem, 3d generation cephalosporin, gentamicin
Escherichia coli (systemic infection)	Ampicillin (amoxicillin); for severe infections, ceftriaxone or cefotaxime	Ampicillin-sulbactam, a cephalosporin, broad-spectrum penicillin,[r] trimethoprim-sulfamethoxazole, aminoglycodes,[s] fluoroquinolone
Francisella tularensis (tularemia)	Streptomycin[t] or gentamicin	Doxycycline, chloramphenicol
Haemophilus influenzae	Cefotaxime or ceftriaxone (for life-threatening infections)	Ampicillin (if beta-lactamase negative), cefuroxime, trimethoprim-sulfamethoxazole, chloramphenicol, amoxicillin-clavulanate
Klebsiella pneumoniae	3d generation cephalosporin for serious infections	Imipenem, aminoglycosides (gentamicin, tobramycin, amikacin), ampicillin-sulbactam, fluoroquinolone, ticarcillin-clavulanate, aztreonam

(continued)

TABLE 194-6 (*Continued*)

Klebsiella pneumoniae subspec *rhinoscleromatis*	Ciprofloxacin	Trimethroprim-sulfamethoxazole + rifampin
Legionella pneumophila	Erythromycin	Add rifampin; fluoroquinolone
Pasteurella multocida	Penicillin G (ampicillin)	A tetracycline, 3d generation cephalosporin, chloramphenicol, fluoroquinolone
Proteus mirabilis	Ampicillin	Cephalosporin, gentamicin, imipenem, aztreonam
Proteus—other species	3rd generation cephalosporin	Ticarcillin or piperacillin, fluoroquinolone, gentamicin, imipenem, aztreonam
Pseudomonas aeruginosa (systemic infection)	Ceftazidime + tobramycin[u]	Ticarcillin (or piperacillin) + gentamicin, amikacin, imipenem, aztreonam, fluoroquinolone
Burkholderia pseudomallei	Ceftazidime + trimethoprim-sulfamethoxazole	Imipenem, amoxicillin clavulanate, chloramphenicol
Salmonella typhi	Ciprofloxacin	Ceftriaxone, chloramphenicol, amoxicillin or ampicillin, trimethoprim-sulfamethoxazole
Salmonella spp.	Fluoroquinolone or ceftriaxone (cefotaxime)	Trimethoprim-sulfamethoxazole, chloramphenicol, ampicillin or amoxicillin
Streptobacillus moniliformis (rat-bite fever)	Penicillin G ± streptomycin	Doxycycline, erythromycin, clindamycin
Yersinia pestis	Streptomycin or gentamicin	Chloramphenicol, doxycycline

[a]Drug susceptibility testing of bacterial isolates should be performed coincident with the initial choice of an antibacterial agent. Dosages of drugs of choice are given in Chaps. 195–200.
[b]Not all drugs are approved by the Food and Drug Administration for treatment of that infection.
[c]When used in low doses, hypersensitivity reactions (5 to 8 percent) are the major problem. Massive therapy (10 to 50 million units daily) for life-threatening gram-positive coccal infections may produce toxicity from hyperkalemia, central nervous system irritation (seizures), and Coombs-positive hemolytic anemia.
[d]A first-generation cephalosporin is preferred. Gram-negative organisms resistant to first-generation cephalosporins *may* be susceptible to second- or third-generation agents. Hypersensitivity reactions, reversible neutropenia, and, very rarely, nephrotoxicity at high doses are chief adverse effects.
[e]Side effects are uncommon except for gastrointestinal disturbances. Rarely, hypersensitivity reactions (fever or rash) and hepatotoxicity occur (with the oral erythromycin estolate preparation). Administered orally or intravenously.
[f]Causes phlebitis and fever, hypersensitivity reactions; and in the presence of renal failure or excessive dosage, ototoxicity. Should be given slowly (~1 h) i.v. to avoid histamine-like systemic effects.
[g]Gastrointestinal irritation (diarrhea) is common; rare pseudomembranous colitis and granulocytopenia.
[h]Gastrointestinal side effects (mainly anorexia and nausea) in 3–13 percent. Headache and mood alterations and interstitial nephritis are uncommon adverse effects. Should not be administered to children because of possible damage to cartilage.
[i]The semisynthetic penicillins (oxacillin, nafcillin, cloxacillin, dicloxacillin) cross-react with penicillin G in evoking hypersensitivity reactions.
[j]Methicillin-resistant strains are *always* cephalosporin-resistant too.
[k]Nephrotoxic and ototoxic, especially in the aged and in the presence of preexisting renal disease. Administered under the closest medical supervision with monitoring of renal (blood levels), auditory, and vestibular function.
[l]Trimethoprim-sulfamethoxazole may cause bone marrow toxicity due to either, or to combined drug effects. Hypersensitivity reactions, gastrointestinal upset, hepatitis, and anemias (megaloblastic and hemolytic) are occasionally encountered.
[m]For endocarditis or other serious infection.
[n]Chloramphenicol may depress bone marrow function, one or all elements being affected. This drug should be given only under close medical surveillance; check differential smear and white blood count; look for a rise in serum iron levels as an indication of toxicity. Associated with the "gray syndrome" when administered without appropriate reduction in dosage to premature infants or neonates.
[o]All the tetracyclines are potent antianabolic drugs, gastrointestinal irritants; potentially hepatotoxic when doses exceed 2.0 g daily parenterally; discolor and alter organogenesis of primary and secondary teeth; photosensitizing. Outdated preparations may be nephrotoxic. All tetracyclines stimulate changes in the indigenous microflora favoring emergence of infections due to yeast and resistant staphylococci and gram-negative bacilli.
[p]Bactericidal for *Bacteroides* and *Clostridia* but variably effective in anaerobic and microaerophilic streptococcal infections.
[q]Second- (cefoxitin) and third- (cefotaxime, ceftazidime) generation cephalosporins are occasionally drugs of choice, guided by susceptibility testing, for selected infections. In addition to cross-hypersensitivity with first-generation agents, they may cause superinfections due to their broad-spectrum activity and some may cause bleeding complications.
[r]Includes carbenicillin, ticarcillin, piperacillin, azlocillin, mezlocillin, which have similar toxic and hypersensitivity effects to penicillin. In addition they may cause bleeding, due to platelet dysfunction, as well as add a significant sodium load.
[s]Gentamicin has been used as a prototype aminoglycoside. In many situations tobramycin (or amikacin) may be selected, depending on the in vitro susceptibility of the organism involved or on known nosocomial patterns of aminoglycoside resistance.
[t]Vestibular toxicity, especially in the aged and those with renal failure, as well as hypersensitivity reactions.
[u]Tobramycin (or gentamicin) and broad-spectrum penicillins should not be mixed in the same intravenous infusion. Tobramycin has toxicity identical to gentamicin.

TABLE 194-7

Oral Cephalosporins Used in Treating Skin Infections

DRUG	ADULT DOSAGE
Cephalexin	250–500 mg q6h
Cefadroxil	500–1000 mg q12h
Cephradine	500 mg q6h
Cefaclor	250–500 mg q8h
Cefprozil	250–500 mg q12h
Cefuroxime	250–500 mg q12h
Cefpodoxime	200–400 mg q12h
Loracarbef	200–400 mg q12h

bacter, may emerge as the dominant potential pathogen of the local flora.

Among the most useful topical antibacterial agents are acetic acid (1 to 5%) for *Pseudomonas* nail and toe web infections and bacitracin (500 units per milliliter or gram) for selected superficial *S. aureus* and streptococcal lesions. Occasionally topical bacitracin may be associated with a cutaneous hypersensitivity reaction. Neomycin (0.5% ointment) and gentamicin (0.17% cream) may be useful in selected patients when mixed gram-negative bacteria require local suppression. Mupirocin (2%) ointment has antibacterial activity against various streptococci and *S. aureus*. It is a safe and effective treatment of impetigo.[42] A number of broad-spectrum antiseptics are also available for topical use, combining antibacterial with nonirritating properties. Povidone-iodine (Betadine) is effective against most gram-positive and gram-negative bacteria but does not persist in the skin to provide a residual action. Chlorhexidine gluconate (4% solution) is an antiseptic that combines broad antibacterial properties with prolonged action due to local accumulation. An alcoholic preparation is especially effective, is not appreciably absorbed into the blood, and generally is not irritating to the skin.[43,44] These broad-spectrum antiseptics can be used prophylactically or to treat local wounds and superficially infected dermatoses.

The topical therapy of burns is discussed in Chap. 129.

REFERENCES

1. Johnson JE II et al: Studies on the pathogenesis of staphylococcal infection. I. The effect of repeated skin infection. *J Exp Med* **113**:235, 1961
2. Leyden JJ et al: Experimental infections with group A streptococci in humans. *J Invest Dermatol* **75**:196, 1980
3. Elek SD: Experimental staphylococcal infections in the skin of man. *Ann NY Acad Sci* **65**:85, 1956
4. Wolfson JS et al: Dermatologic manifestations of infection in the compromised host. *Annu Rev Med* **34**:205, 1983
5. Kligman AM et al: Bacteriology. *J Invest Dermatol* **67**:160, 1976
6. Miller SJ et al: In vitro and in vivo antistaphylococcal activity of human stratum corneum lipids. *Arch Dermatol* **124**:209, 1988
7. Lacey RW, Lord VL: Sensitivity of staphylococci to fatty acids: Novel inactivation of linolenic acid by serum. *J Med Microbiol* **14**:41, 1981
8. Leyden JJ et al: Experimental inoculation of *Pseudomonas aeruginosa* and *Pseudomonas cepaci* on human skin. *J Soc Cosmet Chem* **31**:19, 1980
9. Shinefield HR et al: Bacterial interference, in *Skin Bacteria and Their Role in Infection,* edited by HI Maibach, G Hildick-Smith. New York, McGraw-Hill, 1965, chap 17
10. Fattom A et al: Laboratory and clinical evaluation of conjugate vaccines composed of *Staphylococcus aureus* type 5 and type 8 capsular polysaccharides bound to *Pseudomonas aeruginosa* recombinant exoprotein A. *Infect Immun* **61**:1023, 1993
11. Elin RJ et al: Biology of endotoxin. *Annu Rev Med* **27**:127, 1976
12. Wolff SM: Biological effects of bacterial endotoxins in man. *J Infect Dis* **128**:S259, 1973
13. Young LS et al: University of California/Davis interdepartmental conferences on gram-negative septicemia. *Rev Infect Dis* **13**:666, 1991
14. Tracey KJ et al: Cachectin/tumor necrosis factor. *Lancet* **1**:1122, 1989
15. Dinarello CA et al: New concepts on the pathogenesis of fever. *Rev Infect Dis* **10**:168, 1988
16. Michie HR et al: Detection of circulating tumor necrosis factor after endotoxin administration. *N Engl J Med* **318**:1481, 1988
17. Cannon JG et al: Circulating interleukin-1 and tumor necrosis factor in septic shock and experimental endotoxin fever. *J Infect Dis* **161**:79, 1990
18. Waage A et al: Association between tumor necrosis factor in serum and fatal outcome in patients with meningococcal disease. *Lancet* **1**:355, 1987
19. Girardin E et al: Tumor necrosis factor and interleukin-1 in the serum of children with severe infectious purpura. *N Engl J Med* **319**:397, 1988
20. Tracey KJ et al: Anti-cachectin/TNF monoclonal antibodies prevent septic shock during lethal bacteraemia. *Nature* **330**:662, 1987
21. Fields BN et al: The so-called "paracolon" bacteria: A bacteriologic and clinical reappraisal. *Am J Med* **42**:89, 1967
22. Gold WL, Salit IE *Aeromonas hydrophilia* infections of skin and soft tissue: Report of 11 cases and review. *Clin Infect Dis* **16**:69, 1993
23. Fang FC, Madinger NE: Resistant nosocomial gram-negative bacillary pathogens: *Acinetobacter baumanii, Xanthomonas maltophilia,* and *Pseudomonas cepacia,* in *Current Clinical Topics in Infectious Diseases*-16, edited by JS Remington, MN Swartz. Cambridge, MA, Blackwell Science, 1996, pp 52–83
24. Chuang Y-C et al: *Vibrio vulnificus* infection in Taiwan: Report of 28 cases and review of clinical manifestations and treatment. *Clin Infect Dis* **15**:271, 1992
25. Bornstein DL et al: Anaerobic infections—review of current experience. *Medicine (Baltimore)* **43**:207, 1964
26. Cluff LE: The inflammatory response of skin to bacterial invasion, in *Skin Bacteria and Their Role in Infection,* edited by HI Maibach, G Hildick-Smith. New York, McGraw-Hill, 1965, p 95
27. Thomas L: The effects of cortisone on bacterial infection and intoxication, in *Effects of ACTH and Cortisone upon Infection and Resistance,* edited by G Shwartzman. New York, Columbia Univ Press, 1953, chap 12
28. Lipinski B et al: The organ distribution of ^{125}I-fibrin in the generalized Shwartzman reaction and its relation to leukocytes. *Br J Haematol* **28**:221, 1974
29. Horn RG: Evidence for participation of granulocytes in the pathogenesis of the generalized Shwartzman reaction: A review. *J Infect Dis* **128**:S134, 1973
30. Braude AI et al: Treatment and prevention of intravascular coagulation with antiserum to endotoxin. *J Infect Dis* **128**:S157, 1973
31. Ziegler EJ et al: Treatment of gram-negative bacteremia and shock with human antiserum to a mutant *Escherichia coli. N Engl J Med* **307**:1225, 1982
32. Hook EW III et al: Microbial evaluation of cutaneous cellulitis in adults. *Arch Intern Med* **146**:295, 1986
33. Sachs MK: The optimum use of needle aspiration in the bacteriologic diagnosis of cellulitis in adults. *Arch Intern Med* **150**:1907, 1990
34. Kielhofner MA et al: Influence of underlying disease process on the utility of cellulitis needle aspirates. *Arch Intern Med* **148**:2451, 1988
35. Howe PM et al: Etiologic diagnosis of cellulitis: Comparison of aspirates obtained from the leading edge and the point of maximal inflammation. *Pediatr Infect Dis J* **6**:685, 1987
36. Stamenkovic I et al: Early recognition of potentially fatal necrotizing fasciitis. The use of frozen-section biopsy. *N Engl J Med* **310**:1689, 1984
37. Bernard P et al: Streptococcal cause of erysipelas and cellulitis in adults. A microbiologic study using a direct immunofluorescence technique. *Arch Dermatol* **125**:779, 1989
38. Sanders CC et al: β-lactam resistance in gram-negative bacteria: Global trends and clinical impact. *Clin Infect Dis* **15**:824, 1992
39. Murray BE: New aspects of antimicrobial resistance and the resulting therapeutic dilemmas. *J Infect Dis* **163**:1185, 1991
40. Neu HC: The crisis in antibiotic resistance. *Science* **257**:1064, 1992
41. Editorial: Topical antibiotics. *Br Med J* **1**:1494, 1977
42. Goldfarb J et al: Randomized clinical trial of topical mucopirocin versus oral erythromycin for impetigo. *Antimicrob Agents Chemother* **32**:1780, 1988
43. Editorial: Chlorhexidine and other antiseptics. *Med Lett Drug Ther* **18**:85, 1976
44. Lilly HA et al: Detergents compared with each other and with antiseptics as skin "degerming" agents. *J Hyg (Lond)* **82**:89, 1979

Peter K. Lee
Arnold N. Weinberg
Morton N. Swartz
Richard Allen Johnson

Pyodermas: *Staphylococcus aureus*, Streptococcus, and Other Gram-Positive Bacteria

Normal human skin is colonized soon after birth by a large number of bacteria that live as commensals on the epidermis and epidermal appendages. Coagulase-negative staphylococci (*S. epidermidis*) are inoculated during vaginal passage; coryneform bacteria take up residence on neonatal skin shortly after birth; and within several weeks after birth, the flora of neonatal skin is similar to that of adults (for further reading see Chap. 194).

The majority of the primary and secondary pyodermas (cutaneous bacterial infections) are due to either *S. aureus* or group A streptococcus. *S. aureus* pyodermas occur in individuals who are nasal carriers of the organism, which, when translocated onto the skin, is able to gain access via small breaks in the cutaneous integrity and cause superficial infections. Group A streptococcal pyodermas occur following colonization of the skin either from the skin of another individual colonized with group A streptococci or, less likely, from the patient's nasopharynx. *S. aureus* and group A streptococcus cause a broad clinical spectrum of infection, i.e., superficial pyodermas and invasive soft-tissue infections (see Chap. 197), depending on the organism, on the anatomical location of infections, and on host factors.

STAPHYLOCOCCAL SKIN INFECTIONS

Staphylococci are classified into two major groups: the coagulase-negative staphylococci and coagulase-positive (*S. aureus*) staphylococci. Many different species of coagulase-negative staphylococci are found on the skin, the ratio varying according to the site: *S. epidermidis* (the most common), *S. simulans*, *S. xylosus*, *S. cohnii*, *S. saprophyticus*, *S. hemolyticus*, *S. warneri*, *S. hominis*, *S. capitis*, *S. auricularis*, and *S. saccharolyticus*. Individuals carry a combined minimum of 10 to 24 temporary and resident strains of *S. epidermidis*. The relatively high number of *S. epidermidis* strains is attributable in part to the wide habitat and niche range of this species; this number is usually maintained on the host even though the specific strain composition may change over time. *S. epidermidis* is a reluctant pathogen but is capable of causing superficial and invasive infections (particularly about implanted foreign bodies such as intravascular catheters).[1]

S. aureus is a persistent member of the microbial flora in 10 to 20 percent of the population. Carriage is transient or intermittent in other individuals. Approximately 30 to 50 percent of healthy adults harbor *S. aureus* at some site at any given time. As many as 84 percent of healthy individuals have occasional carriage of *S. aureus* in their anterior nares.[2] Other sites of colonization include the ax-

illae, perineum, pharynx, and hands. Conditions predisposing to *S. aureus* colonization include atopic dermatitis, diabetes mellitus (insulin-dependent), dialysis (hemo- and peritoneal), intravenous drug use, and HIV infection.

S. aureus is an aggressive pathogen and the most common cause of primary pyodermas and soft-tissue infections (STIs) as well as secondary infections on disease-altered skin. *S. aureus* in pyodermas or STIs can invade the bloodstream, producing bacteremia, metastatic infection such as osteomyelitis, and acute infective endocarditis. Some strains of *S. aureus* also produce exotoxins, which cause constellations of systemic symptoms such as staphylococcal scalded-skin syndrome (SSSS), and staphylococcal toxic-shock syndrome (TSS).

General Features

BACTERIOLOGY AND PATHOGENESIS Colonization by *S. aureus* may be transient or represent a prolonged carrier state.[3] In individuals with atopic dermatitis, *S. aureus* was found in the anterior nares and distal subungual spaces of their fingernails 5 and 10 times more frequently, respectively, than in normal subjects.[4] In children and adults with atopic dermatitis, 78 to 100 percent of eczematous lesions (more commonly in exudative lesions than chronic plaques) are colonized with *S. aureus*. Colonization of noneczematous skin is significantly less frequent.[5] Topical glucocorticoid treatment of involved skin reduces the bacterial skin flora in patients with atopic dermatitis.[6]

S. aureus produces many cellular components and extracellular products that may contribute to its pathogenicity. The role of these components in disease is not well understood, except for the variety of exotoxins that are made and secreted extracellularly. The production of coagulase, leukocidin, alpha toxin, etc., may be the same in *S. aureus* strains isolated from staphylococcal cellulitis as in those from normal skin of the carrier. Thus, host factors such as immunosuppression, glucocorticoid therapy, and atopy may also play a major role in the pathogenesis of staphylococcal infections. Preexisting tissue injury or inflammation (surgical wound, burn, trauma, dermatitis, retained foreign body) are of major importance in the pathogenesis of staphylococcal disease. The production of coagulase, a factor capable of clotting plasma, has been employed in the past as the in vitro criterion of the potential pathogenicity of a staphylococcal strain. Coagulase may play a role in the development of the staphylococcal abscess by producing local fibrin thrombi that protect organisms and concentrate toxic factors elaborated by these pathogens. The surface of *S. aureus*, and particularly coagulase-negative staphylococci, may be very mucoid, which facilitates adherence of the organism to surfaces of foreign bodies such as intravascular catheters or prostheses. Increased epithelial-cell adherence is a factor in the increased incidence of *S. aureus* infections in individuals treated with oral retinoids.

Exotoxins elaborated by *S. aureus* (Table 195-1) include enterotoxins and toxic-shock syndrome toxin 1 (TSST-1), involved in TSS and related illnesses, and exfoliative toxins A and B, involved in SSSS (see Chap. 196) and bullous impetigo. These exotoxins, known as superantigens, are characterized by their potent ability to activate a large portion of T lymphocytes by interacting with only the variable region of the β-chain of the T-cell receptor complex outside the antigen-binding groove. The role of these exotoxins in such dermatoses as atopic dermatitis and psoriasis and in Kawasaki's syndrome is being investigated.[7]

Drug resistance One of the major problems in dealing with staphylococcal infections has been the emergence of antibiotic-resistant strains, in particular, to penicillin and the semisynthetic penicillinase-resistant penicillins. Undoubtedly, the initial introduction of the penicillinase-resistant penicillins has altered considerably the prognosis for serious staphylococcal infections. However, with ever-increasing use of such penicillins, methicillin-resistant *S. aureus* (MRSA) strains have become a major epidemiologic problem since the 1980s. Attempts to eradicate MRSA have generally been unsuccessful. Treatment of anterior nares and wounds with mupirocin ointment has been shown to decrease *S. aureus* colonization but has failed to decrease the rate of transmission to a roommate in a long-term-care facility.[8] Although there are many other reports of topical mupirocin being used to reduce colonization of MRSA and methicillin-sensitive *S. aureus* (MSSA) strains, indiscriminate use of topical mupirocin must be avoided because significant mupirocin resistance has already emerged.[9] Interestingly, although the presence of resistance has been of paramount importance in the outcome of infection, there is no evidence that the intrinsic virulence of such strains is any greater than that of penicillin-susceptible organisms.

Epidemiology The ubiquitous presence of *S. aureus* and the difficulty in distinguishing among strains has made understanding the epidemiology of staphylococcal infections difficult. At first glance, the high frequency of staphylococcal colonization of the respiratory tract and the frequency of staphylococci in our immediate environment suggested that their spread from person to person occurred principally via respiratory transmission or fomites. However, careful epidemiologic studies utilizing phage-typing techniques suggest that transfer of organisms to patients occurs predominantly via the hands of personnel rather than through the air. This appears to be particularly true in newborn nurseries, where this route is important in the dissemination of the organisms from nasal carriers and also in the transfer of staphylococci between babies. Individuals, whether infants or adults, with open staphylococcal infections are particularly dangerous potential carriers and transmitters of infection. Nasal carriage of *S. aureus* appears to be a major risk factor for wound infection after cardiac surgery, resulting in

TABLE 195-1

Exotoxins (Superantigens) Produced by *Staphylococcus aureus*

TOXINS	CLINICAL SYNDROME
Enterotoxins B and C	TSS (nearly 50% of nonmenstrual cases)
TSS toxin 1 (TSST-1)	TSS (nearly all menstrual cases)
	Scarlatiniform eruption (staphylococcal scarlet fever)
Exfoliative toxins A and B	SSSS
	Bullous impetigo

higher mortality rates and longer postoperative stays.[10] The rate of *S. aureus* bacteremia is also higher in nasal carriers of *S. aureus*.[11] Good nursery technique, careful handling of patients, strict handwashing procedures, and isolation of patients with open draining staphylococcal infections are important in the reduction of transmission of staphylococci.

Immunity The high prevalence of staphylococci and staphylococcal infections is substantiated by the almost universal presence in adults of circulating antibody to one or more cell-wall antigens or extracellular toxins. The occurrence of staphylococcal infections in the presence of these antibodies suggests that they are not the primary determinants of resistance to such infections. Immunization of experimental animals with alpha toxin does not afford protection against staphylococcal disease following challenge. Hypersensitivity may play a role in recurrent staphylococcal skin infections in humans.

Superficial Staphylococcal Pyodermas

In industrialized nations, *S. aureus* is the most common cause of superficial pyodermas, having more of a "market share" than it did several decades ago. Group A streptococcus continues to be a common cause of pyoderma in developing countries. Pyoderma represents infections in the epidermis, just below the stratum corneum (impetigo) or in hair follicles (folliculitis) (Table 195-2). Untreated, superficial pyodermas can extend into the dermis, resulting in ecthyma and furuncle formation.

IMPETIGO Two clinical patterns of impetigo are recognized: bullous and nonbullous. Bullous impetigo is caused by *S. aureus*. Several decades ago, nonbullous impetigo was most commonly caused by group A streptococcus (see "Streptococcal Impetigo," below). Currently, in industrialized nations, nonbullous impetigo is most commonly caused by *S. aureus*[12] and less often by group A streptococcus, or by both organisms.[13,14] Group A streptococcus remains a common cause of nonbullous impetigo in developing nations.

Nonbullous impetigo This type accounts for >70 percent of cases of impetigo; it occurs in children of all ages as well as in adults. Intact skin is usually resistant to colonization or impetiginization, probably because of absence of fibronectin receptors for teichoic acid moities on *S. aureus* and group A streptococcus. When both organisms are present, group A streptococcus appears to be the primary pathogen and *S. aureus* the secondary invader of the lesions (see "Streptococcal Impetigo," below). Production of bacteriocins, produced by certain *S. aureus* strains (phage group 71) and highly bactericidal to group A streptococcus, may be responsible for the isolation of only *S. aureus* from some lesions due initially to streptococci. The sequence of spread of *S. aureus* is from nose to normal skin (about 11 days later) and to skin lesions (after another 11 days).

Lesions commonly arise on the skin of the face (especially around the nares) or extremities after trauma. Pruritus may be present in some cases. Nasal carriers of *S. aureus* can present with a very localized type of impetigo confined to the anterior nares and the adjacent lip area (Fig. 195-1); soreness of the area is a common complaint (Fig. 195-2). Conditions that disrupt the integrity of the epidermis, providing a portal of entry of impetiginization, include insect bites, epidermal dermatophytoses, herpes simplex, varicella, abrasions, lacerations, and thermal burns. The initial lesion is a transient vesicle or pustule (Fig. 195-2) (usually not seen by the patient or the health care worker) that quickly evolves into a honey-colored

TABLE 195-2

Infections and Toxin Syndromes Involving the Skin and Soft Tissues Caused by *Staphylococcus aureus*

Sites of colonization (carrier state)
  Anterior nares
  Throat
  Axillae, perineum
  Hands
  Involved skin in individuals with atopic dermatitis
Sites of colonization in neonates (and sites of infection)
  Skin
  Umbilicus
  Circumcision site
  Conjunctivae
Superficial pyodermas
  Primary pyodermas
    Skin
      Impetigo
      Bullous impetigo
      Ecthyma
      Botryomycosis
    Hair follicles
      Superficial folliculitis (follicular or Bockhart's impetigo)
      Folliculitis (sycosis barbae)
      Furuncle (boil)
      Carbuncle
    Intertriginous sites
      Perianal "dermatitis"
    Digital infections
      Paronychia
      Blistering distal dactylitis
    Following skin disruption
      Trauma (physical, thermal)
      Foreign body (intravascular catherer, prosthetic device)
  Secondary pyodermas
    Impetiginization of dermatoses such as atopic dermatitis, herpes
      simplex (superinfection)
  Pyodermas associated with systemic disease
    Job's syndrome
    Chédiak-Higashi syndrome
    Chronic granulomatous disease
Invasive infections
  Lymphangitis, lymphadenitis
  Erysipelas
  Cellulitis
  Streptococcal gangrene
  Pyomyositis
  Bacteremia, septicemia
Metastatic skin infections associated with bacteremia (often *S. aureus* acute infectious endocarditis)
  Abscesses (superficial and deep)
  Septic vasculitis (pustular purpura)
Purpura fulminans
  Disseminated intravascular coagulation associated with staphylococcal bacteremia
  Meningococcemia-like syndrome
Staphylococcal toxin-associated syndromes
  Staphylococcal scarlet fever
  Staphylococcal scalded-skin syndrome (SSSS)
  Staphylococcal toxic-shock syndrome (TSS)

crusted plaque that can enlarge to ≥2 cm in diameter (Fig. 195-1*B*). Surrounding erythema may be present. Constitutional symptoms are absent. Regional lymphadenopathy may be present in up to 90 percent of patients with prolonged untreated infection.

The differential diagnosis of nonbullous impetigo includes seborrheic dermatitis, atopic dermatitis, allergic contact dermatitis, epidermal dermatophyte infections, tinea capitis, herpes simplex, varicella, herpes zoster, scabies, and pediculosis capitis. Any of these disorders may occur primarily and become secondarily impetiginized with *S. aureus* or group A streptococcus.

Untreated, the lesions may slowly enlarge and involve new sites over several weeks. In some individuals, lesions resolve spontaneously. In others, the lesions extend into the dermis forming an ulcer (ecthyma).

Bullous impetigo Three types of skin lesions can be produced by phage group II *S. aureus:* (1) bullous impetigo, (2) exfoliative disease (staphylococcal scalded-skin syndrome), and (3) nonstreptococcal scarlatiniform eruption (staphylococcal scarlet fever). All three represent varying cutaneous responses to extracellular exfoliative toxins ("exfoliatin") types A and B produced by these staphylococci (for descriptions of the toxin and the latter two types of lesions see Chap. 196).

In a study of bullous impetigo, 51 percent of patients had concurrent *S. aureus* cultured from the nose or throat; 79 percent of cultures grew the same strain from both sites.[14] Bullous impetigo occurs more commonly in the newborn and in older infants, and is characterized by the rapid progression of vesicles to flaccid bullae (Fig. 195-3). Several decades ago, extensive bullous impetigo (archaic term: pemphigus neonatorum or Ritter's disease) occurred in epidemics within neonatal nurseries.

Bullae usually arise on areas of grossly normal skin. The Nikolsky sign (sheetlike removal of epidermis by gentle traction) is not present. Bullae initially contain clear yellow fluid that subsequently becomes dark yellow and turbid (Fig. 195-3*A*), and their margins are sharply demarcated without an erythematous halo. The bullae are superficial, and within a day or two they rupture and collapse, at times forming thin, light brown to golden-yellow crusts (Fig. 195-3*B*). So-called bullous varicella represents superinfection by *S. aureus* (phage group II) of varicella lesions (bullous impetiginization).

The differential diagnosis is that of blisters localized to one body region and includes allergic contact dermatitis (e.g., poison ivy or oak), pemphigus vulgaris, bullous pemphigoid, erythema multiforme, dermatitis herpetiformis, thermal burns, bullous fixed drug reaction, SSSS, bullous tinea pedis, and bullous insect bites.

Gram's stain of exudates from bullous impetigo reveals grampositive cocci in clusters; *S. aureus* belonging to phage group II can be cultured from the contents of intact bullae. In comparison, Gram's stain of exudates from lesions of SSSS do not show staphylococci, and *S. aureus* are not isolated on culture. Bulla formation in the latter condition is caused by distant production of toxin rather than local infection.

Histologically, the lesions of bullous impetigo show vesicle formation in the subcorneal or granular region, occasional acantholytic cells within the blister, spongiosis, edema of the papillary dermis, and a mixed infiltrate of lymphocytes and neutrophils around blood vessels of the superficial plexus.

Course of staphylococcal impetigo Untreated, invasive infection can complicate *S. aureus* impetigo, including cellulitis, lymphangitis, and bacteremia with resultant osteomyelitis, septic arthritis, pneumonitis, and septicemia.

Management of staphylococcal impetigo Local treatment with mupirocin ointment and removal of crusts and maintenance of cleanliness is sufficient to cure mild cases.[15] However, the results

FIGURE 195-1

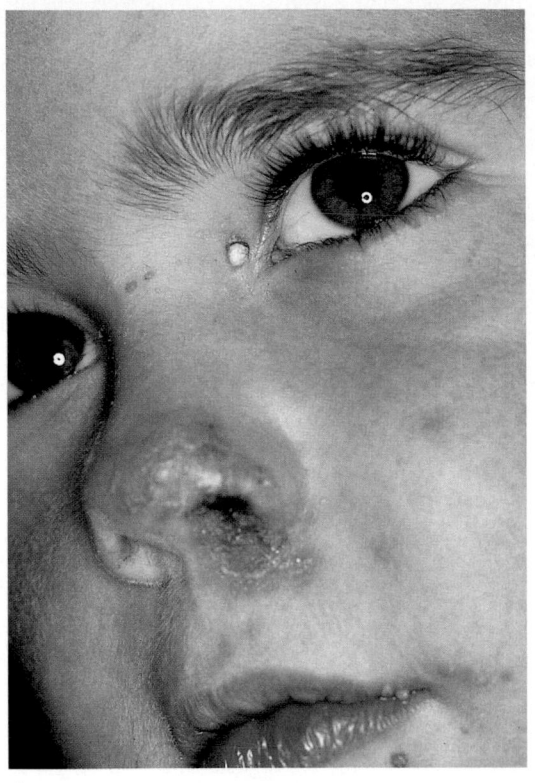

A.

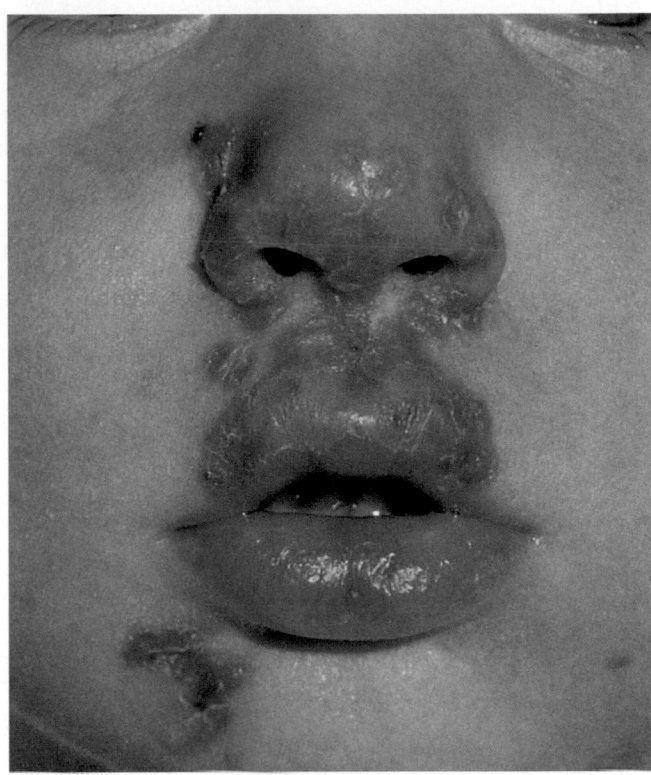

B.

S. aureus: impetigo. Erythema and crusting on the nose and moustache area (*A*), which can spread to involve the entire centrofacial region (*B*).

are further improved, particularly in extensive cases, by the administration of antibiotics. The frequency of isolation of group A streptococcus makes systemic antibiotic therapy a reasonable approach in most patients who have a significant degree of involvement.

FIGURE 195-2

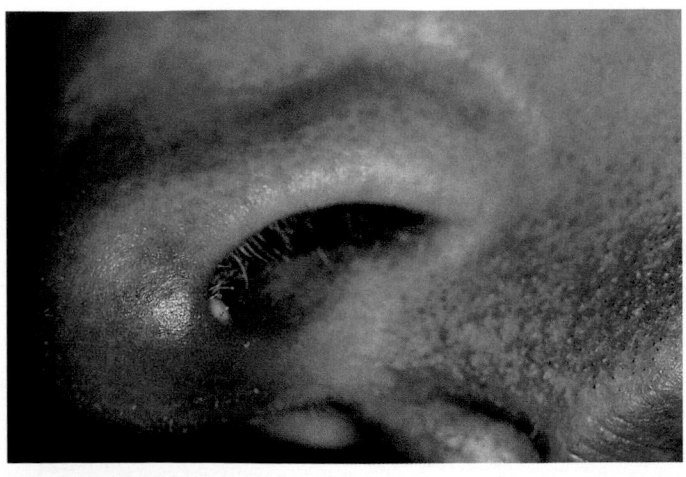

S. aureus: nasal carriage with impetigo. Erythema with a small pustule on the tip of the nose and nares in individual whose nares are colonized by *S. aureus.*

Staphylococcal impetigo responds quite promptly to appropriate treatment. In an adult with extensive or bullous lesions, dicloxacillin (or similar penicillinase-resistant semisynthetic penicillin) (250 to 500 mg PO qid), or erythromycin (in the penicillin-allergic patient) (250 to 500 mg PO qid) should be given. Treatment should be continued for 5 to 7 days (10 days if streptococci are isolated). Also, a single dose of oral azithromycin (in adults 500 mg on the first day, 250 mg daily on the next 4 days) has been shown to be equally as effective as dicloxacillin for skin infections in adults and children. For impetigo due to erythromycin-resistant *S. aureus,* which is commonly isolated from impetigo lesions of children,[16] amoxicillin plus clavulanic acid (Augmentin) (25 mg/kg/day given tid), cephalexin (40 to 50 mg/kg/day), cefaclor (20 mg/kg/day given tid), cefprozil (20 mg/kg once daily), or clindamycin (15 mg/kg/day tid or qid) given for 10 days are effective alternative therapies.

ECTHYMA   Ecthyma is usually a consequence of neglected impetigo. *S. aureus* and/or group A streptococcus can be isolated on culture. Untreated staphylococcal or streptococcal impetigo can extend more deeply, penetrating the epidermis, producing a shallow crusted ulcer (Fig. 195-4). Ecthymatous lesions can evolve from a primary pyoderma or within a preexisting dermatosis or site of trauma (insect bites or excoriations). Ecthyma gangrenosum is a cutaneous ulcer caused by *Pseudomonas aeruginosa* and resembles staphylococcal or streptococcal ecthyma. It usually occurs in individuals with prolonged neutropenia and may be associated with *P. aeruginosa* bacteremia (see Chaps. 197 and 198).

Ecthyma occurs most commonly on the lower extremities of children or neglected elderly patients or individuals with diabetes

FIGURE 195-3

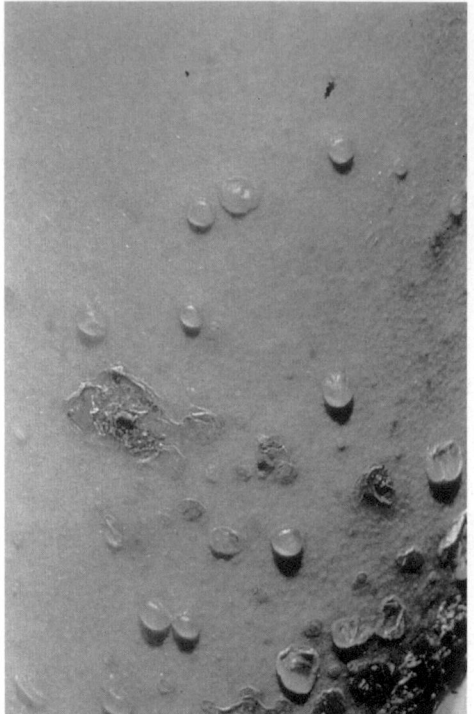

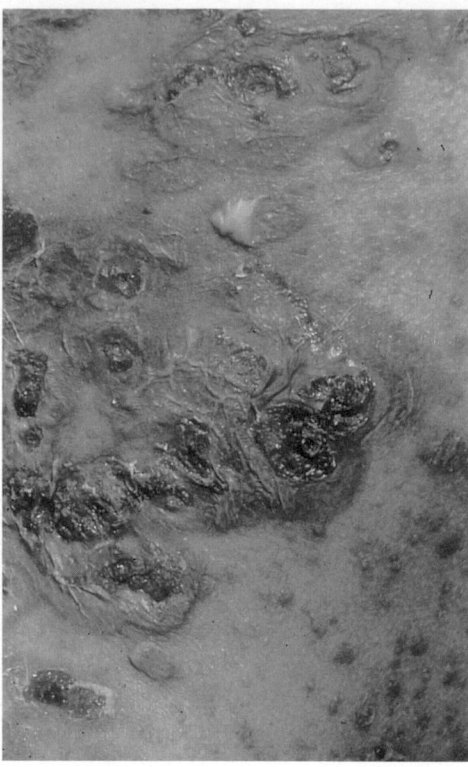

A.

B.

S. aureus: bullous impetigo. A. Multiple vesicles with clear and turbid contents that (*B*) rapidly coalesce to form flaccid bullae.

iporitis staphylogenes" refers to secondary infection of miliaria of the neonate by *S. aureus.* Staphylococcal blepharitis is an *S. aureus* infection of the eyelids presenting with scaling (squamous type) or crusting (ulcerative type) of the eyelid margins, often with associated conjunctivitis; the differential diagnosis includes seborrheic dermatitis and rosacea of the eyelid.

S. aureus folliculitis must be differentiated from other folliculocentric infections (see Table 195-3). Black men are subject to three noninfectious, inflammatory, follicular disorders: pseudofolliculitis barbae, which occurs on the lower beard area (Fig. 195-6); folliculitis keloidalis, on the nape of the neck; and perifolliculitis capitis, on the scalp *S. aureus* can cause secondary infection in these inflammatory disorders. Exposure to mineral oils, tar products, and cutting oils can cause an irritant folliculitis. Acne vulgaris, drug-induced acneform eruptions, rosacea, hidradenitis suppurativa, acne necrotica of the scalp, and eosinophilic folliculitis of HIV disease must be distinguished from infectious folliculitis as well. Also, folliculitis due to *Pseudomonas aeruginosa* may be acquired from exposure in "hot tubs" (see Chap. 198).

Deep folliculitis Sycosis barbae is a deep folliculitis with perifollicular inflammation occurring in the bearded areas of the face and upper lip (Fig. 195-7). If untreated, the lesions may become more deeply seated and chronic. Local treatment with warm saline compresses and local antibiotics (mupirocin) may be sufficient to control infection. More extensive cases require systemic antibiotic therapy. Dermatophytic folliculitis or kerion must be differentiated from *S. aureus* folliculitis. In the latter fungal infection, the hairs are usually broken or loosened, and there are suppurative or granulomatous nodules rather than discrete pustules.

Lupoid sycosis is a deep, chronic form of sycosis barbae associated with scarring, usually occurring as a circinate lesion. A central cicatrix surrounded by pustules and papules gives the appearance of lupus vulgaris (cutaneous *Mycobacterium tuberculosis* infection; see Chap. 201).

ellitus. Poor hygiene and neglect are key elements in pathogenesis. Multiple ecthymatous ulcers on the ankle and dorsum of the foot were the most common pyodermas seen during wartime in tropical climates.[17]

The ulcer has a "punched out" appearance when the dirty grayish-yellow crust and purulent material are debrided. The margin of the ulcer is indurated, raised, and violaceous (see Fig. 195-4), and the granulating base extends deeply into the dermis. Untreated ecthymatous lesions enlarge over weeks to months to a diameter of 2 to 3 cm or more.

The lesions are slow to heal, requiring several weeks of antibiotic treatment for resolution. Problems of spread by autoinoculation or by insect vectors and of poststreptococcal sequela (glomerulonephritis) are the same as with impetigo.

Management of ecthyma Same as for staphylococcal impetigo (see above).

FOLLICULITIS This is a pyoderma beginning within the hair follicle, and is classified according to the depth of invasion, i.e., superficial and deep, and by microbial etiology (Table 195-3).

Superficial folliculitis Superficial folliculitis has also been termed follicular or Bockhart's impetigo. A small fragile dome-shaped pustule occurs at the infundibulum (ostium or opening) of a hair follicle, often on the scalps of children and in the beard area (Fig. 195-5), axillae, extremities, and buttocks of adults. Isolated staphylococcal folliculitis is common on the buttock of adults. "Per-

FURUNCLES AND CARBUNCLES A furuncle or boil is a deep-seated inflammatory nodule that develops about a hair follicle, usually from a preceding, more superficial folliculitis and often evolving into an abscess. A carbuncle is a more extensive, deeper, communicating, infiltrated lesion that develops when suppuration occurs in thick inelastic skin.

Furuncles arise in hair-bearing sites, particularly in regions subject to friction, occlusion, and perspiration such as the neck, face, axillae, and buttocks. They may complicate preexisting lesions such as atopic dermatitis, excoriations, abrasions, scabies, or pediculosis, but occur more often in the absence of any local predisposing causes. In addition, a variety of systemic host factors is associated with furunculosis: obesity, blood dyscrasias, defects in neutrophil function (defects in chemotaxis associated with eczema and high

FIGURE 195-4

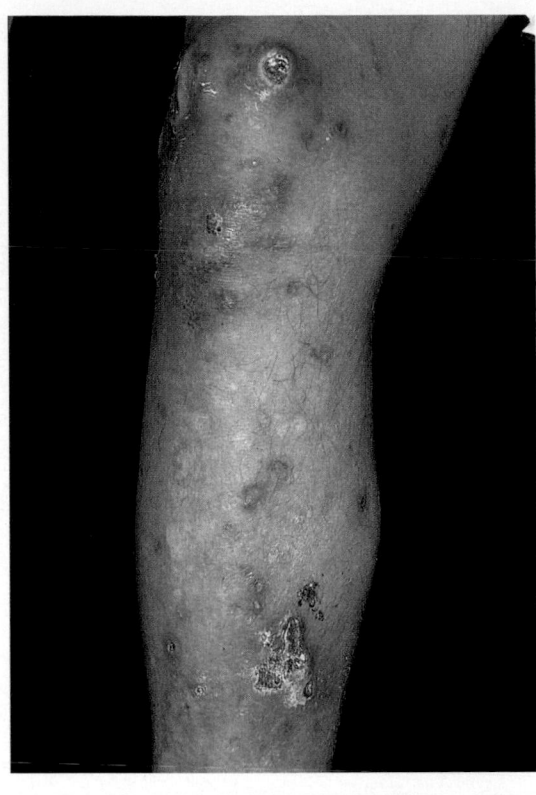

S. aureus: ecthyma. Multiple thickly crusted erosions on the leg of a patient with diabetes and renal failure. Ecthymatous lesions were also present on the other leg, the arms, and the hands.

levels of IgE, defects in intracellular killing of organisms as in chronic granulomatous disease of childhood), treatment with glucocorticoids and cytotoxic agents, and immune globulin deficiency states. Whether diabetes mellitus predisposes to furunculosis is still

TABLE 195-3

Differential Diagnosis of Infectious Folliculitis

Bacterial folliculitis
    S. aureus folliculitis
        Periporitis staphylogenes
        Superficial (follicular or Bockhart's impetigo)
        Deep (sycosis) [may progress to furuncle (boil) or carbuncle]
    Pseudomonas aeruginosa folliculitis ("hot tub" folliculitis)
    Gram-negative folliculitis (occurs at site of acne vulgaris usually the
        face during long-term antibiotic therapy)
    Syphilitic folliculitis (secondary) (acneform)
Fungal folliculitis
    Dermatophytic folliculitis
        Tinea capitis
        Tinea barbae
        Majocchi's granuloma
    Pityrosporum folliculitis
    Candida folliculitis
Viral folliculitis
    Herpes simplex virus folliculitis
    Follicular molluscum contagiosum
Infestation
    Demodicidosis

FIGURE 195-5

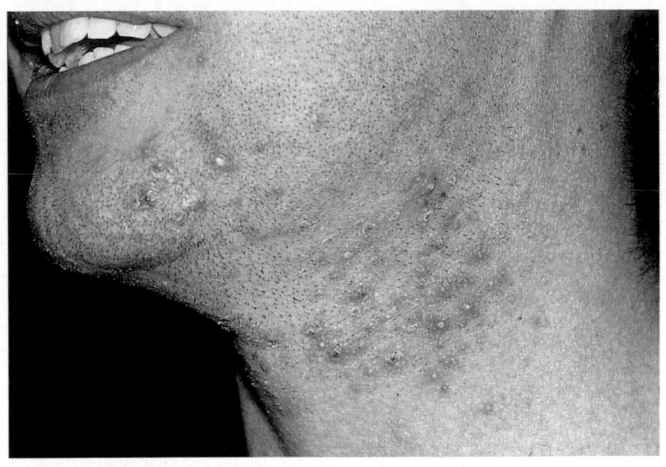

S. aureus: superficial folliculitis. Multiple pustules confined to the beard area.

controversial; once established, however, the process is often more extensive in patients with diabetes. The majority of patients with problems of furunculosis appear to be otherwise healthy.

A furuncle starts as a hard, tender, red folliculocentric nodule in hair-bearing skin, that enlarges and becomes painful and fluctuant after several days (i.e., undergoes abscess formation; Fig. 195-8A). Rupture occurs, with discharge of pus and often a core of necrotic material. The pain surrounding the lesion then subsides, and the redness and edema diminish over several days to several weeks. Furuncles may occur as solitary lesions or as multiple lesions in sites such as the buttocks (Fig. 195-8B).

A carbuncle is a larger, more serious inflammatory lesion with a deeper base, characteristically occurring as an extremely painful

FIGURE 195-6

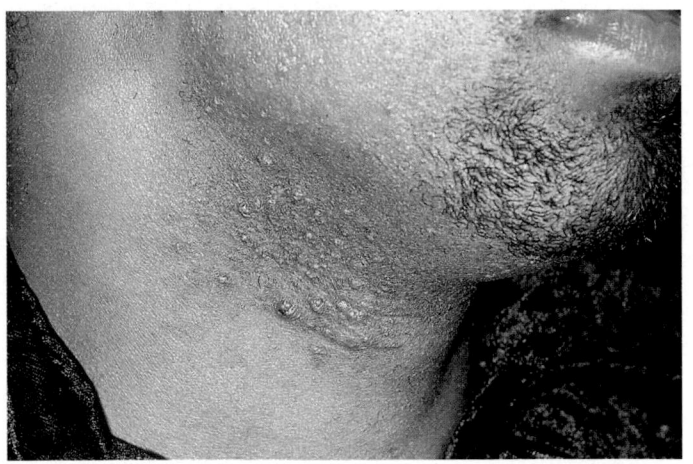

Pseudofolliculitis barbae. Multiple papules in the lower beard area caused by ingrowing of the curved hair shaft in a black male who shaves. If pustules are present, secondary S. aureus infection must be ruled out.

FIGURE 195-7

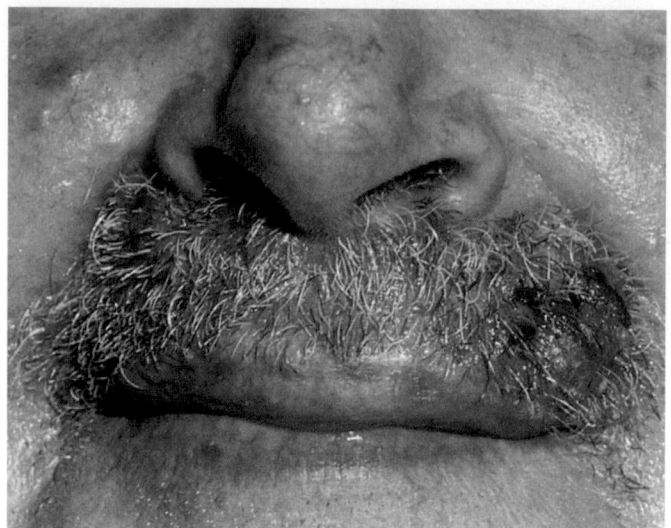

Sycosis barbae. Staphylococcal folliculitis of the mustache region.

lesion at the nape of the neck, the back, or thighs (Fig. 195-9). Fever and malaise are often present, and the patient may appear quite ill. The involved area is red and indurated, and multiple pustules soon appear on the surface, draining externally around multiple hair follicles. The lesion soon develops a yellow-gray irregular crater at the center, which may then heal slowly by granulating, although the area may remain deeply violaceous for a prolonged period. The resulting permanent scar is often dense and readily evident.

The differential diagnosis of furuncles and carbuncles includes "cystic acne," hidradenitis suppurativa (axillae and anogenital region), ruptured epidermal inclusion cyst, furuncular myiasis (e.g., *Dermatobia hominis*) apical (dental) abscess (face), and the external sites (on an extremity of a beginning fistulous track from an underlying osteomyelitis.

Extensive furunculosis or a carbuncle may be associated with a leukocytosis, particularly when there is a large amount of unliberated pus, surrounding cellulitis, or bacteremia. *S. aureus* is almost always the cause of furuncles and carbuncles. Histologic examination of a furuncle shows a dense polymorphonuclear inflammatory process in the dermis and subcutaneous fat. In carbuncles, multiple abscesses, separated by connective-tissue trabeculae, infiltrate the dermis and pass along the edges of the hair follicles, reaching the surface through openings in the undermined epidermis. The diagnosis is made on the basis of the clinical appearance. Gram stain of pus, clusters of gram-positive cocci, or isolation of *S. aureus* on culture confirms the diagnosis.

The major problems with furunculosis and carbuncles are bacteremic spread of infection and recurrence. Lesions about the lips and nose raise the specter of spread via the facial and angular emissary veins to the cavernous sinus. Invasion of the bloodstream may occur from furuncles or carbuncles at any time, in an unpredictable fashion, resulting in metastatic infection such as osteomyelitis, acute endocarditis, or brain abscess. Manipulation of such lesions is particularly dangerous and may facilitate spread of infection via the bloodstream. Fortunately, these complications are not

FIGURE 195-8

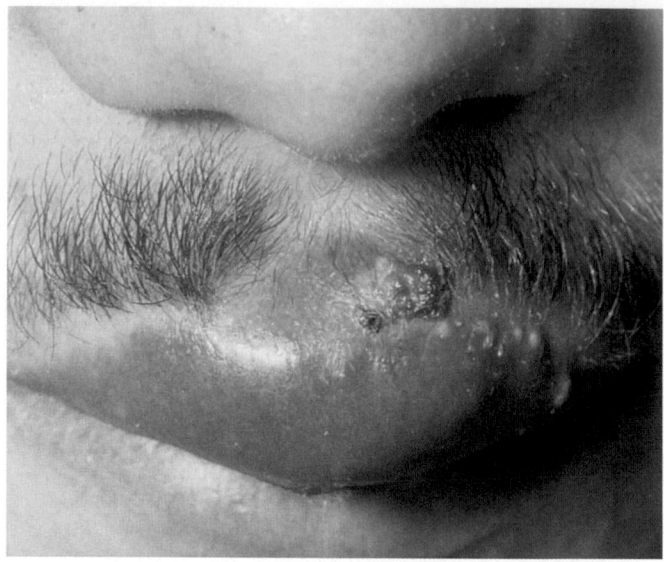

A.

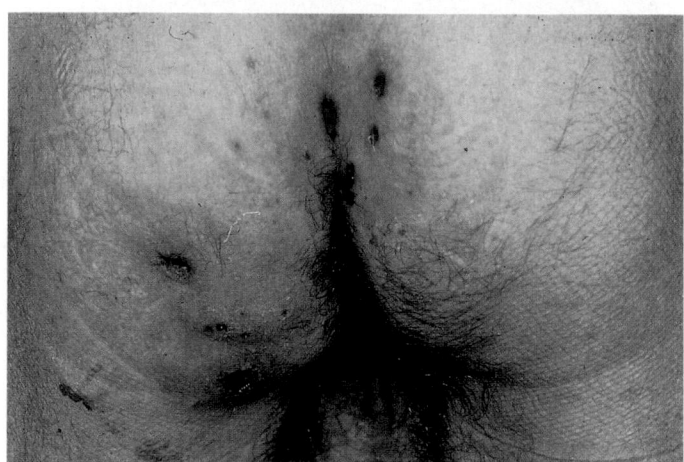

B.

A. Furuncle of the upper lip. The lesion is nodular and the central necrotic plug is covered by purulent crust. Several small pustules are seen lateral to the center of the lesion. *B.* Multiple furuncles. Multiple abscesses on the buttocks of long standing in a young man with inflammatory bowel disease. The lesions healed with scarring after a prolonged course of dicloxacillin.

common. Recurrent furunculosis is a troublesome process that may recur over many years. Most often these lesions are limited to the area of the follicles, but sometimes they extend to produce surrounding cellulitis or bacteremia. Individuals who perspire excessively or who have poor skin hygiene appear more disposed to recurrent furunculosis.

Management of folliculitis, furuncles, and carbuncles Simple furunculosis may be treated by local application of moist heat, which relieves discomfort, aids in the localization of the infection, and promotes drainage. A carbuncle or a furuncle with surrounding cellulitis, or one with associated fever, should be treated with a systemic antibiotic. A semisynthetic penicillin such as dicloxacillin (250 to 750 mg PO q4–6h in the adult) should be used. In the penicillin-allergic adult, clindamycin (150 to 300 mg PO qid) or erythromycin (250 to 500 mg PO qid) may be substituted. For se-

FIGURE 195-9

CHAPTER 195
Pyodermas

2189

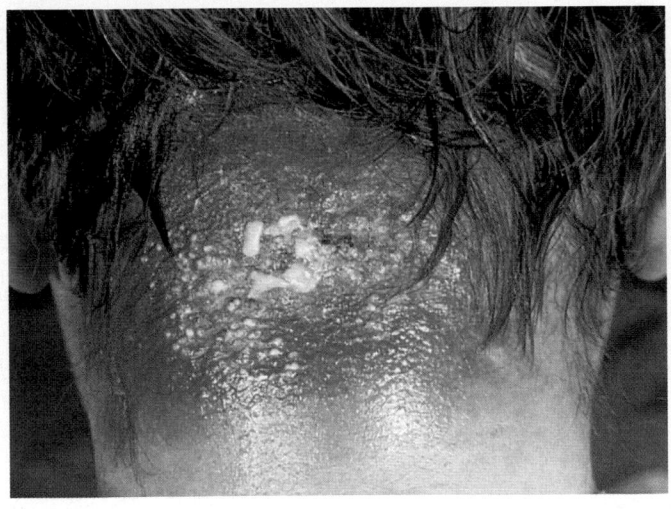

Carbuncle. This lesion represents multiple confluent furuncles draining pus from multiple openings.

vere infections or infections in a dangerous area, maximal antibiotic dosage should be employed by the parenteral route, the patient should be put to bed, and the involved area should be immobilized. If MRSA is implicated or suspected in serious infections, vancomycin (1.0 to 2.0 g IV daily in divided doses) is indicated. Antibiotic treatment should be continued for at least 1 week.

When the lesions are large but localized, painful, and fluctuant, drainage (limited to the necrotic fluctuant area) is indicated. Antimicrobial therapy should be continued until all evidence of inflammation has regressed. After adequate drainage (spontaneous or surgical) has occurred, moist dressings should not be applied because of the danger of local spread enhanced by tissue maceration. Application of a thin layer of 2 percent mupirocin ointment about the lesion protects the surrounding skin. Such draining lesions should be covered with a sterile dressing to prevent autoinoculation. Hands should be thoroughly washed after contact with the lesions.

The treatment of patients with recurrent furunculosis presents a special and frequently exasperating problem (Table 195-4). There is no evidence that this disease is due to any specific staphylococcal strains with special biologic properties. In addition to the treatment

TABLE 195-4

Management of Recurrent Furunculosis

1. Careful evaluation for underlying causes:
   a. Systemic processes: previously discussed.
   b. Specific localized predisposing factors: industrial exposure to chemicals, oils; poor hygiene; obesity; hyperhidrosis; ingrown hairs; pressure from tight clothing or belts.
   c. Sources of staphylococcal contact: pyogenic infections in the family, contact sports such as wrestling, autoinoculation.
   d. Nasal carriage of *S. aureus:* this is the site from which dissemination of the organism may occur to other body sites. The frequency of nasal carriage varies: 10 to 15 percent in infants 1 year of age, 38 percent in college students, 50 percent in hospital physicians and military trainees.[18]
2. General skin care: The aim of these measures is to reduce the numbers of *S. aureus* on the skin. General skin care of both hands and body with water and soap is important (an antimicrobial soap solution, such as 4 percent chlorhexidine solution, may be used to decrease staphylococcal skin colonization). The patient should avoid trauma to the skin as well as potential skin irritants such as strong soaps and deodorants. A separate washcloth (and towel) should be used and carefully washed in *hot* water prior to reuse.
3. Care of clothing: Loose, lightweight, porous clothing should be worn as much as possible. Large numbers of staphylococci are frequently present on the sheets and underclothing of patients with furunculosis and may cause reinfection of the patient and infection of other members of the family. In problem cases it is not unreasonable to recommend that these items be carefully and separately washed in boiling water and changed daily.
4. Care of dressings: Dressings should be changed frequently if purulent drainage collects. They should be carefully discarded into a paper bag that can be sealed and disposed of immediately.
5. General measures: Despite the above measures, some patients continue to have recurrent cycles of lesions. Sometimes the problem can be ameliorated or abolished by removing the patient from the regular routine of work. This is particularly pertinent in individuals who are under considerable emotional stress and physical fatigue. A vacation for several weeks, ideally in a cool, dry climate, may help considerably by providing rest and also the time needed for carrying out the program of careful skin care.
6. Measures aimed at elimination of nasal (and skin) carriage of *S. aureus* (methicillin-susceptible or methicillin-resistant):
   a. Local use of ointment in the nasal vestibule reduces nasal carriage of *S. aureus* and secondarily reduces the "shedding" of organisms on the skin, a process that may contribute to recurrent furunculosis. Intranasal application of a 2 percent mupirocin calcium ointment in a white, soft paraffin base for 5 days can eliminate *S. aureus* nasal carriage in 70 percent of healthy individuals for up to 3 months. In immunocompetent staphylococcal carriers with recurrent skin infections, a 5-day course of nasal mupirocin ointment every month for 1 year resulted in positive nasal cultures in only 22 percent of patients as compared with 83 percent in the placebo group. The nasal culture–negative patients also had significantly fewer skin infections during the treatment period. Staphylococcal resistance to mupirocin was observed in only one patient out of 17.[19] Prophylaxis with fusidic acid ointment in the nares twice daily every fourth week for the patient and family members who are nasal carriers of the infecting strain (along with a peroral antistaphylococcal antibiotic for 10 to 14 days for the patient) has been employed with some success.[20]
   b. Oral antibiotics (e.g., rifampin, 600 mg orally daily for 10 days) have been effective in eradicating *S. aureus* from most nasal carriers for periods of up to 12 weeks.[21] Such a use of rifampin for a brief period to eradicate nasal carriage of *S. aureus* and interrupt a continuing cycle of recurrent furunculosis might be reasonable in a patient in whom other measures have failed. However, selection of rifampin-resistant strains can occur rapidly with such therapy. The addition of a second drug (dicloxacillin, for MSSA; trimethoprim-sulfamethoxazole, ciprofloxacin, or minocycline for MRSA) has been employed to reduce the emergence of rifampin resistance[22] and to treat recurrent furunculosis.

of acute lesions, as above, treatment involves steps in the prophylaxis of recurrent episodes.

ABSCESS   As discussed above, abscesses caused by *S. aureus* commonly occur in folliculocentric infections—i.e., folliculitis, furuncles, and carbuncles. Abscesses can also occur at sites of trauma, foreign bodies, burns, or sites of insertion of intravenous catheters. The initial lesion is an erythematous nodule. Often if untreated, the lesion enlarges with the formation of a pus-filled cavity (Fig. 195-10). In some cases, the portal of entry is apparent.

Management of abscess (see "Management of Folliculitis, Furuncles, and Carbuncles," above)   The initial treatment of an abscess is incision and drainage. If the abscess recurs at the same site, a foreign body should be ruled out by probing or imaging.

BOTRYOMYCOSIS (see also Chap. 202)   This a very rare pyogenic disease, possibly related to a balance between numbers of organisms and host defenses. Predisposing factors include trauma immunosuppression (HIV disease, hyperimmunoglobulin E syndrome), chronic alcoholism, and diabetes mellitus. The lesions (usually solitary) can occur in skin, bone, and liver.

Cutaneous botryomycosis usually presents as a solitary or few lesions, often occurring in the genital area. The lesion has the gross appearance of a ruptured epidermal inclusion cyst (an erythematous circumscribed tender nodule), lichen simplex chronicus, or prurigo nodularis (Fig. 195-11). In the majority of reported cases, a foreign body (fish bone, broom straw, etc.) has played a role in initiating or perpetuating the lesion.

Pinhead-sized, whitish-yellow granules are seen on examination of pus from botryomycotic lesions. When examined under the microscope (fresh mount in saline or in 20 percent potassium hydroxide), these granules appear coarsely lobulated and are seen to contain tightly packed clublike projections (resembling the "sulfur granules" of actinomycosis or a mycetoma). Examination of Gram-stained preparations of crushed granules shows only masses of staphylococci, not the ray fungus appearance of actinomycosis. On

FIGURE 195-10

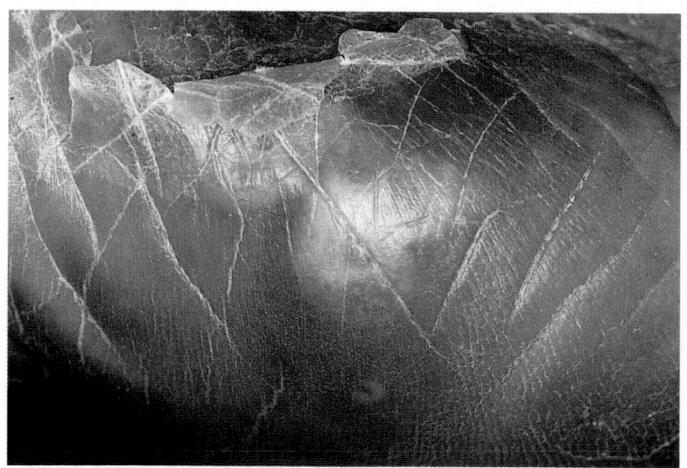

S. aureus: abscess. A large painful abscess on the heel of a patient with diabetes improved clinically, however, the severe pain persisted. X-ray films of the heel revealed a broken off sewing needle. The patient had sensory neuropathy and was unaware of stepping on this foreign body.

FIGURE 195-11

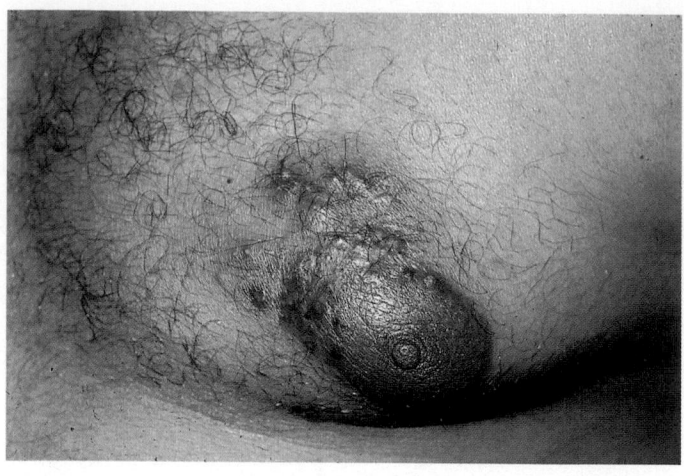

S. aureus: botryomycosis. A plaque on the chest had been present for several months in this HIV-infected individual. The diagnosis was confirmed on lesional biopsy findings and culture.

histologic (hematoxylin-and-eosin stain) section the findings are those of a basophilic granule made up of clusters of cocci (usually within the papillary dermis) surrounded by an amorphous eosinophilic matrix (Splendore-Hoeppli phenomenon); the latter probably represents host immunoglobulin *S. aureus* (40 percent), *P. aeruginosa* (20 percent), coagulase-negative staphylococci, streptococcal species, *Escherichi coli,* and *Proteus* species are the most common pathogens isolated on culture from botryomycosis (see Chap. 202).

Management includes removal of any foreign bodies, surgical drainage of loculated pus, and appropriate systemic antibiotic therapy.

STAPHYLOCOCCAL PARONYCHIA   Individuals exposed to hand trauma or chronic moisture are predisposed to staphylococcal paronychia as well as to other causes of paronychia (e.g., *Candida,* pseudomonas, streptococcus, dermatophytes). *S. aureus* is the major infectious cause of acute paronychia, usually around the fingernails, often originating from a break in the skin, such as a hangnail. Clinically, skin and soft tissue of the proximal and lateral nail fold are red, hot, and tender and, if not treated, can evolve to abscess formation (Fig. 195-12).

In contrast, chronic or recurrent paronychia caused by *Candida albicans* is an infection of the space created by separation of the proximal dorsal nail plate and the undersurface of the proximal nail fold. Candidal paronychia is most common in individuals who have their hands in water for a great deal of time. The predisposing lesion is an inflammatory dermatosis such as an eczematous dermatitis, which causes separation of the nail fold from the nail plate. A potential space is created and *C. albicans* proliferates in it, causing periodic episodes of infection, characterized by recurrent erythema, pain, and swelling, and, in some cases, pus formation. *S. aureus* can cause superinfection in some cases. Chronic or recurrent candidal paronychia is marked by irregular transverse ridging of the dorsal nail plate, originating at the proximal nail fold (see Chap. 207).

Management of paronychia due to *S. aureus* includes oral and topical antibiotics, and incision and drainage of abscesses. Recurrent candidal paronychia should be treated by reducing exposure to moisture, application of topical antifungal cream, possible application of a glucocorticoid if a predisposing inflammatory condition is

FIGURE 195-12

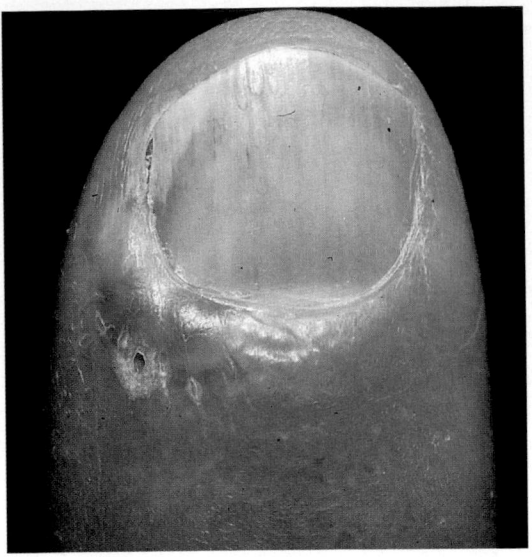

S. aureus: paronychia. An abscess is seen in the dorsum of the finger, beginning in a small break in the cuticle. In contrast, *Candida* paronychia is a space infection, occurring in the space created by the separation of the proximal dorsal nail plate and the overlying proximal nail fold.

present, and intermittent (once weekly) therapy with an oral azole such as fluconazole or itraconazole.

STAPHYLOCOCCAL WHITLOW (FELON) A whitlow is a purulent infection or abscess involving the bulbous distal end of the finger. The most common causes are *S. aureus* and herpes simplex virus. The portal of entry of *S. aureus* is from a traumatic injury or possible extension of an acute paronychia. This infection is usually very painful. Clinically, an obvious portal of entry is often apparent. The finger bulb is red, hot, tender, and edematous, with possible abscess formation (Fig. 195-13). In contrast, individuals with herpetic whitlows usually have a history of prior lesions occurring in the same site, and present with group hemorrhagic vesicles, which may become confluent and form a single bulla. Management of a staphylococcal whitlow requires surgical drainage of loculated abscess(es) within the tissue and intravenous antibiotic therapy. X-ray examination of the involved finger is indicated to determine the presence of osteomyelitis.

STAPHYLOCOCCAL LYMPHOCUTANEOUS SYNDROME
Macronodular sporotrichoid lesions on the forearm (in the distribution of nodular lymphangitis) have been reported very rarely either in the course of *S. aureus* bacteremia[23] or following injury to the hand or with botryomycosis.[24]

Hyperimmunoglobulinemia E Recurrent Infection Syndrome (Hyper-IgE Syndrome) (Job Syndrome)
(See Chap. 117)

Hyper-IgE syndrome is an autosomal dominant primary immunodeficiency characterized by impaired regulation of IgE function, persistently elevated serum IgE levels, and deficiency of neutrophil chemotaxis with resultant recurrent *S. aureus* infections. There is often a history of recurrent bronchitis, pneumonitis (*S. aureus, Hae-*

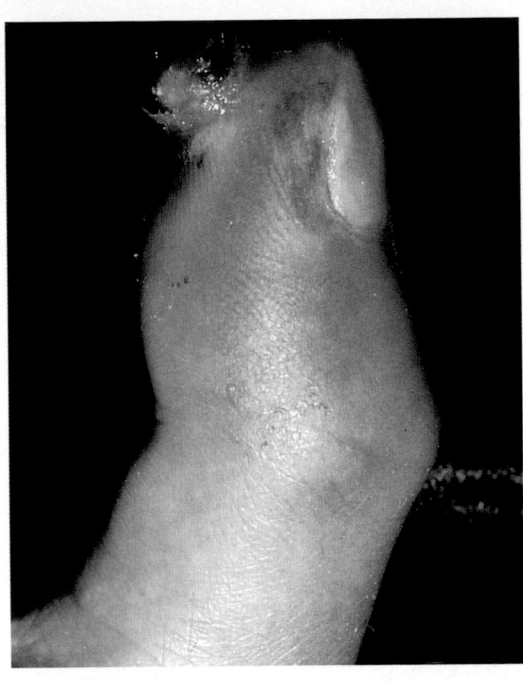

S. aureus: whitlow (felon). A pyogenic granuloma arose 1 week after trauma to the bulb of the thumb. A week later the bulb became swollen, erythematous, and very tender. Abscess formation is seen with loculation of pus. X-ray films showed early osteomyelitis complicating the whitlow.

mophilus influenzae), lung abscesses, pneumatoceles with bacterial or fungal secondary infection, empyemas, recurrent otitis media, or sinusitis. The facies is often coarse, with a broad nasal bridge and prominent nose.

The cutaneous findings often resemble secondarily infected atopic dermatitis (accentuation of dermatitis in flexures, postauricular areas, and the hairline) or a primary pyoderma with excoriated papules, pustules, furuncles, and abscesses (hot and/or cold). The most common pathogen causing the pyoderma is *S. aureus*, but group A streptococcus or *C. albicans* can be causative.

The differential diagnosis of hyper-IgE syndrome includes atopic dermatitis, DiGeorge syndrome, and Wiskott-Aldrich syndrome. Laboratory findings are of markedly elevated serum IgE levels, striking peripheral eosinophilia, clustered gram-positive cocci, and isolation of *S. aureus* on lesional culture. Anti–*S. aureus* IgE antibodies occur at an early age and their detection may be helpful in diagnosis.[25] Management involves use of local and systemic antimicrobial agents for treatment and secondary prophylaxis of *S. aureus* pyodermas.

STAPHYLOCOCCAL BACTEREMIA AND ENDOCARDITIS (See Chap. 166)

S. aureus pyodermas and STIs can invade lymphatics and blood vessels, resulting in bacteremia and metastatic infection at distant sites, causing diverse processes such as acute bacterial endocarditis

(ABE), septic arthritis, or acute osteomyelitis. *S. aureus* infection at internal sites or on the heart valves can result in dissemination to mucocutaneous sites.

Bacteremia with *S. aureus* is defined as seeding of the bloodstream in the presence ("secondary bacteremia") or absence ("primary bacteremia") of a defined peripheral focus of infection. The focus of infection is usually community-acquired (furuncle, carbuncle, wound infection) or nosocomial (intravascular catheter, urinary catheter, or chest tube). In the absence of localizing findings, the clinical presentation may be of a flu-like syndrome and *S. aureus* may be isolated on multiple blood cultures. Presumably in this case, a small unnoticed skin focus has been the initial source of bacteremia. Without an identifiable peripheral focus and in the presence of repeatedly positive blood cultures, endocarditis is assumed and the patient treated accordingly, even in the absence of a heart murmur, demonstrable vegetations, or embolic events.

The risk of endocarditis is probably less than 10 percent in patients with secondary bacteremia (from a defined peripheral site); continued bacteremia increases the risk for endocarditis.[26] Risk factors for *S. aureus* endocarditis include various types of dermatitis, injected-drug use, chronic renal failure, kidney transplantation, chronic active hepatitis, poorly controlled diabetes mellitus, metastatic cancer, cardiovascular disease, and leukemia. Initial bacteremia is usually accompanied by chills and rigors.

In acute *S. aureus* infectious endocarditis, skin and/or mucous membrane lesions occur in 50 percent of patients, and can provide a clue to the diagnosis. These lesions include petechiae on the digits or extremities; a full spectrum of larger skin lesions with elements of infarction (Fig. 195-14), suppuration, and hemorrhage (pustules, subcutaneous abscesses, and purulent purpura); gangrenous symmetric involvement of the extremities; and purpura fulminans (see below) as a manifestation of disseminated intravascular coagulation. The purulent purpura consists of an area of purpura with a white purulent center. (Gram-stained smear of the aspirated contents of the center shows gram-positive cocci in clusters and polymorphonuclear inflammatory cells.)

FIGURE 195-14

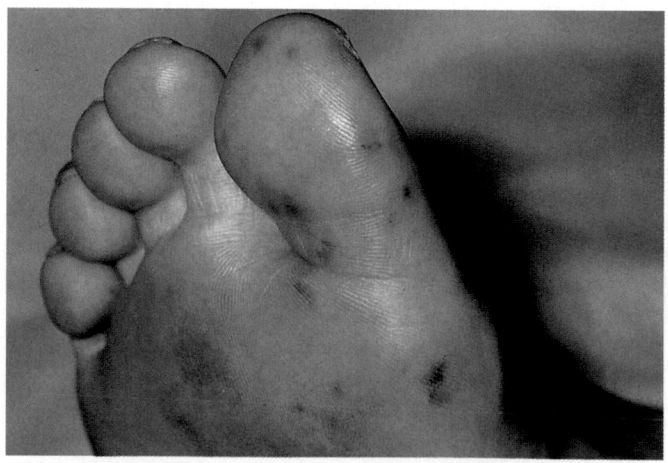

S. aureus: endocarditis and bacteremia with cutaneous infarctions. Multiple cutaneous infarctions are seen on the plantar foot of the injected-drug user with acute infective endocarditis; lesions were also present on the other foot and the palms. (*Courtesy of David N. Silvers, M.D.*)

Multiple tender subcutaneous nodules (2- to 4-cm) with erythema of the overlying skin may occur, with and without abscess formation. Culture of a lesional biopsy specimen often yields the causative *S. aureus*.

Several types of lesions can be seen on the hands of individuals with acute infectious endocarditis. Janeway lesions are typically seen in *S. aureus* endocarditis and appear as nontender small erythematous macules or, more commonly as small hemorrhagic nodules on the palms and soles. Osler's nodes (typically painful, purplish, 4- to 6-mm subcutaneous nodules in the pulp of the fingers and/or toes and thenar and hypothenar eminences) are caused by microemboli leading to vascular occlusion with local vasculitis. Both Osler's nodes and Janeway lesions are described in more detail under subacute infectious endocarditis below. Subungual splinter hemorrhages associated with *S. aureus* acute infectious endocarditis occur in the middle third of the nail bed.

Embolization to the eye results in subconjunctival hemorrhage, petechial and flame-shaped hemorrhages in the retina, cotton-wool exudates in the fundus, Roth spots (oval or boat-shaped white areas in the retina surrounded by a zone of hemorrhage, and endophthalmitis (see Chap. 166).

Syndromes Caused by Staphylococcal Exotoxins

STAPHYLOCOCCAL SCALDED-SKIN SYNDROME (see Chap. 196) ***Definition*** This is the most severe form of skin disease due to the exfoliative exotoxin produced by *S. aureus* of phage group II and is characterized by generalized bulla formation and exfoliation.[27] Unlike bullous impetigo, in which the staphylococcal infection is in the skin at the site of the skin lesion, the infection in SSSS is often at a distant site (umbilical stump, elsewhere on the skin, conjunctiva in neonates) or not in the skin or mucous membrane at all. These extracutaneous infections may consist of bacteremia and a variety of localized abscesses. Thus, SSSS is truly a toxin-mediated disease.

Staphylococcal scarlitiniform eruption This is identical to the generalized scarlatiniform rash with skin tenderness observed in the initial stage of SSSS (Chap. 196). Patients are febrile for the first few days. As in streptococcal scarlet fever (see below), the skin is diffusely erythematous, with a sandpaper roughness. Pastia's lines are present. Pharyngitis, strawberry tongue, and palatal enanthem, typical of streptococcal scarlet fever, are not seen. Bullae and exfoliation do not occur, although Nikolsky's sign may be present in an occasional patient. After 2 to 5 days of erythema, desquamation begins, initially on the face, and extends to involve most of the body. Healing of the skin occurs within 10 days.

Staphylococci belonging to phage group II are recovered from sites of staphylococcal infection (conjunctivitis, abscesses, bacteremia, external otitis). These strains generally produce staphylococcal enterotoxins (SEs) similar to toxins responsible for TSS. Thus, staphylococcal scarlet fever may be a milder form of TSS.

STAPHYLOCOCCAL TOXIC-SHOCK SYNDROME TSS is a multiorgan systemic illness due to exotoxin-producing strains of *S. aureus*. It is characterized by a generalized erythematous eruption and a high fever. Additional elements making up the syndrome include (1) hypotension, (2) functional abnormalities in at least three organ systems, and (3) desquamation following the scarlatiniform eruption. Over 1600 cases occurred in a nationwide outbreak between 1979 and 1982, primarily, but not exclusively, in menstruating women.[28]

Bacteriology and pathogenesis *S. aureus* strains isolated from women with menstrual TSS are usually penicillin-resistant, and over 93 percent of them produce TSS toxin 1 (TSST-1); 62 percent of isolates from women with nonmenstrual TSS produce this toxin, as do 20 percent of randomly tested isolates. Commonly, TSST-1 production by *S. aureus* is associated with tryptophan auxotrophy and with the insertion of a transposon-like segment into several sites on the chromosome.[29] Illness similar to TSS in humans can be produced in animals inoculated with either purified TSST-1 or with TSST-1–producing strains of *S. aureus*. The manifestations of this illness can be prevented by TSST-1 antiserum. Many *S. aureus* isolates from patients with nonmenstrual TSS do not produce TSST-1; enterotoxin B is the only exotoxin produced by at least 38 percent of these non-TSST-1-producing isolates, and a few strains produce a third TSS toxin (enterotoxin C_1).[30] TSST-1 stimulates release of tumor necrosis factor α (TNFα), and the induction of the shock-like state appears to be related to the synergistic action of TNFα with interleukin-1.[31]

In 1980, about 85 to 90 percent of cases of TSS occurred in women at the time of menstruation; almost all had been tampon users (particularly of superabsorbent types). *S. aureus* has been isolated from vaginal cultures of more than 90 percent of menstruating women with TSS, but from only 10 percent of healthy menstruating women. Cervicovaginal ulcerations, possibly produced or aggravated by tampon use, may have provided the initiating infection and the portal for toxin absorption in menstruating women in whom TSS developed. Furthermore, superabsorbent tampons may allow increased oxygen tension, which results in higher amounts of toxin production. Staphylococcal infections (skin, soft tissue, bone, lung) in children, men, and nonmenstruating women have accounted for the remaining 10 to 15 percent of cases of TSS. Minor surgery, burns, trauma, and abrasions are some of the risk factors for nonmenstrual TSS. Two cases of TSS in children with abrasive injuries beneath casts have been reported.[32] Between 1980 and 1990, the number of cases of menstrual TSS declined by over 90 percent, but the number of nonmenstrual cases remained unchanged. The decrease in menstruation-associated TSS cases is directly related to the removal of superabsorbent tampons.

Clinical manifestations Fever, hypotension (or shock), and an erythematous rash are the initial hallmarks of TSS (Fig. 195-15A). The cutaneous findings include a generalized scarlitiniform (resembling scarlet fever) erythema, most intense around an infected site. The rash may be indistinguishable from that of scarlet fever or may be less striking and suggest the flush associated with fever. Nonpitting edema may occur on the face and extremities. The bulbar conjunctivae show intense injection; the mucosa of the oropharynx, tongue (strawberry tongue), vagina, and typmpanic membranes may show intense erythema. Less common findings include petechiae, bullae, subconjunctival hemorrhages, and ulcerations of the mouth, vagina, esophagus, or bladder. Desquamation of palms and soles occurs 1 to 2 weeks later (Fig. 195-15B). Evidence of multiple other organ dysfunctions is seen in TSS: (1) muscular system—myalgias and rhabdomyolysis, (2) central nervous system—toxic encephalopathy, (3) kidney—azotemia, (4) liver—elevated levels of aspartate transaminase and serum bilirubin, and (5) blood—thrombocytopenia.

Differential diagnosis The differential diagnosis include staphylococcal scarlatiniform eruption, SSSS (in which bullae and a positive Nikolsky sign are expected), scarlet fever (not usually associated with hypotension or shock), streptococcal toxic-shock–like syndrome, a febrile drug reaction (not usually associated with hypotension), Kawasaki disease (usually in children, and features prominent lymphadenopathy; see Chap. 205), viral exanthem, systemic lupus erythematosus, acute graft-versus-host disease, and adverse cutaneous drug eruptions (confluent exanthematous, toxic epidermal necrolysis, erythema multiforme).

FIGURE 195-15

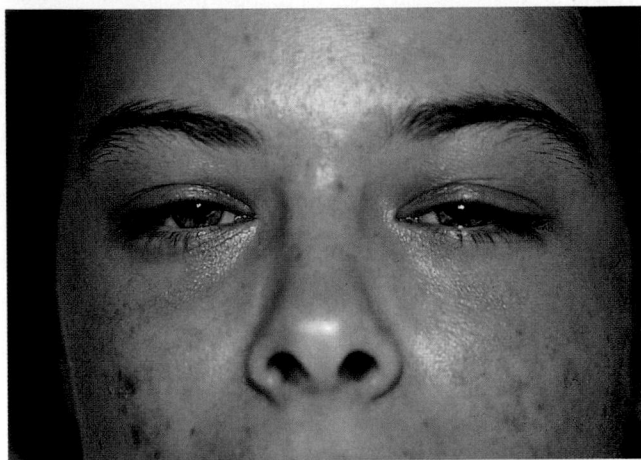

A.

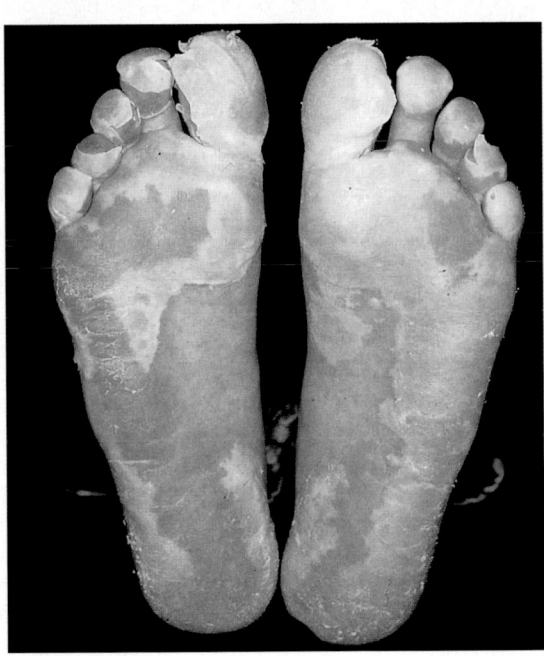

B.

S. aureus: toxic-shock syndrome. *A.* Erythema and edema of the face with conjunctival injection during the acute presentation. *B.* Residual erythema and desquamation occurring 2 weeks after an episode of toxic-shock syndrome; similar findings were also found on the palms. (*Courtesy of Stuart J. Salasche, M.D.*)

Laboratory findings Leukocytosis and thrombocytopenia are usually present. Microscopic hematuria may be present. Elevated blood urea nitrogen and creatinine levels occur in the majority of patients, and liver-function tests are frequently abnormal. Increased serum creatine kinase levels reflect muscle injury, and myoglobinuria occurs in some patients. Hypocalcemia occurs in many patients but the basis is unclear.

Diagnosis Diagnosis is made on the basis of the clinical constellation of findings in a patient who has an *S. aureus* infection or in a menstruating woman, particularly in a tampon user.

Management Treatment of TSS involves (1) immediate institution of vigorous fluid replacement to combat the hypotension, (2) attention to focal staphylococcal infections (drainage of abscesses, removal of tampons), and systemic antimicrobial therapy aimed at penicillinase-producing *S. aureus* (nafcillin 1.0 to 1.5 g intravenously in the adult every 4 h). Intravenous gamma globulin therapy and fresh frozen plasma containing immunoglobulins have been successful, especially when administered early in the disease course.

KAWASAKI SYNDROME This is an acute multisystem vasculitis of infancy and early childhood associated with high fever, mucocutaneous inflammation, and the development of coronary artery abnormalities.[33] Although the etiology of Kawasaki syndrome (KS) is as yet unknown, evidence suggesting that bacterial superantigens from *S. aureus* and group A streptococcus may be important factors in pathogenesis (see Chap. 205).

STREPTOCOCCAL SKIN INFECTIONS

General Features

BACTERIOLOGY AND PATHOGENESIS In view of the association of specific groups of streptococci with certain types of infections and postinfectious sequelae,[34] an understanding of the various categories of streptococci has practical value. The presence of many varieties of streptococci as commensals on mucous membranes, in the intestinal tract, and occasionally on the skin makes the assessment of the significance of their isolation from the skin difficult. Although essentially all group A streptococcal strains are β-hemolytic streptococci (BHS), not all streptococci producing β-hemolysis belong to group A. The Lancefield classification of streptococcal groups (A to T) is based on the C carbohydrate antigens of the cell wall. Because serologic grouping of streptococci is not generally available, a reasonably accurate presumptive test for group A streptococci is necessary. Bacitracin disk ("Taxos S") sensitivity has been widely used; group A streptococci are, almost without exception, susceptible to the low concentration of bacitracin contained in the disk, whereas streptococci of other groups are often resistant. Subtyping of group A streptococci can be performed according to their M protein antigenicity (see below). Certain M protein serotypes appear to correlate with greater virulence of the organism and may act as an important determinant in attachment of the bacterium to epidermal tissue.

The primary invasive streptococcal pyodermas are due almost exclusively to group A streptococcus. The invasive potential of group A streptococcus is usually considerably greater than that of other streptococci. Nonsuppurative postinfectious complications have been limited mostly to those produced by group A streptococcus. Thus, group A streptococcal infections merit antibiotic treatment and eradication.

The hallmarks of invasive group A streptococcal infection (erysipelas, see Chap. 197) are profuse edema, rapid spread through tissue planes, and the relatively thin character of the exudative response. Infection may spread via the lymphatic or hematogenous routes and result in a fulminant clinical course.

The presence of streptococci of groups other than A in skin lesions may represent either surface colonization or actual secondary infection in preexisting dermatoses. Group C and group G streptococci have occasionally been implicated in impetiginous lesions,

secondarily infected dermatitis, wound infections with lymphangitis, and even in erysipelas and cellulitis. Streptococci of groups B and D have been isolated from infections of skin lesions secondary to ischemia or venous stasis and have particularly involved the perineal area and operative wound sites. As with most secondary infections, those due to group B and group D streptococci are frequently mixed infections with enteric bacteria or *S. aureus*. Group B streptococci may cause cellulitis and otitis in neonates and sometimes in adults. Group L streptococci (often carried by pigs, cattle, and poultry) have been responsible for impetigo, secondarily infected wounds, and paronychias in meat handlers.[35]

EPIDEMIOLOGY OF GROUP A STREPTOCOCCAL INFECTIONS Group A streptococci are usually spread by transfer of organisms from an infected person or carrier through close personal contact. The major source of such spread is from patients with infections in the upper respiratory tract. Approximately 10 percent of the normal population carry group A streptococcus asymptomatically—a higher percentage of adults than of children in the oropharynx and less commonly in the nares and anus. While the carriage rate of group A streptococcus on normal skin is less than 1 percent, a variety of skin lesions and puerperal sepsis may also be the source of intrahospital spread of infection. Group A streptococci introduced into the operating room in the form of a minor skin infection, or even through perianal carriage by a surgeon or anesthetist, may be responsible for an epidemic of streptococcal wound infections. In the past, milk- and food-borne epidemics occurred but they no longer represent a major problem in the United States.[36]

Although viable streptococci are found on a variety of articles in the immediate surroundings of a carrier or infected individual, the major factor in spread is not the articles in the contaminated environment but rather proximity to an individual disseminating the organisms. Because many patients with group A streptococcal skin infections harbor the same organism in their pharynxes, they are, for both reasons, potential sources for spread of infection in a hospital. Particular care must be taken to prevent spread of infection, by isolating such patients until antibiotic therapy has rendered them noncontagious.

Despite the salutary effects of penicillin on morbidity and mortality, the overall incidence of streptococcal disease has probably not decreased. Localized epidemics have continued to appear periodically. During such outbreaks, the carrier and infection rates in the community increase. Carriers may then enter the hospital environment. In this way, streptococci can be introduced into surgical incisions and lacerations and initiate infection. Streptococcal operative infections, because of the rapidity with which they progress, may be more severe and dramatic than those caused by staphylococci.

After recovery (without antibiotic treatment) from streptococcal pharyngitis, some individuals may carry the organism for prolonged periods. The carrier state may also occur in the absence of overt antecedent infection. Fifteen to twenty percent of schoolchildren carry group A streptococci in the throat.

DELAYED NONSUPPURATIVE SEQUELAE The incidence of invasive complications (lymphangitis, suppurative lymphadenitis, bacteremia) of streptococcal infections of the skin has decreased in the antibiotic era. Besides these pyogenic complications, a variety of nonsuppurative complications (acute rheumatic fever, acute glomerulonephritis, erythema nodosum) may follow group A streptococcal infections. Distinct differences exist between acute rheumatic fever and acute glomerulonephritis in the site of the antecedent infection, the length of the latent period, and the streptococcal serotypes involved.[37,38] Acute rheumatic fever may be a complication of group A streptococcal pharyngitis or tonsillitis, but it does not occur following streptococcal skin infections. In contrast, acute nephritis may follow infection of either the skin or the upper respiratory tract. The latent period between streptococcal pharyngitis and the onset of rheumatic fever is 2 to 3 weeks; whereas the latent period for pharyngitis-associated nephritis is about 10 days. A longer latent period, about 3 weeks, is characteristic of acute nephritis associated with streptococcal pyoderma.

Group A streptococci are classified into over 80 subtypes, based on the antigenicity of their M proteins (fibrillar structures extending out from the cell surface). While there is as yet no strong evidence of an association between infection with any specific group A serotypes and the subsequent development of rheumatic fever, several serotypes (particularly mucoid strains of types 1, 3, and 18) have been implicated in a few outbreaks of streptococcal sore throat complicated by this sequela.[39] However, there is a clear relationship between infection with certain serotypes and the subsequent occurrence of nephritis—the so-called nephritogenic serotypes. Type 12 is the classic serotype responsible for pharyngitis-associated acute nephritis, but other serotypes such as 1, 4, 25, and 49 have been implicated. The pyoderma-associated nephritogenic strains generally belong to different serotypes: types 2, 49, 55, 57, and 60.[40,41] The skin rather than the pharynx is the principal site of antecedent streptococcal infection causing nephritis, and impetigo is now the most common form of such predisposing skin infections. Major epidemics of pyoderma-associated nephritis have been observed in communities, and multiple cases of overt and subclinical nephritis have occurred within families.

The frequency of acute glomerulonephritis following infection with a known nephritogenic strain is 10 to 15 percent; the frequency of rheumatic fever following an unrecognized or inadequately treated pharyngeal infection by any serotype of group A streptococcus is 2 to 3 percent or less. The distinction between nephritogenic and other strains of streptococci that might be associated with rheumatic fever can be seen in studies from Trinidad, a hyperendemic area for pyoderma-associated nephritis. There, the streptococcal serotypes causing outbreaks of nephritis differed from the serotypes associated with sporadically occurring cases of acute rheumatic fever in the same population.[42]

It has been suggested that several biologic properties are associated with broad categories of group A streptococci. Most M proteins fall into one of two antigenic classes based on the presence (class I) or absence (class II) of a highly conserved antigenic domain. Almost all rheumatic fever outbreak–associated strains belong to serotypes of class I and require a precursor nasopharyngeal infection. However, because many class I serotypes are associated with impetigo as well and because class II serotypes are responsible for both upper respiratory and skin infections, the class of M protein alone is not a determinant of tissue tropism. Current evidence indicates differences among class I organisms that may relate to their capacities to induce rheumatic fever: class I nasopharyngeal isolates appear to lack human IgG-binding activity, whereas nearly all impetigo isolates of the same class bear human IgG receptors.[43]

ANTIBODY RESPONSE AND IMMUNITY The immune response to group A streptococcal infection depends to a large measure on site of infection. Streptococcal infection is usually defined as a positive throat culture with a serologic response to group A streptococcus and the streptococcal carrier state by a positive throat culture and no serologic response.[44] Following streptococcal pharyngitis, specific antibodies develop to many of the extracellular enzymes of the streptococci. Eighty-five percent of patients with acute rheumatic fever and a proven preceding streptococcal infection will have an elevated or increasing antistreptolysin O (ASO) titer. The

serologic demonstration of an antecedent streptococcal infection in this situation can be increased to virtually 100 percent by the simultaneous testing for several other antibodies (antihyaluronidase, anti-DNase B). Antibodies to extracellular products, with the exception of antibody to the erythrogenic toxin of scarlet fever, appear to have no effect on the manifestations of illness. Streptococcal immunity is type-specific (but not group-specific), long-lasting, and depends on the production of bactericidal antibodies to the specific M proteins of the over 80 different serotypes of group A organisms. Although recurrent pharyngeal infections due to the same serotype are most unusual, repeated clinical infections due to different types are not uncommon. Early treatment of streptococcal upper respiratory tract disease with antibiotics may suppress the appearance of type-specific antibody (and immunity) as well as the development of antibody to the extracellular products of the organism.

In contrast to pharyngeal infections, the ASO response with streptococcal skin infections or pyoderma-associated nephritis is weak. To define the latter serologically, anti-DNase B (or antihyaluronidase) titers are much more reliable. Although pyoderma strains of streptococci produce M proteins and although type-specific antibody may develop in patients with pyoderma-associated nephritis, the frequency of production of such antibodies and their role in protection against reinfection are unclear. While pharyngeal reinfection with the same streptococcal serotype is probably unusual, some evidence suggests that the same serotype can be associated with repeated episodes of pyoderma.

Specific Diseases due to Group A (and Other) Streptococci (Table 195-5)

SUPERFICIAL PYODERMA Streptococcal pyodermas include all types of superficial streptococcal skin infections except erysipelas—i.e., impetigo, ecthyma, and secondary infections of preexisting skin lesions (e.g., insect bites, abrasions, eczema). Streptococcal intertrigo such as streptococcal perianal "cellulitis" can occur primarily or secondarily in underlying conditions such as inverse psoriasis.

SUPERFICIAL PYODERMAS IN NONINTERTRIGINOUS SKIN
Impetigo Impetigo caused by group A streptococcus presents as a crusted superficial infection of the skin; an initial vesicular phase has been described but is rarely detected. Lesions are clinically indistinquishable from impetigo caused by *S. aureus*, with the exception of bullous impetigo (see "Staphylococcal Skin Infections," above).

EPIDEMIOLOGY AND BACTERIOLOGY Impetigo caused by group A streptococcus is a highly communicable infection and occurs predominantly in preschool-aged children (usually before the age of 2 except in highly endemic areas). It is more common in warmer, more humid climates than in temperate zones. Its peak seasonal incidence is in the later summer and early fall. Several decades ago, group A streptococcus was the single most common isolate from impetigo in the United States.[45] Mixtures of streptococci and *S. aureus* were isolated from about half the patients with nonbullous impetigo. The relative roles for these two species in any analysis will probably vary, depending on the presence or absence of hyperendemic or epidemic streptococcal disease in the locality and on the nature of the cases selected for study. Overall, the role of *S. aureus* has increased in recent years. Non–group A (groups B, C,

TABLE 195-5

Infections and Toxin Syndromes Caused by Group A Streptococci

Superficial pyodermas
  Nonintertriginous skin
    Impetigo
    Ecthyma
    Blistering distal dactylitis
  Intertriginous skin
    Perianal streptococcal "cellulitis"
    Streptococcal vulvovaginitis
    Streptococcal intertrigo
Invasive infections
  Acute lymphangitis
  Erysipelas
  Cellulitis
  Streptococcal gangrene
  Bacteremia, septicemia
Toxin-associated syndrome
  Scarlet fever
  Streptococcal toxic-shock–like syndrome
  Streptococcal gangrene
Nonsuppurative complications
  Rheumatic fever
  Glomerulonephritis
Other associated cutaneous reaction patterns
  Erythema nodosum
  Erythema multiforme
  Guttate-pattern psoriasis
  Vasculitis

and G) streptococci may be responsible for rare cases of impetigo; group B streptococci are associated with impetigo in the newborn. Whereas many different serotypes of group A streptococci may cause pharyngitis, a limited number of newly described types predominate in impetigo (types 49, 52, 53, 55, 56, 57, 59, and 61).

PATHOGENESIS AND PATHOLOGY   Group A streptococci appear on normal skin of children about 10 days prior to the development of impetigo and they are not recovered from the nose and throat of the same patients until 14 to 20 days after skin acquisition of the organism. Streptococci are recovered from the respiratory tract of about 30 percent of children with skin lesions, but there is no clinical evidence of streptococcal pharyngitis. Thus, the sequence of spread in a given patient is from normal skin to lesions and eventually to respiratory tract.[46] In contrast, the sequence of spread of *S. aureus* (in cases of impetigo in which it is the only organism isolated) is from nose to normal skin (about 11 days later) and to skin lesions (after another 11 days).

Following acquisition of a streptococcal strain on normal skin from another family member or close contact (whose skin was already colonized or contained a pyoderma), minor traumas (insect bites, abrasions) predispose to the appearance of infected lesions. The inflammatory process of impetigo is superficial, with a unilocular vesicopustule located between the stratum corneum above and the stratum granulosum below. This is usually situated near the opening of a hair follicle. Organisms, as well as leukocytes and epithelial cell debris, fill the vesicle.

CLINICAL MANIFESTATIONS   *History:* Crowding, poor hygiene, and neglected minor skin trauma contribute to the spread of streptococcal impetigo in families. Minor outbreaks have also occurred among athletes involved in contact sports. Although the majority of cases occur in children, particularly of preschool age, young adults are also affected. Impetigo may complicate preexisting skin lesions such as scabies, varicella, or eczema. Pruritus and burning may occur, but the lesions are usually painless. Systemic response is minimal unless complications occur.

Cutaneous lesions: Impetigo caused by *S. aureus* and group A streptococci cannot be differentiated on clinical findings. For clinical features see above staphylococcal impetigo, Figs. 195-1 to 195-3).

LABORATORY FINDINGS   A slight leukocytosis may occur. A Gram-stained smear of early vesicle fluid reveals gram-positive cocci in chains. Culture of the weeping area or of the area beneath an unroofed crust reveals group A streptococci or a mixture of streptococci and *S. aureus* (particularly from older crusted lesions). The lesions of bullous impetigo are caused by *S. aureus* of phage group II.

DIAGNOSIS   The diagnosis of impetigo usually presents no difficulties when the lesions are seen at the stage of crusting, but the specific bacteriologic diagnosis requires culture.

COURSE AND PROGNOSIS   Untreated, the process may persist and new lesions may develop over the course of several weeks; thereafter, the infection tends to resolve spontaneously unless there is some underlying cutaneous disorder such as eczema. Untreated some lesions become chronic and deeper, such as, ecthyma. Complicating erysipelas, cellulitis, or bacteremia are unusual. The major serious sequela is acute poststreptococcal glomerulonephritis.

MANAGEMENT   Topical treatment (removal of dirt, crusts, and debris by soaking with soap and water) is a valuable adjunct. Although penicillin treatment will clear the lesions of group A streptococcal impetigo and prevent recurrence for a short time, streptococci can persist on or newly colonize normal skin in spite of this therapy. Mupirocin ointment appears to be as effective as parenteral or oral penicillin for treatment of impetigo.[47,48] However, prophylactic application of mupirocin ointment to insect bites and abrasions in children in an endemic area during the peak season for skin infections may be useful in preventing superficial streptococcal pyodermas.

In superficial pyodermas known to be caused by group A streptococcus, penicillin is the drug of choice, administered either as a single injection of long-acting benzathine penicillin (300,000 to 600,000 units for children; 1.2 million units for adults) or orally (25,000 to 100,000 units/kg per day in divided doses q6h for 10 days). Erythromycin (30 to 50 mg/kg per day by mouth in divided doses q6h for children; 250 to 500 mg by mouth q6h for adults administered for 10 days) is a suitable alternative drug in patients allergic to penicillin. However, it should be noted that 20 percent or more of group A streptococcal strains became resistant to erythromycin in areas (Japan, Finland) where this antibiotic had been extensively used (or overused) for a variety of indications.[49] Whether administration of penicillin is effective in reducing the incidence of pyoderma-associated nephritis remains a moot point. Although the latent period following impetigo is longer than that following pharyngeal infection, the mildness of the illness delays or negates the seeking of medical attention.

Practically, however, the majority of cases of nonbullous impetigo are caused by *S. aureus*, and systemic antimicrobial treatment should be directed at that pathogen (see above, Management of staphylococcal impetigo).

Ecthyma (See above, staphylococcal ecthyma)

STREPTOCOCCAL INFECTIONS IN INTERTRIGINOUS SKIN SITES   Impetigo and ecthyma usually occur on nonoccluded skin sites. Streptococcal pyodermas occur much less commonly in oc-

FIGURE 195-16

CHAPTER 195
Pyodermas   2197

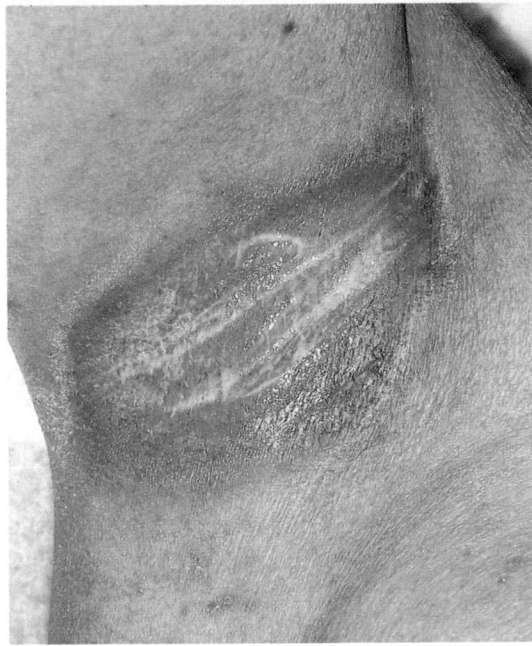

Group A streptococcus intertrigo. A sharply marginated erythematous plaque in the axilla, which was also present in the other axilla, inframammary area, and inguinal folds, was painful in this HIV-infected woman.

FIGURE 195-17

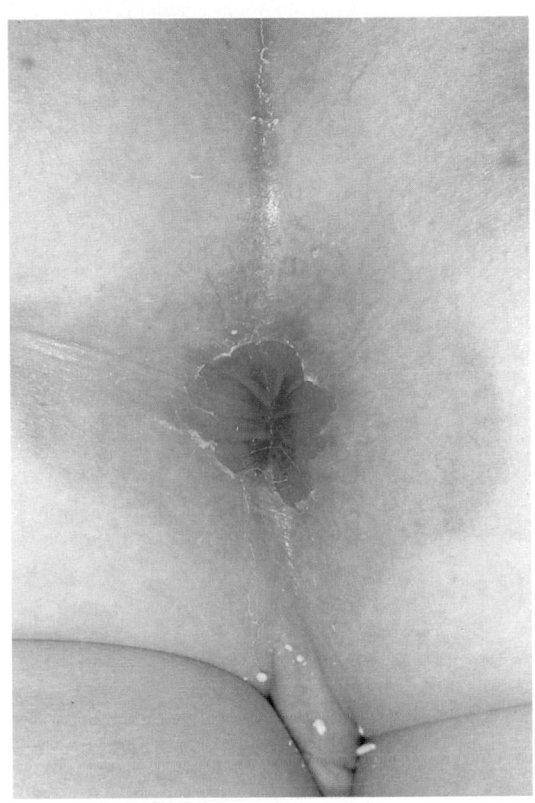

Group A streptococcus: intertrigo—perianal streptococcal "cellulitis." Well-demarcated erythema in the perianal region and perineum in an 8-year-old boy who complained of soreness.

FIGURE 195-18

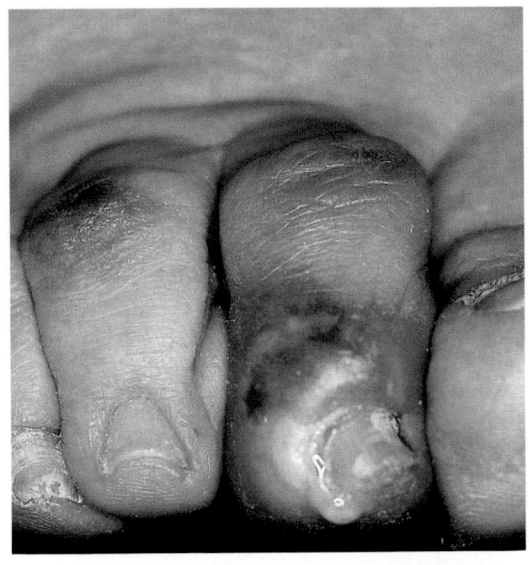

Group A streptococcus: blistering dactylitis. A blister is seen on a toe adjacent to the nail fold; the patient also had group A streptococcal intertrigo of an abdominal skin fold.

cluded sites such as the perineum/perianal region, vulva/vagina, axillae (Fig. 195-16), inframammary region, groin, preputial sac, and web spaces of the feet. Perianal (group A) streptococcal "cellulitis" occurs principally in children, presenting with intense perianal erythema (Fig. 195-17), pain on defecation, blood-streaked stools associated with anal fissures, and chronicity if untreated.[50,51] The infection can also involve the penis and vulva.[52,53] Guttate psoriasis has also occured in children, associated with perianal streptococcal infection.[54]

Blistering distal dactylitis Group A streptococcus is responsible for the majority of cases of this disease, usually occurring in children and adolescents.[55] However, group B streptococcus can also cause this infection.[56] A large, tense blister develops, filled with seropurulent fluid, over the volar skin pad of distal fingers or toes (Fig. 195-18). The blisters are often surrounded by an erythematous base. The lesion may be more proximally located on the finger or extend to involve the nail folds. Group A streptococcus may be cultured from the vesicle fluid. Blistering distal dactylitis may be treated with oral penicillins or erythromycin. Staphylococcal blistering distal dactylitis has been reported with an identical clinical picture as above.[57]

Acute lymphangitis DEFINITION Acute lymphangitis is an inflammatory process involving the subcutaneous lymphatic channels. It is due most often to group A streptococci but occasionally may be caused by *S. aureus*; rarely, soft-tissue infections with other organisms, such as *Pasteurella multocida*, or herpes simplex virus may be associated with acute lymphangitis.

CLINICAL MANIFESTATIONS *History:* The portal of entry is commonly a wound on an extremity, an infected blister, or a paronychia. The systemic manifestations of infection may occur either before any evidence of infection is present at the site of inoculation or after the initial lesion has subsided. The patient may notice pain over an area of redness proximal to the original break in the skin. Systemic symptoms are often more prominent than one might expect from the degree of local pain and erythema.

An unusual spread of streptococcal infection of the thumb (paronychia) or of the interdigital webs between the thumb and index finger may occur occasionally.[58] Lymphatic drainage from this area can bypass the lymph nodes at the elbow and drain into the axillary nodes, which in turn communicate with the subpectoral nodes and the pleural lymphatics. As a consequence, subpectoral abscesses and pleural effusion develop. The subpectoral infection may dissect downward and appear over the lower chest and upper abdomen as an area of cellulitis. This is a very serious illness. The clinical clues to the development of this sequence of events are provided by the location of the original infection on the thumb or medial surface of the index finger and the early occurrence of axillary pain.

Cutaneous lesions: Red linear streaks, which may be a few millimeters to several centimeters in width, extend from the local lesion toward the regional lymph nodes, which are usually enlarged and tender. The lymphangitic streaks are characteristically irregular and tender and may be mistaken for linear excoriations or phytoallergic contact dermatitis (poison ivy or oak). Occasionally, breakdown of overlying skin and ulceration will occur in the course of bacterial lymphangitis, but this is rare in the antibiotic era.

DIFFERENTIAL DIAGNOSIS   In the upper extremities, acute lymphangitis usually can be differentiated from subacute or chronic sporotrichoid syndrome caused by organisms such as *Sportotrix schenckii*. In the lower extremities, superficial thrombophlebitis may produce somewhat similar linear areas of tender erythema. The absence of a portal of entry and of tender regional adenopathy is helpful in distinguishing this process from lymphangitis.

LABORATORY FINDINGS   The peripheral white-blood-cell count is elevated, with a marked increase in polymorphonuclear cells. The offending organism cannot be cultured from the skin, as the infection is restricted to the lymphatic channels. However, the primary portal of entry or a suppurative lymph node, if overt infection is present, may reveal the etiologic agent.

DIAGNOSIS   The combination of a peripheral lesion with proximal red linear streaks leading toward regional lymph nodes is diagnostic of lymphangitis.

COURSE AND PROGNOSIS   The frequent development of bacteremia with metastatic infection in various organs makes this a potentially serious disease. The infection responds readily to penicillin therapy if instituted promptly.

INVASIVE STREPTOCOCCAL INFECTIONS   *Erysipelas*   Erysipelas is a characteristic type of superficial cellulitis of the skin with marked lymphatic-vessel involvement due to group A (or very uncommonly group C or G) streptococci. Group B streptococci may cause erysipelas in newborns. Rarely, a similar clinical picture may be produced by infection with *S. aureus* (see Chap 197).

Cellulitis   This is an acute, spreading inflammation of the skin involving particularly the deeper subcutaneous tissues. *S. aureus* and group A streptococci are by far the most common etiologic agents, but occasionally other bacteria are implicated (see Chap. 197).

Streptococcal gangrene   Gangrene due to group A (occasionally C or G) streptococci is a rare entity, with a high mortality rate, usually developing at the site of a laceration, needle puncture, or surgical wound but sometimes occurring without any obvious portal of entry (see Chap. 197).

STREPTOCOCCAL TOXIN SYNDROMES   *Scarlet fever*   Scarlet fever is a diffuse erythematous eruption resulting from the production and subsequent circulation of pyrogenic exotoxin (erythrogenic toxin) produced by group A streptococci usually located in a pharyngeal infection. The difference between streptococcal tonsillopharyngitis and scarlet fever is the greater toxicity and the cutaneous eruption in the latter.

BACTERIOLOGY AND PATHOGENESIS   Pyrogenic exotoxin is produced by most, but not all, strains of group A streptococci, and its gene is encoded by a lysogenic bacteriophage in the streptococcus. This relationship is very similar to that involving bacteriophage infection and toxin production in *Corynebacterium diphtheriae*. There appear to be three immunologically distinct pyrogenic exotoxins (types A, B, and C) produced by approximately 90 percent of group A isolates. A toxin-producing group A strain may contain the gene encoding for one or more of the exotoxins. In the first half of this century, when scarlet fever was more prevalent and often severe, most scarlet fever strains of group A streptococci produced type A toxin; but in the past three to four decades, strains producing either type B or combinations of type B and C toxins have predominated, perhaps related to the milder course of scarlet fever during this period. More recently, however, there has been a resurgence of severe forms of streptococcal illness resembling scarlet fever, now coined as streptococcal toxic-shock syndrome or toxic-shock–like syndrome (see below).[59] This increase in severity, once again, may be attributed to an increase in exotoxin type A producers.[60]

The streptococcal pyrogenic exotoxins belong to a larger family of exotoxins produced by group A streptococcus and *S. aureus*. These exotoxins are involved in the pathogenesis of toxic-shock–like syndromes and have been implicated in numerous autoimmune and skin disorders, including atopic dermatitis and psoriasis. They have been labeled as superantigens capable of binding to the major histocompatibility complex proteins on the surface of antigen-presenting cells outside the antigen peptide-binding groove. The exotoxin is then recognized by the variable region of the β-chain of the T-cell receptor complex outside the antigen-binding groove on T lymphocytes. This results in massive stimulation of a T-cell repertoire containing the identified Vb T-cell receptor region.[61] Type A toxin is a more potent stimulator of cytokine production (e.g., TNFα) and T-lymphocyte activation, which might explain its association with more severe cases of scarlet fever.

Group A streptococci can cause recurrent infections, but an individual usually has scarlet fever only once because of the development of protective antibody specific to the pyrogenic exotoxins. The few patients with documented recurrent attacks of scarlet fever may represent cases in which the episodes have been due to either of the other two immunologically distinct toxins. The immune status of a patient will determine the response to exposure to a given pyrogenic exotoxin-producing strain of group A streptococcus; it consists of two parts—type-specific antibacterial immunity and antitoxic immunity. The responses fall into three patterns: (1) Patients with type-specific antibacterial immunity (with or without antitoxic immunity) to a given streptococcal type (e.g., type 12) will contract no clinical disease when exposed to that type. (2) Patients with no type-specific antibacterial immunity (but with antitoxic immunity) will contract streptococcal pharyngitis. (3) Patients with neither antibacterial nor antitoxic immunity will contract pharyngitis plus scarlet fever (unless treated early with appropriate antibiotics).

The rash of scarlet fever requires both the presence of pyrogenic exotoxin and the existence of delayed-type skin reactivity to streptococcal products, the latter stemming from prior exposure to the organism. In support of this is the observation that although streptococcal infections are not uncommon in infants and very young children, scarlet fever is rarely seen in this age group, and these infants fail to react to intradermal injection of pyrogenic exotoxin (Dick test). This failure to react correlates with transfer of antibody from the mother. Similarly, infant guinea pigs are not susceptible to intradermal injection of pyrogenic exotoxin. Following immunization with the toxin in Freund's adjuvant, they become sensitized and the Dick test becomes positive.

CLINICAL MANIFESTATIONS *History:* The disease usually occurs in children (the maximal incidence being in the 2- to 10-year age group) and only rarely in adults. The clinical onset of the disease with the appearance of pharyngitis and fever is often abrupt after a 2- to 4-day incubation period. The temperature may be only slightly elevated in mild cases but it often rises rapidly to 38.9 to 40°C (102 to 104°F). Nausea and vomiting, headache, malaise, diffuse abdominal pain, and chilly sensations are prominent initial constitutional manifestations. The fever reaches its peak by the second day, and the temperature gradually returns to normal in 5 to 6 days in the average case. The rash appears 24 to 48 h after the onset of pharyngeal symptoms. Although the streptococcal focus of most patients with scarlet fever is in the pharynx, occasional patients have a form of the disease, surgical scarlet fever, as a consequence of operative or other wound (burn, etc.) infection.

The acute manifestations of scarlet fever consist of those symptoms and signs related to the invasive streptococcal process at the portal of entry and those findings produced by pyrogenic exotoxin (malaise, nausea, vomiting, headache, fever, generalized lymphadenopathy, rash). Rabbits treated with exotoxin alone by either subcutaneous injection or slow-delivery subcutaneous miniosmotic pump develop many classic signs of scarlet fever.[62]

Mucocutaneous lesions: The major physical findings relate to the enanthem and exanthem.

Enanthem: The pharynx is beefy red in color, with edema involving the tonsillar area and extending anteriorly to include the soft palate and uvula. Manifesting the local group A streptococcal infection, the tonsils are enlarged, reddened, and often covered with discrete patches of white or yellow exudate filling the tonsillar crypts. Occasionally, the exudate becomes confluent. Bilateral tender submandibular lymphadenopathy is present, relating to the streptococcal pharyngitis. Pharyngitis and submandibular lymphadenopathy are not seen in individuals with group A streptococcal surgical wound scarlet fever or staphylococcal scarlet fever.

During the first several days of the illness, the tongue is white and furred, but the edges and tip remain reddened. The papillae soon become reddened and hypertrophied and project through the white coating, producing what has been called the "white-strawberry" tongue. By the fourth or fifth day, the white coating has sloughed and the tongue assumes a bright red color punctuated with very prominent papillae, the so-called red-strawberry tongue (Fig. 195-19A). Punctate erythema and scattered petechiae are often present over the soft palate.

Exanthem: The rash usually appears first on the head and neck (Fig. 195-19A), then rapidly encompasses the trunk, and finally spreads to the extremities. The involvement of the body is usually complete within 36 h, but the palms and soles are spared. The rash is a diffuse erythema, blanching on presure, with numerous 1- to 2-mm punctate papular elevations, giving a rough sandpaper quality to the skin (Fig. 195-19B). There are usually no discrete lesions on the face but only a marked flushing of the cheeks and forehead, contrasting quite sharply with the circumoral pallor. On the body the rash is most marked in the skin folds of the inguinal, axillary, antecubital, and abdominal areas and about sites of pressure such as the buttocks and sacrum. The eruption often exhibits a linear

FIGURE 195-19

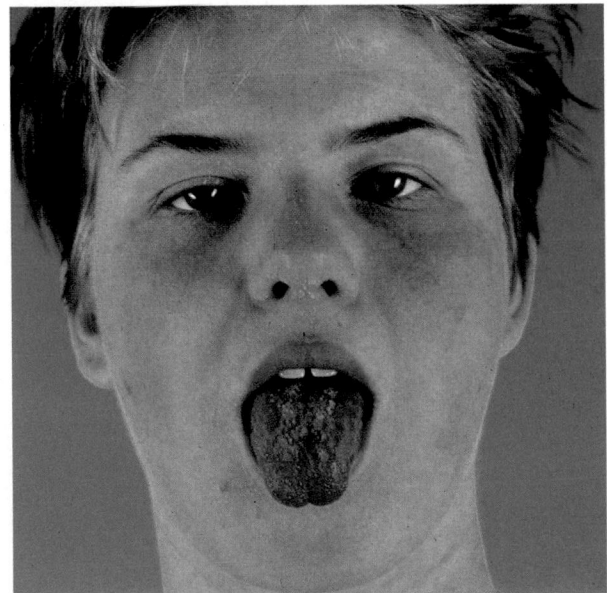

A.

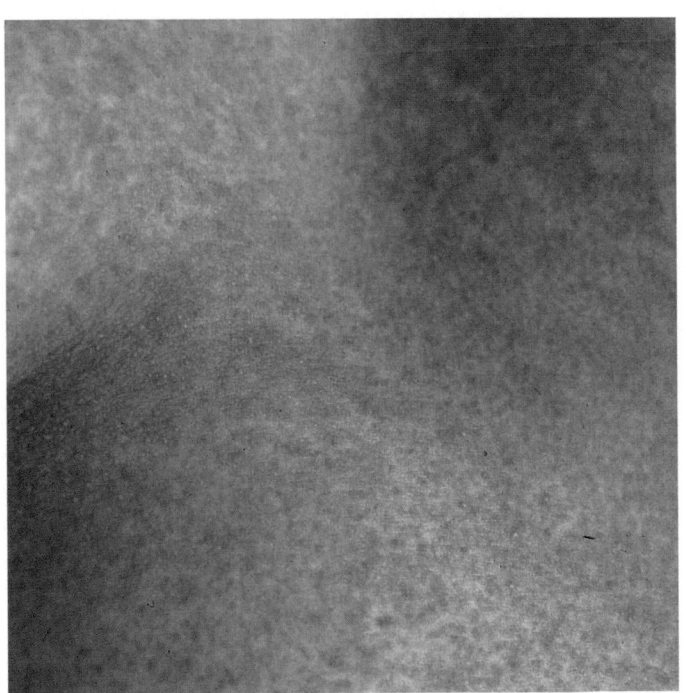

B.

Group A streptococcus, scarlet fever: Exanthem and enanthem. *A.* In this young woman with pharyngitis, the face is erythematous with perioral pallor; the tongue is a beefy or "strawberry" red. *B.* Close-up of scarlatina rash.

petechial character in the antecubital fossae and axillary folds (Pastia's lines). When the eruption is intense, pinhead vesicular lesions (miliary sudamina), seen in a variety of prolonged febrile illnesses, may appear on the abdomen and chest. When the rash is mild, the exanthem may be localized to the trunk and be seen as only a faint erythema. In black patients the rash is often difficult to recognize but may be felt as punctate papular lesions resembling "gooseflesh" or sandpaper. At its peak the rash has a diffuse, bright scarlet appearance. Capillary fragility is increased in the severer cases, and the tourniquet test result is positive. Occasional frank purpura may develop, with or without thrombocytopenia.

The exanthem usually persists for 4 or 5 days but in mild cases may be very transient. One of the most characteristic features of the illness is the desquamation that begins as the rash starts to fade, commencing on the face, usually about the ears, and spreading to the trunk and extremities, involving the hands and feet last (between the second and third weeks of illness). The desquamation on the face and trunk has a brawny character, and frequently a punched-out appearance of the abdomen results from the peeling off of circular areas of skin. Skin on the hands and feet is frequently shed in large sheets. The desquamation is so prominent a feature that it may be helpful in making a retrospective diagnosis in a case in which the eruption was minimal (Fig. 195-20). Similar changes in the nail bed produce a transverse groove in the nails.

Other Physical Findings: Generalized lymphadenopathy is a common finding, and splenomegaly is present occasionally.

DIFFERENTIAL DIAGNOSIS   Although the total clinical picture is highly suggestive of scarlet fever (due to group A streptococci), scarlatiniform eruptions may occur in other conditions and cause confusion in diagnosis. Infection with toxin ("exfoliatin")-producing strains of *S. aureus* belonging to phage group II may produce a rash resembling that of scarlet fever (see above, "Staphylococcal Skin Infections"). Strains of *S. aureus* producing TSST-1 are responsible for TSS (see above). In infants and young children particularly, exanthem subitum and rubella may be mistaken for scarlet fever, but the lack of a pharyngeal focus is important in distinguishing these conditions. Also, neither of these processes is followed by extensive desquamation. Patients with infectious mononucleosis (primary cytomegalovirus or Epstein-Barr virus infection) may have

FIGURE 195-20

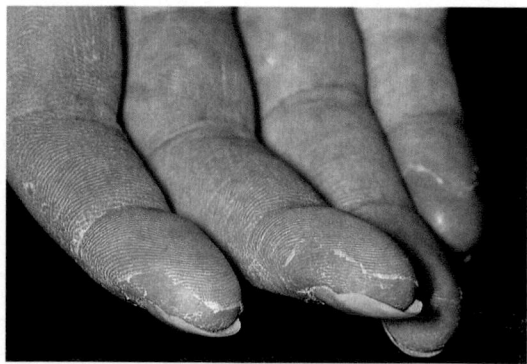

Group A streptococcus, scarlet fever: desquamation. The patient had streptococcal pharyngitis 17 days previously that was successfully treated with ampicillin. The fingertips show the subtle desquamation that occurs in scarlet fever, related to epidermal damage and repair.

an erythematous eruption, and this, together with lymphadenopathy and membranous pharyngitis, may mimic scarlet fever. The typical blood picture and the heterophil agglutination test are helpful in distinguishing between these diseases. Diffuse erythroderma as part of a drug-sensitivity reaction (sulfonamides, streptomycin, penicillin) may be mistaken for scarlet fever, as may the fever and cutaneous blush associated with atropine toxicity. Sunburn in a child with pharyngitis may be a cause of confusion, but the distribution of the lesions is the crucial distinguishing point.

LABORATORY FINDINGS   The hematologic findings in the early stages are of a polymorphonuclear leukocytosis, and later in the illness eosinophilia (5 to 10 percent) is a common finding. Throat culture reveals group A streptococci. If direct bacteriologic confirmation cannot be made during the early phases of the illness, determination of the ASO titer may provide, retrospectively, evidence of a recent streptococcal infection. Slight microscopic hematuria is found not infrequently during the peak of the exanthem and does not represent acute glomerulonephritis. It is usually transient and may be related to a generalized effect of the pyrogenic exotoxin on capillaries.

DERMATOPATHOLOGY   There is an outpouring of polymorphonuclear leukocytes and scattered red blood cells into the skin about small blood vessels. The punctiform lesions are represented by dilated small blood vessels and a focal accumulation of exudate. The suppurative and nonsuppurative sequelae are the same as are seen with any group A streptococcal infection.

The diagnosis is usually made on the basis of clinical features—fever, vomiting, exudative pharyngitis, and an erythematous punctiform eruption going on to desquamation. Confirmatory evidence is provided by isolation of group A streptococci from the pharynx.

CONFIRMATORY TESTS   Two confirmatory tests that have been employed extensively in the past are no longer necessary. The Dick test was performed by an intracutaneous inoculation of 0.1 mL of a standard diluted preparation of pyrogenic exotoxin. The appearance of a 1-cm or greater area of local erythema at 24 h was a positive test result and indicated a lack of antitoxic immunity (i.e., susceptibility to scarlet fever). The Schultz-Charlton phenomenon was observed after the intradermal injection of 0.1 mL of antitoxin into an area of scarlet fever rash that produced "blanching" at the site of injection within 12 to 24 h. The test had to be performed during the very early phase of the eruption before exudation into the lesion made the skin changes irreversible. The blanching test is not used now because of the danger of sensitization to horse serum and because the use of antitoxin of human origin carries the risk of introducing viral hepatitis or HIV infection.

DIAGNOSIS   The typical clinical findings of streptococcal scarlet fever are usually confirmed by isolation of group A streptococcus on throat culture.

COURSE AND PROGNOSIS   The acute febrile course of the untreated, uncomplicated case lasts about 4 to 5 days; desquamation may continue for several weeks thereafter. Many cases seen currently are mild and last only a few days. The course of the illness is dramatically altered by the administration of penicillin, which produces a prompt subsidence of fever and of constitutional symptoms. Adequate, early penicillin treatment eradicates the streptococci from the pharyngeal or other foci, interferes with the development of ASO antibodies, and prevents the development of suppurative and nonsuppurative sequelae. The prognosis is excellent, and today deaths due to scarlet fever are extremely rare.

Group A streptococcus toxic-shock–like syndrome ("toxic-strep syndrome")   Group A streptococci cause an acute multisystem syndrome coined toxic-shock–like syndrome (TSLS) resembling that caused by *S. aureus* (see section on "Staphylococcal Skin Infections," above).[63–65] The initiating streptococcal infection is commonly in soft tissues (cellulitis, necrotizing fasciitis, infection at site of liposuction); other infections include pharyngitis, suppurative phlebitis, peritonitis, osteomyelitis, endophthalmitis, and myometritis.[66] Major differences between staphylococcal TSS and streptococcal TSLS are extensive soft-tissue infection and bacteremia. Staphylococcal TSS does not usually have an obvious cutaneous site of infection, nor is bacteremia common. Streptococcal TSLS usually has an obvious soft-tissue site of infection, and bacteremia commonly occurs.

Clinical features usually include many of the following: hypotension, chills, fever, tachycardia, myalgias, and mental changes as well as manifestations of multiorgan dysfunction (gastrointestinal abnormalities, renal failure, adult respiratory distress syndrome). Localized erythema (usually about the face) is more commonly present than the generalized punctate erythema of scarlet fever. Injection of bulbar and palpebral conjunctivae may be present as well as a strawberry tongue; and skin desquamation may or may not be a later feature.

It is important to recognize as well that "septic scarlet fever" may be reemerging currently, after an absence during the postantibiotic era. Three cases of severe septic scarlet fever with the features of toxic shock has been described in individuals with group A streptococcal cellulitis and bacteremia.[67] Although some clinical distinction could be made, TSLS may be a more severe form or variant of scarlet fever.

Compared to scarlet fever, a smaller number of cases of TSLS have been studied microbiologically. The group A streptococcal isolates produced either type A or a mixture of types B and C pyrogenic exotoxins (also known as erythrogenic toxins). It has been postulated that the attenuated nature of scarlet fever and of nonbacteremic streptococcal infections in recent decades was associated with the virtual disappearance of group A streptococci producing pyrogenic exotoxin A and replacement with strains producing type B (or mixtures of types B and C) toxins. The resurgence of streptococcal strains producing pyrogenic exotoxin A may be responsible for the current outbreak of streptococcal TSLS.

Cutaneous manifestations of subacute bacterial endocarditis A variety of skin lesions have been described in subacute bacterial endocarditis (usually due to viridans streptococci). Although often ascribed to embolic phenomena, it appears that many of these lesions represent local areas of vasculitis.

PETECHIAE AND HEMORRHAGES These are the most common of the skin and mucous membrane lesions in bacterial endocarditis and are found in about half of patients with this disease. These small, reddish-brown, flat lesions do not blanch on pressure. They occur particularly on the extremities and upper chest. Mucous membrane petechiae and/or hemorrhages on the conjunctivae (Fig. 195-21A) or palate is common. The petechiae frequently occur in small crops. Rarely, the lesions may be extremely numerous and involve primarily the lower extremities. They usually deepen in color, last only a few days, and then fade away. It is important to distinguish capillary angiomas, which may be present on the chests of some patients, from petechiae. This can be done by applying pressure with a glass slide and demonstrating blanching of the angiomas.

The limited information on the histology of petechiae in subacute bacterial endocarditis does not suggest local bacterial multiplication or embolization as the basis for the lesions. The endothelial proliferation, hemorrhage, and round-cell infiltration found are consistent with small-vessel inflammation. Increased capillary fragility can be demonstrated in some patients.

SUBUNGUAL "SPLINTER HEMORRHAGES" These small, dark red streaks resembling splinters in the midportion of the nail bed are suggestive of the diagnosis of subacute bacterial endocarditis (Fig. 195-21B). Similar lesions may occur beneath the distal portion of the nail bed as a result of trauma (in dishwashers, carpenters, etc.) or poor hygiene. Splinter hemorrhages may occur as part of the clinical picture in trichinosis and vasculitis. Subungual hemorrhages may occur in acute meningococcemia with extensive petechiae and purpura.

OSLER'S NODES These are split-pea-sized, erythematous, painful, nodular lesions. They appear to be in the skin and in some ways resemble an urticarial wheal, often with a whitish center. The most common location of these swellings is on the pads of the fingers and toes, on the thenar and hypothenar eminences, and over the arms. They are quite transient, lasting 12 to 24 h or perhaps several days. They are not numerous and tend to occur in crops. They may desquamate but do not ulcerate. Currently, they are seen in about 5 percent of patients with bacterial endocarditis.

Histologic examination has not confirmed the suggested embolic nature of the Osler's nodes occurring in subacute bacterial endocarditis. Endothelial swelling and a perivascular inflammatory response have been found at the center of such lesions, but no bacteria or fibrin emboli were observed. Although at first suggested as pathognomonic findings in viridans streptococcal subacute bacterial en-

FIGURE 195-21

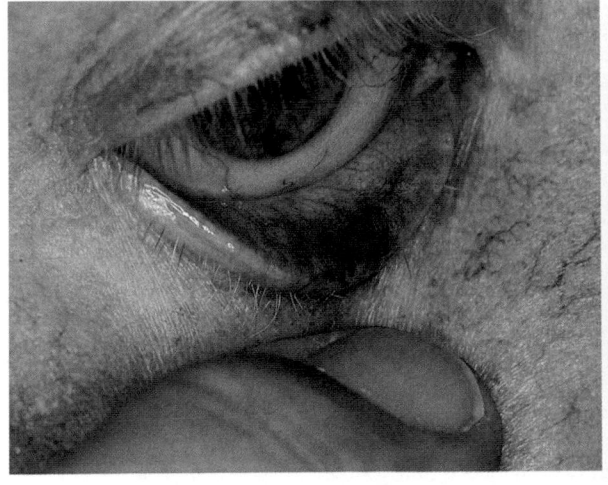

A.

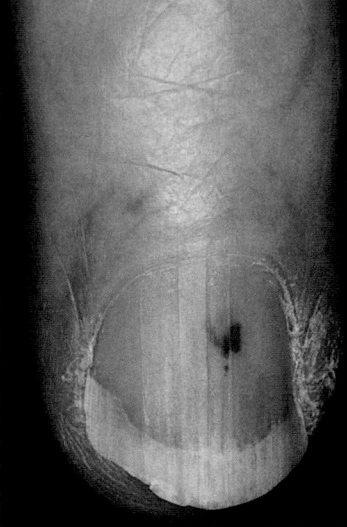

B.

Enterococcal endocarditis with embolization. *A.* Subconjunctival hemorrhage. *B.* Subungual hemorrhages in the midportion of the nail bed. The patient had acute infective endocarditis following an enterococcal urinary tract infection with bacteremia.

docarditis, Osler's nodes have been observed in subacute and acute endocarditis due to a variety of organisms, including *S. aureus.* Histologic examination of Osler's nodes from several patients with acute endocarditis due to *S. aureus* and *C. albicans* has revealed microembolic in dermal arterioles and adjacent microabscesses in the papillary dermis.[68] In these cases the responsible organism has been identified on Gram's stains or cultures of aspirates.

It appears that Osler's nodes in acute bacterial endocarditis may be caused by minute infective emboli; in subacute bacterial endocarditis they may be due to immunologic phenomena resulting in small-vessel arteritis of the skin. (see also Chap. 166).

JANEWAY LESIONS   These lesions, consisting of minimally nodular hemorrhages, or occasionally erythematous macules, in the palms or soles, are seen in acute endocarditis (commonly due to *S. aureus*) or, infrequently, in subacute bacterial endocarditis. They may be rather numerous and, unlike Osler's nodes, are painless. Histologically, there is usually a polymorphonuclear infiltration of the walls of blood capillaries, some extravasation of red blood cells, and microabscess formation in the dermis. Gram-positive cocci in clusters have been demonstrated extracellularly in such a lesion, and *S. aureus* has been isolated on culture of the same lesion in a patient with *S. aureus* endocarditis.[69] Occasional lesions of purulent purpura (lesions with white or dark gray centers with surrounding hemorrhagic halos) may also be seen on the distal extremities in acute *S. aureus* endocarditis, representing progression of Janeway lesions or initial metastatic pustules (see Chap. 166).

POSTSTREPTOCOCCAL (GROUP A) NONSUPPURATIVE CUTANEOUS SEQUELAE   *Erythema nodosum*   See Chap. 111.

Erythema marginatum (cutaneous lesions of acute rheumatic fever)   See Chap. 179.

Purpura fulminans   Purpura fulminans is an uncommon, acute, severe, usually fatal nonspecific hemorrhagic infarction and necrosis of the skin that occurs in the course of, or immediately following, a variety of infections, particularly those due to group A streptococci. Marked depletion of multiple coagulation factors (disseminated intravascular coagulation) is responsible for this condition. Closely related, if not the identical process, is the symmetric peripheral gangrene that is sometimes seen (particularly in infants) during bacteremias.

EPIDEMIOLOGY   Purpura fulminans occurs most often in children but has been seen at all ages. The antecedent or concomitant infections with which it has been associated include those due to bacteria (scarlet fever; group A streptococcal, staphylococcal, pneumococcal, and vibrio bacteremias; and meningococcemia) and, less commonly, those of a viral etiology (varicella). In patients with purpura fulminans after varicella, secondary streptococcal infection may have been an important etiologic factor.

ETIOLOGY AND PATHOGENESIS   Purpura fulminans is one of several cutaneous syndromes whose common feature is a hemorrhagic tendency developing secondary to the acute intravascular activation of the clotting mechanism. The exact means of initiation of the consumption coagulopathy is not yet fully understood. A host of coagulation abnormalities has been noted at one time or another. This variability probably reflects the rapid changes that occur during the evolution of the process and the effects of "secondary" fibrinolysis. The abnormalities more commonly recorded include thrombocytopenia; depression of prothrombin (factor II), fibrinogen (factor I), proaccelerin (factor V), and antihemophilic factor (factor VIII); and findings of secondary fibrinolysis (i.e., increased

plasminogen levels or evidence of fibrinogen or fibrin breakdown products). The coagulopathy and microscopic pathology in purpura fulminans are very similar to those found in rabbits with generalized Shwartzman reaction (see Chap. 194).

CLINICAL MANIFESTATIONS   *History:* The eruption develops during, or on convalescence from, one of the infections noted earlier. Chills and fever usually herald the onset of the hemorrhagic lesions, and the patient appears acutely ill.

Cutaneous lesions: The lesions are localized, massive ecchymoses, often with sharp, irregular ("geographic") borders. They are usually symmetric and on the extremities, particularly in areas of pressure, but may involve the lips, ears, nose, and trunk. There may be a narrow surrounding zone of erythema. Hemorrhagic blebs may develop in the ecchymotic areas associated with edema of the areas (Fig. 195-22). The peripheral ecchymotic lesions, especially of the digits, may rapidly blacken and progress to gangrene.

Other physical findings: The other findings are those of a systemically ill patient with high fever and tachycardia. The disease often rapidly progresses over 48 to 72 h, with peripheral vasoconstriction and shock supervening.

DIFFERENTIAL DIAGNOSIS   All the causes of gross purpura must be considered in the differential diagnosis. The relationship of specific infections, the striking geographic nature of the lesions, and their location on the extremities are suggestive of the diagnosis. Rarely, morphologically similar lesions have been described as complications of coumarin therapy in individuals deficient in coagulation factor protein C.

LABORATORY FINDINGS   There is usually a leukocytosis. The number of platelets is markedly reduced and coagulation factors V, VII, and VIII and prothrombin and fibrinogen are decreased. As a result, the preothrombin time and the partial thromboplastin time are prolonged. Split products of fibrinogen and fibrin may be present.

DERMATOPATHOLOGY   The involved areas show occlusion of arterioles with fibrin thrombi. A dense polymorphonuclear reaction occurs in the dermis in the areas of infarction necrosis. Bacteria are not seen in the lesions. Similar lesions may occur in the viscera, but they are often restricted to the skin.

COURSE AND PROGNOSIS   The mortality rate is extremely high. In patients who survive, amputation of extremities or extensive skin grafting may be necessary to deal with the gangrenous areas.

MANAGEMENT   Treatment includes vigorous antibiotic management of any associated infection. Only if bleeding is significant during the course of diffuse intravascular coagulation in the patient with purpura fulminans is replacement of platelets and coagulation factors undertaken and consideration given to the use of heparin (10 to 15 units/kg per h as a continuous intravenous infusion) to inhibit the intravascular clotting process.

Other skin lesions accompanying or following group A streptococcal infections   ERYTHEMA MULTIFORME–LIKE LESIONS   Round erythematous macules, up to 1.5 cm in diameter, some developing bright borders and subsequently showing clearing in the center, may occur during bacteremia due to group A streptococci (or *S. aureus*) in infants and young children (see Chap. 58).

ACUTE GUTTATE PSORIASIS   Rarely, erythematous, papulosquamous, guttate psoriasiform lesions may develop during or following group A streptococcal pharyngitis or skin infections. Children appear to be most commonly affected. Clearing of the lesions may occur within weeks of antimicrobial therapy of the streptococcal infection. Although the temporal relation of the two processes is striking, a direct causal connection has not been established (see Chap. 43). Superantigens or pyrogenic exotoxins have been investigated as possible agents involved in guttate psoriasis.

FIGURE 195-22

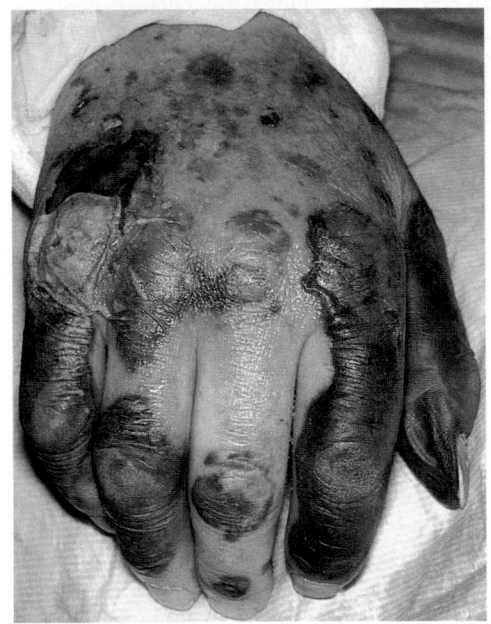

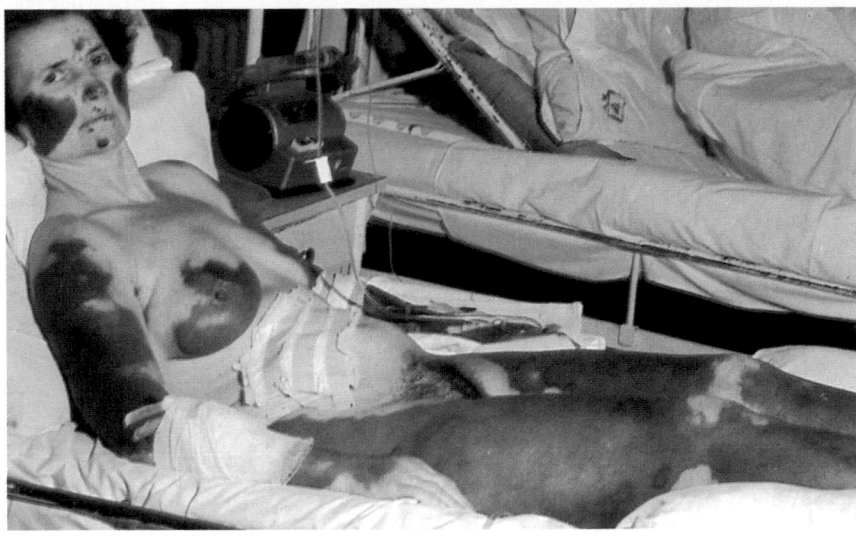

B.

A.

Purpura fulminans. *A.* Hemorrhagic infection in a patient with diabetes with *S. aureus* septicemia and disseminated intravascular coagulation. The patient died within 24 h in spite of therapy. *B.* Purpura fulminans in disseminated intravascular coagulation following abdominal surgery. There are extensive geographic areas of cutaneous infarction involving the face, breasts, and extremities.

MANAGEMENT OF GROUP A STREPTOCOCCAL SKIN INFECTIONS *Antibiotic management* GENERAL PRINCIPLES Penicillin G is the drug of choice in the treatment of known group A streptococcal skin infections. When the etiology is not known immediately (e.g., in cellulitis) and when *S. aureus* is also a distinct consideration, a semisynthetic penicillin (nafcillin or oxacillin) should be employed initially. Penicillin treatment should be continued for at least 10 days to ensure eradication of the infection. Since as many as 40 percent of isolates of group A streptococci may be resistant to the tetracyclines, this group of drugs should not be used in the treatment of known streptococcal disease. Prophylactic penicillin therapy is indicated for close family contacts (particularly children) of patients with streptococcal pharyngitis.

ANTIMICROBIAL THERAPY Mild instances of infections such as impetigo, scarlet fever, or certain cases of erysipelas and cellulitis may be treated with oral penicillin V (250 to 500 mg 4 times daily). When staphylococcal infection is suspected, dicloxacillin (250 to 500 mg orally 4 times daily) should be substituted. In adults allergic to penicillin, erythromycin (250 to 500 mg orally 4 times daily) is a reasonable alternative. Other alternatives include azithromycin, clarithromycin, and clindamycin.

LOCAL THERAPY Superficial lesions (such as ecthyma and secondarily infected dermatoses) benefit from sterile saline dressings. Mupirocin ointment may be of value for softening and removing crusted lesions as well as for its antibacterial effects.

PREVENTION OF SPREAD Patients hospitalized with group A streptococcal infections should be isolated until the organisms have been eradicated by antibiotic treatment. Individuals with recurrent episodes of group A streptococcal infections can be treated with dicloxacillin or erythromycin 250 mg twice daily (penicillin-allergic individuals) as secondary prophylaxis. Where streptococcal infections are highly endemic, prophylactic antibiotics must be administered to all members of the population to reduce the incidence of group A streptococcal infections.[70]

SOFT-TISSUE STREPTOCOCCAL INFECTIONS See Chap. 197.

CUTANEOUS INFECTIONS DUE TO *MICROCOCCUS* *Pitted keratolysis* This bacterial infection involves the stratum corneum of the webspaces and plantar surface. Originally named *keratoma plantare sulcatum* by Castellani in 1910, this disease has become more commonly called by its current name after Taplin and Zaias coined it in 1967.[71,72] The disease was first seen in those who went barefooted during the rainy season.

ETIOLOGY AND PATHOGENESIS The likely causative organism is *Micrococcus sedentarius*, which is a gram-positive staphylococcus-related bacterium that invades the stratum corneum softened by sweat and moisture.[73] There is less convincing evidence that a corynebacterium species or *Dermatophilus congolensis* may be involved. Pitted keratolysis tends to be much more severe in tropical climates than in temperate ones.

Pitted keratolysis occurs in adults and children of both sexes, but adult males with sweaty feet are most susceptible (96 percent of cases).[74] Sliminess of the skin, often manifest by the foot sticking to the socks, is also a common complaint (70 percent of cases). The feet are typically very malodorous (89 percent) and may be mildly pruritic (8 percent).[75]

CLINICAL MANIFESTATIONS Pitted keratolysis presents a superficial erosion of the stratum corneum, composed of numerous small crateriform pits coalescing to form a large discrete defect with serpiginous borders on the plantar surface of the foot. The pits are usually >0.7 mm in diameter but at times the pits are <0.5 mm in diameter. The pits have elongated configurations along the plantar furrows. The pits are located predominantly on the pressure-bearing areas, such as the ventral aspect of the toe, ball of the foot, and the heel, but are also seen on non-pressure-bearing areas. The web spaces between the toes are also commonly involved sites, and may be the only manifestation (Fig. 195-23).

DIFFERENTIAL DIAGNOSIS Interdigital tinea pedis can present with erosive lesions in the web spaces. Erythrasma in the webspaces is usually hyperkeratotic but can be erosive.

LABORATORY FINDINGS Gram-staining of scraping may detect the microorganism more readily than potassium hydroxide examination. Histologically, the organisms are present in the walls and bases of the crateriform defects in the upper layer of the stratum corneum.[76] The organisms appear as coccoid and filamentaous forms with branches and septa, divided only transversely without longitudinal septation.

DIAGNOSIS The diagnosis is made on the unique clinical findings.

MANAGEMENT Prophylactic measures are aimed at keeping the feet as dry as possible. Inert antiseptic foot powders often help. A benzoyl peroxide wash and 5 percent gel are effective therapy in most cases. Other commonly used topical agents include clindamycin, erythromycin, clotrimazole, miconazole, and Whitfield's ointment.

INFECTIONS DUE TO *CORYNEBACTERIUM* *Erythrasma* Erythrasma is a common superficial bacterial infection of the skin characterized by well-defined but irregular reddish brown patches, occurring in the intertriginous areas, or by fissuring and white maceration in the toe clefts.

ETIOLOGY AND EPIDEMIOLOGY *Corynebacterium minutissimum*, the etiologic agent of erythrasma, is a short, gram-positive rod with subterminal granules. The infection is more common in tropical than in temperate climates. In a study in a temperate climate, 20 percent of randomly selected subjects were found to have erythrasma by Wood's lamp examination. The generalized disease is much more common in the tropics. Erythrasma is more common in men, and may occur in asymptomatic form in the genitocrural

area. In obese women with diabetes, extensive erythrasma can occur in the axillae, inframammary folds, groins, and extensive areas of the trunk. It does not appear to be significantly contagious.[77]

CLINICAL MANIFESTATIONS Symptoms vary from a completely asymptomatic form, through a genitocrural form with considerable pruritus, to a generalized form with scaly lamellated plaques on the trunk, inguinal area, and web spaces of the feet. When pruritic, irritation of lesions may cause secondary changes of excoriations and lichenification.

Cutaneous lesions: The most common site of involvement is the web spaces of the feet, where erythrasma presents as a hyperkeratotic white macerated plaque (Fig. 195-24), especially between the fourth and fifth toes. In the genitocrural, axillary, and inframammary regions, the lesions present as well-demarcated, reddish-brown, superficial, finely scaly and finely wrinkled plaques (Fig. 195-25). In these sites, the plaques have a relatively uniform appearance as compared with tinea corporis or cruris, which often have central clearing.

Wood's lamp examination of erythrasma reveals a coral-red fluorescence caused by coproporphyrin III. The fluorescence may persist after eradication of the *Corynebacterium* as the pigment is within a thick stratum corneum. In pityriasis (tinea) versicolor, a yellow fluorescence can be seen on Wood's lamp examination.

DIFFERENTIAL DIAGNOSIS Tinea versicolor is distinguished from erythrasma by the lesions on the trunk being most numerous at nonintertriginous sites. Tinea cruris tends to have an active scaling border with central clearing. Inverse pattern psoriasis usually presents as sharply demarcated plaques with a beefy shiny red color in the intergluteal cleft, inguinal folds, and axillae.

LABORATORY Culture of the specific *Corynebacterium* in abundance from the lesion corroborates the diagnosis. Gram-stained imprints of the horny layer of the skin show rod-like, gram-positive organisms in large numbers. Bacilli have been demonstrated within cells of the horny layer on examination by electron microscope.

DIAGNOSIS The diagnosis is strongly suggested by the location and superficial character of the process, but must be confirmed by demonstration of the characteristic "coral-red" fluorescence with Wood's lamp ilumination.

FIGURE 195-23

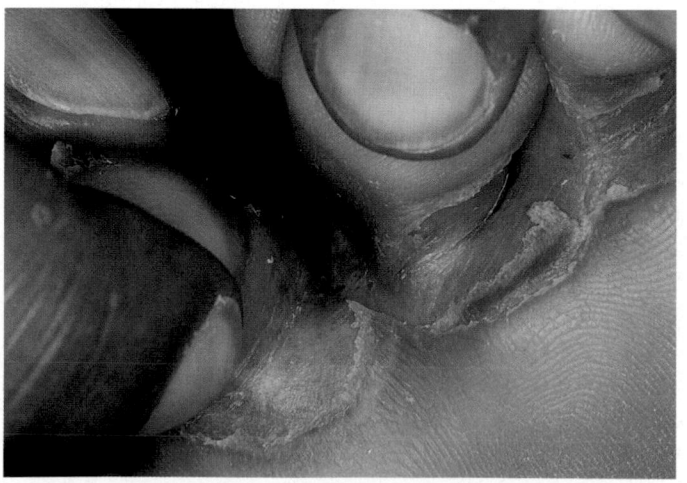

Pitted keratolysis. The web spaces between the toes are sharply eroded. Interdigital tinea pedis and erythrasma may occur concurrently.

FIGURE 195-24

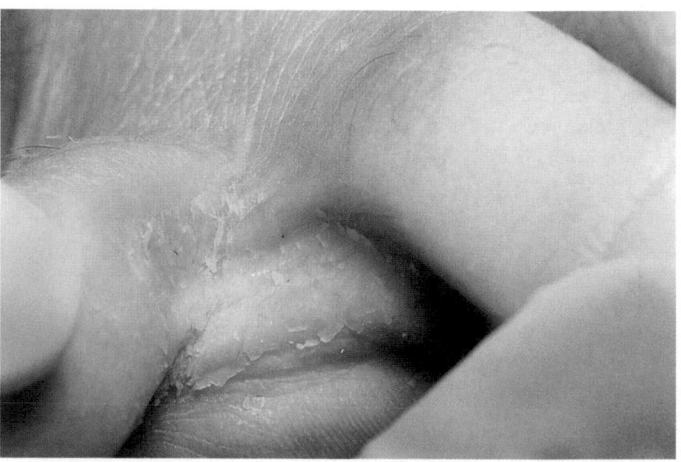

Erythrasma. Hyperkeratosis with a yellowish hue in the web space of the foot. The three lateral web spaces of both feet were involved. The potassium hydroxide preparation was negative; the Wood's lamp examination showed a bright coral red fluorescence.

FIGURE 195-25

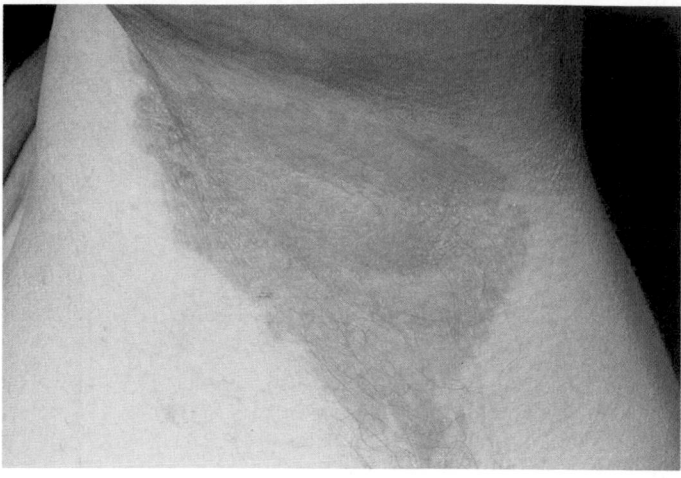

A.

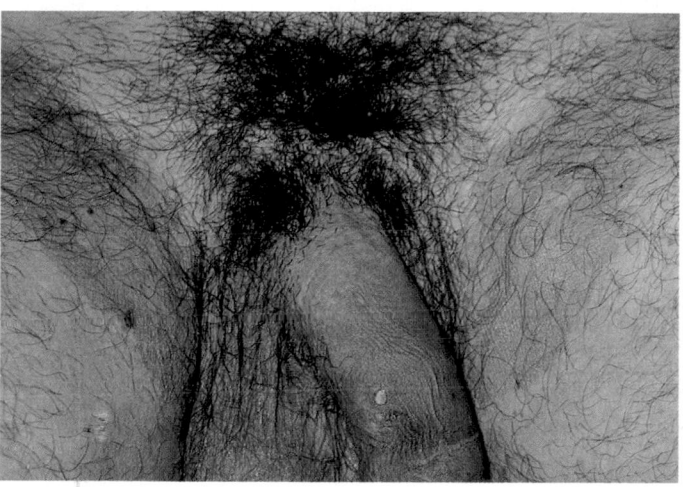

B.

Erythrasma. Well-demarcated erythema in the axilla (*A*) and groin (*B*). The potassium hydroxide preparations were negative; the Wood's lamp examination showed a bright coral red fluorescence.

COURSE AND PROGNOSIS   The disease may remain asymptomatic for years or may undergo periodic exacerbations. Relapses occasionally occur even after successful antibiotic treatment.

MANAGEMENT   For localized erythrasma, especially of the web spaces of the feet, benzoyl peroxide wash and 5 percent gel are effective in most cases. Clindamycin (2 percent solution or azole cream are several of the many effective topical agents.[78] For widespread involvement, oral erythromycin is effective. For secondary prophylaxis, use of an inexpensive antibacterial benzoyl peroxide bar when showering is effective and inexpensive.

Trichomycosis axillaris and pubis   This bacterial infection of the hair shaft (not fungal as the name implies) is characterized by what appears to be nodular thickenings on the hair shaft, composed of colonies of aerobic *Corynebacterium*. The condition occurs both in the axillae and pubic areas, and not just in the axillae, as the name implies. The bacteria produce various pigments, giving the nodules a range of colors. In a study from the United Kingdom, axillary infection was noted in 27 percent of adult male students; in hospitalized mentally retarded patients, the finding was present

FIGURE 195-26

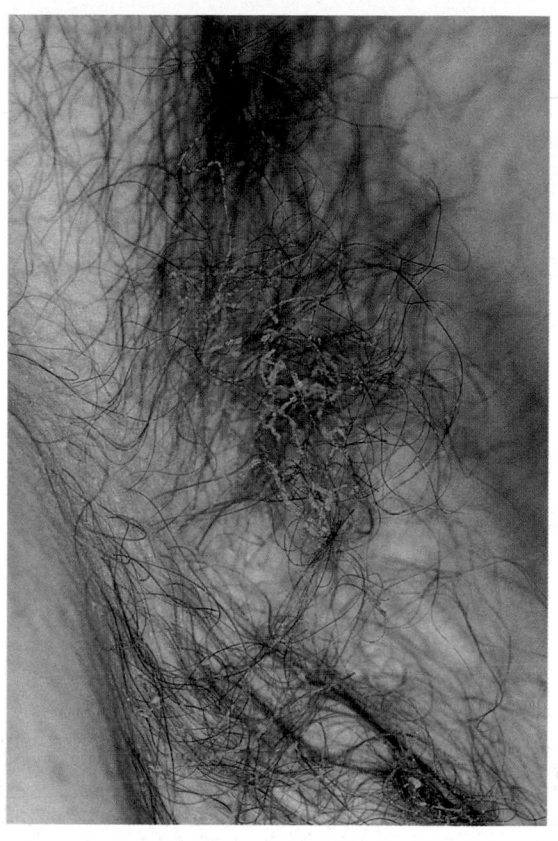

Trichomycosis axillaris. Tan-yellow concretions on the hair shafts of the axilla.

in 42 percent of male patients and in 7 percent of female patients (many of the females had no axillary hair).[79]

Trichomyosis is asymptomatic except for the patient's concern regarding the lesions themselves and because they are malodorous. The concretions on the hair shaft are usually a tan color but may be reddish, yellow, or black (Fig. 195-26). Lesions are most dense in and may be present only in the central portion of the axillary hair. The same lesions may occur in the pubic hair as well.[80]

The diagnosis is usually made on the basis of the physical findings. The concretions can be visualized using a potassium hydroxide preparation. Pediculosis pubis infestation with multiple eggs on the hair shaft should be ruled out.

The involved hair can be removed by shaving. Benzoyl peroxide wash and gel are effective as treatment and prevention against recurrence of trichomycosis.

REFERENCES

1. Hall SL: Coagulase-negative staphylococcal infections in neonates. *Pediatr Infect Dis* **10**:57, 1991
2. Eriksen NHR et al: Carriage of *Staphylococcus aureus* among 104 healthy persons during a 19-month period. *Epidemiol Infect* **115**:51, 1995
3. Tuazon CU: Skin and skin structure infections in the patient at risk: Carrier state of *Staphylococcus aureus*. *Am J Med* **76**(5A):166, 1984

4. Nishijima S et al: *Staphylococcal aureus* in the anterior nares and subungual spaces of the hands in atopic dermatitis. *J Int Med Res* **25**:155, 1997

5. Monti G et al: *Staphylococcal aureus* skin colonization in infants with atopic dermatitis. *Dermatology* **193**:83, 1996

6. Stalder JF et al: Local steroid therapy and bacterial skin flora in atopic dermatitis. *Br J Dermatol* **131**:536, 1994

7. Leung DY, Travers JB, Norris DA: The role of superantigens in skin disease. *J Invest Dermatol* **105**:37S, 1995

8. Kauffman CA et al: Attempts to eradicate methicillin-resistant *Staphylococcus aureus* from a long-term-care facility with the use of mupirocin ointment. *Am J Med* **94**:371, 1993

9. Bradley SF: Effectiveness of mupirocin in the control of methicillin-resistant *Staphylococcus aureus*. *Infect Med* **10**:21, 1993

10. Kluytmans JAJW et al: Nasal carriage of *Staphylococcus aureus* as a major risk factor for wound infections after cardiac surgery. *J Infect Dis* **171**:216, 1995

11. Pujol M et al: Nosocomial *Staphylococcus aureus* bacteremia among nasal carriers of methicillin-resistant and methicillin-susceptible strains. *Am J Med* **100**:509, 1996

12. Barton LL, Friedman AD: Impetigo: A reassessment of etiology and therapy. *Pediatr Dermatol* **4**:185, 1987

13. Mobacken H et al: Epidemiologic aspects of impetigo contagiosa in western Sweden. *Scand J Infect Dis* **7**:39, 1975

14. Dillon HC Jr: Impetigo contagiosa: Suppurative and nonsuppurative complications. *Am J Dis Child* **115**:530, 1968

15. Goldfarb J et al: Randomized clinical trial of topical mupirocin versus oral erythromycin for impetigo. *Antimicrob Agents Chemother* **32**:1780, 1988

16. Dagan R, Bar-David Y: Double-blind study comparing erythromycin and mupirocin for treatment of impetigo in children: Implications of a high prevalence of erythromycin-resistant *Staphylococcus aureus* strains. *Antimicrob Agents Chemother* **36**:287, 1992

17. Allen AM et al: Cutaneous streptococcal infections in Vietnam. *Arch Dermatol* **104**:271, 1971

18. Berkley SF et al: A cluster of blister-associated toxic shock syndrome in male military trainees and a study of staphylococcal carriage patterns. *Milit Med* **154**:496, 1989

19. Reagan DR et al: Elimination of coincident *Staphylococcus aureus* nasal and hand carriage with intranasal application of mupirocin calcium ointment. *Ann Intern Med* **114**:101, 1991

20. Raz R et al: A 1-year trial of nasal mupirocin in the prevention of recurrent staphylococcal nasal colonization and skin infections. *Arch Intern Med* **156**:1109, 1996

21. Wheat LJ et al: Long-term studies of the effect of rifampin on nasal carriage of coagulase-positive staphylococci. *Rev Infect Dis* **5**:S459, 1983

22. Darouiche R et al: Eradication of colonization by methicillin-resistant *Staphylococcus aureus* by using oral minocycline-rifampin and topical mupirocin. *Antimicrob Agents Chemother* **35**:1612, 1991

23. Saenz C et al: Macronodular lesions associated with *Staphylococcus aureus* bacteremia. *Arch Intern Med* **147**:793, 1987

24. Tanaka S et al: Sporotrichoid bacterial infection. *Dermatologica* **178**:228, 1989

25. Lavoie A et al: Anti-Staphylococcus aureus IgE antibodies for diagnosis of hyperimmunoglobulinemia E-recurrent infection syndrome in infancy. *Am J Dis Child* **143**:1038, 1989

26. Sheagren JN: *Staphylococcus aureus:* The persistent pathogen. *N Engl J Med* **310**:1368, 1984

27. Dajani AS: The scalded-skin syndrome: Relation to phage-group II staphylococci. *J Infect Dis* **125**:548, 1972

28. Institute of Medicine, National Academy of Science: Conference on the Toxic Shock Syndrome. *Ann Intern Med* **96**:835, 1982

29. Chu MC et al: Association of toxic shock toxin-1 determinant with a heterologous insertion at multiple loci in the *Staphylococcus aureus* chromosome. *Infect Immun* **56**:2702, 1988

30. Bohach GA et al: Analysis of toxic shock syndrome isolates producing staphylococcal enterotoxins B and C, with use of Southern hybridization and immunologic assays. *Rev Infect Dis* **11**(suppl 1):575, 1989

31. Ikejima T et al: Induction by toxic-shock-syndrome toxin-1 of a circulating tumor necrosis factor-like substance in rabbits and of immunoreactive tumor necrosis factor and interleukin-1 from human mononuclear cells. *J Infect Dis* **158**:1017, 1988

32. Spearman PW, Barson WJ: Toxic shock syndrome occurring in children with abrasive injuries beneath casts. *J Pediatr Orthop B* **12**:169, 1992

33. Leung DY et al: The potential role of bacterial superantigens in the pathogenesis of Kawasaki syndrome. *J Clin Immunol* **15**:11s, 1995

34. Duma RH et al: Streptococcal infections: A bacteriologic and clinical study of streptococcal bacteremia. *Medicine (Baltimore)* **48**:87, 1969

35. Barnham M, Neilson DJ: Group L beta-haemolytic streptococcal infection in meat handlers: Another streptococcal zoonosis? *Epidemiol Infect* **99**:257, 1987

36. Fehrs LJ et al: Group A b-hemolytic streptococcal skin infections in a US meat-packing plant. *JAMA* **258**:3131, 1987

37. Uhr JW (ed): *The Streptococcus, Rheumatic Fever, and Glomerulonephritis.* Baltimore, Williams & Wilkins, 1964

38. Wannamaker LW: Differences between streptococcal infections of the throat and of the skin. *N Engl J Med* **282**:23, 78, 1970

39. Kaplan EL et al: Group A streptococcal serotypes isolated from patients and sibling contacts during the resurgence of rheumatic fever in the United States in the mid-1980's. *J Infect Dis* **159**:101, 1989

40. Wannamaker LW: Differences between streptococcal infections of the throat and of the skin. *N Engl J Med* **282**:23, 78, 1970

41. Dillon HC Jr: Impetigo contagiosa: Suppurative and nonsuppurative complications. *Am J Dis Child* **115**:530, 1968

42. Kaplan EL et al: Group A streptococcal serotypes isolated from patients and sibling contacts during the resurgence of rheumatic fever in the United States in the mid-1980's. *J Infect Dis* **159**:101, 1989

43. Bessen D, Fischetti VA: A human IgG receptor of Group A streptococci is associated with tissue site of infection and streptococcal class. *J Infect Dis* **161**:747, 1990

44. Gerber MA et al: The group A streptococcal carrier state: A reexamination. *Am J Dis Child* **142**:562, 1988

45. Dajani AS et al: Natural history of impetigo. II. Etiologic agents and bacterial interactions. *J Clin Invest* **51**:2863, 1972

46. Ferrieri P et al: Natural history of impetigo. I. Site sequence of acquisition and familial patterns of spread of cutaneous streptococci. *J Clin Invest* **51**:2851, 1972

47. Goldfarb J et al: Randomized clinical trial of topical mupirocin versus oral erythromycin for impetigo. *Antimicrob Agents Chemother* **32**:1780, 1988

48. Britton JW et al: Comparison of mupirocin and erythromycin in the treatment of impetigo. *J Pediatr* **117**:827, 1990

49. Seppälä H et al: The effect of changes in the consumption of macrolide antibiotics on erythromycin resistance in group A streptococci in Finland. *N Engl J Med* **337**:441, 1997

50. Spear RM et al: Perianal streptococcal cellulitis. *J Pediatr* **107**:557, 1985

51. Rehder PA et al: Perianal cellulitis. Cutaneous group A streptococcal disease. *Arch Dermatol* **124**:702, 1988

52. Duhra P, Ilchyshyn A: Perianal streptococcal cellulitis with penile involvement. *Br J Dermatol* **123**:793, 1990

53. Deliyanni VA et al: Balanitis caused by group A beta-hemolytic streptococcus in an 8-year-old boy. *Pediatr Infect Dis* **8**:61, 1989

54. Honig PJ: Guttate psoriasis associated with perianal streptococcal disease. *J Pediatr* **113**:1037, 1988

55. McCray MK, Esterly NB: Blistering distal dactylitis. *J Am Acad Dermatol* **5**:592, 1981

56. Benson PM, Solivan G: Group B streptococcal blistering distal dactylitis in an adult diabetic. *J Am Acad Dermatol* **17**:310, 1987

57. Woroszylski A et al: Staphylococcal blistering dactylitis: report of two patients. *Pediatr Dermatol* **13**:292, 1996

58. Amren DP: Unusual forms of streptococcal disease, in *Streptococci and Streptococcal Diseases,* edited by LW Wannamaker, JM Matsen. New York, Academic, 1972

59. Cone LA et al: Clinical and bacteriologic observations of a toxic shock–like syndrome due to *Streptococcus pyogenes. N Engl J Med* **317**:146, 1987

60. Lee PK, Schlievert PM: Quantification and toxicity of group A streptococcal pyrogenic exotoxins in an animal model of toxic shock syndrome-like illness. *J Clin Microbiol* **27**:1890, 1989

61. Leung DY, Travers JB, Norris DA: The role of superantigens in skin disease. *J Invest Dermatol* **105**:37S, 1995

62. Lee PK, Schlievert PM: Quantification and toxicity of group A streptococcal pyrogenic exotoxins in an animal model of toxic shock syndrome-like illness. *J Clin Microbiol* **27**:1890, 1989

63. Cone LA et al: Clinical and bacteriologic observations of a toxic shock-like syndrome due to *Streptococcus pyogenes. N Engl J Med* **317**:146, 1987

64. Bartter T et al: "Toxic strep syndrome": A manifestation of group A streptococcal infection. *Arch Intern Med* **148**:1421, 1988

65. Jackson MA et al: Multisystem group A β-hemolytic streptococcal disease in children. *Rev Infect Dis* **13**:783, 1991

66. Stevens DL et al: Severe group A streptococcal infections associated with a toxic shock-like syndrome and scarlet fever A. *N Engl J Med* **321**:1, 1989

67. Shaunak S et al: Septic scarlet fever due to *Streptococcus pyogenes* cellulitis. *Q J Med* **69**(new series):921, 1988

68. Alpert JS et al: Pathogenesis of Osler's nodes. *Ann Intern Med* **85**:471, 1976

69. Cardullo AC et al: Janeway lesions and Osler's nodes: A review of histopathologic findings. *J Am Acad Dermatol* **22**:1088, 1990

70. Gray GC et al: Hyperendemic *Streptococcus pyogenes* infection despite prophylaxis with penicillin G benzathine. *N Engl J Med* **352**:92, 1991

71. Taplin D, Zaias N: The etiology of pitted keratolysis. *Proc XIIIth Int Congr Dermatol* **1**:593, 1968

72. Zaias N: Pitted and ringed keratolysis. *J Am Acad Dermatol* **7**:787, 1982

73. Nordstrom KM et al: Pitted keratolysis: the role of *Micrococcus sedentarius*. *Arch Dermatol* **123**:1320, 1987

74. Takama H et al: Pitted keratolysis: Clinical manifestations in 53 cases. *Br J Dermatol* **137**:282, 1997

75. Nordstrom KM et al: The etiology of the malodor associated with pitted keratolysis. *J Invest Dermatol* **87**:159, 1986

76. Tilgren W: Pitted keratolysis (keratolysis plantare sulcatum): Ultrastructural study. *J Cutan Pathol* **6**:18, 1979

77. Sarkany I et al: The etiology and treatment of erythrasma. *J Invest Dermatol* **37**:283, 1961

78. Sindhuphak W et al: Erythrasma: Overlooked or misdiagnosed. *Int J Dermatol* **24**:95, 1985

79. Savin JA et al: The bacterial flora of trichomycosis axillaris. *J Med Microbiol* **3**:252, 1970

80. White SW, Smith J: Trichomycosis pubis. *Arch Dermatol* **115**:444, 1979

CHAPTER 196

Steven D. Resnick
Peter M. Elias

Staphylococcal Scalded-Skin Syndrome

The staphylococcal scalded-skin syndrome encompasses a spectrum of blistering skin disease that ranges in severity from localized bullous impetigo to a generalized syndrome with cutaneous tenderness, widespread blistering, and superficial denudation/desquamation. The disorder is caused by toxigenic strains of *Staphylococcus aureus*, usually belonging to phage group 2.

HISTORY

In 1878, Ritter von Rittershain, director of an orphanage in Prague, described 297 cases of "dermatitis exfoliative neonatorum."[1] Subsequently, a relationship of the disease to staphylococci was appreciated.[2] During the late 1940s and early 1950s, the link between bullous impetigo and phage group 2 staphylococci became evident. The report of toxic epidermal necrolysis (TEN) by Lyell[3] drew attention to the similarity of the condition to the appearance of generalized scalding but also led to a period of confusion between nonstaphylococcal TEN and the bacterial toxin–mediated scalded-skin syndrome.[4] The situation was clarified with the development of a murine model of the staphylococcal disease.[5] The staphylococcal scalded-skin syndrome is now clearly distinguished from other diseases of generalized epidermal necrolysis.[6]

ETIOLOGY AND PATHOGENESIS

Two staphylococcal exotoxins, the epidermolytic toxins A and B (ET-A and ET-B), are responsible for the pathogenic changes of the scalded-skin syndrome. Although most toxigenic strains of *S. aureus* are identified by group 2 phage (types 71 and 55), toxin producers have also been identified among phage groups 1 and 3.[7,8]

TABLE 196-1

Clinical Forms of Staphylococcal Scalded-Skin Syndrome

Disease	Obsolete Name	Intact Bullae	Age Distribution
Bullous impetigo	Pemphigus neonatorum	+	All ages
Bullous impetigo with generalization	Pemphigus neonatorum	+	Biphasic (neonates and immunocompromised adults)
Scarlatiniform eruption	None	−	Neonates and young children
Generalized scalded-skin syndrome (Ritter's disease)	Toxic epidermal necrolysis	−	Neonates and young children

SOURCE: Elias PM et al: *Arch Dermatol* **113**:207, 1977.

Both of the epidermolytic toxins produce blistering and denudation by disruption of the epidermal granular cell layer, apparently by direct effects on desmosomes, leading to interdesmosomal splitting.[9] The toxins appear to bind directly to the desmosomal protein desmoglein-1,[10] but the mechanism of toxin action in the epidermis is not fully understood. In a report of scalded-skin syndrome in a premature infant, acantholysis was seen in association with intercellular edema and separation of ultrastructurally unaltered desmosomes.[11] Although epidermal cell separation appears attributable to epidermolytic toxin, not all of the clinical manifestations of the scalded-skin syndrome are explained by epidermolytic toxin action. Purified epidermolytic toxin does not cause erythema in either neonatal mice or humans, leading some investigators to suggest that the delta-hemolysin toxin may play an important role in the full expression of the syndrome.[12]

The epidermolytic toxins display limited homology to the staphylococcal enterotoxins and toxic shock syndrome toxin 1. Some investigators believe that the epidermolytic toxins share superantigenic activity with these other known staphylococcal superantigens. However, clinical toxic shock–like presentations have not been described in patients with epidermolytic toxin–producing staphylococcal infections. Recombinant epidermolytic toxin A has been shown to possess no superantigenic activity, and it has been proposed that previous reports of superantigenic activity of epidermolytic toxins resulted from the use of preparations contaminated by minute quantities of other staphylococcal exotoxins.[13] Details of the biochemistry, biochemical genetics, and properties of the epidermolytic toxins have been reviewed elsewhere.[6,7,12,14,15]

Children under 5 years of age, and particularly neonates, are most commonly affected by staphylococcal scalded-skin syndrome. This epidemiologic pattern is explained by the importance of mature renal function in the clearance of epidermolytic toxins. The combination of decreased ability to achieve renal clearance of toxin[16] and lack of specific immunity to the toxins makes neonates the highest risk group.

There has been a case report of congenital scalded-skin syndrome in an infant born to a mother with staphylococcal chorioamnionitis.[17] Older children and adults may also develop the disease. In such cases, pathologic renal insufficiency or immunodeficiency appear to explain the susceptibility to the syndrome. Recent reports have highlighted the problem of scalded-skin syndrome in adults, including a case associated with HIV disease[18] and a review summarizing 32 cases in adults.[19] Unlike most cases in young children, adults with scalded-skin syndrome are often found to have positive blood cultures for toxigenic *S. aureus*, and mortality can be significant.

TABLE 196-2

Differentiation of Toxic Epidermal Necrolysis (TEN) and Staphylococcal Scalded-Skin Syndrome (SSSS)

	TEN	SSSS
History	Drug intake; often milder episode preceding	Variable drug intake; first episode
Family history	Noncontributory	Members of family often have impetigo or harbor staphylococci
Epidemiologic features	Cases sporadic	Sometimes linked to epidemics of impetigo
Age predilection	Over 40 years	Under 5 years
Exanthemata	Generalized without clear distribution	Typical distribution pattern and succession of development (face, neck, axillae, groin first)
Cutaneous tenderness	Mild to moderate	Marked
Nikolsky's sign	Positive only in lesions	Positive also in apparently uninvolved skin
Mucous membranes	Severely afflicted	Uninvolved
Course	Protracted (2–3 weeks)	Brief (2–4 days)
Mortality	High (25–50%)	Very low; high incidence of spontaneous recovery
Systemic therapy	Glucocorticoids?	Penicillinase-resistant penicillins; glucocorticoids alone contraindicated
Histologic features	Necrolysis of epidermis, starting in basal layer	Acantholysis; subgranular cleavage
Exfoliative cytologic features*	Necrotic epidermal cells, polymorphs, debris	Normal-appearing acantholytic cells

*Particularly useful for rapid bedside differential diagnosis.
NOTE: This table contains only points where differences exist between the two diseases and only considers the rules, not the exceptions.
SOURCE: Elias PM et al: *Arch Dermatol* **113**:207, 1977.

FIGURE 196-1

CHAPTER 196
Staphylococcal Scalded-Skin Syndrome

2209

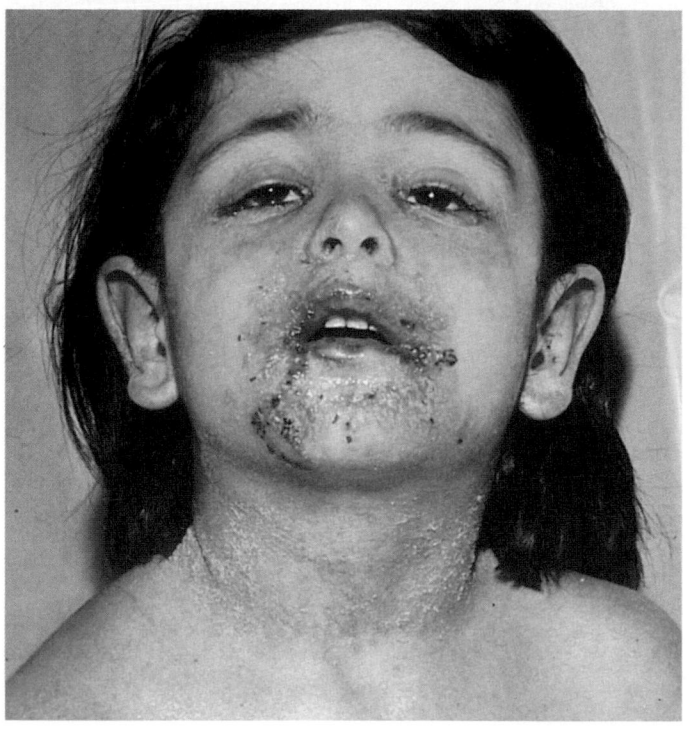

Early stage of generalized staphylococcal scalded-skin syndrome. Initial manifestation may be occult nasopharyngeal, conjunctival, or ear infection, followed by periorificial erythema and crusting.

desquamation (Fig. 196-4), and healing is usually complete within 5 to 7 days. Cultures obtained from intact bullae are usually sterile, consistent with the scenario of hematogenous dissemination of toxin produced at a distant focus of staphylococcal infection. The healing phase may be characterized by very extensive desquamation, with marked perioral crusting and fissuring.

Localized Forms

Bullous impetigo is a localized manifestation of cutaneous staphylococcal infection by toxigenic strains, without hematogenous dissemination of toxin. Presumably, immunity to the toxin plays a crucial role in preventing dissemination, but other factors, including the total burden of toxin and renal clearance of toxin, play a role. As with generalized staphylococcal scalded-skin syndrome, bullous impetigo is predominantly a disease of children, although adult cases also occur.[6] The early lesions are vesicles or bullae filled with cloudy fluid surrounded by an erythematous rim (Fig. 196-5), but more commonly, superficial erosions with a silvery sheen and minimal crusting predominate. The lesions tend to be concentrated on exposed parts of the body and around body orifices. In contrast to generalized scalded-skin syndrome, both Gram stain and cultures of blisters reveal staphylococci, and cutaneous tenderness is absent. Rarely, localized bullous impetigo can progress to generalized scalded-skin syndrome.

Abortive Forms

An abortive form of staphylococcal scalded-skin syndrome, known as the *scarlatiniform variant*, shows the early erythrodermic and final desquamative stages seen in Ritter's disease, but the bullous

CLINICAL FEATURES (See Tables 196-1 and 196-2)

Generalized Form (Ritter's Disease)

Affected children initially have a faint, orange-red macular exanthem, typically associated with purulent conjunctivitis, otitis media, or occult nasopharyngeal infection (Fig. 196-1). Although the rash is not distinctive in appearance, cutaneous tenderness is often apparent at this stage. Periorificial and flexural accentuation may be observed. Also, even prior to the appearance of clinical blisters, a positive Nikolsky's sign can often be elicited (Fig. 196-2). Within 24 to 48 h, the rash progresses from a scarlatiniform to a blistering eruption. Characteristic tissue paper–like wrinkling of the epidermis is followed by the appearance of large, flaccid bullae (Fig. 196-3A) in the axillae, groin, and around the body orifices. Subsequent generalized involvement elsewhere on the body occurs but spares the mucous membranes. As sheets of epidermis are shed, a moist, erythematous base is revealed (Fig. 196-3B). Despite the worrisome appearance of the disease, which at this stage resembles generalized scalding, the entire process usually dries with superficial

FIGURE 196-2

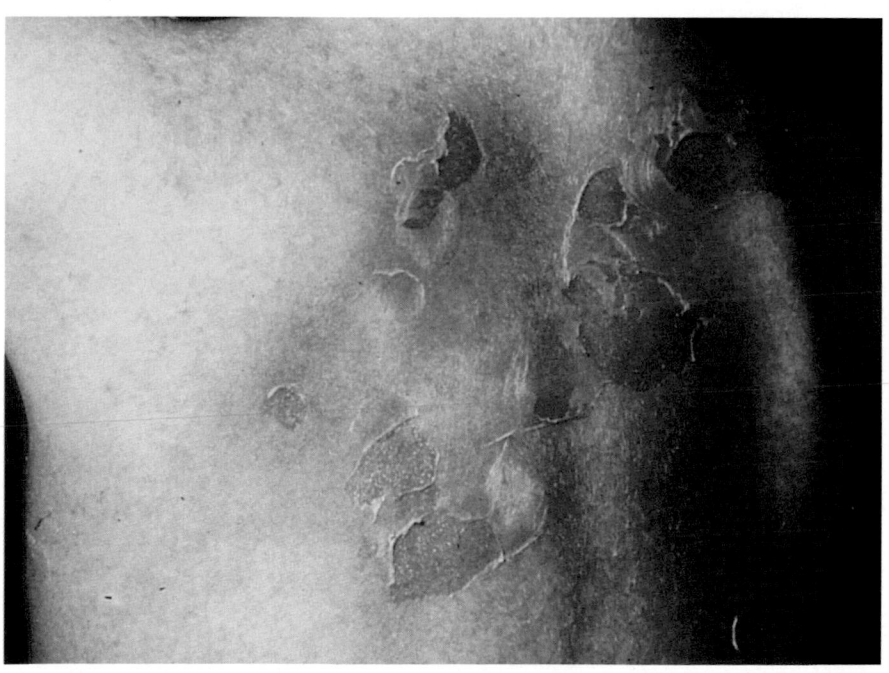

Generalized indistinct erythemas develop, accompanied by a positive Nikolsky's sign and superficial erosions.

FIGURE 196-3

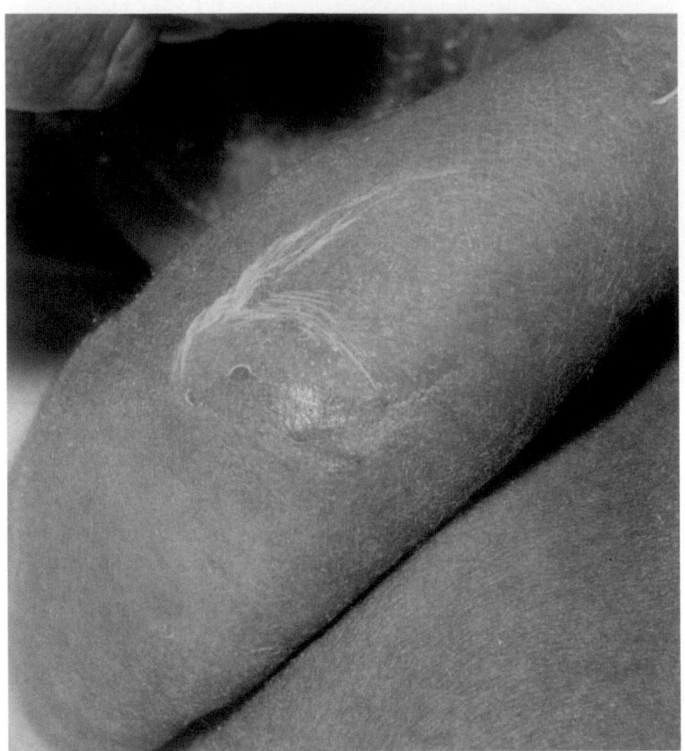

A.

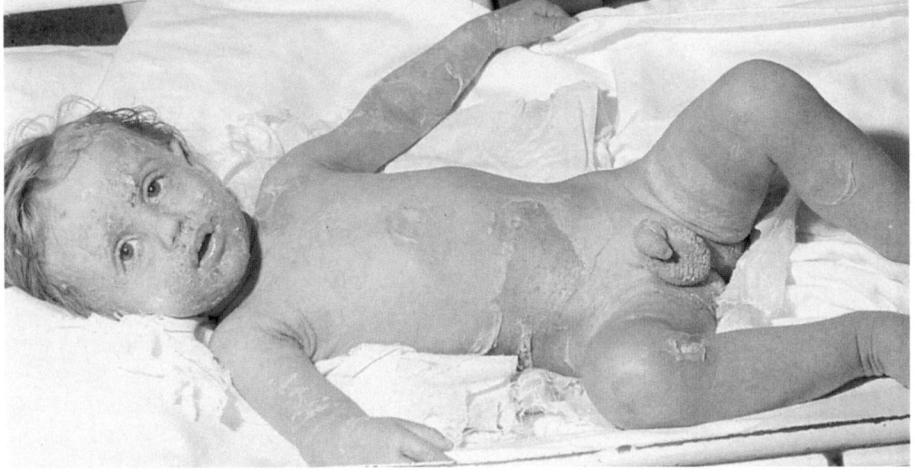

B.

Advanced stages show (*A*) flaccid bullae and (*B*) large denuded areas similar to scalding.

stage does not occur.[20] Such cases may be confused with other toxic exanthems, including toxic shock syndrome. Other intermediate forms of scalded-skin syndrome may be seen that begin as localized bullous impetigo but evolve to produce regionally limited bullae and denuded areas that may or may not harbor staphylococci.

LIGHT MICROSCOPIC AND ULTRASTRUCTURAL PATHOLOGY

All forms of the scalded-skin syndrome are characterized by intraepidermal cleavage, with splitting occurring beneath and within the stratum granulosum.[21] The cleavage space may contain free-floating or partially attached acantholytic cells (Fig. 196-6*A*), but the remainder of the epidermis appears unremarkable and the dermis contains no inflammatory cells, except in cases of localized disease (bullous impetigo). Cells bordering the cleavage space appear uninjured; ultrastructurally, separation seems to occur by simultaneous splitting of the desmosomes and interdesmosomal regions.[22] The noncytotoxicity of the cleavage process has been demonstrated experimentally,[23] and the cell surface target may be desmoglein-1, as noted above.[10]

DIAGNOSIS AND DIFFERENTIAL DIAGNOSIS
(see Table 196-2)

The principal diagnostic problem is distinguishing scalded-skin syndrome from TEN (Table 196-2) (see Chap. 59). Although TEN is rare in infancy and childhood, distinctions based solely on age are risky because TEN can occur in children and scalded-skin syndrome in adults.[4–6,19] Although the use of exfoliative cytology (Fig. 196-7)* and frozen sections (Fig. 196-6*B*) for the rapid bedside differential diagnosis can be particularly

---

*Smears are made from scrapings of Nikolsky-positive areas and after short fixation are stained with methylene blue or Giemsa stain. The test is considered positive when large "fried egg"–like cells are seen.

FIGURE 196-4

CHAPTER 196
Staphylococcal Scalded-Skin Syndrome

2211

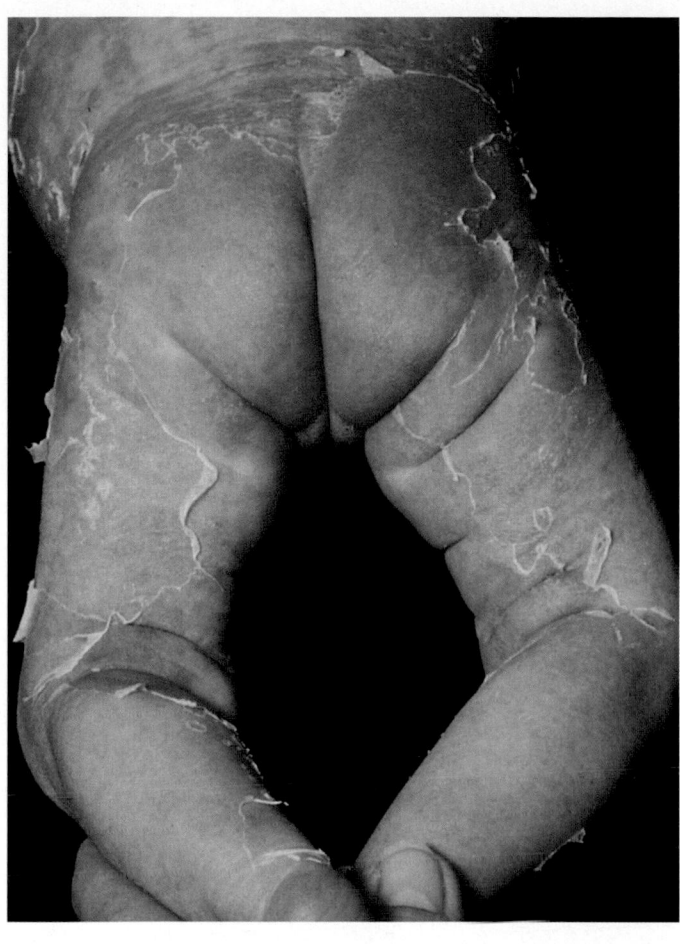

Late stage of generalized staphylococcal scalded-skin syndrome: generalized desquamation with characteristic large sheets.

useful in guiding initial therapy,[24,25] the definitive diagnosis depends on culture and biopsy results. In contrast to the subgranular epidermolysis of the scalded-skin syndrome, TEN produces full-thickness epidermal necrosis and a dermal-epidermal separation.

TREATMENT AND PROGNOSIS

Therapy for scalded-skin syndrome should be directed toward eradication of staphylococci from the focus of infection, which generally requires intravenous penicillinase-resistant antistaphylococcal antibiotics. Usually, oral antibiotic therapy can be substituted within several days or sooner. Antibiotics, supportive skin care, and appropriate attention to fluid and electrolyte management in the presence of disrupted barrier function will usually ensure rapid recovery. The disease still carries a significant mortality (2 to 3 percent), and the morbidity from occasional children who develop cellulitis, sepsis, and pneumonia should not be ignored.[6] Adult patients with scalded-skin syndrome are more likely to be immunosuppressed and suffering from other medical problems. They are much more likely than children to have staphylococcal bacteremia and have a poorer prognosis.[19]

It is important to recognize the potential for epidemic scalded-skin syndrome in neonatal care units.[26] Identification of health care workers colonized or infected with toxigenic *S. aureus* is an integral part of managing the problem. Control measures should be applied, including strict enforcement of chlorhexidine hand washing, oral antibiotic therapy for infected workers, and mupirocin ointment for eradication of persistent nasal carriage.[27]

FIGURE 196-5

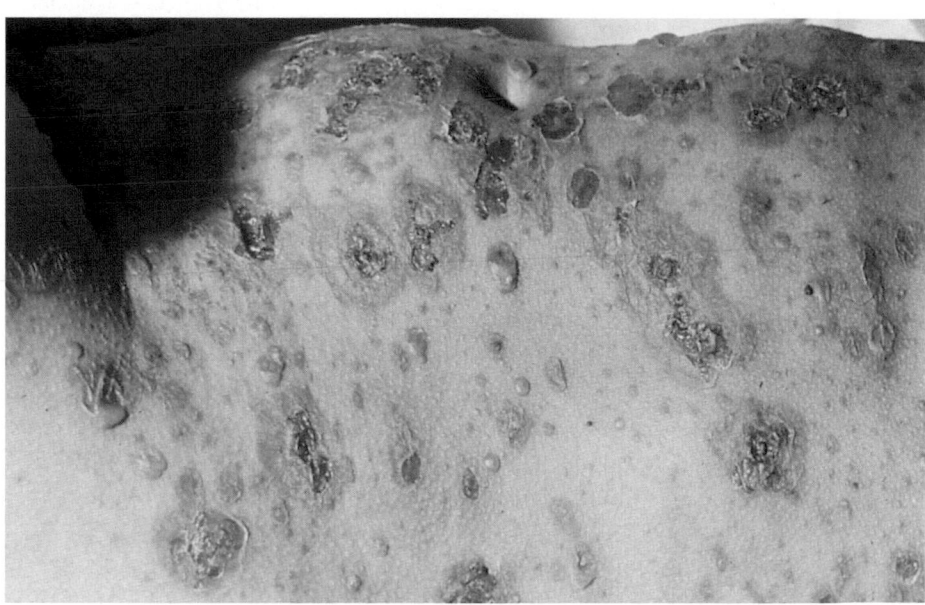

Bullous impetigo due to phage group 2 staphylococci. Blisters are initially filled with cloudy fluid and later rupture, leading to erosions and crusting.

FIGURE 196-6

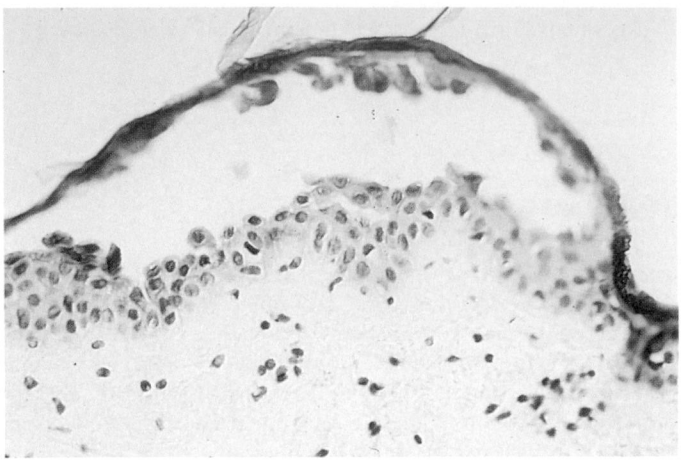

A.

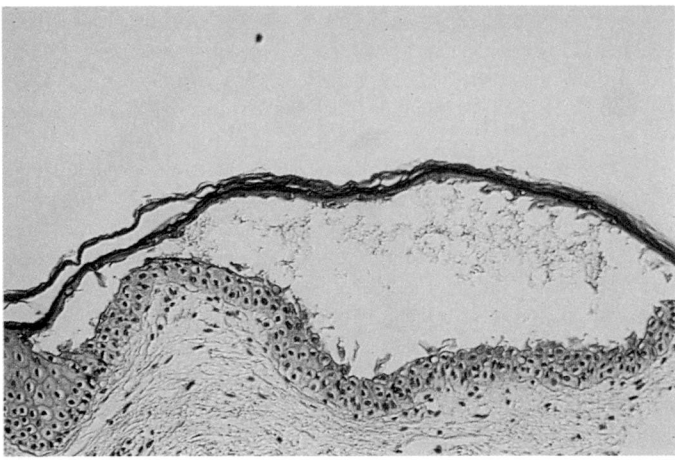

B.

Generalized (*A*) and localized (*B*) staphylococcal scalded-skin syndrome. In both conditions, intraepidermal cleavage occurs within or immediately beneath the stratum granulosum. However, although inflammatory cells are absent in the generalized disease, in the localized form (bullous impetigo) an acute infiltrate impinges and extends from the dermis into the epidermis.

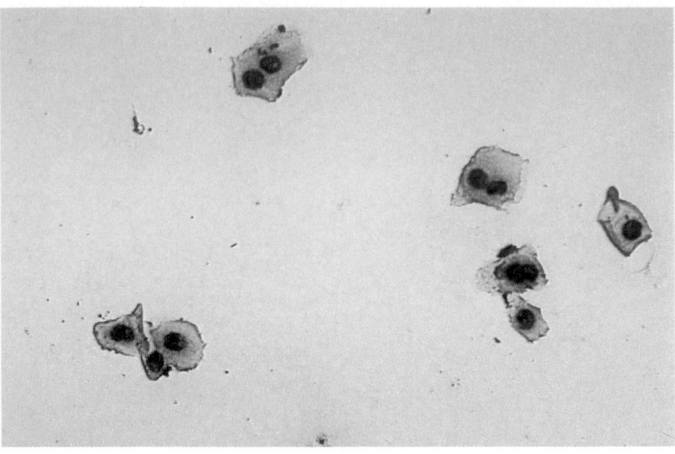

A.

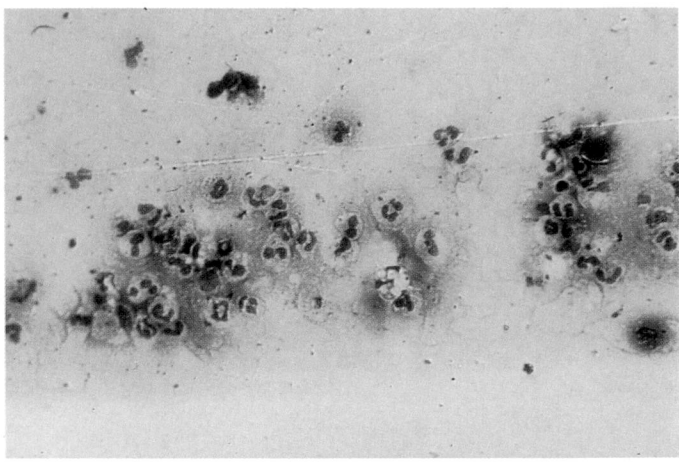

B.

Giemsa-stained exfoliative cytology preparations from lesions of staphylococcal scalded-skin syndrome and drug-induced toxic epidermal necrolysis. In the former (*A*), flattened, fried egg–like nucleated squamae predominate; in the latter (*B*), cellular debris, leukocytes, and occasional cuboidal keratinocytes appear.

REFERENCES

1. Ritter von Rittershain G: Die exfolative Dermatitis jüngerer Säuglinge. *Zentralzeitung fur Kinderheilkunde* **2**:3, 1878
2. Jadassohn J: Die Pyodermien. *Samml Abh Dermatol* **1**:H2, 1912
3. Lyell A: Toxic epidermal necrolysis: An eruption resembling scalding of the skin. *Br J Dermatol* **68**:355, 1956
4. Lyell A: Toxic epidermal necrolysis (the scalded skin syndrome): A reappraisal. *Br J Dermatol* **100**:69, 1979
5. Melish ME, Glasgow A: The staphylococcal scalded skin syndrome: Development of an experimental mouse model. *N Engl J Med* **282**:1114, 1970
6. Resnick SD et al: The staphylococcal scalded skin and toxic shock syndromes, in *Physiology, Biochemistry, and Molecular Biology of the Skin*, 2d ed, edited by LA Goldsmith. Oxford, Oxford University Press, 1992, p 1287

7. Rogolshy M et al: Nonenteric toxins of *Staphylococcus aureus*. *Microbiol Res* **43**:320, 1980
8. Florman A, Holzman RS: Nosocomial staphylococcal scalded skin syndrome. Report of a case. *Am J Dis Child* **134**:1043, 1980
9. Murono K et al: Microbiologic characteristics of exfoliative toxin-producing *Staphylococcus aureus*. *Pediatr Infect Dis J* **7**:313, 1988
10. Takagi Y et al: Action site of exfoliative toxin on keratinocytes. *J Invest Dermatol* **94**:52a, 1990
11. Hoffmann R et al: Staphylococcal scalded skin syndrome and consecutive septicaemia in a preterm infant. *Pathol Res Pract* **190**:77, 1994
12. Gemmell CG: Staphylococcal scalded skin syndrome. *J Med Microbiol* **43**:318, 1995
13. Fleischer B, Bailey CJ: Recombinant epidermolytic toxin A of *Staphylococcus aureus* is not a superantigen. *Med Microbiol Immunol* **180**:273, 1992
14. Resnick SD: Staphylococcal toxin-mediated syndromes in childhood. *Semin Dermatol* **11**:11, 1992
15. Elias PM et al: Staphylococcal toxic epidermal necrolysis: Species and tissue susceptibility and resistance. *J Invest Dermatol* **66**:80, 1976
16. Fritsch P et al: The fate of staphylococcal exfoliation in newborn and adult mice. *Br J Dermatol* **95**:275, 1976

17. Loughead JL: Congenital staphylococcal scalded skin syndrome. *Pediatr Infect Dis J* **11**:413, 1992
18. Farrell AM et al: Staphylococcal scalded skin syndrome in an HIV-1 seropositive man. *Br J Dermatol* **134**:962, 1996
19. Cribier B et al: Staphylococcal scalded skin syndrome in adults: A clinical review. *J Am Acad Dermatol* **30**:319, 1994
20. Melish ME, Glasgow LA: The staphylococcal scalded skin syndrome: The expanded clinical syndrome. *J Pediatr* **78**:958, 1971
21. Koblenzer PJ: Acute epidermal necrolysis (Ritter von Rittershain–Lyell): A clinicopathologic study. *Arch Dermatol* **95**:608, 1967
22. Lillibridge DB et al: Site of action of exfoliative toxin in the staphylococcal scalded skin syndrome. *Pediatrics* **50**:728, 1972
23. Elias PM et al: Staphylococcal exfoliative toxin: Pathogenesis and subcellular site of action. *J Invest Dermatol* **65**:501, 1975
24. Fritsch P: Staphylogene toxische epidermale Nekrolyse: Teil 1. Krankheit und ihre Symptomatik. *Z Hautkr* **59**:477, 1974
25. Amon RB, Diamond RL: Toxic epidermal necrolysis: Rapid differentiation between staphylococcal- and drug-induced disease. *Arch Dermatol* **111**:1433, 1975
26. Dancer SJ et al: Outbreak of staphylococcal scalded skin syndrome among neonates. *J Infect* **16**:87, 1988
27. Hoeger PH, Elsner P: Staphylococcal scalded skin syndrome: Transmission of exfoliatin-producing *S. aureus* by an asymptomatic carrier. *Pediatr Infect Dis J* **7**:340, 1988

CHAPTER 197

Hensin Tsao
Morton N. Swartz
Arnold N. Weinberg
Richard Allen Johnson

Soft Tissue Infections: Erysipelas, Cellulitis, and Gangrenous Cellulitis

Soft tissue infections (STIs), or cellulitides, are characterized by an acute, diffuse, spreading, edematous, suppurative inflammation of the dermis and subcutaneous tissues, often associated with systemic symptoms of malaise, fever, and chills. Nonnecrotizing STIs are treated with antibiotics, drainage of abscesses, and supportive measures. Necrotizing STIs are often life-threatening and require, in addition, extensive surgical debridement.

Erysipelas is a distinct type of superficial cutaneous cellulitis with marked dermal lymphatic vessel involvement due to group A β-hemolytic streptococcus (group A streptococcus; very uncommonly group C or G streptococcus) and rarely due to *Staphylococcus aureus*. Group B streptococci can cause erysipelas in the newborn.

Cellulitis, which may begin as erysipelas, involves more of the soft tissues, extending deeper into the dermis and subcutaneous tissue. *S. aureus* and group A streptococci are by far the most common etiologic agents, but occasionally other bacteria are implicated (e.g., group B streptococci in the newborn, pneumococci, a variety of gram-negative bacilli, and *Cryptococcus*.

Gangrenous cellulitis, characterized by necrosis of the dermis, hypodermis, fascia, or muscle, is classified as necrotizing fasciitis, clostridial STI, and progressive bacterial synergistic gangrene.

ETIOLOGY

See Table 197-1

PATHOGENESIS

Normal skin plays a critical role in the defense against a wide range of pathogens. The details of the host-pathogen interaction are poorly understood but appear to involve barrier function, bacterial factors, and host factors (Fig. 197-1).

Barrier Function

The keratinized epidermis provides physical protection against bacterial entry. STIs often arise at a defect in the integrity of epidermis associated with an underlying dermatosis, traumatic or operative wound, burn, or other cutaneous lesions. STIs occur as pathogens invade the dermis and subcutis; inflammation ensues as a response

TABLE 197-1

Etiology of Soft Tissue Infections

TYPE OF INFECTION	MOST COMMON CAUSE(S)	UNCOMMON CAUSES
I. Erysipelas	Group A streptococcus	Group B, C, and G streptococcus
		S. aureus
II. Cellulitis	S. aureus	Group B, C, and G streptococcus
	Group A streptococcus	Erysipelothrix rhusiopathiae
		Pneumococcus
		H. influenzae (children)
		E. coli
		Campylobacter jejuni
		Moraxella
		Serratia, Proteus, other Enterobacteriaceae
		Cryptococcus neoformans
		Legionella pneumophila L. micdadei
		Bacillus anthracis (anthrax)
		Aeromonas hydrophila
		Vibrio vilnificus, V. alginolyticus
III. Cellulitis in children	S. aureus	Group B streptococcus (neonates)
	Group A streptococcus	
A. Facial/periorbital cellulitis	H. influenzae (young children)	Neisseria meningitidis
B. Perianal cellulitis	Group A streptococcus	S. aureus
IV. Cellulitis secondary to bacteremia	Pseudomonas aeruginosa	V. vulnificus
		Streptococcus pneumoniae
		Group A and B streptococcus
V. Crepitant cellulitis	Clostridia species (C. perfringens, C. septicum)	Bacteroides spp.
		Peptostreptococci
		E. coli, Klebsiella
VI. Cellulitis associated with water exposure	E. rhusiopathiae (erysipeloid)	Seal finger (etiology unknown)
	Vibrio vulnificus	
	Aeromonas hydrophila	
	Mycobacterium marinum (nodular lymphangitis)	
	M. fortuitum complex	
VII. Gangrenous cellulitis (infectious gangrene)		
A. Necrotizing fasciitis (NF)		
1. Streptococcal gangrne	Group A streptococcus	Groups B, C, G streptococcus
2. Nonstreptococcal NF	Mixed infection with one or more anaerobes (Peptostreptococcus or Bacteroides) plus at least one	facultative species (non-group A streptococci; members of the Enterobacteriaceae such as Enterobacter, Proteus, etc.)
	Bacillus cereus (granulocytic patients)	
3. Synergistic necrotizing* cellulitis (necrotizing cutaneous myositis, synergistic nonclostridial anaerobic myonecrosis)	Polymicrobial with aerobic and anaerobic organisms that originate in the intestine; one-third of patients have positive blood cultures, usually a coliform, Bacteroides, or Peptostreptococcus.	
a. Aerobes	Coliforms: E. coli, Proteus, Klebsiella	
b. Anaerobes	Bacteroides, Peptostreptococcus, Clostridium, Fusobacterium	
4. Fournier's gangrene	Similar to nonstreptococcal NF	
B. Clostridial STIs	C. perfringens	
	Other histotoxic clostridial spp.	
1. Anaerobic cellulitis		
2. Anaerobic myonecrosis (gas gangrene)		
3. Spontaneous, nontraumatic anaerobic myonecrosis	C. septicum (bacteremic)	
C. Nonclostridial anaerobic cellulitis	Various Bacteroides spp.	
	Peptostreptococci	
	Peptococci	

(continued)

TABLE 197-1 (*Continued*)

D. Progressive bacterial synergistic gangrene (Meleney's gancrene)	Mixed bacterial infection	
1. Ulcer base	S. aureus	Proteus spp. Other gram-negative bacilli
2. Advancing margin	Microaerophilic or anaerobic streptococci	
E. Gangrenous cellulitis in the immunosuppressed individual	P. aeruginosa (ecthyma gangrenosum)	
Mucoraceae (Mucor, Rhizopus, Absidia)		
		Bacillus spp.

*Essentially the same as nonstreptococcal NF but with some involvement of adjacent skeletal muscle.

to the invasion. Isolation of the organism is not possible in the majority of cases, suggesting that the majority of the clinical findings are mediated by secreted cytokines.[1] The portal of entry can be somewhat remote, such as interdigital tinea pedis giving rise to cellulitis occurring above the ankle or erysipelas of the face occurring in association with colonization of the nasopharynx by group A streptococcus; the route of extension to the soft tissue of the face is unclear. Less commonly, STIs may arise associated with bacteremia and seeding of the skin, as occurs in *Vibrio vulnificus* infec-

tions. In some cases, the portal of entry of infection is not apparent—neither a local nor hematogenous source can be detected.

Bacterial Factors

The normal flora of human skin is composed primarily of aerobic diphtheroids (*Corynebacterium* spp.), anaerobic diphtheroids (*Propionobacterium acnes*), and coagulase-negative staphylococci (see Chap. 195 As in the gastrointestinal tract, when the normal flora is

FIGURE 197-1

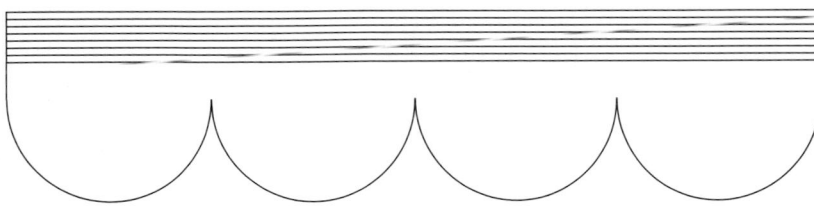

BREACH OF BARRIER FUNCTION
Underlying Dermatoses
• Inflammatory dermatoses: atopic dermatitis, contact dermatitis, stasis dermatitis, psoriasis, chronic cutaneous lupus, pyoderma gangrenosum
• Bullous diseases: pemphigus, bullous pemphigoid, sunburn, porphyria cutanea tarda
• Ulcers: pressure, stasis, ischemic, diabetic
• Umbilical stump (neonates)
• Superficial pyoderma: impetigo, folliculitis, furuncle, carbuncle, ecthyma
• Herpes simplex, varicella, herpes zoster
• Dermatophytosis: tinea pedis, tinea capitis, tinea barbae
Trauma
• Abrasion, laceration, puncture
• Bites: human, animal, insect
• Burns
Surgical wound
• Intravascular catheter
• Surgical incisions

BACTERIAL FACTORS
• Diminished normal flora
• Increased growth of pathogenic species
• Elaboration of toxins and enzymes

HOST FACTORS
Diminished Immune Status
• Diabetes mellitus
• Cancer
• Cancer chemotherapy
• Renal failure
• Nephrotic syndrome
• Alcohol abuse
• Drug abuse
• Malnutrition
• Neutropenia
• Iatrogenic immunosuppression
• HIV disease
• Congenital immunodeficiencies

Circulatory Comprom
• Abnormal lymphatics
• Thrombophlebitis
• Diabetes mellitus
• Lymphedema
• Nephrotic syndrome

Host-pathogen interaction.

eradicated or diminished, pathogenic species may proliferate. Once established, STIs spread via tissue spaces and cleavage planes as hyaluronidases break down polysaccharide ground substances, fibrinolysins digest fibrin barriers, and lecithinases destroy cell membranes. STIs also have a propensity to invade lymphatic and blood vessels, resulting in lymphangitis, lymphadenitis, bacteremia, and septicemia. Local production of exotoxins within the site of infection by *S. aureus* or group A streptococcus may result in staphylococcal scalded skin syndrome (SSSS), toxic shock syndrome (TSS), scarlet fever, or streptococcal toxic shock–like syndrome (STSS).

The strains of group A streptococcus most frequently isolated from invasive infections belong to M types 1, 3, 12, and 28. There is evidence to suggest that the M proteins determine resistance to phagocytosis and invasiveness, while elaboration of streptococcal pyrogenic exotoxin A and B leads to specific clinical syndromes.[2,3]

Host Factors

Two major determinants of the host response to pathogens are the local circulatory physiology and the immunologic status of the patient. Lymphedema associated with abnormal lymphatic drainage (post–radical mastectomy, post–saphenous vein harvest), chronic venous insufficiency, or nephrotic syndrome predisposes to cellulitis. STI of the lower legs can be complicated by thrombophlebitis. Prior cellulitis at a site is often associated with compromise of lymphatic vessels, which predisposes to recurring cellulitis. Many underlying medical conditions can render an individual more susceptible to development of cellulitis by impairing the immune system.

Gangrenous cellulitis (infectious gangrene) occurs as a consequence of thrombosis or occlusion of nutrient dermal and subcutaneous blood vessels. Recent studies have also implicated tumor necrosis factor α as a potential mediator of vascular injury.[4] When the cutaneous sensory nerves are destroyed, local tenderness is replaced by anesthesia. Depending on the pathogen, the host's immune status, and associated medical conditions, the microbes may enter lymphatics (with subsequent lymphangitis and lymphadenitis) or blood vessels (with resultant bacteremia and septicemia).

SUBJECTIVE FINDINGS

In some cases there is a history of an antecedent lesion (stasis ulcer, puncture wound). With onset of the infection, patients experience erythema, local pain, and tenderness and variable degrees of systemic symptoms (fever, chills, and malaise) as the infection spreads. Erythema at the site of infection rapidly intensifies and spreads. Local pain is often marked. In some individuals, systemic symptoms may antedate localizing symptoms and signs of STIs. In a study of 50 patients with cellulitis, only 26 percent had fever $\geq 38°C$.[5] A potential portal of entry was identified in 66 percent of patients: 50 percent of those with upper extremity and 67 percent of those with lower extremity cellulitis. Patients with gangrenous cellulitis may experience severe pain. Postoperative wound infections often arise within 1 to 2 days of the procedure.

OBJECTIVE FINDINGS

ERYSIPELAS This presents as a painful, bright-red, edematous indurated plaque with an advancing raised border, sharply demarcated from the surrounding normal skin (Figs. 197-2 and 197-3). Marking the edge of a cellulitic area with an indelible pen allows extension or regression of the lesion to be observed. The legs (Fig. 197-3) and face are the most commonly involved sites. In cases of facial erysipelas, edema is marked and the eyes are often swollen shut (Fig. 197-2). Erysipelas may extend more deeply into the subcutaneous tissue with resultant cellulitis.

ACUTE CELLULITIS This has many of the features of erysipelas but extends into the subcutaneous tissues. Cellulitis is differentiated from erysipelas by two physical findings: cellulitic lesions are not raised and its demarcation from uninvolved skin is indistinct. In addition, the tissue feels hard upon palpation and is extremely painful. In a study of 50 children with cellulitis, 16 percent of cases had facial infection with the remaining cases on an extremity, the leg being affected three times as often as the arm.[6] In some cases of cellulitis, the overlying epidermis undergoes bulla formation or necrosis, resulting in extensive areas of epidermal sloughing and superficial erosion (Fig. 197-4A). In other cases, with or without antibiotic therapy, infection may localize in the soft tissue, with

FIGURE 197-2

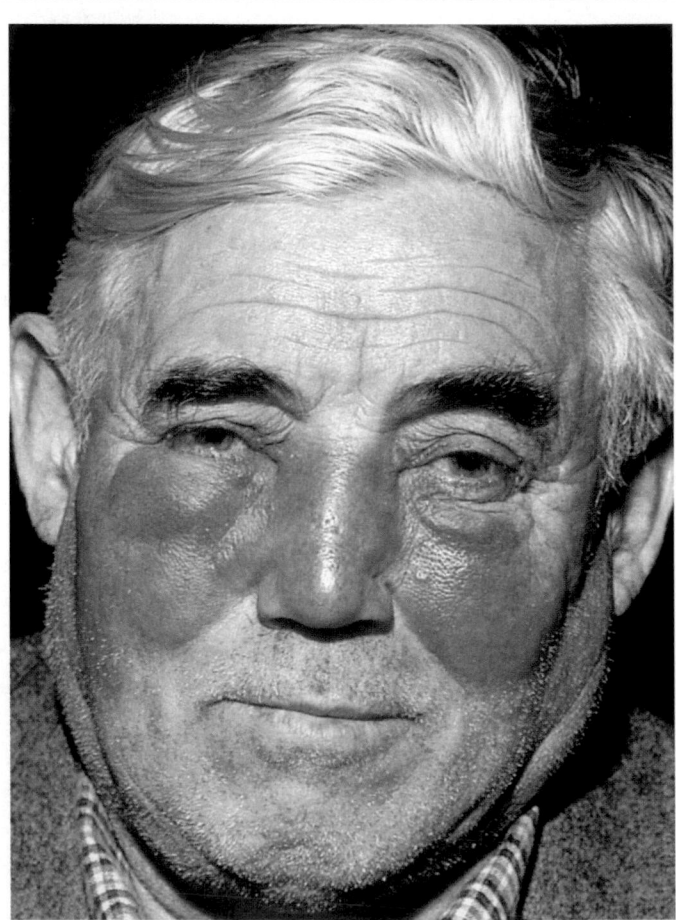

Erysipelas. Painful, edematous erythema with sharp margination on both cheeks and the nose.

FIGURE 197-3

CHAPTER 197
Soft Tissue Infections

2217

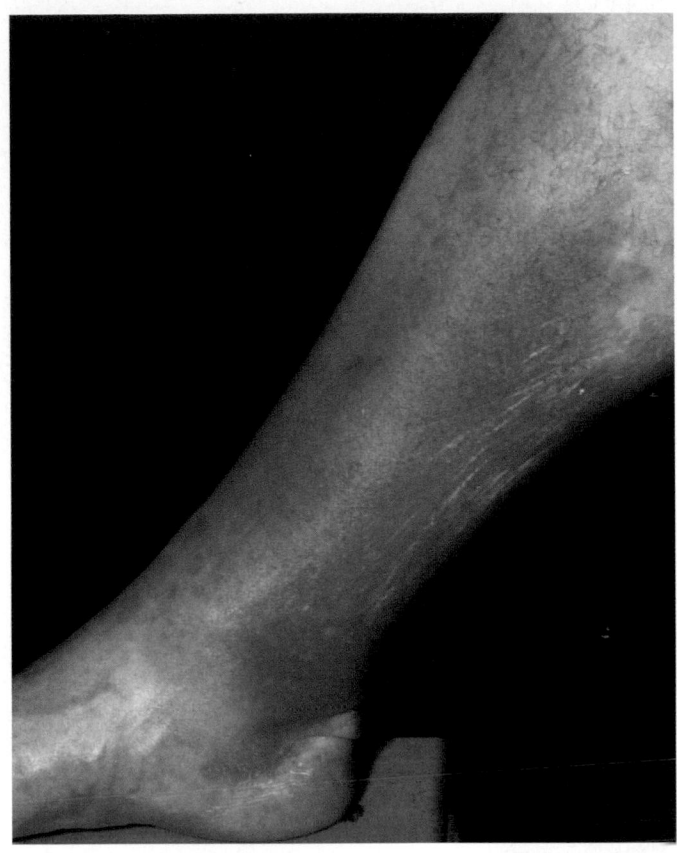

Erysipelas. Fiery-red, brawny, edematous erythema that is sharply and irregularly marginated. There is tenderness, and the patient has fever and chills.

dermal and subcutaneous abscess formation (Fig. 197-4*B*) or necrotizing fasciitis (Fig. 197-5). Regional lymphadenopathy may be associated with cellulitis on an extremity. In older individuals, thrombophlebitis may complicate lower leg cellulitis.

SURGICAL WOUND INFECTIONS   These are classified as incisional (superficial) or deep.[7] Incisional wound infections involve the skin, subcutaneous tissue, and/or muscle located above the fascial layer. Deep wound infections involve structures adjacent to the wound that were entered or exposed during the procedure, such as subfascial layers, viscera, and/or spaces within the peritoneum, thorax, or joints. Up to 80 percent of wound infections are incisional. A wound is considered to be infected if purulent material drains from it, even if cultures are negative or are not taken. Incisional infections present with erythema; pain; tenderness; swelling (Fig. 197-4*B*); fever; a purulent discharge containing neutrophils with, most commonly, gram-positive cocci in clusters (*S. aureus*); separation of the margins of the wound, and peripheral blood leukocytosis. The presentation of deep wound infections may be more subtle and delayed. Progressive bacterial synergistic gangrene and other variants of gangrenous cellulitis can arise in surgical wounds.

The complications of wound infection arise locally (wound dehiscence, fistula formation, failure of the operation, hernia formation, septic thrombophlebitis, pain, and scars) or are systemic (bacteremia, metastatic infection, hypotension, organ failure, and death). Toxin production by *S. aureus* or group A streptococcus wound infection can result in TSS, scarlet fever, or STSS.

INFECTIONS OF INTRAVASCULAR CATHETERS   These are common, with >100,000 cases occurring annually in the United States. *S. aureus*, coagulase-negative staphylococci, and methicillin-resistant S. aureus (MRSA) are the most common etiologic agents. In addition to infection, intravascular catheters are also associated with phlebitis and thrombosis. The most common clinical presentation of catheter-related infection is fever related to bacteremia, without signs localizing to the site of catheter placement. Infection can occur within the lumen of the catheter as well as anywhere along the catheter tunnel. In patients with staphylococcal bacteremia, clinical features suggesting catheter-related infection include local signs of inflammation at the catheter insertion site, lack of another readily identifiable source of bacteremia, sepsis occurring in a patient otherwise not at high risk of bacteremia, embolic phenomena located downstream from an arterial catheter, sepsis refractory to antimicrobial therapy to which staphylococci are susceptible, and prompt resolution of fever following removal of the intravenous device.

CELLULITIS COMPLICATING A PRESSURE ULCER   This is often associated with bacteremia and has a high mortality. Culture of the ulcer surface often fails to reveal the responsible organism(s). Skin biopsy of the margin of the ulcer may be helpful in identifying the etiologic agent. Low-grade infection may extend down into adjacent bone causing osteomyelitis. *S. aureus*, group A streptococcus, and *Pseudomonas aeruginosa* are common pathogens in cellulitis arising within sacral pressure ulcers.

CELLULITIS ARISING AT SITES OF ANIMAL BITES   This is often caused by the oral flora of the animal. Dog and cat bites can give rise to cellulitis caused by *Pasteurella multocida*, *Capnocytophaga canimorsus* [dysgonic fermenter-2 (DF-2)], and a host of other exotic aerobes and anaerobes. *P. multocida* infections have an acute onset, presenting with erythema, pain, and swelling, frequently within hours after the bite (range, ≤12 h to 3 days). Bite wounds are usually located on the hands and arms, legs, or head and neck area. Lymphangitis and lymphadenopathy may also occur. Human bites have a higher incidence of infection than do animal bites and are caused by oral aerobes and anaerobes, most commonly viridans streptococci, group A streptococci, nonhemolytic streptococci, *S. aureus*, peptostreptococci, and *Prevotella* spp.

GANGRENOUS CELLULITIS (INFECTIOUS GANGRENE)   This is characterized by rapid progression of infection with extensive necrosis of subcutaneous tissues and overlying skin[8,9] (Fig. 197-5). Several clinical types of gangrenous cellulitis occur, depending on the causative organism, the anatomic location of the infection, and predisposing conditions (see Table 197-2). Several subtypes of necrotizing fasciitis are recognized. Correct diagnosis is imperative in understanding the pathogenesis and deciding on the appropriate antimicrobial and surgical therapies.

Streptococcal gangrene   This is caused by group A streptococcus (rarely, groups B, C, and G streptococcus); a similar-appearing necrotizing fasciitis is caused by other bacterial species (usually a mixture of anaerobic and facultative organisms). Streptococcal gangrene is a rare entity, with a high mortality rate, usually developing at the site of an injury (minor trauma, laceration, needle puncture, or surgical incision) on an extremity, but it can occur in postoperative abdominal incisions. In some cases, there is no obvious portal of entry. Group B streptococci have caused a similar process post partum secondary to infected episiotomy incisions and unrelated to

FIGURE 197-4

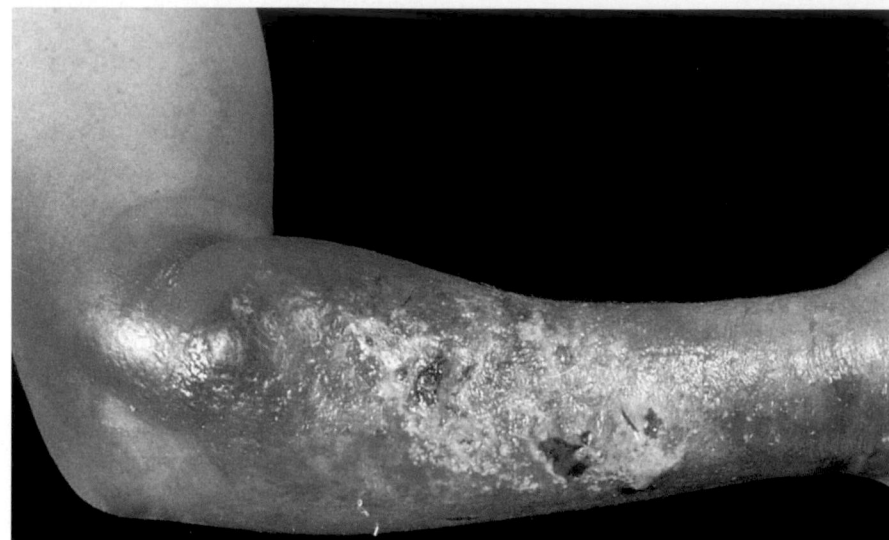

A.

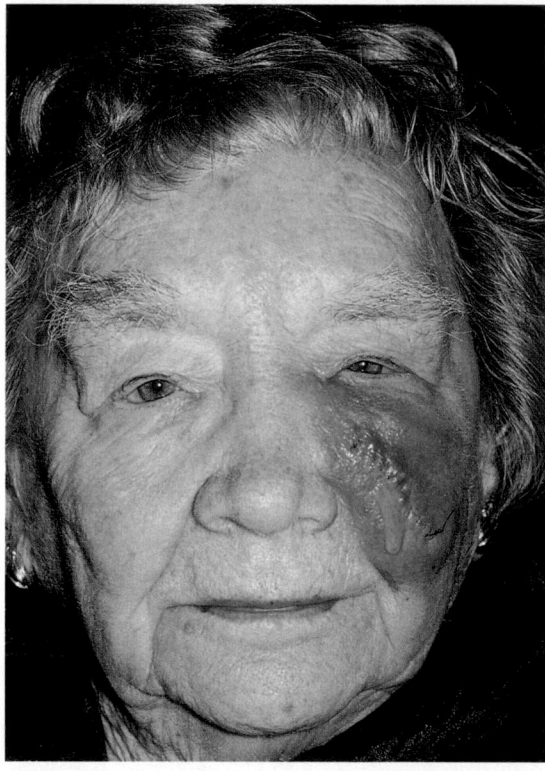

B.

A. Cellulitis following puncture trauma. The forearm is swollen, erythematous, and tender; there is abscess formation, blistering, and crusting. *B.* Cellulitis arising at the site of a surgical excision: *S. aureus.* Note discharge of pus.

obstetric complications, in adult diabetic patients.[10] Group B streptococcal gangrene represents a cellulitis that has progressed rapidly to gangrene of the subcutaneous tissue, with subsequent necrosis of the overlying skin (Fig. 197-5).

Although streptococcal gangrene may be associated with underlying diseases (diabetes, myxedema), the majority of cases have occurred in otherwise healthy persons, often in children and the elderly. Initially there are findings of acute cellulitis (local redness, edema, heat, and pain in the involved area), typically on an extremity. Fever and other constitutional symptoms are prominent as the inflammatory process extends rapidly over the next few days. The characteristic findings of streptococcal gangrene appear within 36 to 72 h after onset: the involved area becomes dusky blue in color; vesicles or bullae containing initially yellowish, then red-black fluid appear. Infection spreads rapidly along fascial planes, resulting in extensive necrotic sloughs. The bullae rupture, and extensive, sharply demarcated cutaneous gangrene develops. At this point the area may be numb, and the black necrotic eschar with surrounding irregular border of erythema resembles a third-degree burn (Fig. 197-5*A*). The eschar sloughs off by the end of a few days (Fig. 197-5*B*). Peripheral areas of involvement develop about the initial site of infection. Metastatic abscesses may occur as a consequence of bacteremia, resembling purpura fulminans but then evolving to dark-colored blebs containing streptococci. Secondary thrombophlebitis is common, but lymphangitis and lymphadenitis are not.

Prior to the availability of antibiotic therapy, streptococcal gangrene commonly progressed and patients developed increasing toxemia and died from metastatic infection or shock. In rare cases, the process became sharply demarcated and self-limited. Even with antimicrobial therapy, the mortality rate remains high.

Necrotizing fasciitis other than that due to group a streptococci This is caused by a mixed infection in which one or more anaerobes (e.g., *Peptostreptococcus, Bacteroides*) are involved together with at least one facultative species (non-group A streptococci; members of the Enterobacteriaceae such as *Enterobacter, Proteus*).[11] Antecedent injury to soft tissues, abdominal surgery, perirectal abscess, decubitus ulcer, and intestinal perforation are common predisposing events. Diabetes mellitus, alcoholism, or parenteral drug abuse are additional contributing factors. The onset is usually acute, and the course is rapidly progressive with high fever and prominent toxicity.

Necrotizing fasciitis other than that due to group A streptococci most commonly occurs on the lower extremities, abdominal wall, perineum, and about operative wounds. Clinically, it is indistinguishable from streptococcal gangrene (Fig. 197-5). It is important to recognize that this infection may present in the thigh (dissection along the psoas muscle) or abdominal wall from an intestinal source (occult diverticulitis, rectosigmoid neoplasm). The involved area is swollen, red, warm, painful, and tender. The process is more extensive than the extent

FIGURE 197-5

CHAPTER 197
Soft Tissue Infections

2219

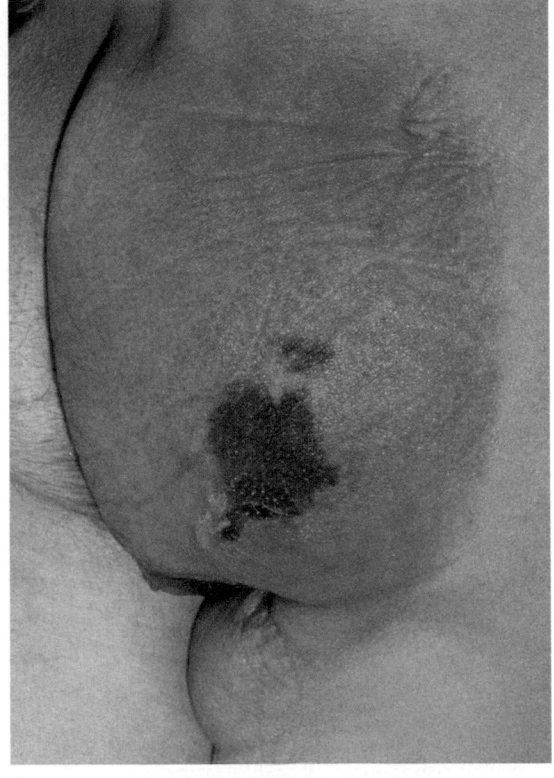

A.

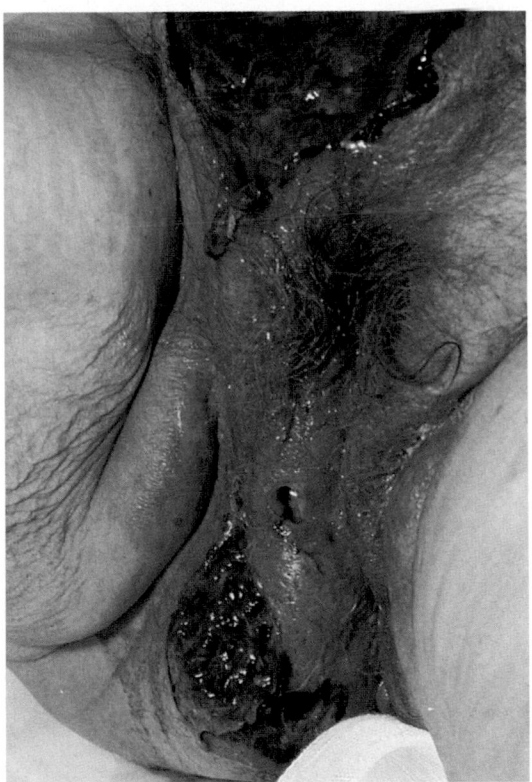

B.

A. Gangrenous cellulitis: necrotizing fasciitis. There is a black necrosis resembling a third-degree burn and an erythematous margin. There is severe systemic toxicity. B. 48 h later, there is progressive gangrene of the pubic, perigenital, and perianal tissue.

TABLE 197-2

Classification of Gangrenous Cellulitis (Infectious Gangrene)

Necrotizing fasciitis
  Streptococcal gangrene
  Necrotizing fasciitis other than streptococcal gangrene
  Synergistic necrotizing cellulitis (necrotizing cutaneous myositis,
    synergistic nonclostridial anaerobic myonecrosis)
  Fournier's gangrene
Clostridial soft tissue infections
  Anaerobic cellulitis
  Anaerobic myonecrosis (gas gangrene)
  Spontaneous, nontraumatic anaerobic myonecrosis
Progressive bacterial synergistic gangrene
Gangrenous cellulitis in the immunosuppressed individual
Localized areas of skin necrosis complicating conventional cellulitis.

of the overlying skin changes would suggest. Within several days, the skin color becomes purple, bullae develop, and frank cutaneous gangrene ensues (Fig. 197-5*B*). At this stage the involved area is no longer tender; it has become anesthetic due to occlusion of small blood vessels and destruction of superficial nerves in the subcutaneous tissues. Crepitus is often present, particularly in patients with diabetes mellitus.

Fournier's gangrene (streptococcal scrotal gangrene, perineal phlegmon)   This is a a variant of necrotizing fasciitis involving the scrotum and penis.[17] It is caused by the same mixture of facultative and anaerobic organisms causing necrotizing fasciitis other than that due to group A streptococci. In rare cases group A streptococci have been implicated. The average age at onset is 50 to 60 years. Most men have underlying disease including diabetes mellitus, ischiorectal abscess, perineal fistula, erysipelas of the perineum, bowel disease (rectal carcinoma, diverticulitis), scrotal trauma, prior urogenital surgery (especially involving the periurethral glands), pressure ulcers of the scrotum and perineum (alcoholics sitting in a drunken stupor), and dissection of pancreatic secretions through the retroperitoneum and into the scrotum.

The onset of Fournier's gangrene can be insidious, with a discrete area of necrosis on the scrotum progressing to advanced skin necrosis rapidly over 1 to 2 days. Pain, swelling, and crepitus in the scrotum are marked. Foul-smelling drainage occurs, and purplish discoloration of the scrotum progresses to frank gangrene. The infection tends to be superficial, limited to skin and subcutaneous tissue and extending to the base of the scrotum, but it may spread to the penis, perineum, and abdominal wall along fascial planes. The testes, glans penis, and spermatic cord are usually spared as they have a separate blood supply. If the process invades the abdominal panniculus of an obese patient, especially one with diabetes mellitus, progression can be extraordinarily rapid.

Synergistic necrotizing cellulitis (necrotizing cutaneous myositis, synergistic nonclostridial anaerobic myonecrosis)   This is another variant of necrotizing fasciitis and is a highly lethal polymicrobial infection, characterized by extensive necrosis of skin and muscle as well as fascia and subcutaneous tissue, with progressive undermining along fascial planes.[13] The process may be rather indolent initially, presenting over 7 to 10 days with mild symptoms. Individuals are often afebrile or have only low-grade fever, lacking systemic toxicity in the early stages. The lower extremities, perineum, and abdominal wall are common sites. The initial skin lesion is a small area of necrosis or reddish-brown blister with extreme local tenderness; the superficial appearance belies the widespread destruction of the deeper tissues. Skin sinuses (with surrounding areas of gangrene) are formed, draining foul-smelling brownish ("dishwater") pus. Between the draining tracts the skin appears uninvolved, even though extensive necrosis of underlying fascia, muscle, and subcutaneous tissues has occurred. Extensive gangrene of the superficial tissues and fat can be visualized by direct inspection through skin incisions, associated with gelatinous necrosis of fascia and muscle. Gas can be palpated in the tissues in 25 patients of patients.

The most common site of involvement of synergistic necrotizing cellulitis is the perineum (half of cases). The major predisposing causes are perirectal and ischiorectal abscesses. These localized infections tract to the deeper structures of the pelvis, leading to a severe infection. A more superficial form involves the buttocks without extension to deeper muscles; 40 percent of individuals have involvement of the thigh and leg. Some infections arise in the adductor compartment of the thigh, often extending from an infected amputation stump or diabetic gangrene. Lesions in the lower leg are usually associated with vascular disease or diabetic foot ulcers. The remaining 10 percent of cases occur in the upper extremities or in the neck, most frequently in patients with vascular disease or diabetes mellitus.

The course can be a rapidly progressive life-threatening infection if the diagnosis is not made promptly and appropriate surgical debridement is not carried out. This applies particularly when the process is secondary to a bowel perforation. Even with treatment, the mortality rate is about 35 percent.

CLOSTRIDIAL SOFT TISSUE INFECTIONS (STI) These are classified as *anaerobic cellulitis*, which involves the subcutaneous tissue, and *clostridial or anaerobic myonecrosis (gas gangrene)*, occurring in the setting of muscle injury and contamination with soil or other foreign material containing spores of *Clostridium perfringens* or other histotoxic clostridial species.[14] *C. perfringens* is an obligate anaerobe usually present in large numbers as normal flora in human feces and thus can contaminate skin surfaces endogenously. In spite of clostridial contamination of major traumatic open wounds, the incidence of gas gangrene is only 1 to 2 percent.

Anaerobic cellulitis This is a clostridial infection of devitalized tissue, usually occurring in a dirty or inadequately debrided wound several days after injury. The onset is more gradual than in anaerobic myonecrosis. The anaerobes are able to grow in the depths of the wound and extend rapidly through tissue planes, with attendant formation of large quantities of gas. A thin, dark gray–brown, foul, serous discharge is produced. Gram-stained smear of the drainage reveals short, plump, blunt-ended, gram-positive rods without spores and with a variable number of polymorphonuclear leukocytes. Unlike anaerobic myonecrosis, there is relatively little local pain or edema, change in overlying skin, toxemia, or extension of the process to involve muscle. At operation, the muscles appear normal, but gas may extend diffusely and is readily evident through the exudate. Anaerobic cellulitis must be distinguished from anaerobic myonecrosis to avoid needless mutilating surgery and amputations. Treatment consists of opening the wound, removing necrotic debris, and administering antibiotics (penicillin preferably, or a broad-spectrum antibiotic, and metronidazole).

Anaerobic myonecrosis (gas gangrene) This is a rapidly progressing, toxemic, potentially lethal infection involving muscle but with secondary changes in the overlying skin. The infection may develop as a complication of a traumatic dirty wound with extensive muscle and soft tissue damage or follow surgery on the bowel or gallbladder.

The incubation period of anaerobic myonecrosis is often short (12 to 24 h) but may be delayed, occasionally developing following anaerobic cellulitis. The first symptom is usually local pain, followed by edema. Gas formation is present but not prominent and may be completely obscured by local swelling of the subcutaneous tissues. The skin often takes on a dark yellow or bronze discoloration, with tense blebs or bullae containing dark brown fluid. A serosanguineous exudate can be expressed from the wound. Gram stain of the exudate reveals plump gram-positive rods and only a few white blood cells. Subsequently, green-black patches of necrosis of the skin at the margin of the wound may develop. Evidences of toxemia are present: high fever, tachycardia, hypotension, and oliguria. Intravascular hemolysis does not usually occur in this type of process, in contrast to septic abortion with septicemia due to this organism.

Spontaneous, nontraumatic anaerobic myonecrosis This occurs in the absence of an external wound and is associated with *C. septicum* bacteremia.[15] *C. septicum* is a relatively aerotolerant species. Intestinal tract abnormalities (especially occult colon cancer) are the major predisposing conditions. Spontaneous *C. septicum* gas gangrene can be fulminant, with a mortality of 67 to 100 percent within 24 h of onset.

NONCLOSTRIDIAL ANAEROBIC CELLULITIS This is very similar to clostridial anaerobic cellulitis. The infection is caused by a variety of non-spore-forming anaerobic bacteria (*Bacteroides* spp., peptostreptococcus, *Prevotella* spp.), either alone or mixed with facultative species (Enterobacteriaceae, various streptococci, staphylococci).

PROGRESSIVE BACTERIAL SYNERGISTIC GANGRENE (MELENEY'S GANGRENE) This is characterized by poor healing with elevation and erythema of the surrounding skin.[16,17] The lesion was designated *synergistic gangrene* in that both microaerophilic streptococci and *S. aureus* are required to produce the infection experimentally. In a rare instance, the picture of progressive bacterial synergistic gangrene following abdominal surgery may be mimicked by postoperative (colonic surgery) amebic abdominal wall infection.

The infection typically occurs in the vicinity of a retention suture or in a drain site following an abdominal operation (ileostomy, colostomy), in an incision in the chest wall, following abdominal or thoracic infection (empyema), at the exit site of a fistulous tract, or in a chronic ulcer on an extremity. The infection is usually recognized 1 to 2 weeks after the operation, when the infection has extended circumferentially.

Progressive bacterial synergistic gangrene usually starts in the first or second postoperative week with local redness, tenderness, and swelling. Early infection shows a local tender area of erythema and swelling, which subsequently forms a small, painful, superficial ulcer that gradually enlarges. In established infections, three zones of involvement are characteristic: a central area of necrosis (ulceration); a middle zone of violaceous, tender edematous tissue; and an outer zone of bright erythema. Local pain and tenderness are nearly always present; fever and systemic toxicity, however, are usually absent. Untreated, the ulceration progressively enlarges, ultimately resulting in enormous ulcerations (Fig. 197-6). *Meleney's ulcer* has the features of progressive bacterial synergistic gangrene (Meleney's gangrene), with associated burrowing necrotic tracts through tissue planes emerging at distant skin sites.

GANGRENOUS CELLULITIS IN THE IMMUNOSUPPRESSED INDIVIDUAL This is caused by the usual agents as well as those

FIGURE 197-6

CHAPTER 197
Soft Tissue Infections

2221

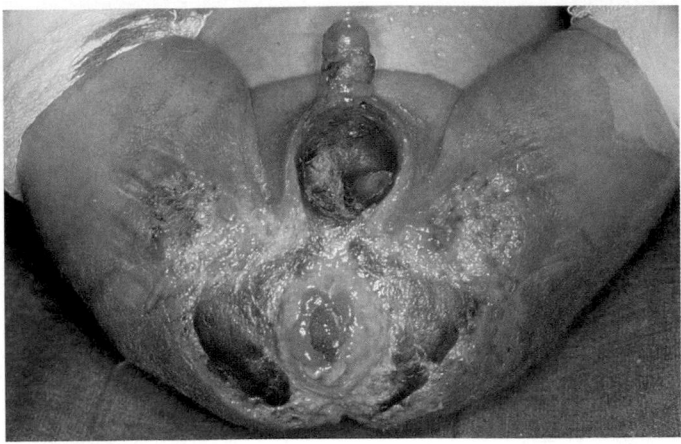

Progressive bacterial synergistic gangrene. Necrosis and deep ulcerations of the genitalia and perineum in a toddler.

not pathogenic in immunocompetent individuals. *P. aeruginosa* primarily infects the skin in persons with prolonged neutropenia. Infection begins at sites where skin integrity is lost or in normal-appearing skin, especially in intertriginous areas. Infection causes a septic vasculitis with resultant infarction of skin; the necrotizing infection is referred to as ecthyma gangrenosum (EG). Cutaneous mucormycosis can occur at a site of cutaneous injury in an individual with or without underlying immunocompromise.[18]

DIFFERENTIAL DIAGNOSIS

The differential diagnosis of erysipelas, cellulitis, and necrotizing cellulitis includes noninfectious inflammatory disorders as well as other infections (see Tables 197-3 and 197-4).

LABORATORY INVESTIGATIONS

Smears of Pus, Exudate, Aspirates

Gram's stain of exudates or pus from the surface of the lesion is often helpful, especially when STIs are associated with a superficial pyoderma. If no obvious portal of entry is detected, nonbacteriostatic saline can be injected into the advancing border of a cellulitis plaque, followed by aspiration of tissue fluid. The infecting bacteria can be visualized on smears or isolated on culture. Immunofluorescent techniques can be used to visualize rare infecting organisms in tissue section.[19]

Hematology

In the report by Hook et al.[5] on cellulitis, only 46 percent of patients had an elevated white blood cell count ($\geq$10,000/mL) and 59 percent had an elevated erythrocyte sedimentation rate ($\geq$25 mm/h).

TABLE 197-3

Differential Diagnosis of Erysipelas and Acute Cellulitis

NONINFECTIOUS DISORDERS

Dissecting cellulitis of the scalp (perifolliculitis capitis abscedens et suffodiens)
Acne conglobata
Hydradenitis suppurativa
Acute allergic contact dermatitis (e.g., to poison ivy or poison oak)
Erythema nodosum
Eosinophilic cellulitis
Giant urticaria and angioedema
Fixed drug eruption
Deep venous thrombosis and lipodermatosclerosis
Vasculitis such as polyarteritis nodosa
Familial Mediterranean fever
Inflammatory breast carcinoma (carcinoma erysipeloides)

INFECTIOUS DISORDERS

Osteomyelitis of the maxillary or frontal bones secondary to paranasal sinusitis
Extension of subperiosteal infection from long bone osteomyelitis
Erythema migrans
Erythema infectiosum (human parvovirus B19 infection with "slapped cheek")
Early prevesicular herpes zoster

Culture

The "gold standard" of etiologic diagnosis of cellulitis is isolation of the infecting organism by culture of the infected site, infected tissue, and/or blood. A pathogen isolated on culture of a likely portal of entry is usually the cause of the STI. In cellulitis arising in a pressure ulcer, however, microorganisms isolated from the surface of the pressure ulcer eschar may not represent the invading pathogen. In a study culturing lesional skin biopsy specimens, aspirate, or blood, a potential pathogen was isolated in only 26 percent of cases of cellulitis in adults.[5] Culture of exudate, erosions, ulcerations, abscesses, or surgical wounds has the highest yield in isolation of the infecting organism.

Needle aspiration has been used in cases of early cellulitis without an apparent portal of entry.[17] Aspiration is attempted with a syringe and needle, placing the needle tip into the advancing edge of the inflamed lesion. If no fluid is obtained by aspiration, 1 to 2 mL of nonbacteriostatic normal saline can be injected into the site

TABLE 197-4

Differential Diagnoses of Necrotizing Soft Tissue Infections

Factitial ulcers
Pyoderma gangrenosum
Purpura fulminans (disseminated intravascular coagulation)
Calciphylaxis
Ischemic necrosis (atherosclerosis obliterans, thromboembolism)
Fixed drug eruption, warfarin necrosis, heparin necrosis
Pressure ulcer
Amebic (*Entamoeba histolytica*) skin gangrene following bowel surgery
Brown recluse spider bite

and aspiration again attempted. The aspirate is streaked on a microscope slide, Gram stained, and cultured. The reported yield of needle aspiration ranges from 5 to 100 percent.[20] Needle aspiration has a higher yield in patients with diabetes mellitus or underlying malignancies. Lesional biopsy specimen culture has been reported to have a higher yield than aspirate or blood culture.

"Touch" Preparation

A lesional skin biopsy specimen is touched to a microscope slide and potassium hydroxide solution applied. The slide is then examined for yeast and mycelial forms of fungi; the technique detects *Candida*, *Cryptococcus*, *Mucor*, and other fungi. A Gram's stain of the touch preparation slide can detect bacteria.

Dermatopathology

Lesional skin punch biopsy is often helpful in ruling out a cellulitis-simulating noninfectious inflammatory lesion such as erythema nodosum, vasculitis, or eosinophilic cellulitis. In ecthyma gangrenosum (caused by *P. aeruginosa*), a septic vasculitis is seen. Direct immunofluorescent techniques have been reported to identify streptococcal pathogens in 19 of 27 cases of erysipelas and in 10 of 15 cases of cellulitis.[21]

Histologically, erysipelas is characterized by intense edema, marked vascular dilatation, and a profuse infiltration of tissue spaces and lymphatic channels with streptococci. The streptococci are not found in the blood vessels themselves, but their presence in the lymphatics produces an inflammatory reaction about these vessels. The dermis is markedly edematous, and there is infiltration with neutrophils and mononuclear cells. The epidermis is only secondarily involved.

Deep incisional biopsy and histopathologic examination on frozen sections has been shown to improve mortality in necrotizing fasciitis by rapidly establishing the diagnosis and thus defining the need for surgical debridement.[22] Indications for an open exploration and a biopsy include confusion, tachycardia, tachypnea, ketoacidosis/hyperglycemia, gangrenous skin changes, bronzing of the skin, severe pain or spreading areas of anesthesia, thin reddish discharge with undermining of wound edges, crepitus, an abscess with multiple tracts, and a cellulitis that either progresses despite antibiotics, has extensive surrounding edema, or complicates a surgical wound.

In streptococcal gangrene, the prominent angiitis and focal dermal necrosis with spread along fascial planes suggest that the disease is fundamentally a gangrene of the subcutaneous tissues followed by necrosis of the overlying skin. Microscopically, fibrinoid necrosis is present in the media of many arteries and veins passing through the destroyed fascia.[23] Fibrin thrombi are present. The epidermis, dermis, and skin appendages in the area of gangrene undergo coagulation necrosis. Numerous polymorphonuclear leukocytes and mononuclear cells infiltrate the lesion, and the upper layers of the dermis contain large numbers of gram-positive cocci.

Imaging

Infections with anaerobic organisms, especially *Clostridia*, may lead to gas formation, which can then be visualized radiographically. Conventional x-ray of anaerobic cellulitis may reveal pockets of gas confined to superficial tissues. True gas gangrene (clostridial myositis) can be distinguished from anaerobic cellulitis by the linear feathery appearance of gas infiltrating through groups of muscle fibers.[24,25]

Magnetic resonance imaging (MRI) has gained momentum as a technique in diagnosing STIs. In a recent study, 23 patients with acute STIs underwent MRI evaluation. T2-weighted images best highlighted the cutaneous disease process. In patients with pyomyositis or subcutaneous abscesses, a spindle-shaped or round, well-defined area of high signal intensity was observed in the muscle or fat, respectively. Patients with necrotizing fasciitis had deep dermal, well-defined dome-shaped areas of increased signal. Patients with nonnecrotizing cellulitis had smaller, heterogeneous areas of increased signal.[26]

DIAGNOSIS

The initial diagnosis of STI is made on clinical findings, identification of pathogenic organisms on Gram's stain of exudates or aspirates, hematologic studies, and possibly imaging studies. The main point of differentiation between erysipelas and acute cellulitis centers on the nature of the margin of the lesion: raised, sharply demarcated from the uninvolved skin in erysipelas; indistinct and gradually blending with uninvolved adjacent areas in cellulitis. The diagnosis is then confirmed by results of microbial cultures.

SPECIFIC BACTERIAL SPECIES ASSOCIATED WITH CELLULITIS

Pathogens Spread from Person to Person

Staphylococcus aureus *S. aureus* causes the majority of all soft tissue infections. Although not one of the cutaneous resident flora, it colonizes the anterior nares in up to 35 percent of healthy individuals at any one time. The incidence of nasal carriage of *S. aureus* is higher in chronically ill individuals, especially those with diabetes mellitus and HIV disease. *S. aureus* colonization on the skin as well as of the nares is very common in individuals with atopic dermatitis. Ensconced in the nares, *S. aureus* is able to colonize and infect superficial skin lesions by entering hair follicles or small breaks in the epidermis, resulting in folliculitis, furuncles, carbuncles, impetigo, and ecthyma.

Once established in the skin, *S. aureus* is able to invade more deeply into the soft tissue with resultant erysipelas (horizontal spread in lymphatics) and cellulitis (vertical spread into subcutaneous fat). An emerging problem is nosocomial spread of MRSA.[27] In one long-term care facility, the monthly MRSA colonization rate was as high as 23 percent.[28] Treatment of active MRSA infection involves use of intravenous vancomycin; mupirocin ointment has also been used with good success in eradicating nasal colonization among health care workers.[29]

S. aureus is the most common cause of wound infections. Staphylococci that cause surgical wound infections originate from the flora of the patient or from that of the health care workers. Risk factors for surgical wound infection are dependent on the following: host factors (immune status, diabetes mellitus); surgical factors (disruption of tissue perfusion that accompanies the surgical procedure, foreign body use); staphylococcal factors (substances that mediate tissue adherence and invasion or that enable staphylococci to survive host defenses and antibiotics in tissues); and antimicrobial prophylaxis.

Various strains of *S. aureus* are capable of producing a variety of toxins, which cause the clinical syndromes of SSSS (rare in infants greater than 2 years of age), staphylococcal scarlet fever, and TSS. TSS is a febrile, multiorgan disease caused by the elaboration of staphylococcal toxins, characterized by a generalized scarlatiniform eruption, hypotension, functional abnormalities of three or more organ systems, and desquamation in the evolution of the exanthem. Cellulitis caused by *S. aureus* that produce TSS toxins can be accompanied by the cutaneous and systemic findings of staphylococcal scarlet fever or TSS.[30]

Beta-hemolytic streptococcus Of the beta-hemolytic streptococci, group A streptococcus (*Streptococcus pyogenes*) is nearly always the species causing erysipelas.[31] Other beta-hemolytic streptococci causing erysipelas include group B streptococcus (*S. agalactiae*), which causes erysipelas in newborns, and group C and group G streptococcus. Other nonstreptococcal organisms occasionally causing erysipelas include *S. aureus*, *Campylobacter jejuni*,[32] and *Moraxella*.[33] The incidence of invasive group A streptococcus infection appears to be increasing in communities, hospitals, and nursing homes.[3,34,35]

Group A streptococci commonly colonize the upper respiratory tract, and secondarily infect (impetiginizes) minor skin lesions from which invasive infection can arise. Certain strains of group A streptococcus have a higher affinity for the skin than the respiratory tract and can colonize the skin, subsequently causing superficial pyodermas or STIs.

Several decades ago, erysipelas occurred most commonly on the face, often associated with an antecedent respiratory tract infection. The exact mode of spread to the skin is not known. Currently, 5 to 20 percent of cases arise on the face (see Fig. 197-2) and 70 to 80 percent on the lower extremities (see Fig. 197-3).[36] Streptococcal bacteremia occurs in 5 percent of individuals with erysipelas.

Lymphatic obstruction/lymphedema predisposes to erysipelas or cellulitis. Individuals at higher risk are those who have had radical mastectomy with axillary node dissection or saphenous vein harvest. STIs occur in the leg from which the saphenous vein has been removed, often with interdigital tinea pedis as the portal of entry.[37] The lymphedema resulting from lymphatic interruption accompanying saphenous vein removal predisposes to the development of cellulitis once organisms reach that area. Symptoms may be quite acute with high fever, prostration, and tachycardia. Erythema and edema extend along the incision; tenderness is marked. Acute lymphangitis and/or thrombophlebitis may complicate the cellulitis. Isolation of group A streptococci from the skin lesions or blood is usually not possible. The appearance of the lesions, the occasional associated lymphangitis, and the response to treatment with penicillin G suggest that the STI is caused by group A or group B, C, or G streptococcus. Because streptococcal infection in an area of lymphedema leads to further lymphedema, episodes of infection tend to recur. Topical treatment of the tinea pedis with topical or systemic antifungal drugs is an important element in management and prophylaxis. Although the cellulitis responds well to penicillin, the response may be slower in patients with peripheral arterial disease. Also, it is important to recognize that the *rubor* of dependency in such a patient may exaggerate the appearance of cellulitis about the saphenous incision. Thus, it is advisable to examine the leg from day to day in the same (horizontal) position. An episode of erysipelas causes lymphatic damage and obstruction; the recurrence rate at the same sites is high, up to 30 percent.[38,39] Injecting drug users are also at increased risk of streptococcal cellulitis at injection sites, often associated with bacteremia, septic thrombophlebitis, and metastatic infection.

Streptococcal cellulitis as an operative wound infection is uncommon today, in contrast to several decades ago. However, in the presence of streptococcal epidemics in the community, these organisms may be carried into the operating room and result in a particularly fulminating type of postoperative wound infection. Such sepsis may be manifest within 6 to 48 h of the procedure, unlike *S. aureus* wound infections, which present after several days. Hypotension (often due to bacteremia) may be the initial manifestation even before local erythema is evident. A thin serous discharge can be expressed from the wound area, and on Gram's stain it shows a myriad of gram-positive cocci in chains. STIs caused by toxin-producing group A streptococci can be complicated by scarlet fever or STSS.[40,41] Acute poststreptococcal glomerulonephritis is an infrequent complication of group A streptococcal STIs.

Group A streptococcus can cause infection at intertriginous sites. The infection is usually superficial but may simulate cellulitis, e.g., perianal streptococcal "cellulitis." Perianal cellulitis occurs principally in children and can be preceded by group A streptococcal pharyngitis or impetigo. *S. aureus* can also cause a similar perianal dermatitis in children.[42] Children present with intense perianal erythema (Fig. 197-7), perianal pruritus, pain on defecation and blood-streaked stools, and the process may become chronic if untreated.[43] Clinically, the perianal skin is erythematous, edematous, painful, fragile, and fissured. The involved tissues have a boggy consistency. *S. aureus* perianal dermatitis may be accompanied by

FIGURE 197-7

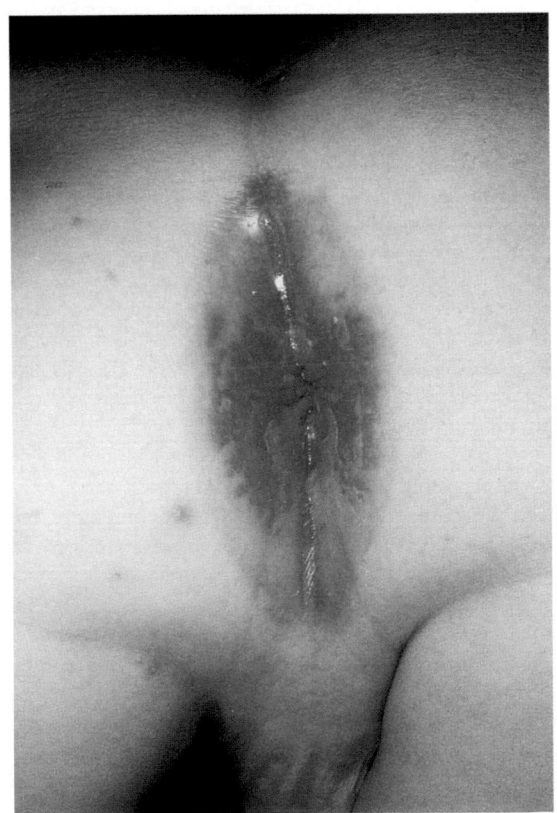

Perianal streptococcal cellulitis. Erythema around the anus and on the perineum. (*Courtesy of Arthur R. Rhodes, MD.*)

distinguishing satellite pustules. The infection can extend to the penis and vulva.[44]

The diagnosis is confirmed by isolation of group A streptococcus (less commonly *S. aureus*) on culture of the erythematous area.[45] Individuals with staphylococcal or group A streptococcal infection respond well to oral amoxicillin with clavulanic acid. Identification of the organism is therapeutically helpful since oral penicillin VK will not be effective in most *S. aureus* infections.

In a report from Sweden of 229 patients with erysipelas, beta-hemolytic streptococci were detected in 34 percent of cases.[46] Group A was the dominant serogroup, but group G was found in about half as many cases. Bacteremia was present in 5 percent. The clinical course was usually benign, with few complications, but recurrences were common, occurring in 21 percent of cases. No cases of STSS were seen. Beta-hemolytic streptococci were isolated on culture of lesional skin biopsy specimens in only 2 of 15 cases.

Group B streptococci commonly colonize the perineum and may cause STIs at this site. Risk factors for group B streptococcus colonization in women include first half of menstrual cycle, intrauterine device use, sexual experience, parity <4, and age <21 years. Infection can occur around the time of delivery in the mother (puerperal sepsis) or the neonate.[47,48] Advanced age, cirrhosis, diabetes, stroke, breast cancer, decubitus ulcer, neurogenic bladder, and foreign bodies (breast or penile implants) have all been associated with a significantly increased risk of acquiring group B streptococcus infection in the community .[49,50] In one series, 7 of 19 patients with group B streptococcus cellulitis were women who had undergone mastectomies for breast cancer.[49] An unusual form of recurrent cellulitis of the lower extremities in women results from impaired lymphatic drainage due to neoplasia, radical vulvectomy or pelvic surgery, or radiation therapy. Such episodes of cellulitis have sometimes occurred temporally in relation to coitus and have been caused by group B or group G streptococci, both colonizers of the perineum and genital tract.[51] Group B streptococcus also causes cellulitis in association with foot and pressure ulcers. Non-group A streptococci can cause cellulitis at sites of saphenous vein harvest.[52] Morbidity and mortality are relatively high for group B streptococcus infections, with a high incidence of bacteremia.[53]

Group C streptococci are common pathogens in animals. These organisms can also cause infections in humans, in rare cases following animal exposure. In a retrospective review of 88 cases of group C bacteremia, endocarditis was the most common presentation, although cutaneous and subcutaneous infections occurred in about 10 percent of the cases.[54] The mortality from group C streptococcal endocarditis was 33 percent.

Group G streptococci most commonly cause skin and STIs as well as puerperal and neonatal infections, septicemia, septic arthritis, endocarditis, meningitis, peritonitis, pleuropulmonary infections, pharyngitis, and otitis media.[55]

In the late 1980s and 1990s, reports of invasive group A streptococcal infection associated with bacteremia, deep STI, shock, and multiorgan failure began to appear, referred to as the *streptococcal toxic shock–like syndrome*, or as infection with "flesh-eating bacteria" in the lay press[2] (Table 197-5). Patients were often young and healthy, unlike previous reports of group A streptococcal bacteremia. The portal of entry was through the skin or mucous membrane at sites of minor trauma, liposuction, hysterectomy, vaginal delivery, bunionectomy, bone pinning, and mouth-to-mouth resuscitation.[3,56] Groups C and G streptococcus can also cause STSS.[57] The streptococcal strains causing STSS are readily transmitted from

TABLE 197-5

Features of Group A Streptococcus Toxic Shock–Like Syndrome

CLINICAL FEATURES	% INVOLVED
Physical Findings	
Cutaneous	
Swelling and erythema	65
Bullae	5
Desquamation (late)	20
Hypotension	100
Tachycardia (>100 bpm)	80
Fever (>38°C)	70
Confusion	55
Outcome	
Renal impairment	80
Transient	70
Permanent	10
Sepsis	60
Acute respiratory distress syndrome	55
Death	30

SOURCE: Modified from Stevens.[2,3]

person to person and have a high propensity to initiate invasive disease in contacts. Numerous clusters of infection in families and nursing homes have occurred.[35,58] For streptococcal toxic shock syndrome, see Chap. 195.

Life-threatening invasive group A streptococcal infections have been associated with varicella in children. In a series of six immunocompetent children, bacteremia ($n = 1$), STSS ($n = 3$), pneumonia ($n = 1$), and pyomyositis ($n = 1$) complicated the typical course of varicella. Intensive care unit management and antibiotic therapy were required; all six children eventually survived.[59]

Streptococcus pneumoniae (pneumococcus) *S. pneumoniae* is a rare cause of cellulitis, occurring in individuals predisposed by connective tissue disease, alcoholism, drug abuse, HIV disease, or glucocorticoid therapy.[60–62] Clinically, infected areas are characterized by bullae, brawny erythema, and a violaceous hue. Approximately 50 percent of cases are the result of pneumococcal bacteremia, often from a pulmonary source. Necrotizing fasciitis due to pneumococcus has been reported.[63] Because of underlying medical conditions, and often pneumonia, the morbidity is high.

Neisseria meningitidis Skin manifestations of meningococcal disease are common, occurring in many patients with meningococcal infection; however, meningococcal cellulitis is very rare. Several cases of periorbital cellulitis in children and a case of cellulitis of the extremities in a patient with endocarditis and connective tissue disease have been reported.[64]

Haemophilus influenzae *H. influenzae* colonizes the upper airways of infants and young children; it is able to pass between epithelial cells and is the most common cause of cellulitis of the face, head, and neck in this age group.[65] Buccal cellulitis occurs in children less than 1 year of age. The *H. influenzae* type b (Hib) vaccine, currently given in infant immunizations, has dramatically reduced the incidence of *H. influenzae* infections in young children.[66,67]

Classically, *H. influenzae* cellulitis occurs with an acute onset on the cheeks. Initially, an erythematous edematous plaque occurs, which enlarges, having a characteristic violaceous or bluish-purple color (Fig. 197-8). *H. influenzae* cellulitis often follows an ear or respiratory infection. Bacteremia is common in children with *H. influenzae* cellulitis; meningitis occurs in 8 percent of cases.

FIGURE 197-8

CHAPTER 197
Soft Tissue Infections

2225

FIGURE 197-9

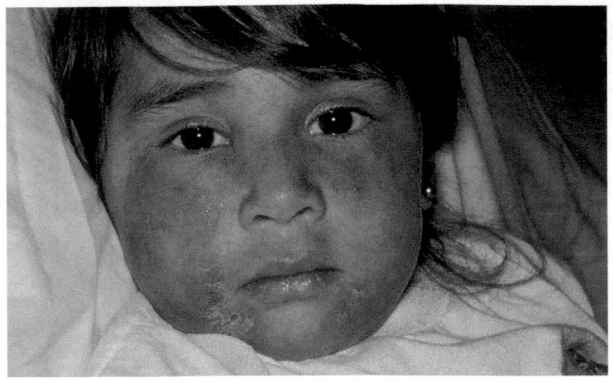

Cellulitis: *Haemophilus influenzae.* Erythema and edema of the face in a child. (*Courtesy of Sandy Urioste, MD.*)

H. influenzae necrotizing fasciitis has been reported in an individual with diabetes mellitus.[68] Children under 4 years of age who are household contacts of children with *H. influenzae* infection should receive chemoprophylaxis if full immunization against *H. influenzae* type b had not already been completed.

    Escherichia coli and other gram-negative bacilli *E. coli* and other gram-negative bacilli rarely cause cellulitis, usually in individuals with cirrhosis, neutropenia, or leukocyte dysfunction (Fig. 197-9).[69] In a report of seven patients with gram-negative bacillary cellulitis and cirrhosis, the STIs that occurred were characterized by bullous lesions, ulcers, abscesses, or extensive cutaneous necrosis. Bacteremia occurred in six patients and these patients eventually died. Isolates from the skin included *Klebsiella pneumonia, E. coli, P. aeruginosa, Proteus mirabilis,* and *Aeromonas hydrophila.*[70]

Pathogens Associated with Aqueous Environments

    Pseudomonas aeruginosa *P. aeruginosa* causes the necrotizing STI ecthyma gangrenosum (Fig. 197-10), which occurs as a primary skin infection or secondary to an underlying pseudomonal bacteremia. Most cases of EG occur with primary STIs that may be complicated by secondary bacteremia.[71,72] EG occurs commonly as a nosocomial infection, especially in immunocompromised patients with diabetes, neutropenia, or poor neutrophil function.[73] *P. aeruginosa* is the most common pathogen causing gangrenous cellulitis in childhood.[74] EG-like infections can be caused by other bacteria such as *K. pneumoniae.*[75] *P. aeruginosa* gains entry into the dermis and subcutaneous tissues via adnexal epidermal structures or areas of loss of epidermal integrity (pressure ulcers, thermal burns, trauma). EG occurring as a primary cutaneous infection arises most frequently in the axillae or anogenital regions; however, it can appear at nearly any cutaneous site.[76]

    EG presents initially as an erythematous, painful plaque or vesicle, which quickly undergoes necrosis and enlarges. Established lesions show hemorrhage, necrosis, and surrounding erythema (see Fig. 197-10). If effective antibiotic therapy is not initiated promptly, the necrosis may often extend rapidly. Bacteremia occurs soon after the onset of EG and may result in metastatic spread of *P. aeruginosa* with subcutaneous nodules and abscesses. Histologically, EG is characterized by a distinctive septic vasculitis. Gram-stained smears of the lesions show thin gram-negative bacilli.

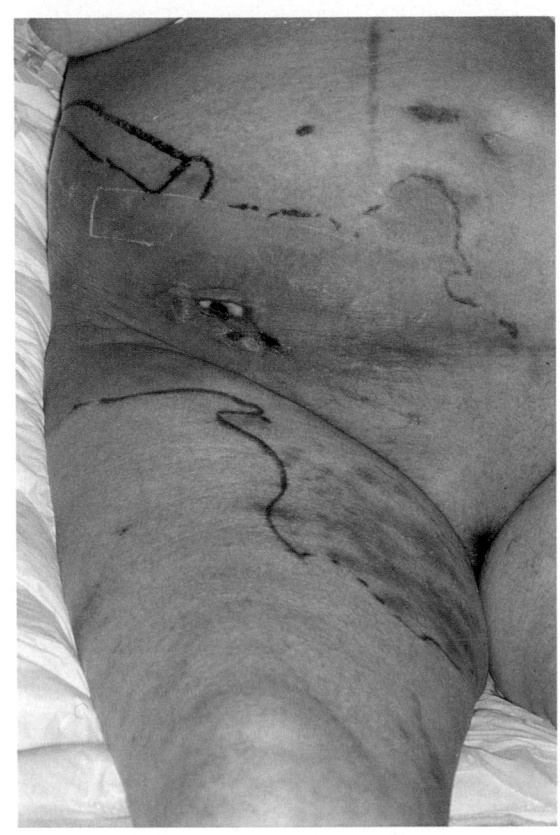

Cellulitis: *E. coli.* Extensive erythema and edema following lymph node biopsy of this elderly woman with lymphoma; *E. coli* was isolated from the wound and blood cultures.

FIGURE 197-10

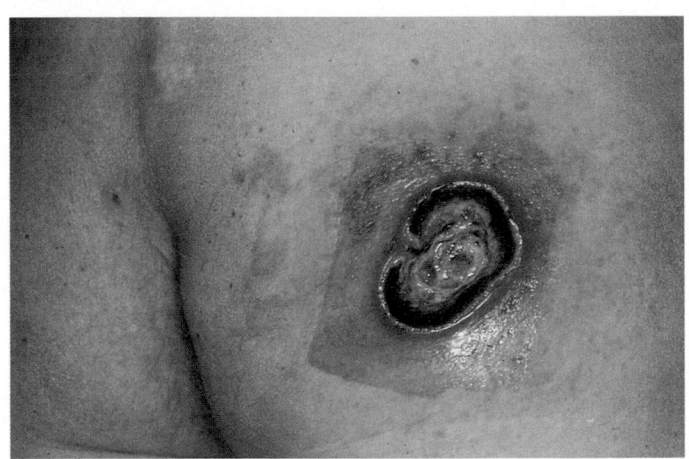

Ecthyma gangrenosum. This ulcer has developed from an extremely painful infarcted area with surrounding erythema on the buttock of a neutropenic HIV-infected male.

Stenotrophomonas maltophilia *S. maltophilia* (formerly classified as *Xanthomonas* or *P. maltophilia*) is a significant cause of morbidity and mortality in hospitalized patients with neutropenia and cancer and undergoing chemotherapy. Primary cellulitis, disseminated cutaneous nodules, and mucocutaneous ulcers caused by *Xanthomonas* are often associated with underlying malignancies.[77]

Aeromonas species *A. hydrophila* is a gram-negative facultative rod that is found naturally in aqueous environments. It causes STIs in healthy individuals and more serious infections in the immunocompromised.[78–81] *A. hydrophila* STIs occur following injuries sustained in a contaminated aquatic environment or the "outdoors." *A. hydrophila* (a normal inhabitant of the foregut of leeches) cellulitis has also followed the therapeutic use of leeches (in 7 to 20 percent of patients) following reimplantation or flap surgery.

Vibrio species (See also Chap. 200) *V. vulnificus* is a free-living gram-negative rod, occurring naturally in the marine environment, occasionally contaminating oysters and other shellfish.[82] Marine *Vibrio* species can cause sepsis and STIs, particularly in patients with cirrhosis and/or diabetes mellitus. *V. damselae* may cause fulminant necrotizing STIs in immunocompetent patients. Either ingestion of raw seafood (Fig. 197-11) or exposure of open wounds to seawater can result in *Vibrio* bacteremia and STIs. Individuals with cirrhosis, hemochromatosis, and diabetes mellitus and other patients with chronic disease are advised to avoid eating raw seafood.[83–87]

Marine *Vibrio* STIs occur by direct inoculation into a superficial wound or by bacteremic spread to the skin (metastatic infection). Following ingestion of *V. vulnificus* in contaminated seafood, the organism is capable of crossing the gut mucosa rapidly, invading the bloodstream without causing gastrointestinal symptoms. The clinical picture is one of abrupt onset of chills and fever, often followed by hypotension, usually complicated by development of metastatic cutaneous lesions within 36 h after onset. The cutaneous lesions begin as erythematous plaques, rapidly evolving to hemorrhagic bullae and then to necrotic ulcers.[83,84,88] The lesions arise commonly on the extremities, occasionally bilaterally (Fig. 197-11). Soft tissue infections can also arise following inoculation of *V. vulnificus* or *V. alginolyticus* directly into a site of soft tissue injury. Infection by either of these *Vibrio* species can be life-threatening in immunocompromised hosts.

Pathogens Associated with Soil Exposure

Clostridium species Crepitant cellulitis is caused by *Clostridium* species: *C. perfringens* infection usually occurs following trauma and tissue damage; *C. septicum* infection occurs in the absence of trauma (spontaneous) following bacteremia from the bowel. Nonclostridial species, such as peptostreptococci or *Bacteroides* can also produce crepitant cellulitis.[94] Diabetes mellitus, along with other underlying conditions, is frequently associated with clostridial infections. Pain is usually mild, and overlying skin changes may be minimal. However, progression may be rapid and tissue gas accumulation may be extensive. Pure clostridial infections only rarely emit foul odors, while other nonclostridial crepitant species are more frequently putrid. The gas is most likely hydrogen, produced by anaerobic organisms through incomplete oxidation.[94] Surgery is critical in the treatment of clostridial crepitant cellulitis, together with antibiotic therapy. Hyperbaric oxygen therapy may be useful.

Cryptococcus neoformans (See Chap. 208) *C. neoformans* cellulitis most often occurs in immunocompromised individuals or in those with immunosuppressed states (systemic lupus erythematosus, chronic lymphocytic leukemia, myeloma, chronic active hepatitis, cervical medullary tumor, congenital lymphedema, congenital lymphedema with lymphopenia, liver transplantation, inflammatory bowel disease, and kidney transplantation).[95–97] Cryptococcal cellulitis has been reported in immunocompetent individuals. STI usually follows dissemination of the yeast to the skin from a primary pulmonary focus of infection. Clinically, well-demarcated edematous plaques with large bullae occur, often resembling bacterial cellulitis.

Pathogens Associated with Animal Exposure

Streptococcus iniae *S. iniae* is a fish pathogen that causes outbreaks of infections in fish on aquaculture farms, characterized by subcutaneous abscesses and meningoencephalitis. In humans, infection has been associated with minor injuries incurred with preparing whole raw fish or puncturing the skin with the dorsal fin, a fish bone, or a knife used in the cleaning or scaling.[98] The most common clinical presentation in humans is cellulitis arising on the hands and bacteremia. Cellulitis develops within 16 to 24 h after injuries. *A. hydrophilia* and *Erysipelothrix rhusiopathiae* can also present with a similar clinical presentation following trauma and cutaneous exposure to raw fish.

Erysipelothrix rhusiopathiae (See Chap. 200) *E. rhusiopathiae* is an aerobic to microaerobic non-spore-forming gram positive bacillus that is widely distributed in the environment. The organism causes erysipeloid, a mild, acute to subacute cellulitis that resolves spontaneously even if untreated with antibiotics. The organism is inoculated into the skin of individuals who prepare foods (saltwater fish, shellfish, meat, poultry).

Bacillus species (See Chap. 200) *B. anthracis* causes anthrax, which occurs most commonly in developing countries. Cutaneous anthrax is primarily a disease of herbivores, which acquire infection after coming into contact with soil-borne spores. Humans become

FIGURE 197-11

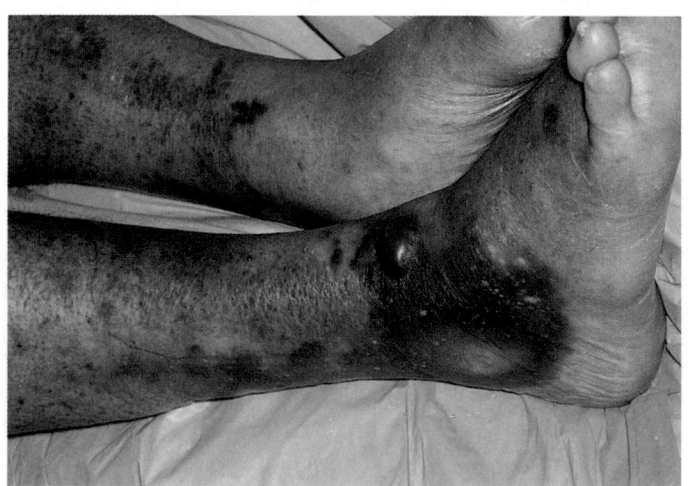

Cellulitis: *Vibrio vulnificus*. Bilateral hemorrhagic plaques and bullae on the legs, ankles, and feet of an older diabetic with cirrhosis who had eaten raw clams. Cellulitis caused by *V. vulnificus* usually follows a primary enteritis with bacteremia and dissemination to the skin.

infected from handling animals or animal products. Cutaneous anthrax usually presents on exposed sites (arms, hands, face, neck).

Pasteurella multocida *P. multocida* is a gram-negative coccobacillus that can be found in the oral cavity of 50 to 70 percent of cats and less frequently in dogs. Cellulitis most frequently follows bites or scratches. Secondary infection of clean wounds can occur after animal licking.[99] *P. multocida* has also been implicated in persistent postoperative wounds.[100] Onset of erythema, pain, and swelling occurs within hours of the bite, with regional lymphadenopathy developing within days.[101]

Miscellaneous Pathogens

Mycobacterium species (See also Chap. 201) *M. fortuitum* complex species are rapid growers and include *M. fortuitum*, *M. chelonae*, and *M. abscessus*. The organisms are widely distributed in soil, dust, and water. Inoculation has occurred via puncture wounds (injection or traumatic) or surgical procedures (augmentation mammoplasty, median sternotomy, percutaneous catheterization) (Fig. 197-12); rarely primary cellulitis occurs without recognizable skin trauma.[89,90] Contaminated gentian violet used for skin marking has been the source in some outbreaks. *M. fortuitum* complex STIs characteristically occur several weeks after the injury and appear as indolent wound infections (nodules, ulcers, granulomatous papules, or verrucous plaques). In immunocompromised individuals, *M. fortuitum* can disseminate hematogenously to skin (multiple recurring abscesses on the extremities) and joints.

Helicobacter cinaedi A syndrome characterized by fever, bacteremia, and recurrent *H. cinaedi* cellulitis has been described in immunocompromised patients. In a series of seven patients (six HIV-infected, one with a history of alcoholism) with *H. cinaedi* STIs, cellulitis with adjacent arthritis occurred in two patients. Ciprofloxacin was effective in treatment in five cases.[91] In a series of 23 febrile patients with *H. cinaedi* bacteremia (11 were HIV-infected; the others had underlying alcoholism, diabetes, or malig-

FIGURE 197-12

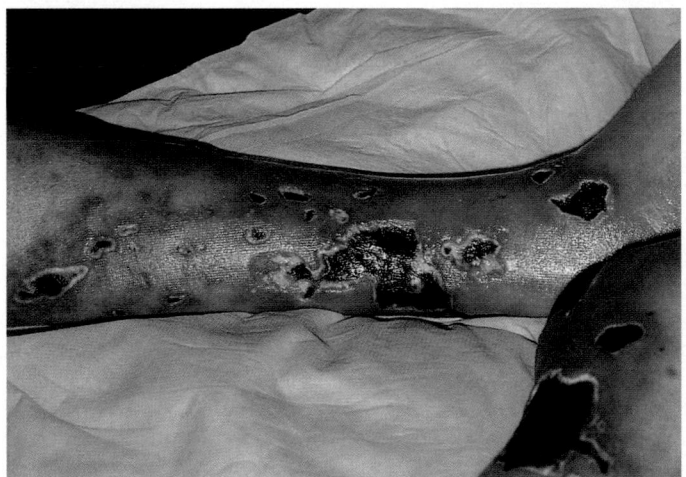

Cellulitis: *Mycobacterium chelonae*. Cellulitis occurred at operative sites following venous harvest and coronary artery bypass in a 37-year-old male with diabetes mellitus. The infection combined with peripheral vascular disease necessitated amputation of both legs above the knees.

nancy), 9 had cellulitis (some with a distinctive red brown or copper discoloration with minimal warmth).[92]

Corynebacterium jeikeium Skin and soft tissue infections due to *C. jeikeium* occur in granulocytopenic patients and take either of two forms: (1) primary infections (cellulitis at bone marrow biopsy sites, infection at insertion sites of intravascular catheters), and (2) secondary infections (erythematous or hemorrhagic papular rash, soft tissue abscess, or necrotic lesions) consequent on bacteremia from primary infection sites.[93] Vancomycin intravenously is the treatment of choice.

COURSE AND PROGNOSIS

Uncomplicated erysipelas remains confined primarily to the lymphatics and subcutaneous tissues. Even in the days prior to antibiotic therapy, it was sometimes a self-limited process, subsiding over 7 to 10 days. Occasionally, the organisms spread beyond the lymphatics, producing cellulitis with hemorrhagic bullae, necrosis, and subcutaneous abscesses. Untreated erysipelas or cellulitis may then be followed by bacteremia with metastatic infection in various organs. Antibiotic therapy produces improvement in the general condition of the patient in 24 to 48 h, but it takes several more days for subsidence of the local lesion to be clearly evident. Prompt treatment prevents both suppurative and nonsuppurative complications. However, in young infants and elderly debilitated patients and in individuals receiving glucocorticoids, the disease may progress with devastating rapidity to a fatal outcome. Erysipelas or cellulitis after saphenous vein harvest may be recurrent, presenting as edema, erythema, and tenderness along the course of the saphenous venectomy.

Erysipelas has a tendency to recur in the same area, perhaps due to the predisposing effects of chronic lymphatic obstruction, edema, and even elephantiasis caused by earlier infections. Such recurrent infections may produce persistent swelling of the lips (macrocheilia), cheeks (particularly the lax tissues beneath the eyes), lower extremities, or even abdomen. Chronic lymphedema of the lower extremities secondary to recurrent erysipelas may result in elephantiasis nostras verrucosa (see Chap. 167). Areas of lymphatic obstruction are predisposed to recurrent infections; for example, following radical mastectomy some patients are liable to recurrent episodes of what appears to be erysipelas in the area of lymphedema.

Acute cellulitis, because of its tendency to spread through the lymphatics and bloodstream, is a serious disease if not treated early. In older patients, involvement of the lower extremities may be complicated by thrombophlebitis. In patients with chronic edema, the process may spread extremely rapidly and recovery may be slow, despite sterilization of the lesions by antibiotics. Occasionally, superinfection of necrotic areas, principally with gram-negative organisms, complicates recovery.

The mortality rate for necrotizing fasciitis is high (reported to be 39 percent); early diagnosis and aggressive treatment of necrotizing fasciitis is the most important factor in determining outcome.[102] Certain risk factors that can impact negatively on outcome have been identified: age > 50, diabetes mellitus, malnutrition, hypertension, and intravenous drug abuse. Premorbid diabetes mellitus, alone, and the presence of three or more of these risk factors

lulitis is 50 percent, the patient usually succumbing to septic shock and circulatory collapse.

TABLE 197-6

Drugs of First Choice and Alternative Drugs for Treatment of Soft Tissue

ORGANISM	DRUG OF FIRST CHOICE	ALTERNATIVE DRUGS
Staphylococcus aureus or epidermidis		
Non-penicillinase producing	Penicillin G or V	A cephalosporin; clindamycin; vancomycin; imipenem; a fluoroquinolone
Penicillinase-producing	A penicillinase-resistant penicillin	A cephalosporin; vancomycin; amoxicillin/clavulanic acid; ticarcillin/clavulanic acid; piperacillin/tazobactam; ampicillin/sulbactam; imipenem; clindamycin; a fluoroquinolone
Methicillin-resistant	Vancomycin ± gentamicin ± rifampin	Teicoplanin, rifampin, trimethoprim-sulfamethoxazole; a fluoroquinolone
Group A, B, C, G streptococcus	Penicillin G or V	An erythromycin; a cephalosporin; vancomycin; clarithromycin; azithromycin; clindamycin
Streptococcus pneumoniae	Penicillin G or V	An erythromycin; a cephalosporin; vancomycin; rifampin; trimethoprim-sulfamethoxazole; azithromycin; clarithromycin; clindamycin; chloramphenicol
Haemophilus influenzae	Cefotaxime or ceftriazone	Cefuroxime; chloramphenicol
Pseudomonas aeruginosa	Ceftazidime + tobramycin	Aminoglycoside (tobramycin, gentamicin, or amikacin) + antipseudomonal penicillin (ticarcillin, mezlocillin, or piperacillin); imipenem + aminoglycoside (tobramycin, gentamicin or amikacin); a fluoroquinolone
Vibrio vulnificus	A tetracycline	Cefotaxime; trimethoprim-sulfamethoxazole; a fluoroquinolone
Aeromonas	Trimethoprim-sulfamethoxazole	Gentamicin or tobramycin; imipenem; a fluoroquinolone
Clostridium perfringens	Penicillin G	Metronidazole; clindamycin; imipenem; a tetracycline; chloramphenicol
Mycobacterium fortuitum complex	Amikacin + doxycycline	Cefoxitin; a sulfonamide; rifampin + ethambutol (for *M. marinum*)
Cryptococcus neoformans	Amphotericin B + flucytosine	Fluconazole

SOURCE: Modified from Med Lett 36:16, 53, 1994.

have been reported to be predictive of a significantly higher mortality rate . Overall, clostridial infections have an attendant mortality of 19 to 70 percent. Of note, spontaneously occurring gas gangrene tends to have a more ominous mortality of 67 to 100 percent due to its rapid onset without an obvious predisposing traumatic or surgical wound and high association with underlying malignancy. Death is usually due to sepsis, multisystem organ failure, or invasion of major vessels. The mortality for synergistic necrotizing cel-

TREATMENT

Antibiotics (See Tables 197-6 and 197-7)

Very mild cases of incipient erysipelas can be treated on an outpatient basis with intramuscular procaine penicillin (600,000 units once or twice daily) or with oral penicillin V, 250 to 500 mg every 6 h. Erythromycin is also effective (250 to 500 mg PO every 6 h) in penicillin-allergic individuals. Some patients with cellulitis without underlying medical problems can be treated with outpatient parenteral antimicrobial-drug therapy.[103]

Individuals with more extensive streptococcal infections and underlying medical problems such as diabetes mellitus should be hospitalized and treated with intravenous aqueous penicillin G (600,000 to 2 million units every 6 h). In severe streptococcal skin infections (e.g., extensive erysipelas, cellulitis, or streptococcal gangrene), parenteral aqueous penicillin G (600,000 to 2 million units every 4 to 6 h) should be given. In the ill patient in whom a staphylococcal etiology might be considered, one of the penicillinase-resistant semisynthetic penicillins (e.g., nafcillin, 1.0 to 1.5 g intravenously every 4 h) should be employed. In the patient with a questionable penicillin allergy, cephalothin (1.0 g intravenously every 3 to 4 h) may be substituted. If the patient has had an immediate type of reaction to penicillin (anaphylaxis or angioneurotic edema, etc.) then vancomycin (1.0 to 1.5 g intravenously daily) would be a reasonable alternative for treatment of a suspected staphylococcal infection.

For individuals with gangrenous cellulitis, broad coverage is recommended until specific pathogens and susceptibilities are available. Ampicillin (or nafcillin), gentamicin, and either metronidazole or clindamycin would be an acceptable initial regimen for treating suspected nonclostridial necrotizing STI pending bacteriologic results (smear, culture). While clostridia are susceptible to penicillin, clindamycin, metronidazole, a combination of beta-lactam and beta-lactamase inhibitor, imipenem, and chloramphenicol, optimal treatment has not been established. High-dose penicillin either alone or in combination with clindamycin, metronidazole, or chloramphenicol should be adequate.

TABLE 197-7

CHAPTER 197
Soft Tissue Infections   2229

Antimicrobial Treatment of Necrotizing Infection of Skin, Fascia, and Muscle

ORGANISM	DRUG OF FIRST CHOICE	ALTERNATIVE DRUGS
Mixed infection	Ampicillin/sulbactam Imipenem/cilastatin Ticarcillin/clavulanate	Cefoxitin, clinda- mycin, or metroni- dazole + an ami- noglycoside
Streptococcus (except en- terococcus)	Penicillin or ampicillin	Cefazolin
	Ampicillin-sulbactam Penicillin + clindamycin for toxic shock syn- drome or necrotizing fasciitis	Vancomycin
Staphylococcus aureus	Nafcillin (or oxacillin) Vancomycin (for methi- cillin-resistant strains)	Cefazolin

SOURCE: Modified from Gorbach.[9]

Local Measures

Care of the local lesion of erysipelas and cellulitis includes immobilization and elevation of the involved area to reduce local edema. Cool, sterile saline dressings decrease the local pain and are particularly indicated in the presence of bullous lesions. The use of a footboard may protect the affected area from trauma. The application of moist heat later may aid in the localization of an abscess in association with cellulitis, but it should not be used in a patient with arterial insufficiency in the involved extremity.

Surgical intervention

Treatment of necrotizing STIs requires early and complete surgical debridement of necrotic tissue in combination with high-dose antibiotics. Surgical management involves debridement of the gangrenous skin and incision and drainage of the surrounding tissues and fascial planes. Pressure on the skin and subcutaneous tissues should be released; incisions should be extended beyond the areas of gangrene and far enough into the superficial fascia to establish good drainage and to reach healthy tissues. Although no discrete pockets of pus are found, there is significant oozing of tissue fluid, which must be replaced by appropriate administration of fluids and colloids. Reexploration and debridement should be performed as necessary to ensure that all necrotic tissue has been removed. In some cases, particularly in clostridial myonecrosis, limb amputations may be necessary to stop the advancement of gangrene.

In synergistic necrotizing cellulitis, the major cause of delay in instituting appropriate therapy is the failure to appreciate involvement of fascia and deep subcutaneous tissue, leading to the misdiagnosis of this infection as cellulitis. Prompt exploration of the involved area is of paramount importance. Easy passage of a hemostat along a plane just superficial to the deep fascia (not expected with early cellulitis) should make the diagnosis. A frozen-section soft tissue biopsy performed deep enough and early in the course of the illness may provide a definitive diagnosis and expedite appropriate treatment. Debridement should be carried out beyond the area of involvement until completely normal fascia is reached. All necrotic fascia and fat should be removed, and the wound should be left open. If there is any question as to the adequacy of the initial de-

bridement, a "second-look" procedure is indicated 24 to 48 h later. Prior to obtaining results from cultures, initial antimicrobial therapy should be based on knowledge of a prominent role of anaerobic bacteria in this infection and on the specific findings on Gram-stained smear of the exudate.

Anaerobic clostridial cellulitis is treated with wide surgical debridement of all devitalized muscle and parenteral administration of penicillin (often with metronidazole) in dosage of about 10,000,000 units daily. The immediate and extensive debridement (or amputation of an extremity) is particularly vital in clostridial myonecrosis. The use of hyperbaric oxygen "drenching," particularly in patients with far-advanced disease involving the trunk in whom surgical excision would be mutilating, appears to have a place in current therapy. Polyvalent gas gangrene antitoxin (40,000 to 60,000 units every 6 h for several doses) has been administered often in the past, but there has been no clear evidence of its efficacy. This antiserum is no longer commercially available.

Although prospective studies are lacking, retrospective data indicate that adjunctive hyperbaric oxygen therapy may reduce morbidity and mortality in both clostridial and nonclostridial necrotizing infections.[104] Proposed mechanisms by which hyperbaric oxygen could improve outcome include enhancement of leukocyte production of bactericidal free radicals, direct inhibition of anaerobic bacterial growth, preservation of poorly perfused tissue, and promotion of wound healing.

Further important considerations in the treatment of these often critically ill patients include nutritional support, fecal diversion, and surgical drains when serosal-lined cavities are involved. Debridement defects should never be repaired primarily. Healing by second intention or delayed closure is acceptable. Secondary plastic surgery should be considered for correction of functional or cosmetic defects.

PREVENTION

Individuals with cellulitis are predisposed to recurrent episodes, especially at sites of chronic lymphedema. Those who have had saphenous vein harvests for coronary bypass grafts are at greatest risk for developing cellulitis in the donor leg; in these patients, eradication of tinea pedis is essential, and topical antifungal therapy, particularly of the toe webs, should be carried out prophylactically. Support stockings and leg elevation are critical for prophylaxis against infections in patients with chronic lymphedema. Secondary prophylaxis with antibiotics such as penicillin V (250 to 500 mg daily) or dicloxacillin (125 to 250 mg daily) on a long-term basis is indicated in some individuals with several episodes of recurring cellulitis in spite of the above recommendations.

REFERENCES

1. Sachs MK: Cutaneous cellulitis. *Arch Dermatol* **127**:493, 1991
2. Stevens DL et al: Severe group A streptococcus infections associated with a toxic shock-like syndrome and scarlet fever toxin. *N Engl J Med* **321**:1, 1989
3. Stevens DL: Invasive group A *Streptococcus* infections. *Clin Infect Dis* **14**:2, 1992
4. Heng MCY et al: Haemorrhagic cellulitis: A syndrome associated with tumor necrosis factor-alpha. *Br J Dermatol* **130**:65, 1994

5. Hook EWI et al: Microbiologic evaluation of cutaneous cellulitis in adults. *Arch Intern Med* **146**:295, 1986

6. Fleisher G et al: Cellulitis: Bacterial etiology, clinical features, and laboratory findings. *J Pediatr* **97**:591, 1980

7. Garner JS et al: CDC definitions for nosocomial infections, 1988. *Am J Infect Control* **16**:281, 1988

8. Swartz MN: Cellulitis and superficial infections, in *Principles and Practice of Infectious Diseases,* 4th ed, edited by GL Mandell, JE Bennett, R Dolin. New York, Churchill Livingstone, 1995, pp 917–919

9. Gorbach SL: IDCP Guidelines: Necrotizing skin and soft tissue infections. Part II: Myositis, Meleney's gangrene, pyomyositis, necrotizing cellulitis, nonclostridial cellulitis, and Fournier's gangrene. *Infect Dis Clin Prac* **5**:463, 1996

10. Riefler JI et al: Necrotizing fasciitis in adults due to group B streptococcus. Report of a case and review of the literature. *Arch Intern Med* **148**:727, 1988

11. Giuliano A et al: Bacteriology of necrotizing fasciitis. *Am J Surg* **134**:52, 1977

12. Laucks SS II: Fournier's gangrene. *Surg Clin North Am* **74**:1339, 1994

13. Salvino C et al: Necrotizing infections of the perineum. *South Med J* **74**:1339, 1994

14. Swartz MN: Cellulitis and superficial infections, in *Principles and Practice of Infectious Diseases,* 4th ed, edited by GL Mandell, JE Bennett, R Dolin. New York, Churchill Livingstone, 1995, pp 917–919

15. Stevens DL et al: Spontaneous, nontraumatic gangrene due to *Clostridium septicum. Rev Infect Dis* **12**:286, 1990

16. Kingston D, Seal DV: Current hypotheses on synergistic gangrene. *Br J Surg* **77**:260, 1990

17. Brook I, Frazier EH: Clinical features and aerobic and anaerobic microbiological characteristics of cellulitis. *Arch Surg* **130**:786, 1995

18. Adam RD et al: Mucormycosis: Emerging prominence of cutaneous infections. *Clin Infect Dis* **19**:67, 1994

19. Shelley WB et al: Occult *Streptococcus pyogenes* in cellulitis: Demonstration by immunofluorescence. *Br J Dermatol* **132**:989, 1995

20. Sachs MK: The optimum use of needle aspiration in the bacteriologic diagnosis of cellulitis in adults. *Arch Intern Med* **150**:1907, 1990

21. Bernard P et al: Streptococcal cause of erysipelas and cellulitis in adults. *Arch Dermatol* **125**:779, 1989

22. Stamenkovic I, Lew PD: Early recognition of potentially fatal necrotizing fasciitis: The use of frozen-section biopsy. *N Engl J Med* **310**:1689, 1984

23. Barker FG et al: Streptococcal necrotizing fasciitis: Comparisons between histological and clinical features. *J Clin Pathol* **40**:335, 1987

24. Swartz MN: Cellulitis and subcutaneous tissue infections, in *Principles and Practice of Infectious Diseases,* 2d ed, edited by GL Mandell, RG Douglas, JE Bennett. New York, Churchill Livingstone, 1985, pp 909–928

25. Swartz MN: Myositis, in *Principles and Practice of Infectious Diseases,* 4th ed, edited by GL Mandell, JE Bennett, R Dolin. New York, Churchill Livingstone, 1995, pp 926–929

26. Saiag P et al: Magnetic resonance imaging in adults presenting with severe acute infectious cellulitis. *Arch Dermatol* **130**:1150, 1994

27. Mulligan ME et al: Methicillin-resistant *Staphylococcus aureus:* A consensus review of the microbiology, pathogenesis, and epidemiology with implications for prevention and management. *Am J Med* **94**:313, 1993

28. Bradley SF et al: Methicillin-resistant *Staphylococcus aureus:* Colonization and infection in a long-term care facility. *Ann Intern Med* **115**:417, 1991

29. Kauffman CA et al: Attempts to eradicate methicillin-resistant *Staphylococcus aureus* from a long-term facility with the use of mupirocin ointment. *Am J Med* **94**:371, 1993

30. DiTomaso A et al: Case report: Toxic shock syndrome arising from cellulitis. *Am J Med Sci* **308**:110, 1994

31. Chartier C, Grosshans E: Erysipelas. *Int J Dermatol* **29**:459, 1990

32. Kerstens PJ et al: Erysipelas-like lesions associated with *Campylobacter jejuni* septicemia in patients with hypogammaglobulinemia. *Eur J Clin Microbiol Infect Dis* **11**:842, 1992

33. Cox NH et al: Pre-septal cellulitis and facial erysipelas due to *Moraxella* species. *Clin Exp Dermatol* **19**:321, 1994

34. Auerbach SB et al: Outbreak of invasive group A streptococcal infections in a nursing home. Lessons on prevention and control. *Arch Intern Med* **152**:1017, 1992

35. Schwartz B et al: Cluster of invasive group A streptococcal infections in family, hospital, and nursing home settings. *Clin Infect Dis* **15**:277, 1992

36. Jorup-Ronstrom C: Epidemiological, bacteriological and complicating features of erysipelas. *Scand J Infect Dis* **18**:519, 1986

37. Baddour LM, Bisno AL: Recurrent cellulitis after coronary bypass surgery: Association with superficial fungal infection in saphenous vein venectomy limbs. *JAMA* **251**:1049, 1984

38. Baddour JM, Bisno AL: Recurrent cellulitis after saphenous venectomy for coronary bypass surgery. *Ann Intern Med* **97**:493, 1982

39. Hurwitz RM, Tisserand ME: Streptococcal cellulitis proved by skin biopsy in a coronary artery bypass graft patient. *Arch Dermatol* **121**:908, 1985

40. Navarro VJ et al: A comparison of *Streptococcus pyogenes* (group A streptococcal) bacteremia at an urban and a suburban hospital. The importance of intravenous drug use. *Arch Intern Med* **153**:2679, 1993

41. Torres-Martînez C et al: Streptococcus-associated toxic shock. *Arch Dis Child* **67**:126, 1992

42. Montemarano AD, James WD: *Staphylococcus aureus* as a cause of perianal dermatitis. *Pediatr Dermatol* **10**:259, 1993

43. Spear RM et al: Perianal streptococcal cellulitis. *J Pediatr* **107**:557, 1985

44. Duhra P, Ilchyshyn A: Perianal streptococcal cellulitis with penile involvement. *Br J Dermatol* **123**:793, 1990

45. Wright JE, Butt HL: Perianal infection with beta hemolytic streptococcus. *Arch Dis Child* **70**:145, 1994

46. Eriksson B et al: Erysipelas: Clinical and bacteriologic spectrum and serologic aspects. *Clin Infect Dis* **23**:1091, 1996

47. Kline A, O'Donnell E: Group B *Streptococcus* as a cause of neonatal bullous skin lesions. *Pediatr Infect Dis J* **12**:165, 1993

48. Barton LL et al: Neonatal Group B streptococcal cellulitis-adenitis. *Pediatr Dermatol* **10**:58, 1993

49. Jackson LA et al: Risk factors for group B streptococcal disease in adults. *Ann Intern Med* **123**:415, 1995

50. Harrison LH et al: Relapsing invasive group B streptococcal infection in adults. *Ann Intern Med* **123**:421, 1995

51. Ellison RT, McGregor JA: Recurrent postcoital lower-extremity streptococcal erythroderma in women. Streptococcal-sex syndrome. *JAMA* **257**:3260, 1987

52. Baddour LMJJ et al: Non-group A beta-hemolytic streptococcal cellulitis: Association with venous and lymphatic compromise. *Am J Med* **79**:155, 1985

53. Schwartz B et al: Invasive group B streptococcal disease in adults. A population-based study in Metropolitan Atlanta. *JAMA* **266**:1112, 1991

54. Bradley SF et al: Group C streptococcal bacteremia: Analysis of 88 cases. *Rev Infect Dis* **13**:270, 1991

55. Butt A, Janney A: Clinical characteristics of group G streptococcal bacteremia. *Infect Dis Clin Prac* **7**:43, 1998

56. Valenzuela TD et al: Transmission of "toxic strep" syndrome from an infected child to a firefighter during CPR. *Ann Emerg Med* **20**:123, 1991

57. Hirose Y et al: Toxic shock-like syndrome caused by non-group A β-hemolytic streptococci. *Arch Intern Med* **157**:1891, 1997

58. Auerbach SB et al: Outbreak of invasive group A streptococcal infections in a nursing home. Lessons on prevention and control. *Arch Intern Med* **00**:1017, 1992

59. Cowan MR et al: Serious group A beta hemolytic streptococcal infections complicating varicella. *Ann Emerg Med* **23**:818, 1994

60. Lawlor MT et al: Cellulitis due to *Streptococcus pneumoniae:* Case report and review of the literature. *Clin Infect Dis* **14**:247, 1992

61. Dinubile MJ et al: Pneumococcal soft-tissue infections: Possible association with connective tissue disease. *J Infect Dis* **163**:897, 1991

62. House NS et al: Acute onset of bilateral hemorrhagic leg lesions. Pneumococcal cellulitis. *Arch Dermatol* **132**:81, 1996

63. Choudhri SH et al: A case of necrotizing fasciitis due to *Streptococcus pneumoniae. Br J Dermatol* **128**:128, 1995

64. Lin VH et al: Meningococcal endocarditis presenting as cellulitis. *Clin Infect Dis* **21**:1023, 1995

65. Israele V, Nelson JD: Periorbital and orbital cellulitis. *Pediatr Infect Dis J* **6**:404, 1987

66. Broadhurst LE et al: Decreases in invasive *Haemophilus influenzae* disease in US army children, 1984 through 1991. *JAMA* **269**:227, 1993

67. Adams WG et al: Decline of childhood *Haemophilus influenzae* type b (Hib) disease in the Hib vaccine era. *JAMA* **269**:221, 1993

68. Stumvoll M, Fritsche A: Necrotizing fasciitis caused by unencapsulated *Haemophilus influenzae. Clin Infect Dis* **25**:327, 1997

69. Castanet J et al: *Escherichia coli* cellulitis: Two cases. *Acta Derm Venereol (Stockh)* **72**:310, 1992

70. Corredoira JM et al: Gram-negative bacillary cellulitis in patients with hepatic cirrhosis. *Eur J Clin Microbiol Infect Dis* **13**:19, 1994

71. Fergie JE et al: *Psaeudomonas aeruginosa* cellulitis and ecthyma gangrenosum in immunocompromised children. *Pediatr Infect Dis J* **10**:496, 1991

72. Huminer D et al: Ecthyma gangrenosum without bacteremia. *Arch Intern Med* **147**:299, 1987

73. Tredget EE et al: Epidemiology of infections with *Pseudomonas aeruginosa* in burn patients: The role of hydrotherapy. *Clin Infect Dis* **15**:941, 1993

74. Boisseau AM et al: Perineal ecthyma gangrenosum in infancy and early childhood: Septic and nonsepticemic forms. *J Am Acad Dermatol* **27**:415, 1992

75. Rodot S et al: Ecthyma gangrenosum caused by *Klebsiella pneumoniae. Int J Dermatol* **34**:216, 1995

76. Sevinsky LD et al: Ecthyma gangrenosum: A cutaneous manifestation of *Pseudomonas aeruginosa* sepsis. *J Am Acad Dermatol* **29**:102, 1992

77. Vartivarian SE et al: Mucocutaneous and soft tissue infections caused by *Xanthomonas maltophilia. Ann Intern Med* **121**:969, 1994

78. Centers for Disease Control and Prevention: *Aeromonas* wound infections associated with outdoor activities—California. *MMWR* **39**:334, 1990

79. Voss LM et al: Musculoskeletal and soft tissue *Aeromonas* infection: An environmental disease. *Mayo Clin Proc* **67**:422, 1992

80. Gold WL, Salit IE: *Aeromonas hydrophila* infections of skin and soft tissue: Report of 11 cases and review. *Clin Infect Dis* **16**:69, 1993

81. Kelly KA et al: Spectrum of extraintestinal disease due to *Aeromonas* species in tropical Queensland, Australia. *Clin Infect Dis* **16**:574, 1993

82. Mouzin E et al: Prevention of *Vibrio vulnificus* infections: Assessment of regulatory educational strategies. *JAMA* **278**:576, 1997

83. Centers for Disease Control and Prevention: *Vibrio vulnificus* infections associated with raw oyster consumption—Florida, 1981–1992. *MMWR* **42**:405, 1993

84. Levine WC, Griffin PM: *Vibrio* infections on the Gulf Coast: Results of first year of regional surveillance. *J Infect Dis* **167**:479, 1993

85. Raza H, Cutrona AF: *Vibrio vulnificus* septicemia should prompt the search for liver disease. *Infect Dis Clin Pract* **2**:273, 1993

86. Rabinowitch BL et al: *Vibrio parahaemolyticus* septicemia associated with waterskiing. *Clin Infect Dis* **16**:339, 1993

87. Perez-Tirse J et al: *Vibrio damsela:* A cause of fulminant septicemia. *Arch Intern Med* **153**:1838, 1993

88. Howard RJ, Bennett NT: Infections caused by halophilic marine *Vibrio* bacteria. *Ann Surg* **217**:525, 1993

89. Lederman C et al: *Mycobacterium haemophilum* cellulitis in a heart transplant recipient. *J Am Acad Dermatol* **30**:804, 1994

90. Torres JR et al: Infection site abscess due to *Mycobacterium fortuitum-chelonae* complex in the immunocompetent host. *Infect Dis Clin Prac* **7**:56, 1998

91. Burman WJ et al: Multifocal cellulitis and monoarticular arthritis as manifestations of *Helicobacter cinaedi* bacteremia. *Clin Infect Dis* **20**:564, 1995

92. Kiehlbauch JA et al: *Helicobacter cinaedi*–associated bacteremia and cellulitis in immunocompromised patients. *Ann Intern Med* **121**:90, 1994

93. Dan M et al: Cutaneous manifestations of infection with *Corynebacterium* group JK. *Rev Infect Dis* **10**:1204, 1988

94. Feingold DS: Gangrenous and crepitant cellulitis. *J Am Acad Dermatol* **6**:289, 1982

95. Sanchez-Albisua B et al: Cryptococcal cellulitis in an immunocompetent host. *J Am Acad Dermatol* **36**:109, 1997

96. Krywonis N et al: Cryptococcal cellulitis in congenital lymphedema. *Int J Dermatol* **29**:41, 1990

97. Gloster HM et al: Cryptococcal cellulitis in a diabetic, kidney transplant patient. *J Am Acad Dermatol* **30**:1025, 1994

98. Weinstein MR et al: Invasive infections due to a fish pathogen, *Streptococcus iniae. N Engl J Med* **227**:589, 1997

99. Yu GVJJ et al: An unusual case of diabetic cellulitis due to *Pasturella multocida. J Foot Ankle Surg* **34**:91, 1995

100. Cook PP: Persistent postoperative wound infection with *Pasturella multocida:* Case report and literature review. *Infection* **23**:252, 1995

101. Brue C, Chosidow O: *Pasturella multocida* wound infection and cellulitis. *Int J Dermatol* **33**:471, 1994

102. Voros D et al: Role of early and extensive surgery in the treatment of severe necrotizing soft tissue infection. *Br J Surg* **80**:1191, 1993

103. Gilbert DN et al: Outpatient parenteral antimicrobial-drug therapy. *N Engl J Med* **337**:829, 1997

104. Mathur MN et al: Cellulitis owing to *Aeromonas hydrophilia:* Treatment with hyperbaric oxygen. *Aust N Z J Surg* **65**:367, 1995

CHAPTER 198

Arnold N. Weinberg
Morton N. Swartz

Gram-Negative Coccal and Bacillary Infections

Many of the characteristic cutaneous manifestations of infection with gram-negative organisms are due to direct microbial invasion of the skin or subcutaneous tissues. In addition, platelet depression, disseminated intravascular coagulation, effects of toxic products of these bacteria, and possibly the dermal or generalized Shwartzman reaction may produce varied hemorrhagic cutaneous manifestations. The typical skin lesions in meningococcal or *Pseudomonas* septicemia, often among the earliest indications of generalized infection, can provide immediate and important clues to early diagnosis.[1]

INFECTIONS DUE TO *NEISSERIA MENINGITIDIS* (MENINGOCOCCUS)

General Features

Three clinical syndromes associated with cutaneous involvement occur in meningococcal disease: meningitis, acute meningococcemia, and chronic meningococcemia. Skin lesions are frequently the most dramatic manifestations and graphically add to the aura of fear attached to these infections. The presence of areas of purpura or gross hemorrhage is generally associated with distinctly poorer prognosis than a local or generalized petechial eruption.

Bacteriology and Pathogenesis

The *Neisseria* are obligate, aerobic, encapsulated gram-negative, kidney bean–shaped cocci that pair with their long axes in parallel. *N. meningitidis* grows well on blood-enriched media (chocolate agar), supplemented by an atmosphere containing 5 to 10% CO_2 and approximately 50% humidity. In potentially mixed bacterial exudates, these organisms should be grown on a selective medium (e.g., modified Thayer-Martin); they can be distinguished from *N. gonorrhoeae* by their fermentation of both glucose and maltose rather than of glucose alone. Meningococci are separable into at least 13 serologic groups on the basis of capsular antigens. Agglutination and capsular swelling reactions identify groups A, B, C, Y, and W-135 as the major pathogens involved in human disease today.[2]

The presence of a virulent strain colonizing the nasal mucous membranes of a nonimmune host precedes clinical disease. Initial colonization may be facilitated by pili that attach to specific receptors on nonciliated columnar mucosal epithelial cells[3,4] and by production of an IgA protease that cleaves host secretory IgA.[5] Encapsulated organisms resist phagocytosis. With the onset of a viral respiratory infection, they may multiply locally and invade the bloodstream or be aspirated into the lower respiratory tract. Men-

ingitis, meningococcemia, or pneumonitis can result. Predisposition to sporadic and occasionally recurrent meningococcal disease occurs in patients with congenital or acquired complement deficiencies, particularly late-acting components C5 to C8.[2,6]

The skin lesions associated with meningococcemia and meningococcal meningitis result from damage to small dermal blood vessels. By light and electron microscopy, bacteria are found within endothelial and polymorphonuclear cells.[7] Organisms can sometimes be seen when needle aspirates or punch biopsies from involved areas of skin are Gram-stained.[8] Local endothelial damage, thrombosis, and necrosis of the vessel walls occur. Immunoglobulins and complement are present, even in early vascular lesions.[2,7] Edema, infarction of overlying skin, and extravasation of red blood cells are responsible for the characteristic macular, papular, pustular, petechial, hemorrhagic, and bullous lesions. Similar vascular lesions occur in the meninges and in other tissues.

In addition to direct involvement of skin vessels by meningococci, many of the cutaneous hemorrhagic lesions may be due to the direct effects of endotoxin or changes via the *dermal* Shwartzman reaction. Data supporting this view have been presented showing that purified meningococcal endotoxin, in contrast to endotoxin derived from *Escherichia coli*, was uniquely potent in production of the dermal Shwartzman reaction in mice.[9] The frequency of hemorrhagic cutaneous manifestations in meningococcal infections, compared to infections with other gram-negative organisms, may be due to increased potency and/or unique properties of meningococcal endotoxins for the dermal reaction. On the other hand, lipopolysaccharide (LPS) endotoxins from meningococci and *E. coli* are equally potent producers of the *generalized* Shwartzman reaction and lethality in mice.[9]

The profound effects on small blood vessels, directly related to bacterial invasion or indirectly due to LPS endotoxin, may lead to diminished blood volume, lowered cardiac output, anoxia in vital organs, myocardial failure, hypotension, acidosis, and diffuse intravascular coagulation.[2,10,11]

Meningococci can be isolated from the blood in chronic meningococcemia, usually during periodic fevers, rash, and joint manifestations. The pathogenesis of this form of disease is less well understood than that of the acute process. This chronic form of meningococcal infection has been linked to absence of terminal components of complement in several patients and recently to a patient with isolated IgA deficiency, associations that may provide insights into pathogenic mechanisms in this unusual host-parasite interaction.[12,13] The absence of bacteria, bacterial antigenic material, and granulocytic inflammation contrasts with the positive findings seen in acute infections. The histopathology of a skin biopsy specimen in an immunocompetent 1½ year-old infant revealed leukocytoclastic vasculitis, an exception to the usual absence of vascular damage found in chronic meningococcemia.[14] The chronic course of the disease, lack of endotoxin-like manifestations (even with demonstrated bacteremia), and the potentiality for metamorphosis to meningitis or endocarditis suggest that an unusual host-parasite relationship is central to this persistent infection.[15]

Epidemiology

Humans are the only known natural hosts, and nasopharyngeal carrier rates vary (5 to 15 percent overall) with age: $\sim$1 percent in children 3 to 48 months of age, 5 percent in those 14 to 17 years of age, and 20 to 40 percent in young adults. In crowded conditions, such as schools or military camps, or when a carrier of a new strain develops disease in a day-care nursery or family setting, carrier rates can increase dramatically, independent of clinical disease.[16]

Asymptomatic exposure to a variety of encapsulated and nonencapsulated *N. meningitidis* strains can stimulate protective bactericidal antibody.[17] In addition, a variety of nonmeningococcal microorganisms, such as *E. coli* K1 strains and *N. lactamica*, stimulate production of cross-reacting protective antibodies to these potential pathogens.[18] Thus, immunity to meningococci increases with age due to subclinical interactions with *N. meningitidis* or to other antigenically related bacteria. As a result, protective bactericidal antibodies, both IgG and IgM, are found in 70 to 95 percent of young adults.[19] Newborn infants are often resistant to meningococcal disease; this protection lasts until approximately 3 to 6 months of age, by which time passively acquired maternal IgG antibody levels have markedly diminished.[17–19] Some young adults with acute meningococcal disease have circulating bactericidal antibody present at the outset. This paradoxical situation may be explained by the finding that such patients can have serum IgA antibody that blocks the bactericidal reaction.[2,20] Even though individuals acquire group-specific antibody from subclinical exposures in youth, the presence of other immunoglobulins may interfere with this protective mechanism. Any endogenous microorganisms that stimulate IgA antibody, such as *E. coli* K1 strains, could paradoxically interfere with the protective effects of bactericidal antibody.[21]

In the past, sporadic cases (or outbreaks) often emerged in the military services in boot camp, where young, susceptible recruits are brought together in situations of overwork, stress, and crowding. This problem has been lessened considerably by the routine use in the military of a quadrivalent vaccine containing polysaccharides of groups A, C, Y, and W-135. Owing to poor immunogenicity and protective efficacy of the group B capsular polysaccharide, current vaccine development has shifted to use of conjugates with outer membrane protein fragments. A number have been in use outside the United States with favorable results, but are not approved in the United States.[22] Unfortunately, little protection is provided the age group at highest risk, children less than 4 years of age.[23,24] There is also concern of possible adverse effects because of the cross-reactivity between group B capsular polysaccharide [(2→8)-linked *N*-acetylneuraminic acid] and central nervous system glycoprotein antigens.

Although the meningococcal polysaccharide vaccines are immunogenic in adults, they do not elicit a good antibody response in children under 2 years of age; newer generations of polysaccharide–protein conjugate vaccines appear to be more immunogenic in this age group, as dramatically demonstrated with the new *H. influenzae* (Hib) conjugates.[25]

In civilian populations, adult family members probably introduce the organism into the household, but secondary cases are most frequently spread from ill children ages 1 through 14 to other family members in the same age group, especially under crowded conditions.[26] Household spread is 500 to 800 times more frequent than secondary cases in the community at large.[27] An exception to this

is the increased incidence of secondary cases in day-care centers where large numbers of susceptible children congregate.[28]

Serogroup A isolates have most often been associated with epidemic disease, but serogroups C and B are also identified in outbreaks, as well as sporadic cases. Isolates belonging to groups Y and W-135 have increased in frequency in the past several decades.[29] Many of these have occurred in cases of respiratory disease in older individuals. Meningococcal disease occurs worldwide, including equatorial Africa (the "meningitis belt," where it is almost always due to serogroup A) and Alaska. Most cases occur in early childhood (to age 4 years) and adolescence, but older individuals also become ill during epidemics. Absence of the spleen has been associated with fulminant meningococcal disease, just as reported for other encapsulated organisms. *N. meningitidis* has been isolated from the genitourinary tract in individuals practicing orogenital sex and in homosexuals.[30]

Acute Meningococcemia and Meningitis

CLINICAL MANIFESTATIONS *History* The disease often follows a mild upper respiratory infection associated with headache, grippelike complaints, nausea and vomiting, and muscle soreness. These symptoms can be so brief that fever, obtundation, and other manifestations of meningitis are the initial findings. In fulminant meningococcemia, vomiting, stupor, hemorrhagic rash, and hypotension may be evident within a few hours of onset of symptoms. Milder cases, developing at a slower pace, also occur.

Cutaneous lesions The skin findings associated with acute meningococcal infections are characteristically petechial, but transient urticarial, macular, or papular lesions (Fig. 198-1A), which can resemble viral exanthems, may be noted initially.[31] The petechiae are small and irregular, have a "smudged" appearance, and are often raised, with pale grayish vesicular centers. While most commonly located on the extremities and trunk, lesions can also be found on the head (Fig. 198-1B), palms, soles, and mucous membranes (including the conjunctivae). Pustular or extensive bullous and hemorrhagic lesions with central necrosis (suggillations) can develop. Gangrenous hemorrhagic areas (indistinguishable from purpura fulminans) (see Chap. 195) can appear in patients with severe meningococcemia, often complicated by disseminated intravascular coagulation (DIC) (Fig. 198-1C). Skin lesions and bacteremia are rarely seen with meningococcal pneumonia.[32]

Other physical findings Patients with meningitis display signs of meningeal irritation and altered consciousness. Occasionally, agitated or maniacal behavior predominates. Cranial nerve palsies, long-tract signs, seizures, and alterations in vital signs associated with changes in intracranial pressure may be present.

Obtundation and hypotension without meningeal signs, associated with the syndrome of DIC, are characteristic features of acute fulminating meningococcemia.[11] Rarely, meningococcemia may result in septic foci in other areas: (1) *septic arthritis* with a pyogenic effusion in one or several joints; (2) *purulent pericarditis* with precordial pain, enlarging cardiac silhouette, and findings of cardiac tamponade; and (3) *bacterial endocarditis*. More commonly, a delayed immune complex–mediated syndrome can result in a sterile arthritis, pericarditis, or episcleritis. The acute arthritis-dermatitis syndrome, characterized by petechiae and nontraumatic arthritis, has traditionally been identified with disseminated *N. gonorrheae*, especially auxotype strains requiring arginine, hypoxanthine, and uracil (AHV⁻) for growth. In recent years, there has been a decline of

FIGURE 198-1

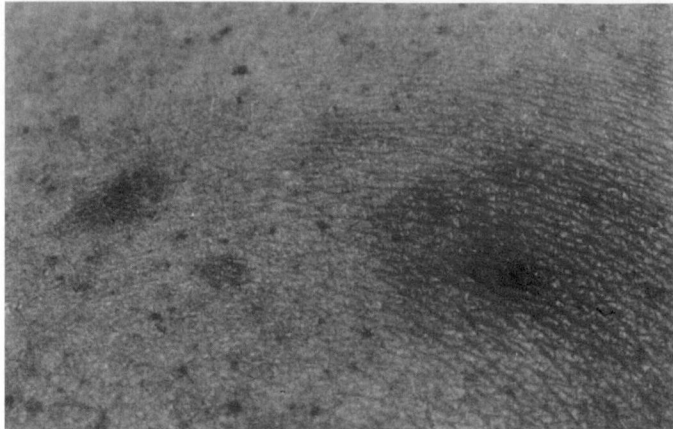

A.

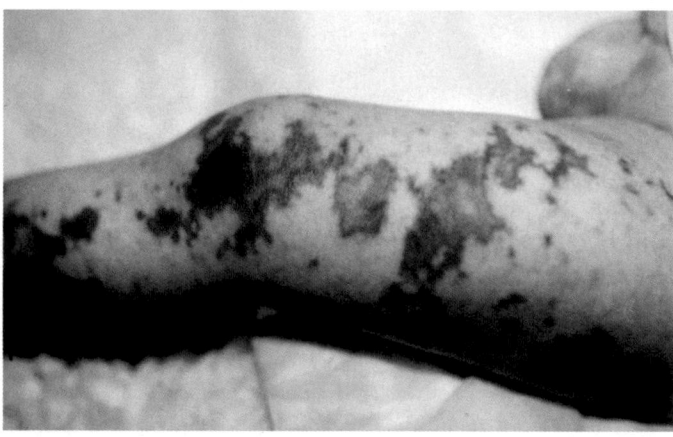

C.

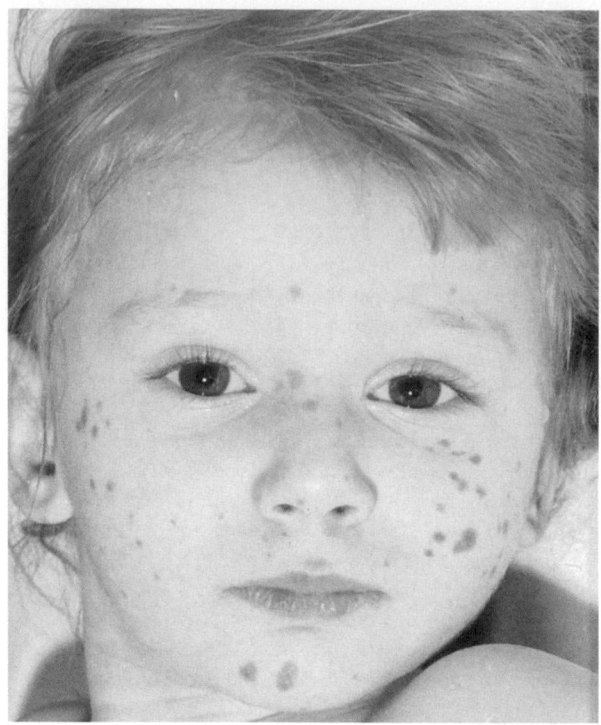

B.

Neisseria meningitidis: Acute meningococcemia. *A.* Transient macular and papular lesions on the upper chest. *B.* Discrete, pink-to-purple macules and papules, as well as purpura, are seen on the face of this young child. These lesions represent early disseminated intravascular coagulation. *C.* Maplike gray-to-black areas of cutaneous infarction are seen in this child with disseminated intravascular coagulation.

gonococcal cases and an increase in this syndrome due to *N. meningitidis.*[33]

LABORATORY FINDINGS With meningitis a polymorphonuclear leukocytosis is present in the peripheral blood and cerebrospinal fluid (CSF). The CSF protein level is increased, and the glucose value is commonly reduced. Characteristic organisms may be seen on Gram-stained smears of fluid, and meningococci are usually isolated from CSF. *Neisseria meningitidis* is isolated from the blood of approximately one-third of patients with meningitis and from almost 100 percent of patients with acute meningococcemia. Demonstration of organisms from cutaneous lesions has been variable and caution must be exercised owing to the presence of gram-negative commensals on the skin. Two recent reports describe positive results in 50 to 80 percent of aspirates, skin films, or punch biopsies of petechial lesions.[8,34] In our experience, aspirates of bullous and pustular lesions often demonstrate characteristic gram-negative diplococci.

The development of rapid, accurate, and inexpensive procedures for detection of soluble antigens in CSF has been a major advance in laboratory methodology. The latex agglutination method is sensitive, and very specific but its clinical usefulness in most situations has recently been challenged.[35] Rapid diagnosis using a modification of the polymerase chain reaction is in development but not available commercially.

PATHOLOGY See "Bacteriology and Pathogenesis," above.

DIFFERENTIAL DIAGNOSIS Meningococcal infection should always be considered in a patient with fever and a petechial or purpuric eruption, especially if meningitis is present. The differential diagnosis should include the following conditions:

1. *Acute bacteremias and endocarditis.* Petechial eruptions may be present, with or without changes in platelet numbers. In endocarditis, mucous membrane and conjunctival lesions as well as subungual "splinter" hemorrhages occur. Very infrequently numerous petechial and purpuric lesions, almost indistinguishable from those of meningococcal bacteremia, occur in patients with acute *Staphylococcus aureus* endocarditis. These patients may also have stiff neck and pleocytosis (usually without bacteria evident on Gram-stained smear of CSF) secondary to cerebral embolization or staphylococcal meningitis, completing the mimicry of systemic meningococcal disease. Usually, a few skin lesions in such a patient with acute *S. aureus* endocarditis are purulent purpura; aspirate from the purulent center of the lesion usually shows gram-positive cocci in clusters (rather than gram-negative biscuit-shaped diplococci) on smear, and subsequently *S. aureus* is isolated on culture. This is a most important distinction to make, because treatment of *S. aureus* endocarditis involves a different antibiotic than would be employed for the treatment of meningococcal meningitis. In acute gonococcemia, the skin lesions are usually nodular, hemorrhagic, few in number, and usually located on the distal parts of the extremities (see Chap. 234). Occasional patients with *H.*

influenzae or *Streptococcus pneumoniae* septicemia will develop petechial eruptions.

2. *Acute "hypersensitivity" vasculitis.* The lesions are usually palpable, present in greatest profusion on the lower extremities, and symmetric. Renal involvement and hypertension may be present. Pathologically, the major focus of inflammation is in postcapillary venules (see Chap. 176).

3. *Enteroviral infections.* Fever, petechial eruptions, and aseptic meningitis are characteristic features of enteroviral disease. Echo- (e.g., type 9) and coxsackieviruses are most often implicated.

4. *Rocky Mountain spotted fever.* The history of exposure to ticks in an endemic area, absence of an antecedent respiratory infection, delay in appearance of the rash, and the location first on the distal parts of the extremities, including palms and soles, are helpful clues (see Chap. 227).

5. *Toxic shock syndrome* (see Chap. 195).

6. *Purpura fulminans* (see Chap. 195).

7. *Weil's disease (leptospirosis)* (see Chap. 200).

COURSE AND PROGNOSIS Untreated, the disease usually ends fatally. The prognosis for treated meningitis or meningococcemia is excellent, with recovery in approximately 90 percent of patients.

In severe meningococcemia, especially with the rapid emergence of cutaneous hemorrhages, hypotension, and DIC, the entire course from onset to death can be measured in hours. These cases are often associated with massive adrenal hemorrhage (Waterhouse-Friderichsen syndrome). The mortality remains close to 100 percent. Gradations in severity of the illness make it difficult to assign an accurate prognosis in an individual case, although a bedside predictive model has been proposed and may prove useful.[36]

Chronic Meningococcemia

CLINICAL MANIFESTATIONS *History* Chronic meningococcemia is a rare disease, occurring much less frequently than the more acute dermatitis-arthritis syndrome of subacute gonococcemia that it resembles.[33] The manifestations of chronic meningococcemia are indefinite and vague at onset but tend to establish a pattern over a period of weeks or months.[14,37] Initially there may be an acute febrile illness, but this wanes and the patient is left with vague, intermittent complaints of muscle aches and pains, joint soreness, mild headache, and anorexia with weight loss. The simultaneous emergence of a localized rash with several days of fever and joint soreness are characteristic symptoms. As the fever recedes, the rash usually fades too, and the patient may be totally free of overt skin manifestations for days at a time. This periodic fever and rash may recur over a period of a few weeks to as long as 6 to 8 months. The average duration of reported cases is 6 to 8 weeks. Untreated cases may eventually evolve into acute meningococcemia, meningitis, or endocarditis. Rare case reports relate this syndrome to absence of a terminal component of complement, a finding also observed in some sporadic and recurrent acute meningococcal infections.[12]

Cutaneous lesions Variability is the hallmark of the eruption associated with chronic meningococcemia. Several different types of skin lesions have been noted, usually distributed about one or more painful joints or on pressure areas, as contrasted with the acral distribution of skin lesions in gonococcemia. They may vary in appearance and in size (1 to 20 mm) from one crop of lesions to the next and include (1) pale to rose-colored macular and papular lesions (the most common type), occurring in about 30 percent of cases; (2) slightly indurated and tender erythema nodosum–like nodules, mainly on the lower extremities; (3) petechiae of variable

size; (4) petechiae with vesicular or pustular centers; (5) hemorrhage (minute) with an areola of paler erythema (very characteristic when it occurs); (6) gross hemorrhagic areas with pale blue-gray centers; or (7) hemorrhagic, tender nodules located deep in the dermis.

Other physical findings Aside from the rash, the physical findings are minimal except for occasional joint swelling and tenderness. If the disease progresses to an acute complication such as meningitis, the new findings will be those of the complicating process.

PATHOLOGY Pathologically, the skin lesions in chronic meningococcemia differ from those in acute meningococcemia. Bacteria are absent, and meningococcal antigens cannot be recognized using fluorescent antibody techniques. In addition to the absence of bacteria or their recognized products, thrombi do not occlude capillaries and venules, endothelial cell swelling is absent, and the perivascular infiltrate consists of mixed polymorphonuclear and mononuclear cells rather than predominantly polymorphonuclear leukocytes, as seen in acute infections. Pathologic findings may be reported as "leukocytoclastic angiitis." An allergic basis for the skin lesions has been suggested in chronic meningococcemia, even though bacterial antigens are not identifiable.[14]

DIAGNOSIS AND DIFFERENTIAL DIAGNOSIS During the febrile periods, blood cultures are frequently positive and provide the specific means of diagnosis. Serologic tests have not proved helpful, and there are no available data for the use of latex agglutination or polymerase chain reaction in chronic meningococcemia.

A number of diseases with periodic fever, skin lesions, and joint involvement resemble chronic meningococcemia, including:

1. *Subacute bacterial endocarditis.* A prolonged febrile course with a pleomorphic petechial rash, joint symptoms, and no overt focus make this an important consideration. A prominent heart murmur, evidence of renal impairment, and positive blood cultures help to establish the diagnosis.

2. *Acute rheumatic fever.* This diagnosis may be suggested when the fever is prolonged, joint findings are prominent, and macular and papular rashes appear (see Chap. 179).

3. *Henoch-Schönlein purpura.* The petechial hemorrhagic rash in association with symptoms of arthritis and fever suggests an illness not unlike chronic meningococcemia; the eruption is more often symmetric, usually on the lower extremities only, and does not have the periodicity of the rash of meningococcemia (see Chap. 176).

4. *Rat-bite fever.* This disease may be acute (mimicking acute meningococcemia) or chronic (resembling chronic meningococcemia). Intermittent fever, rash, and joint manifestations are hallmarks of an illness that follows a rodent bite or ingestion of contaminated milk (see Chap. 199).

5. *Erythema multiforme.* This diagnosis is suggested by the symmetric distribution of the eruption and the iris-type configuration of the lesions (see Chap. 58).

6. *Gonococcemia* (chronic) (see Chap. 234). The cutaneous and joint manifestations may continue for many days or even weeks. The presence of tenosynovitis in gonococcemia, in contrast to its usual absence in chronic meningococcemia, can be an important clue.

COURSE AND PROGNOSIS Some patients with chronic meningococcemia recover spontaneously without specific therapy, whereas others develop serious systemic complications, such as endocarditis or meningitis. The prognosis for treated infection is excellent; almost 100 percent of patients are cured with antibiotic therapy.

Primary Meningococcal Conjunctivitis

The species most commonly involved in acute bacterial conjunctivitis are *S. aureus, S. pneumoniae,* and *H. influenzae; N. meningitidis* is the etiology in up to 2 percent of cases, and the source of infection is most likely direct inoculation of airborne organisms from close contact with carriers or manual contact with secretions from the patient's own nasopharynx.[38] Gram-stained smear of conjunctival exudate commonly reveals gram-negative, biscuit-shaped diplococci, and culture yields *N. meningitidis.* It is important to recognize that several microorganisms that can be found in infected body fluids and blood may appear morphologically similar to *N. meningitidis* on Gram stain: *N. gonorrhoeae, Moraxella* spp., *Acinetobacter calcoaceticus,* and *Pasteurella multocida.* Clinical features of primary meningococcal conjunctivitis include low-grade fever, conjunctival hyperemia, purulent exudate, lid edema, chemosis, photophobia, and preauricular lymphadenopathy. The majority of cases occur in children. Progression to systemic meningococcal disease occurs in about 20 percent of patients within a few hours to 4 days after the initial ocular symptoms. In view of the risk of systemic spread of infection, treatment should include not only topical antimicrobial agents (e.g., sulfonamides) but also systemically administered penicillin. Cellulitis of the cheek has complicated meningococcal conjunctivitis in one child, but meningococcal periorbital cellulitis (and bacteremia) has occurred following an upper respiratory infection in the absence of meningococcal conjunctivitis.[39]

Treatment and Prophylaxis

CHEMOTHERAPY   The therapy of meningococcal infections became complicated by the widespread emergence of sulfonamide-resistant strains over 30 years ago. Initially, these strains belonged predominantly to serogroup B, but in recent years they have been from serogroups A to C, essentially eliminating the sulfonamides as agents for prevention or for treatment.[40] These variations have resulted in penicillin G supplanting the sulfonamides as the treatment of choice for acute meningococcal infections. The usual adult dosage for meningococcal meningitis is 4 million units intravenously every 4 h until approximately 7 days after the temperature has returned to normal. Treatment of chronic meningococcemia does not require "meningeal doses" of penicillin; 6 to 12 million units divided into four to six daily doses, given intravenously for 7 to 10 days, should be effective therapy. In the highly penicillin-allergic patient, chloramphenicol (1.0 g intravenously every 6 h), rather than a third-generation cephalosporin, should be used. In many parts of the world, such as Spain and the United Kingdom, where meningococci that are relatively resistant to penicillin have been isolated,[40] a third-generation cephalosporin (ceftriaxone, cefotaxime) should be considered for initial therapy. All meningococcal isolates from blood, cerebrospinal fluid, or other normally sterile body cavities should be tested for penicillin susceptibility.

SUPPORTIVE THERAPY   Efforts to prevent acute brain swelling are essential in patients with meningitis. These include prevention of overhydration, reduction of body temperature, and employment of agents such as mannitol or dexamethasone (if evidence of rising intracranial pressure develops).

Although it has been postulated that hypotension in acute meningococcemia may be due to adrenal failure associated with the Waterhouse-Friderichsen syndrome (adrenal hemorrhage), blood cortisol levels and corticosteroid secretion rates have been found elevated in this syndrome.

The modern treatment of shock in sepsis begins with a number of well-accepted measures including antibiotic selection, drainage procedures for abscesses, appropriate use of volume expanders, beta-adrenergic–stimulating drugs like dopamine or isoproterenol, correction of severe acidosis and, in selected patients, peripheral vasodilators. Therapies still considered experimental include those directed against cell-envelope components of bacteria (e.g., lipopolysaccharides), those that neutralize host-cell mediated cytokines (e.g., interleukin 1, tumor necrosis factor), and those capable of limiting tissue damage.[41] Although numerous studies have been completed and results have been variable, on balance glucocorticoids do not appear to be indicated for septic shock.

Severe meningococcal infections can be complicated by the syndrome of DIC. The diagnosis is usually made by a composite of associated hematologic abnormalities, including thrombopenia and hypofibrinogenemia, prolongation of the prothrombin time and partial thromboplastin time, and presence of fibrin split products. If clinical bleeding occurs, fresh frozen plasma may be required. Each case must be individualized since therapy may be harmful and produce more problems than the DIC syndrome, especially if acute respiratory distress syndrome is also present. The use of heparin in treating DIC remains unconvincing and inconclusive and, because of potential adverse effects, most septic shock therapists no longer recommend it as routine therapy.

PROPHYLAXIS   Reliance on sulfonamide prophylaxis has been abandoned because of the presence of sulfonamide-resistant meningococcal strains, but the need for reliable chemoprophylaxis continues to exist. In civilian experiences, especially in association with day-care nursery exposures or crowded household contacts, secondary cases can emerge rapidly, often within 24 to 48 h of an index case.[16,28] Currently recommended prophylactic drug regimens in the adult favor rifampin, 600 mg orally twice daily for 2 days.[29] Rifampin resistance has been recognized in the past 10 years, at first in individuals given prophylaxis, but recent reports document failure of rifampin with the development of invasive meningococcal disease.[40] Fortunately the fluoroquinolones, ciprofloxacin and ofloxacin, are effective single-oral-dose substitutes, and ceftriaxone is available for parenteral single-dose use in children and in adults.[40,42] The effectiveness of these agents appears to be due to their presence in adequate concentrations in upper respiratory and salivary secretions.[43]

IMMUNIZATION   Polysaccharide vaccines have been developed from groups A, C, Y, and W-135 *N. meningitidis* and have proved to be safe and effective in preventing meningococcal disease in adults and in children over the age of 2 years.[15,29] Group C vaccine was routinely administered to all U.S. Army inductees and has essentially eliminated group C disease from recruit camps.[15] The development of an effective group B vaccine and improved methods of stimulating protective antibody to other groups and in children (less than 2 years of age) are currently under investigation or in clinical trials.[22–25] Chemotherapy prophylaxis provides immediate potential protection for exposure to all serogroups, but only for a brief period. Immunization protection has a lag of 1 to 2 weeks and remains protective for variable periods, up to 3 years. Indications

INFECTIONS DUE TO *PSEUDOMONAS AERUGINOSA*

General Features

These ubiquitous gram-negative bacilli can cause serious infections, especially in individuals with altered defenses or receiving intense antibiotic therapy or in hospitalized patients. Cutaneous manifestations of *Pseudomonas* infections are common and characteristic. They may represent the only overt findings in septicemias or be the localizing focus in serious infections of the ear. In addition, trivial cutaneous lesions involving nails, toe webs, skin, and the external auditory canal are produced by these organisms.

Bacteriology and Pathogenesis

Pseudomonas aeruginosa is a nonfermentative, obligately aerobic, gram-negative bacillus. Some strains produce a blue pigment (pyocyanin) soluble in chloroform or a water-soluble yellow-green substance (fluorescein). Using Wood's ultraviolet lamp, the presence of organisms in lesions of skin or nails and in the urine can be identified if fluorescein is produced by that particular strain. Either of the pigments or their combination will impart a characteristic greenish color to the surrounding growth media or the tissue substrate involved in clinical disease (e.g., "green nail" syndrome, Fig. 198-2). In addition, growth of these microorganisms is often accompanied by an odor of grapes, characteristic of trimethylamine.

These organisms gain entry through breakdown of the skin or mucous membrane barriers at sites of maceration, dermatophytic foci, trauma, foreign bodies (e.g., indwelling venous or urinary catheters), or via aspiration or aerosolization into the respiratory tract. Infections in otherwise healthy individuals are unusual; when they occur, the involved regions are often areas with increased moisture (toe webs, the external auditory canal). Infection may begin in the base of the nail in persons who frequently have their hands in water. This can progress to paronychia, followed by development of a green-blue discoloration of the nail due to local pigment production. Another example of the ability of this organism to infect healthy but moistened skin are the numerous reports of a diffuse rash on areas of skin of people immersed in public whirlpools, hot tubs (Fig. 198-3), and swimming pools.[44] These organisms can sometimes be aggressive secondary invaders in open wounds, in decubitus and skin ulcerations, or in association with thermal burns. Rarely, a superficial pyoderma due solely to *Pseudomonas* is engrafted upon a generalized or localized dermatitis, such as tinea pedis or eczema, producing irregular pustular areas with macerated and eroded borders.[44]

Serious invasive infections occur in debilitated patients; malnourished infants; individuals whose normal bacterial flora has been suppressed by antibiotics; patients with neoplastic diseases, granulocytopenias of various etiologies, or impaired circulating or cellular immunity, including AIDS[45]; and individuals requiring mechanical respiratory assistance. These organisms frequently colonize body surfaces and survive exposure to antibiotics. *Pseudomonas aeruginosa* can spread widely via the bloodstream, producing a disseminated infective vasculitis in which organisms can be seen in the periadventia, adventitia, and media of vessels without luminal clot. Occasionally, features of the generalized Shwartzman reaction are

FIGURE 198-2

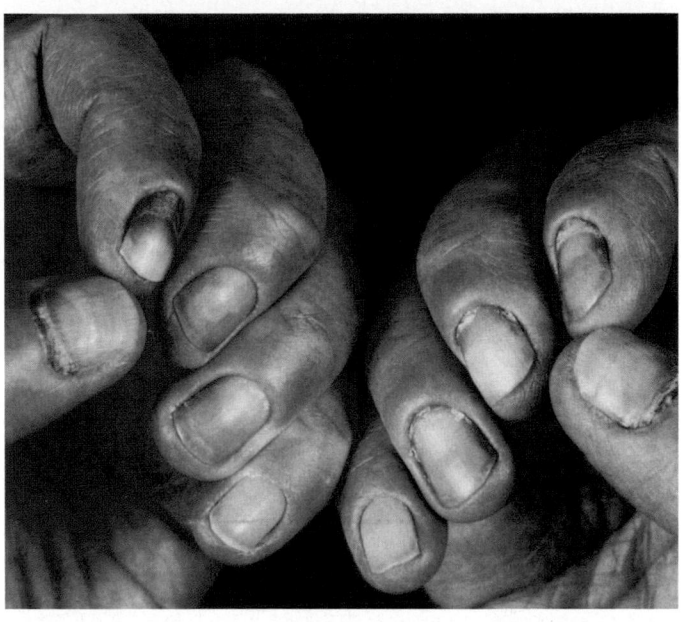

Pseudomonas aeruginosa: "Green nails." This 36-year-old bartender noted a greenish-yellow discoloration of 8 of 10 fingernails during the preceding year. Several of the fingers show chronic candidal paronychia as well.

found, but less frequently than in infections due to *N. meningitidis* or Enterobacteriaceae. Whole dead *Pseudomonas* cells injected into experimental animals produce little if any toxicity compared with the effects of live bacteria. This suggested to Liu and associates that the pathogenicity of this organism might reside in an exotoxin rather than in the classic endotoxin of gram-negative bacteria. Studies during the past 25 years have confirmed the relevance of a number of toxic substances to pathogenesis. Among these, collagenase and elastase may be important determinants for the development of hemorrhagic lesions. A phospholipase similar to the alpha toxin of *Clostridium perfringens* may have a major role in the pathogenesis of respiratory infections through destruction of pulmonary surfactant.[46] Studies have led to the identification and characterization of a potent protein, exotoxin A. The mechanism of action of this cytotoxin is identical to that of diphtheria cytotoxin, but it differs in its cellular specificities, molecular properties, and clinical expression. Among the critical effects of these cytotoxins, the influence on polymorphonuclear leukocyte migration and function is considered vital to pathogenicity.[47] Exotoxin A and other *Pseudomonas* toxins have been reviewed.[48] An antitoxin can neutralize the effects of the toxin in vivo. Efforts to produce a toxoid are in progress. The importance of the contribution of this exotoxin to the pathogenesis of *Pseudomonas* infections has not been definitely established. There is evidence in experimental burn sepsis that synthesis of the exotoxin occurs in local lesions, and the toxin can be identified in the serum.[49]

Epidemiology

Pseudomonas aeruginosa is found widely distributed in nature—in air, water, dust particles, and soil; thus, it is not surprising that it may contaminate plants, vegetables, and occasionally medicinal

FIGURE 198-3

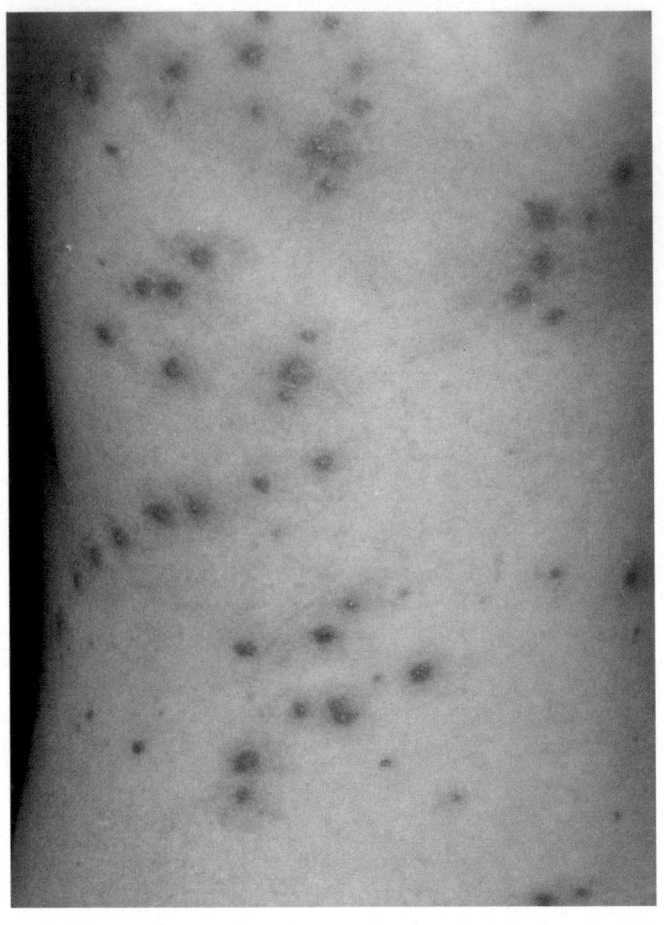

Pseudomonas aeruginosa: "Hot tub folliculitis." This 22-year-old female noted the appearance of erythematous, pruritic papules and pustules on the trunk, buttocks, and upper thighs several days after bathing in a hot tub. The eruption resolved without antibiotic therapy.

preparations such as procaine and fluorescein eye drops. In humans, the moist regions of skin folds and the external auditory canal are the most common sites of natural colonization (approximately 3 to 5 percent of individuals). Any activity that leads to excessive local moisture—such as laundry work, dishwashing, or hiking for long periods in wet terrain—will enhance the presence and growth of these organisms. *P. aeruginosa* is found in small numbers in the feces of 10 to 20 percent of the population but in larger numbers in as many as 35 to 50 percent of patients hospitalized for longer than 1 week. Moist or weeping cutaneous lesions (e.g., thermal burns) encourage the growth of *Pseudomonas* as well as of other gram-negative bacteria. Procedures that increase humidity in the environment are frequently associated with overgrowth of these organisms. Moisture-enhancing bath materials, like loofah or synthetic sponges, easily become contaminated with gram-negative bacteria and have served as vehicles of transmission of *Pseudomonas* to skin.[50] Systemic infection with these indigenous gram-negative bacteria depends primarily on altered susceptibility of the host rather than on spread from individual to individual or on increased pathogenicity. However, there may be exceptions to this in newborn

nurseries, respiratory care units, and, occasionally, urologic wards, where dissemination from a primary source may occur. In hospitalized patients who are neutropenic or immunocompromised, increasing numbers become colonized and a larger number suffer disease due to this organism.

Local and Secondarily Infected Lesions

Pseudomonas produces a number of characteristic lesions. In addition, these organisms contaminate and complicate other skin diseases and open wounds.[51]

CLINICAL MANIFESTATIONS *History* Painful paronychial lesions, with or without characteristic green or blue discoloration of the nails, occur most often in women with a history of chronic immersion of hands in water with soaps and detergents. People with toe-web infection characteristically work or live in an atmosphere of high humidity and often have wet feet. Symptoms usually include slight persistent soreness and scaling of the web tissues. There are a large number of reports of therapeutic recreational whirlpool-, hot tub-, and swimming pool–associated skin rashes developing in healthy individuals within 1 to 5 days after use of public bathing facilities (Fig. 198-3). In all instances, *P. aeruginosa* was isolated in large numbers from the pool water. The skin rash was self-limited, clearing without therapy within 1 week but often accompanied by fatigue, malaise, low-grade fever, external otitis, and mastitis.[44]

Cutaneous lesions In addition to a tender paronychial lesion, patients with "green nail" syndrome may have part or all of the associated nail colored green to blue. The color may be in horizontal bands, representing intermittent activity of the infection at the nail base (see Fig. 198-2). Individuals with toe-web *Pseudomonas* infections have thick, macerated, scaling, slightly green, foul-smelling discolored areas between the toes. External otitis due to any type of bacteria presents a characteristically swollen, macerated appearance in the local area without any specific lesion involving the eardrum. Intense swelling and discoloration with excruciating pain on movement of the pinna are characteristic of external otitis, often referred to as "swimmer's ear." If the skin is traumatized naturally or during a surgical procedure, local infection can spread to the pinna, producing a perichondritis and chondritis with intense tender swelling of the ear. Cartilagenous necrosis may result from pressure effects or inflammatory damage unless immediate drainage with through-and-through incisions and appropriate antibiotics are instituted: Organisms other than *P. aeruginosa* may be causal, including *S. aureus* and streptococci.[52]

The most severe form of this infection, malignant external otitis, has a high mortality if therapy is delayed or inadequate. This serious infection usually occurs in elderly diabetics with significant small-vessel disease but may also be seen in healthy elderly, as a complication of surgical trauma, following minor trauma like water irrigation of the external canal, and in patients with AIDS.[53,54] The onset and early progression are insidious. Swelling, erythema, moderate discharge, and pain are present without fever or constitutional symptoms. As the surface breaks down, invasion of the soft tissues occurs at the junction of cartilage and bone, and the process then advances to involve cartilage, mastoid, and temporal bone. Inflammation at the stylomastoid and jugular foramina can lead to seventh-nerve and ninth- to eleventh-nerve palsies, the seventh-nerve palsy being the earliest objective neurologic defect seen. Diagnosis is made clinically and early if there is adequate visibility, and granulation tissue can be seen erupting at the cartilage-bone interface in the posterior inferior canal wall. The pinna is often swollen and intense pain is present.[55]

Patients who develop folliculitis usually give a history of exposure to warm water in a whirlpool, a public bath like a hot tub, some recreational spa for swimming, or a water slide. The rash can be very local if a limb has been immersed in a whirlpool or generalized in distribution in swimsuit and intertriginous areas. The rash begins as papules, evolves to papulopustules (see Fig. 198-3), and eventually heals with fine desquamation. Pruritus and pain may accompany the lesions and localized areas of mastitis and external otitis.[44] Serotype 0-11 of *P. aeruginosa* is most commonly involved. A small outbreak of *P. aeruginosa* 0-11 folliculitis occurred in granulocytopenic patients in a cancer treatment center; but in these patients, in contrast to normal individuals with swimming pool folliculitis, the lesions rapidly became widespread and progressed to bullae, which became necrotic (ecthyma gangrenosum–like) unless systemic antibiotic treatment was initiated immediately.[56] The development of the changes of ecthyma gangrenosum represented progression of the initial folliculitis rather than the incidental occurrence of superimposed bacteremic *P. aeruginosa* lesions. Sinks and faucets in the patients' rooms were sources of *P. aeruginosa* of identical serotype. In secondarily infected open skin areas, the presence of *Pseudomonas* is sometimes associated with a prominent greenish-blue color to the purulent exudate. Widespread, irregular, superficial pustular lesions may be superimposed on the underlying skin disease; the margins of these regions are usually sharply defined and irregular and may exhibit the characteristic grapelike odor and pigmented exudate.

DIAGNOSIS AND DIFFERENTIAL DIAGNOSIS Nail and skin lesions are recognized by the characteristic pigment and "fruity" odor of the exudate. The organisms can be identified as thin gram-negative rods, or a mixed infection (e.g., with *Candida*) may be observed. Identification of the organism isolated in routine culture is based on pigment production and fermentation reactions. Fluorescence, demonstrated with a Wood's lamp, can help to support the diagnostic impression. Occasionally *Aspergillus* infection of the nails produces a greenish color, but there is usually no associated paronychia and bacteria are not found on careful study of nail clippings. A subungual hematoma may superficially resemble *Pseudomonas* nail infection.

COURSE AND PROGNOSIS Patients with minor *Pseudomonas* infections—such as onychia and paronychia, toe-web inflammation, whirlpool-associated skin rash, and external otitis—usually improve rapidly with topical therapy and drying of the affected area. Malignant external otitis requires systemic antibiotics directed against *Pseudomonas,* utilizing a fluoroquinolone (ciprofloxacin or ofloxacin) with or without imipenam or ceftazidime. High doses and prolonged therapy are combined with local surgical debridement to limit spread to bone, nervous system structures, and the meninges.[55,57]

Septicemia and Cutaneous Involvement

CLINICAL MANIFESTATIONS *History* In individuals ill with *Pseudomonas* septicemia, the history is most frequently centered around the underlying problem and antecedent therapy. A premature infant may have required resuscitation and treatment of a nonspecific pneumonitis prior to developing high fever, obtundation, and macular or hemorrhagic vesicular skin lesions. Infants may present initially with omphalitis or severe diarrhea, followed by septicemia and skin lesions. Urinary tract infections complicating congenital

lesions such as exstrophy of the bladder may predispose to bacteremia. In adults, there is usually a history of antibiotic therapy, treatment with glucocorticoid hormones or antitumor agents, or the use of percutaneous catheters. Frequently, the patient is granulopenic, has already had a significant febrile illness, and may still be receiving antibiotics when one of the characteristic cutaneous manifestations develops. The local lesions are rarely painful, but in the author's experience the patient is usually too sick to focus on the local problem. Occasionally, hemorrhagic manifestations may occur secondary to involvement of small vessels supplying the skin, to platelet reduction, or to DIC.

Pseudomonas involvement of the gastrointestinal tract, particularly in the tropics, may produce the picture of an acute enteric infection, with headache, high fever, diarrhea, and "rose spots"—a syndrome described as *Shanghai fever* and resembling typhoid fever.[58]

Cutaneous lesions The skin lesions, the most characteristic part of the physical findings in *Pseudomonas* septicemia, consist of four types[59]:

1. *Vesicles and bullae.* These occur singly or in clusters and spread in random fashion over the skin, frequently becoming hemorrhagic as they evolve. Occasionally, in infants, they may be surrounded by large erythematous halos and may be mistaken for erythema multiforme.
2. *Ecthyma gangrenosum.* The lesion in this disorder starts with a gunmetal gray, infarcted lesion with surrounding erythema (Fig. 198-4) and evolves into a necrotic black or gray-black eschar and surrounding erythema (Figs. 198-4 and 198-5). This lesion often evolves from a necrotic vesicle. Frequently but not exclusively, the lesion is in the anogenital or axillary region.

FIGURE 198-4

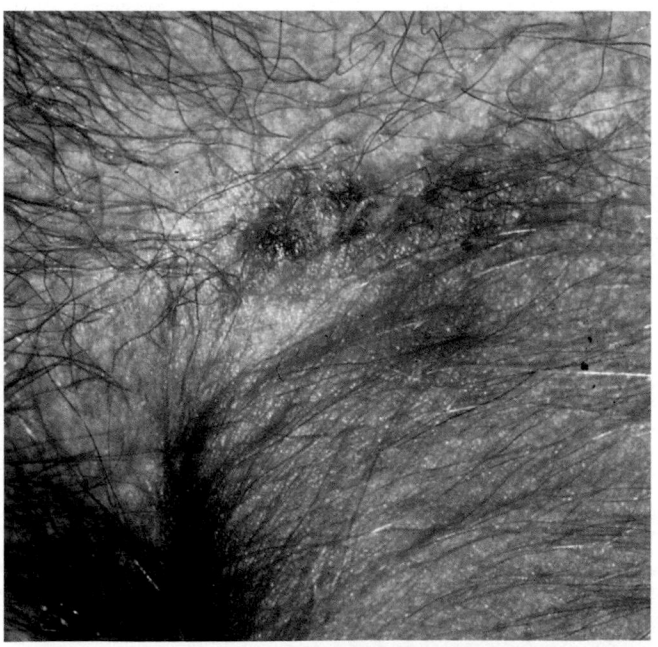

Pseudomonas aeruginosa: Ecthyma gangrenosum. Gunmetal gray, painless, infarcted lesions with surrounding erythema.

FIGURE 198-5

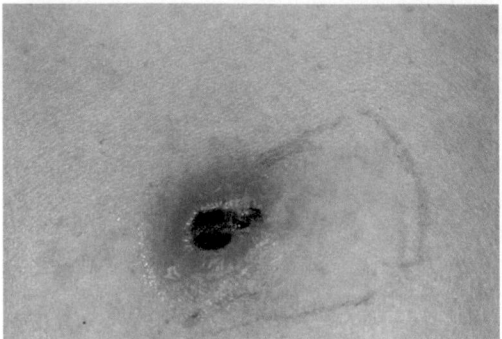

A.

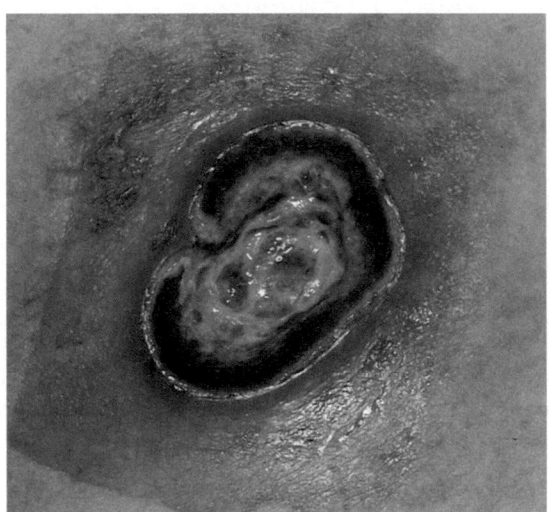

B.

Pseudomonas aeruginosa: Ecthyma gangrenosum. This 32-year-old male with HIV disease noted the onset of a very tender plaque on the right buttock associated with fever and malaise. *A.* Five-day-old lesions with a central infarcted, necrotic area surrounded by erythema. *B.* At 5 weeks, the lesions had initially improved on ciprofloxacin, which was discontinued owing to an adverse drug reaction. Without antibiotic treatment, the necrotic area enlarged and was associated with bacteremia. Eventually, the lesion reepithelialized, but the patient died of pseudomonal pneumonia.

3. *Gangrenous cellulitis.* This may present as a sharply demarcated, superficial, painless, necrotic lesion that may resemble a decubitus ulcer but is located in a nonpressure area and may complicate a prior area of injury such as a thermal burn. Also, it may begin abruptly as an acute infection (with much clinical toxicity), producing local pain, swelling, erythema, and involvement of deep subcutaneous tissue and fascia. Infection may be introduced either by local injury or through bacteremia.

4. *Macular or papular nodular lesions.* These are small, oval, and painless, located predominantly over the trunk, and resemble rose spots of typhoid fever.

Another cutaneous manifestation of *Pseudomonas* septicemia, usually occurring after days or weeks, is nodular cellulitis. The lesions are red, warm, sometimes fluctuant, but often situated deeply

enough to feel solid. Surgical incision reveals suppuration, and *P. aeruginosa* can be cultured from the lesions.[59,60] A variation of this process consists of numerous red, nonfluctuant, hot, nontender, subcutaneous nodules on the trunk and extremities that may be accompanied by other characteristic lesions, such as hemorrhagic bullae and ecthyma gangrenosum.[61] Such lesions may be successfully treated by combination antipseudomonal antibiotic therapy.

Other lesions that have been described include petechiae, ecchymoses, dermal Shwartzman-like reactions, and purpura fulminans. Occasionally, the cutaneous expression of *Pseudomonas* infection may take the form of a typical erythema multiforme reaction. Patients with extensive burns may develop lesions of the above types on areas of normal skin as well as more florid diffuse growth secondarily infecting the burn surface.

Other physical findings Patients with *Pseudomonas* septicemia frequently exhibit physical findings associated with the underlying diseases: malnutrition, mucous membrane ulcerations, glossitis and stomatitis secondary to antibiotics and granulocytopenia, urinary tract infections, proctitis, adenopathy, hepatosplenomegaly, and hemorrhagic bronchopneumonia.

LABORATORY FINDINGS Routine hematologic examination may reveal leukocytosis or leukopenia, with modifications based on underlying illnesses (aleukemic leukemia, leukemia, etc.). Platelets may be diminished and fibrinogen and other clotting factors reduced in association with consumption coagulopathy, liver disease, or profound malnutrition.

Characteristically, in *Pseudomonas* septicemia, aspirated material from bullae, areas of cellulitis, and papular or nodular lesions reveals numerous organisms but few leukocytes even in patients with leukocytosis. Cultures of these lesions and of blood are almost always positive.

PATHOLOGY The distinctive finding in *Pseudomonas* lesions is a necrotizing vasculitis in which the walls of small arteries and veins are invaded by a myriad of bacteria.[62] The internal elastic lamellae may be destroyed by microbial elastase, but the endothelial surface is rarely damaged and thrombosis is unusual.[59] Extravasation occurs around the vessels, the perivascular and adventitial regions are extensively involved with edema and bland necrosis, and blood flow to the region supplied by the affected vessel is curtailed. This, in turn, leads to the formation of cutaneous lesions (bullae, hemorrhagic cellulitis, and gangrenous changes). Organisms tend to spread along the exterior surfaces of vessels and invade the skin. Lungs, liver, kidneys, and brain may be similarly involved by bacterial invasion of their respective blood vessel walls, with the production of characteristic discrete nodular necrotic lesions.

DIAGNOSIS AND DIFFERENTIAL DIAGNOSIS The characteristic ecthyma gangrenosum skin lesions in an acutely ill patient suggests the diagnosis of *Pseudomonas* septicemia. The finding of abundant thin, gram-negative rods with rare granulocytes in vesicle fluid or in association with gangrenous or hemorrhagic cellulitis constitutes further presumptive evidence.

The differential diagnosis of *Pseudomonas* septicemia includes other infections that can produce skin lesions through direct involvement of blood vessels (e.g., those caused by *N. meningitidis*, *Aeromonas hydrophilia*, *E. coli*, *Klebsiella pneumoniae*, and fungi of the *Aspergillus* and *Rhyzopus* groups). In addition, other gramnegative bacteria and *Rickettsiae* may produce petechial, ecchymotic, or gangrenous skin lesions suggestive of the Shwartzman reaction.

COURSE AND PROGNOSIS *Pseudomonas* septicemia is frequently the terminal event in a complex illness involving a patient with malignant disease or altered cellular and humoral defense mechanisms. Therapy may be effective and recovery complete in some instances, especially when the septicemia occurs in patients with more favorable underlying problems like thermal burns, in individuals with urinary tract foci of infection, or in association with the use of percutaneous venous catheters.

TREATMENT *Local infections* Superficial skin and toe-web infections and onychia usually respond to acetic acid, silver nitrate, or gentian violet compresses applied two to three times daily between long periods of drying. Paronychia is best treated by surgical drainage, nail trimming, and 4% thymol in chloroform. Acetic acid in 50% alcohol, polymixin (0.1%) in acetic acid, or glucocorticoids with neomycin are effective for otitis externa. When acetic acid is used topically on chronic ulcers or burns, a 2 to 5% solution is often effective.[63] In addition, topical silver nitrate (0.5%) or silver sulfadiazine has been used to eradicate these organisms in burn patients (see Chap. 129).

Systemic infections *Pseudomonas* septicemia requires early and vigorous systemic bactericidal antibiotic therapy. Effective therapeutic agents include the aminoglycosides gentamicin, tobramycin, and amikacin. One of these drugs is combined with an antipseudomonas penicillin or ceftazidime intravenously in patients who are acutely ill. In the presence of hypotension or of any renal impairment, the dosage of aminoglycoside antibiotics must be drastically reduced; in such circumstances, therapy should be guided by determinations of "peak" and "trough" serum levels of the aminoglycoside drug employed.

In addition to parenteral administration of antibiotics, nodular and fluctuant lesions should be drained surgically. Acute *P. aeruginosa* gangrenous cellulitis/fasciitis requires debridement (often extensive), sometimes with a surgical "second look" 1 or 2 days later. Leukocyte transfusions have been effective in granulopenic infants, and experimental use of human immune globulins with activity against *P. aeruginosa* or specific *Pseudomonas* exotoxin A antibody preparations are under development and in early use.[64] A particularly difficult problem is presented by the markedly granulocytopenic patient with gangrenous cellulitis due to *P. aeruginosa* alone or in polymicrobial combination.[65] Progression of the process can be extremely rapid and thus is an indication for very prompt surgical debridement in addition to antimicrobial therapy and, if indicated, granulocyte colony stimulating factor (G-CSF). Complicating thrombocytopenia and DIC may supervene and add to the urgency.

Prophylaxis Infections caused by *P. aeruginosa* are difficult to treat because they often occur in altered hosts and the organisms are highly resistant to many antibiotics. There is no place for prophylactic antibiotics against *P. aeruginosa* because of drug toxicity and emergence of resistant strains. This reality has led to attempts to develop a polyvalent vaccine against the limited number of serotypes of *P. aeruginosa*. Preliminary clinical trials have been encouraging but variable in patients with thermal burns and cystic fibrosis and in volunteers. Results are less favorable in seriously ill individuals with leukemia or other diseases with impaired host defenses.

Skin Infections Due to Other *Pseudomonas* Species

Pseudomonas putrefaciens, a psychrophilic bacterium, is a rare cause of cellulitis, particularly in the setting of chronic lower extremity infection in ulcers secondary to venous stasis.[66]

SKIN INFECTIONS DUE TO *HAEMOPHILUS INFLUENZAE*

General Features

The characteristic feature of this rare infection of the skin with *H. influenzae* is a cellulitis that usually involves the face, neck, or upper extremities. Most cases occur in young children (6 to 24 months old), but examples in adults have been described in recent years. With the advent of early administration of protective Hib conjugate vaccines, this and other invasive manifestations of *H. influenzae* disease have nearly disappeared.

Bacteriology and Pathogenesis

Haemophilus influenzae is a small coccobacillary, pleomorphic gram-negative organism. It is nonmotile and has fastidious growth requirements, including heme (X factor) and nicotinamide nucleoside (V factor). In mixed cultures the presence of organisms such as *S. aureus* can provide these growth factors, and this allows *H. influenzae* colonies to grow well, as "satellites" of the feeding staphylococcus. There are rough and encapsulated forms, the latter divided into six serologic types (a through f) based on capsular polysaccharide antigens.

Most infections with *H. influenzae*, including meningitis, epiglottitis, and cellulitis, are caused by encapsulated type b strains (Hib). The ribosyl-ribitol phosphate capsule inhibits phagocytosis in nonimmune individuals and allows a period of unchecked bacterial growth and invasiveness to occur. Rough, unencapsulated, nontypable, noninvasive species are commonly found in the upper part of the respiratory tract and are especially incriminated in surface infections such as exacerbations of bronchitis in older individuals with chronic lung disease and in young children with otitis media.

The mechanism involved in the development of cellulitis is uncertain, but in the majority of cases is an antecedent upper respiratory infection (URI) or acute otitis media. The characteristic localization of the cellulitis to the upper part of the body argues for the sequence of URI, fallout onto or invasion of the skin locally, and then bacteremia. This sequence is seen in adult as well as in pediatric cases. The association of otitis media with cellulitis has led to the hypothesis that the ear may serve as the primary focus in cases involving the face.[67] A primary bacteremic mechanism with secondary localization in the skin would be favored by a more random and widespread distribution of lesions than is seen. Localization of a subclinical bacteremia could follow trauma and has been suggested as a possible antecedent predisposing event. The analogy to group A beta streptococcal erysipelas seems relevant. The organisms are usually located in the upper respiratory tract and sometimes produce cellulitis locally; bacteremia is a secondary complication, although less often seen than in Hib cellulitis.

Epidemiology

Humans are the only known natural host for *H. influenzae*. Carrier rates appear to be highest in young children between ages 1 and 5, especially in families and day-care groups with a recent case of Hib disease.[68] These potentially pathogenic bacteria are carried in the oropharynx and nasopharynx as part of the normal indigenous flora.

Early immunization utilizing newly developed conjugate Hib vaccines has resulted in a marked decrease in nasopharyngeal carrier rates, which has probably contributed to the overall decline of clinical disease.[69] Susceptibility to Hib disease appears to be greatest among certain ethnic groups and in socioeconomically disadvantaged populations.[70] Genetic factors, prompt antibiotic treatment of Hib disease, congenital and acquired complement and antibody deficiency, and asplenia may also be responsible for increased susceptibility to disease and to recurrent episodes in traditional age groups as well as in adults. Spread is via droplet aerosol or close contact, and infection frequently occurs in association with a viral URI. Susceptibility to *H. influenzae* disease appears to be greatest between the ages of 3 months and 3 years. Although the early observations of Fothergill and Wright (1933) that this correlated with the absence of significant titers of bactericidal antibody have been questioned,[71] there is general agreement that complement-dependent anticapsular and bactericidal antibodies increase with age and are protective.[72] Paradoxically, Hib disease may occur in individuals endowed with adequate levels of bactericidal antibody. It has been postulated that circulating IgA antibody may block the function of specific IgG,[20] or that assay methodology provides false-positive results in vitro.[73] Although the mechanism of protection in the newborn period remains uncertain, it probably involves transplacental IgG transfer. The majority of adults beyond 15 years likewise have bactericidal and anticapsular antibody, and in this age group *H. influenzae* disease is unusual.[74]

In addition to antibody induction by clinical or subclinical *H. influenzae* disease or by immunization, protective anticapsular antibody may be formed in response to cross-reacting antigens from vegetables, such as legumes, nonencapsulated *Haemophilus* species, other commensals, and enteric bacteria (e.g., *E. coli* K 100).[75]

Clinical Manifestations

HISTORY   Typically, a young infant or child (under age 3) develops an area of swelling and discoloration on the face or arm following several days of coryza and abruptly rising temperature.[76] Rarely, a similar process occurs in adults as a complication of respiratory tract infection involving the upper airway.[77]

CUTANEOUS LESIONS   The typical lesion is a single, circumscribed, indurated area usually located on the face, neck, upper chest, or upper extremity. Although described in infants as characteristically blue-red to purple-red in color and surrounded by a zone of edema, the early lesion may be an area of pale edema or erythema (see Fig. 197-8). The margins are indistinct, in contrast to the sharply defined borders of erysipelas. Regional adenopathy is rarely present. Occasionally, in children with Hib buccal cellulitis, erythematous buccal mucosal lesions are found on the side of the affected cheek, suggesting direct bacterial spread from the oropharynx into buccal soft tissues.[78]

When *H. influenzae* cellulitis occurs in adults, the patients are usually over 50 years of age and the infection follows a striking sequence: marked pharyngitis at first; high fever; then rapidly progressive anterior neck swelling, tenderness, erythema, and dysphagia.[77]

OTHER PHYSICAL FINDINGS   Associated infections of the upper respiratory tract including otitis media, sinusitis or epiglottitis, and pneumonia occur. The patient may appear lethargic; occasionally, metastatic infections such as septic arthritis or meningitis may occur. Fever, in the range of 38.9° to 40°C (102.2° to 104°F) is common.

Laboratory Findings

The white blood cell count is invariably elevated, usually in the 20,000 range. Blood cultures are positive in approximately 50 percent of cases. Aspiration and culture of the margin of the cellulitis has been successful in about half the patients encountered, and Gram-stained smears should be studied.[67] Latex agglutination of soluble Hib capsule material is the method of choice for antigen detection in CSF and other body fluids. It is rapid, easy to perform, and can provide diagnostic information after antibiotic exposure when cultures may be negative.

Pathology

No information is available about the histologic changes associated with this rare lesion, but the inflammatory response is doubtless an acute pyogenic reaction.

Diagnosis and Differential Diagnosis

Haemophilus influenzae cellulitis should be suspected when a child aged 3 to 24 months develops an acute facial (buccal) cellulitis with high fever. There may be concomitant upper airway inflammation. Immediate confirmation of the diagnosis may be possible from inspection of Gram-stained smears of an aspirate of the lesion. Although cellulitis caused by other microorganisms is more common in adults, Hib disease should be considered in patients with respiratory infections and upper body cellulitis, especially in young children not fully immunized with currently available vaccines.[70]

Streptococcal (especially group A) or pneumococcal cellulitis may produce a similar discoloration of the skin. Erysipelas, which rarely occurs in infants, is usually homogeneously erythematous and margins of the plaquelike swelling are distinct compared with the indefinite borders of *H. influenzae* cellulitis. Occasionally, *S. aureus* can produce a similar process, but the presence of pustules or boils is helpful in distinguishing this type of lesion.

Course and Prognosis

Most patients do well with antibiotic therapy even though the disease is usually associated with bacteremia. The patient is often brought to a physician quickly, as the abrupt onset of high fever and easily observed cellulitis indicates the urgency of the situation. Constant vigil must be maintained for suppurative complications in the upper airways, meninges, lungs, bones, joints, or other organs.

Treatment and Prophylaxis

Third-generation cephalosporins (ceftriaxone or cefotaxime) are currently the drugs of choice because of their activity against both ampicillin-susceptible and beta-lactamase-producing strains of *H. influenzae* and because of their efficacy in treating any complicating meningeal spread of infection. Infections caused by beta-lactamase negative isolates can be treated with ampicillin given intravenously in four to six divided doses daily. However, with plasmid-mediated ampicillin resistance at levels of 30 to 45 percent among strains of Hib, initial therapy should be with a third-generation cephalosporin. Chloramphenicol is not recommended owing to its hematologic toxicity, especially in very young children.

Chemoprophylaxis has been studied in a variety of settings, and rifampin appears to be effective in significantly lowering carrier rates in selected populations such as households with an index case of Hib disease. At the present time rifampin is recommended for children and adults (reduced for infants) in doses of 20 mg/kg per day (up to 600 mg maximum) for 4 days, when an index case of Hib invasive disease occurs in a family where other children under age 4 reside.[79] Similar prophylaxis is recommended for nursery and day-care contacts.

With the introduction of Hib conjugate vaccine (capsular polysaccharide covalently linked to a protein moiety) in the past decade, the incidence of invasive Hib disease has declined by over 95 percent in the United States. In addition to their potency these vaccines are effective in stimulating protective antibody when given to infants prior to 6 months of age, a period of great susceptibility to Hib invasive disease.[70,80]

Cellulitis is a rare complication of Hib disease. Scattered case reports continue to appear, mostly from Europe, but there have been no publications in the English literature to accompany the dramatic decline in meningitis and septicemia cases. It is fair to assume that cellulitis, a rare disease prior to effective protective immunization, will become an infection of historic interest only.

CUTANEOUS MANIFESTATIONS OF *SALMONELLA* INFECTION (ENTERIC FEVER)

General Features

Salmonella infections are usually manifest as gastroenteritis, enteric fever (typhoid-like illness), or septicemia. "Rose spots," the classic skin lesions of systemic *Salmonella* infection, have been variably reported (10 to 60 percent) during the natural (untreated) evolution of typhoid fever but less frequently in enteric fevers due to other *Salmonella* species.

Bacteriology and Pathogenesis

Salmonellae are not fastidious organisms, but their isolation from stool is made difficult by the fact that, when present, they represent only a small part of the abundant fecal flora. Extragastrointestinal isolates (abscesses, blood, skin lesions) are easier to identify, as they are usually pure cultures of a given *Salmonella* species. Isolation of the organisms from stool specimens is aided by the use of selective inhibiting media (e.g., MacConkey, SS agar) that decrease the growth of gram-positive organisms as well as many gram-negative species. Salmonellae are motile, gram-negative bacilli that do not ferment lactose. From a practical viewpoint, in stool bacteriology, initial selection of non-lactose-fermenting colonies is followed by biochemical and serologic (agglutination) procedures for identification and serotyping of the organism. There are three primary species: *S. typhi* (1 serotype); *S. choleraesuis* (1 serotype); and *S. enteritidis* (over 1700 serotypes). By habit, organisms are often referred to as *Salmonella* (plus serotype designation—e.g., *typhimurium*) but the correct nomenclature is *S. enteritidis,* serotype *typhimurium,* etc.

There is a latent period of from 3 to as long as 50 days (usually 7 to 14) between ingestion of bacteria and the dramatic onset of clinical symptoms of enteric fever. Shorter latent periods often follow ingestion of larger numbers of organisms. When due to salmonellae other than *S. typhi,* symptoms tend to begin earlier and are milder. During the latent period, organisms multiply in the distal

small bowel and invade and multiply in lymphoid tissues in the area of Peyer's patches in the terminal ileum. Invasion of the bloodstream from this focus heralds the onset of the clinical illness with chills and fever and other constitutional effects of circulating endotoxin. Manifestations of infection occur in many organs and often in a predictable sequence: respiratory and central nervous system symptoms during the first week; skin manifestations during the second week; diarrhea, often following a period of constipation, during the second and third weeks. Bacterial invasion of the skin, liver, gallbladder, bones, and joints as well as manifestations of endotoxemia usually occur during the bacteremic phase of the illness (first 10 days). Organisms are cleared by the reticuloendothelial system (RES), leading to hyperplasia of these elements in the liver, spleen, and lymph nodes. Persistence of organisms in the gallbladder, biliary radicals, bone marrow, or the RES may lead to a chronic asymptomatic carrier state.

Epidemiology

Salmonella typhi and other *Salmonella* species causing enteric fever are acquired by ingestion of contaminated water or food. Travel in developing countries and other areas of marginal sanitation places people in the proximity of enteric pathogens. Rapid transportation can bring them home healthy during an incubation period that can be 5 to 6 weeks long. History of recent travel and unusual or suspicious food or water encounters should be sought in a patient with appropriate clinical manifestations.

Humans are the only hosts for *S. typhi,* and the chronic carrier state that may follow clinical typhoid fever is almost always asymptomatic except for manifestations of gallbladder disease if cholelithiasis and active cholecystitis are present. Other *Salmonellae,* serotypes of *S. enteritidis,*—e.g., *typhimurium, schottmulleri,* and *hirshfeldii*—can produce an enteric fever syndrome similar to but usually milder than, typhoid fever. Unlike *S. typhi,* these other *Salmonella* serotypes are ubiquitous in nature (occurring in animals, birds, reptiles, poultry products) and are difficult to control as sources of human infection.

A number of factors, exclusive of inoculum size, determine whether disease will occur after ingestion of *Salmonella.* Achlorhydria and previous gastric surgery allow organisms to escape destruction by the acid barrier of the stomach. Rapid transit of a smaller inoculum in a liquid vehicle may allow adequate numbers of viable bacteria to reach the distal small bowel. Suppression of competing bowel flora by antimicrobials and gastric acid neutralization by the variety of pharmacologic agents available are unproven but likely contributing factors to the emergence of disease. Underlying illnesses such as Hodgkin's disease, which alters cellular immunity, can interfere with the host defense mechanisms that normally eradicate these pathogens; hemoglobinopathies, such as sickle cell disease, appear to predispose to systemic *Salmonella* infections and osteomyelitis by saturating the protective RES with red cell fragments and occluding small blood vessels, leading to local chronic foci; finally, tumor immunosuppression therapy may be factors predisposing patients to salmonellosis. Infants and young children as well as the very elderly appear to be especially susceptible to serious disease as well as to gastroenteritis.

Clinical Manifestations

HISTORY Symptoms begin several days to several weeks after ingestion of contaminated water or food. Headache, fever, generalized aching, cough, and constipation are often present. Delirium or mental torpor are not unusual, especially when there is a high fever. The pulse rate may be slower than expected for the magnitude of the fever. Symptoms increase in intensity, and the fever often reaches 39.5° to 40.5°C (103.1 to 104.9°F) by the end of the first week. During the second week, rose spots may appear on the trunk and diffuse abdominal cramping becomes prominent, sometimes accompanied by diarrhea. In areas endemic for typhoid fever, the abdominal symptoms may be present from the onset, and diarrhea can also be an early manifestation.[81]

CUTANEOUS LESIONS After about 7 to 10 days of high fever, the characteristic rose spots may appear. These lesions are 2- to 3-mm slightly raised pink papules that blanch on pressure and are nontender. They appear in crops of approximately 10 to 20 lesions and are usually located between the nipple area and the umbilicus on the anterior trunk, rarely on the back or extremities. Without therapy, the crops of spots usually become brownish as they fade and disappear in 3 to 4 days. New lesions emerge over the ensuing 2 to 3 weeks in untreated patients. Their presence in 63 percent of a group of 62 patients in a contemporary study should encourage careful observation for this subtle rash.[82] Antibiotic therapy instituted early in the course of the illness may be responsible for the decreasing incidence of rose spots. The rash is less frequently reported in blacks, but this may be because of difficulty in detecting the small, scarce lesions on dark skin.

Rose spots occur infrequently in enteric fevers caused by other *Salmonella* species, but when they do appear, they may be present in greater numbers and in a more widespread distribution.

A variety of other skin changes have been described in enteric fever during the acute phase of illness. Erythema typhosum, an erythematous rash that is confluent and widely scattered, may occur during the first week of the disease. Erythema nodosum and urticarial lesions have been noted and ascribed to hypersensitivity phenomena. In several recent reports from the Indian subcontinent, subcutaneous and cutaneous abscesses and skin ulcers have been described.[83,84] Transient loss of hair, changes in nails, and posttyphoid anhidrosis reflect the acute catabolic stress.[85] It is distinctly uncommon to observe herpes labialis in enteric fever.

OTHER PHYSICAL FINDINGS During the acute phase of the disease, at the time the cutaneous lesions are appearing, the patient may be disoriented and have signs of pneumonia. The abdomen is often distended, tympanitic, and diffusely tender, with some localization to the right lower quadrant. The spleen is often enlarged but may be difficult to palpate because of abdominal distension and guarding.

Laboratory Findings

Leukopenia or low normal leukocyte counts are often present, but values range from 3000 to 20,000/mm³. The percentage of mononuclear cells may be increased, and atypical lymphocytes can appear in small numbers, suggesting a viral illness. Thrombocytopenia may occur, and rarely hemolysis is observed. During the initial week of illness, blood cultures are usually positive. During the second week, or when diarrhea begins, stool cultures become positive and the white blood cell count may increase. In addition to blood and stool, the typical rose spots should be cultured, preferably using the technique of skin snips.[82] In addition to blood and fecal cultures, bone marrow and skin lesion material may be positive in approximately

65 to 95 percent of cases, even when routine blood cultures simultaneously done are negative or when antibiotics are being administered.[86] Antibodies to somatic ("O") antigens develop after about 2 weeks of illness and rise over the ensuing months. Unfortunately, the serologic tests (Widal agglutination) are positive in about half of patients studied, and antibodies are detected nonspecifically in a variety of other infectious diseases. A more specific and sensitive serologic test for systemic *Salmonella* infections merits development.

Pathology

The rose spot characteristically blanches on pressure, and examination of the lesion histologically reveals gross dilatation of capillaries, described by some pathologists as *capillary atony*. Extravasation of blood is not observed, but there is considerable edema and an abundant pericapillary infiltration with macrophages; organisms may be present within these cells.[87]

Diagnosis and Differential Diagnosis

The diagnosis of *Salmonella* enteric fever may be difficult in a sporadic case, especially if the characteristic rash and gastrointestinal symptoms have not yet appeared and there is no history of travel in an endemic area. Headache, cough, and high fever are not very specific findings. However, when these symptoms are associated with delirium, relative bradycardia, and leukopenia with increased numbers of circulating mononuclear cells, the diagnosis of enteric fever should be considered. The diagnosis is usually made by obtaining blood cultures, which are positive in approximately 80 percent of untreated cases during the first week to 10 days. Serologic tests (Widal) are usually negative during the early phase of the illness and may not be diagnostic later. Likewise, enteric fever due to other *Salmonella* species can usually be diagnosed by blood cultures. Other cultured material (bone marrow, rose spots) may be important, especially in patients who have had prior antibiotic therapy.

The differential diagnosis includes a wide range of diseases. Prominent cough and severe headache in the early phases may suggest a viral or atypical pneumonia (caused by *Legionella pneumophila*, *Chlamydia pneumoniae*, *Mycoplasma pneumoniae*; psittacosis, or Q fever). Typhus and Rocky Mountain spotted fever can usually be excluded by geographic and epidemiologic considerations, serologic studies, the characteristic petechial component to the rash, and, in the case of spotted fever, the distribution of the rash on the distal parts of the extremities. Miliary tuberculosis may begin as an acute febrile illness with similar symptoms, leukopenia, and splenomegaly. The diagnosis may be delayed until a secondary complication such as meningitis occurs or until biopsy material (liver, lymph node) reveals granulomas, sometimes containing acid-fast organisms.

Among the viral diseases, the diagnosis of infectious mononucleosis is suggested by headache, cough, high fever, lymphadenopathy, splenomegaly, and a blood picture with leukopenia and some atypical mononuclear cells.

Malaria and toxoplasmosis are two parasitic illnesses that deserve consideration. Epidemiologic information plus intermittency of symptoms usually suggest the diagnosis of malaria. In generalized toxoplasmosis, the symptoms may be very similar to those of early enteric fever: prominent cough, high fever, a rash that is located on the trunk, and a mononucleosis-like blood picture. The rash tends to be more florid than the crops of 10 to 20 lesions seen in enteric fever and is macular with a petechial component, rather than papular. Diagnosis usually requires identification of *Toxoplasma gondii* in biopsy material or a rising antibody titer (19S fluorescent antibody or hemagglutination inhibition).

Course and Prognosis

The response of patients with enteric fever to antibiotic therapy is usually gradual, taking 3 to 6 days for the temperature to return to normal. With prolonged treatment, the incidence of relapse has been reduced, but this will vary with the age, nutritional condition, and general health of the patient. The major complications in the pre-antibiotic days were perforation and hemorrhage. Although rare, these complications still occur even with prompt, effective chemotherapy and are responsible for approximately 75 percent of the mortality in enteric fever. Deaths have been reduced from approximately 10 percent to 1 to 2 percent with antibiotic therapy. Following typhoid fever, approximately 1 to 2 percent of patients continue to harbor organisms in the gallbladder and excrete them in the stools for an indefinite period, becoming a major potential source for infecting other individuals.

TREATMENT AND PROPHYLAXIS The emergence of multidrug-resistant *Salmonella typhi*—endemic and imported—in many areas of the world has essentially obviated the use of chloramphenicol, ampicillin, and trimethoprim-sulfamethoxazole (TSM) as first-line antimicrobials to treat typhoid fever and other enteric fevers.[88]

The fluoroquinolones (ciprofloxacin, ofloxacin) are active against drug-susceptible and multidrug-resistant (chloramphenicol, TSM, or ampicillin) *S. typhi* or other salmonellae causing enteric fever. Results of clinical trials, involving over 100 patients, indicate that blood cultures become sterile promptly on treatment with ciprofloxacin and that this drug appears to be a safe and effective substitute for chloramphenicol and the treatment of choice of typhoid fever.[88] Ciprofloxacin is administered in 500- to 750-mg dosage orally every 12 h (or 400 mg intravenously every 12 h) in adults for 14 to 21 days. Third-generation cephalosporins, especially ceftriaxone or cefotaxime, are acceptable alternatives for the treatment of typhoid fever if the previously noted antimicrobials cannot be used because of resistance of the infecting strain or because of drug hypersensitivity.[89]

Glucocorticoid therapy for a period of several days has been advocated in addition to antimicrobial treatment for severely toxic and febrile patients, but its efficacy is unproved and prolonged use may increase the relapse rate. A report from Jakarta in 1984 found that high doses of dexamethasone reduced mortality significantly, and a recent review supported the use of glucocorticoids in severe typhoid fever.[90] Among the major complications, hemorrhage usually responds to conservative management, but perforation, often in the ileocecal region, requires immediate surgery.

Identification and eradication of the biliary carrier of *S. typhi* is an important preventive measure for controlling enteric fever. In the presence of stones, antibiotic therapy should be combined with cholecystectomy. In the absence of stones, a prolonged course of treatment with ampicillin or amoxicillin may eradicate the carrier site.[91] Ciprofloxacin has also been reported to be successful.[92]

Individuals traveling to areas of the world endemic for *S. typhi* or *S. paratyphi* A should be instructed in commonsense methods of eating and drinking to avoid potentially contaminated materials. Immunization is available for *S. typhi* and is probably effective for all but massive exposures, but careful personal hygiene and avoidance of suspicious water or foods (e.g., leafy greens) will eliminate most encounters with *S. typhi* and other salmonellae capable of causing enteric fever.

CUTANEOUS MANIFESTATIONS OF INFECTION WITH OTHER GRAM-NEGATIVE BACILLI

General Features

An acute cellulitis, with or without production of gas, may be caused by *E. coli*, *Proteus* spp., *Klebsiella* spp., *Enterobacter* spp., *Serratia marcescens*, a variety of other facultative and nonfermenting bacilli, and members of the obligate anaerobic group of *Bacteroides*. These infections have often but not exclusively been described in the very elderly and in diabetic patients following trauma, surgery, or bowel or perineal inflammation. The infectious process can be limited to the superficial soft tissues or be primarily in the deep fascia, but the extent of the cellulitis is often difficult to establish. Interference with vascular integrity can influence the findings, as can the infecting organism or organisms. Location can be a factor in early diagnosis, extent of spread along fascial planes (e.g., Fournier's necrotizing perineal fasciitis), and treatment decisions (antibiotics and surgery).

Drug addicts may develop mixed infections with these organisms when "skin popping," resulting in lesions such as necrotizing fasciitis.[93] Prior exposure to broad-spectrum antibiotics and altered host defenses can predispose to this type of infection, which is often nosocomial in origin. The finding of gas in the tissues frequently leads to an erroneous provisional diagnosis of clostridial cellulitis or gas gangrene.

Bacteriology and Pathogenesis

The family Enterobacteriaceae is composed of a number of bacilli that grow readily on blood agar and selective media. By means of a number of biochemical reactions and growth characteristics, seven tribes of Enterobacteriaceae have been recognized. *Escherichia coli* is closely related to *Shigella*; *Salmonella* spp. to *Citrobacter*; *Klebsiella-Enterobacter-Serratia* make up a third tribe; and *Proteus-Providencia* comprise a fourth main division. There are a variety of facultative gram-negative bacilli that do not belong to this family, metabolize sugars variably, and can be recognized by utilizing other specialized biochemical tests. In addition, the obligate anaerobic *Bacteroides* spp. reside in the oral cavity, colon, and female vaginal region and are speciated by their anaerobic growth requirements as well as a variety of metabolites that can be identified by gas-liquid chromatography and other methods.

Infection can result from endogenous (host flora) or exogenous (e.g., fresh- or saltwater) contamination of skin or subcutaneous tissues in an area of injury, surgery, or ischemia. Bacteria can also invade the subcutaneous tissues via the circulation from a distinct source or by direct spread from contiguous structures such as the colon. By dissection along fascial planes, cellulitis can erupt in areas removed from the initial focus. The process is often necrotizing, containing a mixture of facultative and anaerobic bacteria and, especially in diabetic individuals, can be associated with gas formation (mainly hydrogen). Edema, bleb formation, ischemia, and gangrene result from thrombosis of nutrient blood vessels.[94] The underlying muscle is almost always spared.[95] Polymorphonuclear leukocytes are abundantly present compared to the relative scarcity of acute inflammatory cells in clostridial infections.

Epidemiology

Cellulitis usually follows contamination of adjacent tissues by bowel contents or a breakdown of skin. The conditions predisposing patients to this type of infection include (1) bowel perforation (appendicitis, neoplasm, diverticulitis, rectal mucosal tear), (2) colon surgery, (3) chronic edema, (4) vascular insufficiency, (5) injection of addictive drugs, (6) decubitus ulcers, (7) percutaneous lines, and (8) superficial perineal dermatitis, including diaper rash. The health of these patients is often further impaired by poorly controlled diabetes, alterations in host defense mechanisms (granulocytopenia, etc.), poor nutrition, or cirrhosis. Crepitant (gas-containing) cellulitis results from infection with gas-forming strains of bacteria (*E. coli, Klebsiella, A. hydrophila*), especially in patients with poorly controlled diabetes or when *Bacteroides* spp. or anaerobic streptococci are present too.[96] Water-related lacerations may cause soft tissue infection with *Edwardsiella tarda*.[97] Similarly, cellulitis, subcutaneous abscess or myonecrosis due to *A. hydrophila* may follow penetrating trauma in either a fresh- or brackish-water environment or associated with fish or other aquatic animals.[98] Halophilic vibrios, including *Vibrio vulnificus*, are responsible for acute infections of traumatized skin or septicemic spread to skin and soft tissues from seawater exposure or ingestion of raw shellfish. (See Chap. 197 for discussion of water-borne cellulitis.) Injuries on farms, particularly from corn-harvesting machinery, have been associated with gram-negative bacilli (*Enterobacter* spp. and *Stenotrophomonas* (formerly *Xanthomonas*) *maltophilia*).[99] Gram-negative bacillary cellulitis (due to *E. coli, Proteus* spp., or *C. freundii*) may occur in immunocompromised patients, including individuals with AIDS, or patients with the nephrotic syndrome.[100] The appearance of the lesions grossly resembles those due to the more common gram-positive pathogens.

Clinical Manifestations

HISTORY Diabetes mellitus, malnutrition, chronic illness (e.g., paraplegia with decubitus ulcers), or several other conditions described under "Epidemiology" are usually present. The onset may be insidious, over 4 to 5 days, or abrupt. Pain, often severe, frequently precedes evidence of local skin changes, especially if the infection is at the level of the deep fascia. High fever, shaking chills, increasing pain, and falling blood pressure may follow. Symptoms of gastrointestinal inflammation such as appendicitis or diverticulitis may precede the cellulitis illness. Rectal or perineal pain can indicate a local process that may be especially devastating in a patient deficient in granulocytes.

CUTANEOUS LESIONS The areas of involvement evolve to the typical findings of cellulitis, with warmth and brawny edema. In the early stages, the skin is rarely discolored beyond a pink hue, and vesicles and blebs or bullae are almost never present. At this juncture, unless pain is present, the process may easily be overlooked, especially if the infection is located in a less obvious area or the patient is obtunded. As the cellulitis progresses, edema and redness increase and areas of gangrene may appear. Palpable tenderness and crepitus, if present, can help define the anatomic extent of the process. The cellulitis may remain localized to the superficial subcutaneous tissues and skin, but progression to the deep fascia with contiguous extension, necrosis of fat, and increasing pain and toxicity suggest a diagnosis of necrotizing fasciitis.[101]

Superficial nasal lesions Several subspecies of *Klebsiella pneumoniae* that infect the upper respiratory tract can produce unique superficial diseases. Ozena is a chronic productive rhinitis caused by infection with *Klebsiella pneumoniae,* ssp. *ozaenae.* The process remains internal without any cutaneous manifestations except a profuse mucopurulent, foul-smelling discharge.[102] *Klebsiella pneumoniae,* ssp. *rhinoscleromatis* is the etiologic agent of a hypertrophic, granulomatous infection of the external nares known as rhinoscleroma. This disease often produces changes in the overlying nasal skin (Fig. 198-6) and the contiguous surfaces of the respiratory and posterior pharyngeal regions. Most cases have been described from very local areas of eastern and central Europe (where the disease is known as "Slavic leprosy"), from Africa, the Near East, and parts of Central and South America.[103] Dissemination of the organism is by prolonged close contact, often in family settings of crowding and poor sanitation. Infected individuals can shed organisms for years, with the result that hyperendemic areas are recognized. As seen in leprosy, the disease rarely becomes clinically apparent in children. Patients complain of chronic nasal and cutaneous discharge, obstructive symptoms, or cutaneous nasal masses. Diagnosis depends upon biopsy identification of characteristic vacuolated Mikulicz cells and isolation of the organism on routine cultures, with biochemical and serologic confirmation.[104] Both *K. pneumoniae,* spp. *ozaenae* and *K. pneumoniae,* spp. *rhinoscleromatis* are susceptible to ciprofloxacin, 500 to 750 mg bid for 1 to 3 months. A recent report describes a successful outcome in all 10 patients treated with this oral regimen.[105] Other successful treatments include a third-generation cephalosporin or rifampin plus TSM.

OTHER PHYSICAL FINDINGS The clinical course is often dominated by systemic manifestations of the underlying illness or decreased mental alertness, hypotension, and dehydration. Abdominal distension and other manifestations of localized or generalized peritonitis may be present. Extreme tenderness of the rectum, with or without a mass, can indicate the local source of a perineal process.

FIGURE 198-6

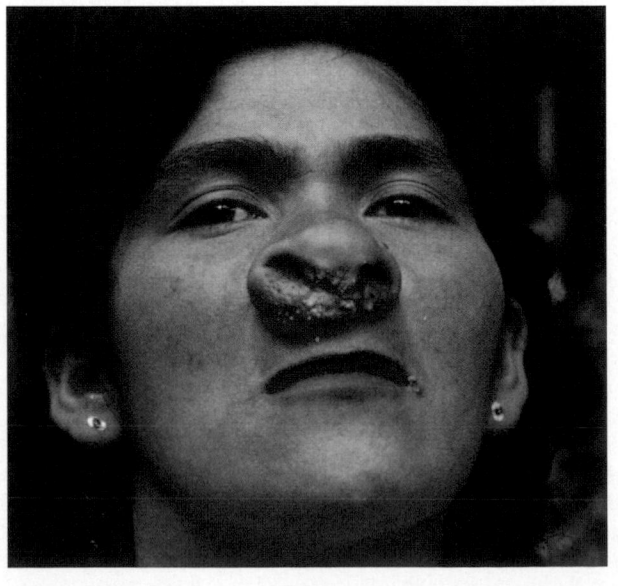

Klebsiella pneumoniae rhinoscleromatis: Rhinoscleroma. The nasal passages and nose are infected, resulting in obstructed respiration.

Laboratory Findings

The leukocyte count is usually elevated, in the range of 20,000 to 30,000/mm^3, but may be markedly diminished in the presence of gram-negative septicemia. Elevated blood glucose values and findings of ketoacidosis are not unusual. In the presence of crepitant cellulitis, roentgenograms or magnetic resonance imaging (MRI) of the soft tissue may show the depth and extent of the gas-forming process.[106] In the absence of palpable gas, a soft tissue x-ray or MRI may indicate gas formation as part of the inflammatory process. Frozen-section biopsy materials in acute soft tissue infection can provide evidence of obliterative vasculitis, a finding suggestive of necrotizing fasciitis.[107]

Pathology

Edema, gangrene of overlying skin, fat necrosis, and a thin exudate containing visible fat droplets and polymorphonuclear leukocytes is usually present. Gas may be seen in the subcutaneous tissues. Blood vessels are often involved in a necrotic, obliterative, thrombotic inflammatory reaction. The underlying muscle is usually not involved unless there is septicemia associated with major vascular thrombosis or there is myonecrosis with an organism like *A. hydrophila.*

Diagnosis and Differential Diagnosis

A specific etiologic diagnosis can be made by needle aspiration of the cellulitis or an overlying bleb. Several morphologic forms of gram-positive as well as gram-negative organisms may be present, and when gas is present, anaerobic cocci and *Clostridia* must also be considered. The presence of anaerobes in the exudate may be accompanied by a foul, fetid odor. Radiologic and surgical evaluation can be helpful in defining a descriptive diagnosis such as crepitant cellulitis or necrotizing fasciitis.

Course and Prognosis

The process may be indolent and may quickly respond to effective antibiotic therapy. Unfortunately, especially in obese diabetic patients with perineal lesions, the progression of necrotizing fasciitis may be astonishingly rapid, even with vigorous antibiotic and surgical therapy. When the process is located centrally, in the perineal-gluteal area, the mortality is often as high as 50 percent. Infection of an extremity is often treated by antibiotics, drainage and debridement, or by amputation, with more favorable results. The course is often prolonged and complex due to metabolic and nutritional complications.[108]

Treatment

Immediate antibiotic therapy and surgical drainage are essential, guided by Gram-stained smears of the exudate and the extent of the process. Extensive debridement is usually unnecessary and hyperbaric oxygen is not indicated in cellulitis or necrotizing fasciitis. Judgment and experience are vital in surgical decisions that include the question of amputation. The existence of a "feeding" source of contamination should be sought, especially with perineal or thigh involvement (e.g., from a ruptured appendix, diverticulum, or rectal tear). If a lower-bowel leak is found, a diverting colostomy should be performed in addition to a local drainage procedure. Decubitus ulcers must be carefully evaluated for undermining necrosis, abscess formation, and cellulitis, since they may be the source of septicemias, including polymicrobial types.[109]

Recent antibiotic usage, status of renal and hepatic function, and prior hospital exposure are factors that will help determine the choice of antibiotics. Single or multiple agents are used initially, depending on the above information and the results of Gram-stained smears of exudate. Hospitalized patients already exposed to antibiotics and acutely ill should be started on a combination of antimicrobials that should include an aminoglycoside if enteric gram-negative organisms are suspected. Crepitant cellulitis with foul exudate suggesting *B. fragilis* should be treated with metronidazole, clindamycin, or chloramphenicol. Selected second- or third-generation cephalosporins or fluoroquinolones can substitute for aminoglycosides in patients with severe renal impairment. If *P. aeruginosa, Klebsiella,* or *Serratia* is suspected in certain hospital-acquired infections, tobramycin or amikacin may be preferred to gentamicin and a broad-spectrum penicillin added if *Pseudomonas* is a major pathogen. The presence of gram-positive cocci on initial stained smears indicates the need for penicillin or ampicillin (for chaining streptococci) or nafcillin (for clusters of staphylococci). If resistant enterococci or methicillin resistant staphylococci are suspected, then vancomycin is the drug of choice for either chaining or clustering gram-positive cocci.

REFERENCES

1. Kingston ME, Mackey D: Skin clues in the diagnosis of life-threatening infections. *Rev Infect Dis* **8**:1, 1986
2. Verheul AFM et al: Meningococcal lipopolysaccharides: Virulence factor and potential vaccine component. *Microbiol Rev* **57**:34, 1993
3. DeVoe IW, Gilchrist JE: Piliation and colonial morphology among laboratory strains of meningococci. *J Clin Microbiol* **7**:379, 1978
4. Pinner RW et al: Evidence for functionally distinct pili expressed by *Neisseria meningitidis. Infect Immun* **59**:3169, 1991
5. Kornfeld SF, Plaut AG: Secretory immunity and the bacterial IgA proteases. *Rev Infect Dis* **3**:521, 1981
6. Figueroa JF et al: Infectious diseases associated with complement deficiencies. *Clin Microbiol Rev* **4**:359, 1991
7. Sotto MN et al: Pathogenesis of cutaneous lesions in acute meningococcemia in humans: Light, immunofluorescent, and electron microscopic studies of skin biopsy specimens. *J Infect Dis* **133**:506, 1976
8. Van Deuran M et al: Rapid diagnosis of acute meningococcal infections by needle aspiration or biopsy of skin lesions. *BMJ* **306**:1229, 1993
9. Davis CE, Arnold K: Role of meningococcal endotoxin in meningococcal purpura. *J Exp Med* **140**:159, 1974
10. DeVoe IW, Gilka F: Disseminated intravascular coagulation in rabbits: Synergistic activity of meningoccal endotoxin and materials egested from leukocytes containing meningococci. *J Med Microbiol* **9**:451, 1976
11. McGehee WG et al: Intravascular coagulation in fulminant meningococcemia. *Ann Intern Med* **67**:250, 1967
12. Adams EM et al: Absence of the seventh component of complement in a patient with chronic meningococcemia presenting as vasculitis. *Ann Intern Med* **99**:35, 1983
13. Farron F et al: Chronic meningococcemia and IgA deficiency in an adolescent. *Arch Pediatr* **3**:149, 1996
14. Ploysangam T, Sheth AP: Chronic meningococcemia in childhood: Case report and review of the literature. *Pediatr Dermatol* **13**:483, 1996
15. Fass RJ, Saslaw S: Chronic meningococcemia: Possible pathogenic role of IgM deficiency. *Arch Intern Med* **130**:943, 1972
16. Zangwill KM et al: School-based clusters of meningococcal disease in the United States. *JAMA* **277**:389, 1997
17. Goldschneider I et al: Human immunity to the meningococcus: II. Development of natural immunity. *J Exp Med* **129**:1327, 1969
18. Robbins JB et al: Enteric bacteria cross-reactive with *Neisseria meningitidis* groups A and C and *Diplococcus pneumoniae* types I and III. *Infect Immun* **6**:651, 1972

19. Goldschneider I et al: Human immunity to the meningococcus. I. The role of humoral antibodies. *J Exp Med* **129**:1307, 1969

20. Griffiss JM, Bertram MA: Immunoepidemiology of meningococcal disease in military recruits. II. Blocking of serum bactericidal antibody by circulating IgA early in the course of invasive disease. *J Infect Dis* **136**:733, 1977

21. Griffiss JM: Epidemic meningococcal disease: Synthesis of a hypothetical immunoepidemiologic model. *Rev Infect Dis* **4**:159, 1982

22. Boslego JB et al: Efficacy, safety, and immunogenicity of a meningococcal vaccine group B (15:P1.3) outer membrane protein vaccine in Iquique, Chile. *Vaccine* **13**:821, 1995

23. deMoraes JC et al: Protective efficacy of a serogroup B meningococcal vaccine in São Paulo, Brazil. *Lancet* **340**:1074, 1992

24. Romero JD, Outschoorn IM: Current status of meningococcal group B vaccine candidates: Capsular or noncapsular? *Clin Microbiol Rev* **7**:559, 1994

25. Lieberman JM et al: Safety and immunogenicity of a serogroups A/C *Neisseria meningitides* oligosaccharide-protein conjugate vaccine in young children. *JAMA* **275**:1499, 1996

26. Munford RS et al: Spread of meningococcal infection within households. *Lancet* **2**:1275, 1974

27. Meningococcal Disease Surveillance Group: Meningococcal disease. *JAMA* **235**:261, 1976

28. Jacobson JA, Holloway JT: Meningococcal disease in day-care centers. *Pediatrics* **59**:299, 1977

29. CDC: Control and prevention of meningococcal disease. *MMWR* **46**:RR-5,1, 1997

30. Salet IE et al: Seroepidemiologic aspects of *Neisseria meningitidis* in homosexual men. *Can Med Assoc J* **126**:38, 1982

31. Feldman HA: Meningoccal infections. *Adv Intern Med* **18**:177, 1972

32. Koppes GM et al: Group Y meningococcal disease in United States air force recruits. *Am J Med* **62**:661, 1977

33. Rompalo AM et al: The acute arthritis-dermatitis syndrome. *Arch Intern Med* **147**:281, 1987

34. Periappuram M et al: Rapid detection of meningococci from petechiae in acute meningococcal infection. *J Infect* **31**:201, 1995

35. Perkins MD et al: Rapid bacterial antigen detection is not clinically useful. *J Clin Microbiol* **33**:1486, 1995

36. Barquet N et al: Prognostic factors in meningococcal disease. *JAMA* **278**:491, 1997

37. Benoit FL: Chronic meningococcemia. *Am J Med* **35**:103, 1963

38. Barquet N et al: Primary meningococcal conjunctivitis: Report of 21 patients and review. *Rev Infect Dis* **12**:838, 1990

39. Ferson M, Shi E: Periorbital cellulitis with meningococcal bacteremia. *Pediatr Infect Dis J* **7**:600, 1988

40. Oppenheim BA: Antibiotic resistance in *Neisseria meningitidis. Clin Infect Dis* **24**:598, 1997

41. Lynn WA, Cohen J: Adjunctive therapy for septic shock: A review of experimental approaches. *Clin Infect Dis* **20**:143, 1995

42. Gilja OH et al: Use of single dose ofloxacin to eradicate tonsillopharyngeal carriage of *Neisseria meningitidis. Antimicrob Agents Chemother* **37**:2024, 1993

43. Darouiche R et al: Levels of rifampin and ciprofloxacin in nasal secretions: Correlation with MIC90 and eradication of nasopharyngeal carriage of bacteria. *J Infect Dis* **162**:1124, 1990

44. Agger WA, Mardan A: *Pseudomonas aeruginosa* infections of intact skin. *Clin Infect Dis* **20**:302, 1995

45. Berger TG et al: Cutaneous manifestations of *Pseudomonas* infections in AIDS. *J Am Acad Dermatol* **32**:279, 1995

46. Liu PV: Extracellular toxins of *Pseudomonas aeruginosa. J Infect Dis* **130**(suppl):S94, 1974

47. Bishop MB et al: The effect of *Pseudomonas aeruginosa* cytotoxin and toxin A on human polymorphonuclear leukocytes. *J Med Microbiol* **24**:315, 1987

48. Pollack M: The virulence of *Pseudomonas aeruginosa. Rev Infect Dis* **6**:S617, 1984

49. Saelinger CB et al: Experimental studies on the pathogenesis of infections due to *Pseudomonas aeruginosa:* Direct evidence for toxin production during pseudomonas infection of burned skin tissues. *J Infect Dis* **136**:555, 1957

50. Bottone EJ et al: Loofah sponges as reservoirs and vehicles in the transmission of potentially pathogenic bacterial species to human skin. *J Clin Microbiol* **32**:469, 1994

51. Noble WC: Gram-negative bacterial skin infections. *Semin Dermatol* **12**:336, 1993

52. Bassiouny A: Perichondritis of the auricle. *Laryngoscope* **91**:422, 1981

53. Ruskin J, Yu VL: Malignant external otitis: Insights into pathogenesis, clinical manifestations, diagnosis and therapy. *Am J Med* **85**:391, 1988

54. McElroy EA Jr, Marks GL: Fatal necrotizing otitis externa in a patient with AIDS. *Rev Infect Dis* **13**:1246, 1991

55. Doroghazi RM et al: Invasive external otitis: Report of 21 cases and review of the literature. *Am J Med* **71**:603, 1981

56. El Baz P et al: *Pseudomonas aeruginosa* 0-11 folliculitis: Development into ecthyma gangrenosum in immunosuppressed patients. *Arch Dermatol* **121**:873, 1985

57. Giamarellou H: Malignant otitis externa: The therapeutic evolution of a lethal infection. *J Antimicrob Chemother* **30**:745, 1992

58. Stanley MM: *Bacillus pyrocyaneus* infections (2 parts). *Am J Med* **2**:253, 1947

59. Bodey GP: Dermatologic manifestations of infections in neutropenic patients. *Infect Dis Clin North Am* **8**:655, 1994

60. Campo RE et al: Subcutaneous nodules as a dermatologic manifestation of bacteremia due to *Pseudomonas aeruginosa. South Med J* **87**:233, 1994

61. Bagel J, Grossman ME: Subcutaneous nodules in *Pseudomonas* sepsis. *Am J Med* **80**:528, 1986

62. Teplitz C: Pathogenesis of *Pseudomonas* vasculitis and septic lesions. *Arch Pathol* **80**:297, 1965

63. Sloss JM et al: Acetic acid used for the elimination of *Pseudomonas aeruginosa* from burn and soft tissue wounds. *J Army Med Corps* **139**:49, 1993

64. Cryz S et al: Production and characterization of a human hyperimmune intravenous immunoglobulin against *Pseudomonas aeruginosa* and *Klebsiella* species. *J Infect Dis* **163**:1055, 1991

65. Kusne S et al: Gangrenous cellulitis associated with gram-negative bacilli in pancytopenic patients: Dilemma with respect to effective therapy. *Am J Med* **85**:490, 1988

66. Chen S et al: Cellulitis due to *Pseudomonas putrefaciens:* Possible production of exotoxins. *Rev Infect Dis* **13**:642, 1991

67. Nelson JD, Ginsburg CM: An hypothesis on the pathogenesis of *Haemophilus influenzae* buccal cellulitis. *J Pediatr* **88**:709, 1976

68. Broome CV: Epidemiology of *Haemophilus influenzae* type b infections in the United States. *Pediatr Infect Dis J* **6**:779, 1987

69. Broadhurst LE et al: Decreases in invasive *Haemophilus influenzae* diseases in US Army children, 1984 through 1991. *JAMA* **269**:227, 1993

70. CDC: Progress toward elimination of *Haemophilus influenzae* type b disease among infants and children—United States, 1987–1995. *MMWR* **45**:901, 1996

71. Shaw S et al: The paradox of *Haemophilus influenzae* type b bacteremia in the presence of serum bactericidal activity. *J Clin Invest* **58**:1019, 1976

72. Robbins JB et al: *Haemophilus influenzae* type b: Disease and immunity in humans. *Ann Intern Med* **78**:259, 1973

73. O'Reilly RJ et al: Circulating polyribophosphate in *Haemophilus influenzae* type b meningitis. *J Clin Invest* **56**:1012, 1975

74. Smith DH et al: Studies on the prevalence of antibodies to *Haemophilus influenzae,* type B, in *Haemophilus influenzae,* edited by S Sell. Nashville, TN, Vanderbilt University Press, 1973

75. Schneerson R, Robbins JB: Induction of serum *Haemophilus influenzae* type b capsular antibodies in adult volunteers fed cross-reacting *Escherichia coli* 075:K100:H5. *N Engl J Med* **292**:1093, 1975

76. Granoff DM, Nankervis GA: Cellulitis due to *Haemophilus influenzae* type b antigenemia and antibody responses. *Am J Dis Child* **130**:1211, 1976

77. McDonnell WM et al: *Haemophilus influenzae* type B cellulitis in adults. *Am J Med* **81**:709, 1986

78. Chartrand S, Harrison C: Buccal cellulitis reevaluated. *Am J Dis Child* **140**:891, 1986

79. *American Academy of Pediatrics Red Book.* Elk Grove Village, IL, 1994, p 206

80. Adams WG et al: Decline of childhood *Haemophilus influenzae* type b (Hib) disease in the Hib vaccine era. *JAMA* **269**:221, 1993

81. Wicks ACB et al: Endemic typhoid fever: A diagnostic pitfall. *Q J Med [New Series XL]* **159**:341, 1971

82. Gilman RH et al: Relative efficacy of blood, urine, rectal swab, bone-marrow, and rose-spot cultures for recovery of *Salmonella typhi* in typhoid fever. *Lancet* **1**:1211, 1975

83. Lalitha MK, John R: Unusual manifestations of salmonellosis—a surgical problem. *Q J Med* **87**:301, 1994

84. Karthikeyan G, Mahadevan S: Cutaneous ulcers in typhoid fever. *J Trop Med Hyg* **97**:298, 1994

85. Raventhiran V: Post-typhoid anhidrosis: A clinical curiosity. *Postgrad Med J* **71**:435, 1991

86. Guerera-Caceres JG et al: Diagnostic value of bone marrow culture in typhoid fever. *Trans R Soc Trop Med Hyg* **73**:680, 1979

87. Litwack KD et al: Rose spots in typhoid fever. *Arch Dermatol* **105**:252, 1972

88. Rowe B et al: Multidrug-resistant *Salmonella typhi:* A worldwide epidemic. *Clin Infect Dis* **24**:S106, 1997

89. Soe GB, Overturf GD: Treatment of typhoid fever and other systemic salmonelloses with cefotaxime, ceftriaxone, cefoperazone, and other newer cephalosporins. *Rev Infect Dis* **9**:719, 1987

90. McGowan JE Jr et al: Guidelines for the use of systemic glucocorticoids in the management of selected infections. *J Infect Dis* **165**:1, 1992

91. Nolan CM, White PC: Treatment of typhoid carriers with amoxicillin. *JAMA* **239**:2352, 1978

92. Asperilla MO et al: Quinolone antibiotics in the treatment of *Salmonella* infections. *Rev Infect Dis* **12**:873, 1990

93. Henriksen BM et al: Soft tissue infections from drug abuse: A clinical and microbiological review of 145 cases. *Acta Orthop Scand* **65**:625, 1994

94. Rubenstein E et al: Severe necrotizing soft-tissue infections: Report of 22 cases. *Conn Med* **59**:67, 1995

95. Culbertson WR: Acute non-clostridial crepitant cellulitis. *Arch Surg* **77**:462, 1958

96. Brook I, Frazier EH: Clinical features and aerobic and anaerobic microbiological characteristics of cellulitis. *Arch Surg* **130**:786, 1995

97. Pitlik S et al: Nonenteric infections acquired through contact with water. *Rev Infect Dis* **9**:54, 1987

98. Gold WL, Salit IE: *Aeromonas hydrophilia* infections of skin and soft tissue: Report of 11 cases and review. *Clin Infect Dis* **16**:69, 1993

99. Agger WA et al: Wounds caused by corn-harvesting machines: An unusual source of infection due to gram-negative bacilli. *Rev Infect Dis* **8**:927, 1986

100. Hick CB, Chulay JD: Bacteremic *Citrobacter freundii* cellulitis associated with tub immersion in a patient with the nephrotic syndrome. *Mil Med* **153**:400, 1988

101. Green RJ et al: Necrotizing fasciitis. *Chest* **110**:219, 1996

102. Goldstein EJ et al: Infections caused by *Klebsiella ozaenae:* A changing disease spectrum. *J Clin Microbiol* **8**:413, 1978

103. Altmann G et al: Rhinoscleroma. *Isr J Med Sci* **13**:62, 1977

104. Malowany MS et al: Isolation and microbiologic differentiation of *Klebsiella rhinoscleromatis* and *Klebsiella ozaenae* in cases of chronic rhinitis. *Am J Clin Pathol* **58**:550, 1972

105. Nielson BC et al: Successful treatment of ozena with ciprofloxacin. *Rhinology* **33**:57, 1995

106. Saiag P et al: Magnetic resonance imaging in adults presenting with severe acute infectious cellulitis. *Arch Dermatol* **130**:1150, 1994

107. Stamenkovic I, Law PD: Early recognition of potentially fatal necrotizing fasciitis: The role of frozen section biopsy. *N Engl J Med* **310**:1689, 1984

108. Sentochnik DE: Deep soft-tissue infections in diabetic patients in infections in diabetes mellitus. *Inf Dis Clin North Am* **9**:53, 1995

109. Galpin JE et al: Sepsis associated with decubitus ulcers. *Am J Med* **61**:346, 1976

CHAPTER 199

George J. Murakawa
Timothy Berger

Bartonellosis

Infections by members of the genus *Bartonella*, which are aerobic, fastidious, gram-negative bacilli, are rapidly emerging. The genus includes, among other species, *B. henselae* (formerly *Rochalimaea henselae*), which causes cat-scratch disease (CSD), bacillary angiomatosis (BA) and peliosis, and endocarditis; *B. quintana* (formerly *R. quintana*), which causes trench fever, urban trench fever, BA, and endocarditis; *B. bacilliformis*, the agent of Oroya fever and verruga peruana; and *B. elizabethae,* which causes endocarditis (Table 199-1). Among bacterial pathogens, a feature unique to *Bartonella* is the ability to induce neoangiogenesis, as is seen in BA and verruga peruana. Infections caused by most of these bacteria are associated with arthropod vectors.

TABLE 199-1

Diseases Caused by *Bartonella*

SPECIES	HUMAN DISEASE	RISK GROUP	RESERVOIR	VECTOR
B. henselae	Cat scratch disease	Immunocompetent	Cat	Cat flea*
	Bacillary angiomatosis	Immunocompromised	Cat	
	Endocarditis	Immunocompromised	Cat	
B. quintana	Trench fever	Immunocompetent	Human	Body louse
	Urban trench fever (including endocarditis)	Immunocompetent alcoholic, homeless	Human	Body louse?
	Bacillary angiomatosis	Immunocompromised	Human?	
B. bacilliformis	Oroya fever and verruga peruana	Immunocompetent, recent travel to Andes	?	Sandfly
B. elizabethae	Endocarditis		?	?
B. clarridgeiae	Cat-scratch disease	Immunocompetent	Cat	?
B. vinsonii	None			
B. talpae	None			
B. peromysci	None			
B. grahamii	None			
B. taylorii	None			
B. doshiae	None			

*Cat fleas have only been shown to transmit *B. henselae* from cat to cat but not to humans.

MICROBIOLOGY

Bartonella organisms are small aerobic, fastidious, pleiomorphic, gram-negative bacteria; they are difficult to culture from clinical samples. This difficulty stems in part from their slow growth rate (doubling time of approximately 10 h) and complex nutritional requirements.[1-2] However, *Bartonella* can be isolated and cultured on blood agar plates or in tissue-culture media using mammalian cell lines. Initial clinical isolates grow slowly and visible colonies may not be detected until weeks later, but subsequent passages grow much more rapidly.[3] The organisms are short rods, ranging from 0.3 to 0.5 μm wide by 1.0 to 1.7 μm long.[3] The genomic size is estimated between 1700 and 2174 kb.[3]

Previously, *B. bacilliformis* and all *Rochalimaea* species were classified in the order Rickettsiales, which contained the families Rickettsiaceae, Bartonellaceae, and Anaplasmataceae. However, unlike the obligate intracellular *Rickettsia*, all *Bartonella* species can be cultured on bacteriologic media. Moreover, sequence analyses of 16s RNA and DNA hybridization data revealed that *Bartonella* are highly related organisms, quite divergent from *Rickettsia*. Thus, these organisms were unified under the common genus, *Bartonella*, including *B. henselae*, *B. quintana*, *B. bacilliformis*, *B. elizabethae*, and *B. vinsonii*.[4] *Grahamella*, bacteria which can be isolated from the blood of small woodland mammals and do not cause human infection, also have been shown to be highly homologous to *Bartonella*, and thus, *B. talpae*, *B. peromysci*, *B. taylorii*, and *B. doshiae* have been added to the genus.[5] Recently, a new species of *Bartonella*, *B. clarridgeiae*, has been isolated from cats.[95]

CAT-SCRATCH DISEASE

Cat-scratch disease (CSD) is a relatively common, benign, self-limited disease caused by *B. henselae*. It is the most common cause of localized chronic lymphadenopathy in children and young adults.[6] The disease is usually transmitted by the bite or scratch of a cat or kitten, although it has rarely been associated with other pets.

CSD was originally reported by Robert Debré in 1931.[7] An infectious etiology was long suspected, but it was not until 1983 that Wear and his colleagues, using Warthin-Starry staining, identified bacteria in 34 of 39 lymph nodes from patients with CSD.[8] Bacilli were also identified in primary cutaneous and ocular lesions of CSD.[9,10] Similar-appearing organisms were identified in lesions of bacillary angiomatosis (BA), and it was suspected that both diseases were caused by the same organism.[11,12] *B. henselae* causes the overwhelming majority of cases of CSD. Significant titers for *B. henselae* were found in 86 of 91 patients (95 percent) who met the clinical definition of CSD.[13] Moreover, by using polymerase chain reaction (PCR) analyses, *B. henselae* DNA sequences can be identified in specimens from CSD patients and in CSD skin test antigens.[14-16] *Afipia felis* causes, at most, a small proportion of CSD cases.[17-19] A single case of CSD caused by *B. clarridgeiae* has been reported.[95]

Epidemiology

Approximately 29.2 million (31 percent) households in the United States own a cat, averaging close to two cats per household, or a total household cat population of 57 million.[20] Given the large population of domestic cats, it is not surprising that over 22,000 cases of CSD are reported annually, resulting in over 2000 hospitalizations and an annual health care cost of over $12 million.[21] Most of these dollars are spent for diagnostic workup of these patients rather than treatment.

CSD affects persons of all ages, although some 60 to 90 percent of cases have been reported in children and young adults.[22,23] CSD is seen worldwide and does not appear to have a racial prevalence. Most patients with CSD can recall a history of cat contact, but this is not absolute, ranging from 90.3 to 99.1 percent.[22,24] The incidence of CSD is slightly higher in males.[22] CSD is seasonal, seen mostly in the second half of the year.[22-24]

Patients with CSD are more likely than others to have at least one pet kitten 12 months old or younger, to be scratched or bitten by a kitten, and to have at least one kitten with fleas.[23] In California, 39.5 percent of cats are bacteremic for *B. henselae*, and bacteremic cats were more likely to be stray cats, young (less than 1 year old), and flea-infested.[25] The seroprevalence of *B. henselae* among pet cats is highly variable throughout regions of North America (overall, 27.9 percent positive); a higher seroprevalence is associated with increasing climatic warmth and annual precipitation.[26] When the geographic seroprevalence of *B. henselae* is compared with predicted estimates of cat flea populations based on temperature and humidity, there is considerable overlap, suggesting a possible role as a vector for the cat flea (*Ctenocephalides felis*). Chomel and coworkers have shown that *B. henselae* can be transmitted from cat to cat via the cat flea.[27]

Clinical Manifestations

The incubation period has been reported to range from 5 to 50 days. However, in a series of 1200 patients, a papule at the site of inoculation developed within 3 to 5 days after exposure to a cat and progressed through a vesicular and crusted stage in 2 to 3 days; within a week or two, lymphadenopathy developed[22] (Fig. 199-1). Lymphadenopathy usually remits spontaneously after several months. Recurrences are uncommon but have been reported. A primary inoculation papule is seen in approximately 60 to 90 percent of patients.[22,28]

Lymphadenopathy is the hallmark of CSD. In one series, 85 percent of patients had single-node involvement.[22] Although unilateral regional lymphadenopathy is the general rule, noncontiguous bilateral lymphadenopathy was detected in 1.9 percent of patients.[22] Lymphadenopathy can occur anywhere, but it is most common on the upper extremities, followed by head, neck, and groin.[22] The lymph nodes either regress over a period of weeks to months or proceed to suppuration and may require aspiration.

Unusual manifestations of CSD have been reported in 2 to 11 percent of cases of CSD.[28] The most common is the oculoglandular syndrome of Parinaud, or granulomatous conjunctivitis and preauricular adenopathy. Other complications include acute encephalopathy and other neurologic manifestations, osteolytic lesions, hepatic and splenic abscesses, and pulmonary manifestations.[6,22,29]

In one study, 5.3 percent of patients had associated skin eruptions, including generalized macular, maculopapular, and morbilliform eruptions and rarely purpuric exanthems.[30] Erythema nodosum is the most common of the skin reactions.[24] Other cutaneous manifestions include leukocytoclastic vasculitis, thrombocytopenic purpura, erythema marginatum, erythema multiforme, and erythema annulare.[22,24,28,30]

In immunosuppressed hosts, infection with *B. henselae*, the CSD bacillus, can produce a spectrum of disease, from classic CSD and complicated CSD to bacillary angiomatosis, peliosis, or septicemia.[31–35]

FIGURE 199-1

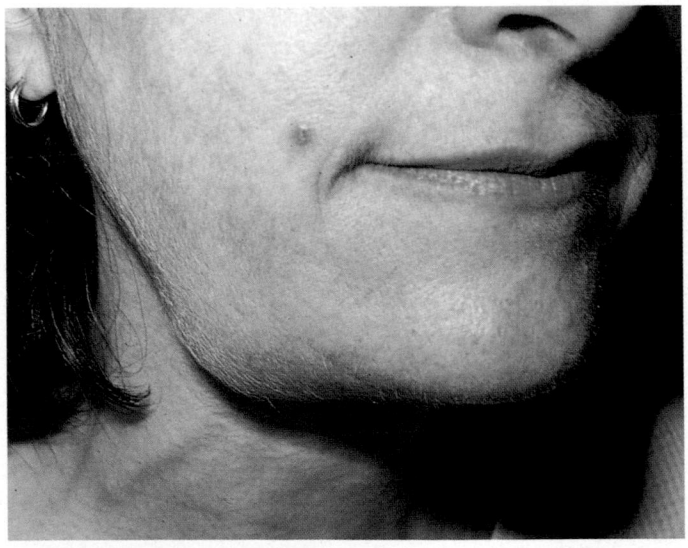

Cat-scratch disease. Primary lesion adjacent to mouth with associated submandibular lymphadenopathy in a woman.

Laboratory Findings

Laboratory findings for CSD are nonspecific and usually not helpful except to exclude other diseases. Patients with CSD may have a slightly elevated white blood cell (WBC) count and elevated erythrocyte sedimentation rate during the acute phase. A variety of radiologic findings may be seen.

Pathology

The histopathology of CSD lymph node lesions is not specific. Lymph nodes undergo three stages in the formation of a granuloma: (1) enlargement with hypertrophy of the germinal centers and thickening of the cortex, (2) formation of granulomas with invasion of lymphocytes and epithelioid cells, and (3) necrosis and infiltration with neutrophils; all of which may be simultaneously present within a single lymph node.[22] Abscess formation may occur.

In primary skin lesions, microscopic examination reveals acute necrosis of the epidermis and upper dermis, ranging from neutrophil and macrophage infiltration to granuloma formation. Organisms observed with Warthin-Starry staining can be solitary or in chains, clumps, or filaments and lie within the areas of necrosis.[28] Conjunctival lesions have similar histologic findings. In a few cases, conjunctival lesions produce proliferating blood vessels and a homogenous eosinophilic to basophilic granular appearance in the background—features similar to those of bacillary angiomatosis.[10]

Diagnosis/Differential Diagnosis

Historically, the diagnosis of CSD was met if three of the following four criteria were fulfilled: (1) a history of animal contact (usually a cat) with the presence of a scratch or primary dermal or ocular lesion, (2) a positive CSD skin test, (3) negative laboratory studies for other causes of lymphadenopathy, and (4) characteristic histopathology of a biopsied lymph node.[8]

CSD Skin Test

The CSD skin test has been the gold standard for diagnosing CSD for many years. It is prepared by aspirating the lymph node of a patient with CSD, heat-inactivating the pus for 3 successive days at 60°C (140°F) to destroy hepatitis B and HIV, diluting the material four- to fivefold with sterile saline, and freezing until use. The mixture is injected intradermally into the forearm of a patient with suspected disease; a raised dermal nodule 48 to 72 h later of over 5 mm is diagnostic. CSD skin tests are positive in 99 percent of immunocompetent patients.[22] Since *B. henselae* has now been identified as the causative agent of CSD, serologic titers, bacterial cultures, an intradermal test using purified *B. henselae* antigens, or PCR analyses will replace the previous clinical criteria.

The differential diagnosis of lymphadenopathy caused by CSD includes other conditions of unilateral or regional lymphadenopathy: other pyogenic infections, tularemia, atypical mycobacteria, and Hodgkin's disease. Rarely, lymphadenopathy may become generalized, and other infectious etiologies must be considered.

Treatment

Most cases of CSD remit spontaneously without therapeutic intervention. Treatment with antibiotics has given variable results. In a retrospective study of 202 patients with CSD treated with 18 different antibiotics, 14 commonly prescribed antibiotics including macrolides, tetracycline derivatives, and cephalosporins were ineffective.[36] However, antibiotic susceptibility studies have shown that *B. henselae* is highly sensitive to macrolides, tetracycline derivatives, and second and third generation cephalosporins, and is variably sensitive to quinolones.[37] The antibiotic susceptibility profiles are more in keeping with therapeutic regimens designed for BA, in which erythromycin, tetracycline, and doxycycline are commonly used. The failure of antibiotics in classic CSD in the immunocompetent host may relate to the small infectious burden and the frequent initiation of therapy once the disease is already improving spontaneously (in its lymphatic phase).

TRENCH FEVER

Bartonella quintana is the etiologic agent of trench fever, a disease that affected over 1 million troops of the German and Allied armies during World War I.[38] This disease is characterized by a fever lasting about a week, followed by recurrent fevers every 4 to 8 days, most commonly every 5 days, hence the name *quintana fever*.[38] Clinically, patients complained of severe headaches and neck, shin, and back pain.[39,40] There are no specific cutaneous manifestations. Although significant morbity is associated with the disease, no fatalities have been recorded. The disease is transmitted by the human body louse (*Pediculus humanus* var. *corporis*). Close body contact and unsanitary conditions have resulted in significant outbreaks. The incubation period ranges from 6 to 25 days, most commonly between 15 and 25 days. The organism has been isolated from patients with the disease and can be transmitted person to person by direct inoculation or through lice.[41] *B. quintana* organisms are found exclusively extracellularly in the louse and multiply within its gut.[42]

Recently, *B. quintana* has been isolated from the blood of patients in the United States and France.[43–45] Most of the patients were homeless alcoholic men, all of whom were HIV-negative. Endocarditis may occur. Moreover, in Seattle, a substantial proportion of the indigent alcoholic inner-city population has serologic evidence of infection with *B. quintana*.[46] Thus, although classical trench fever has presumably disappeared, epidemics of urban trench fever may arise.

Treatment

Treatment for trench fever has not been well established, since most cases were reported prior to the antibiotic era. In vitro antibiotic susceptibility studies show that *B. quintana* is susceptible to a number of agents, including most beta-lactams, aminoglycosides, macrolides, doxycycline, and rifampin. Oxacillin, cephalothin, quinolones, clindamycin, and vancomycin are less effective.[47,48] Several patients were cured using a regimen of ceftriaxone for 7 days followed by oral erythromycin or azithromycin for 3 weeks.[44]

BACILLARY ANGIOMATOSIS AND PELIOSIS

Bacillary angiomatosis (BA) was originally reported in 1983 by Stoler, who described a patient with AIDS and multiple angioproliferative nodules that resolved with erythromycin.[49] Histologic ex-

amination using Warthin-Starry staining revealed small bacillary forms that were confirmed by electron microscopy. In 1987, Cockerell et al. reported five additional cases of BA, two of whom died because of the disease.[50] In the following year, two groups reported similarities between the organisms seen in BA and CSD and proposed that they may be caused by the same bacteria.[11,12] In 1990, Perkocha et al. described eight patients with AIDS with bacillary peliosis hepatitis (BP), large, blood-filled cysts in the liver that contained clumps of bacteria identical to those seen in BA.[51] Patients may have both BA and BP simultaneously. Both *B. henselae* (the CSD bacillus) and *B. quintana* (the agent of trench fever) have been identified as causative agents of BA and BP.[52–57]

B. henselae causes both CSD and BA. At one end of the clinical spectrum, classic CSD is seen in young, immunocompetent hosts. At the other end, BA is seen in patients who are severely immunocompromised. Thus, it is the immunocompetence of the host and the bacterial load that dictates the clinical manifestation of the disease; immunocompetent hosts are able to mount a significant immune response and create a granulomatous response (CSD). Immunocompromised hosts are unable to control the infection and a systemic disease occurs. Moreover, immunocompromised patients with BA develop an angioproliferative response (BA, BP), a feature unique to *Bartonella* infections. Garcia et al. have detected a factor from *B. bacilliformis* that may be responsible for this angioproliferation.[58]

Epidemiology

Bacillary angiomatosis is most commonly seen in patients with advanced AIDS, with CD4 counts less than 50 cells/mm^3. Other immunosuppressed patients with BA, including leukemics, have been reported.[59,60] Several patients with BA who were HIV-negative and nonimmunosuppressed have been reported.[61,62] There is no risk factor predisposition in terms of race, sex, age, or HIV status. BA is not limited to adults.[59,63] A single patient who was pregnant and had AIDS has been reported.[64] Owning a cat and a history of a recent cat lick or trauma (scratch or bite) are significant risk factors for developing BA.[57] BA due to *B. henselae* is acquired from infected pet cats and is a manifestation of infection with the CSD bacillus in the immunocompromised host. Peliosis hepatitis is exclusively associated with *B. henselae*.[96] In contrast, patients with BA caused by *B. quintana* develop subcutaneous and lytic bone lesions, and are associated with low income, homelessness, and exposure to lice. *B. henselae* can adhere to and invade several human cell types, but the mechanisms of pathogenesis are poorly understood.[97]

Clinical Manifestations

The incubation period for BA is unknown but may be years. The clinical characteristics of BA in AIDS patients include fever, a low CD4 lymphocyte count (usually less than 50 cells/mm^3), cutaneous or subcutaneous vascular lesions, lymphadenopathy, and/or abdominal symptoms.[65]

The most common cutaneous morphologies of BA are (1) pyogenic granuloma (PG)-like lesions (Fig. 199-2) (2) subcutaneous nodules, and (3) hyperpigmented indurated plaques. The same patient may have several morphologies.[66] Lesions resembling those of PG can range in size from 1 mm to several centimeters and are dusky-red in color with a collarette of scale and peripheral satellite lesions; they are often indistinguishable from PG (Fig. 199-2). The lesions are firm, bleed easily, and are often tender. Subcutaneous nodules can range from distinct nodules to diffuse swellings

FIGURE 199-2

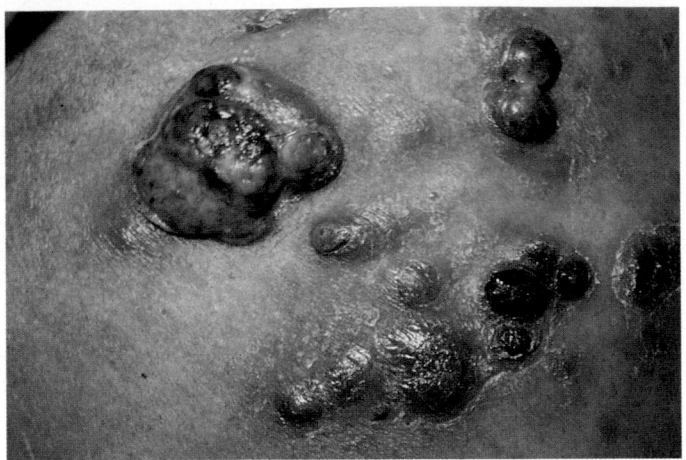

Bacillary angiomatosis. Multiple grouped dusky red and violaceous papules and nodules in a patient with BA.

with or without induration and are also often tender. Hyperpigmented plaques are most commonly seen on African Americans with BA and are oval in shape; they are several centimeters in diameter with indistinct borders. Large, fungating masses rarely occur.[67] Patients with BA may have solitary to thousands of lesions. Oral and other mucosal lesions occur.[68,69]

In addition to cutaneous lesions, BA can affect other organ systems. Hepatic (BP) and splenic lesions can occur concomitantly with or independently of cutaneous lesions.[51] BA can also affect bone and soft tissues.[54,70] Lesions of the central nervous system have been reported and can result in neurologic and psychiatric disorders.[71–73] Bacteremia, chronic fevers, and pulmonary and gastrointestinal lesions have also been reported as manifestations of BA.[74,75] Radiologic findings correlate with vascular lesions in the location of involvement.[76]

There have been several reports of patients with other cutaneous diseases concomitant with BA as well as the simultaneous existence of BA and another disease within the same lesion. Several patients have been reported with both BA and Kaposi's sarcoma (KS).[77] Cytomegalovirus, Epstein-Barr virus, *Cryptococcus neoformans*, and *Mycobacterium avium-intracellulare* have been found within lesions of BA.[78–82] This emphasizes the importance of looking for multiple pathologic infectious processes in patients with advanced HIV disease.

Laboratory Findings

In patients with AIDS and BA, the CD4 T helper cell count is $<200/m^3$ and usually $<50/mm^3$. Patients are anemic and may have elevated liver function tests (characteristically, LDH > alkaline phosphatase > hepatocellular enzymes). Blood cultures are positive for *Bartonella* species in about half of BA patients.[65]

Pathology

Lesions of BA have the general features of a lobular capillary hemangioma (PG) (Fig. 199-3A), but in contrast to a PG, the endothelial cells are often larger and polygonal; they may have marked atypia.[83] There is a prominent inflammatory infiltrate, with significant numbers of neutrophils as well as leukocytoclastic debris (Fig. 199-3B).

FIGURE 199-3

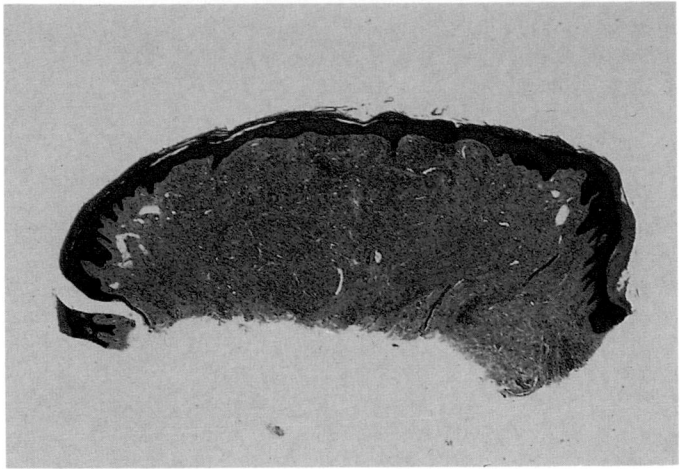

A.

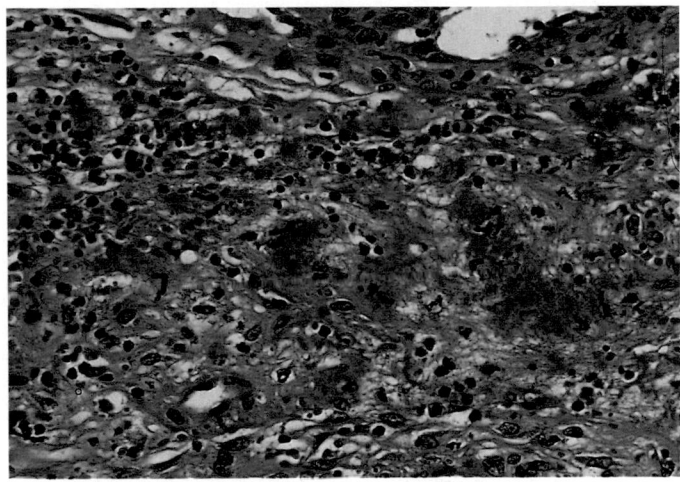

B.

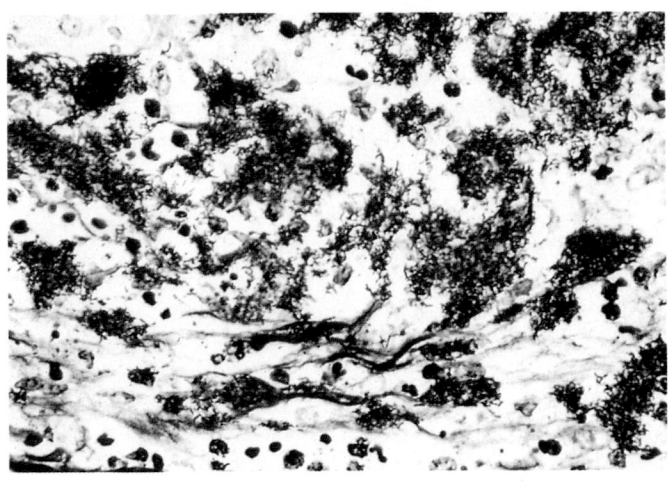

C.

Histology of bacillary angiomatosis. A. Low power magnification showing the architectural features of a lobular capillary hemangioma. B. High power magnification showing new capillary formation and endothelial cells with cytological atypia, a prominent inflammatory infiltrate, and leukocytoclastic debris. C. Warthin-Starry stain showing numerous pleimorphic bacteria. (*Courtesy of P. LeBoit, MD.*)

Polymorphonuclear leukocytes (PMNs) are scattered throughout the lesion, as opposed to classical PG lesions, in which the PMNs are at or near the surface, even if the PG is eroded and impetiginized. There is usually a finely granular pink to purple material in areas of PMN infiltration adjacent to blood vessels (Fig. 199-3*B*). This represents large clumps of bacteria, best visualized with a modified Warthin–Starry stain (Fig. 199-3*C*). A tissue gram stain and the Warthin–Starry stain used for syphilis will *not* stain the organisms. If the diagnosis cannot be confirmed with special stains, electron microscopy may be used. The lack of spindle cells, atypically shaped vascular channels, or hyaline globules distinguish BA from lesions of KS. Lesions of BA in tissues other than liver show similar histologic features.

Diagnosis/Differential Diagnosis

Since BA often resembles PG, solitary lesions must be differentiated from nodular KS and PG. Moreover, most patients with BA are HIV-infected, and ulcerative BA lesions have a broad differential diagnosis including pyoderma, atypical mycobacteria, *Acanthamoeba*, viral, and deep fungal infections. Clinically, widespread lesions may be indistinguishable from disseminated PG or verruga peruana, which can be excluded by travel history. Prior to the discovery of HIV, there were several cases of disseminated PG associated with immunodeficiency; these cases may have been BA.[84,85]

The diagnosis can usually be made histologically. *B. henselae* and *B. quintana* can be cultured from skin lesions and commonly from the blood of BA patients. The organisms grow slowly and may not be detected until prolonged culture (>1 month).[3]

Treatment

Erythromycin 500 mg four times a day or doxycycline 100 mg twice a day are the treatments of choice for BA. Other antibiotics felt to be effective include minocycline, tetracycline, chloramphenicol, azithromycin, and roxithromycin.[86,87] The treatment duration is unknown but should be at least 8 weeks and perhaps 6 months in an HIV-positive individual. Some patients require lifelong suppressive therapy. Relapses have been reported. A Jarisch-Herxheimer reaction not uncommonly occurs after initiation of therapy. Untreated BA is a fatal disease.[50] Most patients respond rapidly to antibiotic therapy.

OROYA FEVER AND VERRUGA PERUANA

Oroya fever (also known as Carrión's disease) and verruga peruana are endemic diseases localized to Peru and a few neighboring countries. The earliest recorded cases date back more than four centuries, and verruga peruana has been identified in a mummy from southern Peru.[88,89] The disease was named after Daniel Carrión, who, as a Peruvian medical student in 1885, inoculated himself with a lesion of verruga peruana and died of the acute phase of Oroya fever, showing that both diseases are caused by the same agent.[90] Oroya fever has a high rate of mortality; during the construction of the Central Railway in Peru in the early twentieth century, over 7000 workers died of the illness. The causative organism of these diseases is *B. bacilliformis*, which is transmitted by an arthropod vector.

Several sandfly vectors have been described, but the main vector is *Lutzomyia verrucarum townsend*.

Epidemiology

Oroya fever and verruga peruana are restricted to the South American Andes, from 5°5″latitude north to 13° south of the equator, including southern Colombia, part of Ecuador, and much of Peru. Most cases have been reported in regions of altitude ranging from 500 to 3200 m above sea level.[91] A recent epidemic of Oroya fever in the Peruvian Andes killed 14 persons and seriously affected 14 others in a small village of 353 people.[92] In this group, 71 percent of patients were male and ranged from 1 to 75 years of age. Humans are the only known reservoir for *B. bacilliformis*, although verruga peruana lesions have been found in dogs, cows, mules, and chickens and can be induced in rhesus monkeys.

Clinical Manifestations

After an incubation period between 1 to 4 weeks (average, 21 days), the acute stage develops, in which patients have severe fevers, headaches, and arthralgias. It is accompanied by a severe hemolytic anemia, in which red blood cell (RBC) counts can reach levels below 10^6/mm^3. Untreated, the mortality is 40 to 88 percent, often from *Salmonella* superinfection.[93] The acute phase is followed by a latency period that is highly variable, ranging from weeks to years. This is followed by the eruptive stage of verruga peruana, during which red angiomatous lesions, very similar to those of BA, develop (Fig. 199-4). Three patterns of cutaneous lesions have been described: miliary, nodular, and mular. In the miliary form, lesions are about 3 mm in diameter and localized mainly to the face and extremities, although they can be generalized. (Fig. 199-4). Mular lesions are larger and pedunculated with a superficial erosion, often disfiguring, and few in number. Nodular lesions are deeper, and may not have overlying erythema. Mucosal lesions may be seen.

Laboratory Findings

During the acute hemolytic phase, a profound anemia may be present. Using Giemsa staining, bacteria may be seen within or attached to 30 to 80 percent of the RBCs on a peripheral blood smear. It is this bacteria-erythrocyte association that is thought to induce hemolysis by the liver and spleen.

Pathology

Lesions of verruga peruana are histologically identical to those of bacillary angiomatosis, showing the distinct angioproliferative pattern. Organisms are stained by techniques similar to those used for BA and are also Giemsa positive. Light microscopy may reveal pink to purple cytoplasmic inclusion bodies within endothelial cells, called *Rocha-Lima bodies*. These correspond to intracellular organisms and extracellular matrix components when visualized with electron microscopy.[94]

Diagnosis/Differential Diagnosis

The differential diagnosis for verruga peruana is the same as that for BA, and includes BA, Kaposi's sarcoma, PG, and angiosarcoma.

FIGURE 199-4

CHAPTER 199
Bartonellosis
2255

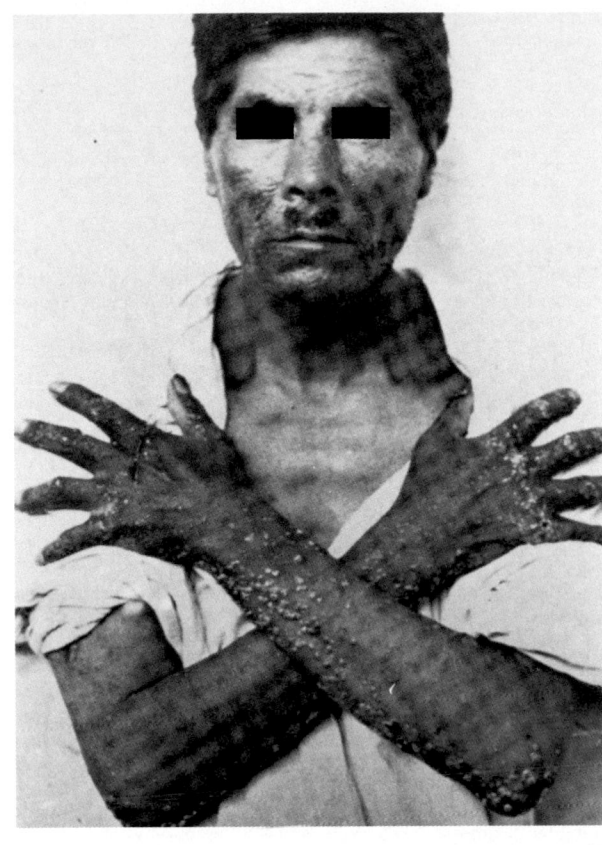

Bartonellosis (verruga peruana). Multiple small papules on the face and extremities. The lesions may ulcerate. (*Courtesy of O. Canizares, MD.*)

Treatment

If untreated, Oroya fever may be a fatal disease. Because of the frequent concomitant infection with *Salmonella*, the treatment of choice for Oroya fever and verruga peruana is chloramphenicol. Tetracycline is also effective.

REFERENCES

1. Myers WF et al: Role of erythrocytes and serum in the nutrition of *Rickettsia quintana. J Bacteriol* **97**:663, 1969
2. Myers WF et al: Nutritional studies of *Rickettsia quintana:* Nature of the hematin requirement. *J Bacteriol* **109**:89, 1972
3. Maurin M, Raoult D: *Bartonella* (*Rochalimaea*) *quintana* infections. *Clin Microbiol Rev* **9**:273, 1996
4. Brenner DJ et al: Proposals to unify the genera *Bartonella* and *Rochalimaea* with descriptions of *Bartonella quintana* comb. nov., *Bartonella vinsonii* comb. nov., *Bartonella henselae* comb. nov., and *Bartonella elizabethae* comb. nov., and to remove the family *Bartonellaceae* from the order *Rickettsiales. Int J Syst Bacteriol* **43**:777, 1993
5. Birtles RJ et al: Proposals to unify the genera *Grahamella* and *Bartonella*, with descriptions of *Bartonella talpae* comb. nov., *Bartonella peromysci* comb. nov., and three new species, *Bartonella grahamii* sp. nov., *Bartonella taylorii* sp. nov., and *Bartonella doshiae* sp. nov. *Int J Syst Bacteriol* **45**:1, 1995
6. Midani S et al: Cat-scratch disease. *Adv Pediatr* **43**:397, 1996
7. Debré R et al: La maladie des griffes de chat. *Bull Mem Soc Med Hôp Paris* **66**:76, 1950
8. Wear DJ et al: Cat scratch disease: A bacterial infection. *Science* **221**:1403, 1983
9. Margileth et al: Cat-scratch disease: Bacteria in skin at the primary inoculation site. *JAMA* **252**:928, 1984
10. Wear DJ et al: Cat scratch disease bacilli in the conjunctiva of patients with Parinaud's oculoglandular syndrome. *Ophthalmology* **92**:1282, 1985
11. LeBoit PE et al: Epithelioid haemangioma-like vascular proliferation in AIDS: Manifestation of cat scratch disease bacillus infection? *Lancet* **1**:960, 1988
12. Angritt P et al: Epithelioid angiomatosis in HIV infection: Neoplasm or cat-scratch disease? *Lancet* **1**:996, 1988
13. Dalton MJ et al: Use of *Bartonella* antigens for serologic diagnosis of cat-scratch disease at a national referral center. *Arch Intern Med* **155**:1670, 1995
14. Anderson B et al: Detection of *Rochalimaea henselae* DNA in specimens from cat scratch disease patients by PCR. *J Clin Microbiol* **32**:942, 1994
15. Anderson B et al: Detection of *Rochalimaea henselae* in cat-scratch disease skin test antigens. *J Infect Dis* **168**:1034, 1993
16. Bergmans AMC et al: Etiology of cat scratch disease: Comparison of polymerase chain reaction detection of *Bartonella* (formerly *Rochalimae*) and *Afipia felis* DNA with serology and skin tests. *J Infect Dis* **171**:916, 1995
17. Alkan S et al: Dual role for *Afipia felis* and *Rochalimaea henselae* in cat-scratch disease. *Lancet* **345**:385, 1995
18. English CK et al: Cat-scratch disease: Isolation and culture of the bacterial agent. *JAMA* **259**:1347, 1988
19. Brenner DJ et al: Proposal of *Afipia* gen. nov., with *Afipia felis* sp. nov. (formerly the cat scratch disease bacillus), *Afipia clevelandensis* sp. nov. (formerly the Cleveland Clinic Foundation strain), *Afipia broomeae* sp. nov., and three unnamed genospecies. *J Clin Microbiol* **29**:2450, 1991
20. Wise JK, Yang J-J: Veterinary service market for companion animals, 1992, part I: companion animal ownership and demographics. *JAVMA* **201**:990, 1992
21. Jackson L et al: Cat scratch disease in the United States: An analysis of three national databases. *Am J Public Health* **83**:1707, 1993
22. Carithers HA: Cat-scratch disease: An overview based on a study of 1200 patients. *Am J Dis Child* **139**:1124, 1985
23. Zangwill KM et al: Cat scratch disease in Connecticut: Epidemiology, risk factors, and evaluation of a new diagnostic test. *N Engl J Med* **329**:8, 1993
24. Warwick WJ: The cat-scratch syndrome: Many diseases or one disease? *Prog Med Virol* **9**:256, 1967
25. Chomel BB et al: *Bartonella henselae* prevalence in domestic cats in California: Risk factors and association between bacteremia and antibody titers. *J Clin Microbiol* **33**:2445, 1995
26. Jameson P et al: Prevalence of *Bartonella henselae* antibodies in pet cats throughout regions of North America. *J Infect Dis* **172**:1145, 1995
27. Chomel BB et al: Experimental transmission of *Bartonella henselae* by the cat flea. *J Clin Microbiol* **34**:1952, 1996
28. Margileth AM et al: Dermatologic manifestations and update of cat scratch disease. *Pediatr Dermatol* **5**:1, 1988
29. Carithers HA, Margileth AM: Cat-scratch disease: Acute encephalopathy and other neurologic manifestations. *Am J Dis Child* **145**:98, 1991
30. Haskes PJ et al: Systemic cat-scratch disease presenting as leukocytoclastic vasculitis. *Pediatr Infect Dis J* **15**:93, 1996
31. Hall AV et al: Cat-scratch disease in patient with AIDS: Atypical skin manifestation. *Lancet* **2**:453, 1988
32. Black JR et al: Life-threatening cat-scratch disease in an immunocompromised host. *Arch Intern Med* **146**:394, 1986
33. Schlossberg D et al: Culture-proved disseminated cat-scratch diseases in acquired immunodeficiency syndrome. *Arch Intern Med* **149**:1437, 1989
34. van der Wouw PA et al: Disseminated cat-scratch disease in a patient with AIDS. *AIDS* **3**:751, 1989
35. Pilon VA, Echols RM: Cat-scratch disease in a patient with AIDS. *Am J Clin Pathol* **92**:236, 1989
36. Margileth AM: Antibiotic therapy for cat-scratch disease: Clinical study of therapeutic outcome in 268 patients and a review of the literature. *Pediatr Infect Dis J* **11**:474, 1992
37. Dolan MJ et al: Syndrome of *Rochalimaea henselae* adenitis suggesting cat scratch disease. *Ann Intern Med* **118**:331, 1993
38. Maurin M, Raoult D: *Bartonella* (*Rochalimaea*) *quintana* infections. *Clin Microbiol Rev* **9**:273, 1996
39. McNee JW et al: "Trench fever": A relapsing fever occurring with the British forces in France. *Br Med J* **1**:225, 1916

40. Hurst A: Trench fever. *Br Med J* **2**:318, 1942
41. Vinson JW et al: Trench fever III: Induction of clinical disease in volunteers inoculated with *Rickettsia quintana* propagated on blood agar. *Am J Trop Med Hyg* **18**:713, 1969
42. Ito S, Vinson JW: Fine structure of *Rickettsia quintana* cultivated *in vitro* and in the louse. *J Bacteriol* **89**:481, 1965
43. Relman DA: Has trench fever returned? *N Engl J Med* **332**:463, 1995
44. Spach DH et al: *Bartonella* (*Rochalimaea*) quintana bacteremia in inner-city patients with chronic alcoholism. *N Engl J Med* **332**:424, 1995
45. Drancourt M et al: *Bartonella* (*Rochalimaea*) quintana endocarditis in three homeless men. *N Engl J Med* **332**:419, 1995
46. Jackson LA et al: Seroprevalence to *Bartonella quintana* among patients at a community clinic in downtown Seattle. *J Infect Dis* **173**:1023, 1996
47. Myers WF et al: Antibiotic susceptibility patterns in *Rochalimaea quintana*, the agent of trench fever. *Antimicrob Agents Chemother* **25**:690, 1984
48. Maurin M et al: MICs of 28 antibiotic compounds for 14 *Bartonella* (formerly *Rochalimaea*) isolates. *Antimicrob Agents Chemother* **39**:2387, 1995
49. Stoler MH et al: An atypical subcutaneous infection associated with acquired immune deficiency syndrome. *Am J Clin Pathol* **80**:714, 1983
50. Cockerell C et al: Epithelioid angiomatosis: A distinct vascular disorder in patients with the acquired immunodeficiency syndrome or AIDS-related complex. *Lancet* **2**:654, 1987
51. Perkocha LA et al: Clinical and pathological features of bacillary peliosis hepatitis in association with human immunodeficiency virus infection. *N Engl J Med* **323**:1581, 1990
52. Relman DA et al: The agent of bacillary angiomatosis: An approach to the identification of uncultured pathogens. *N Engl J Med* **323**:1573, 1990
53. Slater LN et al: A newly recognized fastidious gram-negative pathogen as a cause of fever and bacteremia. *N Engl J Med* **323**:1587, 1990
54. Koehler JE et al: Isolation of *Rochalimaea* species from cutaneous and osseous lesions of bacillary angiomatosis. *N Engl J Med* **327**:1625, 1992
55. Regnery RL et al: Characterization of a novel *Rochalimaea* species, *R. henselae* sp. nov., isolated from blood of a febrile, human immunodeficiency virus-positive patient. *J Clin Microbiol* **30**:265, 1992
56. Welch DF et al: *Rochalimaea henselae* sp. nov., a cause of septicemia, bacillary angiomatosis, and parenchymal bacillary peliosis. *J Clin Microbiol* **30**:274, 1992
57. Tappero JW et al: The epidemiology of bacillary angiomatosis and bacillary peliosis. *JAMA* **269**:770, 1993
58. Garcia FU et al: *Bartonella bacilliformis* stimulates endothelial cells *in vitro* and is angiogenic in vivo. *Am J Pathol* **136**:1125, 1990
59. Myers SA et al: Bacillary angiomatosis in a child undergoing chemotherapy. *J Pediatr* **121**:574, 1992
60. Milde P et al: Cutaneous bacillary angiomatosis in a patient with chronic lymphocytic leukemia. *Arch Dermatol* **131**:933, 1995
61. Cockerell CJ et al: Bacillary epithelioid angiomatosis occurring in an immunocompetent individual. *Arch Dermatol* **126**:787, 1990
62. Tappero JW et al: Bacillary angiomatosis and bacillary splenitis in immunocompetent adults. *Ann Intern Med* **118**:363, 1993
63. Malane MS et al: An HIV-1-positive child with fever and a scalp nodule. *Lancet* **346**:1466, 1995
64. Riley LE, Tuomala RE: Bacillary angiomatosis in a pregnant patient with acquired immunodeficiency syndrome. *Obstet Gynecol* **79**:818, 1992
65. Mohle-Boetani JC et al: Bacillary angiomatosis and bacillary peliosis in patients infected with human immunodeficiency virus: Clinical characteristics in a case-control study. *Clin Infect Dis* **22**:794, 1996
66. Webster GF et al: The clinical spectrum of bacillary angiomatosis. *Br J Dermatol* **126**:535, 1992
67. Fagan WA et al: Widespread cutaneous bacillary angiomatosis and a large fungating mass in an HIV-positive man. *J Am Acad Dermatol* **35**:286, 1996
68. Speight PM et al: Epithelioid angiomatosis affecting the oral cavity as a first sign of HIV infection. *Br Dent J* **171**:367, 1991
69. Glick M, Cleveland DB: Oral mucosal bacillary epithelioid angiomatosis in a patient with AIDS associated with rapid alveolar bone loss: Case report. *J Oral Pathol Med* **22**:235, 1993
70. Herts BR et al: Soft-tissue and osseous lesions caused by bacillary angiomatosis: Unusual manifestations of cat-scratch fever in patients with AIDS. *AJR* **157**:1249, 1991
71. Baker J et al: Bacillary angiomatosis: A treatable cause of acute psychiatric symptoms in human immunodeficiency virus infection. *J Clin Psychiatry* **56**:161, 1995
72. Spach DH et al: Intracerebral bacillary angiomatosis in a patient infected with human immunodeficiency virus. *Ann Intern Med* **116**:740, 1992
73. Harris PJ: Intracerebral bacillary angiomatosis in HIV. *Ann Intern Med* **117**:795, 1992
74. Koehler JE, Cederberg L: Intra-abdominal mass associated with gastrointestinal hemorrage: A new manifestation of bacillary angiomatosis. *Gastroenterology* **109**:2011, 1995
75. Slater LN, Min K-W: Polypoid endobronchial lesions: A manifestation of bacillary angiomatosis. *Chest* **102**:972, 1992
76. Moore EH et al: Bacillary angiomatosis in patients with AIDS: Multiorgan imaging findings. *Radiology* **197**:67, 1995
77. Berger TG et al: Bacillary (epithelioid) angiomatosis and concurrent Kaposi's sarcoma in acquired immunodeficiency syndrome. *Arch Dermatol* **125**:1543, 1989
78. Abrams J, Farhood AI: Infection-associated vascular lesions in acquired immunodeficiency syndrome patients. *Hum Pathol* **20**:1025, 1989
79. Guarner J, Unger ER: Association of Epstein-Barr virus in epithelioid angiomatosis of AIDS patients. *Am J Surg Pathol* **14**:956, 1990
80. Lopez-Elzaurdia C et al: Bacillary angiomatosis associated with cytomegalovirus infection in a patient with AIDS. *Br J Dermatol* **125**:175, 1991
81. Sagerman PM et al: Localization of *Mycobacterium avium-intracellulare* within a skin lesion of bacillary angiomatosis in a patient with AIDS. *Diagn Mol Pathol* **1**:212, 1992
82. LeBoit PE: Bacillary angiomatosis. *Mod Pathol* **8**:218, 1995
83. LeBoit PE et al: Bacillary angiomatosis: The histopathology and differential diagnosis of a pseudoneoplastic infection in patients with human immunodeficiency virus disease. *Am J Surg Pathol* **13**:909, 1989
84. Pembroke AC et al: Eruptive angiomata in malignant disease. *Clin Exp Dermatol* **3**:147, 1978
85. Zak FG et al: Viscero-cutaneous angiomatosis with dysproteinaemic phagocytosis: Its relation to Kaposi's sarcoma and lymphoproliferative disorders. *J Pathol Bacteriol* **92**:594, 1966
86. Adal KA et al: Cat scratch disease, bacillary angiomatosis, and other infections due to *Rochalimaea*. *N Engl J Med* **330**:1509, 1994
87. Cockerell CJ: Bacillary angiomatosis and related diseases caused by *Rochalimaea*. *J Am Acad Dermatol* **32**:783, 1995
88. Strong RP et al: Verruga peruviana, Oroya fever and uta: Preliminary report of the first expedition to South America from the Department of Tropical Medicine of Harvard University. *JAMA* **51**:1713, 1913
89. Allison MJ et al: A case of Carrión's disease associated with human sacrifice from the Huari culture of southern Peru. *Am J Phys Anthropol* **41**:295, 1974
90. Garcia-Caceres U, Garcia FU: Bartonellosis: An immunodepressive disease and the life of Daniel Alcides Carrión. *Am J Clin Pathol* **95**(suppl 1):S58, 1991
91. Caceres-Ríos H et al: Verruga peruana: An infectious endemic angiomatosis. *Crit Rev Oncog* **6**:47, 1995
92. Gray GC et al: An epidemic of Oroya fever in the Peruvian Andes. *Am J Trop Med Hyg* **42**:215, 1990
93. Cuadra M: Salmonellosis complication in human bartonellosis. *Tex Rep Biol Med* **14**:97, 1956
94. Arias-Stella J et al: Histology, immunohistochemistry, and ultrastructure of the verruga in Carrión's disease. *Am J Surg Pathol* **10**:595, 1986
95. Kordick DL et al: *Bartonella clarridgeiae,* a newly recognized zoonotic pathogen causing inoculation papules, fever, and lymphadenopathy (cat scratch disease). *J Clin Microbiol* **35**:1813, 1997
96. Koehler Je et al: Molecular epidemiology of *Bartonella* infections in patients with bacillary angiomatosis-peliosis. *N Engl J Med* **337**:1876, 1997
97. Murakawa GJ: Pathogenesis of *Bartonella henselae* in cutaneous and systemic disease. *J Am Acad Dermatol* **37**:775, 1997

CHAPTER 200

Arnold N. Weinberg
Morton N. Swartz

Miscellaneous Bacterial Infections with Cutaneous Manifestations

This chapter encompasses a group of "exotic" diseases rarely seen in urban practice in the United States. The thread of continuity that can be woven among this miscellaneous group involves epidemiologic considerations. The diagnosis can often be made expeditiously if the following are considered: (1) occupation and travel history; (2) the possibility of animal exposure; (3) the possibility of fresh, brackish, or saltwater immersion; and (4) the duration of the incubation periods. Many of the illnesses described in this chapter, e.g., anthrax and rat-bite fever, are systemic infections having a major cutaneous component that helps to suggest the proper diagnosis.

DISEASES RELATED TO INTIMATE CONTACT WITH ANIMALS, FISH, FOWL, OR THEIR PRODUCTS

Anthrax

The most common form of infection with *Bacillus anthracis* is an acute cutaneous lesion called "malignant pustule."[1] Anthrax is primarily a disease of domestic and wild animals, but humans become accidentally involved through exposure to animals and their products.

BACTERIOLOGY AND PATHOGENIC ASPECTS *Bacteriology* *B. anthracis* is a large, aerobic, encapsulated, gram-positive, square-ended rod that forms central spores in an unfriendly external environment and on culture but not in tissues. Growth occurs readily on blood agar medium without a hemolytic reaction. This characteristic, plus pathogenicity for mice and lack of motility, helps to distinguish this organism from saprophytic *Bacillus* species.

Pathogenic aspects *B. anthracis* has two principal virulence factors. The first is a D-glutamyl polypeptide capsule, the synthesis of which depends on the presence of a specific plasmid.[2] The second is a pair of toxins, designated *edema toxin* and *lethal toxin*. Each of the toxins consists of a pair of noncovalently linked protein components[3]: edema toxin consists of edema factor plus protective antigen (PA), the structural gene of the latter being carried on a second virulence-associated plasmid; lethal toxin consists of lethal factor plus PA. Of the three proteins involved in the two toxins, PA serves as the binding unit for entry of its partner into the cell by receptor-mediated endocytosis. As yet, a catalytic function is known for the toxic moiety of only one of the two toxins. Edema factor (EF) possesses adenylate cyclase activity which, on entry into

cells, is activated by calcium-dependent cellular calmodulin, and this results in conversion of ATP to cAMP.[4] The subsequent supraphysiologic cellular levels of cAMP mediate the toxic consequences of edema toxin. Cutaneous infection usually follows introduction of spores at the site of an abrasion. Following germination, the encapsulated organisms resist phagocytosis and elaborate their toxins. Edema toxin is responsible for the characteristic gelatinous edema of the local lesion. Lethal toxin itself kills several species of experimental animals and is presumed to be the principal cause of shock and death in disseminated anthrax.

Pasteur showed in 1881 that *B. anthracis* grown at elevated temperatures were attenuated and capable of inducing immunity in animals upon subsequent challenge with virulent strains of the organism. Such vaccine strains, avirulent by virtue of their inability to produce toxins, were shown over 100 years later to have become attenuated by virtue of temperature-induced elimination of the plasmid-encoding toxin genes.[2] However, the important protective immunogen is the anthrax toxin because vaccination with anthrax strains containing only the plasmid for capsule production, but lacking the one for toxin production, is not protective. Pasteur's vaccine was effective presumably because his attenuation procedure resulted in cultures with a relatively increased proportion of cells containing only the capsule plasmid and a *relatively decreased* proportion containing both plasmids.[5]

EPIDEMIOLOGY Natural infection occurs in many domestic and wild animals. Highly resistant spores persist for many years in cutaneous products of these animals and in pastures where they live. Vaccination and animal control programs have essentially eliminated reservoirs of infection in the United States, but imported animal products from the Middle and Near East, Africa, India, and South America introduce spores into a selected industrial environment. Worldwide there are estimated to be from 20,000 up to 100,000 cases of human anthrax annually. Outbreaks still occur in endemic areas. In 1979 to 1980, over 6000 cases of anthrax (90 percent involving the cutaneous form, the remainder representing equally pulmonary and gastrointestinal forms) occurred in Zimbabwe.[6] Direct cutaneous contact with carcasses of infected cattle was the major means of infection, but transmission by biting flies, which had earlier fed on carcasses of animals that had died of anthrax, was also likely. Infection in the United States is almost entirely limited to persons working in animal product–associated industries, particularly individuals handling raw materials in wool factories. However, transient exposure to infected animal products (e.g., hair) from abroad through ostensibly unrelated occupations (such as one-time air-conditioning duct repairs in a wool-sorting plant) has been incriminated in acquisition of anthrax. Shaving brushes, imported bongo drums, piano keys (ivory), and raw wool have been implicated in sporadic infections in persons not related to the above industries. In recent years, as regulations to safeguard employees in these plants have been strictly enforced, cases have become extremely rare. The use of protective vaccines, sophisticated ventilation systems, and steam sterilization of hides has drastically reduced cases from the animal product industry. Most often infection occurs on an exposed part (face, neck, or arms) in an area of previous scratch or abrasion, as the organisms cannot penetrate the intact epidermis. In addition to direct inoculation through abrasions, inhalation of spores may rarely result in sinus or pulmonary infection ("woolsorter's disease"). Ingestion of spores may rarely be followed by intestinal anthrax.

CLINICAL MANIFESTATIONS *History* The patient is almost invariably employed in an animal product industry, usually handling wool, goat and other animal hair, hides, bones, etc. The initial symptoms, following a 1- to 3-day incubation period, are usually low-grade fever and malaise. A painless papular lesion is usually noted on an exposed area. Itching or burning may accompany the early lesion; progressive edema, discoloration, and enlargement then occur, but the lesion and surrounding inflammatory edema remains painless. The initial symptoms of inhalation anthrax are insidious, with fever, fatigue, and malaise, but then progress rapidly to chills, high fever, nonproductive cough, dyspnea, cyanosis, and collapse. Chest radiographs characteristically show symmetric mediastinal widening. In this form of the disease, as well as in septicemic anthrax (following cutaneous or ingestion anthrax), meningitis may develop and dominate the clinical picture. Gastrointestinal anthrax following ingestion of contaminated meat is rare in humans and, thus far, has never been reported in the United States. Although vegetative bacteria are killed by acid gastric juice, the anthrax spores are resistant. An uncommon but related form (oropharyngeal) of anthrax also results from ingestion of raw or undercooked meat from infected animals. The epidemiology characteristically involves consumption of tainted meat; not surprisingly, there may be a cluster of cases in a family.[1]

Cutaneous lesion The cutaneous lesion ("malignant pustule") is the classic primary infection in anthrax, occurring in more than 95 percent of cases. It is most often located on an exposed area of the head, neck, or upper extremity (Fig. 200-1), beginning as a pimple or papule. The lesion enlarges and develops into a vesicle or bulla with surrounding brawny, gelatinous, nonpitting edema. During its evolution, the vesicle becomes hemorrhagic and then necrotic and may be surrounded by small satellite vesicles. The area of nonpitting edema increases, an eschar forms, and the red discoloration becomes more intense, *but without pain*. Rarely, the area of necrosis extends over most of the edematous region, or edema may be present without any detectable primary lesion or necrosis. Regional lymph nodes may be slightly enlarged and tender, but there is no lymphangitis.

Other physical findings Systemic manifestations (high fever, tachycardia, hypotension) may accompany either extensive cutaneous involvement or dissemination from a skin site. In woolsorter's disease, tachypnea, stridor, and cyanosis may be prominent. A thick, gelatinous, hemorrhagic nasal discharge may accompany acute sinusitis due to *B. anthracis*.

LABORATORY FINDINGS The white blood cell count is usually elevated, with a preponderance of polymorphonuclear leukocytes.

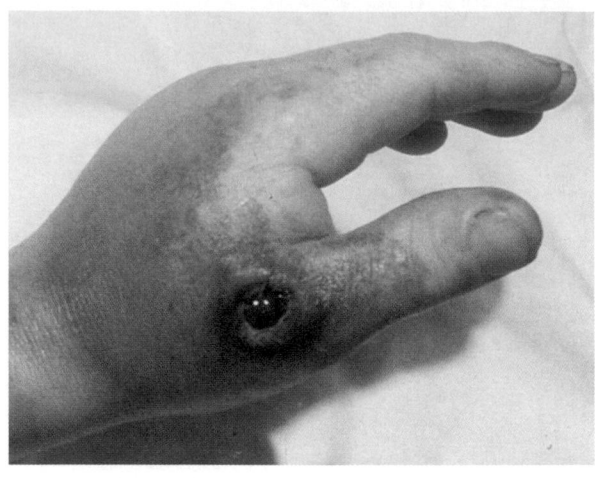

Anthrax. The classic cutaneous lesion of a primary infection in anthrax is a painless papule that evolves into a hemorrhagic bulla with surrounding brawny nonpitting edema. Note typical localization on the hand.

If meningitis is present, the cerebrospinal fluid is characteristically hemorrhagic and gram-positive bacilli may be seen. In inhalation anthrax, the chest x-ray shows significant mediastinal widening and hilar adenopathy due to edema and hemorrhagic necrosis of draining nodes. The pulmonary parenchyma is usually spared.

PATHOLOGY The prominent features are hemorrhagic edema, dilatation of lymphatics, and necrosis of the epidermis in the area of the eschar. Bacteria may be seen in the area of cellulitis.

DIAGNOSIS AND DIFFERENTIAL DIAGNOSIS The diagnosis is usually suspected on the basis of the character of the lesion and the hobby exposure or occupational history. Demonstration of large gram-positive rods in vesicle fluid or upon aspiration beneath the eschar supports the diagnosis. Definitive diagnosis requires culture of the organism and demonstration of its susceptibility to specific bacteriophage lysis. Identification of organisms in smears of exudate or in tissue specimens is possible utilizing a direct fluorescent antibody technique. Occasionally, the organism can be isolated from the blood during the acute cutaneous illness as well as in disseminated anthrax. Retrospective serodiagnosis is possible with the demonstration of a titer rise in an indirect microhemagglutination test. Recently, electrophoretic-immunotransblots for detection of antibody to PA and enzyme-linked immunosorbent assay (ELISA) for detection of anticapsule antibodies have been shown to be helpful in the retrospective diagnosis of anthrax. An anthraxin skin test (that detects cell-mediated immunity) has recently been developed. Results are impressive for its usefulness in early diagnosis (3 days of acute illness) and for identifying cases retrospectively, years after recovery.[7]

Acute staphylococcal cellulitis with a central pustular lesion or a carbuncle with necrotic eschar may be confused with early anthrax. Pyogenic staphylococcal lesions with accompanying gross inflammatory edema are usually very painful and tender, and the etiologic agent is usually present on Gram-stain examination.

TREATMENT Parenteral crystalline penicillin G (2 million units every 6 h) is the treatment of choice. In one study, smears and cultures from vesicles or from the necrotic tissue beneath the eschar became negative within 6 h of initiation of penicillin therapy.[8] For systemic infection (inhalation, gastrointestinal, meningeal), higher doses of penicillin (2 million units every 2 h for the adult) are indicated.

Treatment of cutaneous anthrax should continue until the local edema has disappeared or the lesion has dried up, i.e., for 7 to 14 days. When the edema has almost completely resolved, penicillin therapy may be switched to the oral route to complete the treatment course. In the penicillin-allergic individual, ciprofloxacin, doxycycline, erythromycin, or chloramphenicol are alternatives.[1]

Incision and debridement of the cutaneous lesion should be avoided as this increases the opportunity for bacteremia. The disease does not appear to impart permanent immunity.

Two types of vaccine are available for immunization against anthrax.[5] The first vaccine is licensed for human use in the United States to protect workers in occupations that might expose them to *B. anthracis*. It is supplied by the Michigan Department of Public Health and is an aluminum hydroxide–adsorbed culture supernatant (consisting primarily of PA in a partially purified form) from a nonencapsulated, toxigenic strain. The second vaccine is for immunization of livestock against anthrax and consists of viable spores of an attenuated nonencapsulated, toxigenic strain. A human live anthrax spore vaccine, administered by scarification, by subcutaneous injection, or by aerosol exposure, has been developed in the former Soviet Union.[9]

COURSE AND PROGNOSIS Rapid defervescence and clinical improvement follow the institution of appropriate antibiotic therapy. In pulmonary, intestinal, septicemic, and meningeal anthrax the prognosis is exceedingly grave, even if the disease is recognized promptly.

Brucellosis

Brucellosis is an acute or chronic infection (due to any one of four species of the genus *Brucella*) transmitted to humans from contact with animals or animal products. Such infections may be acute with bacteremia, or chronic with a variety of symptoms and signs.

BACTERIOLOGY AND PATHOGENIC ASPECTS *Bacteriology* The brucellae are nonmotile, coccobacillary gram-negative rods that require enriched media and an atmosphere containing 8 to 10% CO_2 for optimal growth.

Pathogenic aspects Contact with infected animals or contaminated excretions allows organisms to enter through small skin abrasions. Another portal for these organisms is ingestion of contaminated unpasteurized milk or cheese. Inhalation of droplets occurs among abattoir workers employed in or near the killing rooms in the meat industry. The organisms can multiply intracellularly in a variety of tissues and produce acute symptoms. They may persist within cells for prolonged periods, leading to chronic brucellosis. The effects of endotoxin as well as hypersensitivity to brucella antigens appear to contribute to the clinical manifestations.

EPIDEMIOLOGY Domestic animals are the reservoir of brucella; humans are infected primarily by direct contact with animal material or by ingestion of raw milk or unpasteurized cheese. The majority of patients (75 percent) are males employed as abattoir workers in the meat-packing industry, engaged in livestock raising, or are veterinarians. In the past, most infections in the United States were due to *B. abortus* secondary to contact with infected cattle. More recently, 70 percent of blood culture isolates from meat-processing-plant employees with brucellosis have been *B. suis*.[10]

Another important group of patients with brucella infection are travellers who have become infected in endemic areas (countries of the Mediterranean littoral, the Middle East, Mexico) through ingestion of unpasteurized cow's or goat's milk or cheese. Unpasteurized cheese sent from abroad to friends or relatives in the United States may also be a source of infection. In recent years a brucella species, *B. canis*, that produces abortion or prostatitis and epididymitis in dogs has been recognized as a cause of infection in individuals (pet owners, veterinarians) in contact with infected canines.

CLINICAL MANIFESTATIONS *History* In the majority of cases, contact with animals or their products is an essential feature of the history. The incubation period is usually 1 to 3 weeks, followed either by an acute febrile illness with headache (sometimes with involvement of local areas such as liver, joints, or meninges) or an indolent disease with weakness, anorexia, and low-grade fever, which may persist for weeks or months. Brucella involvement of the spine in the form of vertebral body osteomyelitis is not infrequent. Rarer forms of infection include suppurative lymphadenitis and endocarditis.[10] Unlike adults, who often have abdominal pain, children frequently exhibit skin rashes, pharyngitis, and enlarged nodes.[11] Relapses occur in approximately 15 percent of patients. They are often associated with less effective antibiotics, positive blood cultures, and treatment begun too early to allow cell-mediated immunity to develop.[12]

Cutaneous lesions Characteristic cutaneous lesions have been described, especially in children, usually associated with bacteremic disease, including during relapse. The most frequently observed rash is a violet, erythematous, papulonodular eruption that is located primarily on the trunk and lower extremities. Other lesions have included erythema nodosum, purpura, and macular and papular eruptions, some extending into subcutaneous fat and producing a panniculitis. Histology may show dermal perivascular infiltration with histiocytes and lymphocytes arranged into pseudogranulomas. Skin cultures may be positive.[13] Burning, itching, and desquamation have also been described following contact with infected animal products.[14] Rarely, subcutaneous abscesses or cutaneous sinus tracts may develop as a result of extension of suppuration from infected lymph nodes or sites of osteomyelitis, or following introduction of organisms through a skin abrasion. A severe hypersensitivity reaction to brucella antigen may occur among veterinarians and animal handlers exposed directly to infected material. This may be manifested by an acute febrile reaction and the appearance of discrete, elevated, red papules on the hands or arms that may progress to ulceration. Dramatic reactions of this type have occurred in veterinarians who have accidentally inoculated themselves with the attenuated strain of brucella used to immunize farm animals.[15]

Other physical findings Among the characteristic findings may be lymphadenopathy, hepatosplenomegaly, suppurative arthritis, and evidence of osteomyelitis or spondylitis.

LABORATORY FINDINGS The white blood cell count is usually normal or depressed, and anemia is frequently present. Blood cultures may be positive during the acute illness.

PATHOLOGY Lesions in the liver, spleen, and other organs frequently consist of small, noncaseating granulomas. Rarely, larger areas with caseation necrosis and calcification occur in infections due to *B. suis*.

DIAGNOSIS AND DIFFERENTIAL DIAGNOSIS The diagnosis of brucellosis is usually based upon epidemiologic information (animal contact), cultures (blood, bone marrow, organ granulomas), and *rising* serum agglutination titer. A titer of greater than 1:160 should raise the possibility of this disease and warrant repetition of the test 7 to 14 days later. *B. canis* will not be detected by the routine agglutination test for *Brucella* spp. since it lacks smooth lipopolysaccharide. The presence of a prozone phenomenon and the development of "blocking antibody" may occasionally require modifications in the performance of the agglutination test. The antibody response to brucella infection is initially that of IgM followed by IgG antibodies. The IgM response may last for many months up to several years, but the IgG antibodies decrease rapidly following antimicrobial therapy. In patients with chronic symptomatology, the presence of IgG antibodies indicates continuing or recrudescent active infection.[10] Recently, use of IgM and IgG ELISA has suggested that they are very sensitive methods for detecting antibody to *Brucella* and that a secondary increase in IgG, but not IgM, ELISA occurs in patients undergoing clinical relapse.[16] Skin testing with brucella antigen may lead to falsely positive serologic values and should not be performed. Cross-reactions with *Francisella tularensis* occur uncommonly, and vaccination within the year for cholera may stimulate a brucella agglutinin titer.

The differential diagnosis includes other acute bacterial infections such as salmonellosis, listeriosis, tuberculosis, and endocarditis. Hodgkin's disease may mimic many of the findings of brucellosis. Vertebral osteomyelitis may sometimes be the primary or sole manifestation of brucellosis. Occasionally, a prolonged low-grade form of this illness is mistakenly considered as a psychoneurosis.

TREATMENT   Use of antimicrobials that penetrate into cells and treatment prolonged for 6 weeks constitute optimum therapy. A number of equally effective programs, utilizing two drugs, can be recommended. The "gold standard" has consisted of doxycycline and either streptomycin or gentamicin. Equally effective results have been recorded with the combination of doxycycline and rifampin. Trimethoprim plus sulfamethoxazole (TMS) and fluoroquinolones have been useful alternatives, but unacceptable resistance can develop when they are used as monotherapy.[10]

COURSE AND PROGNOSIS   Early treatment results in rapid improvement. Brucellosis relapses in approximately 10 to 15 percent of patients who are treated suboptimally.[12] Chronicity, often in the form of osteomyelitis or joint infection, may lead to more permanent disability.

Erysipeloid

Erysipeloid is an acute infection of traumatized skin caused by a slender, gram-positive rod, *Erysipelothrix rhusiopathiae*, occurring most frequently in fishermen, butchers, and others, such as housewives, handling raw fish, poultry, and meat products.[17]

BACTERIOLOGY   *E. rhusiopathiae* is a thin, gram-positive, straight to slightly curved bacillus that tends to form filaments or "V" configurations in culture. Growth occurs best on media fortified with serum at temperatures between 30 and 37°C and in an atmosphere of 5 to 10% CO_2. The bacillus is microaerophilic and nonmotile and is hardy enough to survive drying, putrefaction of tissue, and saltwater or freshwater exposure.[17] There are certain morphologic and cultural similarities between *E. rhusiopathiae* and *Listeria monocytogenes*.

EPIDEMIOLOGY   *E. rhusiopathiae* is the cause of a cutaneous and systemic infection of swine. It is present as a reservoir in rats and birds and in the slime of saltwater fish, on crabs and other shellfish, or associated with poultry (especially turkeys), meats, and by-products such as hides and bones. Occurrence of the disease is limited almost exclusively to persons handling contaminated products. Most cases occur during summer months. Usually the organisms are inoculated through a break in the skin of the hands. There have been epidemics among crab fishermen (*crab dermatitis*) and bone button makers. Human infection takes one of four clinical forms: (1) localized cutaneous infection (*erysipeloid of Rosenbach*); (2) diffuse cutaneous form, consisting of multiple serpiginous lesions with sharply defined borders; (3) subacute bacterial endocarditis; and (4) bacteremic form without endocarditis, usually in immunocompromised patients.[18] The disease does not seem to confer lasting immunity. A complete discussion and exhaustive reference to the epidemiology are included in a review.[17]

CLINICAL MANIFESTATIONS   *History*   Usually the patient is employed in fishing or animal product industries. Initially, there is burning pain at a site of injury. The incubation period is 2 to 7 days. A violaceous, raised area appears and enlarges. Lymphangitis and regional lymphadenopathy occasionally occur. Constitutional symptoms include low-grade fever and malaise. Occasionally, an adjacent joint is involved. Rarely, bacteremia and even endocarditis may follow.[19]

Cutaneous lesion   The distinctive "erysipeloid" lesion is usually on a finger or hand, is violet or purple-red in color, warm and tender, and has well-defined, raised margins (Fig. 200-2). As the cellulitis advances peripherally, the central region clears without desquamation or ulceration.[20] The lesion may enlarge considerably. Rarely, dissemination occurs with multiple lesions distant from the original site of injury. Brownish discoloration develops as the lesion resolves.[21]

Other physical findings   Arthritis may be associated with the local lesion, and, rarely, distant joints are involved. Bronchitis may follow inhalation of organisms. Conjunctivitis also occurs. Typical peripheral stigmata as well as cardiac findings of endocarditis or septicemia have been reported, including prosthetic valve involvement.[17,19,22]

LABORATORY FINDINGS   There are no characteristic findings, and the organism is seldom seen on Gram's stain of material from the surface of the lesion or from aspirated material. Culture of a biopsy from the advancing edge of the lesion may reveal the organism.

PATHOLOGY   Dilatation of vessels in the papillary and subpapillary areas and perivascular cellular infiltrates deep in the dermis are present. The depth of the process may explain why organisms are rarely seen or cultured from the lesion.

DIAGNOSIS AND DIFFERENTIAL DIAGNOSIS   The character of the local lesion in a person handling fresh meat or fish products suggests the diagnosis. Other forms of bacterial cellulitis or erysipelas may be confused with erysipeloid. There should be little confusion with typical lesions of erysipelas due to *Streptococcus pyogenes*. The lesion of the latter is very superficial with a raised border, there is only moderate pain, and the central area remains the most affected region compared to central clearing in erysipeloid. "Seal finger" may be mistaken for erysipeloid, but there is a history of a recent seal bite. In addition to cultures, the diagnosis can be confirmed utilizing agar-gel diffusion precipitation or fluorescent antibody.[17]

FIGURE 200-2

CHAPTER 200
Miscellaneous Bacterial Infections

2261

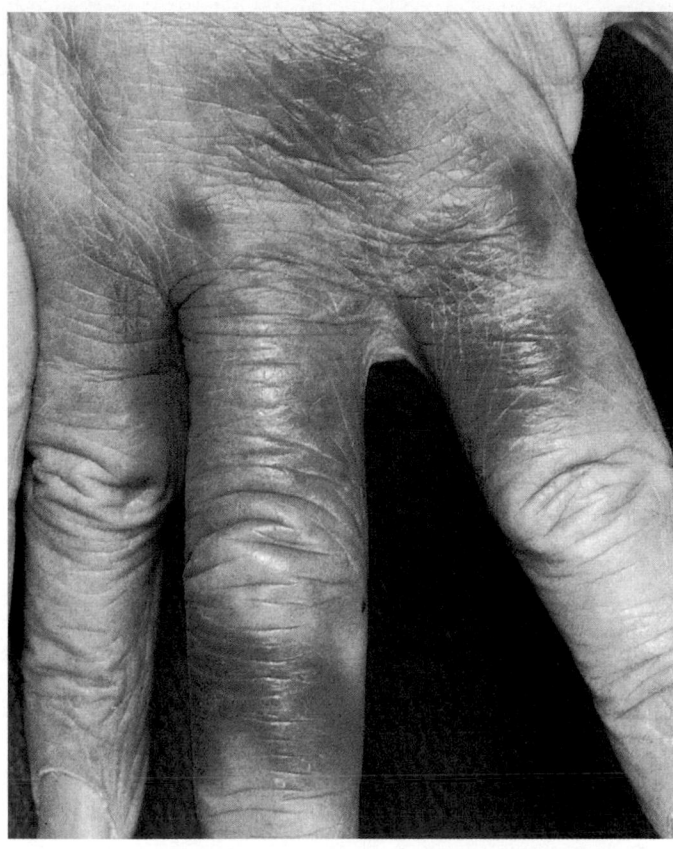

Erysipeloid. Characteristically, the violaceous sharply marginated lesion is composed of macules and plaques and is localized on the hand.

TREATMENT Penicillin, in doses of 2 to 3 million units daily, orally or intramuscularly, for 7 to 10 days, is the treatment for erysipeloid. In the penicillin-allergic patient who has not had a major immediate-type reaction (anaphylaxis, angioedema), a third-generation cephalosporin, imipenem, or ciprofloxacin can be given. This recommendation is based primarily on in vitro studies, not clinical experience.[23] If arthritis, septicemia, or endocarditis is present, the dose of penicillin should be raised to 2 to 4 million units every 4 h, administered intravenously (for 4 weeks in the case of endocarditis). Vancomycin should not be used because most isolates are resistant.

COURSE AND PROGNOSIS In the untreated patient, the lesion usually lasts for 2 to 3 weeks but may persist, with cycles of improvement and worsening over several months. If penicillin is administered, the improvement is dramatic and recurrence is rare. In systemic infection, the course and prognosis depend on early and appropriate treatment.

Glanders

Glanders is an equine disease caused by the bacterium *Burkholderia mallei* (formerly *Pseudomonas mallei*). This infection is rarely transmitted to humans. The clinical picture takes one of two forms: (1) an acute, febrile, disseminated, infectious process whose entire course may encompass only 10 to 30 days; (2) an indolent, relapsing, chronic infection, with multiple cutaneous and subcutaneous abscesses and draining sinuses. "Farcy," the name given to the dis-

ease in horses, refers to the nodular subcutaneous abscesses occurring along the course of lymphatics.

Control measures have almost completely eradicated this previously common equine infection and essentially eliminated transmission to humans in the United States. Occasional cases still occur in Asia, Africa, and South America. Humans are infected by direct contact with horses.

In acute glanders, a nodule or cellulitis appears at the site of inoculation. Local swelling and suppuration occur, and the lesion ulcerates. The ulcer is painful and has irregular edges with a gray-yellow base. Nodular sores rapidly develop along lymphatics draining the lesion; they become necrotic and ulcerated, and sinuses form. Regional lymphadenopathy is present. Widespread dissemination quickly follows, with multiple nodular necrotic abscesses in subcutaneous tissues and muscle. Lesions frequently coalesce into gangrenous areas. During this phase of bacteremic spread, a characteristic eruption appears, which may be generalized or localized to the face and neck. The lesions (papules, bullae, and pustules) appear in crops. Involvement of the nasal mucosa, either initially or by secondary spread, is prominent. Mucopurulent, bloody nasal discharge is commonly noted. Infection may spread to the paranasal sinuses, pharynx, and lung.

In chronic glanders, cutaneous and subcutaneous nodules appear on the extremities and occasionally on the face. The lesions ulcerate, and draining sinuses develop.

The pathologic picture is that of a suppurative, necrotic process, containing numerous intracellular and extracellular bacteria. In the chronic form of glanders, a granulomatous process (with few giant cells) suggesting tuberculosis is usually observed.

The diagnosis is made on the basis of the epidemiologic background, examination of Gram-stained smears of pus, and isolation of the organism from abscesses or blood. Acute glanders may resemble miliary tuberculosis or typhoid fever during the initial stages. The multiple subcutaneous abscesses suggest staphylococcal or mycotic infections or melioidosis. Lymphatic nodularity resembles the lesions of *Mycobacterium marinum*, *Sporothrix schenckii*, and *Francisella tularensis*.

There is no modern collected or controlled experience using contemporary antimicrobial agents for treatment of glanders. Historically, sulfadiazine (100 mg/kg daily in three to four divided doses) has been used successfully in laboratory-acquired and natural infections. The combination of trimethoprim-sulfamethoxazole (TMP-SMX) and ceftazidine, an effective regimen for melioidosis, would be a reasonable choice of agents if faced with a severely ill patient.

Streptobacillus moniliformis Infection ("Rat-Bite Fever")

Rat-bite fever is an acute infection that is usually acquired from rodents and is characterized by fever, polyarthralgias or arthritis, and a rash.[24]

BACTERIOLOGY *S. moniliformis* is a gram-negative, pleomorphic bacillus. Growth in culture occurs as chains of bacilli and filamentous forms, interspersed with swollen bodies that look like *Candida* (*Monilia*), hence the name *moniliformis*. In blood cultures these microaerophilic organisms typically grow as small "puff balls" after prolonged incubation. On occasion, growth may occur as an L form on initial culture.

EPIDEMIOLOGY *S. moniliformis* is found in the nasopharynx of approximately 50 percent of wild and laboratory rats. In recent years, the latter have been an increasing source of infection.[25] Sporadic cases without contact with rats have been reported. Infection may also occur following ingestion of contaminated food. One such milk-borne outbreak occurred in Haverhill, Massachusetts, in 1926, and this illness was designated "Haverhill fever" (erythema arthriticum epidemicum).[26]

CLINICAL MANIFESTATIONS *History* The incubation period averages 1 to 5 days. The rat bite has often healed by the time the illness begins suddenly with fever, chills, headache, and myalgias.

Cutaneous lesions An erythematous macular or papular rash may develop within 2 to 3 days of the onset of symptoms. It is most marked on the extremities (often involving palms and soles), particularly about joints, but may become generalized, resembling measles. Sometimes the lesions are petechial.

Other physical findings Within a week of onset arthritis can develop, involving larger joints such as the knee. This occurs in about half the patients and takes the form of either an asymmetric polyarthritis, resembling rheumatoid arthritis,[27] or a septic arthritis.[28] Regional lymphadenopathy may be present.

LABORATORY FINDINGS Polymorphonuclear leukocytosis is common. *S. moniliformis* can usually be isolated from blood or joint fluid or sometimes from an abscess developing at the bite site. Serologic diagnosis involves use of agglutination, fluorescent antibody, or complement fixation tests.

DIAGNOSIS AND DIFFERENTIAL DIAGNOSIS The skin lesions are not specific. The diagnosis should be suspected in any febrile patient with a history of a recent wild rat bite or exposure to laboratory rats or mice. Blood cultures are the best way to establish the diagnosis. The other form of rat-bite fever (*Spirillum minus*) (sodoku) may cause a similar illness, but several features are helpful in distinguishing between the two conditions[24]:

1. *S. moniliformis* infection has a shorter incubation period (usually less than 10 days).
2. The bite site has usually healed by the time of onset of fever in *S. moniliformis* infection.
3. The incidence of arthritis is low in *S. minus* infection.

The differential diagnosis should also include meningococcemia, gonococcemia, viral exanthems, and Rocky Mountain spotted fever.

TREATMENT Penicillin, 600,000 units intramuscularly every 6 h for 10 to 12 days, is the drug of choice. Doxycycline, erythromycin, or clindamycin are alternatives in the penicillin-allergic patient.

COURSE AND PROGNOSIS Untreated, the disease may last from a few days to several weeks. Rarely, it is complicated by endocarditis. Penicillin produces a prompt clinical response and is often begun immediately in individuals suffering rat or mouse bites. This action and the knowledge that rat-bite fever is not a reportable disease probably means that it is underdiagnosed.

Infections due to *Streptococcus iniae*

S. iniae is a recently recognized fish pathogen that causes cellulitis and invasive infections in individuals handling fish from aquaculture farms.[29]

BACTERIOLOGY *S. iniae* is a beta-hemolytic, nongroupable, streptococcus capable of growth at 10°C (but not at 45°C); most isolates do not grow in 6.5% sodium chloride. It is vancomycin-susceptible and positive on CAMP test. Automated culture systems may not include *S. iniae* in their data bases and report such isolates as *S. uberis* or "unidentified."

EPIDEMIOLOGY *S. iniae* infection occurs in the setting of percutaneous injury while handling fresh aquacultured fish, particularly tilapia (Hawaiian sunfish). *S. iniae* colonizes the surface of aquacultured fish and can cause epizootic meningocephalitis in cultured-fish ponds.

CLINICAL MANIFESTATIONS *History* Cellulitis is initiated by a skin puncture wound (fish bone, fin, or knife for cleaning) while preparing fresh fish from aquaculture ponds. Most reported cases have been in individuals of Asian origin, perhaps related to the volume of tilapia consumed by this population and by the manner in which their fish are prepared (kept at 4°C with fins and scales removed at home).[29]

Cutaneous lesions Characteristically, cellulitis involves the hand and develops within 16 to 24 h after injury. Neither skin necrosis nor bullae occurs, but lymphangitis extending from the site of injury and fever are early features.

Other physical findings Bacteremia is frequent with *S. iniae* cellulitis. Metastatic infections may occur in the form of septic arthritis, meningitis, and endocarditis.[29]

LABORATORY FINDINGS Leukocytosis is usually present (13,000 to 33,000 per mm^3), with neutrophils predominating.

DIAGNOSIS AND DIFFERENTIAL DIAGNOSIS Diagnosis is made on the basis of the setting, clinical findings, and cultures of blood or wound exudate. The common causes of cellulitis (*S. pyogenes*, *Staphylococcus aureus*) as well as other freshwater and fish-borne pathogens (*Aeromonas hydrophila*) should be considered in the differential diagnosis.

TREATMENT *S. iniae* is susceptible to penicillin, cefazolin, ceftriaxone, erythromycin, clindamycin, and TMP-SMX.

COURSE AND PROGNOSIS With prompt initiation of an appropriate antibiotic, the infection responds within 2 to 4 days. Treatment is continued for 10 days for the cellulitis/bacteremia, but longer if extracutaneous complications are present.

DISEASES ASSOCIATED PRIMARILY WITH A SPECIFIC GEOGRAPHIC DISTRIBUTION

Melioidosis

Melioidosis is an infectious disease of animals and humans, endemic in Southeast Asia but also occurring in Africa, the Caribbean, South America, and the Middle East, between 20° north and south latitudes, and caused by the gram-negative bacillus *Burkholderia pseudomallei* (formerly *Pseudomonas pseudomallei*).[30] Apart from rare cases of laboratory-acquired infections, melioidosis has occurred in only those United States residents who have traveled abroad. During the war in Vietnam, extensive exposure to this organism resulted in cases of melioidosis (some fatal) among American servicemen. Melioidosis is very similar to glanders clinically and pathologically but is entirely different epidemiologically. The clinical manifestations of this disease take one of two principal forms: (1) acute melioidosis with suppurative skin infection, pneumonia, or septicemia; (2) chronic melioidosis, the most common form of the disease, which involves the lung (unresolved pneumonia or cavitary lesions), skin (subcutaneous abscesses and draining sinuses), bones, joints, liver, spleen, etc.

BACTERIOLOGY   The etiologic agent is a small, pleomorphic, gram-negative bacillus with bipolar staining that can be grown aerobically on common laboratory media. Colonies tend to wrinkle after a few days, and cultures give off a putrid, pungent odor.

EPIDEMIOLOGY   The etiologic agent of melioidosis can be isolated widely from soil, vegetables, and water in the rice-growing areas of Southeast Asia. Melioidosis appears to be transmitted by contamination of abraded skin with infected soil or water.[31] The prominence of pulmonary findings in many patients, and of diarrhea in some, has suggested the possibility that it may be transmitted by inhalation or ingestion. Person-to-person transmission of melioidosis is rare.[32]

CLINICAL MANIFESTATIONS *History*   The incubation period is variable. It has been as short as 3 days, and the disease has also remained latent for years. The acute pneumonic form may begin with a short prodrome (malaise, anorexia, and diarrhea), but more commonly its onset is abrupt, with chills, fever, cough, dyspnea, and chest pain. The acute septicemic form may start with an ulceration at the site of inoculation, lymphangitis, and regional lymphadenitis. In northeastern Thailand, septicemic melioidosis occurs mainly in the rainy season, primarily in rice farmers or their families. It accounts for about 20 percent of all cases of community-acquired septicemia in this region.[33] Predisposing factors are present in approximately 50 percent of patients and include diabetes mellitus and renal failure but also glucocorticoid therapy, leukemia, cirrhosis, and tuberculosis. In half the patients no source for the bacteremia can be identified on examination, but many have minor abrasions about the feet.[34] Chronic melioidosis may follow the acute disease. More often it develops as an indolent pulmonary infection or as a low-grade febrile illness with multiple superficial abscesses. Recrudescence of a previous latent or clinical infection months or years (as long as 26 years) after initial exposure to the organism may be precipitated by various illnesses (e.g., thermal burns, diabetic ketoacidosis, pneumonia).[35] Recrudescent illness may take the form of localized infections such as splenic abscess, liver abscess, osteomyelitis, septic arthritis, renal abscess, subcutaneous abscesses, or lung abscess, as well as septicemia.[31] It may also take the form of persistent, unexplained fever.[36]

Cutaneous lesions   Cutaneous manifestations are not a specific or diagnostic feature of melioidosis. The acute septicemic form may complicate a superficial ulceration and cellulitis. Multiple superficial pustules may be present or, rarely, ecthyma gangrenosum. In chronic melioidosis, subcutaneous abscesses and draining sinuses (from bone or lymph nodes) are common features and may occur even in the absence of fever.[31]

Other physical findings   In acute pulmonary melioidosis, the findings range from those of bronchitis to those of acute pneumonia or lung abscess. Septicemic spread of the disease leads to jaundice, hepatosplenomegaly, miliary pulmonary densities (secondary bacteremic pneumonia), myocarditis, and severe gastroenteritis. Chronic pulmonary melioidosis produces signs suggestive of fibrocavitary tuberculosis or lung abscess. The disseminated form of chronic disease may extend over many months with septic arthritis, osteomyelitis, suppurative lymphadenopathy, and visceral ab-

scesses. In Thailand, acute suppurative parotitis constitutes 40 percent of cases of localized melioidosis in children.[37]

LABORATORY FINDINGS   The peripheral white blood cell count is usually normal or only moderately elevated.

PATHOLOGY   Sharply circumscribed abscesses are found in many organs and in the subcutaneous tissues. There may be a surrounding granulomatous response.

DIAGNOSIS AND DIFFERENTIAL DIAGNOSIS   The various forms of melioidosis and the multiplicity of organs involved characterize this disease as a great imitator. Acute melioidosis may mimic typhoid fever, staphylococcal pneumonia, mycotic infections, or septicemia. In its chronic form, it must be differentiated from pulmonary tuberculosis, nocardiosis, fungal infections, and lung abscess. Chronic skin infections and draining sinuses in individuals from endemic areas should raise the possibility of melioidosis.

The diagnosis is suspected on epidemiologic grounds and on the finding of bipolar-stained gram-negative bacilli in exudates or pus. Culture of the organism establishes the etiology. Hemagglutination, direct agglutination, and complement-fixation tests are helpful when a rise in titer is demonstrated. A positive serologic test, in the absence of a rising titer, may suggest the diagnosis but it is not definitive. The indirect hemagglutination assay (IHA) is most commonly used in Southeast Asia because it is simple to perform and cheap. An IHA titer of $\geq 1:80$ is 80 to 90 percent sensitive and specific in the diagnosis of active melioidosis, but titers of $1:40$ to $1:160$ (or even above occasionally) are frequently found in healthy individuals in endemic areas.[31]

TREATMENT   Antibiotic susceptibility must be determined on each isolate because of variations from strain to strain. In the past, conventional treatment of melioidosis involved tetracycline (or doxycycline), chloramphenicol, and TMP-SMX (plus kanamycin occasionally) in combination. Due to the bacteriostatic nature of three of these drugs and due to the potentially serious toxicity of this polydrug regimen, other therapeutic programs have been sought. Most strains of *B. pseudomallei* are susceptible to some of the newer antibiotics in vitro: ceftazidime, piperacillin, imipenem, and amoxicillin-clavulanic acid. A recent multicenter clinical trial in Thailand, comparing ceftazidime with amoxicillin-clavulanate favored ceftazidime alone. While the combination of ceftazidime plus TMP-SMX was the therapy of choice as recently as the early 1990s, the emergence of a high percentage of isolates resistant to TMP-SMX has led to the new recommendation.[38]

Surgical drainage of abscesses should be carried out, but only after initiation of appropriate antimicrobial therapy, in order to avoid a sudden septicemic episode.

Antimicrobial treatment should be continued for from 6 to 20 weeks (the longer periods in the case of osteomyelitis or multiple suppurative foci). Following an initial period of intravenous therapy, amoxicillin-clavulanic acid is continued orally.

COURSE AND PROGNOSIS   The mortality rate in melioidosis depends on the clinical form of illness[38]: (1) in disseminated septicemic melioidosis (rapidly fatal bacteremia with shock and evidence of dissemination to skin and viscera), it is approximately 50 percent; (2) in nondisseminated septicemic melioidosis (fairly rapidly progressive bacteremia with only single organ involvement), it is 17 percent; and (3) in localized melioidosis (nonbacteremic slowly progressive focal infection), it is 9 percent.

Plague

Plague is a severe, acute, febrile infection in humans caused by *Yersinia pestis*. Transmission between the natural reservoir of this disease (wild and commensal rodents) and human beings is effected by fleas. Infection occurs in three forms: (1) bubonic plague; (2) bubonic-septicemic plague (a more acute and severe form of bubonic plague with bacteremia and delirium); and (3) pneumonic plague (fulminant form of infection resulting from respiratory spread of *Y. pestis*).[39]

BACTERIOLOGY *Y. pestis* is an aerobic gram-negative bacillus with "safety-pin" bipolar staining. Growth on routine media is not accompanied by motility and, as with other yersiniae and salmonellae, lactose is not fermented. It produces an intracellular toxin (plague toxin) that is plasmid-encoded and an important virulence factor.[40] Two other plasmids encode virulence factors. One plasmid mediates "the low calcium response," which occurs when *Y. pestis* is transferred from the lower temperature of the flea to the 37°C host whose intracellular (leukocytic) environment has a relatively low Ca^{2+} concentration, and which initiates selective synthesis of virulence factors.[41] The second plasmid encodes temperature-dependent coagulase and fibrinolysin activities, which also serve as virulence factors. Most strains produce an antiphagocytic capsule, and all have a potent cell envelope–associated lipopolysaccharide.

EPIDEMIOLOGY Endemic (sylvatic) plague is firmly established among wild rodents in the western United States. In this country, human plague is almost always flea borne and is usually of the bubonic type. Between 1956 and 1983, 231 cases of plague were reported in the United States. Most occurred during the warmer months and were transmitted by flea bites. "Off-season" (October to February) plague occurs during rabbit-hunting season in the western states and is associated with direct contact (skinning, dressing) with animal (rabbits, bobcats) carcasses.[42] In recent years, epizootics have occurred among prairie dogs in the Southwest, and sporadic human cases have been identified on several Indian reservations. Plague has also been transmitted by domestic cats via bites, scratches, or aerosol. Infected fleas can be carried significant distances and into households. Domestic dogs have become infected in endemic areas, but no human cases have resulted.[43,44] The disease is also endemic in Vietnam and Africa (Tanzania, Zaire). Rarely, plague pneumonia secondary to bacteremia complicating bubonic plague may initiate respiratory spread to other persons.

CLINICAL MANIFESTATIONS *History* The incubation period is approximately 1 to 6 days, followed by the sudden onset of malaise, myalgias, backache, tachycardia, and high fever.

Cutaneous lesions In bubonic plague, the initial skin manifestation is related to the flea bite. Usually, this cannot be seen, but occasionally a small papule or vesicopustule persists. Painful, tender, enlarged lymph nodes are present in the area draining the bite site. The nodes become matted (buboes), and there is extensive surrounding subcutaneous gelatinous edema. Bacteremia may supervene and lead to overwhelming systemic illness. In this setting petechiae and ecchymosis often occur due to the effects of plague toxin or to the development of a disseminated intravascular coag-

ulopathy. Eschars and ecthyma gangrenosum can complicate systemic disease or appear at the site of the flea bite.[39,45]

Other physical findings The clinical manifestations (chills, fever, headache, nausea, vomiting, tachycardia, hypotension) of septicemic plague are similar to those of gram-negative bacillemia. Abdominal pain is a feature of almost half the cases.[46] The onset of pneumonic plague is abrupt, with high fever, tachycardia, and tachypnea. Signs of consolidation may appear, and within 24 h of onset the patient is critically ill, raising bloody sputum loaded with *Y. pestis*.[43] Meningitis may complicate all three forms of plague.

LABORATORY FINDINGS Leukocytosis occurs in all forms of the disease. In septicemic plague, bacilli can sometimes be seen on stained smears of venous blood (buffy coat).

PATHOLOGY In the bubonic form, acute inflammatory changes are seen in the involved nodes.

DIAGNOSIS AND DIFFERENTIAL DIAGNOSIS Bubonic plague should be distinguished from tularemia, lymphogranuloma venereum, cat-scratch disease, Eastern Hemisphere spotted fever, and suppurative lymphadenitis. Plague pneumonia must be differentiated from other acute bacterial pneumonias. Epidemiologic considerations and the tempo of the illness are major points in the differential diagnosis. Even minimal epidemiologic information provides sufficient grounds to begin treatment, for delays may be fatal in this rapidly progressive infection. The diagnosis is firmly established by examination of Gram- and Wayson-stained (or specific fluorescent antibody–stained) smears of infected material and by culture of the organism from blood, sputum, or aspirated buboes. Serologic methods can be used for retrospective diagnosis through demonstration of a fourfold or greater difference in titers between acute and convalescent sera. A convalescent passive hemagglutination titer of $\geq 1:16$ is strongly suggestive of the diagnosis.

TREATMENT Streptomycin is the drug of choice, administered intramuscularly (2 g daily in divided doses in the adult) for 10 days. Chloramphenicol or tetracycline are alternatives or may be added initially as strains resistant to streptomycin have been recovered. The dosage of chloramphenicol in the adult is 4 g daily for 2 days, followed by 3 g per day; that of tetracycline, 2.0 g daily intravenously for 1 week, then 1.5 g daily for a second week. Preliminary results suggest that gentamicin may be effective. Strict isolation of pneumonia cases is essential to prevent spread via the respiratory route. Ordinarily, buboes should not be drained until the lesion is well localized and the patient has been treated with antibiotics.

COURSE AND PROGNOSIS Pneumonic and septicemic plague, if untreated, are almost invariably fatal. Untreated bubonic plague has a mortality rate of 30 to 70 percent. Early antibiotic therapy has reduced the mortality rate to 5 to 10 percent. Even the severest forms of the infection respond to antibiotic treatment, if instituted promptly.

DISEASES ASSOCIATED WITH RANDOM ANIMAL CONTACT INDEPENDENT OF GEOGRAPHIC OR OCCUPATIONAL CONSIDERATIONS

Francisella tularensis Infections (Tularemia)

Tularemia is a disease of humans caused by *F. tularensis*, an organism that normally resides in a wide range of animal species and their immediate environments. In humans, most cases follow direct animal contact or transmission by insect vectors. The clinical manifestations fall into eight major patterns: (1) glandular, (2) ulceroglandular (most common form), (3) chancriform, (4) oculoglandular, (5) typhoidal, (6) pulmonary, (7) oropharyngeal,[47] and (8) meningeal.

BACTERIOLOGY *F. tularensis* is a pleomorphic, gram-negative coccobacillus that grows best on cysteine blood agar or in thioglycollate heart infusion medium. Intracellular parasitism of the reticuloendothelial system of humans and experimental animals is characteristic.

EPIDEMIOLOGY Infection in humans, particularly among hunters, most commonly follows contact with infected rabbits but may follow exposure to foxes, squirrels, skunks, and pheasants. Aquatic animals (muskrats, beavers) and mud and water from streams may also be a source of infection. The organisms are commonly introduced through a minimal abrasion or puncture wound. Bites of infected deerflies or ticks are also sources of infection in humans and are responsible for maintaining the disease in animals.[47] Domestic cats may become ill with local abscesses or pneumonia and spread the organism via direct contact, bite, or aerosol.[48] Rarely, ingestion of meat or conjunctival contamination leads to infection.

CLINICAL MANIFESTATIONS *History* After an incubation period of 2 to 10 days, the onset of any of the forms of disease is similar to that of most other acute infections: headache, malaise, myalgias, and high fever. A primary lesion then develops at the site of inoculation (usually on the hand), accompanied by regional adenopathy. Tick-transmitted disease frequently occurs on the head or trunk or may be transmitted to the conjunctivae by careless handling of an engorged arthropod.

Cutaneous lesions In ulceroglandular tularemia, a reddish, tender, painful papule appears at a site of trauma or arthropod bite. Lesions are usually found on a finger or hand when the contact is directly with an animal, hunted or trapped. Arthropod-transmitted lesions are frequently located where ticks feed, on the abdomen or scalp. A small vesicular pustule may develop, and the area rapidly enlarges and becomes necrotic. Nodular lymphangitis may complicate the initial lesion.[49] The lesion then evolves to an ulcer with raised margins, often covered by a black eschar, which later is shed. It appears chancre-like (Fig. 200-3). Regional nodes are enlarged and tender. Systemic signs of toxicity may be marked and pneumonia may accompany dissemination of infection. A macular and papular or petechial exanthem on the trunk and extremities may occur in a minority of patients as the disease progresses. Erythema nodosum and erythema multiforme are occasional manifestations.

In oculoglandular tularemia, the organism is directly introduced via the conjunctivae. The findings are those of a purulent conjunctivitis with marked pain, edema, and congestion. Small yellow nodules may appear on the conjunctivae and ulcerate. Corneal perforation may occur. Preauricular and submaxillary adenopathy is prominent.

Other physical findings Splenomegaly and generalized lymphadenopathy are relatively common, and hepatomegaly may occur. Ulcerative or exudative pharyngotonsillitis with cervical lymphadenopathy may follow ingestion of the organism, which may also be associated with the "typhoidal" form of the disease. Tularemic pneumonia may occur occasionally following inhalation of organisms but is more often secondary to bacteremia. Pleural effusion and mediastinal node enlargement are sometimes evident. Meningitis can occur, and severe muscle tenderness may indicate that rhabdomyolysis is present.

FIGURE 200-3

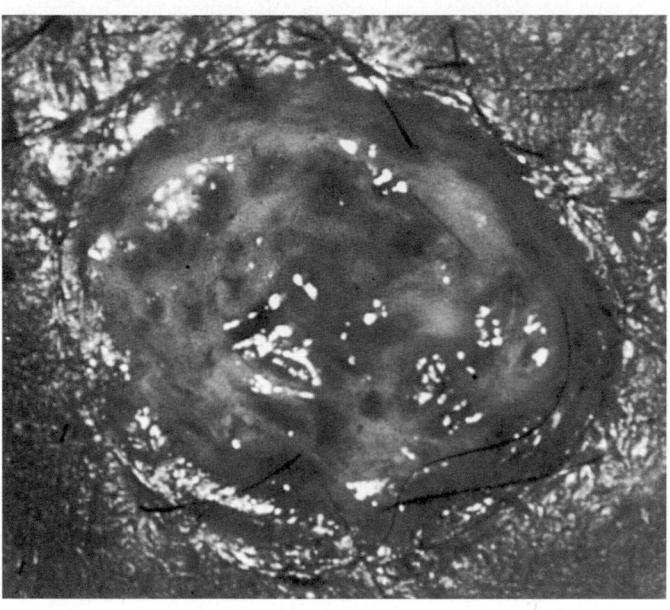

Tularemia. A chancre-like ulcer with raised margins on the back of the hand. There is axillary lymphadenopathy.

LABORATORY FINDINGS The white blood cell count is normal or low, but a polymorphonuclear leukocytosis may be seen. Blood cultures are only rarely positive.[50] Elevated alanine aminotransferase and alkaline phosphatase levels occur in about 10 percent of patients.

PATHOLOGY Following inoculation, the organism progresses through lymphatic channels and nodes to the bloodstream. The pathogen survives intracellularly in phagocytes, and small granulomatous lesions develop in lymph nodes, liver, and spleen. Some of the lesions may caseate, progress to frank abscess formation, or become necrotic.

DIAGNOSIS AND DIFFERENTIAL DIAGNOSIS The primary lesion resembles a furuncle, paronychia, ecthyma, the initial lesion of anthrax, *Pasteurella multocida* infection, or sporotrichosis. The prominent regional adenopathy suggests cat-scratch disease, plague, melioidosis, Eastern Hemisphere spotted fever, or lymphogranuloma venereum. Epidemiologic factors and systemic manifestations are points that suggest tularemia rather than other causes of a chancre-like lesion. A febrile illness occurring after a tick bite might suggest Rocky Mountain spotted fever, but an exanthem is usually present in that condition, without a local chancriform lesion. The skin lesion of Lyme disease, erythema migrans, is an enlarging distinctive lesion that does not ulcerate and occurs after a tick bite in circumscribed geographic regions (see Chap. 204). A febrile illness with hepatomegaly and granulomas (on liver biopsy) resembles tuberculosis, brucellosis, or other causes of granulomatous hepatitis. Isolation of *F. tularensis* from ulcer, blood, or bone marrow requires special (cysteine-containing) media and is difficult to accomplish. The diagnosis is usually made by serologic (agglutination or microagglutination) tests showing a fourfold or greater rise in titer. Cross-reactions occur in brucellosis. A skin test (delayed hypersensitivity), utilizing antigens from *F. tularensis*, becomes positive during the first week of disease and may be helpful in diagnosis.[51] A review of protective immunity in tularemia is useful in considering the host response and how it can be exploited for diagnosis and protective vaccine development.[52]

TREATMENT Streptomycin (1.0 to 2.0 g intramuscularly per day, in adults) is curative in all forms of tularemia if administered early. Gentamicin appears to be an acceptable alternative to streptomycin, but tobramycin is not an effective substitute.[53] Clinical improvement is evident within 24 to 48 h, but treatment should be continued for at least 7 to 10 afebrile days. Tetracycline and chloramphenicol are alternative drugs, but clinical relapses are more frequent, particularly if given for less than 14 days.

COURSE AND PROGNOSIS Untreated, the course may be weeks. Prior to the use of antibiotics, the mortality rate was about 5 percent in ulceroglandular disease and about 30 percent in typhoidal and pulmonary forms. Recovery provides immunity to systemic tularemia, but reinfection may produce a recurrent primary ulcer.

Leptospirosis

Leptospirosis is an acute febrile illness caused by any one of the serovarieties (serovars) of the species *Leptospira interrogans*. Although specific serovars have been reported with specific syndromes (canicola fever, Weil's disease, pretibial fever), any serovar may be responsible for a variety of clinical pictures, and a given clinical picture may be produced by many different serovars.[54]

BACTERIOLOGY These organisms are spirochetes that can be cultured on special (Fletcher semisolid) media. More than 200 antigenically different serotypes have been described. They are now defined as serovarieties of the species *L. interrogans*. Thus, for example, a specific antigenic serotype would bear a designation such as *L. interrogans* serovar *canicola*. The most common serovars in the United States are *canicola*, *icterohaemorrhagiae*, *pomona*, *autumnalis*, and *grippotyphosa*.

EPIDEMIOLOGY The reservoir of leptospira is worldwide in the animal population: farm animals (cattle, swine); laboratory animals (mice); domestic animals (hamsters, dogs); wild animals (squirrels, rats); and reptiles. Infection in humans occurs as a result of direct contact with an animal (either a sick animal or an asymptomatic urinary "shedder") or indirectly through contaminated water or soil. This is especially important considering the urge for travel to exotic places, many of which are in the tropics. The risk of entering contaminated water to "cool off" has recently been emphasized in a report describing leptospirosis in Dutch travelers.[55] Organisms usually enter the body through a break in the skin or, less often, through mucus membranes (including conjunctiva). The disease is most prevalent among children (from playing in contaminated puddles or ponds), farmers, hunters, or abattoir workers.

CLINICAL MANIFESTATIONS *History* The incubation period is usually between 7 and 14 days, and the illness typically has a biphasic course. The onset is sudden, with headache, fever, chills, nausea, vomiting, abdominal pain, and myalgias. This initial nonspecific phase continues for about a week, when defervescence oc-

curs. After several relatively asymptomatic days, the second phase of illness begins with low-grade fever. Meningeal symptoms may begin and persist for another 2 to 4 days or for several weeks. In the initial phase (leptospiremic), leptospiral organisms are present in the bloodstream, cerebrospinal fluid, and other tissues. The second ("immune") phase coincides with the appearance of IgM antibodies. Clinically this phase is characterized by the onset of meningitis, rash, uveitis, and, in more severe cases, by hepatic and renal involvement. Therapy with antimicrobials can be most effective in the initial phase of illness.

Cutaneous lesions Scleral conjunctival injection appears on the third or fourth day of illness. Skin lesions, usually on the trunk (consisting of macules, papules, urticaria, and petechiae), occur in fewer than half the cases. Peripheral desquamation and infarction of portions of the hands and feet have been observed in a few children with leptospirosis.[56] Weil's disease, often but not exclusively due to serovar *icterohaemorrhagiae*, is a form of infection with prominent hepatic (jaundice) and renal (hematuria, azotemia) involvement. Hemorrhagic manifestations occur in a variety of organs, including the skin. Pretibial (*Fort Bragg*) fever is a form of leptospirosis (serovar *autumnalis*) that has a rather distinctive rash occurring on the fourth or fifth day of illness and consisting of slightly raised, 1- to 5-cm, tender, erythematous lesions on the pretibial areas.[57] The rash subsides within 4 or 7 days. Erythema nodosum has occurred in association with infection due to *L. interrogans*.[58]

Other physical findings These depend on the particular syndrome that is presented.

1. Pyrexia of unknown origin—localizing signs lacking; epidemiology critical to diagnosis
2. Aseptic meningitis—nuchal rigidity
3. Weil's disease—jaundice and hepatomegaly; interstitial nephritis; generalized hemorrhagic tendency with epistaxis, hematuria, and gastrointestinal bleeding
4. Pretibial fever—splenomegaly is common

In up to 20 percent of patients with leptospirosis, generalized lymphadenopathy (particularly involving cervical nodes) may be observed. Pulmonary involvement with cough and radiologically demonstrable infiltrates occurs rarely.[59]

In children, acalculous cholecystitis has been observed occasionally as a manifestation of leptospirosis. Rarely, myocarditis is a feature of leptospirosis.

LABORATORY FINDINGS The white blood cell count varies from a leukopenia to a mild leukocytosis, and thrombocytopenia can occur. In Weil's disease, white blood cell count may reach levels of 40,000/mm³. A cerebrospinal fluid pleocytosis, with up to several hundred mononuclear cells, may be present. Abnormalities of liver function are common, even in patients lacking overt jaundice. Azotemia and hematuria occur in patients with renal involvement, and jaundice is usually present.

DIAGNOSIS AND DIFFERENTIAL DIAGNOSIS Skin manifestations are not specific but may suggest leptospirosis in the context of jaundice and aseptic meningitis. Conjunctival suffusion with petechiae or hemorrhages may be helpful clues. The differential diagnosis includes viral hepatitis, all the causes of a lymphocytic aseptic meningitis, nephritis, and the causes of a fever of unknown origin. The diagnosis is established most commonly by serologic means: a fourfold or greater rise in microagglutination titer (to ≧1 : 100), an IHA, or an IgM-specific dot-ELISA.[55] It can also be confirmed by isolation of the organism from blood during the first 10 days of illness. In a series of cases of leptospirosis among military personnel in Panama, leptospires were isolated from blood cultures of 23 of 29 patients studied.[60]

TREATMENT In the past, studies of the effectiveness of antibiotics (tetracyclines, penicillin) in the treatment of leptospirosis have been inconclusive. But in a controlled trial in anicteric leptospirosis, doxycycline therapy, when administered early, has proved effective in reducing the duration of illness and in preventing leptospiruria.[60] Doxycycline, administered orally on a once-weekly basis, has been used successfully by the military as a prophylactic measure for short-term exposure in a hyperendemic area.[61] Penicillin has also been recommended in selected instances of severe illness, but no controlled studies of efficacy are available. The Jarisch-Herxheimer reaction has been reported in several patients treated with penicillin.[62]

COURSE AND PROGNOSIS Recovery is the rule in anicteric cases. In the presence of jaundice, the mortality rate may be as high as 40 percent, although a recent report describes 100 percent survival in 32 patients, only 14 of whom received adequate therapy.[55]

Pasteurella multocida Infections

Infections produced by *P. multocida* follow one of several patterns: (1) local skin infection with adenitis following animal bites (the most common form of infection); (2) septic arthritis and osteomyelitis following an animal bite (usually of the hand); (3) respiratory tract infections or colonization; (4) systemic infections such as meningitis, bacteremia, or spontaneous bacterial peritonitis.[63,64]

BACTERIOLOGY *P. multocida* is a small, ovoid, gram-negative rod. Its prominent bipolar staining may, from time to time, mistakenly suggest *Neisseria* or *Haemophilus influenzae*. It grows readily on nutrient blood agar, but not on MacConkey agar, and can be identified by biochemical tests and agglutination reactions.

EPIDEMIOLOGY Although this organism is primarily a pathogen among birds and animals, causing "hemorrhagic septicemia," it occasionally infects humans. *P. multocida* can be isolated from the upper respiratory tract of healthy cats, dogs, rats, and mice. Animal exposure has occurred in 70 to 80 percent of patients with *P. multocida* bacteremia. Predisposing conditions (alcoholic cirrhosis, neoplastic disease, chronic obstructive pulmonary disease) could be identified in the majority of patients.[65]

CLINICAL MANIFESTATIONS *History* Local pain and swelling occur within a few days of a cat or dog bite. There is little if any fever.

Cutaneous lesions Redness, swelling, ulceration, and seropurulent drainage develop at the bite site. Cellulitis may progress rapidly and extensively, with associated lymphangitis. Local necrosis and abscess formation may follow, and necrotizing fasciitis has been reported, accompanied by septic shock.

Other physical findings Regional adenopathy may be present. Complicating osteomyelitis and septic arthritis may occur as a result of the introduction of organisms beneath the periosteum or into a joint space by the biting animal.

LABORATORY FINDINGS Mild leukocytosis is present. After several weeks, an x-ray of underlying bone may show osteomyelitis.

PATHOLOGY This infection produces an acute pyogenic response.

DIAGNOSIS AND DIFFERENTIAL DIAGNOSIS The diagnosis is suspected when a painful infection develops at the site of an animal bite. It must be distinguished from cat-scratch disease. Local ulceration and proximal lymphadenitis mimic ulceroglandular tularemia, but the lesion is characteristically a necrotizing cellulitis and not chancriform in appearance. The diagnosis is established by isolation of the organism.

TREATMENT Most strains of *P. multocida* are susceptible to penicillin, the drug of choice. In patients with simple cellulitis, oral penicillin (penicillin VK at 500 to 750 mg orally four times daily for adults) or ampicillin or amoxicillin-clavulanate may reasonably be used, but close follow-up is mandatory. Several human isolates have been reported recently to be penicillin-resistant by virtue of plasmid-mediated beta-lactamase production.[66] If the prior animal bite is suspected to have penetrated deeply close to periosteum, parenteral penicillin should be administered until the local lesion is well healed, to avert possible osteomyelitis. *P. multocida* is also susceptible to third-generation cephalosporins. For the penicillin-allergic patient, doxycycline is a suitable alternative, but susceptibility testing must always be performed. Chloramphenicol or TMP-SMX may be effective therapy for the rare patient unable to tolerate either penicillin or doxycycline. Ciprofloxacin has activity against *P. multocida* in vitro. Abscesses should be surgically drained.

COURSE AND PROGNOSIS The infection responds to local measures and antibiotic therapy.

UNCOMMON DISEASES IN WHICH ANIMAL OR WATER CONTACT OR CLIMATOLOGIC FACTORS MAY OCCASIONALLY BE RELEVANT

Listeria monocytogenes Infections (Listeriosis)

Infection with *L. monocytogenes* produces characteristic acute disease in infants (neonatal septicemia, meningitis, and septic granulomatosis) and in both healthy and immunosuppressed adults (septicemia, meningitis, vaginal infection, pneumonitis, and oculoglandular syndrome).[67]

BACTERIOLOGY *L. monocytogenes* is a small, thin, gram-positive rod that often appears coccoid in infected tissues and body fluids. It may resemble a chaining streptococcus or a diplococcus. Its appearance may also mimic that of a diphtheroid and occasionally has been dismissed erroneously as a "contaminant." It is non-spore-forming, beta-hemolytic, and exhibits a characteristic tumbling motility when grown in broth at room temperature. This is the classic facultative intracellular bacteria against which host resistance is mediated by thymus-derived lymphocytes (and macrophages).

EPIDEMIOLOGY *L. monocytogenes* is found in the feces of many wild animals and birds and in soil and vegetation. Approximately 5 percent of humans (this is probably a minimal figure as it is difficult to isolate the organism from stool) appear to be fecal carriers of the organism. Higher rates of carriage have been observed in family contacts of patients with listeriosis. For undetermined reasons, pregnant women may acquire self-limited or asymptomatic genital infections. The highest incidence of infections is in the perinatal period, suggesting that the fetus either becomes infected in utero or on passing through the birth canal. Many but not all adult cases occur on a background of altered cellular immunity (Hodgkin's disease, immunosuppression for organ transplantation, etc.) or cirrhosis. Transfusional iron overload may also be a predisposing factor for listeriosis. *L. monocytogenes* produces a protein in culture supernatants that mobilizes iron from transferrin.[68] Because growth of this organism is stimulated by excess iron and because administration of iron compounds reduces the lethal dose of *L. monocytogenes* in animal models of infection, it is likely that iron overload contributes to the pathogenicity of this organism in humans. Occasionally, veterinarians handling stillborn or ill newborn animals develop cutaneous infections.

Most cases in the United States occur in urban areas without obvious animal contact. The portal of infection is unknown, but introduction through the intestinal tract seems likely. Food-borne (unpasteurized or improperly pasteurized milk or cheese; coleslaw made from cabbage grown on a farm where sheep manure had been used as fertilizer) outbreaks have been described.[68,69]

Immunocompromised individuals and pregnant women (neonatal infection) are at particular risk.[69,70]

CLINICAL MANIFESTATIONS *History* Neonatal listeriosis occurs in two clinical forms—early and late onset.[71] *Early-onset neonatal listeriosis* develops in infants infected in utero from mothers who were undergoing a bacteremic illness with nonspecific symptoms shortly before the onset of labor. The findings of early-onset infection are evident at birth or become apparent within the first several days of life. Widespread granulomas (placenta, liver, spleen, lung, etc.) are characteristic of the syndrome known as *granulomatosis infantiseptica*. Placental, posterior pharyngeal, and multiple small cutaneous granulomas may provide clues as to the specific diagnosis. Neonatal infection, which may be due to any of a variety of agents (*Listeria*, group B streptococci, *Herpes simplex*, etc.) would be suggested in an acutely ill, moribund infant who was meconium-stained at birth and who subsequently exhibited pustular, papular, or petechial skin lesions. *Late-onset neonatal listeriosis* usually occurs several weeks after a normal birth, presumably resulting from postpartum acquisition. Meningitis rather than sepsis is the clinical picture. Listeriosis in the adult may present as a nonspecific acute febrile illness in which the findings of acute or subacute meningitis may predominate. Diarrhea, associated with numerous *L. monocytogenes* in the stool and blood cultures, may predate the onset of meningeal symptoms and findings by several days. *L. monocytogenes* infection in adults is not accompanied by skin lesions. Veterinarians may develop an acute febrile illness with headache, malaise, and rash 2 to 3 days after handling infected bovine fetuses.

Cutaneous lesions In neonatal septicemia and infant granulomatosis, the skin rash consists of generalized erythematous papular or petechial lesions that may become pustular but only rarely vesicular. Veterinarians may develop tender, red papular lesions on the hands and arms, some of which evolve into pustules. Characteristic gram-positive rods can be demonstrated in these skin lesions. Tender axillary adenopathy is frequently present. In oculoglandular infection, there is acute conjunctivitis with preauricular adenitis.

Other physical findings In infants, meconium staining of the skin, hepatosplenomegaly, and lethargy are commonly present. Acute meningitis is accompanied by typical signs in infants and adults.

LABORATORY FINDINGS A significant monocytosis occurs only rarely. In adults with meningitis, the inflammatory reaction is usually a predominantly neutrophilic pleocytosis; in infants, the response in the cerebrospinal fluid may be mononuclear in approximately one-third of cases.

PATHOLOGY Skin lesions show focal necrosis and infiltration by polymorphonuclear leukocytes and monocytes about blood vessels. Abscesses are found in viscera, and granuloma formation may also be evident.

DIAGNOSIS AND DIFFERENTIAL DIAGNOSIS Listeriosis should be suspected in any newborn with meconium-stained skin who exhibits intrauterine growth retardation, fails to thrive, or develops a papular skin eruption. Gram's stain of meconium shows the characteristic gram-positive rods. The skin lesions, cerebrospinal fluid, or blood cultures reveal the etiologic agent.

The differential diagnosis includes other forms of in utero neonatal infection such as toxoplasmosis, cytomegalovirus infection, rubella, disseminated *Herpes simplex* infection, and a variety of disseminated bacterial infections. The latter include those due to group B streptococci, *Escherichia coli*, *Salmonella*, and *Pseudomonas*.

TREATMENT Ampicillin (or penicillin) is the antibiotic of choice, administered by the intravenous route in neonates in two or three divided doses. Care must be exercised in adjusting the dosage of penicillin in the newborn period to 50,000 to 250,000 units/kg per day; ampicillin is administered in a dosage of 100 to 200 mg/kg per day. In adults with meningitis or bacteremia, the dosage of penicillin G should be 12 to 24 million units intravenously daily (in divided doses every 2 to 4 h) and that of ampicillin should be 12 g intravenously (in divided doses every 3 to 4 h). Gentamicin acts synergistically with ampicillin in vitro and is sometimes used in combination with the latter in treatment of *L. monocytogenes* meningitis or endocarditis. In nonpregnant adults who are allergic to penicillin or ampicillin, TMP-SMX is effective therapy.[67] Other possible, but less favored, alternatives for treatment include a tetracycline and erythromycin.

COURSE AND PROGNOSIS In neonatal septicemia and meningitis, morbidity and mortality are high (up to 50 percent). In adult infections, treatment is effective and recovery is the rule, unless the underlying disease prevents this.

Diphtheria

Diphtheria is an acute febrile illness involving primarily the pharynx and mucous membranes of the upper respiratory tract. The major manifestations of this disease are due to (1) local membranous obstruction of the airway, and (2) the effects of a potent cytotoxin on the myocardium and peripheral nervous system. The hallmark of the local lesion is a gray, leathery membrane. Rarely, the primary lesion may be located on the skin, or the infection may complicate a preexisting wound. This is characteristically seen in tropical areas. The early 1990s saw an upsurge of cases of diphtheria, primarily in the New Independent States of the former Soviet Union but also in other areas of the world including the United States. Attention to protecting people from this contagious, potentially lethal disease is essential. An awareness of its epidemiologic features, including cutaneous disease, argues for its inclusion in this chapter.[72,73]

BACTERIOLOGY The causative organism (*Corynebacterium diphtheriae*) is a gram-positive club-shaped rod that exhibits metachromatic bipolar granules on staining with methylene blue. It grows well on ordinary media, but its presence may be obscured by other bacteria in the pharynx or on the cutaneous lesion. For this reason, it is necessary to use selective media such as Loeffler's or tellurite agar to inhibit competing organisms.

Identification of toxigenic strains requires either an Elek plate (agar diffusion precipitin reaction) or demonstration of protection from dermonecrosis in guinea pigs by antitoxin neutralization of a suspension of the isolate of *Corynebacterium*.

EPIDEMIOLOGY Humans are the only natural host for *C. diphtheriae*. The organism is carried in the pharynx of asymptomatic individuals. Infection occurs when a nonimmune person is infected by a toxigenic strain of *C. diphtheriae*; epidemics occur when such a strain becomes widespread in a population of nonimmune individuals. Most commonly, the site of primary infection is the nasopharynx or pharynx.

Cutaneous diphtheria and wound diphtheria occur in tropical areas ("jungle sore") and in association with poor hygiene. There has been an increase in skin diphtheria in the United States in the Pacific northwest and in the south.[74] The contagiousness of cutaneous diphtheria may be greater than that of respiratory infection among school children.[75]

Diphtheria is primarily a disease of young children and the elderly. In the United States most cases occur among poor, crowded, unimmunized individuals. Because of the widespread use and protective effect of toxoid immunization, the disease is rare in this country. It should be stressed, however, that this protection does not prevent the development of the carrier state and subsequent spread of organisms to susceptible individuals. In the past two decades, increasing numbers of cases have occurred in unimmunized migrant farm worker families, in older alcoholics living in "skid row" situations, and among Native Americans in the western United States and Canada. Three outbreaks, involving a total of 1100 infections (40 percent due to toxigenic strains), occurred in Seattle between 1972 and 1982. They occurred almost exclusively in indigent alcoholics, and 86 percent of these infections were cutaneous.[76] Cutaneous infections were much more common in the winter and early spring.

In underdeveloped and overcrowded parts of the world, diphtheria remains an important health problem, with many carriers and susceptible individuals. The majority of cases of cutaneous and wound diphtheria occur in this setting and are associated with poor hygiene and skin trauma.

CLINICAL MANIFESTATIONS *History* Faucial diphtheria usually presents with pharyngitis and low-grade fever. Toxicity is out of proportion to the degree of fever and local findings. As the disease progresses, swelling and pain in the neck, symptoms of airway obstruction, or unilateral nasal discharge may develop. Cutaneous diphtheria occurs in the presence or absence of pharyngeal disease. However, 20 to 40 percent of patients with cutaneous diphtheria carry the identical strain of *C. diphtheriae* in their respiratory tract. The skin lesions are usually indolent but tender and on the extremities. Symptoms of cranial or peripheral neuritis or of myocarditis may complicate the course. The latter usually occurs 5 to 14 days after the onset of the illness, whereas the former may develop any time from 2 weeks to several months after the primary lesion. Myocarditis is extremely rare as a complication of cutaneous diphtheria. Neurologic symptoms such as blurred vision, diplopia, numbness of tongue, palatal paralysis, long-tract sensory and motor findings,

and the Guillain-Barré syndrome have occurred in 3 to 5 percent of patients with ulcerated diphtheritic skin lesions.

Cutaneous lesions There are basically three types of skin involvement[77]: (1) Wound diphtheria is a secondary infection of a preexisting wound, occurs in temperate as well as tropical climates, and may involve any part of the body. This type accounts for almost all cases of cutaneous diphtheria reported in the United States. Underlying (primary) skin lesions include those due to trauma (abrasions, lacerations, burns), chronic dermatitis (eczema, scabies, etc.), and various pyodermas. A latent period of up to 3 weeks transpires between initiation of the primary lesion and evidences of superimposed diphtheritic infection (pain, erythema, tenderness, exudate). The lesion is usually partially covered with a membrane; a purulent exudate is present, and a zone of edema and erythema surrounds the area. In the Seattle outbreak, coinfection with *S. pyogenes* occurred in 73 percent of diphtheritic skin lesions.[76] (2) Primary cutaneous diphtheria begins acutely as a tender, pustular lesion, which then breaks down and enlarges to form an oval punched-out ulcer with a gray membrane at the base. (A similar appearance may be the result of secondary infection by *C. diphtheriae* of a primary lesion of streptococcal ecthyma.) Later the membrane becomes dark brown. This ulcer does not extend below the fascia, has edematous, rolled, bluish margins, is usually located on a lower extremity, and is most often seen in the tropics. (3) Superinfection of eczematized skin lesions by *C. diphtheriae* evokes a more superficial, membranous, tender, edematous reaction.

Skin lesions with the appearance of impetigo, ecthyma, infected insect bites, etc., have been described as yielding *C. diphtheriae* on culture.[74] Whether these represent true infections with *C. diphtheriae* or are the cutaneous equivalent of the respiratory carrier state is unclear.

Other physical findings A membranous pharyngitis may accompany cutaneous diphtheria. Cranial or peripheral nerve palsies may be present.

LABORATORY FINDINGS The organism can be isolated on appropriate media from the skin ulcer or pharyngeal membrane.

PATHOLOGY There is nothing characteristic about the pathologic picture of the diphtheritic lesion. The membrane is composed of coagulation necrosis and inflammatory cells.

DIAGNOSIS AND DIFFERENTIAL DIAGNOSIS A presumptive diagnosis is usually based on the findings of membranous pharyngitis in faucial diphtheria and of a shallow membrane-covered ulcer in cutaneous involvement. In methylene blue–stained smears of material from the edge of the membrane, the characteristic beaded metachromatically stained rods can be seen, but proof of the diagnosis must await culture results and demonstration of toxin production. However, the presence of a pharyngeal membrane, with or without typically appearing organisms, should be presumptive evidence of infection with *C. diphtheriae*, and treatment should be started immediately. Occasionally, membranous infectious mononucleosis can mimic the picture of faucial diphtheria or be complicated by diphtheria.

Tropical ulcers may be confused with diphtheritic skin lesions, but the former usually occur in malnourished individuals and penetrate below the fascia, involving muscle and tendons. Bacterial infections in ulcerated wounds and following trauma are usually purulent and without membrane formation. Cutaneous mycotic infections are frequently more proliferative, and their margins are irregular, without surrounding reactive edema. Nonpathogenic (non-toxigenic) diphtheroids may be present in open skin lesions as superficial contaminants. Impetigo-like lesions and nondistinctive secondary pyodermas should be cultured in any contacts of a patient with diphtheria because of the contagiousness of cutaneous diphtheria.

An organism closely related to corynebacteria, *Rhodococcus equi* (formerly *C. equi*), has been primarily identified as a cause of inhalation lung disease in AIDS patients. Rarely this organism, which resembles *C. diphtheriae* on Gram's stain, can be responsible for skin and subcutaneous infections in healthy individuals, especially those exposed to horse manure or following an injury contaminated with soil.[78]

TREATMENT In faucial diphtheria, treatment consists of both specific equine antitoxin and penicillin. Treatment is initiated on the basis of clinical suspicion without awaiting cultural confirmation, as toxin elaborated in the intervening period could lead to irreversible myocardial damage.

In ulcerative cutaneous diphtheria, bed rest is essential for healing. Antitoxin in doses of 20,000 to 40,000 units is given by the intravenous route after careful testing for horse serum hypersensitivity. As of January, 1997, diphtheria antitoxin is no longer commercially available but may be obtained, in appropriately suspicious or documented cases, through the Centers for Disease Control and Prevention, Child Vaccine Preventable Disease Branch. Injection of antitoxin as well into the subcutaneous area around the ulcer and also the surface application of antitoxin on the lesion have been suggested. Penicillin (2 to 4 million units intramuscularly daily) or erythromycin (2.0 g orally daily) is administered for 7 to 10 days. A few inducible erythromycin- and clindamycin-resistant strains of *C. diphtheriae* have been isolated recently from the lesions of cutaneous diphtheria. The lesion should be debrided and kept clean once antitoxin and antibiotics have been administered.

Close contacts of a case of cutaneous diphtheria should be examined for any skin lesions (which should be cultured for *C. diphtheriae*); the pharynx should be cultured regardless of the presence of pharyngitis or a membrane. While awaiting results of cultures, prophylactic treatment of contacts with erythromycin (or penicillin) should be initiated. In addition, if the immunization status of close contacts is unclear or incomplete, they should receive proper immunization against diphtheria. For children (7 years of age and older) and adults, the adult formulation of the combined diphtheria-tetanus toxoid (Td) preparation should be used rather than the pediatric DPT vaccine, because the latter contains a higher concentration of diphtheria toxoid as well as a pertussis component (both of which produce a higher rate of systemic reactions in older children and adults).

COURSE AND PROGNOSIS If treatment is begun early, the prognosis is excellent for full recovery. In untreated, unimmunized persons with cutaneous diphtheria, ulcers may persist for as long as 6 months. Neuritic symptoms and signs may occur as late as 5 months after the onset of illness. The neurologic defects are almost always completely reversible.

Cutaneous Infections due to *Vibrio* Species

Infections caused by *Vibrio* species produce several different clinical syndromes: (1) gastroenteritis (the most common primarily caused by *V. parahaemolyticus* and *V. cholerae* non-01), (2) wound (and ear) infections, and (3) septicemia (either "primary" or secondary to a wound infection).[79] There has been a recent upsurge of reports of the septicemia syndrome caused by many *Vibrio* species, including their distribution to areas of more temperate climate (e.g., Cape Cod, MA, Denmark). This increase in reports appears to be associated with ingestion of raw shellfish, cutaneous injuries before or during ocean water exposures, and the potential for systemic disease in individuals with cirrhosis and immunodeficiencies.[80]

BACTERIOLOGY AND PATHOGENIC ASPECTS *Bacteriology* Nine *Vibrio* species in addition to *V. cholerae* have been associated with human disease. Five species are capable of producing wound infections: *V. parahaemolyticus*, *V. vulnificus*, *V. alginolyticus*, *V. cholerae* non-01, and *V. damsela*. Of these, *V. vulnificus* is the most pathogenic, causing severe wound infections and a "primary septicemia" syndrome with a mortality rate approaching 50 percent. The *Vibrio* species grow in regular blood culture media and are hemolytic on sheep blood agar; they are curved gram-negative rods. All require added salt in the growth medium, with the exception of *V. cholerae*. Selective media such as thiosulfate-citrate-bile salts-sucrose (TCBS) are necessary to isolate the organisms from stool cultures.

Pathogenic aspects Markers for pathogenicity have been described for some *Vibrio* species. Almost all *V. parahaemolyticus* strains associated with disease (diarrhea) in humans produce a hemolysin (Kanagawa phenomenon). This organism also produces a toxin capable of causing intestinal fluid accumulation in suckling mice and tissue invasiveness, producing a dysentery-like syndrome. *V. vulnificus* produces extracellular collagenolytic, proteolytic, and elastolytic activities that may be important in the aggressive invasiveness of this pathogen. In addition, a metalloprotease exotoxin may be an important factor causing gross edema and cellulitis. *V. cholerae* non-01 secretes a dermonecrotic factor that may be of pathogenic significance in the development of hemorrhagic bullous skin lesions. Among the *Vibrio* species, *V. vulnificus* exhibits a striking pathogenicity when introduced into animal models by either the gastrointestinal or parenteral routes.

EPIDEMIOLOGY *V. parahaemolyticus* and *V. vulnificus* are commonly found in saltwater and estuarine sediments and adherent to fish and concentrated within shellfish. The former has been implicated in 24 percent of reported cases of food-borne gastroenteritis in Japan; it also has been involved in shellfish-associated outbreaks of gastroenteritis in the United States. *V. parahaemolyticus* is responsible for occasional wound infections incurred following lacerations from shellfish or in seawater as well as for septicemia with metastatic skin lesions after ingestion of raw clams.[80,81] Wound infections with *V. vulnificus* typically follow cuts of the hand acquired while cleaning crabs or shrimp, or from entry of the organism through a preexisting open skin lesion exposed to seawater. *V. vulnificus* (and other *Vibrio* species) are endemic along the Gulf of Mexico, to a lesser extent along the Atlantic and Pacific coasts, and in regions of northern Europe (Denmark), particularly in the summer when seawater temperatures exceed 20°C. Primary septicemia due to *V. vulnificus* (and other *Vibrio* species) is associated with the eating of raw oysters and clams and particularly in the setting of hepatic cirrhosis, hemochromatosis, diabetes, glucocorticoid use, or prior gastric surgery.[80,82]

CLINICAL MANIFESTATIONS *History* Gastroenteritis is most commonly associated with *V. parahaemolyticus*. *V. vulnificus* may occasionally cause a similar gastroenteritis. More typically it is responsible for a wound infection with occasional secondary bacteremia occurring several days after a laceration sustained in seawater or brackish inland lakes. Primary septicemia with *V. vulnificus* (or other *Vibrio* species) may follow 24 to 48 h after consumption of raw oysters. This is more likely to occur in individuals with underlying chronic diseases, especially cirrhosis. Fever, chills, nausea, vomiting, abdominal pain, and diarrhea are frequent symptoms in patients with primary septicemia, suggesting an initial gastrointestinal site of infection.

Cutaneous lesions Traumatic wound infections due to *V. vulnificus* may consist of pustular lesions, lymphangitis and lymphadenitis, or cellulitis. These infections may be mild or develop into rapidly progressive, painful cellulitis with myositis, extensive skin necrosis, and gangrene requiring amputation. Secondary bacteremia may ensue, complicated by metastatic cutaneous lesions. Occasionally, cellulitis develops spontaneously without antecedent overt skin trauma but following exposure to seawater.

Skin lesions, in the form of large hemorrhagic bullae on the extremities or trunk, develop commonly in the course of primary *V. vulnificus* septicemia and are seen with other vibrios, including *V. cholerae* non-01.[80,82] These progress to necrotic ulcers and necrotizing fasciitis and can eventuate on the lower extremity in muscle necrosis in the anterior compartment.

Other physical findings Systemic manifestations (high fever, tachycardia, hypotension) are common in *V. vulnificus* septicemia. One-third of patients are in shock on presentation or within the first 12 h of hospitalization.

LABORATORY FINDINGS Although *V. parahaemolyticus* usually produces a watery diarrhea, occasional patients will have a dysentery-like syndrome with leukocytes and blood present in the stool. In *V. vulnificus* primary septicemia, leukopenia is more frequent than leukocytosis. Thrombocytopenia is common and may progress rapidly to disseminated intravascular coagulation. *V. parahaemolyticus*, *V. vulnificus*, and other *Vibrio* species can be grown on blood agar media and isolated from routine blood cultures. Selective TCBS media is used for isolation of *Vibrio* species from stool.

DIAGNOSIS AND DIFFERENTIAL DIAGNOSIS Infection with a pathogenic *Vibrio* species should be suspected when gastroenteritis occurs in the summer months when there is a history of recent ingestion of shellfish (particularly raw oysters, clams, or crabs) or exposure to seawater, especially, but not exclusively, along the Gulf Coast. The development of unexplained fever, shock, and bullous skin lesions in a patient with cirrhosis who has recently eaten raw oysters should alert the physician to the possible diagnosis of limb- or life-threatening primary vibrio septicemia.

Differential diagnosis of the gastroenteritis syndrome includes other causes of watery diarrhea (*V. cholerae*, toxigenic *E. coli*). Wound infections sustained in freshwater would suggest *A. hydrophila* rather than *Vibrio* species, which are typically involved in infected wounds sustained in a saltwater environment. Bullous lesions occurring in a hypotensive febrile patient could be secondary to bacteremic *P. aeruginosa* infection or even clostridial myonecrosis. The latter would be suggested by the presence of crepitus in the involved area and finding typical gram-positive blunt-ended bacilli in the contents of the bullae. *Pseudomonas* bacteremia would be unlikely in a nonleukopenic nonhospitalized patient without a prior history of infection and antibiotic usage.

TREATMENT *V. parahaemolyticus* gastroenteritis is usually a mild to moderately severe form of diarrheal disease that requires no treatment other than oral fluid replacement (e.g., glucose-electrolyte solution). Management of *V. vulnificus* (or other *Vibrio* species) septicemia involves the reversal of hypotension with fluid re-

placement and treatment of systemic infection with both doxycycline (or chloramphenicol) and ceftazidime. There is a role for antimicrobial therapy in infected traumatic wounds due to *V. vulnificus* (or other *Vibrio* species) in view of the potential invasiveness of these organisms. Debridement of necrotic lesions is indicated.

COURSE AND PROGNOSIS *V. parahaemolyticus* gastroenteritis is a self-limited disease. In contrast, the mortality rate for *V. vulnificus* primary septicemia is approximately 50 percent, about three times as high as the mortality for wound infections due to the same organism. In view of the mortality associated with septicemic *Vibrio* infections, patients with cirrhosis, diabetes, AIDS, and other immunocompromising illnesses or treatments should be advised against consuming raw shellfish or exposure of preexisting wounds to contact with warm seawater.

Aeromonas hydrophilia Infections

Clinical infections with aeromonads are usually associated with exposure to contaminated fresh or brackish water. The most common form of disease is gastroenteritis but, during the past several decades, many reports have documented the importance of one species, *A. hydrophilia*, in skin, soft-tissue, and muscle infections as well as in septicemic disease.[83] Except for the freshwater habitat of the causative organism, the diseases and patient population infected resemble those caused by *Vibrio* species.

BACTERIOLOGY AND PATHOGENESIS *Bacteriology* Aeromonads are widespread in nature. The major pathogen, *A. hydrophilia*, is a facultative gram-negative bacillus that grows well on basic blood and MacConkey agar. Beta-hemolysis surrounds colonies, and biochemical reactions place aeromonads in the same family as the vibrios but separated by their lack of a salt requirement.

Pathogenesis In healthy individuals not exposed to trauma in a freshwater setting, acute gastroenteritis is the most common expression of *Aeromonas* infection. Enteropathogenicity is probably due to secretion of an enterotoxin and a cytotoxin, but invasive disease is rarely seen with gastrointestinal infections in immunocompetent individuals. Virulence factors, combined with trauma and fresh- or brackish-water exposure, and cirrhosis, malignancy, or immunodeficiencies can lead to severe soft-tissue and septicemic disease. Virulence factors include cytotoxins, dermonecrotic hemolysins, and other exotoxins. The result of local infection may include necrosis, purulent exudate, and gas formation, localized in healthy individuals, but progressive soft-tissue disease (including myonecrosis and abscess formation) and bacteremia may ensue in debilitated patients.[84,85]

EPIDEMIOLOGY Aeromonads are found worldwide, especially in fresh and brackish water. They are the cause of disease in many aquatic inhabitants, including fish, amphibians, and reptiles. They are part of the normal flora of leeches. The upswing in use of leeches for medical purposes has resulted in a number of cases of soft-tissue disease. Fish tanks, swimming pools, and tap water (including hospital water) have been contaminated with these organisms; common source infections and nosocomial spread and disease have occurred.

CLINICAL MANIFESTATIONS *History* The epidemiology may direct the clinician to consider a water-related disease, especially if there has been some form of laceration or loss of skin cover due to prior trauma or dermatitis. Gastroenteritis is the major clinical complaint associated with *Aeromonas*, but, compared to *V. vulnificus*, it is unusual to have bacteremia and metastatic skin and soft-tissue complications. Fever and hypotension, jaundice, and local disease, such as spontaneous peritonitis, occur in patients with underlying cirrhosis, cancer, and immunocompromising diseases or therapies.

Cutaneous lesions The most common lesion is a cellulitis associated with a laceration, often followed by evidence of an underlying abscess or spread to deeper subcutaneous tissues, with or without palpable gas. The exudate often has a foul or fishy odor. Myonecrosis or necrotizing fasciitis may develop rapidly and mimic clostridial gas gangrene in its rapid onset (24 to 48 h after the initiating wound) and swift progression with severe pain, marked swelling, serosanguineous bullae, crepitation, and systemic toxicity. Occasionally macular, papular, and ecthymatous lesions occur, indistinguishable from those caused by *P. aeruginosa*.

Other physical findings Evidence of cirrhosis or other underlying disease may be present, and jaundice is often apparent. A distended and tender abdomen may indicate spontaneous peritonitis.

LABORATORY FINDINGS Gram's stains of material aspirated from abscesses or bullae may contain gram-negative organisms of one or several morphologic types. Cultures are polymicrobial in over half of the patients; blood cultures may be positive, but less frequently so than in *V. vulnificus* infections. Liver function tests may be abnormal; in the presence of peritonitis, peritoneal fluid shows polymorphonuclear leukocytes, elevated protein concentration, and organisms on Gram's stain or culture. The presence of gas in deeper soft tissues may be appreciated by MRI, CT, or overpenetrated standard radiographic techniques.

DIAGNOSIS AND DIFFERENTIAL DIAGNOSIS The diagnosis is usually suspected from the epidemiologic history of a traumatic or an existing wound exposed to fresh or brackish water, followed by local cellulitis (often with gas formation), increasing pain, and foul discharge. Culture results are confirmatory; bacteremia is rarely demonstrated. The differential diagnosis includes infections due to *Vibrio* species if the water exposure was brackish, streptococcal cellulitis including that due to *S. iniae* if fish culture exposure preceded the infection,[29] and necrotizing fasciitis due to mixed flora in patients with underlying conditions such as diabetes.

TREATMENT Prompt surgical exploration and debridement are essential, often guided by radiologic studies. Most isolates are susceptible to fluoroquinolones and TMP-SMX, either of which can be given as single agents. The third-generation cephalosporins and aminoglycosides other than streptomycin are also effective. Consideration must be given to the polymicrobial nature of these infections, and Gram's stain and culture are essential for antimicrobial decisions.

COURSE AND PROGNOSIS With extensive surgical intervention and appropriate antimicrobial therapy, patients improve rapidly. Prognosis is excellent except when bacteremia is present, which often indicates severe underlying disease and metastatic complications such as peritonitis.

REFERENCES

1. LaForce FM: Anthrax. *Clin Infect Dis* **19**:1009, 1994
2. Green BD et al: Demonstration of a capsule plasmid in *Bacillus anthracis*. *Infect Immun* **49**:291, 1985
3. Singh Y et al: Internalization and processing of *Bacillus anthracis* lethal toxin by toxin-sensitive and -resistant cells. *J Biol Chem* **264**:11099, 1989
4. Gordon VM et al: Adenylate cyclase toxins from *Bacillus anthracis* and *Bordetella pertussis*. *J Biol Chem* **264**:14792, 1989
5. Ivins BE et al: Immunization studies with attenuated strains of *Bacillus anthracis*. *Infect Immun* **52**:454, 1986
6. Knudson GB: Treatment of anthrax in man: History and current concepts. *Military Med* **151**:71, 1986
7. Shlyakhov E, Rubenstein E: Evaluation of the anthraxin skin test for diagnosis of acute and past human anthrax. *Eur J Clin Microbiol Infect Dis* **15**:242, 1996
8. Ronaghy HA et al: Penicillin therapy of human anthrax. *Curr Ther Res* **14**:721, 1972
9. Shlyakhov E, Rubenstein E: Human live anthrax vaccine in the former USSR. *Vaccine* **12**:727, 1994
10. Young EJ: An overview of human brucellosis. *Clin Infect Dis* **21**:283, 1995
11. Yennon AM et al: Effect of age and duration of disease on the clinical manifestations of brucellosis: A study of 73 consecutive patients in Israel. *Isr J Med Sci* **29**:11, 1993
12. Ariza J et al: Characteristics of and risk factors for relapse of brucellosis in humans. *Clin Infect Dis* **20**:1241, 1995
13. Ariza J et al: Characteristic cutaneous lesions in patients with brucellosis. *Arch Dermatol* **125**:380, 1989
14. Berger TG et al: Cutaneous lesions in brucellosis. *Arch Dermatol* **117**:40, 1981
15. Spink WW: The significance of bacterial hypersensitivity in human brucellosis: Studies of infection due to strain 19 *Brucella abortus*. *Ann Intern Med* **47**:861, 1957
16. Ariza J et al: Specific antibody profile in human brucellosis. *Clin Infect Dis* **14**:131, 1992
17. Reboli AC, Farrar WE: *Erysipelothrix rhusiopathiae:* An occupational pathogen. *Clin Microbiol Rev* **2**:354, 1989
18. García-Restoy E et al: Bacteremia due to *Erysipelothrix rhusiopathiae* in immunocompromised hosts without endocarditis. *Rev Infect Dis* **13**:1252, 1991
19. Gorby GL, Peacock JE Jr: *Erysipelothrix rhusiopathiae* endocarditis: Microbiologic, epidemiologic, and clinical features of an occupational disease. *Rev Infect Dis* **10**:317, 1988
20. Nelson E: Five hundred cases of erysipeloid. *Rocky Mountain Med J* **52**:40, 1955
21. Grieco MH, Sheldon C: *Erysipelothrix rhusiopathiae*. *Ann NY Acad Sci* **174**:523, 1970
22. Park C et al: *Erysipelothrix* endocarditis with cutaneous lesion. *South Med J* **69**:1101, 1976
23. Venditti M: Antimicrobial susceptibilities of *Erysipelothrix rhusiopathiae*. *Antimicrob Agents Chemother* **34**:2038, 1990
24. Brown TMcP, Nunemaker JC: Rat-bite fever. A review of the American cases with re-evaluation of etiology. *Bull Johns Hopkins Hosp* **70**:201, 1942
25. Fox JG, Lipman NS: Infections transmitted by large and small laboratory animals. *Infect Dis Clin North Am* **5**:131, 1991
26. Place EH, Sutton LE: Erythema arthriticum epidemicum (Haverhill fever). *Arch Intern Med* **54**:659, 1934
27. Holroyd KJ et al: *Streptobacillus moniliformis* polyarthritis mimicking rheumatoid arthritis: An urban case of rat bite fever. *Am J Med* **85**:711, 1988
28. Anderson D, Marrie TJ: Septic arthritis due to *Streptobacillus moniliformis*. *Arthritis Rheum* **30**:229, 1987
29. Weinstein MR et al: Invasive infections due to *Streptococcus iniae*, a fish pathogen. *N Engl J Med* **337**:589, 1997
30. Dance DAB: Melioidosis: The tip of the iceberg. *Clin Microbiol Rev* **4**:52, 1991
31. Leelarasamee A, Bovornkitti S: Melioidosis: Review and update. *Rev Infect Dis* **11**:413, 1989
32. McCormick JB et al: Human-to-human transmission of *Pseudomonas pseudomallei*. *Ann Intern Med* **83**:512, 1975
33. Chaowogul W et al: Melioidosis: A major cause of community-acquired septicemia in northeastern Thailand. *J Infect Dis* **159**:890, 1989
34. Lumbiganon P, Viengnondha S: Clinical manifestations of melioidosis in children. *Pediatr Infect Dis* **14**:136, 1995

35. Sanford JP, Moore WL Jr: Recrudescent melioidosis: A Southeastern Asian legacy. *Am Rev Respir Dis* **104**:452, 1971

36. Handa R et al: Melioidosis: A rare but not forgotten cause of fever of unknown origin. *Br J Clin Pract* **50**:116, 1996

37. Dance DA et al: Acute suppurative parotitis caused by *Pseudomonas pseudomallei* in children. *J Infect Dis* **159**:654, 1989

38. Suputtamongkol A et al: Ceftazidime vs. amoxicillin clavulanate in the treatment of severe melioidosis. *Clin Infect Dis* **19**:846, 1994

39. Butler T: *Yersinia* infections: Centennial of the discovery of the plague bacillus. *Clin Infect Dis* **19**:655, 1994

40. Portnoy DA et al: Characterization of common virulence plasmids in *Yersinia* species and their role in the expression of outer membrane proteins. *Infect Immun* **43**:108, 1984

41. Mehigh RJ et al: Expression of the low calcium response in *Yersinia pestis. Microbiol Pathogenesis* **6**:203, 1989

42. Centers for Disease Control: Winter plague—Colorado, Washington, Texas 1983–1984. *MMWR* **33**:145, 1984

43. Doll JM et al: Cat-transmitted fatal pneumonic plague in a person who traveled from Colorado to Arizona. *Am J Trop Med Hyg* **51**:109, 1994

44. Orloski KA, Eidson M: *Yersinia pestis* infection in three dogs. *J Am Vet Med Assoc* **207**:316, 1995

45. Centers for Disease Control and Prevention: Fatal human plague—Arizona and Colorado, 1996. *MMWR* **46**:617, 1997

46. Hull HF: Septicemic plague in New Mexico. *J Infect Dis* **155**:113, 1987

47. Markowitz LE et al: Tick-borne tularemia. An outbreak of lymphadenopathy in children. *JAMA* **254**:2922, 1985

48. Capellan J, Fong IW: Tularemia from a cat bite: Case report and review of feline-associated tularemia. *Clin Infect Dis* **16**:472, 1993

49. Kostman JR, DiNubile MJ: Nodular lymphangitis: Distinctive but often unrecognized syndrome. *Ann Intern Med* **118**:883, 1993

50. Evans ME et al: Tularemia: A 30-year experience with 88 cases. *Medicine (Baltimore)* **64**:251, 1985

51. Buchanan TM et al: The tularemia skin test—325 skin tests in 210 persons: Serologic correlation and review of the literature. *Ann Intern Med* **74**:336, 1971

52. Tärnvik A: Nature of protective immunity to *Francisella tularensis. Rev Infect Dis* **11**:440, 1989

53. Enderlin G et al: Streptomycin and alternative agents for the treatment of tularemia. Review of the literature. *Clin Infect Dis* **19**:42, 1994

54. Heath CW Jr et al: Leptospirosis in the United States: Analysis of 483 cases in man, 1949–1961. *N Engl J Med* **273**:857, 915, 1965

55. van Crevel R et al: Leptospirosis in travelers. *Clin Infect Dis* **19**:132, 1994

56. Wong ML et al: Leptospirosis: A childhood disease. *J Pediatr* **90**:532, 1977

57. Daniels WB, Grennan HA: Pretibial fever. *JAMA* **122**:361, 1943

58. Derham RLJ: Leptospirosis as a cause of erythema nodosum. *Br Med J* **2**:403, 1976

59. Turner JS, Willcox PA: Respiratory failure in leptospirosis. *Q J Med* **72**:841, 1989

60. McClain JBL et al: Doxycycline therapy for leptospirosis. *Ann Intern Med* **100**:696, 1984

61. Takafuji ET et al: An efficacy trial of doxycycline chemoprophylaxis against leptospirosis. *N Engl J Med* **310**:497, 1984

62. Emmanouilides CE et al: Leptospirosis complicated by a Jarisch-Herxheimer reaction and adult respiratory distress syndrome. Case report. *Clin Infect Dis* **18**:1004, 1994

63. Weber DJ et al: *Pasteurella multocida* infections. Report of 34 cases and review of the literature. *Medicine (Baltimore)* **63**:133, 1984

64. Koch CA et al: Exposure to domestic cats: Risk factor for *Pasteurella multocida* peritonitis in liver cirrhosis? *Am J Gastroenterol* **91**:1447, 1996

65. Raffi R et al: *Pasteurella multocida* bacteremia: Report of thirteen cases over twelve years and review of the literature. *Scand J Infect Dis* **19**:385, 1987

66. Rosenau A et al: Plasmid-mediated ROB-1 β-lactamase in *Pasteurella multocida* from a human specimen. *Antimicrob Agents Chemother* **35**:2419, 1991

67. Lorber B: Listeriosis. *Clin Infect Dis* **24**:1, 1997

68. Farber JM, Peterkin PI: *Listeria monocytogenes,* a food-borne pathogen. *Microbiol Rev* **55**:476, 1991

69. Schlech WF et al: Epidemic listeriosis—evidence for transmission by food. *N Engl J Med* **308**:203, 1983

70. Stamm AM et al: Listeriosis in renal transplant recipients: Report of an outbreak and review of 102 cases. *Rev Infect Dis* **4**:665, 1982

71. Gellin BC, Broome CV: Listeriosis. *JAMA* **261**:1313, 1989

72. Centers for Disease Control and Prevention: Update: Diphtheria epidemic—New Independent States of the former Soviet Union, January 1995–March 1996. *MMWR* **45**:693, 1996

73. Centers for Disease Control and Prevention: Toxigenic *Corynebacterium diphtheriae*—Northern Plains Indian community, August–October 1996. *MMWR* **46**:506, 1997

74. Belsey MA et al: *Corynebacterium diphtheriae* skin infections in Alabama and Louisiana. A factor in the epidemiology of diphtheria. *N Engl J Med* **280**:135, 1969

75. Koopman JS, Campbell J: The role of cutaneous diphtheria infections in a diphtheria epidemic. *J Infect Dis* **131**:239, 1975

76. Harnish JP et al: Diphtheria among alcoholic urban adults. A decade of experience in Seattle. *Ann Intern Med* **111**:71, 1989

77. Flor-Henry P: Cutaneous diphtheria: Brief historical review qnd discussion of recent literature, with presentation of two cases. *Med Serv J Canada* **17**:823, 1961

78. Adal KA et al: Primary subcutaneous abscess caused by *Rhodococcus equi. Ann Intern Med* **122**:317, 1995

79. Morris JG, Black RE: Medical progress. Cholera and other vibrioses in the United States. *N Engl J Med* **312**:343, 1985

80. Howard RJ, Bennett NT: Infections caused by halophilic marine *Vibrio* bacteria. *Ann Surg* **217**:525, 1993

81. Hally RJ et al: Fatal *Vibrio purahaemolyticus* septicemia in a patient with cirrhosis. A case report and review of the literature. *Dig Dis Sci* **40**:1257, 1995

82. Kontajiannis DP et al: Primary septicemia caused by *Vibrio cholerae* non-01 acquired on Cape Cod, Massachusetts. *Clin Infect Dis* **21**:1330, 1995

83. Gold WL, Salit IE: *Aeromonas hydrophilia* infections of skin and soft tissues: Report of 11 cases and review. *Clin Infect Dis* **16**:69, 1993

84. Ko WC, Chuang Y-C: *Aeromonas* bacteremia: Review of 59 episodes. *Clin Infect Dis* **20**:1298, 1995

85. Janda MJ: Recent advances in the study of the taxonomy, pathogenicity, and infectious syndromes associated with the genus *Aeromonas. Clin Microbiol Rev* **4**:397, 1991

CHAPTER 201

Gerhard Tappeiner
Klaus Wolff

Tuberculosis and Other Mycobacterial Infections

It has been estimated that the genus *Mycobacterium* causes more suffering for humans than all the other bacterial genera combined. Twenty years ago it was assumed that tuberculosis would become extinct in the developed countries, as its incidence decreased at an average rate of 6 percent in the United States and 10 percent in Europe between 1953 and 1985. However, by 1983 it was declared a "global emergency" by the World Health Organization because of a sharp increase (e.g., doubling in sub-Saharan Africa) due largely to the HIV pandemic. One-third of the world's population is estimated to be infected. Currently, it accounts for an estimated 8 to 10 million new cases and 2 to 3 million deaths per year,[1] 98 percent of them in developing countries. It also accounts for 1.5 million new cases and for 500,000 deaths per year among children. It is thought to be responsible for 25 to 30 percent of avoidable deaths and thus has the highest morbidity and mortality of all infectious diseases. In addition, the so-called atypical mycobacteria are increasingly recognized as human pathogens and may be the cause of skin disease more frequently than *M. tuberculosis*.[2]

Obligatory and facultatively pathogenic mycobacteria can be distinguished. In contrast to the obligate pathogens the environmental, facultatively pathogenic mycobacteria do not cause disease by person-to-person spread.[3] Infections due to the latter depend primarily on their occurrence and on individual susceptibility for infection. The immune and tissue responses of the host play a decisive role in determining the type and extent of disease produced by mycobacterial infection. This has been studied extensively in infections with *M. tuberculosis, M. bovis,* and *M. leprae* and, to a lesser degree, with *M. ulcerans.*

CLASSIFICATION OF MYCOBACTERIA

Mycobacteria are acid-fast, weakly gram-positive, nonsporulating, and nonmotile rods. The family Mycobacteriaceae consists of only one genus, *Mycobacteria,* which includes the obligate human pathogens *M. tuberculosis* and the closely related *M. bovis, M. africanum,* and *M. microti* as well as *M. leprae* and a number of facultatively pathogenic and nonpathogenic species, the atypical mycobacteria. Runyon, in the first and still often used classification of atypical mycobacteria, distinguished a slow-growing and a fast-growing group and subdivided the former according to pigment-forming properties in culture: group I—photochromogens, capable of pigment formation upon exposure to light; group II—scotochromogens, capable of pigment production without light exposure; and group III—nonchromogens. Group IV includes all rapid growers.

Today about 60 species are named: 41 of them were included in the Approved Lists of Bacterial Names in 1980.[4] They may be cultivable or not (e.g., *M. leprae, M. genavese*). The main distinction in the group of cultivable mycobacteria, that between the slow growers and the rapid growers, seems to have occurred early in the development of the genus.

For clinical purposes, the organisms may be further subdivided into obligate and facultative pathogens and nonpathogens; a classification scheme of the genus is presented in Table 201-1. *M. leprae* and *M. genavese* have not been included as they have not been grown in culture and thus have not been available for biochemical testing. The listing is not exhaustive, and further mycobacteria may emerge as facultative pathogens.

TABLE 201-1

Classification of Mycobacteria*

SLOW-GROWING MYCOBACTERIA	RUNYON GROUP
Obligate human pathogens[†]	
M. tuberculosis-bovis group including bacillus Calmette-Guérin (BCG) and M. africanum	
Facultative human pathogens	
M. kansasii	I
M. marinum	I
M. simiae	I
M. scrofalaceum	II
M. szulgai	II
M. gordonae	II
M. avium-intracellulare complex	III
M. haemophilum	III
M. ulcerans	III
M. xenopi	III
Nonpathogens	
M. flavescens	II
M. terrae complex	III
M. triviale	III
M. gastri	III

RAPIDLY GROWING MYCOBACTERIA

	RUNYON GROUP
Facultative human pathogens	
M. fortuitum	IV
M. chelonae	IV
M. abscessus	IV
Nonpathogens	
M. smegmatis	IV
M. phlei	IV
M. vaccae	IV
(Others)	

M. leprae and *M. genavese* are not included in this table.
[†]Obligate human pathogens are not included in the Runyon classification.

MYCOBACTERIA AND THE AIDS PANDEMIC

The AIDS pandemic with its profound and progressive suppression of cellular immune functions has led to a resurgence of tuberculosis and to the appearance or recognition of new mycobacterial pathogens. In the United States, the *M. avium-intracellulare* complex is the most common cause of disseminated bacterial infections in AIDS patients, accounting for 20 to 40 percent of cases[5]; it is found much less frequently in European patients. *M. kansasii* is more common than *M. tuberculosis*.[6] Still, the incidence of tuberculosis in AIDS patients is almost 500 times that of the general population.[1]

This sharp increase in pulmonary and bacteremic or disseminated mycobacterial infections has not been paralleled by an equal increase in mycobacterial skin disease, although such cases have been reported. Cutaneous disease in these patients is caused most typically by *M. marinum*, *M. scrofulaceum*, *M. haemophilum*, *M. gordonae*, and the rapid growers.

TUBERCULOSIS OF THE SKIN

Definition and Classification

Tuberculosis of the skin is caused by *M. tuberculosis, M. bovis,* and, under certain conditions, the bacillus Calmette-Guérin (BCG), an attenuated strain of *M. bovis;* the clinical manifestations comprise a considerable number of skin changes, usually subclassified into more or less distinct disease forms. Classification has been attempted according to morphology and, more recently, the mode of infection or the immunologic state of the host, but none of them satisfies completely. The classification used in this chapter distinguishes between exogenous infection and endogenous spread of *M. tuberculosis/bovis;* conditions caused by vaccination with BCG; and a group of eruptions, the tuberculids, which are nosologically and pathogenically less well understood (Table 201-2). Some entities of a nontuberculous nature, which were previously thought to be related to tuberculosis and were thus also termed tuberculids, will be briefly mentioned at the end of this section.

Epidemiology and Incidence

Even though mycobacterial diseases are widespread and serious, the organisms are neither very virulent nor very infectious: only about 5 to 10 percent of infections with *M. tuberculosis* lead to disease; the rate is similarly low for *M. leprae* and is very much lower for the facultative pathogens. Tuberculosis of the skin also has a worldwide distribution; while more prevalent in regions with a cold and humid climate in the past, it now also occurs in the tropics. In European and North American countries, the incidence of skin tuberculosis has shown a steady decline over the past decades. This seems to be true for all countries and parallels the decreasing incidence of pulmonary tuberculosis. A sharp increase of mycobacterial infection has occurred with increasing migrations and with the advent of the AIDS epidemic, but it has not led to a proportional increase of tuberculosis of the skin so far.

In the United States tuberculosis of the skin has always been a rare disease. In Europe it used to be quite common during the first quarter of the twentieth century but now has also become rare. Its two most frequent forms are lupus vulgaris and scrofuloderma; in the tropics, lupus vulgaris is rare, whereas scrofuloderma and verrucous lesions predominate. Lupus vulgaris is more than twice as common in women as in men, while tuberculosis verrucosa cutis is

TABLE 201-2

Classification of Cutaneous Tuberculosis

Exogenous infection	Primary inoculation tuberculosis (infection of the nonimmune host)
	Tuberculosis verrucosa cutis (infection of the immune host)
Endogenous spread	Lupus vulgaris
	Scrofuloderma
	Metastatic tuberculous abscess (tuberculous gumma)
	Acute miliary tuberculosis
	Orificial tuberculosis
Tuberculosis due to BCG vaccination	
Tuberculids	Tuberculids
	Lichen scrofulosorum
	Papulonecrotic tuberculid
	Facultative tuberculids
	Nodular vasculitis
	Erythema nodosum
	Non-tuberculids
	These conditions are not related to tuberculosis but for completeness are discussed in the text

most often found in men. Generalized miliary tuberculosis is seen in infants (and adults with severe immunosuppression or AIDS), as is primary inoculation tuberculosis; scrofuloderma usually occurs in adolescents and the elderly, while lupus vulgaris may affect all age groups.

Etiology and Pathogenesis

M. tuberculosis, M. bovis, and, under certain conditions, the attenuated BCG organism cause all forms of skin tuberculosis. After having gained access to the host's tissues, the mycobacteria multiply intracellularly. Large numbers of mycobacteria are initially found in the tissue. The mere presence of mycobacteria in the skin, however, does not necessarily lead to clinical disease, and it is well to remember that infection with *M. tuberculosis* is not synonymous with tuberculosis.

THE MYCOBACTERIUM Different mammalian species vary in their susceptibility to infection with different mycobacteria. In humans, *M. tuberculosis* and *M. bovis* cause identical skin manifestations. The incidence of skin tuberculosis elicited by these two organisms depends on the exposure to either human or bovine tuberculosis.

In 50 to 90 percent of cases of lupus vulgaris, the bacteria exhibit a virulence that may be as low as that of the attenuated BCG organism. In many forms of skin tuberculosis, the number of bacteria in the lesions is so small that it may be difficult to find them in histologic sections, whereas large numbers of bacteria can be demonstrated in the affected tissues of a primary chancre or of acute miliary tuberculosis.

M. tuberculosis may become dormant in the host tissue. These dormant bacilli are resistant to antimycobacterial drugs and may be responsible for latency and reactivation of mycobacterial disease.[7]

THE HOST   The human species is quite susceptible to tuberculous infections, but differences exist among populations and individuals. Populations whose contact with tuberculosis spans many centuries are, in general, less susceptible than those who have come into contact with mycobacteria recently; genetic factors also play a role. Age, state of health, and somatic type of the individual are of importance, as are environmental factors. In blacks, tuberculosis frequently takes an unfavorable course, but tuberculin sensitivity may be more pronounced than in whites.

After mycobacteria have invaded the host, they may either multiply and lead to progressive disease or their multiplication is checked or completely arrested. The balance between bacterial multiplication and destruction is determined not only by the properties of the invading organisms but also by the ability of the host to control such an infection.

The skin of an individual previously infected with tuberculosis shows an altered inflammatory response upon a second exposure to the organism. An extract containing the specific protein of the mycobacteria (tuberculin) is able to elicit the same, so-called Koch phenomenon, or tuberculin reaction.[8]

THE TUBERCULIN REACTION (THE KOCH PHENOMENON)

The tuberculin reaction is due to delayed-type hypersensitivity, mediated by sensitized T lymphocytes that, when injected into a nonsensitized individual, transfer the hypersensitivity. Sensitization is induced either by the living mycobacterium (e.g., during primary infection with tuberculosis) or, under experimental conditions, with killed bacteria or with bacteria suspended in Freund's adjuvant. The substance that elicited the hypersensitivity reaction in sensitized individuals was designated *tuberculin* by Robert Koch. This "old tuberculin" (OT) was widely used for skin testing but has now been replaced by a purified derivative (purified protein derivative, PPD), which is preferable to OT as its potency and composition are more consistent. Still, even commercial, standardized PPD tuberculins available today are subject to some variation and do not eliminate cross-reactions due to sensitization by other mycobacteria. More recently, a class of tuberculins that are much richer than PPDs in species-specific antigens have been developed and given the generic name *new tuberculins.*

The tuberculin reaction of a sensitized individual may vary in expression, depending on the test dose employed and the route of administration. Local intradermal injection (the method most widely used) leads to the local tuberculin reaction, which usually reaches its maximum intensity after 48 h. It consists of a sharply circumscribed area of erythema and induration and, in highly hypersensitive recipients or after large doses, may lead to a pallid central necrosis.

Tuberculin sensitivity usually develops from 2 to 10 weeks after infection with *M. tuberculosis* and tends to persist throughout life. It may diminish with age or if the infection is treated in its earliest stages. Its intensity may be reduced by conditions that diminish delayed hypersensitivity reactions such as acute viral infections or vaccination with live virus; immunosuppression by drugs, glucocorticoids, disease, or malnutrition; and malignant disease, particularly lymphoma. About 5 percent of individuals with tuberculosis who have none of these conditions still do not react to ordinary intermediate-strength doses of tuberculin.

The state of sensitivity of an individual infected with *M. tuberculosis* is of considerable significance in the pathogenesis of tuberculous skin lesions. Obviously, a primary infection of the skin (tuberculous chancre) will result in clinical manifestations that are quite different from those occurring after inoculation of mycobacteria into the skin of a previously sensitized individual (tuberculosis verrucosa cutis). Similarly, the hematogenous spread of mycobacteria in individuals with low or greatly diminished sensitivity will evolve into a skin disease (miliary tuberculosis of the skin) that is unlike that occurring in persons in whom sensitivity is high (lupus vulgaris).

In patients with clinical tuberculosis, an increase of skin sensitivity usually indicates a favorable prognosis, and in tuberculous skin disease with high levels of skin sensitivity, the number of bacteria within the lesions is small. However, tuberculin sensitivity is not necessary for immunity against *M. tuberculosis,* and sensitivity and immunity do not always parallel each other. There is now sufficient evidence that they are dissociable and that a high degree of tuberculin sensitivity may even be antagonistic to protection. Mycobacterial infection seems to elicit at least two cell-mediated immune responses, both of which produce positive tuberculin tests but vary in their protective efficacy, depending on the site of infection: one is the result of macrophage activation and is protective, while the other is a necrotizing Koch-type reaction that is usually irrelevant or antagonistic to protection.

ROUTE OF INFECTION   The mode of introduction of mycobacteria into the skin and the properties of the tissue components affected are also essential pathogenic factors. The infection may be exogenous (i.e., from an outside source), may occur by autoinoculation, or may be endogenous. Exogenous infection will lead to the tuberculous chancre or to tuberculosis verrucosa cutis, depending on the immunologic state of the host. Lupus vulgaris at the site of BCG vaccination represents another example of exogenous infection, in this instance by attenuated mycobacteria (see below).

Endogenous spread of mycobacteria may occur by continuous extension of a tuberculous process underlying the skin (scrofuloderma), by way of the lymphatics (lupus vulgaris), or by hematogenous dissemination (acute miliary tuberculosis of the skin or lupus vulgaris).

Finally, the structure and vascular supply of the tissue invaded by mycobacteria must also be considered. Lesions developing in the upper dermis assume a clinical appearance and course quite different from those developing in the subcutaneous tissues. Impairment of local blood supply may have an important additive effect, and local injury may act as a localizing factor.

HISTOPATHOLOGY   The hallmark of tuberculosis and infections with some of the slow-growing atypical mycobacteria is the *tubercle.* It consists of an accumulation of epithelioid histocytes with Langhans' giant cells among them and a varying amount of caseation necrosis in the center. This is surrounded by a rim of lymphocytes and monocytes. While this tuberculoid granuloma is highly characteristic of several forms of tuberculosis, it is not pathognomic. Deep fungal infections, syphilis, and leprosy, among other diseases, can produce an identical picture. As in leprosy, the histopathology of skin tuberculosis may be reflective of the host's immune status.

POLYMERASE CHAIN REACTION (PCR)   The detection by PCR of mycobacterial DNA in skin specimens from patients with a variety of tuberculous skin diseases (e.g., lupus vulgaris, papulonecrotic tuberculid, nodular vasculitis) has been used increasingly in recent years to ascertain their mycobacterial etiology.[9–16] While the detection of specific DNA in tissues has yielded valuable information and some surprising results and will conceivably gain im-

portance in the near future,[13] scrupulous interpretation of the results
of these tests in individual patients has yet to be done.[17] In particular, mycobacterial culture will remain the principal method to determine the presence of live mycobacteria and their sensitivity to
antibiotics and to monitor response to therapy.[13]

SKIN DISEASE DUE TO *M. TUBERCULOSIS/ BOVIS* INFECTION

Primary Inoculation Tuberculosis (Tuberculous Chancre; Tuberculous Primary Complex)

Primary inoculation tuberculosis results from the inoculation of mycobacteria into the skin of a host not previously infected with tuberculosis. The tuberculous chancre and the affected regional lymph
nodes constitute the tuberculous primary complex of the skin.

INCIDENCE In 1930 it was estimated to constitute 0.14 percent
of all primary tuberculous lesions; however, it may be not quite as
rare as generally believed. In some regions, particularly in Asia
where the incidence of tuberculosis is still high and where living
conditions and hygiene are poor, primary inoculation tuberculosis
of the skin is not unusual.

Most patients are children, but the lesions may also occur in
adolescents and young adults, particularly in people working in professions related to medicine. All parts of the body may be affected,
but sites of predilection are the face, hands, and lower extremities,
which are readily injured. One-third of the lesions are found on the
mucous membranes of the conjunctiva and oral cavity.

PATHOGENESIS Since tubercle bacilli cannot actively penetrate
intact skin, they are introduced into the tissue at the site of minor
abrasions or wounds. A rare "venereal" inoculation tuberculosis
may occur in healthy individuals after sexual contact with patients
suffering from genitourinary tuberculosis. Lesions in the mouth may
be due to bovine bacilli from nonpasteurized milk and occur after
mucosal trauma or tooth extraction. Primary inoculation tuberculosis following mouth-to-mouth resuscitation has been reported.

The skin lesions appears 2 to 4 weeks after inoculation. Infection
spreads to the regional lymph nodes, producing tuberculous lymphadenitis; with increasing acquired immunity, the process is localized
to the particular region involved.

CLINICAL MANIFESTATIONS The tuberculous chancre initially
presents as a small papule, scab, or wound with little tendency to
heal. A painless ulcer develops, which may be quite insignificant
or may enlarge to attain a diameter of over 5 cm (Fig. 201-1). It is
shallow with a granular or hemorrhagic base studded with miliary
abscesses or covered by necrotic tissue. The ragged edges are undermined and of a reddish-blue hue; as the lesions grow older, they
become more indurated, with thick adherent crusts.

Wounds inoculated with tubercle bacilli may heal temporarily
but break down later, giving rise to granulating ulcers. Mucosal
infections result in painless ulcers or fungating granulomas. Inoculation tuberculosis of the finger may present as painless paronychia; inoculations of mycobacteria in puncture wounds have resulted in subcutaneous abscesses.

A slowly progressing, painless regional lymphadenopathy develops 3 to 8 weeks after the infection (Fig. 201-1) and may rarely
be the only clinical symptom. After weeks or months, cold abscesses may develop that perforate to the surface of the skin and

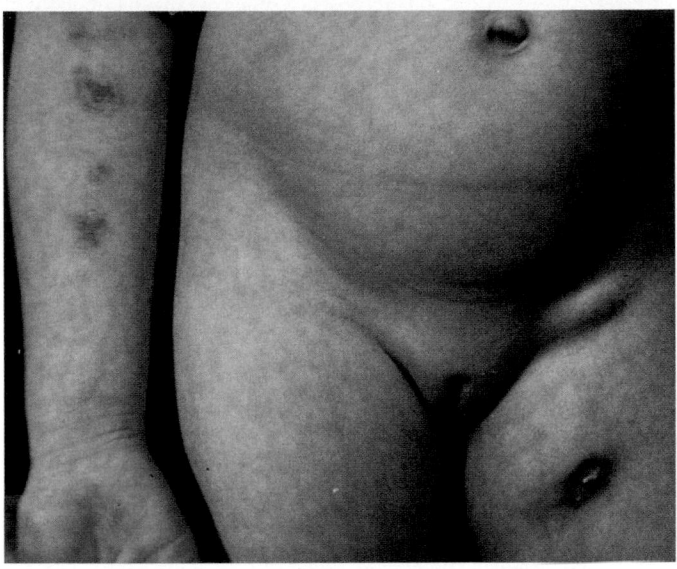

Primary inoculation tuberculosis. Note tuberculous chancre on the
thigh and regional lymphadenopathy. A positive tuberculin test is noted
on the arm.

form sinuses; the lymph nodes draining the primary glands may
also be involved. Body temperature may be slightly raised and,
occasionally, lymph node enlargement, abscess formation, and perforation may take a more acute course. Fever, pain, and inflammatory swelling of the surrounding tissues simulating a pyogenic
infection are present in half the cases.

HISTOPATHOLOGY In the early phase, there is an acute inflammatory reaction and mycobacteria are easily detected. After 3 to 6
weeks, the infiltrate and the regional lymph nodes acquire a tuberculoid appearance.

DIAGNOSIS AND DIFFERENTIAL DIAGNOSIS Lack of awareness of the condition is probably the most common reason for a
diagnostic error. Any ulcer with little or no tendency to heal and
unilateral regional lymphadenopathy in a child should always
arouse suspicion. Acid-fast organisms can be demonstrated in histologic sections or in smears obtained from the primary ulcer and
draining glands in the initial stages of the disease but may be difficult to find in older lesions. The diagnosis is verified by bacterial
culture. The reaction to intradermal PPD is negative in the initial
phases but converts to positive during the course of the disease (Fig.
201-1). A previous tuberculous infection (such as a pulmonary
Ghon focus) should be reasonably well excluded.

The differential diagnosis includes the primary complexes of
syphilis, tularemia, cat-scratch fever, sporotrichosis, and ulcerative
lesions of other mycobacterioses as well as other forms of skin
tuberculosis.

COURSE Without treatment, the condition may last up to 12
months. Lesions heal by scarring, but in rare cases lupus vulgaris
develops at the site of a healed tuberculous chancre. In more than
50 percent of other cases the regional nodes calcify.

Usually, the primary tuberculous complex yields satisfactory immunity, but reactivation of the disease may occur. Hematogenous spread may give rise to tuberculosis of other organs, particularly of the bones and joints. Depending on the size of the inoculum and the age and resistance of the host, primary inoculation tuberculosis may progress to acute miliary disease with fatal outcome. Erythema nodosum is a feature in approximately 10 percent of the cases.

Tuberculosis Verrucosa Cutis (Warty Tuberculosis)

This is a verrucous form of skin tuberculosis due to exogenous reinfection in previously sensitized individuals.

INCIDENCE In western countries, tuberculosis verrucosa cutis is one of the rare forms of skin tuberculosis. It is the most frequent form of tuberculous skin disease in Hong Kong, accounting for more than 40 percent of cases.

PATHOGENESIS This is an inoculation tuberculosis occurring in persons who have acquired a certain degree of immunity. Thus, tests with PPD are highly positive. The inoculation of mycobacteria occurs at sites of minor wounds or abrasions; rarely, inoculation of mycobacteria may occur from the patient's own sputum. In the past, certain professional groups were most liable to acquire warty tuberculosis, particularly physicians, pathologists, medical students, and laboratory attendants, from tuberculous patients or from autopsy material ("verruca necrogenica," "anatomist's wart," "postmortem wart"). Farmers, butchers, and knackers contracted the disease from tuberculous cattle, and in these cases *M. bovis* was responsible. Children can become infected by playing and sitting on ground contaminated with tuberculous sputum.

CLINICAL MANIFESTATIONS Tuberculosis verrucosa usually occurs on the hands, most often on the radial border of the dorsum, and on the fingers. In children, the sites of predilection are the lower extremities. The lesions are asymptomatic and start as a small papule or papulopustule with a purple inflammatory halo; they become hyperkeratotic and are often mistaken for a common wart. Slow growth and peripheral expansion lead to the development of a verrucous plaque with an irregular outline and a papillomatous horny surface (Fig. 201-2). Clefts and fissures discharging pus extend into the underlying infiltrated base, which is brownish-red to purplish. As a rule, tuberculosis verrucosa is solitary, but multiple lesions may occur. The regional lymph nodes are rarely affected. Enlargement of regional lymph nodes may occur after secondary bacterial infection.

HISTOPATHOLOGY (See Fig. 201-3) The most prominent features are pseudoepitheliomatous hyperplasia with marked hyperkeratosis and dense inflammatory infiltrates. Abscesses form in the superficial dermis or within the pseudoepitheliomatous rete pegs. Epithelioid cells and giant cells are found in the midportions of the dermis and beneath the epidermis; typical tubercles may form but are uncommon. Mycobacteria can be demonstrated occasionally. At times, the dermal infiltrate may be nonspecific.

DIAGNOSIS AND DIFFERENTIAL DIAGNOSIS Early lesions resemble warts or keratoses. Hyperkeratotic lupus vulgaris exhibits "apple-jelly" nodules at the periphery and occurs in sites where tuberculosis verrucosa is rare. Blastomycosis, chromomycosis, and

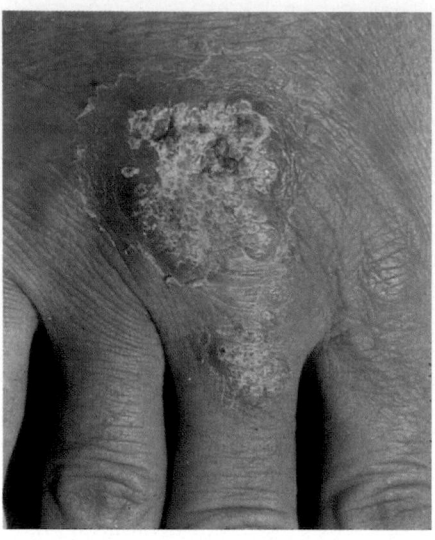

Tuberculosis verrucosa cutis on the back of the hand.

bromoderma may be similar clinically and histopathologically. Negative fungal cultures and small tuberculoid foci are diagnostic aids. Chronic vegetating pyoderma and hyperkeratotic lesions due to other, atypical mycobacteria may be difficult to exclude. Hypertrophic lichen planus is pruritic and more disseminated, and usually other cutaneous and mucosal lesions are found. Tertiary syphilis is not quite as verrucous and is accompanied by diagnostic serologic changes.

COURSE The evolution of the lesions is slow, and, without treatment, the course extends over many years. Secondary pyogenic infection may lead to temporary inflammatory changes of a more acute character, and lymphangitis and regional lymphadenitis ensue. Spontaneous involution does occur and usually results in sunken atrophic scars. Occasionally, ulcerative and sclerotic lesions or fungating granulomas are observed.

FIGURE 201-3

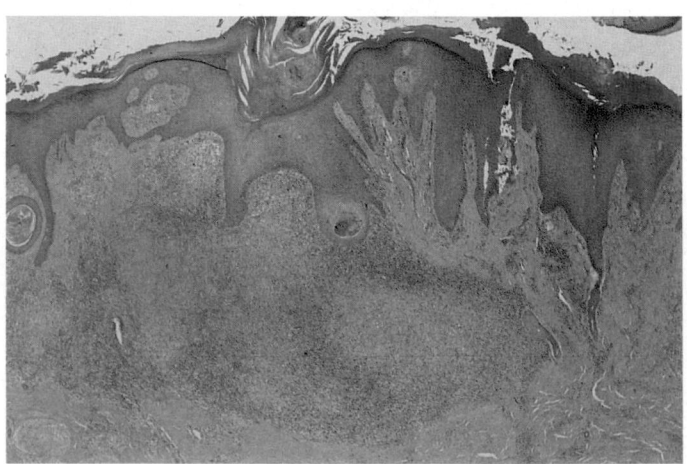

Tuberculosis verrucosa cutis. There is pronounced epidermal hyperplasia. Below the epithelium there is tuberculoid granulation tissue surrounded by lymphocytes.

Lupus Vulgaris

Lupus vulgaris is an extremely chronic and progressive form of tuberculosis of the skin occurring in individuals with moderate immunity and a high degree of tuberculin sensitivity.[18]

INCIDENCE Although the incidence of lupus vulgaris has steadily declined during the past decades, it was estimated in 1960 that some 50,000 new cases occur throughout the world every year. It has always been less common in the United States than in Europe. Females appear to be affected about two to three times as often as males, and all age groups are equally affected.

PATHOGENESIS Lupus vulgaris is a postprimary form of skin tuberculosis arising in previously sensitized individuals with only moderate immunity. The lesions progress steadily and, although spontaneous involution does occur, new lesions arise within old scars. Complete healing is only rarely observed without therapy.

Lupus vulgaris originates from tuberculosis elsewhere in the body by hematogenous, lymphatic, or contiguous spread, most often from cervical adenitis or pulmonary tuberculosis, sometimes from an old, apparently quiescent primary complex. Rarely, it follows primary inoculation tuberculosis or BCG vaccination[19,20] (see below).

CLINICAL MANIFESTATIONS The lesions are usually solitary, but two or more sites may be involved simultaneously; in patients with active pulmonary tuberculosis, multiple foci may develop. In about 90 percent of patients the head and neck are involved. Lupus vulgaris usually starts on the nose or cheek and slowly extends onto adjacent areas. The earlobes are often affected, and solitary patches may be encountered on the scalp. Only a small percentage of the lesions occur on the extremities, and, except for cases with disseminated lupus vulgaris, involvement of the trunk is rare.

In general, lupus vulgaris is asymptomatic. The initial lesion is the lupus macule or papule, characterized by a brownish-red color and a soft, friable consistency. Upon diascopy the infiltrate exhibits a typical apple-jelly color. Early lesions are small, rather ill-defined infiltrates with a smooth surface or covered by a scale. Progression is characterized by an elevation of the lesions and a deeper brownish color (Fig. 201-4). Involution in one area and simultaneous expansion in another result in plaques with a gyrate outline. Its course is

marked by ulceration and scarring; thus, its clinical manifestations are diverse and a number of complications may ensue.

Plane forms manifest as flat plaques with a serpiginous or polycyclic outline and a smooth surface (Figs. 201-4 and 201-5) or psoriasiform scaling; there may be erosions and ulceration. *Hypertrophic forms* appear as soft tumorous growths with a nodular surface (Fig. 201-6) or as epithelial hyperplasia with pronounced hyperkeratosis (Fig. 201-7). Edema, lymphatic stasis, recurrent erysipelas, elephantiasic thickening, and vascular dilation may lead to gross deformity. In *ulcerative forms*, the underlying tissue may be affected by progressive necrosis; when the nasal or auricular

FIGURE 201-5

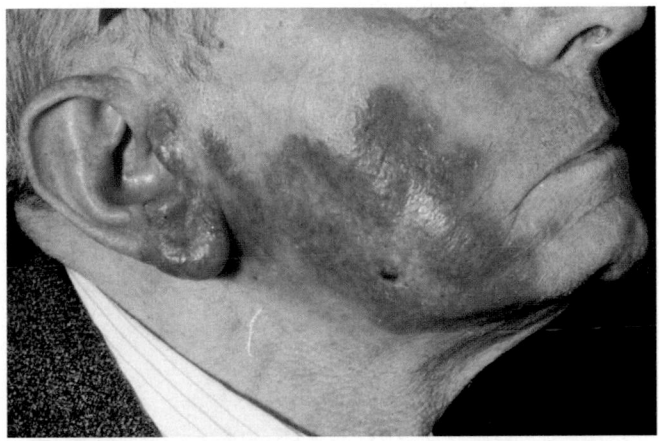

A.

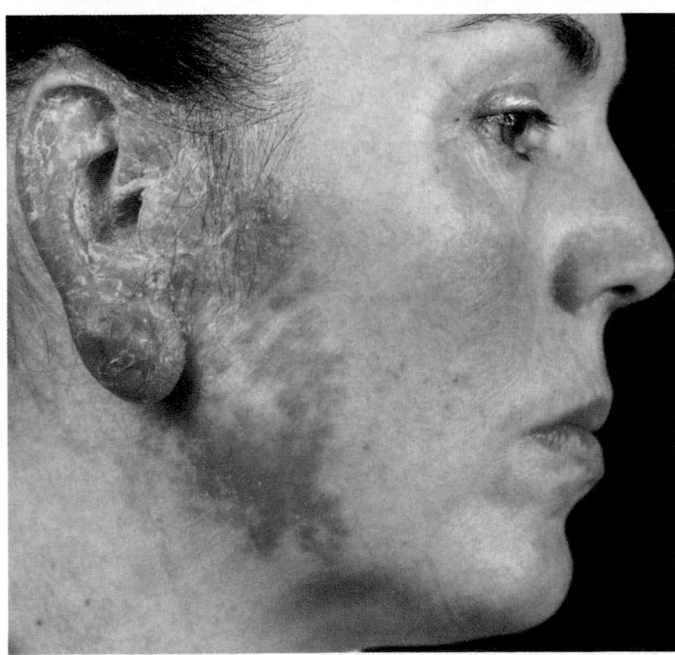

B.

Lupus vulgaris. *A*. Large plaque of lupus vulgaris of 10 years' duration involving the cheek, jaw, and ear. *B*. Reddish-brown plaque which, on diascopy, exhibits the diagnostic yellow-brown color. Note swelling of earlobe and central atrophic scarring on the preauricular lesion.

FIGURE 201-4

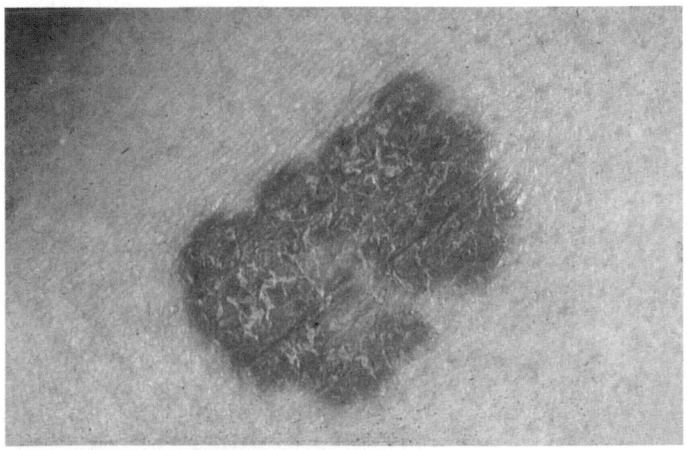

Slightly raised, brownish plaque of lupus vulgaris.

FIGURE 201-6

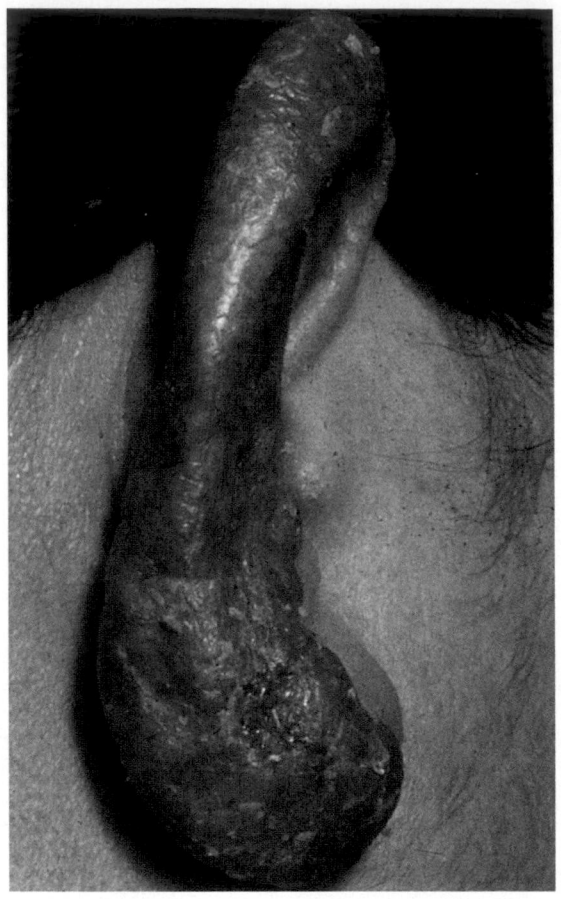

Hypertrophic form of lupus vulgaris involving the ear. There is a soft, brown, tumor-like thickening of the earlobe, which is partially eroded.

FIGURE 201-7

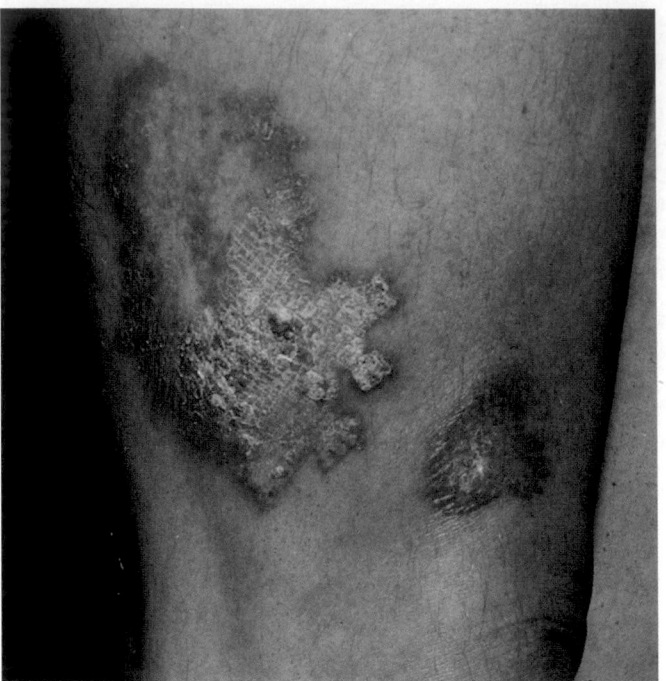

Hyperkeratotic lupus vulgaris on the thigh.

FIGURE 201-8

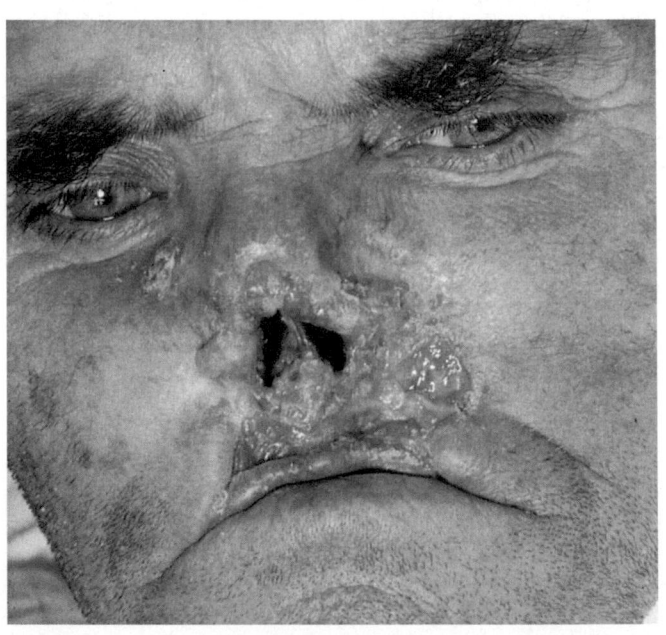

Lupus vulgaris of long duration, having led to the destruction of the nose. Ulcerating squamous cell carcinoma has developed on the upper lip.

cartilage is involved, extensive destruction and disfigurement ensue (Fig. 201-8).

Atrophic scarring, with or without prior ulceration, is a prominent feature of lupus vulgaris. Sometimes, fibrosis is very pronounced and leads to deformations, mutilations and contractures.

Lupus vulgaris of mucous membranes The mucosae may be primarily involved or become affected by the extension of skin lesions. They show small, soft, gray or pink papules, ulcers, or granulating masses that bleed easily. A dry rhinitis is often the only symptom of early nasal lupus, but progressive lesions destroy the cartilage of the nasal septum; cicatricial deformities of the soft palate and stenosis of the larynx may also result.

Lupus postexanthematicus Following a transient impairment of immunity, particularly after measles (thus the term lupus *postexanthematicus*), multiple disseminated lesions may arise simultaneously in different regions of the body due to hematogenous spread from a latent tuberculous focus. During and following the eruption, a previously positive tuberculin test may become negative but will usually revert to positive as the general condition of the patient improves. Clinically and histopathologically, the lesions of postexanthematic lupus are typical for lupus vulgaris, and this distinguishes the condition from acute miliary tuberculosis of the skin.

HISTOPATHOLOGY (See Fig. 201-9) The most prominent feature is the formation of typical tubercles. Secondary changes may be superimposed: epidermal thinning and atrophy or acanthosis with excessive hyperkeratosis or pseudoepitheliomatous hyperplasia. Nonspecific inflammatory reactions may partially conceal the tu-

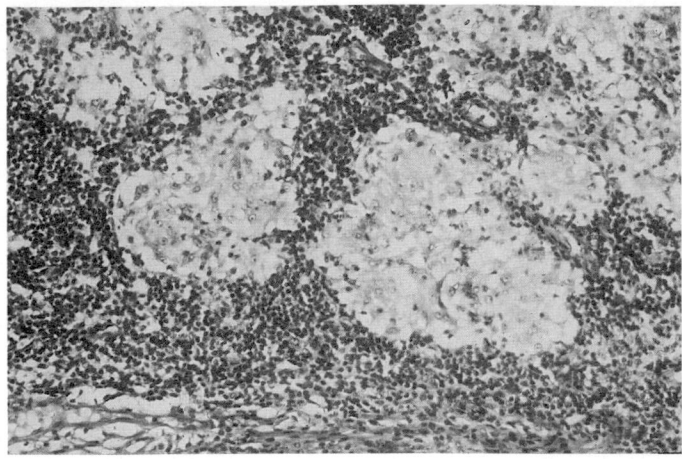

A.

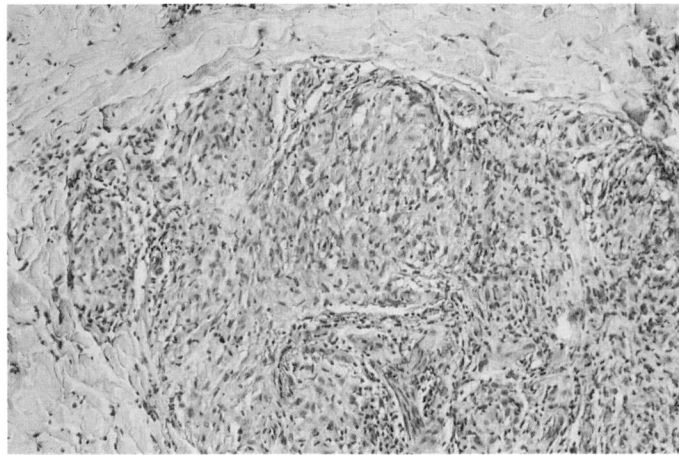

B.

Lupus vulgaris. *A.* Epithelioid cell tubercles surrounded by dense lymphocytic infiltration but without caseation. There are some giant cells of the Langhans type. *B.* Higher magnification of a sarcoid-like epithelioid cell tubercle.

berculous structures. Old lesions are composed chiefly of epithelioid cells and may be impossible to distinguish from sarcoidal infiltrates.

DIAGNOSIS AND DIFFERENTIAL DIAGNOSIS Typical lupus vulgaris plaques do not present diagnostic problems; they have to be distinguished from lesions of sarcoidosis, lymphocytoma, discoid lupus erythematosus, tertiary syphilis, leprosy, blastomycosis or other deep mycotic infections, lupoid leishmaniasis, and chronic vegetating pyodermas. Criteria helpful in the diagnosis are the softness of the lesions, the brownish-red color, and the slow evolution. The apple-jelly nodules revealed by diascopy are highly characteristic; finding them may be decisive, especially in ulcerated, crusted, or hyperkeratotic lesions. Histologic examination and a positive culture for *M. tuberculosis/bovis* confirm the diagnosis. The tuberculin test is strongly positive except for the early phases of postexanthematic lupus.

COURSE Lupus vulgaris is extremely chronic, and without therapy its course usually extends over many years or even decades. Thus, adults or older patients have more extensive lesions than chil-

dren. Although there are periods of relative inactivity, it is progressive and leads to considerable impairment of function and to disfiguration. Contractions result in a reduction of joint mobility, and ulceration and destruction of the cartilaginous structures of the face and scarring lead to cicatricial ectropion with its complications, to microstomia with impairment of speech and food intake, and to other severe mutilations.

The most serious complication of long-standing lupus vulgaris is the development of carcinoma (Fig. 201-8). Early in this century this was estimated to occur in almost 10 percent of patients. Squamous cell carcinomas outnumber basal cell carcinomas by far, and the incidence of metastases is surprisingly high.

THE RELATIONSHIP OF LUPUS VULGARIS TO TUBERCULOSIS OF OTHER ORGANS In 40 percent of patients with lupus vulgaris there is associated tuberculous lymphadenitis, and 10 to 20 percent have pulmonary tuberculosis or tuberculosis of the bones and joints. The morbidity of lupus vulgaris patients from pulmonary tuberculosis is 4 to 10 times higher than in the general population. In some cases, lupus vulgaris may be regarded as a symptom of another tuberculous disease running a serious course.

Scrofuloderma (Tuberculosis Colliquativa Cutis)

Scrofuloderma is a subcutaneous tuberculosis leading to cold abscess formation and a secondary breakdown of the overlying skin.

PATHOGENESIS Scrofuloderma results from contiguous involvement of the skin overlying another tuberculous process, most commonly tuberculous lymphadenitis, tuberculosis of bones and joints, or tuberculous epididymitis. It may affect all age groups, although there is a higher prevalence among children, adolescents, and the aged.

CLINICAL MANIFESTATIONS Tuberculosis colliquativa most often occurs in the parotidal, submandibular, and supraclavicular regions as well as on the lateral aspects of the neck; owing to the involvement of lymph nodes in these areas, the lesions are often bilateral. Lesions on the extremities or on the trunk accompany tuberculous disease of the phalangeal bones, joints, the sternum, and the ribs.

The skin lesions first present as firm, subcutaneous nodules or as a well-defined, freely movable asymptomatic infiltrate. As the infiltrate enlarges it becomes doughy, but it may take months before there is liquefaction with subsequent perforation (Fig. 201-10). Ulcers and sinuses develop and discharge watery and purulent or caseous material. The ulcers are linear or serpiginous with undermined, inverted, bluish edges and uneven, soft, and granulating floors. Sinusoidal tracts undermine the skin, and clefts and dissecting subcutaneous pockets alternate with soft gummatous nodules; scar tracts develop and bridge ulcerative areas or even stretches of normal skin. Tuberculin sensitivity is usually pronounced.

HISTOPATHOLOGY Massive necrosis and abscess formation found in the center of the lesion are nonspecific. However, the periphery of the abscesses or the margins of the sinuses contain tuberculoid granulomas and true tubercles, and *M. tuberculosis* can be found.

DIAGNOSIS AND DIFFERENTIAL DIAGNOSIS *M. avium-intracellulare* lymphadenitis and the more benign *M. scrofulaceum*

FIGURE 201-10

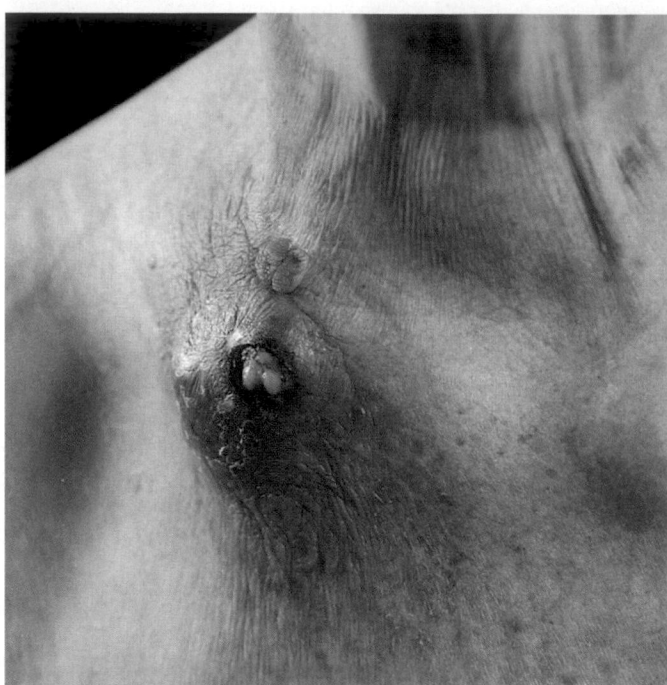

Scrofuloderma in the clavicular region. Note abscess formation, ulceration, and extrusion of purulent and caseous material.

infection have to be excluded by bacterial cultures. If there is an underlying tuberculous lymphadenitis or bone and joint disease, the diagnosis usually presents no difficulty. Syphilitic gums, deep fungal infections, particularly sporotrichosis, actinomycosis, severe forms of acne conglobata, and hidradenitis suppurativa have to be excluded. A confirmation of the clinical diagnosis is achieved by bacterial culture.

COURSE Spontaneous healing does occur, but the course is very protracted and it may take years before the inflammatory and ulcerative lesions have been completely replaced by scar tissue. The typical scars permit a correct diagnosis, even after the process has become quiescent. Lupus vulgaris may develop at the site of scrofuloderma or in its vicinity.

Metastatic Tuberculous Abscess (Tuberculous Gumma)

DEFINITION AND PATHOGENESIS The metastatic tuberculous abscess is due to hematogenous spread of mycobacteria from a primary focus during a period of lowered resistance, resulting in single or multiple cutaneous and subcutaneous lesions. It usually occurs in undernourished children of low socioeconomic status or in immunodeficient or severely immunosuppressed patients; occasionally it may cause a carpal tunnel syndrome.

CLINICAL MANIFESTATIONS Subcutaneous abscesses, which are generally nontender and fluctuant, arise either singly or as multiples on the trunk, extremities, or head (Fig. 201-11*A*); the lesions may invade the overlying skin and break down, forming fistulas

FIGURE 201-11

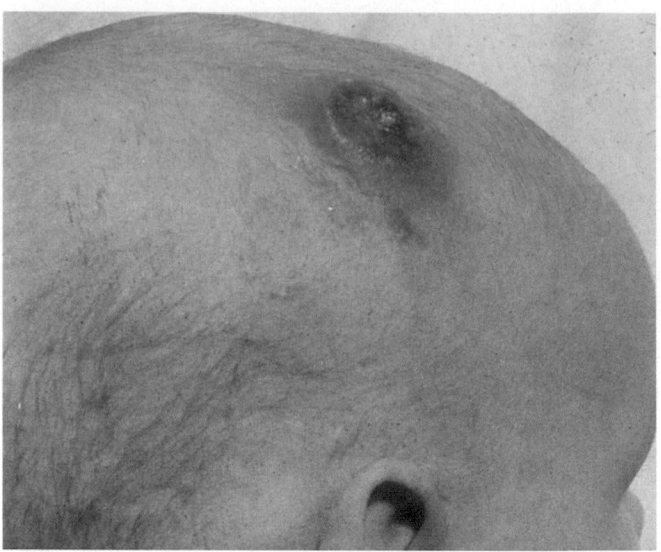

A.

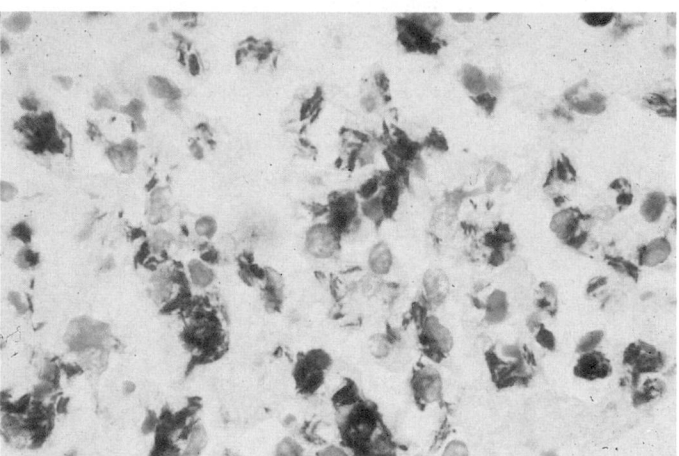

B.

Metastatic tuberculous abscess on the scalp in an infant with combined immunodefiency. *A.* Note abscess formation and discharge of purulent material but little inflammation. *B.* Histopathology of the lesion shown in (*A*) stained for acid-fast bacteria. There are hundreds of intracellular bacteria in this low-power field.

and ulcers. Metastatic tuberculous abscesses may occur with progressive organ tuberculosis or in miliary tuberculosis but may occur without any underlying tuberculous focus. Tuberculin sensitivity is usually lower than in other forms of skin tuberculosis and may be absent in severely ill patients.

HISTOPATHOLOGY As in scrofuloderma, massive necrosis and abscess formation are found. Acid-fast stains usually reveal copious amounts of mycobacteria (Fig. 201-11*B*).

DIAGNOSIS AND DIFFERENTIAL DIAGNOSIS All forms of panniculitis, deep fungal infections, syphilitic gumma, and hidradenitis suppurativa have to be excluded. A confirmation of the clinical diagnosis is obtained by histopathology and bacterial culture.

Orificial Tuberculosis (Tuberculosis Ulcerosa Cutis et Mucosae)

Orificial tuberculosis is a rare form of tuberculosis of the mucous membranes and the skin of the orifices due to autoinoculation of mycobacteria from progressive tuberculosis of internal organs.

PATHOGENESIS   The underlying disease is far advanced pulmonary, intestinal, or, rarely, genitourinary tuberculosis. Mycobacteria shed from these foci in large numbers are inoculated into the mucous membranes of the orifices, usually after trauma. Most patients show a positive intradermal tuberculin reaction, but in terminal stages anergy develops.

CLINICAL MANIFESTATIONS   In orificial tuberculosis of the mouth, the tongue is most frequently affected, particularly the tip and the lateral margins, but the soft and hard palate are also common sites. In far-advanced cases the lips are also involved, and the oral condition often represents an extension of ulcerative tuberculosis of the pharynx and larynx. In cases with intestinal tuberculosis, lesions develop on and around the anus, and in females with active genitourinary disease, the vulva is involved. A small yellowish or reddish nodule appears on the mucosa and breaks down to form a circular or irregular ulcer with a typical punched-out appearance, undermined edges, and soft consistency (Fig. 201-12). Its floor is covered by pseudomembranous material and often exhibits multiple yellowish tubercles and eroded vessels. The surrounding mucosa is swollen, edematous, and inflamed. Lesions may be single or multiple and are extremely painful. The tenderness is often out of proportion to the size of the ulcers and results in dysphagia and inability to eat.

HISTOPATHOLOGY   There is a massive nonspecific inflammatory infiltrate and necrosis, but tubercles with caseation may be found deep in the dermis. Mycobacteria are easily demonstrated.

DIAGNOSIS AND DIFFERENTIAL DIAGNOSIS   Painful ulcers of the mouth in patients with pulmonary tuberculosis should arouse suspicion. Large numbers of acid-fast organisms can be detected in smears, and bacterial culture confirms the diagnosis. Syphilitic lesions, aphthous ulcers, and carcinoma have to be excluded.

FIGURE 201-12

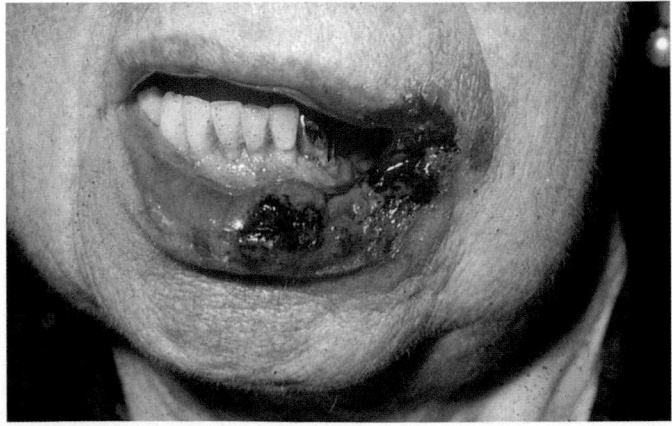

Orificial tuberculosis in advanced cavitary pulmonary tuberculosis.

COURSE   Orificial tuberculosis is a symptom of advanced internal disease with a most unfavorable prognosis. Individuals developing orificial tuberculosis run a downhill course, and as the internal condition progresses, the orificial lesions enlarge and spread.

Acute Miliary Tuberculosis of the Skin (Tuberculosis Cutis Miliaris Disseminata)

DEFINITION AND PATHOGENESIS   Miliary tuberculosis of the skin is an extremely rare skin manifestation of fulminating miliary tuberculosis due to hematogenous dissemination of mycobacteria.[21] The initial focus of infection is either meningeal or pulmonary, and the disease may follow infections such as measles and HIV, which reduce the immunologic defense mechanisms[22]; it most often occurs in babies and infants. Tuberculin sensitivity is usually absent.

CLINICAL MANIFESTATIONS   Disseminated lesions occur on all parts of the body, particularly on the trunk. They consist of minute erythematous macules or papules and purpuric lesions. Sometimes unbilicated vesicles or a central necrosis and crust develop.

HISTOPATHOLOGY   Initially, necrosis and nonspecific inflammatory infiltrates and small abscesses are prominent, and occasionally signs of vasculitis may be seen. Mycobacteria are present both in and around blood vessels. In later stages (if the patient develops immunity), lymphocytic cuffing of the vessels and even tubercles may be observed.

DIAGNOSIS   The eruption occurs in individuals already gravely ill and, because of the severity of the underlying process, often goes unnoticed. A multitude of maculopapular and purpuric rashes must be excluded, but the diagnosis is usually substantiated by the evidence of acute miliary disease of the internal organs.

COURSE   The prognosis is poor, but a favorable outcome after treatment is possible.

BCG Inoculation

Although the effectiveness of vaccination with the attenuated bovine BCG has occasionally been doubted, it has been shown convincingly that it reduces the incidence of childhood tuberculosis substantially, the level of protection being better than 75 percent. Untoward reactions are rare, even in HIV-infected persons[23]; one should nevertheless be aware of these complications.

The normal course of BCG vaccination is as follows: After about 2 weeks, an infiltrated papule develops and, after 6 to 12 weeks, attains a size of about 10 mm, ulcerates, and then slowly heals, leaving a scar. Vaccination may provoke an accelerated reaction if given to a subject previously infected but with a negative tuberculin test. The regional lymph nodes may enlarge but usually heal without breaking down. Tuberculin sensitivity appears 5 to 6 weeks after vaccination.

Nonspecific complications include keloid formation, epithelial cysts, granulomas, eczema, generalized hemorrhagic rashes, erythema nodosum, and other eruptions. After repeated vaccinations, fever, chills, arthralgia, and malaise may occur; anaphylactic shock may be fatal. Hepatic dysfunction and noncaseous granulomas containing the organisms have been observed.

Specific complications comprise tuberculous processes caused by the BCG organism. The large majority of these are lymphoglandular and skin reactions that mimic cutaneous responses to "natural" mycobacterial infection. Their true incidence is difficult to ascertain, but it is extremely low in comparison to the great number of vaccinations performed. Nonfatal generalized complications occur in one or two persons per million; a perforating regional adenitis was seen in 2 percent of vaccinated children in Denmark, and the incidence of postvaccinal lupus vulgaris was estimated to be from five to ten per million. Usually the BCG reactions run a milder course than "spontaneous" tuberculosis of the skin, and they occur more often after revaccination.

Specific lesions following BCG vaccination include the following:

1. Lupus vulgaris may develop at or in the vicinity of the vaccination site after a latency period of several months or after 1 to 3 years.[19,20]
2. Individuals previously sensitive to tuberculin may exhibit a type of Koch's phenomenon. Necrosis and ulceration occur as in normal nonsensitive individuals but with a shorter time course. Regional adenitis is common, and general symptoms may be present.
3. Local subcutaneous abscesses may form if the vaccination material has been injected too deeply into the skin, and excessive ulceration may ensue.
4. Severe regional adenitis is definitely the most common complication and occurs more often in the younger age groups. Scrofuloderma may develop, and suppuration may persist for 6 to 12 months.
5. Generalized tuberculid-like eruptions have rarely been observed.
6. Generalized adenitis, osteitis, and tuberculous foci in distant organs (e.g., the joints) have occurred occasionally.
7. Fatal disease due to generalized BCG tuberculosis is rare— 1 per 10 million vaccinated—and occurs in immunologically compromised individuals.

The Tuberculids

Originally considered to represent recurrent disseminated or systemic skin reactions to toxins of tubercle bacilli, with a tendency to spontaneous involution, the tuberculids were distinguished from "true" cutaneous tuberculosis. They included lichen scrofulosorum, erythema induratum, papulonecrotic tuberculids, lupus miliaris disseminatus faciei, and some other eruptions with rather exotic designations.

During the first half of the twentieth century, tuberculids were eruptions quite familiar to dermatologists, but with the sharp decline and effective chemotherapy of tuberculosis in the developed countries, the tuberculids have also become rare. This does not appear to apply to areas where tuberculosis is still not so uncommon, and with the recent resurgence of tuberculosis in some western countries, some tuberculids have also been observed again.

Their pathogenesis and their relationship to tuberculosis are still poorly understood, and while there is no doubt that for some of them such a relationship exists, there are good reasons to doubt it in others. This relationship is as follows:

1. Mycobacteria. In the early 1900s, "mycobacteria" were "found" in lesions of lupus erythematosus, granuloma annulare, and sarcoidosis. Today, in contrast, it is accepted that mycobacteria cannot be found in tuberculids.

2. Histology. Most tuberculids exhibit tuberculoid features histologically. However, tuberculoid granulomas are produced by a multitude of conditions, and, conversely, "tuberculids" have been described that lacked tuberculoid structures. Therefore, the histologic evidence is of questionable value.

3. Tuberculin sensitivity. The tuberculin reaction is moderate to strong in most patients and in the past was considered positive evidence for the tuberculous nature of the lesions. However, a considerable number of the patients show only low sensitivity, and the reactions may vary within wide limits. Today, it is generally agreed that a positive tuberculin reaction does not establish evidence of the pathogenesis of the tuberculids.

4. Previous and concomitant tuberculosis of other organs. Tuberculous disease was quite common in the first half of the twentieth century, and the chances of finding individuals with evidence of tuberculosis were rather high in the general population. However, in two large series, active tuberculosis was found in only a small percentage of patients with tuberculids and was described to be just as common as, for instance, focal bacterial infections. On the other hand, cases have been published recently in which active tuberculosis and concomitant eruptions satisfying the clinical criteria for tuberculids are documented. The development of lupus vulgaris from lesions of papulonecrotic tuberculid certainly appears to argue in favor of a tuberculous etiology in these cases.

5. Using PCR, *M. tuberculosis* DNA can be detected in skin lesions of erythema induratum (nodular vasculitis) and of papulonecrotic tuberculid.[12] However, a positive PCR result still is rather weak proof for a pathogenic link to *M. tuberculosis*.[17]

6. The therapeutic test. Tuberculostatics have been found beneficial in some cases, and the involution of tuberculid lesions concomitant with the improvement of underlying tuberculosis has been described. However, it should also be kept in mind that some tuberculids tend to involute spontaneously, that some cases do not respond to antituberculous treatment, and that many react equally well to other antibiotics or even to plain rest and nonspecific measures.

In summary, the evidence supporting the tuberculous etiology of tuberculids is largely circumstantial and not always convincing. This term obviously has been used too freely in the past for conditions that are in fact unrelated to tuberculosis; it also is quite clear today that some tuberculids have a multifactorial etiology, and *M. tuberculosis* or its products can, at best, be considered as one of several possible causes. On the other hand, positive evidence disproving the tuberculous nature of some of these eruptions is equally lacking, and in some a relationship to tuberculosis clearly exists.

The following discussion therefore employs a restrictive classification that acknowledges as tuberculids only those conditions for which a reasonable amount of evidence supporting a tuberculous etiopathogenesis exists (Table 201-3). *Tuberculids* comprise only lichen scrofulosorum and papulonecrotic tuberculid. *Facultative tuberculids* are conditions in which *M. tuberculosis* or its antigens can be considered as one of several possible causes: they comprise nodular vasculitis (erythema induratum) and erythema nodosum; finally, *non-tuberculids* are all those conditions that were formerly regarded as tuberculids but are, in fact, unrelated to tuberculosis.

Lichen Scrofulosorum

Lichen scrofulosorum is a lichenoid eruption of minute papules occurring in children and adolescents with tuberculosis.

INCIDENCE AND PATHOGENESIS This uncommon disorder was first recognized by Hebra. It is ascribed to a hematogenous spread of mycobacteria in an individual strongly sensitive to

Tuberculids

Tuberculids (conditions in which *M. tuberculosis/bovis* appears to play a significant role)	1. Lichen scrofulosorum 2. Papulonecrotic tuberculid
Facultative tuberculids (conditions in which *M. tuberculosis/bovis* may be one of several etiopathogenic factors)	1. Nodular vasculitis (erythema induratum) 2. Erythema nodosum
Non-tuberculids (conditions formerly designated tuberculids; there is no relationship to tuberculosis)	1. Lupus miliaris disseminatus faciei 2. Rosacea-like tuberculid 3. Lichenoid tuberculid

M. tuberculosis. Lichen scrofulosorum is usually associated with chronic tuberculous disease of the lymph nodes and bones or with specific pleurisy, but is rare in phthisic patients; it has been observed following BCG vaccination.

CLINICAL MANIFESTATIONS The eruption is asymptomatic and is usually confined to the trunk. The lesions consist of small, firm, follicular or parafollicular papules of a yellowish or pink color; they have a flat top or bear a minute horny spine or fine scales on their surface. Lichenoid grouping is pronounced and results in the formation of rough, discoid plaques that tend to coalesce. The lesions persist for months, but spontaneous involution eventually ensues. Antituberculous therapy results in complete resolution within a matter of weeks.

HISTOPATHOLOGY Superficial tuberculoid granulomas develop around hair follicles but may also occur independent of the adnexae. Mycobacteria are not seen in the sections and cannot be cultured from biopsy material.

DIFFERENTIAL DIAGNOSIS Lichen planus, lichen nitidus, lichenoid secondary syphilis, and micropapular forms of sarcoidosis should be excluded.

Papulonecrotic Tuberculid

This is a symmetric eruption of necrotizing papules appearing in crops and healing with scar formation.

INCIDENCE Reports on papulonecrotic tuberculids were quite common in the older dermatologic and pediatric literature but have become rare. Today the condition still appears to be not so uncommon in populations with a high prevalence of tuberculosis. It occurs preferentially in children or young adults.

PATHOGENESIS As a rule, bacteria cannot be demonstrated in lesions. In a series of 91 cases,[24] lupus vulgaris was seen to evolve from papulonecrotic tuberculids in four patients and *M. tuberculosis* was cultured from two. This suggests that mycobacteria may have been present in the papulonecrotic lesions but does not exclude the possibility that they may have lodged in these lesions secondarily.

In most cases the tuberculin test is positive, and in earlier reports the frequency of associated tuberculous lymph nodes of internal organs has been stressed. In one series, a deep focus of tuberculosis (usually cervical adenopathy—some with scrofuloderma) was found in one-third of patients.[24] A prompt response to antituberculous therapy—irrespective of whether or not a tuberculous focus was known to exist—has been described.

In several studies of skin lesions from patients with papulonecrotic tuberculid,[12,15,25] *M. tuberculosis* DNA has been detected in about 50 percent of patients.

Some forms of papulonecrotic tuberculid have been associated with discoid lupus erythematosus, arthritis, or erythema nodosum and may therefore be triggered by antigens other than those of *M. tuberculosis.*

CLINICAL MANIFESTATIONS Sites of predilection are the extensor aspects of the extremities, buttocks, and lower trunk (Fig. 201-13) with a symmetric distribution. Disseminated crops of dusky red, symptomless, pea-sized papules appear. They may show a central depression and an adherent crust over a crater-like ulcer. If the lesions are seated more deeply, they may enlarge to a diameter of 1 cm and acquire a more livid color. There is spontaneous involution, and pitted scars result. Usually there are no systemic symptoms.

HISTOPATHOLOGY The most characteristic feature is a wedge-shaped necrosis of the upper dermis extending into the epidermis. The inflammatory infiltrate surrounding this necrotic area may be nonspecific but is usually tuberculoid. Involvement of the blood vessels is a cardinal feature and consists of an obliterative and sometimes granulomatous vasculitis leading to thrombosis and complete occlusion of the vascular channels. Recanalization of the vessels may be observed.

DIAGNOSIS AND DIFFERENTIAL DIAGNOSIS The diagnosis should be confirmed by histology. The exclusion of pityriasis lichenoides et varioliformis acuta may present difficulties. Eruptions due to leukocytoclastic necrotizing vasculitis also have to be separated; the history, clinical appearance, and histology help to make the diagnosis. Lichen urticatus, prurigo, and secondary syphilis are easily excluded.

FIGURE 201-13

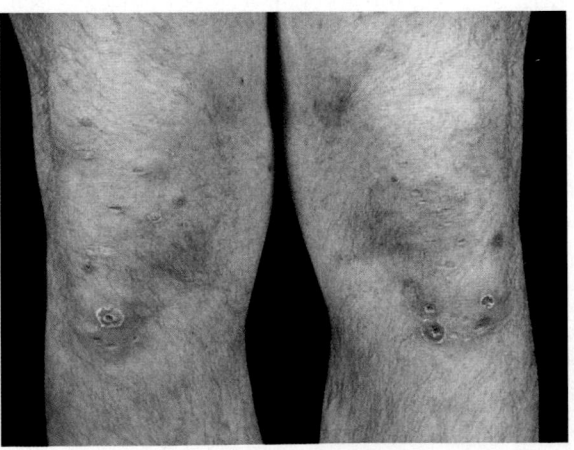

Papulonecrotic tuberculid on the knees.

Nodular Vasculitis (Erythema Induratum of Bazin)
(See Chap. 111)

This is a chronic recurring nodular and ulcerative disorder of the lower legs.

INCIDENCE   Nodular vasculitis is quite common, particularly in Europe. According to one report these cases comprise some 0.1 to 0.2 percent of all dermatologic patients seen at a university hospital. The disease is found predominantly in women; men account only for some 5 to 10 percent of the cases. The age of onset varies from the early teens to old age, but incidence peaks in adolescence and in menopause. There is a seasonal prevalence in winter and early spring.

PATHOGENESIS   Most patients present with erythrocyanotic changes of the lower extremities and have heavy legs, with thick and firm but not edematous skin, and follicular perniosis. Cutis marmorata is common, and the histologic pattern reveals features of vasculitis. The vessels of the patients react abnormally to changes in ambient temperature. Thus, the eruptions are usually associated with exposure to cold.

It has long been thought that transient mycobacteremia produces a reaction that is both induced by and superimposed upon the basic circulatory disorder. However, active tuberculosis is found only rarely in these patients. Similarly, the tuberculin test is of no pathogenic significance; many patients exhibit high sensitivity, but up to 60 percent do not react to a 1:10,000 dilution of OT.

The introductory comments on the relationship of the tuberculids to tuberculosis are particularly relevant to the problem of "erythema induratum." Nodular vasculitis today represents a multifactorial syndrome of lobular panniculitis in which tuberculosis may or may not be one of a multitude of etiologic components. Immune complexes may play a pathogenic role in this condition in which both streptococcal and (in one study) mycobacterial antigens have been found in the lesions. More convincingly, *M. tuberculosis* DNA has been found in about 70 percent of skin specimens from patients using PCR.[10,12,16,26]

Today most authors accept a subdivision of the erythema induratum–nodular vasculitis complex into two groups: one with and one without tuberculous etiology. At the same time, however, it is agreed that the term *erythema induratum* should be reserved for the first group, i.e., for those cases in which the tuberculous origin can be proved. The demonstration of mycobacteria emerges as the only reliable criterion.

Erythema Nodosum (See Chap. 111)

Erythema nodosum is a septal panniculitis of the subcutis; it is associated with a variety of disease processes and results from inflammatory reactions that may be triggered by a multitude of antigenic stimuli including viral, bacterial, and mycobacterial antigens.

"Nontuberculids" (Conditions with Nontuberculous Etiology, Previously Considered Tuberculids)

The older dermatologic literature abounds with entities that were considered tuberculous in nature. Great significance was attached to nomenclature, and the resulting confusion is still reflected in the literature. In none of these conditions has the tuberculous etiology been proved; they all exhibit tuberculoid features histologically; tuberculin sensitivity is low or inconstant; there is no associated tuberculosis; and the incidence of past tuberculous disease among patients with these conditions does not exceed that of the general population. Mycobacteria cannot be recovered from the lesions.

In order to avoid a perpetuation of the terminologic jumble, many of the older designations are not mentioned in this text. Most of them are synonymous.

LUPUS MILIARIS DISSEMINATUS FACIEI   This is a papular eruption of the face, running a chronic course with spontaneous involution. Originally considered a variant of lupus vulgaris or a tuberculid, there is no evidence supporting a link to tuberculosis. The cause and pathogenesis of this condition are unknown, and hence the designation *lupus miliaris disseminatus* is not appropriate. Some cases may represent micropapular forms of sarcoidosis, but most represent a sarcoidal form of rosacea.

The eruption is not uncommon and occurs in adults and adolescents of both sexes. It consists of multiple indolent papules, 1 to 3 mm in diameter, symmetrically distributed in the centrofacial regions (Fig. 201-14), but occasionally more widespread dissemination occurs. The papules develop quite rapidly, may be follicular or nonfollicular, and are distributed at random. Their surface is smooth, their color brownish-red; diascopy reveals an infiltrate similar to the apple-jelly nodules of lupus vulgaris. Histopathology reveals well-defined globular masses of tuberculoid structures in the

FIGURE 201-14

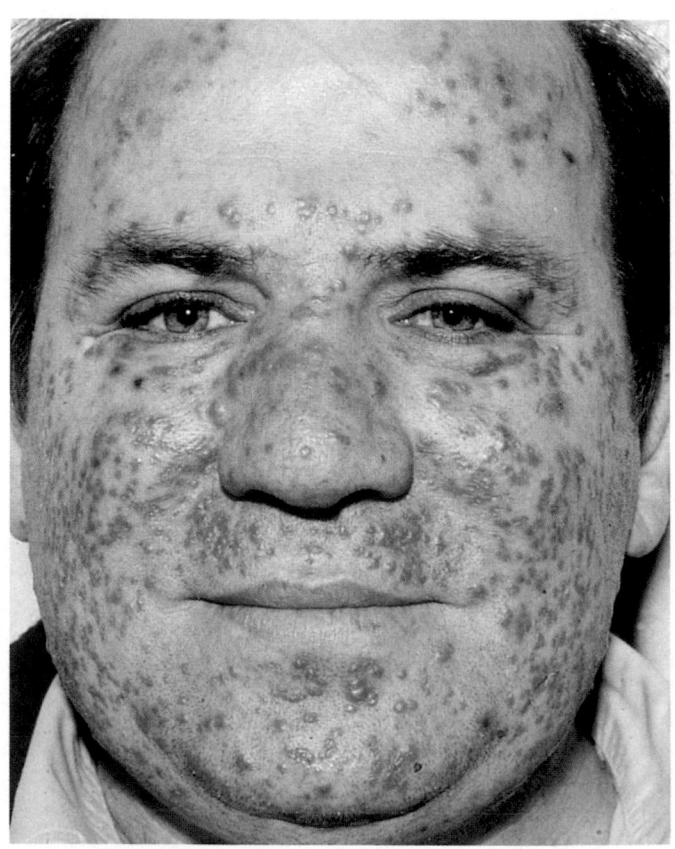

Condition formerly termed *lupus miliaris disseminatus faciei,* with the characteristic distribution of small follicular and nonfollicular papules. This represents a sarcoidal form of rosacea.

upper dermis. In the center there may be frank necrosis, and thus the similarity to true tubercles may be striking. The condition runs a self-limited course. Individual papules regress, leaving pitted atrophic scars, and new crops of lesions arise. After a period of months or up to 2 years, the condition involutes spontaneously. Tetracyclines exert a beneficial effect.

ROSACEA-LIKE TUBERCULID This condition was separated from ordinary rosacea on the basis of its tuberculoid histopathology. It is largely agreed that rosacea-like tuberculid is simply a micropapular form of rosacea with pronounced tuberculoid features.

LICHENOID TUBERCULID[27] This condition probably also represents a sarcoidal reaction. Clinically, there is a sudden symmetric eruption, preferentially localized on the extremities but with a tendency to generalization. The lesions are brown to violaceous papules, with a diameter of 3 to 5 mm. They may be capped by an adherent scale, and teleangiectases are present. Grouping and coalescence are prominent, and annular lesions may be formed. Involution results in brownish macules but no scarring.

Histopathologically, well-demarcated "tubercles" composed chiefly of epithelioid cells are found in the superficial and midportions of the dermis. They show a tendency for perivascular arrangement, and central necrosis is quite common.

Therapy of Skin Tuberculosis

In many respects the management of skin tuberculosis follows the same guidelines and has similar implications as that of tuberculosis of other organs. Chemotherapy is usually the treatment of choice, but ancillary measures may be required to provide the patient with optimal care. The type of cutaneous involvement, the stage of the disease, the level of immunity, and the general condition of the patient are important factors to be considered. Cutaneous tuberculosis associated with mycobacterial disease of internal organs requires a well-coordinated, multidisciplinary plan of therapy.

CHEMOTHERAPY First-line drugs that are highly effective and are used mainly in the initial treatment of susceptible organisms are isoniazid, rifampin, aminoglycosides, and ethambutol. Second-line drugs used mainly in the treatment of patients with drug-resistant mycobacteria are pyrazinamide, ethionamide, viomycin, kanamycin, capreomycin, and cycloserine. The quinolones and particularly their fluorinated derivatives are active against *M. tuberculosis* and a number of other mycobacteria in vitro and thus may gain therapeutic importance in the future.

Isoniazid remains the mainstay of antituberculous therapy. It is both tuberculostatic and tuberculocidal in vitro. It penetrates into all body fluids and cells and also into sclerotic tissue so that it is effective even in old fibrotic lesions. The common daily dose of the drug is 5 mg/kg with a maximum of 300 mg. Side effects seen in 5.4 percent of patients treated include fever (1.2 percent), skin eruptions (2.0 percent), peripheral neuritis (0.2 percent), hepatotoxicity, and hematologic complications (agranulocytosis, eosinophilia, anemia, and thrombocytopenia). Pyridoxine should be given concomitantly to prevent peripheral neuropathy, which may otherwise occur in as many as 20 percent of patients.

Pyrazinamide should be given in a dose of 15 to 30 mg/kg with a maximum of 2 g daily.

Ethambutol, primarily a bacteriostatic drug given in doses of 15 to 25 mg/kg, is always used in combination with other drugs, usually rifampin and isoniazid. It accumulates in patients with impaired renal function and should not be given to children under 13 years of age. The incidence of side effects is low.

Rifampin is one of the most effective drugs for the treatment of tuberculosis. It should not be used alone as mycobacteria rapidly develop resistance in a one-step process. Although it produces a number of side effects, the incidence of these is low, seldom necessitating interruption of treatment. Rifampin is administered as a single oral dose of 600 mg/day, and patients should be warned that the drug may impart an orange stain to excretions, including saliva.

Streptomycin, a time-honored antibiotic in the treatment of tuberculosis, is bactericidal for *M. tuberculosis* in vitro but its activity in vivo is essentially suppressive; it does not penetrate cell membranes (and thus cannot kill intracellular organisms). The toxicity of streptomycin prohibits continuous long-term therapy; nearly 75 percent of patients given 2 g of streptomycin daily for 60 to 120 days develop vestibular disturbances and impairment of hearing. Other side effects include peripheral neuropathy, dysfunction of the optic nerve, rashes, fever, exfoliative dermatitis, and blood dyscrasias, but there is less nephrotoxicity than with other aminoglycoside antibiotics. Streptomycin is never used alone in the treatment of tuberculosis and since other drugs have become available its use has been sharply reduced. It is given in doses of 1 to 2 g/day; it is usually combined with two other drugs and is employed in the more serious forms of tuberculosis.

DRUG COMBINATIONS AND REGIMENS The aim of chemotherapy for tuberculosis is to cure the disease as rapidly as possible, to prevent the emergence of resistant strains, and to prevent relapses. The American Thoracic Society and the Centers for Disease Control and Prevention recommend the following regimen,[28] which comprises an initial, intensive phase and a continuation phase. Phase I is directed towards the rapid destruction of large populations of multiplying mycobacteria and therefore consists of initial, intensive chemotherapy: Daily isoniazid, rifampin, pyrazinamide, and either ethambutol or streptomycin for 8 weeks; ethambutol or streptomycin may be discontinued if the mycobacteria prove susceptible to isoniazid and rifampin or in areas where isoniazid resistance is less than 4 percent. Phase II aims at the elimination of remaining, "dormant" organisms: if they are susceptible to isoniazid and rifampin, these drugs are given either daily, three times weekly, or twice weekly for 16 weeks. If resistant mycobacteria are cultivated, the treatment regimen must be adapted accordingly.

Other treatment options on the basis of drug administration only two or three times weekly are also available but may be instituted only if "directly observed therapy" is possible.

SPECIAL CONSIDERATIONS IN THE THERAPY OF TUBERCULOSIS OF THE SKIN Essentially, the treatment of tuberculosis of the skin is that of tuberculosis in general. A full antituberculous regimen is administered, even in localized forms of skin tuberculosis where a primary focus or evidence of an underlying organ tuberculosis or tuberculosis of lymph nodes exists. Special considerations may apply to tuberculosis verrucosa cutis and localized forms of lupus vulgaris without evidence of associated internal tuberculosis, for which isoniazid has been given alone with a high cure rate. Prolonged treatment, extending up to 12 months, is also necessary in these forms of lupus vulgaris, and total doses of 80 to 140 g may be required. As viable mycobacteria have been cultured from clinically healed lesions, treatment should be continued for at least 2 months after complete involution of the lesions. If, however, there is concomitant internal tuberculosis or if drug resistance emerges, combination therapy is mandatory also in localized lupus vulgaris.

Careful observation and follow-up are essential. Surgical intervention is quite important in the treatment of scrofuloderma. It reduces morbidity and shortens the period necessary for chemotherapy. Small lesions of lupus vulgaris or of tuberculosis verrucosa cutis are also best excised, but tuberculostatics should be given concomitantly. Plastic surgery is important as a corrective measure in long-standing lupus vulgaris with mutilation.

OTHER MYCOBACTERIAL DISEASES

Historic Aspects

Beside the overshadowing problem of infectious disease caused by *M. leprae* or *M. tuberculosis,* probably the largest single cause of infectious disease worldwide, the pathogenic potential of other slow-growing mycobacterial species has only been recognized in the past five decades. The reason for this is in part that these infections usually closely mimic infections with *M. tuberculosis* or, in rare instances, with other organisms, and in part their strict and often unusual culture requirements.

M. ulcerans was identified as the cause of an ulcerating skin condition in Australia in 1948 and in the Buruli district of Uganda (hence the name *Buruli ulcer*) in 1958. *M. marinum,* which has been known since 1926, was isolated from patients with swimming-pool granuloma in 1954. Several other mycobacteria have since been identified as pathogens, producing a wide variety of clinical symptoms,[2,29,30] and further mycobacterial species may be found to cause disease in the future.

The rapid growers have been known as human pathogens since 1938, when Da Costa isolated an organism, which he named *M. fortuitum,* from a postinjection skin abscess.

A current classification of these mycobacteria is found in Table 201-1 and is discussed at the beginning of this chapter.

Identification of Mycobacteria

As in other infectious diseases, the diagnosis of mycobacterial infection depends on the identification of the microorganism isolated from the host. Specimens should be sent to a special laboratory familiar with the culture requirements of mycobacteria, as these vary somewhat from those of other microorganisms; correct incubation temperatures, special media, and prolonged times in culture as well as proper identification procedures are needed.

Antigens for intradermal skin testing (PPDs) of many of the clinically relevant mycobacterial species have been prepared in analogy to PPD from *M. tuberculosis,* but are of very limited use.

Pathology and Pathogenesis

These infections are thought to be the cause of mycobacterial skin disease more often than *M. tuberculosis*[2]; they tend to occur as sporadic cases, but certain types of exposure may lead to small community outbreaks. As in *M. tuberculosis* infection, any organ or organ system may be affected (Table 201-4), but there seems to be much less tendency to dissemination.

Pulmonary infections, which most frequently occur in patients with a ventilatory defect (e.g., after long-term silica exposure), are pathologically indistinguishable from tuberculosis. Only two organ-

TABLE 201-4

Mycobacterial Infections

	ORGAN INVOLVEMENT	
MYCOBACTERIAL SPECIES	**SKIN, SUBCUTIS**	**LYMPH NODES, LUNGS, OTHER**
M. tuberculosis-ovis complex (including *M. africanum* and bacillus Calmette-Guérin)	+	+
M. marinum	+	−
M. ulcerans	+	−
M. kansasii	+	+
M. avium-intracellulare complex (including *M. scrofulaceum*)	+	+
M. gordonae	+	−
M. haemophilum	+	−
Rapid growers		
M. fortuitum, M. chelonae, M. abscessus	+	−

isms, *M. ulcerans* and *M. marinum,* cause a disease with a distinct clinical picture. In contrast to *M. tuberculosis,* atypical mycobacteria are usually acquired from environmental sources (water, soil), and their occurrence reflects their natural distribution. These mycobacteria are widely distributed in different environments and are usually commensals or saprophytes rather than pathogens. An immunosuppressed state of the host or damage to a particular organ (e.g., in *M. kansasii* infection of the lung) facilitates these infections.

In recent years, a number of patients have developed infections with fast-growing mycobacteria after minor or major surgical procedures. Infections with atypical mycobacteria usually run a more benign and limited course than those with *M. tuberculosis.* As a rule, they are much less responsive to antituberculous drugs but may be sensitive to other chemotherapeutic agents.

New mycobacterial pathogens are described from time to time, suggesting that we do not yet appreciate the full pathogenic potential of this genus. It seems desirable to develop a unifying concept of mycobacterial disease and its treatment, but at the present time, our knowledge in this area is not advanced enough to allow us to do so. Thus, mycobacterial skin infections are discussed here according to their causative organisms.

SKIN INFECTIONS WITH ATYPICAL MYCOBACTERIA

M. marinum

This mycobacterium occurs in fresh and salt water, including swimming pools (thus the older name *M. balnei*) and fish tanks.

CLINICAL MANIFESTATIONS The disease begins as a violaceous papule at the site of a trauma about 2 to 3 weeks after inoculation. Patients may present with a nodule or a psoriasiform or verrucous plaque at the site of inoculation, usually the hands, feet, elbows, or knees (Fig. 201-15); the lesions may ulcerate. As a rule they are solitary, but occasionally sporotrichoid spreading occurs. The lesions frequently heal spontaneously within 1 to 2 years, with residual scarring. Sometimes penetration to underlying structures (bursae, joints) may occur. Regional lymph nodes are, as a rule, not involved. Occasionally the lesions are suppurative rather than granulomatous and may be multiple in normal or immunosuppressed hosts. Probably many of the cases described in the older literature and thought to represent "inoculation lupus vulgaris" as well as "swimmer's lupus" have in fact been due to *M. marinum* infection.

HISTOPATHOLOGY   There is a tuberculoid inflammatory infiltrate in the dermis, sometimes with abscess formation.

DIAGNOSIS AND DIFFERENTIAL DIAGNOSIS   As in all mycobacterial diseases, the diagnosis requires a high index of suspicion. An appropriate history (handling of fish, use of swimming pools) and the presence of a tuberculoid granuloma on histopathologic examination are suggestive. Skin testing with PPD is generally not found to be helpful. Many other granulomatous infectious processes of the skin have to be considered in the differential diagnosis; depending on the geographic area, other mycobacterial infections, blastomycosis, coccidioidomycosis, histoplasmosis, and sporotrichosis as well as nocardiosis, tertiary syphilis, and yaws have to be ruled out.

FIGURE 201-15

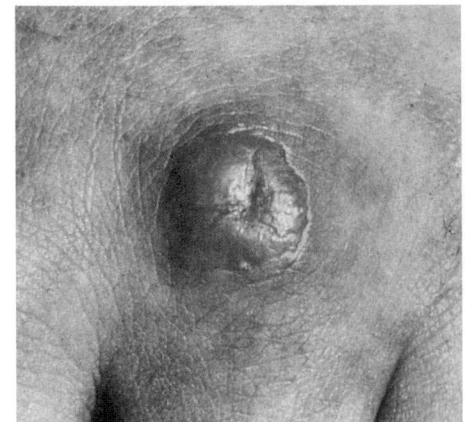
A.

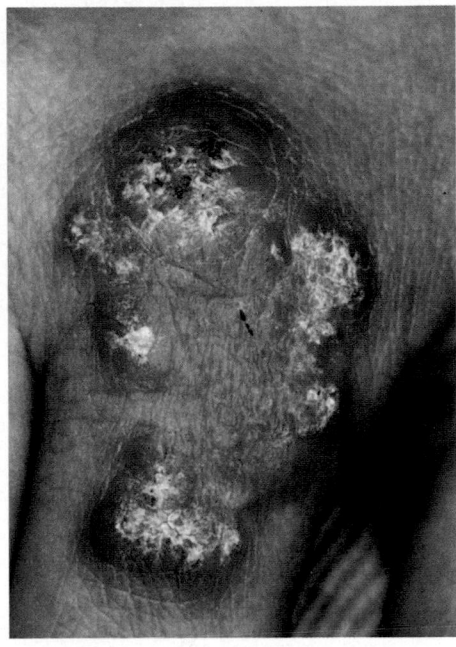
B.

A. *M. marinum* infection on the back of the hand. Granulomatous nodular lesion with central ulceration at the site of inoculation. (*Courtesy of A. Kuhlwein, MD.*) B. Verrucous, violaceous plaque with central spontaneous clearing occurring at the site of an abrasion sustained in a fish tank. The lesion was caused by *M. marinum.*

TREATMENT   Like most atypical mycobacteria, *M. marinum* is poorly susceptible to antituberculous drugs, but spontaneous healing occurs frequently. Minocycline, 200 mg/day for 1 to 2 months, is the treatment of choice. In refractory cases the diagnosis should be reevaluated, and surgical therapy may be considered.

M. ulcerans

The natural habitat of *M. ulcerans* is still not known, and it has never been found outside the human body, but the disease occurs in wet, marshy or swampy areas.

CLINICAL MANIFESTATIONS   The disease is found most often in children and young adults; there is a female prevalence. After an incubation period of about 3 months, a painless subcutaneous swelling develops. The nodule gradually enlarges and eventually ulcerates; a blister may develop before ulceration. The ulcer is deeply undermined, and necrotic fat is exposed (Fig. 201-16). The nodule as well as the ulcer are painless, and the patient continues to feel well. The lesions may occur anywhere on the body but tend to be limited to the extremities in adults; they may be large, involving a whole limb. The ulceration may persist for months and years, and healing and progression of the ulceration may be seen in the same patient. However, this may lead to an appreciable and sometimes disabling amount of scarring and to lymphedema. Neither lymphadenopathy nor any constitutional signs appear at any time of the disease process if it is not complicated by bacterial superinfection.

HISTOPATHOLOGY   Central necrosis, originating in the interlobular septa of the subcutaneous fat, is surrounded by granulation tissue with giant cells but no typical caseation necrosis or tubercles. Acid-fast organisms can always be demonstrated in tissue sections of the lesions.

DIAGNOSIS AND DIFFERENTIAL DIAGNOSIS   Diagnosis is confirmed on the basis of histopathology and microbial culture from a subcutaneous node or an ulcer in an individual with an appropriate history.

The differential diagnosis of *M. ulcerans* infection depends on the stage of the disease. The subcutaneous nodule or node must be distinguished from a variety of processes, such as foreign body granuloma, phycomycosis, nodular fasciitis, panniculitis, nodular vasculitis, sebaceous cysts, or appendageal tumors. When the ulcerative stage is reached, necrotizing cellulitis, blastomycosis and other deep fungus infections, pyoderma gangrenosum, and suppurative panniculitis have to be considered.

TREATMENT   The treatment of choice is simple excision of the early lesion; when ulceration has developed, wide excision and skin grafting are necessary. Local heat therapy, hyperbaric oxygen, and chemotherapy with rifampin and trimethoprim-sulfamethoxazole (TMPS) have been shown to be of some value. BCG vaccination of exposed populations seems to provide about the same amount of protection as in tuberculosis and tuberculoid leprosy. Clofazimine has been shown to be ineffective.

FIGURE 201-16

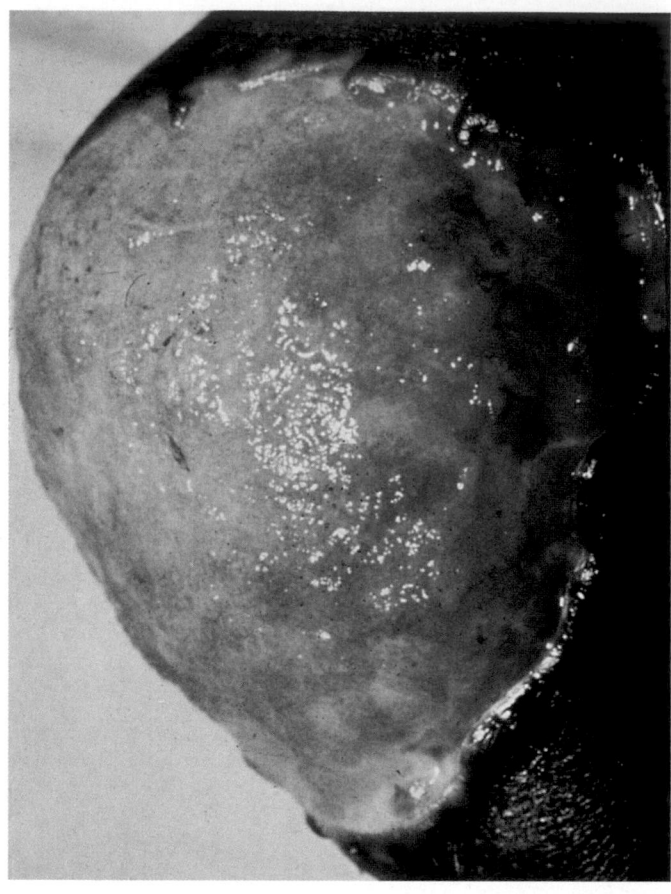

M. ulcerans infection in a child in Uganda. The knee bears an ulcer with an infiltrated undermined margin and a base of necrotic adipose and connective tissue. (*Courtesy of M. Dietrich, MD.*)

M. kansasii

This is the atypical mycobacterium most closely related to *M. tuberculosis*. The organism is usually acquired from the environment; it has been found in tap water and in wild and domestic animals. In the United States, the disease is endemic in Texas, Louisiana, the Chicago area, and California, and it is also endemic in Japan. Skin disease due to *M. kansasii* usually occurs in adults with or without an underlying condition such as Hodgkin's disease, immunosuppression for renal transplantation, or AIDS. The route of entry is usually through minor trauma such as a puncture wound.

CLINICAL MANIFESTATIONS *M. kansasii* infection may present in several forms: most frequently, a sporotrichoid condition develops; sometimes, the subcutaneous tissues and deep structures are affected and this has resulted in a carpal tunnel syndrome or in joint disease; an ulcerated plaque may also develop as a metastatic lesion; disseminated disease due to *M. kansasii* infection occurs in immunosuppressed patients, and such patients have cellulitis and abscesses rather than granulomatous lesions. The most commonly affected organ is the lung, usually in patients with other pulmonary conditions (silicosis, emphysema). It may also cause cervical lymphadenopathy. As with *M. tuberculosis*, *M. kansasii* present in

nasopharyngeal secretions can lead to periorificial cutaneous infection. These infections usually progress slowly, although a chronic persistent lesion or even spontaneous regression may occur. Therefore, drug therapy should be initiated as soon as the diagnosis is made.

HISTOPATHOLOGY *M. kansasii* infection is histopathologically indistinguishable from tuberculosis.

DIAGNOSIS AND DIFFERENTIAL DIAGNOSIS The diagnosis can only be confirmed by the demonstration of *M. kansasii* in bacterial culture. The differential diagnosis includes sporotrichosis, tuberculosis, and other granulomatous infections of the skin (e.g., with *M. marinum* or *M. chelonae*).

TREATMENT *M. kansasii* is more susceptible to antituberculous drugs than other atypical mycobacteria, particularly to streptomycin, rifampin, and ethambutol. Multiple-drug regimens have been of value, and the in vivo response does not always parallel in vitro sensitivities. As in *M. marinum* infection, treatment with minocycline hydrochloride, 200 mg daily, has resulted in complete resolution of sporotrichoid *M. kansasii* infection in one case, but more extensive studies of this regimen are not yet available. In localized skin disease or in cervical lymphadenitis, surgical excision should be performed.

M. scrofulaceum

This organism is widely distributed and has been isolated from tap water, soil, and other environmental sources. Infection probably occurs in children by accidental infestation or inhalation.

CLINICAL MANIFESTATIONS The usual manifestation of *M. scrofulaceum* infection is cervical lymphadenitis in young children, mainly between the ages of 1 to 3 years. Submandibular and submaxillary nodes are usually involved, rather than the tonsillar and anterior cervical nodes characteristic for *M. tuberculosis* infection. The disease is frequently unilateral. There are no constitutional symptoms except mild pain in the neck, but the involved lymph nodes enlarge slowly over several weeks, and eventually ulceration and draining are seen. There is no evidence of lung or other organ involvement, but in older individuals with preexisting lung disease, pulmonary infection may rarely occur; very rarely, there is disseminated infection.[31] Usually, however, the disease is benign and self-limited.

HISTOPATHOLOGY *M. scrofulaceum* lymphadenitis is indistinguishable histopathologically from tuberculous disease.

DIAGNOSIS AND DIFFERENTIAL DIAGNOSIS Unilateral cervical lymphadenitis in a young child with a normal chest roentgenogram should suggest this diagnosis. Skin testing with PPD-S is usually negative. The diagnosis needs confirmation by bacterial culture from a biopsy specimen. Differential diagnoses include all causes of cervical lymphopathy, both infectious and neoplastic.

TREATMENT *M. scrofulaceum* is not very sensitive to antituberculous drugs; the treatment of choice for cutaneous lymph node disease is surgical excision. For more widespread disease, combinations of antituberculous drugs have to be tried until results from bacterial sensitivity testing are available.

M. avium-intracellulare

This species complex encompasses organisms with a wide variety of microbiologic and pathogenic properties. Well over 20 subtypes can be separated by immunologic techniques, although this is not necessary for clinical purposes.

They are usually grouped together with *M. scrofulaceum* in the so-called MAIS (*M. avium-intracellulare–scrofulaceum*) complex but are separated here for clinical reasons. While *M. scrofulaceum* produces only a benign, self-limited lymphadenopathy with no organ involvement, *M. avium-intracellulare* usually causes lung disease or, less frequently, osteomyelitis. It may also cause a cervical lymphadenitis with sinus formation that is clinically indistinguishable from tuberculous scrofuloderma.

CLINICAL MANIFESTATIONS Primary skin disease due to *M. avium-intracellulare* has been reported in rare instances, presenting as single or multiple painless, scaling, yellowish plaques, sometimes resembling lupus vulgaris[32] or subcutaneous nodules,[33] with a tendency to ulceration and a slowly progressing, chronic course. Sometimes, skin involvement occurs secondary to disseminated infection with *M. avium-intracellulare*. Skin lesions have included generalized cutaneous ulcerations, multiple cutaneous granulomas, infiltrated erythematous lesions on the extremities, pustular lesions or soft tissue swelling. *M. avium-intracellulare* infections are an important cause of morbidity in AIDS patients (see Chap. 226).

HISTOPATHOLOGY This shows noncaseating tuberculoid granulomas. Acid-fast bacilli can be found within giant cells and extracellularly.

DIAGNOSIS AND DIFFERENTIAL DIAGNOSIS Demonstration of *M. avium-intracellulare* in bacterial culture is necessary to establish the diagnosis. The differential diagnosis includes all chronic granulomatous conditions of the skin.

TREATMENT Where feasible, surgical treatment of *M. avium-intracellulare* infection is advisable as the organism seems to be poorly susceptible to chemotherapeutic agents. If dissemination of the disease does not allow curative surgery, combination therapy should be tried. Ethambutol, rifampin, amikacin, streptomycin, ciprofloxacin, clofazimine, clarithromycin, azithromycin, and rifabutin are highly active against *M. avium-intracellulare*, while isoniazid and pyrazinamide are not.[34] Experience with AIDS patients suggests that drug regimens including ansamycin and clofazimine may be effective.

M. szulgai

The development of cervical lymphadenitis as well as cellulitis or draining nodules and plaques have been associated with *M. szulgai*. The organism has also been found to cause bursitis and pneumonia; it is more susceptible to antituberculous drugs than most other atypical mycobacteria.

M. haemophilum

This organism was identified as the cause of a subcutaneous granulomatous eruption in several immunosuppressed or HIV-infected patients.[35] Histopathologically, there is a mixed polymorphonuclear and granulomatous inflammation, the so-called dimorphic inflammatory response, with no caseation necrosis, similar to that seen in *M. fortuitum* complex infection. The organism may be sensitive to

p-aminosalicylic acid and rifampin, but further observations of such infections are required.

M. genavese

So far, little is known about the characteristics of this mycobacterium; it causes disseminated disease similar to *M. avium-intracellulare* in HIV-infected patients.[36]

M. fortuitum, M. chelonae, M. abscessus

These three species of rapid-growing, facultatively pathogenic mycobacteria have usually been grouped in the *M. fortuitum* complex. Today, they are recognized as distinct species.[37,38] These organisms seem to be widely distributed and can commonly be found in soil and in water supplies. Contamination of various materials, including surgical supplies, occurs and does not always result in clinical disease.

CLINICAL MANIFESTATIONS These organisms cause similar clinical diseases.[39] Infection usually follows a puncture wound or a surgical procedure. In one large series it was found that cutaneous disease was present in 60 percent of cases; of these, approximately one-half were due to surgery and the other half to accidental inoculation. The disease manifests itself as a painful red infiltrate at the site of inoculation; there are no signs of dissemination and no constitutional symptoms. This type of infection has followed augmentation mammoplasty, median sternotomy, and a variety of other procedures usually involving percutaneous catheterization. Cold postinjection abscesses, especially when occurring in the tropics, may also be due to fast-growing mycobacteria. Recently, an outbreak of localized cutaneous postinjection abscesses or cellulitis in 350 patients was observed in Colombia.[40] It has been suggested that so-called fixation abscesses found in tuberculosis patients after intramuscular injections have frequently been due to inoculation of these organisms.

Primary cutaneous inoculation occurs through skin injuries, in all age groups, without immunosuppression. The lesion presents as a dark red infiltrated node, often with abscess formation and clear fluid drainage. Disseminated disease involving the skin also occurs, usually in hemodialysis or immunologically compromised patients. The skin lesions consist of multiple recurrent episodes of abscesses on the extremities or in a generalized macular and papular eruption. Other manifestations of infection with these organisms include pneumonitis or osteomyelitis, lymphadenitis, and postsurgical endocarditis.

HISTOPATHOLOGY The lesions are characterized by the simultaneous occurrence of polymorphonuclear microabscesses and granuloma formation with foreign body–type giant cells, the so-called dimorphic inflammatory response. There is usually necrosis but no caseation. Acid-fast bacilli may occasionally be demonstrated within microabscesses.

DIAGNOSIS AND TREATMENT Organisms of the *M. fortuitum* complex may be identified by special laboratories. This is of more than epidemiologic interest because *M. fortuitum* is more susceptible to amicacin, cefoxitin, ciprofloxacin, and imipenem; *M. abscessus* is usually sensitive to amikacin, cefoxitin, and clarithromycin[41]; *M. chelnaoe* is usually resistant to cefoxitin, and tobramycin is more effective than amikacin. Thus, a rational treatment has to await the results of identification of the organism and in vitro susceptibility testing. In the Colombian series of 350 patients with postinjection abscesses due to *M. abscessus,* a combination of surgical excision of the lesions and 3 to 6 months of clarithromycin resulted in a 95 percent cure rate, while either measure alone was successful in fewer than 30 percent of patients.[40]

REFERENCES

1. Huebner RE, Castro KG: The changing face of tuberculosis. *Annu Rev Med* **46**:47, 1995
2. Dalovisio JR, Pankey GA: Dermatologic manifestations of nontuberculous mycobacterial diseases. *Infect Dis Clin North Am* **8**:677, 1994
3. Yeager H Jr: Other mycobacterium species, in *Principles and Practice of Infectious Diseases,* 2d ed, edited by GL Mandell et al. New York, Wiley, 1985
4. Skerman VDB et al: Approved Lists of Bacterial Names. *Int J Syst Bacteriol* **30**:225, 1980
5. French AL et al: Nontuberculous mycobacterial infections. *Med Clin North Am* **81**:361, 1997
6. Opravil M: Epidemiological and clinical aspects of mycobacterial infections. *Infection* **25**:56, 1997
7. Wayne LG: Dormancy of *Mycobacterium tuberculosis* and latency of disease. *Eur J Clin Microbiol Infect Dis* **13**:908, 1994
8. Rook GA et al: New insights into the immunopathology of tuberculosis. *Pathobiology* **59**:148, 1991
9. Taniguchi S et al: Scrofuloderma: The DNA analysis of mycobacteria by the polymerase chain reaction. *Arch Dermatol* **129**:1618, 1993
10. Degitz K et al: Successful treatment of erythema induratum of Bazin following rapid detection of mycobacterial DNA by polymerase chain reaction. *Arch Dermatol* **129**:1619, 1993
11. Cormican M et al: Multiplex PCR for identifying mycobacterial isolates. *J Clin Pathol* **48**:203, 1995
12. Degitz K: Detection of mycobacterial DNA in the skin—etiologic insights and diagnostic perspectives. *Arch Dermatol* **132**:71, 1996
13. Butcher PD et al: The application of molecular techniques to the diagnosis and epidemiology of mycobacterial diseases. *J Appl Bacteriol* **81**(suppl):53S, 1996
14. Margall N et al: Detection of *Mycobacterium tuberculosis* complex DNA by the polymerase chain reaction for rapid diagnosis of cutaneous tuberculosis. *Br J Dermatol* **135**:231, 1996
15. Victor T et al: Papulonecrotic tuberculid: Identification of *Mycobacterium tuberculosis* DNA by polymerase chain reaction. *Am J Dermatopathol* **14**:491, 1992
16. Yen A et al: Detection of *Mycobacterium tuberculosis* in erythema induratum of Bazin using polymerase chain reaction. *Arch Dermatol* **133**:532, 1997
17. Trinker M et al: False-positive diagnosis of tuberculosis with PCR. *Lancet* **348**:1388, 1996
18. Marcoval J et al: Lupus vulgaris: Clinical, histopathologic, and bacteriologic study of 10 cases. *J Am Acad Dermatol* **26**:404, 1992
19. Vittori F, Groslafeige C: [Tuberculosis lupus after BCG vaccination. A rare complication of the vaccination]. *Arch Pediatr* **3**:457, 1996
20. Stewart EJ, James MP: Lupus vulgaris–like reaction following BCG vaccination. *Clin Exp Dermatol* **21**:232, 1996
21. Rietbroek RC et al: Tuberculosis cutis miliaris disseminata as a manifestation of miliary tuberculosis: Literature review and report of a case of recurrent skin lesions. *Rev Infect Dis* **13**:265, 1991
22. Libraty DH, Byrd TF: Cutaneous miliary tuberculosis in the AIDS era: Case report and review. *Clin Infect Dis* **23**:706, 1996
23. Felten MK, Leichsenring M: Use of BCG in high prevalence areas for HIV. *Trop Med Parasitol* **46**:69, 1995
24. Morrison JGL, Fourie GD: The papulonecrotic tuberculide. From Arthus' reaction to lupus vulgaris. *Br J Dermatol* **91**:263, 1974
25. Baselga E et al: *Mycobacterium tuberculosis* DNA in papulonecrotic tuberculid. *Arch Dermatol* **132**:92, 1996
26. Baselga E et al: Detection of *Mycobacterium tuberculosis* DNA in lobular granulomatous panniculitis (erythema induratum nodular vasculitis). *Arch Dermatol* **133**:457, 1997
27. Ockuly OE, Montgomery H: Lichenoid tuberculid: A clinical and histopathologic study. *J Invest Dermatol* **14**:415, 1950
28. American Thoracic Society: Treatment of tuberculosis and tuberculosis infection in adults and children. *Am J Respir Crit Care Med* **149**:1359, 1994
29. Watt B: Lesser known mycobacteria. *J Clin Pathol* **48**:701, 1995
30. Mattila JO et al: Slowly growing mycobacteria and chronic skin disorders. *Clin Infect Dis* **23**:1043, 1996
31. Sanders JW et al: Disseminated *Mycobacterium scrofulaceum* infection: A potentially treatable complication of AIDS. *Clin Infect Dis* **20**:549, 1995
32. Kullavanijaya P et al: Primary cutaneous infection with *Mycobacterium avium intracellulare* complex resembling lupus vulgaris. *Br J Dermatol* **136**:264, 1997
33. Ichiki Y et al: Skin infection caused by *Mycobacterium avium. Br J Dermatol* **136**:260, 1997
34. Havlir DV: *Mycobacterium avium* complex: Advances in therapy. *Eur J Clin Microbiol Infect Dis* **13**:915, 1994
35. Strauss WL et al: Clinical and epidemiological characteristics of *Mycobacterium haemophilum,* an emerging pathogen in immunocompromised patients. *Arch Intern Med* **120**:118, 1994
36. Pechère C et al: Clinical and epidemiologic features of infection with *Mycobacterium genavese. Arch Intern Med* **155**:400, 1995
37. Wallace RJ Jr: Recent changes in taxonomy and disease manifestations of the rapidly growing mycobacteria. *Eur J Clin Microbiol Infect Dis* **13**:953, 1994
38. Kusunoki S, Ezaki T: Proposal of *Mycobacterium peregrinum* sp. nov., nom. rev., and elevation of *Mycobacterium chelonae* subsp. *abscessus* (Kubica et al.) to species status: *Mycobacterium abscessus* comb. nov. *Int J Syst Bacteriol* **42**:240, 1992
39. Wallace RJ et al: Skin, soft tissue and bone infections due to *Mycobacterium chelonae chelonae:* Importance of prior corticosteroid therapy, frequency of disseminated infections, and resistance to oral antimicrobials other than clarithromycin. *J Infect Dis* **166**:405, 1992
40. Villanueva A et al: Report on an outbreak of postinjection abscesses due to *Mycobacterium abscessus,* including management with surgery and clarithromycin therapy and comparison of strains by random amplified polymorphic DNA polymerase chain reaction. *Clin Infect Dis* **24**:1147, 1997
41. Wolinsky E: Mycobacterial diseases other than tuberculosis. *Clin Infect Dis* **15**:1, 1992

CHAPTER 202

Mauricio Goihman-Yahr
Michael M. McNeil
June M. Brown

Actinomycosis, Nocardiosis, and Actinomycetoma

INTRODUCTION

Actinomycosis, nocardiosis, and actinomycetoma are chronic infections caused by human pathogenic species of filamentous gram-positive bacteria. These bacteria may develop structures (grains) that are resistant to body defense mechanisms.

Actinomycosis is an infection caused by anaerobic *Actinomyces*, whereas aerobic actinomycete species cause nocardiosis and actinomycetoma. Actinomycosis is a chronic infection, frequently of the cervicofacial area, thorax, or abdomen, and is usually caused by *Actinomyces israelii* and *A. gerencseriae* and only comparatively rarely by other fermentative *Actinomyces* species as well as *Propionibacterium propionicum*.[1] Nocardiosis is primarily an infection of the lungs, with a marked tendency to disseminate to multiple organs, particularly the brain. *Nocardia asteroides* is the most common cause of disease in humans, but other species including *N. brasiliensis* and *N. otitidiscaviarum* may also be etiologic agents. Actinomycetoma is a chronic infection of the subcutaneous tissues, skin, and bone. Actinomycosis, nocardiosis, and actinomycetoma may be occult at onset, progress in a chronic, indolent fashion; and be difficult to diagnose because of the similarity of their clinical features and, in cutaneous disease, their close resemblance to several other chronic dermatologic disorders.

In addition to the patient's clinical presentation, the demonstration of the microorganisms in smears of clinical material or in stained tissue sections may suggest the presumptive diagnosis; however, confirmation of the diagnosis depends upon the culture isolation and identification of the etiologic agents to the genus level (Table 202-1).

The aerobic and facultative anaerobic actinomycetes belong to the order Actinomycetales. No formal subgroups or families of this order exist, but taxonomists have adapted provisional, unofficial, purely descriptive, transitional names for subgroups of the order. However, as more is learned about the similarities between these bacteria, formal taxonomic families will likely be named. The major groups of the order Actinomycetales, actinoplanetes, maduromycetes, nocardioform actinomycetes, streptomycetes, and actinobacteria, probably represent distinct groups.[3]

ACTINOMYCOSIS

Epidemiology

Actinomycosis is a rare infection that is worldwide in distribution; in the United States it is more common in males. The disease's incidence is difficult to estimate, since it is not a reportable disease and there is no skin test available for population surveys. Actinomycosis predominantly affects the cervicofacial area, thorax (Fig. 202-1), or abdomen and is characterized by chronic suppurative fibrosing inflammation, sinus discharge of characteristic "sulfur granules," and direct dissemination via contiguous tissues. The etiologic microorganisms belong to two genera *Actinomyces* and *Propionibacterium*. Besides the most prevalent species, *A. israelii and A. gerencseriae* (formerly *A. israelii* serotype II), the other pathogenic species include in order of frequency: *P. propionicum* (formerly *Arachnia propionicus*), *A. naeslundii*, *A. viscosus*, and *A. odontolyticus*. *A. bovis* causes granulomatous infections in cattle; however, this species is considered to be an unlikely human pathogen and earlier reports of human *A. bovis* infections might in fact have been due to *A. israelii*.[4] Of importance, actinomycosis may be a mixed infection with other anaerobic bacteria such as *Peptostreptococcus* and *Bacteroides* species. In severe and chronic cases, *A. israelii* is usually accompanied by *Actinobacillus actinomycetemcomitans*.[5]

Actinomyces and *Propionibacterium* species are commensals that flourish in regions with anaerobic growth conditions such as peritonsillar crypts, gingivodental crevices, and the lower gastrointestinal tract. They have been implicated as a cause of dental plaque.[5] These microorganisms have only been demonstrated in animal or human hosts, and person-to-person transmission has not been demonstrated. Although these microbes possess low inherent pathogenicity, conditions that result in local tissue ischemia may cause them to proliferate and invade surrounding healthy tissues.[6] Such infections are frequently polymicrobial.

Clinical Disease

Cervicofacial infection is the most frequent clinical presentation. This results when microorganisms invade damaged oral mucosa following dental extraction or other mouth trauma, causing a painful, indurated cutaneous and soft tissue swelling ("woody fibrosis"); the slowly enlarging inflammatory mass is often located at the angle of the jaw ("lumpy jaw") (Fig. 202-2). Direct extension may involve adjacent structures. Thoracic infection involving the lung and pleura is usually secondary to aspiration[78] but rarely may result from bloodstream dissemination. Pleuropulmonary infection may be complicated by mediastinal invasion, with involvement of the pericardium and thoracic vertebrae. Actinomycosis of the gastrointestinal tract most commonly develops in the ileocecal region but may

TABLE 202-1

Presumptive Identification of the Major Medically Important Aerobic and Facultative Anaerobic Actinomycetes to the Genus Level

CHARACTERISTIC	*Actinomyces*	*Propionibacterium*	*Nocardia*	*Streptomyces*	*Actinomadura*
Aerobic growth on SDA	−	−	+	+	+
Anaerobic growth on BAP	+	+	V	−	−
Vegetative filaments					
Aerial	−	−	+	V	V
Substrate	+	+	+	+	+
Metabolism of glucose	F	F	O	O	O
Presence* in whole cells of					
Isomers of DAP	−	*ll*	*dl*	*ll*	*dl*
Sugars	Gal	Gal	Arab,gal	None	Mad
Acid-fast nature	−	−	w	−	
−Granules	+	−	+	+	+
Color	Yellow		White to yellow	Cream to brown	Tan to orange to deep red
Growth in lysozyme	−	+	+	−	−
Catalase	−	+(−)†	+	+	+

*As determined by the methodology of Lechevalier et al.[2]
†*P. propionicum* (formerly *Arachnia propionica*) is catalase negative.
NOTE: SDA, Sabouraud-dextrose agar; BAP, blood agar plate; +, positive; −, negative; V, variable; O,oxidative; F, fermentative; DAP, diaminopimelic acid; gal, galactose; arab, arabinose; mad, madurose; w, weakly or partially acid fast.

also primarily involve the esophageal, gastric, or anorectal areas. Pelvic actinomycosis has been recognized with increasing frequency, and predisposing factors have been identified that include intrauterine devices, contaminated pessaries, prolapse of the uterus, and septic abortion.

Differential Diagnosis

The most important conditions to consider in the differential diagnosis are other diseases that cause fistulae. These include granulomatous diseases, such as Crohn's disease, foreign body granulomas, tuberculosis, and certain pyogenic bacterial infections, such as odontogenic granuloma and fistula on the jaw. *Actinomyces* infections should be considered whenever there are chronic soft tissue orocervical lesions. However, the diagnosis of actinomycosis may be difficult when areas such as the pelvic, perigluteal, or perianal regions are affected. Steps in making the diagnosis include careful clinical examination, stained smear of exudate, and culture isolation of the etiologic agent. In infected patients, the presence of an underlying immunodeficiency state should also be considered, and evidence of polymicrobial infections should also be carefully sought in histologic and microbiologic diagnostic tests.[9–11]

FIGURE 202-1

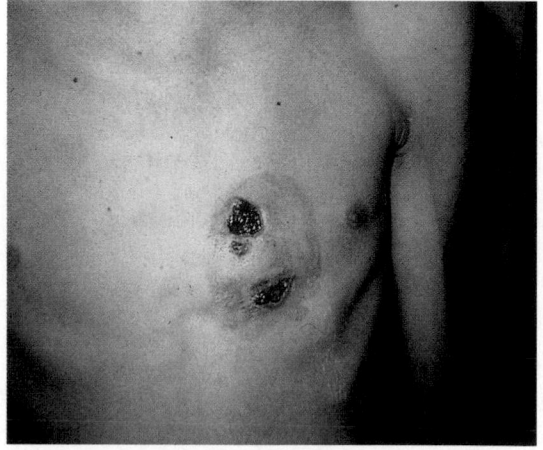

Ulcerated chest wall lesion from a patient who died from invasive actinomycosis. Note minimal drainage. (*Courtesy of María Cecilia Albornoz, MD, Instituto de Biomedicina, Caracas.*)

FIGURE 202-2

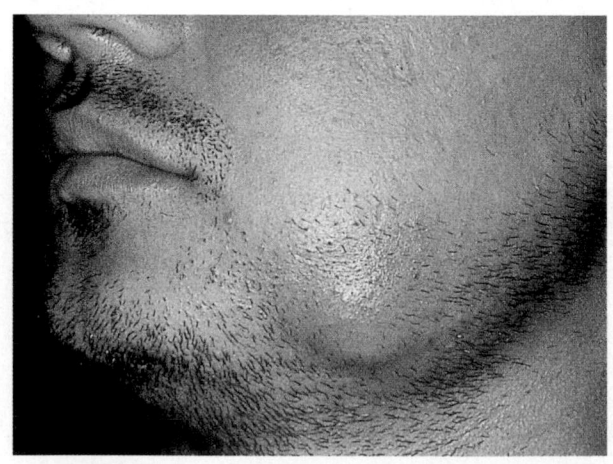

"Lumpy jaw" in a patient with cervicofacial actinomycosis. (Courtesy of María Cecilia Albornoz, MD, Instituto de Biomedicina, Caracas.)

Laboratory Diagnosis

A definitive diagnosis cannot be made solely on clinical grounds. The diagnosis of actinomycosis may be difficult and may depend on a heightened level of clinical suspicion and prior notification of the clinical laboratorian and pathologist. Detection of these microorganisms on Gram stain and culture from an appropriately obtained specimen is needed. Exudates and biopsy material are particularly suitable for laboratory examination. Bronchoscopy and bronchoalveolar lavage fluid smear examination and culture may be important in the diagnosis of thoracic actinomycosis.[6–8] After a sample is obtained, it should be examined by standard histologic methods, anaerobic culture for 2 weeks, and immunofluorescence if available.

CULTURE Culture is the least reliable method of verifying infection (in Fiorino's series only 35 percent of cultures were positive for *Actinomyces*),[12] although an 86 percent success rate has been reported for samples cultured in the presence of metronidazole, which inhibits the growth of faster growing anaerobes[13] Cultures of abscess aspirates and vaginal and cervical swabs frequently grow multiple other species of microorganisms. Both pathogenic *Actinomyces* species and *P. propionicum* are morphologically indistinguishable, anaerobic to facultatively anaerobic, nonsporulating, gram-positive bacilli. Characteristically, they appear as branched filaments (Fig. 202-3); however, fragmentation of these filaments readily occurs, producing bacillary or coccoid forms. They are non-acid-fast and nonmotile. They are best isolated in prereduced anaerobic media such as thioglycolate with 0.5 mL sterile rabbit serum and may require 14 days of anaerobic incubation at 35°C. After initial primary isolation, organisms produce colonies 1 to 2 mm in diameter on solid media after incubation for 3 to 7 days under anaerobic conditions.

BIOCHEMISTRY *A. israelii* differs from the other *Actinomyces* species on the basis of acid production from anaerobic fermentative carbohydrates.[14] *P. propionicum* differs from the *Actinomyces* species biochemically on the basis of production of large amounts of

propionic acid from glucose fermentation, the presence of l-l-diaminopimelic acid in the cell wall, growth in the presence of lysozyme, and acid production from carbohydrates.[15] Differentiation of *Actinomyces* from other anaerobic nonsporulating gram-positive bacilli such as *Bifidobacterium*, *Eubacterium*, and *Propionibacterium* is based on acid production from carbohydrates, hydrolysis of esculin and gelatin, reduction of nitrate, production of indol and catalase, reaction in milk, and gas chromatographic analysis of the organic end products of glucose fermentation (Table 202-2).

Pathology

There is usually a chronic abscess with extensive neutrophil infiltration, granulation tissue, and fibrosis. Filamentous microorganisms may form a matlike colony ("grain"). The organisms stain in tissue with Gomori methenamine silver (GMS) and the Brown and Brenn (B&B) modification of the Gram stain. They are usually pleomorphic, gram-positive bacilli that appear beaded in older cultures, when they take up stain irregularly. The presence of "sulfur granules" is highly suggestive but not diagnostic of actinomycosis. Sulfur granules comprise masses of matted, interconnected bacterial filaments that appear in vivo in a characteristic radial arrangement (see "Actinomycetoma"). Microorganisms may be scarce in pathologic specimens, so detection may require diligent searching of multiple tissue sections.[16]

Serodiagnosis

Serodiagnosis of actinomycosis by detection of precipitating antibodies has not been a particularly useful diagnostic test.[17] However, presumptive identification can be achieved by direct or indirect modification of the immunofluorescence technique.[5,18] Unfortunately, fluorescein isothiocyanate–labeled (direct) and –unlabeled (indirect) antisera needed for these tests and used in research laboratories are not commercially available. Sputum may be culture positive for *Actinomyces* because of contamination from upper airway secretions. In addition, it is important to collect specimens before initiation of antibiotics and to alert the laboratory to the clinical suspicion of actinomycosis so that anaerobic cultures may be observed for an appropriate period.

Therapy

Penicillin is the antimicrobial therapy of choice for deep-seated actinomycosis. Prolonged treatment with large doses of penicillin is required to achieve serum drug concentrations high enough to ensure drug penetration into areas of fibrosis and suppuration and possibly to penetrate the granules themselves.[19] The goal of therapy is to administer intravenous penicillin G (150,000 to 200,000 U/kg per day or 10 to 20 million units per day in divided doses for adults) for 4 to 6 weeks (or for at least 3 to 4 weeks after the patient appears cured), followed by amoxicillin or oral penicillin (e.g., phenoxymethylpenicillin, 2 to 4 g/day, to patient tolerance) for 6 to 12 additional months or even longer to prevent relapse. In a given patient, complications including disseminated infection, critical organ involvement (e.g., central nervous system), and/or associated inability to perform definitive surgery may alter or extend this regimen.[20] Clinical resistance to penicillin may not be a major problem; however, there have been occasional reports of clinical failures following penicillin therapy alone.[21] In addition, there is some in vitro

FIGURE 202-3

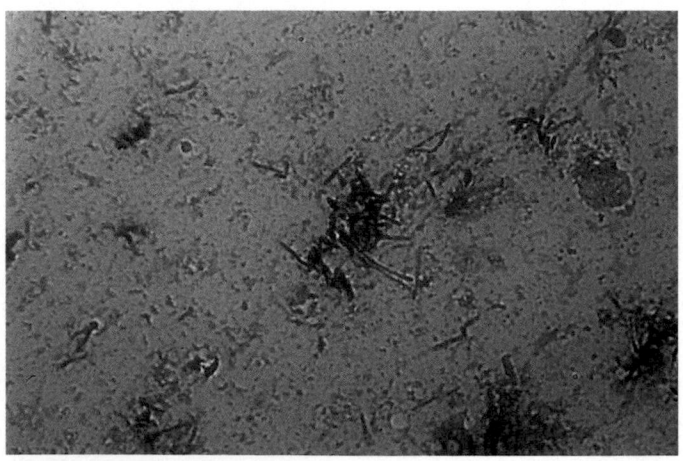

Actinomyces israelii filaments. Gram stain. ×1022. (*Courtesy of María Cecilia Albornoz, MD, Instituto de Biomedicina, Caracas.*)

TABLE 202-2

Comparison of *Actinomyces* and *Propionibacterium* Species to Others of Related Genera*

	SPECIES				
CHARACTERISTIC	*Actinomyces israelii*	*A. gerencseriae*	*A. naeslundii*	*A. odontolyticus*	*Propionibacterium acnes*
Oxygen tolerance	M or an	M or an	F	M or an	An
Acid production from					
D-Glucose	+	+	+	+	+
D-Mannitol	V	V	–	–	V
Lactose	+(–)	+(–)	+(–)	+(–)	–
Sucrose	+	+	+(–)	+(–)	–
Maltose	+	+	+(–)	+(–)	–
Salicin	V	V	V	+(–)	–
Glycerol	–	–	V	V	A
D-Xylose	+(–)	V	–	V	–
L-Arabinose	+	–	V	V	–
Hydrolysis of					
Esculin	+(–)	+(–)	+(–)	V	+(–)
Gelatin	–	–	–	–	+(–)
Reduction of nitrate	V	V	+(–)	+	+
Indol production	–	–	–	–	+(–)
Reaction in milk	(C)	(C)	(C)	(C)	C(G)
Catalase	–	–	–	–	+
Organic acids detected by GLC	A,L,S,	A,L,S,	A,L,S	A,L,S	A,P,(IV)

*Data from Schofield and Schaal.[12]
NOTE: M, microaerophilic; an, anaerobic; F, facultative; +, positive reactions for 90–100%; –, negative reactions for 90–100%; V, variable; ( ), indicates reactions shown in 11–25% of the strains; GLC, gas liquid chromatography; C, clot; G, gas; NC, no change; A, acetic; L, lactic; S, succinic; P, propionic acid; IV, isovaleric acid; B, butyric acid.
SOURCE: Data modified from Dowell and Hawkins.[14]

evidence to support the development of acquired resistance to penicillin.[22] Garrod suggested that unsuccessful penicillin treatment might be accompanied by increased in vitro resistance and reported that the minimum inhibitory concentration for two strains of *A. israelii* increased from 0.03 U/mL to 0.2 U/mL and to >0.5 U/mL, respectively.[23] Boand and Novak reported that four of six strains of *A. bovis* (probably *A. israelii*) developed a two- to fourfold increased resistance with penicillin when tested with this drug at subinhibitory concentrations.[22] In vivo development of acquired antimicrobial resistance by *Actinomyces* species, particularly to penicillin G, has not been reported. If the patient is considered to have a poor clinical response to penicillin therapy, then a search should be made for an undrained abscess, and the possibility of a resistant concomitant bacterial species should also be considered. Lerner has reported that clinical resistance has not been a problem with penicillin G therapy; however, in a patient with penicillin allergy the drug may be contraindicated.[24]

The prognosis of the cervicofacial and abdominal forms of actinomycosis is generally favorable, with a >80 percent survival rate. Survival is less favorable in thoracic actinomycosis because of the greater likelihood that this represents disseminated disease. There is only limited experience with alternative first-line antimicrobial agents, including prolonged courses with tetracycline, erythromycin, and clindamycin.[25] Additional alternative drugs include ciprofloxacin, imipenem, and ceftriaxone; however, evidence for the efficacy of each of these drugs has been limited to single case reports.[26–28] In addition, as previously mentioned, ampicillin (or amoxicillin) has been suggested as an alternative initial therapy because of the likely presence of concomitant bacteria that may be less susceptible to penicillin G in vitro.[29] Despite its excellent activity against other anaerobes, metronidazole is not recommended for the therapy of actinomycosis; however, since concomitant bacteria resistant to

penicillin or other beta-lactam first-line drugs may be present, the combination of ampicillin and metronidazole or clindamycin has been suggested.[30]

In addition to antimicrobial therapy, surgical drainage of empyema and large abscesses and excision of sinus tracts, underlying foreign bodies, necrotic tissues, sequestra, and recalcitrant fibrotic lesions may be indicated in these infected patients.

NOCARDIOSIS

Epidemiology

Nocardia species are aerobic soil bacteria found worldwide as saprophytes on decaying matter and are not normal inhabitants of the respiratory or gastrointestinal tracts. Disease occurs by inhalation, and males are three times more likely than females to become infected.

Nocardia spp. infections are rare in humans, occurring most frequently in patients who are severely immunocompromised.[31,32] The taxonomy of *Nocardia* spp. remains complicated. Most clinical infections in temperate countries have been caused by *N. asteroides* complex, *N. brasiliensis* (Table 202-3), and rarely *N. otitidiscaviarum*. *N. asteroides* complex (including *N. asteroides* sensu stricto, *N. farcinica*, and *N. nova*) has been considered to be responsible for the majority of serious invasive infections. *N. asteroides* sensu stricto continues to demonstrate considerable heterogeneity; and recently, four new unnamed taxa have been characterized.[34] *N. brasiliensis* has been associated particularly with subcutaneous infections and is predominant in tropical countries.[35] A new taxon, *N. pseudobrasiliensis*, was recently separated from

	SPECIES				
P. propionicum	P. Bifidobacterium P. granulosum	Bifidobacterium eriksonii	Eubacterium alactolyticum	E. lentum	E. limosum
M or an	An or F	An	An	An	An
+	+	+	+	−	+
+	−	V	+(−)	−	+(−)
+	−	+	−	−	−
+	+	+	−	−	−
+	+	+	−	−	−
−(+)	−(+)	+	−	−	−
−(+)	+(−)	−	−	−	−
−	−	+	−	−	−
−	−	+	−	−	−
−(+)	−	+(−)	−	−	V
−(+)	V	−	−	−	−
+	−	−	−	−	−
−	−	−	−	−	−
(C)	(C)	(CG)	NC	NC	NC
−	+(−)	−	−	−	−
A,P,L,S	A,P,(IV)	A,L,S	A,B,C	A,L,S	A,B

N. brasiliensis and appears to be generally associated with noncutaneous (pulmonary, central nervous system, or systemic) nocardiosis and differs in susceptibility to ciprofloxacin and resistance to minocycline.[36] *N. otitidiscaviarum* is rare and has no typical geographic distribution.[37] *N. transvalensis* is an unusual emerging human pathogenic *Nocardia* species.[32]

Nosocomial Infection

Although nocardiosis is most often considered a late-presenting, community-acquired infection, nosocomial outbreaks of nocardiosis attributed to airborne bacterial transmission have been reported in immunocompromised patients.[38–41] These outbreaks of nocardiosis have affected patients in a renal transplant unit,[38] children with hematologic malignancies,[39] severely immunocompromised heart transplant patients,[42,43] and patients with acute and chronic liver disease and liver transplants.[40] In addition, in the report by Sahathevan et al., exposure to construction activity was identified as a possible risk factor infection and was present in all cases; however, an extensive environmental investigation, which included environmental cultures, did not reveal any specific environmental source for these microorganisms.[40] Three distinct biotypes were found in the isolates: three patient isolates fit two of the biotype patterns, and one patient isolate fit the third biotype pattern.[40] Thus, available evidence did not support a single source for these infections.

In another report, Schaal suggested that nosocomial airborne transmission, possibly in the operating room environment, was responsible for a cluster of *N. farcinica* postoperative wound infections in patients undergoing cardiac and other vascular surgeries at a university hospital.[41] An environmental investigation did not identify a definite source for these microorganisms; however, outbreak isolates had a characteristic antibiogram, and microorganisms demonstrating this same antibiogram were cultured from air samples from a storeroom in the operating suite.[41] Also Yew et al. reported that during a 3-year outbreak of *Mycobacterium fortuitum* and

M. chelonei postoperative sternal wound infections, two additional patients developed *N. asteroides* infections 2 months and 7 months postoperatively; however, no additional epidemiologic information on these patients was available.[44]

Patterson et al. also reported an episode at a university hospital, in which 18 patient blood cultures were found to be falsely positive for *N. asteroides*.[45] An epidemiologic investigation revealed that the source of contamination was a malfunctioning automated radiometric blood culture machine, and the epidemic strain was confirmed by DNA fingerprinting. Control measures—changing the needle sterilizer and prolonging needle sterilization time on the machine—were instituted and shown to be effective in halting the pseudooutbreak.[45]

An unusual cluster of nocardiosis cases was also reported among cancer patients who had received therapy in a clinic in the Bahamas. An investigation by the U.S. Centers for Disease Control and Prevention determined that the probable cause was contamination of parenterally administered medications.[46] There have also been other reports of cutaneous nocardiosis in patients following intravenous heroin abuse.[47,48]

Clinical Disease

In immunocompromised patients, localized respiratory infection is thought to result from inhalation of *Nocardia* spp. However, in up to half the infected patients, dissemination may occur, with a predilection for the central nervous system and subcutaneous tissues. The clinical manifestations, severity, and prognosis of disease in the infected patient are extremely variable and may be determined by factors such as the route of infection and the presence or absence of a properly functioning immune system. In immunocompetent hosts, localized subcutaneous infection may result. In severely immunocompromised patients, principal predisposing factors include immunosuppressive therapy (particularly steroid drugs), neoplastic diseases, solid organ and bone marrow transplantation, chronic

TABLE 202-3

Distinguishing Features of Systemic and Primary (Cutaneous) Forms of Aerobic Actinomycetes Infections Affecting the Skin

CHARACTERISTIC	DISSEMINATED (SYSTEMIC) NOCARDIOSIS	PRIMARY CUTANEOUS NOCARDIOSIS	*Nocardia* ACTINOMYCETOMA	*Streptomyces* ACTINOMYCETOMA	*Actinomadura* ACTINOMYCETOMA
Geographic distribution	Worldwide	Worldwide	North and South America, Mexico, and Australia	India, Africa, and Saudi Arabia	India, Africa, and Saudi Arabia
Presence of predisposing diseases	Common	Rare	Rare	Rare	Rare
History of trauma	Rare	Common	Common	Common	Common
Other organs involved (besides skin)	Lung, brain, and bone	Lymphatics	Bone	Bone	Bone
Sites on skin	Anywhere	Exposed areas	Exposed areas and back	Exposed areas	Exposed areas
Number of skin lesions	Single or multiple	Usually single	Usually single	Usually single	Usually single
Draining sinuses	Absent	Absent	Present	Present	Present
Growth pattern in vivo	Filamentous	Filamentous	Granules	Granules	Granules
Most common species	*N. asteroides* complex	*N. asteroides* complex *N. brasiliensis*	*N. brasiliensis*	*S. somaliensis*	*A. madurae* *A. pelletieri*

SOURCE: Adapted from Hay.[33]

bronchopulmonary diseases, and AIDS; the most common clinical presentations are invasive pulmonary infection and disseminated disease.[40,42,49,50] However, invasive disease may also occur in non-immunocompromised patients. Underlying pulmonary disorders (e.g., malignancy, tuberculosis) may predispose to respiratory tract colonization by *Nocardia*. In addition, primary cutaneous and subcutaneous infections may develop from inoculation of these microorganisms at the time of surgery or from traumatic inoculation as a result of outdoor activities.

Cutaneous nocardiosis may be subdivided into four clinical types: mycetoma, lymphocutaneous infection, superficial skin infection (abscess or cellulitis), and secondary cutaneous involvement with disseminated disease.

Localized cutaneous nocardial infections may also present as either a chronically draining ulcerative lesion or a slowly expanding nodule and, less commonly, pustules, abscesses, cellulitis, or pyoderma. Frequently, there may be spread beyond the initial cutaneous infective focus to involve the regional lymphatics, and, in up to one-third of cases, the disease may progress to form lymphatic abscesses. When regional lymph node involvement occurs, this form of the disease is referred to as the *lymphocutaneous syndrome*. Since this form of the disease bears a striking clinical resemblance to a superficial infection with the dimorphic fungus *Sporothrix schenckii*, it has also been termed the *sporotrichoid form* of cutaneous nocardiosis. It is necessary to perform an appropriate laboratory diagnostic workup to exclude misdiagnosis of the disease as sporotrichosis (see Chap. 208). More-localized infections may also be misdiagnosed as staphylococcal skin infections. Since skin manifestations may be complications of disseminated disease, the finding of a cutaneous lesion in a patient should not always be attributed to local inoculation.

Differential Diagnosis

The differential diagnosis of cutaneous nocardiosis includes other infections causing granulomas, e.g., eumycotic mycetoma, dermal tuberculosis and cutaneous nontuberculous mycobacterial infections, keloid blastomycosis, mycosis-like pyoderma and certain forms of leishmaniasis, sporotrichosis, and botryomycosis. Nonin-

fectious conditions to consider include foreign-body granulomas, soft tissue sarcomas, and lethal midline granuloma. Clinical history, epidemiologic considerations, and general pathologic features should alert the clinician to include nocardiosis in the patient's differential diagnosis. A confirmation of the diagnosis may be provided by the presence of granules, histopathologic findings, and culture identification of causative microorganisms. Deep organ involvement may pose more of a diagnostic problem, because invasive biopsy procedures may be required and interpretation of the results may be complicated by the occurrence of a mixed infection. Imaging procedures (radiography and computed tomographic and magnetic resonance imaging scans) and invasive procedures (e.g., bronchoscopic biopsy and bronchoalveolar lavage) may be important for making the diagnosis. A heightened level of clinical suspicion and prompt notification of the clinical microbiology laboratory to perform appropriate tests to screen for the causative organisms may provide the key for early diagnosis of nocardiosis.

Pathophysiology

Nocardia infection is usually acquired by inhalation, but, rarely, direct skin inoculation may be implicated. Inhalation allows establishment of a focal pneumonitis that progresses to neutrophilic and histiocytic pneumonias and abscesses. Rarely, colonization of the skin or respiratory tract by *Nocardia* may occur. Invasive infection in an immunocompetent patient may result in a minimal inflammatory response and negligible residual tissue scarring; however, in immunocompromised hosts, particularly those infected by *N. brasiliensis*, there may be a marked tissue response together with true granuloma formation. The immune status of the patient is crucial in determining whether and to what extent disease progression occurs.

Laboratory Diagnosis

Since *Nocardia* spp. are ubiquitous in nature, the isolation of these microorganisms from microbiologic specimens may not be clinically significant. In a patient's sputum culture, their presence may not always indicate invasive infection and may reflect either laboratory contamination or respiratory colonization. The diagnosis of invasive *Nocardia* spp. infection has been hindered by a combination of clinical and microbiologic difficulties, including their often nonspecific clinical presentation, the requirement often for invasive diagnostic biopsy procedures, the difficulty in isolating them, and their imperfect taxonomic classification.

DIRECT EXAMINATION If clumps of bacteria or granules are present in the exudate, these should be selectively removed and crushed between two glass microscope slides. In addition, some of the exudate should be examined in a wet mount to exclude the presence of fungal hyphae. Two smears should be stained prior to microscopic examination of the material; one with Gram stain and the other with modified Kinyoun stain.[51] The presence of gram-positive filaments with some degree of acid fastness is suggestive of *Nocardia*. Although the gross and microscopic characteristics of the granules may suggest the etiologic agent, definitive identification depends upon the culture isolation and identification of the organism involved.

ISOLATION Culture isolation of *Nocardia* may be difficult because growth may take up to 3 weeks on routine culture media and *Nocardia* colonies may be obscured by the rapid overgrowth of concomitant bacterial species. Additionally, *Nocardia* are inhibited by antibiotics in fungal culture media and often do not survive the specimen digestive procedures used in mycobacterial culture isolation. The observation that some nocardial isolates may not survive in respiratory specimens has prompted studies of procedures to facilitate the recovery of aerobic actinomycetes from these sources.[52,53] In 1987, Murray et al. demonstrated that digestion-decontamination of respiratory tract specimens with *N*-acetyl-L-cysteine, sodium hydroxide, and benzalkonium was toxic to *Nocardia*.[54] These same investigators studied the usefulness of Thayer-Martin medium containing vancomycin, colistin, and nystatin, a selective medium commonly used in clinical laboratories for the isolation of *Neisseria* species from contaminated specimens, as a selective medium for the growth of *Nocardia* species. Although this study used seeded sputum specimens and not clinical specimens to evaluate the medium, the results are extremely encouraging for this selective medium.[54] Other promising media include buffered charcoal-yeast extract (BCYE) agar and selective BCYE media containing polymyxin, anisomycin, and vancomycin; these media are commonly used in clinical microbiology laboratories for the isolation of *Legionella* species from respiratory specimens.[55] These investigators also found that pretreatment of clinical specimens with a low-pH (2.2) KCl-HCl solution for 4 min was necessary for adequate isolation of *Nocardia* species.[55] Although no optimal methods for isolating the aerobic actinomycetes from potentially contaminated specimens exist, the methods discussed above likely represent an improvement for these microorganisms' recovery when compared to direct plating of these specimens to conventional media (e.g., Sabouraud-dextrose agar, brain-heart infusion agar, blood agar, or Löwenstein-Jensen).

BIOCHEMICALS The final identification of the aerobic actinomycetes depends upon the results of a battery of tests including the hydrolysis of different substrates (e.g., *N. brasiliensis* hydrolyzes casein and tyrosine but not xanthine, Fig. 202-4), acid production from carbohydrates, production of nitrate reductase and urease, and antimicrobial susceptibility profiles (Tables 202-4 and 202-5). Importantly, routine identification methods in use in many clinical laboratories may often misidentify *N. farcinica* as *N. asteroides* complex, *Rhodococcus/Gordona* complex, or *Mycobacterium* species. Therefore, additional supplemental tests that include compar-

FIGURE 202-4

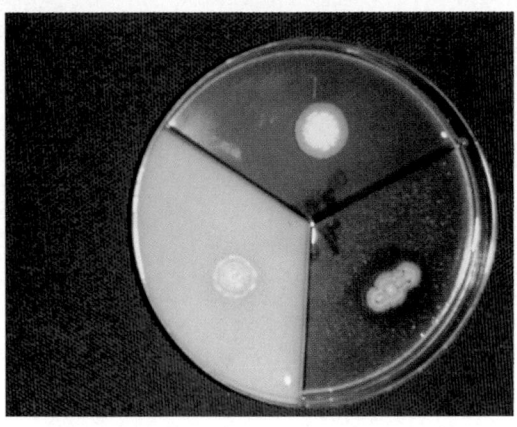

Nocardia brasiliensis is able to hydrolyze casein (*top*), and tyrosine (*right*), but not xanthine (*left*). (*Courtesy of Roberto Arenas, MD, Hospital Manuel Gea González, Mexico City.*)

ison of growth on agar slants at 35° and 45°C, the hydrolysis of acetamide, production of acid from L-rhamnose, arylsulfatase production, and antimicrobial susceptibility testing may be needed for the definitive identification of *N. farcinica* (Table 202-5). In addition, newer rapid, sensitive identification techniques (e.g., use of chromogenic enzyme substrates) are being developed.[61]

Diagnostic Immunology

Diagnosis by immunologic methods[62,63] has been hampered by the antigenic complexity of the aerobic actinomycetes, cross reactivity with other species and genera (including *Mycobacteria*), and development of a generally poor immunologic response against many nocardiae during the infectious process. With the use of affinity chromatography, Boiron and Provost purified a 54-kDa antigen from *N. asteroides* for a Western blot assay and found little cross reactivity with *N. brasiliensis*, *R. rhodochrous*, and *M. tuberculosis* and *M. leprae*.[62] Although there have been many previous immunologic studies with *N. asteroides*, only recently have data on a sensitive *N. brasiliensis* immunodiagnostic assay been published. In 1993, Salinas-Carmona, Welsh, and co-workers[63] described an enzyme-linked immunosorbent assay that used the 26- and 24-kDa proteins for the diagnosis of *N. brasiliensis* mycetoma infections and showed its usefulness in assessing the patient's response to treatment. An additional advantage of this particular assay might be its demonstrated cross-reactivity with *N. asteroides*.

Therapy

Sulfonamides or trimethoprim-sulfamethoxazole (TMP-SMZ) are the therapy of choice for proven or presumed nocardiosis.[31] Recent in vitro and in vivo studies, clinical observations, and taxonomic developments indicate that antimicrobial therapy must be adjusted to the particular species of *Nocardia* present, to individual strain antimicrobial susceptibility patterns, and to the site and type of infection. Certain strains of *N. asteroides* complex may be susceptible to sulfonamides or TMP-SMZ, and response to treatment may be attained in more than 90 percent of cases if the infection is confined

TABLE 202-4

Characteristics Used to Differentiate the Medically Important *Nocardia* Species

CHARACTERISTIC	N. asteroides COMPLEX*	N. brasiliensis	N. pseudobrasiliensis	N. otitidiscaviarum	N. transvalensis
Decomposition of					
Adenine	–	–	+	–	V
Casein	–	+	+	–	–
Hypoxanthine	–	+	+	+	+
Tyrosine	–	+	+	–	–
Xanthine	–	–	–	+	V
Acid produced from					
Adonitol (ribitol)	–	–	–	–	+
L-Arabinose	–	–	–	V	–
i-Erythritol	–	–	–	–	+
D-Galactose	V	+	+	–	+
D-Glucose	+	+	+	+	+
i-myo-Inositol	+	+	+	+	V
D-Mannitol	–	+	+	V	V
L-Rhamnose	V	–	–	–	–
D-Sorbitol (D-glucitol)	–	–	–	–	V
D-Trehalose	V	+	+	V	V
Production of					
Nitrate reductase	+	+	–	+	+
Urease	+	+	+	+	+

The *N. asteroides* complex includes *N. nova*, *N. farcinica*, and *N. asteroides* sensu stricto, four unnamed taxa.
NOTE: +, 90% or more of the strains are positive; v, 11 to 89% of the strains are positive; –, 10% or fewer of the strains are positive.
SOURCE: Data from Steingrube et al.[34] and Ruimy et al.[56]

TABLE 202-5

Characteristics Used to Differentiate the Groups within the *Nocardia asteroides* complex

CHARACTERISTIC	N. asteroides SENSU STRICTO				N. farcinica	N. nova
	I	II	IV	VI		
Resistance* to						
Amikacin (MIC, ≥ 8 µg/mL)	–	–	+	–	–	–
Gentamicin (MIC, ≥ 4 µg/mL)	–	+	+	–	+	±
Kanamycin (MIC, ≥ 16 µg/mL)	–	–	+	±	+	±
Tobramycin (zone < 20 mm)	–	–	+	–	+	±
Ciprofloxacin (MIC,, >4 µg/mL)	+	–	–	+	–	+
Ampicillin (MIC, ≥ 4µg/mL)	±	±	NT	+	+	–
Amoxicillin-clavulanic acid (MIC, ≥ 64/32 µg/mL)	NT	NT	NT	NT	–	+
Cefamandole (zone 20 mm)	–	–	–	–	+	–
Cefotaxime (MIC, ≥ 64 µg/mL)	–	–	–	–	+	–
Ceftriaxone (MIC, ≥ 64 µg/mL)	–	–	–	–	+	–
Imipenem (MIC, ≥ 16 µg/mL)	±	NT	NT	–	±	–
Erythromycin (MIC, ≥ 8 µg/mL)	+	+	+	+	+	–
Growth at 45°C (2 days)	±	–	–	±	+	–
Hydrolysis of acetamide	–	–	–	±	+	–
Arylsulfatase production	–	–	–	–	–	±
Acid production from						
D-Galactose	–	–	+	±	±	±
L-Rhamnose	–	±	–	±	+	–
D-Sorbitol	±	–	±	–	–	–
D-Trehalose	±	±	+	±	–	±
Specific PCR-RFLP pattern	+	+	+	+	+	+
Specific HPLC pattern	–	–	–	–	–	+

*Strains were considered resistant when the MIC was equal to or greater than the breakpoint (NCCLS[60]); strains were considered resistant when the disk zone size was less than 20 mm (Wallace et al.[57]).
NOTE: +, 90% or more of the strains are positive; –, 10% or less of the strains are positive; ±, 11 to 89% of the strains are positive; NT, not tested.
SOURCE: Data reported by Wallace et al.[57–59] and Steingrube et al.[34]

to pleuropneumonia. However, in patients with disseminated disease to the central nervous system and/or renal transplant recipients and HIV-infected patients, optimal drug therapy may be complicated.[31] First, these patients frequently develop side effects (skin rash, fever, neutropenia, hepatotoxicity) with TMP-SMZ that may be aggravated by prolonged use of TMP-SMZ as prophylactic therapy. Second, the infecting microorganism may develop resistance to prolonged therapy with TMP-SMZ, alternative agents, or drug combinations. Third, there are scant data on the efficacy of newer oral alternative antimicrobial agents or combinations that might improve the outcome of patients infected with *Nocardia* species and avoid the problems of TMP-SMZ.

Sulfonamides have good penetration into the cerebrospinal fluid and achieve high concentrations there.[64] Sulfadiazine is the most commonly prescribed, but sulfisoxazole and triple sulfonamide combinations are also effective. Drug therapy should be continued for 6 to 18 months, depending on the extent of the disease, because of the high incidence of relapse and metastatic abscesses with shorter duration of therapy.[31] For most patients with nocardiosis, clinical improvement is expected within 7 to 10 days after the initiation of empiric therapy with sulfonamides (with or without trimethoprim). For infected patients, the exact route of drug administration may be influenced by the assessment of their overall clinical status. In addition, a serum level estimation at least once following institution of antimicrobial therapy may be useful to establish that adequate drug absorption is occurring and to provide a basis for any necessary adjustment of the patient's drug dosage to achieve recommended levels in blood of 100 to 150 μg/mL approximately 2 h after an oral dose. It is recommended that therapy with sulfonamides be given at high doses (3 to 6 g/day) for extended periods of 6 to 12 months. While primary cutaneous nocardiosis may be cured by a 1- to 3-month course of antimicrobial therapy and uncomplicated pulmonary nocardiosis may respond to therapy for 6 months or less, therapy for 12 months or more is usually required for disseminated infection or if the patient is immunocompromised. Alternative antimicrobial agents in patients hypersensitive to sulfonamides include ampicillin, clindamycin, erythromycin, and minocycline. Minocycline reaches excellent concentrations in the brain and can penetrate into phagocytes to kill intracellular organisms.[31] Ampicillin plus erythromycin or sulfonamide have demonstrated synergism in vitro.[31] Although amikacin is an effective agent in vitro, it does not cross the blood-brain barrier and prolonged outpatient therapy is impractical. Surgical drainage of abscesses and debridement of avascular tissue may be important adjuncts in the successful management of infected patients.

ACTINOMYCETOMA

Epidemiology

The word *mycetoma* means a tumor-like lesion produced by a fungus, yet it is accepted to signify a focus of chronic inflammation producing an increase in tissue volume of the affected part. It is caused by *exogenous* organisms that produce *filamentous* grains. Mycetomas may be due to fungi (*eumycetomas*) or bacteria (*actinomycetomas*).[65,66] Patients with these chronic infections may have a history of a specific minor localized traumatic injury. Walking barefoot may be the major mode of acquisition of these infections, since this practice potentially exposes the feet to repeated soil-contaminated puncture wounds. Only actinomycetomas will be discussed further in this chapter.

Microorganisms reported to cause actinomycetomas include *N. brasiliensis*, *Actinomadura madurae*, *A. pelletieri*, *Streptomyces somaliensis*, and, less commonly, *N. asteroides*, *N. otitidiscaviarum*, *Nocardiopsis dassonvillei*, and *N. transvalensis*. In North America, South America, Mexico, and Australia, *N. brasiliensis* is the chief cause of actinomycetomas; however, in Africa, Saudi Arabia, and India, *S. somaliensis* and *A. madurae* predominate. These infections most commonly affect patients in the rural areas in third world countries (see Table 202-3). If the tumescent infection is caused by nonfilamentous bacteria, it is called *botryomycosis*.

Clinical Disease

Actinomycetoma is a chronic, localized, slowly progressive and often painless subcutaneous disease. The foot is the most common site of involvement (Madura foot); however, the hand (Figs. 202-5 and 202-6), face, neck, chest, and upper back (Figs. 202-7, 202-8, and 202-9) may also be involved. The pathology of the disease is characterized by tumefaction, subcutaneous nodules, destructive granulomata, deformity, and discharging sinus tracts with intercommunicating channels that exude pus, often with macroscopically visible granules of various sizes and colors. Macroscopically, the granules of *Nocardia* usually appear white or yellowish in color and those of *A. madurae* tan or orange to deep red; *A. pelletieri* granules appear red, and those of *S. somaliensis* are usually a cream to brown color (see Table 202-1).

Histopathology

Actinomycetomas, eumycotic mycetomas, and botryomycosis are all associated with a similar tissue response. The epidermis is acanthotic, even with pseudocarcinomatous hyperplasia, but absent in ulcerative lesions. Dermis and deeper structures show features related to the age of the individual lesion (not the whole process). Typically, in H&E-stained sections, deeply basophilic granules (grains) may be present. Amorphous, deeply eosinophilic, radially arranged Splendore-Hoeppli material may be present on the periphery of the granule (Fig. 202-10). The latter is surrounded by neutrophils that fail to penetrate the inner parts of the grain. Around the neutrophils there is a variable admixture of lymphocytes, monocytes, and macrophages forming a granuloma. It is uncommon to observe a well-structured tuberculoid granuloma. Areas of fibrosis

FIGURE 202-5

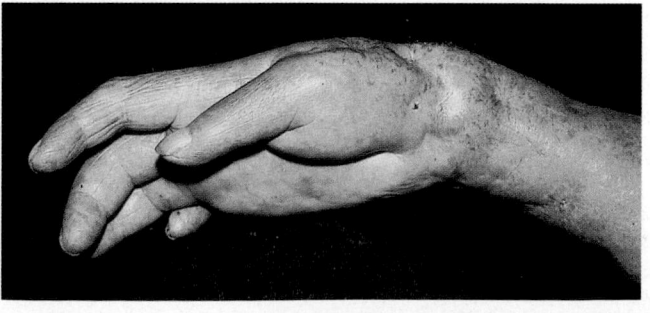

Mycetoma of the hand and wrist caused by *Nocardia brasiliensis.* Note gross deformity. (*Courtesy of Roberto Arenas, MD, Hospital Manuel Gea González, Mexico City.*)

FIGURE 202-6

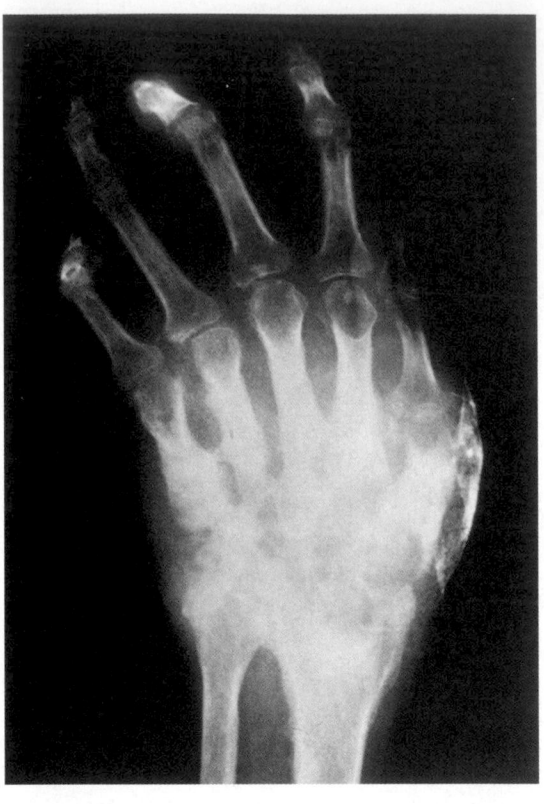

Radiograph from patient in Fig. 202-5 shows associated marked destruction of bones and soft tissues. (*Courtesy of Roberto Arenas, MD, Hospital Manuel Gea González, Mexico City.*)

FIGURE 202-7

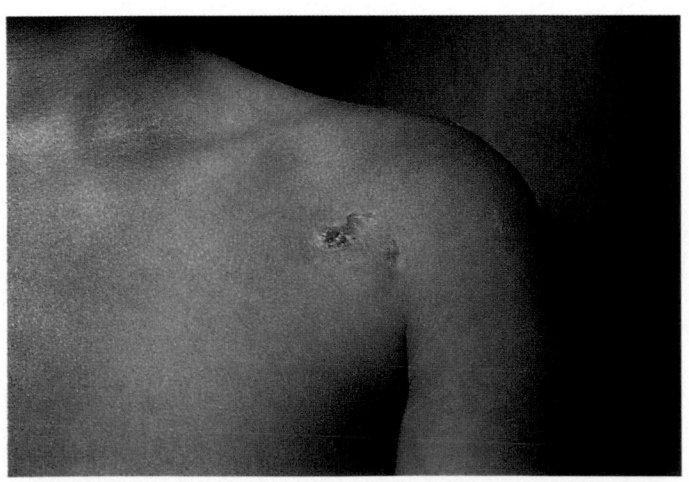

Small mycetoma of the shoulder caused by *Nocardia brasiliensis*. (*Courtesy of María Cecilia Albornoz, MD, Instituto de Biomedicina, Caracas.*)

FIGURE 202-8

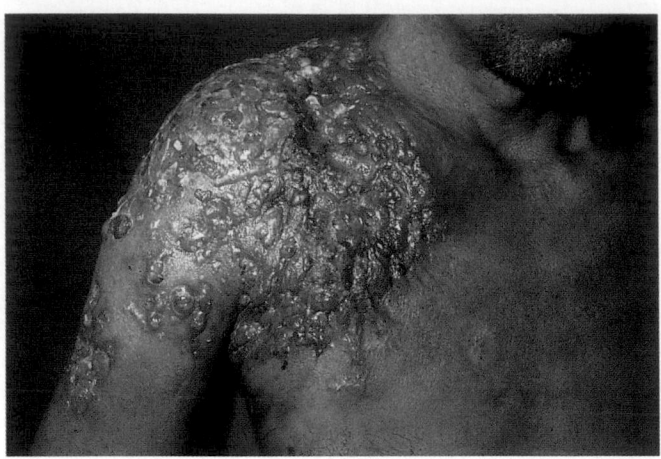

Huge scapulothoracic mycetoma caused by *Nocardia brasiliensis*. Note multiple fistulae. (*Courtesy of María Cecilia Albornoz, MD, Instituto de Biomedicina, Caracas.*)

surround the inflammatory infiltrate. In old lesions, inflammatory foci may be wholly replaced by fibrosis or remain as small islands in a sea of fibrosis.[67]

Usually in H&E-stained tissue sections, neither the filaments of actinomycetoma and eumycotic mycetoma nor the bacterial agents causing botryomycosis are seen. To further define a granule as being actinomycotic or eumycotic, special stains (i.e., B&B stain for bacteria, the GMS method for both bacteria and fungi, and PAS for fungi only) are needed. If either the B&B- or the GMS-stained sections reveal gram-positive branched bacterial filaments ($\leq 1.0\ \mu m$ in width), this finding suggests a diagnosis of actinomycetoma; however, the presence of a pure population of nonfilamentous bacteria (bacilli, cocci, or coccobacilli) suggests the diagnosis of botryomycosis (Fig. 202-11). If either a GMS- or PAS-stained section shows broad (2 to 6 μm) hyphae, often in addition to the presence of numerous chlamydospores in the mycelium, these findings suggest a diagnosis of eumycotic mycetoma.

FIGURE 202-9

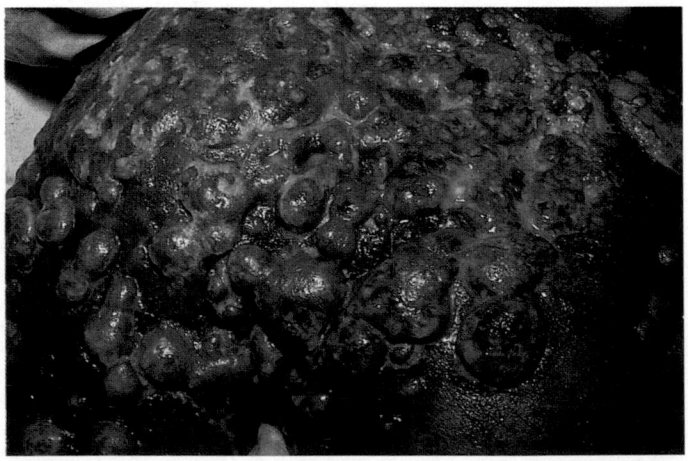

Higher magnification of mycetoma in Fig. 202-8. Note doughnut-shaped masses and purulent drainage. (*Courtesy of María Cecilia Albornoz, MD, Instituto de Biomedicina, Caracas.*)

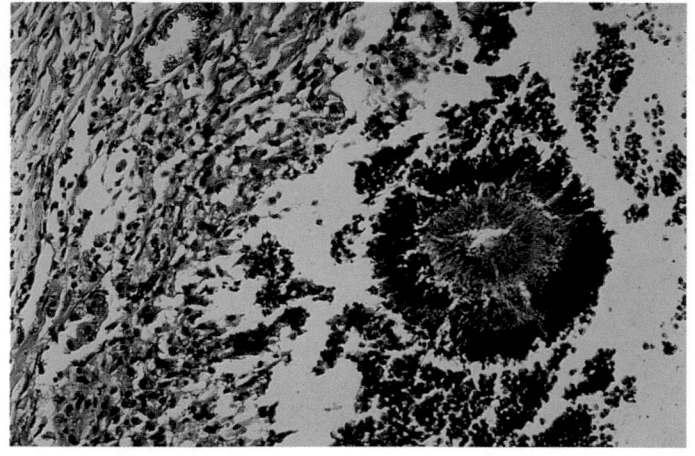

Histopathologic section of mycetoma featuring a granule of *Nocardia brasiliensis*. Note homogeneous center, peripheral clavate area, and surrounding tissue reaction with infiltration by polymorphonuclear leukocytes. H&E stain. (*Courtesy of Oscar Reyes-Flores, MD, Instituto de Biomedicina, Caracas.*)

Among the agents causing actinomycetomas, the granules of *Nocardia* are small (about 100 μm in diameter) and the granules of *A. madurae* are variable in size (0.5 to 5 mm), whereas the granules of *A. pelletieri* and *S. somaliensis* range from 300 to 500 μm and from 0.5 to 5 mm, respectively. Although several earlier references suggested that the histologic appearance may enable a species-specific diagnosis,[68,69] the histopathologic findings (including the appearance of granules, if present), are markedly nonspecific, and culture isolation and identification of the causative agent are essential for confirmation of the diagnosis of aerobic actinomycete infection. This is because recent taxonomic studies (using DNA hybridization and 16S recombinant RNA sequencing) have confirmed marked heterogeneity among the genera of aerobic actinomycetes. In addition, the macroscopic granules that may be seen to emerge in the exudate from the sinus tracts in actinomycetoma patients may

FIGURE 202-11

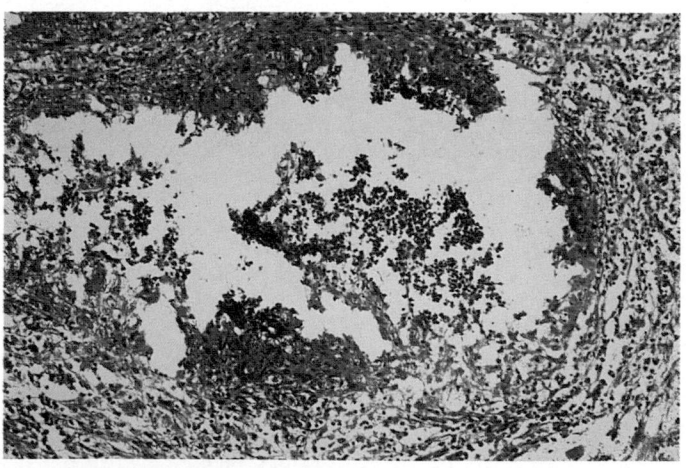

Histopathologic section of botryomycotic granule. H&E stain. (*Courtesy of María Cecilia Albornoz, MD, Instituto de Biomedicina, Caracas.*)

or may not simulate the corresponding microorganism's colonial characteristics on microbiologic culture.

Botryomycosis is usually a chronic or subacute inflammation of the skin and subcutaneous tissues. The bacteria most commonly implicated in causing botryomycosis include *Pseudomonas aeruginosa*, *Actinobacillus lignieresi*, *Staphylococcus aureus*, and *Proteus* and *Escherichia* species.[70]

Diagnosis

Clinical history, epidemiologic considerations, and general pathologic features should alert the clinician to the possible diagnosis of actinomycetoma. The detection of suggestive microorganisms in stained histologic sections obtained by deep wedge-shaped surgical biopsies or preparations from fine-needle aspiration may be of value.[71] Criteria for presumptive microbiologic diagnosis to the genus level are given in Table 202-1. However, it has been suggested that patient isolates should be sent to a specialized reference laboratory for species identification and in vitro susceptibility testing.[31]

Treatment

Therapy for patients with actinomycetoma should be individualized. Economic considerations may influence the choice of therapy, particularly in developing countries. Parenteral treatment is difficult in ambulatory patients. Patient follow-up is always important, and clinical progress may be monitored by biopsy or aspiration and culture. Dapsone (diaminodiphenylsulfone) has been reported to be effective and has been used in combination with other antimicrobials. Dapsone is usually prescribed in an oral daily dosage varying from 1.5 to 5 mg/kg for periods of 1 to 2 years following clinical cure.[72] Presence and levels of glucose-6-phosphate dehydrogenase should be checked before starting dapsone. To prevent methemoglobinemia, 2 g of ascorbic acid or 300 mg of vitamin E should be given daily. In the past two decades, therapy with other sulfonamides (e.g., TMP-SMZ) has been reported to be successful. The recommended therapeutic dose of TMP-SMZ is 8 and 40 mg/kg per day for periods ranging from 6 months to several years, with a reported average success rate of more than 60 percent.[72] This drug should be used with caution in AIDS patients as they may be intolerant of this combination. The use of other agents (e.g., amikacin) has been proposed, but there is no wide-spread consensus on their use. There have been additional reports in patients unresponsive to sulfonamide therapy on the successful use of the combination of amikacin (15 mg/kg per day total dose, divided and administered as two intramuscular injections every 12 h) and oral TMP-SMZ each for a total of 3 weeks followed by oral TMP-SMZ alone for an additional 2 weeks.[72,73] This constitutes a "cycle." One to three cycles are usually required (5 to 15 weeks of treatment).[72] The patient should be monitored for the development of amikacin-associated ototoxicity. Surgery is effective in early or small lesions (minimycetomas) and may be the last recourse in extensive mycetomas. Extension of the infection to involve bone may be an important determinant in deciding the extent of surgical debridement. Medical treatment should precede and continue after surgical treatment. Stopping any immunosuppressant medications and other specific measures to enhance the patient's immune status (e.g., antiviral treatment for HIV infection) and surgery (e.g., removal of prostheses or foreign bodies) may have an important adjunctive role in the patient's therapy.

FUTURE RESEARCH AREAS

The development of modern tools for early and accurate microbiologic diagnosis as well as easier methods for identifying organisms within lesions would seem to be technically feasible, if adequate funds and efforts were available. Diagnosis and management of these often chronic progressive infections are particularly difficult. Newer developments in molecular diagnostics [polymerase chain reaction (PCR) probe technology] may represent an advance that can be effectively utilized, particularly in referral centers in developing countries that manage large numbers of patients with these infections. Selective molecular screening of clinical specimens for the presence of pathogenic bacterial species may overcome the difficulties posed by the routine culture isolation techniques and allow rapid distinction of these pathogens from concomitant colonizing bacteria. In addition, the application of newer molecular typing techniques to the laboratory evaluation of epidemiologically important *Nocardia* isolates will assist in the differentiation of epidemic and endemic or colonizing isolates. In particular, in nosocomial nocardiosis outbreaks, the application of these methods may enable the identification of potential common sources of these microorganisms and aid in the formulation of effective infection control measures.[74] Recently, Steingrube et al. described a PCR–restriction fragment length polymorphism identification schema that used an amplified 439-bp segment of the 65-kDa heat shock protein gene.[75] (Using this method, all clinically significant species and taxa of aerobic actinomycetes, including *Actinomadura, Gordona, Nocardia, Rhodococcus, Streptomyces,* and *Tsukamurella,* were rapidly identified.) This methodology may prove to be sensitive, less time-consuming, and less labor-intensive than traditional biochemical methods.[75] Actinomycetales pose interesting problems in pathogenicity. Grains are microcolonies that evade the host's defense mechanisms. Organisms may produce substances that may attract phagocytes, but at the same time are able to block or evade their action.[37] The occurrence of only a few clinical cases in the face of widespread exposure should stimulate research on the existence of discrete flaws in digestion or lethal capacities of phagocytes, as have been described in paracoccidioidomycosis.[76–78] In addition, effective prophylactic methods, including dental and mouth hygiene as well as wearing of shoes and other mechanical protections, are known and should be put into practice in developing countries, with modest expenditure.

REFERENCES

1. Schaal KP, Hee-Joo Lee: Actinomycete infection in humans—a review. *Gene* 115:201, 1992
2. Lechevalier HA et al: Chemical composition as a criterion in the classification of actinomycetes. *Adv Appl Microbiol* 14:47, 1971
3. Goodfellow M: Suprageneric classification of actinomycetes, in *Bergey's Manual of Systematic Bacteriology,* vol 4, ST Williams, ME Sharpe, JG Holt. Baltimore, Williams & Wilkins, 1989, pp 2333–2339
4. Benhoff DF: Actinomycosis: Diagnosis and therapeutic considerations and a review of cases. *Laryngoscope* 94:1198, 1984
5. Slack JM, Gerencser MA: *Actinomyces, Filamentous Bacteria.* Minneapolis, Burgess Publishing, 1975
6. Pulverer G, Schaal KP: Human actinomycosis. *Drugs Exp Clin Res* X:187, 1984
7. Lenoir P et al: Bronchoscopic diagnosis of an unusual presentation of pulmonary actinomycosis. *Pediatr Pulmonol* 16:138, 1993

8. Coodley EL, Yoshinaka R: Pleural effusion as the major manifestation of actinomycosis. *Chest* 106:1615, 1994
9. Boutbol P et al: Quand penser a l'actinomycose génitale (When to think about genital actinomycosis). *Presse Med* 25:83, 1996
10. Fry RD et al: Actinomycosis as a cause of recurrent perianal fistula in the immunocompromised patient. *Surgery* 111:591, 1992
11. Manfredi R et al: Progressive intractable actinomycosis in patients with AIDS. *Scand J Infect Dis* 27:405, 1995
12. Fiorino AS: Intrauterine contraceptive device–associated actinomycotic abscess and *Actinomycetes* detection on cervical smear. *Obstet Gynecol* 87:142, 1996
13. Traynor RM et al: Isolation of actinomycetes from cervical specimens. *J Clin Pathol* 34:914, 1981
14. Dowell VR, Hawkins TM: *Laboratory Methods in Anaerobic Bacteriology.* CDC Laboratory Manual. US Dept of Health and Human Services, 1990
15. Schofield GM, Schaal KP: A numerical taxonomic study of members of the Actinomycetaceae and related taxa. *J Clin Microbiol* 127:237, 1981
16. Muller-Holzner E et al: IUD-associated pelvic actinomycosis: A report of five cases. *Int J Gynecol Pathol* 14:70, 1995
17. Georg LK et al: Evaluation of an agar gel precipitin test for the serodiagnosis of actinomycosis. *J Immunol* 100:1288, 1968
18. Schaal KP, Gatzer R: Serological and numerical phenetic classification of clinically significant fermentative actinomycetes, in *Filamentous Microorganisms, Biomedical Aspects,* edited by Arai, T. Tokyo, Japan Scientific Societies Press, 1985, pp 85–109
19. Holm P: Some investigations into the penicillin sensitivity of human pathogenic actinomycetes and some comments on penicillin treatment of actinomycosis. *Acta Pathol Microbiol Scand* 25:376, 1948
20. Weese WC, Smith IM: A study of 57 cases of actinomycosis over a 36-year period. *Arch Intern Med* 135:1562, 1975
21. Garland SM, Rawling D: Pelvic actinomycosis in association with an intrauterine device. *Aust NZ J Obstet Gynaecol* 33:96, 1993
22. Boand A, Novak M: Sensitivity changes of *Actinomyces bovis* to penicillin and streptomycin. *J Bacteriol* 57:501, 1949
23. Garrod LP: The sensitivity of *Actinomyces israelii* to antibiotics. *Br Med J* 1:1263, 1952
24. Lerner PI: Susceptibility of pathogenic actinomycetes to antimicrobial compounds. *Antimicrob Agents Chemother* 5:302, 1974
25. Peabody JW Jr, Seabury JH: Actinomycosis and nocardiosis: A review of basic differences in therapy. *Am J Med* 28:99, 1960
26. McFarlane DJ et al: Treatment of recalcitrant actinomycosis with ciprofloxacin. *J Infec* 27:177, 1993
27. Edelmann M et al: Treatment of abdominothoracic actinomycosis with imipenem. *Eur J Clin Microbiol* 6:194, 1987
28. Skoutelis A et al: Successful treatment of thoracic actinomycosis with ceftriaxone. *Clin Infect Dis* 19:161, 1994
29. Schaal KP, Beaman BL: Clinical significance of actinomycetes, in *The Biology of the Actinomycetes,* edited by M Goodfellow, M Mordarski, ST Williams. London, Academic, 1983, pp 389–424
30. Schaal KP, Pape W: Special methodological problems in antibiotic susceptibility testing of fermentative actinomycetes. *Infection* 8:176, 1980
31. Lerner PL: Nocardiosis. *Clin Infect Dis* 22:891, 1996
32. McNeil MM, Brown JM: The medically important aerobic actinomycetes: Epidemiology and microbiology. *Clin Microbiol Rev* 7:357, 1994
33. Hay RJ: Nocardial infection of the skin. *J Hyg (Camb)* 91:385, 1983
34. Steingrube VA et al: DNA amplification and restriction endonuclease analysis for differentiation of 12 species and taxa of *Nocardia* including recognition of four new taxa within the *Nocardia asteroides* complex. *J Clin Microbiol* 33:3096, 1995
35. Smego RD et al: Trimethoprim-sulfamethoxazole therapy for *Nocardia* infections. *Arch Intern Med* 143:711, 1983
36. Wallace RJ Jr et al: New *Nocardia* taxon among isolates of *Nocardia brasiliensis* associated with invasive disease. *J Clin Microbiol* 33:1528, 1995
37. Beaman BL et al: *Nocardia* and nocardiosis. *J Med Vet Mycol* 30(suppl 1):317, 1992
38. Houang ET et al: *Nocardia asteroides* infection—a transmissible disease. *J Hosp Infect* 1:31, 1980
39. Cox F, Hughes WT: Contagious and other aspects of nocardiosis in the compromised host. *Pediatrics* 55:135, 1975
40. Sahathevan M et al: Epidemiology, bacteriology and control of an outbreak of *Nocardia asteroides* infection on a liver unit. *J Hosp Infect* 18(suppl A):473, 1991

41. Schaal KP: Medical and microbiological problems arising from airborne infection. *J Hosp Infect* **18**:451, 1991

42. Krick JA et al: *Nocardia* infection in heart transplant patients. *Ann Intern Med* **82**:18, 1975

43. Simpson GL et al: Nocardial infections in the immunocompromised host: A detailed study in a defined population. *Rev Infect Dis* **3**:492, 1981

44. Yew WW et al: Two cases of *Nocardia asteroides* sternotomy infection treated with ofloxacin and a review of other active antimicrobial agents. *J Infect* **23**:297, 1991

45. Patterson JE et al: Pseudoepidemic of *Nocardia asteroides* associated with a mycobacterial culture system. *J Clin Microbiol* **30**:1357, 1992

46. Anonymous: Cutaneous nocardiosis in cancer patients receiving immunotherapy injections—Bahamas. *Morb Mort Week Rep* **33**:471, 1984

47. Valero-Guillen PL, Martin-Luengo : *Nocardia* in soils of southeastern Spain: Abundance, distribution, and chemical characterization. *Can J Microbiol* **30**:1088, 1984

48. Gaspar G et al: Primary cutaneous nocardiosis and human immunodeficiency virus infection. (letter). *Med Clin (Barc)* **92**:598, 1989

49. Wilson JP et al: Nocardial infections in renal transplant recipients. *Medicine (Baltimore)* **68**:38, 1989

50. Lucas SB et al: Nocardiosis in HIV-positive patients: An autopsy study in West Africa. *Tuber Lung Dis* **75**:301, 1994

51. Berd D: Laboratory identification of clinically important aerobic actinomycetes. *Appl Microbiol* **25**:665, 1973

52. Hosty TS et al: Prevalence of *Nocardia asteroides* in sputa examined by a tuberculosis diagnostic laboratory. *J Lab Clin Med* **58**:107, 1961

53. Krasnow L, Wayne LG: Comparison of methods for tuberculosis bacteriology. *Appl Microbiol* **18**:915, 1969

54. Murray PR et al: Effect of decontamination procedures on recovery of *Nocardia* spp. *J Clin Microbiol* **25**:2010, 1987

55. Vickers RM et al: Clinical demonstration of isolation of *Nocardia asteroides* on buffered charcoal-yeast extract media. *J Clin Microbiol* **30**:227, 1992

56. Ruimy R et al: *Nocardia pseudobrasiliensis* sp. nov., a new species of *Nocardia* which groups bacterial strains previously identified as *Nocardia brasiliensis* and associated with invasive diseases. *Int J Syst Bacteriol* **46**:259, 1996

57. Wallace RJ Jr et al: Antimicrobial susceptibility patterns of *Nocardia asteroides*. *Antimicrob Agents Chemother* **32**:1776, 1988

58. Wallace RJ Jr et al: Cefotaxime-resistant *Nocardia asteroides* strains are isolates of the controversial species *Nocardia farcinica*. *J Clin Microbiol* **28**:2726, 1990

59. Wallace RJ Jr et al: Clinical and laboratory features of *Nocardia nova*. *J Clin Microbiol* **29**:2407, 1991

60. National Committee for Clinical Laboratory Standards: *Methods for Dilution Antimicrobial Susceptibility Tests for Bacteria That Grow Aerobically (M7-A2)*. Villanova, PA, National Committee for Clinical Laboratory Standards, 1990

61. Boiron P, Provost F: Enzymatic characterization of *Nocardia* spp. and related bacteria by API ZYM profile. *Mycopathologia* **110**:51, 1990

62. Boiron P, Provost F: Use of the partially purified 54-kilodalton antigen for diagnosis of nocardiosis by Western blot (immunoblot) assay. *J Clin Microbiol* **28**:328, 1990

63. Salinas-Carmona MC et al: Enzyme-linked immunosorbent assay for serological diagnosis of *Nocardia brasiliensis* and clinical correlations with mycetoma infections. *J Clin Microbiol* **31**:2901, 1993

64. Thea D, Barza M: Use of antibacterial agents in infections of the central nervous system. *Infect Dis Clin North Am* **3**:553, 1989

65. Magaña M: Mycetoma. *Int J Dermatol* **23**:221, 1984

66. Buot G et al: Etude epidemiologique de mycetomas au México. (An epidemiological study of mycetomas in Mexico.) *Bull Soc Pathol Exot* **80**:329, 1987

67. Bueno D et al: Minimicetomas por *Nocardia brasiliensis*. Estudio histológico de 13 casos. (Minimycetomas due to *Nocardia brasiliensis*. Histologic study of 13 cases.) *Med Cut ILA* **15**: 277, 1987

68. Rippon JW: Mycetoma in *Medical Mycology*, 2d ed. Philadelphia, Saunders, 1982, pp 79–114

69. Emmons CW et al: The mycetomas, in *Medical Mycology*, 3d ed. Philadelphia, Lea & Febiger, 1977, pp 437–463

70. Greenblatt M et al: Bacterial pseudomycosis ("botryomycosis"). *Am J Clin Pathol* **41**:188, 1964

71. El Hag IA et al: Fine needle aspiration cytology of mycetoma. *Acta Cytol* **40**:461, 1996

72. Welsh O: Mycetoma: Current concepts in treatment. *Int J Dermatol* **30**:387, 1991

73. Welsh O et al: Amikacin alone and in combination with trimethoprim-sulfamethoxazole in the treatment of actinomycotic mycetoma. *J Am Acad Dermatol* **17**:443, 1987

74. Exmelin L et al: Molecular study of a nosocomial nocardiosis outbreak involving heart transplant recipients. *J Clin Microbiol* **34**:1014, 1996

75. Steingrube VA et al: Rapid identification of clinically significant species and taxa of aerobic actinomycetes, including *Actinomadura, Gordona, Nocardia, Rhodococcus, Streptomyces*, and *Tsukamurella* isolates, by DNA amplification and restriction endonuclease analysis. *J Clin Microbiol* **35**:817, 1997

76. Bujak JS et al: Nocardiosis in a child with chronic granulomatous disease. *J Pediatr* **83**:98, 1973

77. Goihman-Yahr M et al: Defect of in vitro digestive ability of polymorphonuclear leukocytes in paracoccidioidomycosis. *Infect Immun* **28**:557, 1980

78. Goihman-Yahr M et al: Relationship between digestive and killing abilities of neutrophils against *Paracoccidioides brasiliensis*. *Mycoses* **35**:269, 1992

Thomas H. Rea
Robert L. Modlin

Leprosy

Leprosy (Hansen's disease) is a chronic granulomatous infection, primarily of skin and nerves, caused by *Mycobacterium leprae*. It is an important clinical problem, affecting several million people worldwide and imposing a health and economic burden particularly severe on developing countries. Even with the anticipated success of current control programs, the disease will remain a practical problem well into the twenty-first century. Also, despite apparently curative antibacillary therapy, approximately one-third of patients will have a debilitating permanent neurologic deficit. Leprosy is of particular importance to clinicians because the diverse host responses pose a challenging diagnostic problem, and it is of interest to immunologists, because the disease provides an exemplary model for understanding cell-mediated immunity in humans.

HISTORY

Leprosy is an ancient disease; sacred writings from India in the sixth century B.C. give a good description of a similar or identical illness. Greek soldiers returning from Asia in the third century B.C. are thought to have introduced the disease into Europe. From the European pandemic (A.D. 1000 to 1500), stigmatization of patients with leprosy remains an unfortunate but enduring legacy. Hansen's attribution of *M. leprae* as its etiologic agent in 1873 marks the beginning of scientific leprology.[1]

The introduction of sulfones (1943) was the beginning of effective chemotherapy against leprosy.[2] The limited growth of *M. leprae* in the mouse foot pad (1961) provided a way to screen for therapeutic agents and to identify drug resistance.[3] Rifampin was the first drug to be identified as bactericidal for *M. leprae* (1970) and is now the cornerstone of most therapeutic regimens.[4]

The lepromin skin test (1919), as described by Mitsuda, inaugurated systematic study of host resistance as the source of disease diversity,[5] and lymphocyte transformation tests were later established as an in vitro correlate (1960s). The recognition of leprosy in the nine-banded armadillo (1971) provided a source of large quantities of highly purified *M. leprae* for biochemical and immunologic study.[6] The ability to clone and express *M. leprae* genes provided a source of proteins for study of T and B cell responses (1985).[7] More recently, studies of leprosy have illuminated immunoregulation in general, by the initial demonstration in humans of type I (Th1-like) and type II (Th2-like) cytokine patterns (1991),[8] the documentation in humans of γδ T cells as participants in the

response to mycobacteria (1989),[9] and the demonstration that T cells recognize lipoglycan antigens via presentation from CD1b-bearing cells (1995).[10] (See also "Immunology," below, and Chap. 32.)

EPIDEMIOLOGY

Leprosy is primarily a disease of developing countries, although new indigenous cases are reported each year in Louisiana and Texas. The prevalence of leprosy has fallen dramatically in the past decade because patients completing a course of multiple drug therapy are now considered to be cured. As of 1992, the incidence of leprosy was estimated to be 690,000 new cases per year.[11] The preponderance of opinion supports the traditional view that *M. leprae* is transmitted from human to human, but the presence of an *M. leprae*–caused lepromatous-like illness in wild armadillos,[12] evidence of armadillo exposure as a risk factor for leprosy in people,[13] and the presence of an *M. leprae*–like organism in sphagnum moss[14] suggest that nonhuman sources for *M. leprae* may be important. The route of infection is not known, but current evidence favors respiratory transmission; evidence for congenital transmission has been presented, but this route is probably rare.[15] In leprosy-endemic areas, subclinical infection is common, as judged by serologic studies identifying *M. leprae*–specific antibodies.[16] A major drawback of epidemiologic studies is the lack of a reliable skin test to specifically identify infected individuals, such as the tuberculin test that identifies individuals with subclinical tuberculosis.

A twin study has provided compelling evidence that both genetic and environmental factors are important in determining disease susceptibility and disease expression.[17] Major histocompatibility complex class II antigens appear to influence disease expression but not susceptibility.[18] In all populations studied, lepromatous disease is more common in men than in women by a 2:1 ratio. Between different populations, the proportion of tuberculoid to lepromatous patients varies greatly, the tuberculoid form being dominant wherever the disease is common. However, in any given population, the ratio of tuberculoid to lepromatous cases remains constant.[19,20] The median age of onset is less in tuberculoid than in lepromatous patients, but in both groups, leprosy is predominantly a young person's disease, i.e., median age of onset is <35 years of age. Age per se is not protective, however; new cases of both types occur in the eighth and ninth decades of life.

Usually, prolonged close contact appears to be required for transmission. The incubation time for tuberculoid leprosy is up to 5 years and may be 20 years or longer for lepromatous disease.

DIAGNOSIS

Think of Leprosy

The diagnosis begins with a suspicion of leprosy, which should be aroused by the presence of any of several known risk factors, including the following: (1) birth or residence in an endemic area, which is almost a sine qua non for the diagnosis; (2) a blood relative with the disease, which could reflect transmission, common genetic makeup, or common environmental exposure; and (3) armadillo (nine-banded) exposure in North Americans.

The possibility of leprosy should also be suggested by particular clinical constellations, such as: (1) simultaneous skin lesions and peripheral nerve abnormalities; (2) a differential diagnosis that includes granuloma, vasculitis, or lymphoma; (3) a peripheral neuropathy of unknown type in a patient in or from an endemic area, the so-called pure neuritic leprosy; and (4) simultaneous palsies of cranial nerves V and VII, considered to be leprosy until proven otherwise.

Criteria for Diagnosis

Once considered, a firm diagnosis of leprosy requires the presence of a consistent peripheral nerve abnormality or the demonstration of mycobacteria in tissues.

NERVE CHANGES Several kinds of peripheral nerve abnormalities are common in leprosy: (1) nerve enlargement (usually perceived as asymmetry), particularly in those nerves close to the skin, such as the great auricular, ulnar, median, superficial peroneal, sural, and posterior tibial nerves; (2) sensory loss in skin lesions; (3) nerve trunk palsies secondary to granulomatous inflammation within nerves, usually with both sensory and motor loss (weakness and/or atrophy) and, if of long standing, also with contracture; (4) acral distal symmetric anesthesia—a withering away, so to speak, of the type C fibers, involving loss of heat and cold discrimination before loss of perception of pinprick or light touch, beginning in acral areas and, over time, extending centrally but sparing the palms, at least for a while. Uncommon peripheral nerve abnormalities include nerve abscesses (palisading granulomas formed about cutaneous sensory nerves) and the carpal tunnel syndrome. Anhidrosis is a not uncommon manifestation of sympathetic nerve involvement.

IDENTIFICATION AND QUANTITATION OF BACILLI Because *M. leprae* has yet to be grown in cell-free media, demonstration of mycobacteria by their acid-fast property is used almost universally in diagnosis. Acid-fast bacilli in tissue sections are best shown by carbolfuchsin staining, using modifications of the Ziehl-Neelson method, collectively called *Fite-Farraco stains*. *M. leprae*, like *Nocardia* species, is only weakly acid-fast. In smears, either the Ziehl-Neelson method or oramine-rhodamine staining with fluorescent microscopy is satisfactory. Because of characteristic clinical and histologic changes, positive specification of *M. leprae* is rarely required. In tissues, bacilli are usually found in macrophages and nerves.

Bacilli are usually quantified logarithmically by the bacillary index (BI); the numbers of bacilli per oil-immersion field (OIF) or the numbers of OIFs sought to find one bacillus:

	BI
Numbers of bacilli per OIF	
>1000	6
100–1000	5
10–100	4
1–10	3
Number of OIFs per bacillus	
1/1–10	2
1/10–100	1
0/100	0

The BI may be further refined by decimalizing the count according to the log of the number: thus, a count of 74/OIF translates to a BI of 4.7, and a count of 1 in 4 OIFs translates to a BI of 2.6. Because a BI of 6 indicates 10^9 bacilli per gram of granuloma, there may be as many as 10^3 bacilli per gram when the BI is 0.

The morphologic index, referring to the percent of solid-staining organisms, is rarely as large as 10 and usually less than 5, but it is of value because it is predictive of the percent of viable organisms.

Histology in Diagnosis

Characteristic histopathologic changes are very helpful in leading to a diagnosis of leprosy but are usually suggestive, not diagnostic. One exception is the presence of epithelioid cell granulomas within nerves, diagnostic of tuberculoid leprosy or a severe reversal reaction.

False Negatives

There are several errors that lead to missing the diagnosis of leprosy:

1. Failure to consider the diagnosis: often due to ignoring birth or residence in an endemic area.
2. Failure to inform the pathologist of the suspicion of leprosy: a perivascular lymphohistiocytic infiltrate may be so sparse as to mimic normal skin; thus no acid-fast bacilli (AFB) stain will be done by the pathologist, unless warned.
3. Failure to conduct an adequate neurologic examination: in particular, when the patient is not properly instructed to distinguish between dull and sharp. If the patient is not instructable, absence of a histamine-induced axon reflex flare, with a positive symmetric control, is good evidence of type C pain fiber loss.
4. Failure to exclude loss of heat and cold discrimination: presence of pin-prick perception does not exclude this.
5. Improper staining for AFB in biopsy specimens: in a conventional Ziehl-Neelson stain, *M. leprae*, being only weakly acid-fast, may be decolorized altogether.
6. Tissue sampling error: select the advancing border for biopsy, not the clearing center.

False Positives

There are also several errors that lead to improperly diagnosing leprosy:

1. Because of histamine tachyphylaxis, inflammatory lesions may have blunted pain perception, producing a reduction in sensation similar to that seen in some leprosy lesions.

2. Atypical mycobacterial infection may have the abundant AFB and foamy macrophages characteristic of lepromatous disease.

3. Environmental mycobacteria are found in water, including that used to process tissue sections, as suggested by bacilli not associated with cellular infiltrates or bacilli in the embedding medium.

4. From time-to-time, cunning artifacts are interpreted as AFB.

If a patient, suspected of having leprosy, has no history of residence in a known endemic area, then the possibility of one of these errors should be seriously considered.

Other Methods of Diagnosis

Alternative methods of establishing a diagnosis have been pursued but, at present, are of limited value. Antibodies directed against phenolic glycolipid I, evidently *M. leprae* specific, or lipoarabinomannan are most prevalent in multibacillary cases (where the need for better diagnosis is not pressing) and are, in endemic areas, far more prevalent than the disease, thus further restricting their utility.[16] Polymerase chain reaction (PCR) may be negative in up to one-half of paucibacillary cases, making a positive signal of value but a negative signal of no help. PCR should be most helpful in the diagnosis of patients with lesions having AFB, with cultures negative and no other stigmata of leprosy present.[21]

A Clinical Dilemma

One common diagnostic problem is the patient from an endemic area with a cutaneous tuberculoid granuloma, negative for AFB, but having no peripheral nerve abnormality. In such cases, which decision does the clinician prefer to make: treat someone who does not have the disease or not to treat someone with the disease? It is probably best to err on the side of caution and treat such a patient, with the realization that clinical remission does not prove the diagnosis.

CLASSIFICATION

Once a diagnosis of leprosy has been established, then classification is appropriate, often employing one or both of two commonly used systems. The disease forms a spectrum, in which the clinical manifestations correlate with the level of host cell-mediated immunity to the pathogen. A simple classification involves the dichotomy of patients into multibacillary (bacilli detectable in tissue sections or smears, ranging from one to many) or paucibacillary (no bacilli detectable) disease and is useful in determining antibacillary chemotherapy regimens.

A more detailed spectral classification of patients combines clinical and histologic criteria, as best articulated by Ridley and his associates.[22] The Ridley system integrates the clinical and histologic changes of the patient to provide a meaningful representation of the outcome of the host's responses to *M. leprae*. This clinical-histologic classification has been shown to correlate closely with the level of cell-mediated immunity to the pathogen. As it now stands, Ridley's system is a six-membered granulomatous spectrum, a kind of alphabet soup, ranging from high to low resistance: TT (polar

tuberculoid), BT (borderline tuberculoid), BB (borderline), BL (borderline lepromatous), LLs (subpolar lepromatous) and, finally, LLp (polar lepromatous):

$$TT \leftarrow BT \leftrightarrow BB \leftrightarrow BL \leftrightarrow LLs \ LLp$$

The host's position in the spectrum is not static but dynamic, in that the so-called upgrading or downgrading reactions allow patients to move about the spectrum. Conceptually, TT and LLp are clinically stable, but between the poles, the host's granulomatous posture may change (as indicated by the arrows), upgrading (or reversing) to a posture of higher resistance, often with devastating inflammation, or downgrading to a posture of lower resistance, usually silent but occasionally inflammatory. BB is the highly unstable midsection, or midpoint or inflection point of the spectrum. BT patients may upgrade to TT, thus becoming stable, but LLs patients do not downgrade to LLp, nor do LLp patients upgrade (hence no arrow between LLs and LLp) providing a provocative asymmetry. The granulomatous spectrum of leprosy is now functionally attributed to variations in cellular immunity, although originally it was descriptively ascribed to variations in host resistance to bacillary replication.

In a side-by-side comparison of these two classifications, virtually all TT patients are paucibacillary, as are most BT cases. BB, BL, LLs, and LLp are all multibacillary. In side-by-side comparison of pre-Ridley and Ridley terminology, *tuberculoid* corresponds to TT and BT, *borderline* or *dimorphic* to BB and BL, and *lepromatous* to LLs and LLp.

Because of its high rate of positivity in unexposed adults, lepromin skin testing is not useful in diagnosis but is of value in classification of diagnosed patients, all TT and most BT (85 percent in our experience) being positive (≥ 3 mm induration at 21 days) and BB through LLp being negative (< 3 mm). In the evaluation of treated immigrants, whose original biopsy and clinical picture are not known, lepromin skin tests are useful in classifying a patient as to high resistance (> 5 mm induration), low resistance (< 3 mm induration), with 3 to 5 mm being equivocal. This information may be useful in planning further therapy.

CLINICAL AND HISTOLOGIC CHANGES

Polar Tuberculoid Leprosy

In TT leprosy, immunity is strong, as manifested by spontaneous cure and the absence of downgrading to a status of less host resistance. The primary skin lesion of TT is a plaque, often assuming an annular configuration secondary to peripheral propagation and central clearing (Fig. 203-1). The border of the plaque or both borders of the annulus are sharply marginated. Typically, the lesion is firmly indurated, elevated, erythematous, scaly, dry, hairless, and hypopigmented; clinically, however, considerable variation is encountered.

A nearby sensory nerve may or may not be enlarged, but the lesion itself is characteristically anesthetic and anhidrotic. Skin lesions are often solitary, particularly in those patients who are TT de novo, as contrasted to those who upgrade to TT from BT, where several lesions (although usually no more than three) may be found. In both groups, immunity is sufficient to effect cure, thus placing an upper limit of 10 cm on lesion size, but antibiotic therapy is recommended nevertheless. Because of overlapping innervation, facial lesions may not be anesthetic.

FIGURE 203-1

CHAPTER 203
Leprosy

2309

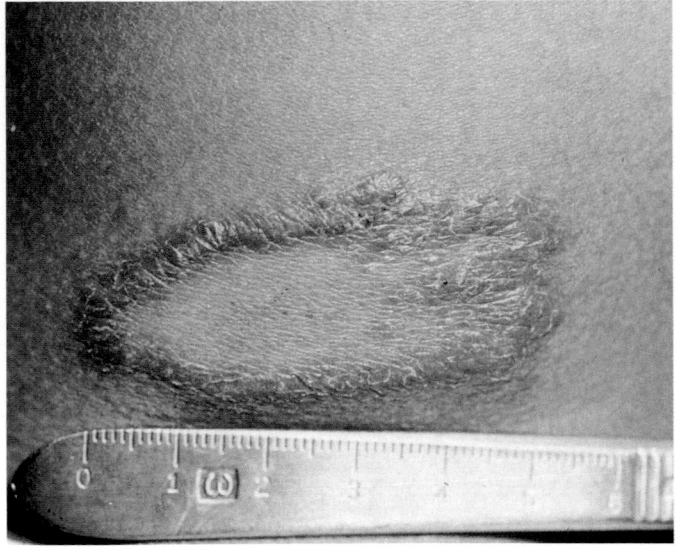

A solitary, anesthetic, and annular lesion of polar tuberculoid leprosy (TT), which had been present for 3 months. Its sharp margins, erythema, and scale are more evident than its elevation. The central red dots are the sequelae or "footprints" of testing for pinprick perception when it is absent. (If present, the patient withdraws, preventing overtly purpuric consequences.)

Histologically, TT disease resembles cutaneous tuberculosis, especially lupus vulgaris, hence the term *tuberculoid* leprosy. Two patterns predominate: (1) mature epithelioid tubercles without giant cells or fibrinoid necrosis and with large lymphocytic mantles but little epidermal exocytosis are associated with de novo TT; and (2) abundant large Langhans' giant cells, somewhat fewer lymphocytes, fibrinoid necrosis, the occasional foci of caseation necrosis, but heavy epidermal exocytosis are associated with TT upgraded from BT.[23] With rare exceptions, tissue is negative for AFB.

Borderline Tuberculoid Leprosy

In BT disease, immunologic resistance is strong enough to restrain the infection, in that the disease is limited and bacillary growth partially inhibited, but the host response is insufficient to self-cure. These patients are somewhat unstable: resistance may increase, upgrading to TT, or decrease, downgrading to BL.

The primary skin lesions of BT are plaques and papules. As in TT, an annular configuration is common and both borders are sharply marginated, but annular lesions or plaques may have satellite papules (Fig. 203-2). Hypopigmentation may be conspicuous in darkly pigmented patients. In contrast to TT, there is typically little or no scaling, less erythema, less induration, and less elevation, but lesions may become

much larger (i.e., well over 10 cm in diameter), and a single lesion may sometimes involve an entire extremity. Multiple, asymmetric lesions are the rule, but solitary lesions are not rare.

Loss of sensation in skin lesions is the rule, and nerve trunk involvement, enlargement, or palsies, usually in no more than two and asymmetric, are not uncommon. Nerve abscesses, when they occur, are most often seen in males with BT disease.

Histologically, BT lesions consist of epithelioid cell tubercules of variable number with fewer lymphocytes than in TT. Epidermal exocytosis, if it occurs, is only focal, and lymphocytic mantles about tubercles may be incomplete or poorly developed. Langhans' giant cells, when present, are smaller than in TT. Necrosis is absent. Most routinely processed tissues are negative for AFB. If AFB or plasma cells are easily found, then upgrading from BL should be considered.

Borderline Leprosy

BB is the immunologic midpoint, or midzone, of the granulomatous spectrum, being its most unstable area, with patients quickly up- or downgrading to a more stable granulomatous posture with or without a clinical reaction. Characteristic skin changes are annular lesions with sharply marginated interior and exterior margins, large plaques with islands of clinically normal skin within the plaque (giving a "Swiss cheese" appearance), or the classic dimorphic lesion. Histologically, the granulomas have epithelioid differentiation and no giant cells and are lymphopenic. AFB are easily found. Because of instability, the BB posture is short-lived, and such patients are evidently rarely seen; for example, the authors have yet to see a nonreactional patient meeting the lymphopenic criterion.

FIGURE 203-2

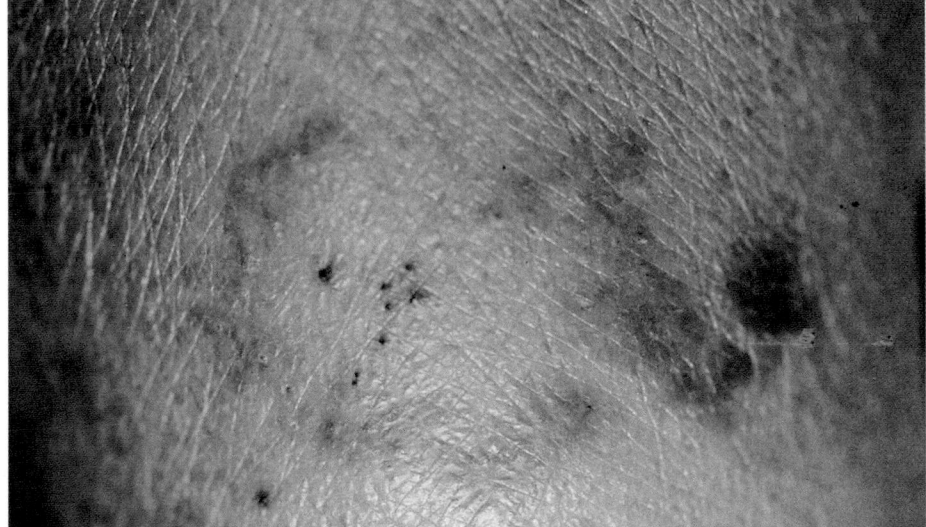

One of several lesions of borderline tuberculoid (BT), which had an incompletely annular configuration with satellite papules. Compared with the TT lesion of Fig. 203-1, there is less erythema, no evident scales, but sharp margination, and the footprints of absent pinprick perception remain.

Borderline Lepromatous Leprosy

In BL disease, resistance is too low to restrain bacillary proliferation significantly but is still sufficient to induce tissue-destructive inflammation, especially in nerves. Thus, patients with BL may have the worst of both worlds.

The BL category is highly variable in its clinical expression. Although seen in only a third of BL patients, the classic dimorphic lesion is the most characteristic, having an annular configuration with a poorly marginated outer border (lepromatous-like) but a sharply marginated inner one (tuberculoid-like; hence, having both morphologies, or dimorphic) (Fig. 203-3). Poorly or sharply marginated plaques with punched-out, or Swiss-cheese, sharply marginated areas of normal skin in the interior of the plaque are also characteristic and can be viewed as a variant of the classic dimorphic lesion. Annular lesions with sharply marginated exterior and interior borders are not uncommon. Lepromatous-like, poorly defined papules and nodules may be numerous but are usually accompanied by some sharply marginated lesions somewhere (Fig. 203-4).

Lesions range in number from solitary (something happens first—the tip of an inapparent iceberg) to numerous and widespread. Generally speaking, the annular and plaque lesions, however numerous, are asymmetric, but the lepromatous-like nodules, if numerous, are symmetric.

Skin lesions are often hypesthetic or anesthetic but not necessarily so. Nerve trunk palsies have their highest prevalence in BL disease but are variable in number, ranging from none to 6 or more, causing serious neurologic deficits, both motor and sensory, in all four extremities. Involvement of both median and ulnar nerves, not infrequently bilateral, is characteristic. When disease is extensive, BL patients may also develop acral distal symmetric anesthesia.

Histologically, the characteristic BL granuloma consists of numerous lymphocytes, confined to the same space as the aggregations of undifferentiated and foamy macrophages. The characteristic

FIGURE 203-3

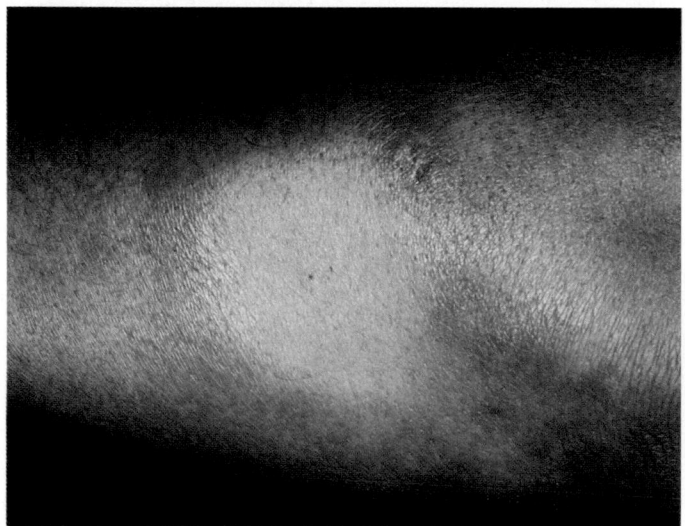

A characteristic borderline or dimorphic lesion, which is an indurated and elevated plaque of borderline lepromatous (BL) leprosy that has sharper margination on the interior than on the exterior border. The footprints of absent pinprick perception are evident.

FIGURE 203-4

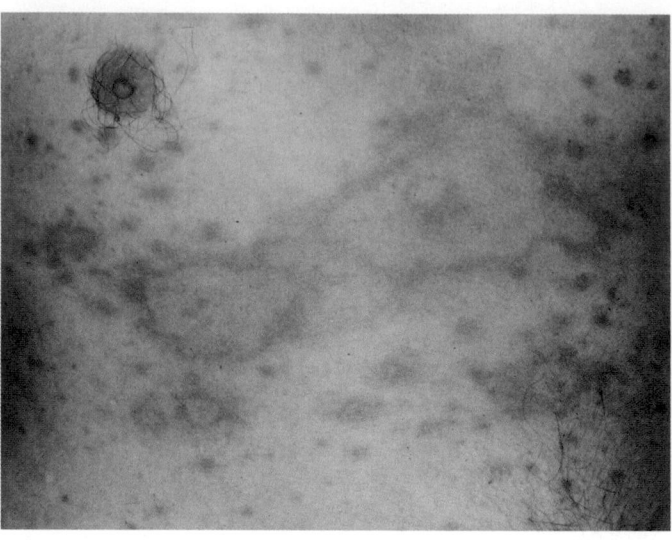

Multiple lesions in a patient with borderline lepromatous (BL) leprosy. The annular lesions vary in size and are asymmetrically distributed. In contrast, the poorly defined papular and nodular lesions are roughly symmetric. Loss of sensation was present in most lesions.

nerve change consists of lamination of the perineurium with inflammatory cell infiltration. Foci of epithelioid differentiation may be seen. However lepromatous the other histologic changes may be, the presence of either of the latter two changes is preemptive, calling for a BL classification. Bacilli are easily found, and globi, (*M. leprae* containing secondary lysosomes within macrophages) are not uncommon. The perivascular (or periappendicular) accumulation of equal numbers of macrophages and lymphocytes may be so mild as to suggest a nonspecific infiltrate or, if even sparser, may mimic that of normal skin, but the numerous AFB, far too many for indeterminate leprosy, call for a classification of BL.

Untreated BL patients have slowly relentless progression of skin and nerve changes. With or without treatment, this course may be altered by a reactional state, upgrading reactions being more common than erythema nodosum leprosum (ENL, see below). Also, BL patients may silently downgrade to a LLs granulomatous posture.

Lepromatous Leprosy

In LL disease, the lack of cell-mediated immunity toward *M. leprae* permits unrestricted bacillary replication and widely disseminated, multiorgan disease. Poorly defined, skin-colored nodules are the most characteristic lesions, usually up to 2 cm in diameter and symmetrically distributed (Fig. 203-5). Dermatofibroma-like or histiocytoma-like lesions, usually multiple, are sharply marginated erythematous papules, sometimes confluent into plaques; they are not rare in untreated Mexican-born patients but are also seen in Filipinos and Samoans (Fig. 203-6). Diffuse dermal infiltration is always present subclinically and may be overtly manifested by widening of the nasal root and fusiform swelling of the fingers, mimicking a rheumatic illness. With progressive bacillary proliferation, further cellular infiltration, and the consequent thickening of the dermis, the skin is thrown into folds, producing the characteristic leonine facies, often in conjunction with nodular lesions. Less common presenting skin lesions include digitate, barely indurated patches of erythema (Fig. 203-7), which in light skin are sometimes followed

FIGURE 203-5

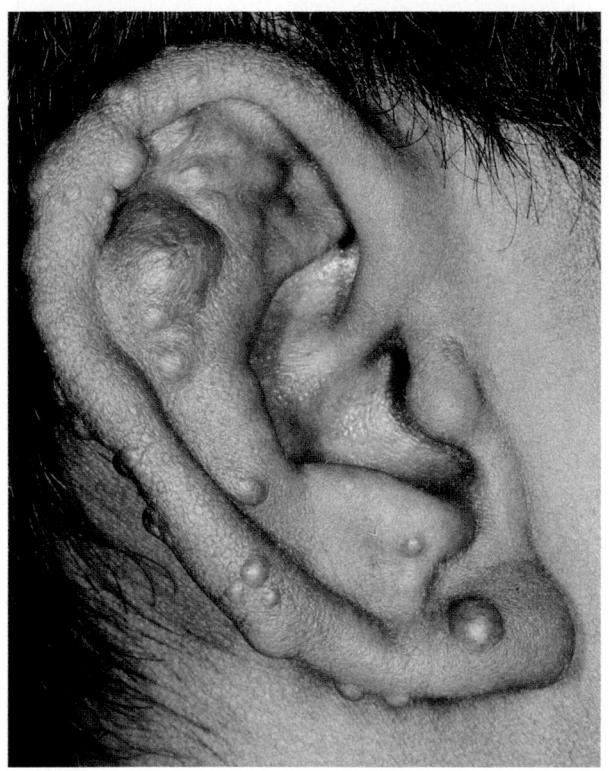

A.

B.

A, B. Multiple, skin-colored, papular and small nodular lesions in a patient with polar lepromatous leprosy (LLp). The margination of the lesions is variable, some being poorly defined. The absence of clinical inflammation is evident. Some distortion of the normal helix is arising from diffuse infiltration as well as from the nodular lesions.

FIGURE 203-6

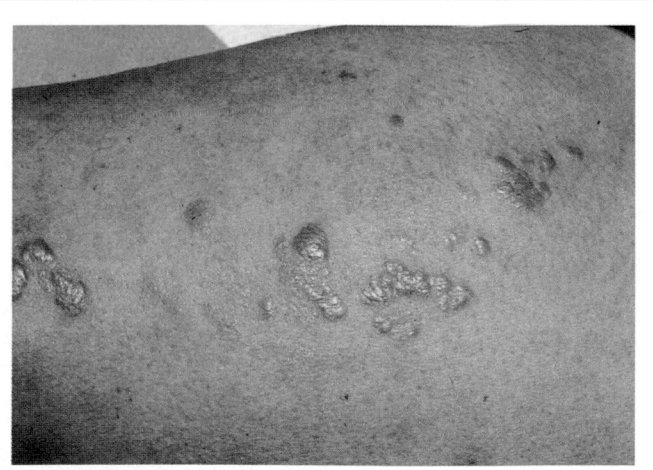

Multiple dermatofibroma-like lesions, which are solitary and confluent, in a patient with subpolar lepromatous leprosy (LLs). Their uniformly sharp margins and erythema are in contrast to the lesions in Fig. 203-5.

FIGURE 203-7

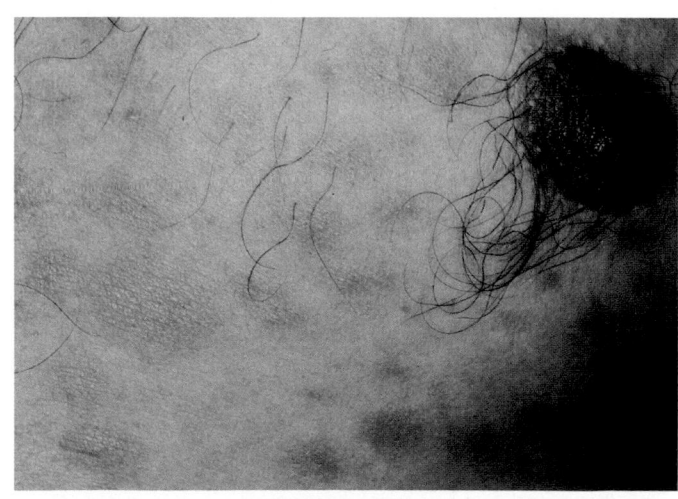

These multiple, barely palpable, erythematous, and asymptomatic lesions had been erupting over the previous 2 months in a subpolar lepromatous (LLs) patient. With treatment, as lesions remitted, they became mildly hyperpigmented. Here, the accentuations of the normal skin markings are in contrast to their effacement in the lesions in Figs. 203-5 and 203-6.

by a mild hyperpigmentation; in dark-skinned patients, multiple hypopigmented macules may originate in such lesions, a veil of melanin concealing the erythema. A clinical clue of LLs is a sharply marginated region in a lesion, perhaps the residual of a BL lesion in a patient who has downgraded to LLs.

Hair loss, common on the eyebrows (where it progresses laterally to medially) but also on the eyelashes and extremities, may be partially reversible if treated early. Scalp involvement is rare. Loss of eccrine sweating from sympathetic nerve involvement is common but rarely so extensive as to lead to heat intolerance.

Any given skin lesion may or may not be hypesthetic, but generally, in each patient, some are. Nerve trunk palsies occur but are less common than in BL. Acral distal symmetric anesthesia is to be expected and may be so severe as to lead to debilitating trophic changes on the hands and feet.

Histologically, in the nodular or papular lesions of LL, there is effacement of the epidermal rete, a grenz zone, virtual replacement of the dermis by foamy macrophages having many globi (some giant—huge secondary lysosomes), and a variable attrition of dermal appendages. In LLp, parasitized nerves have no reaction, whereas in LLs, residual host resistance is manifested by lamination of the perineurium. Lymphocytes are sparsely distributed in LL, LLs having more than LLp, and the former may also have a few dense foci of lymphocytes. Dermatofibroma-like lesions (LLs histologically) also mimic dermatofibromas histologically with collagen trapping, storiform or fascicular patterns, and occasionally, dendritic macrophages. Clinically normal skin shows perivascular and periappendicular macrophages of variable extent, usually with globi.

Untreated LL disease is relentlessly progressive, but this course may be altered by reactional states. LLs and LLp patients frequently develop ENL; LLp patients do not develop reversal reactions, whereas LLs patients may.

LABORATORY CHANGES

Most laboratory changes occur in LL or extensive BL disease. Hyperglobulinemia is the most common, giving an elevated sedimentation rate. A biologic false-positive serologic test for syphilis, anemia of chronic disease, and a mild lymphopenia are also common. If sought, the stained smear of the buffy coat shows AFB up to 10^5/mL. Elevated serum lysozyme and angiotensin-converting enzyme values reflect the extensive accumulation of macrophages synthesizing these proteases. Proteinuria, not uncommon, is associated with focal glomerulonephritis, seen mostly in patients with ENL. As manifested by high serum FSH and LH values, but low testerone levels, LL disease involves the testicles in a majority of LL but a minority of BL males.

OTHER ORGAN INVOLVEMENT

Because of motor or sensory changes in cranial nerve V, the eye may be at risk in paucibacillary as well as in multibacillary leprosy. In the latter, numerous changes in the cornea and anterior chamber are possible; iritis is the most common serious change, occurring de novo or in association with reversal reactions and ENL. Routine ophthalmologic examination is recommended for all patients.

In all LL patients and in BL patients with extensive disease, wide dissemination of the infection is the rule; with the exception of the upper respiratory tract, eyes, and testicles, however, clinically troublesome injury is unusual. With effective chemotherapy, chronic disability from ocular or upper respiratory tract involvement is less common than previously but has not disappeared, making ophthalmologists and otolaryngologists still vital to the successful management of patients with leprosy, to evaluate and treat acute changes and to prevent chronic changes.

PREGNANCY

Pregnancy is a precipitating factor for leprosy in 10 to 25 percent of women patients, presumably because of altered immunity. Pregnant LL and BL patients are predisposed to develop ENL, but in the postpartum period, they are predisposed to develop reversal reactions, putatively due to reduced immunity in pregnancy and restored immunity post partum.[24]

Of the drugs used to treat leprosy, none has been proven to be safe in pregnancy, and one (thalidomide) is clearly contraindicated. Fetal damage attributable to dapsone evidently has not been observed, hence continuation of dapsone in multibacillary patients is usually recommended.

As judged by anti-*M. leprae* IgM antibodies in the cord blood of two patients developing clinical lesions in infancy, congenital transmission of leprosy can occur but is considered to be very rare.[15] Untreated lactating BL and LL patients have viable bacilli in their milk, but no definable risk has been identified in infants ingesting such bacilli.[25]

AIDS

In contrast to the high incidence of tuberculosis and *M. avium-intracellulare* infections in AIDS patients, leprosy does not behave as an opportunistic infection in these individuals. Less certain is a possible influence of HIV infection upon the expression of leprosy, i.e., the position on the granulomatous spectrum or the prevalence of reactional states.[26,27]

INDETERMINATE LEPROSY

Indeterminate leprosy is a term with nearly as many meanings as it has users. The authors prefer the definition of Khanolkar,[28] who assigned it to an early lesion appearing before the host makes a definitive immunologic commitment to cure or to an overt granulomatous response. Clinically, the indeterminate lesion is a hypopigmented macule, with or without a sensory deficit, and AFB, if found, are in very small numbers. Such lesions are rare in the authors' clinic. The term is inappropriately used to describe lesions rich in AFB but having neither a tuberculoid or lepromatous histologic response; such patients usually have BL but occasionally LL disease.

DISABILITY OF HANDS AND FEET

Approximately one-third of newly diagnosed patients with leprosy will eventually have some chronic disability secondary to irreversible nerve injury, usually of the hands or feet. Weakness from loss of innervation of muscles is a self-evident cause of disability. Loss of protective sensation is more subtle but no less real. When a sharp or hot object cannot be perceived as such, injury occurs. Because this injury is more severe than if sensation were normal, infection is apt to occur. Because the infection can produce no painful signal, the part is not rested, allowing the infection to become extensive before help is sought. Repetitive cycles of injury and infection, permitted by loss of protective pain sensation, are the origins of severe tissue destruction in leprosy. Management and prevention of the problems arising from nerve injury require the skills of orthopedic surgeons, podiatrists, plastic surgeons, physical therapists, orthotists, and occupational therapists.

RELAPSING LEPROSY

Multibacillary patients who are noncompliant or who develop drug resistance are prone to relapse. Such individuals present in several ways, including the following: (1) a reprise of their initial presentation; (2) florid dermatofibroma-like lesions (histoid leprosy); (3) a reactional state; and (4) at a posture of higher resistance than their initial presentation, e.g., an initially LLs individual having BL or even BT disease.

REACTIONAL STATES

Generically, the reactional states of leprosy are distinctive, tissue-destructive, inflammatory processes, putatively immunologically driven, greatly increasing the morbidity of the disease. Because of the experience required for optimal patient care, reactional states justify leprology as a clinical subspecialty. When present, the reactional state usually dominates the clinical picture. An analogy with photobiology may be helpful. When the π electron accepts a photon, the molecule goes into an excited state, able to injure tissues in ways it cannot in the ground state. Similarly, when the granulomatous response accepts immunologically driven "energy," the excited granuloma is able to injure tissues in ways that it cannot when in its ground state.

Delayed-Type Hypersensitivity Reaction (Jopling's Type 1 Reaction)

Although the type 1 reaction is widely regarded as a delayed-type hypersensitivity (DTH) response, the nomenclature is not uniform. Reversal reaction, originally synonymous with "upgrading," has come to be used as identical to type 1, probably because most type 1 reactions are associated with reversal or upgrading. DTH reaction, a designation by mechanism, is a rational and acceptable name. DTH reactions are particularly common in BL patients but are not rare in patients with LLs or BT.[29,30] Patients may upgrade to a more resistant granulomatous presentation, remain unchanged, or downgrade to a less resistant disease state.

Clinically, DTH reactions are characterized by the abrupt conversion of previously torpid plaques to tumid lesions and by new tumid lesions arising in clinically normal skin, with or without an abrupt onset of neuritis. Quiescent annular lesions may become indurated throughout, losing their annular configuration. A purplish color is characteristic, and, even if not obvious, the dusky erythema may have a purplish cast (Fig. 203-8). Iritis and lymphedema (elephantiasis graecorum) may be concomitant changes. Lesions are rarely solitary, as can happen in BT upgrading to TT; often multiple; and occasionally myriad, as in BL or LLs upgrading to BT. Neuritis also ranges from mild to severe and is potentially disastrous, particularly if involving multiple nerves.[31] Clinically significant nerve loss may occur in the absence of overt neuritis, i.e., silent neuropathy.[32] DTH reactions may often be a mode of presentation, and DTH reactions occurring soon after presentation and the institution of treatment may well have been DTH reactions from the beginning. DTH reactions may occur up to 3 years after starting therapy and may occur after treatment has stopped.

Although the diagnosis of a DTH reaction is fundamentally clinical, histologic confirmation, if available, should be sought. Epithelioid differentiation of macrophages, edema, and both Langhans' and foreign-body giant cells are characteristic features in upgrading reactions and are easily appreciated if a prereactional specimen is available for comparison. In this instance, bacteriolysis greater than temporally anticipated also is good evidence of an upgrading reaction. Downgrading lesions usually show edema, but no characteristic changes may be found. High serum levels of lysozyme and angiotensin-converting enzyme may occur and, if present, can fall with steroid therapy.

FIGURE 203-8

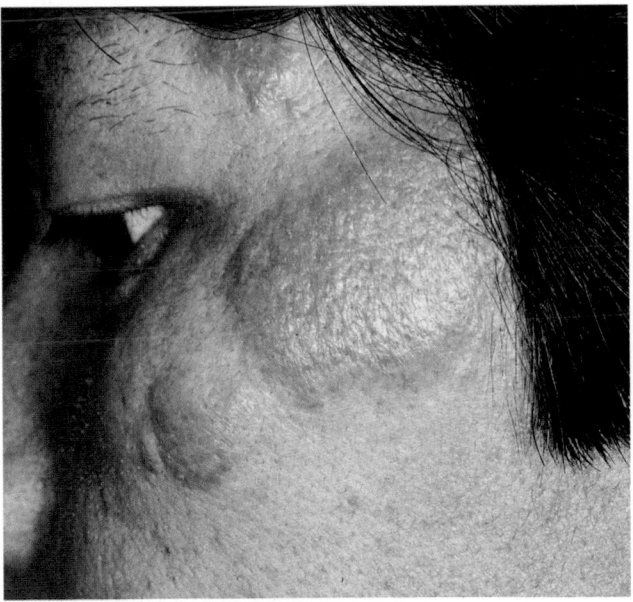

Some of the initial presenting lesions in a patient with a reversal reaction who had borderline lepromatous (BL) leprosy. The tumidity, purplish hues, and sharp margination strongly suggest a reversal reaction. The lesions were neither painful nor tender. The differences between these lesions and those shown in Figs. 203-3 and 203-4 emphasize that the reversal reaction, not the underlying BL disease, dominates the clinical picture. The patient also had an irreversible foot drop of recent onset.

Erythema Nodosum Leprosum

ENL, or Jopling's type 2 reaction (first described by Murata in 1912), occurs most often in LL (in up to 75 percent of cases) but is not rare in BL patients. (ENL is not erythema nodosum occurring in leprosy; it is a leprosy-specific response that has some features in common with erythema nodosum.) It may occur before, during, or after chemotherapy. Clinically, this reaction is characterized by crops of painful and tender, bright pink, dermal and subcutaneous nodules arising in clinically normal skin, in association with fever, anorexia, and malaise (Fig. 203-9). Other organs may be involved; arthralgias and arthritis are more common in ENL than are neuritis, adenitis, orchitis/epididymitis, or iritis, but each of the latter may rarely be the initial mode of presentation. Involvement of both upper and lower extremities is the rule, and facial lesions occur in one-half of patients. A neutrophilic leukocytosis is usual (85 percent) and is occasionally leukemoid in degree. Severe episodes can be associated with an abrupt fall in hematocrit, up to 5 g %, easily mistaken for dapsone-induced hemolysis. The response to thalidomide is dramatic in 90 percent of patients, perhaps qualifying as a diagnostic criterion.

The usual histologic features are small foamy granulomas in the dermis and subcutaneous tissue, with increased numbers of lymphocytes and a variable number of neutrophils, from none to many.[33] The infiltrate preferentially involves the deeper dermis and subcutis (as a lobular panniculitis) with relative sparing of the upper dermis, with or without vasculitis or fibrosis. A less common constellation is profound edema of the papillary dermis with neutrophil and lymphocyte infiltration involving the upper dermis. Extensive fibrosis bridging the dermis and the fascia is rare.[34] AFB are usually found with ease, but in late presentations (after 2 years of treatment) may be rare.

FIGURE 203-9

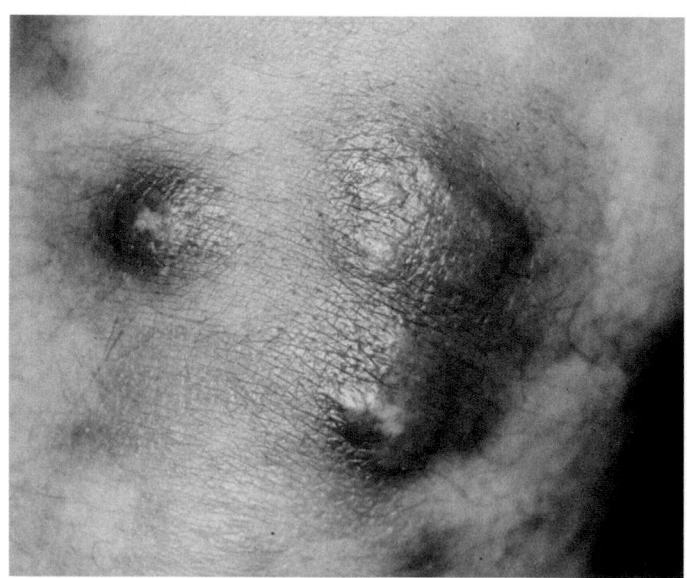

Lesions of erythema nodosum leprosum (ENL) in a patient with lepromatous leprosy (LL). The bright pink color is characteristic. These lesions are edematous, and pustule formation is suggested. The lesions were painful and tender.

When ENL is the presenting mode of leprosy, there may be little or no stigmata of the underlying multibacillary disease; in this case it represents a comparatively early manifestation of the disease. ENL can occur at any time during the course of chemotherapy, after 2 weeks or after 2 years, and can be precipitated by pregnancy or pyogenic infections.

Episodes of ENL may be occasional or sporadic but, in the more severely involved patients, can be frequent to virtually unremitting. In the latter case, brawny induration of the anterior thighs and pre-axial portion of the arms is characteristic, perhaps demonstrating a reversible fibrosis. Other cutaneous variants are annular lesions mimicking erythema multiforme, vesicles or pseudovesicles in association with papillary edema, necrotic lesions, frank subcutaneous abscesses, and pustular lesions mimicking pyodermas. Untreated, severe ENL may be associated with significant loss of protective sensation in the hands and feet, usually without overt neuritis—an example of silent neuritis. The course of ENL, treated or untreated, ranges from sporadic and ephemeral to frequent and persistent, lasting a matter of years.

The diagnosis of ENL, if considered, is usually not difficult because the clinical and histologic features are characteristic and the response to thalidomide dramatic.

The Lucio Reaction

The Lucio reaction, first described by Raphael Lucio in 1853, consists clinically of hemorrhagic infarcts; histologically, these are areas of ischemic necrosis secondary to endothelial proliferation and thrombosis in deep dermal vessels.[35] The Lucio reaction is particularly prevalent in Mexico and the Caribbean region and is restricted to patients with Latapi's lepromatosis, described by Fernando Latapi in 1941, a distinctive form of diffuse nonnodular lepromatous leprosy. In addition to the widening of the nasal root and fusiform enlargement of the fingers, there may be a purplish suffusion of the hands and feet, numerous telangiectatic matts or eruptive telangiectases, nasal septum perforation, total alopecia of the eyebrows and lashes, and a well-developed acral distal symmetric anesthesia. Ocular sparing is the rule.

The Lucio reaction occurs after Latapi's lepromatosis is well developed but before treatment is initiated. The necrotic lesions, arising in crops, have the serrated margins characteristic of septic infarcts and are painful but not tender (Fig. 203-10). Lesions usually crust and heal with scarring. Ulceration is common, especially below the knees. Lesions vary in size and extent, ranging from a few small lesions on the ankles to many large ulcerated lesions, which place life in peril. In the authors' experience, new lesions cease within 1 week of beginning rifampin, but with dapsone alone they may worsen, suggesting a strict requirement for viable organisms. Histologically, both the infarcted and clinically normal skin manifest a rich endothelial cell parasitization by AFB, especially prominent in vessels occluded by proliferating endothelium. Inflammation is scant, making *vasculosis* a better descriptive term than *vasculitis*.

TREATMENT

Medical Management

Medical management is directed at the infection itself or, if present, at a reactional state. For paucibacillary disease (TT or BT), the World Health Organization (WHO) recommends the combination

FIGURE 203-10

CHAPTER 203
Leprosy

2315

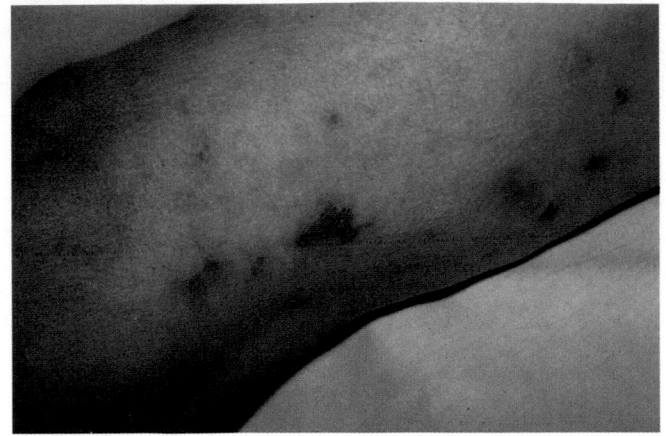

Lesions of the Lucio reaction, which show the characteristic hemorrhagic infarcts and serrated borders. Lesions were painful but not tender. The patient had Latapi's lepromatosis as manifested by diffuse infiltration, total alopecia of the eyelashes and brows, perforation of the nasal septum, no nodular lesions, and severe acral distal symmetric anesthesia.

of unsupervised dapsone (bacteriostatic), 100 mg daily, and supervised rifampin (bactericidal), 600 mg monthly, for a duration of 6 months. The authors prefer dapsone, 100 mg daily, for 3 to 5 years, with or without rifampin, 600 mg monthly, with follow-up examination at 1 and 2 years after discontinuing treatment.

For multibacillary disease (BB, BL, and LL), the WHO recommends unsupervised dapsone, 100 mg daily; supervised rifampin, 600 mg monthly; and clofazimine (bacteriostatic), 50 mg daily, unsupervised, and 300 mg monthly, supervised, for a routine duration of 2 years.[11] The rationale for this regimen is as follows: rifampin will kill all susceptible organisms, including those resistant to dapsone, and dapsone will eventually eliminate all susceptible organisms, including those resistant to rifampin; clofazimine is added to obviate the risk of primary dapsone resistance. This regimen is considered by the WHO to be curative and is the cornerstone of their policy to eliminate leprosy as a public health problem by the year 2000—a laudable goal, but at present its achievement is unproven. The report of a 20 percent relapse rate within 8 years after completion of this regimen indicates a need for alternative approaches.[36]

For the treatment of multibacillary diseases, other regimens may be used. Because the incidence of primary dapsone resistance is low in their patient population, the authors often use the combination of rifampin, 600 mg daily, and dapsone, 100 mg daily, for 3 years, followed by dapsone, 100 mg daily indefinitely. The alternative combination of minocycline (bactericidal), 100 mg daily, and rifampin, 600 mg daily, for 2 to 3 years followed by monotherapy has been well tolerated, excepting for hyperpigmentation from the minocycline. With the recognition that clarithromycin and some fluoroquinolones are also bactericidal for *M. leprae,* other useful regimens are to be anticipated.[37]

In reversal reactions, because of the risk of permanent nerve damage, prompt institution of prednisone therapy (0.5 to 1.0 mg/kg per day) is recommended (but still lacking a controlled trial). The dose of prednisone is titrated against overt nerve tenderness, the patient's symptoms, and careful sensory evaluation of hands and feet, e.g., using graded Weinstein filaments. Once instituted, therapy

should be tapered slowly and continued for a minimum of 6 months. If the response of neuritis to prednisone is not prompt, then rest, enforced with splinting of affected extremities, is also recommended. Because rifampin hastens the catabolism of prednisone, it might be necessary to switch from daily to monthly rifampin.

In ENL, thalidomide use is dramatically effective in a majority of patients, if not interdicted by its teratogenic effects. For outpatients, the authors usually start with 100 to 200 mg nightly and, if the drug is only partially effective, add prednisone, in a 0.5 to 1.0 mg/kg range, tapering the latter over the subsequent 6 to 8 weeks. Higher doses of thalidomide are usually restricted to inpatients, for whom excessive sleepiness is not a problem. If thalidomide is not available, glucocorticoids in conjunction with clofazimine at 200 mg/day may be effective. Thalidomide is slowly tapered to 100 mg and then to 50 mg daily.

The rapid fall in elevated serum levels of tumor necrosis factor (TNF) α in association with thalidomide therapy in ENL patients, and the subsequent in vitro demonstration that thalidomide specifically inhibited (75 percent) TNF-α synthesis by stimulated macrophages, has indicated that TNF-α may be a crucial mediator of ENL and its toxic manifestations.[38]

Adverse reactions to dapsone seen in the near term include the dapsone syndrome, a rare, potentially fatal infectious mononucleosis–like condition, and three kinds of hemolytic anemia, almost universally from a direct membrane effect, uncommonly from a glucose-6-phosphate deficiency, and rarely from an idiosyncratic response. In the long term, dapsone can be associated with peripheral neuropathy, usually motor and rarely bone marrow suppression, especially agranulocytosis. Sulfone therapy is discussed in detail in Chap. 253.

The common serious problem with rifampin is hepatotoxicity. Red urine is alarming but banal. As a P_{450} inducer, rifampin may lessen the effect of other drugs, e.g., oral contraceptive use resulting in pregnancy or reduced anti-inflammatory activity of glucocorticoids. Once-monthly use is rarely associated with severe hemolysis and acute renal failure.

Clofazimine produces skin darkening from the clofazimine itself in the near term and from a ceroid-lipofuscin pigment in the long term.[39] At the usual doses, 50 to 100 mg/day, gastrointestinal intolerance, dry skin, and acquired ichthyosis are common. Prolonged administration of large doses may produce a novel enteropathy secondary to mucosal and enteric lymph node drug accumulation. Accumulation in the spleen may predispose to its rupture.

Thalidomide, infamous for teratogenicity, may also produce constipation, dizziness, and other intolerances. Neuritis, a common side effect in nonleprosy patients, appears to be rare in ENL patients. Thalidomide is discussed in detail in Chap. 262.

Long-term use of minocycline may be limited by hyperpigmentation,[40] much more common in leprosy than in acne and perhaps related to the large accumulation of macrophages in leprosy. The authors have seen both diffuse hyperpigmentation and intense hyperpigmentation at the site of lesions, usually on the legs.

Glucocorticoids, in addition to their well-known side effects, may also exacerbate coexisting diseases, e.g., tuberculosis, hepatitis B, and some gastrointestinal parasites.

Because none of the antibacterial agents used to treat leprosy have been proven to be safe in pregnancy, caution is necessary. In a multibacillary patient who becomes pregnant during treatment, the authors usually recommend continuing dapsone. In all circumstances, the wishes of the patient should be carefully considered.

Management of Disability

Most of the disability in leprosy is due to loss of sensation. Since this can usually not be corrected, the prevention of minor trauma or thermal injury is of major importance, as are wound care and prevention of secondary infection. Patients with claw hand, thenar muscle weakness, drop foot, or paralysis of eye muscles may benefit from physiotherapy and reconstructive surgery.

IMMUNOLOGY

Investigation into the immunology of leprosy offers three promises: (1) a better understanding of the disease itself and, in particular, the immunopathogenesis of the granulomatous spectrum and the reactional states; (2) eradication or control of the disease by vaccination; and (3) illumination of other disease processes, which may arise from intense study of cell-mediated immunity in humans by using the model of leprosy.

Immunogens and Antigens of *M. leprae*

THE ETIOLOGIC AGENT *M. leprae* is a gram-positive, acid fast bacterium. Although still noncultivable in cell-free media, much information has accrued concerning *M. leprae* from the bulk extraction of organisms cultured in the armadillo and from molecular biologic techniques.[41] The bacterial cell wall has a peptidoglycan backbone linked to arabinogalactan and mycolic acids. Phenolic glycolipid I contributes to the waxy exterior of the bacteria and is a target of antibody responses.[42] A lipoglycan, lipoarabinomannan, is inserted into the cell membrane of *M. leprae* and courses through the outer membrane.[43] Lipoarabinomannan is a target of both antibody and T cell responses. Highly immunogenic proteins are located in the cytoplasm and in association with the cell wall. These include highly conserved, immunogenic heat shock proteins, of molecular mass 10 kDa, 65 kDa, and 70 kDa, each bearing *M. leprae*–specific and mycobacterial cross-reactive epitopes.[44,45] The genome of *M. leprae* is being sequenced.

Cellular Immunity

The great diversity of leprosy is exemplified by comparing its two polar forms. The high-resistance tuberculoid form is characterized by few lesions, rare organisms, epithelioid cell granulomas, and a tendency to self-cure. Plaques with sharp margins are the inscription of anti–*M. leprae* DTH on the skin; nerve trunk palsies are its inscription on peripheral nerves. Tuberculoid leprosy appears to be an entirely different disease than the low-resistance lepromatous form, characterized by wide dissemination, abundant organisms, foamy macrophages, and, if untreated, relentless progression. As judged by the scant variation found by restriction fragment length polymorphism analysis of *M. leprae* DNA from a human in India, a monkey in Africa, and an armadillo in Louisiana, strain variation of *M. leprae* cannot explain the diverse host responses[46]; this is a molecular biologic confirmation of a prior epidemiologic study with a similar conclusion.[20]

The observation of a positive lepromin skin test in tuberculoid subjects and unresponsiveness in lepromatous patients (1919) was the first objective and reproducible evidence that host immunity was the mechanism of polar diversity.[5] Lymphocyte transformation tests (1960s) provided an in vitro correlate of the lepromin skin test and substantial evidence that mediation of polar diversity was through the cellular-immune response. On the contrary, antibody responses to *M. leprae* were found to be stronger in lepromatous patients, indicating that humoral immunity does not lead to resistance to disease.

Immunophenotypic studies (1980s) established an important difference between the lymphocyte subsets infiltrating skin lesions; tuberculoid subjects have a predominance of the CD4 subset (CD4 : CD8 = 2 : 1), but lepromatous patients have a predominance of the CD8 subset (CD4 : CD8 = 1 : 2).[47–49] The skewing of T cell subsets in lesions was independent of those in the peripheral blood, since all patients had a normal CD4 : CD8 ratio of 2 : 1 in the blood. Therefore, it is important to study the immune response of patients at the site of disease activity—the skin lesions.

Utilizing the sequential application of reverse transcriptase and PCR techniques to tissue extracts, studies of mRNA cytokine profiles in polar tissues have provided a functional explanation for their immunopathogenesis[8] (see Chap. 32 for more detail). Tuberculoid lesions have a type 1 (T_H1 or T_H1-like) proinflammatory profile, in particular abundant mRNA coding for interleukin (IL) 2, interferon (IFN) γ, and IL-12 but scant mRNA coding for IL-4 or IL-10. In contrast, lepromatous tissues have a type 2 (T_H2 or T_H2-like) anti-inflammatory profile, in particular abundant IL-4 mRNA and IL-10 mRNA but little mRNA coding for the type 1 cytokines. Furthermore, CD4+ T cells in tuberculoid lesions were shown to produce IFN-γ, whereas CD8 T cells in lepromatous lesions accounted for the production of IL-4.[50] The presence of type 1 cytokines likely results in strong T cell and macrophage activation, the result being cell-mediated immunity to localize the infection. On the other hand, the type 2 cytokines found in lepromatous lesions likely lead to the strong antibody responses but concomitantly inhibit T cell and macrophage responses, resulting in progression of the infection. The importance of this paradigm is reflected in experiments designed to augment cell-mediated immunity in lepromatous patients. Administration of recombinant IFN-γ to lepromatous patients reduced the number of bacilli infiltrating tissues.[51,52]

Type 1 reactions and positive lepromin skin tests (Mitsuda reactions), long considered to be DTH responses,[53–57] also have a CD4+ T cell predominance and a type 1 cytokine profile; however, both differ from tuberculoid lesions by having a relative excess of *M. leprae*–reactive $\gamma\delta$ T cells, perhaps related to these being recent lesions.[9] Host cytokine profiles are subject to change, with LLs patients undergoing a reversal reaction switch from a type 2 to a type 1 profile; the mechanism of the switching is yet to be determined.

Antibody Immunity

ENL is widely regarded as being mediated by immune complexes.[58–60] There are large amounts of anti–*M. leprae* antibodies in both LL and BL patients. All classes of antibodies are represented, and their specificities are directed against a number of substrates including specific and cross-reacting peptides and carbohydrates, but these antibodies do not confer disease protection. Also, the blood of BL and LL patients contains abundant antigens including intact bacilli, up to 10^5/mL, as well as various carbohydrates. Therefore, it is readily conceivable that BL and LL patients should be subject to immune complex–mediated tissue injury. The best direct support for the hypothesis that ENL is immune complex–mediated is the presence of split complement products in serum, consistent with extravascular complement activation within tissues. Inferential evidence is that of a histologic pattern consistent with an Arthus phenomenon and an excess of glomerulonephritis in ENL patients. Consistent with an immune complex pathogenesis, the level of cytokines that contribute to immune complex reactions, IL-6, IL-8, and IL-10, are strongly expressed in ENL lesions.[61] Other evidence, however, indicates a role for cellular immunity in the development of ENL.[62,63] CD4+ T cells predominate in lesions and T cell cytokines are abundant.[61,64,65] Additional observations supporting a pathologic role for cellular immunity include HLA-DR framework antigen in lesional epidermis,[66] an increase in IFN-γ-containing cells by hybridization studies,[67] and an excess of IL-2-staining cells compared with LL tissue,[68] collectively suggesting a T cell–mediated component in the pathogenesis of ENL. Perhaps both immune complexes and cellular immunity are important in the pathogenesis of ENL.

Little is known concerning the immunopathogenesis of the Lucio reaction. Extant evidence favors immune complex mediation. The abundant AFB in endothelial cells could be the optimum location for presentation of antigen to antibody. Also, the cryoprecipitate from Lucio serum was more indicative of complement activation than that from ENL patients.[69]

A role for anti–*M. leprae* mucosal IgA conferring protection has not been adequately explored.[70]

Protocols endeavoring to control leprosy by vaccination usually consists of BCG alone, viable BCG in combination with killed *M. leprae*, or killed *M. leprae* alone.[71–73] Most studies support a reduction in leprosy incidence, roughly one-third in tuberculoid cases but considerably less in lepromatous cases. The recent observation that lipid and lipoglycan antigens are presented to T cells (CD4−, CD8−, CD3+) by the CD1+ cells opens the door to entirely new vaccination protocols.[10]

REFERENCES

1. Skinsnes OK: Immunopathology of leprosy: The century in review. *Int J Lepr* **41**:329, 1973
2. Faget GH et al: The promin treatment of leprosy. *Public Health Rep* **58**:1729, 1943
3. Shepard CC: The experimental disease that follows injection of human leprosy bacilli into foot pads of mice. *J Exp Med* **112**:445, 1960
4. Rees RJW et al: Experimental and clinical studies on rifampicin treatment of leprosy. *Br Med J* **1**:89, 1970
5. Mitsuda K: On the value of a skin reaction to a suspension of leprous nodules. *Int J Lepr* **21**:347, 1953
6. Kirchheimer WF et al: Attempts to establish the armadillo (*Dasypus novemcinctus* Linn.) as a model for the study of leprosy. I. Report of lepromatoid leprosy in an experimentally infected armadillo. *Int J Lepr* **39**:693, 1971
7. Young RA et al: Genes for the major protein antigens of the leprosy parasite *Mycobacterium leprae*. *Nature* **316**:450, 1985
8. Yamamura M et al: Defining protective responses to pathogens: Cytokine profiles in leprosy lesions. *Science* **254**:277, 1991
9. Modlin RL et al: Lymphocytes bearing antigen-specific gamma/delta T-cell receptors in human infectious disease lesions. *Nature* **339**:544, 1989
10. Sieling PA et al: CD1-restricted T cell recognition of microbial lipoglycans. *Science* **269**:227, 1995
11. WHO Study Group: Chemotherapy of leprosy. *WHO Tech Rep Ser* **847**:1994
12. Walsh GP et al: Leprosy-like disease occuring naturally in armadillos. *J Reticuloendothel Soc* **18**:347, 1975
13. Thomas DA et al: Armadillo exposure among Mexican-born patients with lepromatous leprosy. *J Infect Dis* **156**:990, 1987
14. Mostafa HM et al: Acid-fast bacilli from former leprosy regions in coastal Norway showing PCR positivity for *Mycobacterium leprae*. *Int J Lepr* **63**:97, 1995
15. Ducan ME et al: A clinical and immunological study of four babies of mothers with lepromatous leprosy, two of whom developed leprosy in infancy. *Int J Lepr* **51**:7, 1983
16. Cho SN et al: Prevalence of IgM antibodies to phenolic glycolipid I
17. among household contacts and controls in Korea and the Philippines. *Lepr Rev* **63**:12, 1992
18. Chakravartti MR et al: A twin study on leprosy, in *Topics in Human Genetics* edited by PE Becher. Stuttgart, Georg Thieme, 1973, p 1
18. de Vries RR et al: HLA class-II immune response genes and products in leprosy. *Prog Allergy* **36**:95, 1985
19. Newell KW: An epidemiologist's view of leprosy. *Bull World Health Organ* **34**:827, 1966
20. Spickett SG: Genetics and the epidemiology of leprosy II: The form of leprosy. *Lepr Rev* **33**:173, 1962
21. Williams DL et al: Detection of *M. leprae* and the potential for monitoring antileprosy drug therapy directly from skin biopsies by PCR. *Mol Cell Probes* **6**:401, 1992
22. Ridley DS: Histological classification and the immunological spectrum of leprosy. *Bull World Health Organ* **51**:451, 1974
23. Ridley DS: *Pathogenesis of Leprosy and Related Diseases*. London, Wright, Butterworth, 1988, pp 157–159
24. Lyde CB: Pregnancy in patients with Hansen's disease. *Arch Dermatol* **133**:623, 1997
25. Pedley JC: The presence of *M. leprae* in human milk. *Lepr Rev* **38**:239, 1967
26. Kawuma HJ et al: Leprosy and infection with the human immunodeficiency virus in Uganda: A case control study. *Int J Lepr* **62**:521, 1994
27. Frommel D et al: HIV infection and leprosy: A four-year survey in Ethiopia. *Lancet* **344**:165, 1994
28. Khanolkar VR: Pathology of leprosy, in *Leprosy in Theory and Practice*, 2d ed, edited by RG Cochrane, TF Davey. Bristol, John Wright and Sons, 1964, p 125
29. Scollard DM et al: Epidemiologic characteristics of leprosy reactions. *Int J Lepr* **62**:559, 1994
30. Lockwood DN et al: Clinical features and outcome of reversal (type 1) reactions in Hyderabad, India. *Int J Lepr* **61**:8, 1993
31. Job CK: Nerve in reversal reaction. *Indian J Lepr* **68**:43, 1996
32. van Brakel WH et al: Silent neuropathy in leprosy: An epidemiological description. *Lepr Rev* **65**:350, 1994
33. Hussain R et al: Clinical and histological discrepancies in diagnosis of ENL reactions classified by assessment of acute phase proteins SAA and CRP. *Int J Lepr* **63**:222, 1995
34. Ridley DS et al: The histology of erythema nodosum leprosum. Variant forms in New Guineans and other ethnic groups. *Lepr Rev* **52**:65, 1981
35. Rea TH et al: Lucio's phenomenon and diffuse non-nodular lepromatous leprosy. *Arch Dermatol* **114**:1023, 1978
36. Jamet P et al: Marchoux chemotherapy study group. Relapse after long-term follow up of multibacillary patients treated by WHO multidrug regimen. *Int J Lepr* **63**:195, 1995
37. Gelber RH: Chemotherapy of lepromatous leprosy: recent developments and prospects for the future. *Eur J Clin Microbiol Infect Dis* **13**:942, 1994
38. Sampaio EP et al: Thalidomide selectively inhibits tumor necrosis factor alpha production by stimulated human monocytes. *J Exp Med* **173**:699, 1991
39. Job CK et al: Skin pigmentation from clofazimine therapy in leprosy patients: A reappraisal. *J Am Acad Dermatol* **23**:236, 1990
40. Fleming CJ et al: Minocycline-induced hyperpigmentation in leprosy. *Br J Dermatol* **134**:784, 1996
41. Gaylord H et al: Leprosy and the leprosy bacillus: Recent developments in characterization of antigens and immunology of the disease. *Annu Rev Microbiol* **41**:645, 1987
42. Hunter SW et al: Structure and antigenicity of the major specific glycolipid antigen of *Mycobacterium leprae*. *J Biol Chem* **257**:15072, 1982
43. Hunter SW et al: Structure and antigenicity of the phosphorylated lipopolysaccharide antigens from the leprosy and tubercle bacilli. *J Biol Chem* **261**:12345, 1986
44. Mustafa AS et al: Human T-cell clones recognize a major *M. leprae* protein antigen expressed in *E. coli*. *Nature* **319**:63, 1986
45. Mehra V et al: A major T cell antigen of *Mycobacterium leprae* is a 10-kD heat-shock cognate protein. *J Exp Med* **175**:275, 1992
46. Clark-Curtiss JE et al: Conservation of genomic sequences among isolates of *Mycobacterium leprae*. *J Bacteriol* **171**:4844, 1989
47. Modlin RL et al: In situ characterization of T lymphocyte subsets in leprosy granulomas (letter). *Int J Lepr* **50**:361, 1982

48. van Voorhis WC et al: The cutaneous infiltrates of leprosy: Cellular characteristics and the predominant T-cell phenotypes. *N Engl J Med* **307**:1593, 1982

49. Modlin RL et al: T lymphocyte subsets in the skin lesions of patients with leprosy. *J Am Acad Dermatol* **8**:182, 1983

50. Salgame P et al: Differing lymphokine profiles of functional subsets of human CD4 and CD8 T cell clones. *Science* **254**:279, 1991

51. Nathan CF et al: Local and systemic effects of intradermal recombinant interferon-gamma in patients with lepromatous leprosy. *N Engl J Med* **315**:6, 1986

52. Kaplan G et al: The reconstitution of cell-mediated immunity in the cutaneous lesions of lepromatous leprosy by recombinant interleukin 2. *J Exp Med* **169**:893, 1989

53. Waters MFR et al: Mechanisms of reaction in leprosy. *Int J Lepr* **39**:417, 1971

54. Godal T et al: Mechanism of reactions in borderline tuberculoid (BT) leprosy. *Acta Pathol Microbiol Scand* **236**(suppl):45, 1973

55. Barnetson RS et al: Cell mediated and humoral immunity in "reversal reactions." *Int J Lepr* **44**:267, 1976

56. Bjune G et al: Lymphocyte transformation test in leprosy: Correlation of the response with inflammation of lesions. *Clin Exp Immunol* **25**:85, 1976

57. Rea TH et al: Serum and tissue lysozyme in leprosy. *Infect Immun* **18**:847, 1977

58. Wemambu SNC et al: Erythema nodosum leprosum: A clinical manifestation of the Arthus phenomenon. *Lancet* **2**:933, 1969

59. Drutz DJ et al: Renal manifestations of leprosy: Glomerulonephritis, a complication of erythema nodosum leprosum. *Am J Trop Med Hyg* **22**:496, 1973

60. Bjorvatn B et al: Immune complexes and complement hypercatabolism in patients with leprosy. *Clin Exp Immunol* **26**:388, 1976

61. Yamamura M et al: Cytokine patterns of immunologically mediated tissue damage. *J Immunol* **149**:1470, 1992

62. Rea TH et al: Variations in dinitrobenzene responsivity in untreated leprosy: Evidence for a beneficial role for anergy. *Int J Lepr* **48**:120, 1980

63. Stach JL et al: Defect in the generation of cytotoxic T cells in lepromatous leprosy. *Clin Exp Immunol* **48**:633, 1982

64. Modlin RL et al: In situ characterization of T lymphocyte subsets in the reactional states of leprosy. *Clin Exp Immunol* **53**:17, 1983

65. Modlin RL et al: In situ and in vitro characterization of the cellular immune response in erythema nodosum leprosum. *J Immunol* **136**:883, 1986

66. Rea TH et al: Epidermal keratinocyte 1a expression, Langerhans cell hyperplasia and lymphocytic infiltration in skin lesions of leprosy. *Clin Exp Immunol* **65**:253, 1986

67. Cooper CL et al: Analysis of naturally occurring delayed-type hypersensitivity reactions in leprosy by in situ hybridization. *J Exp Med* **169**:1565, 1989

68. Modlin RL et al: In situ identification of cells in human leprosy granulomas with monoclonal antibodies to interleukin 2 and its receptor. *J Immunol* **132**:3085, 1984

69. Quismorio FP et al: Lucio's phenomenon: An immune complex deposition syndrome in lepromatous leprosy. *Clin Immunol Immunopathol* **9**:187, 1978

70. Abe M et al: Salivary immunoglobulins and antibody activities in leprosy. *Int J Lepr* **52**:343, 1984

71. Convit J et al: Immunological changes observed in indeterminate and lepromatous leprosy patients and Mitsuda-negative contacts after the inoculation of a mixture of *Mycobacterium leprae* and BCG. *Clin Exp Immunol* **36**:214, 1979

72. Convit J et al: Immunotherapy with a mixture of *Mycobacterium leprae* and BCG in different forms of leprosy and in Mitsuda-negative contacts. *Int J Lepr* **50**:415, 1982

73. Convit J et al: Immunoprophylactic trial with combined *Mycobacterium leprae*/BCG vaccine against leprosy: Preliminary results. *Lancet* **339**:446, 1992

CHAPTER 204

Eva Åsbrink
Anders Hovmark

Lyme Borreliosis

Lyme borreliosis (Lyme disease) is a vector-borne infection primarily transmitted by *Ixodes* ticks and caused by at least three different but closely related species of *Borrelia*. The disease may affect different organs, and the clinical picture and course may be highly variable. Erythema (chronicum) migrans, borrelial lymphocytoma, and acrodermatitis chronica atrophicans (ACA) are the cutaneous hallmarks.

HISTORIC ASPECTS

The three dermatologic conditions—erythema migrans, lymphadenosis benigna cutis (LABC), and ACA—have long been well known to European dermatologists. Both the atrophic and the inflammatory forms of ACA were described by different European authors more than a century ago, but the disease was first named and further characterized by Herxheimer and Hartmann in 1902. The first report of an erythema developing after a tick bite was presented by Afzelius in Sweden in 1909, and he gave it the name *erythema migrans*. A few years later the term *erythema chronicum migrans* was used in an Austrian case report by Lipschütz. The designation *lymphocytoma* was first used by Biberstein in 1923. Bäfverstedt coined the term *lymphadenosis benigna cutis* in his monograph on pseudolymphomas published in 1943.[1]

In 1941 and 1944, the German neurologist Bannwarth described a syndrome, later to be named after him, with focal and often severe radicular pain, lymphocytic meningitis, and cranial nerve paralysis. The association with tick bites and erythema migrans was later observed by Schaltenbrand.

In the United States, erythema migrans was not described until 1970. In 1977, Steere et al. reported on an epidemic form of arthritis occurring in several communities around Lyme on the Connecticut River.[2] Lyme arthritis was soon linked to a preceding erythema migrans, and manifestations in the nervous system and the heart were also found.[2]

In the early 1980s, Burgdorfer et al.[3] showed that Lyme disease was caused by tick-borne spirochetes. With use of modified Kelly medium,[4] cultivation of spirochetes from *Ixodes* ticks, from erythema migrans lesions, and from blood and cerebrospinal fluid specimens from a few patients with Lyme disease was successful. These spirochetes were classified as a new species of *Borrelia* and were named *B. burgdorferi.*[5] Later, spirochetal cultivations and serologic tests also revealed that Bannwarth's syndrome[6] and ACA[7] were caused by *B. burgdorferi* and that these spirochetes may also cause LABC.[8] However, as all cases diagnosed as LABC or pseudolymphomas do not have a borrelial etiology, Weber et al. introduced the term *borrelial lymphocytoma* in 1985.[9]

EPIDEMIOLOGY

Lyme borreliosis is a disease with a wide distribution in the northern hemisphere. Cases have been reported from Canada, 46 of the United States, most European countries, the Federal Republic of China, and Japan. In the former Soviet Union, cases have been recognized from the Baltic republics to the Pacific Ocean. It is the most common vector-borne disease of bacterial origin in the United States and Europe. There have been discussions as to whether the true incidence is rising or whether the reported increase is mainly attributable to greater recognition and awareness of this infection.

ETIOLOGY

The spirochete causing Lyme borreliosis was discovered unexpectedly in conjunction with a tick survey on Long Island, New York, in 1981 and 1982.[3] Studies of the morphology, antigen profile, and DNA indicated that the spirochete named *B. burgdorferi* was a new species in the genus *Borrelia* (order Spirochetales). Antigenic heterogeneity was soon found among different strains of *B. burgdorferi.*[10] The three genospecies of *B. burgdorferi sensu lato,* which have been shown to be human pathogens, have been named *B. burgdorferi sensu stricto, B. garinii,* and *B. afzelii.*[11,12] There are differences in the geographic distribution of these genospecies.[13,14] Thus, until now, only *B. burgdorferi sensu stricto* has been found in the United States. In Europe all three species are present, although at least in the Netherlands, Germany, Austria, Scandinavia, and Russia, *B. garinii* and *B. afzelii* seem to dominate. In the Asian parts of the former Soviet Union and in Japan, Korea, and China, *B. garinii* and *B. afzelii* but not *B. burgdorferi sensu stricto* have been found.

The primary vectors of Lyme borreliosis are hard ticks belonging to the *Ixodes ricinus* complex, i.e., *I. ricinus, I. persulcatus,* and *I. ovatus* in Europe and Asia and *I. scapularis* (*I. dammini*) and *I. pacificus* in North America. They are three-host ticks parasitizing a wide range of animals, including humans. During feeding on a spirochetemic host, the larval or nymphal tick may become infected, and it may then remain infectious throughout the rest of its life by transstadial transmission of spirochetes. The feeding activity of the

different stages is often seasonal during the spring, summer, and autumn. The rate of infection in nymphs and adult ticks ranges from a few percent to more than 50 percent. Transovarial transmission seems to be rare. Instead, the main reservoirs of *B. burgdorferi* are the hosts, mainly considered to be rodents, of the larvae and nymphs. However, birds and many other warm-blooded animals may serve as additional reservoirs. Large animals such as deer may play an important role in feeding adult ticks. In endemic areas, domestic animals are frequently seropositive for antibodies to *B. burgdorferi,* and manifestations of Lyme borreliosis have been demonstrated in such animals.

Tick vectors other than those of the genus *Ixodes* may transmit *B. burgdorferi* but are less efficient vectors. Transmission of *B. burgdorferi* by nontick vectors such as deer flies, horseflies, and mosquitoes or by direct contact with fluids from infected animals has been reported. However, Lyme borreliosis obtained in other ways than through a tick bite is probably very rare.

HUMAN EXPOSURE TO TICK BITES AND B. BURGDORFERI
Many patients with Lyme borreliosis are not aware of a preceding tick bite. The large, blood-sucking, adult female tick is usually easily detected. However, the small nymphal tick, which is considered to be the most important vector for transmitting *B. burgdorferi* to humans, often escapes detection. The tick drops off spontaneously, and the bites are usually painless.

CLINICAL MANIFESTATIONS

CLASSIFICATION OF CLINICAL DISEASE By analogy with syphilis, the natural history of Lyme borreliosis can be divided into three stages based on the clinical manifestations. Because the course in the individual patient does not imply a uniform temporal sequence with development of all the stages and because the infection is sometimes not manifest until stage 2 or 3, many clinicians believe that a staging system with numbers may be misleading. It has therefore been proposed that the terms *early localized infection, early disseminated infection,* and *late* or *chronic infection* should be used instead (Table 204-1). Besides the clinical picture, the duration of the disease is probably also important in therapeutic decisions. A definition of chronic or late infection as persistent infection lasting

TABLE 204-1

Classification of Lyme Borreliosis*

Early Lyme borreliosis
 Localized infection: Erythema migrans and borrelial lymphocytoma without signs or symptoms of disseminated infection. (Regional lymphadenopathy and/or minor constitutional symptoms may be present.)
 Early disseminated infection: Multiple erythema migrans–like skin lesions. Early manifestations of neuroborreliosis, arthritis, carditis, or other organ involvement.
Late Lyme borreliosis
 Chronic infection: ACA. Neurologic, rheumatic, or other organ manifestations—persistent or remitting for at least 12 months.

*The classification provides a guideline for the timing of different disease manifestations.

more than 12 months has been suggested. Because many signs and symptoms of Lyme borreliosis are nonspecific, the cutaneous borrelial manifestations may serve as helpful and important landmarks in the identification of Lyme borreliosis.

GEOGRAPHIC DIFFERENCES IN THE CLINICAL PICTURE The clinical manifestations caused by the different genospecies of *B. burgdorferi sensu lato* are similar but may vary in some respects.[11–14] All three strains may cause erythema migrans, neuroborreliosis, and arthritis. With a few exceptions, analyses of sera or spirochetes isolated from patients with ACA or borrelial lymphocytoma have, however, indicated that these manifestations are associated with infection with *B. afzelii*. *B. burgdorferi sensu stricto* has been associated with a high frequency of articular manifestations. In Europe *B. garinii* has been found to cause neuroborreliosis more often than *B. afzelii*. These findings support the concept of a strain-dependent organotropism of *B. burgdorferi*.

The differences in the geographic distribution of the three genospecies may explain some of the different clinical pictures of Lyme borreliosis described in Europe and the United States. Multiple erythema migrans–like lesions have been found in a higher frequency among American patients (25 to 48 percent)[15,16] than among Europeans (8 percent or less).[17,18] A higher frequency of arthritis has also been reported from the United States. In contrast, only a few cases of ACA and borrelial lymphocytoma have been described in Americans.

Within the last years the risk of concurrent infection with other tick-transmitted agents, such as *Babesia* and *Ehrlichia*, has been described, especially in the northeastern and Great Lakes regions of the United States but also in Europe. In experimentally coinfected animals, disease appears to be more severe than in those infected by *B. burgdorferi* alone, perhaps because babesial as well as ehrlichial infection may lead to immune suppression. Recent data indicate that coinfection may modify the clinical course of human Lyme borreliosis.[19,20] Tetracyclines and clindamycin/quinine, respectively, are the treatments of choice for ehrlichiosis and babesiosis.[21]

CUTANEOUS MANIFESTATIONS

Erythema Migrans

CLINICAL FEATURES[15–18,22–25] Erythema migrans, the principal cutaneous hallmark of Lyme borreliosis, starts at the site of a tick bite, but it is not unusual for the bite to pass unnoticed. The incubation period may vary from a few days to 3 months but is usually 1 to 3 weeks.[15,17,18] In most endemic areas there is a peak in the occurrence during the summer or autumn months. The initial erythema is usually homogeneous (Fig. 204-1), and it sometimes remains so until it heals. However, in the majority of the lesions the center partly or totally fades, leaving an annular erythema that spreads centrifugally (Fig. 204-2). A central reddish patch, representing the site of the tick bite, may sometimes be apparent. The diameter of the erythema migrans ranges from less than one decimeter to several decimeters. The size of the lesion or the distance the erythema has migrated mostly corresponds to the duration of the infection. The peripheral reddish band may be more or less sharply demarcated and is mostly 1 to 2 cm wide. With time the erythematous border often fades; it may wax and wane and is some-

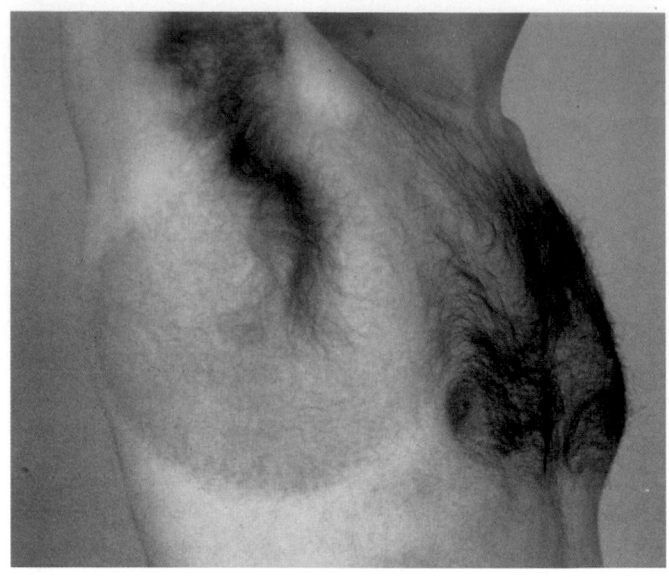

Homogeneous 3-week-old erythema migrans.

times visible only after the skin has been warmed up (for example, in a hot bath). The classic lesion is round, but elliptical or irregular forms may be seen. The duration of an untreated erythema migrans may vary from some days to about a year, but generally it disappears within weeks or months.[15,23] In patients who develop extracutaneous manifestations such as meningitis, the duration of the erythema often seems to be short. Erythema migrans may appear almost anywhere on the skin surface, but the lower extremities are most usually affected.[18,24] Facial involvement is common in children.[22] The clinical spectrum of erythema migrans is wider than has previously been reported. Atypical appearances with blisters or hemorrhagic or scaling lesions may develop.[24] Other variants are small, stationary erythemas or a localized swelling without any obvious erythema at the site of the tick bite.

Erythema migrans may pass unnoticed, as it may be poorly visible and asymptomatic. However, many patients experience local itching or sensations of irritation or heat.[15–17,23] In most cases the local symptoms are mild or moderate, but in a few cases more

FIGURE 204-2

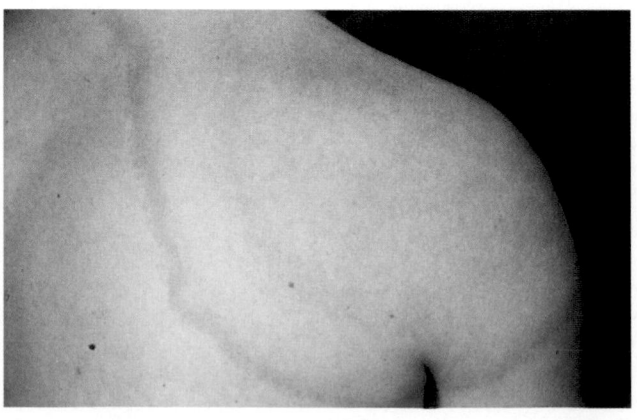

Annular 2-month-old erythema migrans.

intense dysesthesia/hyperesthesia may occur at or near the site of the eruption. Regional lymphadenopathy may be present. In at least half of the patients, constitutional signs or symptoms such as headache, low-grade fever, malaise, gastrointestinal complaints, and/or myalgia/arthralgia accompany the skin lesion or sometimes start before the erythema.[15–17,23–25] Severe fatigue or emotional disturbances such as irritability and depression may develop. Mostly the constitutional reactions are mild or moderate, of an intermittent and changing nature, and last for some days to 1 or a few weeks. If they are more pronounced or long-lasting, they may signal a disseminated infection with meningitis.

Nonspecific cutaneous manifestations such as malar erythema, periorbital swelling, urticaria, maculopapular eruptions, and erythema nodosum have also been described in solitary patients with early Lyme borreliosis.[15,16,18,24]

MULTIPLE ERYTHEMA MIGRANS–LIKE LESIONS The development of secondary erythema migrans–like lesions is the cutaneous sign of hematogenous spread of spirochetes and of disseminated infection, as evidenced by successful spirochetal cultivation from secondary lesions.[16,24] The lesions may follow the initial erythema migrans or sometimes appear almost simultaneously. The multiple lesions may be homogeneous or annular; they are often, but not always, smaller than a solitary erythema migrans and may be non-migrating.

PATHOLOGY The epidermis is usually unaffected and there is a generally sparse dermal lymphocytic infiltrate with an admixture of a few plasma cells. The infiltrate is mainly confined to the perivascular regions.

DIAGNOSIS The clinical picture and the characteristic evolution of the erythema are most often sufficient to make the correct diagnosis. In atypical cases, the seasonal onset, the history of exposure to an area highly endemic for Lyme borreliosis, the history of a tick bite at the site of the lesion, the nonspecific histopathologic features, and/or elevated serum antibodies to *B. burgdorferi* are helpful clues. However, seronegativity does not rule out the diagnosis, as only a minority of the patients with uncomplicated erythema migrans are seropositive. The diagnosis can be confirmed by cultivation of borreliae from a skin biopsy specimen. If the lesion does not resolve after adequate antibiotic therapy, the diagnosis of erythema migrans ought to be reconsidered.

DIFFERENTIAL DIAGNOSIS Important differential diagnoses are granuloma annulare, erysipelas, tinea, fixed drug eruptions, lupus erythematosus, dermatomyositis, erythema gyratum repens, and nonspecific tick or insect bite reactions. In patients with multiple lesions, erythema multiforme and Sweet's syndrome may also be differential diagnoses. Histopathologic examinations are often of help in the differentiation.

Borrelial Lymphocytoma

CLINICAL FEATURES[1,8,9,26] Borrelial lymphocytoma often, but not always, starts at the site of the tick bite. The incubation period may vary from a few weeks to several months.[8,26] Some patients have a history of a preceding erythema migrans, and others may show a concomitant erythema migrans located around or near the lymphocytoma.[1,9,26] That a lymphocytoma may start at a distance from the spirochetal inoculation is obvious in cases where it begins close to the periphery of a large migrating erythema migrans. There are also case reports of concomitant ACA or sclerotic skin lesions.[1,26]

FIGURE 204-3

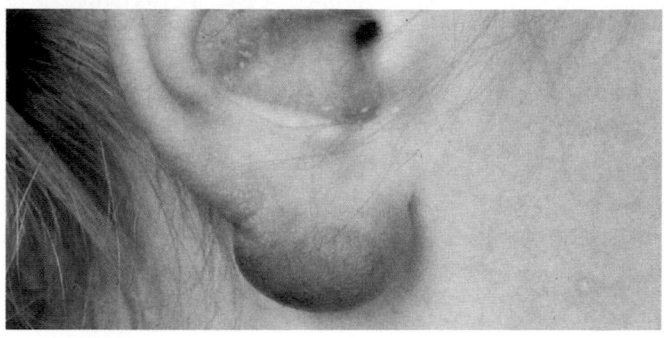

Borrelial lymphocytoma of 3 months' duration.

The classic borrelial lymphocytoma presents as a solitary bluish-red nodule, 1 to 5 cm in diameter, often accompanied by regional lymphadenopathy. Predilection sites are the earlobe (Fig. 204-3) and the nipple/areola mammae region. Other sites of predilection are the scrotum and the nose. Ear lesions are particularly seen in children and breast lesions in adults. In many cases there are no or only slight local symptoms, such as tenderness and itching. However, constitutional symptoms such as headache, fever, and arthralgia/myalgia may occur.

PATHOLOGY Usually the epidermis is unaffected. There is a dense dermal lymphocytic infiltrate, dominated by polyclonal B cells. The presence of germinal centers (Fig. 204-4), similar to those seen in reactive lymph nodes, is a helpful clue but not an obligatory diagnostic sign.

DIAGNOSIS The presence of a bluish-red nodule on the earlobe of a child suggests a borrelial lymphocytoma, as do scrotal nodules. The diagnosis should also be considered in patients with an erythematous swelling of the nipple/areola mammae region. A history

FIGURE 204-4

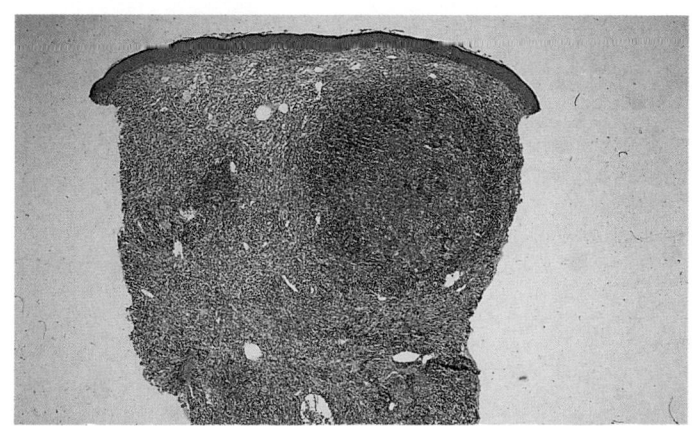

Borrelial lymphocytoma. Punch biopsy specimen from a scrotal lesion. In the dermis and subcutis there is a dense lymphocytic infiltrate displaying a follicular pattern with a huge germinal center. (*Micrograph by Eva Brehmer-Andersson, MD.*)

of a preceding erythema migrans or a tick bite in the vicinity further supports the diagnosis. Histopathologic findings of a dense dermal lymphocytic infiltrate with germinal centers are suggestive of but not specific for borrelial lymphocytoma. Elevated serum antibody titers to *B. burgdorferi* have been found in more than half of the patients.

DIFFERENTIAL DIAGNOSIS Borrelial lymphocytoma of the breast is often primarily suspected of being a malignant tumor. Conventional histopathologic examinations may be decisive in distinguishing a borrelial lymphocytoma from granuloma faciale, granuloma annulare, sarcoidosis, lupus erythematosus, polymorphous light eruptions, and arthropod bite granuloma. Lesions without germinal centers may be difficult to differentiate from malignant lymphoma. In such cases, immunohistochemical characterization of the cell infiltrate is of diagnostic help.

Acrodermatitis Chronica Atrophicans

CLINICAL FEATURES[7,17,22,27–33] A connection between ACA and a preceding tick bite is very seldom suspected by patients. About 20 percent have a history of a preceding untreated erythema migrans, usually on an extremity where ACA lesions developed 6 months to 10 years later.[17,18,31] Some patients also have a history of preceding neurologic and/or rheumatic complaints. Among patients with ACA there is a preponderance of females (about 70 percent), and it is generally a disease of the middle-aged or elderly. It usually starts on the extensor aspect of one extremity. The most common site is the lower leg, with initial involvement of the foot, ankle, or knee region. The dorsal aspect of the hand or the olecranon area are other common sites. The fingers, toes, and soles may become involved. With time, more widespread involvement of the extremity may occur, and the lesions usually spread from distal to proximal sites. Additional limbs may become affected, but sometimes not until after several years. Lesions may also appear on the buttocks. More extensive involvement of the trunk or involvement of the face is uncommon. The first cutaneous sign is a bluish-red discoloration, often with edematous swelling. Sometimes the erythema may be very slight and swelling may dominate the clinical picture, suggesting venous stasis or lymphedema. A typical feature is that one of the feet or just the heel gradually increases in size.[22] ACA lesions often develop slowly and insidiously, and initially both the erythema and the swelling may wax and wane.

Fibrous thickening of the skin in the form of indurated bands or nodules may develop. The most common bands are ulnar bands (Fig. 204-5A). The same area is also the most common site of single or multiple fibrotic nodules. Less often, similar bands and nodules may appear in the knee region, and nodules sometimes also occur adjacent to other joints (Fig. 204-5C). The bands and nodules are generally firm, skin-colored or bluish-red, and not tender. The diameter of the nodules varies from 0.5 cm to 2 to 3 cm and the bands may be of similar width or somewhat wider.

Sclerotic skin lesions that may be clinically and histopathologically indistinguishable from localized scleroderma or lichen sclerosus et atrophicus occur in 5 to 10 percent of patients with ACA.[31] There may be single or multiple sclerotic patches on extremities and/or the trunk. Often the sclerotic lesions develop adjacent to inflammatory or atrophic ACA lesions, or the different types of lesions are mixed in the same regions. The term *pseudoscleroderma*

FIGURE 204-5

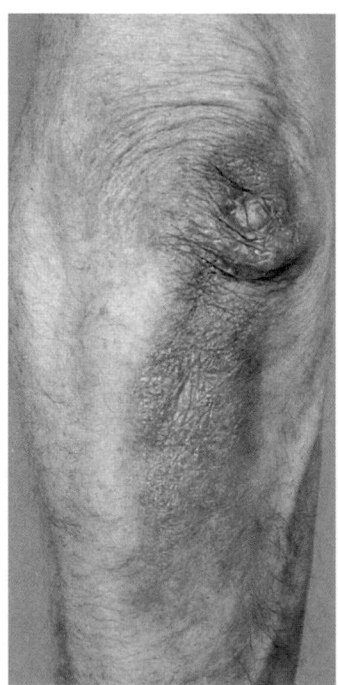

A.

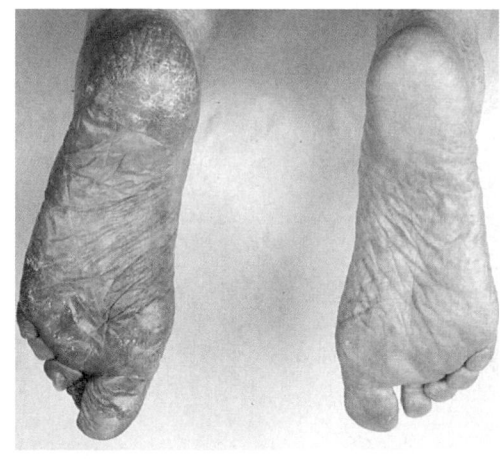

B.

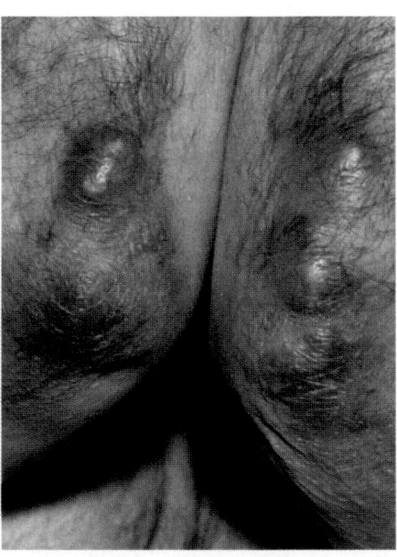

C.

A. Ulnar band in a patient with acrodermatitis chronica atrophicans that has been present for more than 10 years. *B. burgdorferi* has been cultivated from this lesion. *B.* Acrodermatitis chronica atrophicans with bluish-red discoloration and advanced atrophy of the plantar surface of one of the feet. *C.* Acrodermatitis chronica atrophicans with fibrotic nodules on the elbows.

has previously been used for the sclerotic skin lesions that may occur in ACA.[33]

Inflammatory ACA lesions may persist for years or decades, with gradual conversion to atrophic skin lesions (Fig. 204-5B). Both inflammation and atrophy may occur in different regions in the same patient. In the advanced atrophic phase, the skin becomes cigarette paper–like and wrinkled, appendageal structures disappear, and the vessels become prominent (Fig. 204-6). Besides diffuse atrophy, macular atrophy, which has previously been described as *atrophia maculosa cutis* or *dermatitis atrophicans maculosa*, may rarely occur.

Extracutaneous Manifestations in Patients with ACA

Enlarged regional lymph nodes are common, and in rare cases a more widespread lymphadenopathy may develop. Occasionally involuntary loss of weight may occur. Migrating and/or intermittent pains are fairly frequent. A rather common and characteristic feature is pain arising from impacts against bony prominences—such as the knuckles, the olecranon, or the malleolae—underlying ACA skin lesions. As diagnosed by clinical and electroneurographic examinations, more than 50 percent of patients with ACA have peripheral neuropathy, mostly mild or moderate. This neuropathy may be a sensory or motor mono- or polyneuropathy, or patchy dysesthesia, at the sites of the skin lesions. Symptoms such as hyperesthesia, muscular weakness, a feeling of heaviness, and muscle cramps are

FIGURE 204-6

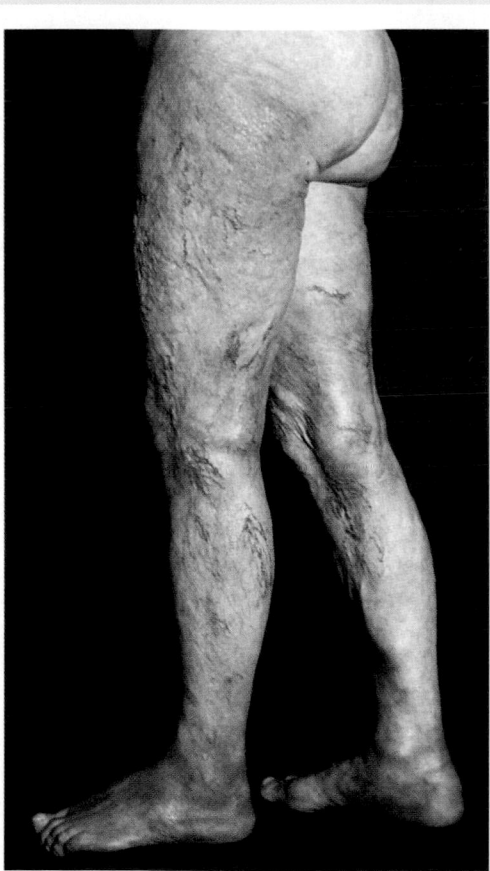

Acrodermatitis chronica atrophicans. Typical end-stage cutaneous atrophy is seen on both legs with prominence of the veins.

common in patients with ACA. These symptoms are mainly located in the limb(s) affected by skin lesions.

Profound fatigue, emotional disturbances, and personality changes may sometimes accompany ACA. Pathologic auditory brainstem responses, similar to those previously described in syphilis, have been found. However, there are usually no cerebrospinal fluid abnormalities in patients with ACA.

Subluxations/luxations of small joints of the fingers or toes and periosteal thickening of bones have been found underneath the skin lesions in patients with long-standing ACA.[30] Periarticular manifestations such as knee or olecranon bursitis and Achilles tendinitis on the same limb as the cutaneous involvement may precede or accompany ACA. Attacks of knee-joint effusions were found to have preceded or to have occurred simultaneously with ACA in about one-fifth of patients studied.[22]

PATHOLOGY[31,34]   There are usually no epidermal changes in the early inflammatory phase of ACA, but sometimes the epidermis is thin and shows liquefaction degeneration. The most common dermal findings are telangiectases in combination with a patchy and/or interstitial, often dense lymphocytic infiltrate with a moderate to rich admixture of plasma cells (Fig. 204-7A and B). This infiltrate may involve the whole or part of the dermis and sometimes also the subcutaneous fat. As the disease progresses, degeneration of elastin and collagen begins. After many years, advanced dermal atrophy develops, including atrophy of hair follicles and of sebaceous glands. In the advanced atrophic phase, the inflammatory cells decrease in number or almost disappear.

Sural nerve biopsies from patients with ACA and polyneuritis, as well as from some cases with early neuroborreliosis, have revealed axonal degeneration and perivascular infiltration with lymphocytes and plasma cells and obliteration of the epineural vasa nervorum.[32]

DIAGNOSIS   The clinical recognition of ACA may be difficult. If a red-violaceous discoloration, with or without swelling, is observed on a foot or heel, the dorsal aspect of a hand, the olecranon area, or, in more advanced cases, on one or more extremities (especially in an elderly woman), a diagnosis of ACA should be considered. Cutaneous atrophy may not appear for several years and is not an obligatory clinical or histopathologic criterion for a diagnosis of ACA. Compared with the prepenicillin era, patients with advanced atrophy are seen less frequently nowadays. Instead, the diagnostic efforts should be concentrated on recognizing inflammatory ACA lesions. The clinical diagnosis should be further verified by the histopathologic pattern and by elevated serum titers of IgG antibodies to *B. burgdorferi*. The diagnosis may be confirmed by spirochetal cultivation, as borreliae may still be present in the skin even after more than 10 years of ACA. Thus, ACA is a cutaneous example of prolonged survival of *B. burgdorferi* in humans.

DIFFERENTIAL DIAGNOSIS   ACA lesions are frequently overlooked by the physician. Acral ACA lesions are often regarded as physiologic changes due to age or occasionally due to cold injury. A discolored, sometimes swollen and painful leg in an elderly woman is very often misdiagnosed as circulatory insufficiency, and different circulatory investigations have frequently been performed in these patients. Erythematous ACA lesions in connection with musculoskeletal pains are sometimes mistaken for a connective tissue disease such as dermatomyositis. Fibrotic nodules may be confused with rheumatic nodules or gouty tophi. Patients with ACA

FIGURE 204-7

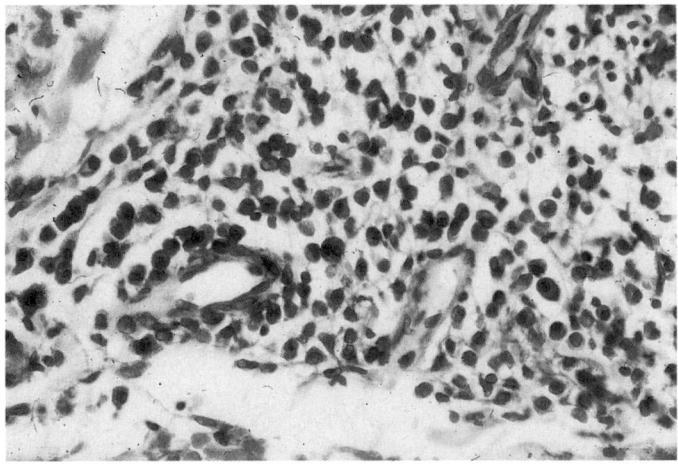

A.

B.

Acrodermatitis chronica atrophicans. Punch biopsy specimen from the dorsal aspect of a foot. *A.* In the dermis there are telangiectases and a patchy cell infiltrate. Epidermis is not involved. *B.* High-power view of the infiltrate, which consists mainly of plasma cells. (*Micrograph by Eva Brehmer-Andersson, MD.*)

often consult different medical specialists about signs or symptoms such as pain, joint manifestations, fatigue, or lymphadenopathy, i.e., unspecific features of Lyme borreliosis. In these cases the cutaneous ACA lesions are often neglected or misunderstood and the diagnosis of Lyme borreliosis is thus missed.

Sclerotic and Other Skin Lesions

Borrelia burgdorferi may cause skin lesions that are clinically and histopathologically indistinguishable from localized scleroderma and lichen sclerosus et atrophicus. A high frequency of elevated serum antibody titers to *B. burgdorferi* has been found in some studies of patients with scleroderma,[35] but this finding could not be confirmed by others.[36] In patients with ACA and pseudoscleroderma, the sclerotic lesions sometimes predominate, the inflammatory ACA lesions are missed, and the patient is diagnosed as suffering from morphea or lichen sclerosus et atrophicus. However, in most cases diagnosed as morphea or lichen sclerosus et atrophicus, there is no evidence of borrelial infection.[31,36]

As with syphilis, *B. burgdorferi* infection may sometimes mimic other conditions in its clinical and histopathologic features. Granuloma annulare, eosinophilic fasciitis, benign lymphocytic infiltration (Jessner-Kanof), and anetoderma have been described in connection with Lyme borreliosis.

EXTRACUTANEOUS MANIFESTATIONS

Lyme borreliosis is a complex multisystem disease that may affect the nervous system, joints, heart, and eyes in addition to the skin.

Neurologic Manifestations

Neuroborreliosis[32,37,38] may involve both the peripheral and the central nervous system (CNS).

EARLY NEUROBORRELIOSIS This usually begins 4 to 10 weeks after the onset of the infection. The triad of lymphocytic meningitis, cranial neuritis, and radiculoneuritis is a typical feature of neuroborreliosis. Compared with many other bacterial meningitides, the symptoms of a borrelial meningitis may often appear mild and fluctuating. Nonspecific signs or symptoms such as fever, fatigue, malaise, vomiting, weight loss, or headache with or without neck stiffness may be the only clinical manifestations. In such cases a history of a preceding tick bite and/or erythema migrans is helpful when considering the possibility of a diagnosis of neuroborreliosis. However, about one-third of the patients lack these important clues.[37]

The most common manifestations from the peripheral nervous system are radicular pains and facial palsy. In patients with a preceding erythema migrans, the skin lesion has often been located in the same part of the body as the subsequent radiculoneuritis or facial palsy. Involvement of other cranial nerves may give rise to eye muscle paresis, blindness, trigeminal neuralgia, hearing impairment, and vestibular neuritis. Paralysis of peripheral nerves in the limbs may also occur. Radicular pains may be intense and give rise to a broad spectrum of clinical features that are often initially misinterpreted. Neck pain may be misdiagnosed as cervical radiculopathy, lumbar pain as lumbago/sciatica, thoracic pain as myocardial infarction, and abdominal pain as gallstones, renal calculi, or gastric ulcers. Untreated early neuroborreliosis generally heals within 3 to 6 months. However, if less than adequate therapy is given, some patients may develop manifestations from other organs or late neuroborreliosis.

LATE NEUROBORRELIOSIS (CHRONIC OR TERTIARY NEUROBORRELIOSIS) This can be defined as neurologic signs and symptoms caused by *Borrelia* infection and occurring ≥1 year after the onset of the disease. One form of late neuroborreliosis is the chronic peripheral neuropathy often associated with ACA.[32] These patients usually lack spinal fluid abnormalities, in contrast to patients with severe CNS syndromes. Progressive encephalomyelitis with hemiparesis, para- and quadriparesis, ataxia, multiple sclerosis–like demyelinating disease, dementia-like deficiencies, mental changes, and/or incapacitating fatigue have been described, but these severe forms of late neuroborreliosis are uncommon.[38]

Rheumatic Manifestations

Reports on Lyme arthritis came first from the United States[2,15,39] and later from Europe.[40] Intermittent episodes of arthralgia or migrating musculoskeletal pain may occur early in the development of Lyme borreliosis. Months after the onset of the infection, a single episode or intermittent attacks of mono- or oligoarthritis may occur. In contrast to the symmetric polyarthritis seen in rheumatoid arthritis, Lyme arthritis characteristically affects only one or a few large joints, most commonly the knee joint. Often the pain is not severe, and swelling of the joint usually dominates the clinical picture. Arthritic attacks can recur for months and even years. In children, Lyme arthritis may sometimes mimic juvenile rheumatoid arthritis. About 10 percent of patients in the United States with Lyme arthritis have been reported to develop chronic arthritis with erosion of cartilage and bone. According to one report, chronic Lyme arthritis is associated with increased frequencies of HLA-DR4, often combined with HLA-DR2.[41]

Cardiac Manifestations

The frequency of cardiac involvement in patients with Lyme borreliosis is not well established. The most common findings have been atrioventricular conduction disturbances, with the majority showing transient first-degree atrioventricular block. Occasionally complete heart block requiring a temporary pacemaker has developed. Other abnormalities are rhythm disturbances, acute myopericarditis, pancarditis, and heart failure.[42]

Ocular Lyme Borreliosis

Early Lyme borreliosis is sometimes accompanied by conjunctivitis. Ocular motor palsies and solitary cases of iritis, iridocyclitis, choroiditis, keratitis, retinal hemorrhage, optic neuritis, ischemic optic neuropathy, and papilledema have been reported.[43]

Gestational Lyme Borreliosis

Most women with documented Lyme borreliosis during pregnancy appear to give birth to normal infants.[44] Solitary cases of fetal death, malformations, and prematurity have been reported.

LABORATORY EXAMINATION

An elevated sedimentation rate, elevated serum IgM levels, circulating immune complexes, and abnormal liver function tests are uncommon in patients with uncomplicated erythema migrans and borrelial lymphocytoma, but they are somewhat more frequent in patients with multiple skin lesions or other signs or symptoms of disseminated infection and in ACA.

Detection of *B. burgdorferi*

CULTIVATION OF SPIROCHETES   In atypical cases, spirochetal cultivation, using modified Kelly medium,[4] is the most specific and reliable way of diagnosing Lyme borreliosis. *B. burgdorferi* requires microaerophilic conditions for growth and reproduces by binary fission. The optimum temperature range for in vitro cultivation is 33° to 37°C (91.4° to 98.6°F). Spirochetal cultivation from human tissue or fluid has not become a routine diagnostic method in most laboratories. It is laborious and mostly a low-yielding process. One exception might be cultivation from skin specimens, as successful cultivation from more than 60 to 70 percent of skin biopsy specimens from patients with erythema migrans has been reported.[14,45]

In addition to cultivation from skin lesions, *B. burgdorferi* has also been cultivated from the blood, the cerebrospinal fluid (CSF), the heart, and synovial fluid from solitary patients with Lyme borreliosis. The cultivation period has usually varied from 1 to 4 weeks.

Animals such as rabbits, Syrian hamsters, rats, and mice have been used for experimental inoculation of *B. burgdorferi* and as animal models for Lyme borreliosis.

DEMONSTRATION OF SPIROCHETES IN TISSUES   Spirochetes may be demonstrated in biopsy specimens with different silver stains. Polyclonal or monoclonal antibodies to borrelial antigens have also been used to demonstrate spirochetes in tissue specimens. These techniques for visualizing spirochetes are difficult to evaluate, however, and there may be a risk of both over- and underdiagnosis.

POLYMERASE CHAIN REACTION (PCR)   Recent studies have reported that the PCR can be used to detect *B. burgdorferi* DNA in CSF, urine, skin, synovial fluid, and blood. In the analysis of skin biopsies from patients with erythema migrans and ACA, PCR has achieved a diagnostic sensitivity at least comparable to that of culture.[46,47] However, further well-controlled clinical studies of the sensitivity and specificity of PCR are needed before the reliability of the PCR method for routine diagnostic use in Lyme borreliosis can be established.

Serology of Lyme Borreliosis

Serologic examination is at present the most important laboratory aid in diagnosing Lyme borreliosis. The serologic results must, however, be interpreted with caution, as false-negative as well as false-positive results are common with the currently used tests. In early Lyme borreliosis, particularly in patients with signs or symptoms of disseminated disease, significantly increasing IgM and/or IgG antibody titers to *B. burgdorferi* may be found in consecutive tests performed at an interval of 2 to 3 weeks. Later on, the IgG titers are often stationary, and finding serologic proof of current infection may be difficult. Because high prevalence of seropositivity has been found among asymptomatic sports enthusiasts, outdoor workers, and other control individuals in endemic areas, the diagnostic value of the serologic findings may be limited, particularly in cases where only slightly elevated titers have been found. The lack of standardization also means that there may be great variations in sensitivities and specificities among different laboratories.

The tests most widely used at present for measuring antibodies to *B. burgdorferi* are the indirect immunofluorescence assay and the enzyme-linked immunosorbent assay (ELISA). Whole cells or sonicated whole cells are used as antigens. Different laboratories use different strains of *B. burgdorferi* as test antigens. The tests are of low diagnostic value in the earliest phase of Lyme borreliosis. Only 20 to 50 percent of patients with uncomplicated erythema migrans have been found to be seropositive in IgM and/or IgG ELISA.[48–51] Patients with multiple erythema migrans–like lesions and those with borrelial lymphocytoma are more often seropositive. In most cases where signs or symptoms of a disseminated infection have been present for several weeks, elevated serum titers to *B. burgdorferi* are found. Almost 100 percent of patients with ACA are seropositive, and they usually show very high serum IgG titers to *B. burgdorferi*.[7,48,50,51] Serologic IgM reactivity in patients with ACA is due to IgM rheumatoid factor activity.[48,51]

B. burgdorferi shares antigenic epitopes not only with other spirochetes but also with many common bacteria, including the normal human flora. Attempts have been made to improve ELISA by replacing the antigens used so far by fractions of spirochetes to eliminate irrelevant cross-reacting antigens. Thus, a purified *B. burgdorferi* flagellum antigen has been found to increase the sensitivity and specificity to some degree when compared with a sonicated whole-cell antigen.[51] An IgM antibody–capture ELISA with whole-cell sonic extracts as antigen has also been reported to be somewhat more sensitive than standard IgM ELISA.

With use of Western blot techniques, IgM and IgG antibodies to a number of spirochetal polypeptides have been found in sera from patients with Lyme borreliosis. Western blotting has also been used as a diagnostic tool with varying criteria for positivity in different investigations. Although it may be a sensitive method, it is difficult to standardize, time-consuming, and nonquantitative.

False-positive serologic reactions may occur in patients with relapsing fever and syphilis. In contrast, patients with high serum titers to *B. burgdorferi,* such as those with ACA, often have cross-reactive antibodies to treponemal antigens that are detectable in the fluorescent treponemal antibody–absorption test. However, the VDRL and Wassermann tests are negative.[7]

CEREBROSPINAL FLUID EXAMINATION IN NEUROBORRELIOSIS The presence of CSF abnormalities with a lymphocytic pleocytosis in combination with the finding of intrathecally synthesized antibodies to *Borrelia* is diagnostic for neuroborreliosis with CNS involvement.[37]

TREATMENT

Since the 1940s European dermatologists have traditionally treated patients with erythema migrans and ACA with oral penicillin. Controversies still exist concerning the most effective antibiotic and the most appropriate duration of treatment for different manifestations of Lyme borreliosis.[23,52–54] Few large, well-controlled treatment studies have been performed on groups of well-defined patients with similar manifestations of Lyme borreliosis. In many treatment trials, patients with uncomplicated erythema migrans have been mixed with patients who, besides erythema migrans, also have signs or symptoms of a disseminated infection, such as multiple erythema migrans–like skin lesions or meningitis.

Many of the minor symptoms that may occur in Lyme borreliosis, such as fatigue and musculoskeletal pain, are common and nonspecific. Thus, the evaluation of such symptoms in follow-up studies after treatment has been difficult in the absence of adequate controls.

As in syphilis, the difficulties of therapy seem to increase with the duration of the disease. The possibility has been considered that the spirochetal division time may be longer in the late than in the early stage of syphilis and that a longer period of therapy will be needed for late cases. The same may be true for late Lyme borreliosis.

Attempts have been made to determine antibiotic sensitivities of *B. burgdorferi* in vitro and in experimental animals. Because the methodology for such studies is not yet standardized, the studies should be interpreted with caution. It is not known whether the antibiotic susceptibility may differ among *B. burgdorferi* strains from different parts of the world.

The recommendations for treatment may be modified in the future, when further treatment trials have been carried out. Current guidelines for treatment of adult patients with different manifestations of Lyme borreliosis are given below.

TREATMENT OF UNCOMPLICATED ERYTHEMA MIGRANS Doxycycline (100 mg orally, qd/bid), phenoxymethyl penicillin (1 g orally, bid/tid), or amoxicillin (500 mg orally, tid) is recommended for 14 days.

In patients with erythema migrans and concurrent manifestations from other organs, the latter may be decisive for the choice of therapy. Such manifestations are particularly common in patients with multiple erythema migrans–like lesions. Before the start of therapy in patients with erythema migrans and signs or symptoms suggestive of neuroborreliosis, a diagnostic spinal tap should be performed. Alternatively, a regimen has to be chosen that gives therapeutic CSF concentrations.

TREATMENT OF BORRELIAL LYMPHOCYTOMA The same treatment regimens as for erythema migrans are proposed. In patients with a disease duration of several months, prolonged courses of antibiotics for up to 20 to 30 days may be required.

TREATMENT OF NEUROBORRELIOSIS OR CARDIAC ABNORMALITIES Penicillin G (3 g intravenously, tid/qid) or ceftriaxone (2 g intravenously, qd) for 14 to 20 days is recommended. In cases of cardiac abnormalities where only first-degree atrioventricular block is present and in early neuroborreliosis, oral regimens with doxycycline (100 mg, bid) have also been used.

TREATMENT OF LYME ARTHRITIS Doxycycline (100 mg orally, bid) or amoxicillin (500 mg orally, tid) for 20 to 30 days is recommended.

TREATMENT OF ACA Doxycycline (100 mg orally, bid) for 20 to 30 days is recommended. In long-standing cases with extracutaneous complications of the joints and/or the nervous system, both intravenous penicillin or ceftriaxone have been used.

Jarisch-Herxheimer Reaction

Mild to moderate Herxheimer reactions may sometimes appear after the institution of antibiotic therapy. Intensification of the current cutaneous rash and of local symptoms or the appearance of new signs or symptoms such as fever have been reported to occur not only during the first 24 h but also later during therapy.[54,55]

CHAPTER 204
Lyme Borreliosis

2327

PREVENTION

Vaccines to protect against Lyme borreliosis are under development and evaluation.

Protection from tick bites by the use of protective clothing in risk areas and body inspection and removal of any attached ticks as soon as possible are the most important prophylactic methods. The best way to remove a tick is with a pair of tweezers; the tick should be grasped as close to the skin as possible and gently pulled off.

Prophylactic antibiotic therapy after a tick bite is generally not recommended in the United States or Europe because it is controversial whether the value of such treatment can balance the risk of adverse reactions to antibiotics. Results of animal tests in the United States have shown that it usually takes at least 24 h of attachment for an infected blood-sucking *I. scapularis* tick to transmit spirochetes to its host.[56] However, data from the former Soviet Union indicate that humans bitten by *I. persulcatus* usually are already infected during the first 24 h of attachment.[57] In this study prophylactic treatment with doxycycline (100 mg bid) for 3 to 5 days was an efficient method for preventing humans bitten by *Borrelia*-infected ticks from contracting Lyme borreliosis.

COURSE AND PROGNOSIS

NATURAL COURSE (Table 204-1) On ethical grounds, the natural history of untreated Lyme borreliosis cannot be studied today, and no prospective investigations on the natural course have been carried out previously on large groups of unselected patients. During the preantibiotic era and the era preceding the discovery of the etiologic agent, many of the cases of early borrelial infection probably healed spontaneously. In 1977 Steere et al. reported on 12 patients in the United States with untreated erythema migrans, 6 of whom had multiple skin lesions. Of those patients, 7 developed arthritis or arthralgia.[2] This study was later expanded to 55 untreated patients. A total of 6 patients (11 percent) developed neurologic abnormalities, 2 (4 percent) developed cardiac involvement, and 28 (51 percent) developed arthritis.[39] Among 16 untreated Swedish patients with solitary erythema migrans, 2 patients developed recurrent erythema migrans lesions, 2 developed meningitis, and 1 developed ankle arthritis during the follow-up period.[23]

POSTTHERAPEUTIC COURSE Treatment failures have been reported with most of the different regimens. However, in the vast majority of patients, antibiotic therapy results in healing of the infection. Convalescence periods of several months, especially with persisting fatigue, are not uncommon in patients treated for Lyme borreliosis.

The resolution time for erythema migrans varies.[23,52,54] In most cases the erythema begins to fade a few days after the start of therapy. In some patients the skin lesion has disappeared when the treatment is terminated, but in others it may persist for some more days. In patients with borrelial lymphocytoma, it might take more than a month after antibiotic therapy before the lesion has disappeared completely.

As a rule, the clinical improvement in ACA after antibiotic therapy occurs gradually and may continue for at least 1 year. The first sign of improvement is an abatement of the swelling. The cyanotic discoloration fades to varying degrees. Histologically there is a reduction in the number of infiltrating cells. Residual erythema, pres-

ent several months after therapy, is generally due to hyperemia resulting from remaining dilated vessels.[27] The least satisfactory results are obtained in patients with advanced atrophy of the skin.

The therapeutic effects on borrelial sclerotic skin lesions are variable.[27,29,33] In some patients the lesions gradually disappear during the months after antibiotic therapy, but in others no beneficial effect is noted.

Serologic follow-up examination after therapy has shown that seroreversal tends to be slower in late than in early Lyme borreliosis. After antibiotic therapy, patients with ACA exhibit gradually decreasing antibody titers to *B. burgdorferi*. However, in only a minority does the titer fall to normal values within 1 year.[50,52] Serologic reactivity after therapy may perhaps persist indefinitely in patients with long-standing ACA, as in patients treated for late syphilis.

In patients with early neuroborreliosis, meningeal symptoms often improve rapidly and the effect on radicular pains is usually dramatic after initiation of therapy. Patients with hemiparesis, paraparesis, or ataxia may improve to varying extents but sometimes there will be residual sequelae.

Some patients with chronic joint involvement do not respond to antibiotic therapy, even after repeated courses of different antibiotics. It has been speculated that *B. burgdorferi* may sometimes initiate immunologic reactions that may continue for varying lengths of time, even in the absence of live spirochetes. The value of additional treatment with glucocorticoids in some cases of neuroborreliosis or Lyme arthritis is still under debate.

Reinfection in patients previously treated for erythema migrans is not unusual.[23,25]

REFERENCES

1. Bäfverstedt B: *Über Lymphadenosis benigna cutis: Eine klinische und patologisch-anatomische Studie.* Stockholm, PA Norstedt, 1943
2. Steere AC et al: Erythema chronicum migrans and Lyme arthritis: The enlarging clinical spectrum. *Ann Intern Med* **86**:685, 1977
3. Burgdorfer W et al: Lyme disease—a tick-borne spirochetosis? *Science* **216**:1317, 1982
4. Barbour A: Isolation and cultivation of Lyme disease spirochetes. *Yale J Biol Med* **57**:521, 1984
5. Johnson RC et al: *Borrelia burgdorferi* sp. nov.: Etiologic agent of Lyme disease. *Int J Bacteriol* **34**:496, 1984
6. Wilske B et al: Antigenic heterogeneity of European *Borrelia burgdorferi* strains isolated from patients and ticks. *Lancet* **1**:1099, 1985
7. Åsbrink E et al: The spirochetal etiology of acrodermatitis chronica atrophicans. Herxheimer. *Acta Derm Venereol (Stockh)* **64**:506, 1984
8. Hovmark A et al: The spirochetal etiology of lymphadenosis benigna cutis solitaria. *Acta Derm Venereol (Stockh)* **66**:479, 1986
9. Weber K et al: Das Lymphocytom—eine Borreliose? *Z Hautkr* **60**:1585, 1985
10. Barbour AG et al: Heterogeneity of major proteins of Lyme disease borreliae: A molecular analysis of American and European isolates. *J Infect Dis* **152**:478, 1985
11. Baranton G et al: Delineation of *Borrelia burgdorferi sensu stricto, Borrelia garinii* sp. nov., and group VS461 associated with Lyme borreliosis. *Int J Syst Bacteriol* **42**:378, 1992
12. Canica MM et al: Monoclonal antibodies for identification of *Borrelia afzelii* sp. nov. associated with late cutaneous manifestations of Lyme borreliosis. *Scand J Infect Dis* **25**:441, 1993
13. Assous M et al: Clinical and epidemiological implications of *Borrelia burgdorferi sensu lato* taxonomy, in *Proceedings of the International Symposium on Lyme Disease,* edited by Y Yanagihara and TM Shizuoka. Japan 1994, p 148
14. Van Dam AP et al: Different genospecies of *Borrelia burgdorferi* are associated with distinct clinical manifestations of Lyme borreliosis. *Clin Infect Dis* **17**:708, 1993

15. Steere AC et al: The early clinical manifestations of Lyme disease. *Ann Intern Med* **99**:76, 1983

16. Berger B: Erythema chronicum migrans of Lyme disease. *Arch Dermatol* **120**:1017, 1984

17. Åsbrink E: Erythema chronicum migrans Afzelius and acrodermatitis chronica atrophicans. Early and late manifestations of *Ixodes ricinus–*borne *Borrelia* spirochetes. *Acta Derm Venereol (Stockh)* **118**(suppl):1, 1985

18. Weber K et al: Erythema-migrans-Krankheit. *Dtsch Med Wochenschr* **108**:1182, 1983

19. Walker DH, Dumler JD: Emergence of the ehrlichioses as human health problems. *Emerg Infect Dis* **2**:1, 1996

20. Krause PJ et al: Concurrent Lyme disease and babesiosis. *JAMA* **21**:1657, 1996

21. Beneson AS: *Control of Communicable Diseases Manual,* 16th ed. Washington DC, American Public Health Association 1995, p 165

22. Åsbrink E, Hovmark A: Early and late cutaneous manifestations in *Ixodes*-borne borreliosis (erythema migrans borreliosis, Lyme borreliosis). *Ann N Y Acad Sci* **539**:4, 1988

23. Åsbrink E, Olsson I: Clinical manifestations of erythema chronicum migrans Afzelius in 161 patients. A comparison with Lyme disease. *Acta Derm Venereol (Stockh)* **65**:43, 1985

24. Åsbrink E et al: Clinical manifestations of erythema chronicum migrans Afzelius in Sweden. A study on 231 patients. *Zentralbl Bakteriol Hygiene* (A) **263**:229, 1986

25. Weber K, Neubert U: Clinical features of early erythema migrans disease and related disorders. *Zentralbl Bakteriol Hygiene* (A) **263**:209, 1986

26. Åsbrink E et al: Lymphadenosis benigna cutis solitaria—*Borrelia* lymphocytoma in Sweden. *Zentralbl Bakteriol Hygiene* **18**(suppl):156, 1989

27. Hauser W: Zur Kenntnis der Acrodermatitis chronica atrophicans. *Arch Dermatol* **199**:350, 1955

28. Hopf HCH: Acrodermatitis chronica atrophicans (Herxheimer) und Nervensystem, in *Monographien aus dem Gesamtgebiete der Neurologie und Psychiatrie.* Berlin, Springer, 1966

29. Åsbrink E et al: Clinical manifestations of acrodermatitis chronica atrophicans in 50 Swedish patients. *Zentralbl Bakteriol Hygiene* (A) **263**:253, 1986

30. Hovmark A et al: Joint and bone involvement in Swedish patients with *Ixodes ricinus–*borne *Borrelia* infection. *Zentralbl Bakteriol Hygiene* (A) **263**:275, 1986

31. Åsbrink E et al: Acrodermatitis chronica atrophicans—a spirochetosis: Clinical and histopathological picture based on 32 patients; course and relationship to erythema chronicum migrans Afzelius. *Am J Dermatopathol* **8**:209, 1986

32. Kristoferitsch W et al: Neuropathy associated with acrodermatitis chronica atrophicans. Clinical and morphological features. *Ann N Y Acad Sci* **539**:35, 1988

33. Jablonska S: Acrodermatitis chronica atrophicans and its sclerodermiform variety; relation to scleroderma, in *Scleroderma and Pseudoscleroderma,* edited by S Jablonska. Warsaw, Polish Medical Publishers, 1975, p 580

34. Brehmer-Andersson E: Histopathologic patterns of acrodermatitis chronica atrophicans. *Clin Dermatol* **11**:385, 1993

35. Aberer E et al: Evidence for spirochetal origin of circumscribed scleroderma (morphea). *Acta Derm Venereol (Stockh)* **67**:225, 1987

36. Halkier-Sörensen L et al: Antibodies to the *Borrelia burgdorferi* flagellum in patients with scleroderma, granuloma annulare and porphyria cutanea tarda. *Acta Derm Venereol (Stockh)* **69**:116, 1989

37. Stiernstedt G et al: Clinical manifestations and diagnosis of neuroborreliosis. *Ann N Y Acad Sci* **539**:46, 1988

38. Ackermann R et al: Chronic neurologic manifestations of erythema migrans borreliosis. *Ann N Y Acad Sci* **539**:16, 1988

39. Steere AC et al: The clinical evolution of Lyme arthritis. *Ann Intern Med* **107**:725, 1987

40. Herzer P et al: Lyme arthritis: Clinical features, serological, and radiographic findings of cases in Germany. *Klin Wochenschr* **64**:206, 1986

41. Steere AC et al: Association of chronic Lyme arthritis with HLA-DR4 and HLA-DR2 alleles. *N Engl J Med* **323**:1438, 1990

42. Van der Linde MR et al: Range of atrioventricular conduction disturbances in Lyme borreliosis: A report of four cases and review of other published reports. *Br Heart J* **63**:162, 1990

43. Winward KE et al: Ocular Lyme borreliosis. *Am J Ophthalmol* **108**:651, 1989

44. Markowitz LE et al: Lyme disease during pregnancy. *JAMA* **255**:3394, 1986

45. Berger BW et al: Cultivation of *Borrelia burgdorferi* from erythema migrans lesions and perilesional skin. *J Clin Microbiol* **30**:359, 1992

46. Schwartz I et al: Diagnosis of early Lyme disease by polymerase chain reaction amplification and culture of skin biopsies from erythema migrans lesions. *J Clin Microbiol* **30**:3082, 1992

47. Stedingk LV et al: Polymerase chain reaction for detection of *Borrelia burgdorferi* DNA in skin lesions of early and late Lyme borreliosis. *Eur J Microbiol Infect Dis* **14**:1, 1995

48. Wilske B et al: Serological diagnosis of erythema migrans disease and related disorders. *Infection* **12**:331, 1984

49. Shrestha M et al: Diagnosing early Lyme disease. *Am J Med* **78**:234, 1985

50. Åsbrink E et al: Serologic studies of erythema chronicum migrans Afzelius and acrodermatitis chronica atrophicans with indirect immunofluorescence and enzyme-linked immunosorbent assays. *Acta Derm Venereol (Stockh)* **65**:509, 1985

51. Hansen K, Åsbrink E: Serodiagnosis of erythema migrans and acrodermatitis chronica atrophicans by the *Borrelia burgdorferi* flagellum enzyme-linked immunosorbent assay. *J Clin Microbiol* **27**:545, 1989

52. Weber K et al: Antibiotic therapy of early European Lyme borreliosis and acrodermatitis chronica atrophicans. *Ann N Y Acad Sci* **539**:324, 1988

53. Berger BW: Treating erythema chronicum migrans of Lyme disease. *J Am Acad Dermatol* **15**:459, 1986

54. Steere AC et al: Treatment of the early manifestations of Lyme disease. *Ann Intern Med* **99**:22, 1983

55. Weber K: Jarisch-Herxheimer-Reaktion bei Erythema-migrans-Krankheit. *Hautarzt* **35**:588, 1984

56. Piesman J: Dynamics of *Borrelia burgdorferi* transmission by nymphal *Ixodes dammini* ticks. *J Infect Dis* **167**:1082, 1993

57. Korenberg EI et al: Prevention of borreliosis in persons bitten by infected ticks. *Infection* **2**:187, 1996

CHAPTER 205

Donald Y.M. Leung
Anne W. Lucky

Kawasaki Disease

DEFINITION

Kawasaki disease (KD) is an acute multisystem vasculitis of unknown etiology that most frequently affects infants and children under 5 years of age. No laboratory test currently exists for the diagnosis of this disease. According to the guidelines set forth by the American Heart Association,[1] the patient with KD should have fever lasting 5 or more days without other reasonable explanation and satisfy at least four of the five following criteria (Table 205-1): (1) bilateral nonexudative conjunctival injection; (2) at least one of the following mucous membrane changes: injected or fissured lips, diffuse injection of the oral and pharyngeal mucosa, or "strawberry tongue"; (3) at least one of the following peripheral extremity changes: erythema of the palms or soles, edema of the hands or feet during the acute phase, or periungual desquamation during the convalescent phase; (4) polymorphous exanthem; and (5) acute nonsuppurative cervical lymphadenopathy (>1.5 cm in diameter). In atypical cases, patients with fever and fewer than four of the principal symptoms can be diagnosed as having KD when coronary artery disease is detected by two-dimensional echocardiography or coronary angiography. Males under the age of 6 months are at particularly high risk for atypical KD. Thus, the diagnosis of atypical KD should be considered in any infant with prolonged fever (>2 weeks).

HISTORIC ASPECTS

KD, originally called mucocutaneous lymph node syndrome, was first recognized and described in Japan in 1967 by Dr. Tomisaku Kawasaki.[2] He reported his experience with 50 children who had been seen during the preceding 6-year period at the Tokyo Red Cross Medical Center. These children appeared to manifest a constellation of findings distinctive from any previously described disease. After this description, numerous cases were reported throughout Japan. Dr. Kawasaki's first description in the English language of the disease appeared in 1974.[3] In 1976, the syndrome was first reported in the United States by Melish, Hicks, and Larson in a group of 12 children from Honolulu seen between 1971 and 1973.[4] Since then, KD has been recognized worldwide in children of every racial group.

EPIDEMIOLOGY

Although KD occurs worldwide in children of all racial groups, it is most prevalent in Japan and in children of Japanese ancestry. KD is primarily an illness of young children, with approximately 80 percent of patients under 5 years of age. The ratio of males to females is about 1.5:1. The incidence rate is the highest for Japanese children between 6 to 12 months of age, with equal numbers in the first and second years of life. KD only rarely occurs in the same school, day care center, or household. Thus, person-to-person transmission of the disease would appear to be unlikely. In Japan, the recurrence rate of KD has been reported to be 3.9 percent and the proportion of sibling cases 1.4 percent.[5] These studies suggest common exposure to an infectious agent in genetically predisposed individuals.

The incidence of KD in Japan increased from 1967 to the mid-1980s. Nationwide epidemics, with wavelike spread of cases, occurred in 1979, 1982, and again in late 1985 to early 1986. Since the mid-1980s in Japan the incidence of KD has plateaued at 5000 to 6000 cases per year. The endemic annual incidence of KD is approximately 67 cases per 100,000 children younger than age 5. Both the endemic and the epidemic form of KD in Japan occur most commonly in the late winter and spring, with another period of slightly increased incidence during late fall. KD has been increasingly recognized in other Asian countries as well.

Epidemiologic findings in the United States and Europe have revealed striking similarities to those in Japan.[6] KD has been reported in all parts of the United States and Europe, occurring sporadically or as temporally limited communitywide epidemic outbreaks. Surveillance studies suggest that approximately 3000 patients with KD are hospitalized annually in the United States. The peak age is 18 to 24 months of age. Males develop KD at a rate that is approximately 1.6 times greater than that in females. The prevalence of KD is highest among Asians, intermediate in blacks, and lowest in whites.[7] Regardless of the racial group affected, however, the clinical picture is similar.

TABLE 205-1

Diagnostic Criteria for Kawasaki Disease

Fever of 5 or more days without other explanation, and at least four of the five following criteria:
  Bilateral nonexudative conjunctival injection
  One of the following changes in the oropharynx: injected or fissured lips, injected pharynx, or "strawberry tongue"
  One of the following extremity changes: erythema of the palms or soles, edema of the hands or feet, or periungual desquamation
  Polymorphous exanthem
  Acute nonsuppurative cervical lymphadenopathy

Because of the striking racial differences in the incidence of KD, potential genetic factors have been investigated. HLA typing studies have yielded conflicting data.[8,9] A ninefold increased prevalence of atopic dermatitis has been reported among children who acquire KD.[10] This observation is intriguing, because patients with atopic dermatitis have underlying immunoregulatory abnormalities and because there is a very high incidence of atopic dermatitis in Japan.[11] Differences have also been reported in immunoglobulin allotypes between white and Japanese KD patients versus appropriate race-matched controls with respect to allotypic frequencies.[12] These observations support the notion that host genetic and immunologic factors play a role in the pathogenesis of KD.

CLINICAL MANIFESTATIONS

General Features

The mucocutaneous manifestations of KD are varied and not all children exhibit each feature. The major diagnostic criteria for KD are listed in Table 205-1 and reviewed in references 13 and 14. KD is a triphasic illness beginning with an acute phase that lasts 7 to 14 days, followed by a subacute phase of approximately 25 days and a convalescent phase that lasts nearly 70 days. The cardinal feature of the acute phase is a prolonged high fever that frequently spikes to 40°C (104°F) and is associated with a toxic appearance in virtually all patients. In the absence of anti-inflammatory therapy, the duration of fever is usually 1 to 2 weeks.

Approximately 90 percent of children with KD develop an exanthem in the first days of their acute febrile illness (Fig. 205-1). The eruption favors the trunk and proximal extremities but can be generalized. It can be quite variable, having been described as macular, papular, morbilliform, urticarial, and even "target-like," resembling erythema multiforme. The initial rash is indistinguishable from an acute viral exanthem or adverse drug reaction and is rarely vesicular or bullous.

One of the earliest signs of KD is a characteristic perineal eruption[15] (Fig. 205-2). In one study of 58 children, 67 percent had the perineal eruption. Onset is usually within the first 6 days of the illness and presents as diffuse macular or plaque-type blanching erythema involving part or all of the perineal skin. These involved areas can be warm and tender. Within 48 h, the erythematous areas begin to desquamate. This desquamation occurs earlier than that of the palms and soles.

In 90 percent of patients, a nonexudative conjunctival injection begins shortly after the onset of fever and generally involves the bulbar conjunctivae more severely than the palpebral conjunctivae (Fig. 205-3). Conjunctival vessels become engorged and dilated. There is no purulent discharge or crusting of the eyelashes, as is seen in bacterial conjunctivitis. Conjunctival injection is associated with anterior uveitis in approximately 83 percent of patients examined within the first weeks of illness.[16]

Oral mucosal findings are very characteristic of KD and occur in almost all cases. The lips become "cherry" red, dry, and often cracked, producing small hemorrhagic fissures (Fig. 205-3). In contrast to staphylococcal scalded skin syndrome, there is no radial crusting of the perioral skin. There are no punctate ulcerations, as are seen in herpes gingivostomatitis or aphthae, and no diffuse erosions with confluent hemorrhagic crusts, as are seen in Stevens-Johnson syndrome. The tongue has been described as "strawberry,"

FIGURE 205-1

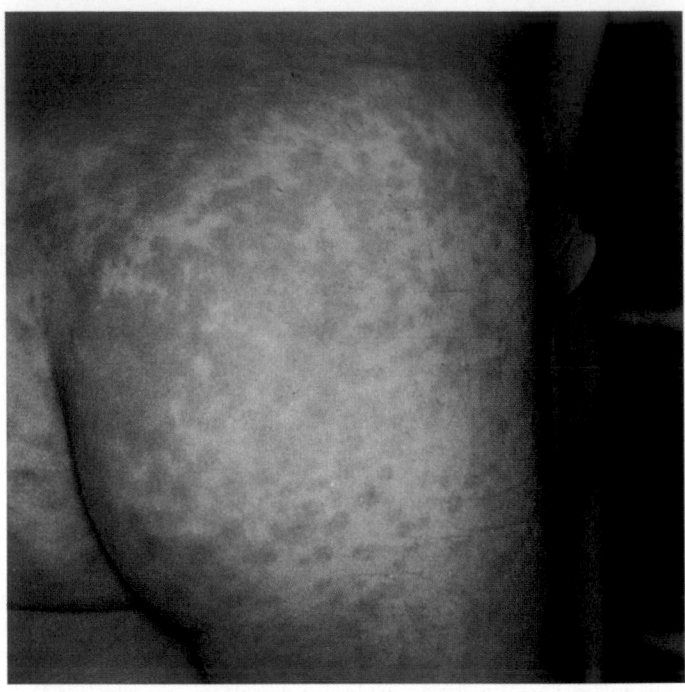

A generalized morbilliform eruption appearing early in the febrile course of this 5-year-old boy with Kawasaki disease.

with hypertrophied papillae and hyperemia, but only about half the cases seem to have this feature.

Profound edema and erythema of the distal aspects of the hands and feet with fusiform swelling of the fingers is also noted in almost all cases (Fig. 205-4). Onset is usually within a few days of the start of illness. These hyperemic areas are subject to desquamation 10 to 18 days later, during the subacute phase. The desquamation characteristically begins at the tips of the fingers and toes and may develop either fine peeling or shedding of thick "casts" of palmar and plantar skin, similar to that seen in scarlet fever (Fig. 205-5).

FIGURE 205-2

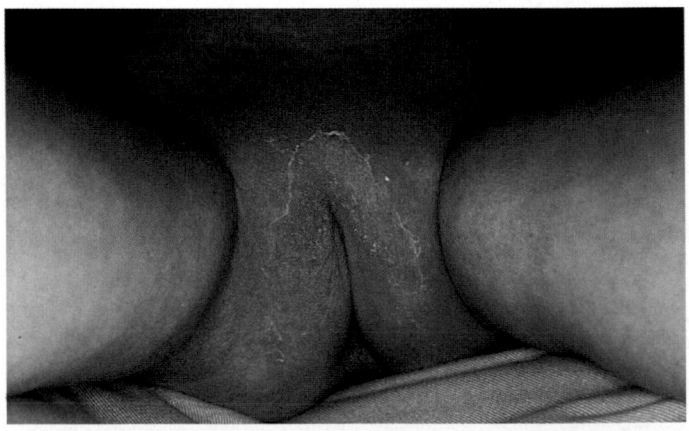

Generalized erythema and early desquamation in the perineal area of a 4-year-old girl with Kawasaki disease. This feature occurs early in the illness and involves 67 percent of affected children.

FIGURE 205-3

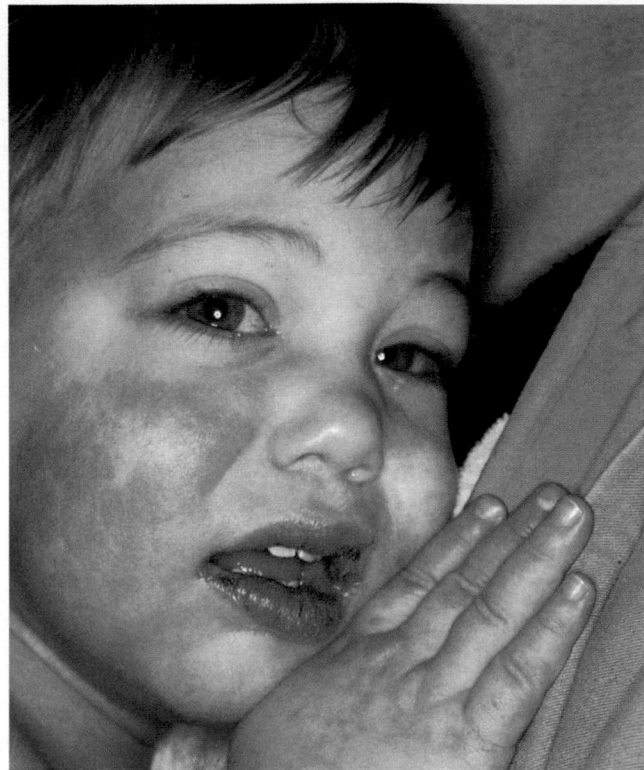

This boy with Kawasaki disease has "cherry red" lips with a few hemorrhagic fissures. His oral mucosa and conjunctivae are injected, and he has a generalized morbilliform eruption.

FIGURE 205-4

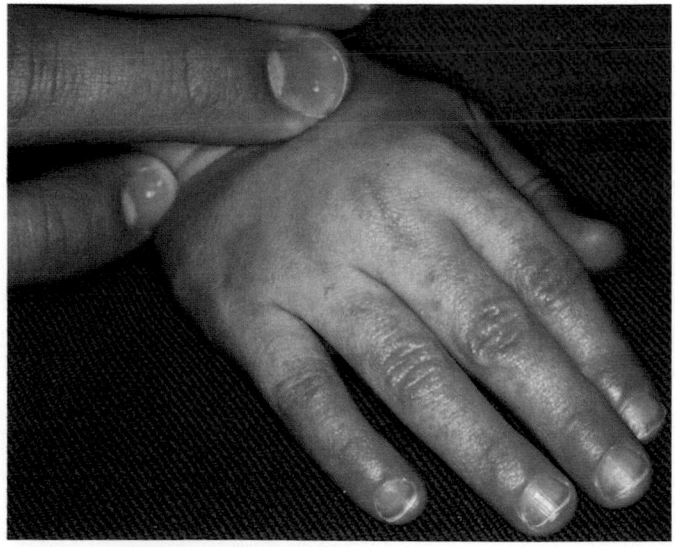

Erythema and edema of the distal fingertips are characteristic of the early phase of Kawasaki disease.

FIGURE 205-5

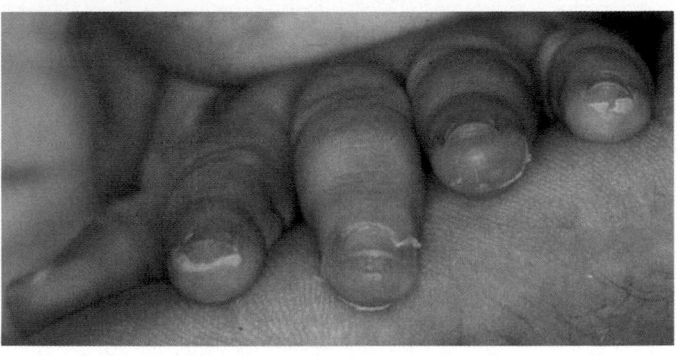

Desquamation starting at the tips of the fingers occurs 10 to 18 days after the onset of illness, as illustrated in this 3-month-old infant with Kawasaki disease.

Generalized fine desquamation, especially in the areas of the skin that had previously been erythematous, is also common at this time. Because of the severe systemic nature of the illness and the prolonged high fever, it is not surprising that some children develop telogen effluvium, with significant but transient hair loss 6 to 12 weeks following the acute phase of the illness. Similarly, Beau's lines of the nails and/or shedding of the nails have been observed weeks to months later. Lymphadenopathy is the least frequent finding and is seen in less than 75 percent of patients. The adenopathy generally consists of a single enlarged, nonsuppurative cervical node measuring at least 1.5 cm.

Other associated clinical features of KD are listed in Table 205-2. Arthralgia and arthritis occur in approximately one-third of patients. During the acute phase, the arthritis usually involves the small joints, whereas involvement of the large weight-bearing joints usually occurs in the second and third weeks of the illness.[8,16] Urethritis associated with sterile pyuria is frequently present in acute KD. Aseptic meningitis is usually associated with mild mononuclear cell pleocytosis of the cerebrospinal fluid and with normal glucose and protein. Hydrops of the gallbladder may be present with or without obstructive jaundice. Diarrhea, vomiting, abdominal pain, cranial nerve palsies, otitis media, and infarction of organs whose vascular supply is compromised by thrombosis may also be presenting symptoms. Sensorineural hearing loss has also been associated with KD.

During the convalescent phase there is generally a paucity of physical findings. Patients who suffer cardiovascular complications

TABLE 205-2

Associated Clinical Features of Kawasaki Disease

Cardiovascular abnormalities, including myocarditis, arterial aneurysms, pericarditis, aortic or mitral regurgitation, ventricular arrhythmias
Arthralgia and arthritis
Urethritis with sterile pyuria
Aseptic meningitis
Hydrops of the gallbladder
Diarrhea, vomiting, or abdominal pain

from this illness may have persistent cardiac abnormalities, including chronic myocardial dysfunction, aortic or mitral regurgitation, and cardiac arrhythmias. Occasionally a patient may experience clinical exacerbation, with recurrence of fever and other acute clinical signs, such as rash and conjunctival injection, after they had appeared to resolve. This occurs most often within a few weeks of onset of illness and may be associated with an increased risk of coronary artery disease.

Cardiac Manifestations

Abnormal cardiac findings are a hallmark of KD.[17] Myocarditis is frequently observed during the first week after onset of fever.[18] Pericardial effusion may develop toward the latter part of the acute phase and is secondary to myopericarditis. It is rare that these patients progress to cardiac tamponade, and the pericardial effusion generally resolves spontaneously. Congestive heart failure may occur due to myocarditis in the acute phase. During the subacute stage, congestive heart failure is usually caused by myocardial dysfunction secondary to ischemia or infarction.

Coronary artery ectasia or aneurysms occur in nearly 25 percent of patients with KD who are not treated with intravenous immunoglobulin.[19] Dilatation of the coronary arteries may be detected by echocardiography beginning 7 days after the onset of fever, usually peaking 3 or 4 weeks into the illness. A minority of patients (~5 percent) may suffer from aortic or mitral regurgitation due to valvulitis, transient papillary muscle dysfunction, or as a complication of myocardial infarction.

On cardiac examination, patients with acute KD often present with tachycardia and gallop rhythms, both in excess of the fever and anemia associated with the illness. In a minority of patients, a pericardial friction rub, dysrhythmias, aortic and mitral regurgitation, the findings of congestive heart failure, and the appearance of peripheral arterial aneurysms appear during the latter part of the acute phase or during the subacute phase.

LABORATORY FINDINGS

During the acute phase of KD, patients develop a leukocytosis with a predominance of neutrophils. A normocytic, normochromic anemia without evidence of hemolysis or reticulocytosis presents during the first week of illness and persists until the inflammatory process subsides. Increased platelet turnover occurs together with marked hypercoagulability in the acute phase. Thrombocytosis peaks typically in the third to fourth week after onset of fever. Elevation of liver transaminases, usually two- to threefold, is common in the acute phase, usually with a cholestatic profile of elevated bilirubin and alkaline phosphatase. Sterile pyuria due to urethritis is observed in up to 75 percent of patients during the first week of illness. Early in the disease, acute-phase reactants such as C-reactive protein and serum α_1 antitrypsin, are increased with the onset of fever and persist for 6 to 10 weeks. Similarly, erythrocyte sedimentation rates are uniformly elevated in patients with acute KD. Elevation of the latter typically persists after resolution of fever, a feature that may help to distinguish KD from common viral illness. Although patients with KD have a polyclonal B cell activation, their sera do not contain the usual autoantibodies associated with

collagen-vascular disease (i.e., no rheumatoid factor or antinuclear or anti-DNA antibodies).

Electrocardiographic changes may be present in over half of patients with acute KD. These abnormalities would include prolonged PR interval, left ventricular hypertrophy, abnormal Q waves, ventricular dysrhythmias, and nonspecific ST-T wave changes. Two-dimensional echocardiography has been used extensively for the assessment of ventricular function, the anatomy of the proximal coronary arteries, and the presence of a pericardial effusion. In general, it is preferable to obtain a baseline two-dimensional echocardiogram before the seventh day of illness (prior to onset of coronary dilation) and a repeat echocardiogram 3 to 5 weeks after illness onset (when coronary artery abnormalities are likely to be detected). Coronary arteriography is generally reserved for the patient with persistent abnormalities on echocardiograms or any patient with symptoms of myocardial ischemia. It is especially useful for visualization of coronary artery stenoses or distal coronary artery lesions that are difficult to define by two-dimensional echocardiography.

DIFFERENTIAL DIAGNOSIS

KD has clinical features compatible with infection, hypersensitivity reactions, or exposure to environmental toxins. The differential diagnosis includes staphylococcal or streptococcal scarlet fever or toxic shock syndrome; staphylococcal scalded skin syndrome; viral exanthem, particularly measles; Rocky Mountain spotted fever; leptospirosis; infantile polyarteritis nodosa; mercury toxicity (acrodynia); Stevens-Johnson syndrome; erythema multiforme; adverse drug reaction; and juvenile rheumatoid arthritis. KD has a variety of mucocutaneous manifestations, some of which are characteristic but many of which are shared with these other infectious and reactive disorders. The correct diagnosis of KD hinges on recognizing the cumulative combination of mucocutaneous, systemic, and laboratory findings.

PATHOLOGY

Extensive gross and microscopic studies have been carried out at autopsy of KD patients who have died in different phases of their illness. The case-fatality ratio for KD is approximately 0.4 percent, with most deaths occurring secondary to the cardiovascular complications of this disease. Fujiwara and Hamashima classified the pathology of this syndrome into four stages, according to the duration of illness at death.[20] Stage 1 (0 to 9 days after onset) is characterized by acute vasculitis and perivasculitis of small blood vessels. Microscopically, the acute vascular lesion in KD is associated with evidence for endothelial activation and endothelial cell damage.[21] The lesion is also associated with the infiltration of both neutrophils and mononuclear cells. The mononuclear cells consist of activated T cells and monocyte/macrophages. A study by Terai and co-workers[22] demonstrated the expression of major histocompatibility class (MHC) II antigens on the coronary arterial endothelium in a patient with KD but not in normal controls. Gamma interferon (IFN-γ) is a potent in vivo inducer of class II MHC antigens, and interleukin 1 (IL-1) as well as tumor necrosis factor (TNF) α plays an important role in the induction of leukocyte adhesion molecules. Thus, the induction of class II MHC antigens on endothelial cells as well as the observation of leukocyte adhesion to endothelial cells in the vascular lesion of KD suggests that cytokine-induced endothelial antigens play an important role in the pathogenesis of this disease.

In the larger arteries, the initial inflammation involves the intima and the vasa vasorum without inflammation of the media.[20] Pericarditis, myocarditis, inflammation of the atrioventricular conduction system, and endocarditis with valvulitis are also present. Stage 2 (12 to 25 days after onset) is characterized by a marked infiltration of inflammatory cells into the media of the coronary arteries as well as other medium-sized arteries, and aneurysms with thrombosis begin to form. At this stage, it is presumed that the formation of aneurysms is occurring as the result of destruction of the blood vessel walls that follows release of proteolytic enzymes and inflammatory mediators into the media. In stage 3 (28 to 31 days), the acute inflammatory process regresses, and granulation of the coronary arteries is noted. In stage 4 (40 days to 4 years), scar formation and organization of thrombi occur. This process can result in severe stenosis of the coronary arteries as well as other medium-sized arteries.

The peak time of death is 3 to 4 weeks after onset of the acute illness. Death can occur as early as during the first week of illness and as late as >10 years after the acute illness. During stage 1 of KD, patients usually die of acute myocarditis or cardiac arrhythmia due to inflammation of the atrioventricular conduction system. In stage 2 of the disease, death can result from rupture of the coronary arteries or myocarditis, including lesions of the atrioventricular conduction system, or myocardial insufficiency due to thrombosis of the coronary arteries. Sudden death late in the illness (stage 3) or years after recovery from acute KD (stage 4) may occur as the result of myocardial infarction in children with residual coronary artery aneurysms and stenoses.

It is worth emphasizing that although coronary arteries are invariably involved in this disease, almost any other medium- or large-sized blood vessel may be involved when examined at autopsy. Aneurysm formation has been reported in the femoral, iliac, renal, axillary, and brachial arteries.[23] KD is a systemic vasculitis that can affect most small- and medium-sized blood vessels. Cutaneous vasculitis, however, is not a prominent feature of KD.

IMMUNOPATHOGENESIS

Although multiple factors are likely to play a role in the pathogenesis of KD, several observations suggest that immune activation is involved in its pathogenesis. First, the acute phase of KD is characterized by an immunoregulatory imbalance that consists of increased numbers of activated helper T cells and monocytes, a deficiency of CD8+ suppressor/cytotoxic T cells, and a marked polyclonal B-cell activation.[24–26] Second, the immune activation associated with acute KD is accompanied by elevated serum levels of IL-1,[27] TNF-α,[25,28] IFN-γ,[29] and IL-6.[30] Furthermore, peripheral blood mononuclear cells from KD patients during the acute but not the convalescent phase spontaneously produce high levels of IL-1[31] and TNF-α.[32] These cytokines elicit an overlapping set of proinflammatory and prothrombotic responses in endothelial cells.[33] Third, the histologic lesion suggests a role for immune-mediated vascular injury. Fourth, the acute phase of KD is associated with the appearance of circulating antibodies that are cytotoxic against vascular endothelial cells prestimulated with IL-1, TNF-α,[34] or IFN-γ[35] but not against unstimulated endothelial cells. Finally, successful treatment of patients with intravenous immunoglobulins (IVIG) plus aspirin reduces the immune activation associated with

this disease.[36] In contrast, KD patients treated with aspirin alone have prolonged T and B cell activation.

EVIDENCE FOR SUPERANTIGEN-MEDIATED IMMUNE ACTIVATION

At present, there is no consensus regarding the etiology of KD. Nevertheless, it is widely agreed that KD is caused by an infectious agent because of the acute, self-limited nature of this disease, seasonal incidence, geographic clustering of outbreaks, and the unique susceptibility of young children. Furthermore, the fever and other clinical findings in acute KD (Table 205-1) significantly overlap with bacterial toxin–mediated diseases such as toxic shock syndrome or scarlet fever.

The activation of T cells and monocytes/macrophages found in the acute phase of KD is characteristic of diseases caused by bacterial toxins that act as superantigens. Staphylococcal enterotoxins (SEs), toxic shock syndrome (TSS) toxin, and streptococcal pyrogenic exotoxins (SPEs) are prototypic *superantigens* that stimulate a large proportion of T cells in an HLA-DR–dependent yet unrestricted manner.[37] These bacterial toxins bind directly to conserved amino acid residues outside of the peptide antigen binding groove on MHC class II molecules and selectively stimulate T cells expressing specific T cell antigen receptor (TCR) β-chain variable gene segments. Other variable elements (Dβ, Jβ, Vα, Jα) of the TCR contribute much less to the recognition of these superantigens. In contrast, nominal peptide antigens generally require all five variable elements for optimal T cell recognition and therefore stimulate only a low number of T cells (<1 in 1000).

To determine whether the immune activation during the acute phase of KD results from stimulation by superantigen(s), T lymphocytes of 19 children were analyzed for evidence of selective TCR Vβ gene usage.[38] Patients with acute KD demonstrated the marked expansion of Vβ2+ and to a lesser extent Vβ8.1+ T cells. In contrast, cells from control subjects showed no evidence for overexpression of TCR Vβs. During the convalescence phase of KD, percentages of Vβ2+ and Vβ8.1+ T cells returned to normal levels. This selective expansion of circulating Vβ2+ T cells is similar to the changes observed in T cells from patients with staphylococcal TSS, an illness with many clinical similarities to acute KD.[39]

Since this initial report, there have been confirmatory and nonconfirmatory reports of Vβ2 expansion in acute KD.[40–45] The ability to find Vβ2+ T cell abnormalities in the peripheral blood of patients with acute KD may depend on the timing of the blood collection, as superantigens stimulate the expression of homing receptors, thereby triggering the migration of T cells into inflamed tissues.[43] Thus, increased Vβ2+ T cells may be observed in the tissue even with normal or decreased Vβ2+ T cell values in the peripheral blood. Indeed, Yamashiro and colleagues[44] have observed a selective expansion of Vβ2+ T cells in the small intestinal mucosa of patients with acute KD. They suggested that the gastrointestinal tract may be the primary site of entry for a superantigen-secreting organism causing acute KD.

To further test the hypothesis that acute KD is triggered by a superantigen, Abe et al.[42] analyzed the sequences of random cDNA clones containing Vβ2 gene segments of T cells from the peripheral blood of patients with acute KD. In patients with a two- to threefold increase in numbers of Vβ2+ T cells, a clonotypic expansion of

Vβ2+ T cells might be expected to result in identical junctional sequences in up to 67 percent of the clones. However, none of the acute KD Vβ2+ T cell clones had the same junctional sequence. In view of the selective expansion of Vβ2+ T cells in acute KD, the extensive β-chain junctional diversity suggests that these Vβs play a dominant role in recognition. This type of recognition is generally not a feature of responses to most peptide antigens. Taken together, this high frequency of response and the prominent role for Vβ2 is most consistent with the hypothesis that T cell activation observed in the peripheral blood of acute KD is mediated by a superantigen that induces Vβ2 expansion.

SUPERANTIGENS RELATED TO ACUTE KD

To further explore the hypothesis that bacterial superantigen(s) are involved in the pathogenesis of KD, Leung et al.[46] analyzed cultures in a blinded manner from the groin, axilla, rectum, and pharynx of 16 patients in the acute phase of KD and 15-age-matched control patients. All group A beta-hemolytic streptococci and coagulase-positive *Staphylococcus aureus* isolates were screened for toxin production. Superantigen-producing bacteria were found in 13 of the 16 patients with acute KD but only in 1 of the 15 control patients ($p < .0001$). Of 13 toxin (superantigen)-positive cultures from patients with KD, 11 were an off-white, nonhemolytic, and coagulase-positive, TSS toxin (TSST)–secreting *S. aureus*, and 2 of 13 were streptococci producing SPEB and SPEC. Importantly, TSST-1 and SPEC are known to possess Vβ2 stimulatory activity whereas SPEC has both Vβ2 and Vβ8 stimulatory activity.

It should be noted that 12 of the 13 culture-positive patients had toxin-producing *S. aureus* isolated from the pharyngeal or rectal cultures. Only 1 of 13 patients had toxin (superantigen) producing bacteria exclusively on the skin. This suggests the primary site of bacterial colonization or infection in KD patients is the mucosal surface of the gastrointestinal tract and is consistent with the observation by Yamashiro et al.[44] that there is a selective expansion of Vβ2+ T cells in the small intestinal mucosa of patients with acute KD. Furthermore, these data suggest that a variety of staphylococcal or streptococcal toxins with superantigenic activity may cause the acute clinical features listed in Table 205-1 by inducing fever and tissue inflammation via the massive release of cytokines. In the future, additional multicenter controlled trials are needed to confirm these observations before there can be general acceptance of the "superantigen hypothesis" of KD.

TREATMENT

Current management is aimed at reducing inflammation in the myocardium and coronary artery wall, and preventing coronary thrombosis. Aspirin (ASA) in combination with high-dose intravenous immunoglobulin (IVIG) is the cornerstone of therapy for acute KD. ASA is administered in doses of 80 to 100 mg/kg of body weight per day to achieve a serum salicylate level of 20 to 25 mg/dL during the acute phase of the illness. At therapeutic doses, ASA has been shown to reduce fever, toxicity, and joint symptoms within 48 h.[47] After defervescence, usually around the 14th day of illness, the ASA dose is reduced to 3 to 5 mg/kg of body weight per day to continue inhibiting platelet activity. ASA is discontinued if no coronary abnormalities have been detected by 6 to 8 weeks after onset of the illness and the platelet count and sedimentation rate have normalized. ASA therapy is continued indefinitely if coronary artery aneurysms develop and persist. Digitalis and diuretics are used as needed in the patient with congestive heart failure. In patients at risk for cardiovascular complications, some physicians add dipyridamole, 1 mg/kg body weight per day, to further inhibit platelet aggregation.[48] Therapy of the mucocutaneous manifestations of the disease is entirely symptomatic and includes emollients for desquamating skin and antihistamines for pruritus.

No definitive prospective study has demonstrated that high-dose ASA therapy prevents coronary artery abnormalities. In contrast, several randomized multicenter studies have demonstrated that high-dose ($>$1 g/kg) IVIG in combination with ASA therapy is safe and effective in reducing the prevalence of coronary artery abnormalities.[49–51] In a single-center study, Rowley et al.[52] demonstrated that IVIG not only reduced the overall prevalence of coronary artery abnormalities but also prevented the formation of giant aneurysms, the most serious form of coronary abnormality caused by KD. Newburger et al.[53] found that abnormalities of left ventricular systolic function and contractility improved more rapidly in children treated in the acute phase with high-dose IVIG together with ASA than in those treated with ASA alone.

At present, the treatment of choice for acute KD is a single high dose of IVIG (2 g/kg) with ASA (80 to 100 mg/kg per day). Compared with multiple-dose regimens of approximately equivalent total dose, this single high dose of IVIG has been associated with a lower incidence of coronary abnormalities, more rapid resolution of fever, laboratory indices of acute inflammation, reduction in the duration of hospitalization, and higher peak serum IgG levels.[51] Of interest, peak adjusted serum IgG levels are lower among patients who subsequently develop coronary artery abnormalities and the levels are inversely related to fever duration and laboratory indices of acute inflammation.

A minority of patients who receive IVIG have persistent fever 48 h after completion of the infusion. A subset of patients may also demonstrate initial defervescence but then have recurrence of their fever after being afebrile for 24 h or more. In both situations, a repeat dose of IVIG may be indicated.

At present, the use of systemic steroids in the treatment of KD is controversial. Several studies from Japan have reported that patients treated with steroids alone or in combination with ASA have a higher frequency of coronary aneurysms and of subsequent myocardial infarction and death.[54] A more recent study of four patients with KD resistant to IVIG suggested a response to high-dose pulse methylprednisolone (30 mg/kg per day for 1 to 3 days) therapy.[55] Controlled studies are needed to determine whether intravenous methylprednisolone should be used in patients who fail to respond to IVIG therapy.

The mechanism(s) by which high-dose IVIG works to reduce the vasculitis associated with acute KD has yet to be established. The observation, however, that IVIG works rapidly in reducing laboratory parameters of the acute-phase response associated with KD suggests a generalized anti-inflammatory effect. In this regard, it has been reported that prior to IVIG therapy peripheral blood mononuclear cells from patients with acute KD secrete high levels of IL-1,[31] an endogenous pyrogen, and tissue vascular endothelial cells express endothelial activation antigens inducible by IL-1. IL-1 secretion remained high in IVIG-treated patients in whom coronary artery abnormalities developed. However, IL-1 secretion levels fell to normal in patients who responded to IVIG therapy and had no coronary artery abnormalities. Furthermore, following IVIG, there was no endothelial cell activation in patients who clinically responded to IVIG therapy. In contrast, patients with persistent fever had evidence of persistent endothelial activation.

These data support the notion that IVIG may work in KD by reducing cytokine-inducible endothelial activation. These observations may be of clinical importance, because duration of fever is a strong risk factor for the development of coronary artery aneurysms.[56] Furthermore, in clinical trials demonstrating that IVIG decreases the prevalence of coronary artery aneurysms in KD, it was also found that the duration of fever is significantly shortened in the IVIG-treated group.[51]

Takei et al.[57] have also demonstrated that IVIG contains high concentrations of neutralizing antibodies that inhibit the T-cell response to eight different staphylococcal superantigens. Using affinity absorption techniques, it was shown that this T cell–inhibitory effect was mediated by antitoxin-specific antibodies in IVIG. Thus, it is possible that the beneficial effect of IVIG in KD is, in large part, due to the presence of antibody that inhibits bacterial toxin-induced stimulation of the immune response.

Patients who develop coronary artery aneurysms must be monitored closely by a cardiologist. Stress echocardiography and coronary angiography may be indicated in patients with evidence of myocardial ischemia. For the KD patients with obstructive changes in one or more coronary arteries, anticoagulant therapy may be required. For more severe cardiovascular symptoms, the options include the use of intravenous streptokinase or urokinase when a thrombus is present, balloon angioplasty, and/or coronary artery bypass grafting. Long-term patency of saphenous vein grafts has been a problem, but recent use of internal mammary artery grafts has been reported to give improved results.[58]

COURSE AND PROGNOSIS

The major long-term morbidity in KD is related to cardiovascular complications from this disease. The majority of children (50 to 67 percent) with arterial aneurysms will show angiographic regression within 6 months to 2 years after onset of their disease.[59,60] The likelihood of resolution of the aneurysms appears to be determined by the initial size of the aneurysm, with smaller aneurysms having a greater likelihood of regression. Patients with giant aneurysms, i.e., those with a maximum diameter greater than 8 mm, have the worst prognosis. Nakano and colleagues have reported that 71 percent of patients with giant aneurysms progress to stenosis or obstruction over an 11-month follow-up period.[61] Tatra and Kusakawa reported that 30 percent of giant aneurysms developed obstruction at a mean follow-up of 32 months. Nearly all late deaths from KD occurred in this subgroup of patients.[62]

Long-term studies are needed to determine whether the intimal damage suffered during acute KD will predispose patients to late cardiovascular complications. Indeed, pathologic examination of regressed arterial aneurysms has revealed fibrous intimal thickening despite normal artery diameters.[63] The histologic abnormalities in arteries with aneurysm regression have raised concerns that such segments may be predisposed to the premature development of other forms of cardiovascular disease, such as atherosclerosis. Furthermore, studies of vascular distensibility in regressed aneurysms have demonstrated reduced vascular reactivity during pharmacologic vasodilation with intravenous nitroglycerin or dipyridamole.[64]

Children without known cardiac sequelae during the first month of KD appear to return to their previous state of health without cardiac impairment. A recent study of patients many years after

resolution of acute KD, however, using high-resolution ultrasound to study endothelium-dependent vascular responses, showed evidence of persistent endothelial dysfunction, even in patients without detectable early coronary artery involvement.[65] Thus, it is generally recommended that children with KD be followed over the long term by a cardiologist to rule out the development of myocardial dysfunction, late-onset valvular regurgitation, or premature coronary artery disease.

REFERENCES

1. American Heart Association Committee on Rheumatic Fever, Endocarditis and Kawasaki Disease: *Diagnostic Guidelines for Kawasaki Disease.* Dallas, AHA, 1989
2. Kawasaki T: Acute febrile mucocutaneous syndrome with lymphoid involvement with specific desquamation of the fingers and toes in children: Clinical observations of 50 cases. *Jpn J Allergol* **16**:178, 1967
3. Kawasaki T et al: A new infantile acute febrile mucocutaneous lymph node syndrome (MLNS) prevailing in Japan. *Pediatrics* **54**:271, 1974
4. Melish ME et al: Mucocutaneous lymph node syndrome in the United States. *Am J Dis Child* **130**:599, 1976
5. Yanagawa H et al: A nationwide incidence survey of Kawasaki disease in 1985–1986 in Japan. *J Infect Dis* **158**:1296, 1988
6. Rauch AM: Kawasaki syndrome: Critical review of U.S. epidemiology. *Prog Clin Biol Res* **250**:33, 1987
7. Shulman S et al: Risk of coronary abnormalities due to Kawasaki disease in urban area with small Asian population. *Am J Dis Child* **141**:420, 1987
8. Kato S et al: HLA antigens in Kawasaki disease. *Pediatrics* **61**:252, 1978
9. Matsuda I et al: HLA antigens in mucocutaneous lymph node syndrome. *Am J Dis Child* **131**:1417, 1977
10. Brosius DL et al: Association of Kawasaki syndrome with atopic dermatitis. *J Pediatr Infect Dis* **7**:863, 1988
11. Ogawa F et al: Investigation of skin diseases: An examination made together with the mass examination of three year old children in Morika City. *J Pediatr Dermatol* **1**:59, 1982
12. Shulman ST et al: Immunoglobulin allotypic markers in Kawasaki disease. *J Pediatr* **122**:84, 1993
13. Hicks RV et al: Kawasaki disease. *Pediatr Clin North Am* **33**:1151, 1986
14. Shulman ST et al: Kawasaki disease. *Pediatr Clin North Am* **42**:1205, 1995
15. Friter BS et al: The perineal eruption of Kawasaki syndrome. *Arch Dermatol* **124**:1805, 1988
16. Burns JC et al: Anterior uveitis associated with Kawasaki syndrome. *Pediatr Infect Dis* **4**:258, 1985
17. Kato H et al: Myocardial infarction in Kawasaki disease: Clinical analyses in 195 cases. *J Pediatr* **108**:923, 1986
18. Yutani C et al: Histopathological study on right endomyocardial biopsy of Kawasaki disease. *Br Heart J* **43**:589, 1980
19. Kato H et al: Fate of coronary aneurysms in Kawasaki disease: Serial coronary angiography and long-term follow-up study. *Am J Cardiol* **49**:1758, 1982
20. Fujiwara H et al: Pathology of the heart in Kawasaki's disease. *Pediatrics* **61**:100, 1978
21. Hirose S et al: Morphological observations on the vasculitis in the mucocutaneous lymph node syndrome: A skin biopsy study of 27 patients. *Eur J Pediatr* **129**:17, 1978
22. Terai M et al: Class II major histocompatibility antigen expression on coronary arterial endothelium in a patient with Kawasaki disease. *Hum Pathol* **21**:231, 1990
23. Fukushige J et al: Spectrum of cardiovascular lesions in mucocutaneous lymph node syndrome: Analysis of eight cases. *Am J Cardiol* **45**:98, 1980
24. Leung DYM et al: Immunoregulatory abnormalities in mucocutaneous lymph node syndrome. *Clin Immunol Immunopathol* **23**:100, 1982
25. Furukawa S et al: Peripheral blood monocyte/macrophage and serum tumor necrosis factor in Kawasaki disease. *Clin Exp Immunol* **48**:247, 1988
26. Leung DYM et al: Immunoregulatory T cell abnormalities in mucocutaneous lymph node syndrome. *J Immunol* **130**:2002, 1983

27. Maury CPJ et al: Circulating interleukin-1 in patients with Kawasaki disease. *N Engl J Med* **319**:1670, 1988
28. Maury CP et al: Elevated circulating tumor necrosis factor-alpha in patients with Kawasaki disease. *J Lab Clin Med* **113**:651, 1989
29. Rowley AH et al: Serum interferon concentrations and retroviral serology in Kawasaki syndrome. *Pediatr Infect Dis J* **7**:663, 1988
30. Ueno Y et al: The acute phase nature of interleukin 6: Studies in Kawasaki disease and other febrile illnesses. *Clin Exp Immunol* **76**:337, 1989
31. Leung DYM et al: Endothelial cell activation and high interleukin-1 secretion in the pathogenesis of acute Kawasaki disease. *Lancet* **2**:1298, 1989
32. Lang BA et al: Spontaneous tumor necrosis factor production in Kawasaki disease. *J Pediatr* **115**:939, 1989
33. Mantovani A et al: Cytokines as communication signals between leukocytes and endothelial cells. *Immunol Today* **10**:370, 1989
34. Leung DYM et al: Two monokines, interleukin 1 and tumor necrosis factor, render cultured vascular endothelial cells susceptible to lysis by antibodies circulating during Kawasaki syndrome. *J Exp Med* **164**:1958, 1986
35. Leung DYM et al: IgM antibodies in the acute phase of Kawasaki syndrome lyse cultured vascular endothelial cells stimulated by γ interferon. *J Clin Invest* **77**:1428, 1986
36. Leung DYM et al: Reversal of immunoregulatory abnormalities in Kawasaki syndrome by intravenous gammaglobulin. *J Clin Invest* **79**:468, 1987
37. Kotzin BL et al: Superantigens and human disease. *Adv Immunol* **54**:99, 1993
38. Abe J et al: Selective expansion of T cells expressing T cell receptor variable regions Vβ2 and Vβ8 in Kawasaki disease. *Proc Natl Acad Sci USA* **89**:4066, 1992
39. Choi Y et al: Selective expansion of T cells expressing Vβ2 in toxic shock syndrome. *J Exp Med* **172**:981, 1990
40. Pietra BA et al: TCR V beta family repertoire and T cell activation markers in Kawasaki disease. *J Immunol* **153**:1881, 1994
41. Curtis N et al: Evidence for a superantigen mediated process in Kawasaki disease. *Arch Dis Child* **72**:308, 1995
42. Abe J et al: Characterization of T cell repertoire changes in acute Kawasaki disease. *J Exp Med* **177**:791, 1993
43. Leung DYM et al: Bacterial superantigens induce T cell expression of the skin-selective homing receptor, the cutaneous lymphocyte-associated antigen (CLA). *J Exp Med* **181**:747, 1995
44. Yamashiro Y et al: Selective increase of Vβ2+ T cells in the small intestinal mucosa in Kawasaki disease. *Pediatr Res* **39**:264, 1996
45. Leung DYM et al: Evidence for superantigen involvement in cardiovascular injury due to Kawasaki syndrome. *J Immunol* **155**:5018, 1995
46. Leung DYM et al: Toxic shock syndrome toxin-secreting *Staphylococcus aureus* in Kawasaki syndrome. *Lancet* **342**:1385, 1993
47. Koren G et al: Probable efficacy of high-dose salicylates in reducing coronary involvement in Kawasaki disease. *JAMA* **254**:767, 1985
48. FitzGerald GA: Dipyridamole. *N Engl J Med* **316**:1247, 1987
49. Furusho K et al: High-dose intravenous gamma globulin for Kawasaki disease. *Lancet* **2**:1055, 1984
50. Newburger JW et al: The treatment of Kawasaki syndrome with intravenous gammaglobulin. *N Engl J Med* **315**:341, 1986
51. Newburger JW et al: A single intravenous infusion of gamma globulin as compared with four infusions in the treatment of acute Kawasaki syndrome. *N Engl J Med* **324**:1633, 1991
52. Rowley AH et al: Prevention of giant coronary artery aneurysms in Kawasaki disease by intravenous gamma globulin therapy. *J Pediatr* **113**:290, 1988
53. Newburger JW et al: Left ventricular contractility and function in Kawasaki syndrome. Effect of intravenous gamma-globulin. *Circulation* **79**:1237, 1989
54. Kato H et al: Kawasaki disease: Effect of treatment on coronary artery involvement. *Pediatrics* **63**:175, 1979
55. Wright DFA et al: Treatment of immune globulin-resistant Kawasaki disease with pulsed doses of corticosteroids. *J Pediatr* **128**:146, 1996
56. Koren G et al: Kawasaki disease: Review of risk factors for coronary aneurysms. *J Pediatr* **108**:388, 1986
57. Takei S et al: Intravenous immunoglobulin contains specific antibodies inhibitory to activation of T cells by staphylococcal toxin superantigens. *J Clin Invest* **91**:602, 1993
58. Kitamura S et al: Severe Kawasaki heart disease treated with an internal mammary artery graft in pediatric patients: A first successful report. *J Thorac Cardiovasc Surg* **89**:860, 1985
59. Takahashi M et al: Regression of coronary aneurysms in patients with Kawasaki syndrome. *Circulation* **75**:387, 1987
60. Kato H et al: Long term consequences of Kawasaki disease: A 10–21 year follow-up study of 594 patients. *Circulation* **94**:1379, 1996
61. Nakano H et al: Repeated quantitative angiograms in coronary arterial aneurysm in Kawasaki disease. *Am J Cardiol* **56**:846, 1985
62. Tatara K et al: Long-term prognosis of giant coronary aneurysm in Kawasaki disease: An angiographic study. *J Pediatr* **111**:705, 1987
63. Tanaka N et al: Pathological study of sequelae of Kawasaki disease (MCLS), with special reference to the heart and coronary arterial lesions. *Acta Pathol Jpn* **36**:1513, 1986
64. Matsumura K et al: Coronary angiography of Kawasaki disease with the coronary vasodilator dipyridamole: Assessment of distensibility of affected coronary arterial wall. *Angiology* **39**:141, 1988
65. Dhillon R et al: Endothelial dysfunction late after Kawasaki disease. *Circulation* **94**:2103–2106, 1996

CHAPTER 206

Ann G. Martin
George S. Kobayashi

Superficial Fungal Infection: Dermatophytosis, Tinea Nigra, Piedra

MYCOLOGY

Background

The dermatophytes are a group of taxonomically related fungi capable of colonizing keratinized tissues such as the stratum corneum of the epidermis, nails, hair, and the horny tissues of various animals. This selective colonization is facilitated by the fact that dermatophytes can use keratin as a source of nutrients.[1]

Systematic study of dermatophytes began 150 years ago when Remak described the mycelial nature of the clinical disease favus. This observation was later supported by Schoenlein. In 1841, Gruby isolated the organism of favus in culture and experimentally produced disease in normal skin. Gruby's studies preceded by almost four decades the work of Koch and his criteria for assessing the etiology of infection. Despite this early start, medical mycology did not witness the accelerated scientific advances seen in bacteriology. At about the turn of the century, Raymond Sabouraud recognized the microscopic and clinical aspects of four genera of dermatophytes. The culmination of this work was his classic treatise, *Les Tiegnes*, in 1910. In 1934, Emmons critically reviewed the taxonomic status of the dermatophytes, accepting only three genera: *Microsporum, Trichophyton,* and *Epidermophyton.*

Other studies have emphasized various epidemiologic and ecologic aspects of the dermatophytes. Those species found only in soil are called *geophilic* and are represented by such organisms as *M. gypseum, M. fulvum,* and *T. terrestre.* Several species found in association with domestic and wild animals are known as *zoophilic.* Species found only in association with human beings are called *anthropophilic.*

Mycologic Procedures

The presumptive diagnosis of dermatophyte infection should be supported by microscopic examination of clinical material and confirmed by culture of the specimen on suitable mycologic media.

Clinical specimens must be properly collected in order to reveal fungal elements.

MICROSCOPIC EXAMINATION

1. *Hair:* When the lesions involve the scalp and beard, examination with a Wood's lamp will occasionally reveal hairs infected with *Microsporum* species. Scalp samples should be picked with the tip of a no. 11 blade scalpel and placed on fungal medium for culture. Suspected hairs are placed on microscope slides with clearing solution,* to be examined by low-power microscopy. One out of three patterns of infection may be seen:
   a. Ectothrix—arthroconidia surrounding the hair shaft as a sheath (Fig. 206-1);
   b. Endothrix—arthroconidia contained within the hair shaft (Fig. 206-2); or
   c. "Favic"—a linear arrangement of hyphal fragments in chains along the longitudinal axis of the hair shaft (Fig. 206-3). The classification of organisms causing tinea capitis is shown in Table 206-1.
2. *Skin and nails:* Skin samples are taken from the advancing margins of the lesion by scraping with the dulled edge of a scalpel. Nail specimens should include clippings of the entire thickness of the nail.

A 10% KOH and ink clearing solution* is used to digest the proteins, lipids, and most of the other epithelial debris present in the samples. The fungal elements will resist this treatment because of the chitin and glycoprotein present in the fungal cell wall. The clearing process can be hastened by gently heating the slide. In a

---

*The clearing solution consists of 10% KOH made up in Parker Super Quink permanent Blue Black Ink. (Swartz JH, Lamkins BE: *Arch Dermatol* **89**:149, 1964.) When KOH is added to the ink, an amorphous precipitate forms. This can be removed by centrifugation (2000 rpm/10 min). The clear supernatant fluid should be stored in a plastic bottle to prevent formation of insoluble carbonates.

FIGURE 206-1

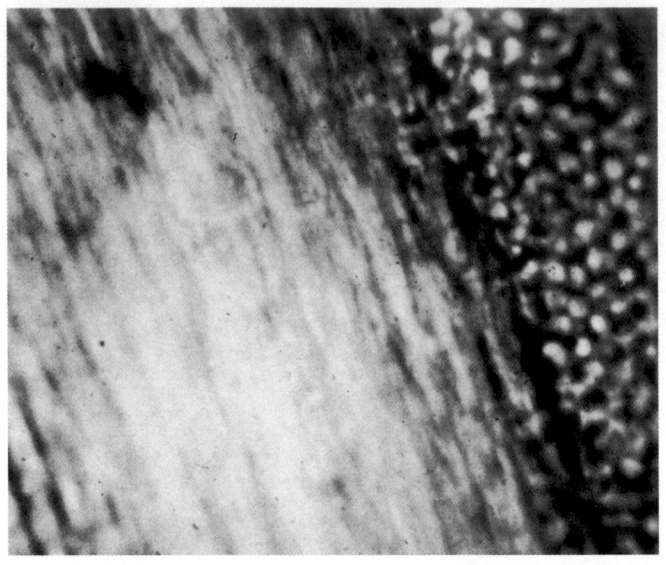

Microscopic examination of ectothrix type hair involvement with arthrospores outside of hair shaft.

positive preparation, fungi will appear as septate and branching hyphal elements (Fig. 206-4). In order to identify the specific agent, the organism must be cultured on suitable medium and examined accordingly.

CULTURE PROCEDURES   Definitive diagnosis of dermatophyte infections rests solely on the macroscopic, microscopic, and, in some cases, the physiologic characteristics of the organism. For these reasons, clinical specimens must be cultured on media suitable

FIGURE 206-2

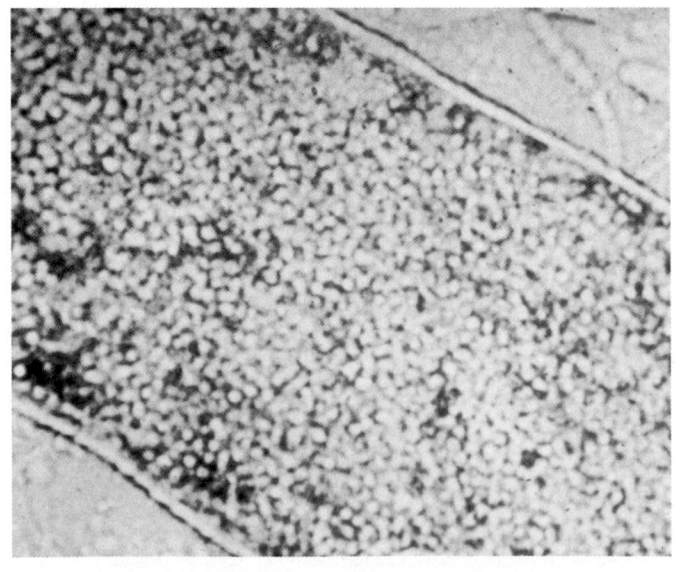

Microscopic examination of endothrix type hair invasion.

FIGURE 206-3

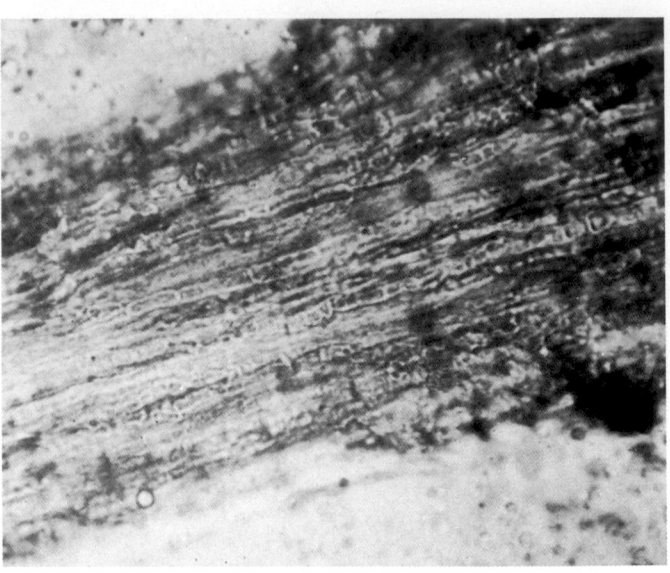

Favic hair invasion due to *T. schoenleinii.*

for growth of these fungi. Sabouraud's dextrose agar* is the most commonly used medium in medical mycology and serves as the basis for most of the morphologic descriptions of these fungi. Unfortunately, saprobes (organisms that feed on dead or decaying organic matter) grow rapidly and well on this medium, and since they frequently contaminate body surfaces from which clinical specimens are taken, they will overgrow any pathogens that may be present, thus making it difficult to isolate and identify pathogens. To circumvent this problem, chloramphenicol (0.05 g/L) and cyclo-heximide (0.4 g/L) may be incorporated into Sabouraud's dextrose agar to make the medium highly selective for the isolation of dermatophytes. The chloramphenicol inhibits bacterial growth, and the cycloheximide inhibits most saprobic fungi. It is imperative that the medium used in a given laboratory is standardized. Several good commercial variants of the standard Sabouraud medium are readily available (Mycosel, Mycobiotic medium). Cultures should be maintained at room temperature (26°C) for up to 4 weeks before they are discarded as showing no growth.

Identification and speciation of the dermatophytes require careful observation of gross colonial morphology and microscopic examination of properly prepared samples. The number of species of dermatophytes is large, and for proper identification one should rely on a suitable reference source.[2]

DERMATOPHYTOSIS

Dermatophytoses are superficial infections of keratinized tissue caused by organisms of three genera of fungi known as the *dermatophytes.*[1,3] In contrast, dermatomycosis represents systemic or deep fungal infections that may have prominent cutaneous and systemic manifestations.

---

*Sabouraud's dextrose agar, formulation: Dextrose 40 g; Peptone 10 g; Agar 20 g; distilled water adjusted to pH 5.5 1000 mL.

The dermatophytes represent more than 40 closely related species classified in three genera: *Microsporum, Trichophyton,* and *Epidermophyton.* Only a few of these species are responsible for most human infections.[1] Thus, knowledge of their ecology is useful for the classification of these organisms (Table 206-2).

Geophilic organisms sporadically infect humans; when they do, the resulting disease is usually inflammatory. *M. gypseum* is the most common geophile isolated in human infections. The strains cultured from humans are more virulent and account for epidemic spread of the infection under appropriate conditions.[4]

Zoophilic species can be transmitted to humans sporadically. Domestic animals and pets are becoming an increasing source of these infections in urban areas[6] (e.g., *M. canis* in cats or dogs). Transmission may occur through direct contact with a specific animal species (Table 206-3) or indirectly by infected animal hair carried on clothing or present in contaminated stalls, barns, or feed. Exposed areas of the body are favored sites of infection (i.e., scalp, beard, face, arms). Although human infections with zoophiles are often suppurative, animal infection may be clinically silent. Under these conditions, animals serve as asymptomatic carriers and underscore the unique adaptation that these organisms have for their animals hosts.[3,4,6]

Anthropophilic species have adapted to infect humans. Unlike the sporadic geophilic and zoophilic infections, anthropophilic infections are often epidemic in nature. They are transmitted from person to person either by direct contact or indirectly through fo-

TABLE 206-1

Classification of Organisms Causing Tinea Capitis

SPECIES	ECOLOGY	GEOGRAPHIC DISTRIBUTION
ECTOTHRIX		
Microsporum		
M. audouinii	Anthropophilic	Sporadic
M. canis	Zoophilic	Worldwide
M. gypseum	Geophilic	Worldwide
M. fulvum	Geophilic	Worldwide
M. ferrugineum	Anthropophilic	Africa, India, Asia, South America
Trichophyton		
T. mentagrophytes	Zoophilic, anthropophilic	Worldwide
T. rubrum	Anthropophilic	Worldwide
T. verrucosum	Zoophilic	Worldwide
T. megninii	Anthropophilic	Europe
ENDOTHRIX		
Trichophyton		
T. tonsurans	Anthropophilic	United States, Central America, Europe, Australia, Caribbean
T. violaceum	Anthropophilic	Africa, Europe, Asia
T. soudanense	Anthropophilic	Central and West Africa
T. gourvilli	Anthropophilic	Central and West Africa
T. yaoundei	Anthropophilic	Central and West Africa
T. schoenleinii	Anthropophilic	Europe, Near East, Mediterranean; rare in United States

mites. Markedly inflammatory reactions can occur because of differences in susceptible hosts or strain virulence. Kerion formation, suppuration, or other manifestations of inflammatory tinea facilitate early diagnoses in these cases. Noninflammatory disease, on the

FIGURE 206-4

TABLE 206-2

Ecology of Dermatophytes

GEOPHILIC	ZOOPHILIC	ANTHROPOPHILIC
(M. boullardii)*	M. canis	E. floccosum
M. cookei	M. distortum	M. audouinii
M. fulvum	M. equinum	M. ferrugineum
M. gypseum	T. equinum	
(M. magellanicum)	T. mentagrophytes	T. concentricum
M. nanum	var. erinacei	T. gourvilii
(M. racemosum)	(T. flavescens)	T. mentagrophytes
(M. ripariae)	M. gallinae	var. interdigitale
M. vanbreuseghemi	T. mentagrophytes	T. megninii
T. ajelloi	T. mentagrophytes	T. rubrum
(T. georgiae)	var. quinckeanum	T. schoenleinii
(T. gloriae)	T. verrucosum	T. soudanense
(T. longifusum)		T. tonsurans
(T. phaseoliforme)		T. violaceum
T. simii		T. yaoundei
(T. terrestre)		
(T. vanbreuseghemii)		
M. amazonicum		
M. praecox		

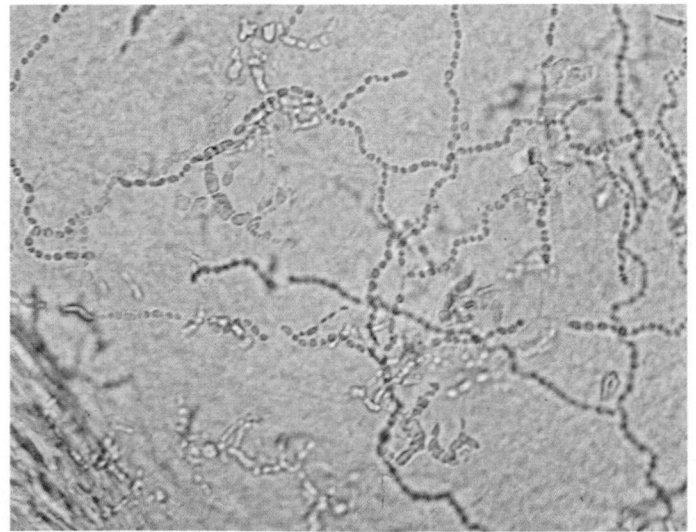

Skin scrapings (scales). This KOH preparation exhibits septate hyphae.

*Organisms in parentheses are not known to cause human disease.
SOURCE: Modified from Otcenasek.[5]

TABLE 206-3

Animal Hosts for Zoophilic Dermatophytes

ORGANISM	ANIMAL HOSTS*
M. canis	Dogs, cats, cattle, sheep, pigs, rodents, monkeys
M. distortum	Dogs, cats, horses, monkeys
M. equinum	Horses
T. equinum	Horses, dogs
T. mentagrophytes var. erinacei	Rodents (hedgehogs)
T. gallinae	Fowl, rodents, cats
T. mentagrophytes var. mentagrophytes	Cats, dogs, cattle, sheep, pigs, horses, rodents, monkeys
T. verrucosum	Dogs, cattle, sheep, pigs, horses

*Italics indicate the usual or preferred host.

other hand, fosters the existence of a clinically silent "carrier" state that serves to delay the diagnosis and propagate the infection.

Host differences and intercurrent diseases play a role in the epidemiology of anthropophilic infections, e.g., dermatophytosis may be severe or recalcitrant to therapy in patients with diabetes mellitus, lymphoid malignancies, immunologic compromise, or Cushing's syndrome.[3,7] Likewise, age, sex, and race differences define populations at risk for these infections. For example, tinea capitis due to anthropophilic organisms (e.g., *T. tonsurans*) is most common in African-American children; when it occurs in adults, it is far more common in women.[6] In contrast, tinea pedis, tinea unguium, and tinea cruris are more common in adults, with the latter occurring predominantly in males.

Certain strains of dermatophytes are endemic to specific geographic areas (Table 206-4). Because of patterns of travel to and from these areas, resident dermatophytes may remain restricted geographically or become more cosmopolitan. Earlier in this century, *M. audouinii* was the predominant cause of tinea capitis in the United States. In the past 15 to 20 years, *T. tonsurans* has assumed that role. The spread of this infection appears to correlate well with the ingress of Mexicans and Puerto Ricans to this country.[6]

TABLE 206-4

Geographically Limited Species

ORGANISM	ENDEMIC REGION
M. nanum	Cuba
T. concentricum	Pacific Islands, Far East, India, Ceylon; areas of North, Central, and South America
T. ferrugineum	Africa, India, eastern Europe, Asia
T. megninii	Portugal, Sardinia
T. soudanense	Central and West Africa
T. yaoundei	Central and West Africa
T. gourvilii	Central and West Africa
M. distortum	New Zealand, United States
T. equinum	Western Europe, Canada, United States
T. ajelloi	Certain areas of North and Central America, Europe, Japan, Australia

SOURCE: Adapted from Ajello.[8]

The location of the dermatophytosis is partially dependent on climatic conditions of the area and the customs of the resident population. Tinea pedis, for example, is more common in areas where occlusive footwear is used.[3] In extremely hot, humid climates, tinea corporis may occur readily under occlusive garments.[7]

Finally, there is some evidence to suggest that certain human populations may be genetically more susceptible to particular dermatophyte infections. *T. concentricum* is not transmitted readily to individuals of different races living with the susceptible population.[9] Likewise, *T. rubrum* infections within a household favor relatives; conjugal pairs, in contrast, are less commonly infected, even though environmental exposure to the organism is equivalent.[3]

In addition to host and geographic factors, the virulence of the infecting organism must be considered. *T. mentagrophytes* var. *mentagrophytes* is a zoophilic organism that produces a marked inflammatory infection in the human host, whereas the variant *interdigitale* does not.

Pathogenesis

The presence of a suitable environment on host skin is of critical importance in the development of clinical dermatophytosis.[1,3,10] In addition to trauma, increased hydration of the skin with maceration is important. Occlusion with a nonporous material increases the temperature and hydration of the skin and interferes with the barrier function of the stratum corneum. Nonporous shoes definitely contribute to the development of tinea pedis.[1,3] In tropical climates, nonacclimatized individuals often develop lesions of tinea corporis, in part because of occlusive clothing.[11–13]

If the host skin is inoculated under suitable conditions, there follow several stages through which the dermatophyte infections progress, including periods of incubation, enlargement followed by a refractory period, and a stage of involution.[1,14,15]

During the incubation period, a dermatophyte grows in the stratum corneum, sometimes with minimal clinical signs of infection. A carrier state has been postulated when the presence of a dermatophyte is detected on seemingly normal skin by KOH examination or culture.

Once infection is established in the stratum corneum, two factors are important in determining the size and duration of the lesion: (1) the rate of growth of the organism, and (2) the epidermal turnover rate. The fungal growth rate must equal or exceed the epidermal turnover rate or the organism will be shed quickly.[7]

Keratinases and other proteolytic enzymes are produced by dermatophytes. The role of these enzymes in the pathogenesis of clinical infection relates to skin colonization and invasion as well as organism virulence. There is evidence that actual enzymatic digestion of keratin may be occurring. Host immunologic response and also enzymes or toxins produced by the organism account for the clinical findings in dermatophytoses.[16–18]

Immunology

Our understanding of the immunology of dermatophyte infections continues to expand. Excellent reviews have been written by Weitzman and Summerbell,[3] Wagner and Sohnle,[1] Jones,[18] Dahl,[16,17,19] Emmons et al.,[20] and Ahmed.[21]

Resistance to dermatophyte infections may involve nonimmunologic as well as immunologic mechanisms,[19] from the increase in saturated fatty acids on the skin that occurs after puberty to the presence of a serum inhibitory factor (SIF) that appears to limit the growth of dermatophytes. Unsaturated transferrin is a likely SIF candidate[22] because it binds the iron that dermatophytes need for continued growth.[23] An alpha$_2$-macroglobulin keratinase inhibitor has also been identified in serum and may modify the growth of the organisms.[24]

The humoral limb of the immune system has a minor role in the development of acquired resistance to dermatophyte infections,[16] while the major immunologic defense mechanism is the type IV delayed-hypersensitivity response.[16] When patients who have not been previously infected with a dermatophyte are experimentally infected with *T. mentagrophytes,* the initial response is one of slight inflammation and scaling. The trichophytin skin test is negative. Between 10 and 35 days into the infection, the site abruptly becomes inflammatory and pruritic and trichophytin skin testing is positive. After the development of cell-mediated immunity, the infected area becomes less inflammatory and eventually spontaneously involutes. If a second infection with the same organism is produced in the same individual, the site becomes inflammatory very early on and resolves relatively quickly. The recall of delayed hypersensitivity to *Trichophyton* is brisk and organisms are less often demonstrated in secondary reactions.[16,25]

A plausible mechanism by which the delayed-hypersensitivity response may cause dermatophyte inhibition has been proposed by Jones[18] and others.[26,27] During the host's first exposure to the *Trichophyton* cell wall glycopeptide antigen, the antigen diffuses from the stratum corneum to stimulate sensitized lymphocytes.[16,17] Inflammatory mediators and lymphokines are produced by these cells and probably act on the host cells rather than on the dermatophyte. Because of this response, the epidermal barrier is abrogated, and SIF gains access to the otherwise privileged layers of the stratum corneum. SIF is fungistatic, and so the cell-mediated immune response typically leads to inhibition but not complete destruction of the dermatophyte. Hence, the organism is still identified in cultures and KOH preparations of the infected area. The greater the inflammation, the fewer the number of organisms that can be found. In most circumstances the cell-mediated immunity that exists is relative rather than absolute.[25,26]

The use of the intradermal trichophytin skin test has identified two groups of patients based on the type of reaction ensuing from this test. Immediate (20 min) and delayed (48 h) reactions have been noted. The latter reaction appears to correlate best with an active delayed-hypersensitivity response resulting from an acute infection with dermatophytes. Patients showing immediate reactions often (75 percent) have chronic infections, most commonly with *T. rubrum.*[16,18,21,27,28]

Chronic dermatophyte infections are characterized by relatively long-standing, widespread disease, often with palmar and plantar involvement, with little or no associated inflammatory response. There is often a negative delayed trichophytin skin test but a positive immediate one. The causative organism is usually *T. rubrum,* typically resistant to therapy with griseofulvin.[3,16,18] When other organisms are found, there may be a higher incidence of serious underlying disease (diabetes, hypercortisolism, lymphoma, etc.).[3,29–31] As many as 50 percent of patients chronically infected with *T. rubrum* have associated atopy[18,30–32]; they usually have an elevated IgE serum level. In vitro lymphocyte transformation studies in these patients often reveal a selective failure to respond to trichophytin, whereas mitogen responses remain intact.[3,16,18,28,31]

There is evidence to suggest that patients with this "atopic–chronic dermatophytosis syndrome" are capable of delayed-hypersensitivity skin test reactions, but these reactions are inhibited by the more sensitive, preceding type I response.[32]

Dermatophytid reactions are secondary inflammatory reactions of the skin at a site distant from the associated fungal infection, occurring in 4 to 5 percent of patients.[33] In contrast to material obtained from the dermatophytosis, cultures and KOH examinations

of the "id" lesions are negative. Id reactions are usually accompanied by a reactive delayed trichophytin skin test. The mechanism responsible for the id response is unknown but may involve a local immunologic response to systemically absorbed fungal antigen.[33,34]

Clinically, id reactions may take several forms, including follicular papules, erythema nodosum, vesicular id of hands and feet, erysipelas-like, erythema annulare centrifugum, and urticaria.[34–39] These reactions tend to occur at the height of the dermatophyte infection, slightly thereafter, or just after initiation of systemic antifungal therapy.[35] Disappearance of the dermatophytid reaction occurs when the dermatophyte infection is successfully treated. Occasionally, concomitant topical or systemic steroid therapy is warranted in addition to griseofulvin—especially if the dermatophytid is extremely widespread or inflammatory.

Clinical Types

TINEA CAPITIS Tinea capitis is a dermatophytosis of the scalp and associated hair that is caused by a variety of species of the genera *Microsporum* and *Trichophyton.* The most common isolated organisms are *T. tonsurans* and *M. canis.* Clinically an inflammatory or noninflammatory alopecia occurs, with a significant preference for children.

Epidemiology The true incidence of tinea capitis is unknown. The source of an infection and the degree of inflammation depend on whether the causative organism is geophilic, zoophilic, or anthropophilic. The patients most commonly affected are children between the ages of 4 and 14 years. In the United States, African Americans and Hispanics have a higher incidence of tinea capitis, especially that caused by *T. tonsurans.*[36,40,41]

After the introduction of griseofulvin in the late 1950s and the immigration of Hispanics and Mexicans to the United States, the local etiologic agent of tinea capitis changed from *M. audouinii* to *T. tonsurans.* This was attributed to the higher antibiotic susceptibility of the former and to improved public health screening and disease control.[36,40,41]

Transmission of certain forms of tinea capitis is fostered by the existence of overcrowding or poor personal hygiene. Low socioeconomic conditions and, in one report, protein malnutrition[42] have also been implicated. It is clear that organisms responsible for tinea capitis can be cultured from brushes, combs, caps, pillow cases, theater seats, and other inanimate objects. The disease can also be transmitted from child to child through exposure at schools or daycare centers. Affected hairs can harbor infectious organisms for a year or more after they have been shed from the host.[41]

The existence of an asymptomatic carrier state in tinea capitis has been repeatedly documented. The finding has important epidemiologic implications, as silent sources of infection are more difficult to detect and eradicate.

Etiology and pathogenesis Virtually any species of *Microsporum* or *Trichophyton* can cause tinea capitis. Exceptions are *T. concentricum* and *E. floccosum.* The causative organisms (see Table 206-1) can be classified according to their host preference (i.e., anthropophilic, zoophilic, geophilic) and according to whether they produce arthroconidia outside or just under the cuticle of the hair (ectothrix) or within the hair (endothrix).

Most of the dermatophytes causing tinea capitis have a ubiquitous geographic distribution. Knowledge of the prevalent organisms responsible for each dermatophytosis in a specific geographic area can facilitate identification of causative agent of disease.

The pathogenesis of tinea capitis has been studied by Kligman[14,15] and by Frieden and Howard.[36,41] Hair appears to be susceptible to ectothrix dermatophytes during mid to late anagen. The infection usually begins in the perifollicular stratum corneum. Following a period of incubation, hyphae generally spread into and around the hair shaft. They descend into the follicle and penetrate the midportion of the hair. Subsequently, hyphae descend within the intrapilary portion of the hair until they reach the border of the keratogenous zone. Here they continue to grow in delicate equilibrium with the keratinization process, so that they proceed no deeper than the upper limit of the keratogenous zone. The hyphae never enter the nucleated zone and, therefore, appear to discern the subtle differences between the partially keratinized and the fully keratinized hair. In this location the terminal tuft of hyphae is termed *Adamson's fringe*. Intrapilary hyphae proliferate and divide into arthroconidia that reach the cortex of the hair and are transported upward on its surface. When the hair is plucked, it breaks at its weakest point, just above Adamson's fringe. When the plucked hair is visualized microscopically, it is the numerous ectothrix spores that are seen, rather than the intrapilar hyphae.

With endothrix infections (e.g., *T. tonsurans*), the same process occurs until the hair is penetrated. The arthroconidia are formed rapidly and in time replace much of the intrapilary keratin, while leaving the cortex intact. The hair is fragile and, with trauma, breaks at its weakest point—the surface of the scalp where it loses the supporting follicular wall. When observed clinically, the remaining hair in this infected follicle resembles a black dot, so endothrix infections are often referred to as "black dot ringworm." A final important difference between endothrix and ectothrix infections is that endothrix infections may continue past the anagen phase of the hair cycle and into telogen. Therefore, these infections tend to be more chronic than those caused by the ectothrix organisms.[4,43]

Clinical manifestations　The different organisms causing tinea capitis may present with several different clinical patterns[40,41] (Table 206-5).

NONINFLAMMATORY, HUMAN, OR EPIDEMIC TYPE　This clinical pattern is produced most commonly by *M. audouinii* or *M. ferrugineum*. The lesion begins as a small erythematous papule surrounding a hair shaft. Subsequently, the lesion spreads centrifugally, involving all hairs in its path. Typically, there is scaling with minimal inflammation. One or more well-demarcated patches are seen usually on the occiput or posterior neck. Hairs in the infected area are gray and lusterless in appearance due to their coating of arthroconidia ("gray patch" ringworm) (Fig. 206-5). They frequently break off just above the level of the scalp, rather than being shed entirely.[41]

INFLAMMATORY TYPE　These infections are caused most commonly by zoophilic organisms (e.g., *M. canis*) or geophilic dermatophytes (e.g., *M. gypseum*).[44] Clinically, a spectrum of inflammatory changes may be seen, ranging from a pustular folliculitis to a kerion (Fig. 206-6), which presents as an inflammatory, boggy mass studded with broken hairs, oozing purulent material from follicular orifices.[40] These infections usually present with pruritus, fever, and pain. There may be associated regional lymphadenopathy. Occasionally, additional lesions are found on glabrous skin. Scarring alopecia is often a sequela due to the degree of inflammation generated.

"BLACK DOT" TINEA CAPITIS　This variety of tinea capitis is most often caused by endothrix organisms such as *T. tonsurans* or *T. violaceum*. Because of the arthroconidia, the hair shaft is extremely brittle and breaks at the level of the scalp. The remnant of hair left behind in the infected follicle appears as a black dot on clinical examination (Fig. 206-7). There may be diffuse scaling with minimal hair loss and inflammation, so that the infection can be confused with seborrheic dermatitis, atopic dermatitis, or psoriasis.[45] When hair loss occurs, the affected areas are characteristically multiple or polygonal in outline with indistinct, fingerlike margins.[46] This is in contrast to *M. audouinii* infections, which usually appear as larger, solitary, annular patches. Within the areas of involvement, black dot infections commonly spare some hairs so that areas of alopecia are sprinkled with a few normal hairs. Black dot infections may also be quite inflammatory, with changes ranging from a pustular folliculitis to furuncle-like lesions or obvious kerions.[40] Finally, black dot tinea capitis may present without obvious black dots, making a high index of suspicion for this infection necessary.[41]

Laboratory findings　Laboratory confirmation of dermatophyte infections is imperative. Wood's lamp examination is valuable in infections caused by *Microsporum* species. A bright green band of fluorescence in the hair just above the level of the scalp is seen. The fluorescence is thought to be produced by pteridines generated as the fungus infects actively growing hairs.[47] *T. tonsurans* infections do not fluoresce. In these instances, careful KOH examination and proper culture techniques are crucial in making the correct diagnosis.

Pathology　In tinea capitis, hyphae are identified around and within the hair shaft. Special stains serve to emphasize their presence (i.e., PAS, methenamine silver). The dermis demonstrates a perifollicular mixed cell infiltrate with lymphocytes, histiocytes, plasma cells, and eosinophils. If follicular disruption has occurred, an adjacent foreign-body giant cell reaction is seen.[48]

In the more inflammatory lesion (i.e., kerions), an intense dermal infiltrate is seen, with polymorphonuclear leukocytes forming abscesses in the dermis and within the follicle.[48] In these markedly inflammatory reactions, fungal organisms are seen with difficulty. Immunofluorescence techniques, however, have demonstrated the presence of fungal antigens.[49]

Diagnosis　The differential diagnosis of tinea capitis includes seborrheic dermatitis, atopic dermatitis,[45] and psoriasis when minimally inflammatory diffuse scaling is the major clinical presentation. When alopecia is more pronounced, diseases such as al-

TABLE 206-5

Organisms Associated with Clinical Types of Tinea Capitis*

INFLAMMATORY	NONINFLAMMATORY	"BLACK DOT"	FAVUS
M. canis	M. audouinii	T. tonsurans	T. schoenleinii
M. gypseum	T. tonsurans	T. violaceum	T. violaceum
T. mentagrophytes	M. canis		M. gypseum
T. tonsurans	M. ferrugineum		
T. verrucosum			
T. schoenleinii			
M. audouinii			
M. nanum			

*Some organisms produce more than one clinical type.

FIGURE 206-5

CHAPTER 206
Superficial Fungal Infection
2343

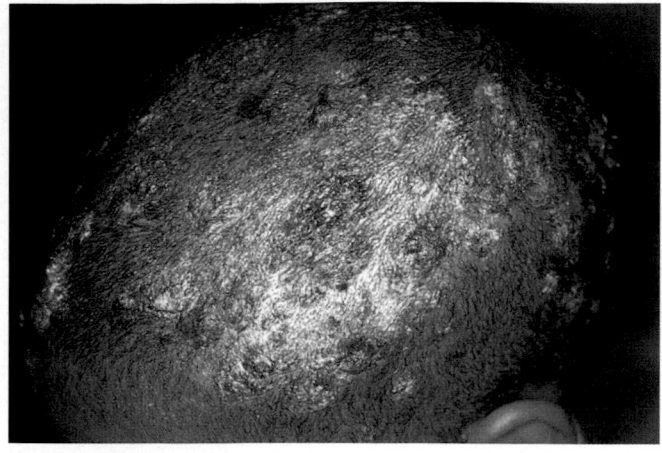

Tinea capitis secondary to *M. audouinii.*

FIGURE 206-6

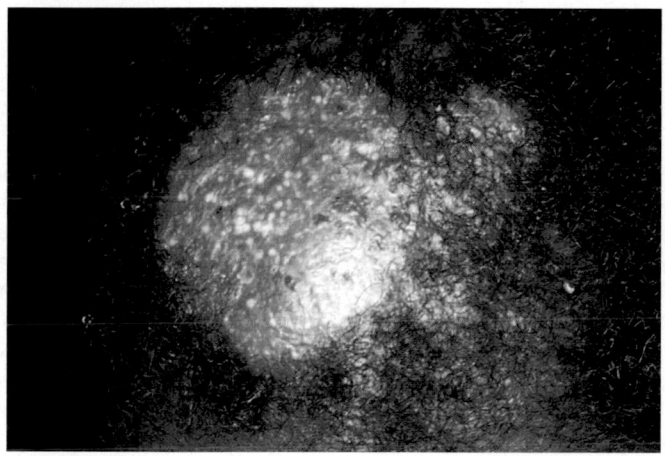

Kerion on scalp.

FIGURE 206-7

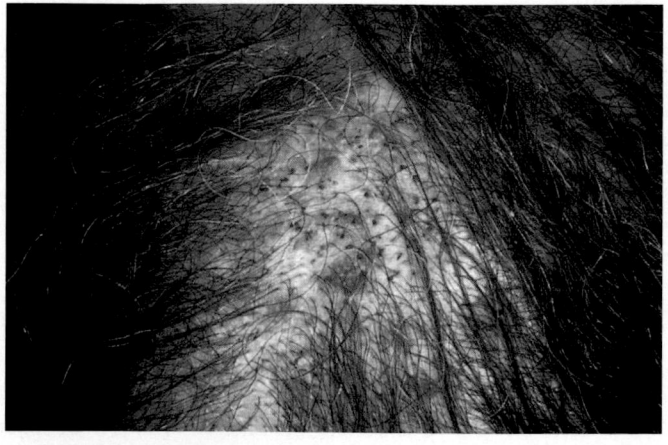

"Black dot" tinea capitis secondary to *T. tonsurans.*

opecia areata, trichotillomania, secondary syphilis, or pseudopelade can be considered. Alopecia due to tinea capitis fails to produce the typical exclamation point hairs seen in alopecia areata or the artefactual-appearing areas with hairs of varying lengths seen in trichotillomania.

In inflammatory tinea capitis, bacterial pyodermas (furunculosis, impetigo) can be simulated. Folliculitis decalvans or perifolliculitis capitis abscedens et suffodiens can also enter into the differential diagnosis. After scarring has occurred, noninfectious processes such as discoid lupus erythematosus, lichen planopilaris, pseudopelade, or radiation dermatitis are often considered in the differential diagnosis.

Treatment   Tinea capitis requires a systemic antifungal such as griseofulvin to penetrate the hair follicle. The usual dose is 1 g/day of the microcrystalline variety or 0.5 g/day of the ultramicrosized drug. For children the dose is 10 to 15 mg/kg per day of the ultramicrosized drug taken with a fatty meal to enhance absorption.[41] Therapy should be continued until both a clinical and mycologic cure are documented, usually in 6 to 8 weeks. The routine monitoring of hepatic and hematologic parameters is normally not necessary in healthy children. Other therapeutic regimens exist for the use of griseofulvin in the treatment of tinea capitis. Occasionally, it is necessary to increase the dose of griseofulvin to 20 to 25 mg/kg per day due to lack of clinical and mycologic response. This may be due to a local defect in individual cellular immunity or to high organism resistance to griseofulvin. In addition, single-dose griseofulvin (2 to 3 g) given monthly has been successful in developing countries. While this may ensure compliance and improve cost effectiveness, further safety studies are needed.[41]

In markedly inflammatory tinea capitis, oral glucocorticoids may be helpful in reducing the incidence of scarring. Although available data have shown no difference in cure rates, the goal of therapy is symptom relief. The usual dose of prednisone is 1 mg/kg per day given at one time in the morning during the first 10 to 15 days of therapy.

Prophylactic measures to prevent transmission of infection include screening and treatment of family members, disinfection of the environment, and identification and proper treatment of infected animals. Adjunct therapy with antifungal shampoos to decrease spore shedding is also advisable.

Individuals who are allergic to, intolerant of, or nonresponsive to griseofulvin require an alternative therapy. The current options are oral ketoconazole, fluconazole, itraconazole, and terbinafine.

Oral ketoconazole is effective in many patients with tinea capitis caused by *Trichophyton.* The risk of hepatotoxicity, the lack of a liquid preparation, and decreased efficacy against other species (e.g., *M. canis*) have not allowed this antibiotic to take precedence over griseofulvin.

Several studies have found itraconazole to be very effective in tinea capitis caused by *Microsporum* or *Trichophyton* species, with an 88 to 94 percent cure rate using a dose of 100 mg daily for 6 to 10 weeks.[50–52] A dose of 3 to 5 mg/kg per day is recommended. The efficacy and safety profile of this new antifungal as well as short duration of therapy makes it a very attractive therapeutic alternative.

Recent studies to evaluate the safety and efficacy of terbinafine in tinea capitis in children has shown encouraging results. A dose of 125 mg/day for 6 weeks has been used.[53] Efficacy has been variable depending on the etiologic agent. Cure rates of 73 to 100 percent have been achieved.[54,55]

Fluconazole has an excellent safety profile, is well tolerated, and has a liquid formulation. To this date there are not enough data to assess its efficacy for tinea capitis.

TINEA FAVOSA   Tinea favosa or favus (Latin, "honeycomb") is a chronic, mycotic infection of the scalp, glabrous skin, and/or nails characterized by the formation of yellowish crusts within the hair follicles (scutula) and eventuating in a cicatrizing alopecia. The only published data over the past 5 years regarding this entity has been from animal studies.

Epidemiology   Favus is typically a chronic infection that begins early in life and commonly extends into adulthood.[56] The disease is seen predominantly in rural areas and is often associated with conditions of poor hygiene, malnutrition, and squalor. Attack rates within families can vary, suggesting that there may be an inherited susceptibility or resistance to the infection.[57] In addition, simple measures to improve personal hygiene in the at-risk population often result in markedly decreased transmission.[58] It is known that *T. schoenleinii* can survive for years on epilated hairs. For this reason, cleanliness with the removal of hairs or other sources of infection is an important factor in controlling the disease.[59]

Although animal favus is known to occur, there is no evidence to substantiate the existence of an animal reservoir to explain human infections.[58]

Etiology   The most common dermatophyte producing favus is *T. schoenleinii*. In some areas, favus is the most common cause of tinea capitis.[60] The infection is endemic in the Middle East and Mediterranean basin area, southeastern Europe, France, southern Asia, and Greenland. In South Africa the disease is quite common.[9] In the Americas, endemic pockets of the disease exist. There are reports from areas of Québec, the United States (Kentucky, West Virginia, Arkansas, New York),[61] Guatemala, and Brazil.

Clinical features   In the early stages of infection, hyphae invade the hair follicle and gradually distend the follicular opening. Clinically, very little is seen within the first 3 weeks of infection except a slight amount of perifollicular scaling.

Scutula are found in most cases of favus. These concentrations of hyphae and keratinous debris take root at the opening of the hair follicle. Here, they gradually expand from a yellowish-red papule to form a yellowish, cup-shaped structure that may become 1 cm or more in diameter. The center of the scutulum is often pierced by a single, lusterless, dry hair (Fig. 206-8). The hair is not as brittle as with *T. tonsurans* endothrix infections, and, for that reason, hairs in favus may frequently attain a normal length. Scutula may expand peripherally and, during the course of the infection, form large, adherent mats of scutula and hair.[9]

In the classic presentation, lesions appear in a patchy distribution on the scalp and coalesce. The borders of the infected lesions represent areas of advancing disease and are often polycyclic in shape.[58] The center of the infected area becomes extensively scarred and almost totally devoid of hair.

Besides scalp involvement, favus may involve glabrous skin and nails. The skin infections may be of various types (i.e., vesicular, papulosquamous, tinea circinata–like), and often true scutula are formed. Nail involvement occurs in 2 to 3 percent of infections[62] and is indistinguishable from onychomycosis due to other organisms.[20]

In some cases, especially when personal hygiene is relatively good, favus lesions may be atypical in appearance. For example, scutula may be small or absent, and the disease may present with diffuse scaling of the scalp.[62] In these instances, the infection is

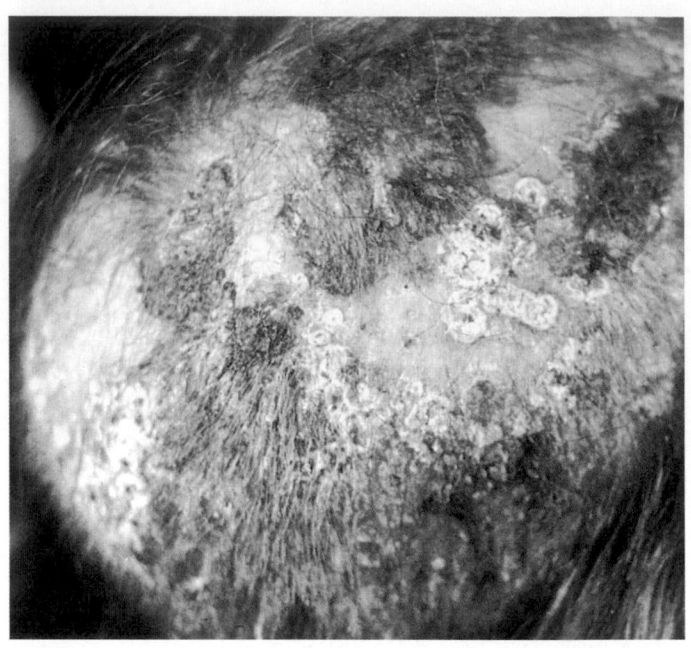

Tinea capitis from *Trichophyton schoenleinii* (favus). Yellowish, adherent crusts and scales, known as scutula. May be complicated by atrophy, scarring, and permanent hair loss.

difficult to distinguish from seborrheic dermatitis, psoriasis, or tinea amiantacea. In later stages of infection, a cicatricial alopecia may be present. In this end-stage presentation, the condition may be identical to that noted in cicatrizing alopecia after radiation or chemical injury or the scarring alopecia seen in some cases of pseudopelade, folliculitis decalvans, lupus erythematosus, or lichen planopilaris.

Laboratory findings   The laboratory diagnosis of favus requires the use of KOH examination and culture techniques discussed previously. On microscopic examination, an endothrix type of hair invasion is seen. The favus hair shows hyphae coursing lengthwise and no arthroconidia.[9] Because of autolysis, vacant tunnels are formed within the hair, and these may appear as air spaces microscopically (Fig. 206-3).[63]

With Wood's lamp examination, a pale green fluorescence is seen along the entire length of the infected hair. The fluorescence may be subtle and can be difficult to appreciate, especially in patients with gray hair.[64]

Histopathology   Degenerating hyphae and necrotic material are seen most typically in the center of the scutulum, whereas the viable organisms reside at the periphery. Under the scutulum there is an atrophic epithelium; acanthosis is noted at the lateral margins.[65] In the dermis, an extensive chronic plasma cell or granulomatous perifollicular infiltrate without organisms is commonly seen and is particularly dense subjacent to the scutulum. Fragments of hair can be seen in the dermis with polarized light. In the later stages of infection, the dermis may simply show fibrosis with a diminished inflammatory cell response.

Treatment   Favus is treated effectively with griseofulvin in the same dosage used in tinea capitis.[66] Nail infections require a longer course of therapy (6 to 12 months). It is important to examine and treat all affected family members simultaneously.[9] Improvement of hygienic conditions is also beneficial, as are efforts at local debridement of areas of extensive crusting.

TINEA BARBAE Tinea barbae (also known as tinea sycosis, "barber's itch") is a fungal infection limited to the coarse hair–bearing beard and moustache area of men. In women and prepubertal boys, infection in the facial areas (tinea faciale) is classified with the other glabrous skin infections.

Epidemiology Tinea barbae is by definition seen only in males. Usually, the infection is contracted by exposure to animals, most commonly cattle and dogs. The infection is most often seen in a rural setting,[9,67] often affecting dairy farmers or cattle ranchers. Prior to the introduction of modern-day antiseptic techniques, tinea barbae—then called barber's itch—was transmitted from person to person by contaminated barbers' razors or clippers.[2]

Etiology and pathogenesis Overall, the most common dermatophytes causing tinea barbae are the zoophilic organisms *T. mentagrophytes* and *T. verrucosum*.[67,68] *M. canis* is causative in a lesser number of cases.[69] Anthropophilic organisms (*T. rubrum, T. violaceum, T. schoenleinii,* and *T. megninii*) have been implicated in urban areas[68] or in areas where these fungi are endemic. In general, the infection caused by the anthropophiles is less inflammatory than that caused by the zoophilic dermatophytes.

The pathogenesis of tinea barbae is thought to be similar to that of the tinea capitis. Coarse hairs are uniquely susceptible; occasionally one may see concurrent involvement of the beard and scalp area.[68]

Clinical manifestations Three clinical types of tinea barbae have been recognized: (1) inflammatory or kerion-like, (2) superficial or sycosiform type,[70] and (3) the circinate, spreading type.

The inflammatory variety is analogous to kerion formation in tinea capitis (Fig. 206-9). In tinea barbae, the lesions are usually unilateral, commonly on the chin, neck, and maxillary or submaxillary areas (Fig. 206-9A). The upper lip is usually spared.[9,67] The inflammatory lesions are most often caused by *T. mentagrophytes* and *T. verrucosum*. Lesions are nodular and boggy; there is often an associated weeping of seropurulent material with subsequent crusting. Perifollicular pustulation is observed; coalescence of these inflammatory areas yields abscess-like collections of pus. The hairs within the infected areas are loose and easily epilated; commonly they are lusterless and brittle as well. Eventually, undermining and sinus tract formation can occur. Scarring and permanent alopecia are the ultimate outcome in severely affected areas.

The superficial type of tinea barbae typically resembles a bacterial folliculitis (Fig. 206-9B). There is a diffuse erythema associated with perifollicular papules and pustules.[70] The organisms causing this clinical picture are the relatively noninflammatory anthropophiles. Hairs may be affected, depending on the organism involved. For example, *T. violaceum* infections commonly result in brittle, lusterless hair due to endothrix invasion. Conversely, *T. rubrum* infections produce hair invasion less often.

The circinate tinea barbae is analogous to tinea circinata of glabrous skin. There is an active, spreading vesiculopustular border with central scaling. There may be a relative sparing of hair in this variant.[70]

Atypical tinea barbae may also be seen, especially if the course of the disease is altered by glucocorticoid or other therapy.[62]

Pathology Histopathologic findings are similar to those seen in tinea capitis. Fungi are seen in the hair keratin and sometimes in the stratum corneum by using special stains. No organisms are seen in the surrounding dermis. Neutrophils may be seen within the hair follicle, but a chronic, sometimes granulomatous inflammatory response is noted perifollicularly. In extremely inflammatory lesions, fungi may be sparse or absent.[48]

Diagnosis Tinea barbae should be differentiated from a bacterial folliculitis (sycosis vulgaris), perioral dermatitis, candidal infection, acneform dermatitis, pseudofolliculitis barbae, contact der-

FIGURE 206-9

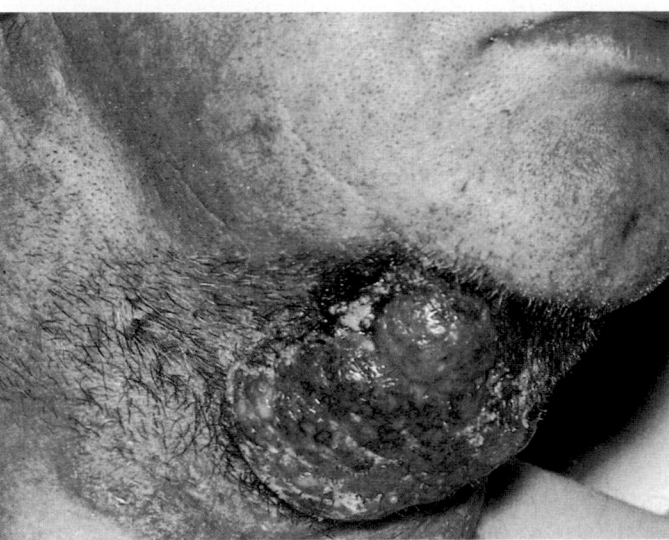

A.

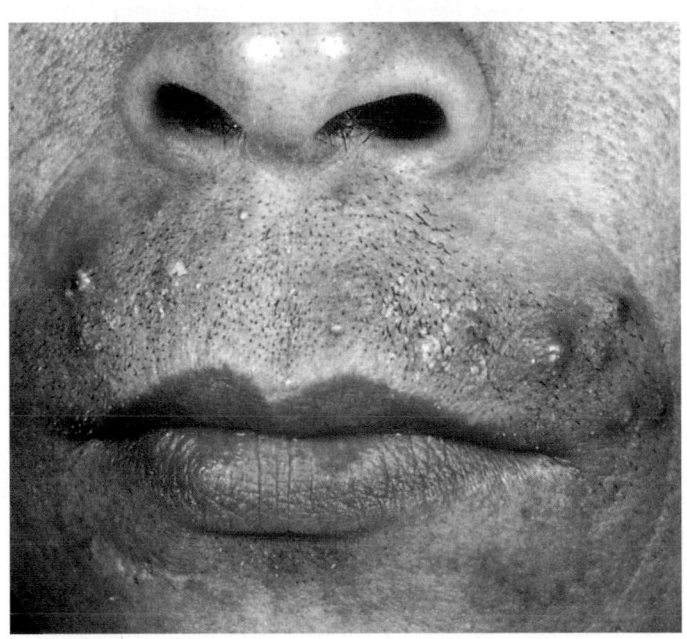

B.

A. Tinea barbae, kerion. Sharply demarcated red nodule (4.0 × 6.0 cm). The surface is moist and studded with multiple yellowish pustules. Regional lymph nodes are not enlarged. B. Tinea barbae. Scattered, discrete, follicular pustules.

matitis, halogenoderma, and herpes simplex. A bacterial folliculitis is usually bilateral and may involve the upper lip. There can be more pain or fever in this instance than in tinea barbae.[67] The other entities mentioned can be differentiated by an accurate history and the use of such diagnostic procedures as patch testing, Tzanck smears, or viral cultures.

Treatment As with tinea capitis, griseofulvin in a dose of 1 g per day (microsized) is used. Therapy is continued for 2 to 3 weeks after clinical resolution has occurred. Local measures such as topical antifungals, wet compresses, and debridement of crusted debris are additive. Occasionally, in severely inflammatory infections, a course of systemic glucocorticoid therapy is helpful. Data are not available on newer antifungal agents.

If no treatment is given, most inflammatory infections resolve spontaneously in a few weeks. Less inflammatory, superficial infections may, in contrast, persist for months.[9,70]

TINEA CORPORIS (TINEA CIRCINATA) Tinea corporis arbitrarily includes all dermatophyte infections of glabrous skin with the exclusion of certain specific locations (i.e., palms, soles, and groin).

Etiology All species of dermatophyte belonging to the genera *Trichophyton, Microsporum,* or *Epidermophyton* are capable of producing tinea corporis. The three most common causative organisms are *T. rubrum, M. canis,* and *T. mentagrophytes;* variations may occur based on the existence of endemic species in specific geographic areas.[6]

Epidemiology The organism responsible for tinea corporis may be transmitted by direct contact with other infected individuals or by infected animals. It may also be transmitted from inanimate fomites such as clothing and furniture. Under appropriate environmental conditions (warmth, humidity), a reservoir of infection on the feet or elsewhere may be the source of tinea corporis.[68] A tropical or subtropical climate is associated with more frequent and severe tinea corporis.[67]

Children appear to have an increased incidence of tinea corporis caused by zoophilic organisms. *M. canis* is transmitted by contact with pets (especially cats and dogs).

Tinea imbricata, caused by *T. concentricum,* is geographically limited to certain areas of the Far East, South Pacific, and South and Central America. Here a large proportion of the native population may be affected, but nonnatives may be spared even though they have resided in endemic areas for long periods. Like favus, tinea imbricata is probably contracted in early childhood and can persist for a lifetime.[71] There is some evidence that the susceptibility to tinea imbricata is hereditarily determined through an autosomal recessive trait.[72]

Pathogenesis The organisms responsible for tinea corporis generally reside in the stratum corneum (Fig. 206-10). Presumably, SIF is responsible for limiting the infection.[17] The pathogenic sequence of events has been outlined previously. The first step involves invasion of the stratum corneum, possibly with the help of warm, moist, occlusive conditions.[17] After a 1- to 3-week incubation period, centrifugal spread occurs. The active, advancing border of infection has an increased epidermal turnover rate.[18] Presumably, the host epidermis is attempting to shed the organism by increasing epidermal turnover to exceed the fungal growth rate. This defense mechanism is successful to a certain extent as there is relative clearing of infection in the center of the annular cutaneous lesion. Temporary resistance to reinfection occurs in this area for a variable time; however, second waves of infection are commonly seen later.[9,17]

Most organisms causing tinea corporis are located superficially in the stratum corneum. Hair follicle involvement can occur—especially with *T. rubrum* or *T. verrucosum*[48]—and seems to be associated with increased inflammation.[70]

Clinical manifestations Tinea corporis may be diverse in its clinical presentation.[70] Table 206-6 summarizes the clinical variants that can be seen, along with distinguishing features of each. The most common presentation is the typical annular lesion with an active, erythematous, and sometimes vesicular border (Fig. 206-11).

FIGURE 206-10

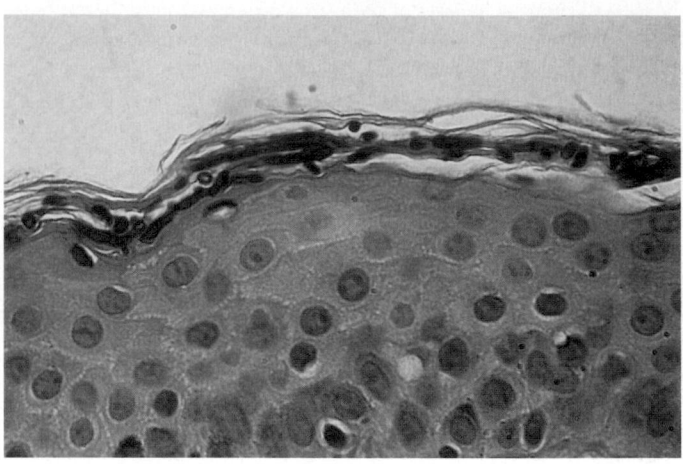

PAS stain of dermatophyte in stratum corneum. (*Courtesy of Sonia Toussaint, MD.*)

Commonly, the center of the lesion shows clearing, but variations may occur. The center often shows concentric rings in tinea imbricata and *T. rubrum* infections. With *T. rubrum* infections, large, confluent plaques of infection may occur. Polycyclic or psoriasiform lesions are also seen frequently (Fig. 206-12). It is clear that a high index of suspicion should exist for tinea corporis. Any red, scaly rash deserves at least a thorough microscopic examination to exclude this entity.

Laboratory findings Specimens for KOH examination should be obtained from the actively spreading border of the lesion, where

FIGURE 206-11

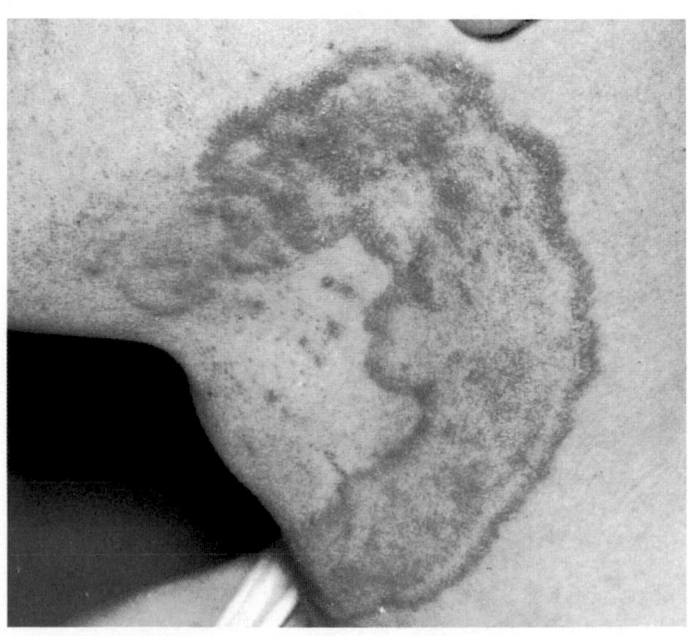

Tinea corporis with typical "ringworm-like" configuration.

TABLE 206-6

Variants of Tinea Corporis

NAME	CAUSATIVE ORGANISM(S)	CLINICAL DESCRIPTION
NONINFLAMMATORY		
Tinea circinata	Any dermatophyte (commonly *T. rubrum*, *T. mentagrophytes*, *M. canis*)	Annular lesions with central clearing and an active, spreading border
Bullous tinea corporis	Usually *T. rubrum*	Spongiotic or subcorneal vesicles/pustules; may be herpetiform
Tinea imbricata	*T. concentricum*	Widespread; multiple concentric, polycyclic scaly lesions with minimal inflammation; there may be an increased immediate hypersensitivity and decreased cell-mediated immunity to trichophytin antigen
INFLAMMATORY		
Kerion of glabrous skin	Zoophilic organisms (e.g., *T. verrucosum* or *T. mentagrophytes*)	Similar to kerion of scalp
Majocchi's granuloma	*T. rubrum, T. violaceum, T. tonsurans, T. mentagrophytes*	Perifollicular, granulomatous nodules mostly on the scalps of children; often painless without pustulation, and associated with underlying disease
Nodular granulomatous perifolliculitis of the legs	*T. rubrum*	Variant of Majocchi's disease. Lesions on the lower two-thirds of women's legs; unilateral; *T. rubrum* is present elsewhere (nails, feet)
Agminate folliculitis	Zoophilic organism	Well-defined, erythematous plaques studed with perifollicular pustules
Subcutaneous abscess (tinea profunda)	*T. mentagrophytes, T. violaceum, T. crateriforme (tonsurans), T. rubrum, M. audouinii*	Deep subcutaneous nodules are present; there is rarely lymph node involvement and associated hematogenous spread
Mycetoma	*M. audouinii, T. verrucosum, T. mentagrophytes, T. violaceum,T. tonsurans, M. ferrugineum, M. canis*	Subcutaneous masses
Tinea faciale	Usually *Trichophyton* species; occasionally *M. canis*	Represents 3 to 4% of tinea corporis; erythematous, scaly plaques with or without active borders are present; telangiectasia, atrophy, and photoexacerbation may mimic lupus erythematosus
Tinea incognito	Any dermatophyte infection modified by glucocorticoid treatment	Atypical appearing lesions; inflammation, scaling, and symptoms may be absent, or kerion-like lesions may occur; dermal nodules present
	M. audouinii	Depressed cell-mediated immunity and a deficient plasma factor needed for lymphocytic blastogenesis

organisms are more numerous and the chances of a positive examination are higher. There are septate, branching hyphae in the stratum corneum (see Fig. 206-4). If bullous lesions are present, the greatest numbers of organisms are found in the roof of the blister. Finally, if dermal granulomatous lesions occur, the greatest positivity on culture is obtained by using biopsy material as the inoculum.

In some reports, the KOH examination is positive in only one-third of patients with tinea corporis.[73] Therefore, fungal culture is imperative for diagnosis. Infected material should be inoculated on Sabouraud's dextrose agar with antibiotics, even when direct KOH examination is negative. Four weeks of incubation at room temperature is required before the culture plates are discarded.

Pathology Histopathologically, fungal organisms can be seen in the stratum corneum in the usual case of tinea circinata. With hematoxylin and eosin, they appear basophilic; with PAS, the fungal elements stain red; with silver methenamine, they stain black.[48]

If organisms are not found, the histopathology is nonspecific and may resemble an acute or chronic dermatitis. If vesiculation is present, it is often seen histologically as a spongiotic vesicle. In the nodular perifolliculitis variant caused by *T. rubrum*, there is a perifollicular granulomatous reaction, often associated with central necrosis and suppuration. Organisms are seen in the hairs as well as in the dermis. Here, spores may be large (6 μm) and located within multinucleated giant cells.[48]

FIGURE 206-12

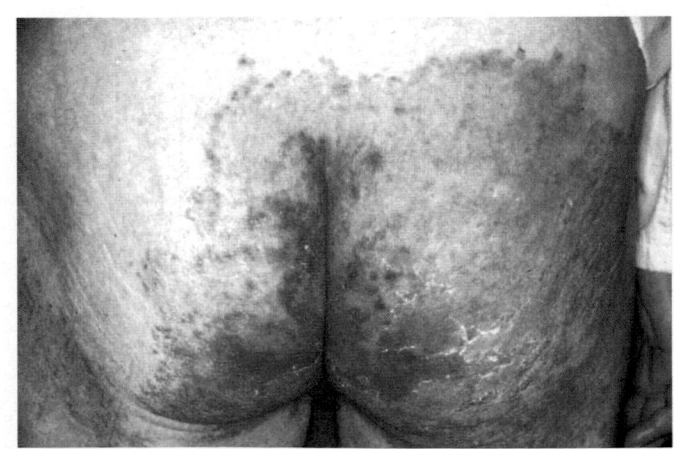

Polycyclic pattern of tinea corporis.

Diagnosis The differential diagnosis of tinea corporis is variable because the clinical findings are variable. In the usual annular ringworm infection, entities such as erythema annulare centrifugum, nummular eczema, and granuloma annulare should be considered. Erythema annulare centrifugum generally shows scaling at the trailing edge of the advancing border, whereas tinea corporis shows scaling over the entire advancing edge. In nummular eczema, lesions show eczematous change or crusting throughout the entire lesion; no central clearing is seen. Furthermore, lesions tend to be more numerous and symmetric than in tinea corporis. In granuloma annulare, intradermal papules without significant epidermal change make up the border of the lesions.

If the clinical lesion is more papulosquamous in appearance, other typically papulosquamous entities can be considered (i.e., psoriasis, lichen planus, secondary syphilis, seborrheic dermatitis, pityriasis rosea, or pityriasis rubra pilaris). Most of the above conditions are readily distinguished by their characteristic clinical features as well as by biopsy.

For the inflammatory variants of tinea corporis, bacterial, candidal, or deep fungal infections enter the differential diagnosis. Verrucous and granulomatous lesions may mimic acid-fast infections or North American blastomycosis. Deeper lesions may resemble bacterial abscesses, panniculitis, or nodular vasculitis.

Tinea faciei may resemble lupus erythematosus or dermatomyositis. The history of photoexacerbation in tinea faciale as well as the absence of a distinct raised scaly border are misleading.[74] Most tinea faciei lesions lack follicular plugging and the true poikiloderma of connective tissue diseases. Other entities to be considered include photodermatoses such as polymorphous light eruption, contact dermatitis, or acne rosacea.

Treatment For isolated lesions of tinea corporis, topical agents such as the allylamines, benzylamine drugs, imidazoles, ketoconazole, and miconazole can be used. For widespread or more inflammatory lesions, griseofulvin is used in a dose equivalent to 1 g/day of the micronized drug. For serious infections not responding to griseofulvin, ketoconazole may be helpful. A recent study showed that a single 400-mg dose of ketoconazole is as effective as 200 mg daily for 10 days, even in tropical environments where there is a higher incidence of tinea corporis. The cost effectiveness and safety profile of this regimen makes it a very attractive alternative.[75]

TINEA CRURIS Tinea cruris is a dermatophytosis involving the groin area and includes infections of the genitalia, pubic area, and perineal and perianal skin.[3]

The transmission of tinea cruris may occur by several mechanisms, e.g., direct contact between infected and noninfected individuals or indirect transmission through contact with nonliving objects that carry infected scales. The causative dermatophytes (especially *E. floccosum*) have been found to survive for long periods on shed squames.[9] These infected scales provide a source for future infections that is difficult to eradicate.

Environmental factors are important in the initiation and propagation of tinea cruris. It is well known that these infections occur more commonly in the summer months or in tropical climates where ambient warmth and humidity are highest. If occlusion from clothing or wet bathing apparel is added, an optimal environment for the initiation or recrudescence of this infection exists.[9]

A final important epidemiologic consideration is the role played by dermatophytoses elsewhere on the body in providing a reservoir for autoinfection in tinea cruris. Other sites of infection may coexist with tinea cruris. The most common associations are the tinea pedis and cruris caused by *T. rubrum*.[43]

Etiology The most common organisms causing tinea cruris are *E. floccosum*, *T. rubrum*, and *T. mentagrophytes*. Differences in the number of infections caused by each organism exist and depend on the prevalence of that organism in the population being surveyed. The groin is by far the most common site for infections caused by *E. floccosum*. The epidemics of tinea cruris reported in some series are caused predominantly by this dermatophyte.[76,77]

Clinical manifestations Pruritus is a common symptom; pain may be present if the involved area is macerated or secondarily infected.

The clinical lesion is characterized by multiple, erythematous papulovesicles with a well-marginated, raised border. The scrotum usually appear completely normal,[43] whereas *Candida* often presents with obvious clinical disease on the scrotum or penis.

The two most common organisms causing tinea cruris may have differences in the clinical lesions they produce. *E. floccosum* typically presents as described above with an active, spreading papulovesicular border and central clearing. The lesions seldom extend beyond the genitocrural crease and medial upper thigh. *T. rubrum* lesions, however, often coalesce and spread to involve wider areas of adjacent skin in the pubic, lower abdominal, buttock, and perianal areas (Fig. 206-13).[9]

Secondary changes may complicate the clinical picture of tinea cruris. Chronic scratching may cause lichenification and present a lichen simplex chronicus–like picture. Secondary bacterial infection may obscure a more chronic tinea cruris. Weeping, maceration, and areas of pustulation may exist. Finally, a secondary allergic or irritant contact dermatitis may be present if sensitizing or irritating topical products have been used in treatment.

Laboratory findings As noted previously, infected scales examined by a 10% to 15% KOH preparation show septate hyphae coursing through infected squames. Cultures inoculated onto Sabouraud's media with antibiotics and incubated at room temperature will grow the responsible organism within 2 weeks.

Pathology The histologic findings are identical to those described with tinea corporis.

FIGURE 206-13

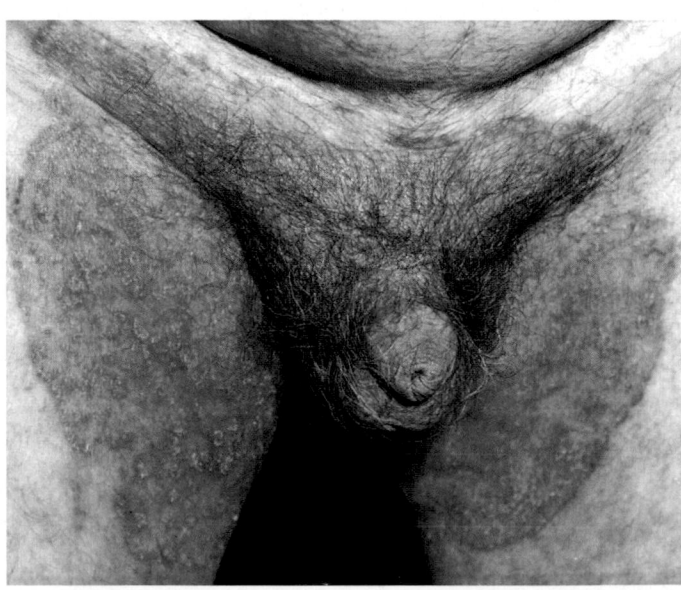

Tinea cruris. Scaling erythematous plaque with sharp margins.

FIGURE 206-14

CHAPTER 206
Superficial Fungal Infection

2349

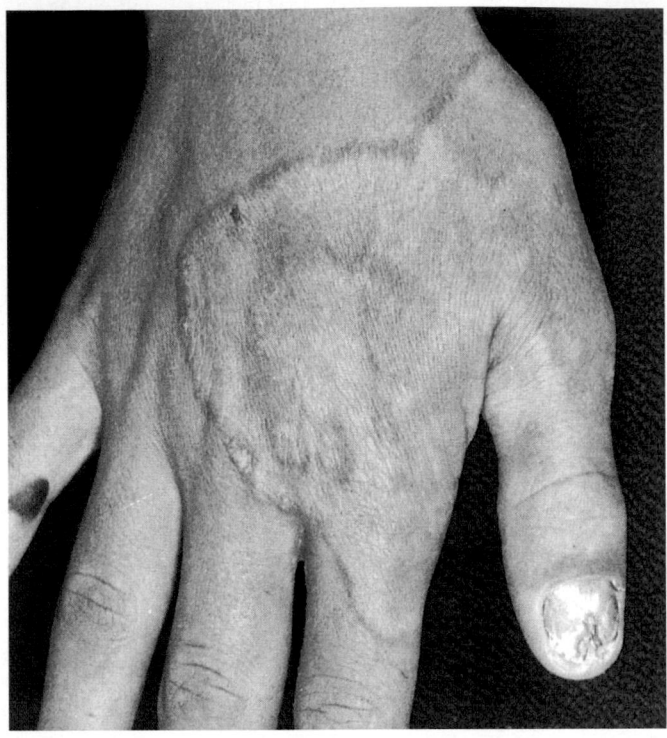

Tinea manus. Polycyclic pattern of an eruption composed of scaling vesicles with involvement of the thumb nail; the nail exhibits destruction of the nail plate.

FIGURE 206-15

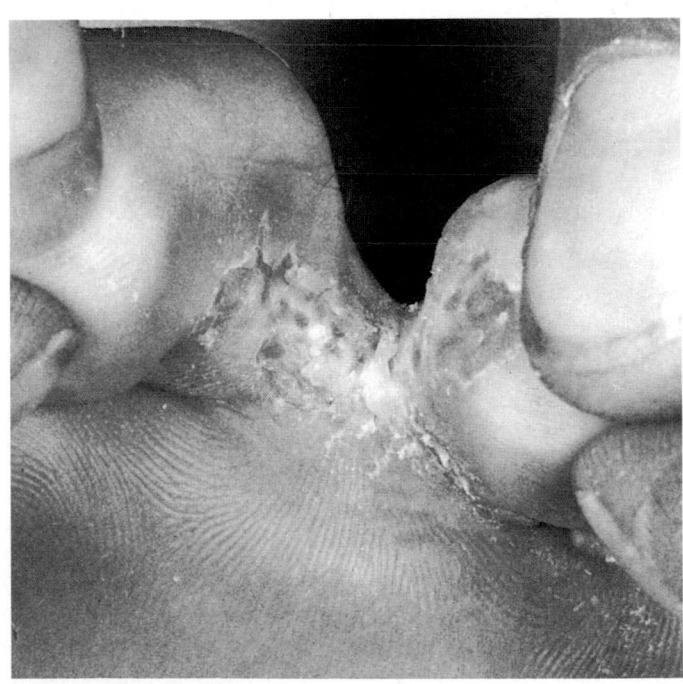

Tinea pedis, interdigital. The area is macerated and has opaque white scales and some erosions.

Diagnosis   The diagnosis is made by the presence of a typical clinical picture associated with positive microscopy or culture. Other dermatoses presenting a similar clinical picture in the crural area are psoriasis, seborrheic dermatitis, candidiasis, erythrasma, lichen simplex chronicus, or even Darier's disease and benign familial chronic pemphigus (Hailey-Hailey).

Candidiasis is distinguished by a greater incidence of obvious scrotal involvement and by the presence of satellite pustules peripheral to brightly erythematous plaques. Erythrasma can be distinguished by examining the suspected lesion under the Wood's lamp. The involved skin in erythrasma shows a coral red fluorescence; lesions of tinea cruris do not. Biopsy may be necessary to totally exclude some of the other diagnoses mentioned.

Treatment   Efforts to decrease occlusion and moisture in the involved area are helpful.[78] In most cases, tinea cruris can be managed by local topical measures. A variety of agents have been used including haloprogin, tolnaftate, and the topical imidazoles (miconazole, clotrimazole, or econazole). A powder or minimally occlusive cream base for these products is recommended.

For more widespread or inflammatory infections, treatment with griseofulvin (500 to 1000 mg/day of the micronized preparation) is indicated. Adequate data on newer antifungal agents are not available.

TINEA PEDIS AND TINEA MANUUM   Tinea pedis is a dermatophyte infection of the feet. Tinea manuum is a dermatophyte infection of the palmar and interdigital areas of the hand.

Epidemiology   Both tinea pedis and tinea manuum are common worldwide; in fact, they represent the most common forms of dermatophyte infections. Approximately 10 percent of the total population can be expected to have a dermatophyte foot infection at any given time. If only closed communities of individuals (athletic teams, military organizations, boarding schools) are considered, the rate of infection is much higher.

The infection is common during the summer months and in tropical or semitropical climates. The incidence of tinea pedis is higher in any population that wears occlusive shoes and in individuals using communal baths or pools. Tinea pedis is an exogenously transmitted infection in which cross infection among susceptible individuals readily occurs.[70]

Etiology   Tinea pedis is caused most commonly by *T. rubrum*, *T. mentagrophytes*, or *E. floccosum*.

T. rubrum commonly produces a dry, hyperkeratotic, mocassin-like involvement of the feet and/or hands (Fig. 206-14); *T. mentagrophytes* often produces a vesicular pattern; and *E. floccosum* may produce either of the two patterns described above. Toenail involvement, however, is less common with *E. floccosum*.

Clinical manifestations   Tinea pedis may present as one of four clinically accepted variants or as an overlap of one or more of these types. The chronic, intertriginous type is the most common and is characterized by fissuring, scaling, and maceration in the interdigital or subdigital areas (Fig. 206-15). The lateral (i.e., 4th to 5th or 3rd to 4th) toe webs are the most common sites of infection. From here infection may spread to the sole or instep of the foot but seldom involves the dorsum. Hyperhidrosis may be an underlying problem for a number of these patients and should be treated along with the dermatophytosis.

The disease we know as "athlete's foot" is not caused solely by dermatophytes. Normal-appearing toe webs have a skin flora consisting of Micrococcaceae (usually *Staphylococcus*), aerobic cory-

FIGURE 206-16

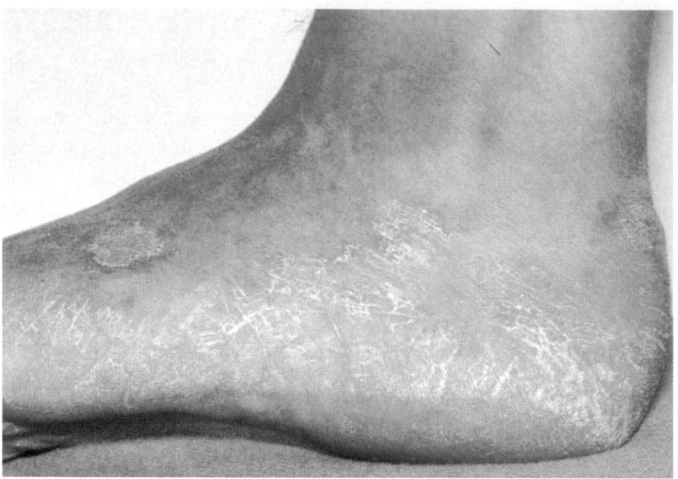

Tinea pedis. Superficial white scales in a moccasin-type distribution. Note arciform pattern of the scales, which is characteristic.

neforms, and small numbers of gram-negative organisms. Dermatophytes can also colonize normal toe webs frequently.[79]

The clinical picture of symptomatic athlete's foot results from the interaction of bacteria and dermatophytes. Overgrowth of bacteria alone or the presence of dermatophytes alone produces a relatively mild clinical picture that is short-lived and relatively asymptomatic.[79]

Another variant of tinea pedis is the chronic, papulosquamous pattern (Fig. 206-16). This is usually bilateral and is characterized by minimal inflammation and a patchy or diffuse mocassin-like scaling over the soles. *T. rubrum* and occasionally *T. mentagrophytes* are the usual causative organisms. In addition to the feet, the hands may be involved as well as multiple toenails. A common but puzzling presentation is the "one hand, two feet" presentation observed frequently with *T. rubrum* infections (Fig. 206-17).

FIGURE 206-17

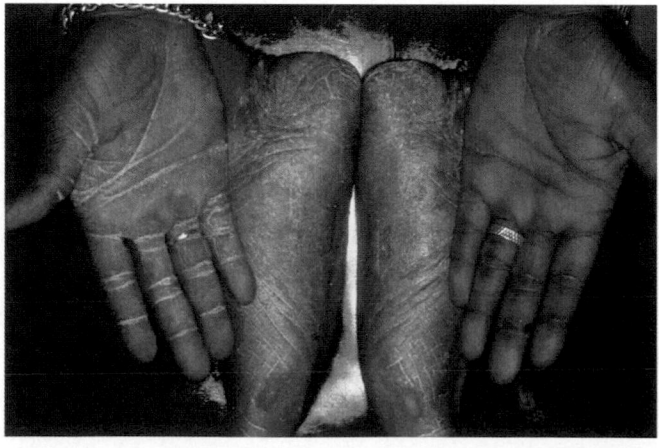

"One hand, two feet" presentation of *T. rubrum.*

The third variant is the vesicular or vesiculobullous type. This is usually caused by *T. mentagrophytes* var. *interdigitale.* Small vesicles or vesicopustules are seen near the instep and on the mid-anterior plantar surface. Usually there is associated scaling in these areas as well as in the toe webs. Larger bullae are more unusual but can be seen. This type of infection may become clinically quiescent during the cooler months of the year only to become symptomatic again in the summer.

The fourth pattern is the acute ulcerative variant commonly associated with maceration, weeping denudation, and ulceration of sizable areas of the sole of the foot. Obvious white hyperkeratosis and a pungent odor are characteristically present. This infection is often complicated by a secondary bacterial (often gram-negative) overgrowth.

The final two variants are commonly seen in conjunction with a vesicular id reaction, either as a dyshidrotic-like distribution on the hands or on the lateral foot or toe area. Cultures of these blisters are by definition sterile.

Laboratory findings KOH examination of scales is positive for septate, branching hyphae in tinea pedis. If vesiculobullous lesions are present, examination of a portion of the blister roof yields the highest rate of positivity. Cultures should be done using Sabouraud's media with cycloheximide and chloramphenicol added.

Pathology Histologic examination reveals different patterns depending on the clinical variant involved. The hyperkeratotic, scaling variety shows acanthosis, hyperkeratosis, and a sparse, chronic superficial perivascular infiltrate in the dermis. On occasion, foci of neutrophils may be seen in the stratum corneum. In the vesicular variant, there is spongiosis, parakeratosis, and subcorneal or spongiotic intraepithelial blisters. Neutrophils are likewise seen in the stratum corneum. In both histologic patterns, special stains (PAS or methenamine silver) show organisms in the horny layer.

Diagnosis With a compatible clinical picture and a positive KOH preparation and/or culture, the diagnosis of tinea pedis can be made comfortably. If these findings are negative, however, there is a sizable differential diagnosis. Interdigital scaling, fissuring, and maceration can be seen with bacterial secondary infection. The more severe the signs and symptoms, the greater is the probability of isolating gram-negative organisms (*Pseudomonas* or *Proteus* spp. in particular). Even if dermatophytes are present, they are more difficult to isolate under these circumstances.[80,81] Other disorders to consider in evaluating an interdigital dermatosis are candidiasis, erythrasma (commonly has a coral red fluorescence with Wood's lamp examination), or soft corns.

In the scaly, hyperkeratotic variety of tinea pedis, confusion can occur with diseases such as psoriasis, hereditary or acquired keratodermas of the palms and soles, pityriasis rubra pilaris, and Reiter's syndrome. In contact dermatitis from shoes, lesions are seen on the dorsum of the foot more commonly than with tinea pedis. In children, peridigital dermatitis or atopic dermatitis is more common than tinea pedis. In the vesicular or vesiculopustular presentation, tinea pedis can be confused with pustular psoriasis, pustulosis palmaris et plantaris, and bacterial pyodermas. In many cases, careful examination of the nails can reveal convincing signs of dermatophytosis that are not seen with many of the above diagnoses.

Prevention and treatment Tinea pedis can be transmitted by contact with infected scales on bath or pool floors as well as on clothing. Laundering of clothing is not always effective in removing infectious material, and it is impossible to prevent most infected individuals from using communal baths or swimming facilities. Control of concomitant hyperhidrosis is important in preventing tinea pedis. Talcum powder or antifungal powders (undecylenic acid or tolnaftate powders) can be used along with absorbent socks and nonocclusive shoes. On occasion, the use of 20% to 25% aluminum chloride hexahydrate topically will help to curb excessive moisture.[70]

Tinea pedis treatment is selected according to the clinical presentation and disease severity.[80] In overt tinea pedis the recently developed oral antifungals are replacing griseofulvin. Their greater affinity for the keratinized areas of the skin, their fungicidal mechanism of action, and their safety profile are expanding the treatment options for clinicians.

There are reports showing an 88.6 percent mycologic cure rate for terbinafine in overt tinea pedis as compared to 50 percent for itraconazole.[82] The newer topical preparations, i.e., terbinafine and butenafine, can be used with or without oral therapy depending on the disease severity.[83–85]

When there is maceration, erythema, or denudation of skin associated with pain, a secondary bacterial infection must be ruled out with cultures and Gram stains. Appropriate systemic antibiotics based on sensitivity studies should be started if bacterial infection is documented. Gram-negative organisms as well as *Staphylococcus aureus* are common pathogens in this area. Adjunctive topical measures such as using antibacterial soaks (e.g., 1/4% acetic acid for *Pseudomonas* overgrowth) are helpful. Colorless Castellani's paint (phenolated resorcinol) is also used frequently.

TINEA UNGUIUM AND ONYCHOMYCOSIS   Tinea unguium is clinically defined as a dermatophyte infection of the nail plate. Onychomycosis, on the other hand, includes all infection of the nail caused by any fungus, including nondermatophytes and yeasts.

Epidemiology   Onychomycosis is a common infection and accounts for 20 percent of all nail disease.[9] Approximately 30 percent of patients with dermatophyte infections on other parts of their body also have tinea unguium. Fungal nail infections are almost exclusively an adult malady. Mold infections usually affect the elderly where underlying nail diseases allow room for these secondary invaders.[67,79]

Although the overall susceptibility to dermatophyte nail infections is higher in men than in women, the number of cases affecting the toenails is increased in women. Paronychial infections caused by *Candida* spp. are also much more commonly seen in the fingernails of women.

The epidemiologic considerations discussed in the section on tinea pedis apply also to tinea unguium. Yet, because fungal nail infections are more chronic and recalcitrant to therapy, these infections provide an endogenous source for reinfection of the feet. This is especially true if a nidus of infection is combined with the environmental conditions of warmth and humidity provided by the climate or by occlusive footwear.[86–88]

Etiology and pathogenesis   Onychomycosis can be caused not only by dermatophytes but also by certain yeasts and nondermatophytic molds.[86] The most common dermatophytes causing tinea unguium worldwide are *T. rubrum, T. mentagrophytes* var. *interdigitale,* and *E. floccosum.* Table 206-7 groups the causative dermatophytes according to other anatomic areas that are often concurrently affected.[86]

Many nondermatophytic fungi have been associated with nail infections (Fig. 206-18).[86] Among the yeasts, *Candida albicans* is found to invade the nail only in chronic mucocutaneous candidiasis. Other species of *Candida* such as *C. parapsilosis* have been isolated from toenails.[86,87] The nondermatophytic molds have also been cultured often from nails clinically thought to be onychomycotic. Strict criteria are necessary, however, to implicate these organisms as primary pathogens as they are often considered to be contaminants when routine cultures are examined.[89,90] English has outlined these criteria as follows[91]: (1) if a dermatophyte is isolated on culture, it is considered to be a pathogen; (2) if a mold or yeast is cultured,

TABLE 206-7

Causative Organisms According to Anatomic Site of Infection

Tinea unguium + tinea pedis and/or tinea manuum
  T. rubrum
  T. mentagrophytes var. *interdigitale*
  E. floccosum
Tinea unguium + tinea corporis + tinea pedis
  T. rubrum
  T. mentagrophytes var. *interdigitale*
  E. floccosum
Tinea unguium + tinea capitis or favus
  T. tonsurans
  T. violaceum
  T. megninii
  T. schoenleinii
Tinea unguium + tinea imbricata
  T. concentricum

it is considered significant only if hyphae, spores, or yeast cells are seen on microscopic examination; and (3) confirmation of an infection by a nondermatophyte requires isolation of the organism on at least 5 out of 20 inocula without concurrent isolation of a dermatophyte. In general, it appears that nondermatophytic onychomycosis favors antecedently diseased nails or aged nails. Toenails are the usual site of involvement.[70]

Zaias[92–94] has divided onychomycosis into four clinical types: (1) distal subungual onychomycosis (DSO), (2) proximal subungual onychomycosis (PSO), (3) white superficial onychomycosis (WSO), and (4) candidal onychomycosis. Characteristically, infected nails coexist with normal-appearing nails.

DSO is the most common type and starts by invasion of the stratum corneum of the hyponychium and distal nail bed. Subsequently, the infection moves proximally in the nail bed and invades the ventral surface of the nail plate. Subungual hyperkeratosis re-

FIGURE 206-18

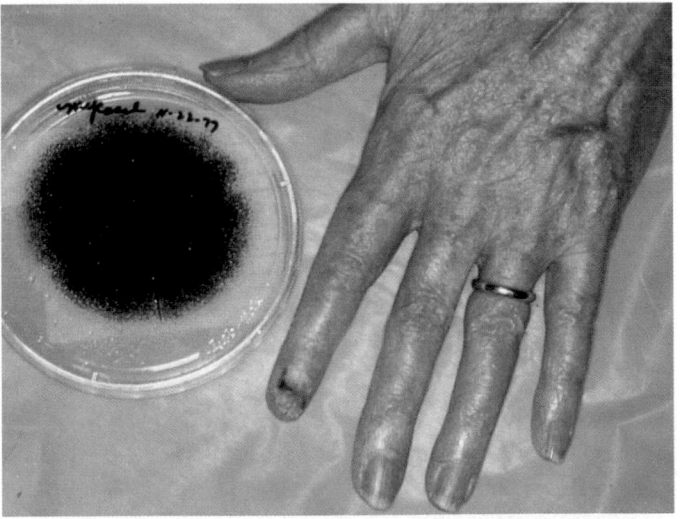

Onychomycosis can be due to nondermatophytic fungi, including *Aspergillus niger.*

TABLE 206-8

Common Causative Organisms for Variants of Onychomycosis

I. Distal subungual onychomycosis (DSO)
  A. Toenails
    1. Dermatophytes: *T. rubrum, T. mentagrophytes, E. floccosum*
    2. Molds: *Scopulariopsis brevicaulis, Aspergillus, Fusarium, Cephalosporium*
    3. Yeasts: *C. albicans, C. parapsilosis, C. tropicalis, Geotrichum candidum, Hendersonula toruloidea*
  B. Fingernails
    1. Dermatophytes: *T. rubrum*
    2. Yeasts and molds: *C. albicans*
II. Proximal subungual onychomycosis (PSO)
  A. Toenails
    1. *T. rubrum, T. megninii, T. schoenleinii, T. tonsurans, T. mentagrophytes*
    2. Molds and yeasts: not documented
  B. Fingernails
    1. Dermatophytes: *T. rubrum, T. megninii*
    2. Molds and yeasts: not documented
III. White superficial onychomycosis (WSO)
  A. Toenails
    1. Dermatophytes: *T. mentagrophytes,* rarely *T. rubrum*
    2. Molds: *Aspergillus, Cephalosporium, Fusarium*
  B. Fingernails: WSO does not occur on fingernails

SOURCE: Modified from Norton[95] and Baron.[96]

sults from a hyperproliferative reaction of the nail bed in response to the infection.[87] As the process continues, invasion of the nail plate results in a progressively dystrophic nail unit.

PSO is the least common variant of onychomycosis. It starts by fungal invasion of the stratum corneum of the proximal nail fold and subsequently the nail plate.

WSO differs from the other variants by primarily invading the dorsal surface of the nail plate. The morphology of the fungus in WSO is typically that of a saprophyte. There are "eroding fronds" or "perforating organs" as seen with in vitro hard keratin invasion.[87,92]

Candidal onychomycosis is seen in patients with chronic mucocutaneous candidiasis. It may affect toenails and fingernails by invasion of the nail plate via the hyponychial epithelium. The entire

thickness of the nail plate is commonly affected.[86,92] The dystrophic nails seen with candidal paronychia do not result from direct fungal invasion and should not be confused with true onychomycosis.

Table 206-8 summarizes the common causative organisms for the different variants of onychomycosis.

Clinical manifestations   The different clinical types of onychomycosis have been described previously. Each type has a rather characteristic clinical picture.

DSO begins as a whitish or brownish-yellow discoloration at the free edge of the nail or near the lateral nail fold. As the infection progresses, subungual hyperkeratosis may lead to a separation of nail plate and nail bed (Fig. 206-19). Fungi invade the nail plate from the ventral surface, and in time the entire nail may become friable and discolored. The subungual debris also provides a site for opportunistic secondary infection by bacteria or other molds and yeasts. A wide spectrum of clinical changes can occur when the infection is advanced.

WSO[87,94] appears as white, sharply outlined areas on the surface of the toenails (Fig. 206-20). The fingernails are not affected. Any area of the nail can be affected initially, and with time much of the nail surface can be involved. The surface of the nail is usually rough and friable as the "eroding fronds" of the organisms remain quite superficial. As discussed previously, *T. mentagrophytes* is the most common organism producing WSO. Recently, *T. rubrum* has been reported as an infrequent cause.[87,97]

The first clinical sign of PSO is a whitish to whitish-brown area on the proximal part of the nail plate (Fig. 206-21). This area may gradually enlarge to affect the entire nail. As in DSO, the organisms invade the ventral surface of the nail plate from the proximal nail fold.

Candida onychomycosis is seen in patients with chronic mucocutaneous candidiasis. Both toenails and fingernails are affected. Clinically, the appearance of these nails resembles DSO with thickening of the nail bed and nail plate, although the entire nail plate is invaded by the organisms. The surface of the nail becomes opaque, rough, and furrowed. It is usually discolored and may be brownish or brownish-yellow in color. Often a surrounding paronychial inflammatory response is present, and the digit tip may become bulbous.

Laboratory findings   Attempts to document fungal infections of the nail involve the use of KOH preparations and fungal cultures. Unfortunately, microscopy is often negative in nails that appear to be infected clinically. Furthermore, nails that are positive by microscopic examination often yield negative cultures.[86,87] A reason for

FIGURE 206-19

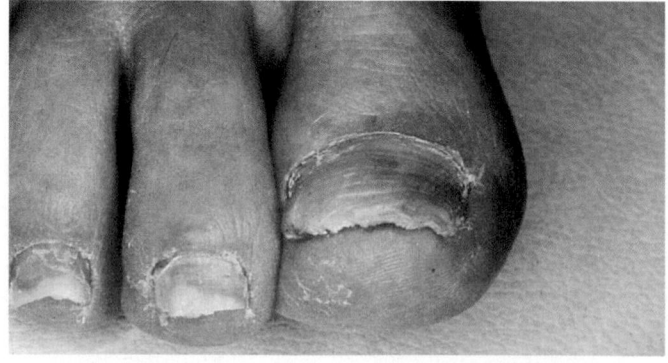

Distal subungual onychomycosis.

FIGURE 206-20

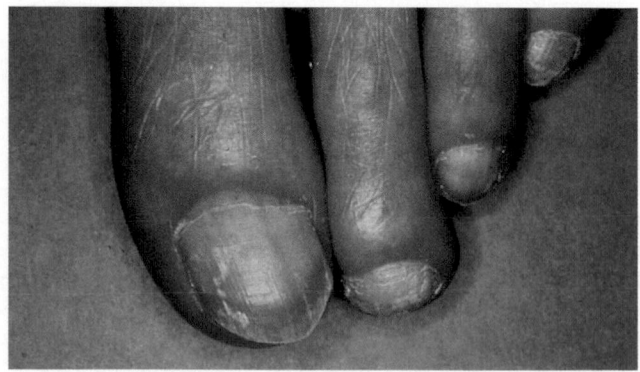

White superficial onychomycosis.

FIGURE 206-21

CHAPTER 206
Superficial Fungal Infection
2353

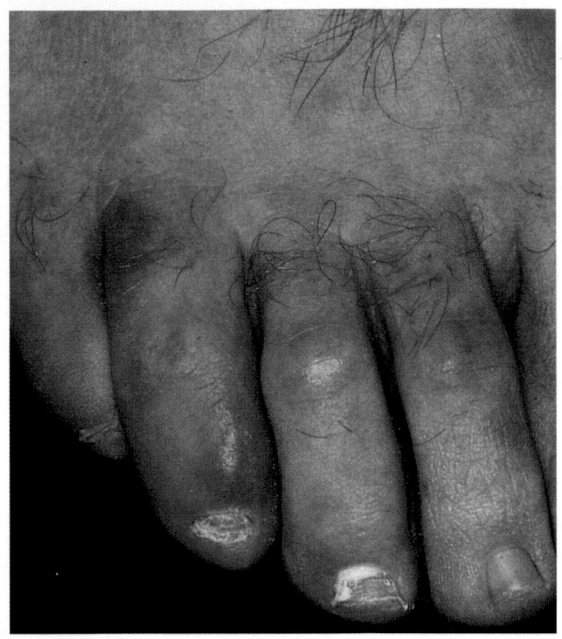

Proximal subungual onychomycosis in a patient with AIDS; Kaposi's sarcoma is also seen on the fourth toe.

this discrepancy is that fungi seen on KOH examination may not be viable and hence do not grow as expected.

Another method of sampling the nail, beyond cutting the distal tip, has been described by Shelley and Wood.[98] Here one selects sites of early, active infection. These appear as whitish areas of discoloration with a normal overlying nail. A razor blade is used to trim away the normal nail and reach the powdery white area of infection. This material is then mounted with xylene and examined microscopically.

Cultures are done on Sabouraud's dextrose agar with and without added chloramphenicol and cycloheximide. Cycloheximide will suppress the growth of nondermatophytic organisms and should not be used if these fungi are suspected.

Pathology Histologically, hyphae are seen lying between the laminae of nail parallel to the surface. The ventral nail and the stratum corneum of the nail bed are preferentially affected.[87] The epidermis may show spongiosis and focal parakeratosis. The inflammatory response in the dermis is minimal.

Diagnosis Onychomycosis can be confused with a variety of nail disorders. The diagnosis is further complicated by the high incidence of false-negative KOH examinations and cultures.

Psoriasis can closely mimic onychomycosis; however, the pitting seen in psoriasis is uncommon in fungal nail infections. The dystrophic nails seen in conjunction with hand eczema are usually transversely ridged, and eczematous changes are apparent in the surrounding skin. Other disorders that can be confused with onychomycosis are the nails of Reiter's syndrome, Darier's disease, lichen planus, exfoliative dermatitis, pachyonychia congenita, and Norwegian scabies. Usually these disorders are separated from onychomycosis by history or evidence of characteristic skin lesions or biopsy findings.

WSO must be distinguished from acquired or congenital leukonychias. Among these leukonychias, those due to trauma are the most common.

Treatment Topical agents are usually of little benefit, and systemic therapy has been less than satisfactory. Prolonged regimens, poor results, and adverse events have affected compliance.[99] The newer antifungals are efficacious and safe and can be administered for shorter periods of time. Several studies have documented the benefits of these agents, particularly itraconazole versus terbinafine (see Chap. 260).[100–103]

Griseofulvin was the standard treatment for onychomycosis until recent years. Poor absorption, side effects, and drug interactions have affected compliance and therefore efficacy. Mycologic cure rates vary between 40 and 80 percent in fingernails and between 3 and 38 percent in toenails.[99,104] A treatment course of 4 to 6 months for fingernails and 10 to 18 months for toenails is required.

Itraconazole has broad-spectrum activity, gets incorporated into the nail, and persists in the nail unchanged for 6 months after discontinuation of therapy.[105] Continuous therapy (200 mg qd for 3 months) and pulse therapy (200 mg twice daily for 1 week per month for 3 consecutive months) are effective, safe treatment modalities. Drug interactions and liver toxicity are the major concerns for clinicians.

Terbinafine is an allylamine fungicidal agent effective against dermatophytes and some molds. Therapeutic levels of drug persist in the nail for 3 to 6 months after therapy is discontinued. Complete cure of toenail onychomycosis has been achieved after 12 weeks of treatment in 82 percent of cases.[99,106] Studies indicate the optimum treatment period is 6 weeks for fingernails and 12 weeks for toenails at a dose of 250 mg daily. Eighty-two percent of toenail infections and 95% of fingernail infections are cured using this regimen.[107]

Some authors have advised chemical removal of nail using 40% urea compounds or surgical avulsion of the nail combined with topical agents and oral griseofulvin.[93] This regimen may increase the cure rate for dermatophyte infections. Avulsion or chemical destruction of the nail in nondermatophytic fungal infections is the only therapy that is effective.[93]

TINEA NIGRA

Tinea nigra is a rare superficial fungal infection of the stratum corneum caused by *Exophiala werneckii*, or, its most recent taxonomic designation, *Phaeoannellomyces wernickii*.[70] Lesions usually appear as brownish-black, velvety macules on the palm.

History

Early reports of tinea nigra were erroneous descriptions of tinea versicolor.[108] The first authentic description was by Cerqueira in 1891. Horta isolated the organism and named it *Cladosporium werneckii*.[109] Subsequently, the name was changed to *Exophiala werneckii* (Horta) v. Arx.[70,110]

Etiology

Although the causative organism is *E. werneckii* in the vast majority of cases, there is some evidence that other species of dematiaceous fungi (*Stenella araguata*) may produce the same clinical picture.[108] The dematiaceous fungi reside in soil, sewage, and decaying vegetation and on wood or shower stalls in very humid environments.[108] Person-to-person transmission has been suspected but occurs only rarely.[111] Inoculation onto the skin of volunteers, however, has resulted in clinical disease; in one case the incubation period may have been 20 years.[112]

The disease is most commonly seen in tropical or subtropical areas (Central and South America, Africa, Asia). About 75 cases have been reported from North America since 1950.[108] Cases from Florida,[113] Texas,[114] and North Carolina[111] are well documented. With increasing awareness of the disease, more North American cases can be expected.

Clinical Manifestations

The clinical lesion appears as a slightly scaly, asymptomatic, mottled brownish- or greenish-black macule on the palm or volar aspect of the fingers (Fig. 206-22). Bilateral plantar involvement as well as concomitant palm and sole involvement have been reported. The lesion gradually spreads centrifugally and may darken, especially at the border. The color resembles a silver nitrate stain.[70,113,115]

Laboratory Findings

Tinea nigra is readily diagnosed by a 10% KOH examination of a scraping from the lesion. On microscopic examination, brownish or olive-colored hyphae and budding cells are seen. The hyphae are septate and freely branching, ranging from 1.5 to 5 μm in diameter.

FIGURE 206-22

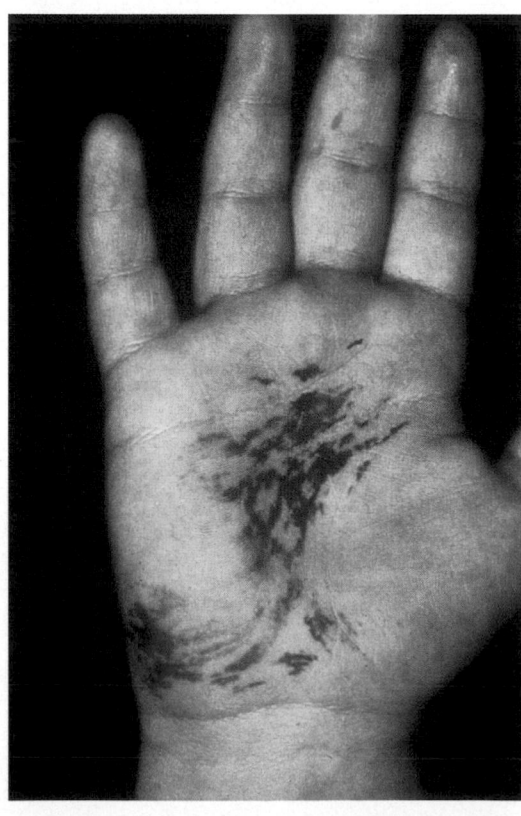

Tinea nigra palmaris showing an irregular, brownish-black macule on the palm. *(Courtesy of Stuart Salasche, MD)*

Oval to spindle-shaped yeast cells, 3 × 10 μm in size, occur singly or paired, separated by a cross wall that is centrally located.

Mycology

The organism can be isolated from clinical specimens on media containing chloramphenicol and cycloheximide on which the growth is initially yeastlike and brownish to shiny black in color. Microscopic examination of these cultures reveals the typical two-celled, yeastlike morphology. As the culture ages, mycelial growth predominates. Aerial hyphae develop on the surface of the pigmented colonies, giving the appearance of a fuzzy, grayish-black growth. Microscopic examination reveals deeply pigmented thick septate hyphal cells, 7 to 10 μm in diameter.

Pathology

Skin biopsy shows hyperkeratosis without dermal inflammation. Hyphae are noted readily by H&E stain but can be stained selectively with a Gomori methenamine silver preparation. Branched, brown hyphae are seen readily in the upper layers of the stratum corneum.

Diagnosis

Tinea nigra may sometimes be confused with melanocytic lesions (i.e., junctional nevi or melanoma). The importance of recognizing this differentiation is underscored by reports of unnecessary surgical removal of lesions in misdiagnosed cases of tinea nigra. Other considerations in the differential diagnosis include pigmentation from Addison's disease, syphilis, or pinta or from a variety of chemicals or dyes. All of these entities are readily excluded by KOH examination.[70]

Treatment and Prognosis

Topical therapy is safe and effective and thus remains the therapeutic route of choice.[116] Cure can be accomplished by the use of keratolytic and antifungal preparations such as Whitfield's ointment, topical 10% thiabendazole, tincture of iodine, or miconazole nitrate.[70,108] Griseofulvin is not effective. Treatment should be continued for 2 to 3 weeks to prevent recurrence.[111]

PIEDRA

Piedra is an asymptomatic fungal infection of the hair shaft caused by *Piedraia hortae* (black piedra) and *Trichosporon beigelii* (white piedra).

History

The disease was reported initially by Beigel in 1865; however, he may have been describing an *Aspergillus* contaminant. The two diseases were distinguished by Horta in 1911.

Etiology

Black piedra is seen commonly in tropical areas of South America, the Far East, and the Pacific Islands. It is seen less frequently in Africa and Asia. In some cultures the infection is encouraged for social or religious reasons.[117] The scalp hair is the most commonly infected area.

CHAPTER 206
Superficial Fungal Infection
2355

White piedra is seen in temperate climates of South America, Europe, Asia, Japan, and the southern United States.[70] Beard, mustache, or pubic hair are more commonly infected than is scalp hair.[70] A recent study in Houston suggests that genital white piedra is more prevalent in Texas than previously suggested and has a variable degree of symptoms and physical findings. Transmission from person to person is felt to be rare, and travel abroad is not the source of infection.[118]

In piedra the source of infection is unknown, but related organisms can be found on animal hair, in soil, or in stagnant water.[117]

Clinical Manifestations

In black piedra, firmly attached, hard, brown-black nodules are present on the hair shaft. They vary in size from microscopic to a few millimeters and are gritty to feel. When the hair is combed, a metallic sound may be heard.[70]

In white piedra, nodules are less firmly adherent and are softer. They may vary in color from light brown to white.

Both forms of piedra may result in weakening of the hair shaft and subsequent breaks. Otherwise, the infections are asymptomatic.

There have been reports of disseminated infections with *T. beigelii* and other *Trichosporon* species.[119-123] These have occurred exclusively as opportunistic infections in an immunosuppressed host. Cutaneous manifestations of dissemination may include erythematous or purpuric papules or papulovesicles. The responsible organism can be cultured from the skin lesions and seen in biopsy material.[119]

Laboratory Findings

When examined microscopically with 10% KOH, black piedra is characterized by nodules largely on the outside of the hair shaft. The periphery of the nodules shows aligned hyphae, whereas the center consists of a packed, well-organized stroma of thick-walled cells (4 to 8 μm in diameter) that house the sexual (ascomycetous) phase of this organism. These are cemented together, and the resultant structure has been termed *pseudoparenchyma* because of its resemblance to organized tissue.[117]

The nodules of white piedra are soft in consistency, commonly intrapilar, and demonstrate less obvious external growth in comparison to black piedra. In contrast to *P. hortae*, *T. beigelii* grows in the asexual phase on infected hairs. The structure shows hyphae that are perpendicular to the hair surface and lack the organized appearance of black piedra.[70,117]

Mycology

P. hortae grows well on most laboratory media, but *T. beigelii* is inhibited by cycloheximide-containing media. Cultures of *P. hortae* grow slowly, have a dark brown to black pigmentation, and initially have a glabrous surface upon which develop aerial mycelia. Microscopic examination reveals septate hyphae, chlamydospores, and irregularly shaped hyphal elements. The asexual phase of this fungus is most frequently cultured from clinical material. The sexual (ascomycetous) phase that occurs on infected hairs can be cultured only under various stringent culture conditions.

Clinical specimens of *T. beigelii* readily grow on Sabouraud's dextrose agar. The yeastlike growth is typically cream colored. As the colony ages, the surface growth develops furrows and convolutions that radiate out from the center. Microscopic examination reveals septate hyphae that readily fragment into arthroconidia, 3 to 7 μm in size. These cells rapidly take on an oval morphology and exhibit budding.

Diagnosis

Microscopic examination readily distinguishes piedra from nits, hair casts, developmental defects of the hair shaft, and trichomycosis axillaris. In the latter case, smaller nodules (<1 μm) are seen, and the hairs may fluoresce under Wood's lamp examination.

Treatment

Shaving the infected hair is curative. Treatment protocols are difficult to assess because of the high frequency of spontaneous remissions. Most authors support shaving the hair alone or shaving the hair in conjunction with oral ketoconazole and/or topical antifungal therapy.[70,118]

REFERENCES

1. Wagner DK, Sohnle PG: Cutaneous defenses against dermatophytes and yeasts. *Clin Microbiol Rev* **8**:317, 1995
2. Rebell G, Taplin D: *Manual of Dermatophytes, Their Recognition and Identification.* Coral Gables, FL, Univ of Miami Press, 1979
3. Weitzman I, Summerbell RC: The dermatophytes. *Clin Microbiol Rev* **8**:240, 1995
4. Greer DL: An overview of common dermatophytes. *J Am Acad Dermatol* **31**:S112, 1994
5. Otcenasek M: Ecology of the dermatophytes. *Mycopathologica* **65**:67, 1978
6. Aly R: Ecology and epidemiology of dermatophyte infections. *J Am Acad Dermatol* **31**:S21, 1994
7. Odom R: Pathophysiology of dermatophyte infections. *J Am Acad Dermatol* **28**:S2, 1993
8. Ajello L: Geographic distribution and prevalence of the dermatophytes. *Ann NY Acad Sci* **89**:30, 1960
9. Rippon JW: Dermatophytosis and dermatomycosis, in *Medical Mycology: The Pathogenic Fungi and the Pathogenic Actinomycetes,* 3d ed. Philadelphia, Saunders, 1988, p 169
10. Knight AG: A review of experimental human fungus infections. *J Invest Dermatol* **59**:354, 1972
11. Allen AM, Taplin D: Epidemic *Trichophyton mentagrophytes* infections in servicemen: Source of infection, role of environment, host factors, and susceptibility. *JAMA* **226**:864, 1973
12. Sanderson PH, Sloper JC: Skin disease in the British army in S.E. Asia III: The relationship between mycotic infections of the body and of the feet. *Br J Dermatol* **65**:362, 1953
13. Taplin D et al: Environmental influences on the microbiology of the skin. *Arch Environ Health* **11**:546, 1965
14. Kligman AM: The pathogenesis of tinea capitis due to *Microsporum audouinii* and *Microsporum canis:* I. Gross observations following the inoculation of humans. *J Invest Dermatol* **18**:231, 1952
15. Kligman AM: Tinea capitis due to *M. audouinii* and *M. Canis:* II. Dynamics of the host-parasite relationship. *Arch Dermatol* **71**:313, 1955
16. Dahl MV: Dermatophytosis and the immune response. *J Am Acad Dermatol* **31**:S34, 1994
17. Dahl MV: Suppression of immunity and inflammation by products produced by dermatophytes. *J Am Acad Dermatol* **28**:S19, 1993
18. Jones HE: Immune response and host resistance of humans to dermatophyte infection. *J Am Acad Dermatol* **28**:S12, 1993
19. Dahl MV: Host defense against dermatophytes. *Adv Dermatol* **2**:305, 1987
20. Emmons CW et al (eds): Dermatophytoses, in *Medical Mycology,* 3d ed. Philadelphia, Lea & Febiger, 1977, p 117

21. Ahmed AR: Immunology of human dermatophyte infections. *Arch Dermatol* **118**:521, 1983

22. King RD et al: Transferrin, iron, and dermatophytes. I. Serum dermatophyte inhibitory component definitely identified as unsaturated transferrin. *J Lab Clin Med* **86**:204, 1975

23. Mosher WA et al: Nutritional requirements of the pathogenic mold: *T. interdigitale. Plant Physiol* **11**:795, 1936

24. Yu RJ et al: Inhibition of keratinases by alpha-2-macroglobulin. *Experientia* **28**:886, 1972

25. Jones HE et al: Acquired immunity to dermatophytes. *Arch Dermatol* **109**:840, 1974

26. Delamater ED, Benham RW: Experimental studies with the dermatophytes. I. Primary disease in laboratory animals. *J Invest Dermatol* **1**:451, 1938

27. Delamater ED, Benham RW: Experimental studies with the dermatophytes. II. Immunity and hypersensitivity in laboratory animals. *J Invest Dermatol* **1**:451, 1938

28. Hunziker N, Brun R: Lack of delayed reaction in presence of cell-mediated immunity in *Trichophyton* hypersensitivity. *Arch Dermatol* **116**:1266, 1980

29. Odom RB: Common superficial fungal infections in immunosuppressed patients. *J Am Acad Dermatol* **31**:S56, 1994

30. Hay RJ: Chronic dermatophyte infections. I. Clinical and mycological features. *Br J Dermatol* **106**:1, 1982

31. Hay RJ, Shennan G: Chronic dermatophyte infections. II. Antibody and cell mediated immune responses. *Br J Dermatol* **106**:191, 1982

32. Jones HE: The atopic-chronic-dermatophytosis syndrome. *Acta Derm Venereol (Stockh)* **92**(suppl):81, 1980

33. Grappel SF et al: Immunology of dermatophytes and dermatophytosis. *Bacteriol Rev* **38**:222, 1974

34. Dahl MV: Host defense: Fungus, in *Clinical Immunodermatology.* Chicago, Year Book, 1988, p 171

35. Martinez-Roig A et al: Erythema nodosum and kerion of the scalp. *Am J Dis Child* **136**:440, 1982

36. Frieden IJ, Howard R: Tinea capitis: Epidemiology, diagnosis, treatment, and control. *J Am Acad Dermatol* **31**:S42, 1994

37. Waisman M: Recurrent, fixed erysipelas-like dermatophytid. *Arch Dermatol* **53**:10, 1946

38. Jillson OF: Allergic confirmation that some cases of erythema annulare centrifugum are dermatophytids. *Arch Dermatol* **70**:355, 1954

39. Weary PE, Guerrant JL: Chronic urticaria in association with dermatophytosis: Response to the administration of griseofulvin. *Arch Dermatol* **95**:400, 1967

40. Smith ML: Tinea capitis. *Pediatr Ann* **25**:101, 1996

41. Howard R, Frieden IJ: Tinea capitis: New perspectives on an old disease. *Semin Dermatol* **14**:2, 1995

42. Vanbreuseghem R: Tinea capitis in the Belgian Congo and Ruanda Urundi. *Trop Geogr Med* **10**:103, 1958

43. Elewski BE: *Topics in Clinical Dermatology: Cutaneous Fungal Infections,* edited by BE Elewski. New York, Igaku-Shoin, 1992

44. Feuerman EJ et al: Kerion-like tinea capitis and barbae caused by *Microsporum gypseum* in Israel. *Mycopathologica* **58**:165, 1976

45. Honig PJ, Smith LR: Tinea capitis masquerading as atopic or seborrheic dermatitis. *J Pediatr* **94**:604, 1979

46. Howell JB et al: Tinea capitis caused by *Trichophyton tonsurans* (sulfureum or crateriforme). *Arch Dermatol* **65**:194, 1952

47. Wolf FT et al: Fluorescent pigment of *Microsporum. Nature* **182**:475, 1958

48. Lever WF, Schaumburg-Lever G: Fungal diseases, in *Histopathology of the Skin,* 7th ed. Philadelphia, Lippincott, 1990, p 364

49. Imamura S et al: Use of immunofluorescence staining in kerion. *Arch Dermatol* **111**:906, 1975

50. Lopez-Gomez S et al: Itraconazole versus griseofulvin in the treatment of tinea capitis: A double-blind randomized study in children. *Int J Dermatol* **33**:743, 1994

51. Legendre R, Esola-Macre J: Itraconazole in the treatment of tinea capitis. *J Am Acad Dermatol* **23**:559, 1990

52. Degreef H: Itraconazole in the treatment of tinea capitis. *Cutis* **58**:90, 1996

53. Nejjam F et al: Pilot study of terbinafine in children suffering from tinea capitis: Evaluation of efficacy, safety and pharmacokinetics. *Br J Dermatol* **132**:98, 1995

54. Haroon TS et al: A randomized double-blind comparative study of terbinafine for 1, 2 and 4 weeks in tinea capitis. *Br J Dermatol* **135**:86, 1996

55. Baudraz-Rosselet F et al: Efficacy of terbinafine treatment of tinea capitis in children varies according to the dermatophyte species. *Br J Dermatol* **135**:1011, 1996

56. Khan KA, Anwar AA: Study of 73 cases of tinea capitis and tinea favosa in adults and adolescents. *J Invest Dermatol* **51**:474, 1968

57. Wilson JW, Plunkett OA: Dermatophytosis, in *The Fungus Diseases of Man.* Berkeley, Univ of California Press, 1965, p 213

58. Hakendorf AJ et al: Favus. *Australas J Dermatol* **8**:22, 1965

59. Guirges SY: Viability of *Trichophyton schoenleinii* in epilated hairs. *Sabouraudia* **19**:155, 1981

60. Malhotra YK et al: A study of tinea capitis in Libya (Benghazi). *Sabouraudia* **17**:181, 1979

61. Rudolph AH et al: Tinea capitis, in *Clinical Dermatology,* edited by DJ Demis et al. Philadelphia, Harper & Row, 1978

62. Rook A, Dawber R: Infections and infestations, in *Diseases of the Hair and Scalp,* 2d ed. Oxford, Blackwell, 1991, p 396

63. Dvoretzky I et al: Favus. *Int J Dermatol* **19**:89, 1980

64. Hopfer RL et al: Antibodies with affinity for epithelial tissue in chronic dermatophytosis. *Dermatologica* **151**:135, 1975

65. Graham JH, Barroso-Tobila C: Dermal pathology of superficial fungus infections, in *Human Infection with Fungi, Actinomycetes, and Algae,* edited by RD Baker et al. New York, Springer, 1971, p 211

66. Sams WM: Favus treated with griseofulvin. *Arch Dermatol* **81**:802, 1960

67. Elewski BE: The dermatophytoses, in *Cutaneous Medicine and Surgery,* edited by KA Arndt et al. Philadelphia, Saunders, 1996, p 1043

68. Pierard GE et al: Treatment and prophylaxis of tinea infections. *Drugs* **52**:209, 1996

69. Loewenthal K: Tinea barbae due to *Microsporum canis. Arch Dermatol* **91**:60, 1965

70. Elgart ML (ed): *Dermatologic Clinics,* vol 14. Philadelphia, Saunders, 1996

71. Hay RJ et al: Immune responses of patients with tinea imbricata. *Br J Dermatol* **108**:581, 1983

72. Ravine D et al: Genetic inheritance of susceptibility to tinea imbricata. *J Med Genet* **17**:342, 1980

73. Emtestam L, Kaaman T: The changing clinical picture of *Microsporum canis* infections in Sweden. *Acta Derm Venereol (Stockh)* **62**:539, 1982

74. Shanon J, Raubitschek F: Tinea faciei simulating chronic discoid lupus erythematosus. *Arch Dermatol* **82**:268, 1960

75. Fernandez-Nava HD et al: Comparison of single dose 400 mg versus 10 day 200 mg daily dose ketoconazole in the treatment of tinea versicolor. *Int J Dermatol* **36**:64, 1997

76. McAleer R: Fungal infection as a cause of skin disease in Western Australia. II. Tinea cruris. *Australas J Dermatol* **21**:33, 1980

77. Blank F, Prichard H: Epidemic ringworm of the groin. *Arch Dermatol* **85**:410, 1962

78. Faegermann TC et al: *Pityrosporum ovale (Malassezia fulfur)* as the causative agent of seborrheic dermatitis: New treatment options. *Br J Dermatol* **134**:12, 1996

79. Leyden JJ: Progression of interdigital infections from simplex to complex. *J Am Acad Dermatol* **28**:S7, 1993

80. Leyden JL: Tinea pedis pathophysiology and treatment. *J Am Acad Dermatol* **31**:S31, 1994

81. Leyden JJ, Kligman AM: Interdigital athlete's foot. *Arch Dermatol* **114**:1466, 1978

82. De Keyser P et al: Two-week oral treatment of tinea pedis, comparing terbinafine (250 mg/day) with itraconazole (100 mg/day): a double-blind, multicentre study. *Br J Dermatol* **130**(suppl 43):22, 1994

83. Evans EGV: A comparison of terbinafine (Lamisil) 1% cream given for one week with clotrimazole (Canesten) 1% cream given for four weeks, in the treatment of tinea pedis. *Br J Dermatol* **130**(suppl 43):12, 1994

84. Tschen E et al: Treatment of interdigital tinea pedis with a 4-week once-daily regimen of butenafine hydrochloride 1% cream. *J Am Acad Dermatol* **36**:S9, 1997

85. Savin R et al: One-week therapy with twice-daily butenafine 1% cream versus vehicle in the treatment of tinea pedis: A multicenter, double-blind trial. *J Am Acad Dermatol* **36**:S15, 1997

86. Midgley G et al: Mycology of nail disorders. *J Am Acad Dermatol* **31**:S68, 1994

87. Scher RK, Daniel CR: *Nails: Therapy, Diagnosis, Surgery,* 2d ed. Philadelphia, Saunders, 1997

88. Clayton YM: Clinical and mycological diagnostic aspects of onychomycoses and dermatomycoses. *Clin Exp Dermatol* **17**(suppl 1):37, 1992

89. Haneke E: Fungal infections of the nail. *Semin Dermatol* **10**:41, 1991

90. Onsberg P: The fungal flora of normal and diseased nails. *Curr Ther Res* **22**:20, 1977

91. English MP: Nails and fungi. *Br J Dermatol* **94**:697, 1976

92. Zaias N: Onychomycosis. *Arch Dermatol* **105**:263, 1972

93. Zaias N: Onychomycosis, in *The Nail: In Health and Disease.* New York, SP Medical & Scientific, 1980, p 91

94. Zaias N: Superficial white onychomycosis. *Sabouraudia* **5**:99, 1966

95. Norton LA: Nail disorders: A review. *J Am Acad Dermatol* **2**:451, 1980

96. Baron R: Onychia and paronychia of mycotic, microbial and parasitic origin, in *The Nail,* edited by M Pierre. New York, Churchill Livingstone, 1981, p 39

97. Reiss F: Leukonychia trichophytica caused by *Trichophyton rubrum.* *Cutis* **20**:223, 1977

98. Shelley WB, Wood MG: The white spot target for microscopic examination of nails for fungi. *J Am Acad Dermatol* **6**:92, 1982

99. Elewski BE, Hay RJ: Update on the management of onychomycosis: Highlights of the third annual international summit on cutaneous antifungal therapy. *Clin Infect Dis* **23**:305, 1996

100. Brautigam M et al: German randomized double-blind multicentre comparison of terbinafine and itraconazole for the treatment of toenail tinea infection. *Br J Dermatol* **134**(suppl 46):18, 1996

101. Havu V et al: A double-blind, randomized study comparing itraconazole pulse therapy with continuous dosing for the treatment of toenail onychomycosis. *Br J Dermatol* **136**:230, 1997

102. De Backer M et al: A 12-week treatment for dermatophyte toe onychomycosis: Terbinafine 250 mg/day vs. itraconazole 200 mg/day—a double-blind comparative trial. *Br J Dermatol* **134**(suppl 46):16, 1996

103. Jones TC: Overview of the use of terbinafine (Lamisil) in children. *Br J Dermatol* **132**:683, 1995

104. Korting HC, Schafer-Korting M: Is tinea unguium still widely incurable? A review three decades after the introduction of griseofulvin. *Arch Dermatol* **128**:243, 1992

105. Gupta AK et al: Current management of onychomycosis. *Derm Clin* **15**:121, 1997

106. Van der Schroeff JG et al: A randomized treatment duration-finding study of terbinafine in onychomycosis. *Br J Dermatol* **126**(suppl 39):36, 1992

107. Roberts DJ: Oral terbinatine in the treatment of fungal infections of the skin and nails. *Dermatology* **194**(suppl 1):37, 1997

108. Rippon JW: Superficial infections: Tinea nigra, in *Medical Mycology: The Pathogenic Fungi and the Pathogenic Actinomycetes,* 3d ed. Philadelphia, Saunders, 1988, p 159

109. Horta P: Sobre un caso de tinha preta e un novo cogumelo *(Cladosporium werneckii). Rev Med Cirug Brazil* **21**:269, 1921

110. McGinnis MR: Taxonomy of *Exophiala werneckii* and its relations to *Microsporum mansonii. Sabouraudia* **17**:145, 1979

111. Van Velsor H, Singletary H: Tinea nigra palmaris: A report of 15 cases from coastal North Carolina. *Arch Dermatol* **90**:59, 1964

112. Blank H: Tinea nigra: A twenty-year incubation period? *J Am Acad Dermatol* **1**:49, 1979

113. Helfman RJ: Tinea nigra palmaris et plantaris. *Cutis* **28**:81, 1981

114. Spiller WF et al: Tinea nigra. *J Invest Dermatol* **27**:187, 1956

115. Isaacs F, Reiss-Levy E: Tinea nigra plantaris: A case report. *Australas J Dermatol* **21**:13, 1980

116. Burke AB: Tinea nigra: Treatment with topical ketoconazole. *Cutis* **52**:209, 1993

117. Rippon JW: Superficial infections: Piedra, in *Medical Mycology: The Pathogenic Fungi and the Pathogenic Actinomycetes,* 3d ed. Philadelphia, Saunders, 1988, p 163

118. Kalter DC et al: Genital white piedra: Epidemiology, microbiology, and therapy. *J Am Acad Dermatol* **14**:982, 1986

119. Manzella JP et al: *Trichosporon beigelii* fungemia and cutaneous dissemination. *Arch Dermatol* **118**:343, 1982

120. Winston DJ et al: Disseminated *Trichosporon capitatum* infection in an immunosuppressed host. *Arch Intern Med* **137**:1192, 1977

121. Rivera R, Cangir A: *Trichosporon* sepsis and leukemia. *Cancer* **36**:1106, 1975

122. Watson KC, Kallinchurum S: Brain abscess due to *Trichosporon cutaneum. J Med Microbiol* **3**:191, 1970

123. Kirmani N et al: Disseminated *Trichosporon* infection: Occurrence in an immunosuppressed patient with chronic active hepatitis. *Arch Intern Med* **140**:277, 1980

CHAPTER 207

Ann G. Martin
George S. Kobayashi

Yeast Infections: Candidiasis, Pityriasis (Tinea) Versicolor

Candidiasis (or candidosis) is an infection with protean clinical manifestations caused by *Candida albicans* or, on occasion, by other yeasts of the genus *Candida.* The infections are usually confined to the skin, nails, mucous membranes, and gastrointestinal tract, but they can be systemic and may infect multiple internal organs.

HISTORIC ASPECTS

Initially classified as a *Sporotrichum* by Gruby, the organism was placed in the genus *Oidium (O. albicans)* by Robin in 1847. Later it was confused with *Monilia candida,* isolated from rotting vegetation. The name *Monilia* was stubbornly defended by Castellani and accounts for the term *moniliasis* being used as a synonym for *candidiasis* even in the relatively modern literature. This term is a misnomer and actually refers to the imperfect stage of certain ascomycetes; it has no relationship to the genus *Candida.*

In 1877, Grawitz described the dimorphic nature of the organism. In 1853, Robin first described systemic candidiasis, whereas cutaneous and chronic mucocutaneous candidiasis were described in 1907 and 1909, respectively. After the genus *Candida* was established in 1923, efforts to speciate yeasts placed in this genus were forged by Martin in 1937. The importance of candidiasis as an opportunistic infection was first appreciated in the postantibiotic era of the 1940s.

Controversy over nomenclature persists, and although *candidiasis* is the accepted term for this infection in the United States, *candidosis* is preferred in Canada, the United Kingdom, France, and Italy.

ETIOLOGY

The genus *Candida* accomodates a heterogeneous collection of yeast species that do not produce ascospores or teliospores. They do not possess morphologic or biochemical characteristics that would classify them in the more homogeneous genera of imperfect yeasts. With the exception of *C. glabrata,* the morphologic feature of this genus is based on the capacity of the yeast to form pseudomycelia (Fig. 207-1). *C. albicans* is the most common cause of superficial and systemic candidiasis, being the causative agent in 85 to 90 percent of yeast infections.[1] Other species classified in this genus can also be responsible for clinical disease under certain cir-

FIGURE 207-1

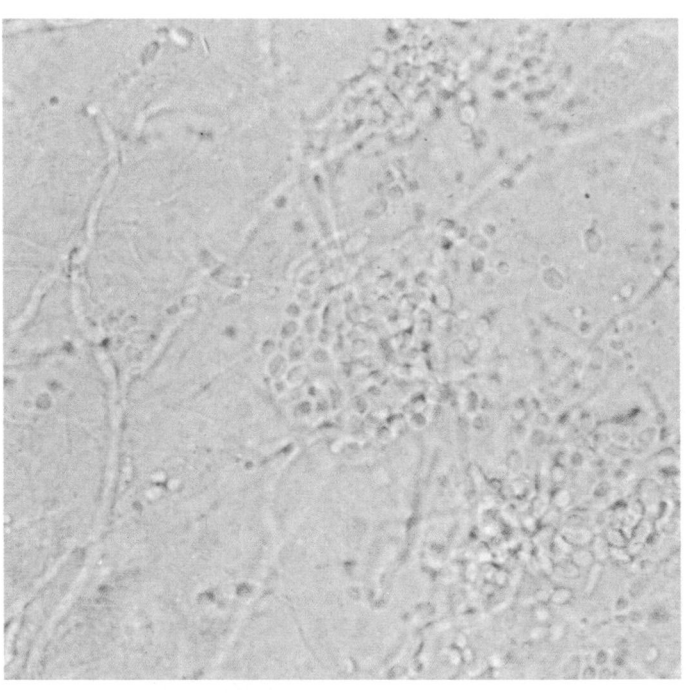

Candida in potassium hydroxide preparation. Pseudomycelia and clusters of grapelike yeast cells.

cumstances (e.g., host immunosuppression, indwelling catheters, intravenous drug delivery). Most of these infections are systemic but can be localized (Table 207-1). The species of *Candida* have been graded by descending degree of pathogenicity as follows: *C. albicans, C. stellatoidea, C. tropicalis, C. parapsilosis, C. kefyr, C. guilliermondii,* and *C. krusei.*

PATHOGENESIS

C. albicans is often found as a saprophyte and colonizes certain mucous membrane surfaces of warm-blooded animals. In 60 percent of normal individuals, colonization of the oropharynx occurs.[2] The organism is rarely isolated from normal human skin except sporadically from certain intertriginous areas. Likewise, the organism is seldom isolated from soil, vegetation, or air samples.

The development of disease due to *Candida* species is dependent on the complex interaction between the innate pathogenicity of the organism and the defense mechanisms of the host. Table 207-2 outlines host factors that predispose to candidal infections.

The intrinsic pathogenicity of *Candida* species as they relate to infections of the skin and mucous membranes are illustrated in an experimental animal model.[3] Using the staphylococcal toxin epidermolysin to cleave the epidermis selectively below the granular layer, Ray et al.[4] demonstrated that only *C. albicans* and *C. stellatoidea* inoculated into this cleft were capable of invading the stratum corneum and eliciting inflammation. Other species were excluded even under occlusive experimental conditions. Maibach and Kligman's experiments in human cutaneous candidiasis also demonstrated differences in virulence among the species of *Candida*.[5]

Other important factors in the initiation of candidal infections include adherence of the organism to epithelial cells and subsequent invasion by elaboration of keratinolytic enzymes, phospholipases, or strain-specific proteolytic enzymes. A clear space is seen around the organisms, suggesting an ongoing process of epithelial tissue lysis. It appears that mycelial growth predominates in invasive disease states, whereas the blastospore growth phase predominates in saprophytic states.[6]

The induction of cutaneous candidiasis in humans under experimental conditions has provided data to elucidate the pathogenic mechanism of the inflammatory response in the disease. Maibach and Kligman[5] noted that the epicutaneous inoculation of *C. albicans* could produce cutaneous disease only if the site of inoculation was occluded. Within 36 to 72 h, typical subcorneal erythematous, pustular lesions developed. The severity of the infection was proportional to the size of the inoculum.[7] Special stains showed organisms in the stratum corneum but not in the pustules. Cutaneous lesions were similarly produced using a sterile extract of disintegrated candidal cells and a sediment of killed ruptured cells. The authors postulated the existence of an endotoxin-like substance that mediated the pustular response.[5] Subsequently, Ray et al.[8] demonstrated that a purified mannan cell-wall polysaccharide from *C. albicans* exhibits endotoxin-like activity in vitro and is capable of activating complement via the alternative pathway, thereby generating products such as C5a, which induce neutrophil chemotaxis. In this way, highly antigenic or toxic products of candidal organisms are able to induce vigorous host response mechanisms that, at the same time, limit infection and produce the typical cutaneous manifestations of the disease. Such a mechanism may explain certain findings in systemic candidiasis. For example, circulating mannan has been demonstrated in systemic invasive candidal infections. By alternative pathway complement activation in this setting, the leukopenia and early neutrophilic tissue response associated with disseminated candidal infections may be partially explained. Furthermore, *Candida* antigen, immunoglobulin, and complement have been found in the nephritic kidney of a patient with *Candida* endocrinopathy syndrome.[9] In contrast, other cell-wall "toxic" products of candidal organisms have been found to interfere with host neutrophil chemotaxis and phagocytosis. Furthermore, cell-wall polysaccharide products may interfere with T lymphocyte–mediated defenses.[6] The

TABLE 207-1

Candidal Isolates Other Than *C. albicans*

CAUSATIVE ORGANISM	CLINICAL DISEASE
C. parapsilosis	Paronychia, endocarditis, otitis externa
C. tropicalis	Vaginitis; intestinal, bronchopulmonary, and systemic infections; onychomycosis; bone and joint disease; central nervous system disease
C. stellatoidea	Vaginitis, systemic disease, bone and joint disease
C. guilliermondii	Endocarditis, cutaneous candidiasis, onychomycosis, bone and joint disease
C. kefyr	Vaginitis, urethritis
C. (Torulopsis) glabrata	Esophagitis, vaginitis, endocarditis
C. krusei	Endocarditis, vaginitis
C. zeylanoides	Onychomycosis
C. viswanathi	Central nervous system disease
C. lusitaniae	Systemic disease

mechanisms of host defense operative during *Candida* infections are complex and still not completely understood. The broad categories include nonimmune and immune factors.

The nonimmune factors include (1) interaction with other members of the microbial flora, (2) the functional integrity of the stratum

TABLE 207-2

Factors Predisposing to Candidal Infections

Mechanical factors
    Trauma (burns, abrasions, etc.)
    Local occlusion, moisture, and/or maceration (dentures, occlusive dressings or garments, obesity)
Nutritional factors
    Avitaminosis
    Iron deficiency (chronic mucocutaneous candidiasis)
    Generalized malnutrition
Physiologic alterations
    Extremes of age
    Pregnancy
    Menses
Systemic illnesses
    Down's syndrome
    Acrodermatitis enteropathica
    Diabetes mellitus and certain other endocrinopathies (Cushing's syndrome, hypoadrenalism, hypothyroidism, hypoparathyroidism)
    Uremia
    Malignancy (especially hematologic, thymoma)
    Intrinsic immunodeficiency states (DiGeorge's syndrome, Nezelof's syndrome, severe combined immunodeficiency syndrome, myeloperoxidase deficiency, Chédiak-Higashi syndrome, hyperimmunoglobulinemia E syndrome, chronic granulomatous disease, AIDS)
Iatrogenic causes
    Barrier-weak factors (indwelling catheters, intravenous drug abusers)
    X-irradiation
    Medications
    Glucocorticoids and other immunosuppressive agents
    Antibiotics (especially broad-spectrum, metronidazole)
    Tranquilizers
    Oral contraceptives (especially estrogen-dominant)
    Colchicine
    Phenylbutazone

corneum, (3) the desquamation process induced by inflammation-induced epidermal proliferation, (4) opsonization and phagocytosis, and (5) other serum factors. The host microbial flora are protective in that they compete with *Candida* for nutrients and epithelial adherence sites and produce by-products toxic to the yeast. Likewise, normal intact skin, with its constant sloughing and regeneration, provides an effective barrier against *Candida*. Skin-surface lipids are partially inhibitory as well. Abrogation of this barrier by mechanical means or occlusion facilitates infection. As with cutaneous dermatophyte infections, the skin increases its turnover rate significantly during the early stages of infection, and this increased desquamation helps shed the organism.[10]

The process of phagocytosis and killing of candidal organisms is accomplished primarily by polymorphonuclear leukocytes (PMNs) and macrophages. Patients with neutropenia or diseases affecting PMN function (Table 207-2) are particularly susceptible to candidal infections. The PMN is the predominant early inflammatory cell seen histologically in candidal infections; it is recruited in part by mannan activation of the alternative complement pathway and the ensuing generation of potent chemotactic factors.[6] The importance of this process to host defense against *Candida* is emphasized in experimental studies on rodents that have been complement-depleted (using cobra venom factor) or on hereditary C5-deficient animals. In this setting, experimental candidal infections do not elicit a PMN response. In addition, the organism invades much more rapidly and extensively in these animals than in normal ones.[3,11] Likewise, macrophages participate in opsonization, phagocytosis, and killing of yeasts. The PMNs and macrophages have C3b surface receptors, and the deposition of C3b opsonins on *Candida* organisms may therefore facilitate phagocytosis.[12,13] The PMNs and macrophages accomplish intracellular killing by both oxidative (myeloperoxidase–hydrogen peroxide–halide system) and nonoxidative means.

Serum factors that may be important in containing candidal infections include the controversial serum "clumping" factor, which reflects the entanglement of hyphal elements grown in serum.[14] Furthermore, transferrin and lactoferrin, by binding iron necessary for fungal growth, may inhibit candidal proliferation.[15,16]

The immune mechanisms responsible for protection against *Candida* infections include both humoral and cell-mediated responses. The latter are considered to be more important. Proof of this assertion comes from experience with chronic mucocutaneous candidiasis and human immunodeficiency virus (HIV) infection, where a defect in cell-mediated immunity leads to extensive superficial candidiasis despite normal or even exaggerated humoral defenses. Serum antibody production to the principal cell-wall glycoprotein antigens of *Candida* occurs in low titers in normal individuals. The protective role of these antibodies reflects a response to colonization of the gastrointestinal tract early in life.[6] It is clear that patients with primarily B cell deficiency states are not at high risk for candidal infections.[17] It is probable that the various innate, nonimmune factors in conjunction with cell-mediated immunity and complement activation contribute more to host defense against candidal infections than does humoral immunity.

CLINICAL MANIFESTATIONS

The cutaneous and mucosal manifestations of candidiasis are varied but in most cases characteristic.

Oral Candidiasis (See also Chap. 114)

Acute pseudomembranous candidiasis or thrush is the most common form of oral candidiasis. Concomitant factors such as diabetes mellitus, systemic steroids, antibiotic use, pernicious anemia, malignancies, and immune deficiency states may also be predisposing factors[18] (Table 207-2). Clinically there are discrete white patches that may become confluent on the buccal mucosa, tongue, palate, and gingivae (Fig. 207-2A). This friable pseudomembrane resembles milk curds and consists of desquamated epithelial cells, fungal elements, inflammatory cells, and food debris. When it is scraped off, a raw, brightly erythematous surface is exposed. Microscopic examination of this material reveals masses of tangled pseudohyphae and blastospores. Severe cases may show ulcerations and necrosis of the mucosal surface.

Acute atrophic candidiasis (the erythematous variant) may occur de novo or after sloughing of the pseudomembrane of thrush.[18] It is commonly associated with broad-spectrum antibiotic administration but can be seen with the use of topical, inhaled, or systemic glucocorticoids.[2] The most common location is on the dorsal surface of the tongue, where there are patchy depapillated areas with minimal pseudomembrane formation.

Chronic atrophic candidiasis (denture stomatitis) (Fig. 207-2B) is a very common form of oral candidiasis. Female patients are affected more commonly than males. Clinical findings of chronic erythema and edema of the palatal mucosa that contacts the dentures as well as angular cheilitis are present. Presumably, the chronic low-grade trauma and occlusion provided by dentures predisposes to candidal colonization and subsequent infection.[18]

Candidal cheilosis or perlèche is characterized by erythema, fissuring, maceration, and soreness at the angles of the mouth (Fig. 207-2C) in habitual lip lickers or in those elderly patients with sagging skin at the oral commissures. The loss of dentition, poorly fitting dentures, malocclusion, and vitamin deficiency may be predisposing factors. It is often associated with chronic atrophic candidiasis due to denture wear.[18]

Chronic hyperplastic candidiasis or candidal leukoplakia is characterized by adherent, firm, raised areas on the buccal mucosa or tongue that are translucent to white in color with surrounding erythema (Fig. 207-2D). This condition can be very resistant to therapy.[18]

Median rhomboid glossitis is a central papillary atrophic condition of the dorsal surface of the tongue. Although it was once thought to be a developmental anomaly, now *Candida* has been recognized as its etiology.[18]

Black hairy tongue has been associated with *C. albicans*. An alteration in normal oral flora allows overgrowth with fungi and bacteria. The filiform papillae hypertrophy and the surface of the tongue cannot undergo normal desquamation (Fig. 207-2E). Factors that may worsen the condition include poor oral hygiene, radiation therapy, and use of antacids. The lesion occurs at the same location as median rhomboid glossitis but can also be generalized to the entire dorsal surface of the tongue. Patients often complain of a tickling sensation due to elongated papillae. Treatment consists of physical debridement and good hygiene.[19]

Oral Candidiasis in Immunocompromised and Cancer Patients

Candida albicans is responsible for mucosal fungal infections in patients immunocompromised by radiation therapy, chemotherapy, transplant therapy, diabetes mellitus, or cell-mediated immune deficiency.[18] The pathogenesis of oral candidiasis is multifactorial and

FIGURE 207-2

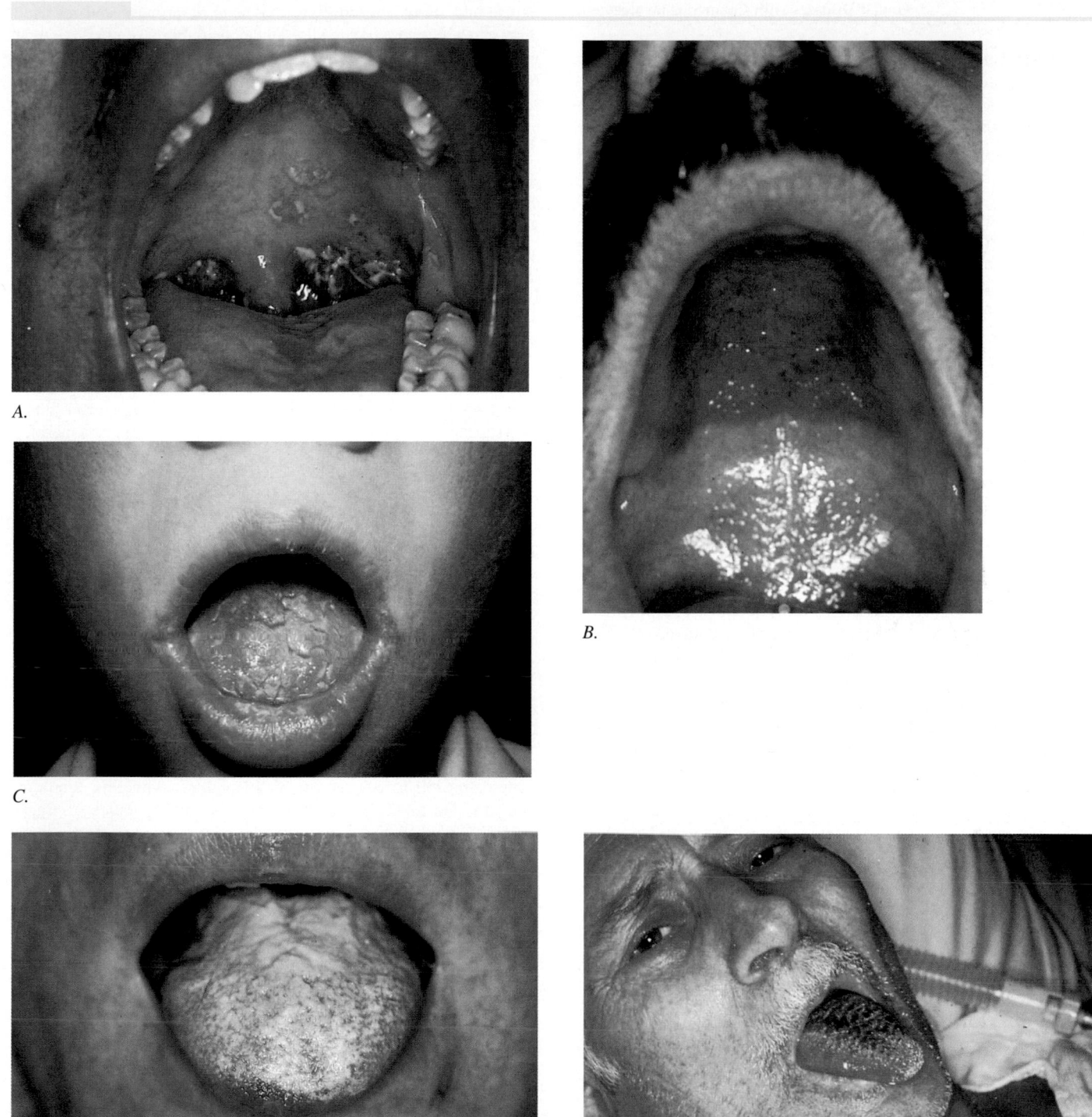

A. Pseudomembranous candidiasis or thrush: note the characteristic white patches on the palate. B. Atrophic candidiasis under dentures. C. *Candida* perlèche with erythema and fissuring at the corners of the mouth. D. Hyperplastic candidiasis of the tongue. E. Black hairy tongue is characterized by pigmented hypertrophied filiform papillae of the dorsum of the tongue and is usually associated with oral antibiotic therapy.

the reported incidence varies between 27 and 100, depending on the type of cancer and treatment.

The soft tissues of the oropharynx are very sensitive to the actions of anti-neoplastic agents. Chemotherapeutics are toxic to the basal cells of the epithelium and directly inhibit cell replication and cytolysis. The result is a thin mucosa that promotes colonization by yeasts.

Severe neutropenia associated with reduced CD4 T cells is the most significant predisposition for oral candidiasis.[20] One study showed the local use of glucocorticoids reduced local CD4 T cells and caused a 400-fold increase in *C. albicans* colonization.[21]

The use of antiseptics such as chlorhexidine and antifungals such as nystatin as mouthwashes to prevent oral candidiasis is controversial. While some studies showed a reduction in the frequency of candidiasis, others showed no significant difference.[20]

Oral Candidiasis and Acquired Immunodeficiency Syndrome (AIDS) (See also Chap. 226)

Oral candidiasis is the most common fungal infection seen at the mucosal surface of HIV-positive patients. This condition occurs in 50 percent of HIV-infected patients and 90 percent of AIDS patients.[22] Oral candidiasis may manifest itself in one of three forms when associated with HIV infection: pseudomembranous, erythematous, or angular cheilitis.[23] More infrequently, palatal papillary hyperplastic lesions have been associated with candidal infections in HIV patients.[24]

The high frequency of oral mucosal infections in HIV patients indicates compromise of mucosal defense mechanisms. Immunoglobulin A, secreted to prevent adherence of microorganisms to the tissue, is the primary protector of the musocal surfaces. Coogan et al. found a significantly reduced parotid saliva flow rate in AIDS patients, which implies decreased total IgA delivery to the mucosa.[22]

Numerous agents are available for the treatment of oral candidiasis. Nystatin oral pastilles, 200,000 U, have been used as oral topical agents in a dose of one to two pastilles by mouth four or five times a day. The drawbacks of nystatin pastilles are poor patient compliance and the tendency to develop dental caries due to the addition of sucrose. Nystatin oral suspension is ineffective owing to its very brief contact time with the oral mucosa. Amphotericin B, another polyene antifungal, has been used against non-*albicans* species of *Candida,* which are often resistant to azole antifungals. *C. glabrata* has responded to the intravenous amphotericin B solution used topically.

Clotrimazole has been used as a 10-mg troche dissolved orally five times a day. Like nystatin, this medication often prompts poor patient compliance. Fluconazole, ketoconazole, and itraconazole have all been used systemically. One study showed that after treatment with fluconazole, there was longer time to relapse as compared with clotrimazole.[23] Fluconazole is often preferred over ketoconazole because of decreased side effects and a once-daily dosing schedule.[25] In recent years, fluconazole-resistant candidal species have emerged, namely *C. glabrata.* In these cases, the choice of therapy is limited. Higher doses of fluconazole have been tried, as have itraconazole and ketoconazole. As a last resort, intravenous amphotericin B has been employed. Studies of itraconazole have shown equivalency to ketoconazole. When compared with clotrimazole, itraconazole showed faster response and longer time to relapse.[23]

Prophylactic use of antifungal medication has been a source of debate and study. Presently, prophylaxis of primary and recurrent disease is not recommended due to the availability of effective treatment, low mortality, low incidence of invasive disease, and the potential for the emergence of drug-resistant organisms.[26]

Vaginal and Vulvovaginal Candidiasis (See Chap. 116)

Approximately two-thirds of all women will experience at least one episode of vulvovaginal candidiasis (VVC) in their lifetimes.[27] Diabetes mellitus, steroid therapy, and any form of immunosuppression are other risk factors for both acute and recurrent VVC.[28] A retrospective study conducted by MacDonald et al. showed a clear relationship between use of oral antibiotics and subsequent VVC.[29] These factors may alter the vaginal microflora, which allows the overgrowth of *Candida.*[30]

Patients generally present with a thick vaginal discharge associated with burning or itching and sometimes dysuria. Examination shows whitish plaques on the vaginal wall with underlying erythema and surrounding edema that can extend to the labia and perineal area.

Recurrent VVC is an ongoing problem for many patients. Changes in the hormonal environment, such as pregnancy and the luteal phase of menstruation, can induce a relapse of VVC. Use of a genital cleansing solution was also associated with recurrent candidiasis. The mechanism for this is thought to be an allergy or hypersensitivity response that increases susceptibility to *Candida.* Sexual promiscuity has been related to recurrent VVC. The etiology of this is related to vaginal abrasions associated with sexual intercourse and to allergy to the partner's semen.[31]

Balanitis or Balanoposthitis (See also Chap. 115)

Candida species are the most common cause of infectious balantis, representing 30 to 35 percent of all patients with this condition. Balanitis due to *C. albicans* presents as small papules or fragile papulopustules on the glans or in the coronal sulcus. These break to leave superficial erythematous erosions with a collarette of whitish scale on thrushlike membrane. Infection may spread to the scrotum and inguinal areas. In diabetics or immunosuppressed patients, a severe edematous, ulcerative balanitis may occur. Occasionally, patients present with a transient erythema and burning occurring shortly after intercourse with partners having candidal vaginitis. This presentation was thought to represent a hypersensitivity response to the organism. Factors predisposing to balanitis include candidal vaginal infection in sexual partners, diabetes mellitus, and an uncircumcised state.[32]

Cutaneous Candidiasis

C. albicans has a predilection for colonizing moist, macerated folds of skin. For that reason, intertrigo in its various forms is the most common clinical presentation of candidiasis on glabrous skin. Common locations for the infection include the genitocrural, subaxillary, gluteal, interdigital (Fig. 207-3*A*), and submammary (Fig. 207-3*B*) areas and between the folds of skin of the abdominal wall. Predisposing conditions include obesity, occlusive clothing, diabetes mellitus, and occupations favoring excessive exposure to moist, occlusive conditions.[33] The clinical appearance consists of pruritic, erythematous, macerated areas of skin in intertriginous areas with satellite vesicopustules. These pustules are fragile and break, leaving a red, macular base with a collarette of easily detachable necrotic epidermis. Several varieties of intertrigo caused by *Candida*

FIGURE 207-3

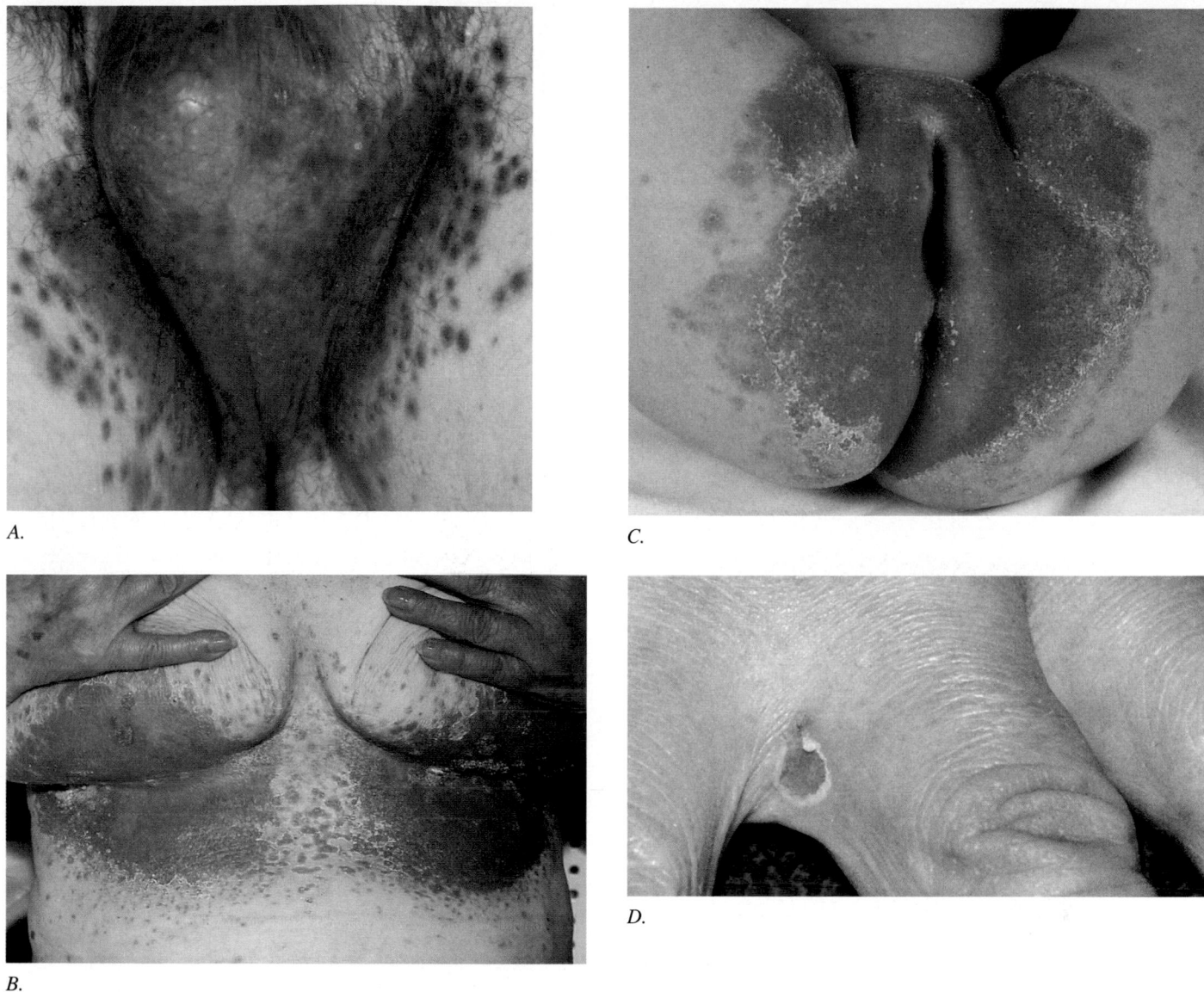

A.

B.

C.

D.

Candidal intertrigo. *A.* Erythematous, eroded plaques involving the scrotum and inguinal area with satellite lesions. *B.* Confluent and discrete erythematous, eroded areas with pustular and erosive satellite lesion. *C.* The infant shows red macular areas on the vulva surrounded by a delicate collar. Outside the main lesions are a few satellite lesions. *D.* Erythematous eroded area between the fingers occurring in a waitress.

deserve special mention. Diaper dermatitis in infants can be of multiple etiologies. However, *Candida* can colonize this area from these infants' gastrointestinal tracts. The chronic occlusive state of diaper wear propagates the infection. Lesions appear first in the perianal area and spread to the perineum and inguinal creases, with pronounced erythema in the latter (Fig. 207-3C). Concomitant thrush or candidal involvement of other intertriginous areas may be present in severe cases.[34] *Erosio interdigitalis blastomycetica* refers to interdigital candidal infection of the hands and usually affects the area between the third and fourth fingers owing to the relative occlusion in the third interspace (Fig. 207-3D). *Candida* miliaria affects the back in bedridden patients, particularly those who are febrile and sweating profusely. Lesions start as isolated vesicopustules that are positive for fungal forms. *Candida* can also colonize and infect the skin around wounds that are being dressed occlusively, especially if broad-spectrum topical antibiotics are being used.[35]

An erythematous pustular folliculitis due to *C. albicans* has been described. Although the lesions are perifollicular in location, true invasion of the hair shaft is usually not observed.[36] A common location for these lesions is in the perioral area.[37] Typical perioral dermatitis presenting as erythematous papulopustules secondary to *C. albicans* has been described as having a more severe pyoderma faciale–like eruption in the perioral area.[38,39]

Candidal paronychia is common in individuals whose hands are chronically involved in wet work (e.g., housekeepers, bakers, fishermen, bartenders). At times the clinical presentation may be complicated by a concomitant bacterial infection. Typically there is redness, swelling, and tenderness of the paronychial area with prominent retraction of the cuticle toward the proximal nail fold (Fig. 207-4). Occasionally, pus can be expressed from beneath this area. Secondary nail changes can occur and include onycholysis and transverse ridging of the nail plate with a brownish or green discoloration along the lateral borders.[40]

The rare syndrome of congenital candidiasis presents in the first 24 h of life and is due to chorioamnionitis acquired through intact membranes. A pink macular and papular eruption progressing to vesicles and pustules with desquamation occurs predominantly on the upper half of the body and on the palms and soles. While most neonates have a benign course of disease, approximately 20 percent have transient respiratory distress or clinical signs of sepsis. Preterm and low-birth-weight infants are at higher risk for fatal dissemination of the disease.[41]

The incidence of disseminated candidiasis is steadily rising as more patients with hematologic malignancies are treated aggressively with potent immunosuppressive drugs and undergo bone marrow and other organ transplants (Table 207-2). The organisms responsible for such infections include *C. albicans*, *C. tropicalis*, *C. kefyr*, *C. krusei*, and *C. parapsilosis*. These organisms may gain hematogenous access from the oropharynx or gastrointestinal tract, when the function of the mucosal barrier is compromised (e.g., mucositis secondary to chemotherapy), or through contaminated intravenous catheters. Organs most commonly involved include the lungs, spleen, kidneys, liver, heart, and brain.[42] The ocular findings include an endophthalmitis, which correlates well with multiple organ involvement.[43] Skin lesions occur in some patients with disseminated infection. The recognition of such lesions may be important in early diagnosis, as antemortem blood cultures are negative in a high percentage of patients with autopsy-proved systemic candidiasis.[42]

The characteristic skin lesions are 0.5- to 1.0-cm erythematous papulonodules that become hemorrhagic in patients with associated thrombocytopenia. The eruption is located on the trunk and extremities and can vary with respect to number of lesions. Associated findings include fever and myalgias.[44,45] Necrotic cutaneous lesions resembling ecthyma gangrenosum (which is caused by *Pseudomonas aeruginosa*) but that are, in fact, due to candidiasis have also been described.[46,47] In intravenous heroin abusers, macronodular and folliculitis-like skin lesions occur in the scalp and other terminal hair-bearing areas when candidal organisms infiltrate the hair follicles.[48]

Chronic Mucocutaneous Candidiasis

Chronic mucocutaneous candidiasis (CMC) is a term used to describe a heterogeneous group of clinical syndromes characterized by chronic, treatment-resistant, superficial candidal infections of the skin, nails, and oropharynx. There is virtually no propensity for disseminated visceral candidiasis. In many cases there are narrow but specific abnormalities in cell-mediated immunity; in others the defects are more global. The clinical findings and immunologic defects have been extensively reviewed.[17]

CLINICAL SYNDROMES Table 207-3 provides an updated categorization of CMC syndromes and a summary of their distinguishing features. In general, the various syndromes may be familial or sporadic in nature. When presenting in childhood, lesions are detected before the age of 3 years. Oral lesions or diaper dermatitis appears first, followed by angular cheilitis (perlèche), lip fissures, nail and paronychial involvement, vulvovaginitis, and cutaneous involvement. In chronic localized mucocutaneous candidiasis, markedly hyperkeratotic, hornlike, or granulomatous lesions may appear (candidal granuloma) on the face, eyelids, scalp, lips, or acral areas (Fig. 207-5). On the scalp they may resemble the lesions of favus and can lead to alopecia. In chronic diffuse candidiasis, lesions may appear atypical for candidiasis in having an erythematous, serpiginous border or areas of brownish desquamation on a background of mild erythema (Fig. 207-5). Concomitant dermatophyte infection of the skin may occur and confuse the clinical presentation.[17]

Nail involvement is characterized by markedly thickened and dystrophic nail plates that are invaded through their entire thickness by *Candida*. The paronychial areas are red and edematous, and the fingertips are often bulbous in appearance (Fig. 207-4).[40]

Conditions that have been associated with CMC include candidal esophagitis or laryngitis, endocrinopathies (usually hypoparathyroidism, hypoadrenalism, hypothyroidism), circulating autoimmune antibodies, diabetes mellitus, vitiligo with antibodies to melanocytes, iron deficiency, chronic active hepatitis, pernicious anemia, malabsorption, alopecia totalis, dental enamel dysplasia, keratocon-

FIGURE 207-4

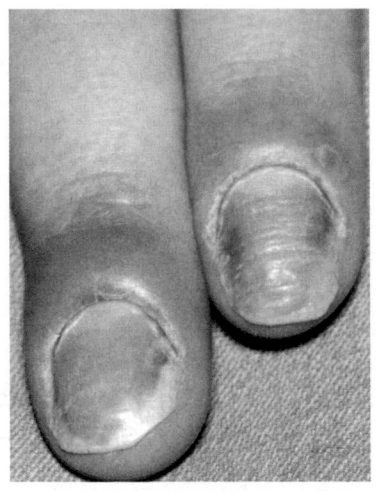

A.

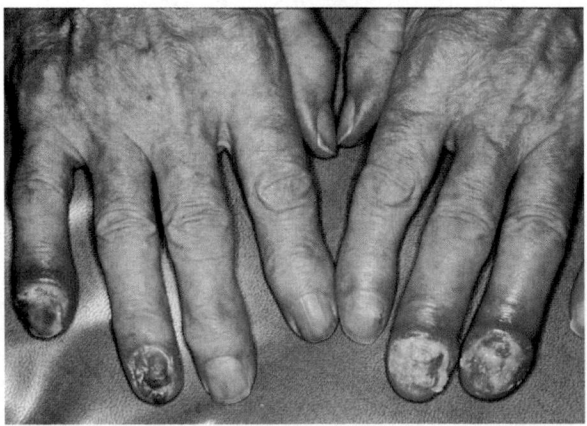

B.

Chronic onychia and paronychia from *C. albicans*. *A.* Note the warm but not hot, slightly tender edematous nail fold with some onycholysis. This is very often misdiagnosed as staphylococcal paronychia. *B.* This is a chronic inflammatory condition of the nail fold that can also involve the nail plate.

TABLE 207-3

Classification of Chronic Mucocutaneous Candidiasis (CMC)

CLINICAL SYNDROME	INHERITANCE	AGE OF ONSET	DISTRIBUTION OF LESIONS	ENDOCRINOLOGY	ASSOCIATED FINDINGS	NOTES
Chronic oral candidiasis	Sporadic	Any	Mucosa of tongue, lips, buccal cavity; perlèche; no skin or nail involvement	None	Esophagitis	Denture stomatitis is a variant
Chronic candidiasis with endocrinopathy	Autosomal recessive	Childhood	Mucous membranes, skin and/or nails	Frequent (hypoadrenalism, hypothyroidism, hypoparathyroidism, or polyendocrinopathy)	Alopecia totalis, thyroiditis, vitiligo, chronic hepatitis, pernicious anemia, gonadal failure, malabsorption, diabetes mellitus	Endocrinopathy may be delayed in onset
Chronic candidiasis without endocrinopathy	Autosomal recessive	Childhood	Mucous membranes, perlèche, and nail involvement; less common skin involvement	None	Blepharitis, esophagitis, laryngitis	
	Autosomal dominant	Childhood		None	Dermatophytosis, loss of teeth, recurrent viral infections	
Chronic localized mucocutaneous candidiasis	Sporadic	Childhood	Mucous membranes, skin, and/or nails	Occasionally	Pulmonary infections, esophagitis	Hyperkeratotic lesions (Candida), granuloma
Chronic diffuse candidiasis	Autosomal recessive	Childhood	Widespread on mucous membranes, skin and nail involvement	None		Erythematous, serpiginous skin lesions
		Adolescence	Widespread on mucous membranes, skin, and nail involvement	None	History of frequent courses of antibiotics	
Chronic candidiasis with thymoma	Sporadic	Adulthood (after third decade)	Mucous membranes, nails, and skin	None	Thymoma, myasthenia gravis, aplastic anemia, neutropenia, hypogammaglobulinemia	CMC often precedes diagnosis of thymoma

junctivitis, pulmonary fibrosis, and keratitis, ichthyosis, and deafness (KID) syndrome and recurrent pyogenic, viral, or other fungal infections. When CMC first appears in adulthood, it is often associated with a thymoma and the other conditions listed in Table 207-3.[49]

IMMUNOLOGY Although no immunologic defect can be found in up to 25 to 30 percent of patients with CMC,[50] numerous immunologic defects have been described. These usually involve abnormalities in cell-mediated immunity (CMI), whereas humoral immunity is largely intact. The following is a listing of some of the commonly described immunologic abnormalities:

1. There may be complete anergy to common skin-test antigens or selective unresponsiveness to *C. albicans* antigen. This group can be further divided based on in vitro lymphocyte transformation and lymphokine production studies to *Candida*.
   a. Lymphocyte transformation negative and lymphokine production positive
   b. Lymphocyte transformation positive and lymphokine production negative
   c. Both lymphocyte transformation and lymphokine production negative
2. Selective IgA deficiency
3. Plasma inhibitor to lymphocyte transformation by *C. albicans*
4. Serum inhibitor of polymorphonuclear leukocyte chemotaxis and killing of *C. albicans*[17]
5. Abnormal monocyte chemotactic and killing responses
6. Combined abnormality of monocyte mobility and phagocytosis killing[51]
7. Abnormal complement function
8. Abnormal macrophage function
9. Hyperimmunoglobulinemia E and impaired granulocyte chemotaxis[52]
10. Defective suppressor T cell function
11. Defective mannan handling by monocytes[53]
12. Impaired generation of helper T cells[51]

In some cases, the observed immunologic defect is reversed after successful antifungal therapy. This suggests that a massive antigenic load (particularly mannan) may interfere with CMI—perhaps by the generation of specific T-suppressor cells.[54]

FIGURE 207-5

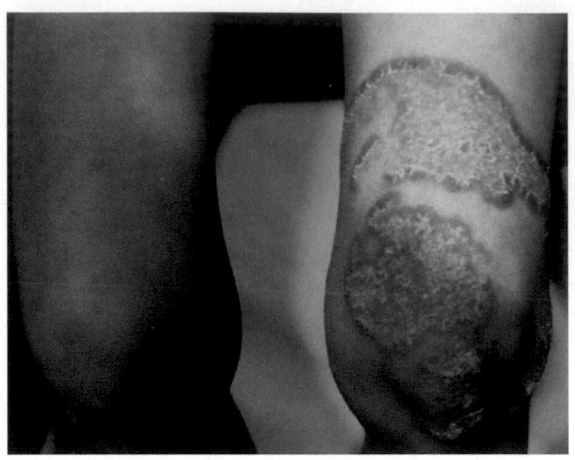

Mucocutaneous candidiasis. Well-demarcated serpiginous border.

There is controversy in the literature about the existence of allergic cutaneous reactions (id reactions) to localized infections with *C. albicans*. Certain recalcitrant cases of erythema annulare centrifugum, chronic urticaria, and groin or hand dermatitis have been attributed to this phenomenon and have cleared with successful therapy of the underlying candidal infection.

LABORATORY FINDINGS

Of the more than 200 species of yeast that have been classified in the genus *Candida,* less than 10 have been identified as capable of producing or contributing to disease in humans.[6] Because of the ubiquity of these unicellular organisms in nature and the fact that they are often found as transient colonizers of the skin and appendages of humans, the clinical diagnosis of candidiasis should be confirmed by laboratory tests for identification of the species of yeast involved. In addition to the clinical evaluation of the patient, direct microscopic examination of specimens for the presence of yeast and isolation of yeast in culture are needed for definitive proof of infection. In superficial candidal infections, the diagnosis can be made by performing an examination of skin scrapings and observing typical budding yeasts with hyphae or pseudohyphae. *C. albicans* grows readily on bacterial media, but Sabouraud's agar with added antibiotics is usually recommended for isolation. Whitish, mucoid colonies grow within 2 to 5 days. Of all superficial infections, chronic paronychiae may have the lowest yield of positive cultures.

In systemic candidiasis with skin lesions, the diagnosis can usually be made from histopathologic examination and culture of appropriate skin biopsy specimens. Blood cultures are often negative in this setting.[42] Serologic studies using immunodiffusion, counterimmunoelectrophoresis, and latex agglutination methods may be somewhat helpful in the diagnosis of systemic candidiasis. However, false-negative and false-positive reactions are common. More promising are techniques to detect circulating candidal antigens (e.g., mannan) or metabolic products (e.g., arabinitol).[55]

Microscopic Studies

Because the clinical manifestations of infections caused by species of *Candida* are protean, the type of specimen taken from patients for laboratory examination will vary from body fluids to surgical biopsy. Direct microscopic examination of these specimens for the presence of yeast forms provides rapid evidence in support of the presumptive clinical diagnosis. Body fluids such as urine and cerebrospinal fluid should be centrifuged and the sediment examined. This procedure increases the probability of finding yeasts. Sputum and other viscous secretions along with surgical biopsies and tissue scrapings must be treated with a clearing agent such as 10% potassium hydroxide (KOH) and ink before the material is examined (see Chap. 206). Yeast forms in the genus *Candida* will appear as oval budding cells, elongated filamentous cells connected in a sausage-like manner (pseudohyphae), or as truly septate hyphae (Fig. 207-1). The presence of such forms in clinical material does not permit species identification but does provide evidence that fungi consistent with the morphology of *Candida* are present. Species identification relies on isolation of the yeast in pure culture and biochemical and physiologic tests.

Culture Methods

Sediment from centrifuged body fluids, tissue from biopsies, and scrapings should be inoculated promptly onto Sabouraud's dextrose agar containing antibacterial antibiotics. Cultures are incubated at room temperature [25° to 27°C (77° to 80.6°F)] and examined periodically for growth of yeast. Negative cultures are discarded after 4 weeks. All colonies of yeast must be subcultured and tested further for identifying morphologic and biochemical characteristics before they can be speciated.

Pathology

Superficial candidiasis is characterized by subcorneal pustules. Organisms are seldom seen within the pustule but can be visualized with the aid of a periodic acid–Schiff (PAS) stain in the stratum corneum. The histology of a candidal granuloma shows marked papillomatosis, hyperkeratosis, and a dense dermal infiltrate consisting of lymphocytes, granulocytes, plasma cells, and multinucleated giant cells.

In systemic candidal infections with skin involvement, biopsies show focal areas in the dermis and within blood vessels, where organisms can be identified using PAS or methenamine silver stains. There may be a surrounding mononuclear cell infiltrate,[56] leukocytoclastic vasculitis, or microabscess formation.

DIAGNOSIS

The diagnosis of most superficial cutaneous candidal infections can be made by the typical appearance of the clinical lesions and the presence of satellite vesicopustules. This can be confirmed by KOH examination and culture of skin scrapings. Nevertheless, intertriginous candidiasis can occasionally be confused with tinea infections, eczema, seborrheic dermatitis, intertriginous psoriasis, erythrasma, bacterial intertrigo, familial benign pemphigus, Leiner's disease, glucagonoma, or flexural Darier's disease.

Candidal paronychia should be differentiated from bacterial paronychia or paronychia associated with hypoparathyroidism, celiac disease, acrodermatitis enteropathica, Reiter's syndrome, acrokeratosis paraneoplastica, or retinoid therapy.

Typical oral thrush is characteristic, but the atrophic or ulcerative forms of oral candidiasis can be confused with mucositis due to chemotherapeutic drugs, herpetic infections, erythema multiforme, pemphigus, lichen planus, histoplasmosis, leukoplakia, secondary syphilis, or an aspirin burn. Perlèche-like lesions may be seen in secondary syphilis, avitaminosis (e.g., riboflavin), glucagonoma syndrome, or iron-deficiency states.

The lesions of CMC should be differentiated from those of tinea (e.g., favus), bacterial pyoderma, acrodermatitis enteropathica, and halogenoderma. The immunodeficiency states listed in Table 207-2 should be considered in evaluating patients with widespread CMC.

Papular cutaneous lesions similar to those seen in systemic candidiasis can be confused with *Pityrosporum* folliculitis,[57] bacterial sepsis (e.g., gonococcal, meningococcal, pseudomonal, staphylococcal), and other disseminated fungal infections (e.g., mucormycosis, aspergillosis). Necrotic cutaneous lesions due to *Candida* may appear identical to *Pseudomonas* ecthyma or deep fungal infections (e.g., cryptococcosis, torulopsosis, or sporotrichosis).

THERAPY (See also Chaps. 247 and 260)

An important aspect in the treatment of candidiasis is the correction of any of the predisposing factors listed in Table 207-2.

For uncomplicated oral candidiasis, topical antifungals have been the first line of treatment.[2] The most commonly used drugs include nystatin suspension (400,000 to 600,000 U qid) held in the mouth and then swallowed, clotrimazole troches (10 mg dissolved in the mouth five times per day), 1 to 2% gentian violet, and chlorhexidine rinse. Nystatin, while safe for long-term use, has the disadvantage of not being as effective as clotrimazole troches. Patients' compliance with the suspension form is also shown to be poor.[18] If reinfection of the oral cavity occurs, systemic therapy is indicated.[2] Ketoconazole is very effective as an antifungal agent in doses of 200 mg/day for 1 to 2 weeks. In AIDS, ketoconazole has been effective in doses of 400 mg/day for 1 to 2 weeks. Ketoconazole, however, can raise liver enzymes and requires periodic evaluation of liver chemistry during treatment.[18] Fluconazole is as efficacious as ketoconazole with a less toxic side-effects profile. It can be used at doses of 50 to 100 mg/day for 1 week.[2] Itraconazole is as effective as clotrimazole troches but showed a faster response time and longer time to relapse than clotrimazole. Itraconazole has been used in doses of 100 mg/day for 3 weeks or 200 mg/day for 3 weeks in AIDS patients.[58] In significantly immunocompromised patients, prophylactic therapy with twice-weekly therapy of ketoconazole or fluconazole has proven effective.[2]

There are numerous vaginal and oral antifungal agents available to treat candidal vulvovaginitis. Many surveys have demonstrated that most women prefer oral therapy. Patients with severe local symptoms may require topical or intravaginal therapy to relieve itching and burning. Some women may find increased vaginal symptoms after using a topical azole. This is due to an allergic contact dermatitis. In general, the physician should inquire about the patient's preference before prescribing.[59] Commonly used topical antifungals include butoconazole, terconazole, tioconazole, miconazole, and clotrimazole.[28] All of these topical agents are safe to use during pregnancy.[59] There are three oral azoles available that have similar efficacy to topical therapy. Fluconazole, itraconazole, and ketoconazole have been compared in many trials.[28] Ketoconazole, while effective, has the undesirable side effect of hepatotox-

icity.[59] Studies have shown better compliance with fluconazole and faster recovery as compared with intravaginal clotrimazole.[60] Itraconazole has also been found to be as effective as clotrimazole.[61] Single-dose therapies have been explored for improved convenience and compliance. One 500-mg clotrimazole suppository as well as one 150-mg fluconazole tablet are two of these options. These drugs have the ability to maintain therapeutic concentrations in the vagina for 5 days. Severe or recurrent candidal vaginitis should not be treated with single-dose therapy. Prophylactic regimens have been used in recurrent VVC.

A weekly intravaginal dose of terconazole[62] or clotrimazole cream[59] has been shown to prevent recurrences. A single 150-mg dose of fluconazole each month has also been used successfully as prophylaxis[63] in women who are HIV-positive with recurrent vaginal candidiasis. A weekly dose of 200 mg of fluconazole has been effective in preventing relapses.[64]

For candidal balanitis, the recommended treatment is clotrimazole topical cream or a single 150-mg dose of fluconazole.[32]

Intertrigo has been successfully treated with one of several topical antifungals. Nystatin has been very effective in cream and powder form. The powder vehicle is especially useful to keep moist, intertriginous areas dry. Any topical imidazole cream can be used to treat intertrigo. Miconazole powder is also available for treating cutaneous candidiasis. Adding a topical steroid to the treatment regimen helps relieve symptoms of itching, burning, and pain.[33]

Chronic paronychial infections due to *C. albicans* are more resistant to therapy. All wet work should be minimized. Topical therapy should be applied and allowed to drain under the proximal nail fold. Occlusion using a finger cot may allow better drug penetration. A topical imidazole in solution form is the ideal treatment.[33] Four percent thymol in chloroform or absolute alcohol has anticandidal activity and is drying. Oral ketoconazole or even surgical marsupialization of the proximal nail fold area has been recommended in resistant cases.[40]

Although congenital cutaneous candidiasis may resolve spontaneously, topical and oral therapy is recommended to prevent disseminated disease. Nystatin is the drug of choice.[41]

The management of disseminated candidiasis includes the early use of amphotericin B. Retrospective studies, however, have shown variable results with regard to benefit of this treatment. Typically, neutropenic patients with fevers who are unresponsive to antibacterial therapy are started on antifungal therapy. Autopsies have shown very small concentrations of amphotericin B in the kidneys and lungs, two common sites of serious candidal infection. 5-Flucytosine is another option in the treatment of disseminated candidiasis. Anaissie and Pinczowski also report success with fluconazole in patients who failed to respond to amphotericin B or had severe dose-limiting toxicities.[42]

In the past, chronic mucocutaneous candidiasis has been notoriously difficult to treat. The best results are seen when a combination of antifungal drugs and immune deficiency correction are used.[49] The most important consideration in the treatment of CMC is the immune deficiency. Although antifungal treatment will clear the lesions quickly, the infection recurs within a few weeks of stopping the drug unless the underlying immune defect is corrected. Patients with CMC have used oral azoles with good efficacy for years.[17] In addition, several different methods of immune regulation have been used. A patient with DiGeorge syndrome received thymic tissue transplantation and had spontaneous clearing of CMC.

The infection of a patient with severe combined immunodeficiency and extensive CMC also cleared after transplantation of cultured fetal thymus donor leukocytes. Infusion with *Candida*-specific cell-mediated immunity has also produced remissions of CMC. The best clinical results have followed treatment with *Candida*-specific transfer factor proteins from donor T lymphocytes.[49]

"*PITYROSPORUM* INFECTIONS" OF THE SKIN: PAPULOSQUAMOUS TINEA VERSICOLOR, "*PITYROSPORUM*" FOLLICULITIS, AND INVERSE TINEA VERSICOLOR

Tinea (pityriasis) versicolor is the most common "*Pityrosporum* infection" of the skin.[65] The disease is seen as a superficial, chronically recurring fungal infection of the stratum corneum characterized by scaly, hypo- or hyperpigmented, irregular macules most often occurring on the trunk and proximal extremities. Tinea versicolor is caused by the fungus *Malassezia furfur*. This organism may also cause a papulopustular folliculitis that resembles the cutaneous lesions of disseminated candidiasis and has been implicated as a cause of fungal sepsis in patients receiving intravenous alimentation, particularly lipid supplementation therapy. There are data that support the concept that *M. furfur* also contributes to the pathogenesis of seborrheic dermatitis.[66]

History

Tinea versicolor was first recognized as a fungal infection of the skin in 1846 by Eichstedt. For several years the disease was considered to be dermatophyte in origin, but Baillon, impressed by the yeastlike nature of the organism, coined the name *Malassezia* in 1889 to distinguish this organism from the *Microsporum* species of dermatophytes.[67] In 1951 Gordon isolated, characterized, and authenticated the organism *M. furfur* and renamed it *Pityrosporum orbiculare*.[68] It is now recognized and accepted that *M. furfur* is the correct name and *P. orbiculare, P. ovale,* and *M. ovalis* are synonyms.

Etiology and Pathogenesis

M. furfur can be cultured from clinically apparent disease and normal skin and is considered part of the normal flora, particularly in sebum-rich areas of the skin.[66] *M. furfur* is a dimorphic, lipophilic organism that grows in vitro only with the addition of C12- to C14-sized fatty acids to the medium. Under appropriate conditions, it converts from the saprophytic yeast to the predominantly parasitic mycelial morphology associated with clinical disease. Factors responsible for mycelial transition include a warm, humid environment, an inherited predisposition, endogenous or exogenous Cushing's disease, immunosuppression, or a malnourished state. There are two species in the genus *Malassezia: M. furfur,* which has an obligate nutritional requirement for fatty acids, and *M. pachydermatis,* which can be isolated from clinical material without addition of fatty acids to the medium.[68]

In its true sense, tinea versicolor represents an opportunistic infection, although specific deficiencies in antibodies or complement components have not been associated with disease. Experimentally,

inoculation of the organism under occlusion can cause infection.[69] The resulting increase in humidity, temperature, and CO_2 tension appear to be important factors that make the skin susceptible to infection.[68] When the occlusive state is terminated, self-healing occurs. The organism is not eradicated from the skin and can be cultured from clinically resolved areas.[69] It may also colonize follicular structures. For these reasons, a high clinical recurrence rate is expected.

Clinical Features

Cutaneous infections with *M. furfur* may take three forms: (1) papulosquamous lesions, (2) folliculitis, and (3) inverse tinea versicolor.

The most common presentation is scaly hypo- or hyperpigmented macules observed in characteristic areas of the body—e.g., the chest, back, abdomen, and proximal extremities (Fig. 207-6). Less common areas of involvement include the face, scalp, and genitalia. The characteristic scale is described as dustlike or furfuraceous. This characteristic feature of the disease can be produced by lightly scraping a scalpel blade over the involved skin.[69] The color of the lesions varies from almost white to reddish-brown or fawn-colored. The presenting complaint is usually a cosmetic one as lesions often fail to tan with sun exposure. Pruritus is mild or absent.

The yeast may filter the rays of the sun and interfere with normal tanning.[68] Also, the metabolites of *M. furfur* can cause depigmentation by inhibiting tyrosinase.[66]

In *Pityrosporum* folliculitis, lesions typically appear on the back, chest, and sometimes the extremities. Pruritus is more common than with typical tinea versicolor. The primary lesion is a perifollicular, erythematous 2- to 3-mm papule or pustule. Only by appropriate culture and KOH examination can it be distinguished from a bacterial folliculitis. Frequently, biopsy with special stains for fungus is necessary (Fig. 207-7*B*). Diabetes mellitus[68] or prior glucocorticoid or antibiotic therapy[66] can predispose one to this disorder.

Inverse tinea versicolor refers to clinical disease located predominantly in flexural areas.[70] In this location, lesions can be confused with seborrheic dermatitis, psoriasis, erythrasma, candidiasis, and dermatophyte infections.

Rarely, *M. furfur* can infect organs other than the skin. A premature infant on total parenteral nutrition with intravenous lipid supplementation has been reported who showed no skin lesions but had an extensive vasculitis of small pulmonary arteries as well as bronchopneumonia. *M. furfur* organisms were seen microscopically in areas of lipid deposition. The organism has been cultured from peritoneal dialysate, blood, and—with increasing frequency—from patients receiving parenteral intravenous lipid supplementation. Presumably, this provides an appropriate culture medium for *M. furfur*.[68]

All of the cutaneous clinical variants have an equal sex distribution and tend to flare during warm weather. Late-adolescent and early adult age groups are predominantly affected. Small children and elderly adults are infected only in unusual circumstances, such as prolonged occlusion or immunosuppression.[68]

Immunology

Immunologic data are scarce in tinea versicolor. No specific deficiencies in antibodies or complement components have been associated with disease. Elevated specific antibody is seen in patients and also in age-matched normal controls.[71] Furthermore, Sohnle and Collins-Lech have shown that *M. furfur* induces IgA, IgG, and IgM

FIGURE 207-6

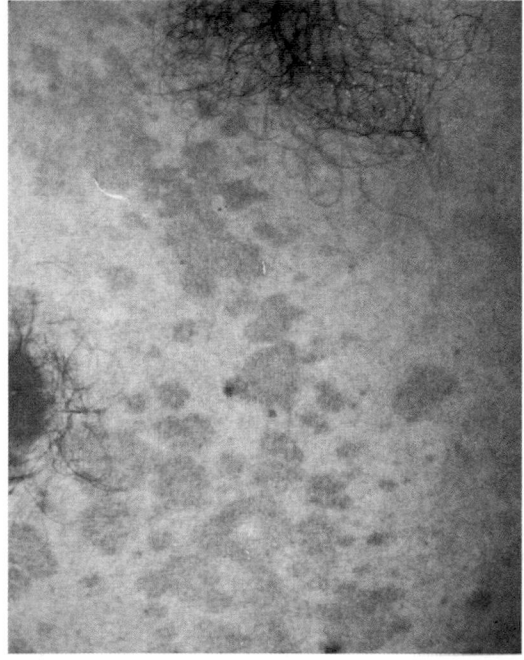

A.

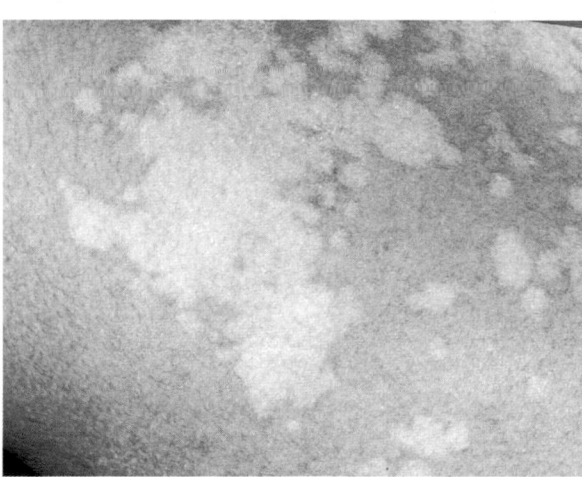

B.

A. Pityriasis versicolor. These lesions are darker because of hyperemia secondary to inflammatory response and increase in melaninization. *B.* Tinea versicolor. There are sharply marginated, uniformly hypopigmented macules with a fine, sometimes barely perceptible scale, but they are easily scraped off with a microscopic slide. When the lesions are very large, as on the left, they can be confused with vitiligo.

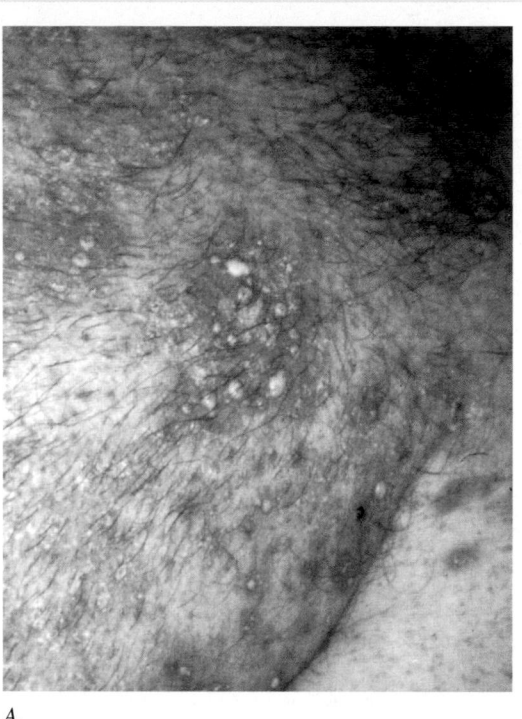

A.

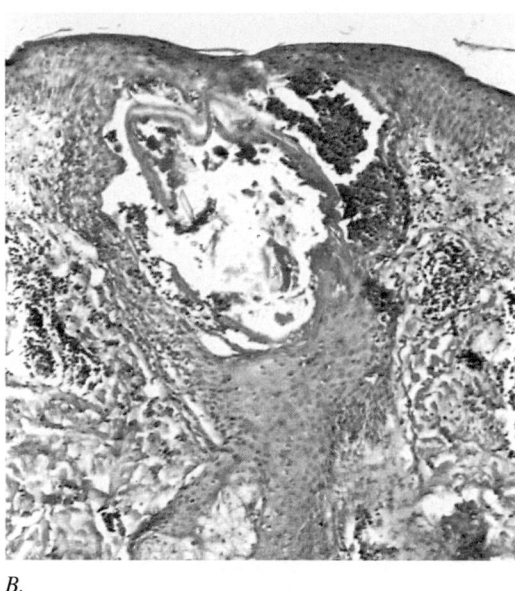

B.

A., B. Pityrosporum folliculitis on the anterior chest. Note the organisms in the follicular ostia on staining with hematoxylin and eosin.

antibodies and that it also activates complement through the alternative and classical pathways.[72] A defect in lymphokine production by patients with chronic tinea versicolor has been demonstrated, but the role that these and other immunologic factors play in the disease process in unknown.[73]

Laboratory Findings

The organism is readily identified in clinical material by treating specimens with 10% potassium hydroxide (KOH). Alternatively, cellophane tape can be used to pick up skin scales from the lesion.

The tape is mounted on a glass slide with methylene blue and the organism is selectively stained.[74] Microscopically, grapelike clusters of yeasts (4 to 6 μm) and short, septate branching hyphal fragments are seen (Fig. 207-8). Cultures are not necessary for diagnosis because of the characteristic "spaghetti and meatballs" appearance of the yeast and hyphal elements seen on microscopic examination of clinical material. A Wood's lamp examination may show yellowish fluorescence of involved skin.

FIGURE 207-8

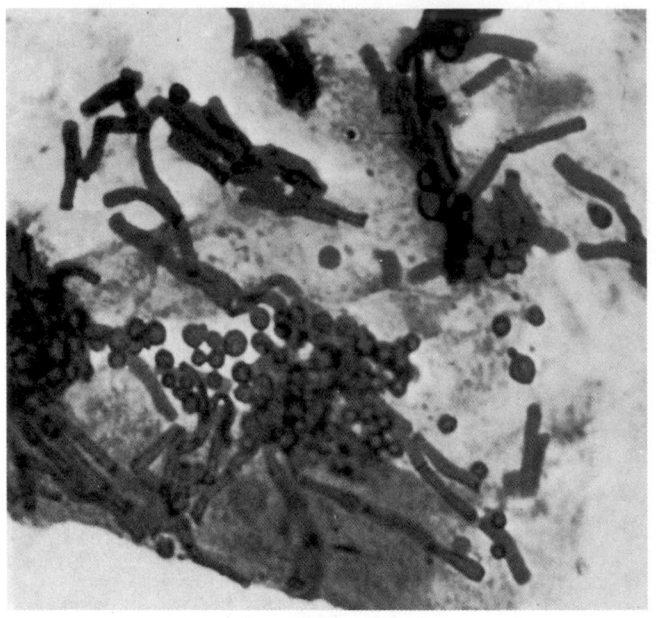

"Spaghetti and meatballs" appearance of tinea versicolor on KOH preparation.

Pathology

In tinea versicolor, the organisms are seen in the stratum corneum. They may be observed with H&E stain alone. PAS staining is confirmatory. There is usually no dermal infiltrate. In *Pityrosporum* folliculitis, organisms are noted in widened follicular ostia admixed with keratinous material (Fig. 207-7*B*). Rupture of the follicular wall can occur, with a resulting mixed inflammatory cell and foreign-body giant cell response. Organisms can occasionally be identified in the perifollicular dermis.

Diagnosis

The clinical appearance of tinea versicolor is usually characteristic, and KOH examination is confirmatory. Occasionally, pityriasis alba, confluent and reticulated papillomatosis of Gougerot and Carteaud, pityriasis rosea, seborrheic dermatitis, vitiligo, or secondary syphilis can enter the differential diagnosis.

For the folliculitis variant, bacterial or candidal folliculitis should be considered. The skin lesions of disseminated candidiasis can sometimes be confused with *Pityrosporum* folliculitis.[75]

Mycology

Sabouraud's dextrose agar overlaid on the surface with sterile olive oil or lanolin readily supports the growth of this lipophilic, yeastlike organism. Antibiotics such as penicillin, streptomycin, and cycloheximide are incorporated into this medium when primary clinical specimens are cultured to reduce growth of contaminating organisms. Microscopic examination reveals oval budding yeast cells ~3.5 × 4.5 μm along with short, septate, and occasionally branching hyphae (Fig. 207-8). In general, cultures are not necessary for diagnosis as the organism can be demonstrated with 10% KOH.

Treatment

There are multiple topical products that are useful in treating tinea versicolor. The most widely used has been 2.5% selenium sulfide shampoo. This should be applied liberally over and beyond the affected areas, left on for 10 min, and then washed off. The cycle is repeated every day for 2 weeks. Subsequently, we recommend applying the drug once or twice per month to prevent recurrence. All the topical azole antifungals have been effective in the treatment of tinea versicolor. While topical therapy is ideal for this condition, which involves the stratum corneum, patients often prefer the convenience of oral therapy. Cure rates range from 90 to 100 percent with ketoconazole and itraconazole and are about 75 percent with fluconazole.[69]

Course and Prognosis

Tinea versicolor is often recurrent. Prophylactic measures, as discussed above, and fastidious cleanliness may lessen the risk of recurrence.

REFERENCES

1. Fidel PL Jr et al: *Candida*-specific cell-mediated immunity is demonstrable in mice with experimental vaginal candidiasis. *Infect Immun* **61**:1990, 1993
2. Fotos PG, Lilly JP: Clinical management of oral and perioral candidosis. *Dermatol Clin* **14**:273, 1996
3. Ray TL, Wuepper KD: Recent advances in cutaneous candidiasis. *Int J Dermatol* **17**:683, 1978
4. Ray TL et al: Experimental cutaneous candidiasis: Role of the stratum corneum. *Clin Res* **24**:495A, 1976
5. Maibach HI, Kligman AM: The biology of experimental human cutaneous moniliasis (*Candida albicans*). *Arch Dermatol* **85**:233, 1962
6. Dupont PF: *Candida albicans,* the opportunist. *J Am Podiatr Med Assoc* **85**:104, 1995
7. Rebora A et al: Experimental infection with *Candida albicans*. *Arch Dermatol* **108**:69, 1973
8. Ray TL et al: Purification of a mannan from *Candida albicans* which activates serum complement. *J Invest Dermatol* **73**:269, 1979
9. Chesney RW et al: *Candida* endocrinopathy syndrome with membranoproliferative glomerulonephritis: Demonstration of glomerular *Candida* antigen. *Clin Nephrol* **5**:232, 1976
10. Odds FC: Pathogenesis of *Candida* infections. *J Am Acad Dermatol* **31**:S2, 1994
11. Ray TL, Wuepper KD: Experimental cutaneous candidiasis in rodents. II. Role of the stratum corneum barrier and serum complement as a mediator of a protective inflammatory response. *Arch Dermatol* **114**:539, 1978
12. Solomkin JS et al: Phagocytosis of *Candida albicans* by human leukocytes: Opsonic requirements. *J Infect Dis* **137**:30, 1978
13. Wilton JMA et al: The role of F_c and $C3_b$ receptors in phagocytosis by inflammatory polymorphonuclear leukocytes in man. *Immunology* **32**:955, 1977
14. Lehrer RT, Cline MJ: Interaction of *Candida albicans* with human leukocytes and serum. *J Bacteriol* **98**:996, 1969
15. Caroline L et al: Reversal of serum fungistasis by addition of iron. *J Invest Dermatol* **42**:415, 1964
16. Boxer LA et al: Lactoferrin deficiency associated with altered granulocyte function. *N Engl J Med* **307**:404, 1982
17. Kirkpatrick CH: Chronic mucocutaneous candidiasis. *Eur J Clin Microbiol Infect Dis* **8**:448, 1989
18. Zegarelli DJ: Fungal infections of the oral cavity. *Otolaryngol Clin North Am* **26**:1069, 1993
19. McNally MA, Langlais RP: Conditions peculiar to the tongue. *Dermatol Clin* **14**:257, 1996
20. Bunetel L, Bonnaure-Mallet M: Oral pathoses caused by *Candida albicans* during chemotherapy, in *Oral Medicine,* edited by J Jacobson, M Van Dis. St Louis, Mosby, 1996
21. Deslauriers N et al: Topical application of a corticosteroid destabilizes the host-parasite relationship in an experimental model of the oral carrier state of *Candida albicans*. *FEMS Immunol Med Microbiol* **11**:45, 1995

22. Coogan MM et al: Immunoglobulin A (IgA), and IgA$_2$ antibodies to *Candida albicans* in whole and parotid saliva in human immunodeficiency virus infection and AIDS. *Infect Immun* **62**:892, 1994

23. Greenspan D: Treatment of oral candidiasis in HIV infection. *Oral Surg Oral Med Oral Pathol* **78**:211, 1994

24. Reichart PA et al: *Candida*-associated palatal papillary hyperplasia in HIV infection. *J Oral Pathol Med* **23**:403, 1994

25. Plettenberg A et al: Fluconazole therapy of oral candidiasis in HIV-infected patients: Results of a multicentre study. *Infection* **22**:118, 1994

26. Reef SE, Mayer KH: Opportunistic candidal infections in patients infected with human immunodeficiency virus: Prevention issues and priorities. *Clin Infect Dis* **21**(suppl 1):S99, 1995

27. McCormack WM et al: The incidence of genitourinary infections in a cohort of healthy women. *Sex Transm Dis* **63**:63, 1993

28. Reef SE et al: Treatment options for vulvovaginal candidiasis, 1993. *Clin Infect Dis* **20**(suppl 1):S80, 1995

29. MacDonald TM et al: The risks of symptomatic vaginal candidiasis after oral antibiotic therapy. *Q J Med* **86**:419, 1993

30. Geiger AM, Foxman B: Risk factors for vulvovaginal candidiasis: A case-control study among university students. *Epidemiology* **7**:182, 1996

31. Spinillo A et al: Epidemiologic characteristics of women with idiopathic recurrent vulvovaginal candidiasis. *Obstet Gynecol* **81**:721, 1993

32. English JC III et al: Dermatoses of the glans penis and prepuce. *J Am Acad Dermatol* **37**:1, 1997

33. Pariser DM: Cutaneous candidiasis. *Postgrad Med* **87**:101, 1990

34. Singalavanija S, Frieden IJ: Diaper dermatitis. *Pediatr Rev* **16**:142, 1995

35. Giandoni MB, Grabski WJ: Cutaneous candidiasis as a cause of delayed surgical wound healing. *J Am Acad Dermatol* **30**:981, 1994

36. Jorizzo JL: The spectrum of mucosal and cutaneous candidosis. *Dermatol Clin* **2**:19, 1984

37. Ray TL: Candidosis, in *Dermatologic Immunology and Allergy*, edited by J Stone. St Louis, Mosby, 1985, p 511

38. Bradford LG, Montes LF: Perioral dermatitis and *Candida albicans*. *Arch Dermatol* **105**:892, 1972

39. Brandrup F et al: Perioral pustular eruption caused by *Candida albicans*. *Br J Dermatol* **105**:327, 1981

40. Hay RJ: Yeast infections. *Dermatol Clin* **14**:113, 1996

41. Santos LA et al: Congenital cutaneous candidiasis: Report of four cases and review of the literature. *Eur J Pediatr* **150**:336, 1991

42. Anaissie E, Pinczowski H: Invasive candidiasis during granulocytopenia. *Cancer Res* **132**:137, 1993

43. Edwards JE et al: Ocular manifestations of *Candida* septicemia: Review of seventy-six cases of hematogenous *Candida* endophthalmitis. *Medicine* **53**:47, 1974

44. Jarowski CI et al: Fever, rash, and muscle tenderness: A distinctive clinical presentation of disseminated candidiasis. *Arch Intern Med* **138**:544, 1978

45. Kressel B et al: Early clinical recognition of disseminated candidiasis by muscle and skin biopsy. *Arch Intern Med* **138**:429, 1978

46. File TM et al: Necrotic skin lesions associated with disseminated candidiasis. *Arch Dermatol* **115**:214, 1979

47. Fine JD et al: Cutaneous lesions in disseminated candidiasis mimicking ecthyma gangrenosum. *Am J Med* **70**:1133, 1981

48. Collignon PJ, Sorrell TC: Disseminated candidiasis: Evidence of a distinctive syndrome in heroin abusers. *Br Med J* **287**:861, 1983

49. Kirkpatrick CH: Chronic mucocutaneous candidiasis. *J Am Acad Dermatol* **31**:S14, 1994

50. Jorizzo JL: Chronic mucocutaneous candidosis: An update. *Arch Dermatol* **118**:963, 1982

51. Herrod HG: Chronic mucocutaneous candidiasis in childhood and complications of non-*Candida* infection: A report of the Pediatric Immunodeficiency Collaborative Study Group. *J Pediatr* **116**:377, 1990

52. Van Scoy RE et al: Familial neutrophil chemotaxis defect, recurrent bacterial infections, mucocutaneous candidiasis, and hyperimmunoglobulinemia E. *Ann Intern Med* **82**:766, 1975

53. Durandy A et al: Mannan-specific and mannan-induced T-cell suppressive activity in patients with chronic mucocutaneous candidiasis. *J Clin Immunol* **7**:400, 1987

54. Rogers TJ, Balish E: Immunity to *Candida albicans*. *Microbiol Rev* **44**:660, 1980

55. Penn RL et al: Invasive fungal infections: The use of serologic tests in diagnosis and management. *Arch Intern Med* **143**:1215, 1983

56. Bodey GP, Luna M: Skin lesions associated with disseminated candidiasis. *JAMA* **229**:1466, 1974

57. Klotz SA et al: *Pityrosporum* folliculitis: Its potential for confusion with skin lesions of systemic candidiasis. *Arch Intern Med* **142**:2126, 1982

58. Blatchford NR: Treatment of oral candidosis with itraconazole: A review. *J Am Acad Dermatol* **23**:565, 1990

59. Sobel JD: Controversial aspects in the management of vulvovaginal candidiasis. *J Am Acad Dermatol* **31**:S10, 1994

60. O-Prasertsawat P, Bourlert A: Comparative study of fluconazole and clotrimazole for the treatment of vulvovaginal candidiasis. *Sex Transm Dis* **22**:228, 1995

61. Stein GE, Mummaw N: Placebo-controlled trial of itraconazole for treatment of acute vaginal candidiasis. *Antimicrob Agents Chemother* **37**:89, 1993

62. Stein GE et al: Prevention of recurrent vaginal candidiasis with weekly terconazole cream. *Ann Pharmacol* **30**:1080, 1996

63. Desai PC, Johnson BA: Oral fluconazole for vaginal candidiasis. *Am Fam Phys* **54**:1337, 1996

64. Schuman P et al: Weekly fluconazole for the prevention of mucosal candidiasis in women with HIV infection. *Ann Intern Med* **126**:689, 1997

65. Roberts SOB: Pityriasis versicolor: A clinical and mycological investigation. *Br J Dermatol* **81**:315, 1969

66. Schmidt A: *Malassezia furfur*: A fungus belonging to the physiological skin flora and its relevance in skin disorders. *Cutis* **59**:21, 1997

67. Baillon H: *Traite de Botanique Medical Cryptoganique*. Paris, Octave Doin Editeur, 1889, p 234

68. Silva-Lizama E: Tinea versicolor. *Int J Dermatol* **34**:611, 1995

69. Savin R: Diagnosis and treatment of tinea versicolor. *J Fam Prac* **43**:127, 1996

70. Burkhart CG et al: An unusual case of tinea versicolor in an immunosuppressed patient. *Cutis* **27**:56, 1981

71. DaMert GJ et al: Comparison of antibody responses in chronic mucocutaneous candidiasis and tinea versicolor. *Int Arch Allergy Appl Immunol* **63**:97, 1980

72. Sohnle RG, Collins-Lech C: Activation of complement by *Pityrosporum orbiculare*. *J Invest Dermatol* **80**:93, 1983

73. Sohnle RG, Collins-Lech C: Cell-mediated immunology to *Pityrosporum orbiculare* in tinea versicolor. *J Clin Invest* **62**:45, 1978

74. Dominguez-Soto L et al: Pigmentary problems in the tropics. *Dermatol Clin* **12**:777, 1994

75. Klotz SA et al: *Pityrosporum* folliculitis: Its potential for confusion with skin lesions of systemic candidiasis. *Arch Intern Med* **142**:2126, 1982

Deep Fungal Infections

Deep fungal infections comprise two distinct groups of conditions, the subcutaneous and systemic mycoses. Neither are common, and the subcutaneous mycoses, with some exceptions, are largely confined to the tropics and subtropics. In recent years the systemic mycoses have become important opportunistic infectious complications in immunocompromised patients, including those with AIDS and patients receiving treatment for malignancies. They also include a group of primary respiratory infections such as histoplasmosis and coccidioidomycosis, which may affect otherwise healthy individuals and those with underlying illness. The fungi that cause these respiratory infections are usually dimorphic or exist in a different morphologic phase, e.g., yeast or mold, at different stages of their life cycle.

Patients with subcutaneous fungal infections usually present to a physician with signs of skin involvement. By contrast, patients with systemic mycoses only occasionally have skin lesions, either following direct involvement of the skin as a portal of entry or after dissemination from a deep focus of infection. There are a number of excellent texts about fungi and the diseases they cause.[1–4]

SUBCUTANEOUS MYCOSES

The subcutaneous mycoses, or mycoses of implantation, are infections caused by fungi that have been introduced directly into the dermis or subcutaneous tissue through a penetrating injury, such as a thorn prick. Although many are tropical infections, some, such as sporotrichosis, are also prevalent in temperate climates; any of these infections may present as an imported disease in a patient who has originated from an endemic area, sometimes after a lapse of many years. The most common subcutaneous mycoses are sporotrichosis, mycetoma, and chromoblastomycosis. Rarer infections include lobomycosis and subcutaneous zygomycosis.

Sporotrichosis

Sporotrichosis is a subcutaneous or systemic fungal infection caused by the dimorphic fungus *Sporothrix schenckii*.[5,6] The fungus occurs in the natural environment, presumably in mold form, but develops in its yeast phase in infections. The most frequent site of this infection is the dermis or subcutis. However, there is also a systemic form of sporotrichosis whose clinical features range from pulmonary infection to arthritis or meningitis. One important characteristic of the diagnosis of cutaneous lesions is the scarcity of organisms in tissue, making confirmation of the diagnosis potentially difficult.[6] Sometimes in tissue, fungal cells are surrounded by an eosinophilic refractile fringe, the asteroid body, which is a characteristic of the organism, although a similar phenomenon may occur with other infections.

HISTORIC ASPECTS The first published case in the western literature was in 1898 by Schenck from the Johns Hopkins Hospital. Subsequently, a series of reports appeared in France from 1903 onwards that described the disease and its treatment with potassium iodide. One important feature of the infection is the development of clusters of cases in defined geographic areas. For instance, there was a major outbreak of sporotrichosis in the South African gold mines from 1941 to 1944.[7]

EPIDEMIOLOGY Infections occur in both temperate and tropical countries. They are seen in North, South, and Central America, including the southern United States and Mexico, as well as in Africa, Egypt, Japan, and Australia.[6] The countries where high rates of infection occur are Mexico, Brazil, and South Africa. In the United States infections are most common in the midwestern river valleys. Infections are now rare in much of Europe. In nature, the fungus grows on decaying vegetable matter such as plant debris, leaves, and wood. Although it is usually a cause of sporadic infection, *S. schenckii* may also affect groups of workers exposed to the organism, such as those using straw as a packing material, gardeners, and forestry workers, and those whose recreational activities may bring them into contact with plant debris. The organism is thought to be introduced into the skin through a local injury.

CLINICAL MANIFESTATIONS The two clinical varieties of sporotrichosis are the subcutaneous and systemic forms of disease.[5,8,9] Subcutaneous sporotrichosis is by far the more common and includes two main forms: *lymphangitic infection* and *fixed infection*. The lymphangitic form is the more common and usually develops on exposed skin sites such as hands or feet. The first sign of infection is the appearance of a dermal nodule that breaks down into a small ulcer. Draining lymphatics become inflamed and swollen, and a chain of secondary nodules develops along the course of the lymphatic (Fig. 208-1); these may also break down and ulcerate. In the fixed variety, which accounts for about 15 percent of cases, the infection remains localized to one site, such as the face, and a granuloma develops that may subsequently ulcerate. Satellite nodules may form around the rim of the primary lesion. Other clinical variants of subcutaneous sporotrichosis may mimic mycetoma, lupus vulgaris, and chronic venous ulceration. In some cases, deep extension of the infection may affect joints or tendon sheaths. Patients with AIDS who develop sporotrichosis often have multiple cutaneous lesions[9] without prominent lymphatic involvement, but deep infections such as arthritis are also reported (see below).

In the much rarer systemic form of sporotrichosis lesions can develop almost anywhere, although chronic lung nodules with cav-

FIGURE 208-1

CHAPTER 208
Deep Fungal Infections

2373

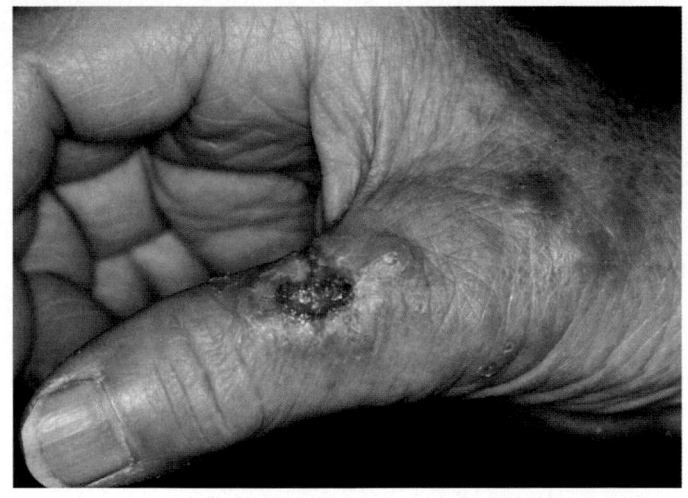

Sporotrichosis. An ulcerated nodule is seen on the thumb with proximal lymphangitic spread represented by subcutaneous nodules. (*Courtesy of Takeji Nishikawa, MD.*)

itation, arthritis, and meningitis have been described most frequently. These may coexist with cutaneous lesions of sporotrichosis.

DIFFERENTIAL DIAGNOSIS Conditions commonly confused with sporotrichosis are mycobacterial infections and leishmaniasis. The nontuberculous mycobacterial infection due to *Mycobacterium marinum* (fish-tank granuloma), in particular, closely resembles lymphangitic sporotrichosis.

LABORATORY DIAGNOSIS The best sources of diagnostic material are smears, exudates, and biopsies. *S. schenckii* is very rarely seen in direct microscopic examination because yeasts are usually present only in small numbers; the organism can be readily isolated on Sabouraud's agar. In primary culture the fungus grows as a mold, with compact, white colonies that darken with age. Microscopically, the hyphae produce small oval or triangular conidia either on specialized hyphae or elsewhere on the mycelium. Ideally, the organism should be converted to yeast phase on enriched media such as brain-heart infusion (BHI) agar at 37°C in order to complete the identification.

Sporotrichosis causes a mixed granulomatous reaction with neutrophil microabscesses. The fungus, if present, is usually in the form of small (3 to 5 μm) cigar shaped or oval yeasts that may, on occasion, be surrounded by a thick, radiating eosinophilic fringe forming the distinctive asteroid body. Organisms are usually sparsely distributed in lesions, and it may be necessary to scan several sections in order to identify one yeast. A sporotrichin skin test is available in many Latin American countries and may have a role to play in allowing the physician to identify the most appropriate laboratory investigations to instigate.

TREATMENT While spontaneous remissions may occur, most patients are treated with antifungal chemotherapy. Potassium iodide (saturated solution), 4 to 6 mL tid, is effective in the cutaneous types of sporotrichosis and should be continued for 3 to 4 weeks after clinical cure. The daily dose is built up slowly from 1 mL tid over 2 to 3 weeks to avoid side effects such as hypersalivation and nausea. This is an inexpensive form of therapy but it is unpalatable.

Alternative treatments include itraconazole, 200 mg[10] daily, or terbinafine, 250 mg daily, which are better tolerated, and intravenous amphotericin B. In all cases treatment is continued for at least 1 week after clinical resolution.

Mycetoma (Maduromycosis, Madura Foot)

Mycetoma is a chronic localized infection caused by different species of fungi or actinomycetes. It is characterized by the formation of aggregates of the causative organisms, known as "grains," that are found within abscesses. These either communicate via sinuses onto the skin surface or involve adjacent bone causing a form of osteomyelitis. Grains are discharged onto the skin surface via these sinuses. The disease advances by direct spread and distant metastatic sites of infection are very rare. Mycetomas caused by species of fungi are known as *eumycetomas*, and those caused by aerobic actinomycetes or filamentous bacteria as *actinomycetomas*. The organisms are usually soil or plant saprophytes[11] that are only incidental human pathogens.

HISTORIC ASPECTS Although this is a disease of great antiquity, the original description of the disease in the western literature was in 1694 by Engelbert Kaempfer, a German physician in southern India. Over a century elapsed before the disease was redescribed by an English army surgeon, called Gill, working in southern India in 1842. Subsequent cases from India, Africa, and South America confirmed the presence of the disease in a wide variety of tropical countries.

EPIDEMIOLOGY Mycetomas are mainly, but not exclusively, found in the dry tropics where there is low annual rainfall.[11,12] They are sporadic infections that are seldom common, even in endemic areas.[13] Occasionally nonimported cases are reported from temperate climates, although in these cases the commonest organism is *Scedosporium apiospermum*. Actinomycetomas due to *Nocardia* species are most common in Central America and Mexico (Table 208-1). In other parts of the world the commonest organism is a fungus, *Madurella mycetomatis*. The actinomycete *Streptomyces somaliensis* is most often isolated from patients originating from Sudan and the Middle East. The causative organisms of mycetoma have been isolated from either soil or plant material, including Acacia thorns, in endemic areas.

The organisms are implanted subcutaneously, usually after a penetrating injury. It is unusual to find any underlying predisposition in patients with mycetoma, and the persistence of the organism after the initial inoculation appears to be related to its ability to evade host defenses through a variety of adaptations such as cell-wall thickening and melanin deposition.[14]

CLINICAL MANIFESTATIONS The clinical features of both fungal and actinomycete mycetomas are very similar.[12] They are most common on the foot, lower leg, or hand, although head or back involvement may also occur. Infection of the chest wall is most characteristic of *Nocardia* infections. The earliest stage of infection is a firm painless nodule that spreads slowly with the development of papules and draining sinus tracts over the surface (Fig. 208-2). Local tissue swelling, chronic sinus formation, and later bone involvement distort and deform the original site of infection (Figs. 208-3 and 208-4). Lesions are seldom painful except in the late stages and where sinus tracts are about to emerge onto the skin

TABLE 208-1

Macroscopic and Histopathologic Features of Mycetoma Grains

ORGANISMS	H&E SECTION APPEARANCES
Eumycetoma	
Dark grains	
Madurella mycetomatis	Cement present, vesicles sometimes prominent
M. grisea	Cement absent, compact outer layer
Leptosphaeria senegalensis	Cement in outer zone, dark periphery with vesicular center
Exophiala jeanselmei	Cement absent, often hollow
Pyrenochaeta romeroi	Cement lacking, compact outer layer
Pale grains	
Fusarium spp.	
Acremonium spp.	Compact, pigment lacking, interwoven fungal filaments (S. apiospermum may have prominent vesicles)
Scedosporium apiospermum	
Aspergillus nidulans	
Neotestudina rosati	
Actinomycetoma	
Pale (white to yellow) grains	
Actinomadura madura	Basophilic-stained fringe in layers
Nocardia brasiliensis	Small, pale blue, eosinophilic fringe
Yellow to brown grains	
Streptomyces somaliensis	Grains fractured, basophilic or pink
Red to pink grains	
A. pelletieri	Small, basophilic layers

NOTE: H&E, hematoxylin/eosin stain.

FIGURE 208-2

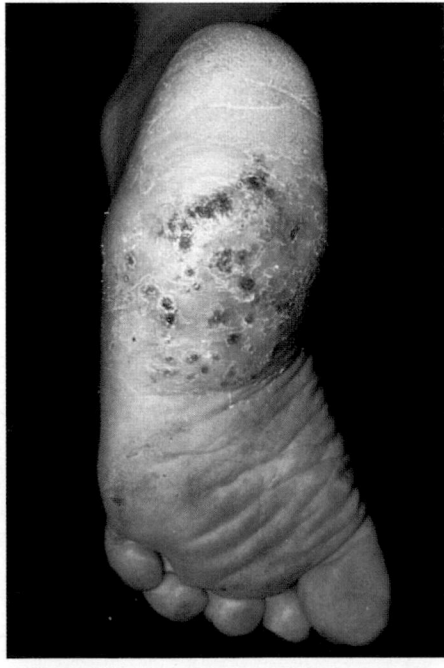

Mycetoma. Brawny edema and crusted papules on the plantar surface.

surface. Dissemination from the initial site is exceptionally rare, although local lymphadenopathy may occur.

X-ray changes include periosteal erosion and proliferation as well as the development of lytic lesions in the bone. Bone scans or magnetic resonance imaging may identify bone lesions at an earlier stage.

DIFFERENTIAL DIAGNOSIS Chronic bacterial or tuberculous osteomyelitis may resemble mycetoma. Actinomycosis (see below) is also similar but usually develops close to certain sites such as the mouth or the cecum where the causative organisms are sometimes commensal.

LABORATORY DIAGNOSIS Finding the mycetoma grains is the key to establishing the diagnosis, and these are generally discharged from the openings of sinus tracts. However, they may also be obtained by removing the surface crust from a pustule or sinus tract with a sterile needle and gently squeezing the edges. Grains are 250- to 1000-μm white, black, or red particles that can be picked out with the naked eye. Direct microscopy of grains is important as it will show whether the grain is composed of the small actinomycete or broader fungal filaments. In general, it is not possible to distinguish the fine actinomycete filaments in KOH mounts or, for that matter, in hematoxylin/eosin-stained material. In addition, black grains are always caused by fungi, red grains by actinomycetes (see Table 208-1).

Final identification requires isolation of the causal agent in culture. In view of the number of possible species, a series of different culture media and conditions of incubation should be employed. Morphologic and physiologic characteristics are used in distinguishing between the genera and species. Serology is only helpful in some cases, e.g., *S. somaliensis,* and even then it is more appropriate as a guide to therapeutic response.

Histologically there is a chronic inflammatory reaction with neutrophil abscesses and scattered giant cells and fibrosis.[11] Grains (50 to 250 μm) are found in the center of the inflammation. Their size and shape may help in the identification, although with nonpigmented fungal causes of mycetoma this is seldom sufficient (Fig. 208-5).

TREATMENT Actinomycetomas generally respond to antibiotics such as a combination of dapsone with streptomycin or sulfamethoxazole-trimethoprim plus rifampin or streptomycin. Amikacin may

FIGURE 208-3

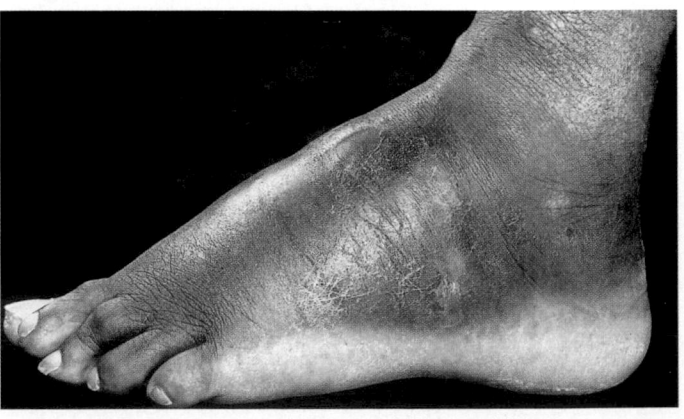

Eumycetoma caused by *Scedosporium.*

also be used in recalcitrant *Nocardia* infections. The responses in all but a few cases are good.[15]

Of the fungal causes of mycetoma, *M. mycetomatis* may respond to ketoconazole, 200 mg daily over several months. For the others, a trial of therapy with griseofulvin or itraconazole is worth attempting. However, responses to chemotherapy are unpredictable, although antifungals may slow the course of infection. Surgery, usually amputation, is the definitive procedure and may have to be used in advanced cases. However, the value of major surgery in a disfiguring but non-life-threatening infection has to be weighed against the availability of appropriate prosthetic limbs.

Chromoblastomycosis (Chromomycosis)

Chromoblastomycosis is a chronic fungal infection of the skin and subcutaneous tissues caused by pigmented or dematiaceous fungi that are implanted into the dermis from the environment. In the ensuing inflammation, they form thick-walled single cells or cell clusters (sclerotic or muriform bodies), and these may elicit a marked form of pseudoepitheliomatous hyperplasia often accompanied by transepidermal elimination of organisms. The infection can be caused by a number of different pigmented fungi, the commonest being *Phialophora verrucosa*, *Fonsecaea pedrosoi*, *F. compactum*, *Wangiella dermatitidis*, and *Cladosporium carrionii*.[16]

HISTORIC ASPECTS The first confirmed case was in a patient from New England described by Lane and Medlar in 1915, although subsequently most of the early reports came from Brazil. There is considerable confusion over the correct designation of the first reported isolates as their names have changed considerably over time. This problem of identification is discussed below.

EPIDEMIOLOGY The fungi that cause chromoblastomycosis can be isolated in the environment from wood, plant debris, or soil.[17] The vast majority of infections are caused by *F. pedrosoi* and *C. carrionii*. As with other subcutaneous mycoses, infection follows implantation through a tissue injury. The infection is found as a sporadic condition in Central and South, although rarely North, America. It occurs in the Caribbean region, Africa (particularly Madagascar), Australia, and Japan. It may also occur as an imported infection outside the usual endemic areas. The disease is most frequent in male rural workers.

CLINICAL MANIFESTATIONS The initial site of the infection is usually on the feet, legs, arms, or upper trunk. The clinical features vary.[17] The initial lesion is often a warty papule that slowly expands over months or years (Figs. 208-6 and 208-7). Alternatively, lesions may be flatter and plaquelike with an atrophic center. The more common verrucous form spreads slowly and locally. Individual lesions may be very thick and often develop secondary bacterial infection. Satellite lesions around the initial site of infection are local extensions of the infection and are usually produced by scratching. Complications of chromoblastomycosis include local lymphedema leading to elephantiasis and squamous carcinomas in some chronic lesions.

DIFFERENTIAL DIAGNOSIS The disease must be differentiated from chronic tropical lymphedema with hyperplasia—mossy foot. Other chronic verrucous lesions such as tuberculosis and blasto-

FIGURE 208-4

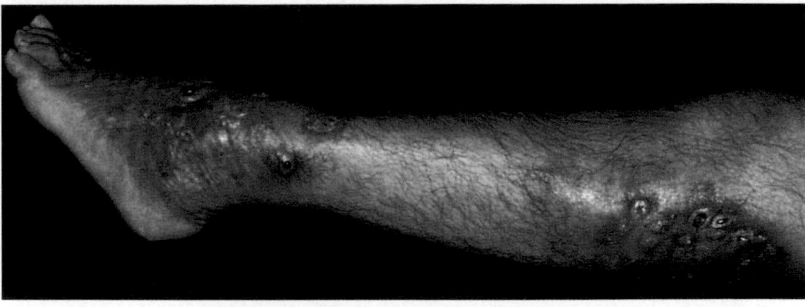

Mycetoma. Chronic fibrotic involvement of the foot with lymphatic spread to the popliteal fossa.

mycosis are often more extensive. The identification of organisms in the lesions of chromoblastomycosis is essential.

LABORATORY DIAGNOSIS The typical sclerotic or muriform fungal cells can be seen in skin scrapings taken from the surface of lesions using KOH mounts. The lesions should also be biopsied, as the pathologic changes and presence of muriform cells are typical. The histology shows a mixed granulomatous response, with small neutrophil abscesses and often exuberant epidermal hyperplasia.[18] The organisms, which are often seen either in giant cells or in neutrophil abscesses, appear singly or in small groups of brown pigmented cells, often with a single or double septum and thick cell wall.

In culture these fungi are very similar in gross macroscopic appearance, producing black colonies with a downy surface. Their cultural identification depends on demonstrating the presence of different but specific types of sporulation, and either single or multiple sporulation mechanisms may be seen in each organism. Accurate differentiation between the different fungi may be difficult. At this stage the choice of treatment does not depend critically on the cor-

FIGURE 208-5

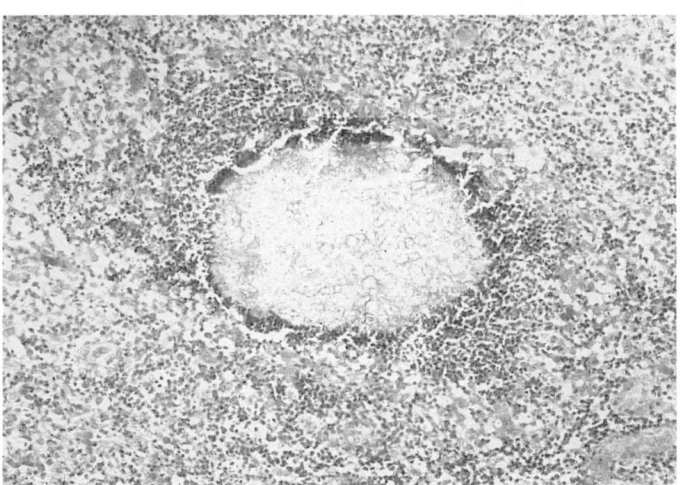

Pale eumycetoma grain. H&E stain.

FIGURE 208-6

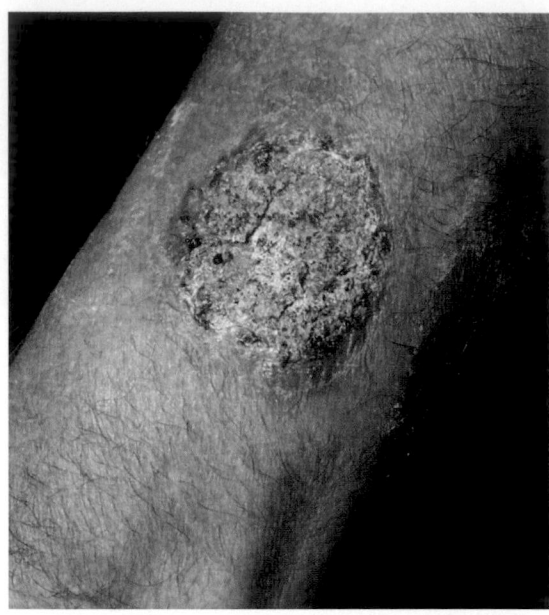

Chromoblastomycosis. A solitary, large verrucous plaque surrounded by a halo of erythema is seen on the calf. (*Courtesy of Ted Rosen, MD, and Howard Rubin, MD.*)

rect identification of the organisms, although there may be differences in the speed of response to azole drugs (see below).

TREATMENT   The main treatments for chromoblastomycosis are itraconazole, 200 mg daily, with or without flucytosine, 30 mg/kg qid (in a patient with normal renal function)[19]; terbinafine, 250 mg daily[20]; and, in extensive cases, intravenous amphotericin B (up to 1 mg/kg daily). Thiabendazole is a further alternative, although nausea and vomiting may limit the use of the drug. Lesions can be

FIGURE 208-7

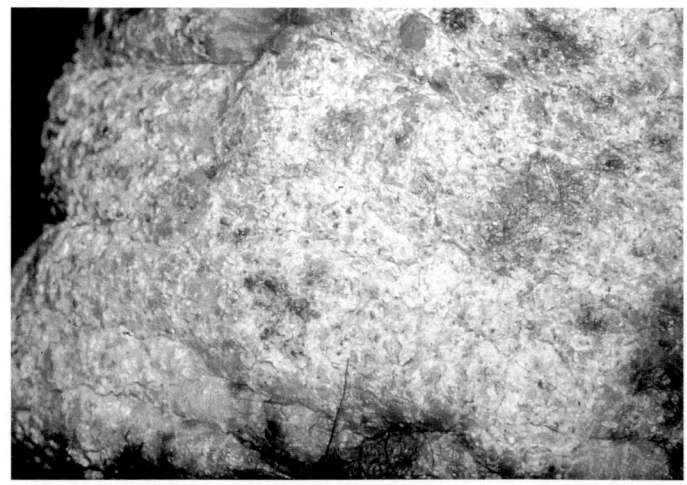

Close-up view of chromoblastomycosis.

spread by surgery, which should only be used as an adjunctive therapy after drug treatment. The local application of heat may be helpful in some instances. The responses of these fungi to different antifungals does not appear to differ significantly, although there is some evidence that *C. carrionii* responds more rapidly to itraconazole. In any event, treatment is continued until there is clinical resolution of lesions, which usually takes several months. Extensive lesions often respond poorly to treatment.

Phaeohyphomycosis (Phaeomycotic Cyst, Cystic Chromomycosis)

Phaeohyphomycosis is a rare infection characterized by the formation of subcutaneous inflammatory cysts. It is caused by dematiaceous fungi, the most common of which are *Exophiala jeanselmei* and *Wangiella dermatitidis,* but some 101 species have been described as causal agents.[21] However, unlike in chromoblastomycosis, these organisms form short irregular pigmented hyphae in tissue. The infection may occur in any climatic area, although it is commoner in the tropics. It may also appear in immunosuppressed patients, particularly those receiving long-term glucocorticoid therapy. The lesions present as cysts and may be mistaken for other similar structures such as Baker's cysts. The diagnosis is usually made after surgical excision. Histologically, the cyst wall consists of palisades of macrophages and other inflammatory cells surrounded by a fibrous capsule, and the fungal hyphae are found in the macrophage zone. Although the fungi in tissue lesions are usually pigmented, this is not always the case; if special melanin stains such as Masson-Fontana are used, the organisms will stain, showing that they can produce melanin in small quantities. The treatment is surgical excision, although relapse can occur, particularly in immunocompromised patients.

Lobomycosis (Keloidal Blastomycosis, Lobo's Disease)

This is an uncommon infection seen in Central and South America, often in remote rural areas. The source of the organism is unknown, although similar lesions have been found on fresh-water dolphins. Lobomycosis is characterized by the appearance of keloid-like skin lesions on exposed sites.[22] Although it cannot be cultured in vitro, it is caused by a fungus that forms chains of rounded cells in tissue, each joined by a small tubule. Lesions may occur anywhere on the body but are usually found on exposed parts such as the legs, arms, and face. They can spread from site to site by autoinoculation. Antifungal drugs are not effective, and surgical removal is the main treatment.

Subcutaneous Zygomycosis [Basidiobolomycosis, Subcutaneous Phycomycosis and Conidiobolomycosis, (Rhino)-Entomophthoromycosis]

This is a rare tropical subcutaneous mycosis characterized by the development and spread of a chronic firm swelling involving subcutaneous tissue. There are two main varieties, caused by different organisms.[23] The first, most often caused by *Basidiobolus ranarum* (*haptosporus*), is more common in children. It occurs in a wide variety of countries and environments from South America to Africa and Indonesia. The organism can be found in plant debris and in the intestinal tract of reptiles and amphibians. Lesions usually develop around limb girdle sites and present with a firm, slowly spreading, woody cellulitis. The second form, caused by *Conidiobolus coronatus*, is seen in adults. The organism can be isolated from soil, plant debris, and some insects. The early infection starts in the region of the inferior turbinates of the nose. Spread involves the central part of the face, and once again the swelling is hard and painless. It may cause very severe deformity of the nose, lips, and cheeks.

Histopathologically, a chronic granulomatous response with large numbers of eosinophils can be seen. The fungi are present as large straplike hyphae without cross walls or septa. They are also often surrounded by refractile eosinophilic material (Splendore-Hoeppli phenomenon). The organisms can be cultured readily on Sabouraud's agar. Lesions usually respond to oral treatment with potassium iodide, given in similar doses to those used in sporotrichosis (see above). Ketoconazole (400 mg daily) and itraconazole (100 to 200 mg daily) may also be useful in this condition, although experience to date is limited to a few cases.

Rhinosporidiosis

Rhinosporidiosis is a chronic infection caused by the organism *Rhinosporidium seeberi*, which causes the development of polyps affecting the mucous membranes. The organism has never been cultured and therefore its status as a fungus has been questioned. Rhinosporidiosis is seldom common but is most often seen in southern India and Sri Lanka. Cases have also been described in South America, the Caribbean, and South Africa. The main area involved is the nasal mucosa, but the conjunctival mucosa may also be affected.[24] The infection causes the development of large polyps that are studded with white flecks; these are small cysts or sporangia containing small spores. These are best seen in histopathologic sections where the large sporangia or spore sacs in different phases of development are readily seen. The only treatment is surgical excision.

SYSTEMIC MYCOSES

The systemic mycoses are fungal infections whose initial portal of entry into the body is usually a deep site such as the lung, gastrointestinal tract, or paranasal sinuses. They have the capacity to spread via the bloodstream to produce a generalized infection. In practice there are two main varieties of systemic mycosis—the opportunistic and endemic respiratory mycoses.

The chief opportunistic systemic mycoses seen in humans are systemic or deep candidiasis, aspergillosis, and systemic zygomycosis. These affect patients with severe underlying disease states, such as AIDS, or with neutropenia associated with malignancy, solid organ transplants, or extensive surgery. In the neutropenic patient, in particular, other fungi may also occasionally cause infection. Different underlying conditions predispose to different mycoses, and a scheme for this is shown in Table 208-2. Generally, skin involvement is not common with these opportunistic infections, which can occur in any climate and environment. The clinical manifestations of the opportunistic mycoses are also variable as they depend on the site of entry of organism and the underlying disease.

The endemic respiratory mycoses are histoplasmosis (classic and African types), blastomycosis, coccidioidomycosis, paracoccidioidomycosis, and infections due to *Penicillium marneffei*. The clinical manifestations of these infections are affected by the underlying state of the patient, and many develop in the presence of particular immunodeficiency states, notably AIDS. However, they follow similar clinical patterns in all infections. These infections may also affect otherwise healthy individuals. They have well-defined endemic areas determined by factors that favor the survival of the causative organisms in the environment, such as climate. The usual route of infection is via the lung.

In practice, because of the tendency for both groups of infections to develop in predisposed patients, the distinction between opportunistic and endemic mycoses is blurred. This is particularly the case with the deep infection cryptococcosis, which shares clinical and pathologic features of the two main types of systemic mycosis but is mainly seen now in AIDS patients.

Histoplasmosis

Fungi of the dimorphic genus *Histoplasma* cause a number of different infections in animals and humans. These range from equine farcy, or equine histoplasmosis, a disseminated infection of horses caused by *H. farciminosum*, to two human infections known as classic or small-form histoplasmosis and African histoplasmosis. These are caused, respectively, by two variants of *H. capsulatum*—*H. capsulatum* var. *capsulatum* and *H. capsulatum* var. *duboisii*. They can be distinguished because their respective yeast phases differ in size, the *capsulatum* variety producing cells from 2 to 5 μm in diameter, the *duboisii* form cells of 10 to 15 μm in diameter. The other important differences are in their epidemiology and clinical manifestations. They also show minor antigenic differences that are apparent in serodiagnosis, but their mycelial phases are identical. The two types of human infections will be referred to as histoplasmosis and African histoplasmosis, as this nomenclature is the most widely used.

HISTOPLASMOSIS (SMALL-FORM OR CLASSIC HISTOPLASMOSIS OR HISTOPLASMOSIS CAPSULATI) Histoplasmosis results from infection with the dimorphic fungus *H. capsulatum* var. *capsulatum*. A sexual state of this fungus, *Ajellomyces capsulatus*, has also been described. The infection starts as a pulmonary infection that, in most individuals, is asymptomatic and heals spontaneously, the only evidence of exposure being the development of a positive intradermal skin test reaction to a fungal antigenic extract, histoplasmin.[25] However, in addition, there is a symptomatic disease that includes respiratory infections and acute or chronic pulmonary histoplasmosis as well as a disseminated infection that may

TABLE 208-2

Underlying Predisposition and Opportunistic Systemic Mycoses

PREDISPOSITION	INFECTION
Neutropenia (whatever cause) or functional neutrophil defects	Aspergillosis, oropharyngeal and systemic candidiasis, zygomycosis, infections due to rare organisms
CD4 lymphopenia (e.g., AIDS)	Oropharyngeal candidiasis, cryptococcosis and endemic respiratory mycoses such as histoplasmosis, nocardiosis
Diabetes mellitus	Zygomycosis
Heart valve surgery	Various but mainly *C. albicans* and non-*albicans Candida* spp.
Abdominal surgery	Candidiasis

spread to affect the skin or mucous membranes. Direct inoculation into the skin may occur as a result of a laboratory accident.

Historic aspects Histoplasmosis was first recognized in Panama by Darling, in 1905, as the cause of death in a patient from Martinique. The proof that this was caused by a fungus rather than a protozoan came in 1929 when de Monbreun, at Vanderbilt University, TN, grew the organism in culture. Even so, its importance as a cause of a wider spectrum of infections including lung disease was not recognized until the 1940s.

Epidemiology Histoplasmosis occurs in many countries from the Americas to Africa, India, and the Far East. In the United States, it is endemic in the Mississippi and Ohio River valleys, where often more than 80 percent of the population may have acquired the infection asymptomatically. Exposure rates are usually lower in all other endemic areas, although high rates are also found in northern South America and some Caribbean islands. Histoplasmosis is not found in Europe. *H. capsulatum* is an environmental saprophyte that can be isolated from soil, particularly when it is contaminated with bird or bat excreta. The disease is acquired by inhalation of spores, and epidemics of respiratory infection may occur in persons exposed to a spore-laden environment when exploring caves or cleaning sites heavily contaminated with bird droppings, such as bird roosts or barns. Although any person can acquire histoplasmosis through inhalation, it may cause a distinctive disseminated infection in patients with disease affecting cellular immune capacity, such as AIDS or lymphoma.[26,27]

Clinical manifestations The spectrum of histoplasmosis includes asymptomatic as well as benign symptomatic infections and a progressive disseminated variety with bloodstream spread to multiple organs.[25] Skin lesions may develop as a result of immune complex formation in the primary infection (erythema multiforme) or from direct spread after dissemination from the lungs; more rarely, infections may develop at a point of inoculation into the skin.

Asymptomatic forms of histoplasmosis are by definition without signs or symptoms, but those exposed usually have a positive histoplasmin skin test. The percentage of skin test reactors in the community indicates the chances of exposure, and in endemic areas this may range from 5 to 90 percent. Occasionally, asymptomatic pulmonary nodules removed at surgical exploration or autopsy are found to contain *Histoplasma*.

ACUTE PULMONARY HISTOPLASMOSIS   In this form, patients are often exposed to large quantities of spores such as may be encountered in a cave or after cleaning a bird-infested area. Patients present with cough, chest pain, and fever, often with accompanying joint pains and rash—toxic erythema, erythema multiforme, or erythema nodosum. These skin rashes are not common, occuring in fewer than 15 percent of patients, but they may be precipitated by treatment of the acute infection. On chest x-ray there is often diffuse mottling, which may calcify with time.

CHRONIC PULMONARY HISTOPLASMOSIS   This usually occurs in adults and presents with pulmonary consolidation and cavitation, closely resembling tuberculosis. Skin involvement is not seen.

ACUTE DISSEMINATED HISTOPLASMOSIS   In these patients there is widespread dissemination to other organs such as the liver and spleen, lymphoreticular system, and bone marrow. Patients present with progressive weight loss and fever. This form is the type that is most likely to occur in AIDS patients, who often develop skin lesions as a manifestation of disseminated infection (Fig. 208-8).[27] These are papules, small nodules, or small molluscum-like lesions that may subsequently develop into shallow ulcers. Diffuse micronodular pulmonary infiltrates may also develop. Patients have pro-

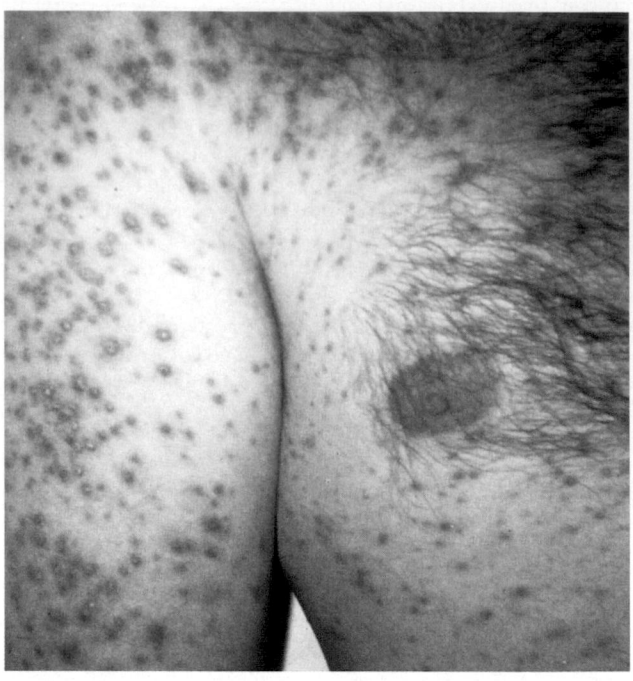

Histoplasmosis, disseminated. Multiple erythematous keratotic papules and small plaques resembling guttate pattern psoriasis are seen on the chest and arm of a male with advanced HIV disease. (*Courtesy of JD Fallon, MD.*)

gressive and severe weight loss, fever, anemia, and hepatosplenomegaly.

The distinction between acute and chronic dissemination in histoplasmosis is somewhat artificial as these merely represent extremes of behavior, with progression occurring over a few months on the one hand and over several years on the other. Intermediate forms occur, and other organs such as the meninges and heart may be affected.

CHRONIC DISSEMINATED HISTOPLASMOSIS   This may appear months or years after a patient has left an endemic area. The most common clinical presenting features are oral or pharyngeal ulceration or adrenal insufficiency (Addison's disease) due to adrenal infiltration. The mouth ulcers are often large, irregular, and persistent and affect the tongue as well as the buccal mucosa. The patients may otherwise appear well, but it is important to investigate them for evidence of infection elsewhere, e.g., by abdominal CT scan. Adrenal infection in particular should be excluded.

PRIMARY CUTANEOUS HISTOPLASMOSIS   This form is rare and follows inoculation of the organism into the skin, for instance, after accidental laboratory- or postmortem room–acquired infection. The primary lesion is a nodule or indurated ulcer, and there is often local lymphadenopathy.

Differential diagnosis The organism is the same size as a number of others causing deep mycoses such as *P. marneffei* and small forms of *Blastomyces* and *Cryptococcus* (see below). It is also similar in size to *Leishmania* species, and, in the tropics, kala-azar is an important part of the differential diagnosis. These observations emphasize the importance of carrying out appropriate laboratory tests to confirm the diagnosis.

Laboratory diagnosis The diagnosis of histoplasmosis is established by identifying the small intracellular yeastlike cells of *Histoplasma* in sputum, peripheral blood, bone marrow, or in biopsy specimens. *Histoplasma* must be separated from *P. marneffei* as the two organisms are of a similar size, although the latter shows characteristic septal formation. The identity of the organism should be confirmed by culture; it grows as a mold at room temperature. The white, cottony colonies develop at room temperature on Sabouraud's glucose agar to produce two types of spore, the larger (8 to 15 μm) rounded tuberculate macroconidia being typical; the smaller microconidia are infectious. Confirmation of the identity should be obtained by demonstrating the production of diffusing exoantigen by an immunodiffusion assay (exoantigen test). Mycelial-phase cultures of *H. capsulatum* are very infectious, and laboratories receiving specimens should be warned about the suspected diagnosis.

The intradermal histoplasmin skin test is an epidemiologic tool that is of no help in diagnosis. In patients with disseminated histoplasmosis it is often negative. By contrast, serology is often useful in diagnosis. A rising complement-fixation titer indicates dissemination. Precipitins detected by immunodiffusion are also valuable since the presence of antibodies to specific antigens, H and M antigens, correlates well with active or recent infection.[28] A new development, particularly helpful in AIDS patients, has been a serologic test for the detection of circulating *Histoplasma* antigen.[29] In histopathologic sections, *H. capsulatum* is an intracellular parasite often seen in macrophages. The cells are small (2 to 4 μm in diameter) and oval in shape with small buds (Fig. 208-9). Mycelial forms are rarely seen in tissue.

AFRICAN HISTOPLASMOSIS (LARGE-FORM HISTOPLASMO-SIS, OR HISTOPLASMOSIS DUBOISII) This infection is sporadic and uncommon.[30] It is seen in patients from areas south of the Sahara and north of the Zambezi river in Africa. Infections seen outside Africa are all imported. The most common clinically involved sites are the skin and bone, although lymph nodes and other organs, including the lungs, may be affected. Skin lesions range from small papules resembling molluscum contagiosum to cold abscesses, draining sinuses, or ulcers. It is not clear if there is an asymptomatic form of African histoplasmosis as in classic histoplasmosis. The diagnosis is confirmed by culture and microscopy (direct microscopy or histopathology). The organisms of *H. capsulatum* var. *duboisii* are different from the smaller *capsulatum* forms. They are usually 10 to 15 μm in diameter, slightly pear-shaped, and clustered in giant cells. *Histoplasma* serology, using conventional tests, is often negative in African histoplasmosis.

FIGURE 208-9

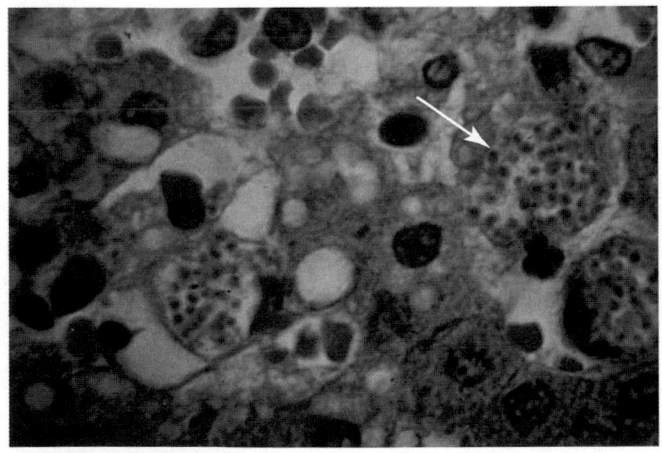

Histoplasmosis, disseminated. Lesional biopsy specimen shows dermal macrophages packed with dozens of tiny yeast forms of *H. capsulatum*.

TREATMENT The choice of therapy for histoplasmosis depends on the severity of the illness. For patients with some disseminated or localized forms of the disease, oral itraconazole (200 to 400 mg daily) is highly effective. It has also been used for long-term suppressive treatment of the disease in AIDS patients after primary therapy either with itraconazole or amphotericin B.[31] Intravenous amphotericin B (up to 1 mg/kg daily) is given to patients with widespread and severe infections and is the main alternative used. Ketoconazole and fluconazole are also effective in many cases. In African histoplasmosis, itraconazole is also the treatment of choice, but once again in severe cases amphotericin B may be used.[30]

Blastomycosis (North American Blastomycosis, Gilchrist's Disease)

Blastomycosis is a chronic mycosis caused by the dimorphic pathogen, *Blastomyces dermatitidis*.[32] Its chief sites of involvement are the lungs, but disseminated forms of the infection may affect skin, bones, central nervous system, and other sites.

HISTORIC ASPECTS The infection was first described by Gilchrist in 1894. Many of the early cases were described from the Chicago area, and originally this disease was called *North American blastomycosis* until, in 1952, the first case was described from north Africa. It is now recognized that this infection has a wider distribution, although it is not common anywhere.

EPIDEMIOLOGY The infection is found in North America and Canada.[33] Most cases, though, come from the Great Lakes region and southern states of the United States. It also occurs sporadically in Africa, with the largest numbers of cases coming from Zimbabwe,[34] and cases have also been reported from the Middle East and India.

It is thought that the natural habitat of *Blastomyces* is in some way related to wood debris and is close to rivers or lakes or in areas subject to periodic flooding. However, it is difficult to isolate *Blastomyces* from the natural environment.[35] Blastomycosis may also affect domestic animals such as dogs.

CLINICAL MANIFESTATIONS As with histoplasmosis, there is a subclinical form of the infection; its prevalence has not been defined in detail because of lack of a commercial *Blastomyces* skin-test antigen and the extent of antigenic cross-reactivity with fungi such as *Histoplasma*. Plasma cutaneous blastomycosis is also very rare and follows trauma to the skin and the subsequent introduction of fungus, for instance, in laboratory workers or pathologists.[36] After inoculation, an erythematous indurated area with a chancre appears in 1 to 2 weeks, with associated lymphangitis and lymphadenopathy.

Pulmonary blastomycosis is very similar in clinical presentation to pulmonary tuberculosis.[33,36,37] There may be no symptoms or there may be low-grade fever, chest pain, cough, and hemoptysis, and unlike histoplasmosis, it often coexists with disseminated disease. Skin lesions are a common presenting feature of disseminated blastomycosis.[36,38] They are often symmetric and usually affect the face and extremities. The early lesion is a papule or nodule, which may ulcerate and discharge pus. With time this enlarges to form a hyperkeratotic lesion, often with central scarring or ulceration (Figs. 208-10 and 208-11). Oral lesions are less common (Fig. 208-12). Multiple skin lesions are often found in disseminated infection.

FIGURE 208-10

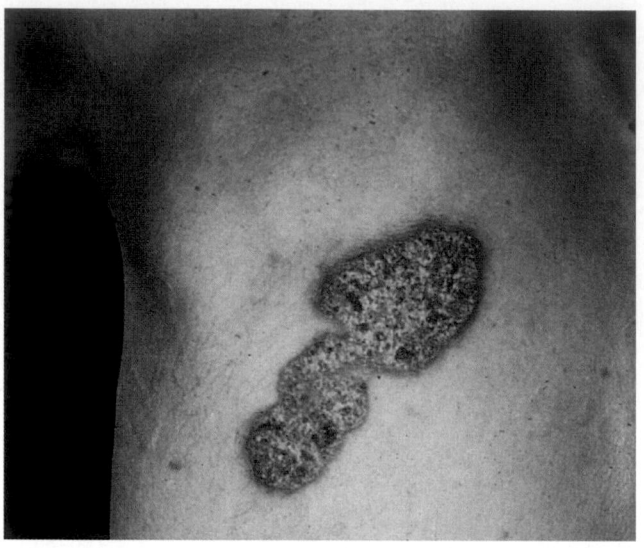

Blastomycosis. Older lesion, appearing as a verrucous plaque.

Other patients may present with nodules and abscesses, and in many patients lesions of different morphologies are present. African patients with blastomycosis have a higher frequency of skin and bone involvement.[34] Although blastomycosis can affect almost any organ, other common sites for dissemination include the bone, the epididymis, and the adrenal gland. Less commonly there is widespread rapid dissemination with multiple organ involvement, and *B. dermatitidis* can produce a form of adult respiratory distress syn-

FIGURE 208-11

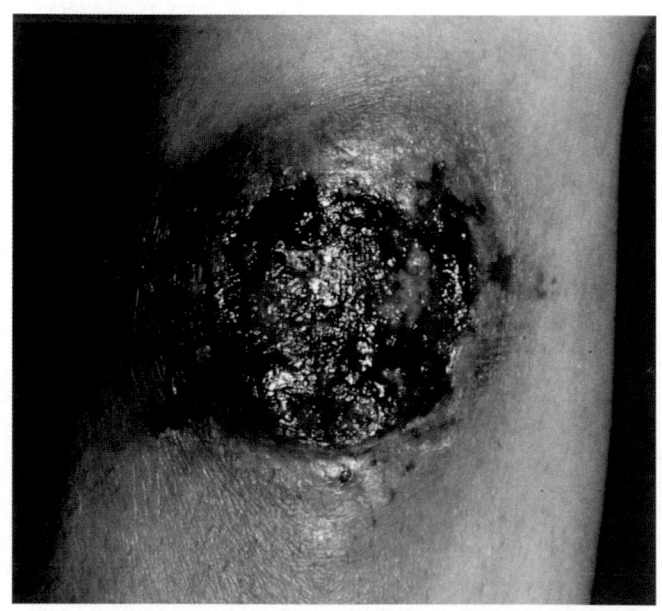

Blastomycosis. Inflammatory plaque with ulceration resembling pyoderma gangrenosum on the calf. (*Courtesy of Elizabeth M. Spiers, MD.*)

FIGURE 208-12

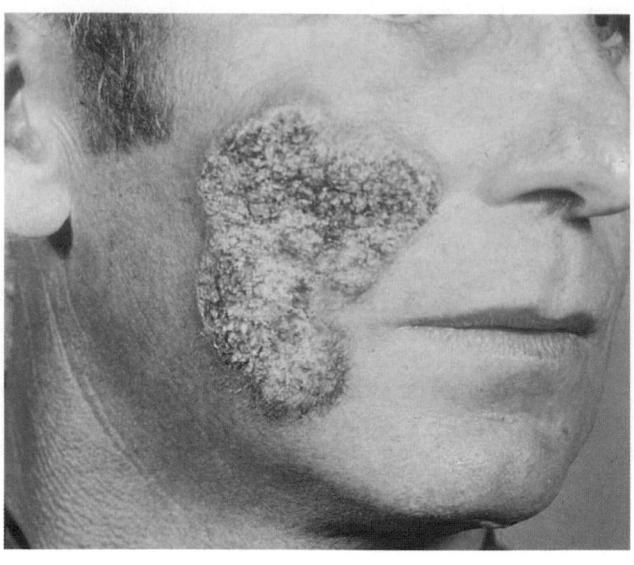

Blastomycosis. Chronic verrucous plaque on the cheek.

drome (ARDS). Skin lesions in widespread disseminated disease are usually papules, abscesses, or small ulcers. Widespread blastomycosis has been described in AIDS patients, but it is not common.[39]

DIFFERENTIAL DIAGNOSIS   The chronic skin granulomas must be differentiated from tuberculosis, other deep mycoses, nonmelanoma skin cancers, pyoderma gangrenosum, and drug reactions due to bromides and iodides.

LABORATORY IDENTIFICATION   The fungus can be found in KOH mounts of pus, skin scrapings, or sputum as thick-walled, rounded refractile spherical cells with broad-based buds (Fig. 208-13). In culture the fungus grows as a mycelial fungus at room temperature. It produces small, rounded or pear-shaped conidia. At higher temperature (37°C) and on enriched media, it produces yeast forms with the characteristic buds. In tissue sections the typical

FIGURE 208-13

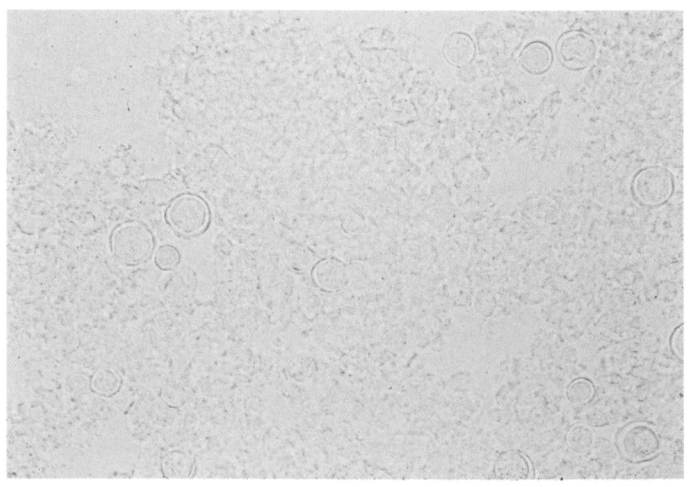

Direct preparation (KOH) of blastomyces.

organisms with broad buds may be found, although it may be necessary to search several fields to find the characteristic cells. These are often found in giant cells or surrounded by neutrophils (Fig. 208-14). Precipitating antibodies to *B. dermatitidis* are often present in the serum of infected patients, and a characteristic precipitin line, the E band, has been described in a high proportion of proven cases; there is also an enzyme-linked immunosorbent assay for blastomycosis. However, one of the problems with serodiagnosis in blastomycosis is the presence of a high number of false-positive reactions in uninfected persons.

TREATMENT   As with histoplasmosis, itraconazole (200 to 400 mg daily) is used in the less severe forms of the infection or where there is only localized spread. Treatment is usually given for at least 6 months. Follow-up surveillance is necessary as relapse can occur, particularly where there are deep sites of infection or the patient is immunosuppressed. Amphotericin B (up to 1 mg/kg daily) is generally used for the treatment of widespread disseminated forms of blastomycosis. Ketoconazole is an alternative therapy.

Coccidioidomycosis (Coccidioidal Granuloma, Valley Fever, San Joaquin Valley Fever, Desert Rheumatism)

Coccidioidomycosis is the infection caused by the fungus, *Coccidioides immitis*. It shows an unusual form of dimorphism, with a mold form at room temperature and the development of large spore-containing structures, spherules, in infected tissue. As with other endemic mycoses, there are asymptomatic, acute and chronic pulmonary and disseminated forms. The disease can affect otherwise healthy individuals or predisposed patients, including those with AIDS.

HISTORIC ASPECTS   Coccidioidomycosis was first described as a disseminated infection in Argentina by Posadas in 1892. Later, this was connected with a benign self-resolving form, valley fever, in California, and in 1938, studies with an antigen from the organism, coccidioidin, confirmed that there was widespread exposure in endemic areas of the United States.

EPIDEMIOLOGY   *C. immitis* is endemic in some semidesert areas of the southwestern states of the United States (e.g., California,

FIGURE 208-14

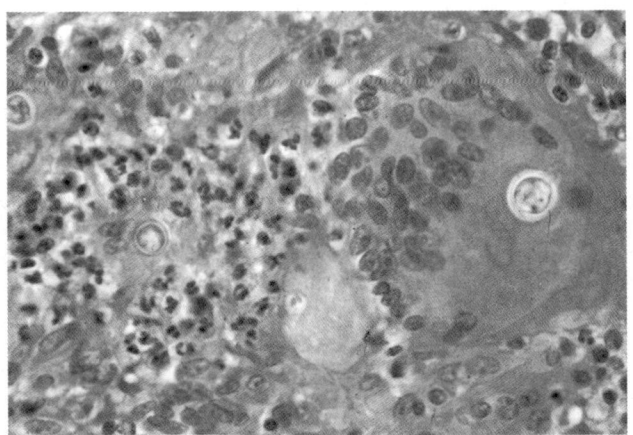

Blastomycosis. Lesional biopsy specimen shows many thick-walled budding yeast forms.

Arizona, New Mexico, and Texas) and in parts of Central and South America. The climate of the endemic areas is marked by very high summer temperatures and low annual rainfall, demonstrated by a characteristic vegetation with cacti and mesquite bushes. Skin tests with coccidioidin show that the incidence of exposure in endemic areas may be as high as 95 percent. The fungus is found in soil and can affect other animals as well as humans. Exposure may result from a brief visit to an endemic area, and local weather can determine exposure rates.[40,41] For instance, dust storms may cause infection in large numbers of individuals. The usual route of infection is respiratory, although direct implantation into the skin can rarely occur.

CLINICAL MANIFESTATIONS   As with other systemic mycoses there is an asymptomatic or subclinical form that is common in endemic areas, judging by the percentages of skin-test reactors to coccidioidin in the healthy population. The primary pulmonary form, which is the most common clinical type, presents as a chest infection with fever, cough, and chest pain. Complications such as pleural effusion may occur. Erythema multiforme or erythema nodosum, often accompanied by arthralgia or anterior uveitis, occurs from the third to the seventh week in about 10 to 15 percent of patients and is more common in females. Sometimes an early, generalized macular and erythematous rash is seen in some patients.

The chronic pulmonary form of the disease presents with chronic cough and resembles tuberculosis. Skin lesions do not normally occur in this phase.

In the rare primary skin infection, following inoculation, there is an indurated nodule that develops 1 to 3 weeks after local trauma. This is followed by regional lymphadenopathy. Disseminated coccidioidomycosis develops in fewer than 0.5 percent of infected individuals. It is mainly seen in patients from certain ethnic backgrounds (American black, Filipino, or Mexican), in pregnant women, and in immunosuppressed patients, including those with AIDS.[42,43] In disseminated disease, lesions may develop in the skin, subcutaneous tissues, bones, joints, and all organs. The skin lesions are abscesses, granulomas, ulcers (Fig. 208-15), or discharging sinuses where there is underlying bone or joint disease. Some lesions appear as flat plaques with central atrophy. Meningitis is a common complication of dissemination and is usually not associated with signs of infection in other sites. In AIDS patients, persistent pneumonia, skin lesions, and widespread dissemination can all occur.

DIFFERENTIAL DIAGNOSIS   Physicians in endemic areas should be aware of the connection between erythema nodosum and coccidioidomycosis. It may also occur in visitors to endemic areas after only a short stay.

LABORATORY DIAGNOSIS   A characteristic of the laboratory findings is the ability of *C. immitis* to form spore-containing spherules. These are large (up to 250 μm) and can be seen in KOH mounts of sputum, cerebrospinal fluid (CSF), or pus. In culture, colonies of *C. immitis* are mycelial, fast-growing, white, and cottony. On microscopy, there are chains of arthrospores at intervals on the older mycelium. *C. immitis* in the mold phase is highly infectious, and cultures should be handled carefully.

Serologic tests are of value in the diagnosis and prognosis of coccidioidomycosis.[44] Precipitins develop in about 90 percent of infected individuals within 2 to 6 weeks but are short-lived; complement-fixing antibodies are characteristic of more severe infections and, in active infection, increase to a maximum after 6 months.

FIGURE 208-15

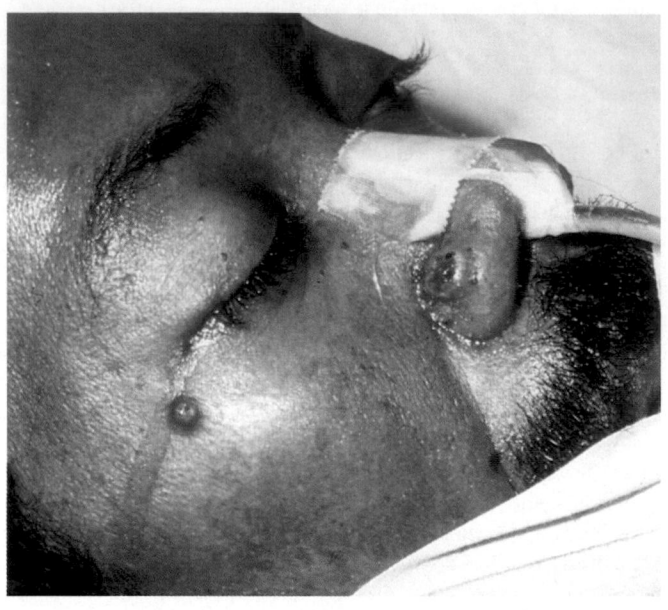

Coccidioidomycosis, disseminated. Intact and ulcerated papules and nodules are seen on the cheek and nose of this comatose patient with coccidioidomycotic meningitis. (*Courtesy of Francis Renna, MD.*)

Skin tests with coccidioidin are of little value in diagnosing infections. Spherulin is an antigen obtained from spherules of *C. immitis* and may be better than coccidioidin for detecting sensitization. However, in severe infections cutaneous anergy to both is common.

Spherules containing large endospores can be seen in tissue sections, although there are a variety of less distinct intermediate stages in spherule formation that can also be seen. Before endospores form, the cytoplasm of the immature spherule is basophilic and subsequently breaks up into spores. Mycelium is rarely seen in histopathologic sections.

TREATMENT No specific therapy apart from rest is necessary in the primary pulmonary infection, and there is little evidence that the symptoms are either improved or shortened by giving an oral azole drug, even though it is widespread practice. For disseminated disease, treatment is still unsatisfactory, but amphotericin B (1 mg/kg daily), itraconazole (200 to 400 mg daily), or fluconazole (200 to 600 mg daily) can all be given.[45] It is important to follow patients carefully, given the frequency of relapse. Meningitis, arthritis, and progressive disseminated infection involving multiple sites are all particularly refractory to therapy. Generally soft tissue coccidioidomycosis (skin and joint) has a better prognosis, and the mortality in patients who present with soft tissue lesions is low. Transfer factor has been used in some patients with coccidioidomycosis with anergy associated with dissemination.

Paracoccidioidomycosis (South American Blastomycosis, Paracoccidioidal Granuloma)

Paracoccidioides brasiliensis is a dimorphic fungus that causes a respiratory infection, with a tendency to disseminate to the mucous membranes and lymph nodes. It is confined to Central and South America.[46]

HISTORIC ASPECTS Paracoccidioidomycosis was first described in Brazil by Lutz in 1908. Although initially thought to be related to coccidioidomycosis, described a few years earlier in Argentina, the organism was isolated in 1912 and shown to be different.

EPIDEMIOLOGY Paracoccidioidomycosis has been reported from most Latin American countries, but the infection is most commonly found in parts of Brazil, Colombia, and Argentina. The infection does not occur in the United States, although it has been reported from Mexico. Exposure rates can be estimated by skin test reactivity and appear to be equal in both males and females, although the prevalence of positive reactors in endemic areas seldom exceeds 25 percent. In contrast, the active infection is predominantly seen in males. The mechanism is thought to be connected to the presence of a cytoplasmic estrogen receptor on the fungus, and, in vitro, estradiol suppresses the conversion of mycelium to yeast.[47] The ecologic niche of the organisms is unknown, but the condition is much more frequent in rural areas; survival of *P. brasiliensis* in nature has been associated with proximity to water or areas of high atmospheric humidity.[48]

CLINICAL MANIFESTATIONS There are a number of different clinical patterns of infection, which depend on the predominant site of clinical involvement. These include the lung (pulmonary form), the mucous membranes (mucocutaneous form), and the lymph nodes (lymphatic form). Many patients have a mixed type of infection with involvement of different organ groups.[46]

Patients rarely present with an acute form of pulmonary infection; rather, it tends to be chronic and slowly progressive with weight loss and chronic cough. The lesions may be bilateral and nodular on chest x-ray, and there is often extensive fibrosis. Other sites of involvement include mucocutaneous areas. Oral or circumoral lesions are common in the mucocutaneous forms of paracoccidioidomycosis; lesions also occur in the nose, conjunctivae, or around the anus. These lesions may be small granulomas or ulcers. They heal with scarring, which may cause considerable deformity.

The cervical lymph nodes are sometimes enlarged, tender, and tethered to the overlying skin; they rarely suppurate. Other systemic sites of involvement include the spleen, intestines, lungs, and liver. Paracoccidioidomycosis is uncommon in AIDS patients, although there is a widespread variety that is a more rapidly progressive form of disseminated infection, occuring in young adults or older children without recognizable predisposition.[49]

DIFFERENTIAL DIAGNOSIS This includes tuberculosis, leishmaniasis, and other deep mycoses.

LABORATORY DIAGNOSIS Sputum, exudates, and scrapings can be screened using KOH. They show numbers of round yeasts with a characteristic form of multiple budding, in which a parent cell is surrounded by large numbers of smaller buds. The organism is dimorphic and produces a cottony mycelial phase growth on primary isolation at room temperature. Once again, the characteristic yeast phase can be induced on enriched media such as BHI blood agar at 37°C. Serology is very helpful in confirming the diagnosis, the main tests being the immunodiffusion assay and a complement-fixation test. Recently, antibodies to a 43-kDa antigen have been found to be highly specific for this infection in immunoblotting. Histopathologically, there is a mixed granulomatous response with fibrosis. The organisms can be seen with special fungal stains such as methenamine silver (Grocott modification). In tissue the characteristic budding pattern can be seen, although it may be necessary to search several fields to find the most typical structures (Fig.

208-16). In widespread infections, masses of small yeast forms may be mistaken for *Histoplasma*.

TREATMENT The treatment of choice in most cases is itraconazole, which can produce remissions in 3 to 6 months.[50] Ketoconazole is an alternative. Relapses can occur, and, where possible, patients should be reviewed periodically after primary therapy. In very extensive infections and in severely ill patients, such as those with the progressive disseminated type of infection, intravenous amphotericin B may be necessary. Severe pulmonary or intraoral fibrosis may remain after treatment.

Infections due to *Penicillium marneffei* (Penicilliosis, Penicilliosis Marneffei)

This infection is a more recently recognized disease found in Southeast Asia. *P. marneffei* is a member of the common genus *Penicillium*. It shows an unusual pattern of dimorphism in that it develops yeastlike cells that reproduce with septal formation dividing the cells into two. It is inhaled via the lungs, and it is not known whether there is a primary cutaneous form of the infection.

HISTORIC ASPECTS This disease was first recognized in 1959 by Segretain in a specimen from Vietnam.[51] Subsequent cases in U.S. veterans from Vietnam and then cases from Thailand and China have confirmed the wide geographic extent of this infection.

EPIDEMIOLOGY The natural source of *P. marneffei* is unknown. Infections are confined to Southeast Asia, particularly Thailand, South China, and Vietnam. However, there are reports in other Asian countries, and imported cases have been seen in Europe and the United States. Natural infections are known to occur in only one group of animals, bamboo rats, which are large burrowing rodents. The infection affects otherwise healthy individuals as well as those with immune defects and is most common after the rainy season.[52] Patients with AIDS appear to be particularly susceptible to this infection.

CLINICAL MANIFESTATIONS There has been no work to demonstrate that there is a subclinical form of *Penicillium* infection,

FIGURE 208-16

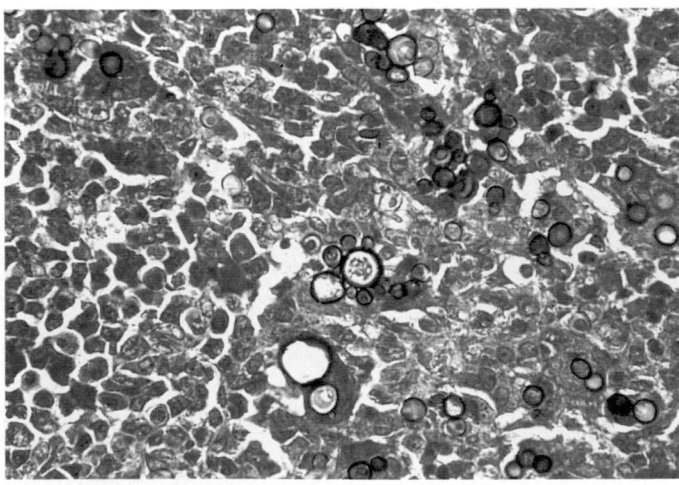

Biopsy of oral mucosal lesion showing multiple budding *Paracoccidioides brasiliensis*.

even though this is likely. Patients usually present with localized pulmonary or disseminated disease. The chest signs are those of chronic pulmonary disease.[53,54] Over 50 percent of patients have multiple skin lesions, which are umbilicated papules that may enlarge and ulcerate. They are usually widely scattered on the face and trunk. Other organs including the liver, gastrointestinal tract, spleen, and bone marrow may be affected.

DIFFERENTIAL DIAGNOSIS The main differential is with other disseminated mycoses such as histoplasmosis and cryptococcosis, which can also be found in the endemic area in AIDS patients. Biopsy and, where necessary, culture will distinguish between the different causes.

LABORATORY DIAGNOSIS *P. marneffei* forms characteristic yeastlike cells that are divided by a septum in tissue and are best seen in histopathologic sections stained with methenamine silver. These cells are small (2 to 4 μm) and difficult to see in blood films or skin or bone marrow smears, but they may be highlighted with stains such as leishmanin. In culture, *P. marneffei* is a green or grayish mold that produces typical *Penicillium* conidiophores and a diffusible red pigment. There is no serologic test as yet.

TREATMENT In severe cases amphotericin B is necessary. In many cases, however, there is a good response to itraconazole, 200 to 400 mg daily. In AIDS patients this is continued after initial therapy to prevent relapse.[54]

Cryptococcosis (Torulosis, European Blastomycosis)

Cryptococcosis is the infection caused by the encapsulated yeast *Cryptococcus neoformans*. Although the main portal of entry is through inhalation into the lungs, the disease usually presents with signs of extrapulmonary dissemination such as meningitis. Cutaneous lesions can develop as a result of dissemination or, rarely, through inoculation.

HISTORIC ASPECTS *C. neoformans* was first demonstrated by Busse and Buschke in a patient with a bone infection in 1894. The capsule was originally misidentified as the result of histolytic action in vivo. In its time this organism has been assigned to a variety of different fungal genera from *Torula* to *Saccharomyces*. Subsequently, other cases showed that *Cryptococcus* could cause a variety of different clinical forms of disease, notably meningitis. The advent of the AIDS epidemic has considerably affected the epidemiology of this infection, and in areas such as northern Thailand, cryptococcosis is one of the main secondary complications of HIV infection.[55]

EPIDEMIOLOGY Cryptococcosis has a worldwide distribution, although exposure rates probably differ markedly in different countries. *C. neoformans* has two variants, *C. neoformans* var. *neoformans* and *C. neoformans* var. *gattii*. These correspond to two clusters of serotypes: (1) A,D, or AD, and (2) B or C.[56] The *neoformans* variety can be isolated from pigeon excreta and is more common in AIDS patients; the *gattii* form is found in the debris of certain eucalyptus trees in the tropics and California, but it is less often isolated from AIDS patients. Two sexual varieties called *Filobasidiella neoformans* and *F. bacillispora* correspond to the *neoformans* and *gattii* varieties, respectively. Patients with certain immunodeficiency states caused by AIDS, malignant lymphomas, sarcoidosis, collagen disease, and carcinoma and those receiving systemic glucocorticoid therapy are particularly susceptible. The incidence of cryptococcosis in patients with established AIDS varies in different countries from 3 to 6 percent in the United States, to 3 percent in the United Kingdom, and over 12 percent in parts of Africa, e.g., Zaire. Strains of serotype D are more likely to be found in skin lesions, which occur in 10 to 15 percent of cases of disseminated cryptococcosis.

CLINICAL MANIFESTATIONS   There is probably a subclinical form of cryptococcosis as unaffected individuals may have positive skin tests. However, the most common clinical manifestation of disease is meningoencephalitis. This presents with classic signs of meningismus, changes in consciousness, mental changes, and nerve palsies. In AIDS patients, these signs may be only weakly expressed. Pulmonary infection can be found in about 10 percent of those with meningitis. Chest signs include the appearance of nodular shadows, cavitation, and pleural effusion. Patients with AIDS often present with fever and mild headache and few other features of infection.[55] Cutaneous lesions may develop in about 10 percent of cases but are seldom pathognomonic.[57–60] Acneiform papules or pustules, progressing to warty or vegetating crusted plaques, ulcers, and hard infiltrated plaques or nodules are characteristic of widespread systemic infection (Fig. 208-17). Cold abscesses, cellulitis, and nodular lesions also occur. In otherwise-healthy patients or those with sarcoidosis, lesions may be solitary, and in such cases they may be the only clinical manifestation of infection.

FIGURE 208-17

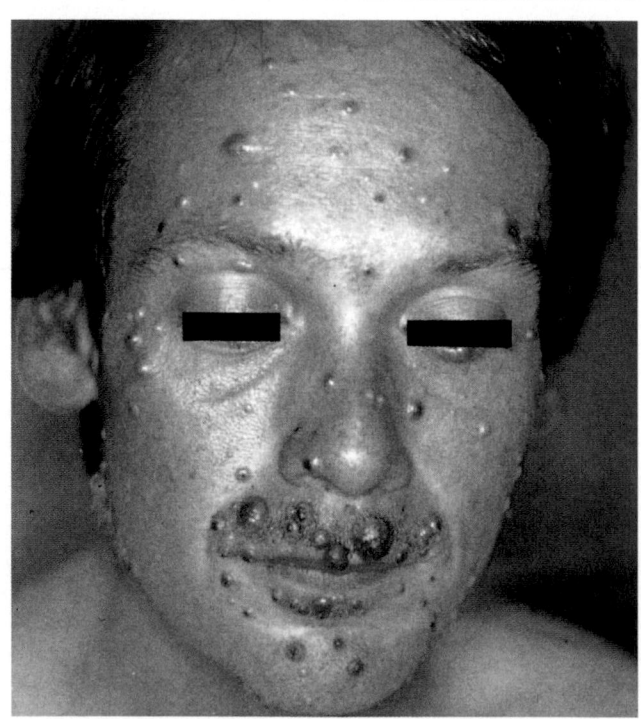

Cryptococcosis, disseminated. Multiple, discrete, skin-colored papules and nodules resembling molluscum contagiosum are seen on the face of a male with advanced HIV disease. (*Courtesy of Loïs Vaillant, MD.*)

In primary cutaneous cryptococcosis with direct inoculation of organisms into the skin, the skin lesions are usually solitary nodules that break down and ulcerate. Local lymphadenopathy also develops. The term *primary cutaneous cryptococcosis* is also used loosely to describe solitary lesions of cryptococcosis, but in many such cases there is also evidence of dissemination to other internal organs. It is important to investigate all patients who present with cutaneous lesions for evidence of dissemination to other sites.[58]

DIFFERENTIAL DIAGNOSIS   Cryptococcal skin lesions may mimic a range of other conditions, particularly other systemic mycoses in AIDS patients. It is important to biopsy and culture suspicious lesions in immunocompromised patients.

LABORATORY DIAGNOSIS   Cryptococci are large (5 to 15 μm), budding cells with capsules, which are best observed by direct microscopy of India ink or Nigrosin mounts (Fig. 208-18). The organism is not difficult to grow in culture. Various biochemical features such as the production of urease and the ability to pigment on Guizotia seed medium are characteristic. Serologic tests are rapid and specific. The main test is an antigen-detection assay using latex agglutination, and this is simple and very rapid to perform on blood or CSF. Very high titers are found in AIDS patients in serum and CSF. Non-AIDS patients with single, localized skin lesions are often antigen-negative.

In tissue sections, the large pleomorphic yeasts stimulate either a granulomatous reaction or very little inflammation. The capsules of the cells can be stained using the mucicarmine or alcian blue stains.

TREATMENT   The most frequently used drug regimen in the non-AIDS patient is intravenous amphotericin B combined with flucytosine. In patients with single skin lesions and no other signs of infection, alternatives such as fluconazole or itraconazole can be used. In AIDS patients there is a very high relapse rate, and the usual policy is to give a 10- to 14-day course of amphotericin B with or without flucytosine, followed by long-term fluconazole.[61] Fluconazole given on its own is an alternative approach.

FIGURE 208-18

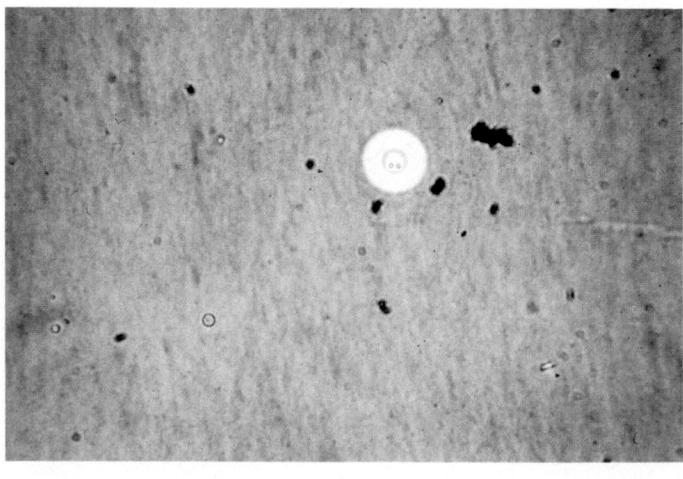

Cryptococcosis. India ink preparation of cerebrospinal fluid.

FIGURE 208-19

CHAPTER 208
Deep Fungal Infections

2385

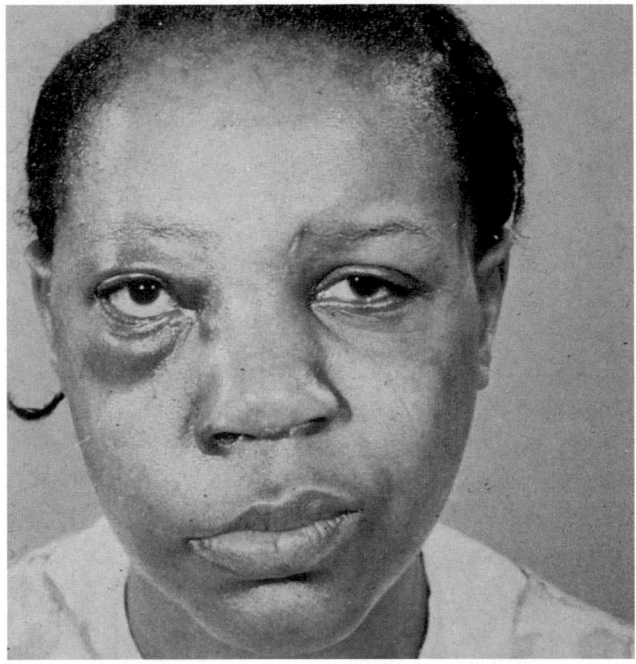

A.

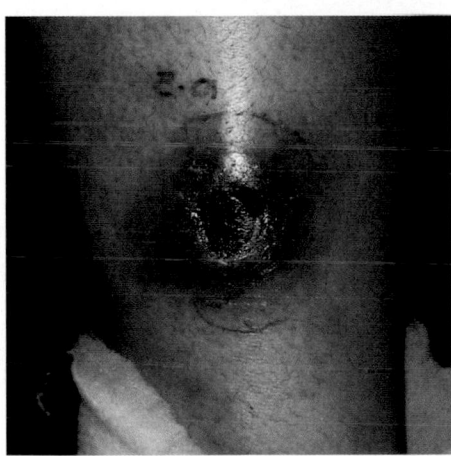

B.

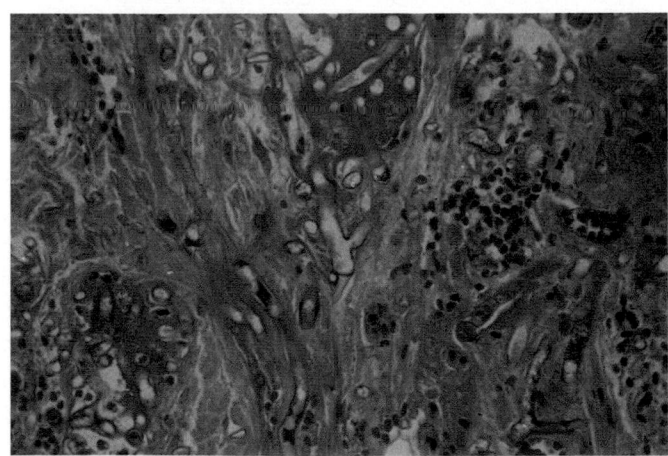

C.

Mucormycosis. *A.* The face of this young woman with diabetes mellitus shows proptosis, unilateral facial edema, and a right-sided facial palsy associated with infection beginning in the right maxillary sinus. *B.* Ulcer. *C.* Hyphae in tissue.

Cutaneous Aspects of Systemic Opportunistic Mycoses

Skin lesions are not common with the opportunistic fungal infections but they can occur in some, particularly in certain predisposed groups. When they occur, their presence may be very helpful as it is possible to biopsy easily accessible lesions in order to establish the diagnosis.

Systemic Candidiasis

This follows dissemination of *Candida* species from the gastrointestinal tract or via the bloodstream. Skin lesions may occur particularly in two situations: (1) In neutropenic patients, there is often a severe disseminated disease with widespread skin nodules, associated with muscle pains[62]; and (2) in intravenous drug abusers, candidiasis may present with a follicular pustular rash in the beard area and scalp. Other lesions include retinal deposits and abscesses around the costochondral junction.[63]

Systemic candidiasis is usually treated with intravenous amphotericin B or fluconazole. Resistance to some azole drugs, such as fluconazole and ketoconazole, is more common with certain non-*albicans Candida* species, and these antifungals should be avoided in infections caused by these species.

Zygomycosis (Mucormycosis, Phycomycosis)

Zygomycosis is a rare disease caused by zygomycete fungi such as *Rhizomucor, Absidia,* and *Rhizopus. Cunnighamella bertollettiae* and *Saksenaea vasiformis* are less common causes. Zygomycetes cause disease in patients with poorly controlled diabetes, neutropenia, or renal disease. They can invade necrotic burned areas or involve the facial skin secondary to invasive infection of the paranasal sinuses (Fig. 208-19). Zygomycete infections have also been associated with close apposition of the skin with contaminated dressing materials in the case of *R. rhizopodiformis*[64] or with wooden tongue depressors in the case of *R. microsporus.*[65] The zygomycete fungi have a tendency to invade blood vessels causing widespread infarction. Infections may respond to intravenous amphotericin, and recent results with lipid-associated amphotericin B formulations have been encouraging.

Other Opportunistic Mycoses

Other fungi causing systemic infections may also produce skin lesions in the process of bloodstream dissemination. The best known of these organisms are *Aspergillus, Trichosporon,* and *Fusarium.* Skin infection is mainly seen in severely immunocompromised patients such as those with neutropenia.

Aspergillus may produce large necrotic lesions such as ecthyma gangrenosum, but smaller papules and cold abscesses can also occur.[66] *Fusarium* infections may produce widely distributed target-like lesions, which may undergo central necrosis, and, in some cases, digital cellulitis and superficial white onychomycosis.[67] Treatment for all these infections is usually amphotericin B.

LABORATORY DIAGNOSIS OF OPPORTUNISTIC MYCOSES
The laboratory confirmation of the diagnosis is fraught with difficulties chiefly because many of the organisms are also commensals in human sites; as they occur in severely ill patients, the capacity

to produce diagnostic antibody titers is compromised. The interpretation of laboratory data is, in consequence, difficult and has to be related to the clinical state of the patient. Ideally, a histologic diagnosis should be made, although biopsy may be impossible because of the risk of bleeding. In many cases the diagnosis of a systemic mycosis is presumptive, and treatment is therefore given empirically.

Actinomycosis

Actinomycosis is an infection caused by filamentous bacteria that form large granules, sulfur granules, in abscess cavities. Draining sinuses communicate from the center of the abscess to the skin or mucosal surface.

HISTORIC ASPECTS The first human case was described by Israel in 1878, 1 year after the disease had been recognized in cattle. Later, in 1910, it was first recognized that the organism, *Actinomyces israelii*, was carried in the oral cavity and tonsils. The early literature is full of reports of this infection, which is fortunately seen much less frequently nowadays.

EPIDEMIOLOGY The main causative organism, *A. israelii,* an anaerobic actinomycete, is a normal inhabitant of the human mouth. Actinomycosis is therefore an endogenous infection. *A. bovis*, *A. naeslundii*, *Arachnia propionica*, and *Bifidobacterium eriksonii*, all inhabitants of the mouth, are rarer causes of human disease. The incidence of the infection is affected by the availability of good dental care, as poor dental hygiene and delayed treatment of intraoral infections lead to a greater risk of actinomycosis. The disease has a worldwide distribution but is not common. Other sites of carriage include the vaginal mucosa, and this may also affect the development of infection. In most cases of actinomycosis, the formation of granules is thought to require cooperation with other bacteria.

CLINICAL MANIFESTATIONS There are five main types of actinomycosis, depending on the primary site of infection.[68,69] Actinomycosis usually remains localized. The infections are cervicofacial, thoracic, abdominal, pelvic, and primary cutaneous.

Cervicofacial actinomycosis is the most common form of this infection. It usually presents with an indurated nodule or plaque on the cheek or submaxillary region. In the later stages, multiple sinuses develop on the surface; these discharge pus and sulfur granules. The initial site of infection is probably a dental abscess, and it is likely that many cases are now treated before the typical features develop. Sulfur granules are sometimes found in tonsillar crypts after elective tonsillectomy, and in this case they do not appear to be causing symptomatic illness.

Thoracic actinomycosis only presents with skin changes if the underlying lung infection, which mimics pulmonary tuberculosis, involves the outer chest wall. Once again, multiple sinuses communicate with the underlying lung infection.

Abdominal actinomycosis usually begins with an abscess in the appendix or cecum. Skin involvement, which is now rare, follows extension of the infection to the anterior abdominal wall with the formation of sinuses.

Pelvic actinomycosis is a distinct form of actinomycosis, associated with the use of intrauterine contraceptive devices. However, the skin is not affected, and the infection presents as an intrapelvic mass associated with signs of chronic pelvic inflammation.

Primary cutaneous actinomycosis is very rare.[70] It occurs on exposed skin and clinically mimics mycetoma; the infection is thought to follow implantation of organisms.

DIFFERENTIAL DIAGNOSIS Actinomycosis has a typical appearance, with draining sinuses related to potential sites of infection. Tuberculosis and mycetoma are the main differentials to be excluded.

LABORATORY DIAGNOSIS The presence of sulfur granules is typical (Fig. 208-20). These are yellow granules up to 1 to 2 mm in diameter, which on Gram staining contain a mixture of thin bacterial filaments. Cultures of *A. israelii* are incubated under anaerobic conditions at 37°C. Histopathologically, there is a suppurative inflammatory process and small abscesses contain the granular colonies of the organism surrounded by neutrophils. With hematoxylin/eosin staining, the outer zone of the granule contains a layer of eosinophilic refractile clublike structures.

FIGURE 208-20

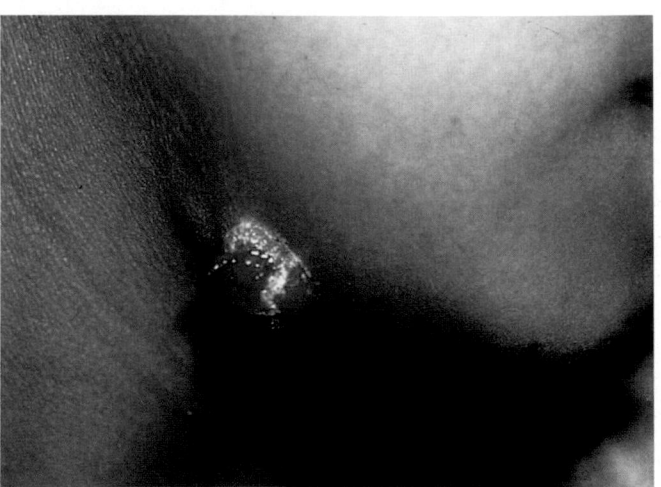

A.

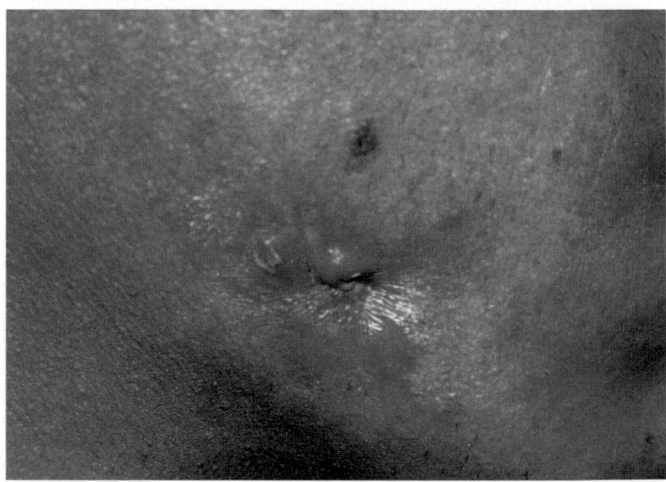

B.

Actinomycosis, cervicofacial form. *A.* Localized lesion with sinus margin. *B.* Chronic cervicofacial, actinomycosis. (*Courtesy of R. Arenas, MD.*)

TREATMENT *A. israelii* is sensitive to sulfonamides, streptomycin, penicillin, chloramphenicol, chlortetracycline, oxytetracycline, tetracycline, rifampicin, and erythromycin.[71] High doses of intravenous or intramuscular penicillin is the usual treatment given for this infection. The course has to be continued for several weeks. Alternative medications include erythromycin, tetracyclines, and imipenem.

Nocardiosis

Nocardiosis is an acute or chronic infection caused by filamentous bacteria of the genus *Nocardia*. These cause localized skin or subcutaneous infections, including abscesses and actinomycetoma, as well as a systemic infection that may disseminate to involve the skin.

HISTORIC ASPECTS As with actinomycosis, nocardial infection was first described in cattle in 1888 by Nocard. The first human patient had a disseminated infection with involvement of the lungs and brain. Nocardiosis has become more common as it is associated with immunosuppression.

EPIDEMIOLOGY The main pathogenic species of *Nocardia* are *N. asteroides*, *N. brasiliensis*, and *N. otitidis-caviarum*. These are soil organisms, but generally *N. asteroides* is environmentally dominant in northern climates, whereas *N. brasiliensis* is more common in the south. *Nocardia* can gain entry through a superficial wound to cause a localized dermal or subcutaneous infection; it can also be inhaled via the lungs to cause a pulmonary infection.

In causing systemic disease, *Nocardia* usually behaves as an opportunistic pathogen causing disease in patients with an underlying predisposition such as AIDS, solid organ transplant, Cushing's syndrome, diabetes, and following the use of glucocorticoids in the treatment of various diseases. Occasionally there are outbreaks of nocardiosis in hospitals, associated with contamination of ventilation systems.[72]

CLINICAL MANIFESTATIONS Rarely *Nocardia* can cause a subcutaneous abscess or a lymphangitic form (see "Sporotrichosis," above), in which multiple suppurative nodules develop along a lymphatic chain.[73–75] Actinomycetoma due to *Nocardia* species has been described earlier. In systemic nocardiosis, the main sites for infection are the lung or the brain. Lung lesions resemble pulmonary tuberculosis, whereas brain lesions present as intracranial space-occupying lesions and with fever. In about 30 percent of cases of systemic infection there are metastatic cutaneous abscesses, which are often multiple.[76]

LABORATORY DIAGNOSIS Although *Nocardia* species form grains in mycetomas, in other infections they are present as fine branching filaments. These can be seen in pus from skin lesions or sputum after staining by Gram stain, methenamine silver, and modified acid-fast techniques, as *Nocardia* are only partially acid fast. The organisms can be cultured on Sabouraud's agar. Serology can be useful in the diagnosis of systemic nocardiosis.

TREATMENT The most widely used treatment is cotrimoxazole. Alternatives include ampicillin, minocycline, amikacin, and, more recently, imipenem. Unfortunately, the results of in vitro testing for antibiotic sensitivity may not accurately reflect the subsequent clinical responses.

REFERENCES

1. Chandler FW et al: *A Colour Atlas and Text Book of the Histopathology of Mycotic Diseases.* London, Wolfe, 1980, pp 92–98
2. Warnock DW, Richardson MD (eds): *Fungal Infection in the Compromised Patient.* Chichester, Wiley, 1991
3. Kibbler CC et al: *Principles and Practice of Clinical Mycology.* Chichester, Wiley, 1996
4. Jacobs PH, Nall L (eds): *Fungal Disease. Biology, Immunology and Diagnosis.* New York, Marcel Dekker, 1997
5. Winn RE: A contemporary view of sporotrichosis. *Curr Top Med Mycol* **6**:73, 1995
6. de Albornoz MCB: Sporotrichosis, in *Tropical Fungal Infections, Bailliere's Clinical Tropical Medicine and Communicable Diseases,* vol 4, edited by RJ Hay. London, Bailliere Tindall, 1989, p 71
7. Findlay GH: The epidemiology of sporotrichosis in the Transvaal. *Sabouraudia* **6**:231, 1970
8. Itoh M et al: Survey of 260 cases of sporotrichosis. *Dermatologica* **172**:203, 1986
9. Bibler MR et al: Disseminated sporotrichosis in a patient with HIV infection after treatment for acquired factor VIII inhibitor. *JAMA* **256**:3125, 1986
10. Restrepo A et al: Itraconazole therapy in lymphangitic and cutaneous sporotrichosis. *Arch Dermatol* **122**:413, 1986
11. Mahgoub ES, Murray IG: *Mycetoma.* London, Heinemann Medical, 1973
12. Hay RJ et al: Mycetoma. *J Med Vet Mycol* **30**(suppl 1):41, 1992
13. Venugopal PV, Venugopal TV: Pale grain eumycetomas in Madras. *Australasian J Dermatol* **36**:149, 1995
14. Wethered DB et al: Ultrastructural and immunogenic changes in the formation of mycetoma grains. *J Med Vet Mycol* **25**:39, 1986
15. Welsh O et al: Treatment of eumycetoma and actinomycetoma. *Curr Top Med Mycol* **6**:47, 1995
16. McGinnis MR: Chromoblastomycosis and phaeohyphomycosis: New concepts, diagnosis and mycology. *J Am Acad Dermatol* **8**:1, 1983
17. Bayles MA. Chromomycosis. *Curr Top Med Mycol* **6**:221, 1995
18. Goette DK, Robertson D: Transepithelial elimination in chromomycosis. *Arch Dermatol* **120**:400, 1984
19. Restrepo A: Treatment of tropical mycoses. *J Am Acad Dermatol* **31**:S91, 1994
20. Esterre P: Treatment of chromomycosis with terbinafine: Preliminary results of an open pilot study. *Br J Dermatol* **134**(suppl 46):33, 1996
21. Matsumoto T et al: Developments in hyalohyphomycosis and phaeohyphomycosis. *J Med Vet Mycol* **32**(suppl 1):329, 1994
22. Baruzzi RG, Marcopito LF: Lobomycosis, in *Tropical Fungal Infections, Bailliere's Clinical Tropical Medicine and Communicable Diseases,* vol 4, edited by RJ Hay. London, Bailliere Tindall, 1989, p 97
23. Drouhet E, Ravisse P: Entomophthoromycosis. *Curr Top Med Mycol* **5**:215, 1994
24. Chitravel V et al: Recurrent rhinosporidiosis in man: Case reports. *Mycopathologia* **73**:79, 1981
25. Goodwin RA et al: Histoplasmosis in normal hosts. *Medicine* **60**:231, 1981
26. Barton EN et al: Cutaneous histoplasmosis in the acquired immunodeficiency syndrome—a report of three cases from Trinidad. *Trop Geograph Med* **40**:153, 1988
27. Wheat LJ et al: Histoplasmosis in the acquired immune deficiency syndrome. *Am J Med* **78**:203, 1985
28. Davies SF: Serodiagnosis of histoplasmosis. *Semin Resp Infect* **1**:9, 1986
29. Wheat LJ et al: Diagnosis of disseminated histoplasmosis by detection of *Histoplasma capsulatum* antigen in serum and urine specimen. *N Engl J Med* **314**:83, 1986
30. Drouhet E: African histoplasmosis, in *Tropical Fungal Infections, Baillieres Clinical Tropical Medicine and Communicable Diseases,* vol 4, edited by RJ Hay. London, Bailliere Tindall, 1989, p 221
31. Wheat J: Endemic mycoses in AIDS: A clinical review. *Clin Microbiol Rev* **8**:149, 1995
32. Domer JE: Blastomyces dermatitidis, in *Fungal Dimorphism,* edited by PJ Szaniszlo. New York, Plenum, 1985
33. Bradsher RW: Histoplasmosis and blastomycosis. *Clin Infect Dis* **22**(suppl 2):S102, 1996
34. Emerson PA et al: North American blastomycosis in Africans. *Br J Dis Chest* **78**:286, 1984

35. Klein BS et al: Isolation of *Blastomyces dermatitidis* in soil associated with a large outbreak of blastomycosis in Wisconsin. *N Engl J Med* **314**:529, 1986

36. Bradsher RW: A clinician's view of blastomycosis. *Curr Top Med Mycol* **5**:181, 1994

37. McAdams HP et al: Thoracic mycoses from endemic fungi: Radiologic-pathologic correlation. *Radiographics* **15**:255, 1995

38. Weil M et al: Cutaneous lesions provide a clue to mysterious pulmonary process. Pulmonary and cutaneous North American blastomycosis infection. *Arch Dermatol* **132**:822, 1996

39. Herd AM et al: Miliary blastomycosis and HIV infection. *Can Med Assoc J* **143**:1329, 1990

40. Standaert SM et al: Coccidioidomycosis among visitors to a *Coccidioides immitis*–endemic area: An outbreak in a military reserve unit. *J Infect Dis* **171**:1675, 1995

41. Olson PE et al: Coccidioidomycosis in California: Regional outbreak, global diagnostic challenge. *Mil Med* **160**:304, 1995

42. Bronniman DA et al: Coccidioidomycosis in the acquired immunodeficiency syndrome. *Ann Intern Med* **106**:373, 1987

43. McNeil MM, Ampel NM: Opportunistic coccidioidomycosis in patients infected with human immunodeficiency virus: Prevention issues and priorities. *Clin Infect Dis* **21**(suppl 1):S111, 1995

44. Martins TB et al: Comparison of commercially available enzyme immunoassay with traditional serological tests for detection of antibodies to *Coccidioides immitis. J Clin Microbiol* **33**:940, 1995

45. Graybill JR: Treatment of coccidioidomycosis. *Curr Top Med Mycol* **5**:151, 1994

46. Del Negro G et al (eds): *Paracoccidioidomicose.* Sao Paulo, Sarvier Editora, 1982

47. Restrepo A et al: Estrogens inhibit mycelium to yeast transformation in the fungus *P. brasiliensis:* Implications for resistance of females to paracoccidioidomycosis. *Infect Immun* **46**:346, 1984

48. Restrepo A: The ecology of *P. brasiliensis:* A puzzle still unsolved. *J Med Vet Mycol* **23**:323, 1985

49. Sugar AM et al: Paracoccidioidomycosis in the immunosuppressed host. Report of a case and review of the literature. *Am Rev Respir Dis* **129**:349, 1984

50. Negroni R et al: Oral treatment of paracoccidioidomycosis and histoplasmosis with itraconazole in humans. *Rev Infect Dis* **9**(suppl):S47, 1987

51. Segretain G: Description d'une nouvelle espece de penicillium: *Penicillium marneffei* n.sp. *Bull Soc Mycol Fr* **75**:412, 1959

52. Chariyalertsak S et al: Seasonal variation of disseminated *Penicillium marneffei* infections in northern Thailand: A clue to the reservoir? *J Infect Dis* **173**:1490, 1996

53. Jayanetra P et al: *Penicilliosis marneffei* in Thailand: Report of five human cases. *Am J Trop Med Hyg* **33**:637, 1984

54. Supparatpinyo K et al: Disseminated *Penicillium marneffei* infection in southeast Asia. *Lancet* **344**:110, 1994

55. Mitchell TG, Perfect JR: Cryptococcosis in the era of AIDS—100 years after the discovery of *Cryptococcus neoformans. Clin Microbiol Rev* **8**:515, 1995

56. Bennett JE et al: Epidemiologic differences among serotypes of *Cryptococcus neoformans. Am J Epidemiol* **120**:582, 1984

57. Manrique P et al: Polymorphous cutaneous cryptococcosis: Nodular, herpes-like, and molluscum-like lesions in a patient with the acquired immunodeficiency syndrome. *J Am Acad Dermatol* **26**:122, 1992

58. Murakawa GJ et al: Cutaneous *Cryptococcus* infection and AIDS. Report of 12 cases and review of the literature. *Arch Dermatol* **132**:545, 1996

59. Manfredi R et al: Morphologic features and clinical significance of skin involvement in patients with AIDS-related cryptococcosis. *Acta Derm Venereol* **76**:72, 1996

60. Pineski R et al: Cutaneous cryptococcosis in a patient receiving chronic immunosuppressive therapy. *Cutis* **57**:229, 1996

61. Dromer F et al: Comparison of the efficacy of amphotericin B and fluconazole in the treatment of cryptococcosis in human immunodeficiency virus–negative patients: Retrospective analysis of 83 cases. French Cryptococcosis Study Group. *Clin Infect Dis* **22**(suppl 2):S154, 1996

62. Bodey G, Luna M: Skin lesions associated with disseminated candidiasis. *JAMA* **229**:1466, 1974

63. Dupont B, Drouhet E: Cutaneous, ocular and osteoarticular candidiasis in heroin addicts: New clinical and therapeutic aspects in 38 patients. *J Infect Dis* **152**:577, 1985

64. Gartenberg G et al: Hospital-acquired mucormycosis (*Rhizopus rhizopodiformis*) of skin and subcutaneous tissue: Epidemiology, mycology and treatment. *N Engl J Med* **299**:1115, 1978

65. Mitchell SJ et al: Nosocomial infection with *Rhizopus microsporus* in preterm infants associated with wooden tongue depressors. *Lancet* **348**:441, 1996

66. Carlisle JR: Primary cutaneous aspergillosis in a leukaemic child. *Arch Dermatol* **114**:78, 1978

67. Rabodonirina M et al: *Fusarium* infections in immunocompromised patients: Case report and literature review. *Eur J Clin Microbiol Infect Dis* **13**:152, 1996

68. Bennhoff DF: Actinomycosis: Diagnostic and therapeutic considerations and a review of 32 cases. *Laryngoscope* **94**:1198, 1984

69. Brown JR: Human actinomycosis. A study of 181 subjects. *Hum Pathol* **4**:319, 1973

70. Reiner SL et al: Primary actinomycosis of an extremity: A case report and review. *Rev Infect Dis* **9**:581, 1987

71. Schlech WF et al: Medical management of visceral actinomycosis. *South Med J* **76**:921, 1983

72. Houang ET et al: *Nocardia asteroides* infection—a transmissible disease. *J Hosp Infect* **1**:31, 1980

73. Kalb RE et al: Cutaneous nocardiosis. *J Am Acad Dermatol* **13**:125, 1985

74. Tsuboi R et al: Lymphocutaneous nocardiosis caused by *Nocardia asteroides. Arch Dermatol* **122**:1183, 1986

75. Freeland C et al: Primary cutaneous nocardiosis caused by *Nocardia otitidiscaviarum:* Two cases and a review of the literature. *J Trop Med Hyg* **98**:395, 1995

76. Smego RA, Gallis HA: The clinical spectrum of *Nocardia brasiliensis* infections in the United States. *Rev Infect Dis* **6**:164, 1984

CHAPTER 209

Douglas R. Lowy

Viral Diseases: General Considerations

Skin lesions are a prominent feature of many viral diseases. In some instances, cutaneous lesions suggest a specific viral illness whose diagnosis can be quickly established by appropriate procedures. At other times, the differential diagnosis includes several viral and nonviral conditions. This situation may require costly, specialized, time-consuming, and possibly nondefinitive diagnostic procedures. However, the application of new techniques for laboratory diagnosis can shorten the time for diagnosis. To complement advances in diagnosis, there are now several effective antiviral agents for treating at least some viral diseases with cutaneous manifestations, and other possible antiviral agents are in clinical trials. Making the correct diagnosis in viral infection may therefore have important implications for therapy as well as for prognosis. It may also contribute to the surveillance and control of infectious disease within the community.

DEFINITION

Viruses form a diverse group of infectious agents that share a distinctive composition and a unique mode of replication.[1-4] Viruses are not cellular organisms. Although certain viruses encode a small number of enzymes, viruses do not possess functional ribosomes or other cellular organelles. These agents therefore lack much of the machinery required for their own multiplication. They multiply only inside cells, where they make use of the cellular synthetic apparatus to produce their components. It is because their replication depends on the host cell that viruses are often referred to as "obligate intracellular parasites."

The most important element of a virus is its genetic information (the viral *genome*), which may be either deoxyribonucleic acid (DNA) or ribonucleic acid (RNA), depending on the type of virus.[5] The life cycle of a virus may be divided into two parts.[6] In one part, the virus exists as an extracellular particle (also called a *virion*), where the viral genetic information is surrounded by a highly organized protein coat that can be seen by electron microscopy. The virion serves to transmit the viral genetic information, functionally intact, to a susceptible host. The second part of the viral life cycle is that period when the viral genetic information is present inside a cell, where it is usually found in a nonparticulate form. Certain pathogenetic aspects of virus infection occur during the nonparticulate portion of the virus life cycle. The duration of this intracellular phase is extremely variable, from a few hours in acute infections, to years when a virus establishes latency.

CLASSIFICATION

All organisms, from bacteria to humans, are susceptible to infection by a range of viruses, but no single virus is capable of infecting all classes of cells. Each virus is broadly classified as a bacterial, plant, or animal virus on the basis of the type of cell it can infect. The animal viruses have been divided into several large families according to the size, shape, and structure of the virion and the type of viral nucleic acid within it, as shown in Table 209-1. In the virion, the viral genome consists of only a single type of nucleic acid, either DNA or RNA. Viruses of a given family can be identified by physical methods, such as the size and shape of their virions by electron microscopy, by antigenic cross-reactivity, or by nucleic acid homology.[5] Although viruses have been grouped principally according to their virion morphology and nucleic acid composition, a given family of viruses usually shares functional, genetic, biochemical, and immunologic features.

As noted above, the virion is composed of the viral genetic core surrounded by a protective protein coat called the *capsid*. The capsids in certain virus families (such as herpesviruses and retroviruses) are located inside a virion *envelope* (composed of lipid, protein, and carbohydrate), which is required for infectivity (Table 209-1). The viral envelope is sensitive to drying, so that infectivity is lost on dry surfaces. The virions of other viruses (such as papillomaviruses) do not possess an envelope, so their capsids are called "naked." Since the capsid proteins are usually stable in dry environments, viruses whose virions lack an envelope typically remain infectious for long periods after drying.

In most viruses, the capsid is arranged in one of two patterns: helical symmetry or icosahedral (cubic) symmetry (Table 209-1). Poxviruses have a more complicated structure, which is classified as "complex." In viruses with helical symmetry, the protein subunits that form the capsid are assembled in an elongated, helical form. The subunits in viruses with icosahedral symmetry are assembled

TABLE 209-1

Selected Animal Virus Groups

GROUP	SIZE, NM	SYMMETRY	ENVELOPE	NUCLEIC ACID	CAPSID ASSEMBLY	EXAMPLES OF VIRUSES
Herpesvirus	120–200	Icosahedral	Yes	DNA	Nucleus	Herpes simplex (types 1 and 2), varicella-zoster, cytomegalo, EB, KHSV/HHV-8
Papovavirus	45–55	Icosahedral	No	DNA	Nucleus	Papillomaviruses
Poxvirus	240 × 300	Complex	No	DNA	Cytoplasm	Molluscum contagiosum, orf, milker's nodules, variola, vaccinia, cowpox
Retrovirus	80–120	?	Yes	RNA	Cytoplasm	HIV, HTLV
Paramyxovirus	150–300	Helical	Yes	RNA	Cytoplasm	Measles, mumps
Togavirus	40–60	Icosahedral	Yes	RNA	Cytoplasm	Rubella, some arboviruses
Parvovirus	20	Icosahedral	No	DNA	Nucleus	Erythema infectiosum
Hepadnavirus	40–50	Icosahedral	No	DNA	Nucleus	Hepatitis B
Adenovirus	70–80	Icosahedral	No	DNA	Nucleus	Multiple human serotypes
Picornavirus	20–30	Icosahedral	No	RNA	Cytoplasm	Entero (coxsackie, ECHO, polio), rhino
Bunyavirus	90–100	Helical	Yes	RNA	Cytoplasm	Some arboviruses
Arenavirus	85–120	?	Yes	RNA	Cytoplasm	Lassa fever
Coronavirus	80–120	Helical	Yes	RNA	Cytoplasm	Several human serotypes
Orthomyxovirus	80–120	Helical	Yes	RNA	Cytoplasm	Influenza types A + B + C
Rhabdovirus	70–80	Helical	Yes	RNA	Cytoplasm	Rabies
Reovirus	50–80	Icosahedral	No	RNA	Cytoplasm	Rotavirus, reovirus

into an icosahedral structure, which is a symmetric polyhedron with 20 equilateral triangular faces. Viruses within a given family may be further classified according to their relatedness at the nucleic acid level, their antigenic cross-reactivity, and the host cells that they infect.

Examples of virions from the three main families of viruses [papovaviruses (papillomaviruses), herpesviruses, and poxviruses] that multiply in the epidermis are shown in Fig. 209-1. The viral genomes of these three families are composed of DNA. As noted above, papillomaviruses possess naked (nonenveloped) capsids, and herpesviruses have enveloped virions. Poxvirus virions are large, have a very complex structure, and are enveloped, but their envelope is not required for their virions to be infectious. Hence, poxviruses can remain infectious after drying.

VIRAL REPLICATION

Viruses replicate inside cells by synthesizing their various structural components separately and then assembling them into multiple virions. This contrasts with cells that multiply by binary fission (the production of two progeny cells from a single parental cell).[6] As noted earlier, viruses utilize the host cell machinery to synthesize and assemble new virions, since these agents do not contain the apparatus required for their own replication.

Viral genomes encode two main classes of proteins. Some virus-encoded proteins are used to form the virions; these proteins are called *structural proteins*, or *virion proteins*. Viral genomes also encode *nonstructural proteins*; as their name implies, these proteins do not participate in forming the structural components of the virion. The nonstructural viral proteins often play key roles in the replication of the virus, although they are not usually incorporated into the virion. Acyclovir inhibits herpesvirus replication because the drug is activated inside herpesvirus-infected cells by virus-encoded nonstructural proteins.[7]

Nonstructural proteins of certain viruses may redirect the cell to synthesize the proteins required by the virus at the expense of those required for normal function of the cell. Many tumor viruses, including papillomaviruses, encode nonvirion proteins that increase cell growth and lead to inappropriate control of cell division (see Chap. 39). The intracellular pathogenicity of a virus may be due partly to effects of nonvirion proteins.[8]

The viral replication cycle, which has been studied in detail in tissue culture, involves several more or less sequential steps: attachment (adsorption), penetration, uncoating, biosynthesis, virion assembly, and release.[6] Attachment of virions to cells involves a specific interaction between the viral capsid or envelope (for those viruses that possess enveloped virions) and receptors on the cell surface. For example, HIV enters cells via an interaction between viral envelope protein and two classes of receptors: cellular CD4 receptors and chemokine receptors.[9] Cells that lack the appropriate cell surface receptors for a particular virus will therefore not be infected by that virus. Although most people are quite susceptible to HIV infection, rare individuals who lack the appropriate chemokine receptors or have modified versions of them may be relatively resistant to HIV infection or the development of AIDS.[10,11]

Following penetration of the virion into the cell, cellular enzymes degrade the envelope and capsid (uncoating), which begins the nonparticulate phase of the virus life cycle. During biosynthesis, the viral genome instructs the infected cell to produce the proteins encoded by the viral genes. Viruses vary in their size and complexity. The genome of poliovirus, which is a small virus with a simple virion structure, encodes a single precursor protein, which is cleaved to give rise to the structural and nonstructural viral proteins. By contrast, poxviruses, whose virions are more than 10 times larger than poliovirus virions and are much more complex, encode dozens of structural and nonstructural proteins.

The virions of most viruses, including papillomaviruses, herpesviruses, and poxviruses, are assembled inside the cell and released following cell death and lysis. However, enveloped viruses whose virions are assembled at the cell surface (such as retroviruses and paramyxoviruses) are released by budding from intact cells; with these viruses, productive infection and release of virions may or may not be accompanied by toxic effects on the infected cell. Each virus has its characteristic site of replication within the cell. Papil-

FIGURE 209-1

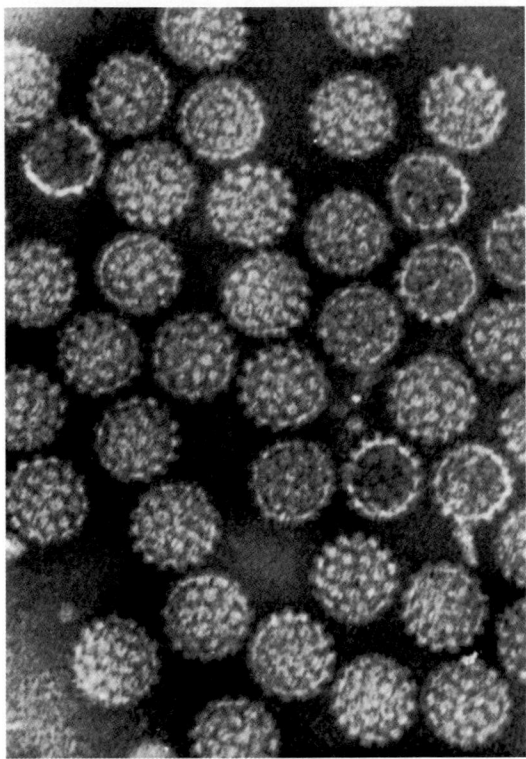

A.

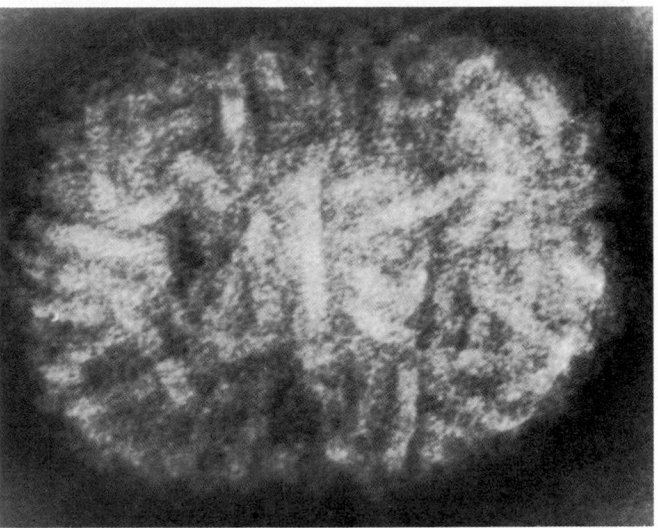

B.

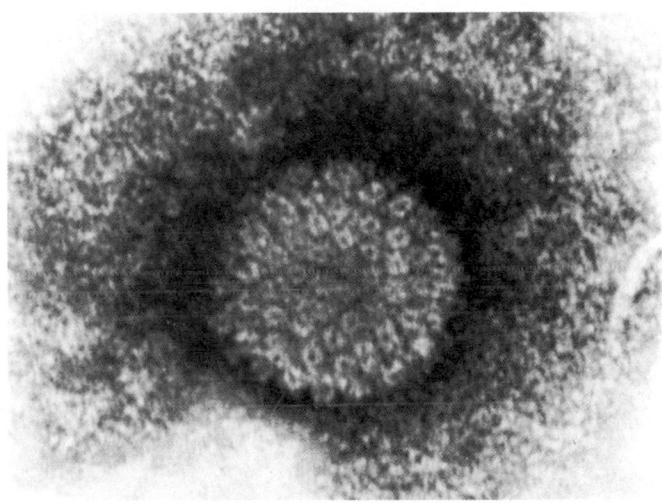

C.

Electron micrographs of negatively stained virions (×200,000). *A.* Papovavirus: multiple nonenveloped human papillomavirus (wart) virions showing capsid subunits (capsomeres). *B.* Poxvirus: single molluscum contagiosum virus virions, showing complex tubular structures. *C.* Herpesvirus: single varicella-zoster virus virion showing capsid inside envelope. [*Parts A and B courtesy of AF Howartson, JD Almeida, and MG Williams. Part C by permission of Almeida JD et al, Virology 16:353, 1962.*]

lomaviruses and herpesviruses are assembled in the nucleus (Figs. 209-2 and 209-3). Poxviruses, which are the only DNA viruses that replicate in the cytoplasm, synthesize their virions in organized cytoplasmic "viral factories" (Fig. 209-4).

Typically, hundreds or thousands of new virions are produced from each infected cell, and they, in turn, infect previously uninfected cells. One cycle of virus replication may last from 3 to 36 h, depending on the virus and cell involved. Interruption of any step will prevent the development of new infectious virions.

Each virus can infect and replicate in only a limited number of cell types. The spectrum of susceptible cells depends on the virus. Human papillomaviruses can infect a very narrow range of cells, namely certain differentiating human epidermal cells. Other viruses can infect a much broader range of cells; herpes simplex viruses can replicate in many different human and nonhuman cell types.

Even within a given tissue, a virus may be infectious only for cells with a specific degree of differentiation. The important role of the differentiated state of the cell in determining whether or not a virus will undergo replication is seen in the skin lesions of molluscum contagiosum. Since molluscum contagiosum virus (MCV) particles are sometimes found in cells of the upper dermis, the virus must be capable of attachment and penetration in these cells. MCV does not, however, replicate in dermal cells, indicating that an intracellular block to MCV synthesis exists in the dermal cells. MCV particles are also found in the basal layer of epidermal cells, but synthesis of new viral components does not begin until the cells reach the suprabasal layers. This observation implies that MCV replication can take place only in partially differentiated epidermal cells.

CELLULAR CONSEQUENCES OF VIRAL INFECTION

Typically, infected cells develop gross and often characteristic cytopathic changes and eventually die. Infections of this type are termed *cytocidal*, or *lytic*. However, some viruses can replicate without causing irreversible damage to the host cell. Noncytocidal infection of this type may occur in tissue culture with measles virus and many other enveloped RNA viruses, leading to a chronically

FIGURE 209-2

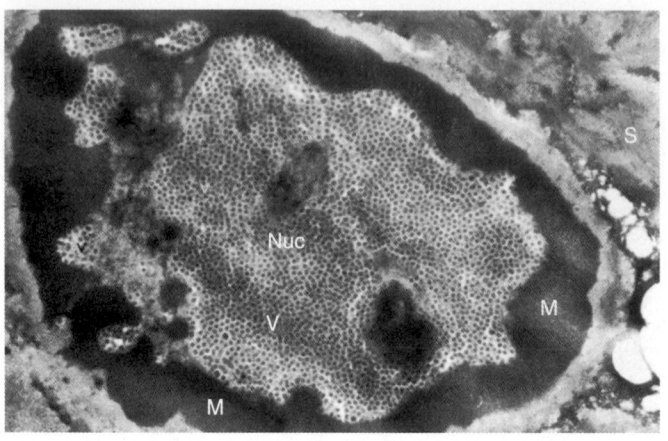

Papillomavirus (a papovavirus). Electron micrograph (×20,000). Nucleus (Nuc) of a stratum corneum cell, filled with papillomavirus virions (V); chromatin is marginated (M). Mature keratin can be seen in an adjacent cell (S).

FIGURE 209-3

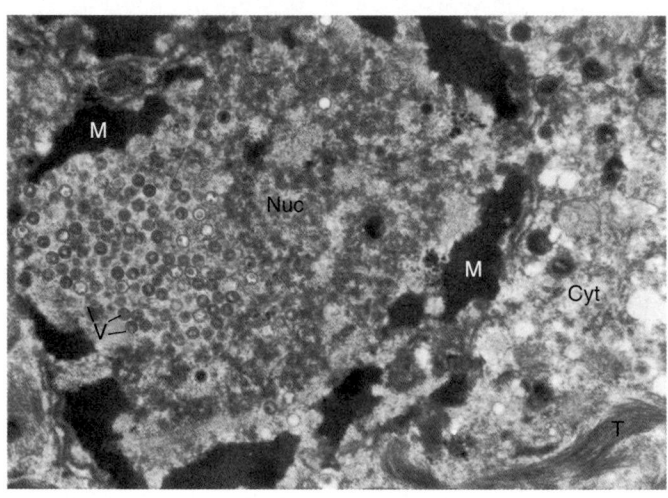

Varicella-zoster virus (a herpesvirus). Electron micrograph (×24,000). Portion of cell of the stratum spinosum. The nucleus (Nuc) contains varicella-zoster virions (V). Chromatin is marginated at (M). Virions (V) and tonofilaments (T) are shown in the cytoplasm (Cyt).

infected culture. While many retroviruses replicate without killing cells, cell lysis plays an important role in the pathogenesis of HIV infection.[9]

Two other types of noncytocidal infection are neoplastic transformation[12,13] and viral latency.[14,15] Tumor viruses, when they transform cells, alter the normal control of cellular proliferation. In general, tumor viruses (such as the papovavirus SV-40) do not synthesize new virions in neoplastically transformed cells, although such transformation requires the continued expression of a portion of the viral genome. It is interesting to note that SV-40 is exclu-

FIGURE 209-4

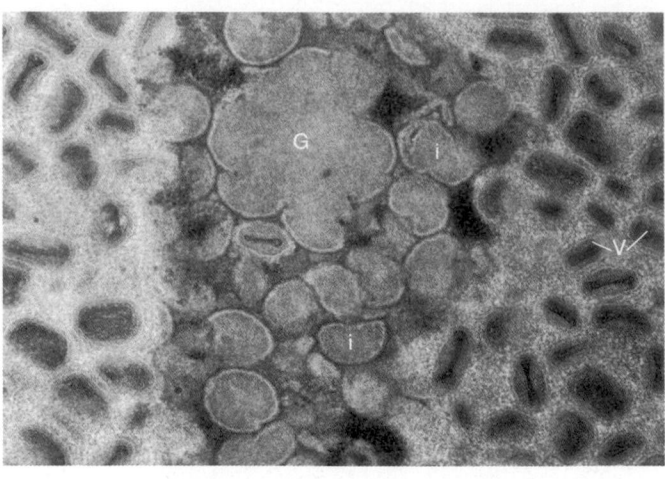

Molluscum contagiosum (a poxvirus). Electron micrograph (×45,000). Cytoplasm of a spinosum cell filled with mature molluscum contagiosum virions (V), immature virus forms (i), and viroplasm in a gyrate pattern (G).

sively cytocidal for some cell types (permissive infection), induces transformation exclusively in other cells (nonpermissive infection), and induces both types of infection in still other cell types (semipermissive infection), again underlining the importance of the host cell in affecting the outcome of infection. Epidermal cells are semipermissive for papillomavirus infection. Virus-induced neoplasia is discussed in greater detail in Chap. 39.

Viral latency, which occurs commonly with herpesviruses and papillomaviruses, represents the other type of noncytocidal infection. Latently infected cells probably either produce very small numbers of new virions so that spread to uninfected cells is minimal or they synthesize no new virus but retain an intact and potentially activable viral genome.

PATHOGENESIS OF VIRAL INFECTIONS IN THE SKIN

There are several general patterns of viral infection.[15] The most typical is that of acute infection followed by viral clearance, usually by immune mechanisms. This pattern occurs frequently with viruses that produce exanthems, such as measles. Another pattern is that of acute infection followed by latent infection, which may then be followed by viral reactivation. In viruses with cutaneous manifestations, this pattern occurs often with herpes simplex virus, varicellazoster virus, and papillomavirus. A third pattern is that of chronic infection, as occurs frequently with HIV infection. Often, active infection with some viruses, such as papillomaviruses and MCV, may persist for months or years even in immunocompetent hosts.

Virus infections may affect the skin by three different routes: direct inoculation, systemic infection, or local spread from an internal focus. In warts, herpes simplex, chickenpox, herpes zoster, molluscum contagiosum, and smallpox, virus shedding from human skin lesions represents an important source in the transmission of virus to other people. Skin lesions may be produced by the direct effect of virus replication on infected cells, the host response to the virus, or the interaction of replication and host response.

The viruses of warts, molluscum contagiosum, vaccinia, orf, milker's nodules, and (primary) herpes simplex, all of which infect the skin by direct inoculation, replicate in the epidermis. Their viral cytopathic effects account for the appearance of early lesions. The immune system presumably contributes to the evolution of those lesions that subsequently develop an inflammatory response. The incubation period is generally short because the lesions develop at the site of inoculation. The incubation period for warts is longer, presumably because the virus replicates slowly or cell-to-cell spread of virus occurs to only a limited extent. Latent papillomavirus infection has been demonstrated in clinically normal laryngeal tissue of patients with a history of laryngeal papillomas, suggesting that host-specific factors may also play a significant role in some papillomavirus-induced lesions.[16]

In systemic infections, the skin is infected during viremia, so that the dermis is generally infected earlier than the epidermis. It is not known how the distribution of viral exanthems is determined. In chickenpox and smallpox, the damage from cytocidal infection of the skin is a prime cause of the lesions. On the other hand, there is suggestive evidence from patients with impaired cellular immunity that the lesions of rubella and measles result in part from a cell-mediated immune response to the virus. The basis of most exanthems associated with enteroviral infections remains to be established; there is significant cytocidal viral replication in the skin in hand-foot-and-mouth disease.

Recurrent herpes simplex and herpes zoster represent the local spread of virus to the skin following reactivation of the latent virus present in peripheral nerves. Cytocidal infection clearly plays an important role in these lesions, although lesions may contain less virus than during primary infection, presumably because of immunity.

HOST RESPONSE

The severity of illness induced by a particular virus varies considerably from person to person. While the size of the viral inoculum and the portal of entry play some role, it is believed that host factors usually account for most of this variation. Both immunologic and nonimmunologic responses appear to be important.[8,15,17,18] Conversely, viral infection may have significant direct and indirect effects on the immune system, especially those viruses that infect lymphoid cells, such as Epstein-Barr virus and HIV.[9]

Antibody responses to viral infection represent the major host defense against reinfection by the same virus[19]; the prophylactic administration of type-specific antibodies can prevent or modify some primary viral infections even in patients with impaired cellular immunity. However, humoral immunity is thought not to contribute to the recovery from most primary viral infections, as viral infection of patients with isolated deficiencies of humoral immunity usually follows a normal course. There are several mechanisms by which antibodies may inhibit the spread of virus. These include neutralization of virus through prevention of viral attachment to target cells (which may be increased by complement); enhancement of viral uptake by phagocytic cells, which then inactivate the virus; and (complement-mediated) immune lysis of infected cells.

Specific cell-mediated immunity (CMI) is also elicited during viral infections and apparently influences the course of many viral infections. CMI is usually protective, although it may sometimes increase the degree of cellular pathology (as in the eruption of measles). Patients with impaired CMI often have difficulty handling primary or recurrent viral infection. Such patients are at risk of developing severe primary virus infections, warts, chronic herpes simplex virus infections, disseminated herpes zoster, and AIDS. The antiviral mechanisms of CMI have not yet been fully established. Sensitized T cells are known to be capable of lysing infected cells and of liberating lymphokines, which attract phagocytic cells. Natural killer cells, virus-specific cytotoxic lymphocytes, and antibody-dependent cell-mediated cytotoxicity can inhibit infection under experimental conditions.

Inflammatory cells may produce some of their antiviral effects via the production of interferons, a unique family of closely related cytokines that are active against viruses.[20] Interferon, which can be induced by foreign RNA or DNA (including viral nucleic acids), is secreted into the extracellular fluid. Resistance to virus infection is induced in those cells that come in contact with the interferon. Virtually all viruses are capable of inducing interferon and are susceptible to its action, but viruses differ greatly in their degree of interferon induction and in their sensitivity to its action. Interferon has been shown to be responsible for recovery in several types of virus infection in mice, and the presence of interferon correlates with the recovery phase of several human viral infections. Genetic factors may also play a role in determining the outcome of viral infections. In animal models, genes can determine the susceptibility to viral infection at several levels, including virion attachment to cells, viral replication, and viral-induced immune responses.[21]

DIAGNOSIS OF VIRAL INFECTIONS

Four major approaches are used in the laboratory to diagnose viral infection: virus isolation, microscopy, detection of viral nucleic acids or viral antigens, and serology.[22–24] As with all laboratory tests, the results must be interpreted in the context of the clinical setting. Fortuitous infection with a virus unrelated to the illness should always be considered. For many viruses, considerable progress has been made in the development of relatively rapid assays that are sensitive and specific.[22,25] Most of these newer assays depend upon the ability to detect small amounts of viral nucleic acids and/or viral antigens.

Cultivation of the virus has represented the traditional "gold standard" for viral diagnosis. Virus isolation is most useful if the suspected pathogen can be readily propagated and positive results can be obtained in a short time. If necessary, more precise identification of the cultured virus can be carried out with specific tests for viral nucleic acid or viral antigen. Culture techniques for herpes simplex virus are quite sensitive, with diagnostic changes in cells often appearing within days of inoculation. The closely related varicella-zoster virus is much more difficult to grow in culture, so false-negative results are extremely common.

When virus isolation is attempted, specimens should be obtained as early in the disease as possible. In vesicular conditions, fluid from an early vesicle is often a good source of virus. Lesional specimens are less likely to be positive with nonvesicular exanthems. Specimens should also be obtained from additional sites as indicated. Each specimen should be placed in a sterile tube with 2 to 5 mL of a buffered isotonic balanced salt solution containing penicillin and streptomycin. Preferably, it should be transported on ice immediately to the laboratory. If this is not practical, the specimen should be frozen (at $-70°C$, if possible). The suspected pathogen(s) should be indicated, since it may determine the type of cell culture or test animal to be inoculated.

The direct identification of a virus in clinical specimens can theoretically be accomplished more quickly than tests that rely on culturing the virus. This approach may be especially useful for detecting those viruses difficult to propagate in culture and those, such as papillomaviruses, for which no reproducible culture system is available. Direct analysis may identify characteristic cells, as with Tzanck smears for herpesviruses (this test will not distinguish between herpes simplex and varicella-zoster viruses) or the histologic appearance of MCV-containing lesions.

The direct identification of virus from clinical material is limited by the sensitivity and specificity of the assay. The use of assays based on detecting viral nucleic acid is having a progressively larger impact on direct identification, initially through molecular hybridization and more recently through application of the polymerase chain reaction (PCR).[22,25] This latter technique, which can specifically amplify minute quantities of viral nucleic acid, is revolutionizing diagnostic virology. Assays based on PCR and related techniques are extremely sensitive, often being able to detect as few as 1 infected cell in 10,000, and highly specific. The main pitfall of PCR is that its great sensitivity makes it very susceptible to yielding false-positive results via cross-contamination with minute quantities of viral nucleic acid. However, meticulous attention to detail and appropriate controls can usually overcome this potential liability.

More traditional techniques are also available. For those lesions that contain large numbers of viral particles, electron microscopy of a lesion or its extract may provide morphologic identification of the virus.[24] The positive identification of specific viral antigen in clinical material through use of immunologic techniques permits a more specific diagnosis than direct microscopy. For example, immunologic techniques can distinguish between herpes simplex virus and varicella-zoster virus. Radioimmunoassay, enzyme-linked immunosorbent assay, immunoelectron microscopy, fluorescent antibody, or immunoperoxidase techniques identify viral antigen by the use of viral-specific antibody.

Serologic studies to detect viral antibodies may be important for epidemiologic purposes, for identifying infection with viruses such as HIV and hepatitis B, and for those situations where acute sera contain diagnostic antibodies, as with heterophile antibodies in infectious mononucleosis. In most acute viral illness, serologic analysis requires acute and convalescent sera, which limits its use in that setting to making a retrospective diagnosis. Paired sera are required because a positive serology during the acute phase may merely mean the individual was infected previously with a member of that virus family, but it does not have implications for the etiology of the current illness. The acute specimen should be taken as early in the illness as possible and the convalescent specimen 2 to 4 weeks later. Serum should be separated immediately from the coagulated blood and refrigerated or preferably frozen at $-20°C$ until antibody tests can be run simultaneously on both specimens. A fourfold or greater rise in antibody titer between the first and second specimen generally indicates recent infection. A variety of assays are used to measure antibody levels, each detecting a certain type of antigen-antibody reaction. The antibody titer of a given serum is defined as the reciprocal of the highest dilution that gives a positive reaction.

THERAPY AND PREVENTION

Prophylaxis of viral infection has thus far proved more successful than the specific treatment of established infection. Vaccines have been extremely useful in the prevention of a variety of viral illnesses.[19,26,27] Recombinant DNA techniques are making it possible to develop effective subunit vaccines composed only of viral protein, rather than traditional vaccines, which represent either an attenuated strain of the pathogen or an inactivated preparation of the entire virus.[28,29] In addition to vaccines that induce active immunity, the passive administration of type-specific antibody soon after exposure can prevent chickenpox in compromised hosts. Sensitive procedures for the detection of hepatitis B and HIV infection in potential blood donors has drastically reduced the incidence of transmission of these agents by transfusion.

Because viruses are adapted to the cells they infect and because they make use of the cellular machinery, many chemotherapeutic agents that have been considered as potential antiviral agents affect cells to about the same extent as they affect viruses. However, this difficulty has already been overcome in several instances, and additional antiviral agents are under development.[1,30,31] Most antivirals seek to exploit a specific property of a particular virus. Azidothymidine (AZT) and several protease inhibitors, which are approved for use in the treatment of HIV infection, interfere with HIV replication by preferentially inhibiting synthesis of the viral genome and the processing of viral proteins, respectively.[9,32,33] Acyclovir, an antimetabolite that has been approved for use in selected herpesvirus infections, is preferentially activated by herpesvirus-infected cells through its affinity for two herpesvirus enzymes involved in DNA synthesis. Interferon is a potentially potent antiviral agent that inhibits most viruses and at low dosages is relatively nontoxic to cells. Interferon has been approved for use in treatment of certain genital papillomavirus infections and has also been helpful in the management of some children with papillomas of the larynx.

REFERENCES

1. Galasso GJ et al (eds): *Antiviral Agents and Viral Diseases of Man,* 4th ed. New York, Lippincott-Raven, 1997
2. Richman DD: *Clinical Virology.* New York, Churchill Livingstone, 1997
3. Fields BN et al (eds): *Fields Virology,* 3d ed. New York, Lippincott-Raven, 1996
4. Volk WA (ed): *Essentials of Medical Microbiology,* 5th ed. Philadelphia, Lippincott-Raven, 1996
5. Mattern CFT: Structure and classification of viruses, in *Medical Microbiology,* 3d ed, edited by S Baron. New York, Churchill Livingstone, 1991, p 559
6. Roizman B: Multiplication of viruses, an overview, in *Fields Virology,* 3d ed, edited by BN Fields, DM Knipe, PM Howley. New York, Lippincott-Raven, 1996, p 101
7. Whitley RJ, Gnann JW: Acyclovir: A decade later. *N Engl J Med* **327:**782, 1992
8. Tyler KL, Fields BN: Pathogenesis of viral infections, in *Fields Virology,* 3d ed, edited by BN Fields, DM Knipe, PM Howley. New York, Lippincott-Raven, 1996, p 173
9. Levy JA (ed): *HIV and the Pathogenesis of AIDS,* 2d ed. Washington, ASM, 1998
10. Dean M et al: Genetic restriction of HIV-1 infection and progression to AIDS by a deletion allele of the CKR5 structural gene. *Science* **273:**1856, 1996
11. Smith MW et al: Contrasting genetic influence of CCR2 and CCR5 variants on HIV-1 infection and disease progression. *Science* **277:**959, 1997
12. Nevins JR, Vogt PK: Cell transformation by viruses, in *Fields Virology,* 3d ed, edited by BN Fields, DM Knipe, PM Howley. New York, Lippincott-Raven, 1996, p 301

13. Bishop JM, Weinberg RA (eds): *Molecular Oncology.* New York, Scientific American, 1996
14. Stevens JG: Overview of herpesvirus latency. *Semin Virol* **5**:191, 1994
15. Ahmed R et al: Persistence of viruses, in *Fields Virology,* 3d ed, edited by BN Fields, DM Knipe, PM Howley. New York, Lippincott-Raven, 1996, p 219
16. Steinberg BM et al: Laryngeal papillomavirus infection during clinical remission. *N Engl J Med* **308**:1261, 1983
17. Whitten L, Oldstone MBA: Immune response to viruses, in *Fields Virology,* 3d ed, edited by BN Fields, DM Knipe, PM Howley. New York, Lippincott-Raven, 1996, p 345
18. Zinkernagel RM: Immunity to viruses, in *Fundamental Immunology,* 3d ed, edited by WE Paul. New York, Raven, 1993, p 1211
19. Murphy BR, Chanock RM: Immunization against virus disease, in *Fields Virology,* 3d ed, edited by BN Fields, DM Knipe, PM Howley. New York, Lippincott-Raven, 1996, p 467
20. Vilcek J, Sen GC: Interferons and other cytokines, in *Fields Virology,* 3d ed, edited by BN Fields, DM Knipe, PM Howley. New York, Lippincott-Raven, 1996, p 375
21. Brinton MA et al: Host genes that influence susceptibility to viral diseases, in *Concepts in Viral Pathogenesis,* edited by AL Notkins, MBA Oldstone. New York, Springer, 1984, p 71
22. Jones-Brando LV, Yolken R: Laboratory diagnosis of viral infections, in *Antiviral Agents and Viral Diseases of Man,* edited by GJ Galasso, RJ Whitley, TC Merigan. New York, Lippincott-Raven, 1997, p 129
23. Lennette EH et al (eds): *Diagnostic Procedures for Viral, Rickettsial, and Chlamydial Infections.* Washington, American Public Health Association, 1995
24. Hsiung GD et al: *Hsiung's Diagnostic Virology: As Illustrated by Light and Electron Microscopy,* 4th ed. New Haven, Yale University, 1994
25. Becker Y, Darai G (eds): *PCR: Protocols for Diagnosis of Human and Animal Virus Diseases.* New York, Springer, 1995
26. Ada GL, Ramsay AJ: *Vaccines, Vaccination, and the Immune Response.* Philadelphia, Lippincott-Raven, 1997
27. Plotkin SA, Mortimer EA (eds): *Vaccines,* 2d ed. Philadelphia, Saunders, 1994
28. Levine MM: *New Generation Vaccines,* 2d ed. New York, Marcel Dekker, 1997
29. Powell MF et al: *Vaccine Design: The Subunit and Adjuvant Approach.* New York, Plenum, 1995
30. Mills J et al (eds): *Antiviral Chemotherapy 4: New Directions for Clinical Application and Research.* New York, Plenum, 1996
31. Jeffries DJ, De Clercq E (eds): *Antiviral Chemotherapy.* New York, Wiley, 1995
32. Sande MA, Volberding P (eds): *The Medical Management of AIDS,* 5th ed. Philadelphia, Saunders, 1997
33. Mohan P, Masanori B (eds): *Anti-AIDS Drug Development: Challenges, Strategies and Prospects.* Chur, Switzerland, Harwood Academic, 1995

CHAPTER 210

Stephen E. Gellis

Rubella (German Measles)

Rubella (German measles) is a common communicable infection of children and young adults characterized by a short prodromal period; enlargement of cervical, suboccipital, and postauricular glands; and a rash of approximately 2 to 3 days' duration. The disease has rare sequelae and, were it not for its devastating effect on the fetus, would be of relatively little significance in terms of morbidity or complications.

tions can be demonstrated by laboratory tests in some "immune" individuals who are subsequently exposed to the wild virus. Two attacks of rubella with rash are most unlikely to be encountered; in such instances, one of the episodes is usually not rubella but is due to another viral infection.

The virus of rubella may be recovered from the pharynx as early as 7 days before and up to 14 days after the onset of the rash. Viremia is rarely demonstrated after the onset of the rash.[1]

EPIDEMIOLOGY

Epidemics of rubella have been noted at 5- to 7-year intervals. The disease is worldwide in its distribution and tends to occur most frequently during the spring months in North America. It is rare in young infants and is most common in school-age children, adolescents, and young adults. It is spread via the respiratory route, and the period of infectivity extends from the end of the incubation period to the disappearance of the rash. A single attack confers lifelong immunity in most individuals, although subclinical reinfec-

CLINICAL MANIFESTATIONS (Table 210-1)

The incubation period ranges between 14 and 21 days and is usually 16 to 18 days. Prodromal signs and symptoms are rare in young children, and the rash usually appears without prior complaint. In older children, adolescents, and adults, low-grade fever, headache, conjunctivitis, sore throat, rhinitis, cough, and lymphadenopathy may precede the rash by 1 to 4 days and disappear rapidly after the rash appears. In some adults, however, these symptoms and signs

arthritis of rubella usually lasts 1 to 2 weeks but occasionally may persist for longer periods or may be recurrent.

TABLE 210-1

Some Distinctive Features of the Rashes of Rubella, Measles, and Scarlet Fever

	RUBELLA	RUBEOLA (MEASLES)	SCARLET FEVER
Prodrome	1–2 days of mild fever and respiratory symptoms	2–4 days of fever with moderate-to-severe respiratory symptoms	1–2 days of fever and sore throat
Duration of rash	Average 1–2 days	Average 3–5 days	Varies with treatment
Color	Pink-red	Purple-red to brown before fading	Yellow-red (may blanch on pressure)
Distribution	Scattered to generalized	Generalized (variable in modified measles) Koplik's spots (early)	Generalized (altered by treatment) Circumoral pallor "Strawberry" tongue
Nature	Macular to macular and papular Discrete with minimal coalescence about thorax	Macular to macular and papular Discrete with marked coalescence about face and thorax	Punctate lesions on erythematous skin Pinhead-sized lesions imparting sandpaper-like texture to skin Accentuation in flexor creases
Postexanthem desquamation	Occasional and branny	Common and branny	Typical and severe, often occurring on the hands and feet

COMPLICATIONS

Rubella is essentially a benign disease. Rarely, it may produce an encephalitis, which tends to be mild and is usually followed by complete recovery and no effect on intellectual function. Thrombocytopenic purpura, which may result from rubella, may be accompanied by epistaxis, petechiae, ecchymoses, intestinal hemorrhage, and hematuria. These manifestations frequently clear within a month of onset but may occasionally persist for longer periods. Rarely, a peripheral neuritis may follow rubella.

LABORATORY FINDINGS

The white blood cell count is usually low but may be normal. Increased numbers of atypical lymphocytes may be noted, and in some cases increased

may persist longer and be more severe, and the infection under such circumstances may be difficult to distinguish from rubeola (measles) unless Koplik's spots, characteristic of measles, are observed. The rash of rubella is first noted on the face (Fig. 210-1) and rapidly spreads to the neck, arms, trunk, and legs. It consists of pink-red macules and papules that are discrete and remain so on the extremities, coalescing on the trunk to give a uniform red blush.

The rash, which usually disappears by the end of 2 or 3 days, clearing first from the face, may occasionally be followed by fine desquamation. This rapid disappearance is in contrast to measles (rubeola), in which the rash persists for longer periods. An enanthem is often seen at the end of the prodromal period or beginning of the rash, consisting of red spots, pinhead in size, scattered over the soft palate. The lymphadenopathy of rubella is striking; it involves all lymph nodes, but enlargement and tenderness are most common in the suboccipital, postauricular, and anterior and posterior cervical nodes. In older children and adults, lymphadenopathy may be noted several days before the rash; but in both children and adults, the enlargement and tenderness are most striking on the first day of the rash. Enlargement of glands may persist for days to weeks but tenderness rapidly subsides. Splenomegaly may occasionally be detected. The fever of rubella is usually of low grade and seldom lasts beyond the first day or two of the eruption except in individuals who have joint involvement, in whom fever may persist. Arthritis due to rubella occurs much more frequently in adults than in children and is usually first noted as the rash fades. Small and large joints may become painful, with or without swelling, possibly simulating rheumatic fever or rheumatoid arthritis. In one epidemic, joint involvement was seen in 25 percent of children under the age of 11 years and in 52 percent of patients 11 years of age or older.[2] Striking effusions into joints have been reported. The

FIGURE 210-1

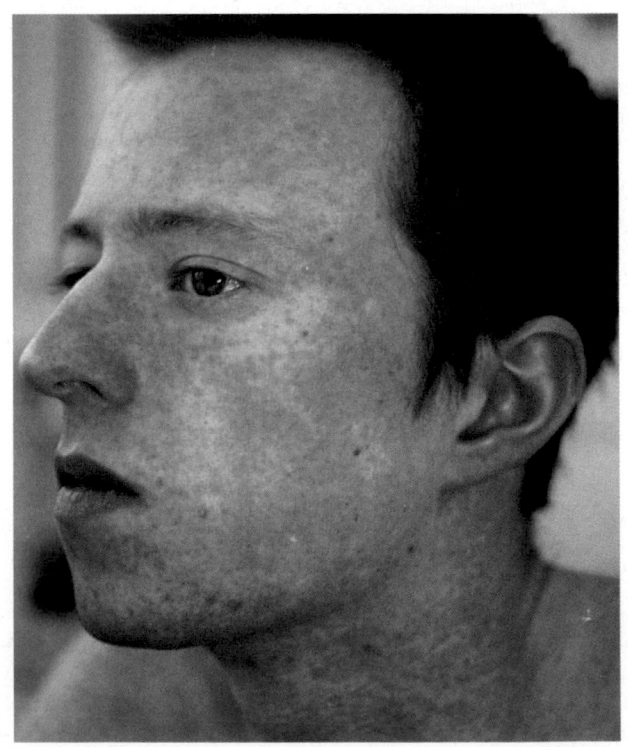

Rubella. Erythematous macules and papules appearing initially on the face and spreading usually within 24 h.

numbers of plasma cells have been reported. Among patients with meningoencephalitis, varying numbers of lymphocytes may be found in the cerebrospinal fluid.

CONGENITAL RUBELLA (Table 210-2)

Gregg in 1941[3] was the first to record the devastating effects of rubella infection in the fetus and to describe the congenital rubella syndrome. Approximately 50 percent of infants who acquire rubella during the first trimester of intrauterine life will show clinical signs of damage from the virus. The earlier the infection, the more severe the fetal damage. In such infants, multiple congenital defects include low birth weight, microcephaly with mental retardation, cataracts, nerve deafness, and congenital heart disease (usually patent ductus arteriosus or ventricular septal defect). Following completion of organ development in the fetus, infection with rubella may produce a variable clinical picture, which may include hepatitis, splenomegaly, pneumonitis, myocarditis, encephalitis, and osteomyelitis. When the bone marrow is affected, the infant may be born with thrombocytopenia and bleeding into the skin, producing a striking picture of petechiae and ecchymoses given the colorful term "blueberry muffin baby." In congenital rubella, a retinopathy consisting of a diffuse deposit of black pigmentation is commonly found.

TABLE 210-2

Some Manifestations of the Congenital Rubella Syndrome

Teratogenic findings—congenital malformations
1. Heart*
    a. Patent ductus arteriosus
    b. Coarctation of pulmonary vessels
    c. Ventricular septal defects
    d. Combination of above
    e. Others
2. Eye*
    a. Cataracts
    b. Microphthalmia
    c. Retinopathy
    d. Glaucoma
    e. Cloudy cornea
3. Hearing defects*
4. Central nervous system*
    a. Microcephaly
    b. Hydrocephaly
5. Bone,* disturbances of growth of skull
6. Abnormal dermatoglyphics
7. Agammaglobulinemia
8. Other organ systems
Other findings
1. Intra- and extrauterine growth retardation*
2. Prematurity*
3. Meningoencephalitis
4. Pneumonitis
5. Hepatitis*
6. Cardiac tissue injury
7. Rarefaction bone*
8. Thrombocytopenia with or without purpura*
9. Anemia
10. Rubelliform skin rash
11. Generalized adenopathy

*More commonly encountered.
SOURCE: Adapted from papers in Rubella Symposium, *Am J Dis Child* 110:345, 1965.

Diagnosis

Infants with congenital rubella may be chronically infected for many months. Virus can be cultured from the nasopharynx, urine, cerebrospinal fluid, and even the lens of infants with congenital cataract. As time passes, the amount of virus shed in the nasopharynx and urine gradually declines and disappears. Approximately 85 percent of infants infected in utero will excrete virus in the first month of life; 1 to 3 percent continue to excrete virus in the second year of life. The large amounts of virus from congenitally infected infants are very hazardous to pregnant women working with such infants who may be susceptible to infection. The infant with congenital infection will usually have elevation of IgM due to antibody produced by the infant itself, together with elevated IgG caused by passive transfer of antibodies in the maternal blood. IgG traverses the placenta, in contrast to IgM, which does not. The IgG antibodies disappear over the first few months of life. Passively acquired IgG by the fetus from an immune mother may explain the rarity of acquired rubella in early infancy. The antibodies against rubella consist of neutralizing, complement-fixing, and hemagglutination-inhibition antibodies. Neutralizing and hemagglutination-inhibition antibodies usually persist for life. The hemagglutination-inhibition antibodies are easily and quickly measured and serve to determine whether a recent infection can be attributed to rubella by an increase in titer in the convalescent period over the titer in the acute stage. A fourfold increase or more is considered diagnostic of the infection. Testing for these antibodies also enables the physician to determine whether a woman of childbearing age is immune or susceptible to German measles.

More sensitive tests are also now available: latex agglutination, fluorescence immunoassay, passive hemagglutination, hemolysis in gel, and enzyme immunoassay tests.

IMMUNITY AND IMMUNIZATION

Lifelong immunity usually follows an attack of rubella. Reinfection can occur but is usually not accompanied by clinical signs and symptoms. A rise in antibody level can occur; viremia from subclinical reinfection is very rare. Thus, congenital rubella is very unlikely in an infant whose mother has had an attack of rubella in the past and acquires a reinfection during pregnancy. In these instances, evaluation of fetal blood obtained by cordocentesis for specific rubella IgM antibodies or for evaluation by newer techniques using polymerase chain reaction (PCR) may help to confirm a diagnosis of fetal infection.[4,5] The availability of rubella vaccine[6,7] and its widespread use has markedly reduced the frequency of congenital infection.

In the United States, rubella vaccine is usually given together with mumps and measles vaccines in a single injection [mumps, measles, rubella (MMR)] at the age of 12 to 15 months and again at school entry (4 to 6 years of age).

Rubella vaccine should not be given to a pregnant woman. If a woman of childbearing age is to be immunized, routine serologic testing is not necessary. However, a sample of blood may be obtained before vaccination and stored for 3 months. This would allow for testing if the woman became pregnant. Pregnancy should be avoided for 3 months after immunization. If the vaccine is inadvertently given to a pregnant woman or to a woman who becomes pregnant within 3 months, there is a theoretical risk to the fetus. Asymptomatic infections have occurred, but no cases of congenital defects have been documented. Interruption of pregnancy is not indicated.

The child or adult to whom rubella vaccine is administered does not shed sufficient virus to infect susceptible individuals in close contact. As a result, it is safe to immunize children in a family in which the mother is pregnant.[8]

REFERENCES

1. Cooper LZ, Krugman S: Clinical manifestations of postnatal congenital rubella. *Arch Ophthalmol* **77**:434, 1967
2. Jedelsohn RG, Wyll SA: Rubella in Bermuda: Termination of an epidemic by mass vaccination. *JAMA* **223**:401, 1973
3. Gregg NM: Congenital cataract following German measles in the mother. *Trans Ophthalmol Soc Aust* **3**:35, 1941
4. Zolti M et al: Rubella-specific IgM in reinfection and risk to the fetus. *Gynecol Obstet Invest* **30**:184, 1990
5. Ho Terry L et al: Diagnosis of foetal rubella virus infection by polymerase chain reaction. *J Gen Virol* **71**:1607, 1990
6. Meyer HM Jr et al: Attenuated rubella virus II: Production of an experimental live-virus vaccine and clinical trial. *N Engl J Med* **275**:575, 1966
7. Meyer HM Jr, Parkman PD: Rubella vaccination: A review of practical experience. *JAMA* **215**:613, 1971
8. American Academy of Pediatrics: Rubella, in *1997 Red Book: Report of the Committee on Infectious Diseases,* 24th ed., edited by G Peter. AAP, Washington, DC, 1997

CHAPTER 211

Louis Z. Cooper

Measles

Measles is a universal, highly contagious, acute viral disease of childhood. It is characterized by high fever, cough, coryza, conjunctivitis, and Koplik's spots, which precede the appearance of a florid, generalized macular and papular rash.

HISTORIC ASPECTS

The term *measles* is thought to come from the Latin *misellus* or *misella*, a diminutive of the Latin *miser*, meaning miserable, which described the inmate of a medieval leper house. *Morbilli*, the diminutive of *morbus*, was introduced to distinguish minor rash disease from bubonic plague, *morbus*, the major disease. *Morbilliform* is a synonym for measles-like; it is still in common use.

No accurate information is available on the early history of measles. The tenth-century Arabian physician Rhazes has generally been credited with distinguishing measles from smallpox, although he cited El Yehudi, a Hebrew physician from the first century, as first describing the disease. However, it was probably not until the severe epidemics of measles during the seventeenth century that these diseases were clearly separated; e.g., the astute clinical and epidemiologic observations by Thomas Sydenham were completed at this time.[1]

In more recent times, transmission of measles to monkeys was first reported by Josias,[2] and other investigators[3,4] demonstrated that monkeys could be infected with blood or nasopharyngeal secretions obtained from patients.

The isolation of measles virus in tissue culture by Enders and Peebles[5] provided the essential techniques for definitive characterization of the virus excretion and antibody response in this disease and for its ultimate control. In 1960, Enders and his co-workers successfully attenuated measles virus,[6] and after extensive field trials, a live measles virus vaccine was licensed for general use in the United States in 1963. Since that time, the administration of approximately 250 million doses of vaccine has significantly decreased the incidence of this infection in this country.

EPIDEMIOLOGY

Measles is a universal illness, worldwide in distribution, that occurs primarily in children. However, the age incidence varies according to the environmental setting. In congested urban areas, the highest attack rate occurs in infancy and early childhood. In rural and less crowded areas, the attack rate is highest in the early school years, at ages 5 to 10 years. When measles has been introduced into isolated communities, the attack rate has approached 100 percent among the susceptible population of all ages. Very young infants, under 4 months of age, are usually protected by the persistence of transplacentally acquired maternal measles antibody.

Neither race nor sex affects the attack rate of measles, but the general state of health and nutrition clearly affects morbidity and mortality rates. Measles is primarily a disease of winter and spring in temperate climates, with the peak incidence of infection usually occurring in March or April.

The epidemiology of measles has changed dramatically because of the impact of massive immunization programs for eradication of the disease. The Measles Elimination Program, aided by a policy of school exclusion for those without proof of measles immunization, reduced the total number of reported cases in the United States to a low of 1497 in 1983. However, social factors and progressively declining immunization rates among urban poor infants and young children have led to increasing rates of measles. During the 3-year period 1989 to 1991, 18,000, 28,000, and almost 10,000 cases, respectively, were reported nationally. Black and Latino infants and preschool children bore the brunt of the epidemic. Hospitalization and death rates were remarkably high. (see "Complications" below). As a consequence of increased efforts targeted at high-risk groups and the requirement that a second dose of measles vaccine be given before school entry, by 1995 the number of confirmed cases of measles in the United States declined to 301. In 1996, the number increased slightly to 508 cases, but the striking finding was that 34 percent of the patients were above 19 years of age. This older group missed the introduction of the second dose of vaccine.[7]

ETIOLOGY AND PATHOGENESIS

Measles virus has been classified as a paramyxovirus. Its structure and many of its biologic properties are similar to those of the larger members of the myxovirus group, i.e., mumps, Newcastle disease virus (NDV), and parainfluenza viruses. It is a heat-labile virus, with an RNA core and an outer envelope of protein and lipoprotein. The virus is stable at low temperatures (especially in the presence of protein) but is rapidly inactivated by ultraviolet radiation, ether, trypsin, acetone, and β-propiolactone. Complement fixation, hemagglutination, and hemolysis are properties of the virus that have been utilized for laboratory diagnosis (see "Diagnosis," below). The virus has been adapted by serial passage to grow well in numerous continuous cell lines.

At the time of the initial isolation of measles virus in tissue culture, certain characteristic cytopathic effects were noted that were strikingly similar to previously well-recognized pathologic changes occurring during natural infection in humans. These included formation of syncytia, or multinucleated giant cells with intranuclear and intracytoplasmic eosinophilic inclusions.

Measles virus is antigenically stable and distinct from mumps virus and the other larger myxoviruses. There is some degree of cross-reactivity with the agents of canine distemper and bovine rinderpest, but these cause no difficulty in serodiagnosis in humans.

The natural route of infection is by droplet spread of infectious secretions from an infected patient to the respiratory tract of a person who is susceptible. It is suspected that after local multiplication at this site of entry, there may be an early viremia; but this has not been documented. During the prodromal period, virus can be detected in nasopharyngeal secretions, lymphatic tissue, blood, and urine,[8] and virus may persist in the urine for 4 days after onset of the rash.[9] However, viremia and pharyngeal shedding of virus cease by the second day of rash, a time when measles antibody reaches detectable levels in the serum.

The mechanism of the rash has not been established; rash may be a direct effect of viral invasion on epithelial and vascular endothelial cells, or it may result from the damaging effects of a virus-antibody complex. In support of the latter theory is the temporal relationship between onset of rash and appearance of antibody (the same is true in rubella, another exanthem) and the absence of rash in the few rare children, usually those with leukemia, who have developed chronic measles infection without rash or antibody production but with fatal giant cell pneumonia.[10] The experience of these children is in sharp contrast to that of children with classic (Bruton-type) agammaglobulinemia, who respond to measles infection in a normal fashion.[11] Delayed allergy (tuberculin-type skin sensitivity) is intact in these children, and they may make small quantities of humoral antibody as well. Similarly, two complications of measles, encephalitis and thrombocytopenia purpura, are suspected of having an allergic basis, but direct evidence is not available to clarify these points.

CLINICAL MANIFESTATIONS

The course of measles may be divided into three distinct phases: (1) an essentially asymptomatic incubation period of 10 or 11 days following exposure; (2) a prodromal phase characterized by fever, malaise, and increasing severe coryza, conjunctivitis, and cough, which persists for 3 or 4 days; followed by (3) onset of the rash, which usually reaches its maximum within several days and rarely persists longer than 5 to 6 days. The pathognomonic Koplik's spots usually appear in the mouth 24 to 48 h before onset of the rash and may remain discrete for 2 or 3 days. A typical clinical course is illustrated in Fig. 211-1.

Prodromal Symptoms

The coryza, conjunctivitis, cough, and fever that characterize the measles prodrome increase in severity until the rash has reached its peak. The coryza is similar to that in a severe common cold. The

FIGURE 211-1

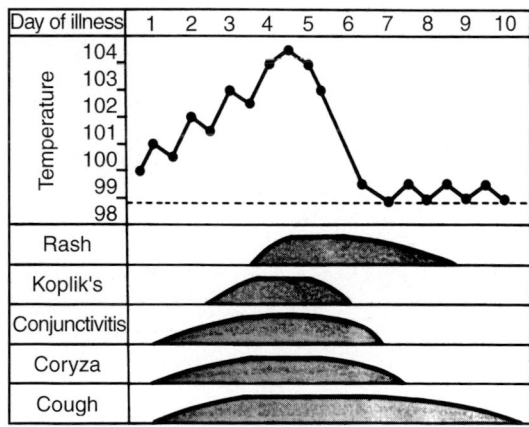

Schematic diagram illustrating the clinical course of typical measles. (*From Krugman S, Ward R: Infectious Diseases of Children, 3d ed. St. Louis, Mosby, 1964, with permission.*)

conjunctivitis is most strikingly palpebral, extending to the lid margin, so that the eyes appear to be red-rimmed. Lacrimation, lid edema, and photophobia accompany the conjunctivitis. A brassy or barking cough, due to the diffuse involvement of the tracheobronchial tree, may be quite severe even in the absence of a complicating pneumonia and may persist for a week after the coryza. The temperature frequently reaches 40° to 40.5°C (104° to 104.9°F) at the peak of the rash but falls promptly to normal in the absence of complications. Generalized adenopathy is common in measles.

Rash

After a prodromal period of 1 to 7 days, an erythematous, discrete, macular and papular rash (Fig. 211-2B and C) appears behind the ears and over the forehead. It spreads down over the neck and trunk and then distally over the upper and lower extremities. The hands and feet are involved. This progression is usually complete, and the rash most intense, within 3 days, which coincides with the peak of the other major clinical signs of fever, cough, and conjunctivitis. Those areas in which the rash appears first tend to be most heavily involved, and confluence of lesions on the face and upper neck is common. Lesions on the legs usually remain discrete and macular and papular. The exanthem begins to fade in the order of its appearance; sometimes clearing of the face begins on the third day while the eruption is still discrete and fresh on the legs. Although the early erythematous rash blanches on pressure, the fading rash consists of a brown staining (inflammatory melanosis with old hemorrhage) that does not blanch.[12] Variable degrees of fine, branny desquamation may be present as the rash clears. In the United States, the desquamation is never as extensive as that which may occur in severe scarlet fever, but desquamation has been described as quite marked in other areas of the world, such as Nigeria.[13]

The severe hemorrhagic measles ("black measles") associated with extreme toxicity, respiratory tract and gastrointestinal bleeding, hyperpyrexia, and a significant mortality rate is now rare and should not be confused with the purpuric lesions that may be seen in fair-skinned children during the course of ordinary measles.

Oral Lesions

The earliest oral lesions, according to Weinstein,[12] are a "series of pin-point elevations connected by a network of minute vessels on the soft palate." These red dots then coalesce as the entire pharynx becomes reddened. Herrman spots, bluish-gray or white areas on the tonsils, may also be present. Neither of these lesions is pathognomonic of measles. The pathognomonic lesions of measles described by Henry Koplik,[14] a New York pediatrician, begin as small, irregular, bright-red spots that usually precede onset of the rash by 24 to 48 h. In the center of each red spot is a minute bluish-white speck. These Koplik's spots are most heavily clustered on the buccal mucosa opposite the second molars (Fig. 211-2A), but oc-

FIGURE 211-2

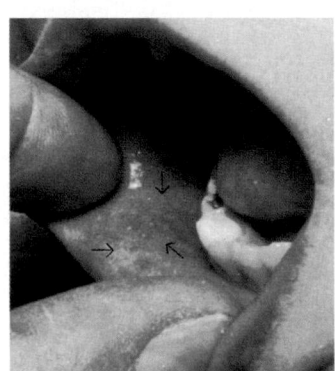

A.

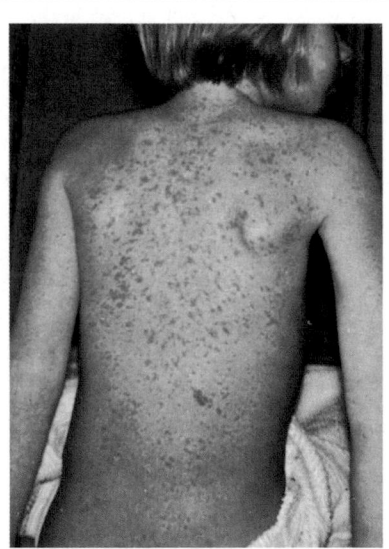

B.

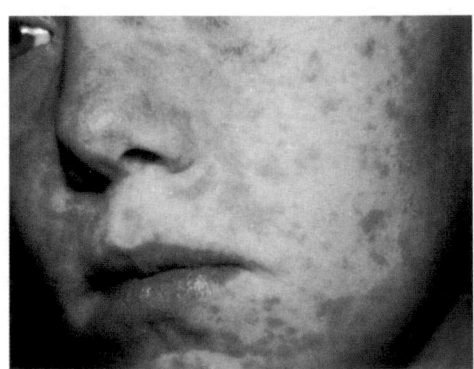

C.

Measles (rubeola; morbilli) has a characteristic prodrome of 3 to 4 days that consists of coryza, a striking palpebral conjunctivitis with photophobia, and a "barking" cough. The first lesions appear on the soft palate as blotchy erythema, but the most pathognomonic lesions of the prodrome, if present, are Koplik's spots (A), which appear as tiny white lesions surrounded by an erythematous ring ("grains of sand"). Koplik's spots precede the onset of the generalized rash by 1 to 2 days, remain for 2 to 3 days, and are usually heavily clustered on the buccal mucosa opposite the second molars. The purplish red rash on the body appears first behind the ears and over the forehead and then spreads slowly to involve the entire body by the third day: the eruption extends downward over the neck, shoulders, and trunk and then distally over the upper and lower extremities; the spread of this rash over the central parts of the trunk (B) first is in contrast with that of German measles, which spreads rapidly to involve the entire body in 1 day. The measles rash remains in its original site while it spreads to the extremities, in contrast with the rash in rubella, which disappears from each site as it spreads. The erythematous macular and papular lesions, which were discrete (C), become confluent on the face and upper part of the neck, whereas they may remain discrete on the legs. As the rash disappears, it becomes brownish yellow, owing to capillary hemorrhages.

casionally they are seen on the conjunctivae at the inner canthus and, at autopsy, in the large intestine.[15] During the first day of rash, Koplik's spots are usually easy to see as a cluster of fine grains of sand on a red background. They normally become less distinct as the rash progresses.

COMPLICATIONS

The complications of measles fall into two categories: those that are due to the measles infection alone and/or the patient's response to the infection and those due to superinfection with pathogenic bacteria. Encephalitis, which occurs in approximately 1 of every 800 cases, is the most dreaded and unpredictable complication of measles. Although most children recover completely, death or permanent brain damage occurs in a significant minority of children who develop measles encephalitis. Purpura, usually associated with thrombocytopenia, may be severe. These complications may be due to a direct effect of measles virus on the target tissues, or there may be an immunologic component. Common bacterial complications are otitis media and pneumonia caused by the pneumococcus, group A hemolytic streptococcus, *Haemophilus influenzae*, or, occasionally, *Staphylococcus aureus*. The onset of these complications is frequently accompanied by a secondary fever spike or prolongation of fever at a time when defervescence would ordinarily be expected.

Complication rates have always been higher among the very young, the malnourished, and those with other underlying diseases. The last serious outbreaks in the United States (1989–1991) were focused in just such inner-city populations. Approximately one-third of cases were in children under 4 years of age. Hospitalization rates of 15 to 20 percent, usually attributed to dehydration and/or respiratory distress, were associated with measles itself or bacterial superinfection. Although most of the deaths occurred in young children, almost one-third of the 97 deaths in 1990 were in adults. Some of the deaths in adults were in individuals known to be immunocompromised (e.g., HIV-infected). Death rates reached almost 4 per 1000 cases, far higher than the less than 1 per 1000 experienced in the United States in the prevaccination era, but still tenfold lower than the rate seen among malnourished children in developing nations.

Measles may aggravate or exacerbate tuberculosis. The reasons for this and for the transient anergy it produces are unknown. Both measles and measles vaccine may depress the tuberculin skin test reaction for 2 or 3 weeks.

A complication, new since the "vaccine era," has been described in children who received killed measles virus vaccine and subsequently were exposed to and infected with natural measles.[16] Some of these children have developed atypical infection characterized by urticarial, vesicular, and petechial rashes, swollen hands and feet, severe pneumonia, high fever, and extreme prostration. Although children may be quite sick with this syndrome, the illness appears to be self-limited. Similarly, administration of the live attenuated measles virus vaccine after prior immunization with the killed vaccine may produce erythema, edema, and even vesiculation at the injection site, with or without fever for several days.

Another late-developing complication of measles is subacute sclerosing panencephalitis (SSPE). Patients with this progressive and usually fatal disease recover uneventfully after acute measles. Months or years later, mental and motor deterioration, often with myoclonic seizures, are associated with a characteristic spike-and-wave pattern of the electroencephalogram, remarkably elevated serum and cerebrospinal fluid (CSF) measles antibody titers, and el-

evated total CSF IgG. In brain tissue, measles virus antigen has been demonstrated by immunofluorescence, measles-like nucleocapsids have been seen on electron microscopy, and infectious virus with the characteristics of measles has been isolated in tissue culture by meticulous techniques of cocultivation and serial passage. Fortunately, this rare complication (estimated at 5 to 10 cases per million cases of measles) appears to be even less common among children protected by attenuated measles vaccines (1 case per million doses of vaccine).

LABORATORY FINDINGS

In uncomplicated measles, routine laboratory tests are unremarkable and not particularly helpful. There is a mild leukopenia, and the chest roentgenogram frequently reveals an increase in bronchovascular markings. Cytologic examination of nasal secretion and sputum may demonstrate characteristic multinucleated giant cells.

Isolation of measles virus from blood, urine, or pharyngeal secretions during the prodromal and early rash period (see "Etiology and Pathogenesis," above) requires virus laboratory facilities, which are available in only a limited number of research and reference institutions.

Serologic tests for measles include measurements of neutralizing, complement-fixing (CF), and hemagglutination-inhibiting (HI) antibodies. Paired serums taken shortly after onset of rash and 2 weeks later will show diagnostic (fourfold or greater) rises in measles antibody measured by each of these tests. Neutralizing and HI antibody persist at detectable levels for many years after natural infection (probably for life in most instances), but CF antibody persistence is not so predictable.[17] The most sensitive and convenient of these serologic tests are the HI technique[18] and the enzyme-linked immunosorbent assay (ELISA).[19] These tests, which are specific for measles, can be most helpful in clarifying the cause of the unusual case of atypical measles. Bacterial superinfections and measles encephalitis are usually associated with a polymorphonuclear leukocytosis.

PATHOLOGY

The measles exanthem begins with hyaline necrosis of epidermal cells, followed by exudation of serum around the superficial vessels in the dermis and by proliferation of endothelial cells.[20] The epithelial cells become necrotic. Intranuclear inclusions may be seen. In the later stages, there is leukocytic infiltration of the dermis and lymphocytic cuffing of vessels. In uncomplicated measles, the invariable presence of multinucleated giant cells in the respiratory tract and lymphoid tissues (Warthin-Finkeldey cells) throughout the body has been accepted as evidence of measles virus invasion of these tissues (see "Etiology and Pathogenesis," above). Tracheobronchitis is as much a part of measles as the exanthem. Rarely, a fatal pneumonia, characterized by the presence of giant cells in the lungs, occurs in children with underlying disease such as leukemia. The histopathologic characteristics of measles encephalitis are similar to those observed in other postviral encephalitides. Early lesions include lymphocytic infiltration of the walls of small veins in gray and white matter, measured cellular infiltration, degeneration of ganglion cells, and microglial proliferation. Perivascular demyelinization follows these initial changes. Adams et al.[21] described intranuclear and intracytoplasmic inclusions and small giant cells in brain tissue obtained from fatal cases of measles encephalitis. Confirmation of these observations by others would add indirect support to the concept that direct invasion of the central nervous system by measles virus is of pathogenic significance in measles encephalitis.

DIAGNOSIS

The clinical course of full-blown measles is so characteristic that diagnosis should represent no problem. The 3- to 4-day prodrome of cough, conjunctivitis, and coryza, with appearance of Koplik's spots, followed by a macular and papular rash, is unambiguous. Laboratory confirmation is usually not necessary. However, when measles has been modified by prophylactic administration of human immunoglobulin at the time of exposure (see "Treatment," below), the disease may be significantly attenuated; it may consist of various combinations of brief fever, cough, and rash, or it may be subclinical.

The unusual clinical picture seen in patients who develop measles despite prior immunization with inactivated (killed) measles vaccine may be diagnosed on the basis of a prior history of such immunization and recent measles exposure (see "Complications," above).

TREATMENT

As in other systemic viral infections, there is no specific therapy for measles. Supportive therapy—consisting of rest, diet, hydration, aspirin, a vaporizer, and mild antitussive agents appropriate for the febrile child with tracheobronchitis—is frequently helpful in management of the self-limited disease. The prophylactic administration of antibiotics is unwarranted, as it does not prevent bacterial complications and, in fact, may predispose the patient to superinfection with a treatment-resistant organism.[22] Antibiotic therapy should be instituted promptly, however, if bacterial complications develop (see "Complications," above). Therapy for measles encephalitis is also supportive.

PREVENTION[23–25]

Measles is preventable. Guidelines for using the highly effective and safe live attenuated measles vaccine (licensed in 1963) have continued to evolve in response to the vaccine-induced changing epidemiology of the disease. A single dose of vaccine produces detectable levels of measles antibody in approximately 95 percent of recipients. Immunity from vaccine is protective against this disease, presumably for life, in most or all of those who seroconvert. However, it has become clear in recent years that the 5 percent of children who fail to respond to an initial dose of measles vaccine have provided a reservoir for continued outbreaks of disease, especially in settings where large numbers of adolescents and young adults congregate (e.g., college and high school campuses).

In 1989, because of the morbidity and costs associated with the outbreaks among young people, public health authorities in the United States adopted a two-dose measles immunization schedule (a practice already in place in 10 European countries). In the United States, the first dose of vaccine is usually given at age 15 months to avoid an interfering effect from maternal measles antibody. The second dose is given prior to school entry or early in elementary school.

The major epidemics of measles experienced in 1990 and 1991 were not due to vaccine failure (i.e., the 5 percent who fail to respond to the first dose of vaccine). The failure has been in distributing vaccine to poor children. Measles vaccination rates for inner-city children 2 years of age dropped to less than 50 percent, setting the stage for epidemics with a lower age distribution and higher complication and death rates than previously experienced in the United States. For control of epidemic measles, the timing and number of subsequent doses of vaccine is now adjusted by local health officials. The first dose may be given as early as 6 months of age. An "extra dose," after age 15 months but before school entry, may be required in certain communities. It is likely that recommendations concerning the timing, number of doses, and perhaps even route of administration of measles vaccine will continue to evolve.

Immune serum globulin (ISG) may be used to modify or prevent measles if given within 6 days of exposure. The recommended dose is 0.25 mL/kg of body weight, given intramuscularly. ISG is especially valuable for infants too young for active immunization. For children and adults who are immunosuppressed, the dose is 0.5 mL/kg. The maximum dose is 15 mL. In contrast to other congenital or acquired causes of immunosuppression, HIV infection is not a contraindication for measles vaccination, but when exposed, such children should still receive ISG.

COURSE AND PROGNOSIS

Uncomplicated measles runs a self-limited course, lasting about 10 days, with no sequelae. However, the prognosis varies greatly with the age of the patient, his or her nutritional and general health status, and, perhaps, access to early and appropriate supportive care. Prior to widespread immunization, approximately 500 deaths were attributed to measles each year in the United States. In the early 1980s, when measles cases dropped to an average of only 3000 yearly, deaths were few. In 1990, with almost 100 deaths, the rate of almost 4 per 1000 greatly exceeded the death rate of 3 per 10,000 that characterized the preimmunization era rate for infants in the United States. Morbidity and mortality in developing nations, where poverty prevents access to care, continues to reflect the general health status of children in these areas, with measles a major contributor to infant mortality. This experience offers ample justification for the World Health Organization's Expanded Program for Immunization.

REFERENCES

1. Katz SL, Enders JF: Measles virus, in *Viral and Rickettsial Infections of Man,* 4th ed, edited by FL Horsfall Jr, I Tamm. Philadelphia, Lippincott, 1965, p 784

2. Josias A: Récherches expérimentales sur la transmissibilité de la rugeole aux animaux. *Med Mod* **9**:158, 1898

3. Anderson JF, Goldberger J: Experimental measles in a monkey: a preliminary note. *Public Health Rep* **26**:847, 1911

4. Blake FG, Trask JD Jr: Studies on measles: I. Susceptibility of monkeys to the virus of measles. *J Exp Med* **33**:385, 1921

5. Enders JF, Peebles TC: Propagation in tissue cultures of cytopathogenic agents from patients with measles. *Proc Soc Exp Biol Med* **86**:277, 1954

6. Enders JF et al: Studies on an attenuated measles-virus vaccine: I. Development and preparation of the vaccine: Technics for assay of effects of vaccination. *N Engl J Med* **263**:153, 1960

7. Centers for Disease Control: Measles. *MMWR* **46**:666, 1997

8. Enders JF: Measles virus: historical review, isolation and behavior in various systems. *Am J Dis Child* **103**:282, 1962

9. Gresser I, Katz SL: Isolation of measles virus from urine. *N Engl J Med* **263**:452, 1960

10. Mitus A et al: Persistence of measles virus and depression of antibody formation in patients with giant cell pneumonia after measles. *N Engl J Med* **261**:882, 1959

11. Janeway CA, Gitlin D: The gamma globulins. *Adv Pediatr* **9**:65, 1957

12. Weinstein L: *The Practice of Infectious Disease*. New York, McGraw-Hill, 1958

13. Morley DC: Measles in Nigeria. *Am J Dis Child* **103**:230, 1962

14. Koplik H: The diagnosis of the invasion of measles from a study of the exanthema as it appears on the buccal mucous membrane. *Arch Pediatr* **13**:918, 1896

15. Corbett EU: The visceral lesions in measles. *Am J Pathol* **21**:905, 1945

16. Rauh LW, Schmidt R: Measles immunization with killed virus vaccine: serum antibody titers and experience with exposure to measles epidemic. *Am J Dis Child* **109**:232, 1965

17. Krugman S et al: Studies on immunity to measles. *J Pediatr* **66**:471, 1965

18. Rosen L: Hemagglutination and hemagglutination-inhibition with measles virus. *Virology* **13**:139, 1961

19. Parker JC et al: Sensitivity of enzyme-linked immunosorbent assay, complement fixation, and hemagglutination inhibition serological tests for detection of Sendai virus antibody in laboratory mice. *J Clin Microbiol* **9**:444, 1979

20. Robbins FC: Measles: clinical features. *Am J Dis Child* **103**:266, 1962

21. Adams JM et al: Inclusion bodies in measles encephalitis. *JAMA* **195**:290, 1966

22. Weinstein L: Failure of chemotherapy to prevent the bacterial complications of measles. *N Engl J Med* **253**:679, 1955

23. Centers for Disease Control: Measles prevention: Recommendations of the Immunization Practices Advisory Committee. *MMWR* **38**(suppl 9): December 1989

24. Markowitz LE, Orenstein WA: Measles vaccines. *Pediatr Clin North Am* **37**:603, 1990

25. National Vaccine Advisory Committee: The measles epidemic, barriers and recommendations. *JAMA* **266**:1574, 1991

CHAPTER 212

Jennifer C. Haley
Antoinette F. Hood

Hand-Foot-and-Mouth Disease

Hand-foot-and-mouth disease (HFMD) is a distinctive clinical syndrome caused by an enterovirus. It is clinically manifested by characteristic vesicular lesions in the mouth and on the extremities.

HISTORIC ASPECTS

In 1957 Robinson et al.[1] described a Canadian epidemic of vesicular stomatitis with an exanthem on the hands and feet from which coxsackievirus type A16 was isolated. In 1959 Alsop et al.[2] coined the term *hand-foot-and-mouth disease* to describe a similar epidemic occurring in England. Subsequently, widespread and individual cases have been reported from around the world.

EPIDEMIOLOGY

Epidemic outbreaks of HFMD tend to occur every three years and are most commonly associated with coxsackievirus A16 or enterovirus 71, although sporadic cases have been associated with coxsackievirus A4–7, A9, A10, B2, and B5.[3-7] The complete nucleotide sequence of the genome of coxsackievirus A16 has been determined. The amino acid sequence differs from most previously sequenced enteroviruses, with the exception of coxsackievirus A2 and enterovirus 71, suggesting that these viruses represent a distinct genetic group of enteroviruses.[8]

As with other enteroviruses, the disease is spread from person to person by the oral–oral and fecal–oral routes and is highly contagious. Typically children under 10 years of age are affected and spread the disease first to other children (horizontal spread) and then to adults (vertical spread). In one study, many asymptomatic family contacts had laboratory evidence of infection, most of them adults.[9] In temperate climates, the disease is seasonal, and it is more common during warmer months. There is a similar seasonal variation in the isolation of the virus from sewage and fecal samples taken from populations where epidemics occur. In tropical and semitropical zones the disease is ubiquitous.

ETIOLOGY AND PATHOGENESIS

Infections due to an enterovirus, a member of the picornavirus group, typically develop according to a basic pathogenic mechanism.[10,11] Initial viral implantation in the buccal mucosa and ileum is followed within 24 h by extension to regional lymphoid tissue. HFMD has a short incubation period of 3 to 6 days. At 72 h, a viremia occurs, followed by the seeding of viruses to the target organs, which in HFMD, are the oral mucosa and the skin of the hands and feet. By the seventh day there is a rise in serum antibodies, and the virus disappears from the blood and other sites of implantation.

FIGURE 212-1

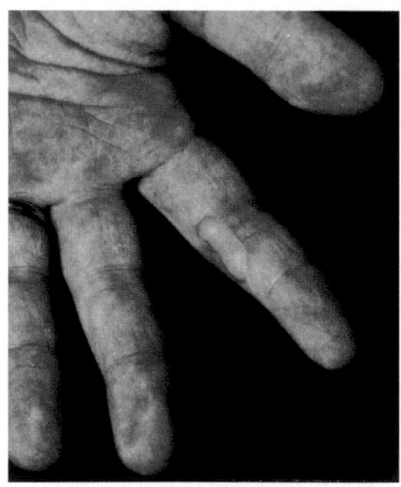

A. *B.*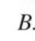

Hand-foot-and-mouth disease is manifested by vesicles, bullae, and pustules, often linear (*A*) on an erythematous base. They are often painful and are usually found on the fingers and toes (*B*). There may be an associated vesicular exanthem. The causative agent is usually coxsackievirus A16, although rarely it may be A5.

CLINICAL MANIFESTATIONS

The typical signs and symptoms of HFMD may be preceded by a brief prodrome of 12 to 24 h characterized by low-grade fever, malaise, and abdominal pain or respiratory symptoms. The most frequent finding of the disease is ulcerative oral lesions. In one series, sore mouth and refusal to eat were the presenting complaints in over 80 percent of laboratory-confirmed cases; oral lesions were present in 100 percent.[12] The number of oral lesions averages between 5 and 10. Although the lesions may be found anywhere within the oral cavity, they appear most frequently on the hard palate, tongue, and buccal mucosa.[9] The oral lesions begin as erythematous macules and papules 2 to 8 mm in diameter, then progress to form gray, thin-walled vesicles surrounded by a zone of erythema. The vesicular stage is short and rarely seen since the vesicles progress to form shallow, yellow-to-gray ulcerations with an erythematous halo. Small lesions may coalesce to form larger ones. The tongue may become red and edematous. These lesions are usually painful and may interfere with eating. In the largest reported epidemic of HFMD in England and Wales to date, the severity of the disease correlated with the degree of oral involvement.[7] In most cases the lesions resolve without treatment in 5 to 10 days.

The cutaneous lesions appear together with or shortly after the oral lesions. They may vary in number from a few to over 100. In general, the hands are more commonly involved than the feet; specifically, the dorsal surfaces and sides of the fingers, hands, toes, and feet are more often involved than the palms and soles. Each lesion begins as an erythematous macule or papule, 2 to 10 mm in size, in the center of which arises a gray, round to oval vesicle.[13] The lesions often run in or parallel to the skin lines (Fig. 212-1). The vesicles are often surrounded by a red areola (Fig. 212-2); they may be asymptomatic, painful, or tender. They crust after a few days and gradually disappear over the course of 7 to 10 days without scarring. Macular and papular erythematous lesions have also been described in association with the more typical lesions of HFMD in infants. This eruption occurs principally on the buttocks but is occasionally generalized.[12–16]

HISTOPATHOLOGY

The characteristic cutaneous lesion is an intraepidermal vesicle containing neutrophils, mononuclear cells, and proteinaceous eosinophilic material. As the lesion ages, there may be focal loss of the basal cell layer resulting in a subepidermal bulla. The roof of the blister is often necrotic with discrete eosinophilic dyskeratotic and acantholytic epidermal cells. The epidermis immediately adjacent to the vesicle exhibits intercellular edema or so-called reticular degeneration (Fig. 212-3). In addition, intracellular edema or ballooning degeneration may be found. Eosinophilic intranuclear inclusions have been described. The dermis beneath a vesicle is edematous and contains a perivascular polymorphous infiltrate composed of lymphocytes and neutrophils. Intracytoplasmic particles in a crystalline array characteristic of coxsackievirus have been observed using electron microscopy.[17] The material obtained by scraping the base of a vesicle, when smeared

FIGURE 212-2

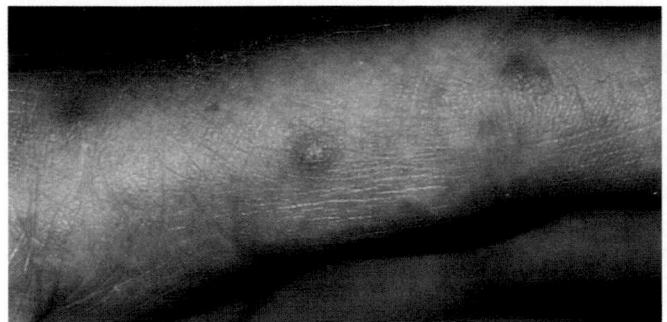

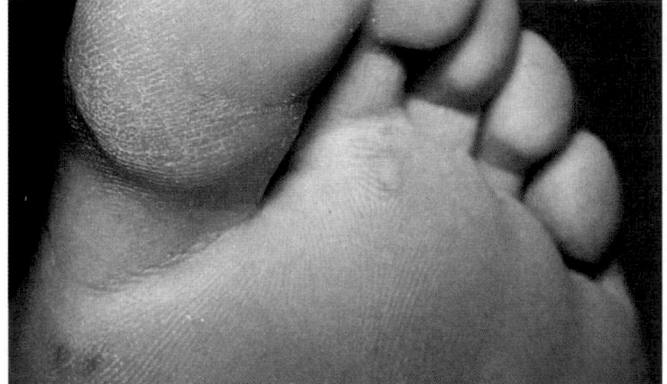

A.

FIGURE 212-3

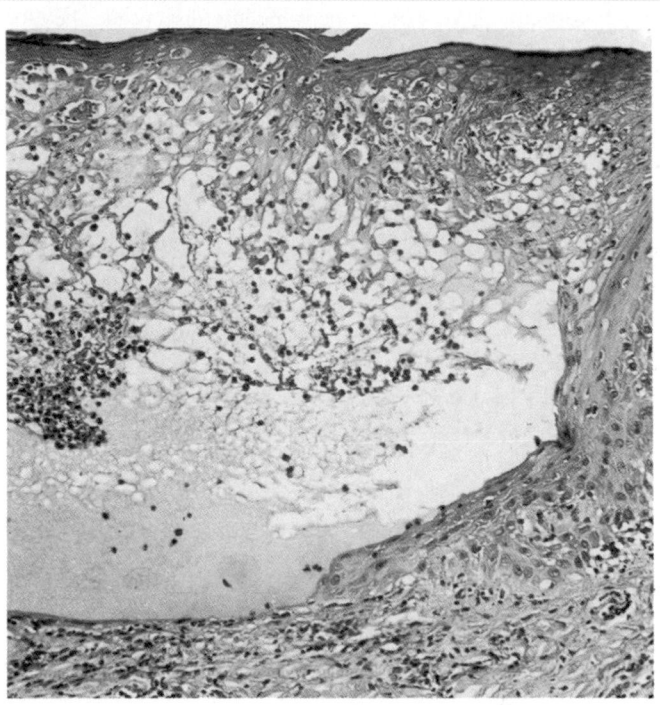

A.

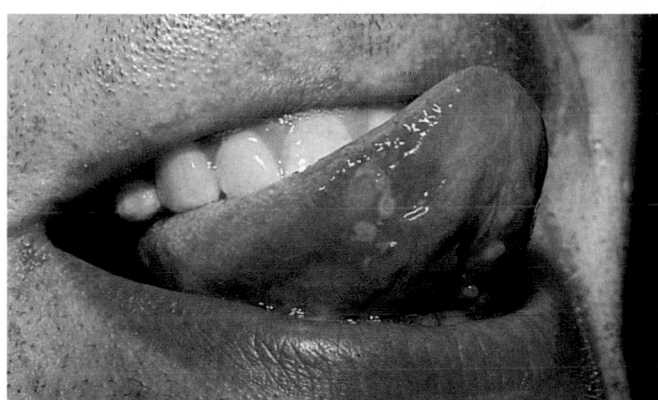

B.

A. Small vesicular and papular lesions distributed on the hands and feet are characteristic of hand-foot-and-mouth syndrome. *B.* Erosions on the tongue may accompany mucosal ulcerations as part of the oral manifestation of coxsackievirus A16 infection.

on a glass slide and stained with Giemsa stain, reveals no multi-nucleated giant cells or inclusion bodies.[18]

DIAGNOSTIC PROCEDURES

The diagnosis of HFMD is usually made on clinical grounds with the observation of ulcerative oral lesions plus an exanthem on the hands and feet occurring in association with a mild febrile illness. Leukocyte counts range from 4000 to 16,000/mm³, occasionally with atypical lymphocytosis.

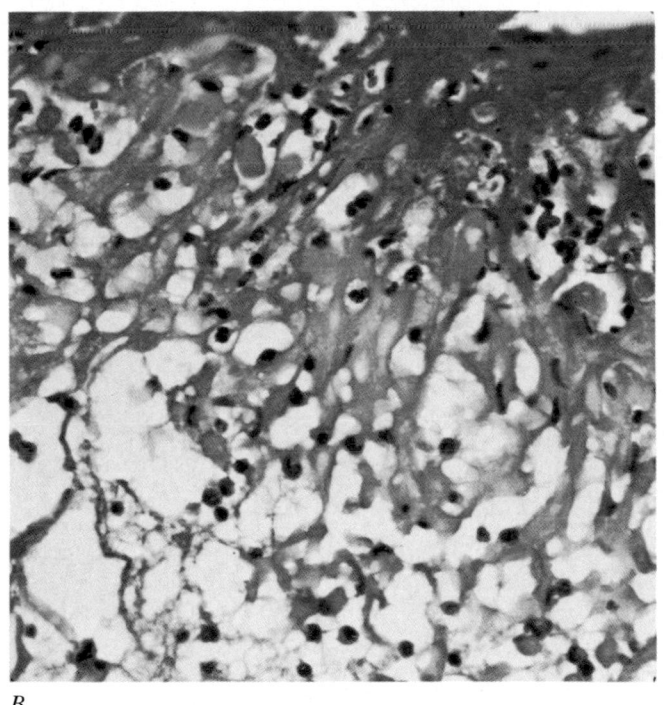

B.

A. An intraepidermal bulla with focal loss of the epidermis at the base. The blister cavity is filled with neutrophils and mononuclear cells. H&E; *B.* Higher magnification of blister roof showing numerous dyskeratotic epidermal cells and exocytosis of mononuclear cells. H&E.

When the diagnosis is in question, a presumptive diagnosis can be made by enzyme-linked immunosorbent assay (ELISA) detection of virus-specific IgM. The antibody rapidly disappears; therefore, serologic examination should be performed during the acute phase of the disease. Elevated titers of complement-fixing antibody may be detected in serum drawn from a patient during the convalescent stage of the illness. These antibodies, however, are usually group-specific, rather than type-specific.

Virus isolation in cell culture remains the only reliable way of demonstrating the virus. Virus culture of specimens from multiple sites with the addition of polymerase chain reaction (PCR) can provide a sensitive, rapid, specific diagnosis. Virus may be recovered from blood, stool, pharyngeal secretions, and vesicular fluid. The most specific sites include blood and fluid from blisters. Fecal specimens are the least specific. Sampling of more than one site is suggested for virus isolation because the various strains of these viruses differ in their ease of isolation.

DIFFERENTIAL DIAGNOSIS

The occurrence of oral and distal-extremity lesions in an outbreak setting is pathognomonic of HFMD. Early nonvesicular lesions may resemble rubella or drug reactions. Both rubella and drug eruptions usually have more extensive cutaneous involvement, and drug reactions tend to be more pruritic than painful. When only oral lesions are present the illness is often mistaken for aphthous stomatitis, herpes simplex virus infections, or herpangina. Aphthae are rarely accompanied by systemic symptoms or fever. Herpesvirus may be accompanied by fever, but perioral areas are often involved and can be distinguished from HFMD by characteristic viral cytopathic changes seen in Tzanck preparations and biopsy specimens. Herpangina, which usually involves the anterior fauces, tonsillar pillars, soft palate, and uvula, does not commonly involve the tongue, buccal mucosa, and gingiva.

Vesicular lesions occurring in the mouth and extremities may also be seen in varicella-zoster virus, exanthems induced by other enteroviruses, erythema multiforme, and sepsis. Skin lesions of varicella are typically more extensive, within different phases of development, and share histologic features of herpes simplex infection. Although other enteroviruses may affect the skin, they are less likely to target the oral mucosa and the distal extremities specifically. Individuals with sepsis usually are more symptomatic with higher fevers and more systemic complaints than those with HFMD. The number of oral ulcerations in erythema multiforme is usually greater than in HFMD and target lesions are frequently present.

The acral vesicles may resemble arthropod bites, acropustulosis of infancy, and tinea infections. Therefore, it is important for the clinician to evaluate the oropharanx to establish the diagnosis of HFMD.

TREATMENT

HFMD tends to resolve spontaneously over the course of a week, therefore treatment is directed toward symptomatic relief of painful lesions. Topical application of dyclonine hydrochloride solution (Dyclone) or lidocaine (Xylocaine, ointment or viscous) may reduce the discomfort that accompanies the oral ulcerations. An open clinical trial of acyclovir in 13 patients resulted in symptomatic relief, defervescence, and involution of lesions within 24 h of initiating therapy. The mechanism of this improvement was not clear.[19]

COURSE AND PROGNOSIS

Patients may present with either enanthem or exanthem, but most patients manifest both aspects of the disease. In general, the disease is accompanied by minimal or mild signs and symptoms, such as low-grade fever, vague malaise, and sore mouth. Some patients, however, are afflicted with high fever, marked malaise, diarrhea, and occasionally even joint pains.[15] In Japan, epidemics of HFMD caused by enterovirus 71 have been associated with an 8 to 24 percent incidence of neurologic signs and symptoms such as headache, nuchal rigidity, hyperreflexia, tremor, ataxia, myoclonus, and central nervous system pleocytosis.[3] Most commonly, however, the entire disease runs its course in 7 to 10 days without the patient's being aware of debility. A few cases of prolonged or recurrent HFMD have been observed.[12,16] Serious sequelae rarely occur; however, coxsackievirus has been implicated as the etiologic agent in cases of myocarditis,[20,21] meningoencephalitis,[20] aseptic meningitis,[20,22] paralytic disease,[23] and a systemic illness resembling rubeola.[24] Infection acquired during the first trimester of pregnancy may result in spontaneous abortion.[25]

REFERENCES

1. Robinson CR et al: Report on an outbreak of febrile illness with pharyngeal lesions and exanthem. Toronto, Summer 1957—isolation of group A Coxsackie virus. *Can Med Assoc J* **79**:615, 1958
2. Alsop J et al: "Hand-foot-and-mouth disease" in Birmingham in 1959. *Br Med J* 2:1708, 1960
3. Ishimaru Y et al: Outbreaks of hand, foot, and mouth disease by enterovirus 71. *Arch Dis Child* **55**:583, 1980
4. Hughes RP, Roberts C: Hand, foot, and mouth disease associated with Coxsackie A₉ virus. *Lancet* 2:751, 1972
5. Duff MF: Hand-foot-and-mouth syndrome in humans: Coxsackie A₁₀ infection in New Zealand. *Br Med J* 2:661, 1968
6. Lindenbaum JE et al: Hand, foot and mouth disease associated with Coxsackie group B. *Scand J Infect Dis* 7:161, 1975
7. Bendig JW, Fleming DM: Epidemiological, virological, and clinical features of an epidemic of hand, foot, and mouth. *Commun Dis Rep CDR Suppl* 6:R81, 1996
8. Poyry T et al: Molecular analysis of coxsackievirus A16 reveals a new genetic group of enteroviruses. *Virology* **202**:982, 1994
9. Adler JL et al: Epidemiologic investigation of hand, foot, and mouth disease: Infection caused by Coxsackie A₁₆ in Baltimore, June through September 1968. *Am J Dis Child* **120**:309, 1970
10. Johnston JM, Burke JP: Nosocomial outbreak of hand-foot-and-mouth disease among operating suite personnel. *Infect Control* 7:172, 1986
11. Cherry JD, Nelson DB: Enterovirus infections: Their epidemiology and pathogenesis. *Clin Pediatr* 5:659, 1966
12. Evans AD, Waddington E: Hand, foot and mouth disease in South Wales, 1964. *Br J Dermatol* **79**:309, 1967
13. Higgins PG, Warin RP: Hand, foot, and mouth disease: A clinically recognizable virus infection seen mainly in children. *Clin Pediatr* 6:373, 1967
14. Meadow SR: Hand, foot and mouth disease. *Arch Dis Child* **40**:560, 1965
15. Fields JP et al: Hand, foot, and mouth disease. *Arch Dermatol* **99**:243, 1969
16. Mihm MC Jr et al: A clinical, epidemiologic, and virologic study of hand, foot, and mouth syndrome. *Proceedings of the Third Joint Meeting of the Clinical Society and Commissioned Officers Association of*

the United States Public Health Service, March 25–29, 1968, San Francisco, California, p 64

17. Kimura A et al: Light and electron microscopic study of skin lesions of patients with the hand, foot and mouth disease. *Tohoku J Med* **122**:237, 1977
18. Cherry JD, Jahn CL: Hand, foot, and mouth syndrome: Report of six cases due to Coxsackie virus group A, type 16. *Pediatrics* **37**:637, 1966
19. Shelley WB et al: Acyclovir in the treatment of hand-foot-and-mouth disease. *Cutis* **57**:232, 1996
20. Wright HT et al: Fatal infection in an infant associated with Coxsackie virus group A, type 16. *N Engl J Med* **268**:1041, 1963
21. Baker DA, Phillips CA: Fatal hand-foot-and-mouth disease in an infant caused by Coxsackie virus A₇. *JAMA* **242**:1065, 1979

22. Froeschie JE et al: Hand, foot, and mouth disease (Coxsackie A₁₆) in Atlanta. *Am J Dis Child* **114**:278, 1967
23. Magoffin RL, Lenette EH: Nonpolioviruses and paralytic disease. *Calif Med* **97**:1, 1962
24. Gohd RS, Faigel HC: Hand-foot-and-mouth disease resembling measles. A life-threatening disease: Case report. *Pediatrics* **37**:644, 1966
25. Ogilvie MM, Tearne CF: Spontaneous abortion after hand-foot-and-mouth disease caused by Coxsackie virus A₁₆. *Br Med J* **281**:1527, 1980

CHAPTER 213

Curtis A. Raskin
Robert H. Parrott

Herpangina

Herpangina[1–5] is a specific infectious disease in which characteristic vesicular lesions develop in the oropharynx. In temperate climates it usually occurs during the summer, and it primarily affects children. The etiologic agent is usually group A coxsackievirus, but it can also be caused by other members of the enterovirus genus of the Picornaviridae.

HISTORIC ASPECTS[1]

Zahorsky first described herpangina as a specific entity in 1920. Outbreaks of an illness similar to what he called herpangina were reported in summer camps and nursery schools in 1939 and 1941. Later, Huebner and his associates recovered group A coxsackieviruses from throat washings and stool from a group of patients with herpangina. This was the first suggestion that specific viruses caused the disease. The clinical association has been confirmed in many reports since that time.

EPIDEMIOLOGY[3,6,7]

Herpangina can occur in any age group but primarily affects infants and young children (typically below the age of 5). Outbreaks of herpangina usually occur during the early summer and may take the form of a mini-epidemic. The viruses that are responsible for herpangina may also cause subclinical infection or febrile illness without typical oropharyngeal lesions, and this situation should be strongly suspected when one finds fever and pharyngitis in siblings

of a patient who has clinically distinct herpangina. These viruses can be isolated from as many as 1.5 to 7.5 percent of persons who are not ill during the summertime in a temperate climate. The group A coxsackieviruses may spread rapidly in a family or neighborhood group and from patient to patient in a hospital or institution. Virus may persist in the feces for up to 47 days after acute infection. In addition to the stool, the herpangina agent can be recovered from saliva, nasal secretions, oropharynx, and stomach washings. Nevertheless, it appears that seasonal outbreaks occur primarily through inhalation of aerosolized drops of saliva (e.g., from sneezing and coughing). The disease is worldwide in distribution.

ETIOLOGY AND PATHOGENESIS[3–9]

Herpangina is classically and usually caused by group A coxsackievirus (typically strains 1 to 6, 8, 10, and 22) but can also be caused by group B coxsackievirus (strains 1 to 4), echoviruses, adenoviruses, and other enteroviruses. Coxsackievirus belongs to the enterovirus genus of the Picornaviridae, which also includes polioviruses, echoviruses, and enteroviruses 68 to 71. As such, it is composed of a single-stranded RNA genome.

Some authors prefer to restrict the diagnosis of herpangina to those cases caused by group A coxsackievirus, but this is not practical as laboratory virus speciation is rarely performed and is not necessary. Further, the subclassification of coxsackievirus into groups A and B is based only on the lesional pathology produced in suckling mice. In actuality, the group A coxsackieviruses are somewhat genetically diverse, with some strains showing significant homology to the polioviruses and the group B coxsackieviruses.

There is no sex difference and no known difference by race or national origin in the occurrence of the disease. In Washington, D.C., 50 percent of cases occur in July, 35 percent in August, 5 percent in June, and 10 percent in September. A strikingly similar pattern of occurrence exists in Japan. The incubation period is approximately 4 days. Permanent immunity occurs to the type-specific agent. However, as multiple viral stains cause herpangina, the clinical syndrome can recur in the same patient in successive years.

CLINICAL MANIFESTATIONS[2]

The child affected with herpangina is usually in good health until a sudden onset of fever. In Zahorsky's description, "The child feels tired and often complains of pain in the back and extremities. Headache and pains in the back of the neck are frequently marked symptoms and lead one to expect poliomyelitis at times. This impression is often accentuated by the tenderness of the extremities on movement."

In 68 cases studied at Children's Hospital in Washington, D.C., temperatures ranging from 38.3° to 40.5°C were found in 89 percent of the patients and lasted for 1 to 4 days. Five percent had febrile convulsions. Seventy percent complained of anorexia, dysphagia, or sore throat. There was vomiting in 38 percent, abdominal pain in 21 percent, and headache in 16 percent.

The characteristic feature of the disease is the presence of gray-white papulovesicular lesions, about 1 to 2 mm in diameter, which progress to slightly larger shallow ulcers. A zone of erythema usually surrounds the lesions (Figs. 213-1. The lesions are distributed, in order of frequency, on the anterior pillars of the tonsillar fauces,

FIGURE 213-1

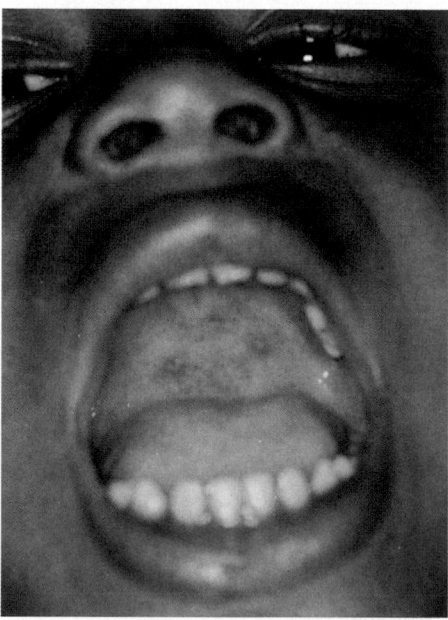

The typical feature of herpangina is the early presence of gray-white papulovesicular lesions on the palate. These progress to slightly larger ulcers as illustrated. A zone of erythema surrounds the lesions.

the soft palate, the uvula, and the tonsils themselves. The lesions may persist for 4 to 6 days. During the illness there is usually a diffuse pharyngeal hyperemia. Occasionally there is a nonpurulent conjunctivitis and, rarely, a rash. Similar lesions have been reported occurring in the vagina in the course of what was otherwise typical herpangina. In the Washington, D.C., series, total peripheral white blood cell counts were under $10,000/\mu L$ in 53 percent of the cases, 20 percent ranged from 10,000 to 15,000, and 27 percent were over 15,000.

PATHOLOGY

The only visible lesions occurring in the course of this disease are the oropharyngeal lesions already described and the diffuse pharyngeal hyperemia. Specific histologic studies of these lesions have not been reported.

DIAGNOSIS AND DIFFERENTIAL DIAGNOSIS[3,5,10,11]

The diagnosis is primarily clinical. Further, laboratory identification of group A coxsackievirus from oropharyngeal or anal swabs is labor-intensive, time-consuming, and expensive. Direct demonstration and serotyping of group A coxsackievirus from clinical samples requires prior amplification in cell culture. However, group A coxsackieviruses are difficult to propagate in cell culture and the "gold standard" technique of infecting suckling mice is rarely performed in diagnostic laboratories. Further, there is no readily available, efficient serodiagnostic test. Clinical testing for group A coxsackieviruses, although not typically necessary, should become simpler once a standardized assay based on the polymerase chain reaction is available.

There are a number of diseases that can be confused with herpangina. Hand, foot, and mouth disease, lymphonodular pharyngitis, and ulcerative oropharyngitis, like herpangina, are all caused by coxsackieviruses. They have in common symptoms of fever, lymphadenopathy (typically cervical), diarrhea, and oropharyngeal lesions. It is the lesion distribution that distinguishes them. Hand, foot, and mouth disease (typically caused by coxsackievirus A16) causes vesiculo-ulcerative lesions on the distal extremities as well as in the oral cavity. In lymphonodular pharyngitis (associated with coxsackievirus A10), the lesions are raised, discrete, white-to-yellow nodules surrounded by erythema. These lesions do not ulcerate. Symptoms and lesions persist somewhat longer than in herpangina. In ulcerative oropharyngitis, aphthous-like lesions develop in the oral cavity. Each of these diseases, like herpangina, is spread through inhalation of aerosolized saliva droplets, and they typically occur as minor endemics.

Infectious gingivostomatitis due to herpes simplex virus is another common childhood illness associated with vesicles and ulcers in the oropharyngeal cavity. However, it occurs throughout the year and the onset is more gradual than that of herpangina. The major symptoms include fever, dysphagia, and sore mouth with a very fetid odor to the breath. There is cervical lymphadenopathy and, unlike herpangina, there can be hyperemia, hypertrophy, and hemorrhage of the gums. The vesicles and ulcers are on the gums, tongue, lips, and buccal mucous membrane as well as occasionally in the location of herpangina lesions. Fever lasts longer, and the oropharyngeal lesions persist for 8 to 14 days. The child with her-petic gingivostomatitis is much more severely ill than the one with herpangina.

In the differential diagnosis of herpangina one must also exclude occasional cases of oral candidiasis; infectious mononucleosis; the enanthems of measles, varicella, scarlatina, and diphtheria; certain heavy metal poisonings; and deficiency diseases and hematologic disorders.

TREATMENT

The major importance of herpangina for the physician is that mak-ing the diagnosis relieves the fear that accompanies sudden fever in children. No specific treatment is available or necessary. Supportive care includes maintaining proper hydration and use of acetamino-phen to control fever. Symptomatic relief from oral lesion pain can be obtained with the use of antihistamine mouth rinses. Rapid res-olution of oral lesions has been reported with the use of allopurinol mouthwashes (3 mg/mL).[12]

COURSE AND PROGNOSIS

Herpangina is a self-limited disease, with the fever rarely lasting more than 4 days and the oral lesions more than a week. With the exception of the occasional child who suffers a febrile convulsion, the prognosis is good and the course benign.

REFERENCES

1. Cole RM et al: Studies of Coxsackie viruses: Observations on epide-miological aspects of group A viruses. *Am J Public Health* **41**:1342, 1951
2. Parrott RH, Cramblett HG: Nonbacterial infections affecting naso-pharynx. *Pediatr Clin North Am* **4**:115, 1957
3. Parrott RH: Clinical importance of group A Coxsackie viruses. *Ann NY Acad Sci* **67**:230, 1957
4. Cherry JD, Jahn CL: Herpangina: Etiologic spectrum. *Pediatrics* **36**:632, 1965
5. Hyypiä T, Stanway G: Biology of Coxsackie A viruses. *Adv Virus Res* **42**:343, 1993
6. Nakamura Y et al: Epidemic patterns of infectious diseases from the results of the surveillance of infectious diseases in Japan. *Pediatr Infect Dis J* **7**:262, 1988
7. Yamadera S et al: Herpangina surveillance in Japan, 1982–1989. *Jpn J Med Sci Biol* **44**:29, 1991
8. Nakayama T et al: Outbreak of herpangina associated with coxsack-ievirus B3 infection. *Pediatr Infect Dis J* **8**:495, 1989
9. Modlin JF, Rotbart HA: Group B Coxsackie disease in children. *Curr Top Microbiol Immunol* **223**:53, 1997
10. Steigman AJ et al: Acute lymphonodular pharyngitis: Newly described condition due to Coxsackie A virus. *J Pediatr* **61**:331, 1962
11. Eversole LR: Inflammatory diseases of the mucous membranes Part 1. Viral and fungal infections. *J Can Dent Assoc* **22**:52, 1994
12. Waldfahrer F, Iro H: Successful treatment of herpangina with allopur-inol mouthwashes. *Laryngoscope* **105**:1405, 1995

CHAPTER 214

Karen Wiss

Erythema Infectiosum and Parvovirus B19 Infection

Erythema infectiosum (fifth disease) is an illness primarily of child-hood that is characterized by a "slapped cheek" appearance of the face and an erythematous, lacy eruption on the trunk and extremi-ties. Parvovirus B19, the etiologic agent, may also cause arthropa-thy, aplastic crisis in patients with increased red blood cell turnover, chronic anemia in immunocompromised persons, and fetal hydrops.

HISTORIC ASPECTS

The first known clinical picture of a patient with erythema infectio-sum is drawn in Robert Willan's book *On Cutaneous Diseases* from 1808. Throughout the 1800s, the disease was thought to be a mild form of rubella or measles. Tschamer described a distinct illness compatible with erythema infectiosum in 1889, although he thought it was abortive rubella.[1] It was designated *fifth disease* in the early 1900s when infectious exanthems were numbered first through sixth.[2]

The first clue to the etiologic agent came in 1975 in England. During routine screening of serum from healthy blood donors for hepatitis B surface antigen, nine samples of blood had false-positive results by counterimmunoelectrophoresis (CIE) but were negative by the more sensitive techniques of hemagglutination and radio-immunoassay (RIA). Electron microscopy of these serum samples demonstrated viral particles that were designated *B19* after a spec-imen label from one of the blood donors.[3] The authors postulated that this was an infectious agent because 30 percent of adults had IgG antibody to the viral antigen. It was later confirmed that B19 was a parvovirus.[4] Parvoviruses had previously been thought to infect only animals. In this manner, the virus was discovered, but association with a clinical illness awaited.

Parvovirus was identified as the etiologic agent of an acute febrile illness in two British soldiers in 1980 and was found in the serum of patients with sickle cell anemia and hypoplastic crisis in 1981. The virus was suggested as a cause of aplastic crisis in sickle cell disease.

In 1983, there was an outbreak of fifth disease among London schoolchildren.[5] Serum samples from 31 schoolchildren as well as 6 exposed adults, all with clinical signs of the disease, contained parvovirus-specific IgM antibody. There was no IgM detected in exposed asymptomatic individuals. These findings suggested parvovirus B19 as the cause of erythema infectiosum.

EPIDEMIOLOGY

Fifth disease is worldwide in distribution, can occur throughout the year, and can affect all ages. It tends to occur in epidemics, especially associated with school outbreaks in the late winter and early spring. Serologic studies have shown increasing prevalence with age. Various studies indicate that from 15 to 60 percent of children 5 to 19 years old and 30 to 60 percent of adults are seropositive.[6] Previous infection with B19 confers lifelong immunity.

The incubation period for erythema infectiosum is from 4 to 14 days.[7] After intranasal inoculation of parvovirus-infected serum to healthy volunteers, low-grade fever and nonspecific complaints occurred at the time of viremia, 6 to 14 days after inoculation, and the rash appeared at day 17 or 18.[8]

Parvovirus B19 is thought to be transmitted primarily by the respiratory route via droplet aerosol during the viremic phase, and B19 DNA has been found in respiratory secretions of viremic patients.[8] After the rash of erythema infectiosum appears, B19 is not found in respiratory secretions and is usually not present in the serum. This suggests that persons with erythema infectiosum are infectious only prior to the onset of the rash.

The virus seems to be effectively spread after close contact. The secondary attack rate among susceptible household contacts is approximately 50 percent. Transmission may occur via blood transfusion, from blood products, and vertically from mother to fetus. The transmission of B19 through blood transfusion is particularly problematic because this nonenveloped virus is not killed by the solvent detergents or heat that are used to inactivate HIV and hepatitis viruses.[9]

ETIOLOGY AND PATHOGENESIS

The B19 virus belongs to the family Parvoviridae and the genus *Erythrovirus*.[9] It has been placed in this genus because of its tropism for red blood cells and is currently the only member of this genus.[9] B19 lacks an envelope and contains single-stranded DNA. It is the smallest DNA-containing virus known to infect humans, measuring 18 to 26 nm in diameter. Parvoviruses are widespread in veterinary medicine, but animal parvoviruses are not transmissable to humans.[9]

The pathogenesis of erythema infectiosum is unknown, but the mechanism may involve immune complexes. The more serious manifestations of parvovirus infection relate to the fact that the virus infects and lyses erythroid progenitor cells. Recent evidence suggests that the blood group P antigen (globoside) is a receptor for parvovirus. Since some individuals lack P antigen, they are not susceptible to infection with B19.[10] In patients with increased red blood cell destruction or loss who depend on compensatory increases in red cell production to maintain stable red cell indices, B19 infection may lead to transient aplastic crisis. Such patients include those with chronic hemolytic anemias and those with anemia associated with acute or chronic blood loss. When parvovirus infects the erythroblasts in a developing fetus with decreased red cell survival, the result may be hemolysis and anemia.[11] Anemia may trigger congestive heart failure, edema (fetal hydrops), and possibly fetal death.

CLINICAL MANIFESTATIONS

Parvovirus B19 in Children

Fifth disease usually begins with nonspecific symptoms such as headache, coryza, and low-grade fever about 2 days prior to the onset of the rash.[12] Patients may have headache, pharyngitis, fever, malaise, myalgias, coryza, diarrhea, nausea, cough, and conjunctivitis coinciding with the rash. Approximately 10 percent of children with erythema infectiosum develop arthralgias or arthritis. Large joints are affected more often than small joints.[13] Occasionally, children may present with chronic joint complaints suggestive of juvenile rheumatoid arthritis.[13]

The characteristic rash begins with confluent, erythematous, edematous plaques on the malar eminences, the "slapped cheeks" (Fig. 214-1). As the facial rash fades over 1 to 4 days, pink to erythematous macules or papules appear on the trunk, neck, and extensor surfaces of the extremities. These lesions have some central fading, giving them a lacy or reticulated appearance[12] (Fig. 214-2). The rash can be morbilliform, confluent, circinate, or annular, and there have been reports of palmar and plantar involvement.[7] The eruption typically lasts 5 to 9 days but can recur for weeks or months with triggers such as sunlight, exercise, temperature change, bathing, and emotional stress. In some outbreaks, pruritus is a major feature of the rash in children.[7]

There have been occasional reports of parvovirus B19 associated with vascular purpura, including Henoch-Schönlein purpura.[14] An enanthem consisting of erythema of the tongue and pharynx and red macules on the buccal mucosa and palate can occur.

Parvovirus B19 in Adults

Acute arthropathy is the primary manifestation of B19 viral infection in adults.[15] It occurs mainly in women and affects the small joints of the hands, the knees, wrists, ankles, and feet. Occasionally other joints such as the spine and costochondral joints are involved. This symmetric polyarthritis is usually of sudden onset and is self-limited but can be persistent or recurrent for months. It may mimic Lyme arthritis and rheumatoid arthritis.

The constitutional symptoms are usually more severe in adults than in children.[16] Fever, adenopathy, and a mild arthritis without a rash is the usual course. Women are more likely than men to have joint complaints and rash, while men often present with only a flulike illness.[15] Some adults may have fatigue, malaise, and de-

FIGURE 214-1

CHAPTER 214
Erythema Infectiosum and Parvovirus B19   2411

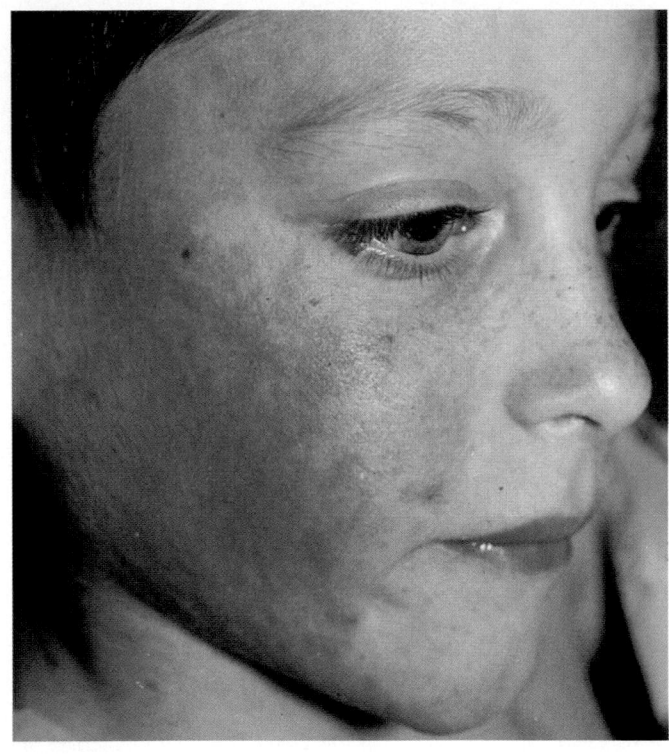

Child with the characteristic "slapped cheeks."

pression for weeks after the infection. Asymptomatic infection can certainly occur in adults as well as in children. Twenty-six percent of adults were reported to be asymptomatic in one outbreak.[15] Parvovirus B19 has been known to cause numbness and tingling of the fingers with or without other features of fifth disease.[17] Pruritus that is sometimes severe can occur with or without a rash. It has been suggested that if pruritus is a complaint in a patient with acute-onset arthritis, parvovirus should be considered as a possible cause.

FIGURE 214-2

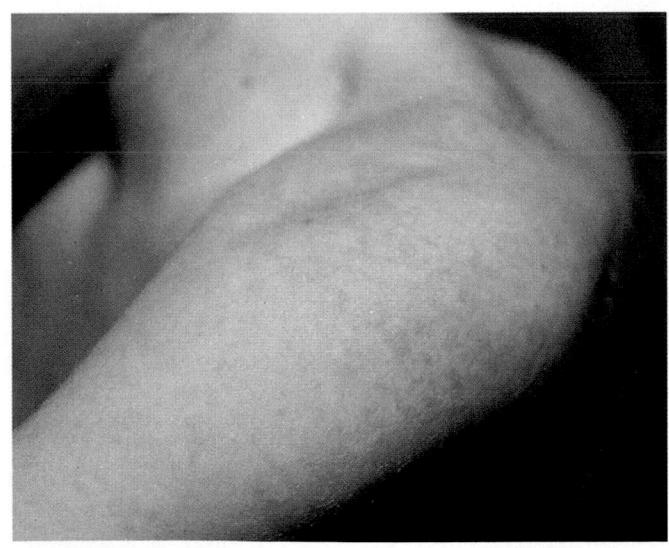

Reticulate erythematous macules on trunk and extremities.

The rash in adults, if present at all, is usually macular or lacy, often on the extremities, and rarely demonstrates the characteristic slapped-cheek appearance.[15] Other cutaneous manifestations associated with B19 infection in adults include purpura, vesicles and pustules, palmoplantar desquamation, a morbilliform exanthem with Koplik spots, and livedo reticularis.

Papular Purpuric "Gloves and Socks" Syndrome

In 1990, Harms et al.[18] described a unique syndrome characterized by pruritic erythema and edema of the hands and feet with petechiae, fever, and oral erosions. This rare exanthem seems to affect teenagers and adults and resolves spontaneously within 2 weeks. Although some reports have not substantiated an association with parvovirus B19, the virus has been implicated by various authors.

COMPLICATIONS

As more attention is focused on parvovirus B19, an increasing number of complications are recognized. Subclinical infection is quite common. However, this virus can be responsible for a variety of hematologic, rheumatologic, and neurologic abnormalities.

Transient Aplastic Crisis

Parvovirus B19 is the most common cause of transient aplastic crisis in patients with chronic hemolytic anemias.[19] This has been demonstrated in sickle cell anemia, hereditary spherocytosis, heterozygous beta-thalassemia, pyruvate kinase deficiency, and autoimmune hemolytic anemia as well as in other conditions of decreased red cell production or increased red cell destruction. The aplastic crisis may be the initial manifestation of the underlying hematologic disease.

Patients typically have fever and constitutional complaints, followed 1 week later by fatigue, pallor, and worsening anemia.[20] Rarely is a rash reported with aplastic crisis. There is an absence of reticulocytes, and the hemoglobin may fall below 4 g/dL. Bone marrow examination shows hypoplasia or aplasia of the erythroid series. Red blood cell transfusion may be necessary and most patients recover in 1 week, although the problem can be fatal if untreated. Transient red cell aplasia can occur in healthy persons without underlying hematologic abnormalities. It is likely that the aplasia is missed in individuals without disorders of shortened erythrocyte survival because the hemoglobin does not drop low enough to cause symptoms.

Chronic B19 Infection

In immunocompromised patients, B19 infection can cause a serious, prolonged anemia from persistent lysis of red blood cell precursors.[21] Parvovirus-related chronic anemia has been reported in HIV-infected patients, with congenital immunodeficiencies, with acute leukemias, in transplant recipients, with lupus erythematosus, and during the first year of life without immunodeficiency. These patients respond dramatically to intravenous gammaglobulin, suggesting that antibody is the main defense to human parvovirus infection.[22]

Fetal B19 Infection

Fetal infection with B19 may result in a normal fetus, spontaneous abortion (especially in the first half of pregnancy), hydrops fetalis in the second half of pregnancy, congenital anemia, and even late fetal death.[23] Nonimmune fetal hydrops is the most common complication of intrauterine infection with B19. Because B19 virus can infect erythroid precursors, extensive hemolysis can occur in the fetus, leading to severe anemia, tissue anoxia, high-output heart failure, and generalized edema. The fetus may show ultrasonographic evidence of subcutaneous edema, ascites, pleural effusion, pericardial effusion, placental edema, and polyhydramnios. The overall risk of fetal death is not clearly known, but recent studies have suggested that this risk is about 6.5 percent with maternal infection.[23] The risk of fetal death for a woman with unknown serologic status is estimated to be less than 2.5 percent after a household exposure and less than 1.5 percent after a significant work exposure. It seems that in B19-infected pregnant women, most fetuses are not infected; if they are infected, usually there is not an adverse outcome.[24] Furthermore, about half of women of childbearing age are immune to parvovirus infection because of prior infection.

Because parvoviruses are known teratogens in animals, there has been much concern about whether they cause birth defects in humans. In sera collected from 253 infants with a wide range of congenital abnormalities, there was no parvovirus-specific IgM detected to suggest recent infection.[25] There has been one report of a B19-infected abortus with eye abnormalities,[26] and another of an infected abortus with cleft lip, cleft palate, and micrognathia.[27] Otherwise, there are no reports of liveborn infants with anomalies linked to B19 infection in utero. It has been concluded from these studies that parvovirus B19 is not a common cause of birth defects.

Other Complications

There have been reports of B19 infection causing encephalitis, meningitis, brachial neuritis, a myasthenia-like syndrome, and motor weakness. Parvovirus infection has been blamed for a Wegener's granulomatosis–like illness,[28] polyarteritis nodosa,[28,29] Kawasaki disease,[30] and a systemic lupus erythematosus–like picture.[31]

In addition, there have been reports of other hematologic complications including idiopathic thrombocytopenic purpura, transient neutropenia, a hemophagocytic syndrome, and Diamond-Blackfan syndrome.

LABORATORY FINDINGS

In patients with erythema infectiosum, laboratory results are usually normal, including reticulocyte count, hematocrit, and tests of liver and renal function. Patients with aplastic crisis have reticulocytopenia and anemia, the severity of which depends on the degree of the underlying anemia. Reticulocytopenia, anemia, lymphopenia, neutropenia, and thrombocytopenia can occur in healthy individuals with B19 infection, although these are usually not significant enough to cause clinical symptoms. The erythrocyte sedimentation rate is rarely elevated, and rheumatoid factor has been positive in some cases of parvovirus-associated arthritis.

PATHOLOGY

Histologic examination of various tissues demonstrates homogeneous, intranuclear inclusions with peripheral condensation of chromatin in erythroid precursor cells.[32] Electron microscopy of these inclusions reveals parvovirus-like particles.[32] In fetal tissues, a leukoerythroblastic reaction may be seen as well. The histologic changes in the skin of patients with erythema infectiosum include a sparse superficial perivascular lymphocytic infiltrate that is not considered diagnostic.

DIAGNOSIS

The diagnosis of erythema infectiosum is usually based on the clinical features. The differential diagnosis includes rubella, measles, scarlet fever, roseola, enteroviral infection, erysipelas on the cheek, and drug hypersensitivity. These other disorders may have more significant systemic illness and lack the progression from the slapped cheeks to the lacy extremities that is so characteristic of fifth disease. Because no animal model or easy tissue culture system exists for the B19 virus, laboratory testing for the antibody or the virus is performed only in a limited number of research laboratories. The Centers for Disease Control and Prevention will currently test the serum of patients with aplastic crisis, immunodeficiency, and chronic anemia; pregnant women with B19 exposure; and fetal hydrops cases in which B19 infection is suspected. The testing is not done on a routine basis and is arranged through state health departments.

Detection of recent infection is usually performed with assays for IgM antibody. RIA or enzyme-linked immunosorbent assay (ELISA) techniques can detect IgM within a few days after onset of illness. IgM can be measured for up to 6 months in many cases, although there is a decline in titer in the second month after onset. IgG can be identified with the same techniques by the seventh day of illness and lasts for years and is therefore best for documenting past infection. Parvovirus antibody is often not detectable in immunodeficient persons. B19 virus can be detected in serum during viremia by a variety of techniques including RIA, CIE, and ELISA. The most specific tests are dot-blot hybridization[33] and the polymerase chain reaction,[34] which may allow identification of B19 DNA in serum, urine, respiratory secretions, cerebrospinal fluid, and bone marrow.

TREATMENT

There is no specific treatment available for parvovirus B19 infection. Erythema infectiosum is a benign condition, and usually no treatment is necessary. Supportive therapy for relief of fatigue, malaise, pruritus, and arthralgia may be needed. The chronic anemia of persistent B19 infection may be treated successfully with commercially available intravenous immunoglobulin, which contains neutralizing anti-B19 antibodies. Aplastic crisis, which can be life-threatening, may require oxygen therapy and blood transfusion.

Serologic testing for B19 IgG and IgM should be offered to pregnant women who are exposed. Infected pregnant women are followed by frequent ultrasonograms. Evidence of hydrops fetalis warrants umbilical cordocentesis to check for anemia, viral DNA,

IgG, and IgM. The management of infected fetuses is controversial. Some physicians advocate observation because spontaneous resolution is common. Fetuses with severe anemia and compromise are usually managed with intrauterine exchange transfusion, but this procedure does carry risk.

PREVENTION

There is currently no vaccine to prevent parvovirus B19 infection. A preparation of recombinant B19 capsid vaccine has been in early clinical trials. It is not known whether immunoglobulin given around the time of exposure will prevent infection or alter the course of the disease. Routine treatment with immunoglobulin is not recommended at the present time.

Since patients with erythema infectiosum are no longer infectious by the time they develop the illness, control measures directed toward these individuals are not likely to be effective. If these persons are hospitalized, no special precautions need to be taken. Because the virus is transmitted before the rash appears, the disease is easily spread in situations of close prolonged contact such as schools, day care centers, workplaces, and homes.

Patients with aplastic crisis or immunosuppression with chronic B19 anemia may have high titer viremia and are particularly infectious. These individuals should be placed in respiratory and contact isolation if hospitalized, and pregnant health care providers should not care for them directly. Hospital workers are at risk of contracting nosocomial infections from these patients[35] and could spread the virus to patients if adequate precautions are not taken.

COURSE AND PROGNOSIS

Parvovirus B19 infection in healthy individuals is self-limited. The rash of erythema infectiosum and the parvovirus arthropathy usually resolve in 1 to 2 weeks but can recur or persist for months. If untreated, transient aplastic crisis can be fatal, but most patients recover in 1 week. Chronic anemia from B19 usually resolves if treated with gammaglobulin. Fetal hydrops can lead to fetal death if not treated.

REFERENCES

1. Tschamer A: Ueber ortliche Rotheln. *Jahrbuch fur Kinderheilkunde* **29**:372, 1889
2. Shapiro L: The numbered diseases: First through sixth. *JAMA* **194**:210, 1965
3. Cossart YE et al: Parvovirus-like particles in human sera. *Lancet* **1**:72, 1975
4. Summers J et al: Characterization of the genome of the agent of erythrocyte aplasia permits its classification as a human parvovirus. *J Gen Virol* **64**:2527, 1983
5. Anderson MJ et al: Human parvovirus, the cause of erythema infectiosum (fifth disease)? *Lancet* **1**:1378, 1983
6. Cohen BJ, Buckley MM: The prevalence of antibody to human parvovirus B19 in England and Wales. *J Med Microbiol* **25**:151, 1988
7. Plummer FA et al: An erythema infectiosum–like illness caused by human parvovirus infection. *N Engl J Med* **313**:74, 1985
8. Anderson MJ et al: Experimental parvoviral infection in humans. *J Infect Dis* **152**:257, 1985
9. Cohen B: Parvovirus B19: An expanding spectrum of disease. *BMJ* **311**:1549, 1995
10. Brown KE et al: Resistance to parvovirus B19 infection due to lack of virus receptor (erythrocyte P antigen). *N Engl J Med* **330**:1192, 1994
11. Anand A et al: Human parvovirus infection in pregnancy and hydrops fetalis. *N Engl J Med* **316**:183, 1987
12. Feder HM, Anderson I: Fifth disease. A brief review of infections in childhood, in adulthood, and in pregnancy. *Arch Intern Med* **149**:2176, 1989
13. Nocton JJ et al: Human parvovirus B19-associated arthritis in children. *J Pediatr* **122**:186, 1993
14. Lefrere JJ et al: Henoch-Schönlein purpura and human parvovirus infection. *Pediatrics* **78**:183, 1986
15. Woolf AD et al: Clinical manifestations of human parvovirus B19 in adults. *Arch Intern Med* **149**:1153, 1989
16. Thurn J: Human parvovirus B19: Historical and clinical review. *Rev Infect Dis* **10**:1005, 1988
17. Faden H et al: Numbness and tingling of fingers associated with parvovirus B19 infection. *J Infect Dis* **161**:354, 1990
18. Harms M et al: Papular-purpuric "gloves and socks" syndrome. *J Am Acad Dermatol* **23**:850, 1990
19. Young N: Hematologic and hematopoietic consequences of B19 parvovirus infection. *Semin Hematol* **25**:159, 1988
20. Ware R: Human parvovirus infection. *J Pediatr* **114**:343, 1989
21. Anderson LJ: Human parvoviruses. *J Infect Dis* **161**:603, 1990
22. Kurtzman G et al: Pure red-cell aplasia of 10 years' duration due to persistent parvovirus B19 infection and its cure with immunoglobulin therapy. *N Engl J Med* **321**:519, 1989
23. Levy R et al: Infection by parvovirus B19 during pregnancy: A review. *Obstet Gynecol Surv* **52**:254, 1997
24. Public Health Laboratory Service Working Party on Fifth Disease. Prospective study of human parvovirus (B19) infection in pregnancy. *Br Med J* **300**:1166, 1990
25. Mortimer PP et al: Human parvovirus and the fetus. *Lancet* **2**:1012, 1985
26. Weiland HT et al: Parvovirus B19 associated with fetal abnormality. *Lancet* **1**:682, 1987
27. Tiessen RG et al: A fetus with a parvovirus B19 infection and congenital anomalies. *Prenat Diagn* **14**:173, 1994
28. Finkel TH et al: Chronic parvovirus B19 infection and systemic necrotising vasculitis: Opportunistic infection or aetiological agent? *Lancet* **343**:1255, 1994
29. Corman LC, Dolson DJ: Polyarteritis nodosa and parvovirus B19 infection. *Lancet* **339**:491, 1992
30. Nigro G et al: Recurrent Kawasaki disease associated with co-infection with parvovirus B19 and HIV-1. *AIDS* **7**:288, 1993
31. Nesher G et al: Parvovirus infection mimicking systemic lupus erythematosus. *Semin Arthritis Rheum* **24**:297, 1995
32. Caul EO et al: Intrauterine infection with human parvovirus B19: A light and electron microscopy study. *J Med Virol* **24**:55, 1988
33. Anderson MJ et al: Diagnosis of human parvovirus infection by dot-blot hybridization using cloned viral DNA. *J Med Virol* **15**:163, 1985
34. Salimans MMM et al: Rapid detection of human parvovirus B19 DNA by dot-blot hybridization and the polymerase chain reaction. *J Virol Methods* **23**:19, 1989
35. Bell LM et al: Human parvovirus B19 infection among hospital staff members after contact with infected patients. *N Engl J Med* **321**:485, 1989

CHAPTER 215

Clyde S. Crumpacker

Herpes Simplex

The human herpes simplex virus (HSV) consists of two closely related viruses designated herpes simplex virus type 1 (HSV-1) and herpes simplex virus type 2 (HSV-2) (Fig. 215-1). The viruses cause a wide variety of mucocutaneous infections and produce both primary and recurrent infections. The primary infection by HSV is more severe and has a different natural history than recurrent disease. Following a primary infection, the virus establishes a latent or dormant state. Recurrent disease is caused by reactivation of this dormant virus, which then travels down the nerve fiber to establish skin infection. The natural history and transmission of these viral infections pose a significant health problem. Effective antiviral therapy for these diseases remains an important medical goal.

EPIDEMIOLOGY

Recurrent oral-facial herpes simplex infection, known commonly as "cold sores" or "fever blisters," afflicts between 25 and 40 percent of the U.S. population and is the most common manifestation of herpes simplex infection. Studies show that 46 percent of graduating college students have serologic evidence of HSV-1 exposure, although only 28 percent report a history of cold sores.[1] In general

FIGURE 215-1

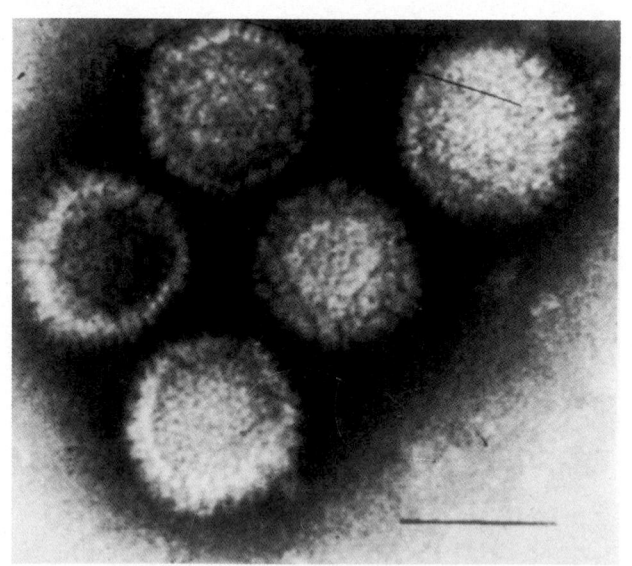

Herpes simplex virion.

in adult populations from city and rural areas throughout the world, >85 percent have serologic evidence of HSV-1 exposure.[2]

Genital infection with herpes simplex virus has increased markedly during the past three decades. Patient consultations with private physicians for genital herpes increased tenfold from 1966 to 1981. Over the same period, the number of new infections increased more than sevenfold.[3]

In the United States, 16 percent of the population age 15 to 74 has serologic evidence of previous exposure to HSV-2. Because nearly 100 percent of positive serologies are due to infections acquired sexually, it is estimated that more than 25 million Americans are infected with genital HSV-2.[4] In one study of women attending family practice clinics, 78 percent of those with serologic evidence of HSV-2 had no historic, clinical, or virologic evidence of genital herpes infection. Of these, 4 percent were asymptomatically shedding herpes simplex virus.[5] Similarly, a study of college students showed that only 25 percent of those exposed had a history of genital herpes.[1] From these studies it is clear that the large majority of HSV-2 infections are clinically inapparent.

The incidence of herpes simplex virus type 2 (HSV-2) infection continues to increase in the United States and in all developed industrial nations. The incidence of infection is increasing most rapidly in the United States among young whites. This increasing incidence is associated with the awareness of subclinical and asymptomatic genital herpes infections.[6]

THE VIRUSES

Herpes simplex virus types 1 and 2 contain a double-stranded linear DNA genome of molecular mass of 160×10^3 kDa surrounded by a protein coat and lipid envelope. The genomes of HSV-1 and HSV-2 have about 50 percent of the nucleotide sequence in common and 50 percent variable. The viral genomes encode for about 50 virus-specific proteins. These include five to six virus-specific glycoproteins that are present on the viral surfaces and on the surface of virus-infected cells. These glycoproteins are important for induction of neutralizing antibodies to the virus and regulate cell fusion exhibited by these viruses. Only one of these surface glycoproteins, gC for HSV-1 and gG for HSV-2, appears to be type-specific. There is significant cross-reactivity of antibodies raised against the other glycoproteins between HSV-1 and HSV-2.

The major glycoproteins that induce neutralizing antibodies, the gD glycoprotein of HSV-1 and HSV-2, share 80 percent of the amino acids in common, and neutralizing antibodies raised against HSV-1 readily neutralize HSV-2. The viral core proteins and structural proteins comprise 20 virus-specific proteins. The viral protein coat consists of protein arranged in 162 capsomeres around the viral nucleic acid.

The herpes simplex virus genome encodes a number of nonstructural proteins that are important for viral DNA replication. These include a viral thymidine kinase, DNA polymerase, ribonucleotide reductase, and alkaline DNase. These enzymes have all been mapped to precise locations on the viral genome, and mutants of herpes simplex virus have been isolated that contain mutations in the genes encoding these viral enzymes. These viral enzymes, which differ in significant ways from cellular enzymes, can be selectively inhibited by antiviral drugs. The development of antiviral drugs that selectively inhibit viral-specific enzyme targets, such as viral DNA polymerase, has progressed rapidly and permitted the successful application of antiviral chemotherapy for the treatment of herpes simplex infections. The use of rapid techniques of viral diagnosis to make an early diagnosis of herpes simplex infection and begin therapy with drugs, such as acyclovir, has made it possible to treat many forms of mucocutaneous infection caused by herpes simplex virus effectively.

PRIMARY INFECTION

A hallmark of infections caused by HSV is that they occur initially in mucocutaneous locations and then remain dormant in neuronal cells located in ganglia before recurring as outbreaks of mucocutaneous infection. The natural histories of primary and recurrent infections differ, the response to treatment may differ, and they need to be considered separately. Primary infection with herpes simplex occurs primarily by direct exposure through mucocutaneous contact with another infected individual. It is estimated that 95 percent of primary genital herpes simplex infection occurs within 2 weeks of sexual contact with an infected sexual partner. In one study, in 70 percent of patients transmission appeared to result from sexual contact during periods of asymptomatic viral shedding.[7] Primary infection is defined as the first infection with herpes simplex virus in a seronegative patient. There are no reliable well-documented examples of herpes simplex virus being transmitted by the respiratory route. Even though some experimental studies have shown that the virus can persist on surfaces like towels, toilet seats, or countertops for as long as 30 min, there is no case of a herpes simplex infection being acquired by contact with such a surface. The virus may persist in water or on a wet surface for a short time also, but the presence of any halogenated compound in the water immediately inactivates the virus infectivity. There is no evidence that herpes simplex infection can be acquired through water transmission.

For primary facial-oral herpes infection, exposure to herpes simplex in a mother's vaginal secretions during delivery can result in a primary neonatal infection in about 50 percent of infants exposed to the virus. This usually is first noted at day 4 to 7 of life by the development of characteristic herpetic skin lesions. The skin infection commonly occurs in areas of trauma on the body and may begin in areas where scalp electrodes were placed to facilitate fetal monitoring during labor. Neonatal infection with herpes simplex virus may also occur in the absence of skin lesions and directly involve the central nervous system and visceral organs such as the liver. In the absence of skin lesions, primary neonatal herpes simplex infection is very difficult to diagnose and remains an important challenge for the pediatric clinician. Primary herpes simplex infection in the neonate is a devastating life-threatening infection that must be diagnosed and treated promptly with antiviral drugs.

Primary facial-oral herpes infection usually occurs as an acute gingivostomatitis, and ulcers may occur throughout the buccal mucosa (Fig. 215-2). Many cases of herpes gingivostomatitis occur early in life and are probably not diagnosed. It is estimated that a great majority (>85 percent) of the worldwide population has evidence of herpes simplex facial-oral infection,[2] whereas only 37 percent of middle-class college-age American students have antibody to herpes simplex infection.[1]

Primary genital herpes infection occurs following sexual exposure in perhaps 95 percent of cases. The usual time for an outbreak of genital herpes is between 3 and 14 days after sexual relations with a person with active genital lesions.

RECURRENT INFECTION

A characteristic feature of all the herpesviruses is that after primary infection occurs, the virus has the ability to establish latent or dormant infection and then to reactivate to produce recurrent disease (Fig. 215-3). The recurrent disease is usually milder and of shorter duration than the primary infection. In the facial-oral herpes simplex infection, the virus is almost always HSV-1 and, following the primary episode of stomatitis, the virus migrates to the trigeminal ganglion. In the ganglion, the viral genome remains in a suppressed state primarily as a circular episome of viral DNA with very few of the viral genes being expressed. Certain triggering events such as exposure to sunlight, severe stress, or neurosurgical manipulation of the ganglia will cause the latent virus to reactivate, express its genome, and produce intact viral particles. The viral particles move down the nerve, probably by axonal flow, and replicate in the epithelial cells of the skin to produce an outbreak of cold sores (Fig. 215-3). Between episodes there is no evidence of viral particles, viral proteins, or viral nucleic acids in the skin at the affected site. These general principles apply to recurrent episodes of herpes infections in all common sites, especially facial-oral herpes, genital

FIGURE 215-2

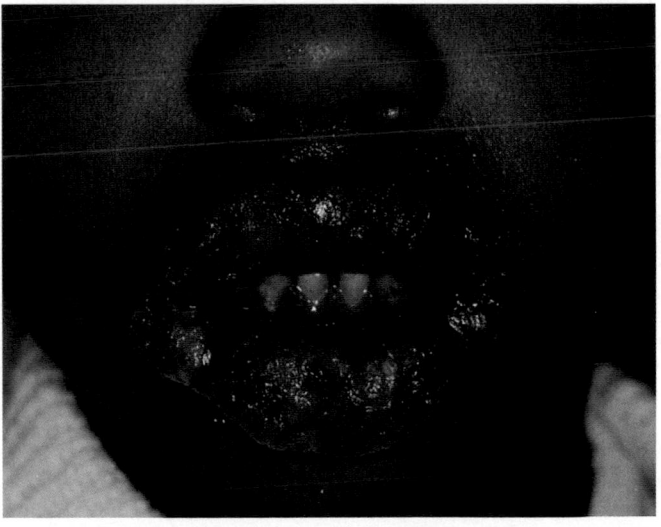

Primary herpetic gingivostomatitis in a child.

FIGURE 215-3

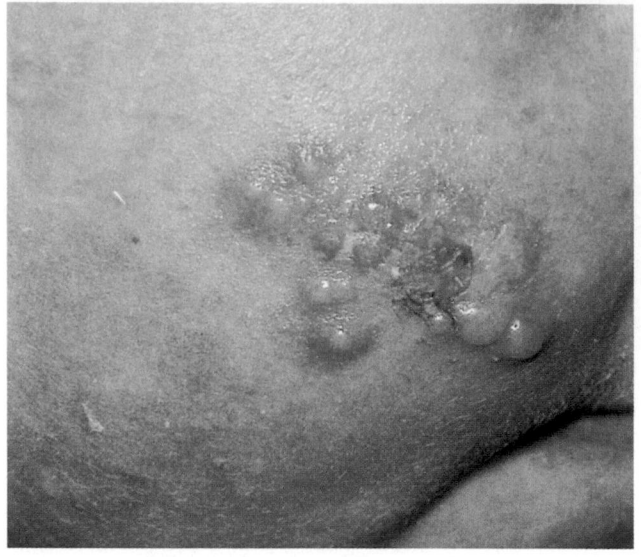

Recurrent facial herpes simplex with grouped vesicles and crusting.

herpes, herpes whitlow, and herpes keratitis. In recurrent herpes infections, patients possess antibody to the virus, and immunologically active mononuclear cells and lymphocytes contribute to the pathogenesis and healing of the outbreak.

CLINICAL MANIFESTATIONS

Primary Gingivostomatitis

Primary herpetic infection of the mouth and pharynx is a disease of children and young adults. The peak years of incidence occur between ages 1 and 5. A study at a large university health service estimated that primary herpes simplex virus infection was a significant cause of sore throats in college students.[8] The infection may be mild and inapparent to severe with high fever. The usual onset is with fever, sore throat and painful vesicles, and ulcerative erosions on the tongue, palate, gingiva, buccal mucosa, and lips. The vesicles on the mucous membranes coalesce to form plaques covered with a gray membrane. Severe oral lesions are associated with drooling, halitosis, enlarged lymph nodes, inability to eat, fever, and generalized complaints. The time from exposure to onset of symptoms is from 5 to 10 days. The diagnosis is suggested by the early onset of lesions in discrete clusters before they spread to involve the entire buccal mucosa extensively. Diagnosis is confirmed by culturing herpes simplex virus from the lesions, or identifying herpes simplex antigens with the use of monoclonal antibodies and immunofluorescence analysis.

The differential diagnosis of primary herpetic gingivostomatitis includes streptococcal pharyngitis, diphtheria, coxsackievirus infection, aphthous ulcers, infectious mononucleosis, severe candidiasis, pemphigus vulgaris, Behçet's disease, erythema multiforme, and primary HIV infection.

Recurrent Facial-Oral Herpes Simplex

After a primary infection with herpes simplex virus, antibody to the virus develops. In one study, 27 percent of college students reported a history of cold sores.[1] It is estimated that about one-third of the population of the United States experiences recurrent episodes of facial-oral infection with HSV, known as *recurrent herpes labialis* or *cold sores*. The incidence of recurrences is variable in different populations, but 15 percent of young adults surveyed had recurrences of at least one lesion per year and in a series of over 1000 young adults, 20 percent had recurrent episodes. The usual number of recurrences is 3 to 4 per year.[9,10]

The onset of a cold sore is heralded by itching and burning at the vermilion border of the lip. This may be associated with an erythematous papule that rapidly goes on to become vesicular and then to ulcerate to produce a sore. The open sore crusts over in about 4 days, the scab falls off, and complete healing occurs in 8 to 9 days. HSV-1 can be isolated from cold sores for about 3.5 days. Neutralizing antibodies do not prevent recurrent episodes, and most patients with recurrent herpes labialis have high levels of neutralizing antibody at the time of recurrence. The most common triggering events for recurrent cold sores are sun exposure, trauma to the lips, emotional stress, and fatigue.[11]

Recurrent herpes labialis must be distinguished from other ulcerative lesions such as aphthous ulcers, erythema multiforme, impetigo, and vaccinia infection. The usual location for recurrent herpes labialis is at the skin-lip junction. Recurrent erosive ulcers inside the mouth are most commonly due to aphthous ulcers or erythema multiforme, rather than herpes simplex infection. An important distinguishing feature of herpes in the mouth from aphthous ulcers (canker sores) is that herpes begins as a few clustered lesions on one part of the buccal mucosa, whereas aphthous ulcers begin as sores on widely separated parts of the buccal mucosa.

Primary Genital Herpes

In industrial countries, herpes simplex virus is the most common cause of genital ulcerations, accounting for 20 to 50 percent of ulcerative lesions in patients attending sexually transmitted disease clinics. It is estimated that 95 percent of episodes of primary genital herpes occur following sexual exposure to a partner with active lesions. The usual period between sexual exposure to a person with active genital herpes and development of an acute episode is from 3 to 14 days. The outbreak begins with small grouped vesicles (Fig. 215-4), which break and progress to ulcerative lesions in 2 to 4 days. Most patients present to the physician with ulcerative lesions. The first episode of genital herpes usually has multiple lesions, which are present bilaterally and coalesce to involve a larger surface. Recurrent genital herpes frequently presents as a single ulcer. Painful enlarged inguinal lymph nodes are common, and the nodes are usually tender on palpation, nonfixed, and slightly firm. About 35 percent of women and 13 percent of men with primary genital herpes will have an aseptic meningitis with fever, stiff neck, headache, photophobia, and pleocytosis in the spinal fluid.[12] The spinal fluid protein may be elevated to near 100 mg/dL, and the glucose may fall below 40 mg. Cells are mainly lymphocytes (200 to 1000/mm³). It is also clear that approximately 20 percent of patients with primary genital herpes will have painful difficulty on urination, which may require catheterization of the urinary tract for relief. This is essentially never present in recurrent genital herpes. The dominant local symptoms of primary genital herpes are pain, itching, dysuria, and vaginal and urethral discharge. The severity of these symptoms increases over the first 6 to 7 days of the illness and peaks at days 8 to 10. New lesions continue to form during the first week of illness in about 75 percent of patients. Both HSV-1 and HSV-2 cause primary genital herpes, with 80 percent being associated with isolation of HSV-2 from lesions. Both produce an identical clinical picture, but HSV-1–induced primary disease is associated with many fewer recurrences than when HSV-2 is isolated from the primary episode. Herpes simplex virus has been isolated from the pharynx of 11 percent of patients with primary genital herpes and in only 1 percent of those with recurrent disease.[12] Clinical signs of herpes simplex virus pharyngitis may be mild erythema or diffuse ulcerative and exudative pharyngitis of the posterior pharynx. This may be associated with tender anterior cervical adenopathy and may mimic streptococcal pharyngitis.

Primary genital herpes may last 18 to 21 days, and virus shedding is present for about 11 days; this correlates with the time from onset of symptoms to the development of crusting. The differential diagnosis of other infections that cause genital ulcers and inguinal lymphadenopathy includes syphilis, chancroid, lymphogranuloma venereum, and granuloma inguinale.

FIGURE 215-4

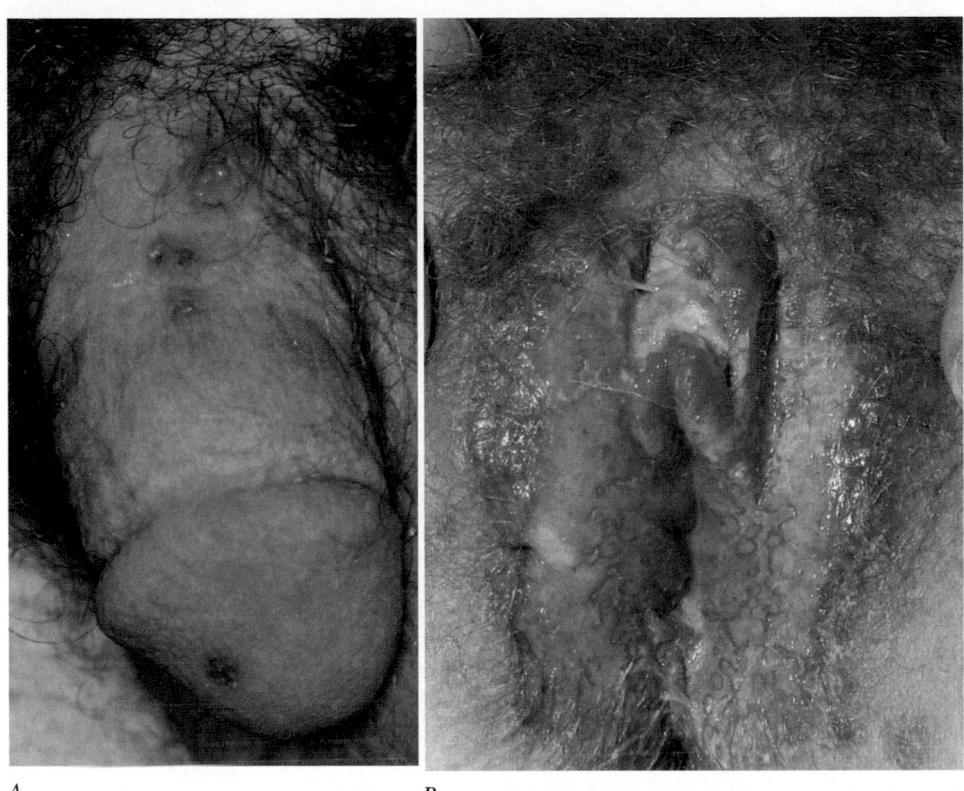

A.   *B.*

A. Primary genital herpes simplex with vesicles. *B.* Primary herpetic vulvitis.

Herpes Simplex Virus Cervicitis

Herpes simplex virus is a common etiology of cervical ulcerations. In women attending a sexually transmitted disease clinic, 88 percent of cervical ulcers were believed to be caused by HSV-2, based on culture and serologic evidence. During the first episode of HSV-2 genital infection, virus may be isolated from the cervix in 59 percent of women. In women with symptomatic recurrences, HSV-2 was isolated from the cervix in only 8 percent.[5]

Of women with cervical cultures positive for HSV-2, 50 percent showed evidence of cervical ulcers on speculum examination, whereas 65 percent had ulcerations seen on colposcopy. Cellular changes indicative of HSV infection were present on cervical cytology in 62 percent of women with positive HSV-2 cultures and in only 0.5 percent of those without positive cultures.[5]

Shedding of HSV is found in patients both with and without symptoms of genital herpes infection. Of women with asymptomatic HSV-2 genital infections, 5 percent actively shed HSV-2, with about 40 percent of those having positive cervical cultures in the absence of symptoms. Acute herpetic cervicitis may be the only manifestation of first-episode genital herpes simplex infection. In one study, 8 percent of women had mucopurulent cervicitis with positive cultures in the absence of external genital lesions.[13]

Because of the high prevalence of genital herpes infection and the amount of asymptomatic HSV-2 shedding, some authors have advocated routine screening for HSV-2 antibodies in high-risk populations to identify and counsel those with subclinical infections.[5]

Recurrent Genital Herpes

It is estimated that recurrent genital herpes infection affects about 25 million adults in the United States.[4] Following the primary infection, about 50 percent of men will have a recurrence in 4 months, whereas 50 percent of women will not have a recurrence until 8 months after the initial outbreak. Recurrent episodes may be more common in men following the initial episode, but the recurrent episodes appear to be more painful in women. The average number of recurrences is 3 or 4 per year, whereas perhaps 15 percent of patients with recurrent disease have 8 or more recurrences per year. The severity of symptoms, duration of symptoms, and duration of viral shedding are all much shorter in recurrent episodes than in primary disease. Virus can be cultured for 3 to 4 days, means time for crusting is 4 to 5 days, and time to complete healing is 9 to 10 days in recurrent genital herpes. The mean lesion area is much smaller in recurrent disease, and new lesion formation is much less. New lesions occur for only 1 to 2 days in recurrent disease as compared with 5 to 6 days in primary disease. Symptoms of fever, aseptic meningitis, and headache are also much less frequent in recurrent disease. With recurrent disease, 40 to 50 percent of episodes have a prodrome consisting of tingling, burning, or dysesthesias that may occur 1 or 2 days to a few hours before the appearance of vesicles. This prodrome may be associated with buttock pain or pain radiating down the back of the thigh and mimicking sciatic pain. In patients with recurrent genital herpes, HSV-1 is isolated much less frequently than in primary episodes. The recurrence rate is definitely much greater with genital herpes associated with HSV-2.

A major cause of morbidity with recurrent genital herpes is the frequency of recurrences and the fear of transmission of disease to infants or to sexual partners. Patients should be instructed to avoid sexual intercourse when prodromal symptoms or lesions occur and to resume sexual activity only when lesions completely reepithelialize. Herpes can be isolated from lesions rarely at the crust stage of disease.

Herpes as a Risk Factor for Human Immunodeficiency Virus (HIV)

Early in the AIDS epidemic, it was noted that genital ulcer disease was more common in HIV-seropositive individuals than in their HIV-negative counterparts. This was first described in East African female prostitutes[14] and men attending African sexually transmitted disease clinics,[15] where the most common etiologies of genital ulcer disease are chancroid and syphilis.

In North America and Europe, where the most common cause of genital ulcer disease is HSV-2, several studies have linked HSV-2 with exposure to HIV. In sexually transmitted disease clinics in Baltimore, HIV-positive men and women more often had a history of genital herpes and showed a higher seroprevalence rate of HSV-2 but not HSV-1 and HIV-negative men and women.[16] In separate cohorts of gay men in San Francisco[17] and Seattle,[18] the presence of HSV-2 antibody was significantly associated with HIV seropositivity. In a Dutch cohort, a history of anogenital HSV infection was more predictive of HIV seroconversion than other sexually transmitted diseases.[19]

Sexual transmission of HIV, both homosexual and heterosexual, is facilitated by genital ulcer disease by the disruption of protective epithelial or mucosal barriers and by the presence of activated T lymphocytes at ulcer bases, which likely serve as reservoirs of virus. In fact, HIV has been cultured from the bases of genital ulcers of both men and women in Africa.[20] Because genital HSV infection is common and may have high rates of recurrence, it may serve as a major cofactor in the sexual acquisition and transmission of HIV in the developed world. This underscores the benefits of preventive "safe sex" measures and early antiviral treatment, which may promote ulcer healing, decrease infectivity, and prevent subsequent recurrences. Clearly, controlling genital ulcer disease, particularly herpes, is an integral part of AIDS prevention efforts.

Herpes Infection in the Immunocompromised Patient

Herpes infections are an important cause of morbidity and mortality in immunocompromised patients. Patients with defects in cellular immunity from hematologic malignancies and HIV infection and those receiving immunosuppressive agents, such as glucocorticoids, or who have undergone organ transplantation are particularly susceptible. Immunocompromised patients infected with herpes simplex may have self-limited, localized disease that varies little from that seen in patients with normal immunity. However, depending on the degree of immunosuppression—either the activity of the underlying disease or the length of immunosuppressive therapy—herpes infection may recur more frequently and have a more severe and prolonged course. Deep, progressive ulcerations of mucocuta-

neous areas of the face, mouth, or anogenital areas (Fig. 215-5) may develop. Lesions may coalesce, becoming much larger than in patients with normal immune function. Lesions may also persist for weeks to months, with continuous shedding of isolable virus. The size and duration of such lesions may also predispose to bacterial or fungal superinfection. Because of the large amount of virus present, patients treated with antiviral agents may be particularly prone to the development of resistant virus.

Oral mucosal lesions can produce an extensive painful stomatitis in immunocompromised patients. The differential diagnosis of oral ulcers in such patients include herpes simplex, cytomegalovirus (CMV), *Candida, Histoplasma,* or primary HIV infection, and chemotherapy or allergic drug reactions. Superficial oral lesions may lead to herpes pharyngitis, esophagitis, or pneumonitis,[21] often after passage of an endotracheal or nasogastric tube. Recurrent orofacial or genital lesions may lead to viremia with subsequent seeding of viscera, including the esophagus, lungs, and liver (Fig. 215-6).

In the presence of a positive HIV serology, definitive evidence of herpes simplex infection causing a mucocutaneous ulcer that persists longer than 1 month, or bronchitis, pneumonitis, or esophagitis of any duration indicates the diagnosis of AIDS (in a patient older than 1 month).[22]

Antiviral therapy can be dramatically effective in reducing morbidity in these patients, both with early recognition and treatment of disease and in the wider use of prophylactic and suppressive therapy.

Herpetic Whitlow

The term *herpetic whitlow* applies to a primary or recurrent herpes simplex infection of the fingers or hands. The disease is a common occupational hazard for medical and dental personnel, who work in and around the mouths of patients shedding the virus. Herpetic whitlow may also complicate recurrent genital herpes infections.[23]

Inoculation may occur on the fingers or hands in areas of abraded or broken skin. Following inoculation, primary infection lasts 2 to 6 weeks and is characterized by painful vesicles (Fig. 215-7), erythema, and edema, often accompanied by erythematous streaking of the forearm and tender axillary lymphadenopathy. Although the process may mimic bacterial infection, there is no evidence of pus formation.

FIGURE 215-5

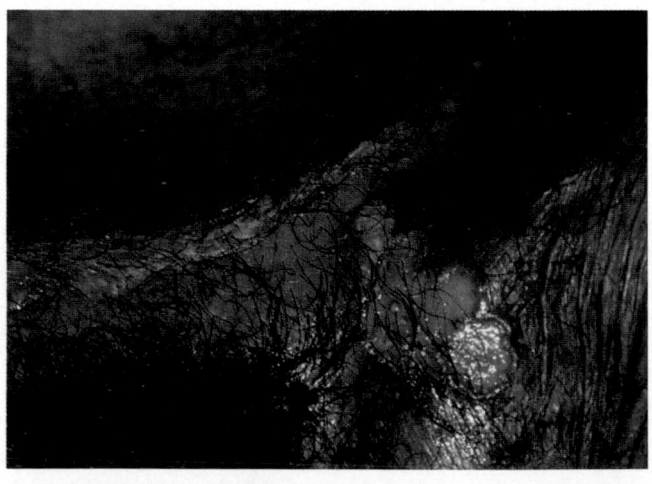

Chronic herpetic ulcer. A 32-year-old male presented with these ulcers of 7 weeks' duration. HIV serology was positive.

The appearance of vesicles with subsequent progression to ulcers at the margin of the skin lesion is highly suggestive of herpetic whitlow. Confirmation by a positive Tzanck smear and viral culture will establish the diagnosis. The lesions resolve spontaneously; however, as with other sites of herpes infection, recurrences are common.

Prevention of contact with saliva and active vesicles or ulcers is an important goal for health care workers. Routine use of latex gloves as part of universal blood and body fluid precautions will likely also reduce the risk of HSV transmission.

Although no controlled studies have been performed, there is anecdotal evidence that acyclovir is successful in the acute treatment of herpetic whitlow and may help to decrease the frequency of recurrences of disease when used prophylactically.[24,25] The latter use may be especially valuable for health care workers who otherwise might need to limit patient care responsibilities during outbreaks. A case report described a 22-year-old man with AIDS and severe herpetic whitlow of his left thumb.[26] The lesion improved during a course of ganciclovir (for presumed CMV pneumonia) then worsened despite lengthy courses of oral and intravenous acyclovir. HSV isolated from the lesion was found to be highly resistant to acyclovir and ganciclovir.

Herpes Gladiatorum

Cases of cutaneous and ocular infections with HSV-1 have occurred among wrestlers and rugby players and have been labeled *herpes gladiatorum.*[27,28] Surveys of high school and college athletic trainers suggest that herpes infection among wrestlers is endemic.[29] An investigation of an outbreak among high school wrestlers attending a training camp supported direct skin-to-skin contact as the primary mode of transmission[30]; nearly half of the affected wrestlers reported an abrasion or break in the skin at the site of subsequent infection. The sites of skin lesions were markedly different from typical orolabial HSV-1 infections and included the head (73 percent), trunk (28 percent), and extremities (47 percent). The attack rate among wrestlers in the same practice groups was as high as 67 percent. Oropharyngeal swabs for HSV-1 culture from affected wrestlers failed to grow HSV-1 in any of those tested, suggesting that saliva was not a major source of transmission. Early identification of skin lesions and the exclusion of infected wrestlers is recommended to decrease the incidence of transmission of herpes gladiatorum.

FIGURE 215-6

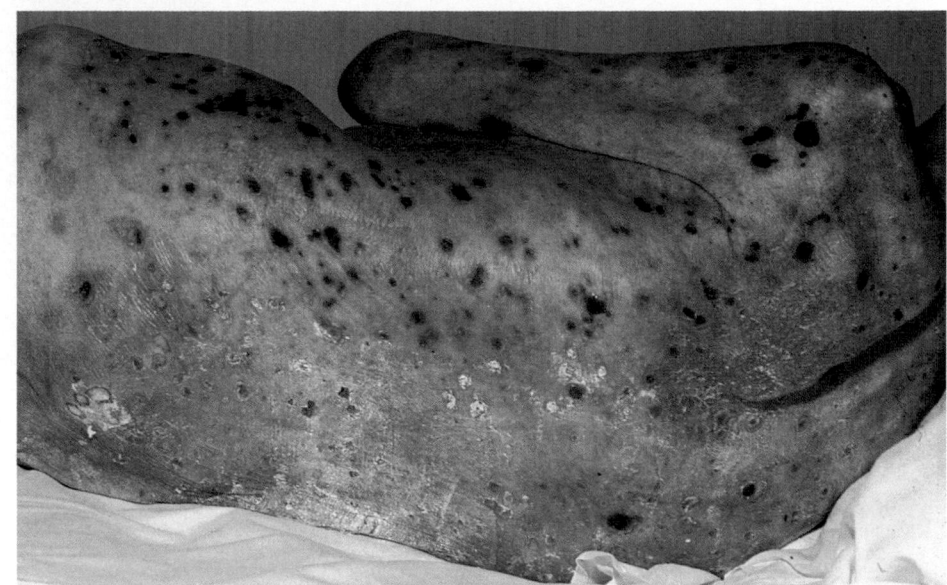

A.

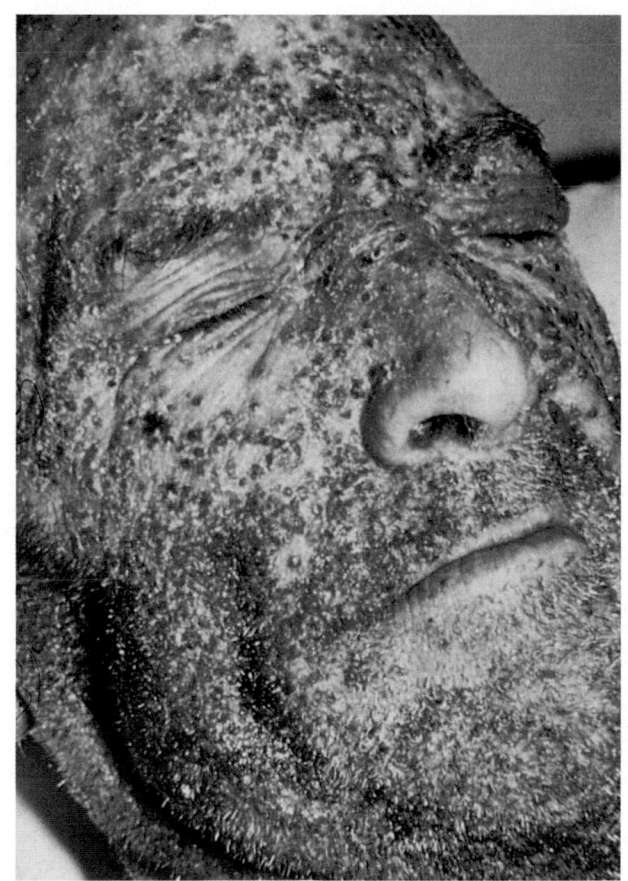

B.

Disseminated herpes simplex infection. *A.* Generalized vesicles and pustules with hemorrhage and necrosis. *B.* Generalized vesicles, pustules, erosions, and ulcerations.

FIGURE 215-7

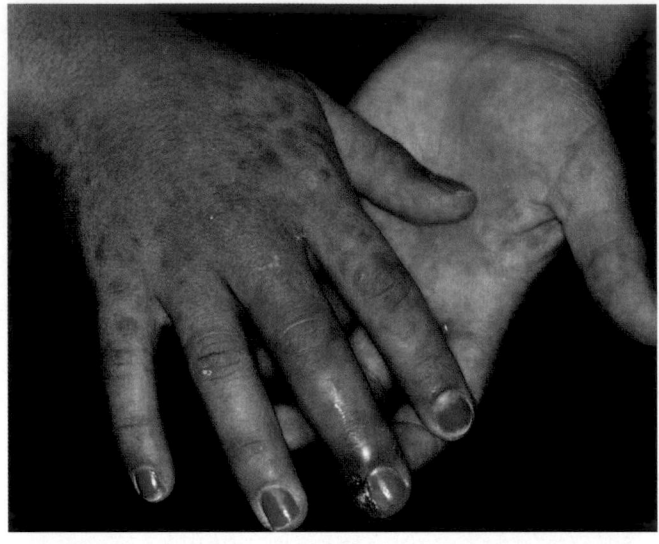

Herpetic whitlow of the middle finger with associated erythema multiforme in a nurse's aide.

FIGURE 215-8

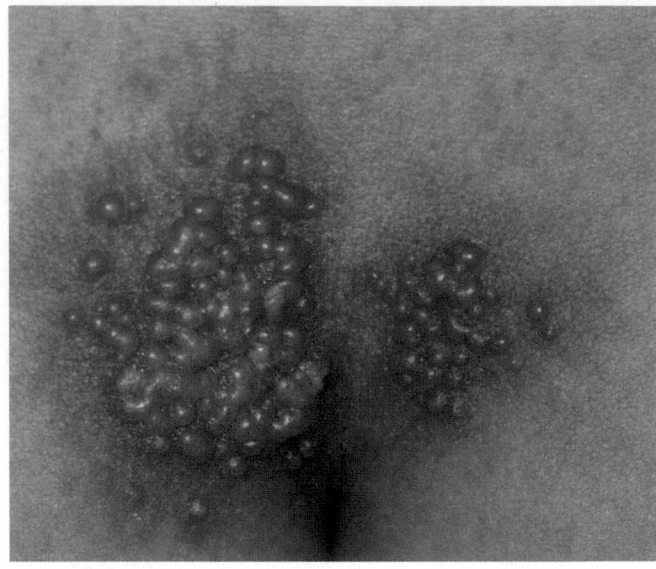

Recurrent lumbosacral herpes simplex.

Herpetic Keratoconjunctivitis

Herpes simplex virus infection of the eye can cause recurrent erosions of the conjunctiva and cornea. The initial phase of the ophthalmologic disease is a superficial corneal ulcer. This is usually specifically diagnosed on slit-lamp examination. With repeated recurrences, deeper ulcers develop and stromal keratitis occurs. With each episode, stromal scarring may progress and blindness may develop. Herpes simplex keratitis is now regarded as the leading cause of infectious blindness in the United States. The differential diagnosis of herpetic keratoconjunctivitis includes herpes zoster, adenovirus infection, vaccinia, and chlamydial conjunctivitis. Early treatment with topical antiviral drugs such as vidarabine or trifluorothymidine can enhance healing and minimize stromal scarring.

Recurrent Lumbosacral Herpes Simplex

Recurrent cutaneous herpetic lesions on the low back and buttocks can occur in the absence of actual genital lesions. Recurrent outbreaks of "buttock herpes" usually occur in men and women over the age of 40 and comprise a small percentage—usually only 10 percent of herpes outbreaks in the pelvic and genital area. The lesions are frequently triggered by stress, fatigue, or the onset of the menstrual cycle. The lesions usually occur on one side of the buttocks or another, begin as clusters on an erythematous base (Fig. 215-8), and heal with hyperpigmentation and minimal scarring. Recurrences can develop on a periodic basis and go on for several years. A central feature of recurrent lumbosacral herpes simplex is the prodrome associated with deep pelvic aching for 1 to 3 days before the cutaneous lesions appear. Some patients may experience pain going down the back of the leg and mimicking "sciatic pain." Patients have even undergone myelography to evaluate this pain. The differential diagnosis of lumbosacral herpes simplex infection must include low back strain, herniated lumbosacral disk, impetigo, and herpes zoster.

Recurrent Herpes Simplex and Erythema Multiforme (See Chap. 59)

In a subset of patients, the development of recurrent herpes simplex infection may be followed in 7 to 10 days by the development of erythema multiforme. The presentation may vary from typical erythematous papules (see Fig. 215-7) evolving into target lesions on the extremities to painful ulcerations of the oral, genital, or conjunctival mucosa. Recurrent lesions may occur as infrequently as once a year or may persist nearly continuously. Spontaneous improvement occurs over about 5 years.

Anecdotal reports suggest that acyclovir may be successful both in aborting attacks of erythema multiforme when given during the prodromal period[31] and in preventing recurrences when given continuously.[32,33] These results suggest that herpes simplex antigens are playing a crucial role in the development of erythema multiforme.

Eczema Herpeticum

Patients with preexisting skin disorders such as atopic dermatitis and Darier's disease may develop widespread cutaneous infections with HSV. Eczema herpeticum (Fig. 215-9) begins as clusters of umbilicated vesicles in areas where the skin has previously been abnormal. The eruption spreads widely over a period of 7 to 10 days and may be associated with fever, malaise, and lymphadenopathy. The vesicular lesions coalesce into large erosions, which frequently become secondarily infected with bacteria. The primary episode of eczema herpeticum will run its usual course and heal in 2 to 6 weeks. Patients with chronic skin damage may have recurrent episodes that are milder and not associated with systemic symptoms. The differential diagnosis of eczema herpeticum includes widespread impetigo and a Kaposi's varicelliform eruption caused by vaccinia virus.

FIGURE 215-9

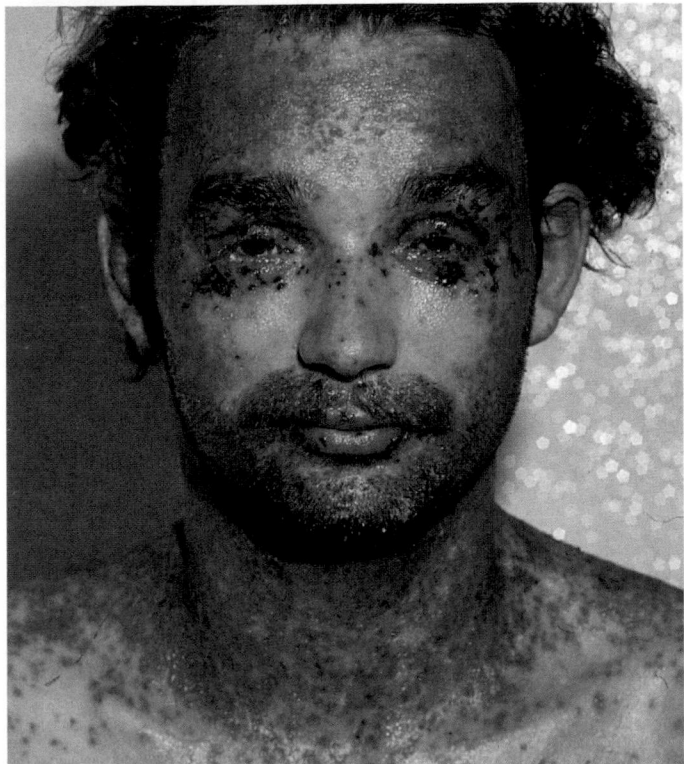

Eczema herpeticum in areas of atopic dermatitis.

Herpes Simplex Encephalitis

Herpes simplex virus is the most common cause of sporadic encephalitis in the developed world. The virus spreads along neural pathways from sites of primary or recurrent herpes infections, causing a necrotizing, hemorrhagic encephalitis, most often of the temporal lobes. It affects men and women of all ages and may occur during all seasons of the year.

A concurrent or prior diagnosis of orofacial or genital herpes simplex infection does not predict the likelihood of developing herpes encephalitis. The disease can occur in healthy adults and children without evidence of previous herpes simplex infection, although 70 percent of cases occur in patients with neutralizing antibody for herpes simplex.[34]

The onset of disease may be sudden, with symptoms of fever, headache, and confusion or temporal lobe signs such as olfactory hallucinations or behavioral changes. The diagnosis is suggested by the clinical presentation, a cerebrospinal fluid (CSF) pleocytosis and elevated protein, and a temporal lobe focus of electroencephalographic signals or focal enhancement on computed tomography or magnetic resonance imaging scans.

Brain biopsy with appropriate histology and cultures remains the definitive way to make the diagnosis. The virus will grow from infected tissue in 95 percent of cases within 5 days. Spinal fluid culture is usually negative for HSV even when tissue culture is positive. Preliminary studies suggest that the use of the polymerase chain reaction for detection of herpes simplex DNA in the CSF may offer an early diagnostic advantage.[35] Untreated, herpes simplex encephalitis has greater than 70 percent mortality. Because antiviral therapy has dramatically altered the course of the disease, the in-

stitution of empiric antiviral treatment while addressing diagnostic procedure options has been recommended.[36]

Caution is advised, however, as one study demonstrated that only 45 percent of patients thought to have HSV encephalitis who had brain biopsy had evidence of HSV infection, whereas another 22 percent of patients had diagnoses other than HSV, including 9 percent with other treatable diseases (including bacterial, mycobacterial, rickettsial, fungal, and malignant processes).[37]

DIAGNOSIS

Viral Culture

The most reliable way to make a precise diagnosis of herpes simplex infection is to grow the virus from skin lesions. The virus obtained from skin lesions can be quantitated by plaque titration, typed, and its sensitivity to antiviral agents determined. When compatible skin lesions are present and viral culture obtained from skin lesions yields herpes simplex virus, this essentially establishes the diagnosis. In the setting of characteristic lesions on the lip-skin junction that progress from papule to vesicle to erosion or ulcer to crusting state, the vast majority of isolates will be HSV. In our clinical trials, lesions that appear to be due to herpes will produce positive virus on culture about 85 to 90 percent of the time.[11] The percent of positive viral cultures obtained from clinical lesions is quite variable but in most large series this has varied between 60 and 90 percent. All other current methods of making a specific viral diagnosis of herpes simplex–induced skin lesions are less sensitive than viral culture.

Tzanck Preparation

A valuable clinical approach to making a rapid diagnosis of herpesvirus infection relies on taking a smear of cells from the base of the skin lesion, spreading the cells on a glass slide, and staining with Wright or Giemsa stain to look for multinucleated giant cells in a Tzanck preparation. Both HSV and varicella zoster virus infection will result in multinucleated giant cells and a positive Tzanck smear. With experience, a clinician can reliably distinguish multinucleated giant cells from cellular debris, crushed cells, and artifacts. In the case of genital herpes, multinucleated giant cells can also be identified on cytologic examination of Papanicolaou smears. A comparison of the yield of positive cultures for HSV with the appearance of multinucleated giant cells obtained from clinical specimens of genital herpes in women revealed that about 60 percent of specimens that grew HSV also possessed multinucleated giant cells on cytologic examination. In another study of biopsy-proved HSV encephalitis, examination of brain tissue by histopathology, immunofluorescence, and electron microscopy demonstrated evidence of HSV infection in 56, 70, and 45 percent, respectively, of cases in which herpes simplex virus was cultured from brain tissue.[34] This study also indicated that false positive results were obtained in 14, 9, and 2 percent of HSV-negative specimens of brain biopsies by histopathology, immunofluorescence, and electron microscopy, respectively. Taken together, these studies document the importance of obtaining a positive culture for HSV in establishing a precise diagnosis.

Monoclonal Antibodies

The use of specific monoclonal antibodies directed against HSV-1 and HSV-2 proteins is currently established as a means of making a rapid and precise viral diagnosis of facial-oral HSV infection and genital herpes simplex. In a study employing monoclonal antibodies to confirm HSV in tissue cultures by immunofluorescence, the monoclonal antibodies for HSV-1 and HSV-2 have proved to be sensitive and specific,[38] with an 88 percent correlation with tissue culture results. The use of monoclonal antibodies has considerable utility in making rapid precise viral diagnosis of herpes infections.

TREATMENT OF HERPES SIMPLEX INFECTION

Acyclovir [9-(2-hydroxyethoxy-methyl)-guanine] is the prototype of a class of antiviral drugs that employ the viral-specific thymidine kinase (TK) enzyme to add a phosphate group to the guanosine analogue (Fig. 215-10). The guanosine analogue acyclovir, utilizes the viral TK enzyme to form the acyclovir monophosphate. Cellular guanylate kinase and guanosine diphosphate kinase then form acyclovir triphosphate, a potent inhibitor of viral DNA polymerase. Acyclovir triphosphate is incorporated as the terminal base in an elongating strand of DNA and functions as a chain terminator to inhibit chain elongation.[39] Acyclovir triphosphate also appears to form an irreversible bond between elongating DNA and viral DNA polymerase, leading to inactivation of the DNA polymerase.[40] This has been described as an example of how acyclovir triphosphate also acts as a competitive inhibitor of guanosine triphosphate on viral DNA polymerase function. In addition to requiring viral TK for activation and inhibition of viral DNA polymerase at a 30-fold less concentration of acyclovir triphosphate than is required to inhibit cellular polymerase functions, acyclovir is taken up preferentially in cells that express a viral TK activity. This third area of specificity, decreased uptake of acyclovir by uninfected cells, probably accounts for the remarkable lack of toxicity associated with high doses of acyclovir.

In carefully randomized placebo-controlled trials, acyclovir is effective in the treatment of mucocutaneous herpes simplex infections.

FIGURE 215-10

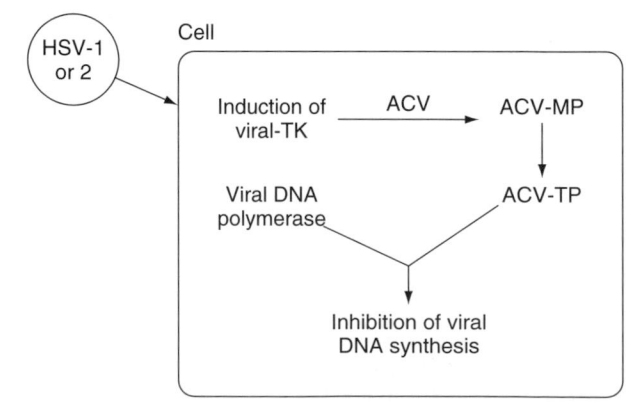

Diagram of mechanism of action of acyclovir.

Penciclovir is an acyclic nucleoside that is activated by the HSV TK enzyme to produce penciclovir triphosphate in infected cells. Penciclovir triphosphate is an effective inhibitor of HIV DNA polymerase and penciclovir is incorporated into elongating viral DNA.[41] Penciclovir is not a rigorous chain terminator as is acyclovir, but viral DNA elongation is greatly slowed. Penciclovir has good activity in tissue culture against HSV-1 and HSV-2 and varicella-zoster virus. Famciclovir is an orally bioavailable prodrug of penciclovir that contains two valine ester moieties. These valine groups are cleaved following absorption from the gastrointestinal tract and one passage through the liver, resulting in plasma levels of penciclovir. The intracellular triphosphate of penciclovir is maintained in vitro inside HSV-infected cells for 10 to 20 h as compared with 0.7 to 1 h for acyclovir. This prolonged half-life represents a pharmacologic advantage for penciclovir over acyclovir.

In addition, other drugs are approved for treatment of HSV infections. These include foscarnet, or phosphonoformic acid, which is a direct inhibitor of the viral DNA polymerase and is effective in the treatment of acyclovir-resistant herpes simplex. Trifluorothymidine, which is phosphorylated by the cellular TK, is an approved drug for HSV keratitis and may be active as a topical treatment for mucocutaneous acyclovir-resistant HSV infection. Ganciclovir, primarily active against CMV infection, also has good antiviral activity against HSV. Adenine-arabinoside, which can be effective therapy against HSV encephalitis, has no activity in the treatment of mucocutaneous infections caused by HSV.

Cidofovir is a nucleotide analogue of cytosine (hydroxyphosphomethyl phosphonocytosine, HPMPC) that contains a single phosphate group and does not require a viral TK for activation. Cidofovir is converted by cellular enzymes to cidofovir triphosphate, the active inhibitor of herpes simplex DNA polymerase. Since cidofovir does not require a viral TK for activation, it is being developed as a topical form for the treatment of acyclovir-resistant, TK-deficient herpes simplex mucocutaneous infections.[42]

Treatment of Facial-Oral Herpes

Therapy of recurrent facial-oral herpes simplex infection with a topical 5% ointment of acyclovir in polyethylene glycol in normal patients has revealed that the early application of the ointment would result in a significant antiviral effect with the virus being eradicated more rapidly from the skin of patients treated in the first 8 h of clinical occurrence of facial-oral HSV.[43] This antiviral effect was not associated with any clinical benefit, and treated cold sores did not heal more quickly nor did pain and discomfort resolve more rapidly. Recurrence rate of facial oral herpes was not affected by acyclovir treatment. In another study in fewer patients employing acyclovir 5% ointment in modified aqueous cream, an increased rate of healing of cold sores was noted in patients treated with acyclovir.[44]

In a randomized, double-blind, placebo-controlled, patient-initiated, multicenter study of topical 1% penciclovir cream for the treatment of recurrent episodes of herpes labialis, 1573 immunocompetent patients were tested and evaluated.[45] The study showed for the first time that a treatment could have an impact on the course of herpes labialis. Healing was 0.7 day faster for penciclovir-treated patients as compared with vehicle control cream—4.8 days versus 5.5 days. (95 percent confidence interval, 1.18 to 1.49 $p < .001$) Pain and lesion virus shedding also resolved more quickly for penciclovir-treated patients. The efficacy of penciclovir cream was apparent whether therapy was initiated early or late. There were no significant adverse effects associated with penciclovir cream. The clinical benefits are small but statistically significant for this rapidly self-healing, recurrent viral infection.

Treatment of Genital Herpes

In primary genital herpes, however, topical acyclovir or oral acyclovir therapy is associated with an antiviral effect and also more rapid healing. Topical acyclovir in a 5% ointment was applied four times a day for 7 days. Topical acyclovir reduced viral shedding from 7.0 days to 4.1 days, and time to complete crusting was reduced from 10.5 to 7.1 days.[46] Intravenous and oral acyclovir treatment of primary and initial genital herpes shortened median healing time by about 50 percent. Treatment with oral acyclovir, 200 mg, five times daily for 10 days, decreased median duration of viral shedding from 9 to 2 days, time for healing from 16 to 12 days, duration of pain from 7 to 5 days, and the number of patients forming new lesions after 48 h in therapy was decreased from 62 to 18 percent.[47] Other studies with patients having true primary disease had similar results. In nonprimary initial disease, the symptoms are intermediate in severity between primary and recurrent disease. Oral acyclovir is probably effective in treatment of nonprimary disease, but sufficient numbers of these patients have not been studied to document efficacy. In all of the studies employing oral acyclovir therapy for 10 days, there was no effect noted in the proportion of patients in whom recurrent disease episodes developed or in the frequency of these episodes. When patients with severe initial cases of genital herpes have an inability to urinate and require urinary catheterization or have severe meningitis with systemic symptoms, they may require hospitalization and treatment with intravenous acyclovir. Oral acyclovir will be the therapy of choice, however, for most patients with initial disease. Oral acyclovir will replace the less-effective topical acyclovir therapy for this indication.

Oral famciclovir has also been effective treatment for recurrent genital herpes. When famciclovir at doses of 125, 250, or 500 mg twice daily was administered within 6 h of the onset of symptoms of recurrent genital herpes, complete healing was more rapid as compared with placebo.[48] The duration of all lesions and associated symptoms, including edema, vesicles, ulcers, and crusting was shortened. Since a superior dose was not identified, a dose of 125 mg twice daily was recommended. As this trial required more observations during the treatment period than other studies, it was not possible to compare this with other antiviral regimens.

Famciclovir also reduced the positivity of viral cultures, and the decrease in viral shedding was the most sensitive statistical marker of efficacy, with a hazard ratio of 2.6 to 4.2 noted. The authors concluded that early patient-initiated antiviral treatment with 125 mg of oral famciclovir twice daily for 5 days was convenient and increased the likelihood that viral shedding would be aborted.

Suppression of Recurrent Disease

In a large double-blind trial comprising 143 patients with a mean of 1.07 recurrences of genital herpes per month, placebo was compared with oral acyclovir (200 mg) five times daily and oral acyclovir twice daily.[49] Patients received the therapy for 4 months, and 94 percent of the placebo patients experienced recurrences during this period as compared with 29 percent of those treated with acyclovir five times daily and 35 percent of those treated with acyclovir twice daily. The recurrences while patients were taking acyclovir were less frequent and of a shorter duration than among placebo recipients, but recurrence rates returned to pretreatment rates once medication was discontinued. In another study, patients taking three or four capsules daily experienced a similar improvement.[50] In the study by Straus et al., three patients in whom recurrences developed while taking acyclovir had acyclovir-resistant HSV isolated from episodes that developed while they were taking the drug.[50]

These episodes were described as "breakthrough recurrences." No other studies in patients with a normal immune system have been able to document the occurrence of acyclovir-resistant HSV. To date, acyclovir-resistant HSV has been detected only in patients with a compromised immune system.

Prolonged, continuous oral acyclovir treatment of normal patients with frequently recurring genital HSV infection has been successful in suppressing recurrences. A 3-year study of patients with six recurrences per year revealed that 400 mg of acyclovir orally twice per day markedly suppressed recurrent episodes.[51] The annual recurrence rate dropped from more than 12 recurrences per year at base line to one recurrence in the third year on suppressive therapy. No significant toxic effects were observed. It was concluded that daily suppressive acyclovir therapy was effective and well tolerated. The study of long-term oral acyclovir suppression is now in the 11th year, and the medication appears to be remarkably safe. The current recommendation of the U.S. Food and Drug Administration suggests the use of oral acyclovir for 1 year in patients with six or more recurrences per year. The long term chronic suppression with oral acyclovir decreases the frequency of asymptomatic HSV shedding also.[52]

Although it has not been studied for a prolonged period, oral valacyclovir is effective in suppressing recurrences of genital herpes outbreaks. Valacyclovir (Valtrex) contains a valine ester and is much better absorbed than is acyclovir from the human gastrointestinal tract: The valine ester is cleaved off by enzymes in the gastrointestinal lining, resulting in high blood levels of acyclovir. For valacyclovir, one 500-mg tablet per day is adequate to suppress recurrences of genital herpes.

Treatment of Recurrent Genital Herpes

The treatment of recurrent genital herpes with acyclovir in any form has been of only limited success. Topical acyclovir treatment did not facilitate healing in women with recurrent disease, but slight beneficial effects were observed in pain reduction and healing in men. Shortened time of virus shedding was observed with topical acyclovir therapy. Due to the slight clinical benefit of acyclovir therapy in recurrent genital herpes, topical treatment of recurrent genital herpes is not justified. In a large multicenter controlled trial, oral acyclovir treatment of recurrent genital herpes was evaluated by comparing patient-initiated therapy with therapy initiated by a physician or placebo.[53] Oral acyclovir capsules (200 mg) were taken five times daily for 5 days. When patients had acyclovir at home and initiated therapy at the onset of a prodrome or at the first sign of lesions, therapy was more effective than when it was initiated by a physician within 48 h of the onset of symptoms. The patient-initiated treatment reduced viral shedding from 3.9 days, in placebo-treated cases, to 2.1 days. Time to healing was reduced from 6.5 days, in placebo-treated cases, to 5.5 days with patient-initiated treatment. New lesions formed in 22 percent of patients on placebo treatment; this incidence was reduced to 7 percent with the patient-initiated treatment. When patients went to a physician and initiated therapy within 48 h of the onset of lesions, new lesion formation was reduced from 22 to 16 percent. The treatment of recurrent episodes with oral acyclovir offers marginal clinical benefit, but the benefit is superior to that obtained with topical acyclovir. Patients with severe recurrent episodes who initiate therapy at the first sign of a recurrence will derive the greatest benefit. Treatment with acyclovir has no effect on the subsequent recurrence rate.

As mentioned above, the use of episodic famciclovir early in recurrent episodes of genital herpes has been successful in reducing the onset and duration of viral shedding, lesion persistence, and symptoms of genital herpes.[48] Famiciclovir was compared with placebo and the authors suggested that this twice-a-day episodic treatment offers an alternative to continuous antiviral suppression.

Treatment of Herpes Infections in the Immunocompromised Patient

In immunocompromised patients with severe herpes simplex infections, the need for effective antiviral therapy is greatest. In these immunocompromised patients acyclovir therapy for mucocutaneous herpes simplex infection can be lifesaving or dramatically successful. Healing of mucocutaneous herpes simplex infection occurs more quickly in those treated with acyclovir because inhibition of HSV replication reduces tissue destruction. In a randomized double-blind trial of intravenous acyclovir for culture-proved herpes simplex infection that followed bone marrow transplantation, 13 of 17 patients who received acyclovir (750 mg/mm^2 per day) for 7 days had a therapeutic response.[54] Only 2 of 17 placebo-treated patients improved. Intravenous acyclovir produced a shorter duration of positive cultures, shortened duration of pain, and hastened healing. These controlled trials have been performed in heart transplant patients and in other immunosuppressed patients. The accumulated data on intravenous acyclovir in immunocompromised patients with mucocutaneous herpes simplex infection indicate that acyclovir shortens the period of viral shedding, shortens the time interval to scabbing and healing, and shortens the duration of pain. On termination of acyclovir, reactivation of herpes simplex infection usually occurs. Intravenous and oral acyclovir are useful in preventing mucocutaneous herpes simplex infection in immunocompromised patients. A double-blind placebo-controlled trial of intravenous acyclovir in bone marrow transplant recipients indicated that herpes infection did not develop in 10 patients who were seropositive for antiherpes antibody and who received acyclovir in a dose of 250 mg per square meter every 8 h for 18 days starting at 3 days before transplantation.[55] Virus-positive lesions developed in 7 of 10 patients who received placebo treatment. When acyclovir treatment was discontinued, however, herpes infection did develop. Oral acyclovir treatment has been found to be effective in preventing reactivation of HSV infections following bone marrow transplantation and in other immunosuppressed patients. Topical acyclovir therapy, however, has not been effective in suppressing recurrence in normal or immunosuppressed patients. In immunocompromised patients, oral acyclovir is more effective than topical acyclovir in treatment of mucocutaneous herpes infections, but severe or life-threatening infections caused by HSV should be treated with intravenous acyclovir. A comparison of the effects of vidarabine and acyclovir in the treatment of a severe mucocutaneous infection caused by HSV in the immunocompromised patient indicates that vidarabine was not very successful. Acyclovir is also much more soluble than vidarabine, and less fluid volume is required for treatment. Vidarabine is also more inhibitory for proliferating granulocytes and bone marrow cells than is acyclovir. At doses of 30 mg/kg per day, adenine-arabinoside therapy will produce a megaloblastic anemia in patients. From the standpoint of efficacy and safety, acyclovir is the preferred therapy for mucocutaneous herpes simplex infections in immunocompromised patients.

Valacyclovir has also been studied as a treatment for herpes infection in immunocompromised patients; but it has not been approved for this indication in the United States. Approval has been under review because of an excessive number of deaths in patients with AIDS who received 8 g per day of valacyclovir as compared with acyclovir treatment. Penciclovir and famciclovir may also be effective in immunocompromised patients, but these drugs have not been adequately studied in this population.

Treatment of Herpes Simplex Encephalitis

Herpes simplex virus is the most common cause of sporadic non-epidemic encephalitis. The disease commonly involves the temporoparietal lobes in a hemorrhagic necrosis, and without treatment has a mortality of greater than 70 percent. In a double-blind, placebo-controlled trial in 1977, treatment of biopsy-proved herpes encephalitis with adenine-arabinoside reduced the mortality from 70 percent in the placebo group to 44 percent survival at 6 months after treatment.[56] In a follow-up study, the mortality was reduced to 39 percent, and one-third of patients who survived had a return to normal function. The level of consciousness and age had the greatest impact on outcome. Patients under 30 years of age, and only lethargic at the beginning of therapy, had the highest recovery. Relapses after vidarabine treatment have occurred.[57]

A comparison of acyclovir at 30 mg/kg per day and vidarabine (15 mg/kg per day) for 10 days as treatment for biopsy-proved herpes encephalitis was carried out by the NIAID (National Institute of Allergy and Infectious Disease) collaborative antiviral study group of the National Institutes of Health, and acyclovir was clearly superior. The mortality of the acyclovir-treated group was 28 percent as compared with 54 percent for vidarabine-treated patients. At 6 months after treatment, 38 percent of acyclovir-treated patients were functioning normally and only 14 percent of vidarabine-treated patients were normal.[58] This study concluded that acyclovir is the preferred treatment for biopsy-proved herpes encephalitis. In another study of 53 patients in whom there was not uniformity of diagnosis for herpes simplex encephalitis, adenine-arabinosine therapy was associated with a mortality of 50 percent and acyclovir mortality at 6 months was 19 percent.[59]

Over two-thirds of the acyclovir survivors returned to normal function. Relapses after acyclovir therapy have also been documented.[60] Both of these studies had remarkably similar outcomes in favor of acyclovir as the preferred treatment for herpes encephalitis.

Treatment of Acyclovir-Resistant Herpes Simplex Infection

The incidence of acyclovir-resistant mucocutaneous HSV infection in immunocompromised patients, especially in AIDS patients, is being increasingly recognized. In the setting of HIV disease or severe immunosuppression, HSV is able to replicate to a high titer. The high replication role in the presence of a highly selective antiviral drug such as acyclovir permits the selection of drug-resistant mutants.[61] Acyclovir is activated by the viral TK enzyme to produce acyclovir triphosphate, a potent inhibitor of the viral DNA polymerase, and acyclovir is the prototype of effective antiviral agents employing the viral TK for activation. In patients with AIDS in whom large mucocutaneous erosions develop due to acyclovir-resistant HSV, the mechanism of resistance is due to TK-deficient mutants of HSV. The mutant strains of HSV do not effectively phosphorylate acyclovir, and there is no inhibition of HSV replication. In bone marrow transplant recipients or patients with leukemia receiving antiviral therapy, the majority of acyclovir-resistant mutants are also due to TK-deficient mutants. In this setting, however, resistance due to an altered viral DNA polymerase or an altered TK enzyme that does not phosphorylate acyclovir has also been reported.[62] In a series of 12 patients with AIDS in whom acyclovir-resistant HSV infection and large mucocutaneous lesions developed in spite of oral and intravenous acyclovir, all the lesions were due to TK-deficient virus.[63] Over half of the TK-deficient mutants were able to establish a latent ganglion infection, and one of the viral isolates produced cerebral infection and death in a murine model following intranasal inoculation.

An effective alternative therapy for acyclovir-resistant HSV has been developed. Foscarnet, or phosphonoformic acid, inhibits viral DNA polymerase activity directly and is an effective agent against TK-deficient HSV. In a controlled clinical trial of foscarnet compared with adenine-arabinoside in patients with AIDS who had acyclovir-resistant mucocutaneous HSV infection, foscarnet was associated with rapid healing and clearing of virus from infected skin lesions.[64] This trial clearly established that mucocutaneous infections with acyclovir-resistant HSV were clinically significant and could be effectively treated with alternative therapy.

Foscarnet is administered intravenously at a dose of 40 mg/kg twice a day for 14 days in patients with previous acyclovir-resistant HSV infection or large mucocutaneous lesions that fail to heal with 10 days of acyclovir. The main side effects of foscarnet are renal failure, hypocalcemia, and seizures. Renal function needs to be carefully monitored in these patients to avoid serious nephrotoxicity. Foscarnet is also effective against ganciclovir-resistant CMV and the drug will also inhibit HIV-1.

Cidofovir gel (forvade) has been effective for topical treatment of acyclovir-resistant herpes mucocutaneous infection in patients with AIDS.[42] When given systemically, intravenous cidofovir must be administered with probenicid and intravenous saline to avoid the possibility of nephrotoxicity. The drug is contraindicated in patients taking other nephrotoxic agents.

Clinical Significance of Acyclovir-Resistant Herpes Simplex Virus

The continuing emergence of HSV infection that exhibits resistance to acyclovir in immunocompromised patients is a clinically significant problem.[65] The lesions caused by these drug-resistant viruses can progress and involve a large area of skin and mucosa. The clearest evidence that these infections are clinically significant was obtained from a randomized clinical trial when acyclovir-resistant HSV infections were treated with either foscarnet or vidarabine.[64] The foscarnet-treated patients showed a dramatic healing in spite of failure of their lesions to resolve after several months of oral and intravenous acyclovir treatment. This intervention study clearly showed that acyclovir-resistant HSV caused clinically important mucocutaneous lesions that healed within 2 weeks of receiving therapy with an antiviral drug that worked by an alternative mechanism on the viral DNA polymerase. In a pediatric tertiary-care hospital, it was estimated that about 10 percent of herpes simplex viral isolates obtained during 1 year showed resistance to acyclovir, and all of these isolates were from clinically important infections.[66] In patients with AIDS, all of the acyclovir-resistant HSV mutants have been TK-deficient mutants. In bone marrow transplant recipients and in patients with leukemia, acyclovir-resistant mutant viruses have been obtained that possess an altered TK or an altered viral DNA polymerase that is not inhibited by acyclovir triphosphate. Significant clinical disease has been attributed to acyclovir-resistant TK-deficient mutants, including fatal HSV-2 meningitis, progressive HSV-1 pneumonia, and progressive HSV-1 disease in newborn infants.[65] Transmission of acyclovir-resistant HSV has not been

documented. With increasing use of antiviral therapy in immunocompromised patients, it is likely that increasing numbers of cases of clinically important acyclovir-resistant infection will be observed.

In patients with a normal immune system, outbreaks of herpes simplex due to acyclovir-resistant virus are very rare. One well-documented report described repeated episodes of recurrent genital herpes due to a strain of herpes simplex virus that exhibited an altered TK enzyme.[67] The first report of chronic vulvar ulceration in an immunocompetent woman due to acyclovir-resistant TK-deficient HSV-2 has also been published.[68] With more widespread use of acyclovir and famciclovir, increasing reports of disease due to acyclovir-resistant HSV may become common.

REFERENCES

1. Gibson JJ et al: A cross-sectional study of herpes simplex virus types 1 and 2 in college students: Occurrence and determinants of infection. *J Infect Dis* **162**:306, 1990
2. Nahmias AJ et al: Sero-epidemiological and sociological patterns of herpes simplex virus infection in the world. *Scand J Infect Dis* **69**(suppl):19, 1990
3. Becker TM et al: Genital herpes infections in private practice in the United States 1966 to 1981. *JAMA* **253**:1601, 1985
4. Johnson RE et al: A seroepidemiologic study of the prevalence of herpes simplex virus type 2 infection in the United States. *N Engl J Med* **321**:7, 1989
5. Koutsky LA et al: Underdiagnosis of genital herpes by current clinical and viral-isolation procedures. *N Engl J Med* **326**:1533, 1992
6. Wald A et al: Virologic characteristics of subclinical and asymptomatic genital herpes infections. *N Engl J Med* **333**:770, 1995
7. Mertz GJ et al: Risk factors for the sexual transmission of genital herpes. *Ann Intern Med* **116**:197, 1992
8. Glezen WP et al: Acute respiratory disease of university students with special reference to the etiologic role of *Herpes-virus hominis*. *Am J Epidemiol* **101**:111, 1975
9. Embil JA et al: Prevalence of recurrent herpes labialis and aphthous ulcers among young adults on six continents. *Can Med Assoc J* **113**:627, 1975
10. Young SK et al: A clinical study for the control of facial mucocutaneous herpes virus infections. I. Characterization of natural history in a professional school population. *Oral Surg* **41**:498, 1976
11. Bader C et al: The natural history of recurrent facial-oral infection with herpes simplex virus. *J Infect Dis* **138**:897, 1978
12. Corey L et al: Genital herpes simplex virus infections: Clinical manifestations, course and complications. *Ann Intern Med* **98**:958, 1983
13. Jeansson SS, Molin L: On the occurrence of genital herpes simplex virus infection: Clinical and virological findings and relation to gonorrhea. *Acta Derm Venereol (Stockh)* **54**:79, 1974
14. Kreiss JK et al: AIDS virus infection in Nairobi prostitutes. *N Engl J Med* **314**:414, 1986
15. Simonsen JN et al: Human immunodeficiency virus infection among men with sexually transmitted diseases. *N Engl J Med* **319**:274, 1988
16. Quinn TC et al: Human immunodeficiency virus infection among patients attending clinics for sexually transmitted diseases. *N Engl J Med* **318**:197, 1988
17. Holmberg SD et al: Prior herpes simplex virus type 2 infection as a risk factor for HIV infection. *JAMA* **259**:1048, 1988
18. Stamm WE et al: The association between genital ulcer disease and acquisition of HIV infection in homosexual men. *JAMA* **260**:1429, 1988
19. Kuiken CL et al: Risk factors and changes in sexual behavior in male homosexuals who seroconverted for human immunodeficiency virus antibodies. *Am J Epidemiol* **132**:523, 1990
20. Kreiss JK et al: Isolation of human immunodeficiency virus from genital ulcers in Nairobi prostitutes. *J Infect Dis* **160**:380, 1989
21. Ramsey PG et al: Herpes simplex virus pneumonia: Clinical, virologic and pathologic features in 20 patients. *Ann Intern Med* **97**:813, 1982
22. Centers for Disease Control and Prevention: 1993 Revised clarification system for HIV infection and expanded surveillance case definition for AIDS among adolescents and adults. *MMWR* **41**:15, 1992

23. Glogan R et al: Herpetic whitlow as part of genital virus infection. *J Infect Dis* **136**:689, 1977

24. Laskin OL et al: Acyclovir and suppression of frequently recurring herpetic whitlow. *Ann Intern Med* **102**:494, 1985

25. Gill MJ et al: Therapy for recurrent herpetic whitlow. *Ann Intern Med* **105**:631, 1986

26. Norris SA et al: Severe, progressive herpetic whitlow caused by an acyclovir-resistant virus in a patient with AIDS. *J Infect Dis* **157**:209, 1988

27. Selling B et al: An outbreak of herpes simplex among wrestlers (herpes gladiatorum). *N Engl J Med* **270**:979, 1964

28. White WB et al: Transmission of herpes simplex virus type 1 infection in rugby players. *JAMA* **252**:533, 1984

29. Beuler TM et al: Grappling with herpes: Herpes gladiatorum. *Am J Sports Med* **16**:665, 1988

30. Belongia EA et al: An outbreak of herpes gladiatorum at a high school wrestling camp. *N Engl J Med* **325**:906, 1991

31. Molin L: Oral acyclovir prevents herpes simplex associated erythema multiforme. *Br J Dermatol* **116**:109, 1987

32. Lemak MA et al: Oral acyclovir for the prevention of herpes associated erythema multiforme. *J Am Acad Dermatol* **15**:50, 1986

33. Leigh IM: Management of non-genital herpes simplex virus infections in immunocompetent patients. *Am J Med* **85**(suppl 2A):34, 1988

34. Nahmias AJ et al: Herpes simplex virus encephalitis: Laboratory evaluations and their diagnostic significance. *J Infect Dis* **145**:829, 1982

35. Aurelius E et al: Rapid diagnosis of herpes simplex encephalitis by nested polymerase chain reaction assay of cerebrospinal fluid. *Lancet* **337**:189, 1991

36. Herpes simplex encephalitis, editorial. *Lancet* **1**:535, 1986

37. Whitley RJ et al: Diseases that mimic herpes simplex encephalitis. *JAMA* **262**:234, 1989

38. Goldstein LC et al: Monoclonal antibodies to herpes simplex viruses: Use in antigenic typing and rapid diagnosis. *J Infect Dis* **147**:829, 1983

39. Elion GB et al: Selectivity of action of an antiherpes agent (9-(2-hydroxyethoxymethyl)-guanine. *Proc Natl Acad Sci USA* **74**:5716, 1978

40. Furman PA et al: Acyclovir triphosphate is a suicide inactivator of herpes simplex virus DNA polymerase. *J Biol Chem* **259**:9575, 1984

41. Vere Hodge RA: Famciclovir and penciclovir: The mode of action of famciclovir including its conversion to penciclovir. *Antiviral Chem Chemother* **4**:67, 1993

42. Lalezari J et al: A randomized double-blind placebo-controlled trial of cidovovir gel in the treatment of acyclovir-unresponsive mucocutaneous herpes simplex virus infection in patients with AIDS. *J Infect Dis* **176**:892, 1997

43. Spruance SL et al: Treatment of herpes simplex labialis with topical acyclovir in polyethylene glycol. *J Infect Dis* **146**:85, 1982

44. Fiddian AP et al: Successful treatment of facial-oral herpes with topical acyclovir. *BMJ* **286**:1699, 1983

45. Spruance L et al: Penciclovir cream for the treatment of herpes simplex labialis: A randomized, multicenter, double-blind, placebo-controlled trial. *JAMA* **277**:1374, 1997

46. Corey L et al: A trial of topical acyclovir genital herpes simplex virus infections. *N Engl J Med* **306**:1313, 1982

47. Bryson Y et al: Treatment of first episode of genital herpes simplex infection with oral acyclovir: A randomized double-blind controlled trial in normal subjects. *N Engl J Med* **308**:916, 1982

48. Sacks SL et al: Patient-initiated, twice daily oral famciclovir for early recurrent genital herpes. *JAMA* **276**:44, 1996

49. Douglas JM et al: A double-blind study of oral acyclovir for suppression of recurrences of genital herpes simplex virus infection. *N Engl J Med* **310**:1551, 1984

50. Straus SE et al: Suppression of frequently recurring genital herpes. *N Engl J Med* **310**:1545, 1984

51. Kaplowitz LG et al: Prolonged continuous acyclovir treatment of normal adults with frequently recurring genital herpes infection. *JAMA* **265**:747, 1991

52. Wald A et al: Frequent genital simplex virus 2 shedding in immunocompetent women—effect of acyclovir treatment. *J Clin Invest* **99**:1092, 1997

53. Reichman RC et al: Treatment of recurrent genital herpes simplex infections with oral acyclovir. *JAMA* **251**:2103, 1984

54. Wade JC et al: Intravenous acyclovir to treat mucocutaneous herpes simplex infection after marrow transplantation: A double blind trial. *Ann Intern Med* **96**:265, 1982

55. Saral R et al: Acyclovir prophylaxis of herpes-simplex virus infections: A randomized double-blind controlled trial in bone marrow transplant recipients. *N Engl J Med* **305**:63, 1981

56. Whitley RJ et al: Adenine arabinoside therapy of biopsy proved herpes simplex encephalitis. *N Engl J Med* **297**:289, 1977

57. Dix RD et al: Recurrent herpes simplex encephalitis: Recovery of virus after Ara-A treatment. *Ann Neurol* **13**:196, 1983

58. Whitley RJ et al: Vidarabine vs. acyclovir therapy in herpes simplex encephalitis. *N Engl J Med* **314**:144, 1986

59. Skoldenberg B et al: Acyclovir versus vidarabine in herpes simplex encephalitis: Randomized multicenter study in consecutive Swedish patients. *Lancet* **8405**:707, 1984

60. VanLandingham KE et al: Relapse of herpes simplex encephalitis after conventional acyclovir therapy. *JAMA* **259**:1051, 1988

61. Schnipper LE, Crumpacker CS: Resistance of herpes simplex virus to acycloguanosine: Role of viral thymidine kinase and DNA polymerase loci. *Proc Natl Acad Sci USA* **77**:2270, 1980

62. Darby G et al: Altered substrate specificity of herpes simplex virus: Thymidine kinase confers acyclovir resistance. *Nature* **289**:81, 1981

63. Erlich KS et al: Acyclovir-resistant herpes simplex virus infections in patients with the acquired immunodeficiency syndrome. *N Engl J Med* **320**:293, 1989

64. Safrin S et al: A controlled trial comparing foscarnet with vidarabine for acyclovir-resistant mucocutaneous herpes simplex in the acquired immunodeficiency syndrome. *N Engl J Med* **325**:551, 1991

65. Chatis PA, Crumpacker CS: Resistance of herpesviruses to antiviral drugs. *Antimicrob Agents Chemother* **36**:1589, 1992

66. Englund JA et al: Herpes simplex virus resistant to acyclovir: A study in a tertiary care center. *Ann Intern Med* **112**:416, 1990

67. Kost RG et al: Recurrent acyclovir resistant genital herpes in an immunocompetent patient. *N Engl J Med* **329**:1777, 1993

68. Sweeter S et al: Chronic vulvar ulceration in an immunocompetent woman due to acyclovir-resistant, thymidine kinase–deficient herpes simplex virus. *J Infect Dis* **177**:543, 1998

CHAPTER 216

Stephen E. Straus
Michael N. Oxman

Varicella and Herpes Zoster

Varicella (chickenpox) and herpes zoster (shingles, zoster) are distinct clinical entities caused by a single member of the herpesvirus family, the varicella-zoster virus (VZV). The particular clinical manifestations of these two diseases are due to differences in the host and in the circumstances of infection, not to differences in their etiologic agent.[1,2]

Varicella, an acute, highly contagious exanthem that occurs most often in childhood, is the result of primary infection of a susceptible individual. It is characterized by a short or absent prodromal period and a generalized pruritic rash consisting of successive crops of lesions that progress rapidly from macules and papules to vesicles, pustules, and crusts. In normal children, systemic symptoms are usually mild and serious complications are extremely rare. In adults and in immunologically compromised persons of any age, varicella is more likely to be associated with an extensive eruption, high fever, severe constitutional symptoms, pneumonia, and other life-threatening complications. With the current prevalence of immune deficiency states including human immunodeficiency virus (HIV) infection, we now recognize that varicella can exhibit a spectrum of complications and presentations.[3]

Herpes zoster is a localized disease characterized by unilateral radicular pain and a vesicular eruption that is generally limited to the dermatome innervated by a single spinal or cranial sensory ganglion. It occurs most often in elderly people. In contrast to varicella, which follows primary exogenous VZV infection, herpes zoster is the result of reactivation of endogenous virus that had persisted in latent form within sensory ganglia following an earlier attack of varicella. As with varicella, the incidence of complicated and atypical herpes zoster has been increasing with the increasing prevalence of HIV infection and other immune-impairing conditions.[3-5]

EPIDEMIOLOGY

Epidemiology of Varicella

Varicella is worldwide in distribution, with no evidence of differing racial or sexual susceptibility. Humans are the only known reservoir, and vectors play no role in transmission. In metropolitan communities in temperate climates, varicella is endemic, with a regularly recurring seasonal prevalence in winter and spring; periodic epidemics depend upon the accumulation of susceptible persons. In Europe and North America, varicella is primarily a disease of childhood; 90 percent of cases occur in children less than 10 years of age and fewer than 5 percent in individuals over the age of 15.[6] In tropical and semitropical countries, infection is delayed and varicella is seen more often in adults. In a serologic survey of parturient women in New York City, only 4.5 percent of those born in the

United States lacked antibody to VZV, whereas 16 percent of those from Latin America were seronegative.[7] The proportion of susceptible adults is even higher in Asia, Africa, and the Middle East. This is an important consideration in delivering health care to immigrant populations and in controlling nosocomial varicella in hospitals with patients and staff from these areas.

Military recruits from Puerto Rico and the Philippines, up to 40 percent of whom are VZV-seronegative, appear to account in part for a recent increase in hospital admissions for varicella at U.S. military facilities.[8] This may also reflect increasing varicella susceptibility in U.S. teenagers and young adults. Delayed acquisition of primary VZV infection may have serious consequences, because the mortality of varicella in adults is 25 times greater than it is in children.[9]

Varicella is highly contagious. Attack rates of 87 percent among susceptible siblings in households and nearly 70 percent among susceptible patients on hospital wards have been reported.[10] Most cases of varicella (i.e., $\geq$ 95 percent) are clinically apparent, although occasionally the exanthem may be so sparse and transient as to pass unnoticed. A typical patient is infectious for 1 to 2 days (rarely, 3 to 4 days) before the exanthem appears and for 4 or 5 days thereafter, i.e., until the last crop of vesicles has crusted. The immunocompromised patient, who may experience many successive crops of lesions for a week or more, is infectious for a longer period of time. The mean incubation period of varicella is 14 or 15 days, with a range of 10 to 23 days. It is often relatively prolonged in patients who develop varicella after passive immunization with varicella-zoster immune globulin (VZIG) or plasma (ZIP) or active immunization with the Oka strain varicella vaccine.[10-12]

The major route by which varicella is acquired and transmitted is thought to be the respiratory tract. Airborne droplets constitute an important mechanism of transmission, but infection may also be spread by direct contact.[13] Varicella crusts are not infectious, and the duration of infectivity of droplets containing virus is probably quite limited. The mechanism by which VZV is shed is unclear. Viremia occurs during the prodromal stage.[14] Although the infectiousness of patients with varicella is thought to depend largely upon virus shed from the mucous membranes of the upper respiratory tract, VZV has only rarely been cultured from pharyngeal secretions; however, it can be detected in the oropharynx of the majority of patients using polymerase chain reaction (PCR)-based assays.[15]

One attack of varicella generally confers lasting immunity to the disease. Reexposure to the virus boosts humoral and cell-mediated immune responses but rarely leads to clinical illness.[16] Most reported second attacks of varicella involve incorrect diagnoses; others may represent cutaneous dissemination in patients with herpes zoster (see below). With the advent of potent immunosuppressive agents, recurrent exogenous VZV primary infections have been observed, and severely immunocompromised patients with HIV infection may also become susceptible to recurrent varicella. In addition, persons who develop modified varicella (e.g., because they are infected early in infancy in the presence of maternal antibody or have been immunized with live attenuated varicella vaccine) may respond to exogenous exposure by developing a second, usually mild episode of "breakthrough" varicella.[17,18]

Epidemiology of Herpes Zoster

Herpes zoster occurs sporadically throughout the year without seasonal prevalence. It affects both sexes and all races equally. As expected with a disease that reflects the reactivation of latent endogenous infection, the occurrence of herpes zoster is independent of the prevalence of varicella, and there is no convincing evidence that herpes zoster can be acquired by contact with other persons with varicella or zoster. Rather, the incidence of herpes zoster is determined by factors that influence the host-virus relationship. One of these is age. The rate of occurrence of zoster is in the range of 1.3 to 5 per 1000 persons per year; although it may be seen in any age group, including children, more than two-thirds of reported cases occur in individuals over 50 years of age and less than 10 percent of cases occur in those under the age of 20 years.[19] Hope-Simpson showed that the annual incidence per thousand rises from 0.74 in children under 10 years of age to a plateau of approximately 2.5 between ages 20 and 50; thereafter, it increases to reach a level of over 10 in octogenarians (Fig. 216-1A).[20] A more recent population-based study in New England involving approximately 500,000 person-years of observation from 1990 to 1996 yielded similar data.[6]

The incidence of herpes zoster among those who have already had an attack appears to be at least as high as that of first attacks in individuals of comparable age. Hope-Simpson estimated that if a cohort of 1000 people were to live to be 85 years old, half would have had an attack of herpes zoster and 10 (1 percent) would have had two attacks.[20] Second attacks make up 4 to 5 percent of reported series, and third attacks are not unheard of. However, patients suffering multiple episodes of zoster-like disease, especially

involving the same anatomic location, are far more likely to be suffering from recurrent zosteriform herpes simplex virus infections.[21] The incidence of herpes zoster in immunosuppressed patients is increased 20 to 100 times, and the severity and likelihood of recurrence of the disease is also increased.

Herpes zoster is rare during the first few years of age. When it occurs in infants, there is usually no history of postnatal varicella, but there is almost always a history of maternal varicella during gestation. Presumably, primary VZV infection and the establishment of ganglionic latency occurred in utero.

Patients with herpes zoster are contagious, but less so than patients with varicella. The rate at which susceptible household contacts develop varicella after exposure to herpes zoster appears to be one-third that of cases following exposure to varicella.[20] Virus can be isolated from vesicles of uncomplicated herpes zoster for up to 7 days after the appearance of the rash and for much longer periods in some immunocompromised individuals. Patients with uncomplicated dermatomal zoster appear to spread the infection by means of direct contact with their lesions. Patients with disseminated herpes zoster may, in addition, transmit the infection in aerosols, so that respiratory isolation is required for such patients.

The increased incidence of herpes zoster in immunocompromised patients with cancer previously led to the incorrect assumption that the occurrence of herpes zoster in an otherwise normal individual might be an indication of an occult malignancy.[22] Nevertheless, herpes zoster is frequently an early manifestation of HIV infection, and thus high-risk individuals who develop herpes zoster should be evaluated for coincident HIV infection.[3–5]

ETIOLOGY

VZV is a member of the herpesvirus family.[1,2] Other members pathogenic for humans include herpes simplex viruses type 1 (HSV-1) and type 2 (HSV-2); cytomegalovirus (CMV); the Epstein-Barr virus (EBV), the cause of infectious mononucleosis; human herpesvirus-6 (HHV-6), the cause of roseola infantum; the related human herpesvirus-7 (HHV-7), which also causes roseola; and the recently described Kaposi's sarcoma–associated herpesvirus, also

FIGURE 216-1

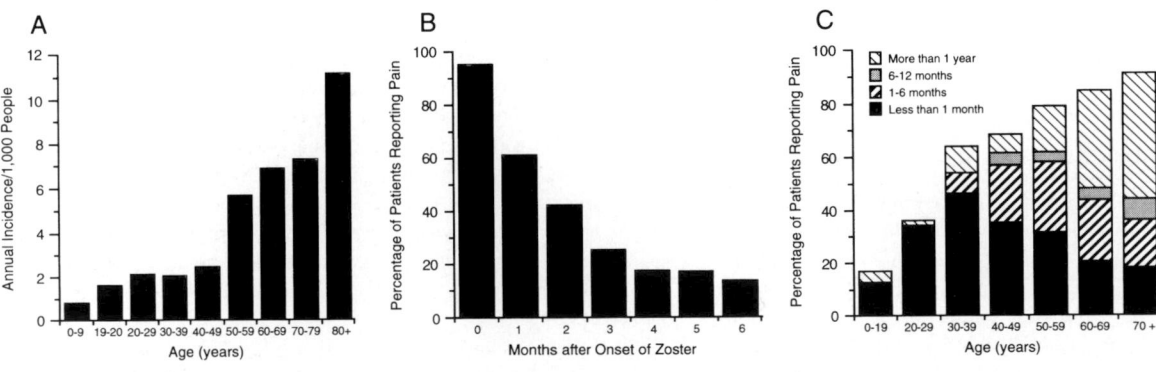

A. The epidemiology of herpes zoster and postherpetic neuralgia. The annual incidence of herpes zoster per 1000 persons in a general medical practice. B. The percentage of patients with pain persisting after the onset of the herpes zoster rash. These data are from the placebo recip-

ients in one large, double-blind treatment study. C. The proportion of patients with postherpetic neuralgia according to age. (*From Kost and Straus,*[50] *with permission.*)

called human herpesvirus type 8.[23] All these herpesviruses are morphologically indistinguishable and share a number of properties, including a propensity for establishing latent infections that persist for life.

VZV consists of an icosahedral capsid 100 nm in diameter that encloses the viral genome, a single molecule of DNA. The genome and capsid (the nucleocapsid) are surrounded by additional layers of protein, termed the *tegument,* and, on the outside, by a loose lipoprotein envelope derived from the nuclear membrane of the host cell (Fig. 216-2).[24] The viral envelope is studded with virally encoded glycoproteins. The complete virion is roughly spherical, with a diameter of 150 to 200 nm. Only enveloped virions are infectious, and this accounts for the lability of VZV; infectivity is rapidly destroyed by organic solvents, detergents, proteolytic enzymes, heat, and extremes of pH. More than 50 virus-specific proteins, including 6 glycoproteins, have been identified in purified virions and in VZV-infected cells. Several of these proteins, especially the glycoproteins, are targets of antibody and cellular immune responses. In addition to structural components of the virion, certain enzymes essential for virus replication, including a virus-specific DNA polymerase and a virus-specific deoxypyrimidine (thymidine) kinase, are synthesized in infected cells. Because these viral enzymes differ in substrate specificity from the corresponding host cell enzymes, they are important targets for specific antiviral chemotherapy.

FIGURE 216-2

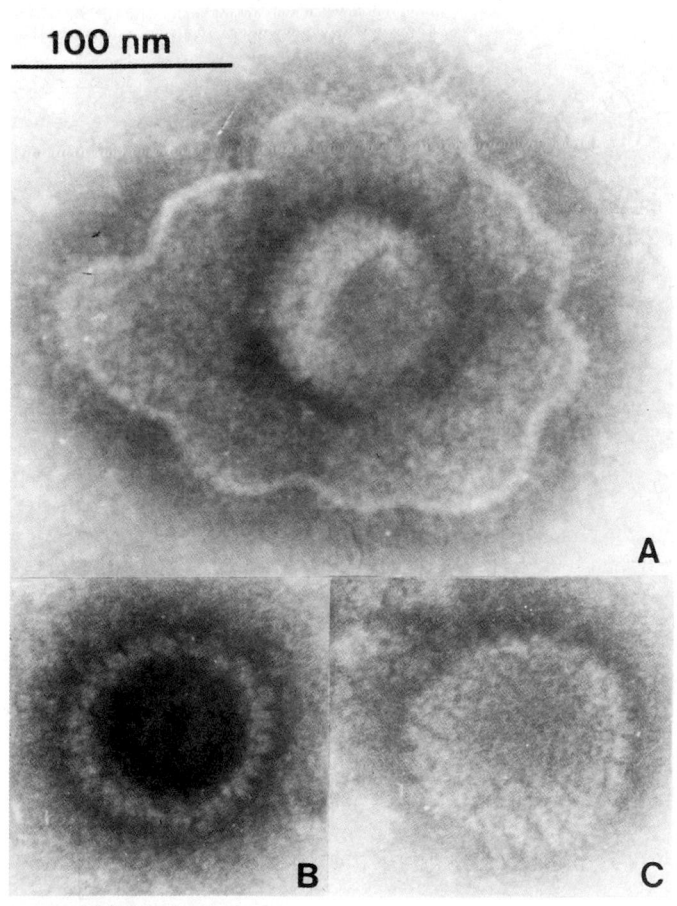

100 nm

A

B   C

Electron micrographs of varicella-zoster virus. *A.* The entire enveloped particle. *B.* A section through the viral nucleocapsid. *C.* The icosahedral structure of the nucleocapsid. (*Courtesy of William Ruyechan.*)

The VZV genome consists of a linear molecule of double-stranded DNA, roughly 125,000 base pairs in length. Like the genomes of HSV-1 and HSV-2, it contains covalently linked long (L) and short (S) segments, each of which consists of a unique DNA segment (U_L and U_S) flanked by internal and terminal inverted repeats (IR_L, TR_L, IR_S, TR_S). In the case of HSV-1 and HSV-2, both the L and S segments can invert with respect to one another to yield four isomers, which are found with equal frequency in mature virions. The genome of VZV, which is about 25,000 base pairs shorter than that of HSV-1 or HSV-2, lacks almost all of the IR_L and TR_L sequences and has a shorter U_S segment. While the S segment inverts freely, the vestigial IR_L and TR_L do not facilitate isomerization, and only two genomic isomers predominate in VZV virions.[1] The complete sequence of the VZV genome has been determined; it contains open reading frames (ORFs) corresponding to 69 distinct genes, many of which have DNA sequence and functional homology to HSV genes, and some of which can even complement their HSV homologs.

VZV gene expression, like that of the other herpesviruses, is coordinately regulated and sequentially ordered in a cascade fashion, with three basic classes of genes: *immediate early* (IE) or *alpha, early* or *beta,* and *late* or *gamma.* IE genes are the first to be expressed and generally encode regulatory proteins that downregulate further IE gene expression and induce the expression of *early* genes. Several of the early genes encode enzymes involved in viral DNA synthesis. Early gene expression is followed by viral DNA replication and by the expression of late genes, most of which encode proteins and glycoproteins destined to become structural components of the virion.

While possessing numerous structural and functional similarities, the HSV and VZV genomes manifest important differences in gene representation, expression, and arrangement, differences that probably determine the distinct behavior of each virus (Table 216-1; see also Chap. 215).[25] Examples include the expression by HSV of latency-associated transcripts (LATs), which have no counterpart in the VZV genome, as well as the expression of IE and early genes during latency by VZV but not by HSV.[26,27]

There is only one VZV serotype. A number of antigens are present in the virion and produced in infected cells, but these are identical in viruses isolated from patients with varicella and herpes zoster throughout the world. Some VZV antigens cross-react with antigens of other members of the herpesvirus family, and this limits the usefulness of certain serologic tests.

The DNAs of viruses isolated from cases of varicella and herpes zoster worldwide are basically similar, but minor variations in nucleotide sequence give the genomes of different clinical isolates of VZV slightly different restriction endonuclease cleavage patterns (i.e., each isolate has a unique pattern or "fingerprint"). More substantial differences distinguish the Oka live attenuated VZV vaccine (see below) from wild-type VZV isolates in the western hemisphere. These differences are epidemiologically useful.[28]

Studies of the molecular biology and pathogenesis of VZV infection have been hampered by difficulty in obtaining adequate quantities of cell-free virus and by the absence of suitable animal models. Some progress has been made in preparing cell-free virus, and the application of molecular cloning procedures has facilitated the physical mapping of the VZV genome. VZV has now been propagated in guinea pig cells, and a guinea pig model of VZV infection and transmission has been established. Some form of VZV latency occurs in experimentally infected rats.[29]

TABLE 216-1

Comparison of Varicella-Zoster Virus (VZV) and Herpes Simplex Viruses (HSV)

Virus	VZV	HSV
Genome size	125,000 base pairs	150,000 base pairs
Percent G + C	46%	68%, HSV-1; 69%, HSV-2
Number of serotypes	1	2
Host range	Narrow	Broad
Cytopathic effect (CPE)	Multinucleated giant cells, eosinophilic intranuclear inclusion bodies	Multinucleated giant cells, eosinophilic intranuclear inclusion bodies
Cell-free virus in tissue culture	No (Focal CPE)	Yes
Acyclovir sensitivity	++	++++
Primary infection		
Epidemiology	Epidemic (winter and spring)	Sporadic
Transmission	Respiratory, direct contact	Direct contact
Incubation period	Long (~14 days)	Short (2–7 days)
Viremia essential	Yes	No
Usual disease location	Distant from portal of entry	At portal of entry
Percent symptomatic	>95%	30–50%
Recurrent infection		
Frequency of symptomatic recurrences in lifetime	Usually once	Up to several hundred
Percent seropositives with symptomatic recurrences	10–20%	20–50%
Prodrome	Prolonged, severe pain	Short, mild dysesthesia
Distribution of lesions	Entire dermatome	Focal within dermatome
Destruction of sensory neurons during a recurrence	Yes	Probably not
Postherpetic neuralgia	Common	Very rare
Risk of recurrence	Increases with age	Decreases over time
Site of latency	Satellite cells; sensory neurons	Sensory neurons
Asymptomatic virus shedding	No	Yes
Serologic response to recurrence	>95%	<10%
Reactivation induced by ultraviolet (UV) light	No	Yes

PATHOGENESIS

Pathogenesis of Varicella

Our present concept of the pathogenesis of varicella is based primarily on circumstantial evidence, analogy with experimental models of other exanthems, and postmortem examination of fatal cases. Entry of the virus is probably through the mucosa of the upper respiratory tract and oropharynx. Initial multiplication at this portal of entry results in dissemination of small amounts of virus via the blood and lymphatics (the primary viremia). This virus is cleared by cells of the reticuloendothelial system, which probably constitutes the major site of virus replication during the remainder of the incubation period.

The incubating infection is partially contained by innate host defenses [e.g., interferon, natural killer (NK) cells] and by developing immune responses. In most individuals, virus replication eventually overwhelms these still undeveloped defenses, so that about 2 weeks after infection a much larger (secondary) viremia occurs. This causes fever and malaise and disseminates virus throughout the body, especially to the skin and mucous membranes, where foci of infection are initiated by the infection of capillary endothelial cells.[30] The skin lesions appear in successive crops, reflecting a cyclic viremia, which in the normal host is terminated after about 3 days by VZV-specific humoral and cellular immune responses. Virus in the blood is cell-associated; it appears to circulate in mononuclear leukocytes, primarily lymphocytes.[31] The frequent observations of elevated serum levels of hepatocellular enzymes in the acute stage of uncomplicated varicella[32] suggest the routine, subclinical involvement of many organs; it is merely the ease with which skin involvement in varicella is recognized that makes it so noteworthy.

Host immune responses terminate viremia and limit the progression of varicella lesions in the skin and other organs. Pneumonia and most other complications of varicella reflect a failure of the immune system to halt virus replication and dissemination and to limit the progression of visceral and cutaneous foci of VZV infection.

IgG, IgM, and IgA antibodies to VZV are detectable within 2 to 5 days after the onset of clinical varicella and reach maximum titers during the second or third week.[33] Thereafter, IgG antibodies decline slowly and persist at low levels for life. IgM and IgA antibodies decline more rapidly and are generally undetectable a year after infection. Cell-mediated immunity to VZV also develops during the course of varicella and persists for many years.[34]

Humoral immunity to VZV protects against varicella. People with detectable serum antibody do not usually become ill after exogenous exposure, whereas those devoid of serum antibody to VZV develop varicella.[33] However, in most individuals, serum antibody to VZV is also indicative of the presence of other immune defenses induced by prior VZV infections, and antibody alone may not be sufficient. Passive immunization with antibody to VZV can prevent varicella in susceptible immunocompetent individuals exposed to exogenous VZV, but it generally does not prevent varicella in susceptible immunocompromised patients.[10,35]

Cell-mediated immunity is more important than humoral immunity in recovery from varicella.[34] The disease is not particularly severe in children with agammaglobulinemia; it is patients with congenital, acquired, or iatrogenic defects in cell-mediated immunity who suffer severe and life-threatening varicella.[3–5,18] Cellular immune responses, especially those mediated by T lymphocytes and cytokines, are critical in limiting the extent and duration of VZV infection.[36] Recovery from varicella is associated with the appearance of circulating T cells that respond specifically to VZV envelope glycoproteins and to the major immediate-early (IE) protein encoded by gene 62.[37] A recent report of a 13-year-old child who lacked natural killer (NK) cells and developed severe varicella with pneumonia, as well as severe infections with other herpesviruses,[38] suggests that these cells may also be important in terminating primary VZV infections.

Pathogenesis of Herpes Zoster

The pathogenesis of herpes zoster is not fully understood, but clinical, epidemiologic, and pathologic data as well as analogy to recurrent herpes simplex virus infections support the following model.[20,25] During the course of varicella, VZV passes from lesions in the skin and mucosal surfaces into the contiguous endings of sensory nerves and is transported centripetally up the sensory fibers to the sensory ganglia. In the ganglia, a latent infection is established and the virus then persists silently and harmlessly; it is no longer infectious and does not multiply but retains the capacity to revert to full infectiousness. Although VZV might also reach the sensory ganglia via the bloodstream during the course of the primary or secondary viremia of varicella, only the neural route can easily explain the coincidence of the anatomic pattern of the incidence of herpes zoster in later life with the distribution of the rash in varicella. Herpes zoster occurs most often in dermatomes in which the rash of varicella achieves the highest density—those innervated by the first (ophthalmic) division of the trigeminal nerve and by spinal sensory ganglia from T1 to L2.[39] Presumably, areas of skin with a denser rash during varicella transmit larger amounts of virus to the corresponding sensory ganglia, thereby endowing these ganglia with a higher concentration of latent VZV. If subsequent reactivation occurs at random, herpes zoster would be expected to occur most frequently in dermatomes innervated by ganglia with the highest concentrations of latent VZV. Also compelling in this regard are the cases of herpes zoster arising at the sites of prior varicella immunization.[40]

Latent VZV persists in sensory ganglia, apparently for life. While infectious VZV has not been recovered from sensory ganglia by cocultivation in vitro (as it has with HSV), VZV DNA has been detected in the majority of sensory ganglia obtained at postmortem examination from seropositive adults.[41] There is controversy as to the precise cellular locus of latency—some studies identified viral nucleic acid sequences only in neurons; others only in satellite cells; still others in both.[26,42] In any event, it is clear that few, perhaps only 4, of the virion's 69 genes are expressed during latency.[25,26,42,43] The role of these genes in latency is not known, but by analogy to other herpesviruses it is probable that they act to maintain the latent carriage of the viral genome, to suppress productive viral replication, and to keep the virus poised to reactivate.

Although the latent virus in the ganglia retains its potential for full infectivity, reactivation is sporadic and infrequent. The mechanisms involved in the reactivation of VZV are unclear, but a number of conditions are associated with the occurrence and localization of herpes zoster. These include immunosuppression in HIV infection and in Hodgkin's disease and other malignancies; administration of immunosuppressive drugs and glucocorticoids; irradiation of the spinal column; tumor involvement of the cord, dorsal root ganglion, or adjacent structures; local trauma; surgical manipulation of the spine; heavy metal poisoning or therapy; and frontal sinusitis as a precipitant of ophthalmic zoster. Most important, though, is the senescence of the cellular immune response to VZV with increasing age. Elderly persons exhibit a selective and gradual decline in cell-mediated immune responses to VZV; this is likely to explain the increased incidence and severity of herpes zoster and its complications in older persons.[44]

It is believed that latent VZV may also reactivate without producing overt disease. HSV reactivates frequently without causing recognizable signs or symptoms.[45] Although the asymptomatic shedding of VZV has not been proven (Table 216-1), it is probable that latent VZV behaves in a similar manner, and the minute dose of infectious virus that reappears is immediately neutralized by circulating antibody or destroyed by cellular immune responses before it can infect other cells and multiply enough to cause perceptible damage. The small quantity of viral antigen released into the bloodstream during such contained reactions would be expected to stimulate and sustain host immune responses. A similar boost in the level of host resistance often follows contact with a patient with varicella, reflecting subclinical exogenous reinfection.[16–18]

When host resistance falls below a critical level, reactivated virus can no longer be contained. Virus multiplies and spreads within the ganglion, causing neuronal necrosis and intense inflammation, a process that is often accompanied by severe neuralgia. Infectious VZV then spreads antidromically down the sensory nerve, causing intense neuritis, and is released around the sensory nerve endings in the skin, where it produces the characteristic cluster of zoster vesicles. The occurrence of neuralgia several days before the rash appears and the presence of degenerative changes in cutaneous nerve fibrils on the first day of the eruption provide additional evidence that infection in the sensory ganglion precedes involvement of the skin. Spread of the ganglionic infection proximally along the posterior nerve root to the meninges and cord results in local leptomeningitis, cerebrospinal fluid pleocytosis, and segmental myelitis. Infection of motor neurons in the anterior horn and inflammation of the anterior nerve root account for the local palsies that may accompany the cutaneous eruption, and extension of infection within the central nervous system may result in rare complications of herpes zoster.

During reactivation, limited hematogenous dissemination of virus from the affected ganglion often produces a few scattered vesicles at a distance from the primary dermatome, even in uncomplicated herpes zoster. Together, the local and disseminated infections stimulate an anamnestic immune response that terminates the infectious process. Sometimes this response is sufficiently rapid to neutralize virus released into the skin and thus prevent the development of recognizable cutaneous lesions; the result is an episode of radicular pain without eruption (zoster sine herpete) and a coincident rise in the titer of antibody to VZV.[46] If the anamnestic host response is delayed or deficient, as it appears to be in many immunosuppressed patients, the duration and severity of the infection are increased.[3–5,47,48]

Pathogenesis of Pain in Herpes Zoster and Postherpetic Neuralgia

Pain is a major symptom of herpes zoster. It often precedes and generally accompanies the rash, and it frequently persists after the rash has healed—a complication known as postherpetic neuralgia (PHN). A number of different but overlapping mechanisms appear to be involved in the sensation of pain in general and in the pathogenesis of pain in herpes zoster and PHN (Fig. 216-3).[49,50] The relative contribution of each of these mechanisms is likely to vary from patient to patient and over time in individual patients.

During the prodrome, the replication and spread of reactivated VZV causes intense inflammation and cell necrosis in the sensory

FIGURE 216-3

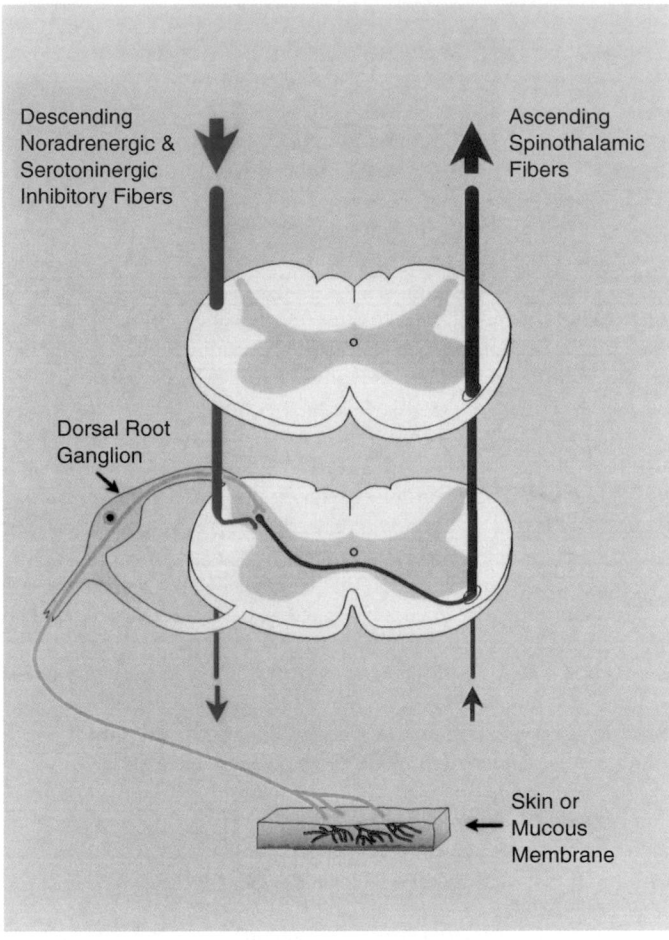

Pathway of normal pain perception. Noxious stimuli activate free nerve endings in the skin to generate signals that are conveyed through unmyelinated C fibers (*red*) and small Aδ fibers to the neuronal bodies in the segmental dorsal root ganglia, then proximally to the dorsal horn of the spinal cord, where they form synapses with second-order neurons. Spinal cord neurons are subject to powerful descending inhibitory signals from the brain (*green*), mediated by the biogenic amines serotonin and norepinephrine. Drugs that potentiate the central effects of biogenic amines, such as tricyclic antidepressant drugs, may act by enhancing these descending pathways. Endogenous opiates also contribute to descending inhibitory input. The net result of peripheral afferent input and descending inhibitory input is projected cephalad, joining other ascending fibers in the contralateral spinothalamic tract (*orange*). Information from the spinothalamic tract is integrated with input from brainstem and cortical areas for the perception of specific aspects of pain as well as more general affective components of pain perception.

ganglion that extends distally to the peripheral nerve and skin and proximally to the dorsal root and spinal cord. Acute injury to the peripheral nerve and to neurons in the ganglion triggers afferent signals perceived as prodromal pain and induces long-lasting changes in the physiology of second-order neurons in the dorsal horn of the spinal cord.

VZV-induced inflammation in the skin itself results in activation and sensitization of peripheral sensory receptors, producing nociceptive signals that further amplify and sustain cutaneous pain. The abundant release of excitatory amino acids and neuropeptides induced by the sustained barrage of afferent inputs during the prodrome and acute phase of herpes zoster may cause excitotoxic injury to and the loss of inhibitory interneurons in the spinal dorsal horn.

Damage to neurons in the spinal cord, the ganglion, and the peripheral nerve has other important consequences. Damaged neurons become spontaneously active and hypersensitive to peripheral stimuli and to sympathetic stimulation. This state persists until the axon is reconnected to the skin, but damage to the nerve sheath may prevent proper healing. The regenerating axons may form neuromas, which also exhibit spontaneous activity and hypersensitivity.

The anatomic and functional changes responsible for PHN appear to be established early in the course of herpes zoster. Consistent with this is the correlation of initial pain severity and the presence of prodromal pain with the subsequent development of PHN, and the failure of antiviral therapy initiated after rash onset to substantially prevent PHN (see below).

CLINICAL MANIFESTATIONS

Clinical Manifestations of Varicella

PRODROME OF VARICELLA In young children, prodromal symptoms are uncommon, and the illness usually begins with the onset of the rash. The rash may be accompanied by a low-grade fever and malaise. In older children and adults, the rash is often preceded by 2 to 3 days of fever, chills, malaise, headache, anorexia, severe backache, and, in some patients, sore throat and dry cough.

RASH OF VARICELLA The rash begins on the face and scalp and spreads rapidly to the trunk, with relative sparing of the extremities (Fig. 216-4). New lesions appear in successive crops, but their distribution remains central. The rash tends to be more profuse in hollows and protected parts of the body than on prominent and exposed parts. Thus it is denser in the small of the back and between the shoulder blades than on the scapulae and buttocks and more profuse on the medial than on the lateral aspects of the limbs. It is not uncommon to have a few lesions on the palms and soles. Vesicles often appear earlier and in larger numbers in areas of inflammation, as in diaper rash, sunburn, or eczema.

The most striking feature of the lesions of varicella is their rapid progression from rose-colored macules to papules, vesicles, pustules, and crusts (Fig. 216-4*A*). The typical vesicle of varicella is superficial and thin-walled, so that it looks like a drop of water lying on rather than in the skin. It is usually 2 to 3 mm in diameter and elliptical, with its long axis parallel to the folds of the skin. The early vesicle is surrounded by an irregular area of erythema, which gives the lesions the appearance of a "dewdrop on a rose petal." The vesicular fluid soon becomes cloudy with the influx of inflammatory cells, which convert the vesicle to a pustule (Fig. 216-4*B*). The lesion then dries, beginning in the center, first producing an umbilicated pustule and then a crust. Crusts fall off spontaneously in 1 to 3 weeks, depending upon the depth of the skin involvement, leaving shallow pink depressions that gradually disappear. Scarring is rare in otherwise uncomplicated varicella unless the lesions were picked at by the patient or superinfected with bacteria. Healing lesions may leave hypopigmented spots that persist for weeks to months.

Vesicles also develop in the mucous membranes of the mouth, occurring most commonly over the palate. Mucosal vesicles rupture

FIGURE 216-4

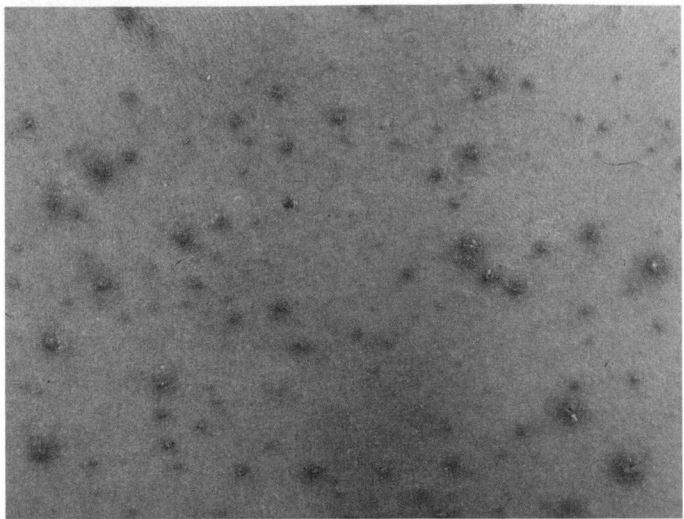

A.

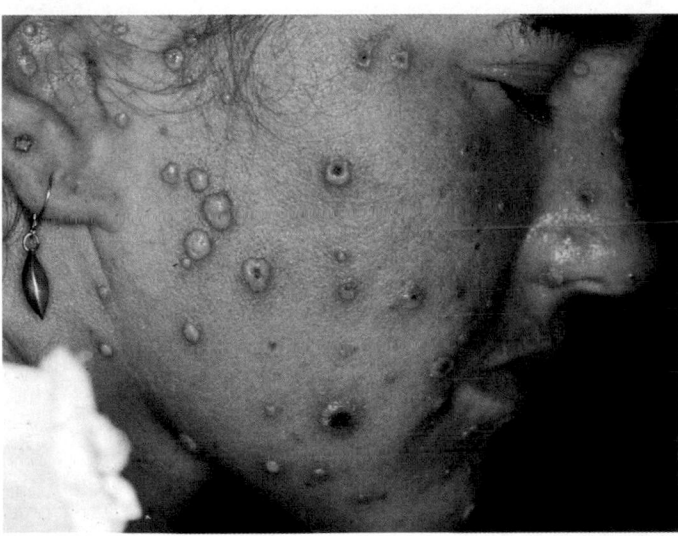

B.

Varicella. *A.* A full spectrum of lesions—i.e., crythematous papules, vesicles ("dewdrops on rose petals"), crusts, and erosions at sites of excoriation—is seen in a child with a typical case of varicella. *B.* A wider range of lesions, including many large pustules, is seen in a 21-year-old female who was febrile as well as "toxic" and had varicella pneumonitis.

so rapidly that the vesicular stage may be missed. Instead, one sees shallow ulcers 2 to 3 mm in diameter. Vesicles may also appear on other mucous membranes, including those of the nose, pharynx, larynx, trachea, gastrointestinal tract, urinary tract, and vagina as well as on the conjunctivae.

A distinctive feature of varicella is the simultaneous presence, in any one area of the skin, of lesions in all stages of development. Careful prospective studies have shown that the average number of lesions in healthy children ranges from 250 to 500; secondary cases resulting from household exposure are more severe than primary cases resulting from exposure at school, presumably because more intense and prolonged exposure at home results in a higher virus inoculum.[9] In general, the mildest cases are seen in younger children. Varicella is more severe in adults and most severe in patients

of any age with impaired cell-mediated immunity (see below). Inapparent infections occur but are rare.

Fever usually persists as long as new lesions continue to appear, and its height is generally proportional to the severity of the rash. In typical cases it rarely exceeds 39°C (102°F); it may be absent in mild cases and rise to 40.5°C (105°F) in severe cases with extensive rash. Prolonged fever or recurrence of fever after defervescence may signify a secondary bacterial infection or another complication. Headache, myalgia, and anorexia generally accompany the fever and are more severe in older children and adults. The most distressing symptom, however, is pruritus, which is usually present throughout the vesicular stage.

COMPLICATIONS OF VARICELLA   In the normal child, varicella is a benign disease rarely attended by secondary complications.[6,9,51] The most common complication is the secondary bacterial infection of skin lesions, usually by staphylococci or streptococci, which may produce impetigo, furuncles, cellulitis, erysipelas, and rarely gangrene.[52] These local infections often lead to scarring and, rarely, to septicemia with metastatic infection of other organs; invasive group A streptococcal infections are particularly virulent. Bullous lesions may be produced when vesicles are superinfected with staphylococci that elaborate exfoliative toxin. Secondary bacterial pneumonia, otitis media, and suppurative meningitis are rare complications that occur mainly in children under 7 years of age and that respond to appropriate antibiotic therapy. Bacterial superinfection is common and life-threatening, however, in leukopenic patients.

Other complications that reflect a basic defect in the capacity of the host to limit VZV dissemination account for the increased morbidity and mortality of varicella in adults, in newborns, in those on high-dose or prolonged glucocorticoids, and in other immunocompromised patients of any age.[3,6,9,51,53]

In adults, fever and constitutional symptoms are more prominent and prolonged, the rash is more profuse, and complications are more frequent.[53] Primary varicella pneumonia is the major complication of adult varicella. It is rarely observed in normal children; adults account for more than 90 percent of reported cases.[54–56]

The incidence of primary varicella pneumonia depends upon the population of patients studied and the diagnostic criteria employed. Radiographic evidence of pneumonia was specifically sought and found in 16 percent of healthy male military recruits with varicella, but clinical signs of pneumonia were present in only 4 percent.[54] In a more recent study, radiographic evidence of pneumonitis was found in fewer than 3 percent of healthy young military personnel with varicella.[56] Pneumonia generally appears 1 to 6 days after the onset of the rash, and the degree of pulmonary involvement correlates best with the severity of the cutaneous eruption. Some patients are virtually asymptomatic, but others develop severe respiratory embarrassment, with cough, dyspnea, tachypnea, high fever, pleuritic chest pain, cyanosis, and hemoptysis. The severity of the symptoms usually exceeds the physical findings, but the roentgenogram typically reveals diffuse, peribronchial nodular densities throughout both lung fields with a tendency to concentrate in the perihilar regions and at the bases. The mortality in adults with varicella pneumonia has been estimated to be between 10 and 30 percent, but it is less than 10 percent if immunocompromised patients are excluded.

Varicella during pregnancy is a threat to both mother and fetus. The disease is more severe in pregnant women than in nonpregnant adults, and mortality from varicella pneumonia and visceral dissemination is increased, especially when varicella occurs in the third trimester.[57] The fetus may die as a consequence of premature labor or maternal death in severe varicella pneumonia, but varicella during pregnancy does not, otherwise, substantially increase fetal morbidity or mortality.[58,59] Nevertheless, even in uncomplicated varicella, maternal viremia can result in intrauterine (congenital) VZV infection.

The spectrum of congenital VZV infection ranges from asymptomatic infection to severe congenital malformations. A characteristic syndrome of developmental abnormalities (including hypoplasia of an extremity, cicatricial skin scarring, cortical atrophy, ocular abnormalities, and low birth weight) has been observed in infants born to women who had varicella between the seventh and twentieth weeks of gestation. This is a rare occurrence, with fewer than 100 cases reported worldwide. In contrast, infants born to women who had herpes zoster during pregnancy do not develop clinical or serologic evidence of intrauterine VZV infection. Infants infected in utero from mothers with varicella harbor latent VZV in their sensory ganglia. Consequently, they frequently develop herpes zoster at an early age without antecedent history of varicella.[58]

Perinatal varicella (i.e., varicella occurring within 10 days of birth) is more serious than varicella in infants infected later, and the severity varies markedly depending upon the proximity of maternal disease to delivery. When an infant acquires VZV infection in utero in the immediate prepartum period but is born before the transplacental passage of sufficient maternal antibody to modify the infection during its incubation period (i.e., when the rash of varicella occurs in the mother less than 5 days before or within 2 days after delivery or begins in an infant between 5 and 10 days of age), the result is often severe disseminated varicella, with mortality as high as 30 percent. When the onset of rash in the mother is 5 days or more before delivery (onset of rash in the infant at 0 to 4 days of age), sufficient maternal antibody has crossed the placenta to modify the infection, and all such infected infants can be expected to survive.

The morbidity and mortality of varicella are markedly increased in immunocompromised patients, including patients with AIDS; patients with leukemia and other malignancies who are receiving glucocorticoids, chemotherapeutic agents, or radiotherapy at the time of infection; patients receiving glucocorticoids for diseases such as nephrotic syndrome and rheumatic fever; and patients with congenital immunologic deficiencies.[3,9,51,60,61] In these patients, continued virus replication and dissemination result in a prolonged high-level viremia, a more extensive rash, and a longer period of new vesicle formation. Immunosuppressed and glucocorticoid-treated patients may develop pneumonia, hepatitis, encephalitis, and hemorrhagic complications of varicella, which range in severity from mild febrile purpura to severe and often fatal purpura fulminans and "malignant" varicella.[60–62]

Central nervous system (CNS) complications of varicella occur in fewer than 1 in 1000 cases; they include several distinct syndromes[63–65]: (1) Reye's syndrome, (2) acute cerebellar ataxia, (3) encephalitis or meningoencephalitis, (4) acute ascending or transverse myelitis, and (5) Guillain-Barré syndrome. Varicella-associated Reye's syndrome (acute encephalopathy with fatty degeneration of the liver) typically occurs 2 to 7 days after the appearance of the rash. It is not discernibly different from Reye's syndrome associated with other viral infections. Although its pathogenesis is not understood, there is no inflammatory response in the CNS, and histopathologic and virologic studies have essentially ruled out direct virus infection of the liver or brain. Instead, Reye's syndrome may be caused by some circulating toxin, perhaps a substance elaborated by virus-infected cells or cells responding to them. From 15 to 40 percent of all cases of Reye's syndrome occur in association with varicella, particularly when aspirin has been taken for fever, and the mortality may be as high as 40 percent.

Varicella-associated Guillain-Barré syndrome is extremely rare, and many of the cases reported are almost certainly examples of varicella myelitis. Apart from the temporal association in the few cases recorded, there is no evidence directly implicating VZV in the pathogenesis of Guillain-Barré syndrome.

Unlike the other neurologic complications of varicella, acute cerebellar ataxia is relatively common and benign.[64] The child may become unsteady or grossly ataxic anywhere from 11 days before to 20 days after the appearance of the rash. Recovery without sequelae is the rule, and no pathologic data are available; however, its occurrence before the onset of rash and the detection of VZV antigens and VZV DNA in the cerebrospinal fluid of patients with this complication[65] suggest that acute cerebellar ataxia is a result of direct invasion of the CNS, presumably as a consequence of viremia and infection of vascular endothelial cells.

The pathogenesis of varicella encephalitis (meningoencephalitis) and myelitis remains obscure. Although many observers favor a postinfectious (autoimmune) demyelinating process like that observed in measles encephalomyelitis, there is increasing evidence that these complications of varicella result from direct VZV infection of the CNS.[65]

Although chemical evidence of mild hepatitis is common in uncomplicated varicella, clinical hepatitis is rare except as a complication of progressive varicella.[30,32] Other rare complications of varicella include myocarditis, glomerulonephritis, orchitis, appendicitis, pancreatitis, gastritis and ulcerative lesions of the bowel, arthritis, Henoch-Schönlein vasculitis, optic neuritis, keratitis, and iritis. The pathogenesis of many of these complications has not been delineated, but direct parenchymal or endovascular infection or vasculitis induced by VZV antigen-antibody complexes appears to be responsible in most cases.

Clinical Manifestations of Herpes Zoster

PRODROME OF HERPES ZOSTER The first symptoms of herpes zoster are usually pain and paresthesia in the involved dermatome. This often precedes the eruption by several days and varies from superficial itching, tingling, or burning to severe, deep, boring, or lancinating pain. It may be constant or intermittent and is often accompanied by tenderness and hyperesthesia of the skin in the involved dermatome. The preeruptive pain of herpes zoster may simulate pleurisy, myocardial infarction, duodenal ulcer, cholecystitis, biliary or renal colic, appendicitis, prolapsed intervertebral disk, or early glaucoma. Thus, quite understandably, it often leads to serious misdiagnosis and misdirected interventions. Constitutional symptoms—including headache, malaise, and fever—occur in about 5 percent of patients, usually in children, and may precede the rash by 1 to 2 days.

A few patients experience acute segmental neuralgia without ever developing a cutaneous eruption—a condition known as *zoster sine herpete*.[46] Although zoster sine herpete may explain some cases of trigeminal neuralgia, most patients with this syndrome do not have serologic evidence of recent herpes zoster. Similarly, although facial palsy frequently complicates cephalic herpes zoster (e.g., the Ramsay-Hunt syndrome), VZV infection does not appear to be responsible for most cases of "idiopathic" facial palsy (Bell's palsy).[66] Recent evidence indicates the HSV-1 is the principal cause of Bell's palsy. Murakami et al. detected HSV-1 DNA in endoneural fluid from the facial nerve or in the posterior auricular muscle innervated by it in 11 of 14 patients with Bell's palsy; they detected VZV

RASH OF HERPES ZOSTER   The most distinctive feature of herpes zoster is the localization and distribution of the rash, which is nearly always unilateral, does not cross the midline, and is generally limited to the area of skin innervated by a single sensory ganglion (Fig. 216-5*A*). As indicated earlier, herpes zoster occurs with great-

est frequency in those areas in which the rash of varicella was most abundant. The area supplied by the trigeminal nerve, particularly the ophthalmic division, and the trunk from T3 to L2 are most frequently affected; the thoracic region alone accounts for more than one-half of reported cases, and lesions rarely occur distal to the

FIGURE 216-5

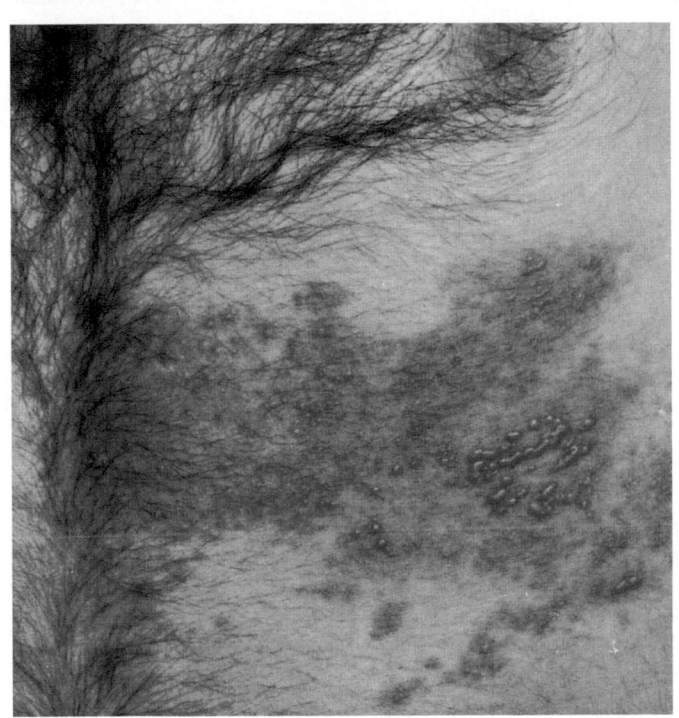

A.

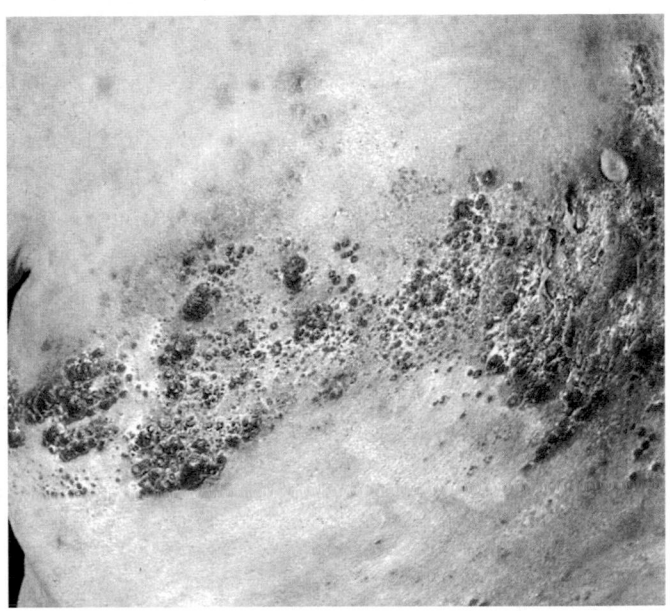

B.

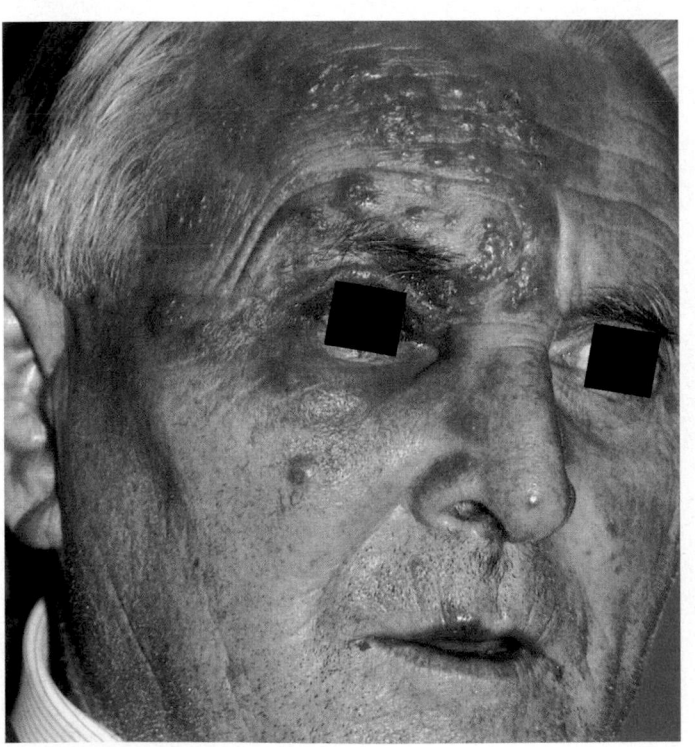

C.

Herpes zoster. *A.* Early involvement of a thoracic dermatome with erythema within the dermatome and areas of grouped vesicle formation. *B.* Later involvement with crusted sites on the back, where the eruption first appeared, and many confluent hemorrhagic vesicles and bullae on the lateral chest wall, where the eruption appeared more recently; some vesicles are also seen outside the involved dermatome, representing hematogenous dissemination, a not uncommon occurrence. *C.* Ophthalmic zoster. Note the involvement of the tip of the nose, which frequently signals involvement of the eye.

elbows or knees.[19,20,68] Regional lymphadenopathy occurs in many cases of herpes zoster.

Although the individual lesions of herpes zoster and varicella are basically indistinguishable, those of herpes zoster tend to evolve more slowly and usually consist of closely grouped vesicles on an erythematous base, rather than the more discrete, randomly distributed vesicles of varicella. This reflects the route of infection of the skin, neural in herpes zoster versus viremic in varicella. Herpes zoster lesions begin as erythematous macules and papules that often first appear where superficial branches of the affected sensory nerve are given off—e.g., the posterior primary division and the lateral and anterior branches of the anterior primary division of spinal nerves. Vesicles form within 12 to 24 h and evolve into pustules by the third day. These dry and crust in 7 to 10 days. The crusts generally persist for 2 to 3 weeks (Fig. 216-5B). In normal individuals, new lesions continue to appear for 1 to 4 days (occasionally for as long as 7 days). The rash is most severe and lasts longest in older people and is least severe and of shortest duration in children.[69]

Between 10 and 15 percent of reported cases of herpes zoster involve the ophthalmic division of trigeminal nerve (Fig. 216-5C).[70] The rash of ophthalmic zoster may extend from the level of the eye to the vertex of the skull, but it terminates sharply at the midline of the forehead. When only the supratrochlear and supraorbital branches are involved, the eye is usually spared. Involvement of the nasociliary branch, as evidenced by a herpetic rash on the tip and side of the nose, occurs in 30 to 40 percent of patients with ophthalmic zoster. Thus, when ophthalmic zoster involves the tip and the side of the nose, careful attention must be given to the condition of the eye. VZV is not, however, as directly pathogenic for the cornea as is herpes simplex virus.

Herpes zoster affecting the second and third divisions of the trigeminal nerve (Fig. 216-6) and other cranial nerves may produce symptoms and lesions in the mouth, ears, pharynx, or larynx. The so-called Ramsay-Hunt syndrome—facial palsy in combination with herpes zoster of the external ear or tympanic membrane, with or without tinnitus, vertigo, and deafness—results from involvement of the facial and auditory nerves.

Complications of Herpes Zoster (Table 216-2)

Most complications of herpes zoster are associated with the spread of VZV from the initially involved sensory ganglion, nerve, or skin, either via the bloodstream or by direct neural extension. Exceptions include bacterial superinfection and, perhaps, postherpetic neuralgia. For example, the infection may disseminate widely from a small, painless area of herpes zoster. In such cases, the initial dermatomal presentation may go unnoticed, and the ensuing disseminated eruption may be mistaken for varicella. This explains some reported second attacks of varicella as well as some of the cases of "atypical generalized zoster" (a disseminated varicella-like eruption without an accompanying dermatomal rash in a person with a history of varicella), which are reported primarily in immunocompromised patients.[71] However, symptomatic reinfections (second episodes of varicella) do occur, especially in immunocompromised patients and in people whose initial infection was modified by passively acquired antibody to VZV.

It is more common for herpes zoster to disseminate after the initial dermatomal eruption has become apparent. When immunologically competent patients are carefully examined, 17 to 35 percent of them are found to have at least a few vesicles in areas distant from the involved and immediately overlapping dermatomes; presumably this is due to hematogenous dissemination of virus from the affected ganglion, nerve, or skin. The disseminated lesions usually appear within a week of onset of the segmental eruption and, if few in number, are easily overlooked. More extensive dissemination (with 25 to 50 lesions or more), producing a varicella-like eruption (generalized herpes zoster; Fig. 216-7), occurs in 2 to 10 percent of unselected patients with localized zoster, most of whom have immunologic defects due to acquired immunodeficiency, as seen with HIV infection, underlying malignancy (particularly lymphomas), or immunosuppressive therapy.[47,48,72,73]

When the dermatomal rash is particularly extensive, as it often is in severely immunocompromised patients, there may be superficial gangrene with delayed healing and subsequent scarring. Secondary bacterial infection may also delay healing and cause scarring. Local bacterial infections may also disseminate, causing septicemia and metastatic foci of infection. Ophthalmic zoster has a relatively high complication rate, especially when involvement of the nasociliary branch provides VZV with direct access to intraocular structures.[70] The eye is involved in 20 to 70 percent of patients with ophthalmic zoster, with a wide range of possible complications. Corneal sensation

FIGURE 216-6

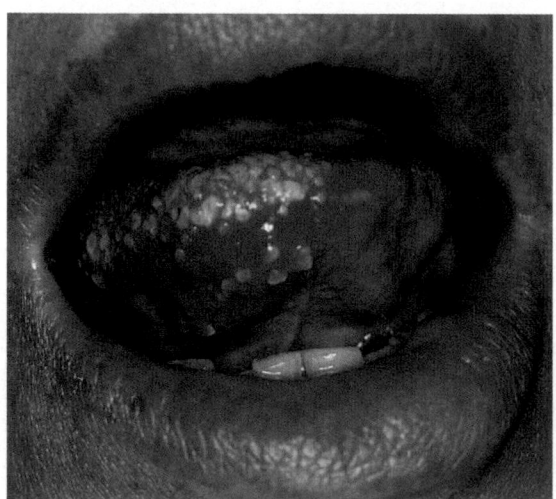

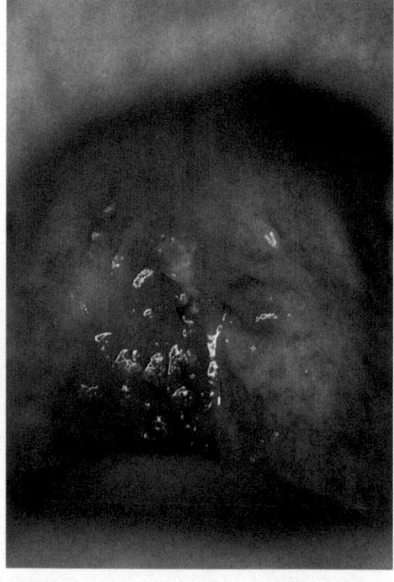

A.

B.

Cephalic herpes zoster with facial palsy (Hunt syndrome). A 60-year-old female with right-sided facial palsy and vesicles on her A. tongue and B. soft palate.

TABLE 216-2

CHAPTER 216
Varicella and Herpes Zoster

2437

Complications of Herpes Zoster

Cutaneous	Neurologic
Bacterial superinfection	Postherpetic neuralgia
Scarring	Meningoencephalitis
Cellulitis	Transverse myelitis
Zoster gangrenosum	Peripheral nerve palsies
Septicemia (with metastatic	Motor
foci of infection)	Autonomic
Cutaneous VZV dissemination	Diaphragmatic paralysis
Visceral	Cranial nerve palsies
Esophagitis	Sensory loss
Gastritis	Granulomatous cerebral angii-
Colitis	tis (causing contralateral
Cystitis	hemiparesis)
Pericarditis	Deafness
Pleuritis	Ocular complications
Peritonitis	Keratitis
Visceral VZV dissemination	Scleritis
Pneumonia	Uveitis
Hepatitis	Chorioretinitis
Myocarditis	Iridocyclitis
Pericarditis	Optic neuropathy
Arthritis	Ptosis
	Mydriasis
	Cicatricial lid scarring
	Secondary glaucoma
	Acute retinal necrosis

is almost always impaired; when the impairment is severe, it may lead to neurotrophic keratitis and chronic ulceration. Rarely, secondary bacterial infection may result in panophthalmitis, requiring enucleation.

VZV is also the principal cause of acute retinal necrosis (ARN), a fulminant sight-threatening disease observed primarily in otherwise healthy individuals.[74] A small number of reported cases have been caused by HSV-1 and HSV-2. Although caused by reactivation of latent VZV, most cases of ARN in immunocompetent persons occur in the absence of cutaneous manifestations of herpes zoster, and the pathogenesis of ARN remains obscure. A high index of suspicion is essential because early initiation of effective antiviral therapy offers the best chance of preserving visual function.

Herpes zoster may be attended by a variety of neurologic complications (Table 216-2), of which postherpetic neuralgia is the most common and important. PHN has been defined in many ways, but the most common definitions involve pain that persists or appears after the rash has healed or at 30 days after onset of the rash. The overall incidence of PHN is 8 to 15 percent (Fig. 216-1B).[19,20,49,50,68,75–78] Age is the most significant risk factor for PHN, which is rare in persons under age 40 but occurs in more than 50 percent of persons with herpes zoster age 60 or older (Fig. 216-1C). Other risk factors for PHN include the presence of pro-

dromal pain, severe pain during the acute phase of herpes zoster, and ophthalmic (as opposed to thoracic or abdominal) herpes zoster. PHN is difficult to treat, but it usually remits spontaneously over several months; the risk of long-lasting PHN also increases with increasing age.

PHN is characterized by three types of pain: (1) spontaneous, constant, deep aching or burning pain; (2) spontaneous intermittent lancinating or jabbing pain; and (3) dysesthetic pain and discomfort provoked by normally innocuous stimuli such as light touch or exposure to cold (allodynia) and often lasting well beyond the duration of the stimulus (hyperpathia).[49,50,75,78]

When patients with PHN are carefully studied, the involved skin almost always shows pigmentary changes and scarring; there are also major local sensory abnormalities that are rarely seen in patients with herpes zoster who recover without developing PHN.

Motor paralysis is reported in 1 to 5 percent of patients with herpes zoster. It results from the direct extension of infection from the sensory ganglion to adjacent parts of the nervous system. Paralysis usually begins within 2 weeks of the onset of the rash and almost always involves muscle groups with innervation that is contiguous with that of the affected dermatome; oculomotor and facial palsies are seen with cephalic zoster, unilateral diaphragmatic paralysis with homolateral cervical herpes zoster, paralysis of the trunk and limbs with herpes zoster involving corresponding dermatomes, and dysfunction of the bladder and anus with sacral herpes zoster. Total or functional recovery occurs in most cases. Rare cases in which the involved myotome and dermatome are widely separated may be the result of more extensive myelitis. Herpes zoster myelitis, with detection of VZV in the spinal cord or cerebrospinal fluid, has been reported both as a complication of typical herpes zoster and of zoster sine herpete.[79]

FIGURE 216-7

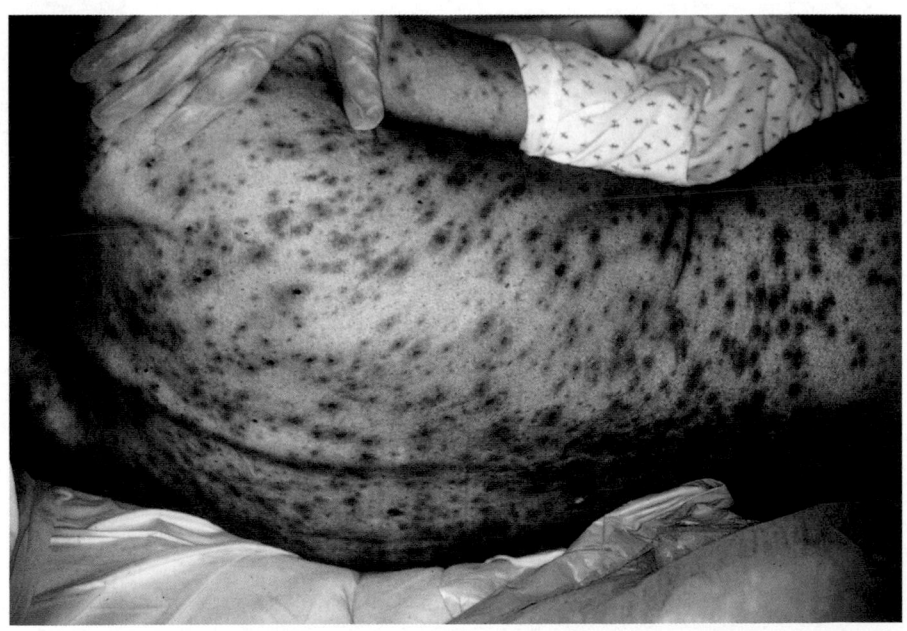

The back of a patient with chronic lymphocytic leukemia and disseminated herpes zoster. (*From Straus et al.,*[24] *with permission.*)

Although lymphocytic pleocytosis, with or without an increase in the concentration of protein in the cerebrospinal fluid, is a regular feature of uncomplicated herpes zoster, the incidence of acute symptomatic meningoencephalitis and myelitis is low (0.2 to 0.5 percent). When these complications do occur, their onset usually follows the onset of rash by 7 to 10 days, but they may precede the rash by a week or more or follow it by up to 2 months. The pathogenesis is not understood, but it may involve both virus-induced and immunopathologically mediated injury. Immunopathology is most likely to be important in cases in which the complication arises long after the cutaneous lesions have fully crusted. Clinical manifestations include fever, altered sensorium (frequently with delirium and hallucinations), headache, meningismus, and cranial or extracranial nerve palsies, often at a cord level corresponding to the rash. There is a lymphocytic cerebrospinal fluid pleocytosis, with the cell count usually ranging from 10 to 500/mm^3; a moderate elevation in protein concentration; and a normal glucose concentration. However, the cell count may occasionally exceed 1000/mm^3, there may sometimes be 30 to 40 percent neutrophils, and the glucose concentration may be low. Most patients recover and return to their preencephalitis cognitive status, but many are left with postherpetic neuralgia, chronic ophthalmologic complications, and motor palsies.

VZV-induced granulomatous angiitis of cerebral arteries is responsible for a syndrome of ophthalmic zoster and delayed contralateral hemiplegia.[80,81] It usually occurs weeks to months after the episode of ophthalmic zoster (average interval about 8 weeks) and may present as an isolated cerebral infarction, multiple cerebral infarctions, stroke in evolution, or transient ischemic attacks. Because the clinical manifestations are similar to those of hypertensive strokes and the delayed onset may obscure the relationship to herpes zoster, the syndrome is probably underdiagnosed. Cerebral arteriograms usually reveal segmental narrowing or occlusion of cerebral arteries ipsilateral to the ophthalmic zoster. Although multiple strokes may occur for several weeks, later recurrences are rare and the disease appears to be self-limited. The mortality in reported cases is about 15 percent.

HERPES ZOSTER IN THE IMMUNOCOMPROMISED HOST

Infection with HIV; certain types of malignancy, especially Hodgkin's disease and lymphocytic leukemia; and the administration of immunosuppressive therapy (e.g., radiation, antimetabolites, antilymphocyte serum, and glucocorticoids) to patients with malignant and nonmalignant diseases markedly increase the incidence and severity of herpes zoster.[4,5,47,48,72,73,82] In fact, except for PHN, most serious complications of herpes zoster occur predominantly in immunocompromised persons.

From 20 to 50 percent of patients with Hodgkin's disease develop herpes zoster within 18 months following diagnosis, with the highest incidence in patients whose disease was far advanced and those receiving radiation and combination chemotherapy. The risk of VZV dissemination was markedly increased in patients with active tumor at the time of infection. When herpes zoster occurred in these patients, it was usually within 1 month of chemotherapy or within 7 months of x-ray therapy.

The severity of herpes zoster and the risk of complications are also increased in immunocompromised patients—necrosis of skin and scarring are fairly common (Fig. 216-8), and the incidence of cutaneous dissemination may be as high as 25 to 50 percent. Approximately 10 percent of patients with cutaneous disseminated le-

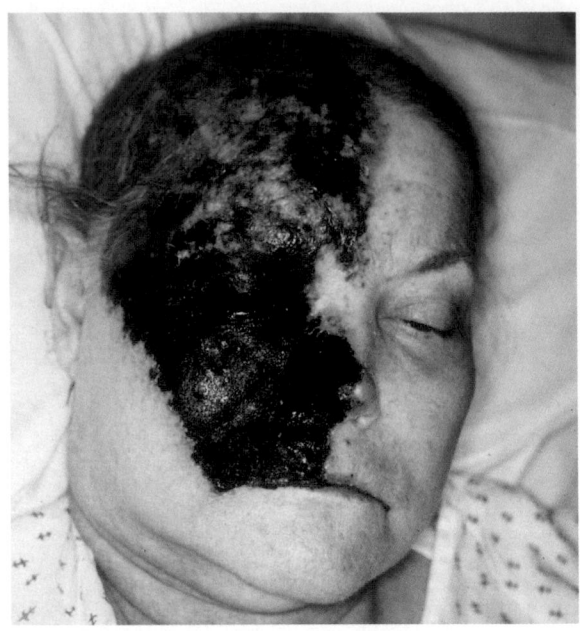

A.

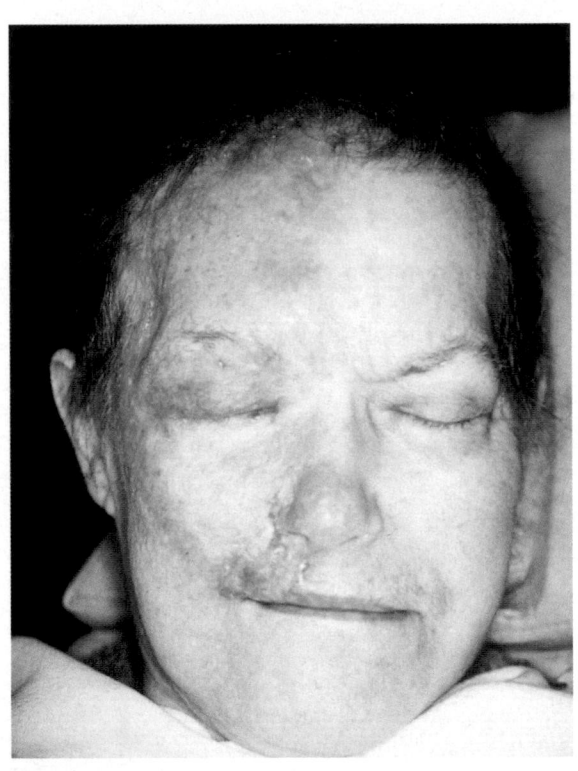

B.

A. Acute, necrotic herpes zoster involving the first and second distributions of the fifth cranial nerve in a woman with lymphoma receiving cytotoxic chemotherapy. *B.* Dense scar formation and temporal muscle wasting several weeks later. (*From Straus et al.,*[24] *with permission.*)

sions manifest widespread, often fatal visceral dissemination as well, particularly to the lungs, liver, and brain.[47,48,72,73,82] The incidence and severity of herpes zoster are also markedly increased in immunosuppressed recipients of solid organ and bone marrow transplants. Some 20 to 40 percent of bone marrow transplant recipients develop herpes zoster within 1 year of transplantation. Disseminated infection, often without a recognizable cutaneous focus of localized herpes zoster, is common, as are postherpetic neuralgia, scarring, and bacterial superinfection.

The incidence of herpes zoster is greatly increased in persons infected with HIV; it tends to occur early in the course of HIV infection and is often the first sign of immune deficiency.[4,5] HIV-infected patients are fairly unique in their tendency to suffer multiple recurrences of herpes zoster as their disease progresses; herpes zoster may recur in the same or different dermatomes or in several contiguous or noncontiguous dermatomes. Patients with AIDS may develop severe herpes zoster with cutaneous and visceral dissemination. They can experience chronic, often acyclovir-resistant cutaneous lesions with unusual verrucous, hyperkeratotic, or ecthymatous features (Fig. 216-9).[10–13] AIDS patients also experience progressive outer retinal necrosis, a blinding infection that can be distinguished from cytomegalovirus retinitis and herpes simplex virus-induced acute retinal necrosis syndrome.[83]

A syndrome resembling progressive multifocal leukoencephalopathy (PML) has been reported following herpes zoster in several immunocompromised patients, mostly ones with advanced AIDS.[84] They exhibit progressive, asymmetric, multifocal neurologic deficits, impaired mental function, and focal seizures and die within months to a year or so. Autopsy reveals multifocal lesions, primarily at the gray-white cortical junction, with demyelination, necrosis, and eosinophilic Cowdry type A intranuclear inclusion bodies in oligodendrocytes, neurons, and astrocytes. These lesions contain abundant viral antigens, particles, and nucleic acids. A remarkable feature of some of these cases has been the long interval (up to 20 months) between the episode of cutaneous zoster and the onset of neurologic symptoms. This observation, as well as the long interval between ophthalmic zoster and the onset of symptoms in patients with segmental granulomatous cerebral angiitis, and the occurrence of chronic cutaneous herpes zoster in patients with AIDS suggest that in addition to established latent infections, VZV can produce chronic, "smoldering" subclinical and clinical infections.

PATHOLOGY

Cytopathology

The cutaneous lesions of varicella and herpes zoster are histologically indistinguishable (Fig. 216-10) and are similar to those produced by herpes simplex virus. The characteristic changes in infected cells, which can be observed in tissue culture as well as in vivo, are "ballooning degeneration," with the formation of intranuclear inclusion bodies and multinucleated giant cells.[20,21] Individual infected cells become greatly enlarged with pale, vacuolated cytoplasm. The nuclei exhibit margination of chromatin and contain inclusion bodies (Fig. 216-10B). Early in infection, these inclusion

FIGURE 216-10

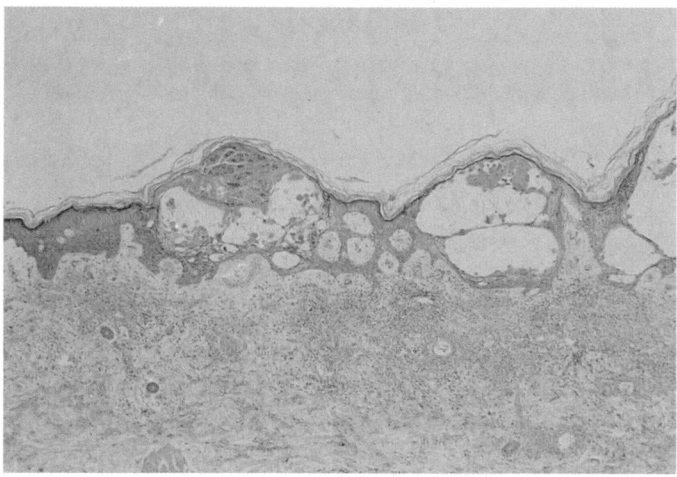

A.

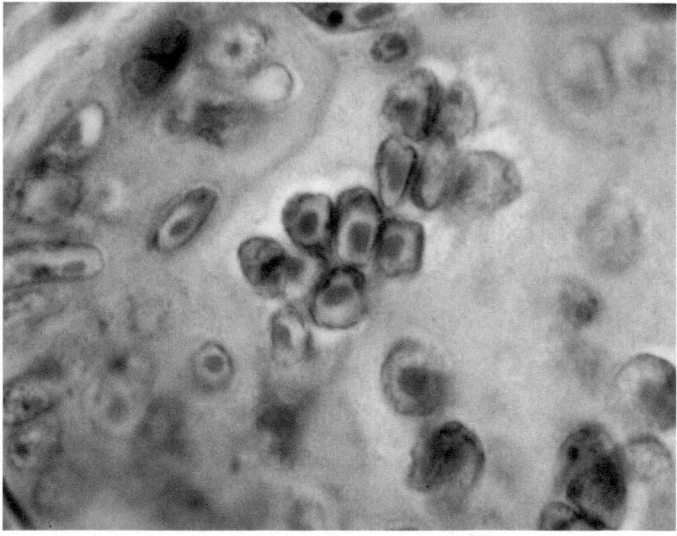

B.

Herpes zoster, histopathology. A. Intraepidermal vesicle, acantholysis, reticular degeneration; underlying dermis shows edema and vasculitis. B. Multinucleated giant cells with characteristic nuclear changes.

FIGURE 216-9

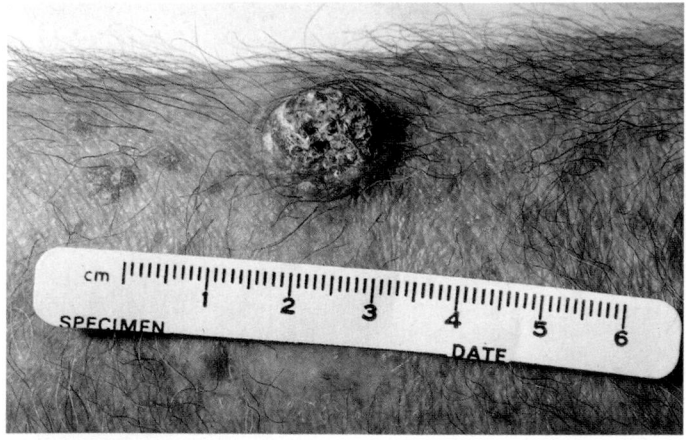

Chronic verrucous lesions of herpes zoster despite long-term acyclovir treatment in a patient with advanced AIDS. (*Courtesy of David Paar, MD.*)

bodies may be homogeneous and moderately basophilic and usually fill the nucleus; however, they rapidly evolve into classical Cowdry type A inclusion bodies—sharply demarcated acidophilic (eosinophilic) inclusions that are separated from the deeply basophilic ring of marginated chromatin at the nuclear membrane by a clear zone or halo. Pairs and groups of adjacent VZV-infected cells fuse to form multinucleated giant cells. Cell fusion is mediated by specific VZV glycoproteins displayed on infected cell membranes. Fusion facilitates cell-to-cell spread of infection, even in the presence of antibody capable of neutralizing extracellular virus.

Pathology of Varicella

The initial event in the formation of cutaneous lesions of varicella is probably infection of capillary endothelial cells in the papillary dermis, with subsequent spread of virus to epithelial cells in the epidermis, hair follicles, and sebaceous glands.[30,85] In early papular lesions, the epithelium is slightly elevated due to swelling of the infected epithelial cells and to edema and vascular congestion of the underlying dermis. In the superficial dermis, capillary endothelial cells are swollen, and their nuclei often contain typical intranuclear inclusion bodies. Similar inclusion bodies may be seen in the nuclei of fibroblasts in the surrounding connective tissue, which is edematous and infiltrated by small numbers of mononuclear cells. Superficial lymphatics are dilated, and cells lining these structures are also swollen and may contain intranuclear inclusion bodies. In the epidermis, the cells initially involved are those of the germinal layer and the deeper portion of the stratum spinosum. These cells show ballooning degeneration with loss of intercellular bridges (acantholysis) and are soon separated by intercellular edema. A few small multinucleated giant cells, containing three to eight nuclei, are usually seen at the base and periphery of these early epithelial lesions. Abundant VZV antigens are evident throughout the affected lesions by immunohistochemical stains.[86,87]

The papular lesions rapidly evolve into intraepidermal vesicles as a result of the infection and degeneration of increasing numbers of epithelial cells, the fusion of adjacent areas of microscopic degeneration, and the continuing influx of edema fluid, which elevates the uninvolved stratum corneum to form a delicate clear vesicle. At this stage, the vesicle fluid contains fibrin, degenerating and "ballooned" epithelial cells, and abundant cell-free infectious VZV. As the lesions progress, polymorphonuclear leukocytes and a small number of macrophages invade from the underlying dermis, and the vesicle fluid becomes cloudy; this transforms the vesicle into a pustule. The fluid is then absorbed, with the formation of a flat, adherent crust that is eventually detached by the regrowth of subjacent epithelial cells. The evolution from papule to early crusting normally occurs over a period of 24 to 48 h. Lesions of uncomplicated varicella heal without scarring. Lesions in mucous membranes develop in the same way, but the thin roof of the vesicle breaks quickly, producing a shallow ulcer that heals rapidly.

In fatal varicella, focal lesions and viral antigens are found in the mucous membranes of the respiratory, gastrointestinal, and genitourinary tracts; in the serosa of the pleural and peritoneal cavities; and in the parenchyma of virtually every organ, the lungs and liver being the most common sites of severe involvement.[88] There is widespread vascular damage, with characteristic acidophilic intranuclear inclusion bodies in the endothelial cells lining small blood vessels and lymphatics; capillaries within individual lesions are often destroyed, resulting in thrombosis and hemorrhage. In varicella pneumonia, the pleura are studded with hemorrhagic nodules, and the lungs show widely disseminated interstitial pneumonia with numerous foci of hemorrhagic necrosis. Alveoli are filled with red blood cells, fibrin, inclusion-bearing mononuclear cells, and occasional multinucleated giant cells. Hyaline membranes are frequently present. Typical acidophilic intranuclear inclusion bodies are also seen within hyperplastic alveolar septal cells, swollen capillary endothelial cells, fibroblasts, and bronchiolar and tracheobronchial epithelial cells. Similar areas of vascular damage and focal necrosis are found in the parenchyma of the liver, spleen, and other organs throughout the body. In some cases, characteristic intranuclear inclusion bodies may be nearly or totally absent, in spite of unmistakable clinical and pathologic evidence of extensive VZV infection and the isolation of VZV from the liver, lungs, brain, and other tissues.

Pathology of Herpes Zoster

Although the histopathology of the skin lesions of herpes zoster and varicella is the same (Fig. 216-10), herpes zoster is accompanied by acute inflammation of the corresponding sensory nerve and ganglion. The ganglion shows intense lymphocyte infiltration, necrosis of nerve cells and fibers, endothelial cell proliferation and lymphocytic cuffing of small vessels, focal hemorrhage, and inflammation of the ganglion sheath.[89] Satellite cells and neurons contain characteristic acidophilic intranuclear inclusion bodies, virus particles visible by electron microscopy, and VZV antigens demonstrable by immunofluorescence. Some degree of neuronal degeneration and lymphocytic infiltration is also generally present in adjacent ganglia on the same side.

The peripheral nerve shows diffuse lymphocytic infiltration and focal hemorrhage, with axonal degeneration and demyelination of sensory fibers. Virus particles and VZV antigens are present in Schwann and perineural cells. These inflammatory and degenerative changes can be traced distally to branches innervating the affected skin. Recent data suggest that reactivated virus may spread from myelinated nerve endings to the dermis to hair follicles and then to surrounding skin.[85] These observations suggest that virus spreads from the sensory ganglion to the periphery by replication in Schwann and perineural cells rather than by axonal transport, a mechanism that would help explain the long prodrome and intense peripheral neuritis that characterize herpes zoster.

The inflammatory reaction in the ganglion also extends proximally to the posterior nerve root and into adjacent regions of the cord or brainstem, producing a segmental myelitis that is predominantly ipsilateral and involves the posterior horn more than the anterior horn. There is degeneration of nerve fibers in the posterior columns and inflammatory changes in the gray matter of the posterior and anterior horns, with perivenous lymphocytic infiltration, scattered neuronal necrosis, and neuronophagia. These changes may extend two or more segments from the one corresponding in the cutaneous eruption. A mild lymphocytic leptomeningitis is generally present and is most intense over the involved segments and nerve roots. Marked inflammation and degeneration of the anterior nerve root within the meninges and in the portion overlying the involved sensory ganglion may also be present, producing a true motor radiculitis. When extensive, the acute inflammatory response is followed by fibrosis of the ganglion and nerve.

Herpes zoster is occasionally complicated by meningoencephalitis or myelitis, in which CNS involvement is not restricted to segments corresponding to the involved dermatome. The pathologic findings in herpes zoster meningoencephalitis vary from focal mononuclear cell infiltration of the leptomeninges to acute necrotizing encephalitis with perivenous encephalomalacia, myelin and axonal degeneration, macrophage infiltration, and typical intranuclear inclusion bodies and virus particles in oligodendrocytes, neurons, and astrocytes.

CLINICAL AND LABORATORY DIAGNOSES

Clinical Diagnosis of Varicella

Varicella can usually be diagnosed quite readily on the basis of the appearance and evolution of the rash (see Fig. 216-4), particularly when there is a history of exposure within the preceding 2 to 3 weeks. Characteristic diagnostic features include (1) the development, after a brief and mild (or absent) prodrome, of a papulovesicular eruption accompanied by fever and mild constitutional symptoms; (2) the appearance of lesions in crops, with a predominantly central distribution including the scalp; (3) the rapid evolution of individual lesions from macules to papules to delicate thin-walled vesicles to pustules and finally to crusts; (4) the presence of lesions in all stages of development in any one anatomic area throughout the acute disease; and (5) the presence of lesions in the mucous membranes of the mouth.

Disseminated HSV infections may occasionally resemble varicella, especially in neonates, pregnant women, immunosuppressed patients, and patients with eczema; however, the distribution of lesions is rarely typical of varicella, and there is often an obvious concentration of lesions at and surrounding the site of the primary or recurrent infection (e.g., the mouth or external genitalia). Marked toxicity and encephalitis are more common in neonatal herpes simplex than in neonatal varicella. The histopathology of lesions caused by HSV and VZV is indistinguishable. Thus, definitive differentiation of the two requires virus isolation or the detection and identification of viral antigens or nucleic acids in the lesions.

Severe varicella resembles smallpox or generalized vaccinia, however, the eradication of smallpox and the consequent cessation of routine smallpox vaccination has virtually eliminated this diagnostic problem. Other diseases that may be confused with varicella include impetigo, the vesicular exanthems of coxsackievirus and echovirus infections (e.g., hand-foot-and-mouth disease syndrome), rickettsialpox, insect bites, papular urticaria, scabies, contact dermatitis, dermatitis herpetiformis, drug eruptions, secondary syphilis, and erythema multiforme. The character, distribution, and evolution of their lesions, together with a careful epidemiologic history, usually differentiate these diseases from varicella. Moreover, the rashes associated with classical measles, rubella, roseola (herpesvirus types 6 and 7 infections), and erythema infectiosum (parvovirus B19 infection) do not vesiculate and should not be mistaken for varicella. When any doubt exists, the clinical impression should receive laboratory confirmation.

Clinical Diagnosis of Herpes Zoster

In the preeruptive stage, herpes zoster is often confused with other causes of localized pain, such as pleurisy, myocardial infarction, cholecystitis, appendicitis, renal colic, collapsed intervertebral disk, glaucoma, or unappreciated trauma. Sometimes the early appearance of regional lymphadenopathy and localized cutaneous sensory abnormalities (e.g., hyperesthesia, dysesthesia) provide a clue to the diagnosis. Once the eruption appears, the diagnosis is almost always obvious (Figs. 216-5 and 216-6).

Lesions outside of the primary dermatome raise the spector of disseminated herpes zoster. Small numbers of lesions outside the primary dermatome (e.g., fewer than 25) are frequently observed in uncomplicated herpes zoster,[70] but many such lesions suggest clinically significant VZV dissemination, especially if they are accompanied by constitutional signs and symptoms. Disseminated herpes zoster may be mistaken for varicella when there is widespread dissemination of VZV from a small, painless area of herpes zoster or from the affected sensory ganglion in the absence of an obvious dermatomal eruption.[71] This is not infrequent in profoundly immunosuppressed seropositive persons (Fig. 216-7).

A cluster of vesicles, particularly at some distance from the mouth or genitals, may represent herpes zoster, but it may also be a recurrent HSV infection.[21] Zosteriform herpes simplex is often impossible to distinguish from herpes zoster on clinical grounds. A history of multiple recurrences at the same site is common in herpes simplex but does not occur in herpes zoster in the absence of profound and clinically obvious immune deficiency. Isolation of virus or the detection of VZV or HSV antigens or DNA in material obtained from the lesions is the only reliable means of differentiating these entities.

Contact dermatitis, burns, vaccinia autoinoculation, and localized bacterial skin infections may occasionally resemble herpes zoster, but a careful history and examination of the lesions (including a Tzanck smear with the identification of multinucleated giant cells and intranuclear inclusion bodies) eliminates any confusion.

Laboratory Diagnosis

Routine blood tests are not helpful or needed in the diagnosis of either varicella or herpes zoster. Asymptomatic elevations in serum levels of alanine aminotransferase (ALT) and aspartate aminotransferase (AST) occur in the majority of children and adults with uncomplicated varicella.[32] They are highest during the first week of illness, rarely exceed five times the upper limit of normal, and resolve in 1 to 4 weeks.

The lesions of varicella and herpes zoster are indistinguishable by histopathology (Fig. 216-10), and both contain VZV virions, VZV antigens, and VZV nucleic acids. The presence of multinucleated giant cells and epithelial cells containing acidophilic intranuclear inclusion bodies (Fig. 216-10B) distinguishes the cutaneous lesions produced by VZV from all other vesicular eruptions except those produced by HSV. These cells can be demonstrated in Tzanck smears prepared at the bedside; material is scraped from the base of an early vesicle and stained with hematoxylin-eosin, Giemsa, Papanicolaou, or Paragon multiple stain.

Punch biopsies provide more reliable material for histologic examination than Tzanck smears and facilitate diagnosis in the prevesicular stage and in atypical lesions such as the chronic verrucous lesions produced by acyclovir-resistant VZV in patients with AIDS[4] (Fig. 216-9). The identification of herpesvirus particles in vesicle fluid or biopsy material by electron microscopy provides another means of diagnosis.[90] However, neither histopathology nor electron microscopy can distinguish VZV from HSV infections.

Sputum from patients with varicella pneumonia may contain desquamated respiratory epithelial cells with acidophilic intranuclear inclusion bodies, but such cells are also found in patients with pneumonia caused by measles virus and in patients with respiratory tract infections caused by HSV.

The definitive diagnosis of VZV infection, as well as the differentiation of VZV from HSV, is accomplished by the isolation of virus in cell cultures inoculated with vesicle fluid, blood, cerebrospinal fluid, or infected tissue or by the direct identification of VZV antigens or nucleic acids in these specimens.[65,91,92] Virus isolation is the only technique that yields infectious VZV for further analysis, such as determination of its sensitivity to antiviral drugs. However, VZV is extremely labile and, except in vesicle fluid, highly cell-associated; this adversely affects the sensitivity of virus isolation procedures; only 30 to 60 percent of cultures from proven cases are positive. To best assure virus recovery, specimens should be inoculated into cell culture immediately. Vesicle fluid is inoculated directly, and tissue specimens are minced or trypsinized, rather than homogenized, to ensure inoculation of viable cells. It is important to select new vesicles containing clear fluid for aspiration because the probability of isolating VZV diminishes rapidly as lesions become pustular. VZV is almost never isolated from crusts. In immunocompetent persons, lesions are typically culture-positive for the first 3 days in varicella and for up to a week in herpes zoster. Virus can be isolated for longer periods in immunocompromised patients.

VZV can be isolated and propagated in vitro in monolayer cultures of a variety of human (and certain simian) cells.[91,92] The cytopathic effect induced by the replicating virus in such cell cultures is characterized by the formation of acidophilic intranuclear inclusion bodies and multinucleated giant cells similar to those seen in the cutaneous lesions of the disease. These changes are indistinguishable from those produced by HSV, but whereas HSV is released into the medium by initially infected cells and rapidly spreads to infect the remaining cells in the culture, the cytopathic effect of VZV remains focal. This is because infectious VZV remains cell-associated and is not released into the medium by the initially infected cells; infection proceeds from cell to cell only by direct contact, and the initial foci of infection gradually enlarge. Serial passage of VZV in tissue culture requires the transfer of infected cells. Special techniques are required to reliably generate infectious cell-free VZV. Cytopathic effects of VZV are generally not apparent until several days after specimen inoculation. Contemporary modifications of the cell culture assays for VZV can greatly speed its detection. Vesicle fluid or lesion scrapings are centrifuged onto cell monolayers growing on coverslips at the bottom of thin, glass-walled "shell" vials. Replicate vials are incubated for 24 to 48 h; the cells are fixed and stained with fluorescein- or enzyme-labeled monoclonal antibodies to VZV proteins. VZV-infected cells can be detected by this technique well before full cytopathic changes are evident.

A specific diagnosis can be achieved more rapidly and with greater sensitivity without resorting to culture techniques by identifying VZV antigens or nucleic acids directly in vesicle fluid, in cells scraped or swabbed from the base of vesicles or ulcers, in crusts, or in tissue obtained by biopsy. Viral antigens can be demonstrated in vesicle fluid or extracts of crusts by countercurrent immunoelectrophoresis (CIE) using antiserum to VZV. Immunofluorescent or immunoperoxidase staining of cellular material from fresh vesicles or prevesicular lesions is a useful diagnostic technique in experienced hands and has become the method of choice in many centers; it can detect VZV significantly more often and faster than virus culture, even relatively late in the disease when cultures are no longer positive. Enzyme immunoassays provide another rapid and sensitive method for antigen detection. Monoclonal antibodies have improved the specificity of these techniques, but it is always important, with all of these methods, to examine aliquots of each specimen with antisera to VZV, HSV-1, HSV-2, and control antigen in parallel, together with positive and negative virus-infected tissue controls.

Detection of VZV nucleic acids in vesicle fluid, cells scraped or swabbed from skin lesions, crusts, respiratory secretions, cerebrospinal fluid (CSF), or tissue obtained by biopsy directly by nucleic acid hybridization or following amplifications by PCR provides an even more sensitive and specific diagnosis.[65] Because of their extraordinary sensitivity, PCR-based techniques are revolutionizing the diagnosis of VZV infections. Restriction fragment length polymorphism analysis of PCR product also permits the identification of epidemiologically linked VZV isolates and can distinguish wild-type VZV from vaccine strains.[28]

Serologic tests can provide a retrospective diagnosis of varicella and herpes zoster reliably when acute and convalescent sera are available for comparison.[33,93,94] They can also identify susceptible individuals who may be candidates for isolation or prophylaxis. The widely available complement fixation (CF) test suffers from two disadvantages: (1) a rise in CF titer to VZV or HSV is not diagnostic if antibody to both viruses increases, because infection by either virus can induce a heterologous anamnestic response, and (2) the CF antibody titer wanes and may disappear within months after varicella infection. Consequently, the CF test is not widely employed today. Indirect fluorescent antibody tests have problems of specificity similar to those of the CF test. VZV neutralization tests are both sensitive and specific but are time-consuming, technically demanding, and expensive. Several more sensitive techniques have been developed to measure humoral responses to VZV. These include an immunofluorescence assay for antibody to VZV-induced membrane antigens (FAMA) that distinguishes immune from susceptible adults[93] and a latex agglutination test that is comparable in sensitivity to FAMA assays but much simpler to perform.[94] The latex agglutination test is the most sensitive commercially available assay for determining immunity to VZV.

Measurement of the in vitro proliferative response of peripheral blood lymphocytes to VZV antigens[34] correlates well with immunity as measured by FAMA, latex agglutination radioimmunoassay (RIA), and enzyme-linked immunosorbent assay (ELISA), and a VZV skin test has been widely and successfully used in Japan to distinguish between immune and susceptible individuals.[95] With all these assays, adequate controls are required to deal with the problem of heterotypic responses to infections by other herpesviruses.

TREATMENT

Antiviral Agents

Several nucleoside analogues—of which acyclovir, famciclovir, valaciclovir, and vidarabine are the best studied—and foscarnet (Fig. 216-11) as well as human interferon-α have shown efficacy in treating VZV infections.[96] Acyclovir is a guanosine analogue that is selectively phosphorylated by HSV and VZV thymidine kinases (it is a poor substrate for cellular thymidine kinase) and is thus concentrated in infected cells. Cellular enzymes then convert acyclovir monophosphate to acyclovir triphosphate, which interferes with viral DNA synthesis by inhibiting viral DNA polymerase. At therapeutic concentrations, acyclovir is remarkably nontoxic, with no observed effects on hematopoietic precursor cells or the immune system.

Two prodrugs, valaciclovir and famciclovir, have substantially greater oral bioavailability than acyclovir, producing higher blood levels and permitting less frequent dosing.[97–99] Valaciclovir is a valine ester of acyclovir that is converted enzymatically to acyclovir after absorption. Famciclovir is a prodrug of penciclovir, a nucleoside analogue similar to acyclovir in mechanism of action and

FIGURE 216-11

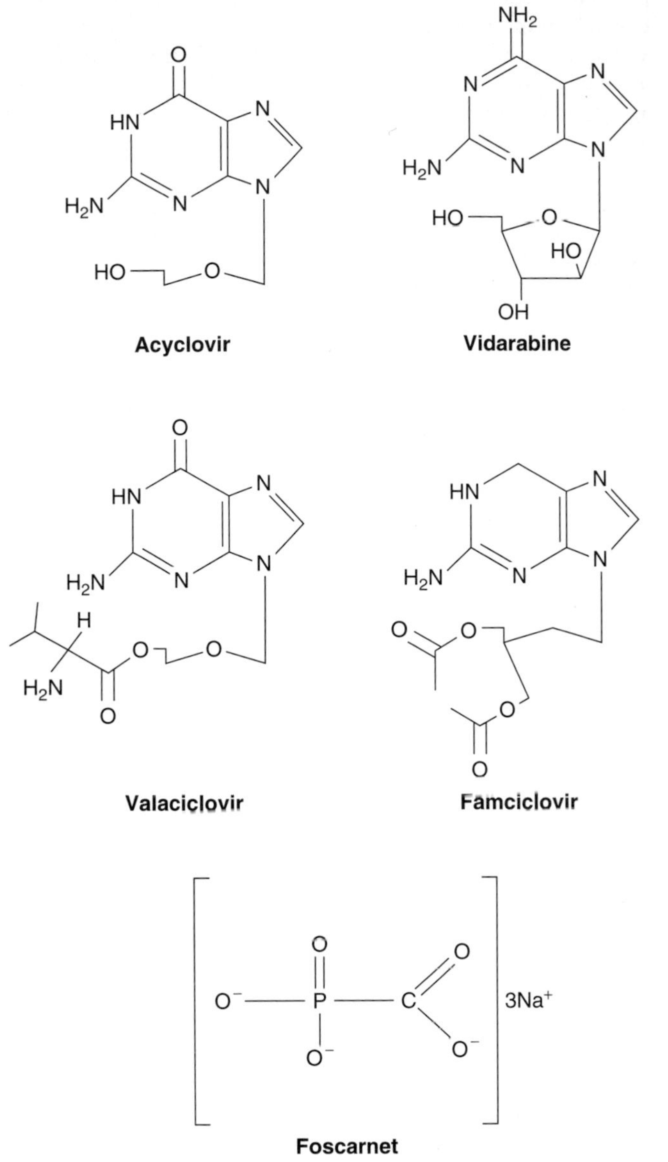

CHAPTER 216
Varicella and Herpes Zoster

2443

Acyclovir

Vidarabine

Valaciclovir

Famciclovir

Foscarnet

The chemical structures of five antiviral drugs proven effective in the treatment of varicella-zoster virus infections.

Foscarnet is an analogue of inorganic pyrophosphate that inhibits the replication of all known herpesviruses in vitro. It exerts its antiviral activity through selective inhibition at the pyrophosphate binding site of virus-specific DNA polymerases and reverse transcriptases at concentrations that do not affect cellular DNA polymerases.[4,5] Foscarnet does not require phosphorylation by thymidine kinase in order to be activated and therefore is active against VZV mutants that lack thymidine kinase activity and are resistant to acyclovir.

Leukocyte and recombinant human interferons have been studied as treatments of VZV infections in the immunocompromised host.[100,101] Their mechanism of action is postulated to include direct antiviral effects as well as augmentation of responses by immune effector cells such as NK cells. Although the interferons are active, their cost, toxicity, and inconvenience have virtually eliminated their use clinically for varicella and zoster.

Treatment of Varicella

In normal children, varicella is generally benign and self-limited. Cool compresses or calamine lotion locally and antihistamines orally may help control the intense pruritus of the rash. Tepid baths with baking soda or colloidal oatmeal (1/4 cup per tub of water) may also relieve itching. Creams and lotions containing glucocorticoids and occlusive ointments should not be used. Antipyretics may be needed, but salicylates must be avoided because of their association with Reye's syndrome.[63] Fingernails should be kept short and clean to minimize secondary skin infections and the scarring that may result from scratching. Other than the use of these practical and nonspecific approaches to uncomplicated varicella, the physician and patient (or parents) are confronted with the choice of whether or not to use acyclovir (Table 216-3). Recent studies of acyclovir treatment of healthy children 2 to 12 years of age found that early treatment (within 24 h of the appearance of rash) with oral acyclovir (20 mg/kg four times a day for 5 days) reduced the duration and severity of chickenpox and led to early defervescence.[102]

antiviral activity against VZV and HSV. Famciclovir is converted enzymatically to penciclovir after absorption, but the intracellular inhibitory concentrations of penciclovir triphosphate persist much longer than those of acyclovir triphosphate. When administered orally, both valaciclovir and famciclovir achieve plasma levels of antiviral activity previously achievable only with intravenously administered acyclovir.

Vidarabine, a purine nucleoside analogue, is phosphorylated by cellular kinases to vidarabine triphosphate, which appears to inhibit herpesvirus DNA polymerases to a greater extent than cellular DNA polymerases.[61,73] Despite its clinical efficacy, vidarabine has drawbacks. It is not a very selective inhibitor of virus replication (vidarabine triphosphate also inhibits cellular DNA polymerases) and thus is potentially cytotoxic. Its low solubility requires that it be administered in large volumes of fluid. Vidarabine is rarely used today.

TABLE 216-3

Treatment of Varicella in the Normal and Immunocompromised Patient

Patient Group	Regimen
Normal	
Neonate	Acyclovir 500 mg/m² q8h × 10 d
Child	Symptomatic treatment alone or acyclovir 20 mg/kg PO qid × 5 d
Adolescent, adult, or glucocorticoids used	Acyclovir 800 mg PO 5×/d × 7 d or valaciclovir or famciclovir
Pneumonia, pregnancy	Acyclovir 800 mg PO 5×/d × 7 d or acyclovir 10 mg/kg IV q8h × 7 d
Immunocompromised	
Mild varicella with mild compromise	Acyclovir 800 mg PO 5×/d × 7–10 d or valaciclovir or famciclovir
Severe varicella with severe compromise	Acyclovir 10 mg/kg IV q8h × 7 d or longer
Acyclovir-resistant (advanced AIDS)	Foscarnet 40 mg/kg IV q8h until healed

Similar but less robust data were obtained in studies of oral acyclovir (800 mg five times daily for 5 days) for treatment of varicella in normal adolescents.[103] Clearly, in children and adolescents, varicella is a relatively benign infection that does not require acyclovir treatment, but many have favored its use where cost is not a concern, where it can be begun in time to benefit the patient (less than 48 to 72 h of rash), and where there is a perceived need to speed resolution of the infection so that parents can comfortably return to work.

The decision regarding treatment of normal adults with varicella is easier. Because they have a relatively higher incidence of visceral involvement and varicella pneumonia, it is reasonable to think that this subset of patients may also benefit from acyclovir therapy. A recent randomized, placebo-controlled trial of oral acyclovir in healthy adults with primary varicella infections showed that early treatment (within 24 h of onset of cutaneous lesions) with oral acyclovir (800 mg five times a day for 7 days) significantly reduced time to crusting of lesions, extent of disease, duration of symptoms, and fever.[56] Thus, routine use in adults is appropriate. Although not tested, it is likely that valaciclovir 1000 mg PO q8h or pamciclovir 500 mg q8h would be convenient and appropriate substitutes for acyclovir in normal adolescents and adults.

Another subset of adults who might benefit from treatment of primary varicella infection is made up of pregnant women; however, data concerning treatment of primary varicella infections in pregnant women are currently unavailable, and treatment guidelines for VZV infections in these patients have not been established. The physician, in weighing the relative risks here, often opts for acyclovir, especially for infections in the third trimester (where organogenesis is complete, there may be a heightened risk of varicella pneumonia, and infection can be spread to the newborn).

Complications of varicella in normal persons are often due to bacterial superinfection. Bacterial infections of local lesions are treated with warm soaks. Systemic antimicrobial drugs are indicated for bacterial cellulitis, otitis media, sepsis, bacterial meningitis, osteomyelitis, septic arthritis, and bacterial pneumonia. The prominence of *Staphylococcus aureus* and group A beta-hemolytic *Streptococcus* as causes of these complications should be recognized, and the choice of antibiotics can be guided by the results of Gram-stained smears and cultures.

Varicella pneumonia usually responds to supportive measures, including positive-pressure ventilation. Nonetheless, antiviral chemotherapy should be used early to inhibit VZV replication. Recent uncontrolled studies of immunocompetent adults with varicella pneumonia demonstrated that early treatment (within 36 h of hospitalization) with intravenous acyclovir (10 mg/kg q 8 h) was useful in reducing fever and tachypnea and improved oxygenation in treated patients versus untreated ones.[55] Antibiotics are indicated only when bacterial superinfection develops. There is no evidence that glucocorticoids are beneficial in this setting, and their use is not recommended.

Reye's syndrome must be considered when a child with otherwise uncomplicated varicella develops lethargy, persistent vomiting, and confusion. Early diagnosis with supportive care and aggressive control of increased intracranial pressure and hypoglycemia should reduce the mortality and morbidity of this mysterious complication.

Varicella encephalitis, meningoencephalitis, and myelitis are very rare complications in normal people; however, the evidence that they are the result of CNS VZV infection rather than of some postinfectious autoimmune mechanism (see above) makes it rea-sonable to treat them with intravenous acyclovir, particularly when lesions are still present on the skin.

Hemorrhagic complications of varicella should be treated on the basis of the results of coagulation studies and bone marrow examination. It is always important to rule out bacterial sepsis. Because of the possible involvement of VZV-induced endothelial damage in purpura fulminans, especially if this complication occurs when new vesicles are continuing to appear, these patients should receive antiviral chemotherapy.

Varicella in immunocompromised children and adults may be severe and life-threatening. Thus, every effort should be made to prevent its occurrence (see "Prevention and Control," below). When this fails, antiviral therapy should be initiated as early in the process as possible and certainly before there is any clinical evidence of disseminated disease. If possible, cancer chemotherapy should be temporarily interrupted; however, treatment of malignancy should take precedence during induction of therapy for disease in relapse. When treatment is stopped, it should be resumed 21 days after exposure or 7 days after complete crusting of all lesions. Steroids should be tapered during the incubation period, and cytotoxic or other immunosuppressive therapy stopped if possible; however, patients who have received prolonged courses of glucocorticoids should continue to receive replacement therapy.

Intravenous acyclovir, intravenous vidarabine (10 mg/kg per day over 12 h for 5 days), and parenteral human interferon-α (3.5 $\times$ 10^5 U/kg per day for 2 days, then 1.75 $\times$ 10^5 U/kg per day for 3 days) have all been shown to decrease the incidence of life-threatening visceral complications when administered within 72 h of onset to immunosuppressed patients with varicella.[60,104] Acyclovir is at least as effective as vidarabine in patients with VZV infections but is free of vidarabine's toxicity and problems of fluid overload. Therefore, current treatment recommendations for primary varicella infection in an immunocompromised host are for intravenous acyclovir at a dose of 500 mg/m^2 in small children or 10 mg/kg for adolescents and adults every 8 h for 7 to 10 days. Treatment must be initiated early in the disease to be effective, and the dosage must be reduced in patients with renal insufficiency.

Immune compromise, after all, is a continuum ranging from minimal to severe. Intravenous acyclovir has been the standard of care for management of varicella in patients with substantive immunodeficiency. The question often arises as to whether high-dose oral acyclovir, or the newer nucleoside analogues, its prodrug valaciclovir, and famciclovir might suffice. While they usually suffice for patients with mild degrees of immune impairment, there are no formal data to guide the decision.

Treatment of Herpes Zoster

During the acute phase of herpes zoster, analgesics and the application of cool compresses, calamine lotion, cornstarch, or baking soda may help to alleviate local symptoms and hasten the drying of vesicular lesions. Occlusive ointments should be avoided, and creams and lotions containing glucocorticoids should not be used. After the acute phase, a bland ointment or olive oil dressings may help to soften and separate adherent crusts. Bacterial superinfection of local lesions is uncommon and should be treated with warm soaks; bacterial cellulitis requires systemic antibiotic therapy.

The major goals of therapy in patients with herpes zoster are to (1) limit the extent, duration, and severity of disease in the primary dermatome; (2) prevent disease elsewhere; and (3) prevent postherpetic neuralgia. Since the pathology in the primary dermatome, as well as that responsible for the visceral and CNS complications of herpes zoster, appears to be the consequence of VZV replication, the first two goals can be addressed by limiting replication and spread. If immunity is intact, herpes zoster is usually self-limited, and there is rarely consequential spread outside of the initially involved dermatome. In contrast, immunocompromised individuals, particularly those with deficiencies in cell-mediated immunity, have more severe and prolonged local disease and a much higher incidence of visceral and CNS complications. Obviously, it is these patients who have the most to gain from effective antiviral therapy.

Acyclovir has proved effective in the early treatment of acute herpes zoster, both in the normal host and in immunocompromised patients. Randomized double-blind, placebo-controlled trials in immunocompromised patients with acute herpes zoster showed that acyclovir (500 mg/m^2 intravenously q 8 h for 7 days) halted progression of herpes zoster, both in patients with localized disease and in those with cutaneous dissemination before treatment.[105] Acyclovir accelerated the rate of clearance of virus from vesicles and markedly reduced the incidence of visceral and progressive cutaneous dissemination. Pain subsided faster in acyclovir recipients, and fewer reported postherpetic neuralgia, but these differences were not statistically significant. No acyclovir toxicity was observed.

The efficacy of vidarabine in immunocompromised patients with acute herpes zoster was established in placebo-controlled studies.[73] Studies comparing intravenous acyclovir therapy with vidarabine therapy for the treatment of herpes zoster infections in immunocompromised patients showed that acyclovir was significantly more effective and less toxic.[82]

Human interferon-α (1.7 or 5.1 × 10^5 U/kg per day intramuscularly for 7 days) has also been shown to reduce new vesicle formation, cutaneous and visceral dissemination, and visceral and CNS complications.[101] Interferon also appears to reduce the incidence of postherpetic neuralgia. Although it was reasonably well tolerated in these trials, interferon appears to be somewhat more toxic, even, than vidarabine.

Immunocompromised patients with herpes zoster who have a deficient or delayed antibody response to VZV have an increased incidence of severe disease and dissemination. This led Stevens and Merigan to conduct a double-blind controlled therapeutic trial of zoster immune globulin (ZIG) in immunocompromised patients with herpes zoster.[106] Despite a much higher titer of antibody to VZV, ZIG did not appear to be superior to the normal immune serum globulin control in preventing dissemination or diminishing postherpetic neuralgia.

Current recommendations for treatment of zoster are listed in Table 216-4. The efficacy of intravenous acyclovir in normal adults with herpes zoster has been evaluated in small controlled trials.[107] Acyclovir (10 mg/kg or 500 mg/m^2 q 8 h for 5 days) shortened the period of virus shedding and of new vesicle formation, accelerated healing, and shortened the duration of pain during the acute phase of the disease; however, no effect on the incidence of postherpetic neuralgia was discerned. Thus, there is no apparent advantage to use intravenous acyclovir to treat uncomplicated herpes zoster in the normal host.

There have been numerous studies to determine the efficacy of oral acyclovir in the treatment of healthy adults with zoster.[50,108] Early studies revealed that doses of 200 or 400 mg orally five times daily were not sufficient. Multiple studies addressed the value of 800-mg doses five times daily, with somewhat conflicting results as regards the therapeutic effects on acute pain and postherpetic neuralgia. Studies of elderly patients treated with 800 mg orally five times a day for 10 days showed significant decreases in healing time, period of viral shedding, and acute pain versus untreated patients when therapy was initiated within 48 h of the appearance of vesicles. Variable effects on postherpetic neuralgia following oral acyclovir therapy have been observed. It is therefore recommended

TABLE 216-4

Treatment of Herpes Zoster in the Normal and Immunocompromised Patient

PATIENT GROUP	REGIMEN
Normal	
Age <50, uncomplicated	Symptomatic treatment only, or acyclovir 800 mg PO 5×/d × 7 d or valaciclovir or famciclovir
Age ≥50 or with ophthalmic involvement	Acyclovir 800 mg PO 5×/d × 7 d, or valaciclovir 1 g PO q8h × 7 d, or famciclovir 500 mg PO q8h × 7 d, and consider a tapering steroid regimen (see text)
Immunocompromised	
Mild compromise or HIV	Acyclovir 800 mg PO 5×/d × 7–10 d or valaciclovir or famciclovir
Severe compromise	Acyclovir 10 mg/kg IV q8h × 7–10 d
Acyclovir-resistant (advanced AIDS)	Foscarnet 40 mg/kg IV q8h until healed

that oral acyclovir therapy be given to healthy adults over the age of 50 with zoster within 48 h of the onset of vesicles. Because of the lower risk of postherpetic neuralgia, antiviral therapy is less valuable or necessary for treatment of uncomplicated zoster in healthy people under age 50. Certainly, there is little reason to consider it if more than 72 h have elapsed since the onset of rash.

Recent studies demonstrated that oral valaciclovir 1000 mg three times daily for 7 days and famciclovir 500 mg three times daily for 7 days are comparable if not superior to treatment with high-dose oral acyclovir five times daily, and with no appreciable toxicity.[97–99]

Topical treatment for zoster has also been attempted with limited success, and no data other than clinical anecdotes justify the use of any antiviral agents for topical treatment of zoster.

Postherpetic Neuralgia

Postherpetic neuralgia, once established, is difficult to treat.[49,50] Fortunately, it resolves spontaneously in most patients—within 3 months in about 50 percent and within a year in 75 percent or more (Fig. 216-1B). Nevertheless, a number of patients are left with persistent, often disabling, pain. Conventional analgesics and even narcotics should be tried but often fail. A wide range of therapies has been advocated, including epidural injection of local anesthetic and glucocorticoid, acupuncture, biofeedback, subcutaneous injections of triamcinolone, and systemic administration of a variety of compounds, but most have not been validated by controlled trials.

The typical dull, persistent, aching pain of postherpetic neuralgia will often respond to tricyclic antidepressants. Newer antidepressants of the serotonin reuptake inhibitor class are not useful. In controlled trials, both amitriptyline and desipramine provided excellent pain relief in about two-thirds of patients with postherpetic neuralgia.[109] These agents must be used with care because of their higher rates of moderate adverse reactions in the elderly. Carbamazepine may also be effective, especially for the lancinating pain that develops in some patients.

Capsaicin (*trans*-8-methyl-*N*-vanillyl-6-nonenamide), an extract of hot chili peppers, is a chemical known to deplete substance P—an important endogenous neuropeptide that acts as a chemomediator of nociceptive impulses from the periphery to the central nervous system. Substance P is found at high levels in sensory nerves supplying sites of chronic inflammation. A small clinical trial of topical capsaicin for 4 weeks in patients with postherpetic neuralgia demonstrated significant effects of this therapy on pain, with 75 percent of patients experiencing substantial pain relief.[110] Capsaicin is the only licensed compound for use in patients with postherpetic neuralgia. Unfortunately, the ointment burns too much to be tolerated by about one-third of subjects. The side effects of capsaicin truly preclude their analysis in any kind of masked fashion, so that the reports of its value must be viewed with a critical eye.

The possibility that postherpetic neuralgia may be caused by inflammation, necrosis, and subsequent scarring of the sensory ganglion and contiguous neural structures has provided the rationale for the use of glucocorticoids during the acute phase of herpes zoster in an attempt to prevent this complication. Two large, randomized, double-blind controlled trials of glucocorticoids for postherpetic neuralgia yielded potentially important but seemingly conflicting results.[111,112] Glucocorticoids afforded no advantage over acyclovir in preventing postherpetic neuralgia in either study, but prednisone alone or in combination with acyclovir sped resolution of acute pain and the impact of zoster on sleep and permitted a sooner return to work or useful activity in the critical early weeks of the infection. Since these studies are unlikely to be repeated, the physician must decide on the basis of current data. The two authors of this review are themselves divided on the issue. One of us believes that prednisone, 60 mg orally for 1 week, 30 mg daily for 1 week, and then 15 mg daily for a final week, together with high-dose oral acyclovir, valaciclovir, or famciclovir for 7 to 10 days is a reasonable regimen for otherwise healthy individuals over age 60 with the new onset of zoster ($\leq$72 h of rash), as long as there are no contraindications to the use of steroids (e.g., hypertension, diabetes, peptic ulcer disease, glaucoma). The other author feels that the potential risks of high-dose glucocorticoids outweigh any benefits they may provide early in the course of zoster.

The advice of an ophthalmologist should be sought in treating all patients with ophthalmic zoster. Therapy of ocular VZV infections is controversial. Mydriatics are used to prevent synechiae, and topical glucocorticoids are frequently recommended for keratitis and uveitis, although their efficacy is unproved.[70] Topical antiviral drugs [IUdR (5'-iodo-2-deoxyuridine), vidarabine, trifluridine] are also frequently recommended and should be included whenever glucocorticoids are used.

Antiviral Drug Resistance

Acyclovir-resistant varicella and zoster infections have been documented in patients with advanced AIDS[4,5,13] (Fig. 216-9). Because of the mechanism of resistance (mutations in the viral thymidine kinase gene), these infections are cross-resistant to ganciclovir, valaciclovir, famciclovir, and penciclovir. They do not respond well to vidarabine. Foscarnet, 40 mg intravenously every 8 h usually resolves the infections, but they commonly recur once treatment has ended.

PREVENTION AND CONTROL

Prevention and Control of Varicella

Varicella is almost always a benign disease in normal children. Because infection results in lifelong immunity, its acquisition in childhood eliminates the problem of varicella in the adult years. Therefore, no preventive measures are recommended for a normal child who has been exposed to varicella.

On the other hand, varicella is potentially fatal in susceptible patients with HIV disease, those undergoing immunosuppressive therapy, those with an immunosuppressive malignancy such as Hodgkin's disease, susceptible newborn infants, and even normal adults. Thus it is desirable to prevent or modify varicella in these high-risk individuals. Potential approaches include passive immunization, active immunization, chemoprophylaxis, and prevention of exposure.

Passive immunization with large doses (0.6 to 1.2 mL/kg) of standard human immune serum globulin (ISG) administered within 3 days of exposure to VZV attenuates but does not prevent varicella in normal children.[10] Passive immunization with zoster immune globulin (ZIG), prepared from the plasma of donors recovering from herpes zoster and containing a high titer of antibody to VZV prevents varicella in susceptible normal children when administered within 3 days of exposure and modifies the disease in immunosuppressed children.[11] One-third of the treated immunosuppressed recipients developed subclinical infection; the disease was mild in most of the others. Similarly, zoster immune plasma (ZIP), obtained from otherwise healthy individuals during convalescence from varicella or herpes zoster, has been shown to modify or prevent varicella in susceptible high-risk children when it is administered within 5 days of exposure.

In order to overcome the relative shortage of zoster convalescent plasma and ZIG for the growing population of immunosuppressed patients, Zaia et al. screened outdated blood from blood banks and used those units with high levels of antibody to VZV to prepare batches of immune globulin (VZIG) with antibody levels equivalent to those in ZIG. In a randomized double-blind trial of their capacity to protect immunosuppressed children from severe varicella, ZIG and VZIG proved comparable.[35] Standard preparations of pooled human immunoglobulins for intravenous administration (IVIG) are probably also acceptable. The incubation period is prolonged in immunoglobulin recipients who develop clinical disease. Recommended criteria for the use of VZIG and related products are listed in Table 216-5. Availability of serologic tests that permit the rapid identification of susceptible individuals and the increased availability of VZIG now make it possible to identify and passively immunize susceptible pregnant[114] and nonpregnant adults with recognized exposure to varicella.

Unfortunately, protection afforded by VZIG is transient, whereas most susceptible people will experience repeated exposures to VZV. Furthermore, exposure to VZV is often unrecognized; thus large numbers of immunocompromised patients will continue to develop unmodified varicella in spite of the availability of VZIG. Continuous prophylaxis by administration of VZIG on a monthly or bimonthly schedule is impractical; what is needed is a safe means of inducing long-lasting immunity to VZV in immunocompromised patients and susceptible adults.

Over two decades ago, Dr. Takahashi and his colleagues in Japan developed a live attenuated VZV vaccine (Oka strain) prepared by serial passage in human and guinea pig cell cultures of a strain of VZV isolated from a varicella vesicle. Despite concerns about its degree of attenuation, capacity to induce latent infections, and safety

TABLE 216-5

CHAPTER 216
Varicella and Herpes Zoster

2447

Criteria for the Use of Varicella-Zoster Immune Globulin (VZIG) for the Prophylaxis of Varicella*

1. Susceptible to varicella
   a. Children <15 years of age with no or unknown history of varicella or herpes zoster
   b. Bone marrow transplant recipients regardless of pretransplantation history of varicella or herpes zoster
   c. Immunocompromised adolescents and adults (≥15 years of age) with no or unknown history of varicella or herpes zoster
   d. Normal adolescents and adults (≥15 years of age) with no or unknown history of varicella or herpes zoster who lack antibody to VZV[†]
2. One of the following underlying illnesses or conditions
   a. Leukemia or lymphoma
   b. Congenital or acquired immunodeficiency
   c. Bone marrow transplant recipient regardless of pretransplantation history of varicella or herpes zoster
   d. Immunosuppressive treatment (including glucocorticoids)
   e. Newborn of mother who had onset of varicella within 5 days before delivery or within 48 h after delivery
   f. Premature infant (≤28 weeks gestation) whose mother lacks a history of varicella or herpes zoster
   g. Any infant ≤14 days of age whose mother lacks a history of varicella or herpes zoster
   h. Susceptible pregnant or nonpregnant adult[†]
3. One of the following types of exposure to person or persons with varicella or herpes zoster
   a. Continuous household contact
   b. Playmate contact (generally > 1 h play indoors)
   c. Hospital contact (in same two- to four-bed room or adjacent beds in a large ward or prolonged face-to-face contact with an infectious staff member or patient)
   d. Intrauterine contact (newborn of mother with onset of varicella 5 days or less before delivery or within 48 h after delivery)
4. Time elapsed after exposure is such that VZIG can be administered within 96 h of exposure (but preferably sooner)

*Patients should fulfill all four criteria.
[†]New serologic tests that permit the rapid identification of susceptible individuals and the increased availability of VZIG now make it possible to passively immunize susceptible pregnant and nonpregnant adults with recognized exposure to varicella. Immunologically normal adults with no history of varicella or herpes zoster are generally considered immune unless it is demonstrated that they lack serum antibody to VZV.[114]

in immunocompromised patients, it has been extensively evaluated and shown to induce high seroconversion rates after one or two administrations in healthy children.[115] Additionally, long-term immunity of recipients of the Oka strain of vaccine has been reported to persist 10 years after vaccination.[116] The vaccine induces a mild papular or papulovesicular rash and slight fever in a small minority of healthy children. Virus is rarely isolated from the rash in normal recipients, and there is no apparent transmission to contacts; however, in contrast to natural varicella, a few of these immunized normal persons have developed very mild varicella on subsequent exposure to VZV. The virus isolated from such patients is wild-type VZV. Herpes zoster has developed in less than 0.3 percent of normal childhood recipients of the vaccine.

When children with leukemia in remission and off chemotherapy are vaccinated, fewer than 10 percent develop a papular or papulovesicular rash, and most develop antibody and cell-mediated immunity to VZV.[117] When children on chemotherapy have it stopped for 1 week before and 1 week after vaccination, up to 40 percent develop rash. When vaccinated leukemic children are exposed to

VZV, most are protected and only 10 to 20 percent develop clinical varicella, which is generally mild. Leukemic vaccinees develop herpes zoster at a lower rate than leukemic patients with a history of natural varicella.[118] It is thought that the lower incidence of zoster in vaccinees may be related to the milder form of varicella that these patients develop, hence the fewer dermatomes affected by vaccine-strain virus or the decreased ability for latent vaccine-strain virus to reactivate. These observations indicate that the Oka VZV vaccine can be safely administered to susceptible immunosuppressed children and will help protect them from the morbidity and mortality that would otherwise result from subsequent exposures to varicella.

Even in normal individuals, the immunity induced by the vaccine is not as solid as that induced in wild-type VZV infection: this is particularly problematic in adults in whom two doses of vaccine are recommended. About 25 percent of vaccinees lost antibodies to VZV over time but continued to experience modified disease and showed partial protection against severe varicella.

The attenuated Oka VZV vaccine has been approved and recommended in the United States for universal childhood use together with or separate from measles, mumps, and rubella vaccine.[119] This represents a tremendous advance in our ability to cope with the problem of varicella.

Acyclovir has been tested and shown to be an effective chemoprophylactic in limiting household spread of varicella.[120] The timing is critical, immunity to varicella may not be achieved, and there are always fears that resistant strains will be selected by promiscuous applications of this approach. Hence it is not recommended.

There is no need to prevent exposure of susceptible normal children to VZV; patients with varicella need only be kept at home until all vesicles have crusted. On the other hand, rigid isolation should be enforced to prevent infection of susceptible immunocompromised patients and newborn infants. Contact with patients with varicella and herpes zoster, and with persons who may be incubating varicella, must be avoided. Exposure of susceptible compromised patients to VZV warrants reduction in the dosage of glucocorticoids to physiologic levels and the elimination or reduction of immunosuppressive drugs until their varicella has resolved or until it is clear that they have escaped infection. Such patients should receive VZIG immediately after exposure. Hospital personnel without a clear history of varicella or herpes zoster should be tested for antibody to VZV so that appropriate leave from work can be instituted following an exposure to VZV. Hospitals should develop and implement effective procedures, including vaccination campaigns to prevent nosocomial varicella. If such exposure occurs or is suspected, susceptible immunocompromised patients and newborn infants should receive prophylaxis with VZIG.

Prevention and Control of Herpes Zoster

Herpes zoster is a sporadic disease that results from reactivation of latent endogenous VZV rather than from exogenous infection. Thus, attempts at prophylaxis must be aimed at preventing the reactivation of endogenous VZV or inhibiting its subsequent replication and spread. One method is to use long-term suppressive acyclovir treatment. This is only practical in immunocompromised patients at proven risk of developing herpes zoster within a defined time frame, as in the year following bone marrow or solid organ transplantation.[121] For the more general population, other strategies are devised. Since the increased incidence and severity of herpes zoster observed in elderly persons appears to be associated with depressed immunity to VZV,[44] primarily depressed cell-mediated immunity, one approach to the prevention of herpes zoster is the stimulation of immunity to VZV in elderly and other high-risk individuals. Healthy adults over 60 years of age who have had zoster develop higher numbers of VZV-specific T lymphocytes after infection than age-matched controls. It is presumed that this increase in cell-specific immunity to VZV affords protection against additional episodes of zoster. Studies of healthy adults over 55 years of age with a history of previous primary VZV infection have demonstrated an increase in VZV-specific T lymphocyte and humoral immunity after vaccination that was similar to the increased immunity to VZV observed after an episode of zoster.[122] These findings suggest that vaccination of this subset of patients may be useful in preventing zoster infections and their complications; however, it remains to be seen whether immunization in such individuals will prove effective.

Patients with herpes zoster are infectious and may transmit varicella to susceptible individuals. Thus, susceptible high-risk patients should be protected from direct contact with individuals with localized herpes zoster. Respiratory isolation is required for patients with disseminated herpes zoster.

REFERENCES

1. Cohen JI, Straus SE: Varicella-zoster virus and its replication, in *Fields Virology,* edited by BN Fields et al. Philadelphia, Lippincott-Raven, 1996, p 2525
2. Arvin AM: Varicella-zoster virus, in *Fields Virology,* edited by BN Fields et al. Philadelphia, Lippincott-Raven, 1996, p 2547
3. Jura E et al: Varicella-zoster virus infections in children infected with human immunodeficiency virus. *Pediatr Infect Dis J* **8**:586, 1989
4. Jacobson MA et al: Acyclovir-resistant varicella zoster infection after chronic oral acyclovir therapy in patients with the acquired immunodeficiency syndrome (AIDS). *Ann Intern Med* **112**:187, 1990
5. Safrin S et al: Foscarnet therapy in five patients with AIDS and acyclovir-resistant varicella zoster virus infection. *Ann Intern Med* **115**:19, 1991
6. Choo PW et al: The epidemiology of varicella and its complications. *J Infect Dis* **172**:706, 1995
7. Gershon AA et al: Antibody to varicella-zoster virus in parturient women and their offspring during the first year of life. *Pediatrics* **58**:692, 1976
8. Gray GC et al: Increasing incidence of varicella hospitalizations in United States Army and Navy personnel: Are today's teenagers more susceptible? Should recruits be vaccinated? *Pediatrics* **86**:867, 1990
9. Preblud SR et al: Varicella: Clinical manifestations, epidemiology and health impact in children. *Pediatr Infect Dis* **3**:505, 1984
10. Ross AH: Modification of chicken pox in family contacts by administration of gamma globulin. *N Engl J Med* **267**:369, 1962
11. Orenstein W et al: Prophylaxis of varicella in high-risk children: Dose-response effect of zoster immune globulin. *J Pediatr* **98**:368, 1981
12. White CJ et al: Varicella vaccine (VARIVAX) in healthy children and adolescents: Results from clinical trials, 1987 to 1989. *Pediatrics* **87**:604, 1991
13. Leclair JM et al: Airborne transmission of chickenpox in a hospital. *N Engl J Med* **302**:450, 1980
14. Asano Y et al: Severity of viremia and clinical findings in children with varicella. *J Infect Dis* **161**:1095, 1990
15. Sawyer MH et al: Detection of varicella-zoster virus DNA in the oropharynx and blood of patients with varicella. *J Infect Dis* **166**:885, 1992
16. Arvin AM et al: Immunologic evidence of reinfection with varicella-zoster virus. *J Infect Dis* **148**:200, 1983
17. Gershon AA et al: Clinical reinfection with varicella-zoster virus. *J Infect Dis* **149**:137, 1984
18. Ljungman P et al: Clinical and subclinical reactivations of varicella-zoster virus in immunocompromised patients. *J Infect Dis* **153**:840, 1986
19. Ragozzino MW et al: Population-based study of herpes zoster and its sequelae. *Medicine (Baltimore)* **6**:310, 1982
20. Hope-Simpson RE: The nature of herpes zoster: A long-term study and a new hypothesis. *Proc R Soc Med* **58**:9, 1965
21. Kalman CM, Laskin OL: Herpes zoster and zosteriform herpes simplex infections in immunocompetent adults. *Am J Med* **81**:775, 1986
22. Ragozzino MW et al: Risk of cancer after herpes zoster: A population-based study. *N Engl J Med* **307**:393, 1982
23. Straus SE: Introduction to Herpesviridae, in *Principles and Practice of Infectious Diseases,* 4th ed, edited by GL Mandell et al. New York, Churchill Livingstone, 1995, p 1336
24. Straus SE et al: Varicella-zoster infections: Biology, natural history, treatment and prevention. *Ann Intern Med* **108**:221, 1988
25. Meier JL, Straus SE: Comparative biology of latent varicella-zoster virus and herpes simplex virus infections. *J Infect Dis* **116**:S13, 1992
26. Croen KD et al: Patterns of gene expression and sites of latency in human nerve ganglia are different for varicella-zoster and herpes simplex viruses. *Proc Natl Acad Sci USA* **85**:9773, 1988
27. Stevens JG et al: RNA complementary to a herpesvirus alpha gene mRNA is prominent in latently infected neurons. *Science* **235**:1056
28. Straus SE et al: Genome differences among varicella-zoster virus isolates. *J Gen Virol* **64**:1031, 1983
29. Myers MG, Connelly BL: Animal models of varicella. *J Infect Dis* **166**:S48, 1992
30. Cheatham WJ et al: Varicella: Report of two fatal cases with necropsy, virus isolation, and serologic studies. *Am J Pathol* **32**:1015, 1956
31. Koropchak CM et al: Investigation of varicella-zoster virus infection by polymerase chain reaction in immunocompetent host with acute varicella. *J Infect Dis* **163**:1016, 1991
32. Myers MG: Hepatic cellular injury during varicella. *Arch Dis Child* **57**:317, 1982
33. Brunell PA et al: Varicella-zoster immunoglobulins during varicella, latency, and zoster. *J Infect Dis* **132**:49, 1975
34. Arvin AM: Cell-mediated immunity to varicella-zoster virus. *J Infect Dis* **166**:S35, 1992
35. Zaia JA et al: Evaluation of varicella-zoster immune globulin: Protection of immunosuppressed children after exposure to varicella. *J Infect Dis* **147**:737, 1983
36. Wallace MR et al: Tumor necrosis factor, interleukin-2, and interferon-gamma in adult varicella. *J Med Virol* **43**:69, 1994
37. Bergen RE et al: Human T cells recognize multiple epitopes of a major tegument/immediate early protein (IE62) and glycoprotein I of varicella-zoster virus. *Viral Immunol* **4**:151, 1991
38. Biron CA et al: Severe herpesvirus infections in an adolescent without natural killer cells. *N Engl J Med* **320**:1731, 1989
39. Donahue JG et al: The incidence of herpes zoster. *Arch Intern Med* **155**:1605, 1995
40. Hardy IB et al: The incidence of zoster after immunization with live attenuated varicella vaccine: A study in children with leukemia. *N Engl J Med* **325**:1545, 1991
41. Mahalingam R et al: Localization of herpes simplex virus and varicella zoster virus DNA in human ganglia. *Ann Neurol* **31**:444, 1992
42. Lungu O et al: Reactivated and latent varicella-zoster virus in human dorsal root ganglia. *Proc Natl Acad Sci* **92**:10980, 1995
43. Cohrs RJ et al: Varicella-zoster virus (VZV) transcription during latency in human ganglia: Prevalence of VZV gene 21 transcripts in latently infected human ganglia. *J Virol* **69**:2674, 1995
44. Berger R et al: Decrease of the lymphoproliferative response to varicella zoster virus antigen in the aged. *Infect Immun* **32**:24, 1981
45. Brock BV et al: Frequency of asymptomatic shedding of herpes simplex virus in women with genital herpes. *JAMA* **263**:418, 1990
46. Gilden DH et al: Varicella-zoster virus reactivation without rash. *J Infect Dis* **166**(suppl 1):S30, 1992
47. Reboul F et al: Herpes zoster and varicella infections in children with Hodgkin's disease. *Cancer* **41**:95, 1978
48. Novelli VM et al: Herpes zoster in children with acute lymphocytic leukemia. *Am J Dis Child* **142**:71, 1988
49. Watson CPN ed: *Pain Research and Clinical Management:* Vol 8. *Herpes Zoster and Postherpetic Neuralgia.* New York, Elsevier, 1993
50. Kost RG, Straus SE: Postherpetic neuralgia—pathogenesis, treatment, and prevention. *N Engl J Med* **335**:32, 1996
51. Fleisher G et al: Life-threatening complications of varicella. *Am J Dis Child* **135**:896, 1981

52. Aebi C et al: Bacterial complications of primary varicella in children. *Clin Infect Dis* **23**:698, 1996

53. Centers for Disease Control and Prevention: Varicella-related deaths among adults—United States. *JAMA* **277**:1754, 1997

54. Triebwasser JH et al: Varicella pneumonia in adults. *Medicine (Baltimore)* **46**:409, 1967

55. Haake DA et al: Early treatment with acyclovir for varicella pneumonia in otherwise healthy adults: Retrospective controlled study and review. *Rev Infect Dis* **12**:788, 1990

56. Wallace MR et al: Treatment of adult varicella with oral acyclovir: A randomized, placebo-controlled study. *Ann Intern Med* **117**:358, 1992

57. Landsberger EJ et al: Successful management of varicella pneumonia complicating pregnancy: A report of three cases. *J Reprod Med* **31**:311, 1986

58. Paryani SG, Arvin AM: Intrauterine infection with varicella-zoster virus after maternal varicella. *N Engl J Med* **314**:1542, 1986

59. Enders G et al: Consequences of varicella and herpes zoster in pregnancy: Prospective study of 1739 cases. *Lancet* **343**:1548, 1994

60. Nyerges G et al: Acyclovir prevents dissemination of varicella in immunocompromised children. *J Infect Dis* **157**:309, 1988

61. Whitley RJ et al: Vidarabine therapy of varicella in immunosuppressed patients. *J Pediatr* **101**:125, 1982

62. Charles ND: Purpuric chickenpox: Report of a case, review of the literature, and classification by clinical features. *Ann Intern Med* **54**:745, 1961

63. Centers for Disease Control: Reye syndrome—United States, 1984. *MMWR* **34**:13, 1985

64. Liu GT, Urion DK: Pre-eruptive varicella encephalitis and cerebellar ataxia. *Pediatr Neurol* **8**:69, 1992

65. Puchhammer-Stöckl E et al: Detection of varicella-zoster DNA by polymerase chain reaction in the cerebrospinal fluid of patients suffering from neurological complications associated with chicken pox or herpes zoster. *J Clin Microbiol* **29**:1513, 1991

66. Adour KK: Current concepts in neurology: Diagnosis and management of facial paralysis. *N Engl J Med* **307**:348, 1982

67. Murakami S et al: Bell palsy and herpes simplex virus: Identification of viral DNA in endoneurial fluid and muscle. *Ann Intern Med* **124**:27, 1996

68. Brown GR: Herpes zoster: Correlation of age, sex, distribution, neuralgia, and associated disorders. *South Med J* **59**:576, 1976

69. Brunell PA et al: Zoster of children. *Am J Dis Child* **115**:432, 1968

70. Liesegang TJ: Diagnosis and therapy of herpes zoster ophthalmicus. *Ophthalmology* **98**:1216, 1991

71. Patterson SD et al: Atypical generalized zoster with lymphadenitis mimicking lymphoma. *N Engl J Med* **10**:848, 1980

72. Locksley RM et al: Infection with varicella-zoster virus after bone marrow transplantation. *J Infect Dis* **152**:1172, 1985

73. Whitley RJ et al: Early vidarabine therapy to control the complications of herpes zoster in immunosuppressed patients. *N Engl J Med* **307**:971, 1982

74. Holland GN: Standard diagnostic criteria for the acute retinal necrosis syndrome. *Am J Ophthalmol* **117**:663, 1994

75. Hope-Simpson RE: Postherpetic neuralgia. *J R Coll Gen Pract* **25**:571, 1975

76. Donahue JG et al: The incidence of herpes zoster. *Arch Intern Med* **155**:1605, 1995

77. Choo PW et al: Risk factors for postherpetic neuralgia. *Arch Intern Med* **157**:1217, 1997

78. Galil K et al: The sequelae of herpes zoster. *Arch Intern Med* **157**:1209, 1997

79. Jacobs A et al: Varicella-zoster-virus myelitis without herpes: An important differential diagnosis of the radicular syndrome. *Dtsch Med Wochenschr* **121**:331, 1996

80. Hilt DC et al: Herpes zoster ophthalmicus and delayed contralateral hemiparesis caused by cerebral angiitis: Diagnosis and management approaches. *Ann Neurol* **14**:543, 1983

81. Gilden DH et al: Varicella-zoster virus, a cause of waxing and waning vasculitis: The *New England Journal of Medicine* case 5-1995 revisited. *Neurology* **47**:1441, 1996

82. Whitley RJ et al: Disseminated herpes zoster in the immunocompromised host: A comparative trial of acyclovir and vidarabine *J Infect Dis* **165**:450, 1992

83. Engstrom RE et al: The progressive outer retinal necrosis syndrome. *Ophthalmology* **101**:1488, 1994

84. Gray F et al: Varicella-zoster virus infection of the central nervous system in the acquired immune deficiency syndrome. *Brain* **117**:987, 1994

85. Muraki R et al: Hair follicle involvement in herpes zoster: Pathway of viral spread from ganglia to skin. *Virchows Arch* **428**:275, 1996

86. Nikkels AF et al: Distribution of varicella-zoster virus gpI and gpII and corresponding genome sequences in the skin. *J Med Virol* **46**:91, 1995

87. Tsukahara T, Horiuchi Y: Immunohistochemical study of cellular events in lesional skin during common virus infections. *J Dermatol* **23**:22, 1996

88. Nikkels AF et al: Distribution of varicella-zoster virus and herpes simplex virus in disseminated fatal infections. *J Clin Pathol* **49**:243, 1996

89. Watson CPN, Deck JH: The neuropathology of herpes zoster with particular reference to postherpetic neuralgia and its pathogenesis, in *Herpes Zoster and Postherpetic Neuralgia,* edited by CPN Watson. New York, Elsevier, 1993, p 154

90. Folkers E et al: Rapid diagnosis in varicella and herpes zoster. Re-evaluation of direct smear (Tzanck test) and electron microscopy including colloidal gold immunoelectron microscopy in comparison with virus isolation. *Br J Dermatol* **121**:287, 1989

91. Cohen PR: Tests for detecting herpes simplex virus and varicella-zoster virus infections. *Dermatol Clin* **12**:51, 1994

92. Coffin SE, Hodinka RL: Utility of direct immunofluorescence and virus culture for detection of varicella-zoster virus in skin lesions. *J Clin Microbiol* **33**:2792, 1995

93. LaRussa P et al: Comparison of five assays for antibody to varicella-zoster virus to the fluorescent antibody to membrane antigen assay. *J Clin Microbiol* **25**:2059, 1987

94. Steinberg SP, Gershon AA: Measurement of antibodies to varicella-zoster virus by using a latex agglutination test. *J Clin Microbiol* **29**:1527, 1991

95. Steele RW et al: Varicella zoster in hospital personnel: Skin test reactivity to monitor susceptibility. *Pediatrics* **70**:604, 1982

96. Hirsch MS et al: Antiviral agents, in *Fields Virology,* 3d ed, edited by BN Fields et al. Philadelphia, Lippincott-Raven, 1996, 431

97. Beutner KR et al: Valaciclovir compared with acyclovir for improved therapy for herpes zoster in immunocompetent adults. *Antimicrob Agents Chemother* **39**:1546, 1995

98. Tyring S et al: Famciclovir for the treatment of acute herpes zoster: Effects on acute disease and postherpetic neuralgia: A randomized double-blind, placebo-controlled trial. *Ann Intern Med* **123**:89, 1995

99. deGreef H: Famciclovir, a new oral antiherpes drug: Results of the first controlled clinical study demonstrating its efficacy and safety in the treatment of uncomplicated herpes zoster in immunocompetent patients. *Int J Antimicrob Agents* **4**:241, 1995

100. Arvin AM et al: Human leukocyte interferon in the treatment of varicella in children with cancer. *N Engl J Med* **306**:761, 1982

101. Winston DJ et al: Recombinant interferon alpha-2a for treatment of herpes zoster in immunosuppressed patients with cancer. *Am J Med* **85**:147, 1988

102. Dunkle LM et al: A controlled trial of acyclovir for chickenpox in normal children. *N Engl J Med* **325**:1539, 1991

103. Balfour HH et al: Acyclovir treatment of varicella in otherwise healthy adolescents. *J Pediatr* **120**:627, 1992

104. Prober CG et al: Acyclovir therapy of chickenpox in immunosuppressed children—a collaborative study. *J Pediatr* **101**:622, 1982

105. Balfour HH Jr et al: Acyclovir halts progression of herpes zoster in immunocompromised patients. *N Engl J Med* **308**:1448, 1983

106. Stevens DA, Merigan TC: Zoster immune globulin prophylaxis of disseminated zoster in compromised hosts. *Arch Intern Med* **140**:52, 1980

107. Bean B et al: Acyclovir therapy for acute herpes zoster. *Lancet* **2**:118, 1982

108. McKendrick MW et al: Oral acyclovir in acute herpes zoster. *Br Med J* **293**:1529, 1986

109. Watson CPN et al: Amitriptyline versus maprotiline in postherpetic neuralgia: A randomized, double-blind crossover trial. *Pain* **48**:29, 1992

110. Bernstein JE et al: Treatment of chronic postherpetic neuralgia with topical capsaicin. *J Am Acad Dermatol* **17**:93, 1987

111. Wood MJ et al: A randomized trial of acyclovir for 7 days or 21 days with and without prednisolone for treatment of acute herpes zoster. *N Engl J Med* **330**:896, 1994

112. Whitley RJ et al: Acyclovir with and without prednisone for the treatment of herpes zoster: A randomized, placebo-controlled trial. The

National Institute of Allergy and Infectious Diseases Collaborative Antiviral Study Group. *Ann Intern Med* **125**:376, 1996

113. Kimberlin DW, Whitley RJ: Antiviral resistance mechanisms, clinical significance, and future implications. *J Antimicrob Chemother* **37**:403, 1996

114. *Report of Committee on Infectious Diseases, Varicella Zoster Infections,* 22d ed. Elk Grove Village, IL, American Academy of Pediatrics, 1991, p 517

115. Weibel RE et al: Live attenuated varicella virus vaccine: Efficacy trial in healthy children. *N Engl J Med* **310**:1410, 1984

116. Asano Y et al: Long-term protective immunity of recipients of the Oka strain of live varicella vaccine. *Pediatrics* **75**:667, 1985

117. Gershon AA, Steinberg SP, and the Varicella Vaccine Collaborative Study Group of the National Institute of Allergy and Infectious Diseases: Persistence of immunity to varicella in children with leukemia

immunized with live attenuated varicella vaccine. *N Engl J Med* **320**:892, 1989

118. Lawrence R et al: The risk of zoster after varicella vaccination in children with leukemia. *N Engl J Med* **318**:543, 1988

119. White CJ et al: Measles, mumps, rubella, and varicella combination vaccine: Safety and immunogenicity alone and in combination with other vaccines given to children. Measles, Mumps, Rubella, Varicella Vaccine Study Group. *Clin Infect Dis* **24**:925, 1997

120. Asano Y et al: Postexposure prophylaxis of varicella in family contact by oral acyclovir. *Pediatrics* **92**:219, 1993

121. Sempere A et al: Long-term acyclovir prophylaxis for prevention of varicella zoster virus infection after autologous blood stem cell transplantation in patients with acute leukemia. *Bone Marrow Transplant* **10**:495, 1992

122. Hayward AR et al: Varicella zoster virus-specific cytotoxicity following secondary immunization with live or killed vaccine. *Viral Immunol* **9**:241, 1996

CHAPTER 217

Kathryn E. Bowers

Cytomegalovirus Infection

In the developed countries, 40 to 80 percent of young adolescents have become infected by the ubiquitous cytomegalovirus (CMV). The gradual rise in the percentage of those seropositive for CMV in subsequent years is most often accounted for by sexual transmission. By old age, nearly everyone has been infected by the virus. After primary CMV infection, which is most often subclinical and asymptomatic, the virus persists in a lifelong latent stage with the omnipresent potential for reactivation. Symptomatic clinical infection in immunocompetent hosts is rare. Clinically apparent disease may manifest itself in neonates and in the immunosuppressed or immunocompromised host. With increasing numbers of organ transplant recipients and individuals infected with the human immunodeficiency virus HIV, the incidence of symptomatic CMV-associated morbidity and mortality has also increased. Unlike herpes simplex virus (HSV) and varicella-zoster virus (VZV) infections, CMV infection only rarely affects the skin.

CMV was first observed in kidney epithelial cells of a stillborn infant in 1881. Weller named the virus in 1960 based on its cytopathic effect.[1] The term *cytomegalic inclusion disease* was coined even before the virus was discovered, based on the large cells with intranuclear inclusions. This double-stranded DNA virus is a member of the Herpesviridae family, which includes HSV types 1 and 2, VZV, Epstein-Barr virus (EBV), and human herpesvirus 6, 7, and 8. The CMV genome is the most complex of all the DNA viruses and is 50 percent larger than that of herpes simplex. Like the other herpes viruses, CMV normally exists in certain tissues in a latent state after the primary infection. CMV can be isolated from urine, breast milk, semen, tears, feces, saliva, blood, cervical secretions, and lymphocytes in healthy persons. Human CMV cannot be readily grown in any experimental animal; many subtypes of CMV exist and are species specific.

EPIDEMIOLOGY

Humans are believed to be the only reservoir of human CMV. Transmission occurs throughout the year via intimate contact with body fluids such as saliva, cervical secretions, semen, breast milk, feces, and blood. Virus excretion may be prolonged in infected individuals, leading to an increased duration of exposure of seronegative individuals to the virus.

CMV seroprevalence varies considerably in different population groups throughout the world. Groups with a poor socioeconomic status have a higher rate of seropositivity, regardless of hygiene practices. In the United States, African Americans, Hispanics, and Native Americans acquire the infection at an earlier age than their Caucasian middle-class counterparts.

Two periods of increased risk for CMV infection occur: the perinatal period (36 to 56 percent of infants are exposed in the first year of life) and the reproductive years. Infants with CMV-seropositive mothers are exposed to the virus during passage through the birth canal and while breast feeding and, later, within their family and while at day care centers. Adolescents have an annual CMV seroconversion rate of 2 to 10 percent.

Primary CMV infection in adults after exposure to children in day care has been well documented. The annual seroconversion rate of seronegative day care workers is >10 percent.[2] As many as 80 percent of toddlers in day care centers have asymptomatic CMV infection with prolonged viral shedding through the urine, saliva, and respiratory tract.[3] Seroconversion of the adults is directly related to the rates of CMV excretion of the children at these centers. When a CMV-infected child returns home, 50 percent of the susceptible family members seroconvert within 6 months.

Sexual transmission in both heterosexual and homosexual populations is the predominant mode of transmission in adults. Outbreaks of CMV mononucleosis have been well documented in sexual partners in college communities. High titers of CMV have been found in semen and cervical specimens of healthy adults attending sexually transmitted disease clinics; a history of multiple sexual partners is the strongest predictor of infection. Eight to ten percent of women shed CMV from the cervix; an association exists between chronic cervicitis and CMV infection.

CMV is transmissible through sexual intercourse in homosexual men; CMV antibodies are present in 94 percent of homosexual men versus 54 percent of heterosexual controls.[4] Using Southern blot hybridization, multiple strains of CMV may be detected in homosexual men with AIDS, a phenomenon not ordinarily observed in a healthy population.[5] Thirty percent of asymptomatic homosexual men have CMV in their semen; CMV seroprevalence increases with age, number of sexual partners, and participation in anal-receptive intercourse. CMV is excreted for a more prolonged period in semen than urine. Reinfection with CMV through passive anal intercourse may account for the high degree of CMV and other infectious gastrointestinal diseases seen in HIV-positive patients. CMV seropositivity is common among African patients with AIDS, but the incidence in hemophiliacs parallels that in the normal population.

CMV was originally thought to be the etiologic agent for AIDS. African patients with Kaposi's sarcoma have an increased incidence of anti-CMV antibodies, and in homosexual men with Kaposi's sarcoma, CMV RNA and early antigens had been demonstrated. However, studies have linked human herpes virus 8 with this disorder.[6]

With an increasing number of heart, lung, kidney, and bone marrow transplant recipients and immunocompromised HIV-infected persons, CMV-associated morbidity and mortality are rising. These patients may become chronic carriers of CMV. The majority of CMV-related morbidity and mortality represents reactivation of the virus in the host; primary infection has been associated with more severe disease. Bone marrow transplant recipients have the highest incidence of CMV-related mortality.[7]

The risk of acquiring CMV from a unit of blood is estimated to be 3 to 4 percent, is highest with fresh blood, and is reduced with leukocyte-depleted or cryopreserved blood, as the leukocyte has been shown to be the vehicle for the transmission of CMV. The exact number of white blood cells needed for transmission is unknown.[8] Fresh frozen plasma does not transmit CMV infection. Infants, in whom primary CMV infection may cause high morbidity and mortality, require as little as 50 to 100 mL of a CMV-seropositive blood transfusion to become infected. CMV infection associated with cardiopulmonary bypass and infusion of a large volume of blood products, the so-called postperfusion syndrome, may develop in as many as 14 percent of patients. CMV-seronegative individuals in certain risk groups, i.e., pregnant women, premature infants, bone marrow recipients, and HIV-infected persons, should be identified and transfused with only CMV-seronegative or specially treated blood products.

CMV has a predilection for all portions of gastrointestinal mucosa, and serious enteric CMV infections may occur in transplant recipients. The virus has been found in the crypts and inflamed mucosa of the gastrointestinal tract of patients with ulcerative colitis.[9] Golden et al.[10] reviewed four cases of gastrointestinal vasculitis secondary to CMV; two of the patients were HIV-positive.

CMV may play a role in atherogenesis. CMV and HSV antigens have been found in arterial smooth muscle cells, where they may induce an inflammatory reaction, proliferation of smooth muscle cells, and accumulation of cholesterol. Heart transplant recipients who develop CMV infection are at higher risk of developing severe coronary artery disease in the transplanted organ.[11]

Nucleic acid sequences specific for CMV have been found localized to the pancreatic Langerhans cells of patients with type 2 diabetes mellitus. CMV antigens have also been detected in peripheral blood monocytes of patients with diabetes; persistent infection may be a factor in the pathogenesis of type 1 diabetes mellitus.[12]

CUTANEOUS MANIFESTATIONS OF CMV INFECTION

Cutaneous lesions associated with CMV are rare and nonspecific. Underlying disorders associated with CMV cutaneous involvement include HIV disease, malignant neoplasms, burns, and iatrogenic immunosuppression occurring with organ transplantation. Most reported patients with cutaneous CMV have evidence of disseminated infection; all patients who died have had either concurrent systemic CMV infection, other overwhelming infections, or systemic diseases.[13]

Multiple morphologic patterns from vesicles to verrucous plaques have been described in the reported cases of cutaneous CMV (Table 217-1). Urticarial and morbilliform eruptions are reported more frequently in healthy patients who have a CMV mononucleosis-like syndrome and have received recent antibiotic therapy

TABLE 217-1

Cutaneous Manifestations of Cytomegalovirus

Papules[14,15]
Verrucous plaques/nodules[16–20]
Vesicles[21–24]
Epidermolysis[25]
Purpura[22,26–29]
Petechiae[27,30–32]
TORCH syndrome[33]
Cutaneous ulcerations[34–40]
Oral ulcerations[41,42]
Pyoderma[18]
Morbilliform rash[18,24,31,38,43]
Urticaria[44]
Granulation tissue/burns[45]
Dermatitis, diaper[46]
Erythema nodosum[47]

NOTE: TORCH, *t*oxoplasmosis, *o*ther (syphilis/bacterial sepsis), *r*ubella, *c*ytomegalovirus, *h*erpes simplex virus.

such as ampicillin. The finding of CMV-induced cytopathic changes in lesional skin biopsies probably indicates widespread tissue infection and does not necessarily mean that the CMV infection is the cause of the cutaneous change (Fig. 217-1).

The most specific cutaneous manifestation of CMV, present in 30 percent of the reported cases of cutaneous CMV,[13] is ulceration, especially in the perianal area. Ulcerations on the buttocks, perineum, and thigh with visceral involvement have also been well described. Horn and Hood[40] demonstrated histologic and immunohistochemical evidence of CMV infection in five consecutive patients with immunosuppression and perineal ulcers. Clinically, these ulcers resembled a chronic herpetic infection. The authors hypothesized that CMV may be a direct cause of the ulcer or evidence of a subclinical infection or it may reflect disseminated CMV infection.

Multiple organisms, including *Staphylococcus aureus* and acid-fast bacilli, as well as HSV, may be found in association with CMV in skin biopsies. Smith et al.[19] reported two patients with concurrent epidermal involvement with both CMV and HSV, documented by both immunohistochemical and DNA hybridization studies, in two HIV-infected patients. Two reported cases have been associated with disseminated intravascular coagulation.[32,38]

FIGURE 217-1

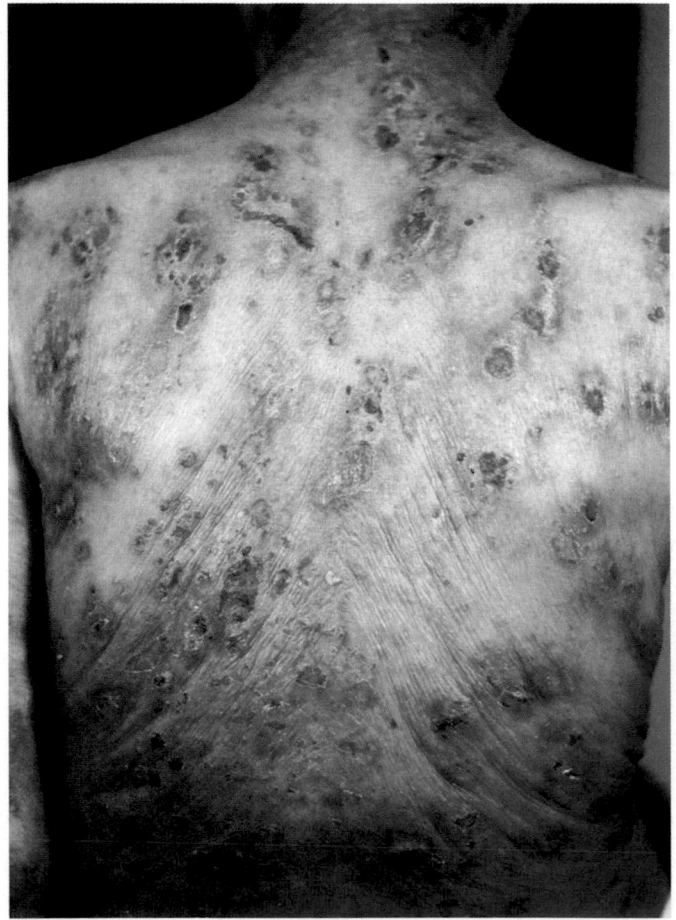

Papules and nodules on the back of a patient with Hodgkin's disease and disseminated CMV. (*From Sugiura,*[17] *with permission.*)

In summary, cutaneous manifestations of CMV infection are usually not distinctive enough to confirm the diagnosis. In contrast to the healthy host, in whom the disease is usually asymptomatic, the immunocompromised host may present with mononucleosis, pneumonitis, hepatitis, encephalitis, gastroenteritis, choreoretinitis, or a cutaneous eruption.

CMV Infection in Pregnancy

Approximately 2 percent of CMV-seronegative pregnant women develop an asymptomatic primary CMV infection during pregnancy. A mononucleosis-like syndrome with a rubelliform or morbilliform rash has been reported. The two principal sources of CMV infection for women of child-bearing age are sexual intercourse and exposure to young children attending day care centers. Intrauterine infection occurs in 55 percent of fetuses whose mothers have a primary CMV infection. Congenital CMV infection is more common in infants of young, single, primigravida mothers who also have other sexually transmitted diseases such as gonorrhea.[48]

Congenital CMV Infection

Primary maternal CMV infection during the first 24 weeks of gestation carries the highest risk of permanent sequelae for the fetus. Infants born of mothers who were infected in the first trimester may be small for gestational age and may have microcephaly, intracranial calcifications, retinitis, and optic nerve malformations (coloboma). Infants infected in later trimesters may have acute visceral disease with hepatitis, pneumonia, purpura, and disseminated intravascular coagulation.

CMV is the major infectious cause of mental retardation and deafness in the United States. CMV infection, part of the TORCH syndrome [*t*oxoplasmosis, *o*ther (syphilis/bacterial sepsis), *r*ubella, *c*ytomegalovirus, *h*erpes simplex virus], is the most common congenital viral infection. One percent of infants born in the United States become infected with CMV in utero and may shed virus in saliva and urine for up to 5 years, although fewer than 10 percent of infected infants have clinical manifestations of the virus. Sixty-five percent of infants with symptomatic CMV infections experience long-term sensorineural hearing loss, mental retardation, learning disabilities, and seizures. The infant mortality rate of congenital CMV infection is 20 to 30 percent; hydrocephalus and intracranial calcification are poor prognostic signs. Demonstration of these on a cranial CT scan is a strong predictor of adverse neurologic outcomes; clinical and laboratory evaluations are poor predictors alone.[49] Involvement of the central nervous system, inner ear, and the choroid of the eye are unique to congenital CMV infection.

The diseases that comprise the TORCH syndrome may each have a similar clinical picture including hepatomegaly, splenomegaly, microcephaly, deafness, chorioretinitis, thrombocytopenia, jaundice, and purpura. The "blueberry muffin baby" has purpuric macules and papules, manifestations of persistent dermal hematopoiesis (Fig. 217-2). The persistence of these blood-forming elements may be the result of tissue hypoxia, chronic anemia, or a direct or indirect effect of the virus on the vascular mesenchyme. These dark blue to violaceous, raised or flat, purpuric lesions present within 24 to 48 h of birth, resolve with a copper color, and are present in 31 percent of infants with the TORCH syndrome.[50]

Recovery of CMV from the urine, throat, or other body fluids during the first week of life is the ideal method for diagnosis since serologic tests are inaccurate because of maternal antibodies and the small amount of IgM produced by the infant. A positive viral culture during the first 3 weeks of life indicates congenital CMV infection.

FIGURE 217-2

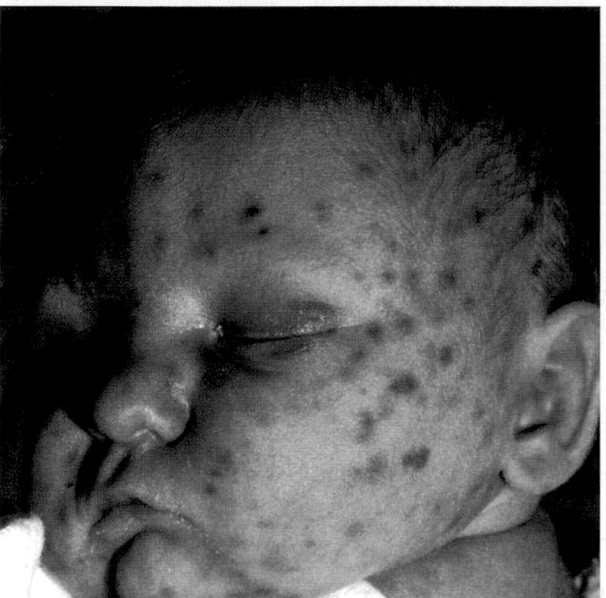

Infant with congenital CMV infection: "blueberry muffin baby." (*From Groark and Jampel,*[33] *with permission.*)

FIGURE 217-3

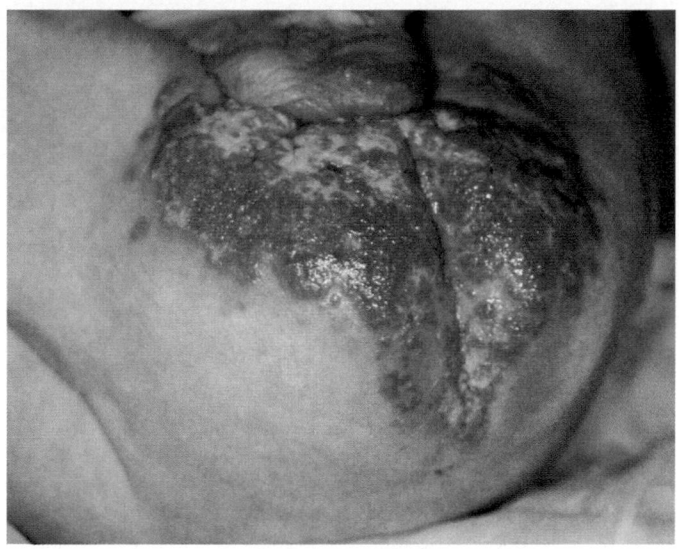

Infant with AIDS and diaper dermatitis secondary to disseminated CMV. (*From Thiboutot et al.,*[46] *with permission.*)

CMV Infection in Children

Acquisition of CMV is common during the first year of life, usually from the infant's mother. Ten to fifteen percent of healthy term infants may be exposed to CMV through the birth canal or from breast milk, but they rarely develop symptomatic CMV infection. Infants who acquire the virus during the perinatal period begin to shed the virus at 4 to 8 weeks and for up to 2.5 years. Preterm or low-birth-weight infants are at greater risk for developing signs and symptoms of infection with CMV and may develop a mononucleosis-like syndrome. Outbreaks of CMV infection have occurred in neonatal intensive care units in high-risk seronegative infants.

Papular acrodermatitis of childhood (Gianotti-Crosti syndrome) is associated with many viral illnesses such as enterovirus, hepatitis B, adenovirus, and CMV. CMV hepatitis may accompany this syndrome, as described by Berant et al.[51]

Viral or bacterial illness may precede the development of scleredema. A preceding CMV illness may have contributed to the development of scleredema in an infant with CMV viruria and pneumonia described by Heilbron and Saxe.[52]

Helm et al.[53] described an infant with disseminated CMV in the KID syndrome (*k*eratitis, *i*chthyosis, and *d*eafness). Multiorgan involvement with CMV inclusions and a lower esophageal ulcer was documented at autopsy. Children with KID syndrome have problems with recurrent bacterial and yeast infections secondary to defective T cell immunity.

A dramatic case of ulcerative perianal diaper dermatitis heralded systemic CMV infection in an infant with AIDS described by Thiboutot et al.[46] The diaper area was covered with vesicles, pustules, and bullae on an erythematous base (Fig. 217-3). Disseminated infection involving the blood, urine, lung, and eyes was subsequently diagnosed. The infant died within 1 month of the diagnosis, despite treatment with ganciclovir.

CMV Infection in Healthy Adults

Most individuals eventually become infected with CMV; primary infection is usually subclinical and asymptomatic. A mononucleosis-like syndrome may develop in healthy adults, usually in an older group than those susceptible to EBV-associated mononucleosis. Women in the third decade are most commonly affected. CMV mononucleosis may also be caused by blood and leukocyte transfusions.

CMV mononucleosis often poses an initial diagnostic problem. The most common presenting signs and symptoms are fever, abnormal liver function tests, a negative heterophile antibody test, and blood smears with an atypical lymphocytosis indistinguishable from that of EBV infectious mononucleosis. These patients tend to have less severe pharyngitis, lymphadenopathy, and splenomegaly than EBV-infected patients. A short-lived rubelliform type rash, lasting from several hours to days, occurs predominantly on the lower extremities, although it may be generalized in 31 percent of patients. This eruption occurs in the majority of patients treated with ampicillin or amoxicillin during the initial phase of the illness; the identical phenomenon occurs in EBV mononucleosis.

Immunologic abnormalities, such as the presence of mixed cryoglobulins, cold agglutinins, rheumatoid factor, and antinuclear antibodies, are observed with both CMV and EBV infection. Although the prognosis is usually excellent, complications of CMV mononucleosis include thrombocytopenia, granulomatous hepatitis, pneumonitis, hemolytic anemia, meningoencephalitis, myocarditis, vasculitis, and the Guillain-Barré syndrome. Spear et al.[47] reported a case of an adult patient with acute CMV mononucleosis and erythema nodosum without viral inclusions in the skin biopsy.

CMV Infection in Immunocompromised Individuals

Prolonged parenteral glucocorticoid therapy alone has a minimal effect on reactivation of CMV. The incidence of CMV reactivation and symptomatic infection is significantly increased in patients with neoplasia, especially lymphoma and leukemia, and in transplant recipients (see below). Patients receiving chemotherapy experience an increase of primary CMV infection, both subclinical and symptomatic. Systemic manifestations of CMV infection include a mononucleosis-like syndrome, pneumonitis, hepatitis, gastroenteritis or gastrointestinal ulcerations, and chorioretinitis. Neutropenia alone does not appear to be an independent risk factor for developing CMV disease.

CMV Infection in HIV-Infected Individuals

The clinical picture of CMV infection is likely to change with the recent introduction of protease inhibitors and triple-drug antiviral therapy. Reactivated latent CMV infection is exceedingly common in HIV-infected individuals. CMV affects more organs in HIV patients than in the transplant population. From 30 to 40 percent of patients with AIDS will develop serious CMV infections, usually when the peripheral CD4 count is less than 100. Concurrent CMV infection may potentiate the immunosuppressive effects of HIV, enhancing HIV replication at the cellular level by transactivation. Dissemination of CMV is associated with fever, wasting, and inanition. A catabolic state in the patient with AIDS can be reversed with therapy for CMV, suggesting that CMV may contribute significantly to the pathology of the overall disease state.

CMV may cause inflammation of the gastrointestinal mucosa with symptoms of esophagitis, colitis, pancreatitis, and cholecystitis. Other pathogens such as *Mycobacterium avium-intracellulare* and *Cryptosporidia* may be cultured as copathogens. The colon is most frequently involved, followed by the esophagus, rectum, and small bowel.

CMV causes five distinct neurologic syndromes in HIV-infected patients: retinitis, myelitis/polyradiculopathy, encephalitis with dementia, ventriculoencephalitis, and mononeuritis multiplex.[54] CMV retinitis occurs in 30 percent of patients with AIDS in the United States and may cause blindness if untreated. Patients with CMV retinitis are usually viremic and have symptoms of decreased visual acuity and multiple spots interfering with vision. The characteristic retinal findings are yellow-white exudates and hemorrhages at the periphery of the fundus, described as resembling "crumbled cheese with ketchup." Viral replication occurs at a very high level, and numerous virions may be detected in the retina by electron microscopy. Ganciclovir and foscarnet are effective in the treatment of CMV retinitis, but therapy must be continued indefinitely because lesions recur if the drug is discontinued. Despite therapy, retinal detachment may occur and is related to extensive viral-induced retinal necrosis.

CMV Infection in Transplant Recipients

Transplanted bone marrow, kidney, heart, lung, and liver are often reservoirs of CMV and may infect the host with a new strain of CMV or cause a primary infection in the seronegative host. Iatrogenic immunosuppression is the most important cause of CMV reactivation; it does not prevent development of an antibody response to the CMV, except in the presence of severe infection. Cyclosporine use is a low risk factor for reactivation but, once it occurs, cyclosporine cripples the host response.

Half of renal transplant recipients experience CMV disease, which is responsible for 25 percent of the deaths in these patients, 20 percent of graft failures, 30 percent of febrile episodes, and 35 percent of leukopenic episodes. A distinct glomerulopathy may occur with renal dysfunction. Fortunately, symptomatic disease occurs 3 to 4 months after transplantation, when immunosuppressive drug doses are being decreased. Fever may be the only manifestation of active CMV infection, although leukopenia, thrombocytopenia, pneumonitis, hepatitis, retinitis, and encephalitis may also occur.

The risk of developing significant CMV-induced disease in solid organ transplant recipients occurs between weeks 4 and 12 after transplantation. CMV disease is associated with a fourfold increase in the relative risk for death within 1 year after transplantation. The highest risk is a CMV-seronegative patient who receives a CMV-seropositive organ.[55] In heart and lung transplant recipients, gastrointestinal disease (gastritis, esophagitis, perforation, and hemorrhage) is the most prominent manifestation of CMV; the overall frequency of severe CMV disease and CMV mycocarditis is higher in this group than in those who receive other organ transplants. CMV hepatitis is a more common complication of liver transplants and is often difficult to distinguish from organ rejection, other than by liver biopsy, in that both are associated with fever and elevated liver function tests. CMV may play a role in hepatic allograft rejection.

CMV-seropositive bone marrow transplant recipients have a higher incidence of subsequent CMV disease related to reactivation of latent virus. Donor marrow and blood product transfusion are important sources of CMV infection in seronegative transplant patients. The major morbidity from CMV disease occurs during the first 40 days after transplantation, before engraftment and resumption of immune function. CMV pneumonia is the most frequent cause of CMV-related morbidity in bone marrow transplant recipients, with a mortality rate approaching 85 percent.[56] The interstitial pneumonia may be an immunopathologic process mediated by a specific T cell response to CMV antigens, enhanced by graft-versus-host disease. Combined therapy with ganciclovir and immune globulin has improved survival in these patients. The CMV virus may also be responsible for a delay in the immunologic recovery of bone marrow transplant patients, with secondary effects on the immune system including leukopenia, decreased cell-mediated immunity with increased risk of other opportunistic infections, and altered macrophage function. The risk of superinfection is directly related to the degree of leukopenia (<3000 leukocytes/μL), decrease in CD4 cell counts, and increase in CD8 cell counts.

DIAGNOSIS

Prompt diagnosis of disseminated CMV is important because of the availability of specific and effective antiviral agents. CMV infection is often asymptomatic and must be distinguished from viral shedding. Cutaneous infection with CMV has a characteristic histopathologic morphology, with preferential involvement of endothelial and ductal cells much more commonly than of epithelium. The characteristic "owl's eyes" basophilic intranuclear inclusion is good evidence of CMV infection (Fig. 217-4). However, there is a false-negative rate of at least 12 percent with light microscopy alone.

Infection can be confirmed by viral culture techniques, traditionally from the urine, blood, and throat. Viremia, diagnosed by buffy-coat cultures, is one of the best indicators of active systemic CMV infection. However, asymptomatic viremia and viruria may occur, especially in patients with advanced HIV disease. CMV grows slowly, and only in fibroblast culture, compared with other herpesviruses, which grow rapidly in both fibroblast and epithelial (amnion) cell cultures. CMV-induced cytopathic effects in conven-

FIGURE 217-4

CHAPTER 217
Cytomegalovirus Infection   2455

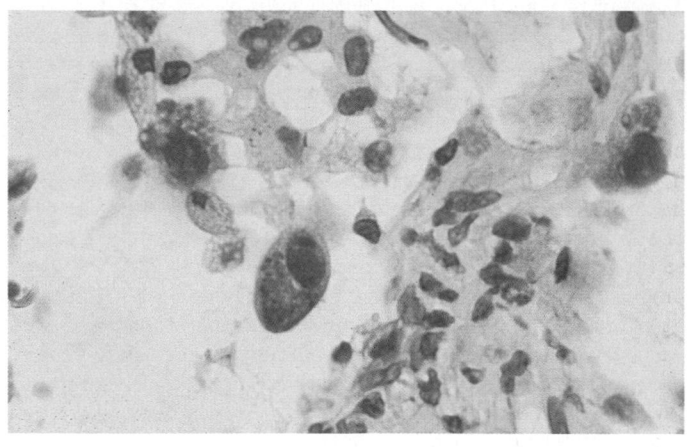

Intranuclear inclusions in a cell infected by CMV. (*From Konstadt et al.,*[30] *with permission.*)

tional cultures are noted within 1 to 2 weeks, although they may be delayed for as long as 6 weeks if viral titers are low. CMV cultured from a skin biopsy specimen indicates the presence of virus either in the tissue itself or in the circulating blood.

Viremia is present long before an anti-CMV IgM immune response. The presence of IgM antibodies indicates infection within the past 12 to 16 weeks; IgM antibodies detected by enzyme-linked immunosorbent assay (ELISA) can occur with primary infection and as a result of reactivation and exogenous reinfection. CMV seroconversion or a fourfold rise in IgG antibody titers in the sera of an acutely ill patient compared with convalescent sera indicates active CMV infection. Both maternal and infant sera should be evaluated in order to diagnose a congenital infection. Antibody production may be decreased in the presence of overwhelming infection.

On histology and electron microscopy, HSV and VZV have only intranuclear inclusions, whereas CMV may have both intranuclear and intracytoplasmic inclusions. Immunohistochemical and immunoperoxidase testing with CMV-specific monoclonal antibodies is rapid, generally available, and may be used on tissue or fluid samples. Early CMV antigens are detectable within hours on flat monolayers of centrifuged samples using monoclonal antibodies. A biotin-labeled CMV probe used for in situ DNA hybridization has little cross-reactivity with the other herpesviruses and can be tested on formaldehyde-fixed or paraffin-embedded samples. Polymerase chain reaction (PCR) may become the "gold standard" for detecting CMV. When PCR is positive, quantitative measures of the CMV-DNA load can be performed on positive leukocytes.[57]

DIFFERENTIAL DIAGNOSIS

CMV infection should be included in the differential diagnosis of an immunosuppressed patient with fever and a generalized or unexplained localized rash, especially if cutaneous ulceration occurs. Because of the multiple case reports of HSV coexisting with CMV, the possibility of an associated HSV or VZV infection must be considered in chronic ulcers and diagnosed by viral culture, immunohistochemistry, or DNA in situ hybridization.

The differential diagnosis of a neonate with purpuric macules and papules should include CMV, the other TORCH infectious agents, lymphoma, leukemia, neuroblastoma with cutaneous metastases, twin transfusion syndrome, hereditary spherocytosis, neonatal systemic lupus erythematosus, and neonatal sepsis.

DERMATOPATHOLOGY

The diagnosis of CMV infection by histologic findings alone is not always possible since the typical CMV-associated inclusions may be subtle and relatively sparse even in highly infected tissues. The typical cytomegalic cell is characterized by the following features: a diameter of 20 to 40 μm; large intranuclear inclusion(s); a clear halo around the nuclear inclusion; a rim of nuclear material; and cytoplasmic inclusions which appear as granular, PAS-positive, perinuclear structures.

The intranuclear inclusions are identical to those seen in HSV or VZV infections, although those occurring with CMV may be larger. The characteristic "owl's eyes" intranuclear inclusion (see Fig. 217-4) indicates CMV infection and often persists for some time. Intraepithelial involvement by CMV occurs in the kidney, lung, salivary gland, gastrointestinal tract, and rarely the skin. CMV usually infects endothelial cells; involvement of the vascular endothelium is specific for disseminated CMV infection. Myerson et al.[58] postulated that the commonly multifocal nature of CMV infection is due to hematogenous dissemination with local spread via infection of the endothelial cells. CMV usually also infects ductal structures and sweat glands.

In three patients with AIDS, CMV was unexpectedly found in biopsy specimens of clinically normal skin. Clinically occult CMV probably occurs more commonly than recognized and may be only an incidental finding in the immunocompromised patient.[59] However, it is important to search for active visceral involvement, especially in the lungs and eyes, if there is evidence of CMV on a skin biopsy specimen in an immunocompromised patient.

PATHOGENESIS

Some strains of CMV are more virulent than others in vivo. The virus infects the vascular endothelium, resulting in an exanthem. As involvement of the vessels increases, vasculitis occurs and the destruction of blood vessels causes secondary ulceration. A prominent neutrophilic perivascular infiltrate may be observed around CMV-infected vessels. Endothelial cells have the ability to phagocytose the virus. The polymorphonuclear leukocyte is the main source of CMV in the blood. Cells that carry latent infection may be present in many organs, and circulating white blood cells or stromal cells may be the source of infection in transplant patients. An oncogenic potential of the virus has been demonstrated in vitro.

Beta$_2$-microglobulin, present in most body fluids, has a high binding affinity for CMV and protects it against immune destruction. CMV also binds nonspecifically to the Fc receptor of immunoglobulins, and that binding provides the virus with another immune protective coat. The finding that lymphocyte proliferative responses to mitogens and viral antigens are decreased in the presence of CMV provides evidence for an immunosuppressive role of CMV in the host.

The most potent reactivator of CMV is exogenous immunosuppressive therapy. Cell-mediated immunity and the activity of cytotoxic T cells are of prime importance in determining the outcome and severity of CMV infection. CMV suppresses functioning of cytotoxic T cells, with decreased CD4 cells and increased CD8 cells leading to an overall depression in cell-mediated immunity. Macrophage phagocytosis and presentation are disrupted, especially in the lung, and immune mediators such as interferon-α are decreased. Natural killer cells and cytotoxic T cells are important not only for recovery from a CMV infection but also for surveillance and prevention of viral reactivation.

CMV encodes for glycoproteins that are homologous to class I major histocompatibility complex (MHC) antigens and causes upregulation of class II MHC antigens in transplanted grafts, which may play a role in allograft rejection. In heart transplant recipients, CMV is associated with early allograft rejection and an increased incidence of graft atherosclerosis. The virus may directly mediate injury to the vascular endothelium with secondary lipid deposition.

Humoral immunity can modify the degree of infection, for example, in newborns who acquire a perinatal CMV infection but have circulating maternal CMV antibodies. The administration of CMV immune globulin decreases the incidence of CMV illness in seronegative transplant recipients.

COURSE AND PROGNOSIS

Early diagnosis and treatment of disseminated CMV may lead to a successful outcome. The treatment of CMV retinitis has been successful with ganciclovir and phosphonoformate (foscarnet), although therapy must be continued for life. The response rates of other manifestations of CMV infection are difficult to assess because of the sporadic case reports and the presence of coinfecting agents. Patients with cutaneous CMV have a very poor prognosis, with a mortality rate that approximates 85 percent within 6 months, although most of these cases were reported before the general use of improved antiviral agents.[13]

TREATMENT

High-dose acyclovir can be used effectively as prophylaxis against CMV infection, although it is ineffective against active viral disease. Ganciclovir is a nucleoside analogue of acyclovir that differs by one hydroxyl side chain. Unlike acyclovir, ganciclovir does not require viral thymidine kinase for phosphorylation and activation. Ganciclovir is 50 times more effective than acyclovir in vitro against CMV and inhibits viral DNA polymerase.

Eighty-five percent of patients with CMV retinitis respond within 2 weeks of therapy with ganciclovir. One-third of patients with AIDS must discontinue therapy because of drug-related adverse side effects such as neutropenia, thrombocytopenia, and central nervous system changes. Significant hematologic toxicity may occur with combination therapy with ganciclovir and zidovudine. Either oral, introcular, or systemic therapy must be continued on a long-term basis since ganciclovir is virostatic and not virocidal. Ganciclovir implants are effective in preventing progression of the

retinitis but are not protective for the contralateral eye. Patients with CMV retinitis will usually relapse within 1 month after discontinuation of therapy. Prophylactic ganciclovir has been used successfully in bone marrow transplant patients to prevent CMV interstitial pneumonia. Ganciclovir-resistant strains of CMV have been reported in as many as 7 percent of patients treated longer than 3 months. PCR techniques are being used to detect specific protein kinase mutations in CMV DNA that confer ganciclovir resistance.[60]

Trisodium phosphonoformate (foscarnet) inhibits DNA polymerase of human herpesviruses and also the reverse transcriptase of HIV in vitro. This drug works at a different site than acyclovir and may be used for acyclovir-resistant HSV and VZV. A more prolonged long-term survival of patients with CMV retinitis has been reported with phosphonoformate treatment compared with ganciclovir treatment.[61] The dose-limiting side effects are nephrotoxicity, transient hypocalcemia, and anemia without neutropenia. A case of a bone marrow transplant patient has been reported in whom three strains of CMV were isolated, one of which was resistant to both ganciclovir and phosphonoformate.[62]

Cidofovir (HPMPC), a potent anti-CMV phosphated nucleoside analogue, has been approved for systemic and implant therapy for CMV retinitis.[63] Saline hydration and high-dose probenecid are required to prevent irreversible nephrotoxicity; iritis, neutropenia, and peripheral neuropathy are other side effects. Clinical isolates resistant to ganciclovir, secondary to a mutation of DNA polymerase, may also be resistant to cidofovir.[64]

Researchers have developed several live attenuated vaccines against CMV for at-risk individuals such as young adults and transplant candidates.[65] Immunity wanes rapidly and there is a theoretical concern regarding the oncogenic potential of a live CMV vaccine. In the future, combination therapy with less toxic antiviral drugs, immunomodulators, and prevention strategies may hold promise in decreasing the morbidity and mortality of severe CMV infections in at-risk groups.

REFERENCES

1. Weller TH et al: Serologic differentiation of viruses responsible for cytomegalic inclusion disease. *Virology* **12**:130, 1960
2. Adler SP: Cytomegalovirus and child day care: Evidence for an increased infection rate among day-care workers. *N Engl J Med* **321**:1290, 1989
3. Murph JR et al: The occupational risk of CMV infection among day care workers. *JAMA* **265**:603, 1991
4. Jacobson MA, Mills J: Serious cytomegalovirus disease in the acquired immunodeficiency syndrome. *Ann Intern Med* **108**:585, 1988
5. Spector SA et al: Identification of multiple CMV strains in homosexual males with AIDS. *J Infect Dis* **150**:953, 1984
6. Chang Y et al: Identification of herpes virus like DNA sequences in AIDS-associated Kaposi's sarcoma. *Science* **266**:1865, 1994
7. Winston DJ et al: Cytomegalovirus infections after allogeneic bone marrow transplantation. *Rev Infect Dis* **12**:S776, 1990
8. Owden RA: Transfusion-transmitted cytomegalovirus infection. *Hematol Oncol Clin North Am* **9**:155, 1995
9. Diepersloot RJA et al: Acute ulcerative proctocolitis associated with primary cytomegalovirus infection. *Arch Intern Med* **150**:1749, 1990
10. Golden MP et al: Cytomegalovirus vasculitis. Case reports and review of the literature. *Medicine* **73**:246, 1994
11. Melnick JL et al: Possible role of cytomegalovirus in atherogenesis. *JAMA* **263**:2204, 1990
12. Lohr JM, Oldstone MBA: Detection of cytomegalovirus nucleic acid sequences in pancreas in type 2 diabetes. *Lancet* **336**:644, 1990
13. Toome BT et al: Diagnosis of cytomegalovirus infection: A review and report of a case. *J Am Acad Dermatol* **24**:857, 1991
14. Kwan TH, Kaufman HW: Acid-fast bacilli with cytomegalovirus and herpes inclusions in the skin of an AIDS patient. *Am J Clin Pathol* **85**:236, 1986
15. Boudreau S et al: Dermal abscesses with *Staphylococcus aureus*, cytomegalovirus and acid fast bacilli in a patient with AIDS. *J Cutan Pathol* **15**:53, 1988

16. Fenoglio CM et al: Kaposi's sarcoma following chemotherapy for testicular cancer in a homosexual man: Demonstration of cytomegalovirus RNA in sarcoma cells. *Hum Pathol* **15**:53, 1982

17. Sugiura H: Successful treatment of disseminated cutaneous cytomegalic inclusion disease with Hodgkin's disease. *J Am Acad Dermatol* **24**:346, 1991

18. Bournerias I et al: Unusual cutaneous cytomegalovirus involvement in patients with acquired immunodeficiency syndrome. *Arch Dermatol* **24**:346, 1989

19. Smith KJ et al: Concurrent epidermal involvement of cytomegalovirus and herpes simplex virus in two HIV-infected patients. *J Am Acad Dermatol* **25**:500, 1991

20. Chiewchanvit S et al: Disseminated cutaneous cytomegalic inclusion diseases resembling prurigo nodules in a HIV-infected patient: A case report and literature review. *J Med Assoc Thai* **76**:581, 1993

21. Blatt J et al: Cutaneous vesicles in congenital cytomegalovirus infection. *J Pediatr* **92**:509, 1978

22. Bhawan J et al: Vesiculobullous lesions caused by cytomegalovirus infection in an immunocompromised adult. *J Am Acad Dermatol* **11**:743, 1984

23. Feldman PS et al: Cutaneous lesions heralding disseminated cytomegalovirus infection. *J Am Acad Dermatol* **7**:545, 1982

24. Lee JY: Cytomegalovirus infection involving the skin in immunocompromised hosts. *Am J Clin Pathol* **92**:96, 1989

25. Muller-Stamou A et al: Epidermolysis in a case of severe cytomegalovirus infection. *Br Med J* **7**:609, 1974

26. Symers WS: Generalized cytomegalic inclusion body disease associated with *Pneumocystis* pneumonia in adults. *J Clin Pathol* **13**:1, 1960

27. Sandler A, Snedeker JD: Cytomegalovirus infection in an infant presenting with cutaneous vasculitis. *Pediatr Infect Dis J* **6**:422, 1987

28. Bamji A, Salisbury R: Cytomegalovirus and vasculitis. *Br Med J* **1**:623, 1978

29. Elenitsas R, Cohen BA: Cutaneous cytomegalovirus in a liver transplant patient. *Transplant Proc* **20**:656, 1988

30. Konstadt JW et al: Disseminated cytomegalovirus infection with cutaneous involvement in a heart transplant patient. *Clin Cases Dermatol* **2**:2, 1990

31. Robson GS, Mackay IR: Generalized cytomegalovirus infection in a patient with lupoid hepatitis. *Aust Ann Med* **18**:147, 1969

32. Tawfik N, Jimbow K: Acute graft-vs-host disease in an immunodeficient newborn possibly due to cytomegalovirus infection. *Arch Dermatol* **125**:1685, 1989

33. Groark SP, Jampel RM: Violaceous papules and macules in a newborn. *Arch Dermatol* **125**:113, 1989

34. Willliams G et al: Cytomegalic inclusion disease and *Pneumocystis* infection in an adult. *Lancet* **2**:951, 1960

35. Minars N et al: Fatal cytomegalic inclusion disease. *Arch Dermatol* **113**:1569, 1977

36. Walker JD, Chesney TM: Cytomegalovirus infection of the skin. *Am J Dermatopathol* **4**:263, 1982

37. Naroneczna I, Kay S: Fatal disseminated cytomegalic inclusion disease in an adult presenting with a lesion of the gastrointestinal tract. *Am J Clin Pathol* **47**:124, 1967

38. Pariser RJ: Histologically specific skin lesions in disseminated cytomegalovirus infection. *J Am Acad Dermatol* **9**:937, 1983

39. Patterson JW et al: Cutaneous CMV infection in a liver transplant patient: Diagnosis by in situ DNA hybridization. *Am J Dermatopathol* **10**:524, 1988

40. Horn TD, Hood AF: Cytomegalovirus is predictably present in perineal ulcers from immunocompromised patients. *Arch Dermatol* **126**:642, 1990

41. Jones AC et al: Cytomegalovirus infections of the oral cavity. A report of six cases and review of the literature. *Oral Surg Oral Med Oral Pathol* **75**:76, 1993

42. Firth NA et al: Oral mucosal ulceration due to cytomegalovirus associated with human immunodeficiency virus infection. Case report and brief review. *Aust Dent J* **39**:273, 1994

43. Lin CS et al: Cytomegalic inclusion disease of the skin. *Arch Dermatol* **10**:524, 1981

44. Humphreys DM, Myers A: Cytomegalovirus mononucleosis with urticaria. *Postgrad Med J* **51**:404, 1975

45. Swanson S, Feldman PS: Cytomegalovirus infection initially diagnosed by skin biopsy. *Am J Clin Pathol* **15**:113, 1987

46. Thiboutot DM et al: Cytomegalovirus diaper dermatitis. *Arch Dermatol* **127**:396, 1991

47. Spear JB et al: Erythema nodosum associated with acute cytomegalovirus mononucleosis in an adult. *Arch Intern Med* **148**:323, 1988

48. Fowler KB, Pass RF: Sexually transmitted disease in mothers of neonates with congenital cytomegalovirus infection. *J Infect Dis* **164**:269, 1990

49. Boppana SB et al: Neuroradiographic findings in the newborn period and long term outcome in children with symptomatic congenital cytomegalovirus infection. *Pediatrics* **99**:409, 1997

50. TORCH syndrome and TORCH screening. *Lancet* **335**:1559, 1990

51. Berant M et al: Papular acrodermatitis with cytomegalovirus hepatitis. *Arch Dis Child* **58**:1024, 1983

52. Heilbron B, Saxe N: Scleredema in an infant. *Arch Dermatol* **122**:1417, 1986

53. Helm K et al: Systemic cytomegalovirus in a patient with the keratitis, ichthyosis and deafness (KID) syndrome. *Pediatr Dermatol* **7**:54, 1990

54. Mcutchan JA: Clinical impact of cytomegalovirus infections of the nervous system in patients with AIDS. *Clin Infect Dis* **21**:S196, 1995

55. Falagas ME et al: Effect of cytomegalovirus infection status on first year mortality rates among orthotopic liver transplant recipients. The Boston Center for Liver Transplantation CMVIG Study Group. *Ann Intern Med* **126**: 275, 1997

56. Schmidt GM et al: A randomized, controlled trial of prophylactic ganciclovir for cytomegalovirus pulmonary infection in recipients of allogeneic bone marrow transplants. *N Engl J Med* **324**:1005, 1991

57. Ehrnst A: The clinical relevance of different laboratory tests in CMV diagnosis. *Scand J Infect Dis Suppl* **100**:64, 1996

58. Myerson D et al: Widespread evidence of histologically occult cytomegalovirus. *Hum Pathol* **15**:430, 1984

59. Horn TD, Hood AF: Clinically occult cytomegalovirus present in skin biopsy specimens in immunosuppressed hosts. *J Am Acad Dermatol* **21**:781, 1989

60. Spector SA et al: Molecular detection of human cytomegalovirus and determination of genotypic ganciclovir resistance in clinical specimens. *Clin Infect Dis* **21**:S170, 1995

61. Jabs DA et al: Mortality in patients with AIDS treated with either foscarnet or ganciclovir for cytomegalovirus retinitis. *N Engl J Med* **326**:213, 1992

62. Knox KK et al: Cytomegalovirus isolate resistant to ganciclovir and foscarnet from a bone marrow transplant patient. *Lancet* **337**:1292, 1991

63. Rahhal FM et al: Treatment of cytomegalovirus retinitis with intravitreous cidofovir in patients with AIDS. *Ann Intern Med* **125**:98, 1996

64. Jacobson MA: Treatment of cytomegalovirus retinitis in patients with the acquired immunodeficiency syndrome. *N Engl J Med* **337**:105, 1997

65. Plotkin SA: Multicenter trial of Towne strain attenuated virus vaccine in seronegative renal transplant recipients. *Transplantation* **58**:1176, 1994

CHAPTER 218

Jeffrey I. Cohen

Epstein-Barr Virus Infections

Epstein-Barr virus (EBV) is the etiologic agent of infectious mononucleosis and is associated with oral hairy leukoplakia and B cell lymphoma in patients with AIDS or acquired immunodeficiencies. EBV is also associated with malignancies including Burkitt's lymphoma, nasopharyngeal carcinoma, Hodgkin's disease, and certain T cell lymphomas.

In 1964, Epstein, Barr, and Achong described the presence of herpesvirus-like particles in Burkitt's lymphoma tissue.[1] In 1968, the Henles reported that EBV was the causative agent of infectious mononucleosis.[2] EBV DNA was demonstrated in biopsy tissues from patients with Burkitt's lymphoma and nasopharyngeal carcinoma in 1970,[3] in AIDS patients with B cell lymphomas in 1982,[4] and in Reed-Sternberg cells from patients with certain subtypes of Hodgkin's disease in 1989.[5]

EPIDEMIOLOGY

Infection with EBV is usually asymptomatic or presents with nonspecific symptoms in infants and young children. In contrast, infection of adolescents and young adults often results in infectious mononucleosis. While most individuals, especially those in developing countries, are infected at a young age and have few symptoms, persons from higher socioeconomic classes are less likely to have been infected during childhood and therefore are more likely to manifest primary EBV infection as infectious mononucleosis.[6] Most adults in the United States are seropositive for EBV by age 25 and are no longer susceptible to reinfection.

EBV is usually spread by contact with salivary secretions from asymptomatic persons shedding the virus. The incubation period of infectious mononucleosis is estimated to be 30 to 50 days. Transmission has been documented from blood transfusion or bone marrow transplantation. EBV can be isolated from saliva of asymptomatic seropositive individuals in 15 to 20 percent of attempts. Higher rates of shedding are seen in immunocompromised patients[7] and in those with infectious mononucleosis.[8]

ETIOLOGY AND PATHOGENESIS

EBV is a member of the herpesvirus family.[9] The receptor for EBV (CD21) is present on B cells and epithelial cells. Infection of epithelial cells results in replication of the virus, lysis of the cell, and release of infectious virus. Infection of B cells in vitro results in transformation and immortalization of the cells. These infected B cells are latently infected and usually do not produce infectious virus.

Humans become infected with EBV from oral secretions. The virus infects epithelial cells in the oropharynx,[10] and B lymphocytes that traffic through the oropharynx become infected either by direct contact with EBV-containing oral secretions or by contact with infected epithelial cells. The infected B cells proliferate and are controlled by an expansion of reactive T cells resulting in enlargement of lymphoid tissues and the symptoms of infectious mononucleosis. Following acute infection, EBV persists for life as a latent infection of B cells. These EBV-infected B cells remain low in number due to continued T cell surveillance. In the setting of cellular immune deficiency disorders, the EBV-infected B cells proliferate and may become clinically significant once again.

CLINICAL MANIFESTATIONS

Infectious mononucleosis is associated with the triad of fever, sore throat, and lymphadenopathy.[11] Erythema of the pharynx occurs in 85 percent of cases, and 20 percent of patients have a grayish-white pharyngeal exudate. Pharyngitis may be accompanied by tonsillar enlargement and may be associated with streptococcal infection. Other frequent signs and symptoms include malaise, headache, anorexia, myalgias, chills, splenomegaly, and hepatomegaly. Less common findings are nausea, abdominal pain, jaundice, and rash. Infectious mononucleosis is usually self-limited and symptomatic for 2 to 4 weeks; however, malaise and fatigue can persist for months. Infrequent complications of infectious mononucleosis include autoimmune hemolytic anemia, thrombocytopenia, upper airway obstruction due to hypertrophy of lymphoid tissue, hepatitis, meningitis, encephalitis, myocarditis, and rupture of the spleen.

Laboratory findings in infectious mononucleosis include lymphocytosis that peaks during the second or third week of illness and ≥10 percent atypical lymphocytes. The atypical lymphocytes are vacuolated with a large cytoplasm. They may have indentations in the cytoplasmic membrane and are predominantly EBV-specific reactive T cells. Neutropenia, thrombocytopenia, and elevated levels of transaminases and alkaline phosphatase are frequent findings during the first month of illness.

Infection with cytomegalovirus, toxoplasmosis, HIV-1, or hepatitis viruses can also produce the symptoms of infectious mononucleosis.

Very rare individuals develop chronic active EBV infection with persistent lymphadenopathy, hepatosplenomegaly, and infiltration of the lungs, eyes, or central nervous system with EBV-infected B cells.[12] EBV-associated lymphoproliferative disease, which presents with fever, lymphadenopathy, and lymphocytic infiltration of tissues, is seen in patients with congenital or acquired immunodeficiency, including transplant recipients and patients with AIDS.[13] The X-linked lymphoproliferative syndrome is a disease of young boys who usually succumb to acute infection with EBV.

DERMATOLOGIC FINDINGS

Infectious Mononucleosis

A morbilliform or papular rash, usually on the arms or trunk, is present in 5 to 15 percent of cases of infectious mononucleosis.[14–16] The rash is more common in young children, is usually present during the first week of the illness, and may persist until the second week. The rash can have atypical features including a vesicular or scarlatiniform eruption, urticaria, or petechiae.

The vast majority (70 to 100 percent) of patients with infectious mononucleosis treated with ampicillin develop a macular and papular eruption (Figs. 218-1 and 218-2).[17] A similar process has been reported with amoxicillin but is less frequent in patients treated with other beta-lactam antibiotics, including penicillin and cloxacillin.[18] The eruption usually begins as erythematous or copper-colored lesions 5 to 10 days after beginning the antibiotic and starts on the trunk and spreads to the face and extremities as it becomes generalized. It may be associated with pruritus and usually resolves within 1 week. The eruption associated with ampicillin differs somewhat from that seen in patients not treated with the antibiotic in that the former usually appears later, is more severe and longer in duration, and more often involves the palms and soles.[17] It can be associated with other features of hypersensitivity reactions such as arthralgia, edema of the face and extremities, and diarrhea.[19] The eruption is not predictive of future positive skin tests or adverse reactions to ampicillin or penicillin.[20]

The etiology of the eruption is thought to be due to formation of antibodies associated with the polyclonal B cell proliferation that occurs with EBV infection, with subsequent immune complex formation and activation of complement. Circulating immune complexes composed of immunoglobulins (IgG, IgA, IgM), complement components (C3, C4, C5), EBV capsid antibody, and viral particles were associated with urticaria in one patient and became undetectable during recovery.[21] Skin reactions (consisting of a wheal ≥3 mm) to ampicillin were detected in two-thirds of patients with infectious mononucleosis, independent of prior ampicillin therapy.[22] Increased levels of serum antibodies (IgG, IgM) reacting to ampicillin were detected in the serum of patients with infectious mononucleosis whether or not they had been treated with the antibiotic. The presence of these antibodies may be important in immune complex formation resulting in an Arthus reaction in the walls of small arterioles.[23]

Urticaria has been reported in 5 percent of patients during the acute stage of infectious mononucleosis in the absence of antibiotic therapy or prior history of allergy.[24,25] Cold-induced urticaria associated with cryoglobulinemia has also been seen during infectious mononucleosis in the absence of ampicillin therapy.[26,27] Cold-induced acrocyanosis, associated with cold agglutinating antibodies to the I and M antigens on red blood cells, was reported in a patient with infectious mononucleosis.[28] Cryoglobulinemia with vasculitis of the small vessels of the skin was noted in one patient.[29]

Case reports of other skin lesions including isolated palmar papules,[30] erythema nodosum,[31] and erythema multiforme[32] have also been reported. Painful, bluish-black genital ulcers have been

FIGURE 218-1

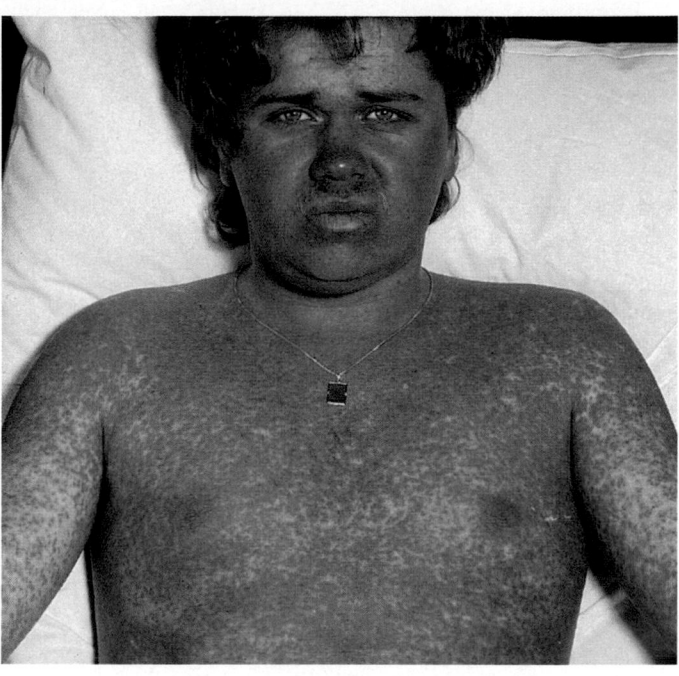

Generalized ampicillin exanthem in a patient with infectious mononucleosis. (*Courtesy of Helmut Hinton, MD, University of Innsbruck.*)

FIGURE 218-2

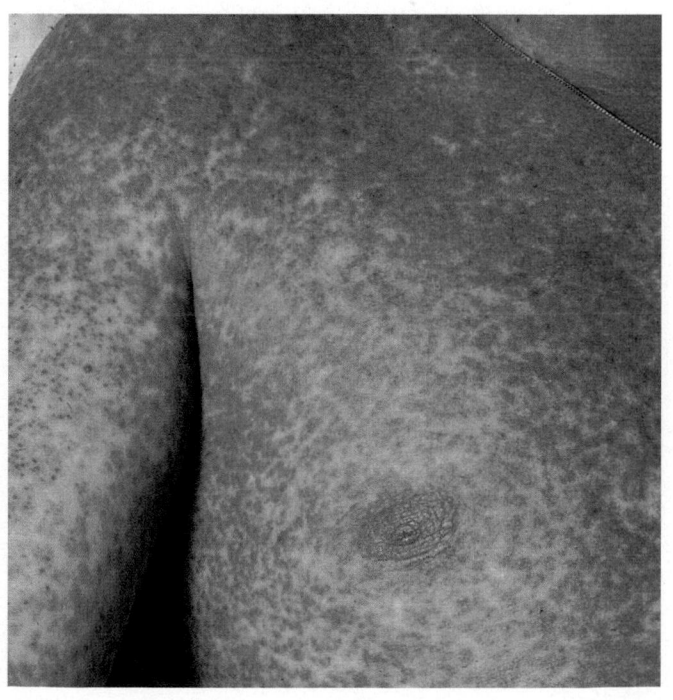

Closeup of ampicillin rash shown in Fig. 218-1. (*Courtesy of Helmut Hinton, MD, University of Innsbruck.*)

reported in patients with acute EBV infection, and EBV was isolated from the ulcers in one case.[33,34]

Periorbital edema is present in 2 to 35 percent of patients with infectious mononucleosis, and palatal enanthem in 3 to 13 percent of cases. The enanthem consists of multiple 0.5 to 1 mm erythematous petechiae, located between the hard and soft palate that can coalesce to form larger lesions.[35,36]

Oral Hairy Leukoplakia

Oral hairy leukoplakia is a nonmalignant hyperplasia of epithelial cells due to active replication of EBV (Fig. 218-3). Lesions are usually present on the lateral surface of the tongue but occasionally involve the dorsal and ventral surfaces of the tongue, buccal mucosa, soft palate, floor of the mouth, or pharynx.[37–39] Patients present with slightly raised white lesions that are not well demarcated and have a corrugated or hairy appearance. The lesions may wax and wane, are not painful, and do not scrape off. Oral hairy leukoplakia is seen predominantly in patients with HIV but has also been found in other immunosuppressed persons, including bone marrow and organ transplant recipients.[40,41] Anecdotal cases have been reported in persons with no known immunodeficiency.[42] The presence of oral hairy leukoplakia is predictive of progression to AIDS.[43] Histologically, the lesions show parakeratosis, acanthosis, intranuclear inclusions, ballooning of the cytoplasm or an eosinophilic "ground glass" appearance, and little inflammation in the subepithelial layer.[44] Dysplasia is usually not seen, and lesions have not progressed to malignancy.

The lesions contain virus in the upper layers of the epithelium but not in the basal layers. Biopsies from oral hairy leukoplakia contain EBV antigens, viral linear DNA (indicative of replicating virus), and large numbers of herpesvirus particles on electron microscopy.[45] EBV viral capsid and early antigens are present, consistent with virus replication. Lesions have been shown to be infected with multiple strains of EBV.[46] While initial reports

FIGURE 218-3

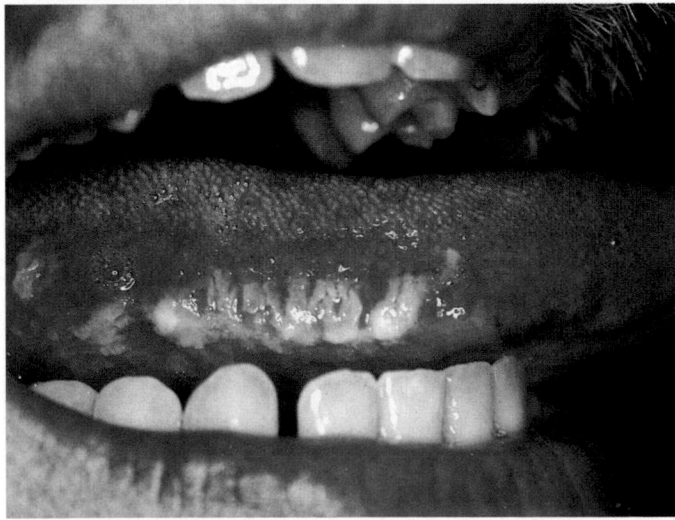

Oral hairy leukoplakia in a patient with HIV. (*Courtesy of James C. Niederman, MD, Yale University*).

suggested that papillomavirus particles and antigens were also present in the lesions, more recent studies indicate that papillomavirus DNA and antigens are absent and that the original observations may have been due to cross-reactivity between EBV and papillomavirus antigens.[44,47]

The differential diagnosis includes candidiasis, lichen planus, idiopathic or tobacco-associated leukoplakia, carcinoma, and geographic tongue. The diagnosis is usually made by the typical clinical appearance in an HIV-infected individual. Biopsy may be appropriate in atypical cases, such as patients not infected with HIV. The presence of intranuclear inclusions with the typical histopathologic findings is considered diagnostic.[44] Confirmation of EBV-associated oral hairy leukoplakia can be obtained by in situ hybridization of cell scrapings for EBV or by demonstration of EBV on a biopsy specimen.[48]

Cutaneous Malignancies

EBV has been detected in skin lesions from patients with cutaneous T cell lymphomas. Most of these lymphomas are termed *angiocentric T cell lymphomas*. They can present with chronic skin ulcers or violaceous papules and may involve the nose.[49–51] Less often, systemic T cell lymphomas or T large cell lymphomas contain EBV DNA and involve the skin.[51] Many patients with EBV-associated cutaneous T cell lymphomas have a poor response to chemotherapy and progress to a hemophagocytic syndrome with pancytopenia and coagulopathy. These lesions differ from adult T cell leukemia/lymphoma since they do not contain human T-lymphotrophic virus (HTLV)-1. A case of cutaneous T cell lymphoma associated with EBV has been reported in a patient with AIDS.[52]

EBV is also associated with posttransplant B cell lymphomas. While most of these patients have lymph node or visceral lesions, some patients present with ulcerated cutaneous nodules containing EBV DNA.[13,53] A patient with Hodgkin's disease who presented with skin nodules containing EBV RNA has been reported.[54] EBV was also detected in epithelial cells in the epidermis in a patient with chronic lymphocytic leukemia and a papular eruption.[55]

Other Skin Findings

Infantile papular acrodermatitis, or the Gianotti-Crosti syndrome, presents with symmetric erythematous lichenoid papules on the face, extremities, and buttocks, usually sparing the trunk. The eruption is not pruritic and may be accompanied by splenomegaly, hepatitis, and lymphadenopathy. The process often occurs in young children after an upper respiratory tract illness. Pathologic specimens show a perivascular infiltration of lymphocytes and histiocytes in the upper portion of the dermis. While the syndrome has been associated with hepatitis B and enterovirus infection, several cases have been associated with acute EBV infection.[56–58] An epidemic of infantile papular acrodermatitis due to EBV was reported in Italy.[59] Kawasaki-like disease[60] and granuloma annulare–like eruption[61] have also been reported in patients with EBV infection.

DIAGNOSIS

Acute infection with EBV is usually diagnosed by a positive heterophile test (e.g., monospot test). Heterophile antibodies agglutinate sheep or horse erythrocytes and do not react with EBV antigens directly. Over 90 percent of patients with the typical findings of infectious mononucleosis, atypical lymphocytes, and a heterophile antibody titer of $\geq 1:40$ have acute EBV infection. Heterophile antibodies may not become elevated until the third week of the illness and usually persist for only 3 months. Heterophile antibodies are less common in patients who do not present with infectious mononucleosis.

EBV-specific antibody tests aid in the diagnosis of patients with negative heterophile antibodies or those with atypical symptoms. IgM antibody to the viral capsid antigen (VCA) is particularly useful for the diagnosis of acute infection since it is elevated only during acute infection. Unfortunately, some commercial assays are too nonspecific and report elevated levels of IgM anti-VCA responses in other settings as well. Antibody to early antigens (EA) are less useful since they are elevated in 70 percent or fewer of patients with infectious mononucleosis. Seroconversion to IgG VCA or EBV nuclear antigen (EBNA) antibody positivity is useful for diagnosis of acute EBV infection; IgG VCA and EBNA antibodies usually persist for life. EBV DNA, RNA, or proteins can be detected in tissues from patients with oral hairy leukoplakia, lymphoproliferative disease, or EBV-associated malignancies. Isolating EBV from oral secretions is of little value, since the virus is shed in a large percentage of healthy persons.

TREATMENT

Infectious mononucleosis is usually self-limited, and therapy for symptoms includes rest and antipyretics. While acyclovir inhibits virus replication in vitro and limits shedding of the virus, acyclovir has been ineffective for reducing the symptoms of infectious mononucleosis.[62] Glucocorticoids are not indicated for patients with uncomplicated illness and may predispose to bacterial superinfection.[63] Glucocorticoids (1 mg/kg per day of prednisone for 2 to 3 days and tapered off over 1 to 2 weeks) may be useful in some patients with airway obstruction, severe hemolytic anemia, or thrombocytopenia or in very selected cases of encephalitis, myocarditis, pericarditis, or debilitating malaise and fever.

Patients with exudative pharyngitis that is accompanied by beta-hemolytic streptococci should be treated with penicillin or erythromycin. Ampicillin or amoxicillin should not be given during the acute phase of infectious mononucleosis.

Treatment for oral hairy leukoplakia is usually unnecessary. The lesions resolve during treatment with oral acyclovir (400 to 800 mg five times daily); however, they usually recur 2 weeks to 2 months after the drug is stopped.[64] Oral hairy leukoplakia has been reported to resolve with antiretroviral therapy,[65] presumably as a result of better control of the underlying HIV infection; these drugs have no activity against EBV per se. Surgical excision has been associated with long-term remissions, but the disease can recur elsewhere on the tongue.[66] Topical tretinoin,[67] podophyllum resin,[68] trichloroacetic acid, and glycolic acid have all been used to remove lesions, but the disease recurs after treatment is discontinued.

REFERENCES

1. Epstein MA et al: Virus particles in cultured lymphoblasts from Burkitt's lymphoma. *Lancet* **1**:702, 1964
2. Henle G et al: Relation of Burkitt's tumor–associated herpes-type virus to infectious mononucleosis. *Proc Natl Acad Sci USA* **59**:94, 1968
3. ZurHausen H et al: EBV DNA in biopsies of Burkitt's tumors and anaplastic carcinomas of the nasopharynx. *Nature* **228**:1056, 1970
4. Ziegler JL et al: Outbreak of Burkitt's-like lymphoma in homosexual men. *Lancet* **2**:631, 1982
5. Weiss LM et al: Detection of Epstein-Barr viral genomes in Reed-Sternberg cells of Hodgkin's disease. *N Engl J Med* **320**:502, 1989
6. Evans AS et al: Epstein-Barr virus, in *Viral Infections of Humans: Epidemiology and Control*, 3d ed, edited by AS Evans. New York, Plenum, 1989, pp 265–292
7. Ferbas J et al: Frequent oropharyngeal shedding of Epstein-Barr virus in homosexual men during early HIV infection. *AIDS* **6**:1273, 1992
8. Golden HD et al: Leukocyte-transforming agent: Prolonged excretion by patients with mononucleosis and excretion by normal individuals. *J Infect Dis* **127**:471, 1973
9. Rickinson AB, Kieff E: Epstein-Barr virus, in *Fields' Virology*, edited by BN Fields et al. Philadelphia, Lippincott-Raven, 1996, pp 2397–2446
10. Sixbey JW et al: Epstein-Barr virus replication in oropharyngeal epithelial cells. *N Engl J Med* **310**:1225, 1984
11. Straus SE et al: Epstein-Barr virus infections: Biology, pathogenesis, and management. *Ann Intern Med* **118**:45, 1993
12. Straus SE: Acute progressive Epstein-Barr virus infections. *Annu Rev Med* **43**:437, 1992
13. Cohen JI: Epstein-Barr virus lymphoproliferative disease associated with acquired immunodeficiency. *Medicine* **70**:137, 1991
14. Contratto AW: Infectious mononucleosis. A study of one hundred and ninety-six cases. *Arch Intern Med* **73**:449, 1944
15. Mason WR, Adams EK: Infectious mononucleosis. An analysis of 100 cases with particular attention to diagnosis, liver function tests and treatment of selected cases with prednisone. *Am J Med Sci* **239**:447, 1958
16. Bernstein A: Infectious mononucleosis. *Medicine* **19**:85, 1940
17. Weary PE et al: Eruptions from ampicillin in patients with infectious mononucleosis. *Arch Dermatol* **101**:86, 1970
18. Patel BM: Skin rash with infectious mononucleosis and ampicillin. *Pediatrics* **40**:910, 1967
19. Pullen H et al: Hypersensitivity reactions to antibacterial drugs in infectious mononucleosis. *Lancet* **2**:1176, 1967
20. Nazareth I et al: Ampicillin sensitivity in infectious mononucleosis—temporary or permanent. *Scand J Infect Dis* **4**:229, 1972
21. Wands JR et al: Circulating immune complexes and complement sequence activation in infectious mononucleosis. *Am J Med* **60**:269, 1976
22. Lund BMA, Bergan T: Temporary skin reactions to penicillins during the acute stage of infectious mononucleosis. *Scand J Infect Dis* **7**:21, 1975
23. McKenzie H et al: IgM and IgG antibody levels to ampicillin in patients with infectious mononucleosis. *Clin Exp Immunol* **26**:214, 1976
24. Cowdrey SC, Reynolds JS: Acute urticaria in infectious mononucleosis. *Ann Allergy* **27**:182, 1969
25. Africk JA, Halprin KM: Infectious mononucleosis presenting as urticaria. *JAMA* **209**:1524, 1969
26. Tyson CJ, Czarny D: Cold-induced urticaria in infectious mononucleosis. *Med J Australia* **1**:33, 1981
27. Lemanske RF, Bush RK: Cold urticaria in infectious mononucleosis. *JAMA* **247**:1604, 1982
28. Dickerman JD et al: Infectious mononucleosis initially seen as cold-induced acrocyanosis. *Am J Dis Child* **134**:159, 1980
29. Hoffman GS, Franck WA: Infectious mononucleosis, autoimmunity, and vasculitis. *JAMA* **241**:2735, 1979
30. Petrozzi JW: Infectious mononucleosis manifesting as a palmar dermatitis. *Arch Dermatol* **104**:207, 1971
31. Bodansky HJ: Erythema nodosum and infectious mononucleosis. *Br Med J* **2**:1263, 1979
32. Williamson DM: Erythema multiforme in infectious mononucleosis. *Br J Dermatol* **91**:345, 1974
33. Portnoy J et al: Recovery of Epstein-Barr virus from genital ulcers. *N Engl J Med* **311**:966, 1986
34. McKenna G et al: Genital ulceration secondary to Epstein-Barr virus infection. *Genitourin Med* **70**:356, 1994
35. McCarthy JT, Hoagland RJ: Cutaneous manifestations of infectious mononucleosis. *JAMA* **187**:153, 1964
36. Caird FI, Holt PR: The enanthem of glandular fever. *Br Med J* **1**:85, 1958
37. Ficarra G et al: Hairy leukoplakia with involvement of the buccal mucosa. *J Am Acad Dermatol* **27**:855, 1992
38. Eversole LR et al: Oral condyloma planus (hairy leukoplakia) among homosexual men. A clinicopathologic study of thirty-six cases. *Oral Surg Oral Med Oral Pathol* **61**:249, 1986

39. Kabani S et al: Oral hairy leukoplakia with extensive oral mucosal involvement: Report of two cases. *Oral Surg Oral Med Oral Pathol* **67**:411, 1989

40. Schmidt-Westhausen A et al: Oral hairy leukoplakia in an HIV-seronegative heart transplant patient. *J Oral Pathol Med* **19**:192, 1990

41. Epstein JB et al: Hairy leukoplakia-like lesions in immunosuppressed patients following bone marrow transplantation. *Transplantation* **46**:462, 1988

42. Eisenberg E et al: Incidental oral hairy leukoplakia in immunocompetent persons. A report of two cases. *Oral Surg Oral Med Oral Pathol* **74**:332, 1992

43. Greenspan D et al: Risk factors for rapid progression from hairy leukoplakia to AIDS: A rested case control study. *J AIDS* **4**:652, 1991

44. Fernandez JF et al: Oral hairy leukoplakia: A histopathologic study of 32 cases. *Am J Dermatopathol* **12**:571, 1990

45. Greenspan JS et al: Replication of Epstein-Barr virus within the epithelial cells of oral "hairy" leukoplakia, an AIDS-associated lesion. *N Engl J Med* **313**:1564, 1985

46. Walling DM et al: Coinfection with multiple strains of the Epstein-Barr virus in human immunodeficiency virus–associated hairy leukoplakia. *Proc Natl Acad Sci USA* **89**:6560, 1992

47. Greenspan D, Greenspan JS: Significance of oral hairy leukoplakia. *Oral Surg Oral Med Oral Pathol* **73**:151, 1992

48. DeSouza YG et al: Diagnosis of Epstein-Barr virus infection in hairy leukoplakia by using nucleic acid hybridization and noninvasive techniques. *J Clin Microbiol* **28**:2775, 1990

49. Park CK, Ko YH: Detection of EBER nuclear RNA in T-cell lymphomas involving the skin—an in situ hybridization study. *Br J Dermatol* **134**:488, 1996

50. Cheng A-L et al: Characteristic clinicopathologic features of Epstein-Barr virus–associated peripheral T-cell lymphoma. *Cancer* **72**:909, 1993

51. Su I-J et al: Cutaneous manifestations of Epstein-Barr virus–associated T-cell lymphoma. *J Am Acad Dermatol* **29**:685, 1993

52. Dreno B et al: Cutaneous anaplastic T-cell lymphoma in a patient with human immunodeficiency virus infection: Detection of Epstein-Barr virus DNA. *Br J Dermatol* **129**:77, 1993

53. McGregor JM et al: Posttransplant cutaneous lymphoma. *J Am Acad Dermatol* **29**:549, 1993

54. Kumar S et al: Primary cutaneous Hodgkin's disease with evolution to systemic disease: Association with Epstein-Barr virus. *Am J Surg Pathol* **20**:754, 1996

55. Fermand J-P et al: Detection of Epstein-Barr virus in epidermal skin lesions of an immunocompromised patient. *Ann Intern Med* **112**:511, 1990

56. Konno M et al: A possible association between hepatitis-B antigen-negative infantile papular acrodermatitis and Epstein-Barr virus infection. *J Pediatr* **101**:222, 1982

57. Iosub S et al: Papular acrodermatitis with Epstein-Barr virus infection. *Clin Pediatr* **23**:33, 1984

58. Lowe L et al: Gianotti-Crosti syndrome associated with Epstein-Barr virus infection. *J Am Acad Dermatol* **201**:336, 1989

59. Baldari U et al: An epidemic of infantile papular acrodermatitis (Gianotti-Crosti syndrome) due to Epstein-Barr virus. *Dermatology* **188**:203, 1994

60. Barbour AG et al: Kawasaki-like disease in a young adult: Association with primary Epstein-Barr virus infection. *JAMA* **241**:397, 1979

61. Spencer SA et al: Granuloma annulare–like eruption due to chronic Epstein-Barr virus infection. *Arch Dermatol* **124**:250, 1988

62. van der Horst C et al: Lack of effect of peroral acyclovir for the treatment of infectious mononucleosis. *J Infect Dis* **164**:788, 1991

63. McGowan JE et al: Guidelines for the use of systemic glucocorticosteroids in the management of selected infections. *J Infect Dis* **165**:1, 1992

64. Resnick L et al: Regression of oral hairy leukoplakia after orally administered acyclovir therapy. *JAMA* **259**:384, 1988

65. Kessler HA et al: Regression of oral hairy leukoplakia during zidovudine therapy. *Arch Intern Med* **148**:2496, 1988

66. Herbst JS et al: Comparison of the efficacy of surgery and acyclovir therapy in oral hairy leukoplakia. *J Am Acad Dermatol* **21**:753, 1989

67. Schofer H et al: Treatment of oral "hairy" leukoplakia in AIDS patients with vitamin A acid (topically) or acyclovir (systemically). *Dermatologica* **174**:150, 1987

68. Gowdey G et al: Treatment of HIV-related hairy leukoplakia with podophyllum resin 25% solution. *Oral Surg Oral Med Oral Pathol* **79**:64, 1996

CHAPTER 219

Sandy Urioste
Mihael Skerlev
Richard Allen Johnson

Human Herpesvirus 6 and 7 Infections and Exanthem Subitum (Roseola Infantum or Sixth Disease)

Human herpesviruses 6 (HHV-6) and 7 (HHV-7) are two newly recognized viruses that share close genetic, biologic, and immunologic features. They differ from all other known human herpesviruses in their primary T cell tropism and their inability to directly induce cellular transformation in vitro. They are present in the normal population in a latent phase and have been implicated as etiologic agents in various conditions, including exanthem subitum.

HISTORIC ASPECTS

Salahuddin and colleagues[1] first isolated HHV-6 in 1986 after identifying herpes-like particles in peripheral blood mononuclear cells (PMBCs) of patients with various forms of lymphoproliferative disorders, some of whom were also infected with human immunodeficiency virus-1 (HIV-1). At the time, only five human herpesviruses were known: herpes simplex virus (HSV- or HHV-1 and 2), varicella zoster virus (VZV or HHV-3), Epstein-Barr virus (EBV or HHV-4) and human cytomegalovirus (CMV or HHV-5). As the virus was initially isolated from B-lymphoreticular disorders, it was named human B-lymphotrophic virus (HBLV). Shortly thereafter, Lusso[2] characterized it as the first preferentially T-lymphotrophic human herpesvirus. HHV-6 has subsequently been found to also infect natural killer cells, monocytes, glial cells, and fibroblasts.[3]

Four years later, using similar culture conditions, Frenkel and colleagues[4] isolated HHV-7, a second human herpesvirus with a predominant T-lymphocyte tropism. The role of these two organisms as etiologic agents in exanthem subitum has been well established.[5,6] Recent observations and in vitro studies have provided a greater insight into other disease states in which they may play a causal role.

EPIDEMIOLOGY

HHV-6 and HHV-7 are ubiquitous in the population. At birth, most children are positive for HHV-6 and HHV-7 IgG antibody because of maternal immunoglobulin.[7] Primary infection is thought to be acquired primarily through oropharyngeal secretions, as suggested by the frequent detection of the virus in salivary secretions.[8] Viral particles have also been recovered from vaginal and cervical secre-

tions. HHV-6 antibody levels reach a nadir at 4 to 7 months and then increase throughout infancy. By 12 months, two-thirds of children have been infected, with peak antibody levels being reached at 2 to 3 years. HHV-7 antibody levels reach a nadir at 6 months, with antibody levels peaking at 3 to 4 years. Adult seroprevalence rates of HHV-6 and HHV-7 show some waning of antibody levels with increased age. Clinical data suggest that HHV-6 and HHV-7 may persist as an active viremia or remain latent in asymptomatic adults.

HUMAN HERPESVIRUSES 6 AND 7

HHV-6 and HHV-7 are members of the beta herpesvirus family. HHV-6 is a double-stranded DNA virus with an enveloped virion[9] and an icosahedral capsid 170 to 200 nm in diameter that encloses the viral genome. The capsid is composed of 162 subunits (capsomeres) resembling tubular structures. The genome and capsid (nucleocapsid) are encapsulated by an amorphous tegument acquired from the nuclear membrane. HHV-6 replicates by a rolling circle mechanism,[10] with the formation of head-to-tail concatamers in infected nuclei. Fusion events with the nuclear membrane result in the release of the tegmented capsid into the cytoplasm of infected cells, where they undergo envelopment in cytoplasmic vacuoles, yielding mature virions. Further fusion with the cell membrane releases completed particles into the extracellular space. More than 30 polypeptides have been identified in virions and infected cells, including 7 glycoproteins. In addition to structural components of the virion, certain enzymes essential for viral replication,[11] including virus-specific DNA-polymerase, are synthesized in infected cells. Thymidine kinase, uracil-DNA-glycosidase, and deoxyuridine triphosphate nucleotidohydrolase, other herpesvirus-specific enzymes, are not synthesized.[12] Ganciclovir kinase, similar to that produced by CMV, has been detected.

The HHV-6 genome is 160 to 170 kbp in length. A central segment containing a unique (UI) sequence, rich in A + T and approximately 140 kbp in length, has been identified. It is flanked by two identical direct repeat (DR) segments, rich in G + C, of approximately 8000 bp each. These direct repeats contain essential elements for viral DNA packaging and replication and possibly for the maintenance of latency.[13,14] They also contain a tandem repetitive sequence (GGGTTA) that is also present in the genome of the

Marek's disease virus. The overall content of G + C is 43 percent, one of the lowest among the herpesviridae. It shares the highest degree of nucleotide sequence homology with HHV-7, while both HHV-6 and HHV-7 are more distantly related to CMV,[15,16] with approximately 65 percent homology. HHV-6 also possesses a gene with striking homology to the *rep* gene of adeno-associated virus type 2 (AAV-2),[17,18] a defective parvovirus dependent on adenovirus for replication. The AAV-2 rep protein inhibits cellular transformation by papillomaviruses. The HHV-6 *rep*-like gene product is functional and has been shown to block H-*ras* cellular transformation, to mediate AAV-2 DNA replication, and to alter HIV-1 transcription[19] via the long-terminal repeat (LTR).

Two major viral subgroups (A and B)[20] have been identified for HHV-6. The overall genetic divergence between the two variants is approximately 5 percent. The prototype of HHV-6 type A is strain GS.[1] The prevalence and time of primary infection are still undefined. It is detected less frequently than type B. To date, no human disease has been definitely linked to this subgroup. However, type A isolates are seen primarily in immunocompromised patients, suggesting a possible role in immunodeficiency states such as AIDS. The prototype of HHV-6 B is strain Z29.[21] It is responsible for most cases of primary infection of early childhood and has been associated with exanthem subitum. Its prevalence in western countries is universal.

Characterization of HHV-7 is not complete to date. The HHV-7 genome is approximately 145 kbp in length. The genome codes for more than seventy proteins, including two major capsid proteins,[22] and shares the greatest nucleotide homology with HHV-6 type A.

PATHOGENESIS

HHV-6 and HHV-7 are believed to establish latent infections, as observed with other herpesviruses, thereby persisting indefinitely in the infected host. Though no in vitro models of latency exist, persistent infection has been documented in cultured monocytes.[23] It is postulated that salivary and bronchial gland epithelial cells and circulating monocytes act as reservoirs for these viruses. HHV-6 is a cytopathic virus. Unlike EBV, HHV-6 does not cause direct immortalization of its target cells. Both viral subgroups preferentially infect CD4+ T cells.[24,25] HHV-6 A is also able to infect cytotoxic effector cells, including CD8+ T cells, natural killer cells, and gamma/delta T cells. HHV-6 can also infect yet ineffectively lyse nonimmune cells such as fibroblasts as well as neural, muscular, and epithelial cells. The receptor for HHV-6 is not known. HHV-6 has been shown to downregulate the expression of CD3 and alpha-beta heterodimers on T cells,[26] thus having a potential immunosuppressive effect. HHV-6 can also transcriptionally activate the expression of CD4 in cells that physiologically do not express it.[27] It is also a powerful inducer of cytokines, including tumor necrosis factor alpha and interleukin 1 beta.

The major receptor for HHV-7 is the CD4 glycoprotein,[28] which also serves as the major receptor for HIV. HHV-7 and HIV-1 compete for CD4 occupancy and reciprocally interfere both in CD4+ T cells and in mononuclear phagocytes. HHV-7 downregulates CD4 expression. The use of its envelope in anti-HIV therapy has been proposed.

CLINICAL MANIFESTATIONS

Cutaneous Manifestations

EXANTHEM SUBITUM This disease was initially described by Zahorsky in 1913 as roseola infantum (Latin, "pink rash of infants"). The name *exanthem subitum* (Greek, "sudden rash") was introduced by Veeder and Hemplemann in 1921 to describe the most characteristic clinical finding, that of the sudden appearance of a rash on the fourth or fifth day of illness.

Exanthem subitum is characterized by a mild, self-limited illness of short duration. The exanthem is commonly mistaken for other causes of fever and rash in children. Exanthem subitum is a nonreportable infection, occurring equally in boys and girls.[11] Though most studies of large groups of affected children found no characteristic seasonal or monthly incidence, Juretic,[29] in a review of 243 cases, noted a peak occurrence in May. The typical age range is between 6 months and 2 years, with occasional cases described in older children and adults. Maternal antibodies play a role in the prevention of clinical infection prior to 6 months of age. The incubation period is estimated to be 5 to 15 days.

Many viruses have been postulated to be the causative agent of exanthem subitum, including echovirus 16, coxsackieviruses, adenoviruses, and parainfluenzavirus type 1. To date, there is no conclusive evidence to support these hypotheses. In 1988 Yamamashi and colleagues[30] provided evidence that HHV-6 was a causal agent of exanthem subitum. HHV-7 has subsequently been shown to play a similar causal role. The virus is present in high concentrations within blood mononuclear cells during the febrile stage of the illness. Subsequent development of HHV-6 and HHV-7 antibodies is seen.

The onset of the disease is abrupt and is characterized by a high fever, ranging from 38.9 to 40.6°C (102.2 to 105.8°F). In spite of this, the child is generally in no distress. A bulging anterior fontanelle, tonsillar and pharyngeal inflammation, tympanic injection, and nodal enlargement have been observed. Other systemic symptoms are generally absent. The fever drops precipitously on the fourth day, coinciding with the rapid onset of a rash.

The exanthem consists of nonpruritic rose-pink macules and papules 2 to 3 mm in diameter, which blanch on pressure and are surrounded by a white halo (Fig. 219-1). The rash characteristically first appears on the trunk and may spread to the neck and the upper and lower extremities. The rash is fully evolved within 12 h and lasts 1 to 2 days. In some cases, it appears suddenly and disappears within a few hours. Resolution occurs without desquamation or hyperpigmentation. Palpebral edema (Berliner's sign, "heavy eyelids") and periorbital edema are quite common.

The differential diagnosis of high fever with sudden defervescence as an evanescent exanthematous eruption appears quite narrow but should include rubella, measles, scarlet fever, erythema infectiosum, other viral infections with exanthems (enterovirus, adenovirus, echovirus, coxsackievirus, rotavirus), and adverse cutaneous drug reactions. The diagnosis is made on the characteristic clinical findings. Laboratory tests may reveal a transient leukopenia with a relative lymphocytosis and occasional atypical lymphocytes.

The course of exanthem subitum is mild, with no sequelae generally observed. The most common complication is seizures. Whether seizures are secondary to fever or infection is unclear. Meningoencephalitis and fulminant hepatitis may occur as complications of exanthem subitum. This has been confirmed by isolation of either HHV-6 or HHV-7 viral DNA from cerebrospinal fluid (CSF) in the febrile phase of exanthem subitum. Thrombocytopenia has also been observed. Intussusception has been reported in three Japanese children with HHV-6 infection.[31] No treatment is generally required, given the self-limited nature of this disease. Primary infection with HHV-6 and HHV-7 confers lasting immunity.

PITYRIASIS ROSEA (see Chap. 47) Recently, Drago and colleagues reported data supporting a role of HHV-7 in patients with pityriasis rosea (PR).[32] For 12 patients with PR, HHV-7 was isolated from sera, PBMCs, and skin biopsies using polymerase chain reaction (PCR) techniques. Weak PCR signals were detected in PBMCs of 11 of 25 control patients. No HHV-7 was detected in control patient sera or skin biopsies. Further studies are needed to establish causality.

Neurologic Manifestations

HHV-6 has also been implicated as a potential trigger for multiple sclerosis (MS). The virus has been detected at high levels in infected oligodendrocytes[33] near plaque formations in the brains of MS patients. As well, elevated IgM titers to an early HHV-6 antigen have been documented during relapses. HHV-6 may act as a cofactor, activating a retrovirus responsible for MS. Both HHV-6[34] and HHV-7[35] have been implicated as causal agents of infant febrile seizures, supported by active viremia and seroconversion in these children, as well as meningitis and meningoencephalitis. This is thought to be due to direct invasion of the central nervous system (CNS) by the virus.

HHV-6 and HIV

HHV-6 is thought to play an important role in the activation and propogation of HIV infection. Given its preferential tropism for CD4+ T cells and its ability to upregulate CD4 expression, HHV-6 is postulated to function as a cofactor for infection of these T cells with HIV. As well, HHV-6 is a potent transactivator of HIV LTR, and the HIV *tat* transactivator enhances HHV-6 replication, each providing a favorable environment for replication. Active HHV-6 has been demonstrated in multiple organs of patients with terminal AIDS at the time of autopsy.[36] In particular, HHV-6 has been localized to the white matter in areas of demyelinization in AIDS patients,[37] sparing areas without pathologic changes. Thus, it is postulated that HHV-6 may play a direct role in the development of AIDS-associated CNS disease. Clinically, HHV-6 has been documented in the CSF of children with AIDS encephalitis.

Neoplastic Disorders

HHV-6 has been suggested as an etiologic factor in neoplastic disorders such as Hodgkin's disease (via IgG serology and PCR),[38] non-Hodgkin's lymphoma[39] (via Southern blot and PCR), Langer-

FIGURE 219-1

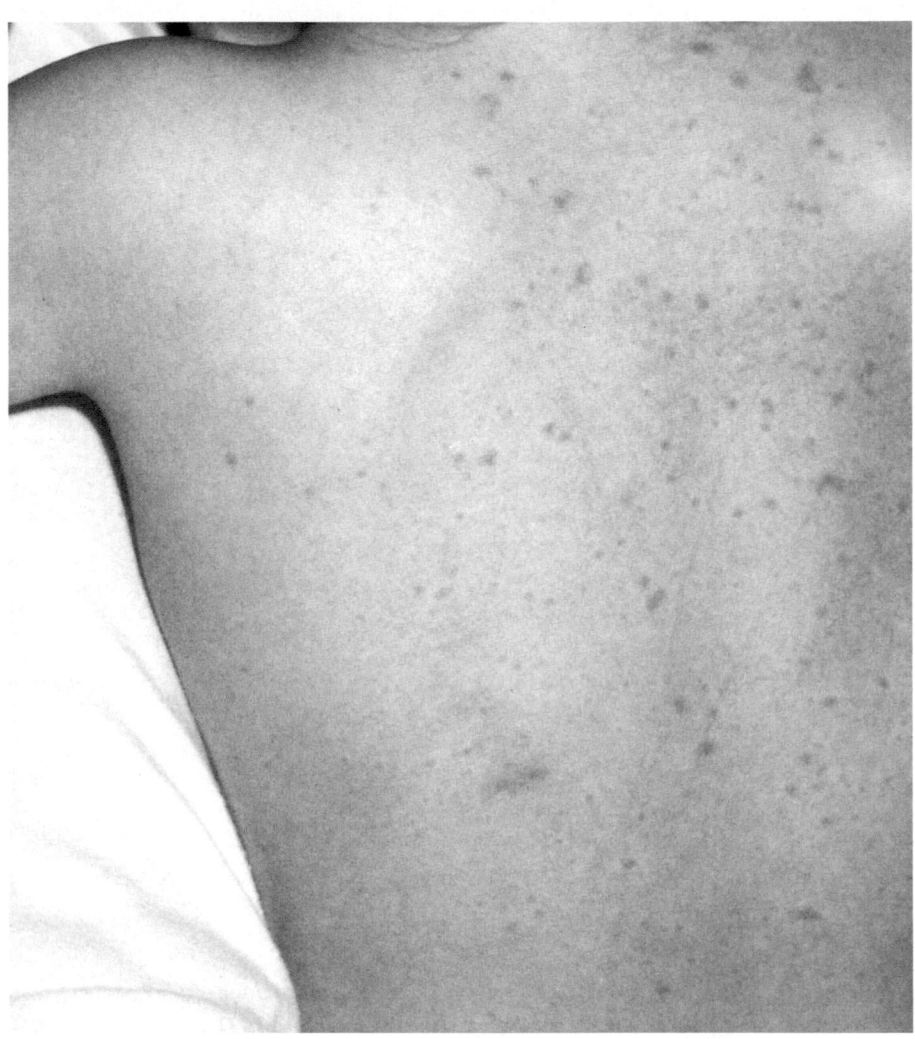

Exanthem subitum. Multiple, blanchable macules and papules on the back of a febrile child, which appeared as the temperature fell. (*Courtesy of Karen Wiss, MD.*)

hans cell histiocytosis[40] (via PCR), Kaposi's sarcoma[41] (via PCR), cervical cancer,[42] and angioimmunoblastic lymphadenopathy with dysproteinemia[43] (via PCR). Unfortunately, no controlled studies have been conducted to support these data. The tumorigenic potential of HHV-6 has nonetheless been well documented in in vitro studies.[44]

Bone Marrow Transplantation

HHV-6 is an important cause of idiopathic bone marrow suppression after bone marrow transplantation,[45] supported by the presence of active viremia at the time of suppression. This marrow-suppressive effect is thought to be partially mediated by cytokine- or virus-produced soluble factors. HHV-6 A produces a more virulent aplastic anemia than HHV-6 B. As well, interstitial pneumonitis,[46] retinitis,[47] and bone marrow graft failure have also been documented in patients with active HHV-6 infections.

Miscellaneous

A putative role of HHV-6 and HHV-7 in the development of chronic fatigue syndrome (CFS) has been questioned. A major impediment is the inability to formulate a precise definition for CFS. Studies have demonstrated higher antibody titers to HHV-6 and HHV-7, as well as EBV, in patients with CFS versus control patients. Confirmation of active viral infection will allow for more supportive data.

LABORATORY TESTS

The most accurate method of detection of HHV-6 and HHV-7 is through the use of PCR evaluation[48] of serum or plasma. IgM antibody reactivity correlates well with active infection. Ig antibody titers do not correlate with actual viral replication. Other methods employed include immunohistochemistry and RNA in situ hybridization, both offering the additional advantage of exact lineage identification.

SUSCEPTIBILITY TO ANTIVIRAL AGENTS

The antiviral susceptibilities of HHV-6 and HHV-7 resemble those of CMV.[49] All three viruses lack a thymidine kinase and encode for ganciclovir kinase. HHV-6 and HHV-7 are susceptible to ganciclovir and foscarnet and show minimal susceptibility to acyclovir. At present, these agents are not routinely utilized for the treatment of HHV-6 or HHV-7. The optimal approach to the prophylactic treatment of transplant patients has yet to be defined. Ganciclovir should be avoided in patients with marrow suppression and foscarnet avoided in patients with renal disease. Other drugs with in vitro activity against these viruses include ampligen and kutapressin.

REFERENCES

1. Salahuddin SZ et al: Isolation of a new virus, HBLV, in patients with lymphoproliferative disorders. *Science* **234**:596, 1986
2. Lusso P et al: In vitro cellular tropism of human B-lymphotropic virus (human herpesvirus 6). *J Exp Med* **167**:1659, 1988
3. Downing RG et al: Isolation of human lymphotropic herpesviruses from Uganda (letter). *Lancet* **2**:390, 1987
4. Frenkel N et al: Isolation of a new herpesvirus from CD4+ T cells. *Proc Natl Acad Sci USA* **87**:748, 1988
5. Takahashi K et al: Human herpesvirus 6 and exanthem subitum. *Lancet* **1**:1463, 1988
6. Tanaka K et al: Human herpesvirus 7: Another causal agent for roseola (exanthem subitum). *J Pediatr* **125**:1, 1994
7. Pietroboni GR et al: Antibody to human herpesvirus 6 in saliva. *Lancet* **1**:1059, 1988
8. Levy JA et al: Frequent isolation of HHV-6 from saliva and high seroprevalence of the virus in the population. *Lancet* **335**:1047, 1990
9. Biberfeld P et al: Ultrastructural characterization of a new human B lymphotrophic DNA virus (human herpesvirus 6) isolated from patients with lymphoproliferative disease. *J Natl Cancer Inst* **79**:933, 1987
10. Martin ME et al: The genome of human herpesvirus 6: Maps of unit-length and concatameric genomes for nine restriction endonucleases. *J Gen Virol* **72**:157, 1991
11. Williams MV et al: Demonstration of the human herpesvirus 6–induced DNA polymerase and DNase. *Virology* **173**:223, 1989
12. Gompels UA et al: The DNA sequence of human herpesvirus 6: Structure, coding content, and genomic evolution. *Virology* **209**:29, 1995
13. Lindquester GJ et al: Properties of the human herpesvirus strain Z29 genome: G + C content, length and presence of variable-length directly repeated terminal sequence elements. *Virology* **182**:102, 1991
14. Thomson BJ et al: Structure and heterogeneity of the sequences of human herpesvirus 6 strain variants U1102 and Z29 and identification of human telomeric repeat sequences at the genomic termini. *J Virol* **68**:3007, 1994
15. Efstathiou S et al: DNA homology between a novel human herpesvirus (HHV-6) and human cytomegalovirus. *Lancet* **1**:63, 1988
16. Berneman ZN et al: Human herpesvirus 7 is a T-lymphotrophic virus and is related to, but significantly different from, human herpesvirus 6 and human cytomegalovirus. *Proc Natl Acad Sci USA* **89**:10552, 1992
17. Thomson BJ et al: Acquisition of the human adeno-associated virus type 2 *rep* gene by human herpesvirus type 6. *Nature* **351**:78, 1992
18. Thomson BJ et al: Human herpesvirus 6 (HHV-6) is a helper virus for adeno-associated virus type 2 (AAV-2) and the AAV-2 rep gene homologue in HHV-6 can mediate AAV-2 DNA replication and regulate gene expression. *Virology* **204**:304, 1994
19. Araujo JC et al: Human herpesvirus 6A *ts* suppresses both transformation by H-*ras* and transcription by the H-*ras* and human immunodeficiency virus type I promoters. *J Virol* **69**:4933, 1995
20. Ablashi DV et al: Genomic polymorphism, growth properties and immunologic variations in human herpesvirus 6 isolates. *Virology* **184**:545, 1991
21. Lopez C et al: Characteristics of human herpesvirus 6. *J Infect Dis* **157**:1271, 1988
22. Ablashi DV et al: Human herpesvirus 7 (HHV-7): Current status. *Clin Diagn Virol* **4**:1, 1995
23. Kondo K et al: Latent human herpesvirus 6 infection of human monocytes/macrophages. *J Gen Virol* **72**:1401, 1991
24. Lusso P et al: In vitro cellular tropism of human B-lymphotropic virus (human herpesvirus 6). *J Exp Med* **167**:1659, 1988
25. Takahashi K et al: Predominant CD4 T-lymphocyte tropism of human herpesvirus 6-related virus. *J Virol* **63**:3161, 1989
26. Lusso P et al: Productive infection of CD4+ and CD8+ mature T-cell populations and clones by HHV-6: Transcriptional down-regulation of CD3. *J Immunol* **147**:2147, 1991
27. Lusso P et al: Induction of CD4 and susceptibility to HIV-1 infection in CD8+ human T lymphocytes by human herpesvirus 6. *Nature* **349**:533, 1991
28. Lusso P et al: CD4 is a critical component of the receptor for human herpesvirus 7: Interference with human immunodeficiency virus. *Proc Natl Acad Sci USA* **91**:3872, 1994
29. Jeretic M: Exanthem subitum: A review of 243 cases. *Helv Pediatr Acta* **18**:80, 1963
30. Yamanashi K et al: Identification of human herpesvirus-6 as a causal agent for exanthem subitum. *Lancet* **1**:1065, 1988
31. Asano Y et al: Simultaneous occurrence of human herpes 6 infection and intussusception in three infants. *Pediatr Infect Dis J* **10**:335, 1991
32. Drago F et al: Human herpesvirus 7 in pityriasis rosea. *Lancet* **349**:1367, 1997
33. Challoner PB et al: Plaque-associated expression of human herpesvirus 6 in multiple sclerosis. *Proc Natl Acad Sci USA* **92**:7440, 1995
34. Kondo K et al: Association of human herpesvirus 6 infection of the central nervous system with recurrence of febrile convulsions. *J Infect Dis* **167**:1197, 1993
35. Torigoe S et al: Clinical manifestations associated with human herpesvirus 7 infection. *Arch Dis Child* **72**:518, 1995
36. Corbellino M et al: Disseminated human herpesvirus 6 infection in AIDS. *Lancet* **342**:1242, 1993
37. Knox KK et al: Active human herpesvirus (HHV-6) infection of the central nervous system in patients with AIDS. *J Acquir Immune Defic Syndr Hum Retrovir* **9**:69, 1995
38. Clark DA et al: The seroepidemiology of human herpesvirus 6 (HHV-6) from a case-control study of leukaemia and lymphoma. *Int J Cancer* **45**:829, 1990
39. Jarrett RF et al: Identification of human herpesvirus 6-specific DNA sequences in two patients with non-Hodgkin's lymphoma. *Leukemia* **2**:496, 1988
40. Leahy MA et al: Human herpesvirus 6 is present in lesions of Langerhans cell histiocytosis. *J Invest Dermatol* **101**:642, 1993
41. Bovensi P et al: Human herpesvirus 6 (variant A) in Kaposi's sarcoma. *Lancet* **341**:1288, 1993

42. Chen M et al: Detection of human herpesvirus 6 and human papillomavirus 16 in cervical carcinoma. *Am J Pathol* **145**:1509, 1994
43. Luppi M et al: Frequent detection of human herpesvirus 6 sequences by polymerase chain reaction in paraffin-embedded lymph nodes from patients with angioimmunoblastic lymphadenopathy and angioimmunoblastic lymphadenopathy-like lymphoma. *Leuk Res* **17**:1003, 1993
44. Razzaque A et al: Oncogenic potential of human herpesvirus-6 DNA. *Oncogene* **5**:1365, 1990
45. Carrigan DR et al: Human herpesvirus 6 (HHV-6) isolation from bone marrow: HHV-6 associated bone marrow suppression in bone marrow transplant patients. *Blood* **84**:3307, 1994
46. Carrigan DR et al: Interstitial pneumonitis associated with human herpesvirus 6 infection after marrow transplantation. *Lancet* **338**:147, 1991

47. Qavi HB et al: Demonstration of HIV-1 and HHV-6 in AIDS-associated retinitis. *Curr Eye Res* **11**:315, 1992
48. Secchiero P et al: Quantitative polymerase chain reaction for human herpesvirus 6 and 7. *J Clin Microbiol* **33**:2124, 1995
49. Burns WH et al: Susceptibility of human herpesvirus 6 to antivirals in vitro. *J Infect Dis* **162**:634, 1990

CHAPTER 220

Vincent A. Fulginiti

Smallpox and Complications of Smallpox Vaccination

SMALLPOX (VARIOLA)

Smallpox is an acute exanthematous disease caused by infection with poxvirus variolae. The significant clinical features include a 3-day prodromal illness and a generalized centrifugal rash with rapidly successive papules, vesicles, pustules, umbilication, and crusting within 14 days. Although the worldwide eradication of smallpox was officially announced in 1979, it is too soon to give up discussion of this disease in medical texts, and it is treated here as though it still existed.

Historic Aspects

The first clinical description of smallpox was by Rhazes, an Arabian physician, in the tenth century A.D. Many curious beliefs concerning the cause and pathogenesis of the disease are recorded in the writings of the early physicians. Frequently smallpox was confused with chickenpox, syphilis, and measles. It is of interest that smallpox was known in China 11 centuries before the birth of Christ, and that inoculation to prevent the disease was described in the sixth century B.C. using dried crusts introduced into the nose. It is likely that smallpox was introduced into the western world in the early centuries after Christ by the migrations of invading armies. Subsequent spread of smallpox in Europe and England is intertwined with the history of these areas. As one reads the various accounts of epidemics of this disease in the fifteenth and sixteenth centuries, and later in the United States, it becomes apparent that smallpox represented a major force in life, often affecting dynasties, determining the outcome of military conflicts, as well as influencing daily life. Until the advent of Jennerian vaccination, its widespread application, and the ultimate eradication of smallpox, this disease continued to be a major threat, with widespread attack rates, persistent infection within a community, and a high mortality rate.

Epidemiology

In the past 20 years, a remarkable event occurred in public health. The efforts of many countries, coordinated by the World Health Organization, resulted in intensive case finding and application of smallpox vaccination across large populations. This resulted in the eradication of smallpox, and there have been no cases since October 1977 anywhere in the world.

Etiology and Pathogenesis

Smallpox is caused by infection with poxvirus variola. The entire DNA genome of the virus has been analyzed, and many of the viral proteins have been sequenced. Many of these share identity with the major gene products of the vaccinia virus. It is believed that infection occurs strictly following contact with another infected human being. Evidence suggests respiratory transmission, and the epidemiologic pattern supports this concept. Skin inoculation and fomite spread may also play a role in some instances.

Following contact, an asymptomatic period of 12 to 13 days follows. Despite the lack of symptoms, viral replication is massive.

The pathogenic events that occur in the human being are suggested by analogy with Jenner's experimental mousepox infection. The virus, following introduction via the respiratory tract, undergoes local multiplication in the respiratory mucosa and regional lymphoid tissue. Primary viremia occurs, which spreads the virus widely throughout the reticuloendothelial system, where a massive multiplication occurs. A secondary viremia heralds the onset of the prodromal illness, resulting in spread to many organs and tissues, with primary manifestations in the skin. It has been postulated that serum antibody is not the significant factor in recovery from initial episodes of smallpox, and it appears likely that both delayed hypersensitivity and interferon production play some role in such recovery. Hemorrhagic forms of the disease are of interest in that a profound coagulation disorder is associated with a decrease in the number of serum platelets. Evidence indicates that depression of platelet formation occurs routinely in smallpox infection and that the hemorrhagic forms of the disease bear some similarity to disseminated intravascular coagulation, which results in reduction in coagulation factors, extensive hemorrhage, and death.

Clinical Manifestations

HISTORY   An influenzal illness shortly after contact has been described ("illness of contact"). A history of contact is essential. Prior vaccination history and interval to symptoms are important, as the disease pattern may be altered. Prior to the onset of the typical cutaneous lesions, a prodromal period of 3 days' duration occurs, characterized by apprehension, sudden prostrating fever, severe headache, back pain, and vomiting. A prodromal rash is not uncommon; it is macular and papular or petechial, and when it occurs in the characteristic "swimming-trunk" distribution, it is felt to be pathognomonic.

CUTANEOUS LESIONS   The disease may take various courses. In the nonvaccinated, a discrete pox eruption is the most frequent form of illness. Severe forms of the disease are associated with confluent eruptions and/or cutaneous hemorrhage. Infrequently variola may occur without eruption, or with just a few pocks. A flat erythematous macular rash may precede the appearance of tense, deep-seated papules which rapidly vesiculate. These lesions are firm and more deep-seated than those of chickenpox. The rash may be very sparse, or individual vesicles may become confluent to form large patches. As the lesions mature, the classic "pustule" occurs (Fig. 220-1). These lesions do not contain bacteria, and the cloudiness represents accumulated white blood cells, debris, and protein. Central umbilication is characteristic (Figs. 220-1 and 220-2), and eventually the lesion crusts over and heals, with scar formation. Although this is the classic evolution of smallpox, many variants are encountered, especially in individuals previously vaccinated. Lesions may present a flat disklike appearance or may undergo resolution without passing through the vesiculopustular stage.

There are two recognized hemorrhagic forms of the disease: one in which hemorrhage occurs in association with prodromal symptoms but death supervenes before any of the characteristic skin lesions can occur; and a second, characterized by hemorrhage into preexisting skin lesions. Both have almost universally fatal outcomes, the first within a week and the second after 8 to 12 days. Bacterial infection of smallpox lesions occurs, and localized abscesses, cellulitis, etc., may result.

OTHER PHYSICAL FINDINGS   Secondary viremia with spread to many organs may result in clinically apparent illness. Particularly common are ulceration of the cornea, laryngeal lesions with symptoms of obstruction in the upper part of the airway, central nervous system involvement with encephalitis or acute psychotic behavior, and, less commonly, osteomyelitis, pneumonia, and orchitis.

LABORATORY FINDINGS   Usual diagnostic laboratory measurements are of little value in smallpox. The white blood cell count may be elevated early in the disease, but this is not of diagnostic significance.

Virus is present in the blood of patients during the prodrome and occasionally thereafter. Virus is uniformly found in the skin lesions; the early papules and vesicles provide the richest source. In hemorrhagic forms of the disease, severe thrombocytopenia occurs; in addition, marked decrease in the level of accelerator globulin (factor V), moderate decreases in the amount of prothrombin and proconvertin, and a circulating antithrombin are noted in early hemorrhagic smallpox. The late hemorrhagic form of the disease is associated with a decrease in platelets without other coagulation disturbances.

Pathology

In the papular stage of the eruption, capillary dilatation and edema of the papillary layer of the dermis are observed. Perivascular inflammatory changes occur, with lymphocytic and histiocytic infiltration. Thickening and vacuolization in the epithelium result in vesicle formation. The vesicle is deep and, because of the destruction of cells, becomes separate. Leukocyte infiltration results in the "pustule formation," which resolves by epithelial migration and crusting. Typical cytoplasmic eosinophilic inclusion bodies have been described (Guarnieri's bodies). Histopathologic changes in the mucosa are similar, with added ulceration.

Diagnosis and Differential Diagnosis

Typical smallpox in endemic areas could usually be diagnosed clinically, and ancillary virologic laboratory aids were usually unnecessary. However, now that smallpox has been eradicated worldwide, if a case arose, it would probably be confused with severe chickenpox or not suspected at all. For this reason virologic diagnosis would be *essential*, with confirmation of variola having global public health implications. Rapid means of laboratory diagnosis include (1) light microscopic identification of elementary bodies with appropriate stains, (2) electron microscopic identification of virus in vesicular fluid or scrapings from the base of a papule or early vesicle, and (3) fluorescent antibody staining of the virus from the same material. All these tests yield rapid, presumptive results in the hands of experienced workers, but definite diagnosis can be achieved only by isolation of the virus in the embryonated egg or in appropriate tissue culture systems and specific identification of the virus by neutralization with variola or vaccinal antiserum. Indirect but rapid methods utilize vesicular fluid as a hemagglutinin, complement-fixing, or precipitating antigen with specific variola vaccinia antiserum. Retrospective diagnosis can be afforded by evaluation of serum antibody rises in a 2- to 3-week interval, utilizing paired sera collected during the acute and convalescent phases of the illness.

In summary, the diagnosis of smallpox is primarily clinical and based upon obtaining an adequate history of exposure, the observation of an approximately 2-week incubation period followed by a severe 3-day prodrome, ultimately terminating in a typical rash with centrifugal distribution and all lesions in the same stage of

FIGURE 220-1

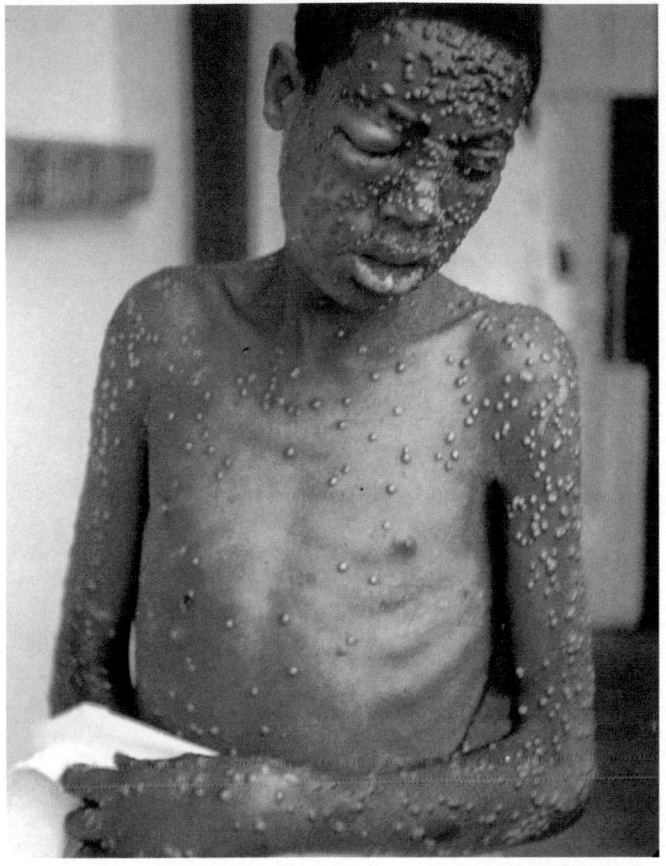

A.

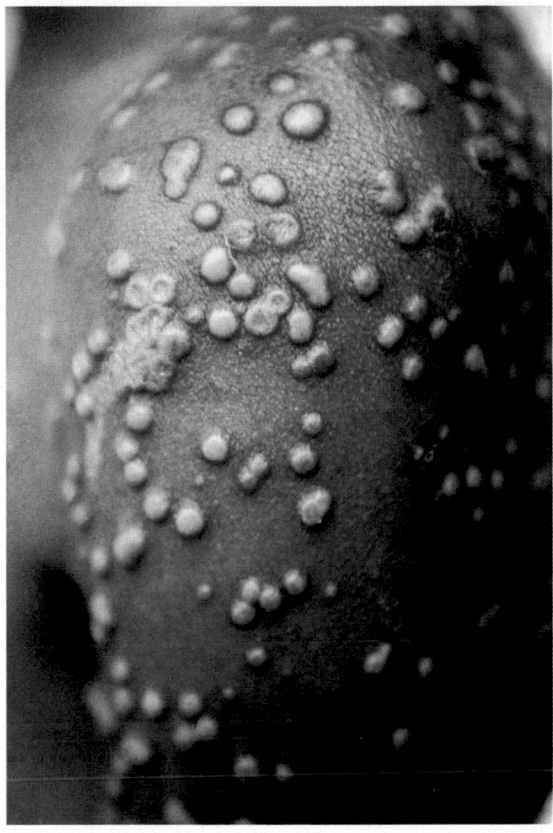

B.

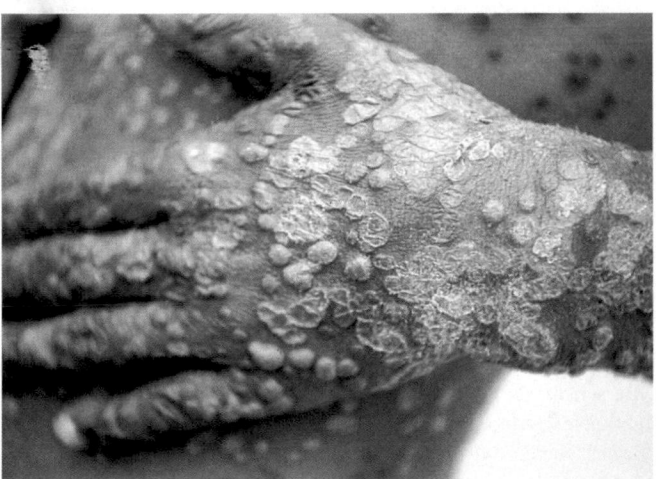

C.

Pustular smallpox: tense, clouded vesicles which maintain firm feel. Note tendency to confluence and beginning central umbilication in some lesions (B,C).

development. One cannot rely on the presence of Guarnieri's bodies to establish the diagnosis, although they may be suggestive.

In the preeruptive phase of smallpox, distinction must be made from dengue, enterovirus infections, and other febrile illnesses. The prodromal rash may be confused with that of measles. History of contact and the appropriate incubation interval should serve to make one suspect smallpox.

Hemorrhagic smallpox may be confused with meningococcal septicemia, coagulation disorders, typhus, and other acute hemorrhagic exanthems. Eruptive smallpox is most frequently mistaken for chickenpox. The lack of prodromal symptoms, the successive appearance of crops of superficial vesicles, the centripetal distribution, and the varying stages of development of chickenpox lesions all serve to distinguish this disease from variola.

Treatment

This disease has now been prevented by Jennerian vaccination, but no effective specific treatment was known. Thiosemicarbazone and antivariola or antivaccinia serum and immune globulin failed in the therapy of established smallpox.

Good nursing care with attention to the prevention of secondary bacterial infection is critical in treatment. Appropriate antimicrobial therapy for bacterial complications should be employed, and attention should be paid to the nutritional, fluid, and electrolyte needs of patients.

Course and Prognosis

The overall mortality rate of smallpox approximates 25 percent, with confluent disease representing a greater risk than discrete eruptions. Fulminant smallpox is universally fatal, as are the hemorrhagic forms of the illness.

FIGURE 220-2

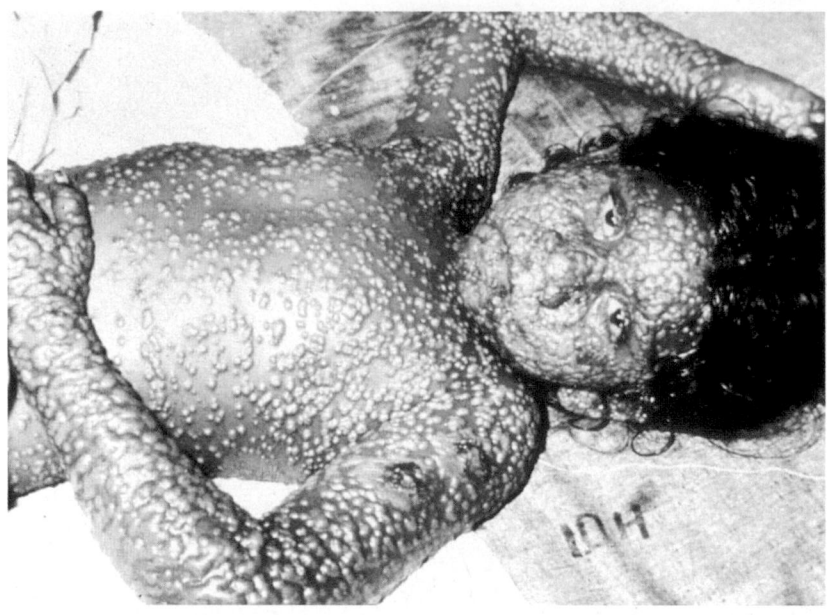

Confluent smallpox. Note massive numbers of lesions, all in same stage of development, and confluency of many.

COMPLICATIONS OF SMALLPOX VACCINATION (VACCINIA)

Definition and Classification

Vaccination against smallpox consists of the introduction of vaccinia virus into the outer layers of the intact skin. Local multiplication of virus occurs, and in some instances regional lymphadenopathy and systemic symptoms ensue. The infection is a localized one which heals by scarring and is limited by host response. A complicated vaccination is one in which any of the above components is altered. Complications may be classified as indicated in Table 220-1.

The vaccinia virus is now being used as a vector to express other genes in mammalian cells, including potential vaccines against other diseases.

Historic Aspects

With the eradication of smallpox in the world, the routine application of infant vaccination has been greatly diminished. As a result, complications of vaccinations are seen infrequently in most countries and not at all in many.

Epidemiology

Most complications may occur at any age, but they are usually seen among young infants and children. Primovaccination is most often administered to this age group, and almost all the significant complications occur most frequently, if not exclusively, after first vaccination. In addition, the infectious complications tend to occur in the immunologically deficient child, which also contributes to the clustering in early childhood. Bacterial superinfection in some instances is related to warm weather, with the opportunity for maceration of skin and with increased exposure of the vaccination site.

Complications are reported more commonly in the western world, despite the prevalence of vaccination in the east. This undoubtedly represents reporting differences, not a true geographic or racial relationship. The incidence of postvaccinal encephalitis appears to be higher in the Netherlands. Whether this represents a true racial difference or simply reflects the fact of primovaccination in the adults is not clear.

Etiology and Pathogenesis

The basic mechanisms of the complications of vaccination may be divided into three categories: (1) bacterial superinfection, (2) abnormal viral replication, and (3) altered reactivity, or "allergy," to some viral component.

Bacteria can invade the vaccination site; indeed, not all vaccine is bacteriologically sterile. That superinfection is not more common is remarkable. Apparently more than contamination is necessary; those factors of greatest importance are concurrent streptococcal infection elsewhere and excessive trauma, maceration, and manipulation of the vaccination site.

Usually the virus remains localized at the site of implantation, but occasionally infection may be transposed to healthy or unhealthy skin elsewhere on the body, or even to another person. Etiologic factors include excessive manipulation, abnormal skin (burns, eczema, etc.), inflammatory lesions (blepharitis, herpes), and abnormal immune mechanisms. Any of these may contribute to spread of the virus away from the intended localized vaccination site.

Among the host factors that are responsible for limitation of viral spread and recovery from vaccination are development of serum antibody, delayed hypersensitivity, and interferon production. Serum antibody and delayed hypersensitivity are specific and are induced soon after infection; antibody would appear to be less important in recovery than delayed hypersensitivity. Interferon is nonspecific and has been found in the skin of animals recovering from vaccinia infection who have been rendered deficient in antibodies and in delayed hypersensitivity. It has also been found in human vaccination crusts. Individuals who lack antibody-synthesizing capacity may develop progressive and widespread vaccinal lesions. However, even these patients, if they retain delayed-hypersensitivity responsiveness, may undergo perfectly normal vaccinations. In addition, patients with normal antibody levels, but with absent delayed-hypersensitivity responsiveness, are susceptible to the progressive form of the disease. As indicated, interferon is also important and may account for recovery of animals in the absence of the other two functions. However, data for human beings are lacking, and the importance of this mechanism of resistance is not known.

Allergy, or presumed altered reactivity, to viral components appears to be responsible for the erythema multiforme type of skin rash observed in some individuals after primovaccination. This mechanism has also been implicated in the pathogenesis of postvaccinal encephalitis; it is assumed the virus or a virus–central nervous system complex invokes an immune response directed against brain antigens, which then results in an antigen-antibody inflammatory reaction and the clinical picture of encephalitis.

Clinical Manifestations

ERYTHEMA MULTIFORME–LIKE ERUPTIONS An intensely erythematous macular rash may follow smallpox vaccination. This rash has the characteristics of erythema multiforme in that iris or bull's eye lesions appear and tend to coalesce. The rash is often symmetric and florid, involving a large portion of the body. This is a totally benign manifestation representing an allergic reaction.

BACTERIAL SUPERINFECTION Purulent complications of smallpox vaccination today involve principally impetiginous infection with *Staphylococcus aureus* or group A beta-hemolytic streptococci. If poultices are employed, tetanus may be introduced by the soil or dung elements incorporated in such primitive techniques.

ACCIDENTAL INOCULATION Vaccinia virus can be implanted from the site of vaccination onto the skin or mucous membrane anywhere on the individual's body. They can also be transferred to another individual. Each of the lesions is characteristic of a primary smallpox vaccination with the exception that they do not tend to scar. Certain implantations may be more hazardous than the occasional single-site inoculation. These include implantation onto large areas of abnormal skin (burns or other dermatoses), into the eye (vaccinal keratitis may result), extensive mucosal lesions, and implantation around various body orifices which may impede certain bodily functions (Fig. 220-3).

TABLE 220-1

Classification of Complications of Vaccination

Major Category	Specific Syndromes	Comment
Noninfectious rashes	Erythema multiforme	Differentiate from generalized
	Macular—toxic eruption	
	Macular and papular	
	Vesicular	
	Urticarial	
Bacterial superinfection	Streptococcal	Often hyperkeratotic
	Staphylococcal	
	Mixed	
	Tetanus	
	Syphilis	Of historical interest in U.S.
Accidental inoculation (may occur in vaccinated individual)	Normal skin	
	Abnormal skin	
	Burns	
	Pyoderma	
	Exanthem	Examples: varicella, herpes
	Eczema	
	Other dermatides:	
	Mucosal	Usually oral or conjunctival
	Corneal	Vaccinal keratitis
Congenital vaccinia		
Generalized vaccinia	Benign becoming malignant with progression	
Progressive vaccinia (vaccinia gangrenosa, vaccinia necrosum)	In immunologically normal persons	
	In hypogammaglobulinemia:	
	Congenital sex-linked	
	Thymic alymphoplasia	
	In dysgammaglobulinemia	
	With malignancies:	
	Chronic lymphatic leukemia	
	Hodgkin's disease	
	Lymphoma	
Encephalitis	Postvaccinal	
Miscellaneous	Hemolytic anemia	
	Arthritis	
	Osteomyelitis	
	Laboratory infections	
	Pericarditis and myocarditis	

CONGENITAL VACCINIA Vaccination of the pregnant woman may result in disseminated disease fatal to the fetus. Congenital vaccination may also occur following exposure to a vaccinated individual. The infant may be stillborn or may develop lesions shortly after birth.

GENERALIZED VACCINIA Generalized vaccinia as used in this classification refers to a benign generalized eruption, each lesion of which is identical to its primary smallpox vaccination. Although little is known of the immunology surrounding such a defect, it is clear that some children with isolated IgM deficiency are liable to this complication. This is not generally a lethal disease.

PROGRESSIVE VACCINIA (VACCINIA GANGRENOSA, VACCINIA NECROSUM) If a smallpox vaccination shows no evidence of normal resolution within 2 weeks of inoculation, a presumptive diagnosis of progressive vaccinia should be made. In this disease, the normal immunologic response to vaccination is impaired. This may occur in an otherwise normal individual or in persons with generalized defects in immunologic capacities.

In its complete form, the site of vaccination fails to heal and continues to enlarge, often for months. Usually, no systemic signs of illness are present and, in the absence of some other disease, physical findings are limited to the vaccination. These lesions differ from normal ones in that little inflammatory response is observed. The vaccination initially has a soft, rubbery appearance with little scabbing (Fig. 220-4). As the lesion progresses in size, considerable central necrosis becomes evident, and thick, dark eschars form (hence the synonym, vaccinia necrosum). The initial lesion may become huge, with the entire upper arm and shoulder involved. In many cases secondary lesions are evident; in some, satellite vaccinations occur close to the primary one, and, in addition, viremic lesions may appear at distant sites. Each of the secondary lesions progresses in the same fashion as the primary one (Fig. 220-5). Variations are observed in that the primary lesion may become ul-

FIGURE 220-3

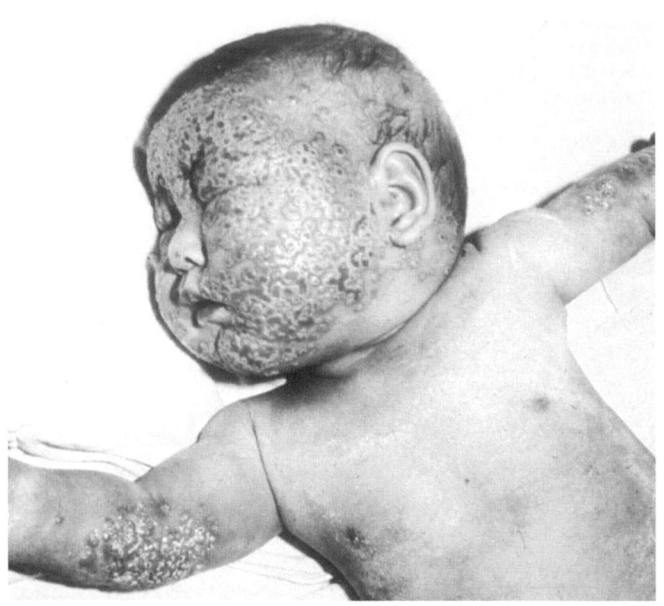

Eczema vaccinatum. Lesions are in areas of active eczema. Note typical vaccinal character of individual lesions.

FIGURE 220-4

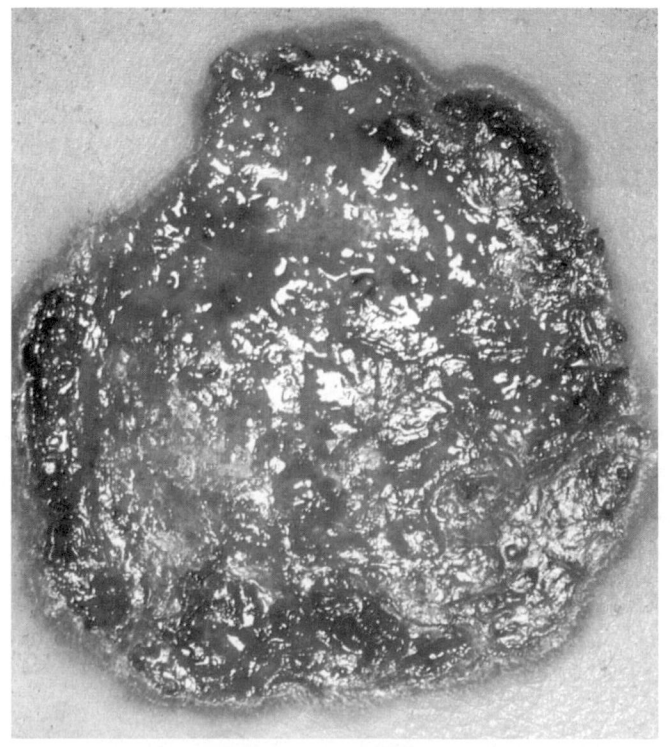

Progressive vaccinia: large, nonhealing vaccination site with "soft, rubbery" border, high virus content, and lack of surrounding inflammatory response; present 4 months in 10-month-old male with variant of thymic alymphoplasia.

FIGURE 220-5

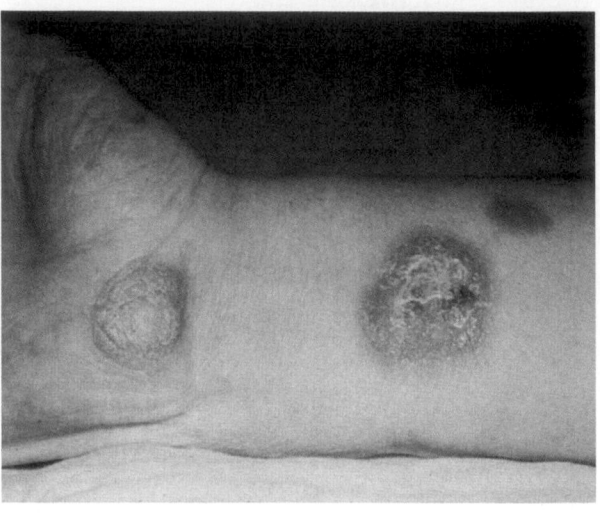

Secondary, viremic lesions in progressive vaccinia. Two lesions on arm, which demonstrate variability, both positive for vaccinia virus, occurred in elderly female with chronic lymphatic leukemia; complete clearing with thiosemicarbazone therapy.

cerative or may have a piled-up appearance, but the progression is characteristic.

Untreated disease or illness failing to respond to treatment may be of long duration, during which extensive tissue destruction, secondary bacterial infection and septicemia, mucosal lesions, pneumonia, and other complications may occur. The course is progressively downhill, although the patient may not manifest correspondingly severe constitutional symptoms until relatively late in the disease.

ENCEPHALITIS A meningoencephalitis syndrome occurs rarely as a complication of smallpox vaccination. The sudden onset of headache and vomiting in the second week after vaccination may herald this illness. Convulsions, lethargy, coma, paralysis, signs of cerebral edema, increased intracranial pressure, and focal neurologic findings may occur. In other instances the disease may resemble aseptic meningitis or myelitis.

Laboratory Findings

VIROLOGIC Specimens from suspected vaccinal lesions can be inoculated into a variety of tissue culture systems or the embryonated hen's egg. Identification is by typical pock formation or by classic cytopathogenic effect with subsequent neutralization by antisera. Additionally, specific vaccinia antigen can be detected by a variety of antibody methods, either from the original specimen obtained from the patient or from the infected cell cultures or egg fluids.

IMMUNOLOGIC AND HEMATOLOGIC Response to vaccinia virus may be critical in determining host susceptibility. Vaccinia-neutralizing antibody can be measured, as can a delayed-hypersensitivity reaction to inactivated vaccinia antigen.

In certain clinical states, total immunologic capacity may need to be surveyed, as the vaccinal infection is simply an indicator of a more comprehensive immunologic defect. Assays for immunoglobulin antibody capacity and for cell-mediated immune function may need to be employed.

Treatment

Complications of vaccination can be reduced by recognizing those predisposing conditions that lead to each of the separate types of complication. Thus, individuals who have eczema or other skin lesions should not be vaccinated or exposed to an individual who is vaccinated. Individuals with immunologic deficiency, receiving immunosuppressive therapy, or suffering from diseases such as lymphatic malignancies that heighten susceptibility should avoid contact with vaccinia virus and should not be vaccinated. If such individuals are exposed, use of either vaccinia immune globulin by injection or methisazone (isatin thiosemicarbazone) can be expected to reduce the risk.

In the past, administration of vaccinia immune globulin (VIG) for complications of vaccination has been facilitated by its ready availability. Currently this product is no longer produced and is in limited supply. As a result, its use should be more stringent than in the past and it should be reserved for those severe complications in which a beneficial effect has been either demonstrated or suspected. Children with erythema multiforme or simple autoinoculation disease and vaccinal encephalitis should not receive this preparation as it is of no benefit. On the other hand, those with extensive intradermal involvement such as eczema vaccinatum or burns should be treated with either VIG or methisazone. VIG should be used in conjunction with methisazone and immunologic therapy in those severe complications such as progressive vaccinia.

Course and Prognosis

As indicated in the separate sections, prognosis is variable. Most complications are self-limited or respond to simple measures; a few require extraordinary forms of therapy, and even with such treatment a small group remains who are unresponsive.

SUGGESTED READINGS

Smallpox (Variola)
Bauer DJ et al: The chemotherapy of variola major infection. *Bull WHO* **26**:727, 1962

Bauer DJ et al: Prophylactic treatment of smallpox contacts with *N*-methylisatin β-thiosemicarbazone. *Lancet* **2**:494, 1963

Bremen JG, Arita I: The confirmation and maintenance of smallpox eradication. *N Engl J Med* **303**:1263, 1980

Dixon CW: *Smallpox*. London, Churchill, 1962

Downie AW: Smallpox, in *Medical History of the Second World War,* edited by Z Cope. London, HM Stationery Office, 1952

Downie AW, MacDonald A: Smallpox and related virus infections in man. *Br Med Bull* **9**:191, 1953

Downie AW et al: Studies on the virus content of mouth washings in the acute phase of smalllpox. *Bull WHO* **25**:49, 1961

Fenner F: Global eradication of smallpox. *Rev Infect Dis* **4**:916, 1982

Kempe CH: Smallpox, in *The Biologic Basis of Pediatric Practice,* edited by R Cooke. New York, McGraw-Hill, 1965

Kempe CH, St Vincent L: Variola and vaccinia, in *Diagnostic Procedures in Viral and Rickettsial Infections,* edited by E Lennette. New York, American Public Health Association, 1964

Kempe CH et al: The use of vaccinia hyperimmune gamma globulin in the prophylaxis of smallpox. *Bull WHO* **25**:41, 1961

Massung RF et al: Analysis of the complete genome of smallpox variola major virus strain Baugladesh-1975. *Virology* **201**:215, 1994

Rao AR et al: A study of 1,000 cases of smallpox. *J Indian Med Assoc* **35**:296, 1960

Wehrle P: A reality in our time—certification of the global eradication of smallpox. *J Infect Dis* **242**:636, 1980

WHO Expert Committee on Smallpox: *WHO Technical Report Series* **283**:1, 1964

Complications of Smallpox Vaccination (Vaccinia)
Adels BR, Oppe TE: Treatment of eczema vaccinatum with *N*-methylisatin beta-thiosemicarbazone. *Lancet* **1**:18, 1966

Barbero GT et al: Vaccinia gangrenosa treated with hyperimmune vaccinal gamma globulin. *Pediatrics* **16**:609, 1955

Daly JJ, Jackson E: Vaccinia gangrenosa treated with *N*-methylisatin β-thiosemicarbazone. *Br Med J* **2**:1300, 1962

Davidson E, Hayhoe FG: Prolonged generalized vaccinia complicating acute leukemia. *Br Med J* **2**:1298, 1962

Dimson SB: Eczema vaccinatum. *Lancet* **2**:73, 1962

Ellis PP, Wenograd L: Ocular vaccinia. *Arch Ophthalmol* **68**:600, 1962

Erichson RB, McNamara MJ: Vaccinia gangrenosa: Report of a case and review of the literature. *Ann Intern Med* **55**:491, 1961

Fekety FR Jr et al: Vaccinia gangrenosa in chronic lymphatic leukemia. *Arch Intern Med* **109**:205, 1962

Flewitt TH, Ker FL: A case of vaccinia necrosum (progressive vaccinia) with severe hypogammaglobulinemia, treated with *N*-methylisatin β-thiosemicarbazone (33T57). *J Clin Pathol* **16**:271, 1963

Fulginiti VA, Kempe CH: Poxvirus diseases, in *Brennemann's Practice of Pediatrics,* vol II, part 1, edited by V Kelley. Hagerstown, MD, Harper & Row, 1937, p 1

Fulginiti VA et al: Therapy of experimental vaccinal keratitis. *Arch Ophthalmol* **74**:539, 1965

Greenberg M: Complications of vaccination against smallpox. *Am J Dis Child* **76**:492, 1948

Kaufman H et al: A cure of vaccinia infection by 5-iodo-2'-deoxyuridine. *Virology* **18**:567, 1962

Kempe CH: Studies on smallpox and complications of smallpox vaccination. *Pediatrics* **26**:176, 1960

Kempe CH, Benenson AS: Smallpox immunization in the United States. *JAMA* **194**:161, 1965

Kempe CH et al: Hyperimmune vaccinal gamma globulin. *Pediatrics* **18**:177, 1956

Moss B: Genetically engineered poxviruses for recombinant gene expression, vaccination, and safety. *Proc Natl Acad Sci USA* **93**:11341, 1996

Naidoo P, Hirsch H: Prenatal vaccinia. *Lancet* **1**:196, 1963

Nanning W: Prophylactic effect of antivaccinia gamma globulin against postvaccinal encephalitis. *Bull WHO* **27**:317, 1962

Neff JM: Smallpox vaccination: Minimal complication rates, United States, 1963. Presentation at Annual Epidemiologic Intelligence Service, Communicable Disease Center, April 1965

O'Connel CJ et al: Progressive vaccinia with normal antibodies: A case possibly due to deficient cellular immunity. *Ann Intern Med* **60**:282, 1964

Sathe PV et al: Prevention of postvaccinal tetanus. *Indian J Pediatr* **31**:306, 1965

Spillane JD, Wells CEC: The neurology of Jennerian vaccination: A clinical account of the neurological complications which occurred during the smallpox epidemic in South Wales in 1962. *Brain* **87**:1, 1964

Sussman S, Grossman M: Complications of smallpox vaccination. Effects of vaccinia immune globulin therapy. *J Pediatr* **67**:1168, 1965

Wielenga G et al: Prenatal infection with vaccinia virus. *Lancet* **1**:258, 1961

CHAPTER 221

Ullin W. Leavell, Jr.
Robert J. Jacob

Contagious Pustular Dermatitis, Contagious Ecthyma: Orf Virus Infection

Contagious ecthyma, or contagious pustular dermatitis, is a disease caused by the orf virus (OV), a member of the Poxviridae family. The disease is endemic among sheep, goats,[1,2] and musk oxen (i.e., ruminants) and can be transmitted to humans.[3–5] Early authors who suggested that the disease was transmitted from animals to humans included Brandenberg,[6] Newsome et al.,[7] and Peterkin.[8] The disease usually develops in the vicinity of the mouth and nose of animals and manifests itself as nodules on exposed areas of the skin. Lesions are similar in humans and animals and heal in about 35 days.[9] The disease is classified as a near-neoplasm, since it stimulates pseudoepitheliomatous hyperplasia and causes a finger-like downward proliferation of the epidermis.

EPIDEMIOLOGY AND ETIOLOGY

The disease has been reported exclusively in whites. Age is not a factor in that the disease has been seen in patients as young as 10 and as old as 72 years.[10] It is commonplace among shepherds in all parts of the world. Not all cases are thoroughly documented because many patients do not seek medical advice. Farmers and veterinarians are most likely to be exposed to the virus, and immunosuppression and skin lesions increase susceptibility in exposed persons. The disease is more prevalent in the spring when newborn lambs, lacking immunity, fall prey to the disease.[11] Infected lambs have lower total serum protein values, hemoglobin concentration, erythrocyte counts, and packed cell volume but higher blood leukocyte counts and increased serum transaminase activity when compared to apparently healthy animals. Individuals feeding milk from bottles to infected, orphaned lambs frequently come in contact with the lamb's sore mouth and may contract the disease. The virus may be acquired indirectly from knives, barbed wire, barn doors, towels, and vehicles that have contacted infected animals.

The virus is sturdy, surviving the winter months on barn doors, feeding troughs, and fences. Susceptible lambs become infected from contact with virus-containing objects. It has been found in goats, camels, bighorn sheep, mountain goats, gazelles,[12] and wild sheep. Pregnancy and fetal development[13] have not been reported to be affected by infection with the virus.

IMMUNITY

Previous cutaneous infection with OV results in lesions that are less pronounced. Recurrences of the eruption have been reported in a patient 8 months after the initial lesion. Response to infection in humans appears to be the same as seen in sheep, including production of interferon and cell-mediated and antibody responses. The lymphoproliferative responses to OV infection are vigorous immediately after infection and then decline rapidly. Antibodies to OV rise during the infection. The antibody produced is against the 40-kDa viral surface tubule protein (see below). Prior exposure to vaccinia or smallpox vaccination does not provide protection against OV infection. Incomplete immunity to OV infection may be explained by the short-lived nature of a local T cell response upon infection. Experimental inoculation of vaccine in animals indicates that reinoculation can take place in 3 to 5 months. The best prevention in animals is vaccination every 6 to 8 months.[14] After vaccination with the OV, mules, deer, musk oxen, moose, and wapiti calves have developed the disease.

MOLECULAR ANATOMY OF OV

OV could be considered a prototype for the genus *Parapoxvirus*. It is an ovoid particle about 250 nm by 160 nm. The surface tubules of parapoxvirus appear as a twinelike structure, 10 nm to 20 nm wide, forming a long crisscross design that extends for up to 1 μm in length.[15] This design is easily seen on negatively stained preparations by electron microscopy (Fig. 221-1). This structure helps distinguish a parapoxvirus from an orthopoxvirus in that orthopoxviruses have an irregular arrangement of tubules in their outer membranes. OV shows serologic cross-reactivity with another parapoxvirus, milker's nodule virus,[16] although it does not appear to be genetically related (see Chap. 223). Parapoxviruses are sensitive to heating at 58°C (136°F) for 30 min and resistant to lipid solvents such as ether and chloroform. The virus's resistance to long-term drying is important for the enzootic spread of infection.

The OV has a linear double-stranded DNA, 140 kbp, that is smaller than that of orthopoxvirus but contains a 64 percent G +

C content that is higher than that of the orthopoxvirus. Nevertheless, the DNA contains an inverted terminal repeat,[17] a crossed-linked terminal region,[18] and sequence patterns reminiscent of orthopoxviruses.[19] Their genomic maps can be tentatively aligned.[20] As with other parapoxviruses,[19] OV has been shown to contain several genes for viral-specific enzymes commonly found in the orthopoxviruses (e.g., vaccinia). These findings suggest a common evolutionary origin for these genera. However, several genes referred to as *virokines*, or viral-encoded analogues of host cytokines (i.e., eosinophil chemotactic factor, transforming growth factor α), that appear to play a role in the pathogenesis of the disease (see below) have been identified for orthopoxviruses but have not yet been identified in the parapoxviruses.

Restriction endonuclease (RE) "fingerprint" analysis of OV DNA reveals heterogeneity in the genome structure that is consistent with reports of antigenic variation in the virus.[21,22] RE analysis could not resolve OV into groups of ovine and human strains. Point mutations, substitutions, and deletions of base pairs; inversions and transpositions; and minor alterations of sequences throughout the DNA are probably responsible for this difference in RE fingerprints. This RE pattern variation is similar to what has been seen in the poxviruses.[23,24] Although Southern blot analysis did not reveal any insertion of host DNA within the OV genome, it did reveal that several field isolates lack a large segment (i.e., 14 to 19 percent) of DNA that is found in the commonly used vaccine strain (i.e., CE vaccine).[25] The right end of the genome is particularly susceptible to variations. The different strains contain sequences that vary from 40 to 63 percent G + C content in this region and often in great variance with the mean genome content, suggesting acquisition from host cell DNA. It is of particular interest in that a viral gene product (14 to 16 kDa) whose amino acid sequence is homologous with a mammalian growth factor, vascular endothelial growth factor (VEGF), maps to this region on the genome.[26,27] VEGF-like genes from the different strains of OV show little DNA homology to each other. At the time of writing, the evidence suggests this to be a virokine that has not been identified in vaccinia infections, the prototype virus of the orthopoxviruses.

MOLECULAR PATHOGENESIS

The virus grows on primary human amnion and other cell cultures, producing cells with pyknotic nuclei and vacuolated cytoplasm. The virus will not produce pocks on the chorioallantoic membrane of fertilized eggs. However, the virus will grow plaques in cultured cells such as bovine and ovine embryonic lung cells,[28] lamb testes,[21] and bovine fetal spleen cells.[29] Plaques form as holes in the monolayer, surrounded by clumps of granular cells. Cytopathic effect is seen during OV replication with complete virions forming at 12 to 16 h after infection. The ultrastructural changes seen are a

FIGURE 221-1

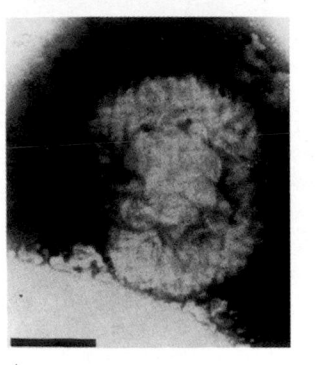
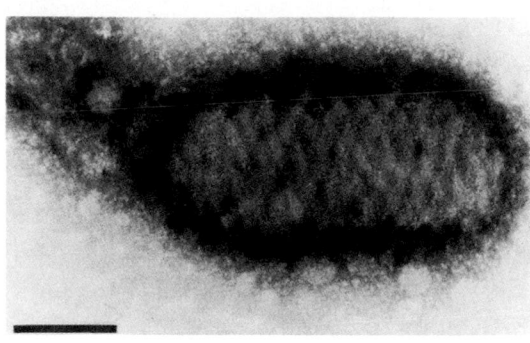

A. *B.*

Electron micrographs of negatively stained preparations of (*A*) orthopox virus and (*B*) parapoxvirus (orf) isolated from vesicular fluid and representing the "M" forms of poxviruses. The bars represent 100 nm. (*Reprinted with permission from "An Atlas of Mammalian Viruses," edited by FL Palmer, ML Martin. Copyright 1982, CRC Press, Inc., Boca Raton, FL.*)

result of focal areas of viral production, which takes place in the cytoplasm in areas called "factories" that are said to contain viroplasm.[15,30] An example of this can be seen in Fig. 221-2. These areas contained immature viral particles in the form of trilamina structures. At this point it is important to remember that the VEGF-like viral gene product (see above) is expressed early during infection and could be indirectly responsible for the induction of epithe-

FIGURE 221-2

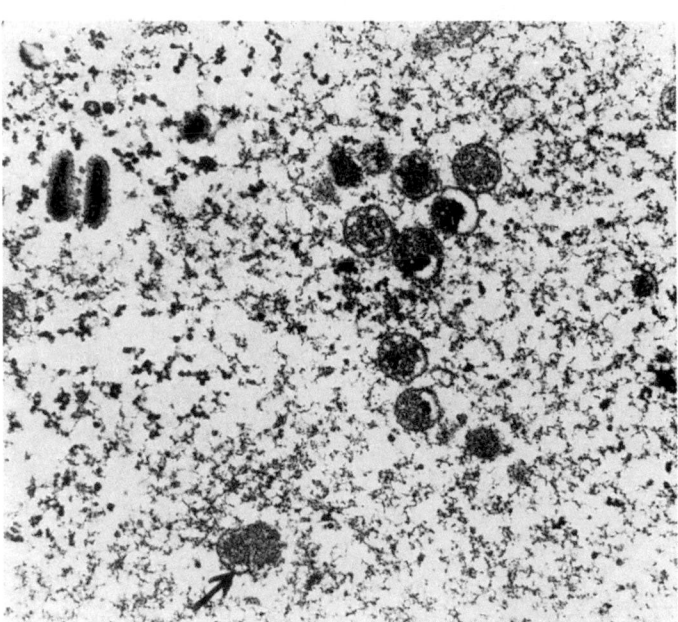

An electron micrograph shows viroplasm, partially encapsulated viroplasm, and mature viral particles. ×36,750. (*Reprinted with permission of Albert J. Dalton, MD, National Institutes of Health, Bethesda, MD.*)

lial proliferation. In any event, it is more likely responsible for dermal capillary endothelial proliferation and dilatation seen at the site of infection.

During the period of viral replication, the nuclear chromatin marginates to the nuclear membrane. Distinct morphologic changes can be seen in the nucleoplasm around 36 h after infection. These changes can be seen as an accumulation of tubules and the formation of fine filaments and appear to be independent of the development of mature virus particles. Accumulation of intranuclear tubules may be a host phenomenon and represents an indirect cellular response to viral infection rather than viral products.[30] This observation is important to note in that an interpretation that this nuclear activity is viral-specific would suggest a nuclear-replicating virus, thus excluding members of poxviridae as etiologic agents.

CLINICAL MANIFESTATIONS

The cutaneous lesions average 1.6 cm in diameter. Usually only one lesion is present, although as many as 10 have been reported. The lesion is most commonly located on the dorsal aspect of the right index finger. Regional lymphadenopathy is common. Lymphangitis and fever may occur,[31] with the fever disappearing within 3 to 4 days and the lymphangitis within 3 to 4 weeks. Toxic erythema, erythema multiforme, and a widespread papulovesicular eruption of the skin and mucosae may occur. Complications may include pain, pruritus, lymphangitis, adenitis, fever, malaise, erythema multiforme, erysipelas, papulovesicular eruption, *Pseudomonas aeruginosa* infection, and bullous pemphigoid.[32,33] Amputation of a finger was necessary in a patient receiving immunosuppressive drugs for lymphoma.

The disease advances through six stages, healing uneventfully in about 35 days. Each stage lasts approximately 6 days. The papular stage shows a red, elevated lesion. The target stage has a nodule with a red center, a white middle ring, and a red periphery (Fig. 221-3). A red, weeping surface is present during the acute stage,

FIGURE 221-3

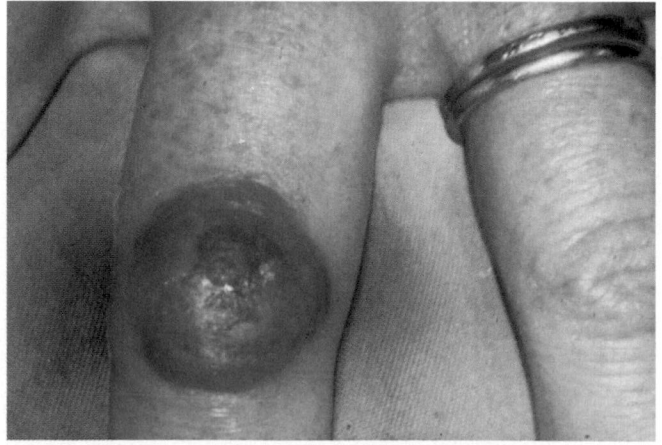

The target phase shows a white circle with central and peripheral erythema.

FIGURE 221-4

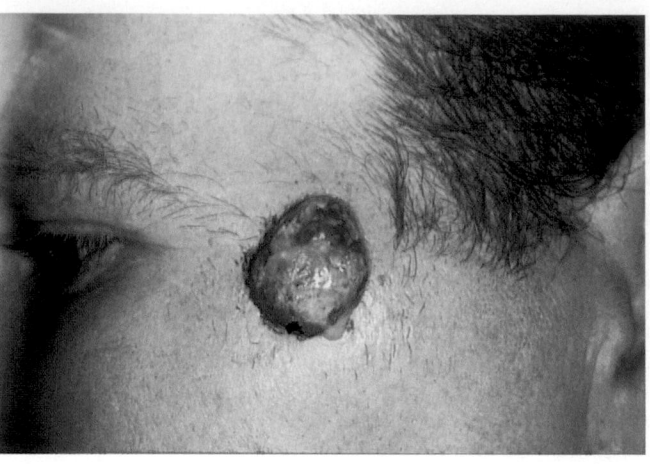

In the acute phase there is weeping of the surface overlying an elevated tumor.

and the lesion may be elevated, appearing to be a rapidly growing infected tumor (Fig. 221-4). In the regenerative stage, a thin, dry crust through which black dots may be seen covers the surface of nodule. Small papillomas appear over the surface of the lesion during the papillomatous stage. In the regressive stage, a thick crust develops over the surface of the lesion, the papillomas decrease in size, and elevation of the lesion subsides.

PATHOLOGY

The papular stage of OV infection has not been studied in humans. In the target stage, intranuclear and intracytoplasmic inclusions are present in superficial, vacuolated epidermal cells in areas corresponding to the white ring (Fig. 221-5). There is an infiltrate of plasma cells, macrophages, histiocytes, and lymphocytes. The acute stage is distinguished by loss of epidermis over the central part of the lesion. Peripherally, there is reticular degeneration. Microvesicles are present. There are distention and loss of the epidermal cells of hair follicles followed by regeneration of the epidermis. The black dots observed clinically correspond to an accumulation of cellular breakdown products in the follicles.

Many papillary elevations and finger-like downward projections of the epidermis are seen in the papillomatous stage (Fig. 221-6). In the regressive stage, the papillomas are reduced in size, and histiocytes, macrophages, lymphocytes, and plasma cells are decreased in number.[34]

Acanthosis within the first week followed by a finger-like downward proliferation of the epidermis are features suggesting neoplasia. Papillomatosis and acanthosis occur within the papilloma. The infiltrate in the dermis contributes to the growing tumor. This suggestive neoplastic pathology and the events of the acute stage of the clinical manifestations are consistent with the most recent findings that identify an early viral gene product to be homologous with mammalian VEGF, an epithelial growth factor described in the previous section.[26,27] However, in the absence of evidence of a VEGF receptor, FLT-1, it is only speculative to suggest that the regressive stage is consistent with the production of a soluble variant of

FIGURE 221-5

CHAPTER 221
Orf Virus Infection

2477

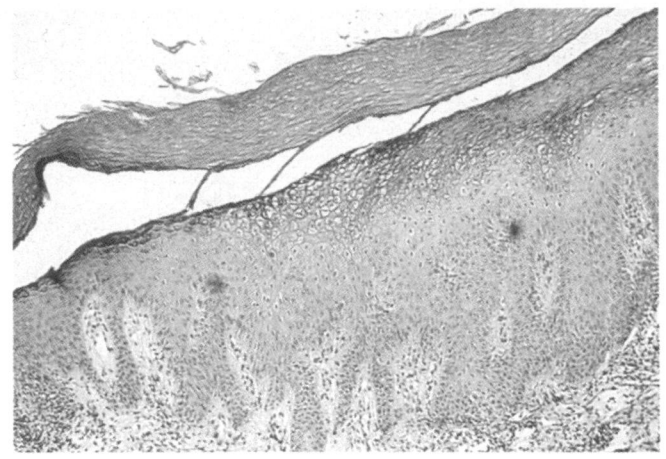

In the target phase vacuolated epidermal cells advance peripherally, leaving behind epidermal thickening and pyknotic epidermal cells.

FIGURE 221-6

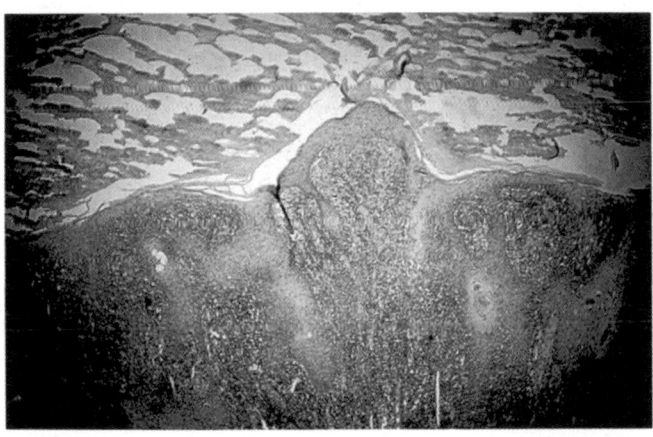

In the papillomatous phase there is a papilloma and finger-like downward projections of the epidermis.

FLT-1 that blocks angiogenesis, leading to a limitation of tumor growth.[37]

The pathology of human regional lymph nodes has not been studied. In sheep, however, there is a progressive increase in the size of the lymph nodes and in the plasma cell infiltrate over a 14-day period.[34,35]

DIAGNOSIS

The diagnosis of contagious ecthyma, OV infection, is established by a history of contact with infected animals, the appearance of the lesions, passage of the virus to sheep cell cultures, fluorescent antibody tests, and electron microscopy (see Fig. 221-2).[36] Electron microscopy of sheep tissue reveals partially and/or totally encapsulated viroplasm and nucleoids and mature oval particles with a

riblike outer structure. Elongated virions with central narrowing and bending of the elementary bodies may be present.[15] As detailed above, structures reminiscent of the virus have been seen in both the nucleus and cytoplasm of epidermal cells. A spiral form in the virus is typical for a member of the parapoxviruses. Complement-fixing antigen has been advanced as the most sensitive technique for diagnosing contagious ecthyma. T cell function, phytohemagglutinin reaction, and natural killer cell activity are interpreted as normal.

TREATMENT

Treatment is not specific. Compresses, culture and sensitivity testing, and appropriate antibiotics are of value for secondary bacterial infection. After excision and cautery, lesions heal uneventfully within 2 to 3 weeks. Glucocorticoids and immunosuppressive drugs should be avoided, inasmuch as acanthosis and pseudoepitheliomatous hyperplasia may appear earlier and be more extensive as a result of their administration. No underlying disease has been found as a predisposition, nor has any residual pathologic change been reported. The prognosis is excellent.

REFERENCES

1. Carr RW: A case of orf contracted by a human from a wild Alaskan mountain goat. *Alaska Med* **10**:75, 1968
2. Guss SB: Contagious ecthyma (sore mouth, orf). *Mod Pract* **61**:335, 1980
3. Cutler TP: Orf: A report of a case. *Clin Exp Dermatol* **6**:205, 1981
4. Erickson GA et al: Generalized contagious ecthyma in a sheep rancher. Diagnostic considerations. *J Am Vet Med Assoc* **166**:262, 1974
5. Leavell UW Jr: Ecthyma contagiosum. *J Ky Med Assoc* **58**:42, 1960
6. Brandenberg TO: Lip and leg ulceration in sheep with report of two cases in man. *JAMA* **8**:818, 1932
7. Newsome IE et al: Sore mouth transmissible to man. *JAMA* **84**:799, 1934
8. Peterkin GAG: The occurrence on humans of contagious pustular dermatitis of sheep ("orf"). *Br J Dermatol* **49**:492, 1933
9. Leavell UW Jr et al: Ecthyma contagiosum (orf). *South Med J* **58**:238, 1965
10. Dupre A et al: Orf and atopic dermatitis. *Br J Dermatol* **105**:103, 1981
11. Gameel A et al: Clinico-pathological observations on naturally occurring contagious ecthyma in lambs in Saudi Arabia. *Rev Elev Med Vet Pays Trop* **48**:233, 1995
12. Yeruham I et al: Parapox infection in a gazelle kid. *J Wildl Dis* **30**:260, 1994
13. Taieb A et al: Orf and pregnancy. *Int J Dermatol* **27**:31, 1988
14. Gourreau J et al: Orf recontamination 8 months after the original infection. Review of the literature apropos of the case (French). *Ann Dermatol Venereol* **113**:1065, 1986
15. Yeh H et al: Ultrastructural studies in human orf. *Arch Dermatol* **109**:390, 1974
16. Gold P et al: Localization of nucleotide phosphorylase within vaccinia virus. *Proc Natl Acad Sci USA* **60**:845, 1968
17. Fraser KM et al: Sequence analysis of the inverted terminal repetitions in the genome of the parapoxvirus, orf virus. *Virology* **176**:379, 1990
18. Garon C et al: Visualization of an inverted terminal repetition in vaccinia virus DNA. *Proc Natl Acad Sci USA* **75**:4863, 1978
19. Grassmann U: Analysis of parapoxvirus genomes. *Arch Virol* **83**:17, 1985
20. Fleming SB et al: Conservation of gene structure and arrangement between vaccinia virus and orf virus. *Virology* **195**:175, 1993

21. Robinson G et al: The genome of orf virus: Restriction endonuclease analysis of viral DNA isolation from lesions of orf in sheep. *Arch Virol* **71**:43, 1982
22. Robinson AJ: Conservation and variation in orf virus genomes. *Virology* **157**:13, 1987
23. Esposito JL et al: Intragenomic sequence transposition in monkey pox virus. *Virology* **109**:231, 1981
24. Holowczak JA et al: Poxvirus DNA. *Curr Top Microbiol Immunol* **17**:27, 1982
25. Rafii F et al: Comparison of contagious ecthyma virus genomes by restriction endonucleases. *Arch Virol* **84**:283, 1985
26. Roberts WG et al: Neovasculature induced by vascular endothelial growth factor is fenestrated. *Cancer Res* **57**:765, 1997
27. Lyttle DJ: Homologs of vascular endothelial growth factor are encoded by the poxvirus orf virus. *J Virol* **68**:84, 1994
28. Mayr A et al: *Virologische Arbeitsmethoden,* vol. 1, *Zellkwturen-Bebrutete Huhnereier-Versuchstire.* Jena, VEB, J. Fisch Verlag, 1974
29. Hessami M et al: Isolation of parapoxviruses from man and animals: Cultivation and cellular changes in bovine fetal spleen cells. *Comp Immunol Microbiol Infect Dis* **2**:1, 1974
30. Pospischil A et al: Nuclear changes in cells infected with parapoxvirus stomatitis papulosa and orf: An in vivo and in vitro ultrastructure study. *J Gen Virol* **47**:114, 1980
31. Wilkinson JD: Orf: A family with unusual complications. *Br J Dermatol* **97**:447, 1977
32. Murphy JK et al: Bullous pemphigoid complicating human orf. *Br J Dermatol* **134**:929, 1996
33. Reymond D et al: Invasive *Pseudomonas aeruginosa* and ecthyma gangrenosum infection in a child without risk factors. *Arch Pediatr* **3**:569, 1996
34. Leavell UW Jr et al: Orf: Report of 19 human cases with clinical and pathological observations. *JAMA* **204**:657, 1968
35. Yirrell DL et al: Response of efferent lymph and popliteal lymph node to epidermal infection of sheep with orf virus. *Vet Immunol Immunopathol* **28**:219, 1991
36. Nagington J et al: The structure of the orf virus. *Virology* **23**:461, 1964
37. Kong HL et al: Regional suppression of tumor growth by in vivo transfer of a cDNA encoding a secreted form of the extracellular domain of the FLT-1 VEGF receptor. *Hum Gen Ther* **9**:823, 1998

CHAPTER 222

Douglas R. Lowy

Molluscum Contagiosum

Molluscum contagiosum is a common, benign, viral disease of the skin and mucous membranes that generally affects children. In adults, the condition may be transmitted sexually. The fully developed lesion is an umbilicated papule, and most patients have multiple lesions. The lesions may be particularly extensive in patients with AIDS or other disorders associated with immunologic dysfunction.

ETIOLOGY

Molluscum contagiosum virus (MCV) is a poxvirus that is distinct morphologically, serologically, and pathologically from other poxviruses.[1-3] It is a large (200 by 300 nm) DNA virus that replicates in the cytoplasm of infected cells and induces hyperplasia, as do other poxviruses. The complete sequence of the MCV DNA genome has been determined.[4,5] It reveals that about two-thirds of the viral genes are similar to those of the orthopoxviruses such as vaccinia virus and variola virus, while about one-third of the MCV genes appear to be distinct. Some of these genes are discussed below, under "Pathogenesis and Pathology."

Unlike most other poxviruses, MCV has not been reproducibly propagated in tissue culture. Some experimental success in reproducing the lesions and inducing MCV replication has been reported by using cell-free lesional extracts to infect human foreskin grafts in nude mice.[6,7] However, serial transmission has not yet been achieved. When viral particles extracted from lesions arising in different patients have been analyzed, some minor differences have been found in viral proteins[8,9] and in restriction endonuclease cleavage patterns of viral DNA. Three different MCV strains (I, II, and III) have been identified, based on restriction endonuclease digestion patterns.[10,11] MCVI is more prevalent than MCVII, with MCVIII being extremely uncommon.[10-12] No clinical differences have been noted between the strains.

Experimental transmission to humans has been achieved, with a reported incubation period of 2 to 7 weeks.[1] Attempts to transmit the disease experimentally in other species have been unsuccessful. MCV infection has been thought to be confined to humans, but

CHAPTER 222
Molluscum Contagiosum

2479

the disease experimentally in other species have been unsuccessful. MCV infection has been thought to be confined to humans, but lesions that are clinically and histologically identical to those in human disease have been reported in the chimpanzee and kangaroo in captivity.[13,14]

FIGURE 222-1

EPIDEMIOLOGY

The disease occurs throughout the world, but its frequency varies considerably.[1-3] It affects mainly children, sexually active adults, and immunocompromised individuals. On some Pacific islands, 5 percent of children under 10 years may be affected. The prevalence rate in the United States is much lower. Although the disease may develop at any age, the vast majority of cases are found in children, with boys being affected more frequently than girls. Multiple familial cases are uncommon.

The disease is believed to be transmitted primarily by person-to-person spread and possibly by fomites, as desiccation does not inactivate poxviruses. Outbreaks have been reported among children attending swimming pools, and genital lesions in adults are probably transmitted sexually.[15,16] As with other sexually transmitted viral diseases, the incidence of genital molluscum increased between the 1960s and 1980s.[17,18] The incidence of subclinical infection is unknown. The role of humoral immunity is unclear, although most patients contain IgG antibodies against viral antigen, and experimental studies suggest that many adults are resistant to infection.[19,20] Individuals with impaired cellular immune function may have widespread lesions.[21,22] Patients with AIDS are at particular risk of MCV infection, with prevalence rates of 5 to 18 percent having been reported[23-26]; the frequency and severity of infection varies inversely with the CD4+ count, and lesions in AIDS patients are often refractory to treatment.

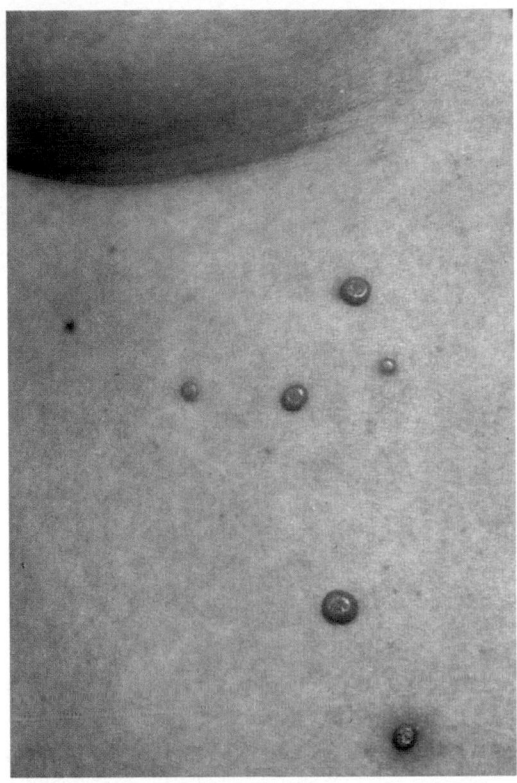

A.

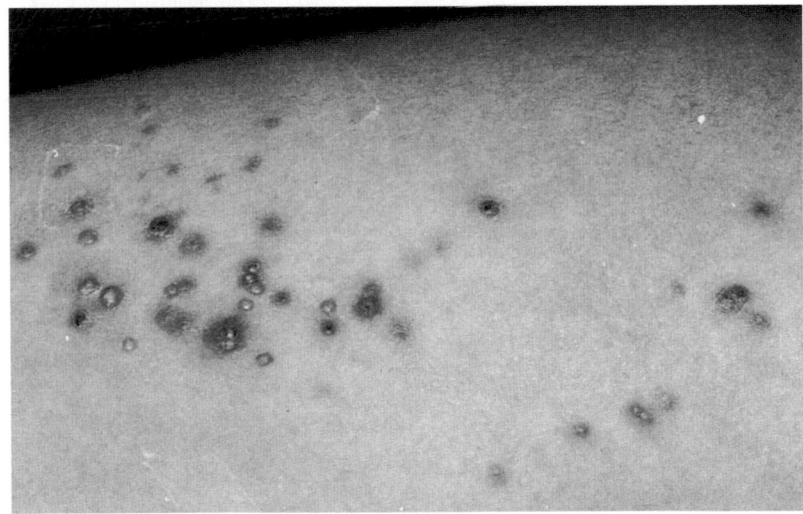

B.

Molluscum contagiosum. *A. Discrete, solid, skin-colored papules, 1.0 to 2.0 mm in diameter with central umbilication. B. Multiple, scattered, and discrete lesions, some of which are inflamed.*

CLINICAL MANIFESTATIONS

The lesions, which begin as minute papules, are usually 3 to 6 mm, although rarely they may be as large as 3 cm in diameter. The individual lesions are discrete, smooth, pearly to flesh-colored, dome-shaped papules, often with central umbilication in which lies a white curdlike core, which may be easily expressed.[27]

Lesions may be located on any area of the skin and mucous membranes. They are usually grouped (Fig. 222-1) in one or two areas but may be widely disseminated. Most patients have fewer than 20 lesions, although some may have several hundred. In temperate climates, the head, eyelids, trunk, and genitalia are affected most often. In the tropics, lesions occur most commonly on the extremities. Lesions in adults are frequently located on the genitalia (Fig. 222-2). In adult patients with AIDS, lesions may often occur exclusively at extragenital sites, although they may be confined to the genitalia. In some AIDS patients, lesions may attain a very large size and mimic cutaneous tumors.[28]

Although lesions are usually asymptomatic, pruritus may be present, and an eczematous reaction may develop around some lesions. Conjunctivitis and keratitis may complicate lesions around

FIGURE 222-2

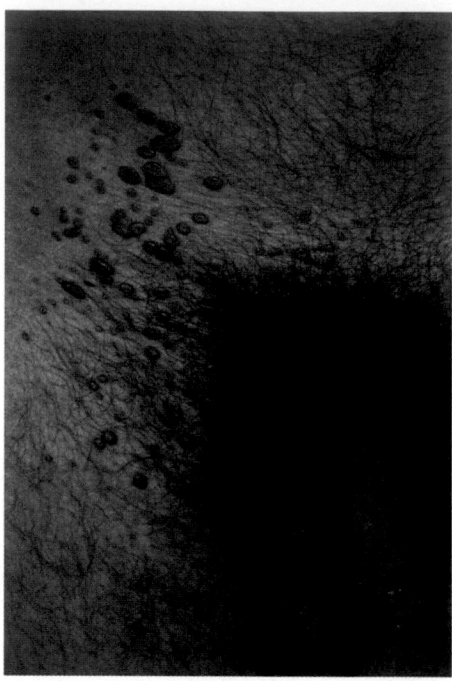

Molluscum contagiosum. Multiple umbilicated papules are seen on the abdomen, thigh, and penis of this 33-year-old HIV-infected male.

FIGURE 222-3

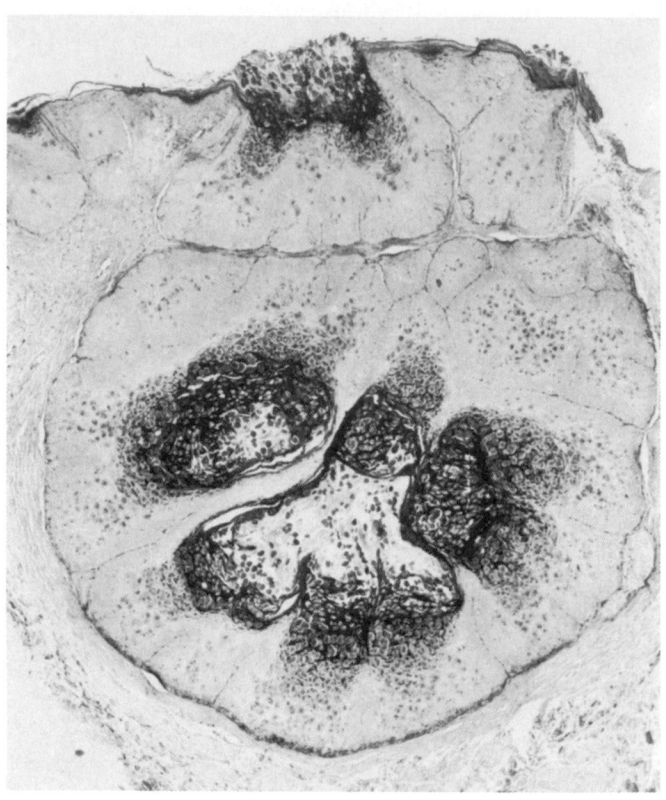

Molluscum contagiosum. Extensive downgrowth of infected cells bearing the large eosinophilic cytoplasmic inclusion bodies. (*Micrograph by Wallace H. Clark, Jr., MD*)

the eyelid. Patients with atopic dermatitis or other conditions with impaired immune function may develop widespread lesions, and secondary bacterial infection also occurs.

PATHOGENESIS AND PATHOLOGY

The rate of cell division in the basal layer of lesional skin is twice that of normal skin.[29] It remains unclear how the MCV infection causes this hyperproliferation. The higher rate may be related to an apparent increase in the number of receptors for epidermal growth factor (EGF) in infected cells.[30] Although indirect evidence that MCV synthesizes an EGF-like growth factor, as do other poxviruses,[31] has not been confirmed by direct sequencing of the MCV genome,[4] it remains possible that the virus activates the EGF receptor indirectly.

Viral growth is confined to the epidermis; virus particles are synthesized in cytoplasmic foci of cells in the malpighian and granular layers.[19,29] The infected cells, which are interspersed with uninfected cells, move more quickly than uninfected cells through the epidermis. Viral antigen is present in infected cells, and 90 percent of patients possess circulating antibody to this antigen. Lesions may resolve spontaneously with or without inflammation.[30,32] Immunocompetent cells are absent from the infected epidermis, even when they are present in the underlying dermis.[30]

The sequencing of the MCV genome has identified several distinct MCV genes that may interfere with immune and other host defense mechanisms.[4,5,33] These include a major histocompatibility complex class I heavy chain homologue that may interfere with

presentation of MCV-specific peptides, a chemokine homologue that may inhibit inflammation, and a glutathione peroxidase homologue that may protect the virus and infected cells from oxidative damage by peroxides, which may be formed in response to infection. A fourth distinct MCV gene may keep MCV-infected keratinocytes viable by interfering with their normally apoptotic differentiation program. These features of the virus, and perhaps other viral genes, may help to explain the paucity of immune response seen even in lesions of immunocompetent patients. They may also account, at least in part, for the difficulties encountered with infection in immunocompromised individuals.

The histologic appearance of the hypertrophied and hyperplastic epidermis is characteristic (Fig. 222-3).[27,34] Above the normal-appearing basal layer are lobules of enlarged epidermal cells that contain multiple Feulgen-positive intracytoplasmic inclusion bodies (*molluscum bodies* or *Henderson-Paterson bodies*). These inclusion bodies, which contain the viral particles, increase in size as the infected cell moves toward the surface. In the horny layer, the molluscum bodies are enmeshed in a fibrous network that dissolves in the center of the lesions, forming the central core, which is composed primarily of molluscum bodies.

DIAGNOSIS AND DIFFERENTIAL DIAGNOSIS

The diagnosis is usually made by the distinctive clinical appearance of the lesions, by stained smears of the expressed core, and by biopsy. Molluscum contagiosum must be differentiated from warts, varicella, pyoderma, papillomas, epitheliomas, basal cell carcinoma, and lichen planus. Cutaneous cryptococcal infection in patients with AIDS may mimic the appearance of MCV infection.[35]

TREATMENT

Since the condition is usually self-limited and lesions heal without scarring in the absence of secondary bacterial infection, treatment is not always mandatory. Removal of lesions with a sharp curette or liquid nitrogen is simple, relatively painless, and usually effective. More than one treatment session is often necessary, either because of recurrence or the development of new lesions. Self-administered topical podophyllotoxin cream has been shown to be superior to placebo in a double-blinded study.[36] In an uncontrolled trial, cimetidine treatment of immunocompetent children with widespread lesions was associated with complete resolution in most patients.[37] Treatment may be especially difficult in patients with impaired immune function. In HIV-infected patients, treatment of the underlying HIV infection may be associated with recovery of immune function and amelioration of the molluscum lesions.[38]

Individual lesions may last 2 to 4 months, but the development of new lesions by autoinoculation is common. Most cases resolve spontaneously in 6 to 9 months, but some may persist for years, especially in immunocompromised patients.

REFERENCES

1. Postlethwaite R: Molluscum contagiosum: A review. *Arch Environ Health* **21**:432, 1970
2. Brown ST et al: Molluscum contagiosum. *Sex Transm Dis* **8**:227, 1981
3. Gottleib SL, Myskowski PL: Molluscum contagiosum. *Int J Dermatol* **33**:453, 1994
4. Senkevich TG et al: Genome sequence of a human tumorigenic poxvirus: Prediction of specific host response-evasion genes. *Science* **273**:813, 1996
5. Senkevich TG et al: The genome of molluscum contagiosum virus: Analysis and comparison with other poxviruses. *Virology* **23**:19, 1997
6. Buller RM et al: Replication of molluscum contagiosum virus. *Virology* **213**:655, 1995
7. Fife KH et al: Growth of molluscum contagiosum virus in a human foreskin xenograft model. *Virology* **226**:95, 1996
8. Oda H et al: Structural polypeptides of molluscum contagiosum virus: Their variability in various isolates and location within the virion. *J Med Virol* **9**:19, 1982
9. Konya J et al: Enzyme-linked immunosorbent assay for measurement of IgG antibody to molluscum contagiosum virus and investigation of the serological relationship of the molecular types. *J Virol Methods* **40**:183, 1995
10. Scholz J et al: Epidemiology of molluscum contagiosum using genetic analysis of the viral DNA. *J Med Virol* **27**:87, 1989
11. Porter CD, Archard LC: Characterization by restriction mapping of three subtypes of molluscum contagiosum virus. *J Med Virol* **38**:1, 1992
12. Porter CD et al: Molluscum contagiosum virus types in genital and non-genital lesions. *Br J Dermatol* **120**:37, 1989
13. Dangall BG, Witson GR: Molluscum contagiosum in a red kangaroo. *Australas J Dermatol* **15**:115, 1974
14. Douglas JD et al: Molluscum contagiosum in the chimpanzee. *J Am Vet Med Assoc* **151**:901, 1967
15. Brown ST et al: Molluscum contagiosum: Sexually transmitted disease in 17 cases. *J Am Vener Dis Assoc* **1**:35, 1974
16. Wilkin JK: Molluscum contagiosum venereum in a women's outpatient clinic: A venereally transmitted disease. *Am J Obstet Gynecol* **128**:531, 1977
17. Becker TM et al: Trends in molluscum contagiosum in the United States, 1966–1983. *Sex Transm Dis* **13**:88, 1986
18. Oriel JD: The increase in molluscum contagiosum. *Br Med J* **294**:74, 1987
19. Shirodaria PV, Matthews RS: Observations on the antibody responses in molluscum contagiosum. *Br J Dermatol* **96**:29, 1977
20. Shirodaria PV, Matthews RS: Virus-specific and anticellular antibodies in molluscum contagiosum. *Br J Dermatol* **101**:133, 1979
21. Solomon LM, Telner P: Eruptive molluscum contagiosum in atopic dermatitis. *Can Med Assoc J* **95**:978, 1966
22. Peachy RDG: Severe molluscum contagiosum infection with T-cell deficiency. *Br J Dermatol* **97**(suppl):49, 1977
23. Goodman DS et al: Prevalence of cutaneous disease in patients with acquired immunodeficiency syndrome (AIDS) or AIDS-related complex. *J Am Acad Dermatol* **17**:210, 1987
24. Matis WL et al: Dermatologic findings associated with human immunodeficiency virus infection. *J Am Acad Dermatol* **17**:746, 1987
25. Coldiron BM, Bergstresser PR: Prevalence and clinical spectrum of skin disease in patients infected with human immunodeficiency virus. *Arch Dermatol* **125**:357, 1989
26. Schwartz JJ, Myskowski PL: Molluscum contagiosum in patients with human immunodeficiency virus infection. *J Am Acad Dermatol* **27**:583, 1992
27. Uehara M, Danno K: Central pitting of molluscum contagiosum. *J Cutan Pathol* **7**:149, 1980
28. Petersen CS, Gerstoft J: Molluscum contagiosum in HIV-infected patients. *Dermatology* **184**:19, 1992
29. Epstein WL, Fukuyama K: Maturation of molluscum contagiosum virus (MCV) in vivo: Quantitative electron microscopic autoradiography. *J Invest Dermatol* **60**:73, 1973
30. Viac J, Chardonnet Y: Immunocompetent cells and epithelial cell modifications in molluscum contagiosum. *J Cutan Pathol* **17**:202, 1990
31. Porter CD, Archard LC: Characterization and physical mapping of molluscum contagiosum virus DNA and location of a sequence capable of encoding a conserved domain of epidermal growth factor. *J Gen Virol* **68**:673, 1987
32. Takematsu H, Tagami H: Proinflammatory properties of molluscum bodies. *Arch Dermatol Res* **287**:102, 1994
33. Bertin J et al: Two death effector domain-containing herpesvirus and poxvirus proteins inhibit both Fas- and TNFR1-induced apoptosis. *Proc Natl Acad Sci USA* **94**:1172, 1997
34. Kwittken J: Molluscum contagiosum: Some new histologic observations. *Mt Sinai J Med* **47**:583, 1980
35. Rico MJ, Penneys NS: Cutaneous cryptoccosis resembling molluscum contagiosum in a patient with AIDS. *Arch Dermatol* **121**:901, 1985
36. Syed TA et al: Topical 0.3% and 0.5% podophyllotoxin cream for self-treatment of molluscum contagiosum in males. *Dermatology* **189**:65, 1994
37. Dohil M, Prendiville JS: Treatment of molluscum contagiosum with oral cimetidine: Clinical experience in 13 patients. *Pediatr Dermatol* **3**:310, 1996
38. Hicks CB et al: Resolution of intractable molluscum contagiosum in a human immunodeficiency virus-infected patient after institution of antiretroviral therapy with ritonavir. *Clin Infect Dis* **24**:1023, 1997

CHAPTER 223

Douglas R. Lowy

Milker's Nodules

Milker's nodule is a benign viral skin disease that generally consists of one or a few nodules on the hand or forearm. The virus is usually transmitted to cattle handlers from infected cows.

ETIOLOGY

The etiologic agent is called *paravaccinia virus*, or milker's node virus (MNV). It is a poxvirus from parapoxvirus subgroup, which also includes orf virus and bovine papular stomatitis virus. MNV is endemic in cattle.[1] Lesions in cows, which may be chronic and recurrent, appear mainly on the teats, although other areas may be affected. In cows the condition is called *pseudocowpox*. There is no cross-immunity with the cowpox, vaccinia, or variola orthopox group of poxviruses. Bovine papular stomatitis virus infection of cattle is characterized by lesions around the mouth[2]; because it induces lesions in humans that are identical to milker's nodules, some investigators believe that the two viruses may be identical.[3]

Paravaccinia virus can be propagated in bovine or human cells in tissue culture.[4,5] It resembles the virus of orf (ecthyma contagiosum) morphologically and serologically (see Chap. 221),[6–8] but the two viruses can be distinguished by viral DNA hybridization.[9] As is true of other poxviruses, paravaccinia is a large (150 by 300 nm) brick-shaped DNA virus that contains many enzymes and replicates in foci in the cytoplasm of infected cells.[10] Infection often induces a mild degree of hyperplasia and increased dermal vascularity. The disease has been transmitted experimentally from human to human and from human to cow.[11]

EPIDEMIOLOGY

Milker's nodule has a worldwide distribution, occurring where cattle are found. Most cases are sporadic, but small epidemics have been reported. Since the disease is usually transmitted to humans by direct contact with infected cattle, milkers are most at risk. Cases also occur among stockyard and slaughterhouse workers. Most cases arise in individuals who have recently become milkers, and infection in humans usually induces lasting immunity. Indirect transmission from virus-contaminated material to patients with burned skin has been reported.[12] The incidence of subclinical infection is not known. Although infectious virus is found in human lesions, person-to-person transmission under natural conditions has not been documented.

CLINICAL MANIFESTATIONS

The typical case consists of a single asymptomatic or slightly painful 1-cm erythematous nodule on a finger (Fig. 223-1).[13,14] There are usually no more than four lesions, and they are generally confined to the hand and forearm. Rarely, other areas of the skin may be involved or numerous lesions may be present. Lymphadenopathy is uncommon.

The incubation period is usually 4 to 7 days but may be as long as 2 weeks. In the absence of secondary bacterial infection, each lesion usually heals spontaneously in 4 to 6 weeks without scar formation. Leavell and Phillips[14] have described six clinical stages, each lasting about a week. Initially, the lesion begins as an erythematous macule, which soon becomes papular. The target stage is next: the lesion, which is papulovesicular, has a red center surrounded by a white ring and a red halo. This stage is followed by a period of weeping and erosion. The lesion then becomes a firm, crusted nodule. Next, small papillomatous elevations develop on the nodule. Finally, during the regressive stage, the lesion darkens and sloughs.

PATHOLOGY

Pathologic changes are present in both epidermis and dermis; the precise histologic appearance depends on the clinical stage.[14,15] The manifestations are similar to those of orf. Epidermal changes include hyperkeratosis, parakeratosis, acanthosis, and striking elongation of the rete ridges. These alterations increase progressively as the lesion develops. In early lesions, the upper portion of the malpighian layer may contain balloon cells and cells with many intracytoplasmic and some intranuclear inclusions. Later, reticular degeneration, multilocular vesicles, spongiosis, and intracellular edema may be the prominent findings. The dermis contains a marked increase in the number of capillaries and a nonspecific inflammatory infiltrate that is most intense during the acute weeping stage. Electron micrographic examination of the superficial portion of a lesion usually reveals the characteristic cytoplasmic viral particles. The hypervascularity in the dermis may be secondary to the production and secretion of a virally encoded homologue of vascular endothelial growth factor (VEGF), a potent stimulator of vascular proliferation. A VEGF homologue has recently been identified in the orf virus,[16] and the close similarity between orf virus and MNV makes it likely that MNV also contains an analogous gene.

FIGURE 223-1

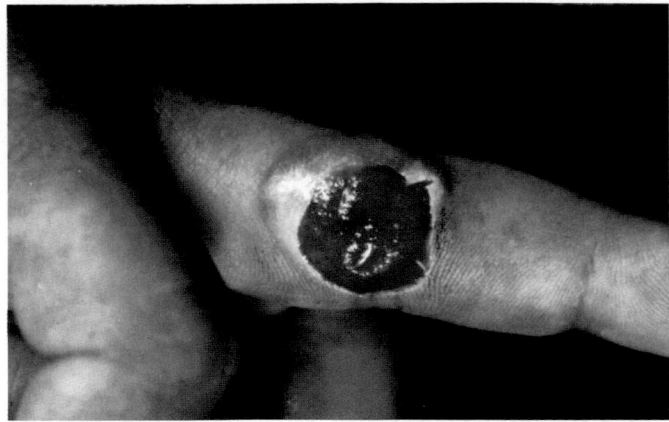

A.

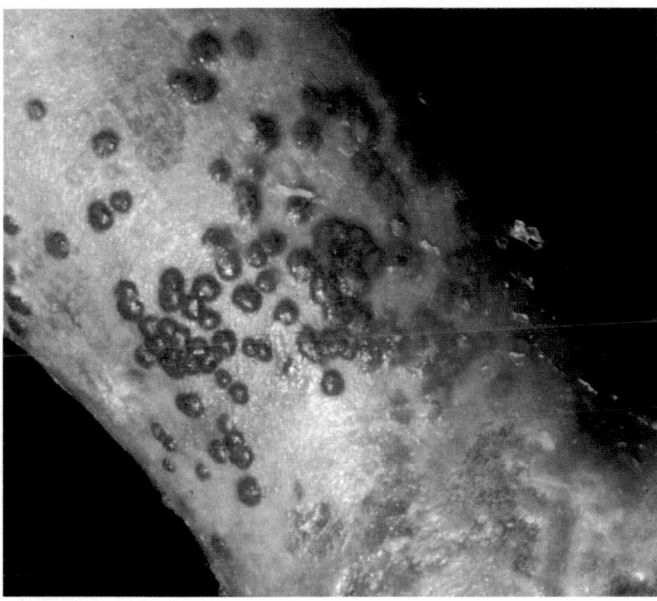

B.

Milker's nodule. *A.* Firm, purple, eroded nodule occurred following milking a cow. *B.* Multiple, purple papules and nodules occurred in a second-degree scalding burn sustained in a milking barn.

DIAGNOSIS AND DIFFERENTIAL DIAGNOSIS

The diagnosis is generally based on the history, clinical appearance, and biopsy. It can be established more definitively by the electron microscopic demonstration of viral particles or by propagation of the virus in tissue culture. Orf and bovine papular stomatitis must be excluded by history.

Milker's nodule must also be differentiated from a large number of other conditions, including true cowpox, herpetic whitlow, pyoderma, anthrax, tularemia, primary inoculation tuberculosis, atypical mycobacterial infection, syphilitic chancre, sporotrichosis, and pyogenic granuloma.

COURSE, PROGNOSIS, TREATMENT, AND PREVENTION

Since the disease is self-limited, only symptomatic therapy is generally indicated. Prevention is limited to the isolation of infected animals.

REFERENCES

1. Moscovici C et al: Isolation of a viral agent from pseudocowpox disease. *Science* **141**:915, 1963
2. Bowman KF et al: Cutaneous form of bovine papular stomatitis in man. *JAMA* **246**:2813, 1981
3. Rossi CR et al. A paravaccinia virus isolated from cattle. *Cornell Vet* **67**:72, 1977
4. Friedman-Kien AE et al: Milker's nodules: Isolation of a poxvirus from a human case. *Science* **140**:1335, 1963
5. Thomas V: Biochemical and electron microscopic studies of the replication and composition of milker's node virus. *J Virol* **34**:244, 1980
6. Nagington J et al: Milker's nodule virus infections and their similarity to orf. *Nature* **208**:505, 1965
7. Leavell UW et al: Orf: Report of 19 human cases with clinical and pathological observations. *JAMA* **204**:657, 1968
8. Lard SL et al. Differentiation of parapoxviruses by application of orf virus–specific monoclonal antibodies against cell surface proteins. *Vet Immunol Immunopathol* **28**:247, 1991
9. Gassmann U et al: Analysis of parapoxvirus genomes. *Arch Virol* **83**:17, 1985
10. Caplen HS, Holowczak JA: Some enzymatic activities associated with purified parapoxvirions. *J Virol* **46**:384, 1983
11. Sonck CE, Penttinen K: Milker's nodules: Transmission from man to man. *Acta Derm Venereol (Stockh)* **34**:420, 1954
12. Schuler G et al: The syndrome of milker's nodules in burn injury: Evidence for indirect transmission. *J Am Acad Dermatol* **6**:334, 1982
13. Wheeler CE, Cawley EP: The etiology of milker's nodules. *Arch Dermatol* **75**:249, 1957
14. Leavell UW Jr, Phillips IA: Milker's nodules: Pathogenesis, tissue culture, electron microscopy, and calf inoculation. *Arch Dermatol* **111**:1307, 1975
15. Groves RW et al: Human orf and milkers' nodule: A clinicopathologic study. *J Am Acad Dermatol* **25**:706, 1991
16. Lyttle DJ et al: Homologs of vascular endothelial growth factor are encoded by the poxvirus orf virus. *J Virol* **68**:84, 1994

CHAPTER 224

Douglas R. Lowy
Elliot J. Androphy

Warts

Warts, or verrucae, are benign proliferations of the skin and mucosa that result from infection with *papillomaviruses* (PVs). These viruses do not produce acute signs or symptoms but induce slow-growing lesions that can remain subclinical for long periods of time. A subset of the human PVs has been associated with the development of epithelial malignancies.

HISTORIC ASPECTS

Cutaneous warts were known to the ancient Greeks and Romans, and until the nineteenth century genital warts were believed to be a form of syphilis or gonorrhea. The viral etiology of warts was implied from the observation that inoculation of wart filtrates from which cellular and bacterial products were removed could induce papillomas at the site of injection. All warts were considered to be derived from a single virus, since isolates from cutaneous, genital, or laryngeal warts could induce papillomas at other sites. However, advances in recombinant DNA technology have now identified more than 80 different human papillomavirus (HPV) genotypes.[1]

ETIOLOGIC AGENT

The PVs comprise a large family of double-stranded DNA viruses found in humans and many other species.[2] They are distantly related to the other members of the Papovavirus class, which includes simian virus 40, polyomavirus, BK virus, and JC virus. All PVs are highly host-specific, which means that PVs from one species do not induce papillomas in heterologous species. HPVs only infect humans. Rabbits, cows, and dogs are the natural host for some PVs, but for unknown reasons PVs are not found in common strains of mice. These limitations place significant restrictions on investigating the mechanism and biologic consequences of PV infection in a laboratory animal model. While it is now possible to cultivate HPVs in normal epithelial cell culture (see below), only minute amounts of virus are produced, and in vitro culture of HPV is not a simple, routine test in any laboratory.

Recombinant DNA technology has enabled the molecular cloning of the complete viral DNA or genome from clinical lesions. The entire nucleotide sequence has been determined for the genomes of many human and animal PVs. Comparison of these PV DNAs reveals that they share a similar genetic organization (Fig. 224-1) and are predicted to encode related protein products.[3] The PV genome is present within the viral particle as a single, supercoiled, cova-

FIGURE 224-1

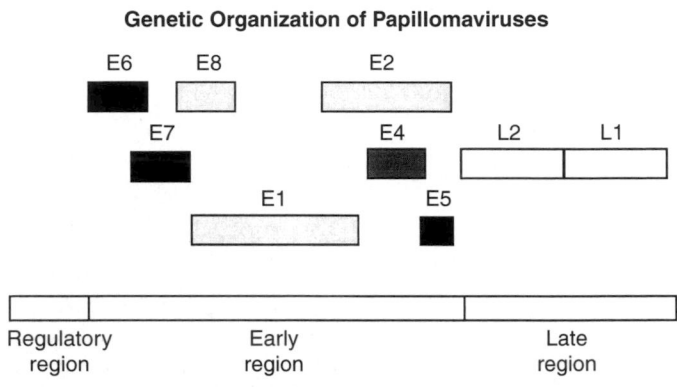

Genetic Organization of Papillomaviruses

All papillomavirus genomes are composed of approximately 8000 nucleotide base pairs, represented as a linear sequence but actually a closed circle of double-stranded DNA. The boxes depict the viral genes, each of which encodes a protein. The regulatory region is a DNA segment that does not encode proteins but has been shown to be involved in the expression of the viral genes and the replication of the viral DNA. In general, E6, E7, and E5 represent transforming genes; E1 and E2 coordinate replication and expression of the viral genome; and the L1 and L2 proteins form the viral capsid. E4 encodes a protein that may be involved in the release of the virus from the cell's keratin framework. For details, see text.

lently closed circle of double-stranded DNA. Each genome is composed of about 8000 nucleotide base pairs, which is about one-twentieth the size of a herpesvirus genome. The PV genome encodes only eight to nine proteins, which are historically separated into two groups, "E" (for "early") and "L" (for "late"). The E proteins, most of which participate in viral DNA replication, are expressed before the L proteins and are not incorporated into the infectious virus particle. The E genes do not encode a DNA polymerase or thymidine kinase, and therefore PVs are not susceptible to inhibition by acyclovir. The L1 and L2 genes encode the structural proteins that form the outer protein shell, called the *capsid* of the viral particle, which is called the *virion*. The spherical virion measures 55 nm in diameter and surrounds the viral DNA.

Until recently, clinical lesions have been the only source of infectious PV particles, except for a limited number of PVs that have successfully propagated in human keratinocytes grown under the renal capsule of athymic nude mice.[4,5] The use of the so-called raft culture system, which forms a stratified squamous epithelium, has now produced limited amounts of infectious HPV.[6,7] In standard tissue culture cells, the application of genetic engineering technology has led to the production of infectious bovine PV.[8] These and related advances make it likely that the number of infectious HPV types produced in the laboratory, as well as the amount of virus, will increase considerably in the near future.

HUMAN PAPILLOMAVIRUS TYPES

While close to 80 HPV types have been completely or partially sequenced,[9] the actual number of types may range between 100 and 150. HPV types are currently discriminated according to the relatedness of their DNA sequence. Until recently, molecular hybridization techniques were used to determine the HPV type of a particular isolate. The ease with which the polymerase chain reaction (PCR), which has both high sensitivity and specificity, can be used to amplify and sequence any viral DNA isolate has now led to HPV types being defined by DNA sequence homology. Fresh tissue is not required, and PCR has been successfully applied to detect and type HPV DNA in paraffin-embedded tissue blocks that are decades old.[10] Two HPV isolates are assumed to be of the same type if the sequences of their L1 genes are at least 90 percent identical.[1] It is likely a new HPV type if, after the viral genome has been molecularly cloned and its L1 gene sequenced, the sequence is less than 90 percent homologous to the closest known HPV type. Using this approach, it has also been possible to study the evolutionary relationships between different HPV genotypes and even within the same HPV type.[11]

HPV types are often associated with distinct regional predilection, histopathology, and biology and are separated on this basis into three categories: cutaneous (nongenital) types such as HPV-1, -2, -3, and -4, genital-mucosal types such as HPV-6, -11, -16, and -18, and those usually isolated from epidermodysplasia verruciformis (EV) such as HPV-5 and -8 (Table 224-1). EV is a rare disease of unique susceptibility to HPV infection (see below). A hypothetical evolutionary tree depicting the relationship among the HPV genotypes shows that those closely related to each other by DNA sequence fit within these categories and tend to induce similar lesions.[11] Examples include highly related types such as 3 and 10,

which induce flat warts, types 6 and 11, which induce genital-mucosal warts (condylomata acuminata), and types 5 and 8, which induce scaly lesions in EV.

Another important distinction is that specific HPV genotypes appear to have malignant potential. The first example of this was noted in EV.[12,13] For example, almost all cutaneous squamous cell carcinomas arise in EV warts that contain specific HPV types such as 5 and 8, while benign lesions, even in the same patient, may harbor many other HPV types. Thus it appears that neoplastic development is restricted to certain HPVs. Similarly, the majority of cervical carcinomas contain HPV-16, -18, or other so-called high-risk types, while the "low-risk" HPV-6 and -11, which are also found in benign cervical disease, are rarely identified in cervical malignancies.[14]

Many other viruses are typed by the ability of antisera to distinguish their capsid antigens, and antisera made by immunization with intact PV virions can generate type-specific antibodies.[15] However, serologic typing requires the generation of specific antisera to each HPV type, which is more cumbersome and less sensitive than DNA sequence analysis and may be subject to greater inter-laboratory variation. Serotyping of HPVs has been studied less extensively because until recently it was usually necessary to obtain virus from lesions. However, it has now been determined that expression of L1 protein molecules of any PV in cultured cells leads to their self-assembly into virus-like particles (VLPs; Fig. 224-2) that exhibit the same type-specific epitopes as the authentic virus. Serologic analyses using antisera obtained by immunization with L1 VLPs have shown an excellent correlation between the serologic results and DNA typing, with little serologic cross-reactivity between different HPV types and considerable cross-reactivity among isolates of the same HPV type.[8,16,17]

Detergent-disrupted PV particles expose common structural antigens shared by all PVs but not by other viruses.[15] Antibodies to such shared antigens can be used to detect structural capsid proteins in clinical materials, including formalin fixed tissue (Fig. 224-3). However, antibodies to structural viral proteins cannot be used to confirm the presence of HPV in cells that do not synthesize large

TABLE 224-1

Clinical Associations of HPV Types

HPV TYPE	MOST COMMON CLINICAL LESION	LESS FREQUENT LESION	POTENTIAL ONCOGENICITY
1	Deep plantar/palmar warts	Common warts	
2, 4, 27, 29	Common warts	Plantar, palmar, mosaic, oral, and anogenital warts	
3, 10, 28, 49	Flat warts	Flat warts in EV	
7	"Butchers" warts		
13, 32	Oral focal epithelial hyerplasia		
5, 8, 9, 12, 14, 15, 17, 19–26, 36, 47, 50	Epidermodysplasia verruciformis (EV); warts in immunosuppression	Normal skin (?)	HPV-5, -8, -9 isolated from SCCs
6, 11	Anogenital warts, cervical condylomata	Bowenoid papulosis; common warts; respiratory papillomatosis	Bushke-Lowenstein tumor; rare in penile, vulvar cervical, and other urogenital tumors; "low risk"
16, 18, 31, 33–35, 39–40, 51–60	Cervical condylomata; anogenital warts; Bowenoid papulosis	Common warts	Genital and cervical dysplasias and carcinomas; rare in cutaneous SCC; "high risk"

NOTE: SCC, squamous cell carcinoma.

FIGURE 224-2

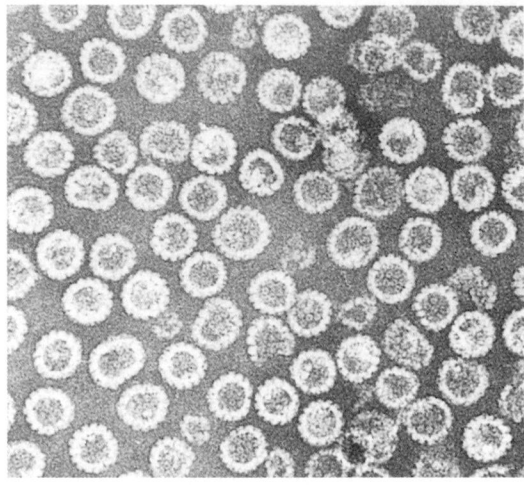

Transmission electron micrograph of HPV 16 virus-like particles composed of the viral L1 and L2 capsid proteins. The L1 and L2 proteins have been expressed in cultured cells and have self-assembled into 55-nm particles that are similar morphologically to infectious virus, except that they do not contain the viral DNA, and then purified from the cells. (*Micrograph courtesy of Heather Greenstone.*)

FIGURE 224-3

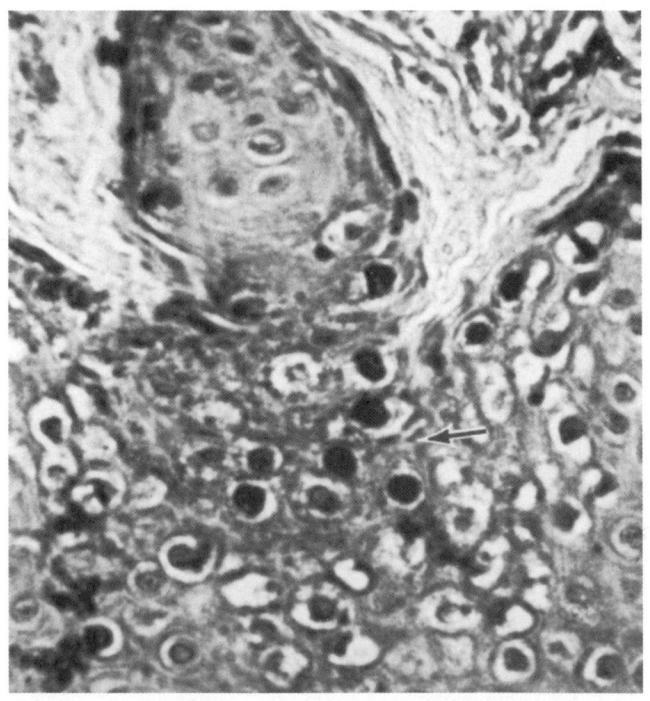

Immunoperoxidase assay of a verruca in which the darkly stained nuclei (arrow) represent cells that contain PV virion structural antigens. The positive nuclei are found in some, but are not limited to, koilocytotic cells.

numbers of virions and are therefore usually negative in genital warts, bowenoid papulosis, dysplasias, and HPV-associated malignancies.

EPIDEMIOLOGY

Contagion of HPV probably depends on several factors, including the location of lesions, quantity of infectious virus present, degree and nature of the contact, and general and HPV-specific immunologic status of the exposed individual. Patients with impaired cell-mediated immunity (CMI) are particularly susceptible to HPV infection, and warts are found in the majority of renal transplant patients on immunosuppressive therapy.[18–23] The source or reservoir for HPV is believed to be individuals with clinical or subclinical infection, as well as infectious virus that may be present in the environment. Using sensitive PCR detection methods, it is becoming increasingly evident that normal skin in immunocompetent individuals can harbor HPVs, including novel types and those found in EV.[24] Therefore, when these sensitive techniques are used to find HPV DNA in a lesion not usually thought to be caused by HPV, additional evidence should be sought to determine whether the virus has contributed to the development of the lesion.

Nongenital warts occur most frequently in children and young adults, in whom the incidence may approach 10 percent.[25] Between 1966 and 1981, there was a sixfold increase in the number of office visits for anogenital warts, which are more frequent than the number of visits for genital herpes.[26] The age-specific incidence of nongenital warts differs from that of anogenital warts. Anogenital warts, which are uncommon in children, behave as a sexually transmitted condition and are transmitted between partners with high efficiency.[27] Penile lesions occur frequently in sexual contacts of women with cervical intraepithelial neoplasia.[28]

Although genital warts in children may be sexually transmitted as a consequence of sexual abuse, such warts in infants and children commonly result from virus inoculation at birth or from incidental spread from cutaneous warts. In contrast to anogenital lesions in adults, a significant proportion of genital warts in children contain HPV types that are usually isolated from nongenital warts.[29–31] Respiratory (laryngeal) papillomas contain the same HPV types as are found in anogenital papillomas.[32] The majority of respiratory papillomas occur in infants and young children. In this age group, the condition is believed to have been transmitted from mothers with genital HPV infection when the infant aspirates infectious virus during birth.[32] The incidence of respiratory papillomas is much lower than that of genital HPV infection, and the factors that predispose to the development of clinical respiratory lesions have not been elucidated.

In addition to causing lesions on the external genitalia, genital-mucosal HPV types also infect the uterine cervix. This sexually transmitted infection, which may involve low- or high-risk HPV types, is especially common in sexually active women younger than 25 years of age, in whom the prevalence of infection may exceed 25 percent.[33] The infection is usually subclinical and self-limited, although the likelihood of persistence is greater with high-risk HPV infection. HPV DNA has also been detected in some clinically normal penile skin.[34] Thus, even normal-appearing genital skin or mucosa may represent a reservoir for contagion.

The most common antibody response to HPV infection is directed against conformational type-specific epitopes present in the

L1 protein of the viral particle. These epitopes are efficiently presented by VLPs, which can be produced in large quantity in cultured cells. The availability of VLPs has facilitated development of HPV type-restricted assays to monitor the seroepidemiology of HPV infection. These assays have been used most extensively to examine the seroprevalence of HPV 16 infection because this is the HPV type that is found most frequently in cervical cancer.[35–37] Most, but not all, infected patients develop low serum antibody titers. The likelihood of becoming antibody positive increases with the duration of the infection. Once an individual becomes antibody positive, the antibodies seem to persist for many years, even if the individual becomes viral DNA negative. Thus, the antibodies detect both past and present infection, and the seroprevalence of HPV 16 antibodies in a given population reflects the relative prevalence of the virus within that population.[38]

PATHOGENESIS

HPV infection is acquired through inoculation of virus into the viable epidermis through defects in the epithelium. Maceration of the skin is probably an important predisposing factor, as suggested by the increased incidence of plantar warts in swimmers who frequent public pools.[39] Recent experimental evidence suggests the cellular receptor for HPV may be the $\alpha_6\beta_4$-type integrin, a cell adhesion molecule found on the surface of basal keratinocytes.[40] It is believed that a single copy or at most a few copies of the viral genome are maintained as an extrachromosomal plasmid within the infected epithelial basal cells. When these basal cells divide, the viral genome is also replicated and transported within the daughter cells as they migrate upward to form the differentiating epithelium.

Once an individual has been infected, new warts may develop in sites of inoculation over a period of weeks to months. Each new lesion probably results either from the initial exposure or spread from other warts. There is no convincing evidence for bloodborne dissemination. Autoinoculation of virus into apposed lesions is commonly seen on adjacent digits (Fig. 224-4) and in the anogenital region.

After experimental PV inoculation, it usually requires from 2 to 9 months for a verruca to become clinically apparent. This observation implies a relatively long period of subclinical infection. This state of inapparent infection represents a potential source of infectious virus. While the epidermis in a wart is acanthotic, hyperplasia of the proliferative basal cell population is not dramatic, in concordance with the observation that warts develop slowly.

HPV DNA has also been detected in normal-appearing mucosa of the larynx of patients with respiratory papillomatosis who were in clinical remission[41] and in normal-appearing skin adjacent to treatment sites of recurrent genital warts.[42] Whether these represent subclinical states rather than true "latency" (i.e., nonreplicating and transcriptionally inactive virus) is unknown. There is also increasing evidence that HPV DNA can be resident in clinically normal skin. Whether HPV DNA persists in the epithelium after successful treatment of immunocompetent individuals remains an unresolved question.

Viral RNA expression (transcription) remains low until the upper malpighian layer, just before the granular layer. There viral DNA

FIGURE 224-4

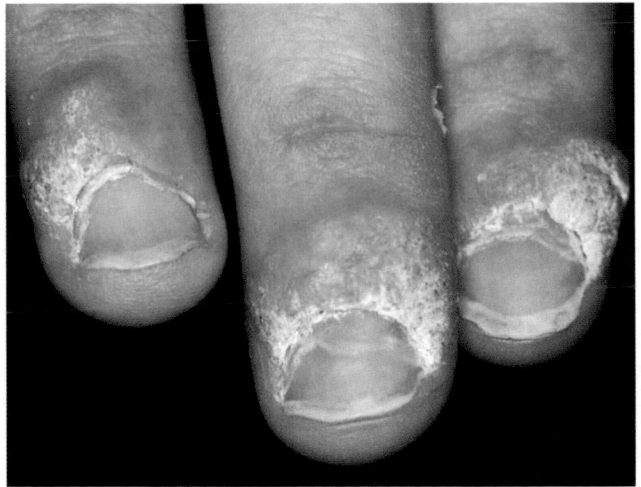

A.

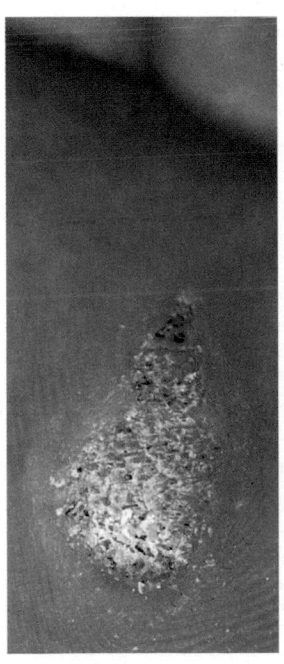

B.

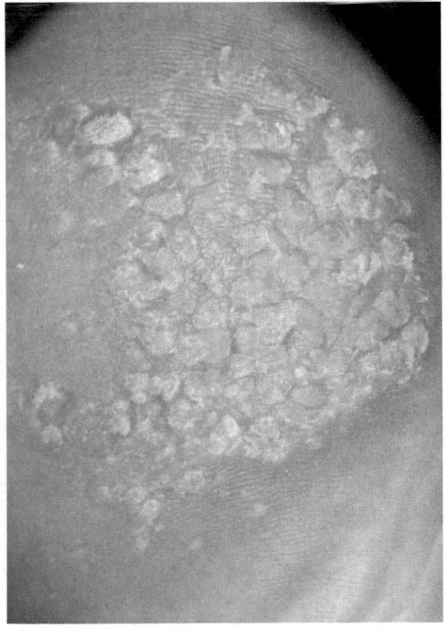

C.

A. Common wart, periungual. Multiple, confluent kerototic papules are seen around the proximal periphery of the fingernails. *B.* Common wart, verruca plantaris. *C.* Common wart, mosaic plantar. A large hyperkeratotic plaque is seen on the heel, made up of multiple small coalescing warts.

replication initiates and may result in hundreds of copies of viral DNA per cell. The viral capsid proteins (L1 and L2, Figs. 224-1 and 224-3) are synthesized and assembled into virions in the nuclei of the cells at this level (Fig. 224-3). The newly synthesized viral DNA is also incorporated into the virions in the nuclei of these differentiated malpighian cells. A viral protein called E1-E4 (it is the product of a spliced RNA from the E1 and E4 genes) may induce collapse of the cytoplasmic keratin filament network.[43] This is postulated to facilitate release of the virions from the cross-linked cytoskeleton so that they can be inoculated into another site or desquamated into the environment.

PVs are not enveloped, since they do not bud from the nuclear or plasma membrane, as do many viruses such as herpes simplex virus or HIV. It is their membrane-derived lipoprotein envelope that causes these latter viruses to be rapidly inactivated by environmental conditions such as freezing or desiccation or chemicals such as ethanol. In contrast, PV virions are resistant to desiccation[44] and to the detergent nonoxynol,[45] although exposure of virions to formalin, mild detergents, or high temperature can reduce their infectivity. They can remain infectious for years when warts are stored in glycerol at room temperature. Indeed, L1 and L2 form a tightly packed protein structure that is even highly resistant to proteases.

The relative abundance of these stable virus particles in a verruca varies with the clinical setting and the HPV type. Newer lesions tend to contain more virions than do older verrucae. Plantar warts containing HPV-1 have a high number of virions, while anogenital verrucae typically have small quantities of mature virus particles, and common warts usually have intermediate numbers. Not only does the quantity of viral DNA present differ among these lesions, but also the proportion that is enclosed within the infectious virions may vary among these verrucae.[46]

Since virions are not detected in the lower epithelial levels in warts, it is believed that viral transcription, DNA replication, and late protein production are coordinated by the state of differentiation of the infected epithelial cell. The recent propagation of limited amounts of HPVs in cultured cells is a consequence of the ability to reproduce the milieu required for physiologic differentiation.[6,7,47,48] Further support for the belief that production of virus particles and virion antigens depends on the state of epithelial differentiation is that as benign papillomas progress toward dysplasia, virion production decreases. Capsid proteins are almost never observed in frank malignancies, although HPV DNA is present. It is also possible to cultivate some HPVs by exposing epithelial cells to infectious virions followed by placement under the renal capsule of an immunodeficient (nude) mouse for prolonged periods. In this system, the epithelial cells differentiate, stratify, and resemble a verruca histologically, and the full virus replication cycle occurs, producing infectious virions.[4,5]

Experimental evidence from cell culture systems has shown that PV genes can alter cell proliferation, a characteristic common to many tumor viruses.[9] Several different transformation assays have been developed to examine the biologic effects of PV genes in vitro.[49] For example, cells may lose contact inhibition and continue to divide, exhibit increased DNA synthesis and replication rates, lose growth factor dependence, or become immortal instead of exhibiting a finite lifespan in vitro. Three different viral genes have been shown to possess some of these properties: E5, E6, and E7 (Fig. 224-1).

These experimental systems have been used to examine and compare the in vitro activities of genital-mucosal HPVs. Their rel-

ative activity varies with the HPV type.[50] In one assay, keratinocytes or cervical cells were grown as a stratified epithelium on a raft that provided an air-media interface. Introduction of high-risk HPV-16 or -18 DNA induced a disorganized pattern of differentiation with suprabasal mitotic figures resembling squamous cell carcinoma in situ, while the cells retained a normal pattern of stratification when low-risk HPV-6 or -11 DNA was used.[51] In other in vitro models, introduction of HPV-16 or -18 DNA into cultured human epithelial cells resulted in an increased growth rate, resistance to differentiation, and the ability to be continuously passaged; HPV-6 and -11 DNA were much less active.[49] Thus, for the genital-mucosal HPVs, there is an excellent correlation between their ability to induce cell transformation in vitro and their association with malignancy.[9,49]

In cutaneous or cervical epithelial cells, transformation is best achieved with both E6 and E7 from HPV-16 or -18. These two HPV genes are preferentially retained and expressed in cervical cancers, implying that these assays measure a property that is closely related to the oncogenic potential of these viruses in cervical infection. One mechanism by which the E6 and E7 proteins exert their effects is by each binding to a different cellular protein that inhibits normal epithelial cell growth. These two cellular proteins, p53 and the retinoblastoma susceptibility protein (Rb), are apparently inactivated by binding to E6 and E7, respectively, thereby relieving infected cells from the normal growth inhibitory activities of p53 and Rb.[52–55] However, the E6 proteins from some HPV types, including those associated with malignancies in EV and immunosuppression do not interact with p53.[56] These observations are supported by several studies that demonstrated that E6 and E7 must have multiple targets in the cell.[57–60] The viral E5 genes encode proteins that appear to activate growth factor receptors.[61] In the bovine (cow) papillomavirus, which induces fibropapillomas, E5 appears to preferentially activate the receptors for platelet-derived growth factor, and HPV-16 E5 may stimulate the epidermal growth factor receptor.[62–65]

The roles of immunity and genetic susceptibility to PV infection are incompletely understood.[66,67] The decrease in the frequency of warts with age implies that resistance to infection develops over time, and much of this resistance may be immunologic. In experimental PV infection in animals, resistance to virus challenge correlates with the presence of neutralizing anticapsid antibodies, and protection can be passively transferred by serum or IgG from resistant animals.[68,69] It is therefore likely that neutralizing antibodies account for at least some of the resistance to reinfection. Serum antibodies to viral capsids can be detected in some patients with current warts or a past history of warts. In patients with warts, these antibodies, as well as other host factors, may help to limit the spread of the warts to new sites.

While humoral immunity may contribute to resistance to infection, most evidence suggests that cellular immune reactivity plays a significant role in wart regression. Individuals with defective CMI are particularly susceptible to PV infection and are notoriously resistant to treatment. In cows, the induction of high levels of neutralizing antibodies, although they can protect against challenge with a PV that causes oral papillomas, do not alter established oral papillomas induced by the same virus.[70] Flat warts in patients may regress spontaneously in association with a mononuclear cell infiltrate.[71,72] There are also instances in which treatment of one or a few warts may lead to resolution of many or all warts in nonimmunosuppressed patients, although this outcome is the exception rather than the rule. In uncontrolled patient studies, vaccination with wart extracts has been reported to be effective in prevention of condylomata acuminata recurrence.[73]

CLINICAL MANIFESTATIONS

Warts are usually classified by their clinical location or morphology and can be separated into cutaneous and extracutaneous PV infections.

Cutaneous Infections (Figs. 224-5 through 224-9)

Common warts (*verruca vulgaris*) are scaly, rough, spiny papules or nodules that can be found on any skin surface (see Table 224-1). They occur often as single or grouped papules on the hands and fingers. Flat warts (*verruca plana*) are 2 to 4 mm, slightly elevated flattopped papules that have minimal scale. These are most frequent on the face, hands, and lower legs. Verrucae may also be filiform or appear as cutaneous horns. Plantar and palmar warts are thick, endophytic, and hyperkeratotic lesions, which may be painful with pressure. *Punctuate black dots* ("seeds") are seen after shaving away the outer keratinous surface and represent thrombosed capillaries in the papilloma. *Mosaic warts* result from the coalescence of plantar or palmar warts into large plaques. Some individuals with an apparently normal immunologic state develop exuberant warts of the palms or soles that are refractory to treatment. *Butcher's warts* are verrucous papules, usually multiple, on the dorsal, palmar, or periungual hands and fingers of meat cutters.[74]

Anogenital warts (also known as *condylomata acuminata*, *genital warts*, or *venereal warts*) consist of epidermal and dermal papules or nodules on the perineum, genitalia, crural folds, and anus. They vary in size and can form large, exophytic ("cauliflower-like") masses, especially in the moist environment of the perineum. Discrete 1- to 3-mm sessile warts may occur on the penile shaft. Lesions that resemble common warts also occur in this region but are unusual. Warts may extend internally into the vagina, urethra, and perirectal epithelium.

Bowenoid papulosis is a clinicopathologic entity in which HPVs have been identified.[75–77] These appear as 2- to 3-mm papules, often multiple, of the external male and female genitalia.[78] Histologically there is cellular atypia resembling Bowen's disease or squamous cell carcinoma in situ. These lesions are usually infected with HPV-16, which suggests that bowenoid papulosis may represent a precursor of penile and vulvar cancer.[79] However, the rate of transition to frank malignancy is much lower for the external genitalia than for the cervix. These small papules should be treated since they may represent a reservoir for transmission of potentially on-

FIGURE 224-6

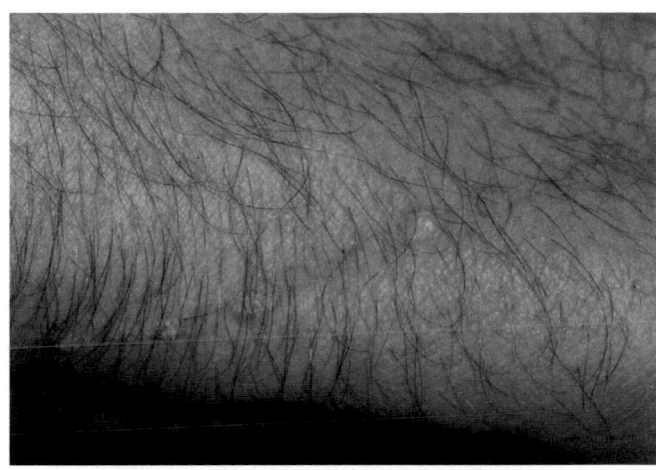

A.

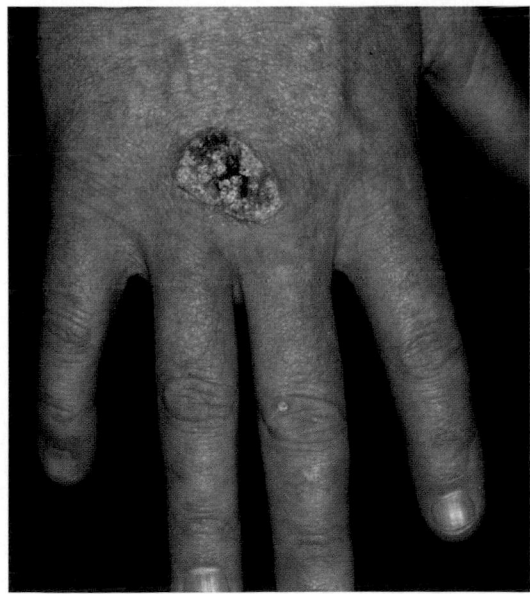

B.

A. Common wart with koebnerization. A linear arrangement of warts is seen on the elbow, arising at the site of an abrasive injury. *B.* Common wart. A giant wart is seen on the dorsum of the hand in a renal transplant recipient; the lesions were resistant to treatment but resolved spontaneously when immunosuppressive therapy was discontinued.

FIGURE 224-5

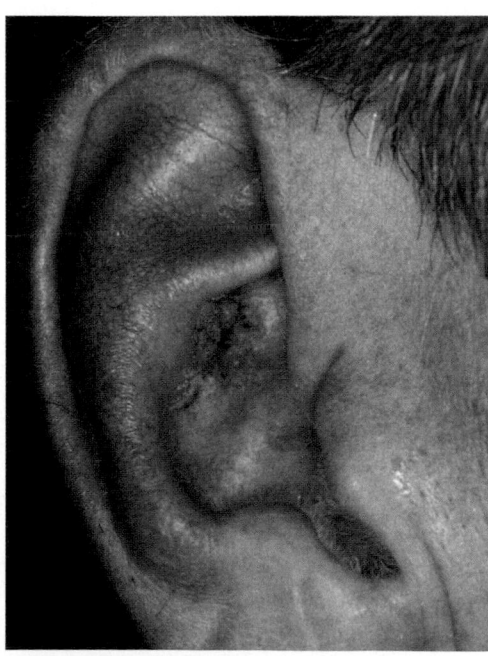

Common wart. A large hyperkeratotic nodule is seen on the ear.

FIGURE 224-7

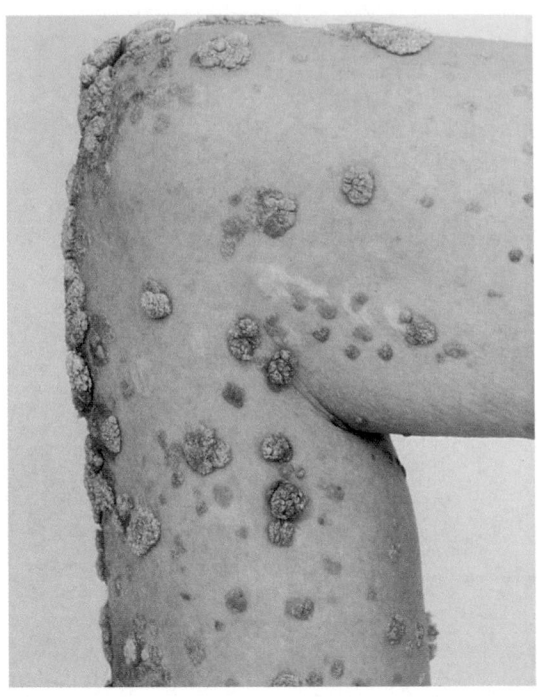

The large, scaly, and horny warts contain HPV-2. The smaller, flatter, less scaly papules are warts that contain HPV-3.

cogenic HPVs.[79] As in all genital warts, virions are difficult to detect in these lesions.[80]

Epidermodysplasia Verruciformis

This disorder represents a unique susceptibility to cutaneous HPV infection.[12,81] Warts in EV usually manifest in childhood and are usually widespread. The individual lesions typically have either the appearance of flat warts or flat scaly red-brown macules, which resemble lesions of pityriasis rosea or tinea versicolor (Fig. 224-10). The first type of lesion is usually caused by the same HPV types as are found in flat warts in the general population (e.g., HPV-3 and -10), while the second are usually caused by EV HPV types (e.g., HPV-5 and -8). Many EV patients are infected with multiple HPV types. The involvement of large areas of the body with warts or the failure to clear lesions despite adequate treatment are the typical setting for this diagnosis to be considered. About 50 percent of EV cases are inherited, usually with an autosomal recessive pattern.[81] An X-linked inheritance has also been reported.[82] Viral studies to identify the HPV genotype in the lesions may be suggestive, although such analyses are still limited to research laboratories. Recent studies suggest that EV HPV types may commensually reside in normal skin at very low levels, and it is not clear that they normally cause disease in this setting, although their association with malignant skin tumors is well substantiated in immunosuppressed individuals.[18,21–24] Warts in EV are usually widespread, although there are some patients with only a few classic lesions limited to one extremity. Mucosal warts of the cervix and oropharynx are rare but can occur. Despite treatment, warts in EV always recur, suggesting failure to mount an effective immune response to the

FIGURE 224-8

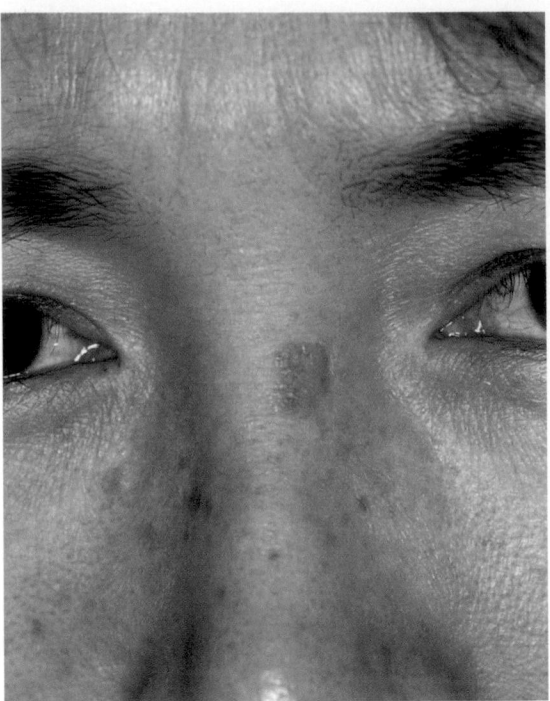

A.

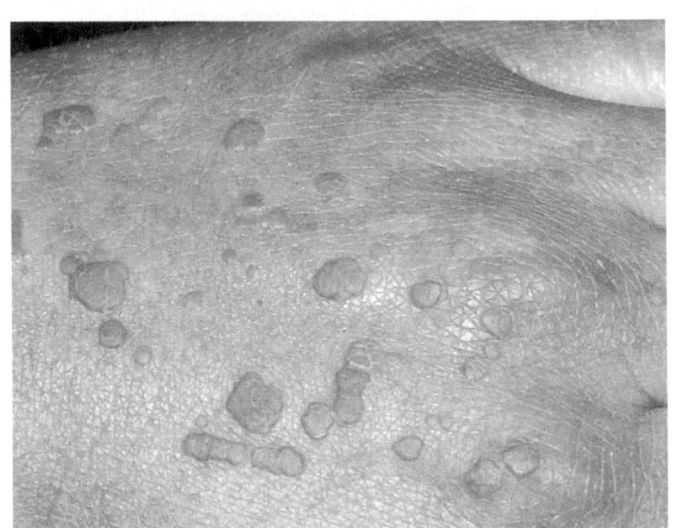

B.

Common wart, verruca plana. *A.* A single pink flat-topped lesion is seen on the nose. *B.* Many flat-topped papules. The linear configuration in the lower part of the picture is due to autoinoculation.

infection. Classically, individuals with EV do not suffer from frequent bacterial or other viral infections. Many EV patients may, however, have readily demonstrable defects of cellular immunity.[67] Immunocompromised individuals may have multiple warts that contain EV types and are difficult to eradicate, but this condition is acquired.

Some EV patients are at high risk of developing cutaneous squamous cell carcinomas.[12,81] These tumors usually arise in pityriasis-like lesions on sun-exposed areas (Fig. 224-11). Most of the malignant tumors remain local, but regional and distant metastases may occur. Although pityriasis-like lesions caused by any EV type may

FIGURE 224-9

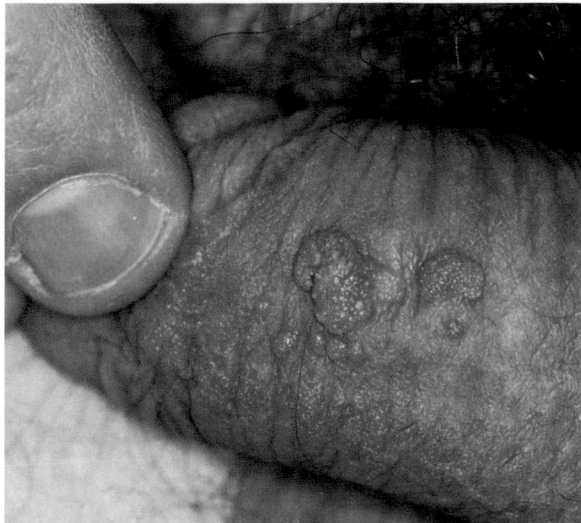

A.

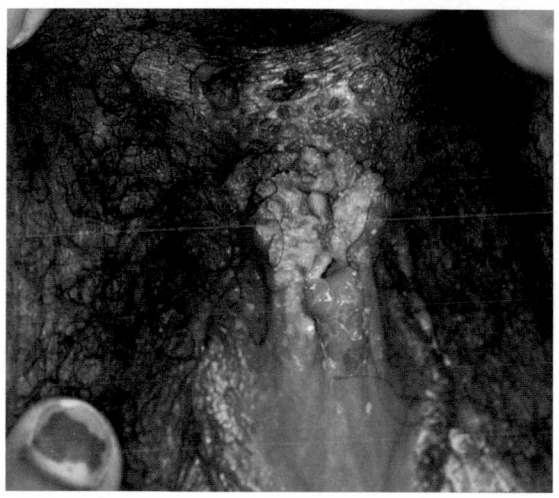

B.

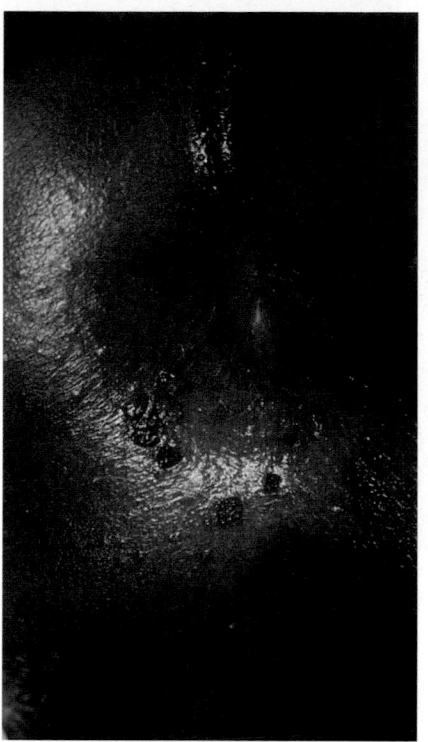

C.

Mucosal wart. *A.* Multiple condyloma acuminata are seen on the shaft of the penis. *B.* Multiple confluent condylomata are seen on the labia minora. *C.* Multiple condylomata are seen on the perineum of this 20-month-old boy, who was infected during vaginal delivery; his mother was not aware of her infection, but on examination was found to have several small condylomata.

be at increased risk of becoming malignant, the risk appears to be greatest for those caused by HPV-5 and -8, as lesions with these two HPV types account for the vast majority of malignancies in EV. Since the malignant tumors develop on exposed areas, it is believed that UV light acts as an important cofactor in the development of the tumors. The lesions of individuals with EV who have only flat warts caused by non-EV HPV types do not seem to be at increased risk of becoming malignant.

Extracutaneous (Mucosal) Infections

Oral warts are small, slightly elevated, soft, often pink or white papules that may be found on the buccal, gingival, or labial mucosa or on the tongue or hard palate. Verrucous, horny papillomas may occur on the palate. Mucosal lesions of the oropharynx, termed *focal epithelial hyperplasia*, have also been demonstrated to contain HPVs.[83] In *oral florid papillomatosis*, which is thought also to be caused by a PV, multiple large verrucae appear within the oral cavity. Progression to verrucous carcinoma may occur. *Oral condylomata acuminata* can result from oro-genital sexual contact. Warts

may also occur in the urethra, usually when meatal warts are present.[84] They may spread to the urinary bladder.

Respiratory (laryngeal) papillomatosis is characterized by the presence of multiple benign, noninvasive warts that usually involve the larynx but may extend to the oropharynx and bronchopulmonary epithelia. Presenting symptoms commonly include hoarseness and stridor. Most cases occur in infants, where the lesions may block the airway, but the condition may develop at any age. These HPV-associated papillomas may spontaneously remit, especially at puberty, but recurrences are frequent, perhaps because of the persistence of viral DNA despite clinical remission.[41] Since the HPVs isolated from these lesions are the same types as those of cervical warts, respiratory papillomatosis is thought to result from seeding of the larynx during parturition by virus present in maternal condylomata acuminata or cervical papillomas.[85] Several studies have demonstrated the epidemiologic correlation of condylomata in mothers of infants with this disease. Nonetheless, cervical and external genitalia warts are common in the child-bearing age bracket, while respiratory papillomatosis of infants is rare. It is controversial whether Cesarean section should be performed in mothers with condylomata, since this procedure itself has some attendant risk.

FIGURE 224-10

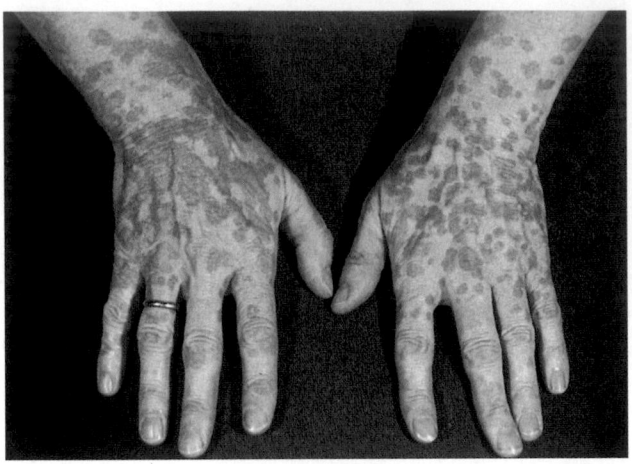

Plane wartlike lesions on the dorsa of the hands and forearms, associated with HPV-5 and -8. The lesions are numerous, flat, reddish, and partly confluent.

FIGURE 224-11

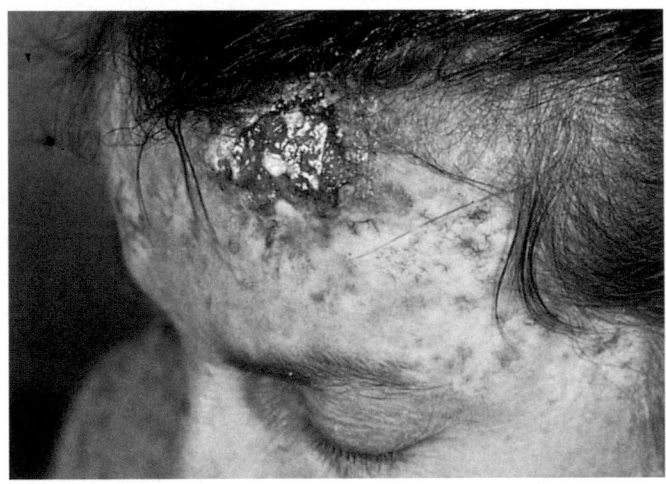

Invasive cancer in a patient infected with numerous EV HPV-5, -8, -9, -14, and others. In the tumor cells, DNA HPV-5 was detected in a high copy number. This large squamous cell carcinoma did not metastasize and did not recur after surgery. There are numerous actinic keratoses on the forehead.

As discussed earlier, the uterine cervix is an important site of HPV infection. Lesions are usually termed *cervical warts* or *atypical condylomata* and are usually flat or slightly elevated. Their visualization may require colposcopy and enhancement following acetic acid application, which makes them appear as white patches (Fig. 224-12). Atypical condylomata may mimic cervical dysplasia or carcinoma in situ histologically, with nuclear atypia and disorganized differentiation. Cells with a central nucleus and a surrounding clear halo (*koilocytotic cells*) may be seen histologically in these lesions as well as in common verrucae and represent a hallmark of HPV infection as visualized in a Pap smear.

FIGURE 224-12

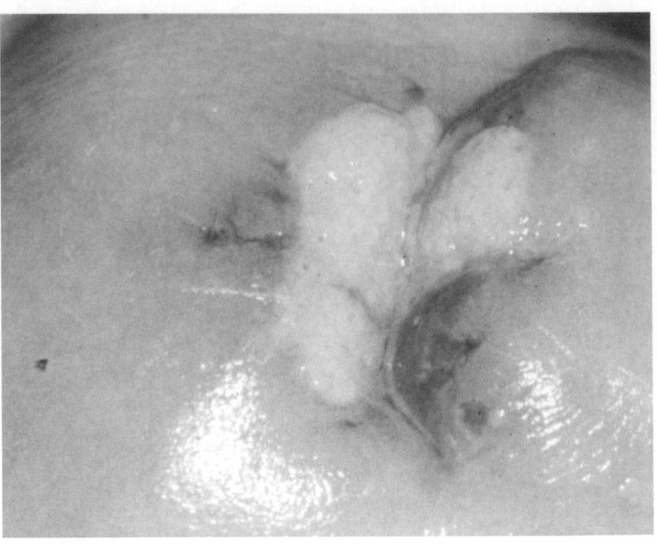

Colposcopic view of cervical condylomata after treatment with acetic acid for visualization as white, elevated patch.

RELATION OF PAPILLOMAVIRUSES AND MALIGNANCY

Although most PVs are associated with and limited to biologically benign lesions, epidemiologic and experimental studies indicate that certain PV genotypes have oncogenic potential.[9,86] In animals, the benign warts induced in rabbits by the (Shope) cottontail rabbit PV can spontaneously convert to invasive squamous cell carcinoma.[87] Small doses of chemical carcinogens induce a high rate of malignant conversion in these lesions. In cattle, esophageal papillomas induced by BPV-4 become malignant if the infected animals graze on bracken fern, which contains a potential carcinogen.[88] These observations and the long latency to malignant progression suggest that PVs do not induce malignant tumors directly; it is more likely that potentially oncogenic PVs act by predisposing the infected cell to become malignant. Similar conclusions seem relevant to human malignancies associated with HPVs.

In humans, the link to infection by specific HPV types was first noted in patients with EV. Squamous cell carcinoma frequently develops in sun-exposed warts in EV lesions and is common with those containing HPV-5 or -8. Metastatic tumors in EV contain the viral DNA, implying its presence is not from skin contamination and that retention of the HPV genome is necessary for maintaining the malignant phenotype. Progression of the verrucae in respiratory papillomatosis to invasive squamous cell carcinoma can occur subsequent to X-irradiation.

There is now compelling evidence that cervical infection with high-risk HPVs is the main cause of cervical cancer.[89] It is important to note, however, that even cervical infection with high-risk HPVs usually has a benign outcome. Patients with impaired cellular immune function, such as in renal transplant recipients or those with HIV infection and AIDS, are at much greater risk of having persistent HPV infection and progressing to severe dysplasia and thus to cancer.[90–92] These observations lead to the conclusion that HPVs usually induce benign lesions, but specific HPV types can induce the development of malignant epithelial tumors. While HPV infection with these high-risk types may be necessary, it is not sufficient and most likely requires other cofactors to alter the cell to a malignant phenotype.

Epidemiologic evidence has also linked some penile, vulvar, and anal carcinomas with HPV infection.[9,33,93–95] As with cervical cancer, these tumors are associated primarily with high-risk HPV types, which is consistent with these HPVs as a cause of the malignancies.[33,93] High-risk HPVs, especially HPV-16, have been identified in some periungual cutaneous tumors.[96,97]

The giant condyloma acuminatum, also called the *Buschke-Lowenstein tumor*, is a low-grade locally invasive squamous cell carcinoma. Low-risk HPVs such as types 6 and 11 are usually found in these tumors.[98,99] Verrucous carcinoma of the penis, however, is not usually associated with HPV infection. *Epithelioma cuniculatum*, another rare type of verrucous carcinoma, is found on the sole and is thought to arise from a plantar wart.

There is also evidence, using very sensitive PCR techniques, that HPVs may be found in a high proportion of nonmelanoma cutaneous tumors in patients without obvious immune impairment as well as in immunosuppressed renal allograft recipients.[21–23] These provocative findings will require careful follow-up to determine the precise relationship between the HPVs and the cutaneous tumors, since the same PCR techniques have also identified small amounts of HPV DNA in normal skin or in dermatologic conditions in which the normal barrier function of the epithelium is impaired.

HISTOPATHOLOGY

Verrucae consist of an acanthotic epidermis with papillomatosis, hyperkeratosis, and parakeratosis (Fig. 224-13); some correlations can be made with HPV type.[100,101] The elongated rete ridges often point toward the center of the wart. The dermal capillary vessels are prominent and may be thrombosed. Mononuclear cells may be present. Large keratinocytes with an eccentric, pyknotic nucleus surrounded by a perinuclear halo (koilocytotic cells or koilocytes), are characteristic of HPV-associated papillomas. Koilocytes do not usually contain keratohyaline granules, although they occur in the malpighian layer. PV-infected cells may have small, eosinophilic granules and dense clumps of basophilic keratohyaline granules. These granules may be composed of or associated with the PV E4 (E1-E4) protein[102] and do not represent conglomerates of virus particles. Flat warts have less acanthosis and hyperkeratosis and do not have parakeratosis or papillomatosis. Koilocytotic cells are usually abundant, indicating the viral origin of the lesion. Anogenital warts may have from slight to extensive acanthosis and parakeratosis: they lack a granular layer since they are within or adjacent to a mucosal surface. The rete ridges often form thick bands extending extensively into the underlying, highly vascular dermis. Koilocytes are often observed in these viral papillomas.

Plane warts, which usually contain HPV-3 or -10, have a similar appearance histologically whether in the general population or in patients with EV (Fig. 224-14). The granular and upper spinous layers contain many cells with perinuclear vacuolization. In EV, many cells from lesions containing HPV-5 or -8 have a characteristic basket-weave-like hyperkeratosis with many large clear cells in the granular and spinous layers (Fig. 224-15).

FIGURE 224-13

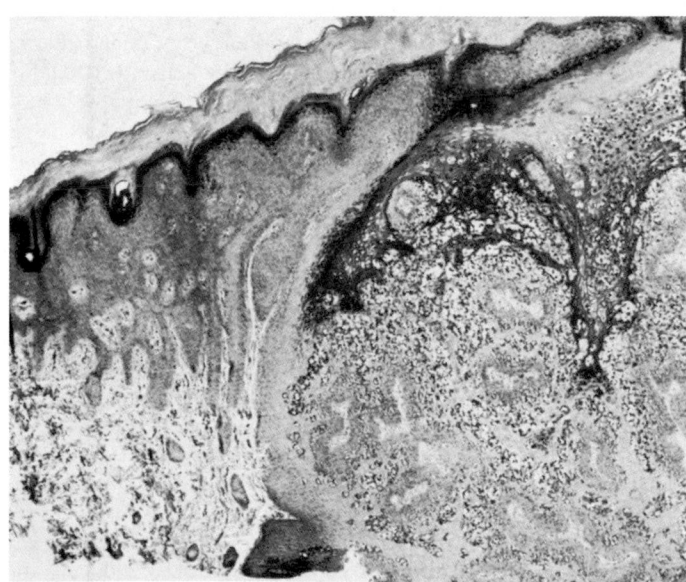

Verruca vulgaris. The process is one of extensive hyperplasia, and the hyperplastic cells contain both intranuclear and intracytoplasmic inclusion bodies. (*Micrograph by Wallace H. Clark, Jr., MD.*)

FIGURE 224-14

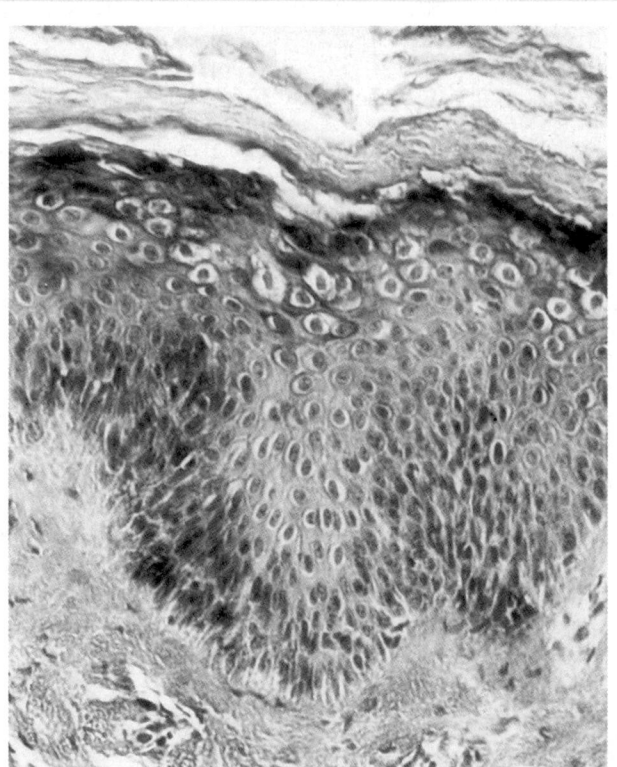

Histology of HPV-3-associated plane wartlike lesion in a patient with EV. The pattern is characteristic of a plane wart with numerous cells showing perinuclear vacuolization in the granular and upper spinous layers. H&E.

FIGURE 224-15

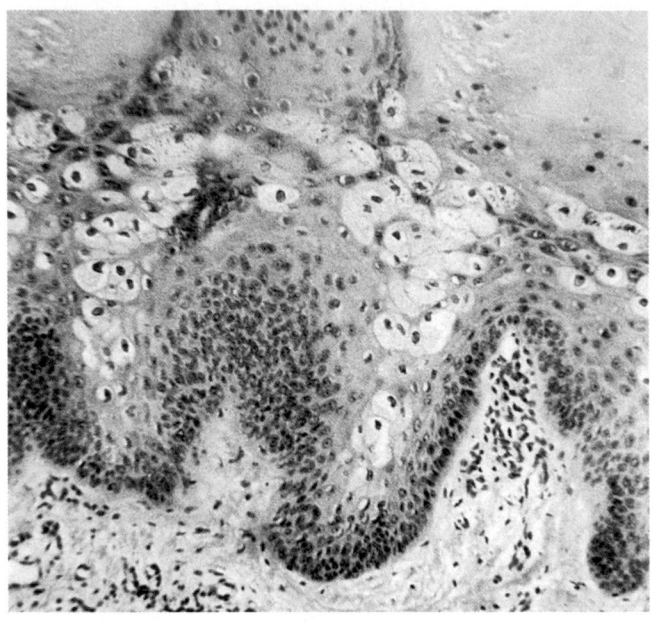

Characteristic cytopathic effect of EV-specific HPV in a patient found to be infected with HPV-5, -8, and -9. Very abundant clear large cells with small pyknotic nuclei replace almost the entire epidermis. H&E.

DIAGNOSIS

The diagnosis of viral wart is usually made by the clinical appearance but can also be suggested by histologic examination. Application of 3 to 5% acetic acid to genital warts enhances detection of these lesions, particularly with colposcopic magnification,[28] although diagnosis should not rest only on the presence of white lesions, since there may be false positives. Immunohistochemical detection of PV structural proteins may confirm the presence of virus in a lesion. DNA hybridization techniques, which are currently limited to research laboratories, may soon be more widely available. Diagnostic tests to identify genital-mucosal HPV type are now commercially available for the common genital HPV types.[103,104]

Cutaneous warts are common in children and young adults but also occur in patients over 40 years of age. Multiple warts that do not spontaneously resolve, always recur after treatment, persist for years, or have an unusual morphology, especially if familial, suggest EV. HPV typing may be of benefit in confirming the diagnosis of EV and will also disclose whether the patient is infected with a type that is associated with malignancy. Immunocompromised patients, such as those with AIDS, lymphoproliferative disorders, or on chemotherapeutic drugs, may have multiple warts.

DIFFERENTIAL DIAGNOSIS

Common lesions such as seborrheic and solar keratoses, nevi, irritated achrocordons, clavi, and squamous cell carcinomas may look like verrucae. Papules of lichen planus may resemble flat warts;

they may be differentiated by the presence of Wickham's striae and buccal involvement. Acrokeratosis verruciformis and epidermolytic hyperkeratosis are characterized by verrucous papules on the extremities. Syphilitic condylomata need to be differentiated from venereal warts.

TREATMENT

The approach to management of warts depends on the age of the patient, the extent and duration of lesions, the patient's immunologic status, and the patient's desire for therapy. Children with common warts may not require therapy. Studies of spontaneous regression of warts in children suggest that two-thirds will remit within 2 years, with remaining verrucae continuing to resolve at this rate.[105] However, new warts may appear while others are regressing.

Current treatments for verrucae involve physical destruction of the infected cells.[106] The existence of multiple treatment modalities reflects the fact that none is uniformly effective or directly antiviral. Choice of treatment depends on the location, size, number and type of wart, as well as the age and cooperation of the patient. Pain, inconvenience, risk of scarring, and experience of the physician are considerations to evaluate prior to treatment. In patients with anogenital warts (including bowenoid papulosis), sexual partners should be examined and treated if necessary. In females, evaluation of the uterine cervix should be performed; male contacts of women with cervical disease should also be examined.[28] Therapy for bowenoid papulosis with standard techniques such as cryotherapy, electrodesiccation, or excision is indicated, for while these may spontaneously remit, HPV-16 is frequently found. Application of 5-fluorouracil has been reported to be effective in some cases of Bowen's disease, flat warts, and condylomata acuminata,[107] and direct instillation has been used for urethral warts.[108]

Cryotherapy utilizing liquid nitrogen applied with a cotton tip or a spray canister is a common and effective treatment for most warts. Caution must be used near the nail matrix when treating periungual warts. Aggressive cryotherapy with a spray canister can injure underlying structures such as nerves and must therefore be used carefully on the lateral surfaces of the digits and genitalia. Warts on the elbows and knees of children may be particularly susceptible to scarring with cryotherapy; although effective, this modality should be used in moderation in these situations.

Warts may be curetted or surgically excised, particularly large anogenital warts unresponsive to topical treatments. Electrodesiccation of condylomata acuminata requires local anesthesia but is effective. The CO$_2$ laser, and potentially other new energy formats, can be of utility for destroying resistant warts or those where careful control of width and depth are necessary, such as in large periungual warts. Use of a surgical mask should be routine since infectious PV has been identified in the vapor plume with laser or with electrocoagulation of warts.[109] Microscopically controlled (Mohs) surgery has been particularly useful in the treatment of verrucous carcinoma. X-irradiation of verrucae is contraindicated because of its association with development of malignancy in respiratory papillomatosis and EV. Avoidance of and protection from sun exposure is also important in EV.

A variety of chemotherapeutic agents are also widely employed. Topical podophyllin resin is a common treatment, particularly for anogenital warts, since it is more effective on mucosal surfaces.[110] However, podophyllin is said to be contraindicated during pregnancy,[111] and the potency of podophyllin preparations may be variable.[112] Purified podophyllotoxin (Condylox) has activity that is uniform from batch to batch, and it is approved for treatment of genital and perianal warts.[113] Intralesional bleomycin may eradicate verrucae but should be used cautiously due to the possibility of extensive tissue necrosis.[114,115]

Caustics and acids such as salicylic acid, lactic acid, and trichloroacetic acid destroy and peel off infected skin. Home use of salicylic acid preparations can be particularly efficacious in young children who cannot tolerate other modalities. Retinoic acid has been used topically for flat warts and probably has a similar mechanism of action. Cantharidin is an extract of the green blister beetle that leads to blistering and focal destruction of epidermis.[116]

Immunotherapies have been attempted in various forms. Induction of allergic contact dermatitis with dinitrochlorobenzene (DNCB) or diphenylcyclopropenone allows localization of inflammation to warts on which the allergen is painted; it has been speculated that this treatment stimulates local immunity.[117,118] DNCB is positive in the Ames bacterial test of mutagenicity, and its utilization remains controversial.[119] Cimetidine has recently gained notoriety in the treatment of cutaneous warts, particularly in children.[120,121] While this regimen has its supporters, a double-blind controlled study showed no beneficial effect.[122] Interferon has been effective in short-term studies in reducing warts in laryngeal papillomatosis and EV, but return of lesions occurs when therapy is stopped.[41,123,124] Recombinant interferon-α was approved for intralesional injection of refractory genital warts in 1989, and several other forms of interferons have shown utility.[125,126] It is not clear that interferon acts through stimulation of immune response. Cytokines were successfully used in the treatment of warts in a patient with cyclic neutropenia.[127] Recently imiquimod (Aldara), a potent stimulator of the release of several proinflammatory cytokines,[106] was approved for treatment of genital warts.

A variety of prophylactic and therapeutic HPV vaccine trials are contemplated or in progress.[128] For animal papillomaviruses, vaccination of rabbits, dogs, and cows with VLPs derived from PVs that can cause lesions in the respective host have shown good protection against subsequent experimental challenge with the authentic virus.[68,70,129] Dogs immunized with formalinized canine oral papillomavirus (COPV), a mucosal PV, were successfully protected from COPV infection under field conditions.[130]

REFERENCES

1. de Villiers EM: Papillomavirus and HPV typing. *Clin Dermatol* **15**:199, 1997
2. Favre M et al: Human papillomaviruses: General features. *Clin Dermatol* **15**:181, 1997
3. Turek LP: The structure, function, and regulation of papillomaviral genes in infection and cervical cancer. *Adv Virus Res* **44**:305, 1994
4. Kreider JW et al: Laboratory production in vivo of infectious human papillomavirus type 11. *J Virol* **61**:590, 1987
5. Howett MK et al: Tissue xenografts as a model system for study of the pathogenesis of papillomaviruses. *Clin Dermatol* **15**:229, 1997
6. Meyers C et al: Biosynthesis of human papillomavirus from a continuous cell line upon epithelial differentiation. *Science* **257**:971, 1992
7. Meyers C et al: Synthesis of infectious human papillomavirus type 18 in differentiating epithelium transfected with viral DNA. *J Virol* **71**:7381, 1997
8. Roden RBS et al: In vitro generation and type-specific neutralization of a human papillomavirus type 16 virion pseudotype. *J Virol* **70**:5875, 1996
9. zur Hausen H: Papillomavirus infections—a major cause of human cancers. *Biochim Biophys Acta Rev Cancer* **1288**:F55, 1996
10. Brandsma JL et al: Detection and typing of papillomavirus DNA in formaldehyde-fixed paraffin-embedded tissue. *Arch Otol Head Neck Surg* **116**:844, 1990
11. Chan SY et al: Analysis of genomic sequences of 95 papillomavirus types: Uniting typing, phylogeny, and taxonomy. *J Virol* **69**:3074, 1995
12. Majewski S et al: Epidermodysplasia verruciformis. Immunological and nonimmunological surveillance mechanisms: Role in tumor progression. *Clin Dermatol* **15**:321, 1997
13. Majewski S, Jablonska S: Human papillomavirus–associated tumors of the skin and mucosa. *J Am Acad Dermatol* **36**:659, 1997
14. Bosch FX et al: Prevalence of human papillomavirus in cervical cancer: A worldwide perspective. *J Natl Cancer Inst* **87**:796, 1995
15. Jenson SB et al: Immunological relatedness of papillomaviruses from different species. *J Natl Cancer Inst* **64**::495, 1980
16. Kirnbauer R et al: Papillomavirus L1 major capsid protein self-assembles into virus-like particles that are highly immunogenic. *Proc Natl Acad Sci USA* **89**:12180, 1992
17. Kirnbauer R et al: Efficient self-assembly of human papillomavirus type 16 L1 and L1-L2 into virus-like particles. *J Virol* **67**:6929, 1993
18. Tieben LM et al: Detection of epidermodysplasia verruciformis–like human papillomavirus types in malignant and premalignant skin lesions of renal transplant recipients. *Br J Dermatol* **131**:226, 1994
19. Shamanin V et al: Specific types of human papillomavirus found in benign proliferations and carcinomas of the skin in immunosuppressed patients. *Cancer Res* **54**:4610, 1994
20. Berkhout RJ et al: Nested PCR approach for detection and typing of epidermodysplasia verruciformis–associated human papillomavirus types in cutaneous cancers from renal transplant recipients. *J Clin Microbiol* **33**:690, 1995
21. de Jong-Tieben LM et al: High frequency of detection of epidermodysplasia verruciformis–associated human papillomavirus DNA in biopsies from malignant and premalignant skin lesions from renal transplant recipients. *J Invest Dermatol* **105**:367, 1995
22. de Villiers EM et al: Prevailing papillomavirus types in non-melanoma carcinomas of the skin in renal allograft recipients. *Int J Cancer* **73**:356, 1997
23. Höpfl R et al: Human papillomavirus DNA in non-melanoma skin cancers of a renal transplant recipient: Detection of a new sequence related to epidermodysplasia verruciformis–associated types. *J Invest Dermatol* **108**:53, 1997
24. Boxman IL et al: Detection of human papillomavirus DNA in plucked hairs from renal transplant recipients and healthy volunteers. *J Invest Dermatol* **108**:712, 1997
25. Laurent R, Kienzler JL: Epidemiology of HPV infections. *Clin Dermatol* **3**:64, 1985
26. Condyloma acuminatum—United States. *MMWR* **32**:306, 1983
27. Kokelj F et al: Study of the partners of women with human papillomavirus infection. *Int J Dermatol* **32**:661, 1993
28. Barrasso R et al: High prevalence of papillomavirus-associated penile intraepithelial neoplasia in sexual partners of women with cervical intraepithelial neoplasia. *N Engl J Med* **317**:916, 1987
29. Cohen BA et al: Anogenital warts in children. Clinical and virologic evaluation for sexual abuse. *Arch Dermatol* **126**:1575, 1990
30. de Villiers EM: Importance of human papillomavirus DNA typing in the diagnosis of anogenital warts in children. *Arch Dermatol* **131**:366, 1995
31. Obalek S et al: Anogenital warts in children. *Clin Dermatol* **15**:369, 1997
32. Kashima HK et al: Recurrent respiratory papillomatosis. *Obstet Gynecol Clin North Am* **23**:699, 1996
33. Schiffman MH, Brinton LA: The epidemiology of cervical carcinogenesis. *Cancer* **76**:1888, 1995
34. Castellsagué X et al: Prevalence of penile human papillomavirus DNA in husbands of women with and without cervical neoplasia: A study in Spain and Colombia. *J Infect Dis* **176**:353, 1997
35. Wideroff L et al: Epidemiologic determinants of seroreactivity to human papillomavirus (HPV) type 16 virus-like particles in cervical HPV-16 DNA-positive and -negative women. *J Infect Dis* **174**:937, 1996
36. Carter JJ et al: The natural history of human papillomavirus type 16 capsid antibodies among a cohort of university women. *J Infect Dis* **174**:927, 1996
37. Olsen AO et al: Seropositivity against HPV 16 capsids: A better marker of past sexual behaviour than presence of HPV DNA. *Genitourin Med* **73**:131, 1997
38. Nonnenmacher B et al: Serologic response to human papillomavirus type 16 (HPV-16) virus-like particles in HPV-16 DNA-positive invasive cervical cancer and cervical intraepithelial neoplasia grade III

patients and controls from Colombia and Spain. *J Infect Dis* **172**:19, 1995

39. Gentles JC, Evans EGV: Foot infections in swimming baths. *Br Med J* **2**:260, 1973

40. Evander M et al: Identification of the alpha 6 integrin as a candidate receptor for papillomaviruses. *J Virol* **71**:2449, 1997

41. Steinberg BM et al: Persistence and expression of human papillomavirus during interferon therapy. *Arch Otolaryngol Head Neck Surg* **144**:27, 1988

42. Ferenczy A et al: Latent papillomavirus and recurring genital warts. *N Engl J Med* **313**:784, 1985

43. Doorbar J et al: Specific interaction between HPV-16 E1-E4 and cytokeratins results in collapse of the epithelial cell intermediate filament network. *Nature* **352**:824, 1991

44. Roden RB et al: Papillomavirus is resistant to desiccation. *J Infect Dis* **176**:1076, 1997

45. Hermonat PL et al: The spermicide nonoxynol-9 does not inactivate papillomavirus. *Sex Transm Dis* **19**:203, 1992

46. Grussendorf-Conen EI et al: Correlation between content of viral DNA and evidence of mature virus particles in HPV-1, HPV-4, and HPV-6 induced virus acanthomata. *J Invest Dermatol* **81**:511, 1983

47. Dollard SC et al: Production of human papillomavirus and modulation of the infectious program in epithelial raft cultures. *Genes Devel* **6**:1131, 1992

48. Frattini MG et al: In vitro synthesis of oncogenic human papillomaviruses requires episomal genomes for differentiation-dependent late expression. *Proc Natl Acad Sci USA* **93**:3062, 1996

49. Mansur CP, Androphy EJ: Cellular transformation by papillomavirus oncoproteins. *Biochim Biophys Acta* **1155**:323, 1993

50. Barbosa MS et al: In vitro biological activities of the E6 and E7 genes vary among human papillomaviruses of different oncogenic potential. *J Virol* **65**:292, 1991

51. McCance DJ et al: Human papillomavirus type 16 alters human epithelial cell differentiation in vitro. *Proc Natl Acad Sci USA* **85**:7169, 1988

52. Vousden KH: Interactions between papillomavirus proteins and tumor suppressor gene products. *Adv Cancer Res* **64**:1, 1994

53. Huibregtse JM, Beaudenon SL: Mechanism of HPV E6 proteins in cellular transformation. *Semin Cancer Biol* **7**:317, 1996

54. Jones DL, Munger K: Interactions of the human papillomavirus E7 protein with cell cycle regulators. *Semin Cancer Biol* **7**:327, 1996

55. Crawford L, Tommasino M: Oncogenes and anti-oncogenes in the development of HPV associated tumors. *Clin Dermatol* **15**:207, 1997

56. Steger G, Pfister H: In vitro expressed HPV 8 E6 protein does not bind p53. *Arch Virol* **125**:355, 1992

57. Jewers RJ et al: Regions of human papillomavirus type 16 E7 oncoprotein required for immortalization of human keratinocytes. *J Virol* **66**:1329, 1992

58. Ishiwatari H et al: Degradation of p53 only is not sufficient for the growth stimulatory effect of human papillomavirus 16 E6 oncoprotein in human embryonic fibroblasts. *J Med Virol* **44**:243, 1994

59. Chen J et al: Interaction of papillomavirus E6 oncoproteins with a putative calcium binding protein. *Science* **269**:529, 1995

60. Nakagawa S et al: Mutational analysis of human papillomavirus type 16 E6 protein: Transforming function for human cells and degradation of p53 in vitro. *Virology* **212**:535, 1995

61. Martin P et al: The bovine papillomavirus E5 transforming protein can stimulate the transforming activity of EGF and CSF-1 receptors. *Cell* **59**:21, 1989

62. Pim D et al: Human papillomavirus type 16 E5 gene stimulates the transforming activity of the epidermal growth factor receptor. *Oncogene* **7**:27, 1992

63. Straight SW et al: The E5 oncoprotein of human papillomavirus type 16 transforms fibroblasts and effects the downregulation of the epidermal growth factor receptor in keratinocytes. *J Virol* **67**:4521, 1993

64. Stoppler MC et al: The E5 gene of HPV-16 enhances keratinocyte immortalization by full-length DNA. *Virology* **223**:251, 1996

65. Petti LM et al: Identification of amino acids in the transmembrane and juxtamembrane domains of the platelet-derived growth factor receptor required for productive interaction with the bovine papillomavirus E5 protein. *J Virol* **71**:7318, 1997

66. Frazer IH: Immunology of papillomavirus infection. *Curr Opin Immunol* **8**:484, 1996

67. Majewski S, Jablonska S: Immunology of HPV infection and HPV-associated tumors. *Int J Dermatol* **37**:81, 1998

68. Breitburd F et al: Immunization with virus-like particles from cottontail rabbit papillomavirus (CRPV) can protect against experimental CRPV infection. *J Virol* **69**:3959, 1995

69. Roden R et al: Papillomavirus L1 capsids agglutinate mouse erythrocytes through a proteinaceous receptor. *J Virol* **69**:5147, 1995

70. Kirnbauer R et al: Virus-like particles of bovine papillomavirus type 4 in prophylactic and therapeutic immunization. *Virology* **219**:37, 1996

71. Rogozinski TT et al: Role of cell-mediated immunity in spontaneous regression of plane warts. *Int J Dermatol* **27**:322, 1988

72. Coleman N et al: Immunological events in regressing genital warts. *Am J Clin Pathol* **102**:768, 1994

73. Abcarian H, Sharon N: Long-term effectiveness of the immunotherapy of anal condyloma acuminatum. *Dis Colon Rectum* **25**:648, 1982

74. Orth G: Identification of papillomaviruses in butcher's warts. *J Invest Dermatol* **76**:97, 1981

75. Zachow KR et al: Detection of human papillomavirus DNA in anogenital neoplasias. *Nature* **300**:771, 1982

76. Ikenberg H et al: Human papillomavirus type-16 related DNA in genital Bowen's disease and in bowenoid papulosis. *Int J Cancer* **32**:563, 1983

77. Bergeron C et al: Human papillomavirus type 16 in intraepithelial neoplasia (bowenoid papulosis) and coexistent invasive carcinoma of the vulva. *Int J Gynecol Pathol* **6**:1, 1987

78. Gross G et al: Bowenoid papulosis. *Arch Dermatol* **121**:858, 1985

79. Obalek S et al: Bowenoid papulosis of the male and female genitalia: Risk of cervical neoplasia. *J Am Acad Dermatol* **14**:433, 1986

80. Guillet GY et al: Bowenoid papulosis: Demonstration of human papillomavirus (HPV) with anti-HPV immune serum. *Arch Dermatol* **120**:514, 1984

81. Orth G: Epidermodysplasia verruciformis: A model for understanding the oncogenicity of human papillomaviruses. *Ciba Found Symp* **120**:157, 1986

82. Androphy EJ et al: X-linked inheritance of epidermodysplasia verruciformis. Genetic and virologic studies of a kindred. *Arch Dermatol* **121**:864, 1985

83. Pfister H et al: Characterization of human papillomavirus type 13 from focal epithelial hyperplasia Heck lesions. *J Virol* **47**:363, 1983

84. Sand PK et al: Evaluation of male consorts of women with genital human papilloma virus infection. *Obstet Gynecol* **68**:679, 1986

85. Puranen MH et al: Exposure of an infant to cervical human papillomavirus infection of the mother is common. *Am J Obstet Gynecol* **176**:1039, 1997

86. Münger K: The molecular biology of cervical cancer. *J Cell Biochem* **23**:55, 1995

87. Kreider JW, Bartlett GL: Shope rabbit papilloma–carcinoma complex. A model system of HPV infections. *Clin Dermatol* **3**:20, 1985

88. Campo MS, Jarrett WF: Papillomavirus infection in cattle: Viral and chemical cofactors in naturally occurring and experimentally induced tumours. *Ciba Found Symp* **120**:117, 1986

89. *Human Papillomaviruses. IARC: Monogr Eval Carcinog Risks Hum* **64**:409, 1995

90. Palefsky JM et al: Anal cytological abnormalities and anal HPV infection in men with Centers for Disease Control group IV HIV disease. *Genitourin Med* **73**:174, 1997

91. Sun XW et al: Human papillomavirus infection in women infected with the human immunodeficiency virus. *N Engl J Med* **337**:1343, 1997

92. Shah KV: Human papillomaviruses and anogenital cancers. *N Engl J Med* **337**:1386, 1997

93. Schiffman MH: New epidemiology of human papillomavirus infection and cervical neoplasia. *J Natl Cancer Inst* **87**:1345, 1995

94. zur Hausen H: Human papillomaviruses in the pathogenesis of anogenital cancer. *Virology* **184**:9, 1991

95. zur Hausen H, de Villiers EM: Human papillomaviruses. *Annu Rev Microbiol* **48**:427, 1994

96. Moy R et al: Human papillomavirus type 16 DNA in periungual squamous cell carcinomas. *JAMA* **261**:2669, 1989

97. McHugh RW et al: Metastatic periungual squamous cell carcinoma: Detection of human papillomavirus type 35 RNA in the digital tumor and axillary lymph node metastases. *J Am Acad Dermatol* **34**:1080, 1996

98. Masih AS et al: Penile verrucous carcinoma: A clinicopathologic, human papillomavirus typing and flow cytometric analysis. *Mod Pathol* **55**:48, 1992

99. Grussendorf-Conen EI: Anogenital premalignant and malignant tumors (including Buschke-Lowenstein tumors). *Clin Dermatol* **15**:377, 1997

100. Gross G et al: Correlation between human papillomavirus (HPV) type and histology of warts. *J Invest Dermatol* **78**:160, 1982

101. Jablonska S et al: Cutaneous warts. Clinical, histologic, and virologic correlations. *Clin Dermatol* **3**:71, 1985

102. Rogel-Gaillard D et al: Human papillomavirus type 1 E4 proteins differing by their N-terminal ends have distinct cellular localizations when transiently expressed in vitro. *J Virol* **66**:816, 1992

103. Bernard C et al: Evaluation of Biohit HPV screening and typing kits in detection of human papillomavirus DNA from lesions of anogenital tract. *Diagn Mol Pathol* **3**:192, 1994

104. Lorincz AT: Molecular methods for the detection of human papillomavirus infection. *Obstet Gynecol Clin North Am* **23**:707, 1996

105. Messing AM, Epstein WL: Natural history of warts: A two year study. *Arch Dermatol* **87**:306, 1963

106. Beutner KR, Ferenczy A: Therapeutic approaches to genital warts. *Am J Med* **102**:28, 1997

107. Goette DK: Topical chemotherapy with 5-fluorouracil. *J Am Acad Dermatol* **6**:633, 1981

108. Carpiniello VL et al: Long-term follow-up of subclinical human papillomavirus infection treated with the carbon dioxide laser and intraurethral 5-fluorouracil: A treatment protocol. *J Urol* **143**:726, 1990

109. Sawchuk WS et al: Infectious papillomavirus in the vapor of warts treated with carbon dioxide laser or electrocoagulation: Detection and protection. *J Am Acad Dermatol* **21**:41, 1989

110. Marcus J, Camisa C: Podophyllin therapy for condyloma acuminatum. *Int J Dermatol* **29**:693, 1990

111. Bargman H: Podophyllin and pregnancy. *Int J Dermatol* **32**:691, 1993

112. Beutner KR et al: Patient-applied podofilox for treatment of genital warts. *Lancet* **1**:831, 1989

113. Baker DA et al: Topical podofilox for the treatment of condylomata acuminata in women. *Obstet Gynecol* **76**:656, 1990

114. Shumer SM, O'Keefe EJ: Bleomycin in the treatment of recalcitrant warts. *J Am Acad Dermatol* **9**:91, 1983

115. Hayes ME, O'Keefe EJ: Reduced dose of bleomycin in the treatment of recalcitrant warts. *J Am Acad Dermatol* **15**:1002, 1986

116. Coskey RJ: Treatment of plantar warts in children with a salicylic acid–podophyllin-cantharidin product. *Pediatr Dermatol* **2**:71, 1984

117. Lee S et al: Therapeutic effect of dinitrochlorobenzene (DNCB) on verruca plana and verruca vulgaris. *Int J Dermatol* **23**:624, 1984

118. Naylor MF et al: Contact immunotherapy of resistant warts. *J Am Acad Dermatol* **19**:679, 1988

119. Wilkerson MG et al: Dinitrochlorobenzene is inherently mutagenic in the presence of trace mutagenic contaminants. *Arch Dermatol* **124**:396, 1988

120. Orlow SJ, Paller A: Cimetidine therapy for multiple viral warts in children. *J Am Acad Dermatol* **28**:794, 1993

121. Karabulut AA et al: Is cimetidine effective for nongenital warts: A double-blind, placebo-controlled study. *Arch Dermatol* **133**:533, 1997

122. Yilmaz E et al: Cimetidine therapy for warts: A placebo-controlled, double-blind study. *Am Acad Dermatol* **34**:1005, 1996

123. Haglund S et al: Interferon therapy in juvenile laryngeal papillomatosis. *Arch Otolaryngol* **107**:327, 1981

124. Androphy EJ et al: Response of warts in epidermodysplasia verruciformis to treatment with systemic and intralesional alpha interferon. *J Am Acad Dermatol* **11**:197, 1984

125. Reichman RC et al: Treatment of condyloma acuminatum with three different interferon-α preparations administered parenterally: A double-blind, placebo-controlled trial. *J Infect Dis* **162**:1270, 1990

126. Baker GE, Tyring SK: Therapeutic approaches to papillomavirus infections. *Dermatol Clin* **15**:331, 1997

127. Gaspari AA et al: Successful treatment of a generalized human papillomavirus infection with granulocyte-macrophage colony-stimulating factor and interferon gamma immunotherapy in a patient with a primary immunodeficiency and cyclic neutropenia. *Arch Dermatol* **133**:491, 1997

128. Frazer IH: The role of vaccines in the control of STDs: HPV vaccines. *Genitourin Med* **72**:398, 1996

129. Suzich JA et al: Systemic immunization with papillomavirus L1 protein completely prevents the development of viral mucosal papillomas. *Proc Natl Acad Sci USA* **92**:11553, 1995

130. Bell JA et al: A formalin-inactivated vaccine protects against mucosal papillomavirus infection: A canine model. *Pathobiology* **62**:194, 1994

CHAPTER 225

Erwin Tschachler
M.S. Reitz, Jr.
Genoveffa Franchini

Human Retroviral Disease: Human T-Lymphotropic Viruses

Viruses have attracted attention as pathogens in malignant and autoimmune diseases in animals ever since the beginning of the twentieth century when Peyton Rous discovered that a virus could cause solid tumors in fowl.[1] The Rous sarcoma virus, named after its discoverer, turned out to contain an RNA genome but appeared to exist as a DNA provirus in infected cells.[1] This paradox was resolved when Baltimore and Temin and Mizutani[1] independently discovered a polymerase that was able to use RNA as a template to produce DNA, i.e., the reverse transcriptase (RT). Viruses that contain an RNA genome and an RNA-dependent DNA polymerase belong to the family Retroviridae (for an extensive review of taxonomy of retroviruses see ref. 1).

The first pathogenic human retrovirus was discovered in 1980. At that time, Poiesz and coworkers isolated a retrovirus from lymphocytes of a patient with cutaneous T cell lymphoma (CTCL)[2] and subsequently from a patient with leukemia classified as Sézary syndrome.[3] Independently of this work, Miyoshi and coworkers later isolated the same retrovirus from a Japanese leukemia patient.[4] The American and Japanese isolates were shown in the following years to be indistinguishable by nucleic acid comparison, and the name *human T cell leukemia virus* (HTLV) type I was proposed[5] for all isolates previously called *adult T cell leukemia virus* (ATLV) in Japan and HTLV in the United States.

In 1982, a second human retrovirus, related to but distinct from HTLV-I, was isolated from a cell line derived from a patient with hairy cell leukemia and was named HTLV-II.[6] Although isolated from a leukemic patient, a clear association to a distinct disease has not been shown for HTLV-II.

VIROLOGY

HTLV-I and -II are related but distinct human retroviruses that together with bovine leukemia virus form a separate genus within the Retroviridae.[1] Many strains of HTLV-I have been isolated from different areas of the world including the United States, the Caribbean islands, Africa, and Japan.[7] From sequencing data it appears that the overall nucleic acid sequence variation among different HTLV-I strains does not exceed 7 percent.[8-10] Although the genomic organization of HTLV-I and -II is quite similar, the nucleotide sequence conservation between these two viruses is only about 55 percent.[11] Like other enveloped retroviruses, the HTLV-I genome consists of a dimer of identical RNA subunits.[1] After infection of host cells, the RNA genome is transcribed into DNA by the viral RT and the viral DNA is integrated into the host cell genome (provirus). The organization of the HTLV-I provirus is depicted in Fig. 225-1; it contains dual long terminal repeats (LTRs) at the 3′ and 5′ ends and *gag, pol,* and *env* genes, which encode integral components of the virions. In addition to these genes, both the HTLV-I and -II genomes contain an extra sequence of about 1.6 kb between the *env* and the 3′ LTR, which was originally called *pX*.[12] While the full-length genomic RNA codes for gag and pol proteins and the env proteins are translated from singly spliced mRNAs, the pX region genes are expressed from RNAs produced mostly by double splicing mechanisms. The pX region codes for at least six proteins. The functions of two of these, i.e., the transregulatory proteins Tax (transactivator in the region x) and Rex (regulator in the region x), have been elucidated in the past few years. The 40-kDa HTLV-I Tax interacts with cellular transcription factors and transactivates the viral LTR, thereby increasing viral RNA synthesis.[13] The 27-kDa Rex protein promotes the export of the viral unspliced and singly spliced, i.e., genomic and enveloped, mRNAs to the cytoplasm where they can be translated. The function of the other proteins of the pX region, i.e., p21Rex, p12I, p13II, and p30II, still awaits elucidation. (For review of regulation of HTLV-I gene expression see ref. 13.)

In contrast to its name, which suggests a limited host cell range, HTLV-I can productively infect a wide variety of cells of different species in vitro.[14] Infection of human, monkey, and rabbit T lymphocytes by HTLV-I in vitro leads to their continuous growth in tissue culture and the development of cell lines with growth characteristics of transformed cells.[14] In infected patients, HTLV-I is mainly present in CD4+ T cells[15] but has also been found in blood dendritic cells[16] and cells from the synovial lining of arthritic joints.[17]

The steps leading from virus infection to the development of the different HTLV-I-associated diseases are still only partly understood. Only a small percentage of patients infected with HTLV-I will ultimately develop adult T cell leukemia/lymphoma (ATL), and the time from infection to leukemia usually lasts several decades.[18] Unlike acute or chronic leukemia viruses, the HTLV-I genome neither contains an oncogene nor does it transduce cellular oncogenes by insertion at critical sites within the host cell genome.[14,18] However, the HTLV-I regulatory gene *tax,* which is necessary for in vitro transformation,[19] is able to transactivate both the viral promoter and certain cellular genes.[13] This assumption is further supported by the fact that mice transgenic for the HTLV-I *tax* gene develop nerve sheath tumors in which the Tax protein is expressed.[20] Transformation of human T cells in vitro is a multistep event that involves selection of infected T cell clones. At first, T cells proliferate in response to exogenous interleukin (IL) (*immortalization*) and, in time, lose growth factor requirement for growth (*transformation*).[21] Tax, the viral transactivator, is necessary but not sufficient to induce T cell transformation in that it interferes with at least two inhibitors of cell cycle progression—the tumor suppressor proteins p16[ink] and p53.[22-24] In the transformed state, HTLV-I-infected T cells proliferate in the absence of exogenous growth factors, and this event correlates with both the constitutive activation of the JaK/STAT signaling pathway[25,26] and the constitutive acti-

FIGURE 225-1

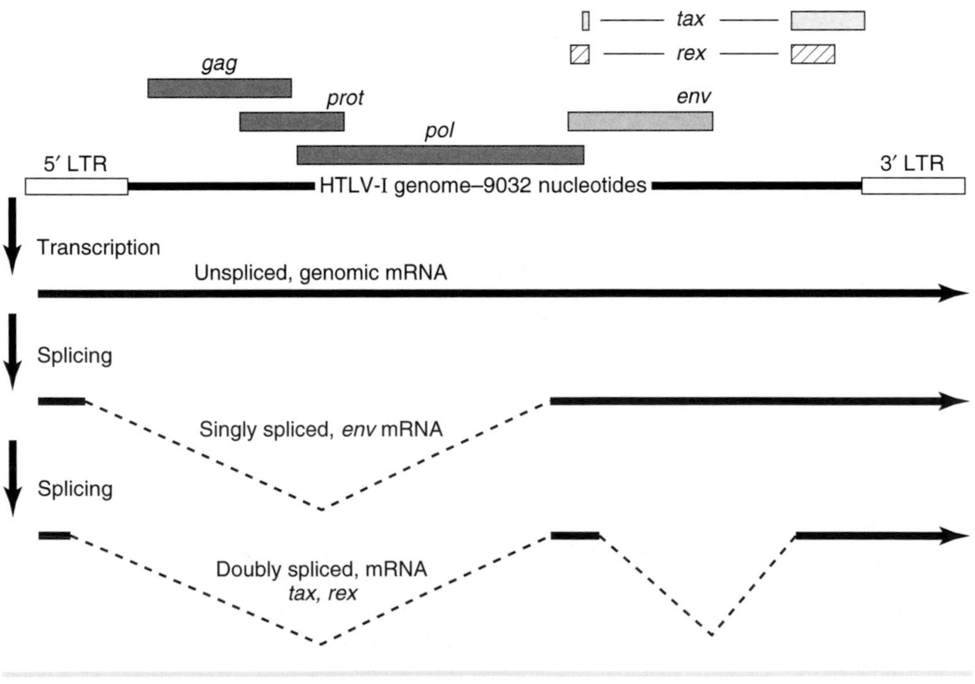

Genomic organization of the HTLV-I provirus and expression of viral structural and regulatory genes.

vation of the cyclin E/CDK2 complex. The in vitro model of T cell transformation appears to mirror the event that leads to leukemogenesis. In most cases of ATL, genetic mutation/deletion of p53 or p16[ink] occur,[27] and the leukemic cells of 70 percent of patients display constitutive activation of the Jak3 and STAT proteins.[28]

Although HTLV-II has been less well studied than HTLV-I, most of the properties described for the latter, including the transformation of T cells in vitro and the presence and importance of transregulatory genes, are true also for the former.[18] To date, however, no disease has been associated with HTLV-II infection.

HTLV-I TRANSMISSION AND EPIDEMIOLOGY

The mode of transmission of HTLV-I appears to be analogous to that of HIV-1. However, HTLV-I, which is mainly infectious by cell-to-cell contact, is less infectious than HIV-1, which can readily be transmitted cell-free. From longitudinal studies it has become well established that sexual transmission of HTLV-I occurs from male-to-female, female-to-male, and male-to-male.[29–32] Although the paths of vertical transmission of HTLV-I are not completely clarified, transmission from mother to child via breast feeding appears to play a more important role than perinatal or intrauterine transmission.[33,34] Programs to eradicate HTLV-I from the endemic areas in Japan by changing the habits of breast feeding are under way.[56]

In parenteral transmission, approximately one-half of patients who receive transfusions from an HTLV-I-infected donor seroconvert,[35,36] whereas cell-free fresh-frozen plasma appears not to be infectious.[36] Transfusion-mediated HTLV-I infection in Japan has been virtually terminated by mass screening of donated blood. In the United States, a screening program for blood units was initiated in 1989. Parenteral transmission via needle sharing very likely accounts for clusters of HTLV-I/II seropositivity in intravenous drug users in certain areas of the United States and Europe.[37–39] There is no indication that arthropod-borne transmission of HTLV-I occurs.

The geographic distribution of HTLV-I and -II has been studied mainly by serologic methods, which cannot distinguish between the two viruses; therefore, seroprevalence data usually refer to both HTLV-I and HTLV-II.[7,18] More recently, molecular methods, which allow the reliable distinction between HTLV-I and -II infection, have led to extensive molecular typing of the viruses.[7,40]

An estimated 10 to 20 million individuals are infected with HTLV-I worldwide.[7] Extensive seroepidemiologic and molecular surveys confirmed an endemic pattern in Southern Japan. In Kyushu, Shikoku, and the Ryuku islands, including Okinawa, seroprevalence ranges from 1 percent up to 36 percent, depending on the location and the age group investigated.[30,41,42] Similar patterns can be found in the Caribbean islands, particularly Jamaica, Trinidad, Tobago, Martinique, Haiti, Guadeloupe, and Barbados,[18,29,30] and in countries of equatorial Africa such as Gabon, Zaire, and the Ivory Coast.[43–46] Small clusters of HTLV-I/II–seropositive populations have been reported from restricted areas in South America,[47,49] among Australian aborigines,[50] and in the Middle East.[51] In the United States, Europe, and Canada, the incidence of HTLV-I infection is low and clusters are found predominantly among immigrants from endemic areas, especially from the West Indies and Africa.[18,52,53] A recent seroepidemiologic survey among 39,898 U.S. blood donors in eight geographically diverse areas showed a

seroprevalence for HTLV-I/II of 0.025 percent.[54] In the United Kingdom, HTLV-I infection among blood donors is similarly low, with a seroprevalence of around 0.05 percent.[55]

THE NATURAL COURSE OF HTLV-I INFECTION AND CLINICAL DISEASE SPECTRUM

Adult T Cell Leukemia/Lymphoma

ATL was first described by Uchiyama and coworkers in 1977 as a distinct malignancy of mature T cells occurring primarily in patients born in southwestern Japan.[56] At the beginning of the 1980s, HTLV-I was linked to ATL by virus isolation from leukemic cells,[4] by the demonstration of oligoclonal or monoclonal integrated HTLV-I provirus in leukemic cells, and by extensive seroepidemiologic studies.[14,18] In 1982, Catovsky and coworkers[57] described ATL in West Indian immigrants in London, which encouraged Blattner and colleagues[58] to investigate the West Indies as a major region where HTLV-I infection and ATL might be endemic.

Although HTLV-I is a prerequisite for ATL development, infection with this virus does not necessarily lead to development of leukemia. More than 90 percent of infected individuals remain asymptomatic carriers.[59] From Japanese epidemiologic studies it appears that the annual incidence rate of ATL among HTLV-I carriers older than 40 years is approximately 0.6 to 1.7 per 1000.[60] The cumulative incidence rate of ATL in HTLV-I carriers is approximately 2 to 5 percent. The latent period from infection to outbreak of leukemia is 20 years or more, as concluded from migrant studies,[61] but the average age of onset of ATL[62] differs in patients from Japan (56 years) and those from the Caribbean (43 years).

Acute, prototypic ATL is a fatal malignancy of adult onset with a clinical presentation that appears to be identical in all endemic areas.[56,57,63–65] It is characterized by the variable combination of multiorgan involvement, including hepatosplenomegaly, systemic lymphadenopathy, central nervous system (CNS) involvement, and skin lesions, with the presence of multilobate leukemic cells in the peripheral blood (Fig. 225-2A). Leukemic infiltrates of different organs may determine the clinical presentation and the morbidity. CNS involvement may alter the mental status of the patient; lymphoma within the liver may lead to abnormalities in liver function tests and jaundice; and lung involvement may lead to tachypnea, cyanosis, and dyspnea.[64–67]

A striking feature in a high percentage of patients with acute ATL is a refractory hypercalcemia that may represent the first sign of the disease and indicates an aggressive course.[63,64,67] Patients may present with weakness, lethargy, polyuria, and polydypsia. Lytic bone lesions resembling those of multiple myeloma are often present at diagnosis, and levels of alkaline phosphatase may be elevated.[57,63–65,67,68] Parathyroid hormone levels and 1,25-dihydroxyvitamin D levels are normal in ATL patients with hypercalcemia, and it had been postulated that factors produced by leukemic cells were involved in osteoclast activation, which led to the clinical symptoms.[69] A variety of cytokines produced by HTLV-I-infected cells or cells derived from ATL patients have been suggested to account for hypercalcemia and bone resorption in ATL patients. Recently, several reports established a link between hypercalcemia

FIGURE 225-2

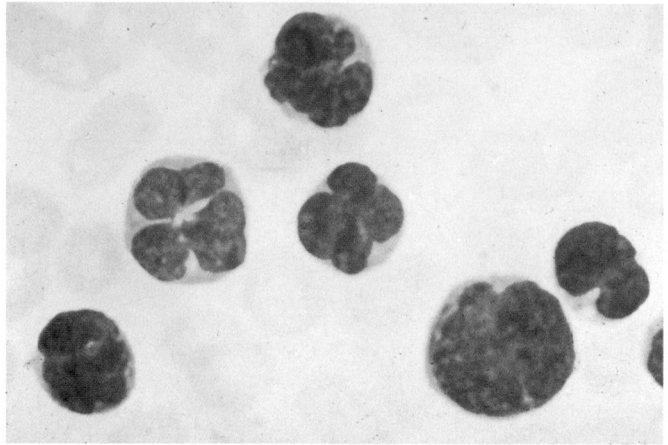

A.

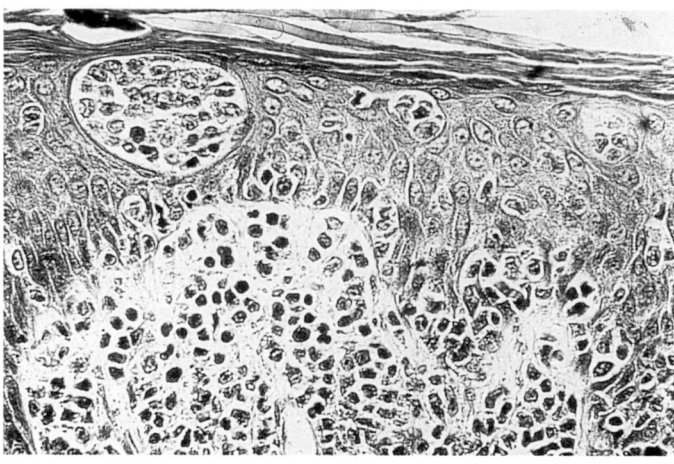

B.

A. Abnormal lymphocyte with multilobate nucleus ("flower cell") from a patient with ATL. (*Courtesy of K. Takatsuki, MD, Kumamoto University, Japan.*) B. ATL tumor cells are infiltrating the epidermis. (*Courtesy of B. Hanchard, MD, University of the West Indies, Kingston, Jamaica.*)

in ATL and augmented serum levels of tumor necrosis factor alpha[70] and beta[71] and parathyroid hormone–like peptide.[72]

Based on the clinical course and laboratory parameters, ATL is classified into four subtypes—smoldering, chronic, lymphoma type, and acute or prototypic—for which diagnostic criteria have been formulated (Table 225-1).[63]

In a large series of 818 patients, 57 percent were classified as acute, 19 percent as lymphoma type, 19 percent as chronic, and 5 percent as smoldering ATL.[63] Smoldering and chronic ATL may convert into acute ATL, which has led some authors to speak of "crisis-type ATL."[64]

The skin involvement in ATL varies considerably among patients but is present to a variable degree in all forms of ATL.[65,67,73–75] Skin lesions may appear as uncharacteristic erythematous patches, as papular and nodular tumors, (Fig. 225-3) and as erythroderma. Nonspecific skin lesions may precede the onset of acute ATL by up to two decades.[76] Specific skin infiltrates may occur as first manifestations of ATL,[76] and these show monoclo-

TABLE 225-1

Distinguishing Features of ATL Subtypes

Smoldering ATL
5% or more abnormal lymphocytes of T cell nature in peripheral blood (PB); normal lymphocyte level ($<4 \times 10^9$/L); no hypercalcemia; LDH value of up to $1.5 \times$ the normal upper limit; no lymphadenopathy; no involvement of liver, spleen, CNS, bone, and gastrointestinal tract; no ascites or pleural effusion. Skin and pulmonary lesion(s) may be present. In cases where there are less than 5% abnormal T lymphocytes in PB, at least one histologically proven skin lesion and/or pulmonary lesions should be present.

Chronic ATL
Absolute lymphocytosis ($\geq 4 \times 10^9$/L) with T lymphocytosis $>3.5 \times 10^9$/L; LDH value up to twice the normal upper limit; no hypercalcemia; no involvement of CNS, bone, and gastrointestinal tract; no ascites or pleural effusion. Lymphadenopathy and involvement of liver, spleen, skin, and lung may be present, and 5% or more abnormal T lymphocytes are seen in PB in most cases.

Lymphoma Type ATL
No lymphocytosis; ≤ 1% abnormal T lymphocytes; and histologically proven lymphadenopathy with or without extranodal lesions.

Acute ATL
Remaining ATL patients who usually have leukemic manifestations and tumour lesions but are not classified as any of the three other types.

nality of skin-infiltrating cells by the criteria both of T cell–receptor rearrangement and integration of HTLV-I DNA. This occurs at a time when circulating T cells of these patients still appear unaffected.[74] For this latter situation the term *cutaneous-type ATL* has been proposed.[77] However, it is questionable whether this form represents an independent course of ATL or whether it should be included with the smoldering form. Alternatively, it may reflect very early diagnosis of prototypic or chronic ATL due to improved diagnostic measures.

DIAGNOSIS AND DIFFERENTIAL DIAGNOSIS OF ATL
Besides the characteristic clinical course of prototypic ATL, examination of the leukemic cells yields a characteristic picture: numerous multilobate cells, called *ATL cells* or *flower cells* (Fig. 225-2A), are present in peripheral blood and can usually be readily distinguished from cells of other T cell leukemias by light microscopy, although sometimes occasional cells indistinguishable from Sézary cells may be present.[63,64,69] In smoldering and chronic ATL, multilobate cells are less frequent, and in lymphoma-type ATL they may comprise fewer than 1 percent of lymphocytes (Table 225-1). Monoclonal or oligoclonal integration of HTLV-I DNA[36,82,83] has been demonstrated in leukemic cells as well as in affected organs. By immunophenotyping, leukemic cells display predominantly a mature CD2+/CD3+/CD4+/CD8−/CD25+ phenotype.[79–82] While most of these T cell markers can be found on other T cell malignancies, the strong expression of the IL-2 receptor α chain (CD25) can be regarded as a distinguishing marker between ATL and Sézary syndrome.[82]

The histopathologic features seen in affected organs and lymph nodes are more variable than the picture encountered in peripheral blood, and ATL is associated with lymphomas of several histologic subtypes. Distinction of ATL from other peripheral T cell lymphomas, especially HTLV-I-positive and -negative cases, cannot be accomplished on morphologic grounds. No specific pathologic finding distinguishes ATL from other forms of non-Hodgkin's lymphoma. Difficulties can also be encountered in differentiating skin involvement of ATL from mycosis fungoides (MF)/Sézary syndrome, since

FIGURE 225-3

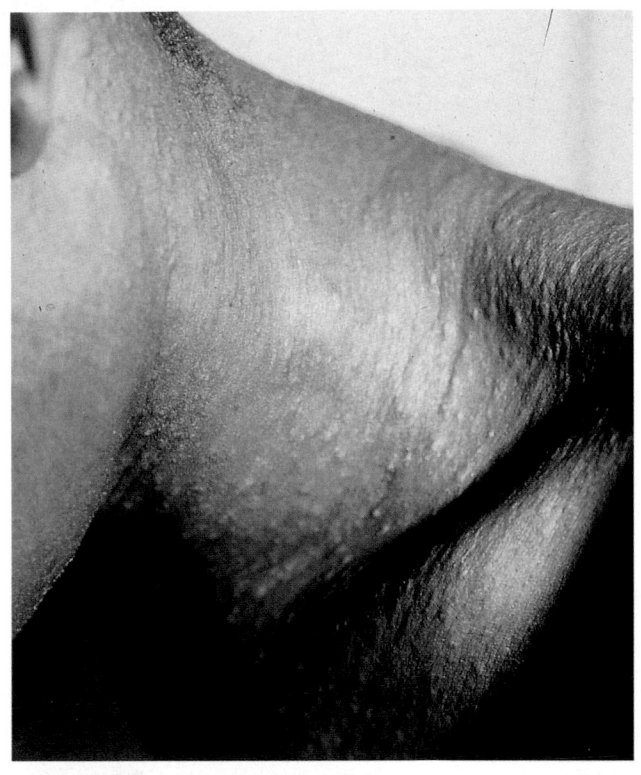

A.

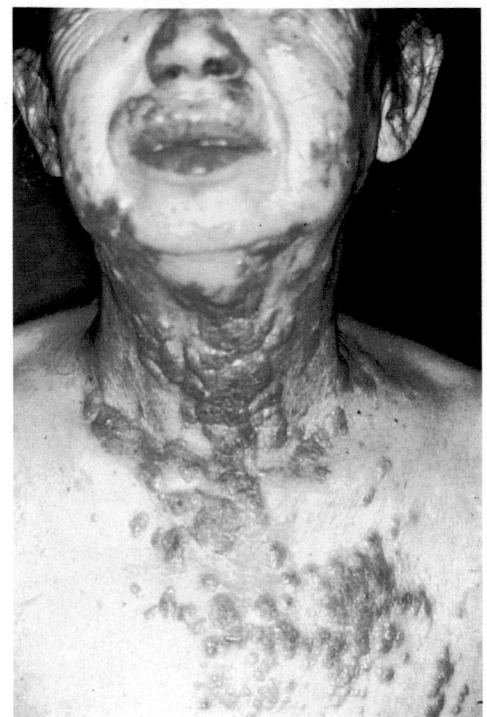

B.

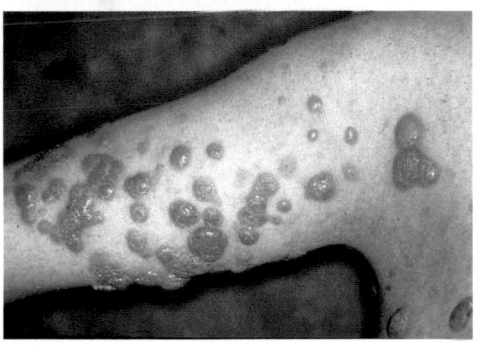

C.

Skin manifestations of ATL. *A.* Generalized papular infiltrates in a patient from Jamaica with prototype ATL. *B, C.* Nodular skin tumors in Japanese ATL patients. (*Courtesy of K. Takatsuki, MD, Kumamoto University, Japan.*)

focal epidermal infiltration by T cells or Pautrier's microabscesses (Fig. 225-2*B*) can be present in skin lesions of ATL.[75,83,84] Indeed, the diseases of patients from whom the original U.S. HTLV-I isolates were obtained were classified as Sézary syndrome[9] and CTLC,[8] respectively. To establish the diagnosis of HTLV-I-associated ATL unequivocally, four diagnostic criteria have been proposed[63,64]: (1) a histologically or cytologically proven lymphoid malignancy with T cell surface antigens; (2) abnormal T lymphocytes in peripheral blood, except in the lymphoma type; (3) anti-HTLV-I serum antibodies; and (4) the demonstration of clonality of HTLV-I proviral DNA.

PROGNOSIS AND THERAPY OF ATL The prognosis of ATL is largely dependent on the subtype. In the most extensive study on the course of ATL to date, 818 newly diagnosed Japanese patients were studied for a median follow-up time of 13.3 months.[62] Median survival time was 6.2 months for acute ATL, 10.2 months for lymphoma-type ATL, 24.3 months for chronic ATL, and not reached at the end of the study for smoldering ATL. Projected 2- and 4-year survival rates were 16.7 and 5.0 percent for acute, 21.3 and 5.7 percent for lymphoma-type, 52.4 and 26.9 percent for chronic, and 77.7 and 62.8 percent for smoldering ATL, respectively. The presence of hypercalcemia, high LDH levels, and an excessively high white blood cell count are bad prognostic factors.[62,85] Controlled, randomized studies comparing different therapeutic protocols have not been performed for ATL. Combination cytotoxic therapy (CHOP, COMLA, VEPA, CAP) has been reported by several groups[56,57,67]; however, long-term remission cannot be obtained with any of these chemotherapeutic approaches and the effects on survival are marginal. Complications of chemotherapy include septicemia and opportunistic infections.[67] Experimental approaches to ATL therapy include an inhibitor of topoisomerase I[86] and antibodies against the CD25 molecule.[87] Recently, the combination of interferon-α and zidovudine, a nucleoside analogue used in anti-HIV-1 therapy, has been reported to be effective in the treatment of ATL.[88,89] In addition, combination chemotherapy together with either hemopoietic growth factors[90] or bone marrow transplantation[91] may represent therapeutic options for the future.

The course of smoldering and chronic ATL is less dramatic, and involvement of inner organs and hypercalcemia are observed less frequently.[67,73] Since patients suffering from smoldering or chronic ATL have a better prognosis[63,67,73] than those with acute ATL, they should not be treated by chemotherapy unless they enter a more aggressive phase of their disease.

The Role of HTLV-I-Related Retroviruses in Cutaneous T Cell Lymphoma

The first HTLV-I isolates were obtained from patients diagnosed as having MF and Sézary syndrome.[2,3] This together with earlier reports about the presence of retroviral particles in skin and lymph nodes of patients with these diseases[92–94] has incited an intensive search for HTLV-I in CTCL. In the past few years it has become clear that subtypes of ATL, i.e., the smoldering and the chronic forms, can mimic CTCL clinically and histologically. In these cases the distinguishing features are the HTLV-I seropositivity and the long-term clinical course. Serologic surveys for HTLV-I in CTCL patients from the United States and Europe revealed HTLV-I seropositivity rates of less than 1 percent[95] and up to 12 percent.[96] Recently, several reports claimed that HTLV-I DNA sequences are detectable by polymerase chain reaction (PCR) in tumor tissue and in cell lines derived from MF patients[97–101] and in peripheral blood mononuclear cells from relatives of patients with MF.[102] In addition, antibodies against the Tax protein were found in an unexpectedly high percentage of intravenous drug addicts who were negative for HTLV-I in conventional serologic tests.[101] In contrast to these findings, other investigators studying patients from the same geographic regions with comparable methods were unable to detect HTLV-I DNA in CTCL samples.[103–109] There are several possible explanations for these contradictory results: (1) technical problems such as contamination of PCR reactions or the presence of inhibitors, (2) differences in the selection of patients, and (3) the involvement of a retrovirus related to but different from HTLV-I. To resolve the controversy about the involvement of a retrovirus, be it HTLV-I or another, isolation and characterization of the agent are warranted.

Neurologic Disease

HTLV-I has been associated with chronic progressive myelopathies, i.e., tropical spastic paraparesis (TSP) in the Caribbean and HTLV-I-associated myelopathy (HAM) in Japan.[110] Since these two conditions appear to be identical, the terms *TSP* and *HAM* are now used synonymously. Patients suffering from TSP/HAM are generally younger than ATL patients, and the latency from infection to development of clinical neurologic symptoms has been described to be very short in individual cases. The lifetime risk to develop TSP/HAM has been estimated at 1 percent.[111] In contrast to ATL, which is associated with HTLV-I infection very early in life, TSP/HAM patients frequently become infected only in adolescence. In particular the acquisition of HTLV-I by blood transfusion has been reported to play an important role for TSP/HAM development.[110]

Concomitant Infectious Diseases

Infective dermatitis (Fig. 225-4) is a severe chronic relapsing eczema in Jamaican children, associated with infection by *Staphylococcus aureus* and beta-hemolytic *Streptococcus*. The association of

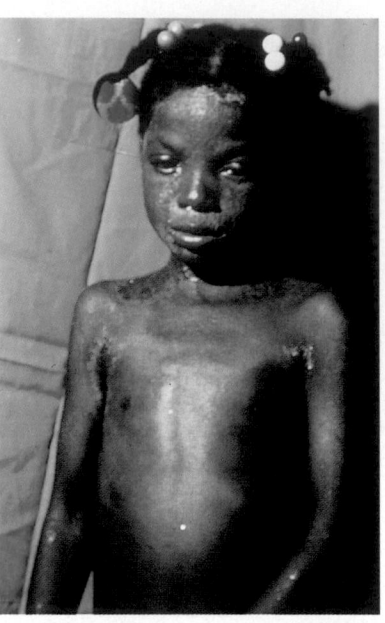

Infective dermatitis in an HTLV-I-infected Jamaican girl. (*Courtesy of L. LaGrenade, MD, University of the West Indies, Kingston, Jamaica.*)

infective dermatitis with HTLV-I infection has recently been reported.[112] Bacterial infection in infective dermatitis is difficult to control, and although it responds to antibiotic treatment, prolonged therapy is necessary and relapses are common after discontinuation.[112] The characteristic clinical picture, the recalcitrant course, and HTLV-I seropositivity set infective dermatitis apart from other forms of recurrent eczema, including atopic eczema. Immunosuppression observed by other investigators in HTLV-I carriers as well as in ATL patients[69,113–115] may play a role in the pathogenesis of infective dermatitis. Whereas HTLV-I-infected individuals have been found to be overrepresented among patients hospitalized for infectious diseases in Japan, infective dermatitis has been reported only rarely from regions outside the Caribbean.[116] Regional, cultural, or genetic factors may play an additive role in the occurrence of infective dermatitis. Future longitudinal epidemiologic and molecular studies should help to elucidate the contribution of disturbances of the immune system to the clinical picture observed in infective dermatitis. Such studies should also help to answer the question raised by LaGrenade and coworkers as to whether infective dermatitis represents a "preleukemic syndrome" that ultimately leads to the development of ATL. Long-lasting (21 years) cutaneous prodromes have been described in a patient who finally developed ATL.[117] Further evidence for infective dermatitis in childhood being associated with subsequent development of ATL comes from a report of a patient who developed ATL 17 years after having been diagnosed in Jamaica as having infective dermatitis.[118]

Other Disorders

Besides the above diseases, a certain type of uveitis,[119] polymyositis,[120] chronic inflammatory arthropathy,[121] and peripheral neuropathy[122] have been associated with HTLV-I infection. However, future epidemiologic and virologic studies will be necessary to establish the causative role of the virus in the pathogenesis of these diseases.

1. Coffin JM: Retroviridae: The viruses and their replication, in *Fields Virology,* edited by B Fields et al. Philadelphia, Lippincott-Raven, 1996, pp 1767–1847
2. Poiesz BJ et al: Detection and isolation of type C retrovirus particles from fresh and cultured lymphocytes of a patient with cutaneous T-cell lymphoma. *Proc Natl Sci* **77**:7415, 1980
3. Poiesz BJ et al: Isolation of a new type C retrovirus (HTLV) in primary uncultured cells of a patient with Sézary T-cell leukemia. *Nature* **294**:268, 1981
4. Miyoshi I et al: Type C virus particles in a cord blood T-cell line derived from cocultivating normal human cord leukocytes and human leukaemic T cells. *Nature* **294**:770, 1981
5. Watanabe T et al: Retrovirus terminology. *Science* **222**:1178, 1983
6. Kalyanaraman VS et al: A new subtype of human T-cell leukemia virus (HTLV-II) associated with a T-cell variant of hairy cell leukemia. *Science* **218**:571, 1982
7. Gessain A: Epidemiology of HTLV-I and associated diseases, in *Human T-Cell Lymphotropic Virus Type I,* edited by P Höllersberg, DA Hafler. Chichester, Wiley, 1996, pp 33–64
8. Ratner L: Molecular variation of human T-lymphotropic viruses and clinical associations, in *Retrovirology: HTLV,* edited by WA Blattner. New York, Raven, 1990, pp 49–64
9. Malik KTA et al: Molecular cloning and complete nucleotide sequence of an adult T cell leukemia virus/human T cell leukemia virus type I (ATLV/HTLV-I) isolate of a Caribbean origin: Relationship to other members of the ATLV/HTLV-I subgroup. *J Gen Virol* **69**:1695, 1988
10. Gessain A et al: Low degree of human T-cell leukemia/lymphoma virus type I genetic drift in vivo as a means of monitoring viral transmission and movement of ancient human populations. *J Virol* **66**:2288, 1992
11. Shimotohno K et al: Complete nucleotide sequence of an infectious clone of human T-cell leukemia virus type II: An open reading frame for the protease gene. *Proc Natl Acad Sci* **82**:3101, 1985
12. Seiki M et al: Human adult T-cell leukemia virus: Molecular cloning of the provirus DNA and the unique terminal structure. *Proc Natl Acad Sci* **79**:6899, 1982
13. Brady JN: Biology of HTLV-I: Host cell interactions and associated diseases, in *Human T-Cell Lymphotropic Virus Type I,* edited by P Höllersberg, DA Hafler. Chichester, Wiley, 1996, pp 79–112
14. Weiss R: Human T-cell retroviruses, in *RNA and Tumor Viruses,* edited by R Weiss et al. Cold Spring Harbor, NY, Cold Spring Harbor Laboratory, 1984, pp 405–485
15. Richardson JH et al: In vivo cellular tropism of human T-cell leukemia virus type 1. *J Virol* **64**:5682, 1990
16. Macatonia SE et al: Dendritic cells from patients with tropical spastic paraparesis are infected with HTLV-I and stimulate autologous lymphocyte proliferation. *AIDS Res Hum Retroviruses* **8**:1699, 1992
17. Kitajima I et al: Detection of human T cell lymphotropic virus type I proviral DNA and its gene expression in synovial cells in chronic inflammatory arthropathy. *J Clin Invest* **88**:1315, 1991
18. Cann AJ, Chen ISY: Human T-cell leukemia virus types I and II, in *Fields Virology,* edited by B Fields et al. Philadelphia, Lippincott-Raven, 1996, pp 1849–1880
19. Grassmann R et al: Role of human T-cell leukemia virus type 1 X region proteins in immortalization of primary human lymphocytes in culture. *J Virol* **66**:4570, 1992
20. Hinrichs SH et al: A transgenic mouse model for human neurofibromatosis. *Science* **237**:1340, 1987
21. Markham PD et al: Infection and transformation of fresh human umbilical cord blood cells by multiple sources of human T-cell leukemia-lymphoma virus (HTLV). *Int J Cancer* **31**:413, 1983
22. Suzuki T et al: HTLV-I Tax protein interacts with cyclin-dependent kinase inhibitor p16^{ink4A} and counteracts its inhibitory activity towards CDK4. *EMBO J* **15**:1607, 1996
23. Low KG et al: Human T-cell leukemia virus type I Tax releases cell cycle arrest induced by p16^{ink4A}. *J Virol* **71**:1956, 1997
24. Pise-Masison CA et al: Inhibition of p53 transactivation function by the HTLV-I Tax protein. *J Virol* **72**:1165, 1998
25. Migone T et al: Constitutively activated Jak-STAT pathway in T cells transformed with HTLV-I. *Science* **269**:79, 1995
26. Xu X et al: Constitutive activation of different Jak tyrosine kinases in human T cell leukemia virus type I (HTLV-I) Tax protein or virus transformed cells. *J Clin Invest* **96**:1548, 1995
27. Franchini G: Molecular mechanisms of human T-cell leukemia/lymphotropic virus type I infection. *Blood* **86**:3619, 1995
28. Takemoto S et al: Proliferation of adult T-cell leukemia/lymphoma cells is associated with the constitutive activation of JAK/STAT proteins. *Proc Natl Acad Sci USA* **94**:13, 897, 1997
29. Tajima K et al: Epidemiological features of HTLV-I carriers and incidence of ATL in an ATL-endemic island: A report of the community-based co-operative study in Tsushima, Japan. *Int J Cancer* **40**:741, 1987
30. Blattner WA: Retroviruses, in *Viral Infections of Humans: Epidemiology and Control,* edited by AS Evans. New York, Plenum, 1989, pp 545–592
31. Brodine SK et al: HTLV-I among U.S. Marines stationed in a hyperendemic area: Evidence for female-to-male sexual transmission. *J Acquir Immune Defic Syndr* **5**:158, 1992
32. Nakashima K et al: Sexual transmission of human T-lymphotropic virus type I among female prostitutes and among patients with sexually transmitted diseases in Fukuoka, Kyushu, Japan. *Am J Epidemiol* **141**:305, 1995
33. Hirata M et al: The effects of breastfeeding and presence of antibody to p40tax protein of human T cell lymphotropic virus type I on mother to child transmission. *Int J Epidemiol* **21**:989, 1992
34. Katamine S et al: HTLV-I proviral DNA in umbilical cord blood of babies born to carrier mothers. *Lancet* **343**:1326, 1994
35. Hino S et al: Transfusion-mediated spread of the human T-cell leukemia virus in chronic hemodialysis patients in a heavily endemic area, Nagasaki. *Gann* **75**:1070, 1984
36. Okochi K et al: A retrospective study on transmission of adult T cell leukemia virus by blood transfusion: Seroconversion in recipients. *Vox Sang* **46**:245, 1985
37. Robert Guroff M et al: Prevalence of antibodies to HTLV-I, -II and -III in intravenous drug abusers from an AIDS endemic region. *J Am Med Assoc* **255**:3133, 1986
38. Lee H et al: High rate of HTLV-II infection in seropositive IV drug abusers in New Orleans. *Science* **244**:471, 1989
39. Schwebke J et al: Prevalence and epidemiologic correlates of human T cell lymphotropic virus infection among intravenous drug users. *J Infect Dis* **169**:962, 1994
40. Kwok S et al: Enzymatic amplification of HTLV-I viral sequences from peripheral blood mononuclear cells and infected tissues. *Blood* **72**:1117, 1988
41. Maeda Y et al: Prevalence of possible adult T-cell leukemia virus carriers among volunteer blood donors in Japan: A nation-wide study. *Int J Cancer* **33**:717, 1984
42. Kajiyama W et al: Seroepidemiologic study of antibody to adult T-cell leukemia virus in Okinawa, Japan. *Am J Epidemiol* **123**:41, 1986
43. Saxinger WC et al: Human T-cell leukemia virus (HTLV-I) antibodies in Africa. *Science* **225**:1473, 1984
44. de Thè G et al: Human retroviruses HTLV-I, HIV-1 and HIV-2 and neurological diseases in some equatorial areas of Africa. *J AIDS* **2**:550, 1989
45. Delaporte E et al: Prevalence of HTLV-I and HTLV-II infection in Gabon, Africa: Comparison of the serological and the PCR results. *Int J Cancer* **49**:373, 1992
46. Garin B et al: HTLV-I/II infection in a high viral endemic area of Zaire, Central Africa: Comparative evaluation of serology, PCR and significance of indeterminate Western blot. *J Med Virol* **44**:104, 1994
47. Trujillo JM et al: Seroprevalence and cofactors of HTLV-I infection in Tumaco, Colombia. *AIDS Res Hum Retroviruses* **8**:651, 1992
48. Tuppin P et al: Risk factors for maternal HTLV-I infection in French Guiana: High HTLV-I prevalence in the Noir Marron population. *J Acquir Immune Defic Syndr Hum Retrovirol* **8**:420, 1995
49. Cortes E et al: HIV-1, HIV-2 and HTLV-I in high-risk groups in Brazil. *N Engl J Med* **320**:953, 1989
50. Bastian I et al: Isolation of a human T-lymphotropic virus type I strain from Australian aboriginals. *J Virol* **67**:843, 1993
51. Meytes D et al: Serological and molecular survey for HTLV-I infection in a high-risk Middle Eastern group. *Lancet* **336**:1533, 1990
52. Blayney DW et al: The human T-cell leukemia-lymphoma virus in the southeastern United States. *J Am Med Assoc* **250**:1048, 1983
53. The HTLV European Research Network: Seroepidemiology of the human T-cell leukemia/lymphoma viruses in Europe. *J Acquir Immune Defic Syndr Hum Retrovirol* **13**:68, 1996
54. Williams AE et al: Seroprevalence and epidemiological correlates of HTLV-I infection in U.S. blood donors. *Science* **240**:643, 1988

55. Brennan M et al: Prevalence of antibodies to human T cell leukaemia/lymphoma virus in blood donors in north London. *BMJ* **307**:1235, 1993

56. Uchiyama T et al: Adult T-cell leukemia in Japan: Clinical and hematologic features of 16 cases. *Blood* **50**:481, 1977

57. Catovsky D et al: Adult T-cell lymphoma-leukemia in Blacks from the West Indies. *Lancet* **1**:639, 1982

58. Blattner WA et al: The human type-C retrovirus, HTLV in Blacks from the Caribbean region, and relationship to adult T-cell leukemia/lymphoma. *Int J Cancer* **30**:257, 1982

59. de Thè G, Bomford R: An HTLV-I vaccine: Why, how, for whom? *AIDS Res Hum Retroviruses* **9**:381, 1993

60. Kondo T et al: Risk of adult T-cell leukemia/lymphoma in HTLV-I carriers. *Lancet* **2**:159, 1987

61. Greaves MF et al: Human T-cell leukemia virus (HTLV) in the United Kingdom. *Int J Cancer* **33**:795, 1984

62. Yamaguchi K et al: Pathogenesis of adult T-cell leukemia from clinical pathologic features, in *Human Retrovirology: HTLV,* edited by WA Blattner. New York, Raven, 1990, pp 163–171

63. Shimoyama M: Diagnostic criteria and classification of clinical subtypes of adult T-cell leukaemia-lymphoma. A report from the Lymphoma Study Group (1984–87). *Br J Haematol* **79**:428, 1991

64. Takatsuki K et al: Adult T-cell leukemia, in *Human T-Cell Lymphotropic Virus Type I,* edited by P Höllersberg, DA Hafler. Chichester, Wiley, 1996, pp 219–246

65. Hanchard B: Adult T-cell leukemia/lymphoma in Jamaica: 1986–1995. *J Acquir Immune Defic Syndr Hum Retrovirol* **13**:S20, 1996

66. Yoshioka R et al: Pulmonary complications in patients with adult T cell leukemia. *Cancer* **55**:2491, 1985

67. Kawano F et al: Variation in the clinical course of adult T-cell leukemia. *Cancer* **55**:851, 1985

68. Blayney DW et al: The human T-cell leukemia/lymphoma virus, lymphoma, lytic bone lesions and hypercalcemia. *Ann Intern Med* **98**:144, 1982

69. Broder S et al: T-cell lymphoproliferative syndrome associated with human T-cell leukemia/lymphoma virus. *Ann Intern Med* **100**:543, 1984

70. Matsuda K et al: Hypercalcemia and serum TNF in T-cell leukemia. *Lancet* **1**:1032, 1990

71. Ishibashi K et al: Tumor necrosis factor-β in the serum of adult T-cell leukemia with hypercalcemia. *Blood* **77**:2451, 1991

72. Yamaguchi K et al: Increased serum levels of C-terminal parathyroid hormone-related protein in different diseases associated with HTLV-I infection. *Leukemia* **8**:1708, 1994

73. Yamaguchi K et al: A proposal for smoldering adult T-cell leukemia (smoldering ATL): A clinicopathologic study of 5 cases. *Blood* **62**:758, 1983

74. Dosaka N et al: Examination of HTLV-I integration in the skin lesions of various types of adult T-cell leukemia (ATL): Independence of cutaneous-type ATL confirmed by Southern blot analysis. *J Invest Dermatol* **96**:196, 1991

75. DiCaudo DJ et al: Clinical and histologic spectrum of human T-cell lymphotropic virus type I-associated lymphoma involving the skin. *J Am Acad Dermatol* **34**:69, 1996

76. Bunker CB et al: Indolent cutaneous prodrome of fatal HTLV-I infection. *Lancet* **1**:426, 1990

77. Jono M et al: ATL (adult T-cell leukemia/lymphoma) and skin eruptions. *Hihubyou-shinryou* (in Japanese) **9**:206, 1987

78. Takatsuki K et al: Adult T cell leukemia: Proposal as a new disease and cytogenetic, phenotypic and functional studies of leukemic cells. *Gann* **28**:13, 1982

79. Hattori T et al: Surface phenotype of Japanese adult T-cell leukemia cells characterized by monoclonal antibodies. *Blood* **58**:645, 1981

80. Uchyama T et al: A monoclonal antibody (anti-Tac) reactive with activated and functionally mature human T cells II. Expression of Tac antigen on activated cytotoxic killer cell, suppressor cells, and on one or two types of helper T cells. *J Immunol* **126**:1398, 1981

81. Yamada Y: Phenotypic and functional analysis of leukemic cells from 16 patients with adult T-cell leukemia/lymphoma. *Blood* **61**:192, 1983

82. Waldmann TA et al: Functional and phenotypic comparison of human T cell leukemia/lymphoma virus positive adult T cell leukemia with human T cell leukemia/lymphoma virus negative Sézary leukemia, and their distinction using anti-Tac. *J Clin Invest* **73**:1711, 1984

83. Chan HL et al: Cutaneous manifestations of adult T cell leukemia/lymphoma. *J Am Acad Dermatol* **13**:213, 1985

84. Maeda K, Takahashi M: Characterization of skin infiltrating cells in adult T-cell leukaemia/lymphoma (ATLL) clinical, histological and immunohistochemical studies on eight cases. *Br J Dermatol* **121**:603, 1989

85. Shimoyama M et al: Major prognostic factors of adult patients with advanced T-cell lymphoma/leukemia. *J Clin Oncol* **68**:169, 1988

86. Tsuda H et al: Treatment of adult T-cell leukaemia-lymphoma with irinotecan hydrochloride (CPT-11). CPT-11 Study Group on Hematological Malignancy. *Br J Cancer* **70**:771, 1994

87. Waldmann TA: The promiscuous IL-2/IL-15 receptor: a target for immunotherapy of HTLV-I-associated disorders. *J Acquir Immune Defic Syndr Hum Retrovirol* **13**:179, 1996

88. Gill PS et al: Treatment of adult T-cell leukemia-lymphoma with a combination of interferon alfa and zidovudine. *N Engl J Med* **332**:1744, 1995

89. Hermine O et al: Brief report: Treatment of adult T-cell leukemia-lymphoma with zidovudine and interferon alfa. *N Engl J Med* **332**:1749, 1995

90. Taguchi H et al: An intensive chemotherapy of adult T-cell leukemia/lymphoma: CHOP followed by etoposide, vindesine, ranimustine, and mitoxantrone with granulocyte colony-stimulating factor support. *J Acquir Immune Defic Syndr Hum Retrovirol* **12**:182, 1996

91. Borg A et al: Successful treatment of HTLV-I-associated acute adult T-cell leukaemia lymphoma by allogeneic bone marrow transplantation. *Br J Haematol* **94**:713, 1996

92. Van der Loo EM et al: C-type virus-like particles specifically localized in Langerhans and related cells of the skin and lymph nodes of patients with mycosis fungoides and Sézary syndrome. *Virchows Arch* **31**:193, 1979

93. Kaltoft K et al: C-type particles are inducible in SE-Ax, a continuous T-cell line from a patient with Sézary's syndrome. *Arch Dermatol Res* **280**:264, 1988

94. Unge T et al: Detection of T-lymphotropic virus-like particles in cultures of peripheral blood lymphocytes from patients with mycosis fungoides. *Proc Natl Acad Sci* **88**:7630, 1991

95. Gallo RC et al: Association of the human C type retrovirus with a subset of adult T-cell cancers. *Cancer Res* **43**:3892, 1983

96. Lange-Wantzin G et al: Occurence of human T cell lymphotropic virus (type I) antibodies in cutaneous T cell lymphoma. *J Am Acad Dermatol* **15**:598, 1986

97. Hall WW et al: Deleted HTLV-I provirus in blood and cutaneous lesions of patients with mycosis fungoides. *Science* **253**:317, 1991

98. Ghosh SK et al: Human T-cell leukemia virus type I tax/rex DNA and RNA in cutaneous T-cell lymphoma. *Blood* **84**:2663, 1994

99. Manca N et al: Persistence of human T cell lymphotropic virus type 1 (HTLV-1) sequences in peripheral blood mononuclear cells from patients with mycosis fungoides. *J Exp Med* **180**:1973, 1994

100. Pancake BA et al: The cutaneous T cell lymphoma, mycosis fungoides, is a human T cell lymphotropic virus-associated disease. A study of 50 patients. *J Clin Invest* **95**:547, 1995

101. Pancake BA et al: Demonstration of antibodies to human T-cell lymphotropic virus-I tax in patients with the cutaneous T-cell lymphoma, mycosis fungoides, who are seronegative for antibodies to the structural proteins of the virus. *Blood* **88**:3004, 1996

102. Zucker-Franklin D et al: Reexamination of human T cell lymphotropic virus (HTLV-I/II) prevalence. *Proc Natl Acad Sci USA* **94**:6403, 1997

103. Capesius C et al: No evidence for HTLV-I infection in 24 cases of French and Portuguese mycosis fungoides and Sézary syndrome. *Leukemia* **5**:416, 1991

104. Chadburn A et al: Detection and characterization of human T-cell lymphotropic virus type I (HTLV-I) associated T-cell neoplasms in an HTLV-I nonendemic region by polymerase chain reaction. *Blood* **77**:2419, 1991

105. Lisby G et al: No detection of HTLV-I DNA in punch skin biopsies from patients with cutaneous T-cell lymphoma by the polymerase chain reaction. *J Invest Dermatol* **98**:417, 1992

106. Bazarbachi A et al: HTLV-1 provirus and mycosis fungoides. *Science* **259**:1470, 1993

107. Bazarbachi A et al: Mycosis fungoides and Sézary syndrome are not associated with HTLV-I infection: An international study. *Br J Haematol* **98**:927, 1997

108. Li G et al: Failure to detect human T-lymphotropic virus type-I proviral DNA in cell lines and tissues from patients with cutaneous T-cell lymphoma. *J Invest Dermatol* **107**:308, 1996

109. Wood GS et al: Evidence against a role for human T-cell lympho-tropic virus type I (HTLV-I) in the pathogenesis of American cuta-neous T-cell lymphoma. *J Invest Dermatol* **107**:301, 1996

110. Gessain A: Virological aspects of tropical spastic paraparesis/HTLV-I associated myelopathy and HTLV-I infection. *J Neurovirol* **2**:299, 1996

111. Kaplan JE et al: The risk of development of HTLV-I-associated my-elopathy/tropical spastic paraparesis among persons infected with HTLV-I. *J Acquir Immune Defic Syndr* **3**:1096, 1990

112. LaGrenade L et al: Infective dermatitis of Jamaican children: a marker for HTLV-I infection. *Lancet* **2**:1345, 1990

113. Tachibana N et al: Suppression of tuberculin skin reaction in healthy HTLV-I carriers from Japan. *Int J Cancer* **42**:829, 1988

114. Funai N et al: Differences in immune functions between human T-lymphotropic virus type I carriers and patients with adult T-cell leukemia/lymphoma. *Clin Immunol Immunopathol* **80**:325, 1996

115. Marsh BJ: Infectious complications of human T cell leukemia/lym-phoma virus type I infection. *Clin Infect Dis* **23**:138, 1996

116. LaGrenade L: HTLV-I-associated infective dermatitis: Past, present, and future. *J Acquir Immune Defic Syndr Hum Retrovirol* **13**:S46, 1996

117. Bunker CB et al: Indolent cutaneous prodrome of fatal HTLV-I in-fection. *Lancet* **1**:426, 1990

118. Hanchard B et al: Childhood infective dermatitis evolving into adult T-cell leukaemia after 17 years. *Lancet* **2**:1593, 1991

119. Mochizuki M et al: HTLV-I uveitis. *J Acquir Immune Defic Syndr Hum Retrovirol* **13**:S50, 1996

120. Morgan OSTC et al: HTLV-1 and polymyositis in Jamaica. *Lancet* **2**:1184, 1989

121. Sato K et al: Arthritis in patients infected with human T lymphotropic virus type I. Clinical and immunopathologic features. *Arthritis Rheum* **34**:714, 1991

122. Vernan JC et al: Pseudo-amyotrophic lateral sclerosis peripheral neu-ropathy and chronic polyradiculoneuritis in patients with HTLV-I as-sociated paraplegias in HTLV-I and the nervous system, in *Neurology and Neurolobiology,* edited by G Roman et al. New York, Alan R. Liss, 1989, pp 361–365

CHAPTER 226

Richard Allen Johnson

Cutaneous Manifestations of Human Immunodeficiency Virus Disease

By 1998, 31 million people throughout the world had become in-fected with the human immunodeficiency virus (HIV), with 16,000 individuals becoming infected daily (1600 children) and 5.8 million annually (350,000 children). More than 90 percent of new infections occur in developing countries. Ninety percent of those infected are unaware of their HIV infection. Globally in 1997, 2.3 million peo-ple died from HIV disease, making it the most common cause of death among the infectious diseases. In the developed nations of Europe and North America, the prognosis of HIV disease has dra-matically improved during the past few years with the advent of highly active antiretroviral therapy (HAART). However, these drugs are not available to 90 percent of HIV-infected individuals in de-veloping nations because of their prohibitive cost.

HIV disease was first described in 1981, a mere two decades ago, following a cluster of cases of a previously unreported acquired immunodeficiency syndrome (AIDS), defined by the opportunistic infections (OIs) *Pneumocystis carinii* pneumonia (PCP) and chronic herpetic ulcers and by opportunistic neoplasia (ON) and Kaposi's sarcoma (KS). The initial case reports were of homosexual men in the United States, followed shortly by cases in persons who injected drugs. Within a year, AIDS was also reported from Europe and Australia in these two groups. Shortly after, the greatest numbers of cases were being reported from Africa. Currently, half the adults in some cities in Botswana, Malawi, and Zambia are infected with HIV.

The demographics of the HIV epidemic are changing rapidly. Globally, the majority of HIV-infected individuals are asympto-matic and are undiagnosed serologically. In developed regions of the world (North America, Europe, Australia), serotesting is readily available for individuals at risk for HIV infection. In developing regions (Africa, South America, and parts of Asia), the health care system is such that HIV serotesting is either not available or is prohibitively expensive, with only 5 percent of HIV-infected indi-viduals aware of their disease; the diagnosis is commonly made on clinical findings. Epidemiologic surveys in these regions are unre-liable.

Within the worldwide HIV pandemic are many different epidem-ics, each with its own dynamics and each influenced by many fac-tors, including time of introduction of the virus into the population, population density, and cultural and social issues.[1] The number of new HIV infections in developed countries are relatively stable. Currently in the United States, 44,000 individuals become infected annually, with the highest numbers of cases of AIDS in the District of Columbia, Puerto Rico, New York, Florida, and New Jersey. In Russia, where the rates of sexually transmitted diseases (STDs) and injected-drug use (IDU) are very high, the HIV epidemic has followed the epidemics of STDs and IDU, the number of HIV-infected persons increasing to approximately 1 million. By year 2000, HIV will have infected 15 to 20 million individuals in Asia, where the dominant mode of transmission is heterosexual.

ETIOLOGY AND EPIDEMIOLOGY OF HIV DISEASE

Etiology

Discovery of a human retrovirus (human T-cell lymphotropic virus [HTLV-I]) was reported in 1980. HTLV-I is also thought to have originated in Africa and to have spread to various geographic locations around the world. HIV (initially human T-cell lymphotropic virus-III [HTLV-III]) was isolated only a few years later, the first cases of HIV disease having been reported in 1981. Two types of HIV have subsequently been identified: HIV-1, the cause of nearly all HIV infection in the North America and Europe; and HIV-2, detected mainly in West Africa, with isolated cases elsewhere. HIV-2 is much less virulent than HIV-1. Individuals infected with HIV-2 are 70 percent less likely to become infected with HIV-1.

HIV-1 has at least 10 subtypes, designated A through J. The B-subtype is prevalent in the United States and Western Europe, found mainly among homosexual men and injected-drug users. The C- and E-subtypes are transmitted efficiently through sexual intercourse. The C-subtype, which is most prevalent in sub-Saharan Africa, has also been detected in North America. The E-subtype, which is responsible for the epidemic in Thailand, has a far greater affinity for epithelial cells that line both the male and female reproductive tracts. In contrast, the B-subtype is not transmitted very easily through these cells, preferring a more direct route into the body through contact with blood. The E-subtype has been found only in isolated instances in the United States and Western Europe. Should the C- and/or E-subtypes, with their enhanced affinity for the reproductive tract, cause significant numbers of cases in the United States and Western Europe, a new HIV epidemic could occur in the heterosexual population. The discovery of highly divergent strains of HIV, not reliably detected by a number of commonly used diagnostic tests, has underscored the need for effective surveillance to track HIV variants and to direct research and prevention activities. Current vaccine research is targeted at development of a vaccine against the B-subtype.

Origins of HIV

The origins of HIV are unclear; however, the most likely explanation is that HIV may have been introduced into human populations from other primates in sub-Saharan Africa. Both HIV-1 and HIV-2 existed in rural Africa prior to the onset of the pandemic, entering the human population several decades ago. Urbanization brought HIV to population centers. In cities, loss of tribal traditions, a migrant worker system that encourages multiple partners and stimulates demand for prostitution, and poverty, which also promotes prostitution, are associated with greater sexual freedom. HIV-2 is still predominantly found in West Africa. In countries outside Africa where HIV-2 infection has been detected, current or historical ties to West African nations exist.

Transmission of HIV

Currently, the major modes of transmission are sexual intercourse, needle sharing during IDU, and perinatal transmission by HIV-infected women. During the first decade of the HIV pandemic (1981–1990), the route of transmission varied greatly between industrialized and developing countries. In the industrialized continents of North America, Europe, and Australia, transmission was most common during male-male sexual intercourse and IDU. In sub-Saharan Africa, transmission has nearly always been by heterosexual intercourse.

HIV is present at contagious levels in blood, genital secretions, and breast milk. HIV transmission occurs most efficiently by injection of a large volume of HIV-infected blood. Rarely, infection has also occurred by spillage of HIV-infected blood on skin or mucosa with breaks in the integrity of the epithelium. Extracellular virus has been found in blood and in seminal fluid, raising the possibility of cell-free transmission. HIV has been demonstrated to infect, multiply, and destroy Langerhans cells of the epidermis and mucosa.

On a population level, host-related factors (susceptibility and infectiousness), environmental factors (the social, cultural, and political milieu), and agent factors (HIV-1) determine HIV infectivity. The variability observed among and within routes of HIV exposure depends partly on the viral dose and also on whether HIV is transmitted directly into the blood or onto a mucous membrane. These differences are influenced by a variety of host factors, including both factors common to all routes of exposure and those unique to sexual transmission.

Transmission through sexual contact accounts for 85 percent of the 31 million HIV infections that have occurred through 1997.[2] The probability of infection through sexual contact varies greatly and appears to be lower than that of infection through other routes of exposure. The HIV-1 C-subtype is most easily transmitted through sexual intercourse. HIV appears to be most contagious during the acute (primary) HIV infection (when viral levels in bodily fluids are high and antibodies absent or just forming) and in late HIV disease (when viral load is high). The rate of HIV transmission is low for each sexual encounter. HIV-2 transmission is 5 to 9 times less efficient than of HIV-1, which may explain the limited geographic distribution of HIV-2.

Risk factors for enhanced sexual transmission of HIV include lack of circumcision in males,[3] lack of condom use, receptive anal intercourse, ulcerative STDs (genital herpes, primary syphilis, chancroid),[4] and nonulcerative STDs (chlamydial infections, vaginal trichomoniasis, gonorrhea).[5] Receptive anal intercourse has the greatest risk of HIV transmission with partners who have primary HIV infection.

In Rwanda, uncircumcised men had a higher prevalence of HIV infection than circumcised men (29 percent versus 21 percent), which was most marked in men reporting ≥5 lifetime sex partners (36 percent versus 23 percent).[6] Uncircumcised men also had a higher rate of genital ulcer disease (GUD), a known risk factor for HIV transmission. Whether the higher risk of HIV transmission is due in part to poor hygiene or to complex mechanisms operating through the acquisition of other STDs is not known. In the United States, uncircumcised males who have sex with other males are also at higher risk for HIV acquisition.

Circumcision may be an appropriate risk-reduction approach for men with known exposures to HIV when there are constraints to alternatives such as condom use. Postexposure prophylaxis of HIV with antiretroviral agents is possible in some instances, the risk of transmission being highest for rectal intercourse, less for vaginal intercourse, and least for orogenital exposure.

Perinatal transmission of HIV from infected women to their children occurs commonly because of the increasing number of HIV-infected females of childbearing age. Through 1993, an estimated 15,000 HIV-infected children were born to HIV-positive women in the United States.[7] Approximately 25 percent of newborns become infected with HIV during gestation, most commonly around the time of delivery. The later pregnancy occurs in HIV disease, the more likely the fetus is to become infected. Transmission of HIV-2 perinatally is uncommon (4 percent). Zidovudine treatment of HIV-infected pregnant women and their infants has resulted in a two-thirds reduction in the risk of perinatal HIV transmission. During pregnancy, antiretroviral agents are prescribed according to the stage of HIV disease of the mother—i.e., dependent on CD4 counts and viral load level. If the mother has previously been untreated, antiviral therapy is usually delayed until the 14 week of pregnancy to minimize teratogenicity of drugs. To prevent perinatal transmission, zidovudine is currently given to the mother as an intravenous bolus and also as a constant infusion; the neonate is then treated with zidovudine for the first 6 weeks of life.

Prior to reliable serotesting, HIV was inadvertently transmitted by the administration of blood or blood products. Transfusion with HIV-infected blood is the most efficient mode of transmission of HIV, with up to 90 percent of recipients becoming infected. Currently, the risk of transmission of HTLV-I/II and HIV-1 in the United States is very low but still exists, calculated as 1 in 60,000 units from donors who are infected with retrovirus but seronegative at the time of donation.[8] HIV has also been transmitted to recipients of tissue transplantation—i.e., kidney, liver, and bone grafts.

HIV transmission occurs in only 1 of 300 skin-piercing injuries when the virus is present on a instrument, more commonly with a hollow needle than a suture needle and more often with a deep injury and a puncture wound. In contrast, 1 of 3 individuals who sustain a puncture wound with an instrument contaminated with hepatitis B virus will become infected. The risk of HIV infection after percutaneous exposure increases with a larger volume of blood and, probably, a higher titer of HIV in the source patient's blood. It should be noted that the great majority of HIV-infected health care workers have become infected through nonoccupational exposures. The current approach to significant occupational HIV exposure (postexposure prophylaxis) is to treat with antiretroviral agents for 4 weeks following the incident.

PATHOGENESIS

Four mechanisms are critical for the establishment and propagation of HIV infection over time and for the progression of HIV disease. HIV is not eliminated after primary infection. Persistent virus replication occurs in lymphoid organs throughout the course of HIV infection. Chronic stimulation of the immune system causes inappropriate immune activation and progressive exhaustion of the immune response. Destruction of lymphoid tissue results in severe impairment of the ability to maintain an effective ongoing HIV-specific immune response and to generate immune responses against new pathogens.

Epidermal Langerhans cells (LC) are antigen-presenting CD4+ dendritic cells that may become infected by HIV. Decreased Langerhans cell function could account for some of the cutaneous manifestations of HIV disease. Studies of epidermal Langerhans cell density in HIV-infected subjects have produced conflicting results, even in advanced HIV disease.

Centers for Disease Control and Prevention (CDC) Classification for HIV Infection and Case Definition for AIDS

The CDC identified and defined the end stage of HIV disease as the acquired immunodeficiency syndrome, or AIDS, in 1982. In industrialized countries, laboratory determinations of HIV serostatus, CD4 cell counts, and viral load levels are used to diagnose HIV infection and to measure disease progression. In developing countries (sub-Saharan Africa and Asia), serologic and other sophisticated testing procedures are not available, and clinical criteria are used to make the diagnosis of AIDS.

AIDS in HIV-infected adolescents and adults aged ≥13 years defined by CDC includes any one of the following criteria: (a) <200 CD4+ cells/μL; (b) a CD4+ cell percentage of total lymphocytes of <14 percent; or (c) any of the following three clinical conditions: pulmonary tuberculosis, recurrent pneumonia, or invasive cervical cancer.

The expanded CDC definition retains the 23 clinical conditions in the AIDS surveillance case definition published in 1987 (Table 226-1),[9] and adds all adults and adolescents infected with HIV with CD4 lymphocyte counts <200/mL. Cohort studies of untreated persons with CD4 lymphocyte counts <200/mL have shown that 80 percent of them will have an AIDS-related OI or malignancy within 3 years.

An alternative to the CDC staging, which defines HIV disease as non-AIDS and AIDS, is a staging system based on the CD4+ cell count as a measure of the degree of destruction of the immune system (Table 226-2). This staging system defines five stages rather than two: acute retroviral syndrome, symptomatic, early symptomatic, late symptomatic, and advanced HIV disease. The combined stages of late symptomatic and advanced HIV disease are similar to the CDC definition of AIDS.

PRIMARY HIV INFECTION

Primary HIV-1 infection is estimated to be symptomatic in up to 80 percent of cases (acute retroviral syndrome [ARS]); presumably primary HIV-2 infection,[10] although less well studied, manifests in a similar manner. The incubation period (from presumed exposure to development of acute febrile illness) ranges from 3 to 6 weeks, varying with the route of infection and the size of the viral inoculum. Symptomatic primary infection is more common in individuals who acquire HIV infection via sexual exposure than by other modes.

Symptoms of ARS include fever, rigors, lethargy, malaise, sore throat, anorexia, myalgia, arthralgia, headache, stiff neck, photophobia, nausea, diarrhea, and abdominal cramps and pain. In a study of 218 patients with documented symptomatic primary HIV-1 infection, the frequency and mean duration of clinical features occurring in more than 50 percent of patients was as follows: fever (77.1 percent, 16.9 days), lethargy (65.6 percent, 23.7 days), rash (56.4 percent, 15 days), myalgia (54.6 percent, 17.7 days), and headache (50.9 percent, 25.8 days).[11] Only 15.6 percent of patients presented with a typical mononucleosis-like illness (fever, pharyngitis or sore throat, and cervical adenopathy); 10 percent had no

TABLE 226-1

1992 Revised Classification for HIV Infection and Expanded Case Definition for AIDS in Adolescents and Adults

CD4 Cell Count	A	B	C
>500/μL (>29%)	A1	B1	C1
200 to 499/μL (14% to 28%)	A2	B2	C2
<200/μL (<14%)	A3	B3	C3

Category A
  Acute retroviral syndrome
  Asymptomatic HIV infection
  Persistent generalized lymphadenopathy
Category B
  Constitutional symptoms (fever of 38.5°C [101.3°F], diarrhea >1 month)
  Idiopathic thrombocytopenic purpura
  Peripheral neuropathy
  Bartonella henselae, B. quintana: bacillary angiomatosis
  Pelvic inflammatory disease
  Listeriosis
  Candidiasis: oropharyngeal or recurrent vulvovaginal
  Varicella-zoster virus infection: herpes zoster
  Epstein-Barr virus infection: oral hairy leukoplakia
  Human papillomavirus infection: Cervical squamous intraepithelial lesion
Category C
  HIV encephalopathy
  Progressive multifocal encephalopathy
  Lymphoma
  Mycobacterium avium-intracellulare complex or *M. kansasii* infection
  M. tuberculosis
  Pneumonia: recurrent with >2 episodes in 12 months
  Salmonellosis
  Candidiasis: esophageal, pulmonary
  Cryptococcosis: extrapulmonary
  Coccidioidomycosis
  Histoplasmosis
  Pneumocystis carinii pneumonia
  Herpes simplex virus infection: esophageal, pulmonary, mucocutaneous ulcers of >1 month duration
  Cytomegalovirus
  Human herpesvirus-8 infection: Kaposi's sarcoma
  Human papillomavirus infection: cervical cancer
  Cryptosporidiosis
  Isosporiasis
  Toxoplasmosis

TABLE 226-2

Stages of HIV Disease

Stage and Clinical Features	Typical Duration	CD4+ Cell Range (Cells/μL)
Acute retroviral syndrome (brief mononucleosis-like illness)	1–2 wk	1000–500
Asymptomatic (no symptoms or signs other than lymphadenopathy)	10+ yr	750–500
Early symptomatic (non-life-threatening infections, chronic or intermittent illness)	0–5 yr	500–100
Late symptomatic (increasingly severe symptoms, life-threatening infections, cancers)	0–3 yr	200–50
Advanced (increasing hazard of death, fewer transferable "opportunistic" infections)	1–2 yr	50–0

features of a mononucleosis-like illness. A meningitis-like syndrome occurred in 9.2 percent.

Cutaneous findings in ARS are not unique, but rather resemble those usually associated with many other acute viral infections.[12] An exanthem occurs in approximately 70 percent of individuals with ARS, characterized by pink-to-red macules and papules, 5 to 10 mm in diameter, which remain discrete and occur on the upper trunk and palms and soles. Genital ulcers occur in 30 to 40 percent of individuals. Oropharyngeal findings occur in 70 percent of cases and include an enanthem, aphthous-like ulcers, and candidiasis; in severe ARS, ulcers and candidiasis may also occur in the esophagus.

The laboratory diagnosis of primary HIV-1 infection is made by four methods: detection of viral antigens, detection of viral nucleic acids, identification of antibodies to viral proteins, and isolation of HIV by viral culture.[13] A delay of 3 to 4 weeks exists between newly acquired HIV-1 infection and development of antibodies, the "window period." The core structural protein p24 antigen can be detected a week before antibodies can be measured. Other laboratory findings during acute infection often include thrombocytopenia, leukopenia, elevated erythrocyte sedimentation rate, and lymphocytic cerebrospinal fluid (CSF) pleocytosis. Isolation of HIV on culture of blood, CSF, or tissue is highly specific but relatively insensitive, due to varying degrees of viremia at different stages of HIV infection. Six months after primary HIV infection, antibodies can be detected in 95 percent of individuals. Antibodies may disappear in patients with advanced HIV-1 infection.

The primary screening test for HIV-1 infection is the enzyme-linked immunosorbent assay (ELISA). If the ELISA test is positive, a Western blot or indirect immunofluorescence assay is performed on the same sample for confirmation. Western blot is considered positive if any two of the p24, gp41, or gp120/gp160 bands are detected. Detection of viral antigen, usually p24, is used as an early diagnostic aid or in infants born to HIV-infected mothers. Viral nucleic acid detection by polymerase chain reaction (PCR) or branched-chain DNA assay has the ability to detect very small quantities of HIV nucleic acids. Plasma viral RNA load levels are used to monitor effectiveness of antiretroviral therapy and progression of disease. Measurement of plasma RNA also permits diagnosis of individuals with advanced HIV disease who may have false negative ELISA and Western blot assays due to severe immunodeficiency, and early diagnosis of infants born to HIV-infected mothers.

Following the initial burst of viral replication and the peak of viremia, the plasma RNA level decreases and then stabilizes to a level called the viral set point.[14] The maximum or peak viral load, the duration of the viral burst, the viral replicative half-life, and the host immune response all influence the viral set point. Antiretroviral intervention has several possible effects on the kinetics of the acute phase of infection. The peak viral load may be reduced without affecting the viral set point, or the peak load might not be affected, but the duration of the viral burst might be shortened with reduction in the viral set point. Cytotoxic T lymphocytes, particularly those specific for Env, help control viral replication and are associated with slower declines in CD4+ cell counts.[15]

The prognosis for patients with prolonged (≥ 14 days) ARS (especially prolonged fever) appears to be significantly poorer, having a much shorter period before progression to AIDS, than for patients with asymptomatic or mildly symptomatic primary infection.[16] These individuals often experience faster disease progression and are candidates for early antiretroviral therapy and possible primary prophylaxis for opportunistic infections. In a study of 134 patients newly infected with HIV-1, 23 were observed to have ARS and 111 were asymptomatic converters. ARS was more frequently observed in subjects who had acquired the infection through sexual transmission; injected-drug users were not commonly affected and presented with milder symptoms. Patients with ARS had a significantly higher risk of AIDS developing than asymptomatic converters (68 percent at 56 months versus 20 percent at 66 months). Low CD4 cell counts at the onset of ARS and delayed seroconversion in ELISA were associated with evolution to AIDS in acute seroconverters.

Approximately 6 months after transmission of HIV, the plasma HIV RNA level reaches a relatively stable set point that dictates the subsequent course. Patients with high viral concentrations ("viral burden"), such as $\geq 100,000$ copies/μL, will have a relatively rapid course, and those with relatively low concentrations, such as 10,000 copies/μL, will have relatively slow progression. Undetectable viral load levels may correspond with nonprogression of HIV disease. The average annual decrease in CD4+ cell count is 50 cells/μL. Early treatment with antiretroviral drugs may reduce the viral set point and alter the prognosis of HIV infection.

NATURAL HISTORY OF HIV DISEASE

Multiple variables are known to influence the rate of progression of HIV disease, contribute to induction of HIV expression, and potentially modify and accelerate the course of HIV disease: size of HIV inoculum, site of infection, immune status of the host, variable virulence of certain HIV strains, and reactivation of latent herpesvirus infection. In a cohort of HIV-infected homosexual males from San Francisco studied prior to effective antiretroviral drug therapy, AIDS developed in approximately 50 percent within 11 years after becoming infected. Similar figures have been reported in other risk groups in the United States. In a cohort of HIV-infected persons from North America, Europe, and Australia whose date of seroconversion was known, the incubation time to the development of an AIDS-defining event varied with the different risk groups, possibly because of different exposures to potential opportunistic pathogens.

The rate of disease progression is more rapid in developing nations than in industrialized countries.

The period of time reported for the development of AIDS following infection by blood transfusion in adults varies from 6.5 to 11 years. In a study of 89 persons infected by contaminated blood products in France, the mean incubation period was 62 months.[17] In children with hemophilia AIDS developed more slowly than in homosexual men, mainly because homosexual men had an added risk factor of KS. Pregnancy does not appear to influence the rate of progression of HIV disease.

HIV disease is a continuum that progresses from primary infection to death, with a sequence of OIs and ONs marking the gradual destruction of the immune system. In a small percentage of individuals, HIV disease does not progress for an extended period of time. The typical course in the absence of treatment (see Table 226-2) is characterized by the following stages: viral transmission; acute retroviral syndrome; a prolonged period of clinical latency accompanied by CD4+ cell decline; and late-stage disease designated at AIDS.

Asymptomatic or early-stage HIV disease (CD4 cell count >500/μL) is characterized by the nearly complete absence of symptoms, with normal laboratory studies, except for serologic and virologic evidence of HIV infection and the gradual decline in the CD4 cell count.

Early symptomatic disease [previously known as AIDS-related complex (ARC)] (CD4 cell count 200 to 500/μL) may be associated with constitutional symptoms (fever, unexplained weight loss, recurrent diarrhea, fatigue, and headache), systemic manifestations (community-acquired pneumonitis, sinusitis, or bronchitis, idiopathic thrombocytopenic purpura, pulmonary tuberculosis, cervical squamous intraepithelial lesions), and/or dermatologic manifestations (seborrheic dermatitis, recurrent vulvovaginal candidiasis, oropharyngeal candidiasis, herpes zoster, recurrent herpes simplex virus (HSV) infection, oral hairy leukoplakia, KS).

Late symptomatic disease (CD4 cell count 50 to 200/μL) or AIDS is defined by two criteria: highly characteristic AIDS-defining diagnoses or a CD4+ cell count of <200/μL. AIDS is recognized as late-stage HIV infection in which there is substantial immunosuppression with vulnerability to a variety of different OIs, ONs, or other complications of HIV infection, such as the wasting syndrome or HIV-associated dementia. In industrialized nations (1996), the most frequent AIDS-defining diagnoses as the initial complication were PCP, HIV wasting syndrome, *Candida* esophagitis, KS, HIV-associated dementia, disseminated cytomegalovirus infection, disseminated *Mycobacterium avium-intracellulare* complex infection, toxoplasmosis, cryptococcal meningitis, chronic (>1 mo) mucocutaneous HSV infection, and tuberculosis.[18]

Advanced HIV disease (CD4 cell count <50/μL) is associated with profound immunosuppression and the occurrence of several coexisting infections or ONs.

MANAGEMENT OF HIV DISEASE

Markers of HIV Disease Progression

The CD4 (helper) lymphocyte count and plasma HIV RNA level[19] are monitored to determine disease progression.[20] The normal CD4 cell count ranges from 31 to 61 percent of the total lymphocyte count. The CD8 (suppressor) lymphocyte count normally ranges from 18 to 39 percent of the total lymphocyte count. The B cells make up the remainder of the blood lymphocytes, ranging from 5 to 20 percent of the total lymphocyte count. Patients with symptomatic or advanced HIV disease usually have CD4 cell counts below 20 percent of the total lymphocyte count.

Changes in the plasma concentration of HIV RNA predict the changes in CD4 cell counts and survival following initiation of HAART. Both the risk of the progression of HIV disease and the efficacy of antiretroviral therapy are strongly associated with the plasma level of HIV RNA and with the viral phenotype.

Antiretroviral Drug Therapy

In the era of HAART, the following principles of management for HIV disease are advocated whenever possible:

- monitor plasma viral load and CD4 count
- initiate treatment before immunodeficiency becomes apparent
- reduce plasma viral load as much as possible for as long as possible
- use combinations of at least two drugs (which maximize antiviral effect, minimize cross-resistance, and avoid overlapping toxicity)
- change to new regimen if plasma viral load rebounds despite continued therapy

The three main groups of antiretroviral drugs are nucleoside analogue reverse transcriptase (RT) inhibitors (NRTIs), nonnucleoside RT inhibitors (NNRTIs), and proteinase inhibitors (PIs).[21,22] Nucleoside analogues that inhibit HIV RT, slow or prevent formation of DNA copies of HIV in infected cells. Like the nucleoside analogues, NNRTIs inhibit RT, but by a different mechanism; their toxicity and resistance patterns do not overlap with those of nucleosides. PIs prevent cleavage of protein precursors essential for HIV maturation, infection of new cells, and replication. PI therapy in individuals with advanced HIV disease has led to marked clinical improvement and prolonged survival. All PIs can cause hyperglycemia and onset or worsening of diabetes mellitus.

NRTIs include zidovudine [ZVD, AZT], didanosine [ddI], zalcitabine [ddC], stavudine [d4T], and lamivudine [3TC]. NNRTIs include nevirapine and delavirdine. PIs include saquinavir, ritonovir, nelfinavir, and indivavir.

Early initiation of more aggressive HAART is currently recommended.[23] Drugs of choice include combinations of 2 NRTIs plus 1 PI or 2 NRTIs plus 1 NNRTI. The recurrent declines in morbidity and mortality of HIV disease are attributable to the use of more-intensive antiretroviral therapies.[24]

The plasma viral load is a crucial element of clinical management for assessing prognosis and the effectiveness of therapy. Treatment failure is most readily indicated by a rising plasma HIV RNA level. None of the currently available antiretroviral drugs has been shown to eradicate HIV infection, but used in combinations they can decrease viral replication, improve immune status, delay opportunistic infections, and prolong life. Therapeutic approaches must be updated as new data continue to emerge, particularly on the long-term clinical effect of aggressive antiretroviral treatment.

Postexposure Prophylaxis

Individuals who are exposed to HIV (occupational or sexual) are advised to seek immediate medical evaluation of the risk of HIV transmission. If the risk of transmission is significant, prophylactic antiretroviral therapy is recommended.

Prophylaxis of Opportunistic Infections

The absolute CD4 count is used as a guideline for several therapeutic interventions. A adequate response to HAART has resulted in an altered course of opportunistic infections in HIV-infected individuals.[25] Primary prophylaxis for PCP is begun when the CD4 cell count is $<200/\mu L$ with either trimethoprim-sulfamethoxazole (TMP-SMX), dapsone, or aerosolized pentamidine. For individuals with IgG antibody to *Toxoplasma* and CD4 count of $<100/\mu L$, TMP-SMX is recommended. Clarithromycin or azithromycin is advised if the CD4 count is $<75/\mu L$ for prevention of *Mycobacterium avium complex* (MAC) infection. Secondary prophylaxis is recommended following infections such as PCP, toxoplasmosis, MAC, and invasive fungal infections.

HIV Vaccine

The prospects for the development of an effective HIV vaccine are poor at present. Six vaccine candidates have been developed but remain untested. Most vaccines have been developed against the B-subtype, which is prevalent in North America, and would probably not be effective against the C- and E-subtypes, which are prevalent in developing nations.

MUCOCUTANEOUS FINDINGS

Opportunistic infections, opportunistic neoplasms, dermatoses, and pruritus involving skin and/or mucosa occur more commonly as immune function deteriorates, being problematic in >90 percent of HIV-infected individuals. Correlated with low CD4 cell counts, cutaneous lesions may become quite atypical, becoming caricatures of presentations in immunocompetent individuals. Certain cutaneous disorders correlate with low CD4 cell counts (200 to 300 cell/μL), including KS, oral hairy leukoplakia, multiple facial molluscum contagiosum, xerosis, and oropharyngeal candidiasis.[26,27]

Mucocutaneous disorders (Table 226-3) are commonly the indication for initial HIV testing.

CUTANEOUS DISORDERS

Pruritic Eruptions

Pruritus, a common complaint in patients with late symptomatic and advanced HIV disease, is a surrogate cutaneous marker for disease progression, occurring commonly in patients with CD4 counts <50 cell/μL as compared with those with counts $>250/\mu L$. In most cases, primary or secondary dermatoses are the cause of pruritus in HIV-infected individuals. The differential diagnosis of primary pruritic skin disorders include atopic dermatitis, xerosis, allergic contact dermatitis, adverse cutaneous drug eruptions, dermatographism, eosinophilic folliculitis, scabies, and insect bites. Less commonly, lymphoma, renal failure, or obstructive liver disease is associated with pruritus in the absence of cutaneous findings, i.e., metabolic pruritus.

An atopic diathesis, which exists in 20 percent of the general population, may become manifest in individuals with advanced HIV

TABLE 226-3

CHAPTER 226
Cutaneous Manifestations of HIV Disease 2511

Mucocutaneous Disorders as Indications for HIV Serotesting

HIGHLY INDICATIVE OF HIV INFECTION

Exanthem of acute retroviral syndrome
Proximal subungual onychomycosis
Chronic herpetic ulcers
Oral hairy leukoplakia
Kaposi's sarcoma
Eosinophilic folliculitis
Multiple facial molluscum contagiosum (in adult)

STRONGLY ASSOCIATED WITH HIV INFECTION

Any sexually transmitted disease (indicative of "unsafe" sexual
practice)
Herpes zoster
Signs of injected-drug use
Candidiasis: oropharyngeal or recurrent vulvovaginal

MAY BE ASSOCIATED WITH HIV INFECTION

Generalized lymphadenopathy
Seborrheic dermatitis (extensive, refractory to therapy)
Aphthous ulcers (recurrent, refractory to therapy)

disease and pruritus. Changes secondary to chronic rubbing and scratching include excoriations, atopic dermatitis, lichen simplex chronicus, and prurigo nodularis. Up to 50 percent of HIV-infected individuals are *Staphylococcus aureus* nasal carriers. Secondary *S. aureus* infection (impetiginization, furunculosis, or cellulitis) is very common in any of these traumatized lesions. Ichthyosis vulgaris and xerosis are common in advanced HIV disease and may be associated with mild pruritus.

Peripheral eosinophilia, which occurs most often in advanced HIV disease, is more common in blacks and is commonly associated with pruritic skin conditions such as adverse cutaneous drug eruptions, eosinophilic folliculitis, atopic dermatitis, and prurigo nodularis.[28] Extensive work-up for asymptomatic eosinophilia in patients with advanced HIV disease and cutaneous disease is not usually indicated.

Exanthematous drug eruptions such as those caused by TMP-SMX occur relatively suddenly and are usually easily linked to a newly prescribed drug. The protease inhibitor indinavir can cause eczematous reactions that are subtle in onset, usually occur relatively soon after initiation of therapy, and may be mild (resembling nummular eczema or widespread xerosis with eczema).

Scabies can present with significant pruritus with few cutaneous findings in HIV disease. Conversely, in individuals with advanced disease, pruritus may be minimal, resulting in delayed diagnosis. In such cases, the clinical presentation is of a generalized eczematous or psoriasiform dermatosis such as hyperkeratotic or crusted (Norwegian) scabies. Mosquito bites can become very large, 1 to 2 cm, presenting as few or multiple pruritic papules or nodules on exposed skin sites.

Eosinophilic Folliculitis

Eosinophilic folliculitis (EF) is a chronic dermatosis occurring in individuals with advanced HIV disease. The condition is distinct clinically from Ofuji's disease (eosinophilic pustular dermatosis), which occurs in non-HIV-infected individuals, has been reported mainly from Japan, and presents as facial plaques. The condition "pruritic papular eruption of HIV disease" previously described in the literature appears to be the same entity as EF. The pathogenesis

of EF is unknown. An infectious agent has been suspected but has not been identified. *Demodex folliculorum*, which is not antigenic in immunocompetent individuals, may trigger the production of *Demodex*-specific IgE antibodies that could bind to Langerhans cell and mast cells in skin, resulting in pruritic follicular lesions. The onset of symptoms usually occurs when the CD4 cell count is <100 cells/μL; however, with HAART, EF has occurred initially, recurred, or flared in association with increasing CD4 cell counts and decreasing viral load levels.

The pruritus associated with EF is intense, more so in individuals with an atopic diathesis. Even early in the course of EF, with few lesions present, pruritus can be the most bothersome symptom, especially by disturbing sleep. Clinically, small pink-to-red, edematous, folliculocentric papules (and much less commonly pustules) occur symmetrically above the nipple line on the chest, proximal arms, head, and neck (Fig. 226-1). The lesions have the appearance of small insect bites (papular urticaria). Rubbing, scratching, and excoriation soon alter primary lesions with the appearance of excoriations, excoriated papules, lichen simplex chronicus, prurigo nodularis, and postinflammatory hyperpigmentation and hypopigmentation. Any of these secondary changes can become infected with *S. aureus,* or less commonly, with group A streptococcus.

Although subjective and objective findings of early EF are nearly pathognomonic, subacute or chronic EF may have many secondary changes that make a clinical diagnosis tentative. In these cases, the diagnosis of EF should be confirmed by the histologic findings. Peripheral eosinophilia is common in HIV-associated EF, up to 35 percent. Diagnostic criteria have been proposed (Table 226-4).[29]

High-potency topical glucocorticoid preparations may reduce the formation of new EF lesions and may cause established lesions to resolve, thus providing symptomatic relief. Sedating antihistamines such as doxepin are most effective for symptomatic control of nocturnal pruritus; nonsedating antihistamines are ineffective. Permethrin cream applied daily may be effective.

Ultraviolet radiation (UVR) (UVB, UVA) is considered to be a safe treatment modality in HIV-infected individuals, and guidelines

FIGURE 226-1

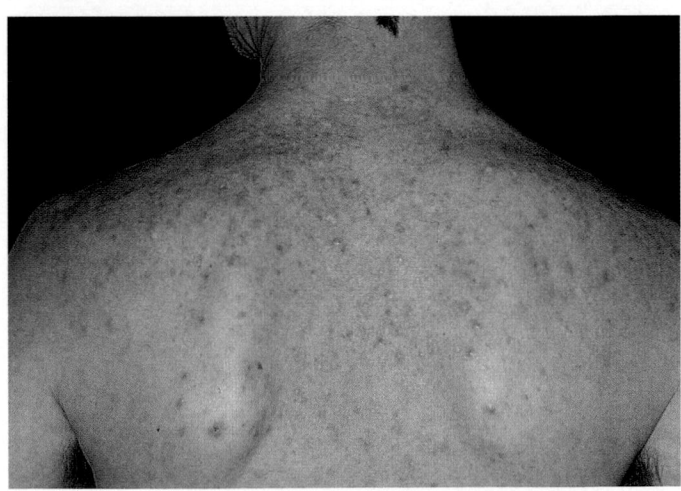

Eosinophilic folliculitis. Multiple erythematous pruritic papules and a few pustules on the upper back in an individual with a CD4 cell count of 50/μL.

TABLE 226-4

Diagnostic Criteria for Eosinophilic Folliculitis

Clinical criteria
   Pruritus (usually severe)
   Follicular urticarial papules
   Head, neck, upper back, and upper arms
   Chronic course that waxes and wanes
Histologic criteria
   Folliculocentric inflammation: predominantly eosinophils, but also
    lymphocytes, histiocytes, and neutrophils
   Follicular spongiosis
   Eosinophilic abscesses in affected follicles
   No bacteria or dermatophytes in affected follicles
Laboratory criteria
   HIV-seropositive
   Culture negative for bacteria and fungi
   Eosinophilia, peripheral
   Elevated serum IgE
   CD4+ cell count <200/μL

have been proposed for its use (Table 226-5).[30] UVR does not appear to have a deleterious effect on the clinical status, CD4 cell counts, or viral load level in treated patients. UVR has been shown, however, to activate HIV and promote its proliferation ex vivo. UVB phototherapy of EF, given by skilled technicians to compliant patients, is effective in suppressing both lesions and symptoms.

Prednisone, given at an initial oral dose of 70 mg and tapered over a 1- or 2-week period, is most effective in treating the cutaneous lesions as well as giving nearly immediate symptomatic relief of EF. If symptoms recur following discontinuation of prednisone, a second course can be given or prednisone 60 mg can be given one day per week.

Oral itraconazole, 200 mg per day, has been reported to be an effective therapy, with symptomatic relief occurring within 2 weeks of therapy; if response is not significant, the dose is increased up to 400 mg/day.[31] Oral isotretinoin has also been reported to be highly effective in treatment of EF, usually 40 mg bid until lesions and symptoms resolve, then tapered to 40 mg daily for several weeks, and then to 20 mg daily or 40 mg qod.[32] Metronidazole,

TABLE 226-5

Proposed Guidelines for Phototherapy of HIV-Infected Patients

Is the skin disease responsive to UVR? If the answer is yes, consider
  phototherapy.
Do alternative therapies offer less risk to the patient? If yes, it may be
  judicious to try alternative treatments first.
Is anticipated improvement in morbidity following phototherapy
  enough to justify potential risks? If yes, proceed with phototherapy.
Is the patient sufficiently reliable to show up for treatment visits? If
  no, consider other treatments.
Are there other contraindications to phototherapy (e.g., medication
  that confers photosensitivity)? If yes, weigh the risk-benefit ratio.

SOURCE: Adams ML et al: Phototherapy of HIV-infected patients: Background, pathomechanisms and proposed guidelines. *Dermatol Ther* **4**:47, 1997, with permission.

250 mg tid for 3 weeks, may be effective. Peripheral eosinophilia usually improves or lessens with prednisone, itraconazole, or isotretinoin therapy.

COMMON DERMATOSES

Psoriasis Vulgaris

The prevalence of psoriasis vulgaris in HIV-infected individuals may be somewhat higher than in the general population; that of psoriatic arthritis, however, is higher, correlating with the presence of HLA-B27. Psoriatic lesions may appear before or after HIV infection. Onset of psoriasis in an individual at risk for HIV disease may be an indication for HIV serotesting. Psoriasis and Reiter's syndrome may coexist in the same patient, suggesting that the two disorders may be part of a spectrum of clinical manifestations of one disease.

In a cohort of 50 HIV-infected individuals with psoriasis, one-third of psoriasis cases were presumed to have occurred prior to HIV infection (group I) and two thirds after (group II).[33] Group I had a lower mean age at onset (19 years versus 36 years) and more commonly had a family history of psoriasis. The clinical patterns of psoriasis have been reported to be plaque type (78 percent), inverse (37 percent), guttate (29 percent), palmoplantar (8 percent), erythrodermic (14 percent), and pustular (8 percent). Palmoplantar and inverse-pattern psoriasis were more common in group II; severe psoriasis occurred in one-quarter of these patients. Psoriasis tended to become more severe as the degree of immunodeficiency increased, but this did not affect survival.

Topical agents are usually effective in management of limited psoriasis, i.e., glucocorticoids, calcipotriene, or retinoids. For more widespread disease, phototherapy with UVB, narrow-band UVB (311 nm), or psoralen UVA (PUVA) is safe and effective. Retinoids (etretinate or acitretin), methotrexate, and cyclosporin also appear to be safe and effective. Zidovudine therapy given for HIV infection may be effective in treatment of psoriasis; whether improvement is a direct result of AZT therapy or of associated improved immune function is not certain. Psoriasis with onset after HIV infection has been observed to improve more with HAART than does psoriasis with onset prior to HIV infection.

Reiter's Syndrome

As with psoriasis, the onset of Reiter's syndrome occurs before or simultaneously with the onset of clinically evident immunodeficiency. Articular symptoms can precede onset of immunodeficiency by up to 14 months, and often may be the first manifestation of HIV infection. Some patients have culture-negative diarrheal illness or culture-negative urethritis at the onset of Reiter's syndrome. In a case study of 21 patients with HIV-associated incomplete or complete Reiter's syndrome, HLA-B27 occurred in 15 (71 percent). Reactive arthritis was associated with antecedent bacterial infections in 30 percent of cases, further emphasizing the similarity of this syndrome with non-HIV-associated Reiter's syndrome. The finding of extensive clinical overlap among psoriatic arthritis, psoriasis, and Reiter's syndrome, the absence of HLA antigens previously found to be associated with psoriasis, and the increased prevalence of HLA-B27 in HIV-infected patients with psoriatic arthritis suggest a close association between psoriasis and Reiter's syndrome in this population.

Erythroderma

Erythroderma in HIV disease may be related to atopic dermatitis, psoriasis vulgaris, photosensitivity dermatitis, the hypereosinophilic syndrome, coexistent HTLV-I infection, and CD8 (cytotoxic T cell) phenotype CTCL.

Xerosis and Ichthyosis

Xerosis and acquired ichthyosis are very common in HIV-infected individuals, occurring in up to 30 percent of those with advanced disease. The pathogenesis is uncertain but may be related to chronic illness, malnutrition, wasting syndrome, or HIV infection itself. In a study of 185 injected-drug users with HIV infection,[34] the prevalence of acquired ichthyosis varied with race (white 6.3 percent, Hispanic 16.4 percent, black 21.7 percent). Ichthyosis was noted only after profound CD4 cell depletion, occurring in association with increasing age and with concomitant HTLV-II infection (22.2 percent versus 6.8 percent in HIV-1 singly infected patients).

Seborrheic Dermatitis (See Chap. 126)

Seborrheic dermatitis is the most common dermatosis occurring in HIV disease, presenting in the usual areas of the scalp, face, and chest. Clinical findings worsen as HIV disease progresses and clear as immune function improves following a response to HAART.

Photosensitivity (See Sect. 19)

Photosensitivity in HIV-infected individuals often occurs as an acute drug-induced reaction; chronic actinic dermatitis is also relatively common. The most common type of drug-induced photosensitivity is the phototoxic reaction, i.e., an exaggerated sunburn response, to TMP-SMX. Photoallergic drug photosensitivity, either in the form of eczematous reactions or lichen planus–like (lichenoid) eruption, are less common, and occur as adverse reactions to sulfonamides as well as many topically applied chemicals. Photoallergic reactions can persist for months or years in the absence of continued exposure to known photosensitizers and are known as chronic actinic dermatitis (older terms include actinic reticuloid, photosensitive eczema, and persistent light reaction).

The diagnostic criteria for chronic actinic dermatitis are as follows: a chronic photodermatitis, in the absence of continued exposure to photosensitizers, abnormal phototest responses, and histologic changes consistent with photodermatosis. Chronic actinic dermatitis occurs more commonly in older men (mean age, 50 years) of skin phototype VI with CD4 cell counts <200/μL, and may be the initial presentation of HIV disease.[35] Chronic actinic dermatitis is associated with decreased minimal erythema doses to UVB, and in some cases UVA. Clinically, an eczematous dermatitis occurs in the sun-exposed sites of the face, neck, arms, and hands (Fig. 226-2). Secondary changes of lichenification and *S. aureus* infection are common. Chronic rubbing and scratching of the skin may result in widespread prurigo nodularis lesions, outside of sites of light exposure. Management is directed at eliminating UVR exposure and treating the eczematous dermatitis with topical, intralesional, or systemic glucocorticoids and antipruritics. Thalidomide has been effective in treatment of prurigo nodularis lesions.

Porphyria cutanea tarda is a hepatic porphyria associated with photosensitivity. Underlying liver disorders are usually attributable to alcohol abuse, viral hepatitis, or HIV infection itself. The usual presentation of porphyria cutanea tarda is blistering on the dorsum of the hands with hyperpigmentation and hypertrichosis of the face;

FIGURE 226-2

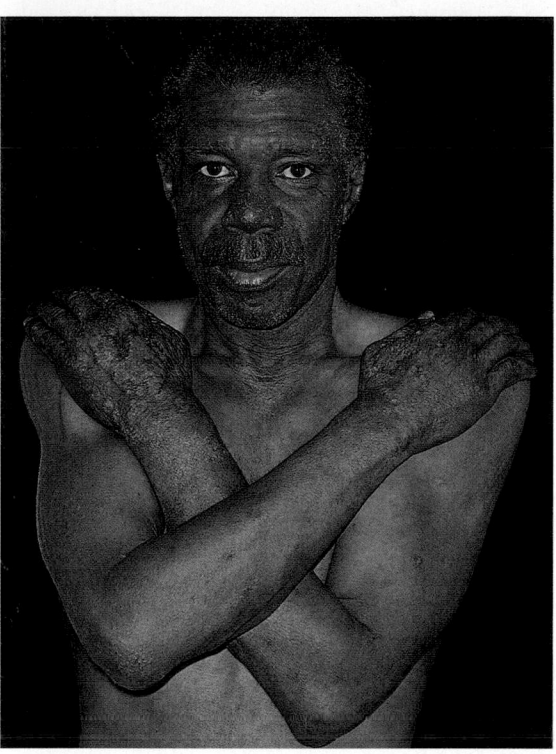

Chronic actinic dermatitis. Eczematous dermatitis and hyperpigmentation in the sun-exposed sites of the face, neck, and dorsum of the hands of a 50-year-old black male; no exogenous photosensitizing agents could be identified.

however, less commonly, a sclerotic or sclerodermatoid presentation with erythema and induration occurs on the dorsum of the hands.

OPPORTUNISTIC NEOPLASMS

The prevalence of the opportunistic neoplasms KS, human papillomavirus (HPV)-induced neoplasia (squamous intraepithelial lesion [SIL], squamous-cell carcinoma (SCC) in situ [SCC IS], invasive SCC of the cervix, external anogenitalia, and perineum), undifferentiated non-Hodgkin's B-cell lymphoma (NHL), and primary central nervous system lymphoma is increased in HIV disease.[36] The incidence of nonmelanoma skin cancer, HPV-induced invasive SCC of the cervix and anus, Hodgkin's lymphoma, T-cell lymphomas, and seminoma may also be increased. Many of these opportunistic neoplasms (NHL, KS, and anogenital in situ and invasive SCC) are associated with oncogenic human viruses and diminished immune-mediated tumor surveillance. HIV-1, through its regulatory protein tat, might also have a direct promoting effect on KS lesions, but it is not essential for their development. The significance of increased frequency of Burkitt's lymphoma and Epstein-Barr virus (EBV)-negative large-cell lymphoma in HIV-infected individuals, but not in immunosuppressed transplant patients, and the increased rate of testicular tumors in HIV-infected patients remains unclear and may indicate either a direct role of HIV or other cofactors. Opportunistic neoplasms may be more aggressive, may respond more poorly to treatment, and may be associated with higher rates of morbidity and mortality as compared with tumors in non-HIV-infected individuals.

Basal-Cell Carcinoma and Squamous-Cell Carcinoma

The prevalence of UVR-induced SCC and basal-cell carcinoma (BCC) appears to be increased in HIV disease, as it is in immunosuppressed renal transplant recipients. In a report from San Francisco,[37] 33 HIV-infected individuals with 97 SCCs were compared with 24 HIV-infected persons with 70 BCCs. Risk factors for the development of both types of carcinoma were fair skin and excessive sun exposure (>6 h per day during the previous 10 years). Those with SCCs tended to have outdoor occupations. SCCs occurred most commonly on the head and neck; BCC, on the trunk. SCCs were diagnosed more commonly in individuals with advanced HIV disease than were BCCs. Human papillomavirus was not an oncogenic factor in the development of these cutaneous tumors; however, p53 overexpression was hypothesized to play an etiologic role.

Clinically, nonmelanoma skin cancers occurring in HIV-infected individuals has the same appearance as in non-HIV-infected persons. Uncommonly, the biologic behavior of BCCs and SCCs may be quite aggressive, with rapid growth of primary lesions, extensive local recurrences, and distant metastasis. Response to therapy is in most cases the same as in the general population; however, aggressive SCCs and BCCs, both UVL- and HPV-induced, have been reported. Frequent follow-up examinations (every 4 to 6 months) for individuals with UVL-associated SCCs or BCCs is recommended, to detect recurrence of treated tumors or development of new lesions.

HIV-Associated Kaposi's Sarcoma (See Chap. 103)

T-Cell Lymphoma

Epidermotropic T-cell lymphoma has been described in HIV-infected individuals. Patients may present with patch, plaque, or tumor stage disease indistinguishable from that typical of mycosis fungoides, with nodular lesions and focal epidermotropism, or with exfoliative erythroderma with large numbers of circulating Sézary cells. HTLV-I serology has been negative in most individuals tested.[38] Immunophenotyping of the lymph nodes and skin infiltrates reveals a suppressor cell (CD8) predominance.

CUTANEOUS MANIFESTATIONS OF SYSTEMIC DISORDERS

Wasting Syndrome

Wasting characterized by weight loss, progressive loss of muscle mass, loss of subcutaneous fat, and severe fatigue occurs commonly in HIV disease. Etiologic factors include loss of appetite, malabsorptive diseases, enterocolitis, and metabolic changes and increased metabolism caused by the production of cytokines such as tumor necrosis factor-α and interleukin-6. Progressive weight loss occurring in HIV-infected sub-Saharan Africans ("slim disease")

has been attributed to *Cryptosporidium* enteritis and may cause death through progressive wasting before opportunistic infections or malignancies occur. Wasting syndrome, which is an AIDS-defining condition, is defined as a weight loss of ≥10 percent in the presence of diarrhea or fever for >30 days that is not attributable to a concurrent condition other than HIV infection itself.

In addition to the generalized loss of subcutaneous fat and muscle, a hollowed-out appearance of the face is common in HIV-infected individuals associated with loss of fat in the cheeks. Despite regain of lost weight, the cheeks often retain this sunken appearance (Fig. 226-3). Enlargement of the parotid glands, which is common in HIV-infected individuals, further accentuates the sunken appearance.

Lipohypertrophy of the upper midback area and neck (dorsocervical fat pad), neck, and preauricular cheeks is being observed more commonly (Fig. 226-4).[39] The clinical findings must be differentiated from the "buffalo hump" of Cushing's syndrome and from scleredema occurring in individuals with diabetes mellitus. The pathogenesis of this lipohypertrophy is uncertain. Although linked to therapy with protease inhibitors,[40] the finding also occurs in persons not treated with this class of antiretroviral agents. The abdominal girth can also enlarge because of accumulation of intra-abdominal fat and may be associated with abdominal fullness, distention, or bloating. The pathogenesis is uncertain but has been linked to treatment with the protease inhibitor indivavir.[41] Wasting syndrome has been treated with appetite stimulants such as megestrol acetate, marijuana derivatives (Marinol), anabolic steroids, and glucocorticoid replacement.

Porphyria Cutanea Tarda (See Chap. 151)

Porphyria cutanea tarda (PCT) occurs in HIV disease, often associated with an underlying hepatopathy and hepatitis C virus infection. HIV or an HIV-associated infectious agent may alter prophyrin metabolism directly, or indirectly by impairment of the cytochrome P-450–dependent mixed-function oxidase system, altering the liver's detoxifying ability and resulting in a heme abnormality. Factors associated with increased serum porphyrin levels include HIV infection, elevated alanine aminotransferase levels, and, to a lesser

FIGURE 226-3

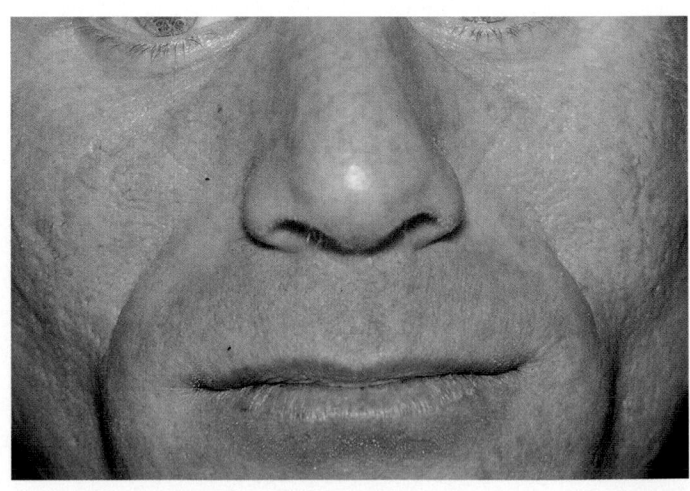

Lipoatrophy. The cheeks are hollowed, secondary to loss of subcutaneous fat, causing a significant cosmetic concern for the patient. The lipoatrophy remained in spite of a 20-lb weight gain.

FIGURE 226-4

CHAPTER 226
Cutaneous Manifestations of HIV Disease

2515

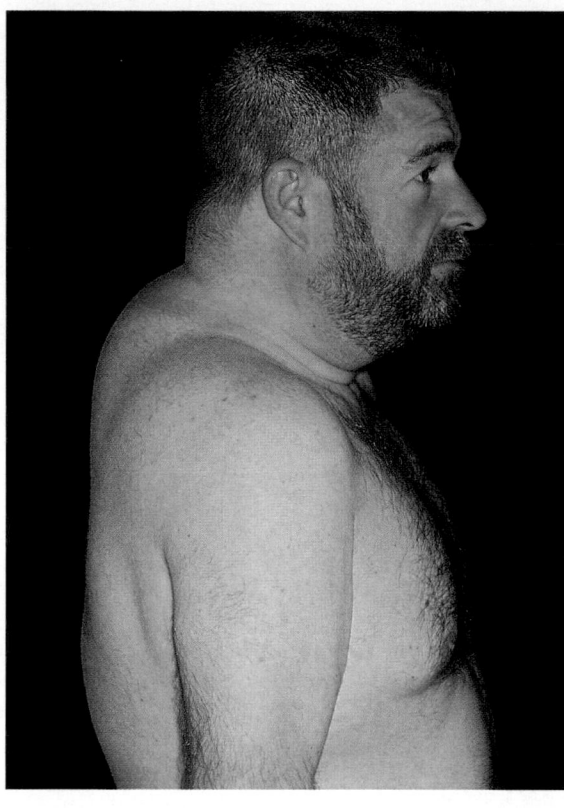

Lipohypertrophy. The subcutaneous fatty tissue of the cervicothoracic region as well as the preauricular cheeks and neck are strikingly enlarged in an otherwise thin male. Liposuction improved his appearance to some degree.

extent, hepatitis C virus infection. Hepatotoxic agents such as alcohol can facilitate the development of symptomatic PCT. In a report of porphyrin abnormalities in advanced HIV disease (33 patients), 40 percent of patients had increased urinary porphyrin excretion and all but 2 were seropositive for hepatitis C virus; 4 patients (12 percent) had urine and stool porphyrin excretion patterns that were classic for PCT.[42] No study patient, however, had clinical evidence of PCT. Porphyrin studies are recommended for HIV-infected individuals with photosensitivity. Some patients may exhibit coproporphyria secondary to underlying hepatic disease.

Thrombocytopenic Purpura

Both idiopathic thrombocytopenic purpura (ITP), characterized by diffuse bruising, petechiae, and hemorrhage, and thrombotic thrombocytopenic purpura have been reported in HIV disease, occasionally as the first manifestation of infection. ITP is treated with HAART, glucocorticoids, intravenous immunoglobulin, or splenectomy.

Vasculitis

Cutaneous (leukocytoclastic) and systemic vasculitis of many etiologies occur in HIV disease, including adverse cutaneous drug reactions, cytomegalovirus infection, polyarteritis nodosa, lymphomatoid granulomatosis, and possibly HIV infection itself.

DISORDERS OF THE OROPHARYNX

Nearly all HIV-infected individuals experience disorders of the oropharynx during the course of the disease.[43] Oropharyngeal disorders have been reported to be the first sign of HIV disease in 10 percent of cases, and their detection may be an indication for HIV serotesting.[44] In a study of oropharyngeal disorders (103 consecutive patients with late symptomatic and advanced HIV disease), candidiasis was the most common finding, diagnosed in more than 90 percent.[45] Other disorders of the lips and oropharynx included herpetic ulcers (10 percent), xerostomia (10 percent), exfoliative cheilitis (9 percent), oral hairy leukoplakia (7 percent), KS (4 percent), patchy depapillation of the tongue (6 percent), and ulcers of uncertain cause (3 percent). Other studies have reported similar oral disorders.

Oropharyngeal Candidiasis (See Candidiasis, below and Chap. 207)

Oral Hairy Leukoplakia) (See Chap. 114)

Epstein-Barr virus selectively infects cells of the B-lymphocyte lineage and certain types of squamous epithelium. The majority of adults have been infected with EBV and harbor the latent virus. With advancing immunodeficiency, EBV replication occurs with the resultant clinical manifestations of oral hairy leukoplakia (OHL),[46] classic Burkitt's lymphoma, and EBV-positive large-cell lymphoma. EBV DNA can be detected in the oral epithelium in HIV-infected patients without clinical signs of OHL, and its detection may be a marker for symptomatic HIV disease.[47] Whether OHL develops after reactivation of latent EBV or superinfection is uncertain.[48]

OHL is a lesion specific to HIV disease. OHL has been reported in up to 28 percent of HIV-infected patients and is more common in males.[49] In a study of OHL as a clinical marker of HIV disease progression, OHL was detected in 9 percent individuals 1 year after seroconversion, in 16 percent at 2 years, 15 percent at 3 years, 35 percent at 4 years, and 42 percent at 5 years.[50] The median CD4 cell count when OHL was first detected was 468/μL. In individuals without an AIDS-defining illness when OHL is first detected, the probability of developing AIDS (without HAART) has been reported to be 48 percent by 16 months after detection, and 83 percent by 31 months.[51] Persons with OHL and a history of hepatitis B virus infection have a fourfold risk for early progression to AIDS; those with syphilis have nearly a threefold risk for early AIDS diagnosis.[52] In a study of HIV-associated mucocutaneous disorders in 456 patients (1982–1992),[53] OHL was diagnosed in 16 percent of cases when the median CD4 cell count was 235/μL. Median survival time after OHL diagnosis was 20 months. In patients with a CD4 cell count of $\geq$300/μL, the detection of OHL was associated with shorter median survival time of 25 months as compared with 52 months in those without OHL.

Clinically, OHL presents as a hyperplastic, whitish epithelial plaque on the lateral tongue. Although described as "hairy," the most characteristic feature is a corrugation with parallel rows arranged nearly vertically, accentuations of the normal tongue ridges (Fig. 226-5). OHL may exist as a single lesion or as three to six discrete plaques separated by normal-appearing mucosa that are usually bilateral but not symmetrical. The most common location is the lateral surface of the tongue, frequently extending onto the

FIGURE 226-5

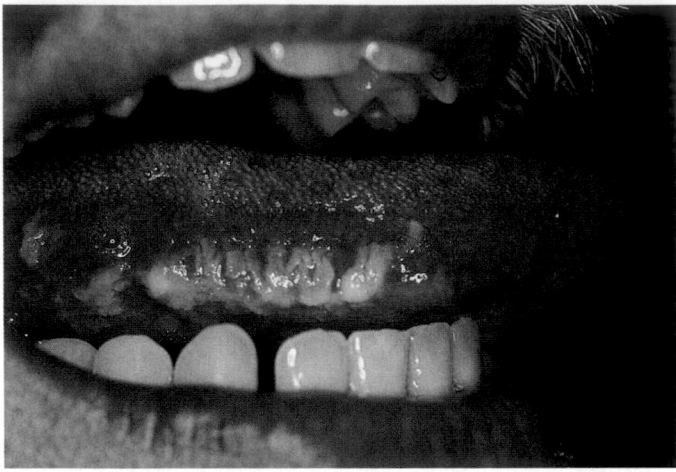

Oral hairy leukoplakia. White plaques with vertical corrugations on the inferolateral aspect of the tongue. The lesions are fixed, as compared with those of thrush, which can be brushed off with a gauze pad.

contiguous dorsal or ventral surfaces; the buccal mucosa and soft palate are much less commonly involved. The clinical appearance of OHL has been noted to change on a day-to-day basis. In comparison with pseudomembranous candidiasis, OHL cannot be removed by rubbing with gauze or resolved with anticandidal therapy.

The differential diagnosis includes hyperplastic oral candidiasis, HPV-induced neoplasia (condyloma acuminatum, SIL, in situ or invasive SCC), geographic tongue, lichen planus, tobacco-associated leukoplakia, mucous patch of secondary syphilis, and occlusive trauma. The histologic findings of OHL are acanthosis, marked parakeratosis with the formation of ridges and keratin projections, areas of ballooning cells resembling HPV-induced koilocytosis, and little or no dermal inflammatory reaction. Electron microscopy demonstrates 100-nm intranuclear virions and 240-nm encapsulated virus particles. Using in situ hybridization, EBV DNA can be demonstrated within nuclei in the upper portions of the epithelium. Keratinocytes are widely infected with EBV; however, expression of viral antigens and replication appears dependent on some process in the epithelial cell maturation-differentiation phase. The diagnosis of OHL is usually made on clinical findings; however, if the diagnosis is uncertain, confirmatory lesional biopsy is advised.

For the most part, OHL is asymptomatic, but its presence may be associated with some degree of anxiety. Patients should be reassured and advised that OHL is not thrush. With HAART, OHL usually resolves without additional interventions. In concerned patients with persistent lesions, topically applied podophyllin in benzoin is effective; recurrence within weeks to months is common. Acyclovir, valcyclovir, famciclovir, ganciclovir, or foscarnet, given for other indications, are often effective therapies for OHL.

Aphthous Ulcers (See Chap. 114)

Minor recurrent aphthous ulcerations (RAUs) are common in all populations, but they tend to occur more often and are larger in persons with advancing HIV-induced immunodeficiency. Major

RAUs are extremely painful ulcerations larger than 1.0 cm in diameter occurring in advanced HIV disease. Ulceration may be extensive, involving the tongue, gingiva, lips, and esophagus; associated odynophagia can be severe, resulting in rapid weight loss (Fig. 226-6).

Diagnosis of large RAU is usually made on clinical findings; however, large persistent ulcers should be biopsied to rule out SCC, lymphoma, herpetic ulcers, and deep fungal infections such as histoplasmosis or cryptococcosis. Ulceration of the gingiva must be differentiated from acute ulcerative necrotizing gingivitis. Lesional biopsy specimens show diffuse inflammation and necrosis affecting the epithelium, submucosa, muscle, and connective tissue.

Major RAUs are most commonly refractory to the usual topical treatments. Intralesional injection of triamcinolone (3 to 5 mg/mL, 0.25 to 0.5 mL) into the ulcer base is effective and safe. Prednisone, 70 mg tapered over 1 or 2 weeks, is very effective, giving prompt symptomatic relief with minimal risk of adverse events.[54] Thalidomide, 100 mg once or twice daily, is effective, with lesions healing within 1 to 2 weeks.[55] Recurrent RAU is common, and can be treated either with another short course of prednisone or thalidomide. Because of the major birth defects associated with thalidomide administration during pregnancy, female patients should be counseled on pregnancy prevention. Common side effects of thalidomide include sedation and constipation; long-term treatment can be complicated by peripheral neuropathy and leukopenia. Granulocyte-colony stimulating factor (G-CSF) (300 mg/day) has been reported to be effective for thalidomide-resistant RAU of the oropharynx and colon in a patient with neutropenia.[56]

Gingivitis

Acute necrotizing ulcerative gingivitis (Fig. 226-7) is a clinical marker for immunocompromise and HIV disease progression. The initial presentation is acute necrosis of the marginal gingiva with loss of the interdental papillae and marked pain. Unless the condition is adequately treated, rapid gingival recession, loss of peri-

FIGURE 226-6

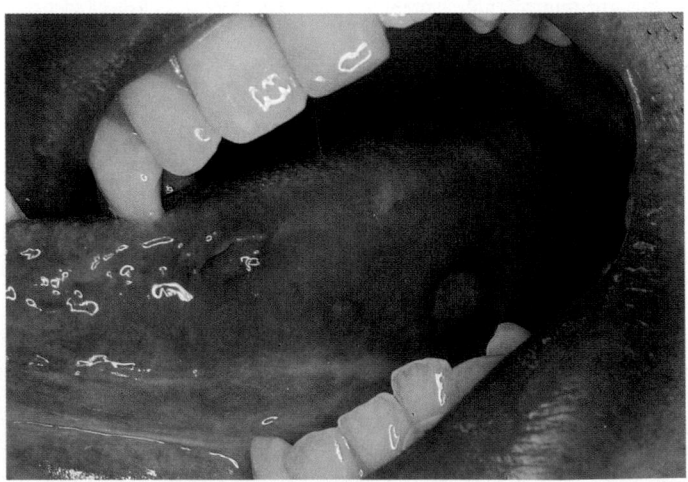

Aphthous ulcers, multiple, chronic. Three sharply marginated, very painful ulcers are seen on the inferior side of the tongue. The lesions had been present for 6 months, resulting in a 50-lb weight loss due to odynophagia, and was the presenting symptom of the patient's HIV disease. The lesions resolved within a few days after intralesional triamcinolone injection and a 1-week tapered course of prednisone.

FIGURE 226-7

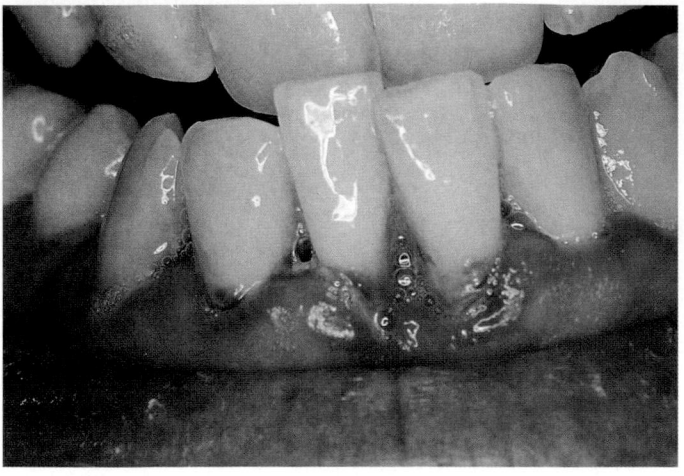

Acute necrotizing ulcerative gingivitis. The gingival margins are necrotic, ulcerated, and receding.

odontal attachment, destruction of alveolar bone, and, in some cases, exfoliation of teeth and necrotic bony sequestra may occur.

Neoplasms

Kaposi's sarcoma commonly occurs on the palate (Fig. 226-8), gingiva, and tongue. Untreated, KS can evolve into large nodular lesions and ulcerate (Fig. 226-8). Oral presentations of non-Hodgkin's lymphoma usually occur on the palate, gingiva, or tonsillar area (Fig. 226-9). HPV-induced SCC, both in situ and invasive, arises on the buccal mucosa (Fig. 226-10), tongue, and palate.

Miscellaneous Disorders

Enlargement of the major salivary glands, especially the parotids, is common, creating a rounded "chipmunk" facies, suggesting a better than actual nutritional status. Xerostomia can be caused by anticholinergic activity of drugs or by sicca-like syndrome. Sugar-containing topical anticandidal therapy (nystatin oral solution, clotrimazole troche), especially with underlying xerostomia, facilitates formation of dental caries. The most common cause of oropharyngeal hyperpigmentation is AZT therapy.

ADVERSE CUTANEOUS DRUG ERUPTIONS

The incidence of adverse cutaneous drug eruptions (ACDE) in response to a variety of drugs is high in HIV disease, and increases with advancing immunodeficiency (Table 226-6).[57] The most common offending agents are sulfonamides and amoxicillin-clavulanate. Although the pathogenesis of the high rates of ACDE in HIV disease is unknown, underlying infections with cytomegalovirus (CMV) or EBV may have a role, as occurs with reactivity to ampicillin and amoxicillin in patients with primary EBV or CMV mononucleosis. Other pathogenetic factors include immune dysregulation with increased B-cell activity with IgE and IgA hyperimmunoglobulinemia and hypereosinophilia.

In a report of 974 HIV-infected individuals followed for 46 months, 283 ACDEs occurred in 201 patients.[58] ACDEs were noted

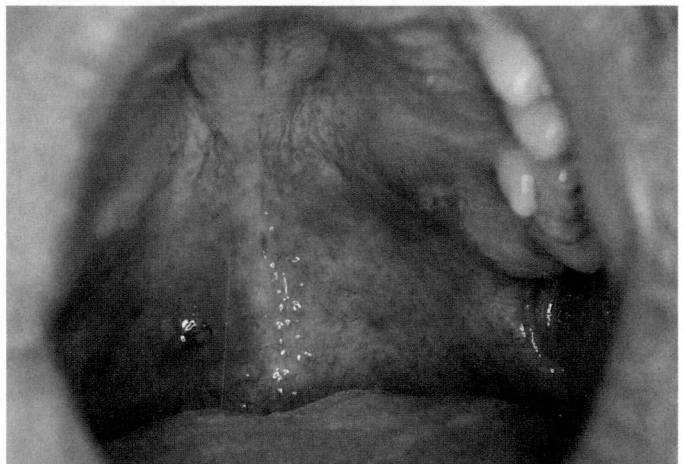

A.

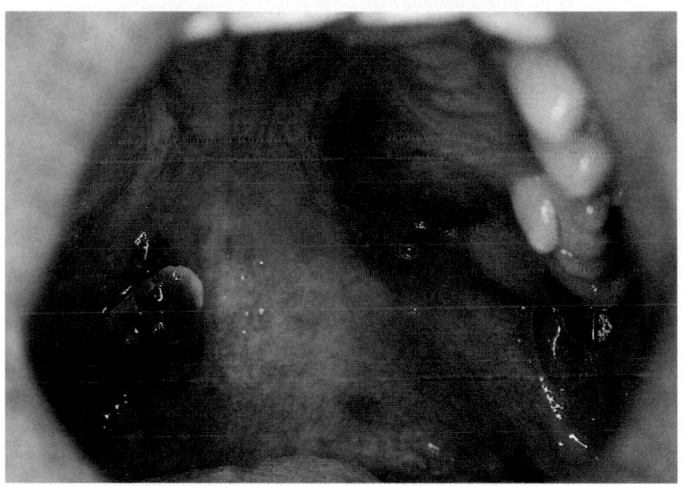

B.

Kaposi's sarcoma: palate. A. Two violaceous nodules are seen on the palate as well as several macular lesions. B. Several months later, the lesions had enlarged manyfold in size in spite of aggressive chemotherapy; the patient died within a few months of disseminated KS.

more commonly in white than in black patients. Acute or reactivated EBV or CMV infections were significantly more common in patients with ACDE. The onset of a majority of ACDE was within 6 to 14 days of the initiation of therapy. TMP-SMX, other sulfonamide drugs, and penicillins were the causative agents in three-quarters of ACDEs. Exanthematous eruptions occurred in 95 percent of cases; other ACDEs observed were urticaria, erythema multiforme, a lichenoid eruption, and fixed drug eruption. Systemic symptoms were reported in 20 percent of cases, including fever, headache, myalgia, and arthralgia.

Trimethoprim-Sulfamethoxazole

Used commonly for the treatment of and prophylaxis for PCP and toxoplasmosis, TMP-SMX is more effective than the alternatives, dapsone or aerosolized pentamidine. Fifty to 60 percent of HIV-

FIGURE 226-9

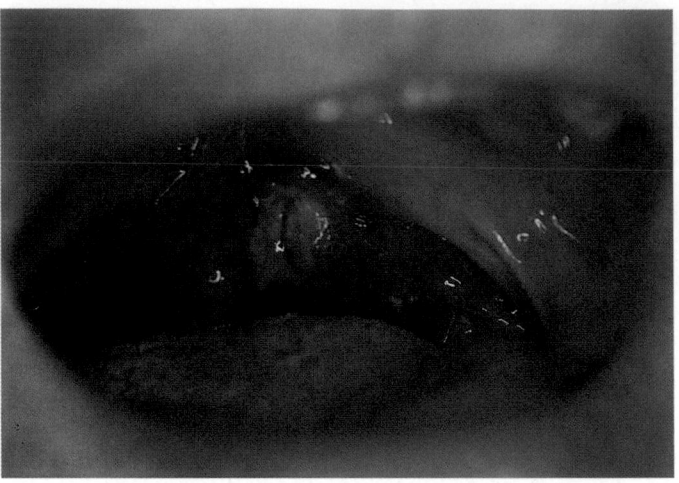

Non-Hodgkin's lymphoma: tonsil. The tonsil is infiltrated by lymphoma, which has caused necrosis and ulceration.

infected individuals treated with intravenous TMP-SMX have an exanthematous eruption (Fig. 226-11) associated with fever 1 to 2 weeks after starting therapy, 10 times more often than in the general population. Successful desensitization has been accomplished in patients with prior exanthematous or urticarial reactions to TMP-SMX, sulfadiazine, and dapsone. Desensitization in patients with prior Stevens-Johnson syndrome has also been reported.[59] Administration of glucocorticoids with TMP-SMX reduced the incidence of adverse cutaneous reactions from 47 percent to 13 percent.[60] The occurrence of adverse reactions to TMP-SMX has also been noted to be associated with more rapid decline in CD4 cell counts.[61]

FIGURE 226-10

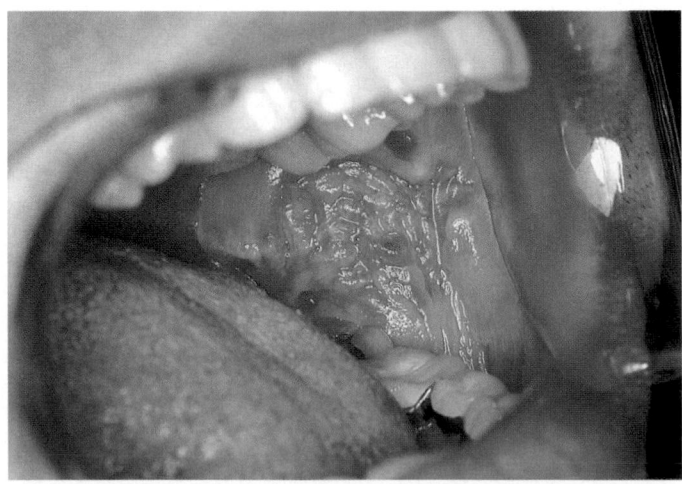

HPV-induced SCC IS. A white plaque covers the buccal mucosa; the involvement was bilateral. HPV-induced SCC IS was also present in the anus and perineum.

Severe bullous eruptions appear to be more common in HIV disease, with sulfa drugs as the most common causative agents.[62] The number of cases of toxic epidermal necrolysis (TEN) was 375 times that expected with a 21 percent mortality rate, which occurred in patients with advanced HIV disease.

Oral Glucocorticoids

Oral glucocorticoid therapy in HIV-infected individuals raises concerns regarding exacerbation of KS or HSV infections. A cohort of 44 asymptomatic HIV-infected individuals (200 to 799 CD4 cells/μL) were treated with oral prednisolone (0.5 mg/kg for 6 months; 0.3 mg/kg thereafter).[63] After 1 year of prednisolone therapy, no major side effects or HIV disease–related events had occurred. Serum p24 antigen and HIV RNA load levels remained stable; CD4 cell counts increased significantly at all time points (median increase at 1 year, 119 cells/μL). Oral glucocorticoid therapy for limited as well as prolonged periods of time appears to be relatively safe in most HIV-infected individuals.

Zidovudine

Although uncommon, adverse drug reactions have been linked to zidovudine AZT, including hyperpigmentation, acne, pruritus, urticaria, and leukocytoclastic vasculitis. Longitudinal melanonychia, brown-black longitudinal streaks in the nail plate (Fig. 226-12), occur in up to 40 percent of AZT-treated individuals, more commonly in blacks than in Latinos or whites. The pigmentary changes are usually noted in the fingernails and/or toenails within 4 to 8 weeks after initiation of AZT therapy but may occur as long as 1 year later. Increased melanogenesis occurs in the nail matrix, pigmentation beginning proximally, progressing distally to occasionally involve the free margin of the nail plate as the nail grows. AZT-pigmented macules of mucous membranes is also common, occurring more frequently in more heavily melanized individuals. Diffuse hyperpigmentation mimicking primary adrenal insufficiency has been reported.

Hypersensitivity to AZT, presenting with symptoms ranging from fever to anaphylaxis, is an uncommon complication of AZT therapy. Although infrequent, severe exanthematous eruptions have been noted in up to 1 percent of AZT-treated patients within 8 to 12 days following initiation of therapy. Successful desensitization has been accomplished in allergic individuals.

Foscarnet

Foscarnet (trisodium phosphonoformate) causes painful, penile erosions and/or ulcers in 30 percent of patients undergoing high-dose induction therapy for cytomegalovirus retinitis, 7 to 24 days after starting treatment. The ulcers are caused by high concentrations of the urinary metabolites of foscarnet. Hyperhydration reduces the risk of ulceration; in some cases, the drug must be discontinued for the ulcers to heal.

OPPORTUNISTIC INFECTIONS

Opportunistic infections of the skin and mucosa occurring in HIV disease, for the most part, represent overgrowth of resident flora (*Candida albicans*), extension beyond sites of colonization (dermatophytosis), reactivation of latent infection (human herpesvi-

TABLE 226-6

Adverse Cutaneous Drug Eruptions in HIV Disease

DRUG	INDICATION	ADVERSE CUTANEOUS DRUG ERUPTIONS
Trimethoprim-sulfamethoxazole (TMP-SMX)	PCP treatment PCP prophylaxis	Exanthematous eruption Erythema multiforme (EM) Toxic epidermal necrolysis (TEN)
Sulfonamides	Toxoplasmosis treatment Toxoplasmosis prophylaxis	Exanthematous eruption Stevens-Johnson syndrome Fixed drug reaction TEN
Dapsone	PCP treatment PCP prophylaxis	Exanthematous eruption Stevens-Johnson syndrome[*] Sulfone syndrome[†] (fever, rash, hemolytic anemia, fulminant hepatitis)
Pentamidine	PCP prophylaxis	Exanthematous eruption[‡][§]
Sulfadoxine-pyrimethamine (Fansidar)	PCP prophylaxis	EM TEN[‖]
Prednisone	Vasculitis PCP NHL	No significant adverse events after 1 yr[¶] Worsening of Kaposi's sarcoma
Methotrexate	Psoriasis	Worsening of Kaposi's sarcoma[*a]
Thalidomide	Aphthous ulcers	Rash[†a] Fever
Foscarnet	Acyclovir-resistant HSV, VZV, CMV	Erosion/ulcers on penis/scrotum[‡a][§a]

Zidovudine	Antiretroviral	Hyperpigmentation
		  Longitudinal nail streaks [‖a][¶a][*b]
		  Lips and oropharynx[†b]
		  Generalized hyperpigmentation
		Exanthematous eruption
		Urticaria
		Anaphylaxis
		Leukocytoclastic vasculitis[‡b]

Lamivudine	HIV infection	Paronychia[§b]
Nevirapine	HIV infection	Stevens-Johnson syndrome[¶b]
Protease inhibitors	HIV infection	Hyperglycemia or diabetes mellitus Lipohypertrophy
Indinavir	HIV infection	Generalized erythema, hypotension, fever[¶b]

[*]Pertel P, Hirschtick R: Adverse reactions to dapsone in persons infected with human immunodeficiency virus. *Clin Infect Dis* **18**:30, 1994
[†]Chalasani P et al: Dapsone therapy causing sulfone syndrome and lethal hepatic failure in an HIV-infected patient. *South Med J* **87**:1145, 1994
[‡]Berger TG et al: Aerosolized pentamidine and cutaneous findings. *Ann Intern Med* **110**:1035, 1989
[§]O'Brien JG et al: A 5-year retrospective review of adverse drug reactions and their risk factors in human immunodeficiency virus-infected patients who are receiving intravenous pentamidine therapy for *Pneumocystis carinii* pneumonia. *Clin Infect Dis* **24**:854, 1997
[‖]Raviglione MC et al: Fatal toxic epidermal necrolysis during prophylaxis with pyrimethamine and sulfadoxine in a human immunodeficiency virus-infected person. *Arch Intern Med* **148**:2683, 1988
[¶]Andrieu J-M et al: Sustained increases in CD4 cell counts in asymptomatic human immunodeficiency virus type 1-seropositive patients treated with prednisolone for 1 year. *J Infect Dis* **171**:523, 1995
[*a]Gill PS et al: Clinical effects of glucocorticoids on Kaposi's sarcoma related to the acquired immunodeficiency syndrome. *Ann Intern Med* **110**:937, 1989
[†a]Haslett P et al: Adverse reactions to thalidomide in patients infected with human immunodeficiency virus. *Clin Infect Dis* **24**:1223, 1997
[‡a]van der Pijl JW et al: Foscarnet and penile ulceration. *Lancet* **335**:286, 1990
[§a]Parry MF: Genital ulceration due to foscarnet: Case report and literature review. *Infect Dis Clin Pract* **3**:453, 1994
[‖a]Don PC et al: Nail dyschromia associated with zidovudine. *Ann Intern Med* **112**:145, 1990
[¶a]Prose NS et al: Disorders of the nails and hair associated with human immunodeficiency virus infection. *Int J Dermatol* **31**:453, 1992
[*b]Gallais V et al: Acral hyperpigmented macules and longitudinal melanonychia in AIDS patients. *Br J Dermatol* **126**:387, 1992
[†b]Greenberger RG, Berger TG: Nail and mucocutaneous hyperpigmentation with azidothymidine therapy. *J Am Acad Dermatol* **22**:237, 1990
[‡b]Torres RA et al: Zidovudine-induced leukocytoclastic vasculitis. *Arch Intern Med* **152**:850, 1992
[§b]Zerboni R et al: Lamivudine-induced paronychia. *Lancet* **351**:1256, 1998
[‖b]Warren KJ et al: Nevirapine-associated Stevens-Johnson syndrome. *Lancet* **351**:567, 1998
[¶b]Rijnders B, Kooman J: Severe allergic reaction after repeated exposure to indinavir. *Clin Infect Dis* **26**:523, 1998

ruses), transformation of subclinical to clinical infection (HPV, molluscum contagiosum virus).

In a report of 46 autopsied patients from the early part of the HIV epidemic (1983–1987), the following infections were noted sometime during the course of their illness: nonmycobacterial bacterial infections (83 percent), parasitic infections (73 percent), viral infections (67 percent), fungal infections (61 percent), and mycobacterial infections (26 percent).[64] *S. aureus* infections occurred in 54%, *Pseudomonas aeruginosa* infections in 15 percent, and enterococcal infections in 13 percent. Undiagnosed bacterial infections were noted in 26 percent of cases at time of autopsy. Nosocomial bacterial infections occurred three times more often in HIV-infected than in non-HIV-infected patients, with intravascular catheters being the most common sites of infection and sources of bacteremia.

The natural history of opportunistic infections in the developed world has changed during the past 5 years, attributable to HAART

FIGURE 226-11

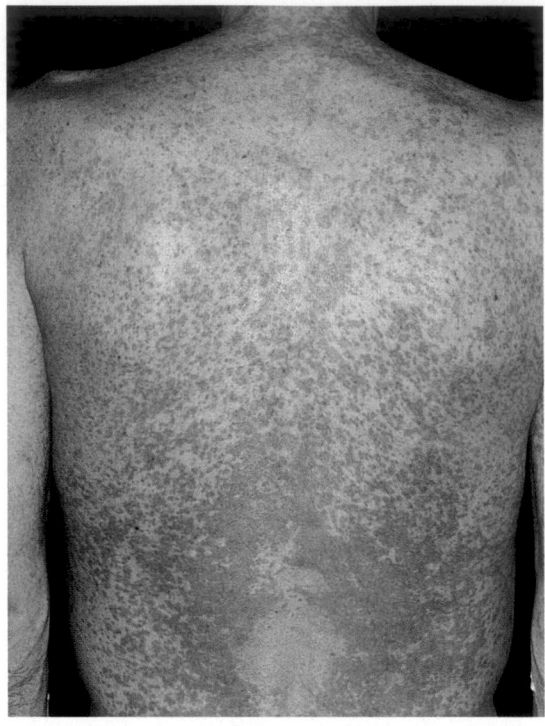

Adverse cutaneous drug eruption: trimethoprim-sulfamethoxazole. A typical exanthematous eruption occurred on the trunk on the 10th day after initiation of therapy with the drug.

and more effective therapies of infections. In individuals responding to HAART, the incidence of *Candida* esophagitis, herpes zoster, and KS has declined; opportunistic infections continue to be frequent but are occurring in more advanced HIV disease.[65]

FIGURE 226-12

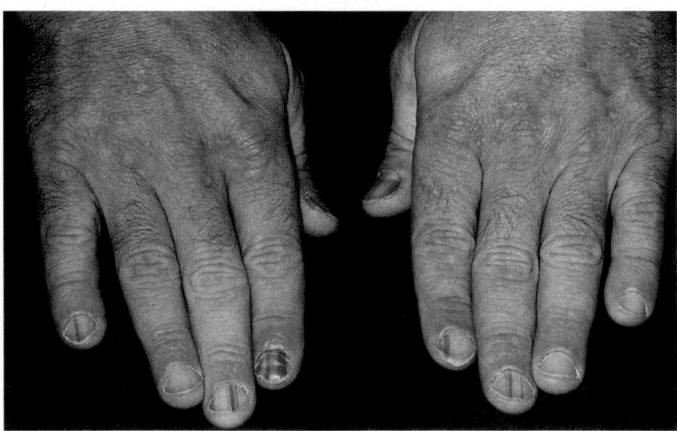

Adverse cutaneous drug eruption: zidovudine nail pigmentation. Longitudinal hyperpigmented brown bands on several fingernails.

BACTERIAL INFECTIONS

Bacterial infections occur commonly in HIV disease, the result of several factors associated with HIV-induced immunodeficiency. A compromised cell-mediated immune system (loss of CD4 cells and diminished cytokine production) and abnormal macrophage function result in loss of protection against some bacterial pathogens such as *Salmonella, Listeria,* and mycobacteria. Altered B-cell function results in reduced specific antibody production against encapsulated organisms such as *Streptococcus pneumoniae* and *Haemophilus influenzae.* Significant neutrophil dysfunction (impaired chemotaxis, phagocytosis, and bacterial killing) in late HIV disease results in functional "neutropenia," which may be combined with absolute neutropenia associated with drug toxicity (zidovudine, ganciclovir), bone marrow dysfunction, or bone marrow infections (*M. avium-intracellulare*).

Loss of integrity of the skin, oral mucosa, gastrointestinal mucosa, and tracheobronchial tree provides portals of entry for organisms into tissue and the bloodstream. Sites of placement of intravascular catheters, frequently used to treat infections such as CMV retinitis, often become colonized and infected by nosocomial pathogens such as methicillin-resistant *S. aureus* and antibiotic-resistant gram-negative rods.

Staphylococcus aureus

S. aureus is the most common bacterial pathogen causing cutaneous and systemic infections in HIV disease. An increased prevalence of *S. aureus* carriage in the nares and perineum has been noted in asymptomatic and symptomatic HIV-infected individuals (up to 50 percent).[66] Prophylaxis with agents such as TMP-SMX and clarithromycin is associated with a decreased nasal carrier rate as well as a reduced rate of infection.

Primary cutaneous infections or secondarily infected dermatoses or breaks in the epidermal integrity usually occur in chronic *S. aureus* carriers. No unique staphylococcal infections occur in HIV disease. Rather a wide range of *S. aureus* pyodermas and soft-tissue infections do occur, the incidence increasing with the degree of immunodeficiency. Primary staphylococcal infections include impetigo, bullous impetigo, and ecthyma; folliculitis, furuncles and carbuncles; cellulitis botryomycosis; and pyomyositis.

Secondary infection of underlying dermatoses and superinfections occur commonly in persons with chronic atopic (eczematous) dermatitis, which may be associated with elevated IgE levels, excoriations, herpetic ulcers, Kaposi's sarcoma, molluscum contagiosum, scabies, injection sites in injected-drug users, and intertrigo.

Staphylococcal bacteremia may complicate either primary or secondary cutaneous infections (psoriasis or scabies); however, the most common site for hematogenous dissemination is the intravenous catheter. Other predisposing factors for staphylococcal bacteremia include injected-drug use, lymphedema secondary to KS, and neutropenia.

The staphylococcal toxin syndromes of nonmenstrual toxic shock syndrome, staphylococcal scalded skin syndrome, and a recalcitrant, erythematous, desquamating disorder associated with toxin-producing staphylococci have been reported.

As with the majority of infections in HIV disease, staphylococcal infections tend to be recurrent. Treatment (see Chap. 195) should be directed at the acute infection, eradication of any underlying dermatoses, eradication of nasal carriage of *S. aureus* with mupirocin (pseudomonic acid) ointment, and chronic oral prophylaxis for recurrent infections. Infection with methicillin-resistant *S. aureus* (MRSA) has been reported and should be treated with appropriate antibiotics. Topical or systemic glucocorticoids may be indicated to treat eczematous dermatitis associated with staphylococcal infection.

Intravascular Catheter–Related Infections

Intravascular catheter–related infections arising along the tunnel created by the device and within its lumen occur commonly, often necessitating removal of the device. The most common etiologic agent is *S. aureus;* however, a number of organisms have been reported to cause infection, including *P. aeruginosa, C. albicans,* and *Stomatococcus mucilaginosus.* Patients may present with fever, phlebitis, a new cardiac murmur, or local tenderness at the insertion site. The infecting agent can be isolated from the catheter and/or blood culture.

Pseudomonas aeruginosa

P. aeruginosa causes primary infections such as cellulitis (i.e., ecthyma gangrenosum), malignant otitis media, infection at catheter sites, and secondary infection of underlying disorders such as molluscum contagiosum and KS in advanced HIV disease.[67] Cutaneous *P. aeruginosa* infection occurs via local invasion, gaining entry through breaks in the skin or by primary infection of skin appendages in the anogenital or axillary regions, or by hematogenous dissemination to the skin. Cutaneous pseudomonal infection may extend into the bloodstream, with resultant bacteremia and seeding of many organ systems. In a report of 73 episodes of community-acquired *P. aeruginosa* infections, 62 percent of cases were bacteremic, associated with central-line catheters and soft-tissue infections as well as pneumonitis and urinary tract infections; the overall mortality rate attributable to pseudomonal infection was 22 percent.

Compresses moistened with 5 percent acetic acid (white vinegar) are effective in treatment of superficially infected lesions such as ulcerated and/or hyperkeratotic KS on the lower legs, feet, and webspaces. Oral administration of ciprofloxacin is recommended for treatment of nonbacteremic pseudomonal infection; intravenous administration with agents such as imipenem are indicated for invasive infections. As with other infections in HIV disease, pseudomonal infections tend to recur. Invasive pseudomonal infections usually have a poor prognosis, with high rates of morbidity and mortality.

Mycobacterium tuberculosis (See Chap. 201)

In developing countries, tuberculosis is the most common opportunistic infection in HIV disease; however, cutaneous tuberculosis is relatively uncommon. As has been true in the past, most cases of symptomatic tuberculosis represent reactivation of latent infection. In non-HIV-infected persons who have tuberculosis in some form, the incidence of extrapulmonary tuberculosis is 15 percent; in HIV disease, 20 percent to 40 percent. In advanced HIV disease, the incidence of extrapulmonary disease increases to 70 percent.

The etiologic agents of human tuberculosis include *M. tuberculosis, M. bovis,* and occasionally bacillus Calmette-Guérin (BCG). Cutaneous tuberculosis is highly variable in its clinical presentation. Cutaneous tuberculosis occurs following *M. tuberculosis* exposure to an exogenous source, or by autoinoculation or endogenous spread from another site. Modes of endogenous spread to skin include direct extension from underlying tuberculous infection, i.e., lymphadenitis or tuberculosis of bones and joints results in scrofuloderma;

lymphatic spread to skin results in lupus vulgaris; hematogenous dissemination results in either acute miliary tuberculosis,[68] lupus vulgaris, or metastatic tuberculosis abscess. In HIV-infected individuals, prior BCG immunization can be followed by reactivation of and infection by BCG at the site of immunization, dissemination of BCG, or lymphadenitis.

Mycobacteria other than tuberculosis, also known as environmental mycobacteria (*M. chelonae, M. fortuitum, M. kansasii, M. malmonense, M. gordonae,* and *M. marinum*) have been reported to cause cutaneous lesions in HIV disease. The most common of these agents in advanced HIV disease is *M. avium-intracellulare complex* (MAC), however, this rarely presents with cutaneous infection.[69] Cutaneous MAC infections are usually complications of disseminated disease; lesions vary from papules, nodules, pustules, and soft-tissue abscesses to ulcerations; localized infection without apparent disseminated infection has been reported.[70] Cutaneous ulcerations have occurred at the sites of underlying MAC-associated lymphadenitis. Subcutaneous abscesses and ulcers due to localized MAC infection have also been described.

Interpretation of isolation of MAC and/or demonstration of acid-fast bacilli in skin biopsy specimens from patients with advanced HIV disease is difficult in that approximately 40 percent have MAC bacteremia. MAC can be detected within lesional skin biopsy specimens from lesions such as KS, but in most circumstances the presence of MAC is incidental, having no part in the pathogenesis of the cutaneous lesion. Following incision and drainage or spontaneous rupture, scrofuloderma occurred with the formation of deep ulcerative lesions; resolution occurred after a short course of routine antituberculous therapy. Subcutaneous masses can also represent underlying osteomyelitis.

Cutaneous *M. haemophilum* infection has been reported to induce erythema, swelling, painful nodules, and abscess formation and disseminated cutaneous lesions (Fig. 226-13) in patients with advanced HIV disease, with systemic involvement of bones, joints, lymphatics, and lungs.[71] Recovery of *M. haemophilum* requires a high level of clinical suspicion and special handling of mycobacterial cultures by the microbiology laboratory, including cultivation on enriched chocolate agar or heme-supplemented media and incubation at 30°C for up to 8 weeks. Response to antimycobacterial therapy has been poor; disease tends to recur and progress.

Mycobacterium leprae (See Chap. 203)

The interrelationship of *M. leprae* and HIV in dually infected persons has not been adequately studied to date. Tropical areas such as Africa and India that have a high prevalence of leprosy are expected to bear the brunt of the HIV epidemic during the next decade. It is probable that leprosy will accelerate the course of HIV disease, and that HIV infection will result in a higher ratio of cases of lepromatous versus tuberculoid leprosy and resistance to antilepromatous therapy.

The natural history of leprosy in HIV disease has been reported in 275 patients from Haiti; 6.5 percent of the entire cohort was HIV-seropositive. No difference in HIV seropositivity was detected in patients with either lepromatous or tuberculoid types of leprosy. Of the HIV-seropositive patients, 22 percent developed new skin lesions and lepromin anergy during the course of dapsone/rifampin leprosy therapy, as compared with 0.8 percent of HIV-seronegative patients.

FIGURE 226-13

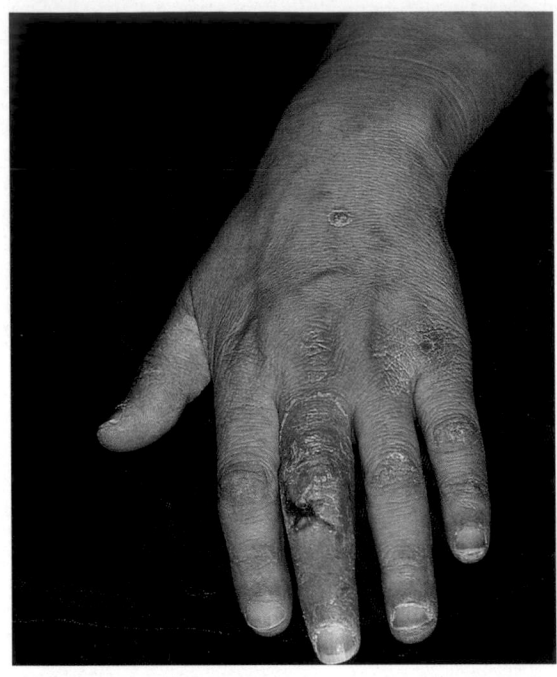

M. haemophilum: disseminated infection. A nodule on the wrist and enlargement of the middle finger were manifestations of hematogenous dissemination.

Bacillary Angiomatosis (See Chap. 199)

Bacillary angiomatosis (BA) and bacillary peliosis (BAP) occur most commonly in the setting of HIV-induced immunodeficiency, characterized by angioproliferative lesions resembling pyogenic granulomas or KS. BAP is caused by infection with fastidious gram-negative bacilli of the genus *Bartonella*—*Bartonella henselae* and *Bartonella quintana*. The vascular lesions are referred to as BA; those occurring in the liver or spleen, as peliosis. In immunocompetent individuals, *B. henselae* also causes cat scratch disease, which is characterized by granulomatous lymphadenitis. HIV-infected individuals with BAP usually have moderate to advanced disease; rarely, BA occurs in immunocompetent, non-HIV-infected individuals. The varied tissue response to *Bartonella* infection in the immunocompetent individual is analogous to the clinical patterns occurring in leprosy. Cat scratch disease or tuberculous leprosy develops in individuals with intact cellular immunity; BAP or lepromatous leprosy develops in those with impaired cellular immunity.

In a study of 49 individuals with BAP, 53 percent were infected with *B. henselae* and 47 percent were infected with *B. quintana*.[72] *B. henselae* and *B. quintana* were equally likely to cause cutaneous BA; only *B. henselae* was associated with hepatosplenic peliosis. Patients with *B. henselae* infection were epidemiologically linked to cat and flea exposure. Those with *B. quintana* infections were linked to low income, homelessness, and exposure to head or body lice. Prior treatment with macrolide (erythromycin, clarithromycin, azithromycin) antibiotics appeared to be protective against infection with either species.

The domestic cat serves as a major persistent reservoir for *B. henselae*. Cats experience prolonged, asymptomatic bacteremia,

and can transmit the infection to humans.[161] The cat flea is the vector of *B. henselae* among cats. The domestic cat, however, appears to be a major vector (by scratch or bite) from cat to humans. Antibiotic treatment of infected cats and control of flea infestation are potential strategies for decreasing exposure to *Bartonella*.

Whether asymptomatic or latent infection occurs in humans is not known. The incubation period is unknown, but is probably days to weeks. Patients with localized infection may be free of systemic symptoms. Cutaneous BA may be painful; in contrast, similar-appearing lesions of KS are usually not painful unless they are ulcerated or secondarily infected. Individuals with more widespread disseminated *Bartonella* infection often experience fever, malaise, and weight loss.

Clinically, the cutaneous lesions of BA are red-to-violaceous, dome-shaped papules, nodules (Fig. 226-14), or plaques resembling KS, ranging in size from a few mm up to 2 to 3 cm in diameter (dermal vascular lesions with thinned or eroded epidermis). Less commonly, domed subcutaneous masses occur without the characteristic red color of more superficial vascular lesions.[74] Lesions are soft-to-firm, and may be tender to palpation. The number of lesions ranges from solitary lesions to more than 100 and, rarely, more than 1000. Nearly any cutaneous site may be involved, but the palms, soles, and oral cavity are usually spared. Following hematogenous or lymphatic dissemination, the spectrum of internal disease caused by *B. henselae* and *B. quintana* includes soft-tissue masses, bone marrow, lymphadenopathy, splenomegaly, and hepatomegaly; internal involvement can occur with or without cutaneous lesions.

The differential diagnosis of the cutaneous papulonodular lesions includes KS, pyogenic granuloma, epithelioid (histiocytoid) angioma, cherry angioma, sclerosing hemangioma, angiokeratomas, and disseminated deep fungal infections. Subcutaneous BA nodules and tumor must be differentiated from enlarged lymph nodes and subcutaneous masses.

The histopathology of lesional skin biopsy specimens of BA is characterized by two patterns of lobular proliferations of capillaries and venules. Pyogenic granuloma–like lesions are characterized by proliferation of small round blood vessels with plump endothelial cells. The stroma is edematous and loose. The inflammatory infil-

FIGURE 226-14

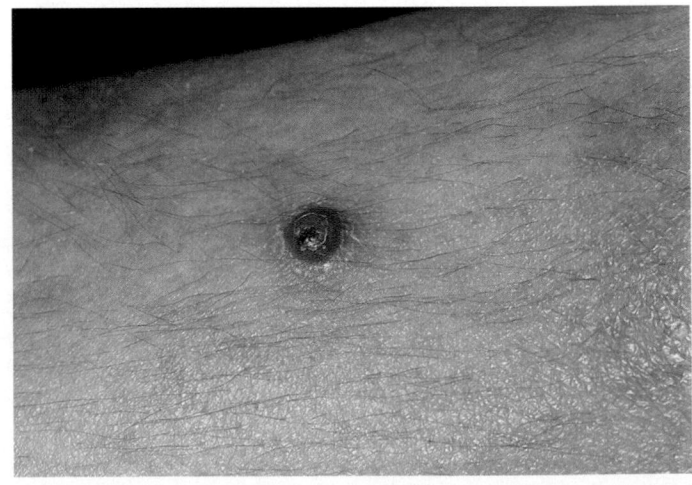

Bacillary angiomatosis. A vascular nodule of the shin was associated with disseminated small red papules and subcutaneous nodules in the inguinal areas bilaterally. The lesions appeared suddenly during a one-week period.

trate is composed of lymphocytes, histiocytes, and neutrophils. The overlying epidermis may show collarette formation, thinning, or ulceration. Few if any bacteria are visualized by silver stain. Lesions arising deeper in the dermis or subcutis appear more cellular, made up of myriad small, round blood vessels lined by plump endothelial cells. The inflammatory infiltrate is composed of neutrophils. The interstitium shows a granular amphophilic material. Abundant clusters of bacilli, corresponding to sites of granular material, are visualized by silver stain.

Percutaneous liver biopsy in patients with peliosis hepatis may be contraindicated because of the vascular nature of the lesions and the risk for uncontrolled bleeding. Histology of liver lesions shows blood-filled cysts with clusters of bacilli in the connective tissue rims of the cysts. The infecting *Bartonella* species can be identified by molecular techniques on tissue samples. Isolation of *Bartonella* is possible from lesional tissue biopsy specimens and/or blood. The diagnosis of BAP is usually made by the demonstration of pleomorphic bacilli on a Warthin-Starry or similar silver stain, or by electron microscopy, and confirmed by detection of anti-*Bartonella* antibodies.

The course of BA is variable. In some patients, lesions regress spontaneously. BA infection may spread hematogenously or via lymphatics to involve bone marrow, bone, spleen, and liver. Death may occur secondary to laryngeal obstruction, liver failure, or pulmonary infection. As with other opportunistic infections in HIV disease, BAP can recur.

BAP is preventable. *B. henselae* is contracted from cats; avoidance should prevent infection. *B. quintana* occurs among homeless people; infection can be prevented by improved hygiene. The antibiotics of choice are erythromycin, 250 to 500 mg PO qid, or doxycycline, 100 mg bid, continued until the lesions resolve, usually in 3 to 4 weeks. Secondary prophylaxis is indicated in patients with recurrent BAP.

FUNGAL INFECTIONS

Superficial Fungal Infections (Dermatomycoses)

Three groups of fungi colonize skin and mucosal sites of many individuals, and are capable of infecting epithelial sites. Dermatophytes infect keratinized structures, i.e., epidermis, nails, and hair. In HIV disease epidermal dermatophytosis can be extensive. Nail infections are commonly associated with tinea pedis, and may involve the proximal subungual nail, i.e., proximal subungual onychomycosis. *Candida* species are common causes of oropharyngeal and vulvovaginal infections in early symptomatic HIV disease, and esophageal candidiasis in advanced HIV disease. The incidence of *Candida* intertrigo appears to be somewhat increased in HIV disease; that of *Candida* paronychia and onychia of the fingers is increased. The incidence of *Pityrosporum* infection, i.e., pityriasis (tinea) versicolor, is probably not increased.

DERMATOPHYTOSES (See Chap. 206)

Although the frequency of dermatophyte infection in HIV disease appears to be no higher than in control groups, the severity and variability of presentation are increased in HIV disease. The inci-

dence of dermatophytoses has decreased during the past decade, inadvertently, in patients with mucosal candidiasis or cryptococcosis who are treated with oral azole antifungal drugs.

Epidermal dermatophytosis occurs most commonly on the feet but may occur at any epidermal site. Scaling erythematous plaques may be extensive, resembling psoriasis or eczema. Tinea facialis mimicking seborrheic dermatitis, and tinea manus and tinea pedis with marked hyperkeratosis, resembling keratoderma blennorrhagicum, and favus-like lesions have been reported.

Onychomycosis (tinea unguium) is common in HIV disease involving the toenails and fingernails. *Trichophyton rubrum* is the most commonly causative agent. Nail infections present clinically as distal and lateral subungual onychomycosis (DLSO) and PSO, which is nearly pathognomonic of HIV infection. In a study of 62 patients with onychomycosis and advanced HIV disease, 87.1 percent had involvement of the toenails, 8 percent of the fingernails, and 4.8 percent of both areas.[75] In 89 percent, the nail involvement was reported to be PSO. DLSO was found in only 3.2 percent of patients, and white superficial onychomycosis (caused by *T. mentagrophytes*) in 4.8 percent. Dermatophytes were the most commonly isolated fungus, *T. rubrum* accounting for 58 percent; *C. albicans* was isolated alone from the nails in 7 patients. PSO presents initially as a chalky white color of the proximal nail bed, more commonly of the toenails but also the fingernails. *T. rubrum* tracks proximally over the dorsal nail plate and infects the proximal nail bed. In time, the entire nail bed is infected, giving the nail a white color. In some cases, the nail matrix is infected and the nail plate is dystrophic.

Dermatophytic folliculitis has been reported to occur on the scalp and other hair-bearing sites, caused by dermatophytes such as *Microsporum canis* and other fungi such as *Scopulariopsis brevicaulis*, and may be associated with erythema, scaling, and alopecia. Complications of dermatophytic folliculitis include Majocchi's granuloma and abscess formation.

Dermatophyte infections in HIV disease are chronic and recurrent. In that many patients are taking oral imidazoles such as ketoconazole, fluconazole, or itraconazole for candidiasis or cryptococcosis, dermatophytoses are inadvertently treated and kept under control. Terbinafine is effective for treatment of dermatophytoses in HIV disease.

CANDIDIASIS (See Chap. 207)

Oropharyngeal candidiasis (OPC) associated with PCP in young homosexual men marked the advent of the HIV epidemic. OPC occurs in the majority of HIV-infected individuals during the natural course of HIV disease as a result of impaired cell-mediated immunity. The oropharynx is the most common site of mucosal candidiasis, which may extend into the esophagus and/or tracheobronchial tree in advanced HIV disease. Candidal vulvovaginitis (VVC) is common in HIV-infected women, and may be the first clinical expression of immunodeficiency. In contrast, *Candida* intertrigo, which is more common than mucosal candidiasis in the normal host, is uncommon in adults with HIV disease. In the 1990s, a diagnosis of oropharyngeal candidiasis in the absence of predisposing local or systemic causes should always raise the issue of HIV serotesting.

Candida colonization of the oropharynx is common in HIV-infected individuals.[76] In a study of HIV-infected outpatients (median CD4 cell count 113/μL), *Candida* species were isolated from the oral swabs in 60 percent of individuals, in the absence of any clinical findings of thrush.[77] *C. albicans* was the most prevalent colonizing species isolated from each individual. Five other species were also isolated, 22 percent of patients were colonized with two different *Candida* species. Isolation of non-*albicans* species alone correlated with advanced HIV diseases with very low CD4 cell counts.

Oropharyngeal candidiasis is a marker of HIV disease progression.[78] In a study of the onset of oropharyngeal candidiasis following documented dates of HIV seroconversion, candidiasis was noted in 4 percent at 1 year after seroconversion, 8 percent at 2 years, 15 percent at 3 years, 18 percent at 4 years, 26 percent at 5 years; the median CD4 cell count was 392/μL when OPC was first detected.

OPC and esophageal candidiasis (EC) have been reported to occur as manifestations of primary HIV infection. Esophageal candidiasis, an AIDS-defining condition, occurs only with advanced CD4 count reduction (<100/μL).

HIV-infected women with CD4 counts 200 to 500/μL had a 33 percent incidence of vaginal candidiasis (VC), and 44 percent if the CD4 count was <200/μL. In a study of 117 HIV-infected women, recurrent candidal vaginitis was the most common initial clinical manifestation of HIV disease (43 of 117 women).[79] In a study of HIV-infected women with vaginal symptoms, 62 percent were documented to have VC by isolation of *Candida* on culture as compared with 32 percent in non-HIV-infected women.[80] Oral and rectal *Candida* colonization was also more common in HIV-infected women. The time to recurrence of VC was significantly shorter in HIV-infected women than in controls and was correlated with severity of HIV-induced immunodepression. Other studies have failed to confirm an increased incidence of VC in HIV-infected women.

OPC is often asymptomatic. Patients may complain of a soreness or burning sensation in the mouth, sensitivity when eating spicy foods, and/or reduced or altered sense of taste. Patients with OPC may also have EC with associated retrosternal burning or odynophagia; however, symptomatic EC may occur in the absence of apparent OPC. OPC presents in four different patterns: atrophic (erythematous), pseudomembranous (thrush), hyperplastic, and as an angular cheilitis. Atrophic candidiasis appears as patches of erythema, most commonly in the vault of the mouth on the hard and/or soft palate, and is easily missed during physical examination. On the dorsal surface of the tongue, atrophic candidiasis appears as depapillated areas with a smooth red glossal mucosa. Pseudomembranous candidiasis or thrush presents as white curd-like colony of *Candida* present in the aerodigestive tract, e.g., oropharynx, esophagus, and/or tracheobronchial tree. The mucosa underlying the white colonies is usually inflamed and appears erythematous. Hyperplastic candidiasis occurs on the dorsum of the tongue, appearing as a white coating. Angular cheilitis is an intertrigo that occurs at the corners of the lips, usually with erythema but at times with a thrush-like membrane.

Documented EC and/or tracheopulmonary candidiasis in a known HIV-seropositive individual is an AIDS-defining condition; EC accounts for 15 percent of AIDS-defining illness in adults and children.[81] Esophagoscopy is advised to document EC in any patient who continues to have esophageal symptoms after adequate anticandidal therapy. In spite of a high prevalence of candidiasis in HIV-infected individuals, disseminated candidiasis is distinctly uncommon, probably because of B-cell activation and the presence of anticandidal protective antibody.

VVC presents as erythema, often with white caseous plaques involving both the vulva and vagina or either site alone, and often associated with a burning or itching sensation. The incidence of VVC and OPC was reduced in women treated with fluconazole, 200 mg daily, after a mean of 29 months; however, the risk of EC was not reduced.

The incidence of cutaneous candidiasis, i.e., *Candida* intertrigo, may be somewhat increased in HIV disease in adults. Fingernail chronic *Candida* paronychia with secondary nail dystrophy (onychia) is common in HIV-infected children.

Candidemia occurs in HIV-infected individuals undergoing total parenteral nutrition, intravenous antibiotic therapy through a central venous catheter, or cancer chemotherapy through a central venous catheter for over 90 days. In a study of HIV-infected children with fungemia, non–*C. albicans* species and *Torulopsis glabrata* were isolated relatively commonly.[82]

Management of mucosal candidiasis should be directed at control of symptomatic candidiasis, which may be followed by secondary prophylaxis. Prophylaxis with topical or systemic agents may be prescribed, primarily or secondarily; however, the risk of azole-resistance increases with usage. Topical treatments rely on high patient compliance in that they require administration 4 to 5 times daily, but they are usually preferred over systemic drugs for initial treatment. Agents for topical therapy of OPC include nystatin (suspension, tablets, pastilles), clotrimazole (troche), itraconazole solution, fluconazole solution, and amphotericin B solution. The imidazoles, ketoconazole (tablets), fluconazole (oral solution, tablets, IV solution), and itraconazole (capsules, oral solution) are available for systemic therapy. Terbinafine is an excellent agent for dermatophytoses, but not for candidal infections. OPC relapses in approximately 40 percent of cases within 4 weeks of discontinuing therapy. Secondary prophylaxis may be indicated in some cases.

EC is usually treated with systemic agents such as fluconazole or itraconazole; cases resistant to fluconazole may respond to itraconazole solution. Fluconazole-resistant candidiasis is defined as persistence of symptoms despite fluconazole administered as 200 mg per day for at least 10 to 14 days. Patients with fluconazole-resistant EC are reported to have had more episodes of EC treated with fluconazole as compared with controls (3.1 versus 1.8), lower mean CD4 cell counts (11/mL versus 71/mL), greater median durations of all antifungal therapy (419 versus 118 days), and greater median durations of systemic azole therapy (272 versus 14 days).[83] Patients with OPC and dysphagia are assumed to have EC, and empirical therapy is begun. If there is no clinical response, endoscopy is advised, with biopsy and cultures obtained to rule out coexisting pathogens or azole-resistant disease. In the cases of resistance to both fluconazole and itraconazole, amphotericin B is given. The EC relapse rate is 84 percent at 12 months if immune function is not improved.

As with most infections in HIV-infected individuals, secondary prophylaxis of OPC and EC is often indicated; however, development of fluconazole-resistant oropharyngeal and/or esophageal candidiasis occurs relatively frequently.[84] Patients taking fluconazole, 200/day, prophylactically experienced reduction in the frequency of cryptococcal infection, EC, and superficial fungal infection, especially those with CD4 cell counts of ≤50/μL; but not they did not experience reduction in the overall mortality rate.[85] Despite fluconazole efficacy in preventing fungal infections, daily routine prophylaxis is not recommended for all individuals with advanced HIV disease because of cost, possible emergence of drug-resistant candidiasis, and potential drug interactions.[86]

PITYROSPORUM INFECTION (See Chap. 207)

Pityrosporum ovale causes pityriasis (tinea) versicolor, pityrosporum folliculitis, and infection of intravascular catheters, and is thought to have a significant role in the pathogenesis of seborrheic dermatitis. The exact relationship of *P. ovale* to the pathogenesis of seborrheic dermatitis in HIV disease is unclear. In most patients with HIV disease and seborrheic dermatitis, the dermatosis is asymptomatic except for its cosmetic appearance. Clinically, seborrheic dermatitis appears as scaling and erythema in the hair-bearing areas such as the eyebrows, nasolabial folds, beard and mustache areas, retroauricular fold, scalp, chest, and pubic area. The main differential diagnosis is with epidermal dermatophytosis (tinea facialis), psoriasis, sebopsoriasis, and Reiter's syndrome. Histology of seborrheic dermatitis occurring in HIV disease differs from that of non-HIV-infected individuals, with added features of spotty keratinocytic necrosis, leukoexocytosis, and superficial perivascular infiltrate of plasma cells and neutrophils with leukocytoclasis. Seborrheic dermatitis in HIV disease remains relatively easy to control. Low-potency topical glucocorticoid or ketoconazole cream is usually effective; however, relapse occurs if treatment is discontinued.

Pityrosporum folliculitis is characterized by numerous pruritic follicular papules and/or pustules occurring on the upper trunk and proximal arms. KOH preparation of lesional scrapings shows yeast forms only in comparison to the spores and hyphal forms seen in pityriasis versicolor. *Pityrosporum* yeasts are also seen in hair follicles in lesional skin biopsy. Pityriasis versicolor can be very extensive, especially in HIV-infected patients living in tropical climates. Both *Pityrosporum* folliculitis and pityriasis versicolor respond to a 10- to 14-day oral course of oral azole drugs.

INVASIVE FUNGAL INFECTIONS (See Chap. 208)

Individuals living in, or having traveled to, geographic regions endemic for coccidioidomycosis, histoplasmosis, and penicilliosis often harbor latent pulmonary infection. Cryptococcosis and aspergillosis are ubiquitous throughout the world. The common scenario of invasive fungal infections (IFIs) in HIV disease is that of reactivated latent pulmonary infection, often with hematogenous dissemination to multiple organs, including the skin. In a report from early in the HIV epidemic, 4 percent of a cohort of HIV-infected individuals had disseminated histoplasmosis and 7 percent had disseminated cryptococcal infection. Cutaneous dissemination may be the presenting finding in IFI.

Lesional skin biopsy, cultured and processed for histology, is often diagnostic of IFI with cutaneous dissemination. A touch smear of the biopsy specimen is often helpful in identifying the fungal pathogen. Histologic sections show fungal pathogens with H&E stains, but often identification is improved with PAS or silver stains. The differential diagnosis of disseminated cutaneous lesions includes molluscum contagiosum, verruca vulgaris, disseminated herpes simplex virus (HSV) or varicella-zoster virus (VZV) infection, bacillary angiomatosis, and furunculosis.

The incidence of disseminated IFIs has decreased during the past decade because of the use of oral azoles to treat candidiasis and dermatophytoses and because of improved immune function related to HAART. IFIs are usually treated with amphotericin B. Itracon-

azole or fluconazole can be used in some cases for short-term therapy but they are usually used in secondary prophylaxis of IFIs.

CRYPTOCOCCOSIS

Cryptococcus neoformans is the second most common fungal opportunist (*C. albicans* is the most common), causing symptomatic cryptococcosis in up to 8.5 percent of HIV-infected individuals. Disseminated cryptococcosis is by far the most common life-threatening fungal infection in HIV disease. Cutaneous cryptococcosis occurs in 5 to 10 percent of individuals with disseminated infection.[87] Cutaneous involvement is essentially always associated with systemic infection, occurring in advanced HIV disease (CD4 cell count $<50/\mu L$). Skin lesions may occur weeks or many months before presentation.

Patients with central nervous system cryptococcosis may present with symptoms that may occur over a few days to several months of malaise, fever, headache, nausea, or vomiting, and with more-specific findings, including personality change, confusion, loss of memory, and symptoms of cranial nerve palsies. Cutaneous manifestations can present 2 to 6 weeks before signs of systemic infection.

Hematogenous dissemination of *Cr. neoformans* to the skin, which occurs in 5 to 10 percent of patients with disseminated infection, results in lesions of various morphologies which are, generally, asymptomatic. Cutaneous lesions occur most commonly on the head and neck (78 percent). The most common morphology of cutaneous cryptococcosis is of molluscum contagiosum–like lesions, i.e., umbilicated skin-colored or pink papules or nodules (54 percent) (Fig. 226-15). Other types of cutaneous lesions include pustules, cellulitis, ulceration, panniculitis, palpable purpura, subcutaneous abscesses, and vegetating plaques.[88,89] Lesions commonly occur on the face, but may be widespread. Oral nodules and ulcers also occur alone or with cutaneous lesions. The papules and nodules of cryptococcosis, ranging from solitary to greater than 100 in number, are usually skin-colored, with little if any inflammatory erythema, and they lack the central umbilication or keratotic plug characteristic of molluscum. Occasionally, crusting or ulceration occurs resembling lesions seen in herpes simplex virus infection. In black or Latino patients, they may be hypo- or hyperpigmented. Cryptococcal cellulitis presenting with a red, hot, tender plaque also occurs in immunodeficient hosts. Cutaneous cryptococcosis may occur in the absence of demonstrable fungal infection in the lung or meninges. Hematogenous dissemination of *Histoplasma capsulatum* or *Coccidioides immitis* can produce identical skin lesions on the face.

Diagnosis can be made by demonstration of cryptococcal yeast forms with H&E, PAS, or methenamine silver stain of the lesional biopsy specimens or of a touch preparation. Tzanck smears obtained by scraping the top of a lesion, placing the material on a glass slide, fixing with methyl alcohol, and staining with rapid Giemsa technique show multiple encapsulated and budding yeast. India ink preparation of lesional skin scraping can also be used to demonstrate encapsulated and budding yeast forms. *Cr. neoformans* can also be isolated on culture of the skin biopsy specimen. Histologically, all lesions revealed numerous encapsulated cryptococcal organisms.

FIGURE 226-15

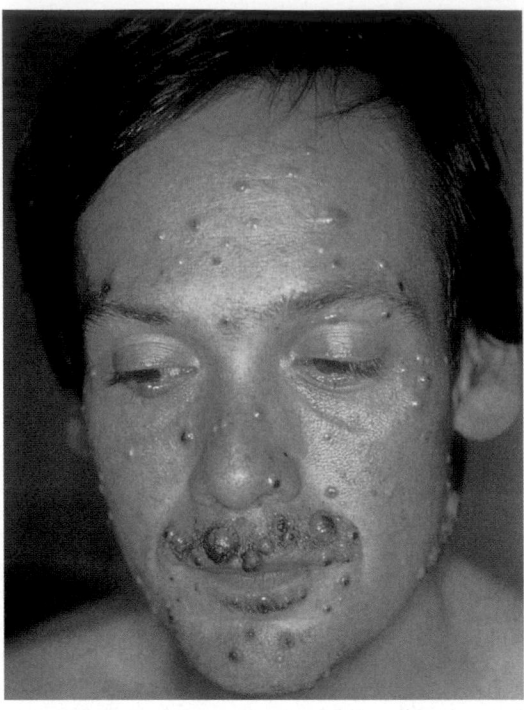

Disseminated cryptococcosis. Multiple skin-colored papules and nodules on the face. At first glance, the lesions mimic molluscum contagiosum, which is very common in advanced HIV disease.

Cryptococcal meningitis is treated with intravenous amphotericin B, which may be given with oral 5-flucytosine or fluconazole. The bone marrow toxicity of 5-flucytosine often precludes its use in HIV-infected patients, especially in patients receiving zidovudine. Cutaneous cryptococcal lesions resolve 2 to 4 weeks after beginning effective primary antifungal therapy, but relapses occur in over 50 percent of patients once primary induction therapy is stopped. Long-term prophylaxis with fluconazole is effective.

COCCIDIOIDOMYCOSIS

C. immitis is limited to the southwestern United States, Mexico, and Central and South America. Latent pulmonary infection may become active and disseminate in advanced HIV disease. Cutaneous lesions of disseminated coccidioidomycosis are usually asymptomatic, beginning as papules, evolving to pustules, plaques, or nodules with minimal surrounding erythema; lesions often resemble molluscum contagiosum. In time, lesions may enlarge and become confluent, with formation of abscess, multiple draining sinus tracts, ulcers, subcutaneous cellulitis, verrucous plaques, granulomatous nodules, and with healing, scars. The oropharynx is usually not involved. Lesional biopsy specimens show sporangia, hyphal forms, and arthroconidia. Disseminated coccidioidomycosis is diagnosed culturally by isolating the fungus from infected tissues. Serum complement fixation titers are often helpful in diagnosis, but may be negative in the setting of HIV disease.

HISTOPLASMOSIS

H. capsulatum is restricted to the Ohio and Mississippi River valleys, Virginia, and Maryland as well as parts of Central America; H. capsulatum var. duboisii occurs in Africa. In endemic geographic areas, e.g., Indiana, disseminated histoplasmosis is the leading opportunistic infection in HIV disease. In a report from Kansas City of HIV-infected individuals, the annual incidence of histoplasmosis was 4.7 percent.[90] The following were associated with an increased risk for histoplasmosis: a history of exposure to chicken coops, a positive base-line serology for complement-fixing antibodies to Histoplasma mycelium antigen, and a base line CD4 of <150/μL.

Disseminated histoplasmosis presents with a variety of cutaneous findings in approximately 10 percent of cases: erythematous macules; necrotic or keratin-plugged molluscum contagiosum–like papules and nodules; pustules, folliculitis, acneform lesions, a rosacea-like eruption, guttate psoriasis-like eruption; ulcers; vegetative plaques; or panniculitis.[91] Several different morphologic lesions may occur on a patient. Lesions occur most commonly on the face, followed by the extremities and trunk. Oral mucosal lesions include nodules and vegetations; ulceration occurs on the soft palate, oropharynx, epiglottis, and nasal vestibule. A subtle, widespread, exanthematous or psoriasiform eruption may occasionally develop in HIV-infected patients already on systemic antifungal therapy, in whom systemic symptoms are completely lacking. Hepatosplenomegaly and/or lymphadenopathy occurs commonly in patients with disseminated histoplasmosis.

Initial induction treatment with intravenous amphotericin, oral itraconazole, or fluconazole is given at a higher dose, followed by oral therapy for up to 8 weeks. Secondary (maintenance) therapy with daily oral itraconazole or fluconazole or weekly amphotericin B infusion is given for one year or longer.

SPOROTRICHOSIS

Sporotrix schenkii is ubiquitous in the environment in rotting organic matter. Percutaneous inoculation results in limited forms of cutaneous sporotrichosis; in HIV disease, dissemination of local infection to other organs occurs from lung or skin foci. A range of cutaneous lesions includes papules-to-nodules, which may become eroded, ulcerated, crusted, or hyperkeratotic (Fig. 226-16). Individual lesions may remain discrete or become confluent. Lesions are often disseminated, but spare the palms soles, and oral mucosa. Ocular involvement results in hypopyon, scleral perforation, and prolapse of the uvea. Joint infection with frank arthritis is also common in the disseminated form of sporotrichosis occurring in HIV disease. Other organs involved in disseminated sporotrichosis in HIV disease include joints, lung, liver, spleen, intestine, and meninges.

BLASTOMYCOSIS

Blastomyces dermatitidis, which is limited to the midwestern and south-central United States, has rarely caused infection in HIV disease, presenting as localized pulmonary infection, or as disseminated or extrapulmonary disease. Crusted papular facial lesions occur in disseminated blastomycosis.

FIGURE 226-16

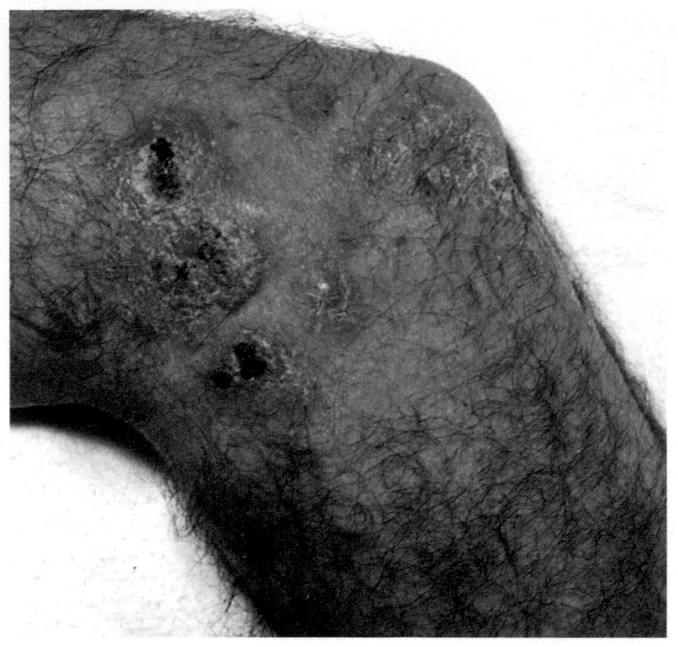

Disseminated sporotrichosis. Multiple crusted ulcers and eroded nodules; the cutaneous lesions were disseminated.

ASPERGILLOSIS

Invasive aspergillosis is rare in HIV diseases, presenting as primary cutaneous infection, occurring under adhesive tape near central venous catheters, or as disseminated infection. Risk factors for invasive aspergillosis in HIV disease included leukopenia and therapy with glucocorticoids, broad-spectrum antibiotics, and antineoplastic agents. Skin lesions appear as skin-colored to pink umbilicated papules resembling molluscum contagiosum. The majority of patients with invasive disseminated aspergillosis die, despite treatment with amphotericin B.

PENICILLIOSIS

The dimorphic fungus *Penicillium marneffei* is the third most common opportunistic infection in HIV-infected residents of countries of Southeast Asia and the southern part of China.[92] In a report of 92 patients,[93] the clinical presentation included fever, weight loss, cough, anemia, and disseminated papular skin lesions (71 percent). The most common skin lesions were umbilicated papules, occurring most frequently on the face, pinnae, upper trunk, and arms. Genital ulcers were also reported, ranging in size from <1 cm to 3 cm in diameter. Oral lesions included papules and ulcers. *P. marneffei* preferentially disseminates to lung and liver as well.

OPPORTUNISTIC VIRAL INFECTIONS

Viruses are major pathogens causing OIs in HIV disease, many of which are manifested at mucocutaneous sites, ranging from cosmetically disfiguring facial molluscum contagiosum to extensive common or genital warts to life-threatening or invasive HPV-induced SCC. In the great majority of cases, viral OIs in HIV disease represent reactivation of latent viral infection, i.e., herpes family of viruses, or of subclinical infection with HPV or MCV. The effect of coinfection of human T lymphotropic virus type I and HIV is not yet determined.

Measles (See Chap. 211)

Measles had been uncommon in the industrialized nations because of childhood immunization; in Third World countries such as in Africa, measles is common and is associated with significant rates of morbidity and mortality. In the United States, focal epidemics have occurred due to failure of immunization. Measles occurring in the setting of HIV disease in unvaccinated persons has high morbidity and mortality rates. The immunogenicity of measles vaccine in children with HIV infection is low, with antibody developing in only 25 percent of immunized HIV-infected children. Clinically, measles occurring in HIV disease may be atypical with prolonged period of rash or absence of exanthem or enanthem. Diagnosis of measles is usually made on clinical findings; however, in cases in which the exanthem is atypical, documentation of seroconversion is helpful. In some cases, seroconversion does not occur due to abnormal B cell function; lesional skin biopsy is helpful, showing multinucleated keratinocytes. Children who develop measles may have severe or occasionally fatal infection.

Herpetoviridae (Human Herpesviruses)

Human herpesviruses (HHVs) share the biological property of being able to establish latency and to cause recurrent infection. Reactivated HHV infection can be particularly severe in individuals with advanced immunodeficiency, resulting in chronic persistent disease, and in some cases, life-threatening disease. Reactivated HHV infections may contribute to increased HIV expression and potentially modify and accelerate the course of HIV disease. Acute or chronic infections caused by HSV and VZV are usually treated until lesions have resolved, secondary prophylaxis not usually being required. CMV infections, especially retinitis, may be devastating and require life-long prophylaxis.

HERPES SIMPLEX VIRUS TYPE 1 AND TYPE 2 INFECTIONS (See Chap. 215) In 1981, chronic perianal herpetic ulcers associated with a severe, previously undetected, acquired immunodeficiency were an early harbinger of the impending HIV epidemic. Genital herpes and other genital ulcerative diseases are risk factors for acquisition of HIV infection during sexual intercourse. The seroprevalence of HSV-2 infection in the United States, which is at an all time high of 20.8 percent (an increase of 30 percent since the onset of the HIV epidemic) is indicative of unprotected sexual intercourse and increased risk of HIV transmission. Reactivated latent HSV infection is one of the most common OIs in HIV disease. Reactivation of latent HSV infection has been documented to increase HIV plasma viral load level[94]; however, acyclovir use was not associated with prolonged survival.[95]

The majority of reactivated HSV infections in early HIV disease heal within 1 to 2 weeks with or without antiviral treatment. Intermittent asymptomatic shedding of HSV is common. In a report of patients with advanced HIV disease, HSV was isolated on periodic culture of the perianal region in 24 percent of patients in the absence of erosive or ulcerative lesions, even among those with no history of perianal HSV lesions.[96] Shedding was short-lived, intermittent, and not associated with early subsequent development of perianal ulcers.

Glucocorticoid therapy in HIV disease is a concern because of the possible risk of reactivation of HHV. In a report of patients treated with prednisone, the incidence of clinically active infections due to CMV, HSV, and VZV that occurred within a 30-day period of therapy was compared for each group; the median total dose of prednisone was 1600 mg.[97] No statistically significant differences between the cases and controls were detected in terms of the incidence of clinically active herpesvirus infections, i.e., CMV infection (2.5 percent versus 5.0 percent), HSV (1.6 percent versus 1.5 percent), and VZV (0 versus 0.3 percent). Only a CD4 cell count of $<50/\mu L$ was a significant risk factor for the development of any herpesvirus infection or for the development of a clinically active CMV infection. The risk of HHV infections was related to the stage of HIV infection and was not influenced by glucocorticoid therapy.

With increasing immunodeficiency, recurrent HSV infection may become persistent and progressive. Erosions occurring at the typical sites (perioral, anogenital, digital) enlarge and deepen into painful ulcers (Fig. 226-17). Oropharyngeal herpetic ulcers can occur alone or in association with lesions of the lip(s). Untreated, these ulcers may become confluent, forming large lesions. Herpetic infection of one or more fingers can form severely painful, large whitlows. HSV can be inoculated into nearly any site, including the ears and toes.[98] In addition to ulceration, chronic HSV infections can also present as proliferative lesions of the epidermis with or without scale. Herpetic ulcers on the buttocks, perineum (Fig. 226-18), and anus can be associated with painful intraanal or rectal HSV ulcerations. Genital herpetic ulcers are common. If left untreated in individuals with advanced HIV disease, the ulcers persist and enlarge. Hematogenous dissemination with visceral infection is rare. Large atrophic scars may follow healing of deep herpetic ulcers.

HSV from labial or oropharyngeal ulcers is swallowed in saliva, and can infect the esophageal epithelium, usually with very low

FIGURE 226-17

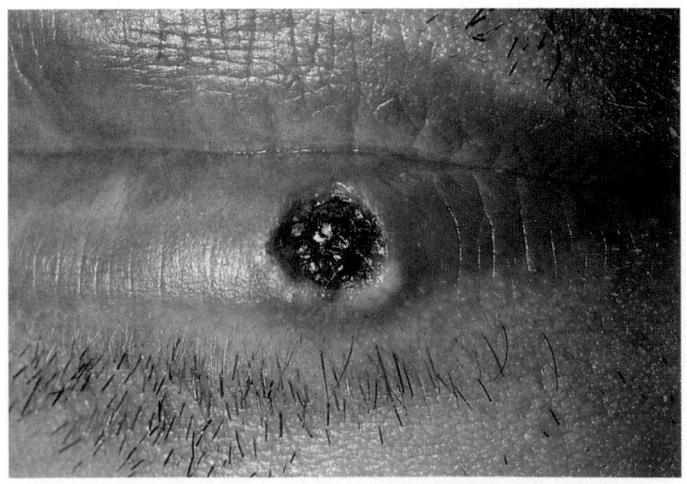

Herpes simplex virus infection: chronic herpetic ulcer of lip. A crusted ulceration has been present on the lip for 2 months, making it an AIDS-defining condition. The lesion resolved promptly with oral acyclovir.

FIGURE 226-18

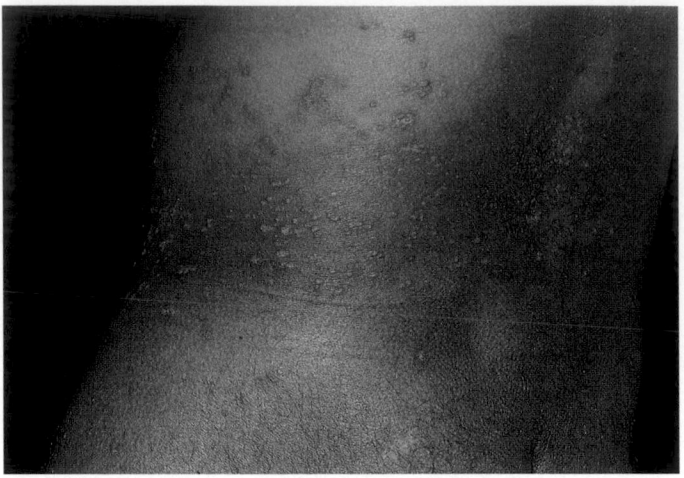

Herpes simplex virus infection: acute extensive ulcers. Large areas of ulcerations are seen on the perineum and buttocks. Although the lesions appear chronic, they had been present for only 1 week.

CD4 counts (<20 cells/μL). Esophageal herpetic ulcers present with odynophagia and/or chest pain.[99] Predisposing factors include nasogastric procedures, glucocorticoid therapy, and cancer chemotherapy. Extraesophageal herpetic lesions (labial, oropharyngeal) are present in one-third of patients with esophageal ulcers.

Herpetic ulcers must be considered in the differential diagnosis of any ulcerative or crusted lesion occurring in HIV disease, especially anogenital or facial. The differential diagnosis includes a wide category of infectious and noninfectious etiologies. HSV infections can be diagnosed by isolation of the virus or identification of HSV antigen in lesional smears or biopsy specimens. If indicated, the isolate can be tested for sensitivity to various antiviral agents. Histology shows multinucleated giant epidermal cells indicative of HSV or VZV infection. The Tzanck test, which looks for giant epithelial or adnexal cells, preferably multinucleated, in smears of lesional exudate, is useful but is not always positive even in frank herpetic lesions; its reliability is completely dependent on the skill of the microscopist. Lesional biopsy is helpful when giant epidermal cells are detected, but cannot distinguish HSV from VZV infection. The polymerase chain reaction can detect VZV and HSV DNA sequences from a variety of sources including formalin-fixed tissue specimens.

Herpetic lesions in early HIV disease usually heal without treatment. Currently, three drugs are available for therapy of HSV infections; famciclovir[100] and valaciclovir are absorbed much better than acyclvoir. These agents can be given to treat reactivated infection or to suppress reactivation. Intravenous acyclovir (5 mg/kg every 8 h) is usually given for severe infections. Foscarnet and cidofovir are administered intravenously for infections caused by acyclovir-resistant HSV. Cidofovir gel has been effective as a topical therapy of acyclovir-resistant HSV infections.[101] The use of long-term HSV suppression is controversial. The oral antiviral agents are indicated for frequently recurring HSV infection. Reactivation of HSV is known to increase the plasma HIV RNA viral load; some care givers recommend chronic HSV suppression for this indication.

VARICELLA-ZOSTER VIRUS INFECTIONS (See Chap. 216) Primary VZV infection is nearly always symptomatic (i.e., varicella or chickenpox)[102]; reactivated infection presents as herpes zoster (HZ). Children with HIV disease represent the largest reservoir of VZV-susceptible immunodeficient children in the world, numbering several million in Africa. Acute varicella does not appear to worsen the course of HIV infection with regard to CD4 or CD8 cell levels.

Varicella occurring in HIV-infected children and adults can be severe, prolonged,[103] and complicated by VZV dissemination (pneumonia, hepatitis, encephalitis, pancreatitis), bacterial superinfection, and death. Primary, recurrent, and persistent VZV infections are a frequent cause of morbidity and hospitalization for HIV-infected children. Rather than resolving, persistent crusted lesions can occur at sites of initial vesicle formation, lasting for weeks or months. In a report of HIV-infected children with varicella, the most common complication was recurrence of VZV infection in 53 percent of cases.[104] Sixty-one percent of children experienced HZ during the first episode of reactivated VZV infection; 32 percent had dissemination of HZ, associated with a low CD4 cell count. A second episode of varicella can occur, presumably following exposure to a different VZV strain than that which caused varicella initially. In a study of 30 cases of varicella in HIV-infected children, HZ developed in 27 percent an average of 1.9 years after varicella (range 0.8 to 3.7).[105] Children with CD4 cell levels of <15% at onset of varicella were at very high risk of reactivation. Recurrent HZ episodes developed in 50 percent of the children with HZ.

Herpes zoster can be the initial clinical presentation of HIV disease. Those who acquire HIV infection sexually are reported to experience HZ more commonly than with those who acquire it by IDU.[106] In a report from Kenya, 85 percent of patients 16 to 50 years old who presented with HZ were HIV-infected.[107] The duration of illness was longer in HIV-infected patients as compared with non-HIV-infected cases of HZ (32 versus 22 days). Seventy-four percent of HIV-infected individuals with HZ had generalized lymphadenopathy as compared with only 3 percent in the noninfected group. Severe pain (69 percent versus 39 percent), bacterial superinfection (15 percent versus 6 percent), more than one affected dermatome (38 percent versus 18 percent), and cranial nerve involvement were all more common in HIV-infected individuals with HZ. The mean CD4 cell count at presentation was $333/\mu L$ in the HIV-infected group and $777/\mu L$ in the HIV-negative group. Recovery was generally complete and uncomplicated. In Ethopia, 95 percent of patients (mean age, 35 years) with HZ ophthalmicus were reported to be HIV-infected.[108] Severe eyelid involvement occurred in 25 percent, ocular involvement in 78 percent, visual loss in 56 percent and postherpetic neuralgia in 55 percent. Severity of HZ ophthalmicus was associated with delay in presentation, lack of antiviral therapy, and advanced HIV disease.

In a report of homosexual men followed after HIV-1 seroconversion, 20 percent had an episode of HZ after a mean follow-up of 54 months; 10 percent of those experienced one recurrence.[109] In a report of patients with advanced HIV disease (CD4 cell count $<25/\mu L$) treated with zidovudine and HZ, 16 percent had a history of HZ on enrollment, and 13 percent of these had a recurrence during the 2-year follow-up.[110] HZ was not associated with a more rapid progression to AIDS.

Major complications of HZ occur in one-quarter of cases and include blindness (HZ ophthalmicus), neurologic complications, chronic cutaneous infection, postherpetic neuralgia, and bacterial superinfection, all of which occur more commonly if the CD4 cell count is $<200/\mu L$.

HZ is a clinical indicator of faltering immunity, and its occurrence should always raise the issue of HIV serotesting. The incidence of HZ in HIV disease is approximately 25 percent. In a cohort study of 287 homosexual men with well-defined dates of HIV seroconversion and 419 HIV-seronegative homosexual men, the in-

cidence of HZ was 15 times greater in HIV-seropositive men (29.4 cases/1000 person-years) than in HIV-seronegative men (2.0 cases/1000 person-years).[111] The overall age-adjusted relative risk was 16.9.

Zoster often occurs early in the course of HIV disease, and in children, it can occur soon after varicella. In several studies, HZ was not predictive of faster progression to advanced HIV disease. Extent of dermatomal involvement, severity of pain, and involvement of cranial or cervical dermatomes have been correlated with a poor outcome of HIV disease.

In a study of men with HZ, the incidence of first episode was 52 per person-year in HIV-infected men and 3.3 in non-HIV-infected men.[112] HZ recurred in 26 percent of HIV-infected men. The incidence of HZ increased by 31.2 per 1000 person-years at CD4 cell counts of $\geq500/\mu L$, 47.2 per 1000 person-years at CD4 cell counts of 200 to $499/\mu L$, and 97.5 per 1000 person-years at CD4 cell counts of $<200/\mu L$. The incidence of HZ increases with the decrease in CD4 cell counts and T-cell reactivity, but HZ is not an independent predictor of disease progression.

Clinically, HZ is typical in most cases. In advanced HIV disease, the spectrum of lesions is much wider. Solitary or a few ulcerations can occur. Epidermal proliferative lesions, either solitary or a few, resemble BCC or SCC.[113] Disseminated or zosteriform verrucous lesions also occur.[114]

In advanced HIV disease, VZV can also infect the neural tissue of the central nervous system (encephalitis), retina (acute retinal necrosis), or the spinal cord, with or without cutaneous lesions.[115] HZ precedes the onset of acute retinal necrosis by several days in 60 to 90 percent of cases.

In that zoster often occurs early in HIV disease, the course is fairly uneventful for the majority of patients. It is most often unidermatomal, but may be multidermatomal, recurrent within the same dermatome, or disseminated. The eruption may be bullous, hemorrhagic and/or necrotic, and accompanied by severe pain. The majority of HIV-infected patients with HZ experience an uneventful recovery, but atypical clinical courses are not uncommon. Limited cutaneous dissemination of zoster secondary to viremia is common in some patients with zoster, but uneventful recovery is the rule. Ophthalmic zoster has the highest incidence of serious complications, which include corneal ulceration, variable decrease of visual acuity, and retinal necrosis. Viral encephalitis can occur via entry into the brain by VZV infection of the optic nerve, or can follow hematogenous dissemination. Systemic dissemination of zoster with hepatitis, encephalitis, or pneumonitis is uncommon.

An uncommon, previously unreported complication of cutaneous VZV infection is VZV lesions that persist for months following either primary or reactivated VZV infection with a pattern of zoster or disseminated infection, referred to as chronic verrucous (Fig. 226-19) or ecthymatous (Fig. 226-20) VZV infection. Lesions may persist for months, either in the localized or disseminated form, appearing as hyperkeratotic, ulcerated, painful nodules often with central crusting and/or ulceration with a border of vesicles. A rare complication of zoster is the occurrence of a granulomatous vasculitis in the involved dermatome, without persistence of the VZV genome, possibly as a reaction to minute amounts of viral proteins.

The diagnosis of varicella and HZ can be confirmed by detection of viral antigen on a smear of the base of a vesicle or erosion or in a section of a lesional biopsy specimen. A positive Tzanck test confirms the diagnosis of either VZV or HSV. Isolation of VZV on culture is more difficult than isolation of HSV. Lesional biopsy is also helpful in establishing a diagnosis, especially in unusual man-

FIGURE 226-19

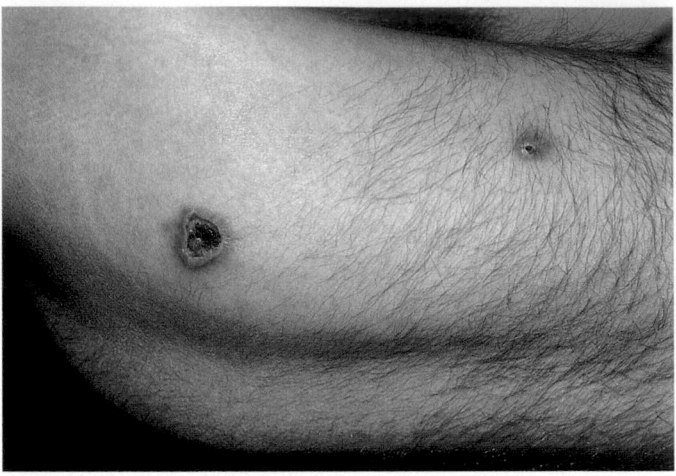

Varicella-zoster virus infection: ecthymatous lesions. Two ulcerated, crusted, painful ulcerations on the hip and lateral thigh had been present for 9 months. The lesions resolved with oral acyclovir therapy.

ifestations of VZV infection such as ecthymatous or chronic verrucous lesions; the diagnosis is confirmed by detection of VZV antigen.

Administration of varicella vaccine in early HIV disease in children appears safe and beneficial. HIV-infected children exposed to

FIGURE 226-20

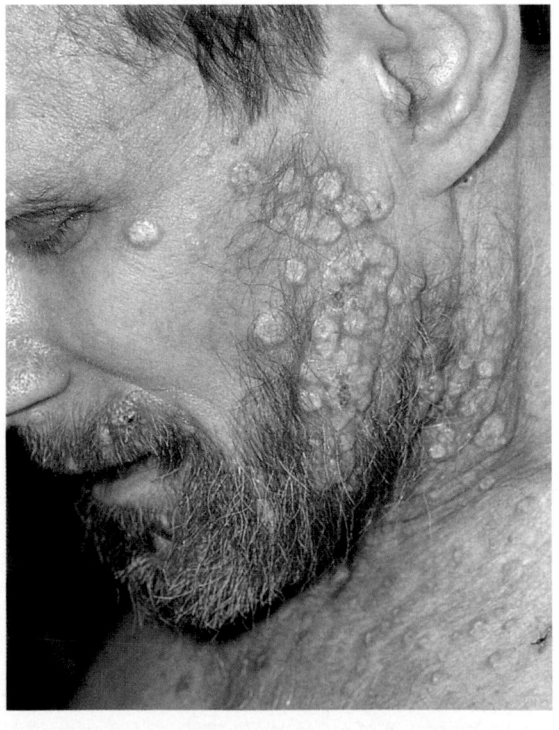

Molluscum contagiosum virus infection: Prior to HAART, multiple facial mollusca would enlarge to cause significant cosmetic disfigurement.

VZV, whether varicella or zoster, may benefit by treatment with varicella-zoster immune globulin prophylactically, as well as acyclovir. Most persons with zoster occurring in early HIV disease do well without antiviral therapy. The same drugs approved for treatment of HSV are approved for treatment of VZV infection: famciclovir, valaciclovir, and acyclovir. Intravenous acyclovir (10 mg/kg every 8 h) is given for severe infections. Because of the risk of visual impairment following ophthalmic zoster, intravenous acyclovir is usually given. As with HSV infections, acyclovir-resistant strains emerge following prolonged acyclovir treatment; most of these resistant strains respond to foscarnet therapy. Secondary prophylaxis is usually not indicated after VZV infection resolves.

CYTOMEGALOVIRUS (See Chap. 217) Seroprevalence studies of CMV infection indicate that nearly 100 percent of sexually active homosexual and bisexual males and injected-drug users are infected with CMV. Most cases of primary CMV infection are asymptomatic; following primary infection, CMV enters a latent phase of infection, during which asymptomatic viral shedding in saliva, semen, and/or urine is extremely common.

CMV is the most common viral pathogen in patients with advanced HIV-induced immunodeficiency. In a study of 82 HIV-1-seropositive persons, 51.7 percent of those with either AIDS-related complex (ARC) or AIDS had evidence of CMV infection of circulating polymorphonuclear cells, whereas no infection was detected among the 50 asymptomatic HIV-infected persons. Manifestations of CMV infection include retinitis, esophagitis, colitis, gastritis, hepatitis, and encephalitis. In a multicenter study of 1002 persons with AIDS or ARC, median survival after diagnosis of CMV disease was 173 days, and CMV was an independent predictor of death.[116] Disseminated CMV has been demonstrated in 93 percent of patients with AIDS; at autopsy, however, association with skin lesions was not reported. CMV reactivation and dissemination are common events as immunodeficiency worsens. As an opportunistic organism CMV commonly infects the retina, causing a sight-threatening retinitis, and the large intestine, causing colitis manifested by intractable diarrhea. Widespread infection is associated with a generalized wasting syndrome, pneumonitis, and encephalitis. CMV infection, although present within various organs as documented by viral culture, is not necessarily the cause of the tissue dysfunction.

Specific CMV-induced skin lesions have not been identified in HIV-infected individuals. Evidence for CMV infection in a variety of mucous membrane lesions, implied by specific cytopathic changes in biopsy specimens by light and electron microscopy, immunofluorescence, immunoperoxidase, and in situ hybridization techniques, has been reported; however, the role of CMV in the pathogenesis of the lesions is not certain. Perianal ulceration caused by CMV occurs as the infection spreads from contiguous gastrointestinal sites. CMV was considered to be the cause of perianal and oral ulceration in five patients with advanced disease, based on typical histologic changes and positive fluorescent monoclonal anti-CMV antibody studies. Empirical treatment with acyclovir failed, but all ulcers healed with either foscarnet or ganciclovir treatment. Other reported presentations of CMV infection in skin of HIV-infected individuals include macular purpura of the extremities associated with leukocytoclastic vasculitis and small, keratotic, verrucous lesions, 1 to 3 cm in diameter, scattered on the trunk, limbs, and face.

MOLLUSCUM CONTAGIOSUM (See Chap. 222) Molluscum contagiosum virus (MCV) infection occurs commonly in keratinized skin, at sites of minor trauma, and in the infundibular portion of the hair follicle.[117] In the immunocompetent host, lesions resolve spontaneously, usually within a year, even in the absence of treatment. Transmission is usually via skin-to-skin contact, occurring commonly in children and sexual partners. The clinical course of MCV infection in HIV disease differs significantly from that in the normal host and is an excellent clinical marker of the degree of immunodeficiency.[118] In adults with multiple mollusca occurring outside of the genital area, especially head and neck lesions, HIV infection should be suspected. Large and confluent lesions cause significant morbidity and disfigurement.

Prior to HAART, MCV infections were detected in 10 percent of individuals with HIV disease and in 30 percent of those with CD4 cell counts of <100/μL; the number of lesions was inversely related to the CD4 cell count.[119] In a study of 27 HIV-infected patients with MCV infection,[120] the mean CD4 cell count was 85.7 cells/μL within 60 days of mollusca diagnosis; 52 percent of patients had facial and neck lesions alone, and 26 percent had lesions in areas associated with sexual transmission. PCP had previously occurred in 30 percent of individuals and Kaposi's sarcoma had been diagnosed in 56 percent.

Clinically, MCV infection presents as skin-colored papules or nodules, often with a characteristic central umbilicated keratotic plug. Lesions are usually 2 to 6 mm in diameter, but may be smaller than 1 cm in diameter (giant molluscum). Large lesions may mimic epidermal inclusion cysts, arising on or about the ear or on the trunk. Shortly after their appearance, lesions may be solitary; in time, multiple lesions are more typical (50+ lesions). With persistent and progressive immunodeficiency, mollusca may continue to enlarge and proliferate, resulting in confluent masses of lesions, e.g., involving the entire beard area (Fig. 226-20). Large and/or multiple confluent facial lesions cause significant cosmetic disfigurement. The most characteristic sites of occurrence in HIV-infected adults are on the face, beard area, neck, and scalp; anogenital and intertriginous (axillae, groins) involvement is also common. In males, lesions are often confined to the beard area, the skin having been inoculated during the process of shaving. Occasionally, lesions become secondarily infected with S. aureus, resulting in abscess formation, or with P. aeruginosa, with resultant necrotizing cellulitis. Significant postinflammatory hyperpigmentation or hypopigmentation, more pronounced in more heavily melanized skin, may occur following cryosurgery of lesions, adding to the cosmetic disfigurement of the mollusca.

The diagnosis of MCV infection in the HIV-infected patient is usually made on clinical grounds, but histologic confirmation is required in some patients. The differential diagnosis of solitary molluscum contagiosum includes a verruca vulgaris, condyloma acuminatum, BCC, keratoacanthoma, and SCC. The differential diagnosis of multiple facial mollusca contagiosa includes hematogenous dissemination to the skin of invasive fungal infections (cryptococcosis, histoplasmosis, coccidioidomycosis, and penicilliosis). Lesional skin biopsy is indicated in patients with sudden appearance of mollusca-like facial papules associated with fever, headache, confusion, or pulmonary infiltrate to rule out deep mycosis with hematogenous dissemination to the skin.

In HIV-infected individuals, MCV infection tends to be progressive, and recurrent after the usual therapies. In HIV-infected individuals, MCV has been demonstrated within clinically normal epidermis surrounding lesions, suggesting the mechanism by which new lesions recur at treatment sites. With the advent of effective antiretroviral therapy, MCV infection regresses or resolves completely, associated with increased CD4 cell counts and reduced viral load level.[121]

Therapeutically, the most efficacious approach toward MCV infection is correction of the underlying immunodeficiency; if this can be accomplished, lesions regress. If correction of immunode-

ficiency is not possible, treatment is directed at controlling the numbers and bulk of cosmetically disturbing lesions rather than at eradication of all lesions. Liquid nitrogen cryospray is the most convenient therapy, and usually must be repeated every 2 to 4 weeks. Electrosurgery is more effective than cryosurgery; local anesthesia is required by most subjects with either injected lidocaine or EMLA cream. CO_2 or pulsed-dye laser ablation is also effective but relatively costly. Cidofovir, a nucleotide analogue with activity against several DNA viruses, given either intravenously or topically as a cream, may be an effective therapy.[122]

HUMAN PAPILLOMAVIRUS INFECTIONS (See Chap. 224)

Subclinical infection with HPV is nearly universal in humans. With increasing immunodeficiency, cutaneous and/or mucosal HPV infection (re)emerges from latency, presenting clinically as verruca, condyloma acumintatum, SIL, SCC IS, or invasive SCC. HPV DNA is 2 to 3 times as frequent in cervicovaginal-lavage specimens and almost 15 times as common in anal-swab specimens from HIV-infected women as in those from HIV-seronegative women.[123] HIV-seropositive women are 5 times as likely as HIV-seronegative women to have vulvovaginal condyloma and oral or anal SIL.[124–126] The increased prevalence of HPV-induced lesions in HIV disease probably is related to deficient cell-mediated immunity rather than to specific antibody formation.[127] Increased HPV replication of the more oncogenic HPV types occurs with more advanced immunosuppression.[128]

In a study of the association between anal SIL, HPV infection, and immunosuppression among HIV-seropositive and HIV-seronegative homosexual men, anal HPV DNA was detected in 55 percent of HIV-seropositive and 23 percent of HIV-seronegative men by Southern transfer hybridization and in 92 percent and 78 percent by PCR.[129] Anal SIL was noted in 26 percent of HIV-seropositive and in 8 percent of HIV-seronegative men; high-grade SIL was noted in 4 percent of HIV-seropositive and in 0.5 percent of HIV-seronegative men. Among HIV-infected men, anal SIL, detection of specific anal HPV types, and detection of high levels of anal HPV DNA were all associated with advanced HIV disease. The risk of anal SIL among HIV-seropositive men with CD4 <500 was increased 2.9-fold over that of HIV-seropositive men with CD4 counts >500/mL.

In a study of HPV infection in HIV-seronegative and HIV-seropositive women, HPV DNA was detected in 83 percent of the seropositive and 62 percent of the seronegative women[130]; 20 percent of seropositive women and 3 percent of seronegative women had persistent infections with HPV-16–associated viral types (16, 31, 33, 35, 58) or HPV-18–associated types (18 or 45), which are most strongly associated with cervical cancer. HIV-infected women were noted to have a high rate of persistent HPV infections with the types of HPV that are strongly associated with the development of high-grade SIL and invasive SCC.

The degree of immunosuppression correlates with the presence of HPV DNA, extent of HPV infection, and potential for malignant transformation, individuals with CD4 cell counts <200/mL being at greatest risk.[131] The potential for malignant transformation varies considerably according to the type and site of HPV-infected epithelium, being greatest for the transitional epithelium of the cervix and anus, lesser for vulvar epithelium, and least for the epithelium of the male genitalia, perineum, inguinal folds, and perianal regions. The immune mechanisms underlying the increased rates of anogenital neoplasia in HIV-infected individuals[132–135] are not well understood, but are thought to be related to a high prevalence of HPV infection, impairment of cellular immunity, activation of latent HPV replication, and local suppression of cytokine production.

In early HIV disease, verrucae are not unusual in morphology, number, or response to treatment; however, with advancing disease, verrucae can enlarge, become confluent, and become unresponsive to therapy. HPV type 5 can cause an unusual pattern of extensive verruca plana and pityriasis (tinea) versicolor–like warts, similar to the pattern seen in epidermodysplasia verruciformis. With moderate or advanced immunodeficiency, warts and condylomata may become much more numerous, confluent, and refractory to usual treatment modalities.

With advanced immunodeficiency, low-grade SIL or high-grade SIL (caused most frequently by HPV types 16 and 18) can arise on the epithelium of the cervix, external genitalia, perianus/perineum, anus, oropharynx, or keratinized skin, especially the nail beds. Although differentiation from condylomata cannot be made on clinical grounds alone, SIL and SCC IS often present as multiple smooth, pink-to-skin-color-to-tan/brown macules or papules, which may form confluent cobblestoned, well-demarcated plaques. Lesions are usually multifocal but may be unifocal. In some cases, multiple foci of epithelial erosion occur, and concomitant herpetic infection must be ruled out. Massive HPV-induced lesions (older terminology giant condyloma of Buschke-Löwenstein) have a much greater chance of showing foci of SIL, SCC IS, or invasive SCC histologically. Extragenital HPV-induced SIL, SCC IS, and invasive SCC also occur in keratinized skin such as the nail beds.[136,137]

Oropharyngeal HPV-induced lesions resemble anogenital condylomata, pink or white in color, but never the tan-to-brown color of some genital lesions. Extensive intraoral condyloma acuminatum (oral florid papillomatosis) presents as multiple large plaques, analogous to anogenital giant condylomata acuminata of Buschke-Löwenstein, and can also transform to verrucous carcinoma.

The diagnosis of verrucae and condylomata is usually made on clinical findings. In individuals with advanced HIV disease, biopsy of suspected HPV infections of the anogenital region is recommended because of the high prevalence of SIL and SCC IS. Exfoliative cytology is very effective at detecting SIL or SCC of the cervix and may also be helpful with anal involvement.[138] External anogenital SIL and SCC IS, unlike cervical and anal lesions, cannot be screened for by the Pap smear using exfoliative cytology. Lesional biopsy specimens should be obtained from several sites, especially in individuals at higher risk for malignant transformation. In most patients, histologic findings are relatively uniform at multiple biopsy sites, ranging from low-grade or high-grade SIL to SCC IS. At one point in time, however, invasive SCC is usually unifocal within a field of SCC IS. A larger nodule within a field of SIL or SCC IS is advised to rule out invasive SCC. Over the course of HPV-induced neoplasia, multiple invasive SCCs may arise at various anogenital epithelial sites.

The natural history of external anogenital HPV-induced neoplasia is probably similar to that of condyloma acuminatum. Prolonged, severe immunodeficiency provides the necessary milieu for the emergence of HPV-induced anogenital neoplasia. The incidence of transformation of SCC IS to invasive SCC appears to be low. The relative risk for HPV-related anal SCC is much higher in HIV-infected than in non-HIV-infected homosexual men, and is more likely in advanced HIV disease.

Invasive cervical SCC is an AIDS-defining condition; however, a documented increase in incidence has not yet been reported. Cervical and anal neoplasias are likely to become more common manifestations of HIV disease as patients with profound immunodeficiency, who would previously have succumbed to OIs, are now surviving for extended periods because of increasingly effective antiretroviral prophylaxis of OIs and newer antimicrobial therapies. External anogenital SIL and SCC IS may also become more common in long-term survivors of HIV disease.

Low-grade or high-grade SIL of the external anogenital epithelium can be treated by several methods: topical chemotherapy (5 percent 5-fluorouracil or 5 percent imiquimod cream, especially for extensive multifocal lesions); surgical excision of single or several lesions; focal destruction of lesions by cryosurgery, electrosurgery, or laser surgery. Unlike topical 5-fluorouracil or imiquimod, surgical methods treat only clinically detectable lesions and not subclinical infection. For minimally invasive SCC arising in an area of external anogenital SCC IS, surgical excision is recommended with adequate borders around the lesion. The role for adjunctive radiotherapy has not yet been defined, nor has the use of combined modality therapy with external beam radiotherapy plus chemotherapy.

Individuals with documented external anogenital SIL or SCC IS should be followed by periodic follow-up examinations (every 3 to 4 months), noting the appearance of new lesions at these sites or an enlarging nodule or ulcerated site; biopsy of these sites is recommended. In that HPV-induced neoplasia may extend to the cervix and/or anus, direct examination by speculum and anoscope should also be performed; Pap smears should be obtained.

The number of individuals with SIL/SCC IS of the external anogenital region is expected to grow with the increasing numbers of long-term survivors of HIV disease.

SEXUALLY TRANSMITTED DISEASES

The great majority of HIV infections are transmitted during sexual intercourse. Individuals presenting with any sexually transmitted disease should be screened for HIV infection, syphilis, *Chlamydia*, gonorrhea, and *Trichomonas*. Possible interrelationships of STDs and HIV disease include: the potential for STDs to increase the rate of both primary HIV acquisition and transmission, the potential for STDs to accelerate the natural progression of HIV infection, and the potential for HIV coinfection to alter critical clinical and/or serologic parameters used to diagnose and treat STDs.[139]

Genital ulcerative diseases such as syphilis, herpes genitalis, and chancroid increase the risk of acquisition of HIV. Gonorrhea and trichomoniasis also increase the risk of HIV transmission.

Syphilis (See Chap. 229)

Individuals with genital ulcer disease such as primary syphilis are at increased risk for becoming HIV-infected if exposed to an HIV-infected sexual partner. Coinfection with both *Treponema pallidum* and HIV may alter the course of either disease. An individual with long-standing HIV infection with some degree of immunodeficiency who becomes infected with *T. pallidum* may experience an altered course of syphilis.

The majority of HIV-infected persons who acquire syphilis have the expected clinical course of disease and the expected serologic findings in serum and CSF, and they respond to the recommended therapeutic regimens. In a small percentage, however, the clinical manifestations, clinical course, serologic response, and response to antibiotic treatment are unusual (Table 226-7), especially with moderate-to-advanced HIV-induced immunodeficiency. Since unusual clinical presentations or failures to treatment are reported as single or a few cases, the actual percentage of cases of syphilis in HIV-infected patients with an unusual clinical course of disease is unknown. An inadequate immune response to *T. pallidum* is considered to cause the various abnormalities in the course of syphilis in the HIV-infected patient.

In a report of syphilis and HIV infection, 23 percent of individuals who presented with syphilis were concurrently HIV-infected.[140] The clinical presentation of syphilis in patients with HIV infection differs from that of patients without HIV infection in that patients with HIV infection present more often in the secondary stage (53 percent versus 33 percent) and those with secondary syphilis are more likely to have chancres (43 percent versus 15 percent).

HIV testing is advised for all sexually active patients with syphilis. Although uncommon, seronegative primary and secondary syphilis have been reported in HIV-infected individuals. Nearly all HIV-infected individuals with symptomatic neurosyphilis have positive syphilis serologies. Normally, treponemal tests remain positive throughout life. However, 7 percent of asymptomatic HIV-infected patients with a history of syphilis and 38 percent of those with symptomatic HIV infection with a history of syphilis have been reported to lose reactivity of treponemal tests.[141]

Neurosyphilis should be considered in the differential diagnosis of neurologic disease in HIV-infected persons. When clinical findings suggest syphilis but serologic tests are negative or confusing, alternative tests such as biopsy of lesions, dark-field examination, and direct fluorescent antibody staining of lesion material should be used.

In comparison with HIV-seronegative individuals, HIV-infected patients who have early syphilis may be at increased risk for neurologic complications and may have higher rates of treatment failure with currently recommended regimens. The magnitude of these risks, although not defined precisely, is probably minimal. No treatment regimens for syphilis are demonstrably more effective in preventing neurosyphilis in HIV-infected patients than the syphilis regimens recommended for HIV-seronegative individuals. Careful follow-up after therapy is essential.

The current CDC recommendations for treating early syphilis appear adequate for most patients, whether or not HIV infection is present.[142] Penicillin regimens should be used whenever possible for all stages of syphilis in HIV: benzathine G penicillin, 2.4 million units intramuscularly, as for HIV-seronegative individuals. Additional treatments (e.g., three weekly doses of benzathine G penicillin as suggested for late syphilis) or supplemental antibiotics in addition to benzathine G 2.4 million units intramuscularly are recommended by some experts. CSF abnormalities often occur among both asymptomatic HIV-infected patients in the absence of syphilis and HIV-seronegative patients who have primary or secondary syphilis. Such abnormalities in HIV-infected patients who have primary or secondary syphilis are of unknown significance. Most HIV-infected patients respond appropriately to the current recommended penicillin therapy; CSF examination before therapy is recommended, with modification of treatment accordingly. Patients should be followed clinically and with quantitative nontreponemal serologic tests (VDRL, RPR) at 1, 2, 3, 6, 9, and 12 months after treatment. Patients with early syphilis whose titers increase or fail to decrease fourfold within 6 months should undergo CSF examination and be re-treated. In such patients, CSF abnormalities could be due to HIV-related infection, neurosyphilis, or both.[143] In that *T. pallidum* may persist in the CNS of the HIV-infected patient in spite of adequate antibiotic treatment, the possibility of chronic maintenance treatment, analogous to secondary prophylaxis of cryptococcal meningitis, has been raised.

TABLE 226-7

Variations in Syphilis Occurring in Individuals with HIV Disease

Clinical findings
Increased severity of clinical findings[*,†,‡,§,||,¶,*a]
The usually painless chancre of primary syphilis may become painful due to superinfection (most often with *S. aureus*)
Lues maligna (secondary syphilis with vasculitis manifested by fever, malaise, headache, and nodules, indurated plaques with or without hyperkeratosis and/or ulceration, sclerosis)
A greater likelihood of ocular (retrobulbar optic neuritis)[†a,‡a] and neurologic disease[§a,||a]
Course of syphilis
Rapid progression to tertiary disease within the first year of infection, i.e., meningovascular syphilis
Serologic response to syphilis
Limited or absent antibody responses to syphilis with repeatedly negative reagin and treponemal antibody testing in serum and CSF
Response to therapy
Greater likelihood of treatment failure [¶a,*b,†b,‡b]
Relapse without reexposure despite "adequate" treatment[§b]

*Rademacher SE, Radolf JD: Prominent osseous and unusual dermatologic manifestations of early syphilis in two patients with discordant serological statuses for human immunodeficiency virus infection. *Clin Infect Dis* 232:462, 1996
†Radolf JD, Kaplan RP: Unusual manifestations of secondary syphilis and abnormal humoral response to *Treponema pallidum* antigens in a homosexual man with asymptomatic human immunodeficiency virus infection. *J Am Acad Dermatol* 18(suppl):423, 1988
‡Johns DR et al: Alteration in the natural history of neurosyphilis by concurrent infection with human immunodeficiency virus. *N Engl J Med* 316:1569, 1987
§Musher DM et al: Effect of human immunodeficiency virus (HIV) infection on the course of syphilis and on the response to treatment. *Ann Intern Med* 113:872, 1990
||Katz DA, Berger JR: Neurosyphilis in acquired immunodeficiency syndrome. *Arch Neurol* 46:895, 1989
¶Hook EW III: Syphilis and HIV infection. *J Infect Dis* 160:530, 1989
*aBerger JR: Spinal cord syphilis associated with human immunodeficiency virus infection: A treatable myelopathy. *Am J Med* 92:101, 1992
†aZaidman GW: Neurosyphilis and retrobulbar neuritis in a patient with AIDS. *Ann Ophthalmol* 18:260, 1986
‡aZambrano W et al: Acute syphilitic blindness in AIDS. *J Clin Neurol Ophthalmol* 7:1, 1987
§aReid SE, Anzarut A: Neurosyphilis and stroke in a patient with antibodies to the human immunodeficiency virus. *Am J Med* 87:119, 1989
||aDiNubile MJ et al: Acute syphilitic meningitis in a man with seropositivity for human immunodeficiency virus infection and normal numbers of CD4 T lymphocytes. *Arch Intern Med* 152:1324, 1992
¶aMatlow AG, Rachlis AR: Syphilis serology in human immunodeficiency virus-infected patients with symptomatic neurosyphilis: Case report and review. *Rev Infect Dis* 12:703, 1990
*bHutchinson CM et al: Characteristics of patients with syphilis attending Baltimore STD clinics: Multiple, high-risk subgroups and interactions with human immunodeficiency virus infection. *Arch Intern Med* 151:511, 1991
†bFiumara N: Human immunodeficiency virus infection and syphilis. *J Am Acad Dermatol* 21:141, 1989
‡bBerry CD et al: Neurologic relapse after benzathine penicillin therapy for secondary syphilis in a patient with HIV infection. *N Engl J Med* 316:1587, 1987
§bGregory N et al: The spectrum of syphilis in patients with human immunodeficiency virus infection. *J Am Acad Dermatol* 22:1061, 1990

PARASITIC INFESTATIONS

Protozoan infections are among the most common opportunistic infections in HIV disease; mucocutaneous involvement, however, is uncommon.

Extrapulmonary Pneumocystosis

P. carinii is a common opportunistic pathogen in individuals with CD4 counts <200 cells/μL, most commonly causing pneumonia (PCP). Primary prophylaxis with TMP-SMX is given when the CD4 cell counts fall below 200/μL, and secondary prophylaxis following an episode of PCP. Other prophylactic regimens include monthly aerosolized or parenteral pentamidine, or orally administered pyrimethamine-sulfadoxine (Fansidar) or dapsone.

Extrapulmonary *P. carinii* infection, pneumocystosis, is uncommon; however, it may be the initial presentation of HIV infection and of AIDS. Pneumocystosis of the external auditory canals presents with formation of unilateral or bilateral polypoid masses, and may be accompanied by loss of hearing. Similar lesions may occur at the tympanic membrane, middle ear, and mastoid air cells, associated with retrograde spread via the eustachian tube. Aerosolized pentamidine prophylaxis reduces the incidence of otic pneumocystosis; however, because the drug is concentrated in the lung, disseminated extrapulmonary pneumocystosis may still occur in patients receiving the drug. Gangrene of the foot has been reported in a patient with widespread pneumocystosis; microemboli containing *P. carinii* were present in small arterioles and capillaries within necrotic skin of the toes. Widespread violaceous papules and nodules arising on the torso, arms, and legs, resembling Kaposi's sarcoma, have been reported.

Leishmaniasis (See Chap. 236)

Following asymptomatic or symptomatic primary infection, *Leishmania* often remains latent in the reticuloendothelial system. Subclinical *Leishmania* infection is common in Mediterranean countries; 5 to 15 percent of adults in parts of Italy have a positive leishmanin skin test.[144] In previously infected individuals, antigen-specific T cells and NK cells interact with parasitized phagocytes in an equilibrium such that only a very low level of replication of *Leishmania* occurs. In HIV-infected persons, the equilibrium is lost. As immunodeficiency progresses, the protozoa may escape confinement by immune surveillance and present with visceral leishmaniasis (VL) (kala-azar).

Coinfection with HIV and *Leishmania* has been reported in more than 700 patients living in the Mediterranean basin, with the greatest number in Spain.[145] In southern Europe, 50 percent of adult VL cases have occurred in HIV-infected individuals; 1.5 percent to 9 percent of HIV-infected individuals have either newly acquired or reactivated VL.[146] More than 400 cases of coinfection with HIV and *Leishmania* have been reported from Spain, 85 percent in injected-drug users. Person-to-person transmission of *Leishmania* as well as HIV has been suggested in injected-drug users. VL may be the presenting manifestation of HIV disease. The course of persons who harbor *Leishmania* as well as HIV remains poorly defined. Coinfection of HIV and *Leishmania* in other sites of endemic leishmaniasis such as Kenya, Sudan, India, and Brazil is poorly understood.

No characteristic skin lesions have been described in HIV disease. Normal skin may also be parasitized. Cutaneous leishmaniasis (CL) usually represents primary infection presenting in multiple crusted papulonodules in sites exposed to insect vectors, as well as an erythrodermic and dermatomyositis-like eruption.[147] A generalized psoriasiform eruption has been reported in a patient with VL.[148] Leishmaniasis can also present at sites of HSV or VZV infection or of KS in HIV-infected individuals with CL or VL.[149] Digital necrosis has been reported associated with leishmanial vasculitis.[150] Diagnosis may be confirmed by demonstration of *Leishmania* on lesional skin biopsy and bone marrow aspiration. Leishmanial serology is often negative. The incidence of relapse of visceral leishmaniasis is high in HIV-infected individuals.

Acanthamoebiasis

Acanthamoebae are free-living amoebae that can enter the upper respiratory tract, disseminate hematogenously, and cause encephalitis and disseminated cutaneous lesions in advanced HIV disease. Cutaneous lesions appear as initially erythematous dermal-to-subcutaneous papules and/or nodules that suppurate, forming abscesses and ulcerations.[151,152] Acanthamoebic cysts and trophozoites, which resemble macrophages, can be visualized in lesional biopsy specimens with PAS or Gomori's methenamine silver stain and immunofluorescence techniques and must be differentiated from *B. dermatitidis*. A leukocytoclastic vasculitis can also occur. The organism can be isolated on culture of a biopsy specimen.

ARTHROPOD INFESTATIONS

Scabies (See Chap. 239)

In early HIV disease, scabies presents as scattered tiny papules and burrows on wrist, ankles, axillae, waist, and genitalia, where scabetic nodules may occur, and is associated with significant symptomatic generalized pruritus. In obtunded or immunocompromised individuals, pruritus may be diminished or absent. In advanced HIV disease, scabetic infestation can be severe, with millions of mites infesting the skin, presenting as a hyperkeratotic dermatitis, i.e., crusted scabies, resembling atopic erythroderma, psoriasis vulgaris, keratoderma blennorrhagicum, keratosis follicularis (Darier's disease), or seborrheic dermatitis (in infants).[153-155] Scabetic infestation usually spares the head and neck in adults but can be generalized in HIV disease. *S. aureus* superinfection is common, which has been complicated by septicemia and death. Because of the number of organisms in crusted scabies, recurrences are common, and hospital epidemics may occur.

Scabies must always be included the differential diagnosis of pruritus in HIV-infected patients, even in those who have experienced prior episodes of exanthematous drug eruptions and/or eosinophilic folliculitis. Use of potent topical glucocorticoids for such previously diagnosed pruritic conditions may mask the presence of scabetic infestation. Topical treatment with gamma benzene hexachloride, permethrin lotion, or 10 percent sulfur ointment is effective; in crusted scabies total-body application may be required. Keratolytic agents may be needed in crusted scabies to debride hyperkeratotic areas, in conjunction with debridement of involved nails. Ivermectin administered orally has been reported to be effective in scabies.[156,157]

HIV DISEASE IN WOMEN

In the United States, AIDS is the third leading cause of death among women 25 to 44 years of age and the leading cause of death among women of color in that age group; women are the population with the fastest growing rate of new HIV infection.[158] In the United States in 1996, AIDS deaths among women increased 3 percent, while among men they declined 15 percent. HIV-1 RNA is present in the vaginal tract as well as in the cervical secretions of HIV-infected women; HIV RNA levels in cervicovaginal lavage correlates with plasma levels. HAART results in marked decrease in HIV RNA levels in vaginal lavage samples.

Gynecologic disease is common in women with HIV disease.[159] The clinical course of HPV-induced condyloma acuminatum, vulvar and cervical SIL, SCC IS, and invasive SCC, pelvic inflammatory disease, syphilis, and vulvovaginal candidiasis may be altered, refractory to standard treatments, especially with increasing degrees of immune deficiency. Weekly fluconazole (200 mg) is safe and effective in preventing vaginal and oropharyngeal candidiasis.[160]

In a report of 82 women (1986–1992), *Candida* esophagitis and PCP were the most common AIDS-defining conditions, accounting for 77 percent of all initial AIDS-defining diagnoses.[161] Gynecologic complications occurred in 41 percent of women, including recurrent *Candida* vaginitis (30 percent), abnormal Pap smear/cervical SIL (22 percent), and recurrent genital herpes disease (8 percent). The overall survival rate was similar to that reported for men. Careful screening for gynecologic disease and vigilant surveillance for treatment failure are recommended.

The prevalence of oral disorders has been reported to vary with gender.[162] The incidence of OHL and candidiasis was higher in men (22 percent and 24 percent, respectively) than in women (9 percent and 13 percent); the odds of having OHL were 2.5 times higher for men than for women.

In a report of 65 HIV-infected women (median CD4 cell count $54/\mu$L) hospitalized for medical (91 percent) and gynecologic (9 percent) indications, 83 percent had gynecologic disease.[163] The diseases and prevalences found were vaginitis (51 percent), cervical SIL (45 percent), genital condylomata (23 percent), genital herpes (20 percent), pelvic inflammatory disease (5 percent), adenovirus infection (3 percent), and foscarnet ulcerations (3 percent).

The incidence of KS in HIV-infected women is much lower than that in men, but, women survived only 9 months following KS diagnosis as compared with a 23-month survival in men.

A higher rate of HPV infection with multiple types has been observed among HIV-infected women than among HIV-seronegative women; infection with multiple HPV types was most common among women with CD4 counts $<200/\mu$L. Although HIV-infected women had an increased incidence of multiple HPV types, their risk of having a high-grade HPV type was no higher than that of seronegative women. HPV type 16, the most virulent type of HPV, was found in 5 percent of HIV-seropositive women and 2 percent of HIV-seronegative women. The presence of HPV 16 in seropositive women was associated with a greater degree of immune impairment. It has been postulated that HPV infection in sexually active HIV-seropositive women reflects an immune-mediated increase in low-level HPV replication rather than recent acquisition of new HPV types through sexual activity.

To date, national data have not shown a greater prevalence of cervical cancer in seropositive women but instead, more aggressive precursor lesions which, if not detected and treated early, could progress to cancer. The impact of HAART regimens on preventing HPV progression through enhancing immune status remains to be determined.

MUCOCUTANEOUS FINDINGS OF HIV DISEASE IN CHILDREN

The clinical presentation of HIV disease in children differs somewhat from that in adults.[164–166] The great majority of HIV disease in children follows perinatal transmission. The majority of HIV-infected children have parents who are injected-drug users or have fathers who are bisexual. Because vertical transmission (transmission from mother to child) accounts for the overwhelming majority of HIV disease in children, a rise in the number of those cases is predicted, associated with the escalating number of young HIV-infected women. Prior to the availability of HIV serotesting of blood, children also became infected through blood and blood product administration, most often in the neonatal period.[167]

In a study of 4480 children hospitalized for the first time, the prevalence of HIV infection was 8.2 percent; the highest age-specific rate (11.2 percent) was in children ages 15 to 23 months.[168] Six clinical syndromes accounted for more than 80 percent of admissions of HIV-positive and HIV-negative children (all ages combined): respiratory infections, malnutrition, malaria, anemia, diarrhea, and meningitis. The dominant syndromic diagnoses in HIV-positive children were respiratory infection (26.1 percent) and malnutrition (25.8 percent); in HIV-negative children they were malaria and respiratory infection. The overall mortality rate in HIV-positive children was 20.8 percent, as compared with 8.7 percent in HIV-negative children; the highest death rate was in children younger than 15 months.

The cutaneous manifestations of pediatric HIV disease differ both in type and in frequency from those seen in the adult. There is no single mucocutaneous disease that is pathognomonic in children with HIV infection. The characteristic opportunistic infections such as PCP and the unusual malignancies such as KS occurring in adults are less common in children.[169,170] Candidiasis of the oral mucosa, skin, and esophagus, herpetic gingivostomatitis, and staphylococcal skin infection are the most common cutaneous manifestations of pediatric HIV disease. These infections are similar to those occurring in nonimmunocompromised children, differing only in severity and frequency of recurrence. Other disorders reported associated with pediatric HIV disease include seborrheic and atopic dermatitis, hypersensitivity vasculitis, nutritional deficiencies, drug eruptions, and pyoderma gangrenosum.[171]

REFERENCES

1. Quinn TC: Global burden of the HIV pandemic. *Lancet* **348**:99, 1996
2. Royce RA et al: Sexual transmission of HIV. *N Engl J Med* **336**:1072, 1997
3. Tyndall MW et al: Increased risk of infection with human immunodeficiency virus type 1 among uncircumcised men presenting with genital ulcer disease in Kenya. *Clin Infect Dis* **23**:449, 1996
4. Nelson KE et al: The association of herpes simplex virus type 2 (HSV-2), *Haemophilus ducreyi,* and syphilis in HIV infection in young men in northern Thailand. *J Acquir Immune Defic Syndr Hum Retrovirol* **16**:293, 1997
5. Bolinger RC et al: Risk factors and clinical presentation of acute primary HIV infection in India. *JAMA* **278**:2085, 1997

6. Seed J et al: Male circumcision, sexually transmitted disease, and risk of HIV. *J Acquir Immune Defic Syndr Hum Retrovirol* **8**:83, 1995

7. Perinatally acquired HIV/AIDS—United States, 1997. *MMWR* **46**:1086, 1997

8. Nelson KE et al: Transmission of retroviruses from seronegative donors by transfusion during cardiac surgery: A multicenter study of HIV-1 and HTLV-I/II infections. *Ann Intern Med* **117**:554, 1992

9. 1993 Revised classification system for HIV definition and expanded surveillance case definition for AIDS among adolescents and adults. *MMWR* **41**:RR-17, 1992

10. Schacker T et al: Clinical and epidemiologic features of primary HIV infection. *Ann Intern Med* **30**:257, 1996

11. Vanhems P et al: Acute human immunodeficiency virus type 1 disease as a mononucleosis-like illness: Is the diagnosis too restrictive? *Clin Infect Dis* **24**:965, 1997

12. Kinloch-de Loës S et al: Symptomatic primary infection due to human immunodeficiency virus type 1: Review of 31 cases. *Clin Infect Dis* **17**:59, 1993

13. Diagnostic tests for HIV. *Med Lett* **39**:81, 1997

14. Schacker TW et al: Biological and virologic characteristics of primary HIV infection. *Ann Intern Med* **128**:613, 1998

15. Musey L et al: Cytotoxic-T-cell responses, viral load, and disease progression in early human immunodeficiency virus type 1 infection. *N Engl J Med* **337**:1267, 1997

16. Vanhems P et al: Severity and prognosis of acute human immunodeficiency virus type 1 illness: A dose-response relationship. *Clin Infect Dis* **26**:323, 1988

17. Msellati P et al: A cohort study of 89 HIV-1-infected adult patients contaminated by blood products: Bordeaux 1981–1989. *AIDS* **4**:1105, 1990

18. Bartlett JG: IDCP guidelines: Management of HIV infection. *Infect Dis Clin Pract* **6**:422, 1997

19. Katzenstein DA et al: The relationship of virologic and immunologic markers to clinical outcomes after nucleoside therapy in HIV-infected adults: With 200 to 500 CD4 cells per cubic millimeter. *N Engl J Med* **335**:1091, 1996

20. Marschner IC et al: Use of changes in plasma levels of human immunodeficiency virus type 1 RNA to assess the clinical benefit of antiretroviral therapy. *J Infect Dis* **177**:40, 1998

21. Drugs for HIV infection. *Medical Lett* **39**:111, 1997

22. Flexner C: HIV-protease inhibitors. *N Engl J Med* **338**:1281, 1998

23. Carpenter CCJ et al: Antiviral therapy for HIV infection in 1997: Updated recommendations of the International AIDS Society—USA panel. *JAMA* **277**:1962, 1997

24. Pelella FJ: Declining morbidity and mortality among patients with advanced human immunodeficiency virus infection. *N Engl J Med* **338**:853, 1998

25. Sepkowitz KA: Effect of prophylaxis on the clinical manifestations of AIDS-related opportunistic infections. *Clin Infect Dis* **26**:806, 1998

26. Reynaud-Mendel B: Dermatologic findings in HIV-1-infected patients: A prospective study with emphasis on CD4+ cell count. *Dermatology* **192**:325, 1996

27. Uhayakumar S et al: The prevalence of skin disease in HIV infection and its relationship to the degree of immunosuppression. *Br J Dermatol* **137**:595, 1997

28. Skiest DJ, Keiser P: Clinical significance of eosinophilia in HIV-infected individuals. *Am J Med* **102**:449, 1997

29. Majors MJ et al: HIV-related eosinophilic folliculitis: A panel discussion. *Semin Cutan Med Surg* **16**:219, 1997

30. Houpt KR et al: Ultraviolet therapy of HIV-infected individuals: A panel discussion. *Semin Cutan Med Surg* **16**:241, 1997

31. Berger TG, Heon V, King C et al: Itraconazole therapy for human immunodeficiency virus-associated eosinophilic folliculitis. *Arch Dermatol* **131**:358, 1995

32. Otley CC, Avram MR, Johnson RA: Isotretinoin treatment for human immunodeficiency virus-associated eosinophilic folliculitis: Results of an open, pilot trial. *Arch Dermatol* **131**:1047, 1995

33. Obuch ML et al: Psoriasis and human immunodeficiency virus infection. *J Am Acad Dermatol* **27**:667, 1992

34. Kaplan MH et al: Acquired ichthyosis in concomitant HIV-1 and HTLV-II infection: A new association with intravenous drug abuse. *J Am Acad Dermatol* **29**:701, 1993

35. Meola T et al: Chronic actinic dermatitis associated with human immunodeficiency virus infection. *Br J Dermatol* **137**:431, 1997

36. Schulz TF et al: HIV infection and neoplasia. *Lancet* **348**:587, 1996

37. Maurer TA et al: Cutaneous squamous cell carcinoma in human immunodeficiency virus-infected patients: A study of epidemiologic risk factors, human papillomavirus, and p53 expression. *Arch Dermatol* **133**:577, 1997

38. Crane GA et al: Cutaneous T-cell lymphoma in patients with human immunodeficiency virus infection. *Arch Dermatol* **127**:989, 1991

39. Lo JC et al: "Buffalo hump" in men with HIV-1 infection. *Lancet* **351**:867, 1998

40. Hengel RL et al: Benign symmetric lipomatosis associated with protease inhibitors. *Lancet* **350**:1596, 1997

41. Miller KD et al: Visceral abdominal-fat accumulation associated with use of indinavir. *Lancet* **351**:871, 1998

42. O'Connor WJ et al: Porphyrin abnormalities in acquired immunodeficiency syndrome. *Arch Dermatol* **132**:1443, 1996

43. Weinert M et al: Oral manifestations of HIV infection. *Ann Intern Med* **125**:485, 1996

44. Itin PH et al: Oral manifestations in HIV-infected patients: Diagnosis and management. *J Am Acad Dermatol* **29**:749, 1993

45. Phelan JA et al: Oral findings in patients with AIDS. *Oral Surg Oral Med Oral Pathol* **64**:50, 1987

46. Walling DM et al: Epstein-Barr virus coinfection and recombination in non-human immunodeficiency virus-associated oral hairy leukoplakia. *J Infect Dis* **171**:1122, 1995

47. Webster-Cyriaque J et al: Epstein-Barr virus and human herpesvirus 8 prevalence in human immunodeficiency virus-associated oral mucosal lesions. *J Infect Dis* **175**:1324, 1997

48. Triantos D et al: Oral hairy leukoplakia: Clinicopathologic features, pathogenesis, diagnosis, and clinical significance. *Clin Infect Dis* **25**:1392, 1997

49. Shiboski CH et al: Human immunodeficiency virus-related oral manifestations and gender: A longitudinal analysis. *Arch Intern Med* **156**:2249, 1996

50. Lifson AR et al: Time from HIV seroconversion to oral candidiasis or hairy leukoplakia among homosexual and bisexual men enrolled in three prospective cohorts. *AIDS* **8**:73, 1994

51. Greenspan D et al: Relation of oral hairy leukoplakia to infection with the human immunodeficiency virus and the risk of developing AIDS. *J Infect Dis* **155**:475, 1987

52. Greenspan D et al: Risk factors for rapid progression from hairy leukoplakia to AIDS: A nested case-control study. *J AIDS* **4**:652, 1991

53. Husak R et al: Oral hairy leukoplakia in 71 HIV-seropositive patients: Clinical symptoms, relation to immunologic status, and prognostic significance. *J Am Acad Dermatol* **35**:928, 1996

54. de Asis MLB et al: Treatment of resistant oral aphthous ulcers in children with acquired immunodeficiency syndrome. *J Pediatr* **27**:663, 1995

55. Jacobson JM et al: Thalidomide for the treatment of aphthous ulcers in patients with human immunodeficiency virus infection. *N Engl J Med* **336**:1497, 1997

56. Manders SM et al: Thalidomide-resistant HIV-associated aphthae successfully treated with granulocyte colony-stimulating factor. *J Am Acad Dermatol* **33**:380, 1995

57. Koopmans PP et al: Pathogenesis of hypersensitivity reactions to drugs in patients with HIV infection: Allergic or toxic? *AIDS* **9**:217, 1995

58. Smith KJ et al: Increased drug reactions in HIV-1-positive patients: a possible explanation based on patterns of immune dysregulation seen in HIV-1 disease. *Clin Exp Dermatol* **22**:118, 1997

59. Douglas R et al: Successful desensitization of two patients who previously developed Stevens-Johnson syndrome while receiving trimethoprim-sulfamethoxazole. *Clin Infect Dis* **25**:1480, 1997

60. Caumes E et al: Effects of corticosteroids on the incidence of adverse cutaneous reactions to trimethoprim-sulfamethoxazole during treatment of AIDS-associated *Pneumocystis carinii* pneumonia. *Clin Infect Dis* **18**:319, 1994

61. Veenstra J et al: Rapid disease progression in human immunodeficiency virus type-1-infected individuals with adverse reactions to trimethoprim-sulfamethoxazole prophylaxis. *Clin Infect Dis* **24**:936, 1997

62. Saiag P et al: Drug-induced toxic epidermal necrolysis (Lyell's syndrome) in patients infected with the human immunodeficiency virus. *J Am Acad Dermatol* **26**:5676, 1992

63. Andrieu J-M et al: Sustain increases in CD4 cell counts in asymptomatic human immunodeficiency virus type 1-seropositive patients treated with prednisolone for 1 year. *J Infect Dis* **171**:523, 1995

64. Nichols L et al: Bacterial infections in the acquired immune deficiency syndrome: Clinicopathologic correlations in a series of autopsy cases. *Am J Clin Pathol* **92**:787, 1989

65. Moore RD, Chaisson RE: Natural history of opportunistic disease in an HIV-infected urban clinical cohort. *Ann Intern Med* **124**:633, 1996

66. Holbrook KA et al: *Staphylococcus aureus* nasal colonization in HIV-seropositive and HIV-seronegative drug users. *J AIDS* **16**:301, 1997

67. Dropulic LK et al: Clinical manifestations and risk factors of *Pseudomonas aeruginosa* infection in patients with AIDS. *J Infect Dis* **171**:930, 1995

68. Antinori S et al: Cutaneous miliary tuberculosis in a patient infected with human immunodeficiency virus. *Clin Infect Dis* **25**:1484, 1997

69. Meadows JR et al: Cutaneous *Mycobacterium avium* complex infection at an intramuscular injection site in a patient with AIDS. *Clin Infect Dis* **24**:1273, 1997

70. Estaban J et al: Localized cutaneous infection caused by *Mycobacterium avium* complex in an AIDS patient. *Clin Exp Dermatol* **21**:230, 1996

71. Strauss WL et al: Clinical and epidemiologic characteristics of *Mycobacterium haemophilum,* an emerging pathogen in immunocompromised patients. *Ann Intern Med* **120**:118, 1994

72. Koehler JE et al: Molecular epidemiology of Bartonella infections in patients with bacillary angiomatosis-peliosis. *N Engl J Med* **337**:1876, 1997

73. Koehler JE et al: *Rochalimaea henselae* infection: A new zoonosis with the domestic cat as reservoir. *JAMA* **271**:531, 1994

74. Schwartz RA et al: Bacillary angiomatosis: Presentation of six patients, some with unusual features. *Br J Dermatol* **136**:60, 1997

75. Dompmartin D et al: Onychomycosis and AIDS: Clinical and laboratory findings in 62 patients. *Int J Dermatol* **29**:337, 1990

76. Carlin EM et al: Nasopharyngeal flora in HIV-seropositive men who have sex with men. *Genitourin Med* **73**:477, 1997

77. McNeil J, Kan V: Oral yeast colonization of HIV-infected outpatients. *AIDS* **9**:301, 1995

78. Lifson AR et al: Time from HIV seroconversion to oral candidiasis or hairy leukoplakia among homosexual and bisexual men enrolled in three prospective cohorts. *AIDS* **8**:73, 1994

79. Carpenter CCJ et al: Human immunodeficiency virus infection in North American women: Experience with 200 cases and a review of the literature. *Medicine (Baltimore)* **70**:307, 1991

80. Spinillo A et al: Clinical and microbiological characteristics of symptomatic vulvovaginal candidiasis in HIV-seropositive women. *Genitourin Med* **70**:268, 1994

81. Reef SE, Mayer KH: Opportunistic candidal infections in patients infected with human immunodeficiency virus: Prevention and priorities. *Clin Infect Dis* **21**(suppl 1):S99, 1995

82. Walsh TJ et al: Fungemia in children infected with the human immunodeficiency virus: New epidemiologic patterns, emerging pathogens, and improved outcome with antifungal therapy. *Clin Infect Dis* **20**:900, 1995

83. Maenza JR et al: Risk factors for fluconazole-resistant candidiasis in human immunodeficiency virus-infected patients. *J Infect Dis* **173**:219, 1996

84. Maenza JR et al: Infection due to fluconazole-resistant *Candida* in patients with AIDS: Prevalence and microbiology. *Clin Infect Dis* **24**:28, 1997

85. Powderly WG et al: A randomized trial comparing fluconazole with clotrimazole troches for the prevention of fungal infections in patients with advanced human immunodeficiency virus infection. *N Engl J Med* **332**:700, 1995

86. Schuman P et al: Weekly fluconazole for the prevention of mucosal candidiasis in women with HIV infection. *Ann Intern Med* **126**:689, 1997

87. Murakawa GJ et al: Cutaneous Cryptococcus infection and AIDS: Report of 12 cases and review of the literature. *Arch Dermatol* **132**:545, 1996

88. Mandredi R et al: Morphologic features and clinical significance of skin involvement in patients with AIDS-related cryptococcosis. *Acta Derm Venereol* **76**:72, 1996

89. Dimino-Emme L, Gurevitch AW: Cutaneous manifestations of disseminated cryptococcosis. *J Am Acad Dermatol* **32**:844, 1997

90. McKinsey DS et al: Prospective study of histoplasmosis in patients infected with human immunodeficiency virus: Incidence, risk factors, and pathophysiology. *Clin Infect Dis* **24**:1195, 1997

91. Bellman B et al: Cutaneous disseminated histoplasmosis in AIDS patients in south Florida. *Int J Dermatol* **36**:599, 1997

92. Chariyalertsak S et al: Case-control study of risk factors for *Penicillium marneffei* infection in human immunodeficiency virus-infected patients in Northern Thailand. *Clin Infect Dis* **24**:1080, 1997

93. Supparatpinyo K et al: Disseminated *Penicillium marneffei* infection in Southeast Asia. *Lancet* **344**:110, 1994

94. Mole L et al: The impact of active herpes simplex virus infection on human immunodeficiency virus load. *J Infect Dis* **176**:766, 1997

95. Torres RA et al: Acyclovir use and survival among human immunodeficiency virus-infected patients with CD4 cell counts of <500/mm^3. *Clin Infect Dis* **26**:85, 1998

96. Pannuti CS et al: Asymptomatic perianal shedding of herpes simplex virus in patients with acquired immunodeficiency syndrome. *Arch Dermatol* **133**:180, 1997

97. Keiser P et al: Prednisone therapy is not associated with increased risk of herpetic infections in patients with human immunodeficiency virus. *Clin Infect Dis* **23**:201, 1996

98. Weaver G, Kostman JR: Inoculation herpes simplex virus infections in patients with AIDS: Unusual appearance and location of lesions. *Clin Infect Dis* **22**:141, 1996

99. Généreau T et al: Herpes simplex esophagitis in patients with AIDS: Report of 34 cases. *Clin Infect Dis* **22**:926, 1996

100. Schacker T et al: Famciclovir for the suppression of symptomatic and asymptomatic herpes simplex virus reactivation in HIV-infected persons: A double-blind, placebo-controlled trial. *Ann Intern Med* **128**:21, 1998

101. Lalezari J et al: A randomized, double-blind, placebo-controlled trial of cidofovir gel for the treatment of acyclovir-unresponsive mucocutaneous herpes simplex virus infection in patients with AIDS. *J Infect Dis* **176**:892, 1997

102. Kelley R et al: Varicella in children with perinatally acquired human immunodeficiency virus infection *J Pediatr* **124**:271, 1994

103. Baran J Jr, Khatib R: Recrudescence of initial cutaneous lesions after crusting of chickenpox in an adult with advanced AIDS suggests prolonged local viral persistence. *Clin Infect Dis* **24**:741, 1997

104. von Seidlein L et al: Frequent recurrence and persistence of varicella-zoster virus infections in children with human immunodeficiency virus type 1. *J Pediatr* **128**:52, 1996

105. Gershon AA et al: Varicella-zoster virus infection in children with underlying human immunodeficiency virus infection. *J Infect Dis* **176**:1496, 1997

106. Alliegro MB et al: Herpes zoster and progression to AIDS in a cohort of individuals who seroconverted to human immunodeficiency virus. *Clin Infect Dis* **23**:990, 1996

107. Tyndall MW et al: Herpes zoster as the initial presentation of human immunodeficiency virus type 1 in Kenya. *Clin Infect Dis* **21**:1035, 1995

108. Bayu S, Alemayehu W: Clinical profile of herpes zoster ophthalmicus in Ethiopians. *Clin Infect Dis* **24**:1256, 1997

109. McNulty A et al: Herpes zoster and the stage and progression of HIV-1 infection. *Genitourin Med* **73**:467, 1997

110. Glesby MJ et al: Herpes zoster in patients with advanced human immunodeficiency virus infection treated with zidovudine. *J Infect Dis* **168**:1264, 1993

111. Buchbinder SP et al: Herpes zoster and human immunodeficiency virus infection. *J Infect Dis* **166**:1153, 1992

112. Veenstra J et al: Herpes zoster, immunological deterioration and disease progression in HIV-1 infection. *AIDS* **90**:1153, 1995

113. Tsao H et al: Chronic varicella zoster infection mimicking a basal cell carcinoma in an AIDS patient. *J Am Acad Dermatol* **36**:831, 1997

114. Nikkels AF et al: Chronic varicella-zoster virus skin lesions in patients with human immunodeficiency virus are related to decreased expression of gE and gB. *J Infect Dis* **176**:261, 1997

115. Manian FA et al: Chronic varicella-zoster virus myelitis without cutaneous eruption in a patient with AIDS: Report of a fatal case. *Clin Infect Dis* **21**:986, 1995

116. Gallant JE et al: Incidence and natural history of cytomegalovirus disease in patients with advanced human immunodeficiency virus disease treated with zidovudine. *J Infect Dis* **166**:1223, 1992

117. Weinberg JM et al: Viral folliculitis: Atypical presentations of herpes simplex, herpes zoster, and molluscum contagiosum. *Arch Dermatol* **133**:983, 1997

118. Myskowski PL: Molluscum contagiosum: New insights, new directions. *Arch Dermatol* **133**:1039, 1997

119. Koopman RJJ et al: Molluscum contagiosum: A marker for advanced HIV infection. *Br J Dermatol* **126**:528, 1992

120. Schwartz JJ, Myskowski PL: Molluscum contagiosum in patients with human immunodeficiency virus infection: A review of twenty-seven patients. *J Am Acad Dermatol* **27**:583, 1992

121. Hicks CB et al: Resolution of intractable molluscum contagiosum in a human immunodeficiency virus-infected patients after institution of antiretroviral therapy with retonavir. *Clin Infect Dis* **24**:1023, 1997

122. Meadows KP et al: Resolution of recalcitrant molluscum contagiosum virus lesions in human immunodeficiency virus-infected patients treated with cidofovir. *Arch Dermatol* **133**:987, 1997

123. Sun XW et al: Human papillomavirus infection in women infected with the human immunodeficiency virus. *N Engl J Med* **337**:1343, 1997

124. Sun XW et al: Human papillomavirus infection in human immunodeficiency virus-seropositive women. *Obstet Gynecol* **85**:680, 1995

125. Hillemanns P et al: Prevalence of anal human papillomavirus infection and anal cytologic abnormalities in HIV-seropositive women. *AIDS* **10**:1641, 1996

126. Chiasson MA et al: Increased prevalence of vulvovaginal condyloma and vulvar intraepithelial neoplasia in women infected with the human immunodeficiency virus. *Obstet Gynecol* **89**:690, 1997

127. Hagensee ME et al: Seroprevalence of human papillomavirus types 6 and 16 capsid antibodies in homosexual men. *J Infect Dis* **176**:625, 1997

128. Palefsky JM et al: Prevalence and risk for human papillomavirus infection of the anal canal in human immunodeficiency virus (HIV)-positive and HIV-negative homosexual men. *J Infect Dis* **177**:361, 1998

129. Kiviat NB et al: Association of anal dysplasia and human papillomavirus with immunosuppression and HIV infection among homosexual men. *AIDS* **7**:43, 1993

130. Sun X-W et al: Human papillomavirus infection in women infected with the human immunodeficiency virus. *N Engl J Med* **337**:1343, 1997

131. Chopra KF, Tyring SK: The impact of the human immunodeficiency virus on the human papillomavirus epidemic. *Arch Dermatol* **133**:629, 1997

132. Palefsky JM et al: Risk factors for anal human papillomavirus infection and anal cytologic abnormalities in HIV-positive and HIV-negative homosexual men. *J Acquir Immune Defic Syndr Hum Retrovirol* **7**:599, 1997

133. Maiman M et al: Human immunodeficiency virus infection and invasive cervical carcinoma. *Cancer* **71**:402, 1993

134. Palefsky JM: Anal human papillomavirus infection and anal cancer in HIV-positive individuals: an emerging problem. *AIDS* **8**:283, 1994

135. Carter PS et al: Human immunodeficiency virus infection and genital warts as risk factors for anal intraepithelial neoplasia in homosexual men. *Br J Surg* **82**:473, 1995

136. Fader DJ et al: Isolated extragenital HPV-thirties-group-positive bowenoid papulosis in an AIDS patient. *Br J Dermatol* **131**:577, 1994

137. Tosti A et al: Human papillomavirus type-16-associated periungual squamous cell carcinoma in a patient with acquired immunodeficiency syndrome. *Acta Derm Venereol* **74**:478, 1994

138. Palefsky JM et al: Anal cytology as a screening tool for anal squamous intraepithelial lesions. *J Acquir Immune Defic Syndr Hum Retrovirol* **14**:415, 1997

139. Rosen T, Spedale JH: Relationships between sexually transmitted disease and human immunodeficiency virus infection. *Curr Probl Dermatol* **9**:242, 1997

140. Hutchinson DM et al: Altered clinical presentation of early syphilis in patients with human immunodeficiency virus infection. *Ann Intern Med* **121**:94, 1994

141. Haas JS et al: Sensitivity of treponemal tests for detecting prior treated syphilis during human immunodeficiency virus infection. *J Infect Dis* **162**:862, 1990

142. Rolfs RT et al: A randomized trial of enhanced therapy for early syphilis in patients with and without human immunodeficiency virus infection. *N Engl J Med* **337**:307, 1997

143. Musher DM: Syphilis, neurosyphilis, penicillin, and AIDS. *J Infect Dis* **163**:1202, 1991

144. Davidson RN: AIDS and leishmaniasis. *Genitourin Med* **73**:237, 1997

145. Alvar J: Leishmaniasis and AIDS co-infection: The Spanish example. *Parasitol Today* **87**:150, 1994

146. WHO: AIDS, leishmaniasis, dangers of clash highlighted. *TRD News* **26**:1, 1991

147. Daudén E et al: Leishmaniasis presenting as a dermatomyositis-like eruption in AIDS. *J Am Acad Dermatol* **35**:316, 1997

148. Rubio FA et al: Leishmaniasis presenting as a psoriasiform eruption in AIDS. *Br J Dermatol* **136**:792, 1997

149. Barrio J et al: *Leishmania* infection occurring in herpes zoster lesions in an HIV-infected patient. *Br J Dermatol* **134**:164, 1996

150. Caballero-Granado JF et al: Digital necrosis due to *Leishmania* species infection in a patient with AIDS. *Clin Infect Dis* **26**:198, 1998

151. Chandrasekar PH et al: Cutaneous infections due to *Acanthamoeba* in patients with acquired immunodeficiency syndrome. *Arch Intern Med* **157**:569, 1997

152. Murakawa GJ et al: Disseminated acanthamebiasis in patients with AIDS: A report of five cases and a review of the literature. *Arch Dermatol* **131**:1291, 1995

153. Donabedian H, Khazan U: Norwegian scabies in a patient with AIDS. *Clin Infect Dis* **14**:162, 1992

154. Portu JJ et al: Atypical scabies in HIV-positive patients. *J Am Acad Dermatol* **34**:915, 1996

155. Arico M et al: Localized crusted scabies in the acquired immunodeficiency syndrome. *Clin Exp Dermatol* **17**:339, 1992

156. Meinking TL et al: The treatment of scabies with ivermectin. *N Engl J Med* **333**:26, 1995

157. Taplin D, Meinking TL: Treatment of HIV-related scabies with emphasis on the efficacy of ivermectin. *Semin Cutan Med Surg* **16**:235, 1997

158. Wortley PM, Fleming PL: AIDS in women in the United States: Recent trends. *JAMA* **278**:911, 1997

159. Korn AP, Landers DV: Gynecologic disease in women infected with human immunodeficiency virus type 1. *J Acquir Immune Defic Syndr Hum Retrovirol* **9**:361, 1995

160. Schuman P et al: Weekly fluconazole for the prevention of mucosal candidiasis in women with HIV infection: A randomized, double-blind, placebo-controlled trial. *Ann Intern Med* **126**:689, 1997

161. Sha BE et al: HIV infection in women: An observational study of clinical characteristics, disease progression, and survival for a cohort of women in Chicago. *J Acquir Immune Defic Syndr Hum Retrovirol* **8**:486, 1995

162. Shiboski CH et al: Human immunodeficiency virus-related oral manifestations and gender: A longitudinal analysis. *Arch Intern Med* **156**:2249, 1996

163. Frankel RE et al: High prevalence of gynecologic disease among hospitalized women with human immunodeficiency virus infection. *Clin Infect Dis* **25**:706, 1997

164. Prose NS: Human immunodeficiency virus infection in childhood: The disease and its cutaneous manifestations. *Adv Dermatol* **5**:113, 1990

165. Straka BF et al: Cutaneous manifestations of AIDS in children. *J Am Acad Dermatol* **18**:1089, 1988

166. Lim W et al: Skin diseases in children with HIV infection and their association with degree of immunosuppression. *Int J Dermatol* **29**:24, 1990

167. Wykoff RF et al: Immunologic dysfunction in infants infected through transfusion with HTLV-III. *N Engl J Med* **312**:294, 1985

168. Vetter KM, Djomand G, Zadi F et al: Clinical spectrum of human immunodeficiency virus disease in children in a West African city. *Pediatr Infect Dis* **15**:438, 1996

169. Gutierrez-Ortega P et al: Kaposi's sarcoma in a 6-day-old infant with HIV. *Arch Dermatol* **125**:432, 1989

170. Connor E et al: Cutaneous acquired immunodeficiency syndrome-associated Kaposi's sarcoma in pediatric patients. *Arch Dermatol* **126**:791, 1990

171. Paller AS et al: Pyoderma gangrenosum in pediatric acquired immunodeficiency syndrome. *J Pediatr* **117**:63, 1990

The Rickettsioses

Rickettsiae are pleomorphic coccobacillary obligate intracellular parasites. Transmitted to humans by arthropods, they produce acute systemic infections of varying severity (Table 227-1).[1]

The most frequent rickettsial infection in the United States is Rocky Mountain spotted fever; reported cases have increased since 1960, predominantly in the southeastern states. Because the dermatologic characteristics of the rickettsioses provide the basis for clinical differential diagnosis and the initiation of proper therapy, they will be emphasized in the discussion that follows.

HISTORIC ASPECTS

Classic louse-borne epidemic typhus has been one of the major scourges of civilization, particularly during periods of famine or war. As Zinsser has dramatically described, typhus—not strategy—has determined the outcome of many military campaigns, thus exerting a direct influence on history. In the epidemics of typhus that swept through Russia and eastern Europe from 1918 to 1922, it is estimated that 30 million persons became ill and 3 million died.

In the 1890s, Wood and Maxcy described an unusual disease of high mortality in Idaho, which was later named Rocky Mountain spotted fever. In the early 1900s, Howard Taylor Ricketts established the tick as the vector of Rocky Mountain spotted fever. The rickettsiae were named for this investigator, who died of typhus while studying that disease in Mexico. In 1910, Brill described a series of patients in New York City who had a disease similar to, but distinct from, typhoid fever. Subsequently, Zinsser correctly postulated that this illness represented a recurrent form of epidemic typhus appearing in patients who had previously had the classic disease. In 1915, two Polish investigators, Weil and Felix, discovered that patients recovering from rickettsial infection had an agglutinin in their serums for certain otherwise unrelated *Proteus* bacteria (the Weil-Felix test). In the 1920s and 1930s, the work of Maxcy, Dyer, and others established the existence of another form of typhus transmitted not by the body louse but by the rat flea, thereby explaining the many cases of mild typhus unassociated with lousiness that had so long puzzled investigators.

PATHOGENESIS

Infected arthropods transmit rickettsiae to humans in two ways: ticks and mites (vectors of spotted fevers and scrub typhus) inoculate rickettsiae directly at the time of the bite, and lice and fleas

TABLE 227-1

Selected Rickettsial Diseases

GROUP	DISEASE	RICKETTSIAL SPECIES	ARTHROPOD VECTOR	RESERVOIR	WEIL-FELIX REACTION
Spotted fever	Rocky Mountain spotted fever	R. rickettsii	Tick	Small mammals, ticks	Positive
	Boutonneuse fever South African tick-bite fever (see Fig. 227-3)	R. conorii	Tick	Dogs, rodents	Positive
	Siberian tick typhus	R. sibirica	Tick	Rodents	Positive
	Queensland tick typhus	R. australis	Tick	Marsupials, rodents	Positive
	Rickettsialpox	R. akari	Mite of house mouse	House mouse	Negative
Typhus	Endemic	R. typhi	Rat flea	Rat	Positive
	Epidemic	R. prowazekii	Human body louse	Humans, flying squirrel	Positive
	Brill-Zinsser disease	R. prowazekii		Recurrence of dormant epidemic typhus	Low or negative
	Scrub	O. tsutsugamushi	Mite	Rodents, mites	
Trench fever	Trench fever	R. quintana	Louse	Humans	Negative
Q fever	Q fever	R. burnetii	Inhalation of dried tick feces	Cattle, sheep, goats	Negative
Ehrlichia	Ehrlichiosis	E. chaffeensis	Tick	Dogs	

(carriers of epidemic and endemic typhus) defecate feces containing rickettsiae into the wound while biting.

After inoculation it is postulated that initial rickettsial multiplication occurs at the site of introduction, and skin lesions at the site of the arthropod bite are the rule in rickettsialpox, scrub typhus, and boutonneuse fever.

Rickettsia rickettsii, the agent causing Rocky Mountain spotted fever, may be considered the rickettsial prototype. It produces the most marked pathologic changes and the most severe disease. The size of the microorganisms (0.2 by 1.0 μm) and their staining characteristics (purple with Giemsa stain or red with Macchiavello stain) enable them to be visualized with the light microscope if they are carefully sought in tissue sections. The members of the spotted fever group of rickettsiae multiply in both the nucleus and the cytoplasm of infected cells. Rickettsiae of the typhus group grow only in the cytoplasm.

Diffuse vasculitis is the pathologic hallmark of rickettsial disease. During the incubation period it is surmised that rickettsemia occurs, seeding the endothelial cells of capillaries, arterioles, and venules. With rickettsial multiplication the endothelial cells proliferate, swell, and degenerate, resulting in partial or complete thrombosis of the vascular lumen. In Rocky Mountain spotted fever, the rickettsiae also invade the smooth muscle wall of arterioles, producing further vascular damage, with resultant microinfarction and extravasation. Accumulations of inflammatory cells surround such areas of vascular injury. These changes occur at intervals along the vessels, leaving normal vascular architecture in intervening areas. In severe cases, thrombosis involves larger vessels, and microinfarction of the affected tissue is extensive (Fig. 227-1).

The vascular lesions account for most of the observed clinical findings, the location of the lesion determining its clinical expression. The skin most directly reflects vascular damage, the rash coinciding with the point and extent of vascular injury. In the brain the glial nodule is its counterpart; in the heart an interstitial myocarditis and microinfarctions are produced. A patchy interstitial rickettsial pneumonitis may occur.

The pathologic changes produced by the rickettsiae causing the typhus fevers closely resemble those described for Rocky Mountain spotted fever, but their extent and severity are usually more limited, there is less tendency to thrombosis, and invasion of the arteriolar smooth muscle almost never occurs.

ROCKY MOUNTAIN SPOTTED FEVER

Rocky Mountain spotted fever, caused by *R. rickettsii* and transmitted via tick bite, is the most severe of the rickettsial infections.[2] The illness ranges from a virtually asymptomatic form to a fulminant disease, with fatality rates ranging from 20 to 80 percent in untreated cases.

The infection is seasonal, the early summer peak of the disease corresponding to the increased seasonal activity of ticks and increased human contact with them. The reservoir of the disease is thought to be in small mammals, but ticks can infect their offspring transovarially, thus also serving as a reservoir. In the western United States the wood tick, *Dermacentor andersoni*, is the vector of the disease; in the eastern United States, however, the dog tick, *D. variabilis*, is the principal vector. Possibly this explains the high incidence in children in the eastern United States and the high in-

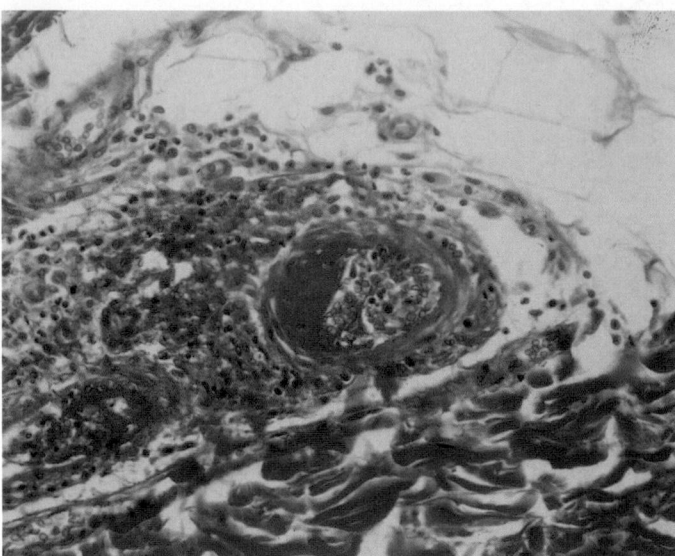

A.

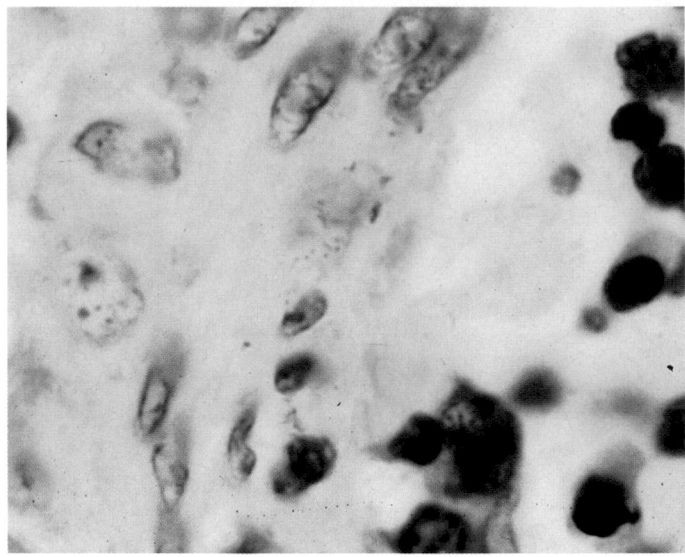

B.

A. The vascular lesion of Rocky Mountain spotted fever as seen in an arteriole in the skin. An early thrombus is present. *B.* Rickettsiae are seen in endothelial cells in a skin biopsy.

cidence in men in the mountain woods of Montana and other western states.

Clinical Manifestations

The incubation period ranges from 3 to 12 days, with a mean of 7 days. The onset is generally abrupt, with the sudden appearance of fever, chills, severe headache, myalgia, and arthralgia. The rash, the most characteristic aspect of the disease, generally appears on the fourth day of fever (range, 2 to 6 days). It goes through a very regular and unique progression, first erupting on the wrists, ankles, and forearms. It is pink and macular, fades on pressure, and is accentuated by warm compresses or a rise in the patient's temperature. After 6 to 18 h, the rash involves the palms and soles and then extends centrally to the arms, thighs, trunk, and face. After 1 to 3 days, the rash becomes macular and papular and a deeper red (Fig. 227-2). After 2 to 4 days, petechiae appear in the rash and the lesions no longer fade on pressure. Pressure from a sphygmomanometer may induce an additional shower of petechiae (Rumpel-Leede test, indicating capillary fragility), and the lesions coalesce and form ecchymoses. Small areas of gangrene may appear over the toes, fingers, earlobes, nose, scrotum, or vulva. Involvement of the scrotum or vulva often serves as a diagnostic clue. The more severe the infection, the more extensive the rash and the more rapid the progression. The rash may not be noticed in black patients. Furthermore, it now is recognized that the disease can involve many organ systems but either spare the skin or present as a rash of atypical distribution. Such illnesses have been called Rocky Mountain "spotless" and "almost spotless" fever.[3]

The diffuse vasculitis of the severe cases results in transudation of plasma, diminishing intravascular volume, falling blood pressure, and rising pulse, and patients appear profoundly ill. These changes are accentuated by the diffuse myocarditis and by the lowered serum albumin level, thought to be a consequence of liver involvement. Such patients, especially children, may appear quite edematous. Impaired circulatory dynamics lead to further diminished renal function.

A firm spleen is palpable in half the cases. Abdominal distention and muscular tenderness may combine to mimic appendicitis or other intraabdominal disease. Severely ill patients may be comatose. Further evidence of neurologic damage, such as seizures or hemiplegia, is associated with a poor prognosis.

On recovery, the areas involved by the rash develop secondary pigmentation, which may persist for some time.

Laboratory Diagnosis

The usual laboratory determinations do not aid in diagnosis. A normochromic, normocytic anemia may develop during the second week of the disease. The white blood cell count is generally within the normal range, although leukopenia or a mild leukocytosis may be observed. Cerebrospinal fluid examination generally reveals only a few red blood cells and lymphocytes. Thrombocytopenia may be a clue to the diagnosis. Various derangements of the blood clotting mechanisms often accompany the moderate and severe forms of the disease as a consequence of diffuse intravascular coagulation. Elevated blood urea nitrogen values usually reflect a prerenal azotemia, and liver function studies show degrees of impairment, especially diminished serum albumin concentrations.

FIGURE 227-2

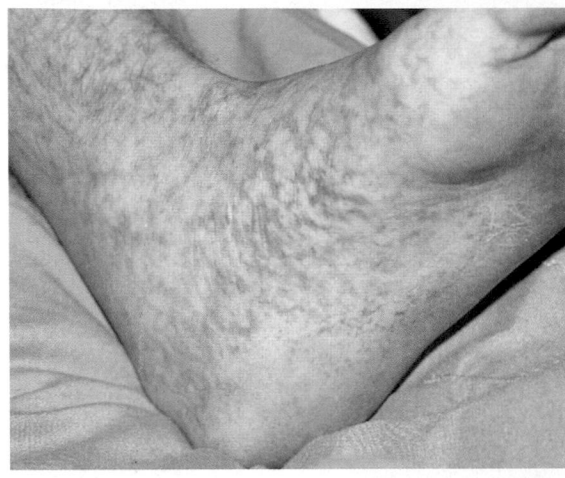

A.

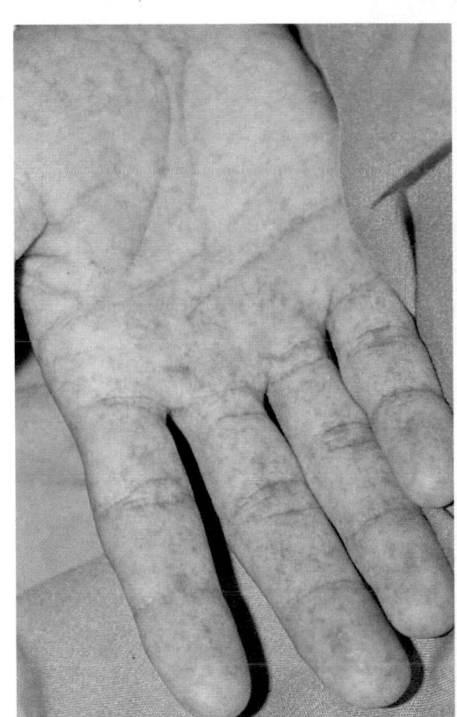

B.

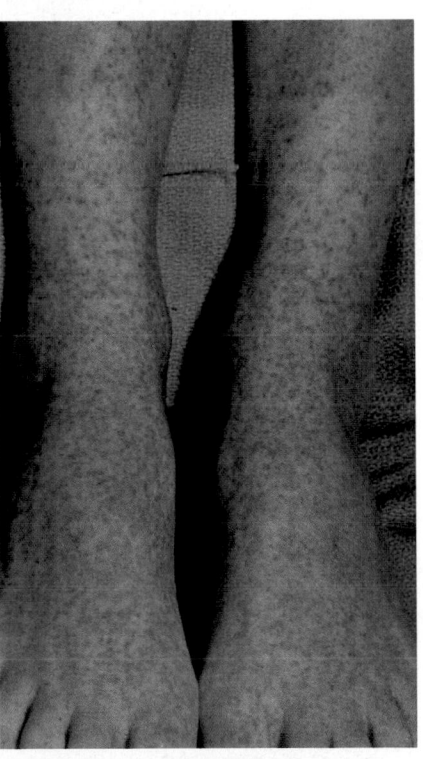

C.

Rocky Mountain spotted fever. *A, B.* Early macular blanchable macules and papules on the palm, soles, and ankles; no trunkal lesions were present at this time. *C, D.* Later lesions on the ankles and palm are hemorrhagic and no longer blanch with pressure; trunkal lesions were present at this time. *E.* Trunkal and facial hemorrhagic macules and papules 7 days after the onset of the rash. *F.* Infarction of fingers in a patient whose course was complicated by disseminated intravascular coagulation. (*C, D, and F, courtesy of Charles W. Stratton, MD.*)

The Weil-Felix test, with OX-K, OX-19, and OX-2 strains of *P. vulgaris*, was once used to help in narrowing diagnostic possibilities to rickettsial disease. It has now been largely abandoned because the test has poor sensitivity and specificity for the diagnosis of Rocky Mountain spotted fever and because it cannot distinguish between the spotted and typhus fevers. It is thus important to have

FIGURE 227-2 (*Continued*)

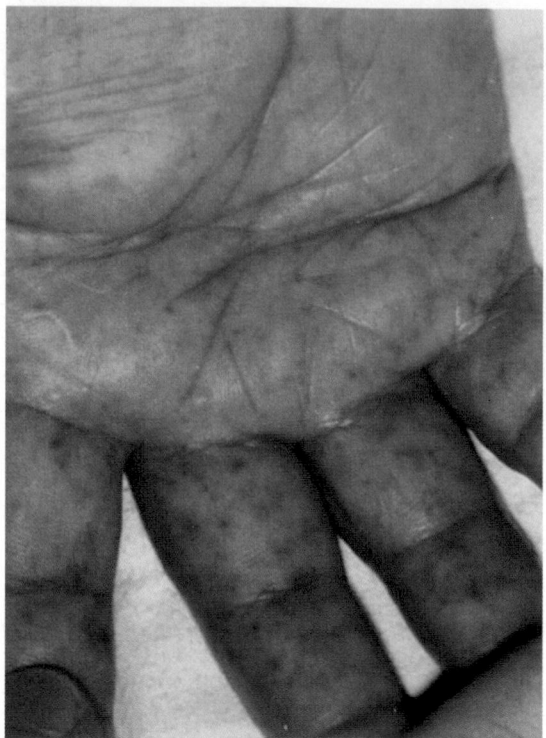

D.

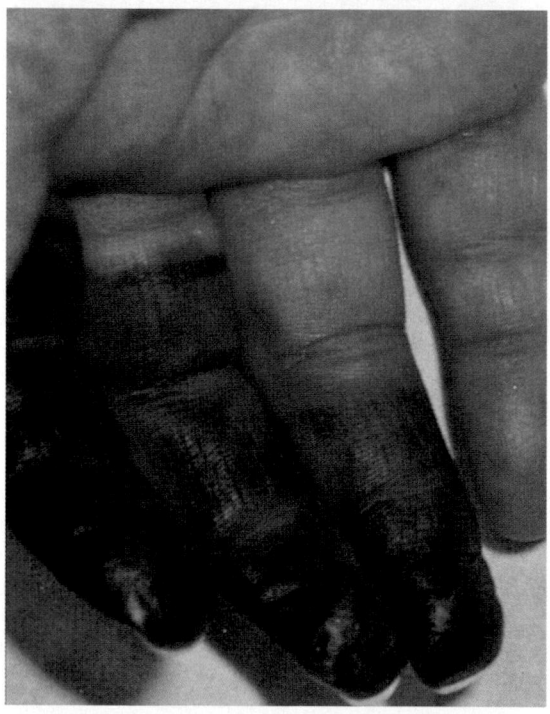

F.

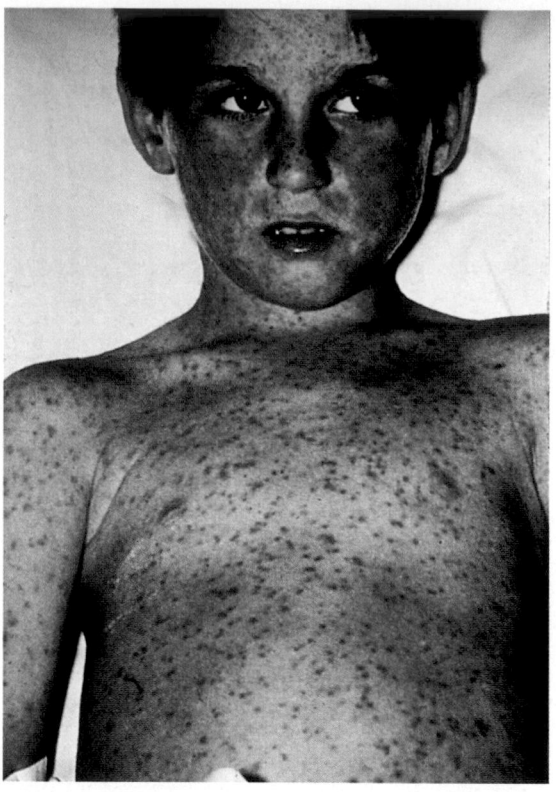

E.

cessed within 8 h is helpful in establishing the diagnosis; the microorganisms are found by immunofluorescent staining in the walls of the small blood vessels of the skin.

Isolation of the microorganism is difficult and dangerous. Unless a laboratory specially equipped to work with rickettsiae is available, serologic methods should be relied upon to establish the diagnosis. Polymerase chain reaction (PCR) methods have been used in research laboratories to identify species-specific rickettsial gene products in acute-phase blood specimens.

Differential Diagnosis

A history of tick bite in a person who has been in an endemic area is helpful but is frequently not available. The two other diseases most frequently considered are meningococcemia and measles. Meningococcemia is the most important as it, too, may kill rapidly. The rash may be entirely similar, ranging from macular to macular and papular to petechial and ecchymotic. In meningococcemia, the rash appears earlier in the course of the illness and does not have the characteristic progression of Rocky Mountain spotted fever rash. A coverslip touch preparation of a lightly scraped meningococcal lesion may reveal the microorganisms on Gram stain. Cultures will reveal the meningococci in petechiae, blood, and cerebrospinal fluid if meningitis is present. In practice, these diseases often cannot be differentiated with certainty. Thus therapy for *both* diseases must often be instituted and subsequently modified when further information becomes available.

Coryza, conjunctivitis, cough, and Koplik spots help to distinguish measles, in which the rash usually starts on the face and only rarely becomes petechial. The presence of edema (a parent's history of a child's puffy eyes, for example) can be very helpful in sug-

specific studies performed with acute and convalescent serums. These tests are available through state health departments and the Centers for Disease Control and Prevention (CDC) in Atlanta, Georgia. Antibiotic therapy, if started early in illness, may delay the appearance of antibodies. Biopsy of skin lesions that can be pro-

gesting Rocky Mountain spotted fever rather than measles. So-called atypical measles (see Chap. 211) may also mimic Rocky Mountain spotted fever. Through the universal use of measles vaccine in childhood this disease has been virtually eliminated in the United States.

The rose spots (papules) of typhoid fever are a delicate pink, are usually few in number, and are found on the abdomen and lower part of the thorax. They do not become petechial.

Some of the enteroviruses produce summer febrile illnesses with a rash. Usually appearing in epidemics, sometimes associated with diarrhea, the illness is short and mild, and the rash only rarely becomes petechial.

Treatment

Tetracycline and chloramphenicol are extremely effective in the treatment of Rocky Mountain spotted fever when administered early in the disease. Tetracycline (10 to 20 mg/kg per 24 h given every 6 h in divided doses) can be used in persons over 9 years of age. In younger children, tetracycline produces permanent discoloration of the teeth. Chloramphenicol (50 mg/kg per 24 h every 6 h intravenously in divided doses) can be used in younger patients. Therapy is continued for about 4 days after the patient has become afebrile, to prevent relapse.

When initial therapy should also be directed against the meningococcus, intravenous cefotaxime should be added to the regimen. Under *no* circumstances should the sulfonamides be employed, as they appear to *enhance* rickettsial infection.

Supportive measures, including intravenous administration of albumin, plasma, plasma expanders, or whole blood, may be of use in the severely ill patient. Glucocorticoids have been employed to reduce fever and toxicity more rapidly, but whether they alter prognosis is unknown. Heparin has been administered to patients with associated disseminated intravascular coagulation, but no definite recommendation can yet be made.

SPOTTED FEVER GROUPS: BOUTONNEUSE FEVER, SOUTH AFRICAN TICK-BITE FEVER, SIBERIAN TICK TYPHUS, AND QUEENSLAND TICK TYPHUS

The rickettsiae producing the milder diseases making up this group are closely related to one another and to *R. rickettsii*, the agent of Rocky Mountain spotted fever. The diseases are transmitted by ticks and occur in various parts of the eastern hemisphere. Boutonneuse fever, caused by *R. conorii*, is the prototype of the group.

Clinical Manifestations

After a 5- to 7-day incubation period, the illness begins with fever and headache. A primary lesion, the *tache noir*, at the site of the tick bite is characteristic of all the eastern hemisphere rickettsioses. It consists of a small ulcer with a black center surrounded by a red halo. It is associated with regional lymphadenopathy. A generalized, red, macular and papular rash erupts on the fourth day (Fig. 227-3). It involves the palms and soles and rarely becomes hemorrhagic. The disease is milder than Rocky Mountain spotted fever, and those who succumb usually have underlying disease. Imported cases occurring in travelers have been described.

FIGURE 227-3

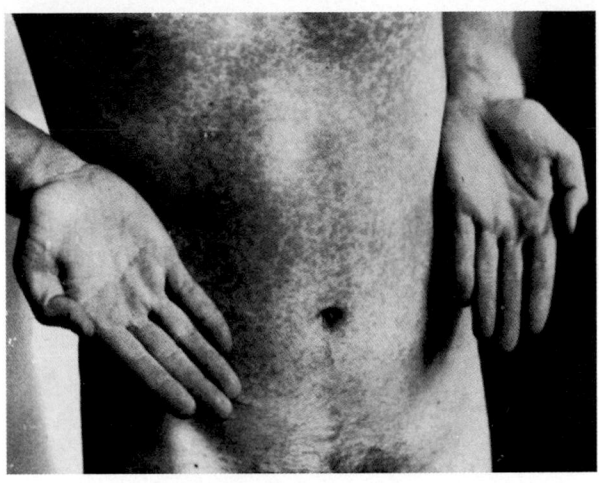

South African tick-bite fever. (*Courtesy of Evelyn Wallace, MD.*)

The diagnosis requires serologic testing of acute- and convalescent-phase serum specimens. Therapy with tetracycline or chloramphenicol is effective.

Tick-borne spotted fever rickettsiae have a worldwide distribution. New rickettsial species are now being identified as contemporary diagnostic testing is being applied to hitherto-remote populations.

RICKETTSIALPOX

Rickettsialpox, a mild disease caused by *R. akari*, was first identified in New York City in 1946. It is transmitted by the mite of the house mouse. It has been recognized in urban locations along the eastern seaboard of the United States and in Russia. It is unusual among rickettsial diseases in that its eruption is vesicular.

Clinical Manifestations

A local lesion at the site of the mite bite appears 1 to 2 days after the bite and precedes the febrile illness. The lesion is a red papule that becomes quite large (1 to 1.5 cm in diameter). A vesicle forms in the center, leaving an erythematous halo. The vesicle dries and a black eschar results that is present when the patient develops systemic symptoms (Fig. 227-4). The febrile illness lasts about a week, during which period the rash appears. It is a generalized macular-papular-vesicular eruption, which is often sparse. Usually on the face, trunk, and extremities, it may involve the palms, soles, and oral mucosa. The lesions develop a scale but no permanent scars. Therapy with tetracycline or chloramphenicol shortens the course.

The Weil-Felix test remains negative after this disease, but specific antibodies do develop.

FIGURE 227-4

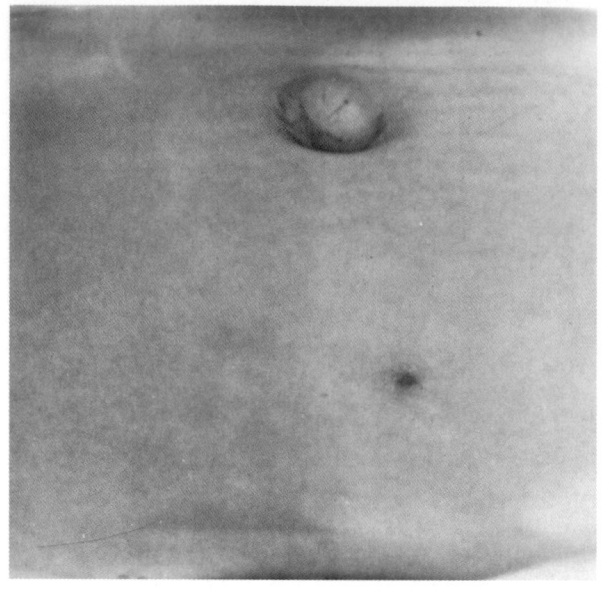

Rickettsialpox. Initial lesion, which is a black eschar resulting from rupture of vesicle. (*Courtesy of F. Daniels, Jr., MD.*)

Differential Diagnosis

Now that smallpox has been eradicated, the major differential diagnosis is with chickenpox. Chickenpox generally occurs in children and has no initial lesion. Its rash appears with the fever, and the whole papule is transformed into a vesicle. In rickettsialpox, fever generally precedes the rash, and the papular base is always discernible under and around the vesicle.

TYPHUS GROUP

Endemic Typhus

Endemic or murine typhus is caused by *R. typhi* (formerly *R. mooseri*), which classically was transmitted to humans by the rat flea. Cases clustered about harbors and granaries where humans were likely to have contact with rats, the reservoir for the disease. More recently in the United States, cat fleas have been implicated as an important vector.

CLINICAL MANIFESTATIONS   After an incubation period of 8 to 16 days, the onset of illness is heralded by chills, fever, severe headache, malaise, nausea, and vomiting. The rash generally appears on the fifth day. It is initially macular, becoming macular and papular. It is not petechial. The distribution of the rash helps to differentiate this disease from Rocky Mountain spotted fever. The lesions are located primarily over the trunk, with limited involvement of the face, extremities, palms, and soles, as opposed to the distal distribution of spotted fever lesions. The rash may be very evanescent and is absent in up to half of cases.

Typhus is generally milder than Rocky Mountain spotted fever, and it has a low mortality rate. One-fourth of patients have a palpable spleen.

Diagnosis is established by serologic testing, and treatment is as for the other rickettsial diseases.

Epidemic Typhus

Classic typhus is caused by *R. prowazekii* and is transmitted by the human body louse. Hence, the disease is easily spread from person to person. The reservoir for the disease is thought to be humans, lice becoming infected from patients with recrudescent typhus (Brill-Zinsser disease). Sporadic cases of classic typhus have recently been reported from rural or suburban areas of the eastern United States. The majority of cases have occurred during the cold months of December, January, and February. Most of the patients have had contact with flying squirrels or their nests. This animal now has been shown to be a sylvatic reservoir of *R. prowazekii*, but the mode of transmission to humans is unknown.

CLINICAL MANIFESTATIONS   The incubation period is about 7 days. As in other rickettsial diseases, the onset is characterized by fever, chills, headache, malaise, and weakness. On the fifth febrile day the rash appears, first in the axillae, then over the trunk, and later on the extremities. The rash initially consists of pink macules, which may become petechial and confluent (Fig. 227-5). The rash does not become papular.

Epidemic typhus is generally at an intermediate level of severity between murine typhus and Rocky Mountain spotted fever. In severe cases of louse-borne typhus, the clinical manifestations detailed for spotted fever, including widespread vascular thrombosis, are also observed (Fig. 227-6). Treatment is as for Rocky Mountain spotted fever. In convalescence, Weil-Felix agglutinins and specific antibodies develop.

FIGURE 227-5

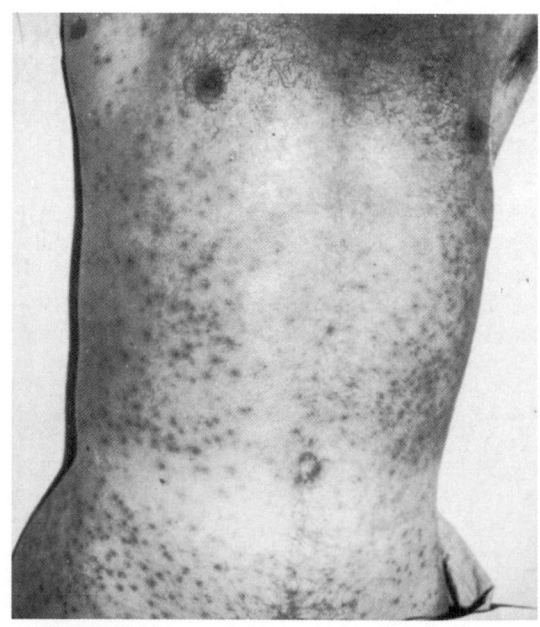

The diffuse macular-petechial eruption of epidemic typhus. The distribution is primarily trunkal. (*From the personal collection of Theodore E. Woodward, MD.*)

FIGURE 227-6

CHAPTER 227
The Rickettsioses

2545

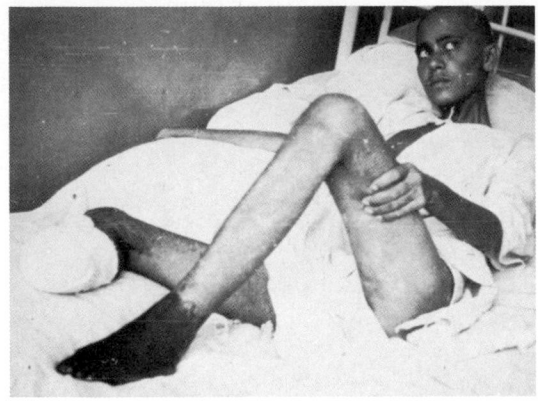

Epidemic typhus. Thrombosis of large vessels may result in significant gangrene. (*From the collection of Theodore E. Woodward, MD.*)

Brill-Zinsser Disease

Individuals who recover from epidemic typhus may continue to harbor small numbers of dormant rickettsiae throughout their lives. For unknown reasons, some patients develop a recurrence of the disease many years later. The clinical manifestations are in all ways similar to those of a mild episode of typhus, and therapy is the same.

The Weil-Felix test is frequently negative or, at best, weakly positive, whereas specific antibodies rise rapidly to high titers in an anamnestic-like response.

Scrub Typhus

Orientia tsutsugamushi, transmitted by the bite of a mite, causes scrub typhus in India, southeast Asia, and Australia.[4] There is marked strain variation in virulence, and mortality rates have varied from 0 to 60 percent.

CLINICAL MANIFESTATIONS   After an incubation period of 6 to 18 days, illness begins suddenly with fever, chills, and headache. The primary lesion, a vesicle or black eschar on an erythematous papular base, can usually be found, associated with local and moderate generalized lymphadenopathy. On the fifth day of fever the red macular and papular rash develops, primarily over the trunk. Unlike the other rickettsial eruptions, it fades within a few days.

The disease resembles the other typhus fevers with two exceptions: early in the disease there is a bradycardia relative to the elevated temperature, and pneumonitis is more frequent. Repeated attacks of scrub typhus are not unusual, as there is considerable antigenic variation in strains.

Therapy is the same as described for the other rickettsial diseases, scrub typhus responding more rapidly than any of the other rickettsial diseases.

TRENCH FEVER

R. quintana, a louse-transmitted microorganism, produces a mild, though sometimes prolonged, illness in humans, characterized by fever, chills, headaches, and a very characteristic myalgia, especially in the lower part of the back and in the legs. The rash consists of red macules confined to the trunk; the extremities and face are infrequently involved. The rash appears during the first day of illness and then waxes and wanes with the height of the fever. The spleen is usually palpable and quite firm. As the disease has been seen only in association with the two world wars, data on the efficacy of therapy are lacking.

Q FEVER

R. burnetii, the agent of Q fever, produces an acute self-limited pneumonitis and hepatitis in humans. It does not produce cutaneous manifestations.

EHRLICHIOSIS

Ehrlichiae are obligate intracellular pathogens that are closely related to rickettsiae. Unlike the rickettsiae, which invade vascular endothelial cells, ehrlichiae have a tropism for leukocytes. Thus, vasculitis and its consequent skin rash occur much less frequently in ehrlichial infection than in Rocky Mountain spotted fever. Indeed, the serologic investigation of Rocky Mountain "spotless" fever often reveals the infection to be ehrlichiosis.[5]

Ehrlichiosis is caused by two species: *Ehrlichia chaffeensis* infects primarily mononuclear cells (human monocytic ehrlichiosis). The other species (still unnamed) invades granulocytes (human granulocytic ehrlichiosis). Although both species are transmitted to humans by the bite of infected ticks, the two species have differing geographic distributions. *E. chaffeensis* occurs primarily in the southeastern and south-central states. Its principal vector is the lone star tick (*Amblyomma americanum*). Human granulocytic ehrlichiosis occurs in Wisconsin and Minnesota as well as in several northeastern states. Its vector is thought to be the deer tick (*Ixodes scapularis*).

The illness produced by the two ehrlichia are indistinguishable and occur primarily from April through September when ticks are active and people are pursuing outdoor activities. After an incubation interval of 1 to 3 weeks, individuals develop fever, chills, muscle aches, and headache. Nausea, vomiting, and anorexia are also common. More severely ill patients may have encephalopathy and renal failure.

Although a rash is usually not present at the time of presentation, approximately a third of adults will develop a macular and papular eruption at some time during their illness. A rash is more likely to be present in children.[6] Petechiae are unusual.

Laboratory abnormalities include thrombocytopenia, leukopenia, anemia, and derangements of liver function. The diagnosis is usually made by detecting an increase in species-specific antibodies in acute- and convalescent-phase serum specimens. The laboratory at the CDC in Atlanta is available to test acute blood specimens using PCR. Therapy must be initiated on clinical suspicion before a specific diagnosis is available. The response to tetracycline is usually quite prompt.

REFERENCES

1. Raoult D, Roux V: Rickettsioses as paradigms of new or emerging infectious diseases. *Clin Microbiol Rev* **10**:694, 1997
2. Kirk JL et al: Rocky Mountain spotted fever: A clinical review based on 48 confirmed cases, 1943–1986. *Medicine* **69**:35, 1990
3. Sexton DJ, Corey GR: Rocky Mountain "spotless" and "almost spotless" fever: A wolf in sheep's clothing. *Clin Infect Dis* **15**:439, 1992
4. Watt G, Strickman D: Life-threatening scrub typhus in a traveler returning from Thailand. *Clin Infect Dis* **18**:624, 1994
5. Dumler JS, Bakken JS: Ehrlichial diseases of humans: Emerging tick-borne infections. *Clin Infect Dis* **20**:1102, 1995
6. Harkess JR et al: Ehrlichiosis in children. *Pediatrics* **87**:199, 1991

CHAPTER 228

Dolores J. Lucas
Denise M. Buntin

Approach to the Patient with Sexually Transmitted Disease

Many of the sexually transmitted disease (STD) syndromes involve the skin and mucous membranes. Dermatologists encounter their share of patients with classic venereal diseases such as syphilis as well as other STDs, including condylomata, molluscum, herpes simplex virus, and scabies. Thus, they play an important role in the management of these highly contagious infections. Of prime importance is not only ensuring proper treatment but also counseling these patients about preventive methods. These include promotion of condoms, abstinence, delay in first intercourse, and sex education, especially for those at highest risk.

In addition, partners of patients with STDs should be referred for evaluation, treatment, and counseling in order to prevent further transmission and reinfection. If these interventions are undertaken, the control of STDs is possible.

CLASSIFICATION

STDs encompass a group of communicable diseases that are acquired predominantly by sexual contact. They are among the most common infectious diseases worldwide, and more than 50 pathogens are currently recognized as being sexually transmitted.[1] Table 228-1 summarizes the most common sexually transmitted pathogens and their related syndromes.

POPULATIONS AT RISK

The worldwide incidence of STDs is estimated to be over 125 million cases a year.[2] In the United States, the incidence is at least 12 million cases per year.[1] The majority of persons at risk of acquiring STDs are young adults. They increase their risk by having multiple sex partners, unprotected coitus, and engaging in the exchange of sex for drugs, especially crack cocaine.[3] Other risk factors include prostitution, inner-city residence, belonging to an ethnic minority,

and poverty. Nevertheless, the prevalence of bacterial STDs, particularly gonorrhea and syphilis, has declined dramatically over the last two decades.[4] This has largely been due to the availability of effective antibiotics, reliable diagnostic tests, and changes in sexual

TABLE 228-1

Classification of Common Sexually Transmitted Diseases

Agent	Disease
Bacteria	
Neisseria gonorrhoeae	Genitourinary tract infection
Chlamydia trachomatis	Genitourinary tract infection
	Lymphogranuloma venereum
Treponema pallidum	Syphilis
Haemophilus ducreyi	Chancroid
Calymmatobacterium granulomatis	Granuloma inguinale (Donovanosis)
Ureaplasma urealyticum	Nongonococcal urethritis
Gardnerella vaginalis	Bacterial vaginosis
Shigella spp.	Shigellosis in homosexual men
Campylobacter spp.	Enteritis in homosexual men
Group B streptococcus	Neonatal sepsis
Viruses	
Herpes simplex virus	Genital herpes
Human papillomavirus	Condyloma acuminatum
Poxvirus	Molluscum contagiosum
Hepatitis B virus	Viral hepatitis
Human immunodeficiency virus	Acquired immunodeficiency syndrome
Protozoa	
Trichomonas vaginalis	Trichomoniasis
Giardia lamblia	Giardiasis in homosexual men
Entamoeba histolytica	Amebiasis in homosexual men
Fungi	
Candida albicans	Vulvovaginitis, balanitis
Ectoparasites	
Phthirus pubis	Pubic lice
Sarcoptes scabiei	Scabies

behavior following the advent of acquired immunodeficiency syndrome (AIDS).[4]

STDS AND HIV INFECTION

Evidence supports the fact that STDs facilitate transmission of the human immunodeficiency virus (HIV), the etiologic agent of AIDS. For example, genital ulcer disease is a risk factor for HIV infection.[5] Conversely, HIV infection may increase the prevalence of genital ulcers and other STDs.[5] In addition, HIV can result in atypical clinical presentations of STDs that include larger, numerous, or persistent lesions (see Chap. 226). As a result, management of these patients becomes difficult, since treatment failures are more likely to be encountered.[5] Nevertheless, the emergence of HIV has greatly accelerated the growth of public concern about STDs as well as motivation for preventive strategies.[6]

MEDICAL AND SEXUAL HISTORY

A complete medical and sexual history is essential in evaluating a patient for STDs. The medical history should include current symptoms and duration, previous therapy, recent travel, and overall general health. The sexual history should include recent sexual contacts and practices, use of preventive methods, past exposure to STDs, and HIV risk factors. In interviewing a patient, a nonjudgmental, straightforward, and sensitive approach is best and generally results in accurate data.

PHYSICAL EXAMINATION

The physical examination of patients with STDs requires inspection of the entire skin surface, with emphasis on pubic and inguinal areas, thighs, abdomen, hands, and forearm. The mouth and throat are also examined, and the cervical, axillary, and inguinal areas are palpated for lymphadenopathy. In men, inspection of the penis requires retraction of foreskin and "milking" the urethra for discharge; the scrotum is palpated and the anus is carefully inspected. In women, the pubic area, external genitals, and anus are inspected; bimanual pelvic and speculum examinations are also performed.

SCREENING

Management of patients with STDs should include screening for other common STDs. Screening should also be performed in persons who are at risk even though they lack specific signs and symptoms of infection. In effect, this will play a role in the prevention and control of certain diseases such as syphilis, gonorrhea, and HIV infection. Routine screening tests should include syphilis serology, tests for chlamydial infection and gonorrhea, and HIV serology with pretest counseling.

GENITAL ULCERS

Genital ulcer disease characterizes a group of STDs that includes herpes simplex virus (HSV) infection, syphilis, chancroid, lymphogranuloma venereum (LGV), and granuloma inguinale (GI). In the United States and western Europe, the most common cause of ulcerative lesions in the genitalia is genital herpes, whereas in developing countries, chancroid is the most common cause.[7] Syphilis is the second most common form in almost all areas of the world. Genital ulcers have been associated with an increased risk for acquiring HIV infection.[8]

In evaluating a patient with genital ulcerations, a complete history and physical examination are sometimes sufficient to make a diagnosis. A clinical diagnosis of genital herpes can be made if typical painful, grouped vesicles or pustules are preceded by a prodrome of stinging or burning. The presence of HSV-infected multinucleated giant cells can rapidly be detected by Tzanck preparation. However, this test is neither specific nor sensitive for HSV infection; definitive diagnosis is achieved by isolation of HSV by culture.

Nevertheless, most cases of genital ulcers cannot be diagnosed accurately based on the clinical findings. If a lesion is not highly characteristic of HSV infection, a dark-field examination or direct immunofluorescence test for *Treponema pallidum* and rapid serologic test for syphilis should be performed. If enlarged lymph nodes are present, these should be aspirated for Gram's staining and culture to detect *Haemophilus ducreyi* and other pathogenic bacteria.

Genital Herpes (See also Chap. 215)

Genital herpes is caused by herpes simplex, a DNA virus. Thus far, only two serotypes of HSV have been identified: HSV-1 and HSV-2, with HSV-2 being responsible for most cases of genital herpes.[9] Over the past two decades, epidemics of genital herpes have occurred, and this has resulted in a steady increase in its incidence.[10] In the United States, it is estimated that approximately 724,000 new cases of genital herpes occur yearly, with a cumulative prevalence of over 20 million infected persons.[2] Clinically, the typical herpetic lesions consist of small, grouped vesicles or pustules that often rupture to form ulcers. These lesions are frequently preceded by a prodrome of paresthesias. Up to 50 percent of infected persons are asymptomatic and recurrences are not uncommon.[9] The recommended treatment by the Centers for Disease Control and Prevention for genital herpes is acyclovir. Newer drugs such as valaciclovir and famciclovir are available for treatment of recurrent genital herpes in the immunocompetent patient. Patients who experience multiple recurrences a year may benefit from suppressive therapy with acyclovir or valaciclovir.[11]

Syphilis (See also Chap. 229)

Syphilis is a sexually transmitted disease caused by the spirochete *Treponema pallidum*. In the 1940s, the annual incidence of syphilis declined dramatically with the introduction of penicillin.[12] However, since the 1980s, there has been a worldwide resurgence of syphilis,[13] and this has partially been attributed to HIV infections.[14] Most cases of syphilis occur in young adults aged 20 to 24 years.[2] Clinically, syphilis is characterized by several stages—primary, secondary, latent, and tertiary. Primary syphilis presents with a painless chancre at the site of inoculation, usually the genitalia. The manifestations of secondary syphilis include a generalized rash, mucocutaneous lesions, fever, malaise, and lymphadenopathy. The tertiary stage consists of destructive gummatous lesions in one or more organ systems. Persons with latent infection have no clinical signs or symptoms but are serologically reactive. The preferred drug for treatment of all stages of syphilis is penicillin.[15]

Chancroid (See also Chap. 231)

The etiologic agent of chancroid is *Haemophilus ducreyi*, a gram-negative bacillus. The worldwide incidence of chancroid exceeds that of syphilis.[2] In the United States, the incidence has been increasing since the 1980s as a result of antibiotic resistance.[16] Prostitution has an important role in the spread of chancroid.[17] The typical lesion is a painful ulcer with ragged, undermined borders and associated tender inguinal lymphadenitis. Recommended treatment regimens include erythromycin, azithromycin, and ceftriaxone.

Lymphogranuloma Venereum (See also Chap. 232)

LGV is an infectious disease caused by *Chlamydia trachomatis* serovars L1, L2, or L3. It is endemic in tropical areas and rare in the United States, with less than 1000 cases reported each year.[16] The primary lesion is a painless papule or ulcer, but the hallmark of LGV is tender inguinal lymphadenopathy, usually unilateral. The preferred treatment is doxycycline or tetracycline.

Granuloma Inguinale (See also Chap. 233)

GI or donovanosis is caused by *Calymmatobacterium granulomatis*, a gram-negative rod. It is endemic in New Guinea, central Australia, the Caribbean, and India but rare in the United States, with fewer than 50 cases occurring per year.[2] Low income and poor hygiene have been associated with donovanosis.[2] Several clinical variants have been described; these include the ulcerative type, the verrucous type, the necrotic type, and the sclerotic type. Inguinal lymphadenopathy is uncommon. The treatment of choice is doxycycline or tetracycline.

LOWER GENITOURINARY TRACT INFECTIONS

Urethritis, epididymitis, cervicitis, and acute pelvic inflammatory disease are most commonly caused by *Neisseria gonorrhoeae* and *C. trachomatis*. Urethritis is more common in men than women and is characterized by a mucoid or purulent discharge. A Gram-stained smear of the discharge is diagnostic of gonorrhea if typical gram-negative diplococci within neutrophils can be demonstrated. If not, a preliminary diagnosis of nongonococcal urethritis can be made. Confirmation studies require isolation of the offending organism by culture. The majority of women infected with *N. gonorrhoeae* or *C. trachomatis* remain asymptomatic, but when symptoms occur, they can present with dysuria, vaginal discharge or bleeding, or salpingitis. Gram's stain and/or culture of vaginal or cervical discharge is warranted. It is also important to exclude the possibility of a bacterial urinary tract infection or acute pyelonephritis, especially in women who present with dysuria.

Gonorrhea (See also Chap. 234)

The etiologic agent of gonorrhea is *N. gonorrhoeae*, a gram-negative diplococcus. The incidence of gonorrhea has steadily been decreasing since the 1970s[18]; this can probably be attributed to a

change in sexual behavior related to the fear of AIDS.[19] The incidence is highest in young adults between the ages of 15 to 34 years.[18] The typical presentation in men is a purulent urethral discharge with dysuria. In women, symptoms include dysuria, increased vaginal discharge, vaginal bleeding, dyspareunia, and acute salpingitis. Recommended treatment regimens include doxycycline, erythromycin, and azithromycin.

Chlamydia (See also Chap. 235)

Genital chlamydial infections are caused by the bacterium *C. trachomatis*. It is the most common bacterial STD in the United States.[2] The incidence rate of chlamydial infections has remained fairly constant at about 4 million cases per year.[1] The symptoms can resemble those of gonorrheal infections, which include dysuria, urethral discharge, vaginal discharge, mucopurulent cervicitis, and pelvic inflammatory disease. The preferred treatment for chlamydial infections is doxycycline.

VULVOVAGINITIS (See also Chaps. 116 and 235)

Vulvovaginal infections are common among young women. Symptoms include vaginal discharge, vulvar pruritus, irritation or burning, vulvar dyspareunia, and vaginal malodor. The three most common diseases characterized by vulvovaginitis are bacterial vaginosis, trichomoniasis, and candidiasis. In evaluating a woman with vaginal discharge, it is important to determine whether the discharge originates from the vagina or cervix. Vaginal discharge, as mentioned above, may be the presenting symptom of mucopurulent cervicitis caused by gonorrhea or chlamydial infection. Thus, a complete pelvic examination is warranted. When it is established that the discharge emanates from the vagina, the diagnosis can usually be made by pH and microscopic examination of the vaginal discharge. A pH < 4.5 suggests candidiasis, whereas a pH > 4.5 is typical of trichomoniasis or bacterial vaginosis.[20] Microscopic examination of vaginal secretions mixed with normal saline can easily demonstrate the clue cells typical of bacterial vaginosis or the motile trichomonads. The yeast or pseudohyphae of *Candida* species are more easily identified using a 10% potassium hydroxide (KOH) preparation. Clue cells and pseudohyphae can also be detected on a Gram-stained smear.[20] Another way to examine the discharge is to perform an amine odor test. A fishy odor detected after the application of 10% KOH suggests bacterial vaginosis or trichomoniasis.

Bacterial Vaginosis (See also Chap. 235)

Bacterial vaginosis is caused by the overgrowth of *Gardnerella vaginalis* and various anaerobic organisms.[21] It is characterized by a vaginal malodor and a scant to moderate, white, homogeneous discharge. It is the most common cause of vaginal malodor. The recommended treatment is oral metronidazole.

Trichomoniasis (See also Chap. 235)

Trichomonas vaginalis, a pear-shaped motile protozoan, is the etiologic agent of trichomoniasis. It is prevalent worldwide, but the overall incidence has been decreasing in the United States, probably owing to a change in sexual behavior.[22] The typical symptoms include a profuse, yellow, purulent, homogeneous discharge and vulvar itching. The amine odor test is positive in about 75 percent of cases.[22] In addition, some women develop petechial lesions on the cervix, which is often described as a "strawberry cervix." The treatment of choice is oral metronidazole.

Candidiasis (See also Chaps. 207 and 235)

Vulvovaginal candidiasis affects approximately 20 percent of women per year.[23] *C. albicans* is responsible for about 80 percent of yeasts isolated from the vagina.[24] The predominant symptom is vulvar pruritus. The vaginal discharge is typically white and cottage cheese–like without a distinct odor. Risk factors associated with the development of vulvovaginal candidiasis include pregnancy, diabetes mellitus, use of systemic glucocorticoids or systemic antibiotics, and tight-fitting clothes. The preferred treatment is with azole drugs.

VIRAL TUMORS

The two most common virally induced tumors of the genitalia are condyloma acuminata, or genital warts, and molluscum contagiosum. Distinction between the two can often be made clinically, but definitive diagnosis requires microscopic examination of a tissue specimen. Histologically, genital warts show marked acanthosis, papillomatosis, hyperkeratosis, and koilocytosis.[25] Molluscum contagiosum show the typical molluscum bodies.[26]

Genital Warts (See also Chap. 224)

Condyloma acuminatum is the most common STD. The incidence has increased over the past three decades, with over a million new cases seen yearly.[27] These warts are caused by the human papillomavirus (HPV), of which more than 70 types are known.[28] Genital warts are most often caused by HPV types 6 and 11, which are associated with benign lesions. HPV types 16, 18, 31, and 33 have been linked with cervical carcinoma. Treatment modalities include podophyllin, cryotherapy, electrocautery, and laser ablation. Intralesional and systemic interferon have been used to treat genital warts with less than satisfactory results and high recurrence rates.[29] Adjuvant therapy with interferon, however, seems to reduce the recurrence rates.[30] Imiquimod, an immune-response modifier that induces interferon-α and other cytokines, has been approved as treatment for condyloma.[31] Another treatment currently under investigation is a 5-fluorouracil/epinephrine injectable gel.[32]

Molluscum Contagiosum (See also Chap. 232)

The causative agent of molluscum contagiosum is a poxvirus that has not yet been identified. The typical lesion is a flesh-colored, firm, smooth, shiny papule with central umbilication. The lesions usually occur in clusters. When they are extensive, however, this condition is a marker for advanced HIV disease.[33] Commonly used destructive methods include curettage, cryotherapy, podophyllin, and cantharidin.

ECTOPARASITES

Parasitic infestations cause extreme pruritus. The two most common sexually transmitted parasites are pediculosis pubis and scabies. A careful examination of the pubic area will often reveal lice or nits on pubic hair or typical burrows of scabies. A skin scraping of the burrow using mineral oil and placing the material on a slide allows microscopic visualization of the scabies mite, its eggs, or its feces (scybala).

Pediculosis Pubis (See also Chap. 239)

Pediculosis pubis is caused by the parasite *Phthirus pubis*, the pubic louse. It is an STD that has become epidemic in the United States. The most commonly affected site is the pubic region, but other hair-bearing areas such as the beard, mustache, and eyelashes can be involved. The main symptom is pruritus. Recommended treatments include permethrin 1% cream rinse or lindane 1% shampoo. Because of its potential for central nervous system toxicity, lindane is not recommended for use on infants, young children, or pregnant or nursing women.[34]

Scabies (See also Chap. 239)

The etiologic agent of scabies is *Sarcoptes scabiei*, an ectoparasite that is acquired by contact with an infected individual. It occurs in epidemics in the United States but is endemic in many third-world countries.[35] The typical lesions are pruritic, erythematous papules and burrows. The classic areas of infestation include the finger webs, axillae, and periumbilical region. Other common sites of involvement are the penis and breasts. The preferred treatment is permethrin 5% cream or lindane 1% lotion.

SUMMARY

STDs remain a common public health issue worldwide. Knowledge of the clinical signs, symptoms, and current diagnostic tests is important in order to ensure proper treatment. Intervention through early sex education at school, condom promotion, routine screening, and wide availability of treatment are keys to prevention and control of STDs.[36]

REFERENCES

1. Kassler WJ, Cates W Jr: The epidemiology and prevention of sexually transmitted diseases. *Urol Clin North Am* **19**:1, 1992
2. De Schryver A, Meheus A: Epidemiology of sexually transmitted diseases: The global picture. *Bull WHO* **68**:639, 1990
3. Wasserheit JN: Effects of changes in human ecology and behavior on patterns of sexually transmitted diseases, including human immunodeficiency virus infection. *Proc Natl Acad Sci USA* **91**:2430, 1994
4. Catchpole MA: The role of epidemiology and surveillance systems in the control of sexually transmitted diseases. *Genitourin Med* **72**:321, 1996
5. Wasserheit JN: Epidemiological synergy: Interrelationships between human immunodeficiency virus infection and other sexually transmitted diseases. *Sex Transm Dis* **19**:61, 1992
6. Laga M: Epidemiology and control of sexually transmitted diseases in developing countries. *Sex Transm Dis* **21**(suppl 2):S45, 1994

7. Mroczkowski TF, Martin DH: Genital ulcer disease. *Dermatol Clin* **12**:753, 1994
8. Mertz GJ: Epidemiology of genital herpes infections. *Infect Dis Clin North Am* **7**:825, 1993
9. Lavoie SR, Kaplowitz LG: Management of genital herpes infection. *Semin Dermatol* **13**:248, 1994
10. Herpes simplex virus infections, in *Atlas of Infectious Diseases: Sexually Transmitted Diseases*, edited by GL Mandell, MF Rein. Philadelphia, Churchill Livingstone, 1996
11. Patel R et al: Valaciclovir for the suppression of recurrent genital HSV infection: A placebo controlled study of once daily therapy. *Genitourin Med* **73**:105, 1997
12. Kilmarx PH, St. Louis ME: The evolving epidemiology of syphilis. *Am J Public Health* **85**:1053, 1995
13. Felman YM: Sexually transmitted diseases: Selections from the literature since 1990. Syphilis: Epidemiology. *Cutis* **52**:72, 1993
14. Hutchinson CM et al: Altered clinical presentation of early syphilis in patients with human immunodeficiency virus infection. *Ann Intern Med* **121**:94, 1994
15. Centers for Disease Control and Prevention: 1993 Sexually transmitted diseases treatment guidelines. *MMWR* **42**:27, 1993
16. Goens JL et al: Mucocutaneous manifestations of chancroid, lymphogranuloma venereum and granuloma inguinale. *Am Fam Phys* **49**:415, 1994
17. Marrazzo JM, Handsfield HH: Chancroid: New developments in an old disease. *Curr Top Infect Dis* **15**:129, 1995
18. Centers for Disease Control and Prevention: Surveillance for sexually transmitted disease. *MMWR* **4**:1, 1993
19. Centers for Disease Control and Prevention: Summary of notifiable diseases, United States. *MMWR* **36**:1, 1997
20. Sobel J: Genital candidiasis, in *Sexually Transmitted Diseases*, 2d ed, by KK Holmes et al. New York, McGraw-Hill, 1990
21. Holmes KK, Handsfield HH: STD: Overview and clinical approach, in *Harrison's Principles of Internal Medicine*, 14th ed, edited by AS Fauci et al. New York, McGraw-Hill, 1998
22. Kreiger JN, Rein MF: Trichomoniasis, in *Atlas of Infectious Diseases: Sexually Transmitted Diseases*, edited by GL Mandell, MF Rein. Philadelphia, Churchill Livingstone, 1996
23. Geiger AM et al: The epidemiology of vulvovaginal candidiasis among university students. *Am J Public Health* **85**:1146, 1995
24. Horowitz BJ et al: Evolving pathogens in vulvovaginal candidiasis: Implications for patient care. *J Clin Pharm* **32**:248, 1992
25. Greene I: Therapy for genital warts. *Dermatol Clin* **10**:253, 1992
26. Gottleib SL, Myskowski PL: Molluscum contagiosum. *Int J Dermatol* **33**:453, 1994
27. McDonald LL et al: Sexually transmitted diseases update. *Dermatol Clin* **15**:221, 1997
28. de Villiers EM: Heterogeneity of the human papillomavirus group. *J Virol* **69**:4898, 1989
29. Stone KM: Human papillomavirus infection and genital warts: Update on epidemiology and treatment. *Clin Infect Dis* **20**(suppl 1):S91, 1995
30. Klutke JJ, Bergman A: Interferon as adjuvant treatment for genital condyloma acuminatum. *Int J Gynaecol Obstet* **49**:171, 1995
31. Beutner KR, Ferenczy A: Therapeutic approaches to genital warts. *Am J Med* **102**:28, 1997
32. Swinehart JM et al: Intralesional fluorouracil/epinephrine injectable gel for treatment of condylomata acuminata: A phase 3 clinical study. *Arch Dermatol* **133**:67, 1997
33. Koopman RJJ et al: Molluscum contagiosum: A marker for advanced HIV infection. *Br J Dermatol* **126**:528, 1992
34. Buntin DM et al: Sexually transmitted diseases: Viruses and ectoparasites. *J Am Acad Dermatol* **25**:527, 1991
35. Rausmussen JE: Scabies. *Pediatr Rev* **15**:110, 1994
36. Piot P, Islam MQ: Sexually transmitted diseases in the 1990s: Global epidemiology and challenges for control. *Sex Transm Dis* **21**:S7, 1994

CHAPTER 229

Miguel R. Sanchez

Syphilis

Syphilis simulates every other disease. It is the only disease necessary to know. One then becomes an expert dermatologist . . . and an expert diagnostician.

Sir William Osler

Syphilis is an infectious disease caused by *Treponema pallidum* (ssp. *pallidum*), a microaerophilic spirochete that is pathogenic only to humans.[1] The organism is too delicate to be grown in vitro, yet so aggressive that it invades almost any organ in the body and so evasive that it can escape a devastating immune attack and, occasionally, even massive doses of antibiotics.[2] The infection is usually contracted through sexual contact with infected lesions or body fluids, less commonly transplacentally from mother to unborn child, and rarely through blood transfusion or accidental inoculation. Despite popular folklore, treponemes are too fragile to be transmitted through contact with toilet seats. Sexually active young adults are the most commonly affected group, followed by adolescents and middle-aged persons.

Dermatologists have a decisive advantage in diagnosing syphilis because of their skill in evaluating skin lesions. However, although the diagnosis is usually made by examination of mucocutaneous lesions, the infection is systemic, even in the absence of symptoms. The highly variable clinical course and diverse manifestations of this "great imitator" were recognized long ago, but much remains to be learned about the pathogenesis of this infection, which continues to baffle and challenge even experienced clinicians, investigators, and epidemiologists.

HISTORY

Syphilis probably evolved from yaws between 15,000 and 3000 B.C.[3] However, it is commonly believed that syphilis was contracted by Spanish sailors from Haitian natives during Columbus' first trip to the New World. Columbus himself reportedly died from syphilitic aortitis. Several infected sailors joined Spanish troops supporting the struggle of Alfonso II of Naples against Charles VIII of France and infected Neopolitan women. The women, in turn, infected mercenaries from different countries fighting for the French army. After the army's disbandment, the mercenaries spread the disease throughout Europe.[4] Portuguese sailors under Vasco da Gama then transported the infection to Asia.

Probably, syphilis was already present in a more attenuated form in several continents. Ancient documents describe "venereal leprosy," an infection that closely resembles syphilis, in the populations of Rome, Greece, and China. Still, scientific publications indicate that a devastating epidemic of a virulent, destructive, and disfiguring form of syphilis (the "Great Pox") swept through Europe at the end of the fifteenth century. In each country the infection was named after a rival nation. The French called it the "Neopolitan itch," the Russians dubbed it the "Polish disease," but the Italian term *morbus Gallicus* (French disease) became particularly popular. In 1530, the physician and poet Girolamo Fracastoro published the third book of his poem *Syphilis sive Morbus Gallicus*, about the affliction of the wealthy and handsome shepherd Syphilus with a repulsive disease as punishment for blasphemy to the Sun God.[4] The poem included a detailed description of the incubation, symptoms, prevention, and treatment, and the name of the shepherd became synonymous with the infection. Fracastoro may have derived the shepherd's name from the mythical Sipylus, a son of the grief-stricken Niobe. The other name by which the disease is commonly known, *lues* (from the Latin for plague or pestilence), was introduced by the sixteenth century physician-poet Jean Fennel, who first differentiated between the primary and secondary stages. By the end of the sixteenth century, the clinical manifestations and treatment with guaiac wood and mercury *("two minutes with Venus, two years with Mercury")* were well documented. But the major contributions were made after the eighteenth century (Table 229-1). None had a greater impact than the introduction of penicillin as treatment for syphilis. Within 10 years, the number of cases had so dramatically declined that the extinction of the disease was predicted, prompting the American Academy of Dermatology and Syphilology to shorten its name.

EPIDEMIOLOGY

In the early part of the twentieth century, 10 percent of the population of the United States and Europe was infected with syphilis.[2] During World War I, the U.S. Congress launched several public health measures after syphilis was detected in 13 percent of military draftees. These included quarantines and compulsory premarital screening. The incidence of syphilis peaked between 1935 and 1947 as efforts to combat the disease were restrained by a "conspiracy of silence." In a statement that is relevant even today, Prince Morrow noted that "social sentiment holds that it is a greater violation

TABLE 229-1

Landmarks in Syphilology

1797	John Hunter concludes that syphilis and gonorrhea are the same disease after developing both infections from a self-administered inoculation of urethral discharge.
1837	Phillipe Ricord distinguishes syphilis from gonorrhea and classifies primary, secondary, and tertiary stages.
1854	John Diday writes popular manual on congenital syphilis.
1856	Ricord generates definitive description of the biology of syphilis.
1880	Jonathan Hutchinson describes triad of congenital syphilis (keratitis, labyrinthitis, and notched teeth).
1891	Caesar Boeck studies the natural course of the disease in 2181 patients who are not treated for fear that complications of mercury are greater than those of syphilis.
1905	Fritz Schaudinn and Erich Hoffman identify treponemes in chancres.
1909	Paul Erlich treats syphilis with a "magic bullet"—arsenic.
1910	August von Wasserman develops complement fixation diagnostic test.
1933	John Nelson generates a treponemal-specific serologic test.
1943	John Mahoney reports that penicillin cures syphilis.

of the properties of life to publicly mention venereal disease than privately to contract it." Surgeon General Thomas Parran, in his ambitious campaign to wipe out the "shadow on the land," called for a "Wasserman dragnet" to screen the population vigorously and to institute partner notification through "shoe leather epidemiology." These aggressive public health policies were largely ineffective.

During World War II, the armed forces instituted successful preventive interventions that included public education, prostitution control, distribution of condoms, and availability of immediate treatment without punitive repercussions. As treatment with penicillin became widely available, the incidence decreased dramatically. The resurgence of sexually transmitted diseases seen in the 1960s was blamed on looser sexual attitudes (permissiveness, promiscuity, and the pill), but in the 1970s, enhanced control efforts lowered the number of syphilis cases. Between 1978 and 1981, the rates of early syphilis increased by 43 percent, declined during the next 5 years, and then began to rise again. In 1990, with a total of 50,223 reported cases of early syphilis and 134,375 cases at any stage, the incidence of syphilis surged to the highest level in 40 years. This resurgence was propelled by the trading of sex for crack-cocaine among heterosexual drug users. Previously, men with same-sex partners constituted a large portion of syphilis cases. However, changes in sexual practices to reduce the risk of HIV infection have dramatically reduced the proportion of syphilis among white gay men from approximately 45 percent to between 10 and 20 percent.

The high number of infected young women resulted in an unprecedented increase in new cases of congenital syphilis, up to a peak of 110 cases per 100,000 births in 1991.[5] Since then, the overall rates of infectious syphilis have dramatically decreased in this country, with new cases concentrated in the southeastern states. Due to aggressive public health intervention the number of reported primary and secondary syphilis cases declined to 8551 in 1997, an 83 percent decrease from the peak of the epidemic in 1990 (Fig. 229-1). This is the lowest incidence since 1959. Although the rates have fallen within all racial and ethnic groups, the rate among non-Hispanic blacks remains 50 times higher than for non-Hispanic whites.[6] The most effective public health strategies have been the

FIGURE 229-1

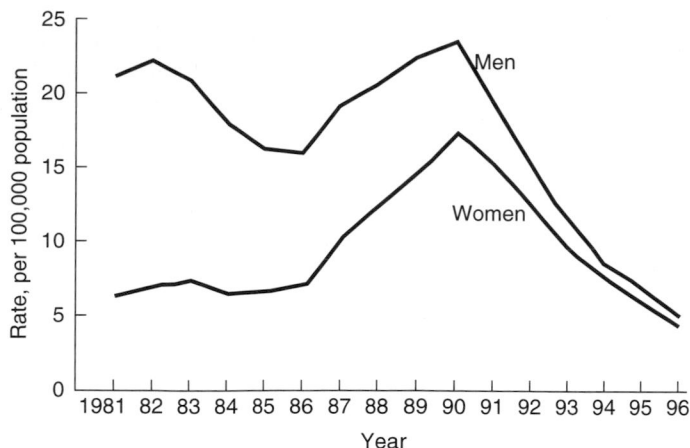

Resurgences of syphilis occur approximately every 10 years.

("coiled hair"). The organism is microscopically indistinguishable from treponemes that cause pinta, yaws, or endemic syphilis and resembles the bacteria that cause Lyme disease, borreliosis, and leptospirosis. Some human or animal nonpathogenic saprophytic treponemes, such as *T. microdentium, T. macrodentium, T. denticola, T. orale,* and *T. vincentii,* are abundant in the oral or anal cavities, making the diagnosis of lesions in these areas unreliable by dark-field microscopy but possible with specific immunoperoxidase stains. *T. pallidum* measures between 6 and 15 μm in length (usually 10 to 13 μm) and 0.10 and 0.18 μm in width (usually 1.5 μm). It has tapered ends between which are 6 to 14 regular tight spiral coils, which are regularly spaced at a distance of 1 μm.[8] When fixed, the spirals impart a wavelike configuration. Its narrow width renders the organism undetectable by light microscopy without silver staining. Under dark-field microscopic examination, the treponemes resemble strings of beads with a characteristic rotatory motion and a flexion and back-and-forth squiggle. This motion is said to be characteristic of virulent treponemes and to facilitate penetration through tissue. However, in fluid medium they lack locomotion, and this distinguishes them from most saprophytic treponemes.

Examination under electron microscopy reveals three main components: the protoplasmic cylinder (protoplast), axial filament, and outer envelope (cell wall). The protoplast is the central part of the treponeme and contains the genetic material and the organelles responsible for metabolism. It is surrounded by a cytoplasmic membrane that regulates absorption and secretion. The axial filament (flagellum) arises at each end of the organism and consists of six to eight elastic fibrils twisted around the protoplast. It imparts a helicoid shape and contributes to the spirochete's mobility. The outer envelope contains the mureine sacculus, a heteropolymer peptidoglycan macromolecule that preserves the organism's shape, protects the fragile cytoplasm against injury, and filters large molecules.[9] An extracellular amorphous slime layer may protect the organism against phagocytosis. The outer envelope contains a paucity of integral transmembrane proteins that stimulate specific antibodies, so the organism more easily evades immune attack.[10] Some of these proteins are proteolipids, which may anchor the membrane and contribute to its rigidity.[11]

Replication occurs through fission, with an interval of 30 to 33 h between divisions. The mureine sacculus is susceptible to damage by antibiotics because growth requires approximately 30 steps and several enzymes.

selection and confidential screening of high-risk populations, partner notification, free treatment of infected persons and partners, and behavior counseling.[7] Now that syphilis has been contained to a relatively small number of communities, strategies for its elimination in this country are being discussed. However, in many parts of the world, the disease continues to be a major public health problem. Despite "therapeutic magic bullets," syphilis has proven to be a formidable opponent. A decline in the number of cases is invariably accompanied by a decrease of funds and public health interest. If history is any indication, syphilis will surge again.

ETIOLOGY

The cause of syphilis is *T. pallidum,* a motile, corkscrew-shaped, gram-negative, prokaryotic bacterium with a flexible, helically coiled cell wall (Fig. 229-2). It belongs to the order Spirochaetales

FIGURE 229-2

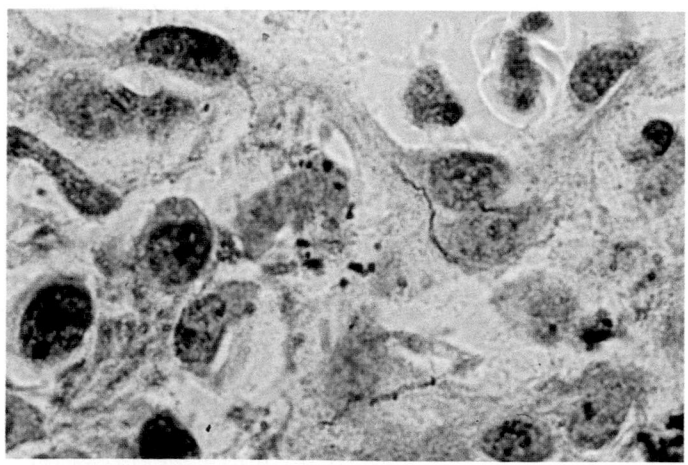

Silver stain of syphilis lesion showing the corkscrew-shaped treponemes.

IMMUNOLOGY

The immune responses in patients with syphilis may differ during the various stages of infection. For this reason, contradictory conclusions have been reported. Our knowledge of the disease has been hampered by the difficulty of growing the organism in culture and the laboriousness involved in growing treponemes in rabbits, the only animal model.

T. pallidum infects the mucosal surfaces and abraded skin of humans. In vitro, the organism penetrates epithelial and endothelial cells as well as connective tissue and muscle layers. Chemotactic factors attract neutrophils to the inoculation site. The neutrophils are replaced by lymphocytes in more mature chancres. Macrophages and plasma cells constitute the remaining cells in the infiltrate. The ratio of CD4-positive T lymphocytes to CD8-positive T-lymphocytes is high in serum and tissue.[12] Lymphocytes secrete lymphokines that attract and activate macrophages, which, in the presence of exogenous antibody, ingest and destroy the organisms. Consistent with a Th1-predominant local cellular response, the lesions contain interleukin (IL) 2, interferon-γ, IL-10, and IL-12.[13] However, not all ingested organisms are destroyed, and some are able to escape phagocytosis. Chondroitin sulfate and hyaluronic acid, which have been reported to modulate immune surveillance, are present in the center of the chancre.

Following tissue penetration, some spirochetes are drained by lymph nodes and the spleen, stimulating antibody formation. A humoral response is elicited, and antibodies to *T. pallidum* are detectable at the time or shortly after the chancre appears. Production of IgM precedes that of IgG.

The combined humoral and cell-mediated immune responses appear to eliminate the spirochetes, resulting in the end of the primary stage. However, after a few weeks the spirochetes proliferate again, and the disease then becomes generalized and systemic. During this stage, called *secondary syphilis*, antibody levels rise in response to the huge numbers of organisms.[1] The antibody response modifies the appearance of the secondary syphilis lesions, which would otherwise resemble primary chancres. At this time, resistance to new infection develops, although delayed-type hypersensitivity to *T. pallidum* becomes inexplicably deficient. The suppression of cell-mediated immunity allows proliferation of the organisms despite rising antibody levels. Such a state predisposes to the formation of immune complexes. Complement may be important as there is evidence that, in its absence, virulent treponemes can resist antibody binding. Also, complement may lyse outer membranes of the treponemes and expose masked antigenic proteins.

The secondary stage is followed by an asymptomatic stage called *latency*. During this period, delayed-type hypersensitivity reappears. In the late stage, the immune response results in the formation of granulomas, although treponemes are rarely detected, even by immunofluorescence.

Immunity to reinfection develops only in untreated patients. After treatment for early syphilis, most patients develop typical chancres when reinfected. However, the majority of patients with untreated latent or congenital syphilis are refractory to reinoculation and do not develop lesions or elevated antibody levels (a few develop dark-field–negative lesions associated with high antibody titers or gummas at the inoculation site). Both humoral and cell-mediated immunity are essential for the development of resistance to reinfection.

The means by which some treponemes resist the immune attack, which effectively clears practically every organism from early lesions, is unknown.[8] Possible explanations include the inhibition of cell-mediated responses, refuge in anatomic sites [central nervous system (CNS), eye, aorta, bone, lymph nodes or perilymph of middle ear] that shield organisms from detection by the immune system, and protection by the slimy mucopolysaccharide coat surrounding the cell wall. Some answers are provided by a study in rabbits. Early on, immunity is normal, resulting in annihilation of most treponemes. However, treponemal products are able to induce the host macrophages to secrete twice as much prostaglandin E_2. As a result, IL-2 synthesis by these cells is halved and, consequently, T cell proliferation is inhibited, leading to suppressed immunity that enables the remaining intact organisms to proliferate, even in the presence of antibody. The suppression persists for at least 1 month and can be reversed by indomethacin or the combination of IL-1 and IL-2.[14]

CLASSIFICATION

Syphilis has been described as an on- and off- and on-again disease. Its course is divided into three clinically distinct stages and two asymptomatic epidemiologic stages. Early syphilis includes the primary stage (chancre), secondary disease (mucocutaneous lesions and/or lymphadenopathy, with or without organ involvement), and clinical relapses. Latent disease is subdivided into early (<1 year) and late (≥1 year) stages. Tertiary (late) disease usually presents with cutaneous, cardiovascular, or neurologic involvement (Table 229-2).

PATHOGENESIS

The natural course of syphilis was studied in three large studies. In the Oslo study conducted in Oslo, Norway, between 1891 and 1910, the records of 953 patients with untreated syphilis were analyzed. The data have been criticized for their emphasis on autopsies, death certificates, and hospital admissions, which biased the results towards a more serious prognosis.[1] In the notorious Tuskegee "experiment,"[15] 412 African-American men with untreated latent syphilis were followed from 1936 to 1972, during which time they were discouraged from receiving treatment. The conclusions of this unethical and racially prejudiced study are limited by its restriction to a single race, sex, and socioeconomic class and by the lack of a protocol. Furthermore, the study has been accused of having as a prime objective the procuring of body tissues and fluids to invent and commercialize serologic tests.[15] The Rosahn study is a review of autopsies and is biased because the population studied obviously had a poor outcome.

TABLE 229-2

Stages of Syphilis

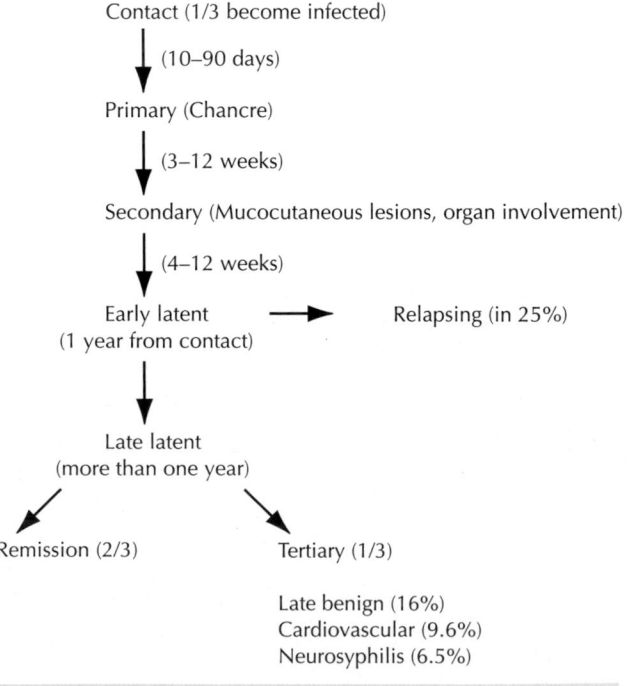

In the Oslo study, the median duration of the primary stage was 30 days in men and 27 days in women. The secondary stage lasted 2.1 months in men and 3.5 months in women. Approximately 25 percent of patients experienced relapsing syphilis, and in this group one-quarter had multiple episodes.

Six months after contracting syphilis, 95 percent of patients become uninfectious, even without treatment. Although the danger of direct transmission is exceedingly low after 5 years of infection, inoculation from gummas has been reported. Latent syphilis follows the secondary stage and may persist for life in an asymptomatic form in about two-thirds of untreated patients. The rest develop tertiary syphilis, which usually becomes manifest as cutaneous (16 percent), cardiovascular (9.6 percent), or CNS (6.5 percent) disease. Syphilis was the cause of death in 11 percent of the patients in the Oslo study. In African-American men with untreated syphilis, the mortality is even higher as cardiovascular disease was found in approximately half of autopsies. As the eminent venereologist Rudolph Kampmeier wrote in 1943, "It would be of great value if the prognosis of untreated syphilis were accurately known (but) this is not known and probably never will be known in these days of more or less universal treatment of the disease."

CLINICAL MANIFESTATIONS

Primary Syphilis

About one-third of persons who come in contact with an early syphilis lesion become infected. At the site of treponemal penetration, after an incubation period that ranges from 10 to 90 days (average 3 weeks), a dusky red macule appears that grows into a papule and becomes a *chancre* by ulcerating in the center (Fig. 229-3). The length of the incubation period varies inversely with the number of inoculated treponemes. The chancre is round or oval, approximately 1 to 2 cm in size, and has sharply defined, regular, raised, indurated borders. The "ham-colored" ulcer base usually has a smooth surface and may be covered with a grayish slough.[16] The lesion feels firm, rubbery, and is painless if uncomplicated by trauma or impetiginization. When squeezed, a thin serous exudate teeming with spirochetes is expressed. Untreated, the chancre persists from 1 to 6

weeks; it resolves within 1 to 2 weeks after treatment and heals without scarring. However, deviation from the above description is common, and the classic "Hunterian" chancre is now seen in only about 60 percent of cases. In 15 to 30 percent, the lesions go unnoticed. In one study, 23 percent of men with primary syphilis had more than one chancre, 8 percent had multiple lesions with edema or phimosis, 4.5 percent erosive balanitis, and 1.1 percent lymphangitis or thrombophlebitis of the dorsal vein (Fig. 229-4). The frequency of multiple lesions has been reported to be as high as 47 percent (Fig. 229-5). A reason for the rising number of multiple chancres may be the increased incidence of herpes genitalis erosions that facilitate treponemal penetration. In men, the commonly involved locations are the glans, the coronal sulcus, and the foreskin. Chancres in the urethral orifice have been reported to cause an inflammatory phimosis that may eventuate in penile gangrene. Retraction of the foreskin with a chancre in its mucosal surface causes the foreskin to flip briskly, a sign dubbed "the dory flop" by John Stokes. In women, the labia, fourchette, urethra, and perineum are affected, in descending order of frequency. *Edema indurativum* describes a unilateral labial swelling with rubbery consistency and intact surface, representing a deep-seated chancre. Chancres develop in the cervix in as many as 44 percent of infected women but are rarely detected. On palpation, chancres in women have edematous induration rather than "cartilaginous" firmness. "Kissing" chancres are common in areas of skin-to-skin contact such as the vulva.

Extragenital chancres have become more common with increased oral sex. About two-thirds occur above the neck, and approximately half of these are seen around the lips or in the oral cavity. The rest appear on the fingers, breasts, trunk, abdomen, and extremities (Fig. 229-6). Chancres of the fingers are often seen in medical or dental personnel and tend to be painful. Anorectal chancres constitute 4 to 10 percent of extragenital primary syphilis cases. Anorectal primary syphilis is underdiagnosed and should be considered in any at-risk person with rectal pain, bloody stools, anal

FIGURE 229-3

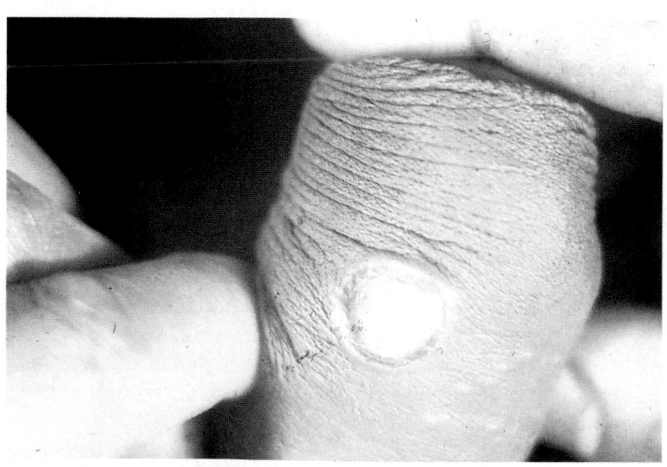

Classic "Hunterian" chancre with raised, indurated borders and a smooth, clean base on the foreskin of a man.

FIGURE 229-4

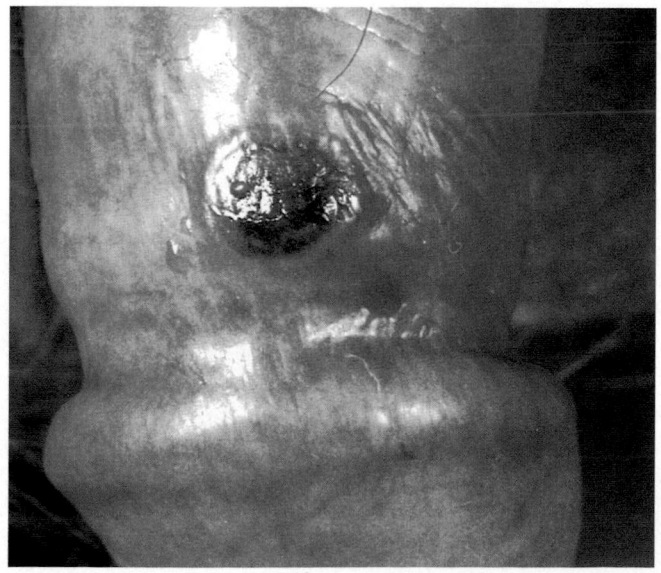

Primary syphilis with chancre.

FIGURE 229-5

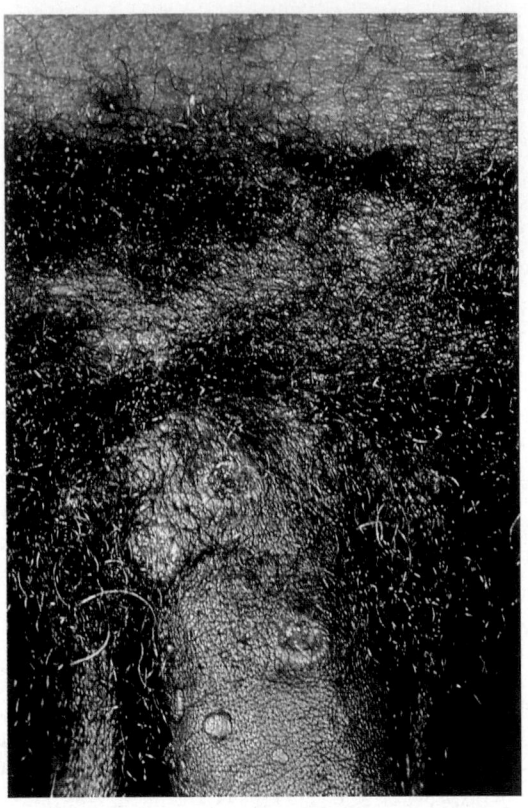

Multiple chancres at the base of the penis and adjacent pubis. Chancres in this location are associated with use of condoms.

fissures, or a precipitously appearing mass or ulcer in the anorectal area.

In 70 to 80 percent of all primary syphilis cases, enlarged, rubbery, movable, nontender, nonsuppurative discrete lymph nodes (*buboes*) appear around the first week of infection. These are usually unilateral at first and most commonly palpated in the inguinal area, although in women the femoral nodes are often enlarged. In

FIGURE 229-6

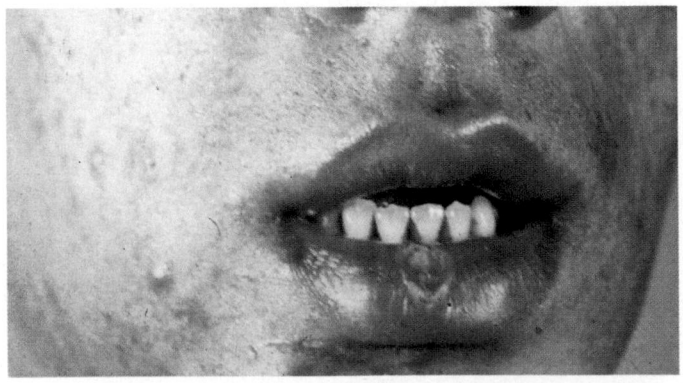

Chancre on the lip, the most common location of extragenital chancres.

one study they were tender in 14 percent of patients. The presence of concomitant sexually transmitted infections, especially chancroid and herpes simplex, is well documented.

Differential Diagnosis

The diseases most frequently misdiagnosed as primary syphilis are chancroid, traumatic ulcers, and herpes genitalis. The differential diagnosis also includes granuloma inguinale, lymphogranuloma venereum, bacterial infections, squamous or basal cell carcinoma, Behçet's disease, lymphoma, aphthous ulcers, fixed drug eruption, and balanitis or vulvitis due to candidiasis, psoriasis, or lichen planus. Relapses of primary syphilis, termed *monorecidive syphilis* or *chancre redux* are rare.

Secondary Syphilis

Lesions of secondary syphilis erupt 3 to 12 weeks after the appearance of the chancre but may develop months later or, in up to 15 percent of cases, before the chancre disappears. The secondary stage usually recedes in 4 to 12 weeks.[16] Not all patients present with the classic textbook presentation. In fact, the symptoms and clinical findings may be subtle, transient, and easily overlooked or so severe that hospitalization is required. Almost 60 percent of patients with latent or late syphilis deny ever experiencing signs or symptoms of secondary disease. One-quarter of these patients cannot recall the appearance of a chancre either. Patients with secondary syphilis may be ill with flulike symptoms that include malaise, appetite loss, fever, headache, stiff neck, lacrimation, myalgias, arthralgias, nasal discharge, and depression. However, the majority of patients present with only an eruption. The frequency of organ involvement differs among studies. In a series of 2269 cases of secondary syphilis, the skin was involved in 81.1 percent, the oral cavity and pharynx in 36.3 percent, the genitalia in 19.9 percent, the CNS in 9.9 percent, the eyes in 4 percent, and visceral organs in 0.2 percent. A wise clinician, possibly once humbled by an earlier misdiagnosis, learns to consider the "great imitator" when challenged by a combination of signs and symptoms that cannot be readily explained.

Skin eruptions develop in 80 to 95 percent of cases. Over 95 percent of the eruptions are macular, maculopapular, papular, or annular. Nodular and pustular eruptions occur infrequently, and vesiculobullous lesions are seen only in prenatal syphilis and not at all in adults. Lesions of secondary syphilis tend to have a symmetric pattern early in the disease and become polymorphic later. According to classic teachings, pruritus is generally not present, but in some reports between 8 and 42 percent of patients experienced itching. Pruritus appears to be more common in African-Americans and immunocompromised patients. As a rule, the secondary lesions heal without scar formation in 2 to 10 weeks, with or without treatment.

MACULAR ERUPTIONS Referred to in old textbooks as "roseola syphilitica," the eruption is seen in about 10 percent of cases. The lesions are pink, discrete, nonscaling, oval macules and patches, about 0.05 to 2 cm in size, which predominantly involve the trunk and flexor aspects of the upper extremities (Fig. 229-7). The face is usually spared, but any area, including the palms and soles, may be involved. The lesions do not tend to follow the lines of cleavage and may become annular or papular.

MACULOPAPULAR ERUPTIONS Reported in between 22 and 70 percent of secondary syphilis cases, this eruption is commonly encountered in practice. It represents an evolution of the macular

FIGURE 229-7

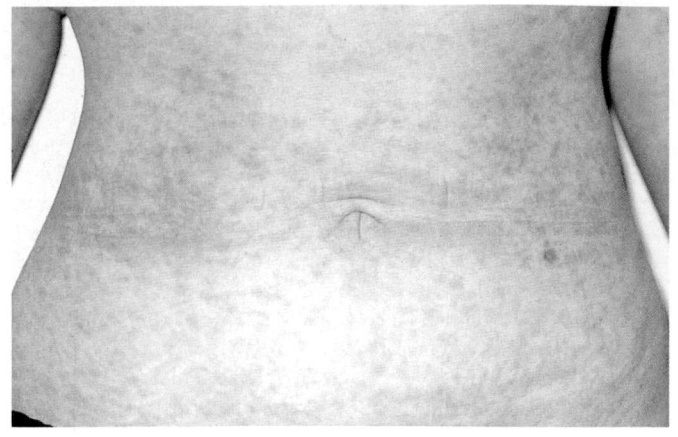

Macular syphilis (roseola syphilitica) with nonscaling, oval pink macules and patches on the chest and abdomen.

FIGURE 229-8

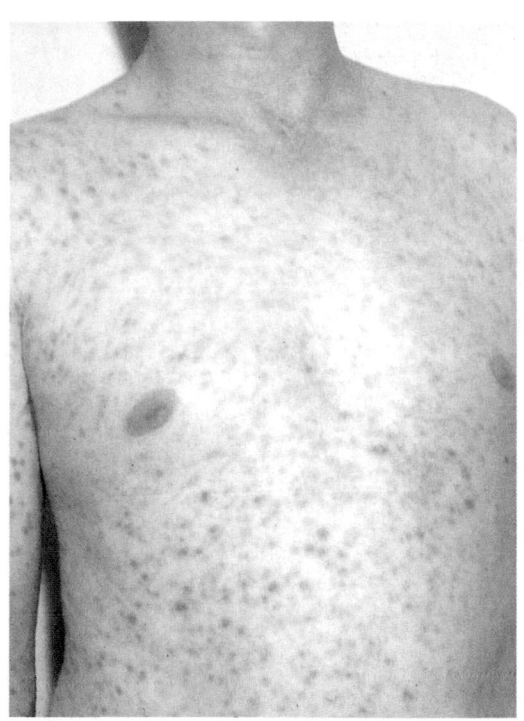

Maculopapular syphilis showing a combination of erythematous macules and papules.

lesions towards papules and plaques, as some macules become thickened and develop a dark coppery hue (Fig. 229-8). Lesions are often present on the genitalia, face, palms, and soles. Lesions around the hairline form a crownlike pattern known as the "corona veneris."

PAPULAR ERUPTIONS This group constitutes about 12 percent of secondary syphilitic eruptions and includes papulosquamous, follicular, lenticular, corymbose, nodular, and annular varieties.

Papulosquamous eruptions have discoid, copper-colored or erythematous, oval or circular, indurated papules or plaques with a

FIGURE 229-9

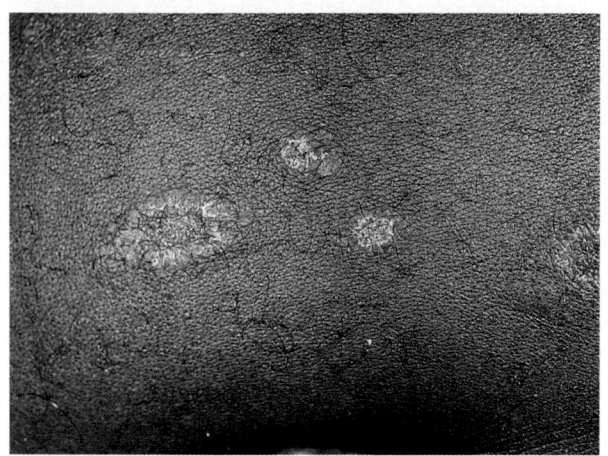

Papulosquamous syphilitic eruption with erythematous, well-demarcated, flattened plaques covered with scales.

FIGURE 229-10

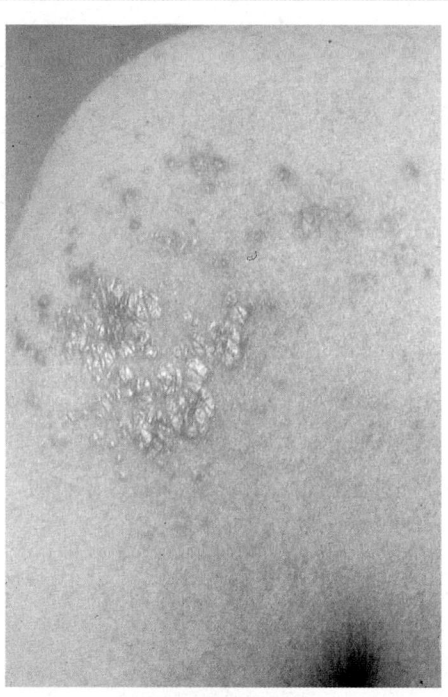

Lichenoid syphilitic eruption with pink to violaceous, planar, polygonal papules resembling lichen planus.

flat, shiny, scaly surface (Fig. 229-9). Annular, serpiginous, concentric (cocarde syphilid), or arcuate configurations may be seen. When the lesions are pruritic and lichenoid, the eruption may be difficult to distinguish from lichen planus (Fig. 229-10) and, when the scaling is thick, from psoriasis. The occasional presence of the Koebner phenomenon further contributes to this confusion. A thin, white ring of scales on the surface of a lesion (Biette's collarette) is a valuable diagnostic sign although, contrary to Dr. Biette's opinion, not pathognomonic. The palms and soles are often involved (Fig. 229-11). On the soles, the lesions may become hyperkeratotic and be mistaken for calluses (clavi syphilitici) or tinea pedis.

Lenticular eruptions consist of pinhead to lentil-size, brown to red papules with smooth surfaces or fine scaling. The face, especially the forehead, oral commissures, nasolabial folds, and the genitalia are favored sites.

FIGURE 229-11

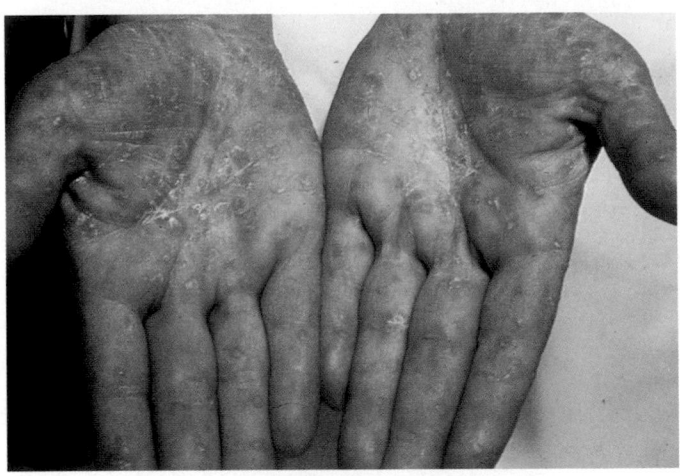

A.

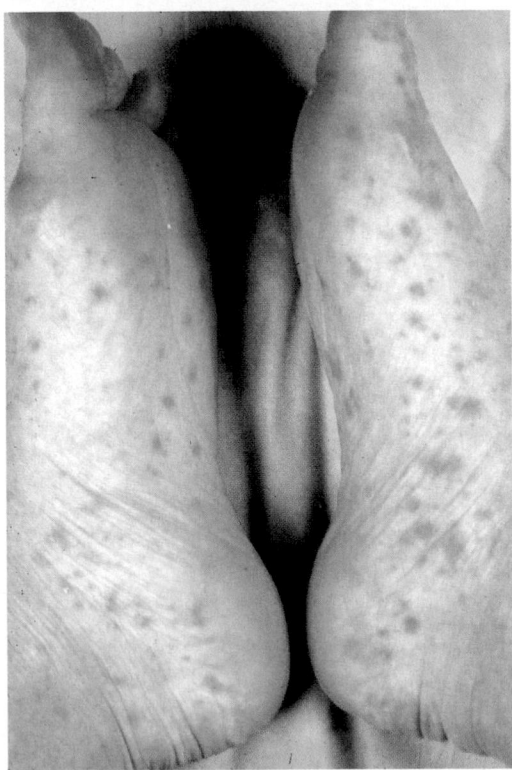

B.

Characteristic secondary syphilis lesions on the palms (*A*) and soles (*B*). Palmoplantar lesions may be macular or papular, discrete or diffuse, and nonscaling, slightly scaly, or hyperkeratotic ("syphilitic corn").

Corymbose ("bombshell") eruptions are rare and seldom occur before 6 to 8 months of infection. Typically a large central papule is surrounded by smaller satellite papules (Fig. 229-12).

Nodular eruptions consist of dermal nodules, which are frequently misdiagnosed as lymphoma or a granulomatous disease (Fig. 229-13).

Annular eruptions consist of oval or round ringlike papules and plaques with a predilection for the face, anogenital area, body folds, palms, and soles (Fig. 229-14). Because the lesions in the face are approximately the size of coins, the eruption has been dubbed the "nickel and dime syphilid." The eruption is often misdiagnosed as sarcoid, granuloma annulare, or tinea corporis.

Follicular eruptions have been called "lichen syphiliticus" or "miliary papular syphilis." The lesions consist of pinpoint, acuminate or rounded, erythematous papules that arise in crops on the torso and extremities. This eruption is uncommon and has been reported predominantly in debilitated persons such as alcoholics.

PUSTULAR SECONDARY SYPHILIS These eruptions include several morphologic variants. In *miliary pustular eruptions*, small acuminate pustules and papules resolve with depressed pigmented scars. In *acneiform*, *varioliform*, or *obtuse eruptions*, there are large, acuminate perifollicular pustules, often with polymorphism (Fig. 229-15). In *impetiginoid* or *ecthymiform eruptions*, flat pustules become confluent and covered with a large crust called a *carapace*. *Malignant syphilis*, also known as "lues maligna," "rupial syphilis," or "pustuloulcerative syphilis," presents with widespread papulopustules that become necrotic and break down into ulcers covered by layers of thick, dirty-looking crust resembling an oyster shell

FIGURE 229-12

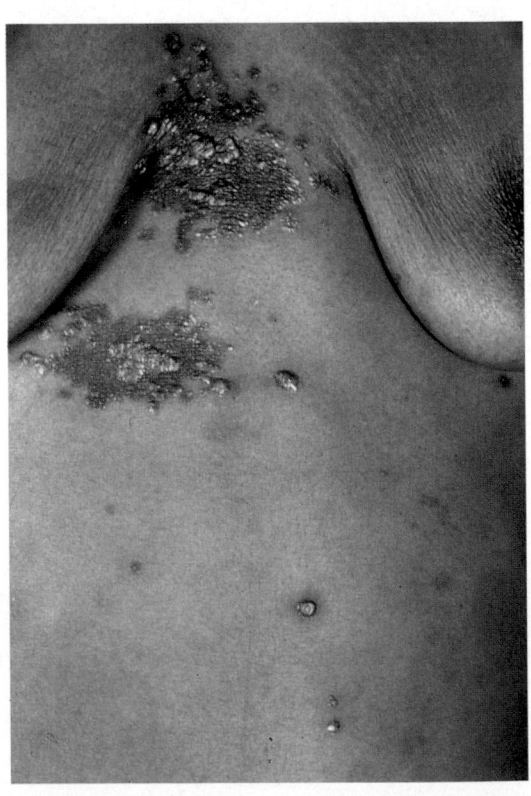

Corymbose syphilitic eruptions occur late in the secondary stage, usually after 6 to 8 months of infection. A larger papule or plaque is surrounded by smaller satellite papules.

FIGURE 229-13

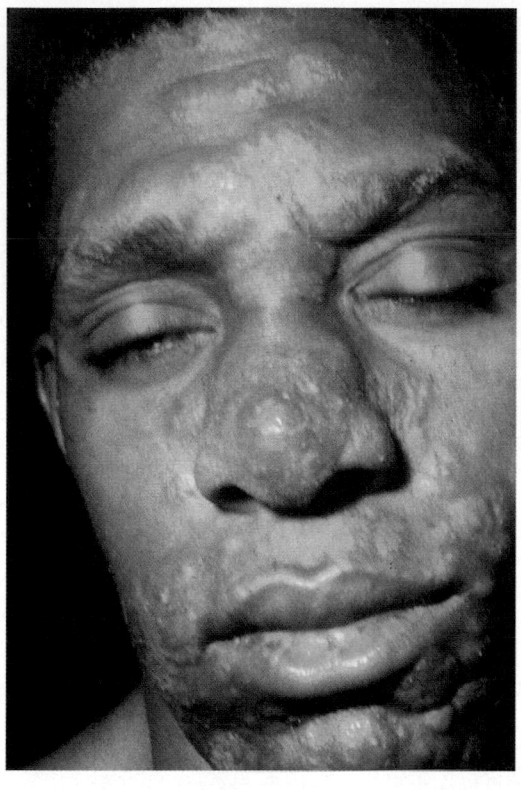

Nodular secondary syphilis in the face of a man. The lesions are frequently misdiagnosed as lymphoma or a granulomatous disease.

FIGURE 229-14

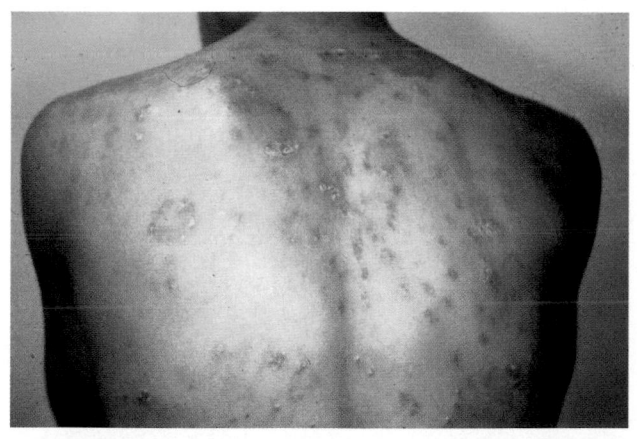

Annular eruption of secondary syphilis. The face and mucous membranes are commonly affected in this variant, which favors dark-skinned patients.

FIGURE 229-15

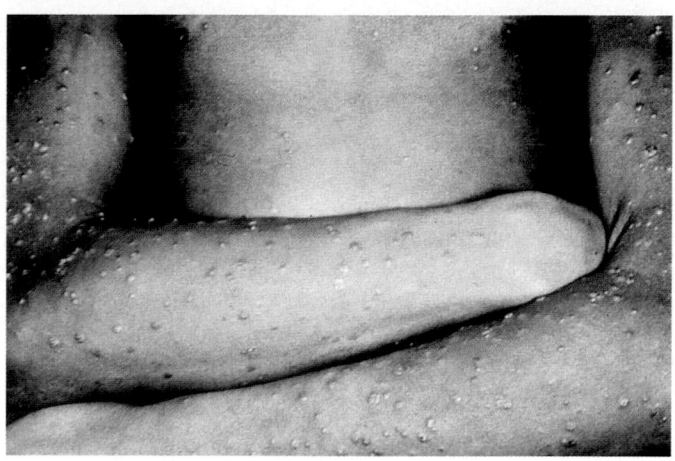

Follicular papulopustular eruptions have been associated with a higher risk of neurosyphilis.

FIGURE 229-16

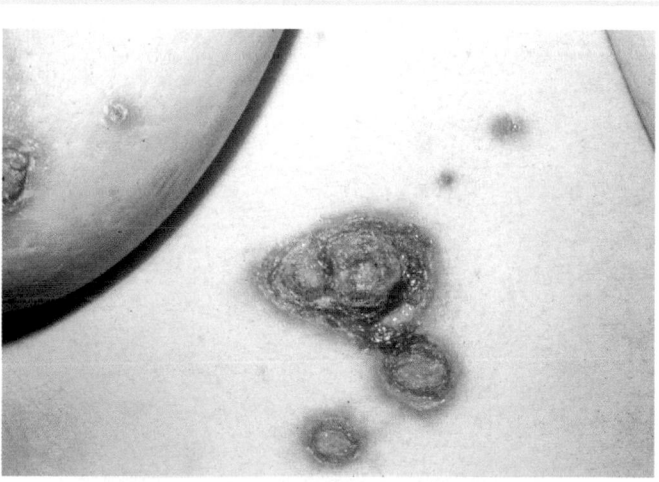

Sharply marginated, necrotic ulcers covered by "rupioid," thick dirty crusts (like oyster shells) are the characteristic lesions of malignant syphilis.

("rupioid") (Fig. 229-16). The eruption, which involves predominantly the face and scalp, is associated with toxicity, fever, arthalgias, and occasionally hepatitis. In some cases, the lesions resemble chancres. Oral ulcers and mucous patches may develop. Most patients have abnormal immune systems or poor health. Infected contacts usually have a more benign course, and there is no evidence that the treponemes causing the infection are more virulent. Apparently, malignant syphilis was more common in the seventeenth century, when it was known as "le grand verole." Noduloulcerative syphilis with or without systemic symptoms is more common in HIV-infected persons.

PIGMENTARY CHANGES   The lesions may heal with postinflammatory hyper- or hypopigmentation. On the sides of the neck an interesting pattern consisting of hypopigmented macules superimposed on linear pigmented reticulated patches is known as "leukoderma colli syphiliticum" or the "necklace of Venus." Similar lesions may occur on the penis as well as on other areas. In dark-skinned individuals, intense loss of pigment within the affected areas may resemble vitiligo. Hypopigmentation in syphilis results from partial inhibition of melanogenesis as the number of melanocytes is normal or only slightly reduced. When dermal atrophy, possibly related to inflammation-induced elastin degradation, is present, the appearance resembles anetoderma.

MUCOUS MEMBRANE LESIONS These lesions are extremely infectious. The three manifestations are condylomata lata, mucous patches, and pharyngitis. The last two heal spontaneously within 2 to 3 weeks, but condylomata may persist for months.

Condylomata lata consist of flesh-colored or hypopigmented, moist, oozing papules that become flattened and macerated (Fig. 229-17). They have been reported in 9 to 44 percent of cases. Their surface may be smooth, papillated, or covered with cauliflower-like vegetations. The common sites are the genital and anal areas and, less frequently, the oral commissures, face, axillae, inframammary folds, and toe webs.[17] Lesions in intertriginous areas may erode or proliferate, forming elevated, brown velvety plaques or grouped hypertrophic, nodular lesions that resemble raspberries ("frambesiform syphilid"). Overgrowth of bacteria produces a foul odor.

Mucous patches are painless, shallow, rounded erosions covered with gray macerated scaling (Fig. 229-18). Present in 7 to 12 percent of secondary syphilis cases, the lesions may appear anywhere in the mouth but are more common on the tongue and lips. The tonsils and epiglottis may be affected, resulting in hoarseness. Confluence of several denuded lesions on the tongue has been termed *plaques fauchées en prairie.* Mucous patches also arise in the glans penis, inner vulva, and anus. In these areas the lesions are more

FIGURE 229-17

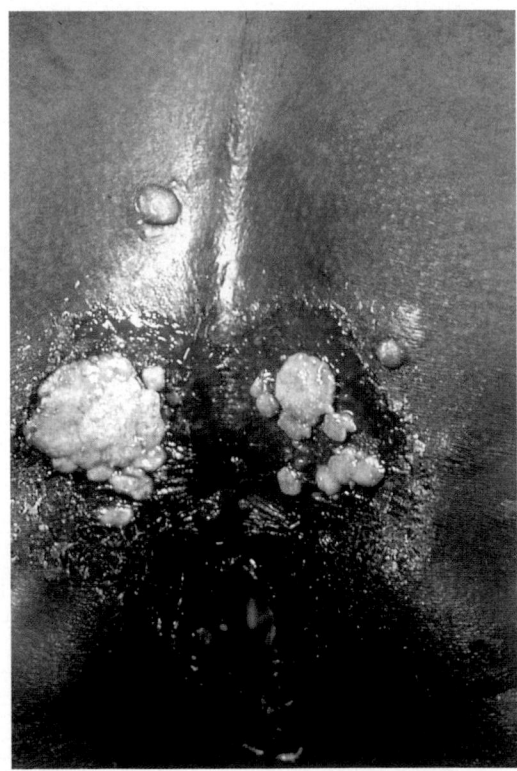

Rounded, gray, moist, vegetating papules (condylomata lata) develop most frequently on the anogenital area but may arise on the lips, groin, and toe webs. The lesions are often confused with condylomata acuminata (venereal warts).

FIGURE 229-18

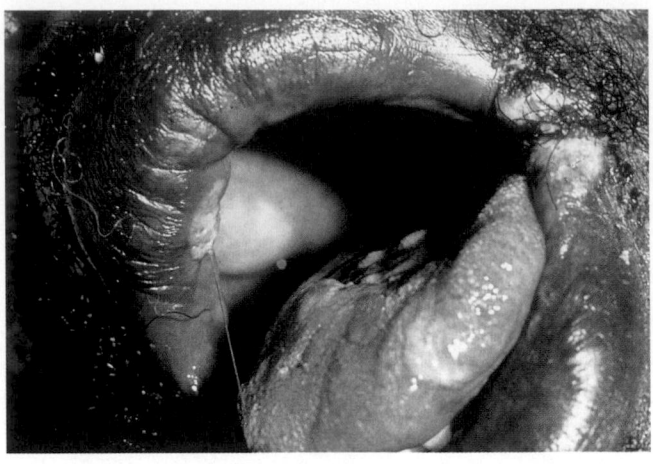

Mucous patches on the lips. These erosions covered with gray-white, macerated scales are seen on the lips, oral mucosa, tonsils, and larynx. Lesions in the buccal commissure are fissured in the center (split papules).

likely to become eroded or ulcerated due to friction. *Split papules* are elevated mucous patches with central fissures in the oral commissures.

Pharyngitis of variable severity may occur in up to a quarter of cases, although soreness is rare. Diffuse redness of the pharynx, palate, and tonsils may be very mild or severe with edema and erosions (Fig. 229-19). Pseudomembranes and necrosis have been reported, and laryngeal involvement may produce hoarseness.

NAIL DISEASE In secondary syphilis, nail changes may be due to involvement of either the nail matrix or the nail folds. In the nail

FIGURE 229-19

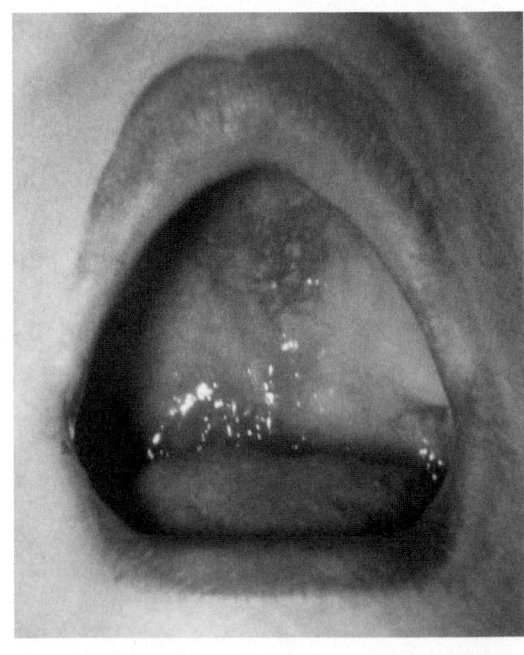

Erythema of the soft palate and pharynx is a commonly missed finding in secondary syphilis.

plate, brittleness, splitting, onycholysis, pitting, lunular elkonyxis with fissuring (onyxis craquelé), and dystrophy have been described. The nail plate growing during the infectious episode may become dull, dry, and thickened or develop Beau's lines and latent onychomadesis. Paronychia of the lateral and proximal nail folds may develop. If prolonged, the skin can break down, leaving a horseshoe ulcer. The nail bed may become ulcerated, producing an exudate that may cause separation, shedding, and even permanent deformity of the nail plate. Amber-colored plates resembling artificial nails have been reported to be characteristic of late syphilis. Cyanotic, painful toes (the "blue toe syndrome") are an unusual manifestation.[18]

HAIR ABNORMALITIES Alopecia may be the only sign of secondary syphilis. It has been described in 3 to 7 percent of cases and may be either patchy, generalized, or a combination.[19] The more characteristic type consists of small irregular patches of nonscarring alopecia throughout the scalp but predominantly on the occipital and parietal regions. Because the margins are not sharp, the term *moth-eaten* is often used descriptively (Fig. 229-20). In some cases, the lesions resemble trichotillomania or alopecia areata.[20] Occasionally the eyebrows, beard, and other hair-bearing areas are affected. Diffuse hair loss may occur as a sign of secondary syphilis or as a telogen effluvium clinically noticeable 3 to 5 months after the infection begins.

OTHER ASSOCIATED CLINICAL MANIFESTATIONS

1. *Lymphoreticular system.* Enlarged lymph nodes are present in 50 to 80 percent of cases. In descending order of frequency,

the inguinal, axillary, cervical, epitrochlear, femoral, and superclavicular chains are involved. Typically the nodes are movable, firm, rubbery, discrete, bilateral, symmetric, and nontender.[16] Mild splenomegaly is common.

2. *Ophthalmologic.* Iritis, which is the most common eye complication, occurs in fewer than 3 percent of all cases and then, late in the disease, usually with relapsing syphilis (Fig. 229-21). Uveitis, chorioretinitis, and, rarely, vasculitic occlusion of the central retinal vein and artery are also observed. A recent report concluded that 4.3 percent of 552 cases of uveitis were syphilitic.[21] Symptoms include photophobia, lacrimation, red painful eyes, and blindness. Topical glucocorticoids without antibiotics are contraindicated.

3. *Auditory.* There are a few reports of sensorineural hearing loss in early acquired syphilis. The condition worsens rapidly and tends to be bilateral. Vestibular involvement with labyrinthitis is uncommon.[22] However, 6 percent of all cases of Ménière's disease are caused by congenital or acquired syphilis.[23] The pathogenesis is usually basilar meningitis with damage to the eighth nerve. Immediate treatment with penicillin antibiotics and a prolonged course of prednisone preserves hearing in almost all cases.

4. *Musculoskeletal.* Because bone and joint involvement are not readily apparent, the impression has been that they are rare. However, different studies have found rates ranging from 0.15 to 4 percent clinically and 9 percent radiologically. The principal symptoms are local pain, erythema, doughy tumefaction, and warmth. Favored affected sites are the long bones of the extremities, especially the tibia, and the skull, with resulting persistent headaches. Radiographs and the more-sensitive bone scans demonstrate any combination of periostitis, osteomyelitis, bone destruction, and sclerosis. Radiographic changes may take up to 11 months for complete resolution. Back pain, arthralgias, arthritis, tenosynovitis, and bursitis may be severe and persist for several months. Patients may experience generalized myalgias and muscle weakness that resembles an inflammatory myopathy.

FIGURE 229-20

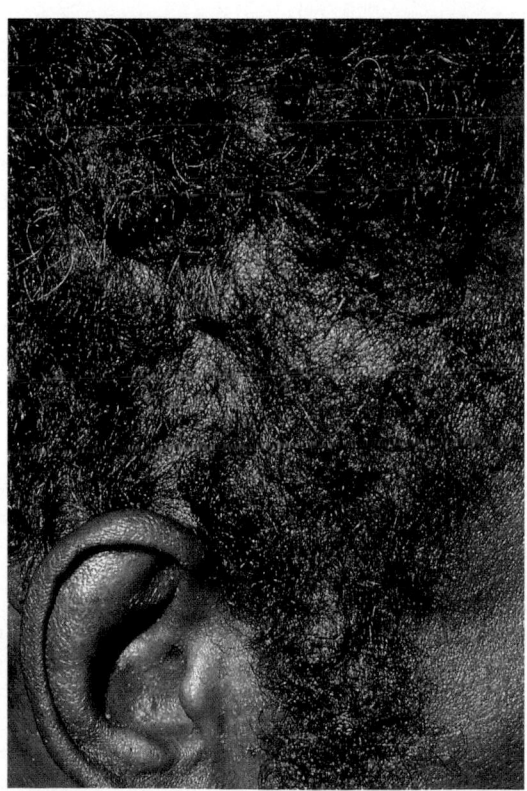

Moth-eaten alopecia is the more common form of hair loss. Irregular, patchy, nonscarring alopecia is present more frequently on the occipital scalp and occasionally affects the eyebrows and beard.

FIGURE 229-21

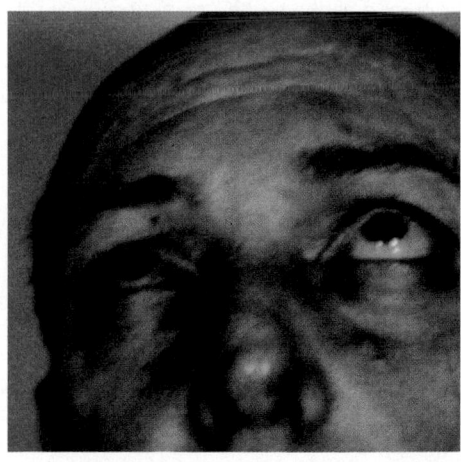

Iritis is the most common eye complication in secondary syphilis. The patient presents with red, injected eyes and complains of pain, lacrimation, and photophobia.

5. *Hematologic.* Abnormalities include anemia, leukocytosis, relative lymphopenia, and elevated sedimentation rate.

6. *Renal.* Acute membranous glomerulonephritis, usually manifested by the nephrotic syndrome, is reversible with treatment.

7. *Hepatic.* Although usually subclinical, the incidence of hepatitis was 9.7 percent in one study. Jaundice is seldom detected.

8. *Gastric.* Epigastric pain and postprandial vomiting may be due to eroded, ulcerated, or polypoidal stomach lesions, which heal with antibiotics.[24] Erosive syphilitic gastritis usually affects the antrum of the stomach.

9. *Cardiopulmonary.* Lesions in the lungs and heart conduction defects have been reported but are extremely rare.

10. *Neurologic.* Abnormal findings in the cerebrospinal fluid (CSF) are common in early syphilis (see "Neurosyphilis," below).

LATENT SYPHILIS

The secondary stage is followed by an asymptomatic stage with no clinical findings in which the only evidence of the disease is reactive serologic testing. Latency may remain indefinitely, be interrupted by a relapse of secondary syphilis, or progress to the tertiary stage. Being a diagnosis of exclusion, careful examination for mucocutaneous lesions and organ involvement is required. Ultrasound evaluation of the aorta to exclude cardiovascular disease should be considered. Although neurosyphilis should be excluded by examination of the CSF, spinal taps are not routinely done due to concern about complications, unless neurologic signs or symptoms are present or the patient is HIV-infected. The duration of infection should be determined by history and previous serologic tests, because, for therapeutic and epidemiologic purposes, the latent stage is divided into early and late stages, as discussed earlier. However, this may not always be possible, and the clinician must settle for a diagnosis of "indeterminate" latency, which is treated in the same manner as late latent disease.

In clinical practice, patients who were adequately treated but continue to have low titers of nontreponemal tests are commonly seen. If previous treatment or lack of reinfection cannot be confirmed, then, from a public health standpoint, these patients should be assumed to be infected and treated. A record of the nontreponemal test titer and the administered therapy should be given to the patient. Too often patients are unnecessarily re-treated over and over again because such records are not readily available.

RELAPSING SYPHILIS

Around 25 percent of untreated patients experience a relapse of secondary lesions despite the absence of reinfection. More than two-thirds of the relapses occur within 6 months, 90 percent within the first year, and 95 percent within 2 years. None occur after 6 years. Relapses may present with the reappearance of chancres or an eruption of secondary syphilis, including mucous patches and condylomata lata. These lesions tend to be less extensive and are frequently confined to the anogenital and oral areas. Because patients may be unaware of the lesions or insufficiently concerned to seek medical help, relapsing syphilis is particularly alarming from an epidemiologic standpoint. Other presentations include periostitis (usually tibial), iritis, and hepatitis.

TERTIARY SYPHILIS

Approximately one-third of patients with untreated latent syphilis develop tertiary syphilis, while the other two-thirds remain in perpetual latency. The three principal presentations during this stage are late benign syphilis, cardiovascular disease, and neurosyphilis.

Late Benign (Tertiary) Syphilis

Late benign syphilis includes any symptomatic syphilitic manifestation after the secondary and relapsing stages that does not involve the cardiovascular or nervous systems. The lesions are caused by a cell-mediated inflammatory response to a few treponemes present in the affected tissue. At the beginning of the twentieth century, the incidence in untreated men and women was 14.4 and 16.7 per 100,000 population, respectively, but now this stage is rare, possibly as a result of widespread use of antibiotics for other infections. The more commonly involved organs are the skin (70 percent), mucous membranes (10.3 percent), and bones (9.6 percent) but gummas may appear in practically any organ, including the brain, parotid glands, thyroid, esophagus, stomach, liver (hepar lobatum), breasts, pancreas, kidneys, adrenal glands, heart, spleen, bladder, and cervix. Chronic iritis, chorioretinitis, interstitial keratitis, and atrophy of the optic nerve are rare. Painless, fibrosing interstitial orchitis can result in atrophy.

LATE BENIGN SYPHILIS OF THE SKIN Tertiary skin lesions can be divided into three types: granulomatous nodules, psoriasiform granulomatous plaques, and gummas. "Precocious" lesions develop within the first 2 years after the resolution of the secondary stage, and "late" lesions at any time after that. Most lesions develop within 3 to 7 years, but gummas have appeared as long as 60 years after infection. The longer the interval before the appearance of the skin lesions, the more solitary and destructive the process.

Even without therapy, there is a tendency to partial healing, but new lesions may develop at the periphery, and spontaneous complete healing is unusual. The lesions may heal with noncontractile, atrophic scars. Noduloulcerative lesions are more superficial than gummas and respond dramatically to penicillin.

Precocious tertiary syphilis develops during the first 2 years of infection and occasionally within weeks. Infiltrated grouped papules that tend to ulcerate may be localized to one site or be more widespread. The papules have features of both secondary stage lesions and tertiary stage granulomas. Treponemes are rarely detected. The lesions heal with little or no scarring.

Nodular and *noduloulcerative lesions* are superficial, firm, painless, dull red, shiny, dome-shaped cutaneous nodules that measure several millimeters to 2 cm in size. The nodules appear in a grouped configuration, rapidly grow horizontally, and become confluent into plaques.[25] The skin overlying the lesions becomes inflamed and breaks down, resulting in crusted superficial ulcers with raised borders. Over weeks or months central healing and advancing borders produce plaques with annular, arciform, serpiginous, or polycyclic configurations that may reach over 30 cm (Fig. 229-22). Some plaques may be psoriasiform (Fig. 229-23). The lesions are most commonly seen on the arms, back, and face. Even without treatment

FIGURE 229-22

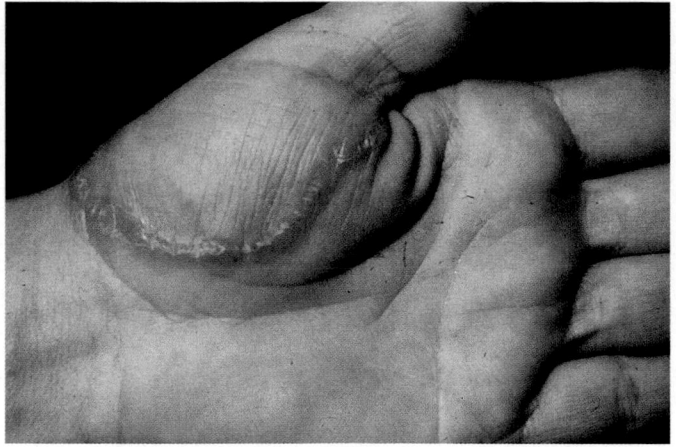

Late benign syphilis presenting with annular plaque involving the thenar eminence.

FIGURE 229-23

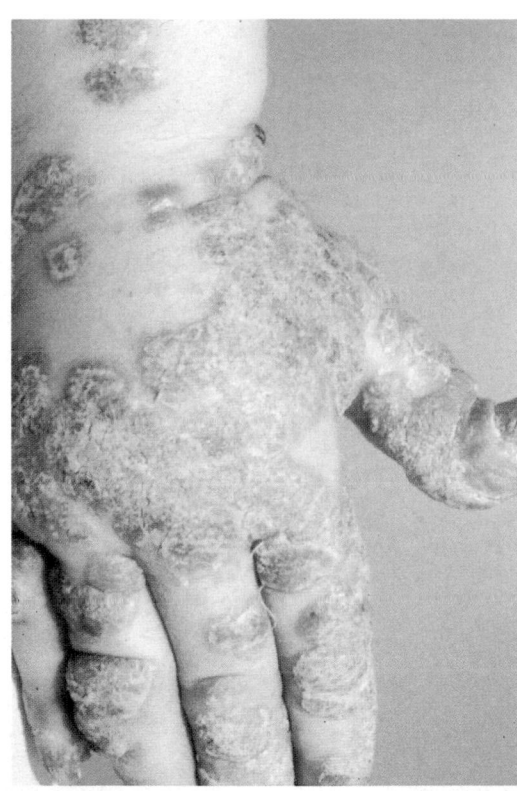

Crusted, psoriasiform noduloulcerative tertiary syphilis plaques with nail dystrophy.

FIGURE 229-24

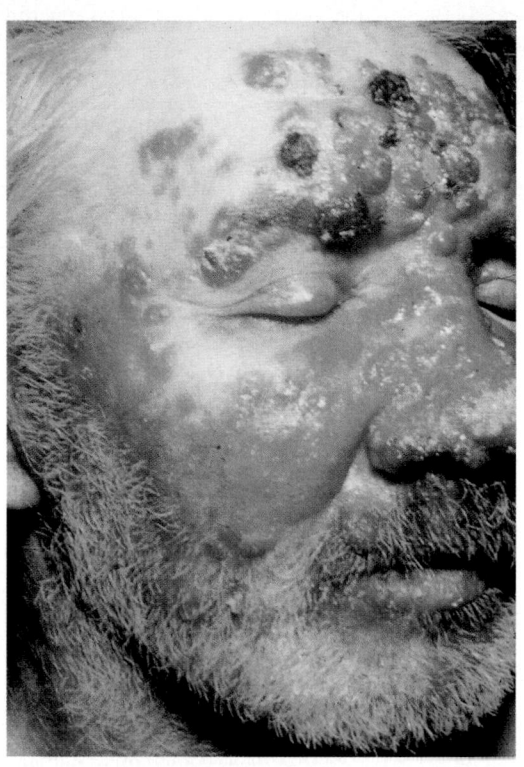

Disfiguring gummatous infiltration of the face with scattered ulcerations and scarring in a man with late benign syphilis.

FIGURE 229-25

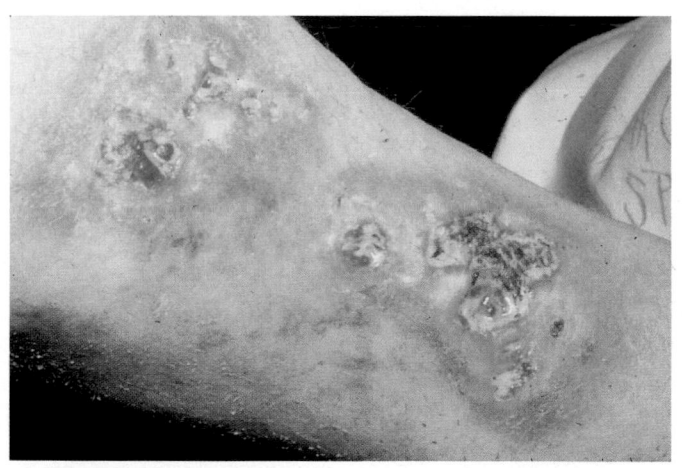

Deep, pretibial gumma showing ulcerations and scarring within the lesion.

the granulomas heal over the years, leaving noncontractile, atrophic scars with increased or decreased pigmentation.

Gummas are nontender pink to dusky red nodules or plaques that vary in size from millimeters to many centimeters in diameter.[26] They favor sites of previous trauma and may arise anywhere in the body but are more common on the scalp, forehead, buttocks, and presternal, superaclavicular or pretibial areas (Fig. 229-24). The

nodule is initially firm but develops a "gum"-like consistency due to accumulation of necrotic tissue; it eventually feels like a cold abscess. In addition to their gummy consistency, gummas differ from noduloulcerative lesions by being more destructive and deeper (Fig. 229-25). Necrosis eventuates in cylindrical, punched-out ulcers with clean granulomatous bases covered with adherent yellow-white slough. The ulcer may enlarge, remain unchanged, or heal spontaneously even as the gumma enlarges. More superficial gummas heal with noncontractile atrophic scars, whereas deeper lesions leave thickened, pitted, ridged scars. Gummas may grow horizontally as well as vertically and have within the lesion small ulcerations and abscesses. Various geometric configurations are assumed. As the central gumma heals, new lesions develop on the periphery, forming scalloped borders. Gummas are rarely contagious, but infection following contact with gummas has been reported.

MUCOUS MEMBRANE LESIONS OF LATE BENIGN SYPHILIS

Discrete gummas or diffuse gummatous infiltration may involve mucous membranes, especially the palate, nasal mucosa, tongue, tonsils, and pharynx (Fig. 229-26). The lesions ulcerate and are disfiguring. Destruction of the nasal cartilage (saddle nose) and perforation of the palate are disease hallmarks (Fig. 229-27). Chronic interstitial glossitis remains premalignant even after penicillin treatment (Fig. 229-28). Gummas of the larynx, trachea, and bronchi are rare. Pulmonary findings include chronic infection with miliary lesions, a nodule, or pleural effusion. *Pseudochancre redux* is a solitary gumma of the penis.

SKELETAL LATE SYPHILIS
Skeletal disease includes gummatous osteitis, periostitis, and sclerosing osteitis. The bones most commonly affected are the tibia, clavicle, skull, fibula, femur, and humerus, but the disease can involve almost any bone. Symptoms include nocturnal pain, swelling, and tenderness. Gummatous bone marrow obliteration (ivory bone) may be confused with tuberculosis or neoplasm. *Sclerosing osteitis* of the skull (caries sicca) is usually a reliable sign of late benign syphilis. *Gummatous osteitis* causes destructive periosteal and/or osteal changes with sclerosis at the periphery. Swelling and sinus tract formation of surrounding soft tissues are commonly observed. A common site is the sternal end of the clavicle. Localized osteoporosis, which is frequently confused with tuberculosis or neoplasm, tends to occur at the diaphysis of long bones and rarely at the shaft. *Periostitis* is characterized by periosteal thickening and a localized density that is similar to cortical bone. It often appears as a laminated periosteal reaction, but a more exuberant lacy pattern or diffuse thickening can be accompanied by destruction of bone. *Bilateral syphilitic bursitis (of Verneuil)* may ulcerate, exposing the gelatinous bursal contents. Juxtaarticular nodes, or *fibroid gummata*, are multilobed, firm nodules

FIGURE 229-26

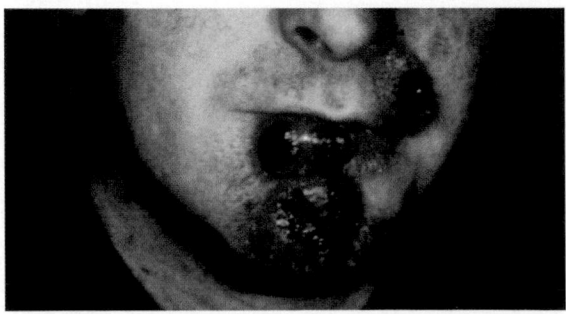

Aggressive gummas of the lower face causing destruction of the lip.

FIGURE 229-27

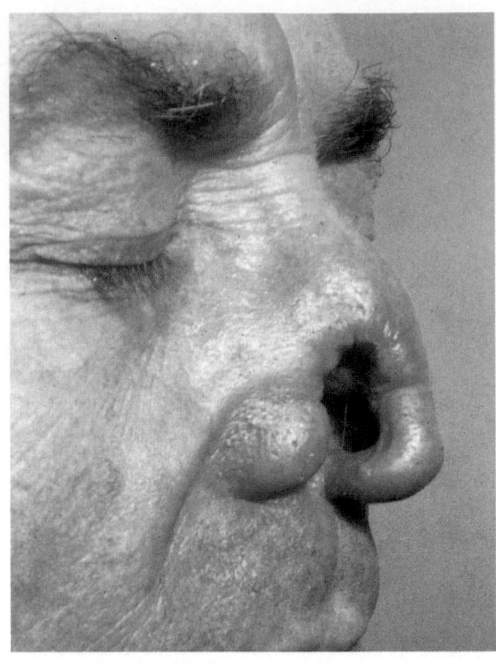

Perforation of the nasal cartilage in tertiary syphilis.

under the skin over joints. The nodes enlarge slowly, sometimes ulcerate, and respond to antibiotics.

Cardiovascular Syphilis

Although currently regarded as a "medical curiosity," cardiovascular syphilis was the cause of death in 1492 persons between 1976 and 1985. The cardiovascular system is not affected in early syphilis. However, there is evidence of infection in up to 80 percent of patients with tertiary syphilis, although most do not have clinically overt disease.[8] In the Oslo study, the disease was clinically apparent in 13.6 percent of men and 7.6 percent of women and was the primary cause of death in 15.1 percent of men and 8.2 percent of

FIGURE 229-28

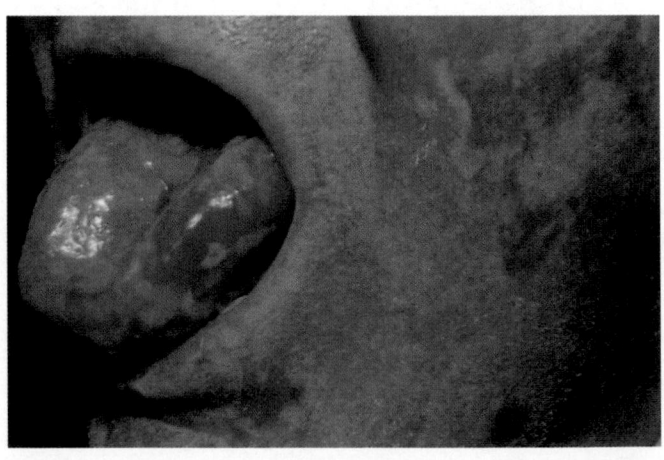

Premalignant, chronic interstitial glossitis secondary to gummatous infiltration of the tongue.

women. Before the availability of penicillin, syphilis constituted 25 to 30 percent and 5 to 10 percent of all cardiac diseases in African-Americans and Caucasians, respectively. Symptomatic cardiovascular disease usually occurs 15 to 30 years after the initial infection, and most patients are between 40 and 55 years old. Only 7 percent of patients with cardiovascular syphilis develop symptoms or signs within 5 years of infection.

Presumably, during the early stages of syphilis, treponemes invade the aortic wall, where they can remain dormant indefinitely. The treponemes have a predilection for the aortic vasa vasorum and produce chronic low-grade inflammation that eventuates in an obliterative endarteritis. This damage to the aortic wall results in necrosis of the muscular and elastic tissues and scarring. Fibrous thickening of the adventitia and atherosclerotic plaques in the intima impart the "tree bark" appearance that is highly suggestive of syphilis. Spotty calcium deposits within the plaques of the descending aorta appear radiologically as "eggshell calcification." The most common complications are aortitis, aortic aneurysm, aortic valve incompetence, coronary ostial stenosis, and myocardial gummatous disease.

Uncomplicated aortitis occurs predominantly in the ascending aorta, with fewer than 10 percent of the cases involving the abdominal aorta and only 2 percent affecting the portion below the renal artery. The disease comprises between 27 and 36 percent of cardiovascular syphilis cases but is asymptomatic and is usually found inadvertently at postmortem examination. The diagnosis is suspected when linear calcifications of the anterolateral aortic wall are present in chest radiographs.

Aortic aneurysms comprise 20 percent of cases of cardiovascular syphilis. The proportion is actually 40 percent if patients who also have coronary ostial or aortic valvular disease are included. Focal weakening of the wall results in a saccular aneurysm, whereas diffuse weakening produces fusiform involvement of the ascending and transverse aorta with subsequent dilation of the aortic ring. More than 60 percent of aneurysms involve the ascending aorta, and 25 percent the transverse arch. Abdominal aneurysms usually form above the renal arteries.

Often the presentation is a palpable pulsating mass or an abnormal mass on a chest radiograph. However, the variety of possible symptoms due to encroachment of surrounding structures or rupture prompted William Osler to warn that "there is no disease more conducive to clinical humility than aneurysms of the aorta." These symptoms include respiratory obstruction, cough, hemoptysis, atelectasis, hoarseness, flushing, distention of the superficial veins of the head and neck, edema, drowsiness, seizures, and symptoms of the superior vena cava syndrome. Direct pressure on the sternum or rib cage produces chest discomfort, while erosion of the vertebrae causes back pain. Undetected, one-third of patients die from spontaneous rupture. The treatment is surgical.

Coronary ostial stenosis constitutes 25 to 30 percent of cases of cardiovascular syphilis. Like ischemic heart disease, the main symptoms are angina pectoris and congestive heart failure. Characteristically, the pain is most intense at night. Clues to the diagnosis are the relative young age of the patient, poor response to vasodilators, and concomitant aortic regurgitation. The diagnosis should be strongly considered in a patient with reactive syphilis serologic tests and angiographic evidence of coronary artery stenosis without arteriosclerotic changes. Acute myocardial infarctions rarely occur because the stenosis is gradual and stimulates the development of an adequate collateral circulation.

Aortic valvular incompetence is found in approximately 30 percent of patients with tertiary disease. It is a late complication caused by aortic ring dilation and stretching of the valve. The soft diastolic blowing murmur of aortic regurgitation is best heard over the sec-

ond right intercostal space. If the pulse pressure is significantly wide, a ventricular diastolic gallop with a tambour-like quality or a diastolic, rumbling "Austin Flint" murmur may be audible at the apex.

The valve should be replaced as soon as there is evidence of cardiac function deterioration, congestive heart failure, or chest pain, especially if the patient is experiencing symptoms. Without surgery, the prognosis is so dismal that in one series more than half the patients died within 3 years after the onset of congestive heart failure.

Myocardial disease occurs in only 2.4 percent of cardiovascular syphilis patients. The gummas may be single or multiple. In diffuse gummatous myocarditis, the most common locations are the left ventricle and septum where gummas can cause heart block and conduction defects. Myocardial aneurysms or cardiac muscle rupture by gummas is rare.

Neurosyphilis

Hematogenous invasion of the meninges by *T. pallidum* occurs early. The resulting infection may resolve spontaneously or proceed to either chronic asymptomatic or acute symptomatic meningitis. Meningitis may progress to involve other areas of the CNS. In one study, *T. pallidum* was recovered from half the patients with secondary syphilis, the only patient with primary syphilis, and none with latent syphilis. In another report, 16 percent of patients with indeterminate latent syphilis had reactive CSF serologies and pleocytosis, and one-quarter of these were asymptomatic.

After resolution of secondary syphilis, the spirochetes presumably remain dormant in the CNS of untreated and even some treated patients. In 9.4 percent of men and 5 percent of women, this asymptomatic state progresses to clinically overt neurologic disease. Symptoms are more common from 5 to 35 years after the initial infection. The clinical manifestations of neurosyphilis are protean, but the clssification (Table 229-3) is useful and widely used. Neurosyphilis is divided into asymptomatic, meningeal, meningovascular, parenchymatous, and gummatous disease.

Asymptomatic neurosyphilis is the presence of CNS infection as indicated by CSF abnormalities in the absence of neurologic signs or symptoms. CSF findings, such as reactive serologic or elevated cell counts and protein, peak at 12 to 18 months after infection but disappear in 70 percent of cases even without treatment. Nontreponemal tests may be nonreactive in up to 39 percent of patients, but treponemal tests are usually positive in the serum as well as in the CSF.[27] Before the introduction of penicillin, between 23 and 87 percent of the cases progressed to clinical neurologic disease.

Meningeal syphilis may occur early or late. Most cases of *acute syphilitic meningitis* occur during the first year of infection. Meningitis is the initial presentation of syphilis in up to 25 percent of patients.[8] Fewer than 10 percent of these patients have skin eruptions at the onset of their meningitis. The symptoms are consistent with any aseptic meningitis and include headache, fever, photophobia, stiff neck (Kernig's sign), confusion, nausea, and vomiting. One-third of patients presents with acute hydrocephalus. These patients complain of headache, nausea, and vomiting due to increased intracranial pressure, and they have low-grade or no fever.[27] Papilledema, usually with little loss of vision, is a principal finding of hydrocephalus.

One-quarter of all cases of syphilitic meningitis have focal involvement of the cerebral vertex (*vertex meningitis*) or posterior fossa, possibly resulting in seizures, aphasia, and hemiplegia.[28] In

TABLE 229-3

Classification of Neurosyphilis

I. Asymptomatic
II. Meningeal
   A. Acute meningitis (headache, fever, photophobia, stiff neck, confusion)
     1. With hydrocephalus (severe headache, nausea, vomiting, papilledema)
     2. With vertex involvement (seizures, aphasia, hemiplegia)
     3. With basilar involvement (tinnitus, deafness, Bell's palsy)
   B. Spinal pachymeningitis (cervical pain, muscle atrophy, sensory loss, spastic paraplegia)
III. Meningovascular
   A. Cerebral (prodromal symptoms, hemiparesis, hemiplegia, aphasia, seizures)
   B. Spinal
     1. Meningomyelitis (paresthesia, spastic weakness of legs, sensory loss, sphincter disturbances)
     2. Acute transverse meningitis (sudden flaccid paraplegia, hemiparesis, sensory loss, urinary retention)
IV. Parenchymatous
   A. General paresis (impaired judgment, irritability, delusions, dysarthria, tremors, incontinence)
   B. Tabes dorsalis (paresthesia, lightning pains, ataxia, incontinence, impotence, pupillary disturbances)
   C. Optic atrophy (visual loss)
V. Gummatous
   A. Cerebral (compression symptoms)
   B. Spinal (compression symptoms)

addition to symptoms of meningeal inflammation and increased intracranial pressure, patients usually experience confusion and delirium. Cranial nerve palsies due to basilar involvement are a common complication of meningitis. The more frequent palsies involve the oculomotor, auditory, and facial nerves. Reversible sensorineural deafness, which characteristically involves the higher frequencies, develops within days in up to 20 percent of patients, even in the absence of meningitis or other signs of secondary syphilis. The hearing loss is often preceded by tinnitus. Response to penicillin is usually good.

Spinal pachymeningitis with inflammation and thickening of the dura mater usually involves the cervical area and causes pain, muscle atrophy, sensory loss, diminished tendon reflexes, and, ultimately, spastic paraplegia with sensory loss.

Meningovascular syphilis constitutes 10 percent of all neurosyphilis cases. The disease may involve the cerebrum (cerebrovascular) or spinal cord (spinal meningovascular).

Cerebrovascular syphilis is caused by endarteritis of the medium and large arteries (Heubner's arteritis) or small arteries and arterioles (Nissl arteritis) that results in thrombotic infarction. The name is partly misleading since the underlying pathogenesis is a chronic meningitis. Because the neurologic signs are focal, the clinical picture resembles atherosclerotic occlusive disease, but the typical patient is a younger adult, 30 to 50 years of age. Symptoms may develop as early as 2 years but usually develop between 4 to 7 years after the initial infection. Weeks to months before the abrupt onset, about half the cases experience prodromes, with symptoms such as dizziness, headaches, insomnia, memory loss, and mood changes.[29] Depending on the artery involved, patients may present with almost any neurologic deficit. The most frequent is hemipa-

resis or hemiplegia, followed in frequency by aphasia and seizures.[29] Therefore, this diagnosis should be considered in anyone with adult-onset epilepsy or strokes. Untreated, the disease can progress to tabes dorsalis or general paresis.

Spinal meningovascular syphilis is divided into meningomyelitis and acute transverse myelitis. *Meningomyelitis,* the more common form, usually begins over 20 years after the initial infection, with paresthesia and spastic weakness of the legs. These symptoms are followed by combinations of sensory loss, sphincter disturbances, pain, and muscular atrophy. *Acute transverse myelitis* produces sudden flaccid paraplegia, sensory deficits, and urinary retention. The presentation may resemble a Brown-Séquard hemisection syndrome.

Parenchymatous neurosyphilis is divided into three well-known syndromes: tabes dorsalis, general paresis, and optic atrophy.[27]

Tabes dorsalis is caused by infection of the parenchyma of the posterior columns and posterior root of the spinal cord. This form of neurosyphilis was once common, developing in 5 percent of patients with untreated syphilis of 20 to 25 years' duration, but is now rare. The three stages are preataxia, ataxia, and paralysis. The early symptoms are recurrent attacks of paresthesia and paroxysms of lightning pain (75 to 90 percent of cases). Stabbing pains in visceral organs such as the abdomen, rectum, and larynx simulate surgical emergencies (10 to 15 percent of cases). As the disease progresses, the patient may develop impotence, urinary retention, visual loss, and rectal incontinence. Locomotor ataxia begins with stumbling and difficulty in walking. Because position sense is lost, the ataxia is more prominent in the dark and is compensated by visual orientation. The Romberg sign is positive, which means that the patient stumbles when the feet are held close together with the eyes closed. Pupil reactivity becomes sluggish early and is seen in 90 percent of cases. The distinctive Argyll-Robertson pupils in which the pupil accommodates (to objects), but does not react (to light) are seen later. Cranial nerves, such as the optic and oculomotor nerves, may be atrophied, and hearing loss due to eighth nerve involvement is found in approximately 25 percent of cases. Charcot joints are enlarged, painless, uninflamed joints, with or without deformity or effusion, in the lower extremities and spine and result from repeated traumatic injury. Serum and CSF serologic tests are reactive in early tabes dorsalis but may be negative late in the course. The disease is rarely fatal, but patients become disabled and dependent.

General paresis, a chronic meningoencephalitis that severely disturbs cerebrocortical function and results in gross atrophy of the frontal and temporal lobes, is characterized by granulations in the ventricles, hydrocephalus, and widened cerebral sulci. Depending on the damaged area, the symptoms may be psychiatric, neurologic, or more commonly both.[27] Untreated, the course of this *dementia paralytica* spirals downward towards death. In the pre-penicillin era, this disease was diagnosed in 5 to 10 percent of psychotic patients admitted for the first time to psychiatric institutions. In the Oslo study, it developed in 2.5 percent of men and 1.4 percent of women. The disease begins about 15 to 20 years after contact. The onset may be sudden but is more commonly insidious, with changes in personality and behavior. Irritability, forgetfulness, inability to concentrate, and headaches are followed by impaired judgement, emotional lability, and inappropriate social or moral behavior.[27] Delusions of grandeur with marked euphoria occur in 20 percent of the cases. It has been pointed out that "everyone in contact with the paretic suffers but the patient." Paranoia, tantrums, and alcohol abuse may appear. Full-blown psychosis is followed by a period of neurologic decline. Tremors of the hands, lips, or tongue; seizures of any type; and incontinence of urine and feces are common. Neurologic signs include monoplegia, speech or handwriting disorders, accentuated tendon reflexes, and irregular, small, unequal pupils that react poorly to light. At this point a paralytic facies devoid of facial expression is typical. Mental and neurologic deterioration progresses to death in an average of 2½ years from pneumonia, infected pressure ulcers, or septicemia. The clinical spectrum is summarized in the clever Holmes mnemonic—*p*ersonality, *a*ffect, *r*eflexes (hyperactive), *e*ye changes, *s*ensorium (delusions), *i*ntellect impairment, and *s*peech dysarthria. Serum and CSF serologic tests are reactive in almost all cases. Adequate antibiotic treatment halts progression of the disease in 80 percent of patients. However, the clinical picture may sometimes worsen due to a "therapeutic paradox."

Optic atrophy may occur as an isolated finding. The visual loss begins in one eye but soon involves the other. Optic atrophy also results from syphilitic optic neuritis. In both conditions the CSF is usually abnormal. Differentiation may be possible through the visual evoked response, since the latency is only abnormal in optic neuritis. Penicillin does not restore vision but prevents further loss.

Focal (gummatous) cerebral meningeal syphilis is caused by compression and invasion of the brain by a gumma, which usually arises from the pia mater. Since serologic tests can be unreactive in the serum and the CSF, a biopsy may be required for diagnosis. The symptoms produced by spinal gummas are caused by compression.[30] Cerebral gummas respond poorly to antibiotics, so surgical resection may be necessary.

Unusual combination of signs and symptoms may be present, resulting in a puzzling neurologic picture. Perhaps as a result of the liberal use of antibiotics, which may partially treat CNS infection, the classic forms of neurosyphilis are becoming less common and the presentations more atypical. There are reports of patients with blurring of vision accompanied by Argyll-Robertson pupils or with isolated bilateral oculomotor nerve paresis or with tinnitus accompanied by variable auditory deficits. The presentation may be ophthalmic symptoms, confusion, personality changes, a Guillain-Barré syndrome, or persistent dizziness. The diagnosis of neurosyphilis should be strongly considered in a young adult with a stroke, new seizure disorder, confusional syndrome or dementia. The diagnosis relies on a combination of clinical manifestations, serum serologic tests, CSF examination, and radiographic scans. MRI findings are not specific for syphilis, but in the presence of other abnormalities they may exclude or confirm the diagnosis.[31]

CONGENITAL SYPHILIS

As early as 1529, Paracelsus recognized that syphilis could infect the fetus, although genetically, "from father to son," rather than transplacentally. At that time, due to another popular misconception, wet nurses were publicly paraded and flogged (with the approval of medical practitioners) for supposedly transmitting the disease to their previously healthy charges. In time, the mode of transmission became clear, but not until the nineteenth century was the disease studied systematically. In 1854, Paul Diday described the syphilitic newborn as a "little wrinkled pot bellied old man with a cold in his head." The definition of congenital syphilis has recently been updated (Table 229-4)[32]; however, some experts argue that because most infants have no clinical or serologic evidence of syphilis at birth and develop abnormalities months to years later, all potentially infected infants should be treated with penicillin.[33] Despite the popularity of the term *congenital syphilis*, prenatal syphilis better indicates that the signs and symptoms may develop before or after delivery rather than always being present at birth, as congenital implies. Mothers usually transmit the infection to the fetus trans-

TABLE 229-4

Definition of Congenital Syphilis*

TYPE	DEFINITION
Confirmed	An infant in whom *T. pallidum* is identified in lesions, placenta, umbilical cord, or autopsy tissue

Presumptive	Any infant whose mother was untreated or treated with antibiotics other than penicillin before delivery, regardless of findings in the infant
	or
	Any infant or child with a reactive treponemal test for syphilis and any one of the following:
	    Evidence of congenital syphilis on physical examination or x-ray of long bones
	    Presence in the CSF of lymphocytosis and elevated protein (without other cause)
	    Reactive CSF VDRL
	or
	Infant RPR fourfold higher than mother (both drawn at birth)
	or
	Reactive IgM-treponemal antibody test in serum

Syphilitic stillbirth	A fetal death in which the mother had untreated or inadequately treated syphilis at delivery of a fetus after a 20-week gestation or of a fetus weighing >500 g

*Congenital syphilis includes cases of prenatally acquired syphilis in infants and children as well as syphilitic stillbirths.

placentally and possibly during delivery through contact with an infectious genital lesion. Syphilis is not transmitted through breast feeding unless an infectious lesion is present on the breast (Fig. 229-29).[34] Many infants are thought to have colonization of *T. pallidum* in the nasopharynx or gastrointestinal tract at birth and develop the infection after birth.

Syphilis may cause preterm delivery, stillbirth, congenital infection, or neonatal death. The shorter the duration of untreated syphilis in the mother, the higher the risk of complication to the unborn infant. Almost all infants born to mothers with untreated secondary

FIGURE 229-29

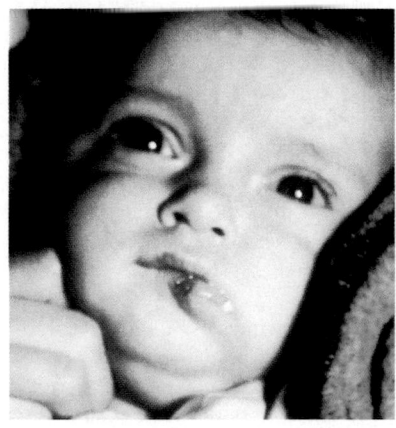

Lip chancre in an infant.

syphilis at any time during gestation become infected, although half of the offspring are asymptomatic. In contrast, the proportion falls to 40 percent with early latent syphilis, and an additional 20 percent are premature, 10 percent stillborn, and 4 percent die perinatally; in late latent syphilis, 10 percent have congenital syphilis and another 10 percent are stillborn or premature.[34] In general, 25 percent of infants from mothers with untreated primary or secondary syphilis die in utero. Of those infants born, almost half develop the disease, another quarter are seropositive without clinical manifestations, and one-quarter are not infected. One-quarter of newborns with signs and symptoms of congenital syphilis die shortly after birth unless treated. Syphilis is the most common cause of nonimmune hydrops fetalis, resulting in pallor, edema, and a bloated abdomen. Treatment of the mother with penicillin prevents prenatal syphilis in at least 98 percent of infants. Syphilis may infect the fetus at any time during gestation.[35] Spirochetes have been detected in fetuses as young as 9 weeks, but before the fifth month of gestation the fetus seems to escape harm, probably due to an inability to mount an inflammatory response. Even at birth, the inflammatory effects on the placenta are more pronounced than those on the infant. A fibrosed, large, thick, and pale placenta may be the only clue to the diagnosis of congenital syphilis. Inflammation of the matrix of the umbilical cord (*necrotizing funisitis*) results in a large number of stillbirths.[36] The diseased umbilical cord resembles a "barber's pole," with alternating streaks of red, pale blue, and chalky white.

Clinical Manifestations

Prenatal syphilis is divided into early (first 2 years) and late (after 2 years) stages. In 80 percent of cases, the diagnosis is missed during the first year of life, and, in one study, the average age at diagnosis was 30 years. Most infants are asymptomatic, and even when manifestations develop, these are often subtle and nonspecific.[37]

EARLY PRENATAL SYPHILIS Clinical manifestations develop within the first 2 years of life. This stage is comparable to the secondary stage of acquired syphilis since treponemes disseminate throughout the fetus. Without treatment almost half of symptomatic infants die. However, with improved perinatal care and treatment, the prognosis is now good. Infants tend to be small for dates or premature, irritable, and cry feebly. In descending order of frequency, the manifestations found are low birth weight, hepatosplenomegaly, anemia, jaundice, thrombocytopenia, skin lesions, respiratory distress, rhinitis, and pseudoparalysis.[1] Rhinitis ("snuffles") has been reported in 73 percent of infants. It usually develops in the second to third week of life and may be the earliest clinical sign. Initially thin, a mucoid nasal discharge, teeming with spirochetes, can become purulent or bloody. The nasal septum may become perforated. If untreated, flattening of the nasal bridge results in the characteristic saddle or "fleur de lis" nose. Within 12 h of penicillin treatment, the discharge is no longer contagious.

Bone disease, although usually asymptomatic, is the most common early manifestation, having been reported in 97 percent of autopsied infants younger than 6 months of age. In many infants, healing occurs regardless of treatment. The long bones are predominantly affected. The most common osseous lesion, osteochondritis, is diagnosed by its characteristic radiographic "sawtooth" appearance in the metaphysis. In the medial aspect of the proximal tibial metaphysis, this defect occurs in one-fifth of early cases and has

been called the *Wimberger* or *cat-bite sign*. Longitudinal lines of rarefaction, like "celery sticks," may expand into the diaphysis. Metaphyseal fractures may occur. Pain from osteochondritis of the long bones, or epiphysitis, is exacerbated by movement, so the child keeps the affected limb still, a sign known as *pseudoparalysis of Parrot*. Painful periostitis, commonly observed in the latter half of the first year, may lead to blunting of the scapular spines and anterior tibial margins in later life. The resulting multiple layers of new bone produce the radiographic "onion-peel periosteum" sign. Osteomyelitis syphilitica is rather rare. Osteitis of the fingers is uncommon but may produce dactylitis during the first 2 years of life. Skull osteitis produces softening, or *craniotabes*, which indents on pressure "like stiff parchment." Even without treatment the osteitis resolves by the end of the first year.

Mucocutaneous manifestations occur in about half of patients under 6 months and, like secondary syphilis lesions, usually consist of an eruption of copper- to red-colored macules and papules, with or without scale, predominantly on the palms, soles, and diaper area. Condylomata lata and mucous patches may also be present. Pustules may appear on the fingers, toes, and at the angles of the mouth. Ulcerations around the mouth, nose, or anus may heal with *rhagades* (Parrot's lines), depressed linear scars that radiate from the orifice like the spokes of a wheel (Fig. 229-30). The eruptions may also be annular or corymbiform. Rare, but characteristic for the disease, are bullae between 1 and 5 cm in diameter. They are highly infectious and may be generalized or, more often, limited to the extremities including the palms and soles. Commonly known as *syphilitic pemphigus*, the blisters are invariably a sign of severe disease. Frequently, the skin of the syphilitic neonate is dry and wrinkled and, in newborns with fair skin, has a café au lait hue.

Lymphadenopathy occurs in half the cases but may not be prominent. The presence of firm, movable, nontender epitrochlear nodes is especially characteristic for prenatal syphilis.

Neurosyphilis occurs in 40 to 60 percent of all syphilitic infants. CSF examination shows lymphocytosis, increased protein, and reactive serology. However, only 10 percent of these infants develop symptomatic neurosyphilis, which does not usually become clinically evident until the third to sixth month of life. It is essentially meningovascular and can present as various neurologic syndromes.

LATE PRENATAL SYPHILIS Manifestations appear after the age of 2 years, but rarely past the age of 30, and can be divided into

FIGURE 229-30

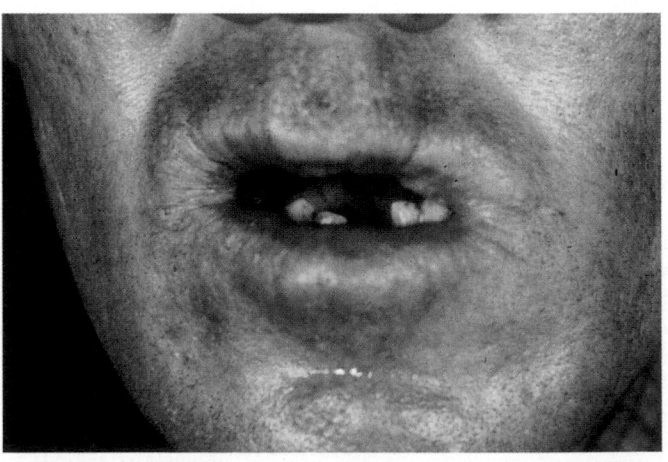

Perioral rhagades are linear scars that result from ulcerations that appear during early congenital syphilis.

two groups: "stigmata," or malformations, and active pathologic processes (Table 229-5). Most manifestations are not specific, with the exception of the "mulberry molars" and the characteristic interstitial keratitis. Late congenital syphilis is not infectious. The order of frequency of late syphilis signs varies in different reports. In the pre-penicillin era, eye lesions constituted the most common finding, followed by frontal bossing, saber shins, dental malformations, saddle nose, and asymptomatic neurosyphilis. However, two more-recent studies reported contradictory findings. In one, frontal bossing was the most common, followed, in descending order, by high arched palate, saddle nose, and tooth abnormalities; whereas in the second series, these signs were infrequently observed. Instead, interstitial keratitis and scaphoid scapula occurred more often.

Interstitial keratitis occurs in 8.8 percent of cases, and the average age of onset is 13.5 years for men and 27.1 years for women. The presenting symptoms are tearing, pain, corneal injection, and photophobia. The course eventuates in corneal clouding (syphilitic nebulae) or glaucoma. Neovascularization of the cornea produces a "salmon" patch appearance. "Ghost vessels" may be noted by slit-lamp examination and represent residual scarring in vessels. Iritis and iridocyclitis may also be found, but usually earlier. Corneal transplantation often restores vision.

Asymptomatic neurosyphilis occurs in 30 to 50 percent of patients and is diagnosed only through abnormal CSF findings. Symptomatic neurosyphilis is rare and usually delayed until puberty. Juvenile paresis, the most common pattern, affects 1 to 5 percent of all patients with congenital syphilis.[38] The presentation often involves personality and behavior changes such as deteriorating school performance and inappropriate emotional responses. Within a year, any combination of ataxia, dysarthria, tremors, and seizures develop. Other CNS complications include mental retardation, and cranial nerve palsies.

Bilateral eighth-nerve deafness has been reported in 3 to 38 percent of patients, usually adolescents. The early symptoms are vertigo, occasionally with nausea and tinnitus. The deafness, which progresses despite antibiotics, is caused by osteochondritis of the otic capsule resulting in cochlear degeneration. High frequencies are lost first. It is one of the few causes of a positive Hennebert's sign. The response to systemic glucocorticoids has been encouraging.

Skin manifestations consist of gummas and gummatous inflammation, just as in late benign syphilis.

Bone manifestations, such as arthritic perisynovitis, epiphysitis, and periostitis, may also occur in late prenatal infection. Chondroosteoarthritis may lead to ankylosis. Fusiform swelling caused by periostitis produces a number of common manifestations. *Frontal bossing of Parrot*—a thickened, prominent forehead produced by lens-shaped bony prominences that develop from localized periostitis of the frontal and parietal bones—is present in approximately 87 percent of patients. A *short maxilla*, with a shallow dish configuration, results from impaired development due to syphilitic rhinitis and is present in up to 83.3 percent of patients. The *Higoumenakis sign*, which is a rather nonspecific finding, is a unilateral, irregular enlargement of the sternoclavicular portion of the clavicle resulting from previous periostitis (Fig. 229-31). Anterior bowing and thickening from periostitis of the midportion of the tibia (*saber shins*) occur in 4 percent. *Scaphoid scapulae*, a concavity of the vertebral border of the scapulae, is observed in 0.7 percent. *Mandibular protuberance*, or bulldog jaw, was found in 25.8 percent. The size is normal but appears proportionally larger in comparison to the size of the small maxilla. *Clutton joints* are symmetric, nontender swelling of the knees, which often follows trauma and produces a bilateral hydrarthrosis. In some cases, however, the condition may be accompanied by fever, redness, warmth, and pain. It represents a synovitis without involvement of bone or cartilage. Systemic glucocorticoids are the preferred treatment. Deformities such as painless perforation of the nasal septum or soft palate and deep ulcers of the pharynx and tongue can result from damage by gummas.

Dental abnormalities are caused by treponemal invasion of the tooth buds. The pathognomonic *Hutchinson's teeth* refer to widely spaced permanent upper incisors which are small, screwdriver- or peg-shaped, wider at the gingival margin, and notched at the biting edge due to defective enamel production (Fig. 229-32). These changes may also be seen in the upper, lower, and lateral incisors. The diagnosis can be made radiologically by the first year of life. *Mulberry* or *Moon's molars*, found in 65 percent of cases, are dome-shaped and have numerous diminutive cusps arrayed in a tight circle

TABLE 229-5

Clinical Manifestations in Late Prenatal Syphilis

Stigmata	Active Disease
Ophthalmic	Interstitial keratitis
	Retinitis
Oral	
Hutchinson's teeth	
Mulberry molars	
High arched palate	
Ears, nose, throat	
Saddle nose	Gummas in nose or palate
Orthopedic	
Frontal bossing	Periostitis
Short maxilla	Dactylitis
Protuberant mandible	Clutton's joints
Saber shins	
Scaphoid scapula	
Thickened medial clavicle	
Neurologic	Eighth nerve deafness
	Neurosyphilis
Mucocutaneous	Gummas
	Gummatous inflammation
Gastrointestinal	Hepatomegaly
	Splenomegaly

FIGURE 229-31

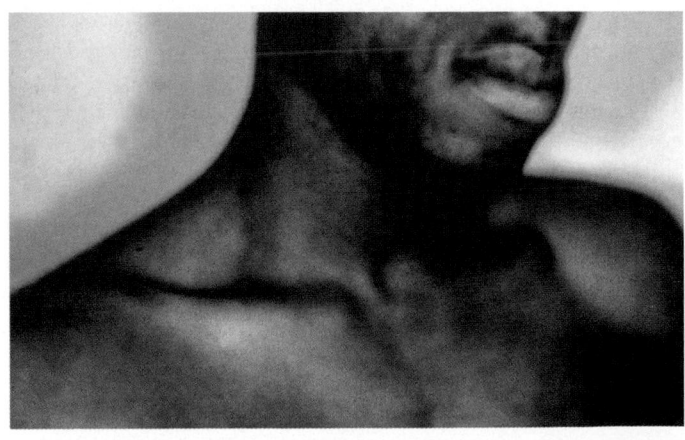

Irregular enlargement of the medial portion of the clavicle (Higoumenakis sign) is a stigmata of late congenital syphilis.

FIGURE 229-32

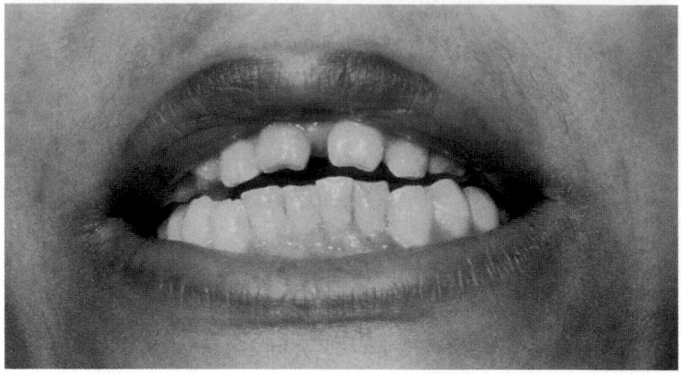

The presence of small, notched, peg-shaped upper incisors (Hutchinson's teeth) is part of the late congenital syphilis triad.

at the top of the dome. Although all the molars may be affected, the diagnostic one is the first lower molar. Due to defective enamel, these teeth are predisposed to caries and are rarely present beyond adolescence. The dental changes can be prevented if treatment is initiated before the third month of age.

Paroxysmal cold hemoglobinuria may occur as the only manifestation. Muscle cramping, chills, and dark red or black urine follows cold exposure. In addition, fever, urticaria, Raynaud's phenomenon, and jaundice may be present. Antibiotics decrease or abolish the episodes.

Congenital syphilis can be a difficult diagnosis in the absence of physical signs and symptoms. Maternal IgG antibodies can cross the placenta, but nontreponemal tests become nonreactive within 3 to 6 months and treponemal tests within 6 to 12 months after birth. There is an interval of 2 to 3 months between the onset of the infection and fetal production of IgM antibodies, so reactivity at birth depends on the time when the fetus became infected. The presence of reactive IgM tests in the serum of newborns is considered to prove the diagnosis of congenital syphilis. The most sensitive test is the Captia (IgM) enzyme immunoassay (EIA). The positive predictive values for IgM-immunoblots are as high as 95 percent. The fluorescence *T. pallidum* antibody with additional absorption step (FTA-ABS) tests are not useful because their positive predictive value is only 73 percent and false-positive results occur in as many as a third of infants. The FTA-ABS IgM may be falsely negative in 35 percent and falsely positive in 10 percent of infants. The umbilical cord should be sent for pathologic examination with special stains for treponemes. Dark-field examination of the umbilical vein will be positive in over half the cases of early prenatal syphilis. Nasal secretions and mucocutaneous lesions should be similarly tested. X-rays showing periostitis of the tibia suggest the diagnosis.

SYPHILIS AND HIV INFECTION

It has been suggested that syphilis may accelerate development of immunodeficiency in HIV-infected persons and, conversely, that HIV infection causes reactivation of dormant syphilis. Infection with syphilis imparts a greater risk of HIV infection, perhaps because the genital ulceration provides an easier entry to the virus into the systemic circulation.[39] Although the same is true for other ulcerated infections, such as herpes simplex and chancroid, numerous studies have demonstrated that syphilis is more common in HIV-infected than in HIV-uninfected gay men and heterosexuals.[40]

HIV infection impairs cell-mediated immunity and, to a lesser degree, humoral immunity. Studies in green monkeys infected with the simian immunodeficiency virus (SIV) found that retroviral-induced immunodeficiency delays the clearance of treponemes from lesions and impairs the humoral response to syphilis.[41] Therefore, alterations in the clinical manifestations and the natural course of syphilis may be anticipated in coinfected patients.[42] Surprisingly, HIV infection does not significantly influence the clinical course, serologic response, or treatment outcome of most patients with early syphilis.[43] The appearance of primary chancres is typical, although their duration may be slightly longer. The course in secondary syphilis is usually unchanged. However, the frequency of nodular and noduloulcerative lesions, while uncommon, is higher (Fig. 229-33). Some of these patients develop symptoms associated with malignant syphilis, but others have no constitutional symptoms.[44] Their rapid plasma reagin (RPR) titers may range from 1:8 to 1:1024.[45] Perforation of the palate has been rarely reported (Fig. 229-34).[46] There are several reports of eye involvement, but syphilis is an uncommon cause of uveitis in HIV infection (0.6 percent).[47]

Although most cases of early syphilis in HIV-positive patients respond to conventional doses of penicillin, serologically defined treatment failures are more common, and for this reason closer post-therapy evaluation is mandatory. In one study, 18 percent of patients treated with intramuscular penicillin had serologically defined treatment failures at 6 months and 14 percent at 12 months. This rate was similar to the HIV-seronegative control group.[48] Clinical relapses occurred in 1 percent of patients in a prospective study and

FIGURE 229-33

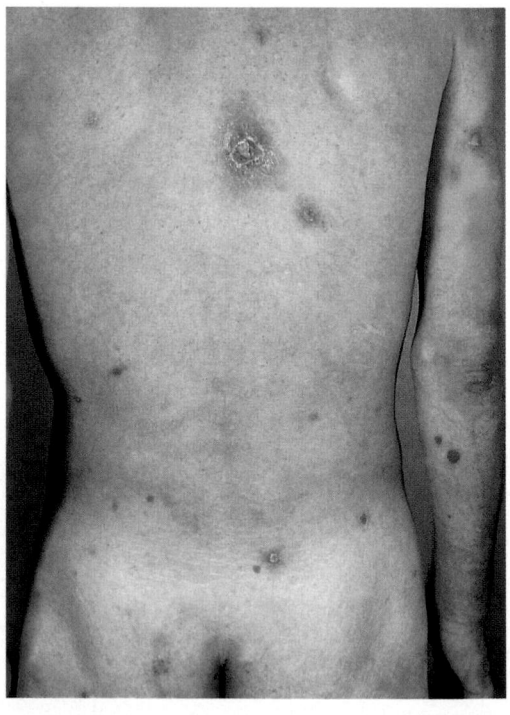

Ulcerated papules in an HIV-infected man. This was the initial presentation of HIV infection.

FIGURE 229-34

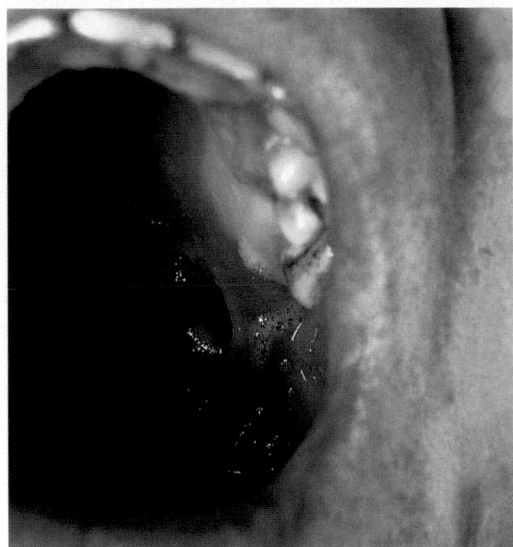

Perforation of the palate has been reported in HIV infection and had been previously associated with late benign syphilis.

more frequently in retrospective studies. There is some evidence that serologically defined and clinical treatment failures are 30 to 50 percent more common in AIDS patients with low percentages of CD4+ T lymphocytes. In 60 percent of these patients, relapses occurred over 1 year after therapy. Patients may experience multiple relapses. There was no association between CD4 lymphocyte counts and relapses, but relapses were more common in patients with reactive CSF Venereal Disease Research Laboratory (VDRL) tests and secondary syphilis eruptions.[49] Unfortunately, enhanced therapy with ampicillin and probenecid after treatment with benzathine penicillin injections did not improve responses.[48]

Neurosyphilis may be the first clinical manifestation of HIV infection. Investigators have recovered *T. pallidum* from the CSF of 26 percent of HIV-infected patients with early syphilis before treatment and 20% after treatment.[48] These are similar percentages to those in HIV-seronegative patients.[48] The presence of *T. pallidum* in the CSF does not differ according to HIV status and is not predictive of treatment failure.[50] In one study conducted over 42 months, 44 percent of neurosyphilis cases occurred in HIV-infected patients. Most cases comprise asymptomatic or meningovascular neurosyphilis, but focal gummas and other types of neurosyphilis have also been reported. Manifestations include cranial nerve palsies, optic neuritis or neuroretinitis, polyradiculopathy, transient ischemic episodes, or strokes. A fulminant form (necrotizing neurosyphilis) has been reported more frequently in AIDS patients.[51]

Not only is the prevalence of neurosyphilis higher in patients infected with both syphilis and HIV, but the progression to asymptomatic forms of neurosyphilis is accelerated, even after conventional therapy.[52] In a small but significant study, which included 15 HIV-infected and 25 HIV-seronegative patients with primary or secondary syphilis, *T. pallidum* was isolated from the CSF by rabbit inoculation in a similar proportion from both groups. Only CSF leukocytosis was more common (67 versus 25 percent) in the HIV-seropositive group. Notably, one injection of benzathine penicillin failed to eradicate the CNS infection in three of the four HIV-infected cases with positive treponeme cultures. Since then, several unsettling reports have alluded to the unexpected frequency of neurorelapse after benzathine penicillin therapy in HIV-infected pa-

tients and suggest that in some patients neurosyphilis is not cured even by the recommended high doses of intravenous penicillin.[53] Serologic response and CSF abnormalities usually resolve successfully in HIV-infected patients with neurosyphilis, but 8 percent may fail therapy the first time, and 23 percent have persistent pleocytoses.[53] CSF examination is recommended for all HIV-seropositive patients with syphilis at any stage. However, patients with CSF abnormalities should be cautiously diagnosed as having asymptomatic neurosyphilis, because CSF leukocytosis or elevated protein is present in up to 60 percent of nonsyphilitic HIV-infected patients.

Dysregulation of the humoral immune response may result in uncontrolled production of antibodies with extremely elevated titers. In a recent study, the median RPR titers were four times higher (1:128 versus 1:32) in HIV-infected than in HIV-uninfected patients with their first episodes of early syphilis.[54] Furthermore, B cell activation occasionally results in a higher rate of biologic false-positive nontreponemal serologic tests.[55] Conversely, an occasional patient may have a nonreactive nontreponemal test during early syphilis, and the sensitivity of treponemal tests appears to be lower in patients treated for past syphilis if they are HIV infected (80 versus 97 percent).[56]

In view of the occasional unreliability of serologic testing, the threshold to biopsy skin lesions is lower. The classic pathologic findings of secondary syphilis are usually present. Occasionally, however, a superficial perivascular mononuclear cell infiltrate with eosinophils may be the only significant finding; in one case, this led to a misdiagnosis of HIV-associated papular dermatosis that was eventually diagnosed as syphilis after detection of treponemes with silver stains.

DIAGNOSTIC TESTS

The definitive test in early syphilis is demonstration of spirochetes in lesional exudate or tissue either by dark-field microscopy or direct immunofluorescence. Unless the diagnosis is unequivocal as a result of these examinations or from clinical evaluation of typical lesions coupled with reactive serologic results, skin biopsy is recommended in primary, secondary, and certainly in tertiary syphilis lesions.

Histopathologic Examination

The epidermis of a chancre is acanthotic at the margins and becomes thinner and more edematous towards the eroded center. A dermal infiltrate, composed predominantly of lymphocytes, plasma cells, some histiocytes, and a few neutrophils, is dense in the central portion and perivascular in the periphery of the chancre. In untreated cases, the spirochetes stain gray with an impregnated silver stain, such as the Warthin-Starry stain. In contrast to immunofluorescence with fluorescein-labeled syphilitic rabbit serum, which requires fresh tissue, immunoperoxidase testing can be done on paraffin-embedded tissue. The spirochetes are more easily found in the epidermis and around dermal capillaries. Under electron microscopy, *T. pallidum* is predominantly found extracellularly; less commonly it is found intracellularly within the endothelial cells of capillaries and inside the vacuoles and phagolysosomes of plasma cells, macrophages, and neutrophils; and, occasionally, within fibroblasts and nerve fibers. Syphilitic bubos show follicular hyperplasia, endothelial proliferation, and a chronic inflammatory infiltrate with plasma cells and many spirochetes. Occasionally, noncaseating sarcoidal granulomas are present at the end of the primary stage.

Characteristically, secondary syphilis lesions show dilatation and thickening of blood vessels with a proliferation of endothelial cells and a superficial and deep perivascular dermal infiltrate containing numerous plasma cells. The infiltrate often becomes lichenoid, may obscure the dermal epidermal interface, and, in a third of cases, surrounds adnexal structures and nerves. Other changes depend on the biopsied lesion. Macules show mild or no epidermal changes.

Papulosquamous plaques show psoriasiform epidermal hyperplasia, parakeratosis and, often, focal spongiosis, basal vacuolar changes, and microabscesses with neutrophils. Other common epidermal changes are epidermal pallor, keratinocyte necrosis, extravasated red blood cells, and exocytosis of mononuclear cells. The dermal vessels show endothelial proliferation and swelling. There is a deep and superficial perivascular infiltrate arranged in a coat-sleeve pattern and composed of lymphocytes, histiocytes, and many plasma cells. The infiltrate assumes a lichenoid pattern that may involve the superficial and deep dermis and, in one-third of the cases, surrounds adnexal, vascular, and neural structures. The infiltrate may also be T-shaped or perivascular. Small epithelioid granulomas, which may have Langhans' or foreign body type giant cells, may be present even in young lesions. In lesions of pustular syphilis, neutrophils within the subcorneal pustules may infiltrate the hair follicles. In ulcerating lesions, there is infarction necrosis of the epidermis and dermis due to occlusion of blood vessels by fibrinoid material. The epidermis may be absent from the specimen.

In nodular tertiary syphilis, there is a dermal lymphohistiocytic and plasma cell infiltrate with small granulomas and islands of epithelioid cells intermingled with some multinucleated giant cells. A mild degree of caseation necrosis may be present. In gummas, the infiltrate contains numerous epithelioid and multinucleated giant cells and extends throughout dermis to the subcutaneous tissues. Extensive caseation necrosis surrounded by epithelioid and giant cells is present in the center of the lesion. Nodular tertiary syphilis may be difficult to differentiate from lupus vulgaris, and gummatous syphilis from scrofuloderma and erythema induratum.

Dark-Field Microscopy

Dark-field examination is the diagnostic test of choice in chancres and some lesions of secondary syphilis, especially condylomata lata and mucous patches. The test is invalid in oral membranes because saprophytic treponemes that cannot be differentiated from *T. pallidum* are common in the mouth.

The surface of the lesion should be cleaned and gently abraded with a sterile gauze soaked in 0.9% sterile saline, carefully avoiding bleeding as blood cells obscure detection of the treponemes. After squeezing the base of the lesion with two gloved fingers, a serous exudate accumulates on the surface and can be scraped off with a scalpel or drawn off with a pipette. The exudate is mixed with one or two drops of saline on a glass slide and covered with a plastic slip. The slide is examined under a dark-field microscope for the presence of "swimming" treponemes. The sensitivity is about 75 percent. Failure to demonstrate treponemes may be due to the resolving state of the lesion, previous treatment with topical or systemic antibiotics, inadequate specimen collection, or inexperience in dark-field microscopy.

Direct Fluorescence Antibody Test

The lesion exudate on the glass slide is stained with fluorescein-labeled anti–*T. pallidum* globulin and examined under a UV light microscope. In contrast to dark-field microscopic examination, the smear can be held for later evaluation and oral or anal lesions can be examined because only *T. pallidum* is stained. The sensitivity of the test is over 90 percent.[59]

Serology

Serologic tests for syphilis are divided into two types. The simpler cardiolipin-based nontreponemal tests are used for screening and to follow therapeutic response. The more elaborate *T. pallidum*—based treponemal tests are used for diagnostic confirmation and to improve diagnosis of early, congenital, and neurosyphilis.[60]

A presumptive diagnosis of syphilis is made by a reactive nontreponemal test (RPR, VDRL) confirmed by a treponemal test [FTA-ABS, microhemagglutination assay with *T. pallidum* antigen (MHA-TP)] (Table 229-6).[61]

Nontreponemal Tests

These tests are inexpensive and are widely used for screening. The antigen (reagent) is a combination of cardiolipin, cholesterol, and lecithin. An antibody (reagin) produced in syphilis reacts with this cardiolipin-lipoprotein complex. The VDRL test is the prototypical nontreponemal test and was the most widely used diagnostic test for 25 years. The test becomes reactive 4 to 5 weeks after infection and reverts to negative in 25 to 30 percent of cases during late latency. Results are reported *qualitatively* as reactive, weakly reactive, or nonreactive or *quantitatively* as a titer of the sample diluted with saline in a geometric progression by a factor of 2 (1:2, 1:4, 1:8, etc.). The highest dilution that gives a positive result is reported as the "titer." A high titer (>1:16) usually indicates active disease, while low titers (<1:8) may remain unchanged for years following therapy of late disease. After treatment, the titers should decline fourfold (a titer of 1:32 decreases to 1:4 or lower) within 6 months in primary or secondary syphilis or within 24 months in latent syphilis. In patients treated for primary syphilis, the tests become nonreactive in 60 percent by 4 months and in all patients by 12 months. In secondary syphilis, the tests become nonreactive in

TABLE 229-6

Interpretation of Serologic Tests

RPR	MHA-TP	CAPTIA (IgM) EIA	
−	−	−	No syphilis (until 3–4 weeks before examination)
−	−	+	Early primary syphilis
+	+	+	Syphilis
+	−	+	Early infection
+	+	−	Late secondary or latent syphilis
+	−	−	Biologic false-positive, late syphilis
−	+	−	Late infection, treated syphilis, or false-positive treponemal test
↑	+	↑	Reinfection, relapse

NOTE: RPR, rapid plasma reagin; MHA-TP, microhemagglutination assay with *T. pallidum* antigen; EIA, enzyme immunoassay; ↑, rising titers.

12 to 24 months after treatment. If therapy is administered in the early latent stage, low titers may remain for up to 5 years. In one study, 18 percent of patients treated for secondary syphilis had reactive tests at low titers after 30 to 35 years, and 44 percent of patients treated during the late latent stage had reactive tests after 35 years. In tertiary syphilis, the tests may revert to nonreactive in 20 to 30 percent of cases, even without treatment. A titer that neither decreases nor increases fourfold after treatment is referred to as "serofast." If an initially high titer ($>1:32$) fails to decrease after treatment, the patient should be evaluated for neurosyphilis and retreated appropriately. A fourfold titer increase indicates reinfection or treatment failure. Weakly reactive qualitative tests should be repeated, because a third will be eventually positive.

False-negative results occur during very early infection or in latent and late syphilis. In 1 percent of secondary syphilis cases, results are falsely reported as nonreactive due to the prozone phenomenon, since, unless the serum is diluted, the high levels of antibody prevent flocculation.[62]

Biologic false-positive results constitute 1 to 2 percent of reactive tests, depending on the population studied. Nonspecific antibodies (reagins) are directed against lipoidal antigens of *T. pallidum* as well as against the mitochondrial and nuclear membranes of human cells (autoantibodies). Lipoidal antigens may be present in normal tissue but are particularly evident in diseases associated with nuclear destruction. These conditions generate autoantibodies that may produce false-positive reactions to nontreponemal tests. Most false-positive results are caused by autoantibodies of the IgM class (rheumatoid factor). In 90 percent, the titers are less than $1:8$. Biologic false-positive results may be transient and "acute" (<6 months) or longer lasting and "chronic" (>6 months) (Table 229-7). False-positive reactions occur frequently in narcotic addicts and may persist even after 14 months of drug abstinence.[56] Patients with chronic biologic false-positive results are at higher risk of developing an autoimmune disease, and an investigation of possible causes such as connective tissue diseases and the antiphospholipid syndrome should be undertaken when titers are high.[63]

The RPR test has become popular because of its simpler technique. It is performed with unheated serum on small plastic cards. Charcoal particles are added to the antigen (as in the VDRL) and cause flocculation of black particles, which can easily be read without a microscope. The specificity, sensitivity, and results are almost identical to the VDRL test.

Other nontreponemal tests include the automated reagin screen test, the unheated serum reagin test, and the reagin screen test.

TABLE 229-7

Causes of Biologic False-Positive Tests

	ACUTE	CHRONIC
Physiologic	Pregnancy	Advanced age
Spirochete infection	Leptospirosis	Endemic syphilis
	Lyme disease	Pinta
	Rat-bite fever	Yaws
	Relapsing fever	
Viral infection	Cytomegalovirus	Human T cell leukemia/lymphoma virus I
	Infectious mononucleosis	HIV-1
	Hepatitis	
	Herpes simplex	
	Herpes zoster—varicella	
	Measles	
	Mumps	
	Mycoplasma pneumonia	
	Toxoplasmosis	
	Viral sepsis	
Bacterial infection	Pneumonia	Lepromatous leprosy
		Lymphogranuloma venereum
		Tuberculosis
Protozoan infection	Malaria	Kala-azar
		Trypanosomiasis
Other		Drug abuse
		Dysproteinemias
		Hepatic cirrhosis
		Malnutrition
		Malignancy
		Lymphoproliferative disorders
Autoimmune disease		Autoimmune hemolytic syndrome
		Autoimmune thyroiditis
		Idiopathic thrombocytopenic purpura
		Mixed connective tissue disease
		Polyarteritis nodosa
		Primary biliary cirrhosis
		Rheumatoid arthritis
		Sjögren's syndrome
		Systemic lupus erythematosus

Treponemal Tests

These tests use whole or fragments of *T. pallidum* as antigen. Compared to nontreponemal tests, they are more cumbersome to perform but have greater sensitivity in the primary and late stages and slightly higher specificity (Table 229-8). They are widely used to confirm reactive nontreponemal test results.[60]

FLUORESCENCE *T. pallidum* ANTIBODY TEST Using indirect immunofluorescence, the first treponemal test, the FTA test was developed in 1957, and its specificity was subsequently improved with an additional absorption step.

FLUORESCENT TREPONEMAL ANTIBODY-ABSORPTION TEST Serum is mixed with an extract of Reiter treponemes to absorb nonspecific treponemal antigens, and the "absorbed" serum is then added to a glass slide containing *T. pallidum* (Nichols strain). If specific antibodies to *T. pallidum* are present in the serum, they will coat the surface of the spirochete. Fluorescent antihuman globulin binds to *T. pallidum* antibody, emitting fluorescence under exami-

TABLE 229-8

Sensitivity and Specificity of Serologic Tests

	SENSITIVITY, %				
	PRIMARY	SECONDARY	LATENT	TERTIARY	SPECIFICITY, %
VDRL	80(74–87)	100	80(75–100)	71(55–94)	98
RPR	86(81–100)	100	80(75–100)	73(55–96)	98
FTA-ABS	98(93–100)	100	95	97(95–100)	99
MHA-TP	82(50–95)	100	99	96(90–99)	99
Captia (IgM) EIA	82	60	53	34	100

NOTE: For explanation of serologic tests, see text.

nation with a UV microscope. Results are reported as nonreactive, borderline, or reactive. A quantitative evaluation can be performed but has little clinical value.

The FTA-ABS test is the most sensitive serologic test in primary syphilis, and reactivity begins during the third week of infection. The test rarely becomes nonreactive in untreated patients, and reactivity usually continues even after treatment. In one study, 87 percent of patients with primary syphilis and all 53 patients with secondary syphilis had reactive FTA-ABS tests 30 years after treatment. The specificity and sensitivity range between 94 and 100 percent during the secondary and the late phases of the disease (Table 229-8). The high sensitivity of these tests permits detection of very small amounts of antibodies, and so the tests are not useful to assess the efficacy of treatment. At present, the FTA-ABS test is the most sensitive serologic test in the early stages of syphilis.

False-negative results are very rare. False-positive FTA-ABS results are usually caused by autoantibodies (rheumatoid factor) or antibodies to spirochetal infections (Table 229-9). Advantages of the FTA-ABS test include detection of early infection 1 to 2 weeks before other assays and high specificity and sensitivity. However, because of higher cost, the test is primarily used to confirm the accuracy of a reactive nontreponemal screening test.

The MHA-TP test is becoming the more widely performed treponemal test. As a variant of the *T. pallidum* hemagglutination assay (TPHA), the test relies on agglutination of sheep erythrocytes coated with *T. pallidum* in the presence of specific treponemal antibodies. The MHA-TP is performed on microtiter plates and requires less serum and reagents. Results are ready in 4 h and can be read in a magnifying mirror. The specificity and sensitivity are comparable to the FTA-ABS, except in primary syphilis, and it is less expensive to perform.

Other assays include the automated microhemagglutination assay with *T. pallidum,* the hemagglutination treponemal test for syphilis, and the microcapsule agglutination test for *T. pallidum* antibodies.

TABLE 229-9

Common Causes of False-Positive Treponemal Tests

Infectious mononucleosis
Lepromatous leprosy
Leptospirosis
Lyme disease
Malaria
Relapsing fever
Systemic lupus erythematosus

ENZYME-LINKED IMMUNOSORBENT ASSAY (ELISA) In this test antibodies to *T. pallidum* react with antigen fixed to the walls of microtiter plates and react in a second incubation with an enzyme-labeled antihuman globulin. A substrate is added for color. There are several variants, which differ in the type of antigen used.[64]

The Captia (IgG) EIA is expected to replace other treponemal tests eventually. The test has higher sensitivity and specificity than the RPR test when used for screening. Used as a screening test, the test is more sensitive (99 percent) and specific (99 percent) than the RPR.[65] It has similar sensitivity to the FTA-ABS in patients treated for past syphilis.[66]

The Captia (IgM) EIA, which detects 19S (IgM) anti–*T. pallidum* antibodies against the 37-kDa major axial filament, is becoming the more widely used IgM-antibody test. IgM antibodies can be detected in the serum towards the end of the second week of infection. The levels decrease after the acute stages of the infection because memory cells do not synthesize IgM antibodies. A reactive IgM test in untreated persons indicates active disease. Reactivity ceases within 3 to 9 months after therapy of early syphilis but may persist for 12 to 18 months after treatment of late disease. In late syphilis, the generation of IgM autoantibodies, directed against antitreponemal IgG, may cause false reactivity. Persistence of reactivity after therapy indicates treatment failure or false-positive results due to autoantibodies of the IgM class.

Due to their large size, IgM antibodies cannot pass through the placenta or the intact blood-CSF barrier. IgM reactivity in the serum of a newborn confirms prenatal infection, and detection of antitreponemal IgM in the CSF indicates neurosyphilis if the blood-CSF barrier function is normal. The Captia (IgM) EIA has high sensitivity and specificity, particularly during the first weeks of infection, but is less sensitive during late disease. It is the first serologic test currently available to become reactive, and it is the serologic test of choice in primary and congenital syphilis. The sensitivity is very high in congenital syphilis (100 percent) and less so in primary (82 percent), neurosyphilis (34 percent), and treated syphilis (11 percent).[67] The test is highly specific because there appears to be no interference by rheumatoid factors or competitive inhibition by antitreponemal IgG. Values below 0.9 are nonreactive, between 0.9 and 1.0 are equivocal, and above 1.0 are reactive.

OTHER TESTS The *IgM solid phase hemadsorption assay* is a simple and inexpensive method for the detection of *T. pallidum*–specific IgM. A titer of 1:4 is borderline; positive is above 1:8. After treatment, the titers drop and reactivity ceases within 3 to 6 months in early syphilis and within 3 to 12 months in late disease. Compared to other IgM tests, the sensitivity is around 96 percent and the specificity is about 97.4 percent. However, false-negative results are seen in about 8 percent of reactive samples, predominantly during the primary and late stages. False-positive findings occur in up to 1 percent. The test is superior to the VDRL in the assessment of treatment and the diagnosis of reinfection. In untreated persons, a reactive result indicates almost with certainty the need for therapy, but a nonreactive result does not exclude infection.

The *solid phase ELISA* (Visuwell test) compares favorably (81 versus 85 percent) with dark-field examinations in verifying the presence of *T. pallidum* in tissue exudate, but monoclonal staining techniques are better (92 percent).[68]

Western blots have a very high sensitivity in primary (97 percent), secondary (100 percent), early latent (100 percent), late latent (98 percent), congenital (83 percent), and neurosyphilis (100 percent).[69] These immunoblots detect antibodies to specific *T. pallidum* antigenic proteins, such as the 15.5- and 45-kDa antigens. The test is particularly valuable in the diagnosis of congenital syphilis and promising as a replacement of other confirmatory treponemal tests due to its near-perfect specificity.[60]

Polymerase chain reaction (PCR) is a promising technique in certain situations. In chancres the test is comparable to direct immunofluorescent staining and has the potential of being better once methods for recovery of DNA become more efficient.[60] More sensitive techniques are being reported. A new reverse transcriptase PCR test could detect 10^{-2} *T. pallidum* equivalents in body fluids.[70]

CSF EXAMINATION   Because no clinical presentation is specific for neurosyphilis, reliable criteria by laboratory examinations are particularly important (Table 229-10).

Elevated cell count [>5 cells per μL (500/mL or 5×10^6/L)] and total protein (>400 mg/L) indicate inflammation and presumed infection. Of course, these findings are found in other types of aseptic meningitis. However, both may be normal or slightly elevated in asymptomatic disease as well as in tabes dorsalis.

A reactive CSF VDRL result indicates neurosyphilis. Blood contamination only occurs when titers are high and the CSF is visibly bloody. Unfortunately, the CSF VDRL is not reactive in up to 70 percent of patients with neurosyphilis, particularly in asymptomatic cases and in tabes dorsalis.[71] The CSF FTA-ABS is unreliable because of false-positive results; however, a nonreactive test virtually excludes CNS involvement.[72] In certain cases the diagnosis of neurosyphilis is particularly challenging. A patient with adequately treated syphilis and no neurosyphilis may have abnormal CSF serology, cell counts, and protein due to nonsyphilitic CNS infection (HIV, malaria) or a neoplasm.

There is intrathecal production of specific *T. pallidum* IgG in 75 percent of neurosyphilis cases and in 25 percent of clinically asymptomatic patients with syphilis. Total intact IgG values are 200 to 500 times higher in the serum than in the CSF, and transudation of IgG from serum to CSF is not uncommon, even when the blood-CSF barrier function is intact. Faced with a positive test, the clinician has to apply specific formulas to differentiate between immunoglobulins produced in the CNS or the serum.[1]

$$\text{Total IgG index} = \frac{\text{Total CSF IgG} \times \text{serum albumin}}{\text{Total serum IgG} \times \text{CSF albumin}}$$

TABLE 229-10

Diagnosis of Neurosyphilis through CSF Testing

Strongly indicative
   Reactive VDRL (or RPR)
   Reactive MHA-TP (or FTA)
   Reactive western blot, PCR, or IgM tests
     TPHA index > 500
Strongly suggestive (in absence of other CNS disease)
   Cell count > 5 cells per μL
   Protein > 40 mg/100 mL
   IgG index > 0.7
Practically excluded
   Nonreactive MHA-TP (or FTA)
   TPHA index < 70

NOTE: For explanation of serologic tests, see text.

A more recently described formula is the "modified" TPHA index (Table 229-11). It is false positive in half of the cases; however, it rarely fails to indicate a case of active neurosyphilis (2.2 percent).

$$\text{"Modified" TPHA index} = \frac{\text{CSF TPHA titer/serum TPHA titer} \times \text{serum albumin}}{\text{CSF albumin}}$$

TREATMENT

Parenteral penicillin is the treatment of choice for all stages of syphilis. Treatment failures are rare and regularly respond to a second course of penicillin at the same or higher doses. The concentration of penicillin in the CSF is less than 10 percent of the serum level. However, even a single injection of benzathine penicillin produces effective levels in the perivascular areas where treponemes are found in the CSF.[73] Parenteral penicillin is the only treatment with documented efficacy in neurosyphilis, HIV infection, and pregnancy. Penicillin is a treponemicidal antibiotic that binds irreversibly to the transpeptidase enzymes required for biosynthesis of the outer envelope and, by so doing, prevents closing of the gaps in the envelope lattice, formed during growth spurts. The resulting high osmotic pressure within the protoplasmic cylinder causes bulging of the inner membrane and bursting of the treponeme. Because penicillin does not interfere with the synthesis of transpeptidases, intact bacteria can resume growth and generate new organisms within 20 min of inadequate, interrupted penicillin levels.

A concentration of penicillin of 0.0025 units/mL kills 50 percent of *T. pallidum* within 16 h. More than 10 times this concentration, or 0.03 units/mL, is recommended for a minimum duration of 7 to 10 days in early syphilis and longer in late syphilis.

Oral penicillin can produce adequate serum and tissue levels but is not recommended because of reduced efficacy due to lack of compliance.

Tetracyclines, macrolides, and third-generation cephalosporins have strong antitreponemal activity in experimental and clinical trials. Clinically, however, their efficacies are less than penicillin, and numerous treatment failures have been reported. Although less investigated and more expensive than tetracycline, doxycycline is preferred because of better compliance and absorption, which is less affected by food.[74] Erythromycin is slightly less effective than tetracycline. However, therapeutic results with another macrolide, azithromycin (500 mg orally daily for 10 days) are very encouraging, and this antibiotic may eventually replace erythromycin and even doxycycline as the alternative treatment of choice.[58,74,75] Ceftriaxone (1 g intramuscularly or intravenously daily for 10 days) is an inferior alternative to penicillin in late latent and CNS syphilis.[76]

TABLE 229-11

Methods to Diagnose Neurosyphilis

	IgG INDEX	MODIFIED TPHA INDEX
Normal	<70	<0.8
Suggestive	70–500	0.8–2
Neurosyphilis	>500	>2

NOTE: TPHA, *T. pallidum* hemagglutination assay.

HIV serology is recommended for all patients with syphilis and should be repeated in 6 months in patients living in areas with high HIV prevalence.

Primary and Secondary Syphilis (without Neurologic, Ophthalmologic, or Auditory Involvement)[77]

A single dose of benzathine penicillin G, 2.4 million units intramuscularly, is the preferred treatment.

Penicillin allergy Patients with uncomplicated syphilis may be treated with doxycycline, 100 mg orally twice daily for 2 weeks. Compliance is better than with tetracycline, 500 mg orally four times daily, or erythromycin, 500 mg orally four times daily. Ceftriaxone, 250 mg daily or 1 g every other day intravenously for 10 days, is an alternative.

Pregnancy Pregnant women should be desensitized and treated with penicillin (see "Treatment in Pregnancy", below).

HIV infection Three doses of weekly injections of benzathine penicillin G are preferred by some experts due to higher prevalence of neurosyphilis in these patients (although there is no evidence that this is more effective).

Children Children should be evaluated for congenital syphilis through examination and review of maternal and prenatal records. If CNS is abnormal, treat for neurosyphilis. If infection was acquired postnatally, consult with child protection agency after treating with a single intramuscular injection of benzathine penicillin G, 50,000 units/kg up to 2.4 million units.

CSF examination If there are signs or symptoms of CNS, eye, or hearing involvement, examine the CSF. Do slit-lamp examination if there is ophthalmologic disease. If CSF findings suggest neurosyphilis, treat accordingly.

Follow-up Patients should be reexamined clinically and serologically at 6 and 12 months (if HIV-seropositive, then at 3, 6, 9, 12, and 24 months).

Treatment failures Patients should be re-treated if there is a fourfold (or greater) increase in RPR titer within 6 months. HIV serology should be repeated. Unless reinfection is definite, CNS examination is indicated. If CSF abnormalities indicate neurosyphilis, treat with intravenous penicillin. If neurosyphilis is excluded, treat with benzathine penicillin G, 2.4 million units intramuscularly for three doses 1 week apart.

The management of patients who remain serofast with RPR titers that do not decline by a fourfold factor in 6 months is unclear. At the very minimum, clinical evaluation and HIV testing are indicated. If the patient is HIV seropositive, do a spinal tap and treat accordingly. If HIV seronegative but compliance cannot be assured, re-treatment (preferably with three injections of benzathine penicillin G 1 week apart) is recommended.

Early Latent Syphilis[77]

A single dose of benzathine penicillin G, 2.4 million units intramuscularly, is the recommended treatment.

Penicillin allergy If the patient is neither pregnant nor HIV-infected, treat with doxycycline, 100 mg orally twice daily for 4 weeks.

Pregnancy Desensitize and treat with penicillin (see "Treatment in Pregnancy," below).

Children The treatment is the same as for primary syphilis.

Follow-up As in late latent syphilis, below.

"Indeterminate" or Late Latent Syphilis[77]

Benzathine penicillin G, 2.4 million units intramuscularly 1 week apart for three doses, is the treatment of choice.

Penicillin allergy Doxycycline, 100 mg orally twice daily for 4 weeks, may be prescribed.

Pregnancy Desensitize and treat with penicillin (see "Treatment in Pregnancy," below).

HIV infection Desensitize and treat with penicillin.

Children After appropriate evaluation to exclude congenital syphilis and sexual abuse, treat with weekly injections of benzathine penicillin G, 50,000 units/kg (up to 2.4 million units) intramuscularly for three doses.

CSF examination In asymptomatic individuals, the yield of positive findings in lumbar punctures is low, but CSF examination is clearly indicated in certain cases:

- Cardiovascular, neurologic, eye, or auditory symptoms or in late benign syphilis
- HIV infection
- RPR titer $\geq 1:32$
- Treatment failure
- Nonpenicillin treatment

If the CSF examination demonstrates abnormal, unexplainable findings, patients should be treated for neurosyphilis. The outcome of treatment has not been conclusively studied, but in 469 treated patients with uncomplicated late latent syphilis who were followed for up to 12 years, the CSF remained normal and no cases of cardiovascular syphilis were reported.

Follow-up Quantitative nontreponemal serologic tests should be repeated at 6, 12, and 24 months (6, 12, 18, and 24 months if the patient is HIV infected). After treatment, the patient should be reevaluated for neurosyphilis and re-treated accordingly if (1) titers increase fourfold, (2) an initially high titer (≥ 32) fails to decrease fourfold within 12 to 24 months, or (3) the patient develops signs or symptoms attributable to tertiary syphilis.

Tertiary Syphilis (Cardiovascular, Late Benign Syphilis)

Benzathine penicillin G, 2.4 million units 1 week apart for three doses, is the recommended treatment.

Penicillin allergy If the patient is not HIV infected and the CSF is negative, treat with doxycycline, 100 mg orally twice daily for 2 weeks.

CSF Examination All patients should have spinal taps, and if abnormalities are found, treat for neurosyphilis.

Prognosis After treatment of late benign syphilis, gummas heal slowly over several months, depending on the extent of tissue destruction. Gummas of the brain or spinal cord may need surgical excision. Because advanced symptomatic disease in cardiovascular syphilis is associated with poor prognosis even with recommended doses of benzathine penicillin, some experts prefer to treat cardiovascular disease with high-dose intravenous penicillin. The evidence suggests that penicillin has a beneficial effect in the majority of patients, although efficacy is difficult to evaluate as most symptomatic patients receive therapy to improve cardiac function. In studies, 63 percent of patients with aortic insufficiency, aneurysms, or both experienced symptomatic improvement from 6 to 12 months after penicillin treatment. The disease progressed in 4 percent of asymptomatic and 4.5 percent of symptomatic patients.

Neurosyphilis[77]

Aqueous crystalline penicillin G, 18 to 24 million units administered daily as 3.5 to 4 million units intravenously every 4 h for 10 to 14 days, is the treatment of choice.

Alternative   Treat with procaine penicillin G, 2.4 million units intramuscularly daily; probenecid, 500 mg orally every 6 h for 10 to 14 days, can be instituted in patients whose compliance can be assured. Treatment of neurosyphilis with ceftriaxone (1 g intravenously daily for 14 days) is not as effective as penicillin.

Penicillin allergy   Desensitize and treat with penicillin.

Follow-up   Reexamine the CSF every 6 months until normal. Cell counts should decrease by 6 months, and CSF VDRL and protein levels by 2 years. If not, re-treat with intravenous penicillin.

Prognosis   In one study, penicillin cured, improved, or stabilized the disease in 91 percent of patients with asymptomatic neurosyphilis, 81 percent with meningovascular disease or meningitis (78 percent cured), 75 percent with general paresis (48 percent cured), 72 percent with tabes dorsalis (47 percent cured), and 88 percent with miscellaneous neurologic abnormalities.

If symptoms worsen during treatment, the dose may need to be increased. Optic atrophy, alone or in conjunction with tabes dorsalis, and eighth-nerve-related deafness are notoriously more resistant to treatment. No case of blindness due to optic atrophy is reversible with penicillin, although lack of progression or improvement occurs in up to 60 percent of cases. Eighth-nerve deafness benefits from the combination of long-term penicillin and prednisone.

Relapse   Neurosyphilis relapses usually respond to additional courses of intravenous penicillin at equal or higher doses.

Treatment in Pregnancy

The penicillin regimen appropriate for the stage of the infection should be used. In primary, secondary, and early latent syphilis, a second benzathine penicillin injection 1 week later is recommended by some experts.

Penicillin allergy   Desensitize and treat with penicillin. Erythromycin's ability to cross the placenta is fair to poor. Infants born to mothers who received erythromycin for syphilis during pregnancy should be thoroughly evaluated for active disease, treated with penicillin, and closely followed. Tetracycline is avoided because of dental staining due to deposition in enamel.

Evaluation   Perform fetal ultrasound, and if signs (hydrops, hepatomegaly) of fetal syphilis are present, consult with an experienced obstetrician.

Screening   Pregnant women should be screened at their initial prenatal visit, and those with seropositive results should be considered infected unless treatment can be verified and sequential serologic antibody titers convincingly demonstrate an appropriate response. In case of doubt, re-treatment is warranted as the potential benefits outweigh the possible risks. Screening should be repeated in the third trimester and again at delivery.

Follow-up   Repeat serologic titers monthly if there is risk of reinfection; otherwise, repeat in the third trimester and at delivery.

Complications   A potential adverse effect of penicillin treatment is the Jarisch-Herxheimer reaction, which may precipitate labor (*placental shock*). However, the association of spontaneous abortion with this phenomenon is debatable and should not delay treatment.

Prognosis   In 414 pregnant women with early syphilis treated with variable doses of penicillin, only 5 percent of their newborns had syphilis and a "normal" rate of stillbirths was reported. The failures were observed in women reinfected or treated late in pregnancy.

Prenatal Syphilis[77]

1. *Newborns*: Aqueous penicillin G, 50,000 units/kg intravenously every 12 h for the first 7 days of life and every 8 h for the next 3 days, or procaine penicillin G, 50,000 units/kg intramuscularly daily for 10 to 14 days.
2. *Post-neonatal period*: Benzathine penicillin G, 50,000 units/kg (up to 2.4 million units) intramuscularly if CSF examination is negative. If neurosyphilis, aqueous penicillin G, 50,000 units/kg every 4 to 6 h intravenously for 10 to 14 days.

Addendum   Infants should be treated for presumed congenital syphilis regardless of evaluation if born to mothers with the following:

- Untreated syphilis at delivery
- Treatment other than with penicillin
- History of treatment before becoming pregnant but no documentation of a fourfold decrease in titers
- Treatment for syphilis within 1 month of delivery
- Inadequate documentation of appropriate treatment
- Serologic evidence of relapse or reinfection after treatment
- No fourfold decrease in RPR titers after treatment during pregnancy

If the infant has signs of congenital syphilis on physical examination or serologic evidence of syphilis (infant's RPR titer is two dilutions greater than mother's), the evaluation should include complete blood count with differential and platelets and CSF examination for cell count, protein, and RPR. Other tests that can be ordered as clinically indicated include long-bone radiographs, chest radiograph, cranial ultrasound, ophthalmologic examination, auditory-brainstem response, and liver function tests.

If the infant's clinical, CSF, serologic, and blood evaluation are normal and compliance is indisputable, the infant may be treated with a single intramuscular injection of benzathine penicillin G, 50,000 units/kg.

If the mother was adequately treated and had an appropriate serologic decline in titers, evaluation of an infant with a nontreponemal titer equal to or less than the mother's titer is not necessary, but a single dose of benzathine penicillin is recommended anyway. If the infant's titer is not reactive, no treatment is necessary.

Follow-up   Seropositive infants (or infants born to mothers who were seroreactive at delivery) must be reexamined clinically and serologically every 2 to 3 months until the test becomes nonreactive or the titer has decreased fourfold. If the reactive test result was caused by passive transplacental transfer, nontreponemal antibody titers should decrease by 3 months and disappear by 6 months of age. If the child was infected and treated, the serologic decline may be slower. If the titers are stable or increasing after 8 to 12 months of age, the child should be reevaluated (including CSF analysis) and retreated with a 10-day course of intramuscular penicillin G. Treponemal tests may remain positive for 15 months if the disease was acquired transplacentally, but if the tests are reactive after 18 months, they indicate congenital syphilis.

Close neurologic follow-up is indicated for infants with initially abnormal CSF examinations. If CSF pleocytosis was present, spinal taps should be done every 6 months until the cell count is normal. If the cell count remains abnormal after 2 years or if a downward trend is not present at each examination, the infant should be re-treated. The CSF-VDRL should also be checked at 6 months, and re-treatment administered if still reactive.

Persons Exposed to Syphilis (Epidemiologic Treatment)

If compliance cannot be assured, examine the patient, do a serologic test, and treat the patient prophylactically for primary syphilis.

If the patient is reliable, examine and do RPR monthly for 3 months from the last exposure.

Syphilis in HIV-Infected Patients

A penicillin regimen should be instituted according to the stage of the disease.

Penicillin allergy Desensitize and treat.

CSF examination Do a spinal tap on patients with indeterminate or late latent disease or with early disease with neurologic symptoms.

Follow-up A closer follow-up with clinical and serologic tests is needed for these patients. CSF examination is indicated if there is serologic evidence of treatment failure at any time or the serofast response continues after 12 months.

Neurosyphilis Treat according to recommended regimens for neurosyphilis. Neurorelapse is more common in these patients, even after adequate treatment.

Penicillin Allergy Testing[77]

About 90 percent of patients with histories of "penicillin allergy" have negative skin tests and can be given penicillin safely, either because their histories were inaccurate or because their expression of penicillin-specific IgE ceased. The other 10 percent with a history of severe reactions are allergic to penicillin and should undergo desensitization. Radioallergosorbent test results are not reliable as penicillin-specific IgE antibodies may be detected in persons without penicillin allergy, and a negative outcome does not definitely exclude penicillin allergy. Testing with only major determinants misses 3 to 10 percent of allergic persons, and fatal reactions can occur. Administration of penicillin to patients who were not also tested with minor determinants must therefore be done with caution (Table 229-12). Patients with a history of penicillin allergy and a negative reaction to penicillin skin testing, who are not taking antihistamines and who had a positive histamine control on skin testing, should be given 250 mg of penicillin orally and observed for 1 h. Patients who tolerate this dose well can then be treated with higher doses of penicillin.

SCRATCH OR PRICK TEST Because serious IgE-mediated allergic reaction can occur, penicillin skin testing should be done in a facility where resuscitative equipment is readily available. The antigens should be diluted 100-fold for preliminary testing if there has been an immediate generalized reaction within the past year. The test is unreliable if antihistamines have been administered within the preceding 48 h. Gently scratch the epidermis in the volar sur-

TABLE 229-12

Reagents for Desensitization

Major determinants
  Benzylpenicilloyl-poly-L-lysine (Pre-Pen)
Minor determinants (difficult to obtain)
  Benzylpenicillin G
  Benzylpenicilloate
  Benzylpenilloate for penicilloyl propylalamine
Controls
  Positive control (histamine, 1 mg/mL)
  Negative control (buffered saline solution)

face of the forearm without drawing blood using a 25-gauge (or higher) needle. Apply one drop of penicillin determinant, saline, and histamine to each linear scratch, and observe for 20 min. If there is no wheal greater than 4 mm, proceed to the intradermal test.

INTRADERMAL TEST Inject 0.02 mL of penicillin determinant, saline, and histamine intradermally with a 27-gauge short-beveled needle and observe for 20 min.

INTERPRETATION The saline control must elicit no reaction, and the positive histamine control must elicit a positive reaction. A positive test is a wheal greater than 4 mm in diameter to any penicillin reagent. In a negative test, the wheals at the site of the penicillin reagents are equivalent to the negative control. All other results are indeterminate.

DESENSITIZATION The protocol for oral desensitization is listed in Table 229-13. The procedure described is not actually a desensitization but rather is an induction of immunotolerance by administration of very small doses of antigen. Hypersensitivity to penicillin still persists, but antibodies of the IgE class bind to scanty amounts of antigen. Therefore, the reaction is faint and remains subclinical.

Complications of Treatment

The Jarisch-Herxheimer reaction is a clinical syndrome consisting of fever, headache, flare of mucocutaneous lesions, tender lymphadenopathy, pharyngitis, malaise, myalgias, and leukocytosis. It occurs within 12 h of therapy for syphilis. The fever peaks in 6 to 8 h usually around 39°C (102.2°F), but it can be as high as 42°C (107.6°F). The reaction is not serious. Patients should be warned about the possibility of developing this reaction prior to receiving treatment. Symptoms are controlled with nonsteroidal anti-inflammatory agents or aspirin.

Patients with neurosyphilis not uncommonly become febrile after treatment with penicillin. Febrile reactions are more common when the CSF contains high numbers of cells and protein. Convulsions, dementia, psychosis, and meningismus have been reported to occur in up to 2 percent of neurosyphilis patients treated with penicillin. Death is rare, occurring only once among 1086 paretic patients. About 50 percent of infants with early and 39 percent of those with late disease develop febrile reactions. Rare cases of elevated liver function tests and the nephrotic syndrome have been reported.

The pathogenesis of the Jarisch-Herxheimer reaction is unknown. It has been proposed that destruction of spirochetes is followed by massive phagocytosis with release of pyrogenic cytokines.

Lesional changes include dilatation of the small dermal vessels, followed by endothelial swelling and migration of leukocytes through the vessel walls into the surrounding edematous tissue. Systemic glucocorticoids modify the febrile reaction without affecting the skin lesions or the leukocytosis; if administered 12 h prior to or at the time of treatment, they suppress or mitigate the reaction.

Therapeutic paradox, or deterioration of tertiary syphilis after therapy, results from rapid decomposition of gummatous tissue. The deterioration may extend to the surrounding tissue, which is histologically but not yet clinically involved. Scarring worsens the appearance of the lesions. Separating these changes, which are by no means limited to the skin, from syphilitic disease becomes a dilemma. For instance, worsening of the aortic insufficiency murmur has been reported from this complication.

Hoigne syndrome (*pseudoanaphylactic reaction*) is a complication associated with intramuscular procaine penicillin treatment and is seen in approximately 1 case per 1000 treated patients. The reaction is characterized by tachycardia, elevated blood pressure, fear of imminent death, violent combativeness, unusual taste sensation, auditory or visual disturbances, neuromuscular twitching, occasional seizures, and even loss of consciousness. It rarely lasts longer than 30 min.

Treatment consists of observation and sedatives or anticonvulsants. Inadvertent intracapillary infusion of procaine or, less likely, penicillin during intramuscular injection resulting in microembolization has been proposed as the mechanism.

VACCINES

Understanding the details involved in the emergence of resistance to *T. pallidum* is integral to the development of a syphilis vaccine. The focus of current syphilis research has centered on the identification and characterization of outer-membrane antigenic polypeptides.[78] Although antigens that can stimulate T cell responses have been found, little is known about their function.

A protective vaccine against syphilis will require considerably more investigation. In one promising study, repeated immunization of rabbits with purified antiendoflagellar antigen over 32 weeks did not prevent reinfection, but the lesions occurred earlier, had a flatter, softer appearance, and resolved more rapidly.

CONCLUSION

The preceding discussion leaves no doubt that syphilis is a disease with an exceptional diversity of possible organ involvement. However, the skin is affected in most cases with active disease. The

TABLE 229-13

Oral Desensitization Protocol

Penicillin V Suspension Dose	Amount, Units/mL, Diluted in 30 mL Water	mL	Units	Cumulative Dose, Units
1	1000	0.1	100	100
2	1000	0.2	200	300
3	1000	0.4	400	700
4	1000	0.8	800	1500
5	1000	1.6	1600	3100
6	1000	3.2	3200	6300
7	1000	6.4	6400	12,700
8	10,000	1.2	12,000	24,700
9	10,000	2.4	24,000	48,700
10	10,000	4.8	48,000	96,700
11	80,000	1.0	80,000	176,700
12	80,000	2.0	160,000	336,700
13	80,000	4.0	320,000	656,700
14	80,000	8.0	640,000	1,296,700

NOTE: Observation period: 30 min before parenteral administration of penicillin; interval between doses: 15 min; Elapsed time: 3 h and 45 min; Cumulative dose: 1.3 million units.
SOURCE: From Wendel, N Engl J Med, with permission.

study and treatment of syphilis had a pivotal influence in the development of dermatology as a specialty. Even today a number of dermatology departments from around the world have retained the word *syphilology* in their names. No practitioner is more capable than a dermatologist of evaluating, diagnosing, or treating syphilis and preventing its daunting complications. The occasional need for consultation with other specialties does not detract from the dermatologist's expertise. In fact, it is appropriate and essential for dermatologists to contribute their experience and skills whenever syphilis is considered as a potential diagnosis by other primary care providers and specialists. The physician who understands syphilis is a more astute and competent clinician. This conclusion was reached long ago by the renowned physician William Osler who wrote, "Know syphilis in all its manifestations and relations, and all other things clinical will be added unto you."

REFERENCES

1. Sanchez MR, Luger A: Syphilis, in *Dermatology in General Medicine*, 4th ed, TB Fitzpatrick et al (eds). New York, McGraw-Hill, 1993, pp 2703–2743
2. Lukehart SA: Modern syphilis—still a shadow on the land. *Western J Med* **163**:587, 1995
3. Rothschild BM, Rothschild C: Treponemal disease revisited: Skeletal discrimination of yaws, bejel and venereal syphilis. *Clin Infect Dis* **20**:1402, 1995
4. Hudson MM, Morton RS: Fracastoro and syphilis: 500 years on. *Lancet* **348**:1495, 1996
5. Nakashima AK et al: Epidemiology of syphilis in the United States, 1941–1993. *Sex Transm Dis* **23**:16, 1996
6. MMWR—Morbidity and Mortality Weekly Report. **47**:493, 1998
7. St. Louis ME, Wasserheit JN: Elimination of syphilis in the United States. *Science* **281**:353, 1998
8. Syphilis in the adult, in *Sexually Transmitted Diseases. Companion Handbook*, edited by A Adimora et al. New York, McGraw-Hill, 1994, pp 63–86

9. Norris SJ: Polypeptides of *Treponema pallidum*: Progress toward understanding their structural, functional, and immunologic roles. *Treponema pallidum* Polypeptide Research Group. *Microbiol Rev* **57**:750, 1993

10. Radolf JD: *Treponema pallidum* and the quest for outer membrane proteins. *Mol Microbiol* **16**:1067, 1995

11. Radolf JD et al: Characterization of outer membranes isolated from *Treponema pallidum*, the syphilis spirochete. *Infect Immun* **63**:4244, 1995

12. Pope V et al: Flow cytometric analysis of peripheral blood lymphocyte immunophenotypes in persons infected with *Treponema pallidum. Clin Diagn Lab Immunol* **1**:121, 1994

13. Van Vorrhis WC et al: Primary and secondary syphilis lesions contain mRNA for Th1 cytokines. *J Infect Dis* **173**:491, 1996

14. Centurion-Lara A et al: Detection of *Treponema pallidum* by a sensitive reverse transcriptase PCR. *J Clin Microbiol* **35**:1348, 1997

15. Roy B: The Tuskegee syphilis experiment: Biotechnology and the administrative state. *J Natl Med Assoc* **87**:56, 1995

16. Sanchez MR: Infectious syphilis. *Semin Dermatol* **31**:134, 1994

17. Templeton SF: Condyloma latum of the toe webs: An unusual manifestation of secondary syphilis. A report of two cases. *Cutis* **57**:38, 1996

18. Federman DG et al: Syphilis presenting as the "blue toe syndrome." *Arch Intern Med* **154**:1029, 1994

19. Cuozzo DW et al: Essential syphilitic alopecia revisited. *J Am Acad Dermatol* **32**:840, 1995

20. Jordaan HF, Louw M: The moth-eaten alopecia of secondary syphilis. A histopathological study of 12 patients. *Am J Dermatopathol* **17**:158, 1995

21. Barile GR, Flynn TE: Syphilis exposure in patients with uveitis. *Ophthalmology* **104**:1605, 1997

22. Chan YM et al: Syphilitic labyrinthitis—an update. *J Laryngol Otol* **109**:719, 1995

23. Peilec JL: Meniere's diseases of syphilitic etiology. *Ear Nose Throat J* **76**:508, 1997

24. Inagaki H et al: Gastric syphilis: Polymerase chain reaction detection of treponemal DNA in pseudolymphomatous lesions. *Hum Pathol* **27**:761, 1996

25. Sule RR et al: Late cutaneous syphilis. *Cutis* **59**:135, 1997

26. Sekkat A et al: Cutaneomucous tertiary syphilis. *Ann Dermatol Venereol* **121**:146, 1994

27. Scheck DN, Hook EW III: Neurosyphilis. *Infect Dis Clin North Am* **8**:769, 1994

28. LoVecchio F: Neurosyphilis presenting as refractory status epilepticus (letter). *Am J Emerg Med* **13**:685, 1995

29. Tyler KL et al: Medical medullary syndrome and meningovascular syphilis: A case report in an HIV-infected man and a review of the literature. *Neurology* **44**:2231, 1994

30. Horowitz HW et al: Brief report: Cerebral syphilitic gumma confirmed by PCR in a man with human immunodeficiency virus infection. *N Engl J Med* **331**:1488, 1994

31. Brightbill TC et al: Neurosyphilis in HIV-positive and HIV-negative patients: Neuroimaging findings. *Am J Neuroradiol* **16**:703, 1995

32. Glaser JH: Centers for Disease Control and Prevention guidelines for congenital syphilis. *J Pediatr* **129**:488, 1996

33. Risser WL, Hwang LY: Problems in the current case definitions of congenital syphilis. *J Pediatr* **129**:499, 1996

34. Sanchez PJ, Wendel GD: Syphilis in pregnancy. *Clin Perinatol* **24**:71, 1997

35. Nathan L et al: In utero infection with *Treponema pallidum* in early pregnancy. *Prenatal Diagn* **17**:119, 1997

36. Rawstron SA et al: Congenital syphilis: Detection of *Treponema pallidum* in stillborns. *Clin Infect Dis* **24**:24, 1997

37. Bennett ML et al: Congenital syphilis: Subtle presentation of fulminant disease. *J Am Acad Dermatol* **36**:351, 1997

38. Goeman J et al: Dementia paralytica in a fifteen-year old boy. *J Neurol Sci* **144**:214, 1996

39. O'Mahony C et al: Rapidly progressive syphilis in early HIV infection. *Int J STD AIDS* **8**:275, 1997

40. Otten MW Jr et al: High rate of HIV seroconversion among patients attending urban sexually transmitted disease clinics. *AIDS* **8**:549, 1994

41. Marra CM et al: Alterations in the course of experimental syphilis associated with concurrent simian immunodeficiency virus infection. *J Infect Dis* **165**:1020, 1992

42. Marra CM et al: Diagnosis of neurosyphilis in patients infected with human immunodeficiency virus type 1. *J Infect Dis* **174**:219, 1996

43. Gourevitch MN et al: Effects of HIV infection on the serologic manifestations and response to treatment of syphilis in intravenous drug users. *Ann Intern Med* **118**:350, 1993

44. Sands M, Markus A: Lues maligna, or ulceronodular syphilis, in a man infected with human immunodeficiency virus: Case report and review. *Clin Infect Dis* **20**:387, 1995

45. Don PC et al: Malignant syphilis (lues maligna) and concurrent infection with HIV. *Int J Dermatol* **34**:403, 1995

46. Balachandran C et al: Perforation of hard palate in lues maligna associated with HIV infection (letter). *Genitourin Med* **73**:225, 1997

47. Shalaby IA et al: Syphilitic uveitis in human immunodeficiency virus–infected patients. *Arch Ophthalmol* **115**:469, 1997

48. Rolfs RT et al: A randomized trial of enhanced therapy for early syphilis in patients with and without human immunodeficiency virus infection. The Syphilis and HIV Study Group. *N Engl J Med* **337**:307, 1997

49. Malone JL et al: Syphilis and neurosyphilis in human immunodeficiency virus type-1 seropositive population: Evidence for frequent serologic relapse after therapy. *Am J Med* **99**:55, 1995

50. Bordon J et al: Neurosyphilis in HIV-infected patients. *Euro J Clin Microbiol Infect Dis* **14**:864, 1995

51. Harris DE et al: Neurosyphilis in patients with AIDS. *Neuroimaging Clin North Am* **7**:215, 1997

52. Gordon SM et al: The response of symptomatic neurosyphilis to high-dose intravenous penicillin G in patients with human immunodeficiency virus infection. *N Engl J Med* **331**:1469, 1994

53. Marra CM et al: Resolution of serum and cerebrospinal fluid abnormalities after treatment of neurosyphilis. Influence of concomitant human immunodeficiency virus infection. *Sex Transm Dis* **23**:184, 1996

54. Yinnon AM et al: Serologic response to treatment of syphilis in patients with HIV infection. *Arch Intern Med* **156**:321, 1996

55. Augenbraun MH et al: Biological false-positive syphilis test results for women infected with human immunodeficiency virus. *Clin Infect Dis* **19**:1040, 1994

56. Nandwani R, Evans DT: Are you sure it's syphilis? A review of false-positive serology (review). *Int J STD AIDS* **6**:241, 1995

57. Genest DR et al: Diagnosis of congenital syphilis from placental examination: Comparison of histopathology, Steiner stain, and polymerase chain reaction for *Treponema pallidum* DNA. *Hum Pathol* **27**:366, 1996

58. Mashkilleyson AL et al: Treatment of syphilis with azithromycin. *Int J STD AIDS* **7**:13, 1996

59. Jethwa HS et al: Comparison of molecular and microscopic techniques for detection of *Treponema pallidum* in genital ulcers. *J Clin Microbiol* **33**:180, 1995

60. Meyer JC: Laboratory diagnosis of syphilis. *Curr Probl Dermatol* **24**:1, 1996

61. Larsen SA et al: Laboratory diagnosis and interpretation of tests for syphilis. *Clin Microbiol Rev* **8**:1, 1995

62. El-Zaatari MM et al: Incidence of the prozone phenomenon in syphilis serology. *Obstet Gyn* **84**:609, 1994

63. Vayssairat M et al: Antiphospholipids—a "guilty ghost" syndrome. *Clin Rev Allergy Immunol* **13**:1, 1995

64. Hooper NE et al: Evaluation of a *Treponema pallidum* enzyme immunoassay as a screening test for syphilis. *Clin Diagn Lab Immunol* **1**:477, 1994

65. Silletti RP: Comparison of CAPTIA syphilis G enzyme immunoassay with rapid plasma reagin test for detection of syphilis. *J Clin Microbiol* **33**:1829, 1995

66. Young H et al: Markers of past syphilis in HIV infection comparing Captia Syphilis G anti-treponemal IgG enzyme immunoassay with other treponemal antigen tests. *Intern J STD AIDS* **6**:101, 1995

67. Spirochetal and Richettsial Infections in Clinical Laboratory Medicine. Clinical application of laboratory data. Ravel R, St. Louis, Mosby, 1995, pp 226–232

68. Cummings MC et al: Comparison of methods for the detection of *Treponema pallidum* in lesions of early syphilis. *Sex Transm Dis* **23**:366, 1996

69. Schmitz JL et al: Laboratory diagnosis of congenital syphilis by immunoglobulin M (IgM) and IgA immunoblotting. *Clin Diagn Lab Immunol* **1**:32, 1994

70. Centurion-Lara A et al: Detection of *Treponema pallidum* by a sensitive reverse transcriptase PCR. *J Clin Microbiol* **35**:1348, 1997

71. MacLean S, Luger A: Finding neurosyphilis without the Venereal Disease Research Laboratory test. *Sex Transm Dis* **23**:392, 1996

72. Marra CM et al: Cerebrospinal fluid treponemal antibodies in untreated early syphilis. *Arch Neurol* **52**:68, 1995
73. Goldmeier D, Hay P: A review and update on adult syphilis, with particular reference to its treatment. *Int J STD AIDS* **4**:70, 1993
74. DeMaria A et al: Minocycline for symptomatic neurosyphilis in patients allergic to penicillin (letter). *N Engl J Med* **337**:1322, 1997
75. Verdon MS et al: Pilot study of azithromycin for treatment of primary and secondary syphilis. *Clin Infect Dis* **19**:486, 1994
76. Marra CM et al: Evaluation of aqueous penicillin G and ceftriaxone for experimental neurosyphilis. *J Infect Dis* **165**:396, 1992
77. 1998 Guidelines for Treatment of Sexually Transmitted Diseases. Centers for Disease Control. *Morb Mort Week Rep* **47**:28, 1998
78. Adimora AA et al: Vaccines for classic sexually transmitted diseases. *Infect Dis Clin North Am* **8**:859, 1994

CHAPTER 230

Miguel R. Sanchez

Endemic (Nonvenereal) Treponematoses

The nonvenereal treponematoses (pinta, yaws, and endemic syphilis) are a group of distinct infections that remain within endemic foci in economically disadvantaged, isolated rural areas of tropical and subtropical countries.[1] In contrast to syphilis, transmission is rarely sexual. Instead, these diseases are transmitted predominantly by children living in unhygienic conditions through direct contact with skin and mucous membrane lesions. Infants contract the infections from their mothers during feeding and children from siblings or playmates. Like syphilis, the diseases have successive clinical stages separated by periods of latency, but neurologic or cardiovascular complications rarely or never occur.[2]

The causative organisms cannot be distinguished from each other or from the organism that causes syphilis with microbiologic, histologic, biochemical, serologic, or even highly sensitive DNA molecular techniques.[3] Most studies using Western blotting, Southern hybridization, and immunoblotting have found no differences, and even DNA sequencing has detected few molecular alterations.

Patients are infectious for long periods of time and may have subclinical or mild disease. Furthermore, they do not develop lifelong immune resistance. Cross-immunity is absent in the early stages of syphilis, yaws, and pinta but is variable in late stages. Patients with late pinta are resistant to syphilis but those with yaws or syphilis at any stage are susceptible to pinta.[3]

The nonvenereal treponematoses are not fatal but are disfiguring and disabling, and patients endure social ostracism. The role of flies and other insects in the transmission of any of these infections remains unproven.

PINTA (MAL DE PINTO, CUTE, PURÚ-PURÚ, ENFERMEDAD AZUL)

Pinta (Spanish, "colored spot") is caused by *Treponema carateum*. The species was named after the Colombian name for the disease (*carate*).

In 1938, Grau Triana and Alfonso Armenteros found treponemes in dark-field examinations of pinta lesions. In 1939, the Cuban physician Leon y Blanco reproduced the disease by inoculating lesional exudate into normal volunteers. Further investigations by Padilha Goncalves determined that pinta was a different treponemal infection than syphilis or yaws. It is probably the oldest treponemal infection affecting humans, but because only the skin is involved, there are no skeletal remains that can be studied and yaws is instead given that distinction.[4] Chimpanzees are the only animals susceptible to infection with *T. carateum*.

The disease typically affects poor, undernourished infants, children, and adolescents who live in small, remote, crowded villages in hot, semiarid coastal areas. Twenty years ago about 750,000 cases were estimated, but now only a few hundred cases are reported each year, mainly from southern Mexico or Central and South America.[1]

Transmission occurs from repeated direct contact of the exposed skin of a healthy person with an infected lesion.

Clinical Course

Pinta is the only treponematosis with clinical manifestations confined to the skin.[1] As in syphilis, there are three distinct clinical stages, but in contrast to syphilis, lesions from different stages may be present in a single patient. Because cell-mediated immunity is not completely effective, the infection persists indefinitely, and people of all ages are infected. However, 40 to 60 percent of patients are under 15 years of age.

PRIMARY STAGE   Between 3 to 60 days (average 1 to 3 weeks) after contact with an infected lesion, one or more small, erythematous papules or desquamating macules develop at the sites of inoculation. These primary lesions may be pruritic, become slightly scaly and enlarge, or coalesce with other lesions to achieve a size of 1 to 3 cm within 3 months and ultimately reach up to 20 cm.[5] These irregular, infiltrated plaques develop a psoriasiform surface. The lesions may become lichenified but never ulcerate (Fig. 230-1). Primary lesions develop more often in the extremities and commonly on the face, neck, and chest. They persist for years and eventually heal with residual hypopigmentation.

SECONDARY STAGE   Secondary lesions (*pintids*) appear 2 to 5 months but sometimes years after the appearance of the primary lesions. They encircle the sites of the primary lesions or, owing to dissemination, arise on any distant sites including the palms, soles and groin.[1] Secondary lesions may be indistinguishable from primary lesions but are smaller and not pruritic. The lesions begin as scaly red to violaceous papules that enlarge to form psoriasiform, dyschromic plaques. These turn brown or copper-colored and eventually slate blue, gray, or black. More than one color may be present within a lesion. Some plaques may be circinate or annular with

raised borders where treponemal activity is highest. Lesions can recur up to 10 years after the initial infection.[6]

TERTIARY STAGE   Late lesions develop between 3 months and 10 years after the appearance of the secondary stage. Typically patients have depigmented patches on their wrists, ankles, and elbows as well as around and within old lesions, imparting a mottled pattern (Fig. 230-2). Patients usually have a combination of dyschromic, hypochromic, and achromic patches, which may be irregular and vary in size.[7] Lymphadenopathy may develop during any stage of pinta.

Depending on the stage of pinta, postinflammatory hypopigmentation, traumatic depigmentation, lichen simplex chronicus, tinea versicolor, psoriasis, deep fungal infections, erythema dyschromium perstans, and other treponematoses are among the diseases that need to be considered in the differential diagnosis. Patients with only late-stage lesions may appear to have vitiligo.

YAWS (PIAN, BUBA, FRAMBESIA, PARANGI, PARÚ)

Yaws is caused by *T. pallidum* (subsp. *pertenue*). Children constitute the primary reservoir. Analysis of skeletal remains of *Homo erectus* in Nairobi suggests that yaws had its origin in Africa during the middle Pleistocene period (1.5 million years ago).[4] The disease was introduced into the Americas by slaves. Yaws is contracted from direct contact with abraded, bitten, or excoriated skin with oozing lesions. Some experts contend that the disease can be transmitted through flies or domestic utensils. Campaigns to eradicate the disease in some countries are hampered by the suspected reservoir of *T. pertenue* in cynocephalic monkeys.[1]

Yaws occurs in countries along the tropical belt in lowlands adjacent to forests characterized by heavy rainfall, high humidity, and hot temperatures that do not fall below 27°C (80.6°F). In 1952, the estimated number of cases was between 25 and 150 million. Owing to mass treatment campaigns and improved living conditions, the disease has been eradicated in many areas and greatly reduced in others. However, foci have recently been reported in several African, South American, and Southeast Asian countries.[8]

FIGURE 230-1

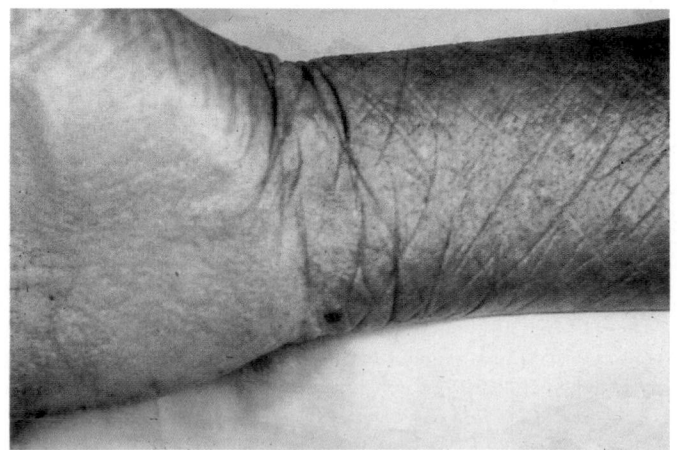

Lichenified patch in primary pinta with dyschromic changes.

FIGURE 230-2

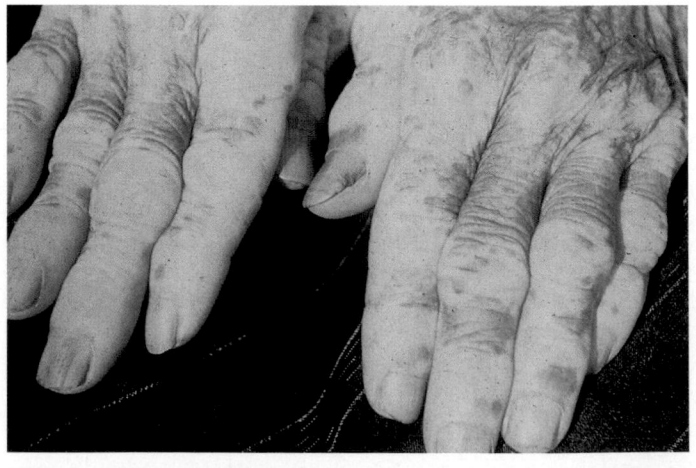

Depigmented, mottled patches in late pinta.

Currently at least 100 million children are estimated to be at risk of becoming infected.[1]

Clinical Course

PRIMARY STAGE After an incubation period of 9 days to 3 months (average 3 weeks), the primary lesion or mother yaw (*buba madre*) appears at the site of inoculation, which is usually an exposed body part such as the face, neck, buttock, legs, feet, arms, or hand. Characteristically the lesion is a nontender, occasionally pruritic, infiltrated, erythematous small nodule that grows horizontally to a size of 1 to 5 cm. Its surface frequently becomes papillomatous. The primary lesion is usually single but satellite papules may be present, becoming confluent into a plaque. The lesion eventually becomes an ulcer with a "raspberry-like" (frambesial) base that may be covered by yellow crust (Fig. 230-3). This mother yaw heals spontaneously in 2 to 6 months with atrophic scarring and central hypopigmentation. Regional buboes are common.[1] Constitutional symptoms are rare.

SECONDARY STAGE Resolution of the primary stage is typically followed by a period of latency, lasting weeks to months, which is then interrupted by an eruption of disseminated skin lesions with or without constitutional symptoms. The lesions (*daughter yaws* or *pianomes*) are soft, warty, or vegetating frambesial, scaly, yellowred papules or plaques not unlike the mother yaws but smaller (up to 2 cm)(Fig. 230-4*A*). As the lesions grow, they become eroded and covered by a highly infectious fibrinous exudate, which dries into a crust (Fig. 230-4*B*). Unfortunately, the exudate attracts flies that torture the afflicted persons.[9]

These *papillomas* may appear in any body area. The term *pianic onychia* refers to paronychial lesions. In addition to the pianomes, dry, papulosquamous patches and plaques (*pianides*), which resemble those of secondary syphilis, may be present on any part of the body. Unless inflamed, the lesions do not itch. In body folds, they resemble condylomata lata, and in mucous membranes, hypertrophic mucous patches. Involvement of the palms and soles with thick hyperkeratotic plaques that become fissured or eroded is called *crab yaws* (Fig. 230-5) because patients walk with a deliberate slow, crustacean gait. The lesions may be annular or circinate (*tinea yaws*). Lesions on the face are often seborrheic or psoriasiform.[10]

Painful osteoperiostitis is common in early yaws. The appearance of turnip-like, fusiform soft tissue swelling of the proximal but not the distal phalanges due to periostitis is classic. The metatarsal and metacarpal bones are also commonly involved. The tibial bones may also be affected.[11] All lesions resolve without scarring, but relapses may develop during the initial 5 years of infection. In relapsing yaws, lesions tend to be confined to the perioral, perianal, and periaxillary areas.

FIGURE 230-3

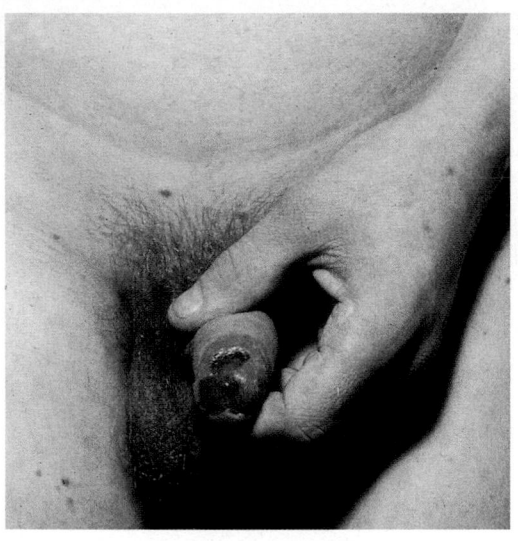

Ulcerated primary-stage nodule ("mother yaw"). The genital location is unusual.

FIGURE 230-4

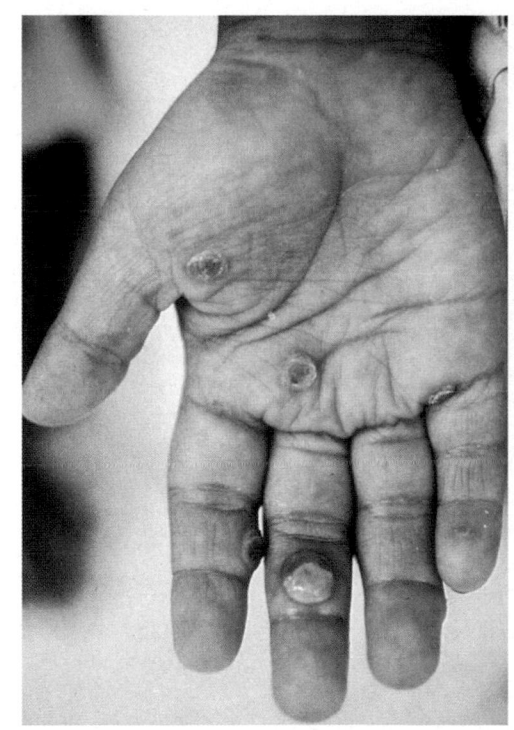

A.

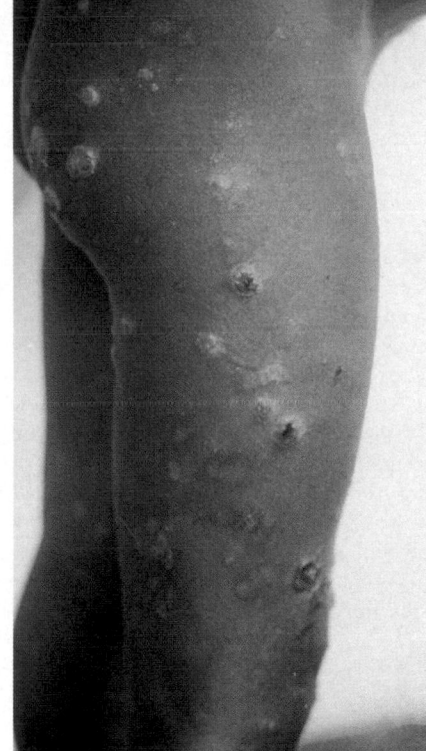

B.

A. Warty secondary-stage papillomas ("daughter yaws"). *B.* Eroded papillomas covered by fibrinous exudate. (*Courtesy of HJH Engelkens, MD, J. van der Stek, MD, and E. Stolz, MD.*)

FIGURE 230-5

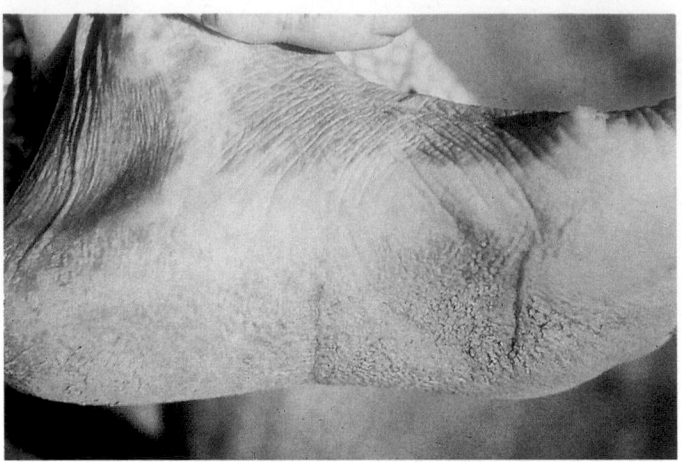

Fissured hyperkeratotic plantar keratoderma in secondary yaws ("crab yaws").

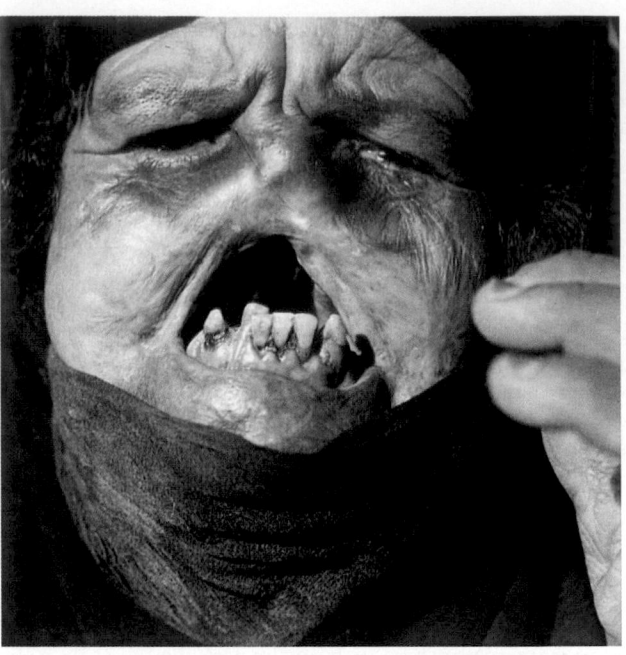

Massive destruction of the maxillary and nasal structures (gangosa) in late yaws.

Most patients then enter a permanent latent period with no signs or symptoms of the disease.

TERTIARY STAGE In approximately 10 percent of cases, latency is interrupted after several years by a late stage with destructive cutaneous and skeletal lesions and possibly ophthalmologic and neurologic involvement. In the late stage, several types of skin lesions may be present. Cutaneous and subcutaneous gummatous nodules necrose centrally and ulcerate, causing deep, mutilating damage. Coalescence of the ulcers may result in formation of circinate, serpiginous tracts that heal with deforming scars and contractures.[2] Palmoplantar hyperkeratosis may lead to keratoderma. Juxtaarticular nodes may form on the elbows and knees. Dyschromic or achromic dry, pintoid patches are seen in the soles and occasionally palms and wrists in some African patients.[3]

Late skeletal changes include hypertrophic periostitis, gummatous periostitis, and osteomyelitis. Considerable bone hypertrophy due to chronic osteitis may result in curvature of the tibia (*saber shins*). Bilateral hypertrophic osteitis of the nasal process of the maxillae with persistent swelling of the nasal bridge (*goundou*) slowly progresses over 5 to 20 years. Massive destruction of the nose, maxillae, upper lip, and central face with eventual perforation of the nose and palate (*gangosa*) occurs in 1 percent of patients (Fig. 230-6).

Although eye and nervous system disease is not usually associated with yaws, some reports have indicated that these systems may be involved. Mild neurologic defects such as disk atrophy were reported in Venezuelan patients. Myeloneuropathy has also been described. Optic atrophy attributed to *T. pertenue* infection has been reported.[1] Treponemes have been detected in the aqueous humor.

A less contagious form of "attenuated" yaws with one or few dry, gray, transient patches predominantly in the axillae and perianal areas has been described.[1]

Because of the diverse appearance of skin lesions in different stages, the differential diagnosis is extensive. Syphilis, the great imitator, must be excluded in any stage of yaws. Other diseases in the differential diagnosis include verruca vulgaris, psoriasis, tinea, eczema, palmoplantar keratodermas, erythema annulare, sarcoid, Hansen's disease, deep fungal infections, rhinoscleroma, rhinosporidiosis, and leishmaniasis.

ENDEMIC SYPHILIS (BEJEL, BELESH, NJOVERA)

Endemic syphilis is a nonvenereal infection caused by *T. pallidum* (*subsp. endemicum*). The disease favors arid climates in rural areas bordering deserts. It has been reported to be a common health problem in children from Burkina Faso and in the Bedouin tribes of the Middle East. Foci persist in the Middle East, in Saharan Africa, and in desert regions north and south of the tropical belt. The infection targets children below the age of 15, but adults may also become infected. Transmission occurs when skin or mucous membranes come in contact with infected skin lesions or saliva. Infection is commonly contracted by drinking from contaminated flasks or from sharing pipes.[1]

Clinical Course

PRIMARY STAGE The incubation period is 10 to 90 days. The lesions resemble the *chancres* of venereal syphilis. The primary lesion is a small eroded or ulcerated papule, which is rarely noted probably because of the small size of the inoculation. Also, it may not be readily detected because it is asymptomatic and usually arises in the oropharyngeal mucosa. A lesion may develop in the nipple of a mother nursing an infected infant. Primary lesions heal in 1 to 6 weeks.[2]

SECONDARY STAGE Usually a few nontender, oval or round, macerated, eroded, mucous patches erupt on the lips, tongue, and tonsils. Vegetating or hypertrophic *condylomata lata* appear in the anogenital area and axillae. Split *papules* are fissured mucous patches in the labial commissures. Occasionally, macular, papular, annular, and circinate eruptions like those seen in secondary syphilis develop. Nontender, generalized lymphadenopathy is common. Nocturnal lower extremity pain is due to osteoperiostitis of the long bones. The secondary stage persists for 6 to 9 months and is followed by a latent period, which may continue for only a few months but usually lasts 5 to 15 years. At this point, a tertiary stage with cutaneous skeletal and systemic manifestations develops.[12]

TERTIARY STAGE Late lesions consist of *gummas* of the skin, bone, nasopharynx, and larynx. The gummas ulcerate and become chronic serpiginous tracts that are destructive but not as mutilating as those of yaws (Fig. 230-7). The ulcerations eventually heal, leaving atrophic, depigmented scars bordered by hyperpigmentation. Saddle-nose deformity, palate perforation, or gangosa are deforming complications.[10]

Skeletal involvement is common, but most patients are not significantly bothered by pain. Clinically apparent tibial bowing or tenderness are exceptions. However, bone defects may be radiologically present, most commonly on the tibia and fibula and sometimes in the ulna and radius. Systemic involvement does not appear to be common. Uveitis, chorioretinitis, and optic atrophy have been observed. Eye disease responds to penicillin except presumably for irreversible atrophy. Aortitis and saccular aneurysms of the aortic arch have infrequently been reported.[3]

An attenuated form of endemic syphilis with fewer lesions that heal more rapidly has been reported. Leg pain due to periostitis was a common manifestation.

FIGURE 230-7

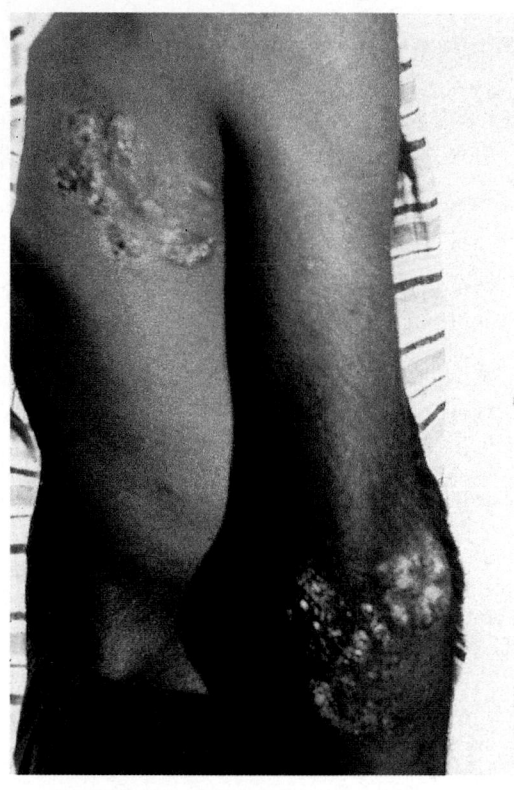

Cutaneous gummas in late endemic syphilis. Note involvement of the elbow.

Diagnosis

The diagnosis of these diseases is made from clinical evaluation of the lesions (Table 230-1) in persons who live or have resided in endemic areas and confirmed by detection of treponemes under dark-field microscopic examination of serum obtained by squeezing the bases of lesions. In the absence of a positive dark-field test, histologic or serologic confirmation is required. In yaws and endemic syphilis, nontreponemal tests [rapid plasma reagin (RPR) and Venereal Disease Research Laboratory (VDRL) tests] are reactive in 2 to 3 weeks after the onset of the primary lesion. In pinta, these tests become reactive in 80 percent of cases 2 to 3 months after the appearance of primary lesions and are reactive in all patients with the late stage of the disease. Other treponemal tests, including enzyme immunoassays (EIA), have not shown greater specificity than the fluorescence treponemal antibody absorption (FTA-ABS) test.[13] A finger-prick indirect hemagglutination test is advantageous for screening children.[14]

TABLE 230-1

Nonvenereal Trepanomatoses—Clinical Manifestations

	PINTA	YAWS	ENDEMIC SYPHILIS
Causative organism	*T. carateum*	*T. pertenue*	*T. pallidum*
Transmission	Skin-to-skin contact	Skin-to-skin contact	Mouth-to-mouth contact, drinking vessels
Peak ages	1–15 years	1–15 years	Months–15 years
Incubation	3–60 days (average 1–3 weeks)	9–90 days (average 3 weeks)	10–90 days
Primary lesions	Erythematous papules become non-ulcerating, psoriasiform plaques	Vegetating, soft, ulcerating papule (*mother yaws*), with satellites	Small eroded papule (often absent)
Secondary lesions	Erythematous scaly and psoriasiform plaques (*pintids*) develop; increased and decreased pigmentation	Warty or framboesiform nodules, papulosquamous plaques, palmoplantar *"crab yaws"*	Mucous patches, condylomata lata, syphilis-like eruptions
Tertiary lesions	Dyschromic, hypochromic, achromic, and polychromic patches	Gummas, pintoid dyschromia, juxtaarticular nodes, gangosa, goundou, keratoderma	Serpiginous gummas, juxtaarticular nodes on elbows only
Reactive serology	2–3 months after primary lesion	2–3 weeks after primary lesion	2–3 weeks after primary lesion
Treatment	Penicillin	Penicillin	Penicillin

Histopathology

In a primary lesion of pinta, epidermal changes consist of mild acanthosis, epidermal edema, exocytosis of lymphocytes, liquification degeneration of the basal cell layer, and loss of melanin. In the upper dermis there is a dense infiltrate of plasma cells, lymphoid cells, some neutrophils and histiocytes, and many melanophages. In contrast to syphilitic chancres, endothelial swelling is minimal or absent.

Histologically, secondary lesions are indistinguishable from primary lesions. In the hyperpigmented patches of tertiary pinta, the epidermis is atrophic and the basal cell layer shows no melanin, but in the upper dermis there is an infiltrate of many melanophages and some lymphoid cells. As the lesions become increasingly depigmented, the infiltrate is milder and treponemes become scarcer to the point that neither is present. Treponemes are found in silver impregnation between epidermal cells in primary, secondary, and late-stage hyperpigmented lesions but not in late hypopigmented patches.

The epidermal changes in a primary lesion of yaws are acanthosis, papillomatosis, edema, and neutrophilic microabscesses. In the dermis, there is a dense mixed cell infiltrate of neutrophils, lymphocytes, histiocytes, fibroblasts, a few eosinophils, and many plasma cells. No endothelial proliferation is seen in the vessels. Secondary yaws lesions have a similar appearance to the primary lesions. In late yaws, the lesions are very similar to late benign syphilitic lesions. In the first two stages, treponemes are easily detected on silver-stained tissue almost exclusively between epidermal cells.[15]

The lesions of endemic syphilis are histopathologically identical to those of venereal syphilis.

Treatment

The recommended treatment for pinta, yaws, and endemic syphilis is a single injection of 1.2 million units of benzathine penicillin in adults or children over 10 years of age and 0.6 million units in younger children. Patients become noninfectious within 24 h. Children older than 8 years of age who are allergic to penicillin may be treated for 15 days with tetracycline 250 mg four times daily, or, if younger, with erythromycin 8 mg/kg four times daily. Penicillin-allergic adults are treated for 15 days with tetracycline 500 mg four times daily, doxycycline 100 mg twice daily, or erythromycin 500 mg four times daily. In pinta, primary and secondary lesions disappear 4 to 12 months after treatment, but achromic patches persist for life. The effect of HIV infection of nonvenereal treponematosis is not known, but based on the experience with venereal syphilis, it appears prudent to screen those persons at risk with HIV serology and consider closer follow-up.[16] Recommendations for epidemiologic treatment depend on the number of seropositive children under 6 years of age (Table 230-2).

CONCLUSION

The means to eradicate the nonvenereal treponematoses are available. However, history has shown that mass treatment campaigns alone are not sufficient.[17] In some areas where the diseases had

TABLE 230-2

Epidemiologic Treatment

AREA (PERCENTAGE OF SEROPOSITIVE CHILDREN)	RECOMMENDATION
Hyperendemic (>50%)	Treat the entire population.
Mesoendemic (10–50%)	Treat all active cases, their contacts, and all children 15 years of age or younger.
Hypoendemic (<10%)	Treat all active cases, their household members, and other obvious contacts.

been thought to be eradicated, new cases are being reported at a surprising rate.[18] Treatment of those infected and those at risk must be followed by such sound public health measures as prolonged serosurveillance and periodic screenings.[19] Resurveys should begin 6 months after initial treatment and continued at least every 2 years. However, such investment is unlikely because these diseases affect impoverished persons who live in remote villages, where they rarely interact with media reporters or political figures. City dwellers are not at risk and the diseases are practically unknown in the West, where a single case usually stimulates a published case report. The western medical establishment regards these diseases as curiosities that are extinct or almost extinct. Since the nonvenereal treponematoses are rarely fatal, are associated with poor hygiene, and are invisible to most of the world, there is little appeal for global and even community support.

REFERENCES

1. Koff AB, Rosen T: Nonvenereal treponematoses: Yaws, endemic syphilis, and pinta. *J Am Acad Dermatol* **29**:519, 1993
2. Arya OP: Endemic Treponematoses, in *Manson's Tropical Diseases,* edited by GC Cook. Philadelphia, Saunders, 1996, pp 940–950
3. Sanchez MR, Luger AFH: Endemic (nonvenereal) treponematoses in *Dermatology in General Medicine,* 4th ed, edited by T Fitzpatrick, AZ Eisen, K Wolff, IM Freedberg, KF Austen. New York, McGraw-Hill, 1993, pp 2743–2748
4. Rothschild BM et al: Origin of yaws in the Pleistocene (letter). *Nature* **378**:343, 1995
5. Engelkens HJ et al: Endemic treponematoses: Part II. Pinta and endemic syphilis (review). *Int J Dermatol* **30**:231, 1991
6. Dominguez-Soto L et al: Pigmentary problems in the tropics. *Dermatol Clin* **12**:777, 1994
7. Fuchs J et al: Tertiary pinta: Case reports and overview. *Cutis* **51**:425, 1993
8. Sehgal VN et al: Yaws control/eradication. *Int J Dermatol* **33**:16, 1994
9. Engelkens HJ et al: Endemic treponematoses: Part I. Yaws. *Int J Dermatol* **30**:77, 1991
10. Hoeprich PD: Nonsyphilitic treponematosis, in *Infectious Diseases,* 5th ed, edited by PD Hoeprich, MC Jordan, et al. Philadelphia, Lippincott, 1994, pp 1018–1028
11. Engelkens HJ et al: Case report: 724 yaws. *Skel Radiol* **21**:194, 1992
12. Yakinci C et al: Bejel in Malatya, Turkey. *J Trop Pediatr* **41**:117, 1995
13. Backhouse JL, Hudson BJ: Evaluation of immunoglobulin G enzyme immunoassay for serodiagnosis of yaws. *J Clin Microbiol* **33**:1875, 1995

14. Backhouse JL et al: Modified indirect hemagglutination test for detection of treponemal antibodies in finger-prick blood. *J Clin Microbiol* **30**:561, 1992

15. Engelkens HJ et al: The localisation of treponemes and characterisation of the inflammatory infiltrate in skin biopsies from patients with primary or secondary syphilis, or early infectious yaws. *Genitourin Med* **69**:102, 1993

16. Noordhoek GT, van Embden JD: Yaws, an endemic treponematosis reconsidered in the HIV era. *Eur J Clin Microbiol Infect Dis* **10**:4, 1991

17. Engelkens HJ et al: The resurgence of yaws: World-wide consequences. *Int J Dermatol* **30**:99, 1991

18. Meheus A, Antal GM: The endemic treponematoses: Not yet eradicated (review). *World Health Stat* **45**:228, 1992

19. Anselmi M et al: Yaws in Ecuador: Impact of control measures on the disease in the province of Esmeraldas. *Genitourin Med* **71**:343, 1995

CHAPTER 231

Alfred R. Eichmann

Chancroid

Chancroid is a sexually transmitted, acute ulcerative disease usually localized at the anogenital area and often associated with an inguinal bubo. The disease is caused by infection with *Haemophilus ducreyi*, a gram-negative, facultative anaerobic bacillus that requires hemin (X factor) for growth.

HISTORIC ASPECTS

Chancroid, or soft chancre (ulcus molle) was first distinguished from syphilis by Basserau in France in 1842. The causative bacillus was discovered and described by Ducrey 1889, a bacteriologist at the University of Naples. Unna described the histology of the chancroidal ulcer and found the chains of gram-negative rods in the lesion. It is still unclear who was the first to culture *H. ducreyi*. In his review, Albritton[1] credited Himmel (1901) with the first convincing isolation of *H. ducreyi,* but other authors in the same period also claimed priority.

EPIDEMIOLOGY

Chancroid is most common in developing countries, especially in tropical and subtropical areas. Soft ulcer is the most common cause of genital ulcer disease in men and women in Africa and many other parts of the developing world.[2] In the United States, chancroid has reemerged during the last decade. After an epidemic in California in 1981, the number of cases increased, peaking in 1987 at approximately 5000. Interpreting chancroid surveillance data is difficult because confirmatory culture media are not commercially available.[3]

The reported cases of chancroid for the entire United States was only 606 in 1995, or 0.2 per 100,000 inhabitants.[4]

The prevalence of chancroid is higher in lower socioeconomic groups. Lower-class prostitutes appear to be a reservoir in all reported outbreaks of this disease. Men have a markedly higher incidence of chancroid than women.[5] Recently, several studies in Africa showed that chancroid-ulcer is an important risk factor for the heterosexual spread of HIV-1.[6] Until now the epidemiology of chancroid has been poorly documented because of low interest and lack of accurate and simple diagnostic tools (phenotypic markers for strain typing). It is still not clear whether there is an asymptomatic reservoir of *H. ducreyi* and what the risks of transmission are.[7]

ETIOLOGY

TAXONOMY *H. ducreyi* is a gram-negative, facultative anaerobic bacillus that requires hemin (X factor) for growth. The organism is small, nonmotile, and non-spore-forming; it shows typical streptobacillary chaining, especially in cultures. The exact taxonomy is still controversial. The current classifications list *H. ducreyi* as a true *Haemophilus* species. Some biochemical properties, however, put this organism close to the Pasteurellaceae.[8]

BIOCHEMISTRY *H. ducreyi* has few distinguishing biochemical features. Nitrate reduction is a characteristic of the genus. All reported strains are oxidase-positive and catalase-negative and have a broad range of phosphatase activity. The alkaline phosphatase reaction is used in its identification.[8] Differentiation from other hemin-requiring strains of *Haemophilus* is made by the lack of requirement for nicotinamideadenine dinucleotide (NAD, V factor) and its failure to produce hydrogen sulfide, catalase, or indole.[8]

GROWTH REQUIREMENTS *H. ducreyi* is a fastidious bacillus. In order to get optimal rates of positive cultures, Nszane et al.[9] recommend the use of two media simultaneously: gonococcal agar supplemented with bovine hemoglobin and Mueller-Hinton agar supplemented with chocolate horse blood, each with 5% fetal calf serum. Growth is best at 30° to 33°C (86° to 91.4°F) in a water-saturated atmosphere.

GENETICS The strains of *H. ducreyi* appear to be serologically and biochemically homogenous. *H. ducreyi* shares a significant gene pool with members of the Pasteurellaceae and the Enterobacteriae. The core plasmid conferring ampicillin resistance in *H. ducreyi* is found in other species of *Haemophilus* and *Neisseria*.[1] Beta-lactamase-production is mediated by plasmids (5000 and 5700 kDa) identical to the two types of *Neisseria gonorrhoeae* beta-lactamase plasmid. A 3200-kDa plasmid mediating beta-lactamase production has also been reported.[10] A 3000-kDa plasmid encoding for beta-lactamase production in *H. ducreyi* was found in isolates from a chancroid outbreak in California in 1983.[10]

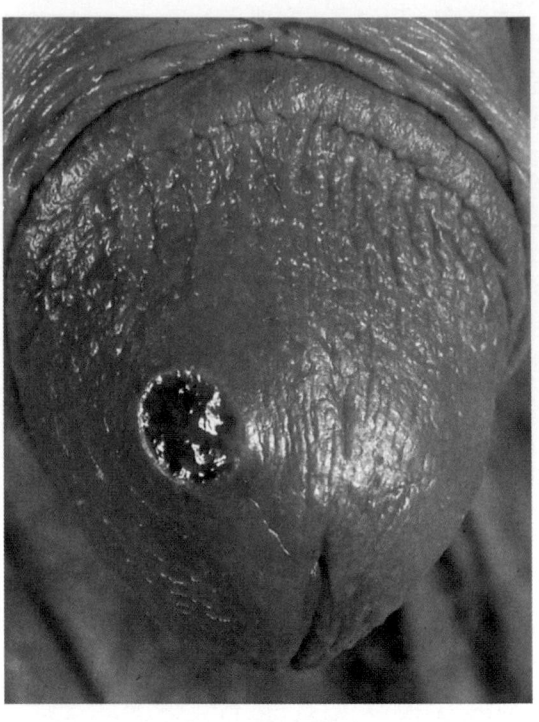

Sharply circumscribed ulcer on the glans.

PATHOGENESIS

Three major problems seem to be important in the pathogenesis of *H. ducreyi* infection: the adherence of *H. ducreyi* to the epithelial surface, the rate of exotoxin production, and the resistance of the host defense mechanism. Many questions about pathogenesis still exist.[7]

CLINICAL MANIFESTATIONS

The incubation period is between 3 and 7 days, rarely more than 10 days. No prodromal symptoms are known.

The chancre begins as a soft papule surrounded by erythema. After 24 to 48 h it becomes pustular, eroded, and ulcerated. Vesicles are not seen. The edges of the ulcers are often ragged and undermined. The ulcer is usually covered by a necrotic, yellowish, gray exudate and its base is composed of granulation tissue that bleeds readily on manipulation. In contrast to syphilis, chancroid ulcers are usually tender and quite painful. Half of the males present with a single ulcer. The diameter varies from 1 mm to 2 cm. Most lesions in males are found on the external or internal surface of the prepuce, the frenulum, and the glans (Fig. 231-1). The urethal meatus, penile shaft, and anal orifice are involved less frequently. Edema of the prepuce is often seen. Rarely, if the chancre is localized in the urethra, *H. ducreyi* causes purulent urethritis.[11]

In females the lesions are mostly localized on the vulva, especially on the fourchette, the labia minora, and the vestibule. Vaginal, cervical, and perianal ulcers have also been described. Extragenital

lesions of chancroid have been reported on the breasts, fingers, thighs, and inside of the mouth. Trauma and abrasion may be important for such extragenital manifestations.

Painful inguinal adenitis (bubo) occurs in up to 50 percent of patients within a few days to 2 weeks (average 1 week) after onset of the primary lesion (Fig. 231-2). The adenitis is unilateral in most

FIGURE 231-2

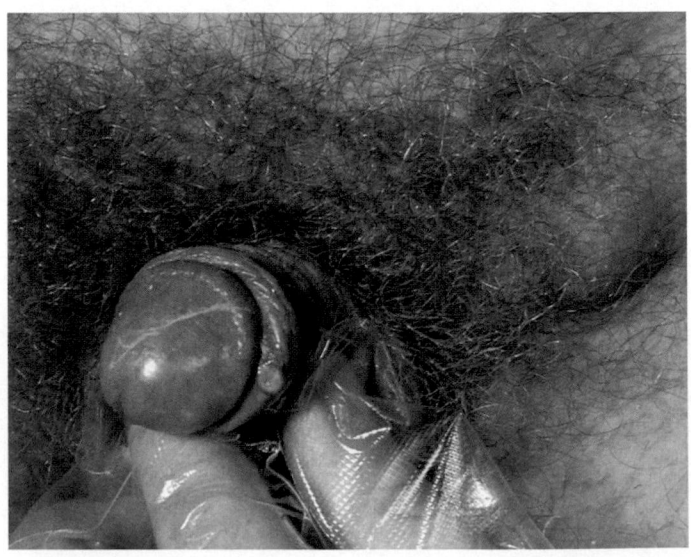

Small chancroid ulcer on the internal suface of the prepuce with inguinal adenitis.

patients and erythema of the overlying skin is typical. Buboes can become fluctuant and may rupture spontaneously. The pus of bubo is usually thick and creamy. Lymphadenitis and buboes are less common in female patients.

CLINICAL VARIANTS OF SOFT ULCER Besides the common types of chancroid described above, a number of clinical variants have been reported:

1. Giant chancroid: a single lesion extends peripherally and shows extensive ulceration.
2. Large serpiginous ulcer: a lesion that becomes confluent, spreading by extension and autoinoculation. The groin or thigh may be involved (ulcus molle serpiginosum).
3. Phagedenic chancroid: a variant caused by superinfection with fusospirochetes. Rapid and profound destruction of tissue can occur (ulcus molle gangrenosum).
4. Transient chancroid: small ulcer that resolves spontaneously in a few days. It may be followed 2 to 3 weeks later by acute regional lymphadenitis (French: chancre mou volant).
5. Follicular chancroid: multiple small ulcers in a follicular distribution.
6. Papular chancroid: a granulomatous ulcerated papule that may resemble donovanosis or condylomata lata (ulcus molle elevatum).

Mild systemic symptoms can rarely accompany chancroid, but systemic *H. ducreyi* infection has never been observed.

LABORATORY AND SPECIAL EXAMINATION

The laboratory diagnosis of chancroid depends on the isolation of *H. ducreyi* from an anogenital ulcer or the direct examination of tissue from an ulcer by Gram or Giemsa stain (Fig. 231-3).[12] The bacilli are usually found in small clusters or parallel chains of two

FIGURE 231-3

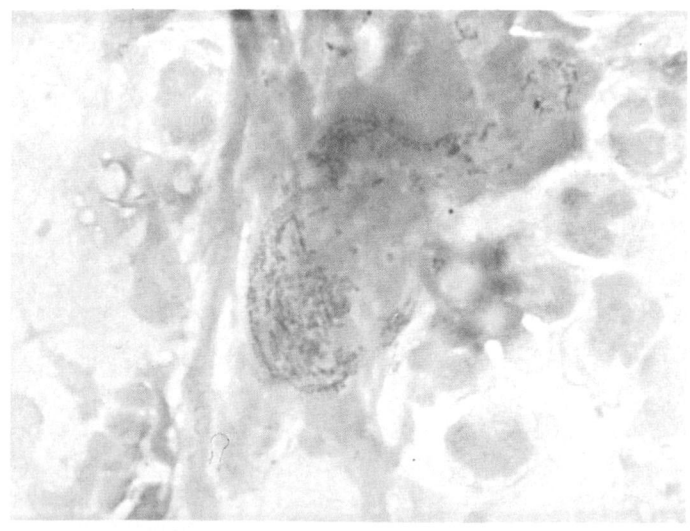

Smear from chancroid ulcer (Giemsa stain).

or three organisms streaming along strands of mucus. This pattern has been described as a "school of fish" or "railroad track" appearance. This arrangement, said to be characteristic of *H. ducreyi,* is nevertheless not pathognomonic, because most genital ulcers have a polymicrobial flora. Cotton or calcium-alginate swabs are recommended for specimen collection.

The bacillus will survive only 2 to 4 h on a swab unless refrigerated. No satisfactory transport system is available.[13]

The simultaneous use of two primary isolation media with a nutritionally rich agar base supplemented with hemoglobin and serum are recommended for high culture sensitivity[9] (see "Etiology," above). Small, nonmucoid, yellow-gray, translucent colonies appear 2 to 4 days after inoculation. Typically, these colonies remain intact when they are pushed across the agar surface. The identification of *H. ducreyi* is performed following the recommendations of Lubwama:[14] demonstration of hemin requirement, oxidase and catalase test, beta-lactamase test, hydrogen sulfide (H_2S), and indole activity. Testing of antibiotic susceptibility is recommended because clinically significant antimicrobial resistance of *H. ducreyi* has become common.

In case of bubo formation, the size of the enlarged lymph nodes can be documented by computed tomography of the groin.[15] In some cases biopsy of ulcers can be a diagnostic aid. The typical histologic findings are three vertically arranged zones: (1) a superficial necrotic zone, (2) a zone of new blood vessel formation, and (3) a deep zone consisting of dense lymphocytic and plasma cell infiltrate. *H. ducreyi* can rarely be demonstrated in tissue sections.[16]

Many attempts have been made to develop serologic tests for chancroid. No reliable test is yet available. Polymerase chain reaction procedures are used for testing and confirming suspected strains, but their usefulness for the clinical routine diagnosis of chancroid remains to be established.[17]

DIFFERENTIAL DIAGNOSIS

The three classic etiologic agents for genital ulceration are *H. ducreyi, Treponema pallidum,* and herpes simplex. The clinical appearance of the diseases caused by these three organisms can be extremely variable in both men and women. The etiology of genital ulcers also differs considerably by geographic region. In a high percentage of genital ulcers no pathogen can be isolated.

Clinical diagnosis alone is inadequate and the majority of authors consider even direct microscopic examination of smears from genital ulcers insufficient for diagnosis of chancroid.[14] Isolation of *H. ducreyi* on appropriate media and subsequent biochemical identification is necessary.

Syphilis may be eliminated by dark-field examination and repeated serologic testing for antibodies. Herpes simplex virus can be diagnosed by culture or by routine electron microscopy of smears from the ulcer base. Lymphogranuloma venereum (LGV) can be eliminated by a negative LGV complement-fixation test (titer less than 1:16) and by failure to demonstrate a significant rise in the titer on repeated testing after 3 weeks. Donovanosis and superinfected traumatic lesions must be considered in the differential diagnosis.

Mixed infections (chancroid and syphilis, chancroid and herpes simplex) are possible.

TREATMENT

The antibiotic susceptibility pattern of *H. ducreyi* has changed, making the treatments previously recommended obsolete. Plasmid-mediated resistance in *H. ducreyi* has been described for ampicillin, sulfonamides, chloramphenicol, tetracycline and kanamycin[20] (Table 231-1).

Based on in vitro susceptibility, the most active drugs against *H. ducreyi* are azithromycin, ceftriaxone, ciprofloxacin and erythromycin.

The quinolones rosoxacin—ciprofloxacin, enoxocin, norfloxacin, and fleroxacin—have all proved to be effective in chancroid.[20]

Local treatment consists of antiseptic dressings (i.e., povidone-iodine). Suppurative nodes should not be incised; if necessary, they can be punctured to prevent spontaneous rupture and sinus tract formation. A large syringe should be used and the fluctuant buboes entered laterally through normal skin. In patients with phimosis, a circumcision may be necessary when all active lesions have healed.

Even after correct treatment, relapses occur in about 5 percent of patients. Retreatment with the original regimen is recommended. If a sexual partner was not treated, reinfection is probably the cause of relapse.

PREVENTION

Patients should be advised to abstain from sexual activity until all clinical lesions have cleared. Sexual contacts of the patient should be examined and treated. Epidemiologic treatment of contacts has been recommended and many authors feel that these persons should be treated even in absence of clinical disease, since asymptomatic carriage of *H. ducreyi* is possible.[21]

TABLE 231-1

Regimens Recommended by the CDC for the Treatment of Chancroid

ANTIBIOTICS	DOSAGE
First-line	
Azithromycin	1 g PO in a single dose
Ceftriaxone	250 mg IM in a single dose
Erythromycin base	500 mg PO four times a day for 7 days
Second-line	
Amoxicillin plus clavulanic acid	Amoxicillin 500 mg plus clavulanic acid 125 mg PO three times a day for 7 days
Ciprofloxacin	500 mg PO twice a day for 3 days

SOURCE: Centers for Disease Control and Prevention.[19]

RELATION BETWEEN HIV-INFECTION AND CHANCROID

Genital ulcers increase the risk for heterosexual transmission of HIV. In many developing countries chancroid is the most common cause of genital ulcer. Therefore it is important to provide effective therapy for chancroid in order to stop the spread of HIV infection.[22] Other observations suggest that HIV-1 can be recovered readily from ulcerous genital lesions of patients infected with HIV-1.[23] Furthermore, it was shown that concomitant HIV-infection has clinically significant effects on the course of the chancroid disease and failure of single-dose[6] or short-course[23] therapy for chancroid in men is associated with HIV-1 seropositivity.[6] A wide variation in the clinical picture of chancroid has been observed in HIV-infected patients.[23]

Epidemiologic control of chancroid may be a very important strategy to interrupt the heterosexual spread of HIV in some parts of the world. Accordingly, patients with chancroid should also be tested for HIV antibodies. HIV-seropositive patients with culture proven chancroid should be treated with a multiple-day regimen.

COURSE AND PROGNOSIS

The disease is self-limited and systemic spread does not occur. Occasionally, without treatment, genital ulcer and inguinal abscess have been reported to persist for years. Local pain is the most frequent complaint. Infections do not confer immunity and reinfections are possible. To avoid reinfections, patients must be instructed to use condoms properly.

REFERENCES

1. Albritton WL: Biology of *Haemophilus ducreyi. Microbiol Rev* **53**:377, 1989
2. Piot P, Meheus A: Epidémiologie des maladies sexuellement transmissibles dans les pays en développment. *Ann Soc Belge Med Trop* **63**:87, 1983
3. Schulte JM et al: Chancroid in the United States, 1981–1990: Evidence for under-reporting of cases. *MMWR* **41**:57, 1992
4. Division of STD Prevention. *Sexually Transmitted Disease Surveillance, 1995.* Atlanta, U.S. Department of Health and Human Services, 1996
5. Ronald AR, Albritton W: Chancroid and *Haemophilus ducreyi,* in *Sexually Transmitted Diseases,* edited by KK Holmes et al. New York, McGraw-Hill, 1990
6. Jessamine PG et al: HIV, genital ulcers and the male foreskin: Synergism in HIV-1 transmission. *Scand J Infect Dis Suppl* **69**:181, 1990
7. Jonasson JA: *Haemophilus ducreyi:* Editorial review. *Int J STD AIDS* **4**:317, 1993
8. Britton WL: Biology of *Haemophilus ducreyi. Microbiol Rev* **53**:377, 1989
9. Nszane H et al: Comparison of media for the primary isolation of *H. ducreyi. Sex Transm Dis* **11**:6, 1984
10. Anderson B et al: Common B-lactamase specific plasmid in *H. ducreyi* and *N. gonorrhoeae. Antimicrob Agents Chemother* **25**:296, 1984
11. Kunimoto DY et al: Urethral infection with *H. ducreyi* in men. *Sex Transm Dis* **15**:37, 1988
12. Joseph AK: Laboratory techniques used in the diagnosis of chancroid, granuloma inguinale and LGV. *Dermatol Clin* **12**:1, 1994
13. Dangor Y et al: Transport media for *Haemophilus ducreyi. Sex Transm Dis* **20**:5, 1993

14. Lubwama SW et al: Isolation and identification of *H. ducreyi* in a clinical laboratory. *J Med Microbiol* **22**:175, 1986
15. Hartmann AA et al: Intravenous single-dose ceftriaxone treatment of chancroid. *Dermatologica* **183**:132, 1991
16. Sheldon WH, Heyman A: Studies on chancroid: Observations on the histology with an evaluation of biopsy as a diagnostic procedure. *Am J Pathol* **22**:415, 1946
17. Chui L et al: Development of polymerase chain reaction for diagnosis of chancroid. *J Clin Microbiol* **31**:659, 1993
18. Dangor Y et al: Antimicrobial susceptibilities of *H. ducreyi*. *Antimicrob Agents Chemother* **34**:1303, 1990
19. Centers for Disease Control and Prevention (CDC): Sexually transmitted disease treatment guidelines 1993: Chancroid. *MMWR* **42**:20, 1993
20. Knapp JS et al: In vitro susceptibilities of *H. ducreyi* from Thailand and U.S. to currently recommended and newer agents for treatment of chancroid. *Antimicrob Agents Chemother* **37**:1552, 1993
21. Hawkes S et al: Asymptomatic carriage of *H. ducreyi* confirmed by the polymerase chain reaction. *Genitourin Med* **71**:224, 1995
22. Wasserheit JN: Epidemiological synergy: Interrelationship between HIV infection and other STDs. *Sex Transm Dis* **19**:61, 1993
23. Abeck D, Ballard R: Chancroid, in *Sexually Transmitted Diseases. Advances in Diagnosis and Treatment,* edited by P Elsner, A Eichmann. Basel, Karger, 1996, p 94

CHAPTER 232

Richard B. Rothenberg

Lymphogranuloma Venereum

Lymphogranuloma venereum (LGV) is a sexually transmitted disease of chlamydial etiology with protean clinical manifestations involving the lymphatic system.[1] It should be considered in the differential diagnosis of benign and malignant lymphadenopathy, genital lesions, proctocolitis, and rectal stricture. LGV, along with other causes of genital ulcer disease, is increasingly important as a potential facilitator of human immunodeficiency virus (HIV) transmission.[2,3]

HISTORIC ASPECTS

The disease has a colorful nosologic history, including such designations as tropical or climatic bubo; third, fourth, fifth, or sixth venereal disease; lymphopathia venerea; and Nicolas-Favre disease. However, the current name is now universally accepted. The first major clinical description appeared in 1913, and inclusion bodies in material from lesions were demonstrated 10 years later. In 1930, the disease was produced experimentally by intracerebral inoculation of monkeys with pus from a bubo of LGV.[4] In 1940 Rake et al.[5] grew the organism, then thought to be a filterable virus, in the yolk sac of embryonated eggs. In the 1960s and 1970s the organism was successfully grown in tissue culture using cyclohexamide-treated McCoy cells,[6] and microimmunofluorescent techniques were developed for speciation and recognition of serovariants.[7] During the 1980s and 1990s, the study of chlamydial infection benefited from the considerable advances in the techniques of microbial genetics and diagnostic methods with the development of polymerase chain reaction and ligase chain reaction techniques for genus identification.[8] No commercial products are yet available for LGV identification, however.

EPIDEMIOLOGY

LGV probably occurs all over the world, with endemic foci in tropical and subtropical countries, but few, if any, systematic data describe incidence or prevalence. Most surveys are actually reports of proportional morbidity in clinic series, and the results are highly variable. The incidence ranges from zero in Paris and Kuala Lumpur[9,10] to 24 percent in Madagascar,[11] with many figures in between.[12–15] In the United States, the number of cases reported yearly declined from 2526 in 1947 to a stable level of 200 to 300 during the 1980s (Fig. 232-1). The chief foci of activity have been the District of Columbia and the southeastern United States, affecting predominantly blacks of low socioeconomic status. Age-specific attack rates are highest in the 20- to 40-year-old group. The disease is spread by direct inoculation from genital fluids, but transmission efficiency is not known. Women may be asymptomatic and culture-positive and may serve as a reservoir for infection,[16] as they do for gonorrhea and other genital chlamydial infections.

ETIOLOGY

The disease is caused by members of the genus *Chlamydia* (previously known as *Bedsonia*) whose structure, metabolism, DNA and RNA content, and method of reproduction make them similar to *Rickettsia*.[17,18] The genus consists of three species: *psittaci, pneumoniae,* and *trachomatis*. The species *Chlamydia trachomatis* has two major biologic varieties (biovars): trachoma or TRIC organisms, and LGV organisms. The latter, in turn, are characterized by three major serologic varieties (or serovars)—L1, L2, L3, and the

FIGURE 232-1

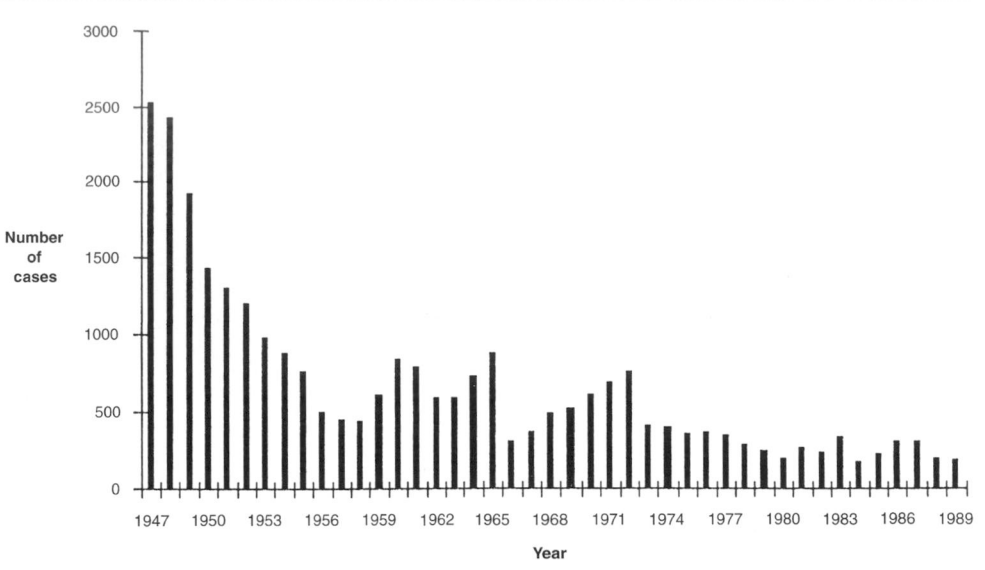

Cases of lymphogranuloma venereum, United States, 1941–1995.

more recently recognized L2'.[19] The LGV serovars are distinguished by their preferential infectivity for lymph nodes, intracerebral lethality for mice, and different behavior in cell culture.[1] Experimentally, the LGV serovars produce severe hemorrhagic proctitis in monkeys and TRIC serovars do not.[20] The two biovars, however, share a major cross-reacting antigen, which complicates serologic distinction between them.

CLINICAL MANIFESTATIONS

LGV is contracted by direct contact with infectious secretions, almost exclusively through sexual activity. The portal of entry and the initial symptoms are determined by the nature of the sex act; inoculation is usually genital, but it may be rectal or pharyngeal.[21] The incubation period varies from 3 to 30 days if primary lesions occur, but it may be longer if adenopathy is the only manifestation.[22] The period of infectiousness and transmission rates are not clearly defined.

Acute and chronic manifestations characterize both the genital (or inguinal) and rectal syndromes. The primary lesion is a 5- to 8-mm soft, erythematous, painless erosion (Fig. 232-2) that heals spontaneously in a few days. Occasionally, a button-like papule may appear, which is also transient. Such lesions are reported by one-fourth to one-third of patients. Secondary inguinal adenopathy begins 1 to 2 weeks after the primary lesion as discrete, movable, tender nodes that later coalesce to form a firm, fist-sized, elongated, immovable mass. These may occur above and below Poupart's ligament, giving rise to the "groove" sign (Fig. 232-3). Nodes are bilateral in one-third of cases.[22] Rupture of fluctuant nodes may lead to chronic sinus formation. Initially, the overlying skin is often slightly reddened and edematous, but it may later become thickened and develop a characteristic purplish hue. Generalized systemic symptoms such as fever, chills, and malaise may be prominent. Meningoencephalitis, hepatosplenomegaly, arthralgia, stiff neck, and headache may also occur.[16] Conjunctivitis with marginal corneal ulceration has been reported as well.[23] In untreated cases, the lymphadenopathy usually subsides spontaneously in 8 to 12 weeks.[22]

Late complications of the male inguinal syndrome are rare. Elephantiasis of the penis and scrotum characterized by infiltrative, ulcerative, and fistular lesions occurs in approximately 4 percent of cases.[24] Recent case reports have highlighted the need to include LGV in general clinical situations in which lymphoproliferation may occur. LGV may mimic cervical lymphoma, as reported in a homosexual male practicing fellatio[25] and a heterosexual male engaging in cunnilingus.[26] In another report, clinical presentation and computed tomography of intrapelvic nodes suggested cervical cancer in a 24-year-old woman with LGV.[27] Finally, LGV has also been shown to be associated with tonsillar infection.[28]

The acute rectal syndrome occurs more frequently in women than in men. In men, direct inoculation of the anal canal is believed to be the mode of entry, whereas the internal lymphatic drainage of

FIGURE 232-2

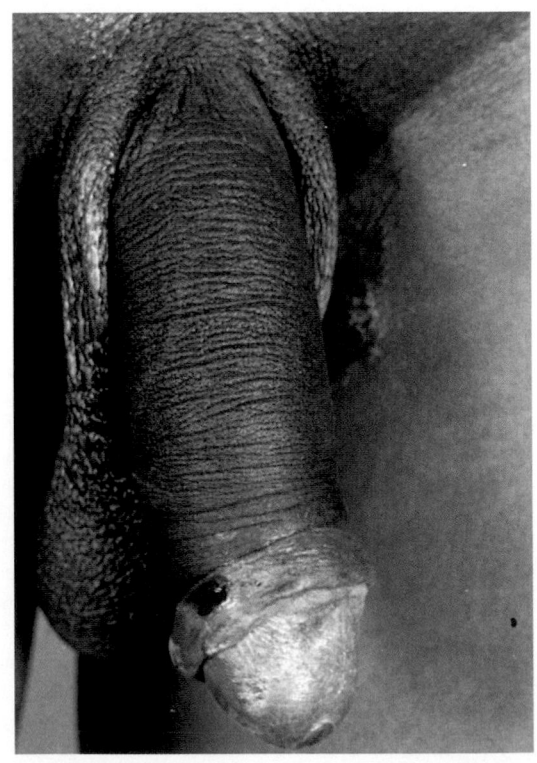

Lymphogranuloma venereum. Soft painless erosion on the prepuce.

FIGURE 232-3

CHAPTER 232
Lymphogranuloma Venereum

2593

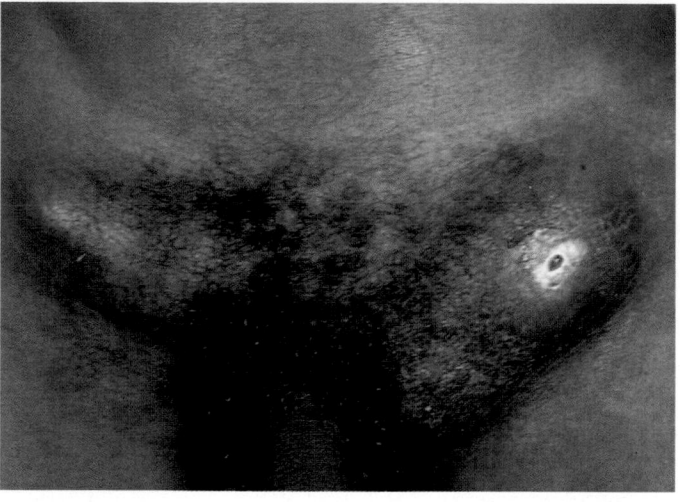

Lymphogranuloma venereum. Bilateral, firm, immovable masses above Poupart's ligament.

the proximal two-thirds of the vagina has been invoked as the source for women. In both sexes, acute manifestations include rectal pain, tenesmus, and mucosanguineous rectal discharge, with typical findings of proctocolitis on sigmoidoscopy. It is important to distinguish LGV from other forms of inflammatory bowel disease, particularly in homosexual men.[29–37] The major late manifestation is rectal stricture. In women, late scarring, fistulas, ulceration, and elephantiasis of the perineum, called *esthiomene*, may require radical surgical intervention.[38]

Various dermatologic conditions have been reported in association with acute manifestations, including erythema nodosum, erythema multiforme, scarlatiniform exanthem, and urticaria.[4] In addition, photosensitivity has been reported in as many as 35 percent of patients, occasionally associated with conjunctivitis, joint involvement, and erythema nodosum.[4] Sonck[39] observed a photosensitivity reaction in 140 of 400 LGV cases studied. This reaction was manifest 1 to 2 months after onset of bubo formation and occurred in 60 percent of the chronic and about 20 percent of subacute cases. Punctiform red papules appeared on the skin 30 min to 3 h after exposure to sunlight. Accompanying this reaction was conjunctivitis in 19 percent, joint involvement in 33 percent, and erythema nodosum in 16 percent of persons with the photosensitivity reaction. The possible allergic or autoimmune nature of these phenomena is supported by the frequent appearance of biologic false-positive tests for syphilis (estimated at 20 percent of cases), the high incidence of cryoprecipitins and rheumatoid factor, and the high serum levels of IgA and IgG in both acute and chronic syndromes.[40]

As noted, as a cause of genital ulceration, LGV may play a role in facilitating transmission of HIV. Because of its lymphatic manifestations and potential effects on the immune system, it may play a role in the differential diagnosis of acquired immunodeficiency syndrome (AIDS) as well. In one reported case, for example, disseminated Kaposi's sarcoma mimicked LGV in its initial presentation.[41] The syndrome of angioimmunoblastic lymphadenopathy has been reported in association with LGV[42] and may, as occurred in one case, lead to progressive immunologic deterioration and rapidly fatal immunoblastic lymphoma.

PATHOLOGY

In general, histopathologic changes of LGV are nonspecific. Primary ulcers are characterized by an exudate of fibrin, polymorphonuclear leukocytes, and cellular debris.[43] Skin test sites or rectal lesions may contain epithelioid nodules, plasma cells, and occasional giant cells, but these changes are not diagnostic. Stellate triangular abscesses may be observed in biopsy specimens of lymph nodes and are characteristic but not pathognomonic of LGV.[44] The pathology of LGV-induced proctocolitis is characterized by crypt distortion, submucosal fibrosis, neuromatous hypertrophy, follicular inflammation, and occasional granuloma formation. It may be difficult to distinguish these changes from those associated with Crohn's disease, although localization of lesions is of considerable help (proximal in Crohn's disease, distal in LGV).[45] It is likely that LGV is not etiologically associated with Crohn's disease.[1]

DIAGNOSIS

One of the earliest diagnostic techniques, the Frei test, used an intradermal inoculation of killed LGV organisms and was important to diagnosis for many years. Its sensitivity and specificity are in serious doubt, however,[46] and the test is now of historic interest only, since the antigen is no longer commercially available. The diagnostic accuracy of the clinical diagnosis is variable. In one study from South Africa, diagnostic accuracy (defined as true positive divided by true positive plus false positive plus false negatives) was found to be 66 percent in men and 40 percent in women, but these figures are based on a small number of cases.[11] In another attempt from South Africa, the diagnostic accuracy was 20 percent overall.[47] Though algorithmic approaches to genital ulcer disease are important in many clinical settings, clinical diagnosis alone may not be dependable.

Clinical diagnosis of LGV is greatly enhanced by laboratory confirmation. Definitive diagnosis is possible through isolation of the organism from tissue or body fluids,[6] and distinction among the four serovars can be made using microimmunofluorescence techniques.[1] Since tissue culture may not be readily available, the clinician must often rely on serologic methods. First developed in the 1930s, the complement fixation test has long been the mainstay of diagnosis of LGV. It suffers from lack of specificity: virtually all members of the genus *Chlamydia* share the target antigen.[48] Although less than 3 percent of the general population has a titer as high as 1:16,[46] 40 to 50 percent of women with uncomplicated TRIC-agent cervical infection had titers of 1:16 to 1:32; similar titers occurred in 15 to 20 percent of men with TRIC-associated urethritis.[3] A titer of 1:64 or greater is, however, highly suggestive of LGV. Coupled with a fourfold change in titer (which is not uniformly detected), a high titer greatly increases diagnostic assurance. The microimmunofluorescence test, originally developed as a guide to identification of organisms, has been successfully adapted as a serologic test. It responds, like the complement fixation test, to the broadly reactive range of antibodies produced by patients with LGV. Again, very high titers of IgG antibody are usual in patients with acute infection. Other tests, including enzyme-linked immunosorbent assay (ELISA) and radioimmunoassay methods, are also available but appear to offer little advantage.[49]

DIFFERENTIAL DIAGNOSIS

In view of the nonspecific nature of signs and symptoms, acute LGV should be considered in the differential diagnosis of syphilis, herpes progenitalis, granuloma inguinale, and chancroid as well as bacterial, fungal, and tuberculous skin infection. Adenopathy may require consideration of benign and malignant lymphoproliferative disorders (e.g., infectious mononucleosis, Hodgkin's disease), particularly in the presence of oral and cervical infection. Late manifestations must be distinguished from neoplastic skin disease, filariasis, rectal cancer, inflammatory bowel disease, and hidradenitis suppurativa.

TREATMENT

Antibiotics are effective in the acute illness but may have little or no effect on late lymphatic pathology. Standard regimens include sulfisoxazole 1 g four times a day for 3 weeks or tetracycline 500 mg four times a day for at least 2 weeks.[50] Other tetracycline derivatives such as minocycline have also been demonstrated to be effective. Fluctuant nodes (buboes) should be aspirated, rather than incised and drained, to avoid formation of fistulous tracts. With treatment, prognosis for avoidance of late complications is excellent.

REFERENCES

1. Schachter J, Osoba AO: Lymphogranuloma venereum. Br Med Bull 39:151, 1983
2. Piot P et al: Retrospective seroepidemiology of AIDS virus infection in Nairobi populations. J Infect Dis 155:1108, 1987
3. Cameron DW et al: Female to male heterosexual transmission of HIV infection, Nairobi. Proceedings of the Third International Conference on AIDS, Washington, DC, June 1–5, 1987
4. Koteen H: Lymphogranuloma venereum. Medicine 24:2, 1945
5. Rake G: Agent of lymphogranuloma venereum in the yolk sac of the developing chick embryo. Proc Soc Biol Med 43:332, 1940
6. Evans RT, Woodland RM: Detection of chlamydiae by isolation and direct examination. Br Med Bull 39:181, 1983
7. Wang SP: Microimmunofluorescence method: Study of antibody response to TRIC organisms, in Trachoma and Related Disorders Caused by Chlamydia Agents, edited by RL Nichols. Amsterdam, Excerpta Medica, 1971, p 273
8. Blanchard TJ, Mabey DC: Chlamydial infections. Br J Clin Pract 94:201, 1994
9. Casin I et al: Microbiological study of male genital ulcers: Apropos of 75 cases. [French]. Pathol Biol (Paris) 90:710–715, 1990
10. Zainah S et al: A microbiological study of genital ulcers in Kuala Lumpur. Med J Malaysia 91:274, 1991
11. Harms G et al: Pattern of sexually transmitted diseases in a Malagasy population. Sex Transm Dis 94:315, 1994
12. Chua SH, Cheong WK: Genital ulcer disease in patients attending a public sexually transmitted disease clinic in Singapore: An epidemiologic study. Ann Acad Med Singapore 95:510, 1995
13. Mulhall BP, Harcourt C: Sexually transmitted diseases in Australia: A decade of change. Epidemiology and surveillance. Ann Acad Med Singapore 95:569, 1995
14. O'Farrell N et al: Genital ulcer disease in men in Durban, South Africa. Genitourin Med 91:327, 1991
15. Bogaerts J et al: The etiology of genital ulceration in Rwanda. Sex Transm Dis 89:123, 1989
16. Becker LE: Lymphogranuloma venereum. Int J Dermatol 15:26, 1976
17. Schachter J: Chlamydial infection. N Engl J Med 298:428, 490, 540, 1978
18. Moulder JW: The relationship of the psittacosis group (Chlamydia) to bacteria and viruses. Annu Rev Microbiol 20:107, 1966
19. Wang SP et al: Immunotyping of Chlamydia trachomatis with monoclonal antibodies. J Infect Dis 152:791, 1985
20. Quinn TC et al: Experimental proctitis due to rectal infection with Chlamydia trachomatis in nonhuman primates. J Infect Dis 86:833, 1986
21. Terho P: Chlamydia trachomatis and clinical genital infections: A general review. Infection 10 (suppl 1):S5, 1982
22. Conizares O: Modern Diagnosis and Treatment of the Minor Venereal Diseases. Springfield, IL, Charles C Thomas 1954
23. Buus DR et al: Lymphogranuloma venereum conjunctivitis with a marginal corneal perforation. Ophthalmology 88:799, 1988
24. Hopsu-Havu VK, Sonck CE: Infiltrative, ulcerative, and fistular lesions of the penis due to lymphogranuloma venereum. Br J Vener Dis 49:193, 1973
25. Thorsteinsson SB: Lymphogranuloma venereum: A cause of cervical lymphadenopathy. JAMA 235:1882, 1976
26. Andrada MT: Oral lymphogranuloma venereum: A cause of cervical lymphadenopathy. Case report. Mil Med 139:99, 1974
27. Zweizig S: Computed tomography of lymphogranuloma venereum mimicking cervical cancer. Comput Med Imaging Graph 91:97, 1991
28. Watson DJ et al: Lymphogranuloma venereum of the tonsil. J Laryngol Otol 90:331, 1990
29. Geller SA: Rectal biopsy in early lymphogranuloma venereum proctitis. Am J Gastroenterol 74:433, 1980
30. Klotz SA et al: Hemorrhagic proctitis due to lymphogranuloma venereum serogroup L2: Diagnosis by fluorescent monoclonal antibody. N Engl J Med 308:1563, 1983
31. Ghinsberg RC et al: Rectal lymphogranuloma venereum in a bisexual patient. Microbiologica 91:161, 1991
32. Quinn TC et al: Chlamydia trachomatis proctitis. N Engl J Med 305:195, 1981
33. Bolan RK et al: Lymphogranuloma venereum and acute ulcerative proctitis. Am J Med 72:703, 1982
34. Quinn TC et al: The etiology of anorectal infections in homosexual men. Am J Med 71:395, 1981
35. Levine JS et al: Chronic proctitis in male homosexuals due to lymphogranuloma venereum. Gastroenterology 79:563, 1980
36. Mindel A: Lymphogranuloma venereum of the rectum in a homosexual man: Case report. Br J Vener Dis 59:196, 1983
37. Bauwens JE et al: Infection with Chlamydia trachomatis lymphogranuloma venereum serovar L1 in homosexual men with proctitis: Molecular analysis of an unusual case cluster. Clin Infect Dis 95:576, 1995
38. Hirschberg SM, Horton CE: Radical perineal resection for far-advanced lymphogranuloma venereum. Plast Reconstr Surg 51:217, 1973
39. Sonck CE: On the occurrence of solar dermatitis in lymphogranuloma inguinale. Acta Derm Venereol (Stockh) 20:529, 1939
40. Sonck CE: Autoimmune serum factors in active and inactive lymphogranuloma venereum. Br J Vener Dis 49:67, 1973
41. Aghadiuno PU et al: Kaposi sarcoma in the acquired immune deficiency syndrome (AIDS), presenting as lymphogranuloma venereum (LGV) in a promiscuous Trinidadian male. Trop Geogr Med 87:88, 1987
42. Senitzer D et al: Infectious antecedent of immunoblastic lymphoma: Progressive immunosuppression in a patient with lymphogranuloma venereum. Am J Med 8:163, 1985
43. Smith EB, Custer RP: The histopathology of lymphogranuloma venereum. J Urol 63:546, 1950
44. Robbins SL, editor: Pathology. Philadelphia, Saunders, 1967, p 366
45. de la Monte SM, Hutchins GM: Follicular proctocolitis and neuromatous hyperplasia with lymphogranuloma venereum. Hum Pathol 16:1025, 1985
46. Schachter J: Lymphogranuloma venereum: I. Comparison of the Frei test, complement-fixation test and isolation of the agent. J Infect Dis 120:372, 1969
47. Dangor Y et al: Accuracy of clinical diagnosis of genital ulcer disease. Sex Transm Dis 90:184, 1990
48. Treharne JD et al: Chlamydial serology. Br Med Bull 39:194, 1983
49. Darougar S: The humoral immune response to chlamydial infection in humans. Rev Infect Dis 7:726, 1985
50. Centers for Disease Control and Prevention: 1998 Sexually transmitted diseases treatment guidelines. MMWR 47(RR-1):27, 1998

Granuloma Inguinale

Granuloma inguinale is an indolent, progressive, ulcerative, granulomatous skin disease caused by *Calymmatobacterium granulomatis*. It is probably spread by both homosexual and heterosexual venereal contact and by nonvenereal means as well.[1] Untreated, it exhibits no tendency to go into spontaneous remission and in later stages may be severely debilitating.

HISTORIC ASPECTS

The first description is credited to McLeod in 1882, who termed the illness *serpiginous ulcer*.[2] Many other names have been suggested, but aside from granuloma inguinale, only the term *donovanosis* persists. Donovan, in 1905, first described the bipolar-staining, intracellular inclusions in macrophages from lesion exudate (termed *Donovan bodies*). These organisms were grown in embryonated eggs in 1943[3]; requirements for growth on artificial media were established in 1959.[4]

EPIDEMIOLOGY

Sporadic cases of granuloma inguinale occur worldwide with recent reports from developed countries such as Canada,[5] Sweden,[6] Italy,[7] France,[8] and Japan.[9] Endemic foci are usually seen only in tropical and subtropical environments, such as New Guinea, Brazil, central Australia, the Caribbean, and parts of India.[10,11] Recently, a focus was recognized in South Africa, after an apparent eclipse of 50 years.[12] Investigators in Durban, S.A., noted a peak in case reports in the late 1980s[13] and recognized that, by 1995, granuloma inguinale accounted for almost 10 percent of cases of genital ulcer disease seen at one clinic in that city.[14] Several large case series[15–17] confirmed a strong association with syphilis and HIV infection, though no change in clinical course or response to drug therapy was noted in those with dual infection.[17]

Since 1970, fewer than 100 cases per year have been reported in the United States; in 1989, there were only 7, and in 1995, no cases were reported.[18] Certain marked racial and ethnic predispositions have been noted—higher incidence in blacks than in whites in the United States; in natives than in Europeans in Papua, New Guinea; in Hindus than in Moslems in India—but there is no evidence for specific racial susceptibility. Rather, socioeconomic status and living conditions may be major risk factors.

The venereal nature of transmission has been debated for many years and is supported by the genital site of early lesions, the prominence of perirectal disease in male homosexuals, and the predominant occurrence of infection in the sexually active group.[19,20] The possibility of nonvenereal transmission is suggested by the occurrence of disease in sexually inactive children, the infrequency of infection in partners repeatedly exposed to open lesions, and the infrequency of infection in sexually active people (e.g., prostitutes) in some endemic areas.[1,20] It seems clear, however, that granuloma inguinale is one of a class of diseases causing genital ulceration that may predispose persons to the transmission of HIV.[21] One investigator has suggested that a global program to eradicate granuloma inguinale could retard the spread of HIV.[22]

ETIOLOGY AND PATHOGENESIS

The causative agent (formerly termed *Donovania granulomatis*) is a gram-negative rod with some antigenic properties in common with the *Klebsiella* group. It has been demonstrated in fecal flora,[23] and there is evidence by electron microscopy that it may share bacteriophage with Enterobacteriaceae.[11,24] Studies by light microscopy of plastic-embedded material with polychromatic staining demonstrate bacteria within vacuoles of cells and thereby fail to corroborate the presence of bacteriophage-like entities.[25] These data support the hypothesis that disease transmission may occur through fecal contamination in environments with lower levels of hygiene and may also explain the occurrence of disease in males practicing rectal intercourse.

Antibody against the organism may be detected by the complement-fixation test, though the test has little diagnostic value. Circulating antibody, which does not affect the relentless course of untreated disease, has raised the possibility that a defect in cell-mediated immunity may predispose the patient to clinical illness, as is the case in the other diseases caused by intracellular organisms (e.g., leprosy and tuberculosis).[26]

CLINICAL MANIFESTATIONS

The primary lesion may be a button-like papule, a subcutaneous nodule, or an ulcer. The incubation period is poorly defined and may range from 2 weeks to 3 months. Experimental human inoculation has produced lesions after latency of 21 days.[19] Papules or nodules are quickly denuded and ulcerate within several days. The subcutaneous nodule, if large enough, may be mistaken for a lymph node, giving rise to the term *pseudobubo*. True adenopathy is rare. In men, the penis, scrotum, and glans are the most common sites of primary lesions; in females, they are the labia minora, mons veneris, and fourchette. Lesions of the cervix may occur in as many as 10 percent of infected women, and the disease may involve the uterus and adnexa as well.[27] Typically, the disease spreads, either by direct extension or autoinoculation, to the inguinal and perineal skin.

Four major clinical varieties are described[28]: the *nodular* variety is characterized by soft red nodules that eventually ulcerate and present a bright-red granulating surface (Fig. 233-1); the *ulcerovegetative* variety (most common) (Fig. 233-2) develops from the nodular type and consists of large, spreading, exuberant ulcers; the *hypertropic* form (relatively rare) exhibits a proliferative reaction and formation of large vegetating masses; and the *cicatricial* type produces spreading scar tissue formation that is a direct consequence of disease spread per se rather than of healing. Superinfection with fusospirochetal organisms may give rise to necrotic lesions with massive tissue destruction, similar to the situation in so-called phagedenic chancroid. The disease may rarely progress to destroy genital and inguinal tissue.[29] Elephantiasis of the penis, scrotum, or vulva may follow involvement with granuloma inguinale.

Extragenital lesions are reported in 6 percent of cases, with occasional systemic involvement, notably in the gastrointestinal tract and bone,[30] including the bony orbit and orbital skin.[31] Chronic ulcerating lesions of the oral mucosa may occur with or without associated genital lesions[32,33] and may resemble actinomycosis.[34] Rarely, granuloma inguinale may affect cervical lymph nodes and resemble tuberculous lymphadenitis.[35] A single case report documented a primary extragenital occurrence of granuloma inguinale in the axilla.[36] The disease shows no tendency toward spontaneous healing, though lesions may be stable for long periods of time. There is believed to be an increased incidence of squamous cell carcinoma of the genital skin in granuloma inguinale.[37]

FIGURE 233-1

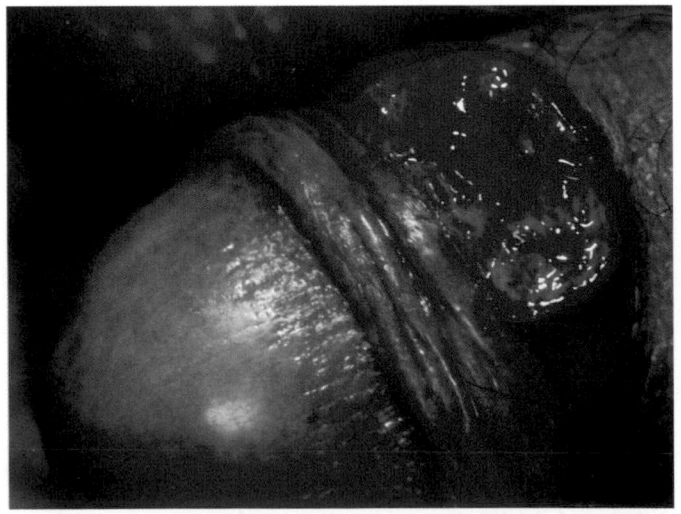

Granuloma inguinale: nodular variety evolving into large, exuberant ulcer. (*Courtesy of A. Eichmann, MD.*)

FIGURE 233-2

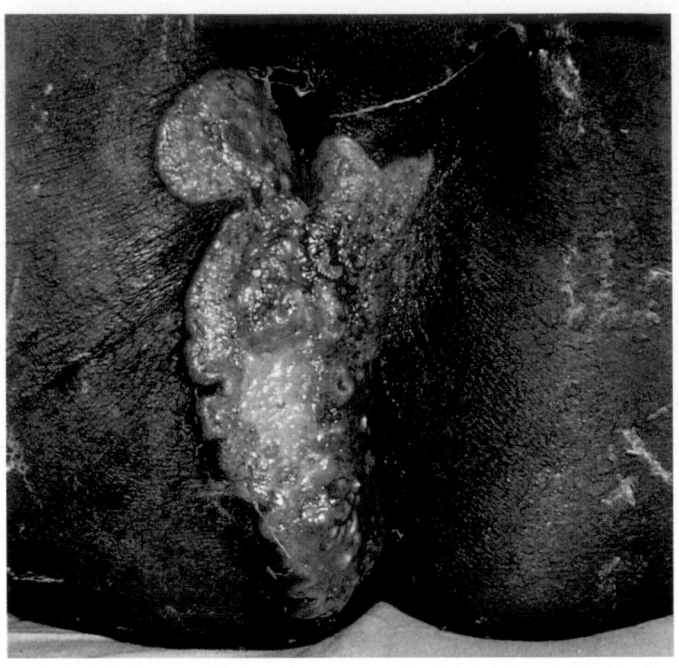

Granuloma inguinale: large ulcerovegetative type.

PATHOLOGY

Histologically, the skin exhibits a massive cellular reaction, predominantly polymorphonuclear, with occasional plasma cells and, rarely, lymphocytes.[10] The marginal epithelium demonstrates acanthosis, elongation of rete pegs, and pseudoepitheliomatous hyperplasia.[25] These latter changes are highly suggestive of early malignancy and squamous cell carcinoma. Hypertropic and cicatricial forms demonstrate the appropriate increase in fibrous tissue. Typically, large mononuclear cells containing numerous cytoplasmic inclusions (the Donovan bodies) are scattered throughout the lesions. These are considered to be diagnostic of granuloma inguinale and are often best demonstrated with special stains, such as Giemsa stain, Delafield hematoxylin, Dieterle silver stain, and the Warthin-Starry stain.[10]

DIAGNOSIS

The clinical diagnosis of granuloma inguinale, based on history and appearance, may be fairly accurate in endemic areas. In one study from South Africa, the diagnostic accuracy was 63 percent and the positive predictive value between 71 and 83 percent.[38] The organism has not been grown in culture media, and laboratory diagnosis requires a crush or touch preparation stained with Wright or Giemsa stain from a punch biopsy specimen.[39] Superficial curettings may be inadequate because of bacterial contamination. The diagnostic Donovan bodies are seen as deeply staining, bipolar, safety pin–shaped rods in the cytoplasm of macrophages (Fig. 233-3). Diagnosis may require multiple specimens, since clinical varieties differ in the quantity of organisms present. Rapid staining techniques [such as the RapiDiff stain (Clinical Science Diagnostics Ltd.)] are now readily available and suitable for use under a variety of field conditions.[40] The use of Warthin-Starry silver impregnation stain is thought to be diagnostic.[39] Serologic tests, such as the use of complement fixation, have evoked some research interest but have little practical application.

In its typical form, granuloma inguinale is easily differentiated from other ulcerative and granulomatous skin diseases, but atypical forms may be difficult to distinguish from syphilis, chancroid, lymphogranuloma venereum, tuberculosis of skin, cutaneous amebiasis, and filariasis. Squamous cell carcinoma with metastases may be closely mimicked by granuloma inguinale and its associated osteolytic bone lesions.

TREATMENT

Numerous drugs have been found useful in treating granuloma inguinale, including streptomycin, chloramphenicol, tetracycline, ampicillin, and gentamicin. Case series, usually assembled over a decade or more, offer a variety of regimens[41–43]; controlled trials are not available. Tetracycline, 500 mg four times a day for 3 to 4 weeks, was a good initial choice, but resistance to this therapy, alone or in combination with sulfisoxazole, was observed in U.S. military personnel in Vietnam. Ampicillin was successful in all but 2 of 31 cases of granuloma inguinale acquired in Vietnam, with complete healing of local lesions occurring primarily on the penis or in the groin. In the same series, lincomycin was successfully used in penicillin-allergic individuals.[44] A preliminary report suggests that the 4-fluoroquinolone antibiotics (norfloxacin) may be effective.[45] Small case series have suggested that azithromycin,[46] ciprofloxacin,[47] and ceftriaxone[48] are effective, although one failure has also been reported on the latter drug.[49] Response may be monitored by clinical appearance and serial biopsy specimens examined for persistent presence of Donovan bodies. In early cases, prognosis for complete healing is good. In late cases, irreparable tissue destruction may have supervened and radical surgery may be required.

REFERENCES

1. Goldberg J: Studies on granuloma inguinale: VII. Some considerations of the disease. *Br J Vener Dis* **40**:140, 1964
2. McLeod K: Precis of operations performed in the wards of the first surgeon, Medical College Hospital, during the year 1881. *Indian Med Gazette* **11**:113, 1882
3. Anderson K et al: An etiologic consideration of *Donovania granulomatis* cultivated from granuloma inguinale (three cases) in embryonic yolk. *J Exp Med* **81**:25, 1943
4. Goldberg J: Studies on granuloma inguinale: IV. Growth requirements of *Donovania granulomatis* and its relationship to the natural habitat of the organism. *Br J Vener Dis* **35**:266, 1959
5. Hacker P et al: Granuloma inguinale: Three cases diagnosed in Toronto, Canada. *Int J Dermatol* **92**:696, 1992
6. Bondeson J et al: Perianal abscess and sinuses caused by granuloma inguinale: Case report. *Acta Chir Scand* **155**:607, 1989
7. Ena P et al: Donovanosis: Presentation of a case. *G Ital Dermatol Venereol* **123**:167, 1988
8. Marchand C et al: Donovanosis, a propos of a new case of granuloma inguinale in France. *Ann Med Interne (Paris)* **137**:656, 1986
9. Fujiwara S et al: A case of donovanosis in Japan. *J Dermatol (Tokyo)* **14**:375, 1987
10. Sehgal VN, Shyam Prasad AL: Donovanosis: Current concepts. *Int J Dermatol* **25**:8, 1986
11. Davis CM: Granuloma inguinale: A clinical, histological, and ultrastructural study. *JAMA* **211**:632, 1970
12. Freinkel AL: The enigma of granuloma inguinale in South Africa. *S Afr Med J* **77**:301, 1990

FIGURE 233-3

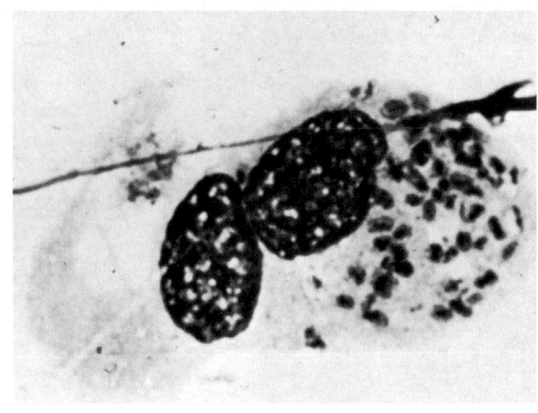

Granuloma inguinale: tissue smear showing Donovan bodies, which are gram-negative and readily stained with Giemsa stain.

13. O'Farrell N: Trends in reported cases of donovanosis in Durban, South Africa. *Genitourin Med* **92**:366, 1992
14. Pham-Kanter GB et al: Sexually transmitted diseases in South Africa. [review]. *Genitourin Med* **96**:160, 1996
15. O'Farrell N: Clinico-epidemiological study of donovanosis in Durban, South Africa. *Genitourin Med* **93**:108, 1993
16. Bassa AG et al: Granuloma inguinale (donovanosis) in women: An analysis of 61 cases from Durban, South Africa. *Sex Transm Dis* **93**:164, 1993
17. Hoosen AA et al: Granuloma inguinale in association with pregnancy and HIV infection. *Int J Gynaecol Obstet* **96**:133, 1996
18. U.S. Department of Health and Human Services. Public Health Service, Centers for Disease Control and Prevention: *Sexually Transmitted Disease Surveillance, 1995*. Atlanta, 1996
19. Rajam RV, Rangiah PN: Donovanosis (*granuloma inguinale, granuloma venereum*). *WHO Monogr Ser* **24**, 1954
20. Kuberski T: Granuloma inguinale (donovanosis). *Sex Transm Dis* **7**:29, 1980
21. Piot P, Laga M: Genital ulcers, other sexually transmitted diseases, and the sexual transmission of HIV. *Br Med J* **298**:623, 1989
22. O'Farrell N: Global eradication of donovanosis: An opportunity for limiting the spread of HIV-1 infection. *Genitourin Med* **95**:27, 1995
23. Goldberg J: Studies on granuloma inguinale: V. Isolation of bacterium resembling *Donovania granulomatis* from the faeces of a patient with granuloma inguinale. *Br J Vener Dis* **38**:99, 1959
24. Kuberski T: Ultrastructure of *Calymmatobacterium granulomatis* in lesions of granuloma inguinale. *J Infect Dis* **142**:744, 1980
25. Dodson RF: Donovanosis: A morphologic study. *J Invest Dermatol* **62**:611, 1974
26. Maddock I et al: Donovanosis in Papua New Guinea. *Br J Vener Dis* **52**:190, 1976
27. Sengupta SK, Das N: Donovanosis affecting cervix, uterus and adnexae. *Am J Trop Med Hyg* **33**:632, 1984
28. D'Aunoy R, Von Haam E: Granuloma inguinale. *Am J Trop Med Hyg* **17**:747, 1967
29. Fritz GS: Mutilating granuloma inguinale. *Arch Dermatol* **111**:1464, 1975
30. Kirkpatrick DJ: Donovanosis (granuloma inguinale): A rare cause of osteolytic bone lesions. *Clin Radiol* **21**:101, 1970
31. Endicott JN: Granuloma inguinale of the orbit with bony involvement. *Arch Otolaryngol* **96**:457, 1972
32. Rao M: Oral lesions of granuloma inguinale. *J Oral Surg* **34**:1112, 1976
33. Garg BR: Donovanosis (granuloma inguinale) of the oral cavity. *Br J Vener Dis* **51**:136, 1975
34. Coovadia YM et al: Granuloma inguinale (donovanosis) of the oral cavity: A case report. *S Afr Med J* **68**:815, 1985

35. Freinkel AL: Granuloma inguinale of cervical lymph nodes simulating tuberculous lymphadenitis: Two case reports and review of published reports. *Genitourin Med* **64**:339, 1988

36. Spagnolo DV et al: Extragenital granuloma inguinale (donovanosis) diagnosed in the United Kingdom: A clinical, histological, and electron microscopical study. *J Clin Pathol* **37**:945, 1984

37. Stewart DB: Ulcerative and hypertrophic lesions of the vulva. *Proc R Soc Med* **61**:363, 1968

38. O'Farrell N et al: Genital ulcer disease: Accuracy of clinical diagnosis and strategies to improve control in Durban, South Africa. *Genitourin Med* **94**:7, 1994

39. Van Dyck E, Piot P: Laboratory techniques in the investigation of chancroid, lymphogranuloma venereum and donovanosis [review]. *Genitourin Med* **92**:130, 1992

40. O'Farrell N et al: A rapid stain for the diagnosis of granuloma inguinale. *Genitourin Med* **66**:200, 1990

41. Rosen T et al: Granuloma inguinale. *J Am Acad Dermatol* **11**:433, 1984

42. Wysoki RS et al: Granuloma inguinale (donovanosis) in women. *J Reprod Med* **33**:709, 1988

43. Latif AS et al: The treatment of donovanosis (granuloma inguinale). *Sex Transm Dis* **15**:27, 1988

44. Breschi LC: Granuloma inguinale in Vietnam: Successful therapy with ampicillin and lincomycin. *J Am Vener Dis Assoc* **11**:118, 1975

45. Ramanan C et al: Treatment of donovanosis with norfloxacin. *Int J Dermatol* **29**:298, 1990

46. Bowden FJ et al: Pilot study of azithromycin in the treatment of genital donovanosis. *Genitourin Med* **96**:17, 1996

47. Ahmed BA, Tang A: Successful treatment of donovanosis with ciprofloxacin [letter]. *Genitourin Med* **96**:73, 1996

48. Merianos A et al: Ceftriaxone in the treatment of chronic donovanosis in central Australia. *Genitourin Med* **94**:84, 1994

49. Evans DT: Failure of single dose ceftriaxone in donovanosis (granuloma inguinale). *Genitourin Med* **92**:146, 1992

CHAPTER 234

David S. Feingold
Monica Peacocke

Gonorrhea

Gonorrhea is a bacterial infection caused by *Neisseria gonorrhoeae*, a gram-negative diplococcus whose only natural reservoir is humans. The infection is almost always contracted during sexual activity.

The usual presentation in males is acute urethritis and, in females, cervicitis, which may be asymptomatic. Other parts of the genitourinary apparatus as well as the rectum, pharynx, and eye may be infected. Occasionally bacteremia occurs, which is regularly associated with arthralgia and skin lesions; metastatic infection in joints or other foci may ensue. Although good treatment is available, the disease remains an important public health problem, causing a large percentage of female sterility and considerable morbidity in both sexes.

Early confusion among the venereal diseases was augmented by the unfortunate experiment of John Hunter in 1767. He inoculated himself with a presumed gonococcal urethral exudate, only to develop syphilis. With isolation of the causative organism of gonorrhea by Neisser in 1879, positive identification of the disease became possible.

Treatment for gonorrhea has progressed from sandalwood oil to urethral irrigations with potassium permanganate to sulfonamides in the 1930s. Resistance to sulfonamides developed rapidly, but, fortunately, in the 1940s the exquisite sensitivity of gonococcal strains to penicillin was discovered. The emerging problem of the organism's resistance to penicillin and other antibiotics is discussed below.

HISTORIC ASPECTS

The name *gonorrhea* is attributed to Galen, who thought the urethritis represented abnormal flow of semen, hence the combination of *gonos*, "seed" and *rhoea*, "flow." The slang name for gonorrhea, *clap*, likely derives from a French word for brothel, *clapoir*.

EPIDEMIOLOGY

The incidence of gonorrhea in the United States increased dramatically in the 1960s and early 1970s to over 1 million reported cases annually. It is estimated that less than one-third of the new cases are reported. In the 1980s there was a slow decline in reported cases to about 700,000 per year. This gradual decline continued into the 1990s, with fewer than 400,000 cases of gonorrhea reported in 1995.[1] Why has this two-phase trend occurred?[2] The epidemic was intensified, first, by behavioral factors, including increased sexual activity, changes in birth control methods, high population mobility, and an increase in repeated infections, and, second, by increased reporting when the federal gonorrhea screening effort was introduced in 1972. The subsequent decrease in incidence in the United States resulted from the herculean efforts of the U.S. Public Health Service through the national control program to detect and treat asymptomatic gonococcal infections. The practice of safer sex in the era of acquired immunodeficiency syndrome (AIDS) had additional impact on decreasing the incidence of all sexually transmitted diseases.

The disease is spread almost exclusively by sexual activity, although newborns may be infected by exposure during parturition. While all age groups are susceptible, infection is more prevalent in the 15- to 35-year-old age group. The disease is concentrated in high-density population centers, with a core group of active transmitters.[3] However, the mobility of individuals results in the occurrence of gonorrhea everywhere.

A signal event that has affected the epidemiology of gonorrhea is the dramatic increase in resistance of N. gonorrhoeae to antibiotics. Since the availability of sulfonamides and penicillin in the 1940s, antimicrobial resistance in N. gonorrhoeae has been evolving. The appearance of penicillinase-producing strains of N. gonorrhoeae in the United States in 1975 accelerated the trend toward greater antibiotic resistance. Penicillinase (beta-lactamase) synthesis in these organisms depends on the presence of plasmids—extrachromosomal packets of DNA—which can be transferred among organisms. At least five beta-lactamase plasmids of N. gonorrhoeae have been reported. Chromosomal resistance to penicillin and tetracycline is also occasionally at levels sufficient to result in treatment failure.[4] The explosive epidemic of antibiotic-resistant cases of gonorrhea in the late 1980s is graphically shown in Fig. 234-1. For all practical purposes, in most areas penicillin is no longer the treatment of choice for gonorrhea.

FIGURE 234-1

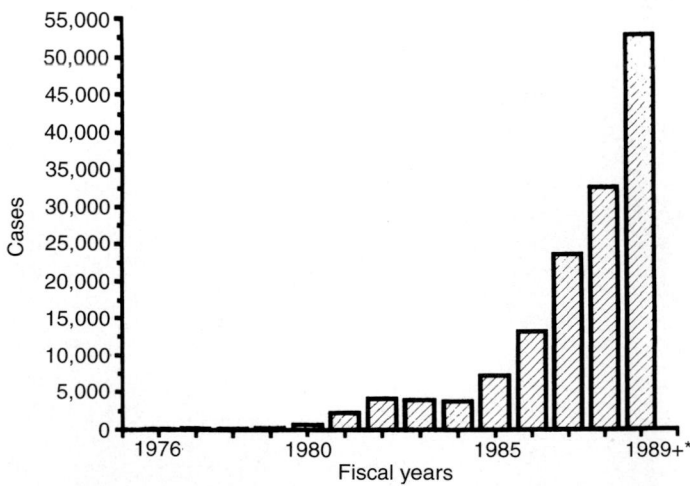

Reported antibiotic-resistant cases of gonorrhea in the United States, fiscal years 1976–1989. *, 95 percent has PPNG strains; +*, estimated. (*From Toomey KE: Sex Transm Dis 17:218, 1990, with permission.*)

In 1996 the Gonococcal Isolate Surveillance Project (GISP) was established by the Centers for Disease Control to monitor, periodically, national trends in N. gonorrhoeae antibiotic resistance.[5] Data analyzed through 1994 confirm penicillin or tetracycline resistance in 31 percent of the isolates. Fluoroquinolone resistance was increasing; most isolates remained highly susceptible to broad-spectrum cephalosporins.[5]

ETIOLOGIC AGENT AND PATHOGENESIS

N. gonorrhoeae is a gram-negative diplococcus with distinctive morphology; the cocci are flattened and the long axes of the bean-shaped organisms are parallel. Gonococci tolerate oxygen but usually require 2 to 10 percent of CO_2 in the growth atmosphere. The organisms have narrow temperature [35° to 37°C (95° to 98.6°F)] and pH (7.2 to 7.6) optima for growth. Although fragile, they have relatively simple growth requirements. Defined media are now available on which the organisms will grow readily. Different strains have somewhat different growth requirements. Careful study of these requirements has led to a system of typing gonococcal isolates called *auxotyping*.[6] Auxotyping was an important advance, since the ability to tell one N. gonorrhoeae isolate from another made epidemiologic studies feasible. Several other systems for typing gonococci have been developed subsequently. These include sensitivity to bacteriocins, the presence of specific lipopolysaccharide antigens, the use of monoclonal antibodies, and identification of specific opa genes.[7,8]

Kellogg and coworkers recognized four colony types of N. gonorrhoeae.[9] Only types 1 and 2 were pathogenic for humans. These types were also found to possess surface hairlike structures termed *pili*. The nature of pili as virulence factors has not been clarified; pili may foster adherence of gonococci to mucosal surfaces or resistance to phagocytosis. Other virulence factors are being identified. These may include capsular production in vivo, resistance to the immune bactericidal action of serum, and the ability of gonococci to survive in the presence of various competing commensal organisms. Griffiss and Artenstein[10] point out that all *Neisseria* are organisms adapted to moist mucous membranes. Of them, the meningococcus and the gonococcus are the ones capable of escaping from host restraints, proliferating rapidly, and even invading the bloodstream. The reason why certain organisms occupy particular ecologic niches and the factors conferring virulence are only beginning to be understood.

CLINICAL MANIFESTATIONS

Signs, symptoms, complications, and the natural history of gonorrhea differ dramatically between males and females. However, careful studies have exposed the myth that males with gonorrhea are symptomatic and females asymptomatic.

Males

After a single exposure to an infected contact, about 25 percent of males will develop gonorrhea. It has been estimated that 85 percent of men with gonococcal urethritis develop an acute process, with discomfort, dysuria, and purulent discharge usually ensuing from 2 to 10 days after exposure. Figure 234-2 shows a typical purulent discharge. Fifteen percent of urethritis in the male is minimally symptomatic or asymptomatic. Since these patients may not receive treatment, they tend to accumulate in the population. The resultant point prevalence of minimally symptomatic or asymptomatic male gonorrhea may be as high as 40 percent.[11] Clearly these men are capable of spreading disease. Untreated symptomatic urethritis subsides over several days to weeks, but occasionally local complications such as epididymitis, seminal vesiculitis, and prostatitis occur. Anorectal[12] and pharyngeal[13] gonococcal colonizations are not common. The incidence of positive cultures correlates with the practices of passive rectal intercourse and fellatio, respectively. Since symptoms of proctitis and pharyngitis correlate poorly with positive cultures, colonization of these areas rather than overt infection is likely to be what occurs.

Females

When an uninfected woman is exposed to an infected man, gonorrhea ensues over half the time. Once infected, the specific symptoms and signs of acute salpingitis may occur (20 to 40 percent) or the less specific symptoms of dysuria, increased discharge, or abnormal bleeding (20 to 30 percent) may be seen within a few days to a few weeks. Thirty to sixty percent of infected women will be minimally affected or asymptomatic yet remain long-term carriers capable of transferring the infection.[14,15] As described for men, these cases will accumulate, since symptomatic gonorrhea is treated preferentially. Since none of the symptoms or signs is diagnostic of gonorrhea, cultures of endocervix, urethra, rectum, and pharynx should be carried out if the disease is suspected or the patient is reported as a contact of gonorrhea.

Pelvic inflammatory disease (PID) is the most important complication of gonococcal infection. PID is the result of ascending infection from the endocervix, causing endometritis and/or salpin-gitis and/or pelvic peritonitis. Clinical findings can vary from crampy abdominal pain with minimal tenderness in mild cases to fever, severe abdominal pain, and exquisite tenderness with adnexal masses in florid cases. Prompt diagnosis and aggressive treatment are mandatory since infertility, ectopic pregnancy, and chronic pelvic pain are frequent complications. Several organisms other than *N. gonorrhoeae* may cause PID. The etiologic diagnosis, which is discussed below, may be difficult. Tragically, the role of "silent" or asymptomatic PID in causing adverse reproductive sequelae is becoming increasingly appreciated.

DISSEMINATED GONOCOCCAL INFECTION (DGI)

Spread of *N. gonorrhoeae* to the bloodstream has been estimated to occur in 1 to 3 percent of patients with gonorrhea,[16] with the majority of cases in females. Although endocarditis and meningitis have been reported, they are rare complications. Arthritis and skin lesions, on the other hand, are regularly associated with DGI. The syndrome is so characteristic that a presumptive diagnosis can usually be made on clinical grounds alone; the syndrome has been labeled the *arthritis-dermatitis syndrome*. The onset of gonococcal bacteremia usually occurs with menstruation or pregnancy in females. In males, DGI is most often seen in association with asymptomatic infection. Fever, chills, polyarthralgias, arthritis, and tenosynovitis are common. In the early stages of the disease, skin manifestations occur that are quite characteristic (Fig. 234-3). The skin lesions typically are few in number (often less than a dozen) and concentrated on the extremities, usually acral, and often around the joints. The lesions may be petechial or papular; however, they usually evolve into vesicles or pustules on an erythematous base, which may become hemorrhagic. Sometimes they present as hem-

FIGURE 234-3

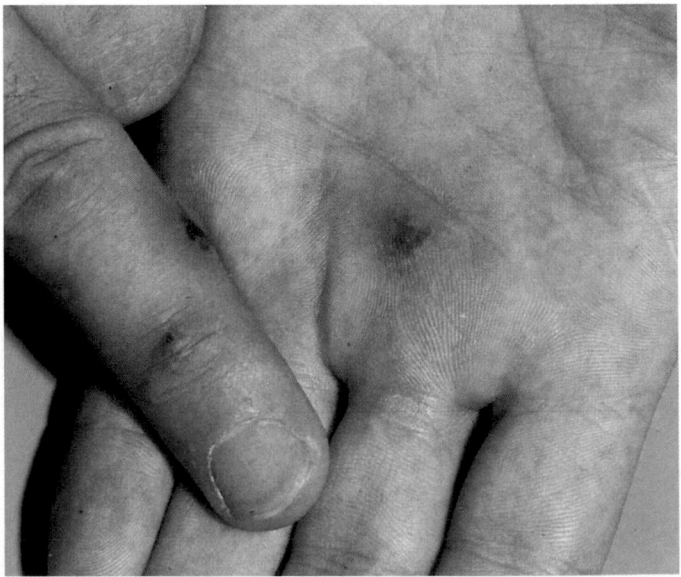

Disseminated gonococcal infection. Lesions on the fingers and palm consisting of pustules and hemorrhagic, necrotic pustules, which are slightly tender.

FIGURE 234-2

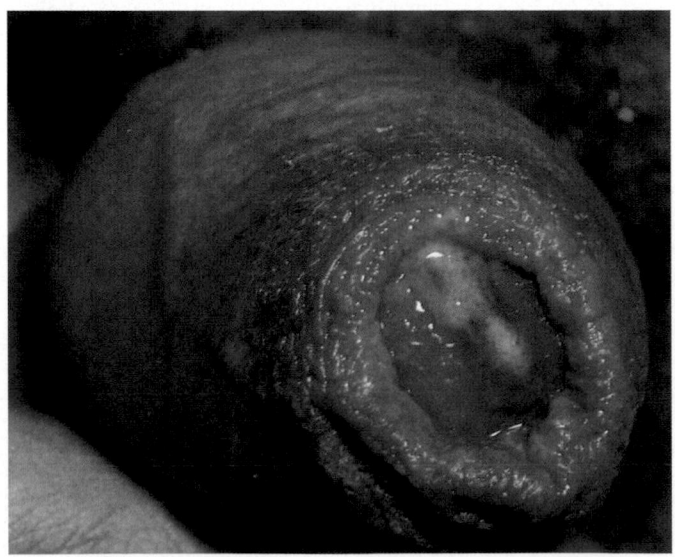

Purulent urethral discharge.

orrhagic bullae. Prompt diagnosis and therapy are mandatory, since delay may result in frank pyogenic arthritis with potential for joint destruction.

It has been recognized that organisms causing DGI often differ from those causing urethritis. Most strains of gonococci are susceptible to the complement-mediated bactericidal action of normal serum; the strains causing DGI are resistant.[16] This important observation may explain why some gonococci are capable of causing bacteremia while others are restricted to mucous membranes. In support of the necessity for serum resistance in strains causing DGI are the reports that patients deficient in the late complement components, which are required for serum killing, are peculiarly susceptible to recurrent neisserial sepsis.[17]

The pathogenesis of the arthritis-dermatitis syndrome is unclear. Bacteremia regularly occurs early in the course of DGI, but it has been suggested that most signs and symptoms of DGI are manifestations of immune-complex formation. (See also Chap. 198.)

MISCELLANEOUS CLINICAL MANIFESTATIONS

In rare cases, an ulcer or abscess may appear on the raphe of the penis. Gonococcal perihepatitis is a complication of gonococcal peritonitis with hepatic capsular fibrosis and adhesions (Fitz-Hugh–Curtis syndrome).[18] Adhesions such as those between the hepatic capsule and the anterior abdominal wall can cause discomfort, which may be persistent and difficult to diagnose.

Gonococcal ophthalmia neonatorum is neonatal purulent conjunctivitis contracted by the newborn in passage through an infected birth canal. Reappearance of this in greater numbers in the 1970s was probably a reflection of the higher incidence of gonorrhea combined with a more casual use of silver nitrate prophylaxis in newborns.[19]

Cornified squamous epithelium is quite resistant to infection with *N. gonorrhoeae*, hence vulvovaginitis is infrequent in adult women. However, in children, the vagina is lined with columnar epithelium; acute vulvovaginitis is the usual manifestation of genital gonococcal infection in the prepubescent female.

PATHOLOGY

The picture of active gonococcal infection is usually that of an acute or subacute inflammatory response with polymorphonuclear leukocytes predominating. The histopathology of the vesiculopustular lesions of DGI consists of infiltrates of neutrophils admixed with some mononuclear cells and red blood cells. Fibrinoid necrosis of vessel walls may be seen. The bullae are subepidermal in location.[20] Bacteria are rarely seen in or grown from the skin lesions.

DIAGNOSIS

Definitive diagnosis of gonorrhea depends upon identification of the organisms by Gram stain and/or culture. A positive Gram stain consists of characteristic gram-negative diplococci in the cytoplasm of

neutrophils (Fig. 234-4). A positive Gram stain from the male urethra is considered diagnostic. Gram stain of endocervical discharge is not usually done, since even a positive smear is not considered diagnostic; culture confirmation is required. In women, endocervical cultures give a higher yield of positives than vaginal cultures. In males without exudate, swabs for culture should be inserted several centimeters into the urethra. In women with gonorrhea, not only endocervical cultures but rectal, urethral, and pharyngeal cultures should be obtained. In DGI, blood, skin lesions, and joint effusions should be cultured. Skin lesions are regularly negative; joint fluid is usually negative until acute purulent arthritis occurs. Blood cultures are positive only early in the disease. Thus, the diagnosis of DGI must frequently be made on clinical grounds only. This rarely presents a problem, since the clinical picture, especially the skin lesions and the tenosynovitis, is quite characteristic.

When culturing an area in which a mixed bacterial flora is unusual, e.g., synovial fluid or male urethra, chocolate agar may be used for isolation. When culturing an area that has an exuberant flora, such as the throat, rectum, or endocervix, one should use selective media containing antimicrobials that inhibit organisms other than *Neisseria*. Modified Thayer-Martin is the medium usually employed. Transgrow is a similar medium, but it also contains CO_2 and is a good transport medium for gonococci.

In addition to *N. gonorrhoeae*, several other organisms cause PID, including *Chlamydia trachomatis*, endogenous anaerobic and aerobic bacteria, and, probably, genital mycoplasmas. It is clearly advantageous for proper therapy to know the causative organism. Endocervical cultures are the only practical way to distinguish between gonococcal and nongonococcal PID; patients in whom gonococci are grown from the cervix are assumed to have gonococcal PID.[21] A DNA probe assay (Gen-Probe) has been tested as an alternative to culture for diagnosis of gonorrhea.[22,23] The DNA probe does not require viable organisms; this is a major advantage that obviates the need for rapid and careful transport of the specimen to the laboratory. Another important advantage of the probe versus culture is that simultaneous testing for *C. trachomatis* on the same specimen is possible. In many institutions the DNA probe assay has replaced culture as the routine screening and diagnostic test for gonorrhea.

FIGURE 234-4

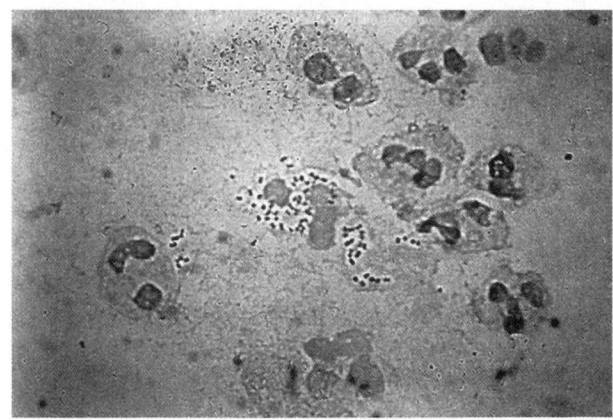

Diagnostic Gram-stained smear of urethral exudate of a man with gonococcal urethritis.

DIFFERENTIAL DIAGNOSIS

The differential diagnosis of genitourinary gonococcal disease in the female includes the following:

1. *Trichomonas vaginalis* infection. This usually presents as a profuse, frothy, foul vaginal exudate, at times with urethritis. A positive saline preparation for the protozoa is diagnostic.
2. *Candida albicans* infection. Often this presents as a pruritic infection with creamy or curdy exudate, and diagnosis depends on identification of the organism by smear and/or culture.
3. *Gardnerella vaginalis* or bacterial vaginosis. There is still dispute about the role of various organisms in bacterial vaginosis. However, the syndrome is well defined, with malodorous, gray, acidic discharge that shows "clue" cells on smear and yields a "fishy" amine odor on alkalinization with potassium hydroxide. All patients with vaginal discharge should be cultured for gonococci. Even though inflammatory vaginitis is rarely seen with gonorrhea alone, mixed infections do occur rather commonly.

In men, urethritis can also be caused by multiple organisms. *T. vaginalis* and *C. albicans* can infect the male and be asymptomatic or cause urethritis or balanitis. Some urethritis has been attributed to *Herpesvirus hominis*. However, even more common than gonorrhea as a cause of urethritis in many populations is so-called nongonococcal or nonspecific or postgonococcal urethritis.

Urethritis with an identified pathogen (except gonococci) is referred to as a *nongonococcal urethritis* (NGU). The term *nonspecific urethritis* describes an urethritis caused by an unidentified organism. NGU may be the most common sexually transmitted disease in humans in most industrialized countries, although reporting is not required in the United States. It is characterized by dysuria, often by urethral discharge or urinary frequency, and by the absence of *N. gonorrhoeae*. In contrast to classic gonococcal urethritis, NGU usually has a longer incubation period, a less acute onset, and scanty urethral discharge; at times, no discharge is evident, only urethral discomfort or tenderness. Occasionally, co-infection with *N. gonorrhoeae* occurs and urethritis remains following effective antibiotic therapy for gonorrhea; this has been labeled *postgonococcal urethritis*.

Until the mid-1970s, causative agents of NGU were not identified; however, it was clear that symptoms usually yielded to therapy with tetracyclines. Now there is good evidence that at least two organisms are responsible for NGU. *C. trachomatis* has been demonstrated convincingly to cause most of the cases of NGU. *Ureaplasma urealyticum* and possibly a few other organisms may be responsible for some of the remaining cases of NGU.

Because NGU has been the subject of such intensive study recently and is so common, it is also discussed separately in the following chapter (Chap. 235).

TREATMENT AND CONTROL

Ideal therapy for gonococcal urethritis would have the following attributes in addition to curing urethritis. It should be given as a single dose; it should abort coincubating syphilis; it should cure coexisting chlamydial infections. No single drug regimen achieves these ideals. Previously recommended penicillin or tetracycline regimens are no longer indicated because of widespread resistance of *N. gonorrhoeae* to these antibiotics.

Multiple regimens have merit: (1) ceftriaxone 250 mg IM in a single dose; (2) cefixime 400 mg PO in a single dose; (3) azithromycin 1 g PO in a single dose; (4) ciprofloxacin 500 mg PO in a single dose; and (5) ofloxacin 400 mg PO in a single dose.

When using a cephalosporin regimen for gonorrhea, additional treatment for coexisting chlamydial infection should be given, often doxycycline 100 mg bid for 7 days. Although the cephalosporins have been used widely to treat gonorrhea, no significant resistance has yet developed. Azithromycin as a single dose effectively treats gonococcal and chlamydial infections. The drawbacks of this regimen are high cost, lack of FDA approval for gonorrhea treatment, and concern regarding increased minimum inhibitory concentrations (MICs) to azithromycin in strains with chromosomal resistance to penicillin or tetracycline.[5] The single-dose fluoroquinolone regimens for gonorrhea treatment may not be adequate for treatment of chlamydial infections. Gonococcal strains with decreased susceptibility to ciprofloxacin have emerged, causing concern about the future efficacy of these agents if widely used.[5] The Gonococcal Isolate Surveillance Project (GISP) of the Centers for Disease Control and Prevention periodically monitors antimicrobial susceptibility of *N. gonorrhoeae*.[5] These surveillance data are valuable for predicting the efficacy of the various antibiotic regimens for gonorrhea treatment.

Control of the gonorrhea epidemic probably depends more on other factors than the details of therapy of acute disease. It is essential to educate the public about venereal disease, including signs and symptoms, methods of prevention, and resources available. Medical personnel must also be made aware of the most effective case-finding techniques, including screening of at-risk populations and aggressive search for contacts of patients with gonorrhea. More controlled sexual activity in the wake of the AIDS epidemic, including widespread use of condoms, will probably help ameliorate the epidemic of gonorrhea.

REFERENCES

1. Centers for Disease Control and Prevention: Summary of Notifiable Diseases, United States 1995. *MMWR* **44**(no. 53):33, 1996
2. Schnell D et al: A time series analysis of gonorrhea surveillance data. *Stat Med* **8**:343, 1989
3. Rothenberg RB, Potterat JJ: Temporal and social aspects of gonorrhea transmission: The force infectivity. *Sex Transm Dis* **15**:88, 1988
4. Johnson SR, Morse SA: Antibiotic resistance in *Neisseria gonorrhoeae*: Genetic mechanisms of resistance. *Sex Transm Dis* **15**:217, 1988
5. Fox KK et al: Antimicrobial resistance in *Neisseria gonorrhoeae* in the United States, 1988–1994: The emergence of decreased susceptibility to the fluoroquinolones. *J Infect Dis* **175**:1396, 1977
6. Carifo K, Catlin BW: *Neisseria gonorrhoeae* auxotyping: Differentiation of clinical isolates based on growth responses on chemically defined media. *Appl Microbiol* **26**:223, 1973
7. Moyes A, Young H: Typing of *Neisseria gonorrhoeae* by auxotype, serovar and lectin agglutination. *Br J Biomed Sci* **50**:295, 1993
8. O'Rourke M et al: Opa typing: A high-resolution tool for studying the epidemiology of *gonorrhoeae*. *Mol Microbiol* **17**:865, 1995
9. Kellogg DS et al: *Neisseria gonorrhoeae*: II. Colonial variation and pathogenicity during 35 months in vitro. *J Bacteriol* **96**:596, 1968
10. Griffiss JM, Artenstein MS: The ecology of the genus *Neisseria*. *Mt Sinai J (NY)* **43**:746, 1976
11. Handsfield HH et al: Asymptomatic gonorrhea in men—diagnosis, natural course, prevalence and significance. *N Engl J Med* **290**:117, 1974

12. Klein EJ et al: Anorectal gonococcal infection. *Ann Intern Med* **86**:340, 1977
13. Wiesner PJ et al: Clinical spectrum of pharyngeal gonococcal infection. *N Engl J Med* **288**:181, 1973
14. McCormack WM et al: Clinical spectrum of gonococcal infection in women. *Lancet* **1**:1182, 1977
15. Weisner PJ, Thompson SE III: Gonococcal diseases. *Disease-a-Month* **26**:2, 1980
16. Schoolnik GK et al: Gonococci causing disseminated gonococcal infection are resistant to the bactericidal action of normal human sera. *J Clin Invest* **58**:1163, 1976
17. Petersen BH et al: Human deficiency of the eighth component of complement. *J Clin Invest* **57**:283, 1976
18. Reichert JA, Valle RF: Fitz-Hugh–Curtis syndrome. *JAMA* **236**:266, 1976
19. Snowe RJ, Wilfert CM: Epidemic reappearance of gonococcal ophthalmia neonatorum. *Pediatrics* **51**:110, 1973
20. Lever WF, Schaumburg-Lever G: *Histopathology of the Skin,* 7th ed. Philadelphia, Lippincott, 1990
21. Eschenback DA et al: Polymicrobial etiology of acute pelvic inflammatory disease. *N Engl J Med* **293**:166, 1975
22. Vlaspolder F et al: Value of a DNA probe assay (Gen-Probe) compared with that of culture for diagnosis of gonococcal infection. *J Clin Microbiol* **31**:107, 1993
23. Schwebke JR, Zajackowski ME: Comparison of DNA probe (Gen-Probe) with culture for the detection of *Neisseria gonorrhoeae* in an urban STD programme. *Genitourin Med* **72**:108, 1996

CHAPTER 235

Alfred R. Eichmann

Other Venereal Diseases

GENITAL CHLAMYDIA INFECTIONS

Eighteen different serotypes of *Chlamydia trachomatis* are presently known: A, B, Ba, and C are considered to be the causative agents of trachoma, D to K the infectious agents of urogenital and other diseases, and L1 to L3 the causative pathogens of lymphogranuloma venereum. Although serotypes E, F, and D account for 60 to 70 percent of urogenital *C. trachomatis* infections, there is no evidence that specific genital syndromes are serotype-specific.[1]

Epidemiology

In the United States half a million cases were reported in 1995, the rate per 100,000 population being 182.[2] In a pan-European study involving 24 centers in 14 countries, the prevalence of genital chlamydial infections was 3.9 percent (range, 1.0 to 7.4 percent). The study population was women aged 16 to 32 years who sought contraceptive advice in family planning clinics.[3]

Etiology and Pathogenesis

Chlamydiae have a cell wall and contain DNA and RNA in their cytoplasm; they are endowed with a characteristic metabolism and are bacteria. However, they are energy-requiring parasites that can multiply only within other cells. The chlamydiae form inclusions in the cytoplasm. Reproduction occurs by binary fission. In cell culture, this cycle of development takes 48 to 72 h.[4] The chlamydial infection leads to an immune response in the form of circulating antibodies and cellular immunity.[4] The major chlamydial antigens are the major outer-membrane proteins (MOMP), the lipopolysaccharides, and the heat-shock proteins (HSP).[5]

Clinical Manifestations

INFECTIONS OF THE FEMALE GENITAL TRACT The most important clinical manifestations include mucopurulent cervicitis, acute urethral syndrome, acute bartholinitis and proctitis, pelvic inflammatory disease (PID), and postpartum endometritis. Sequelae include extrauterine pregnancy, tubal infertility, and cellular atypia of the cervix.

Cervicitis *Chlamydia trachomatis* attacks the cylindrical epithelium of the cervix. This cervicitis cannot be distinguished clinically from other inflammatory processes of the cervix. About 30 to 50 percent of women with proven chlamydial cervicitis show no clinical symptoms. In women who do, the principal symptom is mucopurulent discharge, followed by hypertrophic ectopia, postcoital bleeding, and spotting. Simple objective criteria for the presumptive diagnosis of mucopurulent cervicitis include an increased number ($\geq$10 per high-power field) of polymorphonuclear leukocytes in cervical smears, a positive swab test, erythema, edema, and induced mucosal bleeding in the area of ectopy and the transformation zone.[1]

Pelvic inflammatory disease (PID) PID is the most severe complication of the lower genital tract. The clinical spectrum of chlamydial PID has a wide range: subclinical endometritis, salpingitis, pelvic peritonitis, periappendicitis, and perihepatitis. Therefore the traditional clinical and laboratory criteria for diagnosis of PID are inaccurate. Laparoscopy, endometrial biopsy, transvaginal ultrasonography, or magnetic resonance imaging are recommended to improve the accuracy of the diagnosis. Laparoscopy is generally accepted as the gold standard for diagnosis of PID.[6] Concern about silent PID and its sequelae has led to a change in the recommendations for clinical diagnosis of PID. The minimal criteria for clinical diagnosis of PID are:

Lower abdominal tenderness
Bilateral adnexal tenderness
Cervical motion tenderness
No evidence of a competing diagnosis (e.g., positive pregnancy test, acute appendicitis)

When a proper diagnosis of chlamydial PID is uncertain or delayed, adequate antibiotic treatments should be started if the above mentioned criteria are observed.[1]

Perihepatitis (Fitz-Hugh–Curtis syndrome) Chlamydia can pass from the cervix via the endometrium and the uterine tubes to reach the region of the right diaphragm. There it causes a perihepatitis, which does not involve the liver parenchyma. Clinically it is characterized by piercing pain below the right costal margin. Symptoms are reminiscent of those seen in acute cholecystitis or pleuritis. Perihepatitis appears to be more common in chlamydial infections than in gonorrhea.[7]

INFECTIONS IN MEN The genital manifestations of chlamydial infection are very similar to those of gonococcal infection. Mucous membranes are infected first; later, more invasive infection occurs. Infection by the serotypes D through K can result in the following syndromes in men: nongonococcal urethritis (NGU), postgonococcal urethritis, prostatitis, vas deferentitis, epididimitis, and proctitis. The most frequent clinical symptom in the male is urethritis. In 30 to 50 percent of the patients with NGU, *Chlamydia* can be found. The incubation period ranges from 7 to 21 days. The symptoms are in general the same as in gonococcal urethral infection, but they start later and are milder. Urethritis caused by *Chlamydia* is more often asymptomatic than urethritis caused by *Neisseria gonorrhoeae*. Coinfection with *N. gonorrhoeae* and *Chlamydia* in the male is found in about 15 to 35 percent of patients with gonorrhea. *Chlamydia* causes postgonococcal urethritis in 70 to 80 percent of patients[8] and is the cause of acute vas deferentitis and epididimitis in young men (<35 years of age) in more than 50 percent of cases. Untreated vas deferentitis/epididimitis produces an obliteration of the vas deferens; sterility can result if both sides are affected. Identification of the causative pathogen in an aspirate and increased levels of IgG and IgM antibodies in the serum provide verification of the diagnosis.[9] The role of *Chlamydia* in prostatitis is still controversial. The published data are inconclusive regarding the role of *C. trachomatis* in nonbacterial prostatitis. Chlamydial proctitis is frequently seen in homosexual men, caused by the serotypes D through K. About 50 percent of the men with proctitis present clinical symptoms, including anorectal pain and bleeding, mucous discharge, and diarrhea. Crohn's disease must be excluded in these patients.[10] *Chlamydia* is present in about 80 percent of patients with the genitourinary form of Reiter's syndrome,[11] where it is considered to have a trigger function.

INFECTIONS IN NEWBORN CHILDREN These infections are a direct consequence of a genital chlamydial infection of the mother.

Chlamydial pneumonia in the newborn Chlamydial pneumonia is often afebrile and is accompanied by a pertussis-like cough and mucous sputum. X-ray reveals symmetric interstitial infiltrates. Laboratory findings include marked eosinophilia, hypergammaglobulinemia, and IgM antibodies to *Chlamydia*.[12]

Inclusion-particle conjunctivitis *Chlamydia* can be isolated from 15 to 20 percent of all children with postnatal blennorrhea. The conjunctivitis appears between days 5 to 15 and is often unilateral. The eyelids are edematous and inflamed and a suppurative secretion is observed. For confirmation of the diagnosis, material is taken from the conjunctiva of the lower eyelid.[12]

Laboratory Examinations[12,13]

Several test procedures are available:

Direct visualization of *Chlamydia* in clinical specimens: staining of smears, tissue culture
Serologic tests
Direct isolation of *Chlamydia* from patient's tissue
Detection of specific chlamydial genes or antigens in clinical specimens

The following techniques are used to detect *C. trachomatis:*

Cell culture (cyclohexamide-treated McCoy cells)
Direct fluorescent antibody tests (DFA) (Fig. 235-1)
Enzyme immunoassays (EIA)
Polymerase chain reaction (PCR)
Ligase chain reaction (LCR)

The actual gold standard would be the sum of culture positivity or, if culture negative, a confirmed LCR test.

SEROLOGY All organisms of the genus *Chlamydia* possess a common group-specific antigen that stimulates the formation of IgM, IgA, and IgG antibodies in infected patients. The antibodies can be detected using a microimmunofluorescence test or the enzyme-linked immunosorbent assay (ELISA) technique in the case of invasive forms of the infection. Serologic methods are without significance in localized chlamydial infections. The microimmunofluorescent technique (Micro-IF) is very useful for epidemiologic studies but is particularly useful for diagnosis of genital chlamydial infections.

FIGURE 235-1

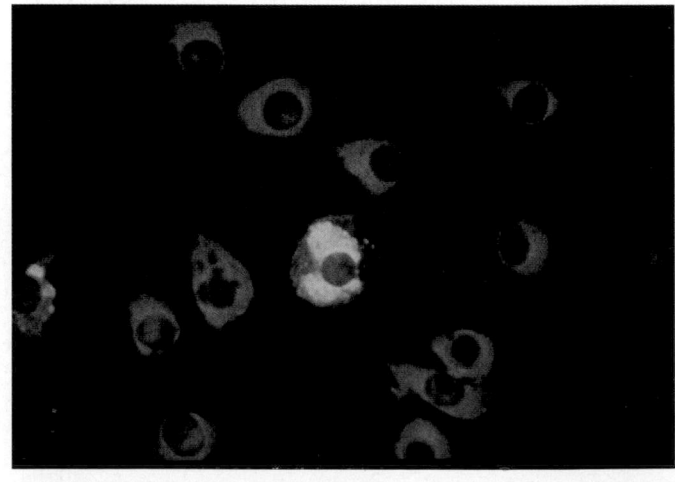

Detection of *Chlamydia trachomatis* by direct immunofluorescence with monoclonal antibodies.

Diagnosis

The definitive diagnosis results from the direct or indirect (serologic) identification of the causative pathogen by one or more of the tests mentioned above.

Treatment

Tetracyclines and the macrolides are the antibiotics of choice for uncomplicated genital chlamydial infections (Table 235-1). Sexual partners and the mothers of infected newborns must be examined and treated. For chlamydial PID and perihepatitis, more extensive treatment regimens are necessary.[1]

Prevention

Effective prevention consists of the careful examination and treatment of all sexual partners. If techniques for appropriate diagnosis are not available, it is recommended that patients with NGU and nongonococcal mucopurulent cervicitis undergo tetracycline or azithromycin therapy just as is used for proven chlamydial infections. Patients at risk during pregnancy must be examined and treated prophylactically when indicated.

GENITAL MYCOPLASMAS

Mycoplasmas are the smallest self-replicating microorganisms. In the genital region, the three species *Mycoplasma hominis, Ureaplasma urealyticum*, and *M. genitalium* have been detected and correlated with genital disease. Whether these mycoplasmas have definite pathogenic properties is still a matter of controversy. Mycoplasmas are found relatively frequently on the genital mucosa in sexually active people without giving rise to any manifest disease. The frequency of the colonization of the genital mucosa increases with sexual experience and the number of partners.[15]

Pathogenesis

It has still not been determined whether *M. hominis* and *U. urealyticum* cause NGU. Many investigations have implicated *Ureaplasma* as a cause of NGU, since clinical improvement of urethritis occurs when therapy is administered. There is some evidence for *M. genitalium* being one of the causes of acute NGU, some evidence

for its role in chronic NGU, but no evidence that it causes chronic prostatitis.[16]

Detection and Treatment

Mycoplasmas can be detected by culture from swabs. Until now, seven serotypes of *M. hominis* and 14 serotypes of *U. urealyticum* are known. Whether a relationship exists between individual serotypes and particular diseases is unknown. In addition to NGU, mycoplasmas have been considered as possible etiologic agents in other diseases: adnexitis, puerperal fever, fever after abortion, natural miscarriage, prostatitis, and bartholinitis.[15] Mycoplasmas are quite sensitive to tetracyclines and erythromycin. Dosage and duration of treatment are the same as those used against chlamydial infections.

TRICHOMONAS VAGINALIS

Since the reporting of sexually transmitted diseases (STDs) is not obligatory in most countries, reliable figures are hard to find. In most western countries, however, trichomonal infections seem to be declining. Transmission results from sexual contact. Perinatal infection is the most frequent nonvenereal form of transmission. The causative pathogen can survive for several hours on moist objects and in body fluids.[17]

Clinical Manifestations

The most common clinical symptoms in women are a yellow vaginal discharge, abnormal vaginal odor, pruritus, reddening and swelling of the vulva, and punctate petechiae of the cervix ("strawberry cervix") (Fig. 235-2). More than half of all infected women show symptoms.[18] The majority of infected men are asymptomatic. In males the most common symptoms are milky discharge and dysuria. Serious complications are unknown.

FIGURE 235-2

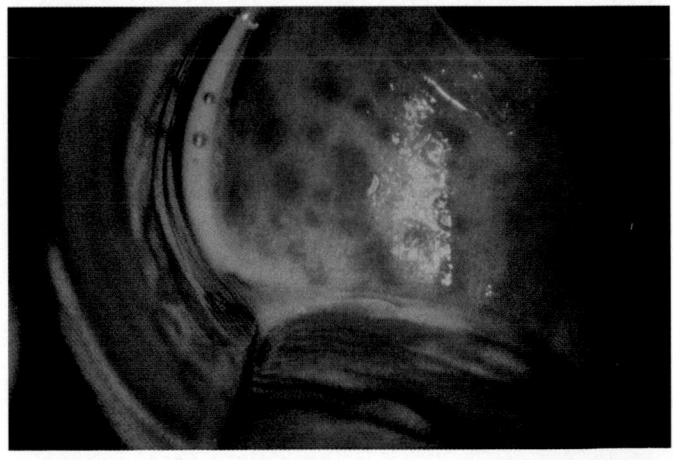

Trichomonas vaginalis infection: "Strawberry" appearance of cervix with punctate bleeding erosions. (*Courtesy of U. Lauper, MD.*)

TABLE 235-1

Center for Disease Control and Prevention (CDC) Guidelines for the Treatment of Chlamydial Infections

CDC-recommended regimens
  Doxycycline 100 mg orally twice a day for 7 days
  Azithromycin 2 g orally in a single dose
Alternative regimens
  Ofloxacin 300 mg orally twice a day for 7 days
  Erythromycin base 500 mg orally four times a day for 7 days
  Erythromycin ethylsuccinate 800 mg orally four times a day for 7 days
  Sulfisoxazole 500 mg orally four times a day for 10 days (inferior in efficacy to other regimens)

SOURCE: Centers for Disease Control and Prevention.[14]

Diagnosis

The 10- to 20-μm protozoan with four to five flagellae can be directly detected on a wet mount. Phase-contrast or dark-field microscopy is helpful (Fig. 235-3). In women, the specimen must be taken from the vagina, since the causative pathogen attacks only the multilayered squamous epithelium. Attempts to demonstrate the causative organism in men are not always successful, but *Trichomonas vaginalis* can be detected in the urinary sediment. Various culture media are available from industrial sources.

Therapy

The therapy of choice is a nitroimidazole, such as metronidazole. This can be given orally as a single 2-g dose or as 250 mg three times daily for 7 days. In some individuals metronidazole has an Antabuse-like effect. Thus, it can produce symptoms like nausea and flushing.

BACTERIAL VAGINOSIS

Bacterial vaginosis (BV) is the most frequent vaginal infection in sexually active women. The prevalence ranges from 5 percent (in women during a routine gynecologic checkup) to 40 percent (in women visiting an STD clinic).[19] BV can be diagnosed by four clinical criteria:

Thin, homogeneous vaginal discharge
Vaginal pH $\geq$ 4.5
Release of a fishy odor from vaginal discharge after alkalinization with 10% potassium hydroxide
Clue cells (see below) on wet mount (Fig. 235-4)

Gram stain gives excellent results with regard to sensitivity and specificity. Routine vaginal microbiologic cultures in women with suspected BV are of no diagnostic value.

FIGURE 235-3

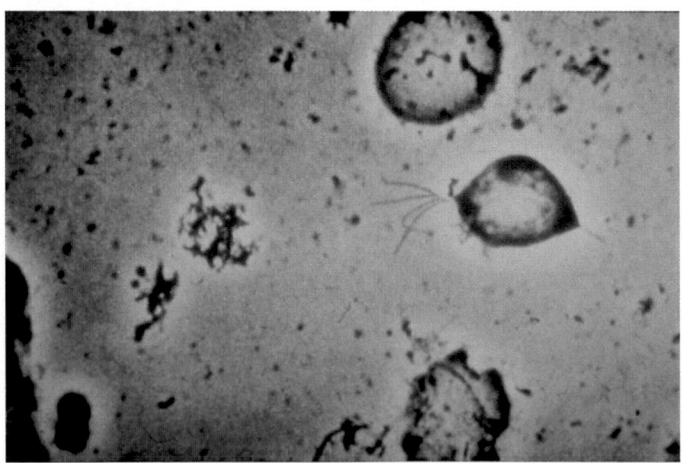

Trichomonas vaginalis, phase-contrast microscopy. (*Courtesy of U. Lauper, MD.*)

FIGURE 235-4

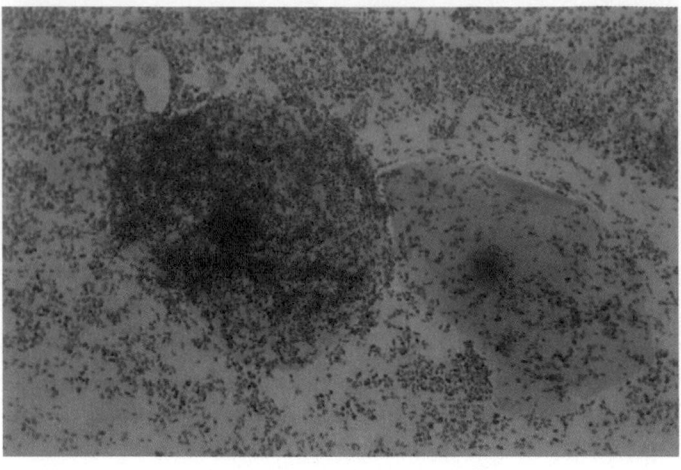

Colpitis due to *Haemophilus vaginalis.* Clue cells, Gram-staining. (*Courtesy of U. Lauper, MD.*)

Clue cells are epithelial cells coated with bacteria (*Gardnerella vaginalis*). *G. vaginalis* is found in high concentrations in the vaginal fluid of more than 90 percent of women with BV. Patients with BV have only few or no lactobacilli in the vaginal flora.[20] BV in nonpregnant women is treated successfully with metronidazole orally or locally. A single oral dose of 2 g metronidazole is as successful as a 5- to 7-day course of 1000 mg daily. Intravaginal clindamycin cream (2%) for 5 to 7 days is the drug of choice in pregnancy.[21]

VIRAL HEPATITIS

At least five different human viruses are now recognized as causative agents of viral hepatitis. Sexual activity influences the transmission of hepatitis A and B virus; hepatitis B virus especially can easily be transmitted by sexual intercourse. It is estimated that every fifth case of hepatitis B in the United States is transmitted heterosexually.[22]

REFERENCES

1. Paavonen J: *Chlamydia trachomatis:* A major cause of mucopurulent cervicitis and pelvic inflammatory disease in women, in *Sexually Transmitted Diseases: Advances in Diagnosis and Treatment,* edited by P Elsner, A Eichmann. Karger, Basel, 1996, p 110
2. Division of STD Prevention: *STD Surveillance, 1995.* U.S. Department of Health and Human Services. Atlanta, Centers for Disease Control and Prevention, 1996
3. Mårdh PA, Genç M: Is Europe ready for screening for genital chlamydial infections? in *Proceedings of 3rd Meeting of European Society for Chlamydial Research,* edited by A Stary. Vienna, 1996
4. Schachter J: Biology of *Chlamydia trachomatis,* in *Sexually Transmitted Diseases,* 3d ed, edited by KK Holmes et al. New York, McGraw-Hill, 1999
5. Stephens RS: Cell biology of *Chlamydia* infection, in *Chlamydial Infections,* edited by J Orfila et al. Bologna, Esculapio, 1994, pp 377–386
6. Weström L et al: PID and fertility: A cohort study of 1844 women. *Sex Transm Dis* **19**:185, 1992
7. Wølner-Hansen P: Perihepatitis in chlamydial salpingitis. *Lancet* **1**:901, 1980

8. Stamm WE, Holmes KK: *Chlamydia trachomatis* infections of the adult, in *Sexually Transmitted Diseases,* 3d ed, edited by KK Holmes et al. New York, McGraw-Hill, 1999

9. Doble A et al: Acute epididymitis: A microbiological and ultrasonographic study. *Br J Urol* **63**:90, 1989

10. Rompalo AM: Potential value of rectal-screening cultures for *Chlamydia trachomatis* in homosexual men. *J Infect Dis* **153**:188, 1986

11. Kousa M et al: Frequent association of chlamydial infection with Reiter's syndrome. *Sex Transm Dis* **5**:57, 1978

12. Schachter J: Evolution of diagnostic tests for *Chlamydia trachomatis* infections, in *Proceedings of 3rd Meeting of European Society for Chlamydial Research,* edited by A Stary. Vienna, 1996

13. Taylor-Robinson D: Tests for infection with *Chlamydia trachomatis. Int J STD AIDS* **7**:19, 1996

14. Centers for Disease Control and Prevention: Sexually transmitted diseases: Treatment guidelines 1993. *MMWR* **42**:17, 1993

15. Taylor-Robinson D: Genital mycoplasma infection. *Clin Lab Med* **9**:501, 1989

16. Taylor-Robinson D: The history and role of *Mycoplasma genitalium* in sexually transmitted diseases. *Genitourin Med* **71**:1, 1995

17. Lossick JS: Epidemiology of urogenital trichomoniasis, in *Trichomonads Parasitic in Humans,* edited by BM Honigberg. New York, Springer, 1989, p 313

18. Wølner-Hansen P et al: Clinical manifestations of vaginal trichomoniasis. *JAMA* **261**:571, 1989

19. Martius J: Bacterial vaginosis, in *Vulvo-vaginitis,* edited by P Elsner, Marlins J. New York, Marcel Dekker, 1993, p 345

20. Martius J: Diagnosis of bacterial vaginosis, in *Sexually Transmitted Diseases: Advances in Diagnosis and Treatment,* edited by P Elsner, A Eichmann. Karger, Basel, 1996

21. Martius J: Bacterial vaginosis, in *Sexually Transmitted Diseases: Advances in Diagnosis and Treatment,* edited by P Elsner, A Eichmann. Basel, Karger, 1996, p 105

22. Centers for Disease Control: Changing patterns of groups at high risk for hepatitis B in the United States. *MMWR* **37**:429, 1988

CHAPTER 236

Sidney N. Klaus
Shoshana Frankenburg

Leishmaniasis and Other Protozoan Infections

Protozoa are unicellar nonphotosynthetic eukaryotic organisms that are microscopic or near microscopic in size. Although most are free-living, some have adapted to a parasitic existence; it is this group that is of major medical importance. Protozoa are ubiquitous, comprising by far the majority of individual animal life forms on earth.

The basic structure of protozoa consists of a cell membrane surrounding cytoplasm in which one or more nuclei are embedded. Each of the major classes of protozoa have evolved distinctive organelles to mediate locomotion and to provide for metabolic activity.

The taxonomy of the protozoa subkingdom is complex. Table 236-1 lists a simplified classification of those protozoan species that cause diseases of dermatologic interest.

LEISHMANIASIS

Leishmaniasis is the result of infection with intracellular protozoan parasites belonging to the genus *Leishmania*. The infections cause a wide spectrum of clinical changes that divide leishmaniasis into four broad divisions based on the extent and severity of involvement in the human host: cutaneous leishmaniasis (CL), diffuse cutaneous leishmaniasis (DCL), mucocutaneous leishmaniasis (MCL), and visceral leishmaniasis (VL).

The prevalence of all forms of leishmaniasis worldwide is in excess of 12 million cases. Movement of new immigrants into endemic areas, an increase in tourism to "exotic" areas of the globe, a decrease in the use of insecticides, and improvement in diagnostic methods have all contributed to raising the incidence of leishmaniasis, which the World Health Organization estimates will soon exceed 400,000 new cases annually. The more serious forms of the disease, such as MCL and VL, cause the death of more than 75,000 persons annually.

Characterization of *Leishmania* Parasites

The protozoan parasites that cause leishmaniasis are members of the order Kinetoplastida, family Trypanosomatidae. The organisms are found in two morphologic forms during their life cycle. In humans and other mammalian hosts, they exist within macrophages as round to oval nonflagellated amastigotes, 2 to 3 μm in diameter. In the arthropod vectors (sandflies belonging to the genus *Phlebotomus* or *Lutzomyia*) the parasites exist as elongated flagellated promastigotes, 10 to 15 μm in length and 2 to 3 μm in width. Both forms of the parasites have a nucleus and a smaller DNA-containing kinetoplast. Although promastigotes of different *Leishmania* species vary slightly in the width-to-length ratio, amastigotes show no significant differences, and it is not possible to distinguish species of *Leishmania* by their morphology in tissue smears.

Until the past decade, different species of *Leishmania* were identified largely by the pattern of their clinical involvement. The old world forms of CL were thought to be caused by *L. tropica*, new world MCL was attributed to *L. braziliensis*, new world CL to *L. mexicana*, and VL to *L. donovani*. Recently, more precise techniques for identifying *Leishmania* species have been developed, such as monoclonal antibodies, isoenzyme characterization, DNA hybridization, and the polymerase chain reaction (PCR). Based on findings using these techniques, the older clinical categories have been subdivided and now include recently identified species. A practical, somewhat simplified classification scheme is found in Table 236-2.

TABLE 236-1

Protozoa Causing Dermatologic Disease

ORGANISM	DISEASE
Flagellates (class Zoomastigophora)	
Leishmania spp.	Cutaneous, mucocutaneous and visceral leishmaniasis
Trypanosoma spp.	African trypanosomiasis, American trypanosomiasis
Ameba-like forms: (class Rhizopodea)	
Entamoeba histolytica	Cutaneous amebiasis
Acanthamoeba spp. (free-living)	Local and disseminated infectious granulomas
Apical-complex forms: (class Sporozoa)	
Toxoplasma gondii	Toxoplasmosis

TABLE 236-2

Classification of Leishmaniasis

CLINICAL FORM	SPECIES	MAJOR LOCALITIES
Cutaneous leishmaniasis (CL):		
Old world	L. major	Near East, Africa
	L. tropica	Near East, former USSR
	L. aethiopica	Ethiopia, Kenya
	L. infantum	Mediterranean rim
New world	L. mexicana complex	Mexico, Central America
	L. braziliensis complex	Brazil, Bolivia
	L. amazonensis	Brazil
Mucocutaneous leishmaniasis (MCL)		
Diffuse (anergic) cutaneous leishmaniasis (DCL):		
Old world	L. aethiopica	Ethiopia
New world	L. braziliensis complex	South America
Visceral leishmaniasis (VL)	L. donovani	India, Kenya
	L. infantum	Mediterranean rim
Uncommon forms of leishmaniasis:		
Leishmaniasis recidivans (LR)	L. tropica	Middle East, former USSR
Post-kala-azar dermal leishmaniasis (PKADL)	L. donovani	India, Nepal, China

VECTORS *Leishmania* parasites are transmitted by phlebotomine sandflies of the genus *Phlebotomus* in the old world and *Lutzomyia* in the new world. Sandflies are small mosquito-like insects 1.5 to 4 mm in length. Their small size allows them to pass through ordinary mesh screens and mosquito netting. Sandflies are widely distributed throughout the tropics and subtropics in a variety of habitats, including deserts, rain forests, and highlands. Only the females are hematophagous (blood sucking).

LIFE CYCLE Parasites, in the form of amastigotes from infected tissue or blood, are taken up from the mammalian host during feeding by female sandflies. Within the midgut of the sandflies, the parasites undergo a change to the promastigote form and multiply. Once the promastigotes are fully developed, they migrate from the gut to the pharynx and proboscis, where they remain until they are injected into a new mammalian host during a subsequent blood meal.[1]

Between 10 and 200 promastigotes enter the dermis during each feeding by an infected sandfly. Many of the "free" promastigotes are thought to be destroyed by polymorphonuclear leukocytes and eosinophils, but the exact details of the early stages of infection are unknown. Some of the promastigotes become attached to receptors on the surface of dermal macrophages and are phagocytosed. It has been shown that sandfly saliva, injected with the parasites, enhances parasite virulence mainly due to its impressive vasodilatory properties.[2] Recent studies suggest that the saliva also has an immunomodulatory effect, delaying a protective cell-mediated response.[3] Within the macrophage, the promastigotes transform into amastigotes (also called Leishman-Donovan bodies) and are incorporated into the cells' phagolysosomes (parasitophorous vacuoles). Within the phagolysosome, the parasites are able to resist destruction and multiply readily by binary fission. When a macrophage becomes filled with amastigotes, the macrophage is disrupted. The amastigotes reenter the extracellular space and are taken up again by other macrophages. The duration of the extracellular stage is unknown.[4]

Dissemination of the parasites from the inoculation site depends in large measure on the species of the parasite.[5] Some species, such as *L. donovani* and *L. infantum*, can spread to macrophages elsewhere in the reticuloendothelial system early in the course of the illness. Other species, such as members of the *L. braziliensis* complex, travel to specific locations in the host, such as the mucosal surfaces of the nose, pharynx, and upper respiratory tract. Amastigotes of dermatotropic species, such as *L. major* and *L. tropica*, generally remain confined to the skin and probably to the draining lymph nodes. The cycle of infection continues when an infected mammal is again bitten, and amastigotes are taken up by a female sandfly.

RESERVOIRS Each species of *Leishmania* favors one or more animal reservoirs, except *L. donovani*, which is thought to be largely anthroponotic. *L. tropica* is probably not anthroponotic, but in many countries the specific animal reservoir has not yet been identified. Identification and control of the reservoir may have a profound influence on the epidemiology of the disease. For example, in southern France and Spain, where dogs serve as the main reservoir for VL (caused by *L. infantum*), destruction of infected animals has led to a marked decrease in the frequency of the disease in humans. In an area of Turkmenistan, as a result of a zoonotic control program, CL was practically eliminated.

Immunobiology

Leishmaniasis can be pictured as an immunologic spectrum that in many aspects parallels leprosy.[6] At one end lies CL, in which the host usually develops a protective immune response; at the other is VL, in which the host shows little evidence of resistance and may show signs of immunosuppression. In the middle are MCL, which provokes an intense inflammatory reaction, and DCL, in which there is extensive and widespread proliferation of the organisms of the skin, but without much inflammation or tendency for visceralization. Unlike leprosy, the extent and pattern of leishmaniasis that develop are strongly influenced by the specific species of *Leishmania* involved.

Additional factors that affect the clinical picture include the number of parasites inoculated, the site of inoculation, the nutritional status of the host, and even the nature of the last non-blood meal of the vector. In some cases the sandfly vector is heavily infected, and a large load of parasites may partially block the insect's pharynx, requiring the sandfly to make multiple probes to obtain an adequate blood meal. This results in a localized cluster of cutaneous lesions in the host. Rather broad differences in the disease pattern may develop from apparently similar or identical strains of *Leishmania*. It is known that some patients who are infected by *L. major* develop inapparent infections, whereas others infected by identical *Leishmania* species show deep or widespread lesions that involve subcutaneous tissue and lymph nodes. Although CL caused by *L. aethiopica* will result in spontaneous cure in 80 percent of patients, widespread diffuse cutaneous lesions will develop in the remaining 20 percent.

Immunologic Response

Cell-mediated immunoregulation plays a central role in the outcome of leishmanial infection. On the one hand, the clinical expression of the disease is due to immunologic processes rather than to the number of parasites in the lesions; on the other hand, cell-mediated immunity is crucial for healing and development of long-lasting immunity. Although antileishmanial antibodies are produced during infection, their presence does not correlate with resolution of the disease. In experimental animals, disease progression is associated with type 2 lymphocytes, which produce interleukin (IL) 4, IL-5, IL-10, and transforming growth factor β; control and resolution of infection are mediated by type 1 lymphocytes, which produce interferon (IFN) γ and IL-2. Experiments using transgenic mice and selective gene disruption have shown that some cytokines, such as IL-4 and IL-12 (produced mainly by macrophages and dendritic cells), play a major regulatory role, although it appears that additional, still undefined, signals are required.[7] For example, inoculation of parasites into the footpad or rump of resistant mice leads to rapid healing (a type 1 response), while inoculation into the dorsal skin leads to progressive disease (a type 2 response), suggesting a local influence on disease outcome.

Parasites are eliminated by an effector mechanism which involves IFN-γ-mediated activation of infected macrophages. Recent evidence suggests that parasite killing within macrophages is mediated largely through the upregulation of nitric oxide synthetase (NOS) and the generation of nitric oxide. The expression of inducible NOS is upregulated by type 1 cytokines and suppressed by type 2 cytokines.[8,9] In general, the murine leishmania model has served as a model for diseases exhibiting the type 1/type 2 dichotomy, such as leprosy.

Although it is suggested that similar mechanisms may be operative in human CL, the picture that emerges from human studies is less clear. Several researchers have measured cytokine production in CL lesions, and mostly a mixture of type 1 and type 2 cytokines has been found, without a clear correlation with healing.[10] Other studies have shown that patients with active CL have circulating lymphocytes that produce IFN-γ in response to leishmanial antigen, thus supporting a role for type 1 lymphocytes in healing. It is not known how parasites are killed in humans. Although it has been shown that human macrophages in vitro can kill parasites by the generation of NO, it is unclear if this represents the operative mechanism during the disease process.

In general, infection and recovery are followed by lifelong immunity to reinfection by the same species of *Leishmania*. In some cases, interspecies immunity has also been reported. An effective vaccine for the prevention of leishmaniasis is still unavailable, but leishmanization, the injection of viable infective parasites in a controlled manner, is being used in some parts of the world as a means of preventing infection upon reexposure under field conditions.

Clinical Patterns

OLD WORLD *CL caused by L. major* CL is found in widely scattered parts of Asia, Africa, and Europe, largely in tropical and subtropical zones, and in much of the Middle East, especially Iran, Iraq, eastern Saudi Arabia, the Jordan Valley (of Israel and Jordan), and the Sinai Peninsula.

The disease begins as a small erythematous papule, which may appear immediately after the bite of the sandfly but usually appears 2 to 4 weeks later. The papule slowly enlarges in size (to 2 cm or more) over a period of several weeks and assumes a more dusky violaceous hue (Fig. 236-1). Eventually the lesion becomes crusted in the center. When the crust is removed, a shallow ulcer is found,

FIGURE 236-1

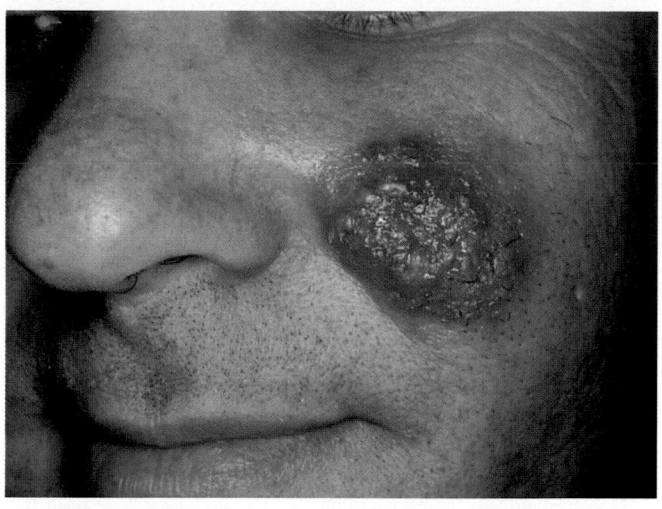

Cutaneous leishmaniasis. Large moist plaque on the cheek caused by *L. major.*

often with a raised and somewhat indurated border. In some cases the central part of the nodule becomes hyperkeratotic, and a firmly adherent horn develops over the lesion. Small satellite papules (Fig. 236-2) may also be found at the periphery of the lesion, and occasionally subcutaneous nodules develop along the course of the proximal lymphatics. Rarely, lesions become locally invasive and extend to subcutaneous tissue and even muscle. This latter occur-

FIGURE 236-2

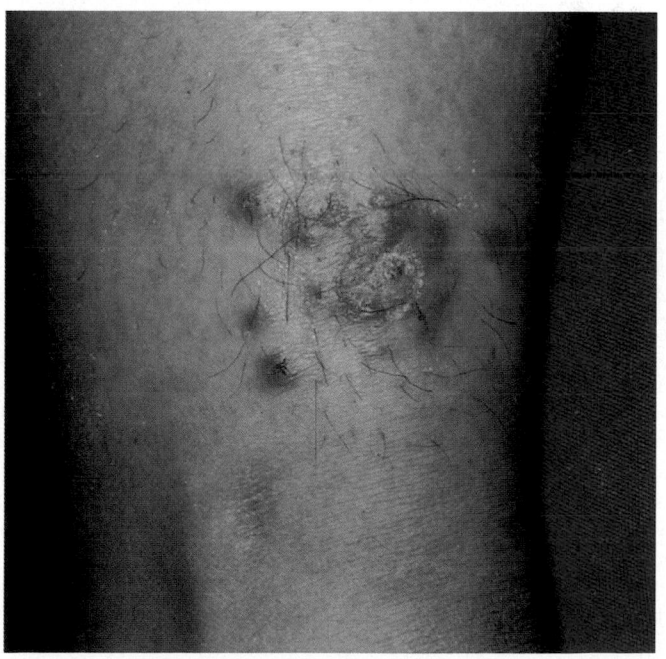

Cutaneous leishmaniasis, late plaque-stage. Central plaque with peripheral satellite papules (*L. major*) is seen near the ankle.

FIGURE 236-3

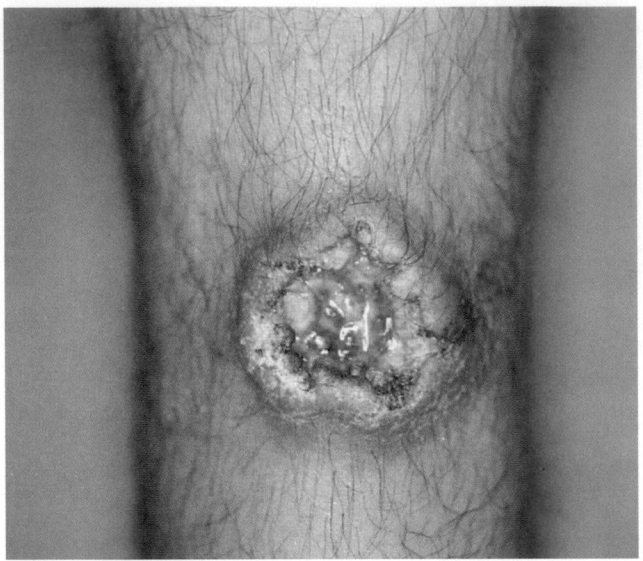

Cutaneous leishmaniasis, old world. A deep ulcerated lesion on the leg, caused by *L. major*, in a man with specific deficit in cell-mediated response to the parasite.

rence may be related to specific deficiencies in the host's immune response.

After the lesion has been present for 2 months or more, peripheral spread stops and the ulcerated nodule remains approximately the same size for another 3 to 6 months, or even longer (Fig. 236-3). The lesion then heals, usually leaving a slightly depressed scar. In some cases CL has been found to remain "active," i.e., with positive smears, for 24 months or even longer. Such cases have been designated *nonhealing chronic cutaneous leishmaniasis.*

The number of lesions that develop in *L. major* CL depends largely on the circumstances of exposure and the extent of the infection within the sandfly vector. Infection with *L. major* may result in multiple lesions (Fig. 236-4); up to 100 or more have been reported in a single individual. The reservoir for *L. major* is desert rodents, and the incidence of the disease is highest in areas close to the burrows of the infected animals.

CL caused by L. tropica CL caused by *L. tropica* is found in parts of southern Europe, Iran, Iraq, the Middle East, and the southern republics of the former USSR. The disease is more common in urban areas than is CL from *L. major*. *L. tropica* is largely a disease of humans, although there is recent evidence suggesting that rats also serve as a reservoir. The clinical pattern of *L. tropica* infection is similar to that of *L. major*, although lesions caused by *L. tropica* are more apt to be solitary and tend to be somewhat more inflammatory. Lesions due to *L. tropica* last longer and are usually more difficult to treat.

CL caused by L. infantum CL caused by *L. infantum* is found in countries bordering the Mediterranean, including southern Europe and northern Africa. The skin lesions are similar to those in the *L. major* form of the disease but their duration is usually shorter. Wild canines and dogs serve as the reservoir for *L. infantum*. Reports from endemic areas in Spain have shown that up to 20 percent

FIGURE 236-4

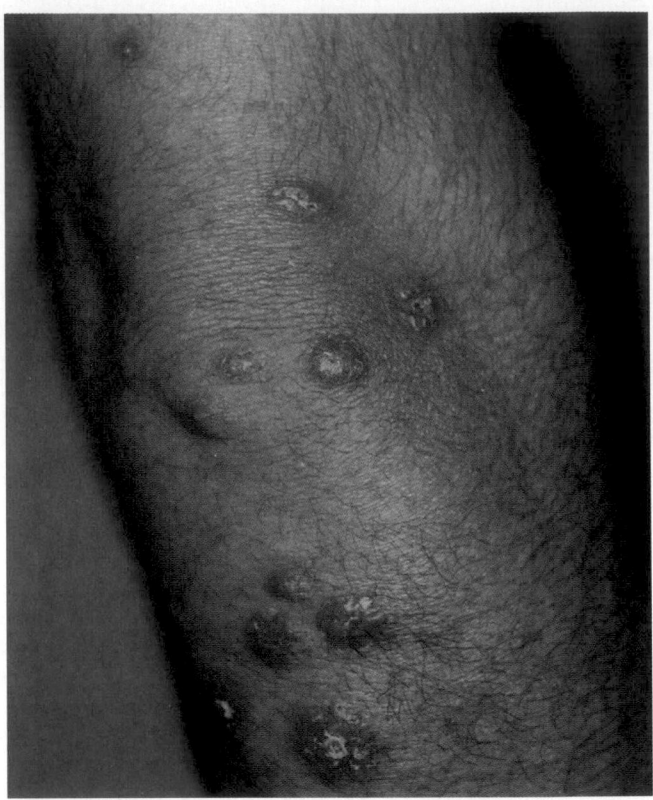

A.

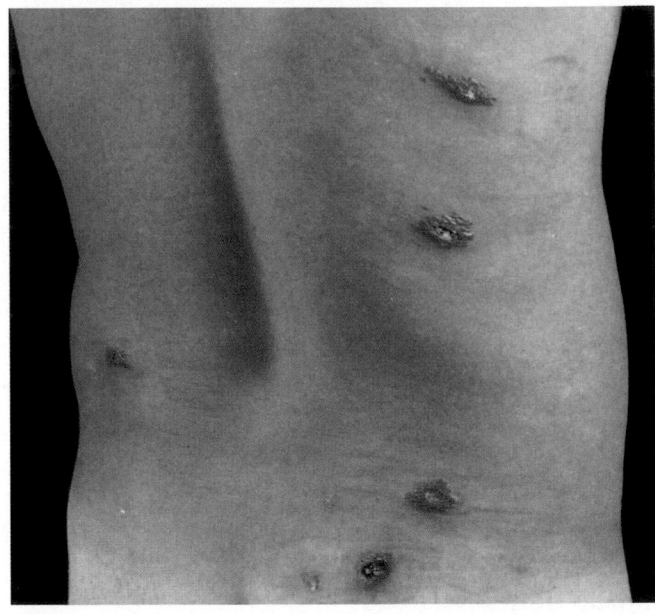

B.

Cutaneous leishmaniasis, multiple lesions. *A.* Multiple nodules on the legs caused by *L. major*. *B.* Multiple, nodular, ulcerated lesions on the trunk at the sites of sandfly bites.

of dogs tested for the presence of *L. infantum* were harboring parasites in the skin and in internal organs.

CL caused by L. aethiopica CL caused by *L. aethiopica* is found in Kenya, the Sudan, and Ethiopia. The common form of the disease seen in these areas is similar to CL caused by *L. major*.

However, in a significant number of patients, widespread skin involvement develops (DCL) that resembles lepromatous leprosy (see below).

NEW WORLD CL *CL caused by L. mexicana complex* In the new world the skin lesions of CL are caused by parasites of the *L. mexicana* complex. The disease is found in Mexico, Central America, as far north as Texas, and as far south as Brazil. The vectors for this form of CL are *Lutzomyia* sandflies. The lesions develop in a similar fashion to those caused by *L. major* in the old world. Generally, a small erythematous papule develops at the site of the bite of an infected sandfly and gradually develops into an ulcerated nodule. Eventually the lesion heals, leaving a depressed scar. Although lesions can develop on any part of the body, in Mexico and Central America sores characteristically involve the pinna of the ears (chiclero ulcers).

CL caused by L. braziliensis Most cases of CL caused by *L. braziliensis* are due to transmission from forest rodent to sandfly to human, with the latter serving as a sporadic host when entering into the habitat of the forest rodent reservoirs. The clinical symptoms of the cutaneous lesions are similar to those caused by the old world species of *Leishmania*, except that some of the strains of the *L. braziliensis* complex can invade the mucous membranes of the mouth, nose, pharynx, and larynx, giving rise to MCL (see below) (Fig. 236-5).

Histopathology[11]

In acute CL the epidermal changes are highly variable and can range from atrophy or ulceration to hyperplasia, which may be pseudo-epitheliomatous. The most constant feature is a diffuse dermal inflammatory cell infiltrate composed of varying proportions of histiocytes, lymphocytes, plasma cells, and neutrophils. Specific diagnosis requires the identification of amastigotes within the cytoplasm of dermal macrophages. In general, the number of parasites

present is inversely proportional to the duration of the lesion. The amastigotes measure from 2 to 4 μm and are a dull blue-gray color with hematoxylin and eosin (H&E) staining. Infected macrophages are usually present in clusters. Although the parasites are more apparent with Giemsa stain, in the authors' experience it is rare to find them with Giemsa stain if they are not visible with H&E. In some laboratories, an immunoperoxidase monoclonal antibody stain can be performed on paraffin sections and is sometimes more helpful than either H&E or Giemsa staining in locating amastigotes. The histology of a long-standing lesion of acute CL may resemble that of the chronic type.

In chronic CL the dermal infiltrate is nodular and is characterized by tuberculoid-type histiocytic granulomas with lymphocytes and plasma cells surrounding them. Amastigotes are usually not detectable. Necrosis rarely occurs. This histology generates a differential diagnosis that includes other causes of tuberculoid type granulomas such as lupus vulgaris, tuberculoid leprosy, and granulomatous rosacea. A specific diagnosis at this stage requires clinicopathologic correlation.

Diagnosis

PARASITOLOGIC DIAGNOSIS[12] The diagnosis of CL rests on finding parasites in the skin. The most effective method for detecting parasites is in a tissue smear from a lesion. Tissue smears are obtained by making a shallow slit in the skin with a no. 11 blade at the edge of the lesion. After staining with Giemsa, the amastigotes are seen as pale-blue oval bodies with a dark-blue nucleus and a small point-shaped kinetoplast within the cytoplasm of tissue macrophages. The organisms are enclosed in a membrane, which may be difficult to see within the histiocyte. Occasionally, abundant organisms are located in an extracellular location. These extracellular amastigotes are generally somewhat larger than the intracellular forms and often have an elongated profile.

Parasites can also be cultured from tissue fluid obtained from a lesion. The material is cultured in a biphasic medium, such as Novy-MacNeal-Nicolle (NNN), or a liquid medium, such as Schneider's insect culture medium, in the presence of fetal calf serum. Promastigote forms appear after several days and can be detected in the culture medium. Cultures should not be discarded as negative before 4 weeks. Strains that do not grow in culture media may be inoculated into susceptible animals, but this method is not very practical for routine diagnosis.

In regions of the world where more than one species of *Leishmania* is found, emphasis should be on species identification, since characterization of the parasite may influence treatment. PCR has proven useful for this purpose, and various groups have developed primers than can detect different parasite species, using very small amounts of tissue material.[13]

IMMUNOLOGIC DIAGNOSIS Although both circulating and cellular responses can be demonstrated during the course of the illness, animal studies have shown that protective immunologic reaction is based solely on cell-mediated immunity. Generally, tests of immune function are of more value in following the course of the disease than they are for diagnosis.

Enzyme-linked immunosorbent assays (ELISA) for circulating antibodies that use purified leishmanial products as the test antigen are available. Antibody levels are often elevated in the early stages of CL, but they are not considered a useful diagnostic sign.

FIGURE 236-5

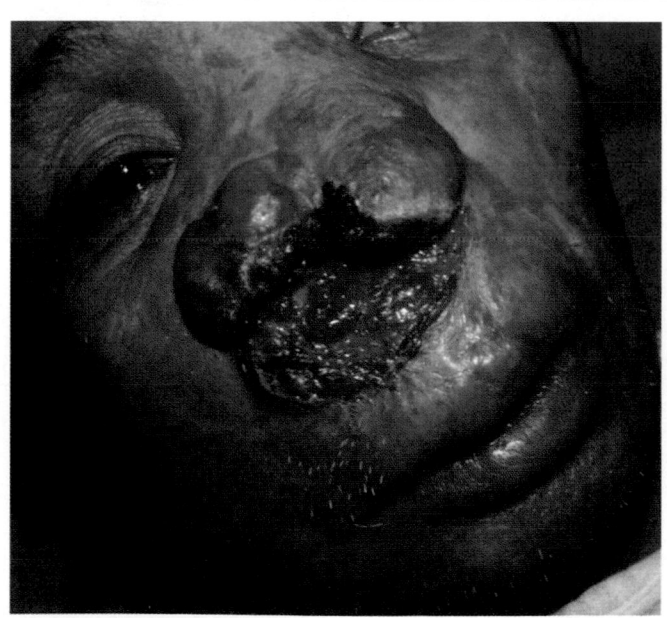

Mucocutaneous leishmaniasis, South American. Painful, mutilating ulceration with destruction of portions of the nose. (*Courtesy of Eric Kraus, MD.*)

The cell-mediated immune response can be measured by the leishmanin (Montenegro) skin test, in which phenol-killed preparations of promastigotes are injected into the dermis; the extent of the inflammatory response is measured at the end of 48 and 72 h. Biopsy of a positive Montenegro test at 72 h shows a diffuse cellular infiltrate in the upper dermis, with occasional histiocytes and eosinophils.

An in vitro lymphocyte proliferation assay for cell-mediated immunity is also available. In this test the proliferation of peripheral blood lymphocytes in response to a crude extract of promastigotes is measured after 6 days of incubation. Like the Montenegro test, this assay reflects both present and past infection.[14] The assay has proved useful in the diagnosis of CL in infants, where it is easier to obtain a drop of blood from a finger prick than a biopsy, especially when the face is involved.

Other Types of Leishmaniasis

DIFFUSE CUTANEOUS LEISHMANIASIS In both the old and new worlds, a form of CL is found in which large areas of the dermis become invaded by leishmania-containing macrophages, without a tendency to visceralization. In the old world, the disease is caused by *L. aethiopica*; DCL is found in 20 percent of leishmaniasis patients in Ethiopia and the Sudan. In South America, DCL is attributed to a poorly characterized member of the

L. braziliensis complex. DCL usually presents as a single nodule, which then spreads locally, often through extension from satellite lesions, and eventually by metastasis. In time, the process becomes widespread, with nonulcerating nodules appearing diffusely over the face and trunk; these lesions show a close clinical resemblance to lepromatous leprosy (Fig. 236-6*A*). DCL usually runs a protracted course but does not visceralize. It responds poorly to treatment. Parasites are abundant in skin smears and skin biopsies from DCL (Fig. 236-6*B*) and circulating antibodies are present, but tests for cell-mediated immune response, such as the Montenegro skin test and lymphocyte proliferation assay, are negative. There is still some question about the pathogenesis of this form of leishmaniasis, but most workers attribute it to deficiencies in the host's immune response, rather than to an especially virulent strain of leishmania.

MUCOCUTANEOUS LEISHMANIASIS MCL is characterized by involvement of both skin and the upper respiratory tract. The disease is caused by parasites of the *L. braziliensis* complex in South America and by *L. aethiopica* in Africa. In the form of the disease caused by *L. braziliensis braziliensis*, mucosal lesions develop from cutaneous lesions in more than 75 percent of those infected. However, in infections caused by less virulent species in the complex, such as *L. braziliensis guyanensis*, nasal involvement develops in only 5 percent of infected cases. In the old world, MCL can be found infrequently in patients infected by *L. aethiopica*. MCL begins with a cutaneous lesion that is identical to that of CL; a small red papule develops at the site of a sandfly bite and gradually enlarges, ulcerates, and finally heals. However, rather than showing

FIGURE 236-6

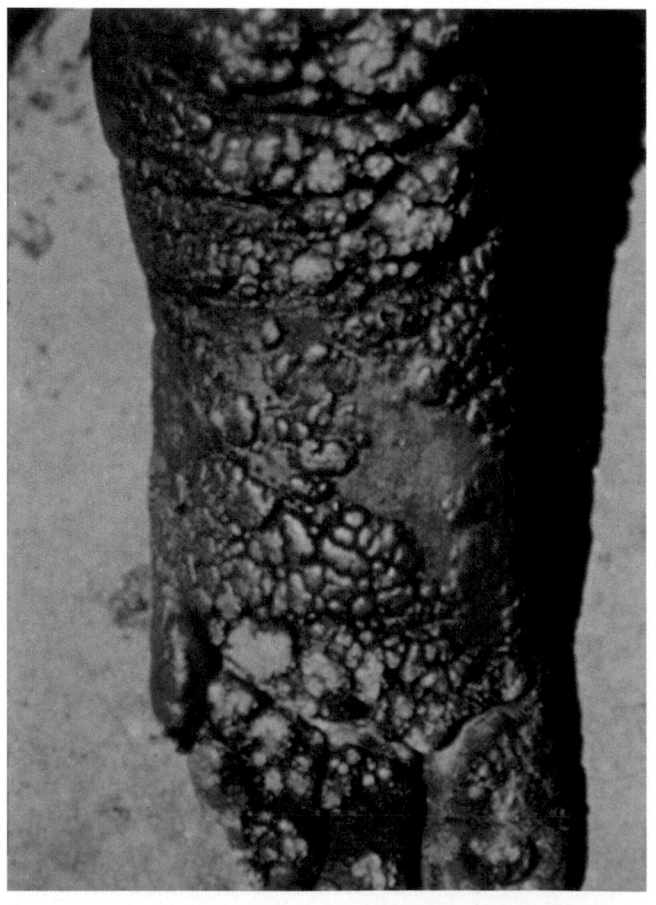

A.

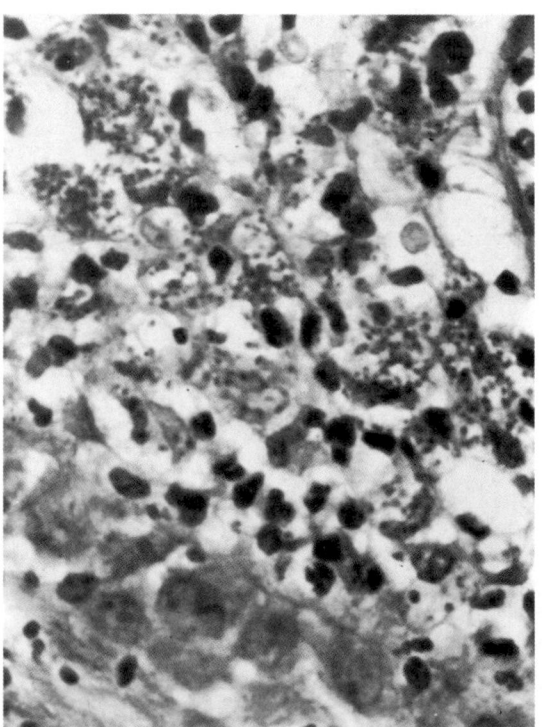

B.

Disseminated anergic cutaneous leishmaniasis. *A.* Confluent nodules on the foot resembling lepromatous leprosy; there was generalized cutaneous involvement as well. (*Courtesy of David Wyler, MD.*) *B.* Section of a nodule showing abundant leishmanial forms.

eventual resolution, as in CL, the infection extends to the mucosa and eventually to the cartilages of the upper respiratory tract, especially the nose, oral pharynx, and, rarely, the larynx (see Fig. 236-5). Edema and inflammatory changes occur that lead to epistaxis and coryzal symptoms. Eventually there is destruction of the cartilaginous structures in the area, including the nasal septum, the floor of the mouth, and the tonsilar areas. Bony structures are usually spared. The disease leads to marked disfigurement, known as *espundia* in South America. If this form of the disease is not arrested, death usually results from superimposed bacterial infection or pharyngeal obstruction leading to acute respiratory failure or malnutrition.

The diagnosis of MCL rests largely on clinical grounds. The parasites are often difficult to demonstrate or isolate from the mucosa of the respiratory tract.

VISCERAL LEISHMANIASIS In VL, also called *kala-azar*, the parasite establishes itself mainly in the bone marrow, spleen, and liver. The disease, if untreated, is often fatal, but in some areas many subclinical cases have been reported. It is a disease of all age groups. The disease is present in China, India, the former USSR, the Middle East, from east Africa through Sudan to west Africa, and across South America. The main *Leishmania* species involved are *L. donovani* in India and Africa, *L. infantum* in the Mediterranean countries, and *L. chagasi* in South America. In India the disease is transmitted directly from person to person by sandflies; post-kala-azar dermal leishmaniasis (PKADL; see below) may represent the human reservoir of the parasite. In other types of VL, foxes, jackals, and dogs are naturally infected, and humans are regarded as accidental hosts. The disease in this case is not believed to be transmitted directly from person to person. In India VL is mostly an urban disease; elsewhere it is mostly rural. As in CL, the incubation period may last from weeks to months; there is often a subacute febrile onset that may be so severe as to be fatal or so slight that it may be little remarked upon. The next symptom to appear is usually splenomegaly, then pancytopenia, fever, wasting, and serious imbalance of serum proteins. There is a high death rate among untreated cases.

Definite diagnosis of VL requires the demonstration of parasites; they can be detected in smears or cultures prepared from bone marrow biopsies or spleen aspirates, or in histologic sections from the spleen. Specific serologic tests are often positive in the acute stage of the disease, but cell-mediated immunity, both specific and nonspecific, are suppressed. This suppression is reversed after treatment and cure. Treatment with pentavalent antimonials (Pentostam) is usually effective against VL.

LESS COMMON FORMS OF LEISHMANIASIS *Leishmaniasis recidivans (LR)* LR is a distinctive form of chronic cutaneous leishmaniasis that is a complication of an *L. tropica* infection. The lesions of LR are characterized by dusky-red plaques, with active, spreading borders and healing centers, giving rise to gyrate and annular forms. LR most commonly affects the face and can cause tissue destruction and severe deformity. Generally, the smear and culture are negative, but the patients have a strongly positive leishmanin test, and tests for cell-mediated immunity are positive.

LR is difficult to treat, although intralesional injections of Pentostam have been reported to give good results in some cases.

Post-kala-azar dermal leishmaniasis PKADL is a sequel to VL that has apparently been cured spontaneously or following adequate treatment. The skin lesions appear a year or so after a course of therapy and consist of macular, papular, and nodular lesions on the face, trunk, and extremities. Many of the lesions take the form of hypopigmented macules and plaques. The nodules rarely ulcerate.

When the lesions are numerous, the clinical picture resembles lepromatous leprosy. *L. donovani* can be recovered from the skin lesions by culture, and smears are usually positive. PKADL develops in almost 20 percent of Indian patients treated for VL and to a lesser proportion among Ethiopian patients treated for VL caused by *L. aethiopica*.

Because there is no known animal reservoir for VL in India, it is thought that patients with PKADL serve as an important human reservoir for this disease.

Treatment

The treatment of leishmaniasis depends on the clinical form of the disease.[15] CL in the old world is usually self-limited and in most cases does not require specific treatment. Treatment in this form of the disease should be given for extensive lesions, especially involving the face, or for those lesions that invade deeper tissues. The most successful therapy consists of intralesional injections of Pentostam, usually administered at weekly intervals. Up to 1 mg/kg body weight of the drug may be injected in the borders of the lesions. For very extensive lesions, Pentostam is administered intravenously. Other measures that have been advocated for the treatment of CL include freezing, local heat, oral ketoconazole, and rifampicin. Trials using these modalities have not been properly controlled, however, and their efficacy is unconfirmed. A topically applied aminoglycoside antibiotic, paromomycin, is sometimes effective for the treatment of CL. Treatment of DCL usually requires parenteral pentostam.

AFRICAN TRYPANOSOMIASIS

Trypanosomiasis, also known as sleeping sickness, is a potentially fatal protozoan infection of the central nervous system that occurs in sub-Saharan Africa, in a band between N15° and S20°. It is estimated that 20,000 persons become infected each year, resulting in an annual death toll of 15,000.

The disease exists in two rather distinct forms: *Gambian trypanosomiasis* (West African sleeping sickness) is caused by the subspecies *Trypanosoma brucei gambiense*. This variety of sleeping sickness is found in the western regions of the continent and is characterized by a relatively slow progression of systemic involvement, leading to mental deterioration, somnolence, and progressive emaciation over a period of months or years. *Rhodesian trypanosomiasis*, caused by *T. b. rhodesiense* is endemic in the eastern regions of Africa and generally follows a more rapid course, with signs of an acute infection (fever, chills, arthralgias, and anemia) overlapping with a diffuse encephalopathy that generally ends fatally within a few months.

The parasites of both forms of trypanosomiasis are transmitted by the bite of male and female tsetse flies (*Glossina* spp.) These insects are vigorous fliers. They are active mainly during daylight hours and are attracted by dark clothing and moving objects.

In the western regions, endemic for *T. gambiense*, humans are the natural hosts. East African trypanosomiasis is a zoonosis, and reservoirs for this form of the disease include wild and domestic animals (such as antelope and cattle) as well as infected humans.[16]

Trypanosomiasis is found mainly in rural sections of Africa. In the west especially, outbreaks have followed periods of civil unrest, where massive displacement of local communities and a breakdown of public health facilities and insect control measures have occurred; during such outbreaks the disease may involve as many as 70 percent of the population in a given region. Because East Africa attracts more tourists than West Africa, visitors from America and Europe are more likely to contract the Rhodesian form of the disease.

Pathogenesis

Parasites that enter the skin following the bite of an infected fly remain within the local area for about 10 days, and then enter the bloodstream as trypomastigotes. In the blood the two subspecies of *T. brucei* are morphologically identical; they have an elongated body, 10 to 30 μm long, with a large central nucleus, a kinetoplast, and an undulating membrane that extends the length of the organism. A single flagellum emerges from the anterior end of the body. Some of the signs and symptoms of sleeping sickness are the direct result of the parasites, while other effects are related to circulating immune complexes.

Researchers have shown that the inability of an infected patient to mount a successful immune response stems from the parasites' ability to express distinct surface antigens (variant surface glycoproteins). Once the parasites enter the host's bloodstream, antibodies are produced that result in the clearing of the majority of trypanosomes. However, the surviving parasites undergo a series of antigenic variations, resulting in subsequent waves of parasitemia. Thus, the host is induced to manufacture antibodies that have little protective value, and the parasites are able to escape total immune elimination.

Clinical Features

GAMBIAN TRYPANOSOMIASIS   Three stages of the infection are recognized, although not all those infected demonstrate the complete range of symptoms. During the early stage, usually within a week after the bite of an infected fly, about one-third or fewer of patients will develop an inflammatory skin lesion at the site of inoculation. The lesion, known as a *trypanosome chancre*, is a local response to the proliferation of parasites in the dermis. It consists of a red or violaceous indurated nodule surrounded by a pinkish halo. It is tender and accompanied by regional adenopathy. Occasionally an eschar develops in the center of the lesion. The chancre persists for a few weeks and then disappears spontaneously.

During the second stage of the disease—6 to 8 weeks later—a transient macular or urticarial eruption develops, often showing an annular or irregular pattern. During this stage the patient begins to show evidence of systemic involvement, including fever, headache, arthralgias, malaise, and dizziness. Facial or peripheral edema may also be present. Winterbottom's sign (enlargement of lymph nodes along the posterior cervical chain) is a characteristic finding during this stage.

The third and final stage of the disease evolves slowly over a period of 2 to 3 years, with signs of central nervous system involvement, including lassitude, weakness, personality change, and apathy, that eventually progress to somnolence, coma, and death.

RHODESIAN TRYPANOSOMIASIS   Trypanosomiasis caused by *T. b. rhodesiense* follows a similar but more fulminant course. Skin involvement, in the early stages of the disease, occurs more commonly and tends to be more severe. A trypanosome chancre is found in more than half of those infected and is often more pronounced than in the Gambian form of the disease. Winterbottom's sign, however, is commonly absent. A transient macular eruption may occur in the second stage of the illness, along with fever, malaise, and headache.[17] There may also be edema of the hands and feet. Disseminated intravascular coagulation may complicate the clinical picture. The major feature characterizing East African sleeping sickness is the rapidity with which the systemic changes develop; trypanosomes enter the circulation within 2 or 3 weeks, and symptoms of central nervous system involvement, such as changes in behavioral and sleep patterns, may appear within 6 to 8 weeks. The Rhodesian form of trypanosomiasis may be fatal within months, even before marked changes of the central nervous system develop.[18]

Mild cases of both forms of trypanosomiasis have been reported among indigenous inhabitants, but generally the course of the disease is progressive and the ultimate prognosis is poor. Without treatment trypanosomiasis is regularly fatal.

Diagnosis

During the early stages the diagnosis of African trypanosomiasis depends on the identification of parasites in blood, bone marrow, or spinal fluid or in material aspirated from the skin lesion at the site of inoculation or from an enlarged lymph node. The parasites may be identified in thick or thin blood films, in tissue aspirates stained with Giemsa, or in unstained wet preparations, using high-power microscopy. Serologic tests, which may provide additional evidence of infection, are available, but are not diagnostic.

The early skin lesion of trypanosomiasis should be distinguished from the skin lesions of other infectious disorders seen in Africa, including tick-borne relapsing fever, cutaneous diphtheria, anthrax, and African spotted fever.[19]

Treatment

Suramin (naphthylamine sulfonic acid) or pentamidine are useful in the early stages of infection. Once central nervous system involvement has been confirmed, specific therapy consists either of melarsoprol B (a trivalent organic arsenical) or eflornithine (an ornithine decarboxylase inhibitor), given by intravenous injection, in slowly increasing doses.

Prior to a lumbar puncture, suramin is given intravenously to clear peripheral parasitemia.

AMERICAN TRYPANOSOMIASIS (CHAGAS' DISEASE)

American trypanosomiasis is a systemic disease caused by the pleomorphic trypanosome *Trypanosoma cruzi*. The disease affects nearly 20 million people, and it is estimated that about 100,000 persons are infected yearly. The annual death toll is over 43,000. The disease is found mainly in rural tropical and subtropical areas of Central and South America.

Chagas' disease is characterized by an acute phase with fever, tissue edema, lymphadenopathy, and diffuse acute myocarditis and by a chronic phase with cardiomyopathy and megacolon. Skin lesions with characteristic features may develop during the early stage of the illness.

Epidemiology

The disease is usually spread by the bite of the reduviid bug (the "cone-nosed" bug), although cases have recently been reported in which the infection was contracted via blood transfusions. The insect vectors (*Reduviidae* spp.) are 3 to 4 cm long and are recognized by their elongated "snout." They inhabit cracks found along the walls and floors of mud or wooden houses in rural areas and come out at night to feed.

Recently, a Chagas' disease control program has achieved remarkable success. The program, which consists of insecticide spraying of thatched and adobe houses, has reduced house infestation in Argentina by 75 percent and in Chile and Uruguay by 90 percent. It is expected that deaths from this disease will continue to drop, and perhaps the disease will be eliminated entirely early in the next century.

Pathogenesis

Trypanosomes exist in the epimastigote form in the gut of the insect vector, as free-living trypomastigotes in the bloodstream of a vertebrate host, and as amastigotes within tissue cells. The organisms are taken up by reduviid bugs during a blood meal and proliferate in the insects' hindgut. When the bugs feed again, epimastigotes are excreted on the skin surface in the insects' feces. From the skin surface, the epimastigotes invade the skin (or conjunctiva) through the bite wound or through an abrasion. Once the parasites invade the host skin, they are taken up by macrophages and other cells in the area. Within a short time, the amastigotes differentiate into trypomastigotes and are spread by way of the bloodstream to other organs and are found in macrophages of the spleen and the Kupffer cells of the liver. Organisms may persist for years in the heart and walls of the gastrointestinal tract, inducing both inflammatory and immunologic disturbances.[20,21]

Clinical Features

The cutaneous lesion that may develop early in the course of the illness at the site of inoculation consists of a small and often painful erythematous nodule, 1 to 3 cm in diameter, surrounded by a halo of edema, and associated with local adenopathy. Occasionally necrosis develops in the skin overlying the lesion, a presentation known as a *chagoma*. If inoculation occurs through the conjunctiva, or nearby on the face (a favorite location for the reduviid bug's blood meal), the resulting conjunctivitis and edema of the orbital area is known as *Romaña's sign*.

Signs of systemic involvement appear about a week after inoculation (between 4 and 12 days) and consist of fever, headache, generalized adenopathy, arthralgias, and malaise. During this stage of the illness a widespread and transient morbilliform eruption may also be seen, along with hepatosplenomegaly. Acute cardiac involvement (giving rise to hypotension and electrocardiographic changes) or acute meningoencephalitis may also be present.

The chronic phase of Chagas' disease may last 20 years or more. During this phase involvement of the heart and gastrointestinal tract is found, eventually leading to congestive failure and/or achalasia of the esophageal sphincter, megaesophagus, and megacolon.

Diagnosis

The diagnosis of American trypanosomiasis is suggested by the appearance of the characteristic chagoma or by Romaña's sign in patients living in endemic areas. The diagnosis is confirmed by finding

parasites in thick or thin blood smears, in material from a lymph node biopsy or aspirate, or in blood cultures. Skin biopsy from an involved area may also reveal amastigotes within macrophages.

Serologic tests for the presence of IgM anti-*T. cruzi* antibodies are positive early in the course of the disease. Complement fixation and hemagglutination tests are also available, but they are more useful in identifying cases during the chronic phase.

Treatment

Treatment during the acute phase consists of either benznidazole (a nitrimidazole) or nifurtimax (a nitrofuran). Both drugs may cause significant side effects. The management of patients with chronic infection is based on individual circumstances.[22]

CUTANEOUS AMEBIASIS

Amebae are unicellular protozoa that belong to the sub-phylum Sarcodina; they are characterized by pseudopod-dependent motility and by reproduction by binary fission. *Entamoeba histolytica*, the causative agent of intestinal amebiasis, occasionally invades the skin, causing cutaneous amebiasis.

It is estimated that as many as 48 million people worldwide (about 1 percent of the world's population) develop intestinal amebiasis each year, although not all cases are symptomatic. The death toll from amebiasis has been estimated at between 50,000 and 70,000 persons annually, mainly infants and children.

Amebiasis is found in all regions of the globe, but its prevalence is higher in the tropics and in rural areas, and especially in areas where sanitary conditions are poor. Skin involvement occurs infrequently, more commonly among malnourished individuals.[23]

Pathogenesis

Intestinal amebiasis is contracted by the ingestion of food or water contaminated with cyst forms of *E. histolytica*. Once inside the bowel, the cysts transform into trophozoites (ameba forms) and invade the intestinal wall, where the organisms may cause little or no irritation or may become invasive, penetrating through the mucosa into the muscular layers. In the cecum, appendix, or ascending colon, the organisms may cause ulcers and eventually perforations into the peritoneal cavity. *E. histolytica* amebae can also penetrate venules and lymphatics and be carried to the liver by the portal circulation to give rise to hepatic amebic abcesses.

If local conditions become unfavorable to the amebae, they encyst and are then capable of survival for long periods. Cysts usually do not induce clinical signs of disease, but they are important in the transmission of the disease by apparently healthy individuals.

Clinical Features

Cutaneous lesions in amebiasis are usually the result of direct invasion of the parasites into the skin from an underlying amebic abcess. Typical sites of involvement include the perianal area (as direct extension of rectal involvement) or the abdominal wall (at the outlet of a sinus draining an abcess in the colon or liver). The penis or vulva may become involved through direct transfer of parasites during intercourse. Amebic skin lesions have also been reported at sites of surgical incisions that were contaminated with amebae during a procedure to remove an abdominal or hepatic amebic abscess. Rarely, cutaneous lesions have been reported in more remote sites, such as the face, spread by autoinoculation.[24–26]

The skin lesion usually begins as an indurated pustule or as a localized area of redness that quickly becomes purulent, breaks down, and develops into a painful ragged ulcer with an erythematous halo. The lesions are often foul-smelling and covered by a layer of pus or necrotic tissue. The borders of the cutaneous lesions are raised and undermined, and regional lymphadenopathy is common. The ulcers tend to expand rapidly and can be especially destructive in children and in poorly nourished adults.

The course of the cutaneous lesions tends to be progressive, and large areas of tissue may be destroyed. Without treatment the disease usually ends fatally.

Diagnosis

The appearance of a rapidly enlarging, painful, and foul-smelling ulcer in a patient with a history of dysentery is suggestive of cutaneous amebiasis, and a careful search for trophozoites (ameba forms) within the border of the skin lesion should be carried out.

The diagnosis of cutaneous amebiasis is made by finding typical trophozoites in tissue scrapings or biopsy material from the border of an ulcer. The tissue is suspended in saline and examined under a microscope for the presence of amebae. The organisms measure 20 to 40 μm and show active movement of pseudopodia in fresh preparations. In biopsy specimens stained with H&E, the organisms are identified by their large size and finely granular pink cytoplasm. *E. histolytica* can be distinguished from nonpathogenic amebae by the presence of ingested erythrocytes within their cytoplasm.

Serologic tests for amebiasis are available, but they may not be positive until several weeks after tissue invasion. The presence of intestinal amebiasis should be confirmed by stool examinations.

Because the clinical features of cutaneous amebiasis are not specific, other causes of ragged-looking skin ulcers must be considered, including other infectious granulomas (such as syphilis, chancroid, and cutaneous tuberculosis) and malignancies.[27]

Treatment

In the past the standard treatment for cutaneous amebiasis has consisted of intramuscular injections of emetine (1 mg/kg daily, not to exceed 60 mg per day), but today newer "mixed" antiamebic agents (effective both in tissues and in the intestinal lumen) are replacing emetine. The most effective of these mixed amebicides are metronidazole and a nitroimidazole derivative, tinidazole.[28]

CUTANEOUS ACANTHAMEBIASIS

Accidental inoculation by free-living amebae (*Acanthamoeba* spp.) may cause granulomatous skin lesions. These parasites are usually introduced at a site of trauma from a contaminated environmental source, including streams, ponds, and swimming pools. Widespread cutaneous involvement may also occur in patients who are immunocompromised and have a disseminated form of the disease.[29]

The skin lesions of acanthamebiasis initially appear as indurated red or violaceous nodules or large pustules, which soon ulcerate. The histologic picture at the border of the ulcer is one of a granulomatous inflammation. The specific diagnosis depends on finding either cysts or trophozoites (ameba forms) in scrapings from the lesions or in biopsy specimens. In wet preparations, the trophozoites of *Acanthamoeba* are actively motile, and show small, pointed pseudopodia that continuously form and disappear.[30]

REFERENCES

1. Walters LL et al: Ultrastructural biology of *Leishmania (Viannia) panamensis (-Leishmania braziliensis panamensis)* in *Lutzomyia gomezi* (Diptera: Psychodidae): A natural host-parasite association. *Am J Trop Med Hyg* **40**:19, 1989
2. Lerner EA et al: Isolation of maxadilan, a potent vasodilatory peptide from the salivary glands of the sand fly *Lutzomyia longipalpis. J Biol Chem* **266**:11234, 1991
3. Hall LR, Titus RG: Sand fly vector saliva selectively modulates macrophage functions that inhibit killing of *Leishmania major* and nitric oxide production. *J Immunol* **155**:3501, 1995
4. Mauel J: Macrophage-parasite interactions in *Leishmania* infections. *J Leuk Biol* **47**:187, 1990
5. Muller I et al: Analysis of the cellular parameters of the immune responses contributing to resistance and susceptibility of mice to infection with the intracellular parasite, *Leishmania major. Immunol Rev* **112**:95, 1989
6. Bryceson ADM: Immunological aspects of cutaneous leishmaniasis, in *Essays on Tropical Dermatology,* edited by J Marshall. Amsterdam, Excerpta Medica, 1972, p 230
7. Reiner SL, Locksley RM: The regulation of immunity to *Leishmania major. Annu Rev Immunol* **13**:151, 1995
8. Stenger S et al: Tissue expression of inducible nitric oxide synthase is closely associated with resistance to *Leishmania major. J Exp Med* **180**:783, 1994
9. Stenger S et al: Reactivation of latent leishmaniasis by inhibition of inducible nitric oxide synthase. *J Exp Med* **183**:1501, 1996
10. Melby PC et al: In situ expression of interleukin-10 and interleukin-12 in active human cutaneous leishmaniasis. *FEMS Immunol Med Microbiol* **15**:101, 1996
11. Kurban AK et al: Histopathology of cutaneous leishmaniasis. *Arch Dermatol* **93**:396, 1966
12. Schnur LF, Jacobson RL: *Parasitological Techniques in the Leishmaniases.* London, Academic, 1987, vol 1, p 499
13. Eresh S et al: Identification and diagnosis of *Leishmania mexicana* complex isolates by polymerase chain reaction. *Parasitology* **109**:423, 1994
14. Frankenburg S: A simplified microtechnique for measuring human lymphocyte proliferation after stimulation with mitogen and specific antigen. *J Immunol Methods* **112**:177, 1988
15. Chong H: A look at trends in and approaches to the treatment of leishmaniasis. *Int J Dermatol* **25**:615, 1986
16. Spencer HC et al: Imported African trypanosomiasis in the United States. *Ann Intern Med* **82**:633, 1975
17. McGovern TW et al: Cutaneous manifestations of African trypanosomiasis. *Arch Dermatol* **131**:1178, 1995
18. Gelfand M: The early clinical features of rhodesiense trypanosomiasis with special reference to the "chancre" (local reaction.) *Trans R Soc Trop Med Hyg* **60**:376, 1966
19. Panosian CB et al: Fever, leukopenia, and a cutaneous lesion in a man who had recently traveled in Africa. *Rev Infect Dis* **13**:1130, 1991
20. DosReis GA: Cell-mediated immunity in experimental *Trypanosoma cruzi* infection. *Parasitol Today* **5**:355, 1997
21. Kierszenbaum F: Chronic chagasic tissue lesions in the absence of *Trypanosoma cruzi:* A proposed mechanism. *Parasitol Today* **12**:414, 1996
22. Luquetti AO: Etiological treatment for Chagas disease. *Parasitol Today* **13**:127, 1997
23. Fujiita WH et al: Cutaneous amebiasis. *Arch Dermatol* **117**:309, 1981
24. Biagi FF, Martuscelli AQ: Cutaneous amebiasis in Mexico. *Dermatologica Tropica* **2**:129, 1963
25. Mendoza JB, Barba EJR: Cutaneous amebiasis of the face: A case report. *Am J Trop Med Hyg* **35**:69, 1986
26. Rimsza ME, Berg RA: Cutaneous amebiasis. *Pediatrics* **71**:595, 1983

27. MhLanga BR et al: Amebiasis complicating carcinomas: A diagnostic dilemma. *Am J Trop Med Hyg* **46**:759, 1992
28. Martinez-Palomo A, Cantellano ME: Update on antiamebic agents development: Clinical results and experience, in *Burger's Medicinal Chemistry and Drug Discovery,* edited by ME Wolff. New York, Wiley, 1997, pp 453–457
29. May LP et al: Diagnosis of *Acanthamoeba* infection by cutaneous manifestations in a man seropositive to HIV. *J Am Acad Dermatol* **26**:352, 1992
30. Wurtman PD: Acanthamoeba infection. *Int J Dermatol* **35**:48, 1996

CHAPTER 237

Leslie C. Lucchina
Mary E. Wilson

Cysticercosis and Other Helminthic Infections

While most parasitic diseases occur sporadically in the United States, parasitic diseases are a common cause of morbidity and mortality worldwide, particularly in tropical and developing countries. Common parasitic infections include ascariasis, cysticercosis (the most common parasitic infection of the central nervous system), enterobiasis, hookworm disease, lymphatic filariasis, onchocerciasis, and schistosomiasis. Because of the increase in global migration of populations—including immigration of persons from tropical countries to the United States, travel, and prolonged visits of people from industrialized to tropical regions—the dermatologist must be familiar with skin manifestations of parasitic diseases (Table 237-1).

For many helminthic infections, skin lesions may provide important diagnostic clues (Tables 237-2 to 237-5). A thorough history taking and physical examination are essential. The patient history

TABLE 237-1

Summary of Helminths Included in this Chapter

Helminth(s)	Disease	Portal of Entry	Source of Infection
Ancylostoma braziliense, other	Cutaneous larva migrans	Skin	Larvae from animal feces in soil
Ancylostoma duodenale, Necator americanus	Hookworm	Skin, usually feet	Larvae in soil
Ascaris lumbricoides	Ascariasis	Gastrointestinal (mouth)	Eggs from contaminated food, soil
Dirofilaria species	Dirofilariasis	Skin	Larvae in mosquito
Dracunculus medinensis	Dracunculiasis	Gastrointestinal	Infective copepods in water
Echinococcus species	Echinococcosis	Gastrointestinal	Eggs from animal (usually dog) feces
Enterobius vermicularis	Enterobiasis (pinworm)	Gastrointestinal	Eggs in environment
Fasciola species	Fascioliasis	Gastrointestinal (mouth)	Metacercariae on plants, in water
Gnathostoma spinigerum, other	Gnathostomiasis	Gastrointestinal (mouth)	Larvae in animal flesh
Loa loa	Loiasis	Skin	Infective fly
Onchocerca volvulus	Onchocerciasis	Skin	Infective *Simulium* fly
Paragonimus westermani, other	Paragonimiasis	Gastrointestinal (mouth)	Metacercariae in seafood
Wuchereria bancrofti, other	Filariasis	Skin	Infective mosquitoes
Schistosoma mansoni, other	Schistosomiasis	Skin	Cercariae in water
Schistosomes, nonhuman	Cercarial dermatitis	Skin	Cercariae in water
Spirometra species	Sparganosis	Gastrointestinal (mouth)	Larvae in copepod or in animal flesh
Strongyloides stercoralis	Strongyloidiasis	Skin	Larvae in soil, feces
Toxocara canis, other	Visceral larva migrans	Gastrointestinal	Eggs in soil
Trichinella spiralis	Trichinosis	Gastrointestinal	Larvae in animal flesh
Taenia multiceps, other	Coenurosis	Gastrointestinal	Eggs (from animal feces) in food, water
Taenia solium	Cysticercosis	Gastrointestinal	Eggs from feces

TABLE 237-2

Helminthic Causes of Dermatologic Nodules and Cysts

Disease	Helminth(s)	Comments
Coenurosis	Several species of *Multiceps*	
Cutaneous larva migrans	Primarily *Ancylostoma braziliense* and *A. caninum*	Larvae of dog and cat hookworms
Cysticercosis	*Taenia solium*	May be multiple
Dirofilariasis	*Dirofilaria immitis* and other *Dirofilaria* species	
Dracunculiasis	*Dracunculus medinensis*	
Echinococcosis	*Echinococcus granulosus* and *E. multilocularis*	
Fascioliasis	*Fasciola hepatica* and *F. gigantica*	
Filariasis, lymphatic	*Brugia malayi*, *B. timori*, and *Wuchereria bancrofti*	Mass in scrotum
Gnathostomiasis	*Gnathostoma spinigerum* and other *Gnathostoma* species	
Loiasis	*Loa loa*	Inflammatory swellings
Onchocerciasis	*Onchocerca volvulus*	Painless, mobile, dermal nodules
Paragonimiasis	Primarily *Paragonimus westermani*	
Schistosomiasis	*Schistosoma haematobium*, *S. intercalatum*, *S. japonicum*, *S. mansoni*, and *S. mekongi*	Verrucous, vegetating
Sparganosis	*Spirometra erinaceri*, *S. mansoni*, *S. mansonoides*, and *S. proliferum*	
Visceral larva migrans	*Toxocara canis* and much less frequently, *Toxocara catis*	

Tables 237-2 to 237-5 are modified and reprinted with permission from: Wilson ME. *A World Guide to Infections: Diseases, Distribution, Diagnosis.* New York, Oxford University Press, 1991

TABLE 237-3

Helminthic Cause of Ulcerative Dermatologic Lesions

Disease	Helminth(s)	Comments
Dracunculiasis	*Dracunculus medinensis*	Ulcer at site of eruption of worm

should include exact geographic location(s) and durations of stay, means of transportation, occupation, lifestyle, housing, dietary habits (food and water), clothing and shoes worn, exposures (beach, fresh or salt water, insects, plants, animals), personal contacts, other family members, fellow travelers or persons in areas previously lived in or visited with similar signs and symptoms, use of preventive measures (insect repellent, mosquito netting), and any known recent outbreaks or diseases endemic to geographic areas previously lived in or visited. The history should also include a thorough review of medications and other preparations (including herbal and local treatments) that the patient may have used. The dermatologic history should include any alterations in skin integrity and underlying skin diseases prior to presentation, description of initial presentation and progression of lesions, time of onset relative to potential exposures, durations of lesions, anatomic distribution and any associated local and systemic signs and symptoms.

The laboratory and diagnostic evaluation of a patient with a suspected helminthic infection is based on the history and clinical findings. Most helminthic infections are associated with a peripheral eosinophilia; however, the peripheral eosinophilia may be low-grade or absent (Table 237-6). Other laboratory (including serology and biopsy of skin lesions for identification of the parasite) and radiologic studies may be warranted depending on the suspected parasite. There are a number of general references for further information.[1-14]

TABLE 237-4

Helminthic Causes of Migratory Dermatologic Lesions

Disease	Helminth(s)	Comments
Cutaneous larva migrans	Primarily *Ancylostoma braziliense* and *A. caninum*	Larvae of dog and cat hookworms
Dracunculiasis	*Dracunculus medinensis*	Movement of worm just below dermis before eruption
Fascioliasis	*Fasciola hepatica* and *F. gigantica*	Migratory areas of inflammation, especially with *F. gigantica*
Gnathostomiasis	*Gnathostoma spinigerum* and other *Gnathostoma* species	Migratory inflammatory lesions, 1 cm/h or faster when subcutaneous
Hookworm	*Ancylostoma duodenale*, *Necator americanus*, and *A. ceylanicum*	
Loiasis	*Loa loa*	Migratory inflammatory swellings; worm may be visible crossing conjunctivae
Paragonimiasis	Primarily *Paragonimus westermani*	Subcutaneous migratory swelling or subcutaneous nodules
Sparganosis	*Spirometra erinaceri*, *S. mansoni*, *S. mansonoides*, and *S. proliferum*	
Strongyloidiasis	*Strongyloides stercoralis*	Migratory, serpiginous lesions (larva currens), 5–10 cm/h

TABLE 237-5

Helminthic Causes of Pruritic Lesions*

DISEASE	HELMINTH(S)	DIAGNOSTIC TEST
Cercarial dermatitis (schistosome dermatitis)	Species of avian and small mammal schistosomes	
Cutaneous larva migrans	Primarily *Ancylostoma braziliense* and *A. caninum*	
Dracunculiasis	*Dracunculus medinensis*	Identification of discharged motile larvae
Enterobiasis	*Enterobius vermicularis*	Identification of eggs and adult worms with perianal tape test
Fascioliasis	*Fasciola hepatica* and *F. gigantica*	Identification of eggs in stool, duodenal contents, and bile. Excision and identification of adult worm in ectopic sites
Gnathostomiasis	*Gnathostoma spinigerum* and other *Gnathostoma* species	Identification of larvae in surgical specimen
Hookworm	*Ancylostoma duodenale, Necator americanus,* and *A. ceylanicum*	Identification of eggs in stool
Loiasis	*Loa loa*	Extraction and identification of adult worm, e.g., from conjunctivae. Serologic tests are also available by special arrangement
Onchocerciasis	*Onchocerca volvulus*	Identification of microfilariae in skin snip or of adult worm in excised nodule
Schistosomiasis	*Schistosoma haematobium, S. intercalatum, S. japonicum, S. mansoni,* and *S. mekongi*	Identification of eggs in urine, feces, or in biopsy specimens, Serologic tests
Strongyloidiasis	*Strongyloides stercoralis*	Identification of larvae in stool, small bowel contents, rarely in sputum, peritoneal fluid, urine, cerebrospinal fluid, or pleural fluid
Visceral larva migrans	*Toxocara canis* and much less frequently, *Toxocara catis*	Identification of larvae in tissue

*In the helminthic infections, parasites and eggs are not often in stool when skin lesions appear. Also, pruritus may be transient or intermittent. All helminthic infections may cause urticaria.

ASCARIASIS[15-17]

Synonyms

Roundworm infection, ascaridiasis

Etiology

Ascariasis is caused by *Ascaris lumbricoides* and occasionally by *Ascaris suum*, the pig roundworm. *A. lumbricoides* is the largest intestinal nematode with the female measuring 20 to 35 cm in length and 3 to 6 mm thick and the male measuring 11 to 22 cm in length.

Life Cycle

Humans are the only host of *A. lumbricoides.* The life cycle is described below.

Pathogenesis

After a human ingests the eggs, larvae emerge from eggs in the duodenum and penetrate the intestinal wall via the mesenteric lymphatics and venules. Five to fourteen days after ingestion, the larvae reach the heart, lungs, trachea, and pharynx. Swallowed larvae reach the intestines (primarily jejunum), and mature into adults (within 60 to 75 days) capable of producing eggs that are passed in the feces. Under the appropriate environmental conditions (temperature, humidity), these eggs embryonate over the course of 2 to 4 weeks. If the infective eggs are ingested by another human, the cycle repeats.

Geographic Distribution

Ascariasis is found worldwide. The number of persons infected may be as high as 1.3 billion. The highest rates of infection are in children, in hot and humid climates, and in areas with crowding and poor sanitation. Clay soils are especially suited for the survival of *Ascaris* species.

Epidemiology

ACQUISITION Infection is acquired by the ingestion of infective eggs in soil contaminated with human feces. Such soil may contaminate fruits, vegetables, water, and hands. Infection may also occur through the inhalation of eggs in dust, carried into homes on footwear, and on dog fur. In some areas prevalence of infection exceeds 90 percent.

INCUBATION PERIOD AND TIME FRAME Pulmonary symptoms and eosinophilia may begin 10 to 14 days after ingestion of eggs. Gastrointestinal symptoms may precede the shedding of eggs in feces, which begins 50 to 75 days after ingestion of infective eggs. Initial symptoms may be noted weeks or months after onset of infection. Most adult worms survive 8 to 12 months, and occasionally as long as 24 months.

Clinical Features

The dermatologic manifestation is urticaria, although the majority of infections are asymptomatic or mild. The rare fatalities occur primarily in children with heavy worm burdens. Patients may have a cough, wheezing, fever, and vague gastrointestinal symptoms. Complications are associated with intestinal obstruction by worms, usually in the terminal ileum. Migration of the adult worm can

TABLE 237-6

Helminthic Infections and Eosinophilia

DISEASE	PRIMARY ANATOMIC LOCATION(S)	COMMENT REGARDING EOSINOPHILIA
Ascariasis	Gastrointestinal; lung (larvae)	Moderate- to high-grade during larval migration, often absent with adult worm
Cercarial dermatitis (Schistosome dermatitis)	Skin	
Coenurosis	Many, including central nervous system	May be low-grade, absent
Cysticercosis	Many, including central nervous system, soft tissues	May be low-grade, absent
Dirofilariasis	Lung, subcutaneous	May be low-grade, absent
Echinococcosis	Liver, lung, central nervous system, other	May be low-grade, absent
Fascioliasis	Hepatobiliary	High-grade early, may wax and wane in chronic infection
Filariasis, lymphatic	Blood, lymphatics	May be low-grade/absent, high-grade in tropical pulmonary eosinophilia
Gnathostomiasis	Subcutaneous, other tissues	May be high-grade, may wax and wane in chronic infection
Hookworm	Skin (transient), gastrointestinal, lung (larvae)	High-grade during larval migration, low/moderate in persistent infection
Loiasis	Subcutaneous, eye	High-grade, especially in expatriates
Onchocerciasis	Skin, subcutaneous, eye	Can be high-grade, normal in up to 30 percent
Paragonimiasis	Lung, central nervous system, subcutaneous	High-grade in early infection, low-grade or absent in late infection
Schistosomiasis	Liver, gastrointestinal, rare central nervous system	May be high-grade in early infection, low-grade or absent in late infection
Schistosomiasis due to S. haematobium	Urinary tract, rare central nervous system	Same as above
Sparganosis	Subcutaneous, multiple sites	May be low-grade, absent
Strongyloidiasis	Gastrointestinal, lung (larvae), skin (episodic)	High-grade during larval migration, low- to moderate-grade in chronic infection
Trichinosis	Gastrointestinal (early), muscle, central nervous system	High-grade during acute infection, absent in late infection
Visceral larva migrans	Liver, eye, lung (larvae)	Moderate- to high-grade, may persist for months or longer

perforate the bowel wall, obstruct biliary or pancreatic ducts, or be associated with acute appendicitis. Cases involving migration of a worm to the eye, brain, and heart have been reported. General anesthesia and fever may precipitate migration of adult worms.

Partial immunity follows infection, but reinfection is common.

Laboratory

A peripheral eosinophilia may accompany the stage of pulmonary migration.

Diagnosis

The diagnosis is usually made by finding eggs in feces. Diagnosis can also follow identification of the adult worm in stool, pharynx, or operative specimen. Rarely, larvae will be found in sputum or on gastric lavage. Transient bilateral infiltrates on chest x-ray films are seen early in infection. Gastrointestinal barium contrast study will reveal a filling defect.

Differential Diagnosis

The differential diagnosis of the skin findings includes causes of acute and chronic urticaria.

Treatment

Treatment options include mebendazole, pyrantel pamoate, or albendazole.

Prevention

Prevention includes proper waste disposal and avoidance of ingestion of fecally contaminated soil. Embryonated eggs can remain viable in soil for years.

CERCARIAL DERMATITIS[18–21]

Synonyms

Clam digger's dermatitis, schistosome dermatitis, sedge pool itch, swimmer's itch

Etiology

Cercarial dermatitis (Fig. 237-1) is caused by infestation of the skin by cercariae (larvae) of nonhuman schistosomes whose usual hosts are birds and small mammals. Many nonhuman schistosomes have been implicated including: *Trichobilharzia, Gigantobilharzia, Or-*

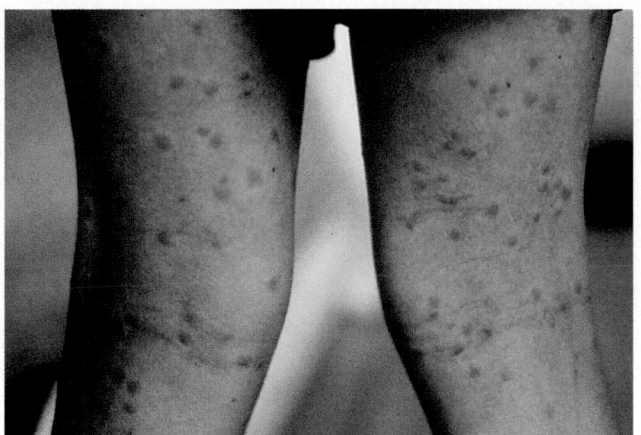

Cercarial dermatitis. (*Courtesy of Jay S. Keystone, MD, FRCPC.*)

nithobilharzia, Microbilharzia, and *Schistosomatium*. Also, see the section on "Schistosomiasis."

Life Cycle

The life cycle includes a primary host (e.g., finch, marshbird, mouse, muskrat, vole, waterfowl) for the adult schistosome. Eggs produced by adult schistosomes living in animals are shed with animal feces into the environment.

On reaching water, the schistosome eggs hatch, releasing miracidia (fully developed larvae). If the miracidia reach appropriate snail hosts (e.g., *Lymnaeidae* and *Physidae*) before dying, they penetrate the snail and mature in its digestive gland as sporocysts. After 4 to 6 weeks of maturation, they emerge from the snail as forktailed cercariae, which must penetrate the skin of a vertebrate host to continue development. Humans cannot support the development of these schistosomes, and hence are incidental, dead-end hosts.

Pathogenesis

The free-swimming, fork-tailed stage of the parasite, the cercariae, penetrate intact human skin and die without invading other tissues. The schistosomes elicit an inflammatory response. Schistosomes capable of causing invasive disease in humans (e.g., *Schistosoma mansoni, S. haematobium*, and *S. japonicum*) may cause a similar skin eruption shortly after penetration as well as late visceral complications as discussed later in this chapter.

Geographic Distribution

The geographic distribution of cercarial dermatitis is worldwide involving fresh and salt water that is inhabited by the appropriate molluscan hosts. Sporadic reports come from all continents.

Epidemiology

ACQUISITION Cercarial dermatitis is acquired by skin exposure to fresh or salt water infested with cercariae. It occurs in swimmers and in people whose occupations lead to water exposures (e.g., paddy workers, rice farmers, clam diggers).

INCUBATION PERIOD AND TIME FRAME Typically, pruritus and skin changes begin within hours of exposure. In persons with previous exposures to cercariae, the rash may begin sooner and may be more severe. The eruption peaks in two to three days and usually resolves over 1 to 2 weeks. Occasionally, lesions first appear days after the exposure.

Clinical Features

A prickling sensation begins during or within minutes of exposure to the cercariae. Approximately 1 hour later, a pruritic, erythematous macular eruption develops that persists for several hours. Ten to fifteen hours after exposure, papular, papulovesicular, and urticarial lesions develop, with marked pruritus. Purpura may develop as well. The distribution of the eruption includes skin surfaces that were exposed to the water and typically spares parts of the body that were covered by clothing. The severity of the eruption increases with repeat exposures. Secondary bacterial infection can complicate the dermatitis.

Laboratory

Laboratory studies are not performed in most instances because process is self-limited. Biopsy of skin lesions will show an inflammatory infiltrate with eosinophils.

Diagnosis

The diagnosis is usually based on characteristic clinical findings and appropriate epidemiologic exposures. Documenting presence of schistosomal cercariae in epidemiologically incriminated water provides supportive evidence.

Differential Diagnosis

The differential diagnosis includes seabather's eruption; contact dermatitis due to marine plants, hydroids and corals; insect bites; and causes of urticaria.

Treatment

Cercarial dermatitis resolves without specific antiparasitic therapy. Systemic antihistamines and topical steroids may reduce the symptoms. Systemic steroids have been used in severe cases.

Prevention

Cercarial dermatitis is prevented by avoidance of contaminated water. If contact does occur, vigorous towel drying as soon as the swimmer leaves the water may reduce the penetration of the cercariae.

COENUROSIS[22,23]

Synonyms

Disease in sheep is named gid and staggers.

Etiology

Coenurosis is caused by the larval stages of several species of *Multiceps*, a cestode (tapeworm). Some authors consider these parasites to belong to the genus *Taenia*. The species most often causing human disease are *M. (Taenia) multiceps, M. (Taenia) serialis*, and *M. (Taenia) brauni*.

Life Cycle

Definitive hosts are the dog, fox, and wolf. Eggs shed in the feces by the infected definitive host are ingested by the intermediate host, herbivorous mammals such as sheep (most commonly), antelope, cattle, gazelle, goat, horse, monkeys, and rarely, humans. In the intermediate host the parasite develops into the larval stage in various tissues that are eaten by the definitive hosts to complete the cycle.

Pathogenesis

In humans, oncospheres hatch from ingested eggs in the intestine, penetrate the intestinal wall, and may reach many parts of the body, including the central nervous system, subcutaneous muscle tissue, and eye. In these tissues, the larval stage (coenurus) develops. Degenerating or dying larvae provoke an inflammatory reaction and fibrosis.

Geographic Distribution

Reported human cases are sporadic and rare, with the majority from Africa. Infections have been described in Asia, Europe, and North America, particularly in areas where sheep are common. In tropical Africa, infections are more commonly located in subcutaneous or muscle tissue, or the eye and orbit (particularly in children). In nontropical Africa, infections occur primarily in the central nervous system of adults.

Epidemiology

ACQUISITION Humans acquire coenurosis by ingesting eggs in water or food or on contaminated fingers.

INCUBATION PERIOD AND TIME FRAME The incubation period is months. The disease may be present for years before the infection is recognized. Limited information suggests that the pathogen may survive in the human for at least 15 years.

Clinical Features

Soft-tissue coenurosis typically presents as a subcutaneous or intramuscular nodule that is a solitary unilocular cyst. Size varies from 2 to 6 cm in diameter. The lesion is often painless. The anatomic locations most commonly include the trunk, intercostal region, and anterior abdominal wall, though cysts on the head, neck, and limbs have been described.

The parasite has a tropism for the eye and central nervous system. In these sites, signs and symptoms reflect the presence of a mass lesion. Systemic signs and symptoms are usually absent.

Laboratory

There is usually no peripheral eosinophilia.

Diagnosis

CT or MRI may be useful to define the exact location of the mass lesion. Definitive diagnosis requires histologic examination of tissues and identification of the parasite. Currently specific serologic tests are not available.

Differential Diagnosis

The differential diagnosis of coenurosis includes cysticercosis, echinococcosis, epidermal inclusion cyst, lipoma, ganglion, and neurofibroma. In the central nervous system, the differential diagnosis includes that of space occupying lesions including neurocysticercosis and cerebral echinococcosis.

Treatment

Complete surgical excision is curative. Follow-up physical examinations for further cysts is important.

The prognosis depends on the location and extent of the cysts.

Prevention

Prevention includes avoiding close contact with infected animals and food contaminated with their feces. Praziquantel may be useful in treating infected sheep.

CUTANEOUS LARVA MIGRANS (CLM)[24-28]

Synonyms

Creeping eruption, creeping verminous dermatitis, sandworm eruption, plumber's itch, duckhunter's itch. Term describes a clinical finding caused by several different parasites.

Etiology

CLM (Fig. 237-2) is caused most often by larvae of hookworms (nematodes) of dogs, cats and other mammals. *Ancylostoma braziliense* is the most common cause. Other skin penetrating nematode larvae that produce CLM include *A. caninum, Uncinaria stenocephala* (hookworm of European dogs), and *Bunostomum phlebotomum* (hookworm of cattle). Filariform larvae of *Strongyloides stercoralis* can penetrate the skin (usually on the buttocks) and cause similar lesions, larva currens. CLM usually refers to lesions produced by nonhuman hookworms, but other parasites, including *Gnathostoma spinigerum, Strongyloides procyonis, Dirofilaria repens, Fasciola hepatica*, and some forms of myiasis can cause migratory skin lesions.

Life Cycle

The human is usually an aberrant, dead-end host who acquires the parasite from an environment contaminated with animal feces. The infective larvae may remain viable in soil for several weeks.

FIGURE 237-2

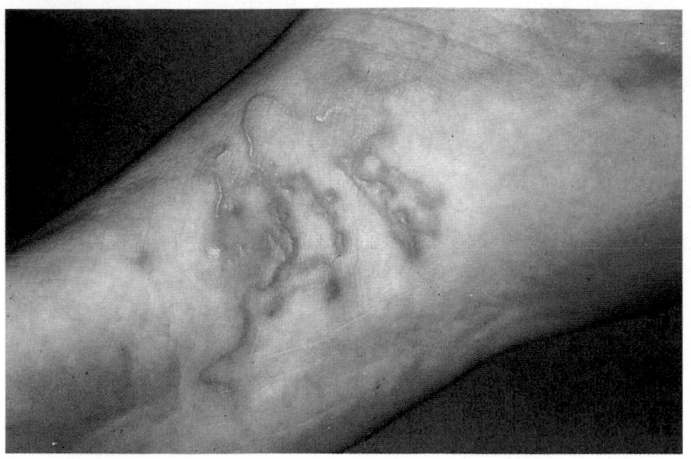

Cutaneous larva migrans. (*Courtesy of Jay S. Keystone, MD, FRCPC.*)

Pathogenesis

Third-stage larvae penetrate human skin and migrate up to several centimeters a day, usually between the stratum germinativum and stratum corneum. This induces a localized eosinophilic inflammatory reaction. Most larvae are unable to undergo further development or to invade deeper tissues and die after days to months.

Geographic Distribution

CLM is widely distributed and most commonly found in tropical and subtropical areas, especially the southeastern United States, Caribbean, Africa, Central and South America, India, and Southeast Asia.

Epidemiology

ACQUISITION CLM is acquired by skin contact with the infective larvae in the soil. Activities that pose a risk include contact with sand or soil contaminated with animal feces, such as playing in a sandbox, walking barefoot on a beach, and working in crawl spaces under houses.

INCUBATION PERIOD AND TIME FRAME The time from exposure to onset of symptoms is usually a few (1 to 6) days. The eruption usually lasts between 2 and 8 weeks, though rarely has been reported to last up to 2 years.

Clinical Features

The lesions are characteristically erythematous, raised and vesicular (Fig. 237-3), linear or serpentine. Lesions are approximately 3 mm wide and may reach 15 to 20 cm in length. Lesions can be single or multiple and are intensely pruritic and may be painful. The hookworm advances a few millimeters to a few centimeters daily. The most common anatomic sites (usually 3 to 4 cm from the penetration site) include the feet, buttocks, and genitalia. Involvement of the oral mucosa has been described. Excoriation and impetiginization are common. Systemic signs and symptoms (wheezing, dry cough, urticaria) have been reported in patients with extensive infection. *A. caninum* larvae can migrate to the small intestine and cause eosinophilic enteritis.

FIGURE 237-3

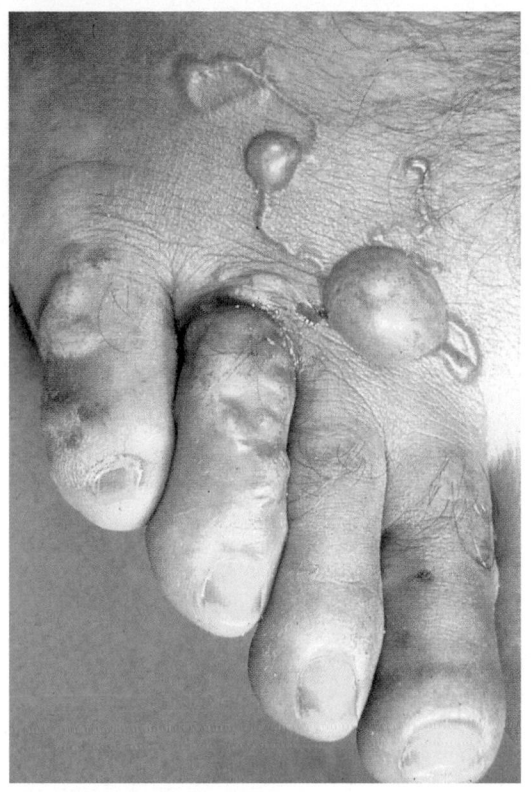

Cutaneous larva migrans. (*Courtesy of Jay S. Keystone, MD, FRCPC.*)

Laboratory

There may be a transient peripheral eosinophilia.

Diagnosis

Diagnosis of CLM is based on characteristic clinical findings as well as known epidemiologic exposure.

Differential Diagnosis

The differential diagnosis includes cercarial or contact dermatitis, bacterial or fungal infection, scabies, myiasis, loiasis, other migratory parasites listed in Table 237-4.

Treatment

Treatment of CLM due to dog or cat hookworm includes topical and/or oral thiabendazole, ivermectin or albendazole. It is important not to attempt to extract the worm, because it has already migrated beyond the visible lesion.

Prevention

Infection with animal hookworms is prevented by avoiding direct skin contact with fecally contaminated soil.

CYSTICERCOSIS[29–35]

Synonyms

Cysticercus cellulosae, larval taeniasis

Etiology

Cysticercosis is caused by the larval stage of the pork tapeworm, *Taenia solium*.

Life Cycle

Humans are the definitive host for *T. solium*. Swine are the intermediate host. Eggs from the adult worm in human small intestine are passed in feces and may remain viable for weeks. If the eggs are ingested by humans or swine, the outer shell disintegrates in the small bowel releasing embryos that penetrate the wall of the small bowel and enter the circulation. They disseminate widely and lodge in tissues, most often subcutaneous tissue, brain, eye, and skeletal muscle and develop into the larval stage (cysticerci), leading to the clinical disease known as cysticercosis.

In humans, *T. solium* infection causes both intestinal taeniasis and cysticercosis. The human host can have either form of infection alone. Intestinal infection with the adult parasites follows eating raw or undercooked pork containing cysticerci. The larval cysts attach to the small bowel mucosa and develop into adult worms.

Pathogenesis

Cysticerci in tissues are surrounded by a connective-tissue membrane and cause little host reaction while they are alive. When the cysticerci die, they may release foreign antigens that provoke granulomatous changes and infiltration of plasma cells, eosinophils, lymphocytes, and macrophages. Calcification may follow. Cysts in muscle collapse and calcify, giving the characteristic spindle shape.

Geographic Distribution

T. solium is a common parasite in Central and South America, Africa, parts of Asia, and eastern Europe. In the United States, this disease is seen primarily in immigrants from endemic areas where poor sanitation and pig farming are common, though acquisition of infection has been well documented in the United States. Cysticercosis is the most common helminthic infection of the central nervous system.

Epidemiology

ACQUISITION Humans acquire cysticercosis by ingesting eggs in food, water, or on fingers contaminated with human feces. Humans infected with adult worms may acquire cysticercosis by ingesting eggs passed in their own feces.

INCUBATION PERIOD AND TIME FRAME The time from infection to the appearance of subcutaneous nodules is highly variable and may be from months to years. Cysticerci can survive in humans for 10 to 15 years. Symptoms may begin or continue long after the parasites are dead.

FIGURE 237-4

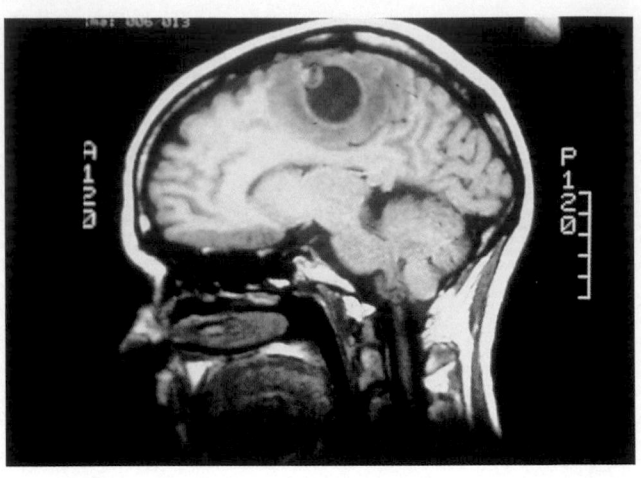

MRI scan of central nervous system cysticercosis. (*Courtesy of Jay S. Keystone, MD, FRCPC.*)

Clinical Features

The clinical features range from asymptomatic to fatal. Fifty-four percent of patients with cysticercosis present with subcutaneous nodules. The skin findings include single or multiple firm, mobile, round, well-circumscribed subcutaneous nodules that may be tender or asymptomatic. The nodules vary in size from millimeters to centimeters, but are commonly about 2 cm in diameter. The most common anatomic locations are the extremities and trunk.

Systemic manifestations reflect the presence of mass lesions. While the central nervous system (Fig. 237-4), subcutaneous tissue, skeletal muscle, and eye (Fig. 237-5) are the most commonly affected sites, there are reports of involvement of the heart, kidneys, liver, lungs, and pancreas. Seizures are the most common manifestation of neurocysticercosis. Almost 50 percent of patients with central nervous system cysticerci found at autopsy had no history of

FIGURE 237-5

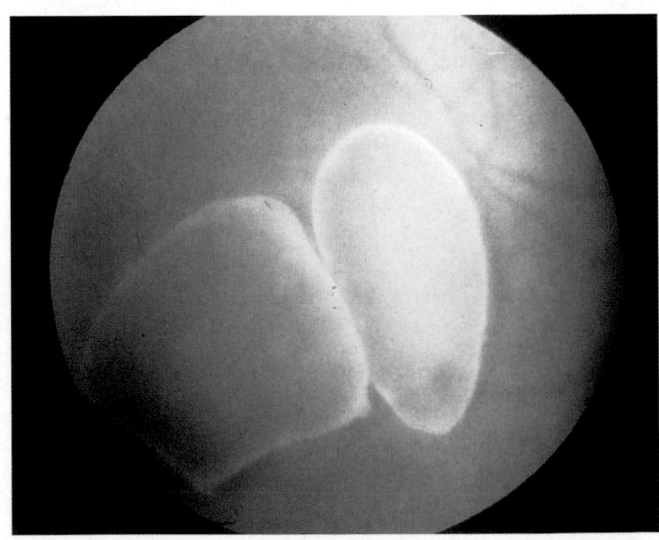

Cysticercosis in retina. (*Courtesy of William S. Kammerer, MD.*)

central nervous system symptoms. Intestinal taeniasis is found in 25 to 50 percent of patients with cysticercosis. Persons with intestinal infection with the adult worms may have abdominal pain, anorexia, constipation, and diarrhea.

Laboratory

Peripheral eosinophilia is absent in 85 percent of patients with neurocysticercosis. High-grade eosinophilia in a patient with cysticercosis should lead clinicians to a search for another process to explain the eosinophilia.

Diagnosis

The definitive diagnosis is made by surgical excision of a nodule and identification of the parasite by characteristic morphology. Serologic tests are also available. High sensitivity and specificity have been reported with an enzyme-linked immunoelectrotransfer blot assay (EITB) and with an enzyme-linked immunoassay (ELISA). Sensitivity is high in patients with multiple lesions, but in one study, only 28 percent of patients with a single lesion had positive EITB results. Other immunologic tests such as complement fixation, direct immunofluorescence, immunoelectrophoresis, and indirect hemagglutination have been less sensitive and less specific.

For neurocysticercosis, MRI allows the evaluation of the developmental stages of larval cysts. Cerebrospinal fluid may be normal or may contain increased protein and cells, including eosinophils and plasma cells.

Differential Diagnosis

The differential diagnosis for subcutaneous lesions includes echinococcosis, onchocerciasis, benign cysts, soft-tissue tumors, and other causes of nodules listed in Table 237-2.

Treatment

Treatment of cysticercosis depends on the location and characteristics of the lesions and may include surgery as well as medical therapy with an anthelmintic drug. If a few subcutaneous lesions are present, they need to be treated only if symptomatic or for cosmetic reasons. If multiple subcutaneous lesions are present, the drug of choice is albendazole or praziquantel. The Food and Drug Administration considers praziquantel an investigational drug for cysticercosis. Concomitant intestinal taeniasis due to *T. solium*, if present, should be treated to eliminate a potential ongoing source of infection for the patient and contacts.

Albendazole should be taken with a fatty meal to increase absorption. When treating neurocysticercosis with praziquantel or albendazole, glucocorticoids should be given two to three days before and during treatment to reduce the inflammatory reaction that may follow death of cysticerci. Plasma levels of praziquantel may decrease by up to 50 percent when given with glucocorticoids.

The prognosis of subcutaneous cysticercosis is excellent. Prognosis involving other organ systems depends on anatomic location of the lesions. Untreated, symptomatic cerebral cysticercosis has a mortality of 10 to 26 percent. Mortality may reach 50 percent in patients with untreated cysticercal meningitis.

Prevention

Preventive measures include proper disposal of feces, avoidance of fecal contamination of food and drink, and treatment of intestinal taeniasis.

DIROFILARIASIS[36–39]

Synonyms

Dog heartworm infection

Etiology

The organisms responsible for dirofilariasis include the filarial nematodes of several species of the genus *Dirofilaria*. These include, most importantly, *D. immitis*, the dog heartworm, as well as *D. tenuis* (raccoon), *D. repens* (dog), and *D. ursi* (bear). *D. immitis* causes pulmonary disease and, rarely, soft-tissue infection.

Life Cycle

D. immitis lives in the right ventricle and pulmonary artery of dogs, producing microfilariae that are ingested with a blood meal by the mosquito. The microfilariae develop into the infective larvae stage in the mosquito.

Pathogenesis

The infective larvae are introduced via the bite of the mosquito (blackfly for *D. ursi*) and undergo a growth period in subcutaneous and deeper tissues. The parasite does not complete its development in humans, so no microfilariae are produced. *D. immitis* may enter the circulation and occlude a small pulmonary artery, resulting in an infarct. The necrotic and granulomatous tissue contains the worm and eosinophils and may calcify.

Geographic Distribution

D. immitis is widespread in dogs, but is thought to be most prevalent in North and South America, Australia, Europe, Japan, India, and China. Sporadic infections with other *Dirofilaria* species have been reported from all continents. In the United States, this infection occurs in the eastern, midwestern, and southern states.

Epidemiology

ACQUISITION Humans are infected when bitten by a mosquito containing infective larvae. The larvae emerge from the mouth parts of the mosquito and enter through the puncture wound.

INCUBATION PERIOD AND TIME FRAME The interval between exposure and development of symptoms is usually at least 2 to 3 months. The parasite occasionally survives for years. Rarely, mature worms have been found in the heart. Dead and calcified worms may be found years after the disease was acquired.

Clinical Features

Soft-tissue dirofilariasis is characterized by erythematous to skin-colored, well-defined, firm subcutaneous nodules that are usually single but may be multiple. The lesion is typically 1 to 2 cm in diameter and may be tender. Some reports describe initial soft tissue swelling, which evolves into a well-circumscribed nodular lesion.

Occasionally lesions are migratory. The most common anatomic sites are the head, neck, breast, arm, leg, and scrotum. Parasites in the conjunctiva and oral cavity have been described. Subcutaneous dirofilariasis has been associated with acute arthritis.

Pulmonary dirofilariasis can cause cough, chest pain, and, rarely, hemoptysis and low-grade fever. More than 50 percent of persons with pulmonary dirofilariasis are asymptomatic.

Laboratory

A peripheral eosinophilia is usually absent or low-grade.

Diagnosis

The definitive diagnosis is made by surgical excision of the nodule and identification of the worm. Serologic studies using ELISA may be positive in 75 percent of patients with pulmonary dirofilariasis. However, cross-reaction with other helminths (strongyloidiasis, toxocariasis, schistosomiasis, and filariasis) may limit usefulness, particularly in tropical locations. Chest x-ray films of pulmonary dirofilariasis show a coin lesion that is usually single and may be calcified.

Differential Diagnosis

The differential diagnosis of subcutaneous dirofilariasis includes loiasis, cysticercosis, onchocercosis, paragonimiasis, as well as epidermal inclusion cyst, lipoma or other benign tumor, and malignant tumor or metastatic disease.

Treatment

Surgical excision of the nodule containing the worm is curative.

Prevention

Dirofilariasis caused by *D. immitis* can be prevented by controlling the heartworm infection in dogs. Prevention of other dirofilarial infections requires avoiding bites of arthropods with infective larvae.

DRACUNCULIASIS[40-43]

Synonyms

Dracunculosis, dracontiasis, Guinea worm disease, Medina worm infection, dragon worm disease, serpent worm disease

Etiology

Dracunculiasis (Fig. 237-6) is caused by the nematode *Dracunculus medinensis*. The female is 70 to 80 cm in length and rarely exceeds 100 cm.

The ancient symbols of medicine, the caduceus and staff of Aesculapius, may have been drawn from the practice of using sticks to extract the *D. medinensis* worm from its host.

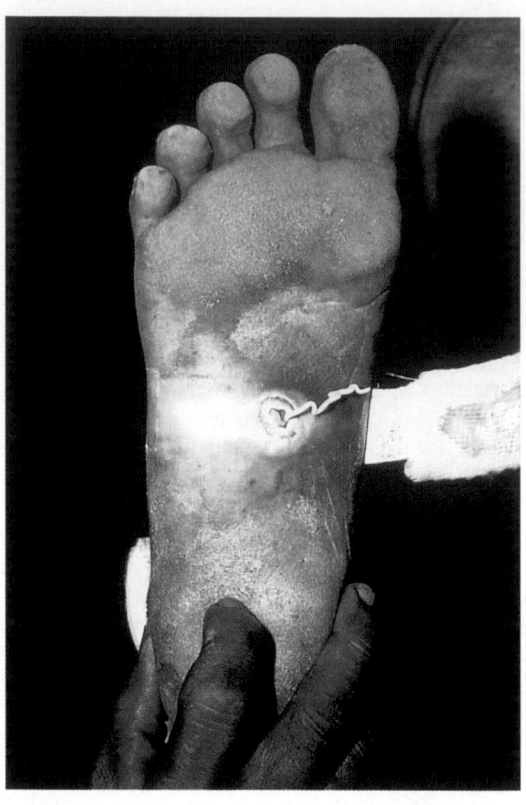

Dracunculiasis. (*Courtesy of Jay S. Keystone, MD, FRCPC.*)

Life Cycle

Larvae are released into water from an infected human and ingested by copepods (tiny aquatic arthropods), in which they develop. Humans ingest the copepods *(Cyclops)* to complete the cycle. Although some animals may be infected, humans are the definitive host and main reservoir of infection.

Pathogenesis

In humans, gastric acid dissolves the ingested copepods which results in release of larvae that then migrate through the stomach wall and reach loose connective tissue. The larvae mature into adult worms over 10 to 14 months without causing a tissue reaction. Migration of the gravid female to skin leads to a localized bulla containing inflammatory cells and many eosinophils. Over a period of four weeks, the worm emerges. The bulla ruptures on contact with water, releasing larvae from the uterus of the female worm, which prolapses through the skin.

Geographic Distribution

As of 1996 endemic transmission continued in India and 16 countries in sub-Saharan Africa. In the past, infection was endemic in Pakistan, Saudi Arabia, and Yemen. Cases reported from Sudan represented 72 percent of all cases reported in the world. Eradication programs are in place in many countries.

Epidemiology

ACQUISITION Humans acquire dracunculiasis by ingesting infected copepods, usually in drinking water taken from shallow lagoons, step wells, and other surface water.

INCUBATION PERIOD AND TIME FRAME The adult worm emerges about 1 year (range, 10 to 18 months) after the larvae are ingested. Symptoms associated with migration of the worm may precede the emergence of the worm. The adult worm typically dies (or is removed) after reaching the skin and releasing larvae. Disabling symptoms may persist for weeks to months. Fatalities rarely result from complications.

Clinical Features

The characteristic clinical findings include a papule, two to seven centimeters in size, that progresses over 1 to 3 days to a vesicle with an indurated border. An intense burning sensation is relieved, at least in part, by submerging the affected body part in water. The bulla ruptures and larvae are ejected into the water. The rupture of the worm in tissues provokes an intense inflammatory response and cellulitis, and may lead to abscess formation. Disruption of the skin by the worm predisposes the person to secondary bacterial infection, including tetanus. One or multiple parasites may be present. The total number is usually fewer than 6 but can exceed 50. The most common anatomic location for the skin lesion is the lower leg or foot, but parasites may emerge on the hands, arms, trunk, and even jaw. Systemic symptoms of nausea, vomiting, diarrhea, urticaria, and pruritus may precede the skin lesion by a few hours. The systemic symptoms improve once the larvae are ejected into the water.

Rarely, worms have been found in the pericardium, spinal canal, eye, broad ligament, testicle, and other deep tissues. Arthritis and ankylosis may result if a joint is infected.

No protective immunity to this parasite develops. Reinfection is common.

Laboratory

Peripheral eosinophilia is common during tissue migration.

Diagnosis

The diagnosis is made by the visual inspection of the morphology of the parasite as it emerges and by identification of the discharged motile larvae.

X-ray examination may reveal dead calcified worms.

Differential Diagnosis

The differential diagnosis includes a carbuncle or cellulitis associated with bacterial infection, onchocerciasis, loiasis, and syphilitic gumma.

Treatment

The treatment of dracunculosis in endemic areas includes extracting the worms by slowly winding them around a stick. This poses the risk of rupturing the worm, resulting in a severe inflammatory reaction.

Medical therapy with some benefit includes metronidazole and thiabendazole. These medications decrease inflammation and may facilitate extraction of the worm. Thiabendazole may actually kill

the adult worm. While both of these drugs are approved by the Food and Drug Administration, they are considered investigational for dracunculiasis.

Prevention

Infection can be avoided by using water that has been filtered or obtained from safe sources. Boiling water or treating water with temephos also renders it safe.

ECHINOCOCCOSIS[44-48]

Synonyms

For *Echinococcus granulosus*—unilocular echinococcosis, hydatid disease caused by *E. granulosus*, classic cystic hydatid disease; for *E. multilocularis*—multilocular echinococcosis, alveolar hydatid disease

Etiology

The larval stages of the cestodes (tapeworms) *E. granulosus* and *E. multilocularis* cause most cases of human echinococcosis.

Life Cycle

The definitive hosts for *E. granulosus* are dogs and other members of the family Canidae. Sheep, moose, horses, and other animals serve as intermediate hosts. The adult worm in the gut of the definitive host produces eggs that are shed into the environment and ingested by the intermediate host, where they develop into hydatid cysts in tissues that are eaten by the definitive host to complete the cycle. Humans are incidental intermediate hosts. The life cycle of *E. multilocularis* is similar to that of *E. granulosus* except that the definitive hosts are foxes and intermediate hosts are small rodents.

Pathogenesis

With *E. granulosus*, the oncosphere (larva) hatches from an ingested egg in the gut, penetrates the intestinal mucosa, and enters the venous and lymphatic pathways then settles in tissue anywhere in the body and begins cystic development. The cyst increases in size at a rate of about 1 to 5 cm per year. The hydatid cyst (metacestode) has an inner germinative layer of cells, surrounded by an acellular, laminated membrane and variable granulomatous reaction. Secondary cysts bud internally from the germinative layer and produce multiple protoscolices, which, if released from the hydatid cyst by rupturing, may establish new sites of infection. The cysts may reach volumes of several liters. The cysts may cause local pressure and mechanical problems due to the large size.

E. multilocularis has no limiting membrane of parasitic or host origin, and the cyst gives rise to new cysts by exogenous budding. This produces an enlarging mass of contiguous vesicles that may invade and replace host tissue (usually the liver). *E. multilocularis* grows more rapidly than *E. granulosus* (commensurate with the short life span of its usual intermediate host, a rodent) and remains in the proliferative stage indefinitely. The mass may undergo central necrosis with cavitation. Hematogenous dissemination leads to metastatic infection.

Geographic Distribution

E. granulosus is present on all continents. Infections are sporadic in North America, Central America, northern South America, northern Europe, Australia, and New Zealand. There is a high prevalence of infection in southern South America, parts of southern Europe, parts of the former Soviet Republics, Middle Eastern countries, and northern and East Africa. The infection is present in most Asian countries.

E. multilocularis is more limited in distribution because of greater host specificity. There are documented cases in North America, Europe, Asia, India, and Iran; one case was reported from northern Africa (Tunisia) in 1981.

Epidemiology

ACQUISITION *E. granulosus* is acquired by the ingestion of infective eggs with food or fluid or on fingers. Eggs are dispersed by wind, water, and arthropods from the site of fecal deposition. Eggs may survive for a year or more in the environment. Transmission by inhalation of infective eggs may account for rare infections. In some highly endemic areas, the prevalence of infection may reach as high as 5 percent or more of the population. In the United States, about 200 cases are diagnosed yearly, with more than 90 percent being acquired outside of the country. Persons at highest risk are those living in endemic areas with close contact with dogs and with poor personal hygiene. Many persons become infected in childhood.

E. multilocularis is acquired by ingestion of infective eggs in food or fluid or on fingers. This is an uncommon infection in humans. In some areas, 40 to 100 percent of foxes are infected. Trappers, hunters, and persons who work with fox fur are at increased infection.

INCUBATION PERIOD AND TIME FRAME The interval between acquisition of infection and onset of symptoms is usually years and may be decades for *E. granulosus*. Both of these parasites live for years, sometimes for the lifetime of the host.

Clinical Features

Most infections with *E. granulosus* are asymptomatic and go unrecognized. Skin and soft tissue manifestations are rare, occurring in <2 percent of infected patients.

Cysts may manifest as firm subcutaneous or intramuscular nodules or masses that are fluctuant and nontender to palpation. There is no epidermal change. Skin fistulas from a hydatid cyst in a patient known to have *E. granulosus* has been reported. *E. multilocularis* has been observed to cause multiple supraumbilical cutaneous and subcutaneous nodules associated with ulceration, surrounding inflammation and painless cutaneous fistulas. Another report described an inflamed epigastric nodule where the mechanism of skin involvement was the progression of larva from the liver to the skin by the falciform ligament.

The clinical features of *E. granulosus* are highly variable and reflect the location and size of cysts (Fig. 237-7, Fig. 237-8). Most symptoms are caused by mechanical pressure of a mass or an allergic reaction to foreign antigens from leaking cyst fluid. Cysts

FIGURE 237-7

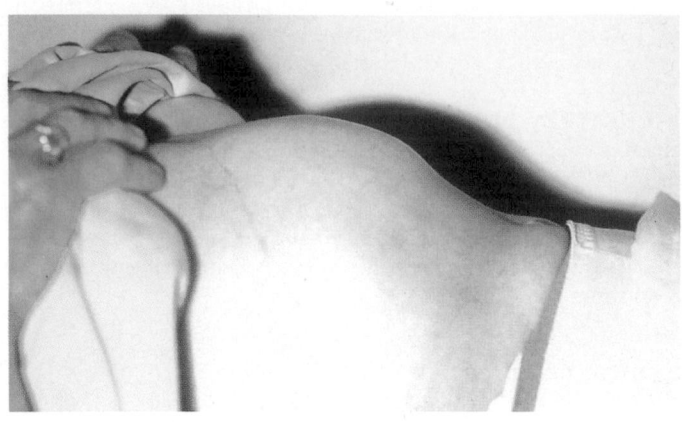

Abdominal bulge from intraperitoneal cyst of echinococcosis. (*Courtesy of Jay S. Keystone, MD, FRCPC.*)

may be single or multiple (at least 25 percent) and infect the liver (50 percent to 75 percent), lung (20 percent to 30 percent), and other sites: kidney, spleen, heart, bones, muscles, and central nervous system (less than 2 percent). The cyst may reach a large size within the abdomen before symptoms develop. If the cyst leaks fluid, the patient may have wheezing, urticaria, or anaphylaxis.

Patients with *E. multilocularis* remain asymptomatic for years. The signs and symptoms are epigastric and right upper quadrant

FIGURE 237-8

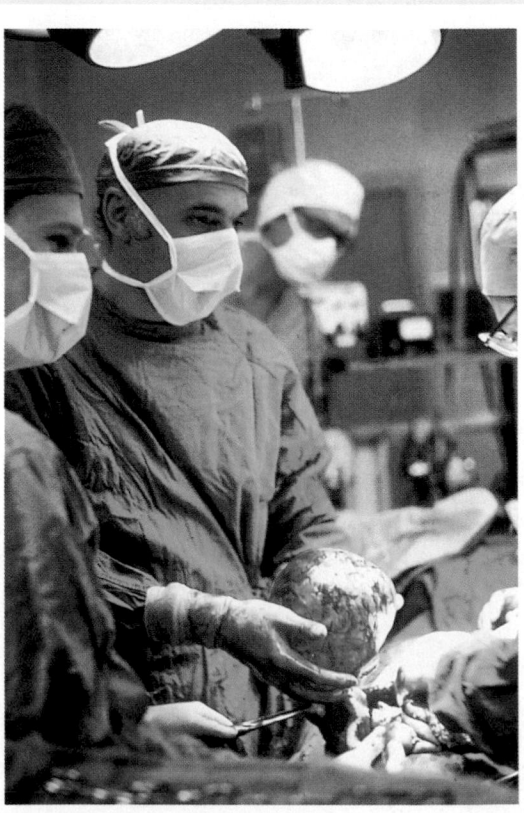

Surgical removal of intraperitoneal echinococcal cyst. (*Courtesy of Jay S. Keystone, MD, FRCPC.*)

Laboratory

Peripheral eosinophilia is present in one-third or fewer of patients with cysts; however, leakage of cyst fluid causes eosinophilia in a higher percentage.

Diagnosis

Diagnosis is confirmed by examination of the contents of the cyst and identification of the parasite. Characteristic morphology of the parasite as seen by imaging (e.g., ultrasound, CT scan, and MRI) can suggest the diagnosis and can detect clinically silent lesions. Serologic studies can aid in the diagnosis and may be used to follow patients after surgical treatment. In echinococcosis granulosus, negative antibody tests do not exclude the diagnosis, as some persons with cysts do not have detectable antibodies. Lesions in the liver are more often associated with positive serologic studies than are lung lesions. A combination of serologic tests may provide the best information. False positive results can occur in persons with other helminthic infections. Tests that assess circulating antigen are also being developed. Serologic tests are usually positive at high titers in patients infected with *E. multilocularis*.

Differential Diagnosis

The differential diagnosis when there is skin involvement includes cysticercosis, paragonimiasis, dirofilariasis, and other cystic lesions of soft tissues.

Treatment

The treatment for *E. granulosus* is surgical resection. An approach that uses chemotherapy and PAIR (puncture-aspiration-injection-reaspiration) is an alternative approach, especially when lesions are inoperable or would pose high surgical risk. It is important to evaluate for silent lesions and follow the patient for recurrence. Albendazole, mebendazole, or praziquantel may be useful if the cysts rupture or leak during surgery, or if surgery is contraindicated. Surgical resection can be curative in *E. multilocularis* if the diagnosis is made early. Albendazole or mebendazole may slow progression of the infection but neither is curative in late infection. Liver transplantation has been used in about 20 patients with inoperable infection. One report describes improvement in a patient with cutaneous alveolar echinococcus after treatment with albendazole.

The operative mortality of *E. granulosus* is 0.9 percent to 3.6 percent, which increases with subsequent surgeries. The mortality for symptomatic patients who are not treated surgically is as high as 22 percent to 60 percent in some series. The clinical outcome depends on the anatomic location, number and size of the lesions.

The mortality rate from *E. multilocularis* has been 50 percent to 75 percent in the past, but may be lower with newer forms of therapy.

Prevention

The incidence of *E. granulosus* may be decreased by preventing dogs and other canines from feeding on infected offal.

ENTEROBIASIS[49–52]

Synonyms

Threadworm, pinworm or seatworm infection, oxyuriasis

Etiology

Enterobiasis is caused by the nematode (roundworm) *Enterobius vermicularis*.

Life Cycle

Humans are the only host for *E. vermicularis*. See below for its life cycle.

Pathogenesis

Humans ingest the infective eggs, which hatch in the intestine and develop into adult worms in the cecum. Female worms migrate out of the anus and deposit eggs in the perianal area. The eggs remain viable for up to 13 days. Worms may be found in surgically resected appendices. The migration of worms to the vagina, uterus, fallopian tubes, and peritoneal cavity may be associated with local granulomatous inflammation and peritonitis.

Geographic Distribution

Enterobiasis is found worldwide. This is a very common infection and the most common helminthic infection in industrialized countries. The highest rates of infection are among children.

Epidemiology

ACQUISITION   Enterobiasis is acquired by the ingestion of infective eggs by direct anus-to-mouth transfer by fingers or sexual activities, contact with contaminated objects (e.g., bed linens, clothing, bathroom fixtures), and the inhalation and ingestion of airborne eggs in dust. Eggs become infective within a few hours of being deposited by the female worm in the perianal area.

INCUBATION PERIOD AND TIME FRAME   A period of 4 to 6 weeks is required before eggs can be found. Symptoms may begin weeks to months after ingestion of infective eggs. The parasite may live months or longer in the human. Autoinfection by anus-to-mouth transfer of eggs by fingers allows infection to continue indefinitely and to amplify.

Clinical Features

The clinical features include nocturnal anal and perianal pruritus. Skin may impetiginize. Other findings have included perianal mass with recurrent cellulitis. Localized urticaria on the buttocks has been reported. In females, vulvovaginitis and vaginal discharge are common, and a nodular lesion of the vulva has been described. Rare complications include appendicitis, inguinal hernia, peritonitis, salpingitis, and urethritis. Reinfection is common.

Laboratory

Laboratory studies are usually normal. Eosinophilia occurs only with tissue invasion (e.g., peritonitis).

Diagnosis

The diagnosis of enterobiasis is made by the identification of the eggs in the perianal area. This is most effectively done by applying transparent tape to the skin in the perianal area, then reviewing it under a microscope for identification of the eggs (Fig. 237-9). Eggs may also be found in stool (<5 percent) and in subungual material. Occasionally the adult worm is found in the perianal area, vagina or underclothes. If ectopic sites are involved, the parasite may be identified in tissue sections.

Differential Diagnosis

Differential diagnosis includes allergic and hypersensitivity reactions, neurodermatitis, and strongyloidiasis.

Treatment

Treatment includes pyrantel pamoate, mebendazole, or albendazole.

Prevention

Prevention includes good personal hygiene.

FASCIOLIASIS[53–55]

Synonyms

Sheep liver fluke disease

FIGURE 237-9

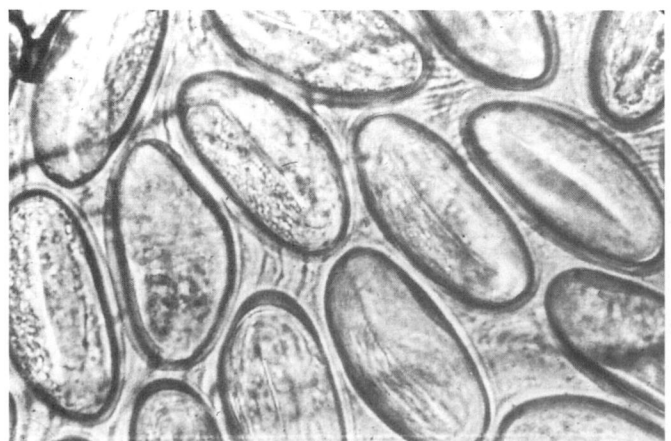

Enterobius vermicularis ova as seen under microscope (collected on transparent tape from perianal area). (*Courtesy of Herman Zaiman, MD.*)

Etiology

Fascioliasis is caused by trematodes (flukes) residing in the human bile ducts. These flukes include *Fasciola hepatica*, the sheep liver fluke, and *F. gigantica*. Human infection is rarely reported with *F. gigantica*.

Life Cycle

In water, miracidia are released from eggs, then penetrate snails and develop into cercariae that encyst on water plants (e.g., watercress) and become metacercariae, which are ingested by herbivores (e.g., sheep and cattle).

Pathogenesis

If metacercariae are ingested by humans, larvae are released from the cyst envelope in the duodenum, and pass through the intestinal wall and peritoneal cavity to penetrate the capsule of the liver. The parasite enters the bile ducts, where it matures and produces eggs that are released into the bile and passed in the feces. The parasite may cause hyperplasia of the bile duct epithelium, periductal fibrosis, and obstruction of the bile ducts. Flukes occasionally migrate to extrabiliary sites, most commonly to subcutaneous tissue.

Geographic Distribution

F. hepatica is found worldwide in sheep- and cattle-raising areas. Sporadic human infections have been reported from all continents.

Epidemiology

ACQUISITION Fascioliasis is acquired by the ingestion of the metacercariae, usually on watercress and other plants (e.g., dandelion leaves and lettuce), or in contaminated water.

INCUBATION PERIOD AND TIME FRAME Eggs are first found in the stool 3 to 4 months after ingestion of metacercariae. The earliest symptoms, which are related to migration of the young fluke in the liver, may occur as early as 2 weeks after exposure. The parasite can survive 10 years or longer in the human host.

Clinical Features

Symptoms may be absent or mild. In a small percentage of patients, more severe disease develops, and these patients may have acute, relapsing, or chronic symptoms. Early changes that begin during liver migration and may persist for weeks to months include hepatomegaly, fever, right upper quadrant pain, nausea, and diarrhea. Jaundice may occur. Patients may have repeated episodes of urticaria, sometimes accompanied by wheezing. Chronic infection is often asymptomatic but may be associated with episodic cholangitis, cholecystitis, and obstructive jaundice.

The most frequent site of ectopic fascioliasis is the subcutaneous tissue. Typical findings are erythematous, painful, and pruritic subcutaneous nodules. The most common anatomic locations include the abdomen, back, and extremities. Migratory tracks cause necrosis, local inflammation, and may be followed by fibrosis. Other documented ectopic sites include the brain, lung, cecum, epididymis, stomach, appendix, pancreas, peritoneum, spleen, skeletal muscle, orbit, and lymph nodes. Ectopic fascioliasis is not always associated with hepatobiliary disease.

Laboratory

Acute infection is characterized by marked leukocytosis and eosinophilia. In chronic infection, eosinophilia may wax and wane. Liver function tests are abnormal.

Diagnosis

The diagnosis is made by the identification of eggs in the stool, duodenal contents, or bile. Eggs are typically present in small numbers in stool, hence may be difficult to find. Adult worms may be recovered during hepatobiliary surgery. When ectopic sites are involved, adult worms can be identified in surgical specimens. Serologic tests may aid in the diagnosis of early infection and ectopic infection, though their value is limited because of cross-reactions with other helminthic infections.

Differential Diagnosis

The differential diagnosis includes viral hepatitis, infection with other liver flukes, schistosomiasis (Katayama fever), toxocariasis, amebiasis, and biliary tract disease. When subcutaneous tissue is involved, the differential diagnosis includes lymphadenitis, epidermal inclusion cyst, abscess, cellulitis, and other parasites causing nodular skin lesions.

Treatment

Fascioliasis is treated with bithionol or triclabendazole. Surgery may also be necessary. In the United States, bithionol is available from the Centers for Disease Control Drug Service, Centers for Disease Control and Prevention, Atlanta, GA 30333. The telephone numbers are (404) 639-3670 during the daytime and (404) 639-2888 in evenings, and on weekends and holidays.

Prevention

Prevention includes avoiding freshwater plants, especially watercress, and untreated water.

FILARIASIS, LYMPHATIC[56–59]

Synonyms and Diseases

Malayan filariasis *(Brugia malayi)*, Timor filariasis *(B. timori)*, Bancroft's filariasis, filariasis bancrofti, and wuchereriasis *(Wuchereria bancrofti)*. Some of these parasites can cause elephantiasis and tropical pulmonary eosinophilia. Disease process depends on the etiologic agent. See Table 237-7 for a summary of filarial parasites.

Etiology

Lymphatic filariasis (Fig. 237-10) is caused by three filarial nematodes: *B. malayi*, *B. timori*, and *W. bancrofti*.

Life Cycle

Microfilariae produced by adult worms in the human are taken up by the mosquito during a blood meal. Over several days, the microfilariae develop into larvae within the mosquito, which can transmit infection to other humans when taking blood meals. *B. malayi* can follow an alternative life cycle that involves the leaf monkey instead of humans as the definitive host.

Pathogenesis

Infective larvae emerge from the mosquito during feeding and migrate through the puncture wound produced by the feeding mosquito. The larvae enter lymphatic vessels, and mature adult worms mate in the lymphatics or lymph nodes and release sheathed microfilariae into the bloodstream. Maturing adult worms provoke an eosinophilic and chronic inflammatory cell infiltrate around lymphatic vessels, producing dilatation and hypertrophy, damage to the lymph valves with eventual scarring, and obstruction of lymphatic flow. Death of worms in lymphatics and lymph nodes results in an intense inflammatory reaction with granulomatous changes and necrosis. Late calcification may result.

TABLE 237-7

Summary of Filarial Parasites*

SPECIES	GEOGRAPHIC DISTRIBUTION	MANIFESTATIONS
Brugia malayi	Southeast Asia	Lymphangitis, lymphadenitis, lymphedema, hydrocele, elephantiasis, tropical pulmonary eosinophilia
Brugia timori	Indonesia	Same as above
Loa loa	Africa	Angioedema, pruritic migratory swellings; migration of worm across eye
Mansonella ozzardi	Central and South America	Pruritus
Mansonella perstans	Africa, South America	Pruritus, angioedema
Mansonella streptocerca	Africa	Pruritius, papular rash, lichenification
Onchocerca volvulus	Africa, Central and South America	Pruritic papules, nodules, lichenification; keratitis, retinitis, blindness
Wuchereria bancrofti	Tropics worldwide	Lymphangitis, lymphadenitis, lymphedema, hydroceles, chyluria, elephantiasis, tropical pulmonary eosinophilia

*Dracunculiasis and dirofilariasis, which are also filarial infections, are covered in separate sections. All filarial infections are transmitted by biting insects, except for dracunculiasis.

FIGURE 237-10

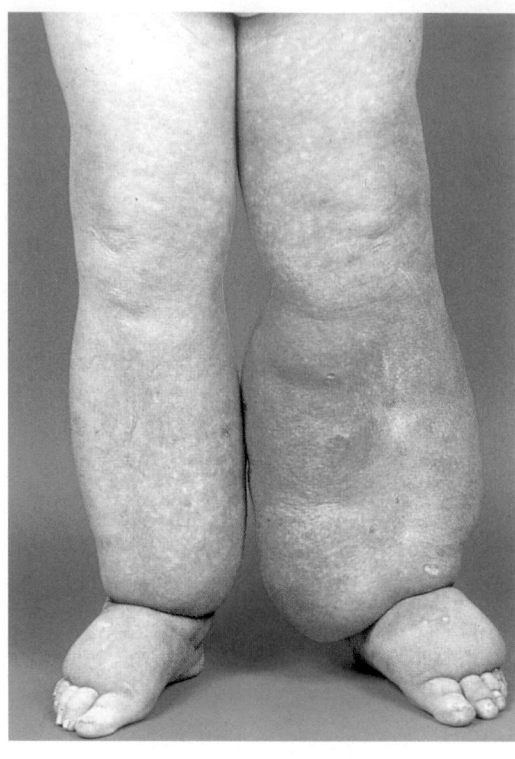

Lymphatic filariasis secondary to *Wuchereria bancrofti*. (*Courtesy of Jay S. Keystone, MD, FRCPC.*)

Geographic Distribution

The geographic distribution for *B. malayi* includes South and East Asia (from India to Korea), as well as adjacent islands. *B. timori* is limited to small volcanic islands of southeastern Indonesia surrounding the Savu Sea (Timor, Flores, Alor, Sumba, Roti, and Savu). *W. bancrofti*, which infects 120 million people worldwide, is found in tropical and subtropical areas of Africa, Asia, Pacific islands, Central and South America, and the Caribbean. Figure 237-11 shows the geographic distribution of *W. bancrofti* in Africa, the Americas, and the Eastern Mediterranean region. Figure 237-12 shows the geographic distribution of *W. bancrofti*, *B. malayi*, and *B. timori* in the Southeast Asian and Western Pacific regions.

Epidemiology

ACQUISITION Lymphatic filariasis is acquired by the bite of an infective mosquito. Microfilariae transfused with blood or those that cross the placenta are unable to develop in humans and disappear within a few weeks. Worldwide the filarial parasites are estimated to infect more than 100 million people.

Infection is uncommon in persons who have spent brief periods in endemic areas. Multiple bites from infective mosquitoes are generally required to establish symptomatic infection. In the United States, infection is seen primarily in immigrants from endemic areas.

INCUBATION PERIOD AND TIME FRAME The incubation period is 5 to 18 months. *B. malayi* microfilaremia may occur as early as 2 to 3 months after exposure. *W. bancrofti* microfilariae first appear in peripheral blood 8 to 12 months after exposure, but symptoms can begin as early as 1 to 3 months after exposure. Adult worms live an average of 10 to 15 years and the microfilariae probably 6 to 12 months. Symptoms and sequelae can persist after the death of all parasites.

Clinical Features

The clinical presentation and course of disease depend on the age at first exposure and the presence of immunity. In endemic areas, the prevalence increases after age 20, with most new cases occurring between the ages of 25 and 40 years old. The clinical course ranges from asymptomatic to severely disabling (<1 percent of those infected). Manifestations may be acute, chronic, and recurrent. Early findings are lymphangitis with a characteristic retrograde progression, lymphadenitis, orchitis, epididymitis and sometimes fever. Lymphangitis is typically recurrent with 6 to 10 episodes per year, usually lasting 3 to 7 days each; the affected body part clinically appears normal between early episodes. Intermittent fevers and lymphangitis can recur for as long as 20 years after an infected person leaves the endemic area.

After 10 to 15 years of infection, chronic disease is manifested by sequelae of lymphatic obstruction including lymphedema, elephantiasis, hydrocele and chyluria. The skin over the involved area is hypertrophic, verrucous, and fibrotic with redundant folds of skin. Fissures, ulceration, and gangrene may occur. Secondary bacterial infection invariably occurs. The anatomic locations most commonly afflicted with elephantiasis include the lower extremity, scrotum, and penis. Less commonly, the upper extremity, breast, and vulva are involved, and rarely, an amputation stump, ears, oral mucosa, periorbital area, and panniculus. The late findings of scarring and lymphatic obstruction are not reversed with treatment. *W. bancrofti* has been reported to cause a skin nodule on the breast.

Tropical pulmonary eosinophilia develops in some patients with filarial infections. Clinical findings include cough, wheezing, dyspnea, chest pain, and fever accompanied by marked eosinophilia and pulmonary infiltrates. Tropical pulmonary eosinophilia may be associated with progressive restrictive pulmonary disease.

In filariasis due to *B. malayi*, the lower extremities are usually involved, lymphangitis is not severe and genital lesions are uncommon. In filariasis due to *B. timori*, lymphatic abscesses are common. Genital lesions, chyluria and tropical pulmonary eosinophilic syndrome are not reported with *B. timori*.

Travelers to endemic areas do not manifest classic findings. Instead, they have a hyperresponsive clinical presentation, with more intense inflammatory reactions to filarial parasites. The clinical findings may include lymphangitis, lymphadenitis, and groin pain from the associated lymphatic inflammation, urticaria, and a peripheral eosinophilia.

Microfilaremic patients have hyporesponsiveness to filarial antigens and a limited host response to the parasite. Persons with a more vigorous immune response may clear the microfilariae from the blood, but have more prominent local pathology and systemic symptoms.

Laboratory

Patients have a peripheral eosinophilia, which may be high grade, and an elevated IgE. More than half of microfilaremic patients with *W. bancrofti* have hematuria and/or proteinuria.

Diagnosis

The diagnosis is made by the demonstration of microfilariae in blood, urine and other body fluids, and tissue or the demonstration of the adult worm in lymphatics or other tissues. The usefulness of serologic tests has been limited by cross-reactions with other antigens, but newer tests with better specificity are becoming available. It is important to note that persons with active filarial infection may not be microfilaremic and persons with microfilaremia may be asymptomatic. Persons with tropical eosinophilic syndrome will have pulmonary infiltrates on chest x-ray films.

Differential Diagnosis

The differential diagnosis depends on the stage of the infection. Acute infection may be confused with a bacterial lymphangitis. The differential diagnosis for the chronic stage includes other filarial infections such as *Onchocerca volvulus*, recurrent bacterial lymphangitis, deep fungal infection, disruption of lymphatic channels due to trauma, chronic venous insufficiency, pretibial myxedema, lymphosarcoma, fibrosarcoma, and congenital diseases such as Milroy's disease and Klippel-Trenaunay-Weber syndrome.

Treatment

The drug of choice for *B. malayi* and *W. bancrofti* is diethylcarbamazine. Diethylcarbamazine is active against microfilariae but has a limited effect on adult worms. A single dose of ivermectin has been reported to be effective for the treatment of microfilariae. Tropical pulmonary eosinophilia syndrome is treated with diethylcarbamazine. When treating filariasis with diethylcarbamazine, antihistamines or glucocorticoids may be used to decrease the allergic reaction that may result from disintegration of microfilariae. Severe reactions may follow the administration of diethylcarbamazine to persons infected with filariasis who also have loiasis or onchocerciasis. Combined therapy with albendazole and ivermectin looked promising in early trials, and additional studies are underway.

Other management strategies include elevation of the affected body part, compression stockings, antiinflammatory drugs, skin care of the affected area, treatment of superficial fungal infections, as well as protection of the affected area from trauma. Surgical treatment includes debulking of the affected area, wide excision of chronic draining areas, and lymphatic shunts.

FIGURE 237-11

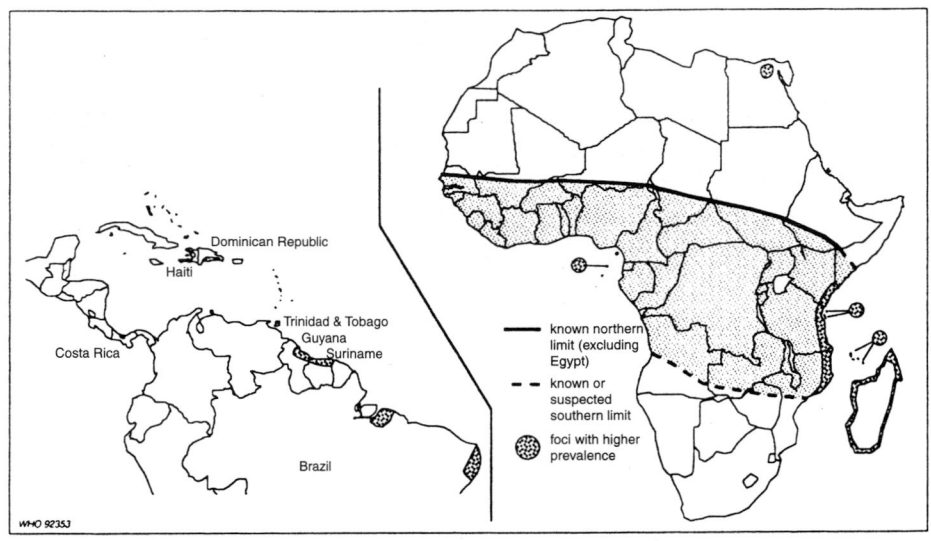

Distribution of *Wuchereria bancrofti* in the African region, region of the Americas, and Eastern Mediterranean region. [*Reprinted from: Lymphatic filariasis: The disease and its control. Fifth report of the WHO Expert Committee on Filariasis. Geneva, World Health Organization, 1992 (WHO Technical Report Series No. 821), with permission.*]

Prevention

Prevention includes the avoidance of mosquito bites in endemic areas. Prophylaxis with diethylcarbamazine (500 mg/d × 2 days each month) is effective for *W. bancrofti* and could be considered

FIGURE 237-12

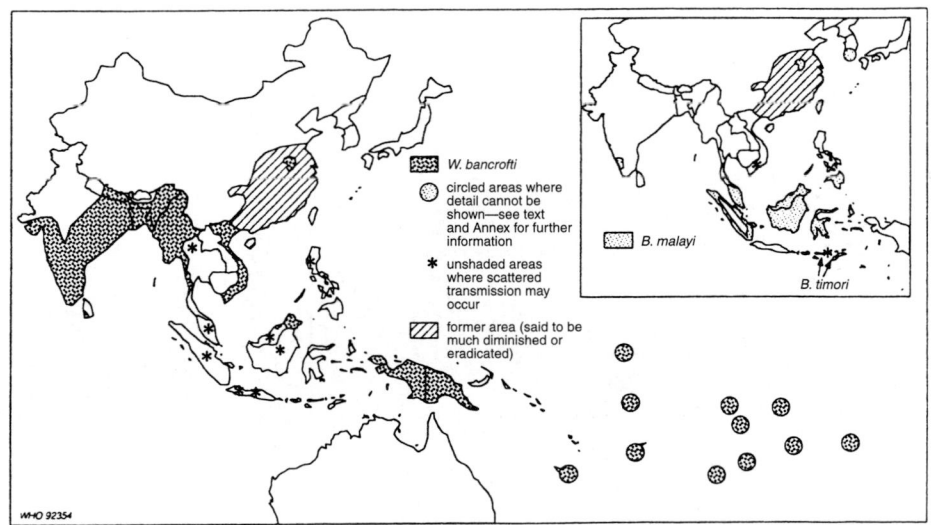

Distribution of *Wuchereria bancrofti, Brugia malayi,* and *B. timori* in the South east Asian and Western Pacific Regions. [*Reprinted from: Lymphatic filariasis: The disease and its control. Fifth report of the WHO Expert Committee on Filariasis. Geneva, World Health Organization, 1992 (WHO Technical Report Series No. 821), with permission.*]

for adults who plan to spend more than a month in endemic areas and are likely to have extensive exposures to mosquitoes.

GNATHOSTOMIASIS[60–62]

Synonyms

Yangtze River edema (China), *tau-chid* (Thailand), *choko-fushu* (Japan), wandering swelling, Consular disease (Nankung), Shanghai's rheumatism, nodular eosinophilic panniculitis (Ecuador), Woodbury bug (Australia)

Etiology

Gnathostomiasis (Fig. 237-13, Fig. 237-14) caused by the nematodes (roundworm) *Gnathostoma spinigerum* and less frequently, *G. hispidum*, *G. nipponicum*, and *G. doloresi*.

Life Cycle

The adult parasite lives in the stomachs of the definitive hosts, cats and dogs. Eggs are passed in the stool and hatch in water. The larvae are then ingested by *Cyclops* (a type of copepod, which are small aquatic arthropods) that are eaten by fish, frogs, and snakes, in which the larvae develop into third-stage larvae. When vertebrates who are unsuited to be definitive hosts (including humans) ingest the third-stage larvae, the larvae do not complete development but encyst or wander in tissues.

Pathogenesis

The ingested larvae penetrate the wall of the stomach and migrate in tissues causing inflammation, edema, hemorrhage, and necrosis. Chronic lesions are associated with eosinophilic and granulomatous inflammation. The parasite may reach any location within the body.

Geographic Distribution

Human gnathostomiasis is endemic in Southeast Asia, especially Thailand and Japan. Imported fish and other flesh can be the source of infection outside of endemic areas. Sporadic cases have been reported in the Americas, Africa, Europe, and Australia.

Epidemiology

ACQUISITION Gnathostomiasis is acquired by ingesting larvae in undercooked or raw flesh (e.g., fish, chicken, duck, pork, and frog). Transmission may also occur by ingestion of infective copepods in water or by skin penetration when handling infected fish.

INCUBATION PERIOD AND TIME FRAME Soft-tissue swellings usually begin 3 to 4 weeks after exposure but may not develop until months or years later. The parasite can survive in the human for 10 years or longer. One report documents recurrences for 20 years.

Clinical Features

The signs and symptoms range from mild to severe. Within 1 to 2 days after ingestion of the larvae, fever, malaise, anorexia, nausea, vomiting, diarrhea, epigastric pain, and urticaria may develop. Migration of the larvae in the skin and subcutaneous tissue results in intermittent, migratory swellings that are associated with erythema, pruritus, and pain. The lesions may be single or multiple, and up to several centimeters in diameter. The swellings develop rapidly, persist for 1 to 4 weeks, then resolve, only to reappear in a different anatomic location after an asymptomatic interval of a week to months. Over time, episodes become less frequent, less intense, and of shorter duration. However, cutaneous gnathostomiasis may continue for months to years. Gnathostomiasis may present as a cutaneous larva migrans-like eruption, and rarely as a skin abscess or nodule. The most common anatomic locations include the trunk, upper body, and thighs.

Visceral gnathostomiasis, involving deeper tissues and organs, has been reported to involve the eye, lungs, gastrointestinal and genitourinary tracts, and the central nervous system. Fewer than 1 percent of patients with cutaneous disease have central nervous system infection. Signs and symptoms reflect the location and activity

FIGURE 237-13

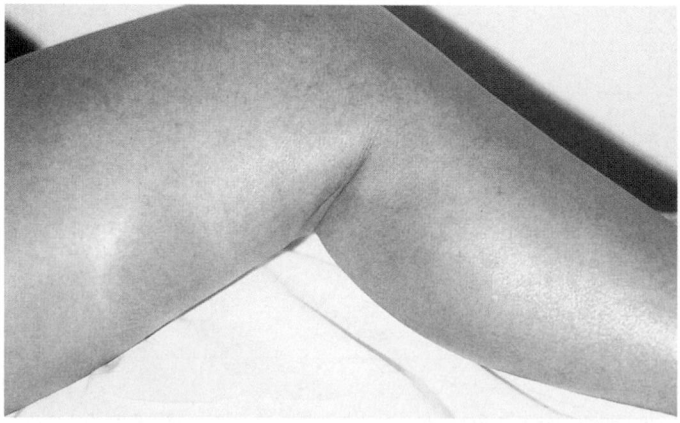

Subcutaneous swellings of gnathostomiasis. (*Courtesy of Jay S. Keystone, MD, FRCPC.*)

FIGURE 237-14

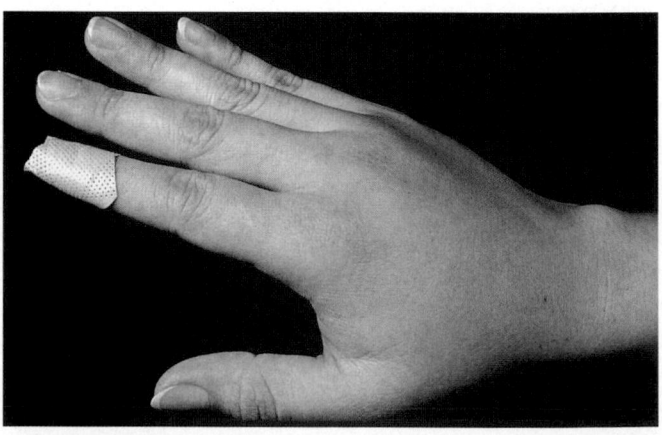

Subcutaneous swellings of gnathostomiasis. (*Courtesy of Jay S. Keystone, MD, FRCPC.*)

of the larvae. Facial migratory swellings are a sign of increased risk for both ocular involvement and possible permanent visual loss as well as central nervous system involvement should the worm migrate through a cranial foramen. Deaths from central nervous system involvement have been reported.

Laboratory

Peripheral eosinophilia may be high grade. Leukocytosis may be present during larval migration. When the central nervous system is infected, the cerebrospinal fluid may be bloody or xanthochromic and contains eosinophils.

Diagnosis

The diagnosis is based on the characteristic morphology of larvae in surgical specimens or at autopsy. ELISA is available in some endemic areas to aid in the diagnosis.

Differential Diagnosis

The differential diagnosis of soft-tissue gnathostomiasis includes loiasis, onchocerciasis, sparganosis, cutaneous myiasis, cutaneous larva migrans, visceral larva migrans, dirofilariasis, cutaneous paragonimiasis, and eosinophilic cellulitis.

Treatment

The treatment of choice is surgical excision plus albendazole. Ivermectin has been shown to be effective in animals.

Prevention

Infection can be prevented by avoiding raw and undercooked flesh of fish, eel, chicken, duck, pork, snake, dogs, cats, and frog; drinking only treated water; and wearing gloves when handling potentially infected flesh.

HOOKWORM DISEASE[63-66]

Synonyms and Diseases

New World hookworm disease, American hookworm disease, uncinariasis, or necatoriasis (for disease caused by *Necator americanus*); Old World hookworm infection or ancylostomiasis (for disease caused by *Ancylostoma duodenale*); ground itch, hookworm folliculitis. See also cutaneous larva migrans

Etiology

The major causes of hookworm disease are *A. duodenale* and *N. americanus*. Pathologic effects show some variation by species. *A. ceylanicum* has a more limited distribution. *A. caninum* causes eosinophilic enteritis as well as cutaneous disease. (See "Cutaneous larva migrans.")

Life Cycle

Eggs embryonate and hatch in the soil and develop into infective larvae over five to ten days. Humans are the main reservoir host for *A. duodenale* and *N. americanus*. Cats and dogs are hosts for *A. ceylanicum* and *A. caninum*.

Pathogenesis

The larvae penetrate the skin, reach superficial venules and enter the circulation. They reach the lungs and penetrate the alveoli. Larvae are carried up the respiratory tract to the pharynx then swallowed. Parasites mature and attach to villi, mainly in the jejunum, where they suck blood and cause bleeding at the site of mucosal attachment. Eggs are shed in the feces. When *A. duodenale* larvae are swallowed instead of entering via the skin, they develop without passing through the lung.

Geographic Distribution

The various species that cause hookworm disease have distinct but overlapping distributions. Hookworm disease is most common in rural tropical and subtropical areas but can also be found in temperate areas when sanitation is poor. In 1996, WHO estimated that hookworm disease affected 151 million persons and caused 65,000 deaths. The majority of persons who harbor hookworms have no or few symptoms; disease develops in about 25 percent as a consequence of infection.

Epidemiology

ACQUISITION   Infection is acquired by penetration of intact skin or mucosa by infective larvae and ingestion of food (e.g., raw vegetables) contaminated by *A. duodenale* larvae. Transmammary infection is possible with *A. duodenale*. There is probable infection in utero by transplacental spread. Skin contact with fecally-contaminated soil poses a high risk. Walking barefoot is the most common way to acquire infection.

INCUBATION PERIOD AND TIME FRAME   Skin changes usually begin 1 to 2 days after skin penetration. Eggs are found in the stool 4 to 6 weeks after skin penetration. Pulmonary symptoms may occur 1 to 3 weeks and gastrointestinal symptoms 1 month after percutaneous penetration. *A. duodenale* survives for approximately 1 year (and up to 5 to 7 years) and *N. americanus* survives for 2 to 6 years (and up to 15 to 20 years) in the human.

Clinical Features

The majority of infections are asymptomatic or mild. Heavy infections are debilitating and can contribute to death. Within 1 to 2 days, the area of skin penetrated by the larvae may have localized erythema, edema, and papular or papulovesicular lesions. This eruption, known as "ground itch," is most commonly located on the feet and lasts 1 to 2 weeks. There may be an associated generalized urticaria. In a minority of patients, the pulmonary migration phase is associated with cough, wheezing, and shortness of breath. Heavy infections are associated with abdominal pain, diarrhea, and gastrointestinal bleeding. Chronic infection is associated with signs and symptoms of hypoproteinemia and chronic anemia: edema, pallor, weakness, shortness of breath, and tachycardia. Hookworm infection in children can retard growth and intellectual development.

Previous infection does not prevent reinfection, but may have a limiting effect on the worm population.

Laboratory

A peripheral eosinophilia begins as early as 2 to 3 weeks after skin penetration and may be high grade during tissue migration. Chest x-ray films may reveal transient pulmonary infiltrates. In chronic infection, abnormal laboratory values include iron deficiency anemia and hypoalbuminemia. There is gross or occult blood in the stool.

Diagnosis

A presumptive diagnosis of "ground itch" is based on characteristic clinical findings in a person with appropriate epidemiologic exposure. At the time a patient presents with skin changes and pulmonary infiltrates, stool examinations will be negative. A period of 4 to 6 weeks after exposure must pass before eggs can be found on stool examination. The eggs of *A. duodenale* and *N. americanus* are indistinguishable by routine light microscopy.

Differential Diagnosis

The differential diagnosis includes other infections, inflammatory diseases, and malignancies of the gastrointestinal tract.

Treatment

In assessing the need for therapy, the worm burden must be estimated by obtaining egg counts. Effective oral medications include mebendazole, pyrantel pamoate (considered investigational by the FDA for this infection) and albendazole. Albendazole appears to be more effective than mebendazole.

Prevention

Hookworm infections can be prevented by the sanitary disposal of human feces.

LOIASIS[67–70]

Synonyms

Calabar swellings, fugitive swellings, loa loa filariasis, African eyeworm infection

Etiology

The filarial nematode (roundworm), *Loa loa*, is the parasite responsible for loiasis.

Life Cycle

The *Chrysops* (a type of fly) bites an infected human and ingests microfilariae along with the blood meal. The microfilariae develop into larvae, which are transmitted when the fly bites another human.

Pathogenesis

Larvae from the biting fly enter the human through the puncture wound. The larvae mature into adult worms that live in subcutaneous tissue and migrate along fascial planes to all parts of the body. The adult worms produce microfilariae that enter the bloodstream during the day and may reside in the lungs when not circulating.

Geographic Distribution

Loiasis is endemic in Central and West Africa.

Epidemiology

ACQUISITION   Loiasis is acquired by the bite of the infective day-biting flies of the genus *Chrysops*. The microfilariae can be transmitted via transfused blood, but will not develop into adult worms in the human host. In endemic areas, infection rates exceed 50 percent in some human populations. Flies live in the canopy of the rain forest and lay eggs in muddy streams and swamps. The flies are attracted by dark clothing, wood smoke, and movement of people or vehicles. Infections in visitors from nonendemic areas occur primarily in persons spending at least 3 months in endemic areas.

INCUBATION PERIOD AND TIME FRAME   Symptoms usually begin one year or longer after exposure, though first findings can appear as early as 4 months or as long as 8 years after acquisition of infection. Microfilariae first appear in the bloodstream 5 to 6 months after the person becomes infected. The adult worm can live longer than 10 years in the human host.

Clinical Features

Loiasis is manifested by pruritus, urticaria, and Calabar swellings (Fig. 237-15), which are localized areas of angioedema associated with the migration of the adult worms through the subcutaneous tissues. Calabar swellings may be erythematous and warm and range from 5 to 10 cm in diameter. They may be associated with pruritus or pain. The lesions last several days and may recur multiple times. The lesions are found predominately on the extremities (upper greater than lower) and especially around joints, such as the wrist or knee. Fatigue, myalgias, arthralgias, and fever may be associated with the lesions. A migrating adult worm may be seen crossing the conjunctivae or the bridge of the nose (hence the term "eyeworm")

FIGURE 237-15

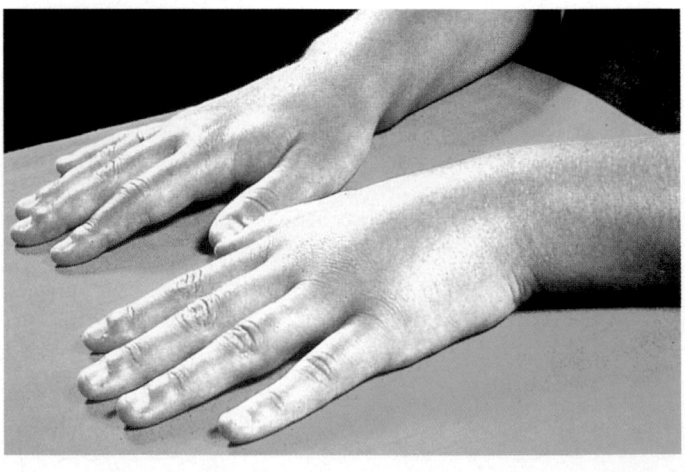

Calabar swelling of loiasis. (*Courtesy of Jay S. Keystone, MD, FRCPC.*)

(Fig. 237-16). This is associated with swellings on the face and particularly of the periorbital region.

Other, less-common systemic findings include arthritis, lymphadenopathy, lymphedema, peripheral neuropathy, cardiomyopathy (endomyocardial fibrosis), hematuria, proteinuria, and encephalopathy.

Individuals living in endemic areas may be microfilaremic, with a wide range of symptoms. Persons from nonendemic regions who become infected often do not have detectable microfilaremia but have prominent symptoms and immunologic hyperresponsiveness.

Laboratory

Findings include a peripheral eosinophilia that may be high grade, leukocytosis, and elevated IgE. *L. loa*–specific IgG4 is elevated. These findings are much less prominent in infected persons who have always resided in endemic areas. While older serologic tests are constrained by cross-reactivity with other parasites, newer approaches are being developed, including the use of polymerase chain reaction (PCR) amplification of *L. loa* DNA from the blood.

Diagnosis

The diagnosis is based on identification of microfilariae in blood (during the day), or occasionally from urine, cerebrospinal fluid, sputum, or other body fluid or by identification of an adult worm removed from the eye or other tissues. Calcified worms may be seen on x-ray films.

Differential Diagnosis

The differential diagnosis includes other filarial infections, gnathostomiasis, and toxocariasis.

FIGURE 237-16

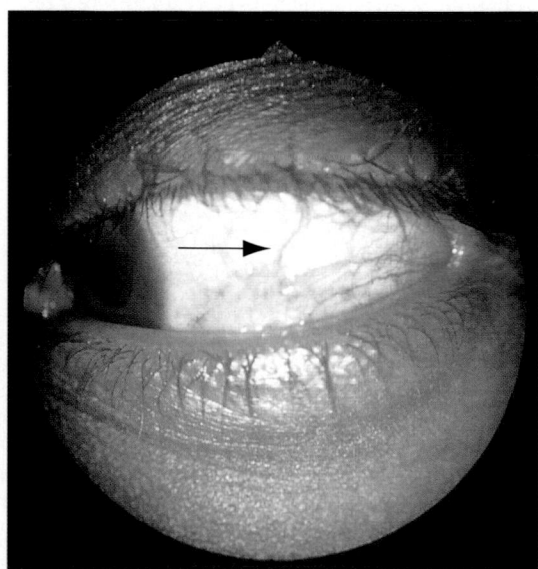

Loiasis. Adult worm crossing eye. (*Courtesy of Murray Wittner, MD, PhD.*)

Treatment

Treatment includes the surgical removal of the worm from the eye or other tissue, if feasible. Patients may be infected with multiple worms (usually not more than 10 to 20 adult worms). Diethylcarbamazine (DEC) is currently the drug of choice for persons who are not microfilaremic. Local inflammatory manifestations may occur within 1 to 2 days of DEC treatment. These include pruritus and subcutaneous nodules, which when biopsied, reveal the adult worm.

Treatment of microfilaremic loiasis patients with DEC can be followed by neurologic complications, including encephalitis and death. Alternative approaches in patients with heavy infections have included use of ivermectin or albendazole or apheresis to reduce microfilaremia.

Prevention

Prevention includes protection from *Chrysops* bites in endemic areas. Prophylaxis with DEC is effective for *L. loa* in adults who may spend more than a month in endemic regions and expect to have frequent exposures to biting flies.

ONCHOCERCIASIS[71–76]

Synonyms

Onchocercosis, blinding filariasis, river blindness, coastal erysipelas, erysipela de la costa (Mexico and Guatemala), onchocercomata, onchodermatitis, sowda (Arabic speaking areas), craw-craw (West Africa)

Etiology

Onchocerciasis is caused by the filarial nematode (roundworm), *Onchocerca volvulus*.

Life Cycle

Blackflies of the genus *Simulium* bite an individual infected with *O. volvulus*. The microfilariae develop into infective larvae within the blackfly, which passes larvae to another human when taking a blood meal.

Pathogenesis

Infective larvae enter the human skin when the blackfly takes a blood meal. The larvae mature to adult worms that are encapsulated in fibrous tissue and reside in nodules in the subcutaneous tissue and deep fascia. Necrosis and calcification may follow the death of the worm. Microfilariae migrate from adult worms and may enter the bloodstream. Presence of microfilariae in the skin, connective tissue, eyes, and lymph nodes is associated with significant pathologic findings.

Geographic Distribution

The greatest concentration of cases is in equatorial Africa. Endemic foci are also found in Latin America, Yemen and Saudi Arabia. Fig. 237-17 shows the geographic distribution of onchocerciasis in Af-

FIGURE 237-17

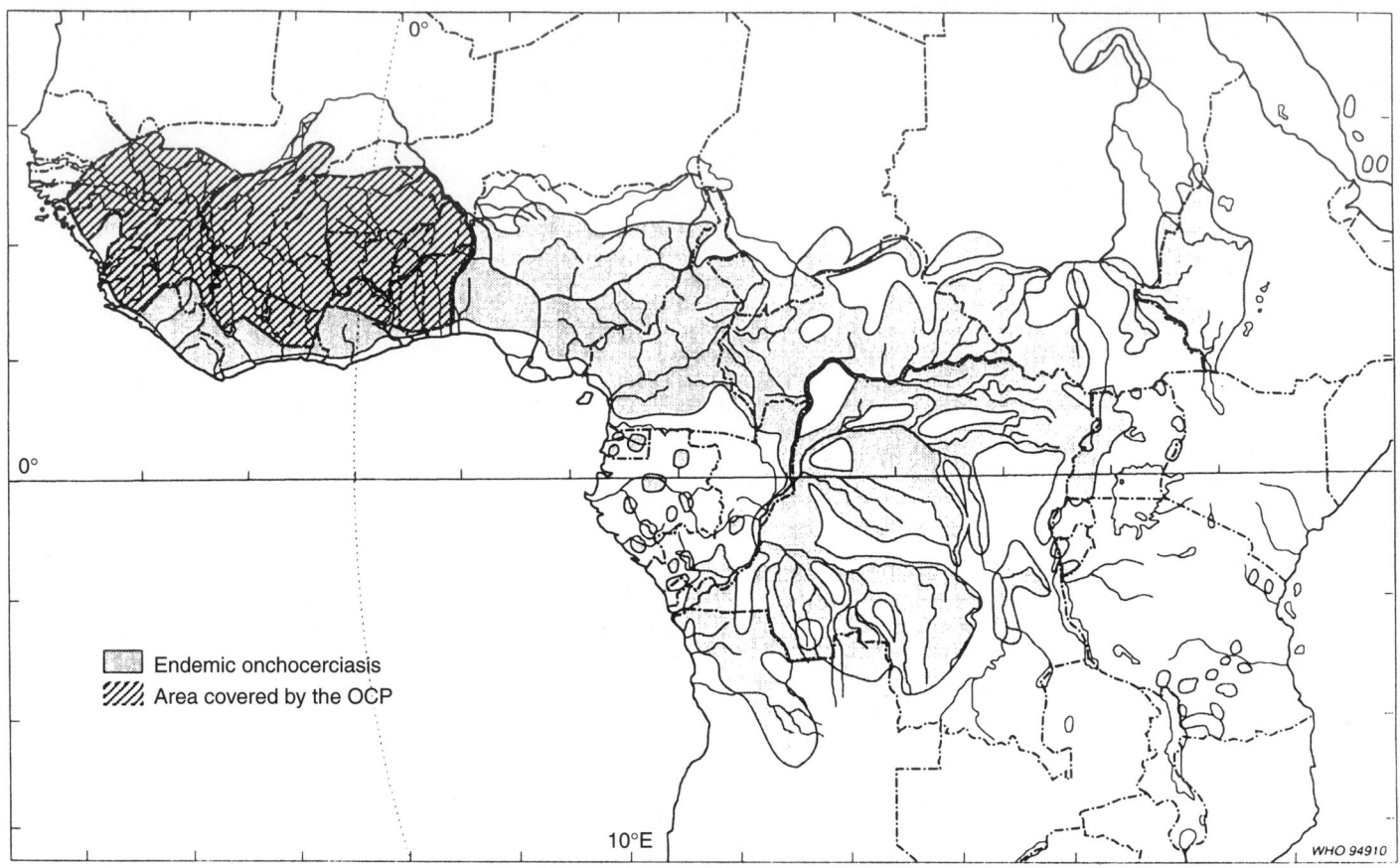

Endemic onchocerciasis

Area covered by the OCP

Geographical distribution of onchocerciasis in Africa and the Arabian peninsula. [*Reprinted from: Onchocerciasis and its control. Report of a WHO Expert Committee on Onchocerciasis Control. Geneva, World* *Health Organization, 1995 (WHO Technical Report Series No. 852), with permission.*]

rica and the Arabian peninsula. Fig. 237-18 shows the geographic distribution of endemic onchocerciasis in the Americas. Onchocerciasis primarily affects people living near fast-flowing rivers where blackflies breed.

Epidemiology

ACQUISITION Onchocerciasis is acquired by the bite of an infective blackfly. Microfilariae can be transmitted to a fetus from an infected mother. The potential exists for transmission of microfilariae by blood transfusion. It is estimated that about 17.5 million persons are infected and 85 million are at risk for infection. An estimated 1 million persons have significant visual impairment due to onchocerciasis, and 3 to 4 million infected persons have onchocercal skin disease. Symptomatic infection generally occurs only in persons who have lived in endemic areas for several months and usually longer. Severe disease requires repeated exposures over many years.

INCUBATION PERIOD AND TIME FRAME The incubation period is usually 1 to 2 years with a range of months to several years. Microfilariae may first appear 3 to 15 months after exposure. The initial symptoms can precede the presence of microfilariae in tissue but often develop only after months or years of infection. The microfilariae can survive in humans for up to 2 to 3 years and the adult worms for 10 to 15 years.

Clinical Features

Persons with onchocerciasis may be asymptomatic or may have severe impairment including loss of vision. The skin and the eye are the two most involved organ systems.

The skin manifestations of onchocerciasis include six different patterns including acute papular onchodermatitis (Fig. 237-19), chronic papular onchodermatitis, lichenified onchodermatitis, atrophy, depigmentation, and palpable onchocercal nodules. More than one pattern of skin involvement may be present simultaneously, or one pattern of skin involvement may evolve into another pattern. Pruritus is often the first symptom of infection. Acute papular onchodermatitis includes widespread small pruritic papules that may progress to vesicles and pustules in the most severe cases. There may be associated erythema and edema. Acute papular onchodermatitis most often involves the face, extremities, and trunk. Ivermectin and DEC can precipitate a rash similar to acute papular

FIGURE 237-18

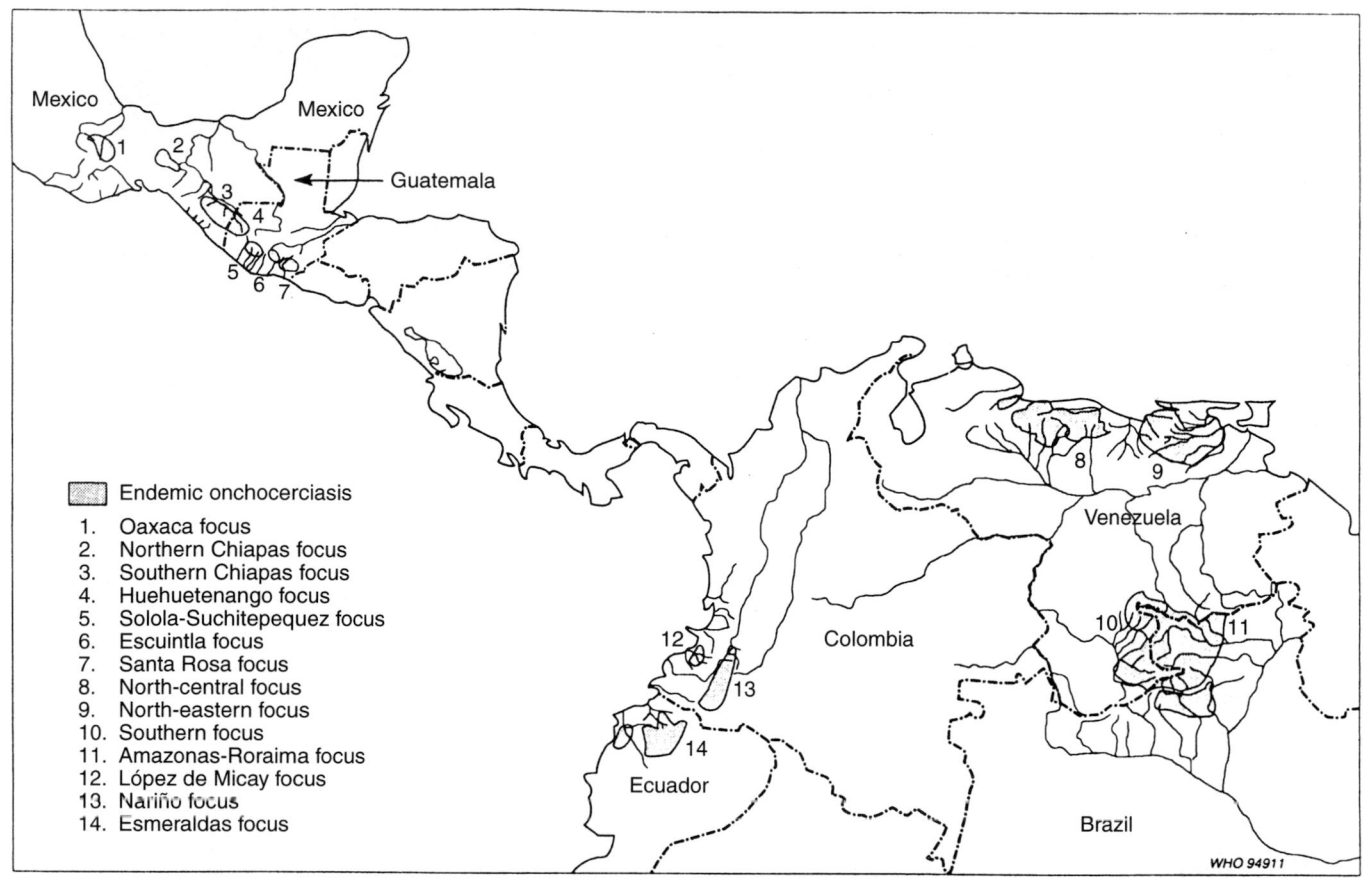

Geographical distribution of endemic onchocerciasis in the Americas. [From: Onchocerciasis and its control. Report of a WHO Expert Committee on Onchocerciasis Control. Geneva, World Health Organization, 1995 (WHO Technical Report Series No. 852), with permission.]

onchodermatitis. In Mexico and Guatemala, erythema, edema and pruritus of the face is known as "erisipela de la costa" and is an acute onchocercal reaction.

The skin lesions of chronic papular onchodermatitis are macules and lichenoid papules varying in size from 3 to 9 mm in diameter. Pruritus is common and post-inflammatory hyperpigmentation may be present. The most commonly affected anatomic areas are the buttocks, shoulders, and waist area.

Lichenified onchodermatitis, also known as "sowda" (Arabic for "black") in Arabic-speaking regions, most commonly affects teenagers and young adults and is most commonly seen in Yemen and Sudan. Hyperkeratotic and hyperpigmented pruritic plaques become more confluent and lichenified with increased severity and time. The plaques have an asymmetric distribution with the lower extremity being the most commonly affected anatomic location. There is often associated lymphadenopathy.

Atrophy, also known as "lizard skin" in its most severe presentation, makes middle-aged persons appear elderly. The anatomic locations most commonly involved are the buttocks and, less commonly, the extremities.

Depigmentation (Fig. 237-20) associated with onchocerciasis is also known as "leopard skin." Depigmentation is associated with perifollicular pigmentation within macular or minimally depressed areas. In black skin, there may be yellow-brown hypopigmentation. Pruritus is rarely seen in this pattern of skin involvement by onchocerciasis. The anatomic location most commonly involved is the skin area bilaterally. A previous report described the depigmentation of the shins as a useful method to screen for onchocerciasis in endemic areas. Less commonly the buttocks, lateral groin, and lower abdomen are involved.

Palpable onchocercal nodules (Fig. 237-21), containing the adult worm, involve the deep dermis and subcutaneous tissue. The nodules are typically asymptomatic and occur over bony prominences such as the skull, iliac crest, knee, rib, sacrum, scapula, and trochanter.

Other clinical findings associated with onchocerciasis include "hanging groin," which consists of folds of inelastic skin in the inguinal area, and associated lymphadenopathy. Other findings include groin hernias, lymphedema of external genitalia or limbs, and lymphadenopathy.

Ocular involvement is the most devastating aspect of this disease with blindness a potential outcome. Ocular findings include chorioretinitis, iritis, optic atrophy, punctate keratitis, and sclerosing keratitis.

FIGURE 237-19

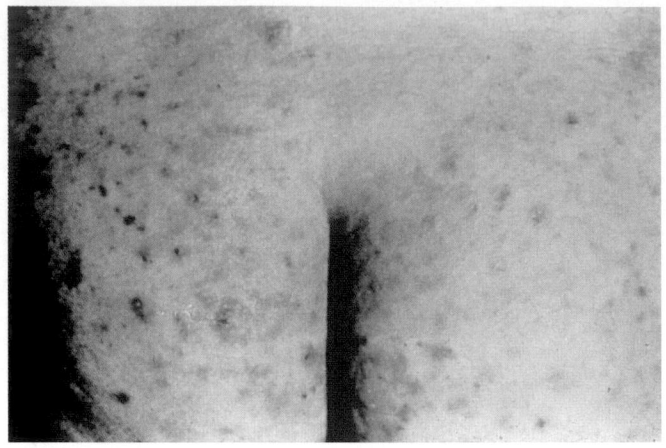

Onchocercal dermatitis. (*Courtesy of Herman Zaiman, MD.*)

FIGURE 237-20

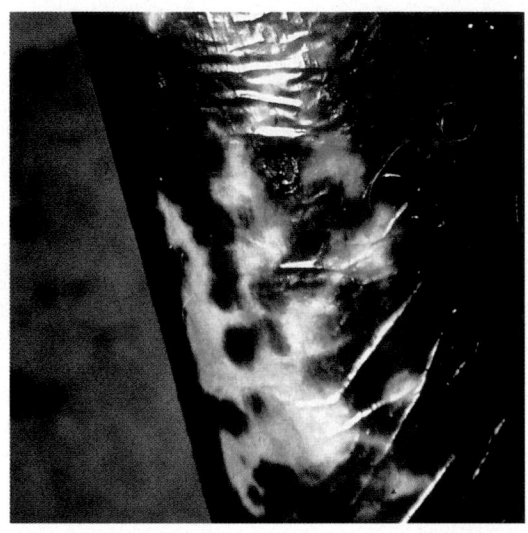

Depigmentation secondary to onchocerciasis. (*Courtesy of Jay S. Keystone, MD, FRCPC.*)

There are many psychosocial issues surrounding onchocerciasis given the potential ocular involvement as well as the obvious skin manifestations that are easily recognizable to those individuals in endemic areas.

The most common presentations in visitors to endemic areas are pruritus and rash. Skin nodules and eye involvement are usually

FIGURE 237-21

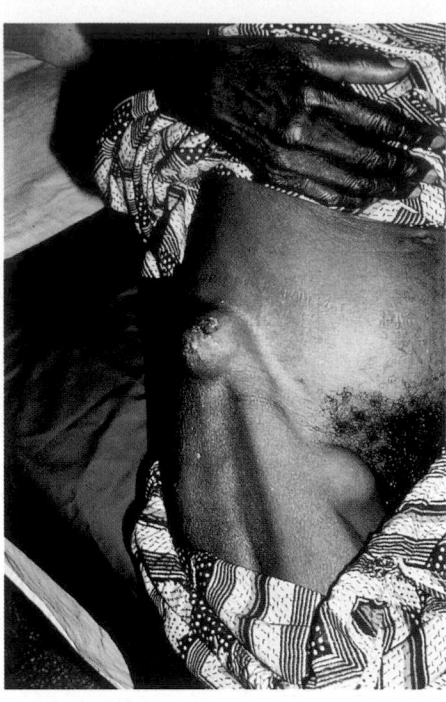

Onchocercal nodule over iliac crest. (*Courtesy of Jay S. Keystone, MD, FRCPC.*)

absent and microfilariae are absent or found in low numbers in the skin.

Laboratory

Peripheral eosinophilia and elevated IgE levels are common findings.

Diagnosis

Onchocerciasis is most commonly diagnosed by the identification of the microfilariae in a skin snip or of an adult worm in an excised nodule. In heavily infected individuals microfilariae may be found in the blood (up to one-third of cases), sputum, cerebrospinal fluid, urine, or other fluids. Microfilariae can easily be seen in the anterior chamber of the eye on slit-lamp examination.

Differential Diagnosis

The differential diagnosis of the skin manifestations of onchocerciasis depends on the skin pattern at presentation. Acute papular onchodermatitis may resemble miliaria, insect bites, or a hypersensitivity reaction. Chronic papular onchodermatitis may resemble a chronic or lichenoid hypersensitivity reaction or atopic dermatitis. The differential diagnosis for lichenified onchodermatitis is broad and includes essentially any diagnosis that involves significant pruritus or rubbing of the involved area. Atrophy associated with onchocerciasis resembles that associated with aging. Onchocercal depigmentation may be confused with postinflammatory hypopigmentation or depigmentation. The differential diagnosis for onchocercal nodules includes cysticercosis, histoplasmosis, paragonimiasis, and epidermal inclusion cysts.

Treatment

The drug of choice is ivermectin. Surgical excision of the nodules, especially if located on the head, is recommended.

Prevention

Prevention of onchocerciasis is primarily through vector control and mass treatment with ivermectin of the population in endemic areas.

PARAGONIMIASIS[77]

Synonyms

Lung fluke infection, oriental lung fluke disease

Etiology

The trematode (fluke) *Paragonimus westermani* and more than 10 species of *Paragonimus* infect humans.

Life Cycle

Eggs hatch in water and release free-swimming miracidia that enter snails and develop into cercariae. The cercariae leave the snail and invade tissues of freshwater crabs, shrimp, or crayfish, where they encyst as metacercariae. The crustaceans are eaten by the definitive host, which may be a human, though other animals are more important in maintaining the life cycle.

Pathogenesis

In humans the ingested metacercariae excyst in the small intestine, migrate through the gut wall, and enter the abdominal cavity, where they remain for several days. They migrate across the diaphragm into the pleural cavity and lungs, where they mature and produce eggs that are expectorated in sputum or swallowed. A fibrous capsule surrounds the flukes, forming a cyst that may rupture, thus releasing ova and necrotic material into the bronchioles. The eggs provoke a granulomatous reaction. Flukes may migrate anywhere within the body, including subcutaneous tissues, and cause an eosinophilic, granulomatous reaction or abscess.

Geographic Distribution

P. westermani is widely distributed in East and Southeast Asia and Africa. Other species of *Paragonimus* are found in Asia, Africa and the Americas.

Epidemiology

ACQUISITION Paragonimiasis is acquired by ingesting metacercariae in raw or undercooked freshwater crayfish, crab, or shrimp or with other foods or fluids contaminated with metacercariae during preparation. Juices from raw crustaceans are used for medicinal purposes in Korea and Japan. Worldwide, more than 10 million persons are estimated to be infected. The rates of infection are high in parts of Asia, where raw, undercooked, salted, pickled, or marinated crustaceans are frequently eaten. Paragonimiasis is also acquired by eating raw or undercooked field rats and wild boar.

INCUBATION PERIOD AND TIME FRAME Urticaria and gastrointestinal symptoms can begin within a few days of ingestion. Migratory subcutaneous nodules may appear as early as 2 weeks, and pulmonary symptoms occur as early as a few weeks. Central nervous system involvement typically manifests 12 to 16 months after the onset of infection. Eggs are first produced approximately 10 weeks after ingestion of metacercariae. The diagnosis may not be made for years. The life span of the fluke within humans is usually 10 years or less, but can be as long as 20 to 30 years.

Clinical Features

The clinical features range from asymptomatic to fatal depending on the intensity of infection and the anatomic location involved.

The acute phase corresponds to fluke migration and tissue invasion. This is manifested by urticaria, abdominal pain, and diarrhea, followed by cough, hemoptysis, production of rusty colored sputum, wheezing, pleuritic pain, and low-grade fever. These findings can continue for weeks.

Patients with chronic infection have pulmonary and sometimes extrapulmonary findings. Ten percent of patients with *P. westermani* and 20 to 60 percent of patients with *P. skrjabini* (*P. szechuanensis*) have subcutaneous swelling or nodules (containing immature flukes). These lesions may be up to 6 cm, migratory, firm, slightly mobile, and tender to palpation. The lesions are most commonly located on the lower abdomen and inguinal region. Cerebral involvement occurs in less than 1 percent of patients and is more common in children. Five percent of central nervous system infections are fatal. Presenting findings include meningoencephalitis (early) and signs and symptoms of a space-occupying lesion (late). Abdominal involvement may result in abdominal pain, bloody diarrhea, and palpable abdominal masses.

Laboratory

A peripheral eosinophilia is seen in 80 percent but may be low grade or absent when the parasites are encysted. Eosinophils may be found in fluids adjacent to the parasite, for example, in cerebrospinal fluid, sputum, pleural, and pericardial fluid.

Diagnosis

The diagnosis is made by the identification of eggs in the sputum, feces, pleural or cerebrospinal fluid or by the identification of the adult parasite or eggs in tissue. An immunoblot serologic test has high sensitivity and specificity. It is available from the Centers for Disease Control and Prevention in Atlanta. Chest x-ray films may reveal many findings, including diffuse infiltrates, nodules, cavities, ring cysts, calcification, and pleural effusions.

Differential Diagnosis

The differential diagnosis for the subcutaneous nodules includes gnathostomiasis, sparganosis, and onchocerciasis. The differential diagnosis of pulmonary involvement includes tuberculosis, lung abscess, fungal infections, malignant tumor, melioidosis, and echinococcosis. The differential diagnosis for central nervous system involvement includes cysticercosis, echinococcosis, angiostrongyloidiasis, gnathostomiasis, fungal infection, tuberculosis, schistosomiasis, and a benign or malignant tumor.

Treatment

The drug of choice is praziquantel. Although it is an approved drug, the Food and Drug Administration considers it investigational for paragonimiasis. When treating cerebral paragonimiasis, glucocorticoids should be given along with praziquantel to blunt the inflammatory reaction that follows release of antigens from the dying worms. Bithionol is an alternative mode of therapy. In the United States, bithionol is available from the Centers for Disease Control Drug Service, Centers for Disease Control and Prevention, Atlanta, GA 30333. The telephone numbers are (404) 639-3670 during the day and (404) 639-2888 on evenings, weekends, and holidays.

Prevention

Paragonimiasis may be prevented by eating only well-cooked crustaceans.

SCHISTOSOMIASIS[78–82]

Synonyms

Bilharziasis, snail fever, Katayama fever

Etiology

Schistosomiasis is caused by trematodes (flukes) that, in the adult stage, live in blood vessels. These include primarily *Schistosoma mansoni*, *S. japonicum*, *S. haematobium*, *S. mekongi*, and *S. intercalatum*. See also cercarial dermatitis for a discussion of disease caused by non-human schistosomes.

Life Cycle

Eggs excreted by a human or animal, hatch in water, releasing free-swimming miracidia that penetrate the intermediate host, the snail, where they develop over 4 to 6 weeks, then emerge as free-swimming cercariae. The cercariae must penetrate the skin of a vertebrate host to continue development to the adult stage. Humans are the only important reservoir for *S. haematobium*. In parts of Africa, baboons are important hosts for *S. mansoni*. Animals (e.g., cows and dogs) are important hosts for *S. japonicum*.

Pathogenesis

Cercariae penetrate the skin over 30 seconds to 10 minutes, become schistosomulae, and may elicit a local inflammatory response. Schistosomulae enter venules and reach pulmonary capillaries in 1 week after skin penetration. Worms mature in the hepatic sinusoids after several weeks, mate, and migrate to the mesenteric venules (*S. intercalatum, S. japonicum, S. mansoni, S. mekongi)* or recto-vesical plexus and branches of the vesical plexus (*S. haematobium),* where the mature worm pairs begin to produce eggs 1 to 3 months after infection. Mature adult females lay eggs daily, of which 60 percent remain in tissues or enter the bloodstream. The remainder of the eggs reach the bowel or bladder and are excreted. Host response to the eggs is characterized by granulomas with epithelioid cells, foreign-body giant cells, and many eosinophils. Necrosis, fi-

brosis, and calcification occur late in the disease. Worms do not multiply in the human host.

Geographic Distribution

S. haematobium is widespread in Africa, western Asia, and possibly a focal area of middle Asia (India). *S. japonicum* is found in several areas in eastern and Southeast Asia. *S. mekongi* is localized to a small area in Southeast Asia. *S. mansoni* is found in more than 50 countries in Africa, tropical South America, the Caribbean, and western Asia (eastern Mediterranean region). *S. intercalatum* has been found in at least six central African countries. Figure 237-22 shows the geographic distribution of schistosomiasis due to *S. haematobium*, *S. japonicum*, and *S. mekongi*. Figure 237-23 shows the geographic distribution of schistosomiasis due to *S. mansoni* and *S. intercalatum*.

Epidemiology

ACQUISITION   Schistosomiasis is acquired by contact with water containing live cercariae (which penetrate intact skin and mucous membranes) and by drinking infested water. An estimated more than 200 million persons in the world are infected and 500 to 600 million live in endemic areas. Infection can be acquired after a brief exposure in an endemic area (e.g., during travel). Activities associated with risk in endemic areas include swimming, wading, rafting, and bathing in infested water. Pools, ponds, shores of lakes, and small dams pose a greater risk than rapidly flowing streams. Invasive schistosomes are not found in saltwater. Chlorination, iodination, and boiling eliminate infective cercariae.

INCUBATION PERIOD AND TIME FRAME   The skin manifestations begin within minutes. Schistosomal fever (Katayama fever), which develops in a minority of those infected, begins 2 to 10 weeks after exposure. Other symptoms may begin after weeks to years. The usual lifespan of the adult worm within the human is 3 to 10 years; but survival of more than 30 years has been documented.

Clinical Features

Schistosomal infections in humans range from inapparent to fatal. Most light infections are asymptomatic and even heavy infections may cause few symptoms. Serious sequelae develop in a small percentage of those who are infected, typically after many years of infection.

Schistosomiasis produces several different cutaneous manifestations. Schistosomal dermatitis occurs shortly after exposure to water infested with cercariae and reflects a hypersensitivity response to the cercariae. An urticarial and erythematous papular eruption associated with pruritus develops in persons who have been previously sensitized. The rash usually resolves over 1 week. In individuals without previous exposure to the parasites, the first exposure results in erythema and pruritus that resolves within hours. A similar rash may appear after exposure to nonhuman schistosomes (sometimes also called schistosomal dermatitis). (See "Cercarial Dermatitis.")

Symptoms of acute schistosomiasis, also known as Katayama syndrome or Katayama fever, are most prominent in primary infection in nonimmune persons. The findings are due to a hypersensitivity response to schistosome antigens as well as circulating immune complexes. Symptoms include fever, myalgias and headache that may persist for 2 to 10 weeks, sometimes longer. Patients may also have lymphadenopathy, abdominal pain, anorexia and diarrhea.

FIGURE 237-22

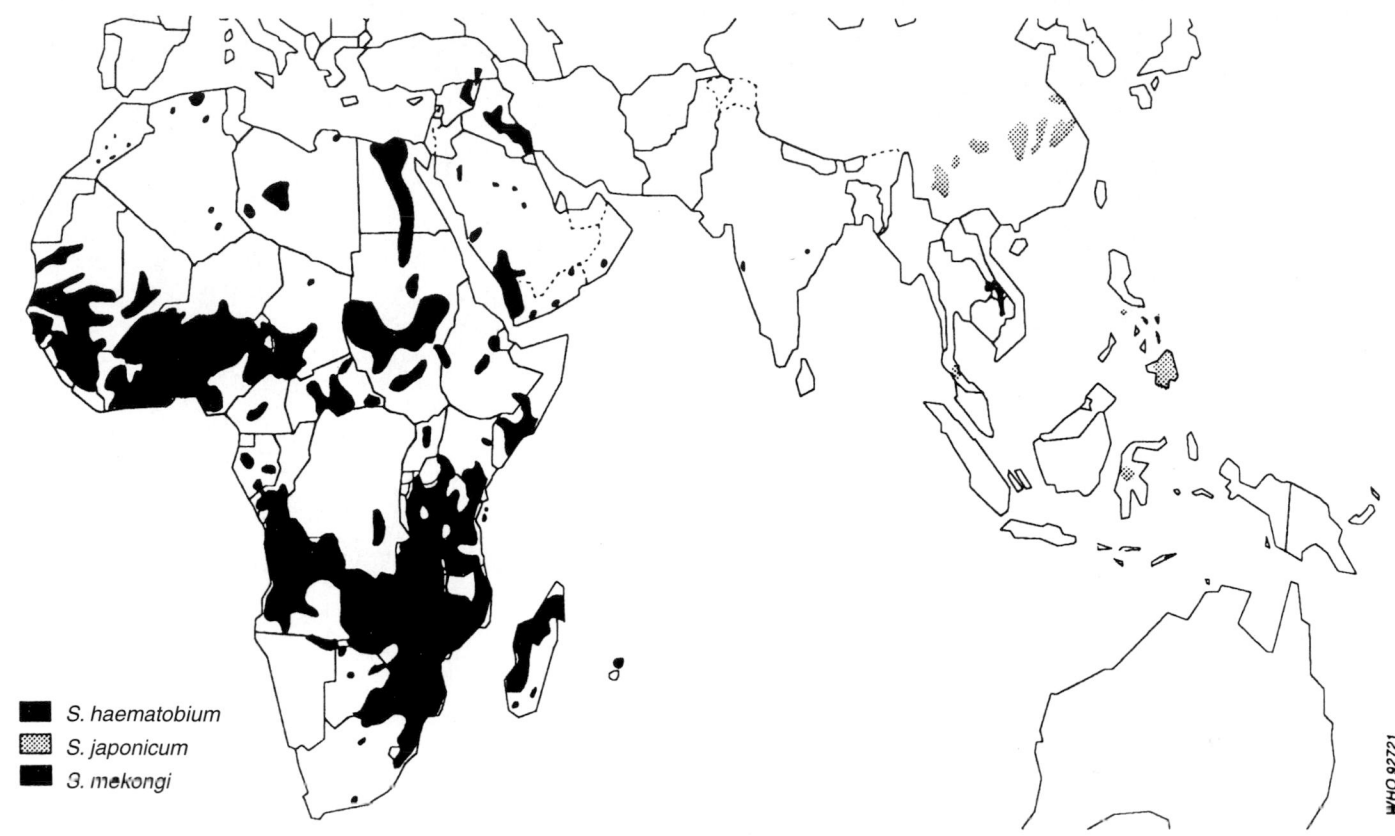

Global distribution of schistosomiasis due to *Schistosoma haematobium, S. japonicum,* and *S. mekongi.* [From: *The control of schistosomiasis. Second report of the WHO Expert Committee. Geneva, World Health Organization, 1993 (WHO Technical Report Series No. 830),* with permission.]

The skin manifestations include urticaria, purpura, and edema of the face and particularly the extremities, genitals, and trunk. Katayama fever occurs with *S. japonicum* and *S. mansoni* but rarely with *S. haematobium.*

Late skin involvement, bilharziasis cutanea tarda, occurs in persons with visceral disease. The cutaneous manifestations are due to the granulomatous, inflammatory reaction to the deposition of eggs in the dermis (Fig. 237-24). This is seen primarily in persons who live in endemic regions. When lesions are present, they manifest as skin-colored or slightly pigmented, 2- to 4-mm, oval papules that may form clusters. The lesions are firm on palpation and are associated with pruritus. The lesions appear in crops, and without treatment remain unchanged. The trunk, particularly the periumbilical region, is the most common anatomic location. A zosteriform distribution has been described. Soft tissue involvement that presented as a breast mass has also been described.

Lesions also appear in the genital and buttocks areas, especially on the vulva in women and the scrotum and penis in men. Early in the disease, the lesions in these locations may also manifest as papules or nodules. The presentation late in the disease is that of painless, skin colored, pink or brown erosive papules and warty, vegetative, polypoid lesions that may be ulcerated and necrotic, with fistulous tracts. Lymphedema and elephantiasis can occur. These lesions may be complicated by secondary bacterial infection and squamous-cell carcinoma.

Ectopic egg deposition can involve many tissues, including the central nervous system, ovaries, fallopian tubes, uterus and cervix, eyes, and gallbladder.

Manifestations of *S. mansoni, S. japonicum, S. mekongi,* and *S. intercalatum,* include hepatomegaly, portal and pulmonary hypertension and complications of such due to fibrosis, and intestinal polyps, fistulae, and strictures. Glomerulonephritis occurs in up to 10 percent of patients with hepatosplenic *S. mansoni.* In *S. haematobium,* patients have dysuria, hematuria, urinary frequency, chyluria, secondary bacterial urinary tract infection, renal calculi, hydroureter, hydronephrosis, renal failure from obstructive uropathy, and bladder carcinoma. Recurrent bacteremia with *Salmonella* species is a frequent complication of schistosomiasis.

Laboratory

Prominent eosinophilia may be present in early infection.

Diagnosis

Schistosomiasis can be diagnosed by identifying viable eggs in the stool (*S. japonicum* and *S. mansoni*), urine (*S. haematobium*), rectal or bladder biopsy, or other tissue. Diagnosis may be difficult to establish in early infection (Katayama fever) before the worms have matured and started to produce eggs. Eggs of *S. haematobium* have

FIGURE 237-23

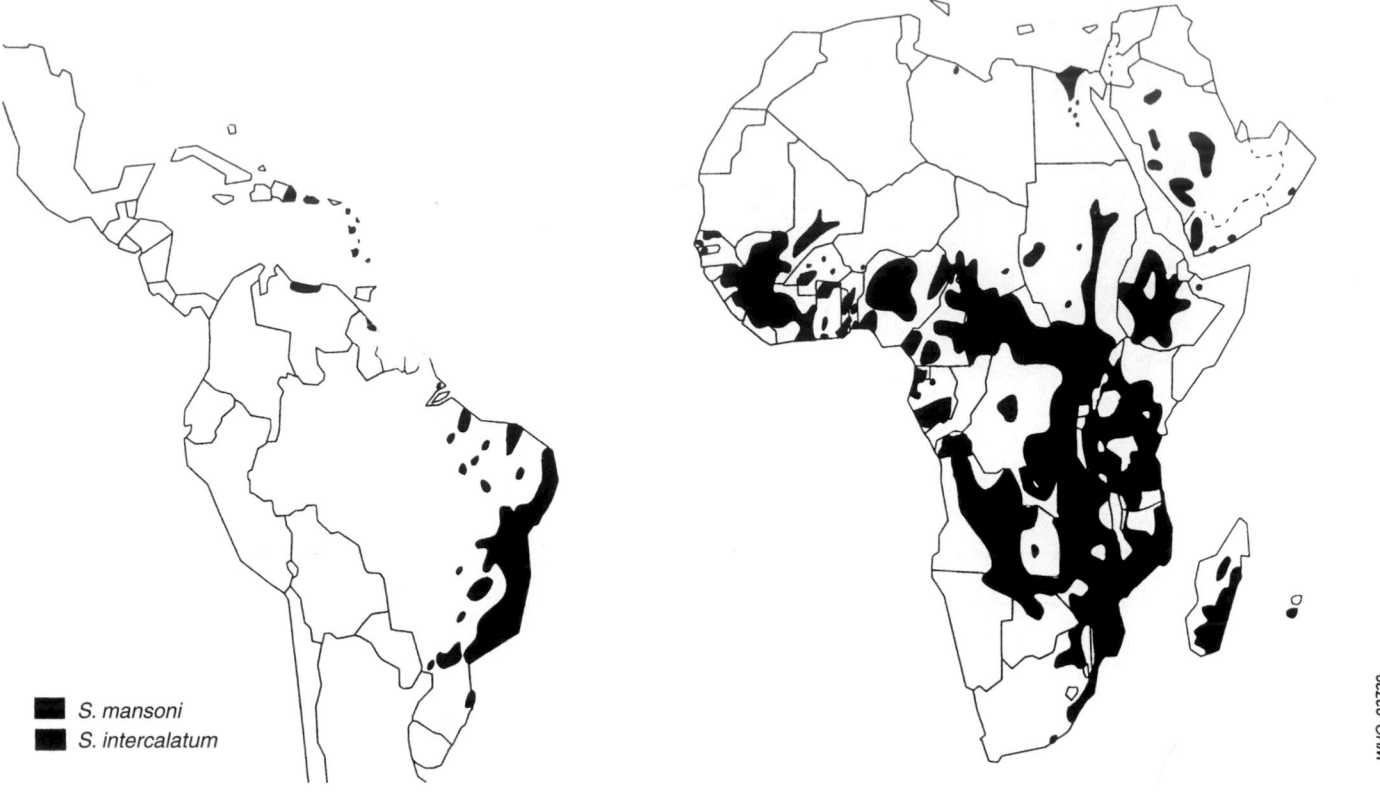

Global distribution of schistosomiasis due to *Schistosoma mansoni* and *S. intercalatum*. [From: The control of schistosomiasis. Second report of the WHO Expert Committee. Geneva, World Health Organization, 1993 (WHO Technical Report Series No. 830), with permission.]

FIGURE 237-24

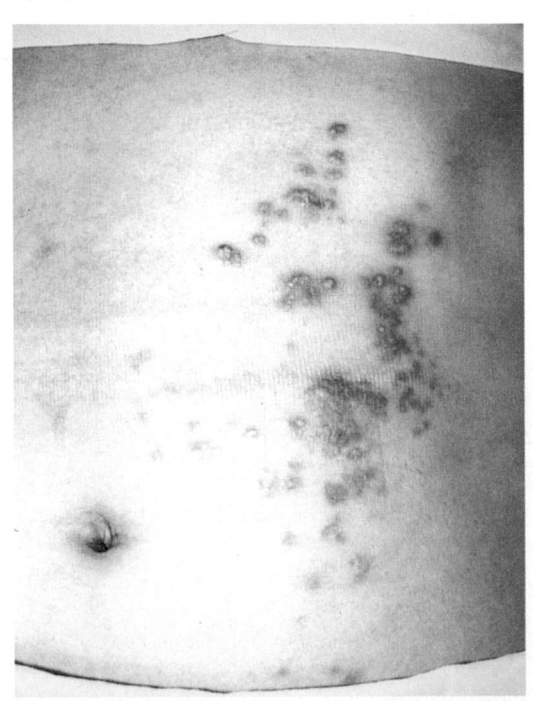

Ectopic deposition of *Schistosoma mansoni* ova.

a terminal spine, *S. japonicum* no spine, and *S. mansoni* a lateral spine (Fig. 237-25).

Several serologic tests are available, though they vary in their sensitivity and specificity. Serologic tests also do not indicate the intensity or duration of infection.

In *S. haematobium*, x-ray films of the pelvis may show linear calcification in the submucosa of the bladder and ureters.

Differential Diagnosis

The differential diagnosis of acute schistosomiasis includes visceral larva migrans, infection with liver flukes, and the migration phase of strongyloides or other helminths.

The differential diagnosis of bilharziasis cutanea tarda of the genital and buttocks area include atypical syphilis or condyloma latum, condyloma acuminatum, elephantiasis and its causes, amebiasis, other granulomatous diseases, malignancy, and hemorrhoids.

Treatment

Praziquantel is the treatment of choice for *S. haematobium*, *S. japonicum*, *S. mansoni*, and *S. mekongi*. Oxamniquine is an alternative treatment for *S. mansoni*.

FIGURE 237-25

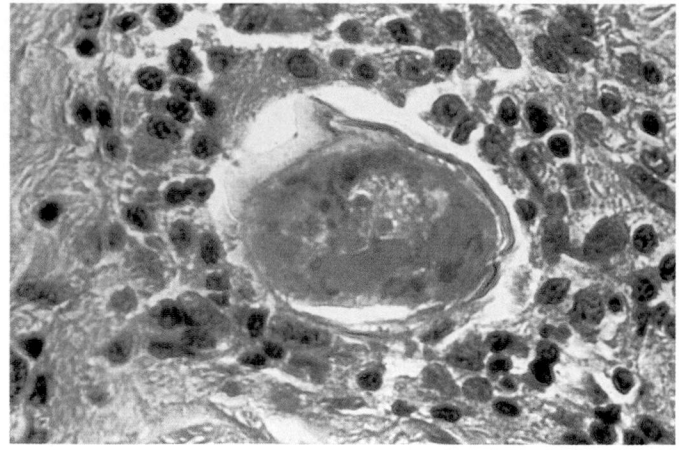

Skin biopsy of patient shown in Fig. 237-24 revealing *Schistosoma mansoni ovum. (Courtesy of Robert F. Cheek, MD.)*

Prevention

The prevention of schistosomiasis includes avoiding contact with infested water in endemic areas as well as snail control. Feces and urine of infected humans should be eliminated in a way that precludes contamination of freshwater.

SPARGANOSIS[83-85]

Synonyms

Spirometrosis, sparganum infection

Etiology

Sparganosis (Fig. 237-26) is caused by the tapeworm larvae of the genus *Spirometra* including *Spirometra mansoni*, *S. erinaceri*, and *S. mansonoides*. At least 10 cases have been caused by *S. proliferum.*

Life Cycle

Development involves definitive hosts (e.g., dogs and cats) and two intermediate hosts, a copepod (a tiny planktonic crustacean) and a vertebrate (e.g., amphibians, reptiles, and birds). Humans are incidental hosts for the second-stage larvae, which do not mature in human tissues.

Pathogenesis

When ingested by humans, the larvae migrate widely and usually lodge in subcutaneous tissue or muscle. They provoke an inflammatory response of lymphocytes, plasma cells, neutrophils, and eosinophils. When the larvae die, there is increased inflammation and tissue eosinophilia as well as tissue necrosis. Usually only one or a few larvae are present. When infected flesh is applied to the skin, the larva migrate directly into the skin or wound, resulting in a localized acute inflammatory reaction.

S. proliferum develops branched proliferating processes that may detach from the parent larva and develop into separate organisms, thus leading to a massive infection.

Geographic Distribution

The parasite is found in animals on all continents but most human cases are from China, Japan and Southeast Asia. Cases have also been reported from Africa, Australia, Caribbean islands, Southern Europe, and the Americas.

Epidemiology

ACQUISITION Sparganosis is acquired by drinking water contaminated with the copepod infected with larvae, ingestion of larvae in raw or undercooked flesh of frog, snake, poultry, or pork, or by the application of flesh containing larvae to human skin or wound when used as a poultice.

INCUBATION PERIOD AND TIME FRAME The incubation period depends on the route of acquisition, with the range being 20 days to 14 months for those eating infected frogs. Symptoms appear much sooner when transmission is via direct larval migration from infected animal flesh into human flesh. The larvae can live in the human for at least 9 years.

Clinical Features

The severity of infection depends on the route of infection, number of parasites, and the anatomic locations involved. Sparganosis caused by ingestion of the infective larvae presents as a slow grow-

FIGURE 237-26

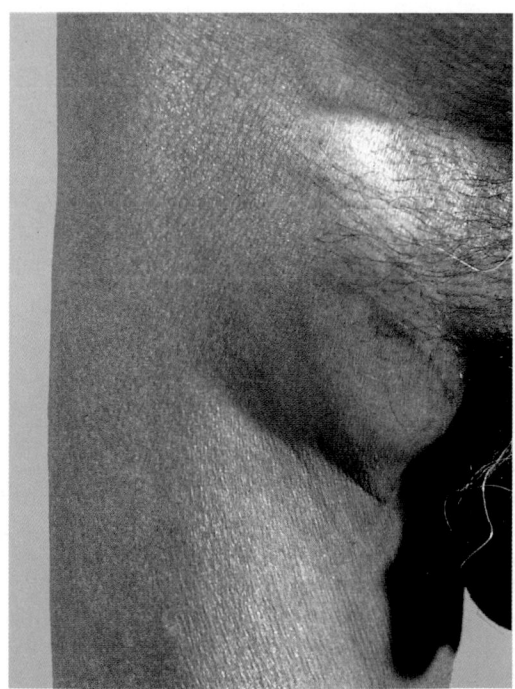

Soft-tissue swelling of sparganosis. (*Courtesy of Jay S. Keystone, MD, FRCPC.*)

ing, subcutaneous nodule that is occasionally migratory. The lesion may be pruritic and either tender or nontender. The infection is located in the subcutaneous tissue or skeletal muscle. Other organs affected include the brain, breast, bowel, eye, epididymis, urethra, and lung.

Sparganosis due to the use of infected flesh results in localized pruritus then erythema, edema and subcutaneous nodules that are painful on palpation.

S. proliferum infection may present as a massive systemic infection with fever and many subcutaneous nodules.

Laboratory

Peripheral eosinophilia and leukocytosis are common during tissue migration.

Diagnosis

The definitive diagnosis is made by the identification of the parasite in the surgically excised tissue.

Differential Diagnosis

The differential diagnosis includes cysticercosis, visceral larva migrans, cutaneous larva migrans, gnathostomiasis, paragonimiasis, as well as a benign or malignant tumor, lipoma, and epidermal inclusion cyst.

Treatment

Treatment includes the surgical excision of the larvae. Only palliative measures are available for *S. proliferum*.

Prevention

Prevention includes boiling or filtering water, avoiding the ingestion of raw or undercooked frog, snake, poultry, or pork, and avoiding the use of raw flesh of such animals for poultices.

STRONGYLOIDIASIS[86–91]

Synonyms

Strongyloidosis, strongyloidal ground itch, larva currens

Etiology

Strongyloidiasis is caused by the nematode (roundworm) *Strongyloides stercoralis*. *S. fuelleborni*, a common parasite of primates, infects humans in limited geographic areas. Other *Strongyloides* species that do not mature in humans affect the skin only.

Life Cycle

The parasite can undergo a full life cycle and multiply in the soil. Although animals can be infected with *S. stercoralis*, humans are the main reservoir host for human infection.

Pathogenesis

Filariform larvae penetrate the skin, enter blood vessels, and then travel to the lungs, where they break into alveoli and migrate up the respiratory tree to the pharynx. When they reach the upper gastrointestinal tract, the females embed in the mucosa, mature, and produce partially embryonated eggs that hatch in the mucosal epithelium. The larvae migrate into the intestinal lumen and are either eliminated in the feces or develop into infective larvae that repeat pulmonary migration, resulting in internal autoinfection. The larvae eliminated in the feces may penetrate the perianal or other skin and reinfect the host resulting in external autoinfection.

Geographic Distribution

The distribution is worldwide but is most common in tropical and subtropical areas. *S. fuelleborni* is endemic in parts of tropical Africa and Asia.

Epidemiology

ACQUISITION   Strongyloidiasis is acquired by the penetration of skin or mucous membranes by the infective larvae, usually in soil. Transmammary infection of *S. fuelleborni* may account for some infections in infants. Transmission also occurs via oral-anal sexual intercourse.

Strongyloidiasis is a common infection with rates as high as 80 percent in some populations in tropical areas. High rates of infection are reported in institutionalized mentally impaired persons and in former prisoners of war. The risk of infection is high for persons with frequent soil contact (e.g., being barefoot) in warm, moist areas where human feces frequently contaminate the soil.

Long-term glucocorticoid and immunosuppressive therapy, malnutrition, and particularly conditions that compromise cell-mediated immunity predispose to hyperinfection and disseminated strongyloidiasis. Slow intestinal transit and achlorhydria may also contribute to an increased risk.

INCUBATION PERIOD AND TIME FRAME   Larvae are found in the stool 2 to 3 weeks after exposure. Skin and pulmonary manifestations can begin within days of exposure. Because autoinfection can occur, infection can persist indefinitely. Infection may first be recognized years after it was acquired.

Clinical Features

Signs and symptoms of strongyloidiasis occur irregularly with prolonged asymptomatic intervals. Nonspecific gastrointestinal complaints include abdominal pain, nausea, vomiting, diarrhea, constipation, malabsorption, and weight loss. Transient pulmonary infiltrates appear during pulmonary migration. Cough and wheezing may be present during this phase.

The characteristic skin manifestation of chronic strongyloidiasis is larva currens, Latin for "racing larva." The filariform larvae invade the perianal skin and travel within the skin resulting in an urticarial serpiginous eruption. Larva currens is associated with intense pruritus. This eruption is unique in that it migrates at a rate of up to 5 to 10 cm per hour. Anatomic locations commonly include the buttocks (Fig. 237-27), groin, and trunk. The duration of the eruption is hours to a few days but may be recurrent over the course of weeks to years. Persons chronically infected with strongyloidiasis may also experience pruritus ani and chronic urticaria consisting of fixed nonmigratory wheals on the trunk, wrists, and ankles.

FIGURE 237-27

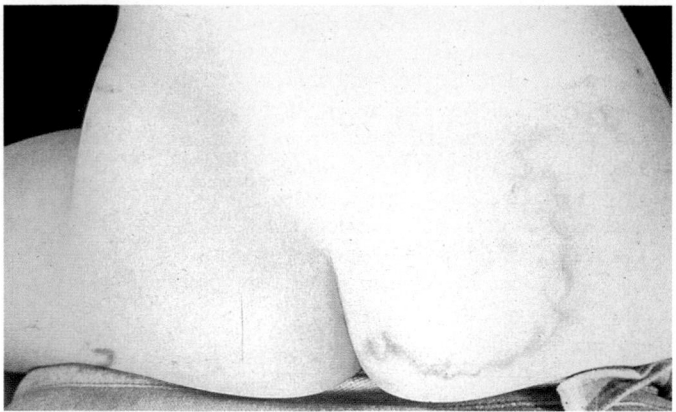

Cutaneous strongyloidiasis. (*Courtesy of Jay S. Keystone, MD, FRCPC.*)

Hyperinfection may cause abdominal pain, nausea, vomiting, diarrhea, and anorexia that are secondary to mucosal edema or ulcers. Malabsorption, ileus, or gastrointestinal bleeding sometimes develops. Pneumonia, adult respiratory distress syndrome, and respiratory failure may develop with disseminated infection. Filariform larvae can penetrate multiple extraintestinal sites such as the brain, liver, and urinary tract. Bacteremia with bowel flora, carried from the gut by the larvae, and meningitis are frequent complications. The mortality rate is high in disseminated strongyloidiasis given the underlying diseases, impaired immune system, damage from the parasite, and bacterial superinfection.

The dermatologic manifestation of hyperinfection and disseminated strongyloidiasis is a rapidly and progressively diffuse petechial and purpuric eruption caused by massive filariform larvae dissemination to the skin (Fig. 237-28). The eruption typically involves the trunk and proximal extremities. The "thumbprint sign" has been used in disseminated strongyloidiasis to describe a unique pattern of periumbilical purpura that resembles multiple thumbprints.

Laboratory

Peripheral eosinophilia is common and may be high grade during larval migration. Eosinophilia may be absent in patients who are on glucocorticoids or are severely immunocompromised.

Diagnosis

The diagnosis is made by identification of larvae in the stool, small bowel contents, and rarely in other body fluids. Multiple stool examinations are often necessary to make the diagnosis. Serologic testing by ELISA has a sensitivity of about 90 percent.

Diagnosis of larva currens is made by its characteristic clinical morphology. Skin biopsy of the larva currens eruption typically fails to reveal larvae. Biopsy of the purpuric and petechial eruption of hyperinfection and disseminated strongyloidiasis will reveal larvae (Fig. 237-29).

Persons with a history of prior residence or activities in areas that place them at an increased risk for strongyloidal infection should be screened for unrecognized infection prior to intentional immunosuppression.

Differential Diagnosis

The differential diagnosis includes other intestinal parasites and other causes of eosinophilic pneumonia. The differential diagnosis for larva currens is cutaneous larva migrans. The differential diagnosis for the petechial and purpuric eruption includes sepsis and causes of diffuse bleeding.

Treatment

Treatment includes thiabendazole or ivermectin. Repeated courses or prolonged therapy may be necessary in patients who are immunocompromised or who have disseminated infection.

FIGURE 237-28

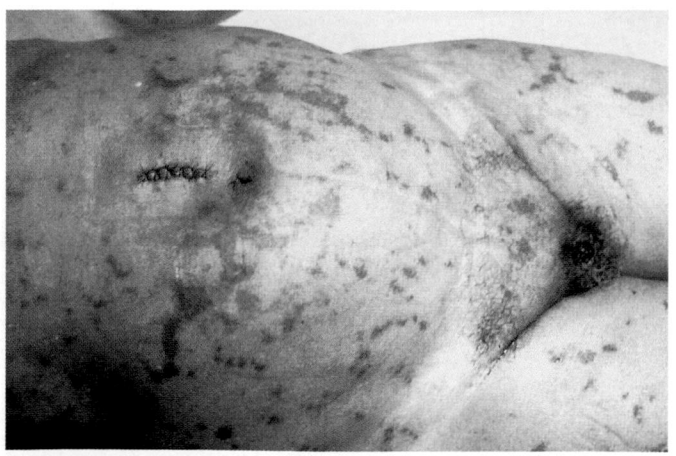

Nonpalpable purpura secondary to disseminated strongyloidiasis. (*Reprinted with permission from: Grossman ME, Roth J: Cutaneous Manifestations of Infection in the Immunocompromised Host. Baltimore, Williams & Wilkins, 1995.*)

FIGURE 237-29

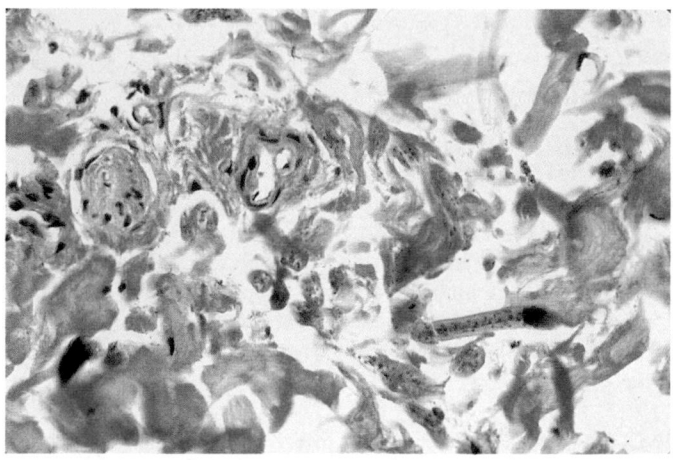

Skin biopsy of patient shown in Fig. 237-28 revealing *Strongyloides stercoralis* larvae. (*Reprinted with permission from: Grossman ME, Roth J: Cutaneous Manifestations of Infection in the Immunocompromised Host. Baltimore, Williams & Wilkins, 1995.*)

Prevention

Prevention includes avoiding skin-soil contact in endemic areas.

TRICHINOSIS[92–95]

Synonyms

Trichinellosis, trichiniasis, trichinelliasis

Etiology

The pathogen in trichinosis is *Trichinella spiralis*, a filiform nematode.

Life Cycle

Animals ingest muscle containing infective larvae and become infected. Humans are incidental deadend hosts.

Pathogenesis

Cysts surrounding larvae are digested in the upper gastrointestinal tract, releasing larvae that attach to villi in the small intestine, where the parasites mature and mate. Over 2 to 4 weeks, each female worm produces 500 to 1500 larvae that penetrate the intestinal wall and enter lymphatics and blood vessels to reach tissues throughout the body. Larvae enter striated muscle cells, where they grow, provoke an inflammatory reaction, followed by the formation of a fibrous capsule surrounding the larvae and an eosinophilic granulomatous infiltrate.

Geographic Distribution

Trichinosis is present in most countries, but there is marked variation in the incidence. The parasite is thought to be absent from Australia and many South Pacific islands. Sporadic infections occur worldwide via shipped meat.

Epidemiology

ACQUISITION Trichinosis is acquired by the ingestion of raw or undercooked infected meat. Sources of human infection have included flesh from swine, bears, wild boars, cougars, walruses, horses, dogs, and cats. Swine fed uncooked scraps are more likely to be infected. Human infection tends to be sporadic and epidemic.

Since 1947, trichinosis has been a reportable condition in the United States. State health departments reported 32 cases during 1994. Laws in the United States prohibit the feeding of offal to swine.

INCUBATION PERIOD AND TIME FRAME The usual incubation period is 10 to 30 days. Gastrointestinal symptoms may begin as early as 1 to 2 days after eating infected meat. Symptoms occur during larval migration, before encystment. The adult parasite is excreted within 2 to 3 months. The encysted larvae may remain viable for 5 to 10 years.

Clinical Features

Trichinosis ranges from being asymptomatic to fatal. The case fatality rate is 1 to 2 percent for recognized infections, usually related to complications of central nervous system or cardiac involvement.

Abdominal pain, diarrhea, and vomiting during the first week of infection are followed by fever, fatigue, myalgias, periorbital edema, and a macular and papular sometimes urticarial rash on the extremities. Subconjunctival and splinter hemorrhages (Fig. 237-30) are common. Headache, cough, and shortness of breath may be reported. The central nervous system is involved in 10 to 20 percent of cases and is manifested by meningitis, encephalitis, paresis and paralysis. Cardiac involvement includes myocarditis that leads to cardiac failure and arrhythmias.

Laboratory

A peripheral eosinophilia may be marked and may persist for months.

Diagnosis

The diagnosis is made by the identification of the parasite in surgically excised tissue (e.g., muscle biopsy) (Fig. 237-31). Serologic testing with ELISA or indirect immunofluorescence is not useful in early infection. Antibody levels are usually low before the third week of the illness.

Differential Diagnosis

The differential diagnosis includes allergic reactions, vasculitis, Katayama fever, visceral larva migrans, and eosinophilia-myalgia syndrome due to ingested tryptophan.

Treatment

The treatment of choice is mebendazole. While mebendazole is an approved drug, the Food and Drug Administration considers it an investigational drug for trichinosis. Albendazole and flubendazole (not available in the United States) may also be effective. Steroids should be given concomitantly when there are severe symptoms.

FIGURE 237-30

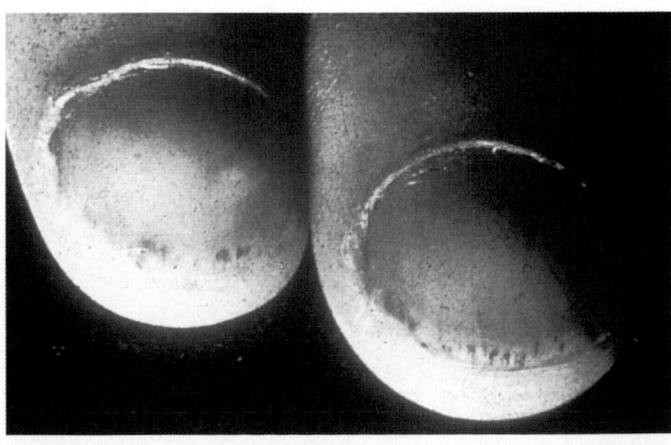

Subungual hemorrhage secondary to trichinosis. (*Courtesy of Herman Zaiman, MD.*)

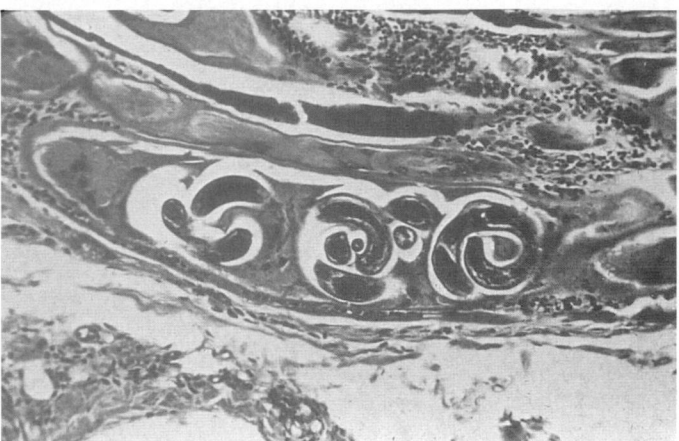

Muscle biopsy showing *Trichinella spiralis* larvae. (*Courtesy of Murray Wittner, MD, PhD.*)

Prevention

Prevention includes avoiding raw and undercooked meat. Cooking the meat to a temperature of 170°F (77°C) will destroy the trichinae. Smoking and drying meat will not result in killing the infective larvae. Salt curing solutions may kill the trichinae, but the temperature and duration are important factors in this method.

VISCERAL LARVA MIGRANS[96–99]

Synonyms

Toxocariasis, toxocaral visceral larva migrans, ocular toxocariasis, ocular larva migrans

Etiology

Visceral larva migrans (VLM) is caused by the common dog roundworm, *Toxocara canis* and much less frequently by the cat roundworm, *T. catis.*

Life Cycle

Dogs become infected by ingesting infective eggs or larvae, by transplacental transmission, or by the transmammary passage of larvae in milk. The eggs are passed in the stool and contaminate soil.

Pathogenesis

In humans, ingested embryonated eggs reach the small intestine and release larvae that penetrate the mucosa and by way of the portal circulation reach the liver, lungs, and systemic circulation. When the larvae reach blood vessels that are too narrow to allow passage, the larvae bore through the vessel wall and migrate in tissues. The organs involved include the liver, heart, brain, spinal cord, eyes, and muscle. The larvae provoke hemorrhage, necrosis, and an eosinophilic and granulomatous tissue response. Because the parasite cannot mature in humans, the larvae may remain dormant or wander in tissues for years.

Geographic Distribution

VLM is a common infection that is found worldwide. It is most common in tropical and temperate climates where both humans and dogs reside.

Epidemiology

ACQUISITION   Humans become infected by ingesting eggs from contaminated soil on fingers, fruits, vegetables, and other foods. Direct contact with dogs is not necessary. Warm, moist clay soil is the most favorable condition for eggs, which must embryonate for 1 to 3 weeks before they become infective. Children and persons with a history of pica are at an increased risk. Toxocara eggs contaminate the soil in 10 to 30 percent of public playgrounds and parks.

Other reported sources of human infection include ingestion of larvae in raw liver from chickens, cattle, sheep, and other animals.

INCUBATION PERIOD AND TIME FRAME   The incubation period is typically 1 month or longer with a range of 1 to 2 weeks to years. The larvae may remain viable in the human for 10 years or longer.

Clinical Features

Most infections are asymptomatic or mild. Occasionally infection leads to a prolonged, debilitating illness, loss of an eye, or death. Clinical findings reflect the intensity and chronicity of infection, and the anatomic location of larvae. Eye involvement is termed ocular larva migrans. Signs and symptoms may include fever, cough, wheezing, abdominal pain, anorexia, arthralgias, myalgias, fatigue, restlessness, and hepatomegaly. Clinical findings usually resolve over time. In heavy infections the heart and central nervous system may be affected.

Skin manifestations may include subcutaneous nodules that may be tender, purpura, urticaria, pruritus, and an erythematous and urticarial eruption that evolves into pruritic papules on the abdomen and extremities. The palms and soles may be involved.

Patients with ocular larva migrans (Fig. 237-32) usually lack systemic symptoms and have findings restricted to the eye. Eye infection typically occurs unilaterally in children or young adults with the subacute presentation of decreased vision, strabismus, leukocoria, a fixed pupil, or a red eye. Clinically, ocular larva migrans can resemble neuroblastoma.

Laboratory

Common findings are peripheral eosinophilia that may be high grade and persistent, leukocytosis, elevated serum IgG, and elevated liver function tests.

Diagnosis

The diagnosis is made by the identification of larvae in tissue or by the combination of serologic evidence of infection and compatible clinical findings. ELISA testing has a sensitivity of 75 to 90 percent. Eggs and larvae are not found in human feces.

FIGURE 237-32

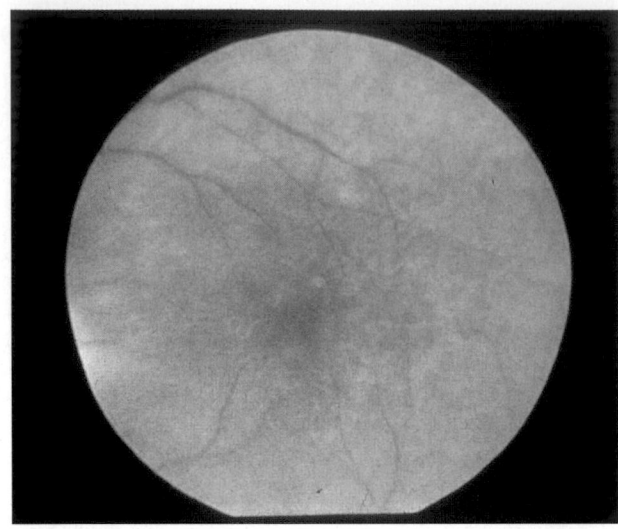

Ocular larva migrans. (*Courtesy of Murray Wittner MD, PhD.*)

Differential Diagnosis

The differential diagnosis includes trichinellosis, schistosomiasis, strongyloidiasis, ascariasis, ancylostomiasis, fascioliasis, gnathostomiasis, filariasis, paragonimiasis, sparganosis, and infection with the raccoon roundworm, *Baylisascaris procyonis*.

Ocular larva migrans may mimic toxoplasmosis, histoplasmosis, diffuse unilateral subacute neuroretinitis, Coats' disease, persistent hyperplastic primary vitreous, and retinoblastoma.

Treatment

The treatment of choice is diethylcarbamazine. Albendazole and mebendazole are alternative treatments. DEC and mebendazole, although approved by the Food and Drug Administration, are considered investigational in the treatment of VLM. It is important to treat infected dogs.

Prevention

Prevention includes avoiding exposure to soil contaminated with animal feces and the treatment of infected dogs.

REFERENCES

GENERAL
1. *Health Information for International Travel.* Washington, DC, Government Printing Office, 1996–1997
2. *International Travel and Health, Vaccination Requirements and Health Advice.* Geneva: WHO, 1998
3. Allen JE, Maizels RM: Immunology of human helminth infection. *Int Arch Allergy Immunol* **109**:3, 1996
4. Beaver PC et al (eds): *Clinical Parasitology,* 9th ed. Philadelphia, Lea & Febiger, 1984
5. Benenson AS (ed): *Control of Communicable Diseases Manual,* 16th ed. Washington, DC, American Public Health Association, 1995
6. Canizares O, Harman R (eds): *Clinical Tropical Dermatology,* 2d ed. Boston, Blackwell, 1992
7. Caumes E et al: Dermatoses associated with travel to tropical countries: A prospective study of the diagnosis and management of 269 patients presenting to a tropical disease unit. *Clin Infect Dis* **20**:542, 1995
8. Chaudhry AZ, Longworth DL: Cutaneous manifestations of intestinal helminthic infections. *Dermatol Clin* **7**:267, 1989
9. de Silva et al: Antihelmintics: A comparative review of their clinical pharmacology. *Drugs* **53**:769, 1997
10. Liu LX, Weller PF: Antiparasitic drugs. *N Engl J Med* **334**:1178, 1996
11. Mahmoud AAF: Tropical medicine: Current problems and possible solutions. *Infect Dis Clin North Am* **9**:265, 1995
12. Ottensen EA, Campbell WC: Ivermectin in human medicine. *J Antimicrob Chemother* **34**:195, 1994
13. Schaller KF (ed): *Colour Atlas of Tropical Dermatology and Venereology.* New York, Springer-Verlag, 1994
14. Wilson ME: *A World Guide to Infections: Diseases, Distribution, Diagnosis.* New York, Oxford University Press, 1991

ASCARIASIS
15. Crompton DWT et al (eds): *Ascariasis and Its Public Health Significance.* Philadelphia, Taylor and Frances, 1985
16. DeSilva et al: Morbidity and mortality due to ascariasis: Re-estimation and sensitivity analysis of global numbers at risk. *Trop Med Int Health.* **2**:519, 1997
17. Khuroo MS: Ascariasis. *Gastroenterol Clin North Am* **25**:553, 1996

CERCARIAL DERMATITIS
18. Centers for Disease Control: Cercarial dermatitis outbreak at a state park—Delaware, 1991. *MMWR* **41**:225, 1992
19. Gonzalez E: Schistosomiasis, cercarial dermatitis, and marine dermatitis. *Dermatol Clin* **7**:291, 1989
20. Hoeffler DF: Cercarial dermatitis: Its etiology, epidemiology, and clinical aspects. *Arch Environ Health* **29**:225, 1974
21. Loken BR et al: Prevalence and transmission of cercariae causing schistosome dermatitis in Flathead lake, Montana. *J Parasitol* **81**:646, 1995

COENUROSIS
22. Benger A et al: A human coenurus infection in Canada. *Am J Trop Med Hyg* **30**:638, 1981
23. Templeton AC: Anatomical and geographical location of human coenurus infection. *Trop Geogr Med* **23**:105, 1971

CUTANEOUS LARVA MIGRANS
24. Caumes E et al: A randomized trial of ivermectin versus albendazole for the treatment of cutaneous larva migrans. *Am J Trop Med Hyg* **49**:641, 1993
25. Davies HD et al: Creeping eruption. A review of clinical presentation and management of 60 cases presenting to a tropical disease unit. *Arch Dermatol* **129**:588, 1993
26. Jelinek T et al: Cutaneous larva migrans in travelers: Synopsis of histories, symptoms, and treatment of 98 patients. *Clin Infect Dis* **19**:1062, 1994
27. Richey TK et al: Persistent cutaneous larva migrans due to *Ancylostoma* species. *South Med J* **89**:609, 1996
28. Wong-Waldamez A, Silva-Lizama E: Bullous larva migrans accompanied by Loeffler's syndrome. *Int J Dermatol* **34**:570, 1995

CYSTICERCOSIS
29. Botero D et al: Taeniasis and cysticercosis. *Infect Dis Clin North Am* **7**:683, 1993
30. De Leon ER, Aguirre A: Oral cysticercosis. *Oral Surg Oral Med Oral Pathol Oral Radiol Endod* **79**:572, 1995
31. Diaz JF et al: Immunodiagnosis of human cysticercosis (*Taenia solium*): A field comparison of an antibody-enzyme-linked immunosorbent assay (ELISA), an antigen-ELISA, and an enzyme-linked immunoelectrotransfer blot (EITB) assay in Peru. *Am J Trop Med Hyg* **36**:610, 1992
32. Falanga V, Kapoor W: Cerebral cysticercosis: Diagnostic value of subcutaneous nodules. Report of two cases. *J Am Acad Dermatol* **12**:304, 1985
33. Jordaan HF et al: Cerebral and subcutaneous cysticercosis treated with albendazole. *Int J Dermatol* **34**:574, 1995
34. Sloan L et al: Evaluation of enzyme-linked immunoassay for serological diagnosis of cysticercosis. *J Clin Microbiol* **33**:3124, 1995

35. Wortman PD: Subcutaneous cysticercosis. *J Am Acad Dermatol* **25**:409, 1991

DIROFILARIASIS

36. Collins BM et al: *Dirofilaria tenuis* infection of the oral mucosa and cheek. *J Oral Maxillofac Surg* **51**:1037, 1993
37. Glickman LT, Magnaval J: Zoonotic roundworm infections. *Infect Dis Clin North Am* **7**:717, 1993
38. Payan HM: Human infection with *Dirofilaria*. *Arch Dermatol* **114**:593, 1978
39. Shenefelt PD et al: Elusive migratory subcutaneous dirofilariasis. *J Am Acad Dermatol* **35**:260, 1996

DRACUNCULIASIS

40. Centers for Disease Control: Progress toward global eradication of dracunculiasis. *MMWR* **44**:875, 881, 1995
41. Okoye SN et al: A survey of predilection sites and degree of disability associated with guineaworm (*Dracunculus medinensis*). *Int J Parasitol* **25**:1127, 1995
42. Pendse AK et al: Testicular dracunculosis—a distinct clinical entity. *Br J Urol* **54**:56, 1982
43. World Health Organization: Dracunculiasis. Global surveillance summary, 1996. *Weekly Epidemiol Rec* **72**:133, 1997

ECHINOCOCCOSIS

44. Ammann RW, Eckert J: Cestodes: Echinococcus. *Gastroenterol Clin North Am* **25**:655, 1996
45. Bresson-Hadni S et al: Skin localization of alveolar echinococcosis of the liver. *J Am Acad Dermatol* **34**:873, 1996
46. Khuroo MS et al: Percutaneous drainage compared with surgery for hepatic hydatid cysts. *N Engl J Med* **337**:881, 1997
47. Webbe G: Recent developments in cestode research. *Trans R Soc Trop Med Hyg* **89**:345, 1995
48. World Health Organization Informal Working Group on Echinococcus: Guidelines for the treatment of cystic and alveolar echinococcosis in humans. *Bull WHO* **74**:100, 1996

ENTEROBIASIS

49. Grencis RK et al: Enterobius, trichuris, capillaria, and hookworm including *Ancylostoma caninum*. *Gastroenterol Clin North Am* **25**:579, 1996
50. Mattia AR: Perianal mass and recurrent cellulitis due to *Enterobius vermicularis*. *Am J Trop Med Hyg* **47**:811, 1992
51. Sun T et al: Enterobius egg granuloma of the vulva and peritoneum: Review of the literature. *Am J Trop Med Hyg* **45**:249, 1991
52. Tornieporth NG et al: Ectopic enterobiasis: A case report and review. *J Infect* **24**:87, 1992

FASCIOLIASIS

53. Arjona R et al: Fascioliasis in developed countries: A review of classic and aberrant forms of the disease. *Medicine* (Baltimore) **74**:13, 1995
54. Harinasuta T et al: Trematode infections: Opisthorchiasis, clonorchiasis, fascioliasis, and paragonimiasis. *Infect Dis Clin North Am* **7**:699, 1993
55. Price TA et al: Fascioliasis: Case reports and review. *Clin Infect Dis* **17**:426, 1993

FILARIASIS, LYMPHATIC

56. Addiss DB et al: Randomized placebo-controlled comparison of ivermectin and albendazole alone and in combination for *Wuchereria bancrofti* microfilaremia in Haitian children. *Lancet* **350**:480, 1997
57. Dey P, Walker R: Microfilariae in a fine needle aspirate from a skin nodule. *Acta Cytol* **38**:114, 1994
58. Ottesen EA: Filarial infections. *Infect Dis Clin North Am* **7**:619, 1993
59. Routh HB, Bhowmik KR: Filariasis. *Dermatol Clin* **12**:719, 1994

GNATHOSTOMIASIS

60. Adame J, Cohen PR: Eosinophilic panniculitis: Diagnostic considerations and evaluation. *J Am Acad Dermatol* **34**:229, 1996
61. Crowley JJ, Kim YH: Cutaneous gnathostomiasis. *J Am Acad Dermatol* **33**:825, 1995
62. Ruiz-Maldonado R: Successful treatment of nodular migratory eosinophilic panniculitis (human gnathostomiasis) with phenylbutazone. *Int J Dermatol* **30**:522, 1991

HOOKWORM DISEASE

63. Albonico M et al: A randomized controlled trial comparing mebendazole and albendazole against ascaris, trichuris and hookworm infections. *Trans R Soc Trop Med Hyg* **88**:585, 1994

64. Chongsuvivatwong V et al: Predictors for the risk of hookworm infection: Experience from endemic villages in southern Thailand. *Trans R Soc Trop Med Hyg* **90**:633, 1996
65. Grencis RK et al: Enterobius, trichuris, capillaria, and hookworm including *Ancylostoma caninum*. *Gastroenterol Clin North Am* **25**:579, 1996
66. Maxwell C et al: The clinical and immunological responses of human volunteers to low dose hookworm (*Necator americanus*) infection. *Am J Trop Med Hyg* **37**:126, 1987

LOIASIS

67. Klion AD et al: Effectiveness of diethylcarbamazine in treating loiasis acquired by expatriate visitors to endemic regions: Long term follow-up. *J Infect Dis* **169**:604, 1994
68. Ottesen EA: Filarial infections. *Infect Dis Clin North Am* **7**:619, 1993
69. Rakita RM et al: *Loa loa* infection as a cause of migratory angioedema: Report of three cases from the Texas medical center. *Clin Infect Dis* **17**:691, 1993
70. Wahl G, Georges AJ: Current knowledge on the epidemiology, diagnosis, immunology, and treatment of loiasis. *Trop Med Parasitol* **46**:287, 1995

ONCHOCERCIASIS

71. Burnham G: Ivermectin treatment of onchocercal skin lesions: Observations from a placebo-controlled, double-blind trial in Malawi. *Am J Trop Med Hyg* **52**:270, 1995
72. Carme B et al: Prevalence of depigmentation of the shins: A simple and cheap way to screen for severe endemic onchocerciasis in Africa. *Bull World Health Organ* **71**:755, 1993
73. Connor DH et al: Pathologic changes of human onchocerciasis: Implications for future research. *Rev Infect Dis* **7**:809, 1985
74. McCarthy JS: Onchocerciasis in endemic and nonendemic populations: Differences in clinical presentation and immunologic findings. *J Infect Dis* **170**:736, 1994
75. Murdoch ME et al: A clinical classification and grading system of the cutaneous changes in onchocerciasis. *Br J Dermatol* **129**:260, 1993
76. Okello DO et al: Dermatological problems of onchocerciasis in Nebbi District, Uganda. *East Afr Med J* **72**:295, 1995

PARAGONIMIASIS

77. Harinasuta T et al: Trematode infections: Opisthorchiasis, clonorchiasis, fascioliasis, and paragonimiasis. *Infect Dis Clin North Am* **7**:699, 1993

SCHISTOSOMIASIS

78. Amer M: Cutaneous schistosomiasis. *Dermatol Clin* **12**:713, 1994
79. Elliott DE: Schistosomiasis: Pathophysiology, diagnosis and treatment. *Gastroenterol Clin North Am* **25**:599, 1996
80. Farrell AM et al: Ectopic cutaneous schistosomiasis: Extragenital involvement with progressive upward spread. *Br J Dermatol* **135**:110, 1996
81. Gonzalez E: Schistosomiasis, cercarial dermatitis and marine dermatitis. *Dermatol Clin* **7**:291, 1989
82. Sloan RS et al: Schistosomiasis masquerading as carcinoma of the breast. *South Med J* **89**:345, 1996

SPARGANOSIS

83. Chung SY et al: Breast sparganosis: Mammographic and ultrasound features. *J Clin Ultrasound* **23**:447, 1995
84. Sarma DP, Weilbaecher TG: Human sparganosis. *J Am Acad Dermatol* **15**:1145, 1986
85. Tsou M, Huang TW: Pathology of subcutaneous sparganosis: Report of two cases. *J Formos Med Assoc* **92**:649, 1993

STRONGYLOIDIASIS

86. Bank DE et al: The thumbprint sign: Rapid diagnosis of disseminated strongyloidiasis. *J Am Acad Dermatol* **23**:324, 1990
87. Chaudhary K et al: Case report: Purpura in disseminated strongyloidiasis. *Am J Med Sci* **308**:186, 1994
88. Gordon SM et al: Disseminated strongyloidiasis with cutaneous manifestations in an immunocompromised host. *J Am Acad Dermatol* **31**:255, 1994
89. Kalb RE, Grossman ME: Periumbilical purpura in disseminated strongyloidiasis. *JAMA* **256**:1170, 1986

90. Mahmoud AAF: Strongyloidiasis. *Clin Infect Dis* **23**:949, 1996
91. von Kuster LC, Genta RM: Cutaneous manifestations of strongyloidiasis. *Arch Dermatol* **124**:1826, 1988

TRICHINOSIS
92. Capo V, Despommier DD: Clinical aspects of infection with *Trichinella* spp. *Clin Microbiol Rev* **9**:47, 1996
93. Centers for Disease Control: Outbreak of trichinellosis associated with eating cougar jerky—Idaho, 1995. *MMWR* **45**:205, 1996
94. Mahannop P et al: Immunodiagnosis of human trichinellosis and identification of specific antigen for *Trichinella spiralis*. *Int J Parasitol* **25**:87, 1995

95. Oppenheim JM et al: Trichinosis: Clinical and laboratory observations in a group of 256 cases. *Milit Surg* **101**:294, 1947

VISCERAL LARVA MIGRANS
96. Boschetti A, Kasznica J: Visceral larva migrans induced eosinophilic cardiac pseudotumor: A cause of sudden death in a child. *J Forensic Sci* **40**:1097, 1995
97. Glickman LT, Magnaval J: Zoonotic roundworm infections. *Infect Dis Clin North Am* **7**:717, 1993
98. Rook A, Staughton R: The cutaneous manifestations of toxocariasis. *Dermatologica* **144**:129, 1972
99. Wolfrom E et al: Chronic urticaria and *Toxocara canis*. *Lancet* **345**:196, 1995

CHAPTER 238

Mark Jordan Scharf
Jennifer Susan Daly

Bites and Stings of Terrestrial and Aquatic Life

The Book of Genesis promised man dominion over the fish of the sea and every living thing that moved on the face of the earth. Unfortunately, it did not guarantee that every encounter between man and beast would be free from harm. The first two sections of this chapter consider the harmful effects of landborne animal bites as well as the bacterial and viral infections they may transmit. The final section reviews bites and stings and other forms of injury that may be inflicted by marine life.

ANIMAL BITES

More than 1 to 2 million animal bites occur yearly in the United States; dog bites constitute the largest group.[1] The human victim is often a 7- to 9-year old boy who is teasing or playing with a dog. Sometimes the bite occurs when a person is trying to break up a pair of fighting dogs, or the victim is the postal delivery person. Most bites are delivered by so called "friendly dogs," known to the victim.[2] The majority are to the upper extremity, especially the hands.[1]

The evaluation and treatment of all bite wounds should include a careful history of the incident, the type of animal, the site of the bite, and the geographic setting. Hand wounds, puncture wounds, and crush injuries most often become infected. Infected bites should be cultured and a Gram-stained smear prepared; the wound should then be washed, well irrigated, and left open. Selection of an antibiotic depends on the bite history and Gram's stain results.[3,4] Most patients with deep cat bites, deep cat scratches, and sutured wounds should be treated with penicillin, amoxicillin-clavulanic acid, cefuroxime, or tetracycline because of the increased incidence of *Pasteurella multocida* infection.[1,5] Tetanus immune status should be evaluated and rabies immunization considered.

Human bites and monkey bites deserve special mention because 30 percent become infected with aerobic or anaerobic mouth organisms. Anaerobic infection may spread through the metacarpal-phalangeal space and cause severe damage. The same procedure as for other animal bites should be followed, that is, culture and Gram's stain, thorough washing, and debridement. Wounds should be left open if possible, especially hand wounds.[3] Patients with human bites should be treated prophylactically with amoxicillin-clavulanate for 7 to 10 days. Clenched fist injuries should be evaluated by a hand surgeon.

Specific Bacterial Infections Caused by Animal Bites

PASTEURELLA MULTOCIDA A common organism infecting bite wounds is *P. multocida*. Disease due to this organism is now diagnosed more frequently; thus, its presence in the nasopharynx in 50 to 66 percent of dogs and 70 to 90 percent of cats is of public health importance.[6]

Most infections in humans fall into one of three clinical patterns.

1. The most common pattern is that of local infection with adenitis after a dog or cat bite or scratch. The infection usually presents within 24 to 48 h, often within several hours.[4] In patients with a cat bite, this may then progress to tenosynovitis or osteomyelitis due to inoculation of the organism into the periosteum by the long, sharp tooth of the animal. Canine teeth are more blunt and less likely to penetrate the periosteum. The onset of infection often occurs within 24 to 48 h, sometimes within several hours, making *P. multocida* the most common organism to be found in patients whose infection presents within the first 24 h.[6,7] *Pasteurella* infections have been reported after bites of large cats, such as lions and tigers.[8]

2. The second pattern is chronic pulmonary infection, in which *P. multocida* may occur as the primary pathogen or in association with other organisms. Bacteria may enter through the respiratory tract by inhalation of barn dust or infectious droplets sprayed by the sneeze of an animal. In such cases, the bacteria probably colonize the respiratory tract and lie dormant in the patient with chronic lung disease. Acute infection occurs only after trauma to the bronchial tree. Bronchiectasis, emphysema, peritonsillar abscess, and sinusitis have all been described with this organism.[6]

3. Finally, systemic infection with bacteremia or meningitis may occur.[9]

The authors wish to thank Dr. Bruce Halstead of the World Life Research Institute, Colton, CA, for allowing us to reprint the photographs from the first and second editions of *Poisonous and Venomous Marine Animals of the World.*

P. multocida is a small, gram-negative, ovoid bacillus that grows well on blood agar but does not grow on selective gram-negative media, such as MacConkey agar. Because of its superficial resemblance to *Haemophilus influenzae* and *Neisseria* organisms, respiratory tract and central nervous system infection with *P. multocida* may be misdiagnosed initially. Failure of growth on routine gram-negative media is an important clue.[6]

Treatment of the patient with presumptive *P. multocida* infection (i.e., any patient with a deep cat bite or scratch or a deep dog bite) should consist of careful washing and an attempt to leave the wound open. The antibiotic of choice is penicillin, orally for 7 to 10 days, with careful follow-up of the wound. In order to treat other possible pathogens in addition to *P. multocida*, amoxicillin-clavulanic acid is the best empirical choice before culture or Gram-stain results are available. Ampicillin, tetracycline, ciprofloxacin, trimethoprim-sulfamethoxazole, or intravenous ceftriaxone are alternatives for *P. multocida*.

STAPHYLOCOCCUS INTERMEDIUS *S. intermedius* is an organism associated with dogs weighing more than 40 pounds. It is more commonly found in canine gingival flora than *S. aureus* (39 percent versus 10 percent).[10,11] It is a gram-positive, coagulase-positive coccus that can be differentiated from *S. aureus* in the laboratory by biochemical testing. In comparison with *S. aureus, S. intermedius* does not produce acetoin from glucose and has β-galactosidase activity. If these tests are not performed, the laboratory may mistakenly report an isolate as *S. aureus*. Antibiotic treatment is the same as that for *S. aureus,* as about 55 percent (slightly less than *S. aureus*) are resistant to penicillin because of production of β-lactamase.[10]

CAPNOCYTOPHAGA CANIMORSUS *Capnocytophaga canimorsus* is a capnophilic, facultatively anaerobic slow-growing, gram-negative rod associated with dog bites.[12–14] The organism has been found in the oral cavity of 17 percent of cats and 24 percent of dogs.[15] Most infections occur in the splenectomized or immunocompromised host and present as overwhelming sepsis. Menigitis has been reported in a child.[9]

PORPHYROMONAS SPECIES *Porphyromonas* species are slow-growing anerobic bacteria that require media enriched with vitamin K and hemin for optimal growth. They are difficult to culture, requiring 4 to 6 days for colony formation and have been recognized as a cause of infection in patients with dog and cat bites.[16] These organisms are found in the deep gingival pockets and cause destructive peridontitis in animals and human. Citron and coworkers found *Porphyromonas* species in 28 percent of culture specimens from patients with infected dog and cat bite wounds.[17]

EDWARDSIELLA TARDA This bacterium is found most frequently in freshwater fish and reptiles, but has been isolated from seals living in saltwater, amphibians, mammals, and birds. It is a gram-negative rod that is a member of the family Enterobacteriaceae, and it resembles salmonella in various biochemical attributes. It is an unusual cause of clinical disease in humans. The most commonly identified infection in humans is gastroenteritis, but soft tissue infection, including cellulitis or abscess have been reported after bites or scratches with animals, including a pet turtle.[18] Osteomyelitis, intraabdominal and pulmonary infections, meningitis, and septic shock have been reported.

MARINE VIBRIOS *Vibrio carachrias*, a saltwater-loving (halophilic) gram negative bacillus, was reported as the cause of a wound infection after a shark bite.[19]

CAT SCRATCH DISEASE *Bartonella henselae* is the most common etiologic agent of cat-scratch disease. *Afipia felis* and other *Bartonella* species may cause some cases (see Chap. 199).

PLAGUE See Chap. 200

TULAREMIA See Chap. 200

RAT-BITE FEVER See Chap. 200

Viral Infections Caused by Animal Bites

RABIES (See Chap. 184) The most notorious viral disease caused by an animal bite is rabies. The epidemiology has changed in the past few years. Now, nonimmune dogs account for only 16 percent of cases, whereas sylvatic animals, such as skunks, raccoons, red and gray foxes, bats, and domestic dogs represent the greatest potential danger; rodents, such as squirrels and hamsters, are probably inconsequential as sources of rabies.[20]

Live virus is introduced into nerve tissue at the time of the bite. The virus multiplies at the site and then spreads to the central nervous system. It replicates in gray matter and then spreads along autonomic nerves to the salivary glands, adrenal glands, and heart. The incubation period varies with the site of the bite, from 5 days to as long as several years.

Clinical features include a prodromal period of 1 to 4 days, followed by high fever, headache, and malaise. Paresthesia at the site of inoculation occurs in 80 percent of patients. The next sequence of events is familiar: agitation, hyperesthesia, dysphagia, excessive thirst, paralysis, and death.

Diagnosis The diagnosis of clinical rabies is difficult and is often not made until after death of the patient.[21] Viral isolation may be positive in specimens of saliva or cerebrospinal fluid during the first 2 weeks of the illness. Serum antibodies may be detected as early as day 6 and usually by day 13. The fluorescent antibody method for the viral antigen is the most rapid and sensitive means of making the diagnosis, and can be used on a biopsy of skin from the highly innervated hair-covered area of the neck or brain tissue.[21]

Prevention and treatment The most effective prevention for rabies is to avoid contact with any wild animal or any unfamiliar domestic animal. Persons at risk of unavoidable contact with rabies, such as spelunkers, veterinarians, virologists, and travelers spending time in countries where rabies is enzootic, should receive preexposure prophylaxis. For people who cannot avoid exposure, the human diploid-cell vaccine series (three intramuscular injections on days 0, 7, and 21 or 28) should be given in the deltoid muscle[20] and repeated every 2 years.[22] In persons vaccinated intradermally, the neutralizing antibody titer should be followed to assess immunity. A case of rabies occurred in a Peace Corps volunteer who had been immunized by the intradermal route.[22] Immunity may or may not be as fully protective after intradermal vaccination as compared to patients vaccinated intramuscularly.[23]

The need for postexposure prophylaxis can be determined by the answers to the following questions: What is the status of animal rabies in the locale where the exposure took place? Was the attack provoked or unprovoked? Of what species and size was the animal? What was the state of health and vaccination record of the animal? Will the brain of the animal be examined with 48 h?

Most animals transmit rabies virus in saliva only a few days before becoming ill themselves (dog and skunk, 5 days; fox, 3 days; cat, 1 day; bats, however, may harbor the virus for many months).

Bites by household pets If the dog or cat is healthy and available for observation for 10 days, the patient should not be treated unless rabies develops in the animal. At the first sign of rabies in the animal, treat the patient with rabies immune globulin (RIG) and human diploid cell rabies vaccine (HDRV). The symptomatic animal should be killed and tested as soon as possible. If the pet is rabid, or suspected of being rabid, or if it is does not have up-to date vaccination records treat the patient with RIG and HDRV.[20] In certain states, ferrets may be kept as pets. These animals should be vaccinated against rabies, as they are large enough to survive a bite by a rabid animal and become infected.

Bites by wild animals All skunks, bats, groundhogs, foxes, coyotes, raccoons, bobcats, and other carnivores should be regarded as rabid unless laboratory tests prove negative. Patients should be treated with RIG and HDRV.

Bites by other animals Consider other animals (livestock, rodents, lagomorphs, e.g., rabbits, hares) individually.[20] Local and state public health officials should be consulted about the need for prophylaxis. Bites by the following almost never call for antirabies prophylaxis: squirrels, hamsters, guinea pigs, gerbils, chipmunks, rats, mice, and other small rodents.

Specifics of treatment The most important step is to cleanse the wound immediately with a brush and soap to remove as much virus as possible. Rinse well, then perform a second scrub with green soap or alcohol, which is rabicidal. If vaccine treatment is indicated, both RIG and HDRV should be given as soon as possible, regardless of the interval after exposure, unless the patient has been previously vaccinated and a serologic assay shows current immunity. In this case, only HDRV is needed and should be given on day 0 and day 3.[20] The administration of RIG is the more urgent procedure. If HDRV is not immediately available, start RIG and give HDRV as soon as it is obtained. RIG (20 IU/kg) should be given to the patient immediately—50 percent around the site of the bite and 50 percent in the thigh or the arm. This passive immunization will result in the early appearance of antibody but will also inhibit development of the active antibody from the human diploid vaccine—thus, the reason for prolonged dosage of the vaccines. Active immunization is accomplished with the HDRV. HDRV is given intramuscularly for a total of five doses. The doses are given on days 0, 3, 7, 14, and 28. Serum for rabies antibody testing should be collected 2 weeks after the fifth dose. If there is no antibody response, an additional booster should be given.

Treatment of the patient with clinical rabies When the rare patient is admitted with the clinical diagnosis of rabies, several steps should be taken immediately. First the diagnosis must be made rapidly by fluorescent antibody staining of various tissues, as well as direct inoculation of a laboratory mouse's brain tissue. Elevated antibody titers in the absence of immunization are clear evidence of infection. The first signs of clinical rabies are usually nonspecific, such as malaise, anorexia, fatigue, headache, and fever. The acute neurologic illness that follows is most commonly characterized by intermittent episodes of hyperactivity. In some cases, however, a progressive paralysis is most common. The usual time from onset of symptoms to onset of coma is 10 days. Risk of exposure for hospital staff includes contamination of open wounds or mucous membranes with saliva or other potentially infectious material such as neurologic tissue, spinal fluid, or urine. Blood, serum, and stool are not considered infectious.[24]

Basic clinical management consists of anticipating and preventing all treatable complications of the rabies infection. Pulmonary hypoxia should be prevented by tracheostomy at the first sign of

respiratory difficulty, monitoring of actual P_{O_2}, and use of supplemental oxygen. Unfortunately there are no specific antiviral treatments for rabies at present. Anticonvulsant therapy should also be instituted. Extreme increases in intracranial pressure may be prevented by insertion of a cerebrospinal fluid reservoir connected to the lateral ventricle, allowing withdrawal of the intraventricular fluid and measurement of intracranial pressure. Cardiac arrhythmias may be anticipated with careful monitoring. Rabies has been regarded as uniformly fatal. There have now been several patients who have survived with prolonged cardiorespiratory support, and there is serologic evidence that some animals have survived. An aggressive approach in the patient with known rabies infection is certainly worthwhile.

LYMPHOCYTIC CHORIOMENINGITIS Lymphocytic choriomeningitis (LCM) virus is an infectious agent common to the house mouse but rarely transmitted to humans. More recently, outbreaks of LCM virus infection in the United States and Germany have been traced to pet hamsters. Hamsters, like mice, may excrete LCM virus for several months and may become lifelong carriers.

When humans are infected, there may be three major manifestations: a grippe-like illness, meningitis, or encephalitis. The cerebrospinal fluid formula usually reveals an increased mononuclear leukocyte count and hypoglycorrhachia. Symptomatic therapy is all that is available.[25]

HERPESVIRUS SIMIAE (B VIRUS) Herpesvirus simiae (B virus) is enzootic in old world monkeys, especially rhesus, cynomolgus, and other macaques. The illness in monkeys is similar to that seen with herpes simplex in humans, and asymptomatic monkeys may shed the virus in saliva. Most cases in humans have occurred after direct exposure to macaque monkeys or monkey tissue through bites, scratches, or cuts.[26–28] A vesicular lesion develops at the wound site with progressive lymphadenitis and fever. Over the next few days to weeks a severe illness develops characterized by rapidly progressive ascending neuropathy and encephalitis.[27] The illness is rare, with only 22 well-documented cases described from 1937 to 1990. Seventy-two percent of cases diagnosed before 1987 were fatal. A cluster of four cases occurring in 1987 in Pensacola, Florida, were treated with acyclovir.[26] The two patients who received acyclovir when their infections were localized responded well to therapy and have been maintained on oral prophylaxis.

The diagnosis can be made by viral culture, serology, or presence of intranuclear inclusion in lymph nodes. All macaques should be presumed to be shedding B virus and should be handled accordingly. All monkey-inflicted injuries should be cleansed, specimens should be collected for viral culture and the patient should be evaluated by a physician. Clinical and serologic monitoring is critical, and high-risk or infected patients should be treated according to established guidelines.[27] The use of acyclovir or ganciclovir initially and acyclovir for years has led to an improved survival in infected patients.

SNAKE BITES

In the United States there are between 1 and 15 fatal snake bites each year, but worldwide the number is as high as 30,000 fatal bites each year. Because of regional differences in varieties of snakes,

FIGURE 238-2

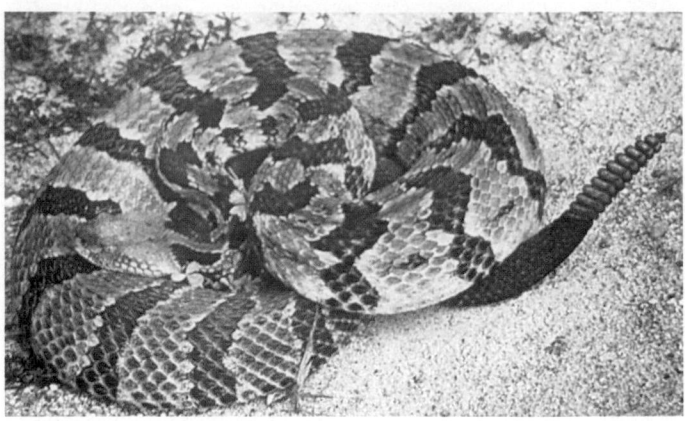

Timber rattler.

management recommendations differ geographically. There are about 7000 poisonous snake bites reported in the United States annually; the largest number occur in the southwestern and Gulf states. The two major poisonous snakes in the Americas are the pit viper (family Viperidae, which includes the rattlesnake, water moccasin, and copperhead) and the coral snake (family Elapidae). Arizona, Florida, Georgia, and Alabama are the states with the highest incidence of snake bites.[29] There are two poisonous snakes native to New England. The northern copperhead, also called the highland moccasin, is pink or reddish brown and is marked with large chestnut-brown barrels resembling dumbbells or hourglasses (Fig. 238-1). The bite is painful but rarely fatal. The timber rattler is dark brown with chevrons of black and brown (Fig. 238-2).

The degree of toxicity of a snake bite depends on the potency of the venom, the amount injected, the size and condition of the snake, and the size of the person bitten.[30] There are immediate clinical manifestations of the pit viper bite. Pain occurs at the site of the bite (usually within 5 minutes). Signs and symptoms of the bite site include wheal with local edema, numbness, and, within moments, ecchymosis and painful lymphadenopathy (Fig. 238-3). Nausea, vomiting, sweating, fever, drowsiness, and slurred speech may then develop. Bleeding of the gums and hematemesis are common hemorrhagic manifestations. If edema and erythema have not developed within 8 hours after the bite, one can assume that significant envenomation did not occur. Death due to untreated snake bites occurs in only 4 percent of patients within the first hour and in the majority 6 to 24 h after the bite.[30] Victims who receive medical care within 2 h generally survive.

For proper treatment, it is extremely important to establish that the bite is from a poisonous snake. The patient should have distinct fang punctures and immediate local pain, followed by edema and discoloration within 30 min. It is helpful to inspect the snake, since those that are poisonous may be differentiated from those that are not by the presence of fangs and the shape of the pupils (Fig. 238-4). A photograph of snakes common to a specific geographic area is important for all hospital emergency wards to aid practitioners in deciding if the patient has been bitten by a poisonous snake.

The patient should be reassured and the affected limb should be immobilized. If the anticipated delay in medical treatment is several hours and evaluation is done within 5 minutes of the bite, a ligature may be applied about 5 cm above the bite or just proximal to the closest joint proximal to the wound. Controversy regarding man-

agement, especially the use of tourniquets, exists. If used, the ligature should be released for 90 s every 15 min and care should be taken not to obstruct arterial or venous circulation. Arterial pulses should be palpable distal to the ligature. The use of ice, incision and suction, or electroshock therapy as part of emergency field therapy should be discouraged. When the patient reaches the physician, he or she should make two longitudinal incisions through the fang marks and apply suction intermittently for the first hour. The erythema and edema should be measured and tracked over time.

Emergency information and specific immune serum can be obtained from the Oklahoma City Poison Control Center (1-405-271-5454, 24 h a day). A polyvalent antiserum used for the bites of North American or South American snakes is available from Wyeth-Ayerst (Philadelphia, Pa). Antivenin is most effective if given within 4 h of the snakebite. The patient should be tested for hypersensitivity to horse serum while reconstituting the antivenom[30,31] so that an attempt can be made to neutralize the venom with immune serum (if the patient does not have a hypersensitivity reaction to horse serum).[29] Polyvalent pit viper antivenin should be used for all severe American snake bites except those of the coral snake. The dosage should be guided by the severity and progression

FIGURE 238-3

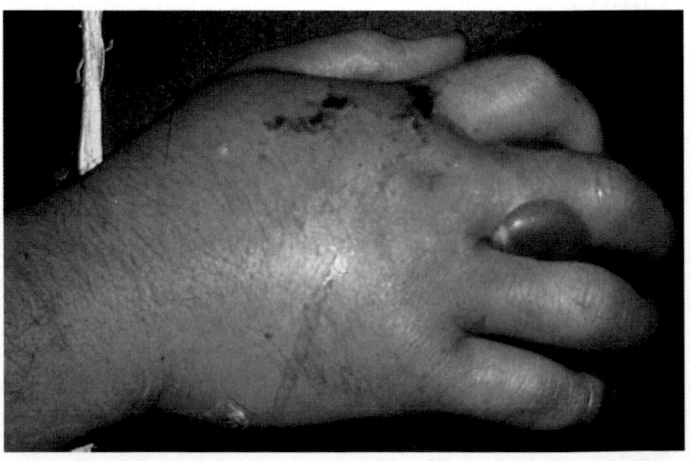

Copperhead snake bite.

FIGURE 238-1

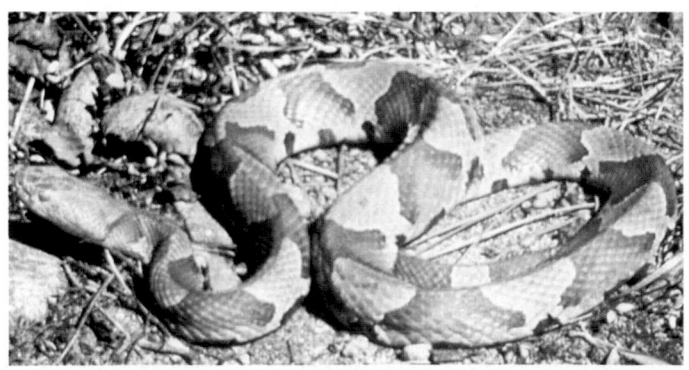

Northern copperhead.

of local changes and systemic clinical signs.[31] The dosage of antivenin for a moderate rattlesnake bite requires 4 to 7 vials (10 mL)—severe cases may require 15 to 20 vials; water moccasin bite requires 1 to 4 vials; for copperhead bites, antivenin is usually necessary only for a child or an elderly patient. The vials should be diluted in 500 mL of normal saline and given intravenously over 30 min. Antitetanus therapy and antibiotic prophylaxis with penicillin, 2 g per day, or tetracycline, 2 g per day, should be initiated for severe bites.

Supportive treatment is important, that is, hospitalization, careful evaluation of base-line hematocrit, platelet count, and prothrombin time. The wound should be cleansed and covered. Surgical debridement of superficial necrosis should be performed between the third and tenth days.

AQUATIC BITES AND STINGS

Seal Bite

Normally, a seal bite occurs on the finger of a trainer or a seal hunter, thus the term seal finger or Spaek finger.[32-34] The etiologic agent is unclear; *Mycoplasma phocedae* has been isolated in one case. The incubation period of 4 to 8 days is followed by throbbing pain, erythema at the site, and swelling of the joint proximal to the bite. Untreated, Spaek finger progresses to cellulitis, tenosynovitis, and arthritis. The treatment before antibiotics were available was amputation of the affected finger to relieve the severe pain and deformity. Tetracycline, 500 mg orally four times a day for 10 days, is now the antibiotic of choice. It is also helpful to immobilize and elevate the finger as well as soak it several times a day.

Injuries Caused by Jellyfish, Portuguese Man-of-War, Sea Anemones, and Corals

Stings due to jellyfish, Portuguese man-of-war, sea anemones, and corals are the most common envenomations encountered by humans in marine environments. All these creatures are members of the phylum Cnidaria, formerly known as Coelenterata. Cnidarians are radially symmetric animals with body walls formed by an inner and outer layer of cells enclosing a jelly-like substance.[35,36] They are divided into three major classes: the first class, Hydrozoa, includes the Portuguese man-of-war, fire corals, and hydroids; jellyfish belong to the second class, called Scyphozoa; sea anemones and true corals are members of the third class, known as Anthozoa.

Almost all cnidarians possess nematocysts, or stinging capsules, which are usually concentrated on some form of tentacle. Each nematocyst contains a toxin or group of toxins and a coiled threadlike apparatus with a barbed end that functions like a flexible hypodermic syringe (Fig. 238-5). When the nematocyst comes into contact with an unwary victim, the barbed end is discharged and the toxin is injected into the skin.

Cnidarian stings may range from mild, self-limited irritations to extremely painful and serious injuries, depending on the toxin of the species involved and the magnitude of the envenomation. In

FIGURE 238-4

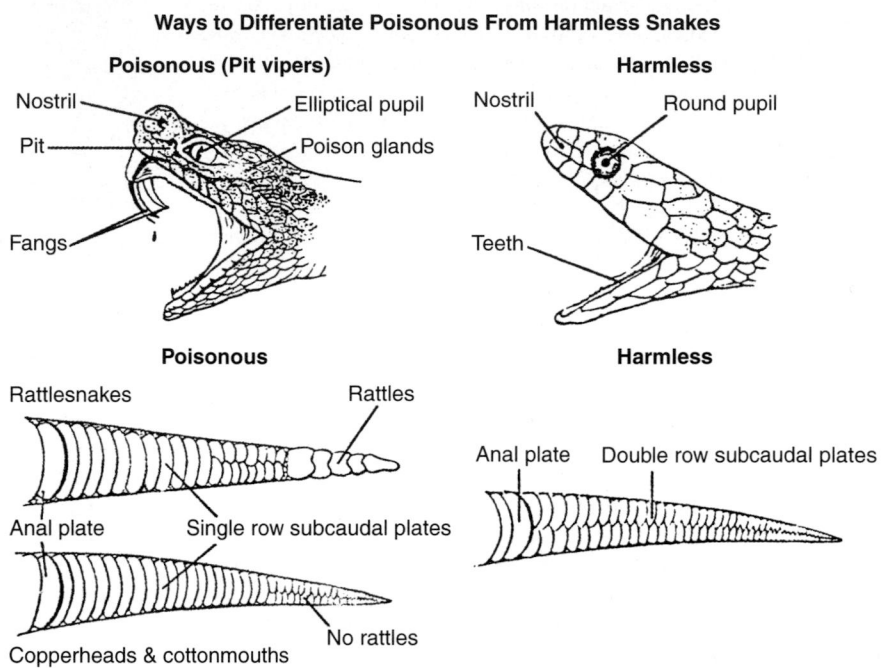

Ways to Differentiate Poisonous From Harmless Snakes

Identification of poisonous and nonpoisonous snakes. (*From Wingert WA, Wainschel W: A quick handbook on snake bites. Resident & Staff Physician, p 56, 1977. Reprinted with permission.*)

certain species such as the cubomedusae, or box jellyfish, stings can be fatal.

In most cases, jellyfish stings elicit toxic rather than allergic types of reactions. These toxic reactions may be localized and/or

FIGURE 238-5

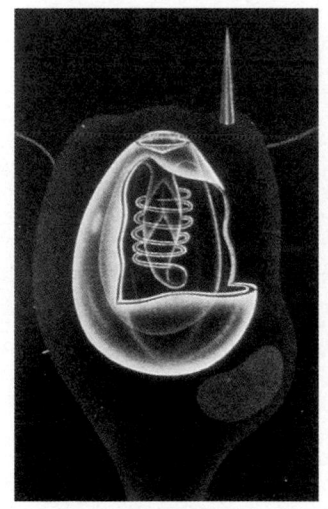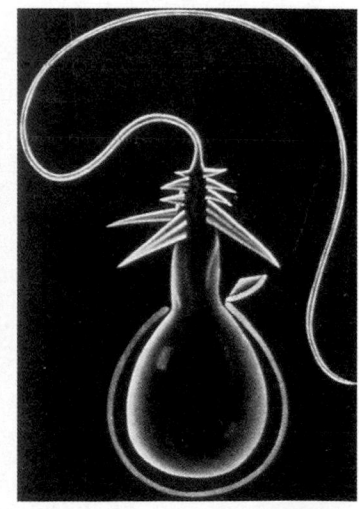

From left to right, a diagrammatic view of an intact and discharged coelenterate nematocyst. (*Courtesy of R. Kreuzinger, World Life Research Institute.*)

systemic in nature and will be discussed in the following sections. Although they occur less frequently, immediate-type hypersensitivity reactions including urticaria, angioedema, and anaphylaxis require prompt medical intervention as shock and death may ensue in highly sensitized individuals. Allergic contact dermatitis, delayed and persistent hypersensitivity reactions,[37] granuloma annulare,[38] and erythema nodosum[39] are several of the possible cutaneous reactions that can occur after jellyfish stings. A summary and classification of reactions to jellyfish stings appears in Table 238-1.[40–45]

INJURIES CAUSED BY JELLYFISH *Sea nettles* Among the most common sources of jellyfish stings are the sea nettles, which comprise two different species, both of which inhabit Atlantic as well as Indo-Pacific waters. *Cyanea capillata* (and its relatives) is the larger of the two species, with a bell measuring up to 1 m and numerous tentacles reaching 30 m in length[40] (Fig. 238-6). *Chrysaora quinquecirrha* is smaller, with a white or rust-colored bell that may reach 30 cm with four digestive tentacles hanging from it.[40]

Although sea nettle stings are seldom lethal, they can be quite painful.[46] Initially the victim experiences a sharp burning pain in the area contacted by the tentacles. Within minutes, the sting area develops a zig-zag-shaped, whiplike pattern of raised red welts 2 to 3 mm wide (Fig. 238-7). The duration of acute pain may vary, but it often begins to subside in 30 min. The wheals usually subside by 1 h, but purplish-brown petechial and postinflammatory pigmentation may persist for several days in the sites of tentacle contact.

Portuguese man-of-war *Physalia physalis* is the species name for the Portuguese man-of-war, which is a member of the class Hydrozoa and is therefore not a true jellyfish. *P. physalis* is encountered in both Atlantic and Mediterranean waters and is easily recognized by its translucent blue to pink or purple, bladder-like float with multiple tentacles suspended from it (Fig. 238-8). Both the floating bell and the tentacles are composed of large colonies of hydroids. *P. physalis* is distinguished from its Pacific ocean relative *P. utriculus*, commonly known as the blue bottle, in that *P. physalis* has a larger bell ranging in size from 10 to 30 cm with

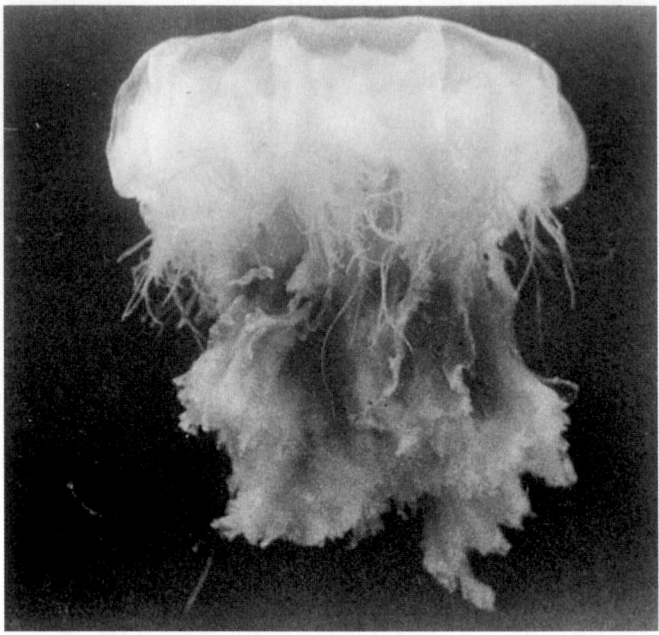

Cyanea capillata, also known as the sea nettle or lion's mane, is a common cause of jellyfish stings. (*Courtesy of B.W. Halstead, World Life Research Institute.*)

multiple fishing tentacles extending up to 30 m, whereas *P. utriculus* has only a single tentacle that rarely exceeds 5 m.[40] These tentacles are armed along their entire length with hundreds of thousands of nematocysts arranged in stinging batteries, with each battery containing hundreds of nematocysts. The nematocysts remain active even after portions of the tentacles are broken off in storms or when these animals are stranded on the shore by high winds or waves. Beached Portuguese man-of-war can cause a severe sting when stepped on or touched. Children who are stung after handling these animals cry and rub their eyes and may develop an acute conjunctivitis.[47]

Stings from *P. physalis* are more painful and severe than those caused by sea nettles and are more extensive and serious than those caused by *P. utriculus*. At the moment of contact with the tentacles of *P. physalis*, the victim experiences a sharp, shocklike, burning pain. There may be painful paresthesias or numbness in the sting area.

Initially the sting area appears as an irregular single line or multiple lines composed of red papules, beaded streaks, or erythematous welts that correspond to the areas of tentacle contact. The wheals resolve in several hours but may progress to vesicular, hemorrhagic, necrotic, or ulcerative stages before healing[36] (Fig. 238-9). Postinflammatory striae may persist for weeks to months. Permanent scarring may occur in some instances.[42] Severe localized complications of

TABLE 238-1

Local and Systemic Reactions to Jellyfish Stings

REACTION	SYMPTOMS
Local	
Immediate onset	Toxin-induced skin changes (wheals, papulovesicles, bullae), allergic reactions (exaggerated local reaction/angioedema)
Delayed onset	Delayed persistent reactions, recurrent reactions, persistent reactions, distant site reactions, contact dermatitis, papular urticaria, acquired cold urticaria[41] granuloma annulare, erythema nodosum
Complications and long term sequelae	Postinflammatory pigmentary changes, scars (pruritic, macular and papular), keloids, Mondor's disease of the breast,[42] fat atrophy, neuropathy, mononeuritis multiplex,[43] limb necrosis due to gangrene secondary to arterial spasm, joint contractions, deep vein thrombosis[44]
Systemic reactions	
Mild to moderate	Nausea, vomiting, diarrhea, headache, malaise, fever, chills, muscle aches, ataxia, muscle weakness, delirium, Irukandji reaction, Guillain-Barré syndrome[45]
Severe or life-threatening	Immediate cardiac arrest, rapid respiratory arrest, intravascular hemolysis, delayed renal failure, allergic reactions, anaphylaxis

SOURCE: Adapted from Burnett et al.[40]

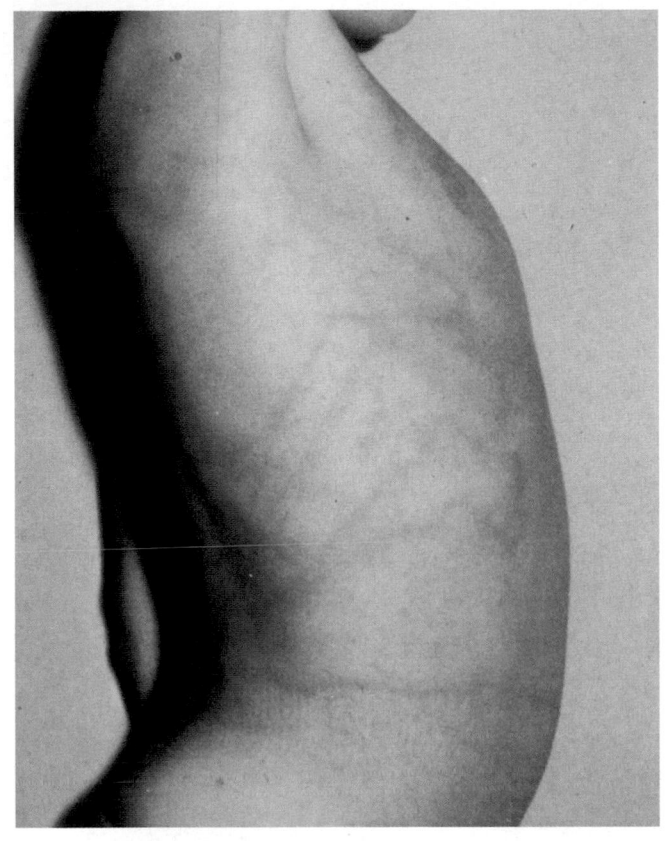

Whiplike sting pattern due to *Cyanea capillata* in a young boy. (*Courtesy of J.H. Barnes, World Life Research Institute.*)

FIGURE 238-8

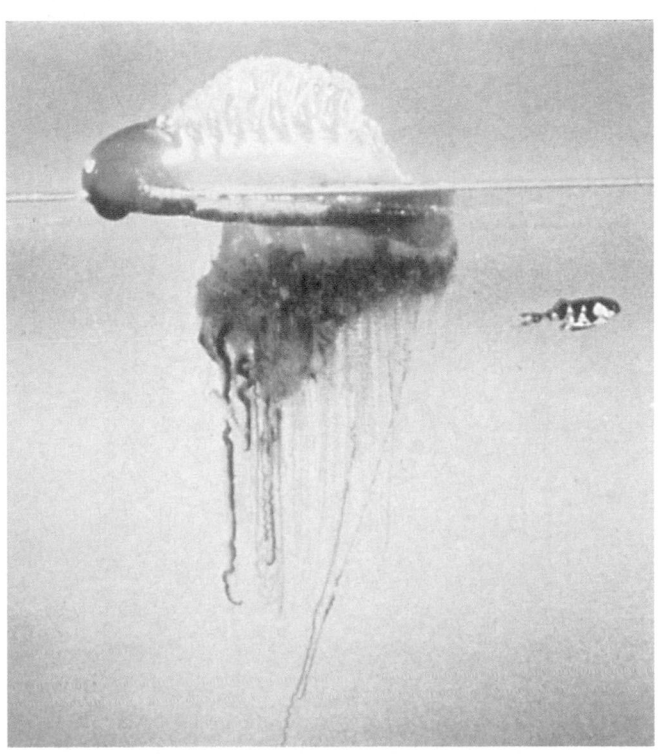

Physalia physalis, the Portuguese man-of-war, is distinguished by its bladder-like float and numerous trailing tentacles. (*Courtesy of B.W. Halstead, World Life Research Institute.*)

P. physalis stings may also include arterial spasm in the sting site, which can result in distal digital gangrene of the affected limb.[48,49]

Within 10 to 15 min of a *Physalia* sting, symptoms of an envenomation reaction may develop, characterized by nausea, abdominal cramps, muscular pains, backache, irritability, dyspnea, and chest tightness. Intravascular hemolysis and acute renal failure have been reported following a severe sting by *P. physalis* in a 4-year-old girl.[50,51] Until recently, reports of fatal stingings due to *P. physalis* were not well documented; however, in 1989 there were two separate well-substantiated case reports of human fatalities caused by *P. physalis* envenomation.[52,53]

Cubomedusae (box jellyfish or sea wasps)   Of all the species of jellyfish that cause painful stings and distress to swimmers, the species with the most established record of lethality is the box jellyfish, *Chironex fleckeri.*[54] Since 1884 it has been responsible for at least 63 confirmed deaths in tropical Australian waters.[55,56] At least one death occurs each year in Australia.[54] The fatality is usually a child, presumably because the size of the victim and the total area of the sting determine the likelihood of mortality.

C. fleckeri (commonly known as the sea wasp) is an advanced species of jellyfish, with a semitransparent cubic bell that may grow to a volume of 9 L and weigh more than 6 kg[54] (Fig. 238-10). Trailing from the bell are up to 60 stinging tentacles, which may reach 2 to 3 m in length.[54] When a human comes into contact with a box jellyfish, some of the tentacles are torn off and adhere to the skin. Rescuers of *C. fleckeri* sting victims must exercise extreme caution, as they too are at risk of envenomation until the tentacles have been neutralized and removed.

FIGURE 238-9

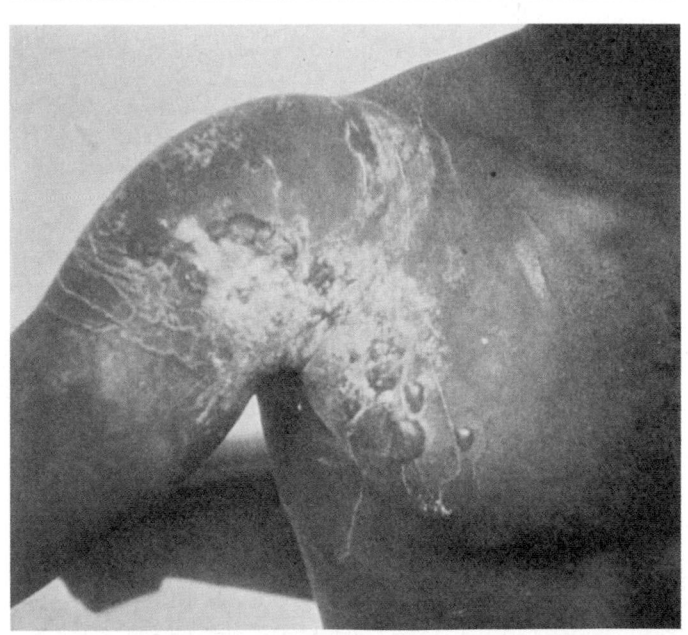

This unfortunate diver surfaced directly under a large Portuguese man-of-war and suffered a severe sting with bulla formation and tissue necrosis. (*Courtesy of S. Anderson, World Life Research Institute.*)

FIGURE 238-10

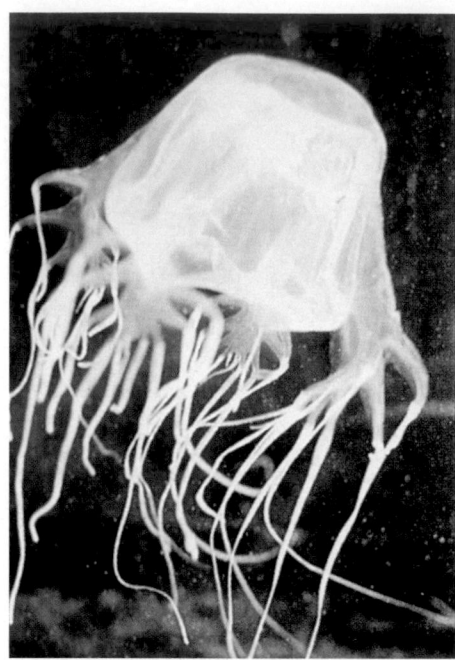

The deadly box jellyfish, *Chironex fleckeri,* is found in Indo-Pacific waters off the coast of Northern Australia. (*Courtesy of R. Hartwick.*[64])

The stings appear initially as linear welts that give the patient the appearance of having been whipped.[54] Fresh stings of *C. fleckeri* are easily recognized because they display a diagnostic frosted cross-hatched or ladder-like appearance[56] (Fig. 238-11). Microscopic diagnosis is also possible from blade scrapings or tape strippings from the sting site.[57] Victims who suffer sublethal stings describe the pain as instantaneous and excruciating.[58] The pain may persist for many hours. Severely stung areas of skin take on a dusky cyanotic appearance and may go on to blister formation and necrosis.[58] The healing process is slow and may be complicated by bacterial superinfection.[58] Permanent scarring is often seen.

Death may ensue within minutes if >6 m of tentacles have made contact with the victim. Pharmacologic analysis of the venom of *C. fleckeri* has resulted in the isolation of dermatonecrotic, hemolytic, and lethal fractions.[56,59] The lethal fractions contain cardiotoxic and neurotoxic agents.[56,59,60] Intravascular hemolysis due to hemolytic fractions in the toxin can precipitate acute renal failure. The potent cardiotoxins can produce ventricular arrhythmias and cardiac arrest, and the neurotoxins lead to respiratory failure. First aid for these victims frequently requires cardiopulmonary resuscitation. Intravenous verapamil has been proposed for both treatment and prophylaxis of ventricular arrhythmias in sting victims.[61,62] Antivenin is available for *C. fleckeri* stings and its early use in severe envenomations may be lifesaving. In addition to blocking or reversing the systemic effects of the toxins, the antivenin has also been shown to significantly reduce the pain and inflammation at the sting site.[54,63]

PREVENTION AND TREATMENT OF JELLYFISH STINGS
Prevention[56,61]

1. Swim only at patrolled beaches with properly trained lifeguards and adequate treatment facilities.

FIGURE 238-11

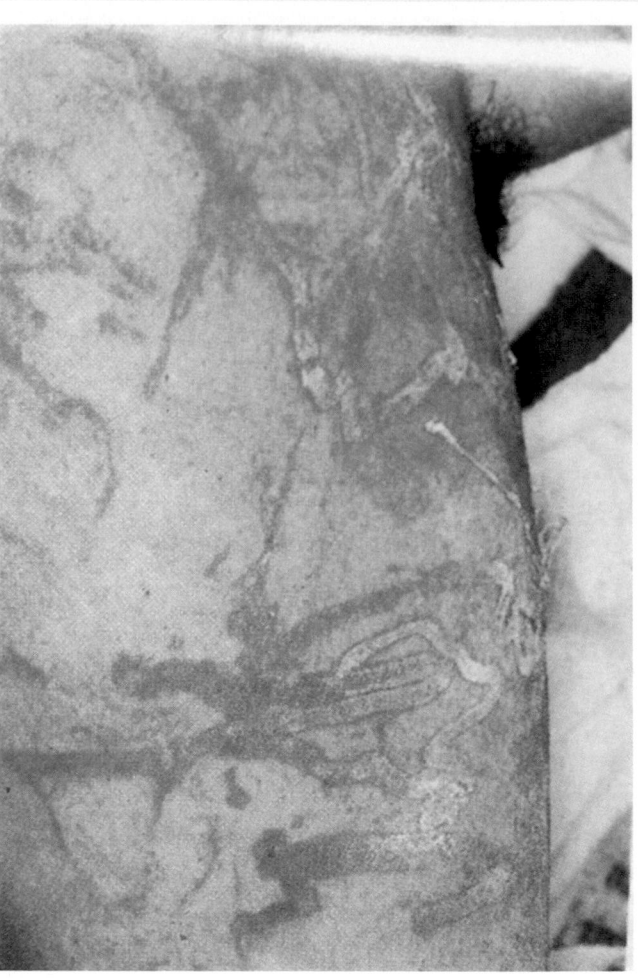

Characteristic frosted cross-hatched tentacle marks are diagnostic of a sting due to *Chironex fleckeri.* (*Courtesy of Townsville General Hospital, Department of Medical Illustration, Townsville, Queensland.*[64])

2. Close bathing beaches during periods of high jellyfish infestation.
3. Avoid swimming in infested waters, especially after a storm, as stings may result from remnants of floating damaged tentacles.
4. Beware of apparently dead or beached jellyfish.
5. Wear protective clothing when snorkeling or scuba diving, such as wet suits, long-sleeved shirts, pants or long woolen underwear, and gloves.

Treatment FIRST AID TREATMENT[35,36,40,63–66]

1. Remove or rescue the victim from the water.
2. Stabilize vital functions: airway, breathing, circulation.
3. Immobilize the affected part to prevent further envenomation by adherent tentacles.
4. Identify the type of jellyfish sting by considering locale, time of year, and indigenous species and by observing the sting pattern. Preserve a portion of the tentacle for future identification. Tape strip or scrape the sting site for microscopic analysis of the pneumatocysts if no tentacles are available.
5. To prevent further envenomation of the victim and to reduce the chance of a sting to the rescuer, disarm the nematocysts before removing the adherent tentacles.

a. If *C. fleckeri* or other box jellyfish species are suspected, douse or spray dilute acetic acid (3 to 10 percent) or household vinegar over all areas of tentacle contact for at least 30 s.[64,67]

b. For sea nettles, mix sodium bicarbonate (baking soda) with water to form a slurry and pour over the affected area or apply the powder directly to the tentacles.[65]

c. For *P. physalis* stings a slurry of baking soda is indicated. Vinegar had been reported to neutralize nematocysts of *P. physalis,* but recent work with species from Australia indicate that it may cause a discharge of nematocysts in some cases.[65,67]

d. If vinegar or baking soda is unavailable, papain, available as a powdered meat tenderizer, may be applied directly as a powder or mixed in water as a slurry to sting areas and tentacles of both sea nettles and Portuguese man-of-war.[35,64]

e. If nothing else is available, the tentacles can be rinsed off with seawater.

f. Do not use freshwater, methylated spirits, or alcohol in any form to deactivate tentacles as these all may cause a rapid massive discharge of nematocysts.[35,36,64]

6. Once the tentacles have been disarmed, they may be carefully removed with a forceps or gently scraped away from the skin with a plastic card, shell, or knife.[36,66]

TREATMENT OF SYSTEMIC REACTIONS

1. Support vital functions with cardiopulmonary resuscitation, oxygen, and intravenous fluids as required.[63]

2. Treat symptoms of anaphylaxis or shock with systemic epinephrine, glucocorticoids, and antihistamines.[39]

3. A proximal venous-lymphatic constriction bandage should be considered in the case of severe stings when systemic reactions are present or likely to occur, when topical deactivation of tentacles is not possible, and when transport to an acute care facility will be delayed.[39,66]

4. Specific antivenin is available for *C. fleckeri* stings. It is prepared by Commonwealth Serum Laboratories, Parkville, Victoria, Australia.[39] The antivenin is prepared from sheep serum and may therefore pose a risk of allergic reaction in sensitive individuals.[39] The preferred route of administration is intravenous, but it may be given intramuscularly. In severe stingings it has proved lifesaving. It is also the only treatment that can alleviate the intense pain (often within minutes of administration).[58] It may also reduce the cutaneous inflammation at the sting site and decrease the chance of scarring.[56]

5. Intravenous verapamil has been advocated both for treatment and prophylaxis of arrhythmias.[61,62]

6. For pain in severe stingings consider parenteral narcotic analgesics, ice packs,[68] and antivenin in cases involving *C. fleckeri.*

TREATMENT OF LOCAL REACTIONS

1. Apply topical anesthetic ointments, creams, lotions, or sprays to relieve itching or burning pain. (Benzocaine preparations should be avoided because of the risk of contact dermatitis.)[35]

2. Cleanse ulcerated or open wounds three times daily, apply a nonsensitizing antiseptic or antibiotic cream or ointment, and cover as needed with a light dressing.

3. Treat secondary infections with the appropriate parenteral antibiotics.

4. For delayed-type hypersensitivity reactions, use topical glucocorticoids, antihistamines, and systemic glucocorticoids if necessary.[40]

5. Antitetanus therapy should be considered, if indicated.

6. Ice or cold packs can relieve the pain of mild to moderate stings from many types of jellyfish.[68]

7. Aspirin or acetaminophen, alone or in combination with codeine, can be used to relieve persistent pain.[36]

SEA ANEMONE DERMATITIS   Sea anemones are members of the phylum Cnidaria, class Anthozoa. They are sessile creatures with graceful flowery tentacles armed with nematocysts (Fig. 238-12). Although stings due to sea anemones are not as common as those due to fire corals and jellyfish, they are a frequent cause of dermatitis in sponge fishermen, sponge divers, and beachcombers who gather snails and crabs from rocky hollows along the shore.[69] Their toxicity to humans depends on the species.

The genus *Sagartia* is worth noting because it is the cause of "sponge fisherman's disease."[35] This anemone lives at the base of sponges sought by commercial fishermen. When they harvest or sort the sponges with their bare hands or forearms, they are likely to come into contact with the tentacles of *Sagartia.* Symptoms of itching and burning occur at the sting site within minutes of the exposure and are accompanied by erythema, edema, and vesicles.[35]

Other species of sea anemones with especially venomous stings include *Actinodendron, Anemonia sulcata,* and *Triactis producta.* Severe stings may progress to vesiculation, ulceration, necrosis, and occasionally abscess formation.[36] Systemic symptoms may follow the exposure and can include headache, nausea, vomiting, fever, chills, muscle spasms, abdominal pain, malaise, thirst, and prostration.[1,2] Fulminant hepatic failure, which resulted in the death of the victim stung by a *Condylactis* species found in the Caribbean Sea, is the only known fatality due to anemone sting.[70]

Treatment for sea anemone stings is similar to that for jellyfish envenomations (see above).[71,72] The tentacles, if still adherent, should be removed carefully with a gloved hand and the sting area rinsed with seawater.[35] Both vinegar and Stingose (an aqueous solution of 20 percent aluminum sulfate and 11 percent surfactant) have been suggested for neutralizing the sting sites of anemones.[71] Sea anemone sting sites often heal slowly and may require treatment with antibiotics.

FIGURE 238-12

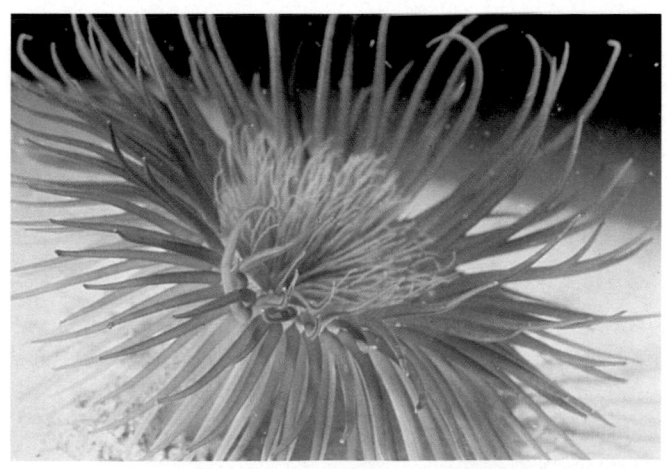

The flowery tentacles of the sea anemone can cause envenomations similar to jellyfish stings. (*Courtesy of Marty Gilman, Worcester, MA.*)

INJURIES CAUSED BY FIRE CORAL AND CORAL CUTS

Corals are colonial organisms belonging to the phylum Cnidaria. They form calcified structures of various sizes and shapes by cementing together their limestone exoskeletons or polyps.[69] True corals are members of the class Anthozoa. Fire corals are members of the class Hydrozoa and are not true corals, although they are similar in many ways.

Coral injuries may be divided into two major types: superficial injuries due to nematocyst stings and lacerations. It is entirely possible for both injuries to occur at the same time. Coral injuries may be complicated by foreign-body reactions, bacterial infections, and localized eczematous reactions.

Nematocyst envenomation in most true corals is a relatively innocuous experience, resulting in mild pruritic erythema that requires little if any treatment.[73] Calamine lotion or antipruritic lotions may bring relief.[74]

In contrast to true corals, the sting from the fire coral, *Millepora alcicornis*, is quite painful, as many scuba divers and snorkelers from the Florida Keys to the Caribbean will attest (Fig. 238-13). The wet mucous membrane surrounding the organism contains numerous nematocysts that readily discharge on contact with the skin, resulting in an immediate burning and stinging pain. Within one to several hours a pruritic erythematous papular eruption appears, which in severe cases may become pustular, and in rare cases may progress to necrosis and eschar formation.[75] Lesions heal in 1 to 2 weeks, often with postinflammatory hyperpigmentation. A delayed and persistent allergic contact dermatitis has also been reported to occur from a fire coral sting from the Red Sea.[76]

The sting may be prevented by wearing protective clothing. Fire coral stings should be rinsed with seawater to remove undischarged nematocysts. The sting area can then be covered with a compress of either acetic acid 5 percent (vinegar), or 40 to 70 percent isopropyl alcohol for 15 to 30 min or until the pain is relieved.[46,77] Seawater compresses, as hot as can be tolerated by the patient, are also reported to inactivate the toxin. A topical steroid cream or ointment may relieve pruritus and promote healing.

Lacerations from the razor-sharp exoskeletons of coral are known collectively as coral cuts. They may be suffered by beach walkers, waders, fishermen, swimmers, surfers, and scuba and skin divers. Coral cuts can be prevented by avoiding dangerous shorelines and by wearing protective clothing such as reef boots, gloves, long pants made of a thick cut-resistant material, or a wet suit.

Coral cuts are notorious for their slow healing and their propensity for secondary infection. Factors that complicate healing in coral cuts include:

1. Wounds often involve the lower extremities and these generally heal more slowly due to decreased tissue blood supply.
2. Wound edges are often irregular, contused, crushed, and abraded.
3. Contamination of wounds is likely, due to pathogenic bacteria found in shore waters.
4. Foreign bodies, including marine algae growing on the coral or portions of the coral itself, may be implanted in the wound.
5. Victims of coral cuts are often actively engaged in water sports and may not comply with optimal wound care.[78]

Treatment of coral cuts[79] should begin with vigorous cleansing of the wound with soap and water with a soft brush or rough towel, followed by copious irrigation with saline to remove foreign bodies. If the wound is extensive, local anesthesia may be required in order to adequately cleanse, explore, debride, and achieve good hemostasis.[78] Washing the wound with hydrogen peroxide before dressing it is recommended.[69]

The decision to close a coral cut wound primarily or to allow it to heal by secondary intention depends on the location of the wound, the degree of tissue trauma at the wound margins, and the likelihood of subsequent infection.[78] Facial and scalp wounds can often be converted to surgically clean wounds by debridement and then closed primarily.[78] Trunk and arm wounds may be closed primarily but require more surgical judgment. Lower-extremity wounds in most cases will heal slowly by secondary intention. Tape stripping is preferable to suturing of leg wounds because sutured leg wounds have a high chance of abscess formation.[78]

Once the wound has been closed, an antibiotic ointment covered with a nonstick dressing, with an outer dressing applying light pressure for 24 to 48 h, is advisable.[78] Rest and elevation will promote healing. It should also be remembered that coral cuts are tetanus prone and require tetanus prophylaxis, depending on the patient's immunization history.[78]

Failure to remove foreign debris following a coral injury may result in foreign-body reactions. Localized episodes of dermatitis have been reported following contact with coral (Fig. 238-14). The lesions may appear within several hours and begin as erythematous papules; these coalesce to form plaques, which may become vesicular. Biopsy of these lesions reveals a superficial and middermal perivascular infiltrate of lymphocytes, eosinophils, and plasma cells resembling an arthropod bite reaction.[73] In some patients these eruptions have been recurrent. Topical steroids may be helpful in treating these eczematous reactions.

Dermatitis from Sponges

Sponges are members of the phylum Porifera, class Desmospongiae. They are simple multicellular animals that live attached to the sea bottom. Sponges grow by forming a series of hollow-centered branching tubes composed of a fibrous material called spongin, which contains spicules of calcium carbonate or silica.[35,80] Spicules from certain species of sponges are capable of penetrating the skin, causing a localized irritant or foreign-body reaction. Treatment of sponge spicule dermatitis involves tape stripping of the affected area.

FIGURE 238-13

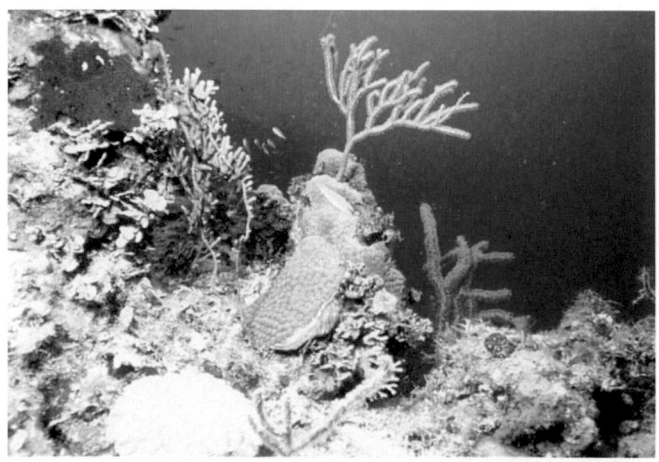

The mustard-colored fingerlike outcropping in the upper left quadrant of this formation of coral and hydroids is a typical example of fire coral.

FIGURE 238-14

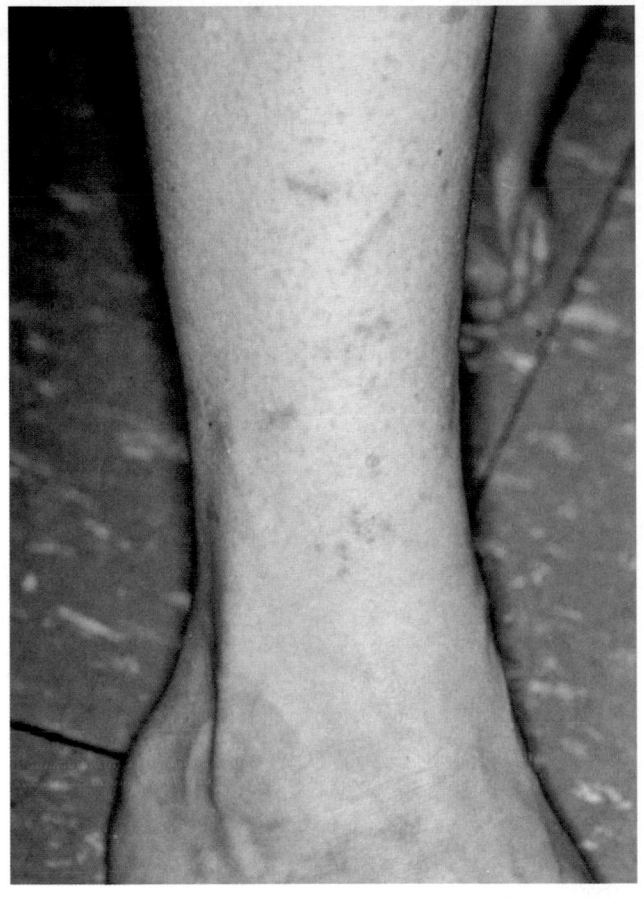

A contact dermatitis-like eruption resembling poison ivy occurred on the unprotected leg of this scuba diver 24 to 48 h after contact with an unknown type of coral. The eruption persisted for several weeks and cleared after treatment with topical steroid creams.

FIGURE 238-15

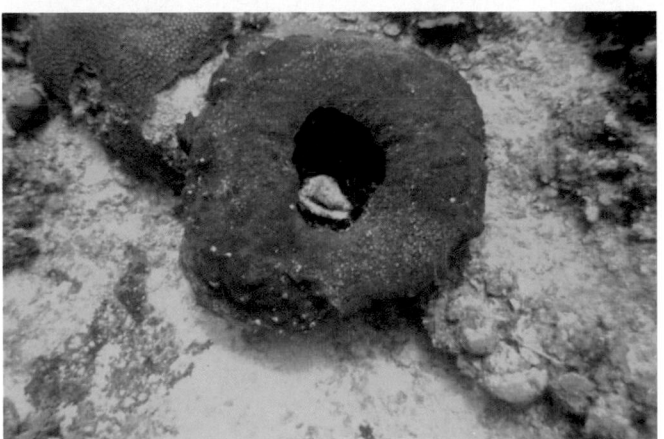

The poison bun sponge, *Fibula nolitangere,* can cause a severe irritant or toxin-induced contact dermatitis.

days. Systemic glucocorticoids may be indicated for severe reactions.[83]

Injuries due to Echinoderms: Sea Urchins, Starfish, and Sea Cucumbers

SEA URCHINS Sea urchins are spiny creatures that belong to the phylum Echinodermata, class Echinoidea. They are encased in a fragile, roughly spherical, calcareous shell, which is protected by a formidable array of mobile spines and pincer-like organs known as *pedicellariae*[84] (Fig. 238-16).

Bathers, surfers, divers, and fishermen are all at risk for sea urchin injuries. These may occur when the victim steps on an urchin, driving the spines into an unprotected foot, or as a result of loss of balance or wave action, in which case the hands or other body parts may be impaled.[85] Injuries from sea urchins may be inflicted either by penetrating wounds from the animal's spines, which often break off and become imbedded in the wound, or by bites from the pedicellariae. In certain species the spines or pedicellariae are venomous. This may explain why the pain of some sea urchin wounds is so excruciating and out of proportion to the apparent injury.

Encounters with sea urchins can result in two types of reactions: immediate and delayed. Immediate reactions are usually localized and are initially manifested by a severe burning pain in the wound site, which quickly becomes red and swollen and may bleed profusely.[81] There may be a black or purple discoloration at the site of the spine penetration, which can represent either retained spines in the wound or a tattoo-like effect from dye released by the spines that have exited intact. Paresthesias may develop in the wound area. Systemic symptoms are not common but can be seen in injuries due to particularly venomous species. Symptoms may include nausea, syncope, paresthesias, ataxia, muscle cramps, paralysis, and respiratory distress.[81,85]

Delayed reactions to sea urchin wounds may be nodular or diffuse; they result from a foreign-body reaction to the retained spine fragments. Delayed type hypersensitivity reactions may occur with erythema and intense pruritus days after the initial injury.[86] In one

There are at least 13 species of sponges that can cause a toxic dermatitis.[81] Of these, the most commonly encountered are the West Indian and Hawaiian fire sponge, *Tedania ignis*; the poison bun sponge, *Fibula nolitangere* (Fig. 238-15); and the red sponge, *Microciona prolifera*, found in the northeastern United States.[81] These creatures are covered by a surface liquid, or slime, that produces an irritant or toxin-induced dermatitis when contacted by bare skin.[80]

Symptoms of itching, prickling, stinging, or burning appear within minutes of exposure and are followed within a few hours by pain, swelling, and stiffness.[35,80,81] If the fingers are involved, they often become immovable within 24 h.[35] The first cutaneous sign of sponge poisoning is local erythema, which progresses to a papular, vesicular, or bullous eruption with weeping of a serous or purulent fluid.[80,81] Desquamation of the site occurs within several days. Erythema multiforme and anaphylactoid reactions have been reported to occur in highly sensitized individuals.[82]

Treatment of sponge dermatitis is similar to that of severe poison ivy. The acute dermatitis can be treated with cool dilute vinegar soaks [30 mL of vinegar per liter of water (2 tbsp/qt water)] several times a day.[81] Soothing lotions, topical steroids, and antihistamines may improve symptoms, which usually begin to subside in several

FIGURE 238-16

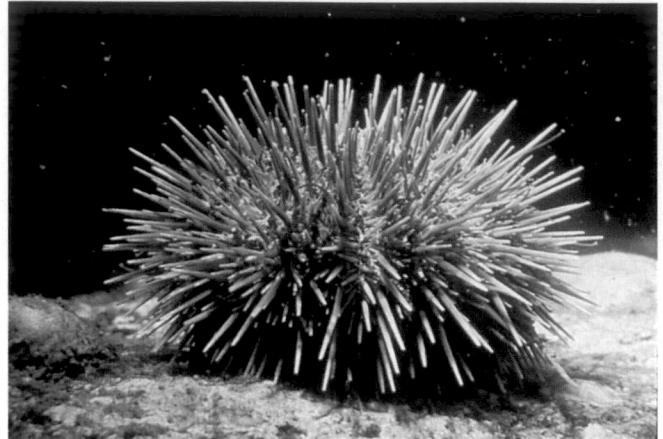

A.

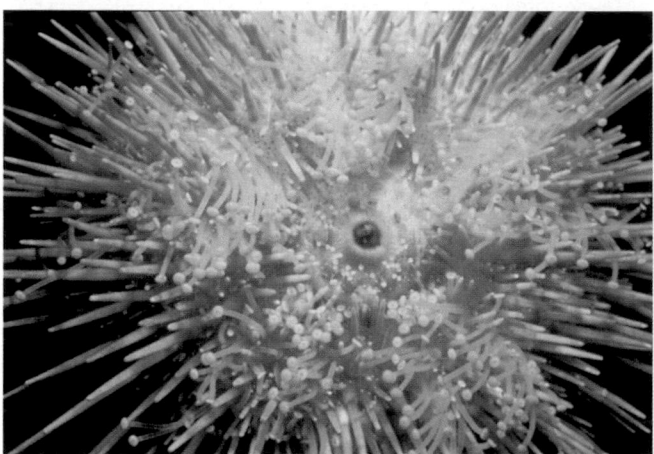

B.

Lateral (*A*) and ventral (*B*) views of a sea urchin demonstrate this animal's protective spines and venomous pedicellaria underneath. (*Courtesy of Marty Gilman, Worcester, MA.*)

of these cases the diagnosis was confirmed by patch testing to extracts of the ground sea urchin spines.[87] A granulomatous response results, which in some cases can resemble sarcoid.[84]

Nodular reactions are not usually painful and are localized to the area of spine penetration. They consist of small firm nodules, which may be flesh colored, pink, or cyanotic or may take on colors from the dye in the spines.[35,88] Nodules may have a central umbilication or a keratotic surface[88] (Fig. 238-17).

The diffuse form more commonly involves the fingers or toes and is manifested by a fusiform swelling of the affected digit with accompanying pain and loss of function.[81,84] Two cases of sea urchin granuloma involving the nail apparatus and resulting in permanent nail deformity have been reported.[89] There may be an associated tenosynovitis and destruction of the underlying bone. Sea urchin spine wounds may also cause direct mechanical injuries to nerves or joints and may be complicated by secondary infection.[81,85]

Initial first aid for the pain from immediate reactions calls for soaking the affected area in hot water [43 to 46°C (110 to 115°F)]

for 30 to 90 min until maximal relief is obtained.[66,81] Infiltration of the wound site with 1 to 2 percent lidocaine without epinephrine may be required in some cases to produce significant pain relief.[66] Spines that are protruding from the wound may be carefully removed. They are very fragile, however, and it is very difficult to extract the entire spine intact, as it is likely to break off at the surface of the skin. More invasive attempts at spine removal should not be performed without the benefit of aseptic surgical facilities and radiography to confirm their location. Removal of the spines may be aided by the use of an operating microscope.[81]

There are anecdotal reports of pounding the wound site with a stone for the purpose of breaking up the spines into smaller fragments, which are more easily absorbed.[90] This practice has been criticized by some authors.[81] The application of ammonia compresses or freshly voided urine has also been recommended, but again these remedies are anecdotal and their value has not been proved.[84,90] Antibiotics are indicated for secondary infections, and tetanus prophylaxis should be given if indicated.

The majority of sea urchin wounds resolve without complications; however, those involving the digits, joint spaces, or nerves will require surgical intervention. Delayed nodular reactions may resolve slowly with time. Topical and intralesional glucocorticoids may be efficacious for nodular reactions, and systemic glucocorticoids have been recommended for diffuse reactions, but their benefit has not been clearly substantiated.[35,81,91,92] Symptomatic nodular or diffuse reactions may not resolve until the spines and granulomatous tissue have been surgically removed.[78]

STARFISH Certain species of starfish may produce puncture wound injuries similar to those caused by sea urchins. The crown-of-thorns starfish, *Acanthaster planci,* accounts for the majority of severe starfish envenomations.[81] The ice pick–like spines of *A. planci,* which may reach 4 to 6 cm in length, are covered with a thin skin and glandular tissue that produce a poisonous slime.[66,92] The resulting wound is quite painful and may be accompanied by numbness and paresthesias.[81] Systemic symptoms including nausea, vomiting, and muscle weakness are infrequent and short-lived.[81] Fragments of spines and their surrounding integument may become imbedded in the wounded area, resulting in granulomatous reactions.

Treatment is similar to that for sea urchin wounds. Initial first aid should include soaking the affected area in hot water for 30 to 90 min until there is maximal pain relief.[66]

In addition to causing spinous injuries, some species of starfish may secrete a toxic substance directly into the water. When these starfish are present in large numbers, there may be sufficient amounts of this toxin to produce a pruritic papulourticarial eruption.[35,81]

SEA CUCUMBER DERMATITIS Sea cucumbers are sausage-shaped bottom-feeding echinoderms that can produce a papular contact dermatitis by means of a toxic liquid substance, known as holothurin, which is secreted from their body walls.[35] Conjunctivitis and even blindness can result from corneal involvement if the toxin comes in contact with the eyes.[81] These animals have also been reported to ingest intact nematocysts from marine coelenterates, which they may later secrete for defensive purposes. Prevention of sea cucumber dermatitis involves protecting the skin and eyes from contact with these creatures and educating children and curious divers about the risk of handling them. Treatment consists of washing the affected area with soap and water to remove the toxin and then treating as for a mild contact dermatitis.[93]

Dermatitis and Bites from Marine Worms

BRISTLEWORM DERMATITIS Bristleworms are multisegemented marine worms of the phylum Annelida, class Polychaeta (which means "many bristles")[93] (Fig. 238-18). Each segment of the worm is armed with rows of silky or bristlelike, hollow, venom-filled setae that can easily penetrate and break off in the unprotected skin of a victim in a fashion similar to cactus spines.[92] Contact with the bristleworm results in an erythematous papular or urticarial eruption at the site, accompanied by symptoms of paresthesias, intense itching, or burning pain.[35,92] The bristles are too small and fragile in most cases to be removed with a forceps; however, tape stripping with cellophane adhesive tape can be effective.[35,93] After the setae have been removed, the application of ammonia soaks or alcohol or water compresses may bring symptomatic relief.[35,93]

LEECHES Leeches are another class of segmental worms whose bites may be encountered in fresh or salt water as well as on land. They are members of the phylum Annelida, class Hirudinea. Leeches have specialized biting jaws that allow them to attach to their host in order to feed on a meal of blood. Although freshwater leeches are capable of attaching painlessly to their human host, saltwater leeches produce pain similar to a bee sting.[35,93] Leeches inject a powerful anticoagulant, hirudin, into the wound, as well as other antigenic substances that are capable of eliciting allergic reactions (including anaphylaxis) in sensitized individuals.[35] Local symptoms of leech bites include bleeding from the puncture sites, pain, swelling, redness, and severe pruritus; urticarial, bullous, or necrotic reactions may occur in sensitized persons.[35,93]

Severe ulcerations may result if the leech is removed forcibly and its mouth parts are left behind in the bite site. Leeches must therefore be removed carefully by inducing them to fall off by applying a noxious agent (such as alcohol, vinegar, brine, or a match flame) to their site of attachment.[35] After the leech has been removed, the wound should be carefully cleansed and minor bleeding controlled by the application of a styptic pencil.[35,93] Secondary infections may be prevented by cleansing the bite site for several days with antiseptic solutions containing alcohol or boric acid.[35]

CERCARIAL DERMATITIS (CLAM DIGGER'S ITCH) Cercarial dermatitis, also known as schistosome dermatitis or swimmer's or clam digger's itch, is an acute pruritic eruption resulting from the penetration of the skin by the cercarial forms of certain parasitic flatworms of the family Schistosomatidae.

Symptoms of cercarial dermatitis begin with urticarial-like lesions and a prickling sensation of the skin, which lasts for about half an hour after exposure to cercaria-infested waters. Severe pruritus of the affected area is seen 10 to 12 h later. Within 24 h, erythematous papules appear that may progress to vesicles and later to pustules. Pain and swelling of the area accompanies the intense itching, which usually peaks in 48 to 72 h. Headache, fever, and superinfection with lymphangitis are occasionally seen.

In the Great Lakes region, several species of schistosome cercariae that cause swimmer's itch have been reported, and many

FIGURE 238-17

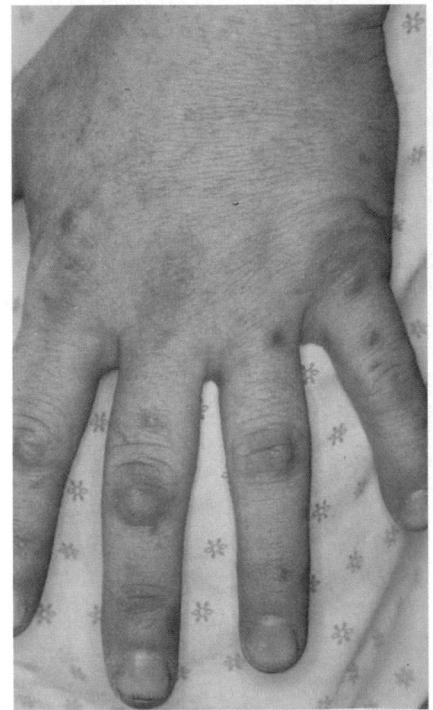
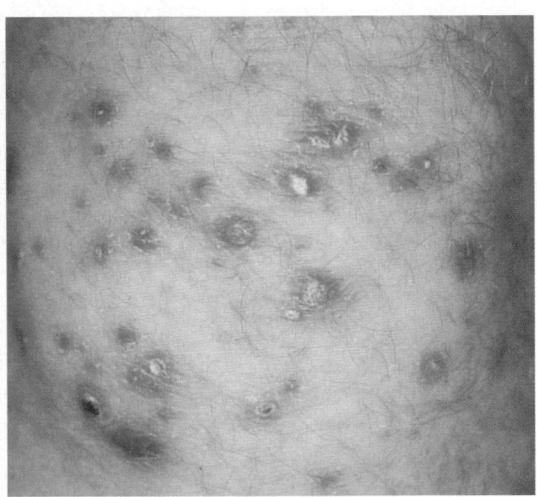

A.

B.

(*A* and *B*) Nodular reactions to imbedded sea urchin spines. (*Courtesy of Karen Rothman, MD.*)

FIGURE 238-18

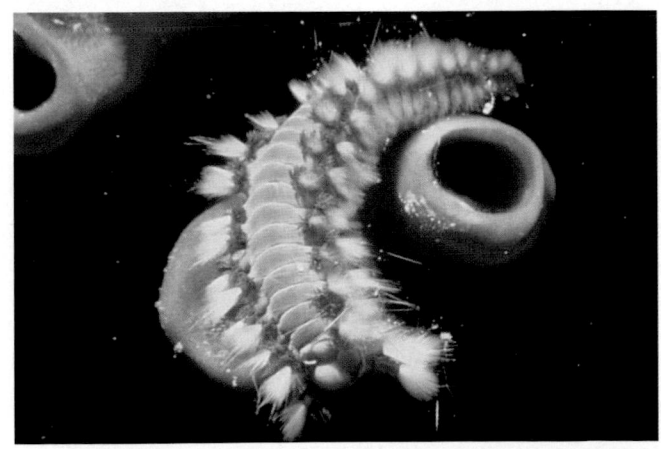

Hermodice carunculata, the West Indian bristleworm, can inflict a painful wound with its hollow, venom-filled bristlelike setae. (*Courtesy of Marty Gilman, Worcester, MA.*)

other species have been discovered throughout the world in fresh as well as salt water.[94,95] The economic impact on regions with recreational lakes in which the parasites are known to occur can be substantial. A severely disabling form of cercarial dermatitis affects the paddy workers and rice farmers of the Far East. Cercarial dermatitis has also been described in shallow coastal waters, notably on Long Island Sound where the condition is known to affect clam diggers, giving rise to the name, "clam digger's itch" (Fig. 238-19).

Humans are accidental hosts in the life cycle of dermatitis-producing schistosomes. The cycle begins when the primary host, a waterfowl, marshbird, finch, muskrat, mouse, or deer, passes schistosomal eggs in its feces into a body of water. Each egg hatches in 10 to 15 min, releasing a secondary-stage miracidium. The miracidia are free-swimming and must locate and infect their definitive snail host within 12 h or they will die. The miracidia migrate to the snail's digestive gland, where they develop into multiple sporocysts. In about 5 weeks the sporocysts give rise to hundreds of fork-tailed cercariae, which measure 0.75 mm in length. The cercariae are released from the snail under favorable conditions

FIGURE 238-19

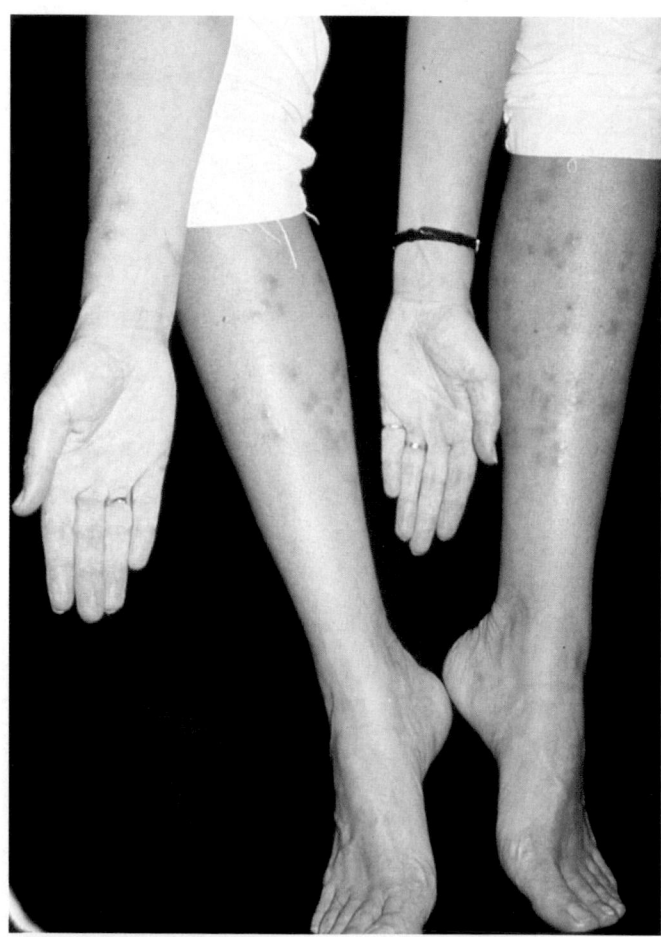

Intensely pruritic papulovesicles suggestive of a severe reaction to flea bites in a patient with clam digger's itch. Note that the left hand, which was not in the water and was holding the pail for collecting the clams, was spared.

of light and heat and are carried toward the shore by prevailing winds and currents.[95] When an appropriate host is encountered, the cercaria attach to the skin with their oral suckers and penetrate the epidermis and dermis by means of histolytic enzymes. They lose their tails in this process and are now called schistosomulae. The schistosomulae migrate via the blood vessels through the heart and lungs to the intrahepatic veins, where they mature into adult male and female trematode flukes. When the worms mate, they pass in pairs through the mesenteric venules of the intestinal wall where the female lays hundreds of eggs.[94] The eggs then penetrate the gut wall and are discharged in the feces, and the cycle is repeated.

When cercariae that do not cause schistosomiasis in humans accidentally attach to the skin, they may penetrate the epidermis but are unable to reach the bloodstream. The organisms die in the superficial papillary dermis and undergo total histolysis within 3 to 4 days. The cercarial protein residua stimulate a delayed-type hypersensitivity response, which may increase in severity with repeated exposures.

Skin biopsies taken at 3 to 4 days reveal an amorphous eosinophilic mass at the site of the dissolved cercaria, with an intense lymphocytic infiltrate. Later, histiocytes appear in the middle and deep papillary dermis.[96]

The differential diagnosis of cercarial dermatitis includes insect bites from chiggers, mosquitoes, and fleas; contact dermatitis from poison ivy; and the stings of other marine coelenterates. In Africa, Asia, South America, and Puerto Rico, swimmer's itch must be distinguished from the dermatitis associated with human schistosomiasis, which produces an eruption with very similar but milder and more transient symptoms.[95,97] Swimmer's itch must also be distinguished from sea bather's eruption, which will be discussed in the next section.

Prevention of cercarial dermatitis in waters where swimmer's itch is known to be a problem is difficult. Avoidance of all aquatic activity is not a reasonable solution, and most swimmers or workers are not willing to apply a protective coat of petrolatum before exposure.[98] Some have advocated a brisk rubdown with a towel immediately after bathing in the belief that the cercaria can be wiped off before they can penetrate the skin, but other investigators have shown that both this and alcohol rubdowns are of little benefit. Various chemical repellents have been tried, including copper sulfate and bathing with hexachlorophene soap before exposure, but these methods remain unproved. Clothing barriers may be of some help, as cercarial dermatitis occurs more commonly on uncovered skin.

Another preventive alternative involves the elimination of the molluscan host. This can be accomplished by a variety of means, including treating the waters with various molluscicides, copper sulfate, or niclosamide. Drainage of lakes or ponds with the removal of aquatic vegetation can deprive the snails of shelter and nourishment.[95] In smaller ponds, hand removal of the snails from the banks of the water may be helpful. The most radical efforts reported involve draining the affected ponds and destroying the snails with flame throwers.[98] Under most circumstances, many of these methods are too expensive or dangerous to the environment to be practical.

Treatment of cercarial dermatitis is largely symptomatic. In mild cases antipruritic or drying lotions, oatmeal or starch baths, and antihistamines may alleviate pruritus. Aspirin may be helpful for the pain and swelling, and a bedtime sedative may be required to allow the patient much-needed sleep. Proper washing and hygiene should be maintained to prevent bacterial superinfection. In severe cases, potent topical steroids and occasionally systemic glucocorticoids may be required.[98]

Sea Bather's Eruption

Sea bather's eruption (SE), also known as marine dermatitis, and more commonly as "sea lice," is an acute dermatitis that begins shortly after bathing in seawater. Seabather's eruption is often confused with swimmer's itch (cercarial dermatitis), not only because they both occur after exposure to water, but also because the common names of these two conditions are easily confused. For many years the cause of SE remained a mystery, but it is now known that the responsible agents in at least two types of SE are the larval forms of marine coelenterates. In waters off the coast of Florida and in the Caribbean, the tiny larvae of the thimble jellyfish, *Linuche unquiculata*, are to blame.[99] Off the coast of Long Island, NY, researchers found that the larval forms of the sea anemone *Edwardsiella lineata* were responsible for the eruption.[100]

In addition to a different etiology, SE can be distinguished from cercarial dermatitis by several other factors (Table 238-2). Sea bather's eruption primarily involves areas of the body covered by bathing suits where water evaporates slowly, as opposed to the uncovered areas typical of swimmer's itch. Most symptoms are not noted until the bather has left the water (although some of those affected have complained of a prickling sensation while still in the water).[101]

The eruption is due to minute stings from the nematocysts of the coelenterate larvae, which become trapped underneath swimwear, or may adhere to hairy areas of the body. Seabather's eruption is believed to be due to an allergic reaction to these nematocyst stings. Factors that may cause the nematocysts to fire include mechanical pressure from a bathing suit or swim cap, or from lying on a surfboard or sitting on a car seat in a wet bathing suit; and changes in osmotic pressure as the swimming suit dries out, or when the bather rinses off with freshwater while wearing the swimwear.[101]

The lesions begin within 4 to 24 h after exposure as erythematous macules, papules, or wheals that may itch or burn (Fig. 238-20).[99] These may progress to vesiculopapules, which crust over and heal in 7 to 10 days.[35,98] Associated systemic symptoms may include chills and a low-grade fever as well as nausea, vomiting, diarrhea, headache, weakness, muscle spasms, and malaise.[101] Febrile and systemic symptoms are more common in children and adolescents.[102] In the presence of such constitutional symptoms, caregivers who do not recognize the pattern of the eruption or who do not take a history of exposure to saltwater may mistakenly make the diagnosis of a viral syndrome.

In waters along the coast of south Florida the season for SE is between March and August with a peak in May. The incidence among bathers during May and June of 1993 in Palm Beach County has been reported to be 16 percent.[102] The strongest risk factor for developing SE is a previous history of the condition, which is consistent with the theory that SE represents a hypersensitivity response to the nematocyst stings.[102] Other risk factors include age less than 16 and surfing.[102] Showering with swimwear removed was found to be a protective measure.[102]

Prevention of seabather's eruption should include the following measures:

1. Bather's should remove their swimwear and shower as soon as possible after leaving the water. Since freshwater may cause discharge of the nematocysts it is important that the suit be removed before showering begins. Showering with saltwater may be preferable, but impractical. Bathing suits should be rinsed out with soap and water and heat-dried, as recurrences of the eruption have occurred after air drying.[101] Persons who have had a severe case of SE may want to consider discarding the suit worn at the time of the exposure.

2. Avoid wearing T-shirts while in the water. Women may consider wearing a two-piece suit to reduce the surface area under which larvae may be trapped. Swimming without a bathing suit has been found to be advantageous (assuming it is permitted and proper care is taken to prevent sunburning), but it should be remembered that the larvae easily attach to hair bearing areas, so that showering after a swim in infested waters is still required.

3. Whole-body Lycra swimsuits or wetsuits with snug-fitting collars and cuffs may be protective, but the eruption may still occur along the collar or cuff edges.[103]

TABLE 238-2

Comparison of Swimmer's Itch and Seabather's Eruption

FACTOR	SWIMMER'S ITCH	SEABATHER'S ERUPTION
Type of water	Fresh and salt	Salt
Part of body involved	Uncovered	Covered or hairy areas
Locale	Northern United States and Canada	Florida and Cuba
Cause	Cercarial forms of schistosomes	Larval forms of marine coelenterates,(*E. lineata,* and *L. unquiculata*)

SOURCE: Modified from Fischer.[35]

FIGURE 238-20

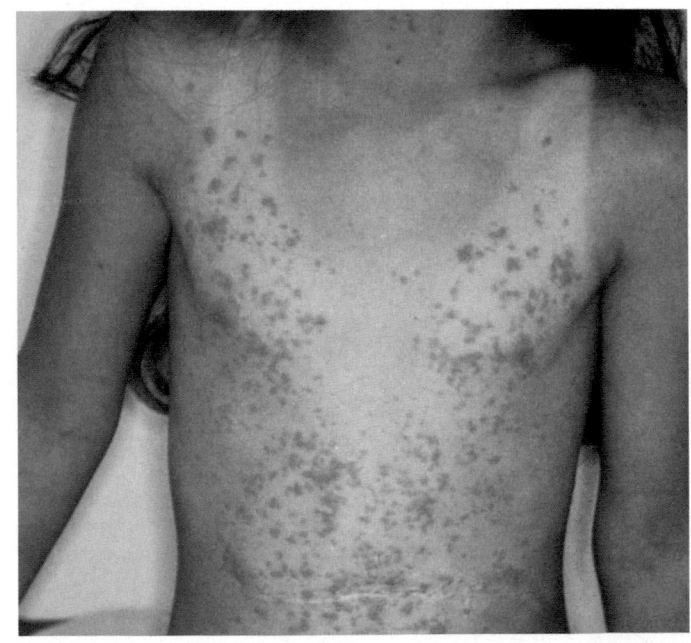

Sea bather's eruption in a young girl; it occurred after a swim at a Florida beach. (*Courtesy of Karen Rothman, MD.*)

4. Highly sensitized individuals should avoid swimming in waters during outbreaks of seabather's eruption.

Treatment of SE is symptomatic, with antipruritic lotions, colloidal baths with starch or oatmeal, antihistamines, and topical glucocorticoids. Severe unremitting cases may warrant systemic glucocorticoids.[99] Secondary bacterial infections may complicate the condition and should be diagnosed and treated appropriately.

Injuries due to Mollusks

CONE SHELL ENVENOMATIONS Cone shells are univalvular gastropods whose ornate cone-shaped shells are highly prized by shell collectors and divers. Unfortunately, a number of species have a highly developed venom apparatus that can inflict a lethal sting. The majority of dangerous cone shell species are found in shallow waters of the Indo-Pacific.[77] Cone shells are carnivorous. They live on the ocean bottom and, depending on the species, may hunt worms, other mollusks, or fish.[104] Cone shells kill their prey by means of a spearlike venomous radular tooth that is thrust out from the animal's proboscis. Cone shell venom contains several different kinds of neurotoxins, and death may result from respiratory paralysis. There is as yet no antivenin for cone shell envenomations, and mortality rates for the more dangerous species (*Conus geographicus* and *C. magus*) may be as high as 15 to 20 percent.[35,104]

Injuries from cone shells are of the puncture wound variety. The degree of pain is variable, ranging from a mild stinging sensation, similar to that of an insect bite, to severe excruciating pain. Early symptoms may include edema, ischemia, numbness, and paresthesias of the wound site. Paresthesias may become widespread, with the lips and mouth commonly affected.[35,81] Localized muscular paralysis may progress to generalized weakness or paralysis with eventual respiratory distress and cardiopulmonary failure. Neurotoxic symptoms that indicate severe envenomations include diplopia, blurred vision, aphonia, dysphagia, and coma.[35,81,104] Rare cases of disseminated intravascular coagulation have been reported after cone shell envenomation.[77]

Great care must be exercised in handling live cone shells. Thick protective gloves should be worn, and the soft underportion of the animal should be avoided. Cone shells should never be placed in pockets of clothing or swimwear as they have been known to sting through clothing.[66]

Treatment of cone shell envenomations is supportive. The victim should be kept at rest, and the sting area kept dependent and immobilized. A compression dressing should be applied to occlude lymphatic-venous, but not arterial, flow.[66] Local suction may be helpful if it can be applied immediately to the wound site with a plunger device, such as the Extractor (Sawyer Products, Safety Harbor, FL).[93] No incision of the wound is required with this device.[93] Compresses or immersion of the sting area in hot water may be indicated in cases in which it is not practical to apply a lymphatic-venous compression dressing or to relieve pain in milder stings.[35,66,81] Advanced life support measures, including artificial ventilation, may be required while victims are being transported to a hospital, where they may require mechanical ventilatory support.[66]

OCTOPUS BITES Octopuses are an advanced class of mollusks belonging to the class Cephalopoda. They are shy and reclusive creatures that tend to avoid encounters with humans; however, bites

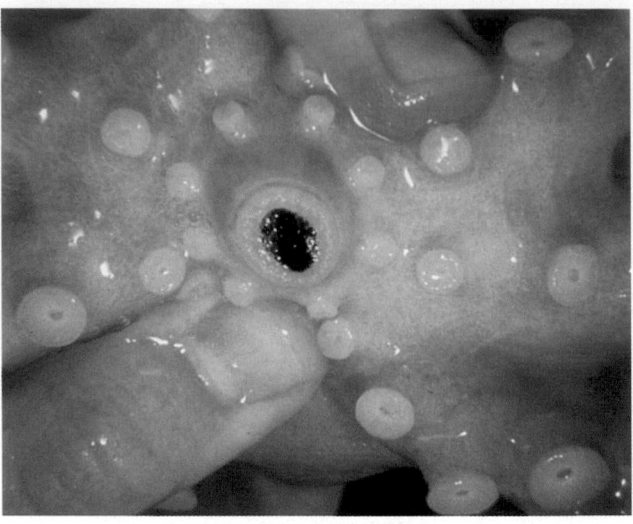

Ventral view of the underside of an octopus exposing the animal's centrally located mouth and parrot-like beak. (*From D. D. Fulghum,*[105] *with permission.*)

can occur when curious divers, fishermen, or beachgoers encounter these animals and handle them carelessly. The octopus bites with a parrot-like chitinous beak located on the ventral side of the head in the middle of its tentacles (Fig. 238-21).

Most octopus bites are not life-threatening to humans. The bite site may be immediately painful, like a bee sting, and is recognized by the presence of two small puncture wounds, which may bleed profusely.[35] Symptoms from octopus bites are usually mild and transient and consist of redness, swelling, and itching.[105] One case of granuloma annulare has been reported to have developed around the site of an octopus bite[105] (Fig. 238-22). Paresthesias and numbness may develop at the site if the species is venomous. In more severe envenomations, these may be followed by more generalized neurologic symptoms similar to those occurring in cone shell stingings.

The most dangerous species of octopus, the Australian blue-ringed octopus, *Hapalochlaena maculosa*, is found in Australian coastal waters. Mortality rates due to bites caused by *H. maculosa* may be as high as 25 percent.[106] *H. maculosa* produces a toxin in its salivary glands, which is introduced into the bite site by the animal's powerful beak. The toxin contains a fraction identical to tetrodotoxin, which blocks peripheral-nerve conduction, resulting in paralysis and subsequent respiratory failure.[93] The bite of the blue-ringed octopus may or may not be painful, so that victims may not realize that they have been bitten until neurologic symptoms develop.[81]

Unfortunately, there is no antivenin yet for bites due to *H. maculosa*. Treatment is supportive and similar to that recommended above for severe cone shell envenomations. Immersion of the wound in hot water does not seem to be beneficial.[81] The use of the pressure-immobilization technique with a lymphatic-venous occlusive pressure dressing or the immediate application of suction to the wound site with a suction device may be of value.[66,93] Excision of the bite site down to fascia has been recommended by some authors, but is of unproved value.[35,81,106]

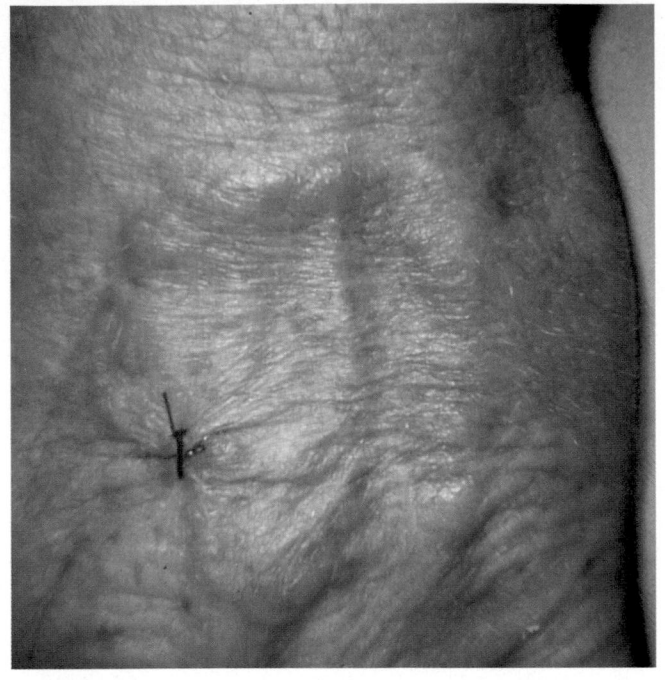

Granuloma annulare, which occurred on the back of the hand of a commercial fisherman several days after being bitten by a small octopus at the same site. (*From D. D. Fulghum,*[105] *with permission.*)

Injuries due to Venomous Fish Spines

Ichthyoacanthotoxicosis is the proper term for envenomations due to puncture wounds or lacerations inflicted by the spines of venomous fish.[107] There are over 200 species of venomous fish in the world that can cause injury to humans.[81] The most notorious of these includes the stingray, catfish, lionfish, scorpionfish, stonefish, weeverfish, toadfish, and spiny dogfish. All of these fish have in common a venom apparatus consisting of a single spine or multiple spines, in various locations, which are covered by an integumentary sheath enclosing various forms of venom glands. When the spine of the animal penetrates the victim, the sheath is torn and the venom glands release their toxins into the wound. The toxins from some of these fish may remain potent for 24 to 48 h after the fish's death.[83,108]

STINGRAYS Stingrays are probably the most common cause of venomous fish stings confronting humans; as many as 1500 stingray attacks are reported each year in the United States alone.[92,107] Rays are grouped into one of four categories; gymnurid (butterfly rays), urolophid (round stingrays), mylobatid (bat or eagle rays), and dasyatid (proper stingrays).[107] The groupings are based on their relative stinging ability, which depends on the size, number, and location of the caudal stinging appendages.[107,109] The most dangerous group, the dasyatid or true stingrays, have the largest spines located further out on their tails, making theirs the most potent striking weapons.[107,109] The spines have retroserrated teeth, which makes removal difficult (Fig. 238-23).

Most stingray injuries occur when bathers, waders, or fishermen accidentally step on rays as they lie partially covered with sand in shallow waters. Severe lacerations and puncture wounds are inflicted by the ray as it defensively whips its tail upward and forward

FIGURE 238-23

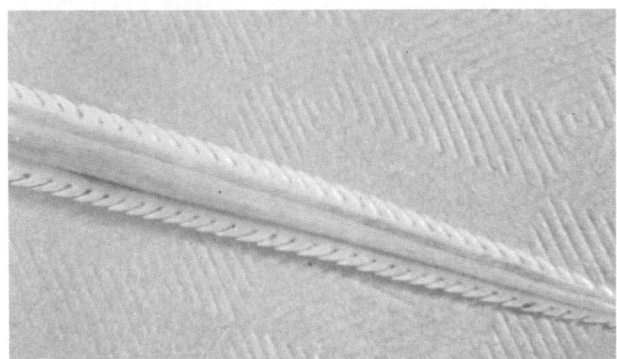

A close-up view of a stingray stinger devoid of its outer membrane and venom glands, demonstrating the retroserrated spine. (*Courtesy of David Fulghum, MD.*)

when stepped on or threatened[110] (Fig. 238-24). The majority of wounds, therefore, are located on the dorsum of the foot or lower leg.[111] Penetrating wounds to other locations have occurred to fishermen stung while attempting to remove rays from their lines or nets; in a freak accident in which a ray leapt from the water, striking a young boy in a small boat; and to divers engaged in feeding rays at popular dive locations.[110,111] When stingray spines penetrate the thorax or abdomen, the resulting wounds may prove fatal.[110,111]

FIGURE 238-24

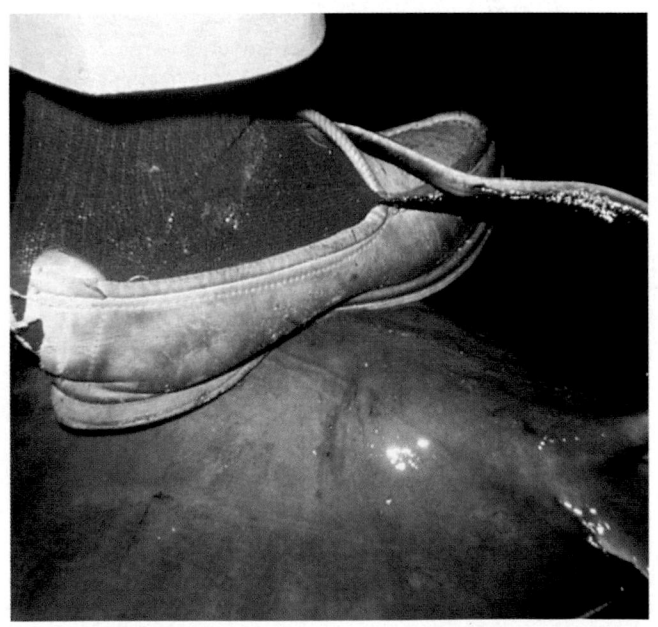

Stingrays reflexively swing their barbed tails up when stepped on, causing painful lacerations and puncture wounds. (The leg used for this photograph was a prosthesis; the stingray was alive.) (*Courtesy of David Fulghum, MD.*)

CATFISH Both fresh and salt water catfish are armed with stout sharp spines located immediately in front of the soft rays of their dorsal and pectoral fins.[107] Catfish defensively lock these spines into an extended position when they are handled or threatened. Bathers may sustain stings on their feet or legs if they step on a catfish, but the majority of catfish stings involve the hand or upper extremity of fishermen or seafood processors.[112,113] Fishermen are commonly stung if they do not take care while attempting to remove catfish from the hooks of their fishing lines.[114] Heavy gloves, pliers, and pincer-like jaws for holding the fish afford some protection.[115] The safest approach in the absence of these devices is to maintain a safe distance from the fish and to cut the line. Fishermen and sea food processors may be stung even by dead catfish while cleaning them.[116] One author has suggested that the offending spines be removed with a pair of pliers before attempting to clean the fish, to prevent these injuries.[115]

Although the majority of catfish stings are mild, they can occasionally result in severe necrosis and even gangrenous tissue loss, which in one case required digital amputation.[112] One of the most dangerous venomous fish in the world whose sting can be fatal is a species of catfish, *Plotosus lineatus*, which is found in waters of Japan, the Philippines, Southeast Asia, East Africa, and Australia.[112,117,118] Swimmers and bathers in the Amazon River are at risk for urologic injuries if they encounter a very small species of catfish called "candiru," which has the ability to enter the human urethra.[114] Barbs on the head of this fish prevent it from swimming backward out of the orifice, and surgical intervention is often required to extract the fish.[114]

SCORPIONFISH Scorpionfish, family Scorpaenidae, are divided into three main groups on the basis of their stinging apparatus. All have venomous spines of varying sizes and toxicity that may be found, depending on the species, on the dorsal, pelvic, and anal locations.

Lionfish, genus *Pterois*, are found in tropical waters and are prized by fish fanciers because of their colorful and ornate fins. The spines of lionfish are long and slender, with small venom glands.[81] Their stings are relatively mild and not life threatening.[92,119] Stings among amateur fish collectors are occurring more frequently because of the increasing popularity of these fish.[119]

Scorpionfish, genus *Scorpaena*, have stings that are of intermediate severity. They are bottom dwellers whose superior camouflage abilities allow them to blend in almost invisibly with their surroundings[102] (Fig. 238-25). Their spines are long and heavy and have moderate-sized venom glands.

Stonefish, genus *Synanceja*, are the most dangerous members of the scorpionfish family. They live in shallow waters, sometimes partially buried in sand or mud or in holes of rocky shoals, reef areas, or tidal pools.[92] Injuries occur when an unsuspecting wader steps on the erect venomous dorsal spine that the stonefish raises in defense. Stonefish spines are short and thick and have very large and well-developed venom glands.[81] The wounds caused by stonefish are quite severe and may be fatal.[107] Fortunately, a stonefish antivenin is available from the Commonwealth Serum Laboratories in Melbourne, Australia.[35,107]

LOCAL AND SYSTEMIC SYMPTOMS OF FISH-SPINE ENVENOMATIONS The toxicity of a given sting depends on a number of factors, including the species of fish involved, the lo-

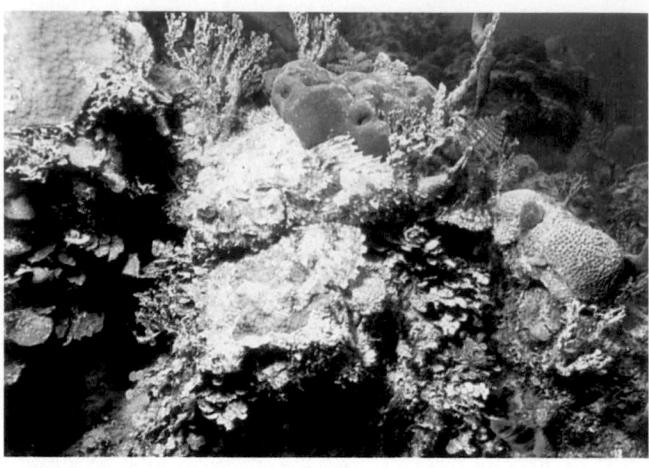

Scopaena plumieri, a species of scorpion fish, is found in the waters of the West Indies. Its camouflage abilities are exceeded only by its painful sting.

cation and severity of the wound, the amount of venom released, and the first aid and subsequent medical care provided to the victim. In general, these wounds produce pain out of proportion to the apparent severity of the injury. The pain is immediate and intense. In the case of scorpionfish stings, the pain may be so severe as to cause the victim to thrash about wildly, scream, and finally lose consciousness.[120]

Initially the sting site may appear pale or cyanotic. The area around the wound may be anesthetic or hyperesthetic.[81] Erythema and edema soon develop, giving the appearance of a cellulitis. Vesicles may form.[93] In severe stingings, especially those due to stonefish, the wounded area may become indurated and develop areas of ischemic necrosis with subsequent sloughing and ulcer formation.

Fish-spine wounds may be complicated by foreign-body reactions to bits of retained spines or remnants of integumentary sheath. Secondary infections from a variety of organisms must be anticipated. Healing is slow, especially in cases plagued by abscess or ulcer formation.

Systemic symptoms from toxic fish spines may range from mild to severe, depending on the species involved and the amount of venom entering the wound. They may include headache, nausea, vomiting, diarrhea, abdominal cramps and pain, fever, local lymphangitis and lymphadenitis, joint aches, muscle weakness, diaphoresis, peripheral neuropathy, limb paralysis, restlessness, delirium, seizures, cardiac arrhythmias, myocardial ischemia, pericarditis, hypotension, respiratory distress, and death.[81,112,119–121]

PREVENTION Prevention of toxic fish–spine wounds begins with a knowledge of and an appreciation for the various venomous species that may be encountered in a given area. Waders and bathers should shuffle their feet in order to scare away and avoid stepping on rays or scorpionfish. Fishermen must exercise care when removing rays or catfish from their fishing lines or when cleaning fish with venomous spines. Fish hobbyists and divers should wear protective clothing and avoid handling venomous species.

TREATMENT Puncture wounds and lacerations from venomous fish spines should be irrigated immediately with sterile saline or water, if available, and with seawater as a last resort.[66] The wounded area should then be soaked as quickly as possible in hot (not scalding) water of approximately 43 to 46°C (110 to 115°F) for 30 to 90 min or until maximal pain relief is achieved. Hot soaks may be repeated if the pain returns. Because the wound or extremity may be partially anesthetic, it is necessary for the person administering first aid to test the water's temperature for the victim.[110] One source of hot water that is often overlooked and may be useful in an emergency is hot seawater from a boat motor's cooling system.[110]

Local infiltration of the wound with 1 to 2 percent lidocaine without epinephrine may bring about significant pain relief and allow for exploration of the wound after x-ray examination has been performed to locate retained portions of spines.[92,110] Longer-acting anesthetics such as procaine and bupivacaine may be chosen to provide a longer period of pain relief.[112] The wound should be thoroughly cleaned to remove any remnants of integumentary sheath. Cleansing with a toothbrush and a solution of hexachlorophene in 70 percent alcohol has been recommended.[110] Abdominal and thoracic wounds and deep wounds to the hands, feet, or fascial compartments of the legs should be explored in the operating room.[92] Debridement of necrotic tissues may be required at the time of exploration, and sequential debridement may be necessary.[92] In general, these wounds should be left open or closed loosely with tape or suture to allow for adequate drainage and to prevent abscess formation.

Tetanus prophylaxis should be administered, if indicated, and antibiotics are recommended if the wound is over 6 h old, is extensive, or involves deep puncture wounds to the hand or foot.[92,110] The initial choice of antibiotic should be based on the bacteriology of the marine environment where the wound occurred and subsequently on deep wound or tissue cultures. A variety of organisms have been reported to cause secondary infections in catfish spine wounds including: *Erysipelothrix, Nocardia, Chromobacterium, Mycobacterium terrae, Sporothrix, Actinomyces, Edwardsiella tarda, Aeromonas hydrophila,* and *Vibrio* species.[122-124] Deep wound or tissue cultures should guide the choice of antibiotic therapy. Empiric therapy for catfish wounds may include cephalosporins or ciprofloxacin.[113]

Stonefish stings complicated by severe reactions may be treated with antivenin by slow intravenous infusion.[107] Antivenin is not usually required for the stings of lionfish and species of scorpionfish other than stonefish.[92] The amount of antivenin given depends on the number of puncture wounds sustained by the victim and the response to treatment.[107] The antivenin is prepared from horse serum and its administration may be complicated by anaphylaxis in sensitized individuals.[107]

Fish Bites

There are many species of fish whose bites are dangerous to humans. Among the best known of these are the sharks, barracudas, and piranha, whose attacks may be lethal. Bluefish, which run in large schools, present a menace to swimmers and surfers and to fishermen who are not wary of their vicious bites.[66] Divers and aquarium hobbyists must be careful when feeding or handling moray eels, which have powerful jaws and knifelike teeth. Although not considered venomous by most sources, they can produce deep puncture wounds and lacerations[66] (Fig. 238-26). Moray eels when biting may tend to lock onto their prey, and this may require decapitation or disarticulation of the eels' jaw in order to release the victim.[125,126] As with all deep puncture wounds or lacerations, moray eel bites should receive tetanus prophylaxis. Empiric antibiotic therapy for prophylaxis or treatment can include ciprofloxacin or cefuroximine for coverage of *Vibrio* or *Pseudomonas* species.[127]

FIGURE 238-26

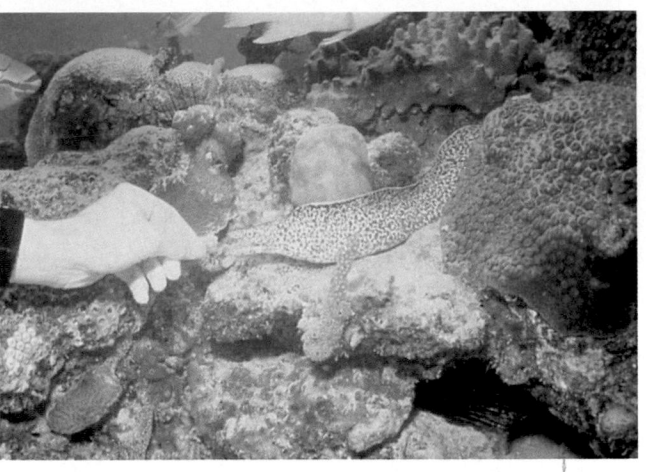

Moray eel bites are uncommon but have increased due to divers feeding these animals at popular dive sites. (*Courtesy of Marty Gilman, Worcester, MA.*)

WATERBORNE INFECTIONS (See also Section 29)

A variety of infections may result from exposures to aquatic environments. Pathogenic organisms may be actively introduced into wounds of the bites, stings, or lacerations caused by marine life;

FIGURE 238-27

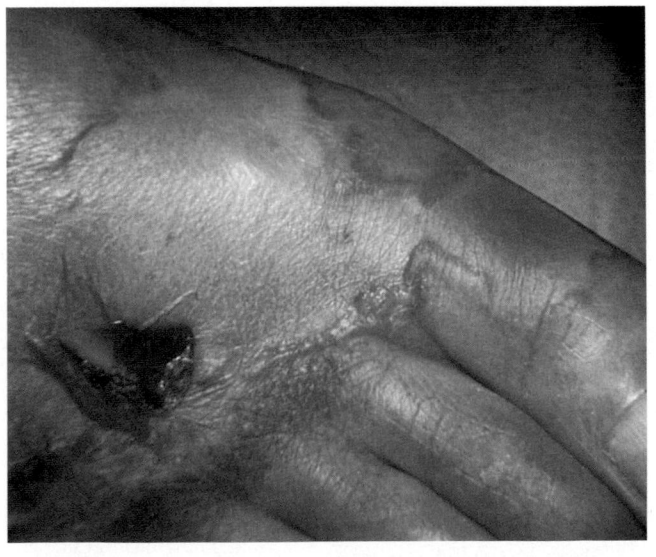

Bullous cellulitis due to *Aeromonas hydrophila;* the cellulitis progressed to ischemic necrosis, requiring amputation. Unfortunately the patient died from the infection. (*From Fulghum D et al: Fatal Aeromonas hydrophila infection of the skin. J South Med Assoc 71:739, 1978, with permission.*)

FIGURE 238-28

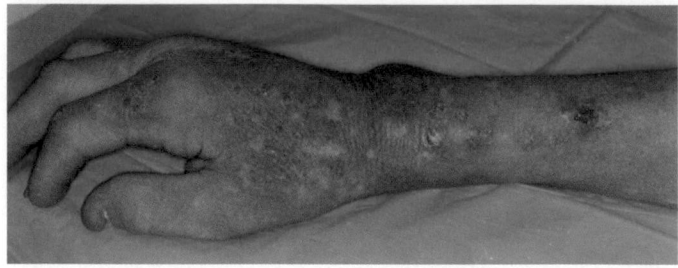

Fish fancier's finger with sporotrichoid spread to the wrist and arm due to a *Mycobacterium marinum* infection, which responded to minocycline. (*Courtesy of Lori Herman, MD.*)

FIGURE 238-29

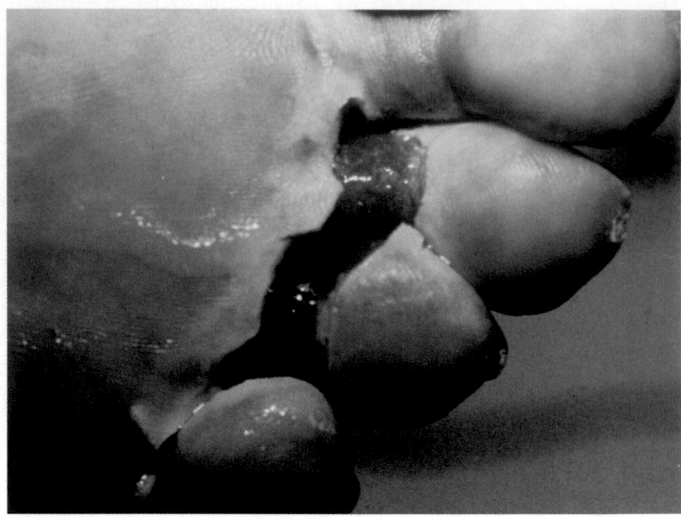

Gram-negative toeweb space infection due to *Pseudomonas*.

preexisting wounds may be passively infected while exposed to contaminated waters. Table 238-3 summarizes those organisms commonly associated with waterborne infections. A host of other agents, such as *Streptococcus* and *Staphylococcus* spp., *Bacteroides fragilis*, *Clostridium perfringens*, *Escherichia coli*, *Salmonella enteritidis*, other marine *Vibrio* species, *Chromobacterium violaceum*, and *Chlorella*, also deserve consideration when dealing with infections derived from aquatic settings.[92]

TABLE 238-3

Wound Infections Associated with Waterborne Organisms

ORGANISMS	CLINICAL FEATURES
Aeromonas hydrophila	Cellulitis (may be bullous) (Fig. 238-27); fasciitis, myonecrosis, bacteremia
Edwardsiella tarda	Cellulitis, absess, osteomyelitis, bacteremia
Erysipelothrix rhusiopathiae	Slowly progressive painful cellulitis without adenopathy or lymphangitis, almost always involving the hand; septic arthritis; subacute bacterial endocarditis
Mycobacterium balnei or *M. marinum*	Swimming pool granuloma; fish fancier's finger (Fig. 238-28); chronic cellulitis and culture-negative ulcers; often the primary lesion is on the hand and then a series of lesions develop in draining lymphatics
Pfisteria piscicida	Raw red pock-marked lesions occur in fish in polluted waterways; rashes, respiratory problems, and memory deficits are possible[128]
Prototechosis	Papular or eczematoid dermatitis in immunosuppressed patients; localized infection of the olecranon bursa
Pseudomonas species	Trench foot; gram-negative toe web space infections (Fig. 238-29); swimmer's ear; hot tub folliculitis
Streptococcus iniae	Cellulitis and bacteremia after skin injuries during the handling of fresh fish grown by aquaculture
Vibrio vulnificus Other *Vibrio* species	Cellulitis sometimes with bulla formation; may progress to septicemia, especially in alcoholics, diabetics, and immunosuppressed patients; metastatic cellulitis, meningitis, and death may result from fulminant infections

CUTANEOUS MANIFESTATIONS OF INGESTING SEAFOOD AND OF SEAFOOD POISONING

There are several dermatologic reactions that may be seen after ingesting seafood. Urticaria, angioedema, and, rarely, leukocytoclastic vasculitis may occur in individuals sensitized to fish or shellfish (Fig. 238-30). Many seafoods, such as kelp, contain large amounts of iodine, which may cause acneiform eruptions.[93]

Scombroid food poisoning involves the ingestion of spoiled fish from the Scombroidae family of fish, which includes tuna, mackerel, bonita, and their relatives.[93] If these fish are not kept cold enough after being caught, their flesh develops scombrotoxins due to the bacterial breakdown of histidine into histamine, saurine, and possibly other toxic byproducts. These can cause striking erythema and flushing of the face, neck, and upper trunk, as well as pruritus and urticarial and angioedematous eruptions. Administration of antihistamines can provide symptomatic relief in severe cases.

Ciguatera toxin, which is produced during blooms of toxic dinoflagellates, is incorporated into the marine food chain and concentrated in the flesh of a variety of fish. Dermatologic symptoms of ingesting these fish may include generalized pruritus and diffuse erythematous macular and papular exanthems that may progress to blister formation and desquamation.[93]

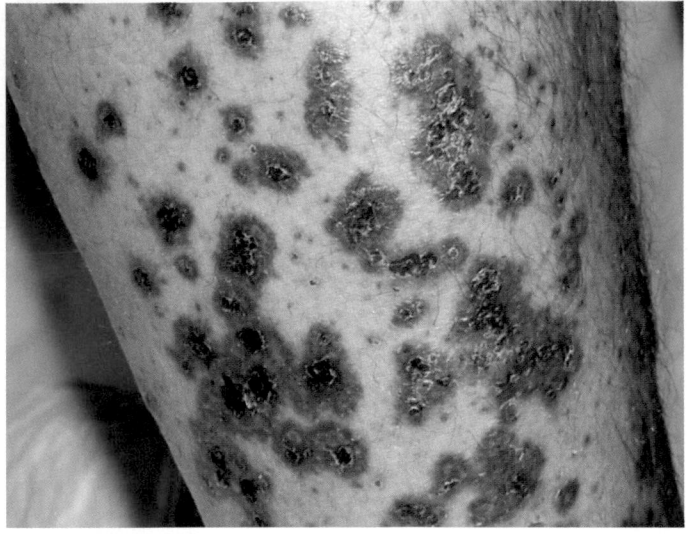

Leukocytoclastic vasculitis occurring in a patient, allergic to shellfish, who consumed a chowder containing quahogs, a type of clam.

REFERENCES

1. Goldstein EJ: Infection secondary to cat and dog bites. *Infect Med* **8**:30, 1991
2. Klein D: Friendly dog syndrome. *NY State Med* **66**:2306, 1966
3. Goldstein EJC: Bite wounds and infection. *Clin Infect Dis* **14**:633, 1992
4. Callaham M: Dog Bite Wounds. *JAMA* **244**:2327, 1980
5. Goldstein E et al: Outpatient therapy of bite wounds: Demographic data, bacteriology and a prospective randomized trial of amoxicillin-clavulinic acid versus penicillin +-dicloxacillin. *Int J Dermatol* **26**:123, 1987
6. Weber DJ et al: "Pasteurella multocida" infections: Report of 34 cases and a review of the literature. *Medicine (Baltimore)* **63**:133, 1984
7. Callahan M: Prophylactic antibiotics in common dog bite wounds: A controlled study. *Ann Emerg Med* **9**:410, 1980
8. Burdge DR et al: Serious *Pasteurella mulocida* infections from lion and tiger bites. *JAMA* **253**:3296, 1985
9. Hsu H, Finberg RW: Infections associated with animal exposure in two infants. *Rev Infect Dis* **11**:108, 1989
10. Talan DA et al: *Staphylococcus intermedius:* Clinical presentation of a new human dog bite pathogen. *Ann Emerg Med* **18**:410, 1989
11. Barnham M, Holmes B: Isolation of CDC group M-5 and *Staphylococcus intermedius* from infected dog bites. *J Infect* **25**:332, 1992
12. Peel MM: Dog-associated bacterial infections in humans: Isolates submitted to an Australian reference laboratory, 1981–1992. *Pathology* **25**:332, 1992
13. Brenner D et al: *Capnocytophagia canimorsus* sp. *nov.* (formerly CDC group DF-2), a cause of septicemia following dog bite and *C. cyodegmi* sp. *nov.,* a cause of localized wound infections following dog bite. *J Clin Microbiol* **27**:231, 1989
14. Blanche P et al: *Capnocytophaga canimorsus* lymphocytic meningitis in an immunocompetent man who was bitten by a dog. *Clin Infect Dis* **18**:654, 1994
15. Westwell AJ et al: DF-2 infection. *BMJ* **298**:116, 1989
16. Hudspeth MK et al: Growth characteristics and a novel method for identification (the WEE-TAB system) of *Porphyromonas* species isolated from dog and cat bite wounds in humans. *J Clin Microbiol* **35**:2450, 1997
17. Citron DM et al: Incidence and characterization of *Porphyromonas* species isolated from infected dog and cat bite wounds in humans by biochemical tests and PCR fingerprinting. *Clin Infect Dis* **23**(suppl 1):S78, 1996
18. Darrow M et al: Zoonotic transmission of turtle-borne *Edwardsiella tarda. Infect Med* **11**:33, 1993
19. Pavia AT et al: *Vibrio carchariae* infection after a shark bite. *Ann Intern Med* **111**:85, 1989
20. Fishbein DB, Robinson LE: Rabies. *N Engl J Med* **329**:1632, 1993
21. Grouleau G: Rabies. *Emerg Med Clin North Am* **10**:361, 1992
22. Elliott DE et al: Pet-associated illness. *N Engl J Med* **313**:985, 1985
23. Kositprapa CC et al: Immune response to simulated postexposure rabies booster vaccinations in volunteers who received preexposure vaccinations. *Clin Infect Dis* **25**:614, 1997
24. Anderson LJ: Human rabies in the United States. *Ann Intern Med* **100**:728, 1984
25. Bigger R et al: Lymphocyctic choriomeningitis outbreak associated with pet hamsters. *JAMA* **232**:494, 1975
26. Holmes GP et al: B virus (herpesvirus simiae) infection in humans: Epidemiologic investigation of a cluster. *Ann Intern Med* **112**:833, 1990
27. Holmes GP et al: Guidelines for the prevention and treatment of B-virus infections in exposed persons. *Clin Infect Dis* **20**:421, 1995
28. Kaplan JE: Herpesvirus simiae (B virus) infection in monkey handlers. *J Infect Dis* **157**:1090, 1988
29. Seiler JG III et al: Venomous snake bite: Current concepts of treatment. *Orthopedics* **17**:707, 1994
30. Gold BS, Barish RA: Venomous snakebites current concepts in diagnosis, treatment, and management. *Emerg Med Clin North Am* **10**:249, 1992
31. Gold BS, Wingert WA: Snake venom poisoning in the United States. *South Med J* **87**:579, 1994
32. Eadie P, Lee T: Seal finger in a wildlife ranger. *Ir Med J* **83**:117, 1990
33. Hilenbrand F: Whale finger and seal finger. *Lancet* **2**:680, 1953
34. Markham RB, Polk F: Seal finger. *J Infect Dis* **1**:567, 1979
35. Fisher AA: *Atlas of Aquatic Dermatology,* New York, Grune & Stratton, 1978
36. Halstead BW: Coelenterate (cnidarian) stings and wounds, aquatic dermatology. *Clin Dermatol* **5**:8, 1987
37. Reed KM et al: Delayed and persistent cutaneous reactions to coelenterates. *J Am Acad Dermatol* **10**:462, 1984
38. Mandojana RM: Granuloma annulare following blue bottle jellyfish (*Physalia utriculus*) sting. *J Wilderness Med* **1**:220, 1990
39. Auerbach Pss, Hays JT: Erythema nodosum following a jellyfish sting. *J Emerg Med* **5**:487, 1987
40. Burnett JW et al: Local and systemic reactions from jellyfish stings. *Clin Dermatol* **5**:14, 1987
41. Mathelier-Fusade P, Leynadier F: Acquired cold urticaria after jellyfish sting. *Contact Dermatitis* **29**:273, 1993
42. Ingram DM et al: Mondor's disease of the breast resulting from jellyfish sting. *Med J Aust* **157**:836, 1992
43. Burnett JW et al: Mononeuritis multiplex after coelenterate sting. *Med J Aust* **161**:320, 1994
44. Al-Ebrahim K et al: Jellyfish-venom induced deep venous thrombosis. *Angiology* **46**:449, 1995
45. Pang KA, Schwartz MS: Guillain-Barre syndrome following jellyfish stings. *J Neurol Neurosurg Psychiatry* **56**:1133, 1993
46. Auerbach PS: Envenomations from jellyfish and related species. *J Emerg Nurs* **23**(6):555, 1997
47. Ionnides G, Davisw JH: Portuguese man-of-war stinging. *Arch Dermatol* **91**:450, 1965
48. Drury JK et al: Jellyfish sting with serious hand complications. *Injury* **12**:66, 1980
49. Adiga KM: Braachial artery spasm as a result of a sting. *Med J Aust* **140**:181, 1984
50. Guess HA, Saviteer PL: Hemolysis and acute renal failure following a Portuguese man-of-war sting. *Pediatrics* **70**:979, 1982
51. Spielman FJ et al: Acute renal failure as a result of *Physalia physalis* sting. *South Med J* **75**:1425, 1982
52. Burnett JW, Gable WD: A fatal jellyfish envenomation by the Portuguese man-o'war. *Toxicon* **27**:823, 1989
53. Stein MR et al: Fatal Portuguese man-o'-war (*Physalia physaslis*) envenomation. *Ann Emerg Med* **18**:312, 1989
54. Sutherland S: Lethal jellyfish. *Med J Aust* **143**:536, 1985
55. Fenner PJ, Williamson JA: Worldwide deaths and severe envenomation from jellyfish stings. *Med J Aust* **165**:658, 1996
56. Williamson JA et al: Serious envenomation by the Northern Australian box-jellyfish (*Chironex fleckeri*). *Med J Aust* **1**:13, 1980

57. Currie BJ, Wood YK: Identification of *Chironex fleckeri* envenomation by nematocyst recovery from skin. *Med J Aust* **162**:478, 1995
58. Williamson JA et al: Acute management of serious envenomation by box jellyfish (*Chironex fleckeri*). *Med J Aust* **14**:851, 1984
59. Chand RP, Selliah K: Reversible parasympathetic dysautonomia following stinging attributed to the box jellyfish (*Chironex fleckeri*). *Aust NZ J Med* **14**:673, 1984
60. Currie B: Clinical implications of research on the box-jellyfish *Chironex fleckeri*. *Toxicon* **32**:1305, 1994
61. Burnett JW, Calton GJ: Response of the box-jellyfish (*Chironex fleckeri*) cardiotoxin to intravenous administration of verapamil. *Med J Aust* **153**:363, 1990
62. Burnett JW: The use of verapamil to treat box-jellyfish stings. *Med J Aust* **153**:363, 1990
63. Fenner PJ et al: Successful use of *Chironex* antivenom by members of the Queensland Ambulance Transport Brigade. *Med J Aust* **151**:708, 1989
64. Hartwick R et al: Disarming the box-jellyfish: Nematocyst inhibition in *Chironex fleckeri*. *Med J Aust* **1**:15, 1980
65. Burnett JW et al: First aid for jellyfish envenomation. *South Med J* **76**:870, 1983
66. Halstead BW, Auerbaach PS (eds): *Dangerous Aquatic Animals of the World: A Color Guide, with Prevention, First Aid, and Emergency Treatment Procedures,* Princeton, NJ, Darwin Press, 1990
67. Fenner PJ et al: First aid treatment of jellyfish stings in Australia: Response to a newly differentiated species. *Med J Aust* **158**:498, 1993
68. Exton DR et al: Cold packs: Effective topical analgesia in the treatment of painful stings by *Physalia* and other jellyfish. *Med J Aust* **151**:625, 1989
69. Massmanian A et al: Sea anemone dermatitis. *Contact Dermatitis* **18**:169, 1988
70. Garcia PJ et al: Fulminant hepatic failure from a sea anemone sting. *Ann Intern Med* **120**:665, 1994
71. Nicholis D: Sea anemone sting while SCUBA diving. *N Z Med J* **105**:245, 1992
72. Maretic Z, Russell FE: Stings by the sea anemone *Anemonia sulcata* in the Adriatic Sea. *Am J Trop Med Hyg* **32**:891, 1983
73. Fisher AAA: Water-related dermatoses, Part II: Nematocyst dermatitis. *Cutis* **25**:242, 1980
74. Weedon D et al: Coral dermatitis. *Aust J Dermatol* **22**:104, 1981
75. Sagi A et al: "The fire coral" (*Millepora dichotoma*) as a cause of burns: A case report. *Burns* **13**:325, 1987
76. Camarasa JG et al: Red Sea coral contact dermatitis. *Contact Dermatitis* **29**:285, 1993
77. McGoldrick J, Marx JA: Marine envenomations, Part 2: Invertebrates. *J Emerg Med* **10**:71, 1992
78. Cangialosi CP: Aquatic contact dermatitis: Report of two cases. *J Am Podiatry Assoc* **71**:21, 1983
79. Cooper MA: Treatment of coral cuts in Hawaii. *Hawaii Med J* **40**:73, 1981
80. Burnett JW et al: Dermatitis due to stinging sponges. *Cutis* **39**:476, 1987
81. Kizer KW: Marine envenomations. *J Toxicol Clin Toxicol* **21**:527, 1983
82. Yaffee HS, Stargardter F: Erythema multiforme from *Tedania ignis*. *Arch Dermatol* **87**:601, 1963
83. Rosson CL, Tolle SW: Management of marine stings and scrapes. *West J Med* **150**:97, 1989
84. Baden HP: Injuries from sea urchins. *Clin Dermatol* **5**:112, 1987
85. Strauss MB, MacDonald RI: Hand injuries from sea urchin spines. *Clin Orthop* **114**:216, 1976
86. Burke WA et al: Delayed hypersensitivity reaction following a sea urchin sting. *Int J Dermatol* **25**:649, 1986
87. Asada M et al: A case of delayed hypersensitivity reaction following a sea urchin sting. *Dermatologica* **180**:99, 1990
88. Baden HP, Burnett JW: Injuries from sea urchins. *South Med J* **70**:459, 1977
89. Haneke E et al: Sea urchin granuloma of the nail apparatus: Report of 2 cases. *Dermatology* **192**:140, 1996
90. Falkenberg P: Sea urchin spines as foreign bodies—an alternative treatment. *Injury* **15**:419, 1985
91. Warin AP: Sea-urchin granuloma. *Clin Exp Dermatol* **2**:405, 1977
92. Auerbach PS: Marine envenomations. *N Engl J Med* **325**:486, 1991
93. Mandojana RM, Sims JK: Miscellaneous dermatoses associated with the aquatic environment. *Clin Dermatol* **5**:134, 1987
94. Hoeffler DF: Cercarial dermatitis. *Arch Environ Health* **29**:225, 1974
95. Hoeffler DF: "Swimmer's itch" (cercarial dermatitis). *Cutis* **19**:461, 1977
96. Kirshenbaum MB: Swimmer's itch: A review and case report. *Cutis* **23**:212, 1979
97. Gonzalez E: Schistosomiasis, cercarial dermatitis and marine dermatitis. *Dermatol Clin* **7**:291, 1989
98. Osment LS: Update: Seabather's eruption and swimmer's itch. *Cutis* **18**:545, 1976
99. Tomchik RS et al: Clinical perspectives on seabather's eruption, also known as "sea lice." *JAMA* **269**:1669, 1993
100. Freudenthal AR, Joseph PR: Seabather's eruption. *N Engl J Med* **329**:542, 1993
101. Russell MR, Tomchik RS: Seabather's eruption, or "sea lice": New findings and clinical implications. *J Emerg Nurs* **12**:197, 1993
102. Kumar S et al: Risk factors for seabather's eruption: A prospective cohort study. *Public Health Rep* **112**:59, 1997
103. Scharf MJ: Aquatic dermatology, in *Cutaneous Medicine and Surgery, an Integrated Program in Dermatology,* edited by KA Arndt et al. Philadelphia, Saunders, 1996, p 793
104. Burnett JW et al: Cone snails. *Cutis* **39**:107, 1987
105. Fulghum DD: Octopus bite resulting in granuloma annulare. *South Med J* **79**:1434, 1986
106. Rosco D: Treatment of venomous and poisonous marine animal injuries. *Int Soc Aquatic Med Newslett* **2**(2), June 1976
107. Halstead BW, Vinci JM: Venomous fish stings (ichthyoacanthotoxicoses). *Clin Dermatol* **5**:29, 1987
108. Soppe GG: Marine envenomations and aquatic dermatology. *Am Fam Physician* **40**:97, 1989
109. Grainger CR: Multiple injuries due to stingrays. *J R Soc Health* **107**:100, 1987
110. Fenner PJ et al: Fatal and nonfatal stingray envenomation. *Med J Aust* **151**:621, 1989
111. Barss PL: Wound necrosis caused by the venom of stingrays: Pathological findings and surgical management. *Med J Aust* **141**:854, 1984
112. Mann III JW, Werntz JR: Catfish stings to the hand. *J Hand Surg* **16A**:318, 1991
113. Das SK et al: Catfish stings in Mississippi. *South Med J* **88**:809, 1995
114. Scoggin CH: Catfish stings. *JAMA* **231**:176, 1975
115. David NR: Still more on catfish stings. *JAMA* **233**:864, 1975
116. Calton GJ, Burnett JW: Catfish (*Ictalurus catus*) fin venom. *Toxicon* **13**:339, 1975
117. Pearn J: The sea, stingers, and surgeons: The surgeon's role in prevention, first aid, and management of marine envenomations. *J Pediatr Surg* **30**:105, 1995
118. Halstead BW: *Poisonous and Venomous Marine Animals of the World,* 2d ed. Princeton, NJ, Darwin, 1988
119. Trestrail JH, Al-Mahasneh QM: Lionfish sting experiences of an in poison center: A retrospective study of 23 cases. *Vet Hum Toxicol* **31**:173, 1989
120. Ell SR, Yate D: Marinefish stings. *Arch Emerg Med* **6**:59, 1989
121. Abdun-Nur D et al: Pericarditis associated with scorpionfish (*Scorpaena guttata*) sting. *Toxicon* **19**:579, 1981
122. Burnett JW et al: Catfish poisoning. *Cutis* **35**:208, 1985
123. Hall JT et al: Chronic tenosynovial hand infection from *Mycobacteerium terrae*. *Arthritis Rheum* **22**:1386, 1979
124. Banks AS: A puncture wound complicated by infection with *Edwardsiella tarda*. *J Am Podiatr Med Assoc* **82**:529, 1992
125. Auerbach PS, Halstead BW: Hazardous aquatic life, in *Management of Wilderness and Environmental Emergencies,* 2nd ed, edited by Auerbach PS, Beehr EC. St Louis, Mosby, 1989, p 933.
126. Auerbach PS: Hazardous marine animals. *Emerg Med Clin North Am* **2**:531, 1984
127. Erickson T et al: The emergency management of moray eel bites. *Ann Emerg Med* **21**:212, 1992
128. Mlot C: *Pfisteria piscicida* puts focus on harmful aquatic microbes. *ASM News* **63**:590, 1997

CHAPTER 239

Milton Orkin
Howard I. Maibach

Scabies and Pediculosis

HUMAN SCABIES

Etiology and Epidemiology

The itch mite, *Sarcoptes scabiei var humanus*, discovered in 1687, makes scabies one of the first diseases with a known cause.[1] Scabies occurs in both sexes and in any age group. It is transmitted by close (not casual) skin-to-skin contact. Sexual transmission is common, as is nonsexual spread in family groups. The more parasites on an individual, the greater the likelihood of transmission. When several members of the family group complain of an itching eruption, scabies is a likely diagnosis.

Clinical Features

CLASSIC SCABIES   Itching is characteristically nocturnal. Lesions are bilateral and often begin on the hands, particularly on the finger webs, and on the sides of the fingers. The flexor surfaces of the wrist, the elbows, and the anterior axillary folds are commonly involved. At most sites, small erythematous, often excoriated papules are present. The pathognomonic burrow (Fig. 239-1) is a short, wavy, dirty-appearing line. The areolas of the female breasts may show eczematous changes; papular lesions are usually present around the umbilicus. Penile involvement is common; especially papules (Fig 239-2), nodules, chancriform ulcers, or pyoderma. The disease may affect the lower buttocks. Secondary eczematization and infection may overshadow other features.

SPECIAL FORMS   Scabies occurs in special forms that may present diagnostic difficulties (Table 239-1) Some special forms are as follows:[2]

Scabies in patients with good hygiene   The disease is easily misdiagnosed because lesions are sparse and burrows are difficult to find.

FIGURE 239-1

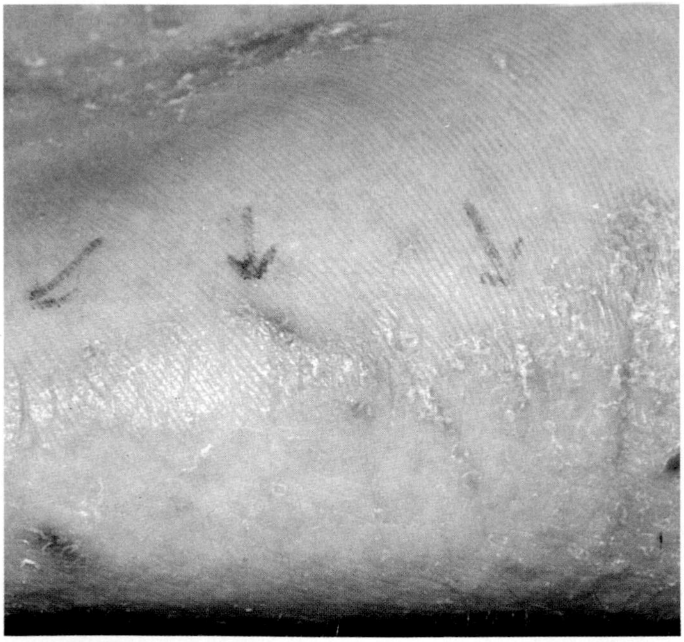

FIGURE 239-2

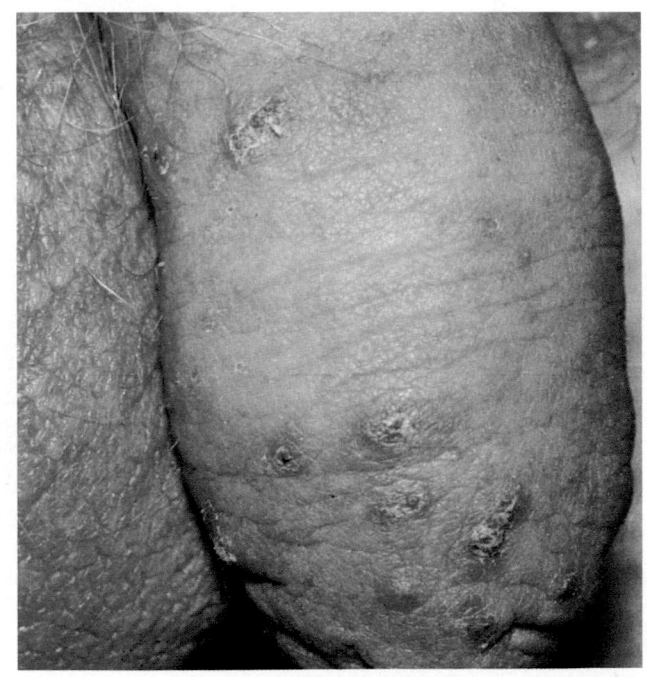

Scabies. Several, slightly scaling, threadlike burrows are seen on the medial aspect of the palm, associated with a more generalized eczematous process; scrapings of a tunnel have the highest yield in detection of a scabietic mite. (*Courtesy of M. Hebert, MD.*)

Scabies. The penis and scrotum are common sites for scabietic infestations; crusted excoriated papules are seen on the prepuce and shaft. (*Courtesy of M. Hebert, MD.*)

TABLE 239-1

Scabies: Special Forms

Scabies in clean persons	Scabies in the atopic
Scabies incognito	Animal transmitted scabies (a
Nodular scabies	zoonosis)
Scabies in infants and small	Scabies of the scalp
children	Dyshidrosiform scabiid
Scabies in the elderly	Urticarial and vasculitic scabies
Crusted (Norwegian) scabies	Bullous scabies
Scabies in HIV/AIDS	

Scabies incognito Glucocorticoid administration (topical or systemic) may mask symptoms and signs of scabies, although the infestation remains freely transmissible. This often results in unusual clinical presentations such as atypical and wide distribution.

Nodular scabies This is characterized by reddish-brown, pruritic nodules (Fig. 239-3) on covered parts (most frequently the male genitalia, groin, and axillary regions) and probably represents a hypersensitivity reaction to retained mite parts or antigens.

Scabies in infants and young children Misdiagnosis is frequent because of a low index of suspicion, secondary eczematous changes, and inappropriate therapy. Scabies in infants and young children presents as a pruritic, often generalized eruption, with frequent involvement of the face, scalp, palms, and soles; the most common presenting lesions are papules, vesiculopustules, and nodules.[3] Secondary eczematization and impetiginization are common, but bur-

FIGURE 239-3

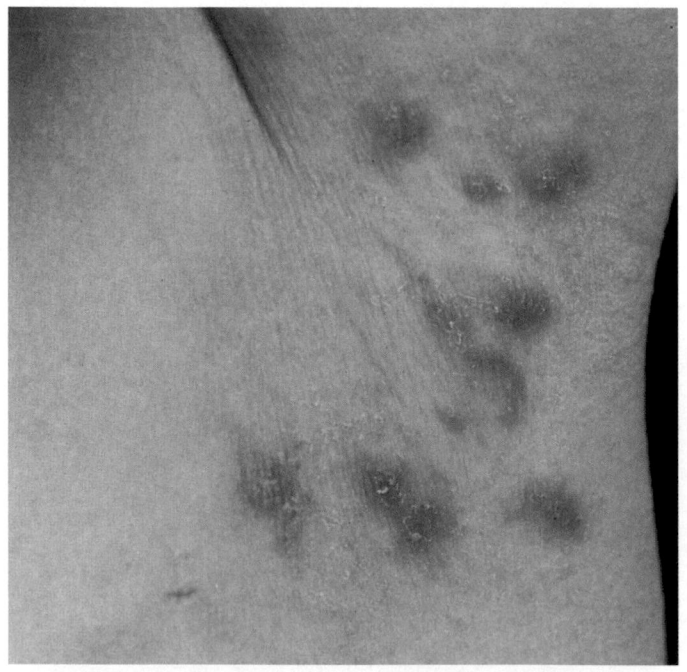

Scabies. Scabietic nodules occur in a minority of persons, especially in the axillae and genitalia; they are pathognomonic and may persist for months after successful eradication of the mite. (*Courtesy of M. Hebert, MD.*)

rows are difficult to find. Involvement of the youngest child in a household is common because these children are frequently carried and hugged by infested adults. The prevalence of scabies is highest in infants less than 2 years of age. The differential diagnosis includes atopic dermatitis, papular urticaria, and pyoderma.

Scabies in the elderly In the elderly, the reaction to the mite is muted, as in allergic and irritant dermatitis, but the patient itches severely. The vivid inflammatory reaction seen in young people is usually absent. Scabies is frequently not recognized; instead, the itching is attributed to "senile pruritus," dry skin, or anxiety. For elderly patients in nursing homes and other extended-care facilities—particularly those who are bedridden for long periods—there may be involvement on the back, which is unique for younger adults.

Crusted (Norwegian) scabies This uncommon condition is highly contagious because of the myriad of mites in the exfoliating scales. Local or regional epidemics of more typical forms of scabies frequently spread from an individual case, usually in hospitals or other institutions. Crusted scabies is a psoriasiform dermatosis on the hands and feet with dystrophy of the nails and an erythematous scaling eruption that may be generalized. Itching in most cases is minimal. Crusted scabies occurs in mentally retarded or physically debilitated persons or those who are immunologically deficient. Crusted scabies may be a marker of human T cell lymphotrophic virus type I (HTLV-I). Some of these patients have adult T cell leukemia/lymphoma (ATL).[4]

Scabies and HIV/AIDS It is not surprising that the expanding epidemic of AIDS has intersected with the scabies pandemic. Scabies occurs in at least 2 to 4 percent of patients with HIV/AIDS. Unusual forms of scabies in HIV/AIDS can be divided into crusted scabies (Fig 239-4) and atypical papular scabies.[5] Most patients early on were considered to have a drug reaction. The drugs were discontinued, but the condition progressed. It was common for individuals to present with ordinary scabies; as their CD4 counts dropped and they were placed on potent systemic medication, this converted into crusted scabies. With this conversion, the pruritus of ordinary scabies decreased or disappeared. Because of the atypical nature of this condition, it was common for the correct diagnosis to be delayed, thereby increasing the potential for spread of scabies to others.

FIGURE 239-4

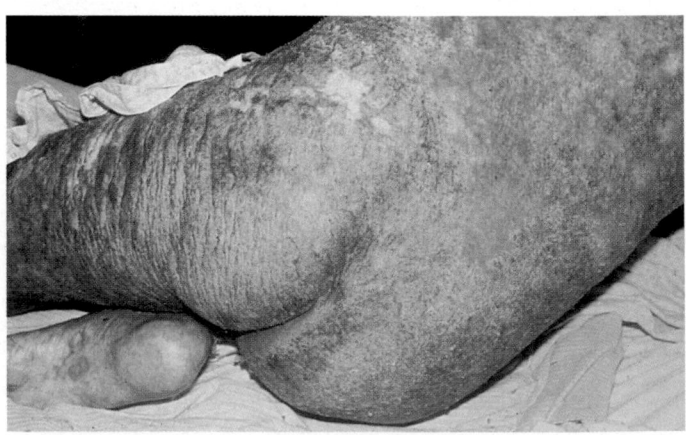

Scabies. Crusted or Norwegian scabies in an HIV-infected person. The clinical presentation of generalized hyperkeratosis and scaling is often misdiagnosed; rather than an infestation with a dozen mites, many thousands are present. (*Courtesy of M. Hebert, MD.*)

Scabies should be suspected in any pruritic (or asymptomatic) rash in patients with HIV/AIDS. It may be the first opportunistic infection in HIV/AIDS, may be combined with other opportunistic infections, or may occur after other opportunistic infections. Ordinary scabies was usually transmitted in hospital settings. Prominent fissures may be the source of bacteremia, resulting in death in several patients. Most of the index patients for hospital epidemics of scabies and all of the patients who developed bacteremia had crusted scabies.

Scabies of the scalp Scabies in infants and children, the elderly, nursing home patients, those residing in tropical areas, immunosuppressed patients having crusted scabies, and scabies in HIV/AIDS patients may include scalp involvement. Aside from these circumstances, scabies rarely involves the adult scalp; when it does, it may simulate or be superimposed on seborrheic dermatitis.[6]

Bullous scabies Vesicles are common in children with scabies but uncommon in adults. Bullous scabies in adults may mimic bullous pemphigoid clinically, pathologically, and immunopathologically.[6] Most patients are over 65 years of age. The duration of the scabies from onset until diagnosis is weeks to months, thereby exposing a number of individuals to the disease. There is no linkage to an underlying disease or immunosuppression except in relation to age. Most patients are treated with oral corticoids for the mistaken diagnosis of bullous pemphigoid. Burrows are present in most cases.

Differential Diagnoses

Scabies can be confused with almost any pruritic dermatosis but most commonly with atopic dermatitis, papular urticaria, pyoderma, insect bites, and dermatitis herpetiformis.

Diagnosis

Definitive diagnosis is made by microscopic identification of the mites, eggs, or fecal pellet. The diagnosis should be verified because scabies may be under- or overdiagnosed. Techniques for diagnoses include the following:

Skin scrapings Burrows or unexcoriated papules are located with the help of the hand lens or loupe. Mineral oil is dropped onto a sterile scalpel blade and allowed to flow onto the lesion, which is vigorously scraped with a blade about six to seven times to remove the tops of the burrows or papules. The oil and scraping material are then transferred to a glass slide, covered with a coverslip, and examined microscopically under low power.

Curettage The long axis of burrows or the center of unexcoriated papules is curetted; the material is deposited on a clean slide; and several drops of mineral oil are placed on the material. It is then covered with a coverslip and examined under low power. This technique is particularly helpful in infants, small children, or anxious or uncooperative patients of any age as well as patients suspected of having HIV/AIDS.

Complications

Secondary bacterial infection may occur. Nephritogenic streptococcal strains may colonize scabietic lesions, leading to acute glomerulonephritis, mainly in tropical areas. The potential for this reaction is universal. Eczema, particularly in atopics, may be prominent in the active scabies infestation and may continue as eczema after the scabies has cleared. The term *acarophobia* (or the more inclusive *delusions of parasitosis*) may characterize individuals who have been successfully treated for scabies or have never had scabies. Successful treatment is difficult (see also Chap. 41).

Treatment

PRINCIPLES The choice of drugs should be based on efficacy and potential toxicity. Patients often apply medications more frequently and longer than prescribed. Limiting the quantity prescribed prevents dermatitis caused by overtreatment, which the patient may mistake for the persistence of scabies. Treatment is traditionally preceded by a tepid bath or shower followed by drying with a towel. Scabicides should be applied thinly but thoroughly to the area behind the ears and from the neck down to all areas, with special attention to the areas between the fingers, the umbilical area, the groin, between the buttocks, between the toes, and particularly under the fingernails and toenails, which should be trimmed short. Medication should be left on for the number of hours suggested, then thoroughly rinsed off with tepid water. At the conclusion of therapy, undergarments, bed linens, and towels should be machine-washed and dried, using the hot cycles.

Selected treatment of asymptomatic family members at high risk for acquiring the infestation from a confirmed case is appropriate—e.g., if the patient shares a bed with another person, has sexual contacts, etc.

SPECIFIC TOPICAL SCABICIDES (Table 239-2)

1. Permethrin 5% cream (Elimite), a synthetic pyrethroid, is an excellent scabicide (equal to lindane), but because of low mammalian toxicity and low potential for toxicity from misuse, it is the first choice.[7] It is minimally absorbed and rapidly metabolized. A single application is removed after 10 h; some prefer to use a second application in 1 week. No resistance (better called "tolerance") has been noted with this product.

   Permethrin should not be used in infants younger than 2 months of age or in pregnant or nursing women. The most common adverse reactions are mild and transient, consisting primarily of burning and stinging (sensory irritation) and exacerbation or recurrence of pruritus. Formaldehyde (0.1%), the preservative in the U.S. formulation, occasionally produces allergic contact dermatitis.

2. Lindane 1% (generic) is easy to use and effective (equal to permethrin). An application is left on for 8 h and then washed off thoroughly; some prefer to use a second application in 1 week. Ten percent of the lindane applied to the skin is absorbed. Central nervous system toxicity has occurred primarily with misuse relating to abuse, overuse, or failure of the patient or parents to comprehend warning instructions.[8] Lindane should not be used in infants, young children, pregnant or nursing women, or in patients with seizure disorders or other neurologic diseases. The scabies mite may develop a tolerance to lindane, but this has not been fully documented.

3. Sulfur, usually prescribed as precipitated sulfur (6%) in petrolatum, is applied nightly for three nights and washed off thoroughly 24 h after the last application. The product has an odor, is messy, and stains, but it is safe and effective in the treatment of scabies.[9] It is appropriate for infants younger than 2 months of age and for pregnant or lactating women.

4. Crotamiton cream (Eurax) is not a highly effective scabicide. Five daily applications may be better than the two currently recommended, but data are inconclusive.

TABLE 239-2

Treatment of Scabies

TREATMENT	USE	DOSING	TOXICITY	TOLERANCE (RESISTANCE)	ACCEPTANCE	COST
Permethrin cream 5%	Do not use in infants younger than 2 months of age, pregnant and lactating women, persons with hypersensitivity.	10 h ×1*	Low	None	Esthetic	Higher
Lindane lotion 1%	Do not use in infants or small children, pregnant or lactating women, persons with significant neurologic disease or those with hypersensitivity.	8 h ×1*	Possible CNS	Alleged	Esthetic	Lower
Precipitated sulfur ointment 6%	Use in infants younger than 2 months of age, pregnant and lactating women.	24-h periods at night ×3	Low	None	Messy	Pharmacist compounded

*There are no controlled studies documenting that two applications are better than one. Repeat in 1 week if there is microscopic and/or morphologic evidence of treatment failure.

IVERMECTIN Ivermectin, an antiparasitic agent used extensively in veterinary practice, is the drug of choice for human onchocerciasis. Macotela-Ruiz and Pena-Gonzalez,[10] in a double-blind study, noted that 23 of 29 patients with scabies were cured 1 week after a single oral dose of ivermectin, 200 μg/kg of body weight, as compared with 4 of 26 in the placebo group. Meinking et al.[11] reported an open-label study with a single oral dose of 200 μg/kg, given to 11 otherwise healthy patients with scabies and to 11 patients with scabies who were also infected with HIV, 7 of whom had AIDS. None of the 11 otherwise healthy patients had evidence of scabies 4 weeks after a single dose. Of the 11 with HIV infection, 10 had no evidence of scabies 4 weeks after the first treatment; 2 of the 10 required a second dose 2 weeks after the first. Meinking et al. concluded that ivermectin given in a single oral dose is an effective treatment for scabies in otherwise healthy patients and in many patients with HIV infections. Additional controlled studies of ivermectin therapy in patients with scabies are indicated. (Ivermectin is not FDA approved.

Antipruritic Medications

Antipruritic medications such as an antihistamine may blunt the itching that characteristically lingers for several weeks after adequate antiscabietic therapy. In young children, application of topical 1% hydrocortisone cream to the most intense rash and a lubricating agent or emollient to the lesser rash may be helpful; in adults triamcinolone cream (0.1%) may be used for relief. In extensive secondary bacterial infections, an oral antibiotic, particularly erythromycin, is indicated.

Treatment of Special Forms of Scabies

CRUSTED SCABIES Therapy for crusted scabies is similar to that for the more common types, although crusted scabies responds more slowly and commonly requires multiple treatments with scabicides, sometimes with the sequential use of several agents. The entire skin should be treated including the scalp, face (exclusive of the areas around the eyes, nose, and mouth), and particularly under the fingernails and toenails, followed by brushing the medication under the free edges of the nails. Treatment is started with permethrin cream followed by lindane and sulfur if necessary. Pretreatment with keratolytic agents may be helpful.

Isolating the index case and treating the environment of patients who have crusted scabies is more important than in ordinary scabies, since the patient with crusted scabies may be laden with mites. Compliance is of concern; the scabicides should be applied under supervision. When sufficient contact justifies it, proplylactic therapy of exposed individuals is indicated.

SCABIES IN HIV/AIDS Management is comparable to that for crusted scabies. The more profound the immunosuppression, the more atypical may be the morphology and the less predictable the response to therapy. Repeated applications of scabicides, sometimes with sequential use of several agents, may be required. Supervision of therapy, isolation of infested patients, and prophylactic treatment of contacts are all important.

Funkhauser et al[12] recommended permethrin as a first-line agent and repeated applications of the permethrin, with treatment to include the head and neck and under the fingernails. A small number of patients with scabies in AIDS developed an intense burning sensation within minutes after application of permethrin.[13] Lindane should not be used daily because of concern about cumulative toxicities, especially neurotoxicity.[14] Some authors have suggested the use of empiric antibiotic treatment in patients with marked fissuring, not restricted to antistaphylococcal coverage but based on the bacterial flora profile of the individual hospital or health care facility.[15]

PEDICULOSIS

Etiology

Lice are wingless, dorsoventrally flattened, blood-sucking insects. Pediculosis is an infestation by *Pediculus capitis* (head louse), *Pediculus humanus* (body or clothing louse), or *Phthirius pubis* (pubic or crab louse). Head and body lice are similar in appearance, but the crab louse is much shorter, being almost as wide as it is long. Lice have three pairs of legs. In the crab louse, the first set of legs terminates in a slender claw, while the second and third pairs have well-developed claws perfectly adapted for grasping the coarse, widely spaced hairs of the pubis, axilla, beard, and eyelashes. Unlike head and body lice, which travel up to 23 cm/min, crab lice are sluggish and travel a maximum of 10 cm/day. The louse egg incubates for 9 to 12 days. Head and body lice develop in adults in 19 to 25 days from the time the egg is laid; crab lice in 22 to 27 days.[16] The nits (egg casings) of head and crab lice are firmly cemented to the hairs of the host. Unlike dandruff, they are difficult to pull from the hair with the fingers.

Clinical Manifestations

The bites of lice are painless and can rarely be detected. Clinical signs and symptoms of infestation arise from the host's reaction to the saliva and/or anticoagulant injected into the dermis by the louse at the time of feeding. Depending on the degree of sensitivity and previous exposure, feeding sites may produce small 2- to 3-mm red macules or papules hours to days after feeding or an acute hivelike immediate reaction with typical flare-wheal formation. Pruritus is the most common symptom in any type of pediculosis. The major louse-borne diseases of the past (epidemic typhus, relapsing fever, and trench fever) have been brought under control by improved hygiene, the ability to wash and change clothes, the development of more effective pediculicides, and the availability of antibiotics for treatment of the rickettsial and borrelial diseases.

HEAD LICE

Etiology

Head lice infestations are a growing problem in the United States and other countries. Official incidence reports are underestimated. No area in the United States is free of head lice, which infest all levels of society and ethnic groups except for the American black population, where the incidence is low. The condition is more common in children. Hair length is not an important factor.

Persons with head lice are seen more commonly by school nurses, public health personnel, and family physicians and less commonly by dermatologists.[17] Patients are frequently treated with over-the-counter medications. Transmission of head lice is most efficient by head-to-head contact. In the tropics and in most of the United States in the summer months, shared towels, brushes, and combs play a significant role.

Clinical Manifestations

Pediculosis capitis is typically confined to the scalp (Fig. 239-5). The hallmark of infestation is intense itching. Detection in schools is usually triggered by the sight of children scratching their heads. Erythema and scaling may be present, as well as pruritic papules on the posterior neck. There may be linear excoriations at the periphery of the hair area. Excoriations frequently lead to pyoderma, with the hairs matted by the exudate. Cervical lymphadenopathy and febrile episodes are not uncommon.

Diagnosis

Diagnosis is confirmed by plucking the hairs, which are placed on a slide and studied microscopically to differentiate the nits from seborrheic scales, hair casts, and artifacts on the hair (e.g., hair

FIGURE 239-5

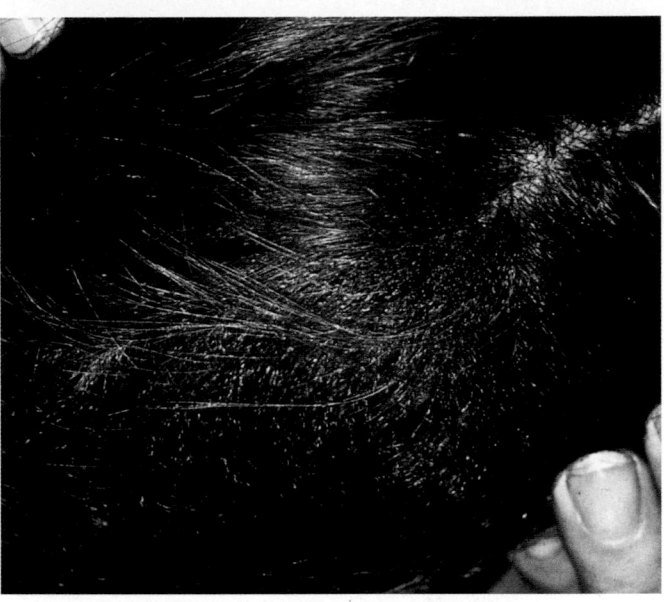

Pediculosis capitis. Myriads of oval, grayish-white egg capsules (nits) are firmly attached to the hair shafts. (*Courtesy of DA Burns, MD.*)

spray) that may be brushed off easily. Active infestation is based on finding live adult lice, immature nymphs, and/or viable-appearing eggs. Empty shells (nits) are not diagnostic of active infestation.

PUBIC (CRAB) LICE

Etiology and Epidemiology

Pediculosis pubis is typically transmitted sexually, frequently coexisting with other sexually transmitted diseases. There is no racial difference in its distribution. This infestation is common and tends to recur in gay men.[18] Patients with pubic lice are seen more commonly by personnel in venereal disease clinics, student health services, and family physicians than by dermatologists; most are self-diagnosed.

Clinical Manifestations

The most commonly affected site is the pubis (Fig. 239-6). Although the organisms do not move far from the initial site of contact, in hairy individuals the short hairs of the thighs, trunk, perianal area, and occasionally the beard and moustache may become involved. Meinking and Taplin,[18] working with a homeless population, observed that 60 percent of their subjects had lice in other areas of the body in addition to or exclusive of the pubis. Infestation of the eyelashes (Fig. 239-7) and periphery of the scalp occur mainly in children. A complete body examination is important on all patients. Excoriations may lead to pyoderma (which may mask the parasites), with lymphadenitis and febrile episodes. Characteristic though not frequently present are *maculae caeruleae* (sky-blue

FIGURE 239-6

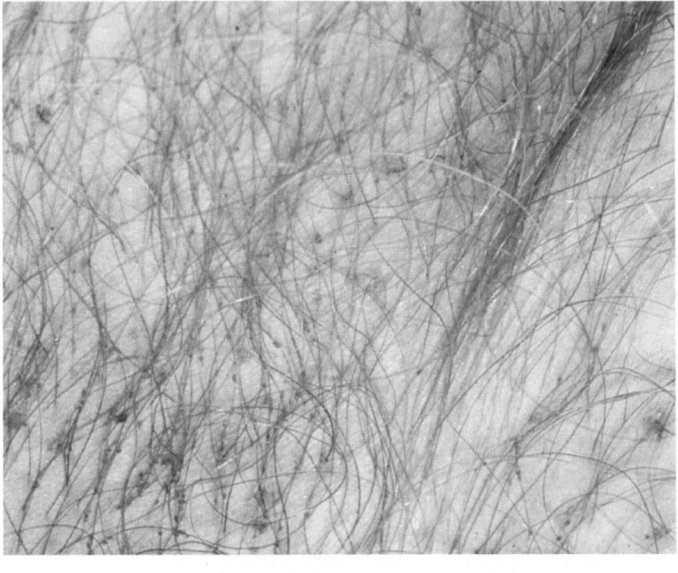

Pediculosis pubis. Dotlike nits attached to the hair shafts as well as several crab lice can easily be seen in the pubic area of this patient. (*Courtesy of DA Burns, MD.*)

FIGURE 239-7

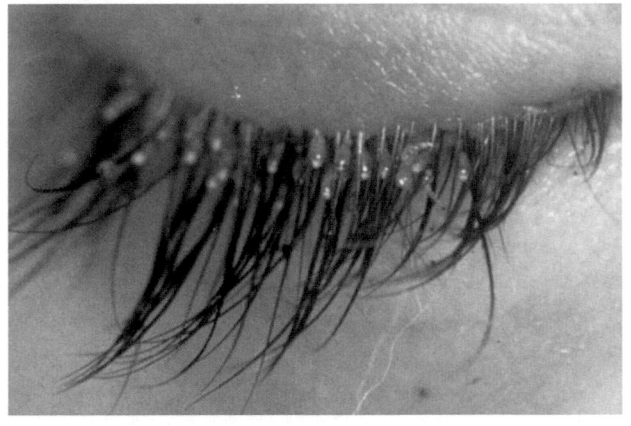

Pediculosis pubis. Eyelash infestation with *Pthirus pubis*. Nits can be seen attached to the eyelashes. (*Courtesy of DA Burns, MD.*)

spots)—unique, asymptomatic bluish or slate-colored macules (Fig. 239-8), located on the trunk and thighs.

Diagnosis

Adult organisms (Fig. 239-9) average 10 to 25 or more on the body; the diagnosis is more frequently made by identifying the more numerous nits cemented to the pubic or perianal hair, initially at the junction with the skin. Since the ova grow out with the hair, as in pediculosis capitis, the duration of infestation can be approximated by the distance of the ova from the skin surface. The diagnosis is confirmed by plucking the hair, placing it on a slide, and viewing

FIGURE 239-8

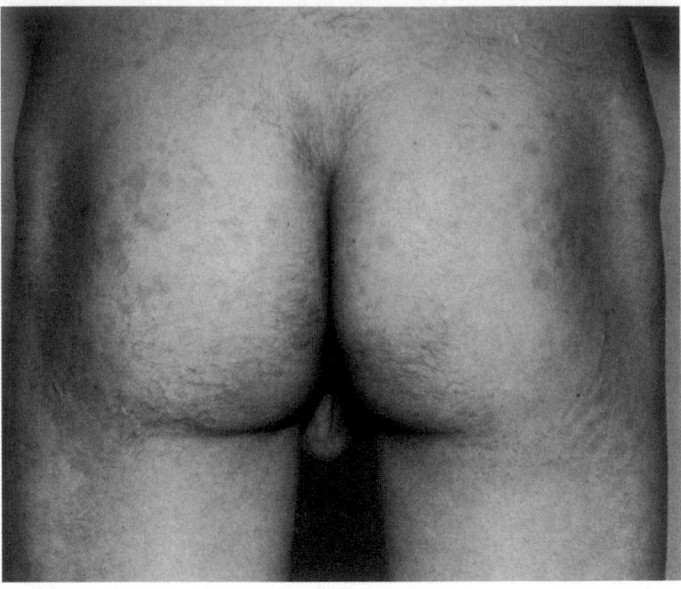

Pediculosis pubis. Maculae caeruleae, slate-gray or blue-gray macules, are seen on the buttocks. (*Courtesy of DA Burns, MD.*)

FIGURE 239-9

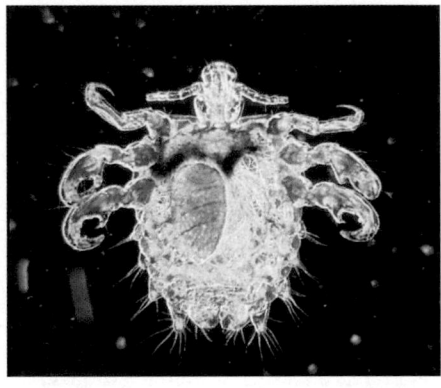

Pediculosis pubis. Microscopic view of an adult female louse containing an egg. (*Courtesy of DA Burns, MD.*)

the eggs under a microscope (Fig. 239-10). Empty eggs are not diagnostic of active infestation.

BODY LICE

Etiology

Infestations of body lice are found mainly in indigent transients, those with low income and poor hygiene, and homeless persons and refugees living in crowded conditions. They are treated mainly in public hospitals. The infestation is transmitted chiefly by contaminated clothing or bedding.

FIGURE 239-10

CHAPTER 239
Scabies and Pediculosis

2683

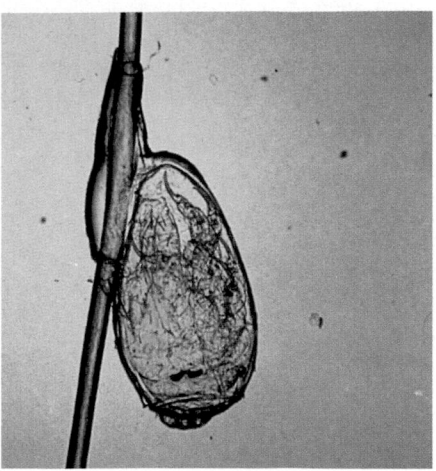

Pediculosis pubis. Microscopic view of an egg, containing an unhatched louse, attached to a hair shaft. (*Courtesy of DA Burns, MD.*)

Clinical Manifestations

Early lesions consist of macules or papules at the site where the louse punctures the skin to obtain blood. The characteristic eruption, however, consists of numerous vertical excoriations, especially on the trunk and neck, caused by intense itching. Crusts and at times pus or serum may stain the underclothing. Transitory wheals and bacterial infections may complicate the process. Postinflammatory pigmentation is common. Few or no adult organisms are seen except in heavily infested persons; numerous nits are found in clothing seams, particularly in contact with the crotch, armpits, belt line, and collar.

TREATMENT AND CONTROL

Pediculosis Capitis

SPECIFIC AGENTS

1. The synthetic pyrethroid permethrin (obtainable over the counter as NIX) is supplied as a 1% cream rinse. Hair is first washed with a regular shampoo, rinsed with water, and towel-dried. Sufficient permethrin cream rinse is supplied to coat the hair and scalp thoroughly. Left on for 10 min and rinsed off with water, a single application is sufficient in over 90 percent of cases. Some dermatologists advise a second treatment 7 to 10 days later. If adult lice are observed 7 to 10 days or more after the first application, a second treatment must be given. The hair is easier to comb and nit removal is facilitated after treatment. Permethrin has low mammalian toxicity and ovicidal (not complete) properties; it has been shown to be as effective or more effective than lindane shampoos in controlled studies. Unlike lindane, permethrin is poorly absorbed and rapidly metabolized and excreted.
2. Synergized pyrethrins (RID and other preparations available over the counter) should be applied undiluted until the scalp is entirely saturated and should be allowed to remain for 10 min; the hair should then be washed thoroughly with warm water and soap or shampoo and dried. Nits should be removed with the fine-toothed comb that accompanies the product. A second application is used in 7 to 10 days to kill any nymphs newly hatched from eggs that survived the first treatment. Synergized pyrethrins have low mammalian toxicity. Individuals allergic to chrysanthemums or ragweed may rarely be allergic to pyrethrins.

    Some natural pyrethrin products contain refined kerosene or petroleum distillates that may cause eye irritation, so care must be exercised in the use of all pediculicide products to avoid contact with the eyes. If accidental contact does occur, the eyes should be washed quickly and thoroughly with tap water.
3. Lindane shampoo (obtainable by prescription) leaves the hair tangled and difficult to comb. Because of potential toxicity, only a single dose should be prescribed. The patient should lather the scalp thoroughly for 4 min with 30 to 40 mL of lindane shampoo (depending on the thickness of the hair). The hair should then be rinsed thoroughly with water and dried. Unnecessary contact of the lindane shampoo with other body surfaces should be avoided. The remaining nits should be removed with a fine-toothed comb. If live lice are observed 7 days or more after the first application, a second treatment is given. Concern has been expressed over the potential for central nervous system (CNS) toxicity from use of topical lindane products; most such reports have related to overuse or accidental ingestion. The likelihood of convulsions or clinical signs of CNS toxicity following a single treatment with lindane shampoo used as directed is remote, but potential for abuse and overuse exists. Blood levels of lindane increase with repeated use. Lindane products should not be used in infants, young children, pregnant or lactating women, or patients with seizure disorders or other neurologic diseases.

TOLERANCE (RESISTANCE) Reports of tolerance of head lice to lindane has been noted from the United Kingdom, the Netherlands, Egypt, Panama, Mexico, Arizona, and California.[19] Mumcuoglu et al.[20] have suggested that resistance to permethrin has developed rapidly among head lice in Israel since permethrin products were introduced in 1991. Since 1994, there has been a growing number of reports throughout the United States of treatment failures following repeated applications of permethrin and synergized pyrethrin products used for head lice infestations.[21] Whether this is due to the emergence of head lice resistant to these agents has yet to be determined. Schachner[22] recently discussed alternative therapies for resistant head lice including petrolatum occlusion.

All children and adults in the household should be examined. Some authors treat only those individuals found to be infested; an exception might be a person who shares a bed with an infested individual. Some authors suggest routinely treating the entire family simultaneously. Cogent evidence of persistent (or recurrent) infestations is the presence of adult organisms; this requires retreatment. Following therapy, infested individuals should put on clean clothing and should machine-wash and dry (hot cycle) all washable clothing, towels, bed linens, and headgear with which they have had contact. Clothing that is not washable should be dry-cleaned. Items that can be taken out of use may be placed in plastic bags and left in a warm place—24° to 29.5°C (75° to 85°F)—for 2 weeks. Combs and brushes may be washed in hot water—54°C (130°F)—for 10 to 20 min; some authors prefer to coat the combs and brushes with the pediculicide for 15 min and then to wash them in hot soapy water. Floors, play areas, and furniture should be thoroughly vacuumed to remove any hairs with viable eggs attached that may have been shed.

Pediculosis Pubis

The preparation is applied to infested and adjacent hairy areas with particular attention to the pubic mons and perianal regions. In hairy individuals, application includes the thighs, the trunk, and axillary regions because of their frequent involvement. A common cause of failure is treating only the pubic area in hairy individuals. Sexual contacts should be treated simultaneously. Other uninfested household members need not be treated. At the conclusion of therapy, previously infested individuals and sexual partners should use fresh underclothing, night wear, sheets, and pillowcases; used articles should be machine-washed and dried (hot cycle) or laundered by boiling and then ironed.

SPECIFIC AGENTS

1. Synergized pyrethrins (RID and other preparations available over the counter) appear to be safe and effective. They are applied undiluted until the infested areas are entirely wet and allowed to remain in place for 10 min. The area is then washed thoroughly with warm water and soap and dried. A fine-toothed comb (provided with some products) facilitates removal of dead lice and eggs. A second application is used in 7 to 10 days to kill any nymphs newly hatched from eggs that survive the first treatment.

2. Lindane shampoo (obtained by prescription) should be lathered into the affected area for 5 min. The area should be rinsed thoroughly and towel-dried. Remaining nits should be removed with a fine-toothed comb or forceps. Some authors routinely prescribe a second treatment in 1 week to kill any newly hatched eggs.

Therapeutic inefficiency is usually due to failure to follow instructions, neglecting to treat sexual contacts, or reinfestation. Persistent itching may be caused by irritation from the pediculicide (usually due to overuse) or patient anxiety. Parasitophobia is fairly common after infestation and is difficult to treat. Therapy for eyelash involvement is petrolatum applied twice daily for 8 days followed by removal of any nits. Patients with HIV/AIDS tend to have more severe infestations with pediculosis pubis and to be unresponsive to conventional therapy.

Pediculosis Corporis

SPECIFIC AGENTS Therapy consists mainly of proper hygiene, bathing, use of clean clothing and bedding, and proper nutrition.

Previously used underclothing and bedding should be laundered with hot water, boiled, or discarded. Dry-cleaning destroys lice on wool garments. Ironing woolens at home is also satisfactory, but special attention must be given to the seams. Following appropriate disposition of clothing, the patient should be treated from head to toe with a single application of permethrin 5% cream (obtained by prescription), which is left on for 8 to 10 h, and then washed off thoroughly.[16]

REFERENCES

1. Orkin M, Maibach HI: Ectoparasitic diseases, in *Dermatology,* edited by M Orkin, HI Maibach, MV Dahl. Norwalk, CT, Appleton and Lange, 1991, p 205
2. Orkin M, Maibach HI: Ectoparasitic infestations, in *Atlas of Infections of the Skin,* edited by R Aly, HI Maibach. Philadelphia, Saunders, 1998
3. Paller AS: Scabies in infants and small children. *Semin Dermatol* **12**:3 1993
4. del Guidice P: Scabies in HTLV-1 seropositive patients. *J Am Acad Dermatol* **36**:134, 1997
5. Orkin M: Scabies in AIDS. *Semin Dermatol* **12**:9, 1993
6. Orkin M: Scabies: What's new, in *Exogenous Dermatology,* edited by C Surber, P Elsner, AS Bircher. Basel, Karger, 1995, p 105
7. Orkin M, Maibach HI: Scabies therapy—1993. *Semin Dermatol* **12**:22, 1993
8. Taplin D et al: Permethrin: 5% Dermal cream: A new treatment for scabies. *J Am Acad Dermatol* **15**:995, 1986
9. Maibach HI et al: Sulfur revisited. *J Am Acad Dermatol* **28**:154, 1990
10. Macotela-Ruiz E, Pena-Gonzalez G: Tratamineto de la escabiasis con ivermectina por dia oral. *Gac Med Mex* **129**:201, 1993
11. Meinking TL et al: The treatment of scabies with ivermectin. *N Engl J Med* **333**:26, 1995
12. Funkhouser ME et al: Management of scabies in patients with human immunodeficiency virus disease. *Arch Dermatol* **129**:911, 1993
13. Meinking TL, Taplin D: Safety of permethrin versus lindane for the treatment of scabies. *Arch Dermatol* **132**:959, 1996
14. Berger TG: HIV infections: Cutaneous manifestations, in *Atlas of Infections of the Skin,* edited by R Aly, HI Maibach. Philadelphia, Saunders, 1998
15. Skinner SM, DeVillez RL: Sepsis associated with Norwegian scabies in patients with acquired immunodeficiency syndrome. *Cutis* **50**:213, 1992
16. Taplin D, Meinking TL: Infestations, in *Pediatric Dermatology,* 2d ed, edited by LH Schachner, RC Hansen. New York, Churchill Livingstone, 1995, p 1465
17. Orkin M, Maibach HI: Louse infestations. *Curr Concepts Skin Dis* **10**:5, 1989
18. Meinking TL, Taplin D: Infestations: Pediculosis, in *Sexually Transmitted Diseases: Advances in Diagnosis and Treatment,* edited by P Elsner, A Eichmann. Basel, Karger, 1996, p 157
19. Meinking TL, Taplin D: Advances in pediculosis, scabies, and other mite infestations. *Adv Dermatol* **5**:131, 1990
20. Mumcuoglu KY et al: Permethrin resistance in the head louse, *Pediculus capitis. Med Vet Entomol* **9**:427, 1995
21. Taplin D, Meinking TL: Permethrin, in *Sexually Transmitted Diseases: Advances in Diagnosis and Treatment,* edited by P Elsner, A Eichmann. Basel, Karger, 1996, p 255
22. Schachner LA: Treatment resistant head lice: Alternative therapeutic approaches. *Ped Dermatol* **14**:409, 1997

Arthropod Bites and Stings

The bites and stings of arthropods cause many patients to consult physicians for relief from these vexatious creatures. Occasionally, death is caused by envenomation, particularly in infants. The clinician primarily diagnoses and treats skin lesions and systemic illnesses produced or transmitted by only five of the nine classes of arthropods: Arachnida, Chilopoda, Diplopoda, Crustacea, and Insecta.[1] All arthropods are invertebrates with a chitinous exoskeleton, bilateral symmetry, true segmentation, and jointed true appendages that vary from few to many (Fig. 240-1 and Table 240-1).

HISTOPATHOLOGY

Most arthropod bites have a similar histologic reaction pattern. In the acute phase, there is variable epidermal necrosis, spongiosis, and parakeratosis with plasma exudate and a dermal inflammatory infiltrate extending upward. Dermal inflammation tends to extend into the deep dermis in a wedge-shaped pattern and surrounds vessels with some extension into dermal collagen. The infiltrate is typically of mixed composition including eosinophils, neutrophils, lymphocytes, and histiocytes in varying proportions. Eosinophils are usually prominent, although neutrophils may predominate in reactions to fleas, mosquitoes, fire ants, and brown recluse spiders. Bullae can form secondary to marked edema, especially in children. Insect parts are rarely seen, except for the burrowed mites of scabies within the stratum corneum and the mouthparts of ticks, which may remain within the dermis after ticks are removed.

Chronic lesions most commonly result when a portion of the arthropod

FIGURE 240-1

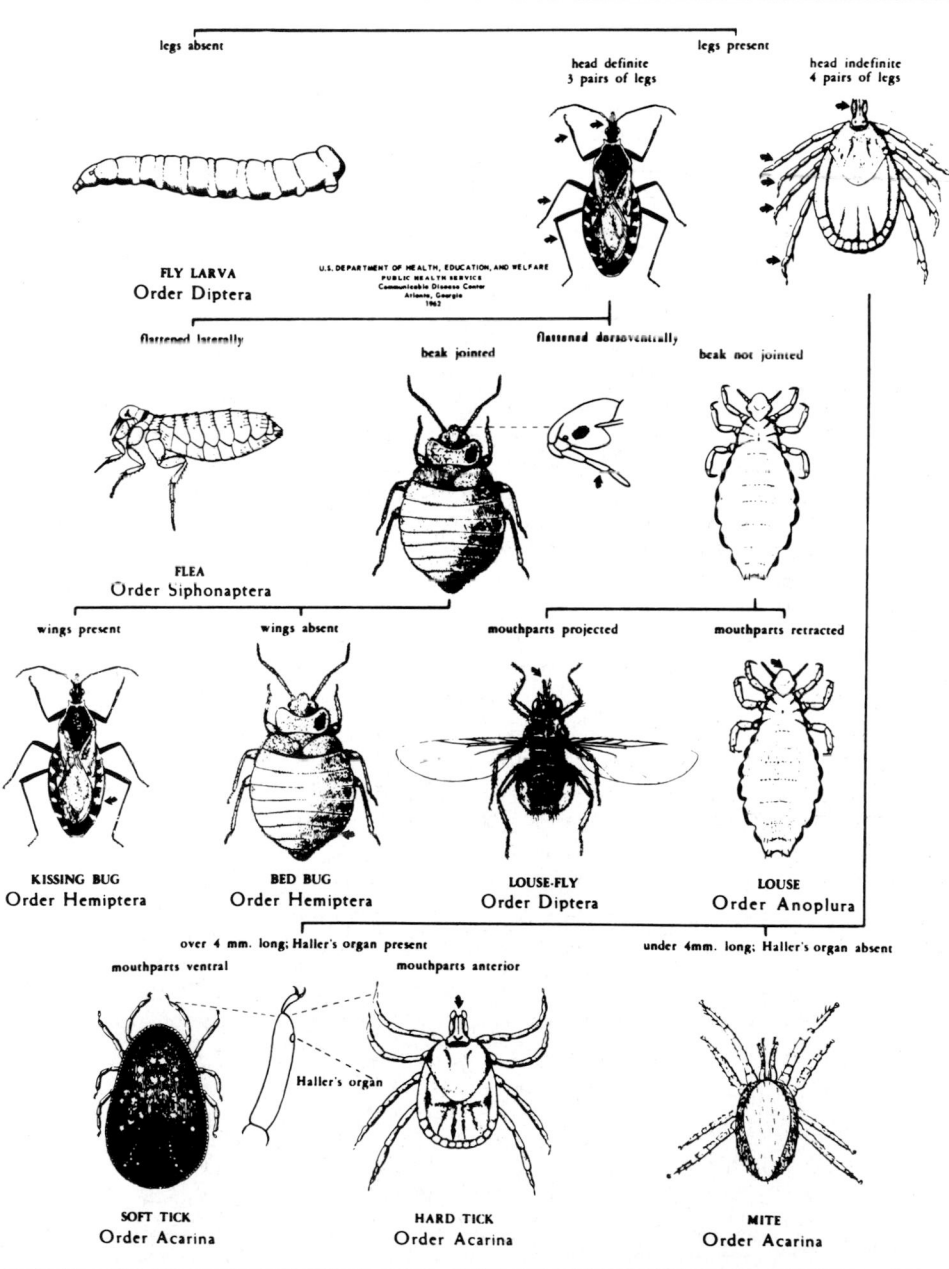

Pictorial key to groups of human ectoparasites. (*CJ Stojanovich and HG Scott, U.S. Department of Health, Education, and Welfare, Public Health Service.*)

TABLE 240-1

Arthropods That Infest, Bite, or Sting Humans

  I. Arachnida—mites, ticks, spiders, scorpions (four pairs of legs)
    A. Acarina
      1. Mites—follicle, food, fowl, grain, harvest, murine, scabies
      2. Ticks
    B. Araneae—spiders
    C. Scorpionida
  II. Chilopoda and Diplopoda—centipedes, millipedes
 III. Insecta (three pairs of legs)
    A. Anoplura—lice
    B. Coleoptera—beetles
    C. Diptera—flies, mosquitoes
    D. Hemiptera—bedbugs, kissing bugs
    E. Hymenoptera—ants, bees, wasps
    F. Lepidoptera—butterflies, moths
    G. Siphonaptera—fleas

lodges within the skin, although hypersensitivity to the bite can be the sole cause. Chronic lesions can present diagnostic problems when they take on a pseudolymphomatous appearance.[2]

ARACHNIDA

The Arachnida class includes three orders of medical interest: Acarina (ticks and mites), Araneae (spiders), and Scorpionida (scorpions). All adults in this class have four pairs of legs; the cephalothorax may vary, but it is typically fused. An exception to this rule is the larval stage of ticks ("seed ticks"), which have only three pairs of legs.

Acarina

The mites in the order Acarina of most interest to the clinician are the follicle mites, food mites, fowl mites, grain mites, harvest mites, murine mites, and scabies. With the exception of *Demodex* and scabies, these mites do not burrow and are known to drop off after feeding.[3] All mites may produce pruritus and/or allergic reactions through salivary proteins deposited during feeding. Although it is not possible to group all mites that cause human diseases into convenient categories, most of the more common mites can be grouped into three suborders:

Trombidiiformes: Harvest/chigger mites, family Trombiculidae; grain mites, family Pyemotidae; follicle mites, family Demodicidae.
Mesostigmata: Bird/rodent mites, family Dermanyssidae; straw mites, family Hemoganasidae.
Sarcoptiformes: Scabies, family Sarcoptidae; food mites, family Acaridae, family Glycyphagidae; mange, family Psoroptidae.

FOLLICLE MITES *Demodex* mites can be detected in sebaceous glands and hair follicles by skin biopsy of symptomatic and asymptomatic humans.[4] Whether *Demodex* is the etiologic agent in rosacea and other dermatoses, or whether its presence reflects asymptomatic parasitosis, is not well documented. Symptoms produced by democidosis, if any, are more likely due to immunologic rather than toxicologic reactions.

FOOD MITES Several species of mites that infest foodstuffs have been described. In their hypopial stage, they may be disseminated on the bodies of insects. The grain mite, *Acarus*, the cheese mite, *Glyciphagus*, and the grocery mite, *Tyrophagus*, produce papular urticaria or vesicopapular eruptions. An occupational history and skin scrapings are frequently required to separate these food mite–induced problems from scabies and other causes of papular urticaria.

FOWL MITES Office workers, homemakers, and bird fanciers are all affected by mites that infest birds, especially pigeons that have nests or roosts near air conditioner intake ducts. *Dermanyssus gallinae* and *D. avium* are the most common fowl ectoparasites identified in the United States. These mites only temporarily infest humans. *Ornithonyssus sylviarum* is an uncommon fowl mite of the northern temperate region that can induce human skin lesions as well as transmit Western equine encephalomyelitis virus.

GRAIN MITES The best studied grain mite of medical importance is the straw itch mite, *Pyemotes ventricosus*. *P. ventricosus* is primarily a parasite of insect larvae that feed on grain, such as the Angoumois grain moth (*Sitotroga cerealella*) and the wheat joint worm (*Harmolita tritici*). The distribution of *P. ventricosus* is worldwide and it has been identified in over half of the United States.

    P. ventricosus infests both animals and humans, occasionally producing unusual epidemics after an exposure to infested hay, grains, grasses, or straw. Affected patients often have systemic symptoms such as fever, diarrhea, anorexia, and malaise. Clinically, the lesions vary from bright red macules to varicelliform eruptions. However, identification of *P. ventricosus* in various infested grain products is often not made because of the low index of suspicion.

HARVEST MITES Perhaps the best known cause of "bites" due to mites in the United States is the chigger, mower, or harvest mite (*Trombicula alfreddugèsi* and *T. splendens*). In other parts of the world, *Trombicula* species are the vectors for *Rickettsia tsutsugamushi* in scrub typhus by *T. deliensis* and *T. akamushi*. Contact with the chigger mite usually occurs during the summer and fall when outdoor activities are maximal. Frequently, the only sign of exposure is intense pruritus on the ankles, legs, or belt line since the bright red mites ("red bugs") typically fall off after feeding or may be scratched off. In nonsensitized individuals, usually only 1- to 2-mm pruritic macules are seen, which require minimal treatment. In sensitized or allergic individuals, the reaction to the chigger infestation may be papular urticaria, vesiculation, or a granulomatous reaction with fever and lymphadenopathy. Clinically, the distribution of the lesions may be confused with other dermatoses since the type of exposure and the clothing worn greatly affect where the mites attach. Occasionally, the mites can be identified by visual inspection.

    Since nonscabetic mites other than *Demodex* do not burrow into the skin, their treatment consists of a warm soapy bath to kill remaining larvae, an important step in the prevention of scrub typhus transmitted by trombiculid mites. The ultimate success of treatment in these nonscabetic cases also depends on treatment of the animal or food sources. Antipruritics are used as needed.

ANIMAL MITES Two species of murine mites are of medical importance throughout the world: *Ornithonyssus bacoti*, tropical rat mite, and *Allodermanyssus sanguineus*, the housemouse mite, a vector of rickettsialpox. *O. bacoti*, a vector of endemic (murine) typhus, has been noted to travel widely to obtain its blood meal if the host rats die or leave the infested nest. Persons working in areas rats commonly inhabit (groceries, granaries, restaurants, storehouses) may be affected without ever finding the mite because it drops off after each feeding.

Cheyletiellid mites are frequently harbored by dogs and cats, producing a condition sometimes referred to as "walking dandruff." Although the pet is usually asymptomatic, the person holding the pet experiences marked pruritus when the mites penetrate clothing and temporarily feed on that individual's skin. Diagnosis depends on finding the mites on the pet by microscopically examining cellophane tape applied to the pet's skin or brushings from the animal. Treatment of the pet by a qualified veterinarian resolves the symptoms.[5]

SCABIES The mite *Sarcoptes scabiei*, var. *hominis*, is the mite in the order Acarina that is of most interest to physicians because of its origin in antiquity and prevalence in modern times (for reviews see Orkin et al.[6]). The diagnosis may be easily missed and should be considered in a patient of any age with persistent generalized severe pruritus. Chronic undiagnosed scabies is the basis for the colloquial term, "the 7-year itch."

Scabies is discussed in greater detail in Chap. 239.

TICKS Ticks are the largest members of the order Acarina. They are important worldwide as vectors of systemic disease. Reactions to tick bites include foreign body reactions, reactions to salivary secretions, reactions to injected toxins, and hypersensitivity reactions.[3]

Ticks are divided into the Argasidae (soft tick) and Ixodidae (hard tick) families[1] (Fig. 240-1). The Ixodidae family is responsible for most tick-related diseases. Ticks are separated from other mites by the presence of a barbed hypostome, which they use for feeding. Using their toothed chelicerae, ticks tear open the epidermis and then insert the barbed hypostome. Salivary secretions are used to soften the epidermis as well. During the insertion process, a cement-like substance is secreted that hardens and firmly anchors the hypostome to the skin. Ticks feed for about 7 days until engorged and then drop off to continue their life cycle.[3]

Tick bites occur most commonly in the spring and summer, coinciding with the life cycle of the tick. Ticks have four stages of the life cycle: egg, larva, nymph, and adult. All stages require a blood meal to advance to the next stage except the egg. Eggs are deposited in early spring and develop to larvae by summer. The larvae feed once on small rodents and then are inactive over winter. The following spring larvae develop to nymphs and again find a suitable host and feed. Generally this host is a small rodent, but larger animals and humans may also become hosts. Nymphs molt to become adults in summer. After finding a suitable host for a blood meal, the adult female survives through the winter to begin the life cycle with egg laying the following spring.

Many different species of ticks are responsible for local tick bite reactions and transmission of diseases in humans. Among those most common in the United States are *Ixodes scapularis*, *I. pacificus*, *Amblyomma americanum* (Lone Star tick), *Dermatcentor andersoni* (American wood tick), and *D. variabilis* (American dog tick). *I. dammini*, the commonly reported vector of Lyme disease, is now felt to be the same species as *I. scapularis*.[7] In Europe, *I. ricinus* and *I. persulcatus* are important vectors of disease, especially Lyme disease. Lyme disease is discussed in greater detail in Chap. 204.

Depending on the species of tick, the bite of the tick may or may not be painful or pruritic. Most bites are not painful. In many

instances, victims are not even aware that they have been bitten and there may be only a red papule at the bite site. This papule can progress to local swelling and erythema. Blistering, severe pruritus, and ecchymosis can be seen. A cellular reaction to the bite can lead to induration and nodularity after a few days. Central necrosis and ulceration rarely occur.[3] The usual bite heals in 2 to 3 weeks, although chronic tick bite granulomas may persist for months to years. Persistent papules respond to intralesional glucocorticoid injections.

Tick paralysis Tick paralysis is thought to be caused by a toxin secreted in the saliva of the tick, although the exact nature of the toxin is unknown. Tick paralysis may be caused by 43 different species of ticks, but most human cases in the United States are attributed to *Dermacentor* species. The paralysis is an acute ascending lower motor neuron paralysis. Typically, the tick is attached from 4 to 7 days before the onset of symptoms. If the tick is found and removed, symptoms disappear rapidly in the reverse order of their appearance. Diagnosis is made by a careful search of the scalp and body for the attached tick. The diagnosis is also suggested if the patient lives in or has traveled to an area where tick paralysis is endemic.[8,9] Treatment, which may require respiratory support, is merely supportive until the symptoms resolve.

Babesiosis Babesiosis is a disease caused by the intracellular red blood cell parasite *Babesia microti*, which is transmitted by the larvae of *I. dammini*. In the United States, eastern Long Island, Martha's Vineyard, and Nantucket are the major endemic areas. There is an increased risk in patients with T lymphocyte depression or after splenectomy. The clinical syndrome of babesiosis includes fever, drenching sweats, myalgia, and hemolytic anemia. Diagnosis is made by observation of the intracellular red blood cell parasite on a Giemsa-stained smear. The tetrad may be confused with the findings in falciparum malaria, but *Babesia*-infected red blood cells do not have pigment granules. Indirect immunofluorescent antibody assays and polymerase chain reaction studies are also helpful in diagnosis.[10] Treatment is symptomatic in the patient with mild infection. In splenectomized patients, exchange transfusions have been helpful. The combination of clindamycin and quinine has also been useful. Atovaquone has shown promise in laboratory studies.[11]

Ehrlichiosis Two new forms of ehrlichiosis transmitted by tick vectors now occur in the United States. Monocytic ehrlichiosis is caused by *Ehrlichia chaffeensis* invading mononuclear white blood cells. The more recently described human granulocytic ehrlichiosis (HGE) is caused by an organism closely related to *E. phagocytophila* and *E. equi*. The invasion of neutrophils in this disorder leads to the characteristic intracytoplasmic inclusions (morulae) in peripheral blood neutrophils. Patients present with nonspecific findings of fever, chills, headache, and myalgias along with leukopenia, anemia, and thrombocytopenia. *I. scapularis* appears to be the vector for HGE. Though HGE may be fatal, early detection and treatment with tetracycline or doxycycline generally lead to recovery.[12]

Preventing bites is the most important measure in controlling both local and systemic tick-related diseases. When exposure is anticipated, proper clothing should be worn and appropriate repellents used. Immediately after potential exposures, the skin should be carefully inspected for ticks in an attempt to remove them before they become embedded or transmit disease. Evidence suggests that the tick must remain attached for more than 24 h in most cases to transmit Lyme disease. Once the tick's hypostome is secure to the skin, the tick must be forced to remove it. A colorful array of remedies has been recommended for removing the tick. These include applying noxious substances such as gasoline and chloroform or burning the tick with a match or other hot object. Suffocating the tick with petrolatum has been recommended. Physical methods such as slow steady pulling on the tick, with or without twisting, have also been advised. If the hypostome is retained in the skin when the tick is extracted, it should be removed surgically. Foreign-body reactions and persistent papules are produced if tick parts remain in the wound.

Ticks are important vectors of many other diseases to humans. They play a role in transmitting viruses, rickettsia, parasites, spirochetes, and bacteria. Those of major importance are summarized in Table 240-2.[13,14]

Araneae

Spiders belong to the class Arachnida and are differentiated from insects by the presence of two separate body parts with five paired appendages and the absence of antennae. Spiders are carnivorous and either capture their prey in webs or attack them and inject venom through their chelicera (mandibles). In the United States, the genera *Loxosceles*, *Latrodectus*, and *Tegenaria* are the only species whose venom produces significant toxic effects in humans. Wolf spiders, tarantulas, jumping spiders, orb weavers, and crab spiders rarely produce cutaneous lesions by other mechanisms, such as the trauma of the bite or secondary infection.[1]

LOXOSCELES There are 13 different species of *Loxosceles* in the United States and five of them, *L. reclusa*, *L. deserta*, *L. arizonica*, *L. laeta*, and *L. refuscens*, have been associated with cutaneous loxoscelism.[1,15] The brown recluse spider, *L. reclusa*, typifies the species and is widely distributed throughout the Southeast and the Midwest. It is often called the violin or fiddleback spider because of the violin-shaped figure on its dorsal cephalothorax (Fig. 240-2). Depending on diet and habitat, it may vary in size from 0.2 to 2.5 cm in diameter. Although its natural habitat is outdoors under dry overhanging rocks and cliffs, human environmental controls have caused it to move indoors and expand its range. Despite its usually timid nature, this spider will bite when trapped or threatened via chance encounters with humans. Since the brown recluse spider hibernates in the winter, most bites occur between March and October when humans disturb their habitat (closets, attics, outbuildings).

The venom of the brown recluse spider contains at least nine protein fractions.[16] One major fraction is a 32-kDa protein with sphingomyelinase D activity. This venom fraction aggregates platelets, generates leukocyte chemoattractants, and liberates thromboxane B_2 in vitro while producing typical skin necrosis when injected into rabbits.

TABLE 240-2

Tick-Borne Diseases in Humans

DISEASE	ORGANISM	VECTOR	GEOGRAPHIC DISTRIBUTION
Lyme borreliosis	*Borrelia burgdorferi*	*Ixodes dammini, I. pacificus, Amblyomma americanum, I. ricinus, I. persulcatus*	Northeast, Midwest, Northwest United States; Europe; Asia; Australia
Relapsing fever	*B. duttonii, B. hermsii, B. turicatae*	*Ornithodoros moubata*	Western mountains, Southern Great Plains, United States
Rocky Mountain spotted fever	*Rickettsia rickettsii*	*Dermacentor andersoni, D. variabilis, A. americanum, Haemaphysalis leporispalustris*	Western hemisphere, especially Southeast United States
Babesiosis	*Babesia microti*	*I. dammini*	Coastal areas, islands off Massachusetts, Rhode Island, New York
Tularemia	*Francisella tularensis*	*D. andersoni, D. variabilis, A. americanum*	South, Southeast, Midwest United States
Ehrlichiosis	*Ehrlichia canis*	*Rhipicephalus sanguineus*	South, Southeast, Midwest United States
	E. sennetsu	*R. sanguineus*	Japan
Monocytic ehrlichiosis	*E. chaffeensis*	*I. scapularis*	Midwest United States
Granulocytic ehrlichiosis	*Ehrlichia* unnamed	*I. scapularis*	Midwest United States
Queensland tick typhus	*Rickettsia australis*	Ixodid ticks	Eastern Australia
Spotted fever groups	*R. conorii*	Ixodid ticks	Worldwide
South African tick-bite fever	*R. conorii*	Ixodid ticks	South Africa
Asia tick fever	*R. siberica*	Ixodid ticks	Central Asia, republics of former Soviet Union
Q fever	*Coxiella burnetii*	All endemic species	Worldwide
Colorado tick fever	Orbivirus	*D. andersoni*	Rocky Mountains, Northern Sierra Mountains, United States; Western Canada
Tick-borne encephalitis	Flavivirus	*I. persulcatus, I. ricinus*	Central Asia; Eastern Europe; republics of former Soviet Union
Tick-bite granuloma	—	All species	—
Tick paralysis	—	*D. andersoni, D. variabilis*	—

SOURCE: Adapted from Jacobs.[14]

FIGURE 240-2

CHAPTER 240
Arthropod Bites and Stings

2689

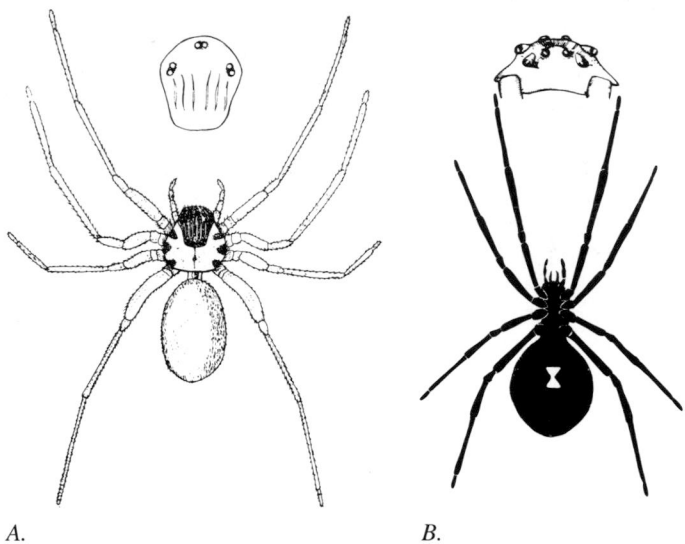

A. B.

A. Brown recluse spider. Characteristically there are six eyes in three pairs and fiddle-shaped markings on the cephalothorax. B. Black widow spider, with eight eyes; it is shiny black, usually with a red hourglass marking on the underside of its abdomen. (*U.S. Department of Health, Education, and Welfare, Public Health Service.*)

Reported responses to envenomation have ranged from a mild local urticarial reaction to full-thickness skin necrosis. This response may be associated with a maculopapular exanthem, fever, headache, malaise, arthralgias, nausea, and vomiting. The bite itself is generally painless, and findings of a central papule and associated erythema may not be seen for 6 to 12 h. Few envenomations, perhaps less than 10 percent, lead to severe skin necrosis or other systemic manifestations. Wounds destined for necrosis generally show signs of progression within 48 to 72 h of the bite.[17] Central blistering with a surrounding gray to purple discoloration of the skin may be seen at the bite site. A surrounding ring of blanched skin is itself surrounded by a large area of asymmetric erythema leading to the typical "red, white, and blue" sign of a brown recluse bite (Fig. 240-3A). At this stage of evolution, these bites may be associated with significant pain related to incipient necrosis of skin and subcutaneous tissues. The resultant necrotic skin ulcer heals slowly (Fig. 240-3B) and may require skin grafts or flaps to reconstruct the defect. Case reports, often unconfirmed, of hemolysis, disseminated intravascular coagulopathy, convulsions, renal failure, or death have been recorded.

The histologic findings of bites are nonspecific, and histologic study should not generally be pursued unless other etiologies are strongly considered. Findings include acute vasculitis, platelet thrombi, and leukocyte infiltrates.[16–19]

Since the clinical appearance of a brown recluse spider bite is nonspecific, diagnosis may be difficult. The potential for exposure to *Loxosceles* spiders, identification of the arachnid, appearance of the lesion, and clinical course must all be considered. Of these, only identification of the captured spider allows for definitive diagnosis of *Loxosceles* envenomation. Laboratory tests for diagnosis are not currently available. Laboratory tests to assess for potential complications such as hemolysis are in order, particularly in children. A broad differential diagnosis must be entertained to include reactions to other biting organisms, allergic reactions, trauma, herpetic eruptions, skin abscesses, and pyoderma gangrenosum.

The treatment of brown recluse spider bites remains controversial. These authors have successfully used, both experimentally and clinically, the leukocyte inhibitor dapsone.[16–19] Ice and elevation are useful in reducing erythema and swelling. Glucocorticoids have not proved useful for the local wound but should be considered for patients with significant systemic symptoms such as hemolysis. Antibiotics are useful in reducing the incidence of abscess formation and secondary infection in large lesions. Acute excision of the bite site should be avoided since the inflammatory reaction produced by the venom will inhibit wound healing and produce an inferior clinical result.[16–18] Surgical management should be postponed until wounds have stabilized with medical management and are no longer progressing.

TEGENARIA The bite of the Hobo spider, *T. agrestis*, has become an important consideration in the differential diagnosis of necrotic skin lesions in the Pacific Northwest regions of the United States. The venom of this spider, the clinical picture related to envenomation, and appropriate treatments have not yet been fully studied.[20,21]

LATRODECTUS Several different species of *Latrodectus* spiders exist in the United States, but the fame and fear of *L. mactans*, the black widow, far exceed the others. *L. mactans* is the most common of the North American "widow" spiders, but *L. variolus* and *L. hesperus* can also be commonly found in a more limited distribution. All three of these spiders have the characteristic red hourglass or double triangle on the ventral surface of the abdomen; the age of the spider determines the relative amount of red on the abdomen (Fig. 240-2B). The red-legged widow, *L. bishopi*, is found only in southern Florida, while the brown widow, *L. geometricus*, is rarely found in the United States. Females are significantly larger than males (leg span up to 40 mm) and are the only spiders capable of envenomation. Black widows spin their large irregular webs close to the ground under debris, over hollow stumps, under woodpiles, or in front of rodent burrows. Clinging upside down to the web, they wait for prey to become entangled in the web and then quickly paralyze the prey with a bite.[22]

The venom of the black widow spider contains a neurotoxin known as alpha-latrotoxin. This toxin acts to destabilize nerve cell membranes by opening ionic channels at the synapses. Acetylcholine is then irreversibly released at motor endplates of neuromuscular synapses. The sympathetic and parasympathetic nervous systems are affected as well, with release of adrenaline and noradrenaline from peripheral nerves.[23]

Clinically, bites may be sensed as a pinprick or a sharp pinch. Dull aching pain or a numb sensation ensues 30 to 40 min after the bite. Skin manifestations are limited to slight erythema, local piloerection, mild edema or urtication, local perspiration, and possibly lymphangitis. Systemic symptoms peak at 1 to 8 h after the bite and may last 24 to 48 h. Severe pain in local muscle groups spreads to regional muscle groups. The characteristic crampy abdominal and chest pain may lead to confusion with acute appendicitis, renal colic, or acute myocardial infarction. Headache, restlessness, anxiety, fatigue, insomnia, salivation, lacrimation, diaphoresis, tremors, tachycardia, bradycardia, hypertension, shock, and coma have all been associated with latrodectism. Death from documented bites occurs in fewer than 1 percent of reported cases.[24]

FIGURE 240-3

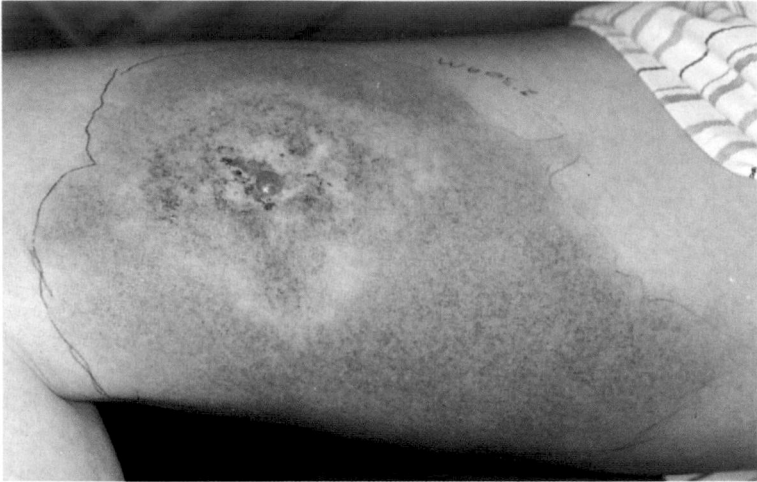

A.

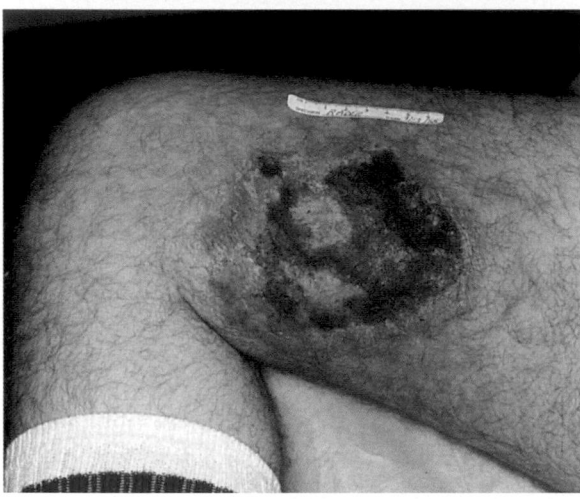

B.

A. Clinically typical brown recluse spider bite showing "red, white, and blue" sign. *B.* Late ulcerative brown recluse spider bite with overlying eschar.

Diagnosis depends on recognition of a consistent history and typical physical findings. Most bites do not result in severe symptoms. In a study of bites of the red-back spider in Australia, 76 percent of victims had only local symptoms.[25] Laboratory evaluation is not helpful, although hemoglobinuria, albuminuria, and leukocytosis may be found.

Treatment of most cases of latrodectism is supportive and generally does not require hospitalization. Exceptions to this rule include the very young and the very old and persons with cardiovascular disease, who are at greater risk for complications. Traditional treatment with intravenous calcium gluconate (10%) and muscle relaxants has proved effective in most patients. Relief of pain with narcotics may reduce the severity of symptoms and muscle spasms.[26] Since antivenom is prepared in horses, it should be used only for severe envenomations in persons not allergic to horse serum.

Scorpions

Scorpions are of medical interest primarily in tropical and/or arid areas such as parts of the southwestern United States, Mexico, India, and the Middle East. Although capable of producing significant local wounds, the primary concern over scorpion envenomation involves the potential for serious cardiovascular complications, which can be lethal. Over 600 species of scorpions have been identified worldwide, with approximately 40 species identified in the United States. The family Buthidae contains almost all the dangerous species. Those of primary concern in the United States are *Centruroides sculpturatus* and *C. gertschi*.[3]

Scorpions are characterized by a body subdivided into an obvious body and tail and five obvious pairs of appendages. The second pair of appendages are quite large and terminate in a powerful pincer used to grasp prey. The tail ends in the stinger, which is brought up over the body to inflict the wound (Fig. 240-4). The venom of scorpions varies from species to species. It is a neurotoxin acting through both adrenergic and cholinergic pathways.

Scorpion stings can produce both local and systemic effects. As with many other venomous arthropods, most stings occur as a result of encounters with the scorpion in a setting where it feels threatened. Most stings occur on the limbs, head, or neck. Initially, there is a sensation of sharp burning pain at the sting site, which may be associated with numbness extending beyond the sting site. Regional swelling can be seen. More rarely, ecchymosis and lymphangitis may occur. Systemic symptoms involve primarily the neurologic, cardiopulmonary, and pancreatic systems. Neurologically, these symptoms may include convulsions, coma, hemiplegia, hyper- or hypothermia, tremor, restlessness, and irritability. Deaths are most commonly related to cardiopulmonary abnormalities, particularly in children. Hypertension, arrhythmias, and pulmonary edema are seen frequently.[27]

Therapy is aimed at inhibiting the effects of the neurotransmitters that are released by the venom. In milder cases with only local effects, therapy is largely supportive and includes local wound care, applications of ice packs, and antihistamines to control inflammation. Local injections of anesthetics may also help to control pain. Systemic effects may require a variety of medical interventions such as antihypertensive agents (hydralazine, nifedipine, or prazosin may be useful) and anticonvulsants (barbiturates). Antivenin is available for some species, but its usefulness has been questioned in the United States, where it is available only in Arizona.[28]

CHILOPODA AND DIPLOPODA

Centipedes and millipedes superficially resemble each other, having one pair of legs and two pairs of legs per segment, respectively. Centipedes are nocturnal carnivores and may produce painful wounds by discharging venom through their claws as they grip the victim. In addition to severe pain, localized sweating, edema, secondary infection, and ulceration may be seen.[29] The *Scolopendra* species is found in Hawaii and the western United States and may attack and produce such lesions when its habitat is disturbed. Local injections of an anesthetic may be used to control pain. Antibiotics

FIGURE 240-4

CHAPTER 240
Arthropod Bites and Stings 2691

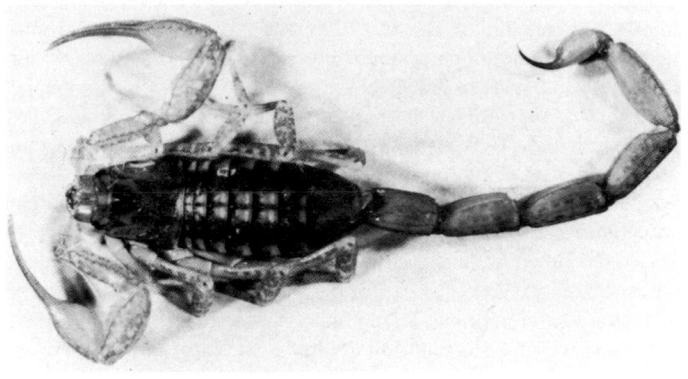

Scorpion. Note the pinching claws, tail, and stinger.

often encountered when the beetle is crushed against the skin. Several other beetle species, which contain chemicals similar to cantharidin, may be the cause of blisters in various geographic areas.[33] A characteristic clinical feature of blisters from beetles is "kissing" or touching lesions, which may produce infection and ulceration. Rove beetles (genus *Paederus*) contain the vesicant paederin. These beetles have been associated with a blistering dermatitis, *Paederus* dermatitis, in various areas of the world.[34] The common carpet beetle (*Anthrenus scrophulariae*) has been associated with a papulovesicular dermatitis. This condition appears to be caused by an allergic response to the larvae of the beetles and not to the beetle itself.[35] If contact with a beetle is suspected early, washing the skin with soap and water may prevent vesiculation. Symptomatic treatment with wet compresses and topical or systemic glucocorticoids may be needed.

to control infection and glucocorticoids to control inflammation may be necessary.

Millipedes are generally harmless vegetarians that neither bite nor envenomate. However, when disturbed or threatened they emit a toxic substance from repugnatorial glands on each side of each segment. This fluid may produce burning, blistering, and pigmentation of the skin. If introduced into the eye, it may cause severe inflammation.[30] For skin contact, no treatment is usually necessary other than thorough washing of the skin as soon as possible.

INSECTA

Anoplura

Blood-sucking lice of the order Anoplura have long been successful obligate ectoparasites of humans. Only two species of Anoplura, *Phthirius pubis* and *Pediculus humanus*, are host-specific parasites of humans (Fig. 240-5).[1,6] Although morphologically very similar, *P. humanus* var. *capitus*, the head louse, is distinct clinically from *P. humanus* var. *corporis*, the body louse. Since interbreeding can occur, it has been speculated that the body louse evolved from the head louse after humans began to wear clothes.[31,32]

Diseases associated with lice are detailed in Chap. 239.

Coleoptera

Since there are over 250,000 species of beetles in the Coleoptera order, the largest order in the animal kingdom, it is not surprising that several species are of medical interest.[1] This section discusses only the beetles whose bodies contain blister-inducing irritants. Five families of Coleoptera produce chemicals that induce blistering or vesiculation upon contact with human skin: Meloidae, Staphylinidae, Paussidae, Coccinellidae, and Edemeridae. The Spanish fly, *Lytta vesicatoria* (family Meloidae), is the most famous of the "blister beetles." Although these beetles neither bite nor sting, they produce blisters because of the chemical cantharidin contained in their bodies. This chemical may be emitted by the beetle, but it is most

Diptera

The order Diptera consists of the two-winged or true flies, and collectively its members are responsible for the transmission of more diseases worldwide than any other arthropod order.[1] At last count, more than 100,000 species in 140 families have been described. The mosquitoes of the family Culicidae are vectors for disease throughout the world. Malaria is transmitted by the *Anopheles* mosquito, while yellow fever and dengue are transmitted by the *Aedes* mosquito. Species of the genus *Culex* transmit filariasis as well as encephalitis viruses. In the continental United States, females of the genus *Aedes* are the most common cause of mosquito bites. The cutaneous reaction is produced when the female mosquito's serrated jaws disrupt the skin and she inserts her blood tube. Irritating salivary secretions are injected to anticoagulate the blood and are responsible for the edema, pruritus, and papular lesions. Mosquito bites may have an urticarial, eczematoid, or granulomatous appearance, depending on the sensitivity of the victim. Mosquitoes prefer blacks to whites, the young to the old, warm to cool skin, and scented to unscented victims. They also are attracted to bright colors and elevated carbon dioxide concentrations in the air, which make summer picnics or gatherings a favorite mosquito haunt.

The black flies of the family Simulidae are also bloodsuckers. Also known as buffalo gnats, these hump-backed insects are found in tremendous swarms near fast-moving water in the late spring and

FIGURE 240-5

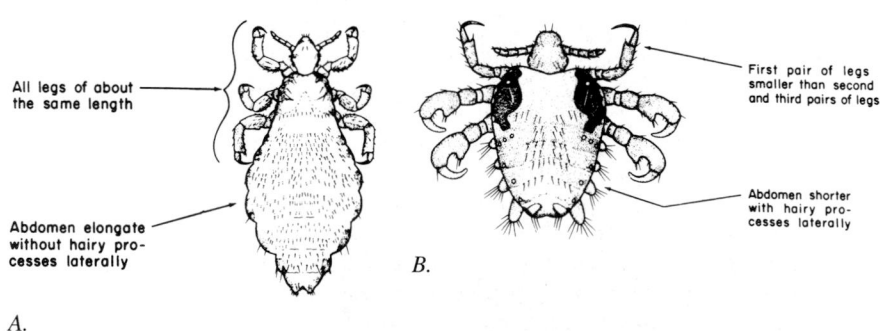

All legs of about the same length

Abdomen elongate without hairy processes laterally

A.

First pair of legs smaller than second and third pairs of legs

Abdomen shorter with hairy processes laterally

B.

Lice commonly found on humans. A. Body louse or head louse, *Pediculus humanus*. B. Crab louse, *Phthirius pubis*. (*U.S. Department of Health, Education, and Welfare, Public Health Service.*)

FIGURE 240-6

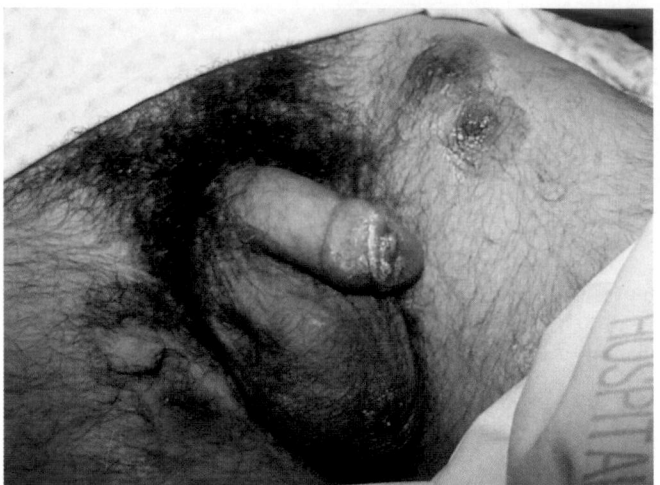

A.

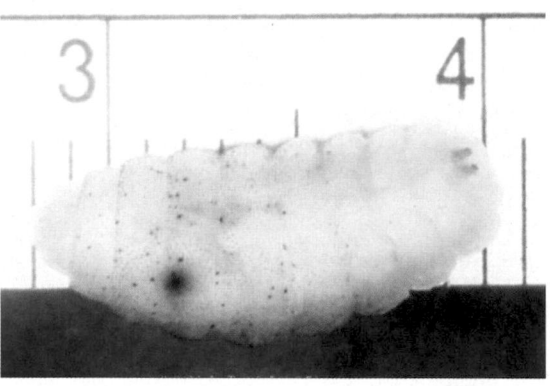

B.

Myiasis. *A.* Abscesses which contain the larval form of *Dermatobia hominis* are seen in the genital area and thighs. *B.* Larva removed from the abscess.

early summer. Because this black fly injects an anesthetic into the wound, the initial bite is painless. However, the bite subsequently becomes extremely painful with itching, erythema, and edema, which may lead to nummular eczema, vesicles, or hard pruritic papules. A systemic reaction termed *black fly fever* producing headache, fever, nausea, and generalized lymphadenitis has been reported.[1] Black flies are vectors in the transmission of onchocerciasis (river blindness) and tularemia.

The biting midges of the genus *Culicoides*, which are also called "punkies," "no seeums," or "sand flies," are another type of bloodsucking arthropod and are known to transmit *Dipetalonema perstans*.[36] Most active in the morning and late afternoon, the female midges are vicious biters and require a blood meal to oviposit. The midge bites produce immediate pain with erythema at the bite site and 2- to 3-mm papulovesicles, followed by indurated nodules of up to 1.0 cm which persist for many months. Unlike black flies and mosquitoes, which pupate in the water, these organisms spend their larval and pupal stages in the ground and metamorphose into adult forms at irregular intervals. Their life cycle makes mass control of this arthropod impossible.

The large family Tabandae are ferocious bloodsucking flies and include horseflies, deerflies, clegs, breeze flies, greenheads, and mango flies. Species of the genus *Chrysops* are known to transmit loiasis and tularemia.[1] Because they are large flies (6 to 25 mm) with bladelike mouth parts, their bite is painful and may bleed vigorously. The cutaneous welt that is produced may be accompanied by urticaria, dizziness, weakness, wheezing, or angioedema. They are a particular problem to campers and hikers in the early spring and summer when the larval forms become adults.

Botfly larvae penetrate the skin or may be deposited onto open wounds to cause cutaneous myiasis. These larvae may be divided into three broad groups as obligatory, facultative, and accidental parasites. Larvae may be fixed to one site or may be migratory, simulating larva migrans. While many species have been described, the screw worm *Callitroga americana* is the most important in the United States. Another important species is *Dermatobia hominis*, a cause of furuncular myiasis in travelers from tropical regions. These painful lesions resemble a pyogenic furuncle, but lack of response to antibiotics points to the correct diagnosis (Fig. 240-6).[37] Phlebotomid sandflies are aggressive biters that produce pruritic, inflamed, indurated lesions. More importantly, however, they are responsible for transmission of leishmanial parasites throughout the world. *Phlebotomus* species are vectors for *Leishmania donovani* and *L. tropica*, while *Lutzomyia* species are vectors for *Leishmania brasiliensis* and *Bartonella bacilliformis*, the agent of Carrión's disease.[3]

The bite of *Glossina*, the tsetse fly, produces minimal cutaneous reaction, yet among the biting flies, it ranks second only to the mosquito as a vector of human disease. Transmission occurs mainly in central Africa where *Glossina* species are vectors for the trypanosomes that cause sleeping sickness.

The treatment of Diptera bites requires meticulous attention to wound care by cleansing with soap or other antiseptics to avoid secondary infection. Local application of steroid ointment and systemic treatment with antihistamines will reduce itching and redness. Although systemic allergic reactions are rare, they should be treated aggressively with epinephrine, fluids, glucocorticoids, and supportive care.

Hemiptera

Most of the Hemiptera order feed on plants. Only the Cimicidae and Reduviidae families commonly feed on animals, including humans.

CIMICIDAE (BEDBUGS) Several genera have members that are commonly grouped as "bedbugs": *Cimex*, *Leptocimex*, *Oeciacus*, *Hematasiphon*. The species most common in each geographic area varies: temperate climates, *C. lectularius*; tropical climates, *C. hemipterus*; Africa and South America, *L. bonati*. Bedbugs are characteristically very flat dorsoventrally and have broad bodies. Bites by these bloodsuckers are usually not noticed immediately unless large numbers of bugs are present. Bedbugs are nocturnal feeders and can travel great distances to reach a suitable host. They may come from unusual locations: bird's nests, poultry houses, bus upholstery, old houses, and furniture. If only a few linear purpuric macules are present, the diagnosis may not be clinically obvious; however, allergic reactions can develop in sensitized individuals.

REDUVIIDAE (KISSING BUGS, ASSASSIN BUGS, CONE-NOSED BUGS) Because several species of Reduviidae transmit *Trypanosoma cruzi*, this family is medically important. Most species are encountered in the Americas with a few in Africa, Asia, and Europe. While many predaceous reduvids produce extremely painful bites, the hematophagus reduvids, the vectors of Chagas' disease, produce painless bites. These vectors typically turn around and defecate immediately after feeding. Subsequent scratching at the bite site inoculates trypanosomes into the wound. Other reduvids defecate at a later time after feeding, reducing the possibility of disease transmission.[3] Genera involved in transmission of Chagas' disease include *Triatoma*, *Rhodnius*, and *Panstrongylus*.

Clinically, the lesions produced by Reduviidae are similar to those from other arthropods and depend on the species, type of exposure, and individual sensitivity. However, predaceous reduvid bites may produce severe local reactions, occasionally resulting in necrosis and ulceration. In some cases, they have been mistaken for spider bites.

Hymenoptera

The general family Hymenoptera includes bees (Apidae and Bombidae), wasps and hornets (Vespidae), and ants (Formicidae).[1] These insects are notorious for their painful stings, which may be associated with an anaphylactic reaction and/or death.

Stings by the female bee, hornet, or wasp from the modified ovipositor (stinger apparatus) produce immediate burning and pain followed by an intense, local, erythematous reaction with swelling and urticaria. The honeybee leaves a barbed ovipositor and paired venom sacs impaled in the victim. The method of removal of the stinger appears less important than the speed with which it is removed.[38] The honeybee dies after stinging. Other Hymenoptera do not lose their stinging units and may use them repeatedly.

Severe systemic reactions occur in 0.4 to 0.8 percent of patients and are divided into three categories: angioedema or generalized urticaria; respiratory insufficiency from laryngeal edema or bronchospasm; and shock. Occasionally, major local reactions may persist at the bite site, presumably mediated by cellular immune mechanisms.[39]

Venom from the honeybee is a highly complex mixture of pharmacologically active agents. Phospholipase A, which comprises 12 percent of honeybee venom, liberates acute inflammatory mediators through the nonspecific membrane damage of its breakdown product, lysolecithin. Other venom constituents include hyaluronidase, histamine, norepinephrine, dopamine, mellitin, apamine, mast cell degranulation peptide, and minimine.[39-41]

The acute treatment of Hymenoptera stings is based on the severity of patient response. Cutaneous reactions may be managed by application of ice and local injection of lidocaine to relieve pain. Hypotension and respiratory failure must obviously be treated vigorously. Systemic reactions require administration of subcutaneous epinephrine, while glucocorticoids and antihistamines may be helpful for urticaria or edema. If a patient experiences an anaphylactic reaction and has a positive skin test, desensitization should be strongly considered.[41]

Fire ants of the genus *Solenopsis* and the harvester ants of the genus *Pogonomyrmex* are aggressive and produce local skin necrosis and systemic reactions when they sting.[42,43] Imported fire ant venom contains a nonproteinaceous, hemolytic factor identified as a dialkylpiperidine derivative, solenopsin D, which induces the lytic release of histamine and other vasoactive amines from mast cells.[44] Clinically, the bite site starts as an intense local inflammatory reaction that becomes a sterile pustule.[40] In contrast, harvester ant venom is proteinaceous and contains histamine, kinins, hyaluronidase, hemolysins, phospholipase, smooth muscle stimulants, and other poorly defined proteins.[40]

The imported fire ants (*S. invicta*) are particularly vicious because they attack in groups. By securing its jaw in the victim's skin, the fire ant is able to pivot, thereby leaving a ring of pustules. Since there is no specific therapy for ant stings, therapy is symptomatic. Systemic reactions occur frequently and may require glucocorticoids or antihistamines. Desensitization may be helpful to protect allergic patients.[45]

Lepidoptera

The Lepidoptera order is medically important solely because of the irritant and allergenic properties of the hairs from caterpillars and moths.[46,47] Contact with caterpillars results in burning and itching or even a stinging reaction in the case of the puss caterpillar (*Megalopyge* species), a common inhabitant in Texas. Skin lesions typically appear as papular urticaria, which can become generalized in severe cases. Systemic reactions to some species have been reported. At least one caterpillar species (gypsy moth, *Lymantria dispar*) may cause irritation due to histamine contained in the lancet hairs, but the allergic potential of the same caterpillar hairs has also been demonstrated.[46] Exposure to the stinging hairs would be expected in people who spend time outdoors such as lumberjacks, farmers, and even campers. Wind-borne dissemination of these hairs may lead to dermatitis as well as keratoconjunctivitis.[48] Whether most "urticating" caterpillar dermatoses are due to histamine, to allergic reactions, or to both is not clear.[46,47] The caterpillars and moths most commonly assumed to cause these problems in the United States and Latin America are the following:

Caterpillars. Brown-tailed moth (*Euproctis chrysorrhoea*); io moth (*Automeris io*); puss or flannel moth (*M. opercularis*); saddleback moth (*Sibine stimulae*).
Moths. Lymantriidae family, tussock moths; brown-tailed moth (*E. chrysorrhoea*); gypsy moth (*L. dispar*); Douglas fir tussock moth (*Hemorocampa pseudotsugata*); silk or peacock moth (Saturniidae family); silk moth (*Hylesia* species); io moth (*A. io*).

As more becomes known about the true allergenic nature of the reactions to the Lepidoptera, as well as about species specificity, some puzzling dermatoses and related mucous membrane reactions may be clarified.

Siphonaptera

Fleas have a unique body shape that is flattened laterally rather than dorsoventrally. Their ability to jump to a height of 18 cm aids in their movement from host to host.

The Pulicidae family is of interest because certain species, most notably the rat fleas (*Xenopsylla cheopis* and *X. brasiliensis*) transmit bubonic plague and endemic typhus. Other species are also capable of transmitting disease. All species bite humans since host specificity is relatively low; severe attacks may occur where the fleas that predominantly bite domestic cats (*Ctenocephalides felis*), dogs (*Ct. canus*) (Fig. 240-7), and birds (*Ceratophyllus gallinae*, *C. columbae*) have recently resided. Survival of adult fleas for months in the absence of host animals makes flea-borne epidemics difficult to detect and eradicate. Usually the bite of the human flea (*Pulex irritans*) causes minimal irritation in a nonsensitized person and produces typically linear or clustered urticarial papules. In allergic individuals, lesions are much more severe, and blisters and even erythema multiforme develop.

In the Tungidae family, only *Tunga penetrans*, the chigoe or sand flea, is well known to produce problems. The female sand flea

FIGURE 240-7

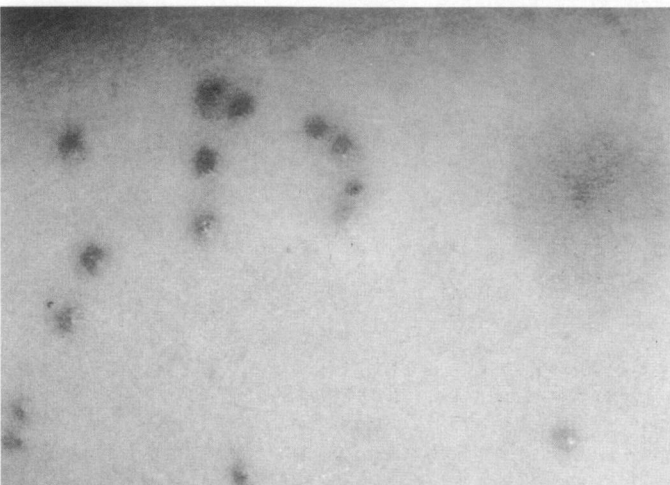

A.

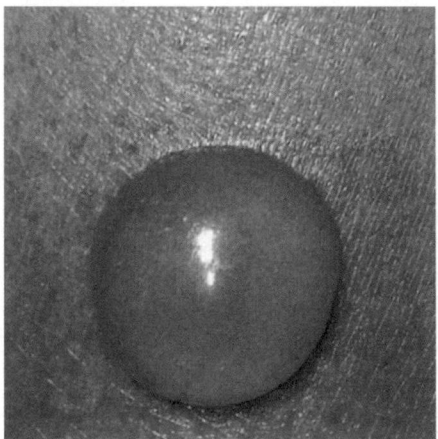

B.

Insect bites. *A.* Papular urticaria. Bites by fleas or bedbugs can present with the clinical picture of multiple, extremely pruritic, edematous papules. *B.* Bullous lesions occur most commonly with flea bites but also occur with bedbugs or contact of blister beetles on the skin.

burrows into the dermis of the animal host. A painful necrotic abscess forms around the site of the female sand flea and her eggs. Secondary infection and scarring are the usual major complications, although tetanus can develop in these wounds. Treatment consists of systemic antibiotics after sterile removal of early lesions, or killing the adult female with a suitable agent. Late lesions resolve by spontaneous ulceration.

PREVENTION

Insect repellents such as diethyltoluamide (DEET) have been the preferred preventive agents for persons bothered by fleas, flies, mites, mosquitoes, and ticks. A variety of concentrations varying from 5 to 100% are available. Although preparations containing less than 50% DEET are almost free of side effects when applied to the skin of adults, encephalopathy in children has followed repeated and extensive application of up to 20% DEET.[49] Passive measures such as screens, nets, and clothing, especially if treated with repellents, are most effective in preventing bites. Permethrin spray, marketed as Permanone in the United States, can be applied to clothing. In contrast to DEET, permethrin is poorly absorbed and rapidly inactivated in mammals. Local reactions are uncommon, and systemic effects have not been reported. Combined use of permethrin-treated clothing with DEET applied to skin gives maximum protection. While the protective effects of permethrin applied to fabrics remains fairly stable over time, DEET efficacy falls over 6 to 8 h. Controlled release formulations of DEET have been studied and appear more effective than simple DEET.[50]

Many other agents are under investigation worldwide, particularly with regard to the protection afforded against mosquitoes. Of interest in countries where malaria is endemic is the efficacy and safety of 2% neem oil (*Azadirachta indica*).[51]

Avon Skin-So-Soft has been of interest in the United States; however; its efficacy is questionable. It seems to function by trapping insects in its film on the skin rather than as a repellent.[52]

Because no preventive measures other than killing the adult or larval forms of bees, spiders, or wasps are currently very effective, future developments are eagerly anticipated.

A variety of insecticides are available for individual or professional use. Proper use of these agents is important in the eradication of field ectoparasites inhabiting inanimate objects such as clothing, furniture, carpets, draperies, and pet bedding. Optimal results from insecticides may require consultation with a professional exterminator.

REFERENCES

1. Harwood RF, James MT (eds): *Entomology in Human and Animal Health,* 7th ed. New York, Macmillan, 1979
2. Ackerman AB: *Histopathological Diagnosis of Cutaneous Inflammatory Skin Disease,* 2d ed. Baltimore, Williams & Wilkins, 1997
3. Alexander JO: *Arthropods and Human Skin.* Berlin, Springer-Verlag, 1984
4. Bonnar E et al: The *Demodex* mite population in rosacea (see comments). *J Am Acad Dermatol* **28**:443, 1993
5. Lee BW: Cheyletiella dermatitis: A report of fourteen cases. *Cutis* **47**:111, 1991
6. Orkin M et al (eds): *Scabies and Pediculosis.* Philadelphia, Lippincott, 1977
7. Oliver JH Jr: Conspecificity of the ticks *Ixodes scapularis* and *I. dammini* (Acari: Ixodidae). *J Med Entomol* **30**:54, 1993
8. Abbott KH: Tick paralysis: A review. *Proc Mayo Clin* **18**:39, 1943
9. Centers for Disease Control and Prevention: Tick paralysis—Washington, 1995. *MMWR* **45**:325, 1996
10. Pruthi RK et al: Human babesiosis. *Mayo Clin Proc* **70**:853, 1995
11. Hughes WT, Oz HS: Successful prevention and treatment of babesiosis with atovaquone. *J Infect Dis* **172**:1042, 1995
12. Bakken JS et al: Clinical and laboratory characteristics of human granulocytic ehrlichiosis. *JAMA* **275**:199, 1996
13. Berger BW et al: Cultivation of *Borrelia burgdorferi* from human tick bite sites: A guide to the risk of infection. *J Am Acad Dermatol* **32**:184, 1995
14. Jacobs RF: Tick exposure and related infections. *Pediatr Infect Dis J* **7**:612, 1988
15. Gertsch WJ: The spider genus *Loxosceles* in North America, Central America and the West Indies. *American Museum Novitates* **1907**:1, 1958
16. Truett AP III, King LE Jr: Sphingomyelinase D: A pathogenic agent produced by bacteria and arthropods. *Methods Enzymol (Adv Lipid Res)* **26**:275, 1993
17. Wilson DC, King LE Jr: Spiders and spider bites. *Dermatol Clin* **8**:277, 1990
18. King LE Jr, Rees RS: Treatment of brown recluse spider bites. *J Am Acad Dermatol* **14**:691, 1986

19. Cole HP III et al: Brown recluse spider envenomation of the eyelid: An animal model. *Ophthal Plast Reconstr Surg* **11**:153, 1995

20. Vest DK: Necrotic arachnidism in the northwest United States and its probable relationship to *Tegenaria agretis* (Walckenaer) spiders. *Toxicon* **25**:175, 1987

21. Necrotic arachnidism—Pacific Northwest, 1988–1996. *MMWR* **45**:433, 1996

22. Gertsch WJ: *American Spiders.* New York, Van Nostrand Reinhold, 1979

23. Binder LS: Acute arthropod envenomation. *Med Toxicol Adverse Drug Exp* **4**:163, 1989

24. Maretic Z: Latrodectism: Variations in clinical manifestations provoked by *Latrodectus* species of spiders. *Toxicon* **21**:457, 1983

25. Jelinek GA et al: Red-back spider bites at Fremantle Hospital, 1982–1987. *Med J Aust* **150**:693, 1989

26. Key G: A comparison of calcium gluconate and methacarbaminol (Robaxin) in the treatment of latrodectism (black widow spider envenomation). *Am J Trop Med Hyg* **30**:273, 1981

27. Ismail M: The scorpion envenoming syndrome. *Toxicon* **33**:825, 1995

28. Groshong TD: Scorpion envenomation in eastern Saudi Arabia. *Ann Emerg Med* **22**:1431, 1993

29. Uppal SS et al: Clinical aspects of centipede bite in the Andamans. *J Assoc Physicians India* **38**:163, 1990

30. Shpall S, Frieden I: Mahogany discoloration of the skin due to the defensive secretion of a millipede. *Pediatr Dermatol* **8**:25, 1991

31. Zinssen RH: *Rats, Lice and History.* Boston, Little, Brown, 1935

32. Buxton PA: *The Louse,* 2d ed. London, Arnold, 1947

33. Nichols DSH et al: Oedermerid blister beetle dermatosis: A review. *J Am Acad Dermatol* **22**:815, 1990

34. Glemetti C, Brimalt R: *Paederus* dermatitis: An easy diagnosable but misdiagnosed eruption. *Eur J Pediatr* **152**:6, 1993

35. Ahmed AR et al: Carpet beetle dermatitis. *J Am Acad Dermatol* **5**:428, 1981

36. Steffen C: Clinical and histopathological correlation of midge bites. *Arch Dermatol* **117**:785, 1981

37. File TM et al: *Dermatobia hominis* dermal myiasis: A furuncular lesion in a world traveler. *Arch Dermatol* **121**:1195, 1985

38. Visscher PK et al: Removing bee stings. *Lancet* **348**:301, 1996

39. Elgart GW: Ant, bee and wasp stings. *Dermatol Clin* **8**:229, 1990

40. Cavagnol RM: The pharmacological effects of Hymenoptera venoms. *Annu Rev Pharmacol Toxicol* **17**:479, 1977

41. Valentine MD et al: The value of immunotherapy with venom in children with allergy to insect stings. *N Engl J Med* **323**:1601, 1990

42. Freeman TM: Imported fire ants: The ants from hell! *Allergy Proc* **15**:11, 1994

43. Pinnas JL et al: Harvester ant sensitivity: In vitro and in vivo studies using whole body extracts and venom. *J Allergy Clin Immunol* **59**:10, 1977

44. Lind NK: Mechanism of action of fire ant (*Solenopsis*) venoms: Lytic release of histamine from mast cells. *Toxicon* **20**:831, 1982

45. Stafford CT: Hypersensitivity to fire ant venom (see comments). *Ann Allergy Asthma Immunol* **77**:87, 1996

46. Allen VT et al: Gypsy moth caterpillar dermatitis—revisited. *J Am Acad Dermatol* **24**:979, 1991

47. Pinson RT, Morgan JA: Envenomation by the puss caterpillar (*Megalopyge opercularis*). *Ann Emerg Med* **20**:562, 1991

48. Vissenberg I et al: Caterpillar induced kerato-conjunctivitis. *Bull Soc Belge Ophthalmol* **249**:107, 1993

49. Brown M, Hebert AA: Insect repellents: An overview. *J Am Acad Dermatol* **36**:243, 1997

50. Rutledge LC et al: Evaluation of controlled-release mosquito repellent formulations. *J Am Mosq Control Assoc* **12**:39, 1996

51. Sharma VP et al: Mosquito repellent action of neem (Azadirachta indica) oil. *J Am Mosq Control Assoc* **9**:359, 1993

52. Magnon GJ et al: Repellency of two DEET formulations and Avon Skin-So-Soft against biting midges (Diptera: Ceratopogonidae) in Honduras. *J Am Mosq Control Assoc* **7**:80, 1991

PART SIX

Therapeutics

CHAPTER 241

Thomas E. Redelmeier
Hans Schaefer

Pharmacokinetics and Topical Applications of Drugs

Pharmacokinetics as it is related to topical applications of drugs describes the time-dependent passage of drugs out of a vehicle or device applied to the skin surface and their subsequent passage through the skin barrier into the underlying skin layers as well as into the general systemic distribution. The subject continues to hold the attention of research scientists and clinicians alike because of its relevance to dermatologic therapy. However, it is fair to say that we may only now be coming to grips with the inherent intricacies and complexities of this subject, despite the early recognition of the principal factors that govern diffusion of a drug into and across the skin.[1]

Difficulties in accurately describing percutaneous absorption are related to the size of the compartments. A topical application of a cream or ointment is routinely spread to a thickness not greater than 10 μm. The stratum corneum is also approximately 10 μm thick; whereas the viable epidermis, dermis, and to a greater extent the systemic compartment represent an effective large sink where absorbed drugs undergo dilution to levels that often remain undetectable to all but the most sensitive techniques. Sampling the time-dependent changes in the concentration of a drug in individual compartments is thus technically challenging. Following application,

1. Topical formulations may undergo radical changes in composition and structure.
2. The effectiveness of the skin barrier often changes with time.
3. The skin barrier is influenced by the type and progression of a disease.
4. There is regional variation in the barrier properties of the skin.
5. The viable tissues themselves respond to topical applications in manners that may either enhance or retard percutaneous absorption.
6. Drugs influence all of these processes in a more or less specific manner.

In view of these facts, the description of pharmacokinetics of topical applications is a complex affair. A number of mathematical models have been developed to describe or define the relative importance of these processes in determining the bioavailability of compounds in a target tissue.[2–6] In this review, we broadly outline the principal factors that determine the pharmacokinetics of a topical application and, where possible, provide the reader with a qualitative feel for their relevance to any particular application.

DIFFUSION

Compounds applied topically to the skin surface migrate down concentration gradients according to well-described laws governing diffusion of solutes in solutions and across membranes. For more complete derivation of relevant equations, interested readers are referred to several comprehensive reviews.[7,8]

Fick's Laws

Diffusion of uncharged compounds across a membrane or any homogenous barrier is described by Fick's first and second laws. The first law [Eq. (241-1)] states that the steady state flux of a compound (J, moles/cm per second) per unit path length (δ, cm) is proportional to the concentration gradient (ΔC) and the diffusion coefficient (D, cm^2/s).

$$J = -D(\Delta C/\Delta \delta) \tag{1}$$

The negative sign indicates that the net flux is in the direction of the lower concentration. This equation holds for diffusion-mediated processes in isotropic solutions under steady-state conditions. Fick's second law predicts the flux of compounds under non–steady state conditions. The solution to these equations depend upon defining appropriate boundary conditions.[6,9,10] However, whether diffusion occurs in a system under steady-state or non–steady state conditions, the principal factors that determine the flux of a compound between two points in an isotropic medium are the concentration gradient, the path length, and the diffusion coefficient.

It is worthwhile to point out that diffusion is a very effective transport mechanism over very short distances but not over long ones. The relationship between the time (Δt) it takes for a molecule to transverse a path length (x) and its diffusion coefficient is governed by

$$\Delta t = x^2/2D \tag{2}$$

For example, the diffusion coefficient for water in an aqueous solution is 2.5×10^{-5} cm^2/s suggesting that a water molecule would transverse a 10-μm path (the equivalent of the width of the stratum corneum) in 0.4 ms. However, since diffusion depends upon the square of the distance, longer path lengths are not efficiently transversed; a 100-μm path would take 40 ms.

The diffusion constant (D) of a solute in solution can be related to its frictional coefficient (f) by the Boltzmann constant (k_B) and temperature (T):

$$D = k_B \ T/f \qquad (3)$$

The frictional coefficient is a function of the molecular size of the compound as well as the viscosity of the medium. Nonspherical particles and molecules have larger frictional coefficients than predicted on the basis of their radius. Moreover, as discussed in more detail elsewhere,[11] diffusion across membranes and within the stratum corneum[12,13] is much lower than predicted on the basis of the radius of the molecule and the viscosity of the medium. In the case of the stratum corneum, this has been attributed to the restricted "tortuous" path that molecules are required to take in transversing the intercellular lipid domains.[14] Notwithstanding these considerations, the general rule governing diffusion in the skin is that it is related to shape and volume of the molecule as well as the properties of the medium (viscosity and structure).

THREE-COMPARTMENT MODEL

Although pharmacokinetic analysis of topical applications may require the description of a relatively large number of compartments, this discussion is confined to the three outlined in Fig. 241-1: the skin surface, the stratum corneum, and the viable tissue. In order to undergo percutaneous absorption, a compound must be released from its formulation, encounter the skin surface, penetrate the stratum corneum, diffuse through the viable epidermis into the dermis, and finally gain access to the systemic compartment through the vascular system. In addition, it may diffuse through the dermal and hypodermal layers to reach underlying target tissues. As summarized in Table 241-1, within each compartment, the compound may diffuse down its concentration gradient, bind to specific components, or be metabolized. The reader should not consider that this is a static model; as suggested previously, the size or characteristics of each compartment may alter with time, and the factors determining diffusion within each compartment may be affected by disease state as well as the nature of the drug or excipient. However, despite this caveat, the properties of these compartments are sufficiently different to make generalizations about their nature relevant to most applications.

FIGURE 241-1

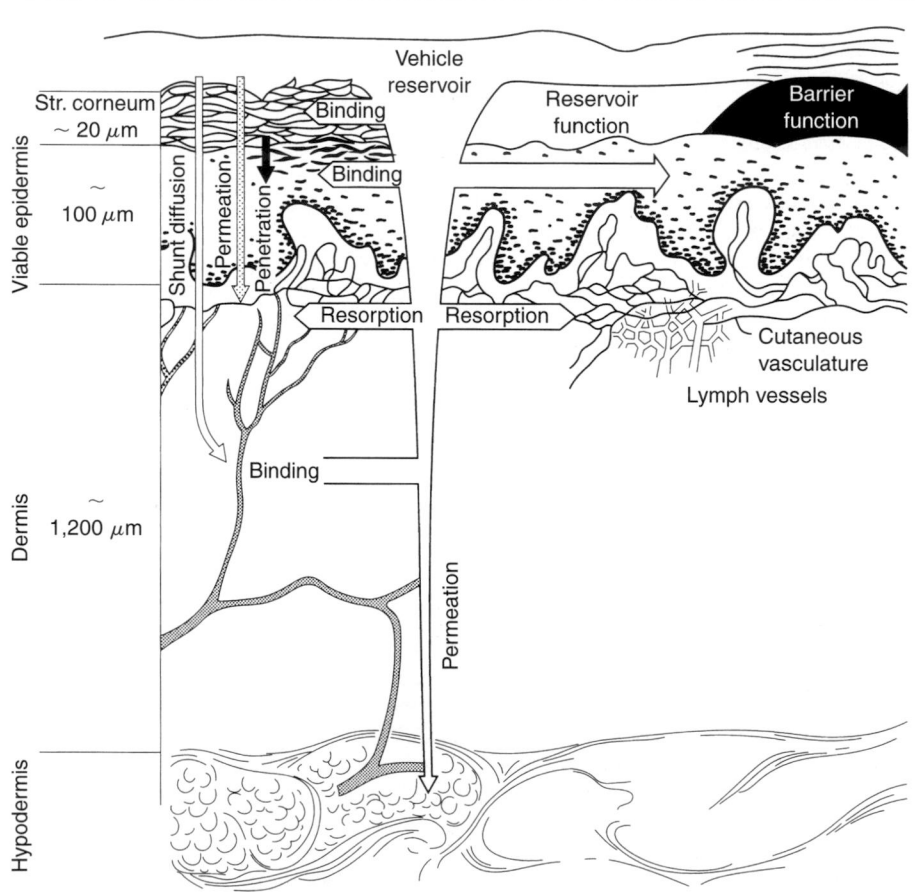

THE SKIN SURFACE

Surface Applications of Formulations

Formulations differ in their physicochemical properties, and, as discussed below, this influences the pharmokinetics of release and/or absorption. However, the principal consideration is that topical applications represent a physically small compartment, which significantly limits the amount of compound that can be applied to the skin surface. When a patient applies a dermatologic preparation, the layer of a formulation covering the skin is very thin (approximately 5 to 10 μm), corresponding to a volume of between 1 and 3 μL/cm^2. Thicker layers are felt as "undesirable" and consciously or subconsciously rubbed or spread to larger surfaces. This restricts the amount of compound that can effectively come in contact with the skin surface to approximately 10 to 30 μg/cm^2 for a 1% (wt/wt) topical formulation.

However, even after being rubbed in, formulations do not remain homogeneous over the time frame of penetration.[15] As discussed in more detail elsewhere, topical applications undergo evaporation, such that even relatively nonvolatile substances such as water are rapidly lost.[16,17] This phenomenon is readily recognized by pa-

Diagrammatic representation of three compartments of the skin: surface, stratum corneum, and viable tissues. Following surface applications, evaporation and structural/compositional alterations in the applied formulation may play an important role in determining the bioavailability of drugs. The stratum corneum, the outermost layer, plays the most significant role in determining the diffusion of compounds into the body. Following absorption, compounds may bind or diffuse within the viable tissues or become resorbed by the cutaneous vasculature.

tients as a cooling sensation. The evaporation results in rapid concentration of nonvolatile substances onto the skin surface, which may result in the formation of supersaturated "solutions" or alternatively, precipitation of active ingredients. Formulations also mix with skin-surface lipids and undergo time-dependent changes in their composition as excipients and drugs undergo absorption. Taken together, these considerations suggest that dramatic changes in the composition and structure of formulations occur following surface application, which determine the subsequent bioavailability of active ingredients.

An additional consideration is that topical formulations are not applied smoothly over the skin[15] and will be deposited in crevices and appendages. This may result in a relative increase in absorption through appendages. This phenomenon may be accentuated in formulations that contain particles or precipitates, since there is evidence that appropriately sized particles can rapidly penetrate along the shafts of hair follicles to a depth of up to 100 to 500 μm.[18,19]

TABLE 241-1

Compartments Encountered by Substances Undergoing Percutaneous Absorption: General Relevance of Processes to Bioavailability

COMPARTMENT	PROCESSES	GENERAL RELEVANCE TO BIOAVAILABILITY*
Vehicle	diffusion	++
	thermodynamic activity	++
	evaporation	+
	precipitation	+/−
Stratum corneum	partitioning	++
	diffusion	+++
	reservoir function	++
	binding	−/+
	metabolism	−
Epidermis	diffusion	+/−
	metabolism	+/−
	binding	++
Cutaneous vasculature	resorption	+
Underlying tissues including dermis	diffusion	+/−
	metabolism	+/−
	binding	−

*−, Though theoretically possible, this process is probably not of general relevance; +/−, this process is of direct relevance, but only in a restricted number of cases; +, the process is generally relevant, but not as important as ++ or +++.

Formulations

A complete discussion of the properties of pharmaceutical formulations is beyond the scope of this chapter, and the reader is referred to several excellent articles.[20-22] Applications can be differentiated on the basis of whether compounds remain on skin surface (cosmetics), are delivered to compartments in the skin (topical formulations), or travel across the skin into the central compartment (transdermal formulations). Formulations determine the kinetics and level of percutaneous absorption and, in turn, influence the onset, duration, and extent of a biological response. In the context of percutaneous absorption, there are several different parameters that should be considered in choosing a formulation: (1) its structure, (2) the thermodynamic activity of the active ingredient, (3) the amount of compound that can be incorporated into the formulation, (4) the stability of the formulation at the skin surface (e.g., emulsions should break easily), (5) the partition coefficient of the active ingredient between the vehicle and the stratum corneum, and (6) the enhancer activity.

In general, percutaneous absorption is proportional to the thermodynamic activity of the compound. Thus, the highest flux is observed at the active ingredient's maximum solubility in a vehicle or, in a few restricted cases, for supersaturated solutions.[23] Vehicles that are very good solvents should be avoided, since they may act to retain the active ingredient on the skin surface. In addition, this may lead to relatively inefficient delivery systems, since high concentrations of the drug are required.

Liposomes as Transdermal Delivery Systems

Liposomes are microscopic spheres comprising a bilayer that encloses an inner aqueous core. A wide variety of cosmetics contain lipids or liposomes. They have proved to be safe, cosmetically attractive, and well accepted. There is considerable evidence that, at least for some preparations, applications of liposomes is mildly occlusive and improves the hydration level of the stratum corneum. Interest in the use of liposomes to enhance the delivery of drugs across the skin has been spurred by several observations in animal models. Liposome formulations have been said to enhance the penetration of compounds across the skin or optimize the retention of bioactive compounds in target tissues.[24-26] However, in contrast to the excitement of these early reports, which rested largely on animal models, there are relatively fewer in vivo studies for humans[27] conducted under standard in-use conditions.

Recent studies using freeze-fracture electron microscopy have elaborated on the interaction of liposomes with the skin surface.[28-30] The most likely scenario is that, following application to a skin surface, liposomes collapse due to evaporation of the vehicle. Vesicle fusion between the liposome and the intercellular lipid domains has been documented, though it is likely to represent only a small fraction of an applied formulation. It is entirely possible that lipids diffuse into the skin and may, under some circumstances, alter the barrier properties. There have been several reports of the appearance of liposome-like particles in underlying skin tissue[28,30]; however, this is unlikely to result from penetration of an intact liposome. An alternative possibility is that the observed liposomes form after the penetration of substantial amounts of lipid monomers. Though available evidence cannot exclude liposomal penetration of skin, it can safely be argued that at most only a very small percentage of an applied formulation can possibly enter in this manner. This effectively limits the usefulness of existing technology to delivery of only the most potent bioactive agents.[31,32]

There are several caveats to these arguments. The first is that there is good evidence that particles can penetrate along the hair shaft and thus may be appropriate systems for delivery of bioactive compounds to sebaceous glands or hair follicles.[33,34] In these particular applications, liposomes and/or other particulates may prove advantageous over more conventional applications that do not target compounds to these sites and are readily removed by surface contact or washing, though this remains to be proven. Second, it is well accepted that the barrier properties of some skin diseases are compromised; it is possible, though perhaps still unlikely, that liposomes can penetrate this diseased skin. Finally, the above argument dismisses the likelihood of the penetration of substantial amounts of intact liposomes; however, the components of the liposome or hydrolytic products thereof may well penetrate as monomers. In turn, like any other excipient, the lipid may increase percutaneous absorption either directly as an enhancer, as in the case of oleic acid or indirectly through occlusion. Alternatively, the deposited lipid film may prove to retain compounds on the skin surface and reduce the percutaneous absorption of hydrophobic compounds. For these reasons, the use of liposomes to deliver bioactive agents across the skin deserves further attention, like other novel excipients or formulations.

THE SKIN BARRIER

The primary compartment that limits the percutaneous absorption of compounds is the stratum corneum. This thin (10 to 20-μm) layer effectively surrounding the body represents a highly differentiated structure that determines the diffusion of compounds across the skin. The physical description of the stratum corneum has now been well documented[35]; and it can be accurately characterized as "bricks" of bundled, water-insoluble proteins, embedded in a "mortar" of intercellular lipid. A model of the organization of the stratum corneum, is presented in Fig. 241-2 (see Chap. 12).

The general consensus today is that the stratum corneum is a highly organized, differentiated structure. In order to participate fully in forming an effective barrier to diffusion, the biogenesis of the corneocytes as well as the synthesis and processing of the intercellular lipid must proceed in an orderly manner. Recent evidence

FIGURE 241-2

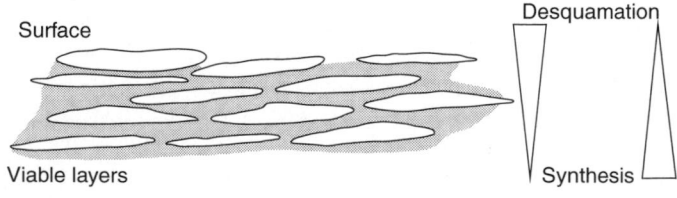

Surface

Desquamation

Viable layers

Synthesis

A schematic drawing of the basic organization of the stratum corneum, indicating the overlapping of the corneocytes and the tortuous path of the intercellular lipid domain (*shaded gray*). Though the corneocytes occupy the bulk of the stratum corneum, the only continuous domain is the intercellular lipid, which is followed by compounds undergoing percutaneous absorption.

suggests that disruption in the kinetics of skin barrier formation by accelerating the division of the keratinocytes found in the underlying layers will lead to a disruption in the barrier properties of the skin.[36,37] Thus the concept of dead or dying skin forming a passive barrier to diffusion is now replaced by a model of the stratum corneum as a highly differentiated structure that has unique properties particularly suited for its role in forming the skin barrier.

Corneocytes

Fully 85 percent of the stratum corneum is protein (as a percentage of dry mass), mostly associated with the cornified cells, termed *corneocytes*. These structures contain a core of keratins surrounded by an envelope made up of cross-linked proteins.[38] The keratins may account for up to 80 percent of the total dry mass of the corneocytes and thus represent the most important constituent. In addition to these fibrous proteins, the core contains low-molecular-weight polar compounds such as amino acids, urocanic acid, and pyrrolidone carboxylic acid. These compounds play a role in maintaining the hydration properties of the stratum corneum. Unlike living cells, which contain approximately 80 to 90 percent water by weight, the corneocytes contain only 15 to 30 percent water by weight.

Recent investigations into the nature of the corneocytes have focused on the role of the corneocyte envelope proteins, since they may be responsible not only for the integrity of the stratum corneum but also for its resistance to irritants. The composition of the envelope has been recently reviewed.[38] It is composed of several proteins termed *loricrin, involucrin*, a family of proline-rich proteins (also termed *cornifin* and *pancornullin*), and *cystatin α* (also termed *keratolinin*) (see Chap. 9). The composition and proportion of the principal components varies only slightly within and between individuals[39] but is altered substantially for several skin diseases[40] with poor skin barrier function.

Intercellular Lipid

Interspersed between corneocytes, the intercellular lipid is organized into sheets, which provide the primary barrier to diffusion across the stratum corneum.[41] This lipid is located in an extracellular domain and thus is not morphologically equivalent to a cellular membrane. The lipid accounts for approximately 15 percent of the dry weight of the stratum corneum or 20 percent of the volume. It is composed of roughly equimolar mixtures of ceramides, cholesterol, and long-chain free fatty acids. There is now substantial evidence that these lipids form structures[42,43] wherein diffusion of the lipids is more than 1000-fold less than that found in cellular membranes.[44,45] This material property of the intercellular lipid is particularly suited to a role as a barrier to diffusion.[35]

Appendages

A variety of appendages penetrate the stratum corneum and epidermis, facilitating thermal control and providing a protective covering. Appendages are potential sites of discontinuity in the integrity of the skin barrier. Appendages account for only 0.1 to 1 percent of the area of the skin and only 0.01 to 0.1 percent of the total skin volume. It can be calculated that in order to significantly influence the flux of compounds across the skin (e.g., by tenfold), the diffusion coefficient would have to be more than three orders of magnitude higher than that across the intercellular lipid domains or corneocytes. For this reason, it is likely that "shunt" pathways are relatively more important for molecules exhibiting relatively slow rates of percutaneous absorption and are of primary importance during early stages after topical application.

CHAPTER 241
Pharmacokinetics and Topical Applications of Drugs   2703

Pathways across the Stratum Corneum

The relevance of the intercellular lipid domain to permeation of compounds across the stratum corneum is inferred from the striking relationship between the hydrophobicity of compounds and their permeability coefficients across the skin.[46] This suggests that the rate limiting step for permeation includes a hydrophobic barrier—i.e., the intercellular lipid. The observation that small polar molecules such as urea exhibit higher permeability coefficients than expected on the basis of their partition coefficient between n-octanol and water has been interpreted to support the presence of polar and apolar pathways.[47] However, alternative single-pathway models have stressed that this observation can be accounted for by considering the influence of molecular volume on the relative diffusivity of compounds in membranes.[48,49] In addition, available evidence suggests that the only continuous domain within the stratum corneum is formed by the intercellular lipid space.[50] This suggests that compounds penetrating the stratum corneum must pass through intercellular lipid, although it does not exclude that compounds can also enter into the inner lumen of corneocytes.

These observations are also consistent with current models of water permeation through the stratum corneum. As discussed in more detail elsewhere,[51] the rate-limiting step for water permeation is through the intercellular lipid. A strong correlation between the membrane order of the intercellular lipid, as determined by Fourier transformed infrared (FTIR) spectroscopy and water permeability of skin, has been observed.[52] Moreover, changes in the composition of the intercellular lipid correlate with increased transepidermal water loss.[35] Taken together, these observations indicate that the principal rate-determining step for water permeation involves the intercellular lipid.

There are several studies that have directly visualized penetration pathways across the stratum corneum with electron microscopy. Osmium vapor can be used to precipitate n-butanol that has penetrated the stratum corneum.[50] Following a brief (5- or 60-s) exposure of murine or human stratum corneum, the alcohol was found enriched in the intercellular spaces (threefold), though significant levels were also found in the corneocytes. Using a different approach involving rapid freezing, water, ethanol, and cholesterol were also found preferentially concentrated in the intercellular lipid spaces.[53] Similarly, the penetration of mercury chloride through the intercellular lipid can be detected following precipitation with ammonium sulfide vapor.[54]

However, in most of these investigations, there was also significant localization of compounds in the corneocytes, more prevalent in the upper layers (stratum disjunctum). Thus, corneocytes undergoing desquamation appear to be relatively permeable, even to rather bulky ions such as mercury. There is additional evidence that other compounds can and do penetrate the corneocytes. It is well established, for example, that occlusion or immersion of skin in a bath leads to swelling of the corneocytes, consistent with the entry of water. Other compounds have also been localized to corneocytes, including the binding of anionic surfactants to keratins. Low-molecular-weight moisturizers like glycerol are likely to partition into the corneocytes and alter their water-binding capacity. Thus, the penetration of compounds into corneocytes cannot be excluded from considerations of percutaneous absorption pathways. The relevance of this step will be related to whether it is rate-determining—i.e., whether the diffusion of compounds within the intercellular lipid is restricted by the corneocytes.

Inter- and Intraindividual Variation in Skin-Barrier Function

Finally, before leaving our description of the skin barrier, it is worthwhile to consider the level of inter- and intraindividual variation in skin barrier activity. The most accurate and reproducible measurement of skin barrier activity is to follow transepidermal water loss (TEWL).[55–57] The extent of inter-individual variation in this parameter for the same individual have been estimated to be 8 percent by site and 21 percent by day to day. The variations between individuals are reported to be somewhat larger, ranging from 35 to 48 percent.[58] There appear to be no significant gender- or ethnic-dependent differences in skin-barrier activity. The skin-barrier activity of premature babies (delivered more than 3 weeks premature) has been demonstrated to be markedly impaired, though skin-barrier function appears normal for full-term infants. There seems to be no significant alteration in skin-barrier activity as a function of age. Better-defined differences in skin-barrier activity between different sites are observed; barrier function can be ranked as arm ≅ abdomen > postauricular > forehead.[55,57]

VIABLE TISSUE

Although the primary barrier to percutaneous absorption lies within the stratum corneum, diffusion within the viable tissue as well as metabolism and resorption will also influence the bioavailability of compounds in specific skin compartments. These processes are interrelated, and factors that increase the rate of one of these processes inevitably influence the others. Since the development of dermatologic formulations is often focused on "targeted" delivery to living tissues, the manipulation of these processes offers a clear-cut rationale for increasing therapeutic efficacy.

The passage of compounds from the stratum corneum into the viable epidermis results in a substantial dilution. This reflects not only the relatively larger size of the epidermis as compared with the stratum corneum but also the lower resistance to diffusion within viable tissues, approximately corresponding to that of an aqueous protein gel.[58] Drug concentrations of 10^{-4} to 10^{-6} M may be attained in the epidermis and dermis for substances that permeate readily (Fig. 241-3). Although the actual concentration gradient of a compound is influenced both by the physicochemical properties of the compounds as well as by the time of application, the presence of a concentration gradient is visible at all times. In other words, strategies to enhance percutaneous absorption generally result in a relatively even increase in the concentration of compounds in all compartments.

Skin Metabolism

The skin contains a wide range of enzymatic activities, including phase I oxidative, reductive, hydrolytic, and phase II conjugative reactions as well as a full complement of drug-metabolizing enzymes.[59,60] Metabolic activity is a primary consideration in the design of prodrugs and may influence the bioavailability of drugs delivered via dermatologic or transdermal formulations. Alterations in skin metabolism have been implicated in a range of diseases including hirsutism and acne, and they may be relevant to risk as-

FIGURE 241-3

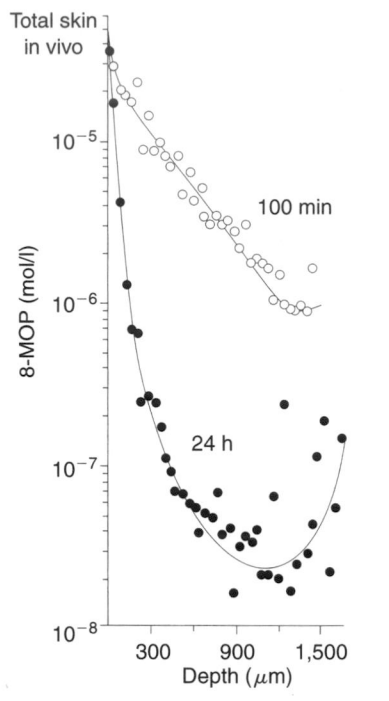

Distribution of 8-MOP in the skin at the indicated time following application. At early times, a steep nonlinear gradient is observed across the whole of the skin. At later periods, the concentration at the dermis has begun to level off.

sessment of carcinogens. Metabolic processing of antigens by Langerhans cells is involved in the presentation of allergens to the immune system. Thus, metabolism in skin compartments plays a significant role in determining the fate of a topically applied compound.

Significant cutaneous metabolism has been demonstrated for a wide variety of compounds of differing physicochemical properties, including the steroid hormones estrone, estradiol, and estriol as well as glucocorticoids, prostaglandins, retinoids, benzoyl peroxide, aldrin, anthralin, 5-fluorouracil, nitroglycerin, theophylline, and propranolol.[59] For example, cutaneous metabolism reduced the systemic bioavailability of nitroglycerin administered in a transdermal drug formulation in rhesus monkeys by 16 to 21 percent[61] and hydrolyzed virtually 100 percent of a salicylate diester.[62] It is convenient to classify metabolic reactions in terms of their cofactor dependence. Processes that require cofactors are likely to be energy-dependent and thus be located within viable tissues. Among the best studied examples are the interconversion of steroids (e.g., estrone and estradiol), and the oxidation of polycyclic aromatic hydrocarbons with mixed-function monooxygenases. In contrast, cofactor-independent processes involve catabolism and may be located outside of viable tissues—i.e., in the transition region between the stratum corneum and stratum granulosum. The best-characterized of these involve hydrolytic reactions such as those described for nonspecific ester hydrolysis.

Metabolic activity is found in: (1) skin-surface microorganisms, (2) appendages, (3) the stratum corneum, (4) the viable epidermis, and (5) dermis. In considering the site of the most significant metabolism, one has to take into account the relevant enzymes and their specific activity as well as their capacity relative to the size of the compartment. Thus, though the level of many enzymes is highest in the epidermis, the relatively large size of the dermal compartment may play a significant role in determining the site of metabolism. A further consideration is that enzymes involved in cutaneous metabolism may be induced upon exposure to xenobiotics. This has been well described for various mixed-function monooxygenases.[60] Finally, the quantitative extrapolation of results from animal models to humans is hazardous owing to the significant species differences in the metabolism of compounds.

Percutaneous absorption and metabolism of compounds can be viewed as two events in kinetic competition with each other.[62,63] Compounds that remain in the skin for longer periods of time are anticipated to undergo significantly more metabolism.[64,65] Further, the type of metabolism of a substance may also be influenced by the nature of its formulation, as illustrated by investigations on metabolism of several transdermal nitroglycerin formulations.[66,67] The inclusion of enhancers in the formulation not only increased the bioavailability of the nitroglycerin but also increased the ratio of one metabolic compound (1,2-glyceryl dinitrate) in relation to another (1,3-glyceryl dinitrate). This may limit the suitability of in vitro experiments for estimating the significance of cutaneous metabolism, since the vasculature is not functional. It further emphasizes that it is difficult to extrapolate quantitatively the level of metabolism obtained for different formulations. This has significant implications for the estimation of bioequivalence.

However, despite the variety of skin-associated metabolic processes, the extent of metabolism is normally relatively modest, perhaps 2 to 5 percent of the absorbed compounds. Metabolism is limited not only by the relatively short period of time that a compound spends in the viable layers of the skin but also by the overall level of enzyme activity. Thus, under many circumstances, the available enzymes are saturated by the level of compound undergoing percutaneous absorption.[59]

Resorption

Resorption, defined as the uptake of compounds by the cutaneous microvasculature, is directly related to the surface area of the exchanging capillaries as well as their blood flow. Total blood flow to the skin may vary up to 100-fold, a process primarily regulated by vascular shunts as well as by recruitment of new capillary beds.[68,69] It has been estimated that under resting conditions, only 40 percent of the blood flow passes via exchanging capillaries capable of acting as a sink for absorbed compounds. However, this value demonstrates considerable variation between body sites, individuals, and species[70] and is influenced by disease states and environmental conditions. In particular, changes in temperature and humidity as well as the presence of vasoactive compounds may directly influence skin blood flow.[71]

For most compounds and situations, resorption does not limit the delivery of compounds to the central compartment after topical applications. This is a result of the relatively high resistance to diffusion within the stratum corneum as compared with uptake by the vasculature. However, for compounds or situations where diffusion across the stratum corneum is rapid, resorption limits the maximum rate of absorption.[71] The evidence that resorption can limit the delivery of compounds to the central compartment has come primarily from studies that examine the influence of blood flow on this process. The percutaneous absorption of methylsalicylate is increased by elevated ambient temperature or strenuous exercise, an observation consistent with increased resorption due to cutaneous blood flow.[73] Moreover, intravenous administered nicotine (which is a vasoconstrictor) reduces the percutaneous absorption of topically applied nicotine.[74] Regional differences in the percutaneous absorption of piroxicam, a nonsteroidal antiinflammatory agent, are dependent upon the local vasculature rather than skin barrier function.[75] However, perhaps the most convincing evidence that resorption can limit delivery to the vasculature has come from in vitro studies on the perfused porcine skin flap.[76] Caffeine (a vasodilator) enhances its own flux.[77] Moreover, vasoactive drugs such as tolazine increase the delivery of lidocaine to the central compartment during iontophoresis.[78]

An additional consideration is that the rate of resorption may indirectly influence the diffusion of compounds to the underlying musculature, tissues, and joints.[79,80] The principle of locally enhanced delivery to underlying musculature has been demonstrated for piroxicam[81] as well as several local anesthetic preparations.[82,83] However, resorption is likely to compete directly with the diffusion of compounds into underlying tissues. In the rat, the clearance of radiolabeled water (1.10 mL/h) and sucrose (0.32 mL/h) from the dermis due to resorption is approximately threefold higher than diffusion (respectively 0.36 and 0.12 mL/h) into underlying tissues.[83] Factors such as vasoconstrictors, which decrease the blood flow to the skin, will lead to increased diffusion of compounds into the underlying tissues. In addition, the physicochemical properties of compounds also determine their penetration rate into underlying tissues. For example, the tissue penetration of the lipophilic, weak base lidocaine is much greater than that of salicylic acid.[83] Thus, blood flow can have a strong influence not only on the kinetics of delivery of compounds to the central compartment but also on diffusion into the underlying tissues.

The Influence of Pathologic Processes on Skin Barrier Function

Reduced skin-barrier function is observed in a number of pathologic conditions including ichthyoses,[86–88] psoriasis,[89–91] atopic dermatitis,[92,93] and contact dermatitis.[94] It is generally accepted that this can be attributed to structural alterations in the stratum corneum.[35] These structural deficiencies may arise from an absence of an enzyme or structural protein in the underlying viable tissues or may be related to the improper formation of the stratum corneum resulting from an increase in keratinocyte proliferation.[84] A consequence of poor barrier function is an increase in keratinocyte proliferation, which may further accentuate the problem. Thus, in individuals predisposed to a defective barrier, a minor perturbation may become amplified as the skin attempts to compensate by increasing keratinocyte proliferation.[84] A further consideration is that the homeostatic mechanisms responsible for recovery of barrier activity after perturbation may be altered for some diseases or physiologic states. For example, whereas the skin of aged people exhibits normal barrier function, the recovery of barrier activity after perturbation is markedly reduced.[85] This kinetic basis for reduced barrier function may also account for interindividual variation in barrier function and/or an apparently increased susceptibility of certain individuals to contact dermatitis.[94]

CONCLUSIONS

The principal factors determining the pharmacokinetics of a topical application are the physicochemical properties of the bioactive molecule. Hydrophobicity, molecular weight, and ionic charge determine the feasibility of transdermal delivery for any particular compound. Formulations influence the pharmacokinetics largely from considerations of the thermodynamic activity of the compound. However, one should not exclude the impact of changes in the formulation that occur following topical application. Evaporation, and changes in the structure of emulsions, may bring dramatic changes in the thermodynamic activity of the compound at the skin surface. Under some circumstances, this may lead to the retention of the drug on the skin surface.

The rate-limiting step for percutaneous absorption of most compounds is penetration through the stratum corneum. There is substantial evidence that this is related to diffusion through a tortuous path around the corneocytes within the highly structured intercellular lipid, the constituents of which exhibit diffusional properties consistent with their role in the skin barrier. For skin diseases exhibiting reduced skin-barrier function, the absence of these critical structures may account for the decreased barrier activity. The progression of a disease and the inherent biological variability makes predictions of percutaneous absorption for diseased skin inherently difficult. This contributes significantly to the challenges of developing topical applications of drugs.

Processes occurring in viable tissues can have a significant though generally less important influence on the bioavailability of compounds undergoing percutaneous absorption. It has been difficult to establish in vivo the level of skin-related metabolism of drugs undergoing percutaneous absorption. Effective manipulation of the rates of resorption with vasodilators or vasoconstrictors offers an attractive opportunity to influence the delivery of compounds to underlying tissues. However, this is likely to be of most importance with those compounds that exhibit rapid rates of percutaneous absorption.

REFERENCES

1. Higuchi T: Physical chemical analysis of percutaneous absorption process from creams and ointments. *J Soc Cosmet Chem* **11**.85, 1960
2. Guy RH, Hadgraft J: Mathematical models of percutaneous absorption, in *Percutaneous Absorption,* edited by RL Bronaugh, HI Maibach. New York, Marcel Dekker, 1989, p 13
3. Guy RH et al: A pharmacokinetic model for percutaneous absorption. *Int J Pharm* **11**:119, 1982
4. Gupta SK et al: Pharmokinetic and pharmodynamic modeling of transdermal products: In vivo methods, problems, and pitfalls, in *Topical Drug Bioavailability: Bioequivalence and Penetration,* edited by VP Shah, HI Maibach. New York, Plenum, 1993, p 311
5. Kuboto K et al: Percutaneous absorption: A single model. *J Pharm Sci* **82**:450, 1993
6. Williams PL, Riviere JE: A biophysically based dermatopharmokinetic compartment model for quantifying percutaneous penetration and absorption of topically applied agents: 1. Theory. *J Pharm Sci* **84**:599, 1995
7. Jain MK: in *Introduction to Biological Membranes,* edited by MK Jain, RC Wagner. Toronto, Wiley, 1980, p 117
8. Gennis RB: *Biomembranes: Molecular Structure and Function,* New York, Springer-Verlag, 1989
9. Barry BW: *Dermatological Formulations: Percutaneous Absorption.* New York, Marcel Dekker, 1983
10. Scheuplein RJ: Mechanism of percutaneous absorption: II. Transient diffusion and the relative importance of various routes of skin penetration. *J Invest Dermatol* **45**:334, 1967
11. Lieb WR, Stein WD: Non-stokesian nature of transverse diffusion within human red blood cell membranes. *J Memb Biol* **92**:111, 1986
12. Hatcher ME, Plachy WZ: Dioxygen diffusion in the stratum corneum: An epr study. *Biochem Biophys (Acta)* **1149**:73, 1993
13. Packer KJ, Sellwood TC: Proton magnetic resonance studies of hydrated stratum corneum: Part 2. Self diffusion. *J Chem Soc Faraday Trans* **2**:1592, 1978

14. Francoeur ML, Potts RO: The perturbation of stratum corneum lipids affects the diffusive but not partitioning aspects of water vapor permeability. *Pharm Res* **5**:S130, 1988

15. Brown S, Diffey BL: The effect of applied thickness on sunscreen protection: In vivo and in vitro studies. *Photochem Photobiol* **44**:509, 1986

16. Flynn GL: General introduction and conceptual differentiation of topical and transdermal drug delivery systems, in *Topical Drug Bioavailability: Bioequivalence and Penetration,* edited by VP Shaw, HI Maibach. New York, Plenum, 1993, p 369

17. Reifenrath WG: Volatile substances. *Cosmet Toil* **110**:85, 1995

18. Rolland A et al: Site-specific drug delivery to pilosebaceous structures using polymeric microspheres. *Pharm Res* **10**:1738, 1993

19. Rolland A: Particulate carriers in dermal and transdermal drug delivery: Myth or reality, in *Pharmaceutical Particulate Carriers: Therapeutic Applications,* edited by KA Walters, J Hadgraft. New York, Marcel Dekker, 1993, p 367

20. Barry BW: *Dermatological Formulations: Percutaneous Absorption.* New York, Marcel Dekker, 1983

21. Bronaugh RL: Diffusion cell design, in *Topical Drug Bioavailability, Bioequivalence and Penetration,* edited by VP Shaw, HI Maibach. New York, Plenum 1993, p 117

22. Hunting ALL, ed: *A Formulary of Cosmetic Preparations: Creams, Lotions and Milks.* Weymouth, Dorset, England, Micelle Press, 1995

23. Davis AF, Hadgraft J: Supersaturated solutions as topical drug delivery systems, in *Pharmaceutical Skin Penetration Enhancement,* edited by KA Walters, J Hadgraft. New York, Marcel Dekker, 1993, p 243

24. Egbaria K et al: Liposomes as topical drug delivery system. *Adv Drug Del Rev* **5**:287, 1990

25. Wohlrab O et al: Distribution of liposome-encapsulated ingredients in human skin ex vivo, in *Liposome Dermatics,* edited by Braun-Falco et al. Berlin, Springer-Verlag, 1992, p 215

26. Mezei M: Liposomes in the topical delivery of drugs: A review, in *Liposomes as Drug Carriers,* edited by G Gregoriadis. 1991, Chichester, England, Wiley, p 663

27. Korting HC et al: Liposome encapsulation improves efficacy of betamethasone diproprionate in atopic eczema but not in psoriasis vulgaris. *Eur J Clin Pharmacol* **39**:349, 1991

28. Junginger HE et al: Liposomes and niosomes: Interactions with human skin. *Cosmet Toil* **106**:45, 1991

29. Hofland HEJ et al: Interaction between liposomes and human stratum corneum in vitro: Freeze fracture electron microscopical visualization and small angle x-ray scattering studies. *Br J Dermatol* **132**:853, 1995

30. Yarosh D et al: Localization of liposomes containing a DNA repair enzyme in murine skin. *J Invest Dermatol* **103**:461, 1994

31. Imbert D, Wickett RR: Topical delivery with liposomes. *Cosmet Toil* **110**:32, 1995

32. Hope MJ, Kitson CN: Liposomes: A perspective for dermatologists. *Dermatol Clin* **11**:142, 1993

33. Lieb LM et al: Topical delivery enhancement with multilamellar liposomes into pilosebaceous units: 1. In vitro evaluation using fluorescent techniques with the hamster ear model. *J Invest Dermatol* **99**:108, 1992

34. Rolland A et al: Site-specific drug delivery to pilosebaceous structures using polymeric microspheres. *Pharm Res* **10**:1738, 1993

35. Schaefer H, Redelmeier TE: *Skin Barrier Principle of Percutaneous Absorption.* Basel, Karger, 1996

36. Williams ML, Elias PM: From basket weave to barrier: Unifying concepts for the pathogensis of the disorders of cornification. *Arch Dermatol* **129**:626, 1993

37. Proksch E et al: Barrier function regulates epidermal lipid and DNA synthesis. *Br J Dermatol* **128**:473, 1993

38. Reichert U et al: The cornified envelope: A key structure of terminally differentiating keratinocytes, in *The Keratinocytes,* edited by M Darmon, M Blumenberg. San Diego, Academic Press, 1993, p 107

39. Legrain V et al: Intra- and inter-individual variations in cornified envelope peptide composition in normal and psoriatic skin. *Arch Dermatol Res* **283**:512, 1991

40. Michel S, Juhlin L: Cornified envelopes in congenital disorders of keratinization. *Br J Dermatol* **122**:15, 1990

41. Elias PM, Menon GK: Structural and lipid biochemical correlates of the epidermal permeability barrier. *Adv Lipid Res* **24**:1, 1991

42. Madison KC et al: Presence of intact intercellular lipid lamallae in the upper layers of the stratum corneum. *J Invest Dermatol* **88**:714, 1987

43. Hou SYE et al: Membrane structures in normal and essential fatty acid-deficient stratum corneum: Characterization by rhuthenium tetroxide staining and x-ray diffraction. *J Invest Dermatol* **96**:215, 1991

44. Bouwstra JA et al: Structure of human stratum corneum by small-angle x-ray scattering. *J Invest Dermatol* **97**:1005, 1991

45. Bouwstra JA et al: Structure of human stratum corneum as a function of temperature and hydration: A wide angle x-ray diffraction study. *Int J Pharm* **84**:205, 1992

46. Flynn GL: Physiochemical determinants of skin absorption, in *Principles of Route-to-Route Extrapolation for Risk Assessment,* edited by TR Gerrity, CJ Henry. New York, Elsevier, 1990, p 93

47. Tayar EL et al: Percutaneous penetration of drugs: A quantitative structure-permeability relationship study. *J Pharm Sci* **80**:744, 1991

48. Kastings GB et al: Effect of lipid solubility and molecular size on percutaneous absorption, in *Skin Pharmakinetics,* vol 1, edited by B Shroot, H Schaefer. Basel, Karger, 1987, p 138

49. Guy RH, Potts RO: Structure-permeability relationships in percutaneous absorption. *J Pharm Sci* **81**:603, 1992

50. Nemaniac MK, Elias PM: In situ precipitation: A novel cytochemical technique for visualization of permeability pathways in mammalian stratum corneum. *J Histol Cytochem* **28**:573, 1980

51. Potts RO, Francoeur ML: The influence of stratum corneum morphology on water permeability. *J Invest Dermatol* **96**:495, 1991

52. Potts RO, Francoeur ML: Lipid biophysics of water loss through the skin. *Proc Natl Acad Sci USA* **87**:3871, 1990

53. Squier CA, Lesch CA: Penetration pathways of different compounds through epidermis and oral epithelial. *J Oral Pathol* **17**:512, 1988

54. Boddé HE et al: Visualization of normal and enhanced $HgCl_2$ transport through human skin in vitro. *Int J Pharm* **53**:13, 1989

55. Pinnagoda J et al: Guidelines for transepithelial water loss (TEWL) measurements. A report from the Standardization Group of the European Society of Contact Dermatitis. *Contact Dermatitis* **22**:164, 1990

56. Lavrijsen APM et al: Barrier function parameters in various keratization disorders: Transepithelial water loss and vascular response to hexyl nicotinate. *Br J Dermatol* **129**:547, 1993

57. Rougier A, Lotte C: Predictive approaches: I. The stripping technique, in *Topical Drug Bioavailability: Bioequivalence and Penetration,* edited by VP Shaw, HI Maibach. New York, Plenum, 1993, p 163

58. Scheuplein RJ: Mechanism of percutaneous absorption: II. Transient diffusion and the relative importance of various routes of skin penetration. *J Invest Dermatol* **45**:334, 1967

59. Kao J, Carver MP: Cutaneous metabolism of xenobiotics. *Drug Metab Rev* **22**:363, 1990

60. Mukhtar H, Khan WA: Cutaneous cytochrome P-450. *Drug Metab Rev* **20**:657, 1989

61. Wester RC et al: Pharmacokinetics and bioavailability of intravenous and topical nitroglycerin in the rhesus monkey. *J Pharm Sci* **72**:745, 1983

62. Guzek DB et al: Transdermal drug transport and metabolism: I. Comparison of in vitro and in vivo results. *Pharm Res* **6**:33, 1989

63. Hadgraft J: Theoretical aspects of metabolism in the epidermis. *Int J Pharm* **4**:229, 1980

64. Santus GC et al: Cutaneous metabolism of transdermally delivered nitroglycerin in vitro, in *Skin Pharmacokinetics,* edited by B Shroot, H Schaefer. Basel, Karger, 1987, p 240

65. Higo N et al: Cutaneous metabolism of nitroglycerin: I. Homogenized versus intact skin. *Pharm Res* **9**:187, 1992

66. Higo N et al: Cutaneous metabolism of nitroglycerin: II. Effect of skin conditions and penetration enhancement. *Pharm Res* **9**:299, 1992

67. Nakashima E et al: Bioavailability and first pass metabolism: A preliminary evaluation with nitroglycerin. *J Pharmokinet Biopharm* **15**:423, 1987

68. Ryan TJ: Cutaneous Circulation, in *Biochemistry and Physiology of the Skin,* vol 2, edited by LA Goldsmith. New York, Oxford University Press, 1983, p 817

69. Riviere JE, Williams PL: Pharmokinetic implication of changing blood flow in skin. *J Pharm Sci* **81**:601, 1992

70. Monteiro-Riviere NA et al: Interspecies and interregional analysis of the comparative histological thickness and laser Doppler blood flow measurements at five cutaneous sites in nine species. *J Invest Dermatol* **95**:582, 1990

71. Riviere JE et al: The effect of vasoactive drugs on transdermal lidocaine iontophoresis. *J Pharm Sci* **80**:615, 1991

72. Anderson BD et al: Heterogenous effects on permeability-partition coefficient relationships in human stratum corneum. *Pharm Res* **5**:566, 1988

73. Danon A et al: Effect of exercise and heat exposure on percutaneous absorption of methylsalicylate. *Eur J Clin Pharmacol* **31**:49, 1986

74. Benowitz NL et al: Intravenous nicotine retards transdermal absorption of nicotine: Evidence of blood flow-limited percutaneous absorption. *Clin Pharmacol Ther* **52**:223, 1992

75. Monteiro-Riviere NA et al: Topical penetration is dependent on the distribution of the local vasculature. *Pharm Res* **10**:1326, 1993

76. Rogers RA, Riviere JE: Pharmacologic modulation of the cutaneous vasculature in the isolated perfused porcine skin flap. *J Pharm Sci* **83**:1682, 1994

77. Carver MP et al: The isolated perfused porcine skin flap: III. Percutaneous absorption pharmokinetics of organophosphates, steroids, benzoic acid, and caffeine. *Toxicol Appl Pharmacol* **97**:324. 1989

78. Riviere JE et al: Determination of lidocaine concentration in skin after transdermal iontophoresis. Effects of vasoactive drugs. *Pharm Sci* **9**:211–214, 1992

79. Auclair F et al: Importance of blood flow to the local distribution of drugs after percutaneous absorption in the bipediculated dorsal flap of the hairless rat. *Skin Pharmacol* **4**:1, 1991

80. Singh P, Roberts MS: Blood flow measurements in skin and underlying tissues by microsphere method: Application to dermal pharmokinetics of polar non-electrolytes. *J Pharm Sci* **82**:873, 1993

81. McNeil SC et al: Local enhanced topical delivery (LETD) of drugs: Does it truly exist? *Pharm Res* **9**:1422, 1992

82. Kushla GP et al: Noninvasive assessment of anesthetic activity of topical lidocaine formulations. *J Pharm Sci* **82**:1118, 1993

83. Singh P, Roberts MS: Effect of vasoconstriction on dermal pharmokinetics and local tissue distribution of compounds. *J Pharm Sci* **83**:783, 1994

84. Williams ML, Elias PM: From basket weave to barrier: Unifying concepts for the pathogenesis of the disorders of cornification. *Arch Dermatol* **129**:626, 1993

85. Ghadially R et al: The aged permeability barrier: Structural, functional, and lipid biochemical abnormalities in humans and a sensecent murine model. *J Clin Invest* **95**:2281, 1995

86. Williams ML: Ichthyosis: Mechanisms of disease. *Pediatr Dermatol* **9**:365, 1992

87. Lavrijsen APM et al: Barrier function parameters in various keratinization disorders: Transepithelial water loss and vascular response to hexyl nicotinate. *Br J Dermatol* **129**:547, 1993

88. Lavrijsen APM et al: Reduced skin barrier function parallels abnormal stratum corneum lipid organization in patients with lamellar ichthyosis. *J Invest Dermatol* **105**:619, 1995

89. Schaefer H et al: *Skin Permeability.* Berlin, Springer, 1982

90. Marks J et al: Clearance of chronic plaque psoriasis by anthralin-subjective and objective assessment and comparison with photochemotherapy. *Br J Dermatol* **105**:96, 1981

91. Takenouchi M et al: Hydration characteristics of pathological stratum corneum: Evaluation of bound water. *J Invest Dermatol* **87**:574, 1986

92. Imokawa G et al: Decreased levels of ceramides in stratum corneum of atopic dermatitis: An etiologic factor in atopic dry skin? *J Invest Dermatol* **96**:523, 1991

93. Werner Y, Linberg M: Transepidermal water loss in dry and clinically normal skin in patients with atopic dermatitis. *Acta Derm Venereol* **65**:102, 1985

94. Wilhelm KP et al: Effect of sodium lauryl sulfate-induced skin irritation on in vivo percutaneous absorption of four drugs. *J Invest Dermatol* **97**:927, 1991

CHAPTER 242

Jerome L. Shupack
Ken Washenik
Grace H. Pak

Principles of Topical Therapy

The use of topical remedies in the treatment of disease is as old as medicine itself. In an eloquent dissertation by Frazier and Blank, entitled "A Formulary of External Therapy of the Skin," may be found the following: "As a dog licks his wounds, so man is inclined to salve his skin."[1] Because the skin is accessible and visible, it is uniquely amenable to external chemical and physical remedies. For the same reason, diseases of the skin also offer the most incontrovertible evidence of therapeutic success or failure to both patients and physicians. When therapeutic failures are encountered, it is often tempting to add other remedies ad infinitum.

The selection and application of appropriate topical remedies are delicate and challenging tasks. Successful dermatologic therapy depends not only on the active drug but also on the physical properties of the formulation applied. The choice of vehicle, the form of medication, the frequency and quantity of application, and the appropriateness of these factors for the anatomic location and the state of the affected skin will often determine the efficacy and tolerability of topical therapy.[2]

Whereas early dermatologic therapy focused on empiric approaches to relieve symptoms (soothing, drying, wetting, antipruritic, protective, antiseptic, etc.), advances in our understanding of pathophysiologic mechanisms underlying disease processes have led to a wide array of therapeutic agents that target diseases by reaction patterns (e.g., inflammatory, psoriasiform, acneiform, neoplastic, infectious). Undoubtedly, dermatologic therapy will continue to advance on the scientific, reductionist path toward correction of disease-specific defects at the cellular, biochemical, and molecular levels.

It is our professional responsibility to maintain a working knowledge of therapeutic advances in dermatology, but we must also be aware of how the treatments we prescribe for our patients affect their quality of life—physically, emotionally, and economically. Choosing the right drug and the right vehicle is of paramount importance, but so is ensuring that the patient knows how and when to apply what is given and that the quantity prescribed is suitable for the area to be treated.

More detailed disease-oriented therapeutic guidelines and discussion of pharmacologically active agents used in topical preparations may be found in monographs.[3–6] In this chapter, some fundamental principles of topical therapy are addressed: (1) classification and clinical application of topical formulations, (2) review of vehicle ingredients commonly used in topical medicaments, and (3) appropriate administration and dosage of topical therapy.

CLASSIFICATION AND CLINICAL APPLICATION OF TOPICAL FORMULATIONS

The term *vehicle* is used for those substances that bring specific drugs into contact with the skin. The vehicle itself may have beneficial nonspecific, or "bland," effects on the skin by possessing cooling, protective, emollient, occlusive, or astringent properties. For any drug to be effective topically, it must be formulated at the proper concentration and in the proper vehicle. An unsuitable combination of drug and vehicle could compromise the effectiveness of the formulation for the following reasons: (1) there may be pharmaceutical incompatibility that inactivates the drug (drug-vehicle interaction), (2) the vehicle may be inappropriate for the skin condition being treated (vehicle-skin interaction), or (3) the vehicle may bind the drug too tightly to permit adequate delivery into the affected layer of the skin (vehicle-drug and drug-skin interactions).

In general, the most important vehicles for topical use may be divided into monophasic, biphasic, and triphasic forms, which can be further classified as shown in Fig. 242-1. For methods of compounding basic materials into monophasic and multiphasic vehicles and rules for the incorporation of specific drugs, Polano's practical and insightful reference is recommended highly.[7]

Monophasic Vehicles

POWDERS In general, powders promote drying. Since they adhere poorly to the skin, their use is almost completely limited to cosmetic and hygienic purposes. Most powders used for skin care consist of zinc oxide or titanium oxide for covering properties, talc (hydrous magnesium silicate) for smooth application, and a stearate (usually zinc or magnesium) for improved adherence to the skin. Powders containing hexachlorophane and zinc undecylenate as disinfectants or antifungal agents such as tolnaftate and nystatin are commonly used in intertriginous areas for hygienic or prophylactic purposes. They provide soothing and cooling effects by virtue of minimizing friction and increasing surface area. However, powders should not be used in the flexures when skin is weeping, as the application may mix with the exudate to form abrasive clumps. Powders containing starch should not be used in intertriginous areas when infection (e.g., *Candida albicans*) is present, because microorganisms can readily metabolize the glycogen in the starch and lead to exacerbation of the condition.

LIQUIDS Liquids are used as solvents for drugs or are made into gels by the addition of thickening agents. Clinical applications of liquid preparations include wet dressings, baths, tinctures, paints, topical solutions, aerosols, and sprays.

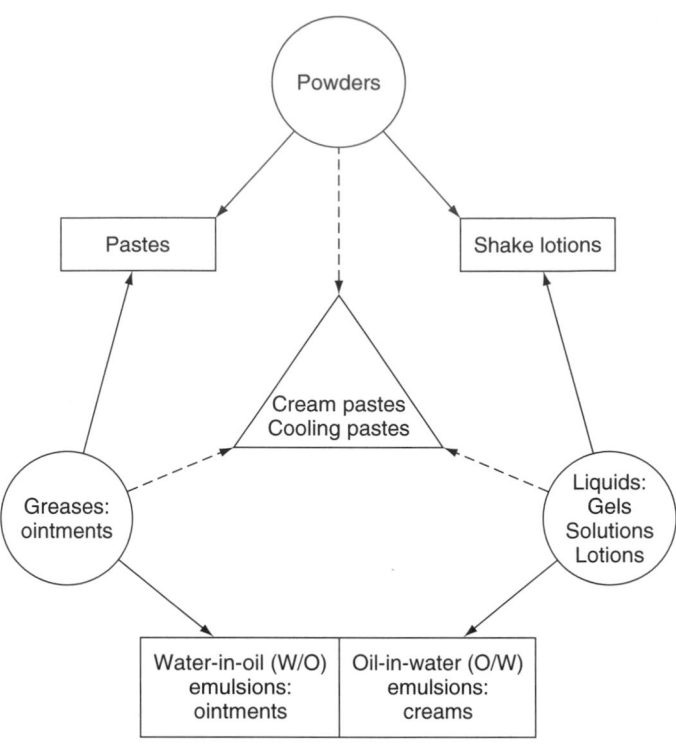

The derivation of basic forms of topical application. ○, Monophasic vehicles; □ biphasic vehicles; △ triphasic vehicles. (*Modified from Polano,[7] with permission.*)

Wet dressings are indicated in the treatment of acute inflammatory states characterized by oozing, weeping, and crusting and in bullous disease, erosions, and ulcers. Solutions of aluminum acetate (Burow's solution; Domeboro) have been used since the nineteenth century for wet dressings. The original Burow's solution was prepared with aluminum and lead acetate, resulting in a solution of aluminum acetate and a sediment of lead sulfate. Burow's solutions in use today are prepared from aluminum sulfate, acetic acid, and calcium carbonate in varying proportions. For wet dressings or compresses, 5% concentration is diluted 1:20 to 1:40 in water. The aluminum acetate in Burow's solution acts as an astringent to decrease exudation by precipitation of protein. For wounds infected with *Pseudomonas*, wet dressings with 0.1 to 0.5% silver nitrate or 5% acetic acid may be helpful. Of historic interest, potassium permanganate wet dressings were used extensively for treating fungal infections, but their use has diminished because of their staining properties.

Baths may cleanse the skin of adherent scale or debris and may be used to deliver medication to the skin in the treatment of widespread, less exudative conditions. Because baths and soaks tend to produce maceration, the duration of immersion should be limited to 30 min. Colloidal oatmeal (Aveeno) or starch may be added for their soothing and antipruritic effects, and bath oils added to prevent drying of the skin. Patients using bath oils should be made aware that these oils cause the bathtub to become slippery and be cautioned against falls. Tar baths, combined with dithranol pastes and UV light, constitute the Ingram regimen for psoriasis. Preparations such as coal tar solutions (3 oz per 1/2 tub of water) or commercial preparations may be used. Bath oils with tar (e.g., Balnetar) are recommended in the treatment of psoriasis and atopic dermatitis.[6]

Tinctures and *paints* are organic solvent solutions that evaporate rapidly after application to the skin, leaving a film of active ingredient. Tinctures were originally alcoholic solutions derived from maceration of herbs.[7] The term *paint* refers to staining solutions such as Castellani's paint. Tinctures and paints are of limited use in modern clinical setting because of their excessive drying and staining properties.

Solutions are solvents in which active ingredients are dissolved to clarity. *Lotions* are liquid preparations in which inert or active medications are suspended or dissolved. As the aqueous phase evaporates, there is drying and cooling of the skin, which are properties desirable in the treatment of exudative dermatoses. All types of lotions are particularly well suited for use in hairy and intertriginous regions, as they are relatively easy to apply and do not predispose to folliculitis.

Lotions and solutions may also be suspended in a propellant to be delivered to the skin in the form of an aerosol or spray. This form of delivery may be useful when the degree of inflammation, tenderness, or oozing makes direct application difficult or painful. However, aerosol systems have the drawbacks of being expensive, ecologically unsound, and not conducive to maintaining the stability of active ingredients.

Gels are transparent, colloidal dispersions that liquefy on contact with skin. They are not greasy and are cosmetically acceptable. When applied to the skin, gels dry as a nonocclusive film and are appropriate for use on hairy areas. Most gels are solutions of solvents such as water, acetone, alcohol, or propylene glycol thickened with organic polymers such as carbopols. While having the advantage of being water-washable, nongreasy, and cosmetically elegant, gels have the disadvantages of being easily removed by perspiration and lacking any protective or emollient properties.

GREASY BASES   Oils are rarely used alone in topical therapy because they do not adhere to the skin. The principal use of oils (mineral oil, cottonseed oil, etc.) is the removal of fat-miscible applications from the skin. Oils added to baths, as mentioned earlier, may function as emollients.

Petrolatum (Vaseline), a purified semisolid hydrocarbon ointment base, and white (decolorized) petrolatum are the most widely used ingredients in water-repellent ointments. Petrolatum is used in dermatology mainly for its emollient properties. It is highly occlusive and water-insoluble and hydrates the skin by preventing water loss. This oleaginous group of bases changes little with time and does not require preservatives and is therefore not associated with allergic contact dermatitis.

Biphasic Vehicles

SHAKE LOTIONS   These are watery lotions to which powder is added so that the area for evaporation is increased. Generally, zinc oxide, talcum, calamine, glycerol, alcohol, and water are used, to which specific drugs and stabilizers may be added. These lotions dry and cool wet, weeping skin. The name *shake lotion* indicates one of the drawbacks of this formulation: a tendency to sedimentation requires shaking prior to each use in order to obtain a homogeneous suspension. In addition, when the water has evaporated from the skin, the powder particles may clump together and become abrasive. For this reason, patients should be instructed to remove such residues carefully prior to reapplication of shake lotions.

CREAMS   Creams are emulsions of oil-in-water (O/W). In a cream, the oil droplets are dispersed in a continuous phase of water or a polar liquid. Emulsifying agents are necessary for such formulations

to increase the surface area of the dispersed phase and that of any therapeutic agent in it. Creams may also contain preservatives, which may produce an allergic contact dermatitis. Creams are used widely for their cooling, moisturizing, and emollient effects.

OINTMENTS   These spread easily to form a protective film on the skin and are more lubricating than creams. Due to their occlusive nature, ointment vehicles generally provide better topical penetration of incorporated drugs than do creams or lotions. Ointment bases used at present in dermatology can be classified into four categories: water-repellent hydrocarbons (e.g., petrolatum, previously discussed under monophasic grease bases), absorption bases, water-in-oil (W/O) emulsions, and water-soluble ointments. Absorbent ointments such as hydrophilic petrolatum and Aquaphor resemble hydrocarbon bases but contain emulsifying agents and *do* absorb water to form W/O emulsions. They are insoluble in water and are difficult to wash off. W/O emulsions spread more easily on the skin and are more cosmetically acceptable than petrolatum or absorbent ointments. W/O emulsions can absorb water into the discontinuous phase, but since oils make up the continuous phase, they are still difficult to wash off. Hydrophilic ointment is a good example of a W/O emulsion. Water-soluble ointments are usually polyethylene glycol preparations (carbowaxes). This group of bases is completely water-soluble and water-washable and lacks an oil phase. Polyethylene glycol ointment is capable of acting as a vehicle for both water-soluble and -insoluble medicaments.

PASTES   Pastes are ointments into which 20 to 50% powder (e.g., zinc oxide, starch) is incorporated. The powders must be insoluble in the ointment base, usually petrolatum or carbowax, in order to exert an absorbent effect. Pastes are more drying, less greasy, and often better tolerated than ointments. They may be useful in the treatment of ulcers and in the management of chronic exudative dermatoses and thick lichenified plaques. In psoriasis therapy, incorporation of anthralin (0.1 to 0.2%) in Lassar's paste (a stiff paste of zinc oxide, cornstarch, and white petrolatum) allows localization of anthralin to the psoriatic plaques.

Triphasic Vehicles

Cooling pastes and cream pastes are triphasic vehicles that consist of oil-water-powder mixtures in varying proportions. The first cooling paste was prepared by Unna in 1900. Cooling pastes are useful for their soothing properties on acutely inflamed and weeping skin, and indications for their use are similar to those for wet dressings. They are less drying than shake lotions and have the added benefit of cooling. Cream pastes are obtained by adding zinc oxide to O/W or W/O emulsions and are comparable to the greasy pastes described earlier. The basic formula for a cooling paste includes zinc oxide, calcium hydroxide solution, and oil.[7]

VEHICLE INGREDIENTS COMMONLY USED IN TOPICAL PREPARATIONS

Table 242-1 lists the general classes of commonly used vehicle ingredients found in topical preparations: emollients, humectants, solvents, emulsifying agents, stabilizers, and thickening agents. It

TABLE 242-1

Vehicle Ingredients Commonly Used in Topical Preparations

Emulsifying agents
  Cholesterol
  Disodium monooleamidosulfo-
    succinate
  Emulsifying wax
  Polyoxyl 40 stearate
  Polysorbates
  Sodium laureth sulfate
  Sodium lauryl sulfate

Auxiliary emulsifying agents/emulsion
  stabilizers
  Carbomer
  Cetearyl alcohol
  Cetyl alcohol
  Glyceryl monostearate
  Lanolin and lanolin derivatives
  Polyethylene glycol (PG)
  Stearyl alcohol

Stabilizers
  Benzyl alcohol
  Butylated hydroxyanisole (BHA)
  Butylated hydroxytoluene (BHT)
  Chlorocresol
  Citric acid
  Edetate disodium
  Glycerin
  Parabens
  Propyl gallate
  Propylene glycol (PG)
  Sodium bisulfite
  Sorbic acid/potassium sorbate

Solvents
  Alcohol
  Diisopropyl adipate
  Glycerin
  1,2,6-Hexanetriol
  Isopropyl myristate
  Propylene carbonate
  Propylene glycol (PG)
  Water

Thickening agents
  Beeswax
  Carbomer
  Petrolatum
  Polyethylene
  Xanthan gum

Emollients
  Caprylic/capric
    triglycerides
  Cetyl alcohol
  Glycerin
  Isopropyl myristate
  Isopropyl palmitate
  Lanolin and lanolin
    derivatives
  Mineral oil
  Petrolatum
  Squalene
  Stearic acid
  Stearyl alcohol

Humectants
  Glycerin
  Propylene glycol (PG)
  Sorbitol solution

should be recognized that many ingredients may serve more than one function in a particular formulation. The information that follows may be considered a time-honored "staple" of vehicle formulation.

Emollients

Emollients are occlusive agents that make the skin soft and pliable by increasing hydration of the stratum corneum. Petrolatum is probably the most occlusive and therefore the best emollient available. Due to its inherent greasy feel, petrolatum is often mixed with other materials to produce a more cosmetically acceptable vehicle. Cetyl alcohol and stearyl alcohol are mixtures of solid aliphatic alcohols that lubricate the skin without being greasy. Isopropyl myristate and isopropyl palmitate are light, mobile liquids that function as emollients without imparting a heavy, greasy feeling on the skin.

Humectants

These are hygroscopic agents that draw moisture into the skin. It should be noted, however, that under dry atmospheric conditions humectants actually withdraw water from the skin. Glycerin, propylene glycol, and sorbitol are examples of humectants used in topical products.

Solvents

Solvents are used to increase the solubility of the active drug in the formulation or to solubilize other necessary ingredients in the product. Water, alcohol, glycerin, and propylene glycol are commonly used solvents.

Emulsifying Agents

These are added to thermodynamically unstable dispersions of two or more immiscible liquid phases (usually an aqueous phase and an oil phase) to improve stability by decreasing surface tension. Synthetic emulsifying agents used in pharmaceutical preparations are anionic, cationic, and nonionic surfactants. Soaps and sodium lauryl sulfate (SLS) are common examples of anionic surfactants. Alkali soaps are stable only at a high pH (>10) because the fatty acid precipitates out of solution at lower pHs. SLS is widely used in topical products as a detergent, wetting agent, and emulsifying agent. Unlike soaps, SLS is compatible with dilute acid and with calcium and magnesium ions. As an emulsifying agent, SLS is usually combined with other emulsifying agents to give more stable emulsions. Sodium lauryl ether sulfate (sodium laureth sulfate) is an ethoxylated agent often used in place of SLS because it is less irritating to the skin.

Cationic emulsifying agents such as quaternary ammonium salts are weak emulsifiers and are generally used in combination with other emulsifying agents. They form emulsions at pHs of 4 to 6. Cationic emulsifiers are physically incompatible with anionic emulsifiers.

By far the most widely used emulsfiying agents are the nonionics. The most commonly used nonionics are combinations of polysorbates and sorbitan esters (Tweens and Spans). Polysorbates are water-soluble polyoxyethylene derivatives of the fatty acid esters of sorbitol. In general, the polysorbates form O/W emulsions, which are stable and little affected by high concentrations of electrolytes or by pH changes. Sorbitans are fatty acid esters of sorbitol and its anhydrides. They are oil-soluble, water-dispersable surfactants. They form W/O emulsions, which have the same stability characteristics as the polysorbate emulsions. Because of their differing solubilities in oil and water and their tendency to form different types of emulsions (O/W versus W/O), the polysorbates and sorbitans are commonly blended to form stable fine-textured emulsions.

In addition to the above emulsifying agents, there are also many chemicals, some of which are weak emulsifiers, that are used as auxiliary emulsifying agents or emulsion stabilizers. Glyceryl monostearate is a poor W/O emulsifying agent used by itself, but it helps to stabilize emulsions when used as an auxiliary agent. Lanolin is a complex mixture of esters of alcohols and acids that has some emulsifying action because it contains cholesterol and aliphatic alcohol. Lanolin alcohol and related semisynthetic molecules impart a high gloss and creamy texture to emulsions and may help to stabilize emulsions by absorption of water. Polyethylene glycols are strongly hydrophilic and useful as emulsion stabilizers.

Stearyl and cetyl alcohols are weak emulsifiers of the W/O type, but, combined with water-soluble surfactant emulsifiers such as SLS, they form powerful emulsifiers of the O/W type. Emulsions formed from such mixed emulsifiers exhibit superior stability and thickening properties compared with emulsions formed with SLS alone.

Stabilizers

Stabilizers include preservatives, antioxidants, and chelating agents. Preservatives are added to prevent or inhibit microbial growth. The parabens, which are esters of *p*-hydroxybenzoic acid, are the most widely used preservatives in topical preparations. Parabens are active against molds, fungi, and yeasts but are less effective against bacteria. Benzyl alcohol, quaternary ammonium surfactants, sorbic acid, potassium sorbate, propylene glycol, and glycerin are examples of other commonly used preservatives.

Antioxidants are used in products in which the drug or the vehicle may deteriorate through oxidation. Butylated hydroxyanisole (BHA) and butylated hydroxytoluene (BHT) are used to retard oxidative degradation in oils and fats. Propyl gallate prevents rancidity in oils and fats and inhibits the development of peroxides in ethers and similar substances. Ascorbic acid, sulfites, and sulfur-containing amino acids are examples of antioxidants used in aqueous phases. Chelating agents, such as citric acid and sodium EDTA, are used to complex heavy metals in aqueous phases and can be considered as synergists for the antioxidants.

Thickening Agents

These include materials used to thicken or increase the viscosity of products or to suspend ingredients in the formulation. They may act as emulsion stabilizers or as ointment bases. Beeswax is used to increase viscosity in ointments and enables the incorporation of water in the formulation to produce W/O emulsions. Carbomers (carbapol or carboxyvinyl polymers) are synthetic, high molecular weight polymers. When dispersed in water as the free acid, they form thin cloudy products. Upon neutralization with alkali hydroxides or amines, carbomers form clear gels of varying viscosities. Carbomers are also used as suspending agents. Petrolatum may be used by itself as an ointment vehicle or in emulsions to increase viscosity and emolliency. Although petrolatum is compatible with most drugs formulated in ointments, it may not release certain drugs readily. Polyethylene, a polymer of ethylene, is resistant to oxidation and is used as a stiffening agent to replace natural waxes.

APPLICATION AND DOSAGE OF TOPICAL THERAPY

The three-phase model of drug action described by Arriens[8] may be applied to topical therapy:

1. The initial *pharmaceutical phase* is represented by application of a drug-vehicle combination to the skin. Studies on the importance of the vehicle deal with this phase.
2. The *pharmacokinetic phase* covers the penetration and permeation of the drug into the skin. After permeation through the skin, no further therapeutic effect in the skin is expected. Systemic effects follow.

3. The *pharmacodynamic phase* refers to the interaction of the drug with receptors in the normal or diseased skin.

These pharmacologic phases of skin therapy are influenced by a myriad of biologic and physiochemical factors, the most pertinent of which include the concentration of the active drug; the amount of the drug-vehicle applied to the skin; and the frequency, mode of application, and regional variation in absorption characteristics of different anatomic sites.[7]

Concentration

The importance of the concentration of active drug was recognized early because most dermatologic drugs have the potential to be irritants at high doses, and some topically applied drugs have systemic toxicity when applied to large areas in high concentrations (e.g., salicylic acid, phenol).

The concentration-response curves for various topical glucocorticoids have been shown to rise steeply to a plateau, above which further increases in concentration do not enhance the effect. However, the concentration at which the response plateaus was found to be different for each glucocorticoid, indicating that the optimal concentration is different for each drug.[9] It is reasonable to assume that the concentration-response curve for other topically applied drugs is similarly nonlinear.

Frequency

It is known that potent fluorinated steroids form reservoirs in the stratum corneum.[10] Although it is possible to elicit vasoconstriction responses for several days after application of these steroids, it is not clear whether or not the reservoirs have therapeutic significance. In a study of 12 patients with steroid-responsive dermatoses, six daily treatments of a topical glucocorticoid were found to be no more effective than three daily applications.[11] When percutaneous absorption of radioactive-labeled hydrocortisone was studied in rhesus monkeys, no significant difference in total absorption was demonstrated for a given amount, whether applied as a single dose or in three divided doses per day.[12] Similarly, one application of fluocinonide ointment was as effective as four applications a day in 52 patients with psoriasis.[13]

It is likely that a single daily application of a drug (at least for glucocorticoids) is a sufficient, if not the most efficient, schedule of delivery to the skin. However, the nonspecific emollient or protective effect of the cream or ointment is likely to be enhanced with more frequent application. This raises the possibility of designing rational, safe, and economical treatment regimens that alternate the use of specific pharmacologic agents with nonspecific remedies.

Quantity of Application

Dosage of topical therapy remains an elusive art form, in marked contrast to scientifically guided dosage for systemic therapy. Quantitative aspects of topical therapy are too often neglected. It must be remembered that the quantity of medication prescribed inevitably influences the way the patient uses the remedy. Insufficient amounts result in too sparing application or interruption of treatment, which may undermine the success of therapy. Excessive amounts pose an unnecessary economic burden on the patient and are simply wasteful. Both physicians and patients should be aware of the approximate cost of generic and trade products. Information regarding the cost of drugs is available in the yearly editions of the American Druggist Blue Book[14] or the Drug Topics Red Book.[15] Whenever possible, the optimum amount of medication needed until the patient's next visit or until the eruption clears should be calculated and prescribed accordingly.

In general, thickness of the layer applied to the skin does not appear to enhance the penetration of a specific drug.[16] Schalla et al. also maintain that a thick layer of an ointment or cream gives no better therapeutic effect than a thin layer.[17] This concurs with the authors' clinical observation that the quantities used by different patients for similar lesions vary greatly without appreciable difference in the therapeutic outcome. The following quantitative recommendations for prescribing topical medications assume that the thickness of application is approximately 0.1 mm.

One gram of cream covers an area approximately 10 by 10 cm. An ointment spreads up to 10 percent further. According to Arndt, the amount needed for the single application of a cream or ointment to the face or hands is 2 g; to one arm or the anterior or posterior trunk, 3 g; to one leg, 4 g; and to the entire body, 30 g. Suggested guidelines (adapted from New York University's Dermatologic Formulary) for amounts of topical medications to dispense, based on the estimated percent body surface area, frequency of application, and duration of therapy, are presented in Table 242-2.

Regional Variations in Penetration

Table 242-3 lists the different regions of the body in order of increasing resistance to penetration by chemical agents. There is marked regional variation in the amount of drug absorbed from different anatomic sites.[18,19] Whereas agents may pass quantitatively through the mucous membrane if they are held in place long enough, penetration through the palms and soles is negligible and for practical purposes insignificant.[20] The stratum corneum is considered to be the rate-limiting barrier to percutaneous absorption. Once the stratum corneum has been removed, there is no essential barrier to the penetration of any chemical agent through the human skin.[20] Hence, the anatomic regional differences in the penetration characteristics essentially represent the variation in the thickness of the stratum corneum. It follows, then, that skin diseases or injuries

TABLE 242-3

Regional Differences in Penetration*

1. Mucous membrane
2. Scrotum
3. Eyelids
4. Face
5. Chest and back
6. Upper arms and legs
7. Lower arms and legs
8. Dorsa of hands and feet
9. Palmar and plantar skin
10. Nails

*Most penetration with number 1 and less penetration with increasing numbers.

that cause damage to the stratum corneum permit increased percutaneous absorption. It should be recognized, however, that as the skin begins to heal, the barrier capacity of the stratum corneum may be restored, and the penetration of drugs decreases accordingly.

The Role of Occlusion in Topical Therapy

When drugs such as glucocorticoids are applied to the skin under an airtight occlusive plastic dressing, their efficacy and absorption are increased 10 to 100 times.[21] Occlusion with a plastic dressing increases the skin surface area that can be treated, increases hydration and temperature, and also appears to induce a reservoir of glucocorticoid in the stratum corneum that lasts for several days after application. The increased absorption of drugs applied under plastic occlusive dressings may also lead more rapidly to the appearance of undesirable side effects such as local atrophy and suppression of the hypothalamus-pituitary-adrenal axis when glucocorticoids are used. Also, greatly enhanced irritant or toxic side effects occur with occlusive dressings when other agents, such as tar, are used. Occlusive therapy can also promote infection, folliculitis, and miliaria and interfere with heat exchange.

A less completely occlusive dressing, the hydrocolloid patch, has recently become available for the treatment of plaques of psoriasis or other chronic recalcitrant disorders.[21] These dressings, used in combination with topical glucocorticoids or other topical medications, have many potential advantages. They are flexible, self-adhesive, skin-colored, and waterproof and can therefore cover up unsightly lesions and allow patients to bathe or shower with the patch in place. The degree of epidermal hydration is sufficient to enhance the effectiveness of topical glucocorticoids to the same degree as plastic film, as measured by the blanching assay, yet because the patches are not completely occlusive, there is no significant bacterial proliferation, skin infection, or irritation.[21] How well these new dressings work in association with various medications will await their widespread use and careful and controlled clinical studies. Simple hydration of skin before application of topical glucocorticoids may increase penetration up to fivefold. The optimal technique for applying topical medications, therefore, is to hydrate the skin by immersion in water for about 5 min, followed immediately

TABLE 242-2

Suggested Amounts of Topical Medications to Dispense—Cream or Ointment

AREA TREATED	ESTIMATED % BODY SURFACE AREA	SINGLE APPLICATION, G	TWICE A DAY FOR 1 WEEK, G	THRICE A DAY FOR 1 WEEK, G
Face	3	1	15	20
Scalp	6	2	30	45
One hand	3	1	15	20
One arm	7	3	45	60
Anterior trunk	14	4	60	90
Posterior trunk	16	4	60	90
One leg including foot	20	5	70	100
Anogenital area	1	1	15	20
Whole body	100	30–40	450–500	600–1000

SOURCE: New York University's Dermatologic Formulary—Skin and Cancer Unit.

by application of the cream or ointment. If occlusion techniques are to be employed, the hydrocolloid dressing, plastic film, or body suit should be put on directly thereafter.

REFERENCES

1. Frazier CN, Blank IH: *A Formulary For External Therapy of the Skin.* Springfield, IL, Charles C. Thomas, 1954, p 3
2. Sulzberger MB et al: *Dermatology: Diagnosis and Treatment,* 2d ed. Chicago, Year Book, 1961, p 39
3. Arndt KA: *Manual of Dermatologic Therapeutics. With Essentials of Diagnosis,* 5th ed. Boston, Little, Brown, 1995
4. Provost TT, Farmer ER: *Current Therapy in Dermatology—2.* Philadelphia, Decker, 1988
5. Landow RK: *Handbook of Dermatologic Treatment.* Greenbrae, CA, Jones Medical, 1983
6. Maddin S (ed): *Current Dermatologic Therapy.* Philadelphia, Saunders, 1991
7. Polano MK: *Topical Skin Therapeutics.* Edinburgh, Churchill Livingstone, 1984
8. Arriens EJ: *Drug Design.* Part IV. New York, Academic, 1973, p 9–10
9. Schlagel CA, Northern JI: Comparative anti-inflammatory efficacy of topically applied steroids on human skin. *Proc Soc Exp Biol* **100**:629, 1959
10. Barry B: *Dermatologic Formulation—Percutaneous Absorption.* New York, Dekker, 1983, p 116
11. Eaglstein WH et al: Topical corticosteroid therapy: Efficacy of frequent application. *Arch Dermatol* **110**:955, 1974
12. Wester RL et al: Frequency of application on percutaneous absorption of hydrocortisone. *Arch Dermatol* **113**:620, 1977
13. Senter RP: Topical fluocinonide and tachyphylaxis. *Arch Dermatol* **119**:363, 1983
14. *1996 Blue Book.* New York, American Druggist, 1996
15. *Drug Topics Red Book.* Oradell, NJ, Medical Economics, 1996
16. Ponec M: Chemical and biochemical aspects of topical psoriasis treatment. Thesis, Leiden, Netherlands, 1977, p 49
17. Schalla W et al: Factors influencing penetration of external steroids. *Aktuelle Dermatol* **6**:3, 1980
18. Feldman RJ, Maibach HI: Regional variation in percutaneous penetration of ^{14}C cortisol in man. *J Invest Dermatol* **48**:181, 1967
19. Feldman RJ, Maibach HI: Percutaneous penetration of steroids in man. *J Invest Dermatol* **52**:89, 1971
20. Christophers E, Kligman AM (eds): *Topical Corticosteroid Therapy: A Novel Approach to Safer Drugs.* New York, Raven, 1988, p 7
21. Ryan TJ (ed): *Beyond Occlusion: Dermatology Proceedings.* No. 137 of International Congress Symposium Series. London/New York, Royal Society of Medicine Series, 1988

CHAPTER 243

Leslie Baumann
Francisco Kerdel

Topical Glucocorticoids

Hydrocortisone, the first topically effective glucocorticoid, was introduced by Sulzberger and Witten in 1952.[1] Subsequently, a succession of ever more potent glucocorticoid preparations have been developed. Currently, topical steroids are the most frequently prescribed of all dermatologic drug products.

PHARMACOLOGY

Steroids can be divided into two classes: fluorinated and nonfluorinated. The term *fluorinated steroid* is used when referring to the steroids that have been chemically altered to increase their potency. The strength of a steroid can be increased by halogenation at the 9α position, which allows improved activity within the target cell and decreased breakdown into inactive metabolites.[2] Halogenation of the compound, however, also increases the mineralocorticoid effects, which leads to more systemic side effects. Addition of a hydroxide or methyl group at the 16 position will increase efficacy without a concomitant increase in the mineralocorticoid effect.[3]

Several factors affect the potency of glucocorticoids regardless of the intrinsic potency of the glucocorticoid molecule. The vehicle in which the steroid is incorporated may be as important as the steroid molecule itself because the vehicle affects the amount of steroid that is released in any given period of time. Very occlusive vehicles, such as ointments, potentiate glucocorticoid effects because they provide increased hydration of the stratum corneum and increase its permeability. By covering the skin with an occlusive dressing such as plastic wrap, this effect can be heightened as much as 100-fold. The solubility of the glucocorticoid in the vehicle also affects penetration into the epidermis. Propylene glycol is one agent commonly used to dissolve the glucocorticoid in the vehicle, and it is found in many topical glucocorticoid preparations.[4] In general, compounds that contain higher amounts of propylene glycol tend to be more potent.

Treatment of the skin prior to application of the topical steroid may also affect the absorption of the compounds into the skin. For example, use of keratolytics or fat solvents such as acetone will allow increased penetration by disrupting the epidermal barrier. Tape stripping of the skin has also been shown to increase the absorption of hydrocortisone by 78 to 90 percent.[5]

Topical glucocorticoid research has focused on strategies to optimize potency while minimizing side effects. One strategy is to develop compounds with enhanced anti-inflammatory effects and minimal unwanted atrophogenic and adrenal suppressive effects. Another strategy is to develop compounds that exert their effects on the epidermis and then are quickly broken down into inactive metabolites. Research to develop a nonsteroidal compound with the same anti-inflammatory effects of glucocorticoids but without the side effects is currently ongoing.[6] Work in the first two areas has led to the development of medium potency topical steroids with less potential for adrenal suppression and less incidence of atrophy. Mometasone furoate (Elocon) and alclometasone dipropionate (Aclovate) are two of the more recently developed products that are potent but have less potential for adrenal suppression.

CLINICAL USES

The clinical effectiveness of glucocorticoids is related to four basic properties: vasoconstriction, antiproliferative effects, immunosuppression, and anti-inflammatory effects. Topical steroids cause capillaries in the superficial dermis to constrict, thus reducing erythema. The ability of a given glucocorticoid agent to cause vasoconstriction usually correlates with its anti-inflammatory potency, and thus vasoconstriction assays are often used to predict the clinical activity of an agent. These assays in combination with double-blind clinical trials have been used to separate the topical glucocorticoids into seven classes based on potency. Class 1 includes the most potent, while class 7 contains the least potent. Table 243-1 lists many of the available topical glucocorticoids according to this classification.

The antiproliferative effect of topical glucocorticoids is mediated by inhibition of DNA synthesis and mitosis. Control of cellular proliferation is a complex process composed of cascades of stimulating influences that are counteracted by multiple inhibitory circuits. Many of these processes are probably influenced by glucocorticoids.[7]

The effectiveness of glucocorticoids in part may also be secondary to their immunosuppressive properties. The mechanism responsible for immunosuppression is poorly understood. Several studies have shown that glucocorticoids can cause mast cell depletion in the skin.[8] This may explain the utility of topical glucocorticoids in patients with urticaria pigmentosa. Experiments have also shown that topical glucocorticoids cause a local inhibition of chemotaxis of neutrophils[9] in vitro, and decrease the number of Ia+ Langerhans cells[10] in vivo. In addition, several cytokines are directly affected by glucocorticoids, including interleukin(IL) 1, tumor necrosis factor α, granulocyte-macrophage colony-stimulating factor, and IL-8.[11] These effects may also be due to the steroid action on AP-1.

It is believed that glucocorticoids exert their potent anti-inflammatory effects by inhibiting the formation of prostaglandins and other derivatives of the arachidonic acid pathway.[12] It is known that glucocorticoids inhibit the release of phospholipase A_2, the enzyme responsible for liberating arachidonic acid from cell membranes, thus inhibiting the arachidonic acid pathway. For many years it was believed that glucocorticoids caused macrophages and other cells to release a specific protein, lipocortin, that was thought to have a direct inhibitory action on phospholipase A_2.[13] Although lipocortins have since been purified and their genes cloned and sequenced,

TABLE 243-1

Potency Ranking of Some Commonly Used Brand-Name Glucocorticoids*

Class 1 (super-potent)
  Temovate cream 0.05%[a]
  Temovate ointment 0.05%[a]
  Diprolene cream[†] 0.05%[b]
  Diprolene ointment 0.05%[b]
  Psorcon ointment 0.05%[c]

Class 2 (potent)
  Cyclocort ointment 0.1%[d]
  Diprolene cream AF 0.05%[b]
  Diprosone ointment 0.05%[e]
  Elocon ointment 0.1%[f]
  Florone ointment 0.05%[g]
  Halog cream 0.1%[h]
  Lidex gel 0.05%[i]
  Lidex cream 0.05%[i]
  Lidex ointment 0.05%[i]
  Maxiflor ointment 0.05%[g]
  Topicort cream 0.25%[j]
  Topicort gel 0.05%[j]
  Topicort ointment 0.25%[j]

Class 3 (potent)
  Aristocort A ointment 0.1%[k]
  Cutivate ointment 0.005%[l]
  Cyclocort cream 0.1%[d]
  Cyclocort lotion 0.1%[d]
  Diprosone cream 0.05%[e]
  Florone cream 0.05%[g]
  Halog ointment 0.1%[h]
  Lidex E cream 0.05%[i]
  Maxiflor cream 0.05%[g]
  Valisone ointment 0.1%[m]

Class 4 (mid-strength)
  Cordran ointment 0.05%[n]
  Elocon cream 0.1%[f]
  Kenalog cream 0.1%[k]
  Synalar ointment 0.025%[o]
  Westcort ointment 0.2%[p]

Class 5 (mid-strength)
  Cordran cream 0.05%[n]
  Cutivate cream 0.05%[l]
  Diprosone lotion 0.05%[e]
  Kenalog lotion 0.1%[k]
  Locoid cream 0.1%[q]
  Synalar cream 0.025%[o]
  Valisone cream 0.1%[m]
  Westcort cream 0.2%[p]

Class 6 (mild)
  Aclovate cream 0.05%[r]
  Aclovate ointment 0.05%[r]
  Aristocort cream 0.1%[k]
  Desowen cream 0.05%[s]
  Synalar solution 0.01%[o]
  Synalar cream 0.01%[o]
  Tridesilon cream 0.05%[s]
  Valisone lotion 0.1%[m]

Class 7 (mild)
  Topicals with hydrocortisone dexamethasone, flumethasone, prednisolone, and methylprednisolone

*Class 1 is the super-potent category; potency descends with each group. There is no significant difference between agents *within* classes 2 through 7; the compounds are simply arranged alphabetically. However, within class 1, Temovate cream or ointment is more potent than Diprolene cream or ointment and Psorcon ointment.
†Diprolene cream has been renamed Diprolene gel (whitener-free reformulation).
[a]Clobetasone propionate
[b]Betamethasone dipropionate (optimized vehicle)
[c]Diflorasone diacetate (optimized vehicle)
[d]Amcinonide
[e]Betamethasone dipropionate
[f]Mometasone furoate
[g]Diflorasone diacetate
[h]Halcinonide
[i]Fluocinonide
[j]Desoximetasone
[k]Triamcinolone acetonide
[l]Fluticasone propionate
[m]Betamethasone valerate
[n]Flurandrenolide
[o]Fluocinolone acetonide
[p]Hydrocortisone valerate
[q]Hydrocortisone butyrate
[r]Alclometasone dipropionate
[s]Desonide

their role in the anti-inflammatory action of glucocorticoids has been questioned.[14] It is the current belief that glucocorticoids inhibit phospholipase A_2 in cells by directly inducing phosphorylation of the enzyme.[15] Other proposed additional mechanisms for the anti-inflammatory effects of glucocorticoids include inhibition of phagocytosis and stabilization of lysosomal membranes of phagocytizing cells.[16]

Certain variables must be considered when treating skin disorders with topical glucocorticoids. For example, the responsiveness of diseases to topical glucocorticoids varies. In this setting, diseases can be divided into the three categories shown in Table 243-2: highly responsive, moderately responsive, and least responsive. Highly responsive diseases will usually respond to weak steroid preparations; less responsive diseases require medium potency steroids; and the least responsive category requires high potency topical steroids.

Before choosing a topical glucocorticoid preparation, one must consider the area of the body that is to be treated because regional differences greatly affect the activity of the topical agent. Penetration of the glucocorticoid varies according to the skin site, and this in turn is related to the thickness of the stratum corneum and the vascular supply to the area. For example, penetration of topical steroids over the eyelids and scrotum is 4 times greater than for the forehead and 36 times greater than for the palms and soles. Inflamed, moist, and denuded skin also shows increased penetration. Areas of the body where the skin is inherently thin not only allow for increased penetration of the drug but are more susceptible to develop side effects than other areas where the skin is thick (see Table 242-3). Potent topical steroids (classes 1 and 2) should rarely, if ever, be used in the areas with the highest level of penetration, such as the eyelids.

Pediatric Uses

Topical glucocorticoids are highly effective, and few side effects are observed when a low potency preparation is used for brief periods of time without occlusion in children. Infants, however, are at an increased risk for side effects for several reasons. They have a higher ratio of skin surface area to body weight, and therefore application to a given area results in a greater potentially systemic dose of steroid. Infants may also be less able to metabolize potent glucocorticoids rapidly.[17] Premature infants are especially at risk because their skin is thinner and the penetration rate of topically applied drugs is greatly increased.[18] Application of topical steroids under the diaper area results in occlusion of the steroid by the diaper, and increased penetration occurs. Excess absorption of topical glucocorticoids can suppress endogenous cortisol production. Subsequent cessation of topical steroid therapy after an extended treatment period can therefore result in an Addisonian crisis characterized by nausea, anorexia, postural hypotension, and vascular collapse. Deaths from Addisonian crisis have been reported with the use of topical steroids,[19] and the risk of this occurring is greater in children. Chronic suppression of cortisol production can also lead to growth retardation. A morning plasma cortisol level can be performed to screen for adrenal suppression. If suppression is present, the child should be slowly weaned from the steroids to prevent an Addisonian crisis.

TABLE 243-2

Responsiveness of Dermatoses to Topical Application of Corticosteroids

HIGHLY RESPONSIVE	MODERATELY RESPONSIVE	LEAST RESPONSIVE
Psoriasis (intertriginous)	Psoriasis	Palmoplantar psoriasis
Atopic dermatitis (children)	Atopic dermatitis (adults)	Psoriasis of nails
Seborrheic dermatitis	Nummular eczema	Dyshidrotic eczema
Intertrigo	Primary irritant dermatitis	Lupus erythematosus
	Papular urticaria	Pemphigus
	Parapsoriasis	Lichen planus
	Lichen simplex chronicus	Granuloma annulare
		Necrobiosis lipoidica diabeticorum
		Sarcoidosis
		Allergic contact dermatitis, acute phase
		Insect bites

Geriatric Uses

Elderly patients can similarly have thin skin, which allows for increased penetration of topical glucocorticoids. They are also more likely to have preexisting skin atrophy secondary to aging and may be diaper-dependent, so the same precautions used in the treatment of infants should be used when treating elderly patients. Topical glucocorticoids should be used infrequently, for brief periods, or under close supervision in those patients with preexisting skin atrophy to avoid unwanted side effects.

Uses in Pregnancy

Appropriate human studies using topical glucocorticoids in pregnancy have never been undertaken. Studies in animals, however, have shown that topical steroids are systemically absorbed and may cause fetal abnormalities, especially when used in excessive amounts, under occlusive dressings, for prolonged periods of time, or when the more potent agents are used. However, numerous studies of pregnant patients taking systemic glucocorticoids throughout pregnancy have shown no increases in the incidence of fetal abnormalities. Most topical steroids are rated by the U.S. Food and Drug Administration (FDA) as category C drugs, which implies that caution must be exercised when used in pregnancy. It is currently unknown whether topical glucocorticoids are excreted in breast milk; however, they should be used with caution in breast-feeding mothers and should never be used on the breasts prior to breast feeding.

DOSAGE SCHEDULES AND FORMULATIONS

Twice-a-day topical application of glucocorticoids is recommended on the labels of most formulations, although no scientific evidence has ever established this schedule as the optimum one. In order to decrease the risks of side effects, it is best to establish, with the aid of the patient, the longest elapsed time between successive applications that still controls the disease. This method may help to decrease the development of side effects and tachyphylaxis. Tachyphylaxis has been demonstrated in experimental conditions by diminished vasoconstriction, rebound of DNA synthesis, and recovery of histamine wheals after application of topical steroids in patients with a history of long-term topical steroid usage.[20]

Topical steroids come in many different vehicles and dosage forms. Ointments are water-insoluble mixtures of oil and petrolatum and are the best preparation when treating dry skin conditions because they provide the most moisture of the available preparations. They are also useful for treating conditions on areas of the body with thick skin, such as the palms and soles. The occlusive nature of the ointment and its ability to moisturize the stratum corneum allow for increased penetration and enhanced potency of the drug. Peanut oil has also been combined with steroids to form a preparation that is thinner and easier to apply while retaining the hydrating capability of ointments. However, patients may feel that ointments and oils are too greasy. New emollient creams have been devised that contain an increased amount of petrolatum but with less greasiness than ointments, and some patients find them more cosmetically appealing.

Creams are suspensions of oil in water. They vary in their composition and generally are far less greasy than ointments but do not provide the same degree of hydration to the skin. Many patients find creams easier to spread on the skin and more cosmetically pleasing than ointments. However, creams may contain emulsifiers and preservatives that can lead to allergic reactions in some patients.

Lotions are suspensions of oil in water and are similar to creams. They contain agents to help solubilize the glucocorticoids and to allow them to be spread more easily on the skin. Solutions contain no oil but are composed of water, alcohol, and propylene glycol. Gels are solid components at room temperature but melt on contact with the skin. Lotions, solutions, and gels have less penetration than ointments but are useful in treating hair-bearing areas such as the scalp where greasiness is cosmetically displeasing to the patient. Steroid-impregnated tapes are useful because they provide occlusion with increased penetration and provide protection of the skin lesion from manipulation, such as scratching, by the patient. Sprays containing steroids are available, and while they represent a convenient mode of applying these agents, the inefficiency of the delivery system is such that they are seldom recommended. (For a more complete discussion of vehicles for topical preparations, see Chap. 242.)

ADVERSE EFFECTS

Side effects from the use of topical steroids have become more prevalent since the introduction of the higher potency topical steroids. Using these products on thin or denuded skin, on the elderly or pediatric population, or under occlusion increases the incidence of side effects. Striae and atrophy, the most commonly observed side effects, occur with prolonged use and are more likely to occur in areas of sweating, occlusion, or high penetration such as the axilla or groin. In general, atrophy does not occur until the agent has been used for 3 to 4 weeks and is usually reversible. Striae, which develop when the weakened skin is stretched, are not reversible. Prolonged treatment can also result in "steroid acne," which is characterized by crops of dense, inflamed pustules in the

same developmental stage. These lesions occur on the face, chest, and back. Perioral and periocular dermatitis have been associated with the use of topical steroids and usually improve with cessation of the steroid. Patients with rosacea who are given topical steroids may initially improve, but a severe rebound phenomenon consisting of edema and pustules may occur. For these reasons, steroid use should be discouraged in the treatment of rosacea and perioral and periocular dermatitis. Purpura, which represents easy bruising, may develop when steroids are used in areas of thin skin.

Topical steroids can also cause suppression of the pituitary-adrenal axis. Growth retardation and iatrogenic Cushing's syndrome are known but rare complications of topical steroid therapy. Morning plasma cortisol serologic tests can be performed to screen for adrenal suppression. If these levels are abnormal, adrenal function can be assessed further by using the cosyntropin stimulation test. Most topical and systemic side effects are readily reversible if recognized early by the clinician. The incidence of side effects, however, can be significantly reduced if appropriate guidelines for topical steroid use are followed.

Patients treated with topical glucocorticoids may develop a contact or irritant dermatitis to the steroid itself or, more commonly, to one of the ingredients used as a preservative. An increase in contact dermatitis due to the steroid component has been reported.[21] Most topical steroid ointments are free of preservatives and are less likely than other topical agents to cause an allergic or irritant contact dermatitis. The most common preservatives that cause allergic contact dermatitis include parabens, polyethylene glycol, and benzyl alcohol (Table 243-3). Fragrance and local anesthetics are also sensitizers that may be included in the topical preparations.

DRUG INTERACTIONS

Topical glucocorticoids have few, if any, known drug interactions. For this reason they are often mixed with other topical medications such as antifungals and antibiotics to form combination products. Although a few combination products are available, development of new combination products has not been encouraged by the FDA. In fact, the FDA has recently rejected new drug applications for combinations of topical antibacterials such as neomycin, bacitracin, and hydrocortisone because the manufacturers were unable to provide proof of effectiveness of each component. However, many of these combination products are found in many countries outside the United States. Theoretically, there should be no need for a combination when each component can be obtained separately.

TABLE 243-3

Common Sensitizers in Topical Steroids

Parabens
Propylene glycol
Benzyl alcohol
Chlorocresol
Ethylenediamine hydrochloride
Isopropyl palmitate
Polysorbate 60
Stearyl alcohol

REFERENCES

1. Sulzberger MD, Witten VH: The effect of topically applied compound 1 in selected dermatoses. *J Invest Dermatol* **19**:101, 1952
2. Brattsand R: Influence of 16α, 17α-acetyl substitution and steroid nucleus fluorination on the topical to systemic activity ratio of corticosteroids. *J Steroid Biochem* **16**:779, 1982
3. Phillips GH: Locally active corticosteroids: Structure-activity relationships, in *Mechanisms of Topical Corticosteroid Activity,* edited by L Wilson, R Marks. Edinburgh, Churchill-Livingstone, 1976, pp 1–18
4. Stoughton RB, Cornell RC: Topical steroids in dermatology, in *Topical Corticosteroid Therapy: A Novel Approach to Safer Drugs,* edited by E Christophers, E Schopf, AM Kligman. New York, Raven, 1988, pp 1–12
5. Hepburn D et al: Topical steroid treatment in infants, children and adolescents in *Advances in Dermatology,* vol 9, edited by J Callen, M Dahl, L Golitz, H Greenway, L Schachner. St Louis, Mosby, 1994, pp 225–254
6. Flower RJ: A molecular biology approach to the design of safer steroid-like drugs, in *Topical Corticosteroid therapy: A Novel Approach to Safer Drugs,* edited by E Christopher. New York, Raven, 1988, pp 27–35
7. Almawi WY et al: Partial mediation of glucocorticoid antiproliferative effects by lipocortins. *J Immunol* **157**:5231, 1996
8. Lavker RM et al: Cutaneous mast cell depletion results from topical corticosteroid usage. *J Immunol* **135**:2368, 1985
9. Norris DA et al: The effect of epicutaneous glucocorticosteroids on human monocyte and neutrophil migration in vivo. *J Invest Dermatol* **78**:386, 1982
10. Furue M, Katz SI: Direct effects of corticosteroids on epidermal Langerhans cells. *J Invest Dermatol* **92**:342, 1989
11. Guyre PM et al: Glucocorticoid effects on the production and actions of immune cytokines. *J Steroid Biochem* **30**:89, 1988
12. Naray-Fejes-Toth A et al: Glucocorticoid effect on arachidonic acid metabolism in vivo. *J Steroid Biochem* **30**:155, 1988
13. Blackwell GJ et al: Macrocortin: A polypeptide causing antiphospholipase effects of corticosteroids. *Nature* **287**:147, 1980
14. Duval D, Freyss-Beguin M: Corticosteroids and prostaglandin synthesis: We cannot see the wood for the trees. *Prostaglandins Leukot Essent Fatty Acids* **45**:85, 1992
15. Bailey JM: New mechanism for effects of anti-inflammatory corticosteroids. *Biofactors* **3**:97, 1992
16. Katchman SD et al: A transgenic mouse model provides a novel biological assay of topical corticosteroid potency. *Arch Dermatol* **131**:1274, 1995
17. West DP et al: Pharmacology and toxicology of infant skin. *J Invest Dermatol* **76**:147, 1981
18. Holbrook K, Sybert V: Basic science, in *Pediatric Dermatology,* edited by L Schachner, R Hansen. New York, Churchill Livingstone, 1995, pp 17–18
19. Cook LJ et al: Iatrogenic hyperadrenocorticism during topical steroid therapy: Assessment of systemic effects by metabolic criteria. *J Am Acad Dermatol* **6**:1054, 1982
20. Singh G et al: Tachyphylaxis to topical steroids measured by histamine-induced wheal suppression. *Int J Dermatol* **25**:324, 1986
21. Lutz ME et al: Allergic contact dermatitis due to topical application of corticosteroids: Review and clinical implications. *Mayo Clin Proc* **72**:1141, 1997

CHAPTER 244

Alexandria S. Kongsiri
Chris Ciesielski-Carlucci
Matthew J. Stiller

Topical Nonglucocorticoid Therapy

Topical nonglucocorticoid therapies are one of the foundations of a dermatologist's therapeutic armamentarium. Several important new topical medications have become available within the past few years. In this chapter we review the latest additions to the dermatologist's repertoire of treatments and reevaluate many of the older therapies that are still highly effective. The drugs in this section are not an exhaustive list. The reader should consult individual chapters for treatment of specific diseases.

ACNE THERAPIES

ADAPALENE   Adapalene, derived from naphthoic acid, has potent retinoid and anti-inflammatory properties. As a 0.1% gel, it was developed for use in acne vulgaris and has slightly lower irritant effects than tretinoin.[1] Adapalene has comedolytic, antiproliferative, and anti-inflammatory activity.[2] It acts on cell proliferation and differentiation via retinoic acid receptor–binding proteins and gene transactivation.[2] Follicular penetration is observed with adapalene, which presents an advantage in treating acne. In 12-week international multicenter studies comparing adapalene gel 0.1% to tretinoin gel 0.025%, adapalene was as effective and in some cases superior to tretinoin.[3] Side effects associated with adapalene 0.1% gel include burning, pruritus, dryness, and scaling.[3]

α-HYDROXY ACIDS   The α-hydroxy acids are keratolytic and as such are discussed below. Their use in the treatment of acne stems from the ability to reduce follicular hyperkeratosis and facilitate stratum corneum desquamation.[4] They have been used in the treatment of acne, but there is currently no well-controlled clinical trial to determine their efficacy compared to other treatment modalities.

AZELAIC ACID   Azelaic acid is a naturally occurring aliphatic dicarboxylic acid that is a competitive inhibitor of tyrosinase. Its use as an acne therapy was serendipitous, since in some patients treated for melasma acne improved.[5] Azelaic acid is a reversible inhibitor of cytochrome P_{450} reductase and 5 α-reductase in microsomes and a reversible inhibitor of some enzymes in the respiratory chain.[6] Its efficacy in acne is attributed to its antimicrobial activity, especially against *Propionibacterium acnes*, and inhibition of comedone formation.[7] Azelaic acid (20% cream) has been reported to be as effective as oral tetracycline in inflammatory acne. A beneficial effect may not be observed until 4 weeks after initiation of treatment, which may need to be continued for several months.

BENZOYL PEROXIDE Benzoyl peroxide rapidly improves both inflammatory and noninflammatory acne lesions. It can be used effectively as monotherapy for mild disease. Benzoyl peroxide has antibacterial activity, reducing the population of *P. acnes* by generating reactive oxygen species.[8] There is a reduction of the fatty acid content in follicles but no effect on sebum production or composition.[9] Benzoyl peroxide can initially irritate skin, and bleaching of skin and hair have been reported.[10] It is available in a variety of formulations, including gels, lotions, creams, and washes with a concentration of 2.5% to 10%, or by prescription in a variety of formulations.

CLINDAMYCIN Clindamycin 1% is available in several topical formulations (gel, solution, lotion). If initial improvement diminishes with prolonged use of topical antibiotics, the development of resistance should be considered. Antibiotic therapy may be discontinued for 1 month then resumed or an alternative agent substituted.

ERYTHROMYCIN Topical erythromycin has been reported to reduce acne lesions by 50 to 60 percent. It decreases comedogenic free fatty acids and exerts an anti-inflammatory effect by suppressing neutrophil chemotaxis. Topical erythromycin has a low potential for sensitization. A combination gel of 3% erythromycin and 5% benzoyl peroxide is more effective than either agent used alone and may inhibit development of resistance.[11]

TAZAROTENE Tazarotene is a synthetic acetylenic retinoid that acts on nuclear retinoic acid receptors. This preferential affinity at the cellular level may result in effects on corneocyte accumulation and cohesion, keratinocyte differentiation, and a blockade of pro-inflammatory and hyperproliferative transcription factors.[11]

TRETINOIN (VITAMIN A ACID) (See also Chap. 245) Vitamin A profoundly affects keratinization. The effective topical use of vitamin A acid was first reported in 1962 and has since found widespread use. The actions of tretinoin include effects on keratinization, epidermopoiesis, DNA synthesis, lysosomal stabilization, and prostaglandin synthesis.[12] By increasing mitotic activity and turnover of follicular epithelial cells and regulating maturation of epidermal cells, tretinoin induces thickening of the granular layer and normalization of parakeratosis. Tretinoin treatment in acne enhances epithelial turnover, loosening keratin debris; it promotes the drainage of preexisting comedones and inhibits formation of new ones. Tretinoin reverses abnormal desquamation and formation of micro-comedones by promoting the shedding of small aggregates of cells rather than sheets of coherent abnormal cells.[9]

Initially, tretinoin may cause erythema and tenderness of the skin, but the comedones then start to extrude[13] and do not usually re-form if therapy is continued. The irritation can be minimized by using the mildest formulation (0.025% cream) first and initiating its use on alternate days. Maximal therapeutic results take up to 6 weeks, and maintenance therapy may be required to prevent exacerbations. Tretinoin is available in cream, gel, and solution formulations in an assortment of concentrations.

Tretinoin may also be effective in other dermatologic conditions including ichthyosis vulgaris,[14] lamellar ichthyosis,[15] Fox-Fordyce disease (apocrine miliaria),[15] solar damage,[16] striae distensae,[17] Darier's disease,[18] and keratosis pilaris.[19]

ANALGESICS

CAPSAICIN Capsaicin, an active ingredient of cayenne peppers and other plants of the Capsicum family, contains about 0.1 to 2.0% of capsaicin.[20] It causes excitation of neural afferent C-fibers and reduction of substance P.[21] The mechanism of pain relief is not known; however, it may be due to reduction in afferent input following depletion of substance P. Consequently, pain impulses cannot be transmitted to the brain. When applied topically, capsaicin causes vasodilatation and a burning sensation. After repeated exposures, the burning sensation may diminish. Capsaicin is applied four to five times per day for 4 to 6 weeks. Patients should be instructed to wash their hands after each application to avoid inadvertent eye contact.[21] Capsaicin has been used to treat postherpetic neuralgia, painful diabetic neuropathy, postmastectomy pain syndrome, notalgia paresthetica, meralgia paresthetica, and cluster headaches.[21] The burning sensation experienced with capsaicin prevents successful blinding of clinical trials. Its effect appears to be modest, but it is quite safe.

EUTECTIC MIXTURE OF LOCAL ANESTHETIC (EMLA) EMLA cream contains a eutectic mixture of 50% lidocaine and 50% prilocaine in an oil-in-water emulsion.[22] EMLA is applied to intact skin and covered with an occlusive dressing. Anesthesia develops in hours at a depth in the skin proportional to the duration of application. Maximal penetration occurs 30 min after the removal of EMLA, and analgesia persists for several hours. Repeated and prolonged exposure to EMLA has not caused irritant effects or delayed hypersensitivity reactions.[23] EMLA is safe and particularly useful in children.

TOPICAL ANESTHETICS Topical anesthetics, such as benzocaine, are sensitizers that should be avoided. Lidocaine (United States) or lignocaine (U.K.) and other "amide" type agents are rare sensitizers and may be used.[24]

ANTIFUNGALS (See also Chap. 247)

ALLYLAMINES This group of topical antifungals includes terbinafine and naftifine. The fungicidal allyamines inhibit ergosterol synthesis, specifically squalene epoxidase, and thus alter the cell wall. They are lipophilic, allowing binding to the stratum corneum layer. Naftifine has similar antifungal potency to tolnaftate and clotrimazole but also exhibits anti-inflammatory activity.[25] Terbinafine remains in skin for up to 7 days after discontinuation of treatment.[26] The side effects of both terbinafine and naftifine include a low incidence of local burning, pruritus, dryness, and erythema.[26]

AZOLES The first- and second-generation imidazoles include clotrimazole,[26] econazole, ketoconazole, miconazole, and sulconazole as topical therapies; they have similar spectrums of efficacy and activity. They function by blocking synthesis of ergosterol, which plays an integral role in cell membrane structure and function. The imidazoles delay or inhibit cellular growth at low concentrations and are fungicidal at 5 to 10 times the minimum inhibitory concentration.

Ketoconazole is available in a shampoo formulation, which has excellent pityrosporicidal activity. It leads to more rapid clearing of lesions in tinea versicolor, with a cure rate greater than other compounds in treating *Pityrosporum* infections.[27]

The triazole terconazole has a wider spectrum and increased potency over imidazoles; terconazole also has fewer side effects.

CASTELLANI'S PAINT Named after Sir Aldo Castellani, this mixture contains resorcinol (8 g), acetone (4 mL), magenta (0.4 g), phenol (4.0 g), boric acid (0.8 g), industrial methylated spirit 90% (8.5 mL), and water (to 100 mL); it is fungicidal and bactericidal with local anesthetic effects.[28] The magenta liquid stains the skin red, but omitting the magenta makes the solution colorless and diminishes its effectiveness only slightly. Castellani's paint, usually applied to the intertriginous areas of the skin, is particularly effective in inflammatory intertriginous tinea and acute *Candida* paronychia. It has also been used to treat seborrheic eczema and tinea pedis. It has drying ability, which makes it useful in treating leg ulcers. It is applied daily for 2 weeks, usually at bedtime.

CICLOPIROX Ciclopirox acts by interfering with the uptake and availability of products required for membrane synthesis. Ciclopirox is fungicidal and fungistatic with anti-inflammatory properties. It is also reportedly effective against certain bacteria, *Actinomyces* and *Eumycetes* species, yeasts, and dermatophytes.[29]

HALOPROGIN Haloprogin exhibits activity against a variety of organisms, including dermatophytes and *Candida*, and against pityriasis versicolor and erythrasma. In yeast infections, it interferes with respiration and disrupts cell membranes. However, its mode of action in dermatophytic infections is not clearly elucidated. Its efficacy is similar to miconazole 2% cream.[29] The side effects associated with its use include local irritation, pruritus, and contact dermatitis.

POLYENES The polyenes, such as nystatin, act by increasing fungal cell membrane permeability by binding to membrane sterol. Nystatin is both fungicidal and fungistatic. It has been the standard therapy for candidiasis, especially oral thrush. Nystatin has limited systemic absorption but can rarely cause nausea, vomiting, and diarrhea.

POTASSIUM PERMANGANATE Potassium permanganate exhibits nonspecific activity against *Candida* species. It is discussed in further detail under the section on astringents.

SELENIUM SULFIDE Selenium sulfide is reported to increase fungal shedding by decreasing corneocyte production through its cytostatic effect on cells. It also has sporocidal activity. It is commonly used as adjunctive therapy in tinea capitis to reduce the period of infectivity[29] and in the treatment of pityriasis versicolor and seborrheic dermatitis. The over-the-counter selenium sulfide (1% concentration) has been reported to be as effective as the prescription 2% concentration in treating tinea capitis.[30] For the treatment of tinea versicolor the solution is applied and left on for 10 min before thoroughly rinsing. This is done on a daily basis for 7 days. There are many other effective regimens for using selenium

sulfide in tinea versicolor. Associated side effects include skin irritation and increased hair loss and discoloration.

TOLNAFTATE Tolnaftate has fungicidal activity. It inhibits squalene epoxidation as do the allylamines. However, it is not as effective as other antifungals in treating dry *Trichophyton rubrum* infections and candidiasis. Uncommon side effects of tolnaftate include contact dermatitis, urticaria, pruritus, and erythema. Stevens-Johnson syndrome and toxic epidermal necrolysis have also been reported.

UNDECYLENIC ACID When combined with zinc, calcium, and sodium, undecylenic acid has fungistatic activity.

WHITFIELD'S OINTMENT Whitfield's ointment, composed of 12% benzoic acid and 6% salicylic acid, is the least expensive preparation to treat dermatophytoses. Effective only against dermatophytes, it is fungistatic and keratolytic. Whitfield's ointment has the ability to kill spores and remove infected debris, although many patients discontinue use because of its local irritant effect.[31]

ZINC PYRITHIONE Zinc pyrithione is a general inhibitor of membrane transport in fungi. It has fungistatic and antimicrobial activity,[32] but its exact mode of action is unknown. Zinc pyrithione has been used to treat dandruff and psoriasis with variable effectiveness. It has been reported to cause allergic contact dermatitis.[33]

ANTI–HAIR LOSS

MINOXIDIL Minoxidil was originally developed as an oral antihypertensive. It is a potent vasodilator that acts directly on peripheral arterioles, decreasing blood pressure with resultant tachycardia. It was serendipitously observed that patients on minoxidil developed hypertrichosis.[34] Subsequently, it has been reformulated into a topical solution, which lacks the systemic effects, to treat alopecia. The exact mode of action of minoxidil is unknown, although it has been postulated that minoxidil increases cutaneous blood flow to the scalp. It is available in a 2% over-the-counter solution and a 5% prescription formulation. Approximately 30 percent of patients with male pattern baldness achieve desirable results. It has also been used in the treatment of alopecia areata with limited efficacy.[35] Minoxidil is reportedly more effective than placebo in the treatment of androgenic alopecia in women.[36]

ANTI-INFLAMMATORY AGENTS

COAL TAR Coal tar is manufactured as the by-product of processing coke and gas from bituminous coal (coal tars). The thick black viscous fluid is a combination of at least 10,000 different chemicals including aromatic hydrocarbons such as benzenes, naphthalenes, creosols, and phenols, of which only about 5 percent have been identified. Different distillation and manufacturing processes produce coal tars of different composition. There is no established method of standardization to determine the biogenic potency of the various coal tar preparations. The cruder the coal tar, the more therapeutically effective it is.

The method by which coal tar exerts its influence is still not well understood. Studies suggest that tars depress DNA synthesis and have an antimitotic effect. Coal tar applied to normal skin produces early suppression of epidermal DNA synthesis followed by a proliferative response.[37] When applications are continued for up to 40 days, there is a cytostatic effect resulting in epidermal thinning.[38] Tars have phototoxic or photodynamic activity, with an action spectrum in the UVA and visible range.

Tar is known to be carcinogenic in animals. Workers in the tar and pitch industry develop skin cancers, but there are very few reports of squamous epithelioma resulting from the therapeutic use of crude coal tar, to which hundreds of thousands of patients have been exposed worldwide. The few reports of cancers resulting from the therapeutic use of crude coal tar suggest that they may develop after application to flexural areas.

The most common adverse effects of tar are folliculitis and irritation. Other side effects include tar acne, phototoxicity, and allergic contact sensitivity.[39]

Efforts to produce cosmetically acceptable and effective formulations have been disappointing; tar application is messy and can stain clothing. Patient compliance is difficult, but therapeutic results in chronic eczema, especially atopic dermatitis, are gratifying. Coal tars are frequently formulated as gels, shampoos, and tar baths. Tar is a key component of the Goeckerman regimen.

SHALE TAR Shale tar (ichthammol) originates from shale oil that undergoes chemical degradation with ammonia and sulfuric acid to form a sulfur-rich substance. It is most often formulated with glycerin and is thought to have both anti-inflammatory and vasoactive properties. Ichthammol has been a time-honored standard in the treatment of eczema, seborrheic dermatitis, and rosacea and has also been used in the treatment of otitis externa when mixed with glycerol. There is little evidence of its pharmacologic activity, but safety is well established. In contrast to coal tar, shale tars are less irritating and are not photosensitizers, but they are also less effective.[40]

WOOD TAR Wood tars are obtained by distilling wood under controlled conditions. Oil of cade from juniper is the most common wood tar and has a strong and distinctive odor. Other wood tars include oil of beech, birch, and pine. They can be added to arachis oil (peanut oil) or simple bases as an application to the scalp in seborrheic dermatitis and psoriasis. Oil of cade is also a major ingredient in the 20-10-5 ointment, which consists of 20% oil of cade, 10% sulfur, and 5% salicylic acid. Like shale tars, wood tars are not photosensitizers.[40]

ANTI-MICROBIAL AGENTS

AMMONIATED MERCURY (UNGUENTUM BOSSI) The first mention of ammoniated mercury in medical therapy was by Daniel Turner in 1714. He subsequently warned of the dangers of its overuse in 1733. Ammoniated mercury was most commonly used to treat psoriasis but has also been used in impetigo, staphylococcal infections, and other infectious or inflammatory diseases.[41] It was not until 1967 that there was any understanding of mercury's mode of action. Lagerholm and Fritz[42] demonstrated in psoriatic plaques that mercury became concentrated in the ribosomes, chromatin, and other nucleolar structures. This led to the inference that mercury

interferes with protein synthesis, subsequently reducing epidermal proliferation. The use of mercury to treat dermatoses is usually ill-advised due to the severity of side effects, especially systemic effects, since mercury is absorbed through the skin. Mercury is deposited in the dermis, around blood vessels, in macrophages, and in elastic and collagen fibrils, resulting in blue-gray discoloration of skin that is largely therapy-resistant.[41] The most frequent adverse effect is allergic contact dermatitis.[41]

CHLORHEXIDINE Chlorhexidine is a bisbiguanide that has bactericidal and fungicidal activity. However, it does not kill bacterial spores[43] or mycobacteria,[44] although it does inhibit their growth. The antimicrobial activities have a rapid onset and persist for several hours after a single application.[45] Since it does not lose its effectiveness in the presence of whole blood, it is an important antiseptic, disinfectant, and preservative.

DYES The two dyes gentian violet (methylrosaniline chloride) and brilliant green (p-diethylamine triphenylmethanol) are both derivatives of triphenylmethane. Gentian violet has been used as a dye for fabrics, wood, and cosmetics and in food. It is also used as a biologic stain (Gram stain, nucleic acid stain), mycostatic agent in poultry feed, antiseptic, antihelminthic, and as a blood additive to prevent the transmission of Chagas' disease by transfusion.[46] Sterling first introduced gentian violet as an antiseptic in 1890.[46] The dyes are effective against *Candida* species, streptococci, and staphylococci, including methicillin-resistant *Staphylococcus aureus*. Additionally, gentian violet is an astringent.

There have been several hypotheses as to gentian violet's mode of antimicrobial activity. These include: (1) inhibition of bacterial cell wall formation at a site different than that of penicillin, (2) inhibition of protein synthesis, (3) alteration of the redox potential by the dye, (4) inhibition of glutamine synthesis, and (5) formation of a dye-bacteria un-ionized complex.[46] Gentian violet is mutagenic in bacteria and may be carcinogenic in mammalian cells due to its clastogenic activity. Gentian violet is most effective at a pH above 6, and brilliant green is most active at a pH below 7.[47] The loss of the antimicrobial activity of brilliant green is associated with decolorization of the dye.

Gentian violet is available in concentrations of 0.5% to 2%. However, it has been reported that a 2% aqueous solution of gentian violet causes severe skin necrosis. The attractiveness in using dyes as topical treatment stems from the fact that they are inexpensive and chemically and physically stable, unlike the modern formulations whose active ingredients are unstable (e.g., nystatin) or whose vehicle is unstable at temperatures above 40°C, a temperature which commonly occurs in developing countries.

HYDROGEN PEROXIDE Hydrogen peroxide has been used for a number of years as a cleansing agent and for the removal of debris. It has antibacterial properties against both gram-positive and -negative bacteria,[48] and its effervescent quality helps to debride wounds. It is useful in the treatment of bacterial infections, because hydrogen peroxide neither induces bacterial resistance nor have there been reports of allergic contact dermatitis.[48]

IODINATED COMPOUNDS Iodine solution is bactericidal and sporicidal at the proper concentration. It is also viricidal as a 1% aqueous solution. Iodophors are complexes of iodine with a carrier that slowly liberates inorganic iodine on contact with reducing substances. This preserves the antimicrobial activities of iodine without the irritant effects of the free tincture. However, their onset of action is slower than iodine solution, and they may be inactivated after contact with whole blood.

Povidone iodine Povidone iodine has a wide spectrum of in vitro activity against gram-negative and -positive bacteria, fungi, and viruses. Wound exudate, however, inactivates povidone. Care must also be taken when using this compound since systemic absorption can occur with resultant renal and thyroid dysfunction.[49]

Clioquinol Clioquinol, 5-chloro-8-hydroxy-7-iodoquinolinol, is weakly antifungal and antibacterial. It is a yellowish-white to brownish-yellow powder available in 1% and 3% cream and ointment bases.[50] It is effective alone or combined with a topical steroid to treat inflammatory dermatoses, especially in intertriginous areas. A yellowish discoloration may occur on clothing or skin with its use. There have been reports of delayed contact hypersensitivity and primary contact dermatitis.[50]

METRONIDAZOLE Metronidazole is an imidazole with the ability to inhibit fungi and *Trichomonas,* an anaerobic bacillus, and is most useful in rosacea. Its mode of action involves the impedance of leukocyte chemotaxis[51] and selective suppression of cellular immunity.[52]

MUPIROCIN Formerly known as pseudomonic acid A, mupirocin is obtained from the fermentation of *Pseudomonas fluorescens.* It is bacteriostatic at low concentration and bactericidal at the higher concentration achieved with topical application to the skin and mucous membranes. Mupirocin is distinct from other antibiotics, since it inhibits bacterial isoleucyl tRNA synthetase, preventing the incorporation of isoleucine into protein chains.[53] It has activity against staphylococci, streptococci, and certain gram-negative bacteria (*Haemophilus influenzae, Neisseria* species, *Pasteurella multocida*) but is inactive against normal skin flora (*Micrococcus, Corynebacterium, Propionibacterium* species). Since mupirocin has a unique structure and mode of action, there is no cross-resistance with other antibiotics. However, bacterial resistance has been reported since 1987.[54]

SILVER NITRATE Silver nitrate has been used for centuries for its strong antiseptic properties and it is effective against *S. aureus, S. epidermidis,* and *P. aeruginosa.* It is bacteriostatic at low concentration (0.5% formulation, used clinically) and bactericidal at higher concentrations (10%). The precise mode of its action is unknown. In its concentrated form, it is extremely toxic to tissues. The adverse effects associated with the use of silver nitrate in burn patients include electrolyte imbalance[55] and methemoglobinemia.

SILVER SULFADIAZINE This compound was originally synthesized in 1968 from silver nitrate and sodium sulfadiazine. It is available as a 1% cream and is effective against a wide spectrum of microbial pathogens. There are two purported mechanisms for its antimicrobial activity: inhibition of DNA replication and modification of the cell membrane. It is largely used to treat burn patients but has been used to treat a variety of other skin conditions including Stevens-Johnson syndrome. Side effects are very few. Of these, transient leukopenia is a side effect encountered with clinical use. It usually commences 2 to 3 days after initiating treatment and is associated with a disproportionate decrease in neutrophils. Early postburn leukopenia is mild and self-limited,[56] and therefore discontinuation of therapy is not usually necessary.[57] After 2 to 4 days of use, silver sulfadiazine can cause formation of a "pseudoeschar," which is due to the interaction of proteinaceous exudate in the wound with the drug.[47]

ANTIPARASITIC AGENTS

CROTAMITON Crotamiton (crotonyl-*N*-ethyl-*O*-toluidine) is a colorless or pale yellow oil used in the treatment of scabies and pediculosis capitis[58] and also as an antipruritic. However, the antipruritic activity of crotamiton has not been proven to be greater than placebo. The first clinical trial involving crotamiton as a scabicide was reported in 1946.[58] Newer antiparasitic formulations such as lindane 1% and permethrin cream 5% are more effective than crotamiton,[59] which is rarely a sensitizer.

GAMMA BENZENE HEXACHLORIDE Gamma benzene hexachloride, a chlorinated hydrocarbon pesticide, is very effective against lice and fleas as a 1% solution. It is amongst the slowest acting ovacides of several antiparasitic agents. Scabies resistant to gamma benzene hexachloride has been reported, as has central nervous system toxicity from systemic absorption.[60] It has been implicated in causing seizures in infants and young children receiving repeated topical applications of a 1% lotion over a prolonged period.[61] Aplastic anemia has also been reported.[62]

MALATHION Malathion is a moderately toxic organophosphate insecticide and is the fastest acting ovacide in comparison with other antiparasitic agents. However, it has only been tested in head lice, and there are no studies assessing its efficacy in scabies. It acts by nonreversibly blocking acetylcholine.[59] Contact dermatitis has been reported with its use.[63]

PERMETHRIN Permethrin [3-phenoxybenzyl($\pm$)-*cis-trans*-3-(2,2-dichlorovinyl)-2,2-dimethylcyclopropanecarboxylate] is a synthetic pyrethroid modeled after the natural insecticide found in the pyrethrum flower, *Chrysanthemum cinerariaefolium,* which has been used for centuries in Iran as an insecticide. It acts on parasitic nerve cell membranes, causing paralysis and death. It is available as a 1% cream rinse, which is left on for 10 min. A single application is effective against head lice and nits, with activity detectable at least 10 days after use. Permethrin as a 5% cream base is an effective scabicide,[64] and is the treatment of choice for children over 2 months of age and pregnant women. Permethrin is also effective against ticks, mites, and fleas and has been used in the treatment of rosacea.[65]

PYRETHRIN Pyrethrin is the naturally occurring ester of chrysanthemumic acid.[66] In combination with piperonyl butoxide, it is an effective alternative to gamma benzene hexachloride in the treatment of head lice[67] and nits. Pyrethrin is a neurotoxin, and piperonyl butoxide inhibits its metabolism, potentiating its effects. This combination has a quicker onset of action than gamma benzene hexachloride in killing head lice and is comparable in ovacidal activity. It is also effective against fleas, mosquitoes, and houseflies.

ANTIPERSPIRANTS

ALUMINUM COMPOUNDS Aluminum chloride, in solution in anhydrous ethyl alcohol (6 to 20%), has been used to treat hyperhidrosis.[68] The solution is applied to the axillae or the palms and soles for at least 6 to 8 h. Shaving of the axillae should be avoided for 24 to 48 h before application of aluminum chloride. Occlusion, used to increase efficacy, increases the likelihood of irritation. Once excessive sweating is under control, use may be decreased to once or twice a week as maintenance therapy. The mechanism of action is controversial and may occur by blockage of the sweat duct or by atrophy of the secretory cells.[69]

ALDEHYDES Gluteraldehyde solution applied to palms or soles has been used to control hyperhidrosis.[70] It may be used on alternate days until desired results are achieved and then decreased to once a week or as needed. Gluteraldehyde as a 10% solution may leave brown pigmentation on the skin. A 2% solution will not produce this discoloration but is less effective. Formaldehyde is a sensitizer and is not commonly used.

METHENAMINE Methenamine is a 6-carbon, 4-nitrogen compound that has been used for a number of years to treat bacterial infections of the urinary bladder. At acid pH, it releases ammonia and formaldehyde. A 10% solution is effective in mild to moderate hyperhidrosis, rarely producing allergic reactions. As a 5% firm gel stick it is effective in reducing palmoplantar hyperhidrosis after 1 month of use, and the effect continues for up to 3 weeks after discontinuation of the product.[71]

ANTIPRURITIC AGENTS

ANTIHISTAMINES Topical antihistamines, such as diphenhydramine, have been associated with a high incidence of contact sensitization[72] and cross-reactivity and rarely with photoallergic reactions.[73] Given the availability of other effective topical agents, topical antihistamines should be avoided.

DOXEPIN Tricyclic compounds, particularly doxepin hydrochloride, given orally are known to have antipruritic properties. Doxepin cream 5% may be used to treat pruritus, although the mechanism of its effect is uncertain. However, doxepin has an affinity for H_1 and H_2 receptors and may also exert its antipruritic effect through the antagonism of α-adrenergic, muscarinic, and serotonergic receptors and through inhibition of norepinephrine and serotonin neuronal re-uptake and the inhibition of platelet-activating factor production.

Topical doxepin has a potential for sensitization.[74] It appears to be effective for atopic dermatitis, lichen simplex chronicus, contact dermatitis, and nummular eczema.[75] Doxepin cream may also be used as an adjuvant to glucocorticoids in treatment of pruritus.

MENTHOL Menthol is a highly lipid-soluble cyclic terpene alcohol, often used interchangeably with or in addition to camphor. It is a naturally occurring plant oil obtained from the *Mentha* species. Brazil is currently the largest producer and supplier of menthol. Menthol is a known chemical activator of cold-sensitive A-delta fibers.[76] Paradoxically, in a recent study, menthol was reported to have a central inhibitory effect on these same fibers. [77] It has also been shown that menthol does not decrease the duration or magnitude of histamine-induced pruritus.[78]

PHENOL Phenol in low concentrations acts as an antipruritic agent through its anesthetic effect. It may be percutaneously ab-

sorbed and should be avoided in pregnant women and infants.[79] It is a common ingredient in over-the-counter preparations for pruritus.

PRAMOXINE HYDROCHLORIDE Pramoxine hydrochloride, a topical anesthetic, is effective in cases of mild to moderate pruritus. It is available in combination with menthol, petrolatum, and hydrocortisone. It is a sensitizer less frequently than other topical anesthetics.

ANTIVIRALS

ACYCLOVIR Acyclovir, 9-(2-hydroxyethoxymethyl) guanine, has specific antiviral activity against herpes simplex virus (HSV), varicella, and Epstein-Barr virus. Acyclovir completely inhibits viral DNA synthesis by inactivating viral DNA polymerase.[80] The highest level of activity is against HSV-1 followed by HSV-2.

Acyclovir is available in a 5% ointment. It has lower efficacy than systemic formulations and is therefore only indicated in initial HSV-2 infections and mucocutaneous HSV infection of immunocompromised patients.[81] Some patients with ulceration may experience pain with application of acyclovir.[81]

ASTRINGENTS

ALUMINUM SALTS Aluminum acetate tablets diluted 1:10 to 1:40 (Burow's solution) are an effective astringent. Over-the-counter aluminum sulfate and calcium acetate (Domeboro) are available and, when dissolved in water, make a modified Burow's solution.[82] These solutions may be used as wet dressings, compresses, or soaks.

POTASSIUM PERMANGANATE Potassium permanganate is a strong oxidizing agent. Solutions of 1:4,000 to 1:16,000 may be used as wet compresses to reduce weeping. Alternatively, a 1:25,000 solution may be used as a medicated bath. Undissolved crystals can burn the skin. The use of this agent is limited because of bright purple staining, which may be removed with a weak solution of oxalic acid or sodium thiosulfate.

SILVER NITRATE Silver nitrate in 0.5% aqueous solution is an astringent and antimicrobial that is valuable in the treatment of infected eczema, gravitational ulcers, and other weeping and/or infected skin lesions. It is applied as a wet dressing and stains the skin black. Its cosmetic disadvantage is often outweighed by the rapid resolution of weeping and superficial infection, often by resistant organisms.[83] A 40% silver nitrate solution in alcohol is helpful in the management of severe folliculitis, and in solid form it may be used as a hemostat.

BLEACHING AGENTS

RETINOIC ACID Retinoic acid is not only an effective acne therapy but has also been used successfully to treat melasma. Retinoic acid combined with 2 to 3% hydroquinone has synergistic effects and causes a rapid decrease in skin pigmentation.[84] It has also been used to treat melasma in black patients effectively.

AZELAIC ACID This agent was discussed under acne treatment. However, it was originally intended for use in disorders of hyperpigmentation. Azelaic acid exhibits antityrosinase activity and is effective in melanosis due to hyperfunction or proliferation of melanocytes. The reduction of hyperpigmentation is superior to 2% hydroquinone[85] and is equivalent to 4% hydroquinone.[86] It has been used to treat melasma, lentigo maligna,[87] and primary cutaneous malignant melanoma.[88] Local irritation with azelaic acid is more common than with hydroquinone. Azelaic acid does not affect normal melanocytes and fibroblasts, and leukoderma and ochronosis are not associated with its use.[86]

HYDROQUINONE A hydroxyphenolic compound, hydroquinone is used extensively as a skin bleaching agent. Its targets tyrosinase, inhibiting conversion of dopa to melanin. It is an effective depigmenting agent in many disorders of hyperpigmentation including melasma, ephelides, and postinflammatory hyperpigmentation.

Hydroquinone has been combined with retinoic acid and/or dexamethasone to enhance efficacy. By far the most worrisome side effect of hydroquinone use is development of ochronosis. This is seen with prolonged use of strong concentrations (6%) of hydroquinone. The first cases of hydroquinone-induced ochronosis occurred in South African Bantu women using 6% hydroquinone for many years.[89] Other adverse events seen with hydroquinone use are development of irritant and allergic contact dermatitis, nail discoloration, and postinflammatory hyperpigmentation.[90] Hydroquinone is available over the counter at concentrations less than 2%.

KOJIC ACID Kojic acid (5-hydroxy-2-hydroxymethyl-4H-pyran-4-one), a pyrone compound, was first isolated from *Aspergillus* in 1907. It can also be obtained from some *Penicillium* and *Acetobacter* species. It is present in many traditional Japanese foods including soybean paste (miso), soybean sauce, and Japanese wine (sake).[91] Mishima et al.[92] initially demonstrated the effects of kojic acid on depigmentation and suppression of melanogenesis. Evidence suggests that it acts by suppressing free tyrosinase through the chelation of the copper moiety in this enzyme.[93]

It is available as a 1% cream in a variety of over-the-counter formulations in Japan as a skin bleaching agent. In a clinical trial in the United States, 1% kojic acid combined with glycolic acid was found to be as effective as 2% hydroquinone in treatment of melasma.[94] Kojic acid reportedly causes contact allergy and has a high sensitizing potential.

KERATOLYTIC AGENTS

α-HYDROXY ACIDS α-Hydroxy acids (lactic acid, glycolic acid, citric acid, glucuronic acid, and pyruvic acid) are found in a variety of natural products including cane sugar, fruits, and yogurt. They are extremely effective keratolytics.[95] α-Hydroxy acids reduce the thickness of hyperkeratotic stratum corneum by reducing corneocyte adhesion in the lower levels. These agents are effective in the treatment of disorders of keratinization (e.g., ichthyosis, hyperkeratotic eczema) and photoaging[96] and have also been used in acne and hyperpigmentation. The pHs of the various α-hydroxy acid preparations including cleansers, moisturizers, and chemical peeling agents are important in determining their efficacy.

PROPYLENE GLYCOL A 40 to 60% aqueous solution of propylene glycol, under occlusion, is effective in softening the skin in cases of ichthyosis.[97] It is also available as a gel containing 6% salicylic acid or combined with lactic acid in a lotion. These are very effective keratolytic agents and are cosmetically acceptable.

SALICYLIC ACID Salicylic acid may be used in concentrations ranging from 0.5 to 60% in almost any base. In concentrations of 3 to 6%, it causes shedding of scales by softening the horny layers. In concentrations higher than 6%, salicylic acid is destructive to tissue. It is for this reason that it is employed in wart therapy. Salicylism has been reported with widespread and prolonged use, especially in children.[79] Sensitization is rare, and irritation can be minimized if introduced at lower concentrations. Its action on hyperplastic keratin is likely twofold. First, it decreases keratinocyte adhesion, thereby promoting desquamation of the horny layer of skin, and second, it increases water binding, thereby hydrating the keratin.[98]

UREA Urea is proteolytic at high concentrations. It has been used as an aqueous solution in the management of black hairy tongue[99] and also to remove nails affected by fungal infections or psoriasis. Urea has been added to some topical glucocorticoid preparations. In various bases, 5 to 10% urea is utilized in the management of ichthyosis. However, some patients experience burning with this therapy.

PSORIASIS THERAPIES

ANTHRALIN Anthralin (USP) or dithranol (BP) is a synthetic derivative of chrysarobin derived from chrysarophanic acid. Chrysarophanic acid is a natural product derived from Goa powder (chrysarobine or yellow araroba), which is extracted from the South American or southern Asian *Vouacopoua araroba* tree.

Anthralin's exact mode of action is unknown. It may affect DNA synthesis (probably mitochondrial DNA), reducing cell turnover, or affect various enzyme systems (e.g., leukotriene synthesis, polyamines, respiratory function).[100] Anthralin is oxidized, and biologically active free radicals are formed. These are most likely responsible for the irritant effects and upon further oxidation form dimers that cause a brownish staining of the skin.[66] The most common adverse events seen with anthralin use are erythema, irritancy, and contact dermatitis.

Anthralin stains normal skin dark brown or black. Consequently, it is usually prepared in a paraffin base so that it does not spread to normal skin. Anthralin is available in pastes, ointments, and creams. Anthralin sticks (not available in the United States) are useful for ease of application. Short-contact therapy (30 min/day), which minimizes irritation, is most commonly used in home treatment.[101] It is a mainstay of topical therapy for the management of psoriasis in the Ingram regimen.

CALCIPOTRIOL Calcipotriol is a vitamin D analogue. Applied topically, calcipotriol has greater efficacy than tars and short-contact dithranol and equal efficacy to betamethasone valerate.[102,103] It possesses the same therapeutic properties as vitamin D_3 including inhibition of epidermal proliferation, induction of differentiation, and anti-inflammatory effects.[104] However, it has a much smaller hypercalcemic effect. Hypercalcemia may occur if more than 100 g is used per week. It is applied initially twice daily, and maximal improvement can be expected within 6 to 8 weeks. Cutaneous irritation may occur in up to 20 percent of patients. This agent should be used cautiously on the face, groin, or intertriginous areas. In view of the risk of hypercalcemia and high cost, this preparation is not recommended for patients with extensive psoriasis. It can be used in conjunction with PUVA but should be applied after exposure to UVA.[105]

TAZAROTENE   Tazarotene is a new synthetic acetylenic retinoid with retinoic acid receptor–specific activity and is useful in treatment of mild to moderate plaque psoriasis. Tazarotene normalizes abnormal keratinocyte differentiation, has antihyperproliferative activity, and is anti-inflammatory.[106] It is nonsensitizing, nonphototoxic, and nonphotoallergenic.[107] Tazarotene is available in a 0.05% and 0.1% gel. It is effective as a once-daily application, and clearing can occur in 12 weeks. The most common side effect is local skin irritation.

WART THERAPIES

DINITROCHLOROBENZENE   Contact immunotherapy with dinitrochlorobenzene (DNCB) was first described in 1973. Cure rates have varied between 70 and 90 percent.[108] DNCB is a potent sensitizer whose exact mechanism of action is not known, but it seems to induce a cell-mediated immune response (type IV hypersensitivity).[109] DNCB is mutagenic and potentially carcinogenic.

DIPHENYLCYCLOPROPENONE   Diphenylcyclopropenone is also used in contact immunotherapy in much the same way as DNCB. However, it is not mutagenic.[110]

5-FLUOROURACIL   5-Fluorouracil is a pyrimidine analogue that inhibits thymidine synthetase, thereby inhibiting DNA synthesis. It has been used successfully in the treatment of flat, mosaic, and genital warts.[111] It may also be very effective in periungual warts resistant to other therapies.[112] Its effectiveness may be heightened by an occlusive dressing or in combination with salicylic acid.

FORMALDEHYDE   Formaldehyde acts similarly to glutaraldehyde. It is useful in the treatment of mosaic plantar warts, which are especially resistant to therapy. A 3% solution is used to soak the infected area for 15 to 20 min daily. The solution can be reused.

GLUTARALDEHYDE   Glutaraldehyde is viricidal. It hardens the wart surface, thereby facilitating paring. It stains skin brown, making it less cosmetically appealing. The benefit to using this agent is that it reduces viral shedding from the wart surface, thus reducing the infectious risk.

IMIQUIMOD   Imiquimod belongs to a class of imidazoquinolinamines that has antitumor and antiviral activity. The mechanism of action is uncertain. It exerts no direct antiviral effect within the mammalian cell in vitro, but does activate the immune system via cytokine induction.[113] Imiquimod is available in a 5% cream.

MONO-, DI-, TRICHLOROACETIC ACIDS   Eighty percent monochloroacetic acid penetrates the skin and may produce necrosis of the epidermis by blister formation. Saturated dichloroacetic acid or trichloroacetic acid in concentrations of 50% to 80% are less powerful but still effective in the management of warts.[114] Occlusive dressings enhance effectiveness. The application needs to be repeated at 1- to 2-week intervals until complete resolution.

PODOPHYLLIN RESIN   Podophyllin is an extract from the dried roots of either *Podophyllum peltatum* or *P. emodi*.[115] It acts as an antimitotic agent by preventing the formation of mitotic spindles. It is available in a range of concentrations in various vehicles such as tincture of benzoin, alcohol, or flexible collodion and is used as a treatment for genital warts.[116]

PODOFILOX   Podofilox is the active ingredient obtained upon purification of the podophyllin resin. It does not contain any of the ingredients responsible for the toxicity of podophyllin.[117]

SALICYLIC ACID   The use of salicylic acid in treating warts lies in the destruction of the epidermis in which the virus is present. Salicylic acid is more irritating than some other over-the-counter preparations.

REFERENCES

1. Caron D et al: Split-face comparison of adapalene 0.1% gel and tretinoin 0.025% gel in acne patients. *J Am Acad Dermatol* **36**:S110, 1997
2. Shroot B, Michel S: Pharmacology and chemistry of adapalene. *J Am Acad Dermatol* **36**:S96, 1997
3. Cunliffe WJ et al: Clinical efficacy and safety comparison of adapalene gel and tretinoin gel in the treatment of acne vulgaris: Europe and U.S. multicenter trials. *J Am Acad Dermatol* **36**:S126, 1997
4. Cargnello JA: Acne: What's new. *Med J Aust* **165**:153, 1996
5. Nazzaro-Porro M et al: Beneficial effect of 15% azelaic acid cream on acne vulgaris. *Br J Dermatol* **109**:45, 1983
6. Nazzaro-Porro M: Azelaic acid. *J Am Acad Dermatol* **17**:1033, 1987
7. King K et al: The effect of azelaic acid on cutaneous microflora in vivo and in vitro. *J Invest Dermatol* **84**:438, 1985
8. Nacht S et al: Benzoyl peroxide percutaneous absorption and metabolic disposition. *J Am Acad Dermatol* **4**:31, 1981
9. Leyden JJ, Shalita AR: Rational therapy for acne vulgaris: An update on topical treatment. *J Am Acad Dermatol* **15**:907, 1986
10. Bleiberg J et al: Bleaching of hair after use of topical benzoyl peroxide acne lotion. *Arch Dermatol* **108**:583, 1973
11. Packman A et al: Treatment of acne vulgaris: Combination of 3% erythromycin and 5% benzoyl peroxide in a gel compared to clindamycin lotion. *Int J Dermatol* **35**:209, 1996
12. Logan WS: Vitamin A and keratinization. *Arch Dermatol* **105**:748, 1972
13. Mills OH et al: Acne vulgaris. Oral therapy with tetracycline and topical therapy with vitamin A. *Arch Dermatol* **106**:200, 1972
14. Peck GL, Yoder FW: Treatment of lamellar ichthyosis and other keratinizing disorders with oral synthetic retinoids. *Lancet* **2**:1172, 1977
15. Tkach JR: Tretinoin treatment for Fox-Fordyce disease (letter). *Arch Dermatol* **115**:1285, 1979
16. Mark R, Lever L: Studies on the effects of topical retinoic acid on photoageing. *Br J Dermatol* **122**(suppl 35):93, 1990
17. Elson ML: Treatment of striae distensae with topical tretinoin. *J Dermatol Surg Oncol* **16**:267, 1990
18. Gunther S: Vitamin A acid in Darier's disease. *Acta Dermatol Venereol Suppl* **74**:146, 1975
19. Goette DK: Keratosis pilaris clearing with topical vitamin A acid. *Acta Dermatol Venereol Suppl* **74**:159, 1975
20. Watson C: Topical capsaicin as an adjuvant analgesic. *J Pain Symptom Manage* **9**:425, 1994
21. Bernstein J et al: Topical capsaicin treatment of chronic postherpetic neuralgia. *J Am Acad Dermatol* **21**:265, 1989
22. Steward D: Eutectic mixture of local anesthetics (EMLA): What is it? What does it do? *J Pediatr* **22**:S21, 1993

23. Evers H et al: Dermal effects of compositions based on the eutectic mixture of lidocaine and prilocaine (EMLA). *Br J Anaesthesiol* **57**:997, 1985

24. Fisher AA: *Contact Dermatitis.* Philadelphia, Lea & Febiger, 1986, p 223

25. Gupta AK et al: Antifungal agents: An overview. Part II. *J Am Acad Dermatol* **30**:911, 1994

26. Clayton YM, Connor BL: Comparison of clotrimazole cream, Whitfield's ointment and nystatin ointment for the topical treatment of ringworm infections, pityriasis versicolor, erythrasma and candidiasis. *Br J Dermatol* **89**:297, 1973

27. Cutsem JV et al: The in vitro antifungal activity of ketoconazole, zinc pyrithione, and selenium sulfide against *Pityrosporum* and their efficacy as a shampoo in the treatment of experimental pityrosporosis in guinea pigs. *J Am Acad Dermatol* **22**:993, 1990

28. Rogers SCF et al: Percutaneous absorption of phenol and methyl alcohol in Magenta Paint B.P.C. *Br J Dermatol* **98**:559, 1978

29. Allen HB et al: Selenium sulfide: Adjunctive therapy for tinea capitis. *Pediatrics* **69**:81, 1982

30. Givens TG et al: Comparison of 1% and 2.5% selenium sulfide in the treatment of tinea capitis. *Arch Pediatr Adolesc Med* **149**:808, 1995

31. Holti G: A double-blind controlled trial of Whitfield's ointment and variotin in ringworm infections with a two year "follow-up." *Acta Dermatol Venereol* **50**:229, 1970

32. Khattar M et al: The influence of pyrithione on the growth of microorganisms. *J Appl Bacteriol* **64**:265, 1988

33. Pereira R et al: Allergic contact dermatitis from zinc pyrithione. *Contact Dermatitis* **33**:131, 1995

34. Burton JL, Marshall A: Hypertrichosis due to minoxidil. *Br J Dermatol* **101**:593, 1979

35. Fenton D, Wilkinson J: Topical minoxidil in the treatment of alopecia areata. *Br Med J* **287**:1015, 1983

36. DeVillez RL et al: Androgenic alopecia in the female: Treatment with 2% topical minoxidil solution. *Arch Dermatol* **130**:303, 1994

37. Walter JF et al: Suppression of epidermal DNA synthesis by ultra violet light, coal tar and anthralin. *Br J Dermatol* **99**:89, 1978

38. Lavker RM et al: The atrophogenic effect of crude coal tar on human epidermis. *Br J Dermatol* **105**:77, 1981

39. Silverman A et al: Tars and anthralins. *Dermatol Clin* **13**:817, 1995

40. Kaidlbey KH, Kligman AM: Clinical and histological study of coal tar phototoxicity in humans. *Arch Dermatol* **113**:592, 1977

41. Aberer W et al: Ammoniated mercury ointment: Outdated but still in use. *Contact Dermatitis* **23**:168, 1990

42. Lagerholm B, Fritz A: Cellular changes in the psoriatic epidermis. *Acta Dermatol Venerol* **47**:222, 1967

43. Russell AD: Bacterial spores and chemical sporicidal agents. *Clin Microbiol Rev* **3**:99, 1990

44. Broadley SJ et al: Anti-mycobacterial activity of biocides. *Lett Appl Microbiol* **13**:118, 1991

45. Peterson AF et al: Comparative evaluation of surgical scrub preparations. *Surg Gynecol Obstet* **146**:63, 1978

46. Docampo R, Moreno SNJ: The metabolism and mode of action of gentian violet. *Drug Metab Rev* **22**:161, 1990

47. Moats WA, Maddox SE: Effect of pH on the antimicrobial activity of some triphenylmethane dyes. *Can J Microbiol* **24**.658, 1978

48. Christensen OB, Anehus SIW: Hydrogen peroxide cream: An alternative to topical antibiotics in the treatment of impetigo contagiosa. *Acta Dermatol Venereol* **74**:460, 1994

49. Rath I, Meissl G: Induction of hyperthyroidism in burn patients treated topically with povidone-iodine. *Burns* **14**:320, 1988

50. Kero M et al: Primary irritant dermatitis from topical clioquinol. *Dermatitis* **5**:115, 1979

51. Esterly NB et al: The effect of antimicrobial agents on leukocyte chemotaxis. *J Invest Dermatol* **70**:51, 1978

52. Grove DI et al: Suppression of cell-mediated immunity by metronidazole. *Int Arch Allergy Appl Immunol* **1**(suppl):107, 1978

53. Hughes J, Mellows G: Inhibition of isoleucyl-transfer ribonucleic acid synthetase in *Escherichia coli* by pseudomonic acid. *Biochem J* **176**:305, 1978

54. Anonymous: Mupriocin-resistant *Staphylococcus aureus* (letter). *Lancet* **2**:387, 1987

55. Moyer CA et al: Treatment of large human burns with 0.5 percent silver nitrate solution. *Arch Surg* **90**:812, 1965

56. Smith-Choban P, Marshall WJ: Leukopenia secondary to silver sulfadiazine: Frequency, characteristics and clinical consequences. *Am Surg* **53**:515, 1987

57. Fuller FW et al: A review of the dosimetry of 1% silver sulfadiazine cream in burn wound treatment. *J Burn Care Rehabil* **15**:213, 1994

58. Karacic I, Yawalkar SJ: A single application of crotamiton lotion in the treatment of patients with pediculosis capitis. *Int J Dermatol* **2**:611, 1982

59. Elgart ML: A risk-benefit assessment of agents used in the treatment of scabies. *Drug Safety* **14**:386, 1996

60. Solomon LM et al: Gamma benzene hexachloride toxicity. *Arch Dermatol* **113**:353, 1977

61. Ginsburg CM, Lowry W: Absorption of gamma benzene hydrochloride following application of Kwell shampoo. *Pediatr Dermatol* **1**:74, 1983

62. Rasmussen JE: The problem of lindane. *J Am Acad Dermatol* **5**:507, 1981

63. Sherma VK, Kaur S: Contact sensitization by pesticides in farmers. *Contact Dermatitis* **23**:77, 1990

64. Schultz M et al: Comparative study of 5% permethrin cream and 1% lindane lotion for the treatment of scabies. *Arch Dermatol* **126**:167, 1990

65. Signore RJ: A pilot study of 5 percent permethrin cream versus 0.75 percent metronidazole gel in acne rosacea. *Cutis* **56**:177, 1995

66. Mitchell JC et al: Allergic contact dermatitis from pyrethrum (*Chrysanthemum* spp.). The roles of pyrethrosin, a sesquiterpene lactone, and of pyrethrin II. *Br J Dermatol* **86**:568, 1972

67. Carson DS et al: Pyrethrins combined with piperonyl butoxide (RID) versus 1% permethrin (Nix) in the treatment of head lice. *Am J Dis Child* **142**:768, 1988

68. Shelley WB, Hurley HJ: Studies on topical antiperspirant control of axillary hyperhidrosis. *Acta Dermatol Venereol* **5**:241, 1975

69. Holzle E, Braun-Falco O: Structural changes in axillary eccrine glands following long term treatment with aluminum chloride hexahydrate solution. *Br J Dermatol* **110**:399, 1984

70. Gordon H: Hyperhidrosis: Treatment with gluteraldehyde. *Cutis* **9**:375, 1972

71. Cullen SI: Topical methenamine therapy for hyperhidrosis. *Arch Dermatol* **111**:1158, 1975

72. Coskey RJ: Contact dermatitis caused by diphenhydramine hydrochloride. *J Am Acad Dermatol* **8**:204, 1983

73. Horio T: Allergic and photoallergic dermatitis from diphenhydramine. *Arch Dermatol* **112**:1124, 1976

74. Taylor J et al: Allergic contact dermatitis from doxepin cream. *Arch Dermatol* **132**:515, 1996

75. Drake L et al: Relief of pruritus in patients with atopic dermatitis after treatment with topical doxepin cream. *J Am Acad Dermatol* **31**:613, 1994

76. Swandulla D et al: Calcium channel current inactivation is selectively modulated by menthol. *Neurosci Lett* **68**:23, 1986

77. Bromm B et al: Effects of menthol and cold on histamine-induced itch and skin reactions in man. *Neurosci Lett* **187**:157, 1995

78. Yosipovitch G et al: Effect of topically applied menthol on thermal, pain and itch sensations and biophysical properties of the skin. *Arch Dermatol Res* **288**:245, 1996

79. Pascher F: Systemic reactions to topically applied drugs. *Int J Dermatol* **17**:768, 1978

80. Furman PA et al: Acyclovir triphosphate is a suicide inactivator of the herpes simplex virus DNA polymerase. *J Biol Chem* **259**:9575, 1984

81. Memer OM, Tyring SK: Antiviral agents in dermatology: Current status and future prospects. *Int J Dermatol* **34**:597, 1995

82. Schmidt LM: Topical dermatologic therapy for the pediatrician. *Pediatr Clin North Am* **25**:191, 1978

83. Cason J, Lowbury E: Mortality and infection in extensively burned patients treated with silver nitrate compresses. *Lancet* **1**:651, 1968

84. Pathak MA et al: Usefulness of retinoic acid in the treatment of melasma. *J Am Acad Dermatol* **15**:894, 1986

85. Verallo-Rowell VM et al: Double-blind comparison of azelaic acid and hydroquinone in the treatment of melasma. *Acta Dermatol Venereol* **143**(suppl):58, 1989

86. Balina LM, Graupe K: The treatment of melasma. 20% azelaic acid versus 4% hydroquinone cream. *Int J Dermatol* **30**:893, 1991

87. Nazzaro-Porro M et al: Effect of dicarboxylic acids on lentigo maligna. *J Invest Dermatol* **73**:296, 1979

88. Nazzaro-Porro M et al: Effect of azelaic acid on human malignant melanoma. *Lancet* **2**:1109, 1980
89. Findley GH et al: Exogenous ochronosis and pigmented colloid millium from hydroquinone bleaching creams. *Br J Dermatol* **93**:613, 1975
90. Engasser PE, Maibach HI: Cosmetics and dermatology: Bleaching creams. *J Am Acad Dermatol* **5**:143, 1981
91. Niwa Y, Akamatsu H: Kojic acid scavenges free radicals while potentiating leukocyte functions including free radical generation. *Inflammation* **15**:303, 1991
92. Mishima Y et al: Induction of melanogenesis suppression: Cellular pharmacology and mode of differential action. *Pigment Cell Res* **1**:367, 1988
93. Kahn V: Effect of kojic acid on the oxidation of DL-DOPA, norepinephrine, and dopamine by mushroom tyrosinase. *Pigment Cell Res* **8**:234, 1995
94. Garcia A, Fulton JE: The combination of glycolic acid and hydroquinone or kojic acid for the treatment of melasma and related conditions. *Dermatol Surg* **22**:443, 1996
95. Smith W: Epidermal and dermal effects of topical lactic acid. *J Am Acad Dermatol* **35**:388, 1996
96. Van Scott E, Yu R: Hyperkeratinization, corneocyte cohesion, and alpha hydroxy acids. *J Am Acad Dermatol* **11**:867, 1984
97. Goldsmith L, Baden H: Propylene glycol with occlusion for treatment of ichthyosis. *JAMA* **220**:579, 1972
98. Davies M, Marks R: Studies on the effect of salicylic acid on normal skin. *Br J Dermatol* **95**:187, 1976
99. Pegum J: Urea in the treatment of black hairy tongue. *Br J Dermatol* **84**:602, 1971
100. Steigleder GK et al: Autoradiographic in vitro examination of psoriatic skin before, during and after dithranol treatment. *Arch Dermatol Res* **246**:231, 1973
101. Lowe NJ et al: Anthralin for psoriasis: Short-contact anthralin therapy compared with topical steroid and conventional anthralin. *J Am Acad Dermatol* **10**:69, 1984
102. Tham S et al: A comparative study of calcipotriol ointment and tar in chronic plaque psoriasis. *Br J Dermatol* **7**:231, 1994
103. Kragballe K et al: Double blind, right/left comparison of calcipotriol and betamethasone valerate in the treatment of psoriasis vulgaris. *Lancet* **337**:193, 1991
104. Kragballe K: Treatment of psoriasis with calcipotriol and other vitamin D analogues. *J Am Acad Dermatol* **27**:1001, 1992
105. Lebwohl M et al: Interactions between calcipotriene and ultraviolet light. *J Am Acad Dermatol* **37**:93, 1997
106. Chandraratna RAS: Tazarotene—first of a new generation of receptor-selective retinoids. *Br J Dermatol* **135**:18, 1996
107. Marks R: Early clinical development of tazarotene. *Br J Dermatol* **135**:26, 1996
108. Naylor MF et al: Contact immunotherapy of resistant warts. *J Am Acad Dermatol* **19**:679, 1988
109. Bucker K, Price N: Immunotherapy of verrucae vulgaris with dinitrochlorobenzene. *Br J Dermatol* **98**:451, 1978
110. Wilkerson MG et al: Diphenylcyclopropenone: Examination for potential contaminants, mechanisms of sensitization, and photochemical stability. *J Am Acad Dermatol* **11**:802, 1984
111. Hursthouse MW: A controlled trial on the use of topical 5-fluorouracil on viral warts. *Br J Dermatol* **92**:93, 1975
112. Goncalves J: 5-Fluorouracil in the treatment of common warts of the hands. A double blind study. *Br J Dermatol* **92**:89, 1975
113. Testerman TL et al: Cytokine induction by the immunomodulators imiquimod and S-27609. *J Leukoc Biol* **58**:365, 1995
114. Baker GE, Tyring SK: Therapeutic approaches to papillomavirus infections. *Dermatol Clin* **15**:331, 1997
115. Baker DA et al: Topical podofilox for the treatment of condylomata accuminata in women. *Obstet Gyn* **76**:656, 1990
116. Beutner K: Therapeutic approaches to genital warts. *Am J Med* **102**:28, 1977
117. Zheng QY et al: Purified podophyllotoxin (CPH-86) inhibits lymphocyte proliferation but augments macrophage proliferation. *Int J Immunopharmacol* **9**:539, 1987

CHAPTER 245

Sewon Kang
John J. Voorhees

Topical Retinoids

The term *retinoid* was coined by Michael Sporn and his colleagues in 1976. The original description referred both to the naturally occurring compounds with vitamin A activity and to synthetic analogues of retinol. Hence, retinoids were defined in both functional (vitamin A activity) and structural (retinol-derivative) terms. The discovery of intranuclear retinoic acid receptors (RARs) in 1987, by two independent groups,[1,2] was pivotal to our understanding of the mechanism of retinoic acid action since it demonstrated for the first time the existence of a retinoid-responsive transcription factor. This also gave rise to the concept that retinoids are like hormones. Therefore, a retinoid can be defined today as any molecule that, by itself or through metabolic conversion, binds to and activates the RARs, thereby eliciting transcriptional activation of retinoic acid–responsive genes that results in specific biologic responses.

PHARMACOLOGY

Nomenclature

Vitamin A is a 20-carbon molecule that consists of a cyclohexenyl ring, a side chain with four double bonds (*all* arranged in *trans* configuration), and an alco*hol* end group. Hence, it is also known

FIGURE 245-1

A. Sequential Oxidation of Retinol

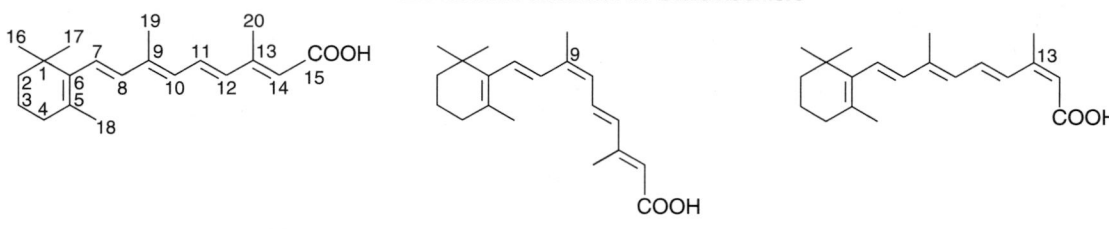

all-*trans* retinol   all-*trans* retinaldehyde   all-*trans* retinoic acid

B. All-*Trans* Retinoic Acid and Its Stereoisomers

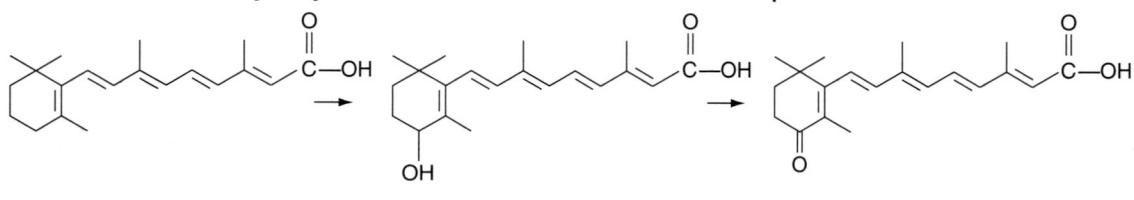

all-*trans* retinoic acid   9-*cis* retinoic acid   13-*cis* retinoic acid

C. Hydroxylation of All-*Trans* Retinoic Acid and Subsequent Oxidation

all-*trans* retinoic acid   4-hydroxy all-*trans* retinoic acid   4-oxo all-*trans* retinoic acid

D. Esterification of Retinol

all-*trans* retinol

H_2O

H_2O

retinyl esters

E. Structural Relationship of β-Carotene and 14-Hydroxy 4,14-*Retro*-Retinol to Retinol

β-carotene

all-*trans* retinol

14-hydroxy 4,14-*retro*-retinol

Nomenclature of natural retinoids.

as all-*trans* retinol. Oxidation of the alcohol end group of all-*trans* retinol results in the formation of an aldehyde (all-*trans* retinaldehyde), which can be further oxidized to carboxylic acid (all-*trans* retinoic acid = tretinoin) (Fig. 245-1A). The numbering of the carbon atoms is as shown in Fig. 245-1B. The terms 9-*cis* and 13-*cis* retinoic acid refer to stereoisomers of all-*trans* retinoic acid in which the double bond that begins with the 9th and 13th carbon atoms, respectively, is in the *cis*- rather than *trans*-configuration. The fourth carbon atom is located in the cyclohexenyl ring of all-*trans* retinoic acid and is involved in a hydroxylation reaction to generate 4-hydroxy-all-*trans* retinoic acid (Fig. 245-1C). The addition of a hydroxyl group to the cyclohexenyl ring renders the molecule more polar, making it more amenable for excretion/elimination from cells and organisms. It is also much less active biologically. 4-Hydroxy-all-*trans* retinoic acid can be further oxidized to 4-*oxo* retinoic acid.

A group of compounds referred to as *retinyl esters* functions as the molecular storage form of retinol. The compounds are formed by esterification of retinol with fatty acids (Fig. 245-1*D*). The fatty acids involved specify the ester. For example, retinyl palmitate is generated when retinol is esterified with palmitic acid. Hydrolysis of retinyl esters regenerates retinol. Beta-carotene is a symmetric 40-carbon molecule (twice the number of retinol or retinoic acid) present in green and yellow-orange fruits and vegetables. As suggested by stoichiometry, one molecule of this carotenoid can potentially generate two molecules of retinol (cleavage of the central double bond) (Fig. 245-1*E*). Finally, 14-hydroxy-4,14-*retro* retinol is a metabolite of retinol originally identified as an inducer of lymphocyte proliferation. In comparison to retinol, the location of double bonds between carbon atoms 4 and 14 is displaced in a retrograde fashion in 14-hydroxy-4,14-*retro* retinol (Fig. 245-1*E*).

Metabolism of Retinoids in Human Skin

As the vitamin designation implies, all-*trans* retinol cannot be synthesized in the body and is thus an essential nutrient. Retinyl esters and beta-carotene are the two major precursors of retinol present in our diet. Once taken in from the diet, retinyl esters and beta-carotene are converted to all-*trans* retinol in the intestine and stored in the liver after reconversion to retinyl esters. Retinol released from the liver is carried in the circulation by plasma retinol-binding proteins. Once transported to target cells, it is taken up apparently through passive diffusion. Consistent with the fact that retinol is a hydrophobic molecule, it associates intracellularly with a ubiquitously expressed binding protein called *cellular retinol-binding protein* (CRBP). In human skin, CRBP-bound all-*trans* retinol (holoCRBP) can be metabolized to at least four important products: retinyl esters, all-*trans* retinoic acid, 14-hydroxy-4,14-*retro* retinol, and all-*trans* 3,4-didehydroretinol (vitamin A$_2$) and its esters. Although critical for lymphocyte growth and proliferation, in normal human skin in vivo and in cultured human keratinocytes, 14-hydroxy-4,14-*retro* retinol elicits no discernible cellular or molecular responses.[3] Therefore, the biologic role of this retinoid in human skin is obscure. Similarly, the functional significance of vitamin A$_2$ formation is unknown.

ESTERIFICATION AND OXIDATION OF RETINOL
Topical treatment of human skin with all-*trans* retinol increases retinyl ester levels in the epidermal layer by more than tenfold.[4] This reaction is catalyzed by two enzymes: lecithin/retinol acyltransferase (LRAT) and acyl CoA/retinol acyltransferase (ARAT). In human keratinocytes, LRAT is the predominant retinol-esterifying activity.[5]

All-*trans* retinoic acid is formed by sequential oxidation of all-*trans* retinol, with all-*trans* retinaldehyde as the intermediate metabolite. The first step (oxidation of all-*trans* retinol to all-*trans* retinaldehyde) is rate limiting for all-*trans* retinoic acid formation. Topical application of all-*trans* retinol to human skin results in histologic and molecular alterations that mimic those following all-*trans* retinoic acid treatment.[4] These include epidermal hyperplasia due to keratinocyte proliferation, epidermal spongiosis, compaction of the stratum corneum, and induction of CRBP, cellular retinoic acid–binding protein (CRABP) II, and retinoic acid 4-hydroxylase.[4,6] In retinol-treated skin, all-*trans* retinoic acid is minimally detectable, which is no different from untreated normal skin.[4] The lack of significant accumulation of all-*trans* retinoic acid in retinol-treated skin is due to the tightly regulated conversion of retinol to retinaldehyde and the effective hydroxylation of all-*trans* retinoic

acid that is formed by retinoic acid 4-hydroxylase. The observation that all-*trans* retinol and retinoic acid elicit similar responses in human skin but that retinol does so without detectable increases in retinoic acid levels indicates that endogenously synthesized retinoic acid is a much more efficient activator of retinoid pathways than exogenously supplied retinoic acid.

Metabolically formed all-*trans* retinoic acid is bound to CRABP. This cytoplasmic protein, of which there are two species (CRABPs I and II), binds all-*trans* retinoic acid selectively and with high affinity. The fact that CRABPs are highly conserved proteins found in multiple species showing distinct patterns of expression in developing embryo and adult organisms suggests that their functions are important in retinoid signaling. In addition to all-*trans* retinoic acid, 9-*cis* and 13-*cis* retinoic acid have been isolated from tissues. It is not known whether the interconversion among the retinoic acid occurs through specific isomerases. When equal amounts (0.1%) of all-*trans*, 9-*cis*, and 13-*cis* retinoic acid are applied topically to human skin, all-*trans* retinoic acid is extracted in significant amounts (36 to 72 percent) regardless of the isomer applied.[6]

HYDROXYLATION OF ALL-*TRANS* RETINOIC ACID
In human skin all-*trans* retinoic acid is catabolized primarily to the more polar 4-hydroxy-all-*trans* retinoic acid, which is further metabolized to 4-*oxo* retinoic acid. 4-Hydroxy retinoic acid is tenfold less potent in inducing retinoid responses in human keratinocytes and mouse skin than all-*trans* retinoic acid.[7] In untreated normal human skin, all-*trans* retinoic acid 4-hydroxylase activity is minimally detectable. Topical administration of all-*trans* retinoic acid or all-*trans* retinol to human skin, however, increases its activity severalfold.[6,8] The 4-hydroxylase is a cytochrome P$_{450}$ enzyme whose activity can be effectively inhibited by ketoconazole and a related azole, liarozole.[8,9] By blocking this major inactivation pathway of all-*trans* retinoic acid pharmacologically, topical liarozole can amplify human skin responses to all-*trans* retinol and retinoic acid.[9] Although this hydroxylase activity is also induced in skin treated with 9-*cis* or 13-*cis* retinoic acid, remarkably it has substrate specificity for the all-*trans* retinoic acid isomer only and does not hydroxylate 9-*cis* or 13-*cis* retinoic acid, retinol, or retinaldehydes.[6] With all-*trans* retinoic acid, the 4-hydroxylase activity is maximally induced after 24 h of occlusive treatment.[6] Recent isolation and molecular characterization of the P$_{450}$ RAI gene, which encodes for retinoic acid–inducible 4-hydroxylase in zebra fish,[10] is expected to lead to the identification of the human counterpart.

The Retinoid Receptors

The landmark discovery of RARs and characterization of their molecular features revealed similarity of RARs to steroid/thyroid hormone receptors.[1,2] A characteristic common to these receptors is that they bind to regulatory regions in DNA called hormone response elements, or target sequences, and activate gene transcription in a ligand-dependent manner. Hence, they are referred to as *ligand (hormone-)-dependent transcription factors*. At the amino acid level, the nuclear receptor superfamily members are organized into six domains, each with a distinct function. Two domains of major importance are the DNA-binding domain and the ligand-binding domain. A short sequence within the DNA-binding domain, called the *P box*, has allowed categorization of the receptors into at least four different subfamilies. RARs, vitamin D receptors (VDRs), and thyroid hormone receptors (TRs) all possess the same P-box amino acid sequence. When their respective ligands are bound, these receptors bind to similar DNA recognition sequences located in the promoter region of target genes. The recognition sequences (hormone-response elements) are composed of two half-sites, each 6-bp long (AGGTCA). The base-pair spacing between the half-sites determines, in part, the specificity of the receptor recognition sequences. The so-called 3-4-5 rule, now considered far too simplified, refers to the number of base pairs that separates the half-sites, which in general is 3 bp for VDR, 4 bp for TR, and 5 bp for RAR. The two half-sites are arranged as direct repeats for RAR, VDR, and TR, whereas for classic steroid hormone receptors (e.g., glucocorticoid, mineralocorticoid, progesterone), the two are in a palindromic (i.e., inverted repeat) configuration. These nuclear receptors bind to their response elements as dimers. Unlike receptors for the steroid hormones, which form homodimers (two identical monomers), RAR, VDR, and TR bind to their elements with greater affinity as heterodimers (two different monomers). The key partner for heterodimerization and ultimate functioning of RAR, VDR, and TR is the retinoid X receptor (RXR).[11] To date, 9-*cis* retinoic acid is the only known physiologic ligand for RXR.[12] In addition to RARs, VDRs, and TRs, RXRs have been found to heterodimerize with other receptors. This ability of RXRs to interact with many receptors suggests its importance as a regulatory protein. There are three different members of RAR (-α, -β, and -γ) and RXR (-α, -β, and -γ), each encoded by different genes. In addition, each of the receptors has isoforms, adding to the diversity of retinoid receptors.

Receptor-Selective Retinoids

Identification and functional characterization of these families of retinoid receptors provided an attractive target for drug discovery. Synthetic molecules could be screened for their ability to bind and activate the specific receptors. Many of these compounds have no structural similarities to all-*trans* retinol or retinoic acid, yet by virtue of their ability to activate the receptor(s), they can mediate the retinoid effect and thus be considered retinoids. A synthetic retinoid that fits this description and has been used topically in humans is adapalene (Fig. 245-2). Adapalene has restricted receptor specificity, possessing poor affinity for RAR-α, higher affinity for RAR-β and -γ, and no interaction with RXR-α.[13] Although adapalene does not bind to CRABPs,[13] it is capable of inducing CRABP II mRNA like all-*trans* retinoic acid.[14,15] Unlike retinoic acid, however, adapalene does not induce clinical erythema, epidermal hyperplasia, or spongiosis following a short-term (4 days) occlusive treatment.[14] Tazarotene is another synthetic molecule that has biologic activity topically. By itself, tazarotene does not bind to RARs or RXRs. However, its acid metabolite (AGN 190299) has a weak but relative receptor selectivity for RARs (RAR-β > RAR-γ > RAR-α)[16] and is felt to be the principal active form.

The Retinoid Receptors in Human Skin

Skin remains the only human tissue in which systematic analysis of the relative levels of each RAR and RXR protein has been made. Human epidermis expresses RAR-α, RAR-γ, RXR-α, and RXR-β mRNAs.[17] RXR-γ mRNA is undetectable, and the transcript for RAR-β is barely detectable. A similar pattern is observed in cultured human keratinocytes and dermal fibroblasts. These relative levels of retinoid receptor mRNA mirror their relative protein levels. In nuclei from human epidermis, there are five times more total RXRs than RARs.[18] For RAR proteins, 87 percent are RAR-γ and 13 percent are RAR-α, with no detectable RAR-β. Of the RXR proteins, 90 percent are RXR-α. In gel shift stud-

ies performed on nuclei isolated from human skin and cultured keratinocytes, which in both cases are expressing their normal endogenous receptors, only RXR-α and RAR (mostly -γ) heterodimers bind to retinoic acid–response elements (RAREs) spaced by two (DR-2) or five nucleotides (DR-5).[18,19] Neither RAR nor RXR homodimers are detectable. Therefore, normal human epidermis is regulated by RXR-α and RAR-γ heterodimers. In terms of the ligands needed to activate RXR/RAR-bound RAREs, based on chloramphenicol acetyltransferase reporter gene activity in keratinocytes, the heterodimer requires only the RAR ligand. Furthermore, the presence of RXR ligand does not confer additional transactivation induced by RAR ligand. Therefore, at their physiologic levels, RARs and RXRs in human skin bind RAREs (DR-2 or DR-5) as heterodimers and transactivate these response elements in response to RAR but not RXR ligands. However, the RXR is key as the heterodimer will not bind to the RARE without the presence of the RXR protein.

Retinoid Target Genes and Their Activation Cascade in Human Skin

Based on current information, retinoid actions are primarily, if not solely, mediated by retinoid receptors. Given that the receptors are transcription factors, the ultimate skin effects of retinoids (phenotypic changes) must be accomplished through regulated gene expression. The best-established mechanism by which retinoid receptors modulate gene expression is activation of retinoid target genes through direct binding to RARE in the gene promoter, thereby stimulating basal transcriptional machinery. In skin, CRABP II, CRBP, and keratin 6, all of which contain RAREs, have been demonstrated to be regulated by all-*trans* retinoic acid.[4,20–22] However, the products of these genes are probably not the effectors of the retinoid response and hence cannot account for the pleiotropic effects of retinoids in skin. Undoubtedly, additional RARE-regulated genes will be identified that encode for proteins that function to modulate cutaneous growth and differentiation directly or indirectly. A likely scenario is that these protein products in turn activate other non-RARE-containing genes in a cascading reaction to produce the clinical features of retinoid action in skin (Fig. 245-3). Since most genes expressed within the cascade would contain no functional RAREs, their activation by retinoids would be indirect. Therefore, the reti-

FIGURE 245-2

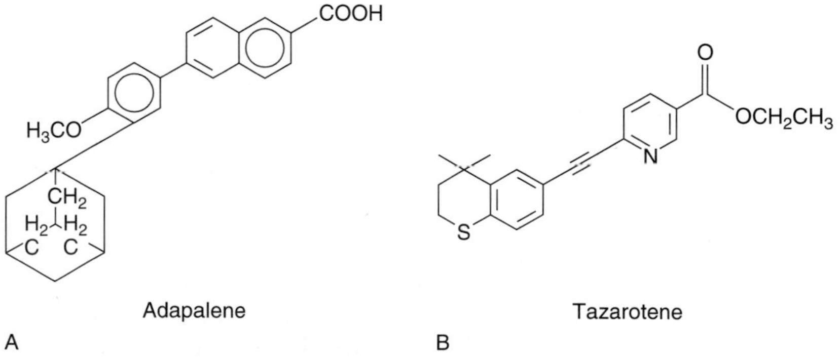

Chemical structures of synthetic retinoids, adapalene and tazarotene.

FIGURE 245-3

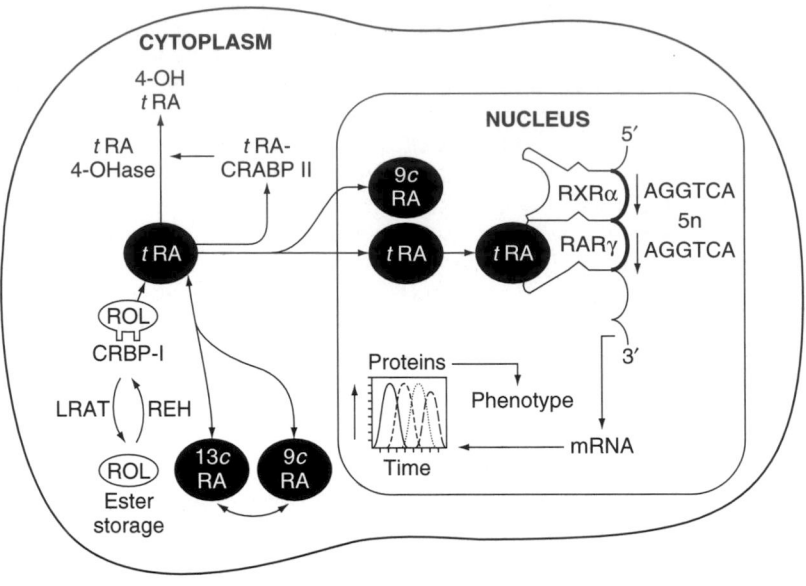

Cellular metabolism of natural retinoids and molecular mechanism of retinoid-specific gene activation.

noid response in human skin is mediated both by direct and indirect activation of genes, initiated by a retinoid signal.

CLINICAL USE

Until very recently, clinical use of topical retinoids has been limited to all-*trans* retinoic acid (tretinoin). Although the initial use of this retinoid was in actinic keratosis, currently the only approved dermatologic indications in the United States are for acne and photoaged skin. For acne therapy, it is widely accepted that, especially for the comedonal variant, topical tretinoin is extremely effective. Of the different classes of antiacne medications, retinoids are felt to be the best, if not the only, agent to normalize the abnormal follicular epithelial differentiation/desquamation viewed to be important in the pathogenesis of acne lesions. Therefore, the use of tretinoin would also provide protection against the development of new lesions. This prophylactic property is the basis for including topical retinoid in almost all antiacne regimens. A potential for aggravating inflammation exists in treating inflammatory acne (i.e., papules and pustules) with topical tretinoin, but when properly administered, this type of acne also responds well to tretinoin (see "Dosage Schedule and Forms"). Topical adapalene has also received approval from the U.S. Food and Drug Administration for acne. Based on published studies, it shows promise as a therapy with a suitable safety profile.[13] Fine wrinkles and dyspigmentation are two salient features of photoaged skin that are improved by topical tretinoin. Several weeks of treatment are required before clinical improvement is appreciated. For the effacement of fine wrinkles, partial restoration of markedly reduced levels of collagen in sun-exposed skin toward those seen in sun-protected skin appears

to be responsible.[23] Tretinoin's ability to improve photoaging is specific and does not result from the irritation or retinoid dermatitis frequently produced by this compound.[24] Although the molecular basis of photoaging prevention by topical tretinoin was recently demonstrated,[25] its value in clinical practice is as yet unstudied.

Besides the two approved indications, topical tretinoin has been demonstrated through well-controlled studies to be effective in the treatment of several other conditions. These include, but are not limited to, postinflammatory hyperpigmentation in blacks,[26] actinic dyspigmentation in Chinese and Japanese,[27] melasma,[28,29] and early stretch marks.[30] These controlled studies have shown more than therapeutic efficacies. They have also provided valuable information to dispel some of the myths about tretinoin use in humans. For example, blacks and Asians tolerate topical tretinoin as well as, if not better than,[26,27,29] Caucasians.[24,28,30] Furthermore, the often observed retinoid dermatitis does not usually lead to postinflammatory hyperpigmentation in those with greater constitutive pigmentation.

Many other skin disorders have been reported to be improved by topical retinoids, but most of these have not been as rigorously studied and their therapeutic claims should thus be interpreted with caution. Molluscum contagiosum, warts, psoriasis, and various forms of ichthyosis may be improved by topical tretinoin to a variable degree. In psoriasis especially, irritation of treated skin has limited the use. Topical tarazotene, which is under development for psoriasis, does not appear to have fully overcome the irritation problem[31]; thus, its usefulness in this disease remains to be seen. The beneficial effects of topical retinoids in treating actinic keratoses have been confirmed through clinical trials. However, there is no role for topical retinoids in the treatment of established cutaneous tumors.

With such a wide variety of skin conditions treatable by topical retinoids, their use has included practically all age groups, perhaps with the exception of neonates. Similar considerations in dose schedule and forms are made in both young and old patients. The use of topical retinoids in pregnancy has become an emotional issue. As discussed below, based on fact teratogenicity is not caused by topical tretinoin (see "Adverse Effects"). However, since no dermatologic conditions seen in pregnancy that may respond to topical retinoids (i.e., acne, melasma, stretch marks) are life-threatening to the mother or the fetus, it seems prudent to delay the treatment until after delivery. In a recent study, which demonstrated that early, inflammatory stretch marks are improved by topical tretinoin, all pregnancy-related stretch marks were treated postpartum.[30] Therefore, even in this pregnancy-associated condition, the therapeutic benefit could still be achieved by instituting the treatment after delivery.

DOSAGE SCHEDULES AND FORMS

Until very recently, tretinoin was the only topical retinoid available for clinical use. Under the trade name Retin-A, three different formulations are available for acne therapy: cream (0.025%, 0.05%, 0.1%), gel (0.01%, 0.025%), and solution (0.05%). For photoaging treatment, tretinoin (0.05%) was introduced as Renova cream. A recent addition to acne therapy, adapalene (Differin) is available in gel formulation (0.1%). Different formulations allow some flexibility in terms of tailoring to an individual's skin dryness or oiliness.

Regardless of the retinoid preparation or the patient's age, the most important element in topical therapy is patient/guardian education. It must be explained clearly to each patient that, as part of the treatment, local skin irritation, characterized by redness and peeling, can be expected. It was once believed, especially for the treatment of photoaged skin, that clinical improvement correlated with the degree of irritation. This concept was erased through a large, controlled clinical study in which 0.025% and 0.1% tretinoin were shown to be equally efficacious but the former was significantly less irritating than the latter.[24] Therefore, unlike most medications for which the dosing schedule may be set as once or twice daily, administration of a topical retinoid should be titrated depending on the skin reaction. For some individuals it may be applied only twice a week, for others four times a week, etc. The frequency of drug application can be increased, as tolerated, to a once-daily regimen. This method of individualizing topical therapy minimizes unwanted acute retinoid dermatitis.

Under the nonprescription category, there are countless "natural retinoid" preparations with various claims (mostly antiaging) being sold throughout the world. Most of these contain retinyl esters, especially retinyl palmitate, retinaldehyde, or retinol. Whether any of these products can deliver retinoid activity to human skin is subject to question. Percutaneous absorption (especially for retinyl esters), adequate concentrations, and stable formulations (especially for retinol) are some of the important unknowns for this group of products. Based on human in vivo work, all-*trans* retinol holds the most promise of these natural retinoids in being biologically active,[4] provided the stability of the compound can be maintained with a proper formulation.

ADVERSE EFFECTS

By far the most common adverse effect associated with topical tretinoin use has been local skin irritation characterized by erythema, peeling, dryness, and pruritus. This is a predictable skin response that is temporary but troubling for many patients. The so-called retinoid dermatitis tends to peak within the first month of treatment and diminishes thereafter. It responds to a temporary reduction in the frequency or amount of retinoid application and to liberal use of emollients.

It has been well documented that the most striking histologic feature of all-*trans* retinoic acid–treated skin is the marked thickening of the epidermis[4,9,24] due to the increased proliferation of basal keratinocytes. An increase is also seen in the number of cell layers expressing the differentiation markers involucrin, loricrin, filaggrin, and epidermal transglutaminase.[22] These epidermal changes collectively translate to clinical desquamation and peeling. This hyperproliferative response of epidermis to retinoic acid is mediated by its nuclear receptor, as was recently demonstrated in transgenic mice expressing a dominant-negative (dn) RXR-α mutant protein targeted to the suprabasal epidermis by the keratin 10 promoter. The mutant protein impaired retinoid signaling by competing with endogenous RAR-γ–RXR-α heterodimers. In these mice, the ability of topically applied retinoic acid to stimulate proliferation of undifferentiated keratinocytes in the basal layer and resultant peeling of stratum corneum from the surface was significantly reduced.[32] Therefore, the peeling component of retinoid dermatitis is a part of

the retinoid-specific skin response. The erythema response, however, appears not to be retinoid-receptor mediated, since all-*trans* retinol, which induces epidermal hyperplasia and CRABP II mRNA like retinoic acid, is unassociated with clinical erythema.[4]

Systemic retinoid exposure has been well documented and established as a cause of embryonic death and congenital malformation. Therefore, concerns about potential teratogenicity from long-term topical retinoid use are completely justified. However, systemic absorption of retinoids from topical application is negligible, and the levels of endogenous retinoic acid in the blood are not increased by twice daily application of 0.025% tretinoin to more than 40 percent of body area over 1 month. Furthermore, controlled topical administration of tretinoin at doses used for acne therapy (2 g of 0.025% gel applied daily to the face, neck, and upper part of the chest for 14 days) has less influence on plasma levels of endogenous retinoids than diurnal and nutritional factors.[33] Indeed, a large population-based study demonstrated no excess risk of birth defects in offspring born to mothers who were exposed to topical tretinoin during pregnancy.[34] Therefore, no evidence exists for teratogenicity of topical tretinoin in humans. As mentioned under "Pharmacology," topical use of tretinoin induces in the skin the enzyme retinoic acid 4-hydroxylase that inactivates it. Therefore, the induction of this enzyme would serve as a protective mechanism to partially reduce the amount of tretinoin for systemic absorption. In this regard, topical use of natural retinoids would be even safer than any of the synthetic compounds, since there already exists a self-inducible enzymatic machinery that will inactivate excess tretinoin, but probably not synthetic retinoids.

"Sun sensitivity" is a frequently discussed subject with topical retinoid use and requires clarification. When formally tested in humans, topical tretinoin does not lower the minimal erythema dose of UVB light.[25] Since its presence in human skin does not increase the likelihood of sunburn reaction, tretinoin is not a phototoxic agent. When one talks to patients who complain of such sun sensitivity, they describe an uncomfortable skin sensation that is felt within minutes of being in the sun rather than hours later. This time line is certainly in disagreement with a typical sunburn reaction which takes longer to be noticed (hours to a day). Furthermore, this sensation is often said to be accentuated in warmer temperatures, which suggests participation of infrared irradiation (heat).

Related to the sun-sensitivity is the issue of photocarcinogenesis. In an animal model of photocarcinogenesis, topical tretinoin has caused skin cancer. However, this seems to be restricted to susceptible animals under contrived experimental conditions, and no evidence exists of a comparable process in humans. Indeed, using a model in which human skin was grafted onto mice with severe combined immunodeficiency disease, gross inadequacy of the commonly used rodent model of photocarcinogenesis has been demonstrated.[35] Specifically, the traditional rodent models significantly overestimate the human carcinogenic potential of tested agents. Topical retinoids, on the contrary, appear to have a protective effect against UV-induced premalignant and malignant lesions. In those predisposed by nevoid basal cell carcinoma syndrome or xeroderma pigmentosum to the development of nonmelanoma skin cancer, systemic retinoids have provided effective protection. These clinically observed anticarcinogenic activities of retinoids are supported by in vitro data demonstrating that tretinoin treatment of human skin upregulates the antigen-presenting activity of Langerhans cells without concomitant increase in autoreactivity.[36] Such a retinoid effect would improve cutaneous immune responsiveness to tumor antigens. Therefore, topical retinoic acid is not a carcinogen in humans.

DRUG INTERACTION AND INCOMPATIBILITIES

Retinoids in general are photolabile and therefore can be photoinactivated. Based on this chemistry, it is prudent to apply the agents in the evening rather than before the start of the day. Since the major avenue of tretinoin inactivation is through a cytochrome P_{450} retinoic acid 4-hydroxylase, drugs that modulate the activity of this enzyme can potentially cause drug interactions. Ketoconazole and liarozole are effective inhibitors of this hydroxylase.[8,9] Therefore, concurrent use of these azoles and topical tretinoin can increase the amount and prolong the half-life of tretinoin locally in the skin, thereby aggravating the local side effect. Indeed, this was observed in one topical tretinoin study when a patient inadvertently started oral ketoconazole for tinea infection and experienced a severe and prolonged dermatitis, which could be reproduced by ketoconazole challenge. If oral liarozole becomes available for psoriasis monotherapy, similar interactions of this medication with topical tretinoin may be more commonly seen. Other than retinoids, no other compounds have been shown to induce the retinoic acid 4-hydroxylase.

The use of vitamin D_3 and its analogues has increased in dermatology. Vitamin D effects in human skin are largely mediated via its nuclear receptor VDR. As previously discussed, VDR is a member of the steroid/retinoic acid/thyroid hormone receptor superfamily. Like RAR, VDR functions in human skin mainly as a heterodimer with RXR (VDR-RXR). In contrast with retinoid signaling via RAR-RXR in which the presence of RXR-ligand confers no additional effect, RXR-ligand provides a synergistic effect with VDR-ligand in vitamin D signaling.[37] Therefore, topical retinoids that possess, or, through metabolic conversion, acquire RXR selectivity can positively influence vitamin D pharmacology in human skin.

REFERENCES

1. Petkovich M et al: A human retinoic acid receptor which belongs to the family of nuclear receptors. *Nature* **330**:444, 1987
2. Giguére V et al: Identification of a receptor for the morphogen retinoic acid. *Nature* **330**:624, 1987
3. Duell EA et al: Extraction of human epidermis treated with retinol yields *retro*-retinoids in addition to free retinol and retinyl esters. *J Invest Dermatol* **107**:178, 1996
4. Kang S et al: Application of retinol to human skin in vivo induces epidermal hyperplasia and cellular retinoid binding proteins characteristic of retinoic acid but without measurable retinoic acid levels or irritation. *J Invest Dermatol* **105**:549, 1995
5. Kurlandsky SB et al: Auto-regulation of retinoic acid biosynthesis through regulation of retinol esterification in human keratinocytes. *J Biol Chem* **271**:15346, 1996
6. Duell EA et al: Retinoic acid isomers applied to human skin in vivo each induce a 4-hydroxylase that inactivates only *trans* retinoic acid. *J Invest Dermatol* **106**:316, 1996
7. Reynolds NJ et al: Retinoic acid metabolites exhibit biological activity in human keratinocytes, mouse melanoma cells and hairless mouse skin in vivo. *J Pharmacol Exp Ther* **266**:1636, 1993
8. Duell EA et al: Human skin levels of retinoic acid and cytochrome P-450-derived 4-hydroxyretinoic acid after topical application of retinoic acid in vivo compared to concentrations required to stimulate retinoic acid receptor-mediated transcription in vitro. *J Clin Invest* **90**:1269, 1992
9. Kang S et al: Liarozole inhibits human epidermal retinoic acid 4-hydroxylase activity and differentially augments human skin responses to retinoic acid and retinol in vivo. *J Invest Dermatol* **107**:183, 1996
10. White JA et al: Identification of the retinoic acid–inducible all-*trans* retinoic acid 4-hydroxylase. *J Biol Chem* **271**:29922, 1996
11. Yu VC et al: RXRβ: A co-regulator that enhances binding of retinoic acid, thyroid hormone, and vitamin D receptors to their cognate response element. *Cell* **67**:1251, 1991
12. Levin AA et al: 9-*cis* retinoic acid stereoisomer binds and activates the nuclear receptor RXRα. *Nature* **355**:359, 1992
13. Bernard BA: Adapalene, a new chemical entity with retinoid activity. *Skin Pharmacol* **6**(suppl 1):61, 1993
14. Griffiths CEM et al: Comparison of CD271 (adapalene) and all-*trans* retinoic acid in human skin: Dissociation of epidermal effects and CRABP-II mRNA expression. *J Invest Dermatol* **101**:325, 1993
15. Elder JT et al: Retinoid induction of CRABP II mRNA in human dermal fibroblasts: Use as a retinoid bioassay. *J Invest Dermatol* **106**:517, 1996
16. Nagpal S et al: Separation of transactivation and AP1 antagonism functions of retinoic acid receptor α. *J Biol Chem* **270**:923, 1995
17. Elder JT et al: Differential regulation of retinoic acid receptors and binding proteins in human skin. *J Invest Dermatol* **98**:673, 1992
18. Fisher GJ et al: Immunological identification and functional quantitation of retinoic acid and retinoid X receptor proteins in human skin. *J Biol Chem* **269**:20629, 1994
19. Xiao JH et al: Endogenous retinoic acid receptor–retinoid X receptor heterodimers are the major functional forms regulating retinoid-responsive elements in adult human keratinocytes. *J Biol Chem* **270**:3001, 1995
20. Aström A et al: Retinoic acid induction of human cellular retinoic acid–binding protein-II gene transcription is mediated by retinoic acid receptor–retinoid X receptor heterodimers bound to one far upstream retinoic acid–responsive element with 5-base pair spacing. *J Biol Chem* **269**:22334, 1994
21. Fisher GJ et al: All-*trans* retinoic acid induces cellular retinol-binding protein in vivo. *J Invest Dermatol* **105**:80, 1995
22. Rosenthal DS et al: Acute or chronic topical retinoic acid treatment of human skin in vivo alters the expression of epidermal transglutaminase, loricrin, involucrin, filaggrin, and keratins 6 and 13 but not keratins 1, 10, and 14. *J Invest Dermatol* **98**:343, 1992
23. Griffiths CEM et al: Restoration of collagen formation in photodamaged human skin by tretinoin (retinoic acid). *N Engl J Med* **329**:530, 1993
24. Griffiths CEM et al: Two concentrations of topical tretinoin (retinoic acid) cause similar improvement of photoaging but different degrees of irritation: A double-blind, vehicle controlled comparison of 0.1% and 0.025% tretinoin creams. *Arch Dermatol* **131**:1037, 1995
25. Fisher GJ et al: Molecular basis of sun-induced premature skin ageing and retinoid antagonism. *Nature* **379**:335, 1996
26. Bulengo-Ransby SM et al: Topical tretinoin (retinoic acid) therapy for hyperpigmented lesions caused by inflammation of the skin in black patients. *N Engl J Med* **328**:1438, 1993
27. Griffiths CEM et al: Topical tretinoin (retinoic acid) treatment of hyperpigmented lesions associated with photoaging in Chinese and Japanese patients: A vehicle-controlled trial. *J Am Acad Dermatol* **30**:76, 1994
28. Griffiths CEM et al: Topical tretinin (retinoic acid) improves melasma: A vehicle-controlled clinical trial. *Br J Dermatol* **129**:415, 1993
29. Kimbrough-Green CK et al: Topical retinoic acid (tretinoin) for melasma in black patients: A vehicle-controlled clinical trial. *Arch Dermatol* **130**:727, 1994
30. Kang S et al: Topical tretinoin (retinoic acid) improves early stretch marks. *Arch Dermatol* **132**:519, 1996
31. Esgleyes-Ribot T et al: Response of psoriasis to a new topical retinoid, AGN 190168. *J Am Acad Dermatol* **30**:581, 1994
32. Feng X et al: Suprabasal expression of a dominant-negative RXRα mutant in transgenic mouse epidermis impairs regulation of gene transcription and basal keratinocyte proliferation by RAR-selective retinoids. *Genes Dev* **11**:59, 1997
33. Bucha P et al: Repeated topical administration of all-*trans*-retinoic acid and plasma levels of retinoic acids in humans. *J Am Acad Dermatol* **30**:428, 1994
34. Jick SS et al: First trimester topical tretinin and congenital disorders. *Lancet* **341**:1181, 1993

35. Soballe PW et al: Carcinogenesis in human skin grafted to SCID mice. *Cancer Res* **56**:757, 1996
36. Meunier L et al: Retinoic acid upregulates human Langerhans cell antigen presentation and surface expression of HLA-DR and CD11c, a β_2 integrin critically involved in T-cell activation. *J Invest Dermatol* **103**:775, 1994
37. Kang S et al: The retinoid X receptor agonist 9-*cis*-retinoic acid and the 24-hydroxylase inhibitor ketoconazole increase activity of 1,25-

dihydroxyvitamin D$_3$ in human skin in vivo. *J Invest Dermatol* **108**:513, 1997

CHAPTER 246

Mark W. Bonner
Paul M. Benson
William D. James

Topical Antibiotics in Dermatology

Topical antibiotics play an important role in the management of many common dermatologic conditions. They are most often prescribed by dermatologists for the management of mild to moderate acne vulgaris or as adjunctive treatment with oral agents. For localized superficial infections, such as impetigo, the use of a topical agent (e.g., mupirocin) may eliminate the need for oral antibiotics and the accompanying problems of compliance, gastrointestinal side effects, and potential drug interactions. Lastly, topical antibiotics are frequently prescribed as prophylactic agents following minor surgery or cosmetic procedures (dermabrasion, laser resurfacing) to reduce the risk of postoperative wound infections and to speed wound healing. The usefulness of topical antibiotics for prophylaxis following such minor procedures has recently been questioned and will be discussed more fully below.

AGENTS USED IN THE TOPICAL TREATMENT OF ACNE

The efficacy of topical antibiotics for treatment of acne vulgaris and acne rosacea may be due to their direct antibiotic effect, but there are some suggestions that many of the topical antibiotics exhibit anti-inflammatory properties by suppressing neutrophil chemotactic factor or by other mechanisms. There are mounting concerns about the use of topical antibiotics in the treatment of acne vulgaris because of the increasing levels of antibiotic resistance to common topicals. This has led investigators to look at combination therapy for acne vulgaris that reduces the development of antibiotic resistance.

Erythromycin

Erythromycin belongs to the group of macrolide antibiotics and is active against both gram-positive cocci and gram-negative bacilli. It is a fermentation product of *Streptomyces erythreus* and is principally used as a topical agent for the treatment of acne. Erythromycin binds to the bacterial 50S ribosome and blocks translocation of the peptidyl-tRNA molecule from the acceptor to the donor site, interfering with the formation of the polypeptide chain and inhibiting protein synthesis.[1] In addition to its antibacterial properties, erythromycin has anti-inflammatory activity, which makes it especially useful in the management of acne.[2]

Erythromycin is available as a 1.5 to 2% solution, gel, pledgets, and ointment as a single agent (see Table 246-1). It is also available in combination with benzoyl peroxide, which may slow the development of antibiotic resistance to erythromycin.[3] The combination of 1.2% zinc acetate and 4% erythromycin may be superior to clindamycin although it is not currently available in the United States.

TABLE 246-1

Topical Antibiotics

NAME	SOURCE	FORM AVAILABLE	MECHANISM OF ACTION	BACTERIA*
Bacitracin	*Bacillus subtilis*	O	Cell wall inhibitor	Gr +
Polymyxin B	*B. polymyxa*	O	Detergent	Gr −
Gramicidin		O	Ion channel	Gr +
Mupirocin	*Pseudomonas fluorescens*	O	tRNA inhibitor	Gr +
Neomycin	*Streptomyces fradiae*	O	30S ribosome inhibition	Gr −
Tetracycline	Semisynthetic[†]	O,S	30S ribosome inhibition	Gr +/−
Meclocycline	Semisynthetic[‡]	C	30S ribosome inhibition	Gr +/−
Erythromycin	*Strep. erythreus*	S,G,P,O	50S ribosome inhibition	Gr +/−
Clindamycin	Semisynthetic	S,G,L	50S ribosome inhibition	
Chloramphenicol	*Strep. venezuelae*[§]	C	50S ribosome inhibition	
Fusidic acid		NA	Interferes with EF-G	
Silver sulfadiazine	Synthetic	C		
Mafenide acetate	Synthetic	C	Enzyme inhibition	Gr +/−
Nitrofurazone	Synthetic	C,S	Enzyme inhibition	Gr +/−
Metronidazole	Synthetic	G,C	Electrochemical	Anaerobes
Clioquinol	Synthetic	C,O	Unknown	Broad spectrum
Azelaic acid	Synthetic	C	Protein synthesis inhibition	Gr +

*Bacteria refers to bacteria usually susceptible to antibiotic; Gr +, Gr −, gram-positive and -negative.
[†]Semisynthetic from chlortetracycline, fermented from some species of *Streptomyces*.
[‡]Semisynthetic from tetracycline.
[§]Now completely synthesized.
NOTE: O, ointment; S, solution; C, cream; P, pledget; L, lotion; NA, not available in U.S.

Clindamycin

Clindamycin is a semi-synthetic lincosamide antibiotic that is derived from lincomycin. The mechanism of action is very similar to erythromycin, with binding to the 50S ribosome and suppression of bacterial protein synthesis.[1] Clindamycin is used topically as a 1% gel, solution, and suspension (lotion) (see Table 246-1) primarily for the treatment of acne. Pseudomembranous colitis rarely has been reported to occur with the topical use of clindamycin.[4]

Tetracycline

Topical tetracyclines, in the form of meclocycline sulfosalicylate and tetracycline hydrochloride solution, have been available in the past for the treatment of acne but have never gained wide acceptance. Meclocycline sulfosalicylate currently is not available, probably because of a lack of efficacy. Undesirable side effects of tetracycline topical solution include odor and yellow staining of skin.

Metronidazole

Metronidazole, a topical nitroimidazole, is currently available as a 0.75% gel and as a 1% cream for the topical treatment of rosacea. In the lower strength, it it applied twice daily, and in the higher strength, it is used once daily. Orally, metronidazole has broad-spectrum activity against many protozoal organisms and anaerobes. The mechanism of action of topical metronidazole in the skin is unknown; however, the anti-rosacea effect may be due to the antibiotic, antioxidant, and anti-inflammatory properties of the drug.[5]

Azelaic Acid

Azelaic acid is a dicarboxylic acid found in food (whole grain cereals and animal products). There is a normal human plasma level (20 to 80 ng/mL), but topical application does not significantly alter the plasma concentration. The mechanism of action is thought to be normalization of the keratinization process (decreased thickness of the stratum corneum, decreased number and size of keratohyaline granules, and decreased amount of filaggrin). There are reports of in vitro activity against *Propionibacterium acnes* and *Staphylococcus epidermidis,* which may be due to inhibition of bacterial protein synthesis (the exact site not known at this time). In aerobic microorganisms, there is inhibition of oxidoreductive enzymes (such as tyrosinase, mitochondrial enzymes of the respiratory chain, 5-alpha-reductase, and DNA polymerases). In anaerobic bacteria, there is disruption of glycolysis. Azelaic acid is used principally in the treatment of acne vulgaris, although there are some advocates for the use of azelaic acid in the treatment of hyperpigmentation (such as melasma). However, this is an off-label use in the United States since the U.S. Food and Drug Administration has not approved the drug for this indication. Azelaic acid is available as a 20% cream preparation.[6]

AGENTS USED FOR THE TOPICAL THERAPY OF SUPERFICIAL BACTERIAL INFECTIONS

Mupirocin

Mupirocin is a topical antibiotic agent derived from *Pseudomonas fluorescens,* which was formerly known as pseudomonic acid A. The drug reversibly binds to iso-leucyl-tRNA synthetase and inhibits bacterial protein synthesis. The activity of mupirocin is limited to gram-positive bacteria, especially staphylococci and most streptococci. Its activity is enhanced in an acid pH environment (5.5), which is the normal pH of the skin. Mupirocin is somewhat temperature-sensitive and thus should not be exposed to high temperatures. Mupirocin ointment 2% is applied three times daily and is principally indicated for the treatment of localized impetigo caused

impetigo or disease occurring in immunocompromised individuals should be treated with systemic therapy to reduce the risk of serious complications. A new formulation that involves the use of the calcium salt of mupirocin (the calcium aids in chemical stability in the intranasal preparation) is available for intranasal use.

AGENTS USED TO PREVENT INFECTION FOLLOWING SURGICAL PROCEDURES OR INJURIES OR TO TREAT CHRONIC DERMATITIS

It is common practice to use topical antibiotics to reduce the potential for wound infections following minor surgical procedures, in cases of chronic dermatitis such as stasis dermatitis or atopic dermatitis, or following minor abrasions of the skin. Recent studies have focused on the incidence of infection after skin biopsy or minor surgery with the use of topical antibiotics or their vehicles. In some cases, the topical antibiotic seemed to decrease the rate of wound healing. In other studies, use of the vehicle alone appeared to be as effective as the topical antibiotic in wound healing without the risk of irritant or allergic contact dermatitis to the antibiotic agent. The results of one large study comparing bacitracin and petrolatum in over 1200 minor surgical procedures and biopsies demonstrated that the active agent, bacitracin, did not statistically decrease the already low rate of infection during such procedures but was associated with a small risk of allergic contact dermatitis.[8]

Bacitracin

Bacitracin is a topical polypeptide antibiotic originally isolated from the *Tracy-I* strain of *Bacillus subtilis,* which was cultured from a patient with a compound fracture contaminated with soil. Thus, the *baci-* portion is derived from *Bacillus* and the *-tracin* from the name of the patient who had the compound fracture (Tracy). Bacitracin is a cyclic polypeptide antibiotic with multiple components (A, B, and C). Bacitracin A is the major component of commercial products and is often used as the zinc salt.[1] Bacitracin interferes with bacterial cell wall synthesis by binding to and inhibiting the dephosphorylation of a membrane-bound lipid pyrophosphate.[9] It is active against gram-positive cocci such as staphylococci and streptococci. Most gram-negative organisms and yeast are resistant to the drug. It is available as bacitracin ointment, 400 to 500 units per gram, and as zinc bacitracin, 400 to 500 units per gram.

Topical bacitracin is effective for the treatment of superficial bacterial infections of the skin such as impetigo, furunculosis, and pyodermas. It is often combined with polymyxin B and neomycin as a triple antibiotic ointment applied several times daily for the treatment of secondarily infected eczematous dermatitis such as atopic dermatitis, nummular dermatitis, or stasis dermatitis.[1] Unfortunately, the topical application of bacitracin carries with it the risk of allergic contact sensitization[8] and, rarely, anaphylactic shock.[10]

Polymyxin B

Polymyxin B is a topical antibiotic, derived from a spore-forming soil aerobe *B. polymyxa,* which was originally isolated from a soil sample in Japan. Polymyxin B is a mixture of polymyxin B_1 and B_2, which are both cyclic polypeptides. They function as cationic detergents that interact strongly with bacterial cell membrane phospholipids, thus disrupting the integrity of the cell membrane.[1]

Polymyxin B is active against a wide range of gram-negative organisms, including *P. aeruginosa, Enterobacter,* and *Escherichia coli.*[1] Polymyxin B is available in ointment form in 5000 to 10,000 units per gram in combination with bacitracin or bacitracin and neomycin. It should be applied one to three times a day.[9]

Topical Aminoglycosides, including Neomycin, Gentamicin, and Paromomycin

The aminoglycosides are an important group of antibiotics used both topically and systemically for the treatment of infections caused by gram-negative bacilli. Aminoglycosides exert their bactericidal effects by binding to the 30S ribosomal subunit and interfering with protein synthesis.[11]

Neomycin sulfate, the aminoglycoside most often used topically, is a fermentation product of *Strep. fradiae*. Commercial neomycin is a mixture of neomycin B and C, whereas framycetin, used in Canada and some European countries, is pure neomycin B.[12] Neomycin sulfate has activity against aerobic gram-negative bacteria and is most commonly used for prophylaxis against infection in superficial abrasions, cuts, and burns.[11] It is available in ointment form (3.5 mg/g) and is found in combination with other antibiotics such as bacitracin, polymyxin, and gramicidin. Other agents, such as lidocaine, pramoxine, or hydrocortisone, may also be found in combination with neomycin.[13]

Neomycin is not recommended by many dermatologists because of the allergic contact dermatitis that occurs after widespread, indiscriminate use of the drug, especially in over-the-counter products.[10] The incidence of contact dermatitis is high, with 6 to 8 percent of patients using topically applied neomycin developing contact sensitivity.[11] Neomycin sulfate (20%) in petrolatum is used to assess for contact allergy.[14]

Gentamicin sulfate is derived as a fermentation product from *Micromonospora purpurea*. Gentamicin is available as a topical 0.1% cream or ointment.[15] It is used by some dermatologic surgeons when operating on the ear, especially in diabetic or other immunocompromised patients, to provide prophylaxis against malignant otitis externa due to *P. aeruginosa.*[16]

Paromomycin is closely related to neomycin and has antibacterial and antiparasitic activities. A topical formulation consisting of paromomycin sulfate and methylbenzethonium chloride is used in Israel to treat Old World cutaneous leishmaniasis.[17]

Miscellaneous Agents

GRAMICIDIN Gramicidin is a topical antibiotic derived from *B. brevis*.[15] The gramicidins are linear peptides that form stationary ion channels in susceptible bacteria. The antibiotic activity of gramicidin is restricted to gram-positive bacteria.[18]

CHLORAMPHENICOL Chloramphenicol is available in the United States with use limited to the treatment of minor bacterial skin infections. Chloramphenicol was originally isolated from *Strep. venezuelae* but is now synthesized because of its simple chemical structure. The mechanism of action is similar to that of erythromycin and clindamycin, with inhibition of the 50S ribosome blocking translocation of peptidyl tRNA from the acceptor to the donor site.[10] Chloramphenicol is available as a 1% cream. It is used infrequently because fatal aplastic anemia or dose-related bone marrow suppression has been reported following topical exposure.[19]

SULFONAMIDES The sulfonamides are structurally similar to para-aminobenzoic acid (PABA) and compete with it during the synthesis of folic acid. Sulfonamides are infrequently used as topical agents with the exception of silver sulfadiazine (Silvadene) cream and mafenide acetate cream. Silver sulfadiazine is thought to release silver slowly. The silver exerts its effect on the bacterial cell walls and membranes.[20] The mechanism of action of mafenide is not the typical sulfonamide mechanism of action because PABA does not antagonize its performance.[21] Mafenide acetate, if used over large areas of skin, has the potential to cause a metabolic acidosis and can cause intense pain upon topical administration. Both agents are broad-spectrum antibacterials useful in the treatment of burns. *Candida* superinfection may be a problem with mafenide cream.[21]

CLIOQUINOL Clioquinol (also known as iodochlorhydroxyquin) is a broad-spectrum antibacterial/antifungal topical that is currently indicated for the treatment of inflammatory skin disorders and tinea pedis and has been used for minor bacterial infections. Clioquinol is a synthetic hydroxyquinoline whose mechanism of action is unknown.[22] The disadvantages of clioquinol include discoloration of clothing, skin, hair, and nails and it may cause irritation. Clioquinol may interfere with thyroid function determination because the iodine moiety interferes with tests that rely upon iodine uptake (this effect can last for up to 3 months after application). However, clioquinol does not interfere with testing for T_3 or T_4.[22]

NITROFURAZONE Nitrofurazone (Furacin) is a nitrofuran derivative used for the treatment of burn patients. The mechanism of action involves the inhibition of bacterial enzymes involved in the aerobic and anaerobic degradation of glucose and pyruvate. Nitrofurazone is available as a 0.2% cream, solution, or soluble dressing, and its spectrum of activity includes staphylococci, streptococci, *E. coli, Clostridium perfringens, Aerobacter enterogenes,* and *Proteus* spp.[23]

FUSIDIC ACID Fusidic acid is a topical preparation that is not currently available in the United States, but is in use in Canada and Europe as an antibacterial available as a cream, ointment, and impregnated gauze.[24] Fusidic acid is a steroidal antibiotic with a mechanism of action that interferes with the function of the elongation factor (EF-G) by stabilizing the EF-G-GDP-ribosome complex, preventing translocation of the ribosomes and EF-G from recycling.[18]

REFERENCES

1. Kapusnik-Uner JE et al: Tetracyclines, chloramphenicol, erythromycin, and miscellaneous antibacterial agents, in *Goodman and Gilman's The Pharmacological Basis of Therapeutics,* 9th ed, edited by JG Hardman et al. New York, McGraw-Hill, 1996, pp 1123–1147
2. Esterly NB et al: The effect of antimicrobial agents on leukocyte chemotaxis. *J Invest Dermatol* **70**:51, 1978
3. Thiboutot DM: Acne: An overview of clinical research findings. *Dermatol Clin* **15**:97, 1997
4. Clindamycin (topical), in *Drug Information for the Health Care Professional (USP DI).* Rockville, MD, United States Pharmacopeial Convention, 1997, pp 854–856
5. Metronidazole (topical), in *Drug Information for the Health Care Professional (USP DI).* Rockville, MD, United States Pharmacopeial Convention, 1997, pp 2028–2029
6. Azelaic Acid (topical), in *Drug Information for the Health Care Professional (USP DI).* Rockville, MD, United States Pharmacopeial Convention, 1997, pp 485–487
7. Mupirocin (topical), in *Drug Information for the Health Care Professional (USP DI).* Rockville, MD, United States Pharmacopeial Convention, 1997, pp 2082–2083
8. Smack DP et al: Infection and allergy incidence in ambulatory surgery patients using white petrolatum versus bacitracin ointment. *JAMA* **276**:972, 1996
9. Neomycin, polymyxin B and bacitracin (topical), in *Drug Information for the Health Care Professional (USP DI).* Rockville, MD, United States Pharmacopeial Convention, 1997, pp 2111–2112
10. Rietschel RL, Fowler JF (eds): Systemic contact-type dermatitis, in *Fisher's Contact Dermatitis,* 4th ed. Baltimore, Williams & Wilkins, 1995, pp 118–119
11. Chambers HF, Sande MA: The aminoglycosides, in *Goodman and Gilman's The Pharmacological Basis of Therapeutics,* 9th ed, edited by JG Hardman et al. New York, McGraw-Hill, 1996, pp 1123–1147
12. Budavari S: *The Merck Index,* 12th ed. Whitehouse Station, NJ, Merck & Co, 1996, p 1108
13. Olin BR (ed): *Drug Facts and Comparisons.* St. Louis, MO, Facts and Comparisons, 1996, pp 2829–2832
14. Marks JG, DeLeo VA: in *Contact and Occupational Dermatology.* St. Louis, MO, Mosby Year Book, 1992, pp 327–328
15. Edwards DI: Biosynthesis of antimicrobial drugs, in *Antimicrobial Drug Action,* Baltimore, MD, University Park Press, 1980, pp 31–32
16. Scherbenske JM et al: Acute *Pseudomonas* infection of the external ear (malignant external otitis). *J Dermatol Surg Oncol* **14**:165, 1988
17. Teva Pharmaceutical Industries, Ltd., package insert for Leshcutan (Paromomycin sulfate, 15%, and Methylbenzethonium chloride, 12%, Ointment), Petah-Tikva, Israel
18. Lancini G et al: in *Antibiotics, A Multidisciplinary Approach,* New York, New York, Plenum, 1995, p 70
19. Chloramphenicol (Topical), in *Drug Information for the Health Care Professional (USP DI).* Rockville, MD, United States Pharmacopeial Convention, 1997, p 795
20. Mandell GA, Petri WA: Sulfonamides, trimethoprim-sulfamethoxazole, quinolones, and agents for urinary tract infections, in *Goodman and Gilman's The Pharmacological Basis of Therapeutics,* 9th ed. edited by JG Hardman et al. New York, McGraw-Hill, 1996, p 1061
21. Mafenide (topical), in *Drug Information for the Health Care Professional (USP DI).* Rockville, MD, United States Pharmacopeial Convention, 1997, pp. 1912–1913
22. Clioquinol (topical), in *Drug Information for the Health Care Professional (USP DI).* Rockville, MD, United States Pharmacopeial Convention, 1997, p 858
23. 1996 Roberts package insert for Furacin (nitrofurazone cream) *Physician Desk Reference,* 51st ed. Montvale, NJ, Medical Economics, 1997, p 3044
24. Additional Products & Indications, in *Drug Information for the Health Care Professional (USP DI).* Rockville, MD, United States Pharmacopeial Convention, 1997, p 3044

CHAPTER 247

James E. Fitzpatrick

Topical Antifungal Agents

Superficial fungal infections such as dermatophytoses, candidiasis, and pityriasis versicolor are typically restricted to epithelial tissues. When presented with such infections, the option is to treat with either systemic or topical antifungal therapy. The decision requires consideration of numerous factors including extent of infection, severity of infection, site of infection (e.g., nails as opposed to glabrous skin), underlying diseases, efficacy of treatment, potential drug interactions, side effects, known allergies, cost, the patient's health care plan, ease of use, patient's preference, and finally the physician's familiarity with different antifungal therapies. In general, patients with limited disease and fungal infections confined to glabrous skin are best treated with topical antifungal therapy. Patients with extensive disease and infections of hair and nails are best treated with systemic therapy. In some cases either option may be utilized. Topical antifungal therapy has numerous advantages over systemic antifungal therapy including the absence of serious side effects (e.g., hepatitis as seen with the oral imidazoles), absence of drug interactions, no requirement to monitor laboratory tests, ability to localize treatment to affected sites, over-the-counter availability of some medications, and ease of use for patients who experience difficulty swallowing pills.

There are numerous topical antifungal drugs available, with many of them becoming available in the past decade (Table 247-1). Prior to 1945, specific antifungal drugs were not available and nonspecific therapies such as keratolytics (e.g., salicylic acid) and antiseptics (e.g., gentian violet, Castellani's paint) were the cornerstones of therapy. Although topical antifungal drugs have been available since the development of undecylenic acid in 1945,[1] there is no consensus as to the best topical antifungal agent. The ideal topical antifungal agent should demonstrate the following properties:

- Fungicidal at therapeutic concentration
- Absence of resistance
- Broad spectrum of action that includes all known superficial fungal pathogens
- Keratinophilic
- Penetrates keratin but is not absorbed systemically
- Hypoallergenic
- Nonirritating
- Anti-inflammatory properties
- Once per day (or less) application
- Short duration of therapy required for cure
- Availability in a wide variety of formulations (e.g., cream, solution) and sizes
- Inexpensive

None of the drugs developed to date fully meets all of the desired properties. Despite the fact that topical antifungal agents have been used for decades and there are numerous studies that demonstrate

TABLE 247-1

Topical Antifungal Agents

CLASS/GENERIC NAME	TRADEMARK NAME	AVAILABILITY
Imidazoles		
Clotrimazole	Lotrimin	Prescription
	Cruex	OTC
	Desenex AF	OTC
	Lotrimin AF	OTC
Clotrimazole/betamethasone dipropionate	Lotrisone	Prescription
Econazole	Spectazole	Prescription
Ketoconazole	Nizoral	Prescription
Miconazole	Monistat-Derm	Prescription
	Micatin	OTC
Oxiconazole	Oxistat	Prescription
Sulconazole	Exelderm	Prescription
Allylamines		
Naftifine	Naftin	Prescription
Terbinafine	Lamisil	Prescription
Polyenes		
Nystatin	Mycostatin	Prescription
Nystatin/triamcinolone	Mytrex	Prescription
Miscellaneous		
Ciclopirox olamine	Loprox	Prescription
Triacetin/sodium propionate/ benzalkonium chloride/ cetylpyridinium chloride/ chloroxylenol	Fungoid	Prescription
Tolnaftate	Equate	OTC
	Tinactin	OTC
Undecylenic acid/zinc undecylenate	Cruex	OTC
	Desenex	OTC

NOTE: OTC, over the counter.

the efficacy of each drug, it remains difficult to compare the efficacy of the various agents. In part this is due to the fact that most antifungal studies are sponsored by the pharmaceutical companies and the antifungal therapy is often compared to the vehicle. Comparing the results between these studies is fraught with error since the studies differ in design, duration of therapy, site of infection, patient selection, method of determining response, and duration of follow-up. There are a number of studies that compare one topical antifungal agent with another, but the conclusions are always limited to that study and the data cannot be compared with data from other studies. Since the two most important medical factors are the type of pathogen and the site of infection, the discussion of topical antifungal therapy that follows is organized in this fashion.

DERMATOPHYTE INFECTIONS

Dermatophyte infections are limited to three genera (i.e., *Trichophyton, Microsporum,* and *Epidermophyton*) that utilize keratin as a substrate. The specific species producing infection is usually not a consideration in the selection of topical therapy, although in vitro studies have shown that *T. mentagrophytes* species are less sensitive to most antifungal drugs than other species.[2] Since the site of infection is critical in selecting therapy, dermatophyte infections may be divided into those of the hair, glabrous skin, and nails.

Dermatophyte infections of hair most commonly present as tinea capitis but may also present as tinea barbae or Majocchi's granuloma. In follicular dermatophyte infections, viable hyphae invade to the bottom one-third of the hair follicle to a region referred to as Adamson's fringe. It is at this level that there is a transition from keratin to viable keratinocytes, which cannot serve as a substrate for dermatophyte growth. Because of the depth of Adamson's fringe, topical antifungal agents should probably not be used as primary therapy, although studies regarding their use in this situation are lacking. Ketoconazole shampoo and selenium sulfide have both been demonstrated to decrease the shedding of viable organisms and are useful adjunctive therapies to prevent the spread of infection to other family members.[3] Neither therapy produces a more rapid clinical response to the primary therapy.

Dermatophyte infections of glabrous skin, which are classified by site of involvement including face (tinea faciei), trunk and extremities (tinea corporis), groin (tinea cruris), hands (tinea manuum), and feet (tinea pedis), are the most common indication for topical antifungal therapy. Topical therapies may be used interchangeably among these sites with the possible exception of tinea cruris, where the skin is sensitive and easily develops an irritant contact dermatitis to some topical antifungals.

Undecylenic acid, which is usually combined with one of its salts (e.g., zinc undecylenate), is the original specific topical antifungal agent. Although the initial study reported a high cure rate in tinea pedis (90 percent), tinea corporis (44 percent), and tinea cruris (100 percent), subsequent studies reported cure rates as low as 27 percent.[1] In addition to its relatively low cure rates, this antifungal also has a disagreeable odor and may require prolonged use (up to 26 weeks in some studies). Despite the advent of newer, more effective antifungal agents, it is still available as an over-the-counter drug.

Tolnaftate was synthesized in Japan and introduced as a topical antifungal agent in 1964. Tolfnaftate is a thiocarbamate derivative, not related to any other antifungal drug. Its mode of action is similar to the allylamines in that it inhibits squalene epoxidase, which results in accumulation of squalene in the fungal cell. Although early studies reported cure rates as high as 73 to 93 percent, at least one study reported a 0 percent cure rate for tinea pedis.[4] This discrepancy in therapeutic response is attributable to different methods for the definition of a "cure." While earlier studies suggested that tolnaftate was superior to undecylenic acid preparations, later studies concluded that the two drugs were equivalent.[5–7] Although definitive comparative studies are lacking, it is probably less effective than newer antifungal agents. Its primary advantage over some of the newer antifungal agents is that it is relatively nonirritating and useful in sensitive areas such as the groin. It has retained a small niche as an over-the-counter antifungal agent.

The advent of the topical imidazoles in the early 1970s produced the class of drugs that are most commonly used on fungal infections of glabrous tissue. The imidazoles are considered to be fungistatic drugs, although at very high levels some imidazoles are fungicidal. The imidazoles act by inhibiting the 14-α-demethylation of lanosterol, which prohibits the synthesis of ergosterol, a fungal cell wall sterol necessary for normal cell membrane permeability and structural integrity. The topical antifungals currently available in this class include miconazole, clotrimazole, econazole, ketoconazole, oxiconazole, and sulconazole. Although all of these drugs have the same mechanism of action, in vitro studies have shown that not all dermatophytes are uniformly susceptible to different imidazoles at identical concentrations.[2] The clinical significance of this finding is not yet resolved.

The reported cure rates for the imidazole class of drugs are highly variable and depend on the design of the study; as stated earlier, it is impossible to compare cure rates between different studies. For example, one may conclude that topical miconazole produces either a 63 percent cure rate[8] or a 100 percent cure rate[9] in dermatophyte infections, depending on the study quoted. A review of the literature of topically applied imidazole agents does not provide convincing evidence that there is a significant difference between any of the members of this group in overall cure rate or relapse rate, although they appear to be marginally superior to both undecylenic acid products and tolnaftate. Miconazole and clotrimazole are the two drugs in the class that are also available over the counter at a considerable savings over their prescription counterparts (Table 247-2). Although mycologic cure rate is not a determining factor in drug selection within this group, there is a difference in irritancy between different preparations, particularly in sensitive areas such as the groin. Comparative data about the potential for irritant reactions are not available, but in at least one study of clotrimazole, it was reported that it produced severe erosive irritant reactions in 4 of 27 patients when used to treat tinea cruris. In the same study, sulconazole did not produce any irritant reactions and was not only well tolerated but also seemed to accelerate healing in denuded areas.[10] In a second study, it was reported that there were severe irritant reactions in miconazole-treated patients but not in sulconazole-treated patients.[9] Until better studies regarding irritant reactions of topically applied imidazoles are available, sulconazole should be considered as the topical imidazole of choice for sensitive skin or macerated areas.

TABLE 247-2

Topical Antifungal Cost

DRUG (CREAM, 15-G TUBE)	RETAIL PRICE, $*
Tolnaftate (OTC)	2.99
Miconazole (OTC)	5.32
Miconazole (prescription)	6.95
Clotrimazole (prescription)	10.45
Sulconazole (prescription)	12.95
Clotrimazole (OTC)	13.09
Ciclopirox olamine (prescription)	15.55
Econazole (prescription)	17.40
Oxiconazole (prescription)	18.45
Ketoconazole (prescription)	19.55
Naftifine (prescription)	24.20
Terbinafine (prescription)	36.25

*Retail price at a retail Pharmacy (NYC October 1998).
NOTE: OTC, over the counter.

Topical imidazoles are available in creams and lotions. Head-to-head comparative studies comparing creams and lotions of the same drug are not available since pharmaceutical companies do not support studies between their own products financially. Limited studies from manufacturers would seem to indicate that creams are more effective than lotions. For example, oxiconazole cream is reported by the manufacturer to produce a clinical and mycologic cure in 52 percent of cases of tinea pedis, whereas oxiconazole lotion only produces a 41 percent cure.[11]

A second issue is that of how often the drug should be applied. Several imidazoles including econazole, ketoconazole, and oxiconazole have received once daily application approval from the U.S. Food and Drug Administration, while the remaining imidazole regimens recommend twice daily application. Sulconazole is recommended by the manufacturer to be applied twice daily, but a study comparing once daily to twice daily application regimens for the treatment of tinea cruris and tinea corporis reported identical cure rates.[10] This result is not unexpected, since all imidazoles have the same mechanism of action. This is an important point since drug companies with once per day indications promote their drugs as being more economical than drugs with twice daily regimens.

A third important issue is the use of topical imidazoles combined with topical glucocorticoids. The combination of clotrimazole and betamethasone dipropionate has gained popularity in recent years, especially among nondermatologists. The rationale for this combination has been that the addition of a topical glucocorticoid will relieve symptoms of pruritus and burning more quickly and produce quicker resolution of erythema and scaling. Early studies reported that the clotrimazole and betamethasone dipropionate combination was more effective than clotrimazole alone in producing resolution of erythema and pruritus.[12,13] The mycologic cure rate was reported to be equivalent to that of clotrimazole, although these studies had short follow-up periods that did not permit proper assessment of the relapse rate. Subsequent striae and persistent dermatophyte infections have prompted many dermatologists to eschew the use of this combination product.[14] In a subsequent study comparing naftifine to clotrimazole/betamethasone diproprionate, it was reported that the combination was less efficacious than naftifine alone. In contrast to prior studies, this study had an 8-week follow-up period that demonstrated a high relapse rate (36 percent) for the antifungal/steroid combination.[15] In sum, based on limited studies and anecdotal reports, this antifungal/steroid combination is more likely to produce permanent side effects and a high relapse rate.

Ciclopirox olamine, a broad-spectrum antifungal agent, is a hydroxypyridone and is not related to any other known antifungal agent. In contrast to the imidazoles, which are fungistatic, ciclopirox olamine is both fungicidal and fungistatic. This antifungal acts by interfering with the uptake of products required for cell membrane synthesis, alters cell permeability, and inhibits respiratory activity. It also demonstrates anti-inflammatory activity by inhibiting prostaglandin and leukotriene synthesis. Ciclopirox olamine also penetrates keratin easily, with cadaveric studies demonstrating levels in the dermis that are 10 to 15 times that of minimum inhibitory concentrations (MICs).[16] In clinical trials, ciclopirox olamine has demonstrated excellent mycologic and clinical response rates.[17] Despite its excellent pharmaceutical properties, its efficacy has not been compared to that of other antifungal agents, and it has been used interchangeably with the imidazoles.

The newest class of drugs are the allylamine antimycotics, with both naftifine and terbinafine being available in topical formations. Allylamines act by specific inhibition of squalene epoxidase. As with the imidazoles, this inhibits ergosterol biosynthesis, which is a fungistatic effect, but it also produces an accumulation of intra-

cellular squalene, which is a fungicidal effect, and this does not happen with the imidazoles. In vitro studies to determine MICs on 80 strains of dermatophytes revealed that naftifine was superior to clotrimazole, miconazole, ketoconazole, and bifonazole as determined by both the dilution method and the disk-diffusion method.[2] In addition to its antifungal effects, naftifine also demonstrates anti-inflammatory activity as measured by its ability to inhibit histamine-induced wheal-and-flare reactions, allergic contact dermatitis, UVB-induced erythema, and neutrophil chemotaxis. Naftifine is also lipophilic and demonstrates penetration to deep portions of the hair follicle. Terbinafine, the newest allylamine, demonstrates properties similar to naftifine except that it demonstrates in vitro activity that is 10 to 100 times greater.[18] There are numerous clinical studies comparing the allylamines to the imidazoles that have often produced conflicting results. Topical naftifine in some studies has been comparable to topical imidazoles,[19–21] whereas in other studies it has demonstrated marginal superiority to topical imidazoles.[22–24] When compared to topical miconazole combined with hydrocortisone cream, naftifine was markedly superior in the treatment of inflammatory dermatophyte infections.[25] The number of studies comparing topical terbinafine to other antimycotics is limited, but in two large multicenter comparisons of topical terbinafine with clotrimazole in the treatment of tinea pedis, a significantly higher cure rate and lower relapse rate for terbinafine was reported.[26,27] In summary, topical allylamines, especially terbinafine, are probably superior to topical imidazoles in cure rates and probably require shorter duration of therapy. However, this is the most expensive class of drugs, and many managed health care plans will not authorize their use.

Tinea unguium is the third major category of superficial dermatophytoses. Although pharmacokinetic studies have demonstrated that imidazoles, ciclopirox olamine, and allylamines are capable of penetrating the nail plate in concentrations sufficient to exceed the MICs of most dermatophytes,[28] they typically fail to produce clinical cures. Topical naftifine gel was reported to produce clinical and mycologic cures in 42 percent of patients with tinea unguium of finger and toe nails. These unexpectedly optimistic results need to be tempered by the fact that the patients were only followed for 6 months and there was no follow-up period.[29] A prescription product composed of triacetin, sodium propionate, benzalkonium chloride, cetylpyridium chloride, and chloroxylenol has been marketed in a tincture base (Fungoid) for the treatment of onychomycosis. An uncontrolled study has reported a 100 percent cure rate after 12 months of treatment; however, treatment also included monthly nail debridement and there was only a 2-month follow-up.[30] In summary, there are limited, often flawed, studies regarding the use of topical antifungal agents in the treatment of onychomycosis. Topical antifungal agents are probably best used on nails to prevent extension of fungal infection onto the hands and feet.

CANDIDIASIS (CANDIDOSIS)

Candida albicans is the primary pathogen in most cases of superficial candidiasis, although other species such as *C. parapsilosis* and *C. guilliermondii* may also produce infection. *Candida* species are commensal organisms that usually require a change in the host milieu, usually alterations in nutrition (e.g., diabetes mellitus), microbial flora (e.g., antibiotic therapy), or host immune defenses (e.g., neutropenia), to produce infections. This is an important consideration in assessing the efficacy of topical therapies, since the recurrence rate is very high if the underlying disease is not corrected.

Before the advent of the imidazoles, the polyenes were the mainstay of topical candidial therapy. There are more than 80 polyene antibiotics, but only nystatin and amphotericin B have been used topically on skin surfaces. Topical amphotericin B has recently been withdrawn from the market, leaving nystatin as the only available topical polyene. Polyene antimycotics are primarily fungistatic at low concentrations and fungicidal at high concentrations. They act by binding irreversibly with ergosterol in the cell membrane, which leads to altered cellular permeability and leakage of cell contents. Nystatin resistance in *Candida* species is increasing and is now seen in up to 20 percent of isolates.[31] Nystatin resistance may be encountered in wild strains (primary resistance) but may also be induced during therapy (secondary resistance). Nystatin is available in powder, suspension, lozenges, and as creams for topical therapy. The suspension and lozenge formulations are used for oral candidiasis, and the powder and creams are used for cutaneous infections. Although there are no recent studies comparing topical nystatin with the imidazoles, older studies demonstrated that the two were comparable.[32] This is an important point since nystatin resistance appears to be increasing, which means that information from the earlier studies cannot be extrapolated to the current time. Nystatin, while effective against candidial infections, is not effective against dermatophytes.

Topical imidazoles are the mainstay of topical therapy for candidiasis. Imidazoles are available as lotions, creams, and troches (clotrimazole). Clotrimazole troches are used for the management of oral candidiasis, and imidazole lotions and creams are used for superficial cutaneous candidiasis.[33] The susceptibility of different strains of *C. albicans* to imidazoles is highly variable (MIC of 0.5 to 100 μg/mL).[31] The implication of this difference in susceptibility to imidazoles has not been studied to determine if it is clinically significant in terms of response rates. All of the topical imidazoles are clinically and mycologicly effective in treating superficial candidial infections and can be used interchangeably.[34] As discussed in the management of dermatophyte infections, there is evidence to suggest that clotrimazole and miconazole are potentially irritating and may not be the preferred imidazoles in sensitive flexural areas infected with *Candida*.

Ciclopirox olamine, like the imidazoles, is a broad-spectrum antimycotic drug that is effective against *Candida* species. Ciclopirox olamine is indicated for the management of cutaneous candidial infections but it does not come in formulations for oral use. Head-to-head studies comparing this drug to the topical imidazoles have not been done, but ciclopirox olamine appears to be equivalent to the topical imidazoles in terms of clinical efficacy.

Topical allylamines (naftifine, terbinafine) demonstrate moderate activity against yeast, including *Candida* species. In vitro studies demonstrate that *Candida* species are more sensitive to the imidazole class of drugs than the allylamines.[31] Despite the higher measured in vitro MICs for yeasts, clinical studies have demonstrated that most cases of cutaneous candidiasis can be successfully treated with topical allylamines; they compare with topical imidazoles in terms of mycologic cure.[35,36] Despite the therapeutic efficacy of the allylamines, they should not be considered as a primary topical therapy for candidiasis since they are expensive, have not received approval for this indication, and demonstrate less favorable MICs.

PITYROSPORUM INFECTIONS

Pityrosporum orbiculare is a lipophilic yeast that produces superficial fungal infections in the form of tinea (pityriasis) versicolor and less commonly as a folliculitis. Since these two forms of infection respond to the same topical therapies, they are discussed together. Since this yeast is a normal component of the skin flora, its total eradication is usually not possible using topical therapies. The ubiquitous nature of the organism also accounts for the high recurrence rate following treatment. For this reason it is difficult to compare different studies since the follow-up periods are usually of different lengths. Patients with extensive involvement are usually best treated with oral antimycotics, whereas patients with limited involvement may be treated with either systemic or topical antimycotics. A number of less conventional agents that are not regarded as antimycotics have been reported in the literature including salicylic acid, propylene glycol, and zinc pyrithione.[37] These are not discussed since they do not appear to offer significant advantages over specific antimycotic agents.

Selenium sulfide (2.5 %) lotion has been shown in uncontrolled and controlled studies to be useful in the management of both tinea versicolor and *Pityrosporum* folliculitis. A variety of different methods and durations of applications have been utilized but one of the most common regimens is to have patients apply the lotion daily for 10 min for 7 consecutive days.[38] Cure rates have been reported to be as high as 87 percent[38] in tinea versicolor and 90 percent in *Pityrosporum* folliculitis.[39] Advantages of this treatment modality include low cost and the ability to treat large areas of the body easily since the lotion is easy to apply. The major disadvantage that limits its use is that the lotion is irritating, with almost one in five patients developing an irritant dermatitis that may range from mild to severe. Some patients also find the odor objectionable.

There are numerous studies that have demonstrated the efficacy of topical imidazoles for the treatment of both tinea versicolor and *Pityrosporum* folliculitis. The clinical and mycologic cure rates vary from 76 to 100 percent in different studies.[40–44] The most common regimen for all imidazoles is a once daily application for 2 weeks. The results of all studies, including those in which there is a head-to-head comparison between different imidazoles, do not demonstrate a significant difference between any of the antifungals in this class. The choice of topical imidazole is primarily based on price. Topical ciclopirox olamine is also effective against *Pityrosporum* species and can be used interchangeably with the imidazoles, although at least one head-to-head study between ciclopirox olamine and clotrimazole demonstrated marginally higher cure rates with ciclopirox olamine.[45]

Topical allylamines have been demonstrated to be clinically and mycologically effective against *Pityrosporum* infections but have not received an indication for use in this disorder. Although in vitro data suggest that allylamines have higher MIC values than imidazoles against yeast, MIC values do not always correlate with clinical efficacy. There are only a limited number of studies using topical allylamines in *Pityrosporum* infections, but the clinical and mycologic cure rates appear to be equivalent to that of topical imidazoles.[46] Despite the clinical efficacy, topical allylamines are not a good choice for the treatment of either tinea versicolor or *Pityrosporum* folliculitis since this is the most expensive class of topical antimycotics and they have not received an indication for treatment of these infections.

REFERENCES

1. Shapiro AL, Rothman S: Undecylenic acid in the treatment of dermatomycosis. *Arch Dermatol Syphilol* **52**:166, 1945
2. Macura AB: *In vitro* susceptibility of dermatophytes to antifungal drugs: A comparison of two methods. *Int J Dermatol* **32**:533, 1993
3. Allen HB et al: Selenium sulfide: Adjunctive therapy for tinea capitis. *Pediatrics* **69**:81, 1982
4. Smith EB: New topical agents for dermatophytosis. *Cutis* **17**:54, 1976
5. Tschen EH et al: Comparison of over-the-counter agents for tinea pedis. *Cutis* **23**:696, 1979
6. Fuerst JF et al: Comparison between undecylenic acid and tolnaftate in the treatment of tinea pedis. *Cutis* **25**:544, 1980
7. Battistini F et al: The treatment of dermatophytoses of the glabrous skin: A comparison of undecylenic acid and its salt versus tolnaftate. *Int J Dermatol* **22**:388, 1983
8. Fredriksson T: Treatment of dermatomycoses with topical tioconazole and miconazole. *Dermatologica* **116**(suppl 1):14, 1983
9. Tanenbaum L et al: Sulconazole nitrate 1.0 percent cream: A comparison with miconazole in the treatment of tinea pedis and tinea cruris/corporis. *Cutis* **30**:105, 1982
10. Tanenbaum L et al: Sulconazole nitrate cream 1 percent for treating tinea cruris and corporis. *Cutis* **44**:344, 1989
11. *Physicians Desk Reference,* 51st ed. Montvale, NJ, Medical Economics Data Production, 1997, pp 1139–1140
12. Katz HI et al: SCH 370 (clotrimazole-betamethasone dipropionate) cream in patients with tinea cruris or tinea corporis. *Cutis* **34**:183, 1984
13. Wortzel MH: A double-blind study comparing the superiority of a combination antifungal (clotrimazole)/steroidal (betamethasone diprprionate) product. *Cutis* **30**:258, 1982
14. Barkey WF: Striae and persistent tinea corporis related to prolonged use of betamethasone dipropionate 0.05% cream/clotrimazole 1% cream (Lotrisone cream). *J Am Acad Dermatol* **17**:518, 1987
15. Smith EB et al: Double-blind comparison of naftifine cream and clotrimazole/betamethasone dipropionate cream in the treatment of tinea pedis. *J Am Acad Dermatol* **26**:125, 1992
16. Gupta AK et al: Antifungal agents: An overview. Part I. *J Am Acad Dermatol* **30**:677, 1994
17. Kligman AM et al: Evaluation of ciclopirox olamine cream for the treatment of tinea pedis: Multicenter, double-blind comparative studies. *Clin Ther* **7**:409, 1985
18. Stiller MJ et al: Treatment of dermatophytoses II: Newer topical antifungal drugs. *Int J Dermatol* **32**:638, 1993
19. Meinike K et al: Treatment of dermatomycoses with naftifine: Therapeutic efficacy on application once daily or twice daily. *Mykosen* **30**(suppl 1):98, 1987
20. Millikan LE et al: Naftifine cream 1% versus econazole cream 1% in the treatment of tinea cruris and tinea corporis. *J Am Acad Dermatol* **18**:52, 1988
21. Nolting S, Weidinger G: Naftifine in severe dermatomycoses: Econazole-controlled therapeutic comparison. *Mykosen* **30**(suppl 1):70, 1987
22. El Darouti MA, Kalinka P: Naftifine cream 1% compared with miconazole cream 2% in dermatophytosis. *Int J Dermatol* **29**:521, 1990
23. Haas PJ et al: Naftifine in tinea pedis: Double-blind comparison with clotrimazole. *Mykosen* **30**(suppl 1):50, 1987
24. Maibach HI: Naftifine: Dermatotoxicology and clinical efficacy. *Mykosen* **30**(suppl 1):57, 1987
25. Nada M et al: Naftifine versus miconazole/hydrocortisone in inflammatory dermatophyte infections. *Int J Dermatol* **33**:570, 1994
26. Bergstresser PR et al: Topical terbinafine and clotrimazole in interdigital tinea pedis: A multicenter comparison of cure and relapse rates with 1- and 4-week treatment regimens. *J Am Acad Dermatol* **28**:648, 1993
27. Evans EGV et al: Comparison of terbinafine and clotrimazole in treating tinea pedis. *BMJ* **307**:645, 1993
28. Stütten G, Bauer E: Bioavailability, skin and nail penetration of topically applied antimycotics. *Mykosen* **25**:74, 1981
29. Klaschka F: Treatment of onychomycosis with naftifine gel. *Mykosen* **30**(suppl 1):119, 1985
30. Meyerson MS et al: Open-label study of the safety and efface of Fungoid tincture in patients with distal subungual onychomycosis of the toes. *Cutis* **49**:359, 1992
31. Macura AB: Fungal resistance to antimycotic drugs: A growing problem. *Int J Dermatol* **30**:181, 1991
32. Clayton YM, Connor BL: Comparison of clotrimazole cream, Whitfield's ointment and nystatin ointment for topical treatment of ringworm infection, pityriasis versicolor, erythrasma, and candidiasis. *Br J Dermatol* **89**:297, 1973
33. Hay RJ: Antifungal therapy of yeast infections. *J Am Acad Dermatol* **31**:S6, 1994
34. Tanenbaum L et al: A new treatment for cutaneous candidiasis: Sulconazole nitrate cream 1%. *Int J Dermatol* **22**:318, 1983
35. Zaias N et al: Naftifine cream in the treatment of cutaneous candidiasis. *Cutis* **42**:238, 1988
36. Paetzold OH et al: Yeast infections in the skin. Comparison of double-blind therapeutic trial with naftifine and clotrimazole. *Mykosen* **30**(suppl 1):112, 1987
37. Silva-Lizama E: Tinea versicolor. *Int J Dermatol* **34**:611, 1995
38. Sànchez JL, Torres VM: Double-blind efficacy study of selenium sulfide in tinea versicolor. *J Am Acad Dermatol* **11**:235, 1984
39. Bäck O et al: *Pityrosporum* folliculitis: A common disease of the young and middle-aged. *J Am Acad Dermatol* **12**:56, 1985
40. Ortiz LG, Papa CM: Topical miconazole nitrate therapy in tinea pedis and tinea versicolor. *Clin Ther* **6**:44, 1978
41. Quiñones CA: Tinea versicolor: New topical treatments. *Cutis* **25**:386, 1980
42. Savin RC, Horwitz SN: Double-blind comparison of 2% ketoconazole cream and placebo in the treatment of tinea versicolor. *J Am Acad Dermatol* **15**:500, 1986
43. Spiekermann PH, Young MD: Clinical evaluation of clotrimazole: A broad-spectrum antifungal agent. *Arch Dermatol* **112**:350, 1976
44. Vicik GJ et al: A new treatment for tinea versicolor using econazole nitrate 1.0% cream once a day. *Cutis* **33**:570, 1984
45. Cullen SI et al: Treatment of tinea versicolor with a new antifungal agent, ciclopirox olamine cream 1%. *Clin Ther* **7**:574, 1985
46. Kagawa S: Clinical efficacy of terbinafine in 629 Japanese patients with dermatomycosis. *Clin Exp Dermatol* **14**:114, 1989

Madhu A. Pathak
Thomas B. Fitzpatrick
Paul Nghiem
David S. Aghassi

Sun-Protective Agents: Formulations, Effects, and Side Effects

PRINCIPLES OF PHOTOPROTECTION

Most of the damaging effects of solar radiation (see Chaps. 134, 136–138) result from primary events following the absorption of UV radiation by DNA, RNA, proteins, enzymes, lipids of cell membranes, and cell organelles present in cells of the epidermis and dermis, including the vascular system. These effects are dose-dependent, relating to factors such as duration of exposure, frequency of exposures, and quality and intensity of radiation. Photoprotection and prevention of such damaging effects of UV radiation can be achieved by attenuation processes that significantly reduce the impact of UV photons impinging on the skin. These are outlined in (Table 248-1 and Fig. 248-1). Attenuation is achieved by providing to the skin certain exogenous photoprotective approaches that are governed by four biophysical principles of attenuation of solar radiation: (1) *absorption and filtration* of UV radiation at the surface of stratum corneum to prevent its further transmission (or penetration) into epidermis and dermis[1]; (2) *scattering* of radiation; (3) *reflection* of radiation impinging on the skin by providing barriers such as molecules of titanium dioxide (TiO_2) and/or zinc oxide (ZnO) on the stratum corneum, which effectively scatter and reflect the UV radiation; and (4) *inactivation or destruction of free radicals* and reactive forms of oxygen species [e.g.,

singlet oxygen ($^1O_2$), superoxide anion ($O_2^{\cdot-}$), hydroxyl radical ($^\cdot OH$)] that are produced in the skin when it is exposed to solar radiation.[1–5] The formation of such UV-induced free radicals and reactive forms of oxygen occurs in the viable cells of epidermis and dermis and can be inhibited or minimized by oral administration or topical application of certain compounds that act as antioxidants or free radical quenchers (or scavengers).[1,2,5–9] In addition, inflammatory mediators (e.g., histamine, prostaglandins, cytokines) formed in response to UV irradiation can be effectively inhibited by specific antagonistic pharmacologic agents administered orally or topically to prevent the inflammatory response (e.g., the action of indomethacin in sunburn reaction).[1,10,11]

The methods for photoprotection include the *topical application of chemical sunscreens* in the form of creams, lotions, gels, or solutions containing a known quantity of UV-absorbing chemical or chemicals that selectively absorb, scatter, or reflect radiation and prevent the penetration of UV radiation into the skin. This is one of the most reliable approaches and is discussed in "Topical Sunscreen Chemicals for Photoprotection of Skin," below. There are many sunscreen chemicals that absorb UV radiation (UVB as well as UVA) and can act as UV filters when used in an appropriate vehicle or base for topical application to the skin. There are, however, very few chemicals that show excellent broad-spectrum absorption characteristics in both the UVB and UVA regions. For this reason, sunscreens are formulated as compounds containing a total of two to six sunscreen chemicals and are designated as *combination sunscreen formulations;* they are enriched with both UVB- and UVA-absorbing chemicals to provide broad-spectrum protection. The UVB- and UVA-absorbing sunscreen chemicals are listed in Tables 248-2 and 248-3 and are discussed in "Topical Sunscreens and the Basis for their Recommendation," below. A few of the sunscreen chemicals (e.g., TiO_2, ZnO) exhibit the properties of scattering and reflection of the impinging UV radiation in both the UVA and UVB regions. These are referred to as *physical sunscreens* or physical blockers of UV radiation and are described separately in "Photoprotection by Physical Sunscreens." Sunscreen chemicals that act as quenchers or scavengers of free radicals are presented in "Antioxidants

TABLE 248-1

General Principles of Photoprotection of Skin against Ultraviolet Radiation*

BIOPHYSICAL PRINCIPLE	SITE OF ACTION	SUGGESTED APPROACHES	EFFECTIVENESS
Absorption of UVR and decreased transmission	Stratum corneum	Topical use of UVB- and UVA-absorbing chemicals	Good to excellent
Enhance scattering of UVR	Stratum corneum and viable epidermis	Topical use of micronized particulate form of TiO_2, ZnO, or melanin	Good to excellent
Enhance reflection of UVR, visible	Stratum corneum	Topical use of micronized TiO_2 and ZnO	Good
Quenching of free radicals and reactive O_2	Viable epidermis, dermis	Use topical or oral antioxidants (free radical quenchers)	Variable, low or fair
Physical blocking of UVR	Skin surface	Use blended fabrics (nylon, polyester, cotton clothing), hats, parasols	Good to excellent

*Avoid exposure to solar radiation (10 A.M.–4 P.M.); block radiation with clothing, broad-brimmed hats, and parasols; use sunscreens on regular basis (sun-protective factor 15–30).

and Other Agents." Additional photoprotective approaches involving the use of synthetic fabrics in the form of clothing are outlined in a section called "Photoprotection by Sun-Protective Clothing." A separate section dealing with artificial tanning of skin by using dihydroxy acetone (DHA) and its protective value appears under "Quick Tanning Lotions and Tanning Accelerators."

FIGURE 248-1

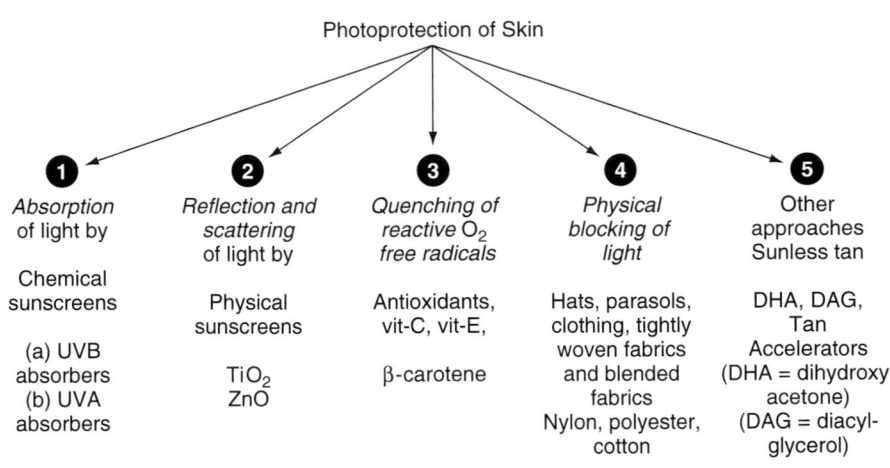

Various approaches useful for photoprotection of skin.

FACTORS INFLUENCING THE EFFECTIVENESS OF SUNSCREENS

Solubility in Lipophilic and Hydrophilic Vehicles

Sunscreens are topical formulations used in the form of lotions, creams, ointments, clear gels, and solutions. Lotions are most popular with consumers. Their effectiveness is influenced by several factors, including the chemical nature of sun-active compounds, their solubility in lipophilic and hydrophilic vehicles used in preparing the formulation for topical use, pH, the UV-absorbing properties in the UVB and UVA range, the concentration of sun-active chemicals used in preparing the formulation, and the amount applied to the skin. Instead of enumerating the importance of each of these several factors, only those that are biologically important and clinically relevant in understanding and determining the effectiveness of topical sunscreens when applied on the epicutaneous surface of the skin will be discussed.

One such factor is the solubility of the UV-absorbing sun-active compound in lipophilic and hydrophilic solvents. Most sun-active and UV-protective chemicals are synthetic organic chemicals; to achieve a high sun protection factor (SPF) of 15 to 30 or higher, two to six such chemicals of varying solubility have to be combined and kept in solubilized form to achieve a total combined concentration up to 20 g/100 mL without precipitation. Thus, the solubility of each compound in lipophilic and hydrophilic solvents plays a major role in formulating the topical preparations for achieving a waterproof and sweat-resistant formulation with high SPF value for smooth and even application to the skin. The solubilized chemicals are incorporated at different concentrations and stabilized to prevent separation or flocculation of each ingredient. Because most sun-active chemicals are synthetic and lipophilic in nature (having an affinity for fat or oils for solubilization), the most popular of all vehicles used in formulating sunscreens are lipophilic stabilized emulsions or lotions. They offer versatility owing to their easy spreadability on the skin and dispensability from bottles in amounts that enable the user to achieve a uniform transparent and colorless thin film without flaking on the large surface area of the skin. For this reason, water-soluble hydrophilic compounds [e.g., para-aminobenzoic acid (PABA)] are less popular than oil-soluble compounds because when applied in hydrophilic emulsions or creams, they can be washed off when the skin is subjected to sweating or water immersion. The range of concentrations of each sun-active ingredient used in making topical sunscreen formulations that have been recommended by the U.S. Food and Drug Administration (FDA) is given in Table 248-2 for UVB-absorbing chemicals and in Table 248-3 for UVA-absorbing chemicals.[12–14] Because sun-active chemicals are recognized by the FDA as drugs, the manufacturers of sunscreens may use only these approved chemicals at the recommended concentrations listed in Tables 248-2 and -3 for formulating any over-the-counter sunscreen product(s).

UV Absorption Property

Photoprotection derived from topical application of sunscreen formulation depends mainly on the UV absorption properties of sunscreen chemicals used in formulating sunscreen products and not the base or vehicle used for dissolving the UV-absorbing chemicals. Because sunscreen chemicals show variable UV absorption properties in the UVB and UVA regions, the second important factor in assessing the photoprotective effectiveness of a sunscreen formulation relates to knowing the absorption spectrum of each UV-absorbing chemical or a composite (compounded) UV absorption spectrum of all chemicals used in preparing the formulation, with emphasis on knowing the absorption peaks and the amplitude of the absorption peak(s). The amplitude is a measure of how intensely the sun-active chemical absorbs UV radiation. This is illustrated in Table 248-4 with extinction coefficient values of some commonly used sunscreen chemicals, giving an important indication why a particular chemical(s) is selected to absorb UVB or UVA radiation preferentially. Chemicals with low molar extinction coefficient values (e.g., octyl salicylate) are less effective in protecting the skin than those with high molar extinction values (e.g., ethyl hexyl p-methoxy cinnamate). The width of absorption bands of sun-active chemicals gives a measure of how broadly across the UV absorption spectrum the sun-active chemical absorbs different wavelengths adjacent to its absorption peak.

Amount and Method of Application

The efficacy of photoprotection or the SPF value of a sunscreen formulation applied to the skin depends in part on the amount of sunscreen applied to the skin per unit area and the uniformity of application.[1,12–15] According to guidelines established by the FDA, the SPF value of any formulation is based on uniform application of 100 μL or 100 mg per 50 cm^2 of skin. This provides at least 2 μL or 2 mg/cm^2 of the product essential for photoprotection. This

TABLE 248-2

UVB-Absorbing Sunscreens Approved by FDA and Examples of UVB-absorptive Compounds Used in Sunscreen Formulation*

GROUP	NAME OF COMPOUND	MAXIMUM CONCENTRATION, %	ABSORBANCE RANGE, NM
Aminobenzoates	Para-aminobenzoic acid (PABA)	5	260–313
	Ethyl-4-[bis(hydroxypropyl)-amino-benzoate	5	280–330
	Glyceryl PABA	5	264–315
	Amyl p-dimethylaminobenzoate* (padimate A)	4–8	260–325
	2-ethylhexyl PABA (padimate O)	1.4–8	264–320
Cinnamates	Diethanolamine p-methoxycinna-mate	8–10	280–310
	2-ethylhexyl p-methoxycinnamate (Parsol MCX)	2.0–7.0%	280–320
Salicylates	2-ethylhexyl salicylate	3.5–5	280–320
	Homosalate (homomenthyl salicy-late)	10	290–320
	Octyl salicylate	3–5	280–320
	Triethanolamine salicylate	5–12	260–320
	Trolamine salicylate	3–0	260–355
Benzophenones	Dioxybenzone	3–0	260–355
	Sulisobenzone	5–10	260–360
	Oxybenzone	2–6	270–360
Miscellaneous	Ethylhexyl, 2-cyano-3, 3-diphenyl-acrylate (octocrylene)	7–10	290–360
	Lawsone and dihydroxyacetone	0.25–5	320–380
	2-phenylbenzimidazole-5-sulfonic acid	1–4	290–320
	Digalloyl trioleate	2–5	270–320
	Red veterinary petrolatum	>30	280–380
	Titanium dioxide	2–2.5	250–380
	Methyl anthranilate	3.5–5	300–370

*This may not be a current list for 1998–1999. Padimate A (amyl-dimethyl PABA) is no longer approved in the United States for over-the-counter products for consumer use. However, avobenzone (butyl-methoxydibenzoyl meth-ane), not listed in the table, is now an approved UVA-absorbing sunscreen. Zinc oxide is also an approved UV-scattering agent. These two agents should be included as category I sunscreens (approved) in the table.

is an average value based on consumer use of lotions and also derived from well-controlled laboratory evaluations of several for-mulations in human subjects.[12,13] If the product were applied in smaller quantities, the SPF value would be lower than the antici-pated value of the product and the user would not be well protected. Likewise, if the product were applied in larger quantities in a thick film as a cream, it would give an erroneously higher SPF value than the true anticipated value. It is essential for achieving optimal sun protection that sunscreens be applied in a smooth and uniform man-ner to achieve a thin film on the surface of the exposed skin.

Substantivity of Sunscreens

Another factor that contributes to the efficacy of protection of a sunscreen is related to the *substantivity* of the formulation.[1,15–17] This reflects the ability of the vehicle or base of the lotion as well as the UV-absorbing chemicals to remain adherent or adsorbed to the skin in a thin film form under conditions of use. Substantivity of sunscreens also reflects the ability of the UV-absorbing chemi-cals to penetrate or diffuse into the stratum corneum through the vehicle (percutaneous absorption) and to remain there to absorb UV

radiation impinging on the skin. Profuse sweating can easily elute or wash off the applied hydrophilic chemical sunscreen and signif-icantly lower the protective value of the formulation. Alternatively, low humidity and high temperature can dry the applied sunscreen product made in a hydrophilic emulsion and cause it to scale or flake off. Immer-sion of skin in water (chlorinated pool or ocean water) can easily wash off the applied sunscreen if the product is not substantive to the skin. To achieve water resistant sunscreens with high SPF value ($\approx$30), water-insoluble lipo-philic sunscreen chemicals are used in a high-level oil phase and emulsified to achieve an oil-in-water emulsion form. Water resistant and water proof (or very water resistant) sun-screens[15–17] adhere well to the skin be-cause of the lipophilic base or the ve-hicle used in formulating the product. Such sunscreens also diffuse or pene-trate into the stratum corneum (Fig. 248-2).

Photostability of Sunscreens

The photoprotective efficacy or the SPF value of a sunscreen is also re-lated to the photostability of the sun-active agent when it is exposed to UV radiation. Photostable compounds re-tain their SPF value and protect the skin when they are subjected to pro-longed exposure to solar radiation.[14] Photolabile compounds partially lose their protective value when exposed to solar radiation and can also become ir-ritating to the skin as a result of pho-tochemical alteration of the sun-active chemical.[14–17] For example, octyl di-methyl PABA exhibits up to a 15.5 percent loss in its photoprotective activity and avobenzone was found to lose up to 36 percent of its activity when subjected to photostability tests.[14–17] Photolabile compounds can at times induce photocontact sensitivity and photoallergic reactions (e.g., padimate-A, or amyl p-dimethyl aminobenzoate,[14–17] and avobenzone). For this reason, padimate A was withdrawn by the FDA from the ap-proved list of UVB-absorbing agents.[13–16]

SELECTING CHEMICAL SUNSCREENS AND SPF VALUES FOR EFFECTIVE PROTECTION

Manufacturers of sunscreens are allowed to formulate and sell sun-screens with only one sun-active ingredient or any combination of two or more sun-active chemicals in a topical formulation with varying SPF values (from 2 to 30 or even higher) as long as the manufacturer complies with certain FDA guidelines or regula-tions,[12,13] provides the SPF value on the label of the product, and lists the approved chemical ingredients used in formulating the product. The SPF value helps the consumer to select the sunscreen appropriate for her or his personal needs and desires. It is essential for physicians to know the extent and limitations of protection of any formulation based on SPF value of the product. Table 248-5 shows the extent of protection in relation to the SPF value of the formulation.[13] A high SPF value gives no assurance of protection against UVA radiation (see sections on types 2, 3, and 4 sunscreens) unless the formulation is enriched with UVA-absorbing chemicals listed in Table 248-3.

Sunscreens with SPF value <12 may provide partial protection and lessen the degree and discomfort of sunburn reaction, but they are likely to be less protective and efficient in preventing other harmful reactions (e.g., DNA damage, protein damage) caused by UVB and UVA radiation that contribute to skin carcinogenesis and photoaging. Such sunscreens should not be recommended for use by any normal individual of SPT I to III. Manufacturers formulate and sell such low SPF value sunscreens for cosmetic and esthetic reasons and for users to achieve a skin-tanning response. Sunscreens in general do not promote or induce a skin-tanning response unless they are enriched with a tan-stimulating chemical such as 5-methoxypsoralen, which is known to stimulate melanogenesis in skin after photosensitization reaction.[18] Such preparations are not only potentially harmful but not approved by the FDA. Although previously tanned skin is less reactive to subsequent exposure to UV radiation, the potential risk of carcinogenesis and malignancy involving keratinocytes and melanocytes outweighs the acquired benefits of enhanced tanning.

After a great deal of deliberation, the FDA has set a cap of 30 as the optimal SPF value recommended for use in ultrahigh-protection formulations.[13] The additional benefit from using sunscreen formulations with SPF > 30 is outweighed by the potential risk of overexposure to UVA radiation and exposure to higher concentrations of sunscreen ingredients, which may also contribute to increasing both the cost of the product and the risk of contact and photocontact sensitization reactions. The calculated increase in protection with products of SPF > 30 is also limited and appears negligible (e.g., a product of SPF-30 blocks 96.7 percent of UV energy from the sun, whereas a product of SPF-40 blocks 97.5 percent of UV energy). Furthermore, a high-SPF product (SPF > 30) tends to give a false sense of security of protection. Frequent sunbathers are tempted to prolong their sunbathing beyond the time when they should be withdrawing from the sun to protect their skin against actinic damage. Although the use of high-SPF sunscreens (SPF > 30) is controversial and the occurrence of irritant, allergic, phototoxic, and photoallergic cutaneous reactions is

not very common, one should not overlook or ignore the photochemical reactions caused by UVA that are potentially harmful.

For best protection, sunscreens should be applied at least 30 min before exposing the skin to the sun.[1,12,17] This assures better diffusion of sun-active chemicals into the stratum corneum to provide a uniform UV-absorbing filter to screen harmful UV rays. It also means that the applied sunscreen should be substantive and adhere well to the skin. For optimal protection after application of the sunscreen, the user should avoid any contact with clothing, which can partially remove the sunscreen film applied to the skin and decrease the protection value of the applied product.

Another misconception involves reapplication of the sunscreen during sunbathing to increase the duration of sun exposure and to gain additional (extra) SPF value. The reapplication of sunscreen, especially after swimming or profuse sweating, assures definite pro-

TABLE 248-3

Sunscreen Chemicals that Absorb UVA Radiation and Protect the Skin against UVA

CHEMICAL	RECOMMENDED CONCENTRATION, %	PROTECTION RANGE, NM	SIDE EFFECTS
Benzophenones			
Oxybenzone	2–6	320–360	Partially effective and irritant to few
Sulisobenzone	5–10	320–360	Partially effective and irritant to few
Dioxybenzone	3.0	320–360	Partially effective and irritant to few
Other chemicals			
Methyl anthranilate	3	300–340	Partially effective
Butylmethoxydibenzoyl methane (avobenzone)	≤3	320–400	Effective up to 400 nm but may be irritant, photolabile
Red veterinary petrolatum	>30	320–370	Smarting and irritant
Titanium dioxide	2–25	300–400	Effective but may be white or occlusive
Zinc oxide	2–20	300–400	Effective but may be white or occlusive

TABLE 248-4

The UV Absorption Characteristics and Extinction Values of Popular Sunscreen Chemicals in the UVB and UVA Range

SUNSCREEN CHEMICAL	ABSORPTION PEAK, NM,* AND SPECTRAL RANGE	EXTINCTION CO-EFFICIENT AT ABSORPTION PEAK
PABA	293, UVB	13,600
Octyl dimethyl PABA	300, UVB	28,400
Octyl salicylate	308, UVB	4,900
Homomenthyl salicylate	310, UVB	4,800
Ethyl hexyl p-methoxy cinnamate	289, UVB	24,200
Methyl anthranilate	324, UVB	5,600
Dioxybenzone	352, UVA	9,400
Sulisobenzone	334, UVA	8,600
Oxybenzone	329, UVA	9,300
Butylmethoxy-dibenzoyl methane avobenzone	360, UVA	31,000

*In nonpolar solvents.

FIGURE 248-2

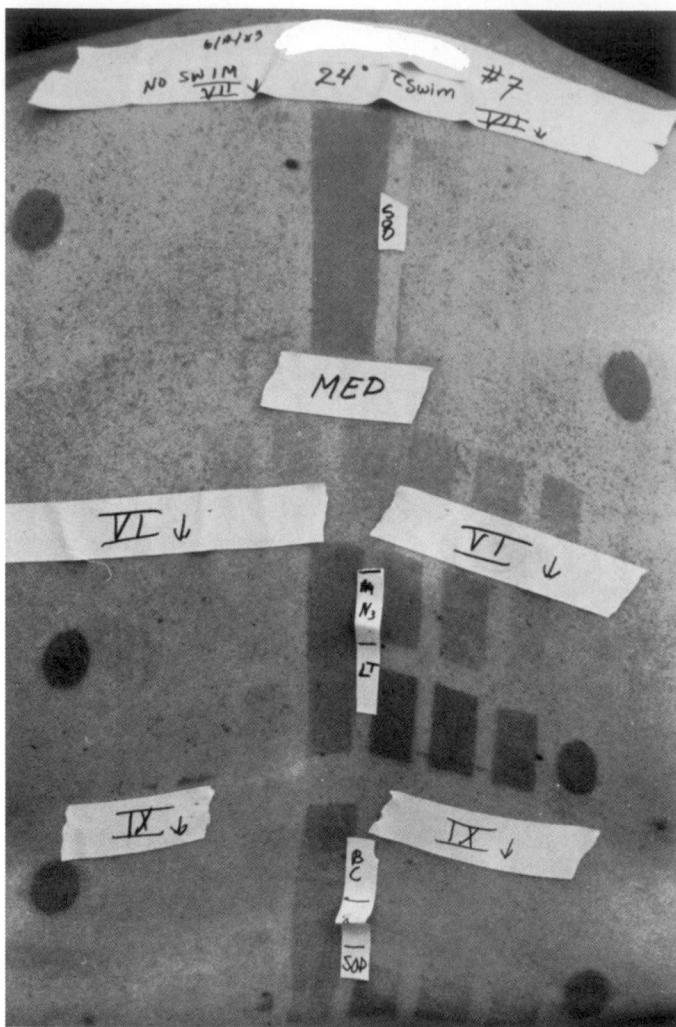

Water resistance of three different SPF 15 sunscreens numbered as VI, VII, and IX. The volunteer was skin phototype II and received sunlight exposure in the prone position under outdoor field conditions between 10:00 A.M. and 3:30 P.M. at San Antonio, TX. The products were evaluated in a randomized, double-blind manner. The right side (marked "swim") of the subject received topical application (2 μL/cm^2) of three coded test products in large areas of the back prior to swimming for 40 min. The subject's back remained under water for 40 min by following a monitored schedule of swimming. The left side (marked "no swim") of the subject received the same coded formulations soon after swimming. The subject's entire back was exposed soon after swimming to solar radiation equivalent to 2.5, 5.0, 7.0, 10, 12.5, and 15 times the MED of the subject between 10:00 A.M. and 3:30 P.M. The exposure row marked "MED" received (left to right) 15, 20, 30, 40, 50, and 60 mJ/cm^2 of UVB radiation at noon time and demonstrates the MED response of the subject at 24 h after UV exposure to be 20 mJ/cm^2. Product VII (top row) was found to be water-resistant and exhibited an SPF value >15. Product VI (center row) was found to be not water-resistant and exhibited an SPF of 2.5 after swimming; the left side ("no swim") treated with product VI showed good protection and SPF value of 15. Product IX (bottom row) applied to the lumbar region was less water-resistant than product VII and exhibited an SPF of 10. The six dark circles on the lateral aspects of the trunk illustrate the uniform sun exposure during the sun-exposure period of testing (to serve as built in control). Water-resistant or waterproof sunscreens should be recommended for effective protection.

tection but does not contribute to increasing the SPF value of the applied product to prolong the extended duration of sun exposure and protection. For example, a product of SPF 6 when reapplied as a second coat during sunbathing will not make that product provide an SPF value of 12.

TOPICAL SUNSCREENS AND THE BASIS FOR THEIR RECOMMENDATIONS

Although sunscreens are recognized and classified as drugs by the FDA[12,13] and promoted by the pharmaceutical industry for topical use as cosmetics for over-the-counter use, they often create confusion in the minds of consumers when they purchase such a product. The statement that the higher the SPF value of the sunscreen the better is the product for photoproduction can be misleading when protection against UVA radiation is objectively examined.

By and large, a consumer buys a sunscreen with the following intentions: (1) to prevent the discomforts of the sunburn reaction (erythema, edema, pain, blistering, and peeling), (2) to facilitate acquiring a healthy looking golden-brown tan, and (3) to protect the normal function of epidermal and dermal cells and minimize the potential risk of skin cancer and photoaging. Many consumers are not aware of the following known biologic facts about sunbathing and tanning:

1. Sunburn (manifest in the form of erythema, swelling, and pain) is principally caused by UVB radiation and to a lesser extent by UVA radiation as a function of UV exposure dose.
2. The intensity of solar radiation, the frequency of sun exposure, and the duration of sun exposure determine the degree of various harmful responses of skin.
3. Sunscreens do not promote or induce the tanning reaction of skin; rather, it is the UV-damaged melanocytic system that is activated to facilitate the tanning response of skin.
4. Skin cancer and photoaging are caused by frequent exposures to solar radiation involving UVB as well as UVA radiation; to prevent these harmful reactions, broad-spectrum UVA- and UVB-absorbing topical sunscreens need to be used on a regular basis and not at sporadic intervals.
5. Only the use of high-SPF products (15 to 30) helps to protect the skin against sunburn, skin hyperpigmentation (or tanning reaction), and the potential problems of skin cancer and photoaging changes.
6. The tanning response is genetically regulated, and only certain individuals of SPTs III to VI can acquire a tan; individuals of SPTs I and II who often indulge in sunbathing do not tan or tan poorly.
7. Products with low SPF values (SPF 2 to 12) will permit a tanning response, but this is preceded by mild, moderate, or sometimes strong harmful sunburn reactions that often contribute to skin cancer and problems of photoaging.[1,12,13,19]

Topical Sunscreen Chemicals for Photoprotection of Skin

The UV-absorbing chemical filters used in formulating sunscreens include certain types of synthetically prepared chemicals (Table 248-6) that can be broadly categorized as UVB- or UVA-absorbing chemicals (e.g., PABA-related chemicals, salicylates, cinnamates, benzophenones). They are colorless and often odorless organic chemicals. Almost all sunscreen products made in the United States,

TABLE 248-5

CHAPTER 248
Sun-Protective Agents 2747

Sunscreen Product Category Designations Based on SPF Values

SPF Value*	Protection Category†
2 to <4*	Minimal
4 to <8*	Moderate
8 to <12*	Good or average
12 to <16*	High
16 to <20	Very high
20 to <30	Ultra-high
>30	Highest

*Based on sunburn reaction at 24 h after exposure.
†Product protection category.

TABLE 248-6

Chemical Components of UVB- and UVA-Absorbing Sunscreens

UV-Absorbing Chemicals	Absorbing Range, UVB/UVA
PABA-related chemicals (see Table 248-2)	UVB
Salicylates (see Table 248-2)	UVB
Cinnamates (see Table 248-2)	UVB
Benzophenones (see Tables 248-2, -3)	UVB and UVA
Butylmethoxy-dibenzoyl methane (avobenzone)	UVA
Anthranilates	UVA
ZnO, TiO$_2$	UVB and UVA*
Camphor derivatives†	UVB

*Reflect and scatter UVB and UVA in addition to absorption.
†These are not contained in products from the United States.

Europe, and Australia contain a mixture of one or more UVB-absorbing chemicals (e.g., cinnamates, salicylates) incorporated in a suitable base for a vehicle. Since very few chemicals effectively absorb UVB as well as UVA radiation, combination sunscreen formulations containing UVB- as well as UVA-absorbing chemicals are combined in an appropriate vehicle or base. To check any sunscreen product for its ability to protect against UVA as well as UVB radiation, one has to read the label to confirm the presence of a benzophenone derivative or dibenzoyl methane (also known as avobenzone, or Parsol 1789) or a physical blocking agent such as ZnO or TiO$_2$.

There are several hundred sunscreen formulations containing different UV-absorbing sun-active chemicals with a wide range of concentrations. For convenience and to simplify the process of selection and avoid recommendation of a specific brand-name, the authors have classified and grouped the chemical components of sunscreens into five identifiable types (see Table 248-7) that are available throughout the United States and in many other parts of the world in the form of lotions, creams, gels, or sprays. The fifth type of sunscreen contains only physical blockers (ZnO, TiO$_2$). A miscellaneous category of sunscreens is also included.

TYPE 1: UVB-ABSORBING SUNSCREEN FORMULATIONS In reality, these products reflect the developmental history of sunscreen chemicals to provide colorless, safe, and effective topical agents to prevent the consequences of acute effects of sunburn reactions. The UVB-absorbing chemicals outlined in Table 248-2 were carefully examined with respect to their safety, efficacy, and potential side effects and were approved by the FDA for use by cosmetic and pharmaceutical companies in formulating over-the-counter sunscreen products for consumer use.[12,13] It should be noted that three benzophenones are listed as UVB-absorbing chemicals,

TABLE 248-7

Classification of Chemical Sunscreen Formulations

	Type 1	Type 2	Type 3	Type 4	Type 5	Miscellaneous*
Type	UVB (290–320 nm)	UVB + UVA (290–360 nm)	UVB + UVA (290–400 nm)	UVB + UVA (290–400 nm)	Physical blockers	
SPF	2–15	12–15	15–20	15–30 or >30	15–30	Variable
Identifying point	Contain only UVB absorbers (see Table 248-2)	Contain UVB + UVA absorbers, e.g., benzophenones (see Tables 248-2, -3)	Contain UVB + UVA absorbers, e.g., benzophenones (avobenzone) (see Tables 248-2, -3)	Contain UVB + UVA absorbers, e.g., benzophenones (avobenzone) TiO$_2$ + ZnO	Contain ZnO + TiO$_2$ (see Tables 248-2, -3)	Contain dihydroxy-acetone, also UVB absorbers (see text)
Effectiveness against UVB	Variable SPF 2–10 poor SPF 12–15 fair	Fair to good	Good	Good to excellent	Good	Poor
Effectiveness against UVA	320–400 nm, poor	Partial, not satisfactory	Satisfactory	Good and satisfactory	Satisfactory	Fair
Strengths or weaknesses	Protection against UVB No protection against UVA	Partial and unsatisfactory protection against UVA	Satisfactory protection against UVB and UVA Problems of photosensitivity	Good and satisfactory protection against UVB and UVA radiation	Nonsensitizing and effective against UVB and UVA May be white or occlusive	Sunless tanning Inadequate protection against UVB

*There are several sunscreen chemicals (dihydroxyacetone, lawsone, precursors of melanin) that have limited use.

although they do absorb some part of the UVA spectrum. The type 1 UVB-absorbing sunscreen formulations do not contain the UVA-absorbing chemicals listed in Table 248-3, and the sunscreen manufacturer may not claim or mention any protection against UVA radiation on the label of the product. The more commonly used UVB-absorbing chemicals are: (1) octyl-dimethyl PABA (padimate-O), (2) glyceryl PABA, (3) 2-ethylhexyl *p*-methoxycinnamate (Parsol MCX), (4) 2-ethoxyethyl, *p*-methoxycinnamate, (5) octyl methoxycinnamate, (6) octyl salicylate, (7) homomenthyl salicylate, (8) triethanol amine salicylate, and (9) 2-ethylhexyl salicylate. European products generally do not contain PABA-related chemicals (see Table 248-2). Products with low SPF values (2 to 10) are intentionally formulated by sunscreen manufacturing companies for achieving a uniform skin tanning response, and they are less effective in protecting the skin than products with SPF 15 to 30. Some European products are cosmetic in nature and generally do not claim any health-related medical benefits of protection against skin cancer, photoaging, or skin diseases caused by or aggravated by sunlight.[19] They are formulated for cosmetic claims of elegance and for prevention of sunburn reaction and achieving tanning reaction. Products sold in the United States but manufactured overseas are required to be in compliance with FDA regulations and can be recommended to consumers.

TYPE 2: UVB- AND UVA-ABSORBING PRODUCTS (See Table 248-7) These are combination sunscreen formulations that contain two or more UVB-absorbing chemicals (e.g., padimate-O, octyl methoxycinnamate, octyl salicylate derivative, or homomethyl salicylate) listed in Table 248-2 and at least one UVA-absorbing chemical listed in Table 248-3. The UVA-absorbing chemicals are invariably benzophenones (either sulisobenzone, dioxybenzone, or oxybenzone). Type 2 formulations are quite effective in protecting skin against UVB radiation but only partially and weakly effective in protecting against UVA radiation (up to 340 to 350 nm). The benzophenones are available in the open market and are not now under U.S. patent restrictions. Therefore, they are widely used by many sunscreen manufacturing companies in formulating over-the-counter sunscreens to provide partial protection against a limited segment of UVA radiation. The ultraviolet A protection factor (APF) value of such sunscreens is less than 3.0 (desired value, 4 to 6). They are not useful or significantly protective against photoaging or to protect patients sensitive to UVA radiation because benzophenones do not effectively absorb and screen UVA radiation beyond 350 to 360 nm. Also, drug-induced phototoxicity reactions and UVA-induced polymorphous light eruptions (PMLE) are not prevented by topical use of type 2 sunscreens.[1,19]

TYPE 3: HIGH-SPF SUNSCREEN PRODUCTS (See Table 248-7) These contain UVB- and UVA-absorbing chemicals plus avobenzone. They are more effective than type 2 sunscreen formulations in protecting individuals against UVA radiation. Such formulations will specify their UVA protection quality on the label as "broad spectrum," although the label will not provide a well-defined APF value. The type 3 formulations contain avobenzone, a specific UVA-absorbing chemical (butylmethoxydibenzoyl methane) used in a 2 or 3% concentration.[20–22] Such formulations are also enriched with one of the three benzophenone derivatives (e.g., oxybenzone) listed in Table 248-2 and two or three other UVB-absorbing chemicals (e.g., padimate-O, cinoxate, octyl methoxycinnamate, octyl salicylate, octocrylene, trolamine salicylate, oxybenzone, or sulisobenzone) in order to provide broad-spectrum protection against

UVB as well as UVA radiation. Although avobenzone was known to have high degree of absorption in the UVA region, it was found to be photolabile and to undergo photoisomerization to compounds that were less protective, occasionally irritating, and the cause of photosensitization reactions (phototoxic and photoallergic).[14,23,24] Fortunately, the FDA has recently approved avobenzone for use in over-the-counter sunscreen products at 2 to 3% concentration when used in combination with certain UVB absorbers listed in Table 248-2.[25] The effectiveness of such UVB- and UVA-absorbing type 3 sunscreens is usually found to be good to excellent provided the duration of sun exposure is not excessive (<3 to 4 h). The SPF value in the UVB spectrum may range from 15 to 30 and the APF in the 320- to 400-nm range may be approximately 4,[20,21,26] a value adequate for protecting most average people against UVA radiation. Some formulations containing avobenzone at a 2% concentration are less irritating and sensitizing than those containing about 3% avobenzone.[27]

TYPE 4: UVB AND UVA COMBINATION SUNSCREENS PLUS PARTICULATE SUNSCREENS WITH HIGH SPF The effectiveness of type 3 sunscreens containing avobenzone plus a benzophenone and other UVB-absorbing sun-active chemicals described above has been further enhanced by enriching the formulations with 1 to 3% concentration of ZnO and TiO_2 or some other protective agent (e.g., octocrylene)[17,28] (see Table 248-7). Such sunscreens protect the skin quite well in UVB and UVA spectral regions.[17,28,29] They provide excellent SPF values of 15 to 30 in the UVB region and APF values of 4 to 6 in the UVA region.[19,26] In addition, the enriched formulations can be made in a water-resistant acrylate polymer base and can protect individuals after immersion for 40 to 80 min in ocean water or chlorinated water of swimming pools. The addition of TiO_2 and ZnO or octocrylene has served some important functions such as enhancing the product's APF, stabilizing photoreactive chemicals such as avobenzone and benzophenones against photodegradation, and improving the overall protective efficacy of the product by reducing potential side effects of sensitization.[14,28] It appears that type 4 sunscreen formulations provide the most effective topical approach for protecting fair-skinned individuals of SPTs I to III against UVB and UVA radiation.[14,19,21,26]

TYPE 5: PHYSICAL OR PARTICULATE SUNSCREENS These formulations (see Table 248-7) are selectively made using particulate and micronized form of TiO_2 and ZnO.[28] They are effective against UVB and UVA radiation and, depending upon the concentration of TiO_2 or ZnO used in formulating the product, the SPF value may range from 6 to 20. The APF value may be around 4, which is quite adequate for protection against UVA radiation. Such formulations are generally safe, effective, and nonsensitizing.

Side Effects of Sunscreen Chemicals

The topical use of sunscreen chemicals listed in Tables 248-2 and 248-3 can cause contact irritation of a nonimmunologic nature or can cause contact sensitization or photocontact sensitization of an allergic nature when the sunscreen-treated skin is exposed to solar radiation (see below).

PHOTOPROTECTION BY PHYSICAL SUNSCREENS

Physical sunscreens such as TiO_2 and ZnO have gained growing acceptance within the past 5 to 7 years[28,30] because of (1) their low toxicity potential with no clinical evidence of phototoxic and photoallergic reactions with their frequent use, (2) their high effectiveness in protecting the skin against UVB and UVA radiation in combination with chemical sunscreens that absorb UVB radiation, and (3) their photostability, cost effectiveness, and applicability to both adults and children. The UVA effectiveness is especially important and highly beneficial for photoprotecting children, in whom photochemically induced sensitization reactions can become a major concern. With increased awareness of the fact that UVA radiation is an important contributing factor to photoaging (dermatoheliosis) and induction of nonmelanoma and melanoma-type skin cancers,[88-90] it is increasingly evident that all fair-skinned individuals (SPTs I to III) should use topical sunscreens containing physical agents on a regular basis, commensurate with their location and lifestyle. The regular use of physical sunscreens is probably the simplest and safest approach for all individuals, including persons with SPTs V and VI, when exposed to unavoidable solar radiation in their daily life.

Detailed information concerning these particulate sunscreens has been reviewed by Fairhurst and Mitchnick[28] and by Anders et al.[30] Unlike chemical sunscreen lotions with solubilized components, the physical sunscreens are essentially particulate and colloidal in nature. Manufacturers advertise these particulate forms of sunscreens as "non-chemical sunscreen, natural in origin," which is actually erroneous and inconsistent with the chemical nature and structural properties of physical sunscreens. The particulate sunscreens may be organic or inorganic in origin or a combination of both. The most commonly recognized inorganic particulate sunscreens include ZnO and TiO$_2$. Other compounds are iron oxide, talc, kaolin, bentonite, silica, or mica.

ZnO and TiO$_2$ are often referred to as *physical blockers* because when used at specified concentrations they provide high-SPF sunscreens that absorb, scatter, and reflect UV radiation in a wide spectral range.[28,30,31] Older physical sunscreens used prior to 1990 as blockers were generally not accepted by consumers because they had to be used in high concentrations (up to 10% or higher) and applied in a relatively thick layer in the form of a cream. This made ZnO- and TiO$_2$-containing creams occlusive, comedogenic, and cosmetically unacceptable.[1,28,30] However, recently developed micronized formulations containing particles of 40 to 100 nm provide translucent or colloidal suspensions of ZnO and TiO$_2$ that are cosmetically very acceptable and need not be applied in thick creamy form; they are efficient in absorbing and scattering UV radiation.[28,30] This has helped to decrease the whiteness of emulsions when applied to the skin significantly and to reduce the occlusive nature and comedogenic properties of ZnO- and TiO$_2$-enriched topical formulations.

The particle size of TiO$_2$ and ZnO in sunscreen formulations is critical for achieving optimal efficacy of protection against the UV radiation range. TiO$_2$ attenuates UV radiation optimally when the particle size is between 40 and 100 nm.[28,30] The commonly used pigmentary grade of ZnO has particle sizes ranging from 200 to 400 nm, but to achieve optimal protection through processes involving absorption as well as scattering, the desired UV-attenuation grade of ZnO should also have particle size between 40 and 100 nm.[28,30] This is in agreement with earlier observations reported by Sayre et al.,[31] who observed that both ZnO and TiO$_2$ have strong absorption bands in the wavelength region of 250 to 400 nm and exhibit a semiconductor property of optical absorption gap, absorbing most radiation at shorter wavelengths than the gap (around 360 nm). At wavelengths longer than the gap, these compounds can mobilize electrons within their atomic structure and scatter the impinging radiation. TiO$_2$ is also an excellent UVB blocker, whereas ZnO is quite effective in scattering UVA radiation. Thus, the combination of these two agents helps to achieve high-SPF products

($\geq$20). Varying possibilities are available for blending TiO$_2$ and ZnO together in a lotion form of a sunscreen formulation. Generally, TiO$_2$ is used in a lower concentration than ZnO (e.g., in a ratio of 1 to 3, or 2.5% TiO$_2$ and 7.5% ZnO). The marked decrease in whitening of emulsions containing ZnO and TiO$_2$ has also been aided by using acetyl dimethicone copolymer, which improves the spreading coefficients of such physical sunscreens, SPF values, and consumer acceptability of the product.[14,28,30] Although TiO$_2$ has been observed to produce hydroxyl radicals when illuminated with UV light and reported to cause oxidative damage in an in vitro system, the benefits of using TiO$_2$ outweigh the potential risk of free radials and oxidative damage.

The second group of inorganic particulate sunscreens referred to earlier includes iron oxide, barium sulfate, mica, and metal powders such as gold. Although iron oxide shows properties of UV absorption and attenuation (scattering), it is not as effective and popular as ZnO or TiO$_2$ because it renders topical formulations a selective color, limiting its usefulness and wide acceptability. However, it is used for making UV-opaque lipsticks in combination with ZnO or TiO$_2$ to achieve high-SPF products (15 to 30) to protect lips against the potentially harmful effects of both UVA and UVB radiation.

The organic particulates comprise such chemicals as charcoal, and melanin and melanin precursors in the form of liposomes.[32] The organic particulates, particularly those incorporating melanin, were formulated only recently for human use, and limited information is available in terms of their effectiveness, safety, and consumer acceptability (or popularity).[32] Melanin, although an effective UV absorber and a stable free radical quencher,[32-34] provides only low SPF value (<6) when used alone as a sunscreen.[32] Limitations resulting from its low solubility, particulate nature, unattractive brownish-black color, and low SPF value has made melanin a less appealing and less popular particulate form of sunscreen than TiO$_2$ or ZnO.

PHOTOPROTECTION BY SUN-PROTECTIVE CLOTHING

The use of sun-protective clothing that can block over 97 percent of harmful UV rays is becoming popular and acceptable for outdoor activities by adults, children, and even teenagers. In the past,[15,35] the medical advice for normal healthy individuals as well as for patients experiencing sun sensitivity problems (e.g., solar urticaria) has been the use of long-sleeved shirts, long pants, and wide-brimmed hats, all made of tightly woven cotton fabrics. However, the availability of synthetic fabrics made from nylon and polyester with a wide choice of color, weave (including tight weaves), and texture, and with documented properties of high SPF (15 to $\geq$45) has made this approach more acceptable.[35-41] With this clothing, sunscreen need only be applied to those areas (e.g., face, chest, neck, arms, and hands) that cannot be shielded by clothing. Children who spend considerable time outdoors and are at greatest risk, teenagers who rarely use any sunscreens, and people frequently engaged in outdoor activities (e.g., golfers, tennis players, roofers, farmers, gardeners) can be well protected by using such clothing. The clothing industry in the United States, in cooperation with the American Society for Testing and Materials, is standardizing methods (both in vitro and in vivo) for determining SPFs of fabrics that are acceptable to the U.S. Federal Trade Commission. It should be emphasized that mere opaqueness to visible light may not ensure the ability of fabrics or clothing to block UV radiation, although a loose weave may enable the passage of UV and visible light and indicate a poor ability to photoprotect. The discomforts of high temperature and high humidity associated with wearing clothing made of synthetic fabrics can be minimized by using tightly knit fabric made of a cotton blend; such fabrics retain high SPF values (>20 to 40). Unblended summer-weight cotton clothing provides low SPF values (6 to 10) and limited protection and cannot be recommended for light-sensitive patients or for high-exposure activities. Wetting of summer-weight fabrics results in less protection. Dermatologists recommending the use of sun-protective clothing to patients with light sensitivity problems should be aware that (1) the weave of some fabrics does appear to affect the transmittance properties and flux of solar radiation through the garments; and (2) some fabrics provide protection by coating applied to fabric, which may lose photoprotective efficacy over time after washing. For this reason, protection standards for clothing need to be developed to protect the consumer.

QUICK TANNING LOTIONS AND TANNING ACCELERATORS

Among fair-skinned Caucasians, tanned skin has been considered good looking and healthy. Although sunbathing and acquisition of a tan are still very popular with fair-skinned individuals, the potentially harmful effects of sun exposure are being recognized by both patients and physicians. For this reason, the possibility of an accelerated tanning reaction without sun exposure has been exploited commercially and has generated a proliferation of several types of consumer products each claiming either to deepen the degree of facultative tanning reaction (acquired tone of increased skin pigmentation over and above the genetically controlled constitutive level of melanin pigmentation) or to accelerate a series of biochemical reactions that contribute to enhancing melanogenesis or the natural process of melanin pigmentation.[42–44]

Dihydroxyacetone (DHA)-Induced Melanoid Staining of Skin

DHA, the active ingredient of sunless tanning preparations, reacts with skin keratins to produce an orange-brown color upon its oxidation. The color remains adherent to the stratum corneum and is not easily washed off.[1,44–47] The applied formulation containing 3 to 5% or more DHA becomes gradually oxidized and polymerized after 3 to 10 h to an orange-brown color. The intensity of the color can vary from light to dark orange-brown, depending upon the concentration of DHA used and the frequency of its application. Repeated (three to five) applications produce a golden-brown color that simulates the tanning reaction. The Maillard browning reaction[48,49] with skin surface proteins, possibly with the amino acids histidine and tryptophan, is central to this process. The browning reaction products were called *melanoidins* by early investigators,[50] because their light-absorbing properties resembled those of the natural pigment—melanin. The authors have examined the photoprotective properties and the SPF value of this staining reaction.[51]

Specimens of human skin obtained at biopsy after six repeated treatments with DHA (5%) decreased the penetration of UV (320 to 380 nm) and visible radiation through the skin and appeared to provide over 50 percent protection against the penetration of long-wave UV and visible radiation. This apparent protection was assessed in vivo by two criteria: (1) the diminution of a phototoxic reaction induced by oral administration of 8-methoxypsoralen (0.6 mg/kg) and exposure to a minimal phototoxic dose of UVA radiation in two patients with psoriasis undergoing PUVA therapy; and (2) protection of the skin of two volunteers with erythropoietic protoporphyria (EPP) who were known to react abnormally to visible radiation (380 to 460 nm) by developing an itching, burning, and swelling reaction. Patients with psoriasis undergoing PUVA therapy showed no evidence of photoxic reactions of stained normal skin treated with DHA lotion when compared to the unstained normal skin, which showed a mild degree of phototoxic reaction. Likewise, two patients with EPP treated with DHA lotion tolerated a fourfold increased exposure dose of visible radiation (400 to 760 nm) without any evidence of the burning, itching, swelling, or redness often experienced by patients with EPP in untreated control skin. Similar observations were reported earlier by Fusaro et al.,[45,46,52,53] who showed protection of DHA-treated skin against longwave UV and visible radiation in normal skin and in patients with polymorphous light eruptions and EPP. DHA-containing products appear to be quite popular in the United States, Europe, and elsewhere, especially during winter and early spring.

Unfortunately, a DHA-induced sunless tanning reaction does not adequately protect against a UVB-induced sunburn reaction. For this reason, cosmetic companies have formulated products containing DHA in combination with UVB-absorbing sunscreen chemicals that provide a high SPF value to protect the skin against UVB, UVA, and visible radiation (see Table 248-7, "miscellaneous"). In terms of practicality and usefulness, this kind of formulation enriched with DHA and UVB-absorbing sunscreen chemicals appears to be better and more useful than DHA formulations without sunscreens for persons of SPTs I to III who often go out in the sun to get a natural tan. Such individuals can also achieve tanned skin or "tanned looks" without any sun or exposure to UV radiation in tanning salons and thus avoid the potential risk of skin damage. Patients with amelanotic macules of vitiligo can also use DHA lotions to color the depigmented skin artificially and protect it against actinic damage.[54]

One cannot equate an artificially induced cosmetic dyeing reaction of skin with the natural process of tanning reaction involving increased proliferation of melanocytes and increased production and transfer of melanin-laden melanosomes to keratinocytes.[55] Histologically and ultrastructurally, the two reactions of skin pigmentation are distinct (in color intensity and appearance) and should not be equated.

The second approach used in acceleration of the tanning reaction involves manipulation of the melanogenic path (tyrosine → dopa → melanin) or modification of the melanogenic support system.[43,44] Recent advances in understanding the factors regulating the process of increased melanogenesis have stimulated investigators to modulate the tanning process of skin via topical application of effector agents, with or without the requirements for damaging UV exposure. One approach is the use of diacylglycerols (DAGs), which activate protein kinase C, thereby increasing the enzymatic activity of skin tyrosinase. Gilchrest and associates have explored the use of DAG to induce increased synthesis of melanin in the presence or absence of UV radiation.[56–58] These findings were further extended by Agin[59] with the addition of riboflavin or riboflavin phosphate to DAG or to other protein kinase C activators, such as triacylglycerols, lipopolysaccharides, unsaturated free fatty acids, and short-chain free fatty acids, that help to hydrolyze glycophospholipids to DAGs and promote a faster, darker, and more effective tan in skin exposed to UV radiation. However, there is at least theoretical concern about the safety of such agents that directly stimulate protein kinase C, as certain tumor promoters such as phorbol ester appear to have this property as their mechanism of action. Perhaps the most interesting exploration of the tanning process relates to some recent observations of Eller et al.,[60] who reported that topical application of UV-damaged DNA fragments to guinea pig skin produced a hyperpigmented tanned skin within 2 weeks which remained pigmented for 2 months. They reported that the DNA repair enzyme T_4 endonuclease catalyzes the repair of pyrimidine dimers that are induced by UV radiation. The presence of this DNA repair enzyme augments melanogenesis. This endonuclease was also delivered in carrier liposomes to enhance repair of UV-induced DNA damage in cultured human cells. Treatment of human melanocytes and S-91 melanoma cells with DNA repair enzyme T_4 endonuclease V was found to enhance melanogenesis after UV irradiation,[60] as evidenced by measuring melanin content, increased tyrosinase activity, and [^{14}C] dopa incorporation. These findings generate promising new methods that may allow alteration and acceleration of the skin tanning reaction process for enhancing photoprotective responses of skin without the requirement for antecedent UV-induced skin damage.

NONCLASSIC SUNSCREENS

Nonclassic sunscreens which protect from the deleterious effects of ultraviolet radiation by mechanisms other than absorption and scattering of UVR are likely to be employed increasingly in the future.

Antioxidants and Other Agents

One prominent class of nonclassic sunscreens is the antioxidant group represented by vitamins C (ascorbic acid) and E (alpha-tocopherol).[61,62] These agents do not possess intrinsic absorptive capacity for UV radiation and are believed to act after UV radiation has penetrated the skin and interacted with resident skin chromophores to generate reactive oxygen radical species. Certain antioxidants then have the capacity to neutralize oxygen radicals partially, preventing damage to tissues. While both vitamins showed efficacy across the UVA and UVB range, vitamin C was most effective in inhibiting UVA damage, whereas vitamin E protected better in the UVB range.

An extract from the plant *Polypodium leucotomos*, which has been used in Spain and Central America for treatment of psoriasis, atopic dermatitis, and vitiligo, has recently been studied for its capacity to ameliorate the effects of UV radiation. In vitro studies showed a highly efficient scavenging capacity of *Polypodium* extract on oxidizing molecules such as singlet oxygen and superoxide anion.[8] In vivo studies in humans pretreated with topical *Polypodium* revealed a block of UVB-induced erythema at up to 10 times the MED. Significant inhibition of PUVA-induced erythema was also observed in *Polypodium*-treated sites on human volunteers when compared with untreated sites.[9] The action of *Polypodium* is not mediated by scattering or absorption as it is effective via the oral route as well and acts as an antioxidant and a free radical quencher.

Silymarin is a flavonoid with strong antioxidant and free radical scavenging properties isolated from the milk thistle of *Silybum marianum* (artichoke).[63] When applied topically in a UVB-induced tumor initiation protocol in mice, it inhibited onset of the first tumor, tumor incidence, number of tumors, and their volume.[63] Silymarin has been used for many years in Europe for treatment of alcoholic liver disease and has been shown to protect against hepatotoxicity from several chemical agents, including carbon tetrachloride. Silymarin's mechanism of action seems to involve inhibition of the UVB-induction of epidermal ornithine decarboxylase and cyclooxygenase as well as edema.

Because of reports of its anti-inflammatory properties and its widespread acceptance in over-the-counter formulas for the palliation of sunburns, aloe (*Aloe barbadensis*) extract was recently investigated for its UV-protective capacity in mice.[64] Although it provided no protection from DNA pyrimidine dimer formation, its effects were significant when applied following UVB exposure. One important photoprotective attribute is the ability to block UVB-mediated immune suppression of Langerhans cells and Thy-1+ dendritic epidermal cells necessary for certain T cell–mediated responses. Aloe extract significantly blocked photoimmune suppression as measured by both contact hypersensitivity (to fluorescein isothiocyanate) and delayed type hypersensitivity (to *Candida*). These effects may have been mediated by aloe's ability to protect in part both the number and morphology of Langerhans cells.[64] Compounds with such properties may prove to be relevant in maintaining effective immune surveillance against UV radiation–induced skin neoplasms.

Prostaglandin Inhibitors and Systemic Agents

The synthesis of prostaglandin via cyclooxygenase is an important step in the induction of erythema and inflammation following solar UV radiation exposure.[11] Indomethacin is a well-known cyclooxygenase inhibitor that has some capacity to penetrate the stratum corneum and diminish post-UV erythema. An investigation into wavelength dependence for the effects of indomethacin on UV-induced erythema revealed surprising results. Application of 1% topical indomethacin significantly blocked redness following UV irradiation at 300 to 320 nm, had no effect in the 330 to 340 nm range, and potentiated erythema following UV irradiation at 350 to 370 nm.[65] These results suggest that prostaglandins may mediate erythema in the UVB range, while a different arachidonic acid metabolite, not dependent on cyclooxygenase for its production (perhaps leukotrienes), may mediate erythema in the UVA range. The utility of indomethacin in protecting against the effects of UV radiation is therefore limited; erythema may not be one of the more serious consequences of UV radiation but may serve as a useful warning of excessive exposure. Furthermore, indomethacin may potentiate erythema following UVA exposure while having virtually no effect on UVC-induced erythema.[65,66] Another cyclooxygenase inhibitor, acetylsalicylic acid (aspirin), has excellent analgesic properties and may influence the early sunburn erythema reaction, but it has failed to provide any significant photoprotective effect against the delayed erythema reaction, which shows a peak response 24 h after sun exposure. Likewise, antihistamines (H_1 histamine antagonists) are not helpful in modifying the delayed phase of sunburn reaction.

A major goal in photoprotection is the development of agents that are orally bioavailable as well as safe and effective. Green tea, which is widely consumed throughout Asia, is a candidate. In the preparation of green (as opposed to black) tea, oxidation of polyphenolic compounds is avoided, preserving a variety of beneficial effects. Hairless mice fed green tea as their sole source of drinking water had a marked decrease in the number, size, and latency of onset of skin tumors induced by UVB plus topical chemical tumor promoters.[63] It remains to be determined whether oral intake of green tea can diminish cutaneous malignancy in humans.

It is likely that nonclassic agents will ultimately be an important complement to standard sunscreens in preventing both the immediate and delayed effects of UV irradiation, but development of these is mostly in the early stage.

Beta-Carotene

Beta-carotene is recommended for the amelioration of photosensitivity reactions caused by visible radiation (400 to 760 nm) in the presence of abnormal levels of porphyrins in patients with EPP and other forms of porphyrias.[67–73] Unless afflicted patients, especially children, avoid exposure to the sun, a severe photosensitivity reaction will occur with painful swelling, itching, erythema, and a burning sensation. Vesicles may develop, often leading to scarring and mutilation. Beta-carotene is a natural constituent of many plants, including common foods such as carrots, tomatoes, green peppers, and oranges; it is nontoxic. Only beta-carotene, which absorbs radiation in the visible spectrum of light (360 to 500 nm) with a maximum absorption at 450 to 475 nm, has been shown to be partially, if not totally, effective as a systemic photoprotective agent, particularly in patients with EPP who are extremely sensitive to visible radiation. In several studies, which eventually included over 133 patients with EPP, all participants showed subjective as well as objective improvement in their tolerance to sunlight and exposure to 400-nm radiation.[67–70]

At the present time, it is recommended that oral ingestion of synthetic beta-carotene be regulated to maintain blood carotene levels between 600 and 800 μg/100 mL (usually a dose of 120 to 180 mg/day for adults). Children under the age of 16 should receive 30 to 120 mg/day. The protective effect of beta-carotene for increased tolerance to sun exposure is evidenced after 6 to 8 weeks of therapy. Many of the patients with EPP receiving oral beta-carotene are able to develop sun tolerance (up to 30 to 60 min during summer months) and can for the first time engage in outdoor activities for a longer time. Even on adequate doses (120 to 180 mg/day), patients with EPP may develop some photosensitivity reactions (e.g., itching, burning, and swelling) after sun exposure, and each patient must carefully establish his or her tolerance limit to sun exposure. An increment in the oral dose of beta-carotene provides increased protection. Also, the concomitant topical application of UVB- and UVA-absorbing sunscreens (SPF 20 to 30, type 4, Table 248-7) is helpful, especially when the patient is likely to be exposed to solar radiation for periods longer than 1 h. Oral beta-carotene is not an effective sunscreen for filtering UVB radiation in sunlight, although it has been shown to slightly increase the MED in healthy individuals.[71] Patients with very noticeable light sensitivity—those with EPP, congenital porphyria, and xeroderma pigmentosum—should employ other photoprotective measures (broad-brimmed hat, long-sleeved clothing, oral beta-carotene, and avoidance of sunlight exposure between 10 A.M. and 4 P.M.) very early in life.

The mechanisms by which beta-carotene is effective in protecting patients with EPP from photosensitivity are unknown.[72] Photoactivated porphyrins (e.g., proto-, uro-, and coproporphyrins) are known to generate singlet oxygen that appears to be implicated in causing cutaneous photosensitivity reactions in different porphyrias; it is unknown how the generation of singlet oxygen can initiate varying forms of cutaneous reactions in different types of porphyr-

ias (vesicular, pruritic, and edematous reactions). Beta-carotene is an effective quencher for singlet oxygen produced by photactivated porphyrins.[1,15,68,73,74] Beta-carotene is photoxidized preferentially and spares the cell components (membrane lipids, cell nuclei, guanine bases of DNA, etc.) from being selectively photodamaged.[69,72]

Beta-carotene, when applied topically, is not an effective agent for preventing sunburn reaction induced by UVB radiation.[71] Upon exposure to sunlight, it is easily photoxidized and degraded. Patients with polymorphous light eruption, actinic reticuloid, solar urticaria, and hydroa aestivale may derive some benefits from systemic beta-carotene; the claims, however, need to be confirmed by well-controlled studies. In the authors' experience, when topical sunscreens do not offer relief to a given patient, it is probably sensible to give a short-term course (3 months) of oral beta-carotene in combination with high-SPF sunscreens (SPF 20 to 30). Beta-carotene is essentially nontoxic and may offer some noticeable relief from photosensitivity.[68,70]

SUNSCREENS AND PREVENTION OF SKIN CANCER

Overview

Since the 1970s, sunscreens have been widely available and promoted for the prevention of skin cancer, especially among those at higher risk. Indeed, sunscreens have been shown to prevent actinic keratoses (AKs) in humans, and there are conclusive studies in rodent species that show that, when applied prior to UV exposure, sunscreens potently block induction of squamous cell carcinoma (SCC).[75] It has become increasingly clear that the relationship of skin cancers and sunscreen usage in humans is complex. Several factors have emerged as relevant in this relationship: (1) sunscreen use may change behavior, causing increased exposure time to UV radiation after applying sunscreens that protect sunburn wavelengths selectively; (2) UV-induced immune suppression can occur at suberythemogenic doses of UV radiation; and (3) evidence in animals and humans now exists for melanoma induction by wavelengths not well protected by most sunscreens.

Sunscreens and Actinic Keratoses

Precancerous AKs are more prevalent and rapid in their onset following UV exposure than are skin cancers. This fact has made it possible for two randomized, blinded, prospective studies in humans to reveal the efficacy of sunscreens in the prevention of AKs. In Australians 40 years or older, the daily application of an SPF 17 sunscreen containing Parsol MCX and avobenzone during a single summer reduced the mean number of AKs present over the following 7 months. The amount of sunscreen usage was related to both the development of new lesions and the remission of existing ones.[76,77] A randomized, double-blind trial in Texas over a 2-year treatment period yielded similar results, with an approximately 36 percent decrease in the annual rate of AKs attributable to the use of an SPF 29 sunscreen as compared with vehicle control.[78] Despite attempts to assess the incidence of skin cancer in the latter study, there was no significant difference between the groups, and the investigators concluded that a longer and larger study would be required to assess the photoprotective efficacy of sunscreens against skin cancer due to its latency. Sunscreens with SPF >15 are therefore effective in decreasing the incidence and promoting the regression of AKs, and these effects are measurable within 1 year of initiating treatment. Hence, regular use of a high-SPF sunscreen is essential in the control of this premalignant condition.

Sunscreens and Basal Cell Carcinomas

Surprisingly, there is no direct evidence in humans that the use of sunscreens decreases either basal carcinomas (BCCs) or SCCs. In fact, in a prospective study of over 70,000 U.S. nurses, those who used sunscreen and spent fewer than 8 h per week outdoors were significantly *more* likely to develop BCC.[76] According to the authors, this may be due to the extensive confounding variables inherent in such a retrospective, self-reported study. Much of the increased risk for the use of sunscreens and avoidance of outdoor activities could be explained by constitutional factors such as skin phototype, family history, and proximity to the equator; that is, women who are most sun-sensitive and presumably have been sunburned many times in the past due to unusually fair skin adopt "preventive" behaviors such as sunscreen use and sun avoidance. These factors are then erroneously associated with risk.

Despite a lack of conclusive data relating sunscreens to BCC risk, suggestions as to the most prudent use of sunscreens can be derived from a population-based retrospective case-control study performed in Canada. This study found that BCC risk was (1) increased with greater recreational sunlight exposure in adolescence and childhood (age 0 to 19 years), (2) most pronounced among sun-sensitive individuals who tended to burn rather than tan, and (3) unrelated to recreational or occupational sun exposure as an adult.[79] A study of two sisters with xeroderma pigmentosum who were subjected to aggressive sun avoidance and sunscreen use (SPF 28) at the time of diagnosis revealed that BCC development is exquisitely sensitive in this disease to early sun exposure. The younger sister, who was 2 years old at diagnosis, was free of skin cancers until age 23, whereas the older sister, who began protection at age 4, developed her first BCC at 13 years of age and had many by age 25.[80] The combination of sunscreen use and sun avoidance in the 0- to 19-year-old age group is most likely to reduce BCC rates, while sun protection later in life appears to have a minimal effect on BCC incidence.

Sunscreens and Squamous Cell Carcinomas

Several lines of evidence suggest that sunscreens may be effective in the prevention of SCCs:

1. Sunscreens are capable of preventing AKs, as noted above, which are precursor lesions to SCCs.
2. The UVB range has been shown to be the most potent in SCC induction in hairless mice,[81] and these wavelengths are best blocked by sunscreens.
3. Sunscreens applied to mouse skin blocked induction of *p53* mutations, a precursor genetic lesion to most AKs and SCCs.[82]
4. Sunscreens potently block UV-induced SCC development in mice.[75]
5. Epidemiologic evidence implicates recent (the 10 years prior to onset of malignancy) sunlight exposure as most relevant in SCC development, suggesting that increased sunscreen usage among adults may lead to reduced rates of SCCs.[83]

Sunscreens and Malignant Melanoma

The relationship of UVR and melanoma is complex and not well understood. Epidemiologic studies link melanoma risk with intermittent recreational exposure and severe sunburns before age 15,

while a mildly protective effect (odds ratio 0.7) was associated with summertime occupational sun exposure in males.[84,85] Moreover, the wavelengths associated with melanoma risk are not known. It has been the policy of dermatologists to recommend sunscreen use (as well as sun avoidance) to those at risk for melanoma. Therefore, great controversy surrounds the findings of several large case-control studies that implicate the use of sunscreens as a risk factor in the development of melanoma, with odds ratios ranging from 1.5 to 1.8.[86,87] Both of these studies stratified subjects and adjusted for confounders such as hair color, freckling, history of sunburn, and sun-exposure habits yet still found increased risk with the use of sunscreens. There are several possible explanations for spurious findings in studies such as these if, in fact, sunscreen usage does *not* increase melanoma risk: (1) There may be other unidentified confounding variables that cannot be eliminated, such as recall bias. For example, sunscreen usage self-reports may be inaccurate as "persons with a history of many sunburn episodes are subsequently likely to use sunscreens more frequently. The ongoing sunscreen use would then appear as a risk factor, while the real cause would be the excessive sun exposure that may have taken place long before."[88] (2) Given the long lag time of 10 to 30 years between sun exposure and appearance of melanoma, the cases identified in these studies during the late 1980s likely stem from sun exposures that occurred when broad-spectrum sunscreens were neither available, recommended, nor regularly used. These results would thus have less relevance to current usage patterns of broad-spectrum sunscreens coupled with increased public awareness of the risks of UV radiation.

On the other hand, sunscreens may in fact be responsible for the reported modest ($\sim$1.5-fold) increased risk of melanoma, and several potential explanations have been proposed:

1. *Altered behavior with sunscreens.* Prolonged or more risky sunbathing may result from the use of sunscreens, permitting increased total exposure time to UV radiation.
2. *Vitamin D.* By absorbing UVB, sunscreens inhibit production of vitamin D, whose intake has been associated with decreased death rates from various cancers, including melanoma. Specific, high-affinity receptors for 1,25-dihydroxyvitamin D_3 have been demonstrated in cultured melanoma cells, whose growth can be slowed by this substrate in vitro and in vivo.[89] Randomized, controlled studies of sunscreen use, however, do not demonstrate significant vitamin D deficiency,[90] and vitamin D intake is more important than sun exposure in predicting serum levels. Furthermore, a large case-control study demonstrated that decreased vitamin D intake was not associated with an increased risk of melanoma.[91]
3. *Increased UVA exposure.* Because sunscreens avert erythema, they allow markedly increased UVA exposure of up to 100 J/cm^2 in a single day.[92] Although UVA is much less efficient than UVB in causing cellular and genetic damage, the flux reaching the earth is orders of magnitude greater than that of UVB. This discrepancy is magnified by UVB-sunscreen use and by the greater fraction of UVA light that penetrates the epidermis. At the basal layer of the epidermis, the ratio of UVA:UVB flux has been estimated to be $\sim$720:1 if a sunscreen of SPF 9 is used. In vitro, human cells undergo approximately equal numbers of DNA mutations by UVA and UVB when the relative flux is in this range.[93] In addition, the DNA mutation characteristics of UVA differ from UVB, with a higher frequency of mutations at A or T base pairs with UVA. A finding

that UVA-specific T to G transversions comprised 25 percent of DNA mutations was used to implicate UVA as a significant mutagen in mammalian cells exposed to simulated sunlight.[94] Other effects of UVA include inhibition of DNA synthesis,[95] DNA fragmentation,[96] pyrimidine dimer formation,[97] DNA strand breaks,[98] chromosomal aberrations,[99] and sister chromatid exchange.[99] The clinical significance of many of these in vitro findings, however, is unclear. In the exquisitely radiation-sensitive *Xiphophorus* fish, the action spectrum for malignant melanoma induction extended past UVA into the visible spectrum, leading Setlow and co-workers to hypothesize that "light energy absorbed in melanin is effective in inducing melanomas in this animal model and that in natural sunlight 90–95% of melanoma induction may be attributed to wavelengths >320—the UVA and visible spectral regions."[100] Although these surprising results from a fish model may not be applicable to humans, multiple, large retrospective studies associate the use of artificial UVA sources, such as sun beds and sunlamps, with an increased risk of melanoma. Relative risks of 1.3- to 1.8-fold for ever having used a sunlamp and 7.7-fold for more than 10 exposures per year among those under age 30 have been reported.[101–104] The association of PUVA therapy with subsequent development of melanoma further supports a role for UVA in the induction of this tumor.[105]

4. *Immune suppression.* The efficacy of sunscreens in blocking UVR-mediated immune suppression is controversial. UV radiation has been shown to affect immune surveillance of skin cancer in several animal models. In mice, UV irradiation of the test animal prior to injection of an established melanoma cell line significantly increases the incidence of tumor growth over the following 5 to 8 weeks. Wolf and co-workers have shown that this facilitation of melanoma growth mediated by UV radiation is not blocked by sunscreens when applied in adequate amounts to block erythema and sunburn cell formation.[106] This suggests that suberythemogenic doses of UV radiation, which are likely to penetrate sunscreens, may have significant immunosuppressive effects.

In summary, the efficacy of sunscreens on melanoma incidence is uncertain. It is clear, however, that sunscreen usage does not provide complete melanoma protection and that UVA may play a role in the etiology of melanoma. Therefore to decrease melanoma risk, exposure should be minimized, and the regular use of broad-spectrum UVA-sunscreens including physical blocks such as TiO_2 should be advocated.

CONTROL OF PHOTOAGING, OR DERMATOHELIOSIS

Photoaging of skin was recognized in the nineteenth century by dermatologists such as Unna[107] and Dubreuilh,[108] who described the damaging effects of sunlight on the sun-exposed skin of farmers and sailors compared with the appearance of indoor workers. Repeated solar exposure over many years (either intentional or unintentional as a consequence of living in areas of high-intensity sunlight) ultimately results in the development of the skin syndrome referred to as *dermatoheliosis* (see Chap. 138).[1] It is more pro-

nounced in white, fair-skinned individuals with ample lifelong sun exposure and is found on the habitually sun-exposed areas (e.g., face, periorbital and cheek areas, neck, V area of chest below the neck covering the sternum, lower arms and hands) (see Chap. 146). These areas exhibit sagging, with a slightly yellowed, rough surface, and facial telangiectases are present. These drastic, visible changes reflect profound epidermal and dermal alterations that are distinctly different from those found in the habitually protected but intrinsically aged skin of the buttock. The severity of photoaging depends principally on the duration and intensity of sun exposure, influenced by the proximity of the place of residence to the equator, and on the constitutive skin color of the individual based on his or her genetic capacity to tan (facultative increased melanin pigmentation resulting from sun exposure). Photoaging is almost invariably and distinctly observed in persons with white skin, especially in individuals of SPTs I to III who sunburn easily and proportionally to the sun exposure dose (see Table 138-5) and show a variable tanning response of skin that is respectively poor, minimal, or moderately low (but not intense or profuse). The Celtic populations of the United Kingdom, Ireland, and Brittany and areas of the world where they have settled, such as Australia, and the United States, tend to show photoaging changes as early as 20 years of age, whereas people of a similar age group with brown and dark-brown (tanned) skin living in India, Ceylon, Mexico, Egypt, the Middle East, Florida, South East Asia, and Central America reveal minimal photoaging changes at age 20 to 30, even though they live in intensely sunny areas. Fair-skinned people who work outdoors (e.g., farmers, telephone linesmen, sailors, outdoor construction workers, lifeguards, sports enthusiasts (amateur and professional) and those who habitually sunbathe invariably show increasing level of photoaging changes of sun exposed skin by 30 to 35 years of age.

Dermatoheliosis reflects a polymorphic response of various components of human skin, especially cells in the epidermis, the vascular system, and dermal connective tissue (see Chap. 146). Specific features include wrinkling (fine surface wrinkles of periorbital areas, deep furrows of forehead and neck),[109,110] shallowness, coarseness, mottled pigmentation, increased translucence, solar keratoses, xerosis, and solar lentigo. The epidermis shows atrophy, guttate hypomelanosis, acanthosis and increased horny layer, atypia of keratinocytes, loss of polarity of keratinocytes, flattening of the dermal-epidermal junction, dermal elastosis, loss of collagen, and increased glycosaminoglycans.[111]

Action Spectrum for Photoaging

Although not established in human skin by exposure to monochromatic radiation, available data obtained from animal experimentation and supporting epidemiologic data indicate that UVB (290 to 320 nm) wavelengths are primarily and predominantly responsible for photaging.[110,111] However, UVA radiation (320 to 400 nm) that penetrates deep into the dermis also plays an important role.[110–114] The UVA radiation generates reactive forms of oxygen (e.g., singlet oxygen, superoxide anion, and hydroxy radicals) that cause an oxidative stress and denaturation of proteins and cross-links (e.g., collagen and elastin).[2,110,115,116] They also cause damage to fibroblasts involving cell membrane lipid peroxidation. Although there is no specific chromophore(s) that selectively absorb UVA radiation, available evidence indicates that non-DNA chromophores, such as flavins, NADPH (reduced form of phosphorylated nicotinamide dinucleotide), and quinones (ubiquinone), absorb UVA radiation and generate reactive forms of oxygen and free radicals.[2,117] The chronic low-grade inflammatory response to repeated UV radiation contributes through repeated and near-continuous release of proteolytic enzymes that induce damage to both cells and extracellular matrix.[110,114] It is also possible that repeated injury to epidermal and dermal cells by UVB and UVA radiation leads to premature senescence of cells known to have a finite replicative capacity.[115,116]

Control or Management of Photoaging

Prior to 1980, photoaging was believed to be an irreversible process, and the use of sunscreens was of limited value because most of the available sunscreens did not filter out the UVB and UVA radiation.[110–112] It is increasingly evident that the process of photoaging, or dermatoheliosis, if not preventable, can at least be slowed or minimized.[116,118,119] The measures listed below can help to minimize the process of photoaging and help to restore the normal appearance of skin.

1. *Avoidance of sunlight:* Individuals living in high-intensity UV light areas (e.g., 0 to 30° N/S) can minimize the progressive increase in structural and cellular changes associated with photoaging of skin by avoiding sunlight between 10 A.M. and 4 P.M. If such individuals can change their habits of performing outdoor activities in the middle of the day, they can help themselves to repair and restore photodamaged skin. The UV intensity of sunlight between 11 A.M. and 2 P.M. is maximum. Evidence of normal repair has been observed in human skin when photodamaged skin was protected and sun exposure was avoided, suggesting that further damage of photoaging skin could be prevented and repaired by avoiding UV radiation.[1,118–121]

2. *Use of protective clothing:* If sunlight cannot be avoided between 10 A.M. and 4 P.M. on a daily basis, other measures should be adopted such as wearing broad-brimmed hats, use of parasols or umbrellas, and wearing sun-protective clothing that covers most of the body (chest, abdomen, arms, and legs).[1]

3. *Regular use of sunscreens:* Sunscreens enriched with UVB- and UVA-absorbing chemicals with SPF value of at least 15 and preferably 30 (e.g., those containing cinnamates, padimate-O, benzophenone, avobenzone, ZnO, and TiO_2) should be recommended.

These protective measures should be advocated and adopted from early age of life. Even brown- or dark-skinned people [blacks, Hispanics, and brown-skinned people from oriental countries (Philippines, Thailand, India, Pakistan, etc.)] should adopt these protective measures to delay the onset of photoaging and increased pigmentary changes of skin. In mouse model experiments and in clinical evaluations involving human volunteers, protection of otherwise habitually sun-exposed skin from further UV damage resulted in clinically and histologically evident improvements of the skin.[121–123] Volunteers using simple regimens of sun protection lotion with moisturizing cream alone experienced a statistically significant improvement in the appearance of facial skin within 24 weeks compared with the volunteers' own baseline appearance, as judged by participants and clinical investigators.[121–124]

ADVERSE EFFECTS OF SUN-PROTECTIVE AGENTS

Since the mid-1970s, the production of sunscreens and their ingredients has tripled to meet demands so that in 1994 67 percent of American adults used sun-protective agents while sunbathing.[125] Moreover, sunscreen chemicals are becoming an important ingredient of many cosmetics and toiletries.

Despite continued advances in the formulation of sun-protective agents, adverse reactions continue to occur, creating barriers to patient compliance. Although, ideally, well-formulated preparations are not irritating or sensitizing, individuals may react idiosyncratically to any of the component chemicals. Now that high-SPF sunscreens dominate the market,[125] sun-active ingredients are being employed in concentrations of up to 26%,[126] increasing the probability of contact irritation and the potential for sensitization reactions. Moreover, many preparations of sunscreen chemicals have been found to contain trace impurities, which can precipitate reactions unexpectedly. In 1978, the FDA redefined sunscreens from cosmetic to drug status, thus requiring tighter regulation over their manufacture and availability, in order to protect consumers against adverse reactions.[12,13]

Most sunscreening agents are low molecular weight compounds, which, after topical application, can diffuse through the stratum corneum, potentially causing both irritant and allergic contact dermatitis. In addition, while physical sunblocks reflect or scatter light, chemical sunscreens absorb UV radiation and can become photoactivated to more reactive states, which create the potential for phototoxic, photoallergic, or mutagenic reactions. Moreover, in order to make their products more stable and aesthetically pleasing for application, sunscreen manufacturers use excipients including preservatives, fragrances, emulsifiers, emollients, antioxidants, solvents, and stabilizers, which can in turn cause any of the above adverse effects. In summary, any sunscreen formulation, and especially those with multiple ingredients, has the potential for generating four types of adverse cutaneous reactions: (1) nonimmunologic contact irritation, (2) nonimmunologic phototoxicity, (3) allergic contact sensitization, and (4) photoallergic contact sensitization. Furthermore, some sunscreening chemicals also exhibit mutagenic properties in cultured cells and in mice.

Contact Irritant Reactions

Over 90 percent of cosmetic side effects are irritant reactions,[127,128] and half of these are completely subjective, with no objective signs of dermatitis.[129] In sunscreens, the likelihood of irritant reactions is even greater, as high-SPF formulations necessitate high concentrations of multiple sun-active ingredients.[128] Moreover, topically applied preparations can aggravate preexisting dermatoses, such as atopic dermatitis, seborrheic dermatitis, AKs, or rosacea.[127,130] "Status cosmeticus" refers to a patient's intolerance of any preparation applied topically to the face, with symptoms out of proportion to signs.[130] In a study population applying either a sunscreen or its vehicle, 114 patients (19 percent) had adverse reactions, but only 6 manifested true allergic sensitization. Of the remainder, 45 developed aggravation of atopic dermatitis, 39 suffered from contact irritation, and 22 exhibited nonspecific cosmetic intolerance.[128]

Phototoxic Reactions

When UV radiation absorbed by the thin film of applied sunscreen chemical is not dissipated harmlessly as heat, it can initiate harmful photobiologic and photochemical cutaneous reactions. The absorbed radiation either can be transferred to vulnerable constituents of epidermal cells, causing an exaggerated sunburn reaction, or it can promote photoexcitation of the sunscreening agent to a reactive singlet or triplet excited state (see Chap. 16). These reactive photoexcited states interact with and damage cell membranes, DNA, enzymes, lysosomes, mast cells, and other crucial epidermal constituents, thus contributing to the phototoxic reaction, with or without involving molecular oxygen. Free radicals and reactive oxygen species, such as singlet oxygen ($^1O_2$), superoxide anion ($O_2^{\cdot -}$), or hydroxy radicals ($^\cdot OH$) may be formed, causing oxidative stress to epidermal cells and resulting in cell death, vesiculation, and epidermal necrosis.

Many sunscreen chemicals are insoluble and diffuse poorly into the epidermis; they remain on the surface of the skin and dissipate the absorbed UV radiation in a harmless manner, without causing phototoxic reactions. In contrast, the photoreactive psoralens, such as 8- and 5-methoxypsoralen (MOP), induce an exaggerated sunburn reaction at low concentrations (<2 to 5 $\mu g/cm^2$), enhanced by effective diffusion of the applied ingredients (see Chap. 264). 5-MOP is occasionally used in combination with UVB-absorbing sunscreens to allow tanning without burning. Padimate A, an ester of PABA, can also be intensely phototoxic and was withdrawn from the market precisely because its phototoxic properties defeated its intended purpose as a sunscreen.

Contact Allergy

Some sunscreen chemicals may become haptens, linking to endogenous proteins and activating afferent pathways of antigen presentation by Langerhans cells to T lymphocytes. On subsequent exposure, a cascade of events mediated by cytokines produces the delayed hypersensitivity reaction, manifest as an acute vesiculated, spongiotic dermatitis with a mononuclear dermal infiltrate, 48 h after the second exposure (Chap. 122).

Sunscreens can also induce an immediate contact urticaria, with a wheal and flare 30 to 60 min after exposure.[131] The diagnosis of contact urticaria is often missed and requires scratch testing. In contact allergy of any type, high concentrations of the inciting chemical are not necessary, and cross-reactions to structurally related antigens may occur.

Photoallergy

In photoallergic dermatitis, the delayed hypersensitivity reaction is equivalent to the contact allergic response, with the exception that UV radiation is required to transform the implicated chemical into a sensitizer. The irradiated hapten, or its photoproduct, is photoconjugated to a membrane-bound epidermal carrier protein,[132] forming a complete antigen recognized by the Langerhans cell (see Chaps. 135 and 137). The hypothesized events in this photochemical reaction, as they occur in vivo, are currently speculative, based on in vitro photochemical reactions involving 6-methylcoumarin, a photosensitizer used as a fragrance in many sunscreen preparations.[132,133] Photoallergy most often involves the UVA portion of the UV spectrum and can be mitigated by incorporating a physical sunblock to minimize UVA absorption by the reactive sunscreen.[134]

Unfortunately, the diagnosis of sunscreen photoallergy is still not well standardized and in most cases is based on history and clinical appearance of the rash. While the standard photocontact tray includes the most widely used sunscreen agents, there are numerous agents it omits. Sunscreen test kits, providing 2% concentrations of the chemicals, are available in Europe but not in the Untied States. Moreover, the maximum nonirritating doses of most sunscreens

have not yet been defined, and when high concentrations are used, the actual allergen may be an impurity or a photoproduct of the original compound.[126] While most sunscreens are tested in petrolatum, this vehicle retards the allergenicity of PABA derivatives, which are both more effective and more sensitizing in alcohol because of enhanced cutaneous penetration.[135] If a false-negative result is suspected in the course of photopatch testing, the clinician can increase the concentration of sunscreen or the dose of UVA, test other components of the sunscreen preparation, or irradiate with a broader spectrum of wavelengths.[126]

Comedogenicity

Of sunscreen ingredients tested, petrolatum is moderately comedogenic, while coconut oil and cocoa butter are strongly comedogenic. Ultraviolet radiation enhances these effects.[136]

Incidence of Sunscreen Allergy

A survey of published reports of contact and photocontact sensitization by sunscreens indicates that the prevalence of such adverse reactions is surprisingly low and manageable. Two large patch test series report sunscreening agents as the cause of between 1 and 3 percent of contact dermatitis cases, translating into approximately 0.01 percent of the population served.[137,138] These figures are consistent with the data reviewed by Nater and DeGroot.[139] In cases of photocontact dermatitis, sunscreens are implicated in 6 to 12 percent and are increasingly important, so that they have now surpassed fragrances as the most frequent photoallergens.[140–143] Published case reports and reviews of contact and photocontact sensitization to sunscreens are summarized in Table 248-8, indicating the wide spectrum of reactions. However, case reports and patch series underestimate the true sensitization rates, as many patients misinterpret sunscreen allergy as inadequate protection from sunburn, and consequently do not report their adverse reactions. However, despite a significant number of adverse events, the benefits of using sun-protective agents significantly outweigh the risks.

SUNSCREEN CHEMICALS IMPLICATED IN BOTH IMMUNE AND NONIMMUNE CONTACT AND PHOTOCONTACT REACTIONS (See Table 248-8)

Para-Aminobenzoic Acid

PABA is one of the oldest sunscreen agents, widely employed in both the United States and Europe from the 1950s through the 1980s, when its use began to decline because of increasing reports of sensitization.[131] Its decreasing popularity over the past 15 years can be attributed to several unacceptable properties: (1) potential sensitization; (2) a photooxidation product, which produces long-lasting yellow stains in both cotton and synthetic fabrics; and (3) its hydrophilic nature, requiring solubilization in irritating alcohol-based formulations.[131] Because of its limited aqueous solubility, the most common adverse event associated with PABA is contact irritation, with subjective sensations of stinging and burning, from the alcoholic base usually required to solubilize the sunscreen chemical.[131] An alcoholic solution is also required for demonstrating al-

TABLE 248-8

Number of Reports of Sunscreen Sensitization Reactions

CHEMICAL	CONTACT SENSITIZATION	PHOTOCONTACT SENSITIZATION	CONTACT AND PHOTOCONTACT	URTICARIAL REACTION	TOTAL
PABA	68	77	2		147
Oxybenzone	16	82	8	1	107
Eusolex 8020 isopropyl dibenzoylmethane	63	19	1	1	84
Glyceryl PABA	30	7	4		41
Parsol 1789	19	15			34
Eusolex 6300 3-(4'-methyl-benzylidene) camphor	24	5	1		30
Padimate A	12	16			28
Padimate O	24	3	1		28
GivTan F 2-ethoxyethyl-p-methoxycinnamate	6	12			18
Mexenone	13	2	1		16
Eusolex 232 2-phenyl-benzimidazole-5-sulfonic acid	5	3			8
Sulisobenzone	3	2		1	6
Benzyl salicylate	6				6
Parsol MCX 2-ethylhexyl-p-methoxycinnamate	4				4
Benzophenone (NOS)	2	2			4
Homosalate	2	2			4
Dioxybenzone	3				3
Witisol	2				2
Bornelone	2				2
Digalloyl trioleate	1				1

SOURCE: Modified from Funk et al.,[126] with adaptations from the literature.

lergic sensitivity to PABA, as patch testing in petrolatum may yield false-negative results.[135]

Up to the 1980s, PABA was the most common cause of allergy to sunscreens.[144] During that decade, two large photopatch series implicated allergy to PABA or its derivatives in 4 to 6 percent of suspected photodermatoses.[140,145] Since 1985, however, the incidence of PABA reactions has decreased, commensurate with its declining use.[142]

Glyceryl PABA

To avoid the pH changes and photochemical reactions induced by PABA, researchers esterified PABA's carboxyl group to a glyceryl moiety. However, the para-amino group remained free in glyceryl PABA and behaved as the source of allergic sensitization and cross-reactivity. Formulated as a creamy white powder, glyceryl PABA has enjoyed longstanding use in both Europe and the United States. It was originally the most common cause of PABA sensitivity[146] since it was implicated in 1948 in the first case report of contact allergy to the PABA family of sunscreens.[147] This landmark patient, in addition, had previously documented contact dermatitis to benzocaine, as well as a systemic hypersensitivity to sulfaguanidine. On further patch testing, he was found to be reactive to aniline, para-phenylenediamine, procaine, sulfanilamide, and sulfadiazine, in addition to PABA, glyceryl PABA, benzocaine, and sulfaguanidine. All of these compounds are related by a common primary amino group in the para position.

Subsequent patients with contact allergy to glyceryl PABA had varying reactions to these structurally related compounds, except benzocaine, which cross-reacted in all cases.[146,148] Chemically, benzocaine is ethyl-aminobenzoate, the ethyl ester of PABA. In 1977, Fisher demonstrated impurities of 1 to 18% benzocaine in Escalol 106, the manufacturer's formulation of glyceryl PABA, thus revealing these "cross-reactions" to be, in actuality, primary reactions to an impurity.[149,150] Of 20 patients reactive to benzocaine, 11 reacted

to glyceryl PABA with a 0.3% benzocaine impurity, while none reacted to a formulation of glyceryl PABA with only 0.001% benzocaine.[151] There are only two reported instances of patients allergic to glyceryl PABA and not to benzocaine.[144] However, when these patients were patch tested to glyceryl PABA purified by high-pressure liquid chromatography, they did not react, implicating some other unknown impurity.[152]

Amyl Dimethyl PABA and Octyl Dimethyl PABA

Padimate A (amyl dimethyl PABA), padimate O (octyl dimethyl PABA), and ethyl dihydroxy PABA were introduced as effective UVB sunscreens intended to replace PABA and glyceryl PABA. The new compounds lack the para-amino moiety and thus should not cross-react with PABA and glyceryl PABA.[147,149] However, impurities of PABA and benzocaine were found by high-pressure liquid chromatography in all analyzed samples of padimate A.[153] Furthermore, a high proportion of patients using padimate A began to complain of burning erythema and pruritus after sun exposure. Padimate A's phototoxicity was demonstrated in the late 1970s both in healthy volunteers and in manufacturers of UV-cured inks containing the compound. Shortly thereafter, padimate A was reclassified as an unapproved sunscreen agent and was taken off the market.

Padimate O, on the other hand, had proven both safe and effective, becoming the most widely used sunscreens. Padimate O is formulated as a viscous liquid, which can be easily incorporated into cosmetic lotions,[131] causing no intermolecular aggregation or unwanted clothing stains. It is not water-soluble and tends to remain on the surface of the stratum corneum, with less than 10 percent penetration over 24 h.[126] Its molar extinction coefficient, reflecting its photoprotective ability, is more than twice that of PABA (23,400) in polar solvents. Finally, it demonstrates a low potential for sensitization, with fewer than 30 reported cases of allergy,[126,154] although personal observations in the authors' laboratories indicate that 5% padimate O causes nonimmunologic contact irritation reactions in fair-skinned individuals.

Cinnamates

Cinnamates are very popular UVB sunscreens. Of the 17 cinnamate derivatives available in European countries, only 5 are approved by the FDA. Of these, Parsol MCX is used most frequently, as it is insoluble in water and thus ideal for waterproof formulations. Moreover, it resists photodegradation and only uncommonly elicits photoallergic sensitization. Octocrylene is the newest cinnamate, developed in Europe and now available in the United States.

Both Parsol MCX and GivTan F (see Table 248-8) have been implicated in allergic reactions. Moreover, cinnamate sunscreens cross-react with several closely related compounds, including balsam of Peru, balsam of Tolu, coca leaves, cinnamic acid, cinnamic aldehyde, and cinnamon oil. These cinnamon derivatives are used in fragrances, cosmetics, medications, flavorings, toothpaste, and are present in tobacco, vermouth, colas, and Xylocaine and should be avoided in patients allergic to cinnamate sunscreens.[155]

Benzophenones

Benzophenones are aromatic ketone derivatives of dibenzoylmethane, exhibiting absorption characteristics not only in the UVC and UVB spectral ranges but also in part of the UVA range, up to 360 nm. For this reason, they are commonly used in combination with UVB sunscreens for extending the spectrum of photoprotection.[156] The benzophenones are the only sunscreens with a photoreactive carbonyl group. Although they do not easily undergo keto-enol tautomerization, they do respond to UVA radiation by the electron resonance delocalization process.[157] This property allows them to become potent allergic and UV-reactive photoallergic sensitizers.[145] One of these, sulisobenzone, has also been found to cause nonimmunologic irritation and contact urticaria.[158]

Benzophenones are extensively incorporated into cosmetics, perfumes, toiletries, accounting for reports of sensitization without knowledge of sunscreen use.[159] In addition, benzophenones have a wide variety of industrial uses: in textiles and plastics for fastness from discoloration by UV radiation; in plastic lens filters for color photography; in aerosol sprays to protect color prints; in polystyrene, acrylic, and rubber products to prevent darkening and loss of strength; and in paints, varnishes, and fluorescent lacquers.[158] Consequently, benzophenone-sensitive patients may face multiple environmental hazards from these industrial uses of this sunscreen.

By 1992, the most popular benzophenone, oxybenzone, had replaced PABA as both the most frequently used sunscreen agent and the most common cause of sunscreen allergy.[160,161] For example, in a large series of 283 patients with suspected photodermatoses between 1982 and 1992, 35 of 46 positive allergic reactions were to oxybenzone (12 percent of all patients photopatch tested).[145] Similar incidences of 13 percent were confirmed in two smaller photopatch series. Oxybenzone rapidly photooxidizes to oxybenzone semiquinone, a potent electrophile that reacts with thiol groups on antioxidant enzymes and substrates, such as thioredoxin reductase and reduced glutathione.[162] Moreover, oxybenzone is metabolized by cytochrome P_{450}, depleting hepatic glutathione.[163] By inactivating these important antioxidant systems, oxybenzone can impair protection from DNA damage.

Dibenzoylmethanes

The dibenzoylmethanes, or substituted diketones, represent a relatively new class of filters with impressive UVA absorption characteristics. As early as 1980, isopropyl dibenzoylmethane (Eusolex 8020) and butyl dibenzoylmethane (avobenzone, Parsol 1789) had been used in Europe as UVA screens, gaining widespread popularity in many countries.[157] Avobenzone, with an absorption maximum at 358 nm,[126,157] exhibits exceptionally high molar extinction values (>30,000). Until April 1997,[125] only one U.S. company had been approved for the manufacture of a sunscreen lotion containing avobenzone, while general FDA approval for its use in over-the-counter sunscreens had been stalled by issues centered around photolability and allergic sensitization potential. Avobenzone demonstrates keto-enol tautomerization and the consequent photolability common to both dibenzoylmethanes.[157] While it can be safe and nonsensitizing in concentrations below 3%, more potent formulations have elicited both irritant and allergic reactions.[164]

Allergic reactions to both avobenzone and Eusolex 8020, as well as cross-reactions between them, have proved exceedingly common. Eusolex 8020 is the more potent allergen, and many reactions to avobenzone have been traced to initial sensitization to the former isopropyl derivative, which had become pervasive in European cosmetics.[165] Because of such frequent adverse reactions, Eusolex 8020 has been withdrawn from the products of several European sunscreen manufacturers.[126] Fortunately, this compound has not been used in the United States.

The camphor derivative 3-(4'-methyl-benzylidene) camphor (Eusolex 6300) is a popular European UVB sunscreen used in combination with Eusolex 8020 to formulate the broad-spectrum dual sunscreen Eusolex 8021. Eusolex 6300 has caused several allergic reactions, cross-reacting invariably with Eusolex 8020.[166] No camphor derivatives have been approved for use in the United States.

Salicylates and Anthranilates

Salicylates and anthranilates are two classes of weak UVB absorbers and are therefore used either in high concentrations or in combination with other UVB sunscreens. However, both classes of compounds are safe and chemically stable.[167] Homomenthyl salicylate (homosalate), which is manufactured as a mixture of cis and trans isomers, has been implicated in fewer than five allergic reactions.[168] Benzyl salicylate has only historic significance as an allergen cross-reactive with balsam of Peru. It is no longer approved as a sunscreen but is used in soaps to solubilize perfumes and impart fragrance.[169]

Anthranilates are derivatives of ortho-aminobenzoic acid, with absorption extending into the UVA spectrum to 360 nm. While homomenthyl-N-acetyl anthranilate and methyl anthranilate are available in Europe, the FDA has approved only methyl anthranilate for over-the-counter use in the United States. As the molar extinction coefficient of anthranilates is much lower (≈6000) than for PABA, cinnamates, or benzophenones, they are not as effective. However, allergic reaction to anthranilates has not yet been reported.[167]

Miscellaneous Sunscreens

Several reports of allergic reactions implicate other chemical sunscreens, including bornelone,[170] digalloyl trioleate (Neo-A-Fil),[171] 2-phenyl-5-methyl benzoxazole (witisol),[172] and 2-phenyl-benzimidazole-5-sulfonic acid.[140] Of these, only 2-phenyl-benzimidazole-5-sulfonic acid has been approved by the FDA as Eusolex

232. It is available as a white, water-soluble powder and absorbs UVB.

Physical Sunblocks

Physical sunblocks, such as TiO_2 and ZnO, have increasingly been used alone or in combination with traditional chemical sunscreens.[28,31] By themselves, physical sunblocks offer both broad-spectrum coverage and unparalleled safety. These compounds are inert and have not been implicated in allergic sensitization. Thus, they are ideal for protecting children and sensitized patients. Unfortunately, they have been found to discolor clothing and can be occlusive, causing acne, folliculitis, and milia.[167]

DHA in combination with lawsone (see Table 248-2) has been used in sunless tanning lotions as an artificial tanning accelerator with physical sunblocking properties.[1,173] Three to four sequential applications impart an orange-brown color to the skin within 10 to 12 h. Its advantages include protection of the skin by a polymerized form of the artificial pigment different from natural melanin. This pigment conjugates with histidine in the stratum corneum and adheres to the skin without washing off. Irritancy or sensitization has not yet been reported.[1]

CHRONIC PHOTOSENSITIVITY

Patients with chronic photosensitivity dermatoses, such as polymorphic light eruption and chronic actinic dermatitis (see Chaps. 136 and 137), have a significantly increased risk of sunscreen allergy, for two reasons: (1) these patients require continual sun protection to mitigate their disease severity, and (2) the sunscreen ingredients more readily penetrate their already inflamed and injured skin, increasing the likelihood of sensitization. Moreover, with increased reactivity comes a greater likelihood of cross-reactivity between sunscreens.[140]

Chronic photosensitivity dermatoses represent an abnormal reaction to UV or even visible light. The action spectrum for polymorphic light eruption generally involves UVA radiation. Thus, the use of UVB screens is counterproductive, in that they provide a false sense of security, encouraging extended exposure to UVA by preventing sunburn. Chronic actinic dermatitis has been hypothesized to begin as a chronic photocontact dermatitis, but the reaction persists longer than 3 months beyond the last exposure to the implicated antigen.[174] Eventually, the photoallergen may alter endogenous proteins, which become "neoantigens" that chronically stimulate the immune system.[175] Thus, chronic photocontact dermatitis becomes persistent light reactivity when the patient develops an abnormal MED. The most extreme variant of chronic actinic dermatitis, actinic reticuloid, is diagnosed when the reactive lymphocytes become atypical.[174]

In a large Scandinavian photopatch study, 16 percent of 745 patients with polymorphic light eruption tested positive for contact or photocontact allergy, with an average of one positive reaction per patient. In contrast, 43 percent of 63 patients with chronic actinic dermatitis had documented allergies, with an average of almost five positive reactions per patient. Thus, chronic actinic dermatitis patients experienced more frequent, multiple sensitizations compared to patients with polymorphic light eruption, but contact allergies were more common than photocontact reactions for both groups.[140] In a smaller study testing specifically for sunscreen allergy, 22 percent of patients with chronic actinic dermatitis and 4 percent of polymorphic light eruption patients reacted. These chronic photosensitivity patients become sensitized to a broad range of sunscreens including PABA, padimate A and padimate O, cinnamates, benzophenones, and dibenzoylmethanes.[140,176–181]

DERMATITIS DUE TO EXCIPIENTS

In addition to their active ingredients, sun-protective agents contain a wide variety of excipients, including alcohols, oils, emulsifiers, preservatives, and fragrances, which serve as a secondary source of allergic reactions.[126] Although these excipients frequently cause contact sensitivity, they only rarely provoke photocontact allergy because they do not absorb UV radiation in most cases. Excipients have also been implicated in nonimmune-mediated irritant reactions. Cosmetic agents exacerbating "status cosmeticus" include benzoic acid, bronopol, cinnamic acid, emulsifiers, formaldehyde, lactic acid, propylene glycol, quaternium-15, sodium lauryl sulfate, sorbic acid, and urea.[130] Alcoholic solutions of PABA can produce severe nonimmune stinging and burning sensations, often with appreciable erythema and edema.[131] Moreover, coconut oil and cocoa butter in sunscreens exert a comedogenic effect exacerbated by ultraviolet light.[136]

Sunscreen allergy may also derive from such base ingredients as emollients and alcohols, including benzyl alcohol, tertiary butyl alcohol, triethanolamine stearate, phenyl dimethicone, avocado oil, dexpanthenol, neopentyl glycol diisooctanoate, PVP/eicosene copolymer, solvent red 1, and solvent red 3. The antioxidant butylhydroxyanisole has also been implicated. Because most manufacturers provide a complete list of sunscreen ingredients, including all excipients, patients should be encouraged to enlist the help of physicians to identify the cause of their allergic reactions. They should subsequently refrain from purchasing those brand-name formulations and specific chemicals implicated in previous episodes of sensitization.

SUNSCREENS AND MUTAGENESIS

Although sunscreens are widely promoted as a preventive measure against sunburn and skin cancer, a number of studies have discovered genotoxic effects for some sun-protective chemicals. Photochemical reactions may involve wavelengths not maximally absorbed by the sunscreen, and extended sunbathing with UVB screens may allow enough absorption of UVA to generate unexpected and harmful reactive species.[182]

UVA is most clearly implicated in the photogenotoxicity of 5-MOP (bergapten), a constituent of oil of bergamot in concentrations of approximately 10 to 50 ppm. Although clearly structurally related to the known carcinogen 8-MOP, 5-MOP was once commonly marketed in French and other European suntan lotions to promote tanning without erythema. 5-MOP enhances melanogenesis, and this upregulation of endogenous melanin pigmentation was thought to provide the best protection against UV-induced harmful effects, including mutagenesis.[183,184] However, 5-MOP has been shown to induce lethal photosensitization of both *Escherichia coli* and Chinese hamster ovary cells, as well as base-pair substitution in *E. coli* and interstrand DNA cross-links.[185] Yeast cells experienced photogenotoxicity when exposed to concentrations of 5-MOP (1 to 4 ng/mL) obtained from suction blisters in human volunteers using a preparation containing bergamot oil.[186] All albino mice repeatedly exposed to 5-MOP and UVA developed persistent skin thickening, dermal cyst formation, atypical squamous papillomas, and invasive SCCs.[187,188] In hairless mice, 5-MOP and only low-dose UVA induced ornithine-decarboxylase activity, a marker for cellular proliferation and tumor promotion in chemical carcinogenesis. Thus, molecular and chromosomal damage can occur at lower doses of UVA than the clinically evident erythema and hyperpigmentation, which require up to 20 J/cm^2 UVA with 5-MOP.[189] Although these experimental studies demonstrate the risk of photocarcinogenesis with 5-MOP to be much smaller than with 8-MOP,[184,188] the potential is still quite significant. Finally, four human patients using a 5-MOP-containing suntan preparation developed the acquired persistent atypical lentigines often seen with PUVA.[190]

While 5-MOP has since fallen into disrepute and is used decreasingly, other sunscreen chemicals have been shown to exert mutagenic effects. PABA interacts with light to generate singlet molecular oxygen and then lipid peroxides, which cause oxidative damage to cells. Oxybenzone rapidly photooxidizes to oxybenzone semiquinone, a potent electrophile that reacts with thiol groups on important antioxidant enzymes and substrates, such as thioredoxin reductase and reduced glutathione. The inactivation of these systems reduces protection against DNA damage.[162]

Padimate O preparations are contaminated with nitrosation derivatives of this sunscreen, which were mutagenic in *Salmonella typhimurium* (Ames test).[191] Yeast cells were also sensitive to lethal mutations induced by Padimate O and UV radiation, an effect more pronounced in rapidly growing or DNA repair–deficient cells. In fact, the very chemical structure of padimate O encourages excited states by the conjugation of an electron-donating dimethylamino group, through the aromatic ring, to an electron-withdrawing carbonyl group.[192]

Another study demonstrated Parsol MCX to be mutagenic in the Ames *S. typhimurium* test and in *Drosophila melanogaster*. However, these results varied according to individual batches of the sunscreen and thus were possibly caused by a contaminant formed in its synthesis. Moreover, 25 other sunscreen ingredients including PABA, padimate O, oxybenzone, dioxybenzone, sulisobenzone, avobenzone, and homosalate were found *not* to be mutagenic in these assays.[193] In another study, Parsol MCX and avobenzone protected *E. coli* and *S. typhimurium* both individually and synergistically from UV-induced genotoxicity.[194] The UVB screen 2-phenylbenzimidazole-5-sulfonic acid proved protective against mutations in Chinese hamster ovary cells.[195] Neither *D. melanogaster* nor the bone marrow of rats suffered mutagenic effects from oxybenzone.[196]

Animal studies showed mice exposed repeatedly to UV light to be protected from AKs and SCCs by glyceryl-PABA, cinnamates, and benzophenone.[197] Padimate O and oxybenzone, when applied to mice, manifested a similar protective effect, which increased with the SPF.[75] However, while Parsol MCX prevented UV-induced cancers in mice, the tumor-promotor croton oil produced cancers in the Parsol MCX–treated mice (including the treated mice that were not irradiated) but not in control mice. Thus, while the sunscreen protects against UV carcinogenesis, it may initiate other tumors sensitive to croton oil promotion.[198]

In a large, randomized, controlled trial in humans, Parsol MCX and avobenzone demonstrated significant suppression of AKs.[199] While several controversial case-control studies appear to imply a higher risk of BCC and melanoma with sunscreens,[86,103,200,201] case-control studies are by nature plagued by confounding factors. Such factors as inherent susceptibility to sunburn (requiring sunscreen use) and justification (by sunscreen use) of prolonged exposure may actually underlie these associations.[86,88,201] Overall, sunscreen photoprotection and defense against UV-induced tumorigenesis in vivo appear to outweigh the mtuagenic effects demonstrated in vitro.

REFERENCES

1. Pathak MA, Fitzpatrick TB: Preventive treatment of sunburn, dermatoheliosis, and skin cancer, in *Dermatology in General Medicine,* 4th ed, edited by TB Fitzpatrick et al. New York, McGraw-Hill, 1993, pp 1689–1717

2. Carbonare DM, Pathak MA: Skin photosensitizing agents and the role of reactive oxygen species in photoaging of skin. *J Photochem Photobiol B* **14**:105, 1992

3. Hruza G, Pentland AP: Mechanisms of UV-induced inflammation. *J Invest Dermatol* **100**(suppl):355, 1993

4. Pentland AP: Active oxygen mechanisms of UV inflammation. *Adv Exp Med Biol* **266**:87, 1994

5. Darr D et al: Topical vitamin C protects swine skin from ultraviolet radiation–induced damage. *Br J Dermatol* **127**:247, 1992

6. Black H, Rajan B: Antioxidants and carotenoids as potential photoprotectants, in *Sunscreens: Development, Evaluation, and Regulatory Aspects,* 2d ed, edited by NJ Lowe et al. New York, Marcel Dekker, 1997, pp 139–153

7. Darr D et al: Effectiveness of antioxidants (vitamin C and E) with and without sunscreens as topical photoprotectants. *Acta Derm Venereol (Stockh)* **76**:264, 1996

8. Gonzalez S, Pathak MA: Inhibition of ultraviolet-induced formation of reactive oxygen species, lipid peroxidation, erythema, and skin photosensitization by *Polypodium leucotomos. Photodermatol Photoimmunol Photomed* **12**:45, 1996

9. Gonzalez S et al: Topical or oral administration with an extract of *Polypodium leucotomos* prevents acute sunburn and psoralen-induced phototoxic reactions as well as depletion of Langerhan cells in human skin. *Photodermatol Photoimmunol Photomed* **13**:50, 1997

10. Snyder DS: Effects of topical indomethacin on UVR-induced redness and prostaglandin E levels in guinea pig skin. *Prostaglandin* **11**:631, 1976

11. Black AK et al: Arachidonic acid and prostaglandin E2, F2a, levels in human skin 24 hrs. after UVB and UVC irradiation. *Br J Pharmacol* **6**:261, 1989

12. Food and Drug Administration: *Sunscreen Drug Products for Over-the-Counter Drugs: Proposed Safety, Effective and Labeling Conditions.* Federal Register, Part II, vol 43, Aug. 25, 1978, pp 38206–38269

13. Food and Drug Administration: *Sunscreen Drug Products for Over-the-Counter Human Use.* Tentative final monograph, Proposed Rule, Federal Register, Part III, vol 58, No 90, May 12, 1993, pp 28194–28302

14. Shaath NA: Evolution of modern sunscreen chemicals, in *Sunscreens, Development, Evaluation and Regulatory Aspects,* 2d ed, edited by NJ Lowe et al. New York, Marcel Dekker, 1997, pp 3–34

15. Pathak MA: Sunscreens: Topical and systemic approaches for protection of human skin against harmful effects of solar radiation. *J Am Acad Dermatol* **1**:285, 1982

16. Klein K: Sunscreen products: Formulation and regulatory considerations, in *Sunscreens: Development, Evaluation and Regulatory Aspects,* 2d ed, edited by NJ Lowe et al. New York, Marcel Dekker, 1997, pp 285–311

17. Lowe NJ, Friedlander J: Sunscreens: Rationale for use to reduce photodamage and phototoxicity, in *Sunscreens: Development, Evaluation and Regulatory Aspects,* 2d ed, edited by NJ Lowe et al. New York, Marcel Dekker, 1997, pp 35–58

18. Pathak MA, Carbonare MD: Melanogenic potential of various furocoumarins in normal and vitiliginous skin, in *Psoralens: Past, Present, and Future of Photochemoprotection and Other Biological Activities,* edited by TB Fitzpatrick et al. Paris, John Libbey Eurotext, 1989, pp 87–101

19. Lowe NJ et al (eds): *Sunscreens: Development, Evaluation and Regulatory Aspects,* 2d ed. New York, Marcel Dekker, 1997

20. Gange W et al: Efficacy of a sunscreen containing butyl methoxylbenzoyl methane against ultraviolet A radiation in photosensitized subjects. *J Am Acad Dermatol* 15:494, 1986

21. Lowe NJ et al: Indoor and outdoor efficacy testing of a broad-spectrum sunscreen against ultraviolet A radiation in psoralen-sensitized subjects. *J Am Acad Dermatol* 17:224, 1987

22. Menter JM: Recent developments in UVA photoprotection. *Int J Dermatol* 29:389, 1990

23. Schauder S, Ippen H: Photoallergic and allergic contact dermatitis from dibenzoylmethanes. *Photodermatology* 3:140, 1986

24. Schauder S, Ippen H: Photoallergic and photoallergic contact dermatitis from dibenzoyl methane compounds and other sunscreens. *Hautarzt* 39:435, 1988

25. Federal Register: Rules and Regulations Notice 21CFR Part 352, vol 62, No 83, April 30, 1997

26. Pathak A: Unpublished, personal observations, 1996

27. Schauder A: UV absorbers: Allergy and photoallergy. A 14-year experience, in Book of Abstracts. International Congress on Photobiology, Vienna, Austria, September 1996, p 216 #078

28. Fairhurst D, Miltchnick MA: Particulate sunblocks: General principles, in *Sunscreens: Development, Evaluation and Regulatory Aspects,* 2d ed, edited by NJ Lowe et al. New York, Marcel Dekker, 1997, pp 313–352

29. Pathak MA: Sunscreens: Progress and perspectives on photoprotection of human skin against UVB and UVA radiation. *J Dermatol* 23:783, 1996

30. Anders MW et al: Broad-spectrum physical sunscreens: Titanium dioxide and zinc oxide, in *Sunscreens: Development, Evaluation and Regulatory Aspects,* 2d ed, edited by NJ Lowe et al. New York, Marcel Dekker, 1997, pp 353–398

31. Sayre RM et al: Physical sunscreens. *J Soc Cosmet Chem* 41:103, 1997

32. Ahene AB et al: Photoprotection of solubilized and micro-dispersed melanin particles, in *Melanin, Its Role in Human Photoprotection,* edited by L Zeise et al. Overland Park, KS, Valdenmar, 1994, pp 255–269

33. Kollias N et al: Photoprotection by melanin. *J Photochem Photobiol B* 9:135, 1990

34. Pathak MA: Function of melanin and protection by melanin, in *Melanin, Its Role in Human Photoprotection,* edited by L Zeise et al. Overland Park, KS, Valdenmar, 1994, pp 125–134

35. Berne B, Fisher T: Protective effects of various types of clothing against UV radiation. *Arch Dermatol* 60:459, 1980

36. Keeling JH et al: Hats: Design and protection from ultraviolet radiation. *Mil Med* 154:250, 1989

37. Welsh C, Diffey B: The protection against solar actinic radiation afforded by common clothing fabrics. *Clin Exp Dermatol* 6:577, 1981

38. Robson J, Diffey B: Textiles and sun protection. *Photodermatol Photoimmunol Photomed* 7:32, 1990

39. Sliney DH et al: Transmission of potentially hazardous actinic ultraviolet radiation through fabrics. *Appl Ind Hyg* 2:36, 1987

40. Sayre RM, Hughes S: Sun protective apparel: Advancements in sun protection. *Skin Cancer* 8:41, 1993

41. Lowe NJ et al: Ultraviolet protection offered by clothing fabrics, in *Sunscreens: Development, Evaluation and Regulatory Aspects,* 2d ed, edited by NJ Lowe et al. New York, Marcel Dekker, 1997, pp 619–629

42. Naeyaert JM et al: Pigment content of cultured human melanocytes does not correlate with tyrosinase message level. *Br J Dermatol* 125:297, 1991

43. Hearing VJ et al: The characteristics of biological melanins are influenced by multiple points in the melanogenic pathway, in *Melanin: Its Role in Human Photoprotection,* edited by L Zeise et al. Overland Park, KS, Valdenmar, 1995

44. Wilmott J et al: Tanning accelerators, in *Sunscreens: Development, Evaluation and Regulatory Aspects,* 2d ed, edited by NJ Lowe et al. New York, Marcel Dekker, 1997, pp 473–495

45. Fusaro RM, Johnson JA: Protection against long ultraviolet and/or visible light with topical dihydroxy acetone. *Dermatologica* 150:346, 1975

46. Fusaro RM et al: Protection against light sensitivity with dihydroxy acetone/naphthoquinone. *Int J Dermatol* 11:67, 1972

47. Fusaro RM et al: Sunlight protection in normal skin. *Arch Dermatol* 93:106, 1966

48. Hodge JE: Chemistry of browing reactions in model systems. *J Agric Food Chem* 1:928, 1953

49. Labuza TB et al: The physical aspects with respect to water and non-enzymatic browning. *Adv Exp Med Biol* 86B:379, 1977

50. Sayre RM et al: Skin optics of melanoid stains versus natural melanin, in *Melanin: Its Role in Human Photoprotection,* edited by L Zeise et al. Overland Park, Valdenmar, 1994, pp 39–47

51. Pathak MA, Fitzpatrick TB: Unpublished observations

52. Fusaro RM, Johnson JA: Dihydroxyacetone naphthoquinone sunscreen. *JAMA* 222:1651, 1972

53. Fusaro RM, Runge WJ: Erythropoietic protoporphyria IV: Protection from sunlight. *Br Med J* 1:730, 1970

54. Mosher DB et al: Vitiligo: Etiology, pathogenesis, diagnosis and treatment, in *Update: Dermatology in General Medicine,* edited by TB Fitzpatrick et al. New York, McGraw-Hill, 1983, pp 205–225

55. Pathak MA et al: Sunlight and melanin pigmentation, in *Photochemical Photobiologic Reviews,* edited by KC Smith. New York, Plenum, 1976, pp 211–240

56. Gilchrest BA et al: Mechanisms of ultraviolet light-induced pigmentation. *Photochem Photobiol* 63:1, 1996

57. Allan AE et al: Topically applied diacylglycerols increase pigmentation in guinea pig skin. *J Invest Dermatol* 105:687, 1995

58. Gilchrest BA et al: Treatment of human melanocytes and S91 melanoma cells with the DNA repair enzyme T4 endonuclease V enhances melanogenesis after ultraviolet irradiation. *J Invest Dermatol* 101:666, 1993

59. Agin PA: World Patent 9,107,167 (1993) and 9,107,168 (1993)

60. Eller MS et al: DNA damage and melanogenesis. *Nature* 372:413, 1994

61. Darr D et al: Topical vitamin C protects porcine skin from ultraviolet radiation-induced damage. *Br J Dermatol* 127:247, 1992

62. Darr D et al: Effectiveness of antioxidants (Vitamin C and E) with and without sunscreens as topical photoprotectants. *Acta Derm Venereol (Stockh)* 76:264, 1996

63. Agarwal R, Mukhtar H: Chemoprevention of photocarcinogenesis. *Photochem Photobiol* 63:440, 1996

64. Strickland FM et al: Prevention of ultraviolet radiation–induced suppression of contact and delayed hypersensitivity by *Aloe barbadensis* gel extract. *J Invest Dermatol* 102:197, 1994

65. Ibbotson SH et al: The effect of topical indomethacin on ultraviolet radiation–induced erythema. *Br J Dermatol* 135:523, 1996

66. Black AK et al: The effect of indomethacin on arachidonic acid and prostaglandins E2 and F2 levels in human skin 24 hr after UVB and UVC irradiation. *Br J Clin Pharmacol* 6:261, 1987

67. Mathews-Roth MM et al: Beta-carotene as an oral photoprotective agent in erythropoietic protoporphyria. *N Engl J Med* 282:1231, 1970

68. Mathews-Roth MM et al: Beta-carotene as an oral photoprotective agent in erythropoietic protoporphyria. *JAMA* 228:1004, 1974

69. Mathews-Roth MM et al: Beta-carotene therapy for erythropoietic protoporphyria and other photosensitivity diseases, in *The Science of Photomedicine,* edited by JD Regan, JA Parrish. New York, Plenum, 1983, p 409

70. Mathews-Roth MM et al: Beta-carotene therapy for erythropoietic protoporphyria and other photosensitivity diseases. *Arch Dermatol* 113:1229, 1977

71. Mathews-Roth MM et al: A clinical trial of the effects of oral beta-carotene on the response of human skin to solar radiation. *J Invest Dermatol* 59:349, 1972

72. Pathak MA: Sunscreens: Topical and systemic protection against solar radiation for human skin, in *Photochemistry and Photophysics, Supplement,* edited by A Favre et al. Amsterdam, Elsevier, 1987, p 447

73. Krook G, Haeger-Aronson B: Erythropoietic protoporphyria and its treatment with beta-carotene. *Acta Derm Venereol (Stockh)* 54:39, 1974

74. Carraro E, Pathak MA: Studies on the nature of in vitro and in vivo photosensitization reaction by psoralens and porphyrins. *J Invest Dermatol* 90:267, 1988

75. Kligman LH et al: Sunscreens prevent ultraviolet photocarcinogenesis. *J Am Acad Dermatol* 3:30, 1980

76. Hunter DJ et al: Risk factors for basal cell carcinoma in a prospective cohort of women. *Ann Epidemiol* 1:13, 1990

77. Thompson SC et al: Reduction of solar keratoses by regular sunscreen use. *N Engl J Med* 329:1147, 1993

78. Naylor MF et al: High sunprotection factor sunscreens in the suppression of actinic neoplasia. *Arch Dermatol* 131:170, 1995

79. Gallagher RP et al: Sunlight exposure, pigmentary factors, and risk of nonmelanocytic skin cancer. I: Basal cell carcinoma. *Arch Dermatol* **131**:157, 1995

80. Kondoh M et al: Siblings with xeroderma pigmentosum complementation group A with different skin cancer development: Importance of sun protection at an early age. *J Am Acad Dermatol* **31**:993, 1994

81. de Gruijl FR et al: Wavelength dependence of skin cancer induction by ultraviolet irradiation of albino hairless mice. *Cancer Res* **53**:53, 1993

82. Ananthaswamy H et al: Sunlight and skin cancer: Inhibition of p53 mutations in UV-irradiated mouse skin by sunscreens. *Nature Med* **3**:510, 1997

83. Gallagher RP et al: Sunlight exposure, pigmentation factors and risk of nonmelanocytic skin cancer. II: Squamous cell carcinoma. *Arch Dermatol* **131**:164, 1995

84. Elwood JM et al: Cutaneous melanoma in relation to intermittent and constant sun exposure—the Western Canada Melanoma Study. *Int J Cancer* **35**:427, 1985

85. Osterind A et al: The Danish case-control study of cutaneous malignant melanoma. II. Importance of UV-light exposure. *Int J Cancer* **42**:319, 1988

86. Autier P et al: Melanoma and use of sunscreens: An EORTC case-control study in Germany, Belgium and France. *Int J Cancer* **61**:749, 1995

87. Westerndahll J et al: Is the use of sunscreens a risk factor for malignant melanoma? *Melanoma Res* **5**:59, 1995

88. Roberts LK, Stanfield JW: Suggestion that sunscreen use is a melanoma risk factor is based on inconclusive evidence. *Melanoma Res* **5**:377, 1995

89. Frampton RJ et al: Inhibition of human cancer cell growth by 1,25-dihydroxyvitamin D$_3$ metabolites. *Cancer Res* **43**:4443, 1983

90. Marks R et al: The effect of regular sunscreen use on vitamin D levels in an Australian population. Results of a randomized controlled trial. *Arch Dermatol* **131**:415, 1995

91. Weinstock MA et al: Case-control study of melanoma and dietary vitamin D: Implications for advocacy of sun protection and sunscreen use. *J Invest Dermatol* **98**:809, 1992

92. Dobak J, F-T Liu: Sunscreens, UVA, and cutaneous malignancy adding fuel to the fire. *Int J Dermatol* **31**:544, 1992

93. Robert C et al: Cell survival and shuttle vector mutagenesis induced by ultraviolet A and ultraviolet B radiation in a human cell line. *J Invest Dermatol* **106**:721, 1996

94. Drobetsky EA et al: A role for ultraviolet A in solar mutagenesis. *Proc Natl Acad Sci USA* **92**:2350, 1995

95. Chew S et al: Longwave ultraviolet radiation (UVA)-induced alteration of epidermal DNA synthesis. *Photochem Photobiol* **47**:383, 1988

96. Boer J et al: Interaction of far- and near-ultraviolet radiation. The occurrence of photo-augmentation and photo-recovery in cultured mammalian cells. *Mutat Res* **125**:283, 1984

97. Freeman SE et al: Production of pyrimidine dimers in DNA of human skin exposed in situ to UVA radiation. *J Invest Dermatol* **88**:430, 1987

98. Roza L et al: The induction and repair of DNA damage and its influence on cell death in primary human fibroblasts exposed to UV-A or UV-C irradiation. *Mutat Res* **146**:89, 1985

99. Lundgren K, Wulf HC: Cytotoxicity and genotoxicity of UVA irradiation in Chinese hamster ovary cells measured by specific locus mutations, sister chromatic exchanges and chromosome aberrations. *Photochem Photobiol* **47**:559, 1988

100. Setlow RB et al: Wavelengths effective in induction of malignant melanoma. *Proc Natl Acad Sci USA* **90**:6666, 1993

101. Autier P et al: Cutaneous malignant melanoma and exposure to sunlamps or sunbeds: An EORTC multicenter case-control study in Belgium, France and Germany. *Int J Cancer* **58**:809, 1994

102. Westerdahl J et al: Use of sunbeds or sunlamps and malignant melanoma in southern Sweden. *Am J Epidemiol* **140**:691, 1994

103. Westerdahl J et al: Is the use of sunscreens a risk factor for malignant melanoma? *Melanoma Res* **5**:59, 1995

104. Walter SD et al: The association of cutaneous malignant melanoma with the use of sunbeds and sunlamps. *Am J Epidemiol* **131**:232, 1990

105. Stern RS et al: Malignant melanoma in patients treated for psoriasis with methoxsalen (psoralen) and ultraviolet A radiation (PUVA). The PUVA follow-up study. *N Engl J Med* **336**:1041, 1997

106. Wolf P et al: Effect of sunscreens on UV radiation–induced enhancement of melanoma growth in mice. *J Natl Cancer Inst* **86**:99, 1994

107. Unna P: *Histopathologie der Hautkrankeiten.* Berlin, Herschwald, 1894

108. Dubreuilh W: Des hyperkeratoses circonscrites. *Ann Dermatol Syphiligr* (set 3) **7**:1158, 1896

109. Gilchrest BA: *Skin and Aging Process.* Boca Raton, FL, CRC Press, 1984

110. Kligman LH, Kligman AM: Ultraviolet radiation–induced skin aging, in *Sunscreens, Development, Evaluation and Regulatory Aspects,* 2d ed, edited by NJ Lowe et al. New York, Marcel Dekker, 1997, pp 117–138

111. Kligman LH, Kligman AM: Photoaging, in *Dermatology in General Medicine,* 4th ed, edited by TB Fitzpatrick et al. New York, McGraw-Hill, 1993, pp 2972–2979

112. Kligman LH: The hairless mouse and photoaging. *Photochem Photobiol* **54**:1109, 1991

113. Bissett DL et al: An animal model of solar aged skin: Histological physical, and visible changes in UV-irradiated mouse skin. *Photochem Photobiol* **46**:367, 1987

114. Werb Z et al: Degradation of connective tissue matrices by macrophages, Proteolysis of elastin, glycoproteins, and collagen by proteinases isolated from macrophages. *J Exp Med* **152**:1340, 1980

115. Gilchrest BA, Rogre GS: Photoaging, in *Clinical Photomedicine,* edited by HW Lim, NA Soter. New York, Marcel Dekker, 1993, pp 95–110

116. Gilchrest BA (ed): *Photodamage.* Cambridge, MA, Blackwell Scientific, 1995

117. Peak MJ, Peak JG: Molecular photobiology of UVA, in *The Biological Effects of UVA Radiation,* edited by F Urbach, RW Gange. New York, Praeger, 1986, pp 42–52

118. Kligman LH et al: Sunscreens promote repair of ultraviolet radiation–induced dermal damage. *J Invest Dermatol* **81**:98, 1983

119. Kligman AM: Perspectives and problems of cutaneous gerontology. *J Invest Dermatol* **73**:39, 1979

120. Stiller MJ et al: Topical 8% glycolic acid and 8% lactic acid creams for the treatment of photodamaged skin. *Arch Dermatol* **132**:631, 1996

121. Kligman AM et al: Topical tretinoin for photodamaged skin. *J Am Acad Dermatol* **15**:836, 1986

122. Rafal ES et al: Topical tretinoin (retinoic acid) treatment for liver spots associated with photodamage. *N Engl J Med* **326**:368, 1993

123. Griffiths CEM et al: Restoration of collagen formation in photodamaged human skin by tretinoin (retinoic acid). *N Engl J Med* **329**:530, 1993

124. Weinstein GD et al: Topical tretinoin for treatment of photodamaged skin: A multicenter study. *Arch Dermatol* **127**:659, 1991

125. Jones PR: Protecting the consumer from getting burned: The FDA, the administrative process, and the tentative final monograph on over-the-counter sunscreens. *Am J Law Med* **20**:317, 1994

126. Funk JO et al: Contact sensitization and photocontact sensitization of sunscreening agents, in *Sunscreens: Development, Evaluation and Regulatory Aspects,* 2d ed, edited by NJ Lowe et al. New York, Marcel Dekker, 1997, pp 631–653

127. DeGroot AC et al: The allergens in cosmetics. *Arch Dermatol* **124**:1525, 1988

128. Foley P et al: The frequency of reactions to sunscreens: Results of a longitudinal population-based study on the regular use of sunscreens in Australia. *Br J Dermatol* **128**:512, 1993

129. Fischer T, Bergström K: Evaluation of customers' complaints about sunscreen cosmetics sold by the Swedish pharmaceutical company. *Contact Dermatitis* **25**:319, 1991

130. Fisher AA: Part I: "Status cosmeticus": A cosmetic intolerance syndrome. *Cutis* **46**:109, 1990

131. Fisher AA: Sunscreen dermatitis: Para-aminobenzoic acid and its derivatives. *Cutis* **50**:190, 1992

132. Kato S et al: Mechanism for 6-methylcoumarin photoallergenicity. *Toxicol Appl Pharmacol* **18**:295, 1985

133. Raugi CJ et al: Photoallergic contact dermatitis to men's perfumes. *Contact Dermatitis* **5**:251, 1979

134. Kaminester LH: Allergic reaction to sunscreen products. *Arch Dermatol* **117**:66, 1981

135. Mathias CG et al: Allergic contact photodermatitis to para-aminobenzoic acid. *Arch Dermatol* **114**:1665, 1978

136. Mills OH, Kligman AM: Comedogenicity of sunscreens. *Arch Dermatol* **118**:417, 1982

137. Adams RM, Maibach HI: A five-year study of cosmetic reactions. *J Am Acad Dermatol* **13**:1062, 1985

138. Gonçalo M et al: Contact and photocontact sensitivity to sunscreens. *Contact Dermatitis* **33**:278, 1995

139. Nater JP, DeGroot AC: *Unwanted Effects of Cosmetics and Drugs Used in Dermatology,* 2d ed. Amsterdam, Elsevier, 1985, p 360

140. Thune P et al: The Scandinavian multicentre photopatch study 1980–1985: Final report. *Photodermatology* **5**:261, 1988

141. Menz J et al: Photopatch testing: A six-year experience. *J Am Acad Dermatol* **18**:1044, 1988

142. DeLeo VA et al: Photoallergic contact dermatitis. *Arch Dermatol* **128**:1513, 1992

143. Trevisi P et al: Sunscreen sensitization: A three-year study. *Dermatology* **189**:55, 1994

144. Thune P: Contact and photocontact allergy to sunscreens. *Photodermatology* **1**:5, 1984

145. Szczurko C: Photocontact allergy to oxybenzone: Ten years of experience. *Photodermatol Photoimmunol Photomed* **10**:144, 1994

146. Fisher AA: Sunscreen dermatitis due to glyceryl PABA: Significance of cross-reactions to this PABA ester. *Cutis* **18**:495, 1976

147. Baer RL, Meltzer L: Sensitization to monoglyceryl para-aminobenzoate: Preliminary report. *J Invest Dermatol* **11**:5, 1948

148. Curtis GH, Crawford PF: Cutaneous sensitivity to monoglyceryl para-aminobenzoate. *Cleve Clin Q* **18**:35, 1951

149. Fisher AA: Dermatitis due to benzocaine present in sunscreens containing glyceryl PABA (Escalol 106). *Contact Dermatitis* **3**:170, 1977

150. Fisher AA: The presence of benzocaine in sunscreens containing glyceryl PABA (Escalol 106). *Arch Dermatol* **113**:1299, 1977

151. Hjorth N et al: Glyceryl *p*-aminobenzoate patch testing in benzocaine-sensitive subjects. *Contact Dermatitis* **4**:46, 1978

152. Bruze M et al: Contact and photocontact allergy to glyceryl para-aminobenzoate. *Photodermatology* **5**:162, 1988

153. Bruze M et al: Occurrence of para-aminobenzoic acid and benzocaine as contaminants in sunscreen agents of para-aminobenzoic acid type. *Photodermatology* **1**:277, 1984

154. Fotiades J et al: Results of evaluation of 203 patients for photosensitivity in a 7.3-year period. *J Am Acad Dermatol* **33**:597, 1995

155. Fisher AA: Sunscreen dermatitis: Part II—the cinnamates. *Cutis* **50**:253, 1992

156. Parrish JA et al: Topical protection against germicidal radiation by benzophenones. *Arch Surg* **104**:276, 1972

157. Shaath NA: Evolution of modern sunscreen chemicals, in *Sunscreens: Development, Evolution and Regulatory Aspects,* 2d ed, edited by NJ Lowe et al. New York, Marcel Dekker, 1997, pp 3–34

158. Ramsay DL et al: Allergic reaction to benzophenone. *Arch Dermatol* **105**:906, 1972

159. Collins P, Ferguson J: Photoallergic contact dermatitis to oxybenzone. *Br J Dermatol* **131**:124, 1994

160. Torres V, Correia T: Contact and photocontact allergy to oxybenzone and mexenone. *Contact Dermatitis* **25**:126, 1991

161. Fisher AA: Sunscreen dermatitis: Part III—the benzophenones. *Cutis* **50**:331, 1992

162. Schallreuter KU et al: Oxybenzone oxidation following solar irradiation of skin: Photoprotection versus antioxidant inactivation. *J Invest Dermatol* **106**:583, 1996

163. Okereke CS et al: Safety evaluation of benzophenone-3 after dermal administration in rats. *Toxicol Lett* **80**:61, 1995

164. Schauder S: UV absorber allergy and photoallergy: A 14-year experience, in *The 12ᵗʰ International Congress on Photobiology,* Book of Abstracts, Vienna, 1996, p 216

165. Motley RJ, Reynolds AJ: Photocontact dermatitis due to isopropyl and butyl methoxy dibenzoylmethanes (Eusolex 8020 and Parsol 1789). *Contact Dermatitis* **21**:109, 1989

166. Marguery MC et al: Photocontact allergy to 3-(4′methylbenzylidene) camphor and contact and photocontact allergy to 4-isopropyl dibenzoylmethane. *Photodermatol Photoimmunol Photomed* **11**:209, 1996

167. Fisher AA: Sunscreen dermatitis: Part IV—the salicylates, the anthranilates, and physical agents. *Cutis* **50**:397, 1992

168. Rietschel MRL et al: Contact allergy to homomenthyl salicylate. *Arch Dermatol* **114**:442, 1978

169. Kahn G: Intensified contact sensitization to benzyl salicylate. *Arch Dermatol* **103**:497, 1971

170. DeGroot AC, Weyland JW: Cosmetic allergy to the UV-absorber bornelone. *Dermatosen Beruf Umwelt* **37**:13, 1989

171. Sams WM: Contact photodermatitis. *Arch Dermatol* **73**:142, 1956

172. Mørk NJ, Austad J: Contact dermatitis from witisol, a sunscreen agent. *Contact Dermatitis* **10**:122, 1984

173. Follett KA et al: Protection of photosensitized rats against long ultraviolet radiation by topical application of compounds with structures similar to that of dihydroxyacetone. *Dermatologica* **175**:58, 1987

174. Lim HW et al: Chronic actinic dermatitis. *Arch Dermatol* **126**:317, 1990

175. Kochevar IE, Harber LC: Photoreactions of 3,3′,4′,5-tetra-chlorosalicylanilide with proteins. *J Invest Dermatol* **68**:151, 1977

176. Green C et al: Chronic actinic dermatitis and sunscreen allergy. *Clin Exp Dermatol* **16**:70, 1991

177. Murphy GM, White IR: Photoallergic contact dermatitis to 2-ethoxyethyl-*p*-methoxycinnamate. *Contact Dermatitis* **16**:296, 1987

178. Millard LG, Barrett PL: Contact allergy from mexenone masquerading as an exacerbation of light sensitivity. *Contact Dermatitis* **6**:222, 1980

179. Murphy GM et al: Immediate and delayed photocontact dermatitis from isopropyl dibenzoylmethane. *Contact Dermatitis* **22**:129, 1990

180. Thune P, Eeg-Larsen T: Contact and photocontact allergy in persistent light reactivity. *Contact Dermatitis* **11**:98, 1984

181. Green C et al: Photoallergic contact dermatitis from oxybenzone aggravating polymorphic light eruption. *Contact Dermatitis* **24**:62, 1991

182. Gasparro FP: The molecular basis of UV-induced mutagenicity of sunscreens. *FEBS Lett* **336**:184, 1993

183. Forlot P: Possible cancer hazard associated with 5-methoxypsoralen in suntan preparation. *Br Med J* **280**:648, 1980

184. Young AR: 5-Methoxypsoralen-containing sunscreens, in *Sunscreens: Development, Evolution and Regulatory Aspects,* 2d ed, edited by NJ Lowe et al. New York, Marcel Dekker, 1997, pp 461–472

185. Ashwood-Smith MJ et al: 5-Methoxypsoralen, an ingredient in several suntan preparations has lethal, mutagenic, and clastogenic properties. *Nature* **283**:407, 1980

186. Moysan A et al: Evaluation of phototoxic and photogenotoxic risk associated with the use of photosensitizers in suntan preparations: Application to tanning preparations containing bergamot oil. *Skin Pharmacol* **6**:282, 1993

187. Cartwright LE, Walter JF: Psoralen-containing sunscreen is tumorigenic in hairless mice. *J Am Acad Dermatol* **8**:830, 1983

188. Young AR et al: A comparison of the phototumorigenic potential of 8-MOP and 5-MOP in hairless albino mice exposed to solar simulated radiation. *Br J Dermatol* **108**:507, 1983

189. Walter JF et al: Psoralen-containing sunscreen induces phototoxicity and epidermal ornithine decarboxylase activity. *J Am Acad Dermatol* **6**:1022, 1982

190. Piérard GE et al: Acquired persistent atypical lentigines as a failure of 5-methoxypsoralen-containing sunscreens in the photochemoprotection from ultraviolet-radiation-induced damage. *Dermatology* **190**:338, 1995

191. Loeppky RN et al: Nitrosation of tertiary aromatic amines related to sunscreen ingredients. *IARC Sci Publ* **105**:244, 1991

192. Knowland J et al: Sunlight-induced mutagenicity of a common sunscreen ingredient. *FEBS Lett* **324**:309, 1993

193. Bonin AM et al: UV-absorbing and other sun-protecting substances: Genotoxicity of 2-ethylhexyl-*p*-methoxycinnamate. *Mutation Res* **105**:303, 1982

194. Chételat A et al: Photomutagenesis test development: I. 8-Methoxypsoralen, chlorpromaxine and sunscreen compounds in bacterial and yeast assays. *Mutat Res* **292**:241, 1993

195. Chételat A et al: Photomutagenesis test development: II. 8-Methoxypsoralen, chlorpromazine and sunscreen compounds in chromosomal aberration assays using CHO cells. *Mutat Res* **292**:251, 1993

196. Robinson SH et al: Assessment of the in vivo genotoxicity of 2-hydroxy-4-methoxybenzophenone. *Environ Mol Mutagen* **23**:312, 1994

197. Wulf HC et al: Sunscreens for delay of ultraviolet induction of skin tumors. *J Am Acad Dermatol* **7**:194, 1982

198. Gallagher CH et al: Ultraviolet carcinogenesis in the hairless mouse skin: Influence of the sunscreen 2-ethylhexyl-*p*-methoxycinnamate. *Aust J Exp Biol Med Sci* **62**:577, 1984

199. Thompson SC et al: Reduction of solar keratoses by regular sunscreen use. *N Engl J Med* **329**:1147, 1993

200. Graham S et al: An inquiry into the epidemiology of melanoma. *Am J Epidemiol* **122**:606, 1985

201. Hunter DJ et al: Risk factors for basal cell carcinoma in a prospective cohort of women. *Ann Epidemiol* **1**:13, 1990

CHAPTER 249

Howard P. Baden
Lynn A. Baden

Keratolytic Agents

The term *keratolysis* describes the shedding of stratum corneum cells from the surface of the skin. This is a continuous process on all body surfaces, but the rate of loss varies depending on location.[1] It is puzzling why the nail surface, which is also cornified, does not shed cells, since at the histologic level it is similar in appearance to stratum corneum and there are no unique intercellular structures.[2] The hair shaft also does not shed from its surface, since it is surrounded by interlocking cuticle cells; these are highly cross-linked, accounting for the maintenance of hair shaft integrity.[3]

The adhesion of viable epidermal cells is primarily a result of the interaction of desmosomes[4] and cadherins,[5] calcium-dependent glycoproteins, on the surfaces of adjacent cells. The intercellular structures of cells change in the stratum corneum, with modification of desmosome morphology and secretion of lamellar bodies rich in nonpolar lipids, giving rise to an orderly layered structure.[6] There is evidence that the lipids are cross-linked to the cornified envelopes by ester bonds.[7] A number of hydrolytic enzymes are also present in the secreted lamellar bodies, and these are thought to play a role in natural keratolysis.[8] The desmosomes undergo a progressive series of morphologic changes in the upper layers of the stratum corneum, leading to their apparent disappearance. In diseases associated with hyperkeratosis, the progressive alteration in desmosome morphology is markedly lessened, pointing to their role in cell adhesion.[9,10]

The mechanism by which the intercellular lipid, covalently linked to the cornified envelope of one cell, is bound to lipids attached to adjacent cells has not been clarified. Extraction of stratum corneum in vitro with organic solvents followed by aqueous solutions, even when they contain a surface-active agent or detergent, does not disperse the tissue into a single cell suspension. This extraction removes considerable intercellular lipid, but it is hypothesized that the residual lipid covalently linked to the envelope alters the configuration of the surface, so that dispersion by aqueous solvents is not possible. However, prolonged treatment of trypsin-treated stratum corneum with an aqueous solution of sodium lauryl sulfate does result in such dispersion. The use of a proteolytic enzyme may alter structural proteins attached to lipids or activate other hydrolytic processes in the intercellular spaces.

In summary, it appears that cell separation in the stratum corneum normally results, at least in part, from degradation of desmosomes as well as alteration of the products of the lamellar bodies. In pathologic states, the desmosomes are retained longer, presumably as a result of the failure of secretion of adequate amounts of hydrolytic enzymes into the intercellular space. The lamellar bodies may also be deficient in their total content of lipid or its composition (e.g., X-linked ichthyosis[11]). It is curious that both topical and systemic keratolytic agents can be extremely effective despite potentially diverse pathophysiologic mechanisms.

GENERAL PRINCIPLES OF KERATOLYSIS

Accumulation of excessive stratum corneum is a common problem; it may be a result of a primary disorder of keratinization such as ichthyosis vulgaris or be a secondary change in the epidermis, as in cutaneous fungal infection. The clinical presentation is a scaly white skin surface often resulting in shedding of stratum corneum when the skin is rubbed. The color is white because of light scattering from air trapped in the scale; the normal skin color can be restored by moistening the skin or rubbing on a lubricant that displaces the air.

Removal of the excess stratum corneum necessitates loosening the cohesive attachment of the cornified cells by topical treatment followed by mechanical debridement. When thickening of the stratum corneum is minimal, this may be accomplished by applying a cream or ointment that moisturizes the skin by the addition of water and/or produces an occlusive film that prevents loss of water, which has diffused outward from below. Numerous products sold as moisturizers or emollients can accomplish this. The increased water content allows the normal mechanism of cell separation described above to occur, and gentle rubbing of the skin during bathing mechanically removes the cornified tissue. Such a treatment is particularly effective for the xerosis that occurs during the winter months in cold regions of the country. Water-binding materials added to moisturizing creams are said to diffuse into the stratum corneum and help bind water. Two common compounds used for this purpose are urea[12] and lactic acid.[13] The latter is much more widely used and is an example of an α-hydroxy acid, discussed below.[14] These are generally well tolerated except in young children where α-hydroxy acids often cause a burning sensation. Although the mechanism for the irritation has not been definitely established, it is likely due to a less impervious stratum corneum barrier. Glycerin has also been used to increase water binding and has been shown to result in enhanced desmosomal degradation.[15]

KERATOLYTIC AGENTS

The oldest keratolytic agent used in dermatology is salicylic acid, which is usually prepared in an ointment or cream base at a concentration of 3 to 6%.[16] Salicylic acid decreases the cell-to-cell cohesion as measured by the ease by which layers of cells can be stripped from the surface of treated skin. Excessive use of ointments containing salicylic acid can result in salicylism and its use should not exceed 30 g of a 6% preparation in a 24-h period. This is especially important in children.

The application of propylene glycol at a concentration of 40 to 60% in water will result in the removal of scales, particularly when used under an occlusive plastic dressing. Although the glycol is not toxic, an occasional patient may develop an unpleasant burning sensation of the skin with its use. Propylene glycol has been used at lower concentrations with organic acids, and that combination has proved effective. The first product was made with salicylic acid in combination with alcohol, water, and hydroxypropylcellulose in a gel formulation. It was extremely effective in removing scales and its effect was markedly enhanced by using occlusion with a plastic wrap such as Saran Wrap.[17]

Lactic acid, in addition to being a humectant, acts as a keratolytic agent and results in the separation of stratum corneum cells as judged by the peeling off of scales from the surface of the skin. Stirring stratum corneum in solutions of lactic acid results in the release of desmogleins, suggesting that its mode of action is breakdown of desmosomes. Lactic acid comes in a variety of commercial preparations and can be sold over the counter at concentration of no higher than 5%. Epilyt, which is a liquid preparation containing 5% lactic acid and propylene glycol as the active agents, is extremely effective relieving the symptoms of dryness and removing scales[18] (Fig. 249-1). Being a liquid preparation, it can be easily

used in the scalp to remove scales and has been a popular treatment for the management of seborrheic dermatitis and psoriasis. It is applied to the scalp at bedtime and shampooed out in the morning. A popular prescription cream preparation of lactic acid (Lachydrin) contains 12% lactate neutralized to pH 5.0 in order to make a stable emulsion possible.[19] There are no data indicating that a neutralized high concentration of lactic acid provides an advantage over a lower concentration of lactic acid that has not been neutralized. One can compound lactic acid at different concentrations in a suitable base such as Aquaphor. Adults will tolerate concentrations up to 12%, and this is very effective in scale removal. If the ointment is applied to moist skin, as after a bath, it spreads much more easily and is more cosmetically acceptable to the patient. Lactic acid in Aquaphor is well tolerated by children, particularly at low concentrations of the acid.

Lactic acid is an α-hydroxy acid, and this family of acids has received considerable attention as peeling agents for sun-damaged skin. The α-hydroxy acids, which are listed in Table 249-1, derive their name from the presence of a hydroxyl group on the α carbon atom. Glycolic acid[20] is probably the most popular as judged from the number of products that have appeared in the last several years.

FIGURE 249-1

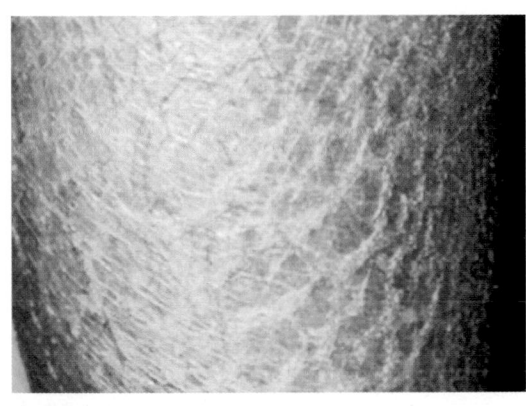

A.

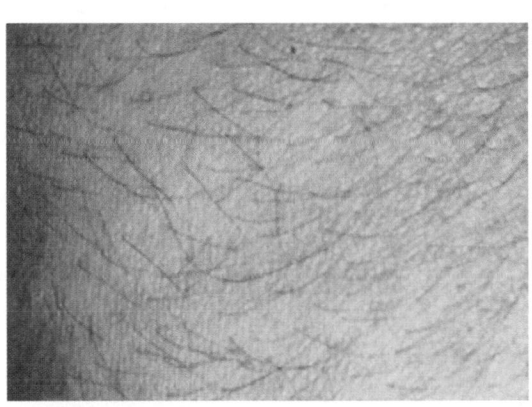

B.

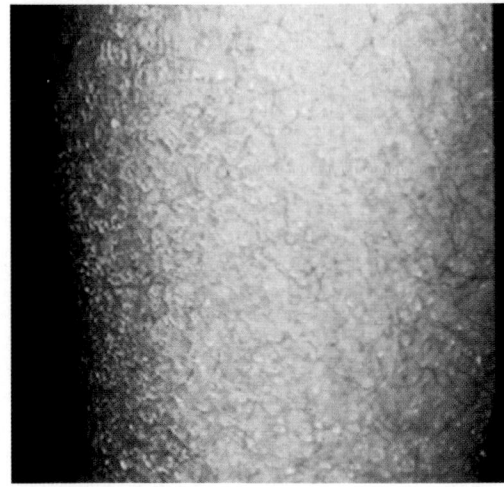

C.

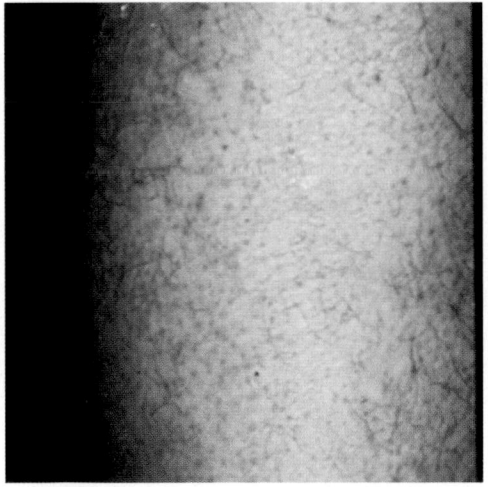

D.

Treatment of lamellar ichthyosis (A and B) and ichthyosis vulgaris (C and D) with Epilyt 2 times a day for 1 week. These conditions before (A and C) and after (B and D) are shown.

TABLE 249-1

Common Organic Acids in Use in Dermatology

	MOLECULAR WEIGHT	DISSOCIATION CONSTANT
Acetic acid	60	1.8×10^{-5}
Citric acid*	210	$8.2 \times 10^{-4\dagger}$
Glycolic acid*	76	1.4×10^{-4}
Lactic acid*	90	1.3×10^{-4}
Salicylic acid	138	—

*α-Hydroxyacids.
†First dissociation constant.

There is no compelling evidence, however, indicating an advantage of one acid over another; the ability of an acid to loosen scales is more related to its concentration and the composition of the base in which it is compounded. As seen in Table 249-1, the molecular weights and dissociation constants of glycolic and lactic acids are almost identical. In general more anhydrous preparations are less irritating and allow the use of higher concentrations of acid without side effects.

Some general principles must be kept in mind in considering the use of keratolytic agents. A plastic occlusive dressing, although not necessary, in many situations will enhance the therapeutic effect and result in more rapid and complete clearing. In treating the palmoplantar surface, occlusive dressings are essential and little effect will be observed without their use. In treating the scalp, wearing a lightweight shower cap enhances the effect of the treatment and prevents staining of the pillow. It is essential not to use a cap lined with cloth. In combining topical corticosteroids with keratolytics, as in the management of psoriasis, it is important to choose a drug that is stable in the presence of acid (e.g., fluocinolone). Although keratolytic agents loosen scales, they do not dissolve them, so that mechanical removal is necessary. Patients should be told to rub the skin with a washcloth or rough sponge while bathing. This will result in the shedding of large quantities of scale after the skin has been treated for several days. Mechanical removal should never be done when the skin is dry, since this traumatizes it.

Children are very sensitive to α-hydroxy acid, and small areas of the skin should be tested before applying it over wide areas. The irritation occurs rather quickly, so it is easy to determine if a particular product is a problem and symptoms can be stopped by wetting the skin thoroughly with water. This sensitivity usually disappears at the time of puberty. It must be remembered that salicylic acid can be absorbed through the stratum corneum, especially so if it is abnormal or thinned by treatment. Not more than 2.0 g of salicylic acid should be applied to a child's skin over a 24-h period.

MECHANISM

The mechanism of action of all organic acids is thought to be the same, and release of desmogleins indicating disintegration of the desmosomes is a consistent finding. It is possible that the acids work directly by solubilizing the protein components of desmosomes. An alternative explanation is that they activate an endogenous proteolytic or other hydrolytic enzyme as a result of a change in pH. However, no acid proteases have been described in the stratum corneum.[21] The desmosome is unlikely to be the only site of action of the acids, since the lipid layer between cells is important in holding cells together. Furthermore, in some of the ichthyoses (e.g., X-linked), it would appear that an abnormality of the lipid layer is responsible for increased coherence of cells, so one would not expect disintegration of the desmosomes by acids to result in cell separation. It seems likely that, in addition to a direct effect on desmosomes, there is an indirect one involving activation of some endogenous pathway responsible for normal cell separation.

FIGURE 249-2

RETINOIDS AS KERATOLYTICS

Retinoids exhibit a keratolytic effect, but this is mediated by alteration in the keratinization pathways in the epidermis. This has been demonstrated for retinoic used topically and etretinate and isotretinoin given orally. The application of retinoic acid to the skin of patients with psoriasis and ichthyosis resulted in shedding of thickened stratum corneum.[22] Later studies using retinoic acid for acne suggested loss of cohesion of cornified cells in the sebaceous duct.[23] A side effect of the treatment was scaling of the skin, indicating loss of cell cohesion in the interfollicular stratum corneum. Retinoic acid has now been approved for the treatment of photoaging, and a number of changes in the epidermis have been reported. The stratum corneum changed from a basketweave structure

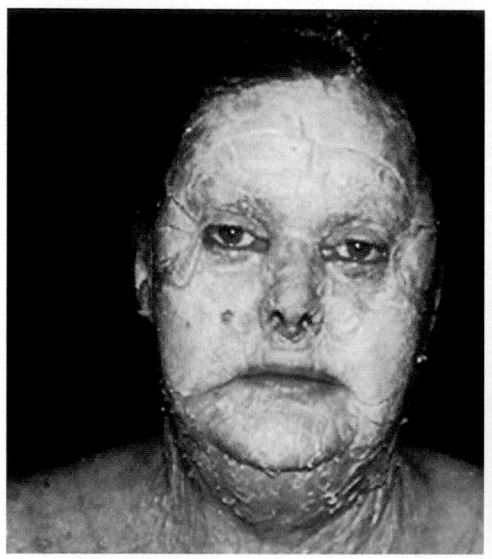
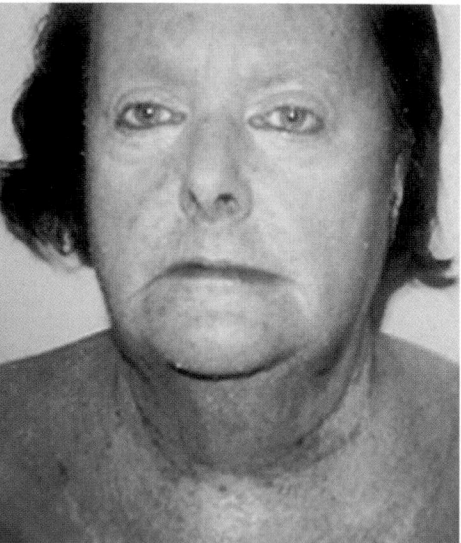

A.　　　　　　　　　　*B.*

Treatment of lamellar ichthyosis (*A*) with isotretinoin at 2 mg/kg/day for 6 weeks (*B*).

to a more compact form.[24] There was a reduction in turnover time of the stratum corneum and an increase in transepidermal water loss. Altered cell surface glycosylation has been reported as well. Patients with photoaging have reported a smoother feel to the skin surface and removal of keratotic lesions.[25]

Isotretinoin is used to treat a number of inherited disorders of keratinization and has proven very effective in reducing the thickness of the stratum corneum in, for example, lamellar ichthyosis (Fig. 249-2).[26] The mechanism for this decrease in cell cohesion is not known, but reduction in the number of desmosomes and altered glycosylation of cell-surface proteins has been mentioned. Etretinate has had a similar effect on the scale of patients with psoriasis and in addition has resulted in clearing of the lesions.

SPECIAL KERATOLYTICS

The hyperkeratosis associated with calluses, clavi, and warts is treated with high concentrations of salicylic and/or lactic acid in a liquid formulation or incorporated into a tape. A 40% salicylic acid preparation in tape is available, which results in marked softening of these lesions. They can then be abraded to remove the hyperkeratotic surface. A personal preference is to mix an equal volume of flexible collodion and 85% lactic acid. After thorough stirring, the solution is applied to the lesion, allowed to dry, and covered with waterproof tape. The lesion is mechanically debrided daily when wet. This is extremely effective in removing thickened stratum corneum but can be very irritating if applied to normal skin. The softened thick skin must be removed with an abrasive such as a pumic stone when wet.

Hyperkeratosis of the nail bed has been treated by an ointment containing 40% urea, 5% paraffin, 20% anhydrous lanolin, 25% white petrolatum, and 10% silica gel type H.[27] The normal skin around the nail is protected by adhesive tape. The urea ointment is applied to the involved nail, covered with an occlusive dressing, and left in place for 1 week. The treated nail is then soaked in water and the keratotic material removed by gentle brushing. A second application may be necessary. Others have modified the ointment without much change in efficacy.

REFERENCES

1. Dover R, Wright NA: The cell proliferation kinetics of the epidermis, in *Physiology, Biochemistry, and Molecular Biology of the Skin,* 2d ed, edited by LA Goldsmith. New York, Oxford University Press, 1991, pp 239–265
2. Hashimoto K: Ultrastructure of the human toenail: II. Keratinization and formation of the marginal band. *J Ultrastruct Res* **36**:391, 1971
3. Montagna W: General review of the anatomy, growth, and development of hair in man, in *Biology and Disease of the Hair,* edited by K Toda, Y Ishibashi, Y Hori, F Morikawa. Tokyo, University of Tokyo Press, 1976, pp 21–31
4. Steinberg MS et al: On the molecular organization, diversity and functions of desmosomal proteins, in *Junctional Complexes of Epithelial Cells,* edited by G Bock, S Clark. New York, Wiley, 1987, p 3
5. Horiguchi Y et al: Ultrastructural localization of E-cadherin cell adhesion molecule on the cytoplasmic memberane of keratinocytes in vivo and in vitro. *J Histochem Cytochem* **42**:1333, 1994
6. Elias PM, Feingold KR: Lipids and the epidermal water barrier: Metabolism regulation and pathophysiology. *Semin Dermatol* **11**:176, 1992
7. Lazo ND et al: Lipids are covalently attached to rigid corneocyte protein envelopes existing predominantly as beta-sheets: A solid-state nuclear magnetic resonance study. *J Invest Dermatol* **105**:296, 1995
8. Menon GK et al: Lamellar bodies as delivery systems of hydrolytic enzymes: Implications for normal and abnormal desquamation. *Br J Dermatol* **126**:337, 1992
9. Suzuki Y et al: The role of proteases in stratum corneum: Involvement in stratum corneum desquamation. *Arch Dermatol Res* **286**:249, 1994
10. Elsayed AH et al: Stereological studies of desmosomes in ichthyosis vulgaris. *Br J Dermatol* **126**:24, 1992
11. Williams ML, Elias PM: Stratum corneum lipids in disorders of cornification. I. Increases sulfate cholesterol content of stratum corneum in recessive x-linked ichthyosis. *J Clin Invest* **68**:1404, 1981
12. Muller KH, Pflugshaupt C: Urea in dermatology I. *Hautarzt* **40**(suppl 9):1, 1989
13. Van Scott EJ, Yu RJ: Control of keratinization with alpha-hydroxy acids and related compounds. I. Topical treatment of ichthyotic disorders. *Arch Dermatol* **110**:586, 1974
14. Van Scott EJ, Yu RJ: Alpha hydroxy acids: Procedures for use in clinical practice. *Cutis* **43**:222, 1989
15. Rawlings A et al: The effect of glycerol and humidity on desmosome degradation in stratum corneum. *Arch Dermatolo Res* **287**:457, 1995
16. Loden M et al: Distribution and keratolytic effect of salicylic acid and urea in human skin. *Skin Pharmacol* **8**:173, 1995
17. Baden HP et al: A new keratolytic gel for the management of hyperkeratosis. *Cutis* **12**:787, 1973
18. Baden HP. Management of scaly skin with Epilyt, in *Seminars in Dermatology, Dermatopharmacology and Therapeutics,* vol 6, edited by HI Maibach. Philadelphia, Grune & Stratton, 1987, pp 55–57
19. Wehr R et al: Controlled two-center study of lactate 12 percent lotion and a petrolatum-based cream in patients with xerosis. *Cutis* **37**:205, 1986
20. Stiller MJ et al: Topical 8% glycolic acid and 8% L-lactic acid creams for the treatment of photodamaged skin: A double-blind vehicle-controlled clinical trial. *Arch Dermatol* **132**:631, 1996
21. Suzuki Y et al: The role of two endogenous proteases of the stratum corneum in degradation of desmoglein-1 and their reduced activity in the skin of ichthyotic patients. *Br J Dermatol* **134**:460, 1996
22. Frost P, Weinstein GD: Topical administration of Vitamin A acid for ichthyosiform dermatoses and psoriasis. *JAMA* **207**:1863, 1969
23. Tagami H et al: Functional assessment of the stratum corneum under the influence of oral aromatic retinoid (etretinate) in guinea-pigs and humans: Comparison with topical retinoic acid treatment. *Br J Dermatol* **127**:470, 1992
24. Ellis CN et al: Sustained improvement with prolonged topical tretinoin (retinoic acid) for photoaged skin. *J Am Acad Dermatol* **23**:629, 1990
25. Griffiths CE et al: Topical retinoic acid changes the epidermal cell surface glycosylation pattern towards that of a mucosal epithelium. *Br J Dermatol* **134**:431, 1996
26. Baden HP et al: Treatment of ichthyosis with isotretinoin. *J Am Acad Dermatol* **6**:716, 1982
27. South DA, Farber E: Urea ointment in nonsurgical avulsion of nail dystrophies: Reappraisal. *Cutis* **21**:609, 1980

CHAPTER 250

Jerome L. Shupack
Irene W. Lai
Ken Washenik

Topical Cytotoxic Agents

5-FLUOROURACIL

5-Fluorouracil (5-FU) has been used in clinical practice since the 1960s and has proved to be efficacious as a topical cytotoxic drug for a variety of diseases. Current developments in the use of this drug focus on different methods of delivery and use in an increasing variety of skin diseases. 5-FU is a structural analogue of thymine, halogenated with fluorine at position 5. It interferes with pyrimidine metabolism and action by conversion to 5-fluoro-2′-deoxyuridine-5′-phosphate (F-dUMP). F-dUMP is a potent inhibitor of thymidylate synthetase; thus, DNA synthesis is blocked. 5-FU itself is also incorporated into RNA and DNA.[1,2]

Systemic absorption of topically applied 5-FU is limited to approximately 6 percent of the applied dose.[2,3] Absorption is selectively higher from abnormal skin than from surrounding normal skin.[4] Normal skin appears to be unaffected clinically, but there are ultrastructural changes.[3] No reports of systemic toxicity after topical application of 5-FU have appeared in the literature to date. Systemic effects of 5-FU include nausea and anorexia, stomatitis, diarrhea, myelosuppression, alopecia, neurological manifestations, and cardiac toxicity. Topical 5-FU is commercially available as a solution (1%, 2%, and 5%) and as a cream (1% and 5%). A 20% ointment can be compounded by using commercially available intravenous 5-FU solution. The intravenous solution can also be used for intralesional injection. A sustained-release preparation of 5-FU for intralesional injection, which combines 5-FU with epinephrine and bovine collagen, is currently undergoing clinical trials. Side effects of the topical preparation are generally local cutaneous reactions of irritation, erythema, pain, swelling, pruritus, hyper- and hypopigmentation, allergic contact dermatitis, and photosensitivity. Unusual reactions may include onycholysis, onychodystrophy, and telangiectasia.[3] The use of injectable preparations may be complicated by local ulceration, erosion, and desquamation.

Successful use of topical 5-FU has been reported in many skin diseases (Table 250-1); however, its use is most established in the treatment of actinic keratoses,[5] particularly in patients with many lesions. It is used twice daily until an inflammatory response is seen, usually 2 to 4 weeks. This inflammation of actinic keratoses is also seen in patients undergoing systemic 5-FU treatment for malignancy and is the observation that initially led to the development of this drug as a topical treatment for actinic keratoses. Pretreatment with a keratolytic agent may be useful for particularly hyperkeratotic lesions. Irritation during treatment sometimes requires reduction or interruption of treatment and the addition of emollients or topical steroids. Another strategy to reduce irritant dermatitis caused by 5-FU is weekly pulse dosing. This involves applying the medication for 1 to 2 days per week for 6 to 7 weeks.[6] During 5-FU treatment,

TABLE 250-1

Diseases in which 5-Fluorouracil Is Useful

Precancerous lesions	Malignant tumors
Actinic keratoses	Basal cell carcinoma
Actinic cheilitis, leukoplakia	Dermatoses
Radiodermatitis	Psoriasis
Xeroderma pigmentosum	Porokeratosis of Mibelli
Bowen's disease	Darier's disease
Bowenoid papulosis	Pityriases rubra pilaris
Erythroplasia of Queyrat	Kyrle's disease
Benign tumors	
Keratoacanthoma	
Warts	

other actinic keratoses may be revealed, and basal and squamous cell carcinomas may become unmasked.[7] Occasionally the therapeutic response is inadequate, and occlusive dressings, more frequent applications, prolonged therapy, or the use of an adjunctive agent such as tretinoin cream is required. Continuous use of 5-FU as a prophylactic measure for actinic keratoses is not of proven benefit,[7–10] although its use in xeroderma pigmentosum has been advocated. There are reports of cutaneous resistance to 5-FU treatment after 18 months of use.[11,12]

Basal cell carcinomas have been extensively investigated for treatment with topical 5-FU.[3] Some researchers have reported adequate tumor clearance,[13–23] but others have found unacceptable recurrence rates and persistence of tumor on biopsy.[24] The 5% cream is approved by the U.S. Food and Drug Administration for treatment of superficial basal cell carcinomas. The sustained-release injectable preparation in an early study produced unacceptably low cure rates of 60 to 80 percent,[25] although it may prove to be of use in selected patients in whom conventional treatment is not possible.

Warts such as verruca vulgaris, verruca plana, plantar warts, and condyloma acuminata can be treated with varying response rates to topical and intralesional injection of 5-FU. Condyloma acuminata have been reported to have response rates to topical 5-FU of up to 69 percent in men and 90 percent in women.[26–31] Most clinicians, however, would reserve this treatment for warts not easily treated with conventional therapy or for recalcitrant or extensive condylomata.[32]

Actinic cheilitis and mucosal leukoplakia have been well managed with topical 5-FU.[33–36] Topical treatment of the lip has the advantage of good cosmetic results, and it may preclude the necessity for surgery.[3] Several reports have shown varying responses to the treatment of radiodermatitis with topical 5-FU.[9,36,37] Bowen's disease, Bowenoid papulosis, and erythroplasia of Queyrat have all been reported as having poor to excellent responses to treatment with topical 5-FU.[38–44] Topical 5-FU as well as intralesional injection have been reported to cure most keratoacanthomas,[45,46] and porokeratosis of Mibelli has reportedly been cured after treatment with topical 5-FU.[47,48] There was some interest in the past in investigating the role of topical 5-FU in lentigo maligna and melanocytic dysplasia,[49,50] but this has not been established.

More recently there are developments in the use of topical and intralesional 5-FU for the treatment of psoriasis. Continuous topical fluorouracil under occlusion can be given for 2 to 3 days per week for about 16 weeks until clearance.[51] Alternatively, weekly intralesional fluorouracil has been tried for treatment of psoriatic papules and portions of larger psoriatic plaques with some effect.[52] The responses observed after injection of 5-FU in a sustained-release gel suggest clinical usefulness in treatment of chronic recalcitrant plaque psoriasis unresponsive to other therapies.[53]

MECHLORETHAMINE (NITROGEN MUSTARD)

Mechlorethamine [methyl-*bis* (2-chloroethyl) amine hydrochloride] was the first nitrogen mustard to be used in clinical medicine. Sulfur mustard, of which mechlorethamine is a nitrogen analogue, is a vesicant and was developed as a chemical warfare agent. Mechlorethamine acts as an alkylating agent and is not cell-cycle specific; however, it has most effect on cells in the late G_1 or S phases.[1] The primary target of mustard is the 7-nitrogen atom of guanine, although other bases may also be alkylated.[1]

Topical preparations of nitrogen mustard are used primarily for cutaneous T cell lymphoma (CTCL). They are generally very well tolerated. *Potential* systemic side effects include nausea, vomiting, myelosupression, menstrual irregularities, oligospermia, alopecia, cardiac abnormalities, hypocalcemia, and central nervous system abnormalities. The drug is also teratogenic. There have been no reports of systemic side effects following topical application.[54] Exposure to vapours released during topical application does not induce pulmonary fibrosis.[55]

The side effects of topical mustard include contact sensitivity, (both immediate and delayed), hyperpigmentation, irritant dermatitis, telangiectases, bullous eruptions, and an increased incidence of skin cancers. Delayed-type hypersensitivity (DTH) may occur in 35 to 60 percent of patients on long-term treatment.[56–58] This reaction consists of erythema and pruritus and histologically is typical allergic contact dermatitis. If hypersensitivity occurs, discontinuation of therapy is not necessarily required. Desensitization has been achieved using intravenous[59] and topical[56,60] methods. UV therapy can delay development of contact sensitization to mustard[61]; however, this modality is not recommended as nitrogen mustard is radiomimetic and coupled with UV will increase the incidence of skin cancers. Although desensitization may be achieved, it may not be desirable as DTH is possibly of therapeutic benefit. CTCL may resolve clinically after the development of DTH, and regression has been reported after application of dinitrochlorobenzene to induce DTH.[54] Most clinicians continue topical mustard in individuals who have developed DTH, employing dilutions below the threshold for clinically observable contact dermatitis. Up to 8 percent of patients may develop an immediate-type hypersensitivity to topical mechlorethamine, manifesting as urticaria. Treatment must be discontinued if this develops to avoid a potential anaphylactic reaction. Desensitization is not achievable. The incidence of hypersensitivity is reported to be less with the ointment preparation than with the aqueous solution of nitrogen mustard.[62]

Changes in pigmentation may also occur secondary to use of topical mechlorethamine. Hyperpigmentation is especially prone to develop in areas of previous CTCL and tends to resolve spontaneously, although slowly.[54,59,60] Hypopigmentation occurs rarely.

A potential troubling property of topical nitrogen mustard is its carcinogenicity.[63,64] It is associated with an increased risk of basal and squamous cell carcinomas and keratoacanthomas, and there is a report of lentigo maligna.[63–66] It is difficult to determine the exact extent of the problem as topical nitrogen mustard is often used with other known carcinogenic therapies such as PUVA. Overall the risk is small,[67] and as the lesions are easily treatable this should not dissuade one from using topical nitrogen mustard. Nevertheless, it is important to advise patients to avoid sun exposure during therapy to minimize the risk.

Not as clear cut is whether topical nitrogen mustard increases the incidence of internal malignancies in patients with CTCL.[68] Some studies have reported an increased risk of colon cancer, whereas others have not. CTCL itself is associated with an increased incidence of systemic lymphoma. High-dose systemic mechlorethamine is not associated with these other malignancies, so perhaps CTCL patients have an underlying increased risk for these second malignancies.[57]

The main role of topical mustard in dermatology is in the treatment of early CTCL.[57,68] There are reports of topical mustard producing complete remission in up to 75 percent of patients,[68] particularly if used in the early stage.[57,69]

Topical mustard is usually dispensed as either an aqueous solution or an ointment preparation. The aqueous solution needs to be prepared daily by the patient. This is done by mixing 10 mg of nitrogen mustard with 60 mL of water. The solution should be applied immediately with a gauze to the entire body but sparingly to intertriginous sites. The genitalia should be excluded. The solution has a shelf life of approximately 1 day. Refrigeration extends the usefulness for up to 6 months. The surrounding environment is minimally contaminated.[62] Those assisting in the application of the drug should limit their exposure by wearing protective gloves, avoiding direct contact, and washing thoroughly after handling the preparation. Effort should be made to dispose of empty vials or unused solution in accordance with Environmental Protection Agency guidelines. An alternative preparation can be made by dissolving the mustard in anhydrous petrolatum. The ointment has a shelf life of approximately 50 days.[70]

Topical nitrogen mustard has also been used with some success in the treatment of psoriasis,[71] alopecia areata,[72] and histiocytosis X.[73]

BCNU (CARMUSTINE)

Carmustine [bischlorethylnitrosourea (BCNU)] is a nitrosourea that acts by alkylation to inhibit DNA, RNA, and protein synthesis.[1] Its action is not cell-cycle specific. The topical formulation, introduced for clinical use in 1971, is used predominantly in the treatment of CTCL. BCNU is effective in patch- and plaque-stage CTCL, with complete clinical response rates of 48 to 86 percent and remission durations of 18 to 66 months.[74,75]

Systemic side effects include profound myelosuppression, renal failure, mucositis, pulmonary fibrosis, alopecia, nausea and vomiting, and azoospermia. These side effects have not been seen resulting from topical treatment, apart from mild myelosuppression. Cutaneous reactions are very common with the topical formulations. Erythema is seen in almost all patients and generally appears after 4 to 8 weeks of therapy. If severe, this may be associated with skin tenderness and telangiectasia. Allergy is uncommon and occurs in fewer than 10 percent of patients, manifesting as DHT. Urticaria is not seen, and an increased incidence of skin cancers is not observed. Mild bone marrow depression can be found, and patients should have regular blood counts while undergoing topical BCNU treatment.

BCNU is available as a powder for reconstitution as a solution or ointment. A 0.2% alcoholic stock solution is made by mixing 300 mg of BCNU with 150 mL of 95% ethanol. This solution is stable for 3 to 12 months if refrigerated. The patient is instructed to mix 5 mL (10 mg) of the stock solution daily with 60 mL of water. This should be applied immediately to the skin, avoiding the face, hands, genitals, and intertriginous areas unless these are directly involved with CTCL. The applications should be continued until clearing is seen, usually in 8 to 16 weeks. If the response to 10 mg daily is inadequate, the dose may be doubled for a further 4 to 8 weeks if tolerated. The ointment is prepared by combining BCNU powder in 95% alcohol and then mixing with white petrolatum USP up to concentrations of 10 mg % (10 mg/100 g base), 20 mg %, and 40 mg %. The ointment is easier for patients to use and leads to fewer cutaneous reactions. However, it is associated with an increased incidence of myelosuppression. The ointment is stable for about 6 months if kept refrigerated.

VINBLASTINE

Vinblastine is a vinca alkaloid. It is an antimitotic agent and acts by disrupting microtubules, blocking cell division in metaphase.[1] In dermatologic practice, this agent is used primarily as an intralesional injection for cutaneous and oral lesions of Kaposi's sarcoma.

Potential systemic side effects are myelosuppression, neuropathy, anorexia, nausea, vomiting and diarrhea, alopecia, mucositis, and dermatitis. Side effects of intralesional injection are usually limited to pain, ulceration, and hyperpigmentation at the injection site.[76] To reduce the pain involved with injection, local anesthesia before injection has been tried,[77] as has mixing lidocaine into the vinblastine solution.[78] This does not reduce postinjection pain, which may persist for up to 48 h. Pain can usually be managed with simple oral analgesics.

The method of intralesional injection generally reported is 0.1 to 0.2 mg of vinblastine per mL of normal saline, with doses escalating up to 0.6 mg/mL. Some authors use one injection only, whereas others recommend injections every 2 to 4 weeks until complete response is seen.[79,80] Complete or partial clinical response is of the order of 88 percent.[78] However, as treatment is local, progression of Kaposi's sarcoma may occur at other sites.

Iontophoresis is under investigation as a method of delivering effective amounts of vinblastine while eliminating the pain associated with intralesional injection.[81] Iontophoresis involves delivering an ionic drug transdermally using a direct electric current through the patient and medication solution. Side effects noted have been a localized papular erythematous eruption. The procedure appears to be well tolerated; however, overall efficacy is not yet established.

BLEOMYCIN

The bleomycins are a group of antibiotics produced by *Streptomyces verticillus*.[1] The drug in clinical use is a mixture of bleomycins A_2 and B_2.[1] Bleomycin acts by disrupting DNA synthesis causing cells to accumulate in G_2, although exactly how it causes its effect in the treatment of warts is unknown. At 48 h after injection, apoptotic keratinocytes are seen in the epidermis.[82] Systemic toxicity from bleomycin includes myelosuppression, hyperpigmentation, hyperkeratosis, ulceration, pulmonary fibrosis, headache, nausea, vomiting, hyperthermia, and hypotension.

Bleomycin has been used successfully as an intralesional injection for recalcitrant warts. Significant systemic exposure does occur, although systemic toxicity has not been found.[82,83] Local side effects of pain, swelling, and Raynaud's phenomenon have been reported.[84,85] Lidocaine may reduce the pain associated with the injection.

Bleomycin is available as a powder. It should be reconstituted with 0.9% sodium chloride into a 1 U/mL solution. Stability in this formulation has been shown at 6 to 8 weeks if the preparation is refrigerated at 4°C, and for several months if stored at −20°C.[82] The solution should be injected intralesionally until the wart blanches; one to two injections may be required. Using this technique, a 77 percent cure rate has been found for warts on extremities; however, the rate falls to about 48 percent for plantar warts.[86] A multiple puncture technique has been employed by one group, which may result in a more uniform distribution of drug into the wart.[87]

PELDESINE (BCX-34)

BCX-34 [9-(3-pyridylmethyl)-9-deazaguanine] is a purine nucleoside phosphorylase inhibitor. It is currently available only as an investigational drug. It was sought after and synthesized in the late 1980s in response to the observation that patients who were deficient in purine nucleoside phosphorylase (PNP) had selectively depressed T cell function without impairment of B cell function.[88] Deficiency of PNP results in elevated levels of 2′-deoxyguanosine, which in T cells is phosphorylated to 2′-deoxyguanosine triphosphate, which blocks DNA synthesis, thereby inhibiting T cell proliferation. Only proliferating T cells are affected.[89] Clinical trials investigating BCX-34 as a topical agent in T cell skin disorders are under way. Phase I/II trials of BCX-34 (5% active ingredient) in CTCL and psoriasis show the drug to be safe, with significant beneficial effect in both diseases.[90]

REFERENCES

1. Chabner BA et al: Antineoplastic agents, in *Goodman & Gilman's The Pharmacological Basis of Therapeutics,* 9th ed, edited by JG Hardman. McGraw-Hill, 1996, pp 1233–1287
2. *Drug Information for the Health Care Professional,* 15th ed. Taunton, MA, Rand McNally, 1995, pp 1359–1360
3. Goette DK: Topical chemotherapy with 5-fluorouracil. A review. *J Am Acad Dermatol* **4**:633, 1981
4. Krebs HB: Treatment of genital condylomata with topical 5-fluorouracil. *Dermatol Clin* **9**:333, 1991
5. Breza T et al: Noninflammatory destruction of actinic keratoses by fluorouracil. *Arch Dermatol* **112**:1258, 1976

6. Pearlman DL: Weekly pulse dosing: Effective and comfortable topical 5-fluorouracil treatment of multiple facial actinic keratoses. *J Am Acad Dermatol* **25**:665, 1991

7. Belisario JC: Topical cytotoxic therapy of solar keratoses. *Med J Aust* **2**:1136, 1969

8. Rossman RE: Topical fluorouracil therapy. *South Med J* **62**:1240, 1969

9. Neldner KH: Prevention of skin cancer with topical 5 fluorouracil. *Rocky Mt Med J* **63**:74, 1966

10. Dillaha CJ et al: Selective cytotoxic effect of topical 5 fluorouracil. *Arch Dermatol* **88**:247, 1963

11. Reed WB et al: Xeroderma pigmentosum. Clinical and laboratory investigation of its basic defect. *JAMA* **207**:2073, 1969

12. Gorlin RJ et al: Xeroderma pigmentosum syndrome. *Modern Med* **38**:223, 1970

13. Klein E et al: Tumors of the skin. IV. Double blind study on effects of local administration of antitumor agents in basal cell carcinomas. *J Invest Dermatol* **44**:351, 1965

14. Klein E et al: Tumors of the skin. VI. Double blind study on effects of local administration of antitumor agents in basal cell carcinomas. *J Invest Dermatol* **47**:22, 1966

15. Stoll HL Jr et al: Tumors of the skin. VII. Effects of varying the concentration of locally administered 5 fluorouracil on basal cell carcinomas. *J Invest Dermatol* **49**:219, 1967

16. Klein E et al: Tumors of the skin. XII. Topical 5 fluorouracil for epidermal neoplasms. *J Surg Oncol* **3**:331, 1971

17. Klein E: Chemotherapy and immunotherapy for cancer involving the skin. Seventh National Cancer Conference Proceedings, Bethesda, MD, 1972. 1973, pp 567–578

18. Litwin MS, Krementz ET: Treatment of basal and squamous cell cancers of the nose and ear with 5-fluorouracil cream. *Laryngoscope* **81**:840, 1971

19. Litwin MS et al: Use of 5 fluorouracil in topical therapy of skin cancer: A review of 157 patients. Seventh National Cancer Conference Proceedings, Bethesda, MD, 1972. 1973, pp 549–561

20. Jansen GT: What are the effects of topical fluorouracil in basal cell carcinoma? *JAMA* **228**:204, 1974

21. Ebner H: Treatment of skin epitheliomas with 5 fluorouracil ointment. *Dermatologica* **140**(suppl):42, 1970

22. Littlewood M, Murray DS: A clinical trial of the use of 5-fluorouracil in the treatment of some cutaneous malignancies. *Br J Plast Surg* **26**:140, 1973

23. Hodge SJ et al: Topical 5-fluorouracil treatment of superficial basal cell carcinoma: A light and electron microscopic study. *J Cutan Pathol* **2**:284, 1975

24. Reymann F: Treatment of BCC with 5FU ointment. A 10-year follow-up study. *Dermatologica* **158**:368, 1979

25. Orenberg EK et al: The effect of intralesional 5-fluorouracil therapeutic implant (MPI5003) for treatment of basal cell carcinoma. *J Am Acad Dermatol* **27**:723, 1992

26. Pareek S: Treatment of condyloma acuminatum with 5% fluorouracil. *Br J Vener Dis* **55**:65, 1979

27. Handojo I, Pardjono I: Treatment of condyloma acuminata with 5% fluorouracil ointment. *Asian Med J* **9**:162, 1973

28. Nel WS, Fourie ED: Immunotherapy and 5% topical 5-fluorouracil ointment in the treatment of condylomata acuminata. *South Afr J Med* **47**:45, 1973

29. Temime P: Treatment of anogenital venereal papillomas by topical application of 5-fluorouracil ointment. *Bull Soc Fr Dermatol Syph* **77**:521, 1970

30. Sanders BB, Stretcher GS: Warts: Diagnosis and treatment. *JAMA* **235**:2859, 1976

31. von Krogh G: 5-Fluorouracil cream in the successful treatment of therapeutically resistant condylomata accuminata of the urethral meatus. *Acta Derm Venereol (Stock)* **56**:297, 1976

32. Kling AR: Genital warts—therapy. *Semin Dermatol* **11**:247, 1992

33. Epstein E: Treatment of actinic cheilitis with topical fluorouracil. *Arch Dermatol* **113**:906, 1977

34. Goldman L: The response of skin cancer to topical therapy with 5-fluorouracil. *Cancer Chemother Rep* **28**:49, 1963

35. Klein E: Tumors of the skin. IX. Local cytostatic therapy of cutaneous and mucosal premalignant and malignant lesions. *NY State J Med* **68**:886, 1968

36. Williams AC: Experiences with local chemotherapy and immunotherapy in premalignant and malignant skin lesions. *Cancer* **25**:450, 1970

37. Dillaha CJ et al: Further studies with topical 5-fluorouracil. *Arch Dermatol* **92**:410, 1965

38. Jansen GT et al: Bowenoid conditions of the skin: Treatment with topical 5-fluorouracil. *South Med J* **69**:185, 1967

39. Knipp TP et al: 5-Fluorouracil topical treatment of carcinoma in situ vulvar cancer. *Obstet Gynecol* **51**:702, 1978

40. Tolia BM et al: Bowen's disease of shaft of penis: Successful treatment with 5-fluorouracil. *Urology* **7**:617, 1976

41. Wade TR et al: Bowenoid papulosis of the penis. *Cancer* **42**:1890, 1978

42. Hueser TN et al: Erythroplasia of Queyrat treated with topical 5-fluorouracil. *J Urol* **102**:595, 1969

43. Goette DK et al: Erythroplasia of Queyrat: Treatment with topically applied 5-fluorouracil. *JAMA* **232**:934, 1975

44. Forney TP et al: Management of carcinoma-in-situ of the vulva. *Am J Obstet Gynecol* **127**:801, 1977

45. Midana A: 5-FU ointment in the treatment of benign and malignant skin lesions. *Dermatologica* **140**(suppl 1):75, 1970

46. Odom RB, Goette DK: Treatment of keratoacanthomas with intralesional 5 fluorouracil. *Arch Dermatol* **114**:1779, 1978

47. Goncalves JCA: Fluorouracil ointment treatment of porokeratosis of Mibelli. *Arch Dermatol* **108**:131, 1973

48. Dupre A, Cvistol B: Mibelli's porokeratosis of the lips. *Arch Dermatol* **114**:1841, 1978

49. Ryan RF et al: A role for topical 5-fluorouracil therapy in melanoma. *J Surg Oncol* **38**:250, 1988

50. Gromet MA: Treatment of lentigo maligna with 5-FU. *Arch Dermatol* **113**:1128, 1977

51. Pearlman DL et al: Weekly pulse dosing schedule of fluorouracil: A new topical therapy for psoriasis. *J Am Acad Dermatol* **15**:1247, 1986

52. Pearlman DL et al: Weekly psoriasis therapy using intralesional fluorouracil. *J Am Acad Dermatol* **17**:78, 1987

53. Lowe NJ et al: Intradermal fluorouracil and epinephrine injectable gel for treatment of psoriatic plaques. *Arch Dermatol* **131**:1340, 1995

54. Ramsay DL et al: Topical treatment of early cutaneous T-cell lymphoma. *Hematol Oncol Clin North Am* **9**:1031,1995

55. Nielsen M et al: Long-term topical nitrogent mustard treatment does not induce pulmonary fibrosis in mf patients. *Acta Derm Venerol (Stockh)* **74**:70, 1994

56. Ramsay DL et al: Topical mechlorethamine therapy for early stage mycosis fungoides. *J Am Acad Dermatol* **19**:684, 1988

57. Vonderheid EC et al: Long-term efficacy, curative potential, and carcinogenicity of topical mechlorethamine chemotherapy in cutaneous T-cell lymphoma. *J Am Acad Dermatol* **20**:416, 1989

58. Ramsay DL et al: Response of mycosis fungoides to topical chemotherapy with mechlorethamine. *Arch Dermatol* **120**:1585, 1984

59. Van Scott EJ et al: Complete remissions of mycosis fungoides lymphoma induced by topical nitrogen mustard (HN2). *Cancer* **32**:18, 1973

60. Constantine VS et al: Mechlorethamine desensitization in therapy for mycosis fungoides: Topical desensitization to mechlorethamine (nitrogen mustard) contact hypersensitivity. *Arch Dermatol* **111**:484, 1975

61. Halprin KM et al: Ultraviolet light treatment delays contact sensitization to nitrogen mustard. *Br J Dermatol* **105**:71, 1981

62. Breneman DL et al: Topical mechlorethamine in the treatment of mycosis fungoides. *J Am Acad Dermatol* **25**:1059, 1991

63. duVivier A et al: Mycosis fungoides, nitrogen mustard and skin cancer. *Br J Dermatol* **99**:61, 1978

64. Lee LA et al: Second cutaneous malignancies in patients with mycosis fungoides treated with nitrogen mustard. *J Am Acad Dermatol* **7**:590, 1982

65. Abel EA et al: Cutaneous malignancies and metastatic squamous cell carcinoma following topical therapies for mycosis fungoides. *J Am Acad Dermatol* **14**:1029, 1986

66. Smith SP, Konnikov N: Eruptive epidermal cysts and multiple squamous cell carcinomas after therapy for cutaneous T-cell lymphoma. *J Am Acad Dermatol* **25**:940, 1991

67. Smoller BR, Marcus R: Risk of secondary cutaneous malignancies in patients with long-standing mycosis fungoides. *J Am Acad Dermatol* **30**:201, 1994

68. Price NM et al: Ointment-based mechlorethamine treatment for mycosis fungoides. *Cancer* **52**:2214, 1983

69. Hoppe RT et al: Mycosis fungoides: Management with topical nitrogen mustard. *J Clin Oncol* **5**:1796, 1987

70. Holloway KB et al: Therapeutic alternatives in cutaneous T-cell lymphoma. *J Am Acad Dermatol* **27**:367, 1992

71. Handler RM, Medansky RS: Treatment of psoriasis with topical nitrogen mustard. *Int J Dermatol* **18**:758, 1979

72. Arrazola JM et al: Treatment of alopecia areata using topical nitrogen mustard. *Int J Dermatol* **24**:608, 1985

73. Berman B et al: Histiocytosis X treated with topical nitrogen mustard. *J Am Acad Dermatol* **3**:23, 1980

74. Zackheim HS: Topical carmustine (BCNU) for patch/plaque mycosis fungoides. *Semin Dermatol* **13**:202, 1994

75. Zackheim HS et al: Topical carmustine (BCNU) for CTCL: A 15-year experience in 143 patients. *J Am Acad Dermatol* **22**:802, 1990

76. Northfelt DW: Treatment of Kaposi's sarcoma: Current guidelines and future perspectives. *Drugs* **48**:569, 1994

77. Epstein JB: Treatment of oral Kaposi sarcoma with intralesional vinblastine. *Cancer* **71**:1722, 1993

78. Boudreaux AA et al: Intralesional vinblastine for cutaneous Kaposi's sarcoma associated with acquired immunodeficiency syndrome. A clinical trial to evaluate efficacy and discomfort associated with infection. *J Am Acad Dermatol* **28**:61, 1993

79. Conant MA: Management of human immunodeficiency virus–associated malignancies. *Recent Results Cancer Res* **139**:423, 1995

80. Epstein JB et al: Oral Kaposi's sarcoma in acquired immunodeficiency syndrome. *Cancer* **64**:2424, 1989

81. Smith KJ et al: Iontophoresis of vinblastine into normal skin and for treatment of Kaposi's sarcoma in human immunodeficiency virus–positive patients. *Arch Dermatol* **128**:1365, 1992

82. James MP et al: Histologic, pharmacologic, and immunocytochemical effects of injection of bleomycin into viral warts. *J Am Acad Dermatol* **28**:993, 1993

83. Shumer SM, O'Keefe EJ: Bleomycin in the treatment of recalcitrant warts. *J Am Acad Dermatol* **9**:91, 1983

84. Epstein E: Intralesional bleomycin and Raynaud's phenomenon. *J Am Acad Dermatol* **24**:785, 1991

85. Gregg LJ: Intralesional bleomycin and Raynaud's phenomenon. *J Am Acad Dermatol* **27**:279, 1992

86. Amer M et al: Therapeutic evaluation for intralesional injection of bleomycin sulfate in 143 resistant warts. *J Am Acad Dermatol* **18**:1313, 1988

87. Shelley WB, Shelley ED: Intralesional bleomycin sulfate therapy for warts: A novel bifurcated needle puncture technique. *Arch Dermatol* **127**:234, 1991

88. Montgomery JA: Purine nucleoside phophorylase: A target for drug design. *Med Res Rev* **13**:209, 1993

89. Kazmers IS et al: Inhibition of purine nucleoside phosphorylase by 8-aminoguanosine: Selective toxicity for T lymphoblasts. *Science* **214**:1137, 1981

90. Montgomery JA et al: BCX-34. Purine nucleoside phosphorylase (PNP) inhibitor. *Drugs Future* **18**:887, 1993

CHAPTER 251

Patricia G. Engasser
Howard I. Maibach

Cosmetics and Skin Care in Dermatologic Practice

Consulting with patients and with the public about cosmetics has become part of a dermatologist's role as a skin care expert. Indeed, the increasing application of biophysical measurement techniques to study skin allows more accurate assessment of the safety and efficacy of cosmetics. Notwithstanding this advance, however, objective information in the form of reliable published clinical data on which dermatologists may safely base this advice are limited, and advertising as well as press reports create unrealistic public expectations. Information technology allows international experts to communicate easily about the dermatotoxicology of cosmetics, and manufacturers frequently sell products internationally; this situation allows global market forces and regulations to determine the nature of available products.

EFFICACY AND SAFETY OF COSMETICS

In response to scientific, economic, and social influences, the definition of cosmetics fluctuates. In the United States, the 1938 Food, Drug and Cosmetic Act defines cosmetics as "articles intended to be rubbed, poured, sprinkled, or sprayed on, introduced into, or otherwise applied to the human body or any part thereof for cleansing, beautifying, promoting attractiveness, or altering the appearance." Drugs in part are defined as "articles . . . intended to affect the structure or any function of the body" (1:510). These definitions are not mutually exclusive, and products such as antiperspirants and bleaching creams are regulated both as over-the-counter drugs and as cosmetics. In Japan, these ambiguities are managed by the classification *quasi-drug*.

In the United States, drugs must meet strict premarket safety and efficacy requirements. Consequently manufacturers, wishing their products to be categorized as cosmetics, make cautious, fanciful, or vague efficacy claims that lead to confusion. Regulatory penalties make cosmetic scientists reluctant to explore the physiologic effects of topical compounds or the nature of their placebo effects as observed in experiments. To deal with these contradictory forces, Kligman[2,3] proposed a separate category—*cosmeceuticals*—for products that have cosmetic purposes but also affect skin structure and function. This term would describe topical minoxidil used to treat physiological balding, topical retinoids that reverse signs of aging, and moisturizers applied to treat xerosis. In the last two decades, dermatologic studies have established that the stratum cor-

neum—the "playground" for cosmetics—has a modifiable meta-
CHAPTER 251
Cosmetics and Skin Care in Dermatologic Practice   2773

bolic activity that influences the structure and function of viable epidermis,[4] making the 1938 definition of a cosmetic outdated. Ver-meer and Gilchrest[5] propose regulatory recognition of these agents, intended for use on normal or nearly normal skin, and suggest pre-market testing appropriate for their risk-benefit ratio. The advancing field of cutaneous biometrics can bring efficacy claims from fan-ciful to provable. Consumers' desire for readily available cosme-ceuticals will ultimately ensure their development.

Physical attractiveness is socially advantageous and results in perceptions of "goodness" and success as well as a sense of well-being. Improvement in both attractiveness and consequent psycho-logical benefit as promoted by effective cosmetic use extends to the elderly.[6] These benefits of cosmetics should be recognized by phy-sicians, who may recommend cosmetics as part of a treatment pro-gram.

An important consideration in cosmetic innovation and toxicol-ogy is the growing concern about the ethics of animal testing.[7] Some manufacturers have voluntarily abandoned testing final prod-ucts on animals. The European Union's Sixth Amendment to the Cosmetic Directive proposed that animal testing of ingredients cease by January 1998.[8] Complete compliance with this ban was unfea-sible because development validation of alternative testing methods is tedious and the pace is slow.

In the United States, manufacturers' reporting of adverse cos-metic reactions to the Food and Drug Administration (FDA) is a voluntary program. The Cosmetic, Toiletries and Fragrance Asso-ciation (CTFA), the manufacturers' trade organization, sponsors the Cosmetic Ingredient Review (CIR) to review the safety of cosmetic ingredients and publishes its findings in the *Journal of the American College of Toxicology*. In the United States, ingredient labeling has been mandated for retail cosmetics since 1978. Ingredients are listed in descending order of amount using nomenclature published in the *International Cosmetic Ingredient Dictionary*.[9] Fragrances (com-plex mixtures) are described simply as fragrance. Voluntary com-pliance with these regulations for cosmetics used or sold in beauty spas and salons was adopted in 1989. Beginning in 1998, European cosmetics are also required to use a similar nomenclature for la-beling. In cooperation with the American Academy of Dermatology (AAD), the CTFA publishes *Cosmetic Industry On Call,* a list of industry scientists who will aid dermatologists in evaluating patients who may have reactions to cosmetics.[10] Irritant, urticarial, allergic, or photosensitive eruptions as well as pigmentary, hair, and nail disorders or systemic reactions can result from cosmetic use. To diagnose affected patients, dermatologists must appreciate the di-versity of these reactions.

ADVERSE REACTIONS TO COSMETICS (See also Chap. 122)

Irritation Syndrome

Previously considered monomorphous, the irritation syndrome (Ta-ble 251-1) now appears to be a heterogeneous process. It often has an eczematous appearance notwithstanding disparate mechanisms. Several clinical and biological entities have been described, and others await clinical or basic science definition.

OBJECTIVE IRRITATION Skin irritation is defined as localized inflammation that is not mediated through the immune system and is caused by endogenous and environmental factors. Hair straight-

TABLE 251-1

Irritation Syndrome Related to Use of Cosmetics

OBJECTIVE IRRITATION	SUBJECTIVE IRRITATION
Acute or corrosive reaction	Sensory irritation
Irritant dermatitis	
Irritant reaction	
Cumulative irritation	
Mechanical irritation	
Acneiform and pustular eruption	
Phototoxic reaction (photoirritation)	

eners, permanents, and depilatories can cause *acute reactions* if di-rections for their safe use are not strictly followed. Cleansers are frequently responsible for causing *irritant dermatitis*. Moisturizers or emollient creams, in which water and oleacous materials are blended, contain surfactants and emulsifiers that are often mild ir-ritants. When these cosmetics are applied to the face or to dry or eczematous skin, where the stratum corneum is a less efficient bar-rier, *irritant reactions* may result. Morphologic features include scaling, which may rapidly clear with avoidance of exposure but becomes erythematous with recurrent dosing and may evolve into chronic irritant dermatitis. Some cosmetics produce irritation only after repeated application; this phenomenon is termed *cumulative irritation*. Friction, injury, and *mechanical irritation* can be caused by popular cosmetics containing granules or by devices (e.g., syn-thetic sponges) used to exfoliate the skin.

Sensitive bioengineering techniques used to evaluate the patho-physiology of irritation include transepidermal water loss, skin im-pedance, conductance resistance, and blood flow velocity.[11,12] Us-ing predictive testing in animals and humans, manufacturers can recognize strong or moderate irritant ingredients or products. In pre-market testing, mild irritants are more difficult to detect and quan-tify.

Some skin and hair care cosmetics cause acneiform eruptions. The term *acnegenicity* encompasses both comedogenicity, which refers to follicular keratin impaction,[13] and papulopustular forma-tion.[14,15] The time course for the appearance of facial papulopus-tules and comedones is different: papulopustules may appear in just a few days, whereas the appearance of comedones is delayed.[16] Considerable confusion derives from the testing techniques: for ex-ample, isopropyl myristate in concentrations as low as 10% in pet-rolatum rapidly induces comedones in the rabbit ear but yields pap-ulopustules in humans. Even common emulsifiers such as sodium lauryl sulfate produce pustules in a dose-related manner. The mech-anisms appear to be related in spite of varied morphology. The European Community's proposed ban on animal testing of final products will result in stronger reliance on human testing, whether this takes the form of use tests, application of a cosmetic under occlusion to the back for 4 weeks and subsequent cyanoacrylate biopsies (to identify microcomedones), or both.[17,18]

The clinical significance of cosmetics in precipitating post-adolescent acne in women has recently been called into question by one of the authors of the original paper on "acne cosmetica."[13,19] To avoid total confusion in light of this development, it seems pru-dent to advise female acne patients to keep their cosmetic regimen of care simple and gentle, using products from manufacturers who test for acnegenicity.

Bergamot oil (5-methoxypsoralen) is a phototoxic fragrance ingredient that was used in cosmetics but has since been removed. As interest in "natural" ingredients increases, new phototoxins may be inadvertently introduced and have serious consequences.

SUBJECTIVE IRRITATION Burning, stinging, or itching caused by application of a cosmetic or topical medicament without detectable visible or microscopic change is termed *sensory irritation*. This reaction usually occurs on the face within an hour of application in susceptible individuals. In a segment of the population, this sensory response is caused by many ingredients in dosages that do not produce clinically *objective irritation*. Examples of such ingredients are propylene glycol, benzoic acid, hydroxy acids, and ethanol.

To identify susceptible persons ("stingers"), Frosch and Kligman[20] applied 5% lactic acid to the nasolabial fold when the subject was sweating profusely; about 20 percent of the population experiences an unpleasant sensation under these circumstances. Some test modifications have recently been introduced to increase reproducibility.[21] Stingers do not have a higher incidence of atopy or dry skin but do report frequent adverse reactions to cosmetics.

Fortunately, sensory irritation can now be inhibited by blockers.[22] These materials will be incorporated into skin care products such as those containing α-hydroxy and β-hydroxy acids.

Contact Urticaria Syndrome

Contact urticaria syndrome typically consists of a wheal-and-flare response developing within 30 to 60 min after the skin is exposed to certain agents. Symptoms range from the mildest manifestations (e.g., itching, tingling, burning, and erythema) to the most severe (e.g., anaphylaxis and death). Diagnosis of immediate contact urticaria is based on a thorough medical history (including notation of burn, sting, or itch resulting from skin contact; urticaria; or respiratory symptoms) and skin testing using suspected substances as summarized by von Krogh and Maibach.[23]

Contact urticaria syndrome is divided into two subtypes—nonimmunologic and immunologic—based on proposed pathophysiologic mechanisms.[24] Nonimmunologic contact urticaria, the most common form, occurs in the absence of previous exposure and remains localized, causing no systemic symptoms. Typically, the strength of the reaction varies by ingredient concentration and location of use. The mechanism is not completely delineated. Benzoic acid, cinnamic acid, and cinnamal are commonly used in cosmetics and are potent substances capable of eliciting this response.

Immunologic contact urticaria is an immediate type I allergic reaction that occurs in sensitized individuals and is induced more frequently in atopic individuals. The eliciting chemicals react with specific IgE molecules on mast-cell membranes. Localized urticaria can extend beyond the site of contact or may be accompanied by other symptoms such as rhinitis, conjunctivitis, asthma, and anaphylaxis. In this manner, methylparaben, ethylparaben, henna, and ammonium persulfate have been associated with systemic reactions.

Delayed Hypersensitivity Reactions

Adverse reactions to cosmetics constitute a small but significant portion of contact dermatitis cases treated by dermatologists. In a study conducted by the North American Contact Dermatitis Group (NACDG), patch testing showed contact dermatitis related to cosmetics in 5% of 13,216 patients evaluated[25]; similar percentages

TABLE 251-2

Cosmetics Not Safely Applied "as Is" in Closed Patch Tests

Shampoos	Cuticle removers
Soaps	Nail polish removers
Detergent foaming cleansers	Nail glues
Foaming bath products	Nail extenders
Shaving lathers	Depilatories
Dentifrices	Bleaching creams
Hair bleach or boosters	Permanent-waving solutions
Straighteners	Hair dyes

Dry thoroughly before covering in closed patch tests:

Mascara	Hair spray
Nail polish	

have been reported from Europe.[26,27] These figures underestimate the total number of cases, because most trivial reactions are not investigated by dermatologists. In the NACDG study, 59 percent of the cosmetic-induced reactions occurred on the face and 79 percent were seen in women, but relation to cosmetics was suspected by the dermatologist or patient initially in fewer than half the cases. Diagnosis of allergic contact dermatitis is based on a compatible history and examination supported by results of patch testing. Most cosmetics are not strong irritants and can be patch-tested closed in the usual manner; however, notable exceptions exist[28] (Table 251-2). Weakly positive reactions should be confirmed by medical history, test repetition, and patch testing of ingredients. Ingredient testing is problematic in the United States because of the limited number of chemicals available on screening trays (Table 251-3). It is important to recognize which of these allergens are found in cosmetics. *Cosmetic Industry on Call*[10] provides information for contacting manufacturers who may provide ingredients for patch testing. De Groot et al.[29] provide reference information on chemical concentrations and vehicles to use in testing cosmetic ingredients.

The Provocative Use Test (PUT), also called the Repeat Open Application Test (ROAT),[30] is a practical way to screen for allergy to cosmetics including fragrances[31] or to confirm the clinical significance of weak positive reactions. The cosmetic is applied twice

TABLE 251-3

Ingredients Found in Cosmetics Included on Screening Trays

	PRESENCE OF INGREDIENT	
INGREDIENT	SCREENING SERIES	T.R.U.E.*
Colophony (rosin)	●	●
Fragrance mix		●
Paraphenylenediamine	●	●
Imidazolidinyl urea	●	
Cinnamic aldehyde (cinnamal)	●	
Lanolin alcohol (wool alcohols)	●	●
Formaldehyde	●	●
Quaternium-15	●	●
Balsam of Peru	●	●
Paraben mix		●
Thimerosal		●
Methylchloroisothiazolinone + methylisothiazolinone		●

*Thin-layer rapid-use epicutaneous test.

Frequently Identified Cosmetic Ingredients Causing Allergic Contact Dermatitis: North American Contact Dermatitis Group (NACDG) Study

Paraphenylenediamine (PPD)
Lanolin and derivatives
Glyceryl thioglycolate
Propylene glycol
Toluene sulfonamide/formaldehyde resin
Sunscreens and other UV absorbers
Methacrylates

SOURCE: Adapted and reproduced by permission of the authors and publisher from Adams and Maibach.[25]

daily for up to 2 weeks to an approximately 5-cm area on the flexor surface of the forearm near the antecubital area.

Most photoallergic ingredients in cosmetics are sunscreening agents or fragrances. To test for photoallergy, the patch site is exposed to between 5 and 10 J of ultraviolet A (UVA) 24 h after application; after 48 h, the photo patch site is compared with a non-irradiated site similarly patch-tested.

Most allergic reactions to cosmetics are caused by fragrances, preservatives, and a small number of other ingredients.[25–27] Familiarity with these allergens will enable clinicians to diagnose most of these cases accurately. Table 251-4 surveys the American experience.[25] Europeans add emulsifiers as significant sensitizers.[27]

FRAGRANCES

Fragrance allergy is common, affecting approximately 1 percent of the general population; dermatitis may develop on the face, neck, hands, and axillae or it may be generalized.[32]

Fragrances are ubiquitous: in addition to cosmetics and toiletries, they are added to household goods or cleansers in the workplace, and some are used as flavorings. Paradoxically, "unscented" cosmetics may contain a masking fragrance. A new method of promoting fragrances is to claim that scents have mood-altering effects—so-called aromatherapy.[33] Inevitably, troublesome sensitization has occurred in consumers who have doused themselves and their surroundings with fragrance.[34] Since 1966, toxicologic information related to fragrance ingredients has been assembled and assessed by the industry-sponsored Research Institute for Fragrance Materials (RIFM).[32,35] Based on this information, the International Fragrance Association (IFRA) publishes guidelines that industry members generally agree to follow.

Photosensitization occurred more commonly before methyl coumarin and musk ambrette were eliminated from fragrances. Sensitization to musk ambrette left an extensive legacy of so-called persistent light eruptions. Because fragrance allergy is frequently not suspected by either the patient or the physician, patch testing is an important tool for reaching this diagnosis. Balsam of Peru, cinnamal, fragrance mix, and colophony are recognized markers for fragrance allergy on patch-test screening series. At present, the fragrance mix [marketed by Hermal and by Chemotechnique and also marketed as T.R.U.E. (Thin-layer Rapid Use Epicutaneous Test) by Glaxo Wellcome] contains eight ingredients: eugenol, isoeugenol, oak moss absolute, geraniol, cinnamal, α-amyl cinnamic aldehyde, hydroxycitronellal, and cinnamic alcohol. In an international study of 165 patients who had probable fragrance allergy, the fragrance mix detected 86 percent of positive reactions.[36] Addition of ylang-ylang oil, narcissus oil, sandalwood oil, and balsam of Peru raised this percentage to 96 percent. Racial and geographic distinctions exist; for instance, Japanese patients tested were more frequently reactive to benzyl salicylate. Such racial differences were highlighted by the epidemic of bizarre facial hyperpigmentation seen in Japanese women in the 1960s and 1970s, which was caused by allergy to fragrances and coal-tar dyes used in some cosmetics; elimination of these allergens solved the problem.[37]

Allergy to fragrance can be tested by using ROAT for 2 weeks.[31] Balsams, cinnamic alcohol, cinnamaldehyde, benzoic acid, and benzaldehyde are fragrance ingredients that can evoke contact urticaria not detected by closed patch testing.

PRESERVATIVES

Preservatives are added to prevent contamination of cosmetics by microorganisms, which degrade the product or cause infection in consumers; but the term *preservatives* may encompass agents that prevent degradation induced by oxidation or ultraviolet light. Approximately 60 chemicals are commonly used as preservatives in cosmetics.[38] Preservatives may consist of a single ingredient or a mixture of ingredients (e.g., methylchloroisothiazolinone and methylisothiazolinone). Use of specific preservatives varies among American, European, and Asian markets; consequently, the incidence of allergic reactions to individual agents also varies. These chemicals penetrate cells and disturb their function; therefore, they not surprisingly cause adverse reactions and so have prompted development of preservative-free cosmetics. Strategies for developing such products include modification of the manufacturing and packaging processes as well as use of botanicals, which have antimicrobial activity. The increasing complexity of cosmetics and their vehicles makes this goal even more difficult to achieve.

Paraben esters, the most popular group of preservatives, are effective against fungi and gram-positive (but not gram-negative) bacteria. Parabens rarely sensitize but may do so when applied to eczematous skin. Sensitized patients frequently tolerate parabens in cosmetics applied to normal skin.[39]

Propylene glycol, a popular solvent and humectant, has antimicrobial properties but is used in some "preservative-free" cosmetics. Interpretation of irritant and sensitization patch test studies of >200 subjects suggests that propylene glycol is a mild irritant that occasionally sensitizes.[40]

Formaldehyde and formaldehyde releasers are widely used.[41] Formaldehyde is formulated in wash-off products such as shampoos. Imidazolidinyl urea is the preservative used third most frequently in American cosmetics and accounts for some reactions, but diazolidinyl urea introduced in the 1980s may elicit more allergic reactions proportionately. DMDM hydantoin and quaternium-15 are frequently classified as sensitizers, but DMDM hydantoin is appearing in more formulations whereas quaternium-15 is appearing less frequently.[38]

When introduced into Europe as a preservative, methylchloroisothiazolinone/methylisothiazolinone was used extensively in concentrations, which frequently caused sensitization.[27] Benefiting from the European experience and in an effort to diminish the problem, CIR set guidelines restricting concentration to ≤15 ppm in wash-off products and to ≤7.5 ppm in leave-on products.

A mixture of methyldibromoglutaronitrile and phenoxyethanol (Euxoyl 400) used initially in Europe has gained popularity and is being reported more frequently as an allergen.[42] Butylated hydroxyanisole (BHA), butylated hydroxytoluene (BHT), tocopherol, propyl gallate, and t-butyl hydroquinone used as antioxidants are sometimes reported as allergens. Other ingredients reported frequently as allergens in cosmetics include paraphenylenediamine, toluenesulfonamide/formaldehyde resin (tolysamide/formaldehyde resin), acrylates, lanolin, glyceryl thioglycolate, and UV light-absorbing agents. These will be discussed below in reviewing cosmetic categories.

Cosmetic Intolerance Syndrome and "Sensitive Skin"

Cosmetic intolerance syndrome is not a single entity but rather a symptom complex of multiple exogenous and endogenous factors (Table 251-5). The syndrome is an uncommon clinical entity in which patients complain bitterly of facial burning and discomfort associated with application of most skin care products. Their skin may show overt inflammatory changes, or symptoms may be only subjective. These patients seriously challenge practitioners' empathy and diagnostic skills because the severity of symptoms does not match objective signs of disease. Many patients affected with this syndrome have tried a myriad of cosmetics and topical medications. Gradually, over the past two decades, most of these individuals have been recognized to have an organic rather than a functional basis for their complaints.

Fisher[43] coined the term *status cosmeticus* for the condition in which patients no longer tolerate use of any facial cosmetic product. Some of these patients initially experience subjective or objective irritation in response to use of cosmetics and become intolerant to many other topical agents during the evolution of this disorder. Other patients have occult allergic contact dermatitis, allergic photocontact dermatitis, contact urticarial reaction, or a combination of these conditions. In this group, causal agents can be documented by careful clinical review and patch testing.

Other patients have a seborrheic-rosacea diathesis which flares and is accompanied by facial erythema and scaling when use of soap and water is abandoned and cleansing creams and emollients are overused. Atopic dermatitis and dry skin are other factors that predispose patients to this condition.

Strictly observing a prolonged program of eliminating cosmetics is an important therapeutic intervention (Table 251-6). Some patients are able to return gradually to using other cosmetics after 6

TABLE 251-5

Types and Causes of Facial Skin Intolerance to Cosmetics

Exogenous causes	Endogenous causes
Subjective irritation	Seborrhea/psoriasis
Objective irritation	Rosacea and perioral dermatitis
Contact urticaria	Atopic dermatitis
Allergic contact dermatitis	Dysmorphobia
Photoallergic contact dermatitis	

SOURCE: Adapted and reproduced by permission of the publisher from Maibach and Engasser.[28]

TABLE 251-6

Diagnosis and Treatment of Patients Whose Skin Is Intolerant to Cosmetics

Examine every cosmetic and skin care product
Administer patch and photo patch test to rule out occult allergic and photoallergic dermatitis
Test for contact urticaria
Do careful repeat open application testing (ROAT)

Treat endogenous inflammatory disease
Limit skin care to
    Water washing without soap or detergent
    Lip cosmetics as desired if lips are clear
    Eye cosmetics as desired if eyelids are asymptomatic
    Face powder
    Glycerin and rose water as a moisturizer if necessary
    Avoiding other cosmetics for 6 to 12 months

to 12 months. Subsequent additions to the skin care regimen can be made one at a time every 2 weeks. For the final regimen, the number of cosmetics and frequency of their use should remain limited.

Other patients experience facial burning continuously without showing objective signs. Cotterill[44] described these patients as having "dermatologic nondisease." Many of these patients have a disturbed body image or dysmorphobia—i.e., they complain of physical defects that lack objective evidence. Many are depressed and require psychiatric help, which they frequently reject.

Sensitive skin covers the same range of pathophysiology as cosmetic intolerance syndrome but it is generally less severe. *Sensitive skin* is a lay term coined to describe the condition of consumers who believe their skin is less tolerant than that of the average person's to environmental conditions and topical preparations. Up to 40 percent of the population believe that they have sensitive skin. The largest segment of these consumers manifest sensory skin irritation.

SKIN CARE COSMETICS

Cleansing Agents

Cleansing the skin removes environmental contaminants, sweat, sebum, desquamated cells, and microorganisms. Soap bars are manufactured by saponification of fat and alkali, and "syndet" bars contain synthetic detergents to emulsify lipids which will then be rinsed off with water. Originally, wipe-off cleansing creams containing mineral oil and borax were commonly used as cleansing agents. Detergents are often used in rinse-off foaming lotions. Lipid-free cleansing lotions contain fatty alcohols and are meant to be wiped or rinsed off. In the 1950s, liquid soaps were developed for cleansing workers' hands and were perceived as harsh; liquid cleansers and gels evolved in the 1970s and 1980s to become popular as gentle hand, face, or body washes using blends of surfactants (including nonionics), which are claimed to be less irritating.[45] Fatty acids and polymers are added to enhance mildness. Antimicrobial agents [chloroxylenol (PCMX) or triclosan] are used in cleansers whose manufacturers make antibacterial claims.

Use of cleansers may cause irritation, to which subsets of the population (such as persons who are elderly or who have atopic

by soap-chamber tests or by use tests, which may be exaggerated.
Visually or with instrumentation, these tests indicate barrier injury,
inflammation, dryness, or skin roughness. Factors that influence irritancy are the structure and quantity of surfactant, mechanical
trauma, water temperature, and duration and frequency of cleansing.

Because wash-off products are in contact with the skin briefly,
they infrequently cause allergic contact dermatitis; however, some
surfactants (cocamidopropyl betaine), preservatives (methylchloro-
isothiazolinone/methylisothiazolinone), antimicrobials (PCMX),
and fragrances have been reported as allergens in these products.

Shaving Products

Foaming shaving creams or gels are designed to wet and soften the
beard hair in order to reduce the friction caused by a metal blade
cutting the hair. Lubricants are added to these fatty acid soaps to
decrease frictional forces as the blade traverses the skin. Preshave
cosmetics for use with electric razors are fragranced alcohol products that dry the skin and reduce friction. Aftershaves are fragrance
cosmetics applied to freshly shaven skin with a compromised barrier, which partially accounts for the frequency of allergic and photoallergic reactions reported in the past when photosensitizers such
as musk ambrette were present.

Hair Removers

Superfluous hair may be disguised by bleaching or removed by
shaving, waxing, plucking, chemical dissolution, or electrolysis.[46]
Laser hair removal is under development. For some patients who
have curly beard hair and are susceptible to pseudofolliculitis barbae, use of barium sulfide depilatories is a helpful but malodorous
and irritating alternative to shaving.

Most modern depilatories contain substituted thiols. Calcium
thioglycolates are favored because they are the least irritating. They
act more slowly than sulfides but are safer. Thioglycolates attack
keratin and may injure the epidermis; manufacturers' directions
should be followed closely.

Deodorants/Antiperspirants

These popular cosmetics are designed for use in the axillae, whose
apocrine sweat glands produce organic chemicals metabolized by
bacteria to produce an odor generally considered undesirable.[47] Eccrine sweat distributes these chemicals more broadly. Deodorants
contain antimicrobial agents (e.g., triclosan) as well as fragrance to
mask odor. Antiperspirants use aluminum salts, which theoretically
cause temporary plugging of the eccrine sweat glands to reduce
their output and decrease the bacterial population. Aluminum salts
may cause irritant reactions, but the allergic reactions associated
with these products are caused by fragrance or by other ingredients.

Moisturizers

Moisturizers improve the appearance and tactile properties of dry
and aging skin by acting on the stratum corneum to diminish scaling
and enhance suppleness, supposedly by increasing its water content.[48,49] Dry skin is dry and not just rough.[50] Traditionally, moisturization is considered to inhibit transepidermal water loss by occlusion. The "bricks and mortar" model illuminates the stratum
corneum's role as an active membrane [51,52] (see Chap. 12). Loss of
intercellular lipids (i.e., ceramides, cholesterol, and fatty acids that

form bilayers) damages the water-barrier function and calls into
play repair mechanisms signaled into action by the stratum corneum. In this way, treating dry skin has consequences in the viable
epidermis.

Usually containing mixtures of water and fatty substances such
as petrolatum, lanolin, lanolin derivatives, and fatty alcohols, moisturizers decrease scale and transiently increase water content in the
stratum corneum. Several theoretical mechanisms are popular:
(1) occlusion—i.e., allowing water to percolate up from the viable
epidermis; (2) replacement or assisted synthesis of lipid mixtures in
the intercellular spaces[6,53]; and (3) use of humectants, which bind
water in the stratum corneum. Success of these maneuvers is determined in the laboratory by measuring transepidermal water loss,
impedance, and conductance[54] as well as by epidermal capacitance
and regression testing.[55] But discerning consumers judge by the feel
and appearance of their skin, which introduces the criterion of es-
thetics. Moisturizers prevent irritant dermatitis caused by detergents,[56,57] and the efficacy of moisturizers is related to their lipid
mass.

A semisolid mixture of hydrocarbons obtained from dewaxed
heavy mineral oils, petrolatum, is a uniquely effective moisturizer
as a result of mechanisms not fully understood. Petrolatum delays
water evaporation from the stratum corneum. In contrast to a vapor-
impermeable membrane (e.g., latex), petrolatum does not impede
barrier lipid repair in acetone-stripped stratum corneum and enhances immediate repair.[4,58] Petrolatum is not a primary or cumulative irritant and can protect against irritant effects of detergents.[59]
The acnegenicity and comedogenicity of petrolatum have been
questioned by Kligman,[19] and high-quality, cosmetic-grade petrolatum appears to be safe in this regard. Unfortunately, large amounts
impart a tacky feel, which consumers do not like.

Lanolin and its derivatives are more esthetically acceptable and
are good emulsifiers. Lanolin is a mixture of esters and polyesters
of high-molecular-weight alcohols and fatty acids. Recent work
studying tape strippings shows that lanolin penetrates the entire stratum corneum and appears to emulsify intercellular water.[60] Although lanolin has been reported to be an allergen in 2 to 5 percent
of patients who received patch tests,[61,62] it infrequently causes reactions on normal skin but can sensitize when applied to eczematous skin, especially in stasis dermatitis. Cronin[62] reported 26 cases
of lanolin-cosmetic facial dermatitis in women, for half of whom
the eyelids were affected to a striking degree. Wool alcohols (30%
in petrolatum) and Amerchol L 101 (50% in petrolatum) are used
in patch tests to screen for allergy.

Three types of lipid—cholesterol, free fatty acids, and ceramides—are required for maintaining the epidermal permeability
barrier. All three lipids in proper molar proportions are alleged to
be necessary. These data are being used to formulate moisturizers.[53]

Glycerin and propylene glycol function as humectants. Studies
of moisturizers containing glycerin showed formation of a glycerin
reservoir in the stratum corneum, suggesting a role in barrier repair
and in preventing transition of stratum corneum lipids to a solid
crystalline state.[63]

The hygroscopic properties of urea allow it to bind water quickly
in the stratum corneum, especially at high humidity.[54] Incorporating
urea in hydrophilic ointment enhances the water binding capacity
for at least several hours, but this function is lost at lowered humidity.

Smoothing rough skin and minimizing signs of aging fit consumers' broad definition of moisturizering. Consequently, kerato-

lytic agents (i.e., α-hydroxy and β-hydroxy acids) have become extremely popular ingredients in skin care products. In 1974, α-hydroxy acids were proposed for treatment of keratinizing disorders,[64] and lactic acid was noted to improve dry skin[65]; however, no major launch of a cosmetic containing α-hydroxy acid occurred until 1992. Hydroxy acids at low concentrations diminish corneocyte adhesion at the lower level of the stratum corneum, stimulate epidermal cell proliferation, and increase the thickness of viable epidermis. The thinner stratum corneum they create is more flexible. The α-hydroxy acids can stimulate glycosaminoglycans and may promote collagen synthesis. Consumers perceive improved skin texture, brightness, and firmness as well as less wrinkling and pigmentation.[66] Like the drug tretinoin, hydroxy acids modify some of the adverse effects of sun exposure (photoaging). If formulated properly, α-hydroxy acids may be useful for treating acne, and salicylic acid—a lipid-soluble β-hydroxy acid—has been used for decades for this purpose.

Improved formulations reduced the irritation and unpleasant odor of skin care products. In general, lower pH and higher concentration increases penetration of these ingredients. The CIR concluded that glycolic acid, lactic acid, and their common salts and esters are safe for use in cosmetics at concentrations $\leq 10\%$ when the product is at pH ≥ 3.5 and formulated to avoid increasing sun sensitivity or when directions for use specify daily use of sun protection.[67] The FDA has proposed further toxicologic study.

Reactive oxygen species (e.g., free radicals) arise from UV light and from other insults that damage cells. Theoretically these chemical species are partly responsible for aging. Antioxidants such as vitamins A, C, and E and their derivatives are added to cosmetics in an attempt to block this injury.[68] To prove that this can be accomplished using any of these agents as currently administered, the complex chemistry of these oxidative processes must be further studied.

Sun-screening agents are added to many cosmetics to prevent photodamage to skin. In the United States, sunscreens are regulated as over-the-counter drugs. The list of permitted ingredients, methods of efficacy testing, and labeling standards are published as regulations in the *Federal Register*.[69]

Self-Tanning Agents

"Sunless" or "self-tanning" lotions containing dihydroxyacetone are regulated as cosmetics, although they do provide some protection from long UVA light.[70,71] Dihydroxyacetone binds to the skin's surface keratin, producing a brown pigment that fades only as corneocytes desquamate. These products have become popular because they can give the illusion of a tan. During the shelf life of these cosmetics, dihydroxyacetone can degrade to form formaldehyde, formic acid, and acetic acid.[72] Adverse contact dermatitis may therefore be irritant as well as allergic.

In 1995, the European Commission ordered the withdrawal of cosmetics containing 5-methoxypsoralen because of possible skin cancer risk. This phototoxin had been added to sun products to enhance tanning.

Bleaching Agents

Hydroquinone inhibits conversion of tyrosine to melanin. Nonprescription bleaching creams containing up to 2.0% hydroquinone are modestly effective in treating some pigmentary disorders.[73] Con-

sumers use these cosmetics to treat postinflammatory hyperpigmentation, lentigines, and melasma. Successful treatment of melasma requires strict protection from UV light. Adverse effects associated with use of bleaching creams include irritant and allergic reactions, hypopigmentation, hyperpigmentation, exogenous ochronosis, and staining of the nails.

Irregular pigmentation is a major cosmetic complaint of consumers worldwide, and chemicals including azelaic acid, kojic acid, antioxidants, and plant extracts are being investigated.

Makeup

Makeup has been used since ancient times to normalize, glamorize, and accentuate features or to create a stylized appearance. Camouflage techniques using specially designed opaque cosmetics have been developed by skilled makeup artists and can be taught to patients with disfiguring disorders, greatly benefiting these patients' psychological well-being.[74]

Sales of ethnic cosmetics have burgeoned in the 1990s, and jet-milled and coated pigments have enabled the development of darker makeup shades, which require more pigment. The most important trend in mass-market color cosmetics is the use of silicone technology to produce long-lasting formulations for lipsticks, foundations, and related products.

To be permitted in makeup, colors must be government-certified for use; consequently, they seldom cause adverse reactions. The United States has certified 34 colors, but only 13 of these are certified in all three major markets (Japan, Europe, and the United States). Most makeup can be tested for allergenicity in the standard manner using a closed patch test. Waterproof mascara is an important exception: it contains volatile solvents and must be dried thoroughly to avoid severe irritant reactions. Upper-eyelid dermatitis syndrome is related to multiple endogenous and exogenous causes. Irritant and allergic contact dermatitis caused by cosmetics accounts for a small percentage of these cases.[28] Mercury preservatives are permitted only in cosmetics designed for use in the eye area owing to the danger of *Pseudomonas* infection. Eye infections are rarely traced to use of eye cosmetics that have not been adequately preserved.

HAIR CARE COSMETICS

Shampoos and Conditioners

Shampoos are cleansing agents designed to remove sebum, scale, microorganisms, and environmental debris. Thorough cleansing can leave hair dry, statically charged, and without luster. Modern shampoos contain single or combined anionic, amphoteric, cationic, or nonionic surfactants that vary in their ability to clean as well as to leave hair manageable. Products designed for use on dry, normal, or oily hair inform consumers regarding cleansing intensity, which is determined by type and concentration of surfactants. Baby shampoos contain amphoteric surfactants that do not sting the eyes and which cleanse moderately well.

Conditioning agents are used in hair care products for many purposes—to enhance combability of wet and dry hair, to neutralize static charges, and to promote the appearance, feel, fullness, luster, and general manageability of hair.[75] Long hair, hair that is frequently shampooed, chemically exposed and treated hair, and dry hair require conditioners to aid grooming, prevent damage, and enhance appearance. Quaternium compounds, hydrolyzed proteins, cationic surfactants, polymers, lipids, glycols, and silicones are the most commonly used conditioners. Some recently marketed shampoos simultaneously cleanse and deposit conditioning agents on the hair shaft. Conditioning can be modified to enhance volume for fine, straight hair without causing buildup. For hair damaged extensively by chemicals, application of conditioner separately after shampooing allows deposition of more material. Shampoos also contain thickeners, foam boosters, colors, and preservatives.

Shampoos and conditioners are only briefly in contact with the skin and infrequently cause adverse contact reactions. Allergic reactions have been reported to occur both in consumers and in beauticians using the "mild" amphoteric surfactant cocamidopropyl betaine.[76] Formaldehyde and a combination of methylchloroisothiazolone and methylisothiazolone are preservatives that have also caused allergic contact dermatitis.

Hair Dyes

Hair coloring has become increasingly popular worldwide: in the United States alone, an estimated 46 million women color their hair. These versatile cosmetics allow men and women to add highlights, change color, or disguise gray hair. In addition to bleaches, hair dyes are classified as temporary, progressive, semipermanent, or permanent.

Temporary colors are deposited on the surface of the hair and are removed by shampooing. They make minor changes in shade or blend gray hair. Dyestuffs used can include basic dyes, indolamine, indophenols, and azo, azine, or thiazine derivatives[77] and are generally harmless.

Progressive lead acetate dyes deposit lead oxides and sulfides, which build on the hair shaft when applied repeatedly. Used almost exclusively by men to conceal graying, these dyes preclude successful perming or use of other color systems. Use of metallic dyes is not considered to put consumers at risk for acute toxicity except when such dyes are accidentally ingested by children.[78] In 1980, the FDA declared these dyes safe after reviewing data on human absorption of lead during simulated use.[79] Recent research has shown that lead from these dyes can contaminate households and therefore might be a special hazard for children who live in these households.[80]

Color from semipermanent dyes lasts through about a dozen shampoos. When used on unbleached hair, these dyes can add new tones to natural hair, cover as much as 50 percent of gray hair, and occasionally improve the appearance of permanently tinted hair. Semipermanent hair-coloring products use low-molecular-weight dyes that penetrate the hair cuticle. These dyes are mostly derivatives of nitroanilines, nitrophenylenediamines, and nitroaminophenols.[81] In the past several years, some of these products have been modified by adding a low percentage of peroxide for a more lasting effect. These formulations have been called *tone on tone*.

Permanent hair dyes contain colorless precursors that react with hydrogen peroxide inside the hair shaft to produce permanent hair colors. Primary intermediates such as *p*-phenylenediamine or *p*-aminophenol are oxidized by hydrogen peroxide and react with many different couplers (e.g., resorcin) to produce a range of shades. Owing to their esthetic appeal, coal-tar hair dyes are popular; however, they can cause allergic reactions (mostly to *p*-phenylenediamine) and satisfactory substitutes are often unavailable. Semipermanent dyes may not induce a cross-reaction, but they do not cover gray nearly as successfully as permanent dyes.

Bleaches

Hair bleaches—hydrogen peroxide solutions that oxidize melanin to a lighter color—may be supplemented with persulfate boosters. Ammonium persulfate does cause types I and IV allergic contact reactions.[24] The type I reaction has rarely progressed to systemic reaction in consumers, whereas type IV can result in hand dermatitis for frequent users such as hairdressers.

Permanents

Permanents allow reconfiguration of the hair fiber while it remains wound around a curling rod. In this process, mercaptans cleave the disulfide bonds in hair so that they can later be reformed in a new configuration when neutralized[82,83]:

$$Ker\text{-}S\text{-}S\text{-}Ker + 2RS\text{-}H \longleftrightarrow 2Ker\text{-}S\text{-}H + R\text{-}S\text{-}S\text{-}R$$

keratin   mercaptan   reduced keratin   disulfide
(cystine)   (cysteine)

$$2Ker\text{-}S\text{-}H + H_2O_2 \longleftrightarrow Ker\text{-}S\text{-}S\text{-}Ker + 2H_2O$$

reduced keratin   hydrogen   new keratin bond
(cysteine)   peroxide   (cystine)

Neutralizers contain hydrogen peroxide, potassium or sodium bromate, perbromates, percarbonates, or sodium borate perhydrate. Curled hair appears more voluminous, so women with fine, thin hair often use permanents to give the illusion of a fuller head of hair.

Ammonium thioglycolate applied improperly can cause extensive hair damage and acute irritant dermatitis, but glyceryl thioglycolate used in "acid" permanents initiates allergic contact dermatitis.[84] Sodium sulfite is used in some home permanent kits, and cystine waving solutions have become popular in Japan.

Ethnic Hair Products

Extremely curly hair may be straightened mechanically by pressing or by using chemical relaxers.[85] After the pressing oils are applied, heated metal combs or round tongs are used to straighten the hair. In the early 1900s, pressing oils consisted of heavy waxes in a petrolatum base; lanolin, phenyldimethicone, and dimethicone now allow production of lighter preparations which leave hair silkier and less greasy.

In the 1940s, sodium and potassium hydroxide containing preparations were introduced as chemical straighteners that permanently changed the configuration of kinky hair, and a petrolatum "base" was applied to the scalp for protection. Gentler to the scalp are "no-lye" relaxers: lithium hydroxide and guanidine hydroxide (made by mixing calcium hydroxide and guanidine carbonate). Neutralizing acid shampoos are applied after the hair has been relaxed; these shampoos contain mixtures of anionic and amphoteric surfactants combined with cationic polymers for conditioning. Relaxing damages the hair; therefore, particular care must be taken when relaxing new growth not to overlap and double-process the hair, causing breakage.

As certain "looks" become popular for ethnic hair styles, the cosmetics necessary to achieve those styles fluctuate in popularity. In the early 1980s, thioglycolate permanents were used on African-American hair to produce "soft curls," and a curl activator—a glycerin spray—was used to condition hair that had been given a permanent. This style had drawbacks because the hair was always moist; it also soiled easily, and therefore soft curls subsequently became less popular. Recently introduced kits combine a no-lye relaxer, conditioner, and color, enabling consumers to combine three processes at one session.

NAIL COSMETICS

Used judiciously, nail cosmetics can protect and enhance the esthetic appearance of nails. Although professional manicures may be complex procedures involving many products, most adverse reactions (aside from mechanical trauma) are caused by nail polish or by acrylates used for nail enhancement.

Nail Polish

Nail polishes, including base and top coats, are of a similar composition, containing the following types of ingredients[86]: (1) a film former of nitrocellulose; (2) resins to improve adhesion and gloss; (3) plasticizers to increase flexibility; (4) solvents and diluents to modify viscosity; (5) colors; and (6) suspending agents to prevent pigments from settling. Most reported allergic reactions to nail enamel have been caused by tolysamide/formaldehyde resin (toluene sulfonamide/formaldehyde resin). In a study of 3549 patients patch-tested between 1992 and 1994, 2 percent of the positive reactions were caused by this resin and 85 percent of these reactions were clinically relevant.[87] Allergic contact dermatitis to nail polish can be misdiagnosed because it frequently affects the face, eyelids, sides of the neck, or mouth and may spare the hands and fingers. In a study of tolysamide/formaldehyde-allergic patients referred to an occupational dermatology clinic, the allergen had not previously been detected; instead the cause was mistakenly attributed to work conditions.[88] The consequences of this mistake were dramatic: 11 of the 18 patients in the study erroneously took sick leave or modified or changed their jobs.[88] Results of patch tests using 10% tolysamide/formaldehyde resin in petrolatum establish the diagnosis, and closed patch tests of dry nail polish were positive in 17 of the 18 patients.[88] New formulations of nail enamels use other resins, so different allergens may emerge.[89]

Nail Elongation Materials

Manicurists enhance natural nails by gluing on preformed prostheses, wrapping and gluing nails with strips of fine cloth, molding acrylic extensions, or adding layers of photodeveloped plastic gels.

Prostheses may consist of plastic nails that cover the entire nail plate, but using cyanoacrylate glue to attach plastic tips to the distal portion of the nail has become popular because their application requires less skill than creating sculptured acrylic extensions. Allergy to instant cyanoacrylate glue can cause nail dystrophy and periungual dermatitis.[90] Acrylics, gels, or wraps are used to smooth and strengthen this form.

Sculptured nails are molded (using liquid acrylic monomers mixed with powdered polymers) onto templates that surround the nail; the sculptured nails are then filed to the desired shape. The liquid may contain a stabilizer such as hydroquinone, plasticizers, and solvents, and the powder contains an initiator (e.g., benzoyl peroxide). Before application, the nail plate is prepared by abrading

it with a file or by painting it with methacrylic acid. As the nail grows out, the base must be filled with new applications of the resin. Infections, paresthesia, nail dystrophies, and allergic dermatitis surrounding the nail and at distant sites have all been reported as a consequence of this procedure.[91,92] Most patients who have inflammatory reactions to sculptured nails are never patch tested, and their reactions are not reported. The chemistry is complex, patterns of cross-reaction are common, and labeling of ingredients in salon products is voluntary and often inadequate. Patch-test data from patients sensitized by the use of acrylic nails suggests that five chemicals may be used as screening patch-test materials: ethyl acrylate, 2-hydroxy ethyl acrylate, ethylene glycol dimethacrylate, ethyl cyanoacrylate, and triethylene glycol diacrylate. In a series of 11 patients, 0.1% ethyl acrylate in petrolatum detected 91 percent of the patients sensitized to these nails.[93]

Ultraviolet light–cured acrylates, known as gels, are also popular for nail enhancement. In studying women sensitized to photobonded acrylic nails, 2-hydroxyethyl methacrylate and ethylene glycol dimethacrylate are useful screening materials for patch testing.[94] Professionals applying these gels had reactions to 15 of the 31 acrylates tested.[95] Complex occupational cases are best evaluated at centers prepared for extended patch testing.

The CIR published a final report on ethyl methacrylate, a frequent ingredient of sculptured nails, and declared it safe as used by professionals; however, it advised against retail sale of products containing ethyl methacrylate because they can sensitize when contacting the skin.[96] However, in a Finnish study, 6 of 23 acrylate-sensitive patients were sensitive to ethyl methacrylate, demonstrating its considerable sensitizing potential.[97]

Despite the adverse reactions seen by dermatologists, the popularity of these cosmetics is great: a myriad of nail salons have opened in the United States during the past decade, supporting the $8-billion-per-year nail care industry.

OCCUPATIONAL HAZARDS

Occupational hand eczema frequently develops in hairdressers. Novice beauticians' hands become dry and chapped from shampooing many clients.[98] Applying moisturizing creams before and after work mitigates this condition. Hairdressers are constantly exposed to sensitizers such as hair dyes, ammonium persulfate, preservatives, amphoteric surfactants, fragrances, and glyceryl thioglycolate.[99] Glyceryl thioglycolate penetrates most protective gloves and remains on customers' hair despite shampooing, making avoidance difficult for the sensitized hairdresser.[84] Rubber gloves worn for protection may prove to be sensitizing. When chronic hand eczema interferes with a beautician's career, patch testing is mandatory to determine if a relevant allergen is causing or aggravating the dermatitis.

Many epidemiologic studies of hairdressers working with coal-tar dyes have looked for a relation between exposure to health hazards and carcinogenesis, but the findings have been equivocal.[78]

CONCLUSIONS

Consumers consider cosmetics useful, industry introduces innovation to enhance their efficacy, and physicians should recognize their functional and psychological importance for patients. Safety considerations must also not be forgotten. We are alerted to this fact by a recent report of mercury poisonings in the United States resulting from use of a mercury-containing cosmetic manufactured in Mexico.[100] Except for small amounts permitted as eye cosmetic preservatives, mercury has long been banned from use in cosmetics sold in major markets. International trade and less stringent laws in some countries can lead unsuspecting consumers to disaster. Skin is not an impermeable membrane, and substances applied for beautification should be monitored carefully.

REFERENCES

1. Kleinfeld VA, Henteleff TO: Legal considerations and regulatory procedures governing cosmetics, in *Cosmetics: Science and Technology,* Vol 3, 2d ed, edited by MS Balsam, E Sagarin. New York, Wiley, 1974, p 503
2. Kligman AM: Why cosmeceuticals? *Cosmet Toiletries* **108**:37, 1993
3. Kligman AM: Cosmeceuticals: Do we need a new category? in *Cosmeceuticals,* edited by P Elsner, HI Maibach. New York, Marcel Dekker, In press
4. Mao-Qiang M et al: Exogenous nonphysiologic vs physiologic lipids: Divergent mechanisms for correction of permeability barrier dysfunction. *Arch Dermatol* **131**:809, 1995
5. Vermeer BJ, Gilchrest BA: Cosmeceuticals: A proposal for rational definition, evaluation, and regulation. *Arch Dermatol* **132**:337, 1996
6. Graham JA, Kligman AM: Physical attractiveness, cosmetic use and self-perception in the elderly. *Int J Cosmet Sci* **7**:85, 1985
7. Goldberg AM et al: The three Rs and biomedical research (editorial). *Science* **272**:1403, 1996
8. Colwell SM: Alternative action. *Soap Cosmet Chem Specialties* **72**:56, 1996
9. *International Cosmetic Ingredient Dictionary,* 6th ed, edited by JA Wenninger, GN McEwen, Jr. Washington, DC, Cosmetic, Toiletry, and Fragrance Association, 1995
10. *Cosmetic Industry on Call 1995–1996,* edited by AS Curry, GN McEwen, F Greene. Washington, DC, Cosmetic, Toiletry and Fragrance Association, 1995
11. *Bioengineering of the Skin: Methods and Instrumentation,* edited by E Berardesca et al. Boca Raton, FL, CRC Press, 1995
12. *Bioengineering of the Skin: Water and the Stratum Corneum,* edited by P Elsner et al. Boca Raton, FL, CRC Press, 1994
13. Kligman AM, Mills OH Jr: "Acne cosmetica." *Arch Dermatol* **106**:843, 1972
14. Bronaugh RL, Maibach HI: Primary irritant, allergic contact, phototoxic, and photoallergic reactions to cosmetics and tests to identify problem products, in *Principles of Cosmetics for the Dermatologist* edited by P Frost, SN Horwitz. St Louis, Mosby, 1982, p 223
15. American Academy of Dermatology invitational symposium on comedogenicity. *J Am Acad Dermatol* **20**:272, 1989
16. Mills OH Jr, Berger RS: Defining the susceptibility of acne-prone and sensitive skin populations to extrinsic factors. *Dermatol Clin* **9**:93, 1991
17. Mills OH Jr, Kligman AM: A human model for assessing comedogenic substances. *Arch Dermatol* **118**:903, 1982
18. Kligman AM, Kwong T: An improved rabbit ear model for assessing comedogenic substances. *Br J Dermatol* **100**:699, 1979
19. Kligman AM: Petrolatum is not comedogenic in rabbits or humans: a critical reappraisal of the rabbit ear assay and the concept of "acne cosmetica." *J Soc Cosmet Chem* **47**:41, 1996
20. Frosch PJ, Kligman AM: A method for appraising the stinging capacity of topically applied substances. *J Soc Cosmet Chem* **28**:197, 1977
21. Christensen M, Kligman AM: An improved procedure for conducting lactic acid stinging tests on facial skin. *J Soc Cosmet Chem* **47**:1, 1996
22. Hahn G: Novel agent that blocks sensory irritation (personal communication).
23. von Krogh G, Maibach HI: The contact urticaria syndrome. *Semin Dermatol* **1**:59, 1982
24. Amin S et al: *Contact Urticaria Syndrome.* Boca Raton, FL, CRC Press, 1997
25. Adams RM, Maibach HI: A five-year study of cosmetic reactions. *J Am Acad Dermatol* **13**:1062, 1985

26. Berne B et al: Adverse effects of cosmetics and toiletries reported to the Swedish Medical Products Agency 1989–1994. *Contact Dermatitis* **34**:359, 1996
27. de Groot AC et al: The allergens in cosmetics. *Arch Dermatol* **124**:1525, 1988
28. Maibach HI, Engasser PG: Dermatitis due to cosmetics, in *Contact Dermatitis,* 3d ed, edited by AA Fisher. Philadelphia, Lea & Febiger, 1986, p 368
29. de Groot AC et al: *Unwanted Effects of Cosmetics and Drugs Used in Dermatology,* 3d ed. New York, Elsevier, 1994
30. Hannuksela M, Salo H: The repeated open application test (ROAT). *Contact Dermatitis* **14**:221, 1986
31. Johansen JD et al: Threshold responses in cinnamic-aldehyde-sensitive subjects: Results and methodological aspects. *Contact Dermatitis* **34**:165, 1996
32. de Groot AC, Frosch PJ: Adverse reactions to fragrances: A clinical review. *Contact Dermatitis* **36**:57, 1997
33. Jackson EM: Aromatherapy. *Am J Contact Dermatitis* **4**:240, 1993
34. Schaller M, Korting HC: Allergic airborne contact dermatitis from essential oils used in aromatherapy. *Clin Exp Dermatol* **20**:143, 1995
35. Opdyke DLJ: Monographs on fragrance raw materials. *Food Cosmet Toxicol* **11**:95–115, 477–495, 855–876, 1011–1081, 1973; **12**:385–405, 517–537, 703–736, Suppl 807–1016, 1974; **13**:91–112, 1975
36. Larsen W et al: Fragrance contact dermatitis: A worldwide multicenter investigation (Part I). *Am J Contact Dermatitis* **7**:77, 1996
37. Nakayama H et al: Pigmented cosmetic dermatitis. *Int J Dermatol* **23**:299, 1984
38. Steinberg DC: Frequency of use of preservatives: A review of the preservatives reported as used in products sold in the United States. *Cosmet Toiletries* **112**:57, 1997
39. Fisher AA: Esoteric contact dermatitis. Part I: The paraben paradox (News). *Cutis* **57**:65, 1996
40. Trancik RJ, Maibach HI: Propylene glycol: Irritation or sensitization? *Contact Dermatitis* **8**:185, 1982
41. Fransway AF: The problem of preservation in the 1990s: I. Statement of the problem, solution(s) of the industry, and the current use of formaldehyde and formaldehyde-releasing biocides. *Am J Contact Dermatitis* **2**:6, 1991
42. de Groot AC, Weyland JW: Contact allergy to methyldibromoglutaronitrile in the cosmetics preservative Euxyl K 400. *Am J Contact Dermatitis* **2**:31, 1991
43. Fisher AA: Cosmetic actions and reactions: Therapeutic irritant, and allergic. *Cutis* **26**:22, 1980
44. Cotterill JA: Clinical features of patients with dermatologic nondisease. *Semin Dermatol* **2**:203, 1983
45. Lundmark L: The evolution of liquid soap. *Cosmet Toiletries* **107**:49, 1992
46. Dawber R: Facial and body hair, in *Cosmetic Dermatology,* edited by R Baran, HI Maibach. London, Martin Dunitz, 1994, p 139
47. Draelos ZD: *Cosmetics in Dermatology,* 2d ed. New York, Churchill Livingstone, 1995
48. Blank IH: Factors which influence the water content of the stratum corneum. *J Invest Dermatol* **18**:433, 1952
49. Rawlings AV et al: Stratum corneum moisturization at the molecular level. *Prog Dermatol* **28**:1, 1994
50. de Rigal J et al: Near infrared spectroscopy: A new approach to the characterization of dry skin. *J Soc Cosmet Chem* **44**:197, 1993
51. Elias PM: Epidermal lipids barrier function and desquamation. *J Invest Dermatol* **80**(suppl):44s, 1983
52. Elias PM, Feingold KR: Lipids and the epidermal water barrier: Metabolism, regulation, and pathophysiology. *Semin Dermatol* **1**:176, 1992
53. Mao-Qiang M et al: A natural lipid mixture improves barrier function and hydration in human and murine skin. *J Soc Cosmet Chem* **47**:157, 1996
54. Obata M, Tagami H: A rapid in vitro test to assess skin moisturizers. *J Soc Cosmet Chem* **41**:235, 1990
55. Kligman AM: Regression method for assessing the efficacy of moisturizers. *Cosmet Toiletries* **93**:27, 1978
56. Hannuksela A, Kinnunen T: Moisturizers prevent irritant dermatitis. *Acta Derm Venereol* **72**:42, 1992
57. Lodén M, Andersson A-C: Effect of topically applied lipids on surfactant-irritated skin. *Br J Dermatol* **134**:215, 1996

58. Ghadially R et al: Effects of petrolatum on stratum corneum and function. *J Am Acad Dermatol* **26**:387, 1992

59. Lui JC et al: The effect of barrier creams on the electrical conductivity of excised skin during exposure to detergents. *J Soc Cosmet Chem* **38**:63, 1987

60. Clark EW, Steel I: Investigations into biomechanisms of moisturizing function of lanolin. *J Soc Cosmet Chem* **44**:181, 1993

61. Henderson CA et al: The frequency of lanolin contact allergy. *Contact Dermatitis* **32**:52, 1995

62. Cronin E: *Contact Dermatitis.* New York, Churchill Livingstone, 1980

63. Froebe CL et al: Prevention of the stratum corneum lipid phase transitions in vitro by glycerol: An alternative mechanism for skin moisturization. *J Soc Cosmet Chem* **41**:51, 1990

64. Van Scott EJ, Yu RJ: Control of keratinization with alpha hydroxy acids and related compounds: I. Topical treatment of ichthyotic disorders. *Arch Dermatol* **110**:586, 1974

65. Middleton JD: Development of a skin cream designed to reduce dry and flaky skin. *J Soc Cosmet Chem* **25**:519, 1974

66. Stiller MJ et al: Topical 8% glycolic acid and 8% L-lactic acid creams for the treatment of photodamaged skin: A double-blind vehicle-controlled clinical trial. *Arch Dermatol* **132**:631, 1996

67. Cosmetic Ingredient Review: *Tentative Report on Glycolic Acid, Lactic Acid.* Washington, DC, Cosmetic Toiletries and Fragrance Association, 1997

68. Werninghaus KI: Role of antioxidants in reducing photodamage, in *Photodamage,* edited by BA Gilchrest. Cambridge, England, Blackwell, 1995

69. *Federal Register* **58**: 28194, May 12, 1993

70. Levy SB: Dihydroxyacetone-containing sunless or self-tanning lotions. *J Am Acad Dermatol* **27**:989, 1992

71. Johnson JA, Fusaro RM: Therapeutic potential of dihydroxyacetone (letter). *J Am Acad Dermatol* **29**:284, 1993

72. Ostrovskaya A et al: Stability of dihydroxyacetone in self-tanning cosmetic products. *J Soc Cosmet Chem* **47**:275, 1996

73. Engasser PG, Maibach HI: Cosmetics and dermatology: Bleaching creams. *J Am Acad Dermatol* **5**:143, 1981

74. Westmore MG: Make-up as an adjunct and aid to the practice of dermatology. *Dermatol Clin* **9**:81, 1991

75. Harusawa F et al: Anionic-cationic ion pairs as conditioning agents in shampoos. *Cosmet Toiletries* **106**:35, 1991

76. de Groot AC et al: Contact allergy to cocamidopropyl betaine. *Contact Dermatitis* **33**:419, 1995

77. Zviak C: Hair coloring: nonoxidation coloring, in *The Science of Hair Care,* edited by C Zviak. New York, Marcel Dekker, 1986, p 235

78. Engasser PG, Maibach HI: Hair dye toxicology, in *Hair and Hair Diseases,* edited by CE Orfanos, R Happle. Berlin, Springer-Verlag, 1990, p 927

79. Lead acetate: Listing as a color additive in cosmetics that color the hair on the scalp. *Federal Register* **45**:72112, 1980

80. Mielke HW et al: Lead-based hair coloring products: Too hazardous for household use. *J Am Pharm Assoc* **NS37**:85, 1997

81. Corbett JF: Hair coloring processes. *Cosmet Toiletries* **106**:53, 1991

82. Wickett RR: Disulfide bond reduction in permanent waving. *Cosmet Toiletries* **106**:37, 1991

83. Manuszak MA et al: The kinetics of disulfide bond reduction in hair by ammonium thioglycolate and dithiodiglycolic acid. *J Soc Cosmet Chem* **47**:49, 1996

84. Storrs FJ: Permanent wave contact dermatitis: Contact allergy to glyceryl monothioglycolate. *J Am Acad Dermatol* **11**:74, 1984

85. Syed AN: Ethnic hair care: History, trends and formulation. *Cosmet Toiletries* **108**:99, 1993

86. Schlossman ML: Modern nail enamel technology. *J Soc Cosmet Chem* **31**:29, 1980

87. Marks JG Jr et al: North American Contact Dermatitis Group standard tray patch test results (1992 to 1994). *Am J Contact Dermatitis* **6**:160, 1995

88. Lidén C et al: Nail varnish allergy with far-reaching consequences. *Br J Dermatol* **128**:57, 1993

89. Kanerva L et al: Methyl acrylate: A new sensitizer in nail lacquer. *Contact Dermatitis* **33**:203, 1995

90. Shelley ED, Shelley WB: Nail dystrophy and periungual dermatitis due to cyanoacrylate glue sensitivity. *J Am Acad Dermatol* **19**:574, 1988

91. Freeman S et al: Adverse contact reactions to sculptured acrylic nails: 4 case reports and a literature review. *Contact Dermatitis* **33**:381, 1995

92. Fisher AA, Baran RL: Adverse reactions to acrylate sculptured nails with particular reference to prolonged paresthesia. *Am J Contact Dermatitis* **2**:38, 1991

93. Koppula SV et al: Screening allergens for acrylate dermatitis associated with artificial nails. *Am J Contact Dermatitis* **6**:78, 1995

94. Hemmer W et al: Allergic contact dermatitis to artificial fingernails prepared from UV light-cured acrylates. *J Am Acad Dermatol* **35**:377, 1996

95. Kanerva L et al: Occupational allergic contact dermatitis caused by photobonded sculptured nails and a review of (meth)acrylates in nail cosmetics. *Am J Contact Dermatitis* **7**:109, 1996

96. Cosmetic Ingredient Review Expert Panel: Final report of safety assessment of ethyl methacrylate. Cosmetic, Toiletry and Fragrance Association, Washington, DC, Sept 12, 1994

97. Kanerva L et al: Statistics on allergic patch test reactions caused by acrylate compounds, including data on ethyl methacrylate. *Am J Contact Dermatitis* **6**:75, 1995

98. Calnan C: Occupational disorders of hairdressers, in *The Science of Hair Care,* edited by C Zviak. New York, Marcel Dekker, 1986, p 425

99. Frosch PJ et al: Allergic reactions to a hairdressers' series: Results from 9 European centres. The European Environmental and Contact Dermatitis Research Group (EECDRG). *Contact Dermatitis* **28**:180, 1993

100. Mercury poisoning associated with beauty cream—Texas, New Mexico, and California, 1995–1996. *Arch Dermatol* **132**:1533, 1996

CHAPTER 252

Victoria P. Werth
Gerald S. Lazarus

Systemic Glucocorticoids

Glucocorticoids are a mainstay of dermatologic therapy because of their potent immunosuppressive and anti-inflammatory properties. In 1949, Hench and co-workers[1] described the beneficial effects of cortisone in patients with rheumatoid arthritis. Since that time, glucocorticoids have been found to be useful in the treatment of numerous skin conditions. By understanding the properties and mechanisms of action of glucocorticoids, one can maximize their efficacy and safety as therapeutic agents.

BIOLOGY

The major naturally occurring glucocorticoid is cortisol (hydrocortisone). It is synthesized from cholesterol by the adrenal cortex. Normally, less than 5 percent of circulating cortisol is unbound; this free cortisol is the active therapeutic molecule. The remainder is inactive because it is bound to cortisol-binding globulin (CBG, also called transcortin) (95 percent) or to albumin (5 percent). The daily secretion of cortisol ranges between 10 and 20 mg, with a diurnal peak around 8 A.M.[2] Cortisol has a plasma half life of 90 min. It is metabolized primarily by the liver, although it exerts hormonal effects on virtually every tissue in the body. The metabolites are excreted by the kidney and the liver.

The mechanism of glucocorticoid action involves passive diffusion of the glucocorticoids through the cell membrane, followed by binding to soluble receptor proteins in the cytoplasm.[3] This hormone-receptor complex then moves to the nucleus and regulates the transcription of a limited number of target genes; some of the most important appear to be inhibitory effects on the transcription factors AP-1 and NF-KB, coupled with increased IKBα, an inhibitor of NF-KB.[4] Glucocorticoids decrease the synthesis of a number of proinflammatory molecules, including cytokines, interleukins, and proteases, largely through their effects on transcription.[5] Similarly, other mediators of inflammation, such as cyclooxygenase-2 and the inducible form of nitric oxide synthase, are inhibited. Glucocorticoids increase the synthesis of other important molecules, such as lipocortin 1, a member of the annexin family of molecules. The mechanism of action of lipocortin is still being investigated, but its biologic consequence is a reduction in phospholipase A$_2$ activity, which reduces the release of arachidonic acid from membrane phospholipids.[6,7] Thus, there is less precursor available for the formation of prostaglandins and leukotrienes.[8,9] There is usually a delay in the onset of pharmacologic activity of glucocorticoids relative to their peak blood concentrations, which is probably consequent to altering the transcription of genes critical to the production of these proteins.[10]

Glucocorticoids profoundly affect the replication and movement of cells. They induce monocytopenia, eosinopenia, and lymphocytopenia and have a greater effect on T cells than on B cells.[11] The lymphocytopenia appears to be due to a redistribution of cells as they migrate from the circulation to other lymphoid tissues, and it has been suggested that glucocorticoids induce apoptosis.[12] The increase in circulating polymorphonuclear leukocytes is related to demargination of cells from the bone marrow and a diminished rate of removal from the circulation; there also appears to be inhibition of neutrophil apoptosis.[13]

Glucocorticoids affect cell activation, proliferation, and differentiation. They modulate the levels of mediators of inflammation and immune reactions, as seen with the inhibition of interleukin 1 (IL-1), IL-2, IL-6, and tumor necrosis factor synthesis (or release).[14-18] Macrophage functions—including phagocytosis, antigen processing, and cell killing—are decreased by cortisol,[19,20] and this decrease affects immediate and delayed hypersensitivity.

Glucocorticoids suppress monocyte and lymphocyte function (both T$_H$1 and T$_H$2 cells) more than polymorphonuclear leukocyte function.[21] This effect is clinically important because granulomatous infectious diseases, such as tuberculosis, are prone to exacerbation and relapse during prolonged glucocorticoid therapy. The antibody-forming cells, B lymphocytes and plasma cells, are relatively resistant to the suppressive effects of glucocorticoids. Very high doses of glucocorticoids are needed to suppress antibody production.[22]

The multiplicity of biologic effects produced by glucocorticoids emphasizes that currently there is no unifying hypothesis to explain the therapeutic efficacy of these extremely potent anti-inflammatory and immunosuppressive agents.

PHARMACOLOGY

When hydrocortisone is given in moderate to high doses, its mineralocorticoid effects can be deleterious, and thus synthetic analogues of cortisol have been developed that have greater anti-inflammatory properties and less sodium retention. Small substitutions on the basic steroid structure of three hexanes and a pentane ring (Fig. 252-1, Table 252-1) account for the differences in plasma half-life and the relative anti-inflammatory and sodium-retaining potencies (Table 252-2). In general, most synthetic analogues bind less efficiently to CBG (about 70 percent binding). This property

FIGURE 252-1

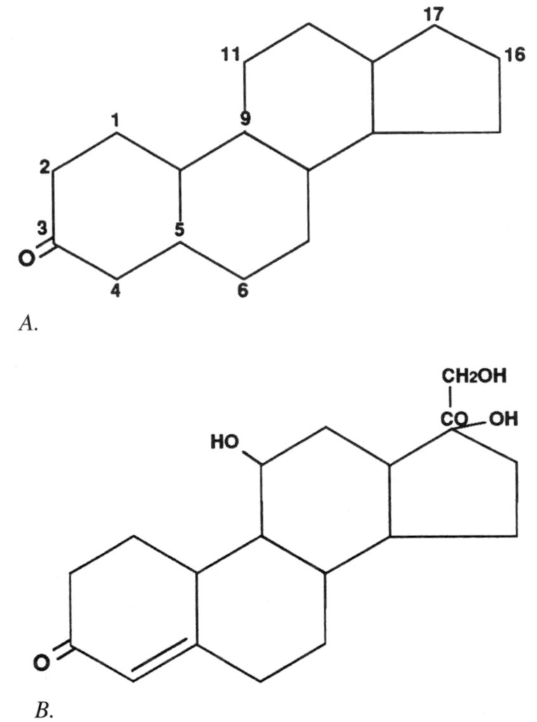

A. Basic steroid skeleton. B. The structure of hydrocortisone (cortisol).

TABLE 252-1

Comparative Structures of Glucocorticoids

| | POSITION | | | | |
	1–2	6	9	11	16
Cortisol	—	—	—	—OH	—
Cortisone	—	—	—	=O	—
Prednisone	Double bond	—	—	=O	—
Prednisolone	Double bond	—	—	—OH	—
Methylprednisolone	Double bond	α-CH3	—	—OH	—
Triamcinolone	Double bond	—	α-F	—OH	α-OH
Dexamethasone	Double bond	—	α-F	—OH	α-CH3

may explain, in part, their tendency to cause side effects at lower dosages. The 11-betahydroxyl group in cortisol is essential for activity. Because cortisone and prednisone are 11-keto compounds, they are active only after being converted in the liver to the corresponding 11-betahydroxyl compounds (cortisol and prednisolone) (Table 252-1). Patients with severe liver disease generally maintain their ability to convert the 11-keto compounds; nevertheless, some authorities suggest that only the converted active compounds should be administered to these patients.[23]

DISEASES TREATED WITH GLUCOCORTICOIDS

Skin diseases commonly treated with oral glucocorticoids include serious blistering diseases (pemphigus, bullous pemphigoid, cicatricial pemphigoid, linear IgA bullous dermatoses, epidermolysis bullosa acquisita, herpes gestationis, erythema multiforme, toxic epidermal necrolysis), connective tissue diseases (dermatomyositis, systemic lupus erythematosus, mixed connective tissue disease, eosinophilic fasciitis, relapsing polychondritis), vasculitis, neutrophilic dermatoses (pyoderma gangrenosum, acute febrile neutrophilic dermatosis, Behçet's disease), sarcoidosis, type I reactive leprosy, capillary hemangiomas, panniculitis, and urticaria/angioedema. Short courses of glucocorticoids, under appropriate conditions, may be used for severe dermatitis (contact dermatitis, atopic dermatitis, photodermatitis, exfoliative dermatitis, erythrodermas). Acne and hirsutism consequent to adrenogenital syndromes can be treated with low doses of glucocorticoids at bedtime if these conditions are unresponsive to more conservative therapy. The use of glucocorticoids is controversial in the treatment of erythema nodosum, lichen planus, cutaneous T cell lymphoma, and discoid lupus erythematosus.

COMPLICATIONS OF SYSTEMIC GLUCOCORTICOID THERAPY

Numerous complications are associated with systemic glucocorticoid therapy (Table 252-3).[4,24,25] Complications increase with higher doses, longer duration of therapy, and more frequent administration. However, osteoporosis and cataracts develop with alternate-day dosing, and avascular necrosis can be seen after only short courses of glucocorticoids.

Osteoporosis

Osteoporosis occurs in 40 percent of people treated with systemic glucocorticoids; it is especially prominent in children, adolescents, and postmenopausal women.[26] Glucocorticoids inhibit osteoblasts, increase calcium excretion by the kidney, decrease intestinal calcium absorption, and concomitantly increase bone resorption by osteoclasts.[27] They also reduce estrogen and testosterone levels, which is likely to be an important factor in the pathogenesis of osteoporosis. Serum osteocalcin, a measure of osteoblast function, decreases within a day after beginning a dosage regimen of as little as 10 mg of prednisone a day; a dosage regimen of 7.5 mg of prednisone a day or more often causes significant bone loss and an increased fracture rate.[28–30] Trabecular bone is primarily affected, leading to painful vertebral fractures.

Avascular Necrosis

Avascular necrosis is manifest by pain and limitation of motion in one or more joints. There is intraosseous hypertension, leading to bone ischemia and necrosis.[31] It is likely that intraosseous lipocyte hypertrophy causes this intraosseous hypertension in persons on glucocorticoids. Underlying diseases, such as systemic lupus erythematosus (SLE), increase the likelihood of steroid-induced avascular necrosis.[32]

Atherosclerosis

Increased risk of atherosclerosis is a concern. A number of factors that increase the risk of atherosclerosis—such as hypertension, hyperglycemia, and hyperlipidemia—are known side effects of glucocorticoids. The bimodal distribution of deaths in patients with SLE treated with glucocorticoids is instructive; the early deaths are caused by active SLE whereas the late deaths are caused by myocardial infarction.[33] A similar pattern with atherosclerosis has been noted in transplant patients receiving glucocorticoids.[34]

TABLE 252-2

Glucocorticoids

	Equivalent Glucocorticoid Potency, mg	Mineralocorticoid Potency	Plasma Half-Life, Minutes	Duration of Action, Hours
Short-acting				
Hydrocortisone (Cortisol)	20	0.8	90	8–12
Cortisone	25	1	30	8–12
Intermediate-acting				
Prednisone	5	0.25	60	24–36
Prednisolone	5	0.25	200	24–36
Methylprednisolone	4	0	180	24–36
Triamcinolone	4	0	300	24–36
Long-acting				
Dexamethasone	0.75	0	200	36–54

TABLE 252-3

Complications of Glucocorticoid Therapy

Central nervous system
  Pseudotumor cerebri and
    psychiatric disorders
Musculoskeletal
  Osteoporosis with spontaneous
    fractures
  Aseptic necrosis of bone
  Myopathy
Ocular
  Glaucoma and
    cataracts
Gastrointestinal
  Peptic ulceration
  Intestinal perforation
  Pancreatitis
Cardiovascular and fluid retention
  Hypertension
  Sodium and fluid retention
  Hypokalemic alkalosis
  Aherosclerosis
Hypersensitivity reactions
  Urticaria
  Anaphylaxis

Endocrinologic
  Suppression of HPA*
  Growth failure
  Secondary amenorrhea
Metabolic
  Hyperglycemia and unmasking genetic predisposition to
    diabetes mellitus
  Nonketotic hyperosmolar states
  Hyperlipidemia
  Alterations of fat distribution (typical cushingoid appearance)
  Fatty infiltration of the liver
  Drug interactions (decreased anticoagulant effect of ethyl
    biscoumacetate)
Fibroblast inhibition
  Inhibition of wound healing
  Subcutaneous tissue atrophy (striae, purpura, ecchymoses)
Suppression of host defenses
Immunosuppression, anergy
  Effects on phagocyte kinetics and function
  Increased incidence of infections

*HPA, hypothalamic-pituitary axis.

Suppression of the Hypothalamic-Pituitary Axis

The hypothalamic-pituitary axis (HPA) is rapidly suppressed after the onset of glucocorticoid therapy. However, if therapy is limited to 1 to 3 weeks, the recovery of the HPA axis is rapid. Longer daily glucocorticoid therapy is associated with suppression of the HPA axis for up to 1 year after therapy is terminated.[35] Symptoms of adrenal suppression include lethargy, weakness, nausea, anorexia, fever, orthostatic hypotension, hypoglycemia, and weight loss.

There also exists a steroid withdrawal syndrome, in which patients experience symptoms of adrenal insufficiency despite having an apparent normal cortisol response to adrenocorticotropic hormone (ACTH). Symptoms most commonly include anorexia, lethargy, malaise, nausea, weight loss, desquamation of the skin, headache, and fever. Less commonly, vomiting, myalgias, and arthralgias occur. These patients have adjusted to high levels of glucocorticoids, and symptoms disappear after the glucocorticoids are restarted. This problem can be treated by slower tapering of the glucocorticoids.[36]

Drug Interactions

Glucocorticoids are associated with a number of important drug interactions. Drugs such as barbiturates, phenytoin, and rifampin, which induce hepatic microsomal enzymes, may accelerate the metabolism of glucocorticoids.[37] Glucocorticoids reduce the serum salicylate level and necessitate a higher dose of warfarin (Coumadin) for anticoagulation.

Immunologic Side Effects

Glucocorticoids impair delayed-type hypersensitivity reactions because of their inhibition of lymphocytes and monocytes. Prednisone at daily doses of 15 mg or more suppresses the response to tuberculin, although it takes an average of 13.6 days for oral prednisone at 40 mg/day to inhibit the response to tuberculin.[38] Thus, even in situations requiring immediate use of prednisone, it is possible to perform simultaneously a PPD and an anergy panel. Overall, there is an increased incidence of infections attributable to both the glucocorticoids and the immunologic changes related to the underlying disease.[39]

Concerns during Pregnancy and Lactation

Glucocorticoids cross the placenta, but they are not teratogenic. Exposed infants as well as breast-fed infants of mothers receiving glucocorticoids should be monitored for adrenal suppression and growth suppression.

THERAPEUTIC USE OF GLUCOCORTICOIDS

Fundamental Principles

Before therapy with glucocorticoids is begun, the benefit that can realistically be expected should be weighed against the potential side effects. In dermatology, this often means assessing whether the disease is serious enough to risk exposing the patient to a toxic drug. Alternative or adjunctive therapies should be considered, especially if long-term treatment is contemplated. Coexisting illnesses such as diabetes, hypertension, or osteoporosis need to be considered before instituting therapy with glucocorticoids. The predisposition of the patient to side effects should be included in an assessment of risk.

Rationale for Choosing among Glucocorticoids

A number of considerations bear on the choice of glucocorticoids. First, a preparation with minimal mineralocorticoid effect is usually picked to decrease sodium retention. Second, the long-term oral use of prednisone or a similar drug, with an intermediate half-life and relatively weak steroid-receptor affinity, may reduce side effects. Long-term use of drugs like dexamethasone, which has a longer half-life and high glucocorticoid-receptor affinity, may produce more side effects without any better therapeutic effects. Third, if a patient does not respond to cortisone or prednisone, the substitution of the biologically active form, cortisol or prednisolone, should be considered. In general, even in severe liver disease, substitution has not proved to be very important. Fourth, methylprednisolone is used

for pulse therapy because of its low sodium-retaining characteristics and high potency.

Route of Administration and Dosage Schedules

Systemic glucocorticoids can be administered intralesionally, orally, intramuscularly, and intravenously. The route and regimen are determined by the nature and extent of the disease being treated.

Intralesional glucocorticoid administration allows direct access to either a relatively few lesions or a particularly resistant lesion. The concentration depends on the site of injection and the nature of the lesion. Lower concentrations (2 to 3 mg/mL) are used on the face to prevent atrophy of the skin, whereas keloids may require concentrations of 40 mg/mL. In conditions requiring sustained effects, such as keloids and alopecia areata, longer-acting glucocorticoids, such as Aristospan, can be administered alone or mixed with the more typically used Kenalog. It is best to limit the total monthly dose of Kenalog to 20 mg to assure that the HPA axis will not be suppressed.[40]

Glucocorticoids are sometimes administered intramuscularly by dermatologists. There are serious drawbacks because of erratic absorption and lack of daily control of the dose. Since Kenalog is longer-acting than prednisone, there are more potential side effects, including increased HPA suppression and myopathy, with serial monthly injections. We rarely if ever use this route of administration.

When oral glucocorticoids are prescribed, prednisone is most commonly selected. Glucocorticoids are usually administered daily or every other day, although for acute disease split daily doses can be administered. The initial dose is most often daily to control the disease process and can range from 2.5 mg to several hundred milligrams daily. As rapidly as possible, the dose should be tapered, as discussed in the section "Adrenal Suppression," below. If used for less than 3 to 4 weeks, glucocorticoid therapy can be stopped without tapering. The lowest possible dose of a short-acting agent every other morning minimizes side effects. Since cortisol levels peak at around 8 A.M., the HPA axis is least suppressed with this morning dosage. Since the drug is administered at the time of the highest level of endogenous cortisol, maximal feedback suppression of ACTH secretion by the pituitary is already occurring. The low levels of glucocorticoids at night allow for normal secretion of ACTH. Low doses of prednisone (2.5 to 5 mg) at bedtime have been used to maximize adrenal suppression in cases of acne or hirsutism of adrenal origin.

Intravenous glucocorticoids are used in two situations. One is for stress coverage for patients who are acutely ill or are undergoing surgery and who have adrenal suppression from daily glucocorticoid therapy. The other is for patients with certain diseases—such as resistant pyoderma gangrenosum, severe pemphigus or bullous pemphigoid, serious SLE, or dermatomyositis—to gain rapid control of the disease and thus minimize the need for long-term, high-dose oral steroid therapy. Methylprednisolone is used at a dose of 500 mg to 1 g daily because of its high potency and low sodium-retaining activity. Serious side effects associated with intravenous administration include anaphylactic reactions, seizures, arrhythmias, and sudden death. Other adverse reactions include hypotension, hypertension, hyperglycemia, electrolyte shifts, and acute psychosis. Slower administration over 2 to 3 h has minimized many of the serious side effects, and as long as vital signs are determined frequently, patients without underlying renal or cardiac disease do not need to be treated in a monitored bed.[41] It is important to monitor serum electrolytes before and after pulse therapy, particularly when patients are on concomitant diuretic therapy.

STRATEGIES TO REDUCE GLUCOCORTICOID SIDE EFFECTS

Evaluation before Treatment

To minimize potential problems, the baseline evaluation should include a personal and family history, with special attention to predisposition to diabetes, hypertension, hyperlipidemia, and glaucoma. All patients should be carefully questioned for associated diseases that could be affected by steroid therapy. As an example, patients with peptic ulcer diseases could be adversely affected by steroids. Baseline blood pressure and weight should be measured. If prolonged administration is anticipated, an eye examination should be performed as well as a purified protein derivative (PPD) test and an anergy panel applied. Examination for other covert infections should be based on history and physical examination. For instance, a stool culture for *Strongyloides* should be performed for immigrants from third-world countries and for Vietnam veterans.[42] If long-term administration of glucocorticoids is anticipated, serious thought should be given to ordering a baseline spinal bone-density measurement, by quantitative computed tomography (CT), dual photon absorptiometry, or dual-energy x-ray absorptiometry (DEXA).

Evaluation during Treatment

At follow-up visits, patients receiving chronic glucocorticoid therapy should be questioned about polyuria, polydipsia, abdominal pain, fevers, sleep disturbances, and psychological effects. There may be serious effects on affect and even psychosis in patients with high doses of glucocorticoids. Weight and blood pressure should be monitored. Serum electrolytes, fasting blood sugar, and cholesterol and triglyceride levels should be measured on a regular basis. Stool examination for occult blood should be performed. Follow-up eye examinations should be performed with careful monitoring for the development of cataracts and glaucoma.

Preventive Measures

GENERAL   A careful initial evaluation and follow up, as discussed in the first two sections above, are mandatory. Exercise should be encouraged.

DIET   Diet should be low in calories, fat, and sodium and high in protein, potassium, and calcium. Protein intake is important to reduce steroid-induced nitrogen wasting.[43] Use of alcohol, coffee, and nicotine should be minimized.

INFECTIONS   Patients with a positive PPD should be given prophylaxis with isoniazid.[44] Anergic patients should have a baseline chest x-ray to search for evidence of previous tuberculosis. Fevers or focal findings should be evaluated with appropriate cultures and diagnostic approaches.

GASTROINTESTINAL COMPLICATIONS   There is ongoing debate over whether the incidence of peptic ulcer disease is increased in otherwise normal patients receiving glucocorticoids.[45] Clearly, patients with a history of peptic ulcer disease or with a new onset of abdominal pain attributable to ulcers during glucocorticoid therapy should be carefully evaluated and treated with an anti-ulcer regimen, which can include antacids, H_2 receptor blockers such as ranitidine or cimetidine, omeprazole, or sucralfate.

ADRENAL SUPPRESSION   Patients receiving daily glucocorticoid therapy for longer than 3 to 4 weeks must be assumed to have adrenal suppression that requires tapering of the glucocorticoids to allow for recovery of the HPA axis. Tapering is best performed by switching from a single daily dose to alternate-day doses, followed by a gradual reduction of the amount of the drug. The daily dose is first gradually tapered to 40 or 50 mg of prednisone. Then one of several approaches can be taken. The prednisone dose can be kept constant on one day and reduced on the alternate day by 5-mg decrements down to 5 mg/day. Alternatively, the steroid dose can be increased on one day and reduced by a similar amount on the alternate day.

After the prednisone dose is tapered to 5 mg on alternate days, the need for maintenance therapy must be assessed. The 8 A.M. plasma cortisol level is measured 4 weeks after the 5-mg dose has been reached. The morning dose of prednisone is held until the plasma cortisol level is determined. If the plasma cortisol level is greater than 10 μg/dL, the alternate-day prednisone dose should be decreased by 1 mg every 1 to 2 weeks to a maintenance dose of 2 mg/day. Then the 8 A.M. plasma cortisol level should be rechecked every month until it is greater than 10 μg/dL, at which point maintenance glucocorticoids can be terminated.[46] At that point and at any point when the patient is receiving tapering doses of steroids, a stress caused, for example, by trauma, surgery, diarrhea, or fever over 38°C (101°F) can precipitate acute adrenal insufficiency related to an inadequate stress response. Patients should wear bracelets or carry cards indicating that they are receiving glucocorticoids. During such stressful situations, it is necessary to give high doses of glucocorticoids, generally 25 to 70 mg/day of prednisone or 100 to 300 mg/day of cortisol in divided doses.[47] Patients must be educated about the need for stress coverage.

In general, adrenal insufficiency resolves within 1 year of the termination of glucocorticoid therapy. An ACTH (cosyntropin) stimulation test may be performed after maintenance glucocorticoids are terminated to assess adrenal reserve. This test is performed in the office by determining a baseline cortisol level, giving an intramuscular injection of 0.25 mg of cosyntropin, and measuring the serum cortisol level again 1 h later.[46] The adrenal response is suppressed if the serum cortisol level fails to increase by at least 5 μg/dL to a stimulated value 60 min later of more than 20 μg/dL. If adequate adrenal response to stress is demonstrated, there is less concern about the endogenous cortisol response to stress. However, such a response is not a guarantee of adequate adrenal reserves if severe stress occurs, and many physicians would choose routine stress coverage with glucocorticoids without performing an ACTH stimulation test.

OSTEOPOROSIS   Attention to the prevention of osteoporosis is becoming increasingly important as newer therapies that may deter bone loss become available. Calcium and vitamin D may decrease the rate of early glucocorticoid-induced bone loss, but its efficacy in long-term glucocorticoid use is unknown.[48] Postmenopausal and premenopausal women who become amenorrheic due to glucocorticoids benefit from hormone replacement therapy. Such therapy helps to reverse the effects of glucocorticoids on bone.[49,50] Simultaneous cycling with medroxyprogesterone (Provera) prevents the increased endometrial carcinoma that occurs in women receiving estrogen alone.[51] Glucocorticoids suppress serum testosterone in men.[52] Low serum testosterone is associated with low bone density in hypogonadal men; bone density increases in these men when they receive supplemental testosterone.[53] One study suggests that testosterone partially reverses the effects of glucocorticoids on bone.[54] Men with low serum testosterone levels who are receiving glucocorticoids should have testosterone supplementation. Calcium and vitamin D supplements, sex hormone replacement, a weight-bearing exercise program, and sodium restriction are suitable first-line therapies.[55] The increased osteolysis caused by steroids has led to the use of a number of agents that inhibit bone resorption, such as calcitonin and the bisphosphonates. Inhibition of bone resorption leads to recoupling of the remodeling unit, thereby preventing further bone loss. In addition, since formation proceeds at a much slower pace than resorption, antiresorptive drugs produce a period of time up to 2 years where formation is greater than resorption. Calcitonin preserves vertebral bone mineral content in patients on steroids, and this result has been demonstrated for up to 2 years of use.[56,57] Several bisphosphonates are now available and have revolutionized the approach to prevention and treatment of steroid-induced osteoporosis. These include alendronate, 10 mg/day; etidronate, 400 mg/day for 2 weeks every 13 weeks; and pamidronate, 30 to 60 mg intravenously every 6 to 12 months; all three agents have been shown to increase vertebral bone mineral density in patients receiving glucocorticoids.[58,59]

Current recommendations include baseline measurements of bone density and sequential study to identify early those who are rapidly losing bone density.[55,60] These individuals can then be targeted for modification of treatment or for newer interventions with calcitonin or bisphosphonates.

Men and premenopausal women should be given elemental calcium, 500 mg twice daily, and vitamin D_2, 400 units twice daily. Vitamin D at a higher dose of 50,000 units once or twice weekly has been used, but patients must be followed very carefully in order not to precipitate hypervitaminosis D.[61] Patients with a history of renal stones should not receive supplemental calcium and vitamin D. Calcium levels should be measured in serum and in 24-h urine collections every 3 months or whenever steroid doses are substantially altered. If the urinary calcium level exceeds 250 to 350 mg/dL, the addition of 12.5 to 25 mg/day of thiazide will reduce the renal excretion of calcium.[62] If thiazide is not added, calcium and vitamin D supplementation should be adjusted. Men with low serum testosterone levels may profit from testosterone supplementation, either by the intramuscular route as testosterone enanthate 100 to 200 mg every 2 to 4 weeks or by newer testosterone scrotal or skin patches.

Postmenopausal women should receive 1500 mg of elemental calcium daily in addition to the dose of vitamin D mentioned above. Women should also receive oral conjugated estrogen (Premarin), 0.625 mg/day. Women with a uterus should also receive medroxyprogesterone, 2.5 mg/day. Women who are to receive hormonal therapy should not have a history of benign or malignant breast disease or other hormone-sensitive tumors, thrombophlebitis, smoking, gallstones, or a family history of breast cancer. Breast and pelvic examinations should be performed initially and at regular 6- to 12-month intervals during hormone therapy.

Calcitonin is often helpful in relieving the pain of compression fractures.[63]

ATHEROSCLEROSIS Blood pressure, serum lipids, and glucose levels should be measured serially. Abnormalities should be treated with dietary manipulation and medication as necessary. Patients who smoke should be encouraged to stop.

AVASCULAR NECROSIS Early detection is important, since early intervention may prevent progression to degenerative joint disease requiring joint replacement. Twenty percent of patients with avascular necrosis have normal x-rays. Bone scan and magnetic resonance imaging (MRI) are more sensitive techniques for evaluating avascular necrosis. Patients should be regularly questioned about pain and limitation of motion of joints. If abnormalities develop, x-ray, bone scan, or MRI should be ordered. If imaging shows avascular necrosis, an orthopedic surgeon skilled in early intervention with core decompression may be able to halt progression of the disease. Patients with avascular necrosis have an increased risk that other joints will also be affected. The progression of avascular necrosis to destructive joint disease may require joint replacement surgery.[64]

REFERENCES

1. Hench PS et al: The effect of a hormone of the adrenal cortex (17-hydroxy-11-dehydrocorticosterone (compound E)) and of pituitary adrenocorticotropic hormone on rheumatoid arthritis. *Mayo Clin Proc* **24**:181, 1949
2. Esteban NV et al: Daily cortisol production rate in man determined by stable isotope dilution/mass spectrometry. *J Clin Endocrinol Metab* **72**:39, 1991
3. Bloom E et al: Nuclear binding of glucocorticoid receptors: Relations between cytosol binding, activation and the biologic response. *J Steroid Biochem* **12**:175, 1980
4. Cato AC et al: Molecular mechanisms of anti-inflammatory action of glucocorticoids. *Bioessays* **18**:371, 1996
5. Boumpas DT et al: Glucocorticoid therapy for immune-mediated diseases: Basic and clinical correlates. *Ann Intern Med* **119**:1198, 1993
6. Flower RJ et al: Lipocortin-1: Cellular mechanisms and clinical relevance. *Trends Pharmacol Sci* **15**:71, 1994
7. Croxtall JD et al: Lipocortin 1 and the control of cPLA2 activity in A549 cells: Glucocorticoids block EGF stimulation of cPLA2 phosphorylation. *Biochem Pharmacol* **52**:351, 1996
8. Pepinsky RB et al: Five distinct calcium and phospholipid binding proteins share homology with lipocortin 1. *J Biol Chem* **263**:10799, 1988
9. Wallner BP et al: Cloning and expression of human lipocortin, a phospholipase A_2 inhibitor with potential anti-inflammatory activity. *Nature* **320**:77, 1986
10. Taylor IK et al: The mechanism of action of corticosteroids in asthma. *Respir Med* **87**:261, 1993
11. Cupps TR et al: Corticosteroid-mediated immunoregulation in man. *Immunol Rev* **65**:133, 1982
12. Lanza L et al: Prednisone increases apoptosis in *in vitro* activated human peripheral blood T lymphocytes. *Clin Exp Immunol* **103**:482, 1996
13. Liles WC et al: Glucocorticoids inhibit apoptosis of human neutrophils. *Blood* **86**:3181, 1995
14. Stosic-Grujicic S et al: Modulation of interleukin 1 production by activated macrophages: In vitro action of hydrocortisone, colchicine and cytochalasin B. *Cell Immunol* **69**:2335, 1982
15. Smith KA: T-cell growth factor. *Immunol Rev* **51**:337, 1980
16. Beutler B et al: Cachectin and tumour necrosis factor as two sides of the same biological coin. *Nature* **320**:584, 1986
17. Amano Y et al: Inhibition by glucocorticoids of the formation of interleukin-1α, interleukin-1β, and interleukin-6: Mediation by decreased mRNA stability. *Mol Pharmacol* **43**:176, 1993
18. Kitajima T et al: A novel mechanism of glucocorticoid-induced immune suppression: The inhibition of T cell-mediated terminal maturation of a murine dendritic cell line. *J Clin Invest* **98**:142, 1996

19. Balow JE et al: Glucocorticoid suppression of macrophage inhibitory factor. *J Exp Med* **137**:1031, 1973

20. Hogan MM: Inhibition of macrophage tumoricidal activity by glucocorticoids. *J Immunol* **140**:513, 1988

21. Parrillo IE, Fauci AS: Mechanisms of glucocorticoid action on immune processes. *Annu Rev Pharmacol Toxicol* **19**:179, 1979

22. Butler WT et al: Effects of corticosteroids on immunity in man: Decreased serum IgG concentration caused by 3 or 5 days of high doses of methylprednisolone. *J Clin Invest* **52**:505, 1973

23. Frey FI: Kinetics and dynamics of prednisolone. *Endocrinol Rev* **8**:453, 1987

24. Werth VP: Management and treatment with systemic glucocorticoids. *Adv Dermatol* **8**:81, 1993

25. Nesbitt LT Jr: Minimizing complications from systemic glucocorticoid use. *Dermatol Clin* **13**:925, 1995

26. Gluck OS et al: Bone loss in adults receiving alternate day glucocorticoid therapy. *Arthritis Rheum* **24**:892, 1981

27. Lukert BP et al: Glucocorticoid-induced osteoporosis. *Rheum Dis Clin North Am* **20**:629, 1994

28. Godschalk MF et al: Effect of short-term glucocorticoids on serum osteocalcin in healthy young men. *J Bone Min Res* **3**:113, 1988

29. Pons F et al: The effect of systemic lupus erythematosus and long-term steroid therapy on bone mass in pre-menopausal women. *Br J Rheumatol* **34**:742, 1995

30. Buckley LM et al: Effects of low dose corticosteroids on the bone mineral density of patients with rheumatoid arthritis. *J Rheumatol* **22**:1055, 1995

31. Solomon L: Idiopathic necrosis of the femoral head: Pathogenesis and treatment. *Can J Surg* **24**:573, 1981

32. Zizic TM et al: Corticosteroid therapy associated with ischemic necrosis of bone in systemic lupus erythematosus. *Am J Med* **79**:596, 1985

33. Urowitz MB et al: The bimodal mortality pattern of systemic lupus erythematosus. *Am J Med* **60**:221, 1976

34. Becker DM et al: Relationship between corticosteroid exposure and plasma lipid levels in heart transplant recipients. *Am J Med* **85**:632, 1988

35. Graber AL et al: Natural history of pituitary-adrenal recovery following long-term suppression with corticosteroids. *J Clin Endocrinol Metab* **25**:11, 1965

36. Dixon RB et al: On the various forms of glucocorticoid withdrawal syndrome. *Am J Med* **68**:224, 1990

37. Gustavson LE, Benet LZ: Pharmacokinetics of natural and synthetic glucocorticoids, in *The Actual Cortex*, edited by DC Anderson, JSD Winters. Cornwall, England, Butterworth, 1985, p 235

38. Bovomkitti S et al: Reversion and reconversion rate of tuberculin skin reactions in correlation with the use of prednisone. *Dis Chest* **38**:51, 1960

39. Aucott JN: Glucocorticoids and infection. *Endocrinol Metab Clin North Am* **23**:655, 1994

40. Firooz A: Benefits and risks of intralesional corticosteroid injection in the treatment of dermatological diseases. *Clin Exp Dermatol* **20**:363, 1995

41. White KP et al: Severe adverse cardiovascular effects of pulse steroid therapy: Is continuous cardiac monitoring necessary? *J Am Acad Dermatol* **30**:768, 1994

42. Genta RM: Global prevalence of strongyloides: Critical review with epidemiologic insights into the prevention of disseminated disease. *Rev Infect Dis* **11**:755, 1989

43. Cogan MG et al: Prevention of prednisone-induced negative nitrogen balance: Effect of dietary modification on urea generation rate in hemodialyzed patients receiving high-dose glucocorticoids. *Ann Intern Med* **95**:158, 1981

44. American Thoracic Society: Treatment of tuberculosis and tuberculosis infection in adults and children. *Am Rev Respir Dis* **134**:355, 1986

45. Conn HO et al: Corticosteroids and peptic ulcer: Meta-analysis of adverse events during steroid therapy. *J Intern Med* **236**:619, 1994

46. Grinspoon SK et al: Laboratory assessment of adrenal insufficiency: Clinical review 62. *J Clin Endocrinol Metab* **79**:923, 1994

47. Baxter JD: Minimizing the side effects of glucocorticoid therapy. *Adv Intern Med* **35**:173, 1980

48. Buckley LM et al: Calcium and vitamin D$_3$ supplementation prevents bone loss in the spine secondary to low-dose corticosteroids in patients with rheumatoid arthritis. *Ann Intern Med* **125**:961, 1996

49. Hall GM et al: Effect of hormone replacement therapy on bone mass in rheumatoid arthritis patients treated with and without steroids. *Arthritis Rheum* **37**:1499, 1994

50. Lukert BP et al: Estrogen and progesterone replacement therapy reduces glucocorticoid-induced bone loss. *J Bone Min Res* **7**:1063, 1992

51. Gambrell RD: Prevention of endometrial cancer with progestogens. *Maturitas* **8**:159, 1986

52. MacAdams MR et al: Reduction of serum testosterone levels during chronic glucocorticoid therapy. *Ann Intern Med* **104**:648, 1986

53. Finkelstein JS et al: Osteoporosis in men with idiopathic hypogonadotropic hypogonadism. *Ann Intern Med* **106**:354, 1987

54. Reid IR et al: Testosterone therapy in glucocorticoid-treated men. *Arch Intern Med* **156**:1173, 1996

55. Recommendations for the prevention and treatment of glucocorticoid-induced osteoporosis *Arthritis Rheum* **39**:1791, 1996

56. Ringe ID et al: Salmon calcitonin in the therapy of corticoid-induced osteoporosis. *Eur J Clin Pharmacol* **33**:35, 1987

57. Luengo M et al: Treatment of steroid-induced osteopenia with calcitonin in corticosteroid-dependent asthma. *Am Rev Respir Dis* **142**:104, 1990

58. Adachi JD et al: Intermittent etidronate therapy to prevent corticosteroid-induced osteoporosis. *N Engl J Med* **337**:382, 1997

59. Struys A et al: Cyclical etidronate reverses bond loss of the spine and proximal femur in patients with established corticosteroid-induced osteoporosis. *Am J Med* **99**:235, 1995

60. Werth VP: Systemic glucocorticoids and the skin: Dermatologists can prevent steroid-induced osteoporosis. *Med Surg Dermatol* **3**:343, 1996

61. Schwartzman MS et al: Vitamin D toxicity complicating the treatment of senile, postmenopausal, and glucocorticoid-induced osteoporosis. *Am J Med* **82**:224, 1987

62. Suzuki Y et al: Importance of increased urinary calcium excretion in the development of secondary hyperparathyroidism of patients under glucocorticoid therapy. *Metabolism* **32**:151, 1983

63. Pun KK: Analgesic effect of intranasal salmon calcitonin in the treatment of osteoporotic vertebral fractures. *Clin Ther* **11**:205, 1989

64. Hungerford DS: Response: The role of core decompression in the treatment of ischemic necrosis of the femoral head. *Arthritis Rheum* **32**:801, 1989

Sulfones

In 1940, Costello[1] first described the dramatic success of sulfapyridine in treating a patient with dermatitis herpetiformis, a disease he believed to be a form of bacterial allergy. Swartz and Lever[2] later reported the regular response of all their patients with dermatitis herpetiformis to sulfapyridine therapy. In the early 1950s, a group of drugs chemically related to sulfapyridine, the sulfones (dapsone and related compounds), were first used in treating patients with this disease.[3,4] Because dapsone is the most widely used drug among these compounds, there has been an enormous amount of research into its metabolism, mechanisms of action, and toxicity.

PHARMACOLOGY

The chemical structure of dapsone (4,4'-diaminodiphenylsulfone, DDS) is shown in Fig. 253-1. Derivatives of dapsone such as sulfoxone (no longer available in the United States) are thought to be metabolized to the parent dapsone structure. Sulfapyridine resembles dapsone in that it has an aminophenyl group attached to a sulfone (SO_2); however, on the other side of the sulfone, there is a pyridine group (Fig. 253-1). Although other sulfonamides have an aminophenyl group attached to a sulfone, they have different groups on the other side of the sulfone, and none is as effective as sulfapyridine in the treatment of inflammatory diseases. The pyridine group was thought to contribute to the beneficial effect of sulfapyridine, and other compounds such as pyribenzamine and nicotinamide were said to be useful in treating patients with dermatitis

FIGURE 253-1

Dapsone

Sulfapyridine

Chemical structure of dapsone and sulfapyridine.

herpetiformis. Because the manufacturer of sulfapyridine in the US has recently changed, the drug is available only under an Investigational New Drug (IND) application.

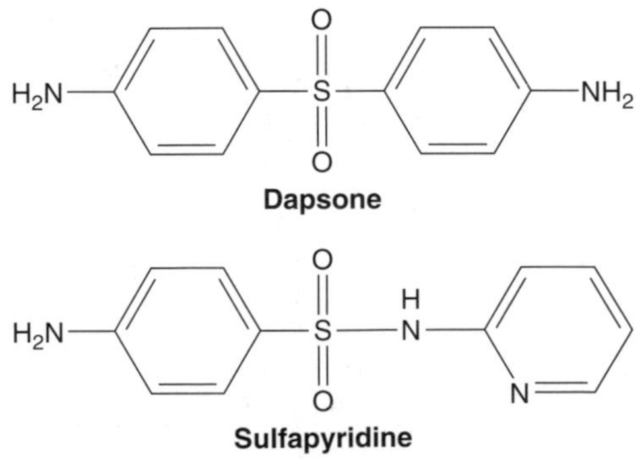

After oral administration of dapsone, approximately 80 to 85 percent is absorbed, with peak levels being reached 2 to 6 h after a single dose. In patients taking 50 to 300 mg/day of dapsone, the peak levels of dapsone and its major metabolite reach 0.5 to 7 mg/L and 0.2 to 5 mg/L, respectively.[5] The half-life of dapsone in the circulation is approximately 30 h.[6] Its retention in the body, however, is prolonged, perhaps because of its enterohepatic recirculation, since high concentrations have been detected in the bile. Dapsone and its metabolites may be transmitted through human milk[7,8] and are excreted by the kidneys.[6]

Dapsone is metabolized in the liver. The two major metabolic pathways involve acetylation and N-hydroxylation (Fig. 253-2). As with isoniazid and certain hydrazides and sulfonamides, dapsone and its derivatives are acetylated polymorphically, i.e., some patients rapidly acetylate dapsone to monoacetyldapsone (MADDS), the major metabolite, whereas in others this process occurs slowly. However, in humans, MADDS is rapidly deacetylated. Thus, an equilibrium is rapidly reached and sustained between MADDS and dapsone. The half-life in the body seems to be unrelated to the rate of acetylation. From a clinical standpoint, it seems that in dapsone's control of symptoms of dermatitis herpetiformis and even in its efficacy as an antileprosy drug, the dapsone dosage requirement is unrelated to acetylator phenotype.[5,9]

The other major metabolic pathway involves hydroxylation of one of the amino groups to form the aminohydroxylamino-diphenylsulfone. This compound is responsible for the methemoglobinemia, hemolysis, and Heinz-body formations that occur regularly when dapsone is administered.[10–12] Thus, these pharmacologic side effects must be anticipated.

Drugs that interfere with the effect of dapsone include probenecid and rifampicin. Probenecid has been reported to block the renal excretion of dapsone; however, serum dapsone levels are not significantly affected.[13] When given concurrently with dapsone, rifampicin increases the rate of dapsone clearance, and this increase is most likely caused by the induction of microsomal enzymes.

INDICATIONS

Since its introduction into clinical medicine, dapsone has had therapeutic trials in a multitude of diseases. Long lists of inflammatory diseases that have responded to dapsone therapy have been generated.[14] Some of the individual reports are difficult to assess critically. Two diseases that invariably respond to dapsone therapy are dermatitis herpetiformis and erythema elevatum diutinum.[15] The dramatic dependence of patients on dapsone is best exemplified by the prompt exacerbations that follow withdrawal of the drug.

Other diseases for which dapsone therapy reportedly has been effective in some patients are rheumatoid arthritis, idiopathic or autoimmune thrombocytopenic purpura, acne conglobata, actinomycetoma, pyoderma gangrenosum, bullous pemphigoid, scarring pemphigoid, relapsing polychondritis, the bullous eruption of systemic lupus erythematosus (SLE), granuloma faciale, subcorneal pustular dermatosis, and certain forms of leukocytoclastic vasculitis. As a unifying feature, most of these diseases have granulocytes (neutrophils or eosinophils) as the predominant infiltrating cell. In most diseases, the neutrophils appear early in the pathologic process. The response to dapsone therapy is not as rapid, regular, or predictable in any of these diseases as it is in dermatitis herpetiformis or erythema elevatum diutinum.

FIGURE 253-2

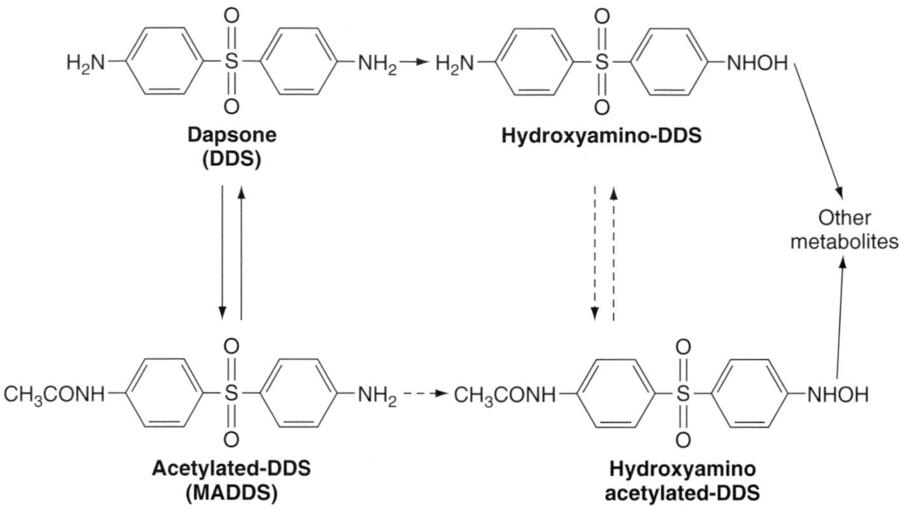

Dapsone metabolism in humans.

Prospective controlled trials show dapsone therapy to be modestly effective in the treatment of some patients with rheumatoid arthritis.[16] Similarly, 40 to 50 percent of patients with thrombocytopenic purpura have been shown to respond to dapsone therapy.[17,18] High dosages (up to 400 mg/day) are usually required in the treatment of otherwise unresponsive patients with cystic acne. With the advent of the synthetic retinoids, however, a trial of dapsone therapy may no longer be necessary. A few patients with bullous pemphigoid have responded fairly dramatically to dapsone therapy.[19] Indeed, some authors have advocated its use as a regularly effective treatment for bullous pemphigoid,[20] while others have found its efficacy in bullous pemphigoid to be limited.[21] Some patients with scarring pemphigoid reportedly have benefitted from dapsone therapy as well.[22] Dapsone and sulfapyridine are effective in ocular cicatricial pemphigoid, particularly in the early inflammatory phases,[23,24] and dapsone is effective in patients with superficial pemphigus who have a low or negative pemphigus antibody titer.[25]

Patients with SLE occasionally have subepidermal vesicular lesions that closely simulate dermatitis herpetiformis histologically.[26] These patients do not have an "admixture" of dermatitis herpetiformis and SLE, although the eruption is extraordinarily responsive to dapsone therapy.[27] A potentially exciting report, which was too brief and could not be evaluated, suggested the efficacy of dapsone therapy in discoid SLE.[28] Dramatic responses to dapsone have occurred in occasional patients with subacute cutaneous lupus erythematosus.[29–31] Granuloma annulare has also been reported to respond to dapsone treatment.[32,33] Some patients with subcorneal pustular dermatosis respond to and become dependent on dapsone, whereas others are unresponsive. This difference may reflect the heterogeneity of this disease, whose nosologic features have been a source of considerable debate.[34]

Although several reports suggest that dapsone therapy is remarkably effective in the treatment of relapsing polychondritis, my experiences with dapsone therapy in several patients with this condition have been uniformly unsuccessful. Occasionally, there are patients with chronic leukocytoclastic vasculitis in addition to those

with erythema elevatum diutinum in whom dapsone therapy induces the prompt cessation of lesions. Since there is no uniformly successful therapy for these patients, many of whom do not seem to have associated internal problems, a short trial of dapsone therapy is warranted. In general, when a pathologic lesion is characterized by a neutrophilic infiltrate and is unassociated with an infectious agent, a trial of dapsone therapy should be considered. Even if a therapeutic trial is successful, the dose of dapsone should be decreased to a point at which lesions recur to be sure that the improvement was indeed due to dapsone and that there is a continuing need for the drug.

In the early 1990s there was considerable enthusiasm for the potential of dapsone as a prophylactic agent for *Pneumocystis carinii* pneumonia (PCP). It is now considered less effective than trimethoprim-sulfamethoxazole (TMP-SMX).[35] Dapsone is a reasonable choice for PCP prophylaxis in patients who are unable to take TMP-SMX.[36]

ADVERSE EFFECTS

Dapsone therapy produces hemolysis and methemoglobinemia. The metabolite responsible for both these pharmacologic effects of sulfones has been identified as aminohydroxylaminodiphenylsulfone. Patients taking more than 50 mg/day of dapsone probably will have some degree of hemolysis that will be reflected in a lowered hemoglobin level. At 150 mg/day, dapsone may produce a decrease of as much as 2 g of hemoglobin. Patients with glucose-6-dehydrogenase deficiency have a greater decrease in the hemoglobin level. Most patients tolerate a 2-g fall in the level of hemoglobin well, but the conditions of older patients or those with cardiopulmonary problems should be closely monitored or they should be given sulfapyridine. An increase in the reticulocyte count accompanies the fall in the hemoglobin level. Several months after treatment has begun, the hemoglobin level may rise almost to pretreatment levels but usually remains about 1 g below the original level.

Methemoglobinemia also regularly occurs in patients treated with sulfones but not as often as in patients treated with sulfapyridine. Methemoglobinemia is not a major problem in most patients. Even in patients taking 200 mg/day of dapsone, the level usually does not exceed 12 percent of the total hemoglobin level and is often less than 5 percent. The methemoglobin level is more pronounced at the onset of treatment and, as with hemolysis, it is dose-dependent. The cyanosis (which may seem more gray than blue) that results from methemoglobinemia may be seen in anyone with a methemoglobin level greater than 3 percent but may not be apparent in some patients with a level as high as 12 percent. Symptoms of methemoglobinemia include weakness, tachycardia, nausea, headache, and abdominal pains, which should not be attributed to methemoglobinemia until levels reach 20 percent or greater. Dapsone-induced methemoglobinemia can be reduced by coadministration of cimetidine.[37]

Other than these pharmacologic side effects, the adverse effects of dapsone may be idiosyncratic or allergic in nature[14,38,39] (Table 253-1). Peripheral neuropathy is one such example and usually occurs at high dosage levels. Loss of motor function is the most common type of neuropathy, and it is reversible by decreasing the dose of dapsone. Sensory neuropathy is rare. Well-known side effects include the induction of acute psychosis[40,41] and a potentially fatal mononucleosis-like syndrome that occurs during the induction of dapsone therapy in patients with leprosy.[42] Severe hypoalbuminemia with anasarca has also been reported.[43]

Agranulocytosis has been estimated to occur in 0.2 to 0.4 percent of patients treated with dapsone.[44] If agranulocytosis occurs, its onset is almost always during the first 3 months of therapy.[44,45] Although it is usually reversible when patients stop therapy, it may be fatal. Patients should be warned to seek medical care immediately if an infection develops during the first several months of therapy. Generally, when adverse reactions occur as a result of therapy with dapsone, dapsone derivatives and even sulfapyridine cause the same types of problems.

Information from two independent studies of carcinogenicity suggests that dapsone is a "weak carcinogen" in rats.[46,47] There is no similar evidence from studies in humans.

TABLE 253-1

Adverse Reactions to Sulfones

Pharmacologic effects	Morbilliform eruptions
Hemolysis	Erythema nodosum
Methemoglobinemia	Erythema multiforme
Headache	Exfoliative dermatitis
Gastric irritation	Toxic epidermal necrolysis
Nausea	Severe hypoalbuminemia
Anorexia	Psychosis
Fatigue	Leukopenia
Hepatitis, infectious mononucleosis-	Agranulocytosis
like with adenopathy	Peripheral neuropathy
Cholestatic jaundice	(almost always motor)

SOURCE: Modified from Lang,[14] Alexander,[38] and Katz et al.[39]

A frequently asked question is whether dapsone is safe to use during pregnancy. In one study, 2 of 56 infants born to patients with leprosy who were being treated with dapsone had congenital malformations.[48] There are no controlled studies in animals or people that address this point.

MONITORING OF DAPSONE THERAPY

Before therapy with the sulfones or sulfapyridine is started, a complete blood cell (CBC) count should be obtained. In addition, Asians, blacks, or persons of Mediterranean descent should be tested for glucose-6-phosphate dehydrogenase deficiency, because sulfones can cause profound hemolysis in persons lacking this enzyme. After therapy is begun, a leukocyte count with a differential and hemoglobin levels should be obtained weekly for the first month and then twice a month during the next 2 months. Thereafter, CBC counts should be done periodically. Liver and renal function should also be tested before therapy starts and periodically thereafter. Once the disease being treated is under control, the dosage of dapsone should be reduced to be sure that the patient is using the minimum amount of drug required. Although in some diseases, such as dermatitis herpetiformis, the patients may alter the drug dosage according to the severity of the disease, they should be reminded not to increase the dosage by large amounts abruptly. Because the blue-gray color of methemoglobinemia may be attributed to other causes by emergency room physicians, patients should be advised to carry a medication card in their wallets.

MECHANISM OF ACTION

The mechanisms of action of dapsone in leprosy and inflammatory diseases have been the subject of considerable study. Dapsone and its derivatives are potent oxidants with a notable influence on glutathione. Interference with the folate biosynthetic pathway of bacteria accounts for their bacteriostatic effect. Less well known activities of dapsone involve its inhibition of choline incorporation into the lecithin of the cell membranes, thereby decreasing phospholipid synthesis.[49] Also, dapsone administered in the diet decreases visceral lesions and mortality in chickens infected with Marek's disease, in which a herpesvirus induces a lymphocytic malignant neoplasm in chickens.[50]

Numerous studies have attempted to determine how dapsone exerts its antiinflammatory effect. Evidence suggests that its antiinflammatory effect is not related to its antibacterial effect. Dapsone inhibits lysosomal enzyme activity,[51,52] interferes with the myeloperoxidase-H_2O_2-halide-mediated cytotoxic system,[53,54] and inhibits the generation of 5-lipoxygenase products in polymorphonuclear leukocytes.[55] Dapsone and its analogues also inhibit the zymosan-mediated human neutrophil respiratory burst.[56] Although these findings may account for the effect of the drug on neutrophils or on their lysosomal enzymes at the site of injury, they probably do not account for the lack of influx of neutrophils into the dermis in treated patients. There is little evidence to support suggestions that dapsone interferes with complement activation and deposition.[57] Some in vivo studies have shown that dapsone at doses of 100 to 200 mg/kg inhibits adjuvant-induced arthritis and carrageenan-induced inflammation in rats.[58]

Several studies have suggested that dapsone and its derivatives do not affect the response of neutrophils to chemotactic stimuli. However, other studies have suggested that dapsone inhibits leukotriene B_4 binding to neutrophils,[59] and yet others have demonstrated that dapsone inhibits the neutrophil response to some chemotactic stimuli.[60,61] More extensive studies with chemotactic stimuli in varied concentrations are required to evaluate the possibility that dapsone may interfere with a specific chemotactic factor or with the response of neutrophils to such a factor. Another possibility for the beneficial effect of dapsone on neutrophil-rich dermatoses may be its ability to inhibit (1) interleukin 1–stimulated neutrophil adhesion to endothelial cells,[56] (2) neutrophil adherence to antibodies deposited in skin,[62] or (3) integrin-mediated neutrophil adherence functions.[63]

REFERENCES

1. Costello MJ: Dermatitis herpetiformis treated with sulfapyridine. *Arch Dermatol Syphilol* **41**:134, 1940
2. Swartz JH, Lever WF: Dermatitis herpetiformis: Immunology and therapeutic considerations. *Arch Dermatol Syphilol* **47**:680, 1943
3. Cornbleet R: Sulfoxone (Diasone) sodium for dermatitis herpetiformis. *Arch Dermatol Syphilol* **64**:684, 1951
4. Kruizinga EE, Hamminga H: Treatment of dermatitis herpetiformis with diaminodiphenylsulphone (DDS). *Dermatologia* **106**:386, 1953
5. Ellard GA et al: Dapsone acetylation in dermatitis herpetiformis. *Br J Dermatol* **90**:441, 1974
6. Zuidema J et al: Clinical pharmacokinetics of dapsone. *Clin Pharmacokinet* **11**:299, 1986
7. Sanders SW et al: Hemolytic anemia induced by dapsone transmitted through breast milk. *Ann Intern Med* **96**:465, 1982
8. Edstein S et al: Excretion of chloroquine, dapsone and pyrimethamine in human milk. *Br J Clin Pharmacol* **22**:733, 1986
9. Ellard GA et al: Dapsone acetylation and the treatment of leprosy. *Nature* **239**:159, 1972
10. McMillan DC et al: Dapsone induced hemolytic anemia: Effect of dapsone hydroxylamine on sulfhydryl status, membrane skeletal proteins, and morphology of human and rat erythrocytes. *J Pharmacol Exp Ther* **274**:540, 1995
11. Grossman SJ, Jollow DJ: Role of dapsone hydroxylamine in dapsone-induced hemolytic anemia. *J Pharmacol Exp Ther* **244**:118, 1988
12. Coleman MD et al: The effect of acetylation and deacetylation on the disposition of dapsone and monoacetyl dapsone hydroxylamine in human erythrocytes in vitro. *J Pharm Pharmacol* **48**:401, 1996
13. Goodwin CS, Sparell G: Inhibition of dapsone excretion by probenecid. *Lancet* **1**:884, 1969
14. Lang P: Sulfones and sulfonamides in dermatology today. *J Am Acad Dermatol* **1**:479, 1979
15. Katz SI et al: Erythema elevatum diutinum: Skin and systemic manifestations, immunologic studies, and successful treatment with dapsone. *Medicine (Baltimore)* **56**:443, 1977
16. Chang DJ et al: Dapsone in rheumatoid arthritis. *Semin Arthritis Reum* **25**:390, 1996
17. Hernandez F et al: Dapsone for refractory chronic idiopathic thrombocytopenia purpura. *Br J Haematol* **90**:473, 1995
18. Godeau B et al: Dapsone for chronic autoimmune thrombocytopenic purpura: A report of 66 cases. *Br J Haematol* **97**:336, 1997
19. Person JR, Rogers RS III: Bullous pemphigoid responding to sulfapyridine and the sulfones. *Arch Dermatol* **113**:610, 1977
20. Venning VA et al: Dapsone as first line treatment for bullous pemphigoid. *Br J Dermatol* **120**:83, 1989
21. Bouscarat F et al: Treatment of bullous pemphigoid with dapsone: Retrospective study of thirty-six cases. *J Am Acad Dermatol* **34**:683, 1996
22. Rogers RS et al: Treatment of cicatricial (benign mucous membrane) pemphigoid with dapsone. *J Am Acad Dermatol* **6**:215, 1982
23. Fern AI et al: Dapsone therapy for the acute inflammatory phase of ocular pemphigoid. *Br J Ophthalmol* **76**:332, 1992
24. Elder MJ et al: Sulphapyridine—a new agent for the treatment of ocular cicatricial pemphigoid. *Br J Ophthalmol* **80**:549, 1996
25. Basset N et al: Dapsone as initial treatment in superficial pemphigus: Report of nine cases. *Arch Dermatol* **123**:783, 1987
26. Penneys NS, Wiley HE III: Herpetiformis blisters in systemic lupus erythematosus. *Arch Dermatol* **115**:1427, 1979
27. Hall RP et al: Bullous eruption of systemic lupus erythematosus: Dramatic response to dapsone therapy. *Ann Intern Med* **97**:165, 1982
28. Coburn PR, Shuster S: Dapsone and discoid lupus erythematosus. *Br J Dermatol* **106**:105, 1982
29. McCormack LS et al: Annular subacute cutaneous lupus erythematosus responsive to dapsone. *J Am Acad Dermatol* **11**:397, 1984
30. Callen J: Treatment of cutaneous lesions in patients with lupus erythematosus. *Dermatol Clin* **12**:201, 1994
31. Fenton DA, Black MM: Low dose dapsone in the treatment of subacute cutaneous lupus erythematosus. *Clin Exp Dermatol* **11**:102, 1986
32. Czarnecki DB, Gin D: The response of generalized granuloma annulare to dapsone. *Acta Derm Venereol* **66**:82, 1986
33. Steiner A et al: Sulfone treatment of granuloma annulare. *J Am Acad Dermatol* **13**:1004, 1985
34. Chimenti S, Ackerman AB: Is subcorneal pustular dermatitis of Sneddon and Wilkinson an entity sui generis? *Am J Dermatopathol* **3**:363, 1981
35. Warnock AC, Rimland D: Comparison of trimethoprim-sulfamethoxazole, dapsone, and pentamidine in the prophylaxis of *Pneumocystis carinii* pneumonia. *Pharmacotherapy* **16**:1030, 1996
36. Beumont MG et al: Safety of dapsone as *Pneumocystis carinii* pneumonia prophylaxis in human immunodeficiency virus-infected patients with allergy to trimethoprimsulfamethoxazole. *Am J Med* **100**:611, 1996
37. Coleman MD, Coleman NA: Drug-induced methaemoglobinemia: Treatment issues. *Drug Saf* **14**:394, 1996
38. Alexander JO: Dermatitis herpetiformis, in *Major Problems in Dermatology*, edited by A Rook. Philadelphia, Saunders, 1975, p 291
39. Katz SI et al: Dermatitis herpetiformis: The skin and the gut. *Ann Intern Med* **93**:857, 1980
40. Fine JD et al: Psychiatric reaction to dapsone and sulfapyridine. *J Am Acad Dermatol* **9**:274, 1983
41. Gawkrodger D: Manic depression induced by dapsone in patient with dermatitis herpetiformis. *Br Med J* **299**:860, 1989
42. Frey AM et al: Fatal reaction to dapsone during treatment of leprosy. *Ann Intern Med* **94**:777, 1981
43. Kingham JGC et al: Dapsone and severe hypoalbuminemia. *Lancet* **2**:662, 1979
44. Hörnsten P et al: The incidence of agranulocytosis during treatment of dermatitis herpetiformis with dapsone as reported in Sweden, 1972 through 1988. *Arch Dermatol* **126**:919, 1990
45. Liozon P et al: Agranulocytoses à la dapsone. *Ann Med Interne (Paris)* **139**:469, 1988
46. *Bioassay of Dapsone for Possible Carcinogenicity*. US Department of Health, Education, and Welfare publication 77-820. National Cancer Institute Carcinogenesis Technical Reports Series, 1977
47. Griciute L, Tomatis L: Carcinogenicity of dapsone in mice and rats. *Int J Cancer* **25**:123, 1980
48. Maurus JM: Hansen's disease in pregnancy. *Obstet Gynecol* **52**:22, 1978
49. Shigeura HT et al: Metabolic studies on dapsone and sulfone derivatives in chick macrophages. *Biochem Pharmacol* **24**:687, 1975
50. Shen TY et al: Read before the American Chemical Society Abstracts Meeting. September 12–16, 1971
51. Barranco VP: Inhibition of lysosomal enzymes by dapsone. *Arch Dermatol* **110**:563, 1974
52. Mier PD, Van Den Hurk JJMA: Inhibition of lysosomal enzymes by dapsone. *Br J Dermatol* **93**:471, 1975
53. Stendahl O et al: The inhibition of polymorphonuclear leukocyte cytotoxicity by dapsone: A possible mechanism in the treatment of dermatitis herpetiformis. *J Clin Invest* **62**:214, 1978
54. Kazmierowski JA et al: Dermatitis herpetiformis: Effects of sulfones and sulfonamides on neutrophil myeloperoxidase-mediated iodinations and cytotoxicity. *J Clin Immunol* **4**:55, 1984
55. Wozel G, Lehmann B: Dapsone inhibits the generation of 5-lipoxygenase products in polymorphonuclear leukocytes. *Skin Pharmacol* **8**:196, 1995

56. Coleman MD et al: Studies of the inhibitory effects of analogues of dapsone on neutrophil function in vitro. *J Pharm Pharmacol* **49**:53, 1997
57. Katz SI et al: Effect of sulfones on complement deposition in dermatitis herpetiformis and on complement-mediated guinea pig reactions. *J Invest Dermatol* **67**:688, 1976
58. Williams K et al: Anti-inflammatory actions of dapsone and its related biochemistry. *J Pharm Pharmacol* **28**:555, 1976
59. Maloff BL et al: Dapsone inhibits LTB$_4$ binding and bioresponse at the cellular and physiologic levels. *Eur J Pharmacol* **158**:85, 1988

60. Anderson R et al: In vitro and in vivo effects of dapsone on neutrophil and lymphocyte functions in normal individuals and patients with lepromatous leprosy. *Antimicrob Agents Chemother* **19**:495, 1981
61. Harvath L et al: Selective inhibition of neutrophil chemotaxis to N-formyl-methionyl-leucyl-phenylalanine by sulfones. *J Immunol* **137**:1305, 1986
62. Thuong-Nguyen V et al: Inhibition of neutrophil adherence to antibody by dapsone: A possible therapeutic mechanism of dapsone in the treatment of IgA dermatoses. *J Invest Dermatol* **100**:349, 1993
63. Booth SA et al: Dapsone suppresses integrin-mediated neutrophil adherence function. *J Invest Dermatol* **98**:135, 1992

CHAPTER 254

Gunnar Swanbeck

Aminoquinolines

The aminoquinolines are derived from quinine, a compound extracted from the bark of the cinchona tree native to South America. They have been used mainly as antimalarials. Even in dermatologic literature, these compounds are generally described under the heading of antimalarials. The antimalarials that are of dermatologic interest may all be regarded as aminoquinolines: chloroquine, hydroxychloroquine, amodiaquine, and quinacrine (Fig. 254-1). The last compound is, of course, more correctly classified as an acridine derivative. These four compounds are all 4-aminoquinolines. In the following discussion, the word aminoquinolines designates the four compounds mentioned above.

FIGURE 254-1

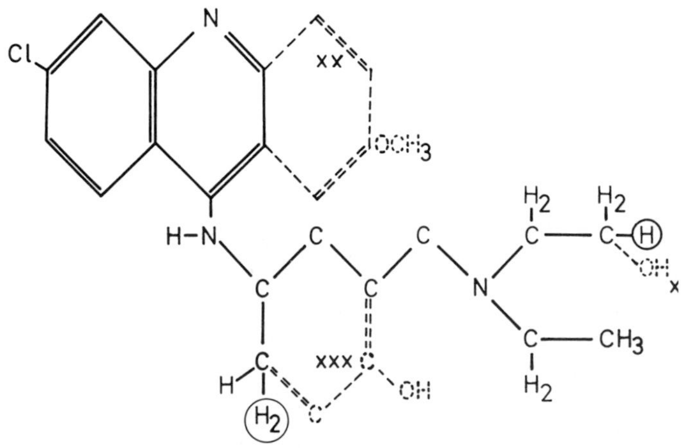

The aminoquinolines used in dermatology are all 4-aminoquinolines and may be regarded as derivatives of chloroquine, which is illustrated by the solid line. The other compounds are indicated by dotted lines: x, hydroxychloroquine; xx, quinacrine; xxx, amodiaquine. The two hydrogens within circles are substituted in the respective derivatives.

MODE OF ACTION

The aminoquinolines have several relatively well-defined effects on biochemical and cellular systems, the significance of which is not fully understood. Some of the more important are mentioned here.

Interactions with Nucleic Acids

Aminoquinolines bind to DNA. They also affect DNA and RNA polymerase activity and inhibit DNA replication and transcription to RNA.[1–3] This process may be directly related to DNA binding and may be involved with the antimalarial properties of these compounds and also with their inhibition of the lupus erythematosus–cell phenomenon and antinuclear antibody reactions.[4,5] This action is one possible explanation for the clinical effect of the aminoquinolines on lupus erythematosus.

Immunologic Effects

The aminoquinolines may suppress lymphocyte transformation in vitro.[6] They may also interfere with complement-dependent antigen-antibody reactions[7] and inhibit superoxide production in stimulated leukocytes.[8] No effect on the development of primary or secondary antibody response has been found.[9]

Anti-Inflammatory Activity

Chloroquine is a lysosomal stabilizer but it also inhibits hydrolytic enzymes.[10] In addition, chloroquine interferes with prostaglandin synthesis.[11] Another important property may be its influence on the chemotaxis of neutrophils, macrophages, and eosinophils.[12,13]

Photodermatologic Properties

There has been much work and speculation concerning the possible sun-screening effect of systemically administered chloroquine. Chloroquine absorbs in the UVA region of the spectrum and is bound in the epidermis in a relatively high concentration; however, there is no effect on the minimal erythematous dose.[14] The clinical action of chloroquine on lupus erythematosus and polymorphous light eruption may very well be explained by its effect on immunologic reactions.

Pharmacokinetics and Distribution

The aminoquinolines are all water-soluble and are readily absorbed in the gastrointestinal tract. The plasma concentration reaches a peak within about 8 h, but plasma is not cleared of the aminoquinoline within 24 h.[15] When daily doses are given, the plasma concentration increases to an equilibrium value after some weeks but remains relatively low, while the concentration in some organs may become many thousand times higher than in the plasma. The liver, spleen, lungs, and adrenal glands store chloroquine in large amounts.[16] Melanin-containing cells have a particular affinity for chloroquine,[17] and chloroquine binds to melanin in vitro.[18] The high uptake of chloroquine in the liver may be important in the use of this drug for porphyria cutanea tarda, and the melanin affinity may be the basis for the ocular side effects.

The equivalent doses of three of the aminoquinolines are 250 mg of chloroquine, 400 mg of hydroxychloroquine, and 100 mg of quinacrine.

SIDE EFFECTS

Side effects that are specific only for the aminoquinolines are discussed here. The acute symptoms resulting from very large doses of chloroquine are weakness, dyspnea, hypotension, tremor, coma, convulsions, and cardiopulmonary arrest.[16] A lethal dose of chloroquine for an adult is 3 to 6 g.

All the aminoquinolines may induce leukopenia within the first few months of treatment. Aplastic anemia has been reported with the use of quinacrine, but it is a very rare side effect.

The aminoquinolines should be regarded as teratogenic. Chloroquine is capable of crossing the placenta, and congenital defects such as deafness, mental retardation, and convulsions have been described in newborn children of women who have taken chloroquine during pregnancy.[19]

Toxic psychosis, headache, and irritability have been reported as consequences of the use of both chloroquine and quinacrine.[20] However, these side effects are usually reversible and disappear when the medication is discontinued.

Among the cutaneous side effects of aminoquinolines, the exacerbation of psoriasis is well known and may lead to a generalized exfoliation. There are conflicting reports in the literature on the actual risk of using aminoquinolines in psoriasis. It is curious that antimalarials are widely used by rheumatologists for the treatment

of psoriatic arthritis and they do not believe that these drugs cause flare-ups of preexisting psoriasis.

Discoloration of the skin may occur as a long-term cutaneous side effect.[16,21] A moderate dose of quinacrine rather regularly causes a yellow discoloration after a few months.

All the aminoquinolines may cause a bluish-black pigmentation of the pretibia, palate, face, and nail beds. These effects on the skin are reversible over time.

Ocular side effects are the greatest problem of the aminoquinolines, especially after long administration. Both chloroquine and hydroxychloroquine may cause deposits in the cornea that are reversible and may produce only slight symptoms in the form of halos around bright objects.[22]

Irreversible retinopathy is probably the factor that most limits use of the aminoquinolines. Most of the cases described involve chloroquine and hydroxychloroquine, although the other aminoquinolines are not safe in this respect. Hydroxychloroquine has been claimed to be safer than chloroquine with regard to induction of retinopathy.[23]

The retinopathy is certainly dose-related. There are two common views about this problem: One is that the accumulated dose of chloroquine should not exceed 200 g, and the other is that the daily dose of chloroquine should not exceed 4.4 mg per kilogram of body weight.[24,25] Some ophthalmologists claim that for an adult a daily dose of about 250 mg of chloroquine is safe if there is a yearly interruption of therapy for about 2 months. The patient should also be seen by an ophthalmologist at regular intervals. An interruption of the medication is, however, no guarantee against progression of the ocular problems. Systemic lupus erythematosus may itself produce ocular changes similar to those seen with aminoquinolines. However, ocular changes have also been observed in patients with rheumatoid arthritis who are taking chloroquine.[26]

INDICATIONS FOR USE

Malaria and rheumatoid arthritis are two of the chief indicators for aminoquinolines. They will not be discussed here because they are outside the field of dermatology. There are positive reports on the use of aminoquinolines for more than a dozen different skin diseases. Some of these findings have withstood the test of time; in other cases a single report on a rare disease has not been verified in spite of a long lapse of time since the original report was published.

Diseases for which the risk/benefit ratio seems to be favorable are lupus erythematosus, polymorphous light eruption, and porphyria cutanea tarda, and these diseases are dealt with in more detail below. Other diseases in which positive results with aminoquinolines have been reported are sarcoidosis, DNA-autosensitivity reaction, solar urticaria, scleroderma, lymphocytic infiltration of the skin, disseminated granuloma annulare, cutaneous cryptococcosis, cutaneous leishmaniasis, epidermolysis bullosa, acrodermatitis chronica atrophicans, and lichen sclerosus et atrophicus.[27]

Lupus Erythematosus (See also Chap. 172)

As early as the nineteenth century, lupus erythematosus was treated with quinine, the forerunner of the aminoquinolines. However, it was not until the 1950s that chloroquine and its derivatives came into more general use for treatment of this disease. The first report was by Page in 1951,[28] but several more followed.

Generally the full effect of the aminoquinolines is obtained within a month. Cutaneous symptoms respond better than do systemic involvements.[29] The seriously ill patient with fever, renal damage, and hematologic abnormalities does not benefit from these compounds.

Today the aminoquinolines are mainly used in combination with glucocorticoids in lupus erythematosus. The clinical effect of glucocorticoids and aminoquinolines seems to be additive. However, their side effects are different, and a more favorable risk/benefit ratio can be achieved by the combined use of the two types of drugs.

Although there are no convincing double-blind studies with aminoquinolines in patients with lupus erythematosus, the clinical evidence for their efficacy in the treatment of this disease is overwhelming. Also the many studies that show a high recurrence rate after discontinuation of treatment strongly support the clinical evidence.[30,31]

Polymorphous Light Eruption (See also Chap. 136)

This disease is confined to the sun-exposed areas of the skin, and the histology of the lesions indicates that there are immunologic factors involved in the pathogenesis. Several reports indicate that chloroquine is effective in patients with this disease.[14,32] In those parts of the world where there is a season with little sun radiation, it is possible for the patient to discontinue aminoquinolines for some months and thereby decrease the risk of long-term side effects. In patients with polymorphous light eruption, aminoquinoline medication is often combined with topical sun-screening agents. PUVA therapy is definitely more effective against polymorphous light eruption than aminoquinolines. Therefore the aminoquinolines are mainly indicated when PUVA cannot be given.[33,34] PUVA can also be given during the dark season to prevent problems during the light season.[35]

Porphyria Cutanea Tarda (See also Chap. 151)

Chloroquine is beneficial in the treatment of porphyria cutanea tarda. Its effect in this disease probably depends on mechanisms other than those in lupus erythematosus and polymorphous light eruption. It is tempting to believe that the high affinity of chloroquine for liver tissue is of primary importance.

When a daily dose of 250 mg of chloroquine is given to a patient with porphyria cutanea tarda, the following effects will be observed on the third to fourth day of medication: headache, nausea, fever, elevated transaminases, and massive excretion of porphyrins in the urine.[36] If the medication is stopped after a week of daily doses of 250 mg, the patient will continue to excrete porphyrins in the urine for 2 months. By the end of the third month, the patient usually has normal excretion of porphyrins, has no other symptoms of disease, and remains symptomless for 2 years or more.

The problem with this type of treatment is the acute reaction and the possible risk to the liver. Two regimens have been proposed to circumvent this problem. One is to give a small dose, 125 mg of chloroquine, twice a week over a long period.[37] The other is to perform phlebotomies three times before 250 mg chloroquine is given daily to the patient for 7 days.[38] Both methods seem to work satisfactorily.

Several theories have been proposed for the mode of action of chloroquine in porphyria cutanea tarda. It seems reasonable to assume, however, that uroporphyrins and chloroquine compete for the same binding sites in liver tissue and that chloroquine is able to displace porphyrins from the tissue. It has also been shown that chloroquine forms complexes with porphyrins.[39,40]

REFERENCES

1. Kurnick NB, Radcliffe IE: Reaction between DNA and quinacrine and other anti-malarials. *J Lab Clin Med* **60**:669, 1962
2. Cohen SN, Yielding KL: Stabilization of the structure of native DNA by chloroquine and observations on the nature of the chloroquine-DNA complex. *Arthritis Rheum* **6**:767, 1963
3. Cohen SN, Yielding KL: Further studies on the mechanism of action of chloroquine: Inhibition of DNA and RNA polymerase reactions. *Arthritis Rheum* **7**:302, 1964
4. Dubois EL: Effect of quinacrine (Atabrine) upon lupus erythematosus phenomenon. *Arch Dermatol Syphilol* **71**:570, 1955
5. Bencze G, Johnson GD: Inhibition of antinuclear factor reaction by chloroquine. *Immunology* **9**:201, 1965
6. Harvitz D, Hirschorn K: Suppression of in vitro lymphocyte responses by chloroquine. *N Engl J Med* **273**:23, 1965
7. Neblett TR et al: Chloroquine: Its mechanism of action upon immune phenomena. *Arch Dermatol* **92**:720, 1965
8. Hurst NP et al: Studies on the mechanism of inhibition of chemotactic tripeptide stimulated human neutrophil polymorphonuclear leucocyte superoxide production by chloroquine and hydroxychloroquine. *Ann Rheum Dis* **46**:750, 1987
9. Kalmanson GM, Guze LB: Studies of the effects of hydroxychloroquine on immune responses. *J Lab Clin Med* **65**:484, 1965
10. Weissmann G: Labilization and stabilization of lysosomes. *Fed Proc* **23**:1038, 1964
11. Greaves MW, McDonald-Gibson WJ: Antiinflammatory agents and prostaglandin biosynthesis. *Br Med J* **3**:527, 1972
12. Ward PA: The chemosuppression of chemotaxis. *J Exp Med* **124**:209, 1966
13. Ganderer CA, Gleich CJ: Inhibition of eosinophilotaxis by chloroquine and corticosteroids. *Proc Soc Exp Biol Med* **157**:129, 1978
14. Cahn MM et al: Polymorphous light eruption—the effect of chloroquine phosphate in modifying reactions to ultraviolet light. *J Invest Dermatol* **26**:201, 1956
15. Rubin M, Zvaifler N: The metabolism of chloroquine. *Clin Res* **10**:22, 1962
16. Dubois EL: Anti-malarials in the management of discoid and systemic lupus erythematosus. *Semin Arthritis Rheum* **8**:33, 1978
17. Zvaifler NJ et al: Chloroquine deposition in ocular tissues. *Arthritis Rheum* **5**:667, 1962
18. Buszman E et al: Electron spin resonance studies of chloroquine-melanin complexes. *Biochem Pharmacol* **33**:7, 1984
19. Lewis R et al: Malaria associated with pregnancy. *Obstet Gynecol* **42**:696, 1973
20. Sapp OL: Toxic psychosis due to quinacrine and chloroquine. *JAMA* **187**:373, 1964
21. Tuffanelli DL et al: Pigmentation associated with anti-malarial therapy. Its possible relationship to the ocular lesions. *Arch Dermatol* **88**:419, 1963
22. Hobbs RF, Calnan CD: Visual disturbances with anti-malarial drugs with particular reference to chloroquine keratopathy. *Arch Dermatol* **80**:557, 1959
23. Finbloom DS et al: Comparison of hydroxychloroquine and chloroquine use and the development of retinal toxicity. *J Rheumatol* **12**:692, 1985
24. Bernstein HN: Chloroquine ocular toxicity. *Surv Ophthalmol* **12**:415, 1967
25. MacKenzie AH: An appraisal of chloroquine. *Arthritis Rheum* **13**:280, 1970
26. Scherbel AL et al: Ocular lesions in rheumatoid arthritis and related disorders with particular reference to retinopathy: Study of 741 patients treated with and without chloroquine. *N Engl J Med* **273**:360, 1965
27. Isacson D et al: Antimalarials in dermatology. *Int J Dermatol* **21**:379, 1982
28. Page F: Treatment of lupus erythematosus with mepacrine. *Lancet* **2**:755, 1951

29. Dubois EL: Quinacrine (Atabrine) in treatment of systemic and discoid lupus erythematosus. *Arch Intern Med* **94**:131, 1954
30. Christiansen JV, Nielsen JP: Treatment of lupus erythematosus with mepacrine. Results and relapses during a long observation. *Br J Dermatol* **68**:73, 1956
31. Merwin C, Winkelmann R: Dermatologic clinics. 2. Antimalarial drugs in therapy of lupus erythematosus. *Mayo Clin Proc* **37**:253, 1962
32. Christiansen JV, Brodthagen H: The treatment of polymorphic light eruptions with chloroquine. *Br J Dermatol* **68**:204, 1956
33. Gschnait F et al: Induction of UV light tolerance by PUVA in patients with polymorphous light eruption. *Br J Dermatol* **99**:293, 1978
34. Parrish JA et al: Comparison of PUVA and beta-carotene in the treatment of polymorphous light eruption. *Br J Dermatol* **100**:187, 1979
35. Murphy GM et al: Prophylactic PUVA and UVB therapy in polymorphic light eruption—a controlled trial. *Br J Dermatol* **116**:531, 1987
36. Cripps DJ, Curtis AC: Toxic effect of chloroquine on porphyria hepatica. *Arch Dermatol* **86**:575, 1962
37. Kordac V et al: Chloroquine in the treatment of PCT. *N Engl J Med* **296**:949, 1977
38. Swanbeck G, Wennersten G: Treatment of porphyria cutanea tarda with chloroquine and phlebotomy. *Br J Dermatol* **97**:77, 1977
39. Moreau S et al: A nuclear magnetic resonance study of the interactions of antimalarial drugs with porphyrins. *Biochim Biophys Acta* **840**:107, 1985
40. Shanley BC et al: Evaluation of the stoichiometry and strength of chloroquine-porphyrin interactions by difference spectroscopy. *Biochem Pharmacol* **34**:141, 1985

CHAPTER 255

Jerome L. Shupack
Jennifer E. Silverman Kitchin
Matthew J. Stiller
Guy F. Webster

Cytotoxic and Antimetabolic Agents

Skin disease refractory to topical therapy can be controlled with systemic cytotoxic and antimetabolic drugs. Several drugs have particular advantages for dermatologists: methotrexate, azathioprine, thioguanine, mycophenolic acid, cyclophosphamide, chlorambucil, and doxorubicin. Cytotoxic and antimetabolic drugs are used in some diseases to modulate the behavior of inflammatory cells. Regardless of the target, these agents primarily exert their effects through the inhibition of cell division, which often leads to cell death. An understanding of the mechanism of action, toxicities, and clinical effects of these drugs is essential for optimal use.

The cell cycle is the sequence of growth phases in which all cells of the body are involved, and effectiveness of cytotoxic drugs depends upon it. During the G_1 phase, cell metabolism is directed toward preparing for DNA synthesis. The S phase of the cell cycle, which follows G_1, is devoted to DNA synthesis. At the end of DNA synthesis, the G_2 phase occurs and precedes cell division, which is termed the M phase. Cells may also enter a resting state, termed G_0, from either the G_1 or the G_2 phase; the length of the G_0 phase is variable (Fig. 255-1) (see Chap. 9).

Most systemic cytotoxic drugs that are useful in dermatology fall into two broad groups, the antimetabolites and the alkylating agents. Antimetabolites mimic natural molecules and are most active while DNA is being synthesized in the S phase. These drugs require a target population that is proliferating in order to exert their effect. A corollary of this principle is that side effects of this class of drugs are most prominent in cells of the body that have an innately high proliferative index, such as visceral epithelium and bone marrow. Alkylating agents exert their effects through an actual physicochemical interaction with preformed DNA molecules. These interactions include alkylation, cross-linking, and carbamylation.

Aalkylating agents not only are effective on proliferating populations of cells but also affect cells that are not actively synthesizing DNA. Their adverse effects are not limited to proliferating cell populations, and they have a greater potential for mutagenicity.

The immunosuppressive potency of cytotoxic drugs has benefits and risks. Infections of lethal proportion may arise quickly and quietly in immunosuppressed patients. Patients should be assessed at each visit for symptoms of infection, including fever, chills, sweats, shortness of breath, cough, headache, dysuria, and arthritis, and they should be instructed to report any new symptoms promptly.

FIGURE 255-1

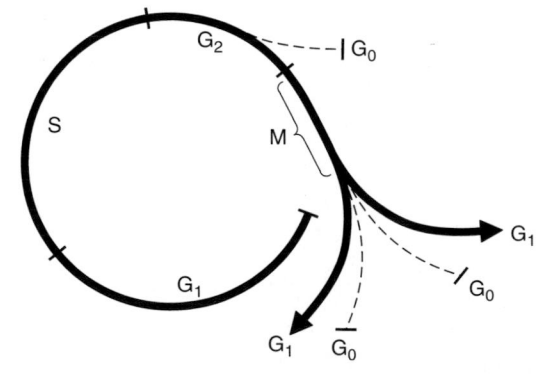

Diagram of the cell cycle.

TABLE 255-1

Potential Mechanisms of Methotrexate Activity in Skin Disease

Folate antagonisms/decreased cell proliferation
Suppression of inflammatory cell chemotaxis
Inhibition of monocyte/macrophage activation
Inhibition of histamine release from basophils (and mast cells?)
Inhibition of lymphocyte function

ANTIMETABOLIC AGENTS

Methotrexate

Methotrexate (amethopterin) was introduced in 1948 and remains one of the most commonly used antimetabolic agents in cancer therapy. It was initially used to treat hematologic malignancies, choriocarcinoma, and various epithelial-derived tumors; but it has been used more recently to treat nonmalignant diseases including rheumatoid arthritis, asthma, graft-versus-host disease, and cutaneous conditions, such as psoriasis and cutaneous sarcoidosis. Dermatologists have judiciously used this drug since the early 1960s and have generated an impressive record of safety.

Methotrexate occurs as a crystalline yellow to brown powder that is nearly insoluble in water or alcohol; methotrexate sodium is a yellow, water-soluble powder used in the preparation of injectable forms of the drug. Methotrexate is a synthetic analogue of folic acid (Fig. 255-2). It differs from folate in two regions, the substitution of an amino for a hydroxyl in the pteridine nucleus and in the methylation of the amino group between the benzoyl and pteroyl moieties. The folate vitamins function as 1-carbon carriers and are essential for the synthesis of purines and thymidylic acid. These products are required for gene synthesis and cell division. Folate exists in two forms in the body, as a monoglutamate in plasma and as a polyglutamate within cells. The polyglutamate is linked by γ-peptide bonds and is preferentially retained within cells. It is a more efficient cofactor than the monoglutamylated precursor. To be active, these folate cofactors must be reduced to tetrahydrofolate by the enzyme dihydrofolate reductase (Table 255-1). Methotrexate enters cells by two mechanisms, active transport and a carrier-independent mechanism that is active only at high methotrexate levels. Inside the cell methotrexate binds to dihydrofolate reductase and inactivates the enzyme. The drug is a competitive inhibitor of the natural substrate dihydrofolate. Synthesis of thymidylate is most sensitive to methotrexate-mediated folate depletion. Purine synthesis is somewhat more resistant.[1-3]

The activity of methotrexate is enhanced by polyglutamylation, just as is the activity of the natural substrate. These derivatives form

FIGURE 255-2

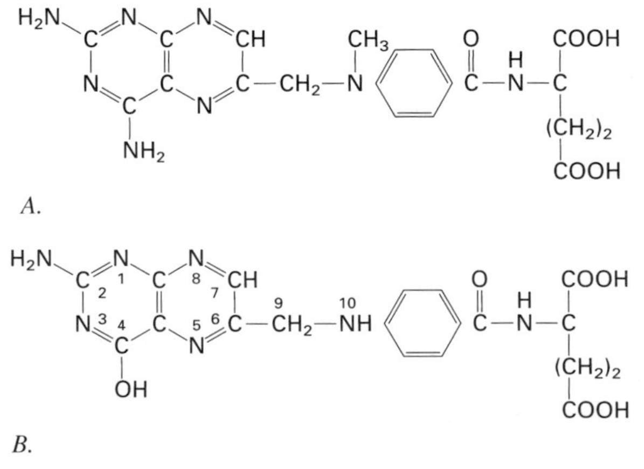

Chemical structure of methotrexate and folic acid. *A.* Methotrexate. *B.* Folic acid.

rapidly within cells and increase with the concentration of the drug and the duration of exposure. This form of methotrexate can persist within cells and bind more tightly to dihydrofolate reductase than does unaltered methotrexate. Glutamylation also broadens the spectrum of enzyme inhibition including thymidylate synthetase and amino imidazolecarboxamide ribonucleoside transferase. Consequently, high methotrexate doses and prolonged exposure produce a greater cytotoxic effect than would be predicted on the basis of drug dose alone. This fact is an important consideration in the design of treatment regimens, adjustment of dosages, and minimization of adverse effects.[3,4]

The mechanism of cytotoxic therapy in nonneoplastic skin disease is poorly understood, as are the diseases themselves. In skin diseases with an apparent inflammatory etiology, methotrexate may suppress white blood cell function. In other diseases, the mechanism is less clear. For example, psoriasis is characterized by excessive growth of the epidermis and supporting vasculature and may be exacerbated by the inflammatory response. The primary defect in psoriasis may either be epidermal or inflammatory. Methotrexate may act directly to inhibit epidermal cell division or may inhibit the effect of inflammatory cells. Van De Putte and colleagues have suggested that methotrexate works on the efferent arc of the immuno-inflammatory process, rather than on T cells.[5] Perhaps, as suggested by Wolff and colleagues,[6] adenosine mediates the methotrexate-induced attenuation of leukocyte adherence and emigration in postcapillary venules. There are few data to prove any of these contentions. High oncologic doses of methotrexate (for example, 100 to 250 mg/m[2] per week) depress the antibody response to common antigens. Lower doses suppress rheumatoid factor production. Low doses of methotrexate suppress division of mononuclear cells and inhibit their response to interleukin 2, suppress neutrophil and monocyte chemotaxis in vitro and in vivo, and depress Langerhans cell activity and leukotriene B$_4$ synthesis by neutrophils.[4,7-12] The mechanisms for most of these effects are not understood.

The proliferation of epidermal cells, a key issue in psoriasis, is also modulated by methotrexate. Strong evidence exists for the direct action of methotrexate on psoriatic epidermal proliferation.[13-16] Psoriatic epidermal cell division is suppressed best with systemic methotrexate. Intralesional or topical methotrexate has much less clinical efficacy despite evidence that local delivery of the drug suppresses the growth of normal animal skin. This discrepancy has been attributed to problems in local penetration and to involvement of a different target for the drug. Suppression of the immune system or of systemic production of a "psoriatic factor" could be such a target.[13-16]

PHARMACOKINETICS Nearly 90 percent of an oral dose of methotrexate can be recovered in the blood, but the time to peak plasma levels can vary from 1 to 5 h.[17-22] Absorption is influenced by food. Milk (and possibly other calcium-containing compounds) decreases bioavailability.[18] In adults, mean bioavailability is 67 percent of the administered dose with plasma peaks between 1 and

3 h after the administration of 10 mg/m^2. Divided oral doses of methotrexate (for example, three 5-mg doses separated by 12 h) result in blood levels ranging from 0.17 to 0.5 μg/mL.

The distribution of methotrexate is determined by its negative charge at neutral pH, which limits its diffusion across biologic membranes.[1] Low central nervous system penetration is a great advantage in the treatment of skin disease. However, the lower membrane transit may also result in a theoretical disadvantage. It follows that a drug that does not penetrate into a third-space collection, such as ascites or pleural effusion, will likewise be delayed in its exit from this area. This delay may be the mechanism for the prolonged blood levels of the drug and, to a degree, may provide the rationale for intermittent methotrexate dosing.

The mean serum half-life of methotrexate depends somewhat on the dose given. At high dosages (e.g., 30 mg/m^2), there is a triphasic elimination curve for the drug and its principal metabolite. Studies of low-dose methotrexate in rheumatoid arthritis and psoriasis show that most patients have a two-phase elimination curve. The mean serum half-life is 6 to 7 h at doses commonly used in dermatology. It should be noted that, although plasma levels fall, intracellular polyglutamylation may stabilize tissue levels of the drug, even in the absence of serum drug levels. The effect of this phenomenon on methotrexate-mediated disease suppression is not clear. Recent studies in rheumatoid arthritis, however, suggest that its effect is negligible.[23]

Methotrexate is 50 to 60 percent bound to serum protein.[1,24] Serum protein binding is decreased in vitro and in vivo by sodium salicylate. One study noted a decrease of 50 to 70 percent. The clinical significance of such displacement is not clear.

Methotrexate is metabolized mainly in the liver. The primary metabolite is 7-OH-methotrexate, which is a weak inhibitor of dihydrofolate reductase; it is about 200 times less potent than methotrexate. Excretion of methotrexate is primarily renal; it is excreted in the renal tubules at a rate that probably exceeds inulin clearance. It is also reabsorbed by a pathway that is not well described. Various weak organic acids, including aspirin, other nonsteroidal agents, and probenccid, interfere with methotrexate excretion. About 80 percent of a single dose of methotrexate eventually appears in the urine, while a smaller fraction is excreted in bile.[25–29]

ADVERSE REACTIONS There is a large collected experience in the rheumatologic and dermatologic literature regarding the toxicity of low-dose methotrexate.[30,31] Adverse reactions (Table 255-2) may be life threatening or trivial. Several principles regarding the side effects of methotrexate are generally applicable. First, higher doses cause more side effects. Second, patients who experience side effects early in therapy will probably continue to do so, whereas patients who are free of early complaints may be more likely to remain so during long-term treatment. Third, sicker, older, or more debilitated patients seem to experience more problems than those who are in good health. Finally, the use of divided drug dosing is often helpful in reducing side effects.

TABLE 255-2

Adverse Reactions to Methotrexate

Gastrointestinal: nausea, vomiting, stomatitis, diarrhea, ulceration

Hepatic: abnormal transaminase levels, hepatitis, fibrosis, cirrhosis

Hematopoietic: anemia, thrombocytopenia, leukopenia, pancytopenia

Pulmonary: acute hypersensitivity, fibrosis

Systemic: anaphylaxis

The most common complaints of patients being treated with methotrexate involve the gastrointestinal tract.[30,31] Nausea and vomiting are the most frequent problems and are largely dose-related. They occur most commonly with oral therapy, but they also occur with intramuscular injection; 10 to 30 percent of all patients experience some difficulty. The administration of antacids, H$_2$ blockers, prochlorperazine, or metoclopramide is often effective in controlling these symptoms. Unusually severe cases may require ondansetron hydrochloride to control the nausea. Diarrhea is relatively infrequent and does not limit methotrexate therapy. Gastric ulceration rarely occurs and is often exacerbated by the concurrent administration of antiarthritic drugs.

Mucocutaneous complaints occur fairly frequently. Oral ulcerations and soreness are most often noted. Skin ulcerations are much less frequent and may herald bone marrow toxicity. When these conditions are severe enough to treat, the authors favor the use of topical anesthetics or low-potency topical glucocorticoids.

A major limitation of methotrexate therapy is the induction of liver fibrosis.[30–39] Methotrexate is clearly a hepatotoxic drug. Elevations in liver enzymes occur frequently in 8 to 67 percent of patients. Although disquieting, these elevations do not seem to have any value in predicting which patients will develop cirrhosis. For unknown reasons, patients with psoriasis seem to have a higher incidence of liver fibrosis than do patients with rheumatoid arthritis who are treated with similar methotrexate regimens. Fibrosis relates to the duration of therapy, total dose, and patient age. Between 0 and 26 percent of patients receiving methotrexate have demonstrated cirrhotic changes. A somewhat larger number may show fatty infiltration and a "trivial" fibrosis.[31] Those receiving total doses of less than 1.5 g have a negligible incidence of fibrosis.[31] The course of methotrexate-induced liver disease is relatively non-aggressive. In fact, several investigators have reported continuation of therapy in these patients with no adverse effects. Since the mechanism by which methotrexate causes liver damage is not known, definitive statements about prevention cannot be made. Patients with prior liver disease, diabetes, obesity, significant alcohol intake, and intravenous drug use are all at increased risk for hepatic fibrosis and cirrhosis.[31]

The only acceptable method for verifying methotrexate-induced cirrhosis is percutaneous needle biopsy of the liver.[32] This procedure is usually safe. The approximate risk of minor bleeding is 1 in 1000, and the risk of death is estimated as 1 in 10,000.[40] Biopsy results are classified according to liver architecture, degree of inflammation and fibrosis, and presence of fat and are graded on a scale of I to IV (Table 255-3). Roenigk and colleagues[31] recommend that patients with grades I and II histology may continue methotrexate therapy, those with grade IIIA histology may continue

TABLE 255-3

Liver Histology Grading Scale

Grade I	Normal to mild fatty infiltration, portal inflammation, and nuclear variability
Grade II	Moderate to severe fatty infiltration, nuclear variability, portal tract expansion and inflammation, and necrosis
Grade IIIA	Mild fibrosis
Grade IIIB	Moderate to severe fibrosis
Grade IV	Cirrhosis

therapy with a repeat liver biopsy in 6 months, and those with grades IIIB and IV histology should discontinue therapy. According to a study published by Newman and colleagues,[41] 8 of 11 patients with fibrosis or cirrhosis secondary to methotrexate therapy showed meaningful improvement in liver histologic findings after methotrexate treatment had been discontinued for 6 months or more; none had progression of abnormalities.

There is conjecture about when a liver biopsy should first be performed. Roenigk and associates,[31] of the Psoriasis Task Force of the American Academy of Dermatology, recommend that liver biopsy be performed after administration of the first 1.5 g of methotrexate. Others contend that the liver should be biopsied once it is clear that the patient is a candidate for long-term methotrexate treatment. Patients may be treated for 1 or 2 months to see if their disease is adequately suppressed and to ensure that any methotrexate-induced side effects are tolerable. Once a commitment to long-term treatment with methotrexate is made by the physician and patient, the liver biopsy should be performed.

Methotrexate-induced bone marrow suppression is not uncommon.[42–45] Marrow cells are rapidly proliferating, and they are particularly susceptible to methotrexate. Severe bone marrow suppression due to low-dose oral methotrexate has been reported. The patients were anemic, neutropenic, and thrombocytopenic, with evidence of sepsis and severe bleeding disorders. Factors that appear to put patients at increased risk for marrow toxicity include advanced age, low creatinine clearance, and concurrent administration of nonsteroidal anti-inflammatory drugs. No single cause has been identified.

Methotrexate can cause mutations in laboratory animals. However, there has been no associated increase in cancer in patients treated with dermatologic doses of methotrexate. Because methotrexate is teratogenic and may act as an abortifacient, administration during pregnancy is absolutely contraindicated. There is no apparent effect on the outcome of pregnancies occurring after the discontinuation of methotrexate therapy. There are no reports of abnormal children fathered by men receiving methotrexate therapy, although sperm motility may be abnormal during treatment.[46–50]

Opportunistic infections have been reported in three otherwise healthy individuals receiving low-dose methotrexate (one case of *Pneumocystis* pneumonia and two cases of cryptococcosis).

Overdosage with methotrexate should be treated promptly with leucovorin (folinic acid).[31] Patients who have episodes of decreased renal function while receiving methotrexate should be treated as they would for an overdosage. An initial dose of 10 mg of folinic acid per square millimeter (about 20 mg) should be given intravenously, followed by oral doses of 20 mg every 6 h (Table 255-4). The blood level of methotrexate should be determined every 12 to 24 h. Leucovorin administration should continue until the level of serum methotrexate falls below 10^{-8} M.

TABLE 255-4

Leucovorin Treatment of Methotrexate Overdosage

SERUM METHOTREXATE LEVEL	LEUCOVORIN DOSAGE*
0.5×10^{-6} M	20 mg q6h
0.1×10^{-5} M	100 mg q6h
0.2×10^{-5} M	200 mg q6h

*Increase proportionately for greater methotrexate levels.

The authors have published[51] two cases supporting leucovorin rescue with oral methotrexate therapy in patients with psoriasis with a history of methotrexate-induced pancytopenia or diminished renal or hepatic function during the period of methotrexate therapy. Leucovorin is metabolized in vivo directly to tetrahydrofolate in the absence of dihydrofolate reductase and acts as an antidote to methotrexate overdose by providing a continued supply of thymidine until the methotrexate is cleared from the body. The optimal dosage and timing of leucovorin rescue for low-dose methotrexate therapy have yet to be established.[51] The authors prefer to measure methotrexate levels in each patient to determine the duration of leucovorin rescue that is necessary, continuing until the concentration decreases below 0.01 μM. Leucovorin doses of 15 mg orally every 6 h, begun within 18 h of methotrexate administration and continued for 36 h to 48 h, appear to be adequate. We conclude that the safety of oral leucovorin and the lack of inhibition of the therapeutic effectiveness of methotrexate suggest that leucovorin rescue following low-dose methotrexate may deserve broad clinical application. Long-term studies have not been carried out.

Several cases of systemic anaphylaxis due to low dose methotrexate have been reported, most recently by Cohn and colleagues.[52] Many of these patients had previously received uneventful methotrexate treatments at comparable doses.

There are three major groups of drug interactions: the first results from alterations in protein binding, the second from altered renal excretion, and the third from hepatotoxicity. Although any drug that may enhance methotrexate toxicity should be avoided, there are several near-absolute contraindications (Table 255-5).

TREATMENT RECOMMENDATIONS Perhaps the most effective way to reduce adverse effects from methotrexate is to exclude inappropriate patients. The ideal patient would have severe skin disease but otherwise would be healthy, young, and compliant. Patients with a history of liver disease, kidney disease, or significant risk factors for such organ impairment are at greater risk. The decrement in renal function that occurs as part of the aging process makes the very old patient less than optimal. Given the tendency of patients to underestimate their alcohol intake, the admission of any ethanol consumption may constitute a relative contraindication. The use of other medications may also predispose patients to drug interactions and so may be a relative contraindication.

The second most effective way to reduce adverse effects is rigorous attention to detail, especially in patients who are less than ideal candidates for the drug. Such attention includes frequent follow-up, detailed review of systems at each visit, the monitoring of appropriate laboratory parameters (Table 255-6), and communication with the patient's general physician at appropriate intervals.

TABLE 255-5

Potential Drug Interactions with Methotrexate

Nonsteroidal anti-inflammatory agents
Sulfonamides
Probenecid*
Ketotifen
Allopurinol
Ethanol*
Penicillins
Cephalosporins
Barbiturates
Phenytoin
Cisplatin and all renal-toxic drugs*

*Near-absolute contraindication.

TABLE 255-6

Premethotrexate Tests

Renal
    Urine analysis
    Creatinine clearance
    BUN/creatinine
Hematopoietic
    Complete blood count
    Folate level
Hepatic
    Transaminase levels
    Alkaline phosphatase level
    Total bilirubin
    Albumin

Most patients receiving antipsoriatic doses of methotrexate experience mild transaminemia for several days after drug administration. The criterion, therefore, for safe use is normal transaminase levels immediately before each weekly pulsed dose.

Optimal patient compliance should be promoted by detailed, clear instructions and reinforced by printed literature (Table 255-7). For particularly noncompliant patients, the physician may elect to require an office visit for parenteral methotrexate administration. This treatment may also be more economical, since injectable methotrexate costs only a fraction of the cost of oral medication.

The authors believe in short-term trials (up to 1 to 2 months) of methotrexate whenever possible. Often a brief administration of methotrexate may allow a patient's disease to be subsequently controlled by less toxic therapy. Using short-term methotrexate to quiet a flare of skin disease is also particularly appropriate in patients with relative contraindications to prolonged therapy such as alcoholism or hepatic disease. Even when therapy is intended to be of short duration, full pretreatment tests should be performed.

While prudent doses of methotrexate produce great improvement, they often do not result in complete clearing of the disease. When doses of methotrexate higher than 25 mg per week are used to treat psoriasis, the side effects may outweigh any benefit. Patients' and physicians' expectations should be for effective control, not complete clearing of disease.

TABLE 255-7

Instructions for Patients Receiving Methotrexate

1. Follow instructions faithfully.
2. Take methotrexate weekly, not daily.
3. Call your physician immediately if overdose is suspected.
4. Notify your physician if fever, cough, or shortness of breath develops.
5. Tell your physician about all side effects.
6. Inform all of your physicians that you are taking methotrexate.
7. Drink no alcoholic beverages and take no other medications without physician approval.
8. Do not take methotrexate while pregnant or while trying to conceive.
9. Do not take methotrexate if you have an active infection (including but not limited to cold/flu, urinary tract infection, pneumonia) without notifying your physician.
10. Allow no one else to take this medication.

SPECIFIC CLINICAL APPLICATIONS *Psoriasis* The largest and most widely accepted dermatologic use for methotrexate in non-neoplastic disease is in the treatment of psoriasis. Such use dates from 1951, when it was reported that a patient's psoriasis unexpectedly cleared during treatment with methotrexate.[53] During the 1950s and 1960s, various treatment regimens were tested.[54] Weinstein and Frost[55,56] related methotrexate dosage to psoriatic cell kinetics and proposed a weekly treatment regimen in which a third of the total methotrexate dose was given every 12 h over a 24-h period to achieve an effective blood level for 36 h. The intent of this regimen was to maximize the exposure of proliferating psoriatic cells to the drug. Currently, the two most common methotrexate regimens are the Weinstein-Frost regimen or a single weekly dose. In 1987, Peckham and colleagues[57] reported that over half of the dermatologists in the United States use methotrexate to treat severe psoriasis. Methotrexate was second only to ultraviolet (UV) radiation as a treatment modality for severe disease.

Current use of methotrexate in psoriasis is usually limited to patients with severe disease that is refractory to conventional topical treatments. When practical, a patient with psoriasis may be allowed to fail a therapeutic trial of UVB phototherapy or photochemotherapy (PUVA)—psoralens plus UVA—before methotrexate is started. The suitability of UVB therapy or photochemotherapy is limited for many individuals, and a trial of this method is often not possible for financial reasons or time considerations.

Patients deemed to be appropriate candidates on the basis of disease severity, general health, and personal habits and whose baseline laboratory results are acceptable may be started on a dose of 2.5 to 5 mg every 12 h for three doses, given by mouth. After 2 to 3 weeks, the patient should return for repeat laboratory tests (CBC, plus differential, BUN/creatinine, liver enzymes), a skin examination, and a review of systems. If all is in order, or if the reported side effects are minor, weekly therapy may be continued at the same dose, or at an increased dose in the absence of a significant response. Concomitant therapy with calcipotriene ointment or with midpotency topical glucocorticoid ointments is usually helpful.

Patients continue periodic visits until their disease is quiescent and their drug dosage is stable (usually 3 to 4 months). At this point the authors continue therapy for several weeks to ensure that the observed improvement has stabilized and then gradually taper the methotrexate dose to the point where the disease flares. This tapering determines the dose for chronic administration. In some cases, the drug may be entirely discontinued and mild recurrences treated with alternate methods. Patients often may need methotrexate for only several months each year because their psoriasis can be well controlled by topical treatment in the interval. There are some patients whose disease does not readily respond to methotrexate. The highest dose of methotrexate that is usually given to patients with psoriasis is a total of 22.5 mg per week, although some patients tolerate higher doses with no apparent problems. Occasional patients with refractory disease respond best to parenteral methotrexate. In refractory cases, combining methotrexate with PUVA photochemotherapy can enhance therapeutic efficacy without significantly increasing toxicity.

Pustular psoriasis is particularly responsive to methotrexate.[58,59] Unfortunately, no large, organized studies can confirm this observation. If a patient with pustular psoriasis qualifies for methotrexate therapy, the authors usually begin treatment with 5 mg every 12 h for three doses every 5 to 7 days until remission is achieved.

The effectiveness of methotrexate in psoriatic arthritis is less clear. Kragballe and colleagues[60] reported a retrospective study of 57 patients with psoriasis who also had seronegative arthritis. The starting dosage was 15 mg per week and the average treatment duration was 3 years. One-half of the patients reported "modest improvement" and one-half reported nearly complete remission. Those patients whose arthritis was of recent onset had the best response. These promising results must be tempered by the fact that accurate grading of the initial level of joint disease may be nearly impossible in a retrospective study. Wilkins and collaborators[61] performed a prospective double-blind, placebo-controlled study of methotrexate in patients with psoriatic arthritis. Doses were 7.5 to 15 mg per week in divided doses. An ongoing stable dose of a nonsteroidal anti-inflammatory drug was permitted. Methotrexate-treated patients improved only in the area of skin involvement and in the physician's global assessment of arthritis activity. Most parameters were unchanged.

More recently, Pigatto and colleagues[62] reported an overall 60 percent satisfactory response, with a 20 percent total remission in 54 patients with psoriatic polyarthritis who were treated with a dose of 10 to 12.5 mg per week of methotrexate. The maximum efficacy was within 6 months, after which there was no further reduction in disease activity. It is not clear why rheumatoid arthritis appears to be more responsive to methotrexate than does psoriatic arthritis, but rheumatologists do view methotrexate as useful in psoriatic arthritis.

The question of whether HIV+ individuals with psoriasis can be safely treated with methotrexate is unsettled. Six HIV+ patients with psoriasis who were treated with methotrexate developed opportunistic infections.[63,64] However, Maurer and colleagues[65] have reported that two of three HIV+ patients with psoriasis treated with methotrexate did not develop opportunistic infections. Because of the theoretical possibility of added immunosuppression by methotrexate in HIV+ patients, the first line of systemic treatment in these patients should be acitretin.[63,64]

Reiter's syndrome Reiter's syndrome is a disease of skin, mucosa, and joints that is very similar to pustular psoriasis. It is often manageable with topical glucocorticoids and oral nonsteroidal anti-inflammatory drugs, but refractory cases may require aggressive therapy. The dermatologic and rheumatologic literature reports various treatment schedules for methotrexate in Reiter's syndrome. Lally and Ho[66] suggest treatment with 10 mg per week by mouth or intramuscular injection. Response usually occurs within weeks, although months may be required for complete clearing.

Sarcoidosis Methotrexate may be useful in cases of refractory sarcoidosis. In 1977, Veien and Brodthagen[67] reported that refractory sarcoidosis in 12 of 16 patients was cleared by 25 mg per week of methotrexate. The authors have had favorable experience with the use of this drug in sarcoidosis.[68] The advantages for patients with severe sarcoidosis include avoidance of the side effects of high-dose or of long-term systemic glucocorticoids. Disadvantages include the potential for kidney, liver, bone marrow, and pulmonary toxicity. In patients with sarcoidosis with hepatic and renal involvement who are receiving methotrexate, it may be difficult to interpret laboratory abnormalities.

Other diseases in which methotrexate is useful include pityriasis lichenoides et varioliformis acuta,[69,70] lymphomatoid papulosis,[71,72] pityriasis rubra pilaris,[73–75] granulomatous vasculitis,[76] rheumatoid vasculitis,[76–78] polymyositis,[79–82] pemphigus vulgaris,[83–85] lupus erythematosus,[86] and pyoderma gangrenosum (G.F.W., unpublished). In severe steroid-responsive cutaneous diseases, the con-comitant use of methotrexate may allow reduction of the systemic dose of the glucocorticoid.

Azathioprine

The thiopurine drugs are synthetic analogues of the natural purine bases. They were first synthesized in the 1950s, and many derivatives have subsequently been produced. The drug most commonly used in dermatology is azathioprine. Azathioprine was first developed as an agent to delay the metabolism of 6-mercaptopurine and is formed by attaching an imidazole ring to the sulfur at position 6 in the parent molecule[87–89] (Fig. 255-3). The drug is a pale-yellow powder that is insoluble in water and is barely soluble in alcohol. It is rendered water-soluble by coadministration with sodium hydroxide. If stored in solution at alkaline pH, azathioprine degrades quickly.

The clinical activity of all the thiopurine drugs is believed to stem from the inhibition of RNA and DNA synthesis and function. Azathioprine is a prodrug that is metabolized to 6-mercaptopurine; 6-mercaptopurine is then activated by hypoxanthine-guanine phosphoribosyl transferase (HGPRT). These monophosphate nucleotide analogues then block purine synthesis at the initial step. Triphosphorylated 6-mercaptopurine is also incorporated into DNA, rendering the molecule susceptible to strand breaks and point mutations. Cells that lack HGPRT—for example, certain tumor lines—are resistant to the cytotoxic effects of azathioprine.[90,91]

Azathioprine and 6-mercaptopurine are equivalent in potency when administered parenterally, but 6-mercaptopurine is much less effective when given by mouth. Azathioprine is readily and fairly completely absorbed after oral administration. Plasma protein binding is about 30 percent. Azathioprine is largely dialyzable and does cross the placenta. Only a small proportion of the thiopurines is excreted intact. Azathioprine is converted into mercaptopurine, which then undergoes oxidations to 6-thiouric acid by xanthine oxidase. Mercaptopurine may also be methylated and sulfated and then excreted in the urine.[90,92]

Genetic polymorphism may contribute to excessive myelosuppression in some patients treated with azathioprine. An unexpected number of patients with thiopurine-induced leukopenia have no detectable levels of thiopurine methyltransferase (TPMT), an enzyme involved in the in vivo catabolism of azathioprine.[93] In addition, levels of 6-thioguanine nucleotide correlate with the degree of myelosuppression in patients with pemphigus treated with azathioprine.[94] There are wide differences among individuals in TPMT levels, which are controlled by a common genetic polymorphism.[95–97] Any episode of leukopenia in an azathioprine-treated patient may indicate a genetically determined sensitivity to the drug. This may require a new, lower maintenance dose of azathioprine, or, alternatively, the substitution of a different oral agent. The complementary DNA for TMPT has been cloned, sequenced, and expressed.[98] This may eventually lead to routine genetic screening of patients before the initiation of azathioprine therapy.

FIGURE 255-3

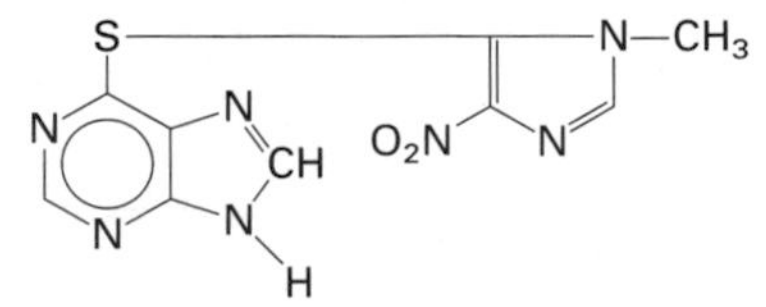

Chemical structure of azathioprine.

ADVERSE REACTIONS (See Table 255-8) Azathioprine is generally a safe drug when used carefully. A comparison of adverse reactions in patients with rheumatoid arthritis treated with methotrexate or azathioprine failed to reveal significant differences.[94]

Myelosuppression is the major toxic side effect of azathioprine administration. A generalized depression of leukocytes is the most common type of myelosuppression, but any cell line may be exclusively suppressed. Because platelets have the shortest life span of all the formed elements, thrombocytopenia is the most common presentation of toxic marrow suppression. Bone marrow suppression usually occurs only at the higher dosage ranges of dermatologic azathioprine therapy.[87,94,99]

Patients receiving high doses of azathioprine may experience nausea, vomiting, and diarrhea.[87] The symptoms are usually not severe and may be minimized by using a divided dose. Toxic hepatitis developed in about 1 percent of patients with rheumatoid arthritis who received azathioprine. This hepatitis is characterized by extremely high alkaline phosphatase levels and is usually reversible. Hepatic venoocclusive disease has also been reported, as has pancreatitis.[100,101]

Patients treated with azathioprine have an increased risk of infection. Most patients treated with this drug also receive large doses of glucocorticoids as part of their treatment regimen, and therefore it is difficult to assess the exact role of azathioprine in predisposing them to infection. Unlike cyclophosphamide-mediated immune suppression, suppression mediated by azathioprine is not proportional to the peripheral leukocyte count. Thus infection may occur at normal white blood cell levels.

Azathioprine infrequently causes a drug fever, often accompanied by chills, headache, and malaise.[102–105] Discontinuation of therapy is indicated.

Azathioprine-induced shock has been reported in dermatology patients.[106] In most cases of azathioprine-induced shock, the hypotensive collapse occurred within hours of the first dose.

Some investigators have found no increased malignancy, while others find a significantly increased azathioprine induction of cancer. The most recent analysis of this problem in a group of patients with rheumatoid arthritis suggests that hematologic malignancies, particularly non-Hodgkin's lymphoma, may be promoted. The relative risk is roughly 10- to 13-fold, or one lymphoma per 1000 patient years of azathioprine treatment.[107] There is an increased incidence of azathioprine-related lymphoma in the renal transplant, the Sjögren's syndrome, and the rheumatoid populations.[87] How patients with skin disease fare is not known. In general, dermatologic doses are lower than those used in patients with renal or rheumatologic disease. Likewise, the duration of therapy for skin disease is usually much shorter than for other diseases. It is the opinion of the authors that the risk of lymphoma in patients with azathioprine-treated dermatologic disease is probably significantly less than in transplant patients or patients with arthritis.

TABLE 255-8

Adverse Reactions to Azathioprine

Myelosuppression
Infection
Drug Fever
Gastrointestinal
  Nausea, vomiting, diarrhea
  Hepatitis
  Pancreatitis
Induction of malignancy
Shock

Roubenoff and associates[108] reviewed the incidence of azathioprine-associated birth defects. The rate of congenital malformation is only 4.3 percent. The prevalance of neonatal immunosuppression may be significant. There appears to be no adverse effect on fertility.

Azathioprine is supplied as 50-mg tablets and in injectable form. Before therapy begins, a baseline blood count, BUN, creatinine, and liver function tests should be performed. Impaired renal function may be associated with greater toxicity even though mercaptopurine metabolites have less activity than the parent drug. During therapy, blood counts and liver function tests should be obtained weekly during the first month and every 2 or 3 weeks thereafter. Dosage increases require more frequent testing.

Some believe that patients who have previously received alkylating agents may have a greatly increased risk for subsequent malignancy after thiopurine therapy. The authors avoid the use of thiopurines in these patients when possible.

CLINICAL APPLICATIONS The autoimmune etiology of the pemphigus group of diseases makes immunosuppressive drugs a logical therapeutic choice. In 1969, Wolff and Schriener[109] reported the successful use of azathioprine in the treatment of pemphigus. Although the drug may be used as a monotherapy, it is most commonly employed as an adjunct to steroid treatment. Other steroid-sparing drugs such as cyclophosphamide, gold, or dapsone are used as well. Bystryn[110] reviewed the literature and found a slightly higher rate of clinical remission in studies using azathioprine or cyclophosphamide. It is widely held that the therapeutic effect of azathioprine in pemphigus is delayed by up to several weeks.

Aberer and colleagues[111] reported a prospective long-term study of patients with pemphigus who were treated with steroids and azathioprine. The starting dose of azathioprine was 2 to 3 mg/kg per day combined with 80 to 200 mg per day of methylprednisolone. The steroid was maintained for several months, then tapered, and eventually discontinued. Azathioprine was withdrawn after 4 disease-free months off steroids. Forty-five percent of patients achieved apparent remission with this drug regimen. Another trial[112] suggests a survival advantage with combined azathioprine-steroid therapy compared either with steroids alone or with methotrexate.

The authors begin azathioprine therapy (1 to 2 mg/kg per day) early in the course of the disease, usually after the first week or two, if 60 to 80 mg of prednisone has failed to control new blister formation. A lower risk of neoplasia with azathioprine than with cyclophosphamide seems to be an advantage. The addition of azathioprine speeds steroid tapering without exacerbating the disease, and several of our patients appear to be in drug-free remission. Azathioprine and other cytotoxic drugs have received little attention as treatment for relatively mild pemphigus. It is not known whether the potential long-term risk of azathioprine outweighs the potential benefits of inducing a long-term remission.

Other bullous diseases respond to azathioprine. Numerous case reports endorse the use of the drug for steroid-resistant bullous pemphigoid.[113,114] Treatment regimens are similar to those used in patients with pemphigus.

The addition of cytotoxic drugs to steroid therapy has been responsible for the greatly increased survival of patients with systemic vasculitis.[115,116] Cyclophosphamide is the cytotoxic drug of choice for this application, but azathioprine is sometimes useful. Azathioprine seems more able to maintain a remission than to induce one. Azathioprine does not induce gonadal dysfunction, and therefore it is sometimes used in patients who wish to conceive after treatment for their disease.

Various other diseases involving uncontrolled inflammation have been targets for azathioprine therapy. They include lupus erythematosus,[117] polymyositis,[118] and various photodermatoses.[119,120] Due to the differences among individuals in azathioprine metabolism (see above), it may be necessary for researchers and clinicians to consider the genetic polymorphism when evaluating the success or failure of the drug.

Thioguanine

Thioguanine, first described by Elion and Hitchings in 1955, is another member of the thiopurine family of drugs. Its metabolism and mechanism of action are similar to those of azathioprine. Thioguanine is a structural analogue of guanine, in which the keto group of carbon 6 of the purine ring is replaced by a sulfur atom. This nucleoside analogue acts as a prodrug and generates guanine analogues in the tissues via the action of purine nucleoside phosphorylase. The guanine analogues must undergo enzymatic conversion to the nucleotide to display cytotoxic activity. The role of the incorporation of thioguanine into cellular DNA in the generation of its cytotoxic and therapeutic effects is not known, although it is likely that this class of drugs acts via multiple mechanisms.

Thioguanine is orally administered. Its absorption is incomplete and unpredictable, and there may be more than a tenfold variation in plasma concentrations. Peak levels occur 2 to 4 h after ingestion. Unlike azathioprine and mercaptopurine, thioguanine may be administered concurrently with allopurinol without a dosage reduction. Adverse effects of thioguanine include bone marrow depression and gastrointestinal disturbances. Kao and colleagues[121] have also described a toxic hepatic venoocclusive disease in association with 6-thioguanine therapy for psoriasis.

Thioguanine is supplied in 40-mg tablets. The authors usually prescribe a dose of 40 mg/day and monitor closely for signs of bone marrow depression. After 1 month, if the clinical response is inadequate, the dose may be increased to 80 to 120 mg/day. At the higher dose levels, significant bone marrow suppression often occurs.

The predominant dermatologic use of thioguanine is in the treatment of psoriasis,[122–124] particularly in patients who have failed other systemic therapies or in whom there is a contraindication to other systemic therapies such as liver disease. When Zackheim and colleagues[124] treated 81 psoriatic patients with thioguanine, they found that 49 percent of the patients with plaques were effectively maintained with 6-thioguanine for a median of 33 months and that 4 of 5 patients with palmoplantar pustular psoriasis experienced a substantial benefit. Molin and Thomsen[122] found thioguanine efficacious for the treatment of psoriasis but reported that bone marrow toxicity was a common problem.

Thioguanine is also used to treat acute granulocytic leukemia, acute lymphocytic leukemia, and chronic granulocytic leukemia.

Hydroxyurea

Hydroxyurea is a low-molecular-weight drug that causes an immediate inhibition of DNA synthesis (Fig. 255-4). The drug inhibits ribonucleotide diphosphate reductase, which converts ribonucleo-

$$H_2N-\overset{\overset{\displaystyle O}{\|}}{C}-NH-OH$$

Chemical structure of hydroxyurea.

tides to their deoxy form. Inhibiting this enzyme limits the supply of DNA bases and thereby decreases the rate of DNA synthesis. Hydroxyurea is most active in cells with a high proliferative index.[125,126]

Hydroxyurea is well absorbed after oral administration. Serum levels peak within 2 h. Eighty percent of an oral dose can be recovered in the urine after 12 h, and at 24 h levels are negligible. Boyd and Neldner[127] recommend that patients should initially receive a dose of 500 mg twice daily and should not exceed a total of 2000 mg/day. Patients should have a baseline chemistry profile, CBC, and urinalysis, with repetition of the CBC at regular intervals.

Hydroxyurea is usually well tolerated.[127] Layton and colleagues[128] found that 57 percent of patients who received 1.5 g/day of the drug experienced no adverse effects and that only 18 percent had to stop hydroxyurea therapy because of side effects. The most significant adverse effects of hydroxyurea are bone marrow suppression and teratogenesis. Bone marrow suppression occurs in nearly all patients who are treated with therapeutic levels of the drug and reflects the susceptibility of proliferating cell populations to hydroxyurea.

Patients taking hydroxyurea may experience adverse cutaneous effects, including but not limited to a lichen planus–like eruption,[129] a benign dermatomyositis-like eruption,[130] and hyperpigmentation of the skin and nails.[130] A rare but important adverse effect of hydroxyurea is fever and a flulike illness.[131] Other reported effects include lupus erythematosus,[132] leg ulcers,[133] mild gastrointestinal effects,[127] and the development of secondary malignancies when used in patients being treated for primary malignancies such as polycythemia vera.[134]

The major dermatologic use of hydroxyurea is for the treatment of psoriasis. Although the drug had been in existence for many years, its effect on psoriasis was not noted until the early 1970s. In a double-blind study of the treatment of psoriasis with hydroxyurea, Leavell and Yarborough[125] found that 9 of 10 patients with severe psoriasis demonstrated clinical and histopathologic responses to hydroxyurea. When Moschella and Greenwald[126] treated 60 patients with psoriasis with hydroxyurea, they achieved a 50 to 60 percent response rate. The authors note that clinical improvement of psoriasis is apparent only if the total white blood cell count is reduced below 4000.

Because hydroxyurea has relatively little hepatic toxicity, it may be a good choice for patients who are excluded from methotrexate therapy because of liver disease. Hydroxyurea seems to be neither as effective nor as rapid in onset of action as methotrexate; however, it is clearly beneficial in some patients. To date no controlled studies have compared the effect of hydroxyurea with that of etretinate or acitretin in severe psoriasis. Such studies would be valuable because the lower side-effect profile of hydroxyurea would seem to make it a superior drug in individuals who cannot tolerate methotrexate. Despite studies indicating the apparent success of hydroxyurea in the treatment of psoriasis, it is believed to be less effective than other oral agents, such as methotrexate and azathioprine.

Mycophenolic Acid

Mycophenolic acid (MPA) is a lipid-soluble, weak organic acid that was named by Alsberg and Black in 1913. MPA is antifungal,[135] antibacterial,[136] antiviral,[137] and immunosuppressive.[138–140] It is well absorbed orally and is quickly converted to its inactive glucuronide in the liver. The inactive glucuronide lacks the ability to penetrate the cell membranes of most tissue types and is subsequently excreted by the kidneys. Certain tissue types, such as the lining of the gastrointestinal tract and the epidermis, have the enzymatic activity of beta glucuronidase, which converts the inactive MPA glucuronide into its active form. MPA can then readily penetrate the eukaryotic cell membrane.[141]

MPA interferes with de novo purine biosynthesis, blocking the production of the necessary precursors of DNA and RNA synthesis. MPA therefore is cytotoxic for cell types that rely predominantly on de novo purine biosynthesis rather than the purine salvage pathway. MPA blocks the proliferative responses of T and B lymphocytes[142] and inhibits antibody formation and the generation of cytotoxic T cells.[43] Specifically, MPA acts as a noncompetitive inhibitor of the eukaryotic inosine monophosphate dehydrogenases by blocking the conversion of inosine-5-phosphate and xanthine-5-phosphate to guanosine-5-phosphate.

ADVERSE EFFECTS *Gastrointestinal* The most common side effects of MPA are related to the gastrointestinal tract, and include nausea, vomiting, diarrhea, anorexia, abdominal cramps, frequent stools, and anal tenderness. These adverse effects are dose-dependent and tolerable for most patients. The incidence of these and other side effects decreases dramatically after the first year of MPA therapy.[144] Ensley[145] and others have shown that there is no clinically significant hepatotoxicity of mycophenolate mofetil (MMF), a morpholinoester derivative of MPA, with greater bioavailability and immunosuppressive capability. MMF is currently marketed for the prevention of renal allograft rejection.

Hematologic There have been reports of reversible, dose-related anemia, neutropenia, and thrombocytopenia,[146–149] although these effects did not contraindicate the administration of the drug.[144] MMF causes less bone marrow toxicity than azathioprine and is safe for long-term therapy.[145]

Infectious The incidence of infectious complications is increased among those receiving MPA therapy. Epinette and others have reported uncomplicated cases of herpes zoster that did not lead to permanent termination of MPA therapy and noted that opportunistic infections have not been associated with MPA.[144] Sollinger and colleagues[150] noted a 40 percent infection rate associated with MMF therapy in transplant recipients being treated concomitantly with other immunosuppressive drugs but felt that this rate was within expectations for that group of patients.

Carcinogenicity The issue of carcinogenicity secondary to therapy with MPA[146] was resolved by a study of 13 years which did not find an increased age-adjusted rate of cancer development.[144]

Azathioprine is metabolized into a purine analogue, with the potential of becoming incorporated into DNA, thus causing chromosome breaks with a potential mutagenic risk.[151] MMF acts as a noncompetitive inhibitor of guanine nucleotide synthesis and has not been shown to cause chromosome breaks.

Teratogenicity MPA has not been used in women of childbearing potential. Its potential teratogenic effect is unknown.

Genitourinary Genitourinary complaints, such as urgency, frequency, dysuria, burning, and a sterile pyuria, are common and dose- and time-dependent. There is no clinically significant nephrotoxicity.[151]

Neurologic Weakness, tiredness, headaches, and tinnitus have been reported. They seem to decrease in incidence after the first several years of therapy and have not been reported to necessitate discontinuation of MPA therapy.

CLINICAL APPLICATIONS *Psoriasis* MPA has been investigated as an oral agent for the treatment of moderate to severe psoriasis since the early 1970s. In a pilot study of MPA in psoriasis, Jones and colleagues[152] demonstrated that it is a safe and effective mode of treatment. This study was then followed by a multicenter, double-blind, placebo-controlled study and a long-term, follow-up study. These investigations have found that MPA is safe and effective at doses ranging from 3000 to 4800 mg/day.

The mechanism by which MPA successfully controls psoriasis is unknown. MPA may act selectively on lymphocytes, the predominant inflammatory cell type found in psoriatic lesions. Lymphocytes rely on de novo purine biosynthesis and are susceptible to the action of MPA. Alternatively, MPA may act via direct antiproliferative effects on keratinocytes. A third possibility is that MPA may exert an antiproliferative effect indirectly through the inhibition of cytokine production.

Alternative clinical applications Topical MPA improved experimental allergic contact dermatitis.[153] The potential application of this therapy includes the treatment of localized psoriasis and other immune-mediated, localized dermatologic diseases. MMF has been successfully used for the treatment of rheumatoid arthritis.[154] Another potential application of MPA is as a steroid-sparing agent, in lieu of azathioprine, in the treatment of dermatologic diseases.

ALKYLATING AGENTS

Cyclophosphamide

Cyclophosphamide is a derivative of nitrogen mustard (Fig. 255-5). As with other nitrogen mustards, cyclophosphamide acts primarily as a DNA cross-linker.[155] Cyclophosphamide is a prodrug that undergoes hepatic conversion to cytoxylamine, which is required for activity. Because the microsomal enzyme systems responsible for this activation are involved in the metabolism of other drugs, there is great potential for drug interaction during cyclophosphamide ther-

FIGURE 255-5

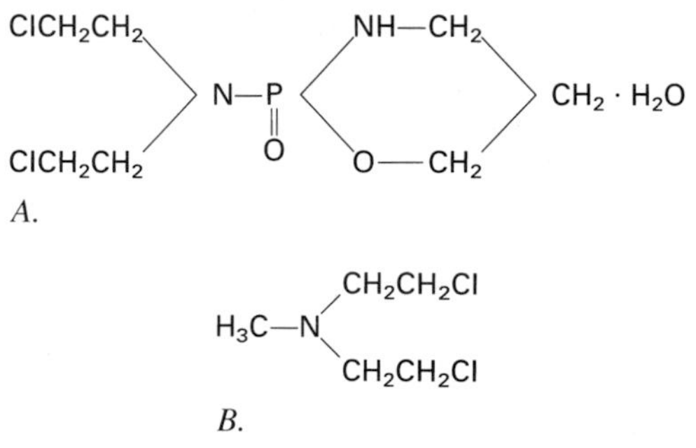

Chemical structure of the alkylating agents (*A*) cyclophosphamide and (*B*) mechlorethamine (nitrogen mustard).

apy. Drugs that induce these enzymes greatly alter the pharmacokinetics of cyclophosphamide. Because cyclophosphamide interacts with preformed DNA and RNA, the drug is active against cells with a low proliferative index.

The side effects of cyclophosphamide are significant. Hematologic disturbances are frequent, especially leukopenia and thrombocytopenia.[155] The leukopenia is proportional to the degree of immune suppression and may be used as an index of the adequacy of the dosage of cyclophosphamide. Cyclophosphamide may also induce hematologic malignancy.[156] Nausea and vomiting are fairly common during cyclophosphamide therapy, especially at higher doses. Alopecia often occurs, as may mucocutaneous ulcerations.[155] There is a clear increase in the incidence of low-grade squamous cell carcinoma of the skin.[115]

A hemorrhagic cystitis occurs in 5 to 10 percent of patients treated with cyclophosphamide. This cystitis is believed to be caused by the metabolite acrolein, and it occurs during therapy.[157,158] A scavenging agent, mesna (sodium 2-mercaptoethanesulfonate), binds acrolein in the bladder and prevents severe bladder irritation. It is used primarily with high-dose cyclophosphamide regimens and is administered intravenously. It is not known whether mesna also prevents the other common genitourinary complication of cyclophosphamide therapy, transitional cell carcinoma of the bladder, which may develop in as many as 5 to 10 percent of patients.[159] No clear relationship exists between cystitis during treatment and the long-term development of cancer. Stein and colleagues[160] reported two cases of cyclophosphamide-induced squamous cell carcinoma of the bladder. This is unusual, because most cyclophosphamide-induced bladder tumors are transitional cell carcinomas. Cancers may arise many years after therapy, and therefore continued monitoring of the lower urinary tract is indicated.[161–164]

Cardiotoxicity is uncommon at the doses of cyclophosphamide typically used in dermatology but has been reported when the drug is used in high doses for antineoplastic purposes, especially when it is combined with radiation or other potentially cardiotoxic drugs (e.g., anthracyclines). The consequences of such toxicity have included debilitating heart failure, arrhythmias, potentially irreversible cardiomyopathy and/or pericarditis, and death.

The use of cyclophosphamide is relatively contraindicated in patients who wish to conceive children. Although the severity of disease may demand treatment with cyclophosphamide, the patient may be rendered infertile by the drug.[108] Infections are easily acquired during cyclophosphamide therapy, particularly after a surgical procedure.[163]

The major dermatologic use of cyclophosphamide is for the treatment of autoimmune diseases. Pemphigus vulgaris in particular may be treated with cyclophosphamide in combination with prednisone.[110,164] The cyclophosphamide is used either to maintain remission following systemic steroid withdrawal, or as a steroid-sparing agent. The latter usage is especially helpful in those patients who have failed azathioprine therapy.[85] Cyclophosphamide is believed to be more effective than azathioprine, although no controlled studies have been performed. Typical regimens are in the range of 1 to 2 mg/kg per day.

There have been recent reports on intravenous pulse therapy of cyclophosphamide in the treatment of pemphigus vulgaris.[165] In addition, there have been case reports[166] that demonstrated a curative effect of dexamethasone-cyclophosphamide pulse therapy for pem-

phigus vulgaris. Side effects of the pulse therapy of cyclophosphamide included facial flushing[167] and hiccuping.[168]

The survival of patients with systemic vasculitis was enhanced with the introduction of combined steroid/cytotoxic therapy.[115,116] Diseases that were lethal in the past are now controllable with such therapy. For example, the 5-year survival of patients with polyarteritis nodosa is 13 percent if the condition is untreated, 48 percent if it is treated with steroid therapy, and 90 percent if cyclophosphamide and prednisone are combined.[115,169,170] Typical doses for systemic vasculitis are 1 mg/kg per day for prednisone and 2 mg/kg per day for cyclophosphamide. Steroids are converted to an alternate-day regimen and tapered over 3 to 6 months. Cyclophosphamide is maintained for one year and then gradually tapered.[115,116] Resistant disease may be treated with higher doses or intravenous pulse therapy.[171]

Granulomatous vasculitis is best treated with combination therapy as well. Wegener's granulomatosis[172] and lymphomatoid granulomatosis[171,173] often require cyclophosphamide therapy for sustained remission.

Other diseases may also respond to cyclophosphamide, including Behçet's disease,[174] pyoderma gangrenosum,[175] lichen planus,[176] and lichen myxedematosus. With the availability of cyclosporine, however, cyclophosphamide may not be the drug of choice for such resistant but nonlethal inflammatory diseases.

Chlorambucil

Chlorambucil (Leukeran) is not cell cycle–specific, and disturbs DNA synthesis and cellular proliferation. It acts most readily on rapidly proliferating tissues, although it also exerts some effects on cells that are not actively synthesizing DNA. The effects of this agent are similar to those seen with the nitrogen mustards. Chlorambucil is well absorbed orally, with a plasma half-life of approximately 1.5 h.

The side effects of chlorambucil include nausea and vomiting, azoospermia, amenorrhea, pulmonary fibrosis, seizures, dermatitis, and, rarely, hepatotoxicity. A large controlled study by the National Polycythemia Vera Study Group showed a marked increase in the incidence of leukemia and other tumors. Chlorambucil also has a myelosuppressive effect, which is usually gradual and readily reversible. This effect is generally seen with excessive doses administered over long periods of time.

In the dermatologic setting, chlorambucil has been anecdotally described for the treatment of granuloma annulare and cutaneous T-cell lymphoma. It is also used in the treatment of chronic lymphocytic leukemia, primary (Waldenstrom's) macroglobulinemia, Hodgkin's disease, and non-Hodgkin's lymphomas. Because of infrequent utilization, dosage schedules of chlorambucil for the treatment of dermatologic disease have not been standardized and must be determined on an individual basis.

Anthracyclines

Anthracyclines are antibiotic molecules with antineoplastic properties. Doxorubicin is cell cycle–specific for the S phase of cell division. Its exact mechanism of antineoplastic activity is unknown but may involve binding to DNA by intercalation between base pairs and inhibition of DNA and RNA synthesis by template disordering and steric obstruction.

Doxorubicin hydrochloride encapsulated in liposomes (Doxil) is approved for the treatment of AIDS-related Kaposi's sarcoma. The cytotoxic mechanism of action of doxorubicin is thought to relate to its ability to bind DNA and inhibit nucleic acid synthesis. The liposomes have been coated with a protective layer of methoxy-polyethylene glycol to protect them from detection by the mononuclear phagocyte system and to increase blood circulation time. These protected liposomes have a 55-h half life, and at least 90 percent of the drug remains encapsulated. Due to their small size and extended persistence in the circulation, the liposomes are able to penetrate the compromised vasculature of the Kaposi's sarcoma, thus accumulating within the tumors. It has been found that the steady-state distribution of doxorubicin remains mostly in the vascular fluid volume.

Doxorubicin is administered intravenously. It is provided as a sterile, translucent, red liposomal dispersion, in 10-mL single-use vials, at a concentration of 2 mg/mL. The recommended dose is intravenous administration of 20 mg/m^2 over 30 min once every 3 weeks, as tolerated by the individual patient.

Adverse reactions include myelosuppression, most commonly presenting as a leukopenia. At the recommended doses, the leukopenia is usually transient. Careful hematologic monitoring (white blood cells, platelets, hemoglobin, and hematocrit) of patients receiving this drug is required. A small percentage of patients may experience an initial infusion reaction, characterized by flushing, shortness of breath, facial swelling, headache, chills, back pain, chest and throat tightness, and/or hypotension. This reaction typically resolves several hours to a day after discontinuation or slowing of the infusion and does not occur in later infusions if not present initially. A palmar-plantar erythrodysesthesia occurred in 3 1/2 percent of the AIDS-related Kaposi's sarcoma patients treated with doxorubicin. In most patients, this reaction was mild and resolved in 1 to 2 weeks. Doxorubicin is embryotoxic and abortifacient and should be avoided in women who plan to conceive. A recurrence of post-radiation skin reaction has occurred in patients receiving this drug.

It should be assumed that doxorubicin will have myocardial toxicity similar to that of other preparations of doxorubicin. In addition, a history of the use of other anthracyclines or anthracenediones will lower the total dose of doxorubicin required to cause cardiotoxicity. Due to hepatic excretion of doxorubicin, caution should be used in patients with prior or concurrent hepatic impairment. Before administration, liver function should be assessed (SGOT, SGPT, alkaline phosphatase, bilirubin).

Other, minor side effects occurred in more than 5 percent of the AIDS-related Kaposi's sarcoma patients on doxorubicin therapy. They include nausea, asthenia, fever, alopecia, increase in alkaline phosphatase, vomiting, diarrhea, stomatitis, and oral moniliasis. These side effects have not been proven to have been directly caused by the drug.

REFERENCES

1. Jolivet J et al: The pharmacology and clinical use of methotrexate. *N Engl J Med* **309**:1094, 1983
2. American Hospital Formulary Service. *Drug Information* **91**:584, 1991
3. Jolivet J et al: The synthesis and retention of methotrexate polyglutamates in cultured human breast cancer cells. *Ann NY Acad Sci* **397**:184, 1982
4. Anderson PA et al: Weekly pulse methotrexate in rheumatoid arthritis. *Ann Intern Med* **103**:489, 1985
5. Van De Putte et al: Methotrexate: Anti-inflammatory or immunosuppressive? *Clin Exp Rheum* **11**(Suppl 8):S97, 1993
6. Wolff R et al: Adenosine mediates methotrexate-induced attenuation of leukocyte adherence and emigration in postcapillary venules. *Arthritis Rheum* **35**:S-35, 1992
7. Weinblatt ME et al: Long term prospective study of methotrexate in rheumatoid arthritis. *Arthritis Rheum* **29**(Suppl):S76, 1986
8. Olsen NJ et al: Immunologic studies of rheumatoid arthritis patients treated with methotrexate. *Arthritis Rheum* **30**:481, 1987
9. O'Callaghan JW et al: The effect of low dose chronic intermittent parental methotrexate on delayed-type hypersensitivity and acute inflammation in a mouse model. *J Rheumatol* **13**:710, 1986
10. Lammers AM et al: Reduction of LTB$_4$-induced intraepidermal accumulation of polymorphonuclear leukocytes by methotrexate in psoriasis. *Br J Dermatol* **116**:667, 1987
11. Ternowitz T, Herlin T: Neutrophil and monocyte chemotaxis in methotrexate treated psoriasis patients. *Acta Derm Venereol (Stockh)* **120**:23, 1985
12. Cream JJ, Pole DS: The effect of methotrexate and hydroxyurea on neutrophil chemotaxis. *Br J Dermatol* **102**:557, 1980
13. Gommans JM et al: Flow cytometric quantification of T6-positive cells in psoriatic epidermis after PUVA and methotrexate therapy. *Br J Dermatol* **116**:661, 1987
14. Weinstein GD, Frost P: Methotrexate for psoriasis: A new therapeutic approach. *Arch Dermatol* **103**:33, 1971
15. Newton JA et al: Study of psoriatic epidermal cell kinetics and cell death after oral methotrexate. *Dermatologica* **171**:469, 1985
16. Weinstein GD et al: Topical methotrexate therapy in psoriasis. *Arch Dermatol* **125**:277, 1989
17. Furst D: Clinical Pharmacology of very low dose methotrexate for use in rheumatoid arthritis. *J Rheumatol* **12**(Suppl):11, 1985
18. Pinkerton DR et al: Can food influence absorption of methotrexate in children with acute lymphoblastic leukemia? *Lancet* **2**:944, 1980
19. Halprin KM et al: Blood levels of methotrexate in the treatment of psoriasis. *Arch Dermatol* **103**:243, 1971
20. Furst DE, Kremer JM: Methotrexate in rheumatoid arthritis. *Arthritis Rheum* **31**:305, 1988
21. Wan SH et al: Effect on route of administration and effusions on methotrexate pharmacokinetics. *Cancer Res* **34**:3487, 1984
22. Edelman J et al: Low dose methotrexate kinetics in arthritis. *Clin Pharmacol Ther* **35**:382, 1984
23. Hanrahan PS, Russel AS: Concurrent use of folinic acid and methotrexate in rheumatoid arthritis. *J Rheumatol* **15**:1078, 1988
24. Taylor JR, Halprin KM: Effect of sodium salicylate and indomethacin on methotrexate-serum albumin binding. *Arch Dermatol* **113**:558, 1977
25. Liegler DG et al: The effect of organic acids on renal clearance of methotrexate in man. *Clin Pharmacol Ther* **10**:849, 1969
26. Nierenberg DW: Competitive inhibition of methotrexate accumulation in rabbit kidney slices by non-steroidal anti-inflammatory drugs. *J Pharmacol Exp Ther* **226**:1, 1983
27. Beach BJ et al: Influence of co-trimoxizole on methotrexate pharmacokinetics in children with acute lymphoblastic leukemia. *Am J Pediatr Hematol Oncol* **2**:115, 1981
28. Evans WE, Christensen ML: Drug interactions with methotrexate. *J Rheumatol* **12**(Suppl):15, 1985
29. Hendwel J, Nyfors A: Nonlinear renal elimination kinetics of methotrexate due to saturation of renal tubular absorption. *Eur J Clin Pharmacol* **26**:121, 1984
30. Weinblatt ME: Toxicity of low-dose methotrexate in rheumatoid arthritis. *J Rheumatol* **12**(Suppl):35, 1985
31. Roenigk HH et al: Methotrexate in psoriasis: Revised guidelines. *J Am Acad Dermatol* **19**:146, 1988
32. Weinblatt ME, Kremer JE: Methotrexate in rheumatoid arthritis. *J Am Acad Dermatol* **19**:126, 1988
33. Coe RO, Bull FE: Cirrhosis associated with methotrexate treatment of psoriasis. *JAMA* **206**:1515, 1968
34. Zachariae H et al: Methotrexate-induced liver cirrhosis: Studies including serial liver biopsies during continued treatment. *Br J Dermatol* **102**:407, 1980
35. Zachariae H, Sogaard H: Methotrexate-induced liver cirrhosis: A follow-up. *Dermatologica* **175**:178, 1987
36. Roenigk HH et al: Hepatotoxicity of methotrexate in the treatment of psoriasis. *Arch Dermatol* **103**:250, 1971

37. Geronemus RG et al: Liver biopsies vs. liver scan in methotrexate-treated patients with psoriasis. *Arch Dermatol* **118**:649, 1982

38. Rademaker M et al: Magnetic resonance imaging as a screening procedure for methotrexate-induced liver damage. *Br J Dermatol* **117**:311, 1987

39. Mitchell D et al: Ultrasound and radionuclide scans poor indicators of liver damage in patients treated with methotrexate. *Clin Exp Dermatol* **12**:243, 1987

40. Tugwell P et al: Methotrexate in rheumatoid arthritis. *Ann Intern Med* **110**:581, 1989

41. Newman MN et al: The role of liver biopsies in psoriatic patients receiving long-term methotrexate treatment. *Arch Dermatol* **125**:1218, 1989

42. Shupack JL, Webster GF: Pancytopenia following low-dose oral methotrexate therapy for psoriasis. *JAMA* **259**:3594, 1988

43. MacKinnon SK et al: Pancytopenia associated with low-dose pulse methotrexate therapy in rheumatoid arthritis. *Semin Arthritis Rheum* **15**:119, 1985

44. Maricic M et al: Megaloblastic pancytopenia in a patient receiving concurrent methotrexate and trimethoprim-sulfamethasoxazole treatments. *Arthritis Rheum* **29**:133, 1986

45. Thomas DR et al: Pancytopenia induced by the interaction between methotrexate and trimethoprim-sulfamethasoxazole treatments. *J Am Acad Dermatol* **17**:1055, 1987

46. Stern RS et al: Methotrexate for psoriasis and the risk of cutaneous and non-cutaneous malignancy. *Cancer* **50**:869, 1982

47. Nyfors A, Jense H: Frequency of malignant neoplasm in 248 long-term methotrexate-treated psoriatics. *Dermatologica* **167**:260, 1983

48. Grunnet E et al: Studies on human semen in topical corticosteroid treated and in methotrexate-treated psoriasis. *Dermatologica* **154**:78, 1977

49. Sussman A, Leonard JM: Psoriasis, methotrexate, and oligospermia. *Arch Dermatol* **116**:215, 1980

50. Krough-Jensen M, Nyfors A: Cytogenic effect of methotrexate on human cells in vivo: Comparison between results obtained by chromosome studies on bone marrow cells and blood lymphocytes and by the micronucleus test. *Mutat Res* **64**:339, 1979

51. Shupack JL et al: Methotrexate with leukovorin rescue: A therapeutic alternative in severe psoriatics with a history of methotrexate-induced pancytopenia and diminished renal or hepatic function. *J Dermatol Treat* **4**:145, 1993

52. Cohn JR et al: Systemic anaphylaxis from low dose methotrexate. *Ann Allergy* **70**:384, 1993

53. Gubner R: Therapeutic suppression of tissue reactivity: II. Effect of aminopterin in rheumatoid arthritis and psoriasis. *Am J Med Sci* **122**:176, 1951

54. Weinstein GD: Three decades of folic acid antagonists in dermatology. *Arch Dermatol* **119**:525, 1983

55. Weinstein GD, Frost P: Abnormal cell proliferation in psoriasis. *J Invest Dermatol* **50**:254, 1968

56. Weinstein GD, Frost P: Methotrexate for psoriasis, a new therapeutic approach. *Arch Dermatol* **103**:33, 1971

57. Peckham PE et al: The treatment of severe psoriasis: A national survey. *Arch Dermatol* **123**:1303, 1987

58. Ryan TJ, Baker H: Systemic corticosteroids and folic acid antagonists in the treatment of generalized pustular psoriasis: Evaluation and prognosis based on the study of 104 cases. *Br J Dermatol* **81**:134, 1969

59. Rosenbaum MM, Roenigk HH Jr: Treatment of generalized pustular psoriasis with etretinate (Ro-10-9359) and methotrexate. *J Am Acad Dermatol* **12**:357, 1984

60. Kragballe KE et al: Methotrexate in psoriatic arthritis, a retrospective study. *Acta Derm Venereol (Stockh)* **63**:165, 1983

61. Wilkins RF et al: Randomized double-blind placebo-controlled trial of methotrexate in psoriatic arthritis. *Arthritis Rheum* **27**:376, 1984

62. Pigatto PD et al: Methotrexate in psoriatic polyarthritis. *Acta Derm Venereol (Stockh)* (Suppl) **186**:114, 1994

63. Duvic M et al: Acquired immunodeficiency syndrome-associated psoriasis and Reiter's syndrome. *Arch Dermatol* **123**:1622, 1987

64. Winchester R et al: The co-occurrence of Reiter's syndrome and acquired immunodeficiency. *Ann Intern Med* **106**:19, 1987

65. Maurer TA et al: The use of methotrexate for treatment of psoriasis in patients with HIV infection. *J Am Acad Derm* **31**:372, 1994

66. Lally EV, Ho GA: A review of methotrexate therapy in Reiter's syndrome. *Semin Arthritis Rheum* **15**:139, 1985

67. Veien NK, Brodthagen H: Treatment of sarcoidosis with methotrexate. *Br J Dermatol* **97**:213, 1977

68. Webster GF et al: Methotrexate therapy in cutaneous sarcoidosis. *Ann Intern Med* **111**:538, 1990

69. Roenigk HH: Pityriasis lichenoides et varioliformis acuta (Mucha-Haberman). *Arch Dermatol* **104**:102, 1971

70. Lynch PJ, Saied NK: Methotrexate treatment of pityriasis lichenoides and lymphomatoid papulosis. *Cutis* **23**:634, 1979

71. Everett MA: Treatment of lymphomatoid papulosis with methotrexate. *Br J Dermatol* **111**:631, 1984

72. Wantzin GL, Thomsen K: Methotrexate in lymphomatoid papulosis. *Br J Dermatol* **111**:93, 1984

73. Brown J, Perry HO: Pityriasis rubra pilaris treatment with folic acid antagonists. *Arch Dermatol* **94**:636, 1966

74. Knowles WR, Chernosky ME: Pityriasis rubra pilaris: Prolonged treatment with methotrexate. *Arch Dermatol* **102**:603, 1970

75. Hanke CW, Steck WD: Childhood onset pityriasis rubra pilaris treated with methotrexate administered intravenously. *Cleve Clin Q* **50**:201, 1983

76. Capizzi RL, Berlino JR: Methotrexate treatment of Wegener's granulomatosis. *Ann Intern Med* **74**:74, 1971

77. Church KS et al: Low-dose methotrexate therapy for cutaneous vasculitis of rheumatoid arthritis. *J Am Acad Dermatol* **17**:355, 1987

78. Espinoza LR et al: Oral methotrexate therapy for chronic rheumatoid arthritis ulcerations. *J Am Acad Dermatol* **15**:508, 1986

79. Fischer TJ et al: Childhood dermatositis and polymyositis: Treatment with methotrexate and prednisone. *Am J Dis Child* **133**:386, 1979

80. Wallace DJ et al: Combined immunosuppressive treatment of steroid resistant dermatomyositis/polymyositis. *Arthritis Rheum* **28**:590, 1985

81. Arnett FC et al: Methotrexate therapy of polymyositis. *Ann Rheum Dis* **52**:536, 1973

82. Tuffanelli DE, Lavoie PE: Prognosis and therapy of polymyositis and dermatomyositis. *Clin Dermatol* **6**:93, 1988

83. Lever WF: Methotrexate and prednisone in pemphigus vulgaris. *Arch Dermatol* **106**:491, 1972

84. Lever WF, Goldberg S: Treatment of pemphigus vulgaris with methotrexate. *Arch Dermatol* **100**:70, 1970

85. Huilgol SC, Black MM: Management of the immunobullous disorders: II. Pemphigus. *Clin Exp Dermatol* **20**:283, 1995

86. Rothenberg RJ et al: The use of methotrexate in steroid resistant systemic lupus erythematosus. *Arthritis Rheum* **31**:612, 1988

87. Nashel DJ: Mechanisms of action and clinical applications of cytotoxic drugs in rheumatic disorders. *Med Clin North Am* **69**:817, 1985

88. Bickers D et al: Cytotoxic and immunosuppressive agents, in *Clinical Pharmacology of Skin Disease*, edited by D Bickers et al. New York, Churchill Livingstone, 1984, chap 5

89. Ahmed AR, Moy R: Azathioprine. *Int J Dermatol* **20**:461, 1981

90. Chabner BA, Myers CE: Clinical pharmacology of cancer chemotherapy, in *Principles and Practices of Oncology*, 2d ed, edited by VT DeVita et al. Philadelphia, Lippincott, 1985, p 287

91. Lee MH et al: Alkaline phosphate activities of 6-thiopurine-sensitive and -resistant sublines of sarcoma 180. *Cancer Res* **38**:2413, 1978

92. Ping TL, Benet LZ: Determination of 6-mercaptopurine and azathioprine in plasma by HPLC. *J Chromatogr* **145**:237, 1978

93. Lennard L et al: Pharmacogenetics of acute azathioprine toxicity: Relationship to thiopurine methyltransferase genetic polymorphism. *Clin Pharmacol Ther* **46**:149, 1989

94. Bacon BR et al: Azathioprine induced pancytopenia: Occurrence in two patients with connective tissue diseases. *Arch Intern Med* **141**:223, 1981

95. Anstey A: Azathioprine in dermatology: A review in the light of advances in understanding methylation pharmacogenetics. *J R Soc Med* **88**:155P, 1995

96. Snow JL, Gibson LE: The role of genetic variation in thiopurine methyltransferase activity and the efficacy and/or side effects of azathioprine therapy in dermatologic patients. *Arch Dermatol* **131**:193, 1995

97. Weinshilboum RM, Sladek SL: Mercaptopurine pharmacogenetics: Monogenetic inheritance of erythrocyte thiopurine methyltransferase activity. *Am J Hum Genet* **32**:651, 1980

98. Honchel R et al: Human thiopurine methyltransferase: Molecular cloning and expression of T84 colon carcinoma cell cDNA. *Mol Pharmacol* **43**:878, 1993

99. Drugs for rheumatoid arthritis. *Med Let Drugs Ther* **31**:61, 1989

100. Kawamski H: Azathioprine induced pancreatitis. *N Engl J Med* **289**:357, 1973

101. McKendry RJ, Cyr M: Toxicity of methotrexate compared with azathioprine in the treatment of rheumatoid arthritis. *Arch Intern Med* **149**:685, 1989

102. Singh G et al: Toxic effects of azathioprine in rheumatoid arthritis. *Arthritis Rheum* **32**:837, 1989

103. Collision DW et al: Azathioprine hypersensitivity in bullous pemphigoid. *J Clin Acad Dermatol* **23**:125, 1990

104. Lipsky BA, Hirschman JV: Drug fever. *JAMA* **245**:851, 1981

105. Pandhi RK et al: Azathioprine-induced drug fever. *Int J Dermatol* **33**:198, 1994

106. Jones JJ, Ashworth J: Azathioprine-induced shock. *J Am Acad Dermatol* **29**:795, 1993

107. Silman AJ et al: Lymphoproliferative cancer and other malignancy in patients with rheumatoid arthritis treated with azathioprine. *Ann Rheum Dis* **47**:988, 1988

108. Roubenoff R et al: Effect of anti-inflammatory and immunosuppressive drugs on pregnancy and fertility. *Semin Arthritis Rheum* **18**:88, 1988

109. Wolff K, Schreiner E: Immunosuppressive therapy for pemphigus vulgaris. *Arch Klin Exp Dermatol* **235**:63, 1969

110. Bystryn JC: Adjuvant therapy for pemphigus. *Arch Dermatol* **120**:941, 1984

111. Aberer W et al: Azathioprine in the treatment of pemphigus vulgaris. *J Am Acad Dermatol* **16**:527, 1987

112. Smolle J: Zur Therapie der Pemphigus krankheiten: Kritische Anmerkungen anhand von 44 faellen. *Hautzart* **36**:96, 1985

113. Pawlofsky C et al: Disseminated cicatrical pemphigoid. *Dermatologica* **171**:259, 1985

114. Korman N: Bullous pemphigoid. *J Am Acad Dermatol* **16**:907, 1987

115. Leavitt RY, Fauci AS: Therapeutic approach to the vasculitic syndromes. *Mt Sinai J Med* **53**:440, 1986

116. Leavitt RY, Fauci AS: Pulmonary vasculitis. *Am Rev Respir Dis* **134**:149, 1986

117. Felson DT, Anderson J: Evidence for the superiority of immunosuppressive drugs and prednisone over prednisone alone in lupus nephritis. *N Engl J Med* **311**:1528, 1984

118. Bunch TW: Prednisone and azathioprine for polymyositis. *Arthritis Rheum* **24**:45, 1981

119. Castro JL et al: Successful treatment of a musk ambrette sensitive persistent light reactor with azathioprine. *Photodermatology* **3**:241, 1986

120. Murphy GM et al: Azathioprine treatment in chronic actinic dermatitis: A double-blind controlled trial with monitoring of exposure to ultraviolet radiation. *Br J Dermatol* **121**:639, 1989

121. Kao NL, Rosenblate HJ: 6-Thioguanine therapy for psoriasis causing toxic hepatic venoocclusive disease. *J Am Acad Dermatol* **28**:1017, 1993

122. Molin L, Thomsen K: Thioguanine treatment in psoriasis. *Acta Derm Venereol* **67**:85, 1987

123. Zackheim HS, Maibach HI: Treatment of psoriasis with 6-thioguanine. *Australas J Dermatol* **29**:163, 1988

124. Zackheim HS et al: 6-Thioguanine treatment of psoriasis: experience in 81 patients. *J Am Acad Dermatol* **30**:452, 1994

125. Leavell VW, Yarborough JM: Hydroxyurea: A new treatment for psoriasis. *Arch Dermatol* **102**:144, 1970

126. Moschella SC, Greenwald MA: Treatment of psoriasis with hydroxyurea—an 18 month study of 60 patients. *Arch Dermatol* **107**:363, 1973

127. Boyd AS, Neldner KH: Hydroxyurea therapy. *J Am Acad Dermatol* **25**:518, 1991

128. Layton AM et al: Hydroxyurea in the management of therapy resistant psoriasis. *Br J Dermatol* **121**:647, 1989

129. Renfro L et al: Ulcerative lichen planus-like dermatitis associated with hydroxyurea. *J Am Acad Dermatol* **24**:143, 1991

130. Richard M: Skin lesions simulating chronic dermatomyositis during long-term hydroxyurea therapy. *J Am Acad Dermatol* **21**:797, 1989

131. Lossos, Najean Y: Unwanted side effect of hydroxyurea. *Ann Hematol* **72**:101, 1996

132. Layton AM et al: Hydroxyurea-induced lupus erythematosus. *Br J Dermatol* **130**:687, 1994

133. Nguyen TV, Margolis DJ: Hydroxyurea and lower leg ulcers. *Cutis* **52**:217, 1993

134. Donovan PB et al: Treatment of polycythemia vera with hydroxyurea. *Am J Hematol* **17**:329, 1984

135. Abrams R, Bentley M: Biosynthesis of nucleic acid purines. *Biochem Biophys* **79**:91, 1959

136. Abraham EP: The effect of mycophenolic acid on the growth of staphylococcus aureus in heart broth. *Biochem J* **39**:398, 1945

137. Cline JC et al: In vitro antiviral activity of mycophenolic acid and its reversal by guanine-type compounds. *Appl Microbiol* **18**:14, 1969

138. Nelson PH et al: Synthesis and immunosuppressive activity of some side-chain variants of mycophenolic acid. *J Med Chem* **33**:833, 1990

139. Mitsui A et al: Immunosuppressive effect of mycophenolic acid. *J Antibiot (Tokyo)* **22**:368, 1969

140. Ohsugi Y et al: Antitumor and immunosuppressive effects of mycophenolic acid derivatives. *Cancer Res* **36**:2933, 1976

141. McDonald CJ: Chemotherapy of psoriasis. *Int J Dermatol* **14**:563, 1975

142. Eugui EM et al: Lymphocyte-selective anti-proliferative and immunosuppressive effects of mycophenolic acid in mice. *Scand J Immunol* **33**:175, 1991

143. Eugui AM et al: Lymphocyte-selective cytostatic and immunosuppressive effects of mycophenolic acid in vitro: Role of deoxyguanosine nucleotide depletion. *Scand J Immunol* **33**:161, 1991

144. Epinette WW et al: Mycophenolic acid for psoriasis: A review of pharmacology, long-term efficacy and safety. *J Am Acad Dermatol* **17**:962, 1987

145. Ensley RD et al: The use of mycophenolate mofetil (RS-61443) in human heart transplant recipients. *Transplantation* **56**:75, 1993

146. Lynch WS, Roenigk HH Jr: Mycophenolic acid for psoriasis. *Arch Dermatol* **113**:1203, 1977

147. Spatz S et al: Mycophenolic acid in psoriasis. *Br J Dermatol* **98**:429, 1978

148. Gomez EC et al: Efficacy of mycophenolic acid for the treatment of psoriasis. *J Am Acad Dermatol* **1**:531, 1979

149. Marinari R et al: Mycophenolic acid in the treatment of psoriasis: Long-term administration. *Arch Dermatol* **113**:930, 1977

150. Sollinger HW et al: RS-61443 (mycophenolate mofetil): A multicenter study for refractory kidney transplant rejection. *Ann Surg* **216**:513, 1992

151. Platz KP et al: RS-61443: A new, potent immunosuppressive agent. *Transplantation* **51**:27, 1991

152. Jones EL et al: Treatment of psoriasis with oral mycophenolic acid. *J Invest Dermatol* **65**:537, 1975

153. Shoji Y et al: Effect of topical preparation of mycophenolic acid on experimental allergic contact dermatitis of guinea pigs induced by dinitrofluorobenzene. *J Pharm Pharmacol* **46**:643, 1994

154. Goldblum R: Therapy of rheumatoid arthritis with mycophenolate mofetil. *Clin Exp Rheum* **11**(Suppl 8):S117, 1993

155. Fosdick WM et al: Long-term cyclophosphamide therapy in rheumatoid arthritis. *Arthritis Rheum* **11**:151, 1968

156. Baker GL et al: Malignancy following treatment of rheumatoid arthritis with cyclophosphamide. *Am J Med* **83**:1, 1987

157. Cox PJ: Cyclophosphamide cystitis: Identification of acrolein as the causative agent. *Biochem Pharmacol* **28**:2045, 1979

158. Townes AS et al: Controlled trial of cyclophosphamide in rheumatoid arthritis. *Arthritis Rheum* **19**:563, 1976

159. Wall RL, Clausen KP: Carcinoma of the urinary bladder in patients receiving cyclophosphamide. *N Engl J Med* **293**:771, 1975

160. Stein JP et al: Squamous cell carcinoma of the bladder associated with cyclophosphamide therapy for Wegener's granulomatosis: A report of 2 cases. *J Urol* **149**:588, 1993

161. Plotz PH et al: Bladder complications in patients receiving cyclophosphamide for systemic lupus erythematosus or rheumatoid arthritis. *Ann Intern Med* **91**:221, 1979

162. Pederson-Bjergaard J et al: Carcinomas of the urinary bladder after treatment with cyclophosphamide for non-Hodgkin's lymphoma. *N Engl J Med* **318**:1028, 1988

163. Bradley D et al: Infectious complications of cyclophosphamide treatment for vasculitis. *Arthritis Rheum* **32**:45, 1989

164. Ahmed AR, Hombal S: Use of cyclophosphamide in azathioprine failures in pemphigus. *J Am Acad Dermatol* **17**:437, 1987

165. Pandya AG, Sontheimer RD: Treatment of pemphigus vulgaris with pulse intravenous cyclophosphamide. *Arch Dermatol* **128**:1626, 1992

166. Pasricha JS, Das SS: Curative effect of dexamethasone-cyclophosphamide pulse therapy for the treatment of pemphigus vulgaris. *Int J Dermatol* **31**:875, 1992

167. Dhar S, Kanwar AJ: Facial flushing: A side effect of pulse therapy (letter). *Dermatology* **188**:332, 1994

168. Kanwar AJ et al: Hiccup: A side-effect of pulse therapy (letter). *Dermatology* **187**:279, 1993
169. Grohnert PP, Sheps SG: Long-term follow-up study of periarteritis nodosa. *Am J Med* **43**:8, 1967
170. Fort JG, Abruzzo JL: Reversal of progressive necrotizing vasculitis with intravenous pulse cyclophosphamide and methylprednisolone. *Arthritis Rheum* **31**:1194, 1988
171. Jenkins TR, Zaloswick AJ: Lymphomatoid granulomatosis: A case for aggressive therapy. *Cancer* **64**:1362, 1989
172. Fauci AS et al: Cyclophosphamide therapy of severe systemic necrotizing vasculitis. *N Engl J Med* **301**:235, 1979
173. Jambrosic J et al: Lymphomatoid granulomatosis. *J Am Acad Dermatol* **17**:621, 1987
174. Fauci AS et al: Cyclophosphamide therapy of severe systemic necrotizing vasculitis. *N Engl J Med* **301**:235, 1979
175. Newell LM, Malkinson FD: Pyoderma gangrenosum response to cyclophosphamide therapy. *Arch Dermatol* **119**:493, 1983
176. Paslin DA: Sustained remission of generalized lichen planus induced by cyclophosphamide. *Arch Dermatol* **121**:236, 1985

CHAPTER 256

Gary L. Peck
John J. DiGiovanna

The Retinoids

The profound clinical impact of the synthetic retinoids was first observed and described in patients with dermatologic disease. Clinical efficacy observed with systemic tretinoin,[1–3] a natural retinoid, preceded the use of the synthetic retinoids. The development of the synthetic derivatives isotretinoin and etretinate, which had less toxicity, generated interest in studies of a variety of dermatologic diseases. Initially, Orfanos and co-workers obtained equivocal results in using isotretinoin for the treatment of psoriasis.[4] Subsequently, etretinate, used either alone[5] or in combination with topical dithranol,[6] was found to be very effective for treating psoriasis. These findings led to the temporary abandonment of isotretinoin. Interest in isotretinoin was rekindled after the discovery that it was effective in the treatment of lamellar ichthyosis and other cutaneous disorders of cornification[7] and in producing complete responses with prolonged remissions in patients with previously treatment-resistant cystic and conglobate acne.[8] It was also found partially effective in the treatment and prevention of basal cell carcinoma.[9–11] Subsequently, isotretinoin and etretinate, used either alone or in combination with other agents, have proven useful in an expanding spectrum of skin diseases, such as lupus erythematosus and cutaneous T cell lymphoma. After their range of clinical efficacy was identified (Table 256-1) and their toxicity elucidated (Table 256-2) in dermatology patients, retinoids became of interest to other medical specialties such as rheumatology and oncology.

Isotretinoin, etretinate, and acitretin, the oral retinoids that are or have been commercially available, differ not only in their spectra of clinical efficacy but also in their observed toxicities and pharmacokinetics. Thus, each retinoid should be studied as a unique drug, and the lack of a disease response to one retinoid does not equate with unresponsiveness to the others. In addition to the synthetic retinoids, tretinoin (all-*trans* retinoic acid), a naturally occurring metabolite of retinol, has been used widely as a differentiation-inducing agent for acute promyelocytic leukemia, leading to renewed interest in this retinoid.[12,13]

This chapter summarizes the efficacy and toxicity of oral synthetic retinoids in dermatology, with emphasis on acne, psoriasis, disorders of cornification, and the prevention and treatment of cancer.

MECHANISMS OF RETINOID ACTION

Retinoids have diverse biologic effects. They affect cell growth and differentiation, morphogenesis, inhibition of tumor promotion and malignant cell growth, immunomodulatory actions, and alterations in cellular cohesiveness.

A major breakthrough in the understanding of retinoid action came from the discovery of nuclear receptors for retinoids.[14] These proteins belong to a superfamily of receptors that act as DNA transcription factors and include, for example, the steroid, vitamin D, and thyroid hormone receptors. These receptors bind to target sequences [hormone response elements (HREs)] on DNA and activate gene transcription. Two classes of nuclear retinoid receptors have been identified, retinoic acid receptors (RARs) and retinoid X receptors (RXRs). RARs bind all-*trans* retinoic acid. Although RXRs do not bind retinoic acid, they do bind 9-*cis* retinoic acid. In the presence of retinoid, the RARs and RXRs can bind specific DNA regulatory sequences and thereby activate specific sets of genes. Some of the genes regulated are other DNA-binding proteins, i.e., other regulatory proteins. According to this paradigm, retinoids may cause changes in the expression of other genes by increasing or suppressing the expression of other regulatory proteins. By altering

TABLE 256-1

Retinoid-Responsive Diseases

Acne
  Cystic acne*
  Papular acne†
  Acne rosacea*
  Gram-negative folliculitis*
  Hidradenitis suppurativa‡
  Steroid acne†
  Oil acne†
Disorders of cornification
  The ichthyoses*
    Ichthyosis vulgaris
    Lamellar ichthyosis
    Nonbullous congenital ichthyosiform erythroderma
    Epidermolytic hyperkeratosis
    X-linked ichthyosis
    Keratoderma palmaris et plantaris
    Mal de Meleda†
    Papillon-Lefevre syndrome†
  Darier's disease*
  Pityriasis rubra pilaris*
  Erythrokeratodermia variabilis*
  Kyrle's disease†
  Pachyonychia congenita†
Skin cancer and precancer chemotherapy and chemoprophylaxis
  Basal cell carcinoma‡
  Squamous cell carcinoma‡
  Actinic keratoses*
  Keratoacanthoma*
  Leukoplakia‡
  Bowen's disease‡
  Mycosis fungoides‡
  Cutaneous metastases of malignant melanoma‡
Psoriasis
  Pustular psoriasis*
  Pustular psoriasis of von Zumbusch*
  Pustular psoriasis of palms and soles*
  Erythrodermis psoriasis*
  Psoriatic arthritis‡
Miscellaneous diseases†
  Subcorneal pustular dermatosis
  Reiter's syndrome
  Epidermodysplasia verruciformis
  Discoid lupus erythematosus
  Lichen planus
  Cutaneous sarcoidosis
  Scleromyxedema

*Very effective
†Reported
‡Somewhat effective

the expression of growth factors, oncogenes, keratins, or transglutaminases, retinoids can exert widespread changes in growth or differentiation, controlling such diverse processes as epithelial differentiation (cornification), embryonic morphogenesis, and carcinogenesis. The RARs and RXRs are complex classes of receptors, each composed of α, β, and γ subtypes. Furthermore, there is more than one isoform of each receptor subtype. These nuclear receptors bind DNA as a pair, either as homodimers (RXR/RXR) or heterodimers (RAR/RXR). RXRs can also heterodimerize with receptors such as vitamin D or thyroid hormone receptors. In adult skin, most of the RAR is RAR-γ subtype. An understanding of the complex interactions among the various nuclear retinoid receptors, including those of other members of this superfamily, will undoubtedly enhance our understanding of retinoid action.

TABLE 256-2

Spectrum of Retinoid Toxicity

Acute
  Mucocutaneous
    Cheilitis
    Facial dermatitis
    Xerosis with pruritus
    Conjunctivitis
    Dry nasal mucosa with minor nosebleeds
    Stratum corneum fragility (peeling from minor trauma)
    Palmoplantar peeling
    Hair loss
    Dry mouth with thirst
    Paronychia; nail plate abnormalities*
    Stickiness of skin*
    Chills*
    Phototoxicity and photosensitivity†
    Inflamed urethral meatus*
    Corneal opacities† (reversible after discontinuation)
    Pyogenic granuloma-like lesions in acne†
  Systemic
    Headache*
    Arthralgias and myalgias*
    Teratogenicity (head, ear, heart, thymus abnormalities)
    Spontaneous abortion; premature births
    Pseudotumor cerebri† (headache, papilledema)
    Mental depression†
    Inflammatory bowel disease†
    Urticaria; vasculitis; erythema nodosum†
    Idiopathic seizures†
  Laboratory
    Hyperlipidemia
      Increased triglycerides, VLDL
      Increased cholesterol, LDL*; decreased HDL*
      Eruptive xanthoma†
      Acute hemorrhagic pancreatitis†
    Elevated liver function tests (transient, minor)
      AST, ALT, alkaline phosphatase, LDH, bilirubin
    Thrombocytosis*; thrombocytopenia,† leukopenia
    Hyperuricemia with gout†; hypercalcemia†
    Elevated CPK and myalgias after exercise†
Chronic
  Mucocutaneous—persistent, post-treatment
    Dry eyes†; hair thinning†
  Systemic
    Vertebral abnormalities resembling diffuse idiopathic skeletal
      hyperostosis
      Osteophyte and bony bridge formation
      Anterior spinal ligament calcification
      Posterior spinal ligament calcification†
    Tendon and peripheral ligament calcification
    Premature epiphyseal closure
    Osteoporosis
  Laboratory: none

*Uncommon
†Rare

CYSTIC ACNE (See Chap. 73)

Cystic acne is unique among the retinoid-responsive diseases in that most cases of even the greatest severity can be successfully treated with only one 4- or 5-month course of isotretinoin at a dosage of

0.5 to 2.0 mg/kg body weight per day (Fig. 256-1).[15] Patients with severe cystic acne located on the trunk, nuchal region, low back, buttocks, and thighs may require higher doses of isotretinoin (up to 2.0 mg/kg per day) and longer treatment periods than do patients with cystic acne limited to the face.

The initial studies of isotretinoin in cystic acne led to several generalizations that were confirmed in subsequent studies. First, a lag period of 1 to 3 months may exist before the onset of the therapeutic effect. Second, continued healing after the discontinuation of therapy is regularly observed. Consequently, it is not required to maintain treatment until total clearance is achieved. Third, most patients whose acne clears completely remain in prolonged remission totally free of cysts. Some patients have an occasional cyst or two and varying amounts of papular acne at follow-up examinations. Approximately one-third of patients with acne require a second course of therapy either for persistent disease or for relapse. Relapses sufficient to require further therapy with isotretinoin are dose-, sex-, age-, and severity-dependent. Thus, young males with extensive truncal acne treated with low doses are most likely to relapse.[16,17] Women whose acne repeatedly relapses after treatment with isotretinoin should be examined for hirsutism, questioned for irregularity of menses, and considered for an endocrinologic consultation for evaluation of ovarian or adrenal dysfunction.

Treatment schedules currently in use were developed in experimental protocols conducted in the late 1970s and early 1980s, before the marketing of isotretinoin, and included patients with the most severe cystic acne. Patients being treated at the present time often have less severe cystic acne and are treated at an earlier age. These patients with comparatively milder cystic acne, particularly if limited to the face, may respond comparably and with less toxicity to lower doses, such as 0.5 mg/kg per day, given for longer periods.[18]

Problems associated with isotretinoin treatment of cystic acne include an initial flare of disease during the first few weeks of treatment; rarely, the evolution of acne cysts into lesions resembling pyogenic granulomas[19]; and *Staphylococcus aureus* impetiginization with colonization of the anterior nares.

The most likely mechanism by which isotretinoin leads to clinical improvement in acne is inhibition of sebaceous gland function with a reduced rate of sebum excretion and alterations in skin-surface lipid film chemistry.[20] In addition, other mechanisms include anti-inflammatory effects, antibacterial effects, inhibitory effects of microbial enzyme activity, and desquamative effects on poral occlusion.[21–24]

PSORIASIS (See Chap. 43)

When retinoids are used as monotherapy for psoriasis vulgaris, etretinate at a dosage of 0.5 to 1.0 mg/kg per day is superior to isotretinoin (Fig. 256-2).[25–28] Approximately 15 to 25 percent of patients fail to have a satisfactory response to etretinate, in some cases owing to a worsening of the disease after therapy is initiated and in others to the development of dose-limiting, unacceptable toxicity.[29]

Etretinate is of particular value in the treatment of pustular and erythrodermic psoriasis, the most severe forms of psoriasis. Isotretinoin is also effective in pustular psoriasis, providing a rapidly excreted, alternative retinoid for women of childbearing potential.[30] Chronic maintenance therapy with etretinate may be necessary for patients with pustular psoriasis, those with erythrodermic psoriasis, and those with severe psoriasis vulgaris who have proved to be resistant to or intolerant of other treatments and who regularly demonstrate relapse on withdrawal of etretinate. Therefore, patients with psoriasis are at greater potential risk of developing chronic retinoid toxicity than are patients with acne.

Combining retinoids with other effective therapies increases effectiveness and minimizes toxicity. Etretinate at lower doses has been used in combination with photochemotherapy (PUVA), anthralin, ultraviolet radiation (UVB, 280 to 320 nm), and topical glucocorticoids.[6,31–36]

Acitretin, the free-acid metabolite of etretinate, has a shorter half-life and decreased potential for posttreatment teratogenicity; it is comparable to etretinate in efficacy and toxicity.[37] However, etretinate is detected in the serum of acitretin-treated patients, raising concerns about prolonged retinoid retention and teratogenic risk.[38] The conversion of acitretin into etretinate may be a consequence of ethanol ingestion.

FIGURE 256-1

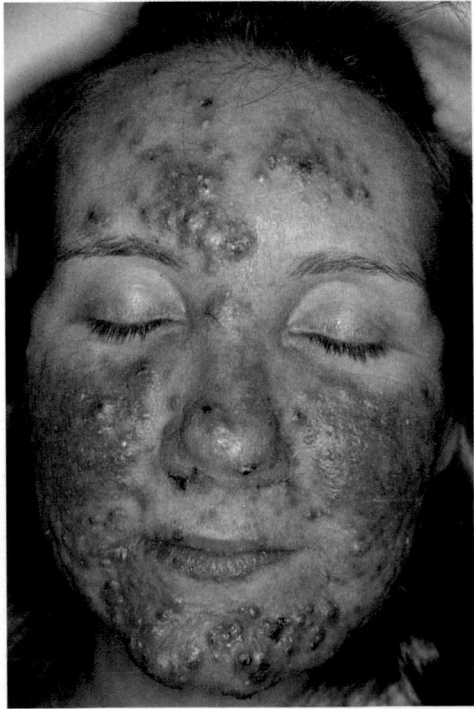

A.

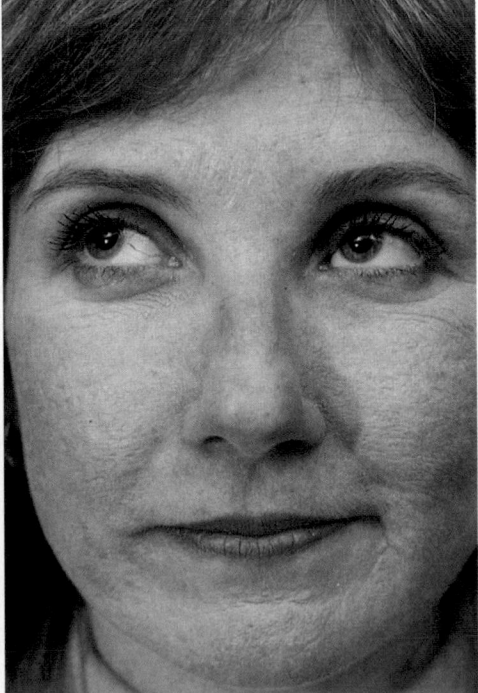

B.

Severe cystic acne in a female before (*A*) and after (*B*) treatment with oral isotretinoin.

FIGURE 256-2

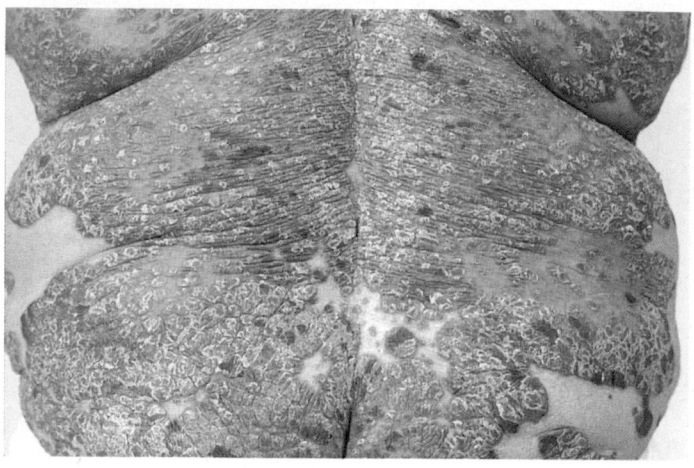

A.

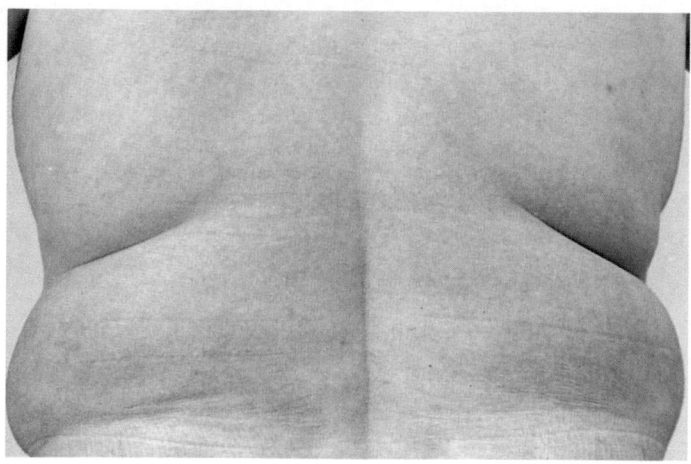

B.

Generalized chronic plaque-type psoriasis before (*A*) and after (*B*) treatment with etretinate.

CUTANEOUS DISORDERS OF CORNIFICATION

In the mid-1970s isotretinoin was demonstrated effective for the treatment of previously recalcitrant cases of disorders of cornification, such as Darier's disease (Fig. 256-3) and pityriasis rubra pilaris (Fig. 256-4).[7,9] Since then, numerous reports have indicated that these and other disorders of cornification respond to isotretinoin, etretinate, acitretin, and newer retinoids such as temarotene (Ro 15-0778)[39–42] (Table 256-1).

Patients with lamellar ichthyosis respond well to retinoids with a reduction in scale, increased heat tolerance and ability to sweat, and improvement of ectropion. Clearing in these patients is usually not complete and may be greater in the summer than in the winter, when their disease is typically more severe.

Because disorders of cornification may require long-term therapy with retinoids, the development of chronic toxicity, particularly skeletal, is a major concern. In children, premature closure of epiphyses[43] and fractures[44] can rarely occur. Changes in the axial skeleton resembling diffuse idiopathic skeletal hyperostosis can occur in both children and adults.[45–47]

CANCER

The synthetic retinoids isotretinoin and etretinate have been used in the treatment and prevention of a variety of cutaneous malignancies.[48] Synthetic retinoids do not often cure cutaneous tumors but usually do produce variable degrees of partial regression when given at high dosage. However, they can have dramatic effects in preventing the formation of new skin tumors. Chemopreventive benefit persists only as long as therapy is maintained, particularly in patients with precancerous genodermatoses (nevoid basal cell carcinoma syndrome, xeroderma pigmentosum).[11,49,50]

Oral isotretinoin was first used in a two-stage trial to treat patients with multiple basal cell carcinomas. In the first treatment stage, high doses (4.5 mg/kg per day for 8 months) were employed as chemotherapy. Only about 10 percent of tumors underwent complete clinical and histologic remission. The second phase successfully used lower doses (0.5 to 1.5 mg/kg per day) for chemoprevention.[11]

Xeroderma Pigmentosum

A controlled prospective study determined that high-dose oral isotretinoin (2 mg/kg per day), given for 2 years, prevented the development of new skin cancers in patients with xeroderma pigmentosum.[49] However, the toxicities observed in some patients during long-term therapy at 2 mg/kg per day were considered significant, and testing with lower doses (0.5 to 1.5 mg/kg per day) was initiated. Compared with the interval without treatment, the frequency of skin cancers occurring during the low-dose treatment decreased in most patients. In some patients, there was an apparent dose response. Furthermore, mucocutaneous toxicity and laboratory abnormalities were less severe with the low-dose treatment. The minimum effective dosage required to prevent the formation of basal cell carcinomas varies among patients and ranges from 0.5 to 1.5 mg/kg per day.

This study, which confirmed that high-dose (2 mg/kg per day) isotretinoin prevents the formation of new skin cancers in patients with xeroderma pigmentosum, represents the first controlled, prospective study to demonstrate cancer chemoprevention in humans. The finding that initiation of therapy decreased tumor incidence and that withdrawal of therapy resulted in a rapid reversal of the chemoprophylactic effect with a significant increase in tumor rates firmly links isotretinoin therapy with tumor suppression. In these patients with xeroderma pigmentosum, isotretinoin seemed to act as a switch, rapidly turning off the appearance of tumors within 2 months of the onset of therapy and quickly losing effectiveness within 3 months of the withdrawal of treatment.

FIGURE 256-3

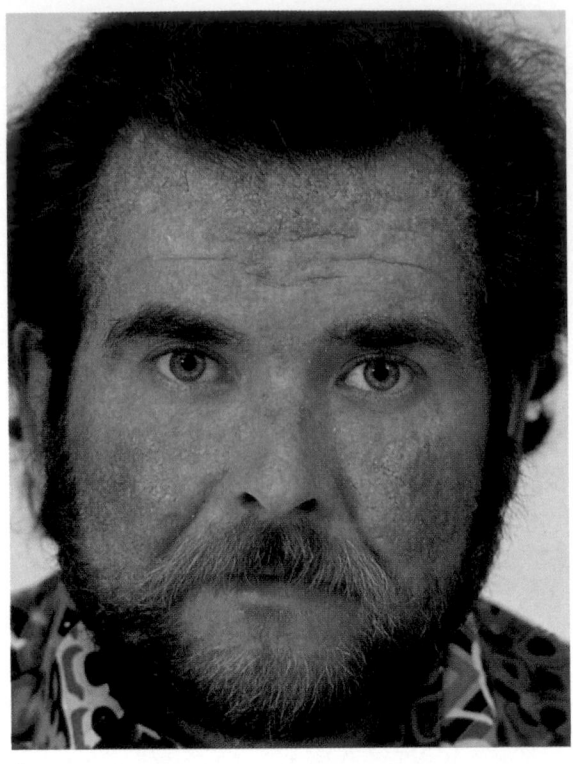

A.

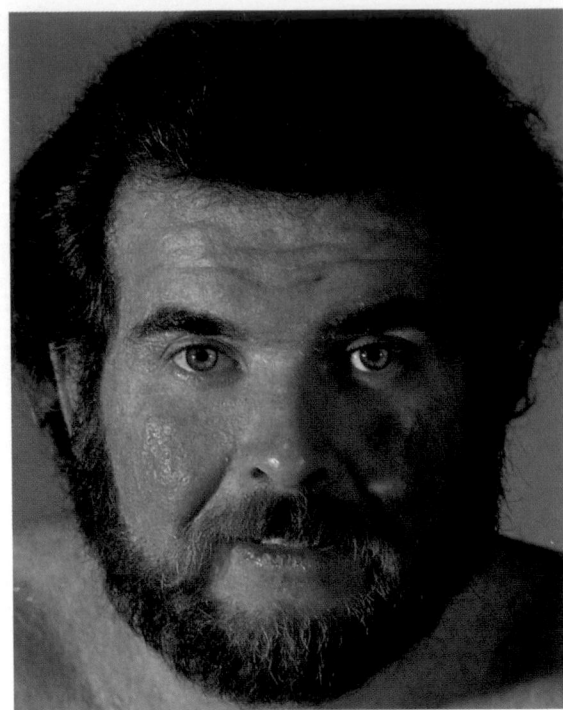

B.

Darier's disease before (A) and after (B) treatment with isotretinoin.

Low-Dose Isotretinoin for Basal Cell Carcinoma

Based on the results of a prior study,[11] the chronic administration of low-dose isotretinoin (10 mg/day or 0.14 mg/kg per day) was evaluated for efficacy in the prevention of new basal cell carcinomas in patients with a history of at least two basal cell carcinomas in the prior 5 years.[51,52]

No significant benefit was observed at the end of the 3-year treatment period. However, even at the low dose of 10 mg/day, isotretinoin produced measurable systemic toxicity. This finding should be weighed in the risk/benefit analysis of the long-term use of isotretinoin. For patients with precancerous genodermatoses (nevoid basal cell carcinoma syndrome, xeroderma pigmentosum) who may develop several dozen skin cancers per year, the potential ben-

FIGURE 256-4

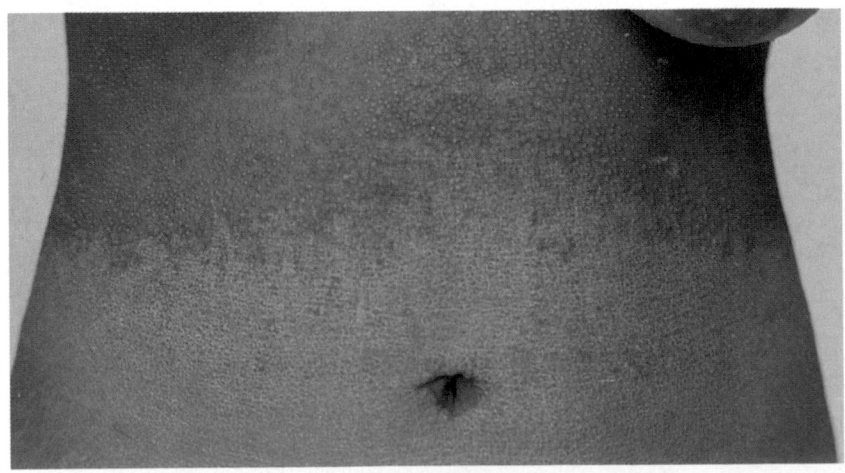

A.

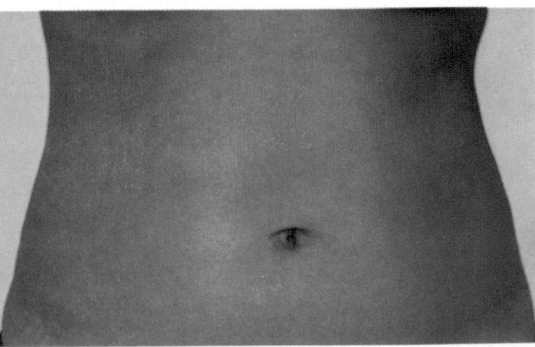

B.

Chronic pityriasis rubra pilaris before (A) and after (B) treatment with isotretinoin.

efit of moderately higher doses of isotretinoin may outweigh the expected detriment of increased toxicity.

Other Studies

There has been a recent expansion of the use of retinoids in oncology.[48] Isotretinoin has been reported to cause regression of squamous cell carcinoma. Complete and partial regressions occurred in four patients with large, recurrent or metastatic squamous cell carcinomas treated with oral isotretinoin, 1.0 mg/kg per day.[53] Isotretinoin given as a chemopreventive agent also lowered the rate of second primary squamous cell carcinomas among patients with previously treated head and neck cancer.[54] Although chemoprevention of potentially lethal cancer occurred, the high dose of isotretinoin used (50 to 100 mg/m^2) resulted in significant participant toxicity with 33 percent of patients dropping out over the 12-month treatment period.

Recent clinical trials have identified clinical responses to combination therapy with retinoids and cytokines. The chemotherapeutic effect of isotretinoin on advanced squamous cell carcinoma of the skin was enhanced by the addition of interferon-α2a. Of 28 patients who were assessed, 7 had complete responses, including 6 patients with advanced local disease and one with distant metastases. The response rate in 14 patients with local advanced disease was 93 percent, roughly twofold higher than that achieved with higher doses of either agent used alone. Although dose reductions were required for most patients, the toxicities of these two agents were reversible and nonoverlapping.[55]

Organ transplant recipients have an increased risk of developing skin cancer. In an Australian series, 44 percent of renal transplant patients had nonmelanoma skin cancer by 9 or more years posttransplant.[56] Even in temperate climates such as the United Kingdom, 40 percent of patients who had their renal transplants more than 9 years had nonmelanoma skin cancer.[57] At a daily dose of 50 mg, etretinate markedly reduced the incidence of squamous cell carcinoma in four renal transplant recipients. In these 4 patients, 23 skin tumors were noted in the 12 months before therapy. Only 6 new lesions developed during the 12-month treatment period and 34 lesions occurred in the 12-month posttreatment period, indicating the need for long-term therapy.[58] Similarly, acitretin (30 mg/day over 6 months) was significantly more effective than placebo in the prevention of squamous cell carcinomas in a group of renal transplant recipients.[59]

ACUTE TOXICITY

The acute synthetic retinoid toxicities (Table 256-2) are well known to dermatologists. Retinoid toxicity mimics many of the findings of vitamin A intoxication but is less severe than toxicities observed with the high doses of vitamin A required for clinical efficacy; it involves primarily the skin and mucous membranes.

The acute toxicities of isotretinoin and etretinate, the two synthetic retinoids, overlap but are not identical. Isotretinoin produces more drying and chapping of skin and mucous membranes than etretinate. Etretinate, however, leads to more hair loss and palmar and plantar peeling than is observed with isotretinoin. It appears that new synthetic retinoids, such as fenretinide, will have unique spectra of clinical toxicity as well as efficacy. For example, drug allergy and nyctalopia are more commonly seen with fenretinide, but the toxicities normally observed with isotretinoin and etretinate are not.[60] Under certain circumstances the differences in relative

toxicity will influence retinoid selection in diseases in which the therapeutic effects are comparable.

Mucocutaneous Toxicities

The acute mucocutaneous toxicities commonly observed with the synthetic retinoids, isotretinoin and etretinate, are well tolerated, not life-threatening, dose-dependent in incidence and severity, treatable with bland therapies, and reversible on dosage reduction or discontinuation of treatment. Cheilitis is the most common toxicity, occurring in almost all patients receiving isotretinoin, even at the low end of the clinically useful dose range. Complete absence of cheilitis when associated with failure of acne to respond at doses of 0.5 mg/kg per day or higher should raise the issue of noncompliance or, rarely, malabsorption of the drug.

Conjunctivitis

Conjunctivitis, which occurs with varying severity in about one-third of patients, may interfere with a patients's ability to wear contact lenses during therapy. *Staphylococcus aureus* has been cultured from the eyelids of patients with isotretinoin-induced blepharoconjunctivitis.[61] If artificial tears and topical ophthalmologic antibiotic therapy fail to relieve the conjunctivitis, then ophthalmologic consultation should be sought. Other ophthalmologic toxicities from retinoids (isotretinoin, etretinate, fenretinide, acitretin) include corneal opacities, decreased night vision with abnormal electroretinograms, transient acute myopia, papilledema secondary to pseudotumor cerebri, cataracts, and teratogenic abnormalities.[62–64] Inhibition of ocular retinol dehydrogenases with decreased formation of 11-*cis* retinal may be the mechanism responsible for retinoid-induced night blindness.[65] Fenretinide may be more likely than other retinoids to interfere with night vision because it markedly reduces plasma concentrations of retinol and retinol-binding protein[66–68]; however, the likelihood of developing this toxicity from fenretinide can be minimized or avoided entirely by scheduling several treatment-free days during each month of therapy.[69] Rarely, dry eyes and decreased night vision have been reported to persist after discontinuation of therapy.

Hair Loss

Hair loss, which is more severe during treatment with etretinate than with isotretinoin, occurs 3 to 8 weeks after beginning treatment and after a minimum total dose of 2 g. It ceases 6 to 8 weeks after discontinuation of therapy, although rare instances of persistent hair loss have been reported.

SYSTEMIC TOXICITY

Teratogenicity

Isotretinoin and etretinate are potent teratogens, and fetal deformities are the major concern in treating fertile women with oral retinoids. The birth defects characteristically induced by retinoids (retinoic acid embryopathy) include central nervous system abnormalities (hydrocephalus, microcephaly), external ear abnormalities, cardiovascular abnormalities, facial dysmorphia, eye abnormalities (microphthalmia), and thymus gland abnormalities.[70,71] The clinical expression of retinoic acid embryopathy may vary with the retinoid; etretinate is less likely to induce cardiac malformations and more likely to induce acral skeletal malformations.[72] In some instances the abnormalities may lead to death. Additional reported defects include premature births, parathyroid hormone deficiency, and cases of low IQ scores in the absence of obvious central nervous system abnormality. The retinoid effects on neural crest cells during the fourth week after fertilization may be responsible for many of the malformations.[73] There is no known safe dose or duration of therapy for avoiding the teratogenicity of retinoids. In summary, isotretinoin and etretinate are contraindicated in pregnant women and in women of childbearing potential who refuse to use or are unreliable in complying with effective contraception. However, several reports indicate that oral tretinoin, when given late in pregnancy for the treatment of maternal acute promyelocytic leukemia, did not adversely affect the fetus.[74–76] Although topical tretinoin had long been considered to be of minimal teratogenic risk, reports of birth defects have led to a recommendation to avoid this agent during pregnancy.[77–79]

Current guidelines are that contraception should be used for 1 month before isotretinoin therapy, during therapy, and for 1 month afterward,[80] and that a negative pregnancy test be obtained 2 weeks before initiating therapy on the second or third day of a normal menstrual period.

Etretinate is stored in body fat deposits, has a terminal elimination half-life in plasma of about 100 days, and can be detected in serum in trace amounts for as long as 3 years after the cessation of therapy.[81] Retinoic acid embryopathy has developed even when conception occurred after the discontinuation of etretinate.[82] Women of childbearing potential should avoid etretinate exposure. It is currently recommended that women who have taken etretinate avoid pregnancy for at least 2 years after the discontinuation of therapy.

Acitretin, the carboxylic acid metabolite of etretinate, is comparable to etretinate in clinical efficacy and toxicity.[37] Initial multiple-dose pharmacokinetic studies indicated that acitretin differs considerably from etretinate by having a terminal elimination half-life in plasma of only 2 days.[38] This rapid clearance after the discontinuation of acitretin therapy would create a potential major clinical advantage of reduced risk of delayed teratogenicity in comparison with etretinate. However, etretinate in small amounts is found in the plasma, most likely as a metabolite, after acitretin administration.[38] Ingested ethanol may play a role in enhancing ethyl ester formation of acitretin.[83] Nonetheless, because the amounts of etretinate formed during acitretin therapy are small, the risk of long-term body storage in women of childbearing potential is almost certain to be less with acitretin therapy than with etretinate. Further research is warranted to determine the degree of advantage in using this agent to reduce the risk of teratogenicity.

The presence of retinoic acid embryopathy may depend on the binding of retinoids to specific retinoic acid nuclear receptors. The spectrum and severity of retinoid-induced birth defects may vary with which RAR (α, β, or γ) the retinoid preferentially binds. Retinoids binding to RAR-α were the most teratogenic in mice and those binding to RAR-γ the least.[84] Thus, retinoids that are RAR-γ ligands, as a class, might have an improved therapeutic ratio and should be explored further for clinical usefulness. Additionally, an RAR-α antagonist effectively reduced the frequency and severity of major malformations induced by an RAR-α agonist (a retinoid binding preferentially to RAR-α) in mice.[85]

Arthralgias and Myalgias

Arthralgias, which disappear after the discontinuation of therapy, occur in only a minority of patients treated with synthetic retinoids. Myalgias, sometimes associated with elevations in CPK, may occur more frequently in physically active patients during retinoid therapy.

Pseudotumor Cerebri

Pseudotumor cerebri has developed rarely during treatment with isotretinoin. If patients receiving isotretinoin develop persistent headache with visual changes, nausea, and vomiting, the drug should be discontinued promptly and the patient should be examined for papilledema possibly in association with retinal hemorrhages. In five such cases, the patients were also being treated with tetracycline or minocycline, drugs that rarely produce increased intracranial hypertension. This finding suggests caution in combining these therapies.

Retinoic Acid Syndrome

Two unusual toxicities not reported in the dermatologic literature were observed in patients with acute promyelocytic leukemia (APL) treated with oral tretinoin. Fever and respiratory distress developed in 9 of 35 patients with APL within 3 weeks of initiating treatment with tretinoin.[86] Additional signs and symptoms of this retinoic acid syndrome included weight gain, lower extremity edema, pleural or pericardial effusions, and episodic hypotension. Three patients died. Early treatment with high-dose intravenous glucocorticoids led to full recovery in three of four patients. The second unique toxicity observed in patients with APL treated with retinoic acid was hyperhistaminemia associated with a marked increase in basophils, leading to shock and severe gastric and duodenal ulceration.[87] The basophilia was consequent to the retinoid-induced differentiation of the leukemic promyelocytes. In addition, an ironic consequence of the successful induction of neutrophilic maturation by tretinoin in a patient with APL was the development of acute neutrophilic dermatosis (Sweet's syndrome).[88]

LABORATORY ABNORMALITIES

Hyperlipidemia

An acute toxicity common to both vitamin A and the synthetic retinoids has been hypertriglyceridemia, probably due to both increased synthesis and decreased elimination of blood lipids. In cases of severe retinoid-induced hypertriglyceridemia, eruptive xanthomas and acute hemorrhagic pancreatitis may occur. The elevations of plasma triglycerides and very low density lipoprotein (VLDL) levels are dose-dependent and reversible on discontinuation of therapy.[89,90] Dosages of isotretinoin of 1 mg/kg per day or higher are usually needed to elevate triglyceride levels markedly beyond the normal range in susceptible individuals. In one report of 20 men with cystic acne of the trunk who were treated with isotretinoin at a maximum dosage of 2 mg/kg per day, the maximum increases from baseline levels were for triglycerides, 67 percent; for VLDL, 56 percent; for LDL, 22 percent; and for cholesterol, 16 percent. The maximum decrease in high-density lipoproteins was 10 percent, leading to an increased LDL/HDL ratio.[89] Hypertriglyceridemia has also occurred with therapy with etretinate and acitretin,[91] particularly in patients with one of the following predisposing factors: obesity, high alcohol intake, diabetes, and pretreatment hypertriglyceridemia.[39] These observations have led to the recommendations to obtain fasting plasma triglyceride levels before initiating retinoid therapy, to monitor levels monthly for the first 2 months and then at 2- to 3-month intervals if values are within normal limits, and to discontinue therapy if triglyceride levels reach 800 mg/dL. Less severe increases may be treated by dose reduction, dietary management (low-fat, high–complex carbohydrate diet), reduction in alcohol and tobacco consumption, and increased physical activity. Supplementation with fish oils containing eicosapentenoic acid and docosahexaenoic acid (MaxEPA) has been reported to reduce triglyceride elevations during retinoid therapy.[92]

The successful use of lipid-regulating agents for the treatment of retinoid-induced hyperlipidemia has been reported.[93] Certainly, if patients with pretreatment elevations in the level of plasma triglycerides are to be treated with retinoids, their condition must be monitored closely to avoid the development of pancreatitis. The effect of retinoid-induced hyperlipidemia and its management during long-term therapy on the development of atherosclerotic cardiovascular disease is unknown.

Liver Toxicity

As with vitamin A, the synthetic retinoids can alter tests of liver function. The transaminases (AST, ALT) are the most commonly elevated tests of liver function, but other tests (alkaline phosphatase, lactic dehydrogenase, bilirubin) can also be abnormal. Elevations of transaminase occur in approximately 15 percent of patients but usually return to normal within 2 to 4 weeks and remain normal even with continued therapy with the retinoids. However, acute hepatotoxic reactions may occur to etretinate, with associated fever and eosinophilia, possibly indicating hypersensitivity.[94] The definitive diagnosis of retinoid hepatitis may require sonography, hepatitis C serology, and a liver biopsy.[95] Although four deaths have been reported due to etretinate-induced hypersensitivity hepatitis, recovery may be complete within 1 to 6 months after discontinuation of the offending retinoid. Case reports have associated the development of chronic active hepatitis[95] and cirrhosis[96] with long-term use of etretinate. However, in prospective studies, long-term therapy with etretinate has not led to chronic liver toxicity[95] measured by liver function tests and by liver biopsies examined by light and electron microscopy, even in patients with preexisting liver disease.[97] Moreover, patients with Gilbert's syndrome have been treated with isotretinoin with an unanticipated normalization of bilirubin level and without evidence of adverse hepatic reaction.[98]

Renal Toxicity

Renal toxicity has not been a characteristic consequence of retinoid administration. Isotretinoin has been safely administered to patients with end-stage kidney disease who were undergoing hemodialysis.[99] However, case reports describing reversible renal function impairment with elevated creatinine levels during etretinate therapy advise monitoring renal function during retinoid therapy, particularly in patients with a history of renal disorders.[100]

Inflammatory Bowel Disease

Synthetic retinoids rarely have been linked with other toxicities, such as inflammatory bowel disease. Of four patients with Crohn's disease or ulcerative colitis treated with isotretinoin for cystic acne, only one had an exacerbation of bowel disease requiring discontin-

uation of isotretinoin. Thus, isotretinoin may be used with caution in the presence of inflammatory bowel disease.[101,102]

CHRONIC TOXICITY

The most common findings in animals and humans during chronic hypervitaminosis A intoxication have been bony changes. Synthetic retinoids induce chronic bone toxicities similar to those of chronic hypervitaminosis A.[103–109]

Bone toxicity was first observed in patients maintained on high-dose, long-term isotretinoin therapy for disorders of cornification. Changes included partial closure of the proximal epiphysis of the tibia, demineralization, and altered bone remodeling.[43] Etretinate produced the following skeletal toxicity: ossification of the interosseous membranes of the forearm, premature epiphyseal closure, fractures secondary to thinning of long bones, periosteal thickening, cortical bone resorption, and osteoporosis.[107]

Synthetic retinoids produce bony changes resembling diffuse idiopathic skeletal hyperostosis (DISH), including anterior spinal ligament calcification, osteophytes, and bony bridges but without narrowing of the disk space. In 50 patients, 37 receiving etretinate and 13 receiving isotretinoin for periods greater than 2 years, 9 had DISH-like changes.[46] The lack of disk-space narrowing eliminates degenerative joint disease as a cause of these changes. Patients treated with isotretinoin for longer than 2 years at a minimum dose of 1.5 mg/kg per day were considered to be at significant risk for developing DISH-like changes of the vertebral column. In a skin cancer prevention study in patients with xeroderma pigmentosum, calcification of the anterior spinal ligament with bony bridging of vertebrae was observed after 2 years of isotretinoin therapy (2 mg/kg per day).[49] Rarely, ossification of the spinal posterior longitudinal ligament has been reported. Unlike involvement of the anterior longitudinal ligament, this change, if progressive, may lead to injury of peripheral nerves exiting from the spinal cord and even to spinal cord compression with signs of partial spastic paraplegia.[103,110,111] Skeletal changes may not require many years of therapy to occur. In a prospective study, vertebral osteophytes formed within 12 months after the initiation of therapy with isotretinoin at 2.0 mg/kg per day.[47,112] Each retinoid may produce a different spectrum of skeletal toxicity. Etretinate produces spinal toxicities similar to but perhaps less severe than those of isotretinoin.[46,107] In a 4-month study employing bone scintigraphy, 3 of 18 patients with acne treated with isotretinoin had pathologic uptake of radiolabel (technetium) in the knee and sacroiliac joints, whereas all 15 patients with psoriasis treated with etretinate had normal examinations.[113]

The skeletal abnormalities in spontaneously occurring DISH (i.e., unrelated to retinoid therapy) includes calcification in tendons and ligaments both in the spine and in extraspinal locations. However, the diagnosis of DISH depends only on the extent of spinal involvement. Several studies in isotretinoin-treated patients have identified radiographic spinal abnormalities that are sufficiently severe to permit a diagnosis of DISH to be made. The increased risk of spinal abnormalities associated with isotretinoin therapy has been identified in controlled studies.[46,114]

Involvement of extraspinal sites has also been identified in individual isotretinoin-treated patients, but the relationship between spinal and extraspinal involvement is not clear. Although spinal involvement has also been observed in etretinate-treated patients, controlled studies have not been done. However, a controlled study of etretinate has found a significant increase in the development of involvement at extraspinal sites. Extraspinal tendon and ligament calcification was identified as a common toxicity in a study of 38 patients who received long-term (average 5 years) etretinate therapy at an average dose of 0.8 mg/kg per day.[108] Radiographic evidence of extraspinal involvement was found in 32 patients (84 percent), but spinal involvement was uncommon. Involvement tended to be bilateral and multifocal. The most common areas of involvement were in the feet (plantar ligament, insertion of Achilles tendon) and in the pelvis (hip joints). Although the presence of radiographic evidence of extraspinal tendon and ligament calcification did not correlate well with the presence of symptoms, those patients with extensive involvement were symptomatic.

The incidence and severity of bony toxicity may depend on the total dose of retinoid received. In patients with acne treated short-term (4 months) with isotretinoin at doses ranging from 1.0 to 2.0 mg/kg per day, only minimal radiographic abnormalities were observed. Small anterior vertebral spurs developed in only 10 of 96 patients. In some instances, the spurs were not visible until 7 to 10 months after treatment.[115]

Skeletal toxicity has been detected even at very low doses. In a placebo-controlled skin cancer prevention trial with isotretinoin at a dose of only 10 mg/day for 3 years, preexisting vertebral osteophytes became enlarged in the retinoid-treated group. At this dose level, only a few patients developed new osteophytes.[114]

Osteoporosis

Osteoporosis was identified by single- and dual-photon absorptiometry in patients who had received long-term therapy with etretinate but not with isotretinoin. Patients with a variety of cutaneous disorders had been treated for at least 2 years with a minimum of 50 g total dose of either retinoid. Bone mineral density was significantly reduced at several anatomic locations.[116] However, no changes in bone mineralization were seen after short-term (20 weeks) therapy of cystic acne with isotretinoin.[117] At the end of the 20-week course of isotretinoin therapy, there was a significant decrease in serum 1, 25 dihydroxyvitamin D without changes in serum osteocalcin, calcium, 25-dihydroxyvitamin D, intact parathyroid hormone, or urine hydroxyproline or calcium.

FACTORS IN THE DECISION TO USE RETINOIDS

As with other medications, a risk/benefit ratio should be used to determine whether or not to treat a dermatologic patient with synthetic retinoids. Factors to be considered include the following:

1. *Responsiveness of the disorder to retinoids.* The treatment of cystic acne with isotretinoin is optimal, with short-term exposure leading to long-term remission.
2. *Dose of retinoid required.* The use of retinoids in combination with other effective treatments, such as RePUVA (combination photochemotherapy) for psoriasis, may allow dose reduction with fewer side effects.
3. *Availability of alternative treatments.* In some diseases (severe Darier's disease, epidermolytic hyperkeratosis) synthetic retinoids may be the only effective treatment.

4. *Chronicity of retinoid therapy.* Diseases that relapse rapidly on withdrawal of synthetic retinoids require continuous retinoid administration and, therefore, are associated with increased risk of chronic skeletal toxicity.
5. *Severity of the disease.* Disease-induced limitations on educational, psychological, or physical development should be considered. For example, early retinoid treatment of lamellar ichthyosis may prevent the development of ectropion.
6. *Age of the patient.* Children with disorders of cornification requiring chronic moderate- to high-dose retinoid therapy are at highest risk of developing bone toxicity. They are at risk of premature epiphyseal closure and, because of longer lifetime exposure to the drug, they are at higher risk for future development of the vertebral changes resembling diffuse idiopathic skeletal hyperostosis.
7. *Sex of the patient.* Retinoid teratogenicity entails special risks for the female patient of childbearing potential. Although isotretinoin and acitretin are rapidly cleared from the body within days, etretinate can be detected in the serum for months or even years after the discontinuation of therapy.
8. *Presence of other disorders that may be aggravated by retinoid use.* Renal or hepatic compromise, preexisting hyperlipidemia, or a family history of hyperlipidemia or premature atherosclerotic cardiovascular disease should be considered in the therapeutic assessment.
9. *Concomitant use of other drugs with similar toxicities.* Other drugs that are hepatotoxic (methotrexate), elevate serum lipids (estrogens, glucocorticoids), or rarely produce benign intracranial hypertension (tetracycline) should be avoided, if possible, or the patient must be carefully monitored during the clinical course.

After more than two decades of experience with isotretinoin and etretinate in the treatment of dermatologic disease and in cancer prevention, synthetic retinoids are firmly established as efficacious therapeutic agents. The recently identified dramatic response of acute promyelocytic leukemia to tretinoin has stimulated renewed interest in the pursuit of new synthetic derivatives[39] and new indications. New retinoids are being designed to interact with selected nuclear retinoic acid receptors (RAR, RXR) to focus on a specific therapeutic goal and to improve the therapeutic index.

REFERENCES

1. Thomson J, Milne JA: The use of retinoic acid in congenital ichthyosiform erythroderma. *Br J Dermatol* **81**:452, 1969
2. Eriksen L, Cormane RH: Oral retinoic acid as therapy for congenital ichthyosiform erythroderma. *Br J Dermatol* **92**:343, 1975
3. Stuttgen G: Oral vitamin A acid therapy. *Acta Derm Venereol (Stockh)* **55**(suppl 74):174, 1975
4. Orfanos CE et al: Effect of vitamin A acid (VAA) on psoriasis: Topical combined therapy using corticoids. Two new VAA preparations for oral administration. *Arch Dermatol Forsch* **244**:424, 1972
5. Ott F, Bollag W: Treatment of psoriasis with an orally administered effective new vitamin A acid derivative: Preliminary report. *Schweiz Med Wochenschr* **105**:439, 1975
6. Orfanos CE, Runne U: Systemic use of a new retinoid with and without local dithranol treatment in generalized psoriasis. *Br J Dermatol* **95**:101, 1976
7. Peck GL, Yoder FW: Treatment of lamellar ichthyosis and other keratinising dermatoses with an oral synthetic retinoid. *Lancet* **2**:1172, 1976
8. Peck GL et al: Prolonged remissions of cystic and conglobate acne with 13-*cis*-retinoic acid. *N Engl J Med* **300**:329, 1979
9. Peck GL et al: Treatment of Darier's disease, lamellar ichthyosis, pityriasis rubra pilaris, cystic acne, and basal cell carcinoma with oral 13-*cis*-retinoic acid. *Dermatologica* **157**(suppl 1):11, 1978
10. Peck GL et al: Treatment of basal cell carcinomas with 13-*cis*-retinoic acid. *Proc Am Assoc Cancer Res* **20**:56, 1979

11. Peck GL et al: Chemoprevention of basal cell carcinoma with isotretinoin. *J Am Acad Dermatol* **6**:815, 1982

12. Breitman TR et al: Induction of differentiation of the human promyelocytic leukemia cell line (HL-60) by retinoic acid. *Proc Natl Acad Sci USA* **77**:2936, 1980

13. Huang M et al: Use of all-*trans* retinoic acid in the treatment of acute promyelocytic leukemia. *Blood* **72**:567, 1988

14. Mangelsdorf DJ et al: The retinoid receptors, in *The Retinoids: Biology, Chemistry, and Medicine,* 2d ed, edited by MB Sporn, AB Roberts, DS Goodman. New York, Raven, 1994, pp 319–349

15. Peck GL et al: Isotretinoin versus placebo in the treatment of cystic acne. *J Am Acad Dermatol* **6**:735, 1982

16. Chivot M, Midoun H: Isotretinoin and acne—a study of relapses. *Dermatologica* **180**:240, 1990

17. Harms M et al: The relapses of cystic acne after isotretinoin treatment are age-related: A long-term follow-up study. *Dermatologica* **172**:148, 1986

18. Layton AM, Cunliffe WJ: Guidelines for optimal use of isotretinoin in acne. *J Am Acad Dermatol* **27**:S2, 1992

19. Exner JG et al: Pyogenic-granuloma-like acne lesions during isotretinoin therapy. *Arch Dermatol* **119**:808, 1983

20. Farrell LN et al: The treatment of severe cystic acne with 13-*cis*-retinoic acid. *J Am Acad Dermatol* **3**:602, 1980

21. Camisa C et al: The effects of retinoids on neutrophil functions in vitro. *J Am Acad Dermatol* **6**:620, 1982

22. Norris DA et al: Isotretinoin produces significant inhibition of monocyte and neutrophil chemotaxis in vivo in patients with cystic acne. *J Invest Dermatol* **89**:38, 1987

23. King K et al: A double-blind study of the effects of 13-*cis*-retinoic acid on acne, sebum excretion rate and microbial population. *Br J Dermatol* **107**:583, 1982

24. Leyden JJ, McGinley KJ: Effect of 13-*cis*-retinoic acid on sebum production and *Propionibacterium acnes* in severe nodulocystic acne. *Arch Dermatol Res* **272**:331, 1982

25. Ward A et al: Etretinate: A review of its pharmacological properties and therapeutic efficacy in psoriasis and other skin disorders. *Drugs* **26**:9, 1983

26. Ehmann CW, Voorhees JJ: International studies of the efficacy of etretinate in the treatment of psoriasis. *J Am Acad Dermatol* **6**:692, 1982

27. Mahrle G et al: Oral treatment of keratinizing disorders of skin and mucous membranes with etretinate. *Arch Dermatol* **118**:97, 1982

28. Goerz G, Orfanos CE: Systemic treatment of psoriasis with a new aromatic retinoid. *Dermatologica* **157**(suppl 1):38, 1978

29. Lowe NJ: When systemic retinoids fail to work in psoriasis, in *Retinoids: 10 Years On,* edited by J-H Saurat. Basel, Karger, 1991, pp 341–349

30. Sofen HL et al: Treatment of generalized pustular psoriasis with isotretinoin. *Lancet* **1**:40, 1984

31. Fritsch PO et al: Augmentation of oral methoxsalen-photochemotherapy with an oral retinoic acid derivative. *J Invest Dermatol* **70**:178, 1978

32. Grupper C, Berretti B: Treatment of psoriasis by oral PUVA-therapy combined with aromatic retinoid (Re-PUVA), in *Retinoids: Advances in Basic Research and Therapy,* edited by CE Orfanos et al. New York, Springer-Verlag, 1981, p 341

33. Lauharanta J et al: Aromatic retinoid (Ro 10-9359, Re-PUVA, and PUVA in the treatment of psoriasis, in *Retinoids: Advances in Basic Research and Therapy,* edited by CE Orfanos et al. New York, Springer-Verlag, 1981, p 201

34. Orfanos CE et al: Oral retinoid and UVB radiation: A new alternative treatment for psoriasis on an outpatient basis. *Acta Derm Venereol (Stockh)* **59**:241, 1979

35. Van der Rhee HJ, Polano MK: Treatment of psoriasis vulgaris with a low-dosage Ro 10-9359 orally combined with corticosteroids topically, in *Retinoids: Advances in Basic Research and Therapy,* edited by CE Orfanos et al. New York, Springer-Verlag, 1981, p 193

36. Honigsmann H, Wolff K: Results of therapy for psoriasis using retinoid and photochemotherapy (REPUVA). *Pharmacol Ther* **40**:67, 1989

37. Gollnick H: Acitretin in psoriasis: An update, in *Retinoids: 10 Years On,* edited by J-H Saurat. Basel, Karger, 1991, pp 204–213

38. Wiegand U-W et al: Pharmacokinetics of acitretin in humans, in *Retinoids: 10 Years On,* edited by J-H Saurat. Basel, Karger, 1991, p 192

39. Orfanos CE et al: The retinoids—a review of their clinical pharmacology and therapeutic use. *Drugs* **34**:459, 1987

40. Blanchet-Bardon C et al: Acitretin in the treatment of severe disorders of keratinization. *J Am Acad Dermatol* **24**:982, 1991

41. Laurberg G et al: Treatment of lichen planus with acitretin—a double-blind, placebo-controlled study in 65 patients. *J Am Acad Dermatol* **24**:434, 1991

42. Bollag W, Ott F: Treatment of lichen planus with temarotene. *Lancet* **2**:974, 1989

43. Milstone LM et al: Premature epiphyseal closure in a child receiving oral 13-*cis*-retinoic acid. *J Am Acad Dermatol* **7**:663, 1982

44. Tamayo L, Ruiz-Maldonado R: Long-term follow-up of 30 children under oral retinoid Ro 10-9359, in *Retinoids: Advances in Basic Research and Therapy,* edited by CE Orfanos et al. New York, Springer-Verlag, 1981, p 287

45. Pittsley RA, Yoder FW: Retinoid hyperostoses: Skeletal toxicity associated with long-term administration of 13-*cis*-retinoic acid for refractory ichthyosis. *N Engl J Med* **308**:1012, 1983

46. Gerber LH et al: Vertebral abnormalities associated with synthetic retinoid use. *J Am Acad Derm* **10**:817, 1984

47. Ellis CN et al: Isotretinoin therapy is associated with early skeletal radiographic changes. *J Am Acad Dermatol* **10**:1024, 1984

48. Peck GL, Coats-Walton DA: Retinoids in dermatology: Current usage, in *The Year Book of Dermatology 1995,* edited by AJ Sober, TB Fitzpatrick. St. Louis, Mosby, 1995, pp 1–32

49. Kraemer KH et al: Prevention of skin cancer in xeroderma pigmentosum with the use of oral isotretinoin. *N Engl J Med* **318**:1633, 1988

50. Peck GL et al: Treatment and prevention of basal cell carcinoma with isotretinoin. *J Am Acad Dermatol* **19**:176, 1988

51. Tangrea JA et al: Isotretinoin—basal cell carcinoma prevention trial: Design, recruitment results and baseline characteristics of the trial participants. *Contr Clin Trials* **11**:433, 1990

52. Tangrea JA et al: Long-term therapy with low-dose isotretinoin for prevention of basal cell carcinoma: A multicenter clinical trial. *J Natl Cancer Inst* **84**:328, 1992

53. Lippman SM, Meyskens FL Jr: Treatment of advanced squamous cell carcinoma of the skin with isotretinoin. *Ann Intern Med* **107**:499, 1987

54. Hong WK et al: Prevention of second primary tumors with isotretinoin in squamous cell carcinoma of the head and neck. *N Engl J Med* **323**:795, 1990

55. Lippman SM et al: 13-*cis*-retinoic acid plus interferon alpha-2a: Highly active systemic therapy for squamous cell carcinoma of the cervix. *J Natl Cancer Inst* **84**:241, 1992

56. Hardie IR et al: Skin cancer in caucasian renal allograft recipients living in a subtropical climate. *Surgery* **87**:177, 1980

57. Glover MT et al: Non-melanoma skin cancer in renal transplant recipients: The extent of the problem and a strategy for management. *Br J Plast Surg* **47**:86, 1994

58. Kelly JW et al: Retinoids to prevent skin cancer in organ transplant recipients. *Lancet* **338**:1407, 1991

59. Bouwes Bavinck JN et al: Prevention of skin cancer and reduction of keratotic skin lesions during acitretin therapy in renal transplant recipients: A double-blind, placebo-controlled study. *J Clin Oncol* **13**:1933, 1995

60. Kelloff GJ et al: Clinical development plan: N-(4-hydroxyphenyl)retinamide (4-HPR). *J Cell Biochem* (suppl 20):176, 1994

61. Blackman HJ et al: Blepharoconjunctivitis: A side effect of 13-*cis*-retinoic acid therapy for dermatologic diseases. *Ophthalmology* **86**:753, 1979

62. Gold JA et al: Ocular side effects of the retinoids. *Int J Dermatol* **28**:218, 1989

63. Safran AB et al: Ocular side effects of oral treatment with retinoids: A review of clinical findings and molecular mechanisms and a prospective study of the influence of acitretin on retinal function, in *Retinoids: 10 Years On,* edited by J-H Saurat. Basel, Karger, 1991, pp 315–326

64. Brown RD, Grattan CEH: Visual toxicity of synthetic retinoids. *Br J Ophthalmol* **73**:286, 1989

65. Law WC, Rando RR: The molecular basis of retinoic acid induced night blindness. *Biochem Biophys Res Commun* **161**:825, 1989

66. Peng YM et al: Pharmacokinetics of N-4-hydroxyphenyl-retinamide and the effect of its oral administration of plasma retinol concentrations in cancer patients. *Int J Cancer* **43**:22, 1989

67. Kaiser-Kupfer MI et al: Abnormal retinal function associated with fenretinide, a synthetic retinoid. *Arch Ophthalmol* **104**:69, 1986

68. Kingston TP et al: Visual and cutaneous toxicity which occurs during N-(4-hydroxyphenyl)-retinamide therapy for psoriasis. *Clin Exp Dermatol.* **11**:624, 1986

69. Costa A et al: Tolerability of the synthetic retinoid fenretinide (HPR). *Eur J Cancer Clin Oncol* **25**:805, 1989

70. Lammer EJ et al: Retinoic acid embryopathy. *N Engl J Med* **313**:837, 1985

71. Stern RS et al: Isotretinoin and pregnancy. *J Am Acad Dermatol* **10**:851, 1984

72. Rosa FW et al: Teratogen update: Vitamin A congeners. *Teratology* **33**:355, 1986

73. Sulik KK, Alles AJ: Teratogenicity of the retinoids, in *Retinoids: 10 Years On,* edited by J-H Saurat. Basel, Karger, 1991, pp 282–295

74. Celo JS et al: Acute promyelocytic leukemia in pregnancy: All-*trans* retinoic acid as a newer therapeutic option. *Obstet Gynecol* **83**:808, 1994

75. Stentoft J et al: All-*trans*-retinoic acid in acute promyelocytic leukemia in late pregnancy. *Leukemia* **8**:1585, 1994

76. Harrison P et al: Successful use of all-*trans* retinoic acid in acute promyelocytic leukaemia presenting during the second trimester of pregnancy. *Br J Haematol* **86**:681, 1994

77. Medicines in pregnancy. *Aust Adv Drug React Bull* **12**:14, 1993

78. Lipson AH et al: Multiple congenital defects associated with maternal use of topical tretinoin. *Lancet* **341**:1181, 1993

79. Camera G, Pregliasco P: Ear malformation in baby born to mother using tretinoin cream. *Lancet* **339**:687, 1992

80. Dai WS et al: Safety of pregnancy after discontinuation of isotretinoin. *Arch Dermatol* **125**:362, 1989

81. DiGiovanna JJ et al: Etretinate: Persistent serum concentrations after long-term therapy. *Arch Dermatol* **125**:246, 1989

82. Lammer EJ: Embryopathy in infants conceived one year after termination of maternal etretinate. *Lancet* **2**:1080, 1988

83. Lambert WE et al: Pharmacokinetics and drug interactions of etretinate and acitretin. *J Am Acad Dermatol* **27**:S19, 1992

84. Elmazar MM et al: Pattern of retinoid-induced teratogenic effects: Possible relationship with relative selectivity for nuclear retinoid receptors RAR alpha, RAR beta, and RAR gamma. *Teratology* **53**:158, 1996

85. Eckhardt K, Schmitt G: A retinoic acid receptor alpha antagonist counteracts retinoid teratogenicity in vitro and reduced incidence and/or severity of malformations in vivo. *Toxicology Letters* **70**:299, 1994

86. Frankel SR et al: The "retinoic acid syndrome" in acute promyelocytic leukemia. *Ann Intern Med* **117**:292, 1992

87. Koike T et al: Brief report: Severe symptoms of hyperhistaminemia after the treatment of acute promyelocytic leukemia with tretinoin (all-*trans*-retinoic acid). *N Engl J Med* **327**:385, 1992

88. Piette WW et al: Acute neutrophilic dermatosis with myeloblastic infiltrate in a leukemia patient receiving all-*trans* retinoic acid therapy. *J Am Acad Dermatol* **30**(2, pt 2):293, 1994

89. Zech LA et al: Changes in plasma cholesterol and triglycerides following treatment with oral isotretinoin—a prospective study. *Arch Dermatol* **119**:987, 1983

90. Bershad S et al: Changes in plasma lipids and lipoproteins during isotretinoin therapy for acne. *N Engl J Med* **313**:981, 1985

91. Vahlquist C: Acitretin and blood lipids, in *Retinoids: 10 Years On,* edited by J-H Saurat. Basel, Karger, 1991, pp 296–301

92. Marsden JR: Lipid metabolism and retinoid therapy. *Pharmacol Ther* **40**:55, 1989

93. Cohen PR: The use of gemfibrozil in a patient with chronic myelogenous leukemia to successfully manage retinoid-induced hypertriglyceridemia. *Clin Invest* **71**:74, 1993

94. Weiss VC et al: Hepatotoxic reactions in a patient treated with etretinate. *Arch Dermatol* **120**:104, 1984

95. Sanchez MR et al: Retinoid hepatitis. *J Am Acad Dermatol* **28**:853, 1993

96. Fallon MB, Boyer JL: Hepatic toxicity of vitamin A and synthetic retinoids. *J Gastroenterol Hepatol* **5**:334, 1990

97. Roenigk Jr HH: Liver toxicity of retinoid therapy. *Pharmacol Ther* **40**:145, 1989

98. Wang JI et al: Isotretinoin-associated normalization of hyperbilirubinemia in patients with Gilbert's syndrome. *J Am Acad Dermatol* **32**:136, 1995

99. Beightler EL, Tyring SK: The use of isotretinoin in a patient undergoing kidney hemodialysis. *J Am Acad Dermatol* **23**:758, 1990

100. Cribier B et al: Renal impairment probably induced by etretinate. *Dermatology* **185**:266, 1992

101. Godfrey KM, James MP: Treatment of severe acne with isotretinoin in patients with inflammatory bowel disease. *Br J Dermatol* **123**:653, 1990

102. MacDonald Hull S, Cunliffe WJ: The safety of isotretinoin in patients with acne and systemic diseases. *J Dermatol Treat* **1**:35, 1989

103. Lawson JP, McGuire J: The spectrum of skeletal changes associated with the long-term administration of 13-*cis*-retinoic acid. *Skel Radiol* **16**:91, 1987

104. Carey BM et al: Skeletal toxicity with isotretinoin therapy: A clinico-radiological evaluation. *Br J Dermatol* **119**:609, 1988

105. Ellis CN et al: Long term radiographic follow-up after isotretinoin therapy. *J Am Acad Dermatol* **18**:1252, 1988

106. Kilcoyne RF: Effects of retinoids in bone. *J Am Acad Dermatol* **19**:212, 1988

107. White SI, MacKie RM: Bone changes associated with oral retinoid therapy. *Pharmacol Ther* **40**:137, 1989

108. DiGiovanna JJ et al: Extraspinal tendon and ligament calcification associated with long-term therapy with etretinate. *N Engl J Med* **315**:1177, 1986

109. Teelmann K: Experimental toxicology of the aromatic retinoid Ro 10-9359 (etretinate), in *Retinoids: Advances in Basic Research and Therapy,* edited by CE Orfanos et al. New York, Springer-Verlag, 1981, p 41

110. Pennes DR et al: Retinoid induced ossification of the posterior longitudinal ligament. *Skel Radiol* **14**:191, 1985

111. Tfelt-Hansen P et al: Spinal cord compression after long-term etretinate. *Lancet* **2**:325, 1989

112. Shalita AR et al: Isotretinoin treatment of acne and related disorders: An update. *J Am Acad Dermatol* **9**:629, 1983

113. Torok L et al: Bone-scintigraphic examinations in patients treated with retinoids: A prospective study. *Br J Dermatol* **120**:31, 1989

114. Tangrea JA et al: Skeletal hyperostosis in patients receiving long-term, very-low-dose isotretinoin. *Arch Dermatol* **128**:921, 1992

115. Kilcoyne RF et al: Minimal spinal hyperostosis with low dose isotretinoin therapy. *Invest Radiol* **21**:41, 1986

116. DiGiovanna JJ et al: Osteoporosis is a toxic effect of long-term etretinate therapy. *Arch Dermatol* **131**:1263, 1995

117. Margolis DJ et al: Effects of isotretinoin on bone mineralization during routine therapy with isotretinoin for acne vulgaris. *Arch Dermatol* **132**:769, 1996

CHAPTER 257

Nicholas A. Soter

Antihistamines

The biologic effects of histamine and its release from tissues during inflammatory reactions were recognized by 1910. In 1927, Lewis suggested that a substance with biologic properties similar to those of histamine accounted for the cutaneous triple-response phenomenon. Also, he showed that the intradermal injection of histamine resulted in the formation of a wheal and erythema. In 1937, Bovet and Staub demonstrated that some of the effects of histamine in experimental animals could be antagonized by amines containing a phenolic ether moiety. Subsequent research yielded a number of related compounds and led to the development of histamine-receptor antagonists, or antihistamines, that became available for clinical use as therapeutic agents in the 1940s.

The fact that antihistamines were unable to block the effects of histamine on the gastric mucosa suggested that histamine might exert its effects via different receptors, which were later designated H_1 and H_2. This observation led to the synthesis of new compounds that selectively blocked histamine at the H_2-receptor site. H_3 receptors have been recognized in brain and peripheral nerve tissue in experimental animals and in the airways in humans; however, clinical therapeutic agents are not yet available to block the H_3 receptor.

All of the clinical blockers, or antagonists, of histamine are competitive inhibitors of the actions of histamine at tissue receptor sites, although some of these therapeutic agents have additional actions.

HISTAMINE

Chemistry and Metabolism

Histamine, β-imidazolylethylamine, which is present in mast cells, basophils, and platelets in association with their granules, in gastric parietal cells, and in nerve endings is formed by the enzymatic decarboxylation of the amino acid histidine by histidine decarboxylase. In mast-cell granules, histamine is stored and bound ionically to a proteoglycan-protein complex. After its release, histamine is catabolized in one of two ways. In the more important pathway in the skin, histamine is catalyzed by histamine methyltransferase to produce methyl histamine, which is converted by monoamine oxidase to methyl-imidazole acetic acid. In the second pathway, histamine undergoes oxidative deamination catalyzed by diamine oxidase to form imidazole acetic acid, which is subsequently conjugated and excreted as riboxylimidazole acetic acid.

Tissue Receptors

The biologic effects of histamine result from its interactions with tissue receptors, designated H_1, H_2, and H_3. Unclassified histamine receptors, which when stimulated are not blocked by H_1, H_2, or H_3 histamine receptor antagonists, have been detected on human peripheral blood lymphocytes and on a human promyelocytic leukemia cell line (HL-60).[1] Heterogeneity in the H_1 receptor is suggested by the detection of H_1 receptors of different molecular weights in various tissues and in cell lines at different stages of maturation and the dissimilar values of binding affinities for H_1 receptor antagonists in multiple cell lines and tissues. Histamine receptor proteins may be specific for a cell type.[1] There may be tissue-specific expression of histamine receptors or receptor subtypes.

The biologic functions mediated by H_1 receptors include contraction of endothelial cells and smooth muscle; increases in venular permeability and airways resistance; stimulation of cutaneous nerves and nasal mucus secretion; and enhancement of chemotaxis of eosinophils and neutrophils. The traditional H_1-type antihistamines bind competitively with histamine at the receptor level, and their binding is reversible. They can be displaced by high levels of histamine, and they dissociate from the receptor. Second-generation H_1-type antihistamines bind in a noncompetitive manner, are not easily displaced by histamine, dissociate slowly from the H_1 receptor, and have a longer duration of action.

The biologic functions mediated by H_2 receptors include dilation of vascular smooth muscle and bronchial smooth muscle; increases in venular permeability, cardiac rate and force of contraction, and airways mucus production; secretion of parietal cell acid; stimulation of CD8+ T lymphocytes with delayed-type hypersensitivity suppression; and inhibition of chemotaxis of neutrophils and eosinophils. Inasmuch as the skin microvasculature contains both H_1 and H_2 receptors, increased venular permeability depends on the interaction of histamine with both of these receptors.

Proposed biologic functions mediated by H_3 receptors include modulation of histamine synthesis and release in cerebral neurons, decreased histamine release from mast cells, and decreased release of tachykinins from unmyelinated C fibers in airways. H_3 receptors also play a role in the modulation of allergic airways disease by acting as autoreceptors for cholinergic neurotransmission at the level of autonomic ganglia in the airways, and they inhibit cholinergic and noncholinergic excitatory nerves in the airways.[2] Blockade of H_3 receptors limits the bronchoconstriction induced by histamine.

ANTIHISTAMINES

Traditional, Classic, or First-Generation H₁-Type Antihistamines

The traditional, classic, or first-generation H_1-type antihistamines have in common with histamine a substituted ethylamine moiety as an integral part of the molecule (Fig. 257-1). The activity of an H_1-type antihistamine is increased by the substitution of a halogen in the *para* position of the phenyl or benzyl group of R^1. For maximum activity, the terminal nitrogen of the ethylamine group should be a tertiary amine with methyl groups or a cyclic moiety in R^2 and R^3. The dextro isomers are more active than the levo isomers. In addition, H_1-type antihistamines have a tertiary amino group linked by a two- or three-atom chain to two aromatic substituents. Traditional H_1-type antihistamines have been divided into six groups (Table 257-1) based on substitution at the X position with nitrogen, oxygen, or carbon. The presence of multiple aromatic or heterocyclic rings and alkyl substituents results in their lipophilic properties.

In addition to their antihistamine actions, the H_1-type antihistamines have a number of effects that include sedation, anticholinergic activity, local anesthesia, antiemetic activity, and anti-motion-sickness effects. Moreover, they have a variety of antiinflammatory and antiallergic properties that are independent of H_1 blockade. Some H_1-type antihistamines possess α-adrenergic receptor or cholinergic muscarinic receptor blocking properties, while others possess antiserotonin effects.

The pharmacokinetics and pharmacodynamics of antihistamines can be studied in the skin in vivo by quantitating the wheal-and-erythema response to the intracutaneous injection of histamine in their presence and absence.

PHARMACOKINETICS H_1-type antihistamines are absorbed from the gastrointestinal tract after oral administration. Their effects can be observed within 30 min of administration, are maximal within 1 to 2 h, and usually persist for 4 to 6 h; however, some of these therapeutic agents may have a longer duration of action. For example, after the oral administration of a single dose, the serum half-lives of brompheniramine, chlorpheniramine, and hydroxyzine exceeded 20 h in adults. The serum half-lives of chlorpheniramine and hydroxyzine are shorter in children and longer in elderly adults. The fact that the half-life of hydroxyzine is prolonged in patients

FIGURE 257-1

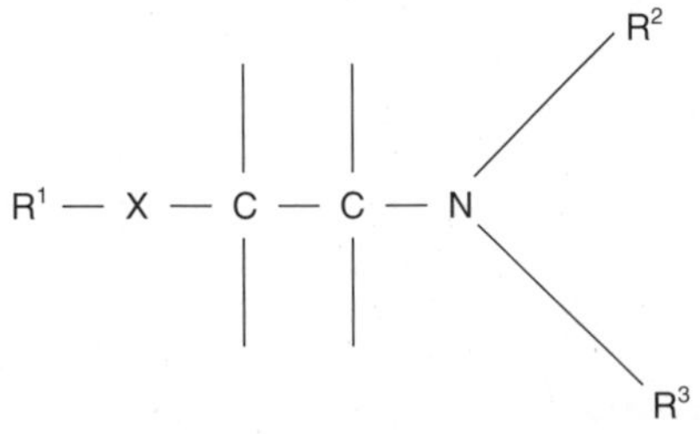

Ethylamine moiety present in H_1 antihistamines. R^1, aromatic and/or heterocyclic groups; X, linkage such as nitrogen, oxygen, or carbon.

TABLE 257-1

First Generation H₁-type Antihistamines

CHEMICAL CLASS	GENERIC NAME
Alkylamine (propylamine)	Brompheniramine maleate
	Chlorpheniramine maleate and tannate
	Dexbrompheniramine maleate
	Dexchlorpheniramine maleate
	Dimethindene maleate
	Pheniramine maleate
	Triprolidine hydrochloride
Aminoalkyl ether (ethanolamine)	Bromodiphenhydramine hydrochloride
	Carbinoxamine maleate
	Clemastine fumarate
	Diphenhydramine citrate and hydrochloride
	Doxylamine succinate
	Embramine hydrochloride
	Mefenidramium methylsulfate
	Phenyltoloxamine citrate
	Trimethobenzamine citrate
Ethylenediamine	Antazoline hydrochloride, mesylate, phosphate, and sulfate
	Mepyramine maleate
	Pyrilamine maleate
	Tripelennamine citrate and hydrochloride
Phenothiazine	Dimethothiazine mesylate
	Mequitazine
	Methdilazine
	Methdilazine hydrochloride
	Promethazine hydrochloride
	Trimeprazine tartrate
Piperidine	Azatadine maleate
	Cyproheptadine hydrochloride
	Diphenylpyraline hydrochloride
	Phenindamine tartrate
Piperazine	Chlorcyclizine hydrochloride
	Hydroxyzine hydrochloride and pamoate

with primary biliary cirrhosis suggests that its pharmacokinetics may be altered in other hepatic diseases. The metabolism of H_1-type antihistamines takes place by the hepatic cytochrome P_{450} system CYA3A3/4, in which they are conjugated to form glucuronides. The H_1-type antihistamines also induce hepatic microsomal enzymes and thus may facilitate their own metabolism. Excretion of these compounds in the urine is almost complete by 24 h after administration.

H_1-type antihistamines achieve different levels in different tissues. For example, hydroxyzine enters the skin rapidly, and sustained high concentrations result after single or multiple doses.[3] The H_1-type antihistamines suppress wheal-and-erythema reactions induced by the intracutaneous injection of histamine for various time intervals depending on the agent studied. A single 50-mg dose of hydroxyzine suppresses the histamine-induced wheal-and-flare reaction for up to 36 h in healthy young adults and up to 144 h in healthy elderly adults.[3,4]

H_1-type antihistamines are conventionally administered in divided doses at intervals between 4 and 6 h. However, the observation that one oral dose of certain of these agents is associated with longer serum half-lives suggests that some H_1-type antihistamines may not require administration as frequently as was previously indicated.

SIDE EFFECTS Approximately 25 percent of patients receiving H_1-type antihistamines experience an adverse reaction. However, there are considerable variations in the responses of individual subjects. Sedation is the most common problem associated with these therapeutic agents. This sedative effect is pronounced with the aminoalkyl ether and the phenothiazine groups. The soporific effect of other groups is less marked, especially the alkylamine group. The sedative effect ameliorates in most individuals within a few days of continuous administration of H_1-type antihistamines. If tolerance to the sedative manifestations does not occur, a trial of an agent from another group should be undertaken. The use of H_1-type antihistamines has been associated with increased occupational injuries at work, and the risk of injury is enhanced with an odds ratio of 1.5.[5] Other central nervous system (CNS) effects include dizziness, tinnitus, disturbed coordination, inability to concentrate, blurred vision, and diplopia. The CNS effects at times may be stimulatory, especially with the alkylamine group; these effects include nervousness, irritability, insomnia, and tremor.

A series of electroencephalographic (EEG) studies have been developed to demonstrate the CNS effects of the traditional H_1-type antihistamines. These include the Multiple Sleep Latency Tests, tests involving brainstem evoked potentials, acuity tests, cognitive skill tests, and driving simulation tests. For example, subjects who received diphenhydramine fell asleep faster than did those who had taken placebo. In brainstem evoked-potential studies, the individual's attention and processing speed are impaired by first-generation H_1-type antihistamines. In multiple studies, driving skills are impaired after the use of first-generation H_1-type antihistamines. A Canadian study on the relation between H_1-type antihistamines and automobile fatalities suggested that antihistamines may affect driving skills sufficiently to result in fatal automobile accidents.

Gastrointestinal complications are the second most frequent side effect and are noted especially with the ethylenediamine group. Anorexia, nausea, vomiting, epigastric distress, diarrhea, and constipation have been reported. The administration of these agents with food may eliminate some of these manifestations.

H_1-type antihistamines have anticholinergic effects, including dry mucous membranes, difficulty in micturition, urinary retention, dysuria, urinary frequency, and impotence. These clinical manifestations have been reported with the administration of therapeutic agents from the aminoalkyl ether, the phenothiazine, and the piperazine groups.

Infrequent side effects of H_1-type antihistamines include headache, a sensation of tightness in the throat, tingling, and numbness. The cardiovascular effects of H_1-type antihistamines are not usually experienced after oral administration. Transient hypotension may develop after intravenous therapy, especially if the administration of the drug is rapid.

Cutaneous reactions occurring after the administration of H_1-type antihistamines are uncommon; they include eczematous dermatitis, urticaria, petechiae, fixed drug eruptions, and photosensitivity.

Acute poisoning may develop, especially in children. Hallucinations, ataxia, incoordination, athetosis, and convulsions are the major features. Anticholinergic effects include flushing, dilated pupils, and hyperthermia. Treatment for poisoning after the ingestion of H_1-type antihistamines is symptomatic and supportive.

CONTRAINDICATIONS AND DRUG INTERACTIONS If patients receiving H_1-type antihistamines become sensitized to the drug, the subsequent systemic administration of the offending agent or a related compound may produce an eczematous dermatitis. An important clinical example is the cutaneous eruption that occurs after the administration of drugs, such as aminophylline, that contain the ethylenediamine moiety. Allergic contact dermatitis may

develop after the topical application of some H_1-type antihistamines.

When H_1-type antihistamines are consumed in combination with alcohol or other therapeutic agents with CNS depressant effects, such as diazepam, there may be an accentuation of the central depressive effects. Antihistamines of the phenothiazine group may block and reverse the vasopressor effect of epinephrine. If individuals receiving a phenothiazine require a vasopressor agent, norepinephrine or phenylephrine should be used. Since monoamine oxidase inhibitors prolong and intensify the anticholinergic effects of antihistamines, the administration of H_1-type antihistamines is contraindicated in patients receiving monoamine oxidase inhibitors.

There are limited guidelines for the use of H_1-type antihistamines in pregnant women. Most drugs are classified as U.S. Food and Drug Administration category B, which is defined as no risk to the human fetus despite possible animal risks, or category C, in which risk cannot be ruled out. Their use during the last 2 weeks before delivery was associated with retrolental fibroplasia in the premature neonate. A neonatal withdrawal syndrome was described in an infant born to a mother receiving 150 mg of hydroxyzine hydrochloride four times a day throughout pregnancy. Teratogenic effects have been observed in experimental animals after the administration of the piperazine group, but fetal abnormalities have not been reported in humans.

Some evidence suggests that the prolonged administration of certain H_1-type antihistamines, for example chlorpheniramine for 3 weeks, may produce subsensitivity, tachyphylaxis, or loss of efficacy; but such observations appear to reflect decreased compliance rather than an increased rate of metabolism.

Low-Sedating or Second-Generation H_1-Type Antihistamines

In recent years low-sedating or second-generation H_1-type antihistamines have been developed (Table 257-2). Low-sedating H_1-type antihistamines have become popular therapeutic agents, owing to their lack of both sedative and anticholinergic side effects. These agents are less lipid-soluble, minimally cross the blood–brain barrier, and preferentially bind to peripheral H_1 receptors. The administration of low-sedating H_1-type antihistamines has not been associated with the development of tachyphylaxis. Some of these agents possess membrane-stabilizing or quinidine-like effects on cardiac muscle and are responsible for a prolongation of the refractory period of the heart and torsade de pointes.[6]

Certain low-sedating H_1-type antihistamines affect the trafficking of cells in the skin and other tissues, the release or generation and release of inflammatory mediators, and the expression of adhesion molecules.[7]

After the administration of cetirizine, the challenge of allergic subjects with grass pollen or 48/80 was associated with a decrease in the influx of eosinophils into the skin, as assessed by a skin-window technique. In a study of pollen-sensitive persons, the oral administration of cetirizine resulted in a decrease in wheal-and-flare reactions, in the immediate release of histamine, in the detection of platelet-activating factor, and in the influx of eosinophils, as assessed by a skin-chamber technique. Moreover, cetirizine was demonstrated to have an inhibitory effect on eosinophil chemotactic responses in vitro to N-formyl-methionyl-leucyl-phenylalanine (FMLP) and platelet-activating factor and in vivo to the influx of eosinophils induced by platelet-activating factor. In skin chambers

TABLE 257-2

Low-Sedating or Second-Generation H$_1$-type Antihistamines

DRUG	CHEMICAL CLASS	ONSET OF ACTION	RESTRICTIONS	SIDE EFFECTS
Terfenadine	Piperidine	Hours	Concomitant use of ketoconazole, itraconazole, erythromycin, clarithromycin, troleandomycin, mibefradil dihydrochloride, indinivir, ritonavir, saquinavir, invirase, nelfinavir, fluvoxamine, nefazodone, sertaline, zileuton, cisapride, sparfloxin, lovastatin	Prolongation of QT interval, torsade de pointes
Astemizole	Piperidine	Days	Empty stomach; concomitant use of ketoconazole, itraconazole, erythromycin, quinine, lovastatin, nefazodone, fluroxamine	Prolongation of QT interval, torsade de pointes, increased appetite
Cetirizine	Piperazine	Hours	None	Sedation
Loratadine	Piperidine	Hours	None	Hepatotoxicity (rare)
Fexofenadine	Piperidine	Hours	None	None
Acrivastine	Alkylamine	Hours	None	Sedation

a decrease in prostaglandin (PG) D$_2$ generation without an effect on histamine release was observed, with an attenuation of the migration of eosinophils, neutrophils, and basophils. Such inhibition of the influx of granulocytes into skin chambers did not occur in experimental studies with terfenadine, promethazine, chlorpheniramine, and diphenhydramine. Cetirizine in vitro inhibited the chemotactic responses of monocytes and T lymphocytes of unspecified types to stimulation with FMLP and leukotriene (LT) B$_4$.[8] After administration of cetirizine to healthy human subjects, peripheral blood monocytes and T lymphocytes showed diminished chemotaxis to the aforementioned stimuli.[8]

High concentrations of certain H$_1$-type antihistamines, including azatadine, oxatomide, and ketotifen, block mediator release from basophils and human mast cells in vitro.[9,10] These antiallergic effects can be seen in vivo in skin, nasal, lung, and ocular challenge studies. In individuals with allergic rhinitis challenged with allergen, azatadine, loratadine, and terfenadine reduced the amounts of histamine and PGD$_2$, and azelastine[11] and cetirizine decreased the amounts of sulfidopeptide leukotrienes. Terfenadine, cetirizine, and loratadine decreased the expression of intercellular adhesion molecule-1 (ICAM-1) on cells obtained from conjunctival or nasal secretions after antigen challenge.[12] In individuals with allergic rhinoconjunctivitis, cetirizine reduced the expression of ICAM-1.[13] In vivo loratadine decreased the expression of ICAM-1 on human keratinocytes,[14] Langerhans cells,[14] and endothelial cells.[13]

Tazifylline, temelastine, noberastine, epinastine,[15,16] mizolastine,[17,18] emedastine, and setastine are investigational agents and will not be discussed further.

TERFENADINE Terfenadine, a piperidine, achieves peak plasma concentrations in 1 h, is metabolized in the liver[19] in the cytochrome P$_{450}$ system CYP3A3/4, and is excreted in the urine and feces. Terfenadine suppresses cutaneous wheal-and-erythema reactions for up to 24 h. Anticholinergic and CNS effects are no greater than those that occur with placebo.

A ventricular tachycardia[20,21] known as torsade de pointes is associated with prolongation of the QT interval. It has been reported to occur after drug overdose and in patients taking concomitant ketoconazole[22] and itraconazole[23,24] but not fluconazole[25]; macrolide antibiotics, such as erythromycin[26] and clarithromycin but not azithromycin[27] or dirithromycin; troleandomycin; lovastatin; pro-

tease inhibitors; and flavonoids, such as naringenin in grapefruit juice.[28] Perhaps individuals with hepatic dysfunction or those susceptible to conditions associated with a prolonged QT interval also may be at risk. There is no interaction between terfenadine and theophylline or between terfenadine and phenytoin. Terfenadine does not enhance the depressant effects of concomitantly administered alcohol or benzodiazepides. There are no restrictions on the ability to take this drug with food except grapefruit juice.[29]

Rare cases of alopecia, urticaria, and morbilliform eruptions have been reported after the administration of terfenadine.

After the recognition of drug interactions and changes in product labeling, a retrospective review of computerized pharmacy claims in New England showed a decline in the concurrent use of terfenadine and contraindicated drugs.[30] The rate of same-day dispensing decreased by 84 percent and of overlapping use declined by 57 percent. Because of its cardiac effects, terfenadine is no longer available in the United States.

ASTEMIZOLE Astemizole, a pipiderine, is a long-acting agent with a slow onset of action and a steady-state concentration reached in 1 week. Its plasma half-life after a single dose is biphasic, with an initial phase of 1.1 days and a second phase of 9.5 days, owing to its metabolite desmethylastemizole. The effects of astemizole are long-lasting, and it suppress the wheal-and-erythema response after its discontinuation. It should be discontinued 4 to 6 weeks before diagnostic prick skin tests are performed.

The sedative effect of astemizole is no greater than that of placebo, but it may stimulate the appetite. The initial suggestion that absorption is decreased with food has not been substantiated. Activated charcoal prevents the absorption of astemizole from the gastrointestinal tract.[31]

Astemizole metabolism studied in human liver microsome preparations in vitro is less sensitive to the effects of ketoconazole than is the metabolism of terfenadine.[32] It is recommended that astemizole not be administered with ketoaconazole, itraconazole, erythromycin, quinine, lovastatin, nefazodone, and fluroxamine. Torsade de pointes has been reported after drug overdosage in both adults[33] and children.

In a prospective trial, astemizole was administered during pregnancy.[34] The use of the drug was not associated with intrauterine growth retardation or perinatal complications. The rate of birth malformations was identical to that of the control group and that of the general population.

CETIRIZINE Cetirizine, a piperizine, is the carboxylic acid metabolite of hydroxyzine and thus is not metabolized in the liver. Peak plasma concentrations are achieved in 1 h and the drug is excreted unchanged in the urine. Cetirizine suppresses cutaneous wheal-and-erythema reactions for as long as 24 h. Cetirizine is less sedating than its parent compound hydroxyzine. When assessed by actual driving, the critical tracking test, and the divided attention test, cetirizine was more sedating than placebo, loratadine, and terfenadine.[35] When assessed by pharmacodymanic comparisons, cetirizine was not more sedating than other second-generation H_1-type antihistamines.[36]

There are no restrictions on the ability to take cetirizine with other medications. Electrocardiographic abnormalities and cardiac side effects have not been reported.[37] Food may decrease the rate of absorption but does not interfere with the extent of absorption.

LORATADINE Loratadine, a piperidine, is related to azatadine. It is metabolized to the metabolite descarboethoxyloratadine.[38] Peak serum concentrations are achieved in 1 to 1.5 h, and it is excreted in the urine and feces. Loratadine causes no greater sedative or anticholinergic side effects than does a placebo. In a study of alertness and performance on a flight simulator, the skills of airline pilots who received 10 mg of loratadine were as unaffected as they were with placebo.[39] A study of the effects of antihistamines on children's learning demonstrated that loratadine caused less learning impairment than did diphenhydramine.[40]

Loratadine is metabolized by cytochrome P_{450} CYP3A4, and it also may be metabolized by cytochrome P_{450} CYP2D6.[41] Although erythromycin and ketoconazole inhibit the metabolism of loratadine,[42,43] electrocardiographic abnormalities and cardiac side effects have not been reported.[37,44] A prolonged QT interval developed in a single patient with coronary artery disease after the administration of loratadine and quinidine. The elimination of loratadine is not decreased in subjects with renal impairment. There are no restrictions on the ability to take this agent with food or other medications. The medication should be discontinued for 1 week before skin tests are performed. Two cases of hepatotoxicity with liver failure have been reported.[45] Small amounts of loratadine are excreted in breast milk.

FEXOFENADINE Fexofenadine, a piperidine, is the carboxylic acid metabolite of terfenadine.[46] It is readily absorbed, and peak plasma concentrations occur at 2.6 h. The plasma half-life is greater in individuals over 65 years of age and in those with renal impairment. The pharmacokinetics in patients with hepatic disease do not differ from those in healthy subjects. Fexofenadine does not have anticholinergic effects. It lacks adverse effects at doses up to 480 mg/day,[47] and the QT interval was not affected when administered with erythromycin or ketoconazole.

ACRIVASTINE Acrivastine, an alkylamine, is a metabolite of triprolidine. It is short-acting, with a rapid onset of action, and peak plasma concentrations are achieved in 1.4 h. Food does not alter its absorption. Sedation is a side effect.[48] Prolongation of the QT interval and other cardiac consequences have not been reported.[49] CNS interactions with alcohol have been observed. In the United States, acrivastine exists in combination with pseudoephedrine hydrochloride for use in allergic rhinitis.

AZELASTINE Azelastine has H_1-type antihistamine activity and inhibits the release of mediators from mast cells and other inflammatory cells. Although available as an oral preparation in other countries, it has been approved in the United States only as a nasal spray for allergic rhinitis.[50,51] Side effects include drowsiness and altered taste perception.

EBASTINE Ebastine, which is a piperidine derivative[52,53] that is detected in plasma as its carboxylic acid metabolite, carebastine, has peak plasma concentrations at 2.6 h. The effects of impaired renal function and hepatic cirrhosis on the pharmacokinetics of carbastine are minimal. It has no sedative[54] or cardiac side effects,[55] nor does it interact with alcohol[56] or diazepam.[57] Ebastine is not available in the United States.

LEVOCABASTINE Levocabastine is a cyclohexylpiperidine derivative[58] that has been developed for nasal and ocular administration.[59] Levocabastine has been detected in the saliva and breast milk of nursing mothers after application to the nasal mucosa or conjunctivae. Levocabastine is not available in the United States.

H_2-Type Antihistamines

H_2-type antihistamines possess an imidazole ring and lack the aryl ring of H_1-type antihistamines. These therapeutic agents are less hydrophilic, which presumably accounts for their lack of CNS effects. H_2-type antihistamines are rapidly absorbed from the gastrointestinal tract and undergo renal clearance with some hepatic metabolism. Although these agents were originally developed to treat peptic ulcer disease, they have been used in the treatment of dermatologic disorders because of the presence of H_2 receptors on the cutaneous microvasculature.

CIMETIDINE Cimetidine was the first widely used H_2-type antihistamine, and the greatest amount of pharmacologic and clinical data has been accumulated with the use of this agent.

Only a small proportion of cimetidine is absorbed from the stomach; most of its absorption occurs in the small intestine. The half-life of cimetidine in plasma is approximately 2 h, with peak levels occurring 80 to 90 min after oral administration; approximately 70 percent is excreted unchanged in the urine. In humans, cimetidine has been recovered from the cerebrospinal fluid of patients with high serum levels, resulting from overdosage or impaired excretion.

A frequently reported side effect of cimetidine is mental confusion, which develops in geriatric patients receiving regular doses and in younger individuals receiving high doses. Hepatic or renal function was impaired in many of the geriatric patients. Other side effects include headache, dizziness, drowsiness, malaise, muscular pain, diarrhea, and constipation. Although cimetidine was initially thought to have no effect on the bone marrow, there are rare reports of granulocytopenia, at times with a fatal outcome.

Uncommon side effects of cimetidine include gynecomastia with or without elevated prolactin levels in men; galactorrhea with elevated prolactin levels in women; and loss of libido, impotence, and reduction of sperm counts in young men. Modest elevations in serum creatinine levels, which may decrease during therapy, are common and are reversible after withdrawal of the drug. Elevated levels of serum transaminases have been reported and are reversible. Interstitial nephritis, fever, and cutaneous eruptions that include urticaria and erythema multiforme syndrome have been observed.

Although a decrease in sebum production in patients with acne who were receiving cimetidine has been described, this observation appears to be of no therapeutic value. The presence of an H$_2$-histamine receptor on CD8+ T lymphocytes may in part explain the augmentation of delayed-type hypersensitivity reactions with increased erythema and induration occurring after the intradermal administration of antigens. In healthy volunteers, the oral administration of cimetidine was associated with an increase in the mitogen-induced proliferation of lymphocytes, a decrease in the number of CD8+ T lymphocytes, and an increase in CD4+ T lymphocytes. Although cimetidine binds to nitrites in the gastrointestinal tract and may yield potential carcinogenic nitroso compounds, the prolonged administration of cimetidine in high doses to rats and dogs failed to result in the development of gastric neoplasms. Cimetidine, however, may mask symptoms associated with gastric carcinoma in humans.

Many drug interactions have been reported with cimetidine therapy and most importantly include prolonged bleeding times and prothrombin times in patients receiving concomitant oral anticoagulants and cimetidine. Cimetidine should be used with caution in patients receiving phenytoin, propranolol, nifedipine, diazepam, and theophylline, since blood levels of these drugs are elevated and their excretion is delayed. Cimetidine increases the concentration of blood alcohol levels due to an inhibitory effect on gastric alcohol dehydrogenase activity.[60]

RANITIDINE Ranitidine achieves peak plasma concentrations in 1 to 2 h. The plasma half-life is 2 to 3 h in adults and is prolonged in older patients and in individuals with liver or kidney diseases. Although ranitidine is metabolized in the liver, the drug and its metabolites are excreted principally in the urine. Ranitidine does not bind to androgen receptors, does not interfere with the hepatic metabolism of other therapeutic agents, and does not enhance cell-mediated immune responses. Ranitidine inhibits gastric alcohol dehydrogenase activity and leads to increased blood alcohol levels.[60] Ranitidine may be preferred to cimetidine for patients taking multiple drugs and for geriatric patients.

Minor adverse effects include headache, dizziness, malaise, nausea, constipation, and abdominal pain. Serum transaminase and creatinine levels temporarily increase but return to base-line levels with continued treatment. Ranitidine appears in breast milk.

Although ranitidine interacts with other medications less frequently than does cimetidine, interactions with fentanyl, metoprolol, midazolam, nifedipine, theophylline, and warfarin have been observed. Ranitidine may decrease the absorption of diazepam and reduce its plasma concentration by 25 percent.

FAMOTIDINE Famotidine differs chemically from cimetidine and ranitidine in that it contains a thiazole ring. Peak plasma concentrations occur 2 h after oral administration, and the plasma half-life is 3 to 8 h. Approximately 25 percent of the drug is excreted in the urine after a single oral dose. In patients with renal failure, the half-life of famotidine may exceed 20 h.

Adverse reactions are infrequent and include headache, dizziness, constipation, and diarrhea. No interference with the hepatic oxidative metabolism of diazepam, phenytoin, theophylline, or warfarin has been observed. Famotidine does not inhibit gastric alcohol dehydrogenase activity[60]; it lacks antiandrogenic side effects.

NIZATIDINE Like famotidine, nizatidine contains a thiazole ring. Its peak serum concentration after oral administration occurs in about 1 h, the plasma half-life is 1 to 2 h, and its duration of action is up to 10 h. Nizatidine is primarily eliminated by the kidneys

within 16 h. The oral bioavailability of nizatidine is not affected by food.

Minor gastrointestinal side effects occur; elevations of serum transaminases and uric acid levels, without adverse clinical consequences, develop; and antiandrogenic effects are absent.

In healthy volunteers, drug interactions were not reported with the concomitant administration of chlordiazepoxide, diazepam, lidocaine, lorazepam, theophylline, or warfarin.

Other Therapeutic Agents with Antihistaminic Activity

TRICYCLIC ANTIDEPRESSANTS Tricyclic antidepressants act on both H$_1$ and H$_2$ receptors. Doxepin, a compound related to amitriptyline, was more potent than chlorpheniramine in inhibiting experimental wheals induced by histamine. Topical doxepin hydrochloride cream can cause allergic contact dermatitis.[61]

KETOTIFEN Ketotifen, a benzocycloheptathiophene derivative, prevents histamine release from mast cells induced by IgE and compound 48/80 in vitro and inhibits passive cutaneous anaphylaxis in experimental animals in vivo. Ketotifen also is an H$_1$-type antihistamine and a calcium-channel blocker. Sedation and weight gain are side effects. Ketotifen is not available in the United States.

OXATOMIDE Oxatomide, a piperidine, is an H$_1$-type antihistamine that also inhibits mediator release. Sedation and weight gain are side effects. Oxatomide is not available in the United States.

ANTIHISTAMINES IN DERMATOLOGY

General Considerations

Antihistamines have been used in dermatology primarily for the relief of pruritus and the treatment of urticaria and angioedema. Not all H$_1$-type antihistamines have similar beneficial therapeutic effects, and nonresponders to one drug may respond favorably to another.[62] Antihistamines are effective in blocking experimental pruritus induced by histamine; however, they are of limited use in many pruritic cutaneous diseases. It has been suggested that the soporific side effect of the traditional H$_1$-type antihistamines plays a role in the treatment of pruritus.

Use in Urticaria/Angioedema

Empiric trials of traditional H$_1$-type antihistamines are used in the treatment of both acute and recurrent episodes of urticaria and angioedema. In double-blind, placebo-controlled studies, traditional H$_1$-type antihistamines were shown to be statistically superior to placebos in the treatment of urticaria and angioedema. However, comparative studies of the groups of traditional H$_1$-type antihistamines have shown them to be of equal efficacy. If an agent from one therapeutic group of H$_1$-type antihistamine proves ineffective, then an agent from another group should be administered. At times, H$_1$-type antihistamines from different groups may be combined. H$_1$-type antihistamines are of benefit to patients with a history of reactions to radiocontrast media to prevent transfusion reactions.

The low-sedating H$_1$-type antihistamines, terfenadine,[63] astemizole,[64] cetirizine,[63–66] loratadine,[65,67] acrivastine, and ebastine,[53] were found in double-blind, placebo-controlled, or parallel studies to be statistically superior to placebo in the treatment of chronic idiopathic urticaria and angioedema. In comparative studies, in which low-sedating H_1-type antihistamines are compared with each other and with traditional H_1-type antihistamines, no single therapeutic agent commands preeminence. Ketotifen[68] and doxepin have been used with therapeutic benefit in chronic idiopathic urticaria.

Traditional and low-sedating H_1 antihistamines also may be used in the treatment of physical urticaria. Doxepin and ketotifen also were used successfully in patients with various types of physical urticaria.

The combination of H_1- and H_2-type antihistamines is of benefit in a few patients with acute and chronic idiopathic urticaria and angioedema as well as certain forms of physical urticaria. Although one double-blind study failed to show a statistically significant advantage when chlorpheniramine and cimetidine were used in combination in the treatment of chronic idiopathic urticaria, the combination of H_1- and H_2-type antihistamines should be considered in patients with refractory chronic idiopathic urticaria, for whom H_1-type antihistamines alone or in combination are ineffective. Although an H_2-type antihistamine alone was claimed to control urticaria in one report, the therapeutic benefit of H_2-type antihistamines when administered as monotherapy has not been demonstrated in controlled trials.

Use in Other Dermatologic Disorders

H_1-type antihistamines have been used in the treatment of pruritus of various causes and especially in patients with atopic dermatitis. The fact that their effectiveness in the control of pruritus is variable suggests that their efficacy may in part be related to the suppression of anxiety and to their sedative effect. Yet, low-sedative H_1-type antihistamines have modified the pruritus in patients with atopic dermatitis. Topical doxepin hydrochloride cream in a double-blind, vehicle-controlled trial reduced the pruritus in patients with atopic dermatitis.[69]

The pruritus and whealing in systemic mastocytosis and urticaria pigmentosa were modified in a double-blind trial of the administration of chlorpheniramine and cimetidine. Ketotifen also has been of benefit in urticaria pigmentosa in a controlled trial. Azelastine suppressed the pruritus in patients with mastocytosis.[70]

Pruritus associated with other conditions, such as allergic contact dermatitis and other forms of eczematous dermatitis, lichen planus, mosquito bites,[71] and infestations, and pruritus secondary to underlying medical disorders or of an idiopathic nature may be controlled by the administration of H_1-type antihistamines.

In anecdotal reports, cimetidine was reported to be of value in the treatment of the pruritus resulting from myelofibrosis, polycythemia vera, and carcinoid flush. Anecdotal reports have also suggested that the combination of H_1- and H_2-type antihistamines was of value in the treatment of carcinoid flush and alcohol-induced flushing.

Cimetidine reversed cutaneous anergy to candida in a group of patients with chronic mucocutaneous candidiasis and was successful in the treatment of verruca vulgaris in some individuals.[72] The immunomodulatory effect of H_2-type antihistamines offers great promise and potential for therapeutic exploration.

In a double-blind, placebo-controlled trial, ranitidine was of value as adjunctive therapy to the use of a topical glucocorticoid cream in the treatment of atopic dermatitis of the hands.[73]

REFERENCES

1. Qui R et al: A histamine derivative increases intracellular calcium mobilization in HL-60 cells. *Immunopharmacology* **26**:213, 1993

2. Arrang JM: Pharmacologic properties of histamine receptor subtypes. *Cell Mol Biol* **40**:273, 1994
3. Simons FER et al: Quantitation of H_1-receptor antagonists in skin and serum. *J Allergy Clin Immunol* **95**:759, 1995
4. Simons FER et al: Effect of the H_2-antagonist cimetidine on the pharmacokinetics and pharmacodynamics of the H_1-antagonists hydroxyzine and cetirizine in patients with chronic urticaria. *J Allergy Clin Immunol* **95**:685, 1995
5. Gilmore TM et al: Occupational injuries and medication use. *Am J Ind Med* **30**:234, 1996
6. Roden DM: Torsade de pointes. *Clin Cardiol* **16**:683, 1993
7. Rihoux JP, Mariz S: Cetirizine: An updated review of its pharmacological properties and therapeutic efficacy. *Clin Rev Allergy Immunol* **11**:65, 1993
8. Jinquan T et al: Cetirizine inhibits the in vitro and ex vivo chemotactic response of T lymphocytes and monocytes. *J Allergy Clin Immunol* **95**:979, 1995
9. Campbell AM et al: Modulation of eicosanoid and histamine release from human dispersed lung cells by terfenadine. *Allergy* **48**:125, 1993
10. Faraj BA, Jackson FT: Effects of astemizole on antigen-mediated histamine release from the blood of patients with allergic rhinitis. *Allergy* **47**:630, 1992
11. Shin M-H et al: The effect of azelastine on the early allergic response. *Clin Exp Allergy* **22**:289, 1992
12. Canonica GW et al: Adhesion molecules of allergic inflammation: Recent insights into their functional roles. *Allergy* **49**:135, 1994
13. Ciprandi G et al: Cetirizine reduces inflammatory cell recruitment and ICAM-1 (or CD54) expression on conjunctival epithelium in both early-and-late phase reactions after allergen-specific challenge. *J Allergy Clin Immunol* **95**:612, 1995
14. Staquet MJ et al: Loratadine downregulates ICAM-1 expression on human keratinocytes and Langerhans cells. *Eur J Dermatol* **6**:369, 1996
15. Kamei C et al: Antiallergic effect of epinastine (WAL 801 CL) on immediate hypersensitivity reactions. I. Elucidation of the mechanism for histamine inhibition. *Immunopharmacol Immunotoxicol* **14**:191, 1992
16. Kamei C et al: Antiallergic effect of epinastine (WAL 801 CL) on immediate hypersensitivity reactions. II. Antagonistic effect of epinastine on chemical mediators, mainly antihistaminic and anti-PAF effects. *Immunopharmacol Immunotoxicol* **14**:207, 1992
17. Rosenzweig P et al: Pharmacodynamics and pharmacokinetics of mizolastine (SL 85.0324), a new nonsedative H_1 antihistamine. *Ann Allergy* **69**:135, 1992
18. Danjou P et al: Assessment of the anticholinergic effect of the new antihistamine mizolastine in healthy subjects. *Br J Clin Pharmacol* **34**:328, 1992
19. Yun C-H et al: Oxidation of the antihistaminic drug terfenadine in human liver microsomes: Role of cytochrome P-450 3A(4): N-dealkylation and C-hydroxylation. *Drug Metab Dispos* **21**:403, 1993
20. Salata JJ et al: Cardiac electrophysiological actions of histamine H_1-receptor antagonists astemizole and terfenadine compared with chlorpheniramine and pyrilamine. *Circ Res* **76**:110, 1995
21. Pratt CM et al: Risk of developing life-threatening ventricular arrhythmia associated with terfenadine in comparison with over-the-counter antihistamines, ibuprofen and clemastine. *Am J Cardiol* **73**:346, 1994
22. Honig PK et al: Terfenadine-ketoconazole interaction: Pharmacokinetic and electrocardiographic consequences. *JAMA* **269**:1513, 1993
23. Pohjola-Sintonen S et al: Itraconazole prevents terfenadine metabolism and increases risk of torsades de pointes ventricular tachycardia. *Eur J Clin Pharmacol* **45**:191, 1993
24. Honig PK et al: Itraconazole affects single-dose terfenadine pharmacokinetics and cardiac repolarization pharmacodynamics. *J Clin Pharmacol* **33**:1201, 1993
25. Honig PK et al: The effect of fluconazole on the steady-state pharmacokinetics and electrocardiographic pharmacokinetics of terfenadine in humans. *Clin Pharmacol Ther* **53**:630, 1993
26. Honig PK et al: Changes in the pharmacokinetics and electrocardiographic pharmacodynamics of terfenadine with concomitant administration of erythromycin. *Clin Pharm Ther* **52**:231, 1992
27. Honig PK et al: Comparison of the effect of the macrolide antibiotics erythromycin, clarithromycin and azithromycin on terfenadine steady-state pharmacokinetics and electrocardiographic parameters. *Drug Invest* **7**:148, 1994

28. Guengerich FP, Kim D-H: *In vitro* inhibition of dihydropyridine oxidation and aflatoxin B_1 activation in human liver microsomes by naringenin and other flavonoids. *Carcinogenesis* **11**:2275, 1990

29. Eller MG et al: Absence of food effects on the pharmacokinetics of terfenadine. *Biopharm Drug Dispos* **13**:171, 1992

30. Thompson D, Oster G: Use of terfenadine and contraindicated drugs. *JAMA* **275**:1339, 1996

31. Laine K et al: The effect of activated charcoal on the absorption and elimination of astemizole. *Hum Exp Toxicol* **13**:502, 1994

32. Lavrijsen K et al: The interaction of ketoconazole, itraconazole and erythromycin with the in vitro metabolism of antihistamines in human liver microsomes. *Allergy* **48**(suppl 16):34,1993

33. Rao KA et al: Torsades de pointes ventricular tachycardia associated with overdose of astemizole. *Mayo Clin Proc* **69**:589, 1994

34. Pastuszak A et al: The safety of astemizole in pregnancy. *J Allergy Clin Immunol* **98**:748, 1996

35. Ramaekers JG et al: Effects of loratadine and cetirizine on actual driving and psychometric test performance, and EEG during driving. *Eur J Clin Pharmacol* **42**:363, 1992

36. Spencer CM et al: Cetirizine: A reappraisal of its pharmacological properties and therapeutic use in selected allergic disorders. *Drugs* **46**:1055, 1993

37. Sale ME et al: Lack of electrocardiographic effects of cetirizine in healthy humans. *J Allergy Clin Immunol* **91**:258, 1993

38. Roman JJ, Danzig MR: Loratadine: A review of recent findings in pharmacology, pharmacokinetics, efficacy, and safety, with a look at its use in combination with pseudoephedrine. *Clin Rev Allergy* **11**:89, 1993

39. Neves-Pinto RM et al: A double-blind study of the effects of loratadine versus placebo on the performance of pilots. *Am J Rhinol* **6**:23, 1992

40. Vuurman EFPM et al: Seasonal allergic rhinitis and antihistamine effects on children's learning. *Ann Allergy* **71**:121, 1993

41. Yumibe N et al: Identification of human liver cytochrome P450s involved in the microsomal metabolism of the antihistaminic drug loratadine. *J Allergy Clin Immunol* **93**:234, 1994

42. Van Peer A et al: Ketoconazole inhibits loratadine metabolism in man. *Allergy* **48**(suppl 16):34, 1993

43. Brannan MD et al: Loratadine administered concomitantly with erythromycin: Pharmacokinetic and electrocardiographic evaluations. *Clin Pharmacol Ther* **58**:269, 1995

44. Van Cauwenberge P: New data on the safety of loratadine. *Drug Invest* **4**:283, 1992

45. Schiano TD et al: Subfulminant liver failure and severe hepatotoxicity caused by loratadine use. *Ann Intern Med* **125**:738, 1996

46. Bernstein DI et al: Fexofenadine: A new nonsedating antihistamine is effective in the treatment of seasonal allergic rhinitis. *J Allergy Clin Immunol* **97**:435, 1996

47. Woosley RL et al: Mechanism of the cardiotoxic actions of terfenadine. *JAMA* **269**:1532, 1993

48. Simons FER: The therapeutic index of newer H_1-receptor antagonists. *Clin Exp Allergy* **24**:707, 1994

49. Sanders RL et al: Cardiac effects of acrivastine compared to terfenadine. *J Allergy Clin Immunol* **89**:183, 1992

50. Davies RJ et al: The effect of intranasal azelastine and beclomethasone on the symptoms and signs of nasal allergy in patients with perennial allergic rhinitis. *Rhinology* **31**:159, 1993

51. Gambardella R: A comparison of the efficacy of azelastine nasal spray and loratidine tablets in the treatment of seasonal allergic rhinitis. *J Int Med Res* **21**:268, 1993

52. Luria X, Bakke O: Ebastine (LAS W-090): Overview of clinical trials. *Drugs Today* **28**(suppl B):69, 1992

53. Simons FER et al: Pharmacokinetics and pharmacodynamics of ebastine in children. *J Pediatr* **122**:641, 1993

54. Hopes H et al: Placebo controlled comparison of acute effects of ebastine and clemastine on performance and EEG. *Eur J Clin Pharmacol* **42**:55, 1992

55. Llenas J et al: Preclinical safety studies with ebastine. II. Pharmacologic effects on the cardiovascular system. *Drugs Today* **28**(suppl B):29, 1992

56. Mattila MJ et al: Lack of pharmacodynamic and pharmacokinetic interactions of the antihistamine ebastine with ethanol in healthy subjects. *Eur J Clin Pharmacol* **43**:179, 1992

57. Mattila MJ et al: Diazepam effects on the performance of healthy subjects are not enhanced by treatment with the antihistamine ebastine. *Br J Clin Pharmacol* **35**:272, 1993

58. Awouters F et al: Levocabastine: Pharmacological profile of a highly effective inhibitor of allergic reactions. *Agents Actions* **35**:12, 1992

59. Heykants J et al: The pharmacokinetic properties of topical levocabastine: A review. *Clin Pharmacokinet* **29**:221, 1995

60. DiPadova C et al: Effects of ranitidine on blood alcohol levels after ethanol ingestion: Comparison with other H_2-receptor antagonists. *JAMA* **267**:83, 1992

61. Shelley WB et al: Self-potentiating allergic contact dermatitis caused by doxepin hydrochloride cream. *J Am Acad Dermatol* **34**:143, 1996

62. Carlsen KH et al: Loratadine and terfenadine in perennial allergic rhinitis: Treatment of nonresponders to the one drug with the other drug. *Allergy* **48**:431, 1993

63. Andri L et al: A comparison of the efficacy of cetirizine and terfenadine: A double-blind, controlled study of chronic idiopathic urticaria. *Allergy* **48**:358, 1993

64. Breneman D et al: Cetirizine and astemizole therapy for chronic idiopathic urticaria: A double-blind, placebo-controlled comparative trial. *J Am Acad Dermatol* **33**:192, 1995

65. Guerra L et al: Loratadine and cetirizine in the treatment of chronic urticaria. *J Eur Acad Dermatol Venereol* **3**:148, 1994

66. Paul E, Paul C: Longterm therapy with cetirizine in chronic urticaria: Results of a multicenter study. *Allergologie* **16**:56, 1993

67. Monroe EW: Loratadine in the treatment of urticaria. *Clin Ther* **19**:232, 1997

68. Egan CA, Rallis TM: Treatment of chronic urticaria with ketotifen. *Arch Dermatol* **133**:147, 1997

69. Drake LA et al: Relief of pruritus in patients with atopic dermatitis after treatment with topical doxepin cream. *J Am Acad Dermatol* **31**:613, 1994

70. Friedman BS et al: Comparison of azelastine and chlorpheniramine in the treatment of mastocytosis. *J Allergy Clin Immunol* **95**:520, 1993

71. Reunala T et al: Treatment of mosquito bites with cetirizine. *Clin Exp Allergy* **23**:72, 1993

72. Orlow SJ, Paller A: Cimetidine therapy for multiple warts in children. *J Am Acad Dermatol* **28**:794, 1993

73. Veien NK et al: Ranitidine treatment of hand eczema in patients with atopic dermatitis: A double-blind, placebo-controlled trial. *J Am Acad Dermatol* **32**:1056, 1995

CHAPTER 258

Jan V. Hirschmann

Overview of Antibiotics

Strictly speaking, antibiotics are chemicals produced by various microbes, such as bacteria, actinomycetes, and fungi, that inhibit the growth of other organisms. In common usage, however, the term *antibiotic* generally refers to a medication that has antibacterial action, whether it is a natural or a synthetic substance. Since the late 1930s, when the sulfonamides emerged as therapeutic agents, and the 1940s, when penicillin came into clinical use, the number and variety of these antibacterial agents have multiplied to the point where the amount of information required to prescribe them intelligently is daunting. Unfortunately, because many of these antibiotics are very expensive and have a wide spectrum of antimicrobial activity, their improper use not only increases the cost of medical care but also encourages the emergence of resistant organisms, which has become a widespread and frightening problem throughout the world. Regrettably, office-based clinicians in the United States (and elsewhere) are prescribing more broad-spectrum, expensive antibiotics than ever before, often from the erroneous belief that the newer agents are necessarily better than the older, cheaper ones.[1] For nearly all skin conditions requiring antibiotic therapy that a dermatologist is likely to encounter, however, inexpensive, generic preparations from one of four categories will suffice: (1) penicillins—penicillin and dicloxacillin; (2) first-generation cephalosporins; (3) tetracyclines, usually doxycycline; and (4) erythromycin. Penicillins, cephalosporins, and erythromycin are alternative options for treating streptococcal and staphylococcal infections. Doxycycline or erythromycin is appropriate for acne or rosacea; penicillin or doxycycline for the cutaneous manifestations of Lyme disease; and erythromycin for bacillary angiomatosis. Other primary infections of the skin are rare. This chapter focuses on these agents, which dermatologists should know thoroughly. Table 258-1 delineates the astonishing differences in price between these medications and some of the newer, more expensive antibiotics for which there are very few dermatologic uses. Table 258-2 lists the antibiotic choices for dermatologic infections.

An understanding of how to prescribe these systemic antimicrobial agents properly, however, first requires an acquaintance with some fundamental concepts, such as mechanisms of action, antibiotic susceptibility testing, drug resistance, and use in special circumstances, such as renal failure and pregnancy.

Mechanisms of Action and Antimicrobial Resistance

Antibacterial agents exert their effects in one of four ways:

1. Some, such as the penicillins and cephalosporins, inhibit cell-wall synthesis, usually leading to the organism's death.
2. By interfering with the 30S or 50S subunit of ribosomes, certain antibiotics impair protein synthesis. The result may be a re-

TABLE 258-1

Costs of Oral Antibiotics for Dermatologic Use

MEDICATION	DOSE	COST (7 DAYS)*
Penicillins		
Penicillin V	250 mg qid	$2.15
Dicloxacillin	250 mg qid	$11.59
Amoxicillin-clavulanate	250 mg qid	$41.38
Cephalosporins		
Cephalexin	250 mg qid	$8.94
Cephradine	250 mg qid	$25.28
Tetracyclines		
Doxycycline	100 mg bid	$3.93
Minocycline	100 mg bid	$27.16
Tetracycline	250 mg qid	$1.12
Macrolides		
Azithromycin	250 mg qd	$42.27
Clarithromycin	250 mg bid	$48.31
Erythromycin	250 mg qid	$7.16
Fluoroquinolones		
Ciprofloxacin	500 mg bid	$47.86
Ofloxacin	200 mg bid	$44.77
Other		
Clindamycin	150 mg qid	$27.21
Trimethoprim-sulfamethoxazole	1 DS tablet bid	$2.30

*Price to the pharmacist based on average wholesale cost in *Red Book 1997*. The cost to the patient is considerably more.

versible inhibition, which temporarily halts growth of the microbe but does not kill it—the mechanism for the tetracyclines and erythromycin—or the effect may be lethal, as with the aminoglycosides, such as gentamicin or amikacin.
3. The agent, such as one of the quinolones (e.g., ciprofloxacin), affects nucleic acid metabolism, typically killing the bacteria.
4. The medication blocks an essential step in the organism's metabolism. This action occurs with sulfonamides and trimethoprim, which interfere with the folic acid metabolic pathway. The process only inhibits some microbes but kills others.

Microorganisms develop resistance against these antimicrobial effects by three general mechanisms:

1. The organism may elaborate substances that inactivate the antibiotic. For example, many bacteria, such as penicillin-resistant *Staphylococcus aureus*, produce beta-lactamases that attack an important ring structure of penicillins and cephalosporins.
2. Changes in the microbe prevent the drug from reaching its target. For instance, an alteration in the organism's outer membrane may make it impermeable to the drug or the microbe

TABLE 258-2

Antibiotic Choices for Dermatologic Infections

ORGANISM	DISEASES	PREFERRED ANTIBIOTIC	ALTERNATIVES
Actinomyces israelii	Actinomycosis	Penicillin V	Clindamycin
Bacillus anthracis	Anthrax	Penicillin G	Erythromycin, doxycycline
Bartonella henselae	Cat-scratch disease	Ciprofloxacin	Trimethoprim-sulfamethoxazole
Bartonella henselae or quintana	Bacillary angiomatosis	Erythromycin	Doxycycline
Borrelia burgdorferi	Erythema migrans (Lyme disease)	Doxycycline or amoxicillin	Penicillin V
Calymmatobacterium granulomatis	Granuloma inguinale	Doxycycline	Trimethoprim-sulfamethoxazole
Chlamydia trachomatis	Nongonococcal urethritis, cervicitis	Doxycycline or azithromycin	Erythromycin
Clostridium perfringens	Gas gangrene	Penicillin G	Clindamycin
Corynebacterium diphtheriae	Diphtheria	Erythromycin	Penicillin V
Erlichia	Erlichiosis	Doxycycline	Chloramphenicol
Erysipelothrix rhusiopathiae	Erysipeloid	Penicillin	Erythromycin, clindamycin
Francisella tularensis	Tularemia	Streptomycin	Gentamicin, doxycycline
Haemophilus ducreyi	Chancroid	Erythromycin or ceftriaxone	Azithromycin, ciprofloxacin
Neisseria gonorrhoeae	Gonorrhea	Ceftriaxone or cefixime	Ciprofloxacin, ofloxacin
Neisseria meningitidis	Meningococcemia	Penicillin G	Ceftriaxone, chloramphenicol
Nocardia asteroides	Nocardiosis	Trimethoprim-sulfamethoxazole	Minocycline
Pasteurella multocida	Dog or cat bites	Penicillin	Doxycycline, amoxicillin-clavulanate
Proprionibacterium acnes	Acne	Doxycycline	Erythromycin, clindamycin
Rickettsia	Rocky Mountain spotted fever, typhus, rickettsialpox	Doxycycline	Chloramphenicol
Staphylococcus aureus	Impetigo, ecthyma, blistering distal dactylitis, carbuncle	Dicloxacillin	First-generation cephalosporin, erythromycin, clindamycin
Streptococcus pyogenes	Cellulitis, impetigo, blistering distal dactylitis	Penicillin V	First-generation cephalosporin, erythromycin, clindamycin
Treponema pallidum	Syphilis	Penicillin G	Doxycycline, ceftriaxone, erythromycin
Vibrio vulnificus	Wound or bacteremia with skin lesions	Doxycycline	Chloramphenicol

may develop a new membrane transport system that actively extrudes the antibiotic from the cell.

3. The site of the drug's action may alter. For example, changes in the organism's ribosomes, to which the antibiotic ordinarily adheres, may prevent the drug from binding to its target and exerting its effect on protein synthesis. Alternatively, by changing its metabolic pathway, the microbe may make the previously effective antimetabolite, such as a sulfonamide, impotent.

These mechanisms of bacterial resistance to antimicrobial agents may arise from random mutations in the organism's chromosomes that are unrelated to drug exposure, with the modified genetic material then passed to its progeny. More commonly, however, the resistance comes from *extrachromosomal* DNA, which other, often unrelated, bacteria transfer to the microbe.[2,3] This genetic material may be in plasmids, autonomously replicating pieces of DNA, or transposons, mobile pieces of DNA that can insert themselves into various locations in the bacterial chromosome or plasmids. Some bacteria have numerous plasmids and transposons that can confer resistance to several different antibiotics, making treatment of infections caused by these organisms difficult or impossible. This multiresistance typically develops in settings of intensive antibiotic use, such as hospital critical care units. Any indiscriminate prescrib-

ing of antimicrobial agents, however, whether in a nosocomial or an outpatient setting, contributes to the emergence and dissemination of these organisms, because the presence of an antibiotic in a patient allows resistant microbes to flourish while it inhibits the competing susceptible ones. Accordingly, all clinicians must use antibiotics wisely, employing them only when necessary and preferentially prescribing an agent with a narrow spectrum of activity—one that inhibits the pathogen without significantly affecting the rest of the patient's flora.

Antimicrobial Susceptibility Testing

After the clinician has submitted an appropriate sample for culture, the laboratory can isolate the infecting organism and determine its susceptibility to a panel of agents likely to have activity against the category of bacteria to which the pathogen belongs.[4] The test employs a concentration of 10^5 to 10^6 organisms per milliliter and assesses the effect of various concentrations of the antibiotics on the bacterium's growth after overnight incubation. The minimum inhibitory concentration (MIC) is the lowest amount of the drug that inhibits growth of the organism. The microbe is "sensitive" or "susceptible" when the MIC is less than a concentration ("breakpoint") of antibiotic ordinarily achievable in the *serum* of patients given conventional doses of the drug. Because the serum level of antibiotic may differ from its concentration at the site of infection and because the susceptibility test may not reflect local factors that affect drug activity there, such as pH, the results of the test are potentially misleading, especially in areas such as the cerebrospinal fluid where some antibiotics penetrate poorly. With dermatologic infections, however, the susceptibility results are very reliable.

Bactericidal versus Bacteriostatic Action

Laboratory tests can also distinguish between antibiotics that temporarily inhibit the growth of organisms (bacteriostatic) and those that kill (bactericidal).[5] After overnight incubation with the drug, an inoculum of organisms is subcultured onto an antibiotic-free medium for 18 to 24 h. By arbitrary definition, a *bactericidal* antibiotic has killed 99.9 percent or more of the original bacteria at that time. In general, antibiotics that interfere with cell-wall synthesis, such as penicillins or cephalosporins, are bactericidal. Those that impair protein synthesis or block steps in metabolic pathways may be either bacteriostatic or bactericidal. Furthermore, some agents may kill certain organisms, but only inhibit others. Usually, bactericidal agents have no clinical superiority over bacteriostatic ones, and for almost all infections that a dermatologist is likely to confront the distinction is unimportant. The special circumstances where killing rather than inhibiting growth is significant are infective endocarditis, bacterial meningitis, infections in neutropenic hosts, and, possibly, osteomyelitis.

Use of Antibiotics during Renal Failure, Pregnancy, and Lactation

For antibiotics eliminated by renal excretion, dose adjustments may be necessary in patients with impaired kidney function to avoid toxic serum levels. Recommended alterations in dose usually depend on an assessment of creatinine clearance. In the absence of a direct measurement, the following formula provides a reasonable estimate for men:

$$\text{Creatinine clearance} = \frac{\text{weight, kg } (140 - \text{patient's age})}{72 \text{ (serum creatinine, mg/dL)}}$$

The value for women is 0.85 of the calculated value for men. These calculations should use the ideal body weight, which for men is 50.0 kg + 2.3 kg/in. over 5 ft and for women is 45.5 kg + 2.3 kg/in. over 5 ft. Patients with creatinine clearances above 50 mL/min require no dose adjustments for any antibiotic, but for lower levels of renal function some medications require either a reduction in the individual amount given or a greater interval between doses. Since hemodialysis removes a substantial portion of some antibiotics from patients, those undergoing this procedure may require an additional dose afterward. Specific recommendations for these adjustments appear in the discussions of the individual antibiotics.

Because of the risk of affecting the fetus or the newborn (for women near term), clinicians should avoid prescribing antibiotics during pregnancy if possible. Those considered safe include the penicillins, the cephalosporins, and erythromycin (except the estolate form). Clindamycin should be used with caution, and contraindicated drugs include the tetracyclines, the fluoroquinolones, and trimethoprim-sulfamethoxazole. Nursing mothers should avoid taking antibiotics, if possible, but especially the tetracyclines, which stain teeth, and the fluoroquinolones, which may damage joint cartilage in newborns.

INDIVIDUAL ANTIBIOTICS

Penicillins

MECHANISM AND SPECTRUM OF ACTIVITY Penicillins,[6] which exert their antimicrobial action by interfering with bacterial cell-wall synthesis, are active primarily against gram-positive organisms. Those most useful to dermatologists include two oral agents, penicillin V and dicloxacillin, and two parenteral preparations, penicillin G and an intravenous penicillinase-resistant drug, such as oxacillin or nafcillin. Penicillin V and penicillin G are effective for skin infections such as cellulitis, blistering distal dactylitis, and impetigo when caused by streptococci and penicillin-sensitive *S. aureus*. As indicated below, however, most strains of *S. aureus* in both the hospital and community settings are penicillin-resistant, and either a penicillinase-resistant penicillin or a cephalosporin is a better choice for infections when *S. aureus* is suspected and its susceptibility to penicillin unknown.

Penicillin G and V are appropriate agents to treat *Pasteurella multocida*, often a cause of infected cat and dog bites; *Streptobacillus moniliformis* and *Spirillum minus*, the two bacteria responsible for rat-bite fever; *Erysipelothrix rhusiopathiae*, the cause of erysipeloid; *Bacillus anthracis*, which causes anthrax; and *Borrelia burgdorferi*, the pathogen in Lyme disease. Penicillin G but not V is the drug of choice for all forms of infection with *Treponema pallidum*, the spirochete responsible for syphilis.

Most strains of *S. aureus* produce penicillinase, a beta-lactamase enzyme that splits the beta-lactam ring of some penicillins, including V and G, producing substances with no antibacterial activity. Certain semisynthetic penicillins, however, are penicillinase-resistant, including dicloxacillin, an oral agent, and both nafcillin and oxacillin, which are primarily used as intravenous medications. These penicillins are also effective against *Streptococcus pyogenes* (group A streptococci) and streptococci of other groups, such as F or G, that are responsible for skin infections like cellulitis. Accordingly, the penicillinase-resistant penicillins are good choices to treat disorders such as impetigo and ecthyma that can be caused by either *S. aureus* alone or a mixture of staphylococci and streptococci. Unfortunately, some isolates of *S. aureus* (methicillin-resistant strains) are impervious to all penicillins.

Alterations of the penicillin molecule have created agents with considerable activity against gram-negative organisms. Such preparations include the aminopenicillins, ampicillin and amoxicillin, which are effective against many isolates of *Escherichia coli* and *Haemophilus influenzae*. These antibiotics have little use in dermatologic practice but are common causes of drug-induced eruptions. Organisms that produce beta-lactamases inactivate amoxicillin and ampicillin. To prevent this effect and thereby increase the spectrum of activity of these agents, drug manufacturers have combined them with beta-lactamase inhibitors (which preferentially and irreversibly bind the enzyme) to produce a parenteral preparation, ampicillin-sulbactam (Unasyn) and an oral formulation, amoxicillin-clavulanic acid (Augmentin).[7] These drugs are active against beta-lactamase–producing stains of *S. aureus, H. influenzae, Neisseria gonorrhoeae, E. coli, Klebsiella* species, and some other gram-negative bacilli. They are also effective against anaerobes that produce beta-lactamase, such as *Bacteroides fragilis*. Despite this increased spectrum of activity, these agents have little application in dermatologic infections. One exception is in the treatment of bite wounds, for these drugs are active against the likely pathogens—oral anaerobes, *Eikenella corrodens*, *H. influenzae,* and *S. aureus* in human bites and *P. multocida,* streptococci, anaerobes, and staphylococci in dog and cat bites.[8] Another use is for serious skin and soft-tissue infections with a complex flora of both aerobic and anaerobic organisms, such as severe diabetic foot infections.

Modifications of the ampicillin molecule have created the carboxypenicillins (carbenicillin and ticarcillin) and the ureidopenicillins (mezlocillin, piperacillin, and azlocillin). These "extended-spectrum" parenteral penicillins have much greater activity against many gram-negative bacilli, including *Pseudomonas aeruginosa*, than other penicillins. Two preparations include beta-lactamase inhibitors: ticarcillin–clavulanic acid and piperacillin-tazobactam. Rarely is any of these agents appropriate for treating dermatologic infections, but they commonly cause drug-induced rashes in hospitalized patients.

DOSAGE AND DRUG INTERACTIONS   The adult dose of penicillin V is 250 to 500 mg by mouth four times a day. No adjustment is necessary in renal failure, but patients undergoing dialysis should receive an extra dose following the procedure. The doses of penicillin G vary according to the infection treated; the reader should refer to the appropriate chapter for details. Patients should receive 75 percent of the recommended dose for glomerular filtration rates between 10 and 50 mL/min and 50 percent of the dose for rates of less than 10 mL/min. Patients undergoing hemodialysis should receive an extra dose after the procedure.

The intramuscular injection of 1.2 to 2.4 million units of benzathine penicillin provides effective serum levels for 2 to 4 weeks and represents a particularly attractive and dependable approach for the therapy or prophylaxis of streptococcal infections in patients who take medicines unreliably. The adult dose of dicloxacillin is 250 to 500 mg orally four times a day. For infections requiring intravenous treatment of infection from penicillinase-producing *S. aureus,* the adult dose of nafcillin or oxacillin is 1 to 2 g four times a day. No adjustment for renal failure is necessary for any of these agents, and they are not significantly removed by hemodialysis. Amoxicillin-clavulanic acid is available in tablets containing 125 mg potassium clavulanate plus either 250 or 500 mg amoxicillin. The usual adult dose is one of the tablets containing 250 mg of amoxicillin three times a day. Patients with creatinine clearances of 10 to 50 mL/min should receive one tablet twice a day and those with clearances less than 10 mL/min should receive one tablet a day. Patients undergoing hemodialysis should receive a supplemental dose following the procedure. The parenteral agent ampicillin-sulbactam contains a 2:1 ratio of the two constituents, respectively. The usual dose is 1.5 g (1 g ampicillin, 0.5 g sulbactam) or 3 g of the combination every 6 h. When the creatinine clearance is 10 to 50 mL/min, the interval should be 12 h; when the creatinine clearance is worse than that, the interval should be every 24 h. Patients undergoing hemodialysis should receive a supplemental dose after the procedure.

ADVERSE EFFECTS   The most serious complication of penicillin use is anaphylaxis, which occurs about 10 times in every 100,000 treatment courses, with about a 10 percent fatality rate.[9] Anaphylaxis is not more frequent in atopic patients than in the general population. It begins within the first hour, usually the first 30 min, after drug administration and is much less common with oral than with parenteral therapy. Clinical features may include hypotension, wheezing, laryngeal edema, and urticaria or angioedema. As opposed to this immediate response, some patients have an "acceler-

ated" allergic reaction from 1 to 72 h after the dose; the characteristics include urticaria or angioedema, wheezing, and laryngeal edema. These are IgE-mediated events in which the antigens are breakdown products of penicillin (not the intact molecule) bound covalently to proteins. One of these is benzylpenicilloyl, also called the *major determinant* because it is the most abundant of the penicillin derivatives; it is the antigen involved in accelerated reactions. Several other breakdown products of penicillin, called *minor determinants*, form in small quantities and are the antigens responsible for anaphylaxis. Penicilloyl polylysine, a manufactured skin-test reagent, tests for IgE against the major determinant; a negative test means that the patient can receive penicillin without developing an accelerated allergic reaction, but it does not exclude the possibility of anaphylaxis. Unfortunately, no commercial preparation of the minor determinants is available in the United States. Studies with noncommercial minor determinant mixtures indicate that a negative skin test predicts that the patient can receive penicillin without developing anaphylaxis. Such skin testing is very safe and quite valuable in assessing the risks of penicillin therapy, since about 80 percent of patients with a history of adverse reactions to penicillin have negative skin tests and can receive the drug without developing anaphylaxis or accelerated reactions.[10] Unless such material is available and the skin testing is negative, however, patients with a history of immediate or accelerated reactions should not receive any kind of penicillin, since the allergic cross-reactivity among all the penicillins appears to be quite high.

Skin testing has no predictive value in reactions not mediated by IgE, which include the remaining major adverse effects. Drug fever tends to occur after the first week of therapy in patients without previous exposure, but it can begin earlier in those who have received penicillin in the past. No characteristic pattern of temperature elevation occurs, and the patient's response may range from an unawareness of fever to shaking chills, hypotension, and delirium. Eosinophilia or a rash accompanies the fever in a minority of cases. The temperature should return to normal within 72 h of discontinuing the medication. Only recurrence of the fever, usually within a few hours, after reexposure to the drug definitively identifies penicillin as the cause, since no reliable laboratory test exists. Such a challenge is safe unless the patient has suffered organ damage, such as nephritis or hepatitis.

Rare reactions include hemolytic anemia, usually only with high-dose intravenous therapy; neutropenia; and interstitial nephritis, which typically causes fever, worsening renal function, a morbilliform rash, and the presence of protein, neutrophils, red cells, and eosinophils in the urine. More frequent are gastrointestinal complaints of nausea, vomiting, and diarrhea, but the last is much more likely with ampicillin or amoxicillin than with penicillin or dicloxacillin. Diarrhea is even more frequent with amoxicillin-clavulanic acid. Occasionally, primarily in hospitalized patients, diarrhea related to amoxicillin or ampicillin arises from colitis due to *Clostridium difficile*.

The mechanism of most of the dermatologic reactions to the penicillins is unknown. Because they are not mediated by IgE, skin tests cannot predict their occurrence, indicate definitively that they are drug-related, or confirm that they arise specifically from penicillins in patients concurrently receiving other medications. The most common type of cutaneous reaction to the penicillins by far is a diffuse erythematous eruption with both macules and papules that usually begins on the trunk and spreads to involve the extremities but typically spares the palms, soles, and mucous membranes. It may begin within hours after the first dose, but most commonly develops about 7 to 10 days later. Occasionally, it starts several days *after* discontinuation of the drug; irrespective of when it begins, however, it usually resolves within 7 days. This kind of eruption is most common and has been most extensively studied in patients receiving amoxicillin and ampicillin. With these agents, the eruptions are especially likely to occur in patients with chronic lymphocytic leukemia, those receiving concurrent allopurinol, and those with infectious mononucleosis and cytomegalovirus infections, where the incidence is nearly 100 percent.[11] It commonly fails to recur when the patient receives the medication again, and its development is not an indication that the patient is "allergic" to penicillin in the sense of being at greater risk for developing life-threatening adverse reactions.

Other skin rashes are distinctly unusual with the penicillins. Serum sickness–like reactions—characterized by fever, arthralgias, lymph node enlargement, and cutaneous eruptions that are morbilliform or urticarial—tend to occur 7 to 10 days after the medication is begun. Other rare skin complications include erythema multiforme, Stevens-Johnson syndrome, toxic epidermal necrolysis,[12] fixed drug eruption,[13] vasculitis,[14] erythroderma, pemphigus,[15] and acute generalized pustulosis.[16]

Cephalosporins

MECHANISM AND SPECTRUM OF ACTIVITY Like the penicillins, the cephalosporins impair cell-wall synthesis and kill susceptible organisms. These agents have been grouped into three "generations" depending on the spectrum of their antibacterial activity. First-generation cephalosporins, which include the parenteral agents cephalothin and cefazolin and the oral preparations cephalexin and cephradine, are active against streptococci (but not enterococci), methicillin-sensitive *S. aureus,* and some gram-negative bacilli, including most *E. coli, Proteus mirabilis,* and *K. pneumoniae.* Second-generation cephalosporins have increased activity against many gram-negative bacilli. Cefamandole, cefaclor, and cefuroxime are effective against *H. influenzae,* and cefoxitin and cefotetan against anaerobic gram-negative bacilli. The third-generation cephalosporins are less active than first- and second-generation agents against gram-positive cocci but are effective against a larger number of gram-negative bacilli, including some that are resistant to many other agents.

DOSAGE AND DRUG INTERACTIONS For dermatologists, cephalosporins are primarily useful for treating infections caused by streptococci and staphylococci in patients with non–life threatening reactions to the penicillins. These patients can receive the parenteral agent cefazolin as 0.5 to 1 g IM or IV q 8 h or the oral preparation cephalexin administered as 250 to 500 mg qid. In patients with renal failure, the appropriate interval between doses of cefazolin is 12 h for those with creatinine clearances between 10 and 50 mL/min and 24 h for those with values less than 10 mL/h. For cephalexin, the interval should be 12 h when the value is less than 10 mL/h. For both agents, a supplemental dose after hemodialysis is advisable.

Two third-generation cephalosporins are useful in treating sexually transmitted diseases. Ceftriaxone given as a single intramuscular dose of 125 mg is effective against urethral, cervical, rectal, and pharyngeal gonorrhea; a single dose of 400 mg of the oral agent cefixime is another option. Ceftriaxone 1 g IV daily, is the agent of choice for gonococcal bacteremia, arthritis, or disseminated disease. A single intramuscular dose of 250 mg is one option for treating chancroid.

ADVERSE EFFECTS Patients with a history of penicillin reactions have a higher incidence of adverse reactions with cephalosporins than do patients without such a history, but the frequency is only about 5 percent, and the manifestations are usually mild, even in patients with positive skin tests to the major and minor determinants

of penicillin.[17] Most importantly, the risk of anaphylaxis or accelerated reaction is extremely low except in patients with a history of such an allergy to penicillin, who should not receive cephalosporins.

Cephalosporins are generally well tolerated. Gastrointestinal symptoms of nausea, vomiting, abdominal cramps, and diarrhea may occur. Sometimes, primarily in hospitalized patients, the diarrhea may arise from *C. difficile* colitis. Candidal vulvovaginitis and pruritus ani are occasional complications, as is blood eosinophilia, which is usually unattended by any other significant findings. Anaphylaxis and urticaria are rare. Macular and papular eruptions, which occur in 1 to 3 percent of patients, resemble those of penicillin, typically beginning on the trunk and extending to the extremities. Serum sickness–like reactions have developed primarily with cefaclor.[18] Other rare cutaneous complications have included toxic epidermal necrolysis, erythema multiforme, Stevens-Johnson syndrome, fixed drug reaction, erythroderma, pemphigus, and acute generalized exanthematous pustulosis.

Tetracyclines

MECHANISM AND SPECTRUM OF ACTIVITY Tetracyclines[19] are bacteriostatic antibiotics that impair protein synthesis by interfering with the 30S subunit of bacterial ribosomes. The most commonly used agents in dermatology are tetracycline, doxycycline, and minocycline. They are active against *Proprionibacterium acnes,* considered the most important bacterial species in the pathogenesis of acne. They are also useful in treating rosacea and perioral dermatitis, although the microbial etiology, if any, of those disorders is unknown. Tetracyclines are important in the therapy of certain sexually transmitted diseases. Because of their activity against *Chlamydia trachomatis,* they are useful for urethritis, cervicitis, epidymitis, and pelvic inflammatory disease caused by this organism and for lymphogranuloma venereum. They are the drugs of choice in treating syphilis for adults (except pregnant or nursing women) unable to tolerate penicillin and for granuloma inguinale, which is caused by *Calymmatobacterium granulomatis.* They are active in primary skin infections due to *Bacillus anthracis* (anthrax), *P. multocida* (infected dog or cat bites), *Vibrio vulnificus* (from wounds contaminated with saltwater), *B. burgdorferi* (the cause of Lyme disease), *Spirillum minus* and *S. moniliformis* (the causes of rat-bite fever), and *Mycobacterium marinum* (the cause of fish-tank granuloma). Tetracyclines are also effective in certain systemic infections that may have cutaneous manifestations, including tularemia, plague, brucellosis, bacillary angiomatosis, psittacosis, erlichiosis, *Mycoplasma pneumoniae* infection causing Stevens-Johnson syndrome, and rickettsial diseases (Rocky Mountain spotted fever, typhus, rickettsialpox).

DOSAGE AND DRUG INTERACTIONS The usual adult dose of tetracycline is 250 to 500 mg qid. Because of its less frequent dosage, only modestly more expensive cost, and fewer side effects, especially diarrhea, doxycycline at 100 mg qd or bid is the tetracycline of choice for most infections. The same dose is used intravenously for patients requiring parenteral therapy. Some dermatologists prefer minocycline for treating difficult acne, but little objective evidence demonstrates any superiority to doxycycline[20] and it is much more expensive. Its usual dose is 100 mg qd or bid. Because they increase azotemia by inhibiting protein synthesis and are eliminated by renal mechanisms, most tetracyclines are not recommended in renal failure; but doxycycline, which is metabolized in the liver, can be given in its usual dose for all levels of kidney function, and no supplemental dose is required after hemodialysis. Metals chelate the tetracyclines, impairing their absorption; patients should therefore avoid concurrent ingestion of medicinal iron or compounds, primarily antacids, containing aluminum, calcium, and/ or magnesium. Sodium bicarbonate, milk, and milk products also decrease absorption of the tetracyclines. Phenytoin, carbamazepine, barbiturates, and alcohol use increase the metabolism of doxycycline; twice-daily dosing is appropriate for patients receiving these substances.

ADVERSE EFFECTS Because they can stain the teeth and impair bone growth in fetuses and in young children, tetracyclines are contraindicated in pregnancy, nursing mothers, and children less than 12 years of age. Otherwise, tetracyclines are generally quite safe. Gastrointestinal complaints of nausea, vomiting, and diarrhea may occur, and *C. difficile* colitis may be a complication, primarily in hospitalized patients. For some, oral or vulvovaginal candidiasis is a problem. Idiopathic intracranial hypertension, pulmonary eosinophilia, and pancreatitis are rare adverse effects. Esophageal ulcerations and strictures occasionally occur from prolonged exposure of the esophageal mucosa to the drug; taking the medication with copious amounts of water and avoiding its ingestion just before the patient is likely to be recumbent, as at bedtime, should prevent these problems. Minocycline can cause unique neurologic complications—consisting of dizziness, vertigo, light-headedness, tinnitus, and imbalance—that usually begin within a few days of treatment. These occur more frequently in women and subside several days after discontinuation of the drug. It has also caused a syndrome that includes autoimmune hepatitis and features of systemic lupus erythematosus.

All the tetracyclines can cause phototoxic eruptions that resemble severe sunburn, and onycholysis may occur in sun-exposed nails of the fingers and toes. Long-term minocycline therapy can result in various forms of pigmentation. Blue-black macules may develop in areas of previous inflammation or in scars, especially those due to acne. Hyperpigmentation, either macular or diffuse, may occur on sun-exposed areas, particularly the extensor surfaces of the legs and forearms. It also occurs on the hard palate. These forms generally abate over a few months after discontinuation of the minocycline. A more persistent type is a brown-gray discoloration, especially in sun-exposed areas, that may also affect the nails, sclera, and teeth.

Other cutaneous reactions to tetracycline are uncommon. Erythema multiforme, erythroderma, Stevens-Johnson syndrome, erythema nodosum, and toxic epidermal necrolysis have been reported, and tetracyclines can cause fixed drug eruptions.

Macrolides

MECHANISM AND SPECTRUM OF ACTIVITY Macrolides—consisting of erythromycin, azithromycin (which belongs to a subclass called *azalides*), and clarithromycin—interfere with protein synthesis by binding to the 50S ribosomal subunit of susceptible organisms. They are generally bacteriostatic. Clarithromycin and azithromycin are structurally similar to erythromycin, but small alterations have created three major differences.[21] They are more stable in gastric acid, promoting better oral absorption and decreasing the degradation of the drugs into inactive metabolites that cause gastrointestinal side effects. Their penetration into cells is superior to erythromycin's, achieving concentrations in most tissues, but not the brain or cerebrospinal fluid, that considerably exceed those in the blood. They also have longer serum half-lives, which allows less frequent dosage. These agents are considerably more expensive than erythromycin, however, and their apparent advantages have little relevance to the treatment of most cutaneous infections.

The macrolides are active against most streptococci and *S. aureus* but not methicillin-resistant strains. Unfortunately, azithromycin and clarithromycin are ineffective against erythromycin-resistant *S. aureus,* which is common in some areas. Because of its action against *P. acnes,* erythromycin is an option for treating acne, and it is effective in rosacea and perioral dermatitis as well. It is useful for erythrasma, an infection caused by *Corynebacterium minutissimum,* and is an option for anthrax, erysipeloid (caused by *E. rhusiopathiae*), and Lyme disease (caused by *B. burgdorferi*). Erythromycin is also useful in sexually transmitted diseases, including chancroid and infections due to *C. trachomatis,* such as nongonococcal urethritis, cervicitis, epididymitis, conjunctivitis, proctitis, and lymphogranuloma venereum. It is the drug of choice for these infections during pregnancy.

Clarithromycin and azithromycin have advantages for two special circumstances of potential relevance to dermatologists. In sexually transmitted diseases, single-dose therapy is ideal, because it can be observed and compliance assured compared with regimens requiring further doses. Azithromycin as a single 1 g dose is effective for chancroid and for infections due to *C. trachomatis,* except lymphogranuloma venereum, which requires protracted therapy (21 days) with erythromycin or doxycycline. The new macrolides are active against various mycobacteria, including *M. leprae* and both rapidly-growing (*M. chelonae, M. abscessus*) and slow-growing species (*M. gordonae, M. szulgai, M. scrofulaceum, M. marinum, M. nonchromogenicum*). Azithromycin and clarithromycin, therefore, may be useful in treating cutaneous mycobacterial infections due to susceptible organisms.

DOSAGE AND DRUG INTERACTIONS The usual adult dose of erythromycin is 250 to 500 mg qid. No changes are necessary in renal failure, and no supplemental doses are required in hemodialysis. Erythromycin increases the levels of several medications, including theophylline, warfarin, carbamazepine, and cyclosporine. All the macrolides increase the levels of terfenadine and astemizole, sometimes causing serious ventricular arrhythmias, and they should be avoided in patients taking those antihistamines. Azithromycin and clarithromycin may increase the blood levels of theophylline and carbamazepine. The usual adult regimen for azithromycin is 500 mg the first day followed by 250 mg daily thereafter. For clarithromycin, the usual adult dose is 250 to 500 mg twice daily. No adjustment is necessary for renal disease.

ADVERSE EFFECTS The most common adverse effects of the macrolides are gastrointestinal, including abdominal cramps, nausea, vomiting, and diarrhea. Occasionally, *C. difficile* colitis occurs, primarily in hospitalized patients. Cholestatic hepatitis rarely develops with erythromycin, almost exclusively with the estolate preparation. Patients typically have nausea, vomiting, and abdominal pain, followed by jaundice and fever. Laboratory findings include abnormal liver tests consistent with cholestatic changes and occasionally eosinophilia. Angioedema and photosensitivity are rare dermatologic complications of azithromycin.

Fluoroquinolones

MECHANISM AND SPECTRUM OF ACTIVITY Fluoroquinolones[22] inhibit DNA gyrase, an enzyme involved in the coiling of the DNA helix, and are usually bactericidal. Ciprofloxacin and ofloxacin, which clinicians extravagantly (and very often inappropriately) prescribe for diverse infections, have few potential uses in dermatology. They are active against *S. aureus,* including some methicillin-resistant strains, but resistance of this organism has emerged from widespread use of these agents. They are not reliable against streptococci. They are active against many gram-negative organisms, including *N. gonorrhoeae,* and against several mycobacteria, such as *M. tuberculosis, M. fortuitum,* and *M. xenopi.* Ofloxacin is also effective against *C. trachomatis.* Ciprofloxacin appears beneficial in treating cat-scratch disease.

The dermatologic use of the fluoroquinolones is primarily as an option for sexually transmitted diseases. Ofloxacin is an alternative but very expensive therapy for urethritis, cervicitis, conjunctivitis, and proctitis due to *C. trachomatis.* The dose is 300 mg bid for 7 days; this is also a reasonable regimen for treating epididymitis. Single-dose ciprofloxacin (500 mg) or ofloxacin (400 mg) is effective for urethral, rectal, cervical, or pharyngeal gonorrhea, and ciprofloxacin 500 mg bid for 3 days is an alternative for treating chancroid.

DOSAGE AND DRUG INTERACTIONS Patients should avoid the concurrent use of sucralfate, supplements containing zinc or iron, and antacids with aluminum, calcium, or magnesium, all of which inhibit the absorption of the fluoroquinolones. The fluoroquinolones can increase the serum levels of warfarin, theophylline, and cyclosporine, and they can alter the blood glucose, causing either hyper- or hypoglycemia in some patients taking oral antidiabetic agents or insulin. The proper adjustment in renal dysfunction for ofloxacin is to give the usual recommended dose every 24 h rather than every 12 h for creatinine clearances of 10 to 50 mL/min and one-half the recommended dose every 24 h for values less than 10 mL/min. For ciprofloxacin, patients with creatinine clearances less than 10 mL/min should receive the usual dose every 24 h rather than twice daily. Neither drug requires a supplemental dose for patients undergoing hemodialysis.

ADVERSE EFFECTS The most frequent adverse effects are nausea, diarrhea, insomnia, headache, and dizziness. Uncommon complications include serum sickness, a morbilliform eruption, anaphylaxis, and vasculitis. Phototoxic reactions can occur, even when patients use a sunscreen. Occasional abnormal laboratory tests include eosinophilia, increased levels of liver enzymes, and leukopenia. Because studies demonstrate cartilage erosions in the joints of young animals given high doses, the fluoroquinolones are not recommended for children. They should not be used in pregnancy or for nursing mothers.

Clindamycin

MECHANISM AND SPECTRUM OF ACTIVITY Clindamycin,[23] a bacteriostatic drug, inhibits protein synthesis by binding to the 50S portion of the ribosome. It is active against streptococci, most *S. aureus,* and most anaerobic bacteria, including *P. acnes.* Its major use in dermatology is as an alternative in treating streptococcal and staphylococcal infections in penicillin-allergic patients and in treating acne. It achieves high levels in the nasal secretions and is one of the most effective agents in eradicating nasal carriage of *S. aureus* and in preventing further episodes in those with recurrent staphylococcal skin infections.

DOSAGE AND DRUG INTERACTIONS The usual adult dose is 150 to 300 mg qid. No adjustment is necessary for renal failure, and no supplemental dose is required for patients receiving hemodialysis. Since clindamycin primarily undergoes hepatic metabo-

lism, it accumulates in patients with severe liver disease, a situation that warrants cautious use, although no specific dose adjustments are available.[24] For preventing recurrent staphylococcal skin infection, a reasonable program is 150 mg qd for 3 months.[25]

ADVERSE EFFECTS Morbilliform rashes are frequent, but anaphylaxis, urticaria, or erythema multiforme are rare. Hepatotoxicity is also very uncommon. The most notorious adverse effect is diarrhea, which may occur in up to 20 percent of recipients. In nearly all outpatients and most inpatients, the cause seems related to the antibiotic itself, and the diarrhea abates after discontinuing the clindamycin. In those in the hospital or recently hospitalized, however, clindamycin, like many other antibiotics, predisposes to colitis due to *C. difficile.* This organism is not part of the normal bowel flora, but it commonly colonizes hospitalized patients, especially those who have received broad-spectrum antibiotics that eradicate the normal intestinal bacteria. The diarrhea may be mild or very severe, accompanied by fever, leukocytosis, and intravascular volume depletion. It usually begins during clindamycin administration but may start days or even weeks after the course has ended. The diagnosis is established by finding *C. difficile* toxin in the stools of symptomatic patients. Mild cases respond to discontinuing clindamycin; more severe ones warrant therapy with oral metronidazole. In general, because of the tendency of this drug to cause diarrhea, either as a direct effect of the antibiotic or through predisposing to *C. difficile* colitis, patients with inflammatory bowel disease should not receive clindamycin.

Trimethoprim-Sulfamethoxazole

MECHANISM AND SPECTRUM OF ACTIVITY This combination of antimicrobial agents,[26] also called *cotrimoxazole,* blocks two separate steps in the folic acid metabolism of susceptible organisms. It is active against a wide variety of gram-negative bacteria and against most *S. aureus,* including many methicillin-resistant strains. Its main use is for urinary tract and respiratory infections, including sinusitis, otitis media, and pneumonia. Because of its activity against *Pneumocystis carinii,* it is effective in treating and preventing pneumonia and other infections due to that organism, and it is widely used for that purpose in patients infected with the human immunodeficiency virus (HIV). It has few indications in dermatology; some experts recommend it for acne refractory to tetracycline, and it may be beneficial in the oral therapy of skin infections caused by methicillin-resistant *S. aureus.* It is effective in treating some patients with mild or moderately severe Wegener's granulomatosis and in preventing recurrent episodes in that disorder. Other agents have replaced it in the therapy of sexually transmitted diseases.

DOSAGE AND DRUG INTERACTIONS The usual adult dose is one double-strength tablet (containing 800 mg of sulfamethoxazole and 160 mg of trimethoprim) bid. It may increase the serum levels of phenytoin and enhance the hypoglycemic effects of chlorpropamide and tolbutamide. It displaces warfarin and methotrexate from their albumin-binding sites, potentiating the effects of these drugs, and it decreases the serum levels of cyclosporine.

ADVERSE EFFECTS Gastrointestinal side effects—including nausea, vomiting, and abdominal discomfort—occur in about 3 percent of patients. Diarrhea develops in fewer than 1 percent, and *C. difficile* colitis is rare. Trimethoprim-sulfamethoxazole can cause mild nephrotoxicity in patients with underlying renal insufficiency, and the drug is not recommended in this circumstance. Hematologic complications include neutropenia, which is more likely in those undergoing hemodialysis and in patients with preexisting folate or vitamin B_{12} deficiency, concurrent phenytoin administration, malnutrition, and alcoholism. Hemolytic anemia can develop in those with glucose-6-phosphate dehydrogenase (G6PD) deficiency. In patients with HIV infection, neutropenia and thrombocytopenia are frequent.

Patients with HIV infection are also predisposed to developing rashes with this medication. Morbilliform eruptions occur in 30 to 85 percent who receive the drug, commonly during the second week of therapy.[27] The findings are itchy or asymptomatic macules and papules that become generalized and usually resolve quickly after discontinuing the agent. A similar rash occurs in about 3 percent of the general population. More severe eruptions develop in about 13 percent of HIV-infected patients, compared to about 1/100,000 of others receiving the drug. These include erythema multiforme, Stevens-Johnson syndrome, and toxic epidermal necrolysis. Indeed, trimethoprim-sulfamethoxazole is one of the most common causes of these drug reactions. Other occasional cutaneous complications include vasculitis, erythema nodosum, erythroderma, fixed drug eruption, and serum sickness.

Systemic Antimicrobial Prophylaxis in Dermatology

Clinicians use antibiotics primarily to treat infections, but a considerable amount of antimicrobial administration is devoted to preventing them. Much of this prophylactic use is unnecessary, and in dermatology only a few indications exist, primarily in patients with recurrent bacterial skin infections. Prophylactic antibiotics are rarely indicated to prevent postoperative infections in cutaneous surgery, which also seldom imposes a risk for hematogenous infection of implanted prosthetic material in patients with such devices as artificial heart valves and joints.

RECURRENT BACTERIAL SKIN INFECTIONS One study of patients with recurrent staphylococcal skin infections demonstrated that oral clindamycin 150 mg qd for 3 months impressively decreased the incidence of further episodes.[25] Among the placebo recipients, 64 percent of patients had a recurrent skin abscess in the 3 months, compared to 18 percent of those receiving clindamycin. Of those who were free of infection while taking the antibiotic, 67 percent had no recurrence for at least 9 months after discontinuing the clindamycin. Although the study did not specifically evaluate this issue, this long-term benefit probably came from eradication of staphylococcal nasal carriage, for which clindamycin is one of the few very effective antimicrobials. No patient had gastrointestinal complaints, including diarrhea. Clinicians considering this prophylaxis should perform appropriate cultures of the skin lesions to ensure that the dermatologic lesions are genuinely due to *S. aureus,* since many cutaneous abscesses and other pustular skin diseases are caused by other organisms or have a noninfectious etiology.

Patients with recurrent bouts of cellulitis typically have predisposing factors including tinea pedis, chronic lymphedema, persistent swelling from other causes, poor hygiene, and trauma. When repeated infections occur despite therapy of these underlying conditions, penicillin or erythromycin given as 250 mg bid is very effective in preventing further episodes. In one study, for example, the recurrence rate over 18 months was 50 percent among patients who received no systemic antibiotics, compared with zero percent

among those taking twice-daily erythromycin.[28] Monthly injections of benzathine penicillin represent another option, particularly in patients who do not take medications reliably.

PREVENTION OF WOUND INFECTIONS FOLLOWING DERMATOLOGIC SURGERY To justify the expense and potential complications of antimicrobials prescribed to prevent postoperative wound infections, such infections should be either quite frequent or very severe. Most dermatologic procedures are "clean" surgery, which involves incisions through uninfected skin without transecting mucosal surfaces. The expected infection rate without antimicrobial prophylaxis is less than 5 percent and in most centers is less than 1 percent. Such infections are rarely severe; consequently, preventive antibiotics are unjustified. Even in surgery that is "clean-contaminated"—involving the transection of mucosal surfaces, such as removing a deep basal cell carcinoma from the nose—the infection rate is low and the infections relatively mild. The 10 percent infection rate quoted for this type of operation derives from studies primarily involving major surgery, such as laryngectomies or gastrointestinal resections, not dermatologic procedures. This kind of skin surgery does not warrant antibiotic prophylaxis. Similarly, in patients with acute nonpurulent inflammation or major breaks in aseptic technique ("contaminated surgery"), where the expected infection rate in major surgery is 20 to 30 percent, the incidence is probably lower in dermatologic procedures, and the infections are usually mild. Even with operations involving purulent lesions ("infected or dirty surgery") in which postoperative infections occur in 30 to 40 percent of patients with major surgery, the risks for patients with cutaneous suppuration are low and the consequences mostly mild. Incision and drainage of skin abscesses, for example, lead to few postoperative infections, and antibiotics seem not only unnecessary but ineffective in this setting.[29,30]

While a procedure with extensive and deep surgery involving a mucosal surface may warrant preoperative antibiotics, such operations are uncommon for most dermatologists. For such procedures one of the most important elements in using antimicrobial agents is the timing of their administration. Since contamination usually occurs only from the beginning of the incision to the time of wound closure, a single preoperative dose of an antibiotic that sustains good tissue levels throughout this interim suffices. Further preoperative or postoperative doses are unnecessary and wasteful. Another important consideration is the choice of the agent; the goal is not to eradicate every microbe that might be present but to reduce the concentration of the most likely contaminating organisms to a level that the host can handle without developing an infection. Most studies on prophylactic antibiotics in surgery have used a parenteral cephalosporin, especially cefazolin, 1 g of which results in good, sustained serum and tissue levels of the antibiotic. Furthermore, it is active against streptococci, staphylococci, and most of the upper respiratory flora that is likely to cause infections in procedures transecting the upper airway mucosa.

ANTIBIOTIC PROPHYLAXIS FOR PATIENTS WITH HEART DISEASE OR PROSTHETIC MATERIAL The transient bacteremia that occurs with various dental and surgical procedures can sometimes lead to infections of abnormal cardiac valves, both native and prosthetic ones, and possibly to infections of such prosthetic devices as artificial joints and vascular grafts. The risk of bacteremia with dermatologic surgery involving incisions through either intact or eroded skin is very low,[31] however, and no prophylaxis is required for patients with either abnormal heart valves or indwelling prosthetic material. Indeed, only with incision and drainage of infected tissue is the frequency of bacteremia likely to be high enough to justify antimicrobial prophylaxis, and even in that or, indeed, any other situation, its efficacy is unknown. A reasonable approach is to give a single dose of an agent about 1 h before the procedure in patients with implanted prostheses. An oral antibiotic is usually feasible, but occasionally a parenteral agent may be required—for example, in patients with nausea or with evidence of systemic infection, in whom blood cultures should precede antimicrobial administration. Appropriate choices include a first-generation cephalosporin (cephalexin 1 g PO or cefazolin 1 g IM or IV), a penicillinase-resistant penicillin (dicloxacillin 1 g PO or nafcillin 1 g IV), or clindamycin for patients with serious penicillin allergies (300 mg PO or IV).

REFERENCES

1. McCaig LF, Hughes JM: Trends in antimicrobial drug prescribing among office-based physicians in the United States. *JAMA* **273**:214, 1995
2. Jacoby GA, Archer GL: New mechanisms of bacterial resistance to antimicrobial agents. *N Engl J Med* **324**:601, 1991
3. Gold HS, Moellering RC: Antimicrobial-drug resistance. *N Engl J Med* **335**:1445, 1996
4. Jorgensen JH: Antimicrobial susceptibility testing of bacteria that grow aerobically. *Infect Dis Clin North Am* **7**:393, 1993
5. Mulligan MJ, Cobbs CG: Bacteriostatic versus bactericidal activity. *Infect Dis Clin North Am* **3**:389, 1989
6. Wright AJ, Wilkowske CJ: The penicillins. *Mayo Clinic Proc* **66**:1047, 1991
7. Sensakovic JW, Smith LG: Beta-lactamase inhibitor combinations. *Med Clin North Am* **79**:695, 1995
8. Goldstein EJC: Bite wounds and infections. *Clin Infect Dis* **14**:633, 1992
9. Lin RY: A perspective on penicillin allergy. *Arch Intern Med* **152**:930, 1992
10. Sogn DD et al: Results of the National Institute of Allergy and Infectious Diseases collaborative clinical trial to test the predictive value of skin testing with major and minor penicillin derivatives in hospitalized patients. *Arch Intern Med* **152**:1025, 1992
11. Sher TH: Penicillin hypersensitivity—a review. *Pediatr Clin North Am* **30**:161, 1983
12. Roujeau JC, Stern RS: Severe adverse cutaneous reactions to drugs. *N Engl J Med* **331**:1272, 1994
13. Korkij W, Soltani K: Fixed drug eruption. A brief review. *Arch Dermatol* **120**:520, 1984
14. Somer T, Finegold SM: Vasculitides associated with infections, immunizations, and antimicrobial drugs. *Clin Infect Dis* **20**:1010, 1995
15. Ruocco V, Sacerdoti G: Pemphigus and bullous pemphigoid due to drugs. *Int J Dermatol* **30**:307, 1991
16. Roujeau JC et al: Acute generalized exanthematous pustulosis. Analysis of 63 cases. *Arch Dermatol* **127**:1333, 1991
17. Saxon A et al: Immediate hypersensitivity reactions to beta-lactam antibiotics. *Ann Intern Med* **107**:204, 1987
18. Platt R et al: Serum sickness-like reactions to amoxicillin, cefaclor, cephalexin, and trimethoprim-sulfamethoxazole. *J Infect Dis* **158**:474, 1988
19. Klein NC, Cunha BA: Tetracyclines. *Med Clin North Am* **79**:789, 1995
20. Webster GF: Acne. *Curr Probl Dermatol* **8**:237, 1996
21. Kanatani MS, Guglielmo BJ: The new macrolides: Azithromycin and clarithromycin. *West J Med* **160**:31, 1994
22. Hooper DC, Wolfson JS: Fluoroquinolone antimicrobial agents. *N Engl J Med* **324**:384, 1991
23. Falagas ME, Gorbach SL: Clindamycin and metronidazole. *Med Clin North Am* **79**:845, 1995
24. Tschida SJ et al: Anti-infective agents and hepatic disease. *Med Clin North Am* **79**:895, 1995
25. Klempner MS, Styrt B: Prevention of recurrent staphylococcal skin infections with low-dose clindamycin therapy. *JAMA* **260**:2682, 1988
26. Cockerill FR, Edson RS: Trimethoprim-sulfamethoxazole. *Mayo Clin Proc* **66**:1260, 1991
27. Zalla MJ et al: Dermatologic manifestations of human immunodeficiency virus infection. *Mayo Clin Proc* **67**:1089, 1992
28. Kremer M et al: Long-term antimicrobial therapy in the prevention of recurrent soft-tissue infections. *J Infect* **22**:37, 1991
29. Meislin HW et al: Cutaneous abscesses: Anaerobic and aerobic bacteriology and outpatient management. *Ann Intern Med* **87**:145, 1977
30. Macfie J, Harvey J: The treatment of acute superficial abscesses: A prospective clinical trial. *Br J Surg* **64**:264, 1977
31. Haas AF, Grekin RC: Antibiotic prophylaxis in dermatologic surgery. *J Am Acad Dermatol* **32**:155, 1995

CHAPTER 259

Raphael Dolin

Antiviral Drugs

Antiviral drugs have been developed at an extraordinary pace during the past decade. As late as the mid-1980s only three antiviral drugs were approved for treatment of systemic viral infections. Currently, there are 20 approved antiviral drugs, and additional ones are likely to be forthcoming. Progress has been accelerated by recent advances in knowledge of the molecular biology and pathogenesis of certain viral infections, of which AIDS has been the most notable. Nonetheless, the field of antiviral drugs still lags considerably behind that of antibacterial antibiotics, both in the numbers of available drugs and in the clinical application of techniques such as pharmacokinetic measurements and in vitro assessment of resistance. These areas are under active development.

This chapter focuses on drugs to treat those viral infections that are most likely to be encountered by dermatologists, such as those caused by herpes simplex virus (HSV) and varicella-zoster virus (VZV). Antiviral drugs used to treat cytomegalovirus (CMV) infections, the interferons, and antiretroviral drugs to combat HIV infection are discussed in less depth, and the reader is referred to reviews of these subjects for more information.

DRUGS FOR THE TREATMENT OF HERPES SIMPLEX VIRUS AND VARICELLA-ZOSTER VIRUS INFECTIONS

Acyclovir

ANTIVIRAL ACTIVITY Acyclovir {9-[(2-hydroxyethoxy) methyl] guanine, Zovirax} (Fig. 259-1) is an antiviral drug widely used for the treatment of HSV and VZV infections.[1] It is highly active against HSV-1, slightly less active against HSV-2, and approximately eightfold less active against VZV in vitro.[2,3] The activity of acyclovir against CMV is variable, and isolates are frequently resistant. Acyclovir has good activity against Epstein-Barr virus (EBV)[4] in vitro, and at higher concentrations it inhibits human herpesvirus (HHV)6.[5] The active antiviral moiety of acyclovir is acyclovir triphosphate, which is a potent inhibitor of certain herpesvirus-induced DNA polymerases but has relatively little effect on host cell DNA polymerase. Acyclovir triphosphate also acts as a terminator of the nascent viral DNA chain, since it lacks the 3′ hydroxyl group. The initial phosphorylation of acyclovir to acyclovir monophosphate is efficiently carried out by herpesvirus-induced thymidine kinases but not by cellular kinases. Thus, acyclovir monophosphate is concentrated in virus-infected cells, which contributes to its highly selective mechanism of action.[6] Resistance to acyclovir in HSV and VZV isolates occurs most commonly by mutations that result in absent or markedly decreased thymidine kinase activity.[7] Less frequent mechanisms of resistance are alterations in substrate specificity of the thymidine kinase or in changes in the viral DNA polymerase.[8] Resistant viruses have been usually, but not invariably, associated with prolonged use of acyclovir in immunosuppressed patients. Viruses that are resistant to acyclovir on the basis of thymidine kinase mutations are also resistant to ganciclovir and famciclovir but are generally sensitive to vidarabine, foscarnet, and cidofovir (see below). Viruses resistant to acyclovir on the basis of a DNA polymerase mutation are also usually resistant to foscarnet and vidarabine but may retain sensitivity to cidofovir.

FIGURE 259-1

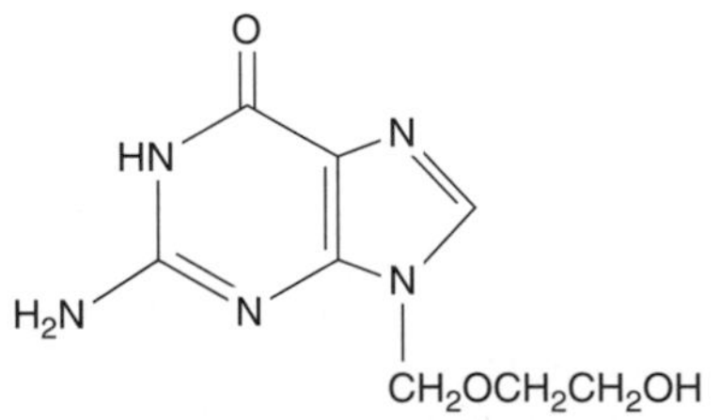

Acyclovir

PHARMACOKINETICS Acyclovir is available in oral, intravenous, and topical formulations. The oral bioavailability of acyclovir is low (15 to 30 percent). A 200-mg oral dose of acyclovir results in a peak plasma concentration of 0.4 to 0.8 μg/mL approximately 1.5 h after administration, while an 800-mg oral dose results in a peak plasma concentration of 1.6 μg/mL.[9,10] Oral absorption may be somewhat less in transplant patients. The plasma half-life of acyclovir is from 2.1 to 3.5 h in patients with normal renal function. Acyclovir is almost entirely eliminated by the renal route, largely unmetabolized (85 percent), while the remainder is metabolized to a 9-carboxymethoxymethylguanine.[11] Therefore, dosage reductions are required for patients with creatinine clearances of <50 mL/min.[12] Acyclovir is widely distributed in body fluids, including cerebrospinal fluid, vesicle fluids, and vaginal secretions. Acyclovir is available as a 5% ointment in a polyethyleneglycol base in the United States, and topical administration results in detectable drug concentrations in lesions but little, if any, systemic absorption.

ADVERSE EFFECTS Acyclovir is generally well tolerated. The major toxicity associated with acyclovir is renal, as a result of crystallization of the drug in renal tubules, which has been reported with high dosage, dehydration, or rapid intravenous administration.[13] Interstitial nephritis associated with acyclovir has also been reported.[14] Central nervous system toxicity has been described, including lethargy, tremors, obtundation, and seizures.[15,16] These side effects have usually been associated with high plasma levels of acyclovir and with underlying diseases involving the central nervous system. The concomitant use of interferon or other nucleoside analogues may contribute to neurotoxicity.

CLINICAL INDICATIONS The efficacy of acyclovir is well established in the treatment of HSV infections in several clinical settings. These include mucocutaneous HSV infections in immunocompromised patients,[17,18] which generally respond to either intravenous administration (5 mg/kg IV q8h) or oral administration (400 mg PO 5 times/day) of acyclovir. These infections are usually treated for 7 to 10 days but may require longer therapy in more severe cases. Acyclovir is also effective as prophylaxis in patients who are seropositive for HSV and who undergo intensive immunosuppression as part of transplantation or chemotherapeutic regimens.[19] Acyclovir administered intravenously or orally to patients with primary genital herpes results in shortened duration of symptoms, acceleration of healing, and reduction of virus shedding.[20,21] Intravenous and oral therapies have similar efficacies, and the choice between routes of administration should be based on the severity of disease, the need for hospitalization, and the ability of the patient to take oral medications. Acyclovir therapy for primary genital HSV does not reduce the frequency or severity of subsequent recurrences. In recurrent HSV genital infections, oral acyclovir has a modest beneficial effect on the length of time to healing and on the duration of viral shedding, particularly when it is initiated within 24 h of the onset of symptoms.[22] Suppressive therapy with 400 mg of acyclovir PO bid reduces the number of recurrences and is recommended for patients with recurrences that are particularly frequent (>six times/year) or troublesome.[23] The need for continuation of suppressive therapy should be assessed on an annual basis by stopping the drug to see whether recurrences develop. Chronic suppressive therapy does not eliminate the latent stage of HSV infection, and asymptomatic shedding of virus can occur.

Acyclovir therapy for orofacial HSV infections has been less extensively studied than for genital infections. Oral therapy for herpes labialis produced a modest beneficial clinical effect, particularly if treatment was started early in the recurrence and if higher doses were used (500 mg PO 5 times/day for 5 days).[24] Primary HSV gingivostomatitis has not been well studied, but anecdotal reports suggest acyclovir may be of some benefit in such cases. The administration of acyclovir prophylactically to patients who experience reactivation of herpes labialis with sunlight may decrease the number of lesions associated with such recurrences but does not appear to have an otherwise beneficial effect.[25]

The topical use of acyclovir as a 5% ointment in polyethylene glycol has been largely supplanted in the United States by oral administration of the drug. Acyclovir ointment is beneficial in the treatment of primary genital infections but less so than oral or intravenous therapy.[26] Topical acyclovir is also modestly beneficial in immunocompromised patients with localized mucocutaneous HSV infections. Topical therapy with acyclovir ointment has not been demonstrated to be of clinical benefit in the treatment of herpes labialis in immunocompetent patients.[27] Intravenous acyclovir is the drug of choice for treatment for life-threatening HSV infections, such as encephalitis[28] or neonatal infection.[29]

Acyclovir is also effective in the treatment of VZV infection. Because VZV is less sensitive to acyclovir than HSV, higher doses of the drug should be used (10 mg/kg IV q8h or 800 mg PO 5 times/day for 7 days). In immunocompromised patients with herpes zoster, intravenous acyclovir reduces the frequency of visceral complications and of cutaneous dissemination.[30] Orally administered acyclovir has a modest beneficial effect on the dermatomal lesions of localized herpes zoster in immunocompetent patients.[31] The effect of acyclovir on postherpetic neuralgia is unclear, and a recently conducted trial suggested that valacyclovir may be more effective in resolution of zoster associated pain[32] (see below). The use of steroids along with acyclovir to prevent the development of postherpetic neuralgia remains controversial. One study showed no benefit from the addition of prednisolone to acyclovir in herpes zoster in immunocompetent patients,[33] whereas another showed a beneficial effect of the combination of prednisone and acyclovir in overall quality-of-life measurements, although not on postherpetic neuralgia specifically.[34] Orally administered acyclovir (600 mg 5 times/day) is effective in the treatment of herpes zoster ophthalmicus.[35]

Intravenous acyclovir has been reported to be clinically beneficial in immunosuppressed patients with varicella (chickenpox) and may reduce the rate of visceral complications.[36,37] Oral acyclovir therapy for varicella in immunocompetent children, adolescents, or adults results in only a modest overall clinical benefit, even if begun within 24 h of onset of lesions.[38,39] Such therapy has not been demonstrated to reduce the rate of serious complications in these patients.

With respect to infections caused by other herpesviruses, acyclovir is not effective in the treatment of CMV infections but has shown efficacy in the prophylaxis of CMV infections in patients undergoing bone marrow, liver, or renal transplantation; it is used in many transplant centers for that purpose.[40] Acyclovir therapy has no clinical benefit for EBV-induced infectious mononucleosis, although shedding of EBV in the oropharynx was reduced during acyclovir administration.[41] Oral hairy leukoplakia in patients with AIDS frequently responds to acyclovir therapy. Anecdotal reports have described the use of acyclovir to treat EBV-associated posttransplantation lymphoproliferative disorders, but the overall effectiveness of acyclovir in that setting is unclear.[42]

Valacyclovir

Valacyclovir {2-[2-amino-1, 6-dihydro-6-oxo-9H-purin-9-yl-methoxy] ethyl-L-valinate hydrochloride, Valtrex} (Fig. 259-2) is the L-valine ester of acyclovir; it was developed to provide increased

FIGURE 259-2

Valacyclovir

oral bioavailability for acyclovir.[43,44] It is rapidly absorbed from the gastrointestinal tract and is converted almost entirely to acyclovir through intestinal and hepatic esterases. Thus, the mechanism of action and spectrum of activity of valacyclovir is that of acyclovir. After a 1-g oral dose of valacyclovir, peak plasma concentrations of acyclovir of 5.7 μg/mL are achieved in 1.75 h, with area under the curve concentrations that are similar to those achieved with 5 mg/kg of acyclovir given intravenously.[45,46] The pharmacokinetics of acyclovir once it has been converted from valacyclovir are those of the parent compound, acyclovir, and adverse effects are those that would be expected with acyclovir. However, severe and even fatal cases of the thrombotic thrombocytopenic purpura/hemolytic uremic syndrome have been reported in patients with AIDS and transplant recipients who were taking high doses of valacyclovir.[47] The basis and causal relationship to valacyclovir of this observation have not been established.

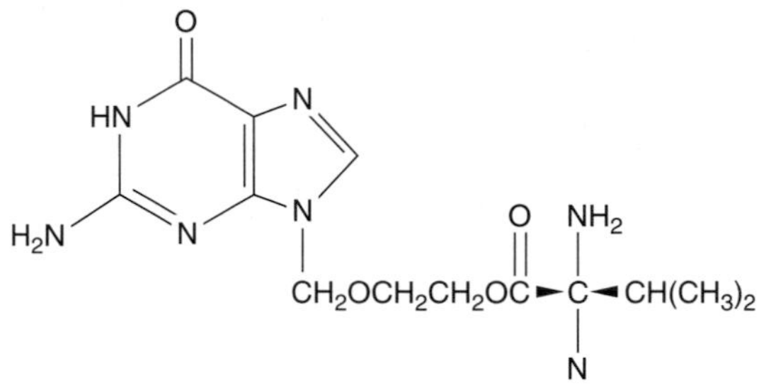

CLINICAL USEFULNESS Valacyclovir is under study for the treatment and prophylaxis of a number of herpesvirus infections. At present, the drug has been approved for treatment of recurrent HSV genital infections[48] (500 mg PO bid for 5 days) and for treatment of herpes zoster in immunocompetent hosts (1 g PO tid for 7 days). In a study of immunocompetent patients with herpes zoster who were treated within the first 72 h of onset of lesions, valacyclovir appeared to be somewhat more effective than acyclovir in the resolution of zoster-associated pain.[32]

Famciclovir and Penciclovir

ANTIVIRAL ACTIVITY Famciclovir [9-(4-hydroxy-3 hydroxymethylbut-1-yl) guanine, Famvir] (Fig. 259-3) is a prodrug of penciclovir [9-(4-hydroxy-3-hydroxy-3-hydroxymethylbut-1-yl) guanine]. Penciclovir is phosphorylated to penciclovir triphosphate, which has antiviral activity against HSV-1, HSV-2, VZV, and EBV and also against hepatitis B virus (HBV).[49–51] The initial phosphorylation of penciclovir to penciclovir monophosphate is carried out by HSV- or VZV-induced thymidine kinases in a manner analogous to that of the initial phosphorylation of acyclovir. Phosphorylation to di- and triphosphate forms of penciclovir is carried out by cellular kinases. Penciclovir triphosphate inhibits viral DNA polymerases and also inhibits extension of the nascent viral DNA chain.[50,51] Because of the presence of the hydroxyl group on the acyclic side chain of penciclovir, some DNA chain extension may occur.

FIGURE 259-4

FIGURE 259-3

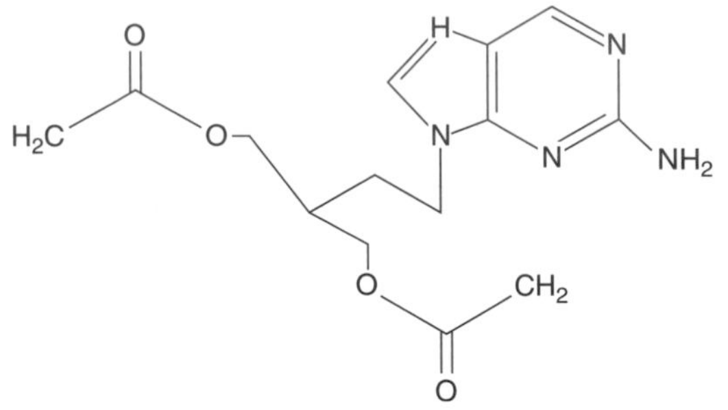

Famciclovir

Idoxuridine

PHARMACOKINETICS Famciclovir is available as an oral formulation, which is converted to penciclovir by deacetylation and oxidation in the liver and intestine.[52] The bioavailability of famciclovir is 77 percent, and a peak penciclovir plasma concentration of 3.3 μg/mL is reached 1 h after oral administration of 500 mg of famciclovir.[53] The plasma half-life of penciclovir is 2 h, and 60 to 70 percent of the drug is excreted unchanged in the urine by both glomerular filtration and tubular secretion. The dose of penciclovir should be reduced in cases of advanced renal dysfunction.[54]

Compared to the intracellular half-life of acyclovir triphosphate, that of penciclovir triphosphate is markedly prolonged in HSV-infected cells (10 to 20 h) and VZV-infected cells (9 h).[49–51] This prolonged intracellular half-life is the rationale for the longer interval of administration of famciclovir (q12h), compared to that recommended for acyclovir (q4h). HSV and VZV isolates that lack thymidine kinases are resistant to penciclovir just as they are to acyclovir. However, some acyclovir-resistant viruses with altered thymidine kinases remain sensitive to penciclovir.[55]

ADVERSE EFFECTS Famciclovir is well tolerated, and serious clinical and laboratory toxicities are uncommon. Prolonged, high-dose administration of famciclovir to rats was associated with an increased incidence of mammary adenocarcinomas in female rats, but the clinical significance of this observation is unknown.[56]

CLINICAL USEFULNESS Famciclovir is approved for the treatment of herpes zoster in immunocompetent patients[57] and for the treatment of recurrent HSV genital infections.[58] In immunocompetent patients with herpes zoster, 500 mg of famciclovir PO for 7 days had a beneficial effect on the resolution of skin lesions and on the duration of postherpetic neuralgia.[57] In a comparative trial, famciclovir was at least as effective as acyclovir given 5 times/day.[59] Famciclovir also had a beneficial effect in recurrent genital HSV infections.[58] Additional clinical trials of famciclovir in herpesvirus infections and in HBV infections are currently underway.

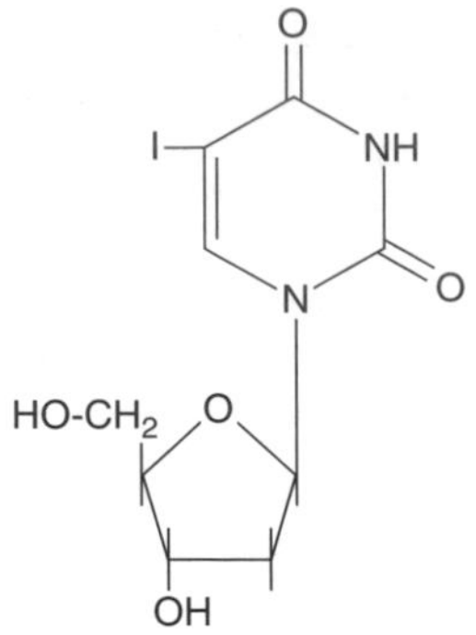

Idoxuridine

Idoxuridine (5-iodo-2'-deoxyuridine, Stoxil, Herplex, Dendrid) (Fig. 259-4) is a nucleoside analogue that has in vitro activity against HSV-1, HSV-2, VZV, and poxviruses.[60] Its antiviral effect is exerted through idoxuridine (IUDR) triphosphate, which inhibits viral DNA polymerases and also acts as a chain terminator.

Idoxuridine is available in the United States as a 1% ophthalmic solution in distilled water and as a 0.5% ophthalmic ointment in a petrolatum base. It is approved for the treatment of herpes simplex keratitis[61] but has been largely supplanted for that use by trifluridine (see below). Topical application of idoxuridine in petrolatum base has not been shown to be efficacious in the treatment of mucocutaneous HSV or VZV infections. In Europe, idoxuridine at varying concentrations is available in dimethyl sulfoxide, and in that vehicle it has been reported to have modest beneficial effects on mucocutaneous HSV and VZV infections.[62] The use of systemic (intravenous) idoxuridine for the treatment of herpesvirus infections has been abandoned because of associated toxicities and lack of efficacy.[63]

Trifluridine

Trifluridine (5-trifluoromethyl-2'-deoxyuridine, Viroptic) (Fig. 259-5) is a pyrimidine nucleoside analogue with activity against HSV-1, HSV-2, CMV, and vaccinia and, to some degree, against certain adenoviruses.[64] Trifluridine monophosphate is an irreversible competitive inhibitor of thymidylate synthetase, and trifluridine triphosphate inhibits HSV DNA polymerase.[64] Trifluridine triphosphate also inhibits cellular DNA polymerases, although to a lesser extent than viral DNA polymerases. Trifluridine shows mutagenesis and teratogenesis in experimental systems.

Because of systemic toxicity, trifluridine is approved only for topical application in the form of a 1% ophthalmic aqueous solution

FIGURE 259-5

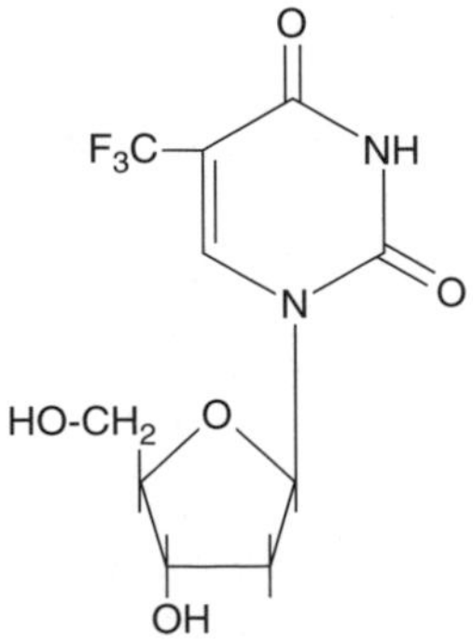

Trifluridine

for the treatment of primary conjunctivitis and recurrent epithelial keratitis caused by HSV.[65] In comparative trials, it was more effective than topical idoxuridine and similarly effective to topical vidarabine (see below).[66] Some patients with herpes simplex keratitis that is unresponsive to idoxuridine or vidarabine have responded to subsequent treatment with topical trifluridine. Topical trifluridine, either alone or in combination with interferon (IFN) α, has been reported to be beneficial in the treatment of acyclovir-resistant mucocutaneous HSV infections in patients with AIDS.[67]

Vidarabine

Vidarabine (9-β-D-ribofuranosyladenine, ara-A, Vira-A) (Fig. 259-6) is a purine nucleoside analogue that is active against HSV-1, HSV-2, VZV, and EBV. The antiviral activity of vidarabine is exerted by its triphosphorylated metabolite through the inhibition of viral DNA synthesis.[68] Vidarabine is administered intravenously, but because of its solubility, it must be administered as a constant 12-h infusion in a dilute solution that can result in a substantial fluid load.[69] At the recommended dosage of 10 to 15 mg/kg per day, vidarabine is generally well tolerated. At higher doses (20 mg/kg per day), vidarabine has been associated with anemia, leukopenia, and thrombocytopenia. Neurotoxicity has been observed at high doses, particularly in patients with hepatic or renal insufficiency.[70] Vidarabine is efficacious in the treatment of mucocutaneous HSV infection in immunosuppressed patients,[71] herpes simplex encephalitis,[72] herpes zoster in immunosuppressed patients,[73] and neonatal HSV infection.[74] However, because of considerations of efficacy, ease of administration, or toxicity, it has largely been supplanted by acyclovir for the above indications. Vidarabine is also available as a 3% ophthalmic ointment in a petrolatum base, which is approved for the treatment of primary HSV keratoconjunctivitis and recurrent HSV epithelial keratitis. Some patients with HSV keratitis who are intolerant or unresponsive to topical idoxuridine therapy have responded to treatment with vidarabine ointment.[75]

DRUGS FOR THE TREATMENT OF CMV INFECTIONS

Ganciclovir

Ganciclovir [9-(1,3-dihydroxy-2 propoxymethyl) guanine, Cytovene] (Fig. 259-7) is a nucleoside analogue that is similar in structure to acyclovir but is markedly more active than acyclovir against

FIGURE 259-6

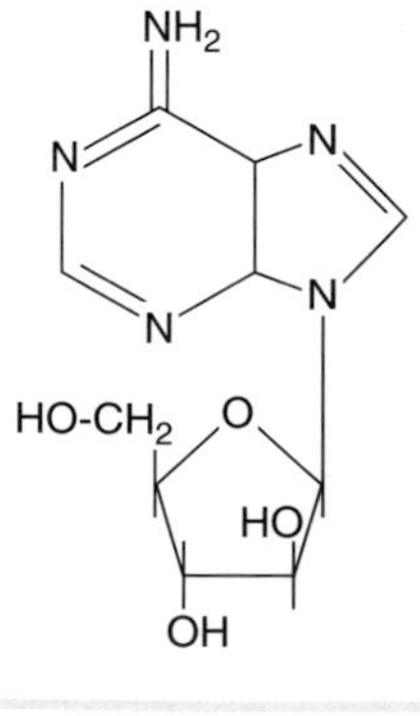

Vidarabine

FIGURE 259-7

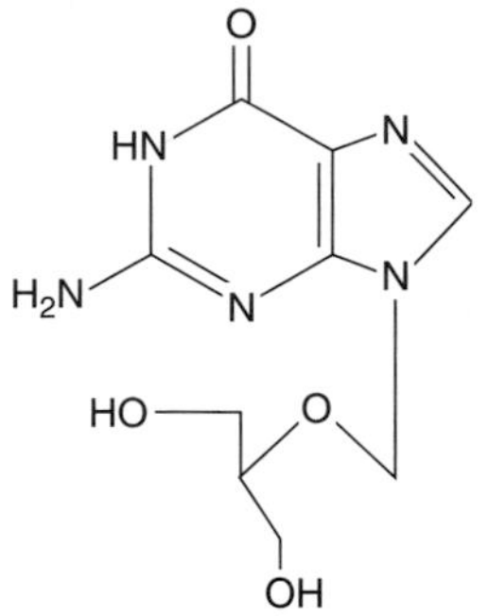

Ganciclovir

CMV.[76,77] Ganciclovir has good in vitro activity against HSV-1, HSV-2, VZV, and EBV and is active against HHV-6 and HBV. The mechanism of action of ganciclovir is similar to that of acyclovir. Ganciclovir is initially phosphorylated by virus-encoded kinases, which, in the case of CMV-infected cells, is a protein kinase encoded by the UL97 gene of CMV.[78,79] Ganciclovir triphosphate competitively inhibits herpesvirus DNA polymerases and also inhibits elongation of the nascent DNA chain. HSV and VZV viruses may be resistant to ganciclovir through thymidine kinase deficiency, and thus would be expected to share cross resistance with viruses that are resistant to acyclovir on the same basis. Ganciclovir-resistant viruses may also arise through mutations in the viral DNA polymerase, which may be at a different locus than that found with acyclovir-resistant DNA polymerase mutants. Thus, viruses resistant to acyclovir on the basis of DNA polymerase mutation may retain sensitivity to ganciclovir. Ganciclovir-resistant CMV isolates may arise through mutations in the UL97 gene, in which case such viruses remain susceptible to foscarnet or cidofovir (see below). CMV isolates that are resistant to ganciclovir on the basis of DNA polymerase mutations may also be resistant to cidofovir and foscarnet.

PHARMACOKINETICS Ganciclovir is available as either an intravenous or an oral preparation. Because of low oral bioavailability (5 to 9 percent), relatively large doses of ganciclovir need to be administered orally (1 g PO 3 times/day) to achieve an effect.[80] Oral bioavailability is improved by administration with food. Intravenous administration of a dose of 5 mg/kg results in a peak plasma concentration of 8 to 11 μg/mL with a serum half-life of 3.5 h.[81] Oral administration of 1 g of ganciclovir results in a peak plasma concentration of 1 μg/mL approximately 4.5 h after administration.[82,83] Ganciclovir is excreted primarily by the kidney unmetabolized, and dosage should be reduced in patients with renal dysfunction. Ganciclovir has also been administered intraocularly by intravitreous injection and by the implantation of sustained-release devices in the eye.

ADVERSE EFFECTS The major toxicity associated with ganciclovir is bone marrow suppression, particularly neutropenia and thrombocytopenia.[83] This effect occurs most frequently in patients with underlying bone marrow compromise and is worsened by concomitant administration of other hematotoxic drugs, such as zidovudine. The oral administration of ganciclovir has lower rates of hematologic toxicity, presumably as a result of poor systemic absorption.

Neurotoxicity, fever, liver function abnormalities, and a variety of gastrointestinal symptoms, especially diarrhea, have also been noted. Gastrointestinal intolerance may be a particular problem in patients taking the drug orally. The risk of seizures may be increased when ganciclovir and imipenem are administered concurrently.

CLINICAL USEFULNESS Ganciclovir is widely used for treatment and, in a more limited way, for prophylaxis of CMV infections in immunosuppressed patients. Its most well-established use is for the treatment of CMV retinitis in patients with AIDS,[84] for whom an initial regimen of 5 mg/kg intravenously twice a day for 14 to 21 days is followed by a maintenance regimen of 5 mg/kg intravenously 5 times/week, indefinitely. The use of oral ganciclovir (1 g PO tid) or ocular ganciclovir implants are alternative modes for maintenance therapy. Ganciclovir is effective for the treatment of gastrointestinal disease caused by CMV in immunosuppressed patients.[85] It is also used for the treatment of CMV-associated pneumonia and neurologic disease, although responses are poor in these cases. Oral ganciclovir has been used in the prophylaxis of CMV disease in patients with AIDS, but two large-scale studies came to different conclusions regarding the benefits of its use for that purpose.[86,87]

Ganciclovir is used for the treatment of CMV infections in patients who are immunosuppressed as a result of organ transplantation. Responses have been variable and, in general, have been better in patients receiving solid organ transplants than in those receiving bone marrow transplants.[88] Various strategies have been employed in attempts to provide prophylaxis against the development of CMV disease in transplant recipients.[89] These have included prophylactic administration of ganciclovir during the time of intensive immunosuppression and "preemptive therapy" when CMV virus is detected in the blood by highly sensitive assays, but before disease is manifested clinically. The use of ganciclovir in combination with anti-CMV immunoglobulin and in combination with other anti-CMV drugs such as foscarnet (see below) is being evaluated.

Foscarnet

ANTIVIRAL ACTIVITY Foscarnet (trisodium phosphonoformate, Foscavir) (Fig. 259-8) is a pyrophosphate-containing compound that is active in vitro against HSV-1, HSV-2, VZV, CMV, EBV, HHV-6, HBV, and HIV. Foscarnet noncompetitively inhibits viral DNA polymerases at the pyrophosphate-binding site.[90] In contrast to the nucleoside analogues discussed above, foscarnet does not require phosphorylation for its antiviral activity and is therefore active against viruses that are resistant to acyclovir, famciclovir, or ganciclovir on the basis of absent or altered kinase activities. CMV isolates resistant to ganciclovir on the basis of DNA polymerase

FIGURE 259-8

Foscarnet

mutations may also be resistant to foscarnet, although foscarnet-resistant HSV and CMV isolates are variable in their sensitivities to ganciclovir. Some isolates that are resistant to both acyclovir and foscarnet may remain sensitive to cidofovir (see below).

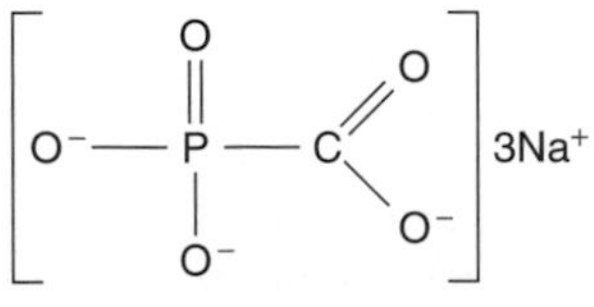

PHARMACOKINETICS Foscarnet is currently available only in an intravenous preparation that has poor solubility and must be administered by an infusion pump in a dilute solution over 1 to 2 h. The plasma half-life of the drug consists of an initial phase of 4 to 8 h and a terminal component of 88 h or more, which reflects a deposition in bone of up to 20 percent of the dose.[91,92] Eighty percent of the dose is excreted unmetabolized by the kidney, and the dosage should be reduced with renal dysfunction.

ADVERSE EFFECTS The major toxicity associated with foscarnet involves the kidney, and its use requires close monitoring of renal function, particularly during the initial phases of therapy.[93] Saline hydration before administration and slow infusion of the drug appear to reduce nephrotoxicity.[94] Electrolyte abnormalities such as hypo- and hypercalcemia, hypo- or hyperphosphatemia, hypomagnesemia, and hypokalemia have been described. Some of these electrolyte abnormalities appear to be related to the ability of foscarnet to bind divalent cations, whereas the mechanism for others may be related to the interaction of foscarnet with renal function or with bone metabolism. Neurologic toxicities, including tremors, seizures, and altered consciousness, have been described. Although anemia and, to a lesser extent, neutropenia have been reported with foscarnet administration, hematologic toxicity is less than that with ganciclovir, and foscarnet can often be administered along with myelosuppressive agents. Genital ulcerations have been noted as a result of high concentrations of foscarnet in the urine.[95]

CLINICAL USEFULNESS The major use for foscarnet is in the treatment of CMV retinitis in patients with AIDS. A comparative clinical trial demonstrated that foscarnet was similarly efficacious to ganciclovir as first-line treatment of CMV retinitis but was associated with longer survival than ganciclovir, perhaps related to the anti-HIV activity of foscarnet.[96] The initial dosage of foscarnet is 60 mg/kg intravenously q8h for 14 to 21 days, followed by a maintenance dose of 120 mg/kg per day. Foscarnet is also used for the treatment of HSV or VZV infection resistant to acyclovir[97] and for ganciclovir-resistant CMV infection.[98] Foscarnet-resistant CMV viruses may emerge on therapy.

Cidofovir

ANTIVIRAL ACTIVITY Cidofovir {(S)-1-[3-hydroxy-2 (phosphonylmethoxy)-propyl] cytosine, Vistide} (Fig. 259-9) is a phosphonate nucleotide analogue, with activity against a broad range of herpesviruses, including CMV, against which is its major use.[99] Cidofovir does not require initial phosphorylation by virus-induced kinases but is converted by host cell enzymes to cidofovir diphosphate, which is a competitive inhibitor of viral DNA polymerases and, to a lesser extent, of host cell DNA polymerases.[100] Cidofovir is usually active against CMV isolates that are resistant to ganciclovir and foscarnet, although viruses that are resistant to all three drugs have been described.

PHARMACOKINETICS Cidofovir is approved for intravenous administration, and a topical formulation and ocular implant are being evaluated. An intravenous dose of 5 mg/kg results in a peak plasma concentration of 11.5 μg/mL.[101] The plasma half-life of cidofovir is 2.6 h, and the drug is excreted almost entirely by the kidney.[102]

FIGURE 259-9

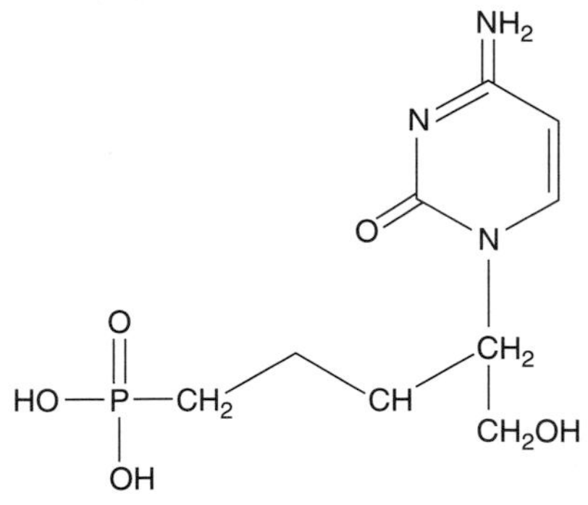

CHAPTER 259
Antiviral Drugs

2843

Cidofovir

Cidofovir diphosphate has a markedly prolonged intracellular half-life (more than 48 h), which is the basis for the recommended dosing regimen of 5 mg/kg twice a week for the initial 2 weeks, followed by one dose every 2 weeks.[103]

ADVERSE EFFECTS   The major toxicity associated with cidofovir is renal tubular damage, manifested by proteinuria and elevated serum creatinine levels.[104] Hydration, along with the administration of probenecid before and after administration, appears to protect against nephrotoxicity. Rashes have been reported in patients receiving cidofovir and probenecid.

CLINICAL USEFULNESS   Cidofovir is approved for the treatment of CMV retinitis in patients with AIDS who have either failed treatment with ganciclovir and foscarnet or are intolerant of them. A study of 60 such patients indicated that a dose of 5 mg/kg resulted in longer time to progression of CMV retinitis than did a dose of 3 mg/kg.[105] Intravitreous administration of cidofovir has also been employed as a maintenance regimen. Topical cidofovir is currently being evaluated as a treatment for acyclovir-resistant HSV infection and for human papillomavirus infections.

INTERFERONS

Interferons are cytokines that have broad antiviral, immunomodulating, and antiproliferative effects.[106,107] The antiviral activities of interferons are multiple and complex and vary according to the cell type and virus being examined. Interferons have been studied in a variety of viral infections as well as in a number of diseases of noninfectious etiology. For viral infections, IFN-α has been studied most extensively, and three such preparations are currently approved for the treatment of certain viral infections: IFN-α2a (Roferon-A), IFN-α2b (Intron-A), and leukocyte-derived IFN-αn3 (Alferon N). Interferon may be administered intravenously, or, more commonly, subcutaneously or intramuscularly. The plasma half-life after intravenous administration of IFN-α is 2 to 3 h and after subcutaneous or intramuscular administration is 4 to 6 h.[108] However, the relationship between conventional pharmacokinetic measurements and the antiviral activities of interferon is unclear.

The most common adverse effects of interferon are fever, chills, headache, myalgia, arthralgia, and gastrointestinal symptoms.[109] These are generally dose-related and are often most prominent with the initial doses of therapy. Granulocytopenia, thrombocytopenia,

various neurotoxicities, alopecia, hepatotoxicity, and autoantibody formation have also been noted.[109]

Recombinant IFN-α2b[110] and leukocyte-derived IFN-αn3[111] have been approved for the intralesional treatment of condylomata acuminata, for which purpose they have proved to be modestly effective in placebo-controlled studies. Interferon is most commonly administered in a volume of 0.1 mL through a 30-gauge needle directly into each wart. The recommended dose of IFN-α2b is 1 million units to each wart three times a week for 3 weeks. Significant systemic absorption and associated side effects can result from the intralesional administration of interferon. Systemic (parenteral) administration of interferon has been evaluated as therapy for extensive and refractory warts. In these studies, parenterally administered interferon was associated chiefly with a reduction in the size of warts but not with a decrease in recurrence rates compared to placebo, although there was some interstudy variability in findings.[112,113]

Interferons have been extensively evaluated in the treatment of chronic HBV and chronic hepatitis C virus (HCV) infection.[109] The administration of recombinant IFN-α2b at a dose of 5 million units per day for 16 weeks resulted in disappearance of HBV DNA in 37 percent of patients and loss of hepatitis B e antigen in 33 percent of patients.[114] Approximately 8 percent of all patients lost hepatitis B surface antigen. In most patients who responded, improvements were sustained for extended periods of time after therapy was discontinued. Predictors of a response to interferon therapy are low HBV DNA levels, high alanine and aspartate aminotransferase levels, short duration of infection, and histopathologic evidence of active hepatitis.[109]

Interferon-α2b has been approved for the treatment of chronic HCV infection. The administration of 3 million units of IFN-α2b three times a week for 24 weeks was associated with a return to normal serum alanine aminotransferase values and improvement in liver histopathology in approximately 40 to 50 percent of patients.[109,115] However, approximately half of such patients relapse after discontinuation of therapy, although some responded to retreatment. Favorable responses were associated with short duration of infection, lower levels of circulating HCV RNA, minimal amounts of hepatic fibrosis, and low hepatic iron stores and with certain HCV genotypes that appear to be more sensitive to interferon.[109] Recently, the addition of ribavirin (Rebetron), 1000–1200 mg PO daily for 24 weeks, to interferon therapy has been demonstrated to be beneficial for patients with HIV infection who relapsed after interferon therapy had been stopped.[116] The FDA has approved the use of combined IFN-α2b and ribavirin for this purpose.

DRUGS FOR THE TREATMENT OF HIV INFECTION

The development of antiretroviral drugs to combat HIV infection has been an area of intense preclinical and clinical research activity. Currently there are eleven approved antiretroviral drugs, and it is likely that additional drugs will receive approval in the near future. Strategies for the use of antiretrovirals have emerged from large-scale clinical trials as well as from advances in our understanding of the pathogenesis of HIV-1 infection. These studies have established two important principles on which recommendations for the use of antiretroviral drugs are based: (1) combination therapy rather than monotherapy should be employed to minimize the emergence of resistant viruses,[117] and (2) virus load should be monitored as an important parameter of the effectiveness of antiviral therapy.[118] Specific recommendations for the use of individual anti-HIV drugs and detailed descriptions of the properties of each drug itself are beyond the scope of this chapter and are reviewed elsewhere.[117,119] Presented below are brief discussions of the major properties of each of the antiretroviral drugs that are currently available.

Reverse Transcriptase Inhibitors

Nucleoside analogues that inhibit HIV-1 and HIV-2 reverse transcriptases have been the most extensively studied antiretroviral drugs. The currently available drugs—zidovudine, didanosine, zalcitabine, stavudine, and lamivudine—require phosphorylation to the triphosphate form to inhibit viral reverse transcriptases. Resistance to each drug can develop by one or more amino acid substitutions in the HIV reverse transcriptase. Each nucleoside analogue has its own pharmacokinetic profile and characteristic set of toxicities, which determine its suitability for use in individual patients and in combination with other antiretrovirals. The major toxic effects of each drug are as follows: zidovudine, myelosuppression; didanosine, pancreatitis and peripheral neuropathy; zalcitabine, peripheral neuropathy, mucosal ulcerations, and pancreatitis; stavudine, peripheral neuropathy and pancreatitis in pediatric patients; and lamivudine, neutropenia at high doses.

Nucleoside analogues are most frequently used in two-drug or three-drug combination regimens. The most common combinations are zidovudine and lamivudine, zidovudine and didanosine, and stavudine and lamivudine. Zidovudine and stavudine appear to be antagonistic in vitro, and probably in vivo; didanosine and zalcitabine are rarely used together because of overlapping toxicities. The most common resistance mutation associated with lamivudine (substitution of isoleucine or valine for methionine at position 184 in the reverse transcriptase) appears to protect against the development of phenotypic resistance to zidovudine and may account in part for the particular efficacy of regimens containing zidovudine and lamivudine.[120]

Nonnucleoside reverse transcriptase inhibitors (NNRTIs) have also demonstrated antiviral efficacy. Of this class of drugs, nevirapine and delavirdine have recently been approved for use against HIV-1.[121] NNRTIs are compounds of diverse chemical structure that inhibit HIV-1 reverse transcriptase at a characteristic region of the enzyme, generally through noncompetitive alosteric binding. These compounds are active against HIV-1 reverse transcriptases but not against HIV-2 reverse transcriptases. NNRTIs have potent HIV-1 activity in vitro and in vivo, but their use as single agents has resulted in the rapid emergence of resistance. Thus, the appropriate use of NNRTIs is as part of combination therapy regimens. The major toxic effect associated with nevirapine has been a nonpruritic maculopapular rash, which occurs in almost half of patients who receive 400 mg/day of the drug. The frequency of the rash may be reduced by beginning at lower initial doses (200 mg/day) and increasing the dose to 400 mg/day after 2 weeks. Rash is also frequently encountered with delavirdine, but lower initial doses are not recommended.

Protease Inhibitors

The protease inhibitors are an important new class of anti-HIV-1 drugs.[119] These compounds inhibit a virus-specific enzyme that is responsible for the proteolytic cleavage of viral polypeptide precursors. Currently, the protease inhibitors that have been approved for use against HIV-1 infections in the United States are saquinavir, indinavir, ritonavir, and nelfinavir. Each protease inhibitor has a unique pharmacokinetic profile, but all are metabolized through the hepatic cytochrome P_{450} system. Thus, they have important interactions with the drugs that induce, inhibit, or are themselves metabolized by cytochrome P_{450}. Saquinavir is well tolerated, and a recently available soft gel capsule has improved bioavailability. Indinavir is poorly soluble and has been associated with both nephrolithiasis and elevated indirect bilirubin levels. The major toxicity associated with ritonavir is gastrointestinal intolerance, which limits its use in some patients. Ritonavir also inhibits the metabolism of saquinavir, and the use of the two drugs in combination is being evaluated to improve blood levels of saquinavir. The molecular basis for resistance to protease inhibitors is complex, but resistance clearly develops when the drugs are used as monotherapy. Therefore, the appropriate use of protease inhibitors is as part of multidrug combination regimens. Several such regimens have been reported to have potent, sustained antiviral and clinical effects.[119]

Other Antiretroviral Drugs

Other steps in the HIV replication pathway have been targeted for the development of antiviral drugs. These include inhibitors of virus-cell fusion, synthesis of virus envelope, and nucleocapsid assembly. It is likely that these and other novel approaches to inhibit virus replication will be entering clinical evaluation in the future.

REFERENCES

1. Whitley RJ et al: Acyclovir: A decade later. *N Engl J Med* **327**:782, 1992
2. Schaeffer HJ: Acyclovir chemistry and spectrum of activity. *Am J Med* **73**:4, 1982
3. Biron KK et al: In vitro susceptibility of varicella-zoster virus to acyclovir. *Antimicrob Agents Chemother* **18**:443, 1980
4. Datta AK et al: Acyclovir inhibition of Epstein-Barr virus replication. *Proc Natl Acad Sci USA* **77**:5163, 1980
5. Russler SK et al: Susceptibility of human herpesvirus 6 to acyclovir and ganciclovir. *Lancet* **2**:382, 1989
6. Elion GB: Mechanism of action and selectivity of acyclovir. *Am J Med* **73**:7, 1982
7. Coen DM et al: Two distinct loci confer resistance to acycloguanosine in herpes simplex virus type 1. *Proc Natl Acad Sci USA* **77**:2265, 1980
8. Schnipper LE et al: Resistance of herpes simplex virus to acycloguanosine: Role of viral thymidine kinase and DNA polymerase loci. *Proc Natl Acad Sci USA* **77**:2270, 1980
9. Van Dyke RB et al: Pharmcokinetics of orally administered acyclovir in patients with herpes progenitalis. *Am J Med* **73**(suppl):172, 1982
10. McKendrick MW et al: Oral acyclovir in acute herpes zoster. *Br Med J* **293**:1529, 1986
11. Laskin OL: Clinical pharmacokinetics of acyclovir. *Clin Pharmacol* **8**:187, 1983
12. Laskin OL et al: Effect of renal failure on the pharmacokinetics of acyclovir. *Am J Med* **73**(suppl):197, 1982
13. Sawyer MH et al: Acyclovir-induced renal failure: Clinical course and histology. *Am J Med* **84**:1067, 1988
14. Rashed A et al: Acyclovir-induced acute tubulointerstitial nephritis. *Nephron* **56**:436, 1990
15. Feldman S et al: Excessive serum concentrations of acyclovir and neurotoxicity. *J Infect Dis* **157**:385, 1988
16. Haefeli WE et al: Acyclovir-induced neurotoxicity: Concentration-side effect relationship in acyclovir overdose. *Am J Med* **94**:212, 1993
17. Wade JC et al: Intravenous acyclovir to treat mucocutaneous herpes simplex infection after marrow transplantation. *Ann Intern Med* **96**:265, 1982
18. Shepp DH et al: Oral acyclovir therapy for mucocutaneous herpes simplex infections in immunocompromised marrow transplant recipients. *Ann Intern Med* **102**:783, 1985

19. Saral R et al: Acyclovir prophylaxis of herpes-simplex virus infections. *N Engl J Med* **305**:63, 1981

20. Corey L et al: Intravenous acyclovir for the treatment of primary genital herpes. *Ann Intern Med* **98**:914, 1983

21. Bryson YJ et al: Treatment of first episodes of genital herpes simplex virus infection with oral acyclovir. *N Engl J Med* **308**:916, 1983

22. Reichman RC et al: Treament of recurrent genital herpes simplex infections with oral acyclovir. A controlled trial. *JAMA* **251**:2103, 1984

23. Straus SE et al: Suppression of frequently recurring genital herpes: A placebo-controlled double-blind trial of oral acyclovir. *N Engl J Med* **310**:1545, 1984

24. Spruance SL et al: Treatment of recurrent herpes simplex labialis with oral acyclovir. *J Infect Dis* **161**:185, 1990

25. Spruance SL et al: Acyclovir prevents reactivation of herpes simplex in skiers. *JAMA* **260**:1597, 1988

26. Corey L et al: A trial of topical acyclovir in genital herpes simplex infections. *N Engl J Med* **306**:1313, 1992

27. Spruance SL et al: Treatment of herpes simplex labialis with topical acyclovir in polyethylene glycol. *J Infect Dis* **146**:85, 1982

28. Whitley RJ et al: Vidarabine versus acyclovir therapy in herpes simplex encephalitis. *N Engl J Med* **314**:144, 1986

29. Whitley RJ et al: A controlled trial comparing vidarabine with acyclovir in neonatal herpes simplex virus infection. *N Engl J Med* **324**:444, 1991

30. Balfour HH Jr et al: Acyclovir halts progression of herpes zoster in immunocompromised patients. *N Engl J Med* **308**:1448, 1983

31. Huff C et al: Therapy of herpes zoster with oral acyclovir. *Am J Med* **85**(A2A):84, 1988

32. Beutner KR et al: Valaciclovir compared with acyclovir for improved therapy for herpes zoster in immunocompetent adults. *Antimicrob Agents Chemother* **39**:1546, 1995

33. Wood MF et al: A randomized trial of acyclovir for 7 days or 21 days with and without prednisolone for treatment of acute herpes zoster. *N Engl J Med* **330**:896, 1994

34. Whitley RJ et al: Acyclovir with and without prednisone for the treatment of herpes zoster. *Ann Intern Med* **125**:376, 1996

35. Cobo LM et al: Oral acyclovir in the treatment of acute herpes zoster ophthalmicus. *Ophthalmology* **93**:763, 1986

36. Prober CG et al: Acyclovir therapy of chickenpox in immunosuppressed children—a collaborative study. *J Pediatr* **101**:622, 1982

37. Nyerges G et al: Acyclovir prevents dissemination of varicella in immunocompromised children. *J Infect Dis* **157**:309, 1988

38. Dunkel L et al: A controlled trial of oral acyclovir for chickenpox in normal children. *N Engl J Med* **325**:1539, 1991

39. Wallace MR et al: Treatment of adult varicella with oral acyclovir. A randomized, placebo-controlled trial. *Ann Intern Med* **117**:358, 1992

40. Myers JD et al: Acyclovir for prevention of cytomegalovirus infection and disease after allogenic marrow transplantation. *N Engl J Med* **318**:70, 1988

41. Andersson J et al: Effect of acyclovir on infectious mononucleosis: A double-blind, placebo-controlled study. *J Infect Dis* **153**:283, 1986

42. Sullivan JL et al: Treatment of life-threatening Epstein-Barr virus infections with acyclovir. *Am J Med* **73**(suppl):262, 1982

43. Beutner KR: Valacyclovir: A review of its antiviral activity, pharmacokinetic properties, and clinical efficacy. *Antiviral Res* **28**:281, 1995

44. Jacobson MA: Valacyclovir (BW256U87): The L-valyl ester of acyclovir. *J Med Virol* **1**(suppl):150, 1993

45. Weller S et al: Pharmacokinetics of the acyclovir pro-drug valacyclovir after escalating single- and multiple-dose administration to normal volunteers. *Clin Pharmacol Ther* **54**:595, 1993

46. Wang LH et al: Pharmacokinetics and safety of multiple-dose valaciclovir in geriatric volunteers with and without concomitant diuretic therapy. *Antimicrob Agents Chemother* **40**:80, 1996

47. Valtrex, package insert, Glaxo Wellcome, Research Triangle Park, NC 27709, March 1995

48. Spruance SL et al: A large-scale placebo-controlled dose-ranging trial of peroral valacyclovir for episodic treatment of recurrent herpes genitalis. *Arch Intern Med* **156**:1729, 1996

49. Weinberg A et al: In vitro activities of penciclovir and acyclovir against herpes simplex virus types 1 and 2. *Antimicrob Agents Chemother* **36**:2037, 1992

50. Earnshaw DL et al: Mode of anitviral action of penciclovir in MRC-5 cells infected with herpes simplex virus type 1 (HSV-1), HSV-2, and varicella-zoster virus. *Antimicrob Agents Chemother* **36**:2747, 1992

51. Vere Hodge RA: Famciclovir and penciclovir. The mode of action of famciclovir including its conversion to penciclovir. *Antiviral Chem Chemother* **4**(2):67, 1993

52. Clarke SE et al: Role of aldehyde oxidase in the in vitro conversion of famciclovir to penciclovir in human liver. *Drug Metab Dispos* **23**:251, 1995

53. Pue MA et al: Linear pharmacokinetics of penciclovir following administration of single oral doses of famciclovir 125, 250, 500 and 750 mg to healthy volunteers. *J Antimicrob Chemother* **33**:119, 1994

54. Boike SC et al: Pharmacokinetics of famciclovir in subjects with varying degrees of renal impairment. *Clin Pharmacol Ther* **55**:418, 1994

55. Talarico CL et al: Analysis of the thymidine kinase genes from acyclovir-resistant mutants of varicella-zoster virus isolated from patients with AIDS. *J Virol* **67**:1024, 1993

56. Famciclovir, package insert, SmithKline Beecham, Philadelphia, PA, June 1994

57. Tyring S et al: Famciclovir for the treatment of acute herpes zoster: Effects on acute disease and postherpetic neuralgia: A randomized, double-blind, placebo-controlled trial. *Ann Intern Med* **123**:89, 1995

58. Sacks SL et al: Patient- and clinic-initiated treatment of recurrent genital herpes with twice daily oral famciclovir. 7th European Congress of Clinical Microbiology and Infectious Diseases, Vienna, March 26–30, 1995

59. Portnoy et al: Famciclovir in the treatment of herpes zoster infection. Abstract 119, Seventh International Conference on Antiviral Research, Charleston, South Carolina, February, 1994

60. Prusoff WH: Idoxuridine or how it all began, in *Clinical Use of Antiviral Drugs*, edited by E DeClercq. Norwell, MA, Martinus Nijhoff, 1988, p 15

61. Pavan-Langston D: Major ocular viral infections, in *Antiviral Agents and Viral Diseases of Man*, 3d ed, edited by GJ Gallaso, RJ Whitley, TC Merigan. New York, Raven, 1990, p 183

62. MacCallum FO et al: Herpes simplex virus skin infection in man treated with idoxuridine in dimethyl sulfoxide. Results of double-blind controlled trial. *Br Med J* **2**:805, 1966

63. Boston Interhospital Virus Study Group et al: Failure of high dose 5-iodo-2'-deoxyuridine in the therapy of herpes simplex virus encephalitis. *N Engl J Med* **292**:599, 1975

64. Carmine AA et al: Trifluridine: A review of its antiviral activity and therapeutic use in the topical treatment of viral eye infections. *Drugs* **23**:329, 1982

65. Kaufman HE: The treatment of herpetic eye infections with trifluridine and other antivirals, in *Clinical Use of Antiviral Drugs*, edited by E DeClercq. Norwell, MA, Martinus Nijhoff, 1988, p 25

66. Van Bijsterveld OP: Trifluorothymidine versus adenine arabinoside in the treatment of herpes simplex keratitis. *Br J Ophthalmol* **64**:33, 1980

67. De Koning EWJ et al: Combination therapy for dendritic keratitis with human leukocyte interferon and trifluorothymidine. *Br J Ophthalmol* **66**:509, 1982

68. Gephart JF et al: Comparison of the effects of arabinosyladenine, arabinosylhypoxanthine, and arabinosyladenine 5'-monophosphate against herpes simplex virus, varicella-zoster virus, and cytomegalovirus with their effects on cellular deoxyribonucleic acid synthesis. *Antimicrob Agents Chemother* **19**:170, 1981

69. Whitley RJ et al: Vidarabine: A preliminary review of its pharmacological properties and therapeutic use. *Drugs* **20**:267, 1980

70. Burdge DR et al: Neurotoxic effects during vidarabine therapy for herpes zoster. *Can Med Assoc J* **132**:392, 1985

71. Whitley RJ et al: Vidarabine therapy of mucocutaneous herpes simplex virus infections in the immunocompromised host. *J Infect Dis* **149**:1, 1984

72. Whitley RJ et al: Adenine arabinoside therapy of biopsy-proved herpes simplex encephalitis. National Institute of Allergy and Infectious Diseases Collaborative Antiviral Study. *N Engl J Med* **297**:289, 1977

73. Whitley RJ et al: Adenine arabinoside therapy of herpes zoster in the immunosuppressed. NIAID Collaborative Antiviral Study. *N Engl J Med* **294**:1193, 1976

74. Whitley RJ et al: Vidarabine therapy of neonatal herpes simplex virus infection. *Pediatrics* **66**:495, 1980

75. Hyndiuk RA et al: Adenine arabinoside in idoxuridine unresponsive and intolerant herpetic keratitis. *Am J Ophthalmol* **79**:655, 1975

76. Field AK et al: 9-{[2-Hydroxy-1(hydroxymethyl) ethoxy] methyl} guanine: A selective inhibitor of herpes group virus replication. *Proc Natl Acad Sci USA* **80**:4139, 1983.

77. Plotkin SA et al: Sensitivity of clinical isolates of human cytomegalovirus to 9-(1,3-dihydroxy-2-propoxymethyl) guanine. *J Infect Dis* **152**:833, 1985

78. Littler E et al: Human cytomegalovirus UL97 open reading frame encodes a protein that phosphorylates the antiviral nucleoside analogue ganciclovir. *Nature* **358**:160, 1992

79. Sullivan V et al: A protein kinase homologue controls phosphorylation of ganciclovir in human cytomegalovirus-infected cells. *Nature* **358**:162, 1992

80. Spector SA et al: Pharmacokinetic, safety, and antiviral profiles of oral ganciclovir in persons infected with human immunodeficiency virus: A phase I/II study. *J Infect Dis* **171**:1431, 1995

81. Yuen GJ et al: Population differences in ganciclovir clearance as determined by nonlinear mixed-effects modeling. *Antimicrob Agents Chemother* **39**:2350, 1995

82. Jacobson MA et al: Human pharmacokinetics and tolerance of oral ganciclovir. *Antimicrob Agents Chemother* **31**:1251, 1987

83. Markham A et al: Ganciclovir: An update of its therapeutic use in cytomegalovirus infection. *Drugs* **48**:455, 1994

84. Masur H et al: Advances in the management of AIDS-related cytomegalovirus retinitis. *Ann Intern Med* **125**:126, 1996

85. Chachoua A et al: 9-(1,3-Dihydroxy-2-propoxymethyl)guanine (ganciclovir) in the treatment of cytomegalovirus gastrointestinal disease with the acquired immunodeficiency syndrome. *Ann Intern Med* **107**:133, 1987

86. Spector SA et al: Oral ganciclovir for the prevention of cytomegalovirus disease in persons with AIDS. *N Engl J Med* **334**:1491, 1996

87. Brosgard CL et al: Randomized, placebo-controlled trial of the safety and efficacy of oral ganciclovir for prophylaxis of cytomegalovirus retinal and gastrointestinal mucosal disease in HIV-infected individuals with severe immunosuppression. Abstracts of the 35th ICAAC, Abstract no. LB-10, San Francisco, CA, 1995

88. Rubin RH et al: Antimicrobial strategies in the care of organ transplant recipients. *Antimicrob Agents Chemother* **37**:619, 1993

89. Goodrich JM et al: Strategies for the prevention of cytomegalovirus disease after marrow transplantation. *Clin Infect Dis* **19**:287, 1994

90. Crumpacker CS: Mechanism of action of foscarnet against viral polymerases. *Am J Med* **92**(suppl 2A):2A, 1992

91. Wagstaff AJ et al: Foscarnet: A reappraisal of its antiviral activity, pharmacokinetic properties and therapeutic use in immunocompromised patients with viral infections. *Drugs* **48**:199, 1994

92. Aweeka F et al: Pharmacokinetics of intermittently administered intravenous foscarnet in the treatment of acquired immunodeficiency syndrome patients with serious cytomegalovirus retinitis. *Antimicrob Agents Chemother* **33**:742, 1989

93. The AIDS Clinical Trials Group: Morbidity and toxic effects associated with ganciclovir or foscarnet therapy in a randomized cytomegalovirus retinitis trial: Studies of ocular complications of AIDS research group. *Arch Intern Med* **155**:64, 1995

94. Deray G et al: Foscarnet nephrotoxicity: Mechanism, incidence and prevention. *Am J Nephrol* **9**:316, 1989

95. Van Der Pijl JW et al: Foscarnet and penile ulceration. *Lancet* **1**:266, 1990

96. Studies of Ocular Complications of AIDS Research Group, in Collaboration with the AIDS Clinical Trials Group: Mortality in patients with the acquired immunodeficiency syndrome treated with either foscarnet or ganciclovir for cytomegalovirus retinitis. *N Engl J Med* **326**:213, 1992

97. Hardy WD: Foscarnet treatment of acyclovir-resistant herpes simplex virus infection in patients with acquired immunodeficiency syndrome: Preliminary results of a controlled, randomized, regimen-comparative trial. *Am J Med* **92**(suppl 2A):30S, 1992

98. Drobyski WR et al: Foscarnet therapy of ganciclovir-resistant cytomegalovirus in marrow transplantation. *Transplantation* **52**:155, 1991

99. Neyts J et al: Mechanism of action of acyclic nucleoside phosphonates against herpes virus replication. *Biochem Pharmacol* **47**:39, 1995

100. Neyts J et al: Particular characteristics of the anti-human cytomegalovirus activity of (S)-1-(3-hydroxy-2-phosphonylmethoxyprophy) cytosine (HPMPC) in vitro. *Antiviral Res* **16**:41, 1991

101. Vistide, Package insert, Gilead Sciences, Foster City, CA, June 1996

102. Cundy KC et al: Clinical pharmacokinetics of cidofovir in HIV-infected patients. *Antimicrob Agents Chemother* **39**:1247, 1995

103. Bronson JJL et al: (S)-1-(3-Hydroxy-2-(phosphonylmethoxy)propyl)cystosine (HPMPC): A potent antiherpesvirus agent, in *Immunobiology and Prophylaxis of Human Herpesvirus Infections*, edited by C. Lopez et al. New York, Plenum, 1991, p 277

104. Polis MA et al: Anticytomegaloviral activity and safety of cidofovir in patients with human immunodeficiency virus infection and cytomegalovirus viruria. *Antimicrob Agents Chemother* **39**:882, 1995

105. Lalezari J et al: A randomized, controlled study of cidofovir for relapsing cytomegalovirus retinitis in patients with AIDS. Abstracts of the 35th ICAAC, Abstract 1, 1995

106. Greenberg SB: Human interferon in viral diseases. *Infect Dis Clin North Am* **1**:383, 1987

107. Sen GC et al: The interferon system. *J Biol Chem* **267**:5017, 1992

108. Wills RJ: Clinical pharmacokinetics of interferons. *Clin Pharmacokinet* **19**:390, 1990

109. Hoofnagle JH et al: The treatment of chronic viral hepatitis. *N Engl J Med* **336**:347, 1997

110. Eron LJ et al: Interferon therapy for condylomata acuminata. *N Engl J Med* **315**:1059, 1986

111. Friedman-Kien A et al: Natural interferon alfa for treatment of condylomata acuminata. *JAMA* **259**:533, 1988

112. Reichman RC et al: Treatment of condyloma acuminatum with three different alpha interferon preparations administered parenterally: A double-blind, placebo-controlled trial. *J Infect Dis* **162**:1270, 1990

113. Condylomata International Collaborative Study Group: Recurrent condylomata acuminata treated with recombinant interferon alfa-2a. A multicenter double-blind placebo-controlled clinical trial. *JAMA* **265**:2684, 1991

114. Wong DKH et al: Effect of alpha-interferon treatment in patients with hepatitis B e antigen–positive chronic hepatitis B: A meta-analysis. *Ann Intern Med* **119**:312, 1993

115. Poynard T et al: Meta-analysis of interferon randomized trials in the treatment of viral hepatitis C: Effects of dose and duration. *Hepatology* **24**:778, 1996

116. Reichard O et al: Randomized, double-blind, placebo-controlled trial of interferon α-2b with and without ribavirin for chronic hepatitis C. *Lancet* **351**:83, 1996

117. Carpenter CCJ et al: Antiretroviral therapy for HIV infection in 1996. *JAMA* **276**:146, 1996

118. Saag MS et al: HIV viral load markers in clinical practice: Recommendations of an International AIDS Society-USA Expert Panel. *Nat Med* **2**:625, 1996

119. Deeks SG et al: HIV-1 protease inhibitors. *JAMA* **277**:145, 1997

120. Larder BA et al: Potential mechanisms for sustained antiviral efficacy of AZT-3TC combination therapy. *Science* **269**:696, 1995

121. Havlir D et al: High-dose nevirapine: Safety, pharmacokinetics, and antiviral effects in patients with human immunodeficiency virus infection. *J Infect Dis* **171**:537, 1995

Oral Antifungal Agents

In order to eliminate refractory dermatomycoses and onychomycosis, physicians must familiarize themselves with the systemic antifungal agents available. Prior to 1990, only two oral antifungal agents had been released over three decades. The first and the only synthetic agent was griseofulvin. Subsequently other drugs, including amphotericin B and ketoconazole, were introduced. Unfortunately, prolonged treatment courses, poor oral bioavailability, and potentially serious side effects discouraged physicians from using these drugs. As a result of recent advancements in antifungal chemotherapy, new drugs with a broad spectrum of activity, high efficacy, tolerability, and with rare and mild side effects are now available.

Three new oral antifungal agents that have been released are the first oral allylamine, terbinafine (Lamisil), and the triazoles fluconazole (Diflucan) and itraconazole (Sporanox). Rational selection of therapy depends on the mechanism of action of each agent and an understanding of tissue pharmacokinetics, spectrum of clinical activity, potential adverse reactions, significant drug interactions, efficacy, and optimal dosage protocols.

TERBINAFINE

Terbinafine hydrochloride (Lamisil) is a synthetic antimycotic agent that belongs to a new family of compounds known as the *allylamines*. All allylamine derivatives, including naftifine, possess a tertiary allylamine, i.e., a nitrogen atom with a neighboring double bond, a structural component crucial for antifungal activity (Fig. 260-1).[1,2] Terbinafine chloride is a white to off-white fine crystalline powder with a molecular weight of 327.90 that is readily soluble in methanol and methylene chloride, soluble in ethanol, and slightly soluble in water.[3] The drug has a broad spectrum and is primarily a fungicidal agent. In vitro it is highly active against dermatophytes but less active against molds, dimorphic fungi, and various yeasts. At clinical concentrations the drug is fungistatic only against *Candida albicans*.[4,5]

MECHANISM OF ACTION Terbinafine blocks the biosynthesis of ergosterol, a sterol essential to the integrity of fungal cell membrane and overall cell growth. In a noncompetitive manner, terbinafine inhibits squalene epoxidase, a complex, microsomal, non–cytochrome P_{450} enzyme catalyzing the first step of the enzymatic pathway, the conversion of squalene into squalene epoxide. Consequently, it causes a concomitant abnormal intracellular accumulation of squalene and deficiency in ergosterol.[6–8] According to previous observations, it is likely that in vitro deficiency of ergosterol is associated with the drug's fungistatic activity or growth arrest, whereas accumulation of squalene accounts for the drug's fungicidal activity, i.e., cellular disruption and cell death.[6]

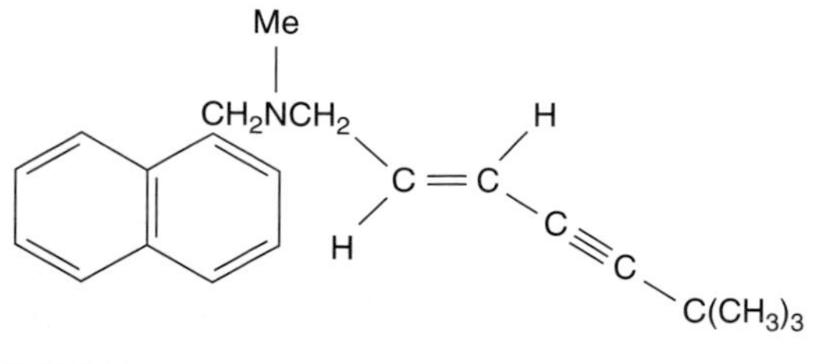

Terbinafine is the most potent inhibitor in its class. Its activity is always reversible and highly selective, with maximal activity at neutral pH. Fungal squalene epoxidase appears to be three to four orders of magnitude more sensitive to the allylamine derivative than the mammalian enzyme, which is essential in cholesterol biosynthesis.[8,9] Terbinafine has little effect on human hepatic cytochrome P_{450} isozymes and therefore does not interfere with synthesis of steroid hormones, prostaglandins, and drug metabolism.[5,10,11]

PHARMACOKINETICS Terbinafine is well absorbed from the gut, mostly in chylomicrons. Following a single oral dose of 250 mg absorption is more than 70 percent, with maximal plasma concentrations of 0.8 to 1.5 $\mu g/mL$ occurring within 2 h of drug administration.[5,12,13] Bioavailability of the drug is linearly dose-dependent and not significantly affected by concurrent intake of food.[5,13] The distribution half-life is 1.5 h, and the elimination half-life is about 22 h.[12] The binding of terbinafine to plasma proteins is nonspecific and extensive with a free fraction of 1 percent. More than 99 percent of terbinafine is evenly bound to plasma proteins, such as albumin and lipoprotein fractions, including low-density lipoprotein (LDL), very low density lipoprotein (VLDL), and high-density lipoprotein (HDL).[5,12]

Terbinafine is highly lipophilic and keratophilic in nature and therefore is widely distributed upon absorption throughout skin and adipose tissue via dermal-epidermal passive diffusion and sebum transport. The concentration of terbinafine was found to be highest in sebum and hair samples when compared to plasma samples.[14]

Terbinafine is extensively biotransformed by the liver, mostly through oxidation by a very small fraction of P_{450} isozymes, into 15 metabolites that do not have the same fungicidal activity as the parent compound. More than 80 percent of the drug is excreted in urine; the rest is eliminated with feces.[5,12]

FIGURE 260-1

Terbinafine.

In patients with hepatic dysfunction, the elimination of terbinafine is slower by 30 percent due to impaired metabolic transformation. In patients with renal insufficiencies, the absorption and distribution of terbinafine are not affected, whereas elimination tends to be slower than in healthy individuals.[12,13]

Terbinafine is indicated for the treatment of onychomycosis of the toenails and fingernails due to dermatophytes (tinea unguium).[15–17] Terbinafine is highly effective in the treatment of tinea corporis, tinea pedis, and, to a lesser degree, cutaneous candidiasis.[5,18]

SIDE EFFECTS Due to its high selectivity, terbinafine is generally well tolerated with a low incidence of adverse side effects. The most common, self-resolving side effects reported by patients following oral administration are of a gastrointestinal nature (3.5 to 5 percent).[4,18,19–21] The symptoms, such as nausea, dyspepsia, and stomach pain, are usually mild and transient. It should be noted that in one study the frequency of the gastrointestinal symptoms reported by patients receiving the drug (250 mg/day) was comparable to that of patients receiving a placebo.[18] Other rare side effects include headache, exanthematous eruption, acute generalized exanthematous pustulosis (AGEP), chest pain, skin reactions, severe neutropenia and pancytopenia (with severe neutropenia), elevated laboratory parameters (LDH, uric acid, triglycerides, and liver enzymes), bitter taste, loss of taste, tiredness and malaise, and Stevens-Johnson syndrome.[4,18–25] A few cases of hepatic injury, including cholestatic liver disease, and severe skin reactions, including toxic epidermal necrolysis and erythema multiforme, were reported as well.[26–30]

DRUG INTERACTIONS Terbinafine does not induce or inhibit hepatic enzymes of the cytochrome P_{450} superfamily and therefore does not produce any clinically significant pharmacokinetic drug interactions with oral or topical administrations.[10] Terbinafine does not interfere with the cytochrome P_{450} enzyme metabolism of antipyrine, a compound used for characterizing hepatic capacity for drug metabolism[11]; nor does it cause an increase in the plasma concentration of cyclosporine, a drug metabolized by cytochrome $P_{450}3A$[31,32]; nor does it significantly change plasma levels of triazolam.[33] Plasma clearance of terbinafine has been shown to be increased by rifampin and decreased by cimetidine,[34] but these changes are clinically insignificant.

Terbinafine is not recommended during pregnancy, and, since it is secreted in breast milk, the drug should not be taken by nursing women.

THE TRIAZOLES

Both itraconazole and fluconazole are triazole antimycotic agents sharing a common structural moiety, a triazole ring, not found in azoles of the imidazole family. The triazole ring contributes to increased specificity for fungal enzymes, thus enhancing the triazoles' efficacy and tolerability.

The azoles impair biosynthesis of ergosterol, the principal structural component of fungal cell membrane, by inhibiting a microsomal cytochrome P_{450} enzyme, 14-α-demethylase, necessary for the conversion of lanosterol to ergosterol.[35–37] Consequently, the accumulation of 14-α-methylsterols leads to the impairment of membrane permeability and membrane-bound enzyme activity and to the arrest of fungal cell growth.[35–37]

Itraconazole

Itraconazole (Sporanox) is a triazole antifungal (Fig. 260-2). The compound is a weak base that can be ionized only in an extremely acidic environment (e.g., stomach acid). It is a highly lipophilic compound, nearly insoluble in water, slightly soluble in acidified polyethylene glycol, and soluble in hydroxyl-β-cyclodextrin.[38]

Itraconazole has a wide spectrum of activity. In vitro it is effective against dermatophytes, yeast, molds, and dimorphic and dematiaceous fungi.[36,39]

PHARMACOKINETICS Serum concentration of itraconazole is influenced by several parameters, including food and gastric acidity. The amount of drug absorbed is markedly increased, approximately twofold, when the drug is administered postprandially in a capsule formulation.[40,41] Absorption and bioavailability of itraconazole nonlinearly depend on the administered dose, presumably due to a saturation of the first-pass metabolism process that takes place in the liver.[42,43] After oral administration of 100 mg, the maximal plasma concentration of 0.13 to 0.16 μg/mL is achieved within 4 h.[43] Almost all (99.8 percent) plasma itraconazole is bound to plasma proteins, mostly to albumin. Only a negligible amount (0.2 percent) is found in body fluids, such as cerebrospinal fluid, eye fluid, and saliva.[13,36,43] Itraconazole binds extensively to tissues, with some tissues demonstrating concentrations of the drug 2 to 20 times higher than the simultaneous concentration in the plasma.[36,43] Itraconazole is extensively metabolized by the liver to more than 30 metabolites. Hydroxy-itraconazole is the only active main metabolite, and its plasma concentration at steady state is twice as high as that of the parent drug.[40,43] About 54 percent of the metabolized drug is excreted in the feces, and 34 percent is excreted in the urine. After single-dose administration, the terminal elimination half-life is 21 h for itraconazole and 12 h for its active metabolite. The pharmacokinetic variables of itraconazole are not affected in patients with renal insufficiency and in those undergoing hemodialysis.[38,43] In patients with liver cirrhosis, the absorption is slightly increased and the half-life is prolonged, due to a reduced first-pass metabolism.[13,38,43] The absorption is decreased in neutropenic patients and in AIDS patients due to gastric hypochlorhydria.[13,38,43,44]

Itraconazole is indicated for the treatment of blastomycosis, histoplasmosis, aspergillosis, candidiasis, cryptococcosis, coccidioidomycosis, paracoccidioidomycosis, sporotrichosis, and phaeohyphomycosis, and superficial infections due to dermatophytes.[43,45–47] Itraconazole has also been approved for the treatment of onychomycosis due to dermatophytes, in which it is effective as continuous or pulse therapy.[48,49]

SIDE EFFECTS The most common reported side effects associated with itraconazole therapy are of a gastrointestinal nature, including nausea and vomiting.[50,51] Less frequent adverse effects are hyper-

FIGURE 260-2

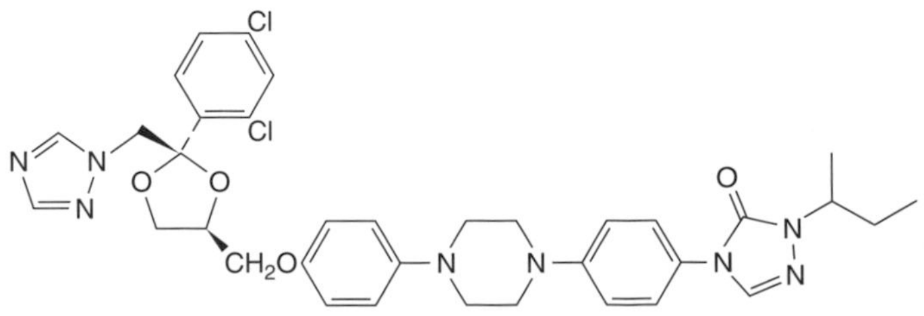

Itraconazole.

triglyceridemia, edema, hypertension, leukopenia, nephrotic syndrome, and mildly elevated liver enzymes.[50,51] Instances of hepatic injury have been associated with the administration of itraconazole but seem to have resolved upon discontinuation of therapy.[52] Patients receiving 600 mg of itraconazole daily have experienced fatigue, weakness, orthostatic dizziness, intolerance to sun and heat, hypokalemia, breast tenderness, and mild maculopapular rash.[44,53] Itraconazole has been implicated in the induction of AGEP in patients with and without a history of psoriasis.[54,55]

DRUG INTERACTIONS Due to its small affinity for the mammalian cytochrome P_{450} isozymes, itraconazole has a low potential to interfere with the metabolism and clearance of concomitantly administered drugs. Itraconazole significantly elevates plasma levels of the following: (1) terfenadine, causing a prolongation of the QT interval; (2) digoxin, leading to digoxin toxicity, manifest by nausea, decreased visual acuity, vomiting, lethargy, and sinus bradycardia; and (3) cyclosporine, resulting in nephrotoxicity.[56–61] In addition, itraconazole causes a significant plasma level elevation of triazolam, felodipine, and midazolam.[62–65] Itraconazole markedly decreases plasma levels of busulfan and cisapride[66,67]; it appears to have an insignificant effect on plasma levels of diazepam and the oral contraceptives ethinyl estradiol and norethindrone.[38,68] Rifampin, phenytoin, phenobarbital, carbamazepine, and rifabutin significantly decrease plasma concentrations of itraconazole during concurrent treatment by inducing the cytochrome P_{450}3A enzyme involved in the metabolism of itraconazole.[38,69,70] Concomitant administration of itraconazole with lovastatin, simvastatin astemizole, cisapride, midazolam, triazolam, or terfenadine is contraindicated.

No congenital abnormalities have been observed in babies of women receiving itraconazole therapy during pregnancy.[71,72] Nonetheless, itraconazole therapy is not recommended during pregnancy and nursing.

Fluconazole

Fluconazole (Diflucan) is a bistriazole antifungal derivative (Fig. 260-3) with a low molecular weight. It is a white crystalline solid that is water soluble in both basic and neutral conditions.[73,74] It is effective against many yeasts (with the exception of *C. krusei*) and dermatophytes.[37,75]

PHARMACOKINETICS The pharmacokinetic parameters of fluconazole are comparable following either intravenous or oral administration.[75] Extensive absorption (>90 percent) of the triazole appears to be similar in both postprandial and fasting states and not dependent on stomach acidity.[41,73,76] The peak plasma concentrations of the compound are linearly dose dependent.[77] The maximum plasma concentration is achieved within approximately 2 h of administration. Fluconazole exhibits a long half-life of 25 to 30 h, and a steady-state level is reached after 7 days of once-daily administrations. Fluconazole is only weakly bound to plasma proteins, with about 90 percent of the drug circulating free in the plasma.[37] The drug is resistant to hepatic metabolism, and hence ~80 percent of fluconazole is excreted unchanged in urine, with 2 percent in feces and about 11 percent as metabolites in urine.[78] Fluconazole is almost minimally lipophilic and penetrates widely into body tissues and fluids. The ability to diffuse substantially into the cerebrospinal fluid (CSF) distinguishes this compound from many other antimycotic agents.[74,79] The levels of fluconazole in cerebrospinal fluid, saliva, vaginal tissue, sputum, skin, and blister fluids have been reported to be comparable with or to exceed simultaneous plasma concentrations.[77]

Altered fluconazole pharmacokinetics, including reduced terminal elimination constant and decreased plasma clearance, are detected in patients with liver cirrhosis, especially those who are receiving concurrent fluconazole and diuretic therapy.[80] The pharmacokinetics of fluconazole are markedly affected by renal impairment as well, leading to protracted (about three times normal) elimination.[81]

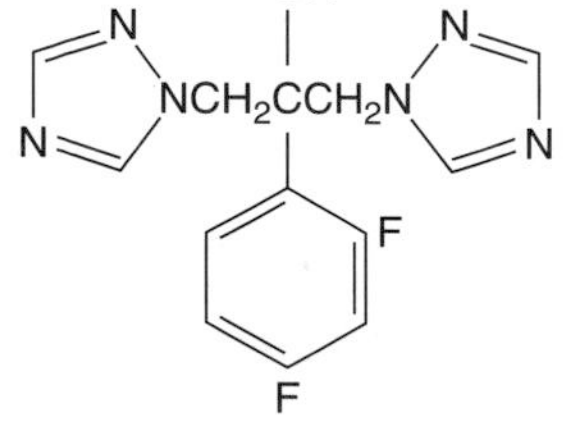

Fluconazole is indicated for the treatment of oral, esophageal, and vaginal candidiasis; cryptococcal meningitis; and prophylaxis of candidiasis in AIDS patients and solid organ transplant recipients.[75,82] It has been found to be effective in the treatment of tinea corporis, tinea cruris, tinea pedis, tinea unguium, histoplasmosis, paracoccidioidomycosis, and sporotrichosis.[75]

SIDE EFFECTS The most common recognized side effects of fluconazole therapy are gastrointestinal, including nausea, vomiting, diarrhea, and abdominal pain.[82] Elevated liver function tests are rarely associated with fluconazole therapy,[79] but in those individuals with elevated liver enzymes, liver biopsy showed either a central lobular cholestasis consistent with drug toxicity or an absence of hepatocyte necrosis.[83,84] Adverse reactions such as fixed drug eruptions, thrombocytopenia, transient amenorrhea, mild increase in levels of serum creatine phosphokinase, dizziness, and anorexia are observed on a single-case basis, and most resolve with continuing fluconazole therapy.[79,85,86] Alopecia, reversible upon dosage reduction or discontinuation of treatment with fluconazole, is reported to be common in patients receiving 400 mg of fluconazole for prolonged periods; however, the condition has been observed in patients receiving a dose as low as 100 mg.[87] Administration of fluconazole has been reported to cause an anaphylactic reaction which presented as pruritus, and paraesthesia with edema of the feet. An allergic reaction was attributed to possible cross-sensitization through an imidazole (ketoconazole or metronidazole).[88]

DRUG INTERACTIONS Fluconazole administration affects neither the plasma concentration nor the half-life of antipyrine, an indicator of the function of some enzymes of the cytochrome P_{450} system.[55] Concurrent administration of fluconazole does not have any significant effect on the pharmacokinetics of the two steroid components of the oral contraceptives ethinyl estradiol and norgestrel.[89] Fluconazole at doses of 200, 300, or 400 mg appears not to affect the level of endogenous testosterone. Continuous therapy with fluconazole significantly elevates plasma levels of phenytoin, warfarin, tolbutamide, nortriptyline, midazolam, triazolam, and FK506 (tacrolimus).[33,89–97] On the other hand, fluconazole has only a minor effect on theophylline disposition.[98] At high doses, fluconazole has been shown to increase the plasma levels of cyclosporine.[89] The

FIGURE 260-3

Fluconazole.

plasma concentration of fluconazole is not significantly affected by phenytoin, rifabutin, and agents that increase gastric pH, such as omeprozole, cimetidine, and Maalox.[70,73,76,89,99] The plasma concentration of fluconazole is decreased by concomitant therapy with rifampin.[69,89,91]

Fluconazole has been reported to be a potent teratogen that produces a characteristic pattern of congenital malformations, including craniofacial, skeletal, and cardiac anomalies, following treatment in the first trimester.[100] However, a lack of a teratogenic effect has been observed after fluconazole therapy during the second trimester.[101] The time period during pregnancy at which fluconazole leads to teratogenicity requires further investigation.

RESISTANCE Resistance to azole drugs is rare. Nonetheless, as a result of severe immunosuppression and prolonged treatment and prophylaxis with fluconazole, strains of yeast resistant to fluconazole have emerged in patients with oropharyngeal candidiasis,[102,103] mucocutaneous candidiasis,[104-107] and esophageal candidiasis[108] who are seropositive for HIV. Resistance of *C. glabrata* and *C. norvegensis* isolates to fluconazole has been reported as well.[109,110]

KETOCONAZOLE

Ketoconazole (Nizoral) is a fungistatic imidazole antifungal agent whose mechanism of action is similar to that of the triazole derivatives. Ketoconazole is a weak base, practically insoluble in water, and dissociable only in highly acidic solutions. Hence, comparably to itraconazole, the absorption of ketoconazole strongly depends on gastric acidity and seems to be enhanced by the concurrent intake of food. Ketoconazole is highly lipophilic and keratinophilic. The drug is highly protein- and erythrocyte-bound, with 1 percent circulating free in plasma; thus only a small amount penetrates into the cerebrospinal fluid. Ketoconazole is extensively metabolized in the liver and mostly excreted in feces. The bioavailability of ketoconazole is impaired in AIDS patients and in patients with neutropenia, but in patients with mild renal and liver impairments it appears to be comparable to that of normal volunteers.[13,111]

Ketoconazole is effective in treatment of histoplasmosis, blastomycosis, esophageal and vaginal candidiasis, oral thrush, coccidioidomycosis, pseudallescheriasis, and paracoccidioidomycosis.[112,113]

The most common side effects associated with ketoconazole therapy are nausea, vomiting, anorexia, and dyspepsia. The drug has the ability to interfere with the production of endogenous steroids and, as a consequence, causes side effects such as irregular menstrual bleeding and decreased levels of testosterone in males, linked to decreased libido and loss of potency.[112,114]

Ketoconazole has been reported to exert uncommon but potentially significant effects on the liver. It has been implicated in the transient asymptomatic elevation of liver function tests in 21 percent of patients and development of overt hepatitis in 5 percent of individuals.[115] Several cases of fatal hepatic failure have been reported.[116]

The concentration of ketoconazole is decreased by antacids and by agents inducing hepatic cytochrome $P_{450}3A4$ enzymes such as rifampin and phenytoin. Ketoconazole inhibits some cytochrome P_{450} isozymes and subsequently increases plasma levels of some antihistamines, including astemizole and terfenadine, possibly leading to abnormal cardiac repolarization. It increases plasma level of cyclosporine and potentiates the anticoagulant effect of warfarin.[61,91]

GRISEOFULVIN

Griseofulvin is an antibiotic with a narrow spectrum of antimycotic activity produced by the penicillin species. It disrupts microtubule mitotic spindle formation, thereby causing mitotic arrest at the metaphase stage.[117-119] The absorption of the compound, which takes place primarily in the duodenum, is enhanced by several factors, including concurrent intake of a fatty meal and a smaller particle size formulation. Griseofulvin demonstrates a weak affinity to keratin. Although the drug is detected in the stratum corneum of the skin 4 to 8 h following oral administration, it is not present at this site 48 to 72 h after discontinuation of therapy. Griseofulvin is mainly metabolized by the liver before excretion.[118,119,120]

Griseofulvin was found to be effective against dermatophytes but not against yeast and bacteria. Although griseofulvin is indicated for the treatment of fingernail and toenail onychomycosis, therapy is prolonged with low cure and high relapse rates, requiring approximately 6 months for the treatment of fingernails and 12 months for toenails.[48,118,119]

The most common side effects are related to the gastrointestinal tract and the central nervous system. Between 20 and 50 percent of patients on griseofulvin experience severe headaches. Visual and psychic impairment are reported as well. As a result of impaired porphyrin metabolism, griseofulvin therapy is associated with photoallergic reactions. The drug has been reported to precipitate lupus erythematosus and severe skin reactions; it is teratogenic and carcinogenic in animal models.[13,61,118,119]

Griseofulvin induces hepatic cytochrome P_{450} enzymes, leading to lower plasma levels of warfarin. Concurrent administration of griseofulvin and oral contraceptives may lead to irregular menstrual bleedings and pregnancy. The compound can potentiate the effects of alcohol. The absorption of griseofulvin is decreased by phenobarbital.[61,91]

REFERENCES

1. Stutz A et al: Synthesis and structure activity relationships of naftifine-related allylamine antimycotics. *J Med Chem* **29**:112, 1986
2. Favre B et al: Characterization of squalene epoxidase activity from the dermatophyte *Trichophyton rubrum* and its inhibition by terbinafine and other antimycotic agents. *Antimicrob Agents Chemother* **40**:443, 1996
3. Sandoz Pharmaceuticals Corporation: *Lamisil Prescribing Information.* East Hanover, NJ, 1996
4. Nolting S et al: Terbinafine in onychomycosis with involvement by non-dermatophytic fungi. *Br J Dermatol* **130**(suppl 43):16, 1994
5. Balfour JA et al: Terbinafine. A review of its pharmacodynamic and pharmacokinetic properties, and therapeutic potential in superficial mycoses. *Drugs* **43**:259, 1992
6. Ryder NS: Terbinafine: Mode of action and properties of the squalene epoxidase inhibition. *Br J Dermatol* **126**(suppl 39):2, 1992
7. Elewski BE: Mechanisms of action of systemic antifungal agents. *J Am Acad Dermatol* **28**:S28, 1993
8. Ryder NS: Specific inhibition of fungal sterol biosynthesis by SF 86-327, a new allylamine antimycotic agent. *Antimicrob Agents Chemother* **27**:252, 1985
9. Ryder NS et al: Inhibition of squalene epoxidase by allylamine antimycotic compounds. A comparative study of the fungal and mammalian enzymes. *Biochem J* **230**:765, 1985

10. Back DJ et al: Comparative effects of the antimycotic drugs keto-conazole, fluconazole, itraconazole and terbinafine on the metabolism of cyclosporin by human liver microsomes. *Br J Clin Pharmacol* **32**:624, 1991

11. Seyffer R et al: Antipyrine metabolism is not affected by terbinafine, a new antifungal agent. *Eur J Clin Phamacol* **37**:231, 1989

12. Jensen C: Clinical pharmacokinetics of terbinafine (Lamisil). *Clin Exp Dermatol* **14**:110, 1989

13. Schafer-Korting M: Pharmacokinetic optimisation of oral antifungal therapy. *Clin Pharmacokinet* **25**:329, 1993

14. Kovarik JM et al: Multiple-dose pharmacokinetics and distribution in tissue of terbinafine and metabolites. *Antimicrob Agents Chemother* **39**:2738, 1995

15. Goodfield MJD et al: Treatment of dermatophyte infection of the finger- and toe-nails with terbinafine (SF 86-327, Lamisil), an orally active fungicidal agent. *Br J Dermatol* **121**:753, 1989

16. Faergemann J et al: Double-blind, parallel-group comparison of ter-binafine and griseofulvin in the treatment of toenail onychomycosis. *J Am Acad Dermatol* **32**:750, 1995

17. Hull PR: Onychomycosis—treatment relapse and reinfection. *Dermatology* **194**(suppl 1):7, 1997

18. Villars V et al: Clinical efficacy and tolerability of terbinafine (Lam-isil)—a new topical and systemic fungicidal drug for treatment of dermatomycosis. *Clin Exp Dermatol* **14**:124, 1989

19. Savin R: Successful treatment of chronic tinea pedis (moccasin type) with terbinafine (Lamisil). *Clin Exp Dermatol* **14**:116, 1989

20. Cole GW et al: A comparison of a new oral antifungal, terbinafine, with griseofulvin as therapy for tinea corporis. *Arch Dermatol* **125**:1537, 1989

21. Roberts DT: Oral terbinafine (Lamisil) in the treatment of fungal infections of the skin and nails. *Dermatology* **194**(suppl 1):37, 1997

22. Kovacs MJ et al: Neutropenia and pancytopenia associated with oral terbinafine. *J Am Acad Dermatol* **31**:806, 1994

23. Dupin N et al: Acute generalized exanthematous pustulosis induced by terbinafine. *Arch Dermatol* **132**.1253, 1996

24. Rzany B et al: Stevens-Johnson syndrome after terbinafine therapy. *J Am Acad Dermatol* **30**:509, 1994

25. Juhlin L: Loss of taste and terbinafine. *Lancet* **339**:1483, 1992

26. Lazaros GA et al: Terbinafine-induced cholestatic liver disease. *J Hepatol* **24**:753, 1996

27. Lowe G et al: Hepatitis associated with terbinafine treatment. *BMJ* **306**:248, 1993

28. van't Wout JW et al: Terbinafine-associated hepatic injury. *J Hepatol* **21**:115, 1994

29. White SI et al: Toxic epidermal necrolysis induced by terbinafine in patients on long-term antiepileptics. *Br J Dermatol* **134**:178, 1996

30. Carstens J et al: Toxic epidermal necrolysis and erythema multiforme following therapy with terbinafine. *Acta Derm Venereol* **74**:391, 1994

31. Jensen P et al: Effect of oral terbinafine treatment on cyclosporin pharmacokinetics in organ transplant recipients with dermatophyte nail infection. *Acta Derm Venereol* **76**:280, 1996

32. Long CC et al: Effect of terbinafine on the pharmacokinetics of cy-closporin in humans. *J Invest Dermatol* **102**:740, 1994

33. Varhe A et al: Fluconazole, but not terbinafine, enhances the effects of triazolam by inhibiting its metabolism. *Br J Clin Pharmacol* **41**:319, 1996

34. Broddell RT et al: Clinical pearl: Systemic antifungal drug interactions. *J Am Acad Dermatol* **33**:259, 1995

35. Grant SM et al: Itraconazole. A review of its pharmacodynamic and pharmacokinetic properties and therapeutic use in superficial and systemic mycoses. *Drugs* **37**:310, 1989

36. Haria M et al: Itraconazole: A reappraisal of its pharmacological properties and therapeutic use in the management of superficial fungal infections. *Drugs* **51**:585, 1996

37. Goa KL et al: Fluconazole: An update of its pharmacodynamic and pharmacokinetic properties and therapeutic use in major superficial and systemic mycoses in immunocompromised patients. *Drugs* **50**:658, 1995

38. Heykants J et al: The clinical pharmacokinetics of itraconazole: An overview. *Mycoses* **32**(suppl 1):67, 1989

39. Van Cutsem J: The in-vitro antifungal spectrum of itraconazole. *Mycoses* **32**(suppl 1):7, 1989

40. Barone JA et al: Food interaction and steady-state pharmacokinetics of itraconazole capsules in healthy male volunteers. *Antimicrob Agents Chemother* **37**:778, 1993

41. Zimmermann T et al: Influence of concomitant food intake on the oral absorption of two triazole antifungal agents, itraconazole and fluconazole. *Eur J Clin Pharmacol* **46**:147, 1994

42. Hardin TC et al: Pharmacokinetics of itraconazole following oral administration to normal volunteers. *Antimicrob Agents Chemother* **32**:1310, 1988

43. Negroni R et al: Itraconazole: Pharmacokinetics and indications. *Arch Med Res* **24**:387, 1993

44. Smith D et al: The pharmacokinetics of oral itraconazole in AIDS patients. *J Pharm Pharmacol* **44**:618, 1992

45. Anonymous: Itraconazole. *Med Lett Drugs Ther* **35**:7, 1993

46. Cleary JD et al: Itraconazole in antifungal therapy. *Ann Pharma-cother* **26**:502, 1992

47. Lesher JL: Recent developments in antifungal therapy. *Dermatol Clin* **14**:163, 1996

48. Anonymous: Itraconazole for onychomycosis. *Med Lett Drug Ther* **38**:5, 1996

49. Bonifaz A et al: Itraconazole in onychomycosis: Intermittent dose schedule. *Int J Dermatol* **36**:70, 1997

50. Graybill JR et al: Itraconazole treatment of coccidioidomycosis. *Am J Med* **89**:282, 1990

51. Tucker RM et al: Adverse events associated with itraconazole in 189 patients on chronic therapy. *J Antimicrob Chemother* **26**:561, 1990

52. Lavrijsen APM et al: Hepatic injury associated with itraconazole. *Lancet* **340**:251, 1992

53. Sharkey PK et al: High-dose itraconazole in the treatment of severe mycoses. *Antimicrob Agents Chemother* **35**:707, 1991

54. Heymann WR et al: Itraconazole-induced acute generalized exan-themic pustulosis. *J Am Acad Dermatol* **33**:130, 1995

55. Park YM et al: Acute generalized exanthematous pustulosis induced by itraconazole. *J Am Acad Dermatol* **36**:794, 1997

56. Honig PK et al: Itraconazole affects single-dose terfenadine phar-macokinetics and cardiac repolarization pharmacodynamics. *J Clin Pharmacol* **33**:1201, 1993

57. McClean KL et al: Interaction between itraconazole and digoxin. *Clin Infect Dis* **18**:259, 1994

58. Kauffman CA et al: Digoxin toxicity associated with itraconazole therapy. *Clin Infect Dis* **15**:886, 1992

59. Alderman CP et al: Digoxin-itraconazole interaction: Possible mechanisms. *Ann Pharmacother* **31**:438, 1997

60. Bickers DR: Antifungal therapy: Potential interactions with other classes of drugs. *J Am Acad Dermatol* **31**:S87, 1994

61. Perfect JR et al: Adverse drug reactions to systemic antifungals: Prevention and management. *Drug Saf* **7**:323, 1992

62. Neuvonen PJ et al: The effect of ingestion time interval on the interaction between itraconazole and triazolam. *Clin Pharmacol Ther* **60**:326, 1996

63. Jalava KM et al: Itraconazole greatly increases plasma concentrations and effects of felodipine. *Clin Pharmacol Ther* **61**:410, 1997

64. von Moltke LL et al: Midazolam hydroxylation by human liver microsomes in vitro: Inhibition of fluoxetine, norfluoxetine, and by azole antifungal agents. *J Clin Pharmacol* **36**:783, 1996

65. Ahonen J et al: Effect of itraconazole and terbinafine on the pharmacokinetics and pharmacodynamics of midazolam in healthy volunteers. *Br J Clin Pharmacol* **40**:270, 1995

66. Buggia I et al: Itraconazole can increase systemic exposure to busulfan in patients given bone marrow transplantation. *Anticancer Res* **16**:2083, 1996

67. Bedford TA et al: Cisapride. Drug interactions of clinical significance. *Drug Saf* **15**:167, 1996

68. Ahonen J et al: The effect of the antimycotic itraconazole on the pharmacokinetics and pharmacodynamics of diazepam. *Fundam Clin Pharmacol* **10**:314, 1996

69. Tucker RM et al: Interaction of azoles with rifampin, phenytoin, carbamazepine: In vitro and clinical observations. *Clin Infect Dis* **14**:165, 1992

70. Strolin Benedetti B: Inducing properties of rifabutin, and effects on the pharmacokinetics and metabolism of concomitant drugs. *Pharmacol Res* **32**:177, 1995

71. Lavalle P et al: Itraconazole for deep mycoses: Preliminary experience in Mexico. *Rev Infect Dis* **9**(suppl 1):S64, 1987

72. Chotmongkol V et al: Itraconazole in cryptococcal meningitis in pregnancy: A case report. *J Med Assoc Thai* **75**:606, 1992

73. Thorpe JE et al: Effect of oral antacid administration on the pharmacokinetics of oral fluconazole. *Antimicrob Agents Chemother* **34**:2032, 1990

74. Sugar AM et al: Overview: Treatment of cryptococcal meningitis. *Rev Infect Dis* **12**(suppl 3):S338, 1990
75. Montero-Gei F: Fluconazole: Pharmacokinetics and indications. *Arch Med Res* **4**:377, 1993
76. Gibaldi M: Drug interactions: Part II. *Ann Pharmacother* **26**:829, 1992
77. Brammer KW et al: Pharmacokinetics and tissue penetration of fluconazole in humans. *Rev Infect Dis* **12**(suppl 3):S318, 1990
78. Dudley MN: Clinical pharmacology of fluconazole. *Pharmacotherapy* **6**:141S, 1990
79. Tucker RM et al: Treatment of coccidioidal meningitis with fluconazole. *Rev Infect Dis* **12**(suppl 3):S380, 1990
80. Ruhnke M et al: Single-dose pharmacokinetics of fluconazole in patients with liver cirrhosis. *J Antimicrob Chemother* **35**:641, 1995
81. Toon S et al: An assessment of the effects of impaired renal function and haemodialysis on the pharmacokinetics of fluconazole. *Br J Clin Pharmacol* **29**:221, 1990
82. Anonymous: Oral fluconazole for vaginal candidiasis. *Med Lett Drugs Ther* **36**:81, 1994
83. Wells C et al: Dose-dependent fluconazole hepatotoxicity proven on biopsy and rechallenge. *J Infect* **24**:111, 1992
84. Trujillo MA et al: Evaluation of hepatic injury arising during fluconazole therapy. *Arch Intern Med* **154**:102, 1994
85. Morgan JM et al: Fixed drug eruption with fluconazole. *BMJ* **308**:454, 1994
86. Mercurio MG et al: Thrombocytopenia caused by fluconazole therapy. *J Am Acad Dermatol* **32**:525, 1995
87. Pappas PG et al: Alopecia associated with fluconazole therapy. *Ann Intern Med* **123**:354, 1995
88. Neuhaus G et al: Anaphylactic reaction after oral fluconazole. *BMJ* **302**:1341, 1991
89. Lazar JD et al: Drug interactions with fluconazole. *Rev Infect Dis* **12**(suppl 3):S327, 1990
90. Levy RH: Cytochrome P450 isozymes and antiepileptic drug interactions. *Epilepsia* **36**(suppl 5):S8, 1995
91. Bickers DR: Antifungal therapy: Potential interactions with other classes of drugs. *J Am Acad Dermatol* **31**:S87, 1994
92. Kerr HD: Case report: Potentiation of warfarin by fluconazole. *Am J Med Sci* **305**:164, 1993
93. Wells PS et al: Interactions of warfarin with drugs and food. *Ann Intern Med* **121**:677, 1994
94. Gannon RH et al: Fluconazole-nortriptyline drug interaction. *Ann Pharmacother* **26**:1456, 1992
95. Olkkola KT et al: The effects of the systemic antimycotics, itraconazole and fluconazole, on the pharmacokinetics and pharmacodynamics of intravenous and oral midazolam. *Anesth Analg* **82**:511, 1996
96. Manez R et al: Fluconazole therapy in transplant recipients receiving FK 506. *Transplantation* **57**:1521, 1994
97. Mignat C: Clinically significant drug interactions with new immunosuppressive agents. *Drug Saf* **16**:267, 1997
98. Konishi H et al: Effect of fluconazole on theophylline disposition in humans. *Eur J Clin Pharmacol* **46**:309, 1994
99. Zimmermann T et al: The influence of gastric pH on the pharmacokinetics of fluconazole: The effect of omeprazole. *Int J Clin Pharmacol Ther* **32**:491, 1994
100. Pursley TJ et al: Fluconazole-induced congenital anomalies in three infants. *Clin Infect Dis* **22**:336, 1996
101. Krcmery V Jr et al: Teratogenicity of fluconazole. *Pediatr Infect Dis J* **15**:841, 1996
102. Revankar SG et al: Detection and significance of fluconazole resistance in oropharyngeal candidiasis in human immunodeficiency virus–infected patients. *J Infect Dis* **174**:821, 1996
103. He X et al: Azole resistance in oropharyngeal *Candida albicans* strains isolated from patients infected with human immunodeficiency virus. *Antimicrob Agents Chemother* **38**:2495, 1994
104. Boken DJ et al: Fluconazole-resistant *Candida albicans*. *Clin Infect Dis* **17**:1018, 1993
105. Smith KJ et al: Azole resistance in *Candida albicans*. *J Med Vet Mycol* **24**:133, 1986
106. Newman SL et al: Clinically significant mucosal candidiasis resistant to fluconazole treatment in patients with AIDS. *Clin Infect Dis* **19**:684, 1994
107. Baily GG et al: Fluconazole-resistant candidosis in an HIV cohort. *AIDS* **8**:787, 1994
108. Kitchen VS et al: *Candida albicans* resistance in AIDS. *J Infect* **22**:204, 1991
109. Warnock DW et al: Fluconazole resistance in *Candida glabrata*. *Lancet* **2**:1310, 1988
110. Sandven P et al: *Candida norvegensis:* A fluconazole-resistant species. *Antimicrob Agents Chemother* **41**:1375, 1997
111. Daneshmend TK et al: Clinical pharmacokinetics of ketoconazole. *Clin Pharmacokinet* **14**:13, 1988
112. Anonymous: Drugs for treatment of deep fungal infections. *Med Lett Drug Ther* **30**:30, 1988
113. Anonymous: Drugs for AIDS and associated infections. *Med Lett Drug Ther* **33**:95, 1991
114. Vidal-Puig AJ et al: Ketoconazole therapy: Hormonal and clinical effects in non-tumoral hyperandrogenism. *Eur J Endocrinol* **130**:333, 1994
115. Chien RN et al: Hepatic injury during ketoconazole therapy in patients with onychomycosis: A controlled cohort study. *Hepatology* **25**:103, 1997
116. Knight TE et al: Ketoconazole-induced fulminant hepatitis necessitating liver transplantation. *J Am Acad Dermatol* **25**:398, 1991
117. De Carli L et al: Griseofulvin. *Mutat Res* **195**:91, 1988
118. Faergemann J et al: Griseofulvin and ketoconazole: A review with special emphasis on dermatology. *Semin Dermatol* **6**:31, 1987
119. Gupta AK et al: Antifungal agents: An overview. Part I. *J Am Acad Dermatol* **30**:677, 1994
120. Meinhof W: Kinetics and spectrum of activity of oral antifungals: The therapeutic implications. *J Am Acad Dermatol* **29**:S37, 1993

CHAPTER 261

Hossein C. Nousari
Grant J. Anhalt

Immunosuppressive and Immunomodulatory Drugs

CYCLOSPORINE

Cyclosporine and tacrolimus (FK506) are effective immunosuppresive agents whose primary mechanism of action is inhibition of T cell responses. Cyclosporine and FK506 also seem to share similar pharmacodynamics.[1] Cyclosporine is a lipophilic and very hydrophobic cyclic undecapeptide, extracted serindipitously from the soil fungi *Tolypocladium inflatum gams* and *Cyclindrocarpon lucidum* by investigators who were searching for antifungal agents. Cyclosporine and FK506, an unrelated fungal product, selectively suppress T cell responses through the inhibition of calcium-dependent signal transmission mechanisms described below (Fig. 261-1). It is known that the T cell proliferation/stimulation process involves the orchestration of complex, interlacing mechanisms, most of which are not completely understood. However, a simplified explanation of the mechanism of action of these drugs is presented in the following sections.

Mechanism of Action

Several T cell activation pathways are recognized, but T cell activation via the T cell receptor (TCR) molecule (TCR-CD3) is the best understood. Other less well understood mechanisms include activation through the CD2 receptor, a mechanism activated by mitogenic lectins, and through a cell membrane receptor–independent mechanism, such as proliferation induced by phorbol-12-myristate-13-acetate (PMA) and the calcium ionophore, ionomycin. Cyclosporine and FK506 inhibit T cell stimulation initiated by the TCR-CD3, CD2, and PMA/ionomycin pathways. Mechanisms involving B7: CD28/CTLA-4, a costimulatory T cell–antigen-presenting cell pathway involved in autoimmunity

FIGURE 261-1

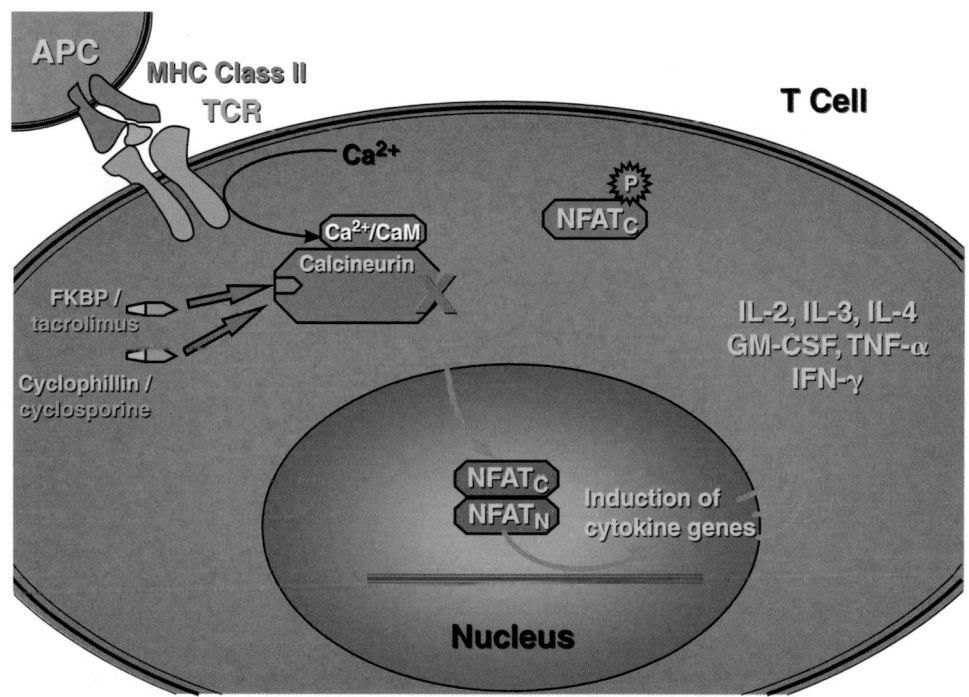

Outline of the key mechanisms by which both cyclosporine and FK506 inhibit T cell activation triggered by presentation of antigen via the T cell receptor. The first step involves presentation of peptide, processed by an antigen-presenting cell (APC), bound within the peptide-binding groove of the MHC class II molecule, and presented to the T cell receptor (TCR). This causes transmembrane signaling that increases intracellular calcium concentrations. The liberated calcium, bound to calmodulin, interacts with calcineurin, a calcium-dependent serine/threonine phosphatase that dephosphorylates $NFAT_C$ (nuclear factor of activated T cells), and this causes NFAT to translocate to the nucleus. There it binds to other nuclear components of NFAT (shown here as $NFAT_N$). This complex regulates the transcription of many cytokine genes, shown in the diagram.

Both cyclosporine and FK506 diffuse freely into the cytoplasm of T cells and bind with their respective immunophillins. This drug-immunophillin complex binds to calcineurin and blocks its ability to dephosphorylate NFAT, and thereby inhibits the production of cytokines that would normally be induced after T cell activation via the TCR.

and infectious diseases,[2] seem not to be affected by cyclosporine or FK506.[3,4]

The first pharmacodynamic step of cyclosporine action involves its binding to a family of cytoplasmic receptors called *immunophillins*. Immunophillins have rotamase (isomerase) activity, which catalyzes the interconversion of peptidyl-prolyl bonds. Cyclosporine binds to a 17-kDa immunophillin called *cyclophillin A* (CyPA), which is the high-affinity receptor for cyclosporine. FK506 binds a 12-kDa immunophillin named *FKBP 12* (FK506–binding protein—12 kDa). These two immunophillins share no structural similarities; however, both have drug-inhibitable rotamase activity. Once cyclosporine and FK506 are bound to their respective immunophillins, rotamase activity is inhibited.

Next, the drug-immunophillin complex binds to calcineurin. *Calcineurin* is a serine/threonine protease composed of two subunits—calcineurins A and B. Calcineurin A constitutes the catalytic unit possessing binding sites for calcineurin B and calmodulin. Calcineurin activity strictly correlates with interleukin (IL) 2 production via CD3 activation. Calcineurin is also involved in the induction of apoptosis and degranulation of cytotoxic T lymphocytes. It is well established that calcineurin activation is not only a rate-limiting step but also a crucial propagating factor in calcium-dependent T cell signaling pathways.

Subsequently, calcineurin regulates the transcription factor *NF-AT* (nuclear factor of activated T cells), which is implicated in the regulation of the cytokine-encoding genes, including the gene regulating IL-2 production. NFAT is a heterodimer complex composed of two molecules: $NFAT_N$ and $NFAT_C$. One of the substrates of calcineurin is the cytoplasmic component of this complex, $NFAT_C$. Once $NFAT_C$ is dephosphorylated by calcineurin, the protein translocates into the nucleus where it binds $NFAT_N$, a nuclear AP-1 family member whose synthesis is induced by protein kinase C–dependent signals. Experimental data have shown that the cyclosporine- and FK506–calcineurin complexes inhibit the nuclear translocation of the $NFAT_C$ by blocking its dephosphorylation. This is thought to be the key step by which these drugs uncouple T cell receptor activation from IL-2 transcription. FK506 is 10- to 100-fold more potent than cyclosporine in in vitro inhibition of calcineurin activity.

There are other actions of these drugs that may be relevant to their behavior. For example, calcineurin (which is complexed and inactivated by cyclosporine) also participates in the regulation of T cell genes coding certain proto-oncogenes (e.g., c-*myc* and H-*Ras*), IL-2 receptors, IL-4, granulocyte-macrophage colony-stimulating factor, tumor necrosis factor α, and interferon-γ, among others. Cyclosporine also dephosphorylates another cytosolic regulatory protein called *octameric activating protein*, which also requires dephosphorylation for transportation into the nucleus to act as a transcription factor. It also decreases IL-2 production via increasing the expression of transforming growth factor β, which is a potent inhibitor of IL-2-stimulated T cell production, and via the generation of antigen-specific cytotoxic T lymphocytes.[5,6] Immunosuppressive and anti-inflammatory activities of cyclosporine can also be mediated via cyclophillin-40 (a 40-kDa cyclophillin), a 70-kDa heat shock protein, and cyclophillin C–related receptors in natural killer cells. Actually, it is postulated that the binding of cyclosporine to cyclophyllin C, P glycoprotein, and actin may be relevant in the pathogenesis of nephrotoxicity and obliterative vasculopathy that can occur with cyclosporine treatment. Cyclosporine and FK506 also inhibit the degranulation of basophils and cytotoxic T lymphocytes through a protein synthesis–independent mechanism. Thus, not all pharmacologic mechanisms of cyclosporine can be explained via calcineurin inhibition.

The beneficial action of cyclosporine in psoriasis seems to be mediated by the drug's inhibition of T cell activation and cytokine and lymphokine production, which would indirectly inhibit keratin-ocyte proliferation. There is controversy about the relevance of any direct and primary effect of cyclosporine on keratinocytes in psoriasis. Although cyclophillins are present in human keratinocytes at levels similar to those found in other tissues, such as T cells, it is not clear if drug binding to cyclophillins in keratinocytes has any role in the beneficial effect of cyclosporine in psoriasis.[7]

There are other potential mechanisms by which cyclosporine may affect keratinocyte kinetics in psoriasis, independent of its effect on T cells. For example, cyclosporine has been shown to block 12-0-tetradecanoyl phorbol-13-acetate–induced cellular mechanisms in in vivo mouse models. These mechanisms include increased activity of ornithine decarboxylase, increased transglutaminase activity, arachidonic acid release, and IL-1B mRNA production. The majority of these are protein kinase C–mediated mechanisms. However, these findings have not been reproduced in human keratinocytes.[8,9]

In summary, cyclosporine inhibits the T cell activation mediated by antigens and lectins. Cyclosporine does not inhibit the early phases of lymphocytic signal transduction occurring after antigen-mediated activation. New cellular mechanisms of action of cyclosporine are being explored and discovered.

Pharmacokinetics

There is remarkably large intra- and interpatient variability in the oral absorption of cyclosporine. In general, bioavailability of ingested drug ranges from 25 to 35 percent. Peak levels occur from 1.3 to 4 h after oral administration. After gaining access to the circulation, cyclosporine has a large apparent volume of distribution (13 L/kg). Cyclosporine is metabolized into more than 30 cyclized metabolites by the liver cytochrome P_{450} 3A enzyme.[10,11] The cyclic subunit of cyclosporine is relatively resistant to degradation, as opposed to its side chains. It is believed that metabolites retain some biologic activities and thus may contribute to immunosuppression and/or toxicity. Cyclosporine's elimination half-life is 6 to 12 h in the absence of severe hepatic disease, and biliary excretion accounts for over 90 percent of its elimination.

Because the primary metabolism of the drug is by hepatic P_{450} 3A enzyme, drugs that compete for binding to P_{450} 3A will increase cyclosporine levels, and drugs that induce P_{450} will accelerate metabolism and decrease blood levels. Cyclosporine activity can be increased or decreased by concurrent administration of drugs listed in Table 261-1. There is a longer list of drugs that may affect the rate of cyclosporine metabolism if cultured human hepatocytes are used as an "in vitro" substrate.[10] Certain foods, particularly grapefruit, seem to increase the drug's bioavailability. Grapefruit's effect on cyclosporine action may be explained by the presence of bioflavonoids, which can inhibit metabolism of the drug by the cytochrome P_{450} 3A enzyme. In renal transplant patients, grapefruit may delay the absorption of cyclosporine and increase its AUC (area under the curve) in comparison with water. The known effect of drugs on cyclosporine activity has been studied in cardiac transplantation. In one carefully performed study, it was found that concurrent administration of ketoconazole, 200 mg/day orally, reduced the amount of cyclosporine required to maintain a therapeutic blood level by 60 to 80 percent.[12] This has been proposed as a way of reducing the cost of the drug in cardiac transplantation. The use of such medications and/or foods such as grapefruit juice to reduce cyclosporine requirements in a setting that is not strictly monitored is not recommended.[13]

The microemulsion-based formulation of cyclosporine (Neoral) has been developed to produce more consistent drug absorption.[14,15] This formulation does not seem to be influenced as greatly by food ingestion and is associated with faster, more extensive, and more predictable absorption.[16] Its absorption is relatively independent of bile production, and it has been demonstrated to be effective even in the presence of malabsorption states. Although more extensive data on efficacy and tolerability are required, its pharmacokinetic properties make the microemulsion-based formulation an attractive option, especially in patients with poor absorption of standard oral formulation and/or in patients with malabsorption states. Cyclosporine can also be administered intravenously as a 50-mg/mL solution made up in an ethanol-polyoxythylated castor oil mixture. Cyclosporine is concentrated in fatty tissues and red blood cells but does not cross the blood-brain barrier. In whole blood, 50 to 60 percent of cyclosporine is accumulated in erythrocytes and 10 to 20 percent accumulates in leukocytes, presumably due to their high cyclophillin content. The accumulation of cyclosporine in erythrocytes and leukocytes is the reason that whole blood monitoring of the drug levels are much more accurate than measurement of plasma levels.

It has not been possible to formulate a preparation of cyclosporine in any topical form that has significant penetration of the epidermal barrier. Cyclosporine solution does have some penetration of mucosal surfaces, but this is not true of cornified epithelium. Intralesional injections of cyclosporine in solution do provide some local effect in psoriasis, but are not widely used.

TABLE 261-1

Medications that Commonly Alter the Metabolism of Cyclosporine through the Cytochrome P_{450} 3A Pathway*

P_{450} 3A INHIBITORS[†]		P_{450} 3A INDUCERS[‡]	
Erythromycin	Methylprednisolone	Rifampicin	Sulfinpyrazone
Triacetyloleandomycin	Ketoconazole	Phenobarbital	Carbamazepine
Doxycycline	Fluconazole	Phenytoin	Trimethoprim-sulfamethoxazole
Midazolam	Itraconazole	Phenylbutazone	Nafcillin
Nifedipine	Bromocriptine		Valproate
Diltiazem	Furosemide		Isoniazide
Verapamil	Thiazides		
Nicardipine	Acetazolamide		
Dihydroergotamine	Colchicine		
Ergotamine	Cimetidine		
Progesterone	Ranitidine		
Ethinyl estradiol	Quinolones		
Danazol	Warfarin		
Cortisol	Amphotericin		
Prednisone	Acyclovir		
Predinosolone	Cephalosporins		

*The number of potential drug interactions emphasizes the need for close monitoring of drug levels and vigilance for potential signs of toxicity during therapy.
[†]Inhibitors have the potential to increase cyclosporine blood levels.
[‡]Inducers will enhance cyclosporine's metabolism and consequently decrease blood levels.

Dosages and Monitoring

Vast experience with cyclosporine dosing schedules can be derived from experience with transplant patients. Oral treatment is commonly initiated 4 to 24 days prior to transplantation at a dose of 15 mg/kg, in a single daily dose. Maintenance doses fall in the 3- to 10-mg/kg range. In dermatologic diseases, recommended doses rarely exceed 8 mg/kg per day, with no initial loading doses. Dosage increases should not exceed 0.5 to 1 mg/kg per day at 2- to 4-week intervals. Patients who are unable to tolerate the oral formulation can receive the diluted intravenous formulation, infused slowly over a period of 2 to 6 h at about one-third of the usual oral dose, or about 2 to 3 mg/kg per day.

The National Academy of Clinical Biochemistry/American Association for Clinical Chemistry Task Force on Cyclosporine Monitoring recommends that whole blood be utilized for cyclosporine assays, that EDTA be the anticoagulant, and that the assay be specific for the parent drug. Trough levels should be used, with samples obtained before the next dose. Timing of trough-level sampling becomes important for patients on a twice-daily regimen, since trough levels are reached at about 12 h. Recommended whole-blood trough levels, using monoclonal antibody assays in renal transplantation, range from 200 to 400 ng/mL. One must remember, however, that trough concentrations do not necessarily correlate well with either toxicity or efficacy in individual patients. Trough-level measurements may be more predictive in patients receiving the microemulsion-based formulation.

The two most common assays are high-performance liquid chromatography (HPLC) and radioimmunoassay.[17] In order to avoid toxicity in the treatment of dermatologic patients, the trough cyclosporine blood levels should generally be less than 250 ng/mL. From a practical standpoint, adequate monitoring of cyclosporine dosage can be achieved by the following: (1) avoidance of cyclosporine doses higher than 5 mg/kg per day; (2) evaluation of clinical response; and (3) vigilance for signs of toxicity by (*a*) detailed physical examination, including blood pressure monitoring with threshold concern triggered by a persistent diastolic blood pressure above 95 to 100 mmHg; (*b*) complete history with emphasis on concomitant drug ingestion and medical conditions that may potentiate cyclosporine toxicity; and (*c*) laboratory evaluations for complete blood count, creatinine and blood urea nitrogen, uric acid, aminotransferases, bilirubin, alkaline phosphatase, electrolytes and serum magnesium, and a urinalysis. In patients receiving long-term cyclosporine therapy (>6 months), the serum creatinine is a poor predictor of altered renal function and potentially irreversible chronic cyclosporine nephrotoxicity.[18–20] In such circumstances, it is recommended that one measure the glomerular filtration rate (GFR) every 4 to 6 months with studies such as isotopic isothalamate 125 or technetium 99 DPTA excretion, or inulin clearance.[21]

Differential Pharmacology

PEDIATRICS Children have comparable bioavailability of orally ingested cyclosporine but have a higher renal drug clearance rate (11.8 mL/min per kg versus 5.7 mL/min per kg in adults) and a correspondingly shorter blood level half-life (7.3 h versus 10.7 h in adults). This may require somewhat higher dosages and/or more frequent administration to achieve comparable trough levels. Preliminary reports have been encouraging, in that they report few significant adverse effects of cyclosporine on growth and development in children receiving transplants. Observed facial changes in children on cyclosporine include retrognathia, prominent supraorbital ridges, coarse skin, and thickening of the lips. Similar changes have not been seen in transplant patients on other immunosuppressive regimens. The use of the microemulsion formulation in children with liver transplantation may improve the efficacy of the drug's immunosuppression in the long term.[22]

GERIATRICS No substantial data exist about differential efficacy and toxicity of cyclosporine in the elderly, although closer monitoring for side effects is strongly advised.

PREGNANCY No significant changes in the dosage and pharmacokinetics have been reported in pregnant women. Adverse effects in the maternofetal period are described in the following section.

Side Effects

RENAL Nephrotoxicity, both acute and chronic, is the main adverse effect of cyclosporine therapy.[23] Acute renal toxicity is generally dose-dependent and reversible upon discontinuation of the drug. Long-term renal toxicity is gradual, progressive, usually irreversible, and is associated with characteristic histologic changes in the kidney. Three types of nephrotoxicity have been described.

The first occurs immediately after renal transplantation and occurs in the context of kidneys already damaged by ischemia. This phenomenon becomes relevant in the design of immunosuppressant protocols that include a delay in administration of cyclosporine until adequate renal function is achieved.[24] Obviously, this type of renal toxicity is not relevant to dermatologic patients.

The second type of nephrotoxicity appears during the first 2 to 3 weeks after transplantation and is usually associated with high cyclosporine blood levels. This type of nephrotoxicity must be differentiated from that due to acute rejection or acute tubular necrosis. An insidious decrease in GFR, hypertension, and tubular dysfunction (renal tubular acidosis, hyperkalemia, hyperuricemia, and decreased fractional excretion of sodium) in association with a recovery of renal function upon lowering the cyclosporine dosage are characteristic features of cyclosporine toxicity. In contrast, fever, graft tenderness, and a relatively rapid deterioration of renal function are more typical features of organ rejection. A fine-needle renal biopsy is often used to further differentiate these. Characteristic histologic findings of this form of cyclosporine toxicity include mild focal infiltrates, tubular vacuolization, and arteriolopathy. However, these histologic changes are not specific, and therefore the diagnosis of cyclosporine toxicity remains one of exclusion.[25,26] This type of nephrotoxicity can also be seen in dermatologic patients within a few weeks of initiation of cyclosporine therapy. Reduction in dosage or cessation of cyclosporine is generally associated with recovery of renal function.

Finally, there is chronic renal toxicity, which is likely due to cumulative subclinical toxicity. This form of toxicity may occur in the absence of any detectable elevation of creatinine or blood pressure. Histologic changes include interstitial fibrosis, tubular atrophy, and some degree of vasculopathy. Although renal function can improve somewhat after discontinuation of the drug, this type of toxicity is generally irreversible. In the treatment of dermatologic diseases, this is the form of toxicity that is most likely to occur. The development of a 50 percent elevation in serum creatinine is a risk factor for persistent renal dysfunction in patients with autoimmune diseases who receive doses above 5 mg/kg per day. In psoriatic patients receiving 5 mg/kg per day of cyclosporine, elevation of serum creatinine may persist for more than 4 months after discontinuation of the drug. Overall, one in four patients on cyclosporine develops clinical and laboratory evidence of altered renal function.

A crucial mechanism of cyclosporine nephrotoxicity in dermatologic and nondermatologic patients appears to be the failure of downregulation of renal vasoconstriction, caused by both an increase in endothelin (ET) 1–mediated vasoconstriction and a decrease of prostaglandin-mediated vasodilatation.[27,28] Elevation of ET-1 is also associated with vasculorejection in renal transplant patients, and ET-1 is produced by both endothelial cells and by graft-infiltrating mononuclear cells. ET-1 decreases the GFR, increases vascular resistance, and possesses mitogenic properties. ET-1 synthesis is regulated in part by T cell and monocyte/macrophage cytokines, and experimental data have shown that cyclosporine stimulates the synthesis of ET-1. Planned future therapeutic strategies include the use of ET-1 receptor antagonists in order to ameliorate or prevent the renal and vascular complications of cyclosporine.[29]

In transplant patients, the use of diltiazem and nifedipine has been associated with a reduction of the incidence of primary nonfunction of the graft, less severe rejection episodes, and a reduction of required cyclosporine dosages. The mechanism of renal protection by these calcium channel blockers seems to be mediated through the inhibition of ET-1 (verapamil is not associated with a reduction in nephrotoxicity or the incidence of rejection).[30–32] Nephrotoxicity can be potentiated by drugs such as aminoglycosides, amphotericin, melphalan, cotrimoxazole, diuretics, and nonsteroidal anti-inflammatory drugs. Hypomagnesemia and isolated hyperkalemia have also been reported to occur.

Hypertension is another very common adverse effect of cyclosporine and occurs in approximately 50 percent of patients overall, although it varies from about 70 percent in transplant patients to 30 percent in psoriatic patients. In nontransplant patients, the highest incidence of hypertension is seen in patients with autoimmune diseases, who carry an intrinsic potential risk for hypertension and renal dysfunction.[33,34] Calcium channel antagonists also exert a beneficial effect on cyclosporine-induced hypertension, presumably through the inhibition of ET-1. On the other hand, angiotensin-converting enzyme inhibitors are not as effective.[35–39] Diuretics should be used with caution because of their potential nephrotoxic effects.[40]

Another uncommon adverse renal complication is the development of hemolytic-uremic syndrome, which is associated with substantial morbidity and mortality. Aggressive therapeutic approaches such as intensive plasmapheresis with fresh-frozen plasma and supportive management are sometimes required. Hemolytic-uremic syndrome seems to be more common in allogeneic bone marrow transplant patients receiving cyclosporine for acute graft-versus-host disease, but this complication has been reported in varied clinical settings.[41–44]

GASTROINTESTINAL Nausea, vomiting, anorexia, and diarrhea are commonly described with the use of cyclosporine. Hyperbilirubinemia and transient mild elevation of liver enzymes are also reported in cyclosporine-treated patients.[45] Elevations of liver enzymes more than 100 percent over baseline should be managed by reduction of the cyclosporine dose by 25 percent weekly, until enzyme levels normalize. Avoidance of drugs with potential hepatotoxicity should be emphasized. Patients with significant liver dysfunction should not receive cyclosporine. An analogue of cyclosporine, cyclosporin G, was developed but had a much higher incidence of hepatoxicity without reduced nephrotoxicity and is not widely used.[46]

NEUROLOGIC Headache is the most common neurologic adverse effect. It is often resistant to regular analgesics, commonly occurs during the first weeks of therapy, and tends to resolve spontaneously as therapy continues. Patients with a history of migraine headaches are especially prone to this complication. Hand tremors, hyperesthesia, and paresthesia of the extremities are also common problems of cyclosporine therapy. Seizures have also been reported, but the vast majority of patients with cyclosporine-induced seizures have had low blood levels of magnesium and were also receiving high doses of intravenous methylprednisolone.[47–49] A form of central nervous system toxicity characterized by lethargy, confusion, seizures, cortical blindness, and hemiplegia has also been described in patients receiving intravenous cyclosporine. Cortical blindness seems to be more frequent in bone marrow transplant recipients.[50]

HEMATOLOGIC Hypercoagulability is a well-known side effect reported to occur in transplant patients receiving cyclosporine. The pathogenesis of this complication is attributed to abnormalities in platelets as well as in coagulation-dependent hemostasis.[51,52] Cyclosporine-treated kidney transplant recipients have shown low levels of tissue plasminogen activator and increased levels of the plasminogen activator inhibitor. There is also evidence of impaired fibrinolysis and endothelial damage associated with cyclosporine.[53–56] Hypercoagulability seems to contribute to the progression of atherosclerosis and gomerular damage in cyclosporine-treated patients. Non-life-threatening cytopenias have rarely been reported. The origin of this hematologic complication may be multifactorial.

METABOLIC Hypercholesterolemia, elevation of low-density lipoproteins, and hypertriglyceridemia may be seen with cyclosporine use[57] and may be contributing factors for the accelerated atherosclerosis and cardiovascular complications seen in transplant patients. Mechanisms such as an increase in lipid synthesis and/or a decrease in catabolism of lipoproteins have been postulated, but the precise mechanism of this adverse effect remains unknown. Preventative measures such as weight reduction, avoidance of alcohol, and increased physical activity should be instituted. Caution should be taken with the use of drugs to treat hyperlipidemias, since bile acid–binding resins may interfere with cyclosporine absorption and the use of HMG-CoA reductase inhibitors such as lovastatin or simvastatin may cause rhabdomyolisis.[58,59] Reversible hyperglycemia has been reported, apparently due to a direct effect of cyclosporine on cells from the islets of Langerhans.

NEOPLASTIC The frequency of Epstein-Barr virus–lymphoproliferative disease in transplant recipients, also known as *posttransplant lymphoproliferative disorder* (PTLD), has been estimated at 1 percent for renal allograft recipients, 2.7 percent for hepatic transplants, 3.3 percent for cardiac transplants, and 3.8 percent for cardiac/lung transplantation.[60] The incidence of this complication in dermatologic patients seems to be much lower than that observed in transplant patients. PTLD frequently fails to respond to chemotherapy but may regress spontaneously after reduction and/or cessation of immunosuppression. For PTLD that fails to regress after discontinuation of cyclosporine, therapies include intravenous immunoglobulin, interferon-α and high doses of intravenous acyclovir.[61]

There is an increased incidence of neoplasms in transplant patients, but this risk does not seem to be greater in patients treated with cyclosporine as opposed to those treated with other immunosuppressive drugs. The relative risk for lymphoma in patients treated with cyclosporine is 27.5, versus a relative risk of 33.8 to 58.6 in patients treated with immunosuppressive regimens that do not include the use of cyclosporine. There are also reports of an increased incidence of non-Hodgkin's B cell lymphomas in patients receiving cyclosporine in conjunction with other immunosuppressants. For example, the incidence of lymphoma in transplant patients receiving cyclosporine alone or in combination with glucocorticoids is less than 1 percent, whereas the incidence in transplant patients receiving cyclosporine in conjunction with other immunosuppressive drugs is as high as 8 percent.[62] In contrast to the high mortality rate attributed to lymphomas arising in immunosuppressed patients, lymphomas developing in cyclosporine-treated patients seem to carry a better prognosis, and the latency period seems to be shorter.

The incidence of lymphoma in cyclosporine-treated dermatologic patients is less than 0.2 percent. Most of these are B cell non-Hodgkin's lymphoma, but T cell non-Hodgkin's and Hodgkin's lymphomas have also been reported.

An increased incidence of skin cancer is a known complication of immunosuppression, and cyclosporine-treated transplant recipients have a relative risk for all skin cancers of 6.8 versus 2.2 to 5.5 in patients receiving other immunosuppressive therapy. Cyclosporine-treated dermatologic patients also have a higher risk of skin cancers, including squamous cell carcinomas (SCC), basal cell carcinomas, Bowen's disease, Kaposi's sarcoma, and perhaps melanoma.[63] There is a high incidence of SCC in psoriatic patients treated with cyclosporine, but this could be biased by previous exposures to PUVA or UVB.[63] Kaposi's sarcoma with visceral involvement that develops during cyclosporine treatment often fails to respond to therapy, but about 25 percent of nonvisceral Kaposi's sarcomas can be expected to undergo complete or partial remission following cessation or reduction of immunosuppresive therapy.

An increased incidence of carcinoma of the penis, vulva, and anus have also been reported, and some of these carcinomas arise from preexisting viral warts. Cessation or reduction of the immunosuppressive regimen as well as retinoid therapy could be worthy therapeutic strategies for prevention and control of viral-induced SCC and dysplastic lesions. Due to the potential carcinogenic potential of viral warts, total eradication of these lesions has been proposed as a way to prevent the future development of SCC, but the validity of this therapy is very controversial.

Other tumors, including endocrine neoplasms, hepatocarcinoma, cancer of the esophagus, and uterine and cervical carcinomas are also reported in cyclosporine-treated patients, although their real incidence is unknown. Pseudolymphoma is another reported complication with the use of cyclosporine.[64–66]

MUCOCUTANEOUS Hypertrichosis is a well-known complication and probably occurs in 100 percent of patients on long term cyclosporine therapy.[67,68] It seems to be more common in dark-skinned patients, is not confined to androgen-dependent hair-bearing areas, and is independent of sex hormone levels.

Hypertrichosis tends to worsen with further treatment and shows no tendency to remit spontaneously. Gingival hypertrophy is reported in 8 to 70 percent of patients on cyclosporine. It tends to develop first on the anterior gingival mucosae, and the peak incidence occurs within 6 months of the initiation of therapy. This complication is more common in children and is found in individuals with poor oral hygiene.[69] Gingival sensitivity is a common complaint. The underlying histologic finding is fibrous hyperplasia, similar to that seen in patients on phenytoin and calcium channel blockers.[70] This is an important issue since calcium channel drugs are important in the management of cyclosporine-induced hypertension, and the risk for development of this side effect may be much higher with the use of this drug combination.[71]

An acneiform eruption, indistinguishable from that seen in steroid-induced acne, is frequently reported. A disseminated comedonal or cystic acneiform eruption can also occur. These side effects can appear at any time during cyclosporine therapy, although it is more commonly described at the time of initiation of therapy.

Keratosis pilaris is reported in 21 percent of cyclosporine-treated patients, sebaceous hyperplasia in 15 percent, and epidermal inclusion cysts in 28 percent. Some of the epidermal cysts are small and located on the face and typically decrease in size and number as time progresses. Flushing, angioedema, urticaria, and anaphylaxis have also been reported with the use of cyclosporine. An increased incidence of keratoacanthomas, sebaceous hyperplasia, and viral warts has also been reported.

MUSCULOSKELETAL Osteoporosis is increased in organ transplant patients receiving cyclosporine and FK506[72] and seems to be the result of actions on osteoblasts and osteoclasts and of alterations in lymphokine release. Cyclosporine can induce hyperuricemia in up to 15 percent of patients, and apparently this is secondary to decreased urate clearance. Gout appears to be more common in men, in patients with preexisting renal impairment, and in those concomitantly using diuretics.[73] Myopathy has been reported in transplant patients receiving high doses of cyclosporine.[74]

REPRODUCTIVE Cyclosporine does not seem to be mutagenic or teratogenic, although there is a high incidence of preterm newborns, fetal growth retardation, abortions, preeclampsia, and hypertension in mothers taking cyclosporine, and these incidences are magnified in transplant patients. There are no reports of neonatal complications in children born to fathers receiving cyclosporine. Adequate contraceptive measures are recommended in women of childbearing potential.[75] Cyclosporine crosses the placenta and is excreted in breast milk. Preexisting conditions such as hypertension, diabetes, and renal dysfunction are risk factors in female transplant patients for the development of cyclosporine toxicity during pregnancy.[76–79] Close monitoring during pregnancy, labor, and post partum is mandatory.

IMMUNOLOGIC There is controversy as to whether there is an increased incidence of infections in nontransplant patients receiving low dose of cyclosporine as sole immunosuppressive therapy. Cyclosporine-treated transplant patients seem to enjoy a relative risk for infectious complications that is lower than that seen in patients receiving azathioprine and prednisolone.[80] However, it is recommended that there be increased vigilance for infectious complications in cyclosporine-treated patients.

Therapeutic Uses

NONDERMATOLOGIC Vast experience has been gained in the use of cyclosporine in organ transplantation and autoimmune disorders. The usual dosage for these indications ranges from 5 mg/kg to 8 mg/kg of the microemulsion-based formulation.

DERMATOLOGIC The medical literature is replete with anecdotal reports of the therapeutic uses of cyclosporine in dermatologic diseases.[81] From a practical standpoint, these can be divided into two groups—psoriasis[82] and nonpsoriatic dermatoses. Within the latter group, the most responsive dermatoses are pyoderma gangrenosum,[83–87] cutaneous[88,89] and oral lichen planus,[90–93] graft-versus-host disease,[94,95] epidermolysis bullosa acquisita,[96–99] Behçet's disease,[100–106] and paraneoplastic pemphigus.[107] Lesser efficacy is reported in atopic dermatitis, dermatomyositis, alopecia areata,[108–113] and disabling morphea,[114] among others.[115,116]

Psoriasis In psoriasis, cyclosporine is indicated as part of a rotational therapeutic regimen for refractory cases. There are anecdotal reports of efficacy in psoriatic arthritis,[117] pustular psoriasis,[118–120] acrodermatitis continua of Hallopeau,[121] nail psoriasis, palmoplantar pustulosis, and psoriatic erythroderma. There is vast experience in the use of cyclosporine in plaque-type psoriasis[122–129]; however, in the United States, cyclosporine is still an off-label drug for psoriasis.

Using the microemulsion-based formulation of cyclosporine (Neoral), the recommended starting dose should be 2.5 mg/kg per day. Dosage increases should be performed after 4 weeks of therapy, and dose reductions are permitted at any time. Doses higher than 5 mg/kg per day are not advisable. In patients going into remissions, defined as PASI (psoriasis area and severity index) reduction greater than 75 percent, the cyclosporine dose should be downtitrated at 4-week intervals, usually starting at week 16. PASI is reduced by 82 to 84 percent in patients on the standard cyclosporine formulation or on a microemulsion-based cyclosporine formulation by week 16 of therapy.

Serum creatinine levels should be carefully monitored during cyclosporine therapy. If creatinine levels increase more than 30 percent above baseline, the dosage should be reduced for 1 to 2 weeks. If after that time the creatinine levels decrease below the 30 percent elevation mark, continuation at the lower dose is advisable. In cases where the creatinine remains elevated by more than 30 percent, discontinuation of cyclosporine is recommended until the creatinine returns to levels within 10 percent of pretreatment levels. More accurate monitoring of the GFR clearance, calculated from the serum creatinine, by 24-h urine collection, or even by radioisotope tests, can be used in individual cases. A short course of cyclosporine (not exceeding 6 months) at an initial dose of 3 mg/kg per day has been shown to be effective and to have a better risk:benefit ratio than 5 mg/kg per day in psoriatic patients.[130] The use of the microemulsion-based formulation of cyclosporine in severe psoriasis has demonstrated better bioavailability and greater efficacy at a lower dose in comparison with the traditional formulation. Long-term cyclosporine therapy, up to 30 months, has been shown to produce significant clinical improvement, although exacerbation was noted in 50 percent of patients after cyclosporine was withdrawn.[131] A randomized, double-blind, placebo-controlled study using low doses of cyclosporine (1.25 to 2.5 mg/kg per day) for 4 weeks in patients with palmoplantar pustulosis has shown significant reduction in pustule formation and few side effects.[132]

Failure of topical cyclosporine to penetrate the epidermal barrier and the problems associated with intralesional injections of cyclosporine in plaque psoriasis discourage topical use.[133]

Nonpsoriatic dermatoses ATOPIC DERMATITIS There is vast European experience in the use of cyclosporine in atopic dermatitis. Its safety and efficacy in children have been studied, and it seems to be a safe, alternative, short-term therapy for severe atopic dermatitis in childhood.[134,135]

In severe and refractory atopic dermatitis in adults, a study comparing two regimens showed that there was no difference in terms of long-term efficacy or safety profile with a starting dose of 3 mg/kg per day and increasing to 5 mg/kg per day as needed, versus starting at 5 mg/kg per day and decreasing to 3 mg/kg per day as needed.[136] Relapses within weeks after discontinuation of cyclosporine are common.[137,138] Topical 10% cyclosporine has been demonstrated to be effective in one trial in atopic dermatitis,[139] but this finding has not been consistent in the medical literature.

DERMATOMYOSITIS Cyclosporine is an adjunctive therapy in refractory cases of juvenile dermatomyositis, used in combination with glucocorticoids alone or with glucocorticoids and cytotoxic drugs.[140-142] It is also a potentially useful agent in refractory polymyositis and dermatomyositis in adults, although several cases report no significant improvement with the use of cyclosporine.[143-145]

OTHER DERMATOSES Refractory cutaneous lichen planus has been reported to respond to 4 weeks of cyclosporine therapy at a dose of 6 mg/kg per day. In oral lichen planus, the use of topical cyclosporine has been demonstrated to be an effective alternative to systemic treatment.[146] In this protocol, cyclosporine is administered as 5 mL of 100 mg/mL oral cyclosporine solution tid, "swish and spit." Patients exhibited improvement in erythema, erosions, reticulation, and pain after 4 to 16 weeks of therapy. Reticulate lesions on the labial and buccal mucosa generally responded better than similar lesions on the tongue and gingivae. In the majority of patients, blood levels due to systemic absorption were very low or undetectable (HPLC and radioimmunoassay, 20–184 ng/mL). Although this regimen is effective, the cost is extremely high.

Topical cyclosporine for oral bullous disorders has been generally discouraging. Aphthous stomatitis has shown inconsistent responses to topical cyclosporine.[147] Pyoderma gangrenosum usually responds to initial doses greater than 3 mg/kg per day, with maintenance therapy at 3 mg/kg per day. Significant improvement is expected within 3 months of initiation of therapy. Cyclosporine seems to be an effective immunosuppressive drug for the treatment of some cases of paraneoplastic pemphigus, at a dose of 5 to 7 mg/kg per day. It is generally more effective when used in combination with prednisone in doses approaching 1 mg/kg per day. Cyclosporine doses, in the range of 5 to 10 mg/kg per day, have been demonstrated to be superior to conventional therapy in controlling ocular (and also, perhaps, extraocular) symptoms in Behçet's syndrome. Refractory cases of epidermolysis bullosa acquisita have been shown to respond to cyclosporine (6 to 9 mg/kg per day), in conjunction with glucocorticoids or as monotherapy. There is controversy about the effects of cyclosporine on circulating autoantibody titers.

Cosmetically acceptable hair regrowth can be achieved in severe alopecia areata using systemic cyclosporine. However, it is expected that rapid hair loss will once again appear within 3 months of discontinuation of the drug. The results of topical cyclosporine in alopecia areata have been disappointing.

TACROLIMUS (FK506)

This immunosuppressant is a macrolide antibiotic that was first isolated from the soil microorganism *Streptomyces tsukubaensis*. FK506 is 100 times more potent than cyclosporine on a molecular basis. This drug is also known to inhibit calcium-dependent events mediated by calcineurin, such as IL-2 gene transcription, nitric oxidase synthase activation, cell degranulation, and apoptosis,[148] but additional molecular mechanisms are being defined. Preliminary results indicate that FK506 and cyclosporine are comparable in safety and efficacy in liver transplantation. FK506 appears to be superior to cyclosporine in the management of acute, steroid-resistant rejection in liver transplantation.[149] A multicenter study has shown that FK506 rescue therapy provides rapid and effective reversal of refractory renal allograft rejection, good long-term allograft function, a low incidence of recurrent rejection, and an acceptable safety profile.[150] It may also constitute a valuable alternative for primary immunosuppression or rescue therapy in other transplant recipients, especially in the pediatric population.[151-154]

FK506 can be administered intravenously or orally. A topical formulation is also being used in clinical trials.[155] The usual adult intravenous dosage is 25 to 50 μg/kg and 50 to 100 μg/kg for pediatric populations. Oral dosages range between 150 and 200 μg/kg for adults and 200 and 300 μg/kg for children.

The pharmakokinetics are characterized by a two-compartment model with a rapid initial drop and a long terminal elimination half-life of 12 to 21 h. Wide oral bioavailability, with a 6 to 60 percent variation, has been observed.[156] FK506 is extensively metabolized in the liver, with less 1 percent of the drug excreted intact.

FK506 has not proved to be more effective than cyclosporine as a first-line agent in renal transplantation. Some minor differences in toxicities are observed. In comparison with cyclosporine, patients on FK506 have a reduced requirement for antihypertensive medications and decreased cholesterol levels. Hypertrichosis, gingival hypertrophy, and coarseness of facial features seem to be less frequent. Major neurotoxicities, such as dysphasia, confusion, psychosis, encephalopathy, and coma, are somewhat higher than with cyclosporine use and have been reported to occur in up to 8 percent of liver transplant patients treated with FK506.[157] Minor neurotoxicities, including tremor, headache, insomnia, and nightmares, are much more frequently observed, occurring in about 20 percent of FK506–treated patients.[158] Glucose intolerance, requiring insulin, is a common side effect, reported in 17 percent of liver transplant patients and developing within the first 30 days post transplant. About half of these patients will remain glucose-intolerant at later stages.[157] This side effect seems to be uncommon in children with transplants.[159] Hyperuricemia and hyperkalemia are also reported. Hypertension seems to be about 50 percent less frequent with FK506, although the lower doses of glucocorticoids used in patients receiving FK506 may contribute to this lower incidence.[160]

Nephrotoxicity seems to be comparable to that seen with cyclosporine use. Around 21 percent of FK506–treated patients have been reported to demonstrate nephrotoxicity 1 year after liver transplantation.[157] In renal transplants, the incidence of nephrotoxicity is similar, at about 27 percent.[161] The onset of nephrotoxicity may be early, correlated with high drug blood levels, but late onset is also reported. The histopathology of the renal toxicity is similar to that seen with cyclosporine nephrotoxicity. The dosage of FK506 should be reduced in the presence of hepatic dysfunction, and close monitoring of whole-blood trough levels should be encouraged. Palpitations and abnormal electrocardiographic findings have also been described as side effects of FK506.

PTLD also occurs in patients receiving FK506.[162] The risk for PTLD seems to be particularly high in children with hepatic transplants who receive both tacrolimus and anti-OKT3.[163,164]

There is a good correlation between enzyme-linked immunosorbent assay (ELISA) and HPLC-MS measurements in the monitoring of blood concentrations of FK506. However, ELISA assays may also detect metabolites of the drug, which could make this method less accurate in conditions with altered metabolism of FK506, such as hepatic disease. Levels greater than 20 ng/mL in whole blood are associated with toxicity, so that 5 to 15 ng/mL blood levels are now widely recommended. The least effective blood level has not been fully defined.[165-167]

Topical FK506 has been used in atopic dermatitis with some benefit. Absorption of topical tacrolimus in eczema seems to occur only in skin that is actively inflamed, presumably due to disruption of the epidermal barrier function.

Systemic FK506 has been shown to be effective for recalcitrant plaque-type psoriasis by the European FK506 Multicenter Psoriasis Study Group. This was a double-blind, placebo-controlled study in which the efficacy and side effects of FK506 in 27 patients were evaluated. An initial dose of 0.05 mg/kg per day for 6 to 9 weeks produced significant improvement in PASI scores, with relatively few side effects—predominantly diarrhea, paresthesia, and insomnia.[168] The use of systemic and topical FK506 in dermatologic diseases still remains to be more deeply explored, although the potential use of FK506 in dermatoses refractory to cyclosporine is promising.

SIROLIMUS (RAPAMYCIN)

Sirolimus is an immunosuppressive macrolide antibiotic with a biochemical structure similar to that of FK506. It was isolated from the fungus *S. hydroscopicus*. Sirolimus binds to the immunophillin FKBP 12. The target of the FKBP 12–sirolimus complex is RAFT-1, a protein kinase that is likely required for T cell proliferation in the presence of IL-2.[169,170] The immediate downstream target of RAFT-1 has not yet been identified. Sirolimus does not block the transcription of the early activation genes but does inhibit cytokine-mediated signal transduction pathways, such as those pathways activated after the binding of IL-2 to its receptor (CD25). Thus, sirolimus inhibits the IL-2-induced phosphorylation and activation of kinases. Sirolimus also inhibits calcium-independent mechanisms responsible for the activation of T cells, acting in the late phases in the cell cycle, specifically between the late phase of G_1 and S. It is a potent T as well as B cell inhibitor and participates in the inhibition of IL-4-driven lymphocyte proliferation.

Sirolimus has some unique properties that differentiate it from cyclosporine and FK506. In addition to its immunosuppressive effects, it has been shown to inhibit smooth muscle cell proliferation and migration. This property may be helpful in preventing the intimal hyperplasia that is characteristic of cyclosporine- and FK506–induced renal vascular toxicity.[171]

The drug is sequestered by erythrocytes. It is metabolized by the same P_{450} 3A enzyme that is involved in the metabolism of cyclosporine and FK506. Its half-life is long, with a 24-h trough concentration, and there is a good correlation between trough levels and administered doses. Further protocols are being explored to delineate its pharmacology and therapeutic uses.[172] There is no significant experience with the use of this drug in dermatologic patients.

OTHER IMMUNOSUPPRESSIVE DRUGS

Mycophenolate Mofetil

Mycophenolate mofetil (MMF) is an ethyl ester of mycophenolic acid, which is metabolized to the active drug—mycophenolic acid (MPA). MPA is a product of several *Penicillium* species. MPA, the active metabolite, was used in the past for the treatment of severe recalcitrant psoriasis. Although MPA was shown to have significant therapeutic efficacy,[173] it was withdrawn because of a high incidence of side effects, primarily infections such as herpes zoster and gastrointestinal side effects. MMF is the reformulated product; it does not have these same drawbacks and has better bioavailability than MPA. This immunomodulatory drug selectively inhibits inosine monophosphate dehydrogenase (IMPDH) in the de novo pathway of purine synthesis. This enzyme converts inosine monophosphate to xanthine monophosphate, an intermediate metabolite in the synthesis of guanosine triphosphate. This drug is more active in its inhibition of the type II isoform of IMPDH, which is found mostly in lymphocytes, and thus inhibits purine synthesis with potent cytostatic effects on both T and B lymphocytes. Lymphocytes are quite susceptible to this drug effect, for they minimally utilize the hypoxanthine-guanine phosphoribosyl transferase salvage pathway for purine synthesis.

Through these actions, MMF inhibits lymphocyte proliferation and antibody formation. This drug also inhibits leukocyte recruitment and glycosylation of lymphocyte glycoproteins involved in adhesion to endothelial cells.[174,175] The drug is rapidly absorbed after oral administration, and antacids and cholestyramine may decrease its absorption. Around 5 percent of the drug is bound to albumin. It is nearly completely metabolized by glucuronyl transferase, and over 90 percent of the drug is eliminated by the kidneys. The MMF glucuronide metabolite, which is increased in renal failure, increases MMF clearance by competing for its binding sites on albumin. MMF pharmacokinetics seem not to be affected by the concomitant administration of cyclosporine.

The usual dose is 1 g every 12 h. Expected toxicities include nausea, stomach upset, vomiting, and diarrhea. There is no increase in nephrotoxicity, hepatotoxicity, hypertension, or neurotoxicity when MMF is used in conjunction with cyclosporine and glucocorticoids. Severe leukopenia has been reported in fewer than 3 percent of MMF-treated patients. An increased incidence of lymphoproliferative diseases and lymphoma is reported with its use, as is some predisposition for infectious complications. Therapeutic drug monitoring measured by IMPDH activity in whole blood could be a viable alternative to assess the overall state of MMF-induced immunosuppression.[176]

This drug is commonly used in combination with cyclosporine and glucocorticoids to prevent renal graft rejection. The role of MMF in immunologic-mediated skin diseases seems to be promising. For example, its therapeutic profile and toxicities make it an attractive substitute for azathioprine in several circumstances. For example, it could be useful in those patients who cannot tolerate azathioprine due to nausea or hepatotoxic reactions, or in those patients who are at risk for azathioprine-induced toxicities due to deficiency of the enzyme thiopurine methyl transferase. Reports of its use in vasculitis and in bullous pemphigoid have been published.[177,178]

Deoxyspergualin

Deoxyspergualin (DSG) is a synthetic analogue of spergualin, a natural product extracted from *Bacillus laterosporus*. DSG strongly suppresses IL-2 receptor expression as well as the generation of cytotoxic T lymphocytes. The mechanism of action is not fully understood, but DSG binds to a heat-shock protein called heat shock cognate 70 (hsp 70). The DSG–hsp 70 complex is thought to bind NF-kB, thus inhibiting its nuclear translocation. NF-kB is a member of the Rel family of transcriptional activation proteins that regulate the transcription of kappa light chains and certain cytokines, including tumor necrosis factor α, IL-6, and IL-8. NF-kB is implicated in the regulation of NO synthase transcription as well as in the modulation of transcriptional factors involved in IL-2 and IL-2R expression.

DSG must be administered intravenously; its pharmacokinetics are first order and linear. Preliminary data show that its metabolism is not affected by cytochrome P_{450}. Clinical trials have demonstrated its efficacy in the reversal of acute renal graft rejection and possibly in the prolongation of pancreatic islet cell allografts. However, additional basic and clinical studies are necessary to delineate its pharmacodynamics and pharmacokinetics.[179]

Leflunomide

Leflunomide is an isoxazole derivative that inhibits the proliferation of T and B cell lines. It is thought to be mediated by the inhibition of pyrimidine biosynthesis, blocking production of uridine monophosphate by the de novo pathway. Tyrosine kinase inhibition may be part of its mechanism of action. Its efficacy in the prevention of heart, kidney, intestine, lung, and skin allograft rejection has been studied in animal models.[180] Since leflunomide is activated by liver metabolism, renal failure has less effects on its kinetics. Its elimination half-life is about 11 days, and its metabolite is mainly excreted by the kidneys. Toxicities that have been observed include the liver, gastrointestinal tract, and morbilliform skin eruptions.

Brequinar Sodium

Brequinar sodium is a novel quinoline carboxylic acid analogue that behaves as a noncompetitive inhibitor of dehydroorate dehydrogenase, an enzyme involved in the de novo synthesis of pyrimidine. Inhibition of the B and T cell proliferation is achieved between G_2 and S in the cell cycle.

REFERENCES

1. Bierer BE et al: Cyclosporin A and FK 506: Molecular mechanisms of immunosuppression and probes for transplantation biology. *Curr Opin Immunol* **15**:763, 1993
2. Reiser H, Stadecker MJ: Costimulatory B7 molecules in the pathogenesis of infectious and autoimmune diseases. *N Engl J Med* **335**:1369, 1996
3. June CH et al: T-cell proliferation involving the CD-28 pathway is associated with cyclosporine resistant interleukin-2 gene expression. *Mol Cell Biol* **7**:4472, 1987
4. Galvin F et al: Effects of cyclosporin A, FK506, and mycalamide A on the activation of murine CD 4+ T cells by the murine B7 antigen. *Eur J Immunol* **23**:283, 1993
5. Suthanthiran M, Strom TB: Renal transplantation. *N Engl J Med* **331**:365, 1994
6. Wiederrecht G et al: The mechanism of action of FK-506 and cyclosporine A. *Ann N Y Acad Sci* **696**:9, 1993
7. Fairley JA: Intracellular targets of cyclosporine. *J Am Acad Dermatol* **23**:1329, 1990
8. Baadsgaard O et al: Interaction of epidermal cells and T cells in inflammatory skin diseases. *J Am Acad Dermatol* **23**:1312, 1990
9. Cooper KD et al: Effects of cyclosporine on immunologic mechanism in psoriasis. *J Am Acad Dermatol* **23**:1318, 1990
10. Watkins PB: The roles of cytochromes P-450 in cyclosporine metabolism. *J Am Acad Dermatol* **23**:1301, 1990
11. Christians U, Sewing KF: Cyclosporin metabolism in transplant patients. *Pharmacol Ther* **57**:291, 1993
12. Keogh A et al: Ketoconazole to reduce the need for cyclosporin after cardiac transplantation. *N Engl J Med* **333**:628, 1995
13. Min DI et al: Effect of grapefruit juice on cyclosporine pharmacokinetics in renal transplant patients. *Transplantation* **62**:123, 1996
14. Furst DE: Innovative treatment approaches for rheumatoid arthritis. Cyclosporin, leflunomide and nitrogen mustard. *Baillieres Clin Rheumatol* **9**:711, 1995
15. Noble S, Markham A: Cyclosporin: A review of the pharmacokinetic properties, clinical efficacy and tolerability of a microemulsion-based formulation (Neoral). *Drugs* **50**:924, 1995
16. Kovarik JM et al: Evidence of earlier stabilization of cyclosporine pharmacokinetics in de novo renal transplant patients receiving a microemulsion fomulation. *Transplantation* **62**:759, 1996
17. Mockli G et al: Laboratory monitoring of cyclosporine levels: Guidelines for the dermatologist. *J Am Acad Dermatol* **23**:1275, 1990
18. Gilbert SC et al: Cyclosporine therapy for psoriasis: Serum creatinine measurements are an unreliable predictor of decreased renal function. *J Am Acad Dermatol* **21**:470, 1989
19. Tomlanovich S et al: Limitations of creatinine in quantifying the severity of cyclosporine-induced chronic nephrotoxicity. *Am J Kidney Dis* **8**:332, 1986
20. Myers BD et al: The long-term course of cyclosporine-associated chronic nephropathy. *Kidney Int* **33**:590, 1988
21. Messana JM et al: Effects of cyclosporine on renal function in psoriasis patients. *J Am Acad Dermatol* **23**:1289, 1990
22. Hoppu K et al: Comparison of conventional oral cyclosporine microemulsion formulation in children with a liver transplant. *Transplantation* **62**:66, 1996
23. Bennett WM: Renal effects of cyclosporine. *J Am Acad Dermatol* **23**:1280, 1990
24. Sheil A GR et al: Australian trial of cyclosporin (CsA) in cadaveric donor renal transplantation. *Transplant Proc* **15**:2485, 1983
25. Neild GH et al: Morphological differentiation between rejection and cyclosporin toxicity in renal allograft. *J Clin Pathol* **39**:152, 1986
26. D'Ardenne AJ et al: Cyclosporin and renal graft histology. *J Clin Pathol* **39**:145, 1986
27. Coffman TM et al: The thromboxane (Tx) synthetase inhibitor CGS 13080 improves renal allograft function in patients taking cyclosporine (CSA). *Kidney Int* **37**:604, 1990
28. Perico N, Remuzz G: Cyclosporin-induced renal dysfunction in experimental animals and humans. *Transplant Rev* **5**:63, 1991
29. Watschinger B, Sayegh MH: Endothelin in organ transplantation. *Am J Kidney Dis* **27**:151, 1996
30. Chrysostomon A et al: Diltiazem in renal allograft recipients receiving cyclosporine. *Transplantation* **55**:300, 1993
31. Donnelly PK et al: Renal transplantation: Nifedipine for the nonstarters? A prospective randomized study. *Transplant Proc* **25**:600, 1993
32. Pirsch JD et al: A controlled double-blind randomized trial of verapamil and cyclosporine cadaver renal transplant patients. *Am J Kidney Dis* **21**.189, 1993
33. Dieterle A et al: Nephrotoxicity and hypertension in patients with autoimmune diseases treated with cyclosporin. *Transplant Proc* **20**(suppl 4):349, 1988
34. Fry L et al: Long-term cyclosporine in the management of psoriasis. *Transplant Proc* **20**(suppl 4):23, 1988
35. Wagner K et al: Interaction of cyclosporine and calcium antagonists. *Transplant Proc* **21**:1453, 1989
36. Magineni CN et al: Cyclosporine A–calcium antagonist interaction: A possible mechanism for nephrotoxicity. *Transplant Proc* **21**:1358, 1987
37. Scoble JE et al: In vitro cyclosporine toxicity: The effect of verapamil. *Transplantation* **47**:647, 1989
38. Bennett WM, Porter GA: Cyclosporine-associated hypertension. *Am J Med* **85**:131, 1988
39. Curtis JJ et al: Hypertension in cyclosporine-treated transplant recipients is sodium dependent. *Am J Med* **85**:134, 1988
40. Deray G et al: Enhancement of cyclosporin nephrotoxicity by diuretic therapy. *Clin Nephrol* **32**:47, 1989
41. Agarwal A et al: Recurrent hemolytic uremic syndrome in an adult renal allograft recipient: Current concepts and management. *J Am Soc Nephrol* **6**:1160, 1995
42. Scantlebury VP et al: Renal transplantation under cyclosporine and FK 506 for hemolytic uremic syndrome. *Transplant Proc* **27**:842, 1995
43. Katznelson S et al: Cyclosporine-induced hemolytic uremic syndrome: Factors that obscure its diagnosis. *Transplant Proc* **28**:2608, 1994
44. Gagnadoux MF et al: Outcome of renal transplantation in 34 cases of childhood hemolytic-uremic syndrome and the role of cyclosporine. *Transplant Proc* **26**:269, 1994
45. Klintmalin GB et al: Cyclosporine A hepatotoxicity in 66 allograft recipients. *Transplantation* **32**:488, 1981
46. Henry ML et al: Trial of cyclosporine vs OG37-325 in cadaveric renal transplantation: A preliminary report. *Transplant Proc* **25**:689, 1993
47. Joss DV et al: Hypertension and convulsions in children receiving cyclosporin A. *Lancet* **1**:906, 1982

48. June CH et al: Correlation of hypomagnesemia with the onset of cyclosporine-associated hypertension in bone marrow transplant patients. *Transplantation* **41**:47, 1986

49. Durrant S et al: Cyclosporin A, methylprednisolone, and convulsions. *Lancet* **2**:829, 1982

50. Edwards LL et al: Neurophysiologic evaluation of cyclosporine toxicity associated with bone marrow transplantation. *Acta Neurol Scand* **92**:423, 1995

51. Vanrenterghem Y et al: Thromboembolic complications and haemostatic changes in cyclosporin-treated cadaveric kidney allograft recipients. *Lancet* **1**:999, 1985

52. Grace AA et al: Cyclosporine A enhances platelet aggregation. *Kidney Int* **32**:889, 1987

53. Cohen H et al: Persistent decreased fibrinolytic activity in cyclosporine-treated renal allograft recipients. *Fibrinolysis* **2**:197, 1988

54. Drouet L et al: Clinical usefulness of plasmatic markers of the endothelial function: Application of cyclosporin nephrotoxicity. *Thromb Haemost* **62**:579, 1989

55. Baker LRI et al: Enhanced in vitro hemostasis and reduced thrombolysis in cyclosporin-treated renal transplant recipients. *Transplantation* **49**:905, 1990

56. Malyszko J et al: The coagulolytic system and endothelial function in cyclosporine-treated kidney allograft recipients. *Transplantation* **62**:828, 1996

57. Ballantyne CM et al: Effects of cyclosporine therapy on plasma lipoprotein levels. *JAMA* **262**:53, 1989

58. Alejandro DS, Petersen J: Myoglobinuric acute renal failure in a cardiac transplant patient taking lovastatin and cyclosporine. *J Am Soc Nephrol* **4**:153, 1994

59. East C et al: Rhabdomyolisis in patients receiving lovastatin after cardiac transplantation. *N Engl J Med* **318**:47, 1988

60. Nalesnik M et al: Experience with posttransplant lymphoproliferative disorders in solid organ transplant patients. *Clin Transplant* **69**:249, 1992

61. Taguchi Y et al: The effects of intravenous immunoglobulin and interferon-alfa on Epstein-Barr virus–induced lymphoproliferative disorder in a liver transplant recipient. *Transplantation* **57**:91, 1994

62. Valdimarsson H: Immunity during cyclosporine therapy. *J Am Acad Dermatol* **23**:1295, 1990

63. Korstanje MJ, Van de Staak WJBM: High cumulative dose of ultraviolet radiation is a contraindication for cyclosporin therapy. *Clin Exp Dermatol* **15**:76, 1990

64. Brown MD et al: Rapid occurrence of nodular T-lymphocyte infiltrates with cyclosporine therapy. *Arch Dermatol* **124**:1097, 1988

65. Bagot M et al: Pseudolymphome induit par la ciclosporine. *Ann Dermatol Venereol* **66**:536, 1989

66. Therstup-Pedersen K et al: Development of cutaneous pseudolymphoma following cyclosporin therapy of actinic reticuloid. *Dermatologica* **177**:376, 1988

67. Bencini PL et al: Cutaneous lesions in 67 cyclosporine-treated renal transplant recipients. *Dermatologica* **172**:24, 1986

68. Wysocki GP, Daley TD: Hypertrichosis in patients receiving cyclosporine therapy. *Clin Exp Dermatol* **12**:191, 1987

69. Daley TD et al: Clinical and pharmacological correlations in cyclosporine-induced gingival hyperplasia. *Oral Surg Oral Med Oral Pathol* **62**:417, 1986

70. Deliliers GL et al: Light and electron microscopic study of cyclosporin A–induced gingival hyperplasia. *J Periodontol* **57**:771, 1986

71. Slavin J, Taylor J: Cyclosporin, nifedipine and gingival hyperplasia. *Lancet* **2**:739, 1987

72. Epstein S et al: Organ transplantation and osteoporosis. *Curr Opin Rheumatol* **7**:255, 1995

73. Lin HY et al: Cyclosporine-induced hyperuricemia and gout. *N Engl J Med* **321**:287, 1989

74. Fernandez-Sola J et al: Reversible cyclosporin study myopathy. *Lancet* **1**:362, 1990

75. Cockburn I et al: Present experience of Sandimmune in pregnancy. *Transplant Proc* **21**:3730, 1989

76. Armenti VT et al: Variables affecting birthweight and graft survival in 197 pregnancies in cyclosporine-treated female kidney transplant recipients. *Transplantation* **59**:476, 1995

77. Bertschinger P et al: Cyclosporine treatment of severe ulcerative colitis during pregnancy. *Am J Gastroenterol* **90**:330, 1995

78. Muirhead N et al: The outcome of pregnancy following renal transplantation—the experience of a single center. *Transplantation* **54**:429, 1992

79. Olshan AF et al for the International Commission for Protection Against Environmental Mutagens and Carcinogens: Cyclosporine A: Review of genotoxicity and potential for adverse human reproductive and developmental effects. Report of a working group on the genotoxicity of cyclosporine A. *Mutat Res* **317**:163, 1994

80. Canadian Multicentre Transplant Study Group: A randomized clinical trial of cyclosporin in cadaveric renal transplantation. *N Engl J Med* **309**:809, 1983

81. Lim KK et al: Cyclosporine in the treatment of dermatologic disease: An update. *Mayo Clin Proc* **71**:1182, 1996

82. Zachariae H, Steen Olsen T: Efficacy of cyclosporin A(CyA) in psoriasis: An overview of dose/response, indications, contraindications and side-effects. *Clin Nephrol* **43**:154, 1995

83. Curley RK et al: Pyoderma gangrenosum treated with cyclosporin A. *Br J Dermatol* **113**:601, 1985

84. Elgart G et al: Treatment of pyoderma gangrenosum with cyclosporin: Results in seven patients. *J Am Acad Dermatol* **24**:83, 1991

85. Shelley ED, Shelley WB: Cyclosporine therapy for pyoderma gangrenosum associated with sclerosing cholangitis and ulcerative colitis. *J Am Acad Dermatol* **18**:1084, 1988

86. Penmetcha M, Navartman A: Pyoderma gangrenosum responsive to cyclosporin A. *Int J Dermatol* **27**:253, 1988

87. Magid ML, Gold MH: Treatment of recalcitrant pyoderma gangrenosum with cyclosporine. *J Am Acad Dermatol* **20**:293, 1989

88. Ho VC et al: Treatment of severe lichen planus with cyclosporine. *J Am Acad Dermatol* **22**:64, 1990

89. Higgins EM et al: Cyclosporin A in the treatment of lichen planus (letter). *Arch Dermatol* **125**:1436, 1989

90. Frances C et al: Effect of local application of cyclosporine on chronic erosive lichen planus of the oral cavity. *Dermatologica* **177**:194, 1988

91. Balato N et al: Dermatological application of cyclosporine. *Arch Dermatol* **125**:1430, 1989

92. Eisen D et al: Cyclosporin wash for oral lichen planus. *Lancet* **335**:535, 1990

93. Eisen D et al: Cyclosporine swish and spit improves oral lichen planus: A double-blind analysis. *N Engl J Med* **323**:290, 1990

94. Harper JI et al: Dermatological aspects of the use of cyclosporin A for prophylaxis of graft-versus-host disease. *Br J Dermatol* **110**:469, 1984

95. Vogersang GB et al: Acute graft-versus-host disease: Clinical characteristics in the cyclosporine era. *Medicine* **67**:163, 1988

96. Connoly SM, Sander HM: Treatment of epidermolysis bullosa acquisita with cyclosporine. *J Am Acad Dermatol* **16**:109, 1987

97. Zachariae H: Cyclosporine A in epidemolysis bullosa acquisita. *J Am Acad Dermatol* **17**:1058, 1987

98. Crow LL et al: Clearing of epidermolysis bullosa acquisita with cyclosporine. *J Am Acad Dermatol* **19**:937, 1988

99. Layton AM, Cunliffe WJ: Clearing of epidermolysis bullosa acquisita with cyclosporine. *J Am Acad Dermatol* **22**:535, 1990

100. Nussenblatt RB et al: Effectiveness of cyclosporin therapy for Behçet's disease. *Arthritis Rheum* **28**:671, 1985

101. Suss R et al: Cyclosporin therapy in Behçet's disease. *J Am Acad Dermatol* **29**:101, 1993

102. Masuda K et al: Double-masked trial of cyclosporin versus colchicine and long-term open study of cyclosporin in Behçet's disease. *Lancet* **1**:109, 1989

103. Nussenblatt RB et al: Treatment of intraocular inflammatory disease with cyclosporin A. *Lancet* **2**:235, 1983

104. Binder AI et al: Cyclosporin A in the treatment of severe Behçet's disease. *Br J Dermatol* **26**:285, 1987

105. Muftuoglu AU et al: Short-term cyclosporin A treatment of Behçet's disease. *Br J Ophthalmol* **71**:387, 1987

106. BenEzra D et al: Revaluation of conventional therapy versus cyclosporin A in Behçet's syndrome. *Transplant Proc* **20**:136, 1988

107. Ståhle-Backdähl M et al: Paraneoplastic pemphigus: A report of two patients responding to cyclosporine. *Eur J Dermatol* **5**:671, 1995

108. Gebhart W et al: Cyclosporin A induced hair growth in human renal allograft recipients and alopecia areata. *Arch Dermatol Res* **278**:238, 1986

109. Gupta AK et al: Oral cyclosporine A for the treatment of alopecia areata: A clinical and immunohistochemical analysis. *J Am Acad Dermatol* **22**:242, 1990

110. Parodi A, Rebora A: Topical cyclosporine in alopecia areata. *Arch Dermatol* **123**:165, 1987

111. Thomson AW et al: Topical cyclosporine in alopecia areata and nickel contact dermatitis. *Lancet* **2**:971, 1986

112. De Prost Y et al: Placebo-controlled trial of topical cyclosporin in severe alopecia areata. *Lancet* **2**:803, 1986

113. Guilhar A et al: Topical cyclosporin A in alopecia areata. *Acta Derm Venereol* **69**:252, 1989

114. Peter RU et al: Low-dose cyclosporin A in the treatment of disabling morphea. *Arch Dermatol* **127**:1420, 1991

115. Ho VC et al: Cyclosporine in nonpsoriatic dermatoses. *J Am Acad Dermatol* **23**:1248, 1990

116. Ruzicka T: Cyclosporin in less common immune-mediated skin diseases. *Br J Dermatol* **135**(suppl 48):40, 1996

117. Ruzicka T: Psoriatic arthritis: New types, new treatment. *Arch Dermatol* **132**:215, 1996

118. Reitamo S et al: Cyclosporin in the treatment of palmoplantar pustulosis. *Arch Dermatol* **129**:1273, 1993

119. Peter RU et al: Low-dose cyclosporin A in palmoplantar psoriasis: Evaluation of efficacy and safety. *J Eur Acad Dermatol Venereol* **3**:518, 1994

120. Meinardi MMHM et al: Generalized pustular psoriasis responding to cyclosporin A. *Br J Dermatol* **116**:269, 1987

121. Peter RU et al: Acrodermatitis continua type of pustular psoriasis responds to low-dose cyclosporine. *J Am Acad Dermatol* **23**:515, 1990

122. Va Joost TH et al: Low-dose cyclosporin A in severe psoriasis. A double-blind study. *Br J Dermatol* **118**:183, 1988

123. Finzi AF et al: Effectiveness of cyclosporin treatment in severe psoriasis: A clinical and immunological study. *J Am Acad Dermatol* **21**:91, 1989

124. Dubertret I et al: Cyclosporin in psoriasis: A long-term randomized study on 37 patients. *Acta Derm Venerol (Stockh)* **146**(suppl):136, 1989

125. Ellis CN et al: Cyclosporin for plaque-type psoriasis: Results of multidose double-blind trial. *N Engl J Med* **324**:277, 1991

126. Griffiths CEM et al: Long-term cyclosporin for psoriasis. *J Dermatol* **120**:253, 1989

127. Mahrle G et al: Low-dose short-term cyclosporin versus etretinate in psoriasis: Improvement of skin, nail, and joint involvement. *J Am Acad Dermatol* **32**:78, 1995

128. Lewis HM et al: Cyclosporin A in the treatment of chronic plaque psoriasis. Six year experience. *J Dermatol Treat* **4**:3, 1993

129. Timonen P et al: Efficacy of low-dose cyclosporin A in psoriasis: Results of dose-finding studies. *Br J Dermatol* **122**(suppl 36):33, 1990

130. Finzi AF: Individualized short-course cyclosporin therapy in psoriasis. *Br J Dermatol* **135**(suppl 48):31, 1996

131. Gulliver WP et al: Increased bioavailability and improved efficacy, in severe psoriasis, of a new microemulsion formulation of cyclosporin. *Br J Dermatol* **135**(suppl 48):35, 1996

132. Reitamo S et al: Cyclosporine in the treatment of palmoplantar pustulosis: A randomized, double-blind, placebo-controlled study. *Arch Dermatol* **129**:1273, 1993

133. Griffiths CEM: Systemic and local administration of cyclosporine in treatment of psoriasis. *J Am Acad Dermatol* **23**:1242, 1990

134. Berth-Jones J et al: Cyclosporin in severe childhood atopic dermatitis: A multicentre study. *J Am Acad Dermatol* **34**:1016, 1996

135. Zaki I et al: Treatment of severe atopic dermatitis in childhood with cyclosporin. *Br J Dermatol* **135**(suppl 48):21, 1996

136. Zonneveld IM et al: The long-term safety and efficacy of cyclosporin in severe refractory atopic dermatitis: A comparison of two dosage regimens. *Br J Dermatol* **135**(suppl 48):15, 1996

137. Motley RJ et al: Resolution of atopic dermatitis in a patient treated with cyclosporin. *Clin Exp Dermatol* **14**:243, 1989

138. Taylor RS et al: Cyclosporine therapy for severe atopic dermatitis. *J Am Acad Dermatol* **21**:580, 1989

139. De Prost Y et al: Randomized double-blind placebo-controlled trial of local cyclosporin in atopic dermatitis. *Acta Derm Venereol (Stockh)* **144**:136, 1989

140. Zabel P et al: Cyclosporin for acute dermatomyositis. *Lancet* **1**:343, 1984

141. Heckmatt J et al: Cyclosporin in juvenile dermatomyositis. *Lancet* **1**:1063, 1989

142. Griadin E et al: Cyclosporine for juvenile dermatomyositis. *J Pediatr* **112**:165, 1988

143. Lueck CJ et al: Cyclosporin in the management of polymyositis and dermatomyositis. *J Neurol Neurosurg Psychiatry* **54**:1007, 1991

144. Levi S, Hodgson HJF: Cyclosporin for dermatomyositis? *Ann Rheum Dis* **48**:85, 1989

145. Borleffs JCC: Cyclosporine as monotherapy for polymyositis? *Transplant Proc* **3**:333, 1988

146. Pigatto PD et al: Cyclosporin A for treatment of severe lichen planus. *Br J Dermatol* **122**:121, 1990

147. Eisen D, Ellis CN: Topical cyclosporine for oral mucosal disorders. *J Am Acad Dermatol* **23**:1259, 1990

148. Thomson AW et al: Mode of action of tacrolimus (FK506): Molecular and cellular mechanism. *Ther Drug Monit* **17**:584, 1995

149. Klintmalm GB: Clinical use of FK506 in liver transplantation. *Transplant Proc* **28**:974, 1996

150. Woodle ES et al: A multicenter trial of FK506 (tacrolimus) therapy in refractory acute renal allograft rejection. *Transplantation* **62**:594, 1996

151. Winkler M, Christians U: A risk-benefit assessment of tacrolimus in transplantation. *Drug Saf* **12**:348, 1995

152. Kelly PA et al: Tacrolimus: A new immunosuppressive agent. *Am J Health Syst Pharm* **52**:1521, 1995

153. Ellis D: Clinical use of tacrolimus (FK506) in infants and children with renal transplants. *Pediatr Nephrol* **9**:487, 1995

154. Peters DH et al: Tacrolimus: A review of its pharmacology and therapeutic potential in hepatic and renal transplantation. *Drugs* **46**:746, 1993

155. Lauerma AI, Maibach HI: Topical FK506—clinical potential or laboratory curiosity? *Dermatology* **188**:173, 1993

156. Wenkataramanan R et al: Pharmacokinetics of FK506 following oral administration: A comparison of FK506 and cyclosporin. *Transplant Proc* **23**:931, 1991

157. Alessiani M et al: Adverse effects of FK506 overdosage after liver transplantation. *Transplant Proc* **25**:628, 1993

158. Eidelman BH et al: Neurologic complications of FK506. *Transplant Proc* **23**:3175, 1991

159. Carroll PB et al: FK506–associated diabetes mellitus in the pediatric transplant population is a rare complication. *Transplant Proc* **26**:3171, 1991

160. Wallemacq PE, Reding R: FK506 (tacrolimus). A novel immunosuppressant in organ transplantation: Clinical, biomedical and analytical aspects. *Clin Chem* **39**:2219, 1993

161. Japanese FK506 Study group: Japanese study of FK506 on kidney transplantation: Result of late phase II study. *Transplant Proc* **25**:649, 1993

162. Deschler DG et al: Posttransplantation lymphoproliferative disorder in patients under primary tacrolimus (FK 506). *Arch Otolaryngol Head Neck Surg* **121**:1037, 1995

163. Malatack J et al: Orthotopic liver transplantation, Epstein-Barr virus, cyclosporin and lymphoproliferative disease: A growing concern. *J Pediatr* **11**:667, 1991

164. Newell KA et al: Posttransplant lymphoproliferative disease in pediatric liver transplantation. *Transplantation* **62**:370, 1996

165. Jusko WJ: Analysis of tacrolimus (FK506) in relation to therapeutic drug monitoring. *Ther Drug Monit* **17**:596, 1995

166. Jusko WJ et al: Consensus document: Therapeutic monitoring of tacrolimus (FK506). *Ther Drug Monit* **17**:606, 1995

167. McMaster P et al: Therapeutic drug monitoring of tacrolimus in clinical transplantation. *Ther Drug Monit* **17**:602, 1995

168. The European FK 506 Multicentre Psoriasis Study Group: Systemic tacrolimus (FK506) is effective for the treatment of psoriasis in a double-blind, placebo-controlled study. *Arch Dermatol* **132**:419, 1996

169. Cardenas ME et al: Molecular mechanisms of immunosuppression by cyclosporine, FK506, and rapamycin. *Curr Opin Nephrol Hypertens* **4**:472, 1995

170. Morris R: Modes of action of FK506, cyclosporin A, and rapamycin. *Transplant Proc* **26**:3272, 1994

171. Pon M et al: Rapamycin inhibits vascular smooth muscle cell migration. *J Clin Invest* **98**:2277, 1996

172. Yatscoff RW et al: Rapamycin: Distribution, pharmacokinetics, and therapeutic range investigations. *Ther Drug Monit* **17**:666, 1995

173. Gomez EC et al: Efficacy of mycophenolic acid for the treatment of psoriasis. *J Am Acad Dermatol* **1**:531, 1979

174. Allison AC et al: Mycophenolate mofetil (RS-61443): Mechanism of action and effects in transplantation. *Transplant Rev* **7**:129, 1993

175. Allison AC et al: Mycophenolate and brequinar, inhibitor of purine and pyrimidine synthesis, block the glycosylation of adhesion molecules. *Transplant Proc* **25**:67, 1993

176. Langman LJ et al: Pharmacodynamic assessment of mycophenolic acid–induced immunosuppression in renal transplant patients. *Transplantation* **62**:666, 1996
177. Nowack R et al: Mycophenolate mofetil for systemic vaculitis and IgA nephropathy. *Lancet* **349**:774, 1997
178. Bohm M et al: Bullous pemphigoid treated with mycophenolate mofetil. *Lancet* **349**:541, 1997
179. Ramos EL et al: Deoxyspergualin: Mechanism of action and pharmacokinetics. *Transplant Proc* **28**:873, 1996
180. Yeh LS et al: Effects of leflunomide and cyclosporine on myocutaneous allograft survival in the rat. *Transplantation* **62**:861, 1996

CHAPTER 262

Gerhard Tappeiner
Klaus Wolff

Thalidomide

HISTORIC BACKGROUND

Thalidomide was marketed in 1957 in Europe, Australia, and several African and Asian countries but never in the United States or Canada. A Japanese pharmaceutical company synthesized and marketed thalidomide independently at the same time in Japan. The drug quickly found wide use as a barbiturate-free sedative with potent antiemetic properties, and it was believed safe even for pregnant women. Thus, it was widely used for emesis and in insomnia during pregnancy.

Beginning in 1961, an increase of cases of severe limb malformations in newborns began to be noted in West Germany; soon, thalidomide was identified as the cause and the drug was taken off the market in Europe in 1961 and in Japan in 1962. A second serious side effect of thalidomide, induction of peripheral neuropathy, was first noted in 1960. Nevertheless, over 10,000 children fell victim to thalidomide embryopathy. Following this tragedy, all civilized countries instituted appropriate procedures to evaluate the safety, efficacy, adverse effects, and risk/benefit ratio of drugs before they were introduced in the market. The thalidomide tragedy was thus a driving force behind the evolution of the ethical principles governing the way clinical studies are undertaken today (Good Clinical Practice; Declaration of Helsinki).

Anti-inflammatory effects of thalidomide were observed early but at first were not followed up. In 1964, Sheskin, a dermatologist at Hansen's Disease Hospital in Jerusalem, noted a rapid anti-inflammatory and analgesic effect of thalidomide in patients with erythema nodosum leprosum (type II leprosy reaction). It was shown subsequently that this beneficial effect occurs in over 90 percent of these patients, which vastly improves the therapeutic options for patients with multibacillary leprosy (see Chap. 203). This (initially, and erroneously, interpreted as immunosuppressive) action of thalidomide has been under investigation since the mid-1960s and is now considered its most relevant activity. Thalidomide has turned out to be an extremely interesting drug for inflammatory skin conditions. Thalidomide has recently been reviewed by the Food and Drug Administration (FDA) and found to be approvable as a therapeutic agent for erythema nodosum leprosum.

CHEMISTRY, PHARMACOLOGY, AND PHARMACOKINETICS

Thalidomide [α-N-phthalimidoglutarimide; 2-(2,6-dioxo-piperidine-3-yl)-isoindole-1,3-dione] is a racemic mixture of its ($-$)(S) and ($+$)(R) isomers. It is poorly soluble in water and in lipids, and this accounts for its very low acute toxicity. Studies on pure isoforms of thalidomide are very much hampered by its rapid racemization ($T_{1/2}$ about 2.25 h). Most of the reliable data on the activities of the isoforms of thalidomide have been obtained using configuration-stable methylated analogues. These studies indicate that the ($-$)(S) form is the active compound and that its beneficial and untoward effects cannot be separated.

In a study of healthy male volunteers,[1] an absorption half-life of 1.7 ± 1.05 h, an elimination half-life of 8.7 ± 4.11 h, and a peak plasma concentration of 1.15 ± 0.2 mg/L at 4.39 ± 1.27 h were seen after a single oral dose of 200 mg thalidomide. The plasma concentration-versus-time curve fit a one-compartment model with first-order kinetics.[1] Excretion was primarily nonrenal. Only weak accumulation of thalidomide has been found except for the kidneys and the hepatobiliary tract; however, this increased accumulation is thought to be related to excretion.

Investigations of the effects of thalidomide in mammals in vitro and in vivo have yielded copious amounts of data, some of which are not easy to interpret; the following activities are rather well established.

Pharmacologic Effects

Thalidomide has potent anti-inflammatory activities, presumably mainly through the inhibition of the pathway of tumor necrosis factor α (TNF-α); in addition, it inhibits HIV replication in vivo. It also inhibits production of interleukin 12 (IL-12) and should thus suppress immunity mediated by T-helper (T_H) cells, but this effect has not yet been unequivocally demonstrated.

Further effects of thalidomide, mainly found in animal models, are a downregulation of certain cell adhesion molecules,[2,3] the extent and importance of which is not yet entirely clear, as well as inhibition of angiogenesis.[3,4] The anti-inflammatory effects of thalidomide may be accounted for by its effects on TNF-α and on angiogenesis, while its teratogenic action could be due to its inhibition of adhesion molecules and angiogenesis.

Adhesion Molecules

Thalidomide has been shown to downregulate β_2-integrin (CD18) and, to a lesser degree, β_1-integrin (CD29) and α_4-integrin on circulating leukocytes of humans; the effect on intercellular adhesion molecule 1 (ICAM-1; CD54) expression was increased on granulocytes but abolished on monocytes.[5,6] A highly teratogenic analogue of thalidomide administered to pregnant mice resulted in a profound and consistent suppression of β_3-integrin (CD61) in the fetus. In this study, β_1- and α_4-integrin subunits were decreased in the limb buds but not elsewhere.[2] If this is representative of the situation in humans, it may offer an explanation for the teratogenic action of thalidomide.

Cytokines

Thalidomide has been shown to be a potent suppressor of IL-12 production by human monocytes; this suppression was dose-dependent, additive to that of dexamethasone, and independent of endogenous inhibitors of IL-12 production; IL-12 stimulates interferon (IFN-γ) production and thus plays a critical role in the development of cellular immune responses mediated by T_H cells. The contribution of IL-12 inhibition to thalidomide's properties is not yet entirely understood; it is not known whether this contributes to its therapeutic activity.[7] However, it may help to explain some of the unexpected phenomena seen when thalidomide is used to treat tuberculosis in HIV-infected patients or chronic graft-versus-host disease.

In cultures of human peripheral blood monocytes, thalidomide inhibited IFN-γ production and enhanced IL-4 and IL-5 synthesis[8]; however, in tuberculosis patients on thalidomide, IL-1 mRNA levels were reduced while serum (but not mRNA) levels of IFN-γ were raised. The effects on other lymphokines have varied, probably because of the different experimental settings in which they were obtained. Furthermore, thalidomide has been demonstrated to be an inhibitor of angiogenesis.[4] In fact, thalidomide analogues for use as antiangiogenic drugs are being developed.

Tumor Necrosis Factor

Thalidomide decreases production of TNF-α in stimulated human monocyte cultures but has no effect on total protein synthesis or the expression of various other cytokines.[9] This decrease in synthesis is caused by a reduction in the half-life of TNF-α messenger RNA[10]; this is a selective and dose-dependent effect but does not lead to a complete arrest of TNF-α production.

Patients with lepromatous leprosy and manifestations of erythema nodosum leprosum have been shown to have high levels of circulating TNF-α and other cytokines. Administration of thalidomide to these patients leads to an often dramatic amelioration of their symptoms and to a concomitant decrease of TNF-α levels.[11] In patients with active tuberculosis with or without HIV-infection, thalidomide treatment likewise results in a decrease of TNF-α and IL-1 levels and an increase in IFN-γ levels. The weight loss often associated with active tuberculosis is probably at least in part due to the high levels of TNF-α in these patients. Not surprisingly, the administration of thalidomide results in a reversal of this weight loss.[12]

Human Immunodeficiency Virus

Thalidomide has a marked effect on the replication of HIV. It has been known for some time that opportunistic infections increase HIV replication. This is very likely due to the induction of TNF-α synthesis which, in turn, activates a nuclear transcription factor (NFκB), a cytoplasmic protein that enhances HIV transcription and is a regulatory component in the gene transcription of several mediators of inflammation, including TNF-α, thus establishing a feedback amplification loop. Tat, a protein initiating HIV replication, also activates NFκB. Viral replication is abolished in tat-defective strains and can be restored by TNF-α; NFκB-defective T cell lines are resistant to infection with HIV. Thus, the pathways for the transcription of TNF-α (and probably other cytokines) and of HIV appear to depend on the same regulatory mechanism.

Thalidomide inhibits TNF-α production; therefore it blocks a pathway for the activation of NFκB and hence the replication of HIV. In addition, it inhibits the synthesis of both TNF-α and NFκB and thus interferes in two places with the positive feedback amplification loop for TNF-α and HIV production.

CURRENT THERAPEUTIC USES OF THALIDOMIDE

Beginning in the mid-1970s, thalidomide's potential as an anti-inflammatory drug began to be recognized for a wide variety of conditions: skin lesions of chronic cutaneous and subacute cutaneous lupus erythematosus, aphthous stomatitis in immunocompetent and immunocompromised patients and in Behçet's disease, chronic graft-versus-host reaction, inflammatory bowel disease, erythema multiforme, pyoderma gangrenosum, postherpetic neuralgia, prurigo nodularis, actinic prurigo, and various problems associated with HIV infection. All of these have been reported to respond to thalidomide therapy. However, most of these observations have been published as case reports or small series and thus await confirmation by larger formal studies. Currently, efforts are being made to make better use of thalidomide's unique properties, to gain approval for the use of thalidomide in selected indications, and to develop analogues—e.g., with more pronounced antiangiogenic properties—for use in a variety of neoplastic and inflammatory diseases.

Erythema Nodosum Leprosum

In a review of 4522 patients with erythema nodosum leprosum (ENL), 99 percent were found to respond to thalidomide. Lesions resolve within 24 to 48 h after treatment is begun; other symptoms (headache, myalgia, anorexia, vomiting, orchitis, leukocytosis, elevated sedimentation rate) also respond quickly. Motor nerve conduction velocity returns to almost normal within 2 weeks. All this is achieved through thalidomide's inhibitory effect on TNF-α; thalidomide has no direct effect on *Mycobacterium leprae*. Because of this impressive efficacy, thalidomide may currently be considered the therapeutic standard for ENL.

HIV Infection

Thalidomide has a beneficial effect on complications of HIV disease. Aphthous ulcers and AIDS wasting associated with tuberculosis[12] have been shown to respond well; other complications such as prurigo nodularis, proctitis, and refractory microsporidial diarrhea may also respond. Furthermore, thalidomide may inhibit HIV replication in AIDS patients with active mycobacterial infections. However, HIV-infected patients are at greater risk for developing untoward effects from this therapy and must be selected and monitored accordingly.[13]

MICROSPORIDIOSIS Microsporidiosis is a common cause of chronic diarrhea in HIV patients, contributing to their often severe wasting problems. In a study of 19 patients with chronic diarrhea due to microsporidiosis, 7 had a complete and 3 a partial clinical remission when given 100 mg of thalidomide daily.[14] Remarkably it was found that all stages of the life cycle of the causative organism, *Enterocytozoon intestinale*, were disrupted.

APHTHOUS ULCERS IN AIDS Patients with advanced HIV disease develop painful aphthous ulcerations of the mouth and the oropharynx resembling the aphthous ulcerations typically found in patients with Behçet's disease. These aphthous ulcers are usually progressive and can be large (over 1 cm^2), deep and destructive, and lead to or aggravate HIV-associated weight loss. These aphthae were usually treated with local or systemic glucocorticoids but have been shown to respond very well to thalidomide at daily doses of 100 to 300 mg.[15] In a recent double-blind, randomized, placebo-controlled study, patients received a 4-week course of either 200 mg of thalidomide or placebo.[16] Complete healing of ulcers after 4 weeks occurred in 55 percent of treated patients as compared with 7 percent in the placebo-treated group; 6 had to discontinue the drug because of toxicity; somnolence and a skin rash were each noted in 7 patients. Interestingly and contrary to expectations,[17] there were increased plasma levels of TNF-α and of HIV-RNA in the thalidomide-treated group; the significance of these findings remains to be studied.

Similarly, 11 of 12 patients with esophageal ulceration had a complete symptomatic remission; in 9 of them there was complete healing[18] after 200 mg thalidomide daily for 4 weeks.

KAPOSI'S SARCOMA As reported recently, a favorable response to thalidomide was seen in two phase II Kaposi's sarcoma trials. In one study, 3 of 5 patients had a greater than 50 percent reduction in the number of lesions; in a second study, a partial response was seen in 5 of 11 evaluable patients. This effect is thought to be related to thalidomide's antiangiogenic properties.

Aphthosis and Behçet's Disease in Immunocompetent Patients

Observations in small series of patients showed that recurrent aphthous stomatitis and Behçet's disease in immunocompetent patients also respond to thalidomide treatment at 100 to 300 mg/day. In one larger study, about one-third of 40 patients with aphthosis of varying severity had full remissions, one-third had improvement with reduction of the severity of aphthous lesions but did relapse after discontinuation of treatment, and the remainder did not benefit from treatment.[19] In a multicenter crossover study of patients with severe aphthous stomatitis, 44 percent of 73 patients receiving thalidomide and 8 percent on placebo achieved complete remissions; almost all patients had some benefit from this treatment, but relapses were common after its discontinuation.[20] In a retrospective study of 25 patients with recurrent aphthous stomatitis followed for 1 year, 6 were able to stop treatment with only minor recurrences, 10 needed further maintenance treatment with low doses of thalidomide, 7 did not respond, 1 had to stop because of side effects, and 1 was lost to follow-up.[21]

In the largest series of patients with Behçet's syndrome, oral and genital lesions of all 22 patients studied healed very rapidly in response to thalidomide 400 mg/day for 5 days, then 200 mg/day for up to 2 months; however, no effect on ocular lesions was seen.[22] After cessation of therapy, recurrences were milder and less frequent. A patient with complete Behçet's syndrome and a severe attack of Behçet colitis in addition to oral ulceration and pleural effusion went into complete remission with thalidomide 300 mg/day and could be maintained with 100 mg daily.[23]

Clearly, patients with HIV-associated oral and esophageal ulceration benefit more from thalidomide therapy than immunocompetent patients with aphthous ulcers with or without Behçet's syndrome; however, thalidomide provides a good and usually well-tolerated therapeutic alternative in these patients. A double-blind, placebo-controlled study of 100 mg thalidomide daily to determine the safety and efficacy of this therapeutic regimen has been instituted.

Lupus Erythematosus

Thalidomide has been found to be an effective and relatively well-tolerated treatment modality for the lesions of chronic cutaneous and subacute cutaneous lupus erythematosus. The value of this therapeutic measure is hardly debated, as the results of the first observations published in the early 1980s[24-27] are essentially the same as those in the larger series published more recently.[28-31] The following facts emerge:

- In a recent survey of 61 lupus centers from 19 countries around the world, 35 percent reported using thalidomide as a therapeutic option.[32]
- When given thalidomide, 50 to 90 percent of patients with subacute or chronic cutaneous lupus erythematosus achieve com-

plete or near complete remissions; in all studies, at least 80 percent of patients responded. Interestingly, the same beneficial effect has been found in one patient with subacute cutaneous lupus erythematosus associated with partial deficiency of the fourth component of complement.[33]

- Thalidomide must be discontinued early owing to unacceptable side effects in 10 to 25 percent of patients.
- Thalidomide dosages used in these studies range from 50 to 300 mg per day, the maximum benefit being achieved within 16 weeks[31]; the higher dosages seem to be associated with somewhat higher response rates but not with lower relapse rates.
- Response may be maintained with 25 to 50 mg/day. Relapses after cessation of thalidomide medication occur in 70 to 75 percent of patients but are usually responsive to a new course of the drug.[31]
- Thalidomide's effect on the skin lesion of lupus erythematosus notwithstanding, it has no influence on the course and severity of the systemic disease.

In some of these studies it is not clear whether concomitant systemic glucocorticoid therapy was given; one of these studies does address the problem, stating that the use of thalidomide allowed the average daily glucocorticoid dose to be reduced from 40 to 17.5 mg.[30] A Ro antibody–positive patient, previously published,[25] exemplifies the effect of thalidomide on the skin lesions of subacute cutaneous lupus erythematosus (Fig. 262-1A): Azathioprine 150 mg/day and 6-methylprednisone 60 mg/day given previously had completely failed to control his rash. Thalidomide at 300 mg/day led to a considerable improvement of the skin disease within 3 weeks and to a complete remission within 10 weeks (Fig. 262-1B), with no additional immunosuppressive/glucocorticoid medication. This remission could be maintained with thalidomide

100 mg/day, and the treatment was tolerated well, with only minor side effects due to sedation.

As with other long-term therapies with thalidomide, women of childbearing age must be exhaustively informed about the necessity of and monitored for the use of reliable contraceptive measures, and all patients must be watched for neuropathy.

In summary, thalidomide is an effective therapeutic alternative for chronic and subacute cutaneous skin lesions of lupus erythematosus that cannot be adequately controlled by more conventional measures provided that it is used by physicians competent to evaluate cutaneous and systemic disease activity in such patients and to treat patients with teratogenic drugs.

Chronic Graft-versus-Host Disease

Apart from uncontrolled case reports, there are two studies of thalidomide in the treatment of chronic graft-versus-host disease (CGvHD) after bone marrow transplantation in adults and one study in children. Vogelsang et al. found a survival rate of 76 percent among patients with GvHD refractory to conventional therapy and of 48 percent of patients with high-risk GvHD[34]; a complete response was observed in 14 patients, a partial response in 12, and no response in 18. They observed only minor side effects. Parker et al. treated 80 patients who failed to respond to conventional therapy (glucocorticoids with or without cyclosporine). A total of 36 percent of their patients had to discontinue thalidomide because of side effects; 20 percent had a sustained favorable response.[35]

Five children with severe glucocorticoid-dependent CGvHD were treated with 12 to 25 mg thalidomide/kg per day.[36] All chil-

FIGURE 262-1

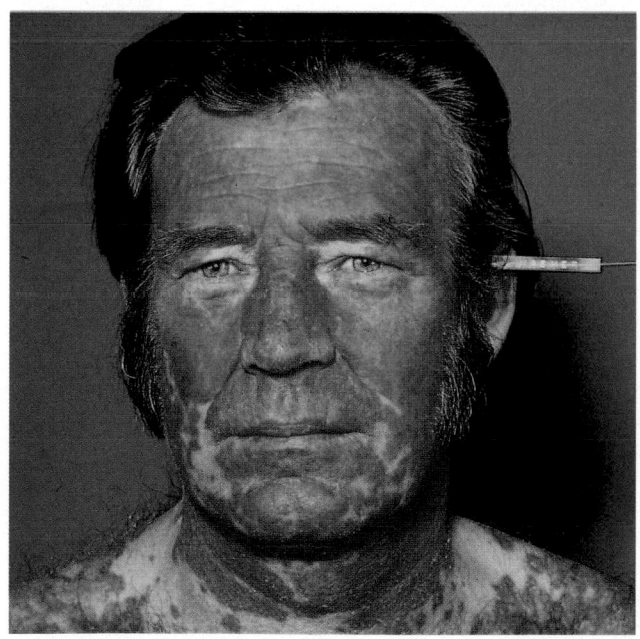

A.

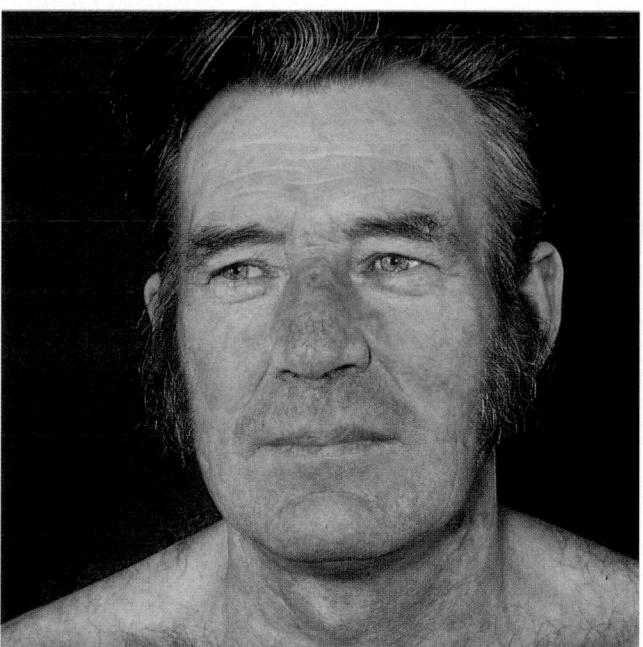

B.

Patient with subacute cutaneous lupus erythematosus unresponsive to treatment with azathioprine/methylprednisone. Skin lesions of the face and neck (*A*) shortly after withdrawal of conventional immunosuppression and at the beginning of thalidomide, 300 mg/day; (*B*) complete resolution of the skin lesions after 10 weeks of therapy.

dren responded to therapy, and concomitant immunosuppressive medication could be reduced. There were only minimal side effects that did not necessitate withdrawal of the drug.

These studies clearly demonstrate that patients with CGvHD refractory to conventional immunosuppressive/glucocorticoid therapy may derive benefit from the additional administration of thalidomide if they can tolerate the side effects. This beneficial effect seems to be even more pronounced in children, possibly because they tolerate the drug better. While thalidomide is an effective therapeutic agent in CGvHD, it cannot be used for its prevention: in a double-blind, randomized trial with 59 patients, both the incidence of CGvHD and the survival rate were unfavorable, as compared with a placebo group, in the group that had received 400 mg of thalidomide starting on day 80 after transplantation.[37] Thus, thalidomide cannot be used for the prophylaxis of CGvHD.

Langerhans Cell Histiocytosis

Langerhans cell histiocytosis is now considered to be a reactive rather than a neoplastic process (see Chap. 160); TNF-α has been shown to play an important role in the induction proliferation of Langerhans cells, and this process can be reversed by thalidomide's inhibition of TNF-α production. So far, six patients with this condition have been treated with thalidomide, all of them responding.[19,38–41] Thus, thalidomide may be considered the treatment of choice for Langerhans histiocytosis even though the condition is so rare that only isolated reports on its treatment exist.

Actinic Prurigo

This condition occurs mainly but not exclusively in Amerindians (see Chap. 136). Over 90 percent of 99 patients responded well to thalidomide at initial doses of 100 to 300 mg/day[42,43] within 3 weeks to 3 months. Some of these patients enjoyed prolonged remissions, but most required maintenance therapy, usually of 50 to 100 mg/day but occasionally as low as 15 mg/day.[43]

Good to excellent results have also been achieved in about 90 percent of patients with polymorphous light eruption, a related condition, in an average of 2 weeks.[44]

Other Dermatoses

Reports on thalidomide treatment of individual patients or small numbers of cases exist for numerous other dermatologic disorders. In all the conditions listed below, more than half of the patients are reported to have benefited from this therapy:

Bullous pemphigoid[45]
Cicatricial pemphigoid[45]
Erythema multiforme[53–55]
Jessner-Kanof disease[59]
Palmoplantar pustulosis[46]
Postherpetic neuralgia[48]
Prurigo nodularis[56,57]
Sarcoidosis[47]
Pyoderma gangrenosum[49–52]
Uremic pruritus[58]
Weber-Christian disease[60]

Although thalidomide cannot currently be prescribed for the treatment of these conditions, it may provide a therapeutic alternative in selected patients who do not respond to more conventional regimens.

Dosage of Thalidomide

The dosage of thalidomide is purely empiric so far; in the absence of acute toxicity, it is determined by clinical effectiveness and limited by the side effects of sedation and constipation. Practical doses range between 100 and 400 mg/day, but they are occasionally as high as 600 mg/day in patients with subacute cutaneous lupus and up to 1200 mg in patients with CGvHD refractory to more conventional anti-inflammatory/immunosuppressive therapy. After a single oral dose, only 0.6 percent of the total could be recovered in the patients' urine, indicating a nonrenal form of excretion[1]; elimination of the drug is thought to be mainly due to hydrolysis. Correspondingly, accumulation does not occur in patients with severely compromised organ function, (e.g., in patients with renal insufficiency). The relation between plasma levels and clinical effects, such as sedation or healing of oral ulcers, may occur at doses that do not produce detectable thalidomide plasma levels.

Side Effects of Thalidomide Therapy

The most important of these is the well-known teratogenic effect of thalidomide; thus, it is mandatory that female patients of childbearing age in whom thalidomide therapy is planned be carefully selected, informed, and monitored and that they should take reliable contraceptive measures.

TERATOGENESIS An estimated 12,000 patients with thalidomide embryopathy have been affected worldwide; over 4000 cases have been reported, 3000 of them in West Germany alone. Malformations due to thalidomide embryopathy are related to the time of exposure to the drug in pregnancy, the sensitive period being the embryonal ages from the third to the fifth week; they may be caused by the action of thalidomide on embryonal adhesion receptors[2] (see above).

Most prominent are malformations of the extremities, including malformations or aplasia of the thumbs, radiate aplasia, phocomelia or amelia of the upper and/or lower limbs, anotia, facial palsy, microphthalmia, and ophthalmoplegia. In addition, neural tube defects, cardiac malformations, renal malformations, esophageal fistulas, duodenal stenosis or atresia, anal atresia, vaginal obstruction, and midline hemangiomas may occur. These malformations must be differentiated from other dysmelic diseases and radial defects, of which Holt-Oram syndrome, an autosomal abdominal disease, is the one most similar to thalidomide embryopathy.

PERIPHERAL NEUROPATHY Another serious side effect is a peripheral sensory neuropathy that may later go on to involvement of motor neurons. Estimates of the incidence of this neuropathy range from more than 60 percent to less than 1 percent of HIV-negative patients. Not much is known about its incidence in HIV patients, but as with other thalidomide side effects, such individuals may be at greater risk. Patients treated for CGvHD may also be at risk because of pretreatment with cytotoxic drugs and the higher doses of thalidomide used in this condition. As this neuropathy can become irreversible, preexistent peripheral neuropathy should be excluded before patients receive thalidomide, and their neurologic status should be assessed frequently.

An erythematous rash with peripheral blood eosinophilia has been observed in two patients with renal insufficiency who received thalidomide for prurigo nodularis.[61] The rash resolved promptly upon withdrawal of the drug. Other dose-related and usually mild side effects are sedation, nausea, mood changes, increased appetite, edema of the face and limbs, menstrual abnormalities, decreased libido, constipation, dizziness, and dryness of the mouth; they tend to disappear with time but can be dose-limiting on occasion.

RASH AND FEVER This occurs predominantly in HIV-infected patients[13] and is similar to the well-known reaction to trimethoprim-sulfamethoxazole in these patients; over 30 percent of such patients, especially those with low CD4+ counts, develop this problem, which requires a cessation of therapy.

REFERENCES

1. Chen TL et al: Plasma pharmacokinetics and urinary excretion of thalidomide after oral dosing in healthy male volunteers. *Drug Metab Dispos* **17**:402, 1989
2. Neubert R et al: Downregulation of adhesion receptors on cells of primate embryos as a probable mechanism of the teratogenic action of thalidomide. *Life Sci* **58**:295, 1995
3. McCarty MF: Thalidomide may impede cell migration in primates by downregulating integrin β-chains: Potential therapeutic utility in solid malignancies, proliferative retinopathy, inflammatory disorders, neointimal hyperplasia, and osteoporosis. *Med Hypotheses* **49**:123, 1997
4. D'Amato RJ et al: Thalidomide is an inhibitor of angiogenesis. *Proc Natl Acad Sci USA* **91**:4082, 1994
5. Neubert R et al: Thalidomide and the immune system. 2: Changes in receptors on blood cells of a healthy volunteer. *Life Sci* **51**:2107, 1992
6. Nogueira AC et al: Thalidomide and the immune system. 3: Simultaneous up- and downregulation of different integrin receptors on human white blood cells. *Life Sci* **55**:77, 1994
7. Moller DR et al: Inhibition of IL-12 production by thalidomide. *J Immunol* **159**:5157, 1997
8. McHugh SM et al: The immunosuppressive drug thalidomide induces T helper cell type 2 (T$_H$2) and concomitantly inhibits T$_H$1 cytokine production in mitogen- and antigen-stimulated human peripheral blood mononuclear cell cultures. *Clin Exp Immunol* **99**:160, 1995
9. Sampaio EP et al: Thalidomide selectively inhibits tumor necrosis factor alpha production by stimulated human monocytes. *J Exp Med* **173**:699, 1991
10. Moreira AL et al: Thalidomide exerts its inhibitory action on tumor necrosis factor α by enhancing mRNA degradation. *J Exp Med* **177**:1675, 1993
11. Sampaio EP et al: The influence of thalidomide on the clinical and immunologic manifestation of erythema nodosum leprosum. *J Infect Dis* **168**:408, 1993
12. Haslett P et al: The metabolic and immunologic effects of short-term thalidomide treatment of patients infected with the human immunodeficiency virus. *AIDS Res Hum Retroviruses* **13**:1047, 1997
13. Haslett P et al: Adverse reactions to thalidomide in patients infected with human immunodeficiency virus. *Clin Infect Dis* **24**:1223, 1997
14. Sharpstone D et al: Thalidomide: A novel therapy for microsporidiosis. *Gastroenterology* **112**:1823, 1997
15. Ghigliotti G et al: Thalidomide: Treatment of choice for aphthous ulcers in patients seropositive for human immunodeficiency virus. *J Am Acad Dermatol* **28**:271, 1993
16. Jacobson JM et al: Thalidomide for the treatment of oral aphthous ulcers in patients with human immunodeficiency virus infection: National Institute of Allergy and Infectious Diseases AIDS Clinical Trials Group. *N Engl J Med* **336**:1487, 1997
17. Moreira AL et al: Thalidomide and thalidomide analogs reduce HIV type 1 replication in human macrophages in vitro. *AIDS Res Hum Retroviruses* **13**:857, 1997
18. Alexander LN, Wilcox CM: A prospective trial of thalidomide for the treatment of HIV-associated idiopathic esophageal ulcers. *AIDS Res Hum Retroviruses* **13**:301, 1997
19. Grinspan D: Significant response of oral aphthosis to thalidomide treatment. *J Am Acad Dermatol* **12**:85, 1985
20. Revuz J et al: Crossover study of thalidomide vs. placebo in severe recurrent aphthous stomatitis. *Arch Dermatol* **126**:923, 1990
21. Bonnetblanc JM et al: Thalidomide and recurrent aphthous stomatitis: A follow-up study. *Dermatology* **193**:321, 1996
22. Saylan T, Saltik I: Thalidomide in the treatment of Behçet's syndrome. *Arch Dermatol* **118**:536, 1982
23. Larsson H: Treatment of severe colitis in Behçet's syndrome with thalidomide (CG-217). *J Intern Med* **228**:405, 1990
24. Scolari F et al: Thalidomide in the treatment of chronic lupus erythematosus. *Dermatologica* **165**:355, 1982
25. Volc-Platzer B, Wolff K: Treatment of subacute cutaneous lupus erythematosus with thalidomide. *Hautarzt* **34**:175, 1983
26. Hasper MF: Chronic cutaneous lupus erythematosus: Thalidomide treatment of 11 patients. *Arch Dermatol* **119**:812, 1983
27. Knop J et al: Thalidomide in the treatment of sixty cases of chronic discoid lupus erythematosus. *Br J Dermatol* **108**:461, 1983
28. Holm AL et al: Chronic cutaneous lupus erythematosus treated with thalidomide. *Arch Dermatol* **129**:1548, 1993
29. Duna GF, Cash JM: Treatment of refractory cutaneous lupus erythematosus. *Rheum Dis Clin North Am* **21**:99, 1995
30. Atra E, Sato EI: Treatment of the cutaneous lesions of systemic lupus erythematosus with thalidomide. *Clin Exp Rheumatol* **11**:487, 1993
31. Stevens RJ et al: Thalidomide in the treatment of the cutaneous manifestations of lupus erythematosus: Experience in sixteen consecutive patients. *Br J Rheumatol* **36**:353, 1997
32. Vitali C et al: International survey on the management of patients with SLE. I: General data on the participating centers and the results of a questionnaire regarding mucocutaneous involvement. *Clin Exp Rheumatol* **14**(suppl 16):S17, 1996
33. Burrows NP et al: Lupus erythematosus profundus with partial C4 deficiency responding to thalidomide. *Br J Dermatol* **125**:62, 1991
34. Vogelsang GB et al: Thalidomide for the treatment of chronic graft-versus-host disease. *N Engl J Med* **326**:1055, 1992
35. Parker PM et al: Thalidomide as salvage therapy for chronic graft-versus-host disease. *Blood* **86**:3604, 1995
36. Cole CH et al: Thalidomide in the management of chronic graft-versus-host disease in children following bone marrow transplantation. *Bone Marrow Transplant* **14**:937, 1994
37. Chao NJ et al: Paradoxical effect of thalidomide prophylaxis on chronic graft-vs-host disease. *Biol Blood Marrow Transplant* **2**:86, 1996
38. Thomas L et al: Successful treatment of adult's Langerhans cell histiocytosis with thalidomide: Report of two cases and literature review. *Arch Dermatol* **129**:1261, 1993
39. Dallafior S et al: Successful treatment of a case of cutaneous Langerhans cell granulomatosis with 2-chlorodeoxyadenosine and thalidomide. *Hautarzt* **46**:553, 1995
40. Meunier L et al: Adult cutaneous Langerhans cell histiocytosis: Remission with thalidomide treatment. *Br J Dermatol* **132**:168, 1995
41. Misery L et al: Remission of Langerhans cell histiocytosis with thalidomide treatment. *Clin Exp Dermatol* **18**:487, 1993
42. Lovell CR et al: Thalidomide in actinic prurigo. *Br J Dermatol* **108**:467, 1983
43. Londono F: Thalidomide in the treatment of actinic prurigo. *Int J Dermatol* **12**:326, 1973
44. Saul A et al: Polymorphous light eruption: Treatment with thalidomide. *Australas J Dermatol* **17**:17, 1976
45. Naafs B, Faber WR: Thalidomide therapy: An open trial. *Int J Dermatol* **24**:131, 1985
46. Hamza M: Behçet's disease, palmoplantar pustulosis and HLA-B27 treatment with thalidomide. *Clin Exp Rheumatol* **8**:427, 1990
47. Carlesimo M et al: Treatment of cutaneous and pulmonary sarcoidosis with thalidomide. *J Am Acad Dermatol* **32**(suppl):866, 1995
48. Barnhill RL, McDougall AC: Thalidomide: Use and possible mode of action in reactional lepromatous leprosy and in various other conditions. *J Am Acad Dermatol* **7**:317, 1982
49. Rustin MH et al: Pyoderma gangrenosum associated with Behçet's disease: Treatment with thalidomide. *J Am Acad Dermatol* **23**:941, 1990
50. Venencie PY, Saurat JH: Pyoderma gangrenosum in a child: Treatment with thalidomide. *Ann Pediatr Paris* **29**:67, 1982
51. Munro CS, Cox NH: Pyoderma gangrenosum associated with Behçet's syndrome—response to thalidomide. *Clin Exp Dermatol* **13**:408, 1988
52. Costa I et al: Aseptic adenitis in pyoderma gangrenosum. *Ann Dermatol Venereol* **21**:550, 1994
53. Moisson YF et al: Thalidomide for recurrent erythema multiforme (letter). *Br J Dermatol* **126**:92, 1992

54. Pinto JS et al: Erythema multiforme associated with autoreactivity to 17 alpha-hydroxyprogesterone. *Dermatologica* **180**:146, 1990
55. Bahmer FA et al: Thalidomide treatment of recurrent erythema multiforme. *Acta Derm Venereol* **62**:449, 1982
56. van den Broek H: Treatment of prurigo nodularis with thalidomide. *Arch Dermatol* **116**:571, 1980
57. Winkelmann RK et al: Thalidomide treatment of prurigo nodularis. *Acta Derm Venereol* **64**:412, 1984
58. Silva SRB et al: Thalidomide for the treatment of uremic pruritus: A crossover randomized double-blind trial. *Nephron* **67**:270, 1994
59. Guillaume JC et al: Crossover study of thalidomide vs. placebo in Jessner's lymphocytic infiltration of the skin. *Arch Dermatol* **131**:1032, 1995
60. Eravelly J, Waters MF: Thalidomide in Weber-Christian disease. *Lancet* **1**:251, 1977
61. Bielsa I et al: Erythroderma due to thalidomide: Report of two cases. *Dermatology* **189**:179, 1994

CHAPTER 263

Jean Krutmann

Therapeutic Photomedicine: Phototherapy

Over the past few years the development of irradiation devices with new emission spectra has led to an expanded role for phototherapy in the treatment of skin disease. This development is best illustrated by the constantly increasing frequency with which 311-nm ultraviolet B (UVB) phototherapy is employed for the treatment of psoriasis.[1] In fact, in Europe, 311-nm UVB is already used more often than psoralens plus ultraviolet A (PUVA) therapy for psoriasis and several other cutaneous diseases. Another example of a new device that has improved and expanded the spectrum of skin diseases amenable to phototherapy is high-dose UVA1.[2] With this modality, doses of UVA1 (340 to 400 nm) up to 130 J/cm^2 are delivered to diseased skin. High-dose UVA1 was first used to treat patients with atopic dermatitis, but it has since been found to be efficacious in several other skin diseases, such as localized scleroderma, where other therapeutic options are limited. These two examples demonstrate that the introduction of new spectra into dermatologic phototherapy has not only broadened and improved phototherapy as it relates to established indications such as psoriasis and atopic dermatitis but, in addition, has fostered the development of new indications for phototherapy such as connective tissue diseases.

PHOTOTHERAPY OF PSORIASIS

One important element in the long-term management of moderate to severe psoriasis is UVB phototherapy. Within recent years the availability of new fluorescent bulbs with an emission spectrum that closely conforms to the peak of the action spectrum for clearing psoriasis has significantly improved the efficacy of UVB phototherapy for psoriasis, making it as efficient as PUVA therapy.

311-nm UVB: The Phototherapy of Choice for Psoriasis

Parrish et al. demonstrated that wavelengths shorter than 295 nm displayed no antipsoriatic effect, even if used at erythemogenic doses, whereas wavelengths between 300 and 313 nm caused the greatest remission of skin lesions.[3] These seminal observations provided the rationale for the development of more selective UVB phototherapy (SUP) irradiation devices. These units have a spectrum that is still broadband UVB but is enhanced in the range of 300 to 320 nm.[4] As predicted, these light sources proved to be superior to conventional UVB phototherapy for clearing of psoriasis. A major breakthrough was achieved shortly thereafter by the development of the Philips TL-01 fluorescent lamp, emitting a narrow UV band at 311 to 312 nm and thereby matching closely the assumed therapeutic optimum for psoriasis.[1] A large number of clinical trials comparing broadband versus 311-nm UVB phototherapy for psoriasis have been conducted since then.[5–8] Based on these studies, it is now generally accepted that 311-nm UVB therapy is superior to broadband UVB therapy for psoriasis. Patients treated with a 311-nm spectrum show faster clearance of skin lesions, fewer episodes of excessive erythema, and a longer period of remission (Fig. 263-1). Even more interesting, comparative studies of 311-nm UVB phototherapy and PUVA have demonstrated that these two

FIGURE 263-1

CHAPTER 263
Therapeutic Photomedicine: Phototherapy

2871

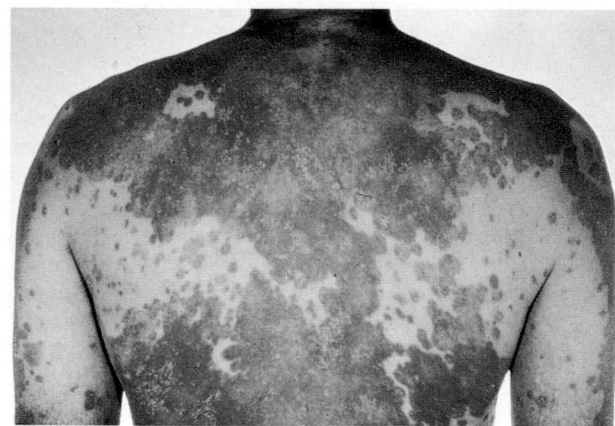

A.

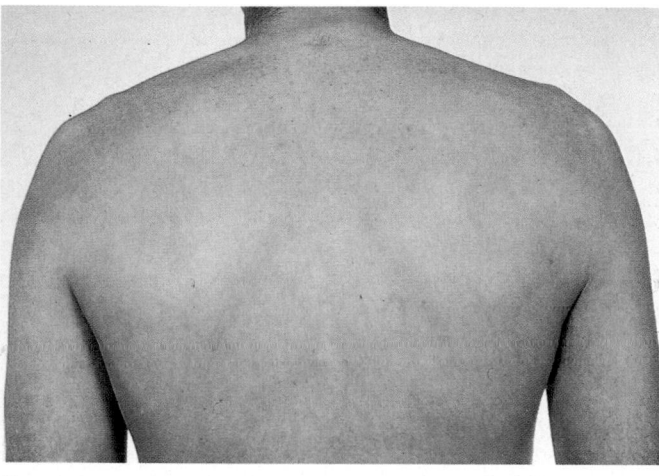

B.

Patient with severe generalized psoriasis before (*A*) and after (*B*) 15 treatments with 311-nm UVB phototherapy. (*Courtesy of J. Ferguson, MD, Dundee, Scotland.*)

nm UVB or conventional broadband UVB from fluorescent bulbs (such as Westinghouse FS, Philips TL12, Sylvania UV21) or medium-pressure mercury arc lamps with or without metal halides[13] are used, a number of guidelines should be followed.

In particular, prior to phototherapy, the patient's minimal erythema dose (MED) must be determined in order to establish the optimal dosage schedule. For determination of the MED and subsequent phototherapy, either the same irradiation device or different devices with identical emission spectra must be used. For 311-nm therapy, the initial dose should equal 0.7 MED (Table 263-1). Patients are treated three to five times per week. If the initial dose is tolerated, a 20 percent incremental increase of the previous dose is used at each visit. When a previous treatment results in erythema, no treatment is given the next day or the dose is decreased, depending on whether the erythema is asymptomatic or severe and painful (Table 263-1). For broadband UVB therapy, one MED is given on the first treatment and is increased by 50 percent, 40 percent, 30 percent, and so on in subsequent treatments. Since ultraviolet radiation is a complete carcinogen,[14] the genitalia and chronically light-exposed areas (e.g., the face, neck, dorsa of hands), if unaffected, should be shielded or protected (with sunscreen) prior to irradiation.[15]

The end point of phototherapy is complete clearance of all psoriatic skin lesions. Psoriasis, however, is a chronic disease and the remission induced by UVB phototherapy is transient. In a randomized, prospective, multicentered trial, postclearing phototherapy was found to significantly increase the disease-free interval, indicating that patients may profit from maintenance phototherapy.[16] On the other hand, maintenance therapy with UVB radiation results in a greater cumulative UVB radiation dose and thereby increases the risk of skin cancer and photoaging. It is therefore preferable to maintain remissions with other antipsoriatic modalities if possible. In order to minimize potential carcinogenic risks from chronic UVB phototherapy, a rotational therapeutic approach including a number of primary and secondary agents has been suggested.[17] Primary agents to treat psoriasis include UVB, PUVA, methotrexate, and etretinate. If the primary agents are no longer effective, then secondary agents such as cyclosporine, hydroxyurea, and low-dose combination regimens (e.g., retinoids + PUVA + topicals) should be considered.

modalities are equally effective.[9–11] This is of particular interest, because 311-nm UVB therapy, in comparison to PUVA, does not require psoralens, is cheaper, can be used in pregnancy and childhood, and does not require posttreatment eye protection. It has also been suggested that 311-nm UVB may be less carcinogenic than PUVA.[12] For these reasons, 311-nm UVB therapy currently represents the phototherapeutic modality of choice for the treatment of psoriasis in Europe and is being used increasingly in the United States as well.

Practical Aspects

For 311-nm UVB therapy, no specific irradiation devices are needed, because the Philips TL-01 fluorescent lamps can be fitted into conventional PUVA cabinets. Regardless of whether 311-

TABLE 263-1

311-nm UVB Phototherapy Regimen

1. Determination of minimal erythema dose (MED)
2. First exposure: 70% of MED
3. Subsequent exposures

a. If no erythema	Increase by 20% at each visit
b. Minimal erythema	Same dose
c. Asymptomatic, well-defined erythema	Postpone exposure until next visit, then same dose and thereafter 10% increments at each visit
d. Painful erythema ± edema or bullae	Omit further exposures until recovery, reduce exposure dose by half, thereafter 10% increments at each visit

SOURCE: According to George et al.[59]

Combination Therapy (See also Chap. 43)

Along the same lines, phototherapy of psoriasis is frequently used in combination regimens in order to achieve higher clearance rates, longer disease-free intervals, and a lower carcinogenic risk.[17] Phototherapy may be combined with topical or systemic agents. Topical agents include anthralin, vitamin D analogues, glucocorticoids, emollients, saltwater baths, and tar. Among these, anthralin and vitamin D analogues constitute the most relevant agents for combination with phototherapy.

Anthralin or dithranol was synthesized by Gallewsky in 1916 and subsequently shown to be effective in the treatment of psoriasis by Unna.[18,19] Anthralin is administered in a petrolatum base containing salicylic acid (concentration should not exceed 3%) in order to stabilize anthralin. Salicylic acid may act as a sunscreen,[20] and anthralin application should therefore follow (not precede) UVB irradiation. Anthralin preparations cause dose-dependent skin irritation (anthralin erythema), which is additive to UVB radiation–induced erythema and may be followed by induction of Koebner's phenomenon and pigmentation of treated skin areas. In addition, the generation of oxidation products from anthralin may stain clothes and bath tubes. For these reasons, the use of anthralin has been mainly limited to the treatment of inpatients in hospitals.[21] A short-term application of anthralin (0.1 to 3% dithranol plus 2% salicylic acid in petrolatum for 10 to 20 min daily) has been developed, which is suitable for treating outpatients or patients in day-care centers.[22]

The combination of phototherapy and administration of anthralin for the treatment of psoriasis was first proposed by Ingram in 1953.[23] This concept has since been confirmed by numerous studies in which topical anthralin treatment was found to enhance the efficacy of either broadband UVB or 311-nm UVB phototherapy for psoriasis.[24,25] In contrast, the combination of UVB irradiation with anthralin short-contact therapy was significantly less effective than the classic Ingram regimen and did not offer an advantage over UVB therapy alone.[26–28]

Antipsoriatic vitamin D analogues include calcipotriol and tacalcitol, which have antiproliferative as well as antiinflammatory effects.[29,30] Local side effects are limited to moderate skin irritation.[31] In order to avoid systemic side effects—in particular hypercalcemia with consequent nephrocalcinosis—from percutaneous absorption, the treated body surface should not exceed 30 percent. Under these conditions, long-term safety may be assured.[32] Main indications are psoriatic plaques of limited extent and lesions on the scalp, face, palms, and soles and in the intertriginous areas.[29,30,33] The combination of either broadband UVB or 311-nm UVB therapy with calcipotriol was shown to increase the therapeutic efficacy of phototherapy alone.[34,35] This observation is of particular interest because UVB therapy reduced the irritation caused by calcipotriol. In contrast to UVB irradiation, a combination of calcipotriol with UVA radiation or a combined UVA/UVB regimen should be avoided, because UVA radiation leads to degradation of vitamin D_3. Vitamin D analogues should therefore be applied after (not before) phototherapy.

Several studies have addressed the question whether the efficacy of UVB phototherapy for psoriasis may be enhanced through combination with topical glucocorticoids. Data from these studies are conflicting and the beneficial effects seem to be limited.[36–39] Topical steroids are useful, however, for treating psoriatic lesions in skin areas not reached by UV irradiation during phototherapy (e.g., scalp, groin, rima ani, perianal area, umbilicus), or for the treatment

of lesions recalcitrant to standard phototherapy. They may also be used in the early, highly inflammatory state of psoriasis to achieve a quick improvement.

Topical application of emollients alters the optical properties of psoriatic lesions.[40] Lubricants improve transmission of UVB, and a combination of topical lubricants with UVB therapy increased efficacy.[41] This is in contrast to thick applications of petrolatum and water-in-oil type creams and salicylic acid, which act as sunscreens.

Balneophototherapy comprises the combination of saltwater baths with UVB phototherapy, which, under natural conditions, has been successfully employed at the Dead Sea for the treatment of patients with recurrent, severe psoriasis.[42,43] Modern approaches to balneophototherapy employing synthetically generated Dead Sea salt or sodium chloride solutions for saltwater baths (usually between 5 to 15%) are hampered by logistics (the requirement for bathtubs) and environmental problems (caused by the salt consumption). The beneficial effects of saline solutions on psoriasis are thought to involve elution of leukocyte elastase from psoriatic skin[44] and anti-inflammatory effects of magnesium ions.[45] Controlled studies demonstrating a synergistic effect between saltwater baths and phototherapy are still lacking. Similarly, the efficacy of balneophototherapy in comparison with established combination regimens for psoriasis remains to be assessed.

The combination of crude coal tar plus UV irradiation has been used in the treatment of generalized psoriasis since 1925.[46] Today, the Goeckerman regimen is no longer considered a standard therapy for psoriasis. Tar has an unpleasant smell, it may lead to discoloration of skin and clothes, it can cause acneiform lesions, and, most importantly, the combination of tar and UVB irradiation may pose an increased carcinogenic risk.[47–51]

Systemic agents that may be used to treat psoriasis include retinoids, glucocorticoids, cyclosporin A, and methotrexate. Retinoids are the most widely used agents for systemic treatment in combination with phototherapy. In contrast, the systemic use of steroids in combination with photo(chemo)therapy is limited to special indications such as generalized pustular psoriasis. Also, combination regimens of UVB therapy with methotrexate or cyclosporin A are not advisable, because both substances increase the possibility of UV-induced skin tumors.

From a theoretical point of view, the advantage of combining retinoids and UVB irradiation is twofold: (1) retinoids exert antipsoriatic effects, which might act synergistically with UVB phototherapy; and (2) they have anticarcinogenic effects and thereby could lower the increased skin cancer risk resulting from long-term UVB therapy. Because of potentially severe side effects, the use of retinoids should be limited to pustular or erythrodermic variants of psoriasis. Combination regimens with broadband UVB or SUP therapy together with etretinate induced improvement in psoriatic patients more quickly than with phototherapy alone and reduced the number of treatments and cumulative UV doses.[52–54] Similar results were obtained when acitretin, the major metabolite of etretinate, was used in combination with broadband UVB or 311-nm UVB therapy.[55–57]

PHOTOTHERAPY OF ATOPIC DERMATITIS
(See also Chap. 124)

In the past few years several new phototherapeutic modalities including UVA/UVB,[58] 311-nm UVB,[59] and high-dose UVA1 phototherapy[60] have been developed to treat atopic dermatitis. As a consequence, dermatologists now have a diverse spectrum of phototherapeutic modalities from which to choose to tailor their treatment to the particular needs of a particular patient. Treatment decisions can now be based on the effectiveness of a given form of phototherapy for a specific stage of atopic dermatitis—i.e., acute and severe versus chronic and moderate disease activity. We have therefore recently developed a phototherapeutic approach for atopic dermatitis[61] that should result in phototherapy for atopic dermatitis that is both as effective and as safe as possible. In general, phototherapy of an acute, severe exacerbation of atopic dermatitis may be achieved with high-dose UVA1 therapy, whereas conventional UVA, UVA/UVB, 311-nm UVB, and low-dose UVA1 phototherapy represent phototherapeutic modalities that are primarily suited for treatment of chronic stages of this disease (Table 263-2).

High-Dose UVA1 Phototherapy for Acute, Severe Atopic Dermatitis

High-dose UVA1 phototherapy is a highly effective modality that can be used as monotherapy for a limited period of time (10 to 15 exposures). It is most effective for the treatment of patients with severe, acute exacerbation of atopic dermatitis (Fig. 263-2). Potential long-term risks of high-dose UVA1 phototherapy are not known; therefore patients should not be treated over extended periods of time—e.g., for maintenance therapy. For the same reasons its use is not recommended for patients younger than 18 years of age. The therapeutic effectiveness of UVA1 irradiation in the management of patients with atopic dermatitis was first evaluated in an open study in patients with acute, severe exacerbations of atopic dermatitis.[62] They were exposed to 130 J/cm^2 UVA1 daily for 15 consecutive days. Its therapeutic effectiveness was assessed by means of a clinical scoring system[63] as well as by monitoring serum levels of eosinophil cationic protein (ECP)—a laboratory parameter that can be measured objectively and has been shown to correlate well with disease activity in atopic dermatitis.[64] In that study, high-dose UVA1 phototherapy was found to be highly efficient in promptly inducing clinical improvement and reducing elevated serum ECP levels. Patients treated with high-dose UVA1 were compared with subjects who had been treated with UVA/UVB phototherapy. Significant differences in favor of high-dose UVA1 therapy were observed.[62] These results were recently corroborated and extended in a multicenter trial in which high-dose UVA1 therapy, as compared with glucocorticoid treatment, was significantly better at day 10 in reducing the clinical score.[65]

The therapeutic effectiveness of UVA1 therapy is dose-dependent. A direct comparison between a low-dose versus a high-dose UVA1 regimen is still missing, but low-dose UVA1 (30 J/cm^2) is less effective than UVA/UVB therapy,[66] whereas high-dose UVA1

FIGURE 263-2

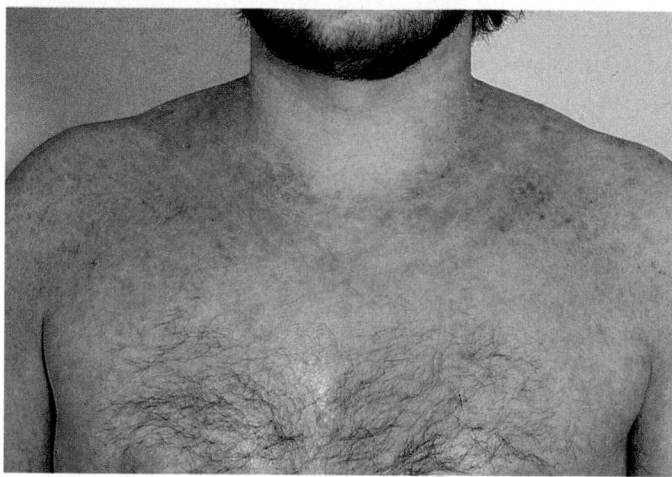

A.

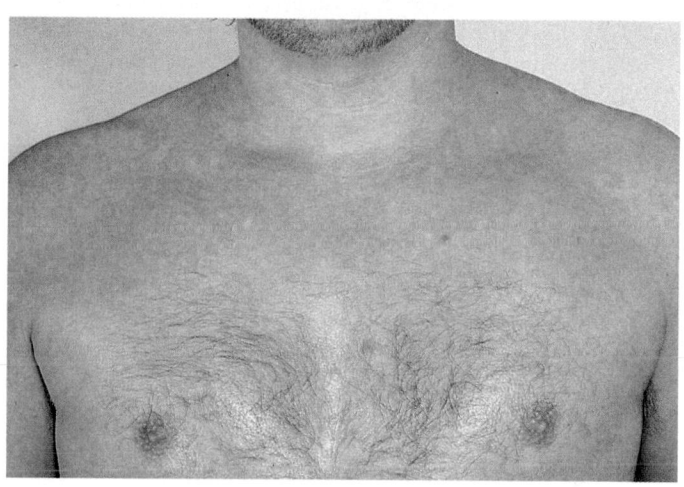

B.

Patient with severe, acute exacerbation of atopic dermatitis before (*A*) and after (*B*) high-dose UVA1 therapy (15 × 130 J/cm^2 UVA1).

therapy (130 J/cm^2) is superior to UVA/UVB phototherapy.[62,65] In addition, a medium-UVA1 dosage schedule (50 J/cm^2) was superior to a low-dose UVA1 regimen (10 J/cm^2).[67]

High-dose UVA1 phototherapy may not be perfomed in patients with UVA-sensitive atopic dermatitis or photodermatoses. It is necessary to exclude these diseases prior to initiation of high-dose UVA1 therapy. This can easily be accomplished by photoprovocation testing. Except for eczema herpeticum, no acute side effects have been observed in any of the patients treated with high-dose UVA1 therapy. No other side effects have been observed, although its potential carcinogenic risk is a theoretical concern. It is important to note that exposure of hairless albino Skh-hr1 mice to high doses of UVA1 radiation has been shown to induce squamous cell carcinoma.[68] The actual contribution of UVA radiation to the development of malignant melanoma in humans is currently under debate and at this point cannot be excluded.[69] Until more is known about high-dose UVA1 therapy, its use should be limited to periods of acute exacerbation of atopic dermatitis and, in general, one treat-

TABLE 263-2

Concept-Linked Phototherapeutic Approach for Atopic Dermatitis

INDICATION	MODALITY	COMMENT
Acute, severe	High-dose UVA1	Monotherapy, alternative to glucocorticoids, long-term side effects unknown
Chronic, moderate	311 nm UVB UVA/UVB Broadband UVB Broadband UVA Low-dose UVA1	Combination therapy to save glucocorticoids, suited for maintenance therapy

ment cycle should not exceed 10 to 15 continuously applied exposures and should not be repeated more than once per year.

Phototherapy of Chronic, Moderate Atopic Dermatitis

Broad-band UVB,[70] combined UVA/UVB,[58,71–73] broad-band UVA,[74] low-dose UVA1,[66,67] and, in particular, 311-nm UVB phototherapy[59] are effective treatments in mild and moderate atopic dermatitis. They are not particularly effective in patients with acute, severe exacerbations of their disease. In contrast to high-dose UVA1 therapy, these forms of UV therapy are usually not employed as monotherapy. Rather, they are used in combination regimens together with topical glucocorticoids in order to reduce the need for glucocorticoid application. All of these therapies are considered to be relatively safe, even if used over extended periods of time, and they should thus be used to induce long-term improvement. Patients do best if severe disease is initially controlled by more potent but also more aggressive modalities. For example, 311-nm UVB phototherapy has proved to be an ideal modality for maintenance therapy once high-dose UVA1 has been used in the initial phase of management of an acute, severe exacerbation of atopic dermatitis.[61] If high-dose UVA1 therapy is not available, severe atopic dermatitis should be controlled prior to start of phototherapy by aggressive topical glucocorticoid therapy or systemic immunosuppressive modalities such as glucocorticoids or cyclosporin A.

Studies directly comparing all the different forms of UV therapy for chronic, moderate atopic dermatitis have not been performed, but recent trials indicate that either UVA/UVB[58,71–73] combination therapy or narrow-band 311-nm UVB therapy[59] is superior to conventional broadband UVB, broadband UVA, or low-dose UVA1 therapy. The actual choice made for a particular patient also depends on what irradiation devices are available. At the moment, UVA/UVB is more widely available than 311-nm UVB therapy. Jekler and Larkö, in a paired comparison study, have observed significant differences in favor of UVA/UVB therapy over broadband UVB therapy.[58] In this trial, patients were allowed to continue the use of topical glucocorticoids and were irradiated three times per week for a maximum of 8 weeks in a UVB MED–dependent manner.

The therapeutic effectiveness of 311-nm UVB therapy for chronic, moderate atopic dermatitis was first reported by George et al.[59] In this well-designed study, patients with chronic, moderate atopic dermatitis were irradiated with 50 100-W TL-01 lamps equipped with reflectors, resulting in a UVB output of 5 mW/cm^2 and maximum treatment times of less than 10 min. The irradiation regimen used with 50 lamps was identical to that previously described for 311-nm therapy of psoriasis (Table 263-1). Patients were monitored for severity of clinical symptoms as well as glucocorticoid use 12 weeks prior to phototherapy, during the 12 weeks of phototherapy, and for another 24 weeks after cessation of phototherapy. The 311-nm UVB phototherapy not only decreased the clinical severity but also significantly reduced the use of glucocorticoids. These beneficial effects were still present in the majority of patients 6 months after cessation of 311-nm UVB therapy. In this study, a specially constructed air-conditioned irradiation unit was used for 311-nm UVB phototherapy. Equivalent therapeutic results could also be achieved if TL-01 lamps were fitted into a conventional PUVA irradiation device, indicating that higher temperatures during 311-nm UVB phototherapy did not lead to heat-induced irritation of eczema.[75] As discussed previously, 311-nm UVB therapy may be associated with a reduced risk of skin cancer compared to broadband UVB or to PUVA therapy.[12] The recent demonstration of 311-nm UVB therapy's effectiveness for treating childhood atopic eczema is therefore of particular interest.[76]

If neither a UVA/UVB nor a 311-nm UVB irradiation device is available, broadband low-dose (0.5-MED) UVB therapy can be used. Placebo-controlled studies have shown it to be effective for this disease.[70]

PHOTOTHERAPY OF OTHER DISORDERS

In addition to psoriasis and atopic dermatitis, UV therapy is increasingly used for a growing number of skin diseases that previously had mainly been treated with PUVA (e.g., polymorphous light eruption and urticaria pigmentosa) or for which no phototherapeutic approach had been available (e.g., localized scleroderma and lupus erythematosus).

Phototherapy of Polymorphous Light Eruption and Other Photodermatoses

Patients with polymorphous light eruption (PLE) respond abnormally to ultraviolet radiation (in particular UVA radiation), resulting in an increased and sustained expression of proinflammatory molecules (cytokines, adhesion molecules) and subsequent development of skin lesions[77] (see Chap. 136). In the majority of PLE patients, exposure to early-season sunlight results in induction of tolerance, a process that has been termed *hardening*. Artificial induction of hardening or artificial photoprotection constitutes the major principle underlying phototherapy of PLE. The precise molecular mechanisms responsible for hardening are not yet known, but it is generally believed that phototherapy-induced photoprotection is based on the induction of epidermal thickening, pigmentation, and as yet to be defined immunologic effects. In order to maintain phototherapy-induced photoprotection, it is important that patients expose themselves to sunlight, because strict avoidance of sunlight exposure will result in a quick loss of the therapeutically induced hardening effect. The use of phototherapy for PLE is restricted to severe cases that fail to respond to more simple measures such as light avoidance, photoprotective clothing, and use of broadband sunscreens. For these patients, broadband UVB and PUVA therapy have previously been found to be effective, with PUVA giving better results than UVB therapy.[78–81] Recent studies, however, indicate that 311-nm UVB therapy represents an effective alternative to PUVA for PLE-induced photoprotection. In a recent study, 25 patients were randomly assigned to either PUVA treatment or 311-nm UVB therapy, which was administered as previously described (Table 263-1). When patients were monitored for 4 months following treatment, there was no difference between PUVA and 311-nm UVB therapy with respect to severity of disease and restriction of outdoor activities. For the reasons given above, 311-nm UVB therapy may therefore be considered the treatment of choice for PLE. The efficacy of 311-nm UVB therapy for photodermatoses other than PLE has not yet been assessed in controlled studies, but observations from a pilot study indicate that patients with actinic prurigo (in particular), hydroa vacciniforme, and erythropoietic porphyria but not with solar urticaria may also benefit from 311-nm UVB therapy.[83]

Phototherapy of Localized Scleroderma

Localized scleroderma has a self-limited course, but skin lesions can cause significant morbidity and discomfort, in particular if they extend over joints and cause flexion contractures or if they lead to muscle atrophy and disfigurement.[84] In the past, numerous modalities including penicillin, penicillamine, antimalarial drugs, cyclosporin A, interferon-γ and topical or systemic glucocorticoids have been employed. In general, the efficacy of each of these agents has been poor. It was therefore of considerable interest to learn that UVA1 phototherapy was of benefit for patients with localized scleroderma[85,86] (Fig. 263-3).

In an open study, 10 patients with histologically proven localized scleroderma were exposed 30 times to a single dose of 130 J/cm^2 UVA1 radiation.[86] In all patients, high-dose UVA1 therapy softened sclerotic plaques. Complete clearance was observed in 4 of 10 patients. High-dose UVA1 therapy significantly reduced thickness and increased elasticity of plaques as assessed by 20-MHz sonography. These changes were not due to spontaneous remissions, because they were present only in UVA1-irradiated but not in unirradiated control plaques in the same patients. Similar therapeutic benefit could also be achieved by employing a low-dose UVA1 regimen.[85]

FIGURE 263-3

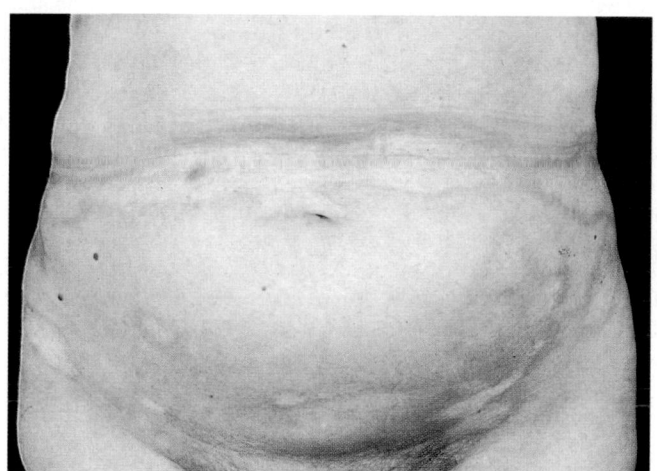

A.

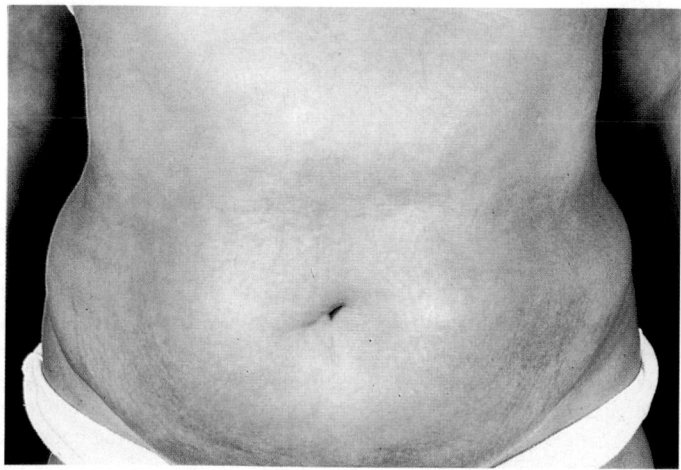

B.

Patient with localized scleroderma before (*A*) and after (*B*) high-dose UVA1 therapy (30 × 130 J/cm^2 UVA1).

Direct comparison of low-dose versus high-dose UVA1 therapy revealed that high-dose UVA1 therapy was superior to low-dose UVA1 therapy, indicating that the therapeutic efficacy is dose-dependent.[86] Patients were followed for 3 months after cessation of UVA1 therapy. Termination of phototherapy was not associated with loss of the beneficial effects achieved by high-dose UVA1 irradiation in 9 of 10 patients, indicating that maintenance therapy may not be required. The precise mechanism by which UVA1 therapy acts in localized scleroderma is not known but most likely involves upregulation of collagenase I expression, which was induced about 20-fold in sclerotic skin lesions after successful UVA1 phototherapy.[86,87]

Phototherapy of Urticaria Pigmentosa

Several studies have demonstrated that PUVA therapy is effective in reducing pruritus and urtication associated with urticaria pigmentosa.[88–90] In the majority of patients, however, cessation of PUVA therapy leads to recurrence of urticaria pigmentosa after 5 to 8 months. A recent study suggests that beneficial effects may also be achieved in these patients by UVA1 phototherapy. In an open study, four adult patients with severe generalized urticaria pigmentosa were treated with high-dose UVA1 phototherapy, which was given as monotherapy once daily five times per week for 2 consecutive weeks.[91] The initial dose was 60 J/cm^2 UVA1, which was subsequently increased to 130 J/cm^2 UVA1. High-dose UVA1 therapy induced reduction of pruritus and loss of urtication from stroking (Darier's sign) after three exposures, whereas hyperpigmented skin lesions faded more slowly. Increased histamine in 24-h urine was reduced to normal levels. In two patients with systemic manifestations of urticaria pigmentosa, such as migraine and diarrhea, relief from systemic symptoms and reduction of elevated serum serotonin to normal levels was observed after 10 exposures. No relapse has occurred in any of these four patients for more than 2 years after cessation of high-dose UVA1 therapy. This is in contrast to PUVA therapy and may be due to the possibility that high-dose UVA1 but not PUVA therapy leads to depletion of dermal mast cells.[90,92]

Phototherapy of Miscellaneous Disorders

It has been suggested that daily low-dose UVA1 irradiation is beneficial to patients with lupus erythematosus (Fig. 263-4). In an open study, 10 patients with systemic lupus erythematosus were treated with low-dose UVA1 irradiation (6 J/cm^2 UVA1 daily) for various time periods (15 days to 8 months).[93] In all patients, a decrease in clinical indices of disease activity was observed, which was most pronounced after 8 months of phototherapy. The UVA1 irradiation decreased fatigue, arthritis, photosensitivity, skin rashes, and often depression, headaches, and sleeplessness. In addition, anti-SSA or antinuclear antibodies decreased or even disappeared in most patients. These promising results have recently been confirmed in an 18 week two-phase study.[94] During the intial 6-week prospective, double-blind, placebo-controlled phase, 26 female patients were divided into two groups. Group A patients were exposed to 6 J/cm^2 UVA1 radiation and group B patients for an equal amount of time to visible light. Each group was subsequently crossed over for 3 weeks. This was followed by a second phase of 12 weeks, in which patients and physicians were unblinded and patients were treated with progressively decreasing levels of UVA1 radiation. In group

FIGURE 263-4

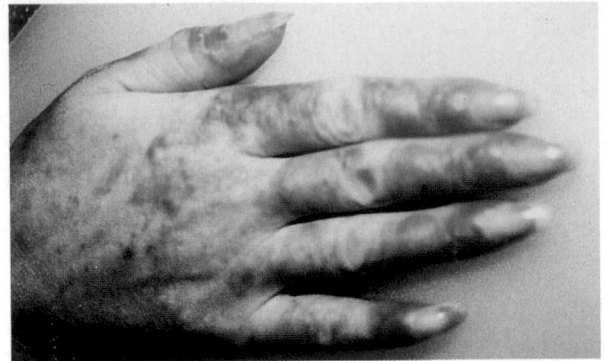

A.

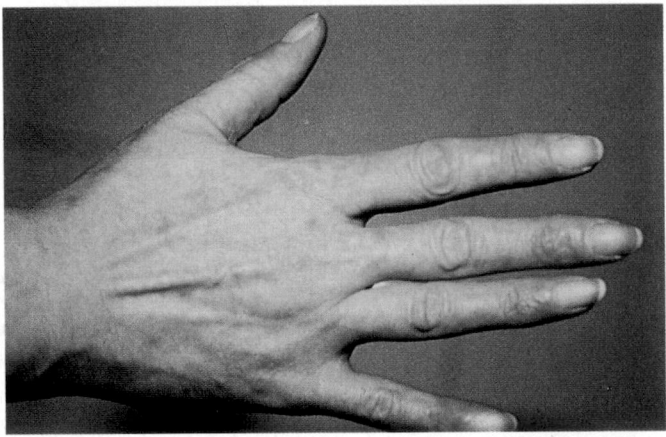

B.

Hand of a 37-year-old woman with subacute cutaneous lupus erythematosus before (*A*) and after (*B*) low-dose UVA1 therapy. Treatment consisted of irradiation daily for 5 days a week with 6 J/cm² UVA1 for three consecutive weeks. (*Courtesy of H. McGrath, Jr., MD, New Orleans, LA.*)

A patients, disease activity was significantly decreased after 3 weeks of UVA1 therapy but relapsed to baseline levels after 3 weeks of visible light treatment. In contrast, group B patients showed no significant response to the initial 3 weeks of visible light treatment nor to the following 3 weeks of UVA1 therapy. In both groups, however, significant improvement of clinical symptoms was detected after 6 weeks of UVA1 phototherapy, which was given under uncontrolled conditions in phase 2. No side effects were noted, although UVA1 irradiation, at least at higher doses, may exert detrimental effects on some lupus erythematosus patients.

Phototherapy with UVB may also be used to treat pityriasis lichenoides acuta et chronica,[95] pityriasis rosea,[96] and early stages of cutaneous T cell lymphoma (parapsoriasis en plaques).

MECHANISMS OF ACTION

Through the induction of DNA photoproducts, UVB radiation transiently inhibits cell proliferation.[97–100] It has therefore been thought that the therapeutic effectiveness of UVB phototherapy in psoriasis is due mainly to its antiproliferative effects. Since the introduction of UVB radiation into dermatologic therapy, however, the number of skin diseases showing a favorable response to phototherapy has grown substantially.[101] The vast majority are immunologic in nature. Studies on the role of UV radiation–induced immunosuppression in photocarcinogenesis[102] and on the effects of UV radiation on the function of epidermal Langerhans cells[103] have provided increasing evidence that UVB but also UVA (and in particular UVA1) radiation exert profound effects on the skin immune system. As a consequence, UVB and UVA phototherapy are currently regarded as modalities whose mechanism of action depends upon the immune system.[104] Most of the immunomodulatory effects that have been described are not specific for a single type of light source. The in vivo relevance of these immunomodulatory effects is dependent on the physical properties of the UV radiation employed. On a per photon basis, wavelengths within the UVB spectrum possess greater energy than UVA radiation, but because of their shorter wavelength, they have a more superficial depth of penetration within the skin.[105] As a result, UVB phototherapy primarily affects the function of epidermal keratinocytes and Langerhans cells, whereas UVA(1) radiation additionally affects dermal fibroblasts, dermal dendritic cells, endothelial cells, T lymphocytes within the dermis, mast cells, and granulocytes (Fig. 263-5). Photoimmunologic effects induced by UVB and UVA(1) radiation fall into three major categories: (1) effects on soluble mediators, (2) modulation of the expression of cell surface–associated molecules, and (3) the induction of apoptosis in pathogenetically relevant cells.

The capacity to affect the production of soluble immunomodulatory mediators has been demonstrated extensively for UVB radiation,[106] but there is growing evidence that UVA(1) radiation may exert quite similar effects.[107] From these studies it is now well established that UVB and UVA radiation can induce the production and secretion of keratinocyte-derived cytokines, neuropeptides, and prostanoides. Some of these factors—e.g., the cytokine interleukin 10,[108] the neuropeptide αMSH,[109] and the prostanoid prostaglandin E_2 (PGE_2)[110]—exert antiinflammatory or immunosuppressive effects and thus may contribute to the efficacy of UV therapy in inflammatory skin diseases. Ultraviolet radiation may also suppress the production of proinflammatory cytokines, e.g., by inhibiting the release and synthesis of interferon γ (IFN-γ) by skin-infiltrating T cells.[111,112]

Studies on the modulation of the expression of cell surface molecules by UV irradiation have mainly focused on adhesion molecules and cytokine receptors. For example, increased expression of intercellular adhesion molecule-1 (ICAM-1) by epidermal keratinocytes is a hallmark of UV-responsive skin diseases such as psoriasis[113] and atopic dermatitis.[111] By serving as a receptor for the lymphocyte function–associated antigen 1 (LFA-1), keratinocyte ICAM-1 molecules play an important role in the generation and maintenance of a variety of inflammatory and immune reactions in the skin. It has therefore been of considerable interest to learn that upregulation of keratinocyte ICAM-1 expression both in vitro and in vivo can be effectively prevented by irradiation with therapeutically relevant doses of either UVB or UVA light.[114–116] This effect is transient in nature but can be reinduced if human skin is reexposed to UVB radiation 24 h after the first irradiation, indicating that maximal antiinflammatory effects require repetitive phototherapy on a daily base. The UVB radiation can also suppress adhesion molecule expression on the surface of antigen presenting cells and thereby alter their costimulatory repertoire, which is required for T cell activation.[117,118]

Keratinocyte-derived interleukin 1 alpha (IL-1 alpha) is one of the key cytokines for initiating cutaneous inflammation.[106] The capacity of UVB radiation to differentially regulate expression of the

IL-1 receptors type I and type II in keratinocytes may therefore represent another mechanism by which UVB phototherapy exerts antiinflammatory effects. IL-1RI and IL-1RII molecules markedly differ from a functional point of view. Only IL-1RI serves as a signaling receptor; IL-1RII does not mediate signals induced by IL-1. By virtue of its capacity to bind IL-1, IL-1RII functions as a decoy receptor in order to limit or inhibit inflammatory responses mediated by IL-1. Upon UVB radiation exposure, expression of IL-1RII is rapidly and dramatically upregulated, whereas at the same time IL-1RI expression is decreased.[119] These observations indicate that UVB therapy may limit potentially exaggerated responses to IL-1 stimulation of keratinocytes by increasing expression of the decoy receptor and decreasing expression of the signaling molecule for IL-1. Decreased expression of the signaling receptor following UVB irradiation has also been reported for the 55-kDa receptor for tumor necrosis factor α, another multifunctional proinflammatory keratinocyte-derived cytokine.[120]

Induction of programmed cell death (apoptosis) in pathogenetically relevant cells is one of the key mechanisms by which antiinflammatory modalities such as glucocorticoids operate. Both UVB and UVA (in particular UVA1) radiation are highly efficient in inducing apoptosis in human cells.[121] T cells, as compared with monocytes or keratinocytes, have an increased susceptibility to UV radiation–induced apoptosis[122]; this mechanism is therefore of particular importance for phototherapy of T cell–mediated skin diseases such as atopic dermatitis[111] and possibly psoriasis.[123] For example, high-dose UVA1 phototherapy of patients with atopic dermatitis was shown to induce apoptosis in skin-infiltrating T helper cells, thereby leading to a gradual reduction of the inflammatory infiltrate and concomitant improvement of patients' skin disease.[124] Similarly, successful UVB phototherapy of psoriasis reduced the number of intraepidermal T cells and subsequently normalized keratinocyte morphology. It was proposed that depletion of T cells was due to UVB radiation–induced T cell apoptosis.[125]

Great progress has been made within recent years to define the mode of action of UV therapy. Continuation of these research efforts will be important for continued progress in the development of new modalities based on a scientific rationale rather than on empiricism.

FIGURE 263-5

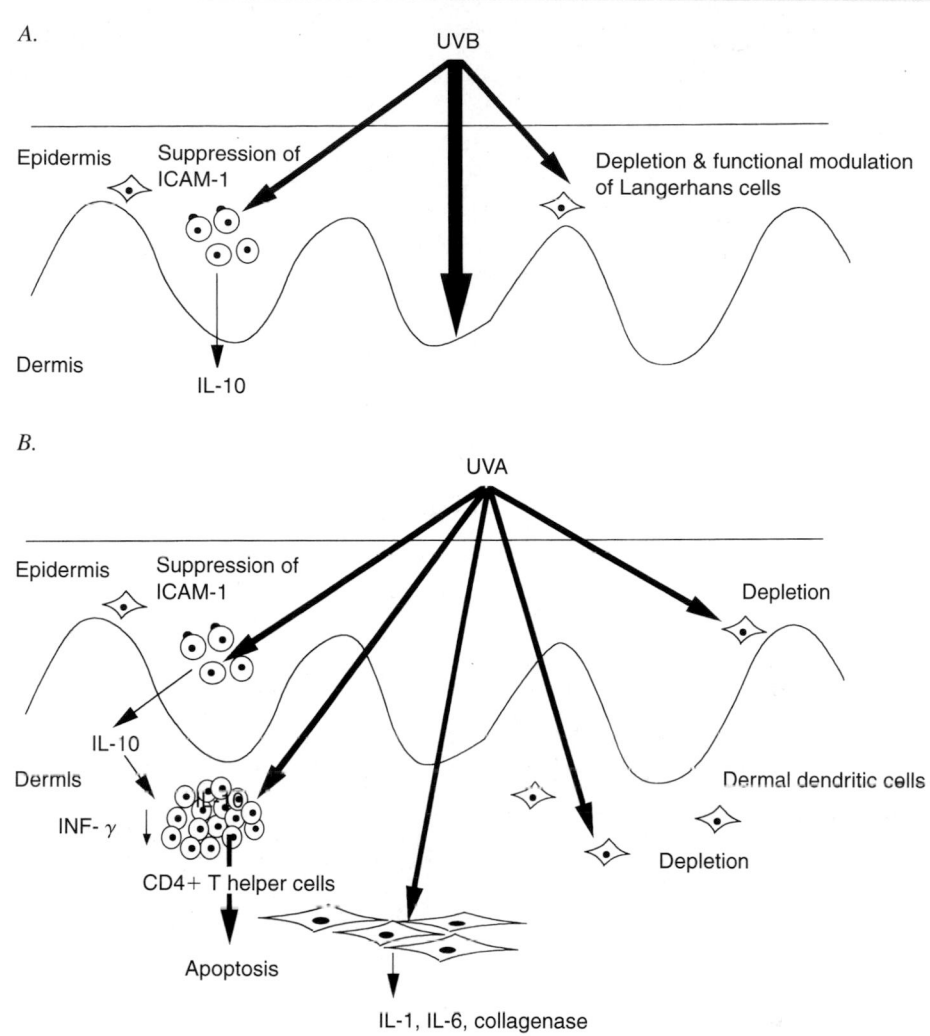

Scheme of immunomodulatory effects induced by UVB or UVA phototherapy. ICAM-1 = intercellular adhesion molecule-1; IFN-γ = interferon-γ; IL-10 = interleukin-10. (*Courtesy of A. Morita, MD, Nagoya, Japan.*)

REFERENCES

1. van Welden H et al: A new development in UVB phototherapy of psoriasis. *Br J Dermatol* **119**:11, 1988
2. Krutmann J: Ultraviolet A1 radiation-induced immunomodulation: High-dose UVA1 therapy of atopic dermatitis, in *Photoimmunology*, edited by J Krutmann, CA Elmets. Oxford, England, Blackwell, 1995, p 246
3. Parrish JA, Jaenicke KF: Action spectrum for phototherapy of psoriasis. *J Invest Dermatol* **76**:359, 1981
4. Pullmann H et al: Praktische Erfahrungen mit verschiedenen Phototherapieformen der Psoriasis—PUVA, SUP, Teer-UV-Therapie. *Z Hautkr* **53**:641, 1978
5. Green C et al: 311 nm UVB phototherapy—an effective treatment for psoriasis. *Br J Dermatol* **119**:691, 1988
6. Larko O: Treatment of psoriasis with a new UVB-lamp. *Acta Derm Venereol (Stockh)* **69**:357, 1989
7. Storbeck K et al: Die Wirksamkeit eines neuen Schmalspektrum-UV-B-Strahlers (Philips TL 01 100 W, 311-nm) im Vergleich zur konventionellen UV-B-Phototherapie der Psoriasis. *Z Hautkr* **66**:708, 1991
8. Picot E et al: Treatment of psoriasis with a 311-UVB lamp. *Br J Dermatol* **127**:509, 1992
9. van Weelden H et al: Comparison of narrow-band UVB phototherapy and PUVA photochemotherapy in the treatment of psoriasis. *Acta Derm Venereol (Stockh)* **70**:212, 1990
10. Green C et al: A comparison of the efficacy and relapse rates of narrow band UVB (TL01) monotherapy vs. etretinate (re-TL-01) vs. etretinate-PUVA (re-PUVA) in the treatment of psoriasis. *Br J Dermatol* **127**:5, 1992

11. Tanew A et al: Halfside comparison study on narrow-band UVB phototherapy versus photochemotherapy (PUVA) in the treatment of severe psoriasis. *J Invest Dermatol* **106**:841, 1996

12. Young A: Carcinogenicity of UVB phototherapy assessed. *Lancet* **346**:1431, 1995

13. Diffey BL, Farr PM: An appraisal of ultraviolet lamps used for the phototherapy of psoriasis. *Br J Dermatol* **117**:49, 1987

14. Elmets CA: Cutaneous photocarcinogenesis, in *Pharmacology of the Skin,* edited by H Mukhtar. Boca Raton, FL, CRC Press, 1992, p 389

15. Stern RS et al: Genital tumors among men with psoriasis exposed to psoralens and ultraviolet A radiation (PUVA) and ultraviolet B radiation. *N Engl J Med* **322**:1093, 1990

16. Stern RS et al: Effect of continued ultraviolet B phototherapy on the duration and remission of psoriasis: A randomized study. *J Am Acad Dermatol* **15**:546, 1986

17. Mentener MA et al: Proceedings of the psoriasis combination and rotation therapy conference. *J Am Acad Dermatol* **34**:315, 1996

18. Gallewski E: Über Cignolin, ein Ersatzpräparat des Chrysarobins. *Dermatol Wochenschr* **62**:113, 1916

19. Unna PG: Cignolin als Heilmittel der Psoriasis. *Dermatol Wochenschr* **62**:113, 1916

20. Kristensen B, Kristensen O: Topical salicylic acid interferes with UVB therapy for psoriasis. *Acta Derm Venereol (Stockh)* **71**:37, 1990

21. Farber EM, Harris DH: Hospital treatment of psoriasis: A modified anthralin program. *Arch Dermatol* **101**:381, 1970

22. Runne U, Kunze JJ: Short-duration ("minutes") therapy with dithranol for psoriasis: A new out-patient regimen. *Br J Dermatol* **106**:135, 1982

23. Ingram JT: The approach to psoriasis. *Br Med J* **2**:591, 1953

24. Karvonen J et al: 311 nm UVB lamps in the treatment of psoriasis with the Ingram regimen. *Acta Derm Venereol (Stockh)* **69**:82, 1989

25. Storbeck K et al: Narrow-band UVB (311 nm) versus conventional broad band UVB with and without dithranol in phototherapy for psoriasis. *J Am Acad Dermatol* **28**:227, 1993

26. Staham BN et al: Short-contact dithranol therapy—a comparison with the Ingram regimen. *Br J Dermatol* **110**:703, 1984

27. Lebwohl M et al: Addition of short-contact anthralin therapy to an ultraviolet B phototherapy regimen: Assessment of efficacy. *J Am Acad Dermatol* **13**:780, 1985

28. Boer J, Smeenk G: Effect of short-contact anthralin therapy on ultraviolet B irradiation of psoriasis. *J Am Acad Dermatol* **15**:198, 1986

29. Menne T, Larsen K: Psoriasis treatment with vitamin D derivatives. *Semin Dermatol* **11**:278, 1992

30. Berth-Jones J, Hutchinson PE: Vitamin D analogues and psoriasis. *Br J Dermatol* **127**:71, 1992

31. Kragballe K et al: Efficacy, tolerability, and safety of calcipotriol ointment in disorders of keratinization: Results of a randomized, double-blind, vehicle-controlled, right/left comparative study. *Arch Dermatol* **131**:556, 1995

32. Ramsay CA et al: Long-term use of topical calcipotriol in chronic plaque psoriasis. *Dermatology* **189**:260, 1994

33. Klaber MR et al: Comparative effects of calcipotriol solution (50 micrograms/ml) and bethamethasone 17 valerate solution (1 mg/ml) in the treatment of scalp psoriasis. *Br J Dermatol* **131**:678, 1994

34. Kragballe K: Combination of topical calcipotriol (MC903) and UVB radiation for psoriasis vulgaris. *Dermatologica* **181**:211, 1990

35. Kerscher M et al: Combination phototherapy of psoriasis with calcipotriol and narrow-band UVB. *Lancet* **342**:923, 1993

36. Petrozzi JW: Topical steroids and UV radiation in psoriasis. *Arch Dermatol* **119**:207, 1983

37. Larko O et al: The effect on psoriasis of clobetasol propionate used alone or in combination with UVB. *Acta Derm Venereol (Stockh)* **64**:151, 1984

38. Dover JS et al: Are topical corticosteroids useful in phototherapy for psoriasis? *J Am Acad Dermatol* **20**:748, 1989

39. LeVine MJ, Parrish JA: The effect of topical fluocinonide ointment on phototherapy of psoriasis. *J Invest Dermatol* **78**:157, 1989

40. Anderson RR, Parrish JA: Optical properties of human skin, in *The Science of Photomedicine,* edited by JD Regan, JA Parrish. New York, Plenum, 1980, p 147

41. Lebwohl M: Effects of topical preparations on the erythemogenicity of UVB: Implications for psoriasis therapy. *J Am Acad Dermatol* **32**:469, 1995

42. Abels DJ et al: Psoriasis treatment at the Dead Sea: A natural selective ultraviolet phototherapy. *J Am Acad Dermatol* **12**:639, 1985

43. Abel EA et al: Psoriasis treatment at the Dead Sea: Second international study tour. *J Am Acad Dermatol* **19**:362, 1988

44. Wiedow O et al: Freisetzung humaner Leukozytenelastase durch hypertone Salzbäder bei Psoriasis. *Hautarzt* **40**:518, 1989

45. Ludwig P et al: Inhibition of eicosanoid formation in human polymorphonuclear leukocytes by high concentrations of magnesium ions. *Biol Chem Hoppe-Seyler* **376**:739, 1995

46. Goeckermann WH: The treatment of psoriasis. *Northwest Med* **24**:229, 1925

47. Stern RS et al: Skin carcinoma in patients with psoriasis treated with topical tar and artificial ultraviolet radiation. *Lancet* **1**:732, 1980

48. Pittlekow MR et al: Skin cancer in patients with psoriasis treated with coal tar. *Arch Dermatol* **117**:465, 1981

49. Wheeler LA et al: Mutagenicity of urine from psoriatic patients undergoing treatment with coal tar and ultraviolet light. *J Invest Dermatol* **77**:181, 1981

50. Larko O, Swanbeck G: Is UVB treatment safe? A study of extensively UVB treated psoriasis patients compared with a matched control group. *Acta Derm Venereol (Stockh)* **62**:507, 1982

51. Pittlekow MR et al: Skin cancer in patients with psoriasis treated with coal tar: A 25-year follow-up study. *Arch Dermatol* **117**:465, 1981

52. Marghescu et al: Die Therapie der Psoriasis mit Retinoiden. *Z Hautkr* **57**:1410, 1982

53. Orfanos CE et al: Oral retinoid and UVB radiation: A new alternative treatment for psoriasis on an outpatient basis. *Acta Derm Venereol (Stockh)* **59**:241, 1979

54. Steigleder G et al: Retinoid-SUP-Therapie der Psoriasis. *Z Hautkr* **54**:19, 1979

55. Lest J, Boer J: Combined treatment of psoriasis with acitretin and UVB phototherapy compared with acitretin alone and UVB alone. *Br J Dermatol* **120**:665, 1989

56. Ruzicka T et al: Efficiency of acitretin in combination with UVB in the treatment of severe psoriasis. *Arch Dermatol* **126**:482, 1990

57. Lowe N et al: Acitretin plus UVB therapy for psoriasis. *J Am Acad Dermatol* **24**:591, 1991

58. Jekler J, Larkö O: Combined UV-A-UV-B versus UVB phototherapy for atopic dermatitis. *J Am Acad Dermatol* **22**:49, 1990

59. George SA et al: Narrow-band (TL01) UVB air-conditioned phototherapy for chronic severe adult atopic dermatitis. *Br J Dermatol* **128**:49, 1993

60. Krutmann J, Schöpf E: High-dose UVA1 therapy: A novel and highly effective approach for the treatment of patients with acute exacerbation of atopic dermatitis. *Acta Derm Venereol (Stockh)* **176**:120, 1992

61. Krutmann J: Phototherapy for atopic eczema. *Dermatol Ther* **1**:24, 1996

62. Krutmann J et al: High-dose UVA1 therapy in the treatment of patients with atopic dermatitis. *J Am Acad Dermatol* **26**:225, 1992

63. Costa C et al: Scoring atopic dermatitis: The simpler the better. *Acta Derm Venereol (Stockh)* **69**:41, 1989

64. Czech W et al: Serum eosinophil cationic protein is a sensitive measure for disease activity in atopic dermatitis. *Br J Dermatol* **126**:351, 1992

65. Krutmann J et al: High-dose UVA1 therapy for atopic dermatitis. *J Am Acad Dermatol* **38**:589, 1998

66. Jekler J, Larkö O: Phototherapy for atopic dermatitis with ultraviolet A (UVA), low-dose UVB and combined UVA and UVB: Two paired comparison studies. *Photodermatol Photoimmunol Photomed* **8**:151, 1991

67. Kowalzick L et al: Low dose versus medium dose UV-A1 treatment in severe atopic eczema. *Acta Derm Venereol (Stockh)* **75**:43, 1995

68. Sterenbroigh HCJM, van der Leun JC: Tumorigenesis by a long wavelength UV-A source. *Photochem Photobiol* **51**:325, 1990

69. Setlow RB et al: Wavelengths effective in induction of malignant melanoma. *Proc Natl Acad Sci USA* **90**:6666, 1993

70. Jekler J, Larkö O: UVB phototherapy of atopic eczema. *Br J Dermatol* **119**:697, 1988

71. Midelfart K et al: Combined UVB and UVA phototherapy of atopic eczema. *Dermatologica* **171**:95, 1985

72. Falk ES: UV-light therapies in atopic dermatitis. *Photodermatol Photoimmunol Photomed* **2**:241, 1985

73. Hannuksela M et al: Ultraviolet light therapy in atopic dermatitis. *Acta Derm Venereol (Stockh)* **114**(suppl):137, 1985

74. Pullmann H et al: Wirkungen von Infrarot- und UVA-Strahlen auf die menschliche Haut und ihre Wirksamkeit bei der Behandlung des endogenen Ekzems. *Z Hautkr* **60**:171, 1985

75. Hudson-Peacock MJ et al: Narrow-band UVB phototherapy for severe atopic dermatitis. *Br J Dermatol* **135**:330, 1996

76. Collins P, Ferguson J: Narrow-band (TL-01) UVB air-conditioned phototherapy for atopic eczema in children. *Br J Dermatol* **133**:653, 1995

77. Hölzle E et al: Polymorphous light eruption. *J Invest Dermatol* **88**:32s, 1987

78. Morison WL et al: UV-B phototherapy in the prophylaxis of polymorphous light eruption. *Br J Dermatol* **106**:231, 1982

79. Ortel B et al: Polymorphous light eruption: Action spectrum and photoprotection. *J Am Acad Dermatol* **14**:748, 1986

80. Addo H, Sharma SC: UVB phototherapy and photochemotherapy (PUVA) in the treatment of polymorphic light eruption and solar urticaria. *Br J Dermatol* **116**:539, 1987

81. Murphy GM et al: Prophylactic PUVA and UVB therapy in polymorphous light eruption. *Br J Dermatol* **116**:531, 1987

82. Bilsland D et al: A comparison of narrow band phototherapy (TL-01) and photochemotherapy (PUVA) in the management of polymorphous light eruption. *Br J Dermatol* **129**:708, 1993

83. Collins P, Fergusson J: Narrow-band UVB (TL-01) phototherapy: An effective preventative treatment for the photodermatoses. *Br J Dermatol* **132**:956, 1995

84. Fleischmajer R: Localized and systemic scleroderma, in *Connective Tissue Diseases of the Skin,* edited by CM Lapiere, T Krieg. New York, Marcel Dekker, 1993, p 295

85. Kerscher M et al: Treatment of localized scleroderma by UVA1 phototherapy. *Lancet* **346**:1166, 1995

86. Stege H et al: High-dose ultraviolet A1 radiation therapy of localized scleroderma. *J Am Acad Dermatol* **36**:938, 1997

87. Takeda K et al: Decreased collagenase expression in cultured systemic sclerosis fibroblasts. *J Invest Dermatol* **103**:359, 1994

88. Christophers E et al: PUVA treatment of urticaria pigmentosa. *Br J Dermatol* **98**:701, 1978

89. Granerus G et al: Decreased urinary histamine levels after successful PUVA treatment of urticaria pigmentosa. *J Invest Dermatol* **76**:1, 1981

90. Kolde G et al: Response of cutaneous mast cells to PUVA in patients with urticaria pigmentosa: Histophotometric, ultrastructural, and biochemical investigations. *J Invest Dermatol* **83**:175, 1984

91. Stege H et al: High-dose UVA1 for urticaria pigmentosa. *Lancet* **347**:64, 1996

92. Grabbe J et al: High-dose UVA1 therapy, but not UVA/UVB therapy, decreases IgE binding cells in lesional skin of patients with atopic eczema. *J Invest Dermatol* **107**:419, 1996

93. McGrath Jr H: Ultraviolet-A1 irradiation decreases clinical disease activity and autoantibodies in patients with systemic lupus erythematosus. *Clin Exp Rheumatol* **12**:129, 1994

94. McGrath Jr H et al: Ultraviolet-A1 (340–400 nm) irradiation in systemic lupus erythematosus. *Lupus* **5**:269, 1996

95. LeVine MJ: Phototherapy of pityriasis lichenoides. *Arch Dermatol* **119**:387, 1983

96. Arndt A et al: Treatment of pityriasis rosea with UV radiation. *Arch Dermatol* **119**:381, 1983

97. Epstein JH: UVL-induced stimulation of DNA synthesis in hairless mouse epidermis. *J Invest Dermatol* **52**:445, 1968

98. Epstein WL et al: Early effects of ultraviolet light on DNA synthesis in human skin in vivo. *Arch Dermatol* **100**:84, 1969

99. Kramer DM et al: Effect of ultraviolet irradiation on biosynthesis of DNA in guinea pig skin. *J Invest Dermatol* **62**:388, 1974

100. Pullmann H et al: Effects of selective ultraviolet phototherapy (SUP) and local PUVA treatment on DNA synthesis in guinea pig skin. *Arch Dermatol Res* **267**:37, 1980

101. Volc-Platzer B, Hönigsmann H: Photoimmunology of PUVA and UVB therapy, in *Photoimmunology,* edited by J Krutmann, CA Elmets. Oxford, England, Blackwell, 1995, p 265

102. Kripke ML: Immunologic mechanisms in UV radiation carcinogenesis. *Adv Cancer Res* **34**:69, 1981

103. Toews G et al: Epidermal Langerhans cell density determines whether contact hypersensitivity or unresponsiveness follows skin painting with DNFB. *J Immunol* **134**:445, 1980

104. Krutmann J, Elmets CA (eds): *Photoimmunology.* Oxford, England, Blackwell, 1995

105. Everett M et al: Penetration of epidermis by ultraviolet rays. *Photochem Photobiol* **5**:533, 1966

106. Luger TA, Schwarz T: Effects of UV light on cytokines and neuroendocrine hormones, in *Photoimmunology,* edited by J Krutmann, CA Elmets. Oxford, England, Blackwell, 1995, p 55

107. Morita A et al: Ultraviolet A1 radiation effects on cytokine expression in human epidermoid carcinoma cells. *Photochem Photobiol* **65**:630, 1997

108. Grewe M et al: Interleukin-10 production by cultured human keratinocytes: Regulation by ultraviolet B and ultraviolet A1 radiation. *J Invest Dermatol* **104**:3, 1995

109. Schauer E et al: Proopiomelanocortin derived peptides are synthesized and released by human keratinocytes. *J Clin Invest* **93**:2258, 1994

110. Grewe M et al: Analysis of the mechanism of ultraviolet B radiation induced prostaglandin E2 synthesis by human epidermoid carcinoma cells. *J Invest Dermatol* **101**:528, 1993

111. Grewe M et al: Lesional expression of interferon-γ in atopic eczema. *Lancet* **343**:25, 1994

112. Morita A et al: Ultraviolet A1 radiation differentially affects cytokine production by atopen-specific human T-helper cells. *J Invest Dermatol* **106**:932, 1996

113. Lisby S et al: Intercellular adhesion molecule-1 (ICAM-1) expression correlated to inflammation. *Br J Dermatol* **120**:479, 1989

114. Norris DA et al: Ultraviolet radiation can either suppress or induce expression of intercellular adhesion molecule-1 (ICAM-1) on the surface of cultured human keratinocytes. *J Invest Dermatol* **95**:132, 1990

115. Krutmann J, Grewe M: Involvement of cytokines, DNA damage, and reactive oxygen intermediates in ultraviolet radiation-induced modulation of intercellular adhesion molecule-1 expression. *J Invest Dermatol* **105**:67S, 1995

116. Roza L et al: Role of UV-induced DNA damage in phototherapy, in *The Fundamental Bases of Phototherapy,* edited by H Hönigsmann, G Jori, AR Young. Milan, OEMF spa, 1996, p 145

117. Krutmann J et al: The cell membrane is a major locus for ultraviolet B–induced alterations in accessory cells. *J Clin Invest* **85**:1529, 1990

118. Weiss JM et al: Low-dose UVB radiation perturbs the functional expression of B7.1 and B7.2 costimulatory molecules on human Langerhans cells. *Eur J Immunol* **25**:2858, 1995

119. Grewe M et al: Interleukin-1 receptors type I and type II are differentially regulated in human keratinocytes by ultraviolet B radiation. *J Invest Dermatol* **107**:865, 1996

120. Trefzer U et al: The human 55-kDa tumor necrosis factor receptor is regulated in human keratinocytes by TNF-α and by ultraviolet B radiation. *J Clin Invest* **92**:462, 1993

121. Godar DE: Preprogrammed and programmed cell death mechanisms of apoptosis: UV-induced immediate and delayed apoptosis. *Photochem Photobiol* **63**:825, 1996

122. Yoo EK et al: Apoptosis induction by ultraviolet light A and photochemotherapy in cutaneous T-cell lymphomas: Relevance to mechanism of therapeutic action. *J Invest Dermatol* **107**:235, 1996

123. Schön P et al: Murine psoriasis-like disorder induced by naive CD4+ T cells. *Nature Medicine* **3**:183, 1997

124. Morita A et al: Evidence that singlet oxygen-induced human T helper cell apoptosis is the basic mechanism of ultraviolet-A radiation phototherapy. *J Exp Med* **186**:1763, 1997

125. Krueger JG et al: Successful ultraviolet B treatment of psoriasis is accompanied by a reversal of keratinocyte pathology and by selective depletion of intraepidermal T cells. *J Exp Med* **182**:2057, 1995

CHAPTER 264

Herbert Hönigsmann
Rolf-Markus Szeimies
Robert Knobler
Thomas B. Fitzpatrick
Madhu A. Pathak
Klaus Wolff

Photochemotherapy and Photodynamic Therapy

PHOTOCHEMOTHERAPY (PUVA)

Psoralen photochemotherapy is a combination of psoralen (P) and long-wave ultraviolet radiation (UVA) that brings about a therapeutically beneficial result not produced by either the drug or radiation alone. This particular form of therapy is currently used in the treatment of several common and uncommon skin diseases. Psoralens can be administered orally or applied topically in the form of solutions, creams, or baths with subsequent UVA exposure.

Historic Aspects

Topical application of extracts, seeds, and parts of plants that contain natural psoralens followed by exposure to sunlight has been used as a remedy for vitiligo for thousands of years by the ancient Egyptian and Indian healers.[1] In modern medicine, the first clinical studies in vitiligo with topical and oral psoralens were performed originally by El Mofty in 1948 and later by Lerner et al.[2,3]

In 1974 it was shown that orally administered 8-methoxypsoralen (MOP) and subsequent irradiation with artificial UVA was a highly effective treatment for psoriasis. This new therapeutic concept was termed *photochemotherapy*, or *PUVA*.[4] In a parallel study the excellent efficacy was confirmed in a large patient cohort.[5] Within a few years the beneficial effects of PUVA were documented worldwide. However, before the development of high-intensity UVA sources, it had already been shown that topically applied psoralens plus irradiation with low-intensity UVA (black light) could clear psoriatic lesions.[6] In recent years the use of psoralen baths and subsequent UVA exposure has become increasingly popular for several reasons that will be detailed later. This type of treatment, termed *bath-PUVA*, originated in Scandinavia.[7] The effectiveness of all variants of PUVA has been widely documented and has profoundly influenced dermatologic therapy in general, providing treatment for a number of diverse disorders besides psoriasis (Table 264-1).

Principles of PUVA Therapy

The rationale of PUVA is to induce remissions of skin diseases by repeated, controlled phototoxic reactions. These reactions occur only when psoralens are photoactivated by UVA. According to the penetration characteristics of UVA, absorption of photons is confined to the skin. However, there is also some evidence that PUVA may exert systemic effects through circulating blood cells. Clinically, PUVA-induced phototoxic reactions are characterized by a

TABLE 264-1

PUVA-Responsive Diseases

THERAPY OF DISEASE	PREVENTION OF DISEASE
Psoriasis	Polymorphous light eruption
Palmoplantar pustulosis	Hydroa vacciniforme*
Mycosis fungoides (stages IA, IB)	Solar urticaria
Vitiligo	Erythropoietic protoporphyria*
Atopic dermatitis	Chronic actinic dermatitis*
Generalized lichen planus	
Urticaria pigmentosa	
Cutaneous graft-versus-host disease	
Generalized granuloma annulare	
Pityriasis lichenoides*	
Lymphomatoid papulosis*	
Pityriasis rubra pilaris*	

*Experience limited to small number of patients.

delayed sunburn-like erythema and skin inflammation that, upon overdosage, may progress to blistering and superficial necrosis. Thus, careful attention to the guidelines for proper dosimetry is essential.

PSORALENS Psoralens are naturally occurring tricyclic furocoumarins present in a large number of plants, but some synthetic psoralen compounds also exist. Most widely used for oral and bath-PUVA is 8-MOP (methoxsalen, xanthotoxin), which is of plant origin but also available as a synthetic drug. 4,5′,8-Trimethylpsoralen (TMP, trioxsalen) is a synthetic compound that is less phototoxic after oral administration but more phototoxic when used for bath-PUVA. It is used primarily in Scandinavia for that purpose. Also 5-MOP (bergapten) has proved to be therapeutically effective by the oral route; it is less erythemogenic in photochemotherapy and does not induce intolerance reactions. It is now used in several European institutions for routine PUVA and experimentally in the United States.

Psoralen photochemistry[8–10] Psoralens intercalate between DNA base pairs without UV radiation. Absorption of photons in the UVA range results in the formation of a 3,4- or 4′,5′-cyclobutane addition product with pyrimidine bases of native DNA. In the first step of this photochemical reaction, a monofunctional adduct with thymine or cytosine is formed. Some psoralens, including 8-MOP, TMP, and 5-MOP, can absorb a second photon, and this reaction leads to the formation of a bifunctional adduct with a 5,6 double bond of the pyrimidine base of the opposite strand, thus producing an interstrand cross-link of the double helix. This conjunction of psoralens with epidermal DNA produces a suppression of both DNA synthesis and cell division,[11–13] and it is generally assumed, although not proved, that this effect may be the therapeutic mechanism in psoriasis. However, cross-linking does not appear to be a prerequisite for the therapeutic effect,[14] and the successful PUVA treatment of other skin diseases is unlikely to be due directly to this molecular reaction; psoralens also react with RNA, proteins, and other cellular components[15] and indirectly modify proteins and lipids via singlet oxygen-mediated reactions or by generating free radicals.[10] Perhaps these mechanisms contribute to the successful use of PUVA in diseases that are not hyperproliferative in nature. More recent data indicate that effects on immunocompetent cells may be a decisive event, possibly also in psoriasis.

The formation of mono- and bifunctional photoadducts in DNA results in the immediate inhibition of DNA synthesis. The interstrand cross-links are believed to be largely responsible for eliciting skin photosensitization reactions of linear psoralens such as 8-MOP. Excessive production of these cyclobutane adducts causes cell death. The events of mutation and skin carcinogenesis appear to be the consequence of photoconjugation of psoralens to DNA. Psoralens that form monofunctional adducts as well as bifunctional adducts (interstrand cross-links) can be carcinogenic because the cells surviving DNA damage and undergoing DNA replication tend to repair DNA damage through an error-prone repair process.[16]

In type II reactions, reactive oxygen species ($^1O_2$, O_2, or OH) induce the oxidation of cellular lipoprotein membrane lipids, destruction of membrane-bound cytochrome P_{450}, and the activation of the cyclooxygenase pathway.[15] The membrane-damaging events activate the arachidonic acid metabolism pathway, which results in an increase of secondary oxidation products that contribute to the increased synthesis of eicosanoids.[17] Furthermore, the reactive oxygen species can directly damage DNA by generating DNA strand breaks.

Mechanisms of photochemotherapy Hypotheses about the mechanism of photochemotherapy of psoriasis are based on the fact that PUVA causes photoconjugation of psoralens to DNA and a subsequent suppression of mitosis, DNA synthesis, and cell proliferation. This would indeed suffice to revert increased cell proliferation rates in psoriasis to normal. On the other hand, PUVA down-regulates certain lymphocyte and antigen-presenting cell functions, influences adhesion molecule expression, and diminishes Langerhans cell numbers within the epidermis (see "Immunologic Effects," below). In addition, PUVA may affect specific cells such as lymphocytes or polymorphonuclear leukocytes. Since there is increasing evidence that psoriasis is caused primarily by the action of blood-derived immunocytes,[18,19] it is reasonable to speculate that PUVA therapy may quite possibly act by an effect on normal or abnormal immune function involving a direct phototoxic effect on lymphocytes in skin infiltrates or on an abnormal immune function. This is in keeping with the observation that several other disorders that are not hyperproliferative in nature respond well to PUVA.

Psoralens also stimulate melanogenesis. This involves the photoconjugation of psoralens to DNA in melanocytes, mitosis and subsequent proliferation of melanocytes, an increased formation and melanization of melanosomes, an increased transfer of melanosomes to keratinocytes, and activation and increased synthesis of tyrosine mediated by stimulation of cAMP activity.

Pharmacokinetics The important steps between the ingestion of a psoralen and its arrival at the site of action include disintegration and dissolution of the drug, absorption, first-pass effect, blood transportation, and tissue distribution.[20] The absorption rate of a psoralen from the gut depends on the physicochemical properties of the molecule, the rate of dissolution, the galenic characteristics

of the preparation, and the fat content of the concomitant food intake.[21] 5-MOP is less water-soluble than 8-MOP, and its absorption rate is approximately 25 percent of that of 8-MOP.[22] Liquid preparations of 8-MOP[23] and 5-MOP[22] give higher and earlier peak serum levels than do crystalline formulations. In addition, peak serum levels are achieved by liquid preparations after a relatively reproducible time interval in all subjects, whereas a wide time variability occurs with crystalline formulations. Before reaching the skin via the circulation, psoralens are metabolized during passage through the liver. Plasma levels of 8-MOP administered orally at different doses show a strong nonlinearity, indicating a saturable first-pass effect.[20] Thus small differences in the ingested doses and absorption rates of psoralens lead to large differences in plasma levels. As a practical consequence, small amounts of the drug are almost completely metabolized by the liver at first pass and therefore may be therapeutically inactive.

Psoralens have a serum half-life of 1 h and are degraded within 12 h. Cytochrome P_{450}–dependent microsomal monooxygenase appears to play a major role in the biotransformation and inactivation of psoralens.[24] Psoralen is distributed by the blood within all tissues and body fluids,[25] including the crystalline lens, which is accessible to UVA.[26] Up to 90 percent of 5-MOP and 8-MOP binds to serum proteins, mainly albumin. 5-MOP has a higher binding affinity than 8-MOP, and the binding sites are different and noninteracting. 8-MOP and 5-MOP serum levels show a wide range of interindividual differences. On different occasions, serum levels also show differences within a single patient[21,23]; however, they are sufficiently constant to provide for relatively reproducible therapeutic results. The unpredictable pharmacokinetic behavior is probably due to inter- and intraindividual variations of intestinal absorption, first-pass effect, blood distribution in the body, metabolism, and elimination of the drug.

Within the same individual, serum levels of 8-MOP correspond fairly well with skin reactivity, the peak of skin phototoxicity coinciding with peak serum levels.[23] However, phototoxic responses to PUVA show large interindividual variations, and the biologic mechanisms of these differences remain to be established. A correlation between 8-MOP and 5-MOP serum levels and epidermal concentrations has been demonstrated. Whether there is a significant correlation between maximum psoralen blood concentrations and the minimal phototoxicity dose remains equivocal.[27,28] The correlation between psoralen blood levels and the therapeutic effect remains to be established, even though individuals with low maximum serum concentration usually show an unsatisfactory therapeutic result.

The pharmacokinetics of 8-MOP following topical treatment depend on the application modalities. Topically applied 8-MOP as a 0.15% emulsion or solution has been shown to lead to plasma levels comparable to those found with oral treatment if large areas of the body are treated.[29] In contrast, plasma levels following bath-PUVA treatment of almost total body surface are very low.[30] Bathwater-delivered psoralens are readily absorbed in the skin but are promptly eliminated without cutaneous accumulation.[31,32]

UVA RADIATION UVA sources commonly used for PUVA therapy are fluorescent lamps or high-pressure metal-halide lamps. The typical fluorescent PUVA lamp has an emission peak at 352 nm and emits approximately 0.5 percent in the UVB range. Another type of lamp that is in use in some centers has an emission peak at 370 nm and less than 0.1 percent UVB output. Recently, tubes with a peak emission at 325 nm with a higher UVB contamination have proved very effective for PUVA therapy.[33]

The choice of the radiation source needs to be made after evaluation of the physical characteristics and practical aspects of each lamp. Major advantages of mercury-halide units are the stability of output and the high irradiance, which permit short treatment times. The use of metal-halide lamps (which have the major part of their UV emission spectrum above 360 nm) and 370-nm fluorescent tubes should perhaps be reconsidered because of the recent observation that the action spectrum of antipsoriatic activity and phototoxic erythema peaks at 335 nm.[33,34] However, longer wavelengths have proved equally effective for clearing psoriasis if delivered in a larger dose to obtain an equal erythemogenic response.[34]

UVA doses are given in J/cm^2, usually measured with a photometer with a maximum sensitivity at 350 to 360 nm. Within the treatment system, the irradiance must be relatively uniform so that the dose will not vary in different anatomic sites of the patient. UVB emission should be kept low enough so as not to reach erythemogenic doses before sufficient UVA is absorbed to produce the psoralen photosensitivity reaction.

Photosensitivity effects of PUVA PUVA treatment produces an inflammatory response that manifests as delayed phototoxic erythema. The reaction is related to the dose of drug and of UVA and to the individual's sensitivity to phototoxic reactions. Though similar in clinical appearance to UVB erythema that appears after 4 to 6 h and peaks 12 to 24 h after exposure, PUVA erythema differs from sunburn in several important respects. Its onset does not appear before 24 to 36 h, and it peaks at 48 to 72 h or even as late as 96 h after irradiation.[35] The erythema dose-response curve is steeper than that of UVB, and thus a relatively small increment of UVA may result in an intense erythema response. The reaction persists for longer periods, lasting up to more than 1 week.[35] PUVA erythema consists of a deeper redness, often exhibiting a violaceous hue. Severe reactions may lead to blistering and to superficial skin necrosis. Overdoses of UVA are frequently followed by swelling, intense pruritus, and sometimes by a peculiar stinging sensation in the affected skin area, possibly due to damage of superficial nerve endings. Erythema is at present the only available parameter that allows an assessment of the magnitude of the PUVA reaction with psoralens and thus represents an important criterion for UVA dose adjustments during the initial treatment phase.[35]

Pigmentation is the second important effect of PUVA. It may develop without clinically evident erythema, especially when oral 5-MOP or TMP is used; this is of particular importance in the treatment of vitiligo and for the preventive therapy of certain photodermatoses. In normal skin, PUVA pigmentation maximizes about 7 days after a PUVA exposure and may last from several weeks to months. As with sun-induced pigmentation, the individual's ability to tan is genetically determined, but the dose-response curve is much steeper. A few PUVA exposures result in a much deeper tan than that produced by multiple exposures to solar radiation.

Treatment Protocols

TOPICAL TREATMENT Application of 8-MOP in creams, ointments, or lotions followed by UVA irradiations is effective in clearing psoriasis but has several disadvantages. The nonuniform distribution on the skin surface induces unpredictable phototoxic erythema reactions and irregular patches of cosmetically unacceptable hyperpigmentation. Furthermore, if numerous lesions are present, the application is laborious and time-consuming, and the treat-

ment does not prevent the development of new active lesions in previously unaffected, untreated areas. Finally, the application of a 0.15% 8-MOP emulsion was found to give rise to plasma levels comparable to those found with oral treatment.[29] Therefore, the use of topical PUVA with psoralen creams, ointments, or lotions is now limited to psoriasis of palms and soles.

ORAL TREATMENT In oral PUVA the general principle is to hold the dose of drug and the interval between drug intake and UVA exposure constant and to vary the UVA dose according to the patient's sensitivity. A dosage of 8-MOP of 0.6 to 0.8 mg/kg body weight is administered orally 1 to 3 h before exposure, depending on the absorption characteristics of the particular drug brand. Liquid drug preparations are absorbed faster and yield higher and more reproducible serum levels than microcrystalline forms.[23] For 5-MOP, the usual dosage is 1.2 to 1.8 mg/kg.[22]

The initial UVA doses are established either by skin typing[36,37] or by minimal phototoxicity dose (MPD) testing.[35,38] In the United States, skin reactivity to solar radiation is evaluated and patients are classified into a skin phototype scheme according to their sunburn history. Therapeutic doses of UVA are then given according to an empirical scheme based on this classification[36] (Table 264-2). In Europe, the most widely used approach consists of MPD determination.[35] The MPD is defined as the minimal dose of UVA that produces a barely perceptible, but well-defined erythema when template areas of the skin are exposed to increasing doses of UVA. The doses range from 0.5 to 5 J/cm^2 if 8-MOP is used and 1 to 10 J/cm^2 if 5-MOP is used.[22] Erythema readings are performed 72 h after testing, at which time the psoralen phototoxicity reaction usually reaches its peak. The MPD test should always be performed on previously nonexposed skin (e.g., buttocks) because this will yield lower values than on previously exposed skin and contributes to a safer initial dosimetry. Although the MPD test is more time-consuming than phototyping, it should be done whenever possible since it allows for more accurate and higher UVA doses during initial treatment.

BATH-PUVA An increasing number of physicians are focusing on bathwater delivery of psoralens because it provides for a uniform drug distribution over the skin surface, very low psoralen plasma levels,[30] and quick elimination of free psoralens from the skin, reducing the risk of accidental sunburns. Bathwater delivery of 8-MOP circumvents gastrointestinal side effects and possible phototoxic hazards to the eyes because there is no systemic photosen-

TABLE 264-2

Skin Phototypes

Skin Phototype*		Recommended Dose, J/cm^2
I	Always burn, never tan†	0.5
II	Always burn, but sometimes tan	1.0
III	Sometimes burn, but always tan	1.5
IV	Never burn, always tan	2.0
V‡	Moderately pigmented	2.5
VI‡	Blacks	3.0

*Types I–IV are determined by history; types V and VI by physical examination (racial descent).
†Patients with erythrodermic psoriasis are to be classified as skin phototype I for determination of UVA dosage.
‡Patients with natural pigmentation of these types should be classified into a lower skin phototype category if the sunburning history so indicates.
SOURCE: Adapted from Melski et al,[36] with permission.

sitization. Skin psoralen levels are highly reproducible, and photosensitivity lasts no more than 2 h. The higher incidence of unwanted phototoxicity can be prevented by a lower starting dose (50 percent of the MPD) and a more cautious dosimetry in the initial treatment phase.[39] Originally, bath-PUVA was performed with TMP, but 8-MOP and 5-MOP[40] are now being used as well. Bath-PUVA consists of 15 to 20 min of whole-body immersion in solutions of 0.5 to 5.0 mg 8-MOP per liter of bathwater. Irradiation needs to be performed immediately, as photosensitivity decreases rather rapidly.[32] TMP is more phototoxic after topical application and is used at lower concentrations than 8-MOP. MPD testing for bath-PUVA must take into account that the phototoxic threshold declines during the early treatment phase, in contrast to oral PUVA. In the authors' experience, the MPD obtained with four consecutive daily determinations is approximately 50 percent of the MPD obtained with only one determination.[39]

Repeated exposures are required to clear PUVA-responsive diseases, with gradual dose increments as pigmentation develops. Lower doses quite frequently result in failure of treatment except in those diseases in which induction of pigmentation is the desired objective. In most dermatoses amenable to PUVA, the frequency of treatments is reduced after satisfactory clearing of disease, and the last UVA dose is used as a maintenance dose if maintenance treatment is planned. The duration of this maintenance phase and the frequency of treatments depend on the particular disease being treated and its propensity to relapse.

PUVA for Psoriasis (See Chap. 43)

The first studies on the use of psoralens in psoriasis therapy involved the topical application of psoralens to psoriatic lesions,[41–43] and in addition to dosimetry problems, the studies revealed that new lesions could develop in previously unaffected, and thus untreated, areas. Topical psoralen photochemotherapy may be indicated only for the treatment of resistant plaques and particularly palmoplantar lesions, in conjunction with total-body oral PUVA. This does not hold for bath-PUVA therapy, which employs whole-body immersion in TMP or 8-MOP baths followed by total-body irradiation[7,44] and which does yield satisfactory results. Bathwater delivery of 8-MOP represents a useful alternative to oral PUVA[44]; because of the higher degree of photosensitivity, the UVA dose can be kept much lower.

The effectiveness of oral PUVA in inducing and maintaining remission of psoriasis has been widely documented and confirmed by large-scale clinical trials both in the United States and in Europe (Figs. 264-1 and 264-2). Bath-PUVA has only recently become quite popular; it is also very successful because there is no systemic phototoxicity and some patients with severe psoriasis recalcitrant to oral PUVA can be cleared.

Two major treatment protocols for oral photochemotherapy have evolved, one in the United States[36,37] and one in Europe[35,38] (Table 264-3). In the U.S. protocol, the first treatment exposure dose is based on skin phototyping and the patients are treated either two or three times a week. Dose increments range from 0.5 to 1.5 J/cm^2, depending on erythema production and therapeutic response. In the European protocol, the initial UVA dose is the patient's MPD. Four treatments are given per week: two exposures on consecutive days followed by a rest on day 3 and on weekends. After clearing, therapy is continued according to a maintenance schedule consisting of two treatments per week for 1 month and one treatment per week for another month.

The first two controlled multicenter clinical trials were conducted between 1975 and 1980 in the United States[36] and Europe.[38] The results of these trials are now the standard of reference for all

FIGURE 264-1

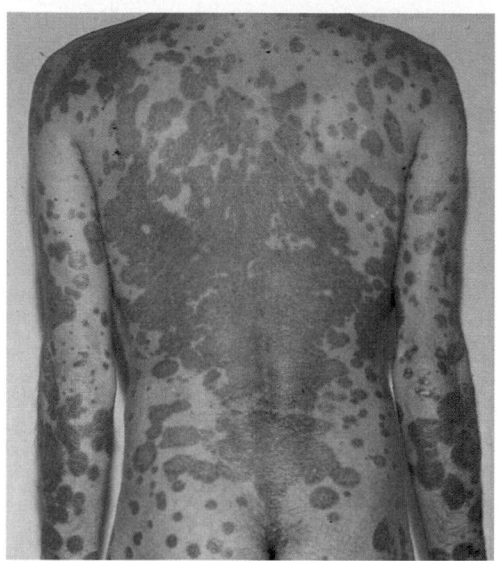

A.

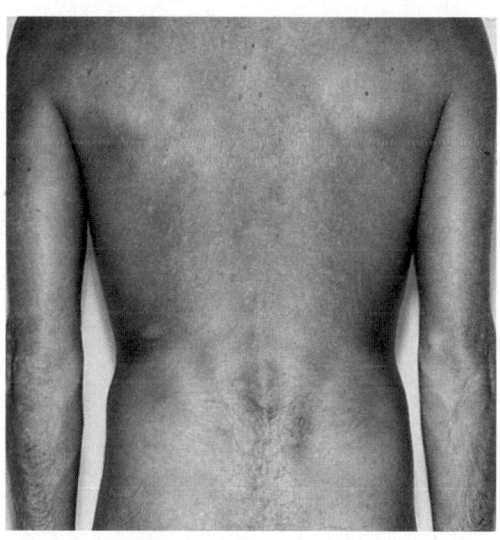

B.

Twenty-three-year-old patient with generalized psoriasis (seborrheic type). *A.* Before PUVA treatment. *B.* After treatment. (*From Wolff et al.,[5] with permission.*)

claims of efficacy of PUVA therapy. Both studies reported similar remission rates, but because of the different treatment schedule in the U.S. Cooperative Clinical Trial,[36] the duration of the clearing phase was twice as long as in the European study.[38] In addition, total UVA requirements in the U.S. study were more than twice as high, and the final single doses differed by about 90 percent (Table 264-4).

Three studies have compared bathwater delivery of 8-MOP with oral administration.[44–46] In two reports, initial doses were determined by skin typing, and treatments were given two to three times weekly.[44,45] Dose increments were instituted with every treatment in one study,[44] whereas smaller increments were given every third treatment in the other.[45] The most recent report, in which patients

FIGURE 264-2

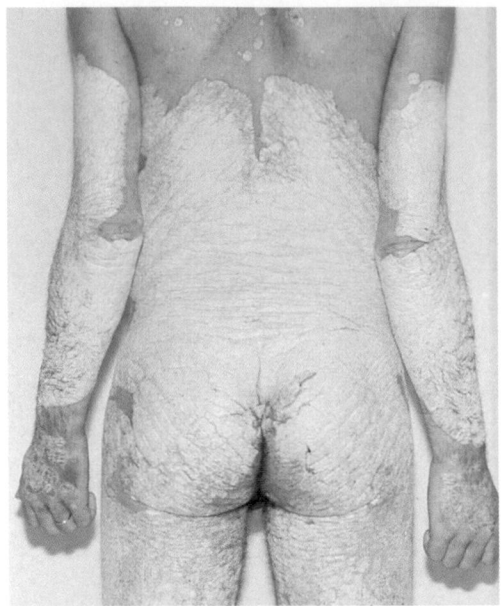

A.

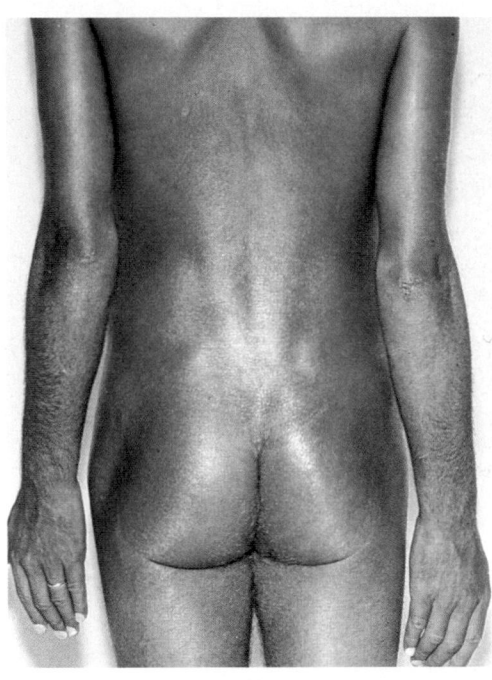

B.

Twenty-three-year-old patient with generalized psoriasis (plaque-type). *A.* Before PUVA treatment. *B.* After treatment. (*From Wolff et al.,*[35] *with permission.*)

were treated according to the guidelines of the standard European regimen for oral PUVA,[38] showed the lowest incidence of treatment failures and overdose episodes.[46] In comparison with the results obtained with oral 8-MOP, bath-PUVA showed equal clearing rates with lower numbers of exposures.[44,46] The greater therapeutic efficacy could be due to a higher penetration of psoralens through the

TABLE 264-3

Differences between U.S. and European Protocols

	UNITED STATES	**EUROPE**
UVA dosimetry	Predetermined dose according to skin phototype	Individualized dose according to MPD determination
Frequency of treatments	Two to three times/week	Four times/week
Dose increments	Predetermined	Individualized
Principle of approach	Rigid, cautious	Flexible, aggressive
Goal	To clear without ponderous testing and acute side effects	To clear rapidly before maximum pigmentation develops

NOTE: MPD, minimal phototoxicity dose.

TABLE 264-4

Treatment Results

	UNITED STATES*	**EUROPE†**
Number of patients	1139	3175
Result better than marked improvement	1005 (88%)	2785 (89%)
Exposures required for clearing (median)	25	20
Duration of treatment (weeks)	12.7	5.3
Cumulative UVA dose (J/cm^2) (all patients and skin phototypes)	245	96

*Adapted from Melski et al.,[36] with permission.
†Adapted from Henseler et al.,[38] with permission.

abnormal stratum corneum overlying psoriatic plaques, as compared with healthy perilesional skin where phototoxicity is monitored during the therapy. The incidences of erythema and pruritus were similar or lower compared to oral therapy. In all investigations, episodes of systemic intolerance such as nausea and vomiting were only recorded with oral PUVA.

Oral 5-MOP–PUVA represents another alternative to 8-MOP–PUVA.[22,47] Psoriatic lesions are cleared with a comparable number of exposures, but 5-MOP requires significantly higher cumulative UVA doses. This difference is due to the lower phototoxicity potential of 5-MOP and to its higher tanning activity. Nevertheless, 5-MOP–PUVA therapy seems particularly valuable because of the absence of nausea and vomiting and the lower incidence of pruritus and severe phototoxic skin reactions.[22,47]

Upon complete clearing, patients are often assigned to maintenance therapy, during which the frequency of treatments is gradually reduced.[48] From several studies it is assumed that the recurrence rate may be significantly higher in patients in whom no maintenance is performed.[49] However, PUVA maintenance does have disadvantages. Patients with a stable remission may be overtreated, and, most significantly, long-term risks of PUVA are related to the total cumulative phototoxic doses delivered to the skin during continuous or long-term treatment.

Erythrodermic and generalized pustular psoriasis (von Zumbusch type) respond to PUVA (Fig. 264-3), but the time required to induce remission is considerably longer, more treatments are needed, and higher failure rates are reported as compared to plaque or guttate

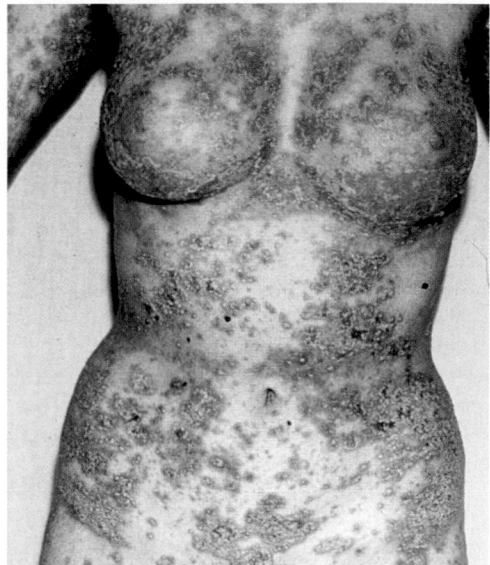

A.

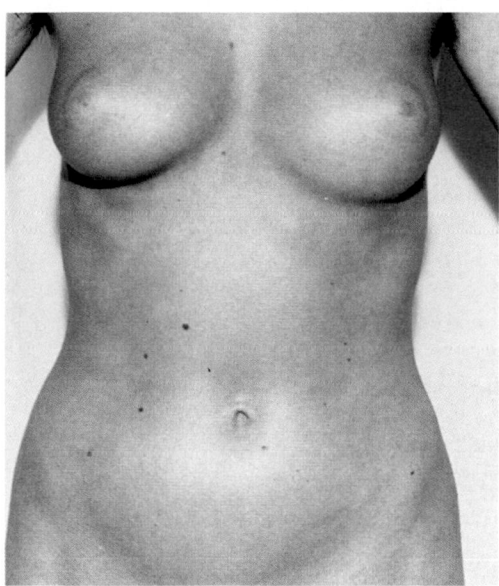

B.

Eighteen-year-old patient with pustular psoriasis (von Zumbusch type). *A.* Before PUVA treatment. *B.* After treatment. (*From Hönigsmann et al., Br J Dermatol 97:119, 1977, with permission.*)

varieties. Pustular eruptions of palms and soles are quite recalcitrant to treatment, regardless of whether they are true localized pustular psoriasis, nonpsoriatic palmoplantar pustulosis or pustular psoriasis, nonpsoriatic palmoplantar pustulosis, or pustular eczema. Oral PUVA alone can produce a slow but definite remission in many cases, but a considerable number of patients require adjunctive therapy for clearing. As mentioned above, the combination with topically applied 8-MOP can be beneficial, but bath-PUVA appears to be also quite effective in such cases. The addition of oral retinoids will help to clear the majority of patients (see below).

COMBINATION TREATMENTS *Topical combination* PUVA has been combined with other treatment forms to improve efficacy

and to reduce possible side effects. Topical adjuvant therapies with glucocorticoids, anthralin, and tar preparations have been tried with some success, and more recently the combination with calcipotriol yielded good results. However, topical therapy is found unacceptable by some patients since it is considered a step backward to conventional treatment.

Methotrexate A combination of PUVA and methotrexate can reduce the duration of treatment, number of exposures, and total UVA dose and is also effective in clearing patients unresponsive to PUVA or UVB alone. However, although methotrexate is delivered at a total dose well below the minimum dose reported for hepatotoxicity, this combination if used for long-term treatment could be potentially hazardous because PUVA and methotrexate may act synergistically in the development of skin cancers.[50,51]

Cyclosporine Cyclosporine plus PUVA therapy and retinoids plus PUVA (RePUVA) therapy cleared widespread plaque-type psoriasis in a comparable time. However, RePUVA was significantly superior regarding the cumulative UVA dose required for clearance and the incidence of severe and early relapses.[52] Particularly in view of possible long-term side effects (immune suppression, skin carcinogenesis), the combination of PUVA plus cyclosporine cannot be recommended.

Retinoids The therapeutic efficacy of PUVA therapy is dramatically increased when combined with daily oral retinoid (etretinate, acitretin, isotretinoin; 1 mg/kg) administration 5 to 10 days before the initiation of PUVA and when this combined treatment is continued throughout the clearing phase.[53–55] RePUVA was reported to reduce the number of exposures by one-third and the total cumulative UVA dose by more than one-half. RePUVA was also shown to clear "poor PUVA responders" who could not be brought into complete remission by PUVA alone.[53,56]

The mechanism of the synergistic action of retinoids and PUVA is unknown but may be due to the accelerated desquamation that optimizes the optical properties of the skin and to the reduction of the inflammatory infiltrate. As an additional beneficial effect, etretinate and other retinoids may theoretically protect against long-term carcinogenic effects of PUVA mainly by reducing the number of exposures and by their potential canceroprotective effect. Short-term side effects of retinoids are completely reversible at discontinuation, and long-term toxicity is not a concern because the administration is limited to the clearing phase. The potential teratogenicity of retinoids represents a serious concern. In Europe, etretinate has been replaced by its active metabolite acitretin because it was believed that its elimination half-life was strikingly shorter than that of etretinate and that it was as effective as etretinate-PUVA.[56,57] Meanwhile, there is now evidence that acitretin is metabolized into etretinate that again accumulates in the body,[58,59] and therefore this substance does not represent an advantage over etretinate. For women of child-bearing age, the use of isotretinoin can be considered because contraception is necessary for only 2 months after discontinuation of therapy, in contrast to etretinate and acitretin, which require 2 years of contraception.

PUVA for Cutaneous T Cell Lymphoma (Mycosis Fungoides) (See Chap. 108)

In the early stages of cutaneous T cell lymphoma (CTCL) (stages IA, IB, IIA), conventional treatment strategy is characterized by topical therapy with increasing stage-dependent aggressiveness. This includes topical steroids, UV radiation, and topical cytotoxic substances such as nitrogen mustard. Later stages are treated with total-body electron beam radiation therapy, x-irradiation, and systemic polychemotherapy. However, there is no information available that clearly proves that any of these therapies leads to permanent remission. Based on the known beneficial effect of natural sunlight on early mycosis fungoides, several prospective studies evaluated the effect of photochemotherapy in this disease.

Since the first promising results with photochemotherapy in 1976[60,61] (Fig. 264-4), numerous investigators from both the United States and Europe have confirmed its efficacy.[62] Treatment schedules and dosimetry in photochemotherapy of CTCL are essentially the same as for psoriasis. The treatment consists of a clearing phase, a maintenance phase, and a follow-up phase without therapy. Remission should be confirmed by histologic examination of previously involved skin sites. The initial treatments are followed by maintenance consisting of two exposures per week for 1 month and one exposure per week for another month. If the patient is then still in remission, therapy is discontinued and the patient monitored monthly and later bimonthly. If a relapse occurs, the patient is again subjected to four PUVA exposures per week until complete clearing.

Several studies on larger patient cohorts have provided data on the rate of initial response to PUVA treatment in relation to the stage of CTCL.[62-65] It should be noted that different treatment protocols, psoralen preparations, and light sources were used in these studies, which may have contributed to the heterogeneity of the published results. Herrmann et al. summarized the treatment results from five of these studies, comprising a total of 244 patients, and calculated average complete initial response rates of 90 percent for stage IA, 76 percent for stage IB, 78 percent for stage IIA, 59 percent for stage IIB, and 61 percent for stage III.[66]

Relapses respond as well as the initial lesions when PUVA is resumed. Clinical remissions appear to be directly related to phototoxic destruction of the malignant infiltrate. Thus complete clearing may be induced when the cells are confined to the epidermis and the superficial dermis and do not exceed the depth of UVA penetration into the skin.

Patients with tumor-stage CTCL exhibit a high rate of early recurrences, which require a permanent maintenance treatment, and only the combination of PUVA with local x-ray treatment and/or systemic chemotherapy can result in complete tumor resolution.[63] There is no uniformly accepted protocol for treating CTCL. Most follow-up studies have demonstrated that the great majority of patients with early disease can be kept in remission with or without maintenance therapy for several years.[62,65,66] Tumor-stage patients (IIB) usually experience multiple recurrences despite aggressive combination therapies and eventually die within a few years.[63,66] Currently, no therapeutic regimen is known to arrest the eventual progression of CTCL to tumor formation, dissemination, and fatal outcome. While PUVA therapy is very effective in inducing remission as long as the lymphoma is confined to the skin, the influence of this therapy on the natural course of CTCL and on patient survival is not yet determined. However, data from Sweden show a significant drop in the death rate of patients since the introduction of PUVA.[67]

Present knowledge indicates that photochemotherapy may induce long-lasting disease-free intervals in CTCL if used in the early stages of the disease.[65,66] In later stages, PUVA may reduce the tumor cell burden and thus may act synergistically with other treatment. It improves the quality of life and may prolong survival when used in combination with more aggressive treatment modalities. Prolonged remissions were observed with combinations of PUVA with retinoids[68] and with interferon-α2a.[69,70] Successful treatment of the erythrodermic type (Sézary syndrome) has been reported with extracorporeal PUVA (photopheresis) (see below). Possible long-term hazards related to frequent PUVA treatments are probably meaningless for patients with CTCL, as compared to patients with benign conditions.

PUVA for Atopic Dermatitis
(See Chap. 124)

Many patients with atopic eczema can benefit from PUVA therapy.[71] The treatment guidelines are essentially the same as for psoriasis. However, the condition is more difficult to treat, and quite often a higher number of treatments are required to clear the eczema. Although the disease may be cleared by PUVA, there is a high and early recurrence rate, requiring frequent maintenance exposures. As the average patient is young, one should hesitate to initiate long-term maintenance therapy until the possible risks of such treatment are better understood. A combination of PUVA with topical glucocorticoids appears to be superior to PUVA alone in

FIGURE 264-4

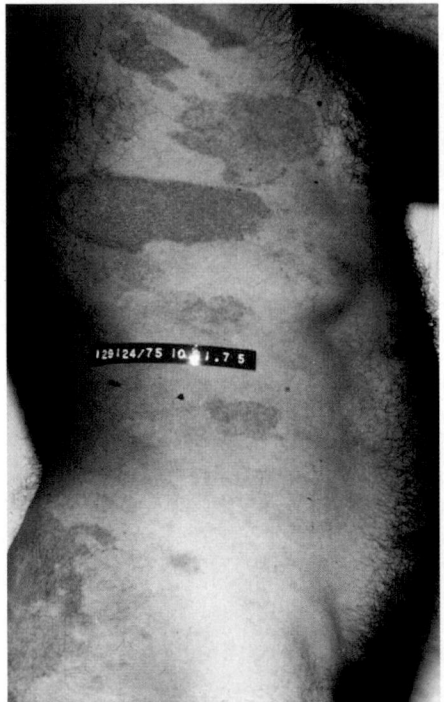
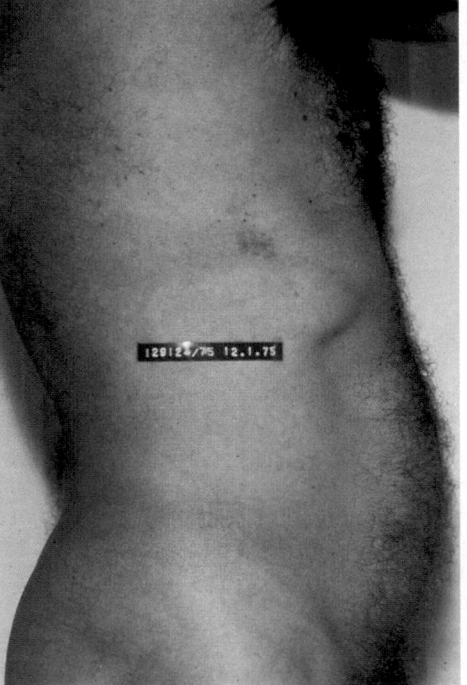

A.   *B.*

Forty-six-year-old patient with cutaneous T cell lymphoma (mycosis fungoides), stage IB. *A.* Before PUVA treatment. *B.* After treatment.

maintaining remissions. The mechanism of action of photochemotherapy in atopic eczema is unclear; current concepts support an alteration of lymphocyte function in the dermal infiltrate.

PUVA for Lichen Planus (See Chap. 50)

In generalized lichen planus, PUVA can provide an effective alternative to systemic glucocorticoid treatment. As indicated by two studies, lichen planus proves to be more resistant to PUVA than psoriasis when treated according to a similar schedule.[72,73] More exposures and higher cumulative UVA doses are required for clearing, and not all patients respond satisfactorily. An exacerbation during PUVA treatment has been reported in a few patients. In patients who have been cleared, relapses respond equally well when PUVA is resumed. Also bath-PUVA can clear lichen planus.[74] A combined PUVA-etretinate regimen may accelerate clearing.

PUVA for Urticaria Pigmentosa (See Chap. 62)

In urticaria pigmentosa (cutaneous mastocytosis), photochemotherapy leads to a temporary involution of skin lesions.[75,76] The treatment results in loss of Darier's sign, relief of itching, and flattening and even complete disappearance of cutaneous papules and macules. Surprisingly, even systemic symptoms such as histamine-induced migraine and flushing fade gradually as treatment is continued.[75] In most patients reported so far, the manifestations of the disease recurred several months after discontinuation of PUVA. The recurrences respond as well as the original lesions, and complete clearing of signs and symptoms can be induced again. Although the clinical response appears to be unequivocal, the mechanisms that lead to this response are a matter of debate. No significant change in either the mean mast cell counts or mast cell ultrastructure was found after clinical clearing of skin lesions,[76] and PUVA did not cause a significant alteration in the histamine content of the skin. Other investigations showed an inhibition of mast cell degranulation in vitro[77] and an increased turnover of mast cells in mouse skin.[78]

Despite this uncertainty concerning its mode of action, PUVA seems to be warranted in patients with urticaria pigmentosa where the disease is causing severe distress. Since the treatment of the cutaneous lesions of mastocytosis has been unrewarding with other modalities, the use of PUVA, though not curative, is at present the only therapy available to control the skin lesions in this condition.

PUVA for Miscellaneous Dermatoses

Both acute and chronic *pityriasis lichenoides*[72,79] respond to photochemotherapy, and favorable results have been reported for *lymphomatoid papulosis*.[72,80] The experience with these conditions is limited to a few anecdotal cases. In *pityriasis rubra pilaris*, the results are quite inconsistent. Some cases seem to respond well,[72] other may flare, and some require combination treatment with retinoid or methotrexate therapy. Generalized *granuloma annulare* has been reported to clear completely, but long-term maintenance treatment was required to maintain remissions.[81] Regrowth of hair was noted in *alopecia areata* with either topical or systemic PUVA exposures localized to the alopecia areas. There was a high variation in the number of treatments required for regrowth, and circumscribed lesions responded better than did total alopecia. Follow-up studies of larger patient groups concluded that PUVA is generally not an effective treatment for alopecia areata.[82,83] The authors' experience has also not been encouraging. *Localized scleroderma* and *pansclerotic morphea* have been successfully treated with bath-PUVA and oral PUVA.[84,85] An indication of increasing importance

may be acute and chronic *cutaneous graft-versus-host disease.* Several studies demonstrated the beneficial effects of PUVA in lichen planus–like eruption[86–89] in patients who had failed with conventional immunosuppressive therapy and even in acute graft-versus-host disease.[87,90] As nonexposed oral lesions also improved, a systemic effect is postulated.[88]

PUVA for Vitiligo (See Chap. 88)

As mentioned above, vitiligo was the first disease treated with an ancient form of psoralen photochemotherapy in folk medicine in India and Egypt. PUVA in its modern form stimulates melanogenesis, melanocyte proliferation and migration and reconstitutes the normal skin color in more than 50 percent of vitiligo patients.

TREATMENT PROTOCOLS AND RESULTS Oral 8-MOP or TMP is the photosensitizer most frequently used, followed by exposure to sunlight or artificial UVA radiation. From a large controlled clinical trial by the Harvard group, detailed information became available on different treatment schedules and efficacy of treatment.[91] Also 5-MOP has been studied in a large trial in India and is routinely used in Vienna with good success (Fig. 264-5).[92] To induce repigmentation, patients need constant long-term therapy (12 to 24 months). Because oral TMP is much less phototoxic than 8-MOP, it is preferred for treatment, with sunlight as the radiation source. Treatments should be given at least twice a week, but not more than three times, with at least 1 day between treatments. If there is no response after 6 months or approximately 50 treatments, PUVA should be terminated. *Responsiveness* is defined as the development of many perifollicular macules of repigmentation. If treatment is discontinued, reversal of acquired repigmentation may occur unless the lesion has completely repigmented. Completely repigmented areas can be stable for a decade or more without relapse.[93]

Another photochemotherapeutic regimen for vitiligo, using khellin (a furanochromone) as photosensitizer and UVA irradiation, was introduced some years ago. This substance does not lead to phototoxic erythema and exhibits a substantially lower mutagenic activity than psoralens. Its efficacy and failure rate in vitiligo treatment are comparable to those of PUVA.[94] The major advantage of khellin is that it does not induce phototoxic erythema and thus can be considered safe for home treatment or treatment with natural sunlight. The treatment schedule is the same as in psoralen photochemotherapy; khellin is administered orally at a dose of 100 mg 2 h before treatment or applied topically as a 5% cream. Khellin is not available in the United States.

Patient selection appears to be particularly important in vitiligo treatment. The patients should be age 12 or over and must be available for 12 to 24 months of continuous therapy. Lips, distal dorsal hands, tips of fingers and toes, areas of bony prominences, palms, soles, and nipples are very refractory to treatment, and patients with involvement limited to these areas should be excluded. Segmental vitiligo tends to show a variable response.

On average, a complete treatment course consists of at least 150 exposures. However, because of the different response in different body areas, total repigmentation is only rarely achieved, and some 30 percent of patients do not respond at all despite many months of therapy.

The mechanisms by which PUVA induces repigmentation in vitiligo skin remain mostly speculative. Bearing in mind the modulating effect of UV radiation on a number of immunologic reactions, one might postulate a hypothetical suppressor cell population gen-

FIGURE 264-5

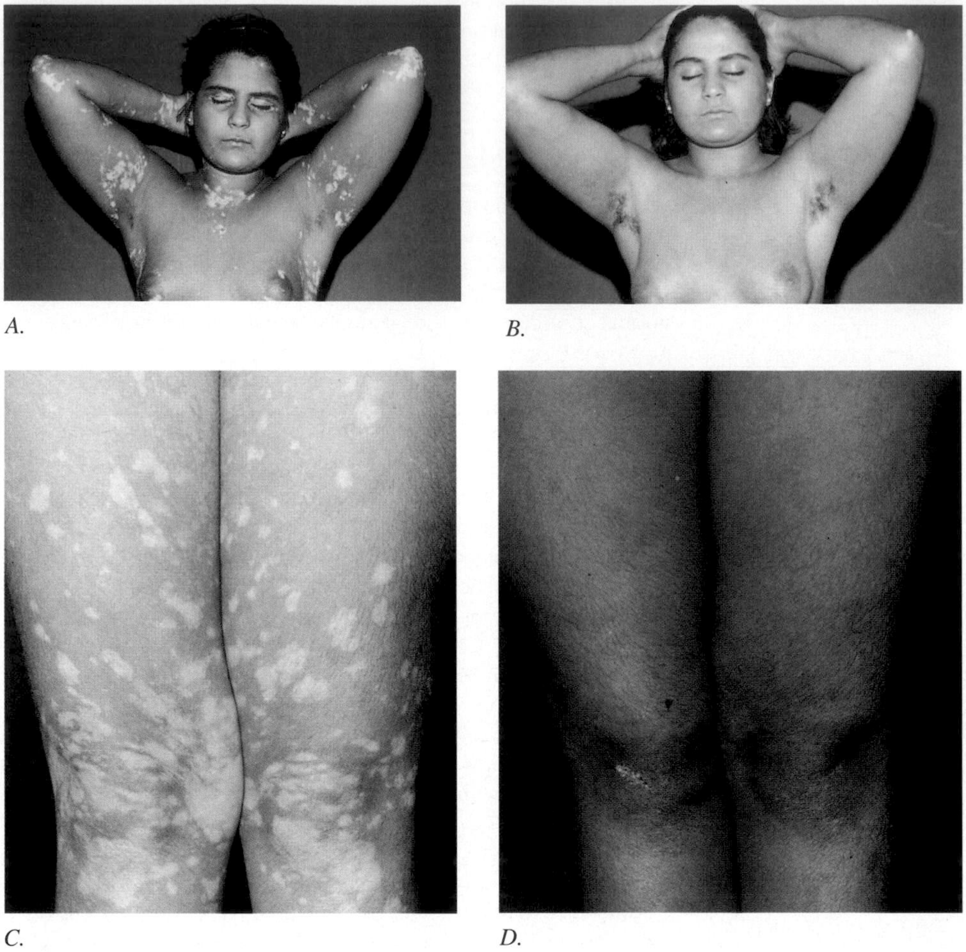

A.

B.

C.

D.

Twelve-year-old patient with generalized vitiligo of 4 years' duration. *A* and *C.* Before PUVA treatment. *B* and *D.* After treatment (8-MOP + artificial UVA) with thrice-weekly exposures for 10 months.

erated by PUVA that suppresses the stimulus for melanocyte destruction during therapy.

PUVA as Preventive Treatment for Photodermatoses

Tolerance to sunlight can be induced in several photodermatoses with PUVA. In *polymorphous light eruption*, the most common photodermatosis, PUVA is the most effective preventive treatment.[95–97] In about 70 percent of patients with this condition, a 3- to 4-week PUVA course of two to three treatments per week suffices to suppress the disease upon subsequent exposure to sunlight.[95] The initial exposure and dose increments during therapy should be performed according to the guidelines outlined above for psoriasis. PUVA has the advantage of a rapid and intense pigment induction at relatively low UVA doses that usually remain well below the threshold doses for eliciting the rash. About 10 percent of patients develop typical lesions during the initial phase of PUVA, but these usually disappear when treatment is continued. The authors' treatment schedule consists of three to four treatments per

week for 3 to 4 weeks in early spring; PUVA preventive treatment protects only temporarily, but regularly repeated sun exposures will maintain protection. However, a considerable number of patients remain protected for 2 to 3 months, even after pigmentation has faded.

The mechanisms by which phototherapy induces tolerance to sunlight are not completely clear. Hyperpigmentation and thickening of the stratum corneum may be important factors for the protective effect. However, other mechanisms may also be involved, since polymorphous light eruption does occur in dark-skinned individuals. In this context, modulations of cutaneous immune functions are being discussed, although there is presently no evidence to confirm the possible role of immune mechanisms.

There is also some experience with PUVA prophylaxis of other photodermatoses. In *solar urticaria*, PUVA therapy appears to be the most effective preventive treatment available and is certainly better than antihistamines. Tolerance to sunlight can be increased tenfold or more after a single treatment course.[96,98,99] The suppressive effect may last throughout the summer if the patients have regular sunlight exposures, which seem to be necessary to maintain tolerance. Problems may arise during the first PUVA exposures, since in some patients the urticaria threshold dose appears to be lower than their MPD. In these cases, careful conditioning by stepwise UVA irradiation of single quadrants of the body surface a few hours before each PUVA treatment have proved useful. Treatments with PUVA are then given during the refractory period.

Successful photochemotherapy has also been reported in some occasional cases of *chronic actinic dermatitis*[98,100] and *hydroa vacciniforme*.[101] Limited experience in patients with *erythropoietic protoporphyria* indicates that, with a very cautious approach and in combination with beta-carotene, PUVA may increase light tolerance considerably.[102,103]

Considerations about long-term hazards are important, especially in benign disorders such as the photodermatoses. However, extended treatment duration is usually not required in polymorphous light eruption, but in solar urticaria and chronic actinic dermatitis, prolonged therapy may be necessary. There exist no ready-to-use schedules for these latter conditions and PUVA is usually just one part of the management.

PUVA in HIV-Infected Patients

The use of phototherapy and photochemotherapy in HIV-infected patients with skin diseases has been a controversial issue. First, both therapies can induce systemic immune suppression and may modify the immune status of the patient in a way that would lead to a worsening of HIV disease.[104] Second, UV radiation as well as psoralen photosensitization were demonstrated to activate the HIV promoter, which could boost viral gene transcription and eventually virus production.[105] In addition, HIV-induced immune suppression could support an accelerated development of skin carcinomas in UVB- or PUVA-treated patients.[106] UVB has been used for psoriasis and proved efficient and safe in the short-term follow-up and has not resulted in worsening of HIV disease or increased complication rates.[107] UVB has also been shown to be very effective in alleviating severe pruritus in patients infected with HIV.[108] With oral PUVA, treatment of psoriasis did not induce progression of HIV disease or an increase in side effects.[109,110] It was concluded from these studies that UVB phototherapy and PUVA may be safe for HIV-positive patients with psoriasis. Theoretical modeling of the UVB- and PUVA-induced HIV promoter activation in human skin indicated that UVB is more likely than PUVA to activate viral transcription in vivo.[111] Data from long-term observations are currently awaited. Thus it is presently impossible to advocate the use of PUVA in (HIV-)immunosuppressed individuals in general, but major hazards are unlikely. The available data and theoretical considerations indicate that UVB is more likely to be a hazard than PUVA in the treatment of an HIV-infected population.[111,112]

Side Effects and Toxicity of PUVA

ACUTE SIDE EFFECTS   The side effects of PUVA include drug intolerance reactions as well as side effects of the combined action of psoralens plus UVA radiation. Oral 8-MOP (0.6 to 0.8 mg/kg) has a high incidence of nausea (30 percent of patients) and vomiting (10 percent of patients), and this may occasionally require discontinuation of the treatment. These side effects are more common with liquid preparations than with crystalline preparations, probably because of higher psoralen serum levels. With 5-MOP, nausea is almost absent, even with doses of up to 1.8 mg/kg body weight.[22] Undesired acute effects of the combined action of psoralens and UVA can range from an increased delayed erythema reaction to severe burns with blistering. Such overdosage phenomena are more common after topical psoralen application because of the high epidermal psoralen concentration. Accumulation of phototoxic effects after several subsequent UVA exposures is also more common with topical PUVA. Some patients experience a persistent pruritus during PUVA treatment, particularly after slight UVA overdosage, and in rare cases a stinging pain may develop in circumscribed areas. The mechanism is unknown, and the symptoms are unresponsive to antihistamines. These complaints usually subside upon continuation of treatment. Overdosage phenomena occur mostly in body areas not usually exposed to natural sunlight. Careful observation of the criteria for dosimetry can minimize these side effects to acceptable levels. The danger of overdosage is much less with 5-MOP.[22]

Very rare side effects of PUVA include polymorphous light eruption–like rashes, acne-like eruptions, subungual hemorrhages due to phototoxic reactions of the nail beds, and occasional hypertrichosis of the face. These are transient and disappear when treatment is discontinued. Single case reports include exacerbation of systemic lupus erythematosus and bullous pemphigoid during photochemotherapy.

LABORATORY DATA   Analysis of laboratory data in several large-scale studies showed no significant abnormal findings in patients receiving PUVA over prolonged periods of time.[36,38,113] Because psoralens can produce liver damage in laboratory animals when given in excessive doses, concern has been expressed in the past about possible hepatotoxic effects in humans. However, serial laboratory examinations performed over a period of several years have not revealed any substantial evidence for an impairment of

hepatic function.[49] Liver biopsies after 1 year of therapy did not reveal signs of hepatotoxicity.[114] Anecdotal case reports of hepatitis during PUVA treatment almost certainly were unrelated to therapy. A slight increase in BUN and creatinine was documented in one series but was considered insignificant; otherwise, no evidence exists suggesting impairment of renal function.[36] Several large-scale studies have negated a possible relation between PUVA therapy and the occurrence of antinuclear antibodies.[115]

POTENTIAL LONG-TERM RISKS OF PUVA   *Chronic actinic damage*   Repeated phototoxic injury to the skin can be expected to result in cumulative actinic damage regardless of whether it is induced by sunlight, artificial UV radiation, or PUVA. Although the precise action spectrum of actinic damage has not been determined, epidermal changes are attributed to UVB and dermal changes to UVA because the latter penetrates more deeply into the skin. Chronic exposure to PUVA may thus produce changes in the skin that resemble photoaging and that may add to the injury induced by sunlight.

PUVA lentigines and generalized PUVA lentiginosis result from repeated and prolonged treatment and are commonly associated with high cumulative doses of UVA and a large number of treatments. They exhibit irregular borders and show uneven pigmentation. So far, no increased risk of cutaneous melanoma associated with these lentigines has been recorded, but the cosmetic effect may be quite disturbing.

Carcinogenesis   Cutaneous carcinogenicity is the major concern about long-term and repeated PUVA treatment associated with high cumulative UVA doses. In laboratory animals, 8-MOP and 5-MOP have been unequivocally shown to induce skin cancer at levels of drug and UVA irradiation comparable to those used in PUVA therapy.[116,117] Obviously the risk is related to DNA damage, but PUVA-induced downregulation of immune responses may play an additional role. Although animal studies provide important evidence for the carcinogenic potential, in the human situation this risk has to be assessed against the potential therapeutic benefit.

All long-term follow-up studies suffer from the fact that patients are likely to have been exposed previously to other carcinogenic treatments such as ionizing radiation, UVB therapy methotrexate, tar, or arsenic. Correct adjustment for all these factors may be quite problematic, particularly because accurate data are often missing.

The first report that provided evidence for the carcinogenic potential of PUVA in treated patients came from the U.S. 16-Center Cooperative Study that is still ongoing.[118] Since this original report, other follow-up studies of the same patient cohort and studies of other U.S. and European investigators have appeared with controversial findings.[119–125] Except for the 16-Center Study, in which the number of treatments is used as parameter, most studies relate carcinoma formation to the cumulative UVA dose, and the existing data show a strong relationship between cancer risk and UVA dose.[126–129] Whereas earlier data indicated an increased risk for basal cell carcinomas (BCC) and squamous cell carcinomas (SCC), more recent findings identified such risk for SCC only.[51,122,125,130]

In several European reports and in one Japanese study, no increased risk for SCC was observed unless the patients had previously received other potentially carcinogenic treatments,[119,121,123,124,130] and uncertainty remains about the magnitude of the contribution of PUVA. The discrepancy between these studies and those of the 16-Center trial has not yet been resolved. Besides other factors, such as ethnic background, skin type, solar exposure, and other treatments, it was speculated that differences in the treatment protocol, which was more aggressive in Europe, could be responsible for the discrepancy.[131] In mouse experiments it has been shown that few but large phototoxic doses are less harmful than frequent small doses, and the question remains whether an aggressive regimen with rest periods is safer than continuous non-aggressive therapy.

However, in the study of Bruynzeel et al.,[125] in which patients with limited exposure to previous risk factors had been treated with the European protocol with higher single doses than in the United States, there was a significant relationship between cumulative UVA dose and SCC incidence. Another European study from Sweden comprising 4799 patients reported an increased risk of SCC, but these patients had been treated in different institutions with quite different protocols.[127] Further evaluation of the various European cohorts is clearly needed to clarify this issue.

In any case, it is wise to keep the cumulative dosages low, and therefore UVA-sparing aggressive regimens without prolonged maintenance therapy appear to be safer than continuous nonaggressive regimens.[131]

An important issue may be therapeutic sun exposure that is common in patients with psoriasis. Bruynzeel et al. noted a trend for nonmelanoma skin tumors on non-sun-exposed areas, but the majority of tumors were on sun-exposed sites. Stern and Laird[51] reported that the incidence of SCC, but not basal cell carcinoma, in usually non-sun-exposed areas was related to a high number of PUVA treatments. However, this does not take into account that psoriasis patients may have a different sun-exposure pattern than others.

Male genitalia (penis, scrotum) appeared to be particularly susceptible to carcinogenic stimuli of long-term PUVA in patients (of the 16-Center Study) previously treated with tar and UVB,[132] but the risk was not increased if only PUVA was used, as revealed in an uncontrolled survey in 11 European institutions.[133] This alarming observation has so far not been documented elsewhere, except for isolated case reports. Further information is clearly required to define the true risk of such tumors.

Carcinogenicity of 5-MOP in PUVA-treated patients is unknown, but 5-MOP has shown a similar activity to 8-MOP in photocarcinogenicity studies in mice.[117,134]

Most studies were performed in patients treated with oral PUVA. Lindelöf et al.[135] compared 572 bath-PUVA patients (observation period >8 years) from one center with 2378 oral PUVA patients from three centers (observation period 6 years). The results showed an enhanced risk of SCC with oral PUVA but no increased risk with bath-PUVA. Similar data came from Hannuksela et al.,[136] who evaluated 527 patients treated with TMP bath-PUVA. However, bath-PUVA results in a much higher epidermal psoralen concentration than with oral PUVA, and the lower UVA dose needed to produce a therapeutic effect may induce an equal or even higher number of mutagenic DNA lesions. Therefore, the reported long-term safety of bath-PUVA may be encouraging, but no premature conclusions should be drawn.

Melanoma Only a few anecdotal cases of malignant melanoma have been observed in long-term PUVA-treated psoriatic patients,[137] and no increased risk of melanoma has been found in all large-scale studies reported so far. However, Stern et al.[138] recently reported 11 melanomas in 9 patients from the cohort of 1380 patients enrolled in the PUVA Follow-up Study (16-Center Study). The authors conclude that about 15 years after the first treatment, the risk increases, particularly in patients with more than 250 treatments. Only four melanomas were observed between 1975 and 1990, and this number equaled the expected incidence (relative risk, 1.1). In the same cohort, seven melanomas were detected from 1991 to 1996 (relative risk, 5.4). This increased incidence is alarming, especially considering the long latency period, which suggests that more cases are to be expected in the future. Also the risk seemed to persist after discontinuation of PUVA. Since there are no data available on dosimetry, it is unclear whether melanomas are associated with a certain cumulative UVA dose or with episodes of phototoxic burns. Moreover, no information is given on other co-carcinogenic factors, on the clinical type of melanoma, and, most importantly, on the patients' history (dysplastic nevi, family history of melanoma). One of the nine patients had three melanomas. If he had familial melanoma or dysplastic nevus syndrome and could be excluded from the cohort, there would be no significant increase in the risk. Despite this lack of important information, this report needs to be taken seriously and emphasizes that the guidelines for PUVA treatment must be rigidly observed. Patients with long-term PUVA must receive life-time monitoring.[139]

Immunologic effects Effects on immunocompetent cells may contribute to the therapeutic efficacy for psoriasis. In PUVA-treated psoriatic skin, the numbers of epidermal and dermal CD3+ T lymphocytes, as well as CD4+, CD8+, and interleukin (IL)2 receptor–positive subsets, are considerably reduced,[140,141] as is HLA-DR expression by epidermal keratinocytes. Langerhans cells do not disappear after PUVA[141] but show a reduction of the expression of immunohistochemical markers.[142,143] Remission of psoriasis seems to be independent of the magnitude of this effect.[144] PUVA treatment reduces lymphocyte responsiveness to mitogen and interleukin stimulation.[145] The ability to alter circulating lymphocytes functionally possibly forms the basis of action in photopheresis. Topical PUVA alters cutaneous lymphocytes in lesional and normal skin of psoriatic patients.[141]

PUVA reverses the pathologic increase in insulin-like growth factor 1 receptors in psoriatic skin, whereas the number of epidermal growth factor receptors, which are increased in psoriasis and can be blocked by psoralens, remains unchanged.[141] PUVA does not affect the total concentration of urocanic acid in psoriatic skin but induces a transient increase in the percentage of the *cis* isomer, which returns to normal 4 weeks after the last treatment.[146] A decrease in the total number of circulating T cells, suppressor T cells, and helper T cells has been reported, but other investigations have challenged these results.[146] Peripheral blood mononuclear cells obtained from psoriatic patients before the start and after completion of PUVA therapy showed an inhibition of the production and release of IL-1β, IL-6, IL-8, and tumor necrosis factor α.[147] PUVA has no measurable effect on complement components and immunoglobulin levels of psoriatic patients.[146]

No substantial adverse reactions have been observed that could be ascribed to altered lymphocyte or leukocyte function in patients during or after photochemotherapy. Besides an increased incidence of recurrent herpes simplex, there is no evidence for an increased risk of bacterial viral or fungal infections in these patients.

The clinical significance of these immunologic effects is unknown, but they suggest that PUVA may suppress immunologic surveillance not only locally in the skin but also systemically. The therapeutic success in some responsive diseases may thus be based on immunosuppression.

Ophthalmologic effects Evidence for the potential ocular toxicity associated with oral PUVA therapy is based mainly on experimental studies. Several studies have determined the effects of photochemotherapy on the human eye, with the result that there is no indication that psoralen-induced cataracts occur in patients undergoing long-term photochemotherapy. The majority of prospective studies did not report an increased incidence of lens opacities in patients who used eye protection following psoralen ingestion.[148] Because some uncertainty remains about the actual risk of eye toxicity, it is recommended that appropriate UVA-opaque spectacles be worn during the entire period of increased photosensitivity after psoralen ingestion. Obviously there is no risk with topical or bath-PUVA.

Patient Selection and Contraindications

In view of the potential long-term hazards, the assignment of patients to photochemotherapy should be based on consideration of the risks and the benefit for the individual patient. If only a short-term course of therapy is planned, as, for example, in prevention of photodermatoses, the benefit outweighs the risk. In the treatment of a malignant condition such as CTCL, long-term risks may be meaningless because other treatment options bear the risk of even greater long-term toxicity. The major concerns relate to long-term treatment of psoriasis because this condition represents by far the most common indication for PUVA. As long as the risks of long-term use are not clearly known, careful patient selection appears to be mandatory. "Guidelines of Care" have been published by the American Academy of Dermatology.[37]

Photochemotherapy should not be used during pregnancy, and women should be advised to use contraceptive measures while on PUVA. This precaution is only for reasons of safety as there exists no evidence that either 8-MOP alone or photochemotherapy is teratogenic. This has been confirmed in a retrospective study in 256 deliveries among the cohort of the 16-Center PUVA Follow-Up Study.[149] However, it has to be emphasized that RePUVA bears the risk of teratogenicity.

Severe impairment of hepatic and renal functions is usually considered a contraindication to PUVA because metabolism and excretion of psoralens may be inadequate. PUVA is also contraindicated in patients with known light-aggravated or light-induced diseases such as lupus erythematosus, porphyria (as mentioned above, light tolerance can be induced by PUVA in erythropoietic protoporphyria), and xeroderma pigmentosum. Pemphigus and bullous pemphigoid may be exacerbated by PUVA. Patients with chronic actinic damage and a history of skin cancers may be at higher risk for the development of new cancers. Previous arsenic intake and previous treatment with ionizing radiation also seem to increase the risk of nonmelanoma skin cancers. Immunosuppressed patients should probably not receive PUVA, although this is not yet clearly defined. As outlined above, PUVA can be used in HIV-positive patients. Cataracts and aphakia are not real contraindications if adequate eye protection is guaranteed.

Conclusions and Perspectives

Photochemotherapy is highly effective treatment for several dermatologic diseases, but it does not lead to permanent cure in most conditions. An exception may be vitiligo, in which PUVA-induced repigmentation may last for many years or even a lifetime. Although there exists comprehensive clinical experience documenting PUVA's short-term safety when used according to standardized methods, as outlined in this chapter, the risk of potential long-term sequelae has still not been clearly determined. Thus, strategies for treatment should take into account whether other forms of therapy are available that carry a lower risk but are equally effective. Risk-versus-benefit decisions should weigh potential long-term hazards against severity and morbidity of the disease and therefore will vary with the disease being treated. In early stages of mycosis fungoides, the risk-versus-benefit ratio will clearly be in favor of PUVA as an

alternative for other treatment options. For polymorphous light eruption, the number of treatments each year necessary to provide relief of discomfort is so small that long-term risks may be negligible. The major concern relates to the treatment of severe psoriasis, as this is the most common indication for PUVA that may require repeated long-term therapy. In many patients with disabling psoriasis, PUVA is more effective than topical therapy, the Goeckerman regimen, or UVB therapy not only in clearing of disease but also in maintaining remission. Regarding chronic toxicity, PUVA appears to be a most valuable alternative to methotrexate and other antimetabolites. Treatment with broadband and narrowband UVB also causes actinic skin changes, alterations of the immune system, and skin carcinomas; and apart from the fact that UVB is not equally effective in all forms of psoriasis, there is no convincing evidence at present that it may be safer than PUVA for long-term use.

Severe widespread psoriasis is a devastating disease that may result in disruption of professional, social, and private life. After almost 25 years of experience with PUVA for the treatment of psoriasis, it has become evident that this therapy offers innumerable patients the chance to resume a normal life. However, in view of the potential risks, careful patient selection should be undertaken before treatment is begun, and the treatment should be limited to those patients with severe recalcitrant psoriasis who can be monitored and thoroughly controlled by an informed, adequately trained, and concerned physician. For disabling psoriasis the choice of therapies lies not between risk and safety but among alternative choices of action (methotrexate, cyclosporine, and UVB), none of which is absolutely safe.

EXTRACORPOREAL PHOTOCHEMOTHERAPY (PHOTOPHERESIS)

In 1987, a new therapeutic approach termed *extracorporeal photopheresis* (ECP), consisting of extracorporeal irradiation of blood fractions in the presence of 8-MOP, was presented for the treatment of erythrodermic CTCL.[150] The initial success in controlling intractable forms of CTCL with minimal side effects and discomfort to the patient was confirmed by subsequent clinical trials, and ECP is now considered a valuable treatment alternative for erythrodermic lymphoma.[151–155]

Based on currently available information, ECP appears to have a very low side-effect and toxicity profile, and this has led to the evaluation of ECP for other indications. The rationale for the additional treatment spectrum was supported by a number of experimental studies evaluating the effect of ECP on the immune system.[156–162] Under the assumption that ECP can suppress pathogenically relevant T cell clones, a number of studies have been performed in order to evaluate the efficacy of ECP in inflammatory diseases other than CTCL where autoreactive T cells may play a causative role. Initial studies have been performed in systemic sclerosis, pemphigus vulgaris, rheumatoid arthritis, and, to a lesser extent, in psoriatic arthritis, systemic lupus erythematosus, dermatomyositis, and atopic dermatitis. Based on recent investigations, it is speculated that ECP may also be valuable in the treatment of acute and chronic organ graft rejection as well as graft-versus-host disease after bone marrow transplantation.

Treatment Method

The procedure involves passage of blood fractions, containing 8-MOP previously ingested by the patient so as to obtain maximum plasma concentrations at the time the procedure is initiated (minimum: 50 μg/mL at 2 h), from one arm vein through a photopheresis machine and back. In the machine, subsequent separation of plasma and the white blood cell fraction (buffy coat, peripheral blood mononuclear cells) from the red cell fraction of nonnucleated cells takes place. The latter is returned to the patient without further treatment. The heparinized 8-MOP–containing plasma and buffy coat fraction is subsequently treated as it flows through a UVA exposure system before it is returned to the patient through another arm vein. In this fashion, 8-MOP can be photoactivated in the bloodstream to cause clinical and immunologic effects on circulating lymphocytes while sparing other body tissues.

Due to problems in obtaining consistently reproducible psoralen levels in the fraction to be irradiated, future treatment units will use extracorporeally administrable 8-MOP. As shown by Knobler et al.,[163] this is a modification that eliminates the known side effects of oral 8-MOP administration and the need for drug-level monitoring. Depending on the various protocols still under evaluation, this treatment is, on average, repeated on two successive days at 3- to 4-week intervals.

The Photopheresis Instrument

The instrument used for the first multicenter international clinical trial integrated an initial discontinuous leuka/plasmapheresis step with subsequent UV exposure in a single unit. After oral administration of 8-MOP, heparinized blood is leukapheresed in six cycles through a continually spinning centrifuge bowl. This permits removal of 240 mL of leukocyte-enriched blood, which is pooled with 300 mL of plasma obtained during the same procedure and 200 mL of sterile normal saline. To activate the 8-MOP, the total volume of 740 mL is then circulated through a sterile cassette and exposed to UVA for a predetermined period. Following exposure to UVA where the average lymphocyte is exposed to approximately 2 J/cm^2, the entire volume is returned to the patient.

With the model (UVAR) currently in use, it is also possible to administer the drug 8-MOP extracorporeally into a collection bag where cells and plasma recirculate during radiation. This has the advantage that psoralen levels can be controlled, and one can achieve predetermined levels to maximize efficacy and reproducibility.[163]

Treatment Results

CUTANEOUS T CELL LYMPHOMA Erythrodermic CTCL (Sézary syndrome) was the first disease for which ECP was evaluated. Its efficacy, confirmed in several clinical studies, led to approval by the U.S. Food and Drug Administration for use of ECP for the palliative treatment of this lymphoma type. In the original study by Edelson et al.,[150] 27 of 37 patients responded with either a partial or a complete remission. In a follow-up study in which ECP was compared to historic controls, ECP appeared to increase survival from a median of 30 months to over 66 months.[153] Subsequent reports confirmed the initially observed efficacy.[152,155,164–166] These studies report a gross response rate in up to 75 percent of the patients, with complete remissions in up to 25 percent and no response in 25 percent. Based on clinical, immunologic, and laboratory data,

the attempt was made to refine the criteria needed to select those patients more likely to respond to ECP. A normal CD4/CD8 ratio, a normal absolute count of CD8-positive cells in the peripheral blood, and short disease duration appear to be predictors of satisfactory therapeutic response.[154,155] Since a subpopulation of Sézary syndrome patients does not respond sufficiently to ECP, studies are currently evaluating possible synergistic effects with other treatments, such as interferon-α and methotrexate.[167]

PEMPHIGUS VULGARIS The first positive treatment results were summarized by Rook et al.,[168] who reported on a therapeutic response in three out of four patients with drug-resistant pemphigus vulgaris. Prolonged remission with concomitant substantial reduction in glucocorticoid and immunosuppressive therapy was obtained. At present, six cases have been treated with ECP with encouraging results.[169,170] Controlled randomized trials in selected therapy-resistant cases are indicated.

PROGRESSIVE SYSTEMIC SCLEROSIS Early T lymphocyte infiltration of affected organs as well as the presence of autoreactive antibodies support the autoimmune concept of progressive systemic sclerosis (PSS), indicating that photopheresis may be useful in PSS. Following a pilot study in two patients with rapidly progressive disease refractory to therapy,[171] a single-blinded, randomized eight-center trial was conducted comparing photopheresis to D-penicillamine. Seventy-nine patients with systemic sclerosis of recent onset (mean symptom duration, 1.8 years) and documented progressive cutaneous involvement 6 months before the study entered this 10-month trial.[172] Following 6 months of treatment, ECP was shown to be superior to increasing doses of D-penicillamine, both in reversing skin changes as well as stopping progression of skin involvement. There was no significant difference between ECP and D-penicillamine at the 10-month evaluation point. All patients on ECP completed the study, while 25 percent of the patients on D-penicillamine had to be dropped due to significant side effects and progression of disease. Thus, ECP may have a beneficial effect at least on the cutaneous manifestations of PSS.[173] A number of trials are presently being performed to determine the potential efficacy and indications for the treatment of PSS.[172,174]

RHEUMATOID ARTHRITIS In an uncontrolled pilot study of seven patients with rheumatoid arthritis resistant to conventional therapy, improvement was noted in four patients after 4 months of treatment. This was taken as evidence that it may be unlikely to represent a placebo effect, not uncommon in patients with this disease.[175] The observation that all patients who did respond experienced a relapse several months after discontinuation of ECP could support this assumption, suggesting that ECP may be of short-term benefit in selected patients with rheumatoid arthritis as it has less toxicity than the drugs currently used for this disease.

TRANSPLANTATION AND GRAFT-VERSUS-HOST DISEASE ECP may prove to be important in organ transplantation. Small clinical trials have demonstrated that ECP can be a valuable adjunct in the control and prevention of heart transplant rejection, with or without immunosuppressive therapy.[176–180] ECP was shown to decrease cardiac rejection episodes significantly without increasing the incidence of infections.[180] Likewise, beneficial effects have been reported in anecdotal studies on patients with other organ transplants[181–184] and graft-versus-host disease, suggesting that ECP may have a possible role in transplantation medicine.[185–187]

SYSTEMIC LUPUS ERYTHEMATOSUS Ten patients who met the criteria of the American Rheumatism Association for lupus erythematosus were treated with ECP.[188] For the purpose of this pilot study the only patients included were those whose systemic involvement was not life-threatening, who had mild to moderate disease adequately controlled with conventional treatment, and who experienced repeat consecutive flares of disease activity upon attempted reduction and/or elimination of medication. In this uncontrolled study, response to treatment was significant in seven of eight patients completing the trial. The clinical activity score decreased from a median of 7 (range 1 to 9) to a median of 1 (range 0 to 5) ($p < .05$), but the laboratory abnormalities did not change significantly. Clinical improvement of arthritis and cutaneous manifestations was noted. It may be interesting that ECP can be used in patients with known photosensitivity without inducing an exacerbation.

Perspectives

Extracorporeal photochemotherapy was originally conceived for the treatment of CTLC, but there are suggestions that this treatment modality may have beneficial effects in a number of other conditions. However, the data available so far are based on uncontrolled studies. A better understanding of the mechanisms of action is desirable.

PHOTODYNAMIC THERAPY

Photodynamic therapy (PDT) aims to destroy the desired target selectively and thus avoid or minimize damage to vital structures. The photodynamic reaction consists of the excitation of photosensitizers (mainly porphyrins) by visible light in the presence of oxygen, resulting in the generation of reactive oxygen species, particularly singlet oxygen. These reactive oxygen species mediate cellular and vascular effects depending on the tissue localization of the photosensitizer. This results in a direct or indirect cytotoxic effect on the target cell.[189] In dermatology, PDT has been used effectively for precancerous and malignant conditions such as actinic keratosis, BCC, Bowen's disease, and superficial SCC but also for inflammatory dermatoses such as psoriasis.

Historic Aspects

In 1904 von Tappeiner coined the term *photodynamic therapy* for the oxygen-dependent destruction of tissue after photosensitization and subsequent irradiation with visible light.[190] Together with Jesionek, a dermatologist, he treated human skin tumors effectively by applying a 5% solution of eosin dye followed by exposure to lamps or sunlight.[191] The first report on successful PDT in psoriasis with oral and intramuscular porphyrin administration appeared in 1937.[192] Systemic PDT with intravenous hematoporphyrin derivative (HpD) of human and animal tumors was originally investigated by Auler and Banzer.[193] The photodynamic properties of this group of substances were defined later.[194] The major breakthrough came with the first systematic study on human tumors with intravenous HpD in 1978.[195] Systemic administration of HpD and subsequent laser irradiation became the standard of PDT because these substances showed a relatively selective accumulation in different tumor tissues and thus led to selective cell destruction. Although PDT is still considered an investigational treatment, it has found its way into the treatment of a variety of internal malignancies and some skin conditions. The main disadvantage of systemic PDT is prolonged cutaneous photosensitivity that may last for several weeks after one single treatment.[196] PDT-treated patients are thus at risk

of severe accidental phototoxic reactions. To avoid generalized photosensitivity, the interest has now focused on the topical application of sensitizers or on the local induction of endogenous porphyrin synthesis in the target tissue.

Principles of Photodynamic Therapy

PHOTOSENSITIZERS The ideal photosensitizer for PDT in dermatology should meet the following criteria: (1) chemical purity, (2) high singlet-oxygen quantum yield, (3) significant light absorption at wavelengths that penetrate the skin sufficiently deeply, (4) high tissue selectivity, and (5) efficacy after topical application.

The only commercially available substance, Photofrin, is a mixture of several HpD ethers and esters. It has a low selectivity to skin tumors and leads to long-lasting photosensitivity; it is thus not ideal for dermatologic use. In contrast, "endogenous" sensitizers such as 5-aminolevulinic acid (ALA), a metabolite of heme biosynthesis, induce the synthesis of the actual photosensitizer (protoporphyrin IX) in the target tissue[197,198] (see Table 264-5 for sensitizers currently under clinical investigation). In this case the concentration of the photosensitizer depends on the metabolic status of the diseased tissue.

Most of the photosensitizers generate singlet oxygen with a quantum yield between 5 and 20%.[199] A high quantum yield means that less sensitizer is required in the target tissue to induce sufficient PDT effects. The absorption maxima of the current sensitizers range from 600 to 700 nm. In this range, light penetration in tissue is only up to 3 mm, limiting PDT to superficial tumors unless interstitial light propagation is used. A high selectivity for sensitizer accumulation in target tissue is necessary to avoid damage to surrounding normal tissue, and this is particularly important when larger areas are treated (e.g., actinic keratoses). So far, only ALA shows reasonably high selectivity after topical application. The ratio of porphyrin induction in skin tumors to the surrounding tissue is higher than 10:1.[200] The reason for this selectivity is unknown.

LIGHT SOURCES AND DOSIMETRY Light penetration into skin increases with longer wavelengths ($\lambda \leq 1100$ nm).[201] To match the absorption maxima of porphyrin-based photosensitizers, wavelengths around 630 nm are necessary. Therefore argon-pumped dye lasers ($\lambda = 630$ nm) or gold vapor lasers ($\lambda = 628$ nm) represent appropriate irradiation sources. However, these laser systems are quite expensive and require regular maintenance. In the near future, laser diodes that are smaller, more powerful, and less expensive will replace these sources. In contrast to other disciplines, dermatologic applications need no fiberoptics for endoscopic treatment and thus simpler incoherent light sources represent a valuable alternative. With regard to therapeutic results, there is no difference between coherent and incoherent light. Slide projectors, equipped with red filters, are frequently used. New lamps are now commercially available with appropriate red light emission designed for treatment of large surface areas. A standardized light dosimetry for PDT does not exist. Dosimetry depends on the photosensitizer used and on the condition to be treated. For PDT of skin tumors and actinic keratoses, light doses of 100 to 150 J/cm^2 are necessary. With current incoherent light sources, the treatment duration is about 20 to 30 min. For treating inflammatory dermatoses (psoriasis), lower doses will suffice because the goal appears not to be tissue destruction but rather sublethal cell damage or perhaps immunomodulation.

TABLE 264-5

Examples of Photosensitizers Presently Under Clinical Investigation for Photodynamic Therapy

COMPANY	PHOTOSENSITIZER	WAVELENGTH FOR PDT, NM	INDICATIONS	ROUTE OF ADMINISTRATION	STATUS
QLT Photo-Therapeutics/Sanofi Winthrop, Ipsen-Bio-tech (USA, Europe)	Porfimer sodium Photofrin	630	Approved for bladder, esophagus, lung cancer Studies for basal cell carcinoma (BCC), cutaneous metastases	IV	Approved in Canada, USA, Japan, Europe
Miravant (USA)	Tin ethyl etiopurpurin (SnET$_2$, Purlytin)	660–665	Cutaneous metastases, Kaposi's sarcoma, macular degeneration	IV, lipid emulsion	Phase II/III
DUSA (USA)	5-Aminolevulinic acid (ALA, Levulan)	635	Actinic keratoses, BCC, cutaneous T cell lymphoma, psoriasis, permanent hair removal	Topical	Phase I–III
Pharmacyclics (USA)	Lutetium texaphyrin PCI-0123 (Lu-Tex)	720–760	Skin cancer	IV	Phase II
Cytopharm Inc. (USA)	9-Acetoxy-2,7,12,17-tetrakis-(β-methoxy-ethyl)-porphycen (ATMPn)	640	Psoriasis	Topical	Phase II
QLT Photo-Therapeutics (Canada)	Benzoporphyrin derivative monoacid ring A (BPD-MA, Verteporfin)	690	BCC, psoriasis, macular degeneration	IV, liposomal formulation	Phase II
Scotia Pharmaceuticals (UK)	Meso-tetra-hydroxy-phenylchlorin (m-THPC, Foscan)	650	BCC, head and neck cancer	IV, topical	Phase I/II
Nippon Petrochemical (Japan)	Mono-L-aspartyl-chlorin e6 (NPe6)	660–665	Skin cancer	IV	Phase I

NOTE: This table is not meant to include all photosensitizers currently under study. The brand names were included because they were reported in published literature or electronic media (Internet).

MECHANISM OF ACTION   PDT-induced effects are mediated by photooxidative reactions. During irradiation, the photosensitizer is absorbing light (energy) and is converted to an excited (triplet) state. The energy can then be transferred to molecular oxygen (type II photooxidative reaction), resulting in the generation of reactive oxygen species, mainly singlet oxygen.[202,203] The biologic effects can be divided into primary cellular and secondary vascular damage. With HpD, early visible damage consists of cell membrane defects as a consequence of lipid peroxidation with consecutive cell lysis. Depending on the intracellular localization of the photosensitizers, damage to subcellular structures such as mitochondria,[204] lysosomes,[205] or endoplasmic reticulum[206] also occurs, whereas DNA is not a primary target.[207] Besides these direct effects, which probably play a key role in topical PDT, vascular effects after systemic application of photosensitizers appear to be the decisive event for the treatment of solid tumors. These effects consist of vasoconstriction, blood stasis, and thrombosis of tumor vessels leading to tumor ischemia and subsequent necrosis.[208–210]

PDT in Dermatology

Potential indications for PDT are listed in Table 264-6. In contrast to other organs, the skin can be sensitized by either intravenous administration or direct topical or intralesional application of the sensitizers.

SYSTEMIC PHOTODYNAMIC THERAPY   So far, HpD and porfimer sodium are the best-studied sensitizers. PDT following systemic application of these dyes has been performed in both skin cancers and inflammatory dermatoses. However, the treatment pro-

TABLE 264-6

Potential Indications for Photodynamic Therapy

Oncologic
  Actinic keratosis
  Bowen's disease
  Superficial basal cell carcinomas (BCC)
  Nevoid BCC syndrome
  Keratoacanthoma
  Superficial squamous cell carcinoma
  Kaposi's sarcoma
  Cutaneous metastases
  (Cutaneous T cell lymphoma)
Nononcologic
  Psoriasis vulgaris
  HPV-associated dermatoses
    Epidermodysplasia verruciformis
    Condylomata acuminata
  (Permanent hair removal)

NOTE: HPV, human papilloma virus.

tocols (dose of sensitizer, time interval between drug application and irradiation, use of laser versus incoherent light, wavelengths, etc.) differ significantly. Thus a comparison of efficacy is difficult. Phase III studies comparing dermatologic PDT with standard therapeutic procedures do not yet exist.

Systemic PDT for oncologic indications Systemic PDT for Bowen's disease has been shown to be very effective. Administration of porfimer sodium (2 mg/kg body weight) and a light dose of 20 to 50 J/cm^2 induced up to 100 percent complete remission.[211–213] A lower sensitizer dose (1 mg/kg) to minimize generalized cutaneous photosensitization also led to complete remission with higher light doses (185 to 250 J/cm^2).[214] In contrast, SCCs respond less well to systemic PDT. Recurrence rates of up to 50 percent were reported within 6 months after HpD-PDT of 32 tumors.[215] Another study reported comparably poor results for HpD and porfimer sodium.[216] However, in both studies the light doses used were very low (30 J/m^2).

Systemic PDT for BCCs with HpD was first employed by Dougherty in 1981.[217] In a recent study, Feyh treated 67 BCCs with HpD (2.0 mg/kg body weight) and an argon-pumped dye laser (100 J/cm^2). Only three recurrences were reported in the 4.5-year follow-up period.[218] In a patient with nevoid BCC syndrome, 40 BCCs were treated with HpD as sensitizer and a dye laser or a lamp as light source. Most tumors resolved clinically within 4 to 6 weeks. During the follow-up period (12 to 14 months), the recurrence rate was 10.8 percent. Crusted and ulcerated tumors did not respond.[219]

Schweitzer and Visscher treated five patients with AIDS-associated Kaposi's sarcoma with 2.0 mg/kg porfimer sodium and red light in the form of surface and interstitial illumination (50 to 200 J/cm^2). Complete or partial remission of cutaneous or mucosal nodular lesions was observed in 54 of 92 lesions.[220] Almost the same results were presented by Hebeda et al. for eight patients with 83 Kaposi's sarcoma lesions. Although the remission rate was 60 to 70 percent, the cosmetic result was rated unsatisfactory because of extensive hyperpigmentation and scar.[221]

A phase I study in 19 patients with BCC, Kaposi's sarcoma, and metastatic malignant melanoma was performed with systemic lutetium texaphyrin, an expanded porphyrin macrocycle with a peak absorption at 732 nm. This sensitizer does not induce significant skin phototoxicity.[222] Benzoporphyrin derivative monoacid ring A (BPD-MA) (see Table 264-5) also offers a significantly shorter cutaneous photosensitization than porfimer sodium (<72 h)[223,224] and is currently being investigated for BCC.

Systemic PDT for nononcologic indications In 1937, Silver reported the use of PDT in the treatment of psoriasis. Six patients received HpD intramuscularly and orally on consecutive days and were irradiated with UV light. After 2 weeks, an improvement of psoriasis plaques was noted.[192] Low HpD doses given intravenously (1.0 mg/kg) and UVA irradiation for 15 days led to 90 percent remission of extensive plaque-type psoriasis in 15 of 19 patients without relevant side effects.[225] Even better results were reported by Weinstein et al. when red light was used instead of UVA.[226] Systemic PDT with BPD-MA is currently being investigated for its efficacy in psoriasis. In a phase I study (using 0.2 mg/kg, irradiation 3 h later, 690 nm, 75 J/cm^2), complete remission of psoriatic plaques was achieved after a single treatment during an observation period of 60 days.[227]

TOPICAL PHOTODYNAMIC THERAPY Topical application of photosensitizers avoids generalized cutaneous photosensitivity. Unfortunately, because of their high molecular weight (~900 g/mol), porphyrins cannot penetrate into the skin in sufficient amounts. In contrast, small hydrophilic molecules such as ALA penetrate well into the skin, particularly if it is covered by a parakeratotic layer as

is the case in some epidermal tumors or in psoriasis.[197] ALA application selectively induces the production of intracellular porphyrins in epidermal cells and the pilosebaceous unit. These structures synthesize porphyrins to a much higher amount than fibroblasts, myocytes, or endothelial cells.[197,228] Epithelial tumors synthesize much higher amounts of protoporphyrin IX than the surrounding tissue and can therefore be destroyed without damage to healthy skin[197,229,230] (Fig. 264-6). Topical ALA-induced photosensitivity is restricted to the target area. Systemic porphyrin induction is not observed following topical application.[231] The only significant acute side effect of ALA-PDT is a stinging pain during and shortly after irradiation.

Topical PDT for oncologic indications[232–251] The first clinical results with topical ALA-PDT were reported by Kennedy et al. in 1990.[232] After application of 20% ALA in a cream formulation and an incubation time of 3 to 6 h, lesions were irradiated with a 500-W slide projector (irradiance, 150 to 300 mW/cm^2; light dose, 15 to 150 J/cm^2). Out of 80 BCCs, 90 percent showed complete remission within 2 to 3 months after therapy.[232] Wolf et al. treated 70 skin tumors with topical ALA-PDT. Five of six superficial SCCs, nine actinic keratoses, and 36 of 37 superficial BCCs showed complete remission.[233] In the only phase III study performed so far, ALA-PDT with a nonlaser light source appeared to be as effective

FIGURE 264-6

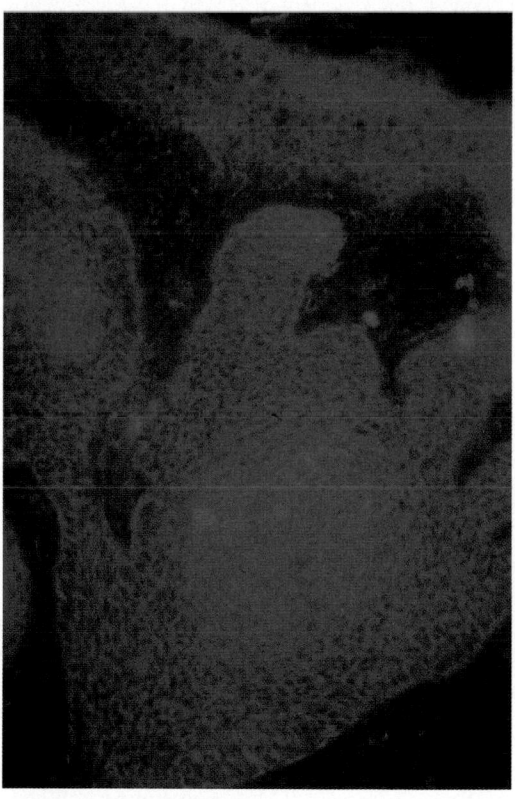

Endogenous porphyrin fluorescence after topical application of 20% ALA formulation to a solid basal cell carcinoma. Twelve hours after ALA application, strong fluorescence of the tumor-bearing areas, weak to no fluorescence of the surrounding dermis. Also visible fluorescence in the overlying epidermis (*marked by white arrows*). (*From Szeimies et al.,*[230] *with permission.*)

FIGURE 264-7

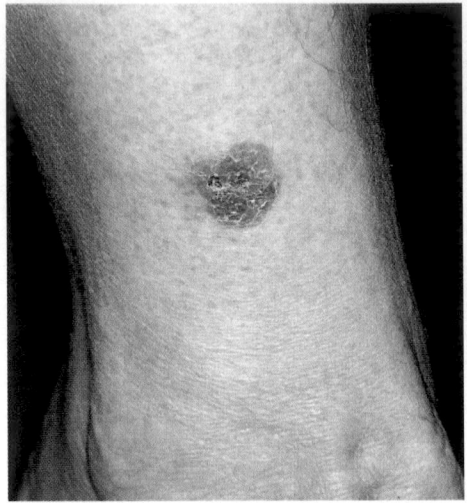

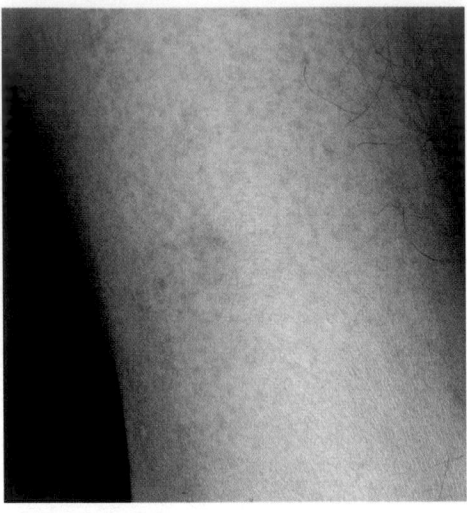

A.

B.

Bowen's disease. Lesion located on the right lower leg (*A*). Twelve months after topical ALA-PDT [10% ALA ointment, application for 4 h, irradiation with argon-pumped dye laser (175 mW/cm²; 180 J/cm²)], clinically and histologically no signs of tumor residue (*B*).

as cryotherapy in the treatment of Bowen's disease, with fewer adverse effects[234] (Fig. 264-7). Topical ALA-PDT is effective, with excellent cosmetic results in patients with nevoid BCC syndrome, arsenic-induced skin cancer, or skin cancer due to immunosuppression after kidney transplantation.[235–237] It is important to note that neither cutaneous metastases of malignant melanoma, pigmented BCC, nor sclerodermiform variants of BCC respond to ALA-PDT,[233,238] probably due to insufficient porphyrin synthesis.[230] Nodular BCC also does not respond sufficiently (response rate 64 percent in 25 lesions), probably because of insufficient light penetration.[239] Tumor thickness appears to be crucial and should not exceed 2 to 3 mm when a single treatment session is planned. Treatment efficacy can be enhanced by repeated treatment sessions.[238] The addition of an iron chelator to the ALA formulation can increase the endogenous porphyrin synthesis.[240]

CTCL (mycosis fungoides) also responded in experimental trials to ALA-PDT after several treatment sessions.[241] Controlled investigations are currently not available, and, as with PUVA treatment of single lesions, this treatment would not be expected to prevent the appearance of new lesions in other areas.

Topical PDT for nononcologic indications   Few data are available regarding the treatment of inflammatory skin conditions. Weinstein and co-workers treated psoriatic plaques once weekly using 10, 20, or 30% ALA and dye laser irradiation (10 to 150 J/cm²). The best results were obtained with 30% ALA and repeated treatments.[242] Boehncke compared the efficacy of ALA-PDT with dithranol in three patients with chronic plaque-type psoriasis with thrice weekly treatments using 10% ALA ointment for 5 h and an incoherent light source (25 J/cm²). In one patient, the PDT-treated side cleared 1 week earlier than the side treated with dithranol.[243]

Other possible indications for topical PDT are human papillomavirus–associated skin diseases. The advantages of PDT for these conditions are the lack of laser plume, in contrast to CO_2 laser treatment, and perhaps a lower recurrence rate due to eradication of subclinical lesions. Complete remission of anogenital condylomata acuminata was achieved in four of seven patients after topical ALA-PDT (20% ALA, 14-h incubation, argon dye laser 100 J/cm²).[244] However, common warts do not respond to ALA-PDT.[245]

Perspectives

The efficacy of PDT in the treatment of superficial neoplastic skin lesion, particularly actinic keratoses, Bowen's disease, and BCCs, has been sufficiently documented. PDT may also find a place in the treatment of selected patients with psoriasis. Nonetheless, the limitations of PDT including its topical variant have to be kept in mind. Crucial parameters are the depth of the penetration of light as well as of the sensitizer into the skin. Moreover, for the treatment of skin cancers with metastatic potential, patients need to be selected carefully, and histologic diagnosis and determination of tumor thickness are a prerequisite. There is still need for controlled studies and for standardized treatment protocols.

REFERENCES

1. Fitzpatrick TB, Pathak MA: Research and development of oral psoralen and longwave radiation photochemotherapy 2000 B.C.–1982 A.D. *Natl Cancer Inst Monogr* **66**:3, 1984
2. El Mofty AM: A preliminary clinical report on the treatment of leukoderma with *Ammi majus* Linn. *J R Egypt Med Assoc* **31**:651, 1948
3. Lerner AB et al: Clinical and experimental studies with 8-methoxypsoralen in vitiligo. *J Invest Dermatol* **20**:299, 1953
4. Parrish JA et al: Photochemotherapy of psoriasis with oral methoxsalen and long wave ultraviolet light. *N Engl J Med* **291**:1207, 1974
5. Wolff K et al: Photochemotherapie bei Psoriasis. Klinische Erfahrungen bei 152 Patienten. *Dtsch Med Wochenschr* **100**:2471, 1975
6. Mortazawi SAM: Meladinine mit UVA bei Vitiligo, Psoriasis, Parapsoriasis und Akne vulgaris. *Dermatol Wochenschr* **158**:908, 1972
7. Fischer T, Alsins J: Treatment of psoriasis with trioxsalen baths and dysprosium lamps. *Acta Derm Venereol (Stockh)* **56**:383, 1976
8. Dall'Acqua F et al: Principles of psoralen photosensitization, in *The Fundamental Bases of Phototherapy,* edited by H Hönigsmann et al. Milan, OEMF SpA, 1996, p 1
9. Schmitt IM et al: Photobiology of psoralens, in *The Fundamental Bases of Phototherapy,* edited by H Hönigsmann et al. Milan, OEMF SpA, 1996, p 17
10. Averbeck D: Recent advances in psoralen phototoxicity mechanism. *Photochem Photobiol* **50**:859, 1989
11. Epstein JH, Fukuyama K: Effects of 8-methoxypsoralen (8-MOP) induced phototoxic effects on mammalian epidermal macromolecular synthesis in vivo. *Photochem Photobiol* **21**:325, 1975
12. Walter JF et al: Psoralen plus black light inhibits epidermal DNA synthesis. *Arch Dermatol* **107**:861, 1973
13. Fritsch PO et al: PUVA suppresses the proliferative stimulus produced by stripping on hairless mice. *J Invest Dermatol* **73**:188, 1979
14. Tanew A, Alsins J: 5-Methoxypsoralen and other furocoumarins in the treatment of psoriasis, in *Light in Biology and Medicine,* edited by RH Douglas et al. New York, Plenum, 1988, p 247
15. Schmitt I et al: Psoralen-protein photochemistry—the forgotten field. *J Photochem Photobiol B:Biol* **27**:101, 1995
16. Averbeck D et al: Mutagenic effects of psoralens in yeast and V79 Chinese hamster cells. *Natl Cancer Inst Monogr* **66**:127, 1984
17. Imokawa G, Tejima T: A possible role of prostaglandins in PUVA-induced inflammation: Implication by organ cultured skin. *J Invest Dermatol* **92**:296, 1989

18. Wrone-Smith T, Nickoloff BJ: Dermal injection of immunocytes induces psoriasis. *J Clin Invest* **98**:1878, 1996

19. Schon MP et al: Murine psoriasis-like disorder induced by naive CD4+ T cells. *Nat Med* **3**:183, 1997

20. Brickl R et al: Pharmacokinetics and pharmacodynamics of psoralens after oral administration: Considerations and conclusions. *Natl Cancer Inst Monogr* **66**:63, 1984

21. Herfst MF, De Wolff FA: Influence of food on the kinetics of 8-MOP in serum and blister fluid in psoriatic patients. *Eur J Clin Pharmacol* **23**:75, 1982

22. Tanew A et al: 5-Methoxypsoralen (bergapten) for photochemotherapy: Bioavailability, phototoxicity and clinical efficacy in psoriasis of a new drug preparation. *J Am Acad Dermatol* **18**:333, 1988

23. Hönigsmann H et al: Serum levels of 8-methoxypsoralen in two different drug preparations. Correlation with photosensitivity and UV-A dose requirements for photochemotherapy. *J Invest Dermatol* **79**:233, 1982

24. Bickers DR, Pathak MA: Psoralen pharmacology: Studies on metabolism and enzyme induction. *Natl Cancer Inst Monogr* **66**:77, 1984

25. Wulf HC, Andreasen MP: Distribution of 3H-8-MOP and its metabolites in rat organs after a single oral administration. *J Invest Dermatol* **76**:252, 1981

26. Lerman S: Psoralens and ocular effects in man and animals: In vivo monitoring of human ocular and cutaneous manifestations. *Natl Cancer Inst Monogr* **66**:227, 1984

27. Treffel P et al: Chronopharmacokinetics of 5-methoxypsoralen. *Acta Derm Venereol* **70**:515, 1990

28. McLelland J et al: The relationship between plasma psoralen concentration and psoralen-UVA erythema. *Br J Dermatol* **124**:585, 1990

29. Neild VS, Scott LV: Plasma levels of 8-methoxypsoralen in psoriatic patients receiving topical 8-methoxypsoralen. *Br J Dermatol* **106**:199, 1982

30. Thomas SE et al: Plasma levels of 8-methoxypsoralen following oral or bath-water treatment. *Br J Dermatol* **125**:56, 1991

31. Calzavara-Pinton PG et al: Phototesting and phototoxic side effects in bath-PUVA. *J Am Acad Dermatol* **28**:657, 1993

32. Degitz K et al: Rapid decline in photosensitivity after 8-methoxypsoralen bathwater delivery. *Arch Dermatol* **132**:1394, 1996

33. Farr PM et al: The action spectrum between 320 and 400 nm for clearance of psoriasis by psoralen photochemotherapy. *Br J Dermatol* **124**:443, 1991

34. Brücke J et al: Relative efficacy of 335 and 365 nm radiation in photochemotherapy of psoriasis. *Br J Dermatol* **124**:372, 1991

35. Wolff K et al: Phototesting and dosimetry for photochemotherapy. *Br J Dermatol* **96**:1, 1977

36. Melski JW et al: Oral methoxsalen photochemotherapy for the treatment of psoriasis: A cooperative clinical trial. *J Invest Dermatol* **68**:328, 1977

37. American Academy of Dermatology Committee on Guidelines of Care: Guidelines of care for phototherapy and photochemotherapy. *J Am Acad Dermatol* **31**:643, 1994

38. Henseler T et al: The European PUVA study (EPS): Oral 8-methoxypsoralen photochemotherapy of psoriasis. Cooperative study among 18 European centres. *Lancet* **1**:853, 1981

39. Calzavara-Pinton PG et al: Phototesting and phototoxic side effects in bath-PUVA. *J Am Acad Dermatol* **28**:657, 1993

40. Calzavara-Pinton PG et al: Bath-5-methoxypsoralen-UVA therapy for psoriasis. *J Am Acad Dermatol* **36**:945, 1997

41. Walter JF, Voorhees JJ: Psoriasis improved by psoralen plus black light. *Acta Derm Venereol (Stockh)* **53**:469, 1973

42. Weber G: Combined 8-methoxypsoralen and black light therapy of psoriasis. Technique and results. *Br J Dermatol* **90**:317, 1974

43. Mortazawi SAM, Oberste-Lehn H: Lichtsensibilisatoren und ihre therapeutischen Fähigkeiten. *Z Hautkr Geschlechtskr* **48**:1, 1973

44. Lowe NJ et al: PUVA therapy for psoriasis: Comparison of oral and bath-water delivery of 8-methoxypsoralen. *J Am Acad Dermatol* **14**:754, 1986

45. Collins P, Rogers S: Bath-water compared with oral delivery of 8-methoxypsoralen PUVA therapy for chronic plaque type psoriasis. *Br J Dermatol* **127**:392, 1992

46. Calzavara-Pinton PG et al: Safety and effectiveness of an aggressive bath-PUVA regimen in the treatment of psoriasis. *Dermatology* **189**:256, 1994

47. Calzavara-Pinton PG et al: A reappraisal of the use of 5-methoxypsoralen in the treatment of psoriasis. *Exp Dermatol* **1**:46, 1992

48. Wolff K et al: Photochemotherapy with orally administered methoxsalen. *Arch Dermatol* **112**:943, 1976

49. Wolff K, Hönigsmann H: Clinical aspects of photochemotherapy. *Pharmacol Ther* **12**:381, 1981

50. Fitzsimons CP et al: Synergistic carcinogenic potential of methotrexate with PUVA in psoriasis. *Lancet* **1**:235, 1983

51. Stern RS, Laird N for the Photochemotherapy Follow-up Study: The carcinogenic risks of treatments for severe psoriasis. *Cancer* **73**:2759, 1994

52. Petzelbauer P et al: Cyclosporin A in combination with photochemotherapy (PUVA) in the treatment of psoriasis. *Br J Dermatol* **123**:641, 1990

53. Fritsch PO et al: Augmentation of oral methoxsalen-photochemotherapy with an oral retinoic acid derivative. *J Invest Dermatol* **70**:178, 1978

54. Hönigsmann H, Wolff K: Isotretinoin-PUVA for psoriasis. *Lancet* **1**:236, 1983

55. Saurat JH et al: Randomized double-blind multicenter study comparing acitretin-PUVA, etretinate-PUVA and placebo-PUVA in the treatment of severe psoriasis. *Dermatologica* **177**:218, 1988

56. Hönigsmann H, Wolff K: Results of therapy for psoriasis using retinoid and photochemotherapy (RePUVA). *Pharmacol Ther* **40**:67, 1989

57. Tanew A et al: Photochemotherapy for severe psoriasis without or in combination with acitretin: A randomized double-blind comparison study. *J Am Acad Dermatol* **25**:682, 1991

58. Chou RC et al: A newly discovered xenobiotic metabolic pathway: Ethyl ester formation. *Life Sci* **49**:169, 1991

59. Maier H, Hönigsmann H: Concentration of etretinate in plasma and subcutaneous fat after long-term acitretin. *Lancet* **348**:1107, 1996

60. Gilchrest BA et al: Oral methoxsalen photochemotherapy of mycosis fungoides. *Cancer* **38**:683, 1976

61. Hönigsmann H et al: Photochemotherapy of mycosis fungoides, in *Book of Abstracts,* VIIth International Congress of Photobiology, Rome, 1976, p 222

62. Tanew A et al: PUVA for cutaneous T-cell lymphoma. 10 years after. *Curr Probl Dermatol* **15**:232, 1986

63. Hönigsmann H et al: Photochemotherapy for cutaneous T cell lymphoma. A follow-up study. *J Am Acad Dermatol* **10**:238, 1984

64. Abel EA et al: PUVA treatment of erythrodermic and plaque-type mycosis fungoides. *Arch Dermatol* **123**:897, 1987

65. Herrmann JJ et al: Treatment of mycosis fungoides with photochemotherapy (PUVA): Long-term follow-up. *J Am Acad Dermatol* **33**:234, 1995

66. Herrmann JJ et al: Ultraviolet radiation for treatment of cutaneous T-cell lymphoma. *Hematol Oncol Clin North Am* **9**:1077, 1995

67. Swanbeck G et al: Indications of a considerable decrease in the death rate in mycosis fungoides by PUVA treatment. *Acta Derm Venereol (Stockh)* **74**:465, 1994

68. Thomsen K et al: Retinoids plus PUVA (RePUVA) and PUVA in mycosis fungoides, plaque stage. A report from the Scandinavian Mycosis Fungoides Group. *Acta Derm Venereol (Stockh)* **69**:536, 1989

69. Kuzel TM et al: Effectiveness of interferon alfa-2a combined with phototherapy for mycosis fungoides and the Sézary syndrome. *J Clin Oncol* **13**:257, 1995

70. Mostow EN et al: Complete remissions in psoralen and UV-A (PUVA)-refractory mycosis fungoides–type cutaneous T-cell lymphoma with combined interferon alfa and PUVA. *Arch Dermatol* **129**:747, 1993

71. Morison WL: *Phototherapy and Photochemotherapy of Skin Disease,* 2 ed. New York, Raven, 1991, p 148

72. Brenner W et al: Erprobung von PUVA bei verschiedenen Dermatosen. *Hautarzt* **29**:541, 1978

73. Ortonne J-P et al: Oral photochemotherapy in the treatment of lichen planus (LP). *Br J Dermatol* **99**:77, 1978

74. Helander I et al: Longterm efficacy of PUVA treatment in lichen planus. Comparison of oral and external methoxsalen regimens. *Photodermatology* **4**:265, 1987

75. Christophers E et al: PUVA treatment of urticaria pigmentosa. *Br J Dermatol* **98**:701, 1978

76. Kolde G et al: Response of cutaneous mast cells to PUVA in patients with urticaria pigmentosa: Histomorphometric, ultrastructural, and biochemical investigations. *J Invest Dermatol* **83**:175, 1984

77. Toda K et al: Effect of 8-methoxypsoralen plus long-wave ultraviolet (PUVA) radiation on mast cells. II. In vitro PUVA inhibits degranulation of rat peritoneal mast cells induced by compound 48/80. *J Invest Dermatol* **87**:113, 1986

78. Toyota N et al: Administration of 8-methoxypsoralen and ultraviolet A irradiation (PUVA) induces turnover of mast cells in the skin of C 57BL/6 mice. *J Invest Dermatol* **95**:353, 1990

79. Honig B et al: Photochemotherapy beyond psoriasis. *J Am Acad Dermatol* **31**:775, 1994

80. Lange Wantzin G, Thomsen K: PUVA-treatment in lymphomatoid papulosis. *Br J Dermatol* **107**:687, 1982

81. Kerker BJ et al: Photochemotherapy of generalized granuloma annulare. *Arch Dermatol* **126**:359, 1990

82. Healy E, Rogers S: PUVA treatment for alopecia areata—does it work? A retrospective review of 102 cases. *Br J Dermatol* **129**:42, 1993

83. Taylor C, Hawk JLM: PUVA treatment of alopecia areata partialis, totalis and universalis: Audit of 10 years' experience at St. John's Institute of Dermatology. *Br J Dermatol* **133**:914, 1995

84. Kerscher M et al: Treatment of localized scleroderma with PUVA bath photochemotherapy. *Lancet* **343**:1233, 1994

85. Scharfetter-Kochanek K et al: PUVA therapy in disabling pansclerotic morphoea of children. *Br J Dermatol* **132**:830, 1995

86. Hymes SR et al: Methoxsalen and ultraviolet A radiation in the treatment of chronic cutaneous graft-versus-host reaction. *J Am Acad Dermatol* **12**:30, 1985

87. Atkinson K et al: PUVA therapy for drug-resistant graft-versus-host disease. *Bone Marrow Transplant* **1**:227, 1986

88. Volc-Platzer B et al: Photochemotherapy improves chronic cutaneous graft-versus-host disease. *J Am Acad Dermatol* **23**:220, 1990

89. Jampel RM et al: PUVA therapy for chronic cutaneous graft-vs-host disease. *Arch Dermatol* **127**:1673, 1991

90. Reinauer S et al: Photochemotherapie (PUVA) der akuten Graft-versus-host-Erkrankung. *Hautarzt* **44**:708, 1993

91. Pathak MA et al: Relative effectiveness of three psoralens and sunlight in repigmentation of 365 vitiligo patients. *J Invest Dermatol* **74**:252, 1980

92. Pathak MA, Fitzpatrick TB: The evolution of photochemotherapy with psoralens and UVA (PUVA): 2000 B.C. to 1992 A.D. *J Photochem Photobiol B: Biol* **14**:3, 1992

93. Ortel B et al: Vitiligo treatment. *Curr Probl Dermatol* **15**:265, 1986

94. Ortel B et al: Treatment of vitiligo with khellin and ultraviolet A. *J Am Acad Dermatol* **18**:693, 1988

95. Ortel B et al: Polymorphous light eruption: Action spectrum and photoprotection. *J Am Acad Dermatol* **14**:748, 1986

96. Addo HA, Sharma SC: UVB phototherapy and photochemotherapy (PUVA) in the treatment of polymorphic light eruption and solar urticaria. *Br J Dermatol* **116**:539, 1987

97. Murphy GM et al: Prophylactic PUVA and UVB therapy in polymorphic light eruption—a controlled trial. *Br J Dermatol* **116**:531, 1987

98. Hölzle E et al: PUVA treatment for solar urticaria and persistent light reaction. *Arch Dermatol Res* **269**:87, 1980

99. Parrish JA et al: Solar urticaria: Treatment with PUVA and mediator inhibitors. *Br J Dermatol* **106**:575, 1982

100. Hindson C et al: PUVA therapy of chronic actinic dermatitis. *Br J Dermatol* **113**:157, 1985

101. Jaschke E, Hönigsmann H: Hydroa vacciniforme Aktionsspektrum. UV-Toleranz nach Photochemotherapie. *Hautarzt* **32**:350, 1981

102. Ros A-M: PUVA therapy for erythropoietic protoporphyria. *Photodermatology* **5**:148, 1988

103. Roelandts R: Photo(chemo)therapy and general management of erythropoietic protoporphyria. *Dermatology* **190**:330, 1995

104. Ullrich SE: Does exposure to UV radiation induce a shift to a Th-2-like immune reaction? *Photochem Photobiol* **64**:254, 1996

105. Morrey JD et al: In vivo activation of human immunodeficiency virus type I long terminal repeat by UV type A (UV-A) light plus psoralen and UV-B light in the skin of transgenic mice. *J Virol* **65**:5045, 1991

106. Wang CY et al: Skin cancers associated with acquired immunodeficiency syndrome. *Mayo Clin Proc* **70**:766, 1995

107. Meola T et al: The safety of UVB phototherapy in patients with HIV infection. *J Am Acad Dermatol* **29**:216, 1993

108. Lim HW et al: UVB phototherapy is an effective treatment for pruritus in patients infected with HIV. *J Am Acad Dermatol* **37**:414, 1997

109. Ranki A et al: Effect of PUVA on immunologic and virologic findings in HIV-infected patients. *J Am Acad Dermatol* **24**:404, 1991

110. Horn TD et al: Effects of psoralen plus UVA radiation (PUVA) on HIV-1 in human beings: A pilot study. *J Am Acad Dermatol* **31**:735, 1994

111. Zmudzka BZ et al: Medical UV exposures and HIV activation. *Photochem Photobiol* **64**:246, 1996

112. Morison WL: PUVA therapy is preferable to UVB phototherapy in the management of HIV-associated dermatoses. *Photochem Photobiol* **64**:267, 1996

113. Hönigsmann H: Psoralen photochemotherapy—mechanisms, drugs, toxicity. *Curr Probl Dermatol* **15**:52, 1986

114. Nyfors A et al: Liver biopsies from patients with psoriasis related to photochemotherapy (PUVA): Findings before and after 1 year of therapy in twelve patients. *J Am Acad Dermatol* **14**:43, 1986

115. Calzavara-Pinton PG et al: Antinuclear antibodies are not induced in uncomplicated psoriatic patients by PUVA treatment. *J Am Acad Dermatol* **30**:955, 1994

116. Dunnick JK et al: Tumors of the skin in the HRA/Skh mouse after treatment with 8-methoxypsoralen and UVA radiation. *Fund Appl Toxicol* **16**:92, 1991

117. Young AR et al: A comparison of the phototumorigenic potential of 8-MOP and 5-MOP in hairless albino mice exposed to solar simulated irradiation. *Br J Dermatol* **108**:507, 1983

118. Stern RS et al: Risk of cutaneous carcinoma in patients treated with oral methoxsalen photochemotherapy for psoriasis. *N Engl J Med* **300**:809, 1979

119. Hönigsmann H et al: Keratoses and non-melanoma skin tumors in long-term photochemotherapy (PUVA). *J Am Acad Dermatol* **3**:406, 1980

120. Stern RS et al: Cutaneous squamous cell carcinoma in patients treated with PUVA. *N Engl J Med* **310**:1156, 1984

121. Tanew A et al: Non-melanoma skin tumors in long-term photochemotherapy treatment of psoriasis. An 8-year follow-up study. *J Am Acad Dermatol* **15**:960, 1986

122. Stern RS et al: Oral psoralen and ultraviolet-A light (PUVA) treatment of psoriasis and persistent risk of nonmelanoma skin cancer. PUVA follow-up study. *Natl Cancer Inst* **90**:1278, 1998

123. Torinuki W, Tagami H: Incidence of skin cancer in Japanese psoriatic patients treated with either methoxsalen phototherapy, Goeckerman regimen or both therapies. A ten-year follow-up study. *J Am Acad Dermatol* **18**:1278, 1988

124. Henseler T et al: Skin tumors in the European PUVA study. Eight-year follow-up of 1,643 patients treated with PUVA for psoriasis. *J Am Acad Dermatol* **16**:108, 1987

125. Bruynzeel I et al: "High single-dose" European PUVA regimen also causes an excess of non-melanoma skin cancer. *Br J Dermatol* **124**:49, 1991

126. Forman AB et al: Long-term follow-up of skin cancer in the PUVA-48 cooperative study. *Arch Dermatol* **125**:515, 1989

127. Lindelöf B et al: PUVA and cancer: A large-scale epidemiological study. *Lancet* **2**:91, 1991

128. Chuang TY et al: PUVA and skin cancer: A historical cohort study on 492 patients. *J Am Acad Dermatol* **26**:173, 1992

129. Lever LR, Farr PM: Skin cancers or premalignant lesions occur in half of high-dose PUVA patients. *Br J Dermatol* **131**:215, 1994

130. Maier H et al: Skin tumours in photochemotherapy for psoriasis. A single centre follow-up of 496 patients. *Dermatology* **193**:185, 1996

131. Gibbs NK et al: PUVA treatment strategies and cancer risk. *Lancet* **1**:150, 1986

132. Stern RS et al: Genital tumors among men with psoriasis exposed to psoralens and ultraviolet A radiation (PUVA) and ultraviolet B radiation. *N Engl J Med* **322**:1093, 1990

133. Wolff K, Hönigsmann H: Genital carcinomas in psoriasis patients treated with photochemotherapy. *Lancet* **1**:439, 1991

134. Young AR: Photochemotherapy and skin carcinogenesis: A critical review, in *The Fundamental Bases of Phototherapy*, edited by H. Hönigsmann et al. Milan, OEMF SpA, 1996, p 77

135. Lindelöf B et al: Comparison of the carcinogenic potential of trioxsalen bath PUVA and oral methoxsalen PUVA. A preliminary report. *Arch Dermatol* **128**:1341, 1992

136. Hannuksela A et al: Cancer incidence among Finnish patients with psoriasis treated with trioxsalen bath PUVA. *J Am Acad Dermatol* **35**:689, 1996

137. Gupta AK et al: Cutaneous melanomas in patients treated with psoralens and ultraviolet A. *J Am Acad Dermatol* **19**:67, 1988

138. Stern RS et al: Malignant melanoma in patients treated for psoriasis with methoxsalen (psoralen) and ultraviolet A radiation (PUVA). *N Engl J Med* **336**:1041, 1997

139. Wolff K: Should PUVA be abandoned? Editorial. *N Engl J Med* **336**:1090, 1997

140. Petzelbauer P et al: Cyclosporin A suppresses ICAM-1 expression by papillary endothelium in healing psoriatic plaques. *J Invest Dermatol* **96**:362, 1991

141. Vallat V et al: PUVA bath therapy strongly suppresses immunological and epidermal activation in psoriasis: A possible cellular basis for remittive therapy. *J Exp Med* **180**:283, 1994

142. Aberer W et al: Effects of physico-chemical agents on murine epidermal Langerhans cells and Thy-1-positive dendritic epidermal cells. *J Immunol* **135**:1210, 1986

143. Koulu LM, Jansen CT: Antipsoriatic, erythematogenic, and Langerhans cell marker depleting effect of bath-psoralens plus ultraviolet A treatment. *J Am Acad Dermatol* **18**:1053, 1988

144. Koulu L et al: Relation of antipsoriatic and Langerhans cell depleting effects of systemic photochemotherapy: A clinical, enzyme histochemical and electron microscopic study. *J Invest Dermatol* **82**:591, 1984

145. Laskin JD et al: Selective inactivation of lymphocytes after psoralen/ultraviolet (PUVA) treatment without affecting systemic immune responses. *J Leukocyte Biol* **54**:138, 1993

146. Gilmour JW et al: The effect of UV therapy on immune function in patients with psoriasis. *Br J Dermatol* **129**:28, 1993

147. Neuner P et al: Cytokine release by peripheral blood mononuclear cells is affected by 8-methoxypsoralen plus UV-A. *Photochem Photobiol* **59**:182, 1994

148. Stern RS: Ocular lens findings in patients treated with PUVA. Photochemotherapy Follow-Up Study. *J Invest Dermatol* **103**:534, 1994

149. Stern RS et al: Outcomes of pregnancies among women and partners of men with a history of exposure to methoxsalen photochemotherapy (PUVA) for the treatment of psoriasis. *Arch Dermatol* **127**:347, 1991

150. Edelson RL et al: Treatment of cutaneous T-cell lymphoma by extracorporeal photochemotherapy. *N Engl J Med* **316**:297, 1987

151. Knobler RM, Edelson RL: Cutaneous T-cell lymphoma. *Med Clin North Am* **70**:109, 1986

152. Armus S et al: Photopheresis for the treatment of cutaneous T-cell lymphoma. *J Am Acad Dermatol* **23**:898, 1990

153. Heald P et al: Treatment of erythrodermic cutaneous T-cell lymphoma with extracorporeal photochemotherapy. *J Am Acad Dermatol* **27**:427, 1992

154. Knobler R: Photopheresis and the red man syndrome. *Dermatology* **190**:97, 1995

155. Zic J et al: Extracorporeal photopheresis for the treatment of cutaneous T-cell lymphoma. *J Am Acad Dermatol* **27**:729, 1992

156. Gasparro FP et al: Effect of monochromatic UVA light and 8-methoxypsoralen on human lymphocyte response to mitogen. *Photodermatology* **1**:10, 1984

157. Gasparro FP et al: Quantitation of psoralen photoadducts in DNA isolated from lymphocytes treated with 8-methoxypsoralen and ultraviolet A radiation (extracorporeal photopheresis). *Curr Probl Dermatol* **15**:67, 1986

158. Perez M et al: Inhibition of antiskin allograft immunity by infusions with syngeneic photoinactivated effector lymphocytes. *J Invest Dermatol* **92**:669, 1989

159. Gasparro FP et al: Cell membrane DNA: A new target for psoralen photoadduct formation. *Phochem Photobiol* **52**:315, 1990

160. Berger CL et al: Inhibition of autoimmune disease in a murine model of systemic lupus erythematosus induced by exposure to syngeneic photoinactivated lymphocytes. *J Invest Dermatol* **94**:52, 1990

161. Vowels BR et al: Extracorporeal photo-chemotherapy induces the production of tumor necrosis factor-α by monocytes: Implications for the treatment of cutaneous T-cell lymphoma and systemic sclerosis. *J Invest Dermatol* **95**:686, 1994

162. Berger CL et al: The immune response to class I-associated tumor-specific cutaneous T-cell lymphoma antigens. *J Invest Dermatol* **107**:392, 1996

163. Knobler RM et al: Parenteral administration of 8-methoxypsoralen in photopheresis. *J Am Acad Dermatol* **28**:580, 1993

164. Zachariae H et al: Photopheresis in the red man or pre-Sézary syndrome. *Dermatology* **190**:132, 1995

165. Duvic M et al: Photopheresis therapy for cutaneous T-cell lymphoma. *J Am Acad Dermatol* **35**:573, 1996

166. Zic J et al: Long term follow-up with cutaneous T-cell lymphoma treated with extracorporeal photochemotherapy. *J Am Acad Dermatol* **35**:935, 1996

167. Gottlieb S et al: Treatment of cutaneous T-cell lymphoma with extracorporeal photopheresis monotherapy and in combination with recombinant interferon alpha: A 10 year experience at a single institution. *J Am Acad Dermatol* **35**:946, 1996

168. Rook AH et al: Extracorporeal photochemotherapy for drug-resistant pemphigus vulgaris. *Ann Intern Med* **112**:303, 1990

169. Liang G et al: Pemphigus vulgaris treated with photopheresis. *J Am Acad Dermatol* **26**:779, 1992

170. Gollnick H et al: Unresponsive severe generalized pemphigus vulgaris successfully controlled by extracorporeal photopheresis. *J Am Acad Dermatol* **28**:122, 1993

171. Rook AH et al: Treatment of autoimmune disease with extracorporeal photochemotherapy: Progressive systemic sclerosis. *Yale J Biol Med* **62**:639, 1989

172. Rook AH et al: Treatment of systemic sclerosis with extracorporeal photochemotherapy—results of a multicenter trial. *Arch Dermatol* **128**:337, 1992

173. DiSpaltro F et al: Extracorporeal photochemotherapy in progressive systemic sclerosis. *Int J Dermatol* **32**:1, 1993

174. Zachariae H et al: Photopheresis and systemic sclerosis. *Arch Dermatol* **128**:1651, 1992

175. Malawista S et al: Treatment of rheumatoid arthritis by extracorporeal photochemotherapy: A pilot study. *Arthritis Rheum* **34**:646, 1991

176. Costanzo-Nordin MR et al: Successful treatment of heart transplant rejection with photopheresis. *Transplantation* **53**:808, 1992

177. Rose EA et al: Photochemotherapy in human heart transplant recipients at high risk for fatal rejection. *J Heart Lung Transplant* **11**:746, 1992

178. Dall'Amico R et al: Extracorporeal photochemotherapy as adjuvant treatment of heart transplant recipients with recurrent rejection. *Transplantation* **60**:45, 1995

179. Meiser BM et al: Reduction of the incidence of rejection by adjunct immunosuppression with photochemotherapy after heart transplantation. *Transplantation* **57**:563, 1994

180. Barr ML: Immunomodulation in transplantation with photopheresis. *Artif Organs* **20**:971, 1996

181. Sunder-Plassman G et al: Renal allograft rejection controlled by photopheresis. *Lancet* **346**:506, 1995

182. Wolfe J et al: Reversal of acute renal allograft rejection by extracorporeal photopheresis: A case presentation and review of the literature. *J Clin Apheresis* **11**:36, 1996

183. Slovis BS et al: Photopheresis for chronic rejection of lung allografts. *N Engl J Med* **332**:962, 1995

184. Andreu G et al: Extracorporeal photochemotherapy treatment for acute lung rejection episode. *J Heart Lung Transplant* **14**:793, 1995

185. Owsianowski M et al: Successful treatment of chronic graft-versus-host disease with extracorporeal photopheresis. *Bone Marrow Transpl* **14**:845, 1994

186. Rosetti F et al: Extra-corporeal photochemotherapy as single therapy for extensive cutaneous, chronic graft-versus-host disease. *Transplantation* **59**:149, 1995

187. Gerber M et al: Complete remission of lichen-planus-like graft-versus-host disease (GVHD) with extracorporeal photochemotherapy (CP). *Bone Marrow Transplant* **19**:517, 1997

188. Knobler RM et al: Extracorporeal photochemotherapy for the treatment of systemic lupus erythematosus. A pilot study. *Arthritis Rheum* **35**:319, 1992

189. Pass HI: Photodynamic therapy in oncology: Mechanisms and clinical use. *J Natl Cancer Inst* **85**:443, 1993

190. Von Tappeiner H, Jodlbauer A: Über die Wirkungen der photodynamischen (fluorescierenden) Stoffe auf Protozoen und Enzyme. *Arch Klin Med* **80**:427, 1904

191. Jesionek A, von Tappeiner H: Zur Behandlung der Hautcarcinome mit fluorescierenden Stoffen. *Dtsch Arch Klin Med* **85**:223, 1905

192. Silver H: Psoriasis vulgaris treated with hematoporphyrin. *Arch Dermatol Syphilol* **36**:1118, 1937

193. Auler H, Banzer G: Untersuchungen über die Rolle der Porphyrine bei geschwulstkranken Menschen und Tieren. *Z Krebsforsch* **53**:65, 1942

194. Lipson RL, Baldes EJ: The photodynamic properties of a particular haematoporphyrin derivative. *Arch Dermatol* **82**:508, 1960

195. Dougherty TJ et al: Photoradiation therapy for the treatment of malignant tumors. *Cancer Res* **38**:2628, 1978

196. Wooten RS et al: Prospective study of cutaneous phototoxicity after systemic hematoporphyrin derivative. *Lasers Surg Med* **8**:294, 1988

197. Kennedy JC, Pottier RH: Endogenous protoporphyrin IX, a clinically useful photosensitizer for photodynamic therapy. *J Photochem Photobiol B:Biol* 14:275, 1992

198. Batlle AM del C: Porphyrins, porphyrias, cancer and photodynamic therapy—a model for carcinogenesis. *J Photochem Photobiol B:Biol* 20:5, 1993

199. Schaffner K et al: Porphycenes as photodynamic therapy agents, in *Biologic Effects of Light,* edited by EG Jung, MF Holick. Berlin, Walter de Gruyter, 1994, p 312

200. Fritsch C et al: *Ex vivo* application of δ-aminolevulinic acid induces high and specific porphyrin levels in human skin tumors: Possible basis for selective photodynamic therapy. *Photochem Photobiol* 66:114, 1997

201. Anderson RR, Parrish JA: The optics of human skin. *J Invest Dermatol* 77:13, 1981

202. Jones LR, Grossweiner LI: Singlet oxygen generation by Photofrin in homogeneous and light-scattering media. *J Photochem Photobiol B:Biol* 26:249, 1994

203. Weishaupt KR et al: Identification of singlet oxygen as the cytotoxic agent in photoinactivation of a murine tumor. *Cancer Res* 36:2326, 1976

204. Kessel D: Sites of photosensitization by derivatives of hematoporphyrin. *Photochem Photobiol* 44:489, 1986

205. Wessels JM et al: Intracellular localization of meso-tetraphenylporphine tetrasulphonate probed by time-resolved and microscopic fluorescence spectroscopy. *J Photochem Photobiol B:Biol* 12:275, 1992

206. Milanesi C et al: Zn(II)-phthalocyanine as a photodynamic agent for tumours. II. Studies on the mechanism of photosensitised tumour necrosis. *Br J Cancer* 61:846, 1990

207. Penning LC, Dubbelman TMAR: Fundamentals of photodynamic therapy: Cellular and biochemical aspects. *Anti-Cancer Drug* 5:139, 1994

208. Castellani A et al: Photodynamic effect of hematoporphyrin on blood microcirculation. *J Pathol Bacteriol* 86:99, 1963

209. Dellian M et al: Effects of photodynamic therapy on leucocyte-endothelium interaction: Differences between normal and tumour tissue. *Br J Cancer* 72:1125, 1995

210. Star WM et al: Destruction of rat mammary tumor and normal tissue microcirculation by hematoporphyrin derivative photoradiation observed in vivo in sandwich observation chambers. *Cancer Res* 46:2532, 1986

211. Robinson PJ et al: Photodynamic therapy: A better treatment for widespread Bowen's disease. *Br J Dermatol* 119:59, 1988

212. Buchanan RB et al: Photodynamic therapy in the treatment of malignant tumours of the skin and head and neck. *Eur J Surg Oncol* 15:400, 1989

213. Waldow SM et al: Photodynamic therapy for treatment of malignant cutaneous lesions. *Lasers Surg Med* 7:451, 1987

214. Jones CM et al: Photodynamic therapy in the treatment of Bowen's disease. *J Am Acad Dermatol* 27:979, 1992

215. Pennington DG et al: Photodynamic therapy for multiple skin cancers. *Plast Reconstr Surg* 82:1067, 1988

216. McCaughan JS Jr et al: Photodynamic therapy for cutaneous and subcutaneous malignant neoplasms. *Arch Surg* 124:211, 1989

217. Dougherty TJ: Photoradiation therapy for cutaneous and subcutaneous malignancies. *J Invest Dermatol* 77:122, 1981

218. Feyh J: Photodynamic treatment for cancers of the head and neck. *J Photochem Photobiol B:Biol* 36:175, 1996

219. Tse DT et al: Hematoporphyrin derivative photoradiation therapy in managing nevoid basal cell carcinoma syndrome. *Arch Ophthalmol* 102:990, 1984

220. Schweitzer VG, Visscher D: Photodynamic therapy for treatment of AIDS-related oral Kaposi's sarcoma. *Otolaryngol Head Neck Surg* 102:639, 1990

221. Hebeda KM et al: Photodynamic therapy in AIDS-related cutaneous Kaposi's sarcoma. *J Acquir Immune Defic Syndr Hum Retrovirol* 10:61, 1995

222. Renschler MF et al: Photodynamic therapy trials with lutetium texaphyrin PCI-0123 (Lu-Tex). *Photochem Photobiol* 65:47S, 1997

223. Lui H, Anderson RR: Photodynamic therapy in dermatology. *Arch Dermatol* 128:1631, 1992

224. Wolford ST et al: Comparative skin phototoxicity in mice with two photosensitizing drugs: Benzoporphyrin derivative monoacid ring A and porfimer sodium (Photofrin). *Fundam Appl Toxicol* 24:52, 1995

225. Berg H et al: Photodynamic hematoporphyrin therapy of psoriasis, in *Photodynamic Therapy of Tumors and other Diseases,* edited by G Jori, C Perria. Padova, Progetto Editore, 1985, p 337

226. Weinstein GD et al: Low-dose photofrin II photodynamic therapy of psoriasis. *Clin Res* 39:509A, 1991

227. Levy JG et al: The preclinical and clinical development and potential application of benzoporphyrin derivative. *Int Photodyn* 1:3, 1994

228. Oseroff AR: Photodynamic therapy, in *Clinical Photomedicine,* edited by HW Lim, NA Soter. New York, Marcel Dekker, 1993, p 387

229. Abels C et al: In vivo kinetics and spectra of 5-aminolevulinic acid–induced fluorescence in an amelanotic melanoma of the hamster. *Br J Cancer* 70:826, 1994

230. Szeimies RM et al: Penetration potency of topical applied δ-aminolevulinic acid for photodynamic therapy of basal cell carcinoma. *Photochem Photobiol* 59:73, 1994

231. Fritsch C et al: Influence of topical photodynamic therapy with 5-aminolevulinic acid on porphyrin metabolism. *Arch Dermatol Res* 288:517, 1996

232. Kennedy JC et al: Photodynamic therapy with endogenous protoporphyrin IX: Basic principles and present clinical experience. *J Photochem Photobiol B:Biol* 6:143, 1990

233. Wolf P et al: Topical photodynamic therapy with endogenous porphyrins after application of 5-aminolevulinic acid. *J Am Acad Dermatol* 28:17, 1993

234. Morton CA et al: Comparison of photodynamic therapy with cryotherapy in the treatment of Bowen's disease. *Br J Dermatol* 135:766, 1996

235. Szeimies RM et al: Topical photodynamic therapy with 5-aminolevulinic acid in the treatment of arsenic-induced skin tumors. *Eur J Dermatol* 5:208, 1995

236. Walter AW et al: Complications of the nevoid basal cell carcinoma syndrome. *J Pediatr Hematol Oncol* 19:258, 1997

237. Fijan S et al: Photodynamic therapy of keratoacanthoma using topical delta-aminolevulinic acid. *J Invest Dermatol* 106:945, 1996

238. Calzavara-Pinton PG: Repetitive photodynamic therapy with topical δ-aminolevulinic acid as an appropriate approach to the routine treatment of superficial non-melanoma skin tumours. *J Photochem Photobiol B:Biol* 29:53, 1995

239. Svanberg K et al: Photodynamic therapy of non-melanoma malignant tumours of the skin using topical δ-aminolevulinic acid sensitization and laser irradiation. *Br J Dermatol* 130:743, 1994

240. Fijan S et al: Photodynamic therapy of epithelial skin tumours using delta-aminolevulinic acid and desferrioxamine. *Br J Dermatol* 133:282, 1995

241. Wolf P et al: Topical photodynamic therapy with endogenous porphyrins after application of 5-aminolevulinic acid. *J Am Acad Dermatol* 28:17, 1993

242. Weinstein GD et al: Photodynamic therapy (PDT) of psoriasis with topical delta aminolevulinic acid (ALA): A pilot dose ranging study. *Photodermatol Photoimmunol Photomed* 10:92, 1994

243. Boehncke WH et al: Treatment of psoriasis by topical photodynamic therapy with polychromatic light. *Lancet* 343:801, 1994

244. Frank RGJ et al: Photodynamic therapy for condylomata acuminata with local application of 5-aminolevulinic acid. *Genitourin Med* 72:70, 1996

245. Ammann R et al: Topical photodynamic therapy in verrucae: A pilot study. *Dermatology* 191:346, 1995

246. Warloe T et al: Photodynamic therapy with 5-aminolevulinic acid induced porphyrins and DMSO/EDTA for basal cell carcinoma, in *5th International Photodynamic Association Biennial Meeting,* edited by DA Cortese. Proc SPIE, 1995, 2371:226

247. Cairnduff F et al: Superficial photodynamic therapy with topical 5-aminolevulinic acid for superficial primary and secondary skin cancer. *Br J Cancer* 69:605, 1994

248. Jeffes EW et al: Photodynamic therapy of actinic keratosis with topical 5-aminolevulinic acid. *Arch Dermatol* 133:727, 1997

249. Szeimies RM et al: Topical photodynamic therapy with 5-aminolevulinic acid in the treatment of actinic keratoses: A first clinical study. *Dermatology* 192:242, 1996

250. Lui H et al: Photodynamic therapy of nonmelanoma skin cancer with topical aminolevulinic acid: A clinical and histologic study. *Arch Dermatol* 131:737, 1995

251. Wennberg AM et al: Treatment of superficial basal cell carcinomas using topically applied delta-aminolevulinic acid and a filtered xenon lamp. *Arch Dermatol Res* 288:561, 1996

CHAPTER 265

Joop M. Grevelink
E. Victor Ross
R. Rox Anderson

Lasers in Dermatology

Lasers operate by the principle for which they are named: *l*ight *a*mplified by *s*timulated *e*mission of *r*adiation. Stimulated emission was predicted by Einstein long before the invention of the first laser, which occurred in 1960 when Maiman produced a ruby laser.[1] Inside a laser, one photon stimulates the emission of another identical photon from molecules that are in an excited metastable state. Two mirrors are placed on each end of the laser in exact parallel alignment so that the photons bounce back and forth through the excited medium. The light is amplified by stimulating more photons with each pass. The front mirror is only partially reflective so that some fraction of the light is transmitted. The result is an impressively bright, monochromatic, highly collimated, coherent, and controllable beam of light. Energy for the whole process is provided by an electrical, chemical, or optical energy "pump" source used to excite the atoms or molecules of the laser medium.

Lasers are truly unique light sources. The monochromaticity of lasers allows precise deposition of energy through absorption by different skin pigments (chromophores). The brightness of lasers far exceeds that of any natural light source. Lasers are now available over the entire optical spectrum, from the vacuum ultraviolet (UV) through the visible and infrared wavelengths. The ability to focus impressive optical power through small, flexible fiber optics has led to endoscopic laser surgical use. A wide range of surgical laser applications has been developed. For example, in laser lithotripsy a pulse of about 100,000 W of light is passed down a fiber only slightly wider than a hair shaft, causing ionization (laser-induced plasma) and fracturing of ureteral or biliary stones.

The history of laser development in dermatology is replete with basic science, clinical art, and serendipity. For several years, the ruby laser, which emits a pulse of deep-red light, was the only laser available. Leon Goldman, who died in 1997, pioneered the use of this and, subsequently, other lasers in dermatology.[2,3] Ruby lasers were essentially abandoned when argon-ion and carbon dioxide (CO_2) lasers were applied for coagulation and cutting during the 1970s. The blue and green light of the argon-ion laser is strongly absorbed by hemoglobins, and this device was shown to be widely useful for superficial coagulation of port-wine stains (PWSs) and other vascular lesions, as detailed below. However, scarring was an occasional and unpredictable side effect, and often operator-dependent.

In the early 1980s, Anderson and Parrish proposed a theory for causing histologically selective injury with pulsed lasers, calling the process *selective photothermolysis*.[4] This led to a new generation of highly selective pulsed lasers in dermatology. A 450-μsec yellow dye laser was initially developed for treating port-wine lesions and was the first laser cavity design intrinsically motivated by a medical need.[5] At present, selective photothermolysis is the basis for lower-risk treatment of microvascular lesions, tattoos, and benign pigmented lesions. The latter two indications have revived the ruby laser as a dermatologic tool.[6]

Lasers emit light either continuously or in pulses. Continuous-wave (CW) laser beams can be interrupted by using a shutter or similar device, some of which are proving to be useful in dermatology. However, CW lasers cannot achieve the impressive instantaneous (peak) power available with pulsed lasers. Thus, the nature of laser-tissue interaction is usually different for CW as compared with high-energy pulsed lasers. The argon-ion (blue/green), argon-pumped dye (tunable), CW neodymium: yttrium-aluminum-garnet (Nd:YAG) (near infrared), and CW CO_2 (far infrared) are CW lasers typically in medical use for coagulation or vaporization of tissue. Some pulsed lasers produce pulses at such a rapid rate, and with such small energy per pulse, that they behave medically like CW lasers. Copper vapor lasers (green/yellow) and so-called KTP lasers, a frequently doubled Nd:YAG green laser, are examples of such quasicontinuous-wave (QCW) lasers that are also useful for coagulation and vaporization of tissue. In contrast, high-energy pulsed lasers can induce selective photothermolysis, a process in which heat injury is confined to microscopic sites of absorption in the skin, such as blood vessels and pigmented cells. Examples of high-energy pulsed lasers in dermatology are pulsed tunable dye (yellow, 585 nm), ruby, and Q-switched Nd:YAG (near infrared, 1064 nm and green, 532 nm) lasers. The term *Q-switch* refers to techniques in which light is blocked from traversing the laser cavity, then suddenly allowed to do so. The result is storage of impressive energy in the laser's metastable excited state, suddenly released in a short, high-intensity pulse.

Table 265-1 lists the types of lasers now used in dermatology, their typical output characteristics, and characteristic effects upon the skin (Fig. 265-1).

The range of laser applications in medicine and surgery is also expanding rapidly. In addition to surgical dermatology, lasers are being used to trigger light-activated photosensitizing drugs for local treatment of cancer. Diagnostic applications of in vivo laser microscopy and spectroscopy have just begun to be explored. At present, there are hundreds of different laser devices used in industrial and military applications. The more recent development of powerful, reliable semiconductor diode lasers is the harbinger of a technological revolution identical to that which computers underwent when bulky vacuum tubes were replaced by transistors and then by electronic microchips. High-power medical semiconductor lasers have just been introduced for clinical use. Based on existing technology, semiconductor medical lasers may conceivably become

TABLE 265-1

Lasers in Dermatology

Laser	Wavelength, nm	Mode	Typical Uses
Alexandrite	755	Q-switched, 50–100 μs Long pulse, 10–50 ms	Epidermal/dermal pigmentation, nevus of Ota, tattoos (black, blue, green), hair removal
Argon, argon dye	488–630	CW	Vascular, light source for photodynamic therapy
CO_2	10,600	CW Pulsed or scanned	Vaporization/ablation rhytides, scars, photodamage
Copper vapor/ bromide	512, 578	QCW	Vascular, epidermal pigment
Diode	800–1000	CW/pulsed	Vascular, hair removal
Erbium:YAG	2940	Pulsed	Rhytides, scars, photodamage
Krypton	520, 568	CW/pulsed	520-pigment, 568-vascular
KTP	532	QCW	Vascular, epidermal pigment (adults > children)
Nd:YAG	532	Q-switched, 10 ns	532-epidermal pigmentation, red tattoos
	1064	Long pulse, 5–50 ms	1064-QS: nonablative dermal remodeling, nevus of Ota, black tattoos, hair removal 1064-long pulse: vascular
Pulsed dye (yellow)	577–600	Pulsed 450 μs–1.5 ms	Vascular (children and adults)
Pulsed dye (green)	510	Pulsed 300 μs	Epidermal pigment, red tattoos
Ruby	694	Q-switched, 20 ns Long pulse, 0.5–3 ms	Epidermal/dermal pigmentation, nevus of Ota, tattoos (black, blue, green), hair removal

NOTE: CW, continuous wave; QCW, quasicontinuous, wave (rapid, low-energy pulses); pulsed, high-energy pulses.

less expensive than electrosurgery machines. There is little doubt that lasers, and probably laser-activated photodynamic drugs, will play an increasing role in dermatology over the next decade.

A broad aim of this chapter is to present a critical rationale for choosing specific laser therapies. Lasers are a unique class of light sources, capable of inducing unique biologic effects. Laser treatment of some skin conditions, such as childhood PWS, is highly compelling. On the other hand, lasers can also mimic the effects of much simpler technology, such as electrosurgery, at greater cost to both physician and patient. The challenge is to understand specific, appropriate uses for available lasers.

OPTICS OF THE SKIN

A brief presentation of cutaneous optics is necessary to understand why certain laser wavelengths are of particular interest in dermatology. The optics of skin are both complex and dynamic, changing literally with each heartbeat, with sun exposure and genetic influences on pigmentation, with aging, and with body site. However, the basic structure of skin and its normal pigments allows a useful model of skin optics to be developed.

Two processes determine the penetration of light into skin: absorption and scattering. With absorption, the photon invests all its energy in the absorbing molecule, called a *chromophore*. Absorp-

tion spectra of the major chromophores in skin throughout the UV, visible, and infrared regions are shown in Fig. 265-2.

With *scattering*, the direction of photon travel is changed. All the light returning from skin is scattered light, the majority of which has penetrated through the epidermis, been scattered by the dermis, and returned again through the epidermis. Together, scattering and absorption limit penetration of light into skin. Across the UV, visible, and near infrared regions to about 1200 nm, longer wavelengths penetrate progressively deeper into skin.

The epidermis and stratum corneum are thin layers in which, at most wavelengths, absorption by melanin and other chromophores dominates over scattering. In the UVC and UVB regions (<320 nm), absorption by proteins and, to a lesser extent, nucleic acids is dominant. Melanin and urocanic acid also contribute significantly to UVC and UVB absorption. In the UVA (320 to 400 nm), visible (400 to 720 nm), and most of the near infrared (720 to 100 nm) regions, melanin is by far the dominant epidermal chromophore. In the mid- and far-infrared (>1000 nm), water is the dominant skin chromophore, with increasingly strong absorption maxima at 970, 1190, 1450, and 2940 nm. Both melanin and water are important chromophores for lasers in dermatology.

In contrast, optics of the dermis are dominated by its scattering properties. The dermis is loaded with light-scattering collagen fibers and appears bright white when blood is removed from it. Scattering by dermal collagen varies inversely with wavelength, which accounts in part for a large increase in optical penetration into the dermis with increasing wavelength from UV through visible and near infrared wavelengths. Throughout this spectrum, normal dermis has very little light absorption other than that by blood. Because of oxyhemoglobin and hemoglobin, vessels strongly absorb UVA, blue, green, and yellow light but are surrounded by a relatively nonabsorbing connective-tissue matrix. Red and near-infrared wavelengths are not strongly absorbed by blood, and penetrate well into the living dermis. Yellow-orange laser energy is selectively deposited in microvessels of the papillary and upper reticular dermis, for treating microvascular malformations.[7,8]

In the red and near-infrared (630 to 1000 nm) part of the spectrum, a so-called window region exists in soft tissue, due to low absorption and low scattering. The ability for light at these wavelengths to penetrate millimeters through tissue makes it attractive for deep treatments, such as photodynamic therapy of tumors and semiconductor diode (800 to 1000 nm) laser, alexandrite (755 nm) laser, and Nd:YAG (1064 nm) laser treatments. All the photosensitizing drugs being developed for tumor treatment are red or near-infrared photosensitizers. In the same 630- to 1100-nm region, melanin is the major absorbing pigment. Thus, even though melanin's absorption is weaker than at shorter wavelengths (Fig. 265-2), the red and near-infrared wavelengths are ideally suited for selective photothermolysis of melanized cells, for example, with ruby

FIGURE 265-1

CHAPTER 265
Lasers in Dermatology
2903

FIGURE 265-2

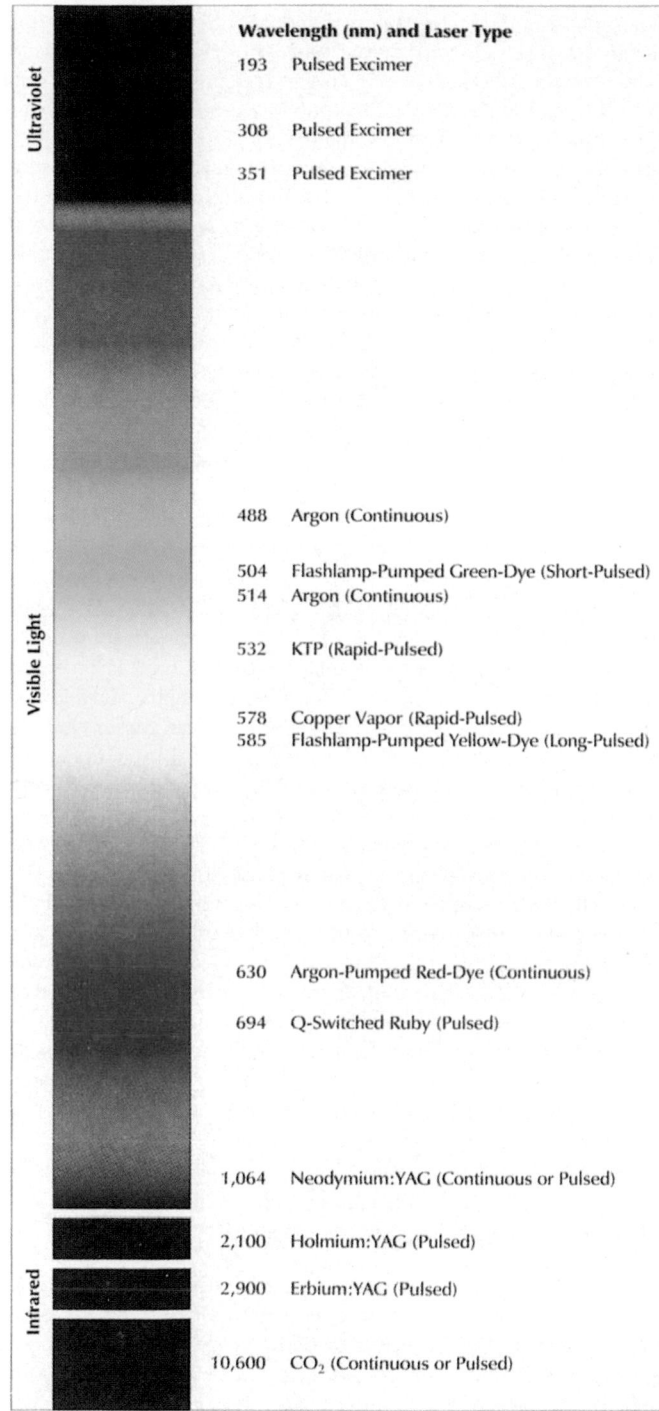

Wavelength (nm) and Laser Type

193	Pulsed Excimer
308	Pulsed Excimer
351	Pulsed Excimer
488	Argon (Continuous)
504	Flashlamp-Pumped Green-Dye (Short-Pulsed)
514	Argon (Continuous)
532	KTP (Rapid-Pulsed)
578	Copper Vapor (Rapid-Pulsed)
585	Flashlamp-Pumped Yellow-Dye (Long-Pulsed)
630	Argon-Pumped Red-Dye (Continuous)
694	Q-Switched Ruby (Pulsed)
1,064	Neodymium:YAG (Continuous or Pulsed)
2,100	Holmium:YAG (Pulsed)
2,900	Erbium:YAG (Pulsed)
10,600	CO_2 (Continuous or Pulsed)

Various medical lasers are plotted according to their wavelengths (nm) within the spectrum of electromagnetic radiation. An attractive feature of many new lasers is pulsed radiation, which permits greater precision than continuous-wave lasers. Of the ultraviolet and infrared lasers, only the CO_2 has widely accepted dermatologic uses. (*From Anderson RR: Lasers and their clinical applications, in Current Challenges in Dermatology. New York, Hospital Practice Publishing Company, Winter 1992. Reprinted with permission.*)

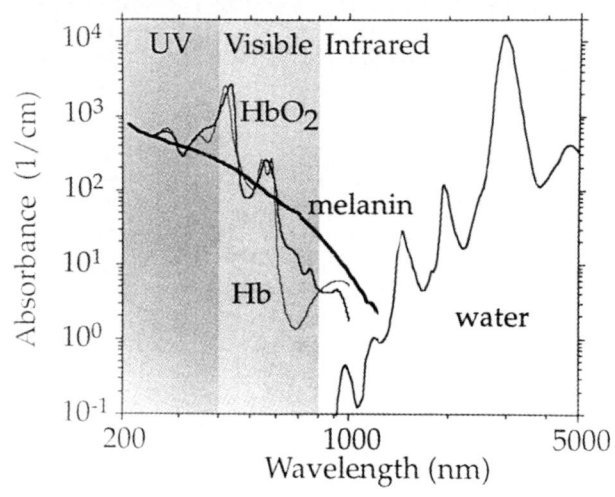

Optical absorption spectra of the major chromophores in skin. (*Courtesy of S. Prahl, PhD.*)

(694 nm), alexandrite (755 nm), or Nd:YAG (1064 nm) laser pulses. CW Nd:YAG lasers are in medical use for treatment of bulky hemangiomas.

Tattoos are an example of grossly altered dermal optics. Strongly absorbing insoluble particles of foreign inks are sequestered in dermal macrophages, fibroblasts, and mast cells. These are sites of strong optical abortion, embedded in a relatively nonabsorbing dermis. Although any tattoo may be removed (with scarring) using CO_2 laser vaporization, the Q-switched pulsed lasers used for lower-risk tattoo removal must be well absorbed by the specific color(s) of ink present. Thus, the deep-red Q-switched ruby laser removes black and green colors well, but often fails to remove red or yellow dyes. The short-pulsed green lasers (e.g., short-pulsed 510-nm dye and 532-nm Q-switched doubled Nd:YAG) remove red inks but usually not green. The near-infrared Q-switched Nd:YAG (1064 nm) removes black ink but usually not green, red, or yellow. Although this provides a nice demonstration of the Grotthus-Draper law (see below), the need for multiple laser wavelengths for proper tattoo removal is unfortunate.

LASER-SKIN INTERACTIONS

The scope of laser applications in dermatology is defined by the primary physical and chemical interactions possible and by subsequent response to these changes. As a photon is absorbed, electronic or vibrational excitation of the chromophore occurs. Planck's law states that the energy carried by a photon is inversely proportional to wavelength. Electronic excitation occurs with UV and visible-wavelength photons, which carry enough energy to promote an electron in the chromophore to a higher, potentially reactive, orbital. Thus, UV radiation can activate many different photochemical reactions, such as the different DNA photoproducts underlying UV mutagenesis and carcinogenesis. Visible light carries sufficient quantum energy for *cis-trans* isomerizations, as in vision and phototherapy of hyperbilirubinemia, and for energy transfer to create excited singlet oxygen, as in the porphyrias. Infrared radiation generally causes no photochemistry, because of its low quantum energy, but causes kinetic excitation leading directly to heat. Even though UV and visible light can activate photochemical reactions, the vast majority of energy absorbed at any wavelength winds up as heat.

Three basic modes of laser effects are possible: *photothermal* effects, which derive directly from heat; *photochemical* effects, which derive from native or photosensitizer-induced photochemical reactions triggered by UV or visible light; and *photomechanical* effects, which result from extremely rapid thermal expansion, pressure waves, shock waves, momentum transfer, or sudden vaporization occurring with pulsed-laser absorption. These three modes of laser interaction frequently coexist, but one or two usually dominate. All are important in dermatology, but photothermal effects are the mainstay of current clinical laser use.

PHOTOTHERMAL INTERACTIONS

Because of their intensity and high average powers, lasers are superb sources for radiant heating of tissue. Thermal effects on tissue are both time- and temperature-dependent. At prolonged temperatures of approximately 40 to 45°C, most cells are injured or killed by denaturation of enzymes and structural proteins. Like most diploid cells, keratinocytes and fibroblasts can mount a protective heat-shock response at these temperatures, which may enhance survival. Serum proteins in blood are coagulated at temperatures above 50 to 60°C, causing hemostasis. Above approximately 65°C, type I collagen in skin undergoes a melt (helix-coil) transition, causing irreversible coagulation and shrinkage of the connective-tissue matrix. The melting of dermal collagen causes immediate shrinkage, visible as local skin contraction, and is associated with later fibrosis and scarring. Above 100°C, tissue water is vaporized (boiled). If desiccated tissue is heated further, carbonization (charring) occurs. All of the above effects of heat on tissue are analogous to grilling a steak: the first effect is browning of the surface, due to thermal denaturation of hemoglobin and other proteins, followed by sizzling as water is vaporized, followed by shrinkage and charring.

Vaporization

Vaporization is the photothermal effect most popularly associated by patients with laser use, which provokes unnecessary anxiety when a nonablative laser procedure is to be used. Laser vaporization, especially with the CO_2 laser, is useful for precise removal of verrucae and other masses. Laser-induced incisions can be hemostatic, due to thermal coagulation at the incision margins. In skin, a thermally coagulated layer of about 50 μm appears to be sufficient for hemostasis. The extent of thermal injury to the remaining skin is a key factor, affecting both hemostasis and wound healing. In general, excessive injury is to be avoided—a deceptively simple statement that impels much of the current development of new medical laser systems.

Two factors dominantly influence laser vaporization or ablation of tissue. The first is the penetration depth for the laser radiation, which depends on wavelength. High absorption coefficients are de-

sirable for producing vaporization because the deposited energy is concentrated near the surface. The 10.6-μm CO_2 laser wavelength is absorbed by water, penetrating only about 20 μm into wet tissue. Thus, CO_2 laser energy in skin is absorbed entirely in the epidermis prior to the onset of vaporization. At 2.94 μm, absorption by water is about 10 times higher, so that energy is deposited in a layer only 1 to 2 μm thick. In addition, absorption by erbium (Er):YAG lasers at the same wavelength makes them very suitable for highly efficient tissue vaporization with minimal residual thermal damage. In the far-ultraviolet region, e.g., at the 193-nm argon-fluoride (ArF) excimer laser wavelength, penetration is less than 1 μm, due to strong absorption by peptide bonds in protein. The 193-nm excimer laser provides the most precise soft-tissue removal of any technique and is currently being used, for example, to reshape the surface of the living human cornea to correct vision. There are as yet no equivalently fine laser surgical techniques in dermatology, although excimer laser ablation of stratum corneum has been demonstrated for the purpose of topical drug delivery.

The second major factor affecting laser tissue ablation is the rate of tissue vaporization. At high temperatures, vaporization occurs suddenly, as with high-energy pulsed lasers designed for tissue removal, e.g., excimer holmium and erbium lasers. With such lasers, a thin, heated surface layer literally explodes away from the tissue, carrying with it most of the energy and leaving minimal thermal injury. In contrast, with CW or QCW lasers, vaporization occurs more slowly, and a greater fraction of the absorbed laser energy enters the underlying tissue to cause thermal injury. In addition, continued exposure of the desiccated tissue surface causes charring. Thus, a seeming paradox exists for tissue removal by lasers: at any given wavelength, higher intensity usually causes less residual tissue injury.

In practice, thermal damage from CW CO_2 laser surgery extends well into the dermis because of thermal conduction. Pulsed CO_2 lasers, which emit short pulses, or rapid scanning of a focused CW CO_2 laser beam may reduce residual thermal damage during laser vaporization surgery by limiting the time available for heat conduction before the heated tissue layer is vaporized. This is the basis for laser skin resurfacing. Using the newer generation of pulsed ablative lasers, one can perform hemostatic debridement of skin, leaving a sufficiently thin layer of thermal injury so that split-thickness grafting is not affected. Thus it is now possible to use lasers for burn, flap, or ulcer debridement.

Selective Photothermolysis

The possibility for exquisite tissue specificity is currently the most compelling reason for laser use in dermatology. The Grotthus-Draper law states that no effect of light occurs without absorption. Conversely, a million watts of laser energy can be delivered through nonabsorbing substances, including much of the skin, without causing damage. Selective photothermolysis uses a combination of selective absorption and thermal energy confinement to yield highly specific damage to pigmented microscopic structures in skin. This process was initially conceived and developed for removing vascular malformations such as PWS and telangiectases, then extended to tattoos, benign pigmented lesions, and hair follicles, all with minimal risk of scarring. The underlying principles are simple and should be familiar to anyone using or about to use a surgical laser system.

Once created within skin, heat flows from the sites of photon absorption by radiation, conduction (diffusion), or transport (such as from blood flow). Therefore, the distribution of laser heating in skin is determined not only by the depth of light penetration and its absorption sites at the particular wavelength used, but also by the time over which the light is delivered. One useful concept is that of the "thermal relaxation time," defined as the time needed for substantial cooling of a given light-absorbing site within skin. If heat is produced in an object faster than it can cool, i.e., within its thermal relaxation time, the object gets very hot relative to its environment. If heat is delivered to the object more slowly allowing it time to cool, then both the object and its surroundings get hot together. Indeed, a continuum of thermal confinement exists, ranging from objects as large as planets to as small as subcellular organelles.

Small objects cool much faster than large ones; the thermal relaxation time varies with the square of size. To a close approximation, the thermal relaxation time in seconds is equal to the object size in millimeters, squared. For example, the thermal relaxation time of a 0.5-mm leg vein is about 0.25 s; the thermal relaxation time of the 30- to 150-μm ectatic venules composing nevus flammeus is a few thousandths of a second (milliseconds); the thermal relaxation time of single cells is tens of millionths of a second (microseconds); and the thermal relaxation time of a subcellular organelle such as the melanosome is a few tenths of a millionth of a second (nanoseconds). The pulse durations shown in Table 265-1 for dermatologic lasers capable of selective photothermolysis derive directly from this logic.

Thermal relaxation is also useful in understanding why most CW lasers produce relatively widespread heat injury. For example, argon-ion laser exposures for photocoagulation of skin lesions are typically in the range of tens to hundreds of milliseconds. During this time, heat can diffuse a hundred microns or more, which is greater than the distance between most blood vessels. Thus, even though the argon laser wavelength of 488 nm is strongly and selectively absorbed by hemoglobin, the entire superficial dermis is heated by heat conduction during the laser exposure.

The biologic consequences of laser-tissue interactions are complex examples of wound healing. CO_2 and other lasers produce superficial thermal burns of skin, which heal in much the same complex manner as other burns at the same depth. Thus, preservation of sufficient follicular epithelium to allow re-formation of the epidermis is critical to healing.

However, healing of laser-induced selective thermal injury strictly *within* the skin is poorly understood and can depend critically on laser-pulse parameters. For example, pulse duration can strongly affect the extent of hemorrhage, vascular wall injury, and clinical efficacy from pulsed-dye lasers used for microvascular injury. The first experimental studies of selective photothermolysis were conducted with submicrosecond, 577-nm pulses that caused extensive hemorrhage. Clinical attempts to treat PWS with these short-pulsed dye lasers gave poor results. With submillisecond pulses ≥ 20 μm, however, hemorrhage was less and vascular wall injury somewhat greater. Greater fluence (energy per unit area) was also needed to achieve vascular injury at the longer pulse durations because thermal confinement was not as great. A pulse duration of several hundred microseconds was therefore tested, proved to be clinically effective, and is now in widespread clinical use[9] (see below). However, the theoretically ideal pulse duration for most PWS is probably in the 1- to 20-ms region. Selective laser microvascular damage involves both photocoagulation and mechanical injury, thrombosis and complement fixation, a necrotizing vasculitis, and, finally, neovascularization without scarring. However, infarction of the skin does not occur, despite the extent of microvascular compromise.

Melanin is a broad-spectrum chromophore that is also amenable to selective photothermolysis. Because melanin absorbs at all visible wavelengths, epidermal pigmentation affects yellow pulsed-dye laser treatment, even though the predominant effect is vascular. Submicrosecond pulses are necessary to rupture melanosomes, the fundamental particle containing melanin, consistent with their short thermal relaxation time. Action spectra for selective photothermolysis of pigmented epidermal cells closely follow the absorption spectrum for melanin. Rupture of epidermal melanosomes occurs at exposures from about 0.1 to 1 J/cm^2, depending on wavelength from 355 nm through 1064 nm. In normal human skin, isolated pigmented keratinocyte and melanocyte-cell necrosis ensues, followed by sloughing of the pigmented cells, epidermal depigmentation, and gradual repigmentation. In guinea pigs, follicular depigmentation leading to permanent leukotrichia occurs for wavelengths >532 nm, consistent with the deep penetration of longer wavelengths. However, laser-induced leukotrichia has not been reported in humans. Selective photothermolysis of melanized cells is useful for the treatment of benign epidermal pigmented lesions, using a Q-switched ruby laser and a short-pulsed 510-nm green dye laser. Nevus of Ota consists of scattered dermal nevus cells, and responds very well to Q-switched ruby or Nd:YAG laser treatment. Laser hair removal is also accomplished by selective melanin absorption, using very high fluence, ms-domain red and near-infrared lasers.

PHOTOMECHANICAL INTERACTIONS

Photomechanical (also called photoacoustic) injury is characterized by immediate disruption of organelles, membranes, and cells. Rapid thermal expansion, high-pressure waves, and local vaporization occur in the setting of high-energy pulsed laser absorption. In selective photothermolysis, the rate of heating can be extreme. Pulsed yellow dye laser treatment of PWS raises the vessel temperature about 100°C in 300 μs, a rate of 300,000°C per second. Mechanical injury and hemorrhage are unwanted side effects during treatment of vascular lesions or during tissue removal.

In contrast, mechanical effects are probably the major therapeutic mechanism for tattoo removal by selective photothermolysis. Tattoos consist of small insoluble ink particles phagocytosed by fixed dermal cells after injection. Q-switched ruby laser treatment raises the pigment granule temperature about 300°C in tens of nanoseconds, a heating rate of 10 billion °C per second. Explosion of the ink granules and the cells containing them appears to play a central role in removal of tattoos by selective photothermolysis.

PHOTOCHEMICAL INTERACTIONS

Classic photobiology of skin is based on photochemical reactions. Indeed, dermatology is foremost among medical specialties in its use of photochemical therapy. Lasers are useful sources for producing photochemical reactions but are not yet as cost effective as phototherapy or photochemotherapy sources. Photochemical interactions of interest to dermatology include both native photobiologic responses to UV radiation and photosensitizer-induced responses.

The major application for laser-induced photochemistry at present is photodynamic therapy of cancer, the development of which emphasizes new photosensitizing drugs rather than new laser devices. Early in this century, it was known that tumors accumulated red-fluorescent compounds, later identified as porphyrins. A derivative of hematoporphyrin synthesized by Lipson and Baldes was extensively developed by Dougherty. This compound, called dihematoporphyrin ether (DHE), is preferentially retained in solid tissue tumors following intravenous injection. DHE can be excited by 630-nm red light to produce an excited triplet state of the drug, which in turn produces singlet oxygen by collision with oxygen molecules, in the process regenerating the ground state of the DHE molecule. The terms *singlet* and *triplet* refer to differences in magnetic spin multiplicity associated with the excited electrons present. Singlet oxygen oxidizes membranes and other sites, leading to cell injury or death. Much of this chemistry is reminiscent of the effects of ionizing radiation, such as x-ray or particle beams, which also involves excited oxygen species. Unlike ionizing radiation, however, mutation is not a major effect of photodynamic therapy.

Photodynamic therapy is an experimental approach to skin cancer. Basal cell and squamous cell carcinomas have been shown to respond to systemic DHE photodynamic therapy. Conceivably, photodynamic therapy may have a role in local eradication of tumors without the induction of radiodermatitis or carcinogenesis. In the case of DHE, extremely prolonged photosensitivity to visible light is produced, which motivates development of other drugs. Other long-wavelength photosensitizers have been studied, such as phthalocyanines, rhodamines, and monoclonal antibody–directed dyes. A precursor to porphyrins, δ-aminolevulinic acid (ALA), can also be used for photodynamic therapy. Provided in excess, ALA bypasses feedback control over heme synthesis, causing cells to overproduce protoporphyrin IX. In the initial clinical study of 80 basal cell carcinomas, topical application of ALA followed by red-light exposure acutely eradicated 90 percent. Subsequent studies have confirmed these results. The efficacy of ALA photodynamic therapy for superficial basal cell and Bowen's tumors appears to be between 80 and 100 percent. A broad range of photosensitizers is under development and it is anticipated that many more compounds will be FDA-approved for systemic and topical photodynamic therapy.

Some examples of laser-skin interaction involve all of the above three classes of effects. For example, Q-switched ruby laser treatment of flesh-colored cosmetic tattoos containing iron oxide results in reduction of the iron to form black iron oxide.[10] This is a photochemical effect; however, the tattoo is removed by photomechanical and photothermal mechanisms.

LASER SAFETY

Mandatory comprehensive laser surgery certification should be obtained prior to performing any laser treatment. The principles of laser safety center around the maintenance of a safe environment and protection of the patient, surgeon, and surgical staff. Potential damage to the skin, eye, and respiratory tract, the risk of fire ignition from a direct or reflected beam, as well as the dangers of electrical malfunctions must be considered.

Biologic hazards include risks to the ocular, respiratory, and skin regions and also risk of transmission of infection. Ocular damage may result from absorption of laser light by the structures in the eye, including the retina, sclera, and cornea. The laser surgeon and staff must wear protective eyewear with an optical density (O.D.) specific for the laser wavelength. In the case of CO_2 laser light, the 10,600 nm wavelength is generally absorbed by water and therefore damage to the cornea and sclera are of greatest concern. For the patient, surgeon, and surgical staff, goggles with side shields must be worn any time the laser is in operation. Each pair of goggles should be marked with the appropriate wavelength of protection and O.D. for the specific lasers in use. Prescription glasses or clear plastic wrap-around goggles made of polycarbonate are also satisfactory when using the CO_2 and Er:YAG lasers. It is important to evaluate these goggles regularly. Check for loose fit or cracked or otherwise damaged filters. Goggles should be replaced as soon as damage is noted.

Both respiratory and infectious disease hazards are addressed by the use of vacuum smoke plume evacuators. Because the smoke plume generated by laser use may contain bacteria, viral DNA, or viable cells, potential infection from laser plume is possible.[11] All lasers used in the treatment of pigmented lesions give rise to plumes as a result of vaporization. Especially, Er:YAG lasers vaporize so efficiently that particulate matter needs to be captured efficiently. In addition, the respiration of these airborne contaminants poses significant risks; particulate matter in the smoke plume can be an irritant to respiratory mucosa. For example, breaking of disulfide bonds with hair removal lasers can lead to pungent noxious smells. Vacuum smoke evacuators with ULPA-rated (ultra low penetration air) filters are necessary. These filters should be checked and replaced on a regular basis to ensure adequate filtration. The surgeon and laser-room staff must also wear specifically designed laser filter face masks with a 0.1-μm-pore diameter during the procedure. Additionally, splatter guards (built-in or mounted on) are needed to prevent debris from flying away from the operating field.

Thermal damage to the skin from lasers can be caused by the conduction of heat from the stratum corneum to deeper layers. Because the beam penetration of the CO_2 laser is shallow, exposure to the high power intensities will generally not result in a deep-tissue burn provided that exposure time is extremely short. In order to mitigate the potential of sudden and unwarranted increases in energy output from the laser, regular calibration is suggested to avoid unnecessary injury to the skin or scarring. Vigilant attention should be paid to correct beam aim and alignment for exact irradiation of the treatment area.

The high voltage requirements for Q-switched and short-pulsed lasers can pose an electrical hazard if accidental discharge of laser power occurs. Electrical risks can persist within the laser itself even after power has been disconnected when the energy-storage capacitator may still hold a substantial charge. A high-energy xenon flashlamp source has been developed for leg vein and hair removal. The flashlamp in this source is potentially explosive and uses lethal voltages, in close proximity to the patient's skin. This source probably has the greatest potential for electrical hazard. Lasers are readily able to cause ignition of tissue, oxygen, volatile solvents such as in hair dyes and hair sprays, gauze, and clothing. The patient should be told not to use hair gel or sprays on the day of the surgery when the scalp area is the target. It is essential that treatment areas are draped with wet gauze and towels when working with the Er:YAG and CO_2 lasers. A basin of water should also be available in case skin, hair, gauze, or drapes catch fire. Drapes should be moistened repeatedly throughout the surgery. Alcohol or flammable skin preparations are prohibited.

Careful attention to safety procedures can significantly minimize potential biologic, electrical, and fire hazards that may accompany laser surgery.

CHAPTER 265
Lasers in Dermatology

2907

LASER TREATMENT OF VASCULAR LESIONS

Port-Wine Stain

The PWS, or nevus flammeus, is a congenital malformation of dermal microvasculature present in 0.3 to 0.5 percent of newborns, which persists throughout life. PWS must be differentiated from hemangiomata, which are common, proliferative vascular lesions occurring with higher incidence but regressing during childhood. In addition, "stork bite" (occipital) or "angel's kiss" (glabellar) telangiectatic midline lesions occur in the majority of newborns. When these persist into later life, they are occasionally referred to as port-wine stains. Unlike PWS, these common lesions fade or regress with time and therefore appear to have a different etiology from PWS.

PWSs have commanded the interest of dermatologists and plastic surgeons because of an often dramatic cosmetic appearance, refractoriness to a variety of treatments, and occasional associations with other underlying syndromes. Approximately 5 percent of PWSs occur in conjunction with vascular defects in the meninges and central nervous system (CNS) with resultant seizures, mental retardation, and/or glaucoma: the Sturge-Weber syndrome. A PWS over an extremity with associated hypertrophy is known as the Klippel-Trénaunay-Weber syndrome.

PWSs range in color from light pink to dark purple and may occur anywhere on the body, with the majority occurring on the face. The histology of PWS reveals an increased number of superficial or superficial and deep ectatic venules compared with normal skin, typically without fibrosis or other abnormality. PWSs darken progressively with age, from pink to red to deep violet, frequently with progressive hypertrophy. The darkening correlates with progressive vessel ectasia and an increase in vessel diameter but not in vessel number. Thus, PWSs are vascular malformations and, unlike hemangiomas, do not actively proliferate but rather progressively dilate.

Treatments of PWS, other than cosmetic camouflage, have relied on destructive methods, which achieve lightening and/or flattening of the lesions, at the risk of surgical disfigurement. These methods include skin grafting, ionizing radiation, cryosurgery, tattooing, dermabrasion, and a variety of laser treatments. At present, lasers clearly offer the treatment of choice. Absorption of blue, green, and yellow light by hemoglobin allows PWSs to be effectively treated with a range of lasers. Different wavelengths have been used for treating nevus flammeus varying from 488 nm (argon) to 532 nm (KTP, frequency-doubled Q-switched Nd:YAG), 568 nm (krypton), 578 nm Cu-vapor/Cu-bromide, 577 to 600 nm (pulsed dye). The disadvantages of shorter wavelengths are their superficial absorption and strong competition with melanin. In addition, a wide range of pulse durations have been tried: from 10 ns (fre-quency-doubled Q-switched Nd:YAG), 450 μs to 1.5 ms (pulsed dye), 5 to 50 ms (KTP, Nd:YAG) to pseudo-CW (Cu-vapor/bromide) to continuous wave (argon-pumped dye, argon). The ideal pulse duration for most PWSs is probably in the 1- to 20-ms range.

The current state of the art is such that children with PWSs are best treated with pulsed dye lasers (585 to 595 nm; 0.4 to 1.5 ms) specifically designed to produce selective photothermolysis of their dermal vessels. Clearing of PWSs can now be achieved by this technique with a low risk of scarring, even in neonates (Fig. 265-3). However, resistant PWS after multiple pulsed dye laser treatments and hypertrophic lesions should be treated by using longer pulsed dye laser (1.5 ms) with cooling of the epidermis or by very cautious treatment with pseudo-CW or CW (copper vapor, KTP, or argon) lasers. PWS should ideally be corrected during infancy or early childhood, when many of the social and psychological consequences of disfigurement can be avoided and the lesions are both smaller and not yet hypertrophic.

In the initial clinical trial, a 577-nm, 300-μs laser producing fluences up to 5 J/cm^2 was used to treat 10 adult patients in PWS test sites. The sites were treated at 1.5$\times$ and 2$\times$, the threshold fluence for causing purpura evident within minutes of exposure. All sites treated at 2$\times$ the purpura dose cleared within 6 weeks, and no scarring was seen. Histologically, epidermal melanocytes and keratinocytes were undamaged, but PWS vessels contained masses of agglutinated erythrocytes with damaged endothelial cells and perivascular collagen. At 24 h, a marked polymorphonuclear leukocyte inflammatory response was noted, mimicking necrotizing vasculitis. A larger study in adults confirmed that a pulse width of 360 μs was superior to a pulsewidth of 20 μs; 52 patients were treated, with 44 percent noted to have greater than 75 percent lightening. No hypertrophic scarring was noted, but small areas of hypopigmentation, epidermal change, or cutaneous depression developed in four patients.

In the first trial of pulsed dye laser for pediatric PWSs, 35 children aged 3 months to 14 years were treated with 577 nm, 360 μs, 1.5$\times$ to 2$\times$ purpura threshold.[12] Total clearing after a mean of 6.5 treatments was reported in 94 percent of children regardless of age, site, or lesion color. Two children (6 percent) had superficial depressed scars, reportedly after traumatizing the areas within 24 h of laser treatment. In this study, 57 percent had transient hyperpig-

FIGURE 265-3

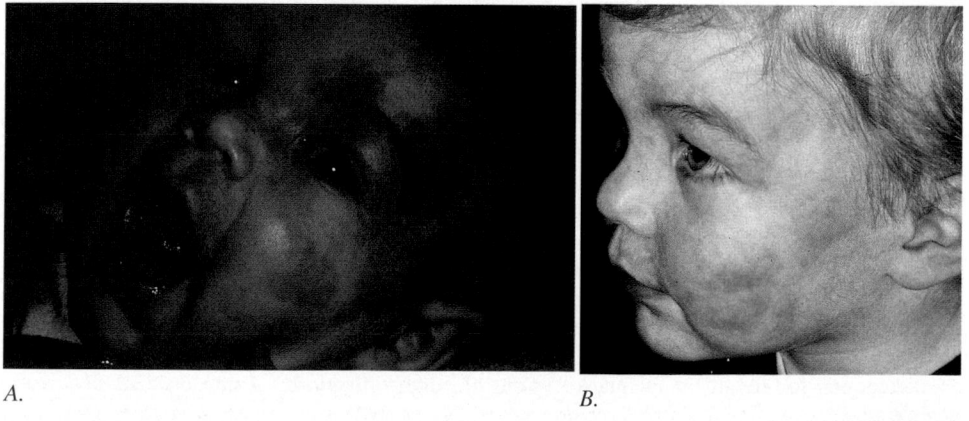

A.　　　　　　　　　　　　　　　　　　　　*B.*

Port-wine stain before (*A*) and after (*B*) six treatments with the pulsed dye laser.

mentation, which cleared in all after 4 months. Although in this study early treatment was advocated to be more beneficial, it is now clear that a favorable response is not age-dependent, as demonstrated in a more recent large clinical trial by Van der Horst et al.[13]

To date, the pulsed dye laser at a wavelength ranging from 577 to 595 nm, with a 450-μs to 1.5-ms pulsewidth, delivering a fluence of between 3 and 10 J/cm^2 (depending on spot size) in contiguous, minimally overlapping 3- to 10-mm exposure spots, is the most efficacious and least scarring method for treatment of pediatric PWSs and most adult PWSs. It appears that this treatment, when performed early in life, arrests the hypertrophy often associated with maturing PWS and prevents significant psychological trauma. Therefore, it is recommended that treatments take place before school age to minimize stigma and prevent future hypertrophy. General anesthesia should be considered in a number of these infants and young children to minimize the risk of eye injury and pain associated with the multiple treatments.[14] However, it is likely that some apparently removed PWSs may recur years after laser treatment. Although transient side effects from proper laser treatment of PWSs are not uncommon, permanent side effects such as depigmentation and scarring are rare.

Strawberry Hemangioma

This lesion, also known as capillary hemangioma of infancy or juvenile hemangioma, is a common lesion of infancy, occurring in up to 2.6 percent of newborns. Histologically, there are dense collections of thin-walled vessels interspersed with sheets of vascular endothelial cells. The number of mast cells is greatly increased, which may play a role in the growth and/or involution of the lesions. The lesions may be apparent at birth, or more commonly in the weeks after birth, starting as a pale macule or group of telangiectatic vessels, and gradually developing into a bright-red or purple nodular mass. The natural history of these lesions is one of more or less rapid growth followed by spontaneous regression in approximately 50 percent of cases within 5 years, regression of 70 percent by 7 years, and eventual regression of 90 percent or more. Ulceration may occur, particularly with trauma during the rapid growth phase. Impairment of visual or respiratory function occurs occasionally due to mass effect, necessitating treatment. Platelet sequestration and sudden-onset coagulopathy with life-threatening disseminated intravascular coagulation may occur; this is known as the Kasabach-Merritt syndrome. Residual cosmetic defects are common and include wrinkled or atrophic skin with hypopigmentation and/or telangiectases.

Because of the usually benign nature of the lesions and the natural course of spontaneous involution, conservative management has been advocated for the majority of these lesions. The specific aims of laser treatment of hemangiomas involve prevention of scarring and infection as a result of ulceration or skin alteration after involution. An additional component of treatment is to provide relief of psychological trauma to both the patient and the family. Although laser treatment of hemangiomas is highly effective for the superficial component, it is nonetheless important to refrain from treating the hemangiomas that present with a more positive prognosis without therapy.

Indications for treatment include recurrent bleeding; infection; ulceration; obstruction of vital structures involved in respiration, vision, and feeding; and extreme familial or patient distress. Treatment methods such as surgery, ionizing radiation, and oral or intra-

lesional steroids have all been associated with scarring. It seems likely that specific medical treatment of hemangiomas will be possible when the events triggering spontaneous involution are understood. Until then, lasers, and especially selective photothermolysis, appear to have a role in the treatment of selected cases.

Because of the success of the 585-nm pulsed dye laser in treating PWSs in children, this laser is used to treat capillary hemangiomas in infancy—either macular or enlarging ulcerated lesions. Almost total lightening leading to normal skin texture and color were reported by Glassberg et al.[15]; a study of 10 children also reported significant lightening of lesions after an average of three treatments. Ulcerated hemangiomas in children have also been reported to heal completely after one to three treatments with a 585-nm pulsed dye laser. However, large controlled trials are lacking at this point. When indicated, selective photothermolysis with pulsed dye laser appears to be effective as an adjunct for limiting the growth phase and has very few complications.

The CW Nd:YAG laser, emitting in the deeply penetrating, near-infrared spectrum at 1060 nm, has also been used on thick hemangiomas and arteriovenous malformations. In the largest study to date, Achauer and van der Kam used the Nd:YAG laser in 25 children with bulky lesions, and analyzed results based on stratifying the lesions by size and height.[16] Seventy-two percent of cases were graded as good-to-excellent response. It was concluded that although the continuous Nd:YAG laser has a significant incidence of side effects, it may be a useful tool in treating bulkier lesions. Photodynamic therapy might offer benefits as well, but is still experimental.

Other Vascular Lesions

A great variety of vascular skin lesions have been treated with the different lasers available. In general, CW argon, CO$_2$, Nd:YAG, KTP, copper vapor/bromide, and krypton lasers provide useful tools for controlled destruction of lesions; the 585-nm pulsed dye lasers offer a somewhat more selective option. Pyogenic granulomas respond to pulsed dye lasers, usually in multiple treatments. Poikiloderma of Civatte responds well to pulsed dye laser, but caution has to be exercised due to the higher incidence of side effects such as hypopigmentation and scarring on neck and chest with any laser system. Cherry angiomas also typically respond well in one or two treatments to various lasers. The vascular component of acne rosacea responds to pulsed dye laser and various CW lasers. Venous lakes, common acquired malformations on the lips, oral mucosa, and ears respond to treatment with copper vapor and pulsed dye lasers. Angiokeratomas and Kaposi's sarcoma have been reported to respond to pulsed dye laser treatment. Adenoma sebaceum for tuberous sclerosis has also been treated successfully with a combination of CO$_2$ and vascular lasers.

Probably the lesions most commonly treated with lasers are essential telangiectasias on the face in adults and spider angiomas in children and young adults. Pulsed dye and copper vapor lasers have been used successfully in a variety of techniques.[17]

Phlebectasias (spider veins) on the legs are extremely common, cosmetically significant lesions that arise from a combination of hormonal, familial, and circulatory factors. By far the most common and successful approach to leg phlebectasias is sclerotherapy. Some vessels are too small or tortuous for injection, however. Attempts to use lasers have met with partial success, hampered by a high incidence of posttreatment hyper- and hypopigmentation. Intense light sources such as the nonlaser flashlamp device have been reported to have some success with treatment of leg veins as well as longer pulsed dye and alexandrite lasers used in conjunction with epidermal cooling. More promising is the use of longer-wavelength (800 to 1100 nm) lasers at longer pulses (5 to 50 ms) due to their relative lack of side effects. A high-power 800-nm diode laser array device with cold-sapphire contact cooling handpiece is now approved for leg vein treatment and hair removal. The successful treatment of atrophic erythematous acne scars and sternotomy scars have been reported using multiple pulsed dye laser treatments alone or combined with intralesional steroid injections. Striae rubra and alba have been treated using the pulsed dye laser with marginal success at this point. Originally, because of the increase in capillary loops in verruca vulgaris, the pulsed dye laser was advocated for the treatment of these viral lesions. Despite initial enthusiastic reports, it is now clear that this treatment is based mainly on nonspecific thermal destruction, but remains a good alternative treatment for lesions resistant to liquid nitrogen. Similarly, the increase of capillaries in the papillary tips as seen in psoriasis has led to the use of the pulsed dye laser for plaque-type psoriasis, with positive results in several studies.

LASER TREATMENT OF PIGMENTED LESIONS

Before the advent of lasers, treatment modalities for pigment abnormalities included benign neglect, surgical excision, dermabrasion and salabrasion, electrodesiccation/fulguration, chemical bleaching, or peeling. These treatments sometimes carry the unwanted side effect of potential scarring or undesired pigmentation changes. Pigment-specific lasers and the newer generation of mid- and far-infrared lasers have emerged in the past decade and have provided a treatment method with a very low risk of side effects for patients with cutaneous pigmentation.

Thus far, a variety of pigmented lesions have been treated with laser, and case reports of successful treatment of rarer pigmented disorders are common. However, controversies still surround the laser treatment of nevomelanocytic lesions, especially congenital and dysplastic nevi.

Superficial pigmented lesions such as lentigines, ephelides, and seborrheic keratoses respond to a variety of pulsed and CW lasers. The most commonly used pulsed lasers are the frequency-doubled Q-switched Nd:YAG at 532 nm, the Q-switched ruby laser (694 nm), alexandrite, and the pulsed dye green laser (510 nm). All these lasers are very effective, and with the exception of the green wavelength lasers causing more purpura, the side effect profiles are similar.[18] However, hypo- or depigmentation appears to be more commonly seen with the Q-switched ruby than with Q-switched alexandrite lasers and the Q-switched Nd:YAG laser. Recurrence of completely treated lentigines and ephelides is uncommon.

All dermatologic lasers are capable of effectively treating simple lentigines. The Q-switched Nd:YAG at 532 nm (2 to 5 J/cm², 3.0-mm spot) or the pulsed dye green at 510 nm (2 to 4 J/cm²) should be considered the first choice for lentigines, especially for non-facial locations (Fig. 265-4).[19] Their relative lack of potential for creating hypopigmentation make them an ideal tool for treating truncal and limb lentigines and flat sebor-

rheic keratoses. The Q-switched ruby (694 nm) and alexandrite (755 nm) lasers are excellent for facial use at fluences between 5 and 7 J/cm² depending on the skin type. In general, lower initial fluences are chosen for darker-complected individuals than for fair-complected patients because postinflammatory hyperpigmentation is more common at higher fluences. The pulsed Er:YAG at 2.94 μm (typical fluence, 0.5 to 0.8 J/cm²) and 60-μs CO$_2$ laser (fluence, 0.25 to 0.4 J/cm²) can be utilized safely as well.[20] Also, a filtered xenon flashlamp has been reported to clear superficial pigmented lesions. CW lasers such as the krypton (520 nm), copper vapor (510 nm), KTP (532 nm), CW dye (504 to 690 nm), and argon (488 to 514 nm) lasers are reasonable alternatives in skilled hands.

Café au lait macules (CALMs) are macular pigmented lesions of varying sizes present in 10 percent of the normal population and can be seen in association with neurocutaneous syndromes such as neurofibromatosis, McCune-Albright syndrome, and tuberous sclerosis. As a sporadic occurrence, they are most commonly found as isolated lesions resulting from increased melanin pigmentation in the skin of healthy individuals. Multiple lesions are especially common in neurofibromatosis of Recklinghausen (NF type 1). Theoretically, CALMs are good candidates for treatment with Q-switched lasers, since submicrosecond laser pulses interact selectively with melanized cells. The target is melanosomes in melanocytes and in keratinocytes, which are of appropriate size and process the appropriate thermal relaxation time for the nanosecond-pulse domain generated with the Q-switched ruby and Q-switched Nd:YAG lasers. In general, treatment with Q-switched lasers does not consistently yield successful results. In adults, complete or partial clearance followed by recurrence appears to be the rule. In some cases, hyperpigmentation may occur and may persist. Three mechanisms may be of importance in the repigmentation of CALM: (1) the melanocyte-keratinocyte melanosome transfer may be temporarily impaired; (2) the pigmented keratinocytes are destroyed and it may take some time before these are replaced; and (3) melanocytes themselves may be damaged or destroyed by the laser, which is followed by a sufficient repopulation of the melanocyte stock. Probably a combination of the mechanisms mentioned above are active.[21]

FIGURE 265-4

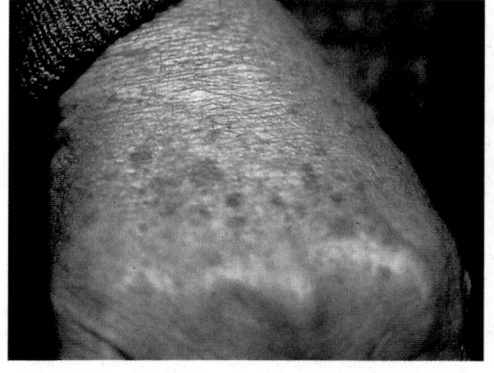 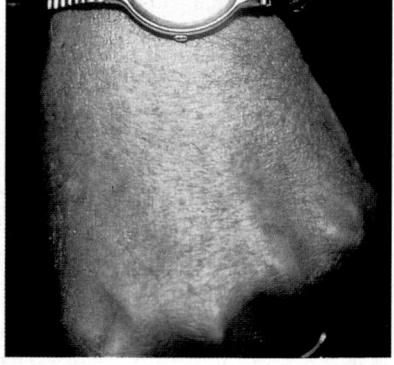

A.   *B.*

Solar lentigines on dorsal hands before (*A*) and after (*B*) treatment with Q-switched Nd:YAG 532-nm laser.

POSTINFLAMMATORY HYPERPIGMENTATION

Treatment by lasers of postinflammatory pigmentation has been disappointing so far. The trauma induced by a laser can itself evoke a hyperpigmentation response in susceptible individuals.[19] Treatment of dark infraorbital circles with the Q-switched ruby laser has been moderately successful. Melanin, hemosiderin, or a combination of both are found in biopsy specimens. Sporadic cases of successful treatment for minocycline-induced hyperpigmentation have been reported.[22] Based on good experiences with treating minocycline pigmentation, other forms of persistent drug-induced hyperpigmentation deserve a test site with a red or near-infrared, pigment-specific laser (e.g., Q-switched ruby or alexandrite) to assess a potential favorable response.

MELASMA

Treatment of melasma centers around the following: sun avoidance, topical retinoids, sunscreens, hydroquinone or other bleaching agents, and time. Superficial, medium, and deep chemical peels (including glycolic acid peels) can be used on lightly complected patients. This treatment option, however, should be used cautiously with dark-skinned individuals. All these treatments for melasma yield mixed results.[23]

Taylor and Anderson assessed the efficacy of Q-switched ruby laser treatment of melasma. Regardless of fluence used, no permanent improvement was observed.[24] In some patients, darkening was noted after laser treatment. No textural changes were seen after healing except for a slight depression at high fluences on black patients. Epidermal and dermal injury was noted immediately after treatment. After several months, epidermal pigmentation returned to base line and dermal macrophages were focally increased.

Since it is most predominant in facial distribution, melasma can be safely treated with a number of pigment-specific and ablative lasers. However, recurrence is the rule, and retreatment on a regular basis is necessary; given the expense and risk for side effects, laser treatment of melasma cannot be generally recommended. When attempted, this should be supported by vigorous use of hydroquinones and broad-spectrum sunscreens. Repeated glycolic acid or Jessner's peeling is helpful as well. Caution should be exercised with darker skin phototypes (IV and higher), since pigment darkening has been observed in several cases.

TATTOOS

Previous treatment methods include excision, dermabrasion, salabrasion, chemical removal, infrared coagulation, cryosurgery, a chemo-laser technique, CO_2 laser vaporization, argon laser, and normal-mode ruby laser pulses. These methods cause either vaporization or necrosis of the epidermis and upper dermis, followed by elimination of tattoo ink, reepithelialization, and typically, some form of scarring.

Q-switched lasers can now be used to remove tattoos with little risk of scarring. Ironically, the development of this new treatment method may have induced an increase in the acquisition of tattoos, since laser treatment is often viewed as the miracle cure (which it is not). The Q-switched ruby laser was initially tested by Leon Goldman and later by Reid et al. for tattoo removal.[25] In a study of amateur and professional tattoos, Taylor et al.[26] showed increased effectiveness at higher fluences up to 6 J/cm². In a prospective study of over 200 tattoos treated with Q-switched ruby laser, amateur tattoos cleared after an average of 4 to 6 treatments at fluences of 4 to 10 J/cm² at treatment intervals of 3 to 4 weeks; in contrast, professional tattoos (including red, green, and bright colors) need an average of 6 to 10 treatments at 8 to 10 J/cm². Common side effects included inflammation, blistering, and transient crusting for up to 2 weeks. Transient hypo- or hyperpigmentation lasting months occurred in up to 50 percent of patients, and transient textural changes were seen in a majority of cases. Permanent textural changes remained in less than 5 percent of patients and hypertrophic scarring was rare, about 0.5 percent of cases. The Q-switched alexandrite laser (50 to 100 ns) can also be used satisfactorily to treat tattoos as was demonstrated by Fitzpatrick et al.,[27] Alster and Williams,[28] and Zelickson et al.[29] The Q-switched alexandrite laser appears to cause less hypopigmentation than the Q-switched ruby laser, but usually requires a few more treatments before clearing is achieved than does the Q-switched ruby and Q-switched Nd:YAG lasers.

A Q-switched Nd:YAG laser at 1064 nm was compared with a Q-switched ruby laser and found to be equally effective for removing black inks when used at equal fluence, but with less epidermal injury and no hypopigmentation. In addition, professional tattoos resistant to a Q-switched ruby laser were shown to respond to subsequent treatment with the more penetrating Q-switched Nd:YAG laser. However, unlike the ruby laser, which is partially effective, the Nd:YAG laser at 1064 nm proved totally ineffective for green inks. Polymer dye technology incorporating handpieces to shift wavelengths are now used in conjunction with Nd:YAG lasers to treat different colors. It is apparent that multiple-wavelength, short-pulse laser systems are needed for removal of the multiple tattoo ink colors. The mechanism of tattoo ink removal by selective photothermolysis is not entirely understood but probably involves a combination of transepidermal elimination, physical alteration of ink granules, transport by phagocytic cells or lymphatics, and possibly an alteration of the dermal stroma. Some tattoos that are "removed" by Q-switched ruby laser treatment still show some dermal pigment granules histologically. Green inks can be particularly difficult to remove. Q-switched ruby and Q-switched Nd:YAG lasers have been used successfully in a minority of cases. Red ink can successfully be removed with a Q-switched Nd:YAG 532-nm laser. Newer fluorescent colors of unclear mixtures can often resist treatment. Flesh-toned tattoos can darken on treatment with a Q-switched laser. A reduction reaction at temperatures exceeding 1400°C from Fe^{3+} to Fe^{2+} might be responsible for this unwanted color change. A test site with a single pulse is recommended with a follow-up visit 2 weeks later to assess the outcome. A similar unusual physicochemical reaction has been reported as localized chrysiasis after Q-switched ruby laser treatment. It was postulated that dermal gold deposits in a patient taking oral gold were altered from a crystalline form to elemental gold (resembling colloidal gold, which has as a blue-purple color). Traumatic tattoos usually contain even less pigment granules than amateur tattoos. Fewer treatments (two to four) are necessary to achieve excellent clearing in most cases. Both Q-switched Nd:YAG and Q-switched ruby lasers have been reported to be effective (Fig. 265-5).

Many treatment methods for tattoos and pigmented lesions for patients with Fitzpatrick skin phototypes V and VI hold a larger potential for complication due to the increased incidence of adverse pigmentary change and keloidal scarring.[23] Q-switched Nd:YAG lasers at 1064 nm are used for darker complected individuals, and Q-switched ruby lasers and alexandrite lasers for fair-complected skin. For green colors, only ruby and alexandrite lasers can occasionally achieve successful clearing. The Q-switched Nd:YAG 532 nm and pulsed dye green laser at 510 nm can be used to treat red and orange colors. Resistant tattoos can be treated with superficially ablative CO_2 lasers such as the TruPulse (Tissue Technologies, Alburquerque, NM) and erbium:YAG. For flesh-toned tattoos, a single pulse test site is advised, with patient returning 2 weeks later for evaluation of the amount of pigment darkening. Traumatic tattoos respond to fluences ranging from 5 to 8 J/cm^2 with Q-switched ruby, Q-switched alexandrite and Q-switched Nd:YAG lasers; fewer treatments (2 to 4) than with regular amateur (4 to 8) or professional (6 to 12) are usually necessary for these accidentally acquired tattoos.

FIGURE 265-5

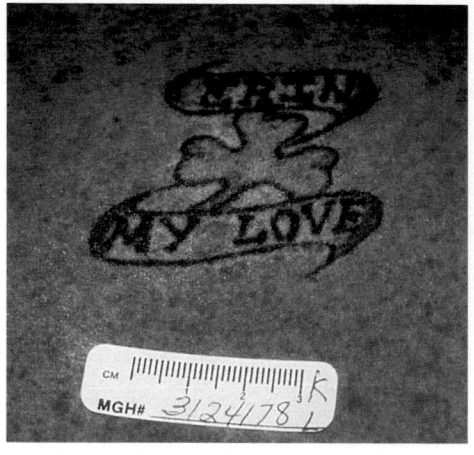 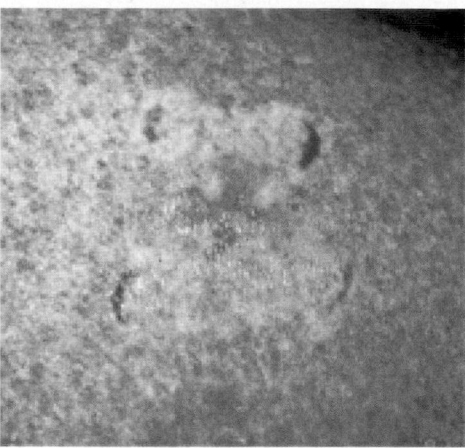

A.   B.

Professional tattoo before (A) and after (B) Q-switched ruby laser treatment. Note resistant green and red colors and mild hypopigmentation.

NEVUS OF OTA, ITO, AND MONGOLIAN SPOT

Prior to the advent of lasers to treat dermal melanocytoses such as nevus of Ota, no effective noninvasive treatment, excluding application of opaque cosmetics, existed. Lasers have provided an optimal and preferential treatment method. In the past 7 years, numerous studies have investigated the use of the Q-switched ruby, Q-switched Nd:YAG 1064 nm, and Q-switched alexandrite lasers to treat these lesions. The Q-switched ruby laser is capable of producing short high-energy pulses and can selectively target cells containing pigments, specifically dermal melanocytes.[26,30] The Q-switched ruby laser became the treatment of choice in the early 1990s. Now satisfactory results can also be obtained with the Q-switched Nd:YAG 1064 and Q-switched alexandrite lasers.[28] Treatment fluences range from 5 to 10 J/cm^2 depending on location and number of treatments, which can exceed 10 for extensive and resistant lesions.

NEVOMELANOCYTIC LESIONS

Q-switched laser treatment of benign pigmented lesions has a low potential for scarring and this has naturally led to an interest in treating nevi with this method. Organelle-specific damage occurs due to selective absorption of high-energy, nanosecond, laser pulses. Selective photothermolysis of melanosomes involves high local temperature gradients leading to melanosome fracture. Melanocyte lethality in vivo correlates with melanosome fracture, and cultured melanocyte lethality is associated with high-pressure acoustic waves. Thus, a combination of microthermal and thermally initiated mechanical injury appears to underlie the biologic effects.

When medically indicated, the current treatment of choice for removing nevi is surgical excision. In the majority of cases, removal of these lesions can be achieved with good lateral margin control. Histologic examination of the tissue may sometimes reveal unexpected cellular atypia.

Because some congenital nevi occur in cosmetically sensitive areas, where a surgical scar might be very noticeable following excision, nonscarring Q-switched lasers have been used for treatment.[31] It is unclear at present whether congenital nevi can be removed entirely by lasers that follow the principle of selective photothermolysis. Although a theoretical concern exists regarding potential "activation" of congenital nevi by selective photothermolysis, there is no clear evidence that laser treatment either increases or decreases the risk of malignant transformation.

Prophylactic removal is often recommended before adolescence for small lesions and in early childhood for giant ones. Despite scarring, surgical excision is still considered the best option once the decision for removal is made. Dermabrasion will often lead to recurrence of the deeper component, and a worse cosmetic result than careful excision. CW lasers such as the argon (488 nm), CO_2 (10,600 nm), and the non-Q-switched ruby (694 nm) lasers have been used in the past to coagulate and/or ablate nevomelanocytic lesions, including congenital nevi. In general, CO_2 laser ablation causes greater scarring than a well-executed surgical excision, and occasional pseudomelanoma can be seen. Pseudomelanoma is a term used by some authors to define atypicality of cells after partial excision and subsequent recurrence. With the emergence of pulsed red and near-infrared lasers and their capability for removing pigmented lesions in a nonscarring fashion, however, it is prudent to reevaluate the efficacy and safety of this treatment method for congenital nevi.

Like the deep melanophages seen in nevus of Ota, congenital nevi also contain deep dermal pigment, mostly in nevomelanocytes.

The Q-switched Nd:YAG laser at 1064 nm has an even deeper penetrating potential, and therefore might be even more suited for treating deep dermal pigmented lesions. Both lasers are now in wide clinical use, and treatment of congenital nevi has been described with Q-switched ruby laser. However, partial effectiveness and recurrence even after multiple treatments was reported by Waldorf et al.[32]

If it is deemed appropriate to treat a congenital nevus, a biopsy is recommended to assess the depth of the nevus cells. This depth is a reliable indicator to evaluate whether total destruction of the nevomelanocytic nests can be achieved. If nests are present beyond 1.0 mm, complete destruction by the Q-switched lasers will not likely occur even with consecutive repetitive treatments. The lasers of promise at present are the long-pulse ruby and long-pulse alexandrite lasers. These will achieve destruction to a depth of 3 to 5 mm. The choice of fluence for the Q-switched lasers should be in the high range (7 to 10 J/cm^2). With appropriate cooling of the epidermis the fluence used with the long-pulse lasers can be from 20 to 80 J/cm^2. Meticulous follow-up of the patients on a yearly basis is mandatory.

The development of melanoma is a discernible risk in patients with atypical (dysplastic) melanocytic nevi. Although not known exactly, the risk for developing melanoma in these lesions is thought to be considerable, depending on the personal and family history of melanoma, total number of nevi, skin type, and lifetime sun exposure. Debate is ongoing as to whether these lesions should be removed prophylactically or followed clinically. Van Leeuwen et al. reported a poor response to three treatments (2-month intervals) using a 50-ns Q-switched alexandrite laser in 55 lesions comparing common nevi with dysplastic nevi.[33] A study by Duke et al. suggested that currently lasers should not be used in the treatment of atypical nevi.[34]

Small nevi can be of cosmetic concern to some persons. The most common treatment methods are elliptical excision or deep saucerization by tangential excision. Unfortunately, this often causes scarring or permanent hypopigmentation. Prior to the advent of the pigment-specific lasers, CW argon laser treatment was successful. Q-switched ruby laser pulses appear to be effective for the removal of small junctional nevomelanocytic nevi. The treatment is brief and well tolerated and requires no anesthesia. Multiple lesions can be treated in a short time. Postoperative care is minimal and a low risk of scarring exists. Treatment failure may be related to inaccurate clinical assessment of pigment depth and reflects the heterogeneity of the population of clinically flat nevomelanocytic nevi, which may represent junctional nevi, flat compound nevi, or lentigo. If the depth of nevomelanocytic nests could be accurately established, a reliable prediction of outcome could be made for all lesions. Shielding by superficial pigmented cells might prevent penetration of the ruby laser light to deeper layers. Possible deleterious long-term effects of laser-induced changes on the remaining nevomelanocytes deserve consideration. In addition, small nevomelanocytic nevi are not thought to carry an intrinsically higher potential for the development of melanoma when compared to large congenital nevomelanocytic nevi.

The long-pulsed ruby and alexandrite lasers might be more effective in the destruction of nevomelanocytic nests, and at depths beyond that observed with the Q-switched ruby laser. In one report, Ueda found complete or nearly complete clearing of large congenital nevi in Asians with long-pulse ruby laser pulses.[35] When the nature or degree of atypicality of a small nevomelanocytic lesion is in doubt, biopsy or excision by conventional methods is indicated

before treatment. If a nevomelanocytic lesion recurs after laser treatment, a biopsy or total excision can be considered.[36]

BECKER'S NEVUS

The color of these lesions may vary from tan to dark brown. They are well demarcated from the normal skin, and range from a few to several hundred square centimeters in diameter. Following onset, a Becker's nevus is likely to grow slowly for a few years producing black terminal hairs that are typical for this lesion. In some cases the color will become lighter with age. Three distinctive types have been described: the melanotic type, the hypertrichotic type, and the mixed type.

Since patients often present with two complaints about their Becker's nevus, hyperpigmentation and hypertrichosis, an ideal laser treatment should be geared toward removing both. With the Q-switched lasers, satisfactory results are not easily obtained. In a small cohort of patients, a variable response was observed. Mottled hypopigmentation, incomplete response, and recurrence were frequent. Decreased hair growth is seen after Q-switched laser treatment, but this effect appears to be of brief duration. In contrast, long-lasting hair removal has been seen after treatment with high fluence, 3-ms ruby laser pulses (40 to 60 J/cm^2). The recurrence can be explained on the basis of the depth of the hair follicle with its pigmented keratinocytes and melanocytes containing larger melanosomes. These act as a reservoir for repigmentation. Interestingly, the long-pulse ruby and Q-switched ruby laser appear to be a perfect match for the treatment of Becker's nevus.

NEVUS SPILUS

Nevus spilus presents as a circumscribed tan-colored macule containing smaller darkly pigmented macules or small papules. The term comes from the Greek word for "spot": spilos. Usually not evident in newborns, nevus spilus typically develop in early childhood. They can appear anywhere on the skin; however, a clear preference can be noted for locations on the chest, back, and extremities. Sizes usually range from 1 to 10 cm in diameter although much larger lesions do exist. The distribution is localized, and sometimes segmental lesions can occur. At first presentation, the dark melanocytic spots are clearly visible. New spots are likely to emerge subsequently.

In theory, the superficial pigment found in nevus spilus provides an excellent chromophore for the laser, and nevus spilus should therefore respond well to treatment.[14] In our opinion, for semantic purposes, a nevus spilus should be considered a combination of a CALM with junctional nevi. Comparable to that of a CALM, the location of the pigment in the macular tan portion of the nevus spilus exists in the epidermis and specifically in the basal cell layer. The location of pigment in the portion of the nevus spilus that contains the small nevi is both in the epidermis and superficial dermis. Careful follow-up is necessary, however, since melanoma has been reported to occur in nevus spilus.

EPIDERMAL NEVI

Epidermal nevi occur in 1:1000 live births and are pigmented hamartomas characterized by hyperplasias of normal epidermal and/or adnexal structures. They are examples of genetic mosaicism, and classification is based on morphology, distribution, and the predominant structure of differentiation. Epidermal nevi may occur with or without extracutaneous defects. Systemic anomalies are more common if the epidermal nevus is extensive. The systems most often involved are ocular (9 to 30 percent), central nervous (15 to 70 percent), and urologic. Their clinical appearance is usually linear, grouped, or in whorls following Blaschko's lines. Consistency may be soft, velvety, or keratotic, and pigmentation is also variable. Malignant changes may also occur rarely with epidermal nevi, most commonly after puberty and especially with nevus sebaceous.

Therapeutic results for verrucous epidermal nevi have been variable. Topical methods have temporary results at best and oral retinoids, although reported to be successful for generalized lesions, are impractical for long-term use because of their toxicity.[37] Surgery by excision, dermabrasion, or grafting have the inherent risk of hypertrophic scarring.[38] Recurrences plague most therapeutic alternatives. The options further narrow for extensive lesions, in which staged treatments are necessary. Reports of successful laser therapy have included the argon (488 to 514 nm) and CO_2 (10,600 nm) lasers in CW modes. In addition, the flashlamp-pumped pulsed dye laser (585 nm) may be useful in the inflammatory linear verrucous epidermal nevus (ILVEN) variant.

Specific clinical characteristics of the epidermal nevus affect response rates to selective lasers. The argon laser was recommended to treat soft, velvety lesions but is unsuccessful with more keratotic or papular lesions. The CO_2 laser, however, is successful with more keratotic nevi but may result in hypertrophic scarring if higher-power outputs are applied (≥ 10 W). This newer generation of pulsed or scanned CO_2 and Er:YAG lasers largely circumvents the scarring that was associated with the CW CO_2 systems. Laser therapy is an attractive alternative for extensive epidermal nevi in which other surgical methods would result in unacceptable cosmetic results (Fig. 265-6).

LASER HAIR REMOVAL

Laser hair removal is mainly based on the fact that hair is the only melanized pigmented structure normally present in the dermis. Hair color is a mixture of eumelanin (brown, black) and pheomelanin (red). Hypertrichosis describes hair density and length beyond the accepted limits of normal for a particular age, race, and sex. Hirsutism refers to excess hair growth in women in anatomic sites under androgen control such as the beard, moustache, and chest areas. Hair removal by laser is currently creating a flurry of excitement in the field of dermatologic laser surgery.

Since the original report by Grossman et al.[39] showing that high-fluence, normal ruby laser pulses could remove pigmented human terminal hair, laser hair removal has become a "hot topic." The most successful approach is based on selective photothermolysis, taking advantage of the fact that hair follicles are the only melanin-containing structures within normal human dermis. Hair follicles cycle through periods of active hair growth (anagen), transition (catagen), and rest (telogen). The length of hair depends on the duration of anagen, which varies from as a short as a month to many years. In catagen, the actively growing and deepest portion of the follicle degenerates by apoptosis, leading to telogen, which may last up to about 1 year (on the lower leg). Most of the melanin in hair follicles exists in the hair shaft and the matrix that produces the hair shaft.

Biologically, there are at least two target structures that can influence hair growth. These are the "bulb," which is responsible for active hair shaft growth, and the "bulge," a region of stem cells in

FIGURE 265-6

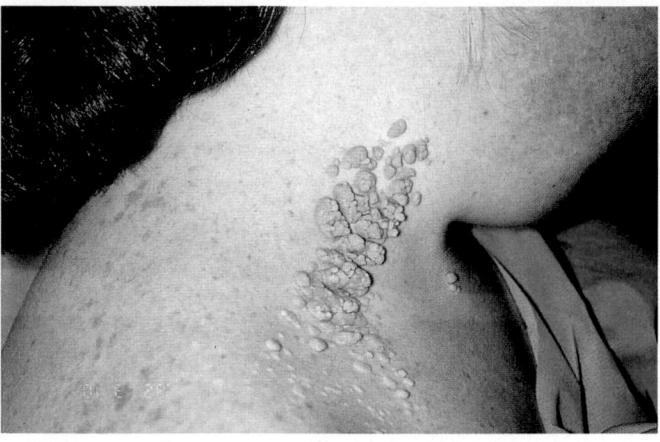

A.

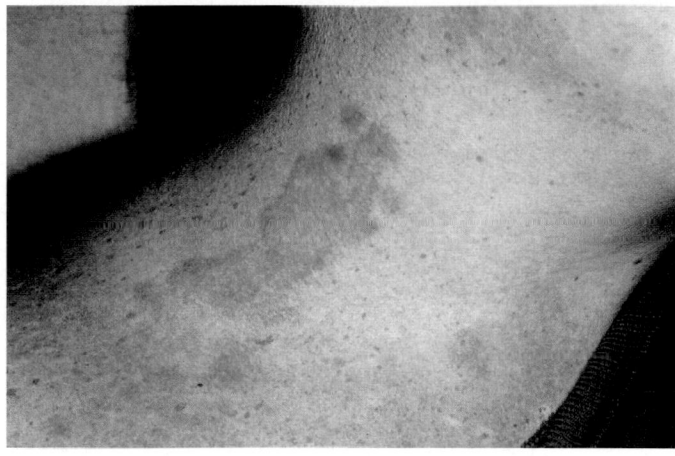

B.

Epidermal nevus in neck before (*A*) and after (*B*) treatment with FeatherTouch CO_2 laser.

the midfollicle. The "bulb" is about 0.5 to 1 mm in diameter for coarse terminal hairs (corresponding to a thermal relaxation time of up to 1 s), and includes both a neurovascular papilla and the rapidly proliferating, heavily pigmented matrix cells that form the hair shaft during anagen. This is the deepest part of the hair follicle, typically at depths of 3 to 7 mm depending on body site. The "bulge" is a poorly localized (in humans) region of stem cells located in the follicular epithelium near the insertion of the arector pili muscle, which appears to provide the cells necessary for formation of a new matrix at the beginning of each anagen phase. Anatomically, the highest concentration of melanin is in the hair shaft and matrix. In contrast, little or no melanin is present in the bulge, approximately 1 mm deep. Irreversible injury to the bulb during the anagen phase would cause arrest of active hair growth until another anagen cycle could begin. Irreversible injury to the bulge alone might not inhibit active hair growth but could potentially prevent formation of a new hair at the subsequent anagen phase. Irreversible injury to both targets may logically lead to both hair growth arrest and permanent inhibition of new hair formation. The most traditional method of "permanent" hair removal is electrolysis (DC current) or electrothermolysis (RF current), in which a fine electrode is inserted into each hair follicle. As the names suggest, electrothermolysis and laser photothermolysis both produce thermal injury.

Selective photothermolysis of pigmented terminal hair follicles is best accomplished using red or near-infrared pulses, because this spectral region is strongly absorbed by eumelanin and penetrates well into the dermis. As discussed above, longer wavelengths penetrate somewhat deeper, but eumelanin's absorption decreases at longer wavelengths. Pheomelanin, which accounts for red hair, has very little absorption in the infrared part of the spectrum. About 10 to 20 percent of incident light from 700 to 1000 nm, respectively, passes through a 3-mm thick human dermis. The spectral region of 700 to 800 nm probably offers the best combination of optical penetration and absorption for hair removal.

Grossman et al. studied skin injury and hair regrowth after 0.3-ms ruby laser (694 nm) pulses delivered at fluences ranging from 30 to 60 J/cm^2, in 6-mm diameter spots delivered through a cold sapphire handpiece designed to reduce epidermal injury.[39] Test sites on the back or thigh were either shaved or wax-depilated, to test the influence of having a pigmented hair shaft present in the follicle at the time of treatment. Selective thermal injury of superficial and deep follicular epithelium was observed histologically. At all fluences, there was a nearly complete arrest of hair growth for 1 to 3 months, as compared with unexposed shaved or wax-depilated control sites. At 6 months after exposure, there was significant, fluence-dependent loss of regrowing terminal hair in sites that were shaved (versus wax-depilated) prior to exposure. A subsequent report noted hair loss up to 2 years after laser treatment in these subjects.[40] Pain, erythema, edema and transient pigmentary changes occurred, but there was no scarring. From this work, there appear to be two distinct follicular responses to laser treatment—immediate arrest of growth anagen hairs and long-term inhibition of new hair growth. Whether these actually correspond to damage at the bulb and bulge, respectively, remains to be seen.

Based on this small but well-controlled study, a host of pulsed lasers including ruby, alexandrite, diode, and a xenon flashlamp have been produced commercially. It must be emphasized that these devices damage any pigmented tissue up to at least several mm below the skin surface. The retinal damage hazard from these sources is therefore extreme—even through the closed eyelid and/or sclera. In general, none of them should be used within the bony orbit.

At the time of this writing, the advantages and disadvantages of different hair-removal light sources are not yet established. However, it is clear that all of them offer at least temporary removal of pigmented terminal hair. Permanent inhibition of hair growth requires the combination of high fluence and large exposure spots (at least 20 J/cm^2 for spots at least 7 mm in diameter, at 694 nm, and probably more at longer wavelengths). Thus, permanent hair removal demands high-energy devices. At present these include alexandrite lasers (755 nm, 2 to 20 ms, 20 to 50 J/cm^2, various pot sizes); ruby lasers (694 nm, 0.7 to 3 ms, 10 to 50 J/cm^2, various spot sizes); diode laser array (800 nm, 5 to 20 ms, 10 to 40 J/cm^2, 9-mm^2 spot), and xenon flashlamp (700 to 1200 nm, 1 to 100 ms, approximately 10 to 100 J/cm^2, 3 $\times$ 35 mm spot). The technology for optical hair removal is likely to evolve rapidly for several years, driven by a largely untapped market. For example, one device now available for hair removal is the first extremely high power diode array laser ever used in medicine. Diode lasers are the world's most efficient light source, which may ultimately replace many other sources. The influence of pulse duration has not been system-

atically determined, but on theoretical grounds the ideal pulse duration probably lies in the region of 10 to 50 ms. Some devices incorporate surface cooling handpieces that use either cold windows, cold lenses, or cryogen spray to limit epidermal injury. Others can be used in combination with topical transparent gels, which also limit epidermal injury.

The best available data at present suggest that the majority of patients with brown or black coarse terminal hair treated at fluences of at least 30 J/cm^2 with ruby, diode array, or alexandrite lasers, using large spot sizes, will experience nearly complete temporary alopecia followed by long-term reduction of hair. Even with aggressive skin cooling, pigmented skin frequently shows epidermal injury with blistering, hyperpigmentation, or hypopigmentation, apparently with all of the sources now available. About one in five patients with dark hair and fair skin respond very well, requiring only one treatment to achieve nearly complete and very long-lasting alopecia. Regrowing hair is reduced in number and tends to be finer and lighter. However, it is not known how many treatments are necessary to achieve alopecia on average, across the wide spectrum of patient hair color, skin color, and laser device parameters. There also appear to be individuals who, despite having dark terminal hair and fair skin, completely regrow hair within 6 months after treatment. Side-by-side prospective comparison to electrolysis has not yet been reported.

The first FDA-approved laser hair removal method involves topical application of a suspension of carbon particles followed by exposure to Q-switched Nd:YAG laser pulses. The carbon is intended to penetrate into hair follicles, allowing specific absorption in the follicle. This technique is capable of temporary hair removal, but has not been reported to induce permanent hair loss despite years of clinical use by private clinics that have licensed the patented method involved. This treatment uses exactly the same combination of chromphore and laser as amateur tattoo removal. It is well established that the injury surrounding carbon particles pumped by Q-switched Nd:YAG laser pulses is very limited spatially, which may explain the poor results of this technique compared with ruby laser hair removal. The technique may be useful for temporary hair control, especially in people with lightly pigmented hair.

Photodynamic therapy has also been reported to inhibit terminal hair growth in human skin.[39] Topical ALA was applied under occlusion for 3 h, followed by exposure to 630-nm argon-pumped dye laser. The highest dose combination of 20 percent ALA and 200 J/cm^2 light fluence led to about 40 percent inhibition of hair growth, which was stable for at least 6 months after treatment. Fluorescence microscopy showed prominent porphyrin fluorescence limited to the epidermis and hair follicles, including the matrix. This interesting observation has not yet been explored, and other photosensitizers have not yet been compared with ALA.

LASER HAIR TRANSPLANTATION

A relatively new application of lasers in aesthetic surgery is their use to create recipient sites for hair transplant grafts.

In actuality, hair transplantation was one of the fields that had long escaped the use of outside innovative technology. Active discussion in the literature has regarded its pros and cons. Laser hair transplantation has been associated with multiple advantages, including control of bleeding, decreased surgical times, less-traumatic graft handling, diminished graft compression, and a more natural appearance. However, these advantages must be weighed against the disadvantages of this procedure, which include increased expense, additional training, safety hazards, and a slight delay in hair growth.

CHAPTER 265
Lasers in Dermatology

2915

Hair transplantation is mostly performed on males. Approximately 200,000 individuals, most with male pattern baldness, undergo hair transplantation annually in the United States. Beginning in the late 1950s, the standard technique involved the use of large punch grafts harvested from the occipital and parietal regions. In more recent years, micrografting techniques involving small round grafts or slit grafts have become the standard of care. Instead of punchgraft harvesting, a stripgraft is obtained, which in turn is dissected into round grafts or slits depending on the preference of the transplant surgeon. Recipient sites for the new grafts are created with trephens, fine blades, or hollow needles in the scalp areas selected to grow new healthy anagen hair. The micrografts usually consist of single, dual, or triple hairgrafts, whereas minigrafts (to attain additional density) usually contain from four to eight hairs. The use of larger grafts often leads to the typical "doll's hair" or "cornrow" appearance, a feature deemed unattractive by most. Refined techniques yield the desired slit and round grafts by diligently and patiently dissecting the stripgraft. Micrografting is also the most commonly used technique for restorative work of "large graft appearance" in the hair transplant practice.

In November 1996 the FDA approved the Sharplan SilkLaser CO_2 laser for round grafts as the first specific system for laser hair transplantation. A rapidly scanning CW laser beam can in a single pulse drill cylindrical holes in the scalp to a depth of 4 to 7 mm. Typical higher average powers are necessary to achieve this (40 to 120 W) with brief scan times (0.05 to 0.25 s) to avoid problems with graft survival. More recently, pulsed Er:YAG lasers (sometimes mixed with CO_2 for good hemostasis) show promise as well.[41]

LASER TREATMENT OF MISCELLANEOUS SKIN LESIONS

Many different exophytic skin lesions have been treated using CO_2 and, more recently, Er:YAG lasers. The newer generation of these controlled ablative lasers are very useful for vaporizing appendageal skin tumors such as syringomas, rhinophyma, trichoepitheliomas, trichilemmomas, xanthomas, xanthelasma, verruca, and molluscum. Also, the destruction of premalignant actinic keratoses and basal cell carcinomas of the superficial type can be performed using these superficially ablative lasers.

LASER SKIN RESURFACING

Although the CO_2 laser had been used for 30 years to vaporize exophytic skin lesions, its use as an "abrading" tool was limited to the lower lip until 1989, when David and co-workers[42] published their observations using 100-ms gated "pulses" from a CW CO_2 laser to "resurface" photodamaged skin with low-power densities ($\sim$50 W/cm^2). In their study, magnification loupes were used to visualize slight graying of the skin as a treatment end point. Long-term wrinkle reduction was demonstrated grossly and microscopically, and most importantly, no clinical scarring was observed. This was attributed to (1) only one pass being made, (2) the clinician's attention to visual feedback from the wound surface, and (3) low total radiant exposures. In addition, the subablative power densities

used in this study have been shown to produce excessive thermal damage that can lead to scarring. These early CO_2 laser skin resurfacing (LSR) attempts depended heavily on operator skill.

The CO_2 laser was the first and continues to be the most popular laser resurfacing tool. The high absorption coefficient for tissue water (800 cm^{-1}) permits precise tissue removal and minimal residual thermal damage (RTD) if power density is sufficient for vaporization to significantly outpace the speed of thermal diffusion, or if the pulse duration is short enough that ablation depth is controlled to within tens of microns per pulse. The minimal RTD is achieved when energy is delivered in less than the thermal relaxation time, τ_r. Although the CO_2 laser beam penetrates only about 20 μm in tissue, the residual thermal damage is at least several times greater due to heat diffusion during and after the laser pulse. *Power density* is the most important parameter in determining residual thermal damage and vaporization depth. This underscores the sensitivity of laser-tissue interactions to the time rate of energy deposition as well as the total radiant exposure. The instantaneous power densities of newer generation pulsed and rapid-scanned CO_2 lasers is about 10,000 W/cm^2.

During high-power laser ablation, high pressures are generated, resulting in superheating to temperatures as high as 200 to 300°C and explosive vaporization. For slower heating with low-power lasers, vaporization is slower and the surface layer can become desiccated. With continued heating of the desiccated surface proteins, charring occurs. This represents temperatures up to 600°C and is akin to placing a red hot coal on the skin. In contrast to explosive surface vaporization, with charring a top-to-bottom temperature gradient is sustained, resulting in thermal damage extending up to several mm into the dermis.

For a CO_2 laser to be considered safe and reliable for resurfacing, it should produce minimal RTD ($<$120 μm). The necessity of tissue vaporization for successful treatment is unclear, as patients showing no dermal tissue removal improve cosmetically so long as there is significant RTD in the dermis ($>$50 μm). A new generation of high-energy pulsed CO_2 lasers has been developed to allow ablation to proceed without significant heat conduction during the pulse. This makes it possible to use the CO_2 laser as a precise heating tool. It was shown that CO_2 pulses around 1 ms, delivered at low repetition rates, are short enough so that RTD is less than 100 μm.[42] This is the approximate theoretical pulse duration for which thermal confinement was predicted for the CO_2 laser. In comparison, the 2.94-μm erbium laser is much more strongly absorbed by water, and penetrates only a few microns into wet skin. For erbium lasers, the thermal relaxation time is τ_r of $\sim$1 to 5 μs for skin.[43]

Conceptually, τ_r is the time it takes for heat to spread over a distance equal to the penetration depth of the beam. Then, if the energy is delivered in $<\tau_r$, heat will only spread outside the beam after the laser pulse. In addition to restricting the pulse duration to τ_r, resurfacing lasers are capable of achieving ablative fluences in this short period with spot sizes practical for clinical applications. This combination of short pulses and high peak powers allows for exquisite control of both vaporization depth and thermal change.

Indications and Patient Selection

The two most popular indications for LSR are photodamage and acne scars. Photodamage, comprised of rhytides, dyschromias, solar lentigines, ephelides, and actinic keratoses, has been shown to respond very favorably to LSR. In particular, perioral and periorbital rhytides are readily reduced. Deeper wrinkles caused by facial expression, for example, the glabella and nasolabial folds, do not respond as well (Fig. 265-7). Deeper wrinkles are often softened, possibly from a general tightening of the entire face. Finer wrinkles resolve more easily. Most wrinkles are associated with solar elastosis, an abnormal deposition of elastic fibers and glycosaminoglycans, which results in dermal mechanical effects ("kinks").[44] Fine wrinkles are not microanatomically distinguishable from adjacent sun-damaged skin, and probably result mainly from redundant skin. A useful comparison is a worn glove. The glove retains the same constituency after multiple wearings, but wrinkles form at areas of material weakness. By replacing the solar elastosis of the upper dermis with new collagen, LSR restores some of the native biochemical and physical features of the skin.[45]

The pathophysiology of acne scarring precludes the procedure from being as effective as for wrinkles; often only modest improvement in scarring is achieved without aggressive therapy. The procedure works best for elevated and shallow distensible scars, in which either fibrotic tissue can be removed or in which the shoulders of shallow depressions can be ablated and remodeled. Deeper scars tend to respond less favorably, most likely because the tethering fibrotic bands persist after treatment; also effacement of the scar requires such aggressive ablation that scarring is likely from the procedure itself. A combined approach incorporating punch excision and/or grafting, and follow-up laser abrasion is acceptable in these cases. One reason LSR, like any resurfacing procedure, improves the appearance of acne scars is that the whiteness of deeper scars is attenuated by a revascularized and replaced papillary dermis. This homogenizes the facial skin hue.

In general, fair-skinned patients can be treated more aggressively with only slightly increased risks of hypopigmentation. In some patients one can actually ablate a superficial scar (noted by the elimination of the gross white color) with marked improvement. The normal surrounding tissue is ablated to reduce any gross stepoff. The level of ablation is important in determining the cosmetic result. If ablation is carried out to where fine yellow stippling appears (representing superficial sebaceous glands about 100 to 200 μm deep in the dermis), healing will be slower, but final improvement will be better than if the wound is carried out more superficially. One must proceed more conservatively with type III to IV

FIGURE 265-7

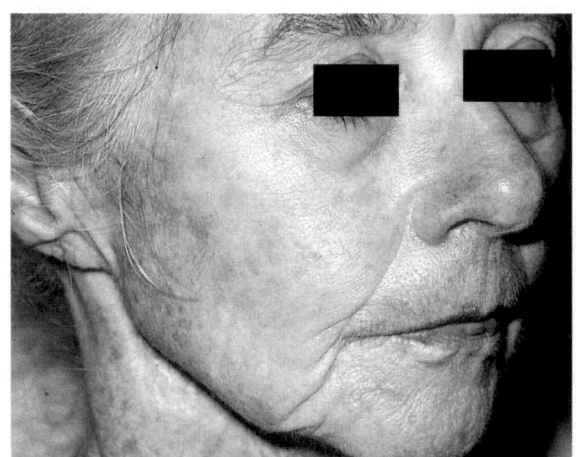

A.

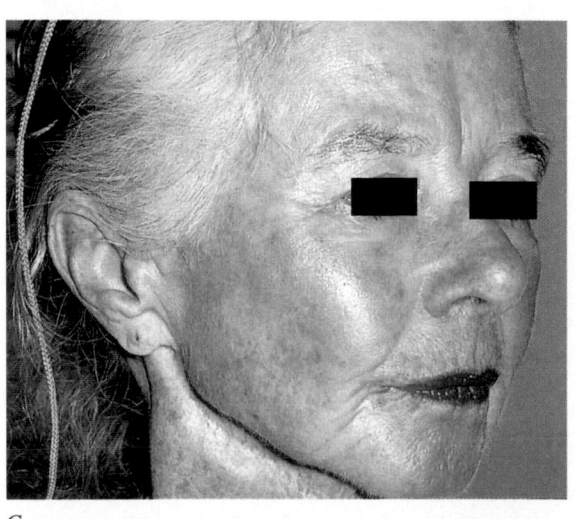

C.

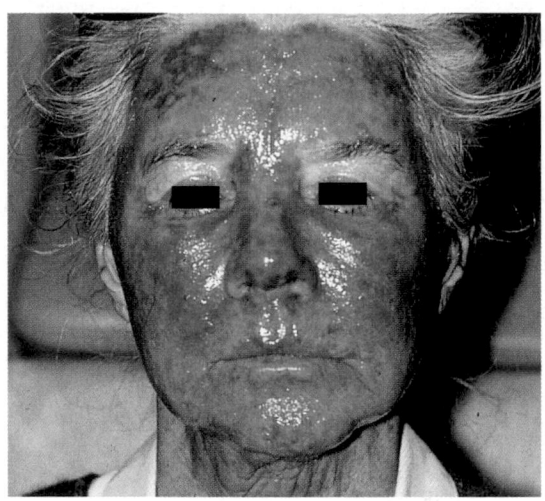

B.

75 year-old woman with dermatoheliosis and rhytides before (*A*), 1 week after (*B*), and 6 months after (*C*) laser skin resurfacing.

skin, or hyperpigmentation is likely. Hyperpigmentation can be minimized by sun avoidance and/or topical hydroquinone before and after treatment.

Other Indications

Almost any skin lesion exhibiting irregular surface topography can be considered for LSR. Like acne scars, varicella scars can be smoothed. Actinic cheilitis can also be treated with decreased postoperative healing time versus CW lasers. Actinic keratoses, Bowen's disease, and superficial basal cell carcinoma are other indications. For the latter two, curettage should be used to increase the rate of cure to that of a standard electrodesiccation and curettage.

Rhinophyma, epidermal nevi, sebaceous hyperplasia, xanthelasma, and benign adnexal tumors can also be treated with resurfacing lasers. The advantage over CW lasers is more precise vaporization with less charring.

Contraindications

Patients who smoke are at greater risk for complications, probably due to vasoconstriction and other factors during healing. Patients in whom keloids form, in general, should not undergo LSR. Also diseases with koebnerizing features are relative contraindications, although microsecond-domain CO_2 lasers might prove useful in treating stable plaque type psoriasis. Any patient with severe systemic disease or diseases complicated by immunosuppression should not be treated, as these may alter wound healing. Isotretinoin has been reported to produce atyical scarring with resurfacing methods, and in one large retrospective study of 1925 LSR patients, two of the four patients in whom severe scarring developed had taken isotretinoin within 2 years. There is no sound scientific recommendation for the length of time required after isotretinoin treatment to proceed with LSR. In any case, the patient should be advised of the possibility of abnormal wound healing after isotretinoin use, and in any condition in which the adnexal structures are compromised (e.g., radiation therapy for acne or resurfacing over large areas of scar or nonsebaceous skin grafts).

Method

The method for CO_2 LSR for wrinkles has become somewhat standardized. Regardless of the specific laser system used, a first pass ("pass" is defined as one contiguous pulse or scan of the laser) is made, resulting in a roughened whitish-yellow surface; this material represents proteinaceous epidermal debris after partial vaporization of intracellular water. After removing this material with wet gauze, the surface reveals a pink color, representing partially denatured papillary dermis. Subsequent passes result in progressive yellowing and visible tissue contraction. With additional passes on the face, the surface reveals fine papillations, which represent exposure of the pilosebaceous units and acrosyringium. Deeper injury may result in delayed healing and scarring. Before each pass, the surface should be blotted dry, since excess water absorbs the laser energy. With multiple passes into the dermis, wiping between passes reduces the variability in RTD across the treated area, decreases the overall depth of heat diffusion, and delays healing. In contrast, if one pass is made (which results in denaturation of the epidermis and slight thermal damage to the dermal papilla), wiping actually increases the degree of inflammation and fibroblast depth 1 day

after injury. Debris remaining on the skin may serve as a natural dressing that impedes water loss and prevents an extension of injury from desiccation. Two to four passes are made over the entire treated area in a normal resurfacing session. In addition, the high points of scars or winkles can be locally removed.

The procedure is somewhat different for acne scars. A deeper injury is necessary to obtain a good result. It is helpful to ablate the edges of scars before treating the whole face, because as surgery proceeds there is generalized facial swelling, and the acne scars become less conspicuous. Because tissue ablation with pulsed or scanned CO_2 lasers is minimal for 5 to 7 J/cm^2, the fluence may be increased by using a smaller spot size, larger pulse energy, or higher power. By doing this, fluences up to 50 J/cm^2 are available and the scar crests can be reduced. Reducing acne scars without treating an entire cosmetic unit can be attempted in fair-skinned patients; however, in others it is better to treat the entire face or at least a cosmetic unit to avoid a conspicuous border between treated and untreated areas.

Adnexal tumors, keloids, and other exophytic lesions can be vaporized. The end point for treatment is gross disappearance of lesions. With keloids, for example, treatment ceases when ropy white collagen is no longer seen. Erbium lasers can ablate exophytic lesions more efficiently with lower fluences; however, there may be more bleeding, particularly with rhinophyma. Warts can be treated by either erbium or CO_2 LSR. The procedure is somewhat different from traditional CW CO_2 treatment, in which the wart is heated until it can be easily separated from the dermis. With high-fluence pulsed LSR, the wart is ablated away like knocking off a stack of coins. At the end of the procedure, a fine white layer of desiccated proteinaceous debris remains.

Perioperative and Anesthesia Considerations

Authors have recommended preoperative treatment with topical tretinoin for all patients, plus topical hydroquinone (HQ) for Fitzpatrick types III to IV patients, beginning 3 to 6 weeks before surgery.[27] Tretinoin has been shown to decrease the healing time and reduce RTD when applied for 30 days prior to surgery. Preoperative HQ is commonly prescribed, although no studies support its efficacy in preventing hyperpigmentation. To prevent HSV infection, acyclovir or another antiviral drug is given, particularly for perioral or full-face cases, regardless of the patient's history of herpes. This is usually begun 2 days before surgery. The need for antibiotic prophylaxis is controversial. Some physicians routinely prescribe a macrolide antibiotic or β-lactamase-resistant penicillin preoperatively; this provides coverage against most gram-positive bacteria, particularly *Staphyloccocus aureus*, which has been implicated in at least one case of toxic-shock syndrome after CO_2 LSR. *S. aureus* proliferates in both wet and dry environments, so that infection can occur without occlusive dressings. *Pseudomonas aeruginosa* and other gram-negative infections have also been reported. One study suggested that the rate of *Pseudomonas* infections was related to the prolonged use (3 to 5 days) of occlusive dressings: the use of open dressing technique (e.g., Aquaphor without long-term occlusive dressings) plus the use of dilute acetic acid perioperatively (0.25 percent), decreased the rate of gram-negative infections. Other physicians continue to use occlusive dressings, citing increased patient comfort and no increased risk of infections, particularly if the dressings are changed during the first 5 days after treatment. Hydrogel, polyurethane, and hydrocolloid dressings have all been used successfully. Some physicians have advocated the use of broad-spectrum antibiotics, but this may increase the emergence of resistant organisms as well as promote the growth of yeasts. Chlorhexidine has been suggested as a general body cleanser 2 to 3 days preoperatively to decrease skin bacterial counts; it should not be used on the face the day of surgery due to the risk of corneal damage. Irgrasan (Septisol, Calgon Vestal Labs, St. Louis) is a good substitute as it is non-alcohol-based (nonflammable), has a good gram-positive and -negative coverage, and has low eye toxicity. Some physicians suggest that because the CO_2 laser sterilizes as it vaporizes, no topical antiseptics are needed; however, preoperative cleansing may decrease the risk of inoculation from the perimeter of the treated area. Topical antibiotics postoperatively would seem to be a logical choice for preventing wound infections after LSR; however, data suggest a higher rate of contact sensitization than with nonthermal resurfacing procedures, particularly in full-face cases. Once wounds have reepithelialized, topical vitamin C and tretinoin have been proposed to accelerate healing and help preserve the effects of LSR. Topical steroids may speed erythema resolution. Topical HQ is effective for hyperpigmentation, which tends to occur between 3 and 8 weeks after treatment and usually resolves within 4 to 6 weeks of application.

Safety

Fire is a major risk for both patients and the operating staff during laser skin resurfacing. Most objects absorb 10.6-μm radiation well. The operative field is one potential source for fires, and all sponges, drapes, or clothing near the operative field should be wet. Topical betadine, chlorhexadine, and other agents in alcohol vehicles can ignite. These agents do not ignite as easily in aqueous solution, which includes most detergent vehicles. The laser surgeon is encouraged to check the alcohol content of any topical agent to be used in the operative field. All instruments on the field should ideally be roughened to prevent inadvertent reflections; this is especially important for lasers with collimated beams. The patient's eyes should be protected with metal shields, and the operating staff should wear safety goggles. One major concern is the endotracheal tube. Polyvinyl chloride (PVC) will ignite in an O_2-enriched atmosphere. Preferably, a laser-safe tube should be used. Another risk of LSR is airborne contamination, which can be minimized by using a smoke evacuator and filtration masks for personnel including the patient when possible. Viral DNA (both human papillomavirus and human immunodeficiency virus) has been detected in the laser plume. Also, the plume itself is carcinogenic and has been shown to cause pulmonary fibrosis in rats. Overall, the risks of erbium laser ablation are similar to those of CO_2. One difference is increased particulate debris in the erbium induced plume.

Anesthesia

The anesthesia requirement for LSR depends in part on the laser used, patient tolerance, and body site. The CO_2 laser generally produces a higher level of discomfort than nonthermal resurfacing; most likely this is due to tissue heating, which stimulates type C pain fibers. These unmyelinated fibers theoretically should be easier to anesthetize than the thicker myelinated fibers responsible for pinprick. The sensation of warmth is more difficult to eliminate, which suggests that receptors may be located in deeper dermal layers. The CO_2 laser generally requires injectable anesthesia for one or two

cosmetic units and systemic agents for full-face cases. For a full-face case, commonly used regimens include: (1) A combination of IM sedation plus nerve blocks and supplemental local anesthesia; (2) IV sedation plus nerve blocks and local anesthesia, with or without tumescence; (3) An inhalational anesthetic; or (4) total intravenous anesthesia (TIVA). TIVA combines propofol, an anxiolytic, narcotic, and laryngeal mask adapter, and has become the anesthetic of choice for office-based CO_2 LSR. Other creative anesthetic regimens have been used with variable success. For example, EMLA cream has been used with preoperative PO sedation (benzodiazapine plus narcotic); the EMLA must be applied after hydration of the epidermis and should be left on until just before resurfacing each cosmetic unit.

After CO_2 LSR, most patients returning to consciousness immediately after general anesthesia report burning and stinging. This is rapidly reduced by application of hydrogel dressing. Regardless of the laser used, postoperative pain usually diminishes 2 days after LSR, although many patients require narcotics for the postoperative night after LSR, after which acetaminophen or a nonsteroidal antiinflammatory drug is adequate. Significant pain, especially if throbbing or focal, usually heralds a wound infection.

Effectiveness of CO_2 LSR

There have been few prospective studies of LSR. Fitzpatrick et al.[46] showed that a short-pulsed laser effectively reduced wrinkles, and Ross et al.[47] showed that scanning laser with a short dwell time performed just as well as a pulsed laser in a side-by-side comparison trial. Clinical results thus far suggest that LSR works best for fine rhytides, especially those around the mouth, and that deeper wrinkles respond less favorably. Wrinkle improvement has been quantified by optical profilometer, a technique in which the severity of shadows is used to examine skin surface irregularities.

Side Effects

Side effects of LSR have been summarized in two recent retrospective studies. Bernstein et al. reported side effects in their own patients and reviewed the literature.[48] They found that their own data and that from other studies ranged as follows for specific side effects: erythema (100 percent of patients, duration of 1 to 4 months), hyperpigmentation (3 to 36 percent of patients), hypopigmentation (0 to 16 percent), acne/milia (30 to 80 percent), scarring (0 to 2.5 percent), pain (3 percent), and infection (0 to 5.6 percent). Weinstein et al.[49] have reported their experience with 1925 patients and found similar percentages of specific side effects. They also reported a 0.1 percent incidence of permanent ectropion and a 2.5 percent incidence of telangiectasias after mild trauma. The telangiectasias appear most often on the lateral cheek. This article addressed other considerations of LSR, one of which was demarcation lines between treated and untreated areas in men. These areas were noted particularly after regional resurfacing, when patients complained because they were unwilling to use makeup to disguise the area. This study also suggested reasons for scars in specific patients. The list included rapid overlapping of pulses, isotretinoin use, bacterial infections, and extensive electrolysis, which may have depleted the patient's reservoir of follicles for reepithelialization. The observation that pulse "stacking" increased scarring is supported by a study that showed that immediate overlapping of as few as two pulses at 5 Hz can increase RTD by as much as $1.25\times$ in live farm pigs. Many of these same side effects are reported after other resurfacing methods; however, erythema duration and time for reepithelialization after CO_2 wounds is probably longer than for nonthermal resurfacing techniques even when the depths of injury are similar. Scarring after LSR is dependent on depth of ablation, depth of thermal damage, and postoperative wound care. It is unclear precisely what depth of total injury is tolerated by human facial skin without clinical scarring; most likely there is regional variation, and the dermal response may be sensitive to factors other than simply depth of tissue necrosis (fibroblast death) immediately after injury. Infection may increase depth of injury, delay healing, and promote abnormal scarring. Generally, dyspigmentation risks are related to the level of injury. A very superficial injury, in which only the epidermis is ablated, usually results in normal pigmentation, although hyperpigmentation can occur. Injury just into the papillary dermis is more likely to cause hyperpigmentation (variably reported as 5 to 35 percent) and is dependent on skin type. With deeper passes, hypopigmentation is possible. Normally, hyperpigmentation is seen 2 to 4 weeks after injury. Hypopigmentation is typically more delayed, sometimes occurring several months after surgery. It is difficult to distinguish genuine laser-induced hyperpigmentation from the patient's constitutive pigment in untreated non-photodamaged skin. The hypopigmentation associated with LSR is of two types. One is a relative hypopigmentation compared to the mottled coloration of background photodamaged untreated skin. Possible remedies include feathering the perimeter of the area or performing a full-face procedure. Another type of hypopigmentation occurs 6 to 12 months after LSR; in these patients there appears to be a return to base-line constitutive pigmentation of the face within 2 months after resurfacing, followed by an unexplained delayed loss of pigmentation.

It is unknown to what degree LSR will replace conventional nonthermal resurfacing methods. Clinicians who are experts in chemical peels and dermabrasion will continue to perform these procedures with good results. Some physicians have creatively combined LSR with chemical peels, using peels for broad expanses of facial skin (cheeks and forehead) and LSR from the more-wrinkled perioral and periorbital areas.

Recent Advances in LSR

Because of prolonged erythema and delayed reepithelialization associated with millisecond-domain CO_2 LSR, alternative wavelengths and pulse durations have been investigated.[50] Accordingly, a CO_2 laser is presently available that uses ~60-μs pulse durations. Because the same fluences are used as in conventional millisecond-domain LSR, higher power densities (peak powers of 70,000 W versus 7000 W for millisecond-domain systems) are achieved so that less thermal diffusion should occur deep to the ablated tissue. These lasers, as theory predicts, do leave less RTD than their 1-ms domain counterparts, but it is suggested that clinical efficacy is compromised as thermal damage is reduced.

Erbium:YAG versus CO_2 Lasers

The Er:YAG laser at a wavelength of 2.94 μm has been used for laser resurfacing.[51] Because of strong water absorption (~10× that of CO_2), the erbium laser is capable of removing tissue with more precision and with lower fluences than CO_2. CO_2 lasers for typically used fluences in the range of 5 to 10 J/cm^2 produce up to 120 μm RTD and only 5 to 10 μm ablation, whereas the erbium lasers ablate approximately 10 to 20 μm of tissue at the same fluence range while leaving only 10 to 50 μm RTD. This RTD is enough to seal off most blood vessels of the upper dermis but not enough to clinically retard wound healing, compared with a mechanically induced wound (dermabrasion). One disadvantage of the erbium laser is that

tissue heating may be insufficient to seal off the vessels of the deeper dermis so that hemostasis may become a problem with an increasing number of passes. In a side-by-side comparison of erbium and CO_2 laser skin resurfacing at similar fluences, it was shown that the erbium laser was capable of achieving results almost equal to those achieved with CO_2, provided that more passes were made with the erbium laser (four to eight versus two to three, respectively).[52] This appeared to be due to the need for a greater depth of tissue removal with the erbium laser to achieve the same level of depth of total injury as the CO_2 (depth of injury = ablation depth + residual thermal damage). Interestingly, even when the total depth of injury was deeper with erbium, the time of reepithelialization was shorter (~3 to 6 versus 6 to 10 days), and the mean duration of postoperative erythema was shorter (2 versus 8 weeks). The authors speculate that the increased thermal damage associated with CO_2 injury might account for the delayed healing. On the other hand, even with aggressive erbium laser resurfacing, the overall cosmetic result as assessed by global wrinkle reduction was better with CO_2 laser. The Er:YAG laser, because of the smaller fraction of absorbed energy converted to heat, normally requires less anesthesia than CO_2. In some patients, cosmetic units may be treated only after the application of topical anesthetic agents such as EMLA. However, for fluences greater than 5 J/cm^2 and faster pulse-repetition rates (10 Hz), injectable anesthesia may be required with or without sedation. The reduced anesthetic requirements may make the erbium laser more acceptable for office practice when a full surgical suite may not be available.

Until the advent of the erbium laser, physicians largely limited the LSR to the face, out of concern that other areas with decreased numbers of adnexal structures might result in scarring. Early results have shown that the erbium laser may prove safe for the neck, arms and hands, and chest.[53] Further studies must be performed to validate the safety and efficacy of erbium LSR for nonfacial areas.

Mechanisms of Action

The mechanisms involved in LSR have only begun to be investigated, but by following wounds grossly and microscopically, some preliminary conclusions can be made. Initially it was proposed that tissue removal (ablation) was the most important mechanism in LSR. This concept was embraced because of its intuitive attractiveness and the observation that wrinkle crests could be gradually sculpted down by multiple passes of the laser. It was later determined, however, that ablation depths into the dermis were often less than the wrinkle depths, and yet marked cosmetic improvement was observed. This led to the proposal of other mechanisms, namely collagen shrinkage and wound healing–induced fibroplasia, as contributing to the final cosmetic improvement. Heating type I collagen over about 70°C causes it to contract, and visible tissue shrinkage occurs during LSR. The shrinkage of collagen, like that of other denaturation processes, is dependent linearly on time and exponentially on temperature. With complete denaturation, collagen loses its native birefringence, the fibrils increase in thickness by a factor of 2 (130 to 280 nm), and can contract in length to one-fourth their original length. Long-term follow-up of wounds in a study of healing and contraction in live pigs showed a correlation between final wound contraction and initial RTD, suggesting a possible role for thermal damage in wrinkle reduction after LSR.

The microscopic changes after LSR aid in understanding the proposed mechanisms. Studies have shown that the epidermis is removed after the first pass of the CO_2 laser if the surface is wiped

FIGURE 265-8

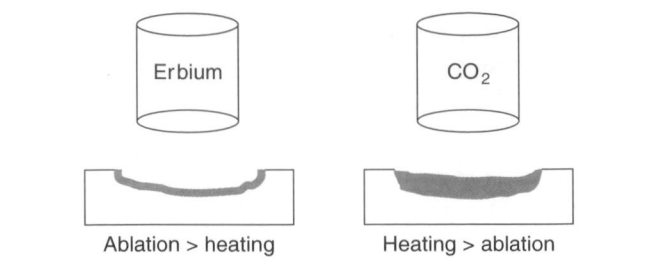

Differences in relative contributions of heating and ablation for erbium and CO_2 lasers for fluences near 5 J/cm².

after irradiation, but that there is little tissue removal after additional CO_2 laser passes at the conventionally applied fluences of ~5 to 7 J/cm². Once the dermis is exposed, additional laser passes do not significantly increase histologically identifiable RTD (between passes four and seven, for example) so long as the passes are delivered in a nonoverlapping fashion. However, using a sensitive thermal camera, Welch et al.[54] have shown that the peak surface temperature increases slightly after successive passes in CO_2 LSR despite wiping and allowing the temperature to return to base line between passes. They suggest that this is from increased absorption or decreased thermal conductivity after each pass. An in vitro study by Gardner et al.[55] summarized the collagen changes and dermal responses to CO_2 pulses and scans. They found that shrinkage increased with pass number and that the temperature rose 15 to 20°C over ambient temperature 500 μm deep in the dermis. They also noted a constant depth of collagen denaturation (~115 μm) regardless of the pass number for two to five passes.

A non-published study of live farm pigs comparing dermabrasion and CO_2 LSR showed that wound healing after LSR occurs as follows for three passes with a 1-ms pulsed CO_2 laser, or scanned CW CO_2 laser, with wiping. After CO_2 LSR there is residual thermal denaturation of collagen seen by histology of 60 to 120 μm and area wound contraction of 10 to 25 percent, depending on the fluence. By 1 day after injury, polymorphonuclear leukocytes (PMNs) line the wound base in "picket fence" fashion. The band of PMNs extends from the histologically altered collagen to the most superficial level of normal-appearing collagen. This level is presumably the site for sloughing (above) and tissue remodeling (below). By 5 to 7 days after injury, there is focal epithelialization with underlying granulation tissue; occasionally, denatured collagen is seen just deep into the new fragile epidermis. At this time fibroblasts are noted within areas of partial collagen denaturation, suggesting that at least part of the shrunken denatured zone has been repopulated by new fibroblasts. By 14 days, a 0.1- to 0.3-mm zone of hypercellular dermis is observed, and the epidermis is completely re-formed. By 4 months, this zone shows horizontally oriented, tightly packed collagen fibers reminiscent of scar histology. It is likely that fibrosis in a narrow band of the upper dermis is responsible for efficacy. Indeed, good results obtained by dermabrasion, chemical peel, or laser resurfacing are almost indistinguishable.

Despite decades of research on cutaneous lesions, at a fundamental level it is unknown how thermal damage modulates wound healing. Margolis et al.[56] showed a greater and more sustained elevation in collagen content after CO_2 laser injury versus 50 percent TCA in mouse skin. Pogrel et al.[57] found that CO_2 laser incision showed earlier, greater, and longer-sustained hyaluronidase activity than scalpel incisions in rats. They suggest that the prolonged activity might be related to the later neovascularization in laser wounds. Smith[58] has shown increased factor 13, vimentin, and actin expression after pulsed carbon dioxide laser injury in a pig. New collagen deposition apparently plays a major role in the final cosmetic result but it is unknown how thermal injury modulates the pattern and quantity of the new collagen deposition.

There are significant differences in laser-tissue interaction between CO_2 and erbium laser ablation for the 5- to 8-J/cm² fluence range. The more explosive vaporization observed with erbium laser ablation is due to a combination of higher absorption coefficient and short micropulses, which sputter tissue from the skin surface. Tissue effects are largely determined by how fast and in what volume the energy is absorbed. The greatest difference is the threshold fluence for ablation, which is about 5 to 10 times higher for the CO_2 laser due to the difference in absorption coefficient. CO_2 lasers in the microsecond or millisecond domain are operating near the tissue ablation threshold, so a large fraction of incident energy is invested in tissue heating. In brief, the CO_2 laser at typical operating parameters performs a self-limited controlled melting of the surface, whereas the erbium laser operates in an almost purely ablation regime (Fig. 265-8).

During skin resurfacing with most erbium lasers, particles are ejected from the surface at supersonic velocities, and it has been suggested that recoil from this explosive vaporization can cause damage to deeper structures. This has been shown for the 193-nm excimer laser, for example, where fibroblasts were selectively damaged over 100 μm deep beyond the ablated surface. However, because of the pulse durations associated with commercially available erbium lasers (~250 μs), pressure waves are not confined during the pulse, so that true shock waves (bulk disruption of the transmitting medium) are probably not generated.

The thermal relaxation time of the thin tissue layer directly heated by erbium laser absorption is ~1 to 5 μs. Because of the pulse duration of clinically available resurfacing erbium lasers, heat diffuses during the laser pulse. This is desirable for hemostasis. High-speed photographs have shown that the erbium laser "burrows" into skin during normal mode operation (the erbium laser is actually a series of twenty 1-μs-long pulses in a train that comprises a 250-μs macropulse). It is how this pulse structure affects the tissue response. However, the depth of residual thermal injury is consistent with the lack of thermal confinement during the 250-μs macropulse.

Future

LSR is likely to be improved by further technical development. However, the clinical outcome is so dependent on wound healing that advances in wound care, growth factor modulation, inhibition of fibrosis, and dressings may play a more significant role. Clinical issues related to LSR also remain to be addressed. For example, the potential of this procedure to affect tumor formation in individuals who are prone to skin cancer remains unknown.

REFERENCES

1. Maiman T: Stimulated optical radiation in ruby. *Nature* **187**:439, 1960
2. Goldman L et al: Pathology of the effect of the laser beam on the skin. *Nature* **197**:912, 1963
3. Goldman L, Hornby P: Radiation from a Q-switched ruby laser. *J Invest Dermatol* **44**:69, 1965
4. Anderson R, Parrish J: Selective photothermolysis: Precise microsurgery by selective absorption of pulsed radiation. *Science* **220**:524, 1983

5. Anderson R, Parrish J: Microvasculature can be selectively damaged using dye lasers: A basic theory and experimental evidence in human skin. *Lasers Surg Med* **1**:263, 1981

6. Anderson R et al: Selective photothermolysis of cutaneous pigmentation by Q-switched Nd:YAG laser pulses at 1964, 532, and 355 nm. *J Invest Dermatol* **93**:28, 1989

7. Agah R et al: Rate process model for arterial thermal damage: implications for vessel photocoagulation. *Lasers Surg Med* **15**:176, 1994

8. van Gemert M et al: Wavelengths for laser treatment of port wine stains and telangiectasia. *Lasers Surg Med* **16**:147, 1995

9. Dierickx C et al: Thermal relaxation of port-wine stain vessels probed in vivo: The need for 1-10 millisecond laser pulse treatment. *J Invest Dermatol* **105**:709, 1995

10. Anderson R et al: Cosmetic tattoo ink darkening: A complication of Q-switched and pulsed laser treatment. *Arch Dermatol* **129**:1010, 1993

11. Baggish M et al: Presence of human immunodeficiency virus DNA in laser smoke. *Lasers Surg Med* **11**:197, 1991

12. Tan O et al: Treatment of children with port-wine stains using the flashlamp-pulsed tunable dye laser. *N Engl J Med* **320**:416, 1989

13. Van der Horst C et al: Effect of the timing of treatment of port-wine stains with the flash-lamp-pumped pulsed dye laser. *N Engl J Med* **338**:1028, 1998

14. Grevelink J et al: Pulsed laser treatment in children and the use of anesthesia. *J Am Acad Dermatol* **37**:75, 1997

15. Glassberg E et al: Capillary hemangiomas: Case study of a novel laser treatment and a review of therapeutic options. *J Dermatol Surg Oncol* **15**:1214, 1989

16. Achauer B, van der Kam V: Capillary hemangioma (strawberry mark) of infancy: Comparison of argon and Nd:YAG laser treatment. *Plast Reconstr Surg* **84**:60, 1989

17. Hruza G: Laser treatment of warts and other epidermal and dermal lesions. *Dermatol Clin* **15**:487, 1997

18. Nehal K et al: The treatment of benign pigmented lesions with the Q-switched ruby laser: A comparative study using the 5.0 and 6.5 mm spot size. *Dermatol Surg* **22**:683, 1996

19. Kilmer S et al: Treatment of epidermal pigmented lesions with the frequency-doubled Q-switched Nd:YAG laser: A controlled, single impact, dose-response, multicenter trial. *Arch Dermatol* **130**:1515, 1994

20. Fitzpatrick R et al: Clinical advantage of the CO_2 laser superpulsed mode: Treatment of verruca vulgaris, seborrheic keratoses, lentigines, and actinic cheilitis. *J Dermatol Surg Oncol* **20**:449, 1994

21. Grossman M et al: The treatment of café-au-lait macules with lasers. *Arch Dermatol* **131**:1416, 1995

22. Knoell K et al: Q-switched ruby laser treatment of minocycline-induced cutaneous hyperpigmentation. *Arch Dermatol* **132**:1251, 1996

23. Grevelink J et al: Laser treatment of tattoos in darkly pigmented patients: Efficacy and side effects. *J Am Acad Dermatol* **34**:653, 1996

24. Taylor C, Anderson R: Ineffective treatment of refractory melasma and postinflammatory hyperpigmentation by Q-switched ruby laser. *J Dermatol Surg Oncol* **20**:592, 1994

25. Reid W et al: Q-switched ruby laser treatment of tattoos: A 9-year experience. *Br J Plast Surg* **43**:663, 1990

26. Taylor C et al: Treatment of tattoos by Q-switched ruby laser: A dose response study. *Arch Dermatol* **126**:893, 1990

27. Fitzpatrick R et al: Preoperative anesthesia and postoperative considerations in laser resurfacing. *Semin Cutan Med Surg* **15**:170, 1996

28. Alster T, Williams C: Treatment of nevus of Ota by the Q-switched alexandrite laser. *Dermatol Surg* **21**:592, 1995

29. Zelickson et al: Clinical, histologic, and ultrastructural treatment of tattoos treated with three laser systems. *Lasers Surg Med* **15**:364, 1994

30. Watanabe S, Takahashi H: Treatment of nevus of Ota with the Q-switched ruby laser. *N Engl J Med* **331**:1745, 1994

31. Grevelink J et al: Clinical and histologic responses of congenital melanocytic nevi after single treatment with Q-switched lasers. *Arch Dermatol* **133**:349, 1997

32. Jaffe B, Walsh JJ: Water flux from partial-thickness skin wounds: Comparative study of the effects of Er:YAG and Ho:YAG lasers. *Lasers Surg Med* **18**:1, 1996

33. van Leeuwen R et al: *Laser Treatment of Common and Atypical Melanocytic Nevi,* Amsterdam: European Society of Dermatologic Research, 1996

34. Duke D et al: Q-switched and long-pulsed ruby laser treatment of nevomelanocytic lesions. *Lasers Surg Med* **22**:58, 1998

35. Ueda S, Imayama S: Normal-mode ruby laser for treating congenital nevi. *Arch Dermatol* **133**:355, 1997

36. Lee P et al: Failure of Q-switched ruby laser to eradicate atypical-appearing solar lentigo: Report of two cases. *J Am Acad Dermatol* 1998 (in press)

37. Nelson B et al: Management of linear verrucous epidermal nevus with topical fluorouracil and tretinoin. *J Am Acad Dermatol* **30**:287, 1994

38. Hohenleutner U, Landthaier M: Laser therapy of verrucous epidermal nevi. *Clin Exp Dermatol* **18**:124, 1993

39. Grossman M et al: Damage to hair follicles by normal-mode ruby laser. *J Am Acad Dermatol* **35**:889, 1996

40. Dierick CC et al: Permanent hair reduction after ruby laser exposures. *Arch Dermatol*, 1998.

41. Grevelink J: Laser hair transplantation, in *Dermatologic Clinics,* edited by T. Alster. Philadelphia: Saunders, 1997, p 479

42. Walsh J et al: Pulsed CO_2 laser tissue ablation: Effect of tissue type and pulse duration on thermal damage. *Lasers Surg Med* **8**:108, 1988

43. Walsh J et al: Er:YAG laser ablation of tissue: Effect of pulse duration and tissue type on thermal damage. *Lasers Surg Med* **9**:314, 1989

44. Ross E et al: Effects of CO_2 laser pulse duration in ablation and residual thermal damage: Implications for skin resurfacing. *Lasers Surg Med* **19**:123, 1996

45. Fitzpatrick R et al: Pulsed carbon dioxide laser resurfacing of photoaged skin. *Arch Dermatol* **132**:395, 1996

46. Fitzpatrick R: Laser resurfacing of rhytides. *Dermatol Clin* **15**:431, 1997

47. Ross E et al: Long-term results after CO_2 laser resurfacing: A comparison of scanned and pulsed systems. *J Am Acad Dermatol* **37**:709, 1997

48. Bernstein L et al: The short- and long-term side effects of carbon dioxide laser resurfacing. *Dermatol Surg* **23**:519, 1997

49. Weinstein C et al: Complications of carbon dioxide laser resurfacing. *Aesthet Surg J* **17**:216, 1996

50. Duke D et al: Comparison of a 60 microsecond pulse duration to a one millisecond pulsed duration CO_2 laser in skin resurfacing (abstract). *Lasers Surg Med Suppl* **9**:30, 1997

51. Kaufmann R, Hibst R: Erbium:YAG laser ablation in cutaneous surgery. *Lasers Surg Med* **19**:324, 1996

52. Khatri K et al: Comparison of erbium:YAG and CO_2 lasers in skin resurfacing. *Lasers Surg Med Suppl* **9**:37, 1997

53. Teikemeier G, Goldberg D: Skin resurfacing with the erbium:YAG laser. *Dermatol Surg* **23**:685, 1997

54. Welch A et al: Infrared imaging of CO_2 laser resurfacing. *Proc SPIE* **2970**:305, 1997

55. Gardner E et al: In vitro changes in non-facial human skin following CO_2 laser resurfacing: A comparison study. *Lasers Surg Med* **19**:379, 1996

56. Margolis RJ et al: Quantitative comparison of CO_2 laser and TCA peel in skin resurfacing. New England Society of Plastic Surgery Annual Meeting, 1996.

57. Pogrel MA et al: Profile of hyaluronidase activity distinguishes carbon dioxide laser from scalpel wound. *Ann Surg* **217**:196, 1993

58. Smith KG et al: Depth of morphologic skin damage and viability after one, two, and three passes of a high-energy, short-pulse CO_2 laser (Tru-Pulse) in pig skin. *J Am Acad Dermatol* **37**:204, 1997

CHAPTER 266

George J. Hruza

Dermatologic Surgery: Introduction and Approach

During the past 25 years, dermatology has evolved from a primarily medical specialty to a combined medical and surgical specialty.[1] Dermatologists have been in the forefront of cutaneous laser surgery, Mohs micrographic surgery, and cosmetic surgery development,[1,2] and now dermatologic surgery is a required component of dermatology residency training. This chapter deals with the basics of dermatologic surgery and serves as an introduction to subsequent chapters that deal with more advanced dermatologic surgery techniques.

PATIENT SELECTION

Prior to dermatologic surgery, a careful history, review of systems, and focused physical examination are essential. Special attention should be paid to atherosclerotic heart disease, hypertension, presence of cardiac pacemaker, renal disease, diabetes, immunosuppression, healing ability (poor healing, keloids, or hypertrophic scars), bleeding tendency, allergies to systemic antibiotics, local anesthetics or topical antibiotics, pregnancy, and history of syncope, especially from injections or phlebotomy. A detailed medication history should be obtained, with special attention to platelet inhibiting agents such as aspirin, nonsteroidal anti-inflammatory drugs, and dipyridamole; coagulation-inhibiting agents, such as coumadin; beta-blocking agents, phenothiazines, tricyclic antidepressants, thyroid hormones, and monoamine oxidase inhibitors. A history of abnormal heart valves, heart murmur, or prosthetic joints or vessels should be ascertained, as some of these patients may require preoperative prophylactic antibiotics to prevent bacterial endocarditis or prosthesis infection.[3] Smoking may interfere with the survival of skin grafts or flaps because of vasoconstriction[4] while alcohol ingestion may increase the patient's bleeding tendency by causing qualitative platelet inhibition.

Aspirin, nonsteroidal anti-inflammatory drugs, and warfarin increase intraoperative bleeding[5] but have not been clearly demonstrated to increase postoperative bleeding.[5,6] If the patient's medical condition allows and these medications are stopped, warfarin and nonsteroidal anti-inflammatory drugs should be held for 3 days preoperatively, while aspirin should be held for at least 10 days because it causes irreversible inhibition of platelet function.[7–9] Alcohol and cigarettes should be stopped during the perioperative period. Epinephrine should be used with caution in patients taking beta-blocking agents,[10] tricyclic antidepressants, thyroid hormones, and monoamine oxidase inhibitors because of the risk of severe hypertension. However, in routine dermatologic surgery where small amounts of local anesthetic with epinephrine are used, the risk of hypertension is remote.[11] A detailed oral and written informed consent discussing the potential benefits, risks, and alternative treatments should be obtained from the patient or, if the patient is mentally incompetent or under age 18, from the patient's legal guardian.

INFECTION CONTROL

Skin preparation before surgery is designed to reduce but not eliminate the extensive bacterial flora present on intact skin. For minor procedures such as biopsies, cleansing with isopropyl alcohol and the use of nonsterile gloves is sufficient. As the procedure increases in complexity and duration, more elaborate skin preparation is warranted. The skin should be prepared with a povidone-iodine (Betadine) or chlorhexidine scrub followed by the placement of sterile towels or drapes around the surgical field. Hair in the surgical field should be left intact or clipped with scissors. Preoperative shaving of hair has been associated with an increase in wound infections.[12]

Povidone-iodine acts by releasing free iodine onto the skin, with bactericidal activity against most bacteria. Its onset of action is within a few minutes, but once it has dried, is wiped away, or comes in contact with blood, it loses its bactericidal activity, and some patients are allergic to the iodine.[13] Chlorhexidine attacks cell membranes and is bactericidal for most bacteria, with a rapid onset of action. It binds to cell membranes, with bactericidal activity lasting several hours after application. However, it is toxic to the cornea[14,15] and tympanic membrane. Therefore, its use around the eyes and ears should be avoided. As povidone-iodine and chlorhexidine are toxic to tissue in open wounds, they should not be used within such wounds.[16] As hexachlorophene and quaternary ammonium compounds are not bactericidal against many gram-negative organisms,[17] they are rarely used for skin preparation. In addition, hexachlorophene is absorbed through intact skin and is potentially neurotoxic, especially in neonates.[18]

All patients must be thought of as being potentially infected with HIV, hepatitis B or C, or some other blood-borne agent. Therefore, universal precautions must be adhered to in order to protect the surgical staff as well as patients against cross-contamination from other patients.[19] For skin surgery, this means wearing sterile surgical gloves, masks, and protective eyewear. Double gloving reduces the risk of glove perforation during surgery by a factor of 3 to 8.[20,21] If significant exposure to bodily fluids is anticipated, waterproof gowns and caps should be worn as well. Healthcare workers are most commonly exposed to blood by needle sticks. To reduce the risk of needle-stick injury, needles should never be recapped, suture needles should be handled only with instruments, and all sharps should be disposed of in punctureproof containers immediately after use. All instruments that come in contact with a patient's blood must be carefully sterilized or discarded.[22]

The risk of wound infection after skin surgery is quite small.[23] Therefore, routine prophylactic antibiotics are usually not indicated except for patients or anatomic sites at greatest risk for infection. If antibiotics are given, they must be in the bloodstream at the time surgery starts in order to be effective.[24] Infections are more likely to develop in patients who are immunosuppressed or debilitated or who have reduced blood flow to the surgical site, such as the legs in patients with peripheral vascular disease or diabetes. Anatomically, the ears,[23] perineum, legs, and feet seem to be the areas at greatest risk for postoperative wound infection. Open wounds almost never become infected, while closed wounds with hematomas or a large amount of necrotic tissue are at increased risk for infection. For surgery around the lips, prophylactic antiherpesvirus medications are indicated to prevent activation of herpes labialis by the surgery.[25]

The risk of bacteremia after skin surgery of intact skin using proper sterile technique is slight; this risk is similar to that among normal human volunteers not undergoing surgery.[26,27] Recommendations for the use of prophylactic antibiotics in skin surgery have been extrapolated from situations with a much higher incidence of bacteremia, such as urologic or dental procedures. One approach has been to recommend prophylactic antibiotics for patients with eroded skin lesions who the American Heart Association (AHA) has identified as being at high risk for developing bacterial endocarditis (e.g., patients with artificial heart valves, mitral valve prolapse with regurgitation, congenital cardiac malformations, rheumatic or other valvular dysfunction, and history of previous endocarditis).[3] However, according to the AHA, if the skin is intact and surgically scrubbed prior to incision, antibiotic prophylaxis is not indicated.[28] If the skin lesion to be surgically manipulated is infected or the patient has active infection elsewhere on the skin, prophylactic antibiotics should be given to the AHA's high-risk groups as well as to patients with orthopedic prostheses or internal shunts.[3] Antibiotics such as dicloxacillin, with good coverage for gram-positive organisms, and especially *Staphylococcus aureus,* should be given 1 to 2 h before surgery, with a second dose given 6 h after the first.

SURGICAL ANATOMY: DANGER ZONES

Fortunately, dermatologic surgery usually involves tissue layers above the level of the superficial fascia, while, with a few significant exceptions, most structures at risk for damage from surgery, such as motor nerves, lie deep to the fascia. Muscles of facial expression are innervated by the facial nerve, which exits the base of the skull through the stylomastoid foramen and enters the deep lobe of the parotid gland. Within the parotid gland, the facial nerve divides into five major branches that travel within the parotid gland, between the superficial and deep lobes. Once the branches have left the parotid gland and before they have significantly arborized, they are at risk during surgery, as transection of one of these branches will result in permanent motor paralysis of the related muscle group. This danger zone is approximately between the anterior surface of the parotid gland and a vertical line drawn from the lateral canthus to the inferior border of the mandible at the insertion of the masseter muscle.[29]

The temporal (frontal) branch of the facial nerve is at risk as it crosses the temple after having left the parotid gland and before it has entered the deep surface of the frontalis muscle. It is very superficial, being located within or on top of the superficial fascia.[30] Transection of the temporal nerve may result in unilateral eyebrow ptosis. This deficit, if permanent, can be corrected through a unilateral eyebrow lift.[31] Undermining in the temporal and zygomatic region should be carried out in the superficial fat. The temporal artery is a useful guide to depth of undermining, as it lies superficial to the temporal nerve.

The zygomatic branch of the facial nerve is at greatest risk as it crosses the zygoma after exiting the parotid gland and before entering the deep surface of the orbicularis oculi muscle. Transection of the zygomatic nerve may result in unilateral inability to close the eyelid and ectropion, with resultant exposure conjunctivitis. Partial correction of the deficit can be achieved by placing gold weights into the upper eyelid, which will allow the eyelids to close properly.[32]

The buccal branch of the facial nerve is at risk as it crosses the masseter muscle in the middle of the cheek after leaving the parotid gland parallel with the parotid duct. It is located on top of the masseter muscle fascia, which is covered by a thick fat pad in most patients. Therefore, injury to this nerve during dermatologic surgery is quite rare. If the nerve is severed, the patient will develop significant facial asymmetry and an inability to pucker his or her lips, with a resultant difficulty in keeping fluids in the mouth. Nerve grafting and/or repair offer the best chance for restoring function.[33]

The marginal mandibular branch of the facial nerve is at risk as it crosses the mandible at the insertion of the masseter muscle, where it is located within the subcutaneous fat in close proximity to the facial artery. Injury to the marginal mandibular nerve may result in facial asymmetry. Nerve grafting or repair may be necessary in order to restore normal muscle function.[33] The cervical branch of the facial nerve exits the inferior pole of the parotid to innervate the platysma. Injury to this branch is not usually associated with any functional impairment.

The spinal accessory nerve traverses the posterior triangle of the neck deep to the superficial cervical fascia, from the posterior surface of the sternocleidomastoid muscle to the anterior surface of the trapezius muscle. The posterior triangle of the neck is bounded by the sternocleidomastoid muscle anteriorly, the trapezius muscle posteriorly, and the clavicle inferiorly. The spinal accessory nerve exits the posterior surface of the sternocleidomastoid muscle at the junction of the superior and middle thirds of the sternocleidomastoid muscle. Injury to the spinal accessory nerve will cause weakness of the shoulder and winged-scapula deformity.[34]

Transection of sensory nerves may result in permanent anesthesia of the denervated area. However, most of the anesthetic area usually regains some sensation over 2 to 3 years. Occasionally, a painful traumatic neuroma develops at the site of nerve injury. The possibility of permanent sensory loss in an area of surgery should be included in the informed consent prior to surgery.

The blood supply of the face has extensive anastomoses between the various arteries. Therefore, cutting any of the facial arteries has no clinical significance as long as effective hemostasis is achieved. Small vessels can be electrocoagulated. But larger, named vessels, such as the temporal artery, should usually be tied off with a suture to reduce the risk of delayed bleeding, which can develop after the vasoconstricting effect of epinephrine has dissipated. The external and internal carotid systems communicate in the periorbital and perinasal areas via anastamoses between the angular artery (external carotid system) and branches of the ophthalmic artery (internal carotid system).[34] Therefore, injection of any material, such as a sclerosant, has the potential to be carried back into the internal carotid system, with the possibility of cavernous sinus thrombosis. Interruption of lymphatic drainage with dermatologic surgery in the head and neck area causes only brief periods of edema. The one exception is the infraorbital region, where a long horizontal incision may lead to lymphedema of the lower eyelid lasting several months and, in rare cases, years. On the extremities, incisions should involve less than 50 percent of the circumference of the limb in order to prevent distal lymphedema.

LOCAL ANESTHESIA

Mechanism of Action

Local anesthetics diffuse through the tissue to the nerves and pass through the nerve cell membrane to block Na^+ influx during depolarization. This blocks action potentials from occurring. Smaller unmyelinated C-type nerve fibers that conduct temperature and pain sensation are blocked more easily than myelinated A-type nerve fibers, which carry pressure sensations and motor fibers.[35]

Local anesthetics are weak organic bases that, to be water-soluble and injectable, require the addition of a hydrochloride salt. In aqueous solution, the salt equilibrates between the ionized and nonionized form. The ionized form is water-soluble and allows injection into the tissues, but it is the nonionized, lipid-soluble base that diffuses through the tissue to the nerve cell membrane, where the ionized cation is responsible for blocking nerve conduction. At physiologic pH of 7.4, some 80 percent or more of most local anesthetics is in the cationic ionized form. Cocaine is vasoconstricting, but all other local anesthetics are vasodilating.

Types of Anesthetics

Local anesthetics consist of a hydrophobic aromatic end and a hydrophilic secondary or tertiary amine end. The two ends are joined together by an ester or amide linkage (Table 266-1). Esters include benzocaine, chloroprocaine, cocaine, procaine, and tetracaine. They are hydrolyzed in plasma and liver by cholinesterases and subsequently excreted by the kidneys. Amides include bupivacaine, dibucaine, etidocaine, lidocaine, mepivacaine, and prilocaine. They are N-dealkylated and subsequently hydrolyzed by microsomal liver enzymes.

Lidocaine 1% with 1:100,000 epinephrine is the standard local anesthetic used for skin surgery. This mixture is very acidic in order to keep the epinephrine component from becoming inactivated. The addition of 1 mL of 1 meq/mL $NaHCO_3$ to 10 mL of lidocaine with epinephrine before injecting it neutralizes the anesthetic solution, reducing burning on injection and facilitating anesthetic diffusion but also somewhat reducing the hemostatic effect.[36] For anesthetic effects that are to last more than 1 to 2 h, bupivacaine or etidocaine can be used.[35,37]

TABLE 266-1

Local Anesthetics

Generic Name	Trade Name	Primary Use	Relative Potency	Onset	Duration* Plain	Maximum[†] Dose Plain	Maximum[†] Dose with Epinephrine
Amides							
Bupivacaine	Marcaine	Infiltration	8	2–10 min	3–10 h	175 mg	250 mg
Dibucaine	Nupercaine	Topical		Rapid	Short		
Etidocaine	Duranest	Infiltration	6	3–5 min	3–10 h	300 mg	400 mg
Lidocaine	Xylocaine	Infiltr./Topical	2	Rapid	1–2 h	300 mg	500 mg (3850 mg dilute)
Mepivacaine	Carbocaine	Infiltration	2	3–20 min	2–3 h	300 mg	400 mg
Prilocaine	Citanest	Infiltration	2	Rapid	2–4 h	400 mg	600 mg
Prilocaine/Lidocaine	EMLA	Topical		30–120 min	Short		
Esters							
Benzocaine	Anbesol, etc.	Topical		Rapid	Short		
Chloroprocaine	Nesacaine	Infiltration	1	Rapid	0.5–2 h	600 mg	
Cocaine		Topical		2–10 min	1–3 h	200 mg	
Procaine	Novocaine	Infiltration	1	Slow	1–1.5 h	500 mg	600 mg
Proparacaine	Ophthaine	Topical		Rapid	Short		
Tetracaine	Pontocaine	Infiltration	8	Slow	2–3 h	20 mg	
Tetracaine	Cetacaine	Topical		Rapid	Short		

*In clinical practice the duration of anesthesia appears to be less than stated above, especially for head and neck areas, and addition of epinephrine prolongs anesthesia by a factor of two.
[†]Maximum doses are for a 70-kg person.

Side Effects

Contraindications to local anesthetics include severe blood pressure instability, history of true allergy to the anesthetic, psychological instability, severe liver compromise (for amide-type anesthetics), and severe renal compromise (for ester-type anesthetics). The most frequent side effect encountered is a vasovagal reaction manifest by hypotension and bradycardia. Injecting with the patient recumbent or in the Trendelenburg position will usually keep the vasovagal reaction from becoming symptomatic. Local side effects include bruising and edema, especially in the periorbital area, and transient motor nerve paralysis. Prolonged paresthesia from sensory nerve injury can occur with nerve blocks if the needle traumatizes the nerve being anesthetized.

Overdosage is rarely a problem in dermatologic procedures as long as the maximum recommended doses of 5 mg/kg of 1% lidocaine or 7 mg/kg of 1% lidocaine with 1:100,000 epinephrine are respected. For tumescent anesthesia, the maximum safe dose appears to be at least 55 mg/kg of 0.05 to 0.1% lidocaine with 1:1,000,000 epinephrine.[38] Signs of overdosage start with circumoral numbness and tingling and can progress to seizures and cardiovascular collapse with severe overdosage.[39] Toxic effects are exacerbated by acidosis and hypoxia.

Local anesthetic allergic reactions are usually IgE-mediated type I reactions that are manifest by urticaria, angioedema, or anaphylaxis with hypotension and tachycardia. True allergic reactions to ester anesthetics are infrequent, but there is cross-reactivity with paraamino benzoic acid, sulfonamides, sulfonylureas, thiazides, and paraphenylene diamine. Patients who are allergic to one of the ester anesthetics can cross-react with other ester anesthetics but not with the amide anesthetics. Amide anesthetics do not cross-react with other drugs and true allergic reactions are extremely rare. Many multidose bottles of local anesthetics contain methylparaben and/or bisulfite preservatives, which can cause allergic reactions and may be the most frequent cause of local anesthetic "allergy." Management of patients with local anesthetic allergy includes skin testing, use of a preservative-free anesthetic, or substitution of amide for ester or vice versa.[40] Diphenhydramine hydrochloride (Benadryl) 12.5 mg/mL can be used for local anesthesia, but the patient may develop systemic antihistamine side effects. Normal saline injected intradermally can achieve very brief anesthesia.

Prilocaine metabolizes to ortho-toluidine. This is an oxidizing agent capable of converting hemoglobin to methemoglobin—an effect that can be significant with large doses of >500 mg. Bupivacaine poses a greater risk of cardiac toxicity—with ventricular arrhythmias and cardiovascular collapse—than lidocaine.

Epinephrine

Epinephrine prolongs the duration of anesthesia by 100 to 150 percent and decreases the anesthetic's systemic toxicity by slowing its absorption. It is hemostatic in a dilution of up to 1:1,000,000. It is absolutely contraindicated in patients with hyperthyroidism and pheochromocytoma. Relative contraindications include hypertension, severe cardiovascular disease, pregnancy, and narrow-angle glaucoma as well as in patients taking beta blockers, phenothiazines, monoamine oxidase inhibitors, or tricyclic antidepressants. Injection of epinephrine into digits and the penis should be avoided, especially in patients with peripheral vascular disease. When a relative contraindication is present, epinephrine should be used with caution by diluting it to 1:500,000 and using it sparingly.

Side effects of epinephrine include self-limited palpitations, anxiety, fear, diaphoresis, headache, tremor, weakness, and tachycardia. Serious side effects include arrhythmias, ventricular tachycardia, ventricular fibrillation, cardiac arrest, and cerebral hemorrhage. Serious side effects are extremely rare when appropriate dosages are used in patients without significant contraindications. Skin necrosis can occur in patients with poor perfusion or in anatomic sites with limited perfusion or limited collateral circulation, such as the digits.

Topical Anesthetics

The conjunctiva can be anesthetized with proparacaine or tetracaine eyedrops. Superficial mucous membrane anesthesia can be achieved with various topical anesthetics including Surfacaine, Topicale, Dyclone, Anbesol, viscous lidocaine, and lidocaine jelly. For more thorough anesthesia, especially of the intranasal mucosa, a 4 to 10% cocaine solution is effective, with the added benefit of being hemostatic. Partial anesthesia of intact skin can be achieved with eutectic mixture of local anesthetics (EMLA) cream[41] or 30 to 40% lidocaine in acid-mantle cream applied under occlusion 1 to 2 h before the procedure. The resulting anesthesia is variable and in general effective only for very superficial surgery and some laser procedures.[42–45] Iontophoresis of lidocaine can also achieve superficial skin anesthesia.[46] Cryoanesthesia with Fluoroethyl or Frigiderm can achieve sufficient anesthesia for superficial procedures and is especially useful for dermabrasion.

"Painless" Local Anesthesia

Minimizing the pain of anesthetic infiltration is for many patients the most important part of the procedure. Minimizing pain starts with verbal reassurance and distraction, accompanied by mechanical distraction through pinching at the injection site, using small, 30-gauge needles and small 1- to 3-mL syringes to reduce the pressures generated on injection. A buffered anesthetic solution is helpful to reduce the burning sensation of the anesthetic being injected. Injections should be made very slowly, with additional sticks through already anesthetized tissue. Injection into the subcutis is less painful than into the dermis. Injection is started on the side where the sensory innervation originates and proceeds distally. Cryoanesthesia or EMLA is used before injecting sensitive areas or in children. Before injection, oral sedatives such as diazepam can be useful for very anxious patients. Long-acting local anesthetics may serve as supplements for prolonged procedures.[47,48]

Large areas such as the scalp for hair transplantation can be anesthetized with field-block anesthesia, in which infiltration is into the tissues surrounding the surgical field. In certain areas a specific nerve can be blocked by injecting 1 to 2 mL of anesthetic into its vicinity. Blocks of the supraorbital and supratrochlear nerves anesthetize the central forehead and frontal scalp.[49] Block of the infraorbital nerve anesthetizes the medial cheek, upper lip, and nasal ala, and block of the mental nerve anesthetizes the lower lip.[50] The entire foot can be anesthetized with nerve blocks of the tibial, sural, superficial peroneal, and deep peroneal nerves.[51]

SUTURING TECHNIQUES

Correct suturing technique[52] is crucial for functionally and cosmetically outstanding results from skin surgery. In addition to approximation of wound edges, properly placed sutures are important for skin-edge eversion, minimization and redistribution of tension, elimination of dead space, and maintenance or restoration of natural anatomic contours while avoiding the formation of permanent suture marks on the skin surface. The suturing technique chosen for a specific wound closure will depend on which of the above functions are most important as well as the anatomic location and thickness of the wound edge.

Suture Materials

The two main characteristics differentiating suture materials are the suture configuration and its absorbability (Table 266-2). Sutures can have either monofilament (single-strand) or multifilament (braided) construction. Advantages of monofilament sutures include decreased tendency of infection or suture reaction and ease of passage through tissue, including easy removal. The main advantage of braided sutures is low memory. Memory is the tendency of the suture to retain its original shape. Low suture memory increases knot security and ease of handling. Monofilament suture, with its high memory, has reduced knot security and less ease of handling. Braided sutures pose a greater risk of causing suture reactions and infections and are more difficult to pass through tissue and remove.

Sutures that lose at least 50 percent of their tensile strength within 2 months are considered absorbable, even though such sutures may not dissolve completely for many months. Absorbable sutures are used mainly as buried sutures. They can also be used as surface sutures in cases when suture removal is impractical, as in the case of patients who live far away from the surgeon's office; those who are difficult to treat, such as young children; and in the case of skin grafts, where the wound bed should not be disturbed. Nonabsorbable sutures maintain their tensile strength for more than 2 months and are used mainly on the surface, with the intention of removing them as soon as the wound edges have fully reepithelialized. They are used for skin-edge approximation and exact alignment, with any tension across the wound having been eliminated by the deeper absorbable sutures. Occasionally, permanent sutures

are used as buried sutures that are left in place indefinitely in order to provide long-lasting support, as in rhytidectomy.

Synthetic sutures have almost entirely replaced natural sutures in dermatologic surgery. Because natural sutures—including silk and catgut—are much more reactive than synthetic sutures, they are used only in very limited situations. Silk, a nonabsorbable braided natural suture, is useful near mucous membranes, as it is a very soft and pliable suture with low memory. This makes it much less irritating to the mucous membrane than a stiff monofilament suture. Fast-absorbing catgut or mild chromic catgut suture is a monofilament suture that is rapidly absorbed; it is useful for securing skin grafts and for eyelid skin closure.

Selection of suture size depends on skin thickness, body site, and amount of tension across the wound. Small-gauge 5-0 and 6-0 sutures should be used on facial skin, with eyelid skin receiving only 6-0 sutures. The trunk, extremities, and scalp can be sutured with 3-0 and 4-0 sutures and the neck, digits, and genitals with 4-0 and 5-0 sutures. If a larger suture than that recommended above is needed to close a defect, the wound is under too much tension and additional manipulation is in order, such as increased undermining, relaxing incisions, or redesign of the closure plan.

Interrupted Sutures

The simple interrupted suture is the most basic and versatile suture used by dermatologic surgeons. If the suture is placed close to the wound edges, very precise coaptation of the wound edges can be achieved, even in wounds with edges of unequal thickness. If it is placed further from the wound edges, deeper tissues can be pulled in with redistribution of tension across the wound. When the suture is properly placed in a flask-shaped configuration, eversion of the wound edges can be achieved (Fig. 266-1).[53] Wounds in which the edges are of unequal thickness can be aligned by taking a larger

TABLE 266-2[131,132]

Suture Materials

	Type	Memory	Tissue Reactivity	Tensile Strength Half-Life
Nonabsorbable				
Cotton	Twisted	Low	Very high	—
Nylon (Ethilon, Dermalon)	Monofilament	High	Low	—
Nylon (Nurolon, Surgilon)	Braided	Low	Low	—
Polybutester (Novafil)	Monofilament	High	Low	—
Polyester, uncoated (Mersilene)	Braided	Low	Low	—
Polyester, coated (Ethibond)	Braided	Low	Low	—
Polypropylene (Prolene, Surgilene) Surgilene)	Monofilament	Very high	Very low	—
Silk	Braided/twisted	Very low	High	—
Stainless steel	Monofilament/braided/twisted	Very high	Very low	—
Absorbable				
Catgut, fast absorbing/mild chromic	Twisted	Very high	High	2 days
Catgut	Twisted	Very high	High	4 days
Catgut, chromic	Twisted	Very high	High	1 week
Polyglactin 910 (Vicryl)	Braided	Very low	Low	2 weeks
Polyglycolic acid (Dexon)	Braided	Very low	Low	2 weeks
Poliglecaprone 25 (Monocryl)	Monofilament	Low	Very low	1 week
Polyglyconate (Maxon)	Monofilament	Low	Very low	1 month
Polydoxanone (PDS)	Monofilament	High	Very low	1 month

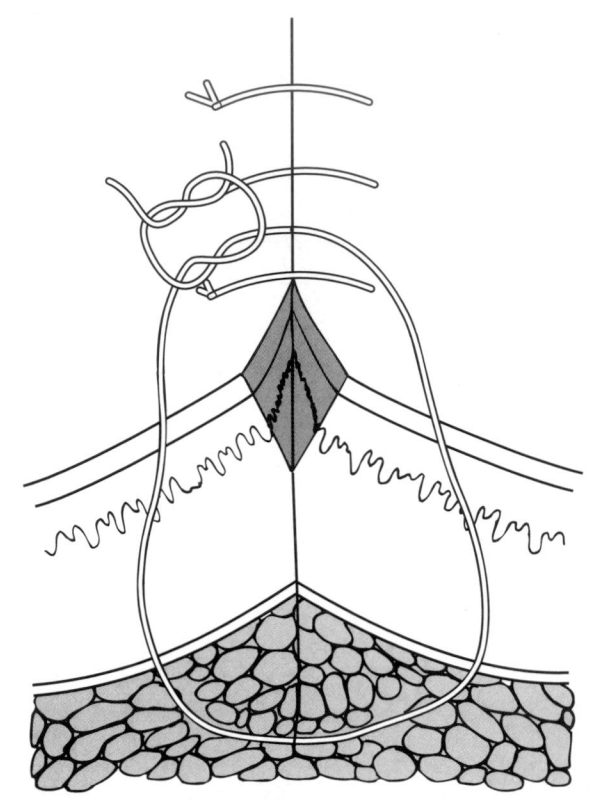

"Flask-shaped" simple interrupted suture.

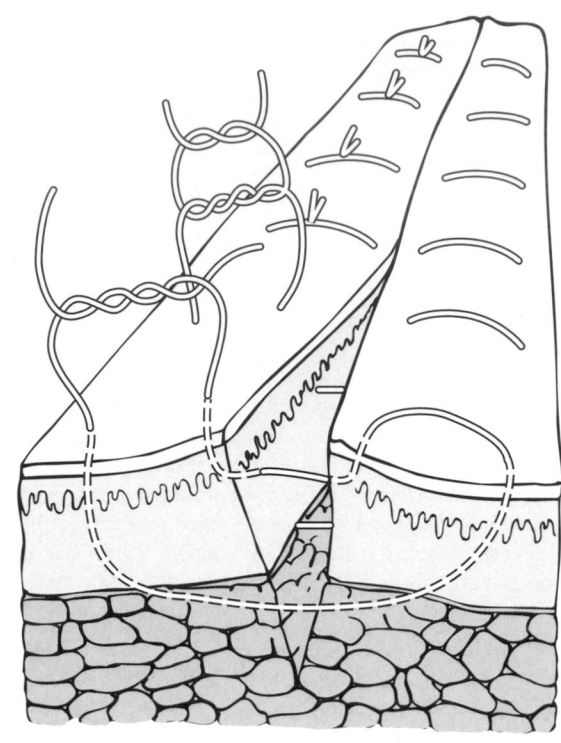

Vertical mattress suture.

bite from the thinner edge and a smaller bite from the thicker edge. Wounds in which one edge appears higher than the other can be similarly aligned. The simple interrupted suture can also be used as a temporary tacking suture to align complex wound edges or position a flap properly.[54]

The main disadvantage of the simple interrupted suture is the risk of crosshatch marks across the suture line. This problem can be minimized by removing the sutures within 5 to 7 days before the formation of epithelial suture tracks is complete, using minimally reactive monofilament suture such as polypropylene and eliminating tension across the wound with appropriate planning of wound closure, adequate undermining, and the use of buried sutures. A minor problem as compared with a running suture is that the simple interrupted suture is more time-consuming to place and remove, especially for long suture lines. In settings where wound healing may be impaired due to the patient's advanced age or underlying disease, interrupted suture techniques may be preferred, as interrupted sutures may have, with all other factors being equal, greater tensile strength and less potential to cause edema, induration, and impaired microcirculation than running sutures.[55]

The vertical mattress suture is one of the best sutures for wound-edge eversion, and this is the main indication for its use by dermatologic surgeons (Fig. 266-2). It also reduces dead space and minimizes tension across the wound, doing the job of both a buried dermal suture and a skin suture. Because this suture requires four entry points in the skin, significant crosshatching can be expected if the suture is not removed within 5 to 7 days. Even though the

vertical mattress suture can be used anywhere on the body, its use on the trunk and extremities results in significant suture marks because it must be left in place longer than 7 days. On the face, some surgeons use vertical mattress sutures instead of a two-layer closure. Even when deep dermal sutures are used, a few vertical mattress sutures can be placed along the wound for maximal wound-edge eversion,[56] while the intervening areas can be precisely approximated with simple interrupted sutures.[53]

The half-buried vertical mattress suture is a modification of the standard vertical mattress suture; it is designed to eliminate half of the four suture marks in areas such as the face, where minimal scarring is important. This suture is intermediate between a simple interrupted and standard vertical mattress suture in terms of relieving tension across the wound and achieving eversion of the wound edges. It is sometimes used along the hairline, where the buried component is placed on the face and the exposed part of the suture is placed in the hairline.[54]

Classically, the horizontal mattress suture has been used for reducing tension across wound closures under significant tension (Fig. 266-3). This suture can be placed as an initial tension-reducing or holding suture and to bring the wound edges closer together, so that subcutaneous sutures can be placed to distribute tension and close the wound. At this point, if the tension has been adequately distributed, the horizontal mattress suture may be removed. If tension across the wound persists, the horizontal mattress suture may be left in place for a few days while early wound healing proceeds and removed before suture tracks have had a chance to form. In areas at high risk for wound dehiscence, such as the lower extremities, the horizontal mattress suture may even be left in place for a few days after the skin sutures have been removed. However, when left in place for more than 7 days and sometimes even less time, significant suture tracks are almost certain to form.[53]

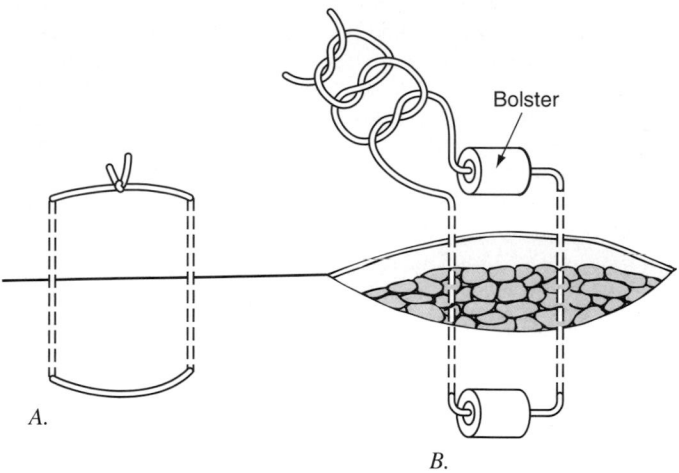

FIGURE 266-4

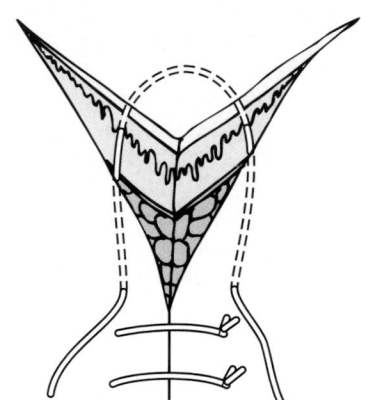

Horizontal mattress suture (*A*) without and (*B*) with a bolster.

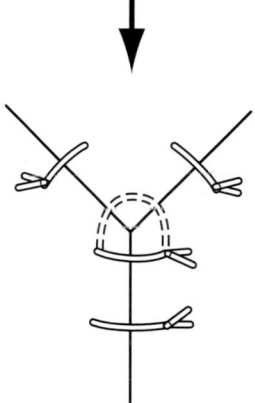

Half-buried horizontal mattress suture.

Alternatively the horizontal mattress suture may be used to pre-suture 12 to 24 h before a proposed excision that may be under considerable tension. This short-term tissue expansion may allow as much as 30 percent more tissue to be removed at the time of definitive excision.[57] Presuturing has been used successfully in alopecia reduction, rhytidectomy, and congenital nevus excision.[57-59]

The main disadvantage of this suture is the possibility of wound-edge necrosis, as this suture can easily strangulate the dermal plexus between its limbs. This problem is minimized by taking large bites with the needle to encompass large amounts of tissue, by using bolsters, by tying the suture only as tight as necessary to accomplish the task of bringing the wound edges together, and by removing the suture as soon as possible, ideally within 2 days of wound closure. Prior to contemplating the use of a horizontal mattress suture for tension reduction, the surgeon should consider other means of reducing tension across the wound, including appropriate use of undermining and closure orientation, flaps from areas of tissue excess, preoperative or intraoperative tissue expanders, serial excisions, and subcutaneous sutures.

Another effect of the horizontal mattress suture is prominent wound-edge eversion. This property can be utilized by using a relatively fine suture material and taking relatively small bites when placing the suture across a tension-free wound that has been closed with buried sutures. This achieves wound-edge eversion and, if the suture is not tied too tightly, wound-edge necrosis is unlikely to develop.[60]

The half-buried horizontal mattress suture is primarily indicated for the positioning of various corners and tips including flap tips, M-plasty tips, and V-Y closure tips (Fig. 266-4). It can also align the edges of tangential flaps and flaps with ischemic wound edges. The buried limb of this suture is placed in the potentially ischemic area in order to minimize interference with the dermal vascular plexus.[60] This reasoning has been challenged, since a superficial simple interrupted suture through a flap tip does not appear to result in increased risk of flap tip necrosis.[61]

A wound gains only 7 percent of its final strength after 2 weeks.[62] As most skin sutures are removed within 1 week of placement, absorbable buried sutures are used as part of layered wound closure. This provides support for the wound until tensile strength has increased sufficiently to prevent wound dehiscence. Deep, bur-

ied sutures are placed into wounds to reduce or eliminate tension on the wound edges. On the trunk and extremities, where tension across wounds is greatest, the use of buried sutures may reduce the amount of scar spread. Buried sutures can align the wound edges, so that the skin edges are closely approximated even before the placement of skin sutures. Deep sutures can eliminate dead space and align deep structures such as skeletal muscle or fascia. Deep sutures can also be used to anchor overlying tissue to underlying fixed structures, such as periosteum, to maintain proper facial contour and function. This is exemplified by the anchoring to the maxillary periosteum of a melolabial flap used to close a nasal defect.

The buried dermal suture is used routinely as part of layered closures in dermatologic surgery to eliminate tension across the superficial wound edges and align the wound edges properly. A properly placed buried dermal suture will allow the easy placement of skin sutures without tension. As this suture is placed at the junction of dermis and fat, the knot must be buried so as to minimize tissue reaction to the suture and extrusion through the wound.

The deep subcutaneous suture is entirely subcutaneous. It is used to decrease the amount of dead space, to anchor flaps, and to align deep structures. Because it is deep, tissue reaction to the suture or suture extrusion through the wound is very unlikely even if nonabsorbable suture material is used. Therefore the knot need not be buried.

The buried horizontal mattress suture is a "purse-string" suture that is occasionally used to eliminate dead space or reduce tension across wounds in areas where there is not enough room to place vertical sutures, as in defects on the nose, with its stiff dermis and minimal subcutaneous tissue. Also, this suture can be used to close off dead space in other areas, such as after the removal of an epidermal cyst. It must be placed deeply and not tied too tightly, as the enclosed tissue can easily become strangulated.[63]

One disadvantage of the standard buried dermal suture is that the wound edges are pulled flat without significant wound-edge eversion.[64] The buried vertical mattress suture incorporates a modification of the buried dermal suture, which maximizes prolonged wound-edge eversion with resulting improved wound healing.[65] The buried vertical mattress suture can be visualized as a standard vertical mattress suture that is completely moved below the skin surface while maintaining its shape. The suture is more superficial further from the wound edge than at the wound edge.[64,66]

Running Sutures

The simple running suture can be used in situations where the wound edges are of equal thickness without tension, closely approximated, and with an absence of subcutaneous dead space (Fig. 266-5). This suture is most useful for wounds that have already been closed by buried sutures, for the attachment of full-thickness or split-thickness skin grafts, and in areas of thin skin such as the eyelids, ears, neck, and scrotum.[67] By eliminating all but two knots, there is less suture material resting against the skin, resulting in the

development of fewer scars from suture marks. However, fine adjustments along the suture line are difficult to make and the suture has a tendency to pucker when very lax and thin skin, such as eyelid skin, is being sutured. In thin skin, the knots at each end may be tied over small bolsters to prevent them from cutting into the tissue.[53,54,56]

The running locked suture is a variant of the simple running suture in which, after the placement of each loop, the needle is passed through the previous loop prior to starting the next loop. It is intended for the closure of well-vascularized wounds under a moderate amount of tension. The wound edges should be stiff and of equal thickness without a tendency for inversion. It is stronger than a simple running suture. However, if it is placed too tightly or if significant postoperative swelling develops, tissue strangulation with wound-edge necrosis may ensue. It is used primarily on the scalp for the closure of scalp reduction defects and hair transplant donor sites. This suture is strong but should be used sparingly and only when clearly indicated because of the potential for tissue strangulation if it is not placed properly.[53,56]

The running horizontal mattress suture is primarily a skin-edge-everting suture. It is the ideal suture for closure of wounds with a significant tendency for wound-edge inversion. In addition, by pulling in additional tissue to the wound edge, spreading of facial scars (as seen in young patients) can be minimized. If it is tied too tightly, wound-edge strangulation and necrosis may develop.

The running subcuticular suture is basically a buried running horizontal mattress suture (Fig. 266-6). It is ideal for the closure of wounds in areas such as the trunk and extremities where the suture must remain in place for more than 7 days.[68] As the suture is buried, there are no suture marks and the suture may be left in place for several weeks; when absorbable suture material is used, it may be left in place until it is absorbed.[69,70] As this suture is capable of only modest wound-edge alignment, it should be reserved for wounds in which the tension has been eliminated with deep sutures

FIGURE 266-5

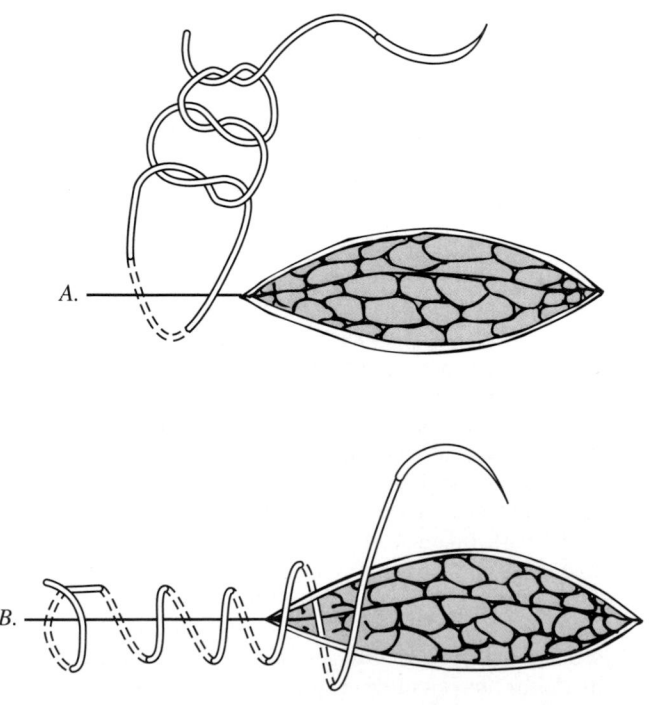

Simple running suture.

FIGURE 266-6

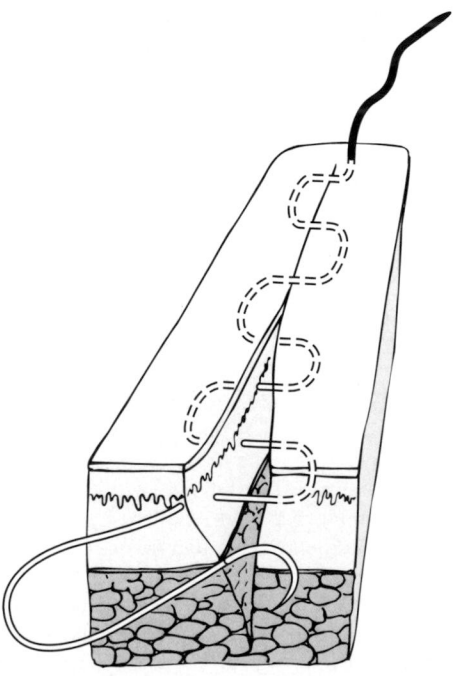

Running subcuticular suture.

and the wound edges, of approximately equal thickness, are closely approximated. The running subcuticular suture should be placed with a nonreactive monofilament suture such as polypropylene to facilitate suture removal and prevent suture breakage within the wound.[71] Some surgeons advocate the use of permanent sutures left in place indefinitely, as this can reduce scar stretching.[72] If nonabsorbable sutures are to be used and to be totally buried, clear, nonreactive suture material such as polypropylene should be used.[53,56]

The running subcutaneous suture is designed for the closure of the deep component of relatively long surgical defects that are under only moderate tension. It replaces the buried dermal interrupted suture in selected situations. The main advantage of this suture over interrupted sutures is the speed of placement. However, if the suture material were to rupture anywhere along the suture line, the entire wound might dehisce or a subcutaneous dead space could form under the skin edge without being apparent at the surface.[53,73]

Suture Removal

Suture marks are due to epidermal downgrowth along the suture track seen within 5 to 7 days of suture placement and aggravated by sutures that have been tied too tightly.[56,60] Sutures should be removed at the earliest possible time to prevent or minimize suture reaction, infection, and suture marks. However, they should remain in place long enough to prevent wound dehiscence and scar spread. In general, the less blood supply to an area and the greater the tension across a wound, the longer the sutures should be left in place. On the face and ears, most skin sutures should be removed within 5 to 7 days, with eyelid sutures being removed in 3 to 5 days. Neck sutures should be removed in 7 days and scalp sutures in 7 to 10 days. On the trunk and extremities, risk of wound dehiscence takes precedence over suture marks. Sutures on the trunk and upper extremities should be left in place for 10 to 14 days. Lower extremities may require 14 to 21 days of suture support.[74]

Absorbable sutures are left in place. However, some patients develop suture reactions, consisting of suture abscesses and suture extrusion through the wound. If this happens, the suture should be picked up carefully with small forceps and cut out of the wound. Any purulent material should also be drained.

Stainless Steel Staple Closure

Staple closure of wounds is an alternative to suture closure. The staples have the advantage of very quick placement, minimal tissue reaction, and a very strong wound closure.[75,76] This type of closure is most often used with long wounds, especially on the scalp, where the suture line is hidden by scalp hair. Potentially contaminated wounds that are closed with staples appear to be more resistant to infection than wounds closed with sutures.[77] Staples provide efficient wound closure; but when exact wound-edge alignment is required, sutures should be used. Also, surgical staples are far more expensive than suture material.[76] Staples are removed with a staple remover or hemostat.

Wound Closure Tapes

Wound closure tapes are used to provide additional support to a suture line, especially when a running subcuticular suture has been used.[56] In addition, they are helpful in supporting the wound edges after the skin sutures have been removed. Wounds closed with wound closure tapes have a lower risk of wound infection than sutured wounds.[78,79] However, as they fail to achieve adequate

wound-edge eversion and tension reduction, wound closure tapes are rarely used as primary wound closure materials.[80] Keeping them in place for several weeks may reduce the amount of scar spreading.[81]

EXCISIONAL SURGERY

A fusiform (elliptical) excision is indicated for the removal of small to moderate-size benign or malignant neoplasms as well as for excisional biopsy. Fusiform closure can be utilized wherever there is sufficient skin laxity to allow direct side-to-side closure of the defect, after adequate undermining, under minimal tension, and without distortion or functional impairment of surrounding structures. For optimal cosmetic results, the long axis of the fusiform excision should be oriented along the relaxed skin tension lines, which are generally perpendicular to the muscle pull in the area, without crossing over cosmetic unit boundaries, such as the nose-cheek concavity.[82] If relaxed skin tension lines are not obvious, manipulation of the skin will indicate the direction of least tension. An alternative to fusiform excision is disk excision. The lesion is excised as a circle with adequate margins and the wound is either allowed to heal by second intention or the defect is closed into a straight line with excision of the resulting bilateral standing cones of excess tissue.[83]

ELECTROSURGERY

Electrosurgery is a simple, quick, and effective technique for the treatment of various benign and malignant lesions. Electrosurgery is often combined with curettage to help in debulking of the lesion and removing charred tissue. The main disadvantage of electrosurgery is that there is no histologic confirmation of the lesion having been destroyed. Therefore, if there is any doubt as to the diagnosis of a lesion, a biopsy should be performed prior to destroying it with electrosurgery. Also, when used to destroy malignant lesions, electrosurgery does not provide tissue for histologic checking of margins. If tissue is obtained from an area subjected to significant electrosurgery, significant tissue artifact is generated, making reliable histologic interpretation very difficult.

Electrodesiccation and electrocoagulation are the most frequently used forms of electrosurgery. They both consist of a high-frequency, high-voltage, low-amperage damped current.[84] The main difference is that in electrodesiccation, there is no dispersive electrode, and the voltage, frequency, and current damping are all greater, while amperage is lower than with electrocoagulation. The observed tissue effect is from contact of the treatment electrode with tissue, generating resistive heating of tissue with resultant tissue dehydration and coagulation. Electrodesiccation is less destructive than electrocoagulation, as less current passes into the tissue and there is less channeling of current along conductive structures such as blood vessels and nerves.[85] Electrodesiccation is most often used for the destruction of verrucae, superficial nonmelanoma skin cancer, and actinic keratoses. Epidermal lesions can be effectively removed by electrodesiccating their surface. This causes dermal-epidermal separation, which can be taken advantage of with a dermal curette to scrape the lesion away. Electrocoagulation, with its affinity for tracking along blood vessels, is ideally suited for achieving hemostasis during scalpel surgery. In bipolar electrocoagulation, there is no dispersive electrode; instead, both electrodes are part of a forceps. The tissue to be coagulated, usually a blood vessel, is gently picked up by the forceps and current is applied to coagulate it.[86]

Electrofulguration uses a current of very high voltage, very high frequency, and very low amperage that is highly damped without a dispersive electrode.[84] Treatment is performed by holding the electrode tips slightly above the lesion surface in order to generate a spark that carbonizes the surface through resistive heating. The carbonized surface protects deeper tissue from additional fulguration. Therefore, this modality is ideal for very superficial benign lesions, such as dermatosis papulosa nigra and skin tags. Healing is rapid and scarring rare.

Electrosection uses a high-voltage, low-amperage, high-frequency undamped current to cause tissue separation with extremely localized molecular oscillations and heat generation. As the effect is very localized, there is minimal tissue damage; consequently, no hemostasis is achieved with a pure undamped current. To make electrical cutting more practical by achieving hemostasis as the tissue is separated with the current, most devices deliver a blended current that damps the current slightly with increased tissue coagulation and hemostasis.[84] Electrosection is useful in patients with bleeding disorders or on anticoagulants that cannot be stopped before the procedure. By this method, as compared with scalpel surgery, the wound heals more slowly with decreased tensile strength early on, due to the thermally coagulated tissue left in the wound.

In electrocautery, a high-amperage, low-voltage direct or alternating current is passed through a treatment tip that becomes red hot through resistive heating. The heated tip is applied to tissue to coagulate it through direct conduction of heat. As compared with electrodesiccation, electrocautery can cause greater tissue damage through heat conduction from the treatment site. One advantage of electrocautery is that it can work in a bloody surgical field and on nonconductive surfaces such as cartilage, bone, or nails.

Galvanic current is a direct low-voltage, low-amperage current in which the treatment electrode is negative and the dispersive electrode positive. The negative polarity of the treatment electrode generates hydroxides and hydrogen gas in the tissue. These hydroxides liquefy the tissue. Only very small areas can be destroyed with galvanic current, minimizing the risk of scarring but slowing the treatment process down significantly.[87] The most frequent use of galvanic current is for electrolysis of unwanted hair and destruction of small facial telangiectasias. However, as this technique is so slow, it has generally been replaced by electrodesiccation and electrocoagulation, which is referred to as *thermolysis*.[87]

Modern pacemakers are very well shielded from standard electrosurgical current. However, it is prudent not to use electrosurgical current near the heart or the pacemaker; when the current is used, it should be applied in short bursts so that any interference would be limited in duration.[88] The best option is to use bipolar electrocoagulation where the current passes between the two forcep tips or electrocautery where no current enters the body.

Electrosurgery can cause fire, especially in an oxygen-enriched environment or in the perianal area from the release of methane gas.[89] Electrosurgery generates a significant amount of smoke, which is not only carcinogenic[90] but may contain viable tissue fragments containing infectious particles, such as human immunodeficiency virus (HIV). Therefore, the use of smoke evacuators is ad-visable when electrosurgery is being performed. Electrode tips should be changed after each patient, as electrodes can transmit viral particles.[91]

HEALING BY SECOND INTENTION

Healing of full-thickness skin wounds by second intention is indicated for patients who are poor surgical risks for reconstructive surgery and those who refuse reconstructive surgery. It is also used for infected wounds, to allow observation of the wound bed after resection of tumors at high risk for recurrence, for selected pathologic ulcers, and when the anticipated cosmetic result is at least as good as that achieved by reconstruction.[92] Wounds that are allowed to granulate are very resistant to infection and cannot form a hematoma. The locations that lend themselves best to wound healing by second intention, with superior cosmetic results, are concave areas such as the nose-cheek junction, medial canthus, ear concha, preauricular cheek, and retroauricular scalp.[93] Wounds allowed to heal by second intention may decrease in size as much as 50 percent or more.[94] Superficial wounds heal with less wound contraction, since there is less deposition of collagen. Therefore a superficial wound, even on a convex surface such as the forehead or the nose, will usually heal well. Because all wounds contract to some degree, it is important that there be no "free" margin along one side of the wound that can be pulled up during wound contracture and cause distortion at the site. This may be encountered along the eyelid margins, ear margins, eyebrow, nasal ala, and lip vermilion border. These areas are better managed with appropriate reconstructive surgery.[93] Disadvantages of healing by second intention include prolonged healing time of several weeks, the need for daily wound care by the patient, and the somewhat unpredictable cosmetic results.[95]

LOCAL SKIN FLAPS

When simple primary closure cannot be done because a wound is too large, there is too much tension on the wound edges, or an unacceptable functional or cosmetic result would ensue, a tissue-movement procedure such as a flap or a graft should be considered. A local skin flap is a portion of full-thickness skin transferred from a donor site into a surgical defect while maintaining its blood supply from the donor site via a random or axial vascular pedicle that remains attached to the donor site.[53] The point of attachment or pedicle is critical for the survival of the flap, since it is through this area that the flap will receive its blood supply. Therefore, for random flaps, the length-to-width ratio should not exceed 3:1 or 4:1 on the face and 2:1 on the trunk and extremities. The thickness of flaps also varies depending on location and should be adjusted for the site into which it will be placed.[96] Flap incisions should, whenever possible, be made so that they fall into relaxed skin tension lines.[97] Care should be taken not to include hair in a flap to be placed in an area that is not naturally hair-bearing. If hair is intentionally included in the flap, the direction of hair growth should be the same as that in the area of the defect. There are two movements occurring in a flap. The action of placing the flap into the defect is the primary movement. There is also secondary movement of tissue in the donor area needed to close the secondary defect and to facilitate primary flap movement. Both movements are important in terms of distributing tension in the proper direction and over a larger area so as to minimize tension on the flap itself, which might compromise its survival.[98]

There are various kinds of flaps. In an advancement flap, the tissue movement is in a straight line from the donor area to the recipient site, and it may be unilateral or bilateral. A classic example is a bilateral advancement flap to close a moderate-size defect on the forehead with incision lines made in natural furrows of the forehead and with tissue advancement in the horizontal plane.[96] The rim of the ear helix can be advanced to close defects of the helical rim, relying on excess tissue present in the earlobe.[99] Another bilateral advancement flap is an A-to-T flap, in which incisions extend from the base of a triangular defect and the two sides are slid together along this baseline. A third similar advancement flap is a Burrow's triangle single-advancement flap.[100] Common areas for the use of advancement flaps include defects of hair-bearing skin in the eyebrow[101] (Fig. 266-7) or mustache area, where orientation of the hair shafts is critical. The rotation flap slides skin into the defect by rotating it on its axis. This is classically used to close relatively large defects on the cheek,[102] forehead, or scalp. A rotation flap with a back cut can increase tissue movement in areas of limited tissue laxity, such as the nose.[103] A double-rotation or an O-to-Z flap can also increase the amount of tissue rotated into the defect.

Transposition flaps belong in a different category, since they transpose skin from one site to another, crossing normal, non-flap skin in between. The classic transposition flap is the rhombic flap with its exact geometric design (Fig. 266-8). The defect is visualized in the shape of a rhombus with equal sides and angles opposite each other of 60 and 120 degrees, respectively. The flap is then created by drawing a line out from and bisecting either of the 120-degree angles equal in length to one side. The next line creates a 60-degree angle with that line and is parallel to and equal to the side of the rhombus.[104] Other transposition flaps include the note flap,[105] banner flap, nasolabial (melolabial) flap,[106] bilobed flap,[107] Webster's 30-degree modified rhombic flap,[108] and Z-plasty.[109] Transposition flaps are very versatile, being useful for the repair of various facial defects.[96] A subcutaneous island pedicle flap has had all of its connections to the epidermis and dermis severed, maintaining its blood supply only through a subcutaneous tissue pedicle (see Fig. 266-7).[110,111] This flap is usually slid from the defect apex into the center to close an area that would be under great tension if closed side-to-side.[112] It is often used to close defects on the side of the nose and in the melolabial fold.[113]

The most commonly used axial vascular pedicle flap on the face is the paramedian forehead two-stage transposition flap[114] (Fig. 266-9). Tissue is mobilized from the forehead, based on one of the supratrochlear arteries, and transposed to repair large distal nasal defects with the pedicle remaining attached in the glabellar region. Division of the pedicle is performed in 2 to 3 weeks after the flap has established a local blood supply from the original defect's wound bed.[115] Another useful flap is the nasolabial two-stage flap, in which a flap based on the angular artery is mobilized and used for repair of nasal ala and tip defects of moderate size. The advantage over the one-stage nasolabial fold transposition flap is the complete preservation of the nose-cheek concavity, which is often distorted or obliterated with the one-stage flap.[116] Finally, larger ear helix full-thickness defects can be repaired with a two-stage flap raised from the postauricular sulcus.

Flaps are more delicate and therefore require more careful postoperative wound care than simple excisions. Tightly applied bandages may compromise the blood supply to the flap and cause necrosis. The area under the flap must be free of any bleeding or oozing as hemorrhage or hematoma formation may jeopardize flap

FIGURE 266-7

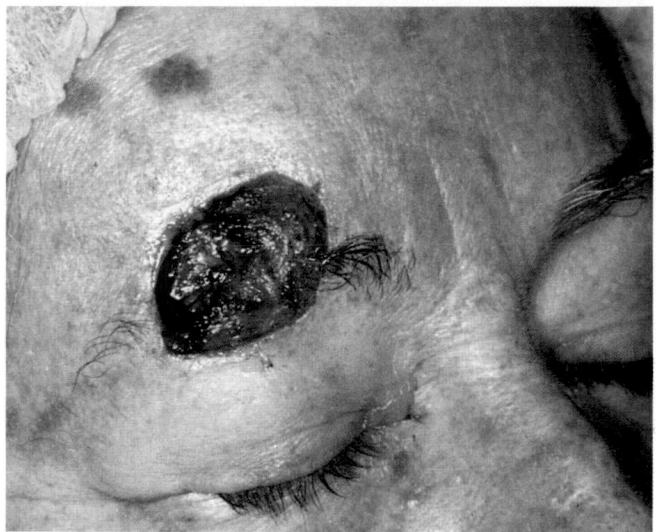

A.

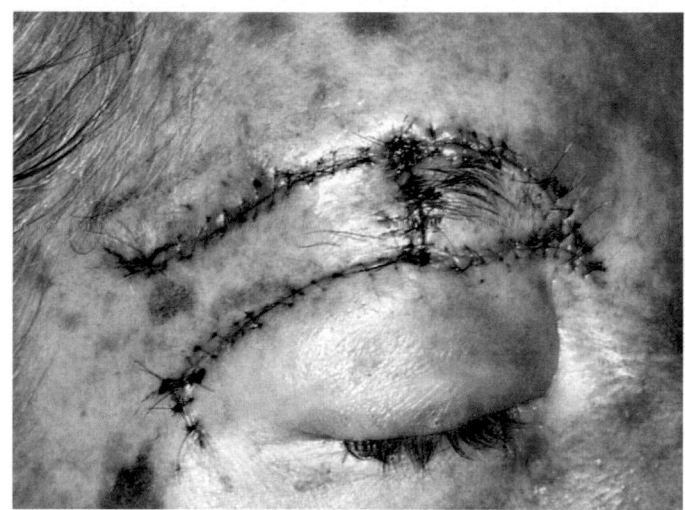

B.

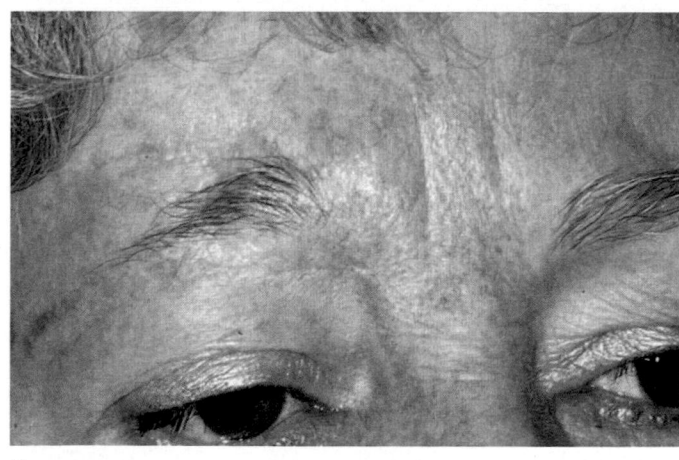

C.

A. Right eyebrow surgical defect after tumor resection. B. Immediately after repair with a laterally based advancement flap and a medially based island pedicle flap. C. Final result (7 months postoperative).

FIGURE 266-8

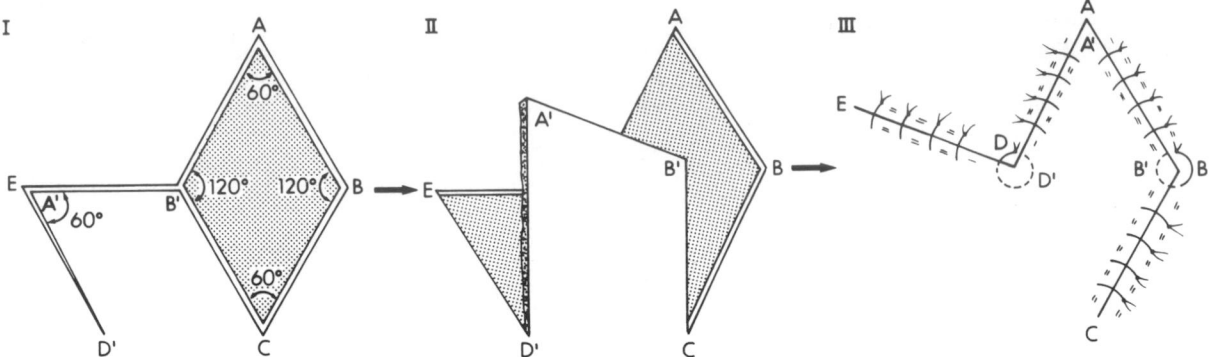

Rhombic transposition flap: (I) Design with shaded area representing surgical defect, (II) transposition after undermining, and (III) final suture line.

survival and increase the risk of infection. Patients who smoke may compromise the blood supply to the flap, and large flaps should be reconsidered in such patients.[117] The "trapdoor" effect occurs with some flaps when the center of the flap becomes elevated and the suture line becomes depressed. This is most often seen with curved transposition flaps and is probably due to centripetal contraction of the scar at the suture line and under the flap. It may resolve spontaneously over a period of 6 to 12 months. However, if it fails to resolve spontaneously, it may respond to intralesional glucocorticoids and/or flap elevation with flap thinning, possibly combined with multiple Z-plasties to break up the curved scar line.[118] The trapdoor effect may be prevented with wide undermining around the primary defect, proper thinning of the flap, proper size of the flap, and the use of a geometric shape for the flap.[106,118]

SKIN GRAFTS

Grafts are totally detached from the donor site and receive all nutrients from the wound bed of the recipient site. They are named after the harvesting method (punch, pinch, dermatomal) and/or their composition (epidermis, dermis, fat, hair, cartilage, bone). Full-

FIGURE 266-9

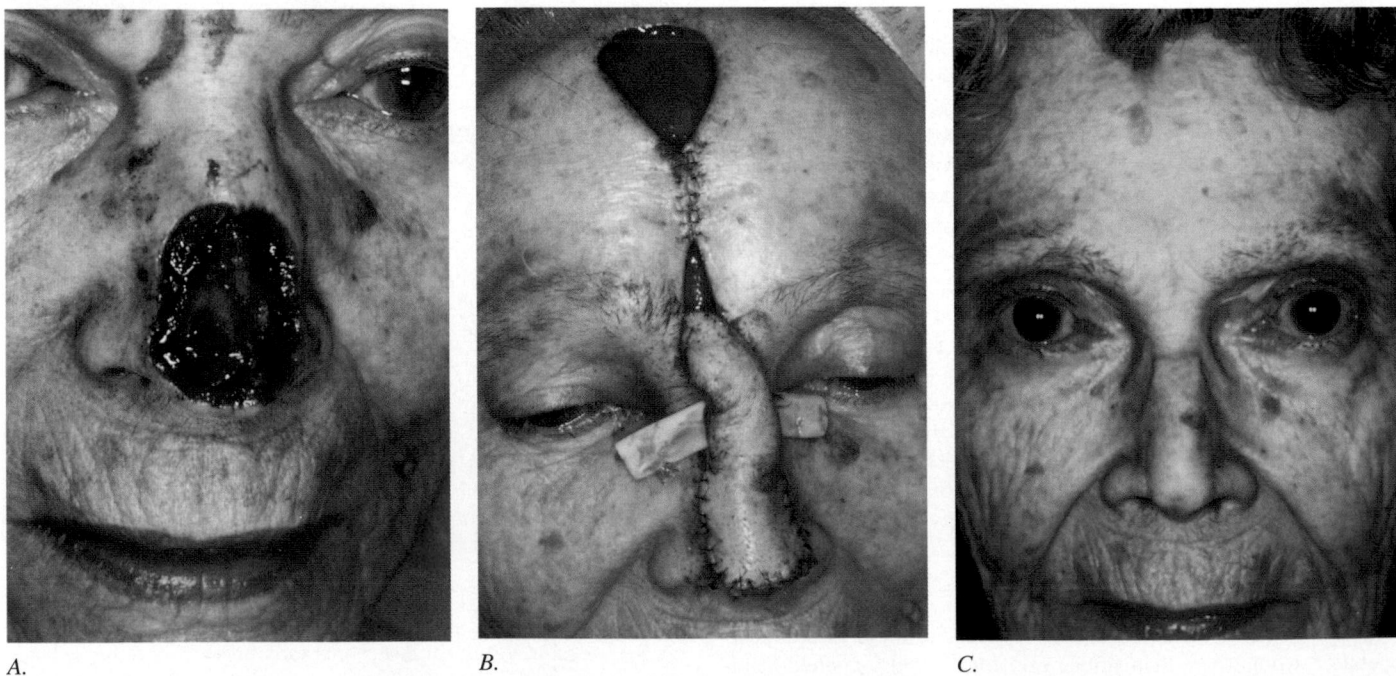

A. *B.* *C.*

A. Dorsal nose surgical defect after tumor resection. *B.* Immediately after first stage of paramedian forehead flap with upper forehead donor area to heal by second intention healing. *C.* Final result 8 months after flap division and inset.

thickness skin grafts (FTSG) consist of epidermis with full-thickness dermis, while split-thickness skin grafts (STSG) consist of epidermis with a varying thickness of dermis.

A STSG is used to cover large defects, to allow better wound bed surveillance, to line a large pedicle flap or cover the donor site of a large FTSG, or to resurface mucosa.[119] It is usually harvested from the thigh, buttock, scalp, or abdomen using a manual or power dermatome set to the desired thickness. The STSG is placed on the wound and fixed in place with absorbable sutures or staples. The main advantage of a STSG is that it will survive even in a relatively hostile environment, such as a leg ulcer. Cosmetically, this graft is suboptimal, with absent appendages, poor color match, and frequent wound contracture under the graft. For very large recipient sites, STSGs may be meshed.[120] These meshed grafts are useful for coverage of lower leg ulcers because they also allow for drainage, with less chance of seroma formation underneath the graft.[121] The donor site will reepithelialize rapidly and relatively painlessly with the use of bioocclusive dressings.[122,123]

A FTSG is generally indicated for relatively shallow full-thickness facial defects that may not be amenable to primary closure or local flap repair or to temporarily cover a defect that needs to be observed for possible tumor recurrence. It is usually harvested from the preauricular, nasolabial, postauricular, conchal bowl,[124] supraclavicular, or eyelid areas. The donor site is chosen so as to match the recipient site skin texture, thickness, color, and appendiceal structure density.[125] Burrow's triangle FTSGs are harvested in contiguity with the graft recipient site from areas of tissue excess, achieving superior skin color and texture match.[126] A FTSG will contract less than a STSG. Appendiceal structures are retained and skin color match is better than with a STSG. A FTSG is harvested with a fusiform excision, often with use of a template of the recipient defect. The graft is then trimmed to exactly fit the defect and defatted. The donor site is closed with a primary side-to-side closure or second intention healing; if it is too large, a STSG may be used to cover it. The graft is sutured onto the recipient site, including basting sutures[127] as needed. A bolster dressing may be placed over the graft to keep it in place and to prevent fluid accumulation underneath it. For the bolster, a traditional tie-over dressing can be used. Alternatively, the graft can be secured with a Reston foam dressing secured with staples or an Aquaplast thermoplastic heat-moldable dressing.[128] Because skin grafts do not bring any blood supply with them, they are more vulnerable to necrosis than simple closures or well-designed flaps. Skin color match is difficult to predict. Fairer-skinned individuals with even pigmentation and less sun damage do well with FTSGs. The more darkly pigmented or mottled the surrounding skin, the less likely a good color match will be. Uneven edges around the graft may be smoothed out with dermabrasion 6 to 8 weeks after surgery.[129]

Composite grafts include a component in addition to the epidermis and dermis. The most common composite graft includes cartilage and is used for the correction of full-thickness nasal ala defects. The graft is harvested from the ear helix so that it contains a sandwich of skin surrounding a piece of cartilage. After being sutured in place, the graft receives its blood supply only from its lateral margins. Therefore, only up to 1 cm of nasal ala rim can be replaced with a composite graft, as a larger graft will not receive sufficient nutrients to allow its central portion to survive.[130]

REFERENCES

1. Bennett RG, Krull EA: ASDS 20th anniversary: The history of dermatologic surgery. *J Dermatol Surg Oncol* **16**:384, 1990
2. Hanke CW: The literature of dermatologic surgery 1970—present. *J Dermatol Surg Oncol* **16**:202, 1990

3. Haas AF, Grekin RC: Antibiotic prophylaxis in dermatologic surgery. *J Am Acad Dermatol* **32**:155, 1995
4. Goldminz D, Bennett RG: Cigarette smoking and flap and full-thickness graft necrosis. *Arch Dermatol* **127**:1012, 1991
5. Billingsley EM, Maloney ME: Intraoperative and postoperative bleeding problems in patients taking warfarin, aspirin and nonsteroidal antiinflammatory agents. *Dermatol Surg* **23**:381, 1997
6. Otley CC et al: Complications of cutaneous surgery in patients who are taking warfarin, aspirin, or nonsteroidal anti-inflammatory drugs. *Arch Dermatol* **132**:161, 1996
7. Goldsmith SM et al: Management of patients taking anticoagulants and platelet inhibitors prior to dermatologic surgery. *J Dermatol Surg Oncol* **19**:578, 1993
8. Patrono C: Aspirin as an antiplatelet drug. *N Engl J Med* **330**:1287, 1994
9. Salasche S: Acute surgical complications: Cause, prevention, and treatment. *J Am Acad Dermatol* **15**:1163, 1986
10. Foster CA, Aston SJ: Propranolol-epinephrine interaction: A potential disaster. *Plast Reconstr Surg* **72**:74, 1983
11. Dzubow LM: The interaction between propranolol and epinephrine as observed in patients undergoing Mohs' surgery. *J Am Acad Dermatol* **15**:71, 1986
12. Alexander JW et al: The influence of hair-removal methods on wound infections. *Arch Surg* **118**:347, 1983
13. Brown TR et al: A clinical evaluation of chlorhexidine gluconate spray as compared with iodophor scrub for preoperative skin preparation. *Surg Gynecol Obstet* **158**:363, 1984
14. Hamed LM et al: Hibiclens keratitis. *Am J Ophthalmol* **104**:50, 1987
15. Nasser RE: The ocular danger of Hibiclens. *Plast Reconstr Surg* **89**:164, 1992
16. Lineaweaver W et al: Cellular and bacterial toxicities of topical antimicrobials. *Plast Reconstr Surg* **75**:394, 1985
17. Sebben JE: Sterile technique and the prevention of wound infection in office surgery: Part 2. *J Dermatol Surg* **15**:38, 1989
18. Shuman RM et al: Neurotoxicity of hexachlorophene in humans: A clinicopathologic study of 46 premature infants: Part 2. *Arch Neurol* **32**:320, 1975
19. CDC: Update: Universal precautions for prevention of transmission of human immunodeficiency virus, hepatitis B virus, and other blood-borne pathogens in health-care settings. *MMWR* **37**:377, 1988
20. Greco RJ, Garza JR: Use of double gloves to protect the surgeon from blood contact during aesthetic procedures. *Aesthetic Plast Surg* **19**:265, 1995
21. Gross DJ et al: Surgical glove perforation in dermatologic surgery. *J Dermatol Surg Oncol* **15**:1226, 1989
22. Hruza GJ: Infection control precautions for surgical personnel in the surgery unit and for laboratory personnel in the Mohs surgery unit areas. *Semin Dermatol* **14**:228, 1995
23. Futoryan T, Grande D: Postoperative wound infection rates in dermatologic surgery. *Dermatol Surg* **21**:209, 1995
24. Classen DC et al: The timing of prophylactic administration of antibiotics and the risk of surgical wound infection. *N Engl J Med* **326**:281, 1992
25. Perkins SW, Sklarew EC: Prevention of facial herpetic infections after chemical peel and dermabrasion: New treatment strategies in the prophylaxis of patients undergoing procedures of the perioral area. *Plast Reconstr Surg* **98**:427, 1996
26. Sabetta JB, Zittelli JA: The incidence of bacteremia during skin surgery. *Arch Dermatol* **123**:213, 1987
27. Wilson WR et al: Incidence of bacteremia in adults without infection. *J Clin Microbiol* **2**:94, 1975
28. Dajani AS et al: Prevention of bacterial endocarditis: Recommendations by the American Heart Association. *JAMA* **277**:1794, 1997
29. Bernstein L, Nelson RH: Surgical anatomy of the extraparotid distribution of the facial nerve. *Arch Otolaryngol* **110**:177, 1984
30. Campiglio GL, Candiani P: Anatomical study on the temporal fascial layers and their relationships with the facial nerve. *Aesthetic Plast Surg* **21**:69, 1997
31. Grabski WJ, Salasche SJ: Management of temporal nerve injuries. *J Dermatol Surg Oncol* **11**:145, 1985
32. Freeman MS et al: Surgical therapy of the eyelids in patients with facial paralysis. *Laryngoscope* **100**:1086, 1990
33. Conley J, Baker DC: The surgical treatment of extratemporal facial paralysis. *Head Neck Surg* **1**:12, 1978

34. Otani A et al: The superficial neurovasculature of the head and neck. *Semin Dermatol* **13**:43, 1994

35. Auletta MJ: Local anesthesia for dermatologic surgery. *Semin Dermatol* **13**:35, 1994

36. Stewart JH et al: Neutralized lidocaine with epinephrine for local anesthesia. *J Dermatol Surg Oncol* **15**:1081, 1989

37. Arpey CJ, Jynch WS: Advances in local anesthesia. *Clin Dermatol* **10**:275, 1992

38. Ostad A et al: Tumescent anesthesia with a lidocaine dose of 55 mg/kg is safe for liposuction. *Dermatol Surg* **22**:921, 1996

39. deJong RH: Toxic effects of local anesthetics. *JAMA* **239**:1166, 1978

40. Glinert RJ, Zachary CB: Local anesthetic allergy. *J Dermatol Surg* **17**:491, 1991

41. Hruza GJ: EMLA cream: Painless local anesthesia? *Fitzpatrick's J Clin Dermatol* **2(1)**:50, 1994

42. Sherwood KA: The use of topical anesthesia in removal of port-wine stains. *J Pediatr* **122**:S36, 1993

43. Gupta AK, Sibbald RG: Eutectic lidocaine/prilocaine 5% cream and patch may provide satisfactory analgesia for excisional biopsy or curettage with electrosurgery of cutaneous lesions. *J Am Acad Dermatol* **35**:419, 1996

44. Raveh T et al: Efficacy of the topical anesthetic cream, EMLA, in alleviating both needle insertion and injection pain. *Ann Plast Surg* **35**:576, 1995

45. Lubens HM, Sanker JF: Anesthetic skin patch. *Ann Allergy* **22**:37, 1964

46. Maloney JM: Local anesthesia obtained via iontophoresis as an aid to shave biopsy. *Arch Dermatol* **128**:331, 1992

47. Randle HW: Reducing the pain of local anesthesia. *Cutis* **53**:167, 1994

48. Arndt KA et al: Minimizing pain of local anesthesia. *Plast Reconstr Surg* **72**:676, 1983

49. Pay AD, Kenealy J: The use of nerve blocks in the laser treatment of cutaneous lesions. *Br J Plast Surg* **50**:132, 1997

50. Randle HW et al: Know your anatomy: Local anesthesia for cutaneous lesions of the head and neck—practical applications of peripheral nerve blocks. *J Dermatol Surg Oncol* **18**:231, 1992

51. Cohen SJ, Roenigk RK: Nerve blocks for cutaneous surgery on the foot. *J Dermatol Surg Oncol* **17**:527, 1991

52. Hruza GJ: Suturing techniques, in *Principles and Techniques of Cutaneous Surgery,* edited by GP Lask, RL Moy. New York, McGraw-Hill, 1996, p 171

53. Stegman SJ et al: *Basics of Dermatologic Surgery.* Chicago, Year Book, 1982

54. Lober CW: Suturing techniques, in *Dermatologic Surgery: Principles and Practice,* edited by RK Roenigk, HH Roenigk Jr. New York, Marcel Dekker, 1989, p 205

55. Speer DP: The influence of suture technique on early wound healing. *J Surg Res* **27**:385, 1979

56. Stegman SJ: Suturing techniques for dermatologic surgery. *J Dermatol Surg Oncol* **4**:63, 1978

57. Meirson D et al: Presuturing in alopecia reductions. *J Dermatol Surg Oncol* **16**:818, 1990

58. Liang MD et al: Presuturing: A new technique for closing large skin defects: Clinical and experimental studies. *Plast Reconstr Surg* **81**:694, 1988

59. Hedén P: Presuturing in rhytidectomy: A case report. *Aesthetic Plast Surg* **15**:161, 1991

60. Perry AW, McShane RH: Fine tuning of the skin edges in the closure of surgical wounds: Controlling inversion and eversion with the path of the needle: The right stitch at the right time. *J Dermatol Surg Oncol* **7**:471, 1981

61. McQuown SA et al: Gillies' corner stitch revisited. *Arch Otolaryngol* **110**:450, 1984

62. Harris DR: Healing of the surgical wound: I. Basic considerations. *J Am Acad Dermatol* **1**:197, 1979

63. Presser SE: The subcutaneous stitch revisited. *J Dermatol Surg Oncol* **15**:342, 1989

64. Davidson TM: Subcutaneous suture placement. *Laryngoscope* **97**:501, 1987

65. Zitelli JA: TIPS for a better ellipse. *J Am Acad Dermatol* **22**:101, 1990

66. Zitelli JA, Moy RL: Buried vertical mattress suture. *J Dermatol Surg Oncol* **15**:17, 1989

67. McLean NR et al: Comparison of skin closure using continuous and interrupted nylon sutures. *Br J Surg* **67**:633, 1980

68. Clayer M, Southwood RT: Comparative study of skin closure in hip surgery. *Aust N Z J Surg* **61**:363, 1991

69. Sanders RJ: Subcuticular skin closure: Description of technique. *J Dermatol Surg* **1**:61, 1975

70. Herron J: Skin closure with subcuticular polyglycolic acid sutures. *Med J Aust* **2**:535, 1974

71. Pham S et al: Ease of continuous dermal suture removal. *J Emerg Med* **8**:539, 1990

72. Elliot D, Mahaffey PJ: The stretched scar: The benefit of prolonged dermal support. *Br J Plast Surg* **42**:74, 1989

73. Ftaiha Z, Snow SN: The buried running dermal subcutaneous suture technique. *J Dermatol Surg Oncol* **15**:264, 1989

74. Chernosky ME: Scalpel and scissors surgery as seen by the dermatologist, in *Skin Surgery,* 6th ed, edited by E Epstein, E Epstein Jr. Philadelphia, Saunders, 1987, p 88

75. Roth JH, Windle BH: Staple versus suture closure of skin incisions in a pig model. *Can J Surg* **31**:19, 1988

76. Gatt D et al: Staples for wound closure: A controlled trial. *Ann R Coll Surg Engl* **67**:318, 1985

77. Stillman RM et al: Skin wound closure: The effect of various wound closure methods on susceptibility to infection. *Arch Surg* **115**:674, 1980

78. Moy RL et al: Commonly used suturing techniques in skin surgery. *Am Fam Pract* **44**:1625, 1991

79. Edlich RF et al: Wound healing and wound infection, in *Wound Healing and Wound Infection: Theory and Surgical Practice,* edited by TK Hunt. New York, Appleton-Century-Crofts, 1980

80. Bunker TD: Problems with the use of Op-Site sutureless skin closures in orthopaedic procedures. *Ann R Coll Surg Engl* **65**:260, 1983

81. Hodges JM: Management of facial lacerations. *South Med J* **69**:1413, 1976

82. Meirson D, Goldberg LH: The influence of age and patient positioning on skin tension lines. *J Dermatol Surg Oncol* **19**:39, 1993

83. Swanson NA: *Atlas of Cutaneous Surgery.* Boston, Little, Brown, 1987

84. Sebben JE: Electrosurgery: High frequency modalities. *J Dermatol Surg Oncol* **14**:367, 1988

85. Sebben JE: *Cutaneous Electrosurgery.* Chicago, Year Book, 1989

86. Bodian EL: Electrosurgery by bipolar modalities. *J Dermatol Surg Oncol* **4**:325, 1978

87. Wagner RFJ et al: Electrolysis and thermolysis for permanent hair removal. *J Am Acad Dermatol* **12**:441, 1985

88. Sebben JE: Electrosurgery and cardiac pacemakers. *J Am Acad Dermatol* **9**:457, 1983

89. Miller JM: Explosion in sigmoid colon during colonoscopic polypectomy. *V A Med* **107**:296, 1980

90. Tomita Y et al: Mutagenicity of smoke condensates induced by CO_2-laser irradiation and electrocauterization. *Mutat Res* **89**:145, 1981

91. Sheretz EF et al: Transfer of hepatitis B virus by reusable needle electrodes after electrodesiccation in simulated use. *J Am Acad Dermatol* **15**:1242, 1986

92. Levin BC et al: Healing by secondary intention of auricular defects after Mohs surgery. *Arch Otolaryngol Head Neck Surg* **122**:59, 1996

93. Zitelli JA: Wound healing by secondary intention: A cosmetic appraisal. *J Am Acad Dermatol* **9**:407, 1983

94. McGrath MH, Simon RH: Wound geometry and the kinetics of wound contraction. *Plast Reconstr Surg* **72**:66, 1983

95. Reed BR, Clark RA: Cutaneous tissue repair: Practical implications of current knowledge II. *J Am Acad Dermatol* **13**:919, 1985

96. Tromovitch TA et al: *Flaps and Grafts in Dermatologic Surgery.* Chicago, Year Book, 1989

97. Stroud MB: Design of skin flaps with a new technique using templates. *J Dermatol Surg Oncol* **13**:1171, 1987

98. Dzubow LM: Flap dynamics. *J Dermatol Surg Oncol* **17**:116, 1991

99. Calhoun KH et al: Biomechanics of the helical rim advancement flap. *Arch Otolaryngol Head Neck Surg* **122**:1119, 1996

100. Gromley DE: Use of Burrow's wedge principle for repair of wounds in or near the eyebrow. *J Am Acad Dermatol* **12**:344, 1985

101. Whitaker DC, Birkby CS: Mohs surgery report: An approach to cutaneous surgical defects of forehead and eyebrow following Mohs micrographic surgery. *J Dermatol Surg Oncol* **13**:1312, 1987

102. Katz AE, Grande DJ: Cheek-neck advancement-rotation flaps following Mohs excision of skin malignancies. *J Dermatol Surg Oncol* **12**:949, 1986

103. Wee SS et al: The frontonasal flap: Utility for distal nasal defects and technical refinements. *Br J Plast Surg* **44**:201, 1991
104. Borges AF: Choosing the correct Limberg flap. *Plast Reconstr Surg* **62**:542, 1978
105. Walike JW, Larrabee WF: The note flap. *Arch Otolaryngol* **111**:430, 1985
106. Zitelli JA: The nasolabial flap as a single-stage procedure. *Arch Dermatol* **126**:1445, 1990
107. Zitelli JA: The bilobed flap for nasal reconstruction. *Arch Dermatol* **125**:957, 1989
108. Webster RC et al: The thirty degree transposition flap. *Laryngoscope* **88**:85, 1978
109. Bernstein L: Z-plasty in head and neck surgery. *Arch Otolaryngol* **89**:36, 1969
110. Hruza GJ: Subcutaneous island pedicle flap revisited. *Fitzpatrick's J Clin Dermatol* **2(2)**:35, 1994
111. Tomich JM et al: Subcutaneous island pedicle flaps. *Arch Dermatol* **123**:514, 1987
112. Dzubow LM: Subcutaneous island pedicle flaps. *J Dermatol Surg Oncol* **12**:591, 1986
113. Wee SS et al: Refinements of nasalis myocutaneous flap. *Ann Plast Surg* **25**:271, 1990
114. Quatela VC et al: Esthetic refinements in forehead flap nasal reconstruction. *Arch Otolaryngol Head Neck Surg* **121**:1106, 1995
115. McGregor IA: Local flaps in facial reconstruction. *Otolaryngol Clin North Am* **15**:77, 1982
116. Barlow RJ, Swanson NA: The nasofacial interpolated flap in reconstruction of the nasal ala. *J Am Acad Dermatol* **36**:965, 1997
117. Salasche SJ, Grabski WJ: Complications of flaps. *J Dermatol Surg Oncol* **17**:132, 1991
118. Koranda FC, Webster RC: Trapdoor effect in nasolabial flaps. *Arch Otolaryngol* **111**:421, 1985
119. Wheeland RG: Skin grafts, in *Dermatologic Surgery: Principles and Practice,* edited by RK Roenigk, HH Roenigk Jr. New York, Marcel Dekker, 1989, p 323
120. Davison PM et al: The properties and uses of nonexpanded machine-meshed skin grafts. *Br J Plast Surg* **39**:462, 1986
121. Berretty PJ et al: Treatment of ulcers on legs from venous hypertension by split-thickness skin grafts. *J Dermatol Surg Oncol* **5**:966, 1979
122. Weber RS et al: Split-thickness skin graft donor site management: A randomized prospective trial comparing a hydrophilic polyurethane absorbent foam dressing with a petrolatum gauze dressing. *Arch Otolaryngol Head Neck Surg* **121**:1145, 1995
123. Smith DJJ et al: Microbiology and healing of the occluded skin-graft donor site. *Plast Reconstr Surg* **91**:1094, 1993
124. Rohrer TE, Dzubow LM: Conchal bowl skin grafting in nasal tip reconstruction: Clinical and histologic evaluation. *J Am Acad Dermatol* **33**:476, 1995
125. Hruza GJ: Guide to full-thickness skin grafts. *Fitzpatrick's J Clin Dermatol* **2(5)**:35, 1994
126. Zitelli JA: Burrow's grafts. *J Am Acad Dermatol* **17**:271, 1987
127. Adnot J, Salasche SJ: Visualized basting sutures in the application of full-thickness skin grafts. *J Dermatol Surg Oncol* **13**:1236, 1987
128. Fish FS, Hilger PA: Aquaplast thermoplastic (Opti-Mold): A unique moldable tie-down dressing for full-thickness skin defects. *J Dermatol Surg Oncol* **20**:239, 1994
129. Katz BF, Oca MAGS: A controlled study of the effectiveness of spot dermabrasion ("scarabrasion") on the appearance of surgical scars. *J Am Acad Dermatol* **24**:462, 1991
130. Konior RJ: Free composite grafts. *Otolaryngol Clin North Am* **27**:81, 1994
131. Melton JL, Hanke WC: Wound closure materials, in *Principles and Techniques of Cutaneous Surgery,* edited by GP Lask, RL Moy. New York, McGraw-Hill, 1996, p 77
132. Garrett AB: Wound closure materials, in *Cutaneous Surgery,* edited by RG Wheeland. Philadelphia, Saunders, 1994, p 199

CHAPTER 267

Harold J. Brody

Skin Resurfacing: Chemical Peels

Chemical peeling is also called *chemical resurfacing, chemexfoliation,* or *chemosurgery.* The process involves the application of one or more exfoliating agents to the skin, resulting in the destruction of portions of the epidermis and/or dermis with subsequent regeneration. These application techniques produce a controlled wound and reepithelialization.

HISTORIC ASPECTS

Dermatologists pioneered skin peeling for therapeutic benefit. In 1882, P.G. Unna, a German dermatologist, described the properties of salicylic acid, resorcinol, phenol, and trichloroacetic acid (TCA);

and during the first half of the twentieth century, phenol and TCA were used in several centers. The combination of two agents, solid carbon dioxide followed by TCA, to produce the first medium-depth combination peel was reported in 1986. These peels have replaced the more risk-prone 50 percent TCA peel. The alpha-hydroxy acids (AHAs) as peeling agents became available in the late 1980s and the 1990s as superficial peeling agents. Presently, resurfacing lasers can be used in combination with or in addition to peeling agents.

HISTOLOGIC CLASSIFICATION

Based on the study of histologic changes in wound depth, a classification of peels can be developed (Table 267-1). The strength of a dermal wounding agent is based on evaluating the reaction at its peak by noting the depth of the wound as opposed to the depth of inflammation. Examination of the wound at 90 days to evaluate the middermis is imperative for proper evaluation of dermal collagen remodeling.[1]

Epidermal injury (superficial wounding) without clinical vesiculation results from Jessner's solution (JS), the AHAs[2-7] and solid carbon dioxide (CO_2), with results similar to those from tretinoin application.[8,9]

Upper dermal injury (medium-depth wounding) follows the use of 40 to 60% trichloroacetic acid (TCA) and the medium-depth 35 percent TCA peeling combinations. Ninety days after peeling, a normal-appearing zone of expanded papillary dermis referred to as a *Grenz zone* is seen. The thickness of this zone varies with the strength of the wounding agent used and the depth of the wound. A band of thick, amorphous brown fibers in the middle to upper dermis is composed of elastotic fibers and glycosaminoglycans (GAGs). The thickness and depth of staining of this band increases with the strength of wounding agents[10,11] (Fig. 267-1).

Middermal injury (deep wounding) with phenol formulas results in a deeply stained elastotic dermal band. The new subepidermal,

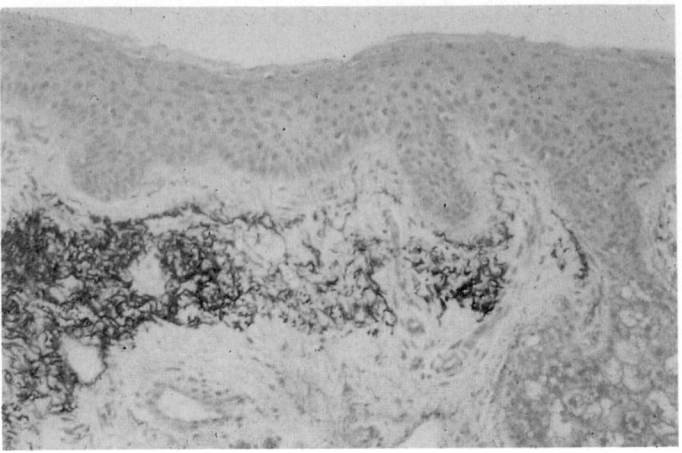

Elastic staining 90 days after CO_2 (hard pressure) plus 35% TCA. Peel shows a return to a normal epidermal pattern and the appearance of a papillary dermal Grenz zone with a middermal elastotic band.

horizontally arranged collagen band in the papillary dermis is probably responsible for the lessening of wrinkles.[12,13]

Dermal peeling can be compared with CO_2 laser treatment. A single or double pass with a superpulse laser at 400 mJ, 10 W, 0.33-s interval in sun-protected and sun-exposed periauricular skin produces a depth of injury approximating that seen with medium-depth chemical peels. Healing at 90 days occurs in a similar fashion as with chemical peeling but perhaps with less inflammation.[14,15]

INDICATIONS FOR CHEMICAL PEELING

Actinic keratoses and sun-induced rhytids respond to chemical peeling. Medium-depth peels will reduce the number of visible actinic keratoses by 75 percent with results sustained for as long as 30 months in a majority of patients. This is comparable to 5-fluorouracil (5-FU).[1,16] Regeneration of the actinic damage may occur and necessitate repeat treatment after 2 to 4 years. *Pigmentary dyschromias* in the form of melasma or postinflammatory hyperpigmentation also respond. Serial repetitive peels of increasing strength are used to treat melasma. In a study of 70% glycolic acid compared with Jessner's solution in the treatment of melasma resistant to medical therapy, there was a 63 percent reduction in the patients' melasma area and severity index, statistically significant lightening on colorimetry, and equal response to both agents.[17] Glycolic acid caused mild irritancy. Topical glycolic acid can be utilized between peels but is not imperative for good results. *Depressed scarring* responds variably to chemical peeling. Dermabrasion or the resurfacing laser are generally more effective. Medium-depth peeling with solid CO_2 to efface the rims or the edges of depressed scars combined with the immediate repetitive application of TCA 35 to 50% to the rims has resulted in substantial improvement.[11,15] *Acne vulgaris* may be improved by superficial chemical peeling, although medium peeling can aggravate or actually produce acne. In rosacea the existing erythema of the disease makes medium peeling more risky due to persistent tenderness or erythema.

TABLE 267-1

Chemical Peeling Wounding Classification*

Superficial wounding—to the stratum granulosum/papillary dermis
  Very light—stratum corneum exfoliation or stratum granulosum
    depth
      10–25% trichloroacetic acid (TCA), resorcinol, Jessner's solution,
      salicylic acid, solid carbon dioxide, alpha-hydroxy acids, tretinoin
  Light—basal layer or upper papillary dermal depth
      35% TCA, unoccluded, single or multiple applications
Medium-depth wounding—through the papillary dermis to the upper
  reticular dermis
  Combination peels, single or multiple applications
      CO_2 + 35% TCA, Jessner's solution + 35% TCA, glycolic acid
      + 35% TCA, 50% TCA unoccluded (TCA, deep), single
      application
  Full-strength phenol, 88% unoccluded
Deep-depth wounding—to the midreticular dermis
  Baker's phenol, unoccluded
  Baker's phenol, occluded

*Depth is dependent on the prepeel skin-defatting preparation, strength of the wounding agent, amount applied, and skin thickness or location.

PATIENT SELECTION—RELATIVE CONTRAINDICATIONS

Prior to peeling patients must be evaluated for relative contraindications (Table 267-2).[15,18,19] Fitzpatrick's classification measures pigmentary responsiveness of the skin to ultraviolet light, most often based on the ethnic background. Skin types I to III are ideal for peeling. Types IV through VI can also be peeled with all peeling agents, but the risk of unwanted pigmentation is greater. A classification of photoaging is helpful in assessing sun damage (Table 267-3).[20] The past or present use of systemic isotretinoin must be ascertained, since retinoids may be associated with a greater risk of scarring after peeling. If the patient has a past history of superficial x-ray treatment for acne, the adnexal structures should be assessed by observing the presence of vellus hairs or by punch biopsy to ensure adequate reepithelialization. Smoking may multiply the wrinkling effects of sunlight. There are few absolute contraindications to the entire spectrum of chemical peeling, since superficial peeling may be tolerated with little risk in all patients of all skin types regardless of their general state of health. Postmenopausal estrogens and oral contraceptives may sensitize the skin to the sun or may produce postinflammatory splotching. Patients infected with HIV may experience delayed healing or be at risk for secondary infection after peeling. If the patient has a history of recurrent herpes simplex, he or she may be given prophylactic acyclovir, valacyclovir, or famciclovir during medium-depth or deep peeling. True hypertrophic scar or keloid formers may be at greater risk to scar with deep as opposed to medium-depth peeling. A method to document the evaluation prior to peeling includes the mapping and detailing of the defects on a diagram as well as good photography (Fig 267-2). A time interval of 4 to 12 weeks is recommended between peeling and procedures involving undermining such as rhytidectomy, a coronal brow lift, or blepharoplasty. Following peeling, patients must use sunscreens to prevent continuing damage.

Rejuvenation Regimen for the Skin before and after Peeling

The daily, morning use of a sunscreen and the nightly application of tretinoin will reduce solar pigmentation as well as promote faster healing in the immediate postpeel period. Tretinoin application be-

fore and after TCA does not significantly enhance the efficacy of the peel; it potentiates the action of hydroquinone, although the role of hydroquinone in prepeel treatment to prevent pigment return after peeling is unsubstantiated.[19] Hydroquinone gel, 4%, for example, may be used twice daily for at least a month prior to peeling to test the patient's reactivity to the product and begin bleaching of epidermal pigment. It can be reinstituted after reepithelialization. Prolonged use of high concentrations of hydroquinone may paradoxically produce ochronosis in Fitzpatrick types V and VI skin. This is much more common in South African black skin. Kojic acid has a similar tyrosinase-suppressive mechanism and may be used in the program.

TABLE 267-3

Photoaging Groups—Glogau's Classification

Group I: Mild, usually age 28–35
  No keratoses
  Little wrinkling
  No scarring
  Little or no makeup
Group II: Moderate, usually age 35–50
  Early actinic keratoses—slight yellow skin discoloration
  Early wrinkling—parallel smile lines
  Mild scarring
  Little makeup
Group III: Advanced, usually age 50–65
  Actinic keratoses—obvious yellow skin discoloration
  Wrinkling—present at rest
  Moderate acne scarring
  Makeup always worn
Group IV: Severe, usually age 60–75
  Actinic keratoses and skin cancers have occurred
  Wrinkling—actinic, gravitational, and dynamic
  Severe acne scarring
  Makeup is worn; does not cover but cakes on skin

TABLE 267-2

Factors in the Assessment for Relative Contraindications

Fitzpatrick skin type
Degree of actinic damage and photoaging
Philosophy of sun exposure
Present and past sebaceous gland density; previous isotretinoin or radiation
Prior cosmetic surgery
Philosophy of smoking
General state of physical and mental health
Medications
Pregnancy history
History of herpes simplex
History of hypertrophic scarring
Realistic expectations

FIGURE 267-2

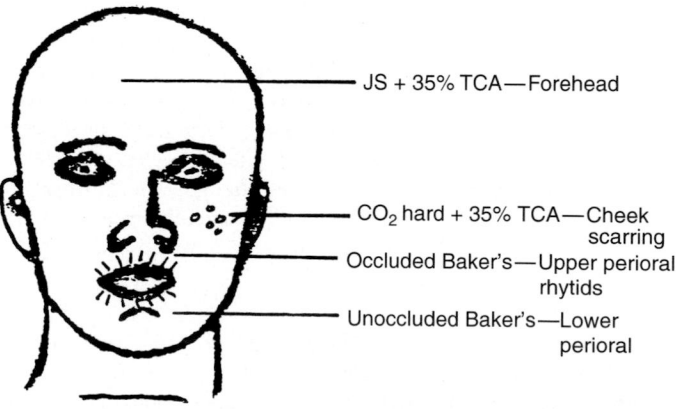

Example of rubber-stamp diagram mapping the defects and types of peels performed on a given patient.

PRINCIPLES OF WOUNDING AGENT APPLICATION

Prior to the application of all wounding agents, cutaneous lipids are removed by cleansing with alcohol or acetone-soaked sponges.[15] Excessive defatting prior to 70% glycolic acid peels may cause untoward peeling erythema or pigmentation. The amount of wounding agent applied, the degree of rubbing, and the duration of skin contact must be carefully monitored to ensure good results. Documentation of application with one or two cotton-tipped applicators, with a more aggressive 4- by 4-in. gauze sponge, or with a sable brush should be written into the patient's record. Frosting with different wounding agents is variable in rate and appearance and depends on the preexisting degree of photodamage, the choice of applicator, and the adequacy of defatting. Observation of the frost itself as a measure of depth is not as valuable as the actual selection of proper wounding technique or wounding agent.[21] The appearance of the frost does give an index of protein agglutination and indicates how evenly the agent has been applied. "Neutralization" of TCA with alcohol or water immediately after frosting is useless to reverse the effect of the application of the wounding agent. Once complete frosting has occurred, penetration is already achieved, and dilution with water is not necessary. Alpha-hydroxy acids are dependent upon the contact time with the skin, and washing them from the skin after a given amount of time is important.

Superficial Peeling

Superficial peels, which are generally epidermal and pose little risk of scarring, usually require multiple weekly or monthly applications for effectiveness.[15] They do not vesiculate, and patients generally continue normal activities. They can be used on all Fitzpatrick skin types, skin colors, and body areas. These agents may amplify 5-fluorouracil and are preparatory agents to make papillary dermal peeling agents (e.g., TCA 35%) penetrate deeper. It has been postulated that superficial peeling agents induce upper dermal increased collagen production in response to repeated epidermal sloughs. Minimal postoperative care is needed for superficial peels, and patients may return to their normal daily activities immediately, wearing cosmetics to conceal erythema.

TRICHLOROACETIC ACID 10 TO 35% TCA should be prepared by the weight to volume (wt/vol) method, mixing the desired concentration in grams of United States Pharmacopeia (U.S.P.) TCA crystals with the appropriate volume of distilled water to make 100 mL.[15] Although TCA is marketed as a paste mask application, it is more expensive in this form and offers no clear therapeutic advantage over the aqueous application. Strengths of TCA from 10 to 35% are used to accomplish superficial chemical peeling on facial and nonfacial areas; such peels may be repeated every 7 to 28 days.

MODIFIED UNNA'S RESORCINOL PASTE Unna described the use of resorcinol paste as a peeling agent in concentrations of 10 to 30% in the late 1800s. Letessier's modified formula to treat acne, melasma, and sun damage avoids excessive erythema by using axungia, a derivative of pig fat or lard added to a clay-bearing soil with 40% resorcin.[22]

JESSNER'S SOLUTION Jessner's combination of resorcinol, salicylic acid, and lactic acid in ethanol was formulated to lower the concentration and toxicity of any one agent and to enhance the keratolytic effects (Table 267-4). Application can be light or heavy, and may be repeated after 3 to 4 min.[16,23] The advantages of Jessner's solution are that only a single solution is needed, timing the duration of application is unnecessary, and dilution or "neutralization" is not performed. The lactic acid in Jessner's solution is an alpha-hydroxy acid, and it is very effective in the treatment of melasma (Fig. 267-3). The combination in which Jessner's solution or glycolic acid amplifies the effects of 5-FU is called the *fluorhydroxy pulse peel.*

SALICYLIC ACID Salicylic acid, a beta-hydroxy acid, can be used as a 50% ointment under occlusion to peel lentigines, pigmented keratoses, and actinically damaged skin from the dorsa of the hands and forearms.[24] The dressing is removed after 48 h, and mild salicylism with tinnitus and headache is expected. A peeling solution of 35% salicylic acid in ethanol (Beta-lift, Medicis) has been applied to the face with cotton-tipped applicators for improvement of comedones. Erythema and edema are minimal, and the peel can be repeated every 2 to 4 weeks.

SOLID CARBON DIOXIDE Solid CO_2 (dry ice) is a physical modality for peeling and not a true chemical peeling agent. It may be used alone or to amplify TCA as a medium-depth peel.[15] The dry ice is wrapped in a small hand towel and dipped as needed in a solution of approximately 3:1 acetone and alcohol, which serves to facilitate application to the skin. A moderate application of 8 s to excoriated areas will serve to improve acne excoriee (Fig. 267-4).

ALPHA-HYDROXY ACIDS Alpha-hydroxy acids (AHAs) are naturally occurring but synthetically mass-produced carboxylic acids normally found in many foods. The AHAs include glycolic, lactic, malic, citric, and tartaric acids. The two acids with the shortest carbon chains, glycolic and lactic, are most commonly used in dermatology and are naturally found in sugar cane and sour milk, respectively. Though irritancy of a product is often directly related to lower pH, vehicle irritancy must be considered also. The available free acid, which is difficult to ascertain, is the best method to judge concentration and irritancy.[2,5]

The factors that determine whether AHA peels result in desquamation or epidermolysis are the concentration of the acid, the pH, the degree of buffering or neutralization with sodium bicarbonate, the vehicle formulation, the frequency of application, the conditions of delivery, the amount of acid delivered to the skin over a given period, and, most importantly, the length of time that the acid remains on the skin. Glycolic acid peels become more unpredictable following overzealous scrubbing. The agent is applied in any cosmetic unit order, rapidly—covering the entire face within about 20 s—with a large cotton applicator. A starting application time for weekly or monthly application with 50 or 70% unbuffered glycolic acid is generally in the range of 3 min, and the time is increased

TABLE 267-4

Jessner's Solution

Resorcinol	14 g
Salicylic acid	14 g
Lactic acid (85%)	14 mL
Ethanol (95%) qs ad*	100 mL

*Quantity sufficient to add up to.

FIGURE 267-3

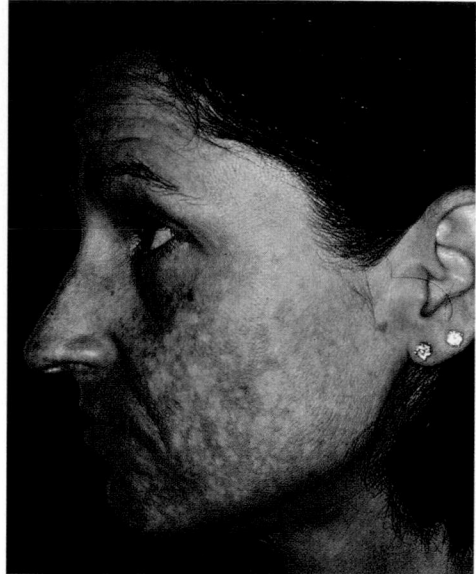

A.

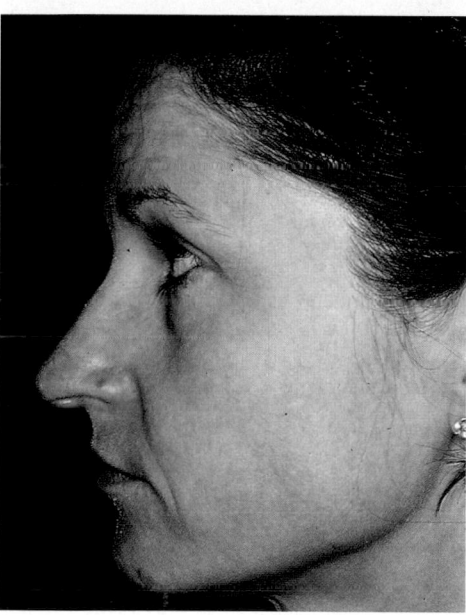

B.

A. Melasma on cheek prior to the application of Jessner's solution. B. Improvement after three monthly peels, allowing increased penetration of hydroquinone. (*Photos courtesy of Sue Ellen Cox, MD, and Naomi Lawrence, MD.*)

with subsequent peels. Neutralizers with sodium bicarbonate marketed to the physician have no advantage over water rinsing as long as all acid is removed thoroughly from all rhytids and cosmetic units. This peeling is very forgiving, complications are very rare, and results are slow to appear. Patients should be realistic about subtle results.[25,26]

TRETINOIN Topical tretinoin, all-*trans*-retinoic acid, is a supplement to most peel regimens along with daily application of sunscreen.[9,19] Daily application of 0.1% tretinoin cream for 2 weeks prior to a 35% TCA peel significantly enhanced the healing time

FIGURE 267-4

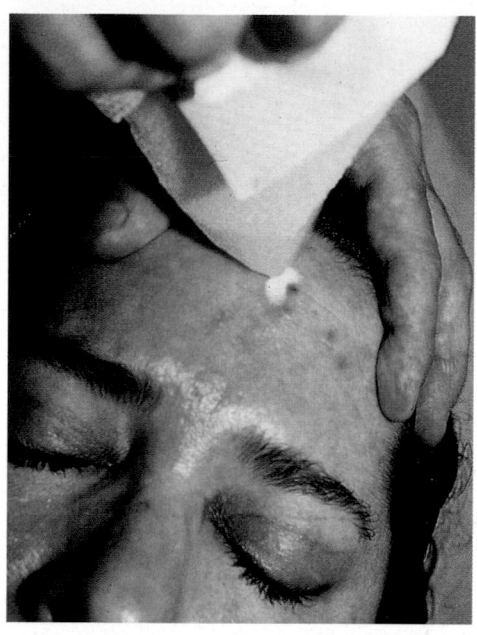

Application with moderate pressure of solid CO_2 slushed in acetone and alcohol to excoriations and with mild pressure to surrounding skin of the cosmetic unit will promote healing and discourage excoriation.

of the facial, forearm, and hand skin in a double-blind, placebo-controlled study. Tretinoin application before and after TCA does not significantly enhance the efficacy of the peel.[19,27,28]

Medium-Depth Peeling

Medium-depth peels are usually performed as a single procedure to remove actinic keratoses, mild rhytids, or pigmentary dyschromias or to flatten depressed scars. They may be repeated approximately every 3 to 12 months based on the amount of actinic damage still remaining or recurring after the peel or for continued scar effacement. The classic peel for this depth category was the 50% TCA peel. Since TCA is prone to produce increased scarring and hypopigmentation with higher concentrations, the use of a more superficial epidermal peeling agent such as solid CO_2,[1,11,15] Jessner's solution,[16,21,23] or glycolic acid[29] prior to the application of 35% TCA will produce a wound equivalent in depth to the higher-strength 50% solution or full strength 88% phenol. This technique is called *combination medium-depth peeling* (Figs. 267-5 through 267-9).

The addition of emulsifiers or additives to TCA may increase its penetration to the lower dermis, leading to overtreatment and scarring. Combinations of medium-depth peels to effectively blend cosmetic units are effective and useful. Resurfacing of the perioral region with the laser, dermabrasion, or deep phenol peel and blending the rest of the face with combination medium-depth peeling is very effective and is discussed below. Wet to dry soaks of tap water or povidone-iodine skin cleanser twice daily in the shower, followed by application of an occlusive ointment such as bacitracin or petrolatum to minimize crusting, is the optimal aftercare for rapid healing.

FIGURE 267-5

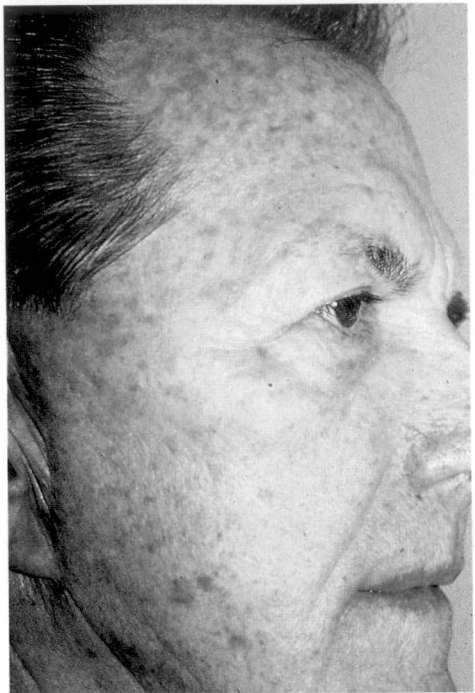

A.

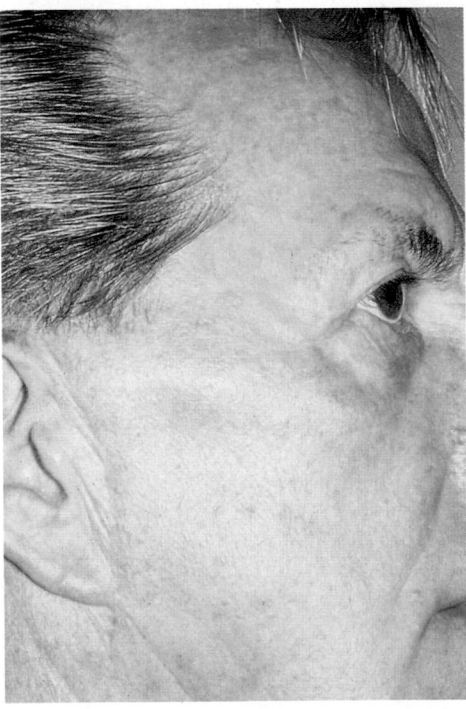

B.

Improvement in actinic keratoses in a male patient with Fitzpatrick skin type II—Glogau photoaging type IV, severely actinically damaged and very sebaceous. Hard CO_2 was used in all areas, followed by TCA 35% applied twice with a single gauze sponge and applied three times to the forehead. *A.* Before peeling. *B.* Three months after treatment. (*From Brody,*[15] *with permission.*)

FIGURE 267-6

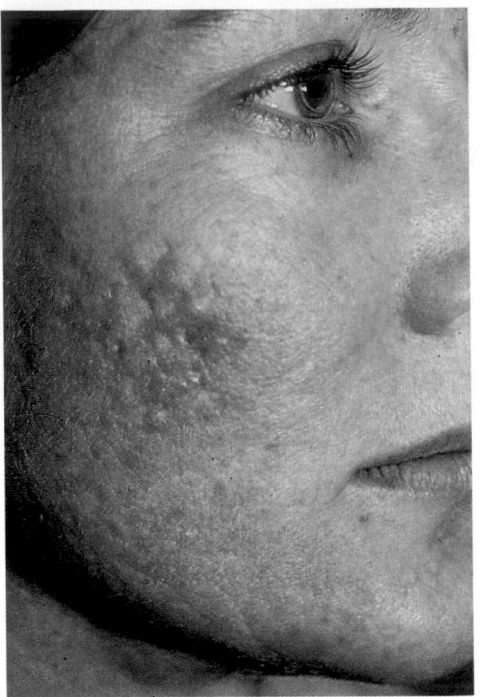

A.

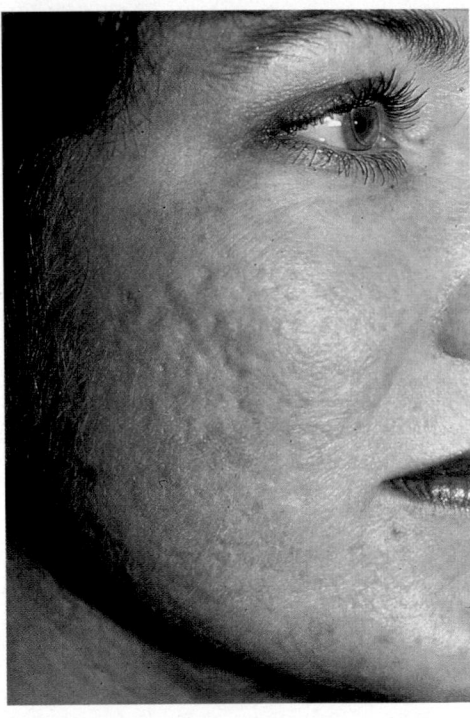

B.

This patient with Fitzpatrick type II skin has depressed scarring on her cheeks without any pitted component. *A.* Her skin is peeled with hard carbon dioxide immediately electrodesiccating the edges of the scars; then 50% TCA is applied to the edges with the broken end of a wooden cotton-tipped applicator. The 35% TCA was then applied liberally to the entire face with a single 4- by 4-in. gauze pad. Improvement is substantial 3 months later. *B.* The combination of carbon dioxide and TCA peel is the only effective treatment for scarring because it employs a physical modality. (*From Brody,*[15] *with permission.*)

FIGURE 267-7

CHAPTER 267
Skin Resurfacing: Chemical Peels

2943

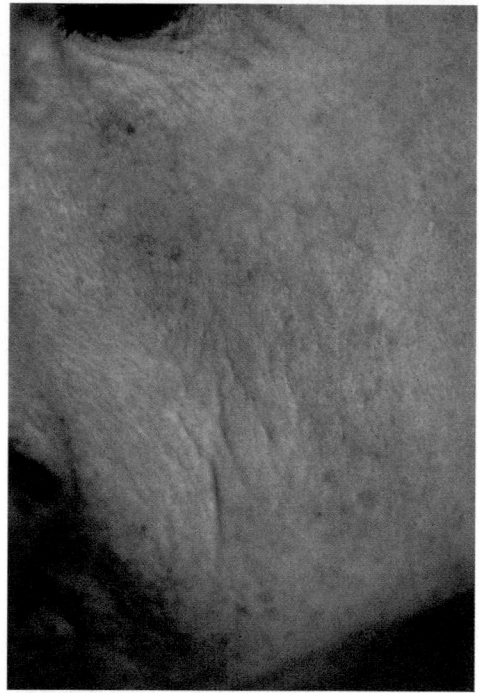

A.

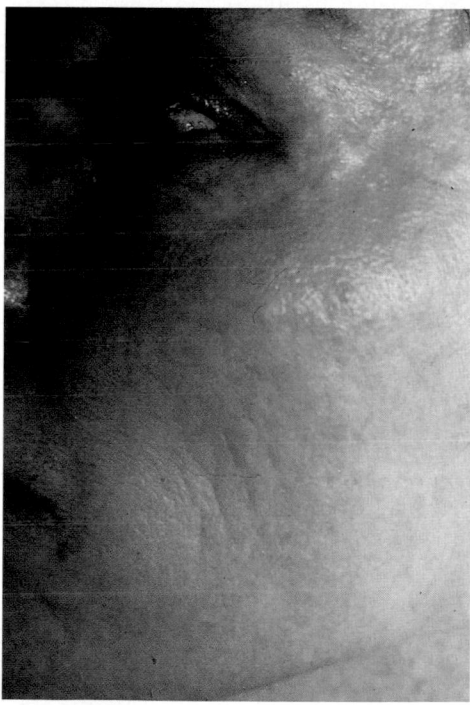

B.

A. Before the application of hard CO_2 plus TCA 35%, with 50% to cheek rhytids in Fitzpatrick type III, Glogau photoaging group III skin. *B.* Ninety days after peeling, there is easing of the rhytids and improvement of mottled pigmentation. (*From Brody and Hailey,*[11] *with permission.*)

FIGURE 267-8

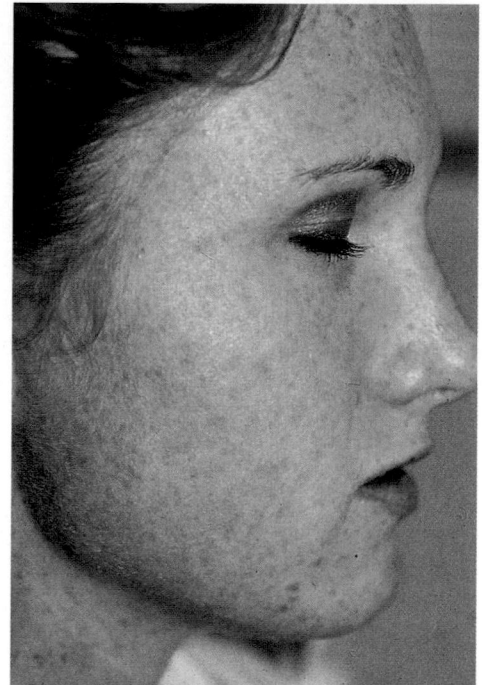

A.

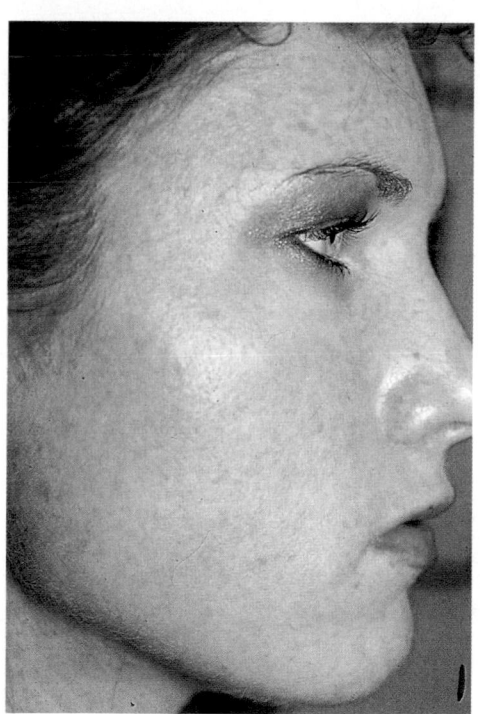

B.

A. Before the application of Jessner's solution plus TCA 35% for splotchy increased pigmentation in Glogau photoaging II and Fitzpatrick type II skin. *B.* Three months later, pigment remains eliminated.

FIGURE 267-9

The Baker-Gordon Formula

Phenol U.S.P.	3 mL
Tap water or distilled water	2 mL
Septisol liquid soap	8 drops
Croton oil	3 drops

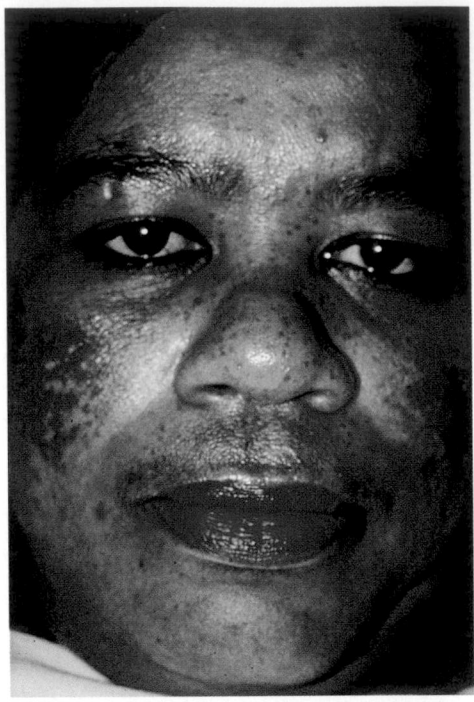

A.

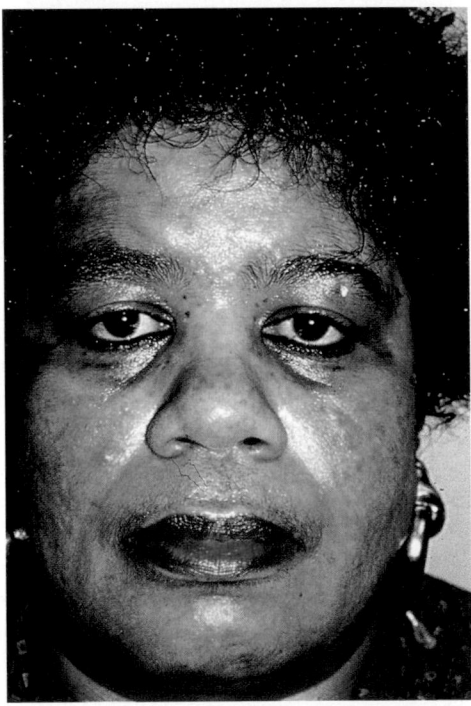

B.

A. Patient with Fitzpatrick type VI skin with melasma. Skin was peeled with unbuffered glycolic acid 70% for 2 min, followed by trichloroacetic acid 35%. *B.* Four weeks later. (*Courtesy of William P. Coleman, MD.*)

Deep Peeling

The traditional chemical peel formula with phenol was described in 1961 by Baker and Gordon (Table 267-5). The application of waterproof tape for 48 h will increase penetration. More aggressive cleaning of the skin prior to application of the wounding agent and the application of more peel solution may eliminate taping. Occlusive petrolatum may be substituted for the tape. The 55% phenolic Baker-Gordon formula penetrates further into the dermis than full-strength undiluted phenol because the latter causes immediate coagulation of epidermal keratin proteins and blocks further penetration of phenol.[10,12,13]

For full-face application, regional nerve blocks or preoperative sedatives and analgesics such as diprivan and midazolam are employed. Because phenol is partially detoxified in the liver and excreted by the kidney and because phenol may induce cardiac arrhythmias, hydration with 500 mL of lactated Ringer's solution prior to the procedure and 1000 mL during and after the peel will prevent phenol toxicity on these organ systems.

The face is degreased prior to the application of the wounding agent and divided into six esthetic units: forehead, perioral, right and left cheeks, nose, and periorbital areas.[15,20] Peel solution is usually applied in this order, allowing 10 to 15 min between units to minimize renal and cardiac toxicity; thus the entire procedure would take 60 to 90 min. If indicated, tape is applied to each segment. After 48 h, the exudate has lifted the tape considerably, with drainage from the mask's lower edge, and it is easily removed. Wet-to-dry soaking three to five times daily in the shower using tap water, half-strength boric acid, or dilute antiseptic povidone-iodine skin cleanser will dry the exudative edema. An occlusive moisturizer (e.g., petrolatum) should then be used. (Fig. 267-10).

Application of Baker's phenol to one cosmetic unit or less does not require intravenous hydration or cardiac monitoring. The amount of phenol applied to the skin in this fashion is equivalent to or less than that applied for a phenol nail matrixectomy. Oral hydration may be given in the form of 8 to 16 oz of water prior to the peel if patients have not been drinking much fluid on the day of the procedure. After phenol has been applied to the perioral area, for example, medium-depth peeling or other resurfacing modalities may be utilized on other cosmetic units[30] (Fig. 267-11).

COMPARISON OF DEEP PEELING WITH CO₂ RESURFACING LASER

Preliminary clinical comparison between the laser and Baker's solution reveals that the laser improves severe photodamage by approximately 50 percent.[14] The laser may eliminate mild wrinkles in

FIGURE 267-10

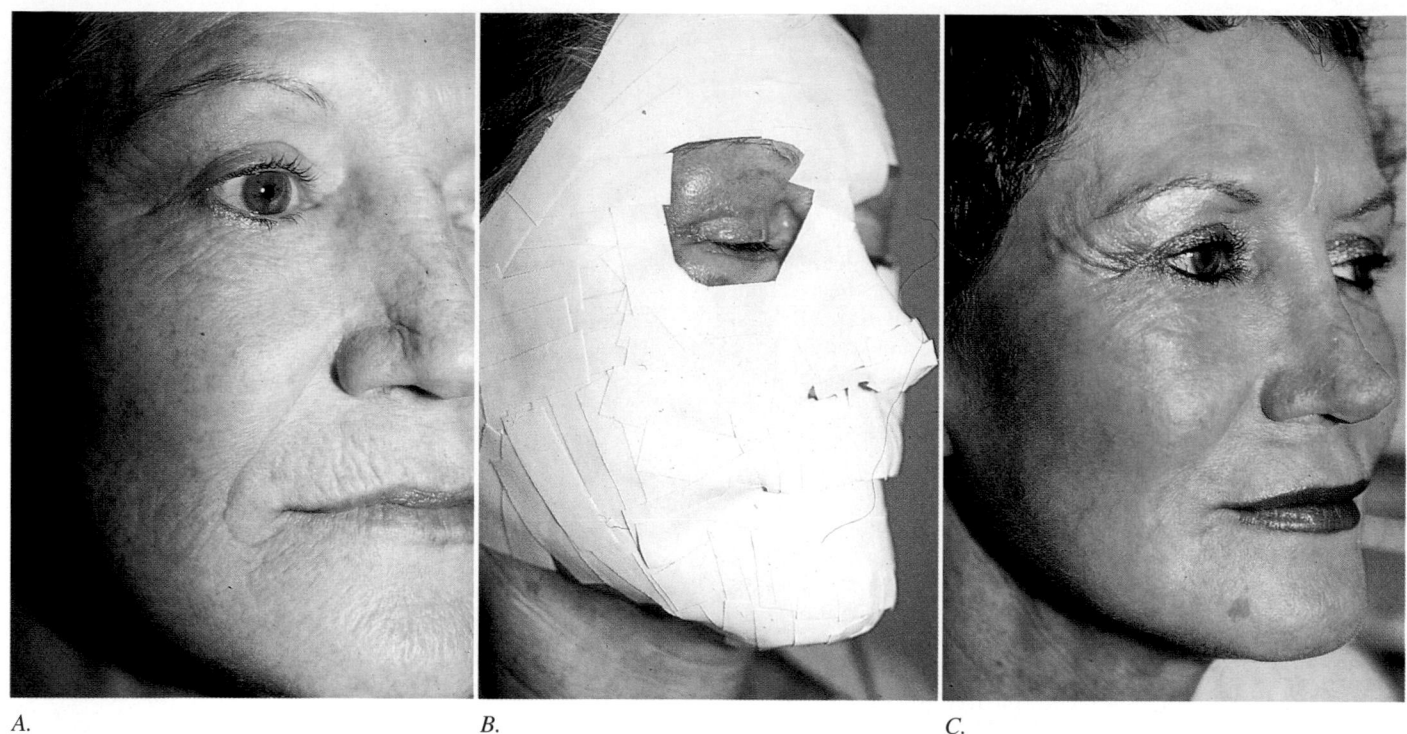

A. *B.* *C.*

A. Fitzpatrick type II, Glogau photoaging types III and IV skin before Baker-Gordon phenol formula peel. *B.* Immediately after taping.

C. Three months after peeling.

one treatment with little risk of pigmentary change. The peel does the same but may be more likely to cause slight hypopigmentation. In contrast, very severe rhytids may require multiple touchups by the laser for adequate treatment. However, the Baker's peel can eliminate the vast majority of deep rhytids in one treatment.[30] Neither procedure for severe rhytids leaves bothersome residual hypopigmention, but mild pigment loss is not unexpected with both peel and laser for this indication.

FIGURE 267-11

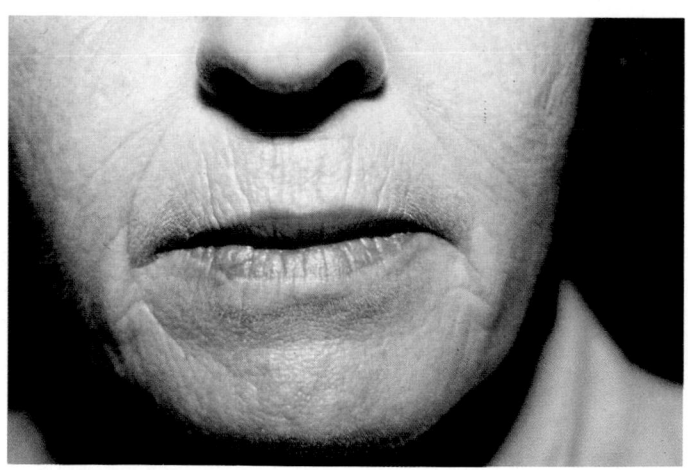 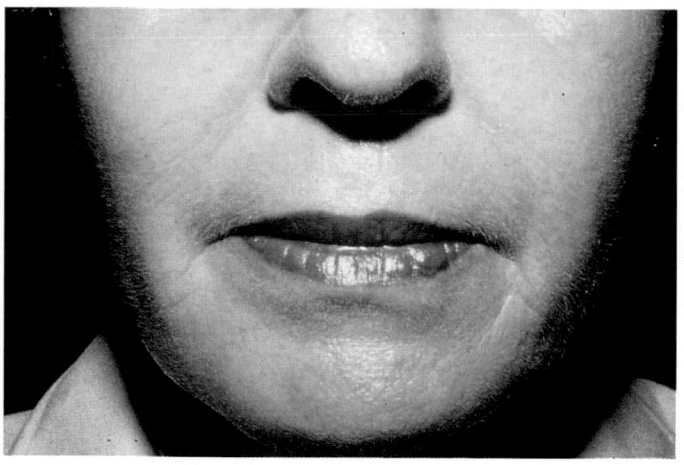

A. *B.*

Fitzpatrick type II and Glogau photoaging type IV skin with the most severe defects in the perioral area (*A*). Three months later, there is no perceptible color change after application of perioral occluded Baker-

Gordon formula and CO_2 plus TCA 35% on the remainder of the face (*B*). (*From Brody,[15] with permission.*)

COMPLICATIONS ARISING FROM CHEMICAL PEELS

A favorable test spot result in patients at higher risk for pigmentation or scarring does not guarantee the behavior of the rest of the facial skin, but it may ease the patient's fears.[15,20]

Pigmentary changes in the form of hyperpigmentation may occur in darker skin types and is caused by sunlight, estrogens, photosensitizing drugs, or pregnancy.[31] Hypopigmentation after Baker's phenol application is a function of patient selection and mode of application as well as subsequent wound care. The hypopigmentation is proportional to the amount of phenol applied, and a small loss of pigment is an expected result and not a complication. The rate of hypopigmentation with laser resurfacing is not uncommon, depending on depth and skin type, and can be as high as 16 percent. Treatment of such hyperpigmentation with hydroquinone regimens is effective.

The risk of hypertrophic scarring is less than 1 percent with the three combination medium-depth peels. By itself, 50% TCA is capable of unpredictable hypertrophic scarring while 35% TCA is relatively safe. The incidence of scarring with the traditional Baker's phenol formula in the series of over 1000 patients peeled by Dr. Baker and Dr. Gordon was less than 2 percent. The rate of scarring may increase with deviations in technique, the use of preliminary treatments or topicals to increase absorption, recent isotretinoin use, or improper patient selection. Comparison with the CO_2 laser reveals comparable safety with less than 3 percent complications. The delayed healing syndrome, probably due to a defect in transepidermal water loss, has been noted after TCA and phenol peeling as well as laser resurfacing.[15,32] The constellation of symptoms includes friable, stellate, nonindurated painful unhealed erosions with serous granulation tissue persisting for 10 days after peeling. The areas may heal with hypopigmented flat scars and should be treated with artificial semipermeable dressings or very dilute triamcinolone injections into the wound margins. Other treatments for scars include topical, intralesional, or tape-impregnated glucocorticoids, silicone gel sheeting, or the 585-nm flash lamp–pumped pulsed dye laser (FLPDL).[33]

Bacterial, viral, or fungal *infection* may occur after peeling. Toxic shock syndrome, induced by *Staphylococcus aureus* exotoxin, has been reported rarely following Baker's phenol face peels. Patients with a positive history of herpes should be treated prophylactically during healing with therapeutic doses of acyclovir, valacyclovir, or famciclovir beginning on the day of the peel. Unusual and unexpected postpeel pain may reflect the onset of herpes viral infection. Candidiasis has been reported more frequently after dermabrasion and CO_2 laser resurfacing, probably because of the partially protective presence of a nonviable epidermis remaining after peeling and because of the lack of occlusive dressings.[15]

Prolonged erythema, which may occur after peeling, may be treated with topical hydrocortisone. Isotretinoin administration prior to peeling, atopic problems in the patient, rosacea, contact dermatitis, or minimal amounts of alcoholic beverages may also affect redness. *Textural changes* in the form of large pores may occur temporarily after peeling. *Milia* or *acne* occurring after peeling may be aggravated by thick ointments. A poor physician/patient relationship in the face of minor, manageable complications can result in a loss of follow-up and litigation.

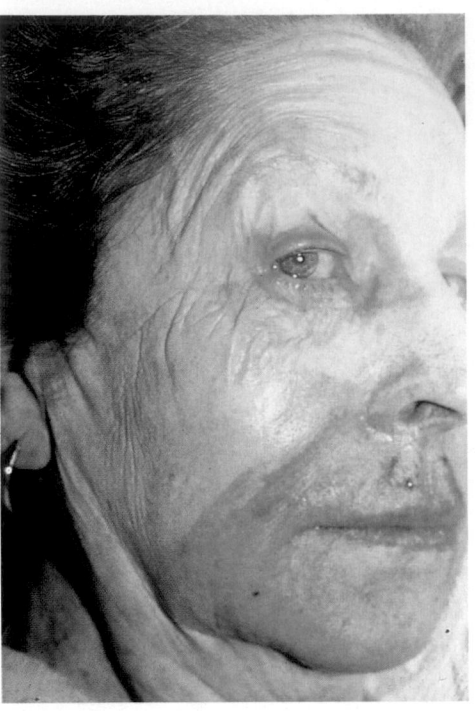

Combination skin resurfacing shown immediately after using the CO_2 resurfacing laser to correct the wrinkles in the perioral area and combination medium-depth TCA peeling elsewhere on the less photodamaged parts of the face.

Skin atrophy, cardiac arrhythmias, laryngeal edema, and exacerbation of a Köbnerizing pemphigus-like disease may occur with phenol peels.[34]

COMBINATION SKIN RESURFACING—COMBINING CHEMICAL RESURFACING WITH LASER OR DERMABRASIVE RESURFACING

As discussed above, deep phenol peeling will eliminate rhytids in the perioral area and medium peels can be used on the remainder of the face if warranted.[15] The resurfacing CO_2 laser or dermabrasion can also be used to eliminate rhytids or reduce scars in the perioral, periorbital, or cheek areas.[14,36] The remainder of the face can be blended with chemical peeling. Operator-sensitive differences in technique in the three modalities make comparison of the three resurfacing modalities difficult (Fig. 267-12).

REFERENCES

1. Brody HJ: Variations and comparisons in medium depth chemical peeling. *J Dermatol Surg Oncol* **15**:953, 1989
2. Moy LS et al: Glycolic acid peels for the treatment of wrinkles and photoaging. *J Dermatol Surg Oncol* **19**:243, 1993
3. Moy L et al: Comparison of the effect of various chemical peeling agents in a mini-pig model. *Dermatol Surg* **22**:429, 1996
4. Moy L et al: Glycolic acid modulation of collagen production in human skin fibroblast cultures in vitro. *Dermatol Surg* **22**:439, 1996

5. Becker FF et al: A histological comparison of 50% and 70% glycolic acid peels using solutions with various pHs. *Dermatol Surg* **22**:463, 1996

6. Ditre CM et al: The effects of alpha hydroxy acids on photoaged skin: A pilot clinical, histological and ultrastructural study. *J Am Acad Dermatol* **34**:187, 1996

7. Griffin TD et al: Increased factor XIIIa transglutaminase expression in dermal dendrocytes after treatment with alpha hydroxy acids: Potential physiologic significance. *J Am Acad Dermatol* **34**:196, 1996

8. Bhawan J et al: Reversible histologic effects of tretinoin on photodamaged skin. *J Geriatr Dermatol* **3**:62, 1995

9. Griffiths CEM et al: Two concentrations of topical tretinoin (retinoic acid) cause similar improvement of photoaging but different degrees of irritation. *Arch Dermatol* **131**:1037, 1995

10. Stegman SJ: A comparative histologic study of the effects of three peeling agents and dermabrasion on normal and sun-damaged skin. *Aesthet Plast Surg* **6**:123, 1982

11. Brody HJ, Hailey CW: Medium-depth chemical peeling of the skin: A variation of superficial chemosurgery. *J Dermatol Surg Oncol* **12**:1268, 1986

12. Kligman AM et al: Long-term histologic follow-up of phenol face peels. *Plast Reconstr Surg* **75**:652, 1985

13. Brown AM et al: Phenol-induced histologic skin changes: Hazards, technique and uses. *Br J Plast Surg* **13**:158, 1960

14. Fitzpatrick RE et al: Pulsed carbon dioxide laser, trichloroacetic acid, Baker-Gordon phenol and dermabrasion: A comparative clinical and histologic study of cutaneous resurfacing in a porcine model. *Arch Dermatol* **132**:469, 1996

15. Brody HJ: *Chemical Peeling and Resurfacing,* 2d ed. St Louis, Mosby–Year Book, 1997

16. Lawrence N et al: A comparison of the efficacy and safety of Jessner's solution and 35% trichloroacetic acid vs 5% fluorouracil in the treatment of widespread facial actinic keratoses. *Arch Dermatol* **131**:176, 1995

17. Lawrence NL, Cox SE, Brody HJ: A comparison of Jessner's solution versus glycolic acid: A comparison of clinical efficacy. *J Am Acad Dermatol* **36**:589, 1997

18. Brody HJ: The art of chemical peeling. *J Dermatol Surg Oncol* **15**:918, 1989

19. Humphreys TR et al: Treatment of photodamaged skin with trichloroacetic acid and topical tretinoin. *J Am Acad Dermatol* **34**:638, 1996

20. Glogau RG, Matarasso SL: Chemical peels. *Dermatol Clin* **13**:263, 1995

21. Brody HJ: Trichloroacetic acid application in chemical peeling. *Oper Tech Plast Reconstr Surg* **2**:127, 1995

22. Letessier SM: Chemical peel with resorcin, in *Dermatologic Surgery: Principles and Practice,* 2d ed. edited by RK Roenigk, HH Roenigk. New York, Marcel Dekker, 1996, pp 1115–1119

23. Monheit GD: The Jessner's + TCA peel: A medium depth chemical peel. *J Dermatol Surg Oncol* **15**:945, 1989

24. Swinehart JM: Salicylic ointment peeling of the hands and forearms. *J Dermatol Surg Oncol* **18**:495, 1992

25. Newman N et al: Clinical improvement of photoaged skin with 50% glycolic acid: A double-blind vehicle-controlled study. *Dermatol Surg* **22**:455, 1996

26. Brody H et al: Round table discussion of alpha hydroxy acids. *Dermatol Surg* **22**:475, 1996

27. Kimbrough-Green CK et al: Topical retinoic acid (tretinoin) for melasma in black patients. *Arch Dermatol* **130**:727, 1994

28. Hevia O et al: Tretinoin accelerates healing after trichloroacetic acid chemical peel. *Arch Dermatol* **127**:678, 1991

29. Coleman WP, Futrell JM: The glycolic acid + trichloroacetic acid peel. *J Dermatol Surg Oncol* **20**:76, 1994

30. Matarasso SL, Brody HJ: Deep Chemical Peeling. *Semin Cutaneous Med Surg* **15**:155, 1996

31. Brody HJ: Complications of chemical peeling. *J Dermatol Surg Oncol* **15**:1010, 1989

32. Szachowicz EH, Wright WK: Delayed healing after full-face chemical peels. *Facial Plast Surg* **6**(1):8, 1989

33. Goldman MP, Fitzpatrick RE: Laser treatment of scars. *Dermatol Surg* **21**:685, 1995

34. Detwiler SP, Saperstein HW: Physically induced pemphigus after cosmetic procedures. *Int J Dermatol* **32**:100, 1993

35. Bernstein LJ et al: The short- and long-term side effects of carbon dioxide laser resurfacing. *Dermatol Surg* **23**:519, 1997

36. Hruza GJ, Dover JS: Laser skin resurfacing. *Arch Dermatol* **132**:451, 1996

CHAPTER 268

Christopher B. Harmon
John M. Yarborough, Jr.

Skin Resurfacing: Dermabrasion

Over the past decade, the availability of many pulsed and shuttered CO_2 lasers has rekindled an interest in resurfacing treatments of the skin. Many of the current laser surgery practices—such as patient selection, postoperative dressings, and management of complications—are based on years of experience with dermabrasive resurfacing and chemical peeling. While chemical peeling utilizes the application of exfoliating chemicals to remove epidermal and dermal layers of the skin, dermabrasion surgically abrades or planes the epidermis and dermis with the use of a rapidly rotating wire brush or diamond fraise. A working knowledge of the limitations and advantages of each of these resurfacing options is requisite in optimizing surgical outcomes for the entire spectrum of clinical presentations.

Historic Factors

Armed with the success of 200 cases performed over a two-year period, Dr. Abner Kurtin presented "corrective surgical planing of skin" to the Dermatologic Section of Mount Sinai Hospital in January 1953.[1] His technique combined the use of high-speed rotary dermabraders, intraoperative freezing, and various cutting end pieces for resurfacing facial skin.[2] This office-based surgical procedure laid the groundwork for modern dermabrasion and introduced the subspecialty of cosmetic dermatologic surgery.

Indications

The indications for dermabrasion include those lesions and defects of the epidermis, papillary dermis, and upper reticular dermis that can be partially or completely removed by surgically planing to the level of the reticular dermis. Wound healing by second-intention allows reepithelialization to occur from the underlying adnexal structures. During the maturation phase of wound healing, fibroblasts replace and remodel collagen bundles in the papillary and upper reticular dermis.[3] These mechanisms allow the superficial and saucer-shaped scars of facial acne to be greatly improved, while ice-pick scars and deep postvaricella scars may require elevation or punch grafting prior to dermabrasion.[4]

Programmed dermabrasion of surgical and traumatic scars performed 6 to 8 weeks following injury frequently yields a complete elimination of visible evidence of scar formation.[5] While the cellular mechanisms of this phenomenon are not completely understood, ultrastructural studies have demonstrated an increase in collagen bundle density and size with a tendency toward a more normal unidirectional fiber orientation parallel to the epidermal surface. Furthermore, immunohistochemical assays have shown a postabrasive upregulation in tenascin expression in the papillary dermis and an alteration in integrin expression in the spinous layer of the epidermis (Fig. 268-1A and B). These observations suggest that dermabrasive scar revision produces a less perceptible scar by modifying the extracellular ligand expression of the primary cicatrix, thereby influencing epithelial cell-cell interaction and the reorganization of underlying connective tissue.[6]

As a resurfacing treatment for photoaging, dermabrasion can be used to treat actinic keratoses, solar elastosis, and wrinkles (Fig. 268-2A and B).[7] Benign conditions—such as rhinophyma, adenoma sebaceum, epidermal nevi, syringomas, small cysts, milia, and seborrheic keratoses—can easily be removed with planing. Abrasion can also be used to eradicate superficial malignancies, including Bowen's disease and superficial basal cell carcinomas.[8] Pigmentary disorders such as melasma, tattoos, and lentigines can be improved with dermabrasion when used in conjunction with bleaching and tretinoin creams.[9]

Patient Selection

In evaluating patients for dermabrasive procedures, a complete history and comprehensive consultation are paramount. A review of "before" and "after" photographs is often helpful in preparing the patient and providing realistic expectations of improvement. The risks of preoperative, intraoperative, and postoperative care should be discussed in obtaining informed consent. A recent history of isotretinoin therapy is a contraindication because of many reports of hypertrophic scarring and poor healing attributed to concomitant or recent isotretinoin usage. Generally, 6 months is considered an adequate interval between isotretinoin treatment and any abrasive surgery.[10-13] Similarly, dermabrasions should not be performed for at least 6 months following any extensive undermining (i.e., face lifts, brow lifts, etc.), to allow re-establishment of the vascular bed of the area to be abraded.[14]

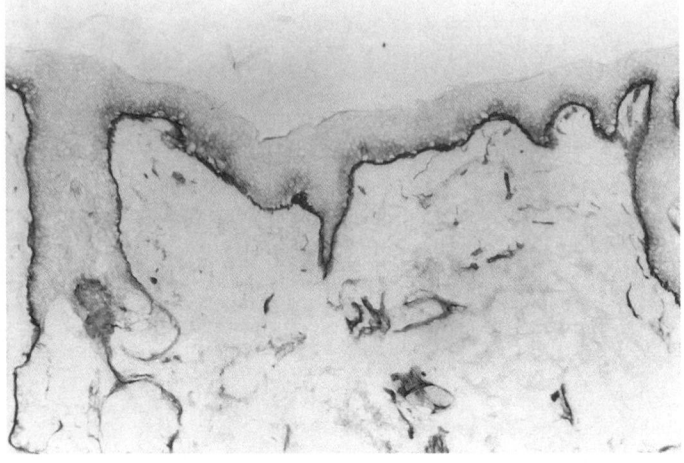

A.

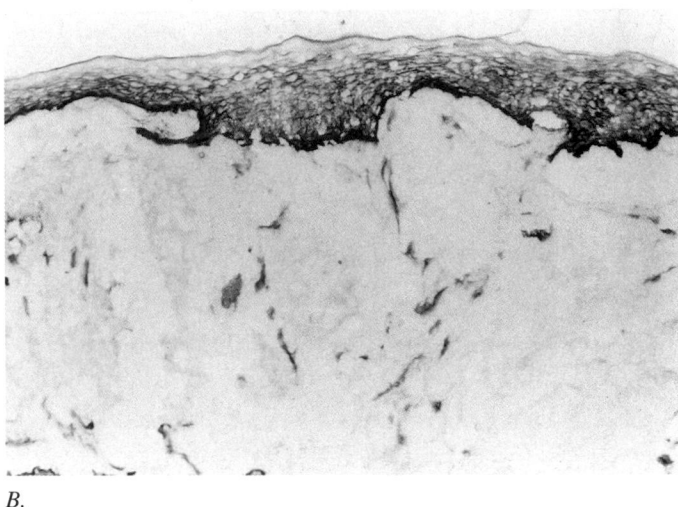

B.

A. This immunoassay demonstrates alpha-6 integrin subunit staining along the basement membrane prior to dermabrasion. *B.* Six weeks after dermabrasion, the immunoassay shows a dispersion of alpha-6 integrin subunits throughout the papillary dermis.

Drug allergies, clotting disorders, abnormal scarring, cold intolerance, pigmentary disorders, or Koebnerizing skin conditions are other important historical factors to be considered. Preoperative antiviral prophylaxis obviates the great potential for activation of herpes simplex with perioral or full-face abrasions. Furthermore, the risk of aerosolization of viral particles mandates universal precautions.[15-16]

Equipment

Various manufacturers produce hand engines capable of providing 15,000 to 60,000 rpm for driving the cutting end pieces. The wire brush and diamond fraise are the most commonly used. The fraises come in a variety of shapes, sizes, and grades of coarseness. Pear-shaped fraises and cones are often used around the nose and oral commissure, whereas the wheels can be used over broad, flat surfaces. Diamond fraises can be used without cryogenic spray and offer a broader safety margin than the wire brush.

FIGURE 268-2

CHAPTER 268
Skin Resurfacing: Dermabrasion

2949

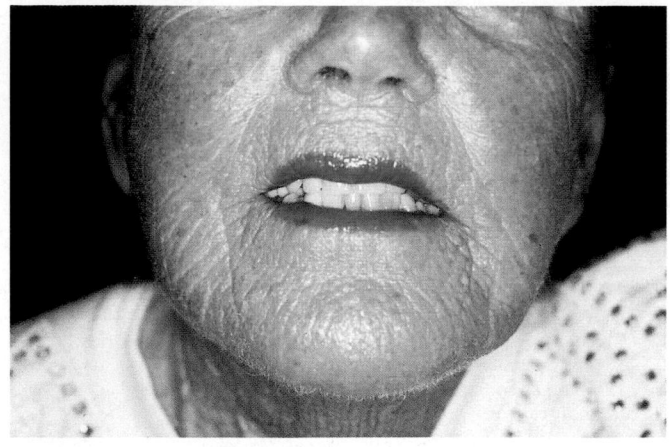

A.

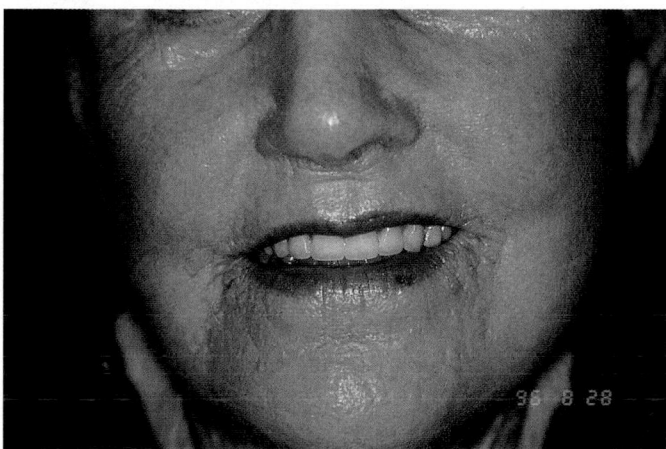

B.

A. Perioral rhytides prior to wire brush dermabrasion. *B.* Improved perioral rhytides 6 months following wire brush dermabrasion.

The wire brush removes greater amounts of tissue with less thermal injury, thereby allowing the surgeon to plane deeply into the midreticular dermis with less risk of scarring. For more aggressive abrasions with a wire brush or a coarse diamond fraise, the use of intraoperative cryogenic sprays provides a firm surface on which to work and prevents the skin from grabbing or gouging. However, excessive freezing or the use of sprays with extremely low boiling points can produce unwanted tissue damage and scarring. The products containing freon 114 and freon 114-ethylchloride mixtures are safe, while products using freon 11 and freon 12, which lower skin temperatures more, may cause excessive skin damage.[17,18]

Anesthesia

Today, most dermabrasions are performed as outpatient procedures in offices, ambulatory surgery facilities, or hospital operating rooms. Regional or spot dermabrasions can usually be performed with local anesthesia and no additional analgesia. However, full-face abrasions may require oral or IM sedation in conjunction with cryoanesthesia, local or tumescent anesthesia, or nerve blocks. Intravenous sedation or general anesthesia is rarely necessary. Like cryoanesthesia, the tumescent technique offers local anesthesia and

a solid surface for planing. Some surgeons prefer the increased hemostasis of tumescence and choose to eliminate the refrigerant spray because of the chance of unintended tissue damage.[19] A topical eutectic mixture of local anesthetic (EMLA) may provide supplemental surface anesthesia, but its use should be limited to less than 10 g.[20] The controversial and potential benefit of abrading scars frozen into place may be lost with the distention of tumescence.

Wound Care

Following dermabrasion, white petroleum ointment (Aquaphor) or an antibiotic ointment is applied to the abraded area. Significant advances have been made in the development of semipermeable hydrogel dressings that can be applied directly on top of the ointment. By maintaining a critical plane of humidity for epithelial cell migration, these dressings have reduced the time of reepithelialization to only 5 or 6 days.[21–22] During this time the ointment and dressing can be changed daily. A mild soap or nonmentholated shaving cream can be used to clean the area and prevent any buildup or crust formation. Once the treated area has been reepithelialized, the new skin is pink to red in color and requires the frequent application of moisturizer. The pinkness can be covered with makeup and usually fades over a period of 6 to 12 weeks.

Complications

Postoperative complications include scarring, pigmentary changes, persistent erythema, and infection. The deeper the dermabrasion, the greater the risk of scarring, especially over the upper lip, mandible, and bony prominences. Because of the decreased number of adnexal structures in nonfacial skin, dermabrasions performed away from the face are also more likely to produce scarring. Hypertrophic scars and keloids may be treated with topical flurandrenolide tape, intralesional steroids, or silicone gel sheeting.[23] Some 30 to 50 percent of all patients may experience some degree of hypopigmentation following dermabrasion. The chance of hyperpigmentation is greatest during the first six weeks after surgery, especially in skin types III and IV, and can often be prevented with the postoperative use of hydroquinone and retinoic acid creams. Because of the low incidence of bacterial infections following dermabrasion, prophylactic antibiotics can produce more harm than good by promoting gram-negative superinfections. Primary bacterial infections are extremely rare and best managed with culture-directed antibiotic regimens. Antiviral prophylaxis, on the other hand, should be performed on a routine basis for full-face abrasions and perioral treatments (see Chap. 259). Careful patient selection, attentive surgical technique, state-of-the-art postoperative dressings, and prompt management of any developing problem can greatly reduce the risk of postabrasive complications and significantly enhance surgical outcomes.

REFERENCES

1. Robbins N: Dr. Abner Kurtin, father of ambulatory dermabrasion. *J Dermatol Surg Oncol* **14**:425, 1988
2. Kurtin A: Surgical planing of the skin. *Arch Dermatol Syphilol* **68**:389, 1953
3. Burks JW: *Wire Brush Surgery.* Springfield, IL, CC Thomas, 1956
4. Yarborough JM: Dermabrasion by wire brush. *J Dermatol Surg Oncol* **13**:610, 1987
5. Yarborough JM: Ablation of facial scars by programmed dermabrasion. *J Dermatol Surg Oncol* **14**:292, 1988

6. Harmon CB et al: Dermabrasive scar revision: Immunohistochemical and ultrastructural evaluation. *Dermatol Surg* **21**:503, 1995

7. Benedetto AV et al: Dermabrasion: Therapy and prophylaxis of the photoaged face. *J Am Acad Dermatol* **27**:439, 1992

8. Roenigk HH: Dermabrasion for miscellaneous cutaneous lesions (exclusive of scarring from acne). *J Dermatol Surg Oncol* **3**:322, 1977

9. Mandy SH: Tretinoin in the preoperative and postoperative management of dermabrasion. *J Am Acad Dermatol* **15**:878, 1986

10. Roenigk HH et al: Acne, retinoids, and dermabrasion. *J Dermatol Surg Oncol* **11**:396, 1985

11. Rubenstein R et al: Atypical keloids after dermabrasion of patients taking isotretinoin. *J Am Acad Dermatol* **15**:280, 1986

12. Katz BE et al: Atypical facial scarring after isotretinoin therapy in a patient with previous dermabrasion. *J Am Acad Dermatol* **30**:852, 1994

13. Stegman SJ et al: Dermabrasion, in *Cosmetic Dermatologic Surgery,* edited by SJ Stegman, TA Tromovitch, RG Glogau. Chicago, Year Book, 1990, p 59

14. Kamer FM et al: Injectable collagen, chemical peeling, and dermabrasion as an adjunct to rhytidectomy. *Facial Plast Surg* **8**:89, 1992

15. Vaughn RY et al: HIV and the dermatologic surgeon. *J Dermatol Surg Oncol* **16**:1107, 1990

16. Kemsley GM: Transmission of hepatitis B in dermabrasion. *Plast Reconstr Surg* **56**:440, 1975

17. Hanke CW et al: Complications of dermabrasion resulting from excessively cold skin refrigerant. *J Dermatol Surg Oncol* **11**:896, 1985

18. Hanke CW et al: Laboratory evaluation of skin refrigerants used in dermabrasion. *J Dermatol Surg Oncol* **11**:45, 1985

19. Coleman WP et al: Use of the tumescent technique for scalp surgery, dermabrasion, and soft tissue reconstruction. *J Dermatol Surg Oncol* **18**:130, 1992

20. Goodman G: Dermabrasion using tumescent anesthesia. *J Dermatol Surg Oncol* **20**:802, 1994

21. Pinski JB: Dressings for dermabrasion: New aspects. *J Dermatol Surg Oncol* **13**:673, 1987

22. Mandy SH: A new primary wound dressing made of polyethylene oxide gel. *J Dermatol Surg Oncol* **9**:2, 1983

23. Gold MH: Topical silicone gel sheeting in the treatment of hypertrophic scars and keloids. *J Dermatol Surg Oncol* **19**:912, 1993

CHAPTER 269

Robert Herd
Jeffrey S. Dover
Kenneth A. Arndt

Skin Resurfacing: Laser

Expectations of modern medicine are high. As people live longer and healthier lives, they want their outward appearance to match their inward perception of youth and vitality. For some, a lasting youthful appearance is genetic; for others, it must be engineered. This wish and the public's willingness to pay for treatment have driven the development of skin rejuvenation therapies. The skin of the present adult population has had more sun exposure than that of previous generations, causing an acceleration of the aging process. Topical preparations such as alpha hydroxy acids and retinoic acid and treatments like chemical peels and dermabrasion have been used with some success, but the most efficacious of these carry the highest risk of complications.

The latest and most successful method of rejuvenation is laser resurfacing. High-energy pulsed CO_2 lasers have now been joined by erbium:yttrium-aluminum-garnet (Er:YAG) lasers as the principal tools for laser resurfacing.[1,2]

THEORETICAL CONSIDERATIONS

The CO_2 Laser

The CO_2 laser, first developed in 1964, has an emission wavelength of 10,600 nm in the infrared part of the electromagnetic spectrum, where the major chromophore is water. The CO_2 laser was originally operated in a focused mode as a cutting tool, but it is now most often used in a defocused mode for tissue ablation and resurfacing. Three modes of delivery of CO_2 light are used for resurfacing: pulsed, superpulsed, and continuous wave (CW). Pulse duration of pulsed lasers conforms to parameters considered appropriate for ablating tissue. Superpulsed lasers emit a train of pulses at 100 to 5000 Hz, which can be gated to produce a tissue effect equivalent to that of a pulsed laser. Finally, CW lasers are scanned to give a dwell or tissue exposure time that results in a tissue effect similar to that of pulsed lasers.

Erbium:YAG Laser

Among alternative lasers being developed, the Er:YAG laser is the most useful to date. Its emission wavelength of 2940 nm is close to an absorption peak of H_2O 16 times greater than that of CO_2 laser light.[3] Shallower skin penetration (1 μm as compared with 20 μm for CO_2 laser light) allows more precise ablation with less thermal damage.[4]

Er:YAG lasers have been used for ablation of superficial skin lesions as well, but it is too early to make definitive clinical comparisons. This laser may well become an important instrument for skin resurfacing.[5]

LASER-TISSUE INTERACTION

The high intra- and extracellular water content of the epidermis and dermis ensures that most CO_2 laser light is absorbed rather than scattered and that penetration is shallow. The precise tissue effect is dictated by the energy per pulse and the pulse duration.

When the pulse duration is sufficiently long, there is a zone of black material called *char*. There is an area below this where the fibrillar appearance of the collagen is lost. The third zone of thermally altered material shows stronger hematoxylin staining than normal but less than the second zone. The ideal laser would ablate a small amount of tissue and leave a very narrow zone of thermal damage.

When CO_2 laser energy impacts the skin, it causes a predictable and reproducible tissue effect. Absorption by water converts the light to heat, which vaporizes or ablates tissue if the temperature is above 100°C (212°F). Accounting for the penetration depth of the CO_2 laser light, the estimated ablation threshold is 5 J/cm^2. The energy per pulse must be above this level for the CO_2 laser to have a clinical effect. Less energy would not heat tissue enough to cause vaporization, leaving a wider zone of thermal necrosis, and more energy would produce a rate of tissue ablation linearly related to the energy per pulse up to a ceiling of 19 J/cm^2.[6–8]

The pulse duration should be equivalent to or less than the thermal relaxation time of the target. It is impossible to define a precise thermal relaxation time for a volume of tissue that varies according to the energy imparted, but it is thought that the thermal relaxation time for the irradiated layer of tissue is about 1 ms. The ablation threshold increases for pulse widths over 1 ms.[9] When the energy is above ablation threshold, pulse widths below 1 ms limit the thermal damage induced by CO_2 lasers down to a minimum of about 50 μm at 600 μs.[10] Any reduction below 600 μs is thought to result in very little further reduction in the zone of thermal damage.

Therefore a pulse duration of less than 1 ms with a fluence of above 5 J/cm^2 gives a predictable zone of ablation with minimal collateral damage. Similar effects can be achieved by CW lasers using scanning devices with dwell times and energies conforming to these parameters.

Measurements on the Er:YAG laser predict an ablation threshold of 0.6 to 5 J/cm^2.[4,11] Although absorption takes place in the first 1 to 2 μm of tissue, fluences of 80 J/cm^2 can ablate 400 μm of tissue, a finding that cannot be explained. The Er:YAG laser has been tested in quasicontinuous (normal) mode with a pulse width of 200 μs and in Q-switched mode with a pulse width of 90 ns. At fluences below 25 J/cm^2, 2.5 to 30 μm of tissue is ablated and the zone of

damage is limited to 10 to 40 μm with the quasicontinuous laser and 5 to 10 μm with the Q-switched laser when tested in guinea pig skin.[12] In the Q-switched mode, residual thermal damage is insufficient to coagulate blood vessels, leaving a bloody surgical field that limits its clinical utility. In the normal mode, skin vaporization leaves a relatively bloodless field after two or three passes. Bleeding becomes a greater problem with successive passes.

HISTOLOGY

Resurfacing lasers are designed to ablate a superficial zone of skin, leaving minimal thermal damage. Macroscopically, shrinkage is seen during CO_2 laser treatment and appears to be directly proportional to the number of passes.[13] Contraction has not been measured in photoaged human skin, but shrinkage in pig skin was proportional to the number of passes and to fluence, resulting in a 10 to 30 percent reduction in area.[9]

A study of porcine skin compared the Ultrapulse CO_2 laser (Coherent, Palo Alto, CA) with trichloroacetic acid and phenol peels and dermabrasion.[14] The depth of residual thermal necrosis was <40 μm, but it was up to 53 and 106 μm with second and third passes and increased with increased pulse energy. Dermal vaporization plus necrosis depth was directly proportional to pulse energy; i.e., with each pass, the depth of vaporization decreases while the residual thermal damage increases.

One study examined the depth of ablation and residual damage with each pass.[15] Three different laser systems, the Ultrapulse (Coherent, Palo Alto, CA), Silktouch flashscanner (Sharplan, Allendale, NJ), and Surgilase 150XJ (Sharplan, Allendale, NJ), were compared with a continuous wave CO_2 laser as a control. The Ultrapulse is a pulsed laser with a computerized scanner; the Silktouch is a scanned CW laser; and the Surgilase is a superpulsed laser. At the settings used, which were those proposed for optimal response to each laser, the CW laser caused a zone of thermal necrosis 400 to 500 μm thick. The flashscanner and superpulsed laser ablated 30 to 50 μm of tissue and completely removed the epidermis. One pass with the Ultrapulse vaporized a 20 to 30-μm layer, and the second pass reached the papillary dermis. Subsequent passes with these last three lasers ablated into the dermis. The zone of coagulation necrosis also increased with each pass. The CW laser left 400 μm of damage with one pass, the Silktouch and Surgilase left 150 μm after three passes. Another report of 40 patients tested the flashscanner and superpulsed lasers and confirmed that the first pass ablated the epidermis, the third pass removed the papillary dermis, and the fourth pass penetrated into the reticular dermis.[16]

A study of a superpulsed laser (Surgilaser XJ 150, Sharplan, Allendale, NJ) in four patients assessed treated preauricular and postauricular skin and examined biopsies at days 1, 3, and 90.[17] Increased doses of laser energy vaporized more tissue per pass. At day 1, there was a mononuclear cell infiltrate with added neutrophils and eosinophils. At day 3, 78 percent of specimens had reepithelialized and there was an infiltrate of eosinophils and mononuclear cells. At day 90, half showed a return to a rete ridge pattern. Most showed a dermal repair zone composed of dense, compact collagen bundles in parallel alignment, well demarcated from underlying collagen. There was alteration in the density, distribution, and orientation of elastic fibers. Findings were similar to those after medium-depth peels.

In summary we can make the following statements about CO_2 laser resurfacing:

1. With each laser pass, there is a reproducible tissue effect with three distinct zones.

2. The depth of tissue vaporization increases with each pass.
3. The residual thermal damage increases with each pass.
4. A repair zone with new collagen is seen in follow-up biopsies.

Whether the histologic changes with the Er:YAG are similar remains to be determined. It appears that the depth of ablation increases with fluence up to 80 J/cm^2. Residual damage also rises with increasing fluence and with increasing pulse width.[11,12] There is insufficient thermal damage to produce immediate tissue contraction. Whether long-term wound healing is associated with contraction of collagen, which improves sagging skin, remains to be seen.

CLINICAL RESULTS

The original CO_2 lasers used for resurfacing were gated CW lasers. These were superseded by a pulsed and scanned CO_2 laser, on which there is a growing body of published clinical results.

Results of treatment of wrinkles and acne scarring with the UltraPulse CO_2 laser have been impressive (Fig. 269-1).[18–22] Assessment has not always been blinded, but all reported series show a marked improvement in the appearance of photoaged skin with associated tightening of sagging skin. There was a significant reduction in perioral and periorbital wrinkles. The treatment of acne scars was found to be less effective.[20,23] Mild to moderate acne scarring is improved significantly more than severe scarring.[24] Similar results have been achieved with the Silktouch flashscanner laser,[16,20,25] which improved perioral and periorbital wrinkles more than glabellar and nasolabial folds. Recent presentations demonstrated no long-term difference in clinical outcome after resurfacing of photoaged skin with the UltraPulse, Feathertouch, Silktouch, Novapulse (Luxar), or True Pulse (Palomar Technologies, Beverly, MA).

Results of resurfacing with the Er:YAG are encouraging. More passes than with the CO_2 lasers are required to ablate to the same depth. The CO_2 lasers ablate more tissue per pass and leave a large zone of thermal damage, with associated immediate collagen contraction. Whether the final clinical results with the Er:YAG laser will be as impressive in the absence of this effect remains to be seen.

SIDE EFFECTS/ COMPLICATIONS

Side effects following CO_2 laser resurfacing are frequent and predictable. They are similar to those following chemical peels and

FIGURE 269-1

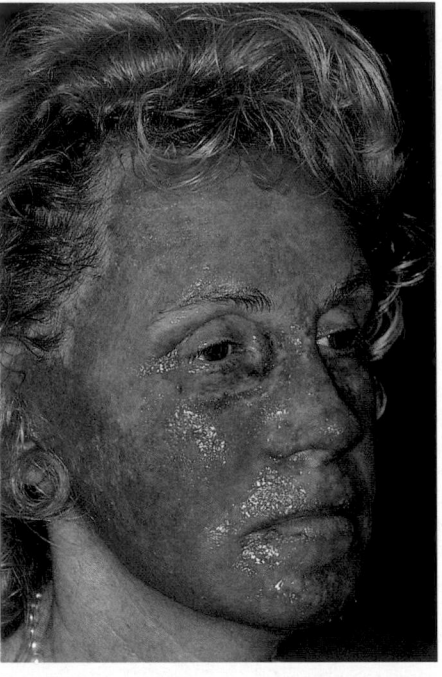
A.

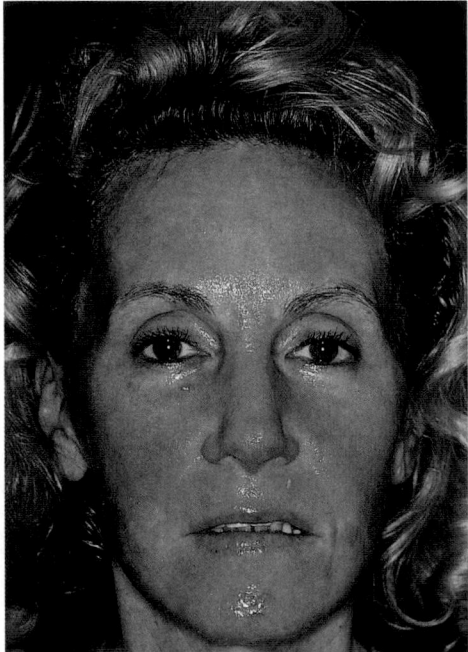
C.

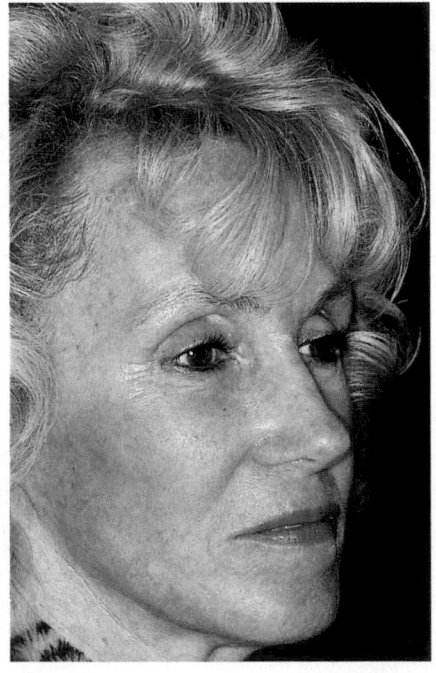
D.

A. Prior to CO_2 laser resurfacing. *B.* Three days after full-face laser skin resurfacing. *C.* Ten days after full-face laser skin resurfacing. *D.* Three weeks after full-face laser skin resurfacing.

dermabrasion, but they are less common and can be prevented if excellent technique is followed and postoperative management is fastidious. They can be divided into six categories: immediate, predictable effects; pigmentary changes; infection; follicular effects; eczematous effects; and scarring (Table 269-1).

Erythema is universal and is considered part of the normal healing process. It lasts on average of 6 to 12 weeks, while erythema and flushing, which develop in the treated site with exertion or emotional upset, are frequent for a year after resurfacing. Some individuals do have persistent continual erythema lasting up to 12 months; this may be related to the depth of ablation.[16,22,25,26]

The most frequent complication is pigmentary alteration. Transient hyperpigmentation has been reported in up to 36 percent of patients, mainly affecting those with types III and IV skin.[23] More recent studies demonstrate rates of hyperpigmentation as low as 2.8 percent. Pretreatment with tretinoin and hydroquinone may account for the lower incidence. Hyperpigmentation can last up to 6 months. Resolution may be hastened by treatment with tretinoin and hydroquinone.[20,26] Permanent hypopigmentation has also been reported in 16 percent of individuals.[27] It is most frequent in patients with skin bronzing induced by actinic drainage; it is more common in patients who have previously been treated with dermabrasion[21,23] and appears to be related to depth of treatment.

Milia are a result of follicular reepithelialization compounded by the use of occlusive moisturizers. Acne is a frequent postoperative event, especially in patients with a past history of acne. It usually develops in the first few weeks after resurfacing and responds to usual acne treatments.

Contact dermatitis, noted with the use of some topical anesthetic preparations, does not correspond with patch-test findings but resolves with appropriate treatment.[18,25] This occurrence increases the chances of postoperative erythema and hyperpigmentation.[26]

Eczematous dermatitis occasionally develops in the first 4 weeks after treatment. It responds rapidly to moisturizers and topical midpotency glucocorticoids.

Hypertrophic scarring is seldom seen following laser resurfacing.[21,25,27] It results from a large number of passes or use of excessive energy and from pulse stacking (overlap of laser-irradiated sites, especially after the first pass), resulting in excessive thermal damage (personal communication, RE Fitzpatrick).

In a procedure that removes the epidermis and part of the dermis, infection is a concern.[26] Laser surgeons have learned from past experience with dermabrasion and have avoided bacterial infection through the judicious use of antibacterials. Antiviral chemoprophylaxis was originally confined to those with a history of herpes simplex infection, but results suggest that subjects with no past history of infection frequently develop activation of herpes simplex in treated areas.[18,25] It is now standard practice to use antiviral prophylaxis in all laser resurfacing treatments. Yeast infections have also occurred, but they respond well to treatment.[25]

The main advantage of the Er:YAG is thought to be the improved side-effects profile. The procedure is less painful and may be completed under topical anesthesia. There is less oozing and crusting and the subsequent erythema, although dependent on the number of passes, lasts a shorter time than that following CO_2 laser treatment.[28]

FUTURE CONSIDERATIONS

As CO_2 laser technology is refined, the side effects and complication profiles of CO_2 laser resurfacing will improve. The place of the Er:YAG laser in the resurfacing armamentarium has yet to be decided. New approaches to laser resurfacing include the use of a carbon black topical suspension followed by low-fluence neodymium:YAG (Nd:YAG) laser irradiation for limited epidermal resurfacing and the use of a midinfrared (1.32 μm) pulsed (20 ms) light to produce dermal shrinkage while the epidermis is protected with cooling.[29]

REFERENCES

1. Dover JS: CO_2 laser resurfacing—why all the fuss? *Plast Reconst Surg* **98**:506, 1996
2. Hruza GJ, Dover JS: Laser skin resurfacing. *Arch Dermatol* **132**:451, 1996
3. Hale GM, Querry MR: Optical constants of water in the 200-nm to 200-μm wavelength region. *Appl Optics* **12**:555, 1973
4. Vogler K, Reindl M: Improved Erbium laser parameters for new medical applications. *Biophotonics International* November/December 1996, pp 40–47
5. Kaufmann R, Hibst R: Pulsed erbium:YAG laser ablation in cutaneous surgery. *Lasers Surg Med* **19**:324, 1996
6. Walsh JT, Deutsch TF: Pulsed CO_2 laser tissue ablation: measurement of ablation rate. *Lasers Surg Med* **8**:264, 1988
7. Green HA et al: Pulsed carbon dioxide laser ablation of burned skin: in vitro and in vivo analysis. *Lasers Surg Med* **10**:476, 1990
8. Green HA et al: Middermal wound healing: a comparison between dermatomal excision and pulsed carbon dioxide laser ablation. *Arch Dermatol* **128**:639, 1992
9. Ross EV et al: Effects of CO_2 laser pulse duration in ablation and residual thermal damage: implications for skin resurfacing. *Lasers Surg Med* **19**:123, 1996
10. Walsh JT et al: Pulsed CO_2 laser tissue ablation: effect of tissue type and pulse duration on thermal damage. *Lasers Surg Med* **8**:108, 1988
11. Walsh JT, Deutsch TF: Er:YAG laser ablation of tissue: measurement of ablation rates. *Lasers Surg Med* **9**:327, 1989
12. Walsh JT et al: Er:YAG laser ablation of tissue: effect of pulse duration and tissue type on thermal damage. *Lasers Surg Med* **9**:314, 1989
13. Gardner ES et al: In vitro changes in non-facial human skin following CO_2 laser resurfacing: a comparison study. *Lasers Surg Med* **19**:379, 1996
14. Fitzpatrick RE et al: Pulsed carbon dioxide laser, trichloroacetic acid, Baker-Gordon phenol, and dermabrasion: a comparative clinical and histological study of cutaneous resurfacing in a porcine model. *Arch Dermatol* **132**:469, 1996
15. Kauvar ANB et al: A histopathological comparison of "char-free" carbon dioxide lasers. *Dermatol Surg* **22**:343, 1996
16. Lask G et al: Laser skin resurfacing with the SilkTouch flashscanner for facial rhytides. *Dermatol Surg* **21**:1021, 1995
17. Cotton J et al: Histological evaluation of preauricular and postauricular human skin after high-energy, short-pulse carbon dioxide laser. *Arch Dermatol* **132**:425, 1996

TABLE 269-1

Side Effects and Complications Associated with Laser Resurfacing

Predictable	Erythema, pruritus, swelling, oozing, crusting
Pigmentary	Hyperpigmentation
	Permanent hypopigmentation
Infection	Bacterial
	Viral
	Yeast
Dermatitis	Eczema
Scarring	Atrophic, hypertrophic, keloidal
Follicular	Acne
	Acneiform eruption
	Milia

18. Fitzpatrick RE et al: Pulsed carbon dioxide laser resurfacing of pho-toaged facial skin. *Arch Dermatol* **132**:395, 1996
19. Lowe NJ et al: Skin resurfacing with the ultrapulse carbon dioxide laser: observations on 100 patients. *Dermatol Surg* **21**:1025, 1995
20. Ho C et al: Laser resurfacing in pigmented skin. *Dermatol Surg* **21**:1035, 1995
21. Weinstein C: Ultrapulse carbon dioxide laser removal of periocular wrinkles in association with laser blepharoplasty. *J Clin Laser Med Surg* **12**:205, 1994
22. Alster TS, Garg S: Treatment of facial rhytides with a high-energy pulsed carbon dioxide laser. *Plast Reconstr Surg* **98**:791, 1996
23. Alster TS, West TB: Resurfacing of atrophic facial acne scars with a high-energy, pulsed carbon dioxide laser. *Dermatol Surg* **22**:151, 1996
24. Apfelberg DB: A critical appraisal of high energy pulsed CO_2 laser facial resurfacing for acne scars. *Ann Plast Surg* **38**:95, 1997
25. Waldorf HA et al: Skin resurfacing of fine to deep rhytides using a char-free carbon dioxide laser in 47 patients. *Dermatol Surg* **21**:940, 1995
26. Lowe NJ et al: Laser skin resurfacing: pre- and posttreatment guide-lines. *Dermatol Surg* **21**:1017, 1995
27. Bernstein LJ et al: The short- and long-term side effects of carbon dioxide laser resurfacing. *Dermatol Surg* **23**:519, 1997
28. Teikemeir G, Goldberg D: Skin resurfacing with the erbium YAG laser. *Dermatol Surg* **23**:685, 1997
29. Nelson JS et al: Clinical study of non-ablative laser treatment of facial rhytids. *Lasers Surg Med* **20**(suppl 9):32, 1997

CHAPTER 270

Michelle Choucair
Tania J. Phillips

Wound Dressings

An "occlusive" or moisture-retentive dressing is one that maintains its moisture vapor transmission rate (MVTR) to permit optional healing for a given wound. Moisture-retentive dressings maintaining MVTRs of less than 35 g/m^2 per hour in partial-thickness wounds such as donor sites permit moist wound healing.

HISTORIC ASPECTS

Prior to the twentieth century, wounds were left open to dry, allow-ing the wound to "breathe."[1] In 1958 Odland first observed that a blister healed faster when left unbroken.[2] In 1962 a landmark article by Winter demonstrated the beneficial effect of a polyethylene film on wounds in domestic pigs.[3] This study, which showed that wounds in pigs reepithelialize faster under occlusion, revolutionized the approach to wound care and paved the way for the development of occlusive dressings. The first experimental work performed on human volunteers, conducted by Hinman and colleagues in 1963, established the beneficial effect of occlusion on wounds.[4] Since then, a large number and variety of wound dressings have become available, accounting for over $200 million in sales in 1987, as compared with practically no sales in 1980.[5]

EFFECT OF MOIST ENVIRONMENT ON ACUTE WOUNDS

Acute wounds are wounds with no underlying healing defect that proceed to heal in an orderly and timely fashion. The beneficial effects of a moist environment have been well studied in this type of wound.

Enhancing Debridement/Reepithelialization

A moist environment enhances the rate of epithelialization. Covered wounds resurface up to 40 percent faster than those exposed to air.[6] Enzymes that debride wounds of necrotic tissue or fibrin need water to become active. Thus water retained at the wound surface plays a vital role in enhancing debridement and subsequent reepithelial-ization. Rovee and co-workers stressed that greater epidermal cell movement rather than mitosis accounts for the faster healing time.[7] Keratinocyte migration is facilitated by the absence of necrotic tis-sue. However, the formation of a functional stratum corneum is delayed under occlusion, as demonstrated by an elevated transepi-dermal water loss (TEWL) in epithelialized wounds as compared with unwounded skin.[8]

Keeping a wound moist maintains a lateral voltage gradient that aids the repair process.[5] Fibroblasts exposed to electrical energy proliferate and increase the synthesis of collagen by increasing the number of growth factor receptors.[9]

Dermal Effect

The beneficial effects of occlusion extend to the dermis. The dermis of occluded acute wounds—as opposed to the dermis of air-exposed wounds—demonstrates a modified cell infiltrate.[10] Occlusion seems to accelerate the transition from a predominantly neutrophilic to a macrophage-rich infiltrate. In pigs, full-thickness wounds demonstrated an acceleration of the inflammatory and proliferative phases of dermal repair under moist as compared with dry conditions.[11] Initial breaking strength in a wound, which is largely related to collagen tissue deposition, is delayed under occlusion. Interstitial collagenase, a crucial enzyme for initiating collagen degradation, is increased under occlusion and is closely associated with keratinocyte migration and reepithelialization.[12] True in vivo collagen deposition has not been measured, and the exact relationship between the rate of epidermal resurfacing and dermal collagen synthesis remains to be determined. However, occluded wounds remain cosmetically superior, suggesting a modulation of the inflammatory process and accelerated remodeling and wound contraction.

Angiogenesis

Oxygen is both stimulatory and inhibitory to the wound-healing process. Nucleated cells require oxygen for cellular activities such as mitosis or migration, and it is well established that hypoxia is a potent stimulus of angiogenesis. The oxygen gradient between the wound's edge and its center stimulates capillary ingrowth toward the relatively hypoxic center of the wound.[13] The accumulation of factors stimulating angiogenesis under occlusion, such as heparin or tumor necrosis factor (TNF), may partly account for this enhanced angiogenesis.

In vitro trials have demonstrated that optimal growth of fibroblasts in tissue culture occurs at a low P_{O_2} (5 to 10 mmHg), and that epidermal cell growth is inhibited at an O_2 level higher than that of the surrounding air. Thus a delicate O_2 balance is reached under occlusion which may facilitate the formation of granulation tissue.

Retention of Wound Fluid

Acute wound fluid beneath occlusive dressings stimulates the proliferation of the various cells involved in wound healing. Katz and co-workers have demonstrated that acute wound fluid obtained up to 3 days postoperatively stimulates the in vitro growth of both human dermal fibroblasts and umbilical vein endothelial cells.[14] Identified growth factors included platelet-derived growth factor (PDGF), basic fibroblast growth factor (bFGF), epidermal growth factor (EGF), transforming growth factor β (TGF-β), and interleukin 1 (IL-1).[15] PDGF and PDGF-like peptides may be particularly involved in fibroblast stimulation as well as being chemotactic to neutrophils and mononuclear cells.[16] Other growth factors important for cell migration and matrix formation are TGF-β and EGF.[17] TGF-β stimulates the production of fibronectin by fibroblasts and keratinocytes, promotes angiogenesis, and regulates collagen synthesis. EGF stimulates keratinocyte proliferation and locomotion and inhibits fibroblast proliferation. Alteration of the expression or action of endogenous growth factors occurs within 24 h after wounding. The dressing may be removed between 24 to 48 h without loss of rapid reepithelialization.[18]

Protection Against Infection

The presence of either aerobic or anaerobic organisms does not influence wound healing, and there is no relationship between the rate at which the ulcer heals and the appearance or disappearance of the organisms. Although there might be an increased rate of bacterial colonization of occluded wounds, the rate of infection remains lower than in nonoccluded wounds.

Hutchinson, in his extensive review of clinical and research studies, reported an infection rate of 7.1 percent with conventional dressings, compared with 2.6 percent with occlusive dressings ($p < .001$).[19] Hydrocolloids fostered the lowest infection rate, followed by the foams and the hydrogels. In vivo hydrocolloids have been shown to prevent the invasion of a heavy external inoculum of Staphylococcus aureus and Pseudomonas aeruginosa applied to the outer surface of the dressing and the skin around it. A polyurethane foam dressing prevented wound contamination by organisms applied to the dressing but not by those inoculated around it.

Several mechanisms account for the low infection rate under occlusion.[20] First, there are enhanced defense mechanisms, as demonstrated by enhanced phagocytic and lysosomal activity under occlusion. Neutrophils infiltrate moist wounds more easily than dry wounds and their presence may be bactericidal. Second, necrotic tissue, which may act as a foreign body predisposing to wound infection, is absent under occlusion. Third, the dressing acts as a physical barrier against exogenous bacteria and viruses. Fourth, the relatively hypoxic environment under occlusion results in an acidic pH that inhibits bacterial growth, particularly of Pseudomonas.

EFFECT OF MOIST ENVIRONMENT ON CHRONIC WOUNDS

Chronic wounds are wounds with an underlying pathology that do not heal in a timely fashion. The effect of occlusion on chronic wounds is less well studied due to the paucity of good animal models and well-controlled clinical trials. Chronic wound fluid, unlike acute wound fluid, was found to be inhibitory to cell proliferation and contained fibronectin and vitronectin degradation products, which are inhibitory to keratinocyte migration.[21]

In venous ulcers, occlusive dressings may increase the rate of healing over the first month of treatment; but at the end of 12 weeks, controlled studies failed to show any difference between compression plus occlusion versus compression alone.[20] In clinical trials comparing moist saline gauze and other types of moist wound dressings in the treatment of pressure ulcers, no significant differences in healing outcomes were noted.[22]

For patients with chronic wounds, occlusive dressings offer the advantage of pain relief, painless wound debridement, containment of wound exudate, reduction in incidence of complications, and improved quality of life.

DRESSING CATEGORIES

There are five basic types of occlusive dressings: the hydrogels, alginates, foams, films, and hydrocolloids (Table 270-1). New categories of dressings are emerging that combine some of the above

the mannuronic acid, the greater the speed of absorption, resulting in the formation of a soft gel that can be irrigated from the wound for complete removal (Fig. 270-1).

When in contact with a small volume of sodium-rich solution, such as saline or wound exudate, calcium alginate fibers gel at the interface, owing to ion-exchange of sodium for calcium-generating free calcium ions; this amplifies the clotting cascade and creates a gel-like substance that conforms to the wound and provides a soft, moist healing environment.[1] Some alginates can absorb up to twenty times their weight, allowing the wound to remain undisturbed for several days at a time and minimizing dressing changes.

Being nonadherent, alginates require a secondary dressing over them. They are useful in heavily exudating wounds and can be packed into deep wounds and sinuses. They are also used as hemostatic dressings and are to be avoided on dry wounds.

Hydrocolloids

Hydrocolloids consist of a mixture of adhesive, absorbent polymers and a gelling agent (sodium carboxymethyl cellulose). They are opaque and impermeable to gas and water. In the presence of wound exudate, they interact with wound fluid to form a gel over the wound (Fig. 270-2).

TABLE 270-1

Wound Dressings

Products	Advantages	Disadvantages	Indications
Hydrogels	Semitransparent, soothing, do not adhere to wounds, absorbent	Require secondary dressing, frequent dressing changes	Painful wounds, postdermabrasion, laser wounds, chemical peels, partial-thickness wounds
Alginates	Absorbent, hemostatic, non-adherent, fewer dressing changes	Require secondary dressing; foul smell of the gel	Highly exudative wounds, partial- or full-thickness wounds, post-operative wounds
Hydrocolloids	Fibrinolytic, enhance angiogenesis, absorbent, bacterial and physical barrier	Opaque, foul-smelling gel	Partial- or full-thickness wounds, stage 1 to 4 pressure ulcers
Foams	Absorbent, conform to body contours	Opaque, require secondary dressing, may adhere to wounds	Partial-thickness exudative wounds, pressure relief
Films	Transparent, bacterial barrier, adherent	May adhere to wounds, can cause fluid collection	Donor sites, superficial burns, partial-thickness wounds with minimal exudate

characteristics. The choice of a dressing is dictated by the location of the wound, the nature of the wound bed, the amount of exudate, the surrounding skin, and the patient's comfort level.

Hydrogels

Hydrogels consist of a matrix of polymers with up to 96 percent water content.[23] They are semitransparent, nonadherent, and semipermeable to gas and water vapor. These dressings have a soothing and cooling effect when placed over a wound, reducing the temperature by up to 5°C (9°F) for up to 6 h. Hydrogels interact with aqueous solutions by swelling (at 200 to 300 percent saline absorption, their absorbing capacity is high), but their rate of absorbency is low. They are not good bacterial barriers. A secondary dressing is usually needed to secure them in place. They are primarily indicated for treatment of dry to mildly exudating wounds and second-degree burns, split-thickness skin grafts, donor sites, and chronic wounds.

Alginates

Alginates are naturally occurring polysaccharides found in the cell walls of brown seaweeds (*Phaeophyceae*). The principal constituent is isomeric alginic acid present in varying proportions, depending on the seaweed source. The building blocks are mannuronic and guluronic acids. They occur in different ratios and with different structures, depending on the algal species. The higher the amount of guluronic acid in the fiber, the greater its integrity or the tendency to remain in one piece. This characteristic allows for easy removal of the hydrated dressing with a forceps. In comparison, the higher

FIGURE 270-1

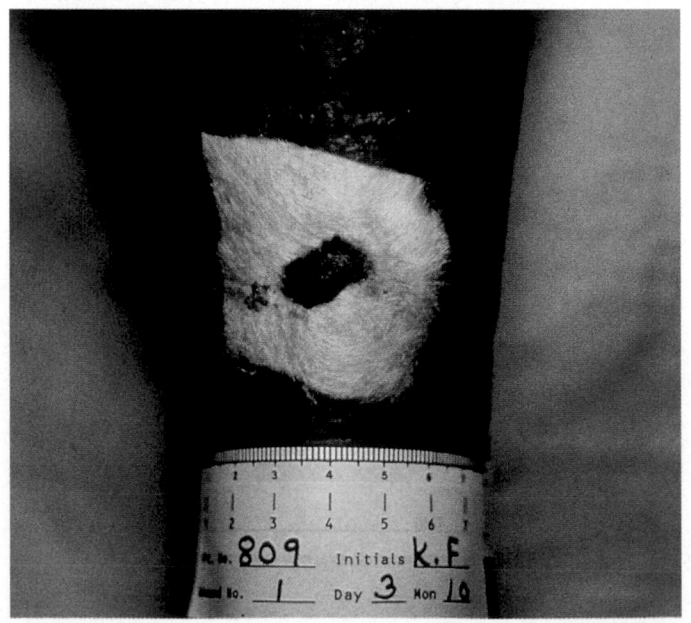

An alginate dressing on a wound. The alginate forms a gel over the wound surface but stays dry around the wound margins.

FIGURE 270-2

CHAPTER 270
Wound Dressings

2957

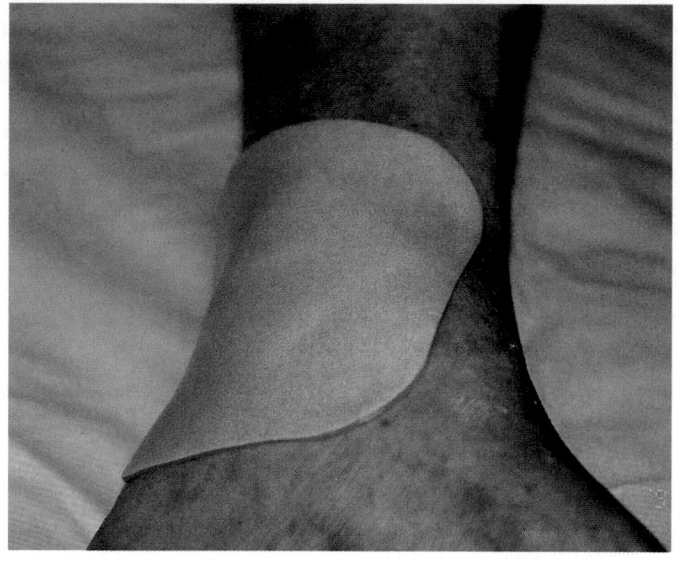

An opaque hydrocolloid dressing placed over a chronic wound.

Hydrocolloids have been well studied in vivo and in vitro. When factor VIII–related antigen antibodies were used to stain sections of tissue from porcine full-thickness wounds, there was significant enhancement of angiogenesis under DuoDerm (Convatec, Princeton, NJ) compared with both Opsite (Smith and Nephew, Hull, England) and a dry dressing on days 3, 6, and 9 after surgery.[24] Macrophages in wounds have been shown to elicit an angiogenic response through the release of growth factors, and hydrocolloid dressings stimulate macrophages. Furthermore, the relatively hypoxic environment under hydrocolloids is another potent stimulus for angiogenesis. The hydrocolloids have fibrinolytic activity, as demonstrated by the promotion of clot dissolution in a lysis assay in vitro and resolution of ^{131}I-labeled clots in experimental wounds.[25]

Some of the therapeutic benefits of the hydrocolloid dressings in the treatment of chronic wounds may be related to their ability to suppress excessive keratinocyte proliferation and activation and stimulation of epidermal migration. Hydrocolloids inhibit bacterial overgrowth by their physical barrier properties and by their provision of an acidic microenvironment.

Hydrocolloid dressings are convenient to use, offering infrequent dressing changes, ease of application, and a water-resistant surface that lets patients bathe or take showers. They may cause maceration of the surrounding skin, and patients should be warned about the malodorous, yellow-brown exudate that can form underneath them. In wounds heavily contaminated by anaerobes or caused by hemoglobinopathies such as sickle cell anemia, oxygen-permeable dressings rather than hydrocolloids should be used.

Hydrocolloids are used to treat mild to moderate exudating wounds, pressure ulcers, venous ulcers, donor sites, ulcerative lesions of scleroderma, and epidermolysis bullosa.

Foams

Polyurethane foam dressings contain a hydrophilic surface that comes into contact with the wound and a hydrophobic backing to prevent leakage. They are semiocclusive and permeable to both gas and water vapor.[23] Their absorptive ability varies with the manufacturer and depends partly upon agents impregnated in the dressing. Being nonadherent, they are good alternatives for wounds with surrounding dermatitis and on bony prominences. They are used for mild to moderately exudating wounds and after dermabrasion or Mohs surgery.[1] They are opaque, can adhere to wounds if exudate dries, and sometimes require a secondary dressing to keep them in place. Foams with adhesive borders are now commercially available.

Films

These are clear polyurethane dressing materials with an acrylic adhesive that facilitates adherence to the wound margins. They are thin and transmit moisture vapor and gases but are impermeable to fluid and bacteria. Being transparent, they allow the physician to inspect the progress of healing without disturbing the dressing or the wound. Clinical trials on surgical incisions have demonstrated that film dressings offer advantages over conventional postoperative dressings in reducing discomfort, edema, redness, and discharge and facilitating wound maturation.[26] They are used in the treatment of skin donor sites, stasis and decubitus ulcers, and superficial burn wounds (Fig. 270-3).

Films require frequent dressing changes. The problem with leakage primarily depends on the amount of fluid accumulated and the technique of application. Needle puncture to aspirate large amounts of fluid and careful observance of the recommended technique of application on the package insert will reduce the incidence of leakage.[27] Good preparation of the surrounding skin by cleaning with hydrogen peroxide and thorough drying with a dry gauze pad helps to assure good adhesion. As secondary dressings, films may be used as waterproof coverings over polyurethane foams, alginates, and hydrogels.

FIGURE 270-3

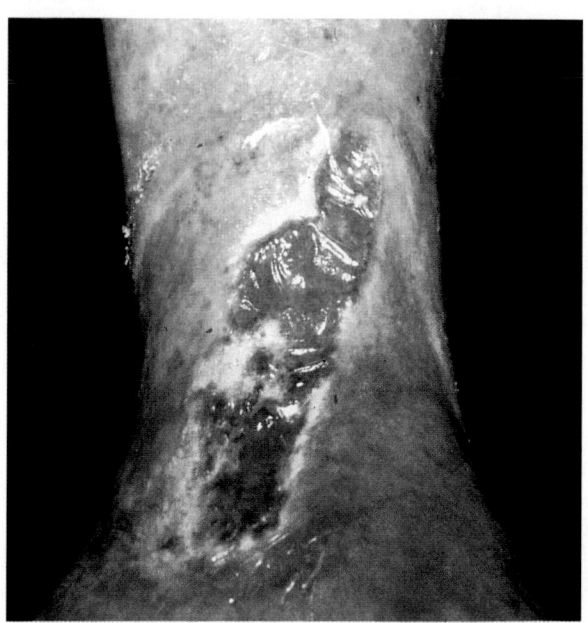

A transparent film dressing on a wound.

New dressings that combine characteristics of the categories mentioned above are emerging. A new nonadhesive, hydrophilic film dressing has been developed with a very high permeability to moisture vapor, allowing topical delivery of many drugs or antibiotics without disturbing the wound bed.[28] "Smart dressings" have been designed to adjust their rate of moisture vapor transmission according to how wet the wound is. The wetter the wound, the more moisture is transmitted through the dressing. An adhesive foam is now available with the capacity to handle high levels of exudate, and because of the dressing's waterproof backing and adhesive margins, patients can bathe and shower without any liquefaction of gel from around the edges. Collagen-alginate wound dressings combine the structural support of collagen and the gel-forming properties of alginates into sterile, soft, absorbent, and comfortable topical wound dressings. Dressings based on a superabsorbent "diaper" technology keep excessive exudate away from the wound yet keep the healing environment moist.

The choice of an appropriate dressing for a wound depends on the nature of the wound, the amount of exudate, the condition of the skin around the wound, and the patient's history. Treatment of the underlying cause is paramount, particularly in the case of chronic wounds.

REFERENCES

1. Kannon GA et al: Moist wound healing with occlusive dressings: a clinical review. *Dermatol Surg* **21**:583, 1995
2. Odland G: The fine structure of the interrelationship of cells in the human epidermis. *J Biophys Biochem Cytol* **4**:529, 1958
3. Winter GD: Formation of a scab and the rate of epithelialization of superficial wounds in the skin of the young domestic pig. *Nature* **193**:293, 1962
4. Hinman CD et al: Effect of air exposure and occlusion on experimental human skin wounds. *Nature* **200**:377, 1963
5. Eaglstein WH et al: Wound dressings: Current and future, in *Clinical and Experimental Approaches to Dermal and Epidermal Repair. Normal and Chronic Wounds.* 1991, pp 257–265
6. Eaglstein WH: Experiences with biosynthetic dressings. *J Am Acad Dermatol* **12**:434, 1985
7. Rovee DT et al: Effect of local wound environment on epidermal healing, in *Epidermal Wound Healing,* edited by HI Maibach, DT Rovee. Chicago, Year Book, 1972, pp 159–181
8. Silverman RA et al: Effects of occlusive and semiocclusive dressings on the return of barrier function to transepidermal water loss in standardized human wounds. *J Am Acad Dermatol* **20**:755, 1989
9. Falanga V et al: Electrical stimulation increases the expression of fibroblast receptors for transforming growth factor beta. *J Invest Dermatol* **88**:488, 1987
10. Falanga V: Occlusive wound dressing: Why, when, which? *Arch Dermatol* **124**:872, 1988
11. Dyson M et al: Comparison of the effects of moist and dry conditions on dermal repair. *J Invest Dermatol* **91**:434, 1988
12. Inoue M et al: Collagenase expression is rapidly induced in wound edge keratinocytes after acute injury in human skin, persists during healing, and stops at re-epithelialization. *J Invest Dermatol* **104**:479, 1995
13. Field CK et al: Overview of wound healing in a moist environment. *Am J Surg* **167**:2s, 1994
14. Katz MH et al: Human wound fluid from acute wounds stimulates fibroblast and endothelial cell growth. *J Am Acad Dermatol* **25**:1054, 1991
15. Bolton LL et al: Occlusive dressings: Therapeutic agents and effects on drug delivery. *Clin Dermatol* **9**:573, 1992
16. Deuel TF et al: Growth factors and wound healing: Platelet-derived growth factor as a model cytokine. *Annu Rev Med* **42**:567, 1991
17. King LE et al: Epidermal growth factor, in *Biochemistry and Physiology of the Skin,* edited by LA Goldsmith. New York, Oxford University Press, 1983, pp 269–281
18. Eaglstein WH: Occlusive dressings. *J Dermatol Surg Oncol* **19**:716, 1993
19. Hutchinson JJ: Prevalence of wound infection under occlusive dressings: A collective survey of reported research. *Wounds* **1**:123, 1989
20. Cordts PR et al: A prospective, randomized trial of Unna's boot versus Duoderm CGF hydroactive dressing plus compression in the management of venous leg ulcers. *J Vasc Surg* **15**:480, 1992
21. Grinell F et al: Degradation of fibronectin and vitronectin in chronic wound fluid: Analysis by cell blotting, immunoblotting and cell adhesion assays. *J Invest Dermatol* **98**:410, 1992
22. U.S. Dept of Health and Human Services. *Treatment of Pressure Ulcers:* Clinical Practice Guideline No. 15: AHCPR Publication No. 95-0652. Washington, DC, USDHHS, December 1994
23. Choucair M et al: A review of wound healing and dressing materials. *Wounds* **8**:165, 1996
24. Pickworth JJ, De Sousa N: Angiogenesis and macrophage response under the influence of Duoderm, in *Fibrinolysis and Angiogenesis in Wound Healing.* Amsterdam, Excerpta Medica 1988, pp 45–48
25. Lydon MJ et al: Dissolution of wound coagulum and promotion of granulation tissue under Duoderm. *Wounds* **1**:95, 1989
26. Holland KT et al: A comparison of the in vitro antibacterial and complement activation effect of Opsite and Tegaderm dressing. *J Hosp Infect* **5**:323, 1984
27. Gardezi SAR et al: Role of polyurethane membrane in postoperative wound management. *J Pakistan Med Assoc* **33**:219, 1983
28. Limova M et al: Clinical experience with a new, non-adherent film dressing. *Wounds* **2**:213, 1990

CHAPTER 271

Robert A. Weiss
Margaret A. Weiss

Sclerotherapy for Varicose and Telangiectatic Veins

Bulging varicose veins and unsightly "road-map" telangiectatic webs affect millions of patients. Telangiectases represent the most common of cosmetic complaints, affecting up to 50 percent of women, while larger varicose veins affect up to 20 percent of the American population.[1] Varicose veins may cause significant morbidity, including chronic stasis dermatitis, ankle edema, spontaneous bleeding, superficial thrombophlebitis, recurrent cellulitis, lipodermatosclerosis, and skin ulceration on the ankle and foot.

The incidence of varicose veins increases with each decade of life. As the age of the U.S. population grows, there will be increased demand for treatment of varicose and telangiectatic veins. While 41 percent of women in the fifth decade have varicose veins, this number rises to 72 percent in the seventh decade.[2] Statistics for men are a 24 percent incidence in the fourth decade, increasing to 43 percent by the seventh decade. Six million workdays per year may be lost in the United States due to complications of varicose veins.[3]

Sclerotherapy, defined as the intravascular introduction of a sclerosing substance, is the most widely employed procedure for the treatment of superficial telangiectases, superficial venulectases, and mid-size varicose veins. Sclerotherapy has gained increased acceptance as a markedly effective treatment in the last decade.[4] It serves as an adjunct to modern-day surgical techniques such as ambulatory phlebectomy or ligation of the saphenofemoral junction.[5,6] Venous anatomy and physiology, principles of venous insufficiency, methods of diagnosing venous abnormality, uses and actions of sclerosing solutions, and proper use of compression are essential elements of successful therapy.

HISTORIC ASPECTS

Hippocrates, in the fourth century B.C., mentions compression and a bloodletting technique utilized until the Middle Ages. Primitive stripping and cauterization were practiced by Celsus, while ligation was mentioned by Antillus (A.D. 30). In the second century, Galen proposed tearing out the veins with hooks, foreshadowing the modern-day technique of ambulatory phlebectomy originated by Swiss dermatologist Robert Muller.

A crude concept of sclerotherapy appeared in 1682, as Zollikofer described injection of acid into a vein to create a thrombus. By the late 1700s the critical role of saphenofemoral reflux in the pathogenesis of varicose veins had been recognized by the Swiss surgeon Rima. Reports of use of absolute alcohol as a sclerosing agent appeared in 1835–1840. In 1851 Pravaz attempted sclerotherapy with ferric chloride using the hypodermic syringe, his new invention.

The foundation of modern sclerotherapy was laid during World War I when Linser and Sicard both noticed the sclerosing effect of intravenous injections against syphilis, which they extended to varicose veins. Tournay greatly refined the sclerotherapy technique in Europe. It was not until 1946, when a safe sclerosant, sodium tetradecyl sulfate (Sotradecol) had been tested and described, that sclerotherapy began to be seriously studied in the United States.[7]

Another key to success and acceptance of the treatment of varicose veins by sclerotherapy was the addition of compression. Sigg and Orbach in the 1950s and Fegan in the 1960s emphasized the importance of combining external compression immediately following injections. Starting in the 1980s, Duffy promoted the technique among dermatologists and advocated the use of polidocanol and hypertonic saline as safe and effective sclerosing solutions.[8] Goldman's first American textbook of sclerotherapy integrated the world's phlebology literature, introduced new sclerosing solutions, and validated dermatology's claim to expertise in vein treatment.[9]

PATIENT SELECTION—VENOUS ANATOMY AND PHYSIOLOGY, SYMPTOMS, AND CONTRAINDICATIONS

The venous system is made up of a primary deep venous compartment and a superficial compartment with thousands of small veins (perforating veins) connecting the two systems. The deep compartment, "the muscle pump," normally acts as a conduit for 85 to 90 percent of venous return from the leg. During contraction of the calf muscles, the valves of the perforating veins and associated superficial veins close, allowing blood to flow only proximally at high pressures through the deep system. This generates primary propulsive force in returning venous blood to the heart (Fig. 271-1).

The superficial venous system consists of three primary territories: the greater saphenous vein, the lesser saphenous vein, and the subdermic lateral venous system (Fig. 271-2). Comprising the three major patterns are multiple collateral veins (accessory) and multiple tributary veins, emptying into each respectively. The points of connection (perforating veins) between the superficial and the deep system play important roles, as these are sites through which reflux or reverse flow often develops (Fig. 271-3). Owing to gravitational hydrostatic pressure, sequential retrograde breakdown of venous valve function often follows a leak at one point, leading to propagation of a varicosity. Increased diameter between valve leaflets with failure to oppose properly (caused by a genetically weak venous wall or venous valve structure) may initiate these events. Calf muscle pump pressure plus gravitational hydrostatic forces are transmitted directly via the incompetent perforating vein or communicating veins to the surface veins. Venous hypertension may reach a level as high as 300 mmHg in the cutaneous venules with

FIGURE 271-1

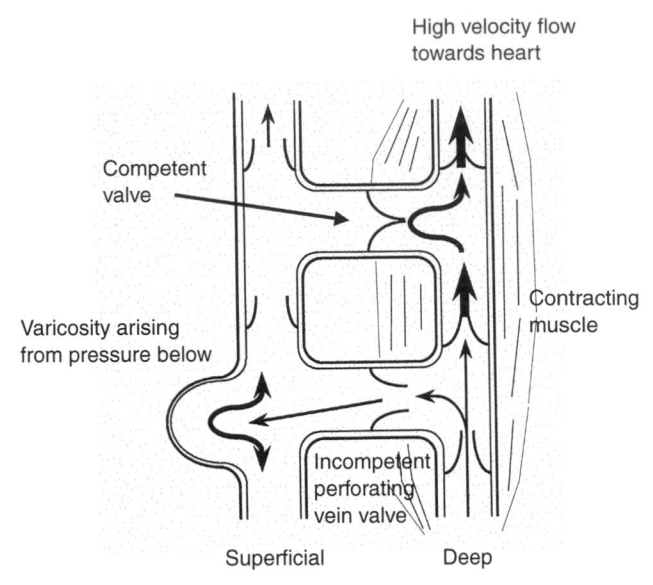

High velocity flow
towards heart

Competent
valve

Varicosity arising
from pressure below

Contracting
muscle

Incompetent
perforating
vein valve

Superficial   Deep

Schematic of the calf muscle pump with malfunctioning perforating vein connecting the superficial and deep systems. High pressures are generated when the gastrocnemius muscle contracts to pump blood proximally. A malfunctioning valve is shown diverting pressure to the skin surface. Competent valve directs flow proximally.

FIGURE 271-2

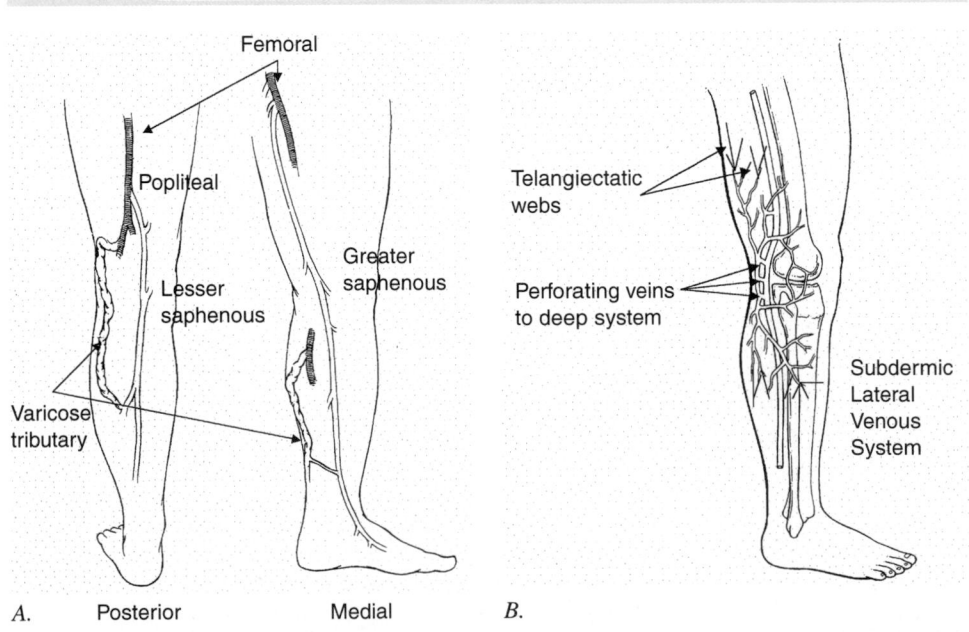

Femoral

Popliteal

Lesser
saphenous

Greater
saphenous

Varicose
tributary

Telangiectatic
webs

Perforating veins
to deep system

Subdermic
Lateral
Venous
System

A.   Posterior   Medial   *B.*

Schematic of the major portions of the superficial venous system. *A.* Greater saphenous vein and lesser saphenous vein. *B.* Subdermic lateral venous system. When varicosities or telangiectatic webs are present within the distribution of these saphenous veins, the source of pressure must be elucidated. The lateral venous system is the most common source of telangiectasias.

FIGURE 271-3

Saphenofemoral
Junction

Hunterian
perforator

Dodd's
perforator

Boyd's
perforators

Saphenopopliteal
Junction

Cockett's
perforators

Submalleolar
perforator

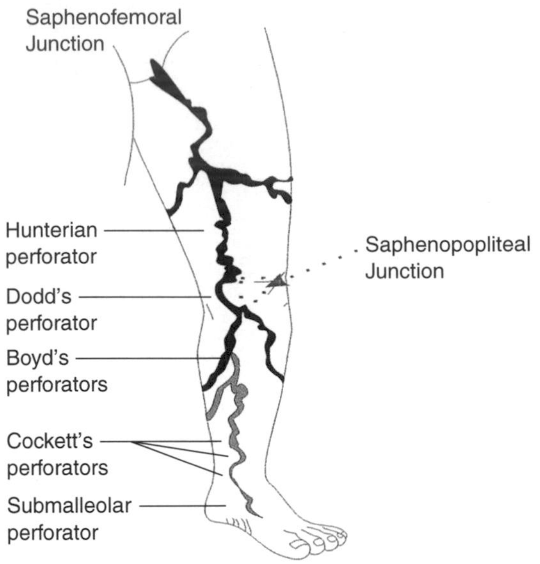

Diagram indicating major junctions points of the superficial venous system with the deep venous system. Larger varicose veins may originate from any of these points.

the patient erect. Transmission of pressure may result in venular dilatation over a wide area of skin, including the formation of telangiectatic webs.

When present in significant quantity, the volume of blood sequestered and stagnant in reticular veins and associated telangiectatic webs (particularly of the lateral venous system) may cause enough distention to produce symptoms.[10] Symptoms are relieved by the wearing of support hose or with rest and elevation of the legs. Prolonged standing or sitting worsens symptoms. The diameter of the vessels causing moderately severe symptoms may be as little as 1 to 2 mm. Sclerotherapy has been reported to yield an 85 percent reduction in these symptoms as well as superb cosmetic results.[10]

Contraindications (Table 271-1)

Sclerotherapy may be performed safely and effectively in virtually all types of veins except when reflux exists at the saphenofemoral junction. Since the goal of sclerotherapy is to eliminate reflux at its origin, the goal of noninvasive diagnostic evaluation is to uncover primary sources of high reverse flow pressure. A high rate of recurrence for sclerotherapy is commonly seen when reflux originates at the major saphenous junctions. A surgical consultation is important in these situations.[11]

Sclerotherapy is contraindicated in a bedridden patient, since ambulation following sclerotherapy is important

Indications and Contraindications for Sclerotherapy

INDICATIONS	CONTRAINDICATIONS
Pain	Reflux at saphenofemoral or saphenopopliteal junction*
Major tributaries of greater and lesser saphenous veins	Nonambulatory patient
Major perforator reflux	Obesity
Lateral venous system varicosities	Deep venous thrombosis
Cosmetic	Known allergy to sclerosing agent
	Arterial obstruction
	Pregnancy

*Relative contraindication; success has been reported under the right conditions, proper sclerosing solutions (not available in the United States) and/or the use of duplex-guided sclerotherapy.

for minimizing risks of thrombosis. Similarly, patients under general anesthesia for unrelated procedures should not undergo simultaneous sclerotherapy. Severely restricted arterial flow to the legs necessitates postponement of vein treatment. A history of deep venous thrombosis (DVT) or previous trauma to the leg (e.g., a vehicular accident) should preclude sclerotherapy until the patient is adequately evaluated by duplex ultrasound. Previous urticaria or suspected allergy to a sclerosing agent should serve as a relative contraindication to use of that particular sclerosing agent.

Pregnancy should be considered a contraindication during the first and second trimesters, although extremely painful or bleeding varices may be treated in the last trimester. Treatment is typically postponed, since many varicosities and telangiectasias will resolve spontaneously 1 to 6 months postpartum.

Obesity should be considered a relative contraindication, since maintaining adequate external compression is difficult. Sclerotherapy of larger varicosities should be postponed until weight reduction is achieved. During hot summer months, heat-induced vasodilatation and inability to comply with wearing of compression hose may require postponement of treatment.

TECHNIQUE

Pretreatment Evaluation

Previous venous surgery may warrant further testing before proceeding. Those patients with a family history of large varicose veins are more likely to have early axial (saphenous) reflux even when presenting with telangiectasias alone.[5]

Physical examination is performed by viewing the patient's legs in a 360 degree rotation. Palpation is performed along the saphenous vein distributions to rule out early large axial varicosities that cannot be seen. Based on the history and physical examination, noninvasive diagnostic vascular tests are performed as necessary.[12] Once the patient is judged to be a candidate for sclerotherapy, informed consent is obtained. The necessity of multiple treatment sessions is emphasized.

Any veins visible or palpable suggestive of saphenous system involvement should be minimally evaluated by hand-held Doppler ultrasound, which is equivalent to using an enhanced "stethoscope" to hear vein flow. In order to generate or augment an audible signal of flow, a maneuver such as manual compression of the calf must

be performed by the examiner. When compression is released, gravitational hydrostatic pressure causes reverse flow to cease within 0.5 to 1 s when valves are competent, but a long flow sound is audible when valves are incompetent.

The most essential part of the Doppler examination is the examination of the saphenofemoral junction below the inguinal fold just medial to the femoral arterial signal. During a Valsalva maneuver, a continuous and pronounced reflux signal is a reliable sign of valvular insufficiency. An equivocal result may require a duplex ultrasound examination for a definitive answer. Methods of complete Doppler examination are detailed elsewhere.[5]

Another noninvasive method used to quantify reflux is photoplethysmography (PPG). PPG permits assessment of the physiologic significance of anatomic Doppler findings. Digital (quantitative) PPG measures total venous insufficiency as well as changes in venous function after treatment and allows evaluation of deep venous function (venous ejection fraction) during a defined series of calf muscle movements.[13]

The gold standard of noninvasive examination of the venous system is duplex ultrasound. This allows direct visualization of the veins and identification of flow through venous valves. An image is created by an array of Doppler transducers, which are switched on and off sequentially. This is combined with a second method to echo pulse a Doppler signal. The duplex examination is often used to uncover hidden sources of reflux prior to beginning any method of treatment or to delineate reflux sources when patients experience poor results from sclerotherapy.

Sclerosing Solutions

Sclerosing solutions have been classified into groups based on chemical structure and effect: hyperosmotic, detergent, and corrosive agents (chemical toxins or salts, alcohols, and acid or alkaline solutions). Commonly employed sclerosing solutions are summarized in Table 271-2.

HYPERTONIC SALINE Although approved by the FDA only for use as an abortifacient, hypertonic saline (HS) is a commonly employed solution in the United States. Used at a concentration of 23.4%, a theoretical advantage of HS is its total lack of allergenicity when unadulterated. HS has been commonly used in various concentrations from 10 to 30%, with the occasional addition of heparin, procaine, or lidocaine. Additional agents typically provide no benefit. Therefore, HS is used either unadulterated or diluted to 11.7% with sterile water for smaller telangiectasias.[14]

With hypertonic solutions, damage of tissue adjacent to injection sites may easily occur. Skin necrosis may be produced by extravasation at the injection site, particularly when injecting very close to the skin surface. Injection of hyaluronidase into sites of extravasation may significantly reduce the risks of skin necrosis with HS.[15]

HYPERTONIC SALINE AND DEXTROSE Hypertonic saline and dextrose (HSD) (Sclerodex, Omega Laboratories Ltd., Montreal, Canada) is a viscous mixture of dextrose 250 mg/mL, sodium chloride 100 mg/mL, propylene glycol 100 mg/mL, and phenethyl alcohol 8 mg/mL. It is a relatively weak sclerosant for local treatment of small vessels, with a total volume of injection not to exceed 10 mL per visit with 0.1 to 1.0 mL per injection site. HSD is marketed predominately in Canada. Although a slight burning sensation occurs, pain is far less than with HS.

TABLE 271-2

Comparison of Commonly Employed Sclerosing Agents

Sclerosing Solution	Category	Advantages	Disadvantages	Vessels Treated	Concentrations, %
Sodium tetradecyl sulfate (Sotradecol)	Detergent	FDA-approved Painless unless injected extravascularly	May cause skin breakdown at higher concentrations	All sizes	0.1–0.2 telangiectasias 0.2–0.5 reticular 0.5–1.0 varicose 1.0–3.0 axial varicose
Polidocanol	Detergent	Painless Low ulceration risk at low concentrations	Not FDA-approved	Small to medium	0.25–0.5 telangiectasias 0.5–1.0 reticular 1.0–3.0 varicose
Hypertonic saline	Hyperosmolar	Low risk of allergic reactions	Ulcerogenic Painful to inject	Small	23.4–11.7 telangiectasias 23.4 reticular
Hypertonic saline plus dextrose (Sclerodex)	Hyperosmolar	Low risk of allergic reaction Mild stinging Low ulcerogenic potential	Not FDA-approved Relatively weak sclerosant	Small	Undiluted; telangiectasias Undiluted; reticular
Sodium morrhuate (Scleromate)	Detergent	FDA-approved	Allergic reactions highest	Small	Undiluted; telangiectasias Undiluted; reticular
Chromated glycerin (glycerin with 6% chromium salt) (Scleremo)	Chemical irritant	Low skin ulcer potential	Not FDA-approved Very weak sclerosant	Smallest	Undiluted to half strength; telangiectasias
Polyiodinated iodine (Varigloban)	Chemical irritant	Highly corrosive; allows treatment of largest veins	Not FDA-approved Avoid in iodine allergic patients	Largest	1–2 for up to 5-mm veins 2–6 for the largest veins

POLIDOCANOL Polidocanol (POL) (Aethoxysklerol, Chemische Fabrik Kreussler & Co, Wiesbaden-Biebrich, West Germany) is a detergent-based urethane compound. It was originally developed as an anesthetic but was found to have the property of sclerosing small-diameter vessels after intradermal injection. POL contains hydroxypolyethoxydodecane dissolved in distilled water with 5% ethanol as a stabilizer. First used as a sclerosing agent in the late 1960s in Germany, POL is popular worldwide for smaller vessels owing to its painless injection and lowest incidence of cutaneous necrosis with intradermal injection. Lower concentrations of POL were initially suspected to produce a lower incidence of hyperpigmentation than HS or sodium tetradecyl sulfate (STS), but recent clinical trials indicate that a significant percentage of hyperpigmentation occurs.[16] The U.S. FDA has not yet approved POL, although clinical trials are completed with availability in the United States anticipated shortly.

SODIUM TETRADECYL SULFATE STS (Sotradecol, Wyeth-Ayerst Laboratories, Philadelphia; S.T.D. Injection, S.T.D. Pharmaceuticals, United Kingdom) is a long-chain fatty acid salt with strong detergent properties; it is a highly effective sclerosing agent used worldwide. Approved for use in the United States since 1946,

it has been popular with vascular surgeons since the 1960s and was first described for use in telangiectasias in the 1970s. A relatively high incidence of postsclerosis pigmentation was reported at inappropriately high doses (1% STS). More appropriate concentrations for superficial telangiectasias are 0.1 to 0.2%. Other concentrations are 0.2 to 0.5% in reticular veins or small varicosities (1 to 3 mm in diameter) and 0.5 to 3% in larger varicosities related to major sites of valvular reflux.

SODIUM MORRHUATE Sodium morrhuate (Scleromate, Palisades Pharmaceuticals, Inc., Tenafly, NJ) is a 5% solution of the salts of saturated and unsaturated fatty acids in cod liver oil. Approximately 10 percent of its fatty acid composition is unknown, and its use is limited by reports of fatalities secondary to anaphylaxis.[9] Although sodium morrhuate is approved by the FDA for the sclerosis of varicose veins, its use in the treatment of telangiectasias is not common because of its caustic qualities, with potential for cutaneous necrosis and higher risks of allergy. This agent is reserved primarily for sclerosis of esophageal varices.

CHEMICAL IRRITANTS The chemical irritants include polyiodinated iodine (very caustic) and chromated glycerin (very weak); they are believed to have a direct toxic effect on the endothelium. After injection of polyiodinated iodine salt, the endothelium near the site of injection is destroyed within seconds. The corrosive action is limited owing to rapid inactivation by blood proteins. At the sites of endothelial destruction the chemical can penetrate further and diffuse into deeper layers of the vessel wall, causing further destruction.

Technique

A basic principle of treatment is to begin at the largest (reflux sources) and progress to the smallest varicosities. Sclerotherapy of telangiectasias is approached by combined injection of visibly connected reticular veins, venulectases, and telangiectatic webs or networks. Progression from proximal to distal regions will focus initial treatment on vessels most likely to be proximal pressure sources.

Reticular veins are treated only after all sources of reflux from major varicosities have been treated by sclerotherapy and/or surgery. When no clear feeder vessel is seen or identified by Doppler, transillumination (Venoscope, Applied Biotech Products, Inc., Lafayette, LA) is another method which may be used to identify the "feeding" reticular vein (Fig. 271-4). When one is unable to locate an associated reticular vein, then the point at which the telangiectasias begin to branch out is the site at which to begin injection. Injection of telangiectasias is simultaneously performed with injection of reticular veins in the hope of decreasing the number of treatments.[17]

FIGURE 271-4

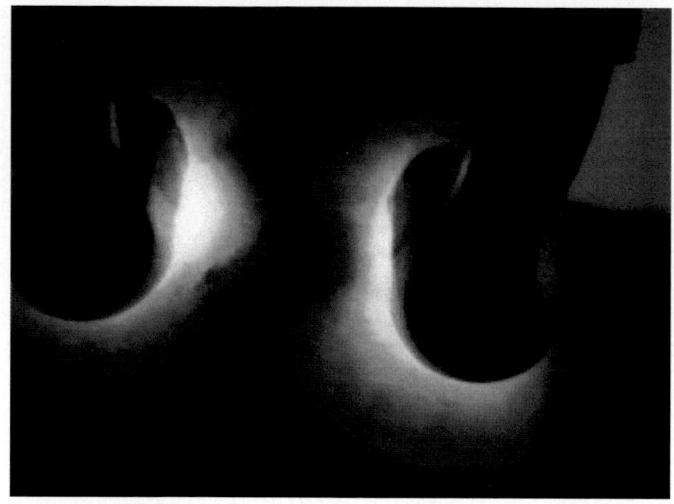

Transillumination of a reticular vein. The reticular vein shows up as a dark, curvilinear object against a light background.

The injection method for telangiectasia is basically as previously described by Duffy and Goldman.[8,18] The sclerotherapy tray is prepared with the necessary equipment (Table 271-3). A 30-gauge needle, bent to an angle of 10 to 30 degrees with the bevel up, is placed on the skin so that the needle is parallel to the skin surface. A 3-mL syringe filled with 1.5 to 2 mL of solution is held between the index and middle fingers while the fourth and fifth fingers support the syringe against the leg in a fixed position, facilitating accurate penetration of the vessel. The nondominant hand is used to stretch the skin around the needle and may offer additional support for the syringe (Fig. 271-5). Magnifying lenses or operating loops on the order of 1.5 to 3× may help in cannulation of the smallest telangiectasias.

The initial treatment of telangiectatic webs begins with the minimal effective concentration (FDA-approved) of sclerosing solution.[14] When ineffective sclerosis occurs as judged at a subsequent visit, the concentration, *not* the volume per site, of sclerosing solution is increased. Posttreatment compression consists of graduated 20 to 30-mmHg or 30- to 40-mmHg support hose for 2 weeks for larger veins and OTC 15-mmHg compression for smaller veins.

TABLE 271-3

The Sclerotherapy Tray

Cotton balls soaked with 70% isopropyl alcohol
Protective gloves
3-mL disposable syringes
30-g disposable transparent hub needles
Cotton balls or STD* pads for compression
Transpore and/or paper tape
Nitroglycerin paste (for prolonged blanching or extravasation)
Sclerosing solutions
　1. Sodium tetradecyl sulfate (ranging concentrations 0.1–0.5%)
　2. Hypertonic saline (11.7–23.4%)
　3. Hypertonic saline (10%) and dextrose (25%) (may be mixed by local pharmacy)
　4. Polidocanol (0.25–1%) (pending FDA clearance)

*STD pad, is a brand name of specially shaped foam rubber pads (STD Pharmaceutical, Hereford, England).

FIGURE 271-5

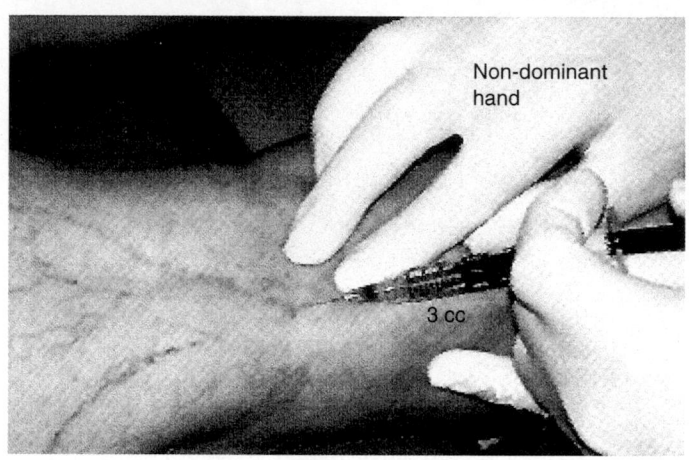

Position of the hands for sclerotherapy. While the dominant hand holds the syringe and creates a platform with the fifth digit, the nondominant hand stretches the skin and acts as a support for the needle hub so that fine changes in position are permitted.

Treatment intervals vary, but allowing 4 to 8 weeks between treatments helps to minimize the number of necessary sessions. Typical results are shown in Fig. 271-6.

SIDE EFFECTS AND COMPLICATIONS

POSTSCLEROTHERAPY HYPERPIGMENTATION Postsclerosis pigmentation is defined as the appearance of increased visible pigmentation along the course of a treated vein of any size. Initially perivascular hemosiderin deposition and not increased melanin production causes this appearance.[19] The incidence of pigmentation is related to dilution and type of sclerosing agent as well as the diameter of the treated vessel.[20] Pigmentation incidence ranges from 11 to 30 percent using HS,[21] 11 to 30 percent with POL,[22,23] and up to 30 percent with STS. The incidence of pigmentation may be reduced in varicose veins by expressing the dark, viscous blood—thought to be a liquefied coagulum or intravascular hematoma—which may accumulate 1 to 4 weeks following sclerotherapy.

Pigmentation clears in 70 percent of patients within 6 months but rarely persists for more than a year.[20] Attempts to hasten resolution of pigmentation have been mostly unsuccessful, as the pigment is dermal hemosiderin and not epidermal melanin. Bleaching agents, exfoliants such as trichloroacetic acid or phenol, cryotherapy, various lasers, and intense pulsed light have achieved limited success.[24,25]

TELANGIECTATIC MATTING Telangiectatic matting is defined as the appearance of groups of new, fine (<0.2-mm diameter) telangiectasias surrounding or replacing a previously treated area in a blushlike manner. A retrospective analysis of over 2000 patients reports an incidence of 16 percent in patients treated with HS and POL.[26] Resolution usually occurs spontaneously within a 3- to 12-month period, with 70 to 80 percent spontaneous resolution within the first 6 months.[27]

FIGURE 271-6

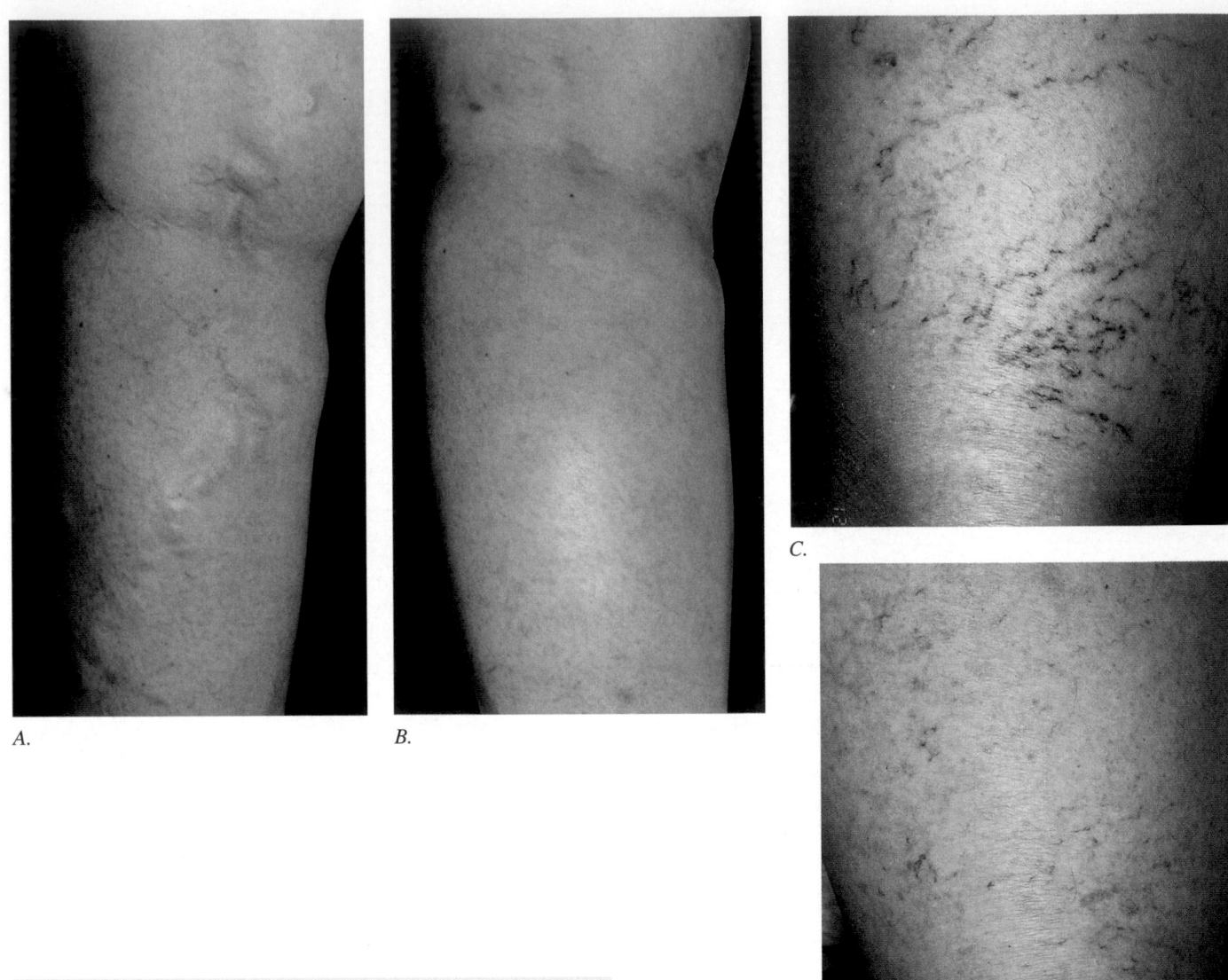

Typical results following sclerotherapy. *A.* Large varicose vein treated twice with 0.5% sodium tetradecyl sulfate (STS). *B.* Excellent clinical results at 15-month follow-up. *C.* A 62-year-old patient with focal burning symptoms on the anterior thigh. *D.* Results 5 months later, after three treatments with 0.1% STS and 0.5% polidocanol.

Matting may also occur as a result of trauma to the leg, in association with pregnancy or hormonal therapy, or in scars around previous sites of surgical stripping. Predisposing factors include predilection for certain areas of the leg, such as the medial lower thigh; obesity; hormonal therapy with estrogen; family history; and a longer history of telangiectasias.[26] The relative risk factor for development of telangiectatic matting is 3.17 times greater for female patients taking hormonal supplements.[28] Successful treatment of matting with the flash-lamp pumped-dye laser (FLDL) is reported accompanied by temporary hyperpigmentation.[29] Treatment is typically not required, since most matting will resolve spontaneously.

CUTANEOUS NECROSIS/ULCERATION Cutaneous ulceration may occur with all sclerosing solutions in spite of the most skilled technique. Unavoidably, a tiny amount of sclerosing solution may be left along the needle tract as the needle is withdrawn. Sclerosing solution may also leak out into the skin through the small puncture sites of vessel cannulation. The varicose vein may have a fragile, thin wall, with the injection causing rapid injury, leading to sudden unexpected rupture with perivascular accumulation of sclerosant. Additionally, injection may inadvertently occur into a small arteriole associated with telangiectatic varicosities, with resultant necrosis and ulceration.

When the dermatologic surgeon recognizes that extravasation has occurred, the risk for necrosis can be minimized by injecting normal saline in a ratio of 10:1 into the extravasation site.[27] Extensive massage of small subcutaneous blebs to spread the trapped sclerosing agent as quickly as possible will minimize prolonged blanching of the area. An anecdotal report of topical nitroglycerin paste applied immediately to the extravasation site indicates that necrosis may be reduced or prevented (M. Goldman, personal communication).

SUPERFICIAL THROMBOPHLEBITIS This complication is most commonly mistaken for the normal nodular fibrosis (endosclerosis) that occurs with proper sclerotherapy. A nontender, nonpigmented, nonerythematous fibrotic cord may normally be palpable along the course of a treated 4- to 8-mm vein. In contrast, superficial thrombophlebitis is characterized clinically by a very tender, indurated, linear erythematous swelling. Incidence is quite variable being estimated at 1 to 0.01 percent following sclerotherapy,[30] although a recent report indicates that the incidence is higher than previously suspected.[31] A liquefied coagulum usually accompanies the presence of superficial thrombophlebitis and should be evacuated. Treatment also consists of leg elevation and/or compression and regular administration of aspirin or other nonsteroidal anti-inflammatory drugs. Extension of superficial thrombophlebitis into the deep system is extremely rare.

PULMONARY EMBOLISM Pulmonary emboli probably occur from extension of a superficial thrombus into the deep venous system. Evidence of extension from superficial thrombus to deep thrombophlebitis should be treated promptly by anticoagulation. The incidence of pulmonary embolism has been associated with injection of large quantities of sclerosant at a single site. The incidence is extremely low (less than 1 in 40,000).

ARTERIAL INJECTION This dreaded medical emergency is fortunately extremely rare. Warning signs include immediate intense pain far beyond the normal discomfort at the initiation of injection. Continuous, intense burning pain with immediate bone-white cutaneous blanching over a large area is the usual initial sign. Progression to a sharply demarcated cyanosis within minutes is typical for arterial injection. Emergency treatment involves immediate application of ice, attempts to flush the inadvertently injected artery with normal saline and/or heparin, injection of 3% procaine to inactivate STS, and consultation for intravenous anticoagulation. Rarely, arterial injection may not be accompanied by the usual signs of immediately intense pain and discoloration.[32] Arterial injection may lead to wide areas of skin necrosis and damage to subcutaneous tissue and muscle.

ALTERNATIVE APPROACHES

Surgical Ligation and Limited Stripping

For larger varicose veins, particularly originating from an incompetent valve at the saphenofemoral junction, ligation of the greater saphenous vein with short stripping of its proximal end in the thigh is the presently favored vascular surgery method. After proximal ligation without stripping of the saphenous vein, varicography has shown persistent midthigh perforator incompetence in 34 percent, a patent portion of saphenous vein in 54 percent, and residual or recurrent femorosaphenous communication in 80 percent of patients.[33] High ligation combined with sclerotherapy or with varicosity excision was inferior to high ligation and stripping of the saphenous vein.[34]

Ambulatory Phlebectomy

This technique, originally described by Robert Muller and further refined by Albert-Adrien Ramelet, another Swiss dermatologist, involves the use of tiny incisions through which the varicose vein is removed by a small hook.[35,36] This technique is safe when done on an outpatient basis with local anesthesia. It allows removal of almost any varicose vein except the saphenofemoral or saphenopopliteal junction. Areas or veins that are resistant to sclerotherapy (axial) are particularly indicated for ambulatory phlebectomy (Fig. 271-7). Risks minimized compared with sclerotherapy are deep venous thrombosis, postsclerotherapy pigmentation, skin necrosis, and superficial phlebitis. In many cases larger varicose veins coexist with smaller reticular veins and associated telangiectatic webs. It is reasonable to treat larger varicose veins by various surgical techniques and to follow up with sclerotherapy of the remaining reticular networks.

Intense Pulsed Light Source

An intense pulsed light source (IPLS) (PhotoDerm VL, ESC, Inc., Needham, MA) uses a pulsed flash lamp–generated wavefront to generate fluences in the range of 3 to 90 J/cm^2 on the skin in single, double, or triple pulse modes for photocoagulation of telangiectasias up to 2 mm (Fig. 271-8). The duration of each pulse can be varied from 0.6 to 20 ms and the delays between pulses can be varied from

FIGURE 271-7

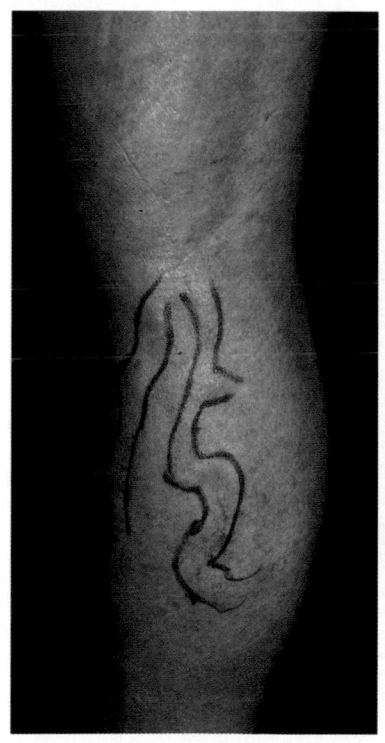
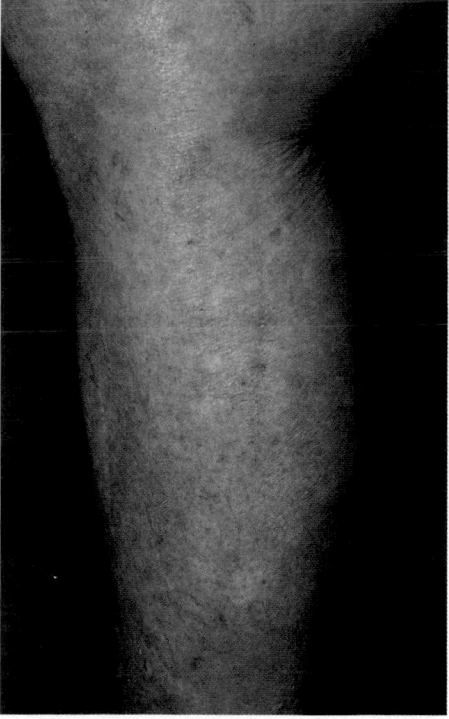

A.   *B.*

Ambulatory phlebectomy of a large truncal varicose vein. *A.* Marked just prior to surgery. *B.* Clinical results with complete disappearance at 6 weeks. Bruising usually lasts no longer than 2 weeks. This vein was previously resistant to treatment by sclerotherapy.

REFERENCES

1. Biegeleisen K: Primary lower extremity telangiectasias relationship of size to color. *Angiology* **38**:760, 1987
2. Engel A et al: Health effects of sunlight exposure in the United States: Results from the first national health and nutrition examination survey, 1971–1974. *Arch Dermatol* **124**:72, 1988
3. Lofgren KA: Varicose veins: Their symptoms, complications, and management. *Postgrad Med* **65**:131, 1979
4. Weiss RA et al: Physicians' negative perception of sclerotherapy for venous disorders: Review of a 7-year experience with modern sclerotherapy. *South Med J* **85**:1101, 1992
5. Goldman MP et al: Diagnosis and treatment of varicose veins—a review. *J Am Acad Dermatol* **31**:393, 1994
6. Weiss RA, Weiss MA: Ambulatory phlebectomy compared to sclerotherapy for varicose and telangiectatic veins: Indications and complications. *Adv Dermatol* **11**:3, 1996
7. Cooper WM: Clinical evaluation of sotradecol, a sodium alkyl sulfate solution, in the injection therapy of varicose veins. *Surg Gynecol Obstet* **83**:647, 1946
8. Duffy DM: Small vessel sclerotherapy: An overview. *Adv Dermatol* **3**:221, 1988
9. Goldman MP: *Sclerotherapy: Treatment of Varicose and Telangiectatic Leg Veins.* St. Louis, Mosby–Year Book, 1991
10. Weiss RA, Weiss MA: Resolution of pain associated with varicose and telangiectatic leg veins after compression sclerotherapy. *J Dermatol Surg Oncol* **16**:333, 1990
11. Bergan JJ: Surgical procedures for varicose veins: Axial stripping and stab avulsion, in *Atlas of Venous Surgery,* edited by JJ Bergan, RL Kistner. Philadelphia, Saunders, 1992, pp 61–77
12. Weiss RA: Vascular studies of the legs for venous or arterial disease (review). *Dermatol Clin* **12**:175, 1994
13. Kerner J et al: Quantitative Photoplethysmographie bei gesunden Erwachsenen, Kindern und Schwangeren und bei Varizenpatienten. *Phlebology* **21**:134, 1992
14. Sadick NS: Sclerotherapy of varicose and telangiectatic leg veins: Minimal sclerosant concentration of hypertonic saline and its relationship to vessel diameter. *J Dermatol Surg Oncol* **17**:65, 1991
15. Zimmet SE: The prevention of cutaneous necrosis following extravasation of hypertonic saline and sodium tetradecyl sulfate. *J Dermatol Surg Oncol* **19**:641, 1993
16. Conrad P et al: The Australian polidocanol (aethoxysklerol) study: Results at 2 years. *Dermatol Surg* **21**:334, 1995
17. Weiss RA, Weiss MA: Painful telangiectasias: Diagnosis and treatment, in *Varicose Veins and Telangiectasias: Diagnosis and Treatment,* edited by JJ Bergan, MP Goldman. St. Louis, Quality Medical Publishing, 1993, pp 389–406
18. Goldman MP, Bennett RG: Treatment of telangiectasia: A review. *J Am Acad Dermatol* **17**:167, 1987
19. Goldman MP et al: Postsclerotherapy hyperpigmentation: A histologic evaluation. *J Dermatol Surg Oncol* **13**:547, 1987
20. Weiss RA, Weiss MA: Incidence of side effects in the treatment of telangiectasias by compression sclerotherapy: Hypertonic saline vs. polidocanol. *J Dermatol Surg Oncol* **16**:800, 1990
21. Weiss RA, Weiss MA: Resolution of pain associated with varicose and telangiectatic leg veins after compression sclerotherapy. *J Dermatol Surg Oncol* **16**:333, 1990
22. Duffy DM: Small vessel sclerotherapy: An overview. *Adv Dermatol* **3**:221, 1988
23. Goldman PM: Sclerotherapy for superficial venules and telangiectasias of the lower extremities. *Dermatol Clin* **5**:369, 1987
24. Thibault P, Wlodarczyk J: Postsclerotherapy hyperpigmentation: The role of serum ferritin levels and the effectiveness of treatment with the copper vapor laser. *J Dermatol Surg Oncol* **18**:47, 1992
25. Goldman MP: Postsclerotherapy hyperpigmentation: Treatment with a flashlamp-excited pulsed dye laser. *J Dermatol Surg Oncol* **18**:417, 1992
26. Davis LT, Duffy DM: Determination of incidence and risk factors for postsclerotherapy telangiectatic matting of the lower extremity: A retrospective analysis. *J Dermatol Surg Oncol* **16**:327, 1990
27. Goldman MP et al: Cutaneous necrosis, telangiectatic matting, and hyperpigmentation following sclerotherapy: Etiology, prevention, and treatment (review) *Dermatol Surg* **21**:19, 1995
28. Weiss RA, Weiss MA: Incidence of side effects in the treatment of telangiectasias by compression sclerotherapy: Hypertonic saline vs. polidocanol. *J Dermatol Surg Oncol* **16**:800, 1990

FIGURE 271-8

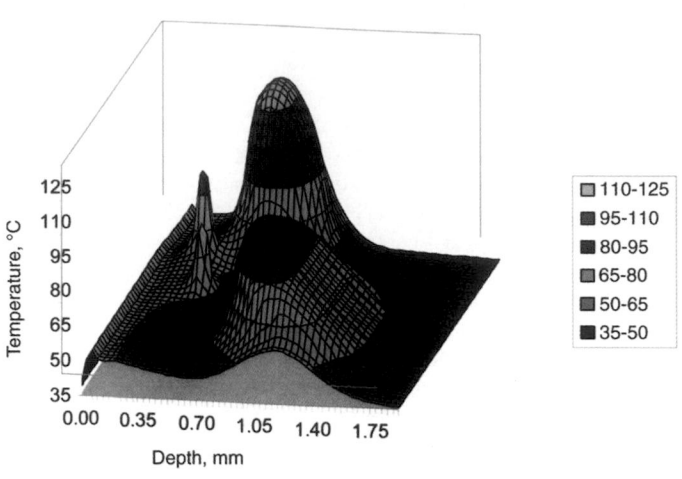

Light interaction with blood vessels. Temperature distribution for 1-mm vessel, 1 mm below skin surface following a triple pulse of noncoherent intense pulsed light with total fluence of 50 J. In this mathematical model, temperature reaches a peak of 125°C (257°F), which is necessary for photocoagulation. Smaller vessels at 0.3-mm depth reach 100°C (212°F).

10 to 200 ms. Noncoherent light output is varied within the 515- to 1000-nm range. A large rectangular spot size of 8 by 35 mm allows much larger areas to be treated with a single pulse than is possible with laser devices. Selectivity is achieved by combining the optimal spectrum that will have a high interaction with oxyhemoglobin or deoxyhemoglobin, minimal interaction with melanin, and adequate depth penetration. A recent multicenter study demonstrated 70 percent of patients responding with up to five treatments per region.[37]

Lasers

Many trials of lasers have occurred on leg telangiectasias with less than optimal results. The flash-lamp pumped-dye laser (FLPD) at 585 nm is highly efficacious on facial vascular lesions, but lower extremity telangiectasias have not responded as well. Pigmentation changes, approximately 50 percent incidence of both hyperpigmentation and hypopigmentation, persisting for several months have been the primary problem. Hyperpigmentation is believed to result from thermal rupture of superficial vessels and hypopigmentation from nonspecific melanin absorption. Efficacy rates in the smallest of telangiectasias (0.2 mm) have been reported ranging from 25 to 70 percent.

New technology includes a longer pulse width and longer wavelengths for the FLPD (Sclerolase, Candela Corp., Wayland, MA) and the use of longer-pulsed, skin-cooled Nd:YAG (532 nm) (Versapulse, Coherent, Palo Alto, CA). Preliminary results indicate that the success rates for superficial leg telangiectasias are improved over those obtained with previous lasers. With all lasers or light sources, larger sources of reflux must be eliminated initially before success on smaller vessels can be achieved.

29. Goldman MP, Fitzpatrick RE: Pulsed-dye laser treatment of leg telangiectasia: With and without simultaneous sclerotherapy. *J Dermatol Surg Oncol* **16**:338, 1990

30. Goldman MP: Sclerotherapy treatment for varicose and telangiectatic leg veins, in *Cosmetic Surgery of the Skin,* edited by WP Coleman. Philadelphia, Decker, 1991, pp 197–211

31. Feied CF: Deep vein thrombosis: The risks of sclerotherapy in hypercoagulable states. *Semin Dermatol* **12**:135, 1993

32. Biegeleisen K et al: Inadvertent intra-arterial injection complicating ordinary and ultrasound-guided sclerotherapy. *J Dermatol Surg Oncol* **19**:953, 1993

33. Corbett CR et al: Reasons to strip the long saphenous vein. *Phlebology* **41**:766, 1988

34. Neglen P: Treatment of varicosities of saphenous origin: Comparison of ligation, selective excision, and sclerotherapy, in *Varicose Veins and Telangiectasias: Diagnosis and Management,* edited by JJ Bergan, MP Goldman. St. Louis, Quality Medical Publishing, 1993, pp 148–165

35. Ramelet AA: Le Traitement des telangiectasies: Indications de la phlebectomie selon muller. *Phlebolology* **47**:377, 1995

36. Ramelet AA: Muller phlebectomy: A new phlebectomy hook. *J Dermatol Surg Oncol* **17**:814, 1991

37. Goldman MP, Eckhouse S: Photothermal sclerosis of leg veins. *Dermatol Surg* **22**:323, 1996

CHAPTER 272

Arnold William Klein
Rhoda S. Narins
Jeffrey A. Klein

Tumescent Liposuction

HISTORY

Liposuction as we know it today was first described by Dr. Yves Illouz in Paris in the late 1970s. The innovations that made this procedure possible were the development of a blunt cannula and the injections of small amounts of a hypotonic saline solution into the subcutaneous tissue, both of which diminished bleeding.[1] Over the next several years various amounts of lidocaine and epinephrine were added to these solutions, and in 1985 Dr. Jeffrey Klein introduced the technique of tumescent liposuction. In this form of liposuction, a dilute concentration of lidocaine and epinephrine is infused into the fatty tissue in large enough quantities to tumesce this tissue, enabling the procedure to be done under local anesthesia alone with minimal blood loss compared with the other forms of liposuction. With this technique the patient avoids general anesthesia and thus has a milder postsurgical course. Additionally, during the procedure the patient can get into any position necessary for exact removal of fat, thus making the procedure more precise. Thus, tumescent liposuction is the most evolved form of liposuction.[2,3]

Presently, the available techniques for liposuction are (1) the dry technique (using general anesthesia without preinfiltration of a vasoconstrictive solution), which is rarely used[4–6]; (2) the wet technique (using general anesthesia and preinfiltration with a low volume of vasoconstrictive solution), which is commonly used[7,8]; and (3) the tumescent technique (no general anesthesia and the preinfiltration of a high volume of vasoconstrictive anesthetic solution). It is this latter technique, described herein, which has essentially revolutionized the liposuction process and is the current state of the art for this procedure.[9–13]

CONSULTATION

Liposuction surgery is done to improve the contour of the patient's body and to rearrange deposits of adipose tissue without changing the surface of the skin. It is not a treatment for obesity, striae, spider veins, or cellulite, nor does it tighten the overlying skin. It is important to choose a patient with realistic expectations from the procedure and do an extensive preoperative evaluation and consultation.[14,15]

ANESTHESIA

The hallmark of the tumescent technique is the concentration of lidocaine, which is usually 0.05%, 0.075%, or 0.1%, and the concentration of epinephrine, which is usually 1/1 million. The formulas for these solutions are given in Table 272-1. For smaller areas, a 250-mL bag of saline can be used rather than a 1000-mL bag. The total safe concentration of lidocaine is based on the published figure of 35 mg/kg. Thus, if a patient weighs 150 lb, this is divided by 2.2, giving 68 kg. Multiplying 68 kg by 35 mg/kg would allow the safe use of approximately 2400 mL of a 0.1% solution, which would add up to 2400 mg of a 0.1% solution in this 150-lb subject (2400 mg of lidocaine). If greater amounts of fluid are necessary for the surgery (a large number of treatment areas), then up to 4500 mL of the 0.05% solution can be utilized. Indeed, any mixture of solutions that totals 2400 mg of lidocaine is acceptable

Tumescent Liposuction Solutions

		0.5%	0.1%	SMALLER AREAS
Normal saline	0.9%	1000 mL	1000 mL	250 mL
Lidocaine	2%	25 mL	50 mL	12.5 mL
Epinephrine	1/1000	1 mL	1 mL	0.25 mL
Bicarbonate	8.4%	12.5 mL	12.5 mL	4 mL
Total		500 mg lidocaine = 0.05% 1/1 million epinephrine	1000 mg lidocaine = 0.1% 1/1 million epinephrine	250 mg lidocaine = 0.1% 1/1 million epinephrine

in a patient who weighs 150 lb. The preceding calculations and formulas can easily be extrapolated to determine the "safe" amount and concentration that can be utilized in a given patient. A report stating that 55 mg/kg is safe is expected to be published in the near future. Intravenously, however, the usual maximum dose for lidocaine is 4.5 to 7 mg/kg.

In the tumescent technique, the anesthesia is delivered in a three-step procedure wherein the incision sites—the openings through which the cannulas are inserted—are first injected with a small amount of local anesthetic using a syringe and a 30-gauge needle. The second stage is the delivery of a small amount of anesthetic solution through a spinal needle radially through these incision sites, fanning out to achieve preliminary anesthesia. This preliminary anesthetic can be pushed in with a pressure cuff around a bag of saline or by the use of an infiltration machine on settings 1 to 3. Finally, the initial incision sites are slightly enlarged with an 11 blade and the tumescent anesthetic is delivered through an infiltration cannula with multiple openings. During this final step in the anesthetic process, the infiltration machine is on settings 7 to 9 and the tissue is infiltrated ("tumesced") until firm. After the fatty tissue has been tumesced, it is necessary to wait 30 min or so for the full vasoconstricting effect of the epinephrine solution. The anesthesia is injected at deep as well as intermediate levels to obtain a full effect.

SURGERY

Liposuction surgery is the removal of fatty tissue through tiny excisions in the skin using small, blunt cannulas.[16] It is remarkably safe and should be performed using a sterile technique. The surgery is done using cannulas of various sizes and designs, which are introduced into the incision sites and criss-crossed to produce the result. Suction is utilized at many levels throughout the fatty tissue during the procedure. Suction can be obtained with an aspiration machine or with syringes.[17–19] Sometimes, especially if the area of surgery is very large or very fibrous (male breasts, back, anterior thighs, areas of previous liposuction, etc.), special "ultrasonic" cannulas may be used prior to the regular liposuction cannulas. The ultrasonic devices (ultrasonic liposuction) cavitate the fat, liquefying it and enabling it to be extracted more easily.

AREAS AMENABLE TO LIPOSUCTION

Liposuction surgery is a procedure that can be performed on many areas of the body. The lateral cheeks, jowls, and upper neck are common areas for liposuction that respond beautifully in both men and women.[20,21] The most common body areas in younger women are the lateral thighs with or without the hips and buttocks and in older women the abdomen. In addition to the waist, back, breast fat, inner and anterior thighs, calf and ankle fat can be treated. The most common body areas in men are the flanks and the abdomen. Also, gynecomastia and pseudogynecomastia can be treated in males, as can disorders such as lipomas, lipodystrophy, and axillary hyperhidrosis. Liposuction can also be utilized in association with skin reconstruction. It can be employed to assist in flap elevation and movement and can also serve as means of subcutaneous debulking.

RESULTS AND COMPLICATIONS

While the results from fat removal are almost immediate, subsequent normal elastic retraction of the skin may take up to 6 months to occur. Complications from tumescent liposuction are extremely rare, with the usual postoperative sequelae.[22–25] Occasionally dysesthesia and ecchymosis may occur, with the former lasting a few months and the latter 2 to 3 weeks. With the tumescent technique there have been rare reports of seroma, infection, and hematoma, but no deaths or serious complications have been observed and no transfusions have been required, as reported in two surveys by Hanke et al. on 15,336 patients.[24]

SUMMARY

Tumescent liposuction is a safe and effective technique for removing adipose tissue to effect a change of contour using local anesthesia.

REFERENCES

1. Illouz Y: Body contouring by lipolysis: A 5-year experience with over 3,000 cases. *Plast Reconstr Surg* **72**:591, 1983
2. Klein JA: Anesthesia for liposuction in dermatologic surgery. *J Dermatol Surg Oncol* **14**:1124, 1988
3. Narins RS: Liposuction and anesthesia. *Dermatol Clin* **8**:421, 1990
4. Elam M, Fournier P: *Liposuction: The Franco-American Experience.* Beverly Hills, CA, Medical Aesthetics, 1986
5. Fischer A, Fischer G: Revised techniques for cellulitis fat reduction in riding breeches deformity. *Bull Int Acad Cosmet Surg* **2**:40, 1977
6. Fournier P, Otteni F: Lipodissection in body sculpturing: The dry procedure. *Plast Reconstr Surg* **72**:598, 1983
7. Courtiss EH et al: Large-volume suction lipectomy: An analysis of 108 patients. *Plast Reconstr Surg* **89**:1068, 1992

8. Teimourian B: *Suction Lipectomy and Body Sculpturing.* St. Louis, Mosby, 1987
9. *Am J Cosmet Surg* (special liposuction issue) 1986
10. Field LM: Liposuction surgery: A review. *J Dermatol Surg Oncol* **10**:530, 1984
11. Hanke CW: Liposuction under local anesthesia (editorial). *J Dermatol Surg Oncol* **15**:12, 1989
12. Newman J, Dolsky R: Liposuction surgery: History and development. *J Dermatol Surg Oncol* **10**:467, 1984
13. Stegman S, Tromovitch T: Liposuction, in *Cosmetic Dermatologic Surgery.* Chicago, Year Book, 1983, pp 226–224
14. Cook W Jr: Preoperative consultation and evaluation. Paper given at American Society of Dermatological Surgery (ASDS), 1996.
15. Field L, Narins R: Liposuction surgery, in *Skin Surgery,* 6th ed, edited by E Epstein, E Epstein, Jr. Philadelphia, Saunders, 1987, pp 370–378
16. Cook W Jr: Technical aspects of liposuction. Paper given at American Society of Dermatological Surgery (ASDS), 1996.
17. Field LM: The dermatologic surgeon and liposculpting, in *Liposculpture: The Syringe Technique,* edited by PF Fournier. Paris, Arnette Blackwell, 1991, pp 265–266
18. Fournier P: *Body Sculpturing through Syringe Lipo-Extractions and Autologous Fat Reinjection.* Solana Beach, CA, Samuel Rolf International, 1988
19. Fournier PF: *Liposculpture: The Syringe Technique.* Paris, Arnette Blackwell, 1991, p 163
20. Cook W Jr: Regional liposuction face/neck and arms. Paper given at American Society of Dermatological Surgery (ASDS), 1996.
21. Narins RS: Liposuction of the face and neck, in *Evaluation and Treatment of the Aging Face,* edited by ML Elson. New York, Springer-Verlag, 1995
22. Coleman WP III: The history of dermatologic liposuction. *Dermatol Clin* **8**:381, 1990
23. Dillerud E: Suction lipoplasty: A report on complications, undesired results, and patient satisfaction based on 3511 procedures. *Plast Reconstr Surg* **88**:239, 1991
24. Hanke C et al: Safety of tumescent liposuction in 15,336 patients. *Dermatol Surg* **21**:459, 1995
25. Hetter G: *Lipoplasty, The Theory and Practice of Blunt Suction Lipectomy.* Boston/Toronto, Little, Brown, 1984

CHAPTER 273

Arnold William Klein

Substances for Soft Tissue Augmentation

Many implantable substances and devices have been utilized to improve soft tissue defects and deficiencies. Some, such as adulterated silicones and impure paraffins, invariably produce cosmetic disasters.[1,2] Others, such as pure injectable-grade liquid silicone, while historically extremely useful in the hands of certain experienced physicians, have been declared illegal by the Food and Drug Administration (FDA) and are not available to the practitioner. A substance or device for soft tissue augmentation must have certain intrinsic properties. It must have both a high "use" potential, producing pleasing cosmetic results with a minimum of untoward reactions, and a low "abuse" potential, such that widespread and possibly incorrect or indiscriminate use would not result in significant morbidity.[3] Additionally, it must be nonteratogenic, noncarcinogenic, and nonmigratory. Moreover, the agent must provide predictable persistent correction through reproducible implantation techniques. If not autologous, the substance, agent, or device must be FDA-approved. FDA approval assures purity, accessibility, as well as information regarding use. Currently, in the United States the most commonly utilized injectable filling agents include autologous fat, Fibrel (Mentor H/S, Inc., Santa Barbara, CA), and Zyderm/Zyplast collagen (Collagen Corporation, Palo Alto, CA). Furthermore, this chapter will discuss Botox (Allergan, Irvine, CA).

While not approved for cosmetic indications and not an injectable "filling" agent per se, its judicious use has been shown to address certain age-related rhytides.

INJECTABLE BOVINE COLLAGEN

Injectable bovine collagen, Zyderm collagen implant, has been in use since 1977, receiving FDA approval in 1981. This was the first approved injectable xenogenic agent in the United States for soft tissue augmentation, and its approval reawakened interest in the entire field of filling agents. At present an estimated 1.5 million individuals worldwide have received injectable collagen implants. Following the release of Zyderm I (ZC-I), two additional forms, Zyderm II (ZC-II) and Zyplast (ZP), were approved. Zyderm Collagen Implants (ZC-I, ZC-II, and ZP) are all suspensions of bovine dermal collagen. Processing of the material involves purification, pepsin digestion, and sterilization. Pepsin digestion removes the more antigenic end portions of the bovine collagen molecule (the telopeptides) without disturbing the natural helical structure. Zyderm Collagen Implants are all 95 to 98 percent type I collagen, with the remainder type III.[4] The products are suspended in phosphate-buffered physiologic saline containing 0.3% lidocaine. In ZP, bovine dermal collagen is lightly cross-linked by the addition of 0.0075% glutaraldehyde. As a result of this cross-linkage, ZP is more resistant to proteolytic degradation and less immunogenic.[5,6] It is applicable for deeper contour defects unresponsive to ZC-I or ZC-II.

Treatment with injectable collagen requires an initial screening skin test. A positive test consists of redness, swelling, or both which occurs 6 h or more after test implantation. This is an absolute contraindication to treatment and occurs in 3 to 3.5 percent of individuals.[7–9] Despite one negative skin test, 1.3 to 2 percent of patients will have treatment-associated hypersensitivity responses.[7–10] While the majority of these treatment-associated hypersensitivity reactions resolve within 11 months, occasionally they can persist for a longer period, lasting more than 24 months in isolated situations. To reduce the possibility of these reactions, which usually occur shortly after the first treatment, it is advisable to turn the first treatment exposure into a second test.[3,11–13]

Correction of defects with bovine collagen is highly technique-dependent and requires two to three treatment sessions at 2- to 4-week intervals.[14,15] This correction is temporary and requires periodic maintenance at 4- to 12-month intervals.[16] In the human, while histologic studies of ZP as opposed to ZC-I/ZC-II have revealed some deposition of host collagen, there is no convincing evidence that this deposition contributes to longevity of correction.[17,18] Indeed, correction with all forms of bovine collagen appears to be lost as the material is displaced in the human from its site of implantation in the dermis into the subcutaneous space.[19]

Indications for ZC-I/ZC-II include horizontal forehead lines, glabellar lines, crow's-feet, nasolabial lines, fine lip lines, marionette lines, acne scars, excisional scars, and the like. Deep nasolabial folds, marionette grooves, deep acne scars, and the like respond best to ZP with or without ZC-I/ZC-II overlay. ZP is also best suited to resurface the vermilion border between the lip and skin for lip enhancement.

Adverse treatment responses to injectable collagen can be divided into nonhypersensitive and hypersensitive reactions. Nonhypersensitive reactions include bruising, reactivation of herpetic eruptions, and bacterial infection. Additionally, local necrosis due to vascular interruption at the treatment site has been noted with ZP and rarely ZC-I/ZC-II.[20] Since 56 percent of these locally necrotic events occur in the glabellar area, physicians are cautioned against using ZP at this site. Two reports of partial vision loss after ZC therapy have been noted.[21] These are probably the result of an occlusive event involving the retinal artery. These serious consequences of a cosmetic procedure underscore the need to remember that the dermal site is the proper locale for collagen implantation. Treatment-associated hypersensitivity reactions to bovine collagen implants are, for the most part, cosmetic and consist of redness and swelling at the treatment site. Rarely, mild systemic symptoms can accompany these reactions. Hypersensitive reactions are almost uniformly associated with anti-Zyderm antibodies. These antibodies do not cross-react with human collagen.[10,22] "Cyst-abscess" formation is a rare but severe hypersensitivity response occurring at a rate of 4 in 10,000 treated individuals.[20] Clinically, individuals develop painful, swollen cysts at the sites of treatment. These reactions are usually associated with ZP and rarely ZC-I/ZC-II. Furthermore, 86 percent of these individuals have associated anti-Zyderm antibodies. Incision and drainage, as well as intralesional steroids, have been advocated to manage this most undesirable sequela. This severe hypersensitive response can persist for more than 2 years. As to the possibility of bovine collagen inducing connective tissue disease in the human host, retrospective studies as well as an expert panel convened by the FDA have found no supporting evidence.[22]

FIBREL

Bailey and Ingraham first used "fibrin foam" as a surgical hemostatic agent in 1944. In 1957 Spangler reported the efficacy of fibrin foam in treating depressed scars in 23 patients. Subsequently, he reported good to excellent results in treating 7000 patients with this substance.[23] The composition and fabrication of Fibrel, the modern descendant of fibrin foam, was delineated by Gottlieb.[24] It is composed of porcine gelatin powder and epsilon-amino caproic acid that is reconstituted with the patient's plasma and 0.9% sodium chloride. Fibrel works by creating a clot that becomes colonized by host collagen. The gelatin provides the framework on which a clot forms, and aminocaproic acid is added to prevent lysis of this clot. In this situation the patient's plasma serves as a supplemental source of clotting factors.[25,26]

Recently, some investigators have advocated deleting the patient's plasma and replacing it in the fabrication process with lidocaine or a greater quantity of 0.9% sodium chloride to make the product's implantation less painful and associated with less inflammation. This alteration in fabrication appears not to affect the longevity of correction.[25]

Prior to Fibrel implantation, the subject must undergo skin testing. A skin test is performed by intradermally placing 0.05 mL of reconstituted gelatin matrix implant diluted with 0.9% sodium chloride. The patient's plasma is not added to the suspension during testing. A positive test is defined as swelling, tenderness, redness or inflammation that lasts for more than 5 h or appears more than 24 h after implantation.[27] Treatments are begun 4 weeks after skin testing.

Indications for Fibrel include acne scars, surgical scars, and age-related rhytides such as the glabellar furrows, horizontal forehead lines, nasolabial and meilolabial folds/lines and the oral commissures (marionette lines). Fine lines, such as the small lines on the lips and crow's-feet, usually are not amenable to correction with Fibrel and have an increased propensity for morbidity with implantation.

Injection techniques for Fibrel are less standardized than those of bovine collagen.[27,28] It can be molded upon injection, and postimplantation ice packs are an excellent treatment adjunct. Since Fibrel produces a clot with a subsequent healing response, a certain degree of swelling and inflammation will occur with its use. Bruising, swelling, redness, pain, or induration are usual expected local effects and not adverse reactions. These inflammatory reactions are usually of 3 to 4 days duration though prolonged inflammation for 4 to 6 weeks has been noted. Additionally, the use of Fibrel can be uncomfortable, and local anesthesia prior to its application is frequently utilized.[29]

It appears that one to two treatments are necessary in most applications of Fibrel for complete correction. These data are based on treatment of scars, and prospective studies on the treatment of rhytides are not available. In a study of 840 acne scars treated with Fibrel, physicians found a 65 percent or greater improvement in almost 50 percent of the scars at 52 weeks.[28] Subsequent studies have supported these results as well as shown good long term persistence of correction (2 to 5 years) in treated individuals.[29,30]

As to adverse reactions, several instances of embolic necrosis have been seen with Fibrel (as with Zyplast), and these appear to be technique-dependent.[3] While some individuals have shown Fibrel to be safe and effective in Zyderm-allergic patients, Zyderm-allergic patients should be approached with caution.[31]

FAT TRANSPLANTATION

Injectable fat (autologous fat transplantation) is the oldest material utilized for tissue augmentation. Indeed, Neuber reported almost 100 years ago the technique of free fat grafts for tissue augmentation. Although Brunings, in 1919, reported on fat injection as a technique for soft tissue augmentation, it was ignored in favor of pedicle flaps and the use of paraffin and silicone as filling agents at that time.[32] In the late 1950s, Peers utilized free fat grafts, though their loss of volume upon transplantation made many question their efficacy.[33]

In the 1980s a dramatic change occurred. With the advent of liposuction, Drs. Georgio, Fisher, Illouz, and Fournier all felt that it was possible to return the viable fat to the body. Nevertheless, the best mode of fat removal and the best mode of fat implantation are still not known.[34,35] Furthermore, the longevity of correction achieved with fat implantation is not clear. Pinski and Roenigk noted that only about 25 to 30 percent of original transplanted fat remained at 1 year in the forehead, nasolabial folds, and cheeks.[34] In regard to longevity of correction in relationship to the etiology of lesions treated, these investigators found that linear scleroderma provided the most persistence, with 55 percent correction at 1 year, while wrinkles and acne scars provided only about 30 percent and discoid lupus lesions only 10 percent at 1 year. In another excellent study, Gormley and Eremia found microlipoinjection of fat unpredictable, yet a good result at 6 months usually was maintained at 1 year.[37] The exact mechanism by which transplanted fat augments defects is not fully understood. Does it survive as a viable fat transplant or does it correct by producing fibrosis?[37,38]

There is a great deal of individual physician variation in techniques employed for fat transplantation.[31,35,38,39,40] The thighs, buttocks, knees, and abdomen are the donor sites most often utilized. Individual preference and donor fat availability appear to be directing forces in choosing the proper donor site. After adequate anesthesia, the fat is removed as atraumatically as possible either by syringe extraction or a machine-assisted method. Once the fat is extracted, its treatment appears to vary greatly; in general, however, individuals appear to use either gentle centrifugation or gravity to separate the extracted fat from the fluids present. For implantation, a scalpel is employed to prick the skin and a syringe containing the fat is then inserted at this recipient site and the material injected at the level of the subcutaneous space. Molding after implantation is frequently utilized. Sites most amenable for correction with microlipoinjection, by consensus, appear to be the dorsal hand, depressed temples, hollow cheeks, deep nasolabial grooves, and defects due to liposuction or lipodystrophy. Fat implantation has also been advocated for malar and chin augmentation.[31,38,39,40] Evolving techniques in microlipoinjection include flash freezing fat for subsequent injection at 1- to 12-month intervals, injection of fat with small gauge needles, lysis of the fat with intradermal implantation, and separation of "autologous collagen" from fat prior to injection.[41]

With the recent resurgence of fat transplantation, it is expected that complications will be reported. While swelling and bruising are fairly common and usually minor at the recipient site, persistent edema, asymmetry, punctate scarring, lumping and bleeding can occur occasionally. Infection is a rare occurrence. There has also been a single case of unilateral blindness reported following autologous fat transplantation. This is obviously the most serious adverse consequence reported to date.[39]

BOTOX

Botox is a sterile, vacuum-dried purified form of botulinum toxin type A indicated for the treatment of strabismus, blepharospasm, and related conditions.[42] It is a highly potent neurotoxin that acts by inhibition of acetylcholine release at the motor endplates. Its judicious use to predictably temporarily denervate specific muscles responsible for certain facial rhytides including the glabellar furrow, horizontal forehead lines, horizontal neck lines, and crow's-feet has become a superb adjunct for the treatment of the aging face. Nevertheless, one must remember this is an off-label use of this substance.[43–45]

Botox is injected into the involved muscles to create the desired effect. Electromyographic guidance can be employed to assure accuracy of placement.[46] In addressing the frown the target muscles are the corrugator supercilii as well as the procerus, depressor supercilii and portions of the upper medial orbicularis oculi. For horizontal forehead lines the upper frontalis is the target muscle and for crow's feet the lateral orbicularis oculi. With horizontal neck lines and platysmal bands the involved muscle is the platysma. In addition to these sites Botox has many other potential cosmetic applications.[47] For example, in individuals with flaring ala nasi the dilator nari muscles can be treated. Effective therapy with Botox should result in significant cosmetic improvement for a period of 3 to 6 months. Furthermore, retreating the same area may result in a prolongation of this response. Botox treatments have not been associated with any permanent clinical effects though histologically there are reversible and rarely irreversible histologic changes in muscles that have been injected.

In addition to the above agents, there are numerous products and techniques whose position and value in the field of soft tissue augmentation has not been fully defined.

REFERENCES

1. Urbach F et al: Generalized paraffinoma (sclerosing lipogranuloma). *Arch Dermatol* **103**:277, 1971
2. Klein JA et al: Paraffinomas of the scalp. *Arch Dermatol* **121**:382, 1985
3. Klein AW, Rish DC: Injectable collagen: An adjunct to facial plastic surgery. *Facial Plast Surg* **4**:87, 1987
4. Wallace DG et al: Injectable collagen for tissue augmentation, in *Collagen:* vol III. *Biotechnology,* edited by ME Nimmi. Boca Raton, FL, CRC Press, 1988, pp 117–144
5. McPherson JM et al: The preparation and physiochemical characterization of an injectable reconstituted glutaraldehyde crosslinked, bovine corium collagen. *J Biometer Res* **20**:79, 1986
6. Elson ML: Clinical assessment of Zyplast implant: A year of experience for soft tissue contour correction. *J Am Acad Dermatol* **116**:707, 1988
7. Castrow FF II, Krull EA: Injectable collagen implant—update. *J Am Acad Dermatol* **9**:889, 1983
8. Cooperman LS et al: Injectable collagen: A six-year clinical investigation. *Asthet Plast Surg* **9**:145, 1985
9. Kamer FM, Churukian M: The clinical use of injectable collagen: A three-year retrospective study. *Arch Otolaryngol* **110**:93, 1984

10. Siegle RJ et al: Intradermal implantation of bovine collagen: Humoral responses associated with clinical reaction. *Arch Dermatol* **120**:183, 1984

11. Klein AW: In favor of double testing. *J Dermatol Surg Oncol* **15**:263, 1989

12. Elson ML: The role of skin testing in the use of collagen injectable materials. *J Dermatol Surg Oncol* **15**:301, 1989

13. Klein AW, Rish DC: Injectable collagen update. *J Dermatol Surg Oncol* **10**:519, 1984

14. Klein AW: Implantation techniques for injectable collagen: Two-and-one-half years of personal clinical experience. *J Am Acad Dermatol* **9**:224, 1983

15. Bailin PL, Bailin MD: Collagen implantation: Clinical applications and lesion selection. *J Dermatol Surg Oncol* **14**(suppl 1):49, 1988

16. Klein AW: Indications and implantation techniques for the various formulations of injectable collagen. *J Dermatol Surg Oncol* **14**(suppl):27, 1988

17. Kligman AM, Armstrong RC: Histologic response to intradermal Zyderm and Zyplast (glutaraldehyde cross-linked) collagen in humans. *J Dermatol Surg Oncol* **12**:351, 1986

18. Kligman AM: Histologic responses to collagen implants in human volunteers; Comparison of Zyderm Collagen with Zyplast implant. *J Dermatol Surg Oncol* **14**(suppl):35, 1988

19. Stegman SJ et al: A light and electron microscopic evaluation of Zyderm Collagen and Zyplast Implants in aging human facial skin: A pilot study. *Arch Dermatol* **123**:1644, 1987

20. Hanke CW et al: Abscess formation and local necrosis after treatment with Zyderm or Zyplast collagen implant. *J Am Acad Dermatol* **25**:319, 1991

21. DeLustro F et al: Reaction to injectable collagen: Results in animal models and clinical use. *Plast Reconstruct Surg* **79**:581, 1987

22. Klein AW: "Bonfire of the wrinkles." *J Dermatol Surg Oncol* **17**:543, 1991

23. Spangler AS: Treatment of depressed scars with fibrin foam—Seventeen years of experience. *J Dermatol Surg Oncol* **1**:65, 1975

24. Gottlieb S: "GAP Repair Technique." Poster exhibit. Annual meeting of the American Academy of Dermatology, Dallas, December 1977

25. Gold MH: The Fibrel mechanism of action study: A preliminary report. *J Dermatol Surg Oncol* **20**:586, 1994

26. Millikan L: Fibrel and wound healing. *Clin Dermatol* **9**:569, 1991

27. Millikan L et al: Treatment of depressed cutaneous scars with gelatin matrix implant: A multicenter study. *J Am Acad Dermatol* **16**:1155, 1987

28. Cohen IS: Fibrel. *Semin Dermatol* **6**:228, 1987

29. Millikan L: Long-term safety and efficacy with Fibrel in the treatment of cutaneous scars. *J Dermatol Surg Oncol* **15**:837, 1989

30. Millikan L et al: A 5-year safety and efficacy evaluation with Fibrel in the correction of cutaneous scars following one or two treatments. *J Dermatol Surg Oncol* **17**:223, 1991

31. Stegman SJ et al: *Cosmetic Dermatologic Surgery,* Chicago, Year Book, 1990

32. Bruning P: Cited by Broeckaert JJ: *Bull Acad R Med Belaiaue* **28**:440, 1919

33. Peer LA: *Transplantation of Tissues, Transplantation of Fat.* Baltimore, Williams & Wilkins, 1959

34. Pinski KS, Roenigk HH: Autologous fat transplantation. *J Dermatol Surg Oncol* **18**:179, 1992

35. Asken S: Autologous fat transplantation, in *Dermatologic Surgery, Principles and Practices,* edited by RK Roenigk, HH Roenigk. New York, Marcel Dekker, 1988

36. Gormley DE, Eeremia S: Quantitative assessment augmentation therapy. *J Dermatol Surg Oncol* **16**:12, 1990

37. Sergott TJ et al: Human adjuvant disease, possible autoimmune disease after silicone implantation: A review of the literature, case studies, and speculation for the future. *Plast Reconstr Surg* **78**:104, 1988

38. Pinski KS, Roenigk HH: Microlipoinjection, in *Surgical Dermatology: Advances in Current Practice,* edited by RK Roenigk, HH Roenigk. London, Martin Dunitz, 1993, pp 451–460

39. Guidelines of care for soft tissue augmentation: Fat transplantation. *J Am Acad Dermatol* **34**:690, 1996

40. Monheit GD: Soft Tissue Augmentation, in *Cutaneous Surgery,* edited by RG Wheeland. Philadelphia, Saunders, 1994, pp 446–462

41. Coleman WP et al: Autologous collagen? Lipocytic dermal augmentation: A histopathologic study. *J Dermatol Surg Oncol* **19**:1032, 1993

42. Jankovic J, Hallet M (eds): *Therapy with Botulinum Toxin.* New York, Marcel Dekker, 1994

43. Blitzer A et al: Botulinum toxin for the treatment of hyperfunctional lines of the face. *Arch Otolaryngol Head Neck Surg* **1018**:22, 1993

44. Carruthers JDA, Carruthers JA: Treatment of glabellar frown lines with C. botulinum-A exotoxin. *J Dermatol Surg Oncol* **18**:17, 1992

45. Carruthers A: Botulinum A exotoxin use in clinical dermatology. *J Am Acad Dermatol* **34**:788, 1996

46. Klein AW: Cosmetic therapy with botulinum toxin: Anecdotal memoirs. *Dermatol Surg* **22**:757, 1996

47. Carruthers A, Carruthers J: Cosmetic uses of botulinum A exotoxin. *Adv Dermatol* **12**:325, 1997

CHAPTER 274

Walter Unger

Hair Transplantation and Alopecia Reduction

The first written account of autografting of hair occurred in a doctoral thesis by Dieffenbach in 1822 at Königsberg, Germany[1]; however, the concept did not really capture the medical profession's imagination or the general public's enthusiasm until 1959, when Norman Orentreich published an article including an account of successful hair transplantation in male-pattern baldness (MPB).[2] In addition, in the late 1970s, the concept of alopecia reduction (AR) or serial excision of areas of alopecia was introduced by the Blanchards and Ungers.[3,4] This chapter summarizes the present state of graft hair transplantation and AR. Controversial aspects and alternative approaches cannot be dealt with here but are available in detailed form elsewhere.[5]

HAIR TRANSPLANTATION

Patient Selection and Planning

Hair transplantation is based on the concept of "donor dominance" in MPB.[2] If a graft is taken from an area destined to be permanently hair-bearing and transplanted into an area of MPB or future MPB, it will, after an initial short effluvium, continue to grow in its new site for as long as it would have in its original one. Thus, all planning is predicated on an accurate assessment of the eventual extent of MPB and conversely the permanent donor rim. A careful family history, physical examination, and consideration of the patient's age are all important.

One can try to treat all of the anterior half of the present as well as future area of MPB[6] or, alternately, create only an "isolated frontal forelock" (IFF), which will look natural standing on its own (Fig. 274-1).[7] This latter objective avoids any need for an accurate prognosis of the eventual boundaries of the area of MPB and is most suitable for those who are likely to develop type VI or VII MPB (see Chap. 71). However, less than 24 percent of men who reach the age of 80 years will develop type VI or VII MPB.[8,9] In addition, a donor area only 44 to 50.75 mm high, extending approximately from ear to ear, is sufficient to produce 500 or more minigrafts in each of six sessions (see below). Even men with type VI and VII MPB can usually be expected to maintain substantially wider donor areas. In this light, limiting most patients to an IFF seems excessively conservative. A more reasonable course is to attempt to transplant all present and future areas of at least the anterior half of MPB but to complete the borders of the entire area with small grafts (Fig. 274-2). If hair loss does eventually exceed the estimated extent of MPB, one can treat the new areas or leave them as empty "alleys"

adjacent to a relatively large IFF. With today's techniques, few patients are totally unacceptable candidates.

It is not necessary to wait until an area is totally alopecic before transplanting is begun. Existing hair allows for better postoperative camouflage and longer—often more convenient—intervals between sessions that are timed to keep pace with the rate of hair loss. Transplanting probably does not accelerate future hair loss, but the more hair is present, the more skill the physician needs; incisions must be made in the same direction and at the same angle as the original hair, or MPB will be accelerated.[6] Similarly, no absolute rules apply to the correct age at which to begin—experience and skill extend the limits, although it is very uncommon to begin before age 21 or after age 80.[6]

In women, transplanting should be limited to those who appear likely to maintain a sufficiently large area of reasonably dense hair. Some women develop diffuse thinning that affects all areas of the scalp hair; therefore they are not candidates for hair transplanting. Others maintain relatively dense rim hair in parietal and/or occipital areas and are excellent candidates.[10]

The less contrast between the color of the hair and skin, the better. Light colored hair is advantageous if the patient is Caucasian. Darker colors are ideal in darker skinned individuals such as African Americans. Other advantageous hair characteristics are good density, frizziness, curl or wave, and fine texture. In particular, the latter allows transplanted hair to blend in less perceptibly in areas of moderate or advanced thinning without contrasting too much against hair that gradually becomes finer as MPB progresses.

AR can be used to decrease not only the width of an area of MPB but also its length; both of these reductions will result in substantial graft "savings."[6] Potentially negative sequelae of AR, such as significantly decreased hair density in future donor areas, disorientation of hair direction, permanently noticeable and/or poor scars, and partial loss of initial gains or "stretchback" are minimal or can be totally avoided by appropriate planning and technique.[11–15] AR can usually be done prior to any transplanting or between sessions.

GRAFT TYPES Grafts are obtained by sectioning strips of donor tissue. They are classified as follows:

1. *Micrografts* are 1- to 2-hair grafts that are placed into holes prepared with a 16- to 19-gauge needle or Nokor needle.
2. *Beaver grafts* are 2- to 3-hair grafts that are placed into incisions made with a "Beaver ES mini-blade" (Ellis Instruments, Inc., 21 Cook Ave., Madison, NJ 07940).
3. *Minigrafts* contain 2 to 6 hairs; if they are placed into slits made with a scalpel blade or laser, they are referred to as *slit grafts* or *laser slit grafts* respectively, and if they are placed into holes made with a round trephine or laser, they are referred to as *round* or *laser minigrafts.*
4. *Small minigrafts,* whether they are round minigrafts or slit grafts, contain 3 to 4 hairs.
5. *Large minigrafts,* whether they are round minigrafts or slit grafts, contain 5 to 6 hairs.
6. Standard grafts are 3.5 to 4.5 mm or larger in diameter; they are round or square grafts containing 8 to 30 hairs and are placed into holes made with slightly smaller round trephines or square punches.

Three variables are considered in choosing the type of graft to be employed: hair characteristics, density objectives, and the amount of persisting recipient area hair: (1) The finer and lighter-

FIGURE 274-1

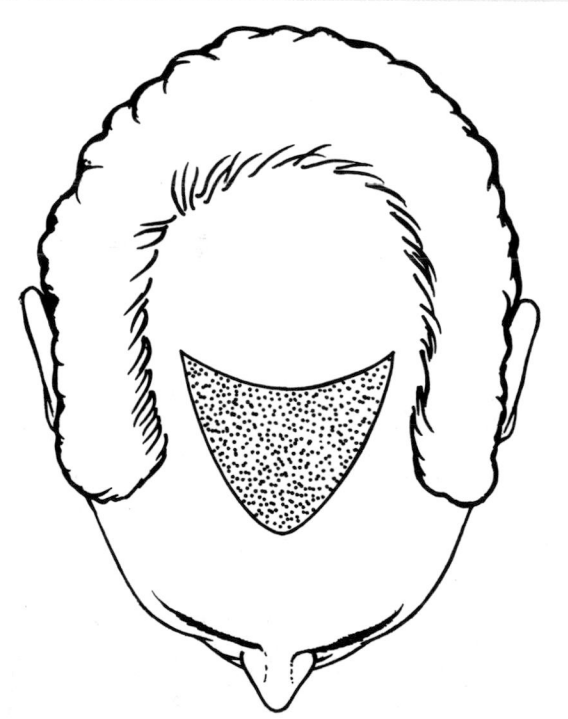

Pattern of an "isolated frontal forelock." Grafts are progressively larger as one moves toward its center.

FIGURE 274-2

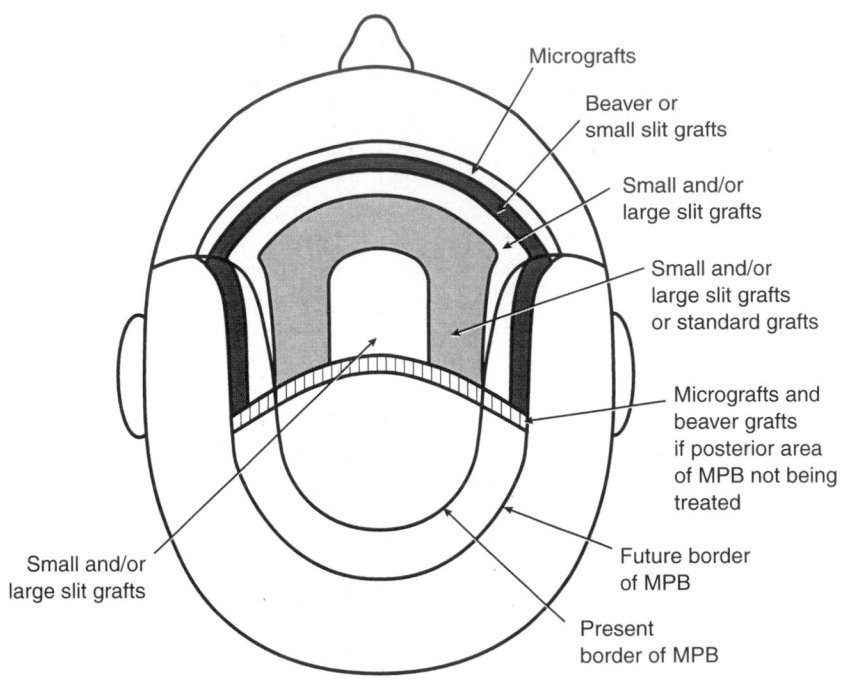

Micrografts

Beaver or
small slit grafts

Small and/or
large slit grafts

Small and/or
large slit grafts
or standard grafts

Micrografts and
beaver grafts
if posterior area
of MPB not being
treated

Future border
of MPB

Present
border of MPB

Small and/or
large slit grafts

Round minigrafts may be added to areas
treated with slit grafts in any sessions *after* the first,
in order to increase density

Schematic drawing of the distribution of various types of grafts utilized in frontal hair transplantation. The periphery of this area is composed of small grafts. If MPB progresses beyond the anticipated extent of MPB, one can either treat the new areas or leave them as empty "alleys" adjacent to a relatively large "isolated frontal forelock."

colored the hair, the less plugginess will be noticed with larger grafts. (2) Micrografts, Beaver grafts, and minigrafts are ideal for producing light to moderate density (Fig. 274-3). (3) However, initially, micrografts and slit grafts of whatever type will produce a greater increase in hair density than will round or laser slit graft sites in a recipient area with persisting hair. This is because in preparing round or laser slit graft sites, any existing hair at those sites is removed, so that the net gain in hair will be equal only to the difference between how many hairs have been removed and how many have been added. With micrografts and slit grafts, the net gain will be equal to the number of hairs being transplanted, as no hair is removed when slits and micrograft holes are correctly made between them. In the long term, however, the more round grafts or laser slit grafts that are used, the greater the density that will be achieved, because bald or potentially bald skin is also being removed.

To add to the complexity, the more hair that remains in the recipient area, the less noticeable will be any temporary tendency to a pluggy appearance (Fig. 274-4). Thus patients for whom maximum ultimate density is of paramount concern might reasonably decide to choose more laser slit grafts or round grafts—even standard-sized round grafts—despite the fact that they would temporarily have had a greater increase in hair density if they had chosen all micrografts and slit grafts instead. Notwithstanding this, hairline

zones—the anterior 2 cm or more—are always constructed with micrografts and minigrafts.

It is popular to assume that the use of standard-sized grafts posterior to the hairline zone will always produce noticeable plugginess. This is not so if patients are properly selected and a combination of grafts of proper types and sizes are utilized (Fig. 274-4). It is also important to note that the use of mixed graft types (micrografts, minigrafts, and standard round grafts) in the anterior half of any new area of MPB results in the transfer of more hairs per session than sessions made up entirely of micrografts and minigrafts (Table 274-1). In addition, any time I use standard grafts, I plan on ultimately completely filling that area with transplanted hair, so that when all of the original hair has finally been lost and the hair is wet or windblown, no plugginess will be seen.

Sessions entirely devoted to micrografts should only be used if the donor hair is fine and density objectives are quite low. Micrografts are the least efficient in producing substantial hair density. On the other hand, micrografts also produce the least temporary "plugginess." From the preceding discussion it should be clear that each graft type has advantages as well as disadvantages and that using only one or two types of grafts for all patients and circumstances is not wise or true state-of-the-art.

"Megasessions," involving thousands of micrografts in a single session, and "dense packing," have been suggested as means of producing more density in less time.[16,17] Unfortunately sessions of 8 h or longer are necessary and may be medically unwise for some individuals. There is also considerable concern as to whether hair survival is as good as it is with sessions of the usual length.[18–21] Statements that a single session of 3000 or more micrografts can produce significant density in the entire alopecic area of type V or greater MPB should be viewed skeptically. In the author's experience, between 5500 and 6500 hairs are necessary to produce good density in either the anterior or posterior half of most areas of MPB. Achieving this density in a single session of micrografts only may be an attractive idea for advertising purposes but is technically impossible.

TECHNIQUE

Anesthesia

Diazepam (Valium) 20 mg is given orally 30 min before surgery to minimize anxiety and the possibility of anesthetic toxicity. Oral meperidine hydrochloride (Demerol) 50 mg can be added to the diazepam for patients with low pain thresholds. For patients with extreme anxiety, premixed and self-administered nitrous oxide and oxygen 50%/50% or intravenous propofol—the latter administered by a fully qualified anesthetist—can also be employed as the local anesthetic is being injected. Field blocks are utilized in both donor and recipient areas and are produced, respectively, with buffered 1% and 2% lidocaine with 1/100,000 epinephrine in order to minimize pain. A "tumescent" anesthetic technique[22] is used superior to the donor area field block and a 1/50,000 solution of epinephrine

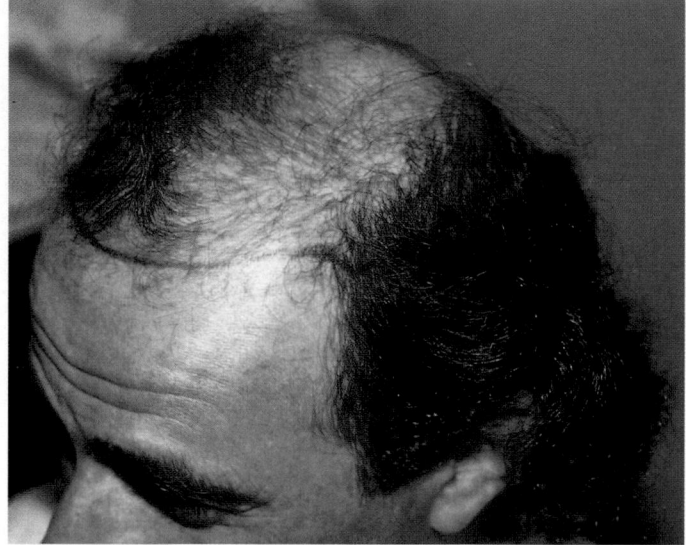

A.

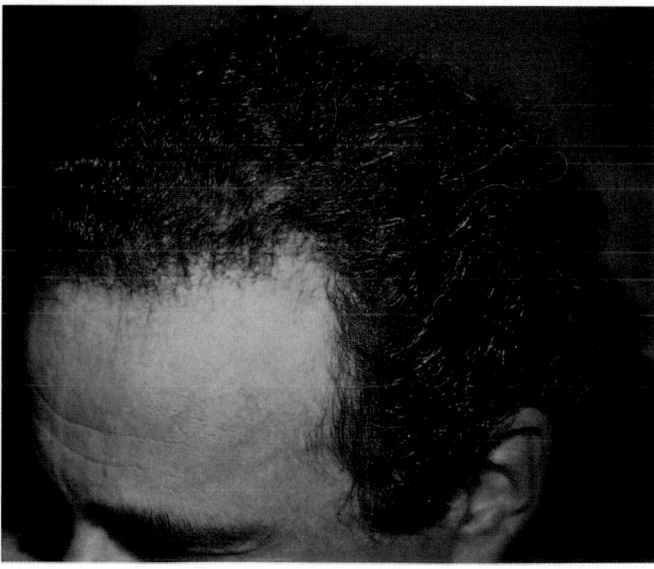

B.

A. Before transplanting. *B.* Nine months after the third session of micrografts, Beaver slit grafts, and small slit grafts. Note light to moderate coverage rather than dense hair. This is characteristic of results seen with these types of grafts unless hair characteristics are better than average (e.g., high density, light coloring, fine or curly texture).

is used superior to the recipient area block. Each area is prepared separately with at least a 30-min interval between them in order to minimize epinephrine/lidocaine toxicity.

The Donor Area

Improved donor area harvesting technique has revolutionized what can be accomplished with hair transplanting.[23] Conceptually one excises a donor area of appropriate size and sections it into the desired number and types of grafts. The author employs two donor zones in most patients—one inferiorly in the occipital area and the other more superiorly, extending from the midline into the parietal

area and as far as 28 mm anterior to a line drawn perpendicularly from the tragus. The former is taken from an area with the finest-caliber hair that is judged to be permanent and is ideal for use in the hairline zone. The superior donor zone contains hair that is coarser and can be used to produce greater density posterior to the hairline zone. Using figures obtained in a study of 328 men 65 years of age or older, a donor area that is "safe" for 80 percent of the patients under the age of 80 was established and is shown in Fig. 274-5.[9]

The hair in the donor zones is clipped to approximately 2 mm in length and a povidone-iodine (Betadine) solution is applied. Four no. 11 Personna Plus blades are employed in a multibladed scalpel handle (Universal handle, straight, Robbins Instruments, 2 North Passaic Ave., Box 441, Chatham, NJ 07928). A no. 15 scalpel blade is then used to produce a triangular tapering of both ends. Incisions are made into the midsubcutaneous tissue and the blades are always held parallel to the angle of exiting hair. After removing the strips of tissue, any vessels that are bleeding excessively are cauterized and the wound is closed with a running continuous 2-0 Supramid suture; this is removed in 7 to 10 days. Appropriate spacing of blades and donor sites is an important consideration. Any scar tissue left from previous sessions is excised at the same time as the new harvesting, so that only one or two scars will ultimately be left no matter how many operations are carried out.

The Recipient Area

Beaver grafts or small slit grafts are used in a 2.0- to 2.5-cm wide "hairline zone" during the first session and 200 or more micrografts are scattered anterior to this zone as well as within it. After 4 or more months have elapsed, slit grafts and micrografts are placed between those transplanted during the first session. If hair characteristics are good and greater density is preferred in the hairline zone, some large slit grafts and/or small round minigrafts may be used during the second session. Four or more months later a third session is held; in most cases it will complete the hairline and other peripheral zones. (In some patients—for example, those with coarser and/or darker hair—a fourth session of primarily micrografts may be utilized to further refine the hairline.) Although one is ultimately looking for a random and therefore natural-looking distribution of hair in the hairline zone, the author has found that a careful "organized disorganization" will produce a better short-term as well as long-term appearance.[24–27]

A similar distribution and types of grafts are used in many patients for the entire recipient area. However, in 10 to 25 percent of male patients, if the objective is greater hair density, an organized pattern of standard-sized grafts may be employed posterior to the hairline zone and medial to the peripheral grafts described earlier (Fig. 274-2). As a rule, I currently use rectangular grafts 3.5 × 3.0 mm placed into round recipient sites made with a 3.25-mm punch and grafts 3.75 × 3.25 mm placed into round recipient sites made with a 3.5-mm punch. Any given area of alopecia can be solidly filled with either three or four sessions of standard-sized grafts, though I am most comfortable with the latter. The intervals between sessions of standard grafts should be the same as those employed for slit grafts. In the author's view, reports of the demise of the standard graft are premature. Such grafts are appropriate for most patients who want more than light to moderate hair density (Fig. 274-4).

The need for consistent direction and angling of recipient sites (mimicking the original direction and angle) cannot be overempha-

FIGURE 274-4

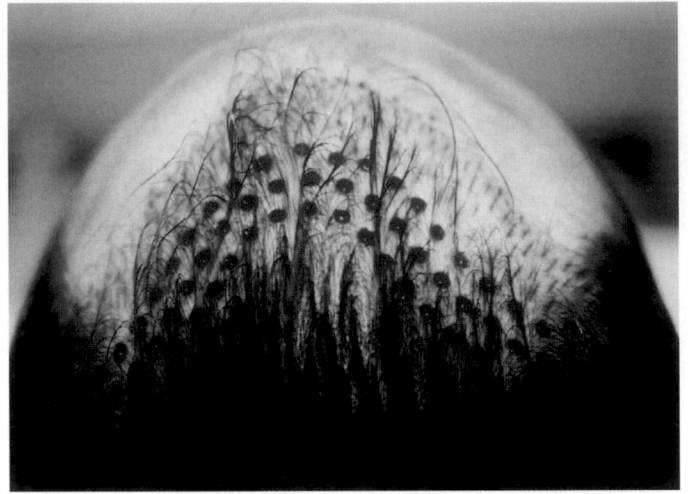

A.

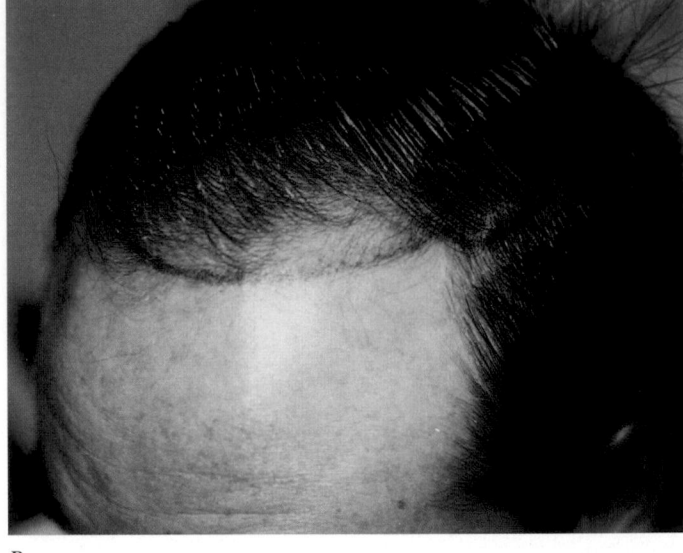

B.

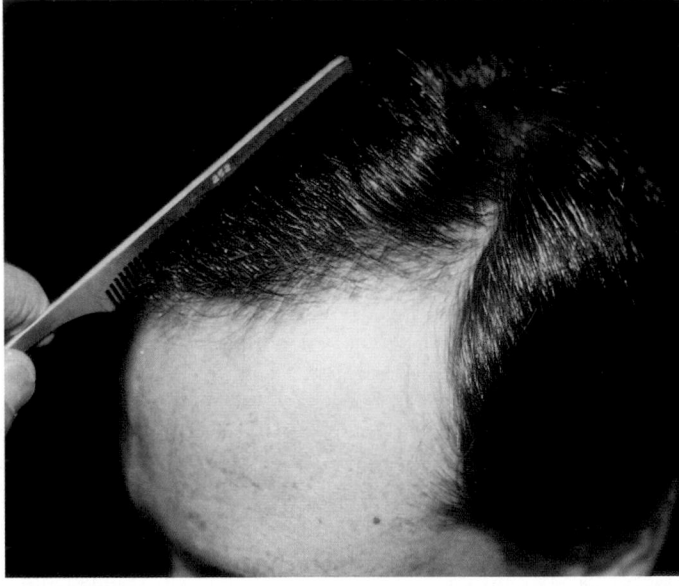

C.

A. Pattern of first transplanting session consisting of 48 micrografts, 108 large slit grafts, and 68 standard round grafts. B. The patient shown in (A) before transplantation. C. Seven months after the first transplanting session, with the hair combed back for critical evaluation. A combination of fine hair and enough original hair in that part of the recipient area treated with standard round grafts avoided any noticeable plugginess despite the use of standard grafts.

sized. Slight changes in the angle at which one prepares a recipient site, especially for standard grafts, can result in injury to or excision of adjacent original or previously transplanted hair matrices and the creation of new small areas of alopecia.

For African-American patients, a combination of micrografts and slit grafts for the hairline zone and round grafts of various sizes posterior to the hairline zone should be used. For all other races (as described earlier), the use of this combination of graft types is optional.

Laser Transplanting

An Ultrapulse or Silktouch CO_2 laser can be used to make recipient sites for slit grafts (preferably an Ultrapulse laser) or for round grafts (preferably a Silktouch laser). These lasers produce less bleeding and probably less edema and postoperative pain. The use of a laser to produce round holes will not result in superior cosmetic results but will eliminate the need to remove tissue from the hole.

The chance that some of it may be left behind to cause epidermal cysts is thus eliminated, and the time consumed in removing recipient-site plugs is also saved. When slits are made with a laser, tissue is ablated. Thus the density and absence of compression of round grafting are combined with the cosmetically superior linear shape of a slit graft. Extremely natural-looking results are possible with only one session.[28–30] On the other hand, there is usually some additional crusting over the grafts and a delay of 2 to 6 weeks before hair growth begins. When a laser is not employed, there is less crusting and delay. Optimum laser settings have not yet been established, but it is likely that lasers will play an increasingly important role in hair transplanting.

Graft Preparation and Insertion

After donor strips have been excised, they are carefully separated from each other and oriented on a moistened tongue depressor, so that a clear view of hair follicles is possible. Then, utilizing a small forceps and Personna super stainless shaper blades, the strips are carefully sectioned into pieces containing the desired number of hairs and placed in a petri dish filled with saline.[31] The use of binocular stereoscopic dissecting micrografts to effect a more precise preparation of grafts is growing in popularity.[32,33] It is likely, however, that a true need for these instruments will vary with the visual acuity and skill of the staff preparing grafts. Prepared grafts are gently eased into the recipient sites using small serrated forceps or jewelers' forceps. Two or three droplets of an ethyl cyanoacrylate glue (Loctite 15494) are applied to the edge of any standard grafts that does not sit flush with the surrounding skin.[34]

Bandaging

Most physicians use a small turban-like postoperative overnight dressing.[35] However, if there is no more than the usual amount of bleeding, many patients can leave without a bandage. All patients should ideally return the next day to confirm that the grafts are still positioned properly as well as to carefully clean away any blood clots that may have developed overnight, using hydrogen peroxide–soaked gauze and Q-tips. Properly trained assistants then carefully wash, style, and dry the hair.

Postoperative Course

Patients are supplied with three analgesics to be used as required: acetaminophen tablets with 30 mg of codeine (Tylenol-3), oxycodone (Percocet), and meperidine hydrochloride (Demerol) 50 mg. Most patients use only the acetaminophen and codeine tablets and only for the first night. If more than the usual amount of pain is expected, intramuscular ketorolac tromethamine (Toradol) 30 to 60 mg generally eliminates all postoperative pain for 6 to 8 h. Most physicians inject a glucocorticoid such as 80 mg of methyl prednisolone acetate (DepoMedrol) intramuscularly just prior to beginning surgery to reduce postoperative edema.

A small amount of crusting forms over the grafts. Most of this is removed during the first cleaning and washing the day after surgery. Patients use an antibiotic ointment or any other sterile moisturizing ointment three times daily until all of the crusting is gone (in 7 to 14 days). The grafts will usually lose their hair in 2 to 6 weeks while new hair growth normally begins 10 to 20 weeks after surgery and grows approximately 1.5 cm per month. The ultimate cosmetic effect of any given session is therefore not

TABLE 274-1

Characteristics of Various Types of Hair Transplantation Grafts

TYPE OF SESSION	NUMBER OF EACH GRAFT TYPE	NUMBER OF HAIRS TRANSPLANTED	NUMBER OF GRAFTS TRANSPLANTED
All micrografts (average of 1.6 hairs each)	1000 grafts 2000 grafts 3000 grafts	1600 hairs 3200 hairs 4800 hairs	1000 2000 3000
All micrograft and small (3- to 4-) minigrafts	200 micro = 320 hairs 400 small minigrafts 200 × 3 hairs = 600 hairs 200 × 4 hairs = 800 hairs	1720 hairs	600
All micrografts, small and large (5- to 6-hair) minigrafts	200 micro = 320 hairs 200 small minigrafts 100 × 3 hairs = 300 hairs 100 × 4 hairs = 400 hairs 200 large minigrafts 100 × 5 hairs = 500 hairs 100 × 6 hairs = 600 hairs	2120 hairs	600
Mixed micrograft Beaver, small minigraft, standard graft (average hair count in three of author's recent patients was 23 hairs per 3.5 mm² graft)	200 micro = 320 hairs 150 Beaver 75 × 2 hairs = 150 hairs 75 × 3 hairs = 225 hairs 260 small minigrafts 100 × 3 hairs = 300 hairs 100 × 4 hairs = 400 hairs 60 × 3.5 mm² = 1380 hairs	2775 hairs (equivalent to 1609 micrografts)	610

FIGURE 274-5

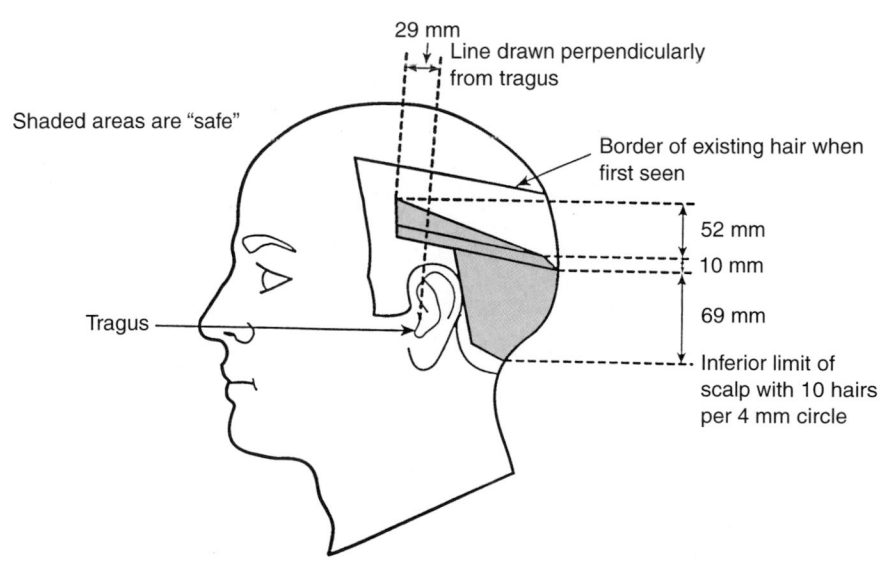

A safe donor area for 80 percent of patients under the age of 80 years. These boundaries were arrived at by studying 328 men 65 years of age or older.

clearly perceived until 9 months after surgery. A 3% solution of minoxidil used twice daily for 5 to 6 weeks postoperatively will often accelerate regrowth. Some hypesthesia of the scalp can be expected to occur postoperatively in nearly everyone. This is usually temporary, but it may sometimes persist in one or more small areas.

Complications

True infection in the recipient area occurs in fewer than 0.1 percent of patients, while a few usually self-resolving ingrown hairs are seen in 1 to 5 percent. Hot compresses and topical as well as systemic antibiotics are prescribed if pathogens grow from the exudate or if there is clearly infection present. Grafts may be slightly elevated ("cobblestoning") or slightly depressed. Cobblestoning can be treated with light electrodesiccation, while depressed grafts should be excised and repositioned at that site or replaced with new grafts that lie flush with the skin. Other complications include epidermal cysts, keloids, hypertrophic scars, minimal growth, arteriovenous fistulas, osteomyelitis, telogen effluvium, chronic follicullitis, accelerated hair loss, temporary curly or lusterless hair, indented "grooves" in the recipient area, "hyperfibrotic healing," and wound dehiscence. These are either rare, temporary, or minor sequelae of hair transplanting and should be viewed from that perspective.[36]

ALOPECIA REDUCTION

Alopecia reduction (AR) or scalp reduction can be defined as the excision of an area of alopecia or future alopecia. The larger the area that can be removed, the smaller the remaining area of alopecia will be, with the result that fewer grafts will be required to produce the same hair density. In general, the author recommends that one or more ARs be employed any time the objective of the patient is maximum coverage of frontal and vertex alopecia.

In some individuals, a second very important function of AR is raising of the superior border of the hair-bearing temporoparietal area with each AR. If the patient intends to part his hair, for aesthetic reasons the AR should begin at a line drawn vertically from the lateral canthus of the eye or at some point medial to this. AR will effectively move the superior border of the temporal parietal area and the anterior superiormost point of the temporal hair more superiorly, so that if a part is used, it will pass through intact original temporoparietal hair instead of transplanted areas.[6]

A variety of AR patterns have been described, but the most common patterns employed are the ellipse, inverted Y, and, more recently, the "lazy-S" shape.[37] The inverted Y pattern should be used if one anticipates insufficient donor tissue to transplant the entire bald area even after AR. This design avoids a scar in areas that cannot later be covered with transplanted hair.

Technique

AR is usually carried out on an outpatient basis under sterile conditions. The patient is given 15 to 20 mg of oral diazepam 30 min before surgery with or without meperidine 50 mg orally or intramuscularly. The procedure begins with drawing in the chosen pattern, using a marker. Two percent lidocaine with 1/100,000 epinephrine is utilized to produce a circle of anesthesia around the

circumference of the head inferior to the expected extent of undermining. In addition, it is injected along the proposed lines of incision to minimize bleeding.

If the pattern is an ellipse, a variant of an ellipse, or a "lazy S," an incision is made down to and through the galea along one side of its entire length, usually in a staged fashion, stopping to control bleeding with cautery where required. Care is taken to angle the blade so as to not injure any adjacent follicles. If previously transplanted grafts are nearby, a 2-mm margin of safety is observed. Mayo scissors are used to begin the undermining between the periosteum and galea aponeurotica. It is then completed to at least 10 cm or more on either side by blunt finger dissection.

The amount of redundant scalp tissue is estimated by overlapping the tissues, followed by perpendicular incisions made through the top flap, stopping at the points where the flaps meet.[37] The perpendicular cuts are then joined and the excess tissue is thereby removed. If the AR is done in the shape of an inverted Y, each "arm" of the Y is treated as a separate ellipse. ARs are closed in two layers and an overnight dressing is applied.

Complications

Complications of AR include postoperative bleeding, infection, nerve damage, persistent hair thinning or loss in the fringe areas, disorientation of hair direction, and poor scars. All of these occur infrequently or not at all if the procedure is carried out properly.[6]

Major Reductions

"Major" reductions have been described by numerous authors. Brandy has suggested calling them *bilateral occipital parietal flaps* and *bilateral temporal flaps*.[38] Major reductions are distinguished from standard ARs by more extensive undermining involving the severing of temporal and/or postauricular and/or occipital arteries and nerves bilaterally. The efficacy of these procedures in excising substantial areas of alopecia is beyond question. However, potential complications include wound dehiscense, permanent hypesthesia, persisting marked thinning of existing scalp hair, and necrosis of large areas of the scalp. Although they are infrequent, they are serious enough that the author does not recommend major reductions. Vertical scars in the temporal area and raising of the inferior border of supraauricular and occipital hair, which always accompanies major AR, can also lead to cosmetic difficulties.

Scalp Extension

Scalp extension was first described by Frechet in 1993. As part of a conventional AR, he inserted a thin stretched sheet of silicone elastomer in the subgaleal space. Rows of titanium hooks attached to the lateral ends of this extender were hooked into the galea. The wound was then sutured closed in two layers. The extender has a natural tendency to return to its original size, thus stretching of the tissue located lateral to the hooks and contracting the scalp between them. After a period of approximately 30 days, the extender is removed. Substantial scalp laxity is then present and another AR is carried out.[39] Frechet's studies revealed that if the extender had been stretched to twice its original length, approximately twice the expected area of alopecia could have been removed on this second occasion and as soon as 30 days after the first (instead of the more usual 2 to 3 months between ARs). Another extender can be inserted at the time of the second and even a third AR. Remarkable results can be achieved very quickly (Fig. 274-6). Disadvantages include additional discomfort during the postoperative period, last-

FIGURE 274-6

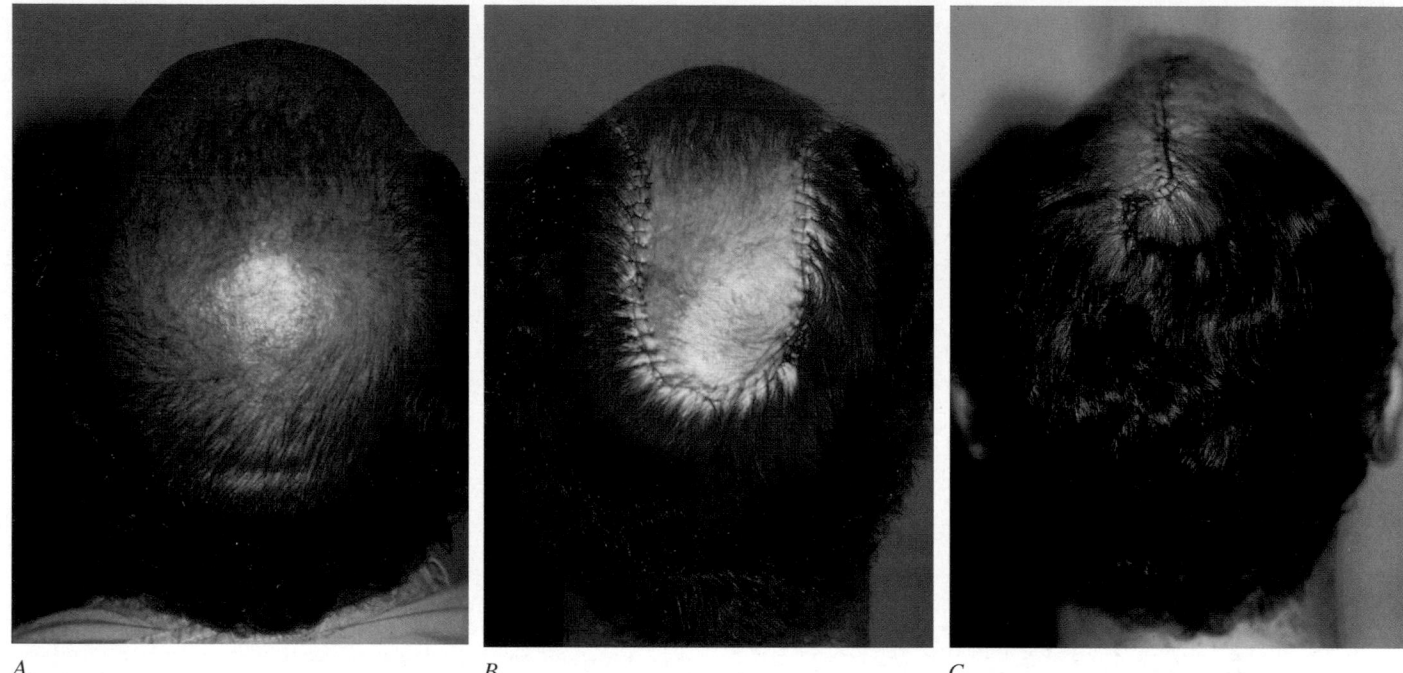

A.   B.   C.

A. Before reduction. B. Immediately after the second alopecia reduction (AR), 30 days after the first AR, during which a Frechet extender was inserted. C. Immediately after a third AR, which was done 60 days after the first and 30 days after the second and included a three-flap corrective procedure for the slot that would have otherwise been present. (*Courtesy of Patrick Frechet, MD.*)

ing anywhere from 1 to 2 weeks, an infection rate of approximately 0.5 percent and a "slot" defect that must be repaired if the entire area of alopecia is excised.

Alopecia Reduction Preceded by Soft Tissue Expansion

Tissue expansion has been used prior to AR for over a decade. In brief, a specially designed surgical "balloon" is inserted as a separate procedure prior to a planned AR. It is gradually inflated with injections of saline every 1 or 2 weeks for 6 to 12 weeks. The expander is then removed and an AR is carried out.[40] The use of such expanders has enabled physicians to excise as much as 10 to 12 cm of alopecia in one AR. An infection rate of less than 0.5 percent is the only complication "price" over the complications that can occur with modified major AR. Anderson has described elegant procedures that utilize soft tissue expansion prior to *bilateral advancement transposition* (BAT) and *triple advancement transposition* (TAT) flaps that produce excellent cosmetic results.[41] Despite this, the cosmetic disability caused by the gradually inflated expanders, which produce a hydrocephalic appearance toward the end of the inflation period, has to a large extent limited this technique to individuals with cicatricial alopecia. Unger has recently described the use of what he terms *prolonged acute tissue expansion* (PATE) during the course of a conventional modified major AR.[42] A "U" shaped expander is inserted under the hair-bearing skin and is expanded over 2 to 3 h while the patient remains in the operating room under local anesthesia. Then AR is carried out and generally will result in the removal of approximately twice the area that would have been removed with a conventional modified major AR. This technique offers a reasonable compromise approach to the advantages of tissue expansion while eliminating most of its disadvantages. Complications are similar to those of a modified major AR.

REFERENCES

1. Dieffenbach JF: Nonnulla de regeneration et transplantation. Dissertation inauguralis, Königsberg, Germany, 1822
2. Orentreich N: Autografts in alopecias and other selected dermatological conditions. *Ann NY Acad Sci* **83**:463, 1959
3. Blanchard G, Blanchard B: Obliteration of alopecia by hair lifting: A new concept and technique. *J Nat Med Assoc* **69**:639, 1977
4. Unger MG, Unger WP: Management of alopecia of the scalp by a combination of excisions and transplantations. *J Dermatol Surg Oncol* **4**:670, 1978
5. Unger WP: *Hair Transplantation,* 3d ed. New York, Marcel Dekker, 1995
6. Unger WP, Knudsen R: General principles of recipient site organization and planning, in *Hair Transplantation,* 3d ed, edited by W Unger. New York, Marcel Dekker, 1995, pp 105–158
7. Marritt E, Dzubow L: Re-assessment of male pattern baldness: A re-evaluation of treatment, in *Hair Replacement,* edited by D Stough. St Louis, Mosby, 1995, pp 30–41
8. Norwood OT: Senile alopecia, in *Hair Transplant Surgery,* edited by OT Norwood, R Shiell. Springfield, IL, CC Thomas, 1984, pp 10–14
9. Unger W: Delineating the "safe" donor area for hair transplanting. *Am J Cosmet Surg* **11**:239, 1994
10. Cotterill P: Hair transplanting in females, in *Hair Transplantation,* 3d ed, edited by W Unger. New York, Marcel Dekker, 1995, pp 287–292
11. Marritt E: "Yes, Virginia, you can remove all the baldness . . . but." *Hair Transpl Forum* **3**:3, 1995
12. Unger MG: Alopecia reduction and stretchback. *Clin Dermatol* **10**:345, 1992
13. Hitzig GC, Sadick NS: A new technique for curvilinear scalp reduction. *J Dermatol Surg Oncol* **15**:1108, 1989
14. Nordstrom R: "Stretch-back" in scalp reductions for male pattern baldness. *Plast Reconstr Surg* **73**:422, 1984

SECTION THIRTY-SEVEN
Surgery in Dermatology

15. Nordstrom R: Alopecia reduction, paper delivered at the Annual Meeting of the International Society of Hair Restoration Surgery, Las Vegas, 1995
16. Rassman W: Megasessions: Dense packing. *Hair Transpl Forum* **4**:5, 1994
17. Stough D: Editor's note, in *Hair Replacement, Surgical and Medical,* edited by D Stough, R Haber. St Louis, Mosby, 1995, p 162
18. Pomerantz M: More problems with megasessions. *Hair Transpl Forum* **5**:4, 1995
19. Unger W: Micrografting, in *Hair Transplantation,* 3d ed, edited by W Unger. New York, Marcel Dekker, 1995, pp 804–807
20. Greco J: The H-factor in micrografting procedures. *Hair Transpl Forum Int* **6**:8, 1996
21. Shiell R: Editor's notes. *Hair Transpl Forum Int* **4**:12, 1996
22. Unger W: Anesthesia, in *Hair Transplantation,* 3d ed, edited by W Unger. New York, Marcel Dekker, 1995, pp 165–181
23. Unger W: The donor site, in *Hair Transplantation,* 3d ed, edited by W Unger. New York, Marcel Dekker, 1995, pp 183–214
24. Unger W: The recipient area, in *Hair Transplantation,* 2d ed, edited by W Unger, R Nordstrom. New York, Marcel Dekker, 1988, pp 211–328
25. Unger W: Hair transplantation, in *Recent Advances in Skin Surgery,* edited by E Epstein, Sr. New York, Elsevier. In press
26. Unger W: Surgical approach to hair loss, in *Disorders of Hair Growth: Diagnosis and Treatment,* edited by E Olsen. New York, McGraw-Hill, 1994, pp 353–374
27. Unger W: The recipient area, in *Hair Transplantation,* 3d ed, edited by W Unger. New York, Marcel Dekker, 1995, pp 215–322
28. Unger W, David L: Laser hair transplanting. *J Dermatol Surg Oncol* **20**:515, 1994
29. Unger W: Laser hair transplantation II. *Dermatol Surg* **21**:759, 1995
30. Unger W: Laser hair transplantation, in *Hair Transplantation,* 3d ed, edited by W Unger. New York, Marcel Dekker, 1995, pp 323–330
31. McKeown M: Preparation and insertion of grafts, in *Hair Transplantation,* 3d ed, edited by W Unger. New York, Marcel Dekker, 1995, pp 331–348
32. Limmer R: Elliptical donor harvesting, in *Hair Replacement Surgical and Medical,* edited by D Stough, R Haber. St Louis, Mosby, 1995, pp 142–147
33. Seager D: Binocular stereoscopic dissecting microscopics: Should we all be using them? *Hair Transpl Forum Int* **6**(4):2, 1996
34. Morrison J: Tissue adhesives in hair transplant surgery. *Plast Reconstr Surg* **68**:491, 1981
35. Unger W: Bandaging, in *Hair Transplantation,* 3d ed, edited by W Unger. New York, Marcel Dekker, 1995, pp 349–352
36. Unger W: Complications of hair transplantation, in *Hair Transplantation,* 3d ed, edited by W Unger. New York, Marcel Dekker, 1995, pp 363–374
37. Unger M: Scalp reduction, in *Hair Transplantation,* 3d ed, edited by W Unger. New York, Marcel Dekker, 1995, pp 509–569
38. Brandy N: Scalp lifting, in *Hair Transplantation,* 3d ed, edited by W Unger. New York, Marcel Dekker, 1995, pp 594–614
39. Frechet P: Scalp extension, in *Hair Transplantation,* 3d ed, edited by W Unger. New York, Marcel Dekker, 1995, pp 625–642
40. Argenta LC et al: Treatment of male pattern baldness by tissue expanders, in *Male Aesthetic Surgery,* 2d ed, edited by EH Courtiss. St Louis, Mosby, 1991, pp 212–225
41. Anderson R: New expanded scalp flap techniques for elimination of male pattern baldness, in *Hair Transplantation,* 3d ed, edited by W Unger. New York, Marcel Dekker, 1995, pp 673–691
42. Unger M, Solish N: Prolonged acute tissue expansion (Pate). *Am J Cosmet Surg* **12**:231, 1995

CHAPTER 275

Gloria F. Graham

Cryosurgery

HISTORY

Cold has been an important adjunct in medicine since the Egyptians around 2500 B.C. used it to treat injuries and inflammation.[1] Even Hippocrates (460–370 B.C.) used cold to relieve the pain of injury and illness.[2] Baron Dominique Jean Lorrey used cold to stop hemorrhage after amputations done in Napoleon's historic retreat from Moscow.[3] Using a brine solution, Arnott,[4] a London physician, lowered temperatures to −24°C (−11°F) for treatment of neuralgia and as palliation in terminally ill cancer patients.

New York became the "cradle of cryosurgery" in the United States in 1899 when White, a dermatologist, first dipped a cotton-tipped applicator into liquid air and successfully treated warts, nevi, keratoses, and skin cancers.[5,6] Whitehouse, another New York dermatologist, developed a spray from a laboratory wash bottle in 1907.[7] In the mid 1960s, Zacarian used this concept to develop a spray of liquid nitrogen after first working with copper probe tips.[8] Around the same time, Torre, another New York dermatologist, used an instrument developed by Cooper for use in the brain. He treated multiple types of skin lesions with this instrument.[9]

Carbon dioxide was the primary cryogen used from the early 1900s until Allington, in 1948, introduced liquid nitrogen applied with a cotton swab.[10] This technique is still in wide use.

Cryosurgery, a technique utilizing heat removed from tissues by application of cold, is effective in treating a wide array of skin conditions including many benign, premalignant, and malignant skin lesions. Because it also offers partial anesthesia, numerous lesions may be treated at one sitting. This efficient, effective, and economical method is now widely used by physicians who manage skin lesions.

TABLE 275-1

PATIENT SELECTION

Dermatologists now have a variety of treatment methods available for skin lesions including excision, electrodesiccation, chemical peeling, laser, the Mohs technique, radiation, and topical agents such as 5-fluorouracil, glycolic acid, and retinoids. The selection will depend on the patient as well as his or her skin type, general health, and overall expectations. Not all methods are available in every office, but freezing and electrodesiccation are extensively used by many dermatologists.

Cryosurgery is unique in its versatility for treatment of multiple warts or keratoses in fair-skinned patients. Patients allergic to local anesthesia or anticoagulants or with anticipated poor wound healing are excellent candidates for freezing. For lesions over 3 to 4 mm in size, cryosurgery is often selected, while for multiple 1- to 2-mm lesions, electrodesiccation may be preferable. Laser is preferred over freezing for port-wine stains and some other vascular lesions, but freezing may be more cost-effective for treatment of multiple lentigines.[11] For physicians managing patients with HIV infection, cryosurgery, which is "blood-free," has unique advantages, especially in the treatment of warts, molluscum contagiosum, and Kaposi's sarcoma.[12]

CRYOBIOLOGY

Cryosurgery involves removing heat from the skin by applying a cryogenic agent. The mechanism of injury involves the direct effect of freezing on the cells as well as vascular stasis, which develops after thawing. These changes are dependent on several factors, including the rate of temperature fall, the rate of rewarming, solute concentration, the length of time cells are exposed to a below-freezing temperature in the $0°$ to $-50°C$ (32 to $-58°F$) range, and the coldest temperature reached in the target tissue.[13,14] Slow cooling produces extracellular ice formation and rapid cooling leads to intracellular ice formation. The later results in more cellular damage, since the cells are ruptured during the thawing process. Slow thawing also causes an increased concentration of electrolytes. The recrystallization that takes place is damaging to cells.[15] The local inflammatory response adds to the final cellular destruction.[16] The vascular stasis that occurs assures greater cell destruction.

EQUIPMENT

Cryosurgery can be performed with a number of cryogens (Table 275-1) and various forms of equipment. The Kidde apparatus utilizing carbon dioxide is rarely used today, but some offices still use dry ice slush with a combination of pulverized carbon dioxide (dry ice), sulfur, and acetone. Liquid nitrogen applied with a cotton swab is still in use, but in the United States as well as numerous foreign countries liquid nitrogen is frequently applied by using a small hand-held spray unit. These units come equipped with interchangeable apertures and probe tips of varying size. Some of the units

Cryogens and Their Temperatures

CRYOGENS	BOILING POINT STP (C°)
Carbon dioxide (solid)	-78.5 ($-109.3°F$)
Nitrous oxide (liquid)	-89.5 ($-129.1°F$)
Liquid nitrogen	-195.8 ($-320.4°F$)

available include the Frigitronics Cryo-Surg and the Brymill Cry-AC units, nitrospray, and Wallach Ultra Freeze.

Liquid nitrogen may be purchased from many welding supply companies at a cost of about $2.50/L. It is stored in 20- to 30-L Dewar flasks.

There is evidence that viral contamination of liquid nitrogen may occur when warts are treated by the dipstick method.[17] Use of a Styrofoam or stainless steel cup is recommended for holding liquid nitrogen prior to dipping the cotton swab in order to avoid this possible complication.

TREATMENT OF BENIGN LESIONS

Many benign tumors and conditions may be managed by cryosurgery and a number of factors must be considered before deciding that cryosurgery is the treatment of choice. These include the depth of the lesion, the location, the skin type, the total number of lesions anticipated, cosmetic results, and the anticipated discomfort that might result in certain locations, such as the plantar surface of the foot.

Technique

In general, freezing a benign tumor until a 1- to 2-mm rim of normal tissue has been frozen is sufficient. Some lesions, such as the seborrheic keratosis, may be especially stubborn to eradicate and longer freeze times are needed (Table 275-2). The use of intermittent freezing allows for better control than one would have using a continuous spray, especially for small lesions. Probes are advantageous for small vascular lesions and sebaceous hyperplasia. The approximate freeze times for eradication of common benign lesions and the anticipated cosmetic results are given in Table 275-3.

PREMALIGNANT LESIONS

The actinic keratosis is one of the most widely treated lesions by cryosurgery. The type of keratosis and its size determines the duration of freeze. A relatively macular lesion with a thin scale may be eradicated by a 5- to 7-s freeze, whereas a thicker hypertrophic lesion may require up to 20 or 30 s of freezing (Table 275-2). The comedonal type of actinic keratosis may require at least 20 s. Outlining the lesion with a marking pen prior to freezing is helpful in making certain the entire lesion is treated adequately. A cryopattern develops with freezing keratoses, and this is useful in determining lesion size. Prethinning of lesions with emollients and especially

TABLE 275-2

Treatment Chart—T Table*

Type	Treatment	Tip	Time, s	Target, mm	Technique	Thermocouple	Turnout
Actinic keratosis	√Choice	B or C	F = 5–10 T = 10–20	2	√Cryospray √Cotton swab √Cryoprobe 1 Cryocycle	No	Excellent to good
Hypertrophic actinic keratosis	√Choice Alternate √Adjunct (with curettage)	B	F = 20–30 T = 30–40	2	√Cryospray Cryoprobe 1 Cryocycle	No	Excellent to good
Seborrheic keratosis	Choice √Alternate √Adjunct	B	F = 8–15 T = 15–30	2.5	√Cryospray Cryoprobe 1 Cryocycle	No	Good
Dermatofibroma	√Choice √Alternate √Adjunct (with shave)	B or probe	F = 20–30 T = 30–40	3–4	√Cryospray √Cryoprobe 1 Cryocycle	No	Good
Basal cell carcinoma (BCC)	√Choice √Alternate √Adjunct (with shave or curettage)	>1 cm(A) <1 cm(B) Small, deep BCC (probe)	F = 60–120 T = 60–180	3–4	√Cryospray √Cryoprobe 2–3 Cryocycles	Yes	Good Good
Lentigo maligna	√Choice Alternate Adjunct	A or B	F = 60–120 T = 90–120	3–4	√Cryospray √Cryoprobe 2–3 Cryocycles	Yes	Good to fair (hypopigmentation)

*Using Brymill Cry-Ac intermittent spray.
√ Under Treatment is treatment of choice, alternate or adjunct; F, freeze time; T, thaw time; √ under Technique is preferred or acceptable technique.

glycolic acid compounds results in an even shorter freeze time of 4 to 6 s in some patients.

A 2- to 4-mm margin or lateral spread of freeze around the lesion should be sufficient. Thermocouple monitoring is not necessary when treating benign lesions.

TABLE 275-3

Comparison of Freeze Times for Benign and Malignant Lesions and Range of Expected Cosmetic Results*

Lesion	Freeze Times, s	Range of Expected Cosmetic Results
Acne scarring	10	Good to fair
Actinic keratoses	5–10	Excellent to good
Cherry angioma	15–20 (probe)	Good to fair
Chondrodermatitis	30	Good to fair
Granuloma faciale	30	Good to fair
Hemangioma	60+	Good to fair
Hypertrophic scarring	20	Good to fair
Keloidal scarring	30	Excellent to good
Keratoacanthoma	30	Excellent to good
Lentigines	10	Excellent to good
Lentigo maligna	60–120	Good to fair
Morphea-type basal cell	90–120	Good to fair
Nevi	10	Excellent to good
Nodular basal cell	60–90	Excellent to good
Sebaceous hyperplasia	5–10 (spray or probe)	Good to fair
Seborrheic keratoses	10	Excellent to good
Superficial basal cell	60	Excellent to good

*Using intermittent spray (unless otherwise specified).

MALIGNANT LESIONS

Sufficient experience has been gained by numerous cryosurgeons who agree that a freeze time of approximately 60 s utilizing an intermittent spray is adequate for many skin malignancies such as basal cell carcinoma and squamous cell carcinoma, especially those arising from an actinic keratosis. To measure the depth of freeze by thermocouple monitoring requires inserting a needle beneath the tumor. While this is no longer done by many experienced cryosurgeons, it can be quite advantageous for learning the technique.

Technique

The tumor is frozen with an intermittent spray until a zone of 5 mm of frozen tissue is reached around the lesion (Figs. 275-1 to 275-3). This usually requires about 60 s of freezing. If a neoprene or other type of cone is used, this may shorten the freeze time to 45 s or less. The halo thaw time will be approximately 60 s, and the complete thaw time for the entire lesion is 2 to 5 min. If a thermocouple is used, freezing should continue until the monitor registers around −50°C (−58°F). The thaw time to 0°C (32°F) is often around 1 min. For the greatest destruction, a double freeze-thaw cycle is used.

Mallon and Dawber[18] have found that for facial lesions, a double freeze-thaw cycle yields a higher cure rate; but for superficial basal cell carcinomas on the trunk, a single freeze-thaw cycle is sufficient to yield a 95.5 percent cure rate. Recording of the freeze and thaw times in the medical record is prudent.

Debulking of the tumor by curettage or razor blade saucerization prior to freezing is a technique preferred by many (Fig. 275-2).[19] This provides an adequate specimen for the pathologist and allows for better judgment in terms of tumor depth and lateral extent of

FIGURE 275-1

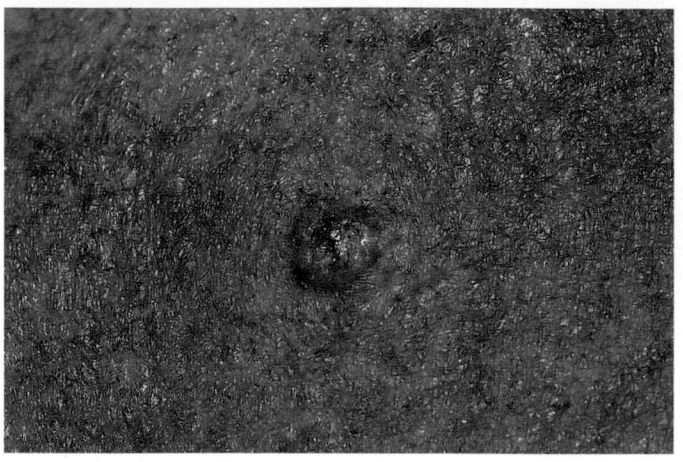

An actinic keratosis with squamous cell carcinoma on the cheek. Lesion size 0.6 cm.

the tumor. Freezing is performed on the tumor bed (Fig. 275-3). Lesions 3 to 4 cm in size may be divided into 1- to 2-cm portions but may be treated at one visit. More extensive lesions may be treated over several months.

Cryosurgery is especially effective in treating lesions overlying cartilage, as on the ear. The external auditory canal may be protected with a cotton pledget or with one's hand. When treating the nose or eye, protection with a tongue blade or a Jaegher retractor for the eye is useful.

Postoperative Management

The care of the cryosurgical wound, while simple, requires specific instructions to the patient. Washing the lesion with soap and water once to twice daily is the most useful approach. While some locations will need a dressing because of the bullous reaction and the drainage, most sites may be left open and actually seem to heal better that way, since the eschar is not inadvertently removed by adherence to dressings. The cryowound is its own biologic dressing

FIGURE 275-2

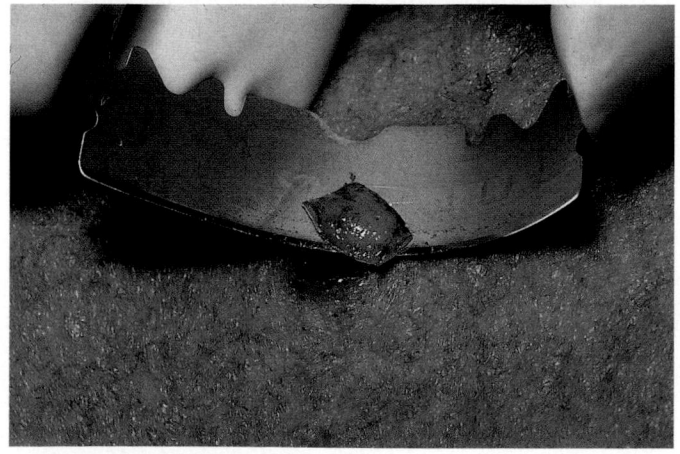

After debulking by saucerized razor blade removal and curettage.

FIGURE 275-3

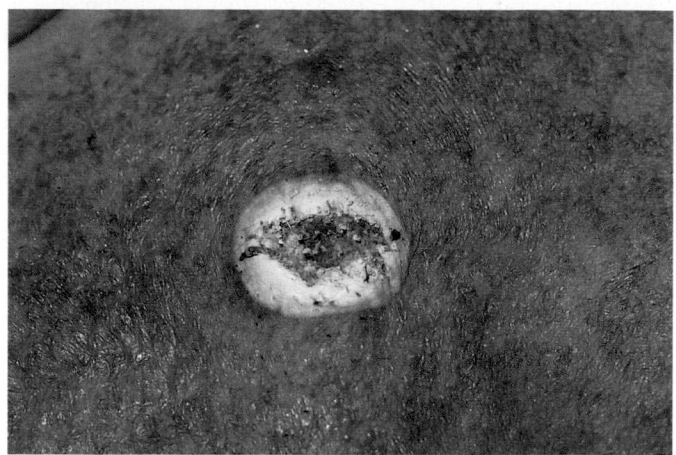

The tumor bed and surrounding skin are shown after freezing. A 5-mm halo of normal skin is frozen around the tumor. A double freeze-thaw cycle is used.

(Fig. 275-4). It is wet from its inception, and benign and premalignant lesions heal in 10 days to 2 weeks. The final eschar separates and comes off in about 1 month for most skin cancers. Those on the back and leg, especially if over 1 to 2 cm in diameter, may require 6 weeks to 3 months to heal. If the eschar becomes dry and adherent, it may be removed and the base treated with antibiotic ointment twice daily until healed. Duoderm or a similar dressing may be used if upon removal of the eschar an ulcer is present.

SIDE EFFECTS AND COMPLICATIONS

The expected effects following freezing are edema, vesicles, bullae, weeping, and eschar formation. Periorbital edema may be lessened by the use of systemic steroids[20] or potent topical steroids twice

FIGURE 275-4

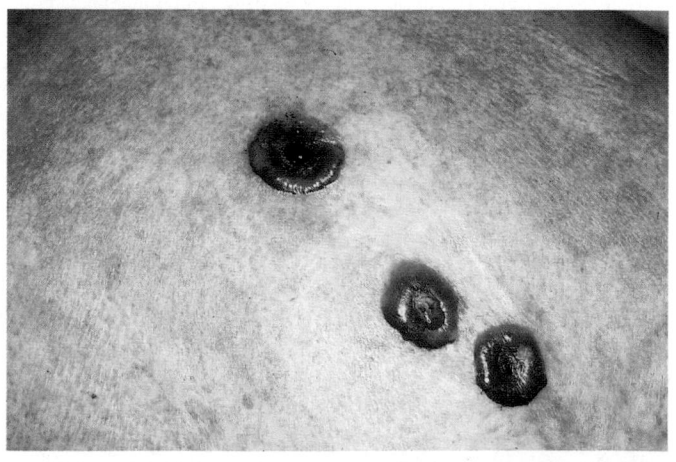

The bulla resulting from freezing is its own biologic dressing and heals in 10 to 14 days when 10 to 20 s of intermittent freeze time is used.

daily[21] for 3 to 4 days. Pain following freezing is more likely to occur when lesions on the palms, soles, fingers, toes, scalp, and temple are treated. Rarely are analgesics other than aspirin or acetaminophen required. Bleeding following freezing is uncommon but should be considered in patients taking anticoagulants. Syncope occurs infrequently but should be anticipated after freezing warts on the digits.

Infection

The incidence of infection following freezing is very low, probably due to destruction of skin flora, maintenance of the basement membrane, and the rapid reepitheliazation that occurs after treatment of benign and premalignant lesions. Patients should be cautioned that if increased heat, redness, or purulent drainage develops they should return to see the physician promptly.

Abnormal Scarring

The maintenance of a normal dermal fibrous network after freezing allows many wounds to heal with little or no scarring. The most common scar is soft and hypopigmented. Linear hypertrophic scarring may be seen following treatment of cancers on the nose, upper lip, and chest. Ectropion may result following freezing of eyelid carcinoma, but this is rare. Loss of eyelashes is routine. Notching of the ala of the nose and helix of the ear is seen when large tumors are treated.

Pigment Alteration

Pigment loss due to sensitivity of the melanocytes, which are destroyed at $-4°C$ (24.8°F) is common after freezing,[22] but when freezing times under 20 to 30 s are used, this pigment loss is often temporary. Peripheral hyperpigmentation may be noted especially on the leg and back. Use of topical steroids, glycolic acids, and retinoids as well as hydroquinones may decrease this effect.

Nerve Damage

Damage to nerves is rare following freezing of benign and premalignant lesions and is uncommon in treating malignancies. Digital neuropathy after treating a wart on the finger has been reported.[23] Sensory loss following freezing usually resolves in 6 to 12 months. The sense of touch recovers more quickly than the sensations of pain and cold.[24]

Insufflation of Soft Tissue

Nitrogen gas may escape into perilesional skin when freezing follows a biopsy. Pressure on the crepitant area will result in expulsion of the gas. The use of a cone surrounding the biopsy site can prevent this from occurring.

Alopecia

Freeze times longer than 20 s may result in alopecia of the scalp hair, eyebrow, eyelashes, or beard. Alopecia is more common after freezing skin cancer than after treating benign lesions.

Miscellaneous

Adherence of probes to mucous membranes can result in loss of mucosa upon removing the probe. This can be prevented by prechilling the probe or applying K-Y jelly. If the probe does adhere, it should be allowed to defrost so it pulls away from the mucosa without tearing it.[19] Pseudotumor recidive and exuberant granulation tissue are occasionally seen.

RECENT ADVANCES IN CRYOSURGERY

Full-Face Cryosurgical Peels

Full-face cryopeeling was carried out for over 40 years using dry-ice slush made by mixing carbon dioxide, acetone, and sulfur and applying it with a gauze ball. Graham first used liquid nitrogen for spraying acne and acne scarring and did full-face peeling instead of dermabrasion for scarring.[25]

Chiarello used a similar technique with several modifications, calling it a *cryopeel*, for the treatment of sun-damaged skin, actinic keratoses, seborrheic keratoses, lentigines, and wrinkles (Figs. 275-5 to 275-7).[26] He has since combined freezing and dermasanding with tumescent anesthesia as modified by Goodman[27] and achieves excellent, consistent, and reproducible results with minimal complications in the treatment of rhytids.[28]

Ultrasound

The use of ultrasound in determining depth and lateral extent of tumor aids in the decision-making process with regard to the type of procedure to be used for the treatment of a particular cancer. If the tumor has indefinite margins, a procedure such as Mohs surgery should be selected over cryosurgery. The dermatopathologist can aid in this determination by describing the location of the tumor on biopsy—i.e., upper, mid, or lower dermis.[19,29]

Abramovits et al.[30] found ultrasound useful for the accurate placement of thermocouples. They located the thermocouples using ultrasound and accurately measured their distance from the skin

FIGURE 275-5

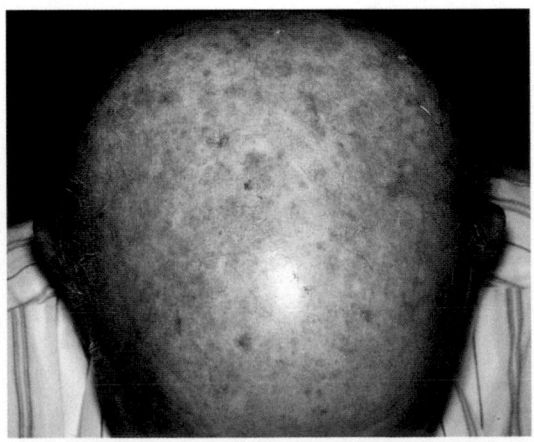

A patient with severe photo damage and multiple actinic keratoses of the scalp prior to cryopeeling. (*Photograph courtesy of Stephen Chiarello, MD.*)

FIGURE 275-6

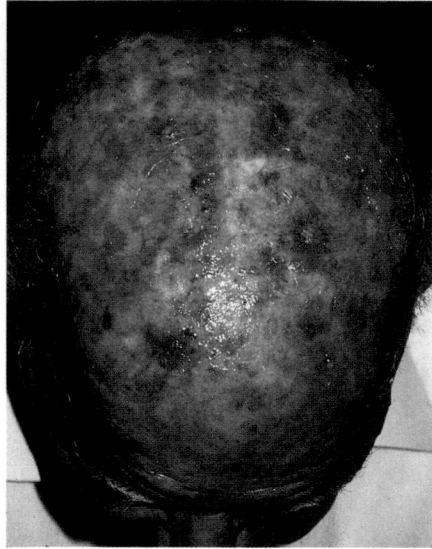

An exudative reaction is noted on the scalp one day after freezing of the entire involved area. (*Photograph courtesy of Stephen Chiarello, MD.*)

surface. This will be a significant advantage to the cryosurgeon who uses thermocouples routinely for the treatment of skin malignancies.

Granuloma Annulare

While cryosurgery has been used for years in the treatment of granuloma annulare, a prospective trial carried out in Germany in 1993 found that using liquid nitrogen or nitrous oxide applied with one freeze-thaw cycle for 10 to 60 s produced excellent results. A total of 25 of 31 lesions (80.6 percent) resolved after one treatment. One patient relapsed during a 2-year follow-up.[31]

FIGURE 275-7

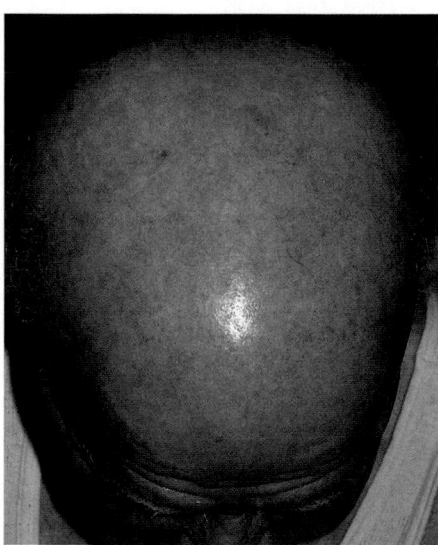

The skin of the scalp is well healed 15 days later and the patient is free of actinic keratoses. (*Photograph courtesy of Stephen Chiarello, MD.*)

Lentigines

These common hyperpigmented macules on the hands and face may be satisfactorily removed by freezing. Pretreating the skin with topical tretinoin, hydroquinone, or glycolic acid helps to thin these lesions prior to freezing and makes the final cosmetic result much better. About 5 to 7 s of intermittent freeze will clear a significant portion of the lesions. Cryopeeling works well on these.[26]

Stern et al. compared laser therapy with cryotherapy and found that freezing worked as well as or better than laser and was more cost-effective.[11]

Keloids

Freezing may be very effective in some keloids.[25] The variability in size, age, consistency, skin color, and location play a role in deciding which treatment to use. Numerous modifications have been added, such as freezing and intralesional steroid with or without prior debulking. The addition of an Epiderm dressing for a few weeks prior to the freezing is helpful. Some have used radiation therapy for treatment prior to freezing. Comparison of intralesional steroid and cryosurgery in acne keloids was carried out by Layton et al.[33] (1994) and showed an average of 80 percent improvement in early lesions treated with cryosurgery.

Psoriasis

While there are few publications attesting to its effectiveness, freezing is used widely by clinicians in treating small and medium-sized plaques of psoriasis.[19,33,34]

Nouri[35] report success in using average freeze times of 12 s/cm^2. There was complete resolution of lesions in 5 of 9 subjects. Two others improved substantially and one worsened. Graham[25] has noted koebnerization in one patient with a brief freeze of only 5 s on an elbow. With freeze times of 10 to 15 s, this did not occur.

Seborrheic Keratosis

Cryosurgery alone or followed by curettage is an effective form of therapy for this lesion, whose treatment is covered by only few insurance companies. The pruritus is disabling in some patients, who may be helped by using alpha-hydroxy body cleanser applied with a polyethylene sponge and followed by an alpha-hydroxy lotion. Castor oil applications are also helpful. Thin lesions are treated with 10 to 15 s of freeze. Some very thick lesions may be treated successfully by curettage and cryosurgery.[19,36]

Prurigo Nodularis

Cryosurgery is one of the treatments of choice for recalcitrant lesions. The C fibers of the nerves are altered by freezing, thereby decreasing pruritus and ameliorating the itch-scratch cycle.[19] Due to differences in lesion size, shape, and thickness, freeze times vary from 15 to 30 s. Spray or a contact probe may be used. Topical and oral antipruritic agents and topical steroids help to prevent recurrence.[37]

Neurodermatitis also responds to freezing.[38] Freon 12 from a 12-oz aerosol can was sprayed onto a 2 cm lesion in the occipital area through an applicator tube held 5 cm from the skin surface.

Myxoid Cyst

There are numerous reports of resolution of myxoid cysts following cryosurgery with a single double freeze-thaw cycle.[39–42] Healing occurs in 2 to 3 weeks and the cosmetic results are good.

Verruca

The treatment of verruca may be the most frustrating of dermatologic conditions.[43,44] Pretreatment of warts with topical salicylic acids[45] results in a higher cure rate.[19] Also giving acetaminophen or aspirin before freezing reduces pain after the procedure. The dipstick method is preferred by some, while many others prefer the spray technique. Kuflik[46] was able to eradicate 97.4 percent of 80 periungual warts with the dipstick technique. While the spray technique alone will cure some plantar warts, combining spray with salicylic acid pads and paring will clear more. Failures may respond to bleomycin.[47]

Condylomata Acuminata

Complete cure of these lesions is difficult if not impossible despite use of freezing, surgical excision, laser surgery, and interferon. The use of Podofilox[48,49] with reliable patients enhances the resolution. Damstra and Van Vloten[50] did a controlled study of 64 patients with small penile and vulvar condylomas. They used a fine needlespray technique and achieved 92 percent remission rate after 3 months.

Kaposi's Sarcoma

Cryosurgery is frequently used to treat Kaposi's sarcoma. A spray using a double freeze-thaw cycle every 3 weeks usually for three treatments was found effective by Tappero et al.[12] Freezing may be combined with vinblastine or other therapies.[12,51]

Basal Cell Carcinoma

The virtues of one versus two freeze-thaw cycles for treatment of basal cell carcinoma (BCC) was studied by Mallon and Dawber.[18] They treated 84 facial BCCs with a single or double 30-s freeze-thaw cycle. The double freeze-thaw cycle on the face achieved a 95.3 percent cure rate, while the single one had a 79.4 percent cure rate. Twenty-nine superficial BCCs on the trunk achieved a 95.5 percent cure rate with the single freeze-thaw cycle. Graham et al.[52] and Torre[53] have used a single freeze-thaw cycle successfully for BCCs at 3 mm or less in depth, whether on the trunk or face. The size and depth of the lesions should be defined with reasonable certainty.

Kuflik and Gage reported a 5-year cure rate of 99 percent for 628 BCCs ranging from <0.5 to 2 cm in diameter using a double freeze-thaw cycle.[54,55]

Zacarian has consistently achieved cure rates around 97.3 percent over 32 years of performing cryosurgery.[56] He has steadfastly maintained that double freeze-thaw cycles were necessary. Graham has compared shave excision/or curettage plus cryosurgery with single and double freezes (Fig. 275-1 to 275-3), achieving a higher cure rate with the combination. A double freeze coupled with curettage yielded a 98.4 percent cure rate. Her freeze times are usually 60 s or longer, while Dawber's were for 30 s.[52] This may account for the lower cure rate in his series.

The use of ultrasound for depth determination and placement of a thermocouple needle would probably improve the cure rates in most series.[29,30] Patient selection is of paramount importance. The cure rate in our series[52] improved over a 30-year period, especially after a Mohs surgeon was available in North Carolina and larger, more difficult tumors could be referred. This is an agricultural area where many patients spend their lives in the sun during the entire year. Despite the severe sun damage, healing after freezing has been remarkable. Treating tumors with indefinite borders is discouraged unless the treatment is used in a palliative way, as may effectively be done in the nursing home setting.

There is increasing use of cryosurgery in the management of some larger tumors. Biro,[57] Kuflik,[58,59] Gage,[60] Goncalves,[61] and Spiller and Spiller[62] reported on the eradication of large tumors by freezing. Stolar and Turjansky in Argentina have managed many large tumors effectively and their series supports the effectiveness of this procedure for both therapy and palliation.[63]

REFERENCES

1. Squazzi A, Bracco D: A historical account of the technical means used in cryotherapy. *Minerva Med* **65**:3718, 1974
2. Hippocrates: *Greek Medicine.* Translated by AJ Brock. Dent, London, 1929
3. Lorrey DJ: *Memoires de Chirurgie Militaire et Campagnes.* Philadelphia, Carey & Lea, 1832, pp 1812–1817
4. Arnott J: *On the Treatment of Cancers by Regulated Application of an Anaesthetic Temperature.* London, Churchill Livingstone, 1855
5. White AC: Liquid air in medicine and surgery. *Med Rec* **56**:109, 1899
6. White AC: Liquified oxygen and x-ray treatment of malignant growths. *Interstate Med J* **9**:657, 1902
7. Whitehouse HH: Liquid air in dermatology: Its indications and limitations. *JAMA* **49**:371, 1907
8. Zacarian SA, Adham MI: Cryotherapy of cutaneous malignancy. *Cryobiology* **2**:212, 1966
9. Torre D: Cradle of cryosurgery. *NY State J Med* **67**:465, 1967
10. Allington HD: Cryosurgery. *Calif Med* **72**:153, 1950
11. Stern RS et al: Laser therapy versus cryotherapy of lentigines: a comparative trial. *J Am Acad Dermatol* **30**:985, 1994
12. Tappero JW et al: Kaposi's sarcoma. *J Am Acad Dermatol* **28**:371, 1993
13. Shepherd J, Dawber R: The historical and scientific basis of cryosurgery. *Clin Exp Dermatol* **7**:321, 1982
14. Zacarian SA: *Cryosurgery for Skin Cancer and Cryogenic Techniques in Dermatology.* Springfield, IL, CC Thomas, 1969, pp 11–21
15. Gage AA: Experimental cryogenic injury of the palate; observations pertinent to cryosurgical destruction of tumors. *Cryobiology* **15**:415, 1978
16. Johnson JF: Immunologic aspects of cryosurgery: Potential modulation of immune recognition and effector cell maturation, in *Clinics in Dermatology: Advances in Cryosurgery,* edited by EW Breitbart, E Siwiec. New York, Elsevier, 1990, pp 39–47
17. Jones SK, Darville JM: Transmission of virus by cryotherapy and multi-use caustic pencils: A problem to dermatologists? *Br J Dermatol* **121**:481, 1989
18. Mallon E, Dawber R: Cryosurgery in the treatment of basal cell carcinoma: Assessment of one and two freeze-thaw cycle schedules. *Dermatol Surg* **22**:854, 1996
19. Graham GF: Cryosurgery for benign, premalignant and malignant lesions, in *Cutaneous Surgery,* edited by RG Wheeland. Philadelphia, Saunders, 1994, pp 835–867
20. Kuflik EG, Webb W: Effects of systemic corticosteroids on post-cryosurgical edema and other manifestations of the inflammatory response. *J Dermatol Surg Oncol* **11**:464, 1985
21. Holt P: Cryotherapy for skin cancer: Results over a 5-year period using liquid nitrogen spray cryotherapy. *Br J Dermatol* **119**:231, 1988
22. Gage AA, Meenaghan M: Sensitivity of pigmented mucosa and pigmented cells in skin due to freezing injury. *Cryobiology* **16**:348, 1979
23. Nix TW Jr: Liquid nitrogen neuropathy. *Arch Dermatol* **92**:185, 1965
24. Dawber RPR: Cold kills! *Clin Exp Dermatol* **13**:138, 1988
25. Graham GF: Cryotherapy in the treatment of acne, in *Skin Surgery,* edited by E Epstein, E Epstein, Jr. Springfield, CC Thomas, 1982, pp 680–697

26. Chiarello SE: Cryopeeling. *J Dermatol Surg Oncol* **18**:329, 1992

27. Goodman G: Dermabrasion using tumescent anesthesia. *J Dermatol Surg Oncol* **20**:802, 1994

28. Chiarello SE: Tumescent dermasanding with cryospraying: a new wrinkle on the treatment of rhytids. *Dermatol Surg* **22**:601, 1996

29. Graham GF: High cure rates reported with cryosurgical methods. *Cosmet Dermatol* **7**:43, 1994

30. Abramovits W et al: Ultrasound-guided thermocouple placement for cryosurgery. *Dermatol Surg* **22**:771, 1996

31. Blume-Peytavi U et al: Successful outcome of cryosurgery in patients with granuloma annulare. *Br J Dermatol* **130**:494, 1994

32. Layton AM et al: A comparison of intralesional triamcinolone and cryosurgery in the treatment of acne keloids. *Br J Dermatol* **130**:495, 1994

33. American Academy of Dermatology, Committee on Guidelines of Care: Guidelines of Care for Cryosurgery. *J Am Acad Dermatol* **31**:648, 1994

34. Scoggins RB: Cryotherapy of psoriasis. *Arch Dermatol* **123**:427, 1987

35. Nouri K et al: Cryotherapy for psoriasis. *Arch Dermatol* **133**:1608, 1997

36. Smoller BR, Graham G: Benign neoplasms of the epidermis, in *Cutaneous Medicine and Surgery,* vol I, edited by KA Arndt, PE LeBoit, JK Robinson, BU Wintroub. Philadelphia, Saunders, 1996, pp 1441–1449

37. Stoll DM et al: Treatment of prurigo nodularis: Use of cryosurgery and intralesional steroids plus lidocaine. *J Dermatol Surg Oncol* **9**:922, 1983

38. McDow RA, Wester MM: Cryosurgical treatment of nodular neurodermatitis with refrigerant 12. *J Dermatol Surg Oncol* **15**:621, 1989

39. Bardach HG: Managing digital mucoid cysts by cryosurgery with liquid nitrogen: Preliminary report. *J Dermatol Surg Oncol* **9**:455, 1983

40. Dawber RPR et al: Myxoid cysts of the finger: Treatment by liquid nitrogen spray cryosurgery. *Clin Exp Dermatol* **8**:153, 1983

41. Bohler-Sommeregger K, Kutschera-Hienert G: Cryosurgical management of myxoid cyst. *J Dermatol Surg Oncol* **14**:1405, 1988

42. Kuflik EG: Specific indications for cryosurgery of the nail unit: Myxoid cysts and periungual verrucae. *J Dermatol Surg Oncol* **18**:702, 1992

43. Keefe M, Dich DC: Cryotherapy of hand warts—a questionnaire survey of "consumers." *Clin Exp Dermatol* **15**:260, 1990

44. Hopkins P: Treatment of warts with liquid nitrogen. *J R Coll Gen Pract* **59**:173, 1989

45. Mottaz JH et al: Transdermal delivery of salicylic acid in the treatment of viral papillomas. *Int J Dermatol* **27**:596, 1988

46. Kuflik EG: Cryosurgical treatment of periungual warts. *J Dermatol Surg Oncol* **10**:673, 1984

47. Shumer SM, O'Keefe EJ: Bleomycin in the treatment of recalcitrant warts. *J Am Acad Dermatol* **9**:91, 1983

48. Greenberg MD, Rutledge LH: A double-blind, randomized trial of 0.5% Podofilox and placebo for the treatment of genital warts in women. *Obstet Gynecol* **77**:735, 1991

49. Stone KM et al: Treatment of external genital warts: A randomized clinical trial comparing podophyllin, cryotherapy and electrodesiccation. *Gentourin Med* **66**:16, 1990

50. Damstra RJ, van Vloten WA: Cryotherapy in the treatment of condylomata acuminata: A controlled study of 64 patients. *J Dermatol Surg Oncol* **17**:273, 1991

51. Tappero JW et al: Cryotherapy for cutaneous Kaposi's sarcoma (KS) associated with acquired immune deficiency syndrome (AIDS): A phase II trial. *J AIDS* **4**:839, 1991

52. Graham GF, Clark LC: Statistical analysis in cryosurgery of skin cancer, in *Clinics in Dermatology: Advances in Cryosurgery,* vol 8, edited by EW Breitbart, E Dachow-Siwiec. New York, Elsevier, 1990, pp 101–107

53. Torre D: Cryosurgery of basal cell carcinomas. *J Am Acad Dermatol* **15**:917, 1986

54. Kuflik EG, Gage AA: Results, in *Cryosurgical Treatment for Skin Cancer,* edited by EG Kuflik, AA Gage. New York, Igaku-Shoin, 1990, p 243

55. Kuflik EG, Gage AA: The five-year cure rate achieved by cryosurgery for skin cancer. *J Am Acad Dermatol* **24**:1002, 1991

56. Zacarian SA: Cryosurgery for cancer of the skin, in *Cryosurgery for Skin Cancer and Cutaneous Disorders,* edited by SA Zacarian. St Louis, Mosby, 1985, pp 96–162

57. Biro L, Price E: Cryosurgery for benign and malignant skin tumors, in *Skin Surgery,* edited by M Harahap. St Louis, Green, 1985, pp 767–821

58. Kuflik EG: Debulking large tumors. *J Dermatol Surg Oncol* **8**:431, 1982

59. Kuflik EG: Cryosurgical treatment for large malignancies on the upper extremities. *J Dermatol Surg Oncol* **12**:575, 1986

60. Gage AA: Cryosurgery of advanced tumors, in *Clinics in Dermatology: Advances in cryosurgery,* edited by EW Breitbart, E Dachow-Siwiec. New York, Elsevier, 1990 pp 86–95

61. Goncalves JA: Cryosurgery of advanced cancer of the extremities. *Skin Cancer* **1**:211, 1986

62. Spiller WF, Spiller RF: Cryosurgery in dermatologic office practice with special reference to basal cell carcinoma. *Texas Med* **68**:84, 1972

63. Turjansky E, Stolar E: Our experience in the treatment of cancer of the skin, in *Cryomedicine.* Montserrat, Argentina, 1996, pp 187–198

CHAPTER 276

Bruce A. Russell
Rex A. Amonette
Neil A. Swanson

Mohs Micrographic Surgery

HISTORY

As a medical student at the University of Wisconsin, Dr. Frederic Mohs observed that 20% zinc chloride behaved as an in vivo fixative when injected into tissues. Histologic features of the tissue were preserved after this fixation and could be assessed microscopically. This discovery was seminal to the development and evolution of what we know today as Mohs micrographic surgery. Initially, Mohs termed his technique *chemosurgery*, because of the chemical paste used as the in situ fixative.[1] This paste contained zinc chloride, *Sanguinaria canadensis*, and stibinite, a granulated mineral. Typically, it was applied to the neoplasm and allowed to fix the tissue for 12 to 24 h. After this period of in situ fixation, the tissue was surgically excised and submitted for histopathologic review using horizontal sections.

Chemosurgery was a labor-intensive process, requiring rigorous adherence to the protocol for it to be effective. For instance, stratum corneum is impermeable to zinc chloride and dichloroacidic acid had to be applied first to the surface of the neoplasm to allow transepidermal absorption of the paste. After fixation, a detailed map of the tumor was drawn. As individual pieces of tissue were excised from the tumor, their position on the map was carefully noted and marked. The corresponding site from which the tissue was taken was also marked by the surgeon and, to prevent errors in orientation, the edges of the tissue were inked with two or three different colors. This process was repeated until the entire neoplasm had been removed.

The sine qua non of Mohs' technique was that the tissue was removed in a manner that would allow histologic examination of 100 percent of the margin. This required that the peripheral epidermal margin be incised with a 45° blade bevel, rather than the traditional 90° scalpel-to-skin angle. Horizontal sectioning of tissue excised in such a manner could then yield an en bloc view of both the peripheral, epidermal, *and* deep (dermal/subcutis) margin. Referring to the carefully constructed color-coded map, the surgeon could then review the histologic sections in the on-site laboratory, mark on the map where tumor remained, return to apply fixative, and excise only tissue that harbored residual neoplasm. This process was repeated until all tumor-involved tissue had been removed.

Unfortunately, this method was so labor-intensive that very few surgeons were able to devote the necessary time and resources to carry it out. The art of judging the appropriate length and depth of fixation accurately took considerable experience and, even then, was still somewhat unpredictable. The fixative paste was frequently painful—a major problem. The surgeon was also required to have dedicated on-site space for preparation and review of the histology specimens, which were often densely inflamed as a result of the

fixative. Finally, the neoplasm had to be excised in a manner contrary to a fundamental surgical principle: it required a tangential incision peripherally and precise maintenance of a horizontal plane (parallel to the skin) across the perceived deep margin of the tumor. Although this technique allowed examination of 100 percent of the surgical margin, due to the time needed for repeated applications of fixative, it could sometimes take several days to clear a large, complex tumor.

Because of these disadvantages, Mohs tried doing without the zinc chloride paste in selected cases, often eyelids, reducing treatment time greatly. Although others repeated these efforts, it was not until 1970 at a meeting of the American College of Chemosurgery that Tromovitch reported a series of patients treated without paste. Tromovitch and Stegman then reported a large group of patients treated without in situ fixation but with the other critical features of chemosurgery maintained. They termed this method *chemosurgery: fresh-tissue technique*. Many incarnations of this approach have been variously named *Mohs surgery*, *microscopically controlled surgery*, *Mohs micrographic surgery*, and others. Although the American College of Chemosurgery changed its name to the American College of Mohs Micrographic Surgery and Cutaneous Oncology in 1987, it is crucial to note that the essential features of the physician serving as both surgeon and pathologist and on-site horizontal tissue sectioning are identical in both techniques; only the fixative is omitted in the fresh-tissue technique.[2]

The fresh-tissue technique of Mohs micrographic surgery is outlined as follows (see Fig. 276-1)[3]:

1. The neoplasm is identified and its apparent border marked.
2. Local anesthetic is infiltrated into the area.
3. A curette is applied to delineate the extent of the tumor.
4. Using a tangential incision circumferentially around the tumor, the neoplasm is removed, with the deep margin excised horizontally, parallel to the skin surface.
5. The specimen is divided into small pieces, its sides are carefully color-coded, and a map created, duplicating the tissue orientation and color locations.
6. The tissue is presented to the technician, inverted, and sectioned on a microtome, on-site.
7. The surgeon reviews the sections microscopically, marking the areas of residual tumor precisely on the map.
8. The surgeon repeats the above process until the tumor has been extirpated.
9. Reconstruction of the defect is addressed.

It is imperative to note that the central guiding principle of this process is that the Mohs surgeon personally handles the tissue from incision to the time it is presented to the technicians and reviews the histology him- or herself. This tenet is crucial to prevent orientation errors or mislabeling of tissue specimens, either of which can result in a poor outcome.

INDICATIONS

Mohs micrographic surgery is indicated primarily for the treatment of difficult basal cell carcinomas (BCCs) and squamous cell carcinomas (SCCs), and this continues to be its main application.[4] However, as this technique has evolved, it has been applied to other challenging cutaneous neoplasms, in many cases with results superior to these using previously published methods. Although an exhaustive discussion is beyond the scope of this chapter, the list of neoplasms and nonneoplastic disease states treated with this technique continues to grow.

Basal Cell Carcinoma

There are approximately 1 million BCCs diagnosed each year in the United States. Because of the incidence and prevalence of this disease, therefore, inadequate or incomplete treatment techniques can have major public health implications. Mohs micrographic surgery has had its greatest success in the treatment of BCCs that are either recurrent or, as primary tumors, display one or more criteria of size, location, or aggressive histology or are otherwise difficult to treat adequately by other techniques (Fig. 276-2). This is primarily due to the extremely high recurrence rate of standard techniques in the treatment of these recurrent or aggressive tumors. Additionally, smaller BCCs of the nodular type located in high-risk areas of embryonic fusion planes, often referred to as the "H-zone" of the face, are best treated with Mohs, in view of their frequent deep extension and propensity for recurrence (Fig. 276-3).

For primary tumors, size can play a role. Tumors >2 cm in diameter can have a higher recurrence rate unless treated with the Mohs technique. It has been well documented that sclerosing BCCs represent a disproportionate percentage of lesions in surveys of recurrent tumors.[5,6] In the aggressive growth pattern of BCCs, there may be areas in which traditional evaluation yields a falsely negative histologic margin (when horizontally sectioned, the same tissue reveals discontinuous small islands or nests of tumor cells). BCCs displaying such histologic features of aggressiveness may have significant subclinical extension; spread along deep fascial planes; involve deep soft tissues; or track along periosteum, perichondrium, or perineurium. Hence, Mohs micrographic surgery is the treatment

FIGURE 276-1

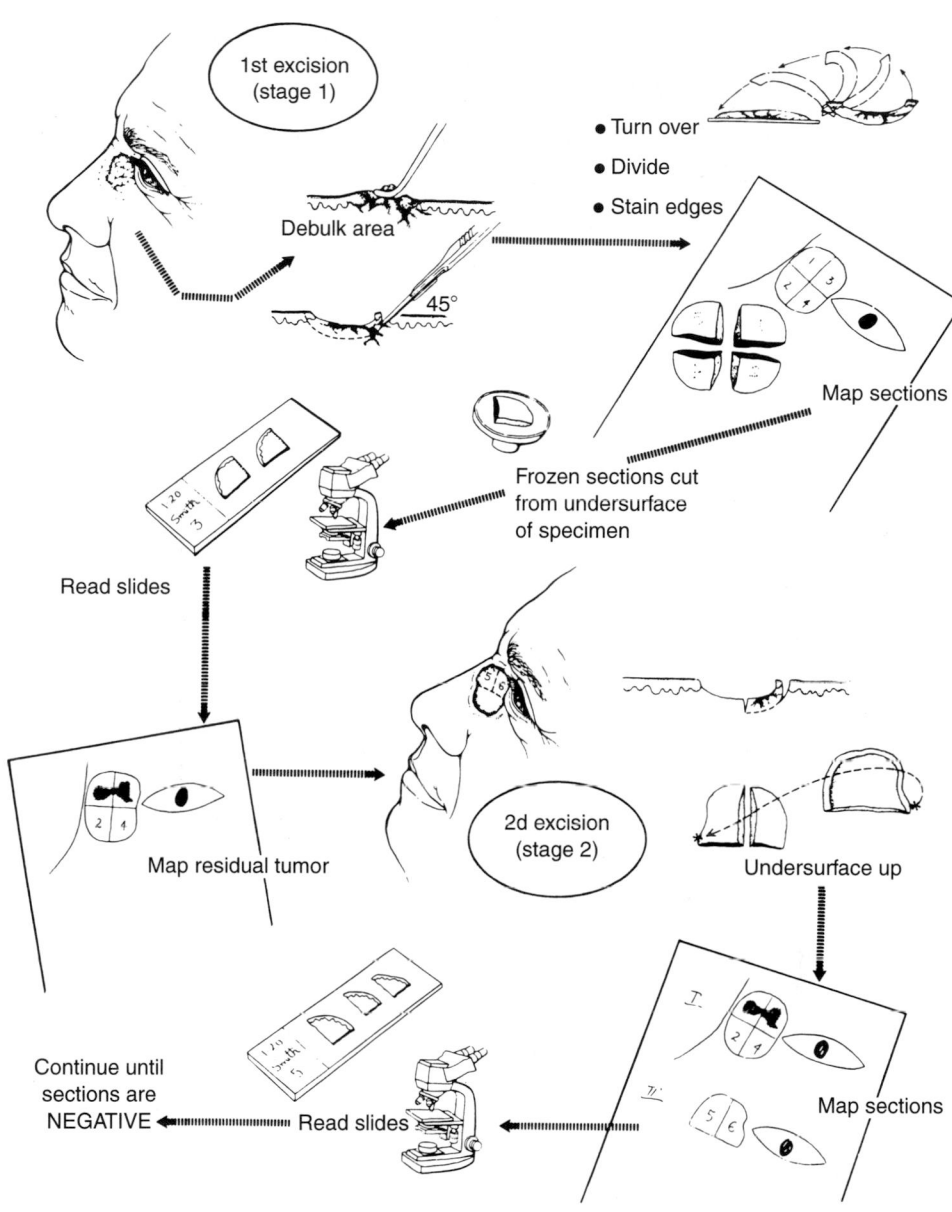

Schematic representation of technique of Mohs surgery. See text for detailed explanation.

of choice for these histologic subtypes. The clinical nature of the tumor (ill-defined margins, multicentric) and/or host (immunosuppression-iatrogenic or disease) are also important in the treatment decision-making process.

Recurrent BCCs are often clinically subtle lesions in which the actual extent of the neoplasm is frequently difficult to assess.[7] Because of this, the recurrence rates of BCC after 5 years of follow-up are 18 percent for excision, 10 percent for radiation therapy, 40 percent for electrodesiccation and curettage, and 12 percent for cryotherapy (this, with follow-up of <5 years). In contrast, the recurrence rate for BCCs treated with Mohs micrographic surgery after 5 years of follow-up are between 3.4 and 7.9 percent.[8,9] Therefore, Mohs micrographic surgery is the treatment of choice for recurrent BCCs.[10]

FIGURE 276-2

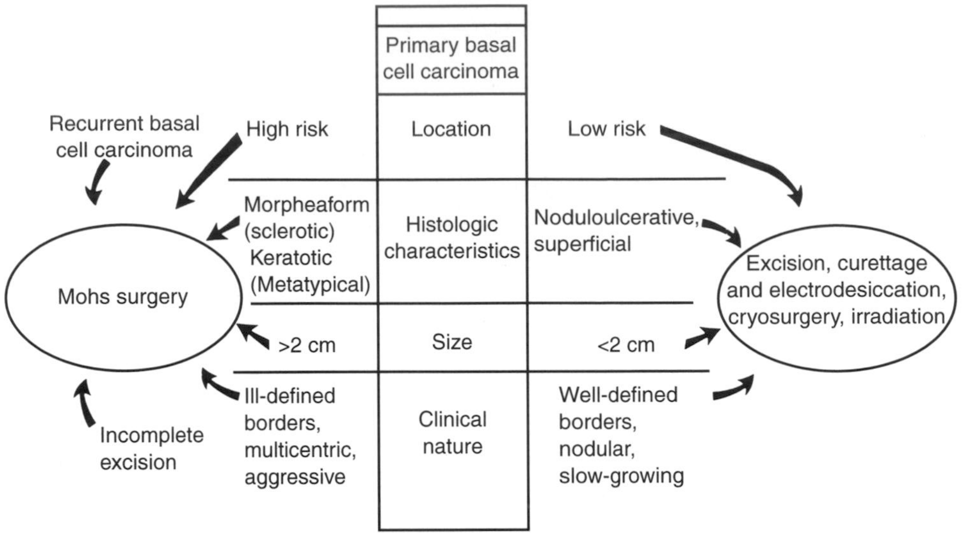

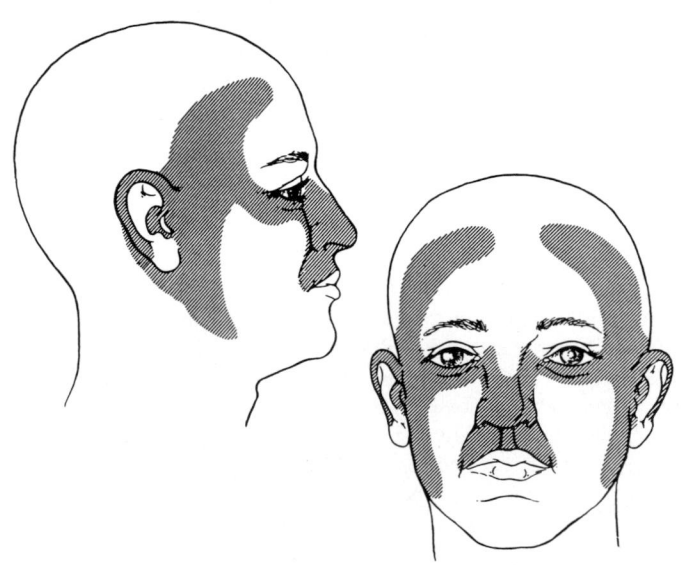

	Primary basal cell carcinoma	
High risk	**Location**	Low risk
Morpheaform (sclerotic) Keratotic (Metatypical)	**Histologic characteristics**	Noduloulcerative, superficial
>2 cm	**Size**	<2 cm
Ill-defined borders, multicentric, aggressive	**Clinical nature**	Well-defined borders, nodular, slow-growing

Recurrent basal cell carcinoma

Mohs surgery

Incomplete excision

Excision, curettage and electrodesiccation, cryosurgery, irradiation

Indications for consideration of Mohs surgery.

Incompletely excised BCCs with positive histologic margins may persist and "recur" in between 33 and 43 percent of cases with follow-up of 2 to 5 years.[11,12] Studies focusing on high-recurrence areas such as the central face show "recurrence" rates of up to 82 percent after incomplete excision of BCCs. Although there is great variation from one study to another, it is clear that excision of BCCs with positive margins by traditional techniques results in a high recurrence rate. Because these recurrences may not be noted until

FIGURE 276-3

Tumor location plays an important role in treating basal cell carcinoma. In the schematic presentation, shaded areas represent "H" zone on face, including periauricular area, which warrants special consideration for Mohs surgery.

many years after the initial excision, they may be large and extensive, requiring complex excision and reconstruction. Therefore, in the authors' view, adequate treatment of such incompletely excised BCCs should be appropriately addressed with the Mohs technique to ensure their adequate extirpation.[13]

Squamous Cell Carcinoma

Although SCCs that have arisen in actinically damaged skin have traditionally been felt to be nonaggressive, a number of such lesions do metastasize. Therefore, Mohs micrographic surgery should be considered in the following circumstances:

1. SCCs in the periauricular, lip, temple, and nose areas
2. Lesions >2 cm in diameter
3. SCCs that are poorly or moderately differentiated
4. A scar-, burn-, or radiation-associated SCC
5. SCCs with neurotropic spread
6. Lesions with increased depth of extension
7. SCCs in patients who are immunosuppressed either from intercurrent illness or as a consequence of medications

In addition to the above considerations, review of the literature regarding the effectiveness of Mohs micrographic surgery for incompletely excised or recurrent SCCs has shown Mohs to result in cure rates in excess of 94 percent, clearly superior to any other treatment method. Therefore, Mohs remains the treatment of choice for incompletely excised or recurrent tumors, independent of any of the above features.

Other Malignant Epithelial Neoplasms

Verrucous carcinoma occurs most commonly in the oral cavity, on the plantar surface of the foot, or on the genitalia. It has been demonstrated to be treated far more effectively with Mohs micrographic surgery than with standard, local excision.[14] The reported cure rate with Mohs approaches 98 percent, whereas the cure rate with excision is approximately 80 percent. Other malignant epithelial neoplasms including some keratoacanthomas (giant, central facial) and extramammary Paget's disease have been reported to be treated successfully with the Mohs technique, with cure rates exceeding those of traditional therapies.[15] Both microcystic adnexal carcinoma, more recently referred to as sclerosing sweat duct carcinoma, and sebaceous carcinoma have been shown to have been treated successfully with the Mohs technique.[16] The former, a rare tumor, has a propensity for neurotropic spread and thus is ideally treated with Mohs. The sebaceous carcinoma, occurring most commonly on the lower eyelid, has an alarming metastatic rate and may, therefore, be best treated with microscopically controlled excision.

FIBROHISTIOCYTIC TUMORS A number of fibrohistiocytic tumors have been treated with the Mohs technique, with varying degrees of success. Certainly the most impressive and well-documented improvements over standard therapy have been in the management of dermatofibrosarcoma protruberans (DFSP). Traditional excisional methods with frozen section control have had recurrence rates of up to 60 percent. Several studies documenting the long-term lack of recurrence of DFSP in patients treated with the Mohs technique have been published in the past several years. A recent review of the world literature shows a total recurrence rate of 1.6 percent for Mohs surgery–treated DFSP versus 20 percent for wide excisions.[17] Atypical fibroxanthomas have also been successfully treated with Mohs.[18] Because of the low numbers of such cases, no statistically significant studies in these tumors with respect to the effectiveness of Mohs in their management are available at this time.

OTHER TUMORS Leiomyosarcoma, angiosarcoma, liposarcoma, neuroendocrine carcinoma of the skin (Merkel cell carcinoma), to name a few, have all been reported to be treated successfully with the Mohs technique. Again, the small numbers of such cases preclude any conclusions about the utility of this technique for these unusual neoplasms. However, reports suggest that Mohs surgery may offer superior cure rates, while sparing normal tissue, for some of these neoplasms.

MALIGNANT MELANOMA The role of Mohs micrographic surgery in the management of melanoma continues to be the subject of much discussion and controversy among those who treat a large number of such patients. In particular, treatment of melanoma in situ of the face, with its propensity for sometimes dramatic subclinical extension, has been discussed extensively in the literature. Its hallmark, clinically indistinct margins in cosmetically and often functionally vital areas, would suggest this tumor as an ideal candidate for the Mohs technique. Problems with precise identification of melanocytes in frozen sections have hampered the widespread adoption of this method, however. Some have argued for the use of special stains such as HMB-45 and S-100, while others recommend formalin-fixed final margins to ensure that the tumor has been cleared prior to reconstruction.[19,20]

ISSUES AND CONTROVERSIES IN MOHS SURGERY

The theory and practice of Mohs surgery have evolved dramatically since Mohs first performed chemosurgery. Knowledge about tumor biology and histologic nuances has expanded geometrically. At the same time, reconstructive surgery for Mohs-related defects has become extraordinarily sophisticated, whereas "chemosurgery" mandated wound healing by secondary intention. Cases that formerly required the assistance of general or facial plastic surgeons are now routinely handled by the properly trained Mohs surgeon.

Mohs surgery has been demonstrated to be a cost-effective means of treating appropriate tumors. Its cost compares favorably with that of an excision with frozen-section interpretation; the difference is in the superior cure rates obtained with Mohs. The American Academy of Dermatology has recently published guidelines of care for Mohs micrographic surgery; these, along with a critical review of the evolving literature, should serve as a template for the proper utilization of Mohs surgery.[21] A recent study in a system in which the Mohs providers had no economic incentive to operate found that the overall percentage of nonmelanoma skin cancer treated by Mohs surgery was 32.7 percent.[22] These data provide some perspective when assessing what the role of Mohs surgery should be.

REFERENCES

1. Mohs FE: Chemosurgery: A microscopically controlled method of skin cancer excision. *Arch Surg* **42**:279, 1941
2. Tromovitch TA, Stegman SJ: Microscopic-controlled excision of cutaneous tumors: Chemosurgery; fresh tissue technique. *Cancer* **41**:653, 1978
3. Swanson NA: Mohs surgery: Technique, indications, applications, and the future. *Arch Dermatol* 119, 1983
4. Albom MJ, Swanson NA: Mohs micrographic surgery for the treatment of cutaneous neoplasms, in *Cancer of the Skin*. Philadelphia, Saunders, 1991
5. Freeman RH, Duncan WC: Recurrent skin cancer. *Arch Dermatol* **107**:395, 1973
6. Freeman RH: Histopathologic correlates in the management of skin cancer. *J Dermatol Surg Oncol* **2**:215, 1976
7. Salasche SJ, Amonette RA: Morpheaform basal cell epitheliomas. A study of subclinical extensions in a series of 51 cases. *J Dermatol Surg Oncol* **7**:387, 1981
8. Rowe DE et al: Long-term recurrence rates in previously untreated (primary) basal cell carcinoma: Implications for patient follow-up. *J Dermatol Surg Oncol* **15**:315, 1989
9. Mohs FE: *Chemosurgery and Microscopically Controlled Surgery for Skin Cancer*. Springfield, IL, Charles C Thomas, 1978
10. Cottell WI, Proper S: Mohs surgery, fresh-tissue technique: Our technique with a review. *J Dermatol Surg Oncol* **8**:576, 1982
11. Dellon AL et al: Prediction of recurrence in incompletely excised basal cell carcinoma. *Plas Reconstr Surg* **75**:860, 1985
12. Gooding CA et al: Significance of marginal extension in excised basal cell carcinoma. *N Engl J Med* **273**:923, 1965
13. Swanson NA et al: A novel method of reexcising incompletely excised basal cell carcinomas. *J Dermatol Surg Oncol* **6**:438, 1980
14. Swanson NA, Taylor WB: Plantar verrucous carcinoma: Literature review and treatment by the Mohs' Chemosurgery Technique. *Arch Dermatol* **116**:794, 1980
15. Mohs FE et al: Microscopically controlled surgery for extramammary Paget's disease. *Arch Dermatol* **115**:706, 1979
16. Yount AB et al: Mohs micrographic excision of sebaceous carcinoma of the eyelids. *J Dermatol Surg Oncol* **20**:523, 1994
17. Gloster HM Jr et al: A comparison between Mohs micrographic surgery and wide surgical excision for the treatment of dermatofibrosarcoma protuberans. *J Am Acad Dermatol* **35**:82, 1996
18. Zalla MI et al: A comparison of Mohs micrographic surgery and wide excision for the treatment of atypical fibroxanthoma. *Dermatol Surg* **23**:105, 1997
19. Zitelli JA et al: Mohs micrographic surgery for the treatment of primary cutaneous melanoma. *J Am Acad Dermatol* **37**:236, 1997
20. Stonecipher MR et al: Management of lentigo maligna and lentigo maligna melanoma with Paraffin-embedded tangential sections: Utility of immunoperoxidase staining and vertical sections. *J Am Acad Dermatol* **29**:589, 1993
21. Drake LA et al: Guidelines of care for Mohs micrographic surgery. *J Am Acad Dermatol* **33**:271, 1995
22. Welch ML et al: How many nonmelanoma skin cancers require Mohs micrographic surgery? *Dermatol Surg* **22**:711, 1996

CHAPTER 277

Paul Kechijian

Nail Surgery

Nail surgery is an indispensable diagnostic and therapeutic tool. Diagnoses of inflammatory and hereditary dystrophies, nail infections such as tinea unguium, and benign and malignant neoplasms are made by biopsy. Nail surgery relieves pain; facilitates drainage of liquid, purulent material and blood; removes benign and malignant neoplasms; and corrects anatomic deformities and repairs injuries. Minimizing intraoperative trauma and postoperative dystrophy are important concurrent goals of nail surgery.

Because the nail plate grows slowly, postoperative recovery is often prolonged. On average, a new fingernail grows within 4 to 6 months and a toenail within 1 year following complete removal. Depending on the procedure performed, it is possible to predict recovery time and likelihood of postoperative dystrophy—i.e., intact, absent, split or thin nail plate. A candid preoperative discussion enables the patient to better anticipate postoperative discomfort, extent of recovery, and prognosis. A phone call on the evening following or the day after surgery is also therapeutic.

Certain caveats apply. Underlying problems such as valvular heart disease, peripheral vascular disease, cigarette smoking, and diabetes mellitus increase the risk of operative complications. Drug allergies, systemic glucocorticoid therapy, and chronic or concomitant infection pose potential problems. Under supervision of the patient's primary physician, anticoagulants should be stopped prior to surgery (coumarin, 4 days; aspirin, 1 week). Prophylactic antibiotics should be considered when surgery is performed under suboptimal conditions—i.e., in patients with concomitant infection or compromised circulation or when surgery is performed on the toes. Because dermatophyte infections of the nail unit are common, a periodic acid–Schiff (PAS) stain should be requested whenever onychomycosis is even a remote diagnostic possibility.

GENERAL CONSIDERATIONS

Draping

Draping is accomplished by removing the corresponding digit from a sterile glove. The glove is placed over the involved hand, leaving the affected digit exposed (Fig. 277-1). Supplemental draping is performed as desired.

Instruments

Instruments play a crucial role in nail surgery (Fig. 277-2). Nail elevators facilitate relatively atraumatic separation not only of nail plate from nail bed but also of proximal/lateral nail folds from nail plate. The nail extractor, a "platypus-like" instrument, has two flat

FIGURE 277-1

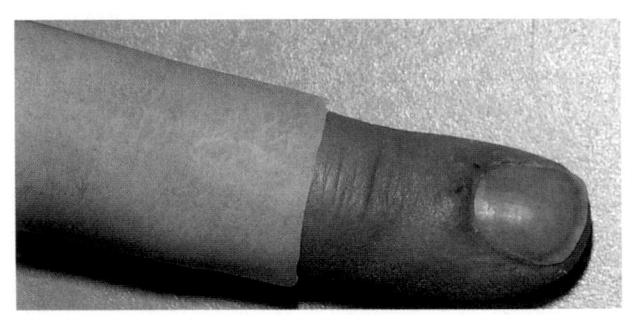

Draping. The tip of a sterile glove is removed to provide exposure of the involved digit.

surfaces with approximating toothlike structures. It is indispensable when the nail is being tightly secured for avulsion. Double-action nail clippers complete the trio of essential instruments. The clipper's fine tip makes difficult dissections and extractions easier and less painful. The clipper's dual action (double fulcrum) greatly magnifies the force that is applied at the tip of the clipper; because of it, an "impossibly thick" nail plate cuts with relative ease. Parenthetically, nail splitters, while theoretically useful, have two important disadvantages relative to clippers. Splitters are single action (single

FIGURE 277-2

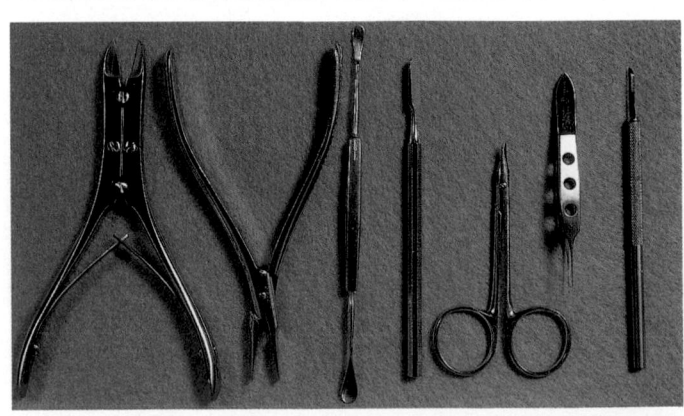

Instruments in nail surgery. From left to right: Double-action nail clipper, nail extractor, nail elevators (two), fine Gradle scissors, Bishop-Harmon forceps, and Beaver scalpel.

fulcrum) in design and offer no mechanical advantage; great force is necessary to split thick nails. The handles are relatively weak and break when sufficient force (necessary to cut thick nails) is exerted. Beaver scalpels, Bishop-Harmon forceps, skin hooks, and fine Gradle scissors are also helpful. The nail unit is relatively delicate and the risk of trauma to small specimens is great. With these instruments, surgery is performed with precision, relative ease, and minimal trauma.

Anesthesia

AGENTS Local anesthetics have important vasoactive effects. Because the nail unit is acral, the extent of vasodilation/vasoconstriction is important. Depending on the type of surgical procedure, the volume of anesthetic injected, and individual patient parameters, either vasoconstriction or vasodilatation may be preferable. Lidocaine 2%, a smooth muscle relaxant and vasodilator, is the most commonly used anesthetic. Vasodilation is generally desirable in digital surgery. In young, healthy patients or patients with small operative sites, vasoconstriction may be preferable provided that there are no vascular contraindications. Vasoconstriction reduces intraoperative and postoperative bleeding (shortening operative time) and prolongs postoperative anesthesia. Vasoconstriction is achieved with epinephrine dilutions of 1:100,000 or 1:200,000 in lidocaine. Lidocaine with epinephrine may be administered distally, *never proximally* (see below).

Bicarbonate, another supplement, raises the pH of lidocaine and diminishes the burning discomfort associated with injection. The densely innervated, pain-sensitive digit responds favorably to buffered lidocaine; one part 7.5% bicarbonate (44.6 meq/50 mL) mixed with nine parts plain lidocaine or lidocaine with epinephrine raises the pH nearer to physiologic levels.

Bupivacaine 0.5% is another useful adjunct. Too slow in onset of action and too painful to administer initially, it is useful postoperatively. Injected after completion of surgery, it extends the duration of anesthesia by several hours, significantly diminishing patient discomfort.

METHODS OF ADMINISTRATION Anesthetics are administered via 30-gauge needle on a Luer-lock syringe. Lidocaine may be injected either proximally at the base of the digit or distally and periungually at the operative site. Both locations present inherent advantages and disadvantages. *Proximal* anesthesia usually achieves a digital block that is less painful to administer and slower in onset of action. Because the needle delivers anesthetic in close proximity to delicate digital arteries and nerves on the dorsal and ventral sides of the digit, it poses a risk to these structures (see below). *Distal* administration, while more painful, is more rapid in onset of action; the risk of injury to nerves and vessels is negligible because the digital tip is rich in vascular and neural anastomoses.

A proximal digital nerve block is accomplished by injecting lidocaine slightly distal to the web space in the middle of the finger (Fig. 277-3A). Initially, 0.1 mL of lidocaine is injected locally into the epidermis. The needle is then advanced dorsally and ventrally and 0.5 mL is injected in close proximity to the respective dorsal and ventral nerves on the medial and lateral sides of the digit. The nerves lie deep in close proximity to the phalanx; larger volumes of anesthetic are unnecessary when anesthetic is injected near the nerve. To prevent injury to the fragile dorsal and ventral nerves and vessels, the needle is *always* withdrawn between dorsal and ventral injections (Fig. 277-3A). Failure to withdraw the needle completely to the superficial dermis increases the possibility of tearing nerves and arteries. Briefly retracting the plunger prior to injecting will

FIGURE 277-3

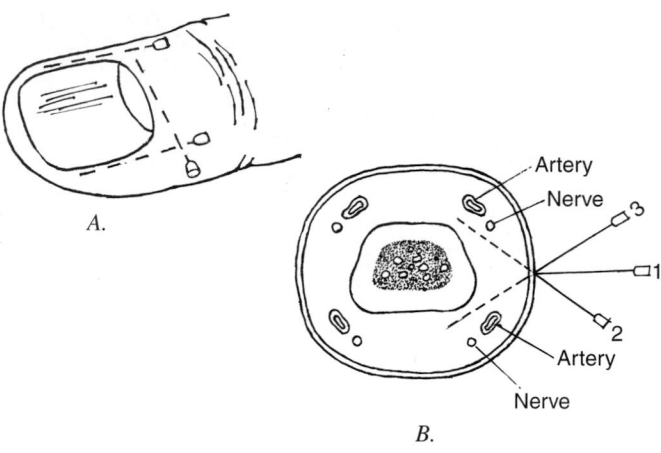

Digital anesthesia. *A.* In proximal nerve blocks, the needle is inserted at the base of the digit. Anesthetic is injected in close proximity to the dorsal and ventral digital nerves. *B.* In periungual blocks, anesthetic is injected into both lateral nail folds and the adjoining proximal nail fold.

diminish the risk of intravascular injection. Anesthesia occurs within 15 to 20 min.

Distal anesthesia is achieved by three methods:

Periungual administration (Fig. 277-3B) begins by introducing the needle at the junction of the proximal and lateral nail folds on one side of the digit. From this point of entry, anesthetic is injected at multiple sites along the lateral nail fold. To minimize discomfort, the needle is slowly advanced as lidocaine is injected slightly ahead of the needle. Once the lateral nail fold is anesthetized, the contiguous proximal nail fold is injected perpendicularly across the proximal fold. The opposite lateral nail fold is subsequently injected in a similar manner. Ultimately, both lateral nail folds and the adjoining proximal nail fold are completely infiltrated. Supplemental hyponychial administration completes a full circle of anesthesia when surgery on the distal nail unit is performed. While more painful to administer than proximal anesthesia, digital injection usually achieves rapid and complete anesthesia.

Median distal administration is performed quickly and relatively simply (Fig. 277-4). The needle is introduced at a 30-degree angle into the middle of the proximal nail fold and advanced distally into the underlying matrix. Anesthetic is injected slowly as the needle first pierces the nail plate, then the matrix, and finally the adjacent nail bed. The nail plate is soft and offers little resistance. Blanching confirms delivery of anesthetic to the nail matrix and bed. Pain is brief and anesthesia nearly instantaneous. This method is suitable for most procedures performed in the proximal half of the nail unit; it is not suitable for matricectomy or complete nail avulsion (see below).

Direct local administration is performed preoperatively on soft tissue components of the nail unit. The hyponychium as well as the lateral and proximal nail folds lend themselves well to local injection. In the absence of nail plate, the nail bed and matrix may also be injected. Small amounts of anesthetic achieve rapid and complete local anesthesia. This method is useful for partial matricectomies (see below).

Supplemental distal administration is used intraoperatively as an adjunct to digital and distal blocks when anesthesia is incomplete.

FIGURE 277-4

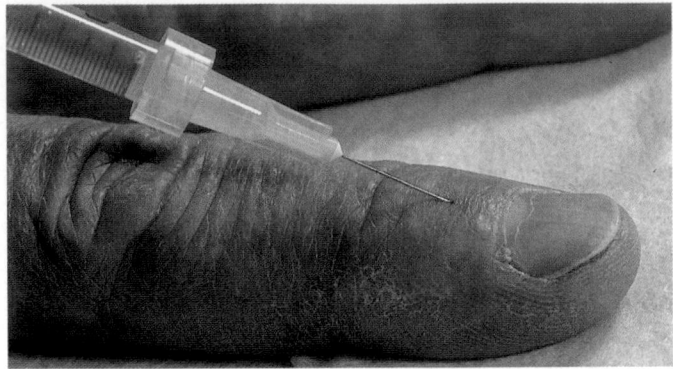

A.

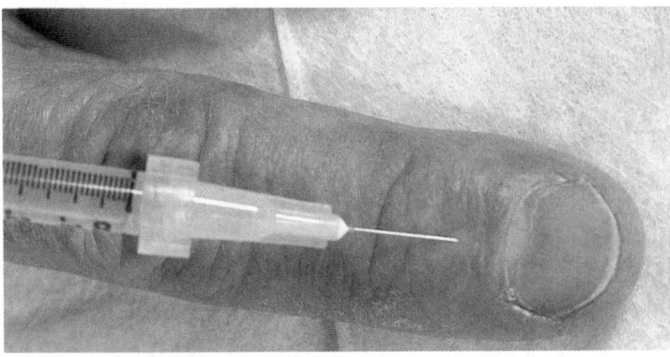

B.

Median distal anesthesia. A single injection into the proximal nail fold, underlying matrix, and adjacent nail bed achieves rapid anesthesia.

Anesthetic may be injected into perioperative soft tissues or directly into the operative site. After the nail is incised, the needle is inserted (through the surgically induced cleft in the nail plate) into the matrix or bed. Rapid additional pain relief is achieved with small amounts of anesthetic.

While most authorities discourage the use of epinephrine with lidocaine, small amounts judiciously administered distally are useful for median distal, direct local, supplemental, and periungual administration. In spite of epinephrine-induced vasoconstriction, circulation is usually not compromised in the digit. Because epinephrine may cause vasospasm of the digital arteries, *lidocaine with epinephrine is not injected proximally.* Vascular collapse of primary and collateral vessels could lead to digital necrosis.

Tourniquets

Nail surgery is optimally performed in a bloodless operative field. Brief intraoperative hemostasis is achieved by squeezing the sides of the digits. A tourniquet provides prolonged hemostasis. Tourniquet pressure should be moderate, not excessive—just enough to stop arterial blood flow. Many authorities still recommend a maximum tourniquet time of 15 min, interrupting tourniquet application for a few minutes during longer procedures. This time limitation is of historical interest only. Digits are viable hours after microsurgical

attachment. Hand surgeons routinely apply arm tourniquets for periods of 2 h; the limiting factor is tourniquet-induced (neural) paresthesias, not (vascular) ischemia.

METHODS The *nonexsanguinating method* is simplest. A thin rubber hose or 3/8-in. Penrose drain is secured around the base of the digit with a hemostat. A small piece of gauze placed circumferentially under the tourniquet distributes pressure evenly and minimizes trauma to nerves and vessels (Fig. 277-5A). Similar cushioning is helpful whenever tourniquet width is less than 1 in. Because small amounts of blood are trapped in the digit when the tourniquet is applied, momentary bleeding occurs after the first incision.

In the *exsanguinating method*, a 1-in. Penrose drain is wrapped circumferentially around the tip of the digit, leaving the distal end of the drain exposed (Fig. 277-5B–5F). Wrapping is continued proximally as overlapping segments of drain squeeze blood from the digit. Enveloping is continued to the base of the digit. This step completed, the distal end is unwound proximally toward the base of the digit. At the final loop, the ends of the tourniquet are firmly secured with a hemostat. A wide drain assures an even distribution of pressure that minimizes the risk of injury to underlying nerves and vessels. Thin drains (less than 1 in. wide) exsanguinate less efficiently and should be cushioned *prior* to wrapping.

Dressing and Postoperative Care

Dressings are best applied when hemostasis is complete. If bleeding does not stop, absorbable gelatin sponge (Gelfoam) may be placed within the surgical site. Bactroban is a useful antibacterial that may be applied under a Telfa pad. To help control bleeding, several layers of gauze may be wrapped around the digit, then covered with tape alone or with Surgitube gauze dressing (Fig. 277-6). Gentle pressure is applied as tape is circumferentially wrapped around the nail unit. Patients with postoperative bleeding should return the day following surgery for examination and dressing change. When hemostasis is not a concern, simple adhesive bandages offer the advantage of easy application. During the first postoperative week, the surgical site is cleaned daily with hydrogen peroxide; Bactroban is reapplied under the adhesive bandage.

Elevating the extremity during the immediate 24- to 48-h postoperative period helps minimize pain and swelling.

PROCEDURES

Avulsion

PARTIAL AVULSION Partial nail avulsion is an important diagnostic and therapeutic tool. It may be performed *without anesthesia* when the nail is already separated. Avulsing unattached nail prevents inadvertent tearing. When significant subungual hyperkeratosis is present, the nail plate and adherent hyperkeratosis may be removed for biopsy and PAS stain. This method is particularly useful when onychomycosis is suspected, and 10% potassium hydroxide (KOH) examinations and cultures are negative—more proximal material yields the best results. Onycholysis, a common problem, is often the result of a concomitant bacterial and candidal infection. Avulsing onycholytic nail provides access to the nail bed for KOH and fungal cultures. Avulsion is therapeutic; it eliminates nail bed maceration and provides access for application of topical therapy in

FIGURE 277-5

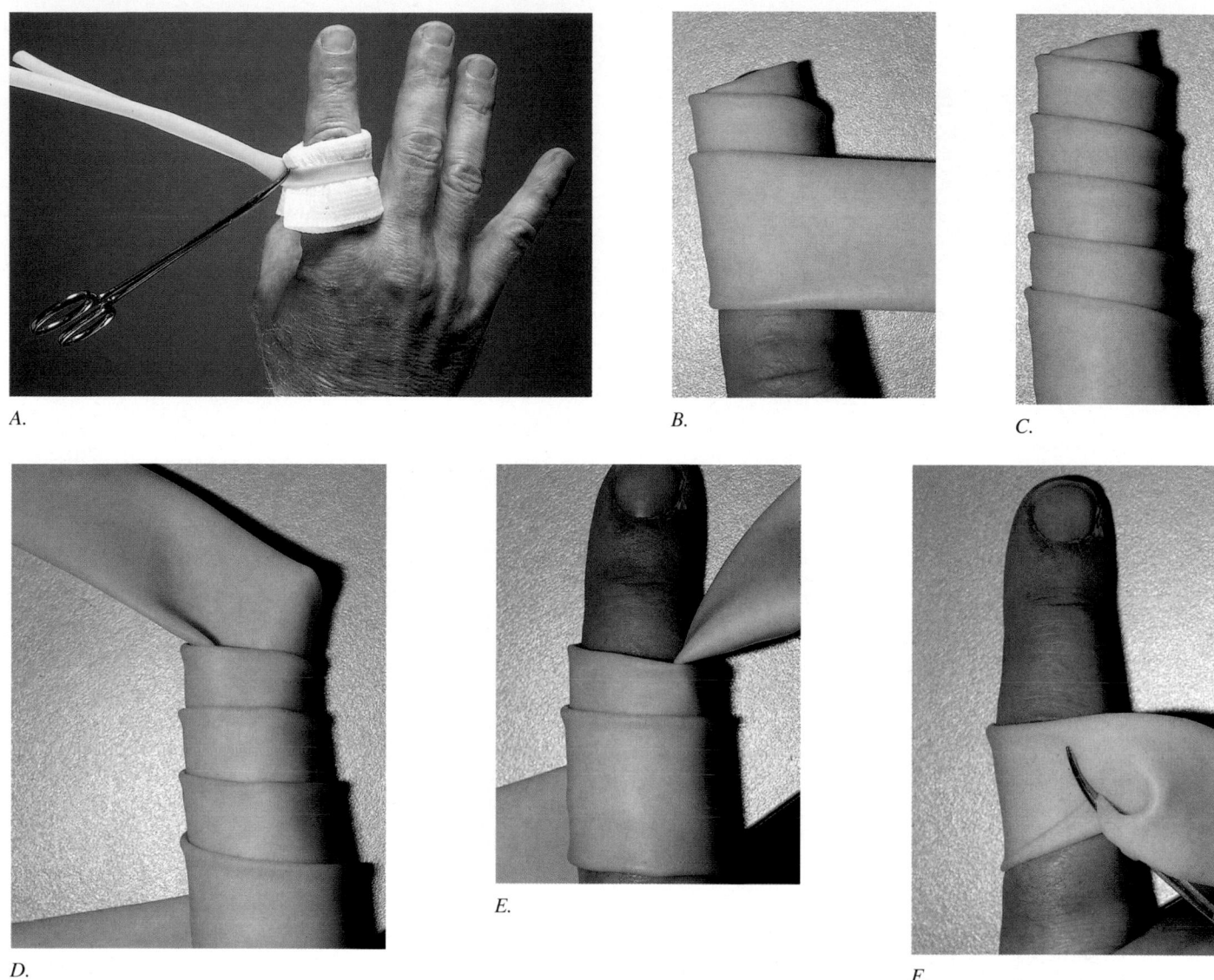

A.

B.

C.

D.

E.

F.

Tourniquet. Nonexsanguinating (*A*) and exsanguinating methods (*B–F*).

onycholytic nails. The tip of the double-action nail clipper is placed under the separated nail; the nail is then cut and removed (Fig. 277-7). Small pieces of nail are removed sequentially until all unattached nail is avulsed. Performed with patience and care, the procedure is virtually painless.

Partial avulsion may be performed to attached nail *with anesthesia* to expose the full dimensions of an underlying wart or to remove symptomatic portions of onychomycotic, onychogryphotic, or ingrown nail. The nail is separated with an elevator, as in complete avulsion (see below). Avulsion is confined to affected nail; clippers are employed to separate intact from involved nail. Small pieces may be removed sequentially or larger pieces en bloc.

COMPLETE AVULSION Complete avulsion, which usually requires anesthesia, may be performed to expedite resolution of an infection or hematoma or to provide access to the nail bed for surgical or exploratory purposes. When partial hemostasis with lateral digital pressure is insufficient, complete hemostasis is achieved with a tourniquet.

The nail elevator is wedged distally between the nail plate and bed. With proximal force, the elevator finds the natural cleavage plane between plate and bed. When the elevator reaches the matrix, resistance dissipates. The elevator is pushed a bit further to completely separate the plate and then withdrawn. Contiguous *parallel* tracts of nail are separated across the nail plate (Fig. 277-8). The elevator should *not* be fanned "like a windshield wiper" along the surface of the nail bed; side-to-side movements tear the longitudinal grooves in the nail bed (Fig. 277-9). Similarly, thick, blunt instruments (e.g., hemostats) are best avoided. Wedged under the nail, they concentrate great pressure focally and injure the nail bed; thin, broad nail elevators distribute pressure more evenly and less traumatically. Once loosened, the plate is grasped with the nail extractor and dislodged with a side-to-side "alligator" motion and then removed (Fig. 277-10); hemostats are less effective in securing and rotating the nail. The proximal nail fold and plate are separated in like manner with the elevator. To completely free the nail, adherent pieces of nail may be cut with scissors or nail clippers and trimmed away after the nail is removed.

FIGURE 277-6

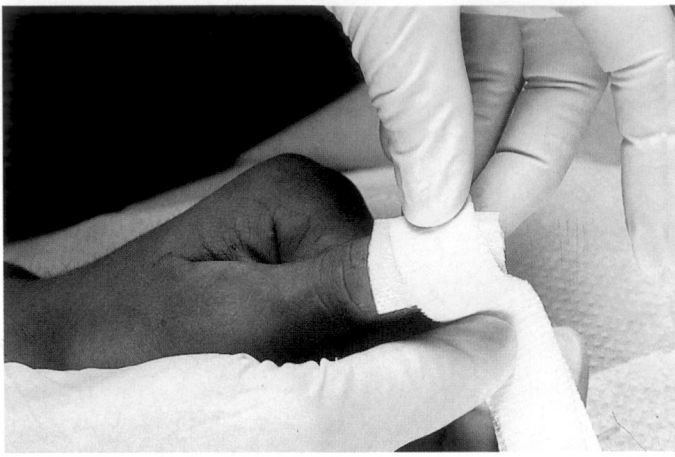

A.

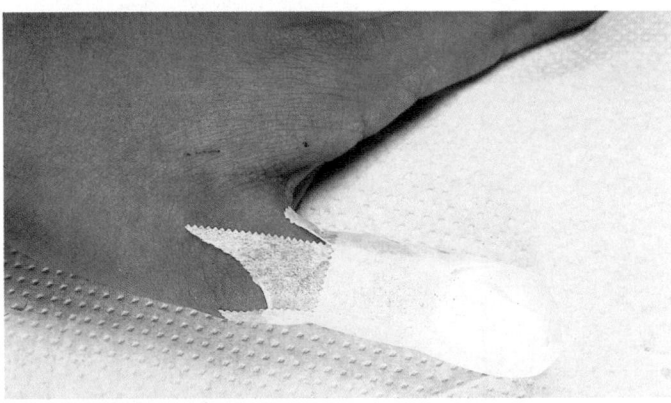

B.

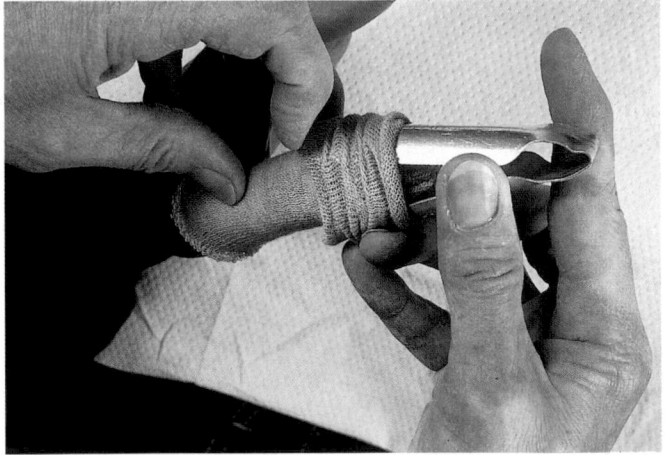

C.

Dressing. Gauze wrapped around the finger is secured with tape. A tubal gauze dressing may be applied.

FIGURE 277-7

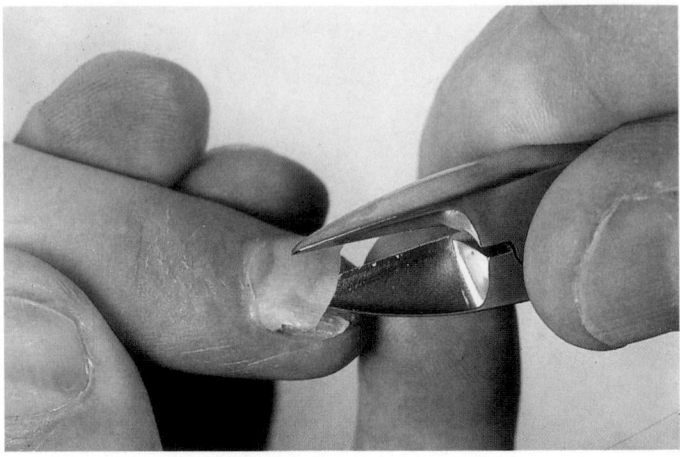

A.

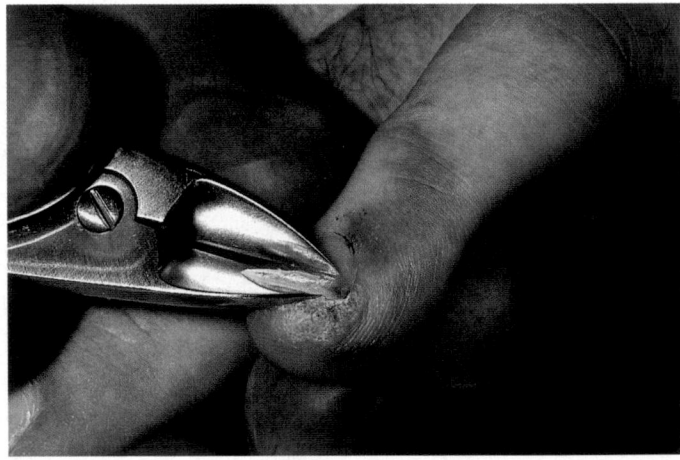

B.

Partial avulsion. The clipper's fine tip facilitates precise placement for avulsion.

Hematoma Drainage

Subungual hematomas result from crush injuries or blunt trauma to the highly vascular nail bed. Blood accumulates between the nail plate and periosteum. With sufficient volume, blood produces intense pressure and pain. Drainage affords immediate relief. When significant soft tissue injury or lacerations are visible or when the hematoma extends periungually, it is prudent to consider the possibility of fracture or substantive injury. Appropriate radiographs are obtained.

When pain is present, the hematoma is drained. When pain is absent, treatment is expectant. As new nail pushes the injured nail distally, partial nail separation may eventuate. To prevent loose nail from tearing, partial avulsion or debridement is performed as needed.

PUNCTURE A paper clip or 18-gauge needle is heated with a butane lighter until red hot. With moderate pressure, the probe easily penetrates the nail plate. Under significant pressure, blood may spray into the air upon decompression; one should be mindful of this eventuality. The tip is best inserted at a 45° angle to the plate. Perpendicular insertion is more likely to injure the bed. Once the

FIGURE 277-8

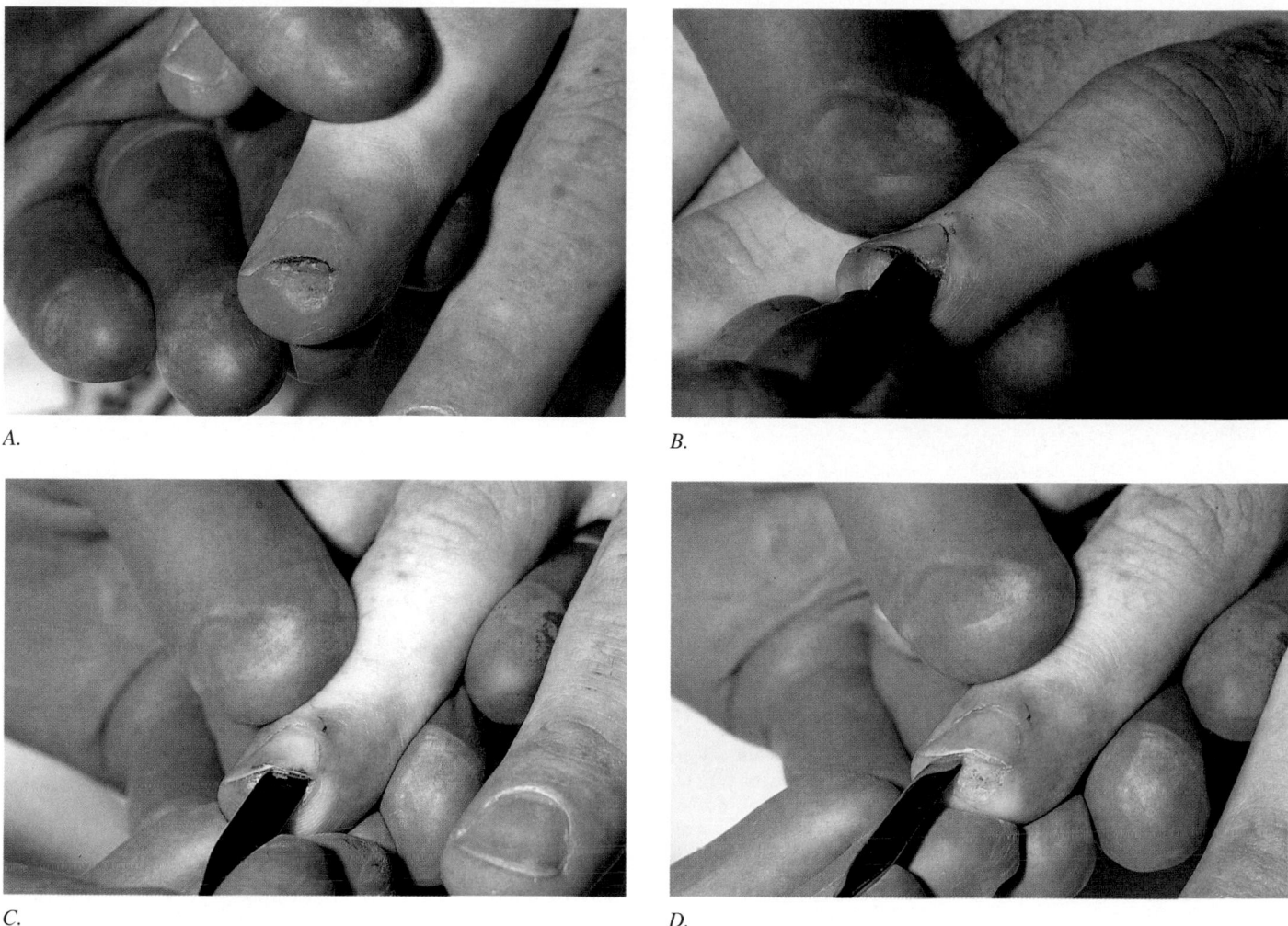

A.

B.

C.

D.

Complete avulsion. The nail plate and bed are separated along adjacent parallel tracts; the nail elevator is not "fanned" across the nail bed.

probe penetrates the nail, there is a sudden "give" as inertia carries the hot probe to the bed. The hole may be enlarged by making "supplemental" holes with the probe, then removing interconnecting nail remnants with nail clippers.

PARING   Horizontal paring with a scalpel offers an alternate method of evacuation. Nail overlying the hematoma may be pared down with a #15 scalpel as if paring a wart or callus. After a few thin pieces of nail are removed, blood erupts through the slit in the nail plate. The space between the plate and bed is usually wide enough to allow insertion of the tip of nail clippers to "snip away" affected nail and enlarge the hole. The paring method, while slightly more difficult, achieves more complete evacuation and better exposure of the nail bed.

AVULSION   When a hematoma occupies more than 50 percent of the nail bed, total avulsion is indicated (Fig. 277-11). Depending on the extent of nail separation, anesthesia may not be necessary. The entire hematoma is evacuated and the bed explored for laceration and injury.

Biopsy

The diagnosis of hereditary, inflammatory, infectious, and neoplastic disorders often mandates a biopsy. Whichever biopsy method is selected, it is important to bear in mind that *biopsy is necessary but not sufficient* for diagnosis. The tissue sample must be adequate, representative of the underlying problem, and accompanied by a complete history and clinical description to facilitate histologic interpretation. The skill of the dermatopathologist ultimately determines diagnostic accuracy.

NAIL CLIPPER BIOPSY   Specimens of nail plate and bed may be obtained by clipping or partial avulsion. Biopsies may be submitted to confirm the diagnosis of onychomycosis or subungual hematoma, even psoriasis. When longitudinal melanonychia and subungual hematoma are a concern, partially removing the plate with clippers may confirm the presence of blood, thus sparing the patient a more invasive surgical procedure (see below).

SHAVE AND INCISIONAL BIOPSY   Shave and incisional biopsies are performed in like manner to those of the skin. Suspected warts or other soft periungual tumors are removed with scissors or

FIGURE 277-9

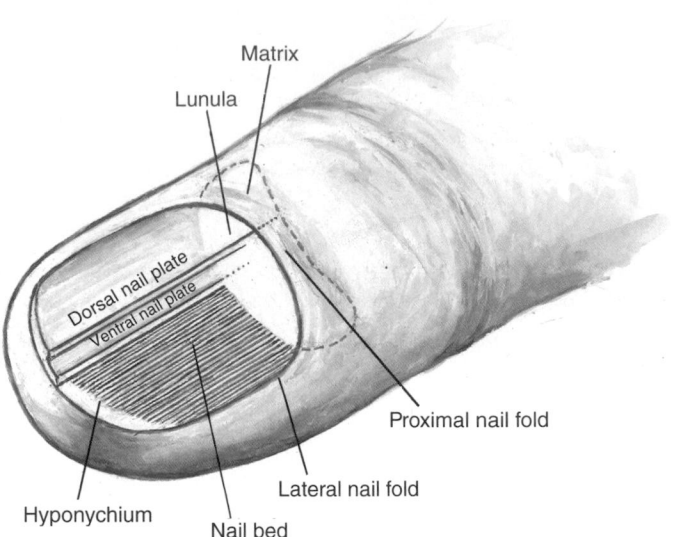

Normal nail unit. The nail plate is formed by the nail matrix, a boomerang-shaped structure that may be partially visible (distally) as the lunula or "half moon"; the proximal half of the matrix lies under the proximal nail fold. Proximal matrix forms the dorsal half of the nail; distal matrix forms the ventral half of the nail. The nail bed is composed of parallel longitudinal epidermal ridges that interface with and adhere to the overlying nail plate. Proximal and lateral nail folds surround the nail plate. The hyponychium, the most distal component of the nail unit, is usually covered by the distal tip of the nail plate; the nail plate and bed first separate at the hyponychium.

scalpel. A 2-mm wedge incision of the proximal nail fold is often helpful in the diagnosis of collagen vascular disease. Depending on clinical circumstances and surgical expertise, the wedge can be allowed to heal by secondary intention or undermined and sutured. Suturing may require the placement of relaxing incisions in the nail fold (see below).

PUNCH BIOPSY   An understanding of nail unit anatomy and nail formation (Fig. 277-9) is important in selecting the most appropriate biopsy site and surgical approach. *The nail is formed by the matrix.* Matrix biopsies may cause permanent nail alterations because the matrix generates nail plate. *Nail is not generated by nail bed.* Although nail bed biopsies may cause permanent onycholysis, they have no direct effect on nail formation and do not produce dystrophies. *Dorsal nail plate is formed by proximal matrix; ventral nail is formed by distal matrix* (Fig. 277-9). The lunula, when present, is the visible portion of the matrix and comprises the distal matrix. Biopsies from the proximal matrix may cause a longitudinal depression in the nail plate. Distal matrix biopsies may cause longitudinal onycholysis; they do not affect the nail plate surface. Biopsies that include confluent areas of proximal and distal matrix are likely to cause a permanently split nail. Biopsies that remove less than 3 mm of matrix usually cause no permanent dystrophy. However, matrix "size" affects the likelihood of post-operative dystrophy; in larger nails, proportionately less matrix is removed. A 3-mm biopsy from the thumb, which has a relatively large matrix, is less likely to heal with dystrophy than a biopsy from the fifth finger, which has a small matrix.

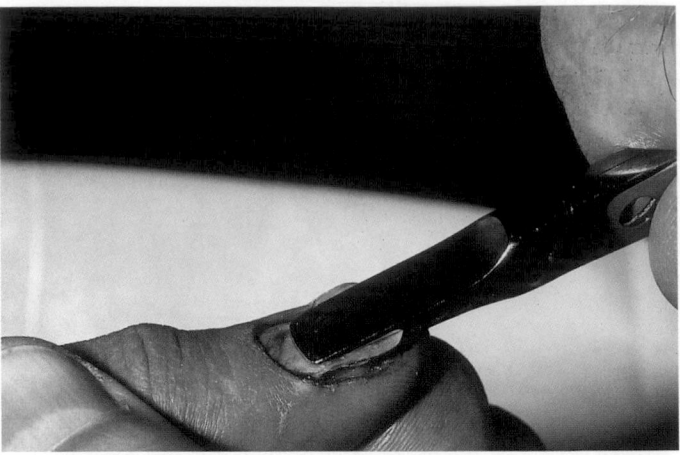

A.

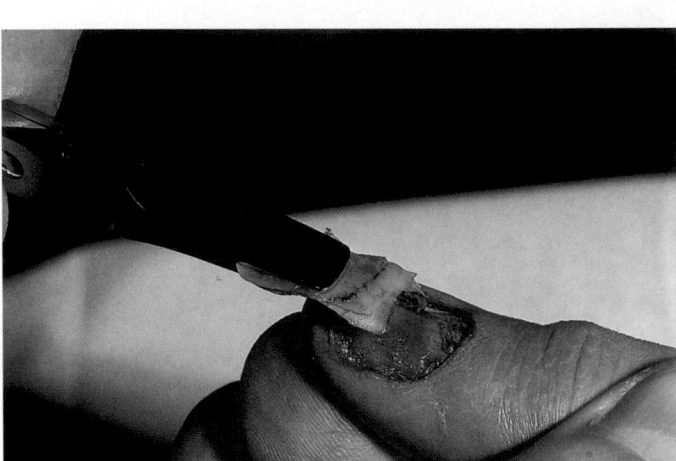

B.

Nail extractor. The nail is first loosened by twisting the nail with a side to side rotational movement; once free, the plate is removed.

Matrix biopsies are performed following matrix exposure—never "blindly" through intact proximal nail fold. Two parallel relaxing incisions transect the cuticle and proximal nail fold to expose the matrix (Fig. 277-12A). Incisions need be only wide enough to visualize the affected area. Under gentle retraction with a skin hook, the transected flap is undermined with scalpel or fine Gradle scissors. During surgery, the operative field is maintained with the skin hook (Fig. 277-12B). After biopsy is completed, two 6-0 nylon sutures are placed at the distal margin of the proximal nail fold to return the nail fold to its original smooth contour.

Single-punch method   With the proximal nail fold retracted, biopsies of the matrix and bed may be performed in an identical manner. With firm pressure, a 3-mm punch is rotated clockwise-counterclockwise through the plate. Gradually, the punch transects the plate. The nail overlying the matrix is soft and easily incised; over the bed, the nail is thicker and more difficult to incise. A (sharp) replacement punch may be substituted for the "primary" punch, when the latter becomes dull cutting the plate. The punch will suddenly "give" when the nail is transected. Because transected nail invariably becomes "trapped" in the punch, it is advisable to complete the matrix/bed biopsy with a different (replacement) punch; otherwise, the nail, wedged in the primary punch, tends to

FIGURE 277-11

CHAPTER 277
Nail Surgery   2999

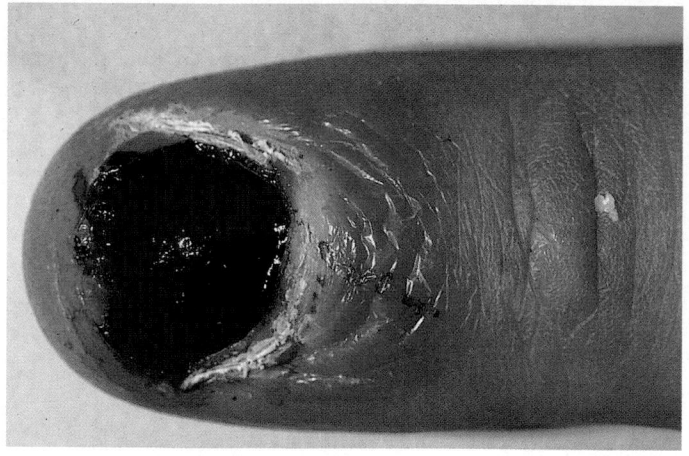

Subungual hematoma. The nail was completely avulsed from this subungual hematoma. Because the nail was completely detached by the
hematoma, anesthesia was unnecessary. The nail bed is hemorrhagic
and edematous.

FIGURE 277-12

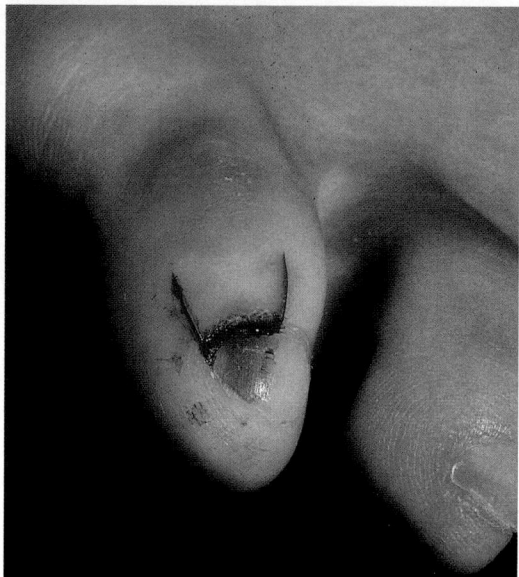

A.

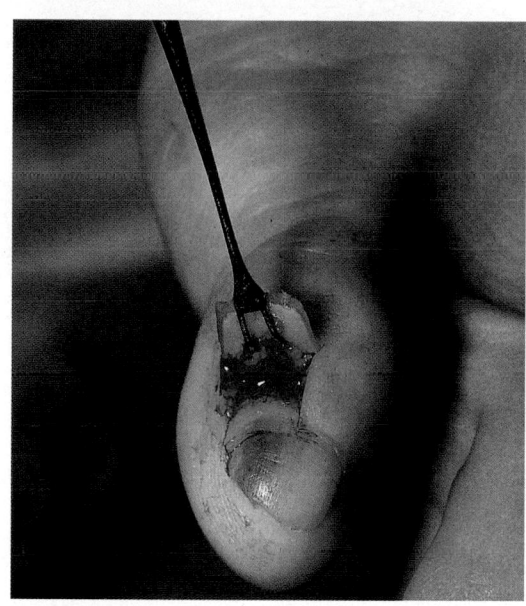

B.

Relaxing incisions. Bilateral incisions free a flap of proximal nail fold,
which is retracted with a skin hook to reveal underlying matrix.

crush underlying tissue as the punch is forced into the matrix/bed.
Trapped nail can be released from the punch by forcing a stick
(from a cotton swab) through the plastic handle into the metal barrel
of the punch; if the punch handle is not hollow, the punch is removed with a hemostat.

   Double-punch   method   Executing   biopsies   atraumatically
within the confines of the nail unit is difficult. This method employs
a larger-diameter punch to transect the nail and a smaller (3-mm)
punch to biopsy the matrix or bed (Fig. 277-13). With no risk to
the integrity of the matrix or bed, larger-diameter (4-, 5, or even
6-mm) punches provide a larger "window" within which to dissect
the biopsy specimen free. Absent the plate, a 3-mm punch is rotated
through the bed/matrix until it reaches underlying periostium. With
the lateral nail margins freed by the punch, the more difficult dissection of adherent bed or matrix is undertaken. The biopsy cylinder
may be atraumatically lifted by "spearing" the biopsy cylinder with
a 30-gauge needle, thus averting crush artifact (Fig. 277-13). At
greater risk for crush artifact, the specimen may be held, albeit more
securely, with Bishop Harmon forceps. After the specimen is secured, it is elevated and the fibrous periosteal attachment transected
with fine Gradle scissors—the thin convex tip snipping along the
periosteal surface. A careful and patient dissection yields the best
biopsy results.

Ingrown Nail

Ingrown nail is a common disorder that occurs most frequently in
the great toe. Among its many causes, the most frequent are improper trimming and tight-fitting shoes. When the lateral nail is cut
at an angle, a spicule of nail remains (Fig. 277-14). As the nail
regenerates, the spicule lacerates the lateral nail fold and (by its
persistence) causes a foreign-body reaction. Tearing rather than cutting the nail leads to similar spicule formation. Trimming the nail
straight across and slightly distal to the hyponychium prevents spicule formation. Tight-fitting shoes squeeze the nail into the lateral
nail fold, causing similar pain and inflammation. Properly fitting
footwear is important in preventing recurrences.

   Two common complications of ingrown nail are infection and
pyogenic granuloma. Clearing infection with appropriate antibiotics

is important not only for its own sake but also because a persistently
edematous nail fold is continuously transected by regrowing nail.
Pyogenic granulomas develop in association with the chronic inflammation, edema, and foreign-body reactions that occur with ingrown nails. The ingrown nail and pyogenic granuloma perpetuate
each other; the ingrown nail and granuloma must each be removed
to achieve resolution. Under direct local anesthesia, the granuloma
is destroyed by desiccation and curettage or carbon dioxide laser;
antibiotic therapy is instituted in conjunction with destruction.

FIGURE 277-13

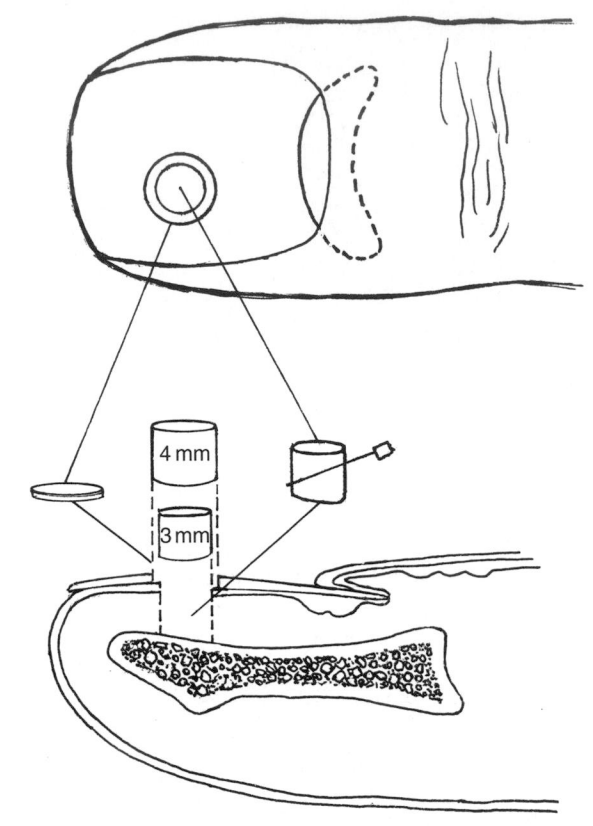

Double-punch biopsy. A 4-mm punch is used to remove a larger disk of nail plate. A smaller 3-mm punch is used to biopsy the nail bed or matrix. The biopsy specimen is "speared" with a needle to prevent crush artifact during removal.

Several therapeutic options are available for managing ingrown nails. The underlying principle in each is to remove ingrown nail and simultaneously facilitate nail regrowth by preventing further lateral nail fold injury. Treatment is best accomplished by first

FIGURE 277-14

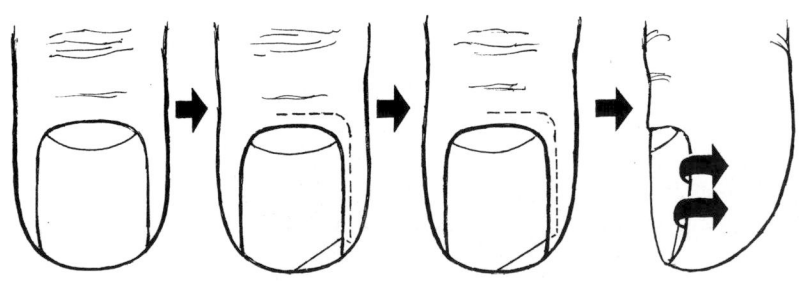

Ingrown nail. Ingrown nail often develops as a result of improper clipping. Cutting the nail proximal to the edge of the lateral nail fold leads to spicule formation. The spicule grows into the lateral nail fold as new nail is generated, causing infection, inflammation, and pain. Removing the spicule allows the nail to grow back unimpeded. The latter is facilitated by pulling the nail fold away as the nail regenerates, allowing new nail to "track" back without interference.

avulsing the ingrown spicule under local anesthesia. Under direct visualization (retracting the affected nail fold), the spicule and adjacent nail are transected with nail clippers (Fig. 277-14). Beveling the cut facilitates unimpeded growth; new nail glides over the lateral nail fold as it elongates. A cotton swab (saturated with hydrogen peroxide) is gently wedged into the groove between the nail plate and fold to maintain separation of plate and fold and a clear path for the new nail. Bactroban ointment applied twice daily after swabbing helps maintain nail fold pliability and prevent reinfection. During recovery, the lateral fold is gently pulled away from the nail to help maintain an unimpeded path for regrowing nail. In the absence of underlying problems such as bone abnormalities or overly curved, deformed, or widened nails, conservative therapy usually leads to resolution. If conservative management fails, lateral matricectomy is performed with phenol, laser, or scalpel surgery.

Matricectomy

Matricectomy is performed when the nail plate must be permanently removed, either partially or completely. Indications include (1) thickened, onychogryphotic nails that are painful and/or infected; (2) pincer nails (not caused by subungual exostosis) that squeeze the nail bed, causing pain; (3) overly curved nails that incise the nail bed or lateral nail fold; (4) onychomycotic nails that cause discomfort and fail conventional therapy; and (5) ingrown nails that persist. Prior to matricectomy, the affected nail is avulsed partially (e.g., ingrown toenail) or completely (e.g., onychogryphotic nail).

Unless the matrix is completely destroyed, a new nail will regrow. Accordingly, it is important to remove the lateral portions ("horns") of the matrix that underlie the proximal nail fold (Fig. 277-9). Several methods of matrix destruction are available. The "easiest" is phenol destruction. Prior to treatment, petroleum jelly is applied (for protection) to all nontreated areas. A bloodless field is secured with an exsanguinating tourniquet to assure the phenol will not be "diluted" or inactivated. In partial matricectomy, visible matrix and residual nail plate are removed with a curette following avulsion; then 88% phenol is applied with a cotton swab to the lateral horn(s) of matrix under the proximal nail fold. The swab is pushed deep under the lateral recesses of the nail fold and rotated clockwise/counterclockwise for 1 to 3 min, depending on the amount of matrix to be destroyed. Subsequently, the phenol is neutralized with 70% isopropyl alcohol. Because phenol produces an anesthetic effect, postoperative pain is minimal. However, phenol also produces considerable postoperative sloughing and drainage and the wound takes several weeks to heal. Phenol may be applied in a similar manner to the entire boomerang-shaped matrix (Fig. 277-9) to achieve complete matricectomy. Drainage will be extensive and daily dressing changes and hydrogen peroxide cleaning will be required.

The other methods of matrix destruction are performed under *direct visualization* of the matrix, not "blindly" as in phenol destruction. More "skill" is required to identify and successfully remove the matrix. Although operative time is longer, recovery is faster and easier because drainage and inflammation are minimized. For *partial matricectomy*, a single relaxing incision (Fig. 277-15) is made in the proximal nail fold to expose the lateral matrix. The involved matrix, once exposed, may be excised with a scalpel or vaporized with a carbon dioxide laser; electrodessication and curettage is more likely to cause excessive inflammation. After the matrix is removed, the margins of the nail fold are approximated with 6-0 nylon suture. Successful extirpation is not method-dependent; rather, success depends on properly identifying the matrix and effectively removing it by the method that works best for the operator. *Complete matricectomy* may be performed under direct visualization by scalpel or carbon dioxide laser. Bilateral relaxing incisions in the corners of the lateral nail folds allow complete exposure for matricectomy. Because the extensor tendon attaches to the dorsal phalanx just proximal to the matrix, care must be exercised to prevent injury during matricectomy.

SPECIAL PROBLEMS

Longitudinal Melanonychia

Longitudinal melanonychia—a tan, brown, or black pigmented band—results from melanin deposition in the nail plate. It may be caused by subungual melanoma, benign melanocytic alterations, or benign or malignant nonmelanocytic neoplasms; simulants of longitudinal melanonychia include subungual hematoma and bacterial, yeast, and fungal infections. Often, biopsy is the only way to make the correct diagnosis.

Longitudinal melanonychia originates in the matrix (Fig. 277-16); the origin is identified by exposing the matrix with relaxing incisions in the proximal nail fold (Fig. 277-12). Based on the likelihood of subungual melanoma, band width, and the risk of postoperative dystrophy, the origin, once identified, may be *completely* or *partially* removed. *Thin* band origins are readily removed in their entirety; *wide* bands may be biopsied (in part) or removed in their entirety. It is important to remember (whatever biopsy method is selected) that when the origin is not completely removed, postoperative pigment recurrence or persistence will occur. Postoperative longitudinal melanonychia is usually unacceptable, particularly when the original pathology is equivocal or residual pigmentation changes months or years following biopsy.

While no single biopsy method is universally satisfactory, punch biopsy is the most popular. However, punch biopsy, while performed with relative ease, is disadvantageous for a variety of reasons: (1) a *circular* piece of tissue is removed when a *rectangular* configuration is more appropriate (Fig. 277-16); (2) once removed from the matrix, a round specimen is not easily oriented, and biopsies of longitudinal melanonychia are best sectioned along the proximal distal axis—the direction of nail growth; (3) the rotational forces of punches are traumatic—additionally, the punch traps nail within its opening, producing crush artifact on the underlying tissue. Modified longitudinal biopsy, while slightly more difficult to perform, offers several advantages: (1) a more complete rectangular biopsy is removed, one that correctly reflects the vertical and horizontal growth pattern of longitudinal melanonychia (Fig. 277-16); (2) longitudinal biopsies provide flexibility in length and width of tissue removed; (3) absent shearing/rotational punch dynamics, longitudinal biopsy is more likely to remove the plate and matrix en bloc without trauma or crush artifact; (4) orientation for sectioning is easily accomplished. Modified longitudinal biopsy is a useful,

FIGURE 277-15

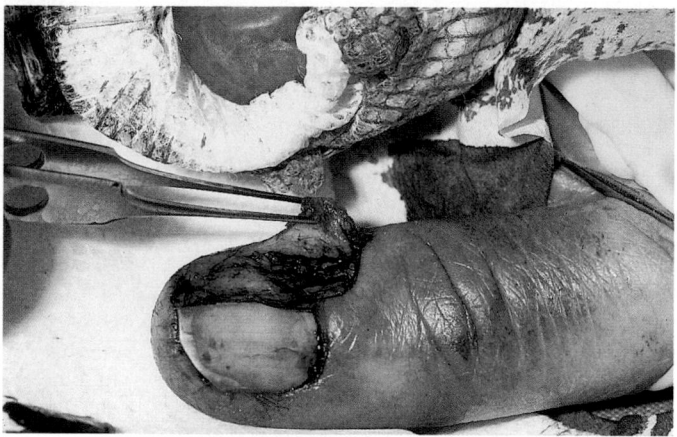

A.

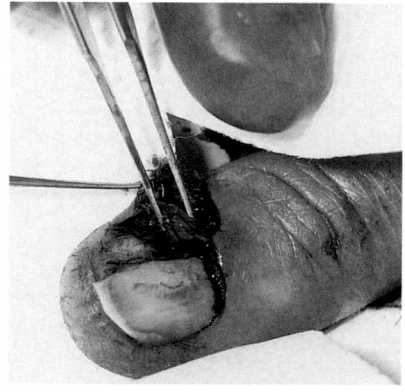

B.

C.

Lateral (partial) matricectomy. A single semicircular incision is made in the proximal nail fold. The lateral "horn" of the matrix is visible. Thus exposed with a skin hook, the lateral matrix is dissected free, effectively preventing it from generating new nail plate. The nail fold margins are approximated postoperatively with 6-0 nylon suture.

FIGURE 277-16

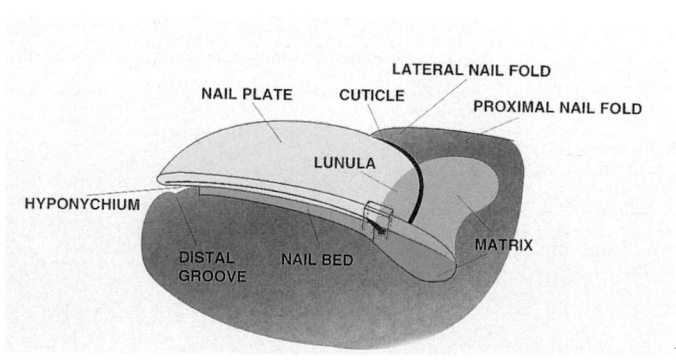

Longitudinal melanonychia. Longitudinal melanonychia originates within the matrix. When longitudinal melanonychia begins in the distal matrix, a portion of the origin may extend into the adjacent nail bed; accordingly, it is best to include the proximal nail bed in biopsies of longitudinal melanonychia. Because the origin grows vertically (distally) *and* horizontally, a rectangular configuration is the logical biopsy method.

practical, and preferable method for biopsying longitudinal melanonychia.

With the origin exposed, rectangular incisions (Fig. 277-16) are made with a #15 scalpel or Beaver scalpel. In bands 3 mm or less in width, thin portions of normal matrix are included in the lateral biopsy margins to prevent postoperative pigment recurrence/persistence. The lateral margins of bands wider than 3 mm may be biopsied completely or partially. Anterior and posterior incisions define the proximal and distal margins of the rectangle (Fig. 277-16). Because the *distal* origin may extend into adjacent nail bed, the distal incision should include a *thin margin of proximal nail bed.* The *proximal* incision should include a thin margin of *uninvolved matrix* (proximal to the origin). The resulting rectangular biopsy includes all or part of the lateral origin; the proximal-distal ends include thin margins of normal nail bed and matrix. If the band originates in the proximal matrix, a permanently split nail will develop postoperatively—an unavoidable (but necessary) outcome if one wishes to obtain a representative and adequate biopsy. The rectangle is dissected free in a manner similar to a punch biopsy. To facilitate extraction, a 4-, 5-, or 6-mm punch may be used to incise nail around the biopsy site after the rectangular incisions are made. The surrounding nail plate is removed first, leaving the (rectangular) biopsy site intact; the biopsy is then extracted more easily—in a manner similar to that of the double punch method.

Verruca vulgaris

Nail unit verrucae are vexing for many reasons: (1) verrucae are "benign" and will (eventually) resolve spontaneously; prolonged, painful treatment is not easily justified; (2) verrucae are often multiple and arise in locations (periungual and subungual) that are difficult to access; (3) the full extent of subungual warts often remains undefined because the nail is not adequately removed to provide satisfactory exposure; (4) because periungual epidermis is thick, verrucae usually extend more deeply than is clinically apparent; (5) because verrucae often arise near germinative tissue, viable wart is often not removed completely for fear of resultant dystrophy. In the absence of compelling reasons, *most periungual and subungual verrucae are probably best left to resolve spontaneously.*

With the decision to treat, the first task is to define the full extent of the wart(s)—whether subungual and periungual. Avulsing all nail in proximity to the wart achieves this goal (Fig. 277-8). The next decision is how best to remove the wart. Cryotherapy, a popular and simple modality, has important disadvantages: (1) at best, the cure rates are modest; (2) after freezing deeply enough to reach the wart's base, postoperative pain and swelling are significant; and (3) the limited confines of the digit and nail unit magnify discomfort and swelling. Electrodesiccation and curettage is a preferable option. After the full extent of the the wart is defined by avulsion, all visible wart is lightly desiccated. Heat causes the wart to retract from dermal tissues, facilitating its removal by curettage. Depending upon the wart's dimensions, further electrodessication and curettage may be necessary. *If* no virus persists in "involved" epidermis surrounding the wart and *if* destruction has been largely confined to the epidermal component (i.e., not dermis, nail bed, and matrix), minimal scarring and cure are likely. The greater the number of warts, the less likely it is that cure will be achieved. It is probably best to confine treatment to no more than five warts at one time. The carbon dioxide laser offers another method of destruction, "vaporizing" the wart. Whether vaporizing with laser or removing by electrodesiccation and curettage, therapeutic success is determined by the experience of the surgeon and the care with which the procedure is performed. Two caveats: (1) no therapeutic method is foolproof—all fail to achieve consistent cures, and (2) the possibility of squamous cell carcinoma must be always be considered in verrucae that fail conventional therapy.

CONCLUSION

A number of problems not considered here include exostoses, glomus tumors, acute and chronic paronychias, myxoid cysts, pincer nails, and repairs of dystrophies and lacerations. These topics and further discussion of the subjects considered in this chapter are given more detailed consideration in specialized textbooks.[1,2,3] With time and experience, nail unit anatomy becomes more familiar. As easier procedures are mastered and the clinician's confidence builds, all the procedures discussed in this chapter can be successfully performed. The results for patient and physician alike will be gratifying.

REFERENCES

1. Baran R, Dawber RPR (Eds): *Diseases of the Nails and Their Management,* 2d ed. Oxford, England, Blackwell, 1994
2. Zaias N: *The Nail in Health and Disease,* 2d ed. Norwalk, CT, Appelton & Lange, 1990
3. Scher RK, Daniel CR (Eds): *Nails: Therapy–Diagnosis–Surgery,* 2d ed. Philadelphia, Saunders, 1997

NOTE: Bold number indicates the start of the chapter that contains the main discussion of the topic; numbers followed with "f" and "t" refer to figure and table pages.

ISBN 0-07-912938-2

90000

9 780079 129383

FREEDBERG/DIGM5
(US SET)

ISBN 0-07-021943-5

90000

9 780070 219434

FREEDBERG/DIGM5
(US VOL. II)